EQUINE INTERNAL MEDICINE

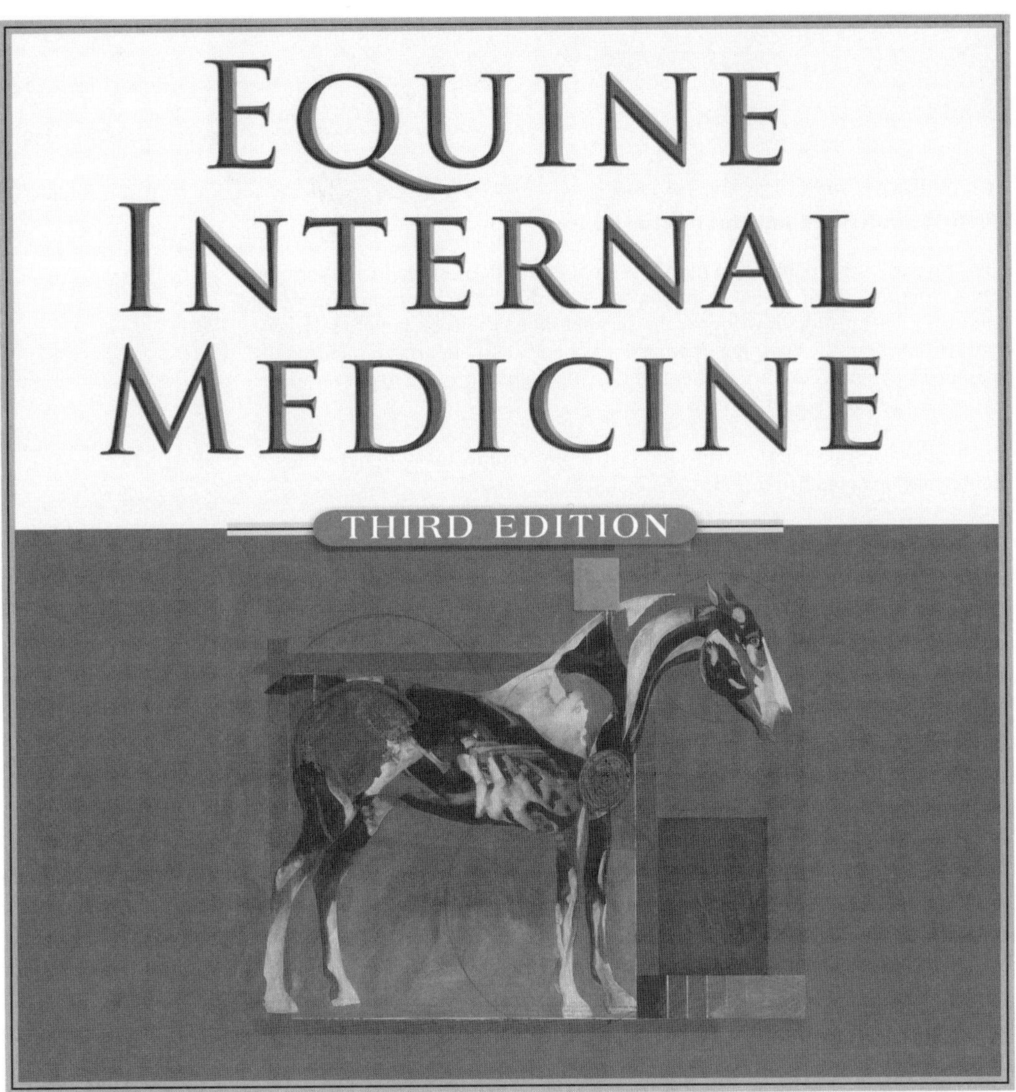

EQUINE INTERNAL MEDICINE

THIRD EDITION

Stephen M. Reed, DVM, Dipl ACVIM

Associate • Rood & Riddle Equine Hospital • Lexington, Kentucky

Warwick M. Bayly, BVSc, MS, PhD, Dipl ACVIM

Provost and Executive Vice President • Washington State University • Pullman, Washington

Debra C. Sellon, DVM, PhD, Dipl ACVIM

Professor, Department of Veterinary Clinical Sciences • College of Veterinary Medicine

Washington State University • Pullman, Washington

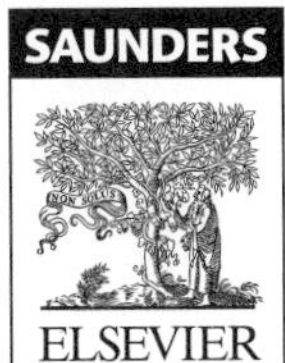

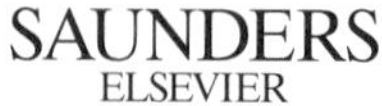

3251 Riverport Lane
St. Louis, MO 63043

EQUINE INTERNAL MEDICINE

ISBN: 978-1-4160-5670-6

Notices

Knowledge and best practice in this field are constantly changing. As new research and experience broaden our understanding, changes in research methods, professional practices, or medical treatment may become necessary.

Practitioners and researchers must always rely on their own experience and knowledge in evaluating and using any information, methods, compounds, or experiments described herein. In using such information or methods they should be mindful of their own safety and the safety of others, including parties for whom they have a professional responsibility.

With respect to any drug or pharmaceutical products identified, readers are advised to check the most current information provided (i) on procedures featured or (ii) by the manufacturer of each product to be administered, to verify the recommended dose or formula, the method and duration of administration, and contraindications. It is the responsibility of the practitioner, relying on their own experience and knowledge of their patient, to make diagnoses, to determine dosages and the best treatment for each individual patient, and to take all appropriate safety precautions.

To the fullest extent of the law, neither the Publisher nor the authors, contributors, or editors, assume any liability for any injury and/or damage to persons or property as a matter of products liability, negligence or otherwise, or from any use or operation of any methods, products instructions, or ideas contained in the material herein.

The Publisher

Previous editions copyrighted 2004, 1998

Library of Congress Cataloging-in-Publication Data

Equine internal medicine/[edited by] Stephen M. Reed, Warwick M. Bayly, Debra C. Sellon. -- 3rd ed.

p. ; cm.

Includes bibliographical references and index.

ISBN 978-1-4160-5670-6 (pbk. : alk. paper) 1. Horses--Diseases. 2. Veterinary internal medicine. I. Reed, Stephen M. II. Bayly, Warwick M. III. Sellon, Debra C.

[DNLM: 1. Horse Diseases. SF 951 E638 2010]

SF951.E565 1998
636.1'0896--dc22

2009036106

Vice President and Publisher: Linda Duncan
Acquisitions Editor: Penny Rudolph
Associate Developmental Editor: Lauren Harms
Publishing Services Manager: Patricia Tannian
Project Managers: Jonathan Taylor, Sharon Corell
Design Direction: Karen Pauls

Printed in the United States of America

Last digit is the print number: 9 8 7 6 5 4 3 2 1

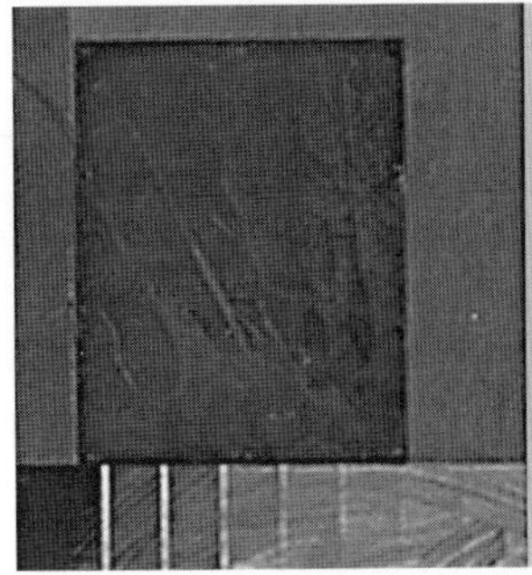

Contributors

Dorothy M. Ainsworth, DVM, PhD, DACVIM
Professor of Medicine
Department of Clinical Sciences
College of Veterinary Medicine
Cornell University
Ithaca, New York

Frank M. Andrews, DVM, MS, DACVIM
LVMA Equine Committee
Professor and Director
Equine Health Studies Program
School of Veterinary Medicine
Louisiana State University
Baton Rouge, Louisiana

Bonnie S. Barr, VMD, DACVIM
Department of Internal Medicine
Rood and Riddle Equine Hospital
Lexington, Kentucky

Michelle Henry Barton, DVM, PhD, DACVIM
Fuller E. Callaway Chair and Professor
Department of Large Animal Medicine
University of Georgia
Athens, Georgia

Warwick M. Bayly, BVSc, MS, PhD, Dipl ACVIM
Provost and Executive Vice President
Washington State University
Pullman, Washington

Laurie A. Beard, DVM, MS, DACVIM
Clinical Associate Professor
Department of Clinical Sciences
Veterinary Medical Teaching Hospital
Kansas State University
Manhattan, Kansas

Joseph J. Bertone, DVM, MS, DACVIM
Professor
College of Veterinary Medicine
Western University of Health Sciences
Pomona, California

Anthony T. Blikslager, DVM, PhD, DACVS
Professor
Department of Clinical Sciences
College of Veterinary Medicine
North Carolina State University
Raleigh, North Carolina

John D. Bonagura, DVM, MS, DACVIM
Professor
Department of Veterinary Clinical Sciences
College of Veterinary Medicine
The Ohio State University
Columbus, Ohio

Barbara A. Byrne, DVM, PhD, DACVIM
Assistant Professor
Department of Pathology, Microbiology, and Immunology
College of Veterinary Medicine
University of California
Davis, California

Elaine M. Carnevale, DVM, PhD
Department of Biomedical Sciences
Animal Reproduction and Biotechnology Laboratory
Colorado State University
Fort Collins, Colorado

Jonathan Cheetham, VetMB, PhD, DACVS
Department of Comparative Biomedical Sciences
College of Veterinary Medicine
Cornell University
Ithaca, New York

John B. Chopin, BVSc, MACVSc (Equine Medicine), PhD, FACVSc (Equine Reproduction)
Coolmore Stud
Jerry's Plains, New South Wales, Australia

Noah D. Cohen, VMD, MPH, PhD, DACVIM
Professor
Department of Large Animal Clinical Sciences
College of Veterinary Medicine and Biomedical Sciences
Texas A&M University
College Station, Texas

Marco A. Coutinho da Silva, DVM, PhD, DACT
Assistant Professor
Department of Veterinary Clinical Sciences
College of Veterinary Medicine
The Ohio State University
Columbus, Ohio

Mark V. Crisman, DVM, MS, DACVIM
Professor
Department of Large Animal Clinical Sciences
College of Veterinary Medicine
Virginia Maryland Regional College of Veterinary Medicine
Blacksburg, Virginia

Jennifer L. Davis, DVM, PhD, DACVIM, DACVCP
Assistant Professor
Department of Clinical Sciences
College of Veterinary Medicine
North Carolina State University
Raleigh, North Carolina

Patricia M. Dowling, DVM, MSc, DACVIM, DACVCP
Department of Veterinary Biomedical Sciences
Western College of Veterinary Medicine
Saskatoon, Saskatchewan, Canada

Susan C. Eades, DVM, PhD, DACVIM
Professor
Department of Veterinary Clinical Sciences
School of Veterinary Medicine
Louisiana State University
Baton Rouge, Louisiana

Jonathan H. Foreman, DVM, MS, DACVIM
Associate Dean for Academic and Student Affairs
Professor
Department of Veterinary Clinical Medicine
Veterinary Teaching Hospital
University of Illinois
Urbana, Illinois

Nicholas Frank, DVM, PhD, DACVIM
Associate Professor
Department of Large Animal Clinical Sciences
University of Tennessee
Knoxville, Tennessee
Associate Professor
School of Veterinary Medicine and Sciences
University of Nottingham
Sutton Bonington, United Kingdom

Grant S. Frazer, BVSc, MS, MBA
Director
Veterinary Medical Teaching Hospital
College of Veterinary Medicine
The Ohio State University
Columbus, Ohio

Martin Furr, DVM, PhD, DACVIM
Adelaide C. Riggs Professor of Medicine
Virginia-Maryland Regional College of Veterinary Medicine
Leesburg, Virginia

Katherine S. Garrett, DVM
Department of Diagnostic Imaging
Rood & Riddle Equine Hospital
Lexington, Kentucky

Ray J. Geor, BVSc, MVSc, PhD, DACVIM
Professor and Chairperson
Department of Large Animal Clinical Sciences
College of Veterinary Medicine
Michigan State University
East Lansing, Michigan

Caroline N. Hahn, DVM, MSc, PhD, DECVN, DECEIM, MRCVS
Director
Neuromuscular Disease Laboratory
Royal (Dick) School of Veterinary Studies
Easter Bush Veterinary Centre
University of Edinburgh
Midlothian, United Kingdom

Bernard D. Hansen, DVM, MS, DACVIM, DACVECC
Associate Professor
Department of Clinical Sciences
College of Veterinary Medicine
North Carolina State University
Raleigh, North Carolina

Joanne Hardy, DVM, PhD, DACVS
Clinical Associate Professor
Department of Large Animal Clinical Science
College of Veterinary Medicine
Texas A&M University
College Station, Texas

Kenneth W. Hinchcliff, BVSc, PhD, DACVIM
Dean of Veterinary Science
University of Melbourne
Werribee, Victoria, Australia

Melissa T. Hines, DVM, PhD
Associate Professor
Department of Veterinary Clinical Sciences
College of Veterinary Medicine
Washington State University
Pullman, Washington

Siddra A. Hines, DVM
Equine Internal Medicine Resident
Veterinary Teaching Hospital
Washington State University
Pullman, Washington

David W. Horohov, MS, PhD
William Robert Mills Chair and Professor
Department of Veterinary Sciences
University of Kentucky
Lexington, Kentucky

Laura H. Javsicas, VMD, DACVIM
Lecturer
Department of Large Animal Medicine
College of Veterinary Medicine
University of Florida
Gainesville, Florida

Samuel L. Jones, DVM, PhD, DACVIM
Professor
Department of Clinical Sciences
College of Veterinary Medicine
North Carolina State University
Raleigh, North Carolina

Eduard Jose-Cunilleras, DVM, DACVIM
Clinical Instructor
Department of Veterinary Clinical Science
College of Veterinary Medicine
The Ohio State University
Columbus, Ohio

Thomas R. Klei, BS, PhD
Boyd Professor of Parasitology and Veterinary Science
Associate Dean for Research and Academic Affairs
Louisiana State University
Baton Rouge, Louisiana

Catherine W. Kohn, VMD, DACVIM
Professor
Department of Veterinary Clinical Sciences
College of Veterinary Medicine
The Ohio State University
Columbus, Ohio

Katharina L. Lohmann, Dr.med.vet., PhD, DACVIM
Associate Professor
Department of Large Animal Clinical Sciences
Western College of Veterinary Medicine
University of Saskatchewan
Saskatoon, Saskatchewan, Canada

Maureen T. Long, DVM, PhD, DACVIM
Associate Professor
Department of Infectious Disease and Pathology
College of Veterinary Medicine
University of Florida
Gainesville, Florida

D. Paul Lunn, BVSc, MS, PhD, MRCVS, DACVIM
Professor and Head
Department of Clinical Sciences
James L. Voss Veterinary Teaching Hospital
College of Veterinary Medicine and Biomedical Sciences
Colorado State University
Fort Collins, Colorado

Jennifer M. MacLeay, DVM, PhD, DACVIM
Associate Professor
Department of Clinical Sciences
Colorado State University
Fort Collins, Colorado

Peggy S. Marsh, DVM, DACVIM, DACVECC
Internist
McGee Medicine Center
Hagyard Equine Medical Center
Lexington, Kentucky

Dianne McFarlane, DVM, PhD, DACVIM
Assistant Professor
Department of Physiological Sciences
Center for Veterinary Health Sciences
Oklahoma State University
Stillwater, Oklahoma

Robert H. Mealey, DVM, PhD, DACVIM
Associate Professor
Department of Veterinary Microbiology and Pathology
College of Veterinary Medicine
Washington State University
Pullman, Washington

Elizabeth S. Metcalf, MS, DVM, DACT
Owner
Honahlee, PC
Sherwood, Oregon

Rustin M. Moore, DVM, PhD, DACVS
Bud and Marilyn Jenne Professor and Chair
Department of Veterinary Clinical Sciences
College of Veterinary Medicine
The Ohio State Unviersity
Columbus, Ohio

Peter R. Morresey, BVSc, DACT, DACVIM
Department of Internal Medicine
Rood and Riddle Equine Hospital
Lexington, Kentucky

William W. Muir, DVM, PhD, DACVA, DACVECC
Regional Director
American Academy of Pain Management
Veterinary Clinical Pharmacology Consulting Services
Columbus, Ohio

Yvette S. Nout, DVM, MS, PhD, DACVIM, DACVECC
Assistant Researcher
Department of Neurosurgery
College of Veterinary Medicine
University of California
San Francisco, California

J. Lindsay Oaks, DVM, PhD, DACVM
Associate Professor
Department of Veterinary Microbiology and Pathology
College of Veterinary Medicine
Washington State University
Pullman, Washington

Dale L. Paccamonti, DVM, MS, DACT
Professor and Head
Department of Veterinary Clinical Sciences
School of Veterinary Medicine
Louisiana State University
Baton Rouge, Louisiana

Nigel R. Perkins, BVSc (Hons), MS, PhD, DACT, FACVSc
Director
AusVet Animal Health Services
Toowoomba, Queensland, Australia

Carlos R. F. Pinto, DVM, PhD, DACT
Associate Professor
Department of Veterinary Clinical Sciences
College of Veterinary Medicine
The Ohio State University
Columbus, Ohio

Michael B. Porter, DVM, PhD, DACVIM
Clinical Assistant Professor
Department of Large Animal Clinical Sciences
College of Veterinary Medicine
University of Florida
Gainesville, Florida

Nicola Pusterla, DVM, DACVIM
Associate Professor
Department of Medicine and Epidemiology
College of Veterinary Medicine
University of California
Davis, California

Stephen M. Reed, DVM, Dipl ACVIM
Associate
Rood & Riddle Equine Hospital
Lexington, Kentucky

Virginia B. Reef, DVM
Director of Large Animal Cardiology and Diagnostic Ultrasonography
Executive Board Member, Center for Equine Sport Medicine
Chief, Section of Sports Medicine and Imaging
Mark Whittier and Lila Griswold Allam Professor of Medicine
Department of Clinical Studies
School of Veterinary Medicine
New Bolton Center
University of Pennsylvania
Kennett Square, Pennsylvania

Christine A. Rees, DVM, DACVD
Veterinary Dermatology
Veterinary Specialists of North Texas
Dallas, Texas

Bonnie R. Rush, DVM, MS, DACVIM
Professor
Department of Clinical Sciences
College of Veterinary Medicine
Kansas State University
Manhattan, Kansas

Juan C. Samper, DVM, MSc, PhD, DACT
Veterinary Reproductive Services
Abbotsford, British Columbia, Canada

L. Chris Sanchez, DVM, PhD, DACVIM
Assistant Professor
Department of Large Animal Clinical Sciences
University of Florida
Gainesville, Florida

William J. Saville, DVM
Professor and Chair
Department of Veterinary Preventative Medicine
College of Veterinary Medicine
The Ohio State University
Columbus, Ohio

Harold C. Schott II, DVM, PhD, DACVIM
Professor
Department of Large Animal Clinical Sciences
College of Veterinary Medicine
Michigan State University
East Lansing, Michigan

Colin C. Schwarzwald, Dr.med.vet., PhD, DACVIM
Senior Lecturer
Internal Medicine Section
Equine Department
Vetsuisse Faculty
University of Zurich
Zurich, Switzerland

Kathy K. Seino, DVM, MS, PhD
Assistant Professor
Department of Veterinary Clinical Sciences
College of Veterinary Medicine
Washington State University
Pullman, Washington

Debra C. Sellon, DVM, PhD, Dipl ACVIM
Professor, Department of Veterinary Clinical Sciences
College of Veterinary Medicine
Washington State University
Pullman, Washington

Daniel C. Sharp III, BS, MS, PhD
Professor Emeritus
Department of Large Animal Medicine
College of Veterinary Medicine
University of Florida
Gainesville, Florida

Carla S. Sommardahl, DVM, PhD, DACVIM
Assistant Professor
Department of Large Animal Medicine
College of Veterinary Medicine
University of Tennessee
Knoxville, Tennessee

Ashley M. Stokes, DVM, PhD
Associate Professor and Extension Veterinarian
Department of Human Nutrition and Food and Animal Sciences
College of Tropical Agriculture and Human Resources
University of Hawaii
Honolulu, Hawaii

Patricia Ann Talcott, MS, PhD, DVM, DABVT
Associate Professor
Department of Veterinary and Comparative Anatomy, Pharmacology and Physiology
College of Veterinary Medicine
Washington State University
Pullman, Washington
Veterinary Diagnostic Toxicologist
Washington Animal Disease Diagnostic Laboratory
Pullman, Washington

Ramiro E. Toribio, DVM, MS, PhD, DACVIM
Assistant Professor
Department of Veterinary Clinical Sciences
College of Veterinary Medicine
The Ohio State University
Columbus, Ohio

Bryan M. Waldridge, DVM, MS, DACVIM, DABVP
Department of Internal Medicine
Rood & Riddle Equine Hospital
Lexington, Kentucky

David A. Wilkie, DVM, MS, DACVO
Professor
Department of Veterinary Clinical Sciences
The Ohio State University
Columbus, Ohio

Pamela Anne Wilkins, DVM, PhD, DACVIM-LA, DACVECC
Professor and Section Head
Veterinary Teaching Hospital
College of Veterinary Medicine
University of Illinois
Urbana, Illinois

W. David Wilson, BVMS, MS
Professor
Director of the William R. Pritchard Veterinary Medical Teaching Hospital
Associate Dean for Clinical Programs
School of Veterinary Medicine
University of California
Davis, California

L. Nicki Wise, DVM
Resident
Department of Veterinary Clinical Sciences
College of Veterinary Medicine
Washington State University
Pullman, Washington

Dana N. Zimmel, DVM, DACVIM, ABVP
Clinical Assistant Professor
Associate Chief
Department of Large Animal Clinical Sciences
College of Veterinary Medicine
University of Florida
Gainesville, Florida

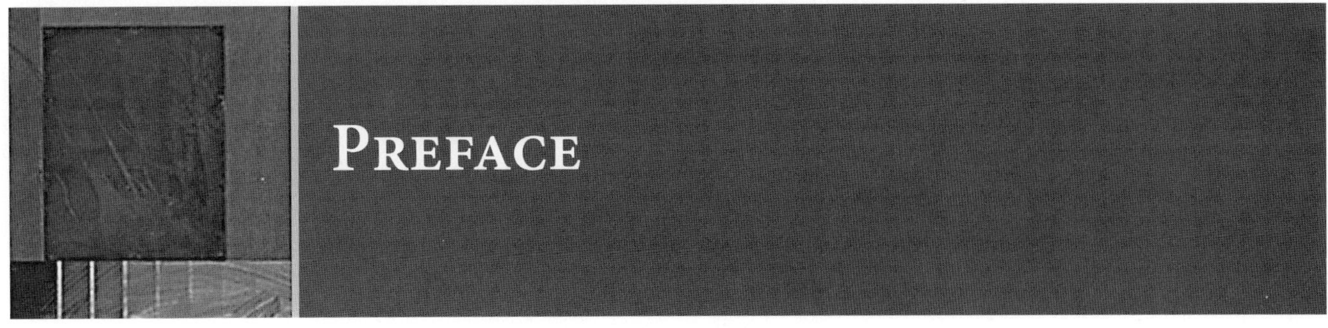

PREFACE

This is the third edition of *Equine Internal Medicine.* Like its two predecessors, it has been written and edited with the aim of promoting a clearer comprehension of the principles of medical disease and/or problem development by focusing on the basic pathophysiologic mechanisms that underlie the development of various equine diseases. As with previous editions, basic information is presented and then related to the clinical characteristics of each disease and its therapy and management.

All the chapters that appeared in the first two editions have been updated, and a number of them have been extensively revised or rewritten. Although the bulk of the chapters address specific diseases along systems-based lines, we realize that the practitioner is initially confronted with a specific problem that may have its origin in one or more of the body's systems. The first section of the book is therefore devoted to an in-depth discussion of the basic mechanisms by which problems might develop and the principles underlying the treatment of many of them. The reader can build on this foundation by reading about specific disorders in the second section of the book, which is divided into chapters dealing with problems of a particular body system or of a specific nature.

Many true experts have contributed to this text. Their depth of knowledge about all aspects of equine internal medicine is encyclopedic and daunting. We are grateful for their efforts and diligence in helping us to produce what we hope will come to be regarded as the definitive text on medical diseases of horses. We are indebted to them for their efforts. We trust that they derive a sense of pride from the part they have played in producing what we hope represents the gold standard in equine medical textbooks.

In these days of progressive globalization of the world's societies and associated growth in the international movement of horses for breeding, recreational, and competitive purposes, there has also a worldwide increase in expectations relating to the standard of veterinary care and evaluation of sick horses. The sophistication of specialist training programs and the increased number of equine internists also taking advantage of postgraduate doctoral opportunities have resulted in a wealth of new information and the maturing of an increasingly complex and challenging discipline—equine internal medicine. The delivery of superior health care and increased client expectations that have been associated with the growth of this discipline have led to the appearance of extremely well-informed and astute equine general practitioners everywhere and specialist equine internists on most continents. More than ever before, equine internal medicine now stands as an autonomous specialty in the veterinary profession. We trust that the third edition of *Equine Internal Medicine* will prove to have as much universal appeal and application as those that preceded it.

Finally, we would be remiss if we did not thank the many people at Elsevier for their persistence and efforts. Penny Rudolph and Lauren Harms in particular deserve our gratitude. They and many others have assisted in manuscript preparation, correspondence, and all the other tasks that must be accomplished to get a book like this into print. Without them and the generosity of our colleagues, this book would not have been published. We think that everyone's efforts have been worthwhile.

Stephen M. Reed, DVM, Dipl ACVIM
Warwick M. Bayly, BVSc, MS, PhD, Dipl ACVIM
Debra C. Sellon, DVM, PhD, Dipl ACVIM

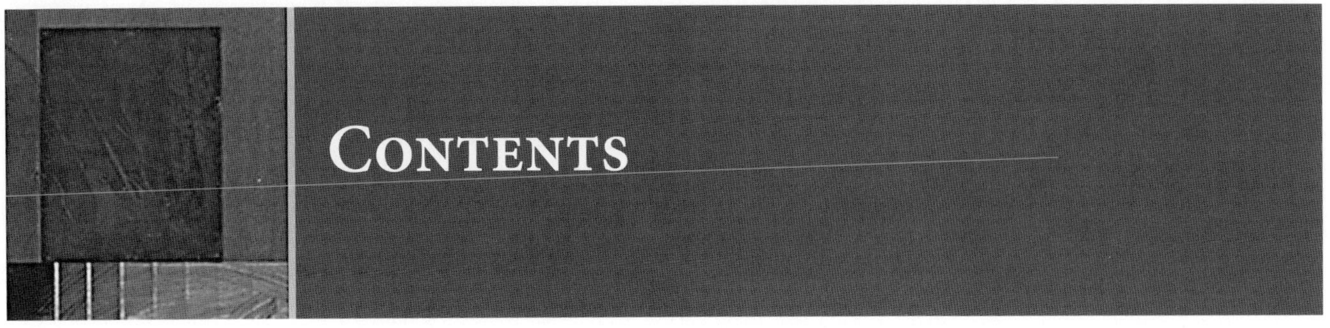

Contents

EQUINE INTERNAL MEDICINE

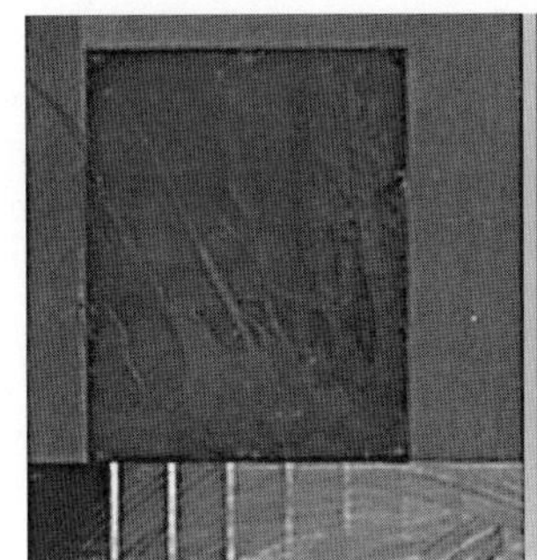

PART I

Mechanisms of Disease and Principles of Treatment

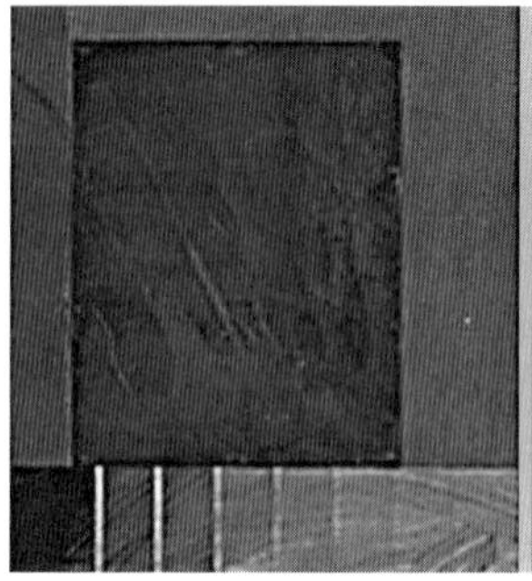

The Equine Immune System

CHAPTER 1

Paul Lunn, David Horohov

EQUINE IMMUNOLOGY

Although much of modern immunology has focused on humans and murine models of human diseases, the horse has played a significant role in our understanding of immunologic processes. These contributions include the earliest work on serotherapy and passive transfer; immunoglobulin structure and function; immunity to infectious agents; immunodeficiencies; and, more recently, reproductive immunology. Work in the horse continues in many of these areas to the benefit of equine medicine and comparative immunology. The overall organization and function of the equine immune system are similar to those of other mammalian species, although there are differences. The reader is referred to any one of a number of texts[1-3] for a more in-depth review of basic immunology. Here we shall focus on those aspects of the immune system that may be of most interest to equine researchers and clinicians. When possible, pertinent references to equine work will be provided.

INNATE IMMUNITY AND THE ACUTE INFLAMMATORY RESPONSE

Immune defenses include both *innate responses* and *adaptive responses,* each of which is mediated by cellular and soluble components. Although we often regard the innate and adaptive responses as separate, they are in fact intimately related, sharing many of the same processes and components. The major difference lies in the specificity and recall capability that characterizes the adaptive response. It is both the specificity of adaptive responses, mediated by antibodies or by effector cells such as cytotoxic T-lymphocytes (CTLs), and the phenomena of immunological memory that are responsible for the capacity to completely protect an animal against a particular pathogen. Nevertheless, the role innate responses play in both prompting the adaptive response as well as providing valuable time for specific adaptive responses to develop cannot be overstated.

The horse, like every other species, is under constant assault from a variety of microbes that share its living space. Although most of these organisms are thought to be harmless, their disease-causing potential is evident when they cause opportunistic infections in individuals with compromised immune systems.[4] Mammals, in general, have evolved a variety of defensive measures to prevent infections. The first line of defense includes the physical barriers provided by the skin and the mucosal surfaces of the digestive, respiratory, and urogenital tracts. In addition to providing a barrier to penetration, the surface of the skin contains various enzymes, fatty acids, and oils that inhibit the growth of bacteria, fungi, and viruses. Mucous membranes and mucosal secretions contain bacteriolytic enzymes, bacteriocidal basic polypeptides, mucopolysaccharides, and antibodies that prevent colonization and penetration of these surfaces. Mucus also provides a physical barrier that entraps invading organisms and leads to their eventual disposal.[5] Particles trapped in the mucous secretions of the respiratory tract, for example, are transported upwards through the action of ciliary cells to the trachea, where they are swallowed.[6] Once they are swallowed, the acidic secretions and digestive enzymes of the stomach destroy most organisms. Normal epithelial and tissue architecture is essential for successful exclusion of bacteria, and the disruption of this mechanism makes the host susceptible to infection by bacteria that normally colonize the upper airway.[7,8]

Acute Phase Proteins, Pro-inflammatory Cytokines, and Complement

Once breached, the host presents a variety of internal defenses to contain and eliminate the invaders. Invading organisms can initiate an inflammatory response either via the activation of plasma protease systems directly, such as by bacterial cell wall components, or by the secretion of toxins or other proteins that can directly activate the inflammatory response.[9] The cell walls and membranes of bacteria contain various proteins and polysaccharides with characteristic, often repeating, molecular structures. These pathogen-associated molecular patterns (PAMPs) include such molecules as lipopolysaccharides (LPSs), peptidoglycans, lipoteichoic acid, and flagellins.[10] Other PAMPs include single- and double-stranded ribonucleic acid (RNA) found on viruses and unmethylated deoxyribonucleic acid (DNA) characteristic of bacteria. These PAMPs are recognized by a class of receptors known as *toll-like receptors* (TLRs), initially identified in *Drosophila melanogaster* (the fruitfly).[10] This ancient family of receptors recognizing different PAMPs is widely distributed on the various cells of the body. Not surprisingly, a number of different TLRs are found on the cells of the immune system, particularly those cells involved in the initial encounter with invading microbes. The binding of a PAMP to its specific TLR leads to an intracellular signaling event, culminating in the expression of various accessory proteins that provide the co-stimulatory signals for the developing adaptive immune response. Injured cells also release products that initiate plasma protease cascades or produce pro-inflammatory cytokines that augment the inflammatory process. Resident macrophages that encounter the invader add to the genesis of the inflammatory response through the production of pro-inflammatory cytokines such as interleukin (IL)-1, IL-6, and tumor necrosis factor alpha (TNF-α).[9] Cytokines are hormonelike proteins that mediate a variety of cellular responses. A vast number of cytokines are involved in the regulation of innate and adaptive immune responses. IL-1, for example, is a pleiotropic mediator of the host response to infections and injurious insults (Box 1-1). Many of the effects of IL-1 are mediated through its capacity to increase the production of other cytokines, such as granulocyte colony-stimulating factor (G-CSF), TNF-α, IL-6, IL-8, platelet-derived growth factor (PDGF), and IL-11 (cytokines, chemokines, and interleukins are discussed later). IL-6 is responsible for the increased production of *acute phase proteins* (Table 1-1) by hepatocytes. Although the function of some of the acute phase proteins remains unclear, many of these proteins and the cytokines that elicited them are responsible for the characteristic physical signs of inflammation, including increased blood flow and vascular permeability, migration of leukocytes from the peripheral blood into the tissues, accumulation of leukocytes at the inflammatory focus, and activation of the leukocytes to destroy any invading organisms.[11] The acute phase proteins include a number of *complement* proteins. The complement system is an interacting series of proteases and their substrates, resulting in the production of physiologically active intermediaries that can damage membranes, attract neutrophils and other cells, increase blood flow and vascular permeability, and opsonize bacteria and other particles for phagocytosis.[12] The complement cascade can be activated in two ways (Figure 1-1). The *classical pathway* involves the recognition and binding of C1 to antigen-antibody complexes. Bound C1 is proteolytic and cleaves C4. This cleavage of C4 leads to the binding of C2 to C4b. C2 is in turned cleaved by C1 into C2a. The C4bC2a complex is referred to as the *classical pathway* C3 convertase because it is a protease capable of cleaving C3 into C3a and C3b. Another C3 convertase is generated via the alternate pathway. The activation of complement via the *alternate pathway* does not involve antibodies; instead, certain microbial products (zymosan and LPS) stimulate the association of Factor D, a proteolytic enzyme, with the complex of Factor B and C3b leading to the formation of the C3bBb complex, which is the alternative pathway C3 convertase. C3a, produced by the cleavage of C3 by the C3 convertases can bind to mast cells, causing them to degranulate, and is thus referred to as an *anaphylatoxin,* as is C4a. C3b serves as an opsonin for C3b receptor-bearing phagocytic cells. C3b is also required for the formation of the membrane attack complex by the terminal complement components, C5 through C9. In this process C5 is cleaved by either the C4b2a3b (Classic pathway C5 convertase) or C3b, Bb, and properidin (alternate pathway C5 convertase). C5 is cleaved into C5a and C5b. C5a is a chemoattractive factor for neutrophils and monocytes.[13] C5b forms a complex with C6, C7, and C8 on cell surfaces. This leads to the insertion and polymerization of C9 that forms a pore in the membrane, leading to cell lysis.

BOX 1-1

BIOLOGIC ACTIVITIES OF INTERLEUKIN 1

Activates T cells	Induces fever
Activates B cells	Cytotoxic for some tumor cells
Enhances NK cell killing	Cytostatic for other tumor cells
Fibroblast growth factor	Stimulates collagen production
Stimulates PGE synthesis	Stimulates keratinocyte growth
Stimulates bone resorption	Stimulates mesangial cell growth
Chemotactic for neutrophils	Activates neutrophils
Activates osteoclasts	Induces IL-6 production

NK, Natural killer; *IL,* interleukin.

TABLE 1-1

Acute Phase Proteins

Name	Function
C3, C4, and Factor B	Opsonins
C-reactive protein	Opsonin and complement activator
Fibrinogen	Fibrin precursor, clotting factor
Kininogen	Kinin precursor
Alpha$_1$-acid glycoprotein	Function unknown, immunomodulatory
Ceruloplasmin, Ferritin	Iron restriction
Haptoglobulin	Binds free hemoglobulin
Hemopexin	Binding free heme
Serum amyloid A (SAA)	Lipid transporter, inhibitor of neutrophil function
Serum amyloid P (SAP)	Lipid transporter, inhibitor of neutrophil function
α_1-antichymotrypsin	Protease inhibitor
α_2-macroglobulin	Protease inhibitor
Cysteine protease inhibitor	Protease inhibitor

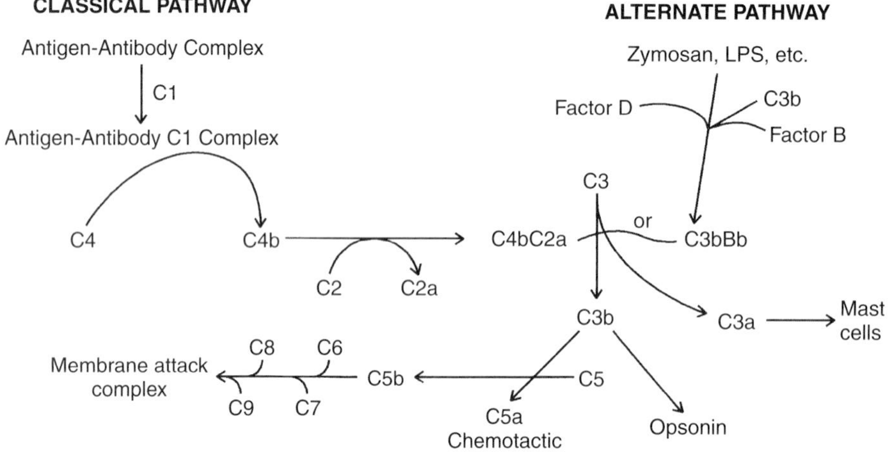

FIGURE 1-1 Classical and alternate pathways of complement activation (see text for explanation). *LPS*, Lipopolysaccaride.

Lipid Mediators

Prostanoids are lipid mediators that regulate the inflammatory response.[14,15] The prostanoids group includes the prostaglandins (PGs), leukotrienes (LTs), and prostacyclin (PGI_2), and they are the product of cyclooxygenase cleavage of arachidonic acid followed by endoperoxidation (Figure 1-2). The major sources of prostanoids in acute inflammation are the phagocytes, endothelial cells, and platelets. Prostanoids, in general, mediate the cardinal effects of pain, fever, and edema characteristic of the acute inflammatory response, but their particular roles are somewhat confounding and can be either pro- or anti-inflammatory (Table 1-2).[16] Prostanoid production depends on the activity of the two isoforms of the cyclooxygenase enzymes within cells: COX-1, which is present in most cells and its expression is generally constitutive, and COX-2, whose expression is low or undetectable in most cells, but its expression increases dramatically upon stimulation, particularly in cells of the immune system. Increased COX-2 expression by inflammatory stimuli likely accounts for the high levels of prostanoids found in chronic inflammatory lesions and is the basis for the development of COX-2–specific inhibitors for treating chronic inflammatory diseases.[17] However, studies using mice have indicated that the earliest prostanoid response to deleterious environmental stimuli depends on COX-1, and only as the inflammatory process progresses does COX-2 become the major source of prostanoids.[18] Further, evidence for increased cardiovascular risk associated with COX-2 inhibitors has called into question the use of COX-2 inhibitors as treatments for inflammatory diseases.[19,20]

Both COX isoforms produce PGH_2, which is the common substrate for a series of specific synthase enzymes that produce PGD_2, PGE_2, PGF_2, PGI_2, and TXA_2 (see Figure 1-2). It is the differential expression of these enzymes within cells present at sites of inflammation that will determine the profile of prostanoid production. For example, mast cells predominantly generate PGD_2, whereas resting macrophages produce TXA_2 in excess of PGE_2, although this ratio changes to favor PGE_2 production after activation. Likewise, the biological effect of a prostanoid depends on its binding to G protein–coupled cell surface receptors. The receptors for PGF_2, PGI_2, and TXA_2 are called FP, IP, and TP, respectively. In contrast, PGD_2 acts through two receptors, the DP receptor and the recently identified CRTh2 receptor, and there are four subtypes of receptors for PGE_2, termed *EP1–EP4*. The prostanoid receptors themselves are coupled to various G protein–coupled intracellular signaling pathways. The DP, EP2, EP4, IP, and one isoform of the EP3 receptor can couple to G_s and thus increase intracellular cAMP concentration, which in T cells and other inflammatory cells is generally associated with inhibition of effector cell functions. By contrast, the EP1, FP, IP, and TP receptors, as well as other EP3 isoforms, couple to G_q, and activation of these receptors leads to increased intracellular calcium levels and immune cell activation. Finally, TP, CRTh2, and yet another EP3 receptor isoform can each couple to G_i, causing cAMP levels to decline while also mobilizing intracellular calcium. Many cells of the immune system express multiple receptors that couple to these apparently opposing pathways. The impact of prostanoids present during an inflammatory response is thus determined by the array of receptors the cells express and the intracellular pathways to which they are coupled. Activation of these receptors, even when coupled to similar pathways, might evoke different responses because of differences in the levels of expression (both constitutive and induced) or in the patterns of desensitization. The role of prostanoids in a given inflammatory response depends not only on the presence of the lipid mediators in the lesion but also on the receptor profile on immune cells and the biochemical signaling pathways of these receptors.[18] Thus PGE_2 is considered proinflammatory because it promotes vasodilation by activating cAMP-coupled EP2 receptors on vascular smooth muscle and increases vascular permeability indirectly by enhancing the release of histamine and other mediators from tissue leukocytes such as mast cells. PGE_2 is also the prostanoid responsible for fever production. However, as inflammation progresses, PGE_2 synthesis by macrophages is enhanced as a result of increased expression of COX-2 and PGE-synthase, and the resulting increased levels of PGE_2 inhibit leukocyte activation, mast cell degranulation, and relax smooth muscle contractions. In the lung PGE_2 promotes bronchodilation through activation of Gs-coupled EP2 and EP4 receptors. Thus in these situations PGE_2 may be considered anti-inflammatory.

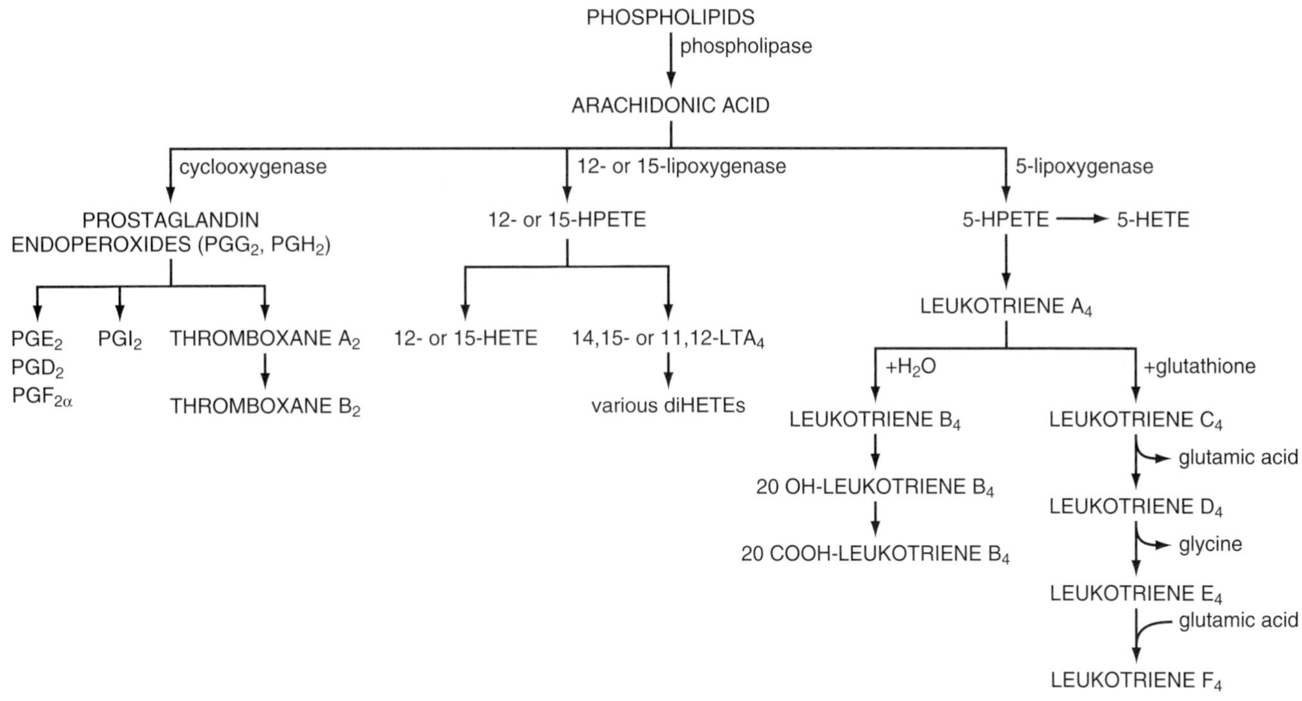

FIGURE 1-2 Lipid mediators of inflammation (see text for explanation). *HPETE*, Hydroperoxyeicosatetraenoic acid; *HETE*, hydroxyeicosatetraenoic acid; *LTA*, leukotriene A (From Davies P, Bailey PJ, Golderberg MM, et al: The role of arachidonic acid oxygenation products in pain and inflammation, *Annu Rev Immunol* 21:337, 1984).

Chemotaxis and Leukocyte Trafficking

One of the initial and most crucial aspects of the acute inflammatory response is the recruitment of leukocytes (primarily neutrophils) to the site of injury. Neutrophils constitute the first line of the cellular defense and are the initial cells involved in an inflammatory response. These phagocytic cells are derived from multipotent stem cells located chiefly in the bone marrow. Under the influence of a variety of signals provided from both within and outside of the bone marrow, these stem cells become committed to developing into cells of the granulocyte lineage. The critical signal is provided by a family of growth factors known as *colony-stimulating factors* (CSFs) that provide both proliferative and differentiative signals leading to the development of granulocytes and other leukocytes. Once released into the circulation, these cells must find their way to the site of the inflammatory response. The production of various chemotactic factors by host cells, bacteria, and other invaders causes various leukocytes to enter the circulation and be carried to the site of the injury.[21] Chemokines are soluble proteins produced by host cells that induce the directional migration and activation of leukocytes, as well as other somatic cell types, and thus play a major role in the inflammatory response.[22] Interleukin 8 (IL-8) plays a central role in this process. Other chemokines promote humoral and cell-mediated immune reactions; regulate cell adhesion, angiogenesis, leukocyte trafficking, and homing; and contribute to lymphopoiesis and hematopoiesis.[23]

The specific trafficking of leukocytes from the blood to inflammatory sites depends on both the production of chemotactic factors and the interaction of specific receptors on the leukocytes with corresponding adhesion molecules on the endothelial surface of the blood vessels. Neutrophil adherence is a two-step process first involving endothelial cell surface molecules known as *selectins*.[9] Small venular endothelium overlying a site of inflammation and exposed to thrombin, platelet activating factor (PAF), IL1, histamine, or other mediators released by clotting, platelet activation, or mast-cell activation express P-selectin.[24] P-selectin mediates the process in which neutrophils initially interact with the endothelial surface in a process known as "rolling," in which the circulating neutrophil interacts with the endothelial cell before the actual adherence.[25] Selectins function by binding to carbohydrate ligands present on the cell surface. In the case of neutrophils, the ligand is sialylated Lewis-X antigen for the endothelial E-selectin. The second part of the adherence process is the tight binding of *integrins* on the neutrophil surface with intracellular adhesion molecules (ICAMs) on the endothelial cell surface. Leukocyte integrins are heterodimeric proteins with distinct α and shared β polypeptide chains. The α and β chains can combine in different heterodimers to form multiple shared and unique specificities. Neutrophil expression of αMβ2 and αXβ2 is activation dependent. Neutrophils can be activated by a number of soluble proteins, including formylmethionylleucylphenylalanine (fMLP), *N*-formulated peptides present in bacterial but not eukaryotic proteins. Host factors present at the site of inflammation can also activate neutrophils, notably the complement proteins (C5a, C3a) and cytokines such as IL-8 and tumor necrosis factor (TNF), and immune complexes.[26] Expression of integrins by activated neutrophils allows them to become tethered to the endothelial surface. The migration of neutrophils through the vascular wall is less well understood than these initial events leading to firm adhesion. The β2 integrins, as well as αvβ3, PECAM-1 and integrin-associated protein (IAP), appear to play a role in this process. Endothelial

TABLE 1-2

Physiologic Effects of Lipid Mediators

Effect	LIPID MEDIATOR									
	PGD_2	PGE_2	$PGF_{2\alpha}$	PGI_2	TXA_2	LTB_4	LTC_4	LTD_4	LTE_4	PAF
Constricts smooth muscle	X		X	X	X	X	X	X	X	X
Dilates systemic vasculature	X									
Increases vascular permeability	X			X		X	X	X	X	X
Inhibits platelet aggregation	X			X						
Aggregates platelets					X					X
Increases vasodilation									X	
Arteriolar constriction and vasodilation							X	X		
Increases mucus production							X			X
Chemoattractant for neutrophils						X				
Inhibits leukocyte chemotaxis		X								
Relaxes smooth muscles		X								
Inhibits mediator release		X								
Stimulates mediator release						X				X

PGD_2, Prostaglandin D_2; *PGE_2*, prostaglandin E_2; *$PGF_{2\alpha}$*; prostaglandin $F_{2\alpha}$; *PGI_2*, prostaglandin I_2; *TXA_2*, thromboxane A_2; *LTB_4*, leukotriene D_4; *LTC_4*, leukotriene C_4; *LTD_4*, leukotriene D_4; *LTE_4*, leukotriene E_4; *PAF*, platelet-activating factor.

cell–produced IL-8 also is believed to have a critical role in this process. Once through the endothelium, the phagocytes will follow chemotactic signals and migrate toward the point of injury. They may adhere to other cells during migration to the site of inflammation, and these interactions also depend on αMβ2 and αXβ2 integrins. Migration through the extracellular matrix is mediated by β1, β3, and β5 integrins recognizing specific protein ligands.

Neutrophils recruited and activated in this manner will actively phagocytose microscopic invaders and attempt to destroy them using reactive oxygen products generated via an NADPH-oxidase–dependent "respiratory burst."[25,27] In the process the neutrophils release additional pro-inflammatory mediators, thus amplifying this response. Among those cells attracted to the area are *natural killer (NK)* cells capable of lysing virus-infected and other abnormal cells. The production of interferon-α/β by macrophages and other cells enhances the cytolytic activity of the NK cells. The NK cells themselves can be the source of interferon-γ, another pro-inflammatory cytokine. Depending on the magnitude of the initial insult and the susceptibility of the invader to neutophil-mediated destruction, the inflammatory response may be either acute or chronic.

Acute inflammation is thus a rapid response to an injury that is characterized by accumulations of fluid, plasma proteins, and neutrophils that rapidly resolves once the initial inflammatory stimulus is removed. Deactivation signals include PGE_2, cortisol, IL-10, and transforming growth factor-β (TGF-β). Some of those chemotactic agents responsible for initiating the response (IL-8, FMLP, C5a, LTB4, and PAF) also serve to downregulate its intensity by inducing the shedding of IL-1 receptors from neutrophils.[28] The shedding of this decoy receptor may have anti-inflammatory effects as it effectively binds and neutralizes this cytokine. Likewise, many of the acute phase proteins are thought to have immunomodulatory activity downregulating neutrophil function.[29] Acute inflammatory responses may often be subclinical and resolve without complications. However, if the invader is resistant to neutrophil-mediated destruction or the degree of injury is large, the response may become more chronic with the added recruitment of macrophages and lymphocytes, and fibroblast growth.

The essential characteristic of the innate immune response is that it does not exhibit specificity for the invading organism. Thus the induction of an innate immune response does not require prior exposure to the invading organism nor is it augmented by repeated exposure to the same organism. Whereas resistance may be genetically controlled, the genes encoding resistance are not found within the gene complex that controls adaptive immune responses. In most instances these mechanisms are adequate for eliminating casual invaders. However, pathogenic organisms have evolved various methods for avoiding elimination. In response to these organisms, the specialized cells and products of the adaptive immune response are mobilized.

ADAPTIVE IMMUNITY

The adaptive immune response is initiated in response to an encounter with a foreign agent and depends on antigen-specific immune responses mediated by different divisions of the lymphocyte family (Figure 1-3). In contrast to the nonspecific nature of the innate immune response, an important characteristic of the adaptive immune response is the specificity of this interaction. Thus exposure of the host to a particular microbe or parasite results in the induction of immune responses that are directed against specific components of the invading organism that do not affect unrelated organisms. The specificity of the adaptive immune response is the result of the interaction of specific molecular structures or *antigens* of the invader with antigen-specific receptors on lymphocytes. All types of chemical structures can serve as antigens, but not all antigens can induce an immune response. *Immunogens*, those antigens that can stimulate an immune response, are usually high molecular–weight, chemically complex molecules. Proteins, nucleic acids, lipids, and polysaccharides can all serve as immunogens. Large immunogens, such as proteins, contain multiple *antigenic determinants* or epitopes, which interact with lymphocytes via their antigen-specific receptors. Haptens consist of single antigenic determinants and can effectively combine with the binding site of antibody molecules. However, because they consist only of a single antigenic determinant, they cannot cross link B-cell receptors (antibody molecules), and they are also unable to stimulate T cell responses. Haptens therefore cannot stimulate an immune response unless multiple haptens are physically attached to a larger molecule, known as a *carrier*. Although these distinctions between antigens, haptens, and immunogens appear minor, they provide the underlying basis for our understanding of many allergic and autoimmune responses.

Like the innate response, the adaptive immune response to a specific antigen consists of both humoral and cellular effector mechanisms. The humoral component is mediated by immunoglobulins or antibodies found in plasma and tissue fluids. Antibodies are produced by B lymphocytes, small lymphoid cells characterized by the cell surface expression of immunoglobulin molecules. B cells represent fewer than 15% of the circulating peripheral blood mononuclear cells but are present in higher proportions in lymph nodes and the spleen. B cells are derived from the fetal liver and bone marrow of mammals and the bursa of Fabricius of birds. In the bone marrow B cells are the products of a putative lymphoid stem cell derived from the pluripotent stem cell. Under the influence of various cytokines produced by bone marrow *stromal* cells, the B cell precursor undergoes its 3-day development into a mature B cell. Upon stimulation with specific antigen, B cells differentiate into *plasma cells* that produce enormous quantities of specific antibody. The activation, proliferation, and differentiation of B lymphocytes into plasma cells depends on other cells, including T lymphocytes, which represent the cellular component of the adaptive immune response. The T lymphocyte is also derived from the multipotent stem cell and lymphoid precursor in the bone marrow, although its subsequent development into the mature T cell occurs in the *thymus*. Within the thymic environment the prothymocyte undergoes a developmental and selective process while emigrating through the cortex into the medullary region of the thymus. Fewer than 3% of all the immature thymocytes found in the cortex survive to become peripheral T cells.

Although the induction of an antibody response requires the interaction of B and T lymphocytes, these cells recognize

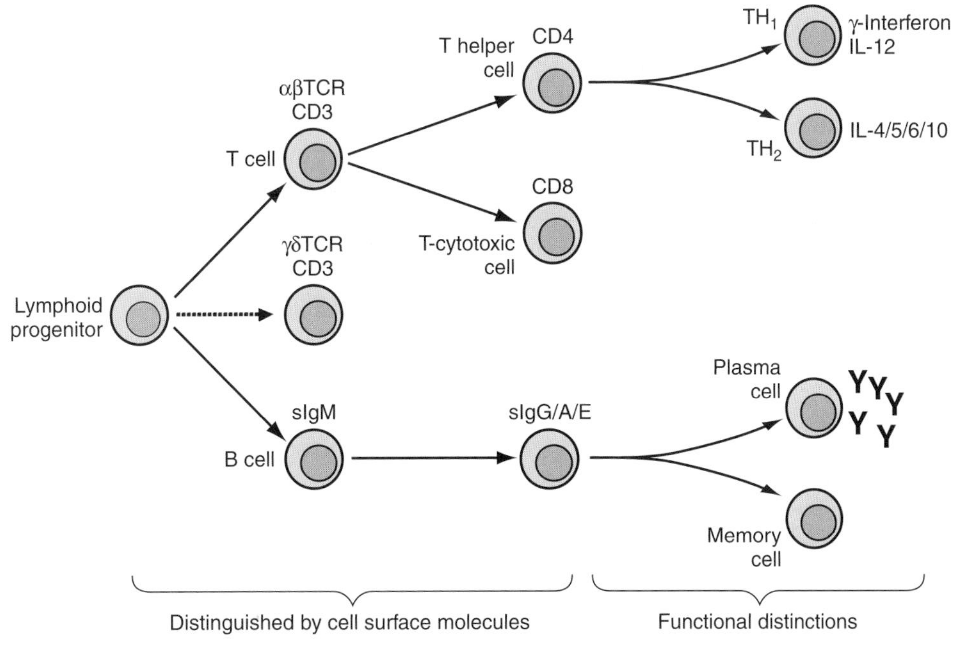

FIGURE 1-3 Major divisions of the lymphocyte family. To the left of the diagram, different populations of lymphocytes are distinguished by expression of different cell surface molecules. To the right of the diagram, the distinctions are functional.

different epitopes on the same antigen. Indeed, antigen recognition by B cells and T cells is fundamentally quite different. B cells, and antibodies, recognize antigens in solution or on cell surfaces in their native conformation, whereas T cells recognize antigen only in association with self molecules known as *major histocompatability complex* antigens found on most cells' surfaces. The adaptive immune response thus differs from innate immunity in that it is antigen driven and those cells that mediate the adaptive immune responses, T and B lymphocytes, express specific receptors for the antigen. Because the immune system will respond to the antigens of both live and killed pathogens, it is possible to stimulate immunity without causing infection, which is the basis of vaccination. Although this principle appears to be straightforward, vaccination does not always yield the expected result. Why some vaccines work and others fail is a complex issue, a major component of which is the nature of the antigen-specific receptors of lymphocytes.

Immunoglobulin: Antigen-specific Receptor of B Lymphocytes

The antigen-specific receptor of the B cell is cell surface–bound antibody. An antibody molecule is composed of two identical light chains and two identical heavy chains that form a disulfide-linked Y-shaped molecule (Figure 1-4). The light chain can be divided into two domains, a conserved carboxy-terminal domain and a highly variable amino-terminal domain. Analysis of heavy chains reveals a similar domain structure, with the amino-terminal domain being highly variable and the presence of three constant domains. The antigen-binding region of an antibody molecule is formed by the association of the amino ends of a light and a heavy chain, whereas the carboxyl end of the heavy chain determines the isotype of the molecule. Five different *isotypes,* or classes, of antibody molecules have been identified in most species, including the horse: IgD, IgM, IgG, IgA, and IgE (Table 1-3).[30,31] Additionally, the IgG isotype can be subdivided into subclasses based on physico-chemical properties. Analysis of equine genomic DNA has indicated the existence of one IgM, one IgD, one IgE, one IgA, and seven IgG genes.[31] Before the availability of genetic characterization of the equine immunoglobulin heavy chain gene loci, at least four IgG subclasses were identified by physico-chemical means and defined serologically by monoclonal antibodies as IgGa, IgGb, IgGc, and IgG(T).[32] Each of these "classical" (older) IgG subclasses has been identified as a gene product of one or more of the equine heavy chain gene loci.[30,31] It appears that both IgGb and IgG(T) are encoded by two loci each, raising the possibility that these classical subclasses may each comprise two distinct subclasses. At the time of writing, this remains uncertain, although ongoing studies are starting to resolve the issue.[30] The gene product of at least one IgG heavy chain locus is not defined by the classical IgG subclasses, and it remains to be determined whether it is expressed as a protein and what its role may be.[31] Given the current remaining uncertainties as to the role of equine IgG subclasses as defined by nomenclature based on heavy chain gene locus, this edition of this text will continue to use the classical nomenclature.

Membrane-bound IgM and IgD serve as the antigen-specific receptors for B lymphocytes. Each contains a membrane-spanning region near its carboxy end that is inserted into the mRNA during differential splicing of the heavy chain exons. Although rarely detectable in the circulation, IgD is

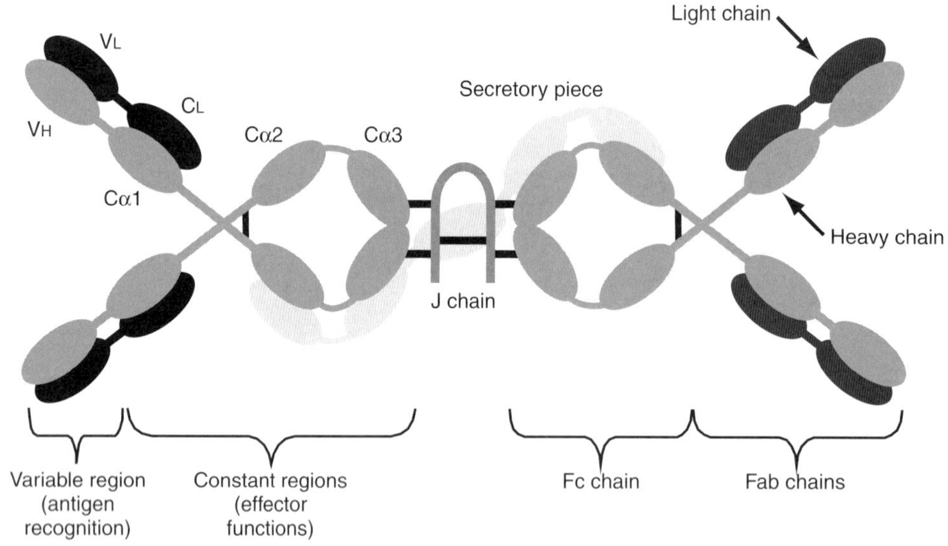

FIGURE 1-4 Molecular structure of secretory immunoglobulin (Ig) A. This schematic illustrates the major features of immunoglobulin molecules. The illustrated IgA molecule is dimeric, with the two immunoglobulin units joined by a "J-chain" and a series of disulphide bonds, and IgG molecules are monomeric. Each immunoglobulin unit consists of two heavy chains and two light chains. The heavy chains have four subunits and the light chains two. One end of the immunoglobulin unit has a highly variable protein structure and is involved in antigen recognition, whereas the remainder of the immunoglobulin unit has a constant structure in each immunoglobulin class and subclass and determines the functional characteristics of the molecule, such as binding complement, or recognition by macrophages or neutrophil Fc receptors. This specialized dimeric IgA molecule also has a secretory piece that increases its stability in the harsh mucosal environment.

TABLE 1-3

Immunoglobulin Isotypes	
Isotype	**Immunologic Function**
IgD	Antigen receptor of naïve B lymphocytes. An IgD heavy chain gene has been identified in the horse, and it is probably expressed.
IgM	Surface IgM is found on naïve, activated, and memory B cells. Secreted IgM is a pentamer and represents the major antibody produced during a primary response. IgM efficiently mediates agglutination, neutralization, opsonization, and complement activation.
IgG	The principle immunoglobulin found in plasma representing up to 80% of the total immunoglobulin concentration. Various subclasses of IgG have been identified (see text). The classical view is that there are four IgG subclasses in the horse (IgGa, IgGb, IgGc, and IgG(T)) defined by physicochemical properties and monoclonal antibodies, although seven IgG heavy chain genes have been identified and there is evidence that all are expressed. The major functions of IgG include opsonization and neutralization reactions. IgGa and IgGb are effective in fixing complement and participates in antibody-dependent cellular cytotoxicity (ADCC) while IgGc and IgG(T) are not, although they appear to play an important role in exotoxin neutralization and immunity to parasites. As our understanding of IgG heavy chain gene expression and function increases, a new nomenclature (i.e., IgG1–7) will replace the classical nomenclature (i.e., IgGa).
IgA	IgA, the most abundant antibody in secretions (e.g., tears, mucus, saliva, colostrum) is a dimer composed of two IgA molecules joined by a J chain. IgA in the plasma is predominantly monomeric. IgA antibodies can be neutralizing but only activate complement via the alternative pathway.
IgE	Most IgE is found associated with the surface of mast cells and basophils and only very small amounts are present in the plasma. The cross-linking of two IgE moleulces with specific antigen results in the degranulation of the mast cells and basophils. Thus IgE is the primary antibody responsible for Type I hypersensitivity reactions and appears to play a central role in immunity to parasites.

Data from Wagner B. Immunoglobulins and immunoglobulin genes of the horse. *Dev Comp Immunol* 2006;30:155-164; Lewis MJ, Wagner B, Woof JM. The different effector function capabilities of the seven equine IgG subclasses have implications for vaccine strategies. *Mol Immunol* 2008;45:818-827; and Wagner B, Miller DC, Lear TL, Antczak DF. The complete map of the Ig heavy chain constant gene region reveals evidence for seven IgG isotypes and for IgD in the horse. *Journal of Immunology* 2004;173:3230-3242.
Ig, immunoglobulin.

present in large quantities on the surface of naïve B lymphocytes. Following activation, the surface expression of IgD is lost, although the cell may continue to express the membrane form of IgM. Early in an immune response, the B cell secretes large amounts of the pentameric form of IgM. As the immune response proceeds, the B cell will switch the isotype of its heavy chain. Isotype switching involves the substitution of one heavy chain–constant region in place of another. The genes encoding the five different constant regions of the heavy chain are sequentially arranged on the chromosome (C_δ, C_μ, C_γ, C_ε, and C_α). Initially, the first two constant region genes encoding the δ and μ constant regions are used to form the heavy chain. The 5′ region of each constant region gene segment contains repetitive regions of DNA known as *switch sequences*.[33] The switch sequences appear to play a role in this rearrangement and may serve as the target for specific recombinases. When switching occurs, a new constant region segment is selected and the intervening genes are removed either by splicing or looping out. Isotype switching affects only the heavy chain–constant domains and has no effect on the antigen specificity of the immunoglobulin molecule. The signal for B cells to undergo isotype switching is provided by T lymphocytes in the form of various cytokines.[34] For example, IL-4 induces isotype switching to the IgE isotype, whereas interferon-γ blocks this induction and augments IgG production.[35,36] IgA is produced in response to the combination of the cytokines IL-4, IL-5, and transforming growth factor-ß (TGF-β).[37]

The antigen specificity of a particular antibody molecule (and the B cell that produces it) is determined by the combination of the variable domains of the light and heavy chains. The association of these two domains results in the formation of an antigen-binding groove or pocket that contains regions of hypervariability that define the specificity of a particular antibody molecule. It has been estimated that more than 10^8 different antibody specificities are possible. The generation of this tremendous amount of diversity in antibody specificity occurs during B cell ontogeny in the bone marrow.[38] Within a given B cell, the genes encoding the heavy and light chains of an antibody molecule are organized into specific gene segments. Thus the light chain is formed from variable (V_l), joining (J_l), and constant (C_l) gene segments that together form the variable and constant domains of the light chain. In the germ line of an undifferentiated cell, several hundred different V_l and several dozen J_l gene segments can be found. Likewise, the heavy chain of a B lymphocyte is composed of V_H, diversity (D), and J_H segments that form the variable domain, and these join to the constant region genes to form the complete heavy chain molecule. Similarly, in the germ line a large number of V_H gene segments and a smaller number of D and J_H segments are found. During the differentiation of a B cell (Figure 1-5), there is the sequential selection and rearrangement of a V_L segment with a J_L segment and the accompanying deletion of intervening V_L and J_L segments (Figure 1-6). The rearranged VJC sequence is then transcribed into mRNA and translated into the light chain. A somewhat similar sequence follows for

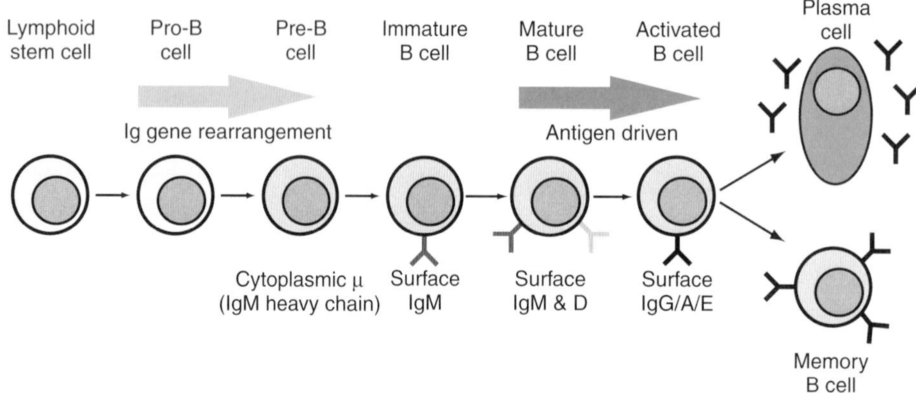

FIGURE 1-5 B cell differentiation. Different stages of B lymphocyte development can be recognized by expression of immunoglobulin molecules. This maturation requires a series of gene rearrangements in order to select the genes that will encode the antigen binding part of the immunoglobulin molecule (variable region) and subsequently to select the genes that determine the class or subclass of the antibody molecule. Initially immature B cells express IgM (the majority of peripheral blood B cells), but after antigen exposure the B cell becomes activated and may express any of the immunoglobulin classes or subclasses. This decision depends in large part on cytokine signals from T-helper cells. Finally activated B cells either mature into short-lived antibody secreting plasma cells or become long-lived memory B cells.

heavy chains except that two rearrangements are necessary, a D to J_H rearrangement followed by a V_H to DJ_H rearrangement. Once completed, the VDJ segment is brought into the proximity of the appropriate C_H segment and transcribed. Not all of the gene segment rearrangements produce functional genes. Because a B cell has two sets of heavy chain genes, one on each chromosome, and most species, including the horse, have two different sets of light chain genes,[39,40] there are several chances to form appropriate heavy and light chains. Once the heavy and light chain gene segments are successfully recombined, the genes on the sister chromosome neither recombine nor are they expressed. This process of allelic exclusion ensures that the B cell produces antibodies of a single specificity. Although this random assortment of gene segments accounts for much of the diversity in antibody specificity, additional mechanisms are also involved, including junctional diversity, which results from the imprecise joining of gene segments and somatic mutations. Somatic mutations are point mutations in the hypervariable region of either the heavy or light chain that occur during the proliferation of antigen-activated B lymphocytes. Such mutations appear to play a role in increasing antibody affinity for its antigen. Thus fewer than 1000 genes can give rise to more than 10^8 molecules of the various specificities needed to recognize the vast number of antigens the host may encounter.

TcR and CD3 Complex: Antigen-specific Receptor of T Cells

T lymphocytes can be differentiated from B lymphocytes in that they do not express surface immunoglobulins but instead express the T cell receptor (TcR). T cells also express another antigen called *CD3*. (The designation *CD* stands for *cluster designate* and is the result of an international workshop to standardize the terminology used to describe leukocyte surface antigens recognized by monoclonal antibodies.) The TcR and CD3 form a multimeric complex on the T cell surface, and this complex is involved in antigen-specific recognition.[41] The TcR structure was first identified using antibodies that recognized a surface antigen expressed on a cloned T lymphoma cell line. This antibody recognized a disulfide-linked heterodimer composed of an acidic (α) and a basic (β) protein of 40 to 45,000 molecular weight. Similar heterodimers were found on a variety of antigen-specific T cell lines but not on B cells. Peptide mapping studies of the α and ß chains from many different T cell lines demonstrated that they contained variable and constant domains reminiscent of immunoglobulin structure. Further analysis indicated that, like immunoglobulin genes, the TcR genes underwent gene rearrangements during T cell development. Subsequently, two additional TcR genes were identified, the γ chain and δ genes corresponding to a second heterodimer. Thus two TcR exist, an α/β heterodimer that constitutes the TcR on almost 90% of all T cells and a γ/δ heterodimer present on approximately 10% of the peripheral T cells. The significance of these two different TcR heterodimers has not yet been determined. It should be noted that γ/δ T cells have not yet been identified in the horse. It is clear that γ/δ T cells represent a functionally distinct population of T cells typically associated with mucosal surfaces.[42] As such they are thought to play an important role in immunologic surveillance.

Analysis of the predicted amino acid sequences for the TcR proteins confirmed a structural similarity with antibody molecules. One peculiarity in the structure of the TcR was observed from the amino acid sequence analysis. Whereas both the α and β chains of the TcR contained a transmembrane region, both proteins had very short cytoplasmic tails. It therefore seemed unlikely that TcR itself could transmit any cytoplasmic signal in response to antigen binding. This led to the search for other proteins associated with the TcR. Solubilization of the T cell membranes revealed that five other proteins could be immunoprecipitated with the TcR. Similar results were obtained when anti-CD3 antibodies were used. Thus the TcR heterodimer is noncovalently associated with

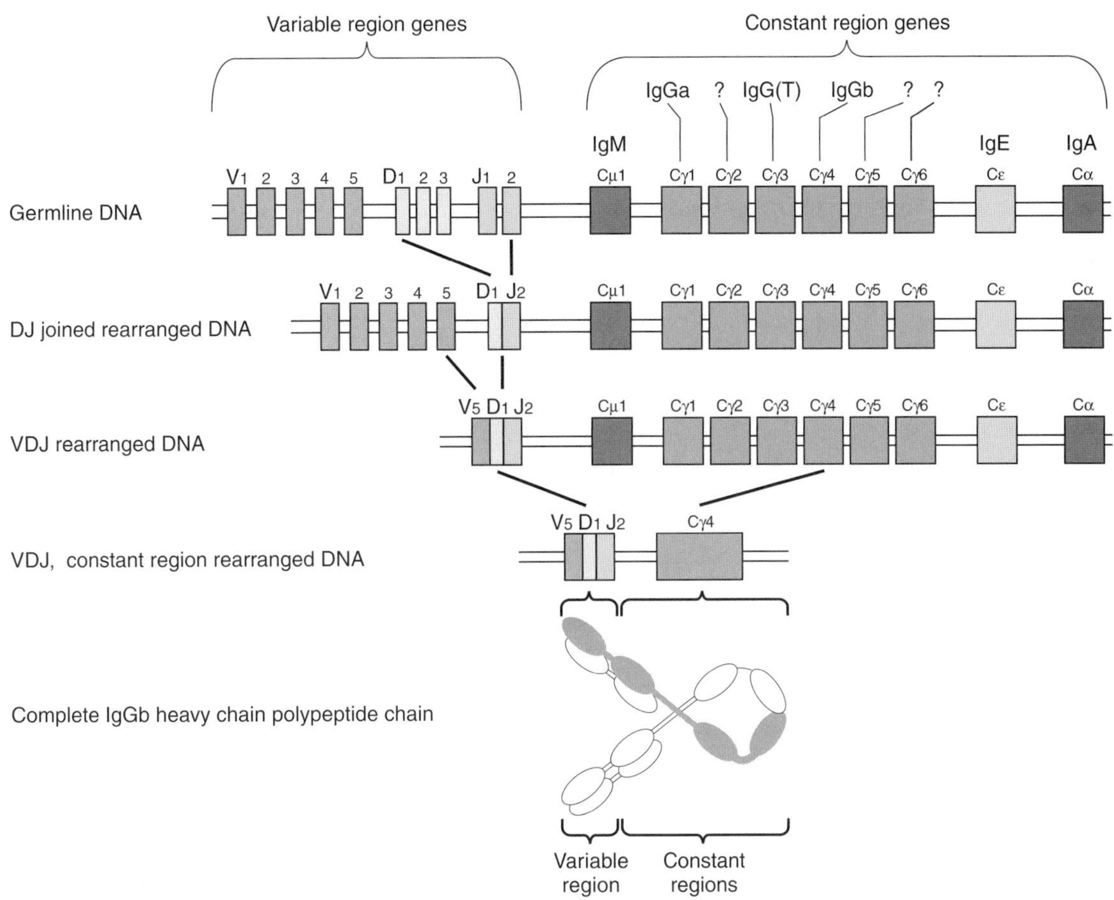

FIGURE 1-6 Immunoglobulin gene rearrangement–somatic recombination process for production of an immunoglobulin heavy chain. The figure shows a hypothetical series of V, D, and J variable heavy chain genes, positioned 5′ to the known equine heavy chain constant region gene loci. In the first step in somatic recombination a D and a J gene segment are joined, and in the second step a V gene segment is joined to complete the VDJ recombination and form a gene capable of encoding the variable region. Subsequently one of the seven equine γ heavy chain constant regions, labeled with their corresponding IgG subclass when known, was selected to complete the gene rearrangement. Because the Cγ4 heavy chain constant region gene was selected, this leads to production of an IgGb heavy chain.

the CD3 complex of proteins. The five proteins of the CD3 complex (γ, δ, ε, ζ, and ξ) are involved in signal transduction following TcR binding to antigen.[43] Unlike the TcR α and β proteins, the CD3 proteins have large intracellular domains, some of which are phosphorylated in response to stimulation of the TcR. In addition to providing a signaling mechanism for the TcR, the CD3 complex is also required for the expression of the TcR heterodimer on the cell surface.[41]

The generation of diversity in the TcR during T cell ontogeny employs a mechanism quite similar to that used to generate immunoglobulin diversity. The TcR α and γ chains resemble immunoglobulin light chains in that they are composed of V, J, and C gene segments. The particular V, J, and C segments used are selected from a germ line configuration containing a few (C region) to several hundred (V region) gene segments. The selection and rearrangement of the gene segments are similar to those employed by the immunoglobulin light chain and appear to involve the same recombinase. Likewise, the β and δ chains resemble heavy chains, each being composed of V, D, J, and C gene segments, and their selection and rearrangement from germ line genes also parallel immunoglobulin heavy chain rearrangement. Thus the generation of diversity is the result of the combination of multiple gene segments and junctional diversity. However, unlike immunoglobulins, the TcR genes do not undergo somatic mutations.

T Lymphocyte Subsets

Mature thymocytes and T lymphocytes can be further divided into two distinct populations on the basis of their expression of either the CD4 or CD8 antigen.[44] The expression of these antigens is directly correlated with the specificity of the T cell. The expression of either CD4 or CD8 also correlates to some extent with the T cell's function. Thus those cells that express the CD8 antigen are typically CTLs, whereas those that express the CD4 antigen are typically helper cells that produce those cytokines that enhance antibody and cell-mediated immune responses. Whereas the T lymphocytes in the periphery express either CD4 or CD8 antigens, cortical thymocytes express both antigens. During the process of thymic selection, these cells convert to either $CD4^+$ or $CD8^+$ cells or they are eliminated (Figure 1-7). It is at this stage of their development that T cells are said to "learn" to recognize antigen. It is also at this stage

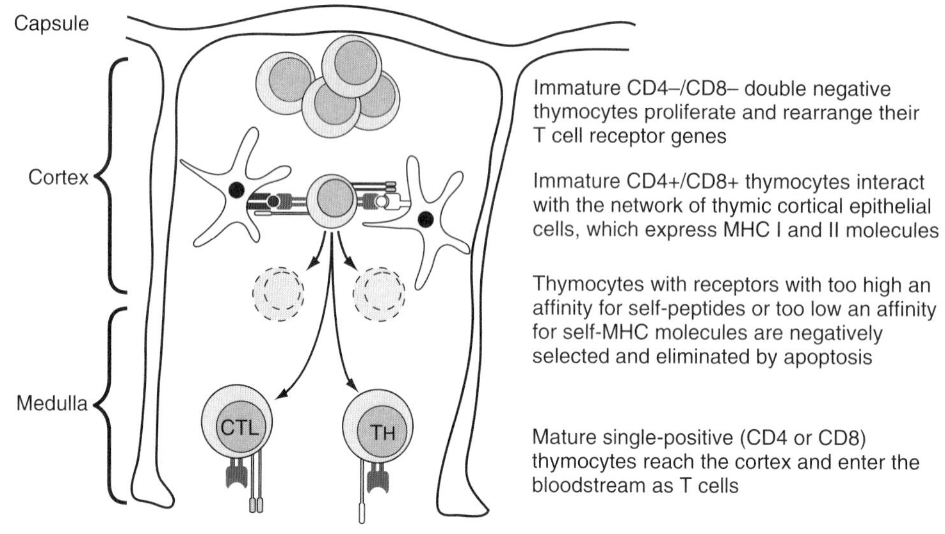

FIGURE 1-7 Thymic development.

that autoreactive T cells are eliminated. Although experimental studies have shown that both positive and negative selection of the T cells is occurring, the exact mechanism of these selective processes remains unknown. Interestingly, although T cells expressing the α/β heterodimer of the TcR can be either $CD4^+$ or $CD8^+$, γ/δ cells are either $CD8^+$ or $CD4^-$ CD8. These results suggest that the γ/δ cells undergo a different developmental process than do the α/β cells. Like the CD3 complex, both the CD4 and the CD8 antigen are involved in the intracellular signaling event following TcR engagement with its specific antigen. Unlike B cells, and antibodies, that recognize antigens in solution or on cell surfaces in their native conformation, T cells recognize only *processed* antigen in association with self molecules known as *major histocompatability complex* (MHC) antigens.

Major Histocompatibility Antigens and Antigen Presentation

The MHC was originally defined in terms of its role in allograft rejection. Following the rejection of a primary allograft, antibodies that reacted with the allograft could be found in the recipient's sera. These antibodies could be used to identify or type tissues to determine the suitability of a donor for transplantation. It was also determined that multiparous females had similar antibodies in their sera as a result of the exposure to paternal MHC antigens on the fetus.[45] Through the use of these sera, it was possible to identify a large number of serologically defined transplantation antigens. Subsequent genetic analysis of the MHC region demonstrated that there were a number of closely linked genes encoding several different, though related, antigens that were involved in allograft rejection. These closely related genes are collectively referred to as *MHC I genes* and their products as *MHC I antigens*. In addition to the serologically defined MHC I antigens, another group of antigens was identified within the MHC; these antigens were involved in the stimulation of mixed lymphocyte responses and the control of immune responsiveness. These MHC II antigens are structurally and functionally distinct from the MHC I antigens, except that both are involved in T cell recognition of antigen.

MHC I antigens are cell surface glycoproteins consisting of two noncovalently associated proteins, an MHC-encoded transmembrane protein of approximately 44 kd (α chain) and $ß_2$-microglobulin, a 12 kd protein encoded outside of the MHC.[3] MHC I antigens are expressed on the surface of most nucleated cells. The highest level of expression is on lymphoid cells with lower expression on fibroblasts, muscle cells, and neural cells. MHC I antigens are not detectable on early embryonal cells, placental cells, and some carcinomas. The level of expression of MHC I antigen can be modified by treatment with cytokines or infection with viruses. Interferons and TNF-α augment MHC I antigen expression. This augmented expression is the result of increased production of MHC I mRNA, and the regulatory region of the MHC I antigen genes has been shown to contain interferon and TNF-α responsive elements that control the transcriptional activity of these genes.

The MHC I region of most animal species, including the horse, contains a number of MHC I α chain genes, some of which are pseudogenes and are not expressed.[46] The known total of different equine MHC class I genes (loci) expressed as mRNA is seven.[47] In the horse these genes are located on chromosome 20, and those genes that are expressed exhibit a great deal of polymorphism.[48,49] Much of this polymorphism is localized in the α_1 and α_2 domains, the α_3 domain being more conserved. The polymorphism of these two domains is related to their role in presenting antigen to T cells. The physiologic role of MHC I antigens was defined when it was discovered that cytotoxic T cell (CTL) lysis of virus-infected cells was restricted to target cells expressing the same MHC I antigen as the CTL.[50] This observation led to the realization that T cells recognized the combination of self-MHC and foreign antigen. Furthermore, those T cells that recognized MHC I antigens invariably expressed the CD8 co-receptor. The nature of the association between MHC I and the foreign antigen remained unclear until X-ray crystallographic studies of human MHC I antigen were performed.[51,52] In addition to revealing the structural organization of the domains of the MHC I antigen, the image also revealed a cleft that lay between the α_1 and α_2 domains. It was proposed that this cleft binds the processed peptide epitopes for presentation to the T cell receptor. Indeed, the cleft of the cyrstalized protein used for the X-ray diffraction studies was found to contain a contaminating peptide.[51] Other experiments showed that the incubation of cells with purified viral peptides resulted in the lysis of the cells by virus-specific, MHC I–restricted CTL.[52] Together these results support the notion that the *endogenous processing* of viral antigens leads to the association of viral peptides with MHC I antigens on the surface of the infected cell, and this is recognized by the TcR-CD3 complex in association with CD8.[52] How these viral antigens get to the cell surface is the result of a peptide transport system whose function is to transport processed peptides from the cytosol to the ER.[53] Once in this compartment, peptides are handed off to newly formed MHC class I molecules and stabilize a trimolecular complex with β2 microglobulin. This complex is then transported to the cell surface, where antigen presentation occurs. Because this is a normal cellular process for eliminating degraded proteins from the cell, it is not surprising that MHC I antigens are normally loaded with these self-peptides. Indeed, it is this encounter with MHC I loaded with self-peptides in the thymus that is responsible for the deletion of autoreactive clones during T cell ontogeny. This unique peptide-binding characteristic of MHC-I molecules has led to their use as immunologic reagents (tetramers) for the identification and enumeration of antigen-specific $CD8^+$ T cells.[54] In the horse tetramers based on the equine MHC class I molecule 7-6, associated with the ELA-A1 haplotype, have been used to identify and enumerate equine infectious anemia virus (EIAV)–specific cytotoxic T cells.[55] In the future similar approaches may be used to analyze CTL responses to a variety of viruses and provide important information on the role these cells play in protection from these infections.

MHC II antigens are heterodimeric, transmembrane glycoproteins composed of an acidic α chain (25 to 35 kd) and a basic β chain (25 to 30 kd).[56] A third chain, the invariant chain, is associated with the MHC II antigen during assembly in the endoplasmic reticulum but is not expressed on the cell surface. Both the α and β polypeptides are encoded within the MHC region. Both polypeptides possess two extracellular domains. The α chain has a single disulfide bond located in its membrane proximal (α_2) domain, and the β chain has a disulfide bond in both of its extracellular domains. Structurally, the MHC II antigens resemble MHC I antigens and are also members of the immunoglobulin superfamily, a group of proteins that have structural similarities to immunoglobulin molecules (Figure 1-8).[57]

The MHC II genes are functionally and structurally distinct from the MHC I genes. Unlike MHC I antigens, the MHC II antigens are restricted in their expression to certain cells of the immune system: B lymphocytes, dendritic cells, macrophages, and activated T lymphocytes of some species. Other cells may also express MHC II antigens after treatment with various cytokines.[58-60] Interferon-γ, TNF-α, 1,25-dihydroxyvitamin-D3, and granulocyte-macrophage colony stimulating factor can induce MHC II antigen expression on monocytes and macrophages and other cells. IL-4 enhances MHC II antigen on B cells. A number of agents downregulate MHC II antigen expression, including glucocorticoids, prostaglandins, and α-fetoprotein. Although MHC II antigen expression is also regulated at the transcriptional level, no interferon or TNF-α response elements have been identified in the regulatory regions of MHC II genes. In fact, the regulatory region of MHC I and MHC II genes are quite different, and this fact is probably responsible for the differences in tissue distribution for these two MHC antigens.[46]

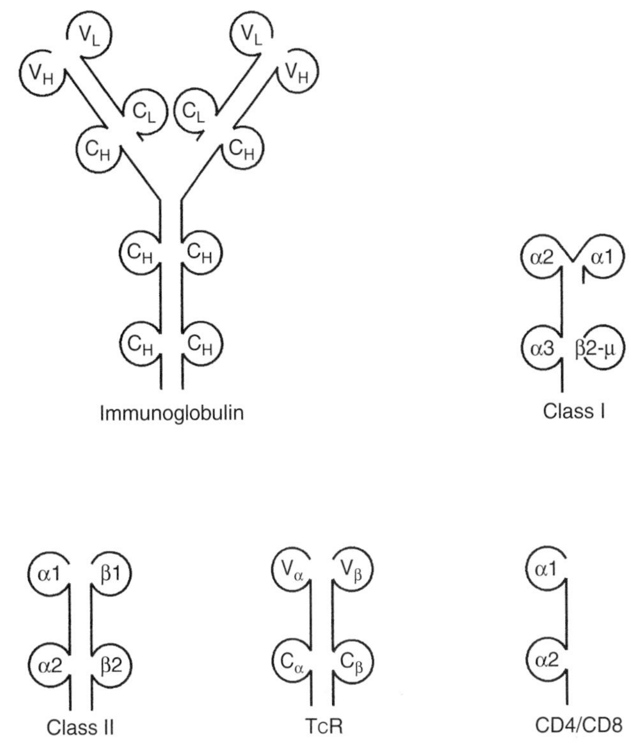

FIGURE 1-8 The immunoglobulin superfamily. Immunoglobulin serves as the prototype model for the superfamily. Both the heavy and light chains of an immunoglobulin molecule can be divided into variable (V_H and V_L) and constant domains (C_H and C_L). Analogous regions have been identified on a variety of other molecules involved in immune recognition including class I and class II antigens, the T cell antigen receptor (TcR), and the CD4 and CD8 antigens found on T cells (see text). Disulfide bonds forming the domains are not shown.

Like the MHC I genes, the MHC II region contains genes for multiple MHC II antigens, some of which appear to be pseudogenes and are not expressed. Those α and β chains that are expressed exhibit a high degree of allelic variability, although typically the β chain exhibits the most polymorphism. Unlike the MHC I genes, the variability in the MHC II genes is the result of point mutations. There is also correspondingly less polymorphism in the MHC II genes when compared with the MHC I genes. The MHC II region of other species, including the horse, have been studied using human DNA probes, and extensive polymorphism involving several genes has been identified.

Whereas antigens processed via the endogenous pathway are associated with MHC I antigens, antigen processed via the *exogenous pathway* is associated with MHC II antigens (Figure 1-9).[52] Here endocytosed antigen, such as that phagocytosed by a macrophage, is partially degraded in a prelysosomal compartment of low pH and limited proteolytic activity. The processed protein associates with a peptide binding site at the junction of the α_1 and β_1 domains of the MHC II molecule. This association of the epitope with the MHC II molecule protects it from further degradation. The MHC II molecule is then re-expressed on the cell surface for subsequent presentation to the T cell. The immune system contains a distinct group of antigen-presenting cells called *dendritic cells* (DCs) that are specialized to capture antigens and initiate T cell immunity

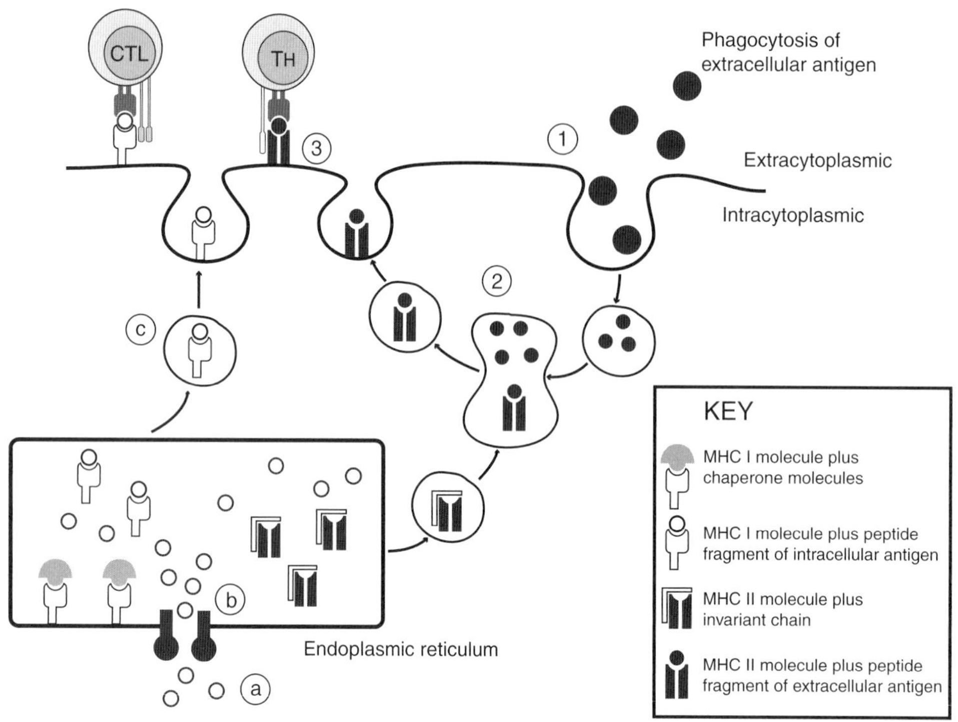

FIGURE 1-9 Antigen processing pathways. This figure depicts major histocompatibility complex (MHC) I antigen presentation to the left of the diagram and MHC II antigen presentation to the right. In MHC I antigen presentation (a) peptides generated by degradation of proteins in the cytoplasm are transported into the endoplasmic reticulum (b). In this location MHC I molecules bound by a membrane protein calnexin bind the peptides, which allows release of the MHC I molecules by the calnexin and transport through the Golgi complex to the cell surface (c). In MHC II antigen presentation antigen is taken up by phagocytosis (1) into the endosome compartment and routed to lysosomes for degradation. Vesicles containing MHC II molecules produced in the endoplasmic reticulum fuse with the endosomes (2) and the MHC II molecules bind with the degraded peptides for transport back to the cell surface (3). The MHC II molecules are prevented from binding the endogenous peptides in the endoplasmic reticulum by the presence of invariant chain, which is only lost in the acidic endosomal environment.

and move freely from epithelial surfaces to adjoining lymph nodes.[3] DCs can be found in a variety of locations in the body and are often named according to their microscopic appearance. Hence interdigitating cells found in lymph nodes, veiled cells in lymphatics, and Langerhan's cells in skin are all DCs. Immature DCs can take up antigens by micropinocytosis using their extensive cellular processes or receptor mediated phagocytosis. This results in activation and migration to a regional lymph node where antigen presentation to T lymphocytes occurs. Mature DCs have high levels of MHC II expression on their surfaces and are no longer phagocytic but are extremely efficient stimulators of both MHC I– and MHC II–restricted T cell responses in the draining lymph node (Figure 1-10).

In a complex immunogen certain antigenic determinants are particularly effective at stimulating an antibody response. These *immunodominant* epitopes are often located at exposed areas of the antigen such as in polypeptide loops. These types of structures are often quite mobile and may allow for easier access to the antibody binding site. T cell epitopes possess a particular structural characteristic of amphipathic helices. However, structure alone does not determine the immunogenicity of a particular antigen, and T cell recognition of foreign antigen requires more than just the expression of the processed antigen on the surface of the antigen presenting cell. Additional signals provided by the antigen presenting cell are also required for the activation of the T lymphocytes. Among these are signals provided by other accessory molecules found on the antigen presenting cell and various cytokines present in the extracellular environment.

Signaling Through the Antigen-specific Receptors

The encounter of specific antigen either by a T cell or a B cell's antigen-specific receptor results in an intracellular signaling cascade that eventually leads to the production of various proteins and the proliferation of the stimulated cell. T cell recognition of antigen involves the engagement of a TcR-CD3-CD4 or TcR-CD3-CD8 complex with processed peptide in the cleft of a MHC II or MHC I molecule (Figure 1-11).[3] The engagement of the TcR-CD3 complex with the appropriate MHC antigen containing peptide results in the binding of CD4 or CD8, depending on the MHC antigen, with the TcR-CD3 complex. In doing so the Lck protein tyrosine kinase associated with the cytoplasmic tail of CD4/CD8 phosphorylates the cytoplasmic regions of the CD3 proteins in regions known as *immunoreceptor tyrosine-based activation motifs* (ITAMs; Figure 1-12). These ITAMs serve as docking sites for other kinases, including

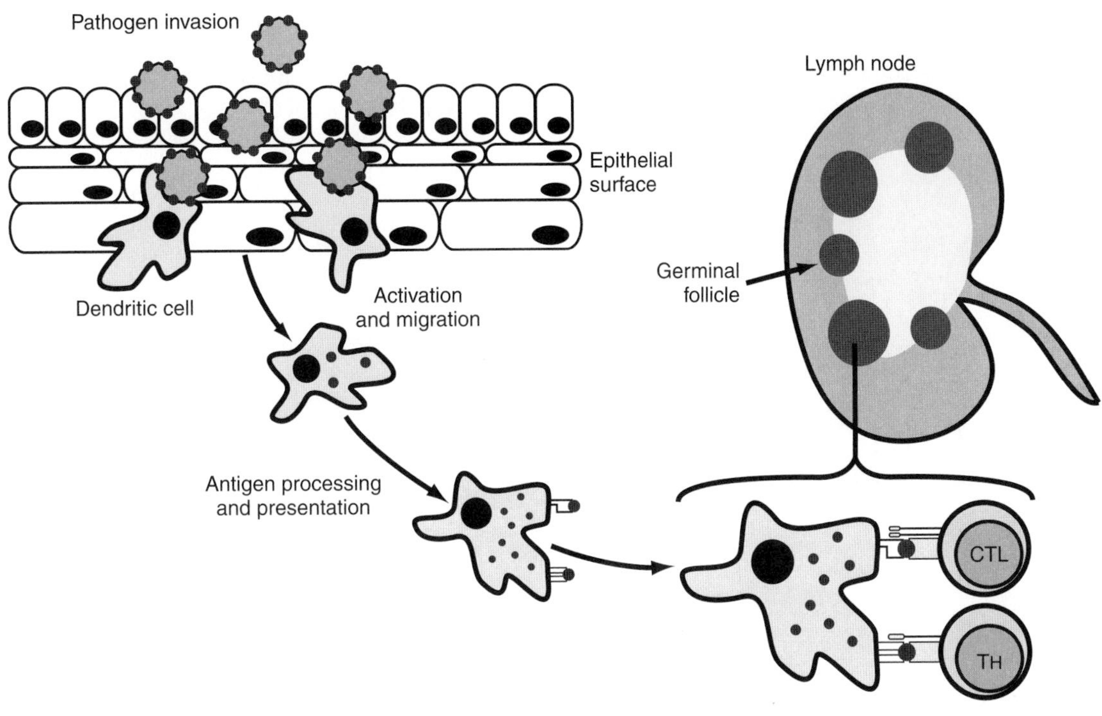

FIGURE 1-10 The role of professional antigen-presenting cells (APCs). In this figure pathogen invasion is followed by antigen uptake by a dendritic cell, the most potent of the APC family. The dendritic cells become activated and migrate to a local lymph node, where they are extremely effective at stimluating naïve T cells including both T helper cells and CTLs.

ZAP70 and Fyn. Recruitment of ZAP70 to CD3 results in its subsequent phosphorylation and activation by Lck. Once activated, the ZAP70 can subsequently phosphorylate other signal proteins, including phospholiase C (PLC; Figure 1-13). Activation of PLC leads to the cleavage of phosphatidylinositol bisphosphate (PIP_2) into inositol 3-phosphate (IP_3) and diacylglycerol (DG). Both IP3 and DAG are second messengers with IP_3, causing the release of stored CA^{2+} from the endoplasmic reticulum and DAG-activating protein kinase C. The increase in intracellular Ca levels and the activation of protein kinase C lead to the phosphorylation of various transcriptional factors. These transcriptional factors regulate the expression of the genes for various cytokines and/or their receptors (see Figure 1-13). The process is subsequently downregulated by various phosphatases that are recruited to and subsequently dephosphorylate the CD3 ITAMs. A similar process occurs in a B cell when its surface immunoglobulin receptor is cross-linked upon binding to specific antigen.

Co-stimulatory Signals

In addition to the interaction of TcR-CD3 and CD4/CD8, other cell surface antigens are involved in the signaling pathways.[3] Of greatest importance is the interaction of CD28 on the T cell with B7 on the antigen presenting cell. In the absence of CD28/B7, co-stimulation T cells are rendered functionally inactive or anergic. Upon restimulation, these anergic T cells failed to proliferate or produce cytokines such as IL-2. The induction of anergy can be prevented either by the addition of exogenous IL-2 or, more important, by interaction of the CD28 cell surface antigen with its ligands, B7-1(CD80) and B7-2(CD86). Stimulation of CD28 appears to be necessary for subsequent intracellular signaling events following TcR stimulation as CD28 cross-linking enhances various biochemical events triggered by TCR-mediated signaling, including the activation of PLC, Lck, and Raf-1 kinase, as well as inducing the influx of Ca^{2+} and generation of phosphoinositides. Other molecules, including the TNF-receptor family member CD40, regulate either T cell growth or cell death. The engagement of CD40 on the T cell with its ligand, CD40L, on the antigen presenting cell leads to NF-κB activation and thus promotes cell survival and cell cycle progression. The binding of other members of this family, notably TNF-α, to their receptor on activated T cells typically results in the activation of a biochemical cascade of caspases that lead to apoptosis. The cytocidal activity of these receptors is the result of their intracytoplasmic portion of the receptor containing death effector domains. By contrast, CD40 lacks the intracellular death domains and instead has amino acid motifs that bind TNF-R–associated factors (TRAFs) and promote NF-kB activation. In addition to their role in promoting T cell activation and growth, both the CD28/B7 and TNF-receptor pathways may also play a dominant role in the induction of specific T helper cell subsets.

CYTOKINES, CYTOKINE RECEPTORS, AND T HELPER CELL SUBSETS

Frequent mention has been made in this chapter of the role of cytokines in regulating immune responses. Indeed, this particular area of immunology has seen impressive growth over the past several years. This rapid acquisition of knowledge is the result of the application of modern molecular biology techniques to the identification and characterization of specific cytokines. Initial studies of the role of soluble factors in the regulation of immune responses were often confounded by the heterogeneous nature of the culture supernatants used as the source of the cytokine activity. Furthermore, the use of biological assays to identify specific cytokines resulted in the practice of assigning descriptive names to newly discovered cytokines (e.g., lymphocyte activating factor, T cell growth factor).[61] This quickly led to confusion because individual cytokines often exhibited multiple biological activities and the biological assays were not specific for a particular cytokine. Once the genes for the cytokines had been cloned and the resulting proteins identified, it was possible to eliminate much of this confusion. The adoption of the interleukin (IL) terminology for naming cloned immunoregulatory cytokines has further clarified the biological function and role of particular cytokines.[62] Once a new cytokine's gene is identified and the biological activity of the purified protein characterized, it is assigned an interleukin designation. To date, more than 50 different cytokines and chemokines have been cloned, sequenced, and synthesized in bacterial and eukaryotic expression systems. This has led to both a better understanding of cytokine function and to their application in a variety of clinical settings. Table 1-4 contains a list of interleukins and their known biological activity. Not all cytokines have been given interleukin designation. Interferons, certain growth factors (platelet derived growth factor, TGF-β), and TNF-α have retained their original names. It should also be emphasized that other cells besides T cells produce cytokines and interleukins. For example, monocytes and macrophages are the major source of IL-1, IL-6, and TNF-α. Thus the term *lymphokine,* which was originally used to describe immunoregulatory products of lymphocytes, has been replaced with *cytokine,* which denotes the more varied sources of immunoregulatory molecules.

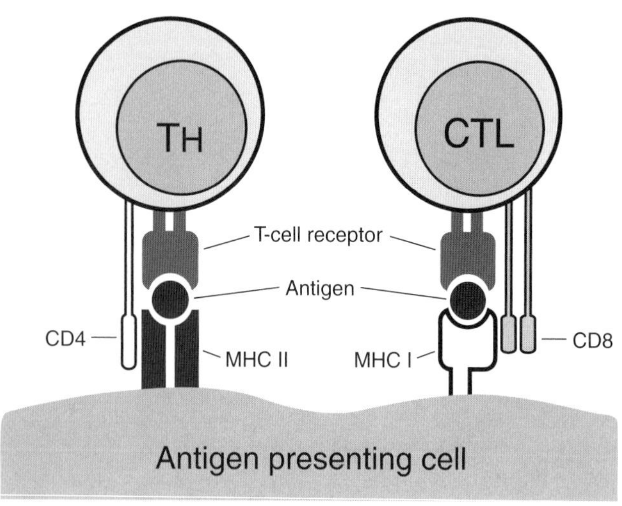

FIGURE 1-11 Class I and class II restricted T cell recognition: the role of T cell CD4 and CD8 molecules. T cell use their T-cell receptors to recognize processed antigen presented in combination with either MHC I or MHC II molecules. T cells exclusively express either CD4 (T-helper cells) or CD8 (cytotoxic lymphocytes; CTLs), and the CD4 molecule is required for interaction with MHC II molecules, whereas CD8 is required for MHC I interaction. As a result, T-helper cells recognize antigen presented by MHC II, and CTLs recognize only antigen presented by MHC I molecules.

Many cytokines have similar structures and can be grouped into like families. Hence helical cytokines have alpha helices as the predominant structure with IL-2 serving as the prototypical cytokine for this family (Figure 1-14). This family can be further divided into two subclasses according to the length

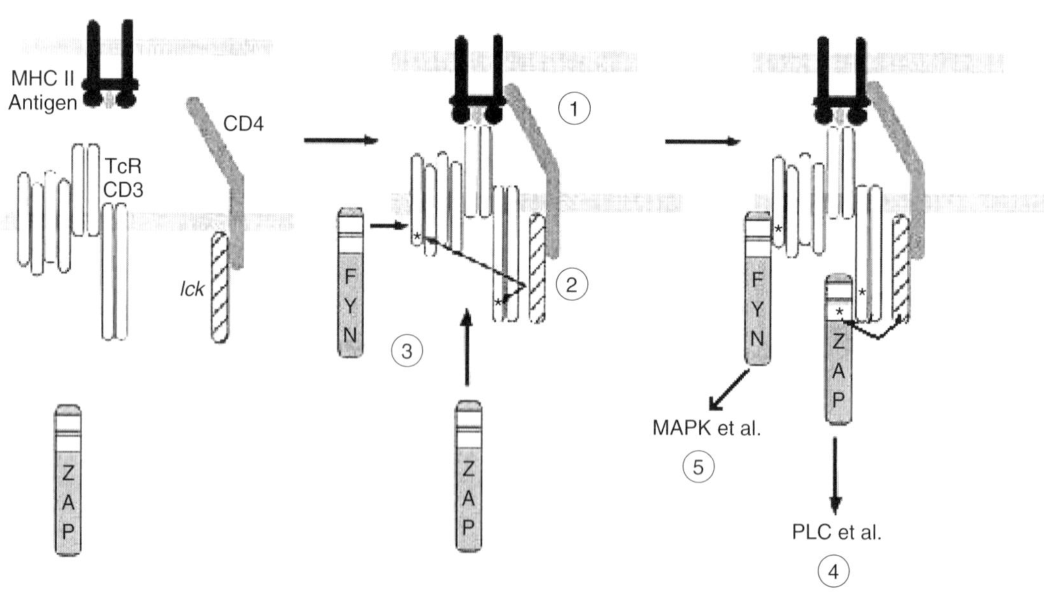

FIGURE 1-12 Intracellular signaling by the TcR-CD3 receptor. TcR recognition of its specific peptide in the peptide binding groove of a MHC molecule on an antigen-presenting cell results in the attraction of CD4/CD8 to the complex (1) and the phosphorylation of CD3 proteins by *lck* associated with CD4/CD8 (2). The phosphorylation of these sites (*) on CD3 leads to the attraction and binding of other kinases (fyn and ZAP 70) to CD3, where they are in turn phosphorylated and activated. Activation of ZAP70 leads to the subsequent activation of phospholipase C (4), and activation of *fyn* ultimately leads to the MAP kinases pathway and cell division (5) (see also Figure 1-13).

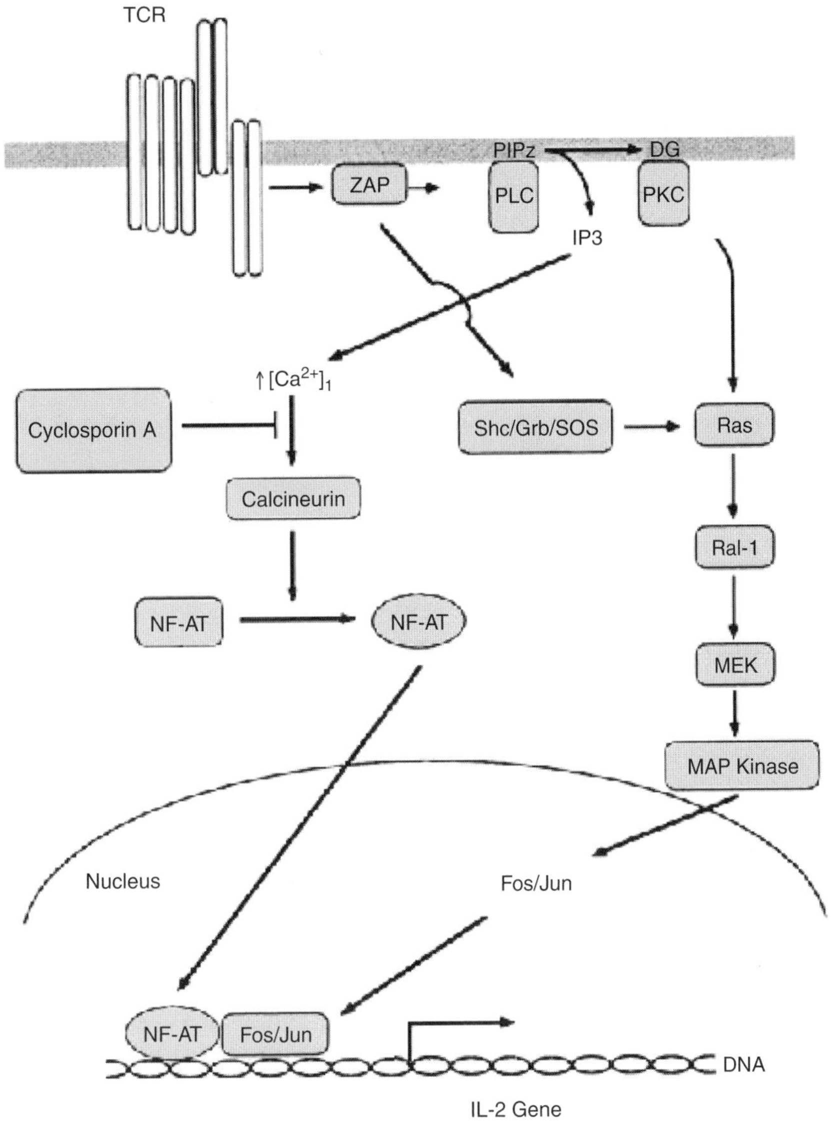

FIGURE 1-13 Intracellular signaling pathway. Following activation of ZAP70, and other receptor-associated kinases, there is a subsequent propagation of the signal as subsequent kinases and target proteins are phosphorylated. Increases in intracellular CA^{2+} lead to the activation of calcineurin that is necessary for NF-AT activation. This step is the target for cyclosporin A, a potent and specific immunosuppressive agent. Activation of the transcriptional factors NF-AT and *fos/jun* leads to their translocation into the nucleus and the binding to regulatory DNA sequences upstream of the promoter for the IL-2 gene.

of the helices: long helical (many growth factors including IL-3 and IL-7) and short helical (IL-2, IL-4, and IL-13). IL-1 is a β-trefoil cytokine whose overall structure is composed of 12 antiparallel β strands that form a bowl-like structure. Most chemokines and other smaller cytokines contain both α helices and β sheets, typically a single α helix and more than two β sheets. TNF-α is the prototype for the β-sandwich family whose structure characteristic consists of five antiparallel strands with an overall jelly roll structure.

The availability of cloned cytokines has also permitted the subsequent identification and characterization of cytokine-specific receptors. Cytokine receptors can also be grouped into major families: Class I or Class II receptor families, immunoglobulin superfamily receptors, the TNF receptor family, and TLRs (IL-1, IL-18).[63] The best characterized of these is the Class I receptor for IL-2, which is composed of three subunits: α, β, and γ. Whereas the α and β subunits are involved in specific binding to IL-2, the γ chain is involved in signal transduction once IL-2 is attached to the receptor. Five different immunologically important cytokines share this common cytokine receptor γ chain, though each has its own unique α and/or αβ binding subunits (Figure 1-15). Other common signaling chains of this type of receptor include βc (IL-3, IL-5, and GM-CSF) and gp130 (IL-6 and IL-11). Class II receptors are illustrated by the interferons whose receptors consist of at least two chains. In contrast to the chains being denoted α and β, analogous to the nomenclature for type I cytokine receptors, the chains are called *IFNAR-1* and *IFNAR-2* for α/β interferons and *IFNGR-1* and *IFNGR-2* for interferon-γ. A third receptor, CRF2-4, is a component of the IL-10 receptor.

TABLE 1-4

Interleukins

IL	Biologic Activities and Source
1	Lymphocyte activating factor; multiple biologic activities affecting a variety of lymphoid and nonlymphoid cells
2	T cell growth factor; provides proliferative signal for T cells; also affects B cells, macrophages, and NK cells; high concentrations of IL-2 stimulate cytolytic activity in NK cells and T cells; produced by activated Th1 and some $CD8^{+}$ cells
3	Multi-CSF; promotes the growth of various hematopoietic cell precursors; produced by T cells and myelomonocytic cell lines
4	B cell stimulatory factor 1; stimulates growth, maturation, and differentiation of B cells; also provides proliferative and differentiation signals for some T cells; produced by Th2 cells
5	T cell–replacing factor; stimulates B cell proliferation and immunoglobulin synthesis; also stimulates T cell proliferation and differentiation as well as eosinophil formation in the bone marrow; produced by Th2 cells
6	B cell differentiation factor; promotes maturation and immunoglobulin production by B cells; stimulates T cell growth and IL-2 synthesis; induces the production of acute phase proteins by hepatocytes; produced by macrophages, T cells, stromal cells, fibroblasts, and a variety of other cell lines
7	Pre-B cell growth factor; stimulates proliferation and maturation of early B and T cells as well as mature T cells; produced by bone marrow–derived stromal cells
8	Neutrophil chemokine produced by monocytes and hepatocytes
9	Also known as *P40;* supports the growth of certain T cell clones; produced by $CD4^{+}$ T cells
10	Cytokine synthesis inhibitory factor; inhibits the production of IL-2 and interferon-γ by Th1 cells; produced by Th2 cells
11	An IL-6–like factor produced by bone marrow stromal cells
12	NK cell differentiation factor; augments NK cell function and stimulates generation of Th1 cells; produced by macrophages
13	Produced by Th2 cells; downregulates cytokine production by macrophages/monocytes while activating B cells
14	A high-molecular-weight B cell growth factor produced by T cells and some B cell lines
15	A T cell growth factor similar in function to IL-2
16	Chemokine for $CD4^{+}$ T cell subset; produced by T cells, mast cells, and eosinophils
17	A family of related cytokines; enhances expression of the ICAM-1 on fibroblasts; also stimulates epithelial, endothelial, or fibroblastic cells to secrete IL6, IL8, and G-CSF and PGE_2
18	An inducer of IFN-gamma production by T-cells
19	A homolog of IL-10
20	An autocrine factor for keratinocytes that regulates their participation in inflammation
21	Stimulates proliferation of B-cells stimulated by cross-linking of the CD40 antigen, bone marrow progenitor cells, and naïve T cells
22	A proinflammatory cytokine that increases the production of acute phase proteins
23	Produced by dendritic cells; stimulates the production of IFN-γ by T-cells
24	Selectively suppresses the growth of tumor cells by promoting cell death by apoptosis
25	Produced by stromal cells and supports proliferation of cells in the lymphoid lineage
26	Induces the expression of IL6, IL8, and ICAM-1 in primary bronchial epithelial cells
27	Similar to IL-17; expressed in brain
28	Type III interferons; similar to Type I interferons in function and induction
29	Another Type III interferon
30	Similar to IL-27, an early product of antigen presenting cells that stimulates IFN-γ production
31	Produced by Th2 cells and is related to the IL-6 family of cytokines; possible role in pruritis, alopecia, and other allergic skin lesions
32	Inducer of inflammatory cytokine production by monocytes; highly expressed in synovial tissue of rheumatoid arthritis
33	Inducer of Th2 cytokines

IL, Interleukin; *NK,* natural killer; *CSF,* colony-stimulating factor; *ICAM-1,* intracellular adhesion molecule-1.

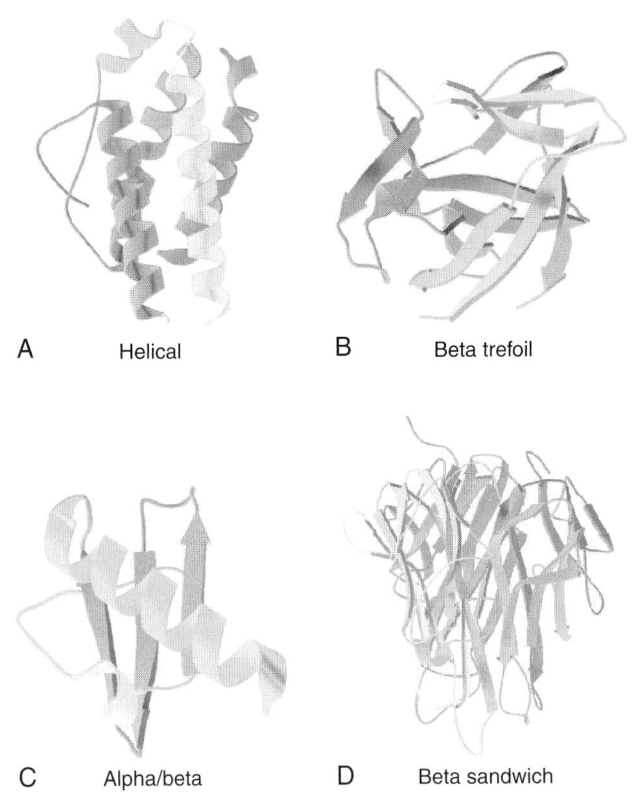

FIGURE 1-14 Cytokine structural families. (a) helical cytokine, (b) β-trefoil, (c) α/β, and (d) β sandwich.

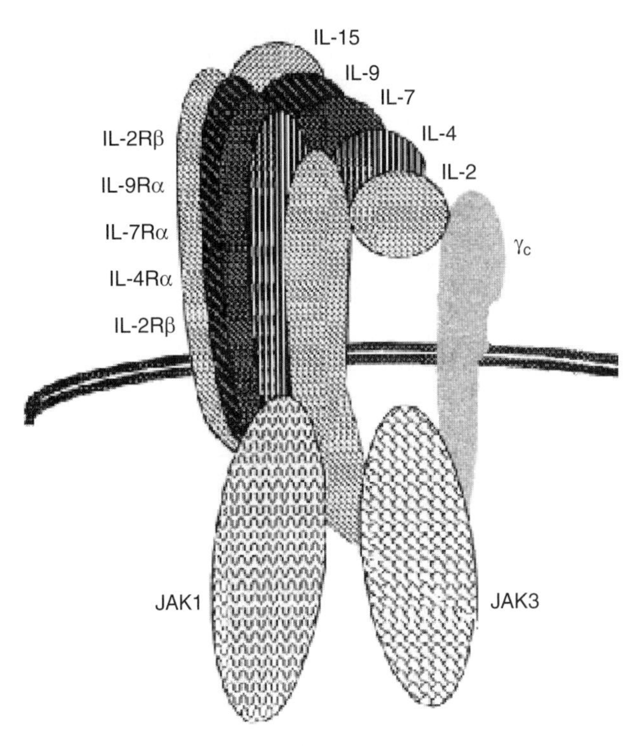

FIGURE 1-15 Type I cytokine receptors. These receptors are characterized as having a cytokine specific α and β chain involved in ligand binding and a shared or common γ chain that is used for intracellular signaling. The Janus kinases (JAK) are associated with the cytoplasmic tails of these receptors and are responsible for the signal transmission.

The TNF receptor family is composed of two separate receptors, TNF-RI and TNF-RII. Though both can bind TNF, no structural homology is found in their intracellular domains, indicating that they signal by distinct mechanisms. TNF-RI is thought to be the main signaling receptor because many biological actions of TNF, including cytotoxicity, fibroblast proliferation, and the activation of NF-κB, can be elicited in the absence of TNF-RII. The IL-1 receptor is a member of the Toll-like receptor family. As discussed previously, this receptor superfamily represents an ancient signaling system that was initially identified in *Drosophila melanogaster*. The introduction of a pathogen into *Drosophila* spp. leads to the activation of proteases that cleave a precursor and generates an extracellular ligand of a receptor called Toll, the intracellular part of which is homologous to the IL-1 receptor cytoplasmic tail. Other Toll-like receptors are involved in other signaling pathways involved in innate immune and inflammatory responses, indicating that this receptor superfamily represents an ancient signaling system.[64]

A common feature of all these receptor families is that signaling is initiated through the recruitment of protein tyrosine kinases and other cytosolic proteins to the receptor.[65,66] Although most cytokine receptors lack intrinsic kinase activity, they do have a family of Janus protein tyrosine kinases (JAKs) associated with their cytoplasmic tails. Following binding of a ligand to its cognate receptor, receptor-associated JAKs are activated. A family of transcriptional factors known as STAT (signal transducers and activators of transcription) are in turn activated by tyrosine phosphorylation by the activated JAKs, allowing the STAT to dimerize. After dimerization the STATs translocate into the nucleus and bind to the DNA sequence it recognizes via a DNA binding domain on the protein. The binding of the STAT proteins to DNA subsequently modulates gene expression. It is the sharing of receptor subunits, combined with a similar sharing of JAKs and STATs, that accounts for similar biological functions of many cytokines (see Table 1-4).

In addition to the JAKs and STATs, other transcriptional factors can activate multiple genes involved in inflammatory responses and apoptosis. One of these transcriptional factors, NF-κB, regulates many pro-inflammatory cytokines, including TNF-α, IL-1, and IL-8. NF-κB itself is activated by a number of cytokine receptor–signaling cascades, including TNF receptors.[67] In the cytoplasm NF-κB is associated with an inhibitory protein, IκB, which prevents its translocation to the nucleus. Phosphorylation of IκB leads to its degradation and the translocation of NF-κB to the nucleus, where it binds to its corresponding DNA motif, altering gene transcription. NF-kB activation is also associated with resistance to apoptosis, probably as the result of its effect on IL-8 transcription because this chemokine is anti-apoptopic.[68] Increased levels of IL-8 in inflammatory lung lesions and the increase in NF-κB activation likely account for the neutrophil accumulation seen in some forms of human asthma[69] and equine recurrent airway obstruction.[70]

Immunoregulation

The generation of an immune response requires the interaction of multiple leukocyte subsets, including macrophages, dendritic cells, B cells, and both CD4+ and CD8+ T cells.

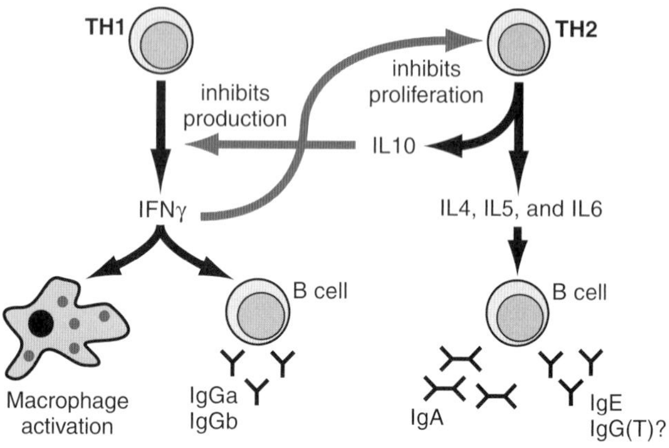

FIGURE 1-16 Th1and Th2 regulation. The Th1 lymphocyte subsets provide help for macrophage activation, cytolytic activity, and production of a subset of IgG subclasses. The Th2 promotes antibody responses, including IgA, IgE, and the remainder of the IgG subclasses. This is mediated by production of cytokines, which have a regulatory effect on each other.

Whereas the initial interactions of B and T cells involves the recognition of specific epitopes, which in the case of the T cell are presented in the context of MHC antigens, subsequent interactions are mediated by the cytokines produced by the various cells. Although macrophages, B cells, and even nonhematopoietic cells produce a variety of cytokines with immunoregulatory activity, it is the T helper cell that plays a central role in regulating immune responses. Much effort over the past decade has focused on the characterization of helper T cells and the soluble factors they produce. It is now apparent that $CD4^+$ helper cells may be further divided into distinct helper cell subsets on the basis of the cytokines they produce (Figure 1-16). Thus Th1 cells produce interferon-γ and IL-2, two cytokines involved in the induction of cell-mediated immune responses. Th2 cells, on the other hand, produce IL-4, IL-13, and IL-5, cytokines involved in the induction of antibody responses. The best evidence for separate T helper cell populations comes from the study of intracellular parasite infections in mice. Those strains of mice resistant to *Listeria donovani* infection develop a cell-mediated immune response characterized by activated macrophages and Th1 helper cells. By contrast, the susceptible BALB/c strain of mice generates a vigorous antibody response and Th2 helper cells. Th1 cells have also been implicated in various autoimmune diseases characterized by the induction of self-reactive cytotoxic cells. Th2 cells in turn play a central role in the resistance to extracellular parasites, such as intestinal helminthes, and in the induction of allergic diseases. A similar contribution of Th1 and Th2 responses in protective and pathologic responses in the horse has been described.[71,72] Regulatory T cells (Tregs) are specialized subsets of T cells that play a central role in the prevention of hyperimmune responses and autoimmunity and are thought to represent traditional suppressor cells.[73] Although naturally occurring Tregs constitute 5% to 10% of the $CD4^+$ T cell population, antigen-specific or adaptive Tregs, also known as Th3 cells, are also present. These different Tregs subsets can be identified on the basis of the expression of cell surface markers, production of cytokines, and mechanisms of action. Most Tregs express the CD25 surface antigen and produce various immunoregulatory cytokines and growth factors, including IL-10 and/or TGF-β.[74] Besides CD25, Tregs can express several other activation markers, such as the glucocorticoid-induced TNF-receptor–related protein (GITR), OX40 (CD134), L-selectin (CD62 ligand [CD62L]), and cytotoxic T lymphocyte-associated antigen 4 (CTLA-4 or CD152).[74] However, it should be noted that these markers can also be expressed to various degrees on activated T cell subsets and various antigen-presenting cells.[74] A specific subpopulation of Tregs can be identified on the basis of the expression of the transcriptional factor FoxP3. The FoxP3+ Tregs are thought to be important regulators of autoimmunity insofar as loss of function or mutation in this factor leads to the development of autoimmune disease.[74] A population of NK cells and natural killer T (NKT) cells with regulatory function has also been described whose immune suppressive function is mediated by secretion of various cytokines (IL-13, IL-4, IL-10) or by direct cell-cell contact. [74] Although the suppressive function of most Tregs is likely mediated by the production of suppressive cytokines, direct contact with Th1 cells, which limits interaction with dendritic cells, is another mechanism.[74,75]

Although it remains unclear as to what determines whether a helper cell will be a Th1or Th2 cell, it has been proposed that it is the initial encounter with the antigen during the innate immune response that may determine its fate. Multiple factors are probably involved in this process, but the single most important factor is the type and amounts of cytokines present at the time of the initial encounter with the antigen. Among the cytokines that may play a role, IL-12 and interferon-γ are the main inducers of Th1 responses, and IL-4 and IL-10 play a similar role for Th2 responses. IL-12, produced by macrophages and dendritic cells, is a potent inducer of interferon-γ that inhibits Th2 cell induction. The evidence from a variety of models to date suggests that IL-12 is the single most important factor in regulating the differentiation and magnitude of the Th1 response; however, this should not preclude the possibility that additional factors, such as IL-18, may have an equally important role in regulating Th1 responses in some situations. It is also apparent that IL-4 plays a similar crucial role in the induction of Th2 immune responses. IL-4 production by mast cells and IL-10 production by macrophages favor Th2 development in part by inhibiting Th1 cells. Other signals (e.g., PGE_2) can induce differentiation of potent antigen presenting cells with dendritic morphology that produce low levels of IL-12 and high levels of IL-10 preferentially inducing Th2 differentiation.

In addition to cytokines, another influence on T helper cell differentiation is the interaction of the B7/CD28 and CD40/CD40L co-stimulatory pathways.[3] In particular, these co-stimulatory pathways may regulate the differentiation of Th1 and Th2 cells by affecting the intensity and the strength of signals through the CD3/TCR complex and those provided through the co-stimulators. High-intensity stimulation favors Th2 development, whereas lower intensity signals favor Th1 cells. The association of stronger co-stimulation with Th2 responses contrasts with the ability of higher concentrations of antigen to mostly induce Th1 responses, whereas lower doses induce Th2 responses suggesting that Th differentiation may be influenced quite differently by the strength of signals through the CD3/TCR complex versus signals delivered through co-stimulators and their associated enzymes.[3]

Th Paradigms

The role of cytokines in regulating immune responses can best be illustrated in two scenarios, the first involving the induction of a Th1 immune response in response to viral infection and the second an allergic response to inhaled mold antigens. In the first scenario, viral antigen present at the site of an ongoing infection in the respiratory tract is processed by a resident macrophage via the exogenous pathway. The processed epitope is presented on the surface of the macrophage or a dendritic cell in the context of a MHC II antigen to a $CD4^+$ T cell in a regional lymph node. Additionally, these cells produce IL-12 that induces NK cells, attracted to the site of the infection, to produce interferon-γ that, along with antigen presentation, activates the T cell and drives it toward a Th1 phenotype. Meanwhile, $CD8^+$ T cells encounter viral antigen on the surface of virus-infected cells that has been processed via the endogenous pathway and is now associated with the MHC I antigens on the infected cell's surface. Once antigen-activated, these T cells express the high affinity form of the IL-2 receptor. The CD4+ Th1 cell produces IL-2 and interferon-γ. The interaction of IL-2 with its receptor drives the clonal proliferation of the activated $CD8^+$ T cells. The interferon-γ also stimulates the $CD8^+$ cell to differentiate into CTLs that produce additional interferon-γ. These CTLs can lyse the target cells either through the production of TNF-α or via the activation of the *fas* receptor on the target cell via the *fas* ligand (*fas*L) expressed on the activated CTL. Both pathways lead to target cell apoptosis via the activation of cytoplasmic caspases in the target cell. Meanwhile, virus-specific B cells have also encountered antigen and in the presence of interferon-γ differentiate into IgG-secreting plasma cells. This combination of IgG antibodies and CTL cells serves to eliminate the virus. PGE_2 and IL-10 production by macrophages exert anti-inflammatory effects on the response, and that, coupled with the production of soluble cytokine receptors, dampens the immune response as the invader is eliminated.

In the second scenario, the introduction of mold antigens into the respiratory tract leads to the processing of the antigen by macrophages and dendritic cells, as before. However, in the absence of IL-12 and interferon-γ, and perhaps the presence of IL-3, IL-4, IL-9, IL-10, or PGE_2, there is the induction of Th2 cells that produce additional IL-4 and IL-13. These cytokines cause those B cells recognizing the allergens to isotype switch to IgE antibodies that bind to mast cells. Subsequent degranulation of these mast cells ensues, as the result of antigen binding to the IgE, leading to the production of other mediators, including IL-4 and PGE_2 that exacerbate this response. In the continued presence of the allergen, a secondary inflammatory response characteristic of recurrent airway obstruction occurs.

The Role of Cytokines in the Horse

The field of equine immunology continues to expand with the development of better reagents. Recent advances in gene cloning technology have led to the cloning and expression of a number of equine cytokines. Thus the cDNA sequences for a number of equine cytokines are known, and specific protocols are now available to measure their expression (Table 1-5). Through use of these procedures, it has been possible to identify the role of Th1 and Th2 cells in both protective and pathologic responses in the horse (Table 1-6).[71,76,77] The results from these and other studies confirming the role of inflammatory cytokines in equine sepsis and in joint and airway diseases emphasize the similarities between equine and human immune systems. As such, the potential for manipulating these responses using recombinant cytokines or anticytokine reagents is as applicable to equine medicine as it is to human medicine.

Lymphocyte Trafficking Pathways

Leukocyte trafficking has been reviewed previously, with a particular emphasis on the innate immune response. Lymphocytes involved in adaptive immune responses differ in their migration from most other cells in that they recirculate instead of making one-way trips. Memory and naïve T lymphocytes, with their different capacities for response to antigens, differ also in their migration pathways through the body. Two general pathways of lymphocyte recirculation have been demonstrated. Naïve T lymphocytes take the most common route, which involves entry into the lymph node by extravasation from the high endothelial venule (HEV) and return to the peripheral circulation via the efferent lymphatic. The endothelial cells of HEVs have a distinctive appearance and specialized receptors and can support a great deal of lymphocyte migration. This allows rapid repeated circulation of naïve lymphocytes through lymph nodes where there is the greatest chance of exposure to their specific antigens. Memory lymphocytes, on the other hand, leave the bloodstream in peripheral vascular beds, particularly in inflamed tissues, and return to lymph nodes via afferent lymphatics. This leads to the exposure of primed memory lymphocytes to the most likely early sites of antigenic encounter and allows for an early response to recall antigens. Thus memory lymphocytes are most common in inflammatory lesions and in the epithelial surfaces of the lung and gut wall. Differing expression of the adhesion and homing molecules may play an important role in mediating these different migration pathways.

For lymphocytes to follow the previously outlined maturation and migration pathway, the first step is for the naïve lymphocyte to get into a lymph node so that it can meet its antigen on a professional antigen-presenting cell. To achieve this, the T-lymphocyte needs to exit in the HEV. The naïve lymphocyte expresses L-selectin, and this can bind to the vascular addressins GlyCAM-1, CD34, and MAdCAM-1, which are expressed on HEVs and promote rolling similar to that mediated by P- and E-selectin when they bind to phagocytes. These molecules are expressed on a variety of tissues, but in HEVs they have specific patterns of glycosylation that makes them bind L-selectin. These differences represent the key to the specificity of the migration of lymphocytes to HEVs. This weak interaction initiates the process of extravasation that is promoted by locally bound chemokines (e.g., IL-8), which increase the affinity of the lymphocyte integrins for their ligands.

Approximately 25% of lymphocytes passing through an HEV leave, and this could mean 1.4×10^4 cells in a single lymph node every second, and in the body 5×10^6 lymphocytes may extravasate through HEVs every second (human). The "sticking" process (rolling, activation, arrest) takes a few seconds, with transendothelial migration and passage through the HEV basement membrane occurring in about 10 minutes. After leaving the blood, most T cells travel through the lymph node uneventfully and leave via efferent lymphatics; however,

TABLE 1-5

Cloned Equine Cytokines

Cytokine*	GeneBank Accession	References	RT-PCR†	
			ABI No.	Order Name
IL-1α	D42146, E13117,U92480	(Howard et al., 1997; Howard et al., 1998; Kato, 1994; Kato et al., 1995; Katou et al., 1997; Takafuji et al., 2002)		
IL-1β	D42147, D42165, E13118, U92481	(Howard et al., 1997; Howard et al., 1998; Kato, 1994; Kato et al., 1995; Kato et al., 1996; Katou et al., 1997; Takafuji et al., 2002)	1749300	EQIL-1B-JN2
IL-1ra	U92482, D83714	(Howard et al., 1997; Howard et al., 1998; Kato, 1996; Kato et al., 1997)		
IL-2	L06009, X69393	(Dohmann et al., 2000; Tavernor, 1992; Tavernor, 1993; Vandergrifft and Horohov, 1993)	1918058	EquineIL-2-JN2
IL-4	L06010, AF035404, AF305617	(Hammond et al., 1999; Dohmann et al., 2000; Schrenzel et al., 1997; Schrenzel et al., 2001; Steinbach and Mauel, 2000; Vandergrifft et al., 1994)	1798106	EQIL4IS-JN2
IL-5	U91947	(Cunningham et al., 2003; Vandergrifft and Horohov, 1997)	50442836	EQIL5IS-JN1
IL-6	U64794, AF005227, AF041975	(Lai, 1998; Leutenegger et al., 1997; Swiderski and Horohov, 1996; Swiderski et al., 2000)	50414323	EQIL-6
IL-8	AF062377, AY184956	(Capelli et al., 2002; Franchini, 1998; Nergadze et al., 2006)	1833786	EQIL-8IS-JN1
IL-10	U38200	(Swiderski et al., 1995)	50442836	EQIL10IS-JN2
IL-12p35	Y11130	(McMonagle et al., 2001; Nicolson, 1997; Nicolson et al., 1999)		
IL-12p40	Y11129	(McMonagle et al., 2001; Nicolson, 1997; Nicolson et al., 1999)	1649196	IL-12
IL-13	DQ889711		50442836	EQIL13IS-JN1
IL-15	AY682849	(Cook et al., 2004)	1833786	EQIL-15IS-JN1
IL-17	AY014959	(Joubert et al., 2000)		
IL-18	Y11131	(Nicolson, 1997; Nicolson et al., 1999)	1833786	EQIL-18IS-JN3
IL-23	AY704416	(Kralik, 2004; Kralik et al., 2006; Musilova et al., 2005)		
GM-CSF	AY040203, AF448481	(Mauel et al., 2001; Mauel et al., 2006; Vecchione et al., 2001; Vecchione et al., 2002)		
IFN-α 1	M14540	(Himmler et al., 1986; Steinbach et al., 2002)		
IFN-α 2	M14541	(Himmler et al., 1986; Steinbach et al., 2002)	1947516	EQIFNA-4-SITER
IFN-α 3	M14542	(Himmler et al., 1986; Steinbach et al., 2002)		
IFN-α 4	M14543	(Himmler et al., 1986; Steinbach et al., 2002)		
IFN-β	M14546	(Adolf et al., 1990; Himmler et al., 1986; Steinbach et al., 2002)	1947516	EQIFNBETA-SITER
IFN-γ	M14544, D28520, U04050	(Curran et al., 1994; Grunig, 1993; Grunig et al., 1994; Himmler et al., 1986; Nicholson, 1994; Steinbach et al., 2002)	50442836	EQIFNGIS-JN3
TGF-β	X99438, AF175709	(Nixon et al., 1999; Penha-Goncalves, 1996; Penha-Goncalves et al., 1997)		
TNF-α	M64087	(Su et al., 1991; Su et al., 1992)	1787254	EQTNFAIS-JN2

IL, interleukin

*Coligan JE, Kruisbeek AM, Margulies DH, et al. (editors). *Current protocols in immunology.* September, 2004.

†*RT-PCR,* Real time PCR primers and probes available as Assay-by-Design kits from Applied Biosystems (ABI). Each intron-spanning primer/probe combination amplifies cDNA but not chromosomal DNA with the exception of IFN-α and IFN-β, which lack introns (see figures).

Modified from http://www.ca.uky.edu/gluck/HorohovDW_EIRClonedCytokines.asp.

TABLE 1-6

T Helper Cell Paradigm in the Horse

Protection	Immunopathology
Th1	*Rhodococcus equi*
	Equine recurrent uveitis
Th2	*Strongylus vulgaris*
	Insect bite hypersensitivity

Th, T helper cell.

in rare events a naïve T cell recognizes its specific peptide/MHC complex and becomes activated, eventually leading to formation of effector and memory T-cells. That process takes 4 or 5 days, and, once activated, the migration pathway of memory T cells differs considerably from naïve cells. All activated T cells lose the L-selectin molecules that mediated homing to lymph nodes and increase the expression of other adhesion molecules. The homing of individual lymphocytes to specific sites is regulated by expression of specific adhesion molecules. Memory cells are specifically attracted to areas of inflammation as a result of the increased levels of adhesion receptor ligands expressed on vascular endothelium in these regions. This is typically a result of TNF-α production by regional macrophages encountering infections. Sometimes infections do not result in TNF-α production, but memory cells also migrate randomly throughout the body. When they encounter their antigens, they can produce cytokines like TNF-α themselves, which in turn causes local endothelial cells to increase expression of E-selectin and VCAM-1 and ICAM-1. This will subsequently recruit more effector and memory cells to the region.

Mucosal Immunity

The mucosal immune system comprises a series of distinct compartments within the imune system, which are adapted to immunologic response in unique environments such as the gut or respiratory or urino-genital tract. The mucosal immune system is perhaps the most important component of our adaptive immune system, and the reader is referred elsewhere for an appropriately detailed description of its general features,[1] and of its role in equine immunity in the context of respiratory disease.[78] The mucosal immune system may represent the original vertebrate immune system, and it certainly protects the largest vulnerable area of the mammalian body and composes a large proportion of the total lymphocyte populations and immunoglobulin pool.[79,80]

The mucosal immune system consists of organized and dispersed lymphoid tissues that are closely associated with mucosal epithelial surfaces, and mucosal immune responses generated in one location are transferred throughout the mucosal immune system by lymphocytes programmed to home to regional effector sites. The principal immunoglobulin produced by the mucosal immune system is secretory IgA, which in humans is the most abundant immunoglobulin class in the body. Secretory IgA has unique adaptations that promote transport out onto mucosal surfaces, where it protects the body from bacteria and viruses principally by immune exclusion (i.e., by physically preventing attachment to mucosal surfaces). The importance of mucosal IgA has already been demonstrated in immunity to numerous equine diseases.[78] Secretory IgA (sIgA) is formed by dimerization of two IgA monomers, which are attached by means of disulphide bonds to a J-chain also produced by the same plasma cell that secretes the IgA. This confers the advantage of increased valency to sIgA, which can bind up to four of its targets, thus increasing its agglutinating ability. Secretory IgA protects the body from bacteria and viruses principally by immune exclusion (i.e., by physically preventing attachment to mucosal surfaces). Immunoglobulin A is relatively noninflammatory (i.e., it does not fix complement as effectively as IgGa or IgGb), consistent with a role in defense by immune exclusion.[3] Similarly, although myeloid cells possess Fc receptors for IgA, it is not clear that IgA functions as an efficient opsonin or promotes phagocytosis.

Coordination of the mucosal immune response depends on organized mucosal-associated lymphoid tissue (MALT) principal examples of which are the pharyngeal tonsils and the intestinal Peyer's patches. In the gastrointestinal tract MALT is distributed throughout the gut, but in the respiratory tract these tissues are found only in the nasopharynx and oropharynx. MALT consists of lymphoid follicles containing IgA-committed B cells, surrounded by interfollicular T cell areas with APCs and high endothelial venules (HEVs), with an overlying follicle-associated epithelium (FAE). Naïve lymphocytes enter the MALT by extravasation from the HEVs (there are no afferent lymphatics in MALT), and, after antigen encounter in the MALT, they leave through efferent lymphatics. The FAE is specialized for antigen sampling, by having reduced secretion of mucus, and through the presence of specialized antigen uptake cells termed *microfold* or *M cells.* These M cells are typically closely associated with underlying aggregates of lymphocytes, often within large basolateral membrane pockets, and play a critical role in mucosal immune surveillance. Adherent macromolecules or particles bound to the apical M cell membrane undergo endocytosis or phagocytosis and are released at the pocket membrane, where antigen presentation is initiated by dendritic cells resulting in activation of antigen-specific B cell (Figure 1-17). Subsequent trafficking and recirculation of memory IgA-positive B cells to the other components of the mucosal immune system (e.g., respiratory tract, intestinal tract), is responsible for the dissemination of local mucosal IgA responses throughout what is termed the common *mucosal immune system.* After homing of these B cells to effector sites, such as the lamina propria of the gut and respiratory tract, and extravasation into the lamina propria from HEVS, further antigen encounter and second signals from antigen presentation cells and from T helper cells result in further differentiation into IgA producing plasma cells. The short half-life of IgA secreting plasma cells requires a constant generation of precursors in induction sites and flow to effector sites. Antigen sampling and presentation are not restricted to organized MALT because throughout the mucosal surfaces dendritic cells play a key role in antigen uptake and presentation, subsequently migrating to local lymph nodes or MALT to initiate immune responses.

After release of secretory IgA by plasma cells into the interstitium, it is bound by the polymeric Ig receptor on the abluminal surface of epithelial cells. Subsequently, the sIgA is transported across the epithelial cell and released at the luminal surface together with secretory component formed by cleavage of part of the polymeric Ig receptor. Secretory component can also be found in a free form in mucosal secretions. Secretory

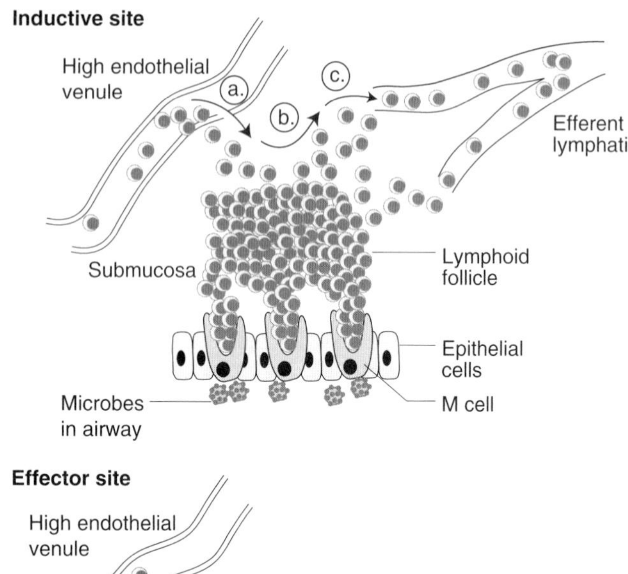

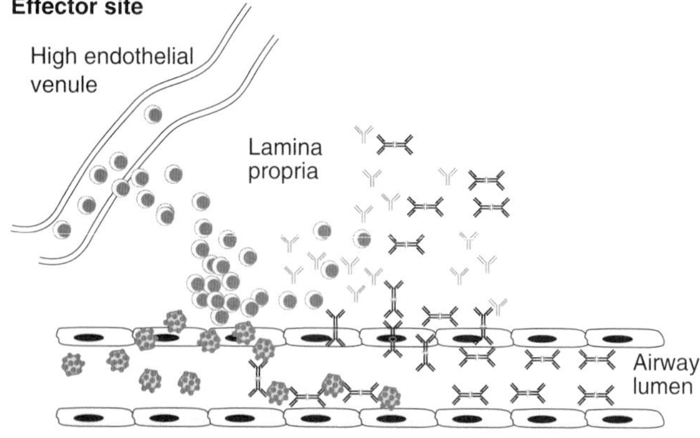

FIGURE 1-17 Initiation of mucosal immune responses. Respiratory mucosal immune responses typically originate after antigenic encounter at inductive sites, which are the tonsils of the nasopharynx and oropharynx in the horse. Naïve lymphocytes enter the inductive sites from high endothelial venules (HEV) via the specialized cuboidal endothelium of those vessels in response to specific molecular signals. Antigens, such as microbes, are taken up by microfold or M cells, which are part of the highly specialized follicle associated epithelium present at these sites. Antigenic material is transported across the M cell, and antigen presentation to B and T lymphocytes is accomplished by dendritic cells in the underlying tissues. The underlying lymphoid follicle is composed primarily of B lymphocytes, surrounded by T lymphocytes areas. Antigen-specific B lymphocytes become committed primarily to IgA production at these sites, although some IgG B lymphocytes are also generated. Subsequently, the primed lymphocyte populations exit the inductive site via efferent lymphatics, eventually reaching the blood circulation through the thoracic duct. Then these cells traffic to HEVs of effector sites throughout the respiratory epithelium and extravasate to make up the intraepithelial lymphocyte and lamina propria lymphocyte population and to give rise to lymphoid aggregates. Subsequent antigen encounter results in terminal differentiation to plasma cells, primarily IgA producing, although some IgG plasma cells are also formed. IgG is largely restricted to tissues, but secretory IgA is transported to the respiratory epithelial surface, where it can aggregate infectious organisms. (From McGorum BC, Dixon PM, Robinson NE, et al. *Equine respiratory medicine and surgery,* Edinburgh, Saunders, 2007).

component confers resistance to proteolytic enzymes found in the respiratory and gastroenteric environment, some of which are secreted by pathogens, and prolongs the longevity of sIgA. During its transit through the epithelial cell sIgA can neutralize intracellular infections encountered in the endosomal compartments of cells.[81] In addition, sIgA can bind antigens in the submucosa and literally transport or excrete them to the mucosa by this mechanism. The majority of the IgA in the mucosa is dimeric sIgA, whereas the bone marrow–derived IgA in circulation is predominantly monomeric.

In the horse our understanding of the architecture and functions of the mucosal lymphoid system is best developed for respiratory lymphoid tissues.[78] Although lymphoid tissues are distributed throughout the respiratory tract, the greatest masses comprise the nodular lymphoid tissue of the nasopharynx and oropharynx, which can have an overlying lymphoepithelium specialized for antigen uptake and processing, as in the case of tonsillar tissues. Additional nodular lymphoid tissues are typically present at sites where antigen-laden mucus and air currents converge throughout the trachea and bronchi and are called *bronchus-associated lymphoid tissue* (BALT). Tonsils represent the most complex mucosal nodular lymphoid tissues. Horses possess all of the various tonsillar tissues that are recognized in other species, and they are anatomically complex.[78] The nasopharyngeal tonsil is the largest mass of lymphoid tissue in the respiratory tract of horses of all ages, and its epithelium has been extensively characterized.[82] This epithelium has a classical FAE and is heavily folded, forming crypts; it also contains M cells. The nasopharyngeal tonsil exists in the dorsal recess of the nasopharynx, and extends ventrally toward the opercula on either side of the nasopharynx. Therefore it is ideally placed for the sampling of antigens before entry to the airways or alimentary tract and may serve as an important target for intranasal vaccines. This tissue appears to be most abundant in young foals and atrophies with age, though many lymphoid follicles remain throughout the nasopharynx.

The nasopharyngeal epithelium also contains numerous lymphocytes. Immmunohistochemical studies indicate that the majority of these lymphocytes are $CD8^+$ T lymphocytes, although B lymphocytes are also present.[82] The contribution of these lymphocytes to mucosal cellular immune defenses of the upper respiratory tract is poorly studied. However, following intranasal challenge of yearling and 2-year-old horses with EHV-1, virus-specific cytotoxic activity is detectable in several mucosal lymphoid tissues of the upper respiratory tract, as well as the local draining lymph nodes, and is particularly evident in the nasopharyngeal lining.[83] This cellular immune response is presumably mediated by $CD8^+$ T lymphocytes found in the nasopharyngeal epithelium and underlying lamina propria and may provide an important contribution to the clearance of infectious virus from the upper respiratory tract.

Ontogeny of the Equine Immune System

Few studies of the prenatal development of the equine immune system have been conducted. As in other species, the thymus is the first lymphoid organ to develop, and mitogen responsive cells can be identified there from day 80 of the 340 day gestational period of the horse.[84] Subsequently, these cells appear in peripheral blood at 120 days, lymph nodes at 160 days, and the spleen at 200 days. Cells responsive in mixed lymphocyte reactions are detectable in the thymus from 100 days and in the spleen at 200 days. Immunoglobulin production is detectable before 200 days, and newborn foals typically have IgM concentrations in their serum of approximately 165 μg/ml. Overall, it appears that functional T lymphocytes are present by day 100 and B lymphocytes by day 200 of gestation. Immunologic competence of the equine fetus has been assessed in terms of specific antibody responses. In utero immunization of foals in late gestation with keyhole limpet hemocyanin in an alum adjuvant results in detectable specific antibody production and T cell responsiveness at the time of birth.[85] In addition, the equine fetus can respond to coliphage T2 at 200 days, and Venezuelan equine encephalitis virus at 230 days.[86,87]

Detailed studies of the appearance of lymphocyte subpopulations defined by monoclonal antibodies have not been performed in the equine fetus. However, some information regarding the maturation of thymocytes in young horses is available. During thymic maturation of T cells, stem cells migrate into the thymus and mature into T cells under the influence of the epithelial microenvironment.[88,89] In this process different patterns of cell surface differentiation and antigen expression distinguish successive stages of thymocyte maturation. In humans the earliest thymic precursor cells express low levels of CD4.[90] This CD4 expression is lost as early thymocytes become double negative CD4-CD8-cells and then demonstrate their T cell commitment by TCRβ gene rearrangement, which is an essential trigger for subsequent events and leads to low levels of expression of a cell surface TCRβ-CD3 complex.[91] Intermediate thymocytes are $CD4^{lo}CD8^{lo}$, but after TCRα gene rearrangement and expression of cell surface TCRαβ, they rapidly become $CD4^{hi}CD^{hi}TCR\text{-}CD3^{hi}$.[90] Subsequently, thymocytes selected on the basis of productive TCR gene rearrangement and lack of self-reactivity become mature T cells expressing either CD4 or CD8 (single positive) in combination with high levels of TCR-CD3. Using two-color FACS analysis, it is possible to demonstrate similar patterns of EqCD3, EqCD4, and EqCD8 antigen expression in the equine thymus.[92,93]

Immunocompetence in Foals

Infectious disease in neonatal foals is associated with high morbidity and mortality. Although failure of passive transfer is a major cause of this problem, immaturity of the immune system has also been considered a potential contributing factor. As a result, a number of studies of neonatal immunocompetence have been completed and reviewed.[94]

INNATE IMMUNE RESPONSES IN FOALS

A number of studies have reported neutrophils to be fully functional from birth,[95-97] but their function is significantly impaired before absorption of colostral antibodies, which are required for opsonization.[97,98] A recent study of foal neutrophil development over the first 8 months of life demonstrated killing (measured by chemiluminescence) to be reduced in the first 2 weeks of life, as was phagocytic ability when assays were performed using autologous serum.[99] When serum from adult horses was used, neutrophil phagocytic ability in foals was normal. This latter difference may have been due to absence of either adequate immunoglobulin or complement in foal serum. A similar study of foals younger than 7 days of age confirms that phagocytosis and oxidative burst activity of neutrophils is reduced in foals of this age, although the use of adult serum did not improve phagocytosis.[100] Similarly, alveolar macrophages recovered from bronchoalveolar lavages may be low in number in foals up to 2 weeks of age and have impaired chemotactic function.[101]

The importance of complement in foals is illustrated by the finding that the opsonic capacity of foal serum for bacteria is halved by heat inactivation.[12] Interestingly, complement activity in the first week of life is considerably elevated in colostrum-deprived foals, possibly as an alternative defense mechanism.[102] In bovine colostrum–fed foals, serum complement levels reach adult levels by 1 to 3 weeks of age.[103]

ADAPTIVE CELL-MEDIATED IMMUNITY IN FOALS

Recent studies have measured lymphocyte numbers and subpopulations in foals.[104-106] Foals are born with B and T lymphocytes and with CD4+ and CD8+ T lymphocyte subsets. Lymphocyte counts rise in the first 4 months of life, and the proportion of B lymphocytes increases. A comprehensive study of lymphoproliferative responses in foals from the day of birth through 4 months of age found no difference between foals and adults.[106] Another study reported foal lymphoproliferation as low on the day of birth, possibly as a result of high serum cortisol levels.[107] Foals do exhibit reduced levels of IFNγ production throughout the prenatal period, which could account for their susceptibility to *Rhodococcus equi* and other intracellular pathogens.[108] Decreased production of this cytokine could be due to dysregulation of its production or reflect the fact that most T lymphocytes in the foal are naïve. Currently, markers for the development of memory lymphocytes are unavailable in horses, although increased expression of MHC II antigen on T lymphocytes throughout the first year of life may identify a developing population of memory cells.[59] Although there is evidence for the capacity of foals to mount immune responses in utero,[85-87] there have been few studies of antigen specific immune responses in the first days of life, except in the context of the immunosuppressive effect of passive transfer of immunity.[109] When foals are immunized with antigens against which they have no maternally derived specific antibodies, it is clear that they can mount immune responses from at least 3 months of age, and possibly sooner.[110]

ANTIBODY-MEDIATED IMMUNITY IN FOALS

Passively Transferred Maternal Antibody During the first 1 to 2 months of life, foals depend on passively transferred immunity for protection from infectious disease. The diffuse epitheliochorial nature of the equine placenta does not allow for in utero immunoglobulin transfer to foals. Although minor concentrations of some immunoglobulins can be detected at birth, the foal is born essentially agammaglobulinemic and acquires passive immunity by the ingestion and absorption of colostrum from the dam.[111,112] Colostrum is a specialized form of milk containing immunoglobulins, which are produced during the last 2 weeks of gestation under hormonal influences.[113] Colostrum contains primarily IgGa, IgGb (IgGa plus IgGb is the equivalent of IgG), and IgG(T), with smaller quantities of IgA and IgM, all of which have been concentrated into mammary secretions from the mare's blood.[114,115] Colostrum is produced only one time each pregnancy and is replaced by milk that contains negligible immunoglobulins within 24 hours of the initiation of lactation.[111,114] This extremely rapid decline in immunoglobulin concentrations in mammary secretions is consistent with equine colostrum production ending at or even before parturition.[115] The absorptive capacity of the foal's gastrointestinal tract for immunoglobulins is greatest during the first 6 hours after birth, and then steadily declines until immunoglobulins can no longer be absorbed when the foal is 24 hours old. This "closure" of the gut to absorption of large intact molecules is due to replacement of specialized enterocytes by more mature cells.[116]

De Novo Antibody Production in Foals

Few studies of *de novo* antibody production have been conducted in foals without the effect of passively transferred maternal antibody. In a study of 10 pony foals fed only bovine colostrum, endogenous equine antibody production measured by radial immunodiffusion (RID) resulted in serum concentrations of IgG of 200 mg/dl by 2 weeks of age, 400 mg/dl by 1 month, and 1000 mg/dl by 3 months of age.[117] In a smaller study of two colostrum-deprived pony foals, comparing them with 18 colostrum-fed foals, and measuring serum γ-globulin levels by immunoelectrophoresis, very similar results were obtained, although it was apparent that the colostrum-deprived foals achieved higher serum γ-globulin levels between 6 weeks and 3 months of age than did colostrum-fed foals.[111] In a third study, antibody concentrations in six colostrum-deprived foals were substantively higher than in five control foals between 3 and 5 months of age.[102] These three studies provide evidence for substantial endogenous production of IgG in the first month of life in foals deprived of equine colostrum and suggest that the onset of production is earlier, and the rate is higher, in foals deprived of colostrum. This observation is consistent either with nonspecific immunosuppression in colostrum-fed foals or to stimulation of immunoglobulin production in colostrum-deprived foals. In another study of foals from mixed breed horses fed only bovine colostrum, endogenous IgG production started later and was first detected at 1 month of age in the majority of foals, reaching similar levels to foals fed equine colostrum by 2 months of age.[118]

In colostrum-fed foals, serum IgG concentration falls to its lowest level at 1 to 2 months of age as a result of catabolism of maternally transferred immunoglobulin, subsequently rising toward adult levels as a result of endogenous immunoglobulin production.[99,105,106,112] A study by Sheoran et al.[114] extended these observations and extensively documented changes in serum IgG subclass concentrations in five Quarter Horse foals in the first 9 weeks of life. This study showed that IgG (the equivalent of IgGa plus IgGb) concentrations were lowest at 1 month of age. However, the subsequent increase in IgG concentration was due to de novo IgGa production, not IgGb. At the end of this study at 9 weeks of age, there was still no clear evidence of IgGb production, although IgGa and IgG(T) concentrations had reached or exceeded adult levels. In adult horse serum, IgGb comprises more than 60% of total serum IgG and is by far the dominant subclass in foal serum after passive transfer of immunity.[114] IgGb has also been shown to have a critical role in immunity to a variety of pathogens,[119,120] and it is possible that the naturally late onset of endogenous production may be a factor in the increased susceptibility of foals to infections such as bacterial respiratory disease at this age.[121,122] This possibility was investigated in a study by Grondahl et al.,[12] in which the opsonic capacity of foal serum was measured during the first 42 days of life using the foal pathogens *Escherichia coli* and *Actinobacillus equuli*. No differences were detected over time, and foal serum was as effective as adult horse serum. Although this study did not provide evidence of decreased opsonization in serum of older foals, the studies were extended only to samples from 42-day-old foals, and in this in vitro system immunoglobulin concentrations may not have been rate limiting. Finally, Holznagel et al.[123] studied immunoglobulin concentrations throughout the first year of life in foals and demonstrated that all foal immunoglobulin concentrations measured showed decreasing serum levels at 4 weeks of age, after which point all but IgGb began to rise. This pattern was the result of catabolism of maternal immunoglobulins and the different times and rates of onset of endogenous production of immunoglobulin classes and subclasses; IgA and IgG(T) levels stabilized at 8 to 12 weeks of age. IgGa levels peaked at 8 weeks of age and then slowly declined throughout the duration of the study. IgGb levels reached their nadir at 2 to 5 months of age and did not begin to rise until after 16 weeks of age. This factor could provide a basis for reduced endogenous antibody-mediated immunity in the first year of life. This study also showed that at 1 year of age, serum immunoglobulin concentrations had still not yet reached adult levels.

A factor that significantly affects de novo immune responses in foals is the suppressive effect of passively transferred antigen-specific maternal antibodies. The rate of decline of these antibodies varies for both individuals and different infectious agents. The half life for maternal IgG in foals is estimated at 20 to 30 days.[111] Studies of antigen specific antibodies demonstrated similar half lives for anti-influenza virus and antitetanus antibodies of 27 to 29 days for IgGa, 35 to 39 days for IgGb, and 35 days for IgG(T).[124] For many important pathogens the concentration of maternal antibodies in foals falls to nonprotective levels by 2 to 3 months of age.[125,126] However, the remaining antibody can still render the foal unresponsive to vaccination for weeks or even months to come. In the case of equine influenza virus[127,128] and tetanus toxin, maternal antibodies can persist until 6 months of age and prevent immune responses in foals vaccinated before reaching that age.[124] When foals are vaccinated against antigens against which they have no passively transferred antibody, normal antibody responses have been documented from at least 3 months of age.[110]

IMPLICATIONS FOR IMMUNOCOMPETENCE IN FOALS

The previously presented evidence suggests that the foal's immune system is competent in many regards, with the innate immune system completely functional at least by the second week of life and with the full complement of lymphocytes present from birth. Antibody is entirely provided by passive transfer at first, although endogenously produced immunoglobulin is detectable within a few weeks of birth and predominates from 1 to 2 months of age. Nevertheless, there are some key features of the foal immune system that can limit its ability to defend against infection. A critical factor is antigen specific and nonspecific immunosuppression resulting from transferred maternal antibody. As the foal ages, the continuing immunomodulatory effect of maternal antibody may limit foal immunoresponsiveness while no longer providing comprehensive protection itself. Of similar importance is the fact that although the lymphocytic immune system is complete from the time of birth, it is naïve. Neonates can mount normal immune responses but require appropriate presentation of antigen and co-stimulatory signals.[129] Antigen presentation in the absence of co-stimulatory second signals (e.g., T helper cells) can induce immune deviation or a failure to mount the appropriate immune response, and particularly so in neonates.[130-132] The absence of memory responses and a well-developed repertoire of immune responses is a serious handicap that only appropriate antigenic encounters can overcome. Most important, recent studies have documented that maturation of the adaptive immune system of the foals in terms of both the humoral[123] and cellular arms[108,133] is incomplete throughout the first year of life.

HYPERSENSITIVITY AND AUTOIMMUNITY

Hypersensitivity refers to an altered state of immunoreactivity resulting in self-injury. Four different types of hypersensitivity can be defined by the type of immunologic process underlying the tissue injury, as was originally proposed by Gell and Coombs.[1] The general features of this classification system are presented in Table 1-7. The most common and important type of hypersensitivity disease, at least in humans, is Type I hypersensitivity, mediated by IgE. In these diseases some individuals produce IgE antibodies against a normally innocuous antigen, which is called an *allergen*.[2] Exposure to the allergen triggers mast cell degranulation as described later, and a series of responses result that are characteristic of *allergy*. Allergic diseases are so important that more is known about the function of IgE in this hypersensitivity disease than about its normal role in host defense. In this definition, and throughout this chapter, the term *allergy* refers only to Type I hypersensitivity diseases mediated by IgE,[2] whereas in other definitions *allergy* can refer to the entire spectrum of hypersensitivity diseases.[3] Other forms of hypersensitivity disease depend on IgG antibodies (Types II and III hypersensitivities) or T cells (Type IV hypersensitivity). Each of these disease processes can play a role in the immunopathogenesis of *autoimmune disease*, in which the body mounts an adaptive immune responses to self tissue antigens.

Clinical hypersensitivity diseases, such as recurrent airway obstruction (RAO) or purpura hemhorrhagica, can involve more than one type of hypersensitivity reaction simultaneously, which limits the utility of this classification for clinical diagnosis. Alternative strategies for classifying these diseases may have greater clinical utility. For example, antibody mediated hypersensitivity diseases (Types I, II, and III) are *immediate* in onset if preformed antibody exists in circulation or tissues, with some variation in time course dependent on the antibody isotype involved. Cell mediated hypersensitivity (Type IV) is delayed, even in sensitized individuals, for 1 to 3 days, while effector cells are recruited to the site of antigen exposure.[3] The goals of this section are as follows:

- Review the classical hypersensitivity types in order to explain the immunopathogenesis of hypersensitivity diseases.
- Describe immediate and delayed hypersensitivities of horses and their immunologic basis.
- Identify autoimmune conditions of horses with a known immunologic basis.

Detailed descriptions of clinical aspects of hypersensitivity and autoimmune diseases and their diagnosis and management are presented elsewhere in this book. Detailed explanations of many immunologic mechanisms involved in these disease processes are provided previously in this chapter.

TABLE 1-7

Four Types of Hypersensitivity*

	TYPE I	TYPE II	TYPE III	TYPE IV		
	IgE	IgG	IgG	Th1	Th2	CTL
Antigen	Soluble antigen	Cell or matrix associated antigen	Soluble antigen in excess (immune-complex formation)	Soluble antigen	Soluble antigen	Cell-associated antigen
Effector mechanism	Mast cell degranuation	Fc-receptor positive cells (phagocytes of reticulo-endothelial system)	Fc-receptor positive cells, complement	Macrophage activation	Eosinophil activation	Cytotoxicity
Examples of hypersensitivity reaction	Systemic anaphylaxis, *Culicoides* hypersensitivity	Penicillin-associated hemolytic anemia	Purpura hemorrhagica	Equine recurrent uveitis	Chronic *Culicoides* hypersensitivity	Contact dermatitis

Ig, Immunoglobulin; *Th,* T helper cell (type 1 or 2); *CTL,* cytotoxic T lymphocyte.
*The four types of hypersensitivity can be differentiated by the immune mediator involved, the form of antigen recognized, and the effector mechanism elicited in producing pathology. Equine examples of each condition are given when available.

CLASSICAL TYPES OF HYPERSENSITIVITY REACTION

Type I Hypersensitivity

As described previously, Type I hypersensitivity, or allergy, is mediated by IgE antibody specific for allergens, which are extrinsic antigens normally not recognized by the healthy immune system.[2] IgE is predominantly found in tissues, where it is bound to mast cells through the *high-affinity IgE receptor*, which is called *FcεRI* and has been identified in the horse.[4] When antigen binds to IgE on the surface of mast cells, cross-linking two or more IgE molecules and their FcεRI receptors, this triggers the release of chemical mediators from the mast cells, which cause Type I hypersensitivity reactions. Basophils and eosinophils (when activated) also possess FcεRI receptors and therefore can participate in the same process. In addition to FcεRI receptors, there is an unrelated *low-affinity IgE receptor* called *CD23*, which is present on many lymphocytes, monocytes, eosinophils, platelets, and follicular dendritic cells. The role of CD23 appears to be to enhance IgE responses to specific antigens when those antigens are complexed with IgE. Thus CD23 on antigen presenting cells can capture IgE bound antigens. In the horse CD23 has been identified, and its expression is upregulated by equine IL-4.[5]

The selective stimulation of IgE responses depends on characteristics of the antigen (allergen), the individual affected (genetic factors such as MHC antigens), and the mechanism of antigen presentation. The antigen must be capable of eliciting a Th2 immune response in order to stimulate IgE production. Small, soluble proteins, frequently enzymes, containing peptides suitable for MHC II antigen presentation and presented to mucosal surfaces at low doses, are particularly efficient at generating IgE responses. Low doses of antigen specifically favor Th2 over Th1 responses, and exploiting this relationship is the basis of some therapeutic hyposensitization strategies (see under Immunomodulators). These processes are thought to be regulated by regulatory T cells (Tregs). Natural Tregs are CD4/CD25 positive, and in healthy individuals they suppress Th2 cytokine production.[2] When Tregs are deficient, atopy can result. When CD4 T helper cells are exposed to IL-4, as opposed to IL-12, during antigen presentation by dendritic cells, they are driven toward becoming Th2 cells. This process is critical to promoting IgE responses and may be favored at enteric and respiratory mucosal surfaces, or skin, where parasite invasion typically occurs. This makes teleologic sense insofar as IgE responses are very important for antiparasitic immunity.[6] The dendritic cells at such locations are frequently programmed to stimulate Th2 responses.[2] Cross-linking of FcεRI receptors on granulocytes also results in CD40L expression and IL-4 secretion, which further promotes IgE production by B lymphocytes and sustains allergic reactions.

Some individuals maintain IgE responses to a wide variety of allergens, a condition called *atopy*. Affected individuals have high levels of IgE in the blood and increased eosinophil populations. In humans this condition depends partly on genetic factors, including genetic variations in the IL-4 promoter sequence or association with particular MHC II genes. Nevertheless, environmental factors are also important, as atopy is increasingly common in humans in economically developed parts of the world. Four possible explanations for this are decreased exposure to infectious disease during childhood, environmental pollution, allergen levels, and dietary change. The first explanation is currently favored, and its basis is the proposal that many infectious diseases bias the immune system toward Th1 responses[2] and that their decreased prevalence results in an increased tendency to mount Th2 responses, which may be the natural bias of the neonatal immune system.[7]

EFFECTOR MECHANISMS IN TYPE I HYPERSENSITIVITY ALLERGIC REACTIONS

When triggered by antigen cross-linking of IgE bound to FcεRI cell surface receptors, activated mast cells release chemical mediators stored in preformed granules and synthesize leukotrienes and cytokines. In Type I hypersensitivity reactions the outcome of this reaction can vary from anaphylactic shock to minor localized inflammation. Mast-cell degranulation causes an *immediate allergic reaction* within seconds, but there is also a sustained *late-phase response* that develops up to 8 to 12 hours later as a result of recruitment of Th2 lymphocytes, eosinophils, and basophils.

Mast cells are highly specialized cells of the myeloid lineage that are common in mucosal and epithelial tissues near small blood vessels. The range of inflammatory mediators released by degranulating mast cells is wide and includes enzymes that can remodel connective tissues; toxic mediators such as histamine and heparin; cytokines such as IL-4, -5, -13, and TNF-α; and lipid mediators, including leukotrienes and PAF.[2] Histamine causes an increase in local blood flow and permeability. Enzymes activate matrix metalloproteinases that cause tissue destruction, and TNF-α increases expression of adhesion molecules and attracts inflammatory leukocytes. These reactions are all appropriate when the mast cell is reacting to an invasive pathogen, but in allergy this is the basis of the immediate inflammatory response and also the initiating step in the late-phase response.

The role of *eosinophils* in inflammation is tightly controlled at several levels. Synthesis in the bone marrow depends on IL-5 produced by Th2 cells in the face of infection or other immune stimulation. Transit of the eosinophils to tissues depends on two chemokines, *eotaxin 1* and *eotaxin 2*. Activation of eosinophils by cytokines and chemokines induces them to express FcεRI and complement receptors and primes the eosinophil to degranulate if it encounters antigen that can cross-link IgE on its surface. Mast cell degranulation and Th2 activation recruit and activate large numbers of eosinophils at the site of antigen encounter. Basophils are similarly recruited, and together their presence is characteristic of chronic allergic inflammation. Eosinophils can trigger mast cells and basophil degranulation by release of major basic protein. This late-phase response is an important cause of long-term illnesses such as chronic asthma in humans.

CLINICAL MANIFESTATIONS OF TYPE I HYPERSENSITIVITY REACTIONS DEPEND ON THEIR SITES

The clinical outcome of Type I hypersensitivity reactions depends on the amount of IgE present, doses of allergen, and the sites of allergen introduction. Direct introduction of allergen into the bloodstream or rapid enteric absorption can lead to widespread activation of connective tissue mast cells associated with blood vessels. This potentially disastrous event is called *systemic anaphylaxis* and can cause catastrophic loss of blood pressure and airway obstruction owing to bronchoconstriction and laryngeal swelling. This leads to anaphylactic shock and can follow administration of drugs against which an individual has an established IgE response. Treatment with epinephrine can control these potentially fatal events.

Penicillin is one example of a drug that can cause Type I hypersensitivity reactions in humans, although it is less certain that it can induce this type of hypersensitivity reaction in the horse. Penicillin can act as a hapten (see the section on equine immunology). Penicillin alone can elicit antibody formation by B cells but cannot elicit T helper cell responses because it is not a protein. However, the β-lactam ring of penicillin can react with amino groups on host proteins to form covalent conjugates, and the modified self-peptides can generate Th2 responses in some individuals. The Th2 cells can in turn release cytokines, which activate penicillin-binding B cells to produce IgE. In this scenario penicillin is a B cell antigen and becomes a T cell antigen by modifying self-peptides. Intravenous penicillin results in protein modification and recognition and cross-linking of mast cell IgE, leading to anaphylaxis.[2]

Allergen inhalation, in contrast, induces local inflammation of the respiratory tract—for example, in the upper airways, as in allergic rhinitis, or in the lower airways, as in human asthma. Similarly, allergen introduction into the skin causes local histamine release initially and a wheal-and-flare reaction, followed by a late-phase response several hours later. When allergens are ingested and reach the skin from the bloodstream, a disseminated form of the wheal-and-flare reaction occurs that is called *urticaria* or *hives*. Prolonged inflammation of the skin results in *eczema* or *atopic dermatitis* in some individuals. Ingestion of allergens causes activation of gastrointestinal mast cells, resulting in fluid loss across the bowel and smooth muscle contraction. The clinical presentation is diarrhea and vomiting. Sometimes ingestion of allergens can lead to systemic anaphylaxis, if they are absorbed rapidly, or urticaria, as is sometimes seen after oral penicillin administration.

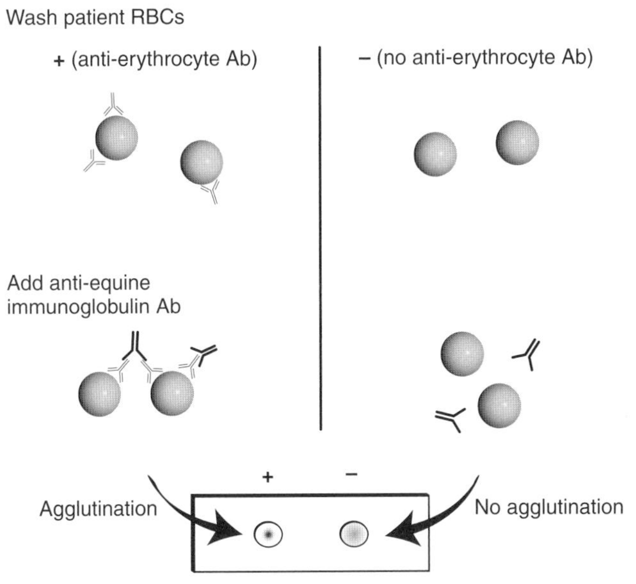

Wash patient RBCs
+ (anti-erythrocyte Ab)
– (no anti-erythrocyte Ab)
Add anti-equine immunoglobulin Ab
Agglutination
No agglutination

FIGURE 1-18 Direct Coombs' test. *Ab,* Antibody; *RBCs,* red blood cells.

Type II Hypersensitivity

Type II hypersensitivity disease occurs when the causal antigen is associated with cells or tissue components of the body and there is an IgG antibody response to this antigen. Phagocytes, or other cells expressing Fcγ receptors, mediate destruction of the affected tissue or removal from the circulation by the reticulo-endothelial system in the case of antibody-positive erythrocytes or platelets. Antibody-mediated hemolytic anemia and thrombocytopenia are examples of drug-associated Type II hypersensitivities. In the case of the horse, penicillin is an established cause of hemolytic anemia.[8] Diagnosis can be accomplished using a Coombs' test (Figure 1-18). Penicillin binds to the erythrocyte surface and is targeted by antipenicillin antibodies of the IgG isotype. Interestingly, quite large numbers of horses have antipenicillin antibodies of the IgM isotype, but this does not lead to disease.

Type III Hypersensitivity

In Type III hypersensitivity the antigen is soluble and present in the circulation. Disease results from formation of antibody-antigen aggregates or *immune complexes* under certain specific conditions.[2] Although immune complexes are generated in all antibody responses, they are generally harmless. Large complexes fix complement and are removed from circulation by the reticulo-endothelial system. However, small complexes can form at antigen excess (Figure 1-19), and these can deposit in blood vessel walls and tissues, where they ligate Fc receptors on leukocytes, causing an inflammatory response, increased vascular permeability, and tissue injury. Complement activation also contributes to this process. Local injection of antigen can sometimes lead to a necrotizing skin lesion caused by Type III hypersensitivity, and this is called an *Arthus reaction*.

The classical example of a Type III hypersensitivity reaction is *serum sickness*, which is seen after administration of horse antiserum in humans (e.g., in treating snake bites). After an IgG response to the horse, serum is generated (7-10 days), and signs of fever, urticaria, arthritis, and sometimes glomerulonephritis result. The foreign antigen is cleared as part of this process, which makes this condition ultimately self-limiting. Alternative scenarios for induction of Type III hypersensitivity reactions include persistent infectious diseases in which pathogens are not completely cleared from tissues or

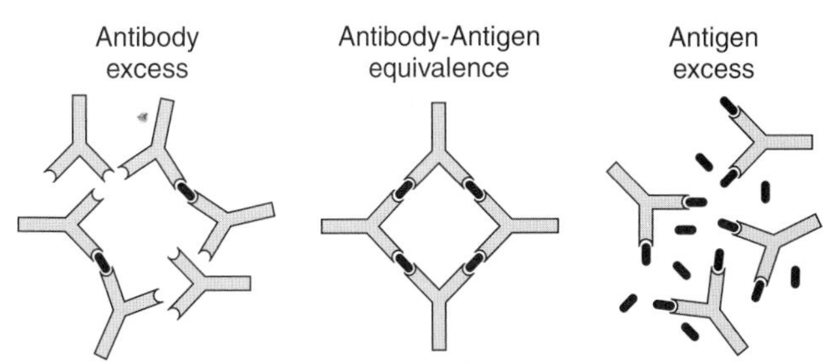

FIGURE 1-19 Antibody-antigen precipitation. Antibody can precipitate soluble antigen in the form of immune complexes. This is most efficient when concentrations of antibody and antigen reach equivalence, and large immune complexes are formed. However, when antigen is in excess some immune complexes are too small to precipitate and can produce pathologic changes such as are seen in Type III hypersensitivities.

autoimmune diseases in which antigen persists. Inhaled antigens that induce IgG responses can lead to immune complex formation in the alveolar wall, as occurs in *farmer's lung*, compromising lung function.[2] Any such circumstance in which immune complexes are deposited in tissues can lead to this type of pathology.

Type IV Hypersensitivity

Cell-mediated Type IV hypersensitivities cause delayed hypersensitivity reactions. A variety of cutaneous hypersensitivity reactions are seen, such as the contact hypersensitivity seen after absorption of haptens such as pentadecacatechol in poison ivy or the local Th1 response seen in the diagnostic tuberculin reaction. When Type IV hypersensitivity results in a Th2 response, the principle outcome is eosinophil activation and recruitment such as in chronic asthma.

IMMEDIATE HYPERSENSITIVITY DISEASES IN THE HORSE

Previously, a major limitation of our ability to study hypersensitivity disease in the horse has been the lack of reagents capable of detecting equine IgE. Although equine IgE has long been known to exist,[9,10] and the genetic sequence has been known since 1995,[11-13] the only reagents for studying it have historically been conventional polyclonal antisera produced by vaccination with physico-chemically purified IgE[14,15] or made in chickens after vaccination with recombinant fragments of the IgE heavy chain.[16] Although many valuable studies have been performed using these reagents,[17-20] the recent availability of well-characterized monoclonal antibodies recognizing equine IgE holds much promise for future studies.[21,22] It has already been demonstrated that the onset of IgE production in horses does not occur before 9 to 11 months of age and does not reach adult levels before 18 months.[23] This may help explain why hypersensitivity disease is uncommon in horses before puberty.

The following section describes a series of equine diseases with characteristics of immediate hypersensitivity disease. This is not an exhaustive list of equine hypersensitivity diseases, and additional examples will be found throughout this book.

Systemic Anaphylaxis

The incidence of true systemic anaphylaxis in horses is unknown, although the condition has been reported in association with administration of a wide range of compounds, including serum, vaccines, vitamin E–selenium preparations, thiamine, iron dextrans, and antibiotics such as penicillin.[24,25] Target organs in experimental equine anaphylaxis are the lung and the intestine.[24] Sudden dyspnea; hypotension, as evidenced by poor peripheral pulse character; rapid onset of urticaria; and collapse are cardinal signs of the onset of systemic anaphylaxis.

The therapeutic goals in treating systemic anaphylaxis are to (1) prevent or reverse the complications caused by mediator release, (2) maintain respiratory integrity, and (3) maintain cardiovascular stability. Not all anaphylactic reactions require therapy. However, rapid recognition of those that do is critical to patient survival. Intravenous access via an indwelling intravenous catheter and airway patency should be established immediately because cardiovascular collapse and upper airway obstruction caused by angioedema can occur rapidly. Because the conscious horse does not tolerate tracheal intubation, emergency tracheotomy may be required. Oxygen should be administered if available because bronchoconstriction and cardiovascular collapse result in hypoxemia. The fluid requirement of horses in anaphylactic shock is not known, but large volumes of balanced polyionic fluid should be administered rapidly.

The principal therapeutic agent is epinephrine, which is a potent sympathetic stimulant. Epinephrine administration may cause excitement in the horse. Epinephrine should be administered intramuscularly (10 to 20 μg/kg, equivalent to 5 to 10 ml of 1:1000 dilution of epinephrine for a 450-kg horse) if dyspnea or hypotension are mild. Epinephrine should not be administered subcutaneously because its potent vasoconstriction can lead to poor absorption and tissue necrosis. If dyspnea or hypotension is severe, epinephrine should be administered intravenously or endotracheally if there is no venous access (3 to 5 μg/kg or 1.5 to 2.25 ml of 1:1000 dilution of epinephrine for a 450-kg horse). Epinephrine doses can be repeated every 15 to 20 minutes until hypotension improves. The side effects of epinephrine therapy are tachyarrhythmias and myocardial ischemia, which can be life threatening. Alternatively, an epinephrine or norepinephrine drip can be instituted for cases of refractory hypotension. Other therapeutic agents, such as antihistamines, β-agonists, or other pressors, may be indicated, although their value is less certain. Though its effects may be delayed, glucocorticoid therapy is indicated to help reverse persistent bronchospasm and angioedema and break the cycle of mediator-induced inflammation triggered during hypersensitivity reactions. Ideally, a rapid acting glucocorticoid should be used, such as prednisolone sodium succinate 0.25 to 10.0 mg/kg, administered intravenously. Glucocorticoid therapy during the acute phase will aid in preventing the late-phase reaction.

Insect Bite Hypersensitivity

Horses commonly suffer from hypersensitivity to salivary antigens of *Culicoides* and *Simulium* species leading to an intensely pruritic skin disease with characteristics of both immediate and delayed-type hypersensitivity.[26] The clinical sign of urticaria, combined with the presence of increased numbers of IgE positive cells in the skin and high levels of *Culicoides*-specific IgE in serum are all evidence of immediate (Type I) hypersensitivity in the immunopathogenesis of this disease.[17,18] This pathogenesis has received further support from studies employing the newly available monoclonal antibodies to equine IgE.[22] Interestingly, one recent study demonstrated that in addition to IgE, the IgG(T) subclass can also bind skin mast cells and elicit clinical signs consistent with hypersensitivity.[27] It remains to be seen if IgG(T) plays a role in the pathogenesis of naturally occuring insect bite hypersensitivity. In some breeds a genetic predisposition based on an MHC-linkage has been demonstrated.[28,29]

Recurrent Airway Obstruction

Recurrent airway obstruction is a severe inflammatory disease of middle-aged and older horses induced by exposure of susceptible horses to inhaled organic dust, generally from hay, although a summer pasture-associated form is also observed in the southern United States.[30] Hay dust contains a mixture of mold spores, forage mites, particulates, and endotoxins, which can induce and exacerbate airway inflammation. Removal of the hay dust by returning the horse to pasture leads to decreased inflammation within a few days. In RAO-susceptible horses, exposure to hay dust leads to invasion of the lungs and airways by neutrophils within 4 to 6 hours and concurrent airway obstruction resulting from bronchospasm, inflammation, and increased mucus viscosity, which principally affect the bronchioles. RAO-affected horses develop nonspecific airway hyperresponsiveness, which is a bronchospasm in response to a wide variety of stimuli, including inflammatory mediators and neurotransmitters. Horses affected by RAO demonstrate increased histologic lesions and worsening airway function with increasing age. In addition, significant histopathologic changes are present before abnormal airway function can be detected.

The immunologic basis of RAO remains poorly elucidated. Two pieces of evidence suggest a role for Type I hypersensitivity in this disease. First, IgE levels are increased in bronchoalveolar (BAL) fluid of RAO-affected horses,[14] and second, allergen-specific IgE is increased in affected horses.[20,31,32] However, the immediate onset of airway obstruction typical of a Type 1 reaction to exposure to allergens is rarely observed because clinical signs of RAO only develop several hours after antigenic exposure.[30] A study of immunoregulatory cytokines in RAO demonstrated evidence for a Th-2 bias in RAO, with increased levels of IL-4 and IL-5 and decreased IFN-γ mRNA in BAL cells.[33] However, other investigators have documented increased IFN-γ levels in RAO.[34] It seems likely that a number of immunologic processes, including IgE mediated pathology, increased expression of Toll-like receptor 4,[35] and dysregulation of cytokine responses,[36] may be involved in this disease.

IgG-Mediated Diseases

IgG-mediated diseases, which broadly correspond to Type II and III hypersensitivities, have also been termed *immune-complex diseases* in the horse.[3] The examples described here are distinguished from the other immediate hypersensitivities of the horse described previously in that there is no evidence for the involvement of IgE in their pathogenesis.

NEONATAL ISOERYTHROLYSIS AND ALLOIMMUNE THROMBOCYTOPENIA

Neonatal isoerythrolyis is a common condition of foals and is extensively reviewed elsewhere in this text. The condition results from the passive transfer of maternal antibodies in colostrum that recognize allogenic foal erythrocyte antigens principally of the Aa and Qa haplotype inherited from the sire. A similar condition occurs in mules as a result of the inheritance of a donkey-specific erythrocyte antigen.[37,38] A severe, potentially life-threatening anemia results as the antibody-positive erythrocytes are removed by the reticulo-endothelial system or, less commonly, lysed by complement. A similar condition less commonly affects platelets, causing severe neonatal thrombocytopenia in horses[39] and mules.[40] These conditions are typical of Type II hypersensitivities and are mediated by circulating IgG recognizing cell surface antigens on erythrocytes. Diagnosis can be performed using a variation of the Coombs' test (Figure 1-20).

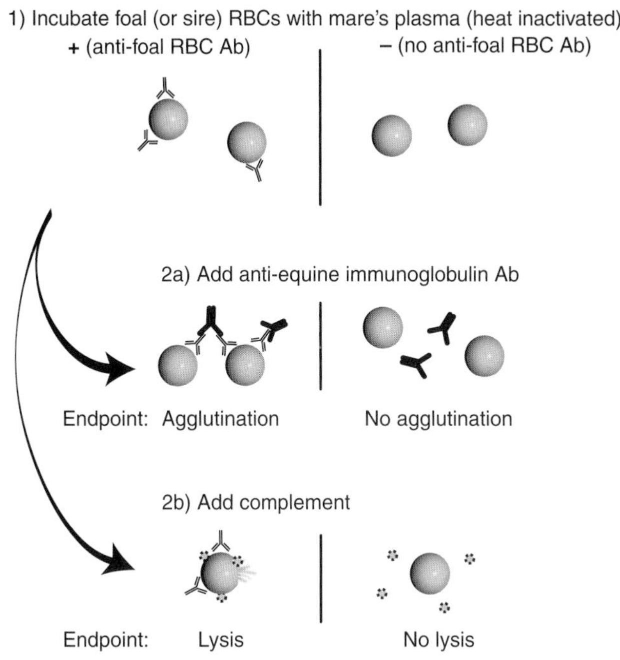

FIGURE 1-20 Neonatal isoerythrolysis test. *Ab,* Antibody; *RBCs,* red blood cells.

PURPURA HEMORRHAGICA

Purpura hemorrhagica is an acute disease of the horse characterized by edema of the head and limbs; leucocytoclastic vasculitis; petechial hemorrhages in mucosae, musculature, and viscera; and sometimes glomerulonephritis.[41] It is usually associated with *Streptococcus equi* subsp. *equi* infection of the upper respiratory tract disease. Serum of affected horses contains immune complexes of *S. equi* subsp. *equi*–specific antigens with equine IgA.[41] The glomerulonephritis sometimes seen in association with purpura has been attributed to deposition of similar immune complexes containing streptococcal antigens and IgG.[42]

DELAYED HYPERSENSITIVITY DISEASES IN THE HORSE

Documented immunologic characterization of delayed hypersensitivity conditions of the horse are lacking, although contact hypersensitivities have been reported in horses.[3] One very well-characterized example of this type of condition is recurrent uveitis.

Equine Recurrent Uveitis

Equine recurrent uveitis (ERU), also known as *moon blindness* or *periodic ophthalmia,* is the most important cause of blindness in horses.[43] The disease results in both acute and chronic ocular inflammatory disease, and chronic sequelae include development of posterior and anterior synechiae, cataracts, lens opacities, secondary glaucoma, and blindness. Eyes of affected horses contain IgG antibodies and autoreactive T cells specific for retinal antigens.[44] A specific cause has not been identified. However, sensitization to a variety of pathogens, and in particular to *Leptospira* spp.,[45,46] is thought to induce the immune mediated pathology that is central to the disease.[47] Treatment with corticosteroids and other anti-inflammatory agents is essential to prevent visual debility or blindness. However, treatment failures are common, and the disease frequently recurs with further ocular damage months after the initial event, commonly leading to euthanasia.[43]

Our understanding of the immunologic basis of ERU has been extended by studies of the immunoregulatory events in the eyes of affected horses. It has been shown that the T lymphocytes that invade the iris-ciliary body during this disease produce a pattern of IFN-γ cytokine production typical of a T helper 1 (Th1) response.[48] These studies indicate that ERU is an equine example of a Type IV hypersensitivity disease mediated by Th1 cells.

AUTOIMMUNITY

Although a number of equine diseases are considered to be autoimmune in etiology, few have been extensively studied.[49] Much of the explanation given in the previous sections for the immunopathologies involved in hypersensitivity disease can be applied to autoimmune disease. Well-described equine autoimmune diseases include neonatal isoerythrolysis and alloimmune thrombocytopenia, which are described previously and have characteristics of Type II hypersensitivities, as does immune-mediated anemia in adults.[50] Less well-described entities include systemic lupus erythematosus[51] and pemphigous foliaceus,[52] which have characteristics of both Type II and III hypersensitivity diseases. As described previously, equine recurrent uveitis appears to represent a Type IV hypersensitivity, and there is some morphologic and immunologic evidence for similarly classifying cauda equine syndrome (polyneuritis equi).[53-55]

With the exception of a few conditions, such as neonatal isoerythrolysis and penicillin-associated hemolytic anemia, there are few autoimmune conditions in which the cause is well understood. One exception, however, is the anemia that can develop subsequent to administration of human recombinant erythropoietin to horses.[56,57] There is substantial evidence that horses mount an antibody response to the exogenous erythropoietin that cross-react with the endogenous hormone and result in erythroid hypoplasia. The lesson of this example may be that in the modern world, with increasing availability of recombinant drugs that mimic natural biologic compounds, we would do well to remember that the immune system has an exquisite ability to distinguish what is foreign and to reject it vigorously.

IMMUNODEFICIENCY

Immunodeficiencies occur in both primary and secondary forms and have been extensively reviewed.[1,2] Primary immunodeficiencies have a genetic basis, whereas secondary immunodeficiencies result from failure of passive transfer in foals, immunosuppressive infections or drug treatments, neoplasia, or malnutrition. Immunodeficiencies can affect specific components of the immune system, such as the lymphoid or phagocytic system. Typically, immunodeficiency is suspected in any of the following circumstances:[3]

- Onset of infections in the first 6 weeks of life
- Repeated infections that are poorly responsive to therapy
- Infections caused by commensal organisms or organisms of low pathogenicity
- Disease resulting from the use of attenuated live vaccines
- Failure to respond to vaccination
- Marked neutropenia or lymphopenia that persists for several days

Equine immunodeficiency is most commonly suspected on the basis of the first three reasons—that is, because of increased susceptibility to infection. The most common immunodeficiency recognized in clinical practice is failure of passive transfer in foals.[4-6] Other causes of immunodeficiency vary from well-defined clinical entities, such as severe combined immunodeficiency of Arabian foals,[7] to cases in which immunodeficiency is suspected on clinical grounds, but the specific cause or nature of the problem is difficult or impossible to define.[8] Regardless of their cause, immunodeficiencies result in increased susceptibility to infections, which are in turn poorly responsive to appropriate therapy. Defects in antibody production tend to predispose to pyogenic infection, whereas deficiencies in cell-mediated responses lead to infections with organisms normally nonpathogenic in horses such as *Candida albicans, Cryptosporidium* spp., or adenovirus. When any immunodeficiency is suspected, specific diagnostic tests are indicated to define the deficiency. The aim of the next section is to identify tests that clinicians can apply practically in such cases and to explain their merits and limitations.

TESTS OF EQUINE IMMUNE FUNCTION

Tests of components of the immune system (e.g., lymphocytes, immunoglobulins) generally can either quantitate that component or measure its functional capacity. In Table 1-8 the components of the immune system that currently can be analyzed in this manner are identified, and corresponding quantitative and functional tests are listed. The table also identifies those tests that are likely to be commercially available, and it should be noted that few of the functional tests are available unless the clinician is able to identify a sympathetic and capable equine immunologic research laboratory. Despite these limitations, the available tests do permit the identification of many of the well-defined causes of immunodeficiency in horses.

Tests of Antibody-mediated Immunity

Some assays of B lymphocyte function and number are described later, but the principal tests of humoral immunity are quantitative assays of immunoglobulin concentration and measurements of specific antibody responses to vaccination. The variety of classes of immunoglobulins in the horse is complex and reviewed earlier in this chapter.[9] For practical purposes our attention is generally focused on IgG (representing the combination of two subclasses: IgGa and IgGb), IgG(T), IgA, and IgM.

The current gold standard for measurement of concentrations of immunoglobulin classes is the RID assay. The disadvantage of this test is its cost and the time required to perform the assay (24 hours or more), which makes it generally unsuitable for screening for failure of passive transfer of immunity in foals. Nevertheless, this form of test remains the single most valuable assay available to the clinician trying to measure total antibody concentrations in the horse. Currently, test kits are available for IgG, IgG(T), IgA, and IgM (VMRD Inc., Pullman, Wash.), although specific IgG subclass RID tests are available

TABLE 1-8

Components of the Immune System and Tests for Quantitative or Functional Analysis*

Components of the immune system that can be evaluated in horses and appropriate tests for quantitative or functional analyses of each component. The list of tests is not exhaustive but restricted to tests of likely practical value for which normal data are available. Tests listed in bold are routinely available to clinicians.

Component	Quantitative Tests	Functional Tests
Immunoglobulin	**Radial immunodiffusion, membrane-ELISA, electrophoresis, precipitation tests**†	Response to vaccination
Lymphocytes	**Complete blood cell count, DNA-PK$_{cs}$ genetic evaluation,**‡ FACS analysis of lymphocyte subsets using monoclonal antibodies	Response to vaccination, intradermal PHA test, in vitro lymphoproliferation assays
Neutrophils and macrophages	**Complete blood cell count**	Chemiluminesence and bactericidal assays, flow cytometric evaluation of phagocytosis and oxidative burst
Eosinophils and basophils	**Complete blood cell count**	No commonly available tests
Complement	No commonly available tests	No commonly available tests
Acute phase proteins	**Electrophoresis**	No commonly available tests

ELISA, Enzyme-linked immunosorbent assay; *DNA-PK,* DNA-protein kinase catytic subunit; *FACS,* florescence-activated cell sorter; *PHA,* phyohemagglutinin.

*Components of the immune system that can be evaluated in horses and appropriate tests for quantitative or functional analyses of each component. The list of tests is not exhaustive but restricted to tests of likely practical value for which normal data are available. Tests listed in bold type are routinely available to clinicians.

†Zinc sulfate turbidity and glutaraldehyde coagulation.

‡See SCID for description of DNA protein kinase catalytic subunit genetic testing.

for research use only that extend this range to include all the well-characterized IgG subclasses (i.e., IgGa, IgGb, IgGc, and IgG(T); Bethyl Laboratories, Montgomery, Tex.). The RID test is based on the ability of antigen and antibody to precipitate at equivalence when combined in proportion in agar gel plates. The serum being tested is added to punched-out wells in agar, impregnated with antibody to the specific immunoglobulin class being measured, and allowed to diffuse outward and bind with the anticlass-specific antisera. A precipitate forms when equivalence is reached and the area within the precipitate ring is directly proportional to the concentration of the patient's immunoglobulin class. Normal ranges of serum immunoglobulin concentrations are typically provided with commercial kits, and normal serum, milk, and colostrum concentrations of equine immunoglobulins have been described in numerous published studies. These results have been summarized and are available in tabular form in two sources.[3,10] More recent studies of foal and adult horse serum IgG and IgM concentrations using currently available RID assays measured considerably higher normal values in some instances.[11,12] In addition, an extensive study of immunoglobulin concentrations in adult and foal serum and nasal secretions and in colostrum and milk using an experimental monoclonal antibody based–system has been reported.[13]

By far the most common question that a clinician seeks to answer with regard to a horse's immune status is whether a foal has achieved adequate passive transfer of immunity. Whatever test is chosen must be able to distinguish serum concentrations of IgG of <200 mg/dl, 200 to 400 mg/dl, 400 to 800 mg/dl, and >800 mg/dl in order to permit diagnosis of total or partial failure of passive transfer. The test should be rapid, in order to allow early initiation of therapy, which decreases the utility of the RID test. A wide variety of tests have been used for this purpose: zinc sulfate turbidity, latex bead agglutination tests, ELISA assay, turbidometric analysis, glutaraldehyde coagulation, or infrared spectroscopy.[14-17] Addition of serum to zinc sulfate solution causes precipitation of immunoglobulins, principally IgG. Although the degree of resultant turbidity is usually proportional to the IgG concentration, turbidity may be increased by hemolysis in the sample, poor operating conditions, and poor-quality reagents. In the glutaraldehyde coagulation test, glutaraldehyde forms insoluble complexes with basic proteins in the serum.[18] Gel formation in 10 minutes or less is equated with a serum IgG concentration of 800 mg/dl or greater, whereas a positive reaction in 60 minutes is indicative of at least 400 mg IgG/dl serum. Like the zinc sulfate turbidity test, hemolysis may falsely overestimate the IgG concentration. In the latex agglutination test (Foalcheck, Haver Mobay Corp., Shawnee, Kan.), the patient's serum is mixed with the anti-equine IgG absorbed to latex particles. Macroscopic agglutination is proportional to serum IgG. Currently, for rapid diagnosis, the most convenient test system may be membrane filter–based ELISA systems (e.g., SNAP, Idexx, Westbrook, Me.; Figure 1-21). This test can be performed "foal-side" with whole blood. Tests such as the glutaraldehyde coagulation test are simpler and cheaper, although they have the disadvantage that serum is required. While some data suggest that the glutaraldehyde coagulation test may be more sensitive than membrane-filter ELISAs in detecting

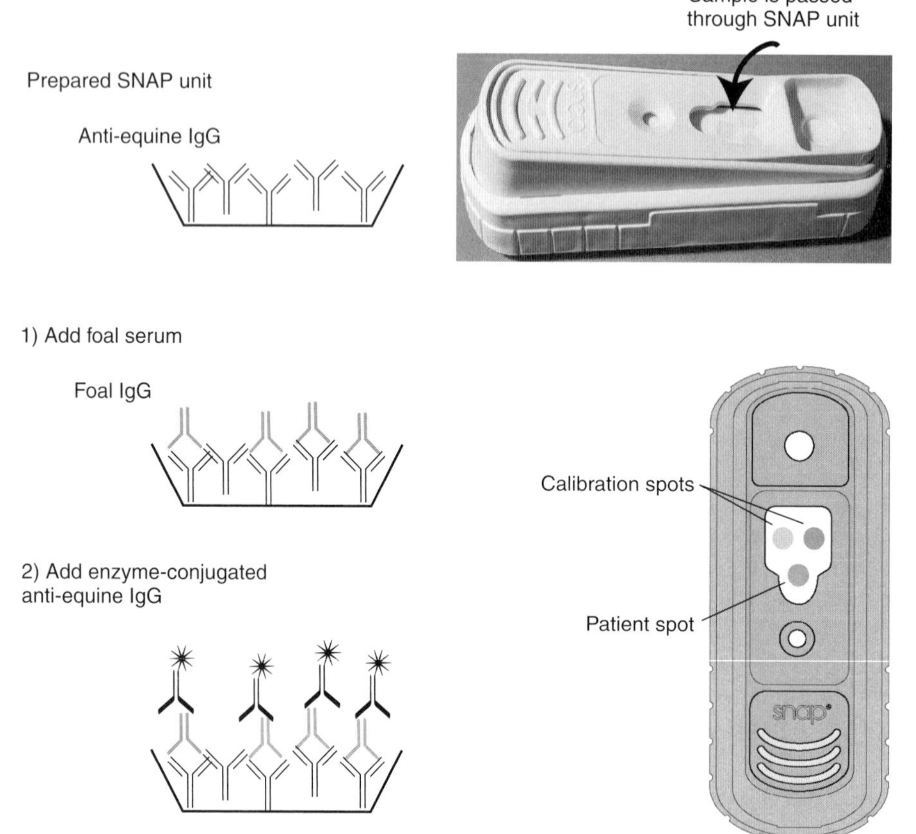

FIGURE 1-21 Membrane-based ELISA system (SNAP; Idexx, Westbrook, Me.) for measuring serum IgG concentration. The diluted test equine serum sample is applied to a "patient spot" on a membrane impregnated with a capture antibody recognizing equine IgG. Calibration spots corresponding to specific concentrations of equine IgG (400 and 800 mg/dl) are adjacent to the patient spot. An enzyme-conjugated second antibody against equine IgG is applied to the entire membrane, and finally the device is triggered to release an enzyme substrate that produces a colored reaction corresponding to the amount of enzyme-conjugated antibody on the membrane. By comparison with the calibration spots, the test sample IgG concentration can be estimated.

failure of passive tranfer,[15,22] particularly in differentiating normal foals (>800 mg/dl IgG) from partial failure of passive transfer (400 to 800 mg/dl), specificity can be relatively poor. The latter problem affects many of the rapid diagnostic tests for failure of passive transfer, and a more extensive discussion of test selection for this condition is presented later in the section covering this disease.

Alternative available tests that give information about serum immunoglobulin content include electrophoresis and immunoelectrophoresis (IEP). IEP analysis can demonstrate the presence of all the currently recognized equine immunoglobulin classes. However, the test has a relatively poor sensitivity and gives no quantitative information, as might be obtained from rocket electrophoresis.[23] Serum electrophoresis gives quantitative information about albumin and α, β, and γ globulin concentrations (Figure 1-22), and its utility is demonstrated when detecting the monoclonal gammopathies that accompany plasma cell myelomas.[24] Nevertheless, in the diagnosis of immunodeficiencies electrophoresis should be seen as an adjunct to RID assays, which are superior in terms of specificity and sensitivity.

Tests of Cellular Immunity

The simplest test of the cellular arm of the immune response is a total and differential white blood cell count, and this should be the starting point for any evaluation. Identification of an absolute lymphopenia, for example, is a critical finding in a suspected case of severe combined immunodeficiency (SCID) in an Arabian foal, although the result must be repeatable in a series of tests given the variability of blood lymphocyte counts. Such a finding would logically lead to genetic testing to confirm the diagnosis.[7] The evaluation of a lymph node biopsy for normal architecture, including the presence or absence of cells in either the B lymphocyte– or T lymphocyte–dependent areas, is another powerful test of the immune system. However, in profound immunodeficiencies such as SCID, lymphoid organs may be impossible to locate ante mortem. Beyond these readily available conventional techniques, three other more complex types of analysis can be of value: flow cytometric analysis (primarily of lymphocytes, although other cell types can be analyzed), lymphocyte function testing, and functional analysis of phagocytic cells.

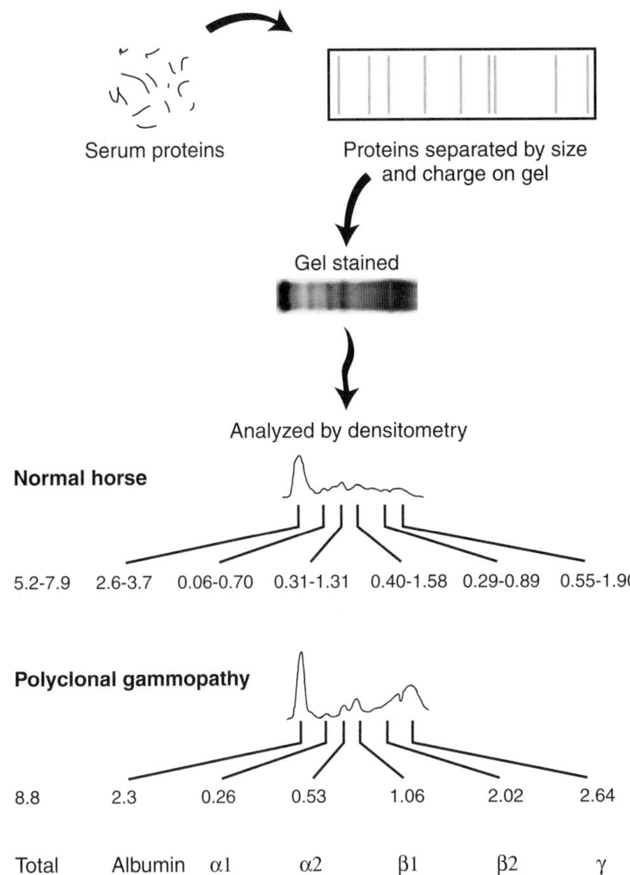

FIGURE 1-22 Serum protein electrophoresis. The complex mixture of serum proteins are separated by migration through[19-21] an agarose gel slab in response to an electric field. Proteins are stained, and the intensity of staining of different bands is measured by densitometric scanning. These measurements are used to identify different types of globulins and albumin corresponding to stained bands.

FLOW CYTOMETRY

It is currently feasible to take the equine differential white blood cell count a step further, because monoclonal antibodies are now available that can differentiate the morphologically identical equine lymphocyte family into distinct subsets with specific functions (Table 1-5).[25] Flow cytometry allows rapid measurements to be made of individual cells in a fluid stream. Flow cytometers utilize lasers to measure multiple parameters, including light scatter and fluorescence characteristics of cells, and are complex instruments to construct, but the principles of their operation are relatively simple (Figure 1-23). The fluidics system of the flow cytometer delivers cells one by one to a point in space intersected by a laser beam. The laser beam emits light of a defined wavelength to illuminate the cell, which results in both scattered light of the same wavelength and fluorescent light of a different wavelength that is collected by photodetectors and converted into electronic signals.

Light is collected by the forward collection lens on the other side of the flow chamber from the laser source. Here light scattered from 1 to 20 degrees from the laser-beam axis is collected as "forward scatter," and its amount depends on the size of the cell being analyzed. At 90 degrees (orthogonal) to the laser beam, path light is collected for the purpose of measuring "side scatter" and fluorescent emission. Optical filtration separates scattered light and fluorescent light to permit their independent measurement. Side scatter light depends on the granularity of cells. Fluorescent light can be detected independently for a number of fluorochromes of different wavelengths, and typical examples would be fluorescein (FITC) or phycoerythrin (PE).

Signals from the different detectors can be processed directly or after logarithmic amplification. The advantage of log amplification for the fluorescent signals is that it amplifies weak signals and compresses large signals, allowing their simultaneous display. By these means signals with a 10,000-fold difference in intensity can be displayed. Signals are typically displayed as either histograms or dual parameter correlated plots (dot plots), and statistical analysis is completed by computer. Histograms are analyzed by setting markers in particular channels and dot plots by drawing rectangular or polygonal boxes around data points. The software also allows the setting of "gates" for determining which events are collected in the first instance or which events are to be included in later analyses. Typically, these gating techniques are employed using forward and side scatter to differentiate cell types, such as lymphocytes, monocytes, and granulocytes. The final key characteristic of flow cytometers is their capacity to analyze large numbers of "events" (cells) in a short time, making it possible to analyze many thousands of cells in a matter of seconds.

An example of such an analysis is shown in Figure 1-23. In this instance the goal was to identify lymphocytes expressing the equine homologs of the CD4 and CD8 molecules using two monoclonal antibodies independently labeled with the FITC (CD4) and PE (CD8) fluorochromes. For this analysis a peripheral blood leukocyte population was prepared by simply lysing the erythrocytes in a blood sample using distilled water. Subsequently, the whole leukocyte population was stained in solution using the monoclonal antibodies. Alternatively, lymphocytes could have been purified from blood using differential centrifugation techniques before staining. However, identical analytical results are obtained in the horse using the more rapid technique of whole leukocyte preparation and exploiting the capacity of the flow cytometer to distinguish lymphocytes from other cells.[26] During the flow cytometric analysis the first step was to identify the lymphocytes using the different forward and side scattering characteristics of different leukocyte populations. Panel A in Figure 1-23 shows a dot-plot of forward scatter versus side scatter, with each dot representing a cell. Granulocytes (G) can be distinguished from lymphocytes (L) by their greater granularity (side scatter) and size (forward scatter). The dotted line is a "gate" drawn around the lymphocyte population. Subsequent analysis of fluorescence is directed toward only those cells that fall within this gate. After establishing the physical characteristics of the cells to be analyzed, their fluorescence can be examined. In Panel B of Figure 1-23, a histogram is shown depicting CD4 (FITC) staining. A vertical marker identifies a gate set based on staining by a negative control antibody. Therefore all cells to the right of this marker are staining positively for CD4. For two-color staining dot plots are again used. In Panel C each dot represents a cell, and its position relative to the two axes illustrates its

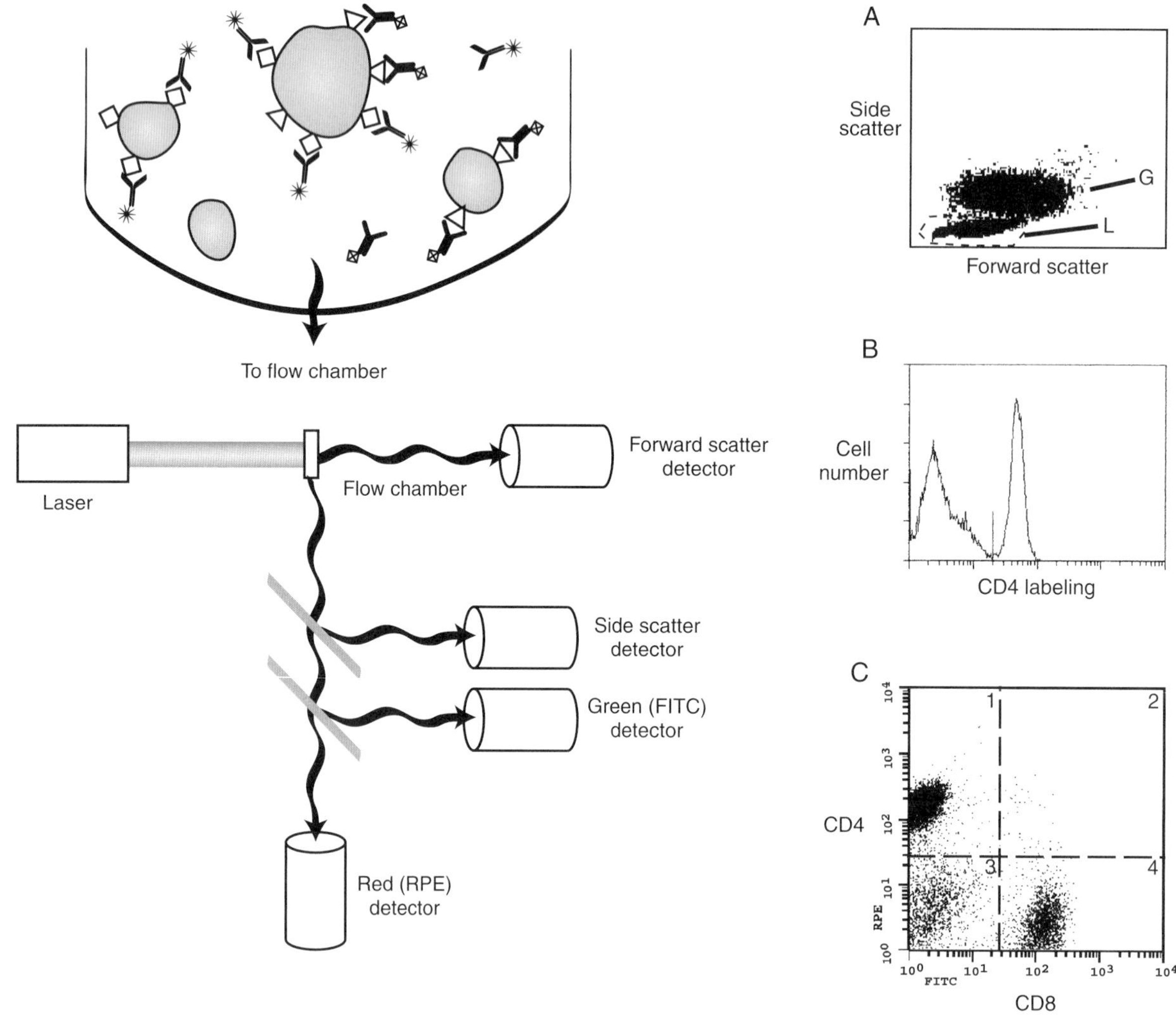

FIGURE 1-23 Flow cytometric analysis (see text for key); *FITC,* Fluoroscein isothiocyanate; *RPE,* R-phycoerythrin.

staining characteristics; the dotted lines represent the cutoff points for negative or positive staining. Therefore all cells in quadrants 1 and 2 are positively stained for CD4, and all cells in quadrants 2 and 4 are positively stained for CD8. Effectively, quadrant 1 contains all the helper T lymphocytes (CD4 positive), quadrant 4 contains all the cytotoxic T lymphocytes (CD8 positive), quadrant 3 contains the B lymphocyte population, and quadrant 2 is empty because there are no "double-positive" T lymphocytes in the blood of horses. The sum of the cells in quadrants 1 and 4 represents the T lymphocyte population.

This technique has revolutionized immunobiologic studies in recent years, finding its most obvious clinical application in enumerating human CD4-positive lymphocytes in cases of acquired immune deficiency[27] and in classifying leukemias and lymphomas.[28,29] A large number of antibodies are now available for use in the horse[25] (see Table 1-5), and recent reports describe the use of this approach in charting the response to microbial infection,[11,30,31] and in differentiating equine leukemia.[29,32,33] Several recent studies provide examples of normal values for peripheral blood analysis.[11,12,34,35]

LYMPHOCYTE FUNCTION TESTING

Unfortunately, tests of lymphocyte function are generally limited in their availability in the field. In vitro tests of lymphocyte function include lymphocyte proliferation responses to mitogens such as pokeweed (B cell dependent), phytohemagglutinin (T cell dependent), or concanavilin A (T and B cell dependent). These assays are generally not commercially available, although they are commonly performed by immunologic researchers. In addition, some caution should be used because it may not always be valid to draw inferences about the intact animal from the results of these in vitro tests,[3] and because of significant variability in results, it is essential to perform parallel studies on suitable age-matched control horses. The end point of these tests is usually read by determining the incorporation of radioactive ^{3}H-thymidine into the total population of proliferating cells. Nonradioactive alternatives exist, and one strategy uses intracellular labeling of lymphocytes with 5-carboxyfluorescein diacetate-succinimidyl ester (CFSE). Labeled cells fluoresce, and after subsequent divisions in response to mitogens, this fluorescence decreases by half for each cycle of cell division. This allows for measurement of equine lymphocyte proliferation using flow cytometry, and simultaneous two-color staining allows for measurement of proliferation in specific lymphocyte subsets.[36]

Two tests that can be of value and are readily available in practice are response to vaccination, as measured by rising serum titers, and response to intradermal phytohemagglutinin, which is dependent on a delayed-type hypersensitivity T lymphocyte response and develops in normal animals without prior sensitization.[37] A 50-μg dose of phytohemagglutinin (PHA) in 0.5 ml of phosphate-buffered saline is injected intradermally while 0.5 ml of phosphate-buffered saline is administered intradermally at a distant site. At the PHA site an increase in wheal size of 0.6 mm or less indicates a defect in cell-mediated immunity. Response to vaccination has proved to be a potent means of identifying immunodeficiency in such conditions as juvenile llama immunodeficiency syndrome.[38] Similarly, the equine immune response to a polyvalent inactivated bovine vaccine has been used to document the immunosuppressive effects of corticosteroid administration.[39] For practical purposes, response to rabies or tetanus vaccination may be the most suitable available tests provided that no routine vaccination had been administered in the immediate past. Equine rabies or tetanus antibody titer determination is typically commercially available, and the majority of available vaccines are sufficiently potent to provoke a fourfold increase in titer in normal horses.

PHAGOCYTE FUNCTION TESTING

Testing of equine neutrophil migration, phagocytic function, and bactericidal activity has been reported by several investigators.[40-43] The techniques employed are typically only available in research laboratories and are not well adapted to investigations of individual animals unless adequate age-matched control animals are also examined. More quantitative information can be obtained by adapting assay systems to flow cytometric analysis. Two reports describe flow cytometric analysis of neutrophil phagocytosis of either fluorescent microspheres[44] or yeast cells.[45] Raidal et al. have described testing of alveolar macrophage and blood neutrophil phagocytic function using fluorescent-labeled bacteria and oxidative burst activity using oxidation of dichlorofluorescein.[46-49] These flow cytometric approaches have great promise and have been applied to various studies, including measurements of the effect of age [48-50] and of exercise[51] on neutrophil function.

TESTS OF INNATE IMMUNITY

Components of the innate immune response that have been measured in the horse include the numbers of granulocytes and monocytes in peripheral blood and their phagocytic function (see previous discussion); natural cytotoxicity in terms of lymphokine-activated killer (LAK) cell activity;[41,52,53] and measurement of soluble factors, including several acute-phase proteins, [54-58] and complement. Equine complement activity can be measured using a hemolytic assay in which antibody sensitized chicken erythrocytes are used as target cells, and the amount of serum required to lyse 50% of these targets is expressed as CH_{50} units.[59] More recently, a flow cytometric assay has been described.[60] These tests have been used in some instances to detect relative immunodeficiency in terms of LAK cell activity in exercised horses[53] or complement activity in foals.[61] Currently, these techniques have very limited availability.

PRIMARY IMMUNODEFICIENCIES

SEVERE COMBINED IMMUNODEFICIENCY

SCID is a lethal primary immunodeficiency, affecting Arabian foals, humans, mice, and dogs, characterized by failure to produce functional B and T lymphocytes, and resulting in lack of any antigen-specific immune responses.[1,62-64] The vast majority of affected foals are Arabians, in which the condition is inherited as an autosomal recessive trait, and results from a lack of DNA protein kinase activity that prevent V(D)J recombination.[7,65] In studies conducted in the United States and reported in 1977, the incidence of SCID among Arabian foals was at least 2% to 3%,[66] suggesting a carrier prevalence rate between 25% and 26%. However, in more recent studies conducted in the United States using a precise molecular diagnosis of the carrier state, carrier prevalence was consistently 8%.[67,68]

CLINICAL SIGNS AND LABORATORY FINDINGS

Affected foals are clinically normal at birth but develop signs of infection during the first 1 to 3 months of life. The age of onset of infection depends on the adequacy of passive transfer and degree of environmental challenge. As maternal antibodies are catabolically eliminated, SCID foals are increasingly susceptible to infections with bacterial, viral, fungal, and protozoal agents. Bronchopneumonia is a common disease, often caused by adenovirus, which is the most significant pathogen of SCID foals, affecting two thirds of all animals.[69] Adenoviral infection frequently extends to the gastrointestinal and urogenital system and causes pancreatic disease, leading to loss of endocrine and exocrine tissue and possibly contributing to the impaired growth and weight loss observed in SCID foals.[1] Other common infections in SCID foals include *Pneumocystis carinii* pneumonia; *Rhodococcus equi* infections; enteritis, frequently caused by *Cryptosporidium parvum*[70]; arthritis; and omphalophlebitis.

Clinical signs in SCID foals may include nasal discharge, coughing, dyspnea, diarrhea, fever, and weight loss. Although antibiotics, plasma, and supportive care prolong the course of disease, death invariably occurs before 5 months of age. The only exception to this rule was a single foal experimentally treated with a bone marrow transplant from a histocompatible donor that lived until 5 years of age before dying of an unrelated cause.[71] A consistent hematologic finding is absolute lymphopenia (<1,000 μ/L), with neutrophilia a variable finding resulting from bacterial infection. Total serum globulins and serum IgG can be normal in the first weeks of life if passive transfer is adequate but decline as maternal immunoglobulins are catabolized. Normal foals synthesize IgM from 180 days of gestation and have detectable IgM at birth in presuckle samples, whereas SCID foals have no IgM.[72] After colostral ingestion SCID foals also have IgM, although with its relatively short half life it is undetectable by 2 to 4 weeks of age.[1]

ETIOLOGY AND PATHOGENESIS

Normal maturation of T and B cells requires rearrangement of a series of germ line genes in order to create genetic sequences that can encode the wide diversity of antigen receptors required by these lymphocytes (the T cell receptor or immunoglobulin antigen binding sites, respectively, as described under Equine Immunology). These genes are called the V, D, and J genes, and the overall process is called *V(D)J recombination*. This process depends on two groups of enzymes, the recombinase activating gene (RAG) products and DNA-protein kinase (DNA-PK), which is critical for DNA double-stranded break repair. In SCID foals a component of DNA-PK called *DNA-PK catalytic subunit* (*DNA-PK*$_{cs}$) is defective, and consequently V(D)J recombination events do not occur, lymphocytes do not mature, and the immature lymphocytes are eliminated.[7,65] The defect is a five nucleotide deletion in the DNA-PK$_{cs}$ gene that produces a premature stop codon and prevents formation of the complete enzyme.

DIAGNOSIS

Antemortem diagnosis of SCID is suggested by appropriate clinical signs in a foal of Arabian breeding with persistent marked lymphopenia (usually <500/μl) and the absence of serum IgM by RID. If presuckle serum is unavailable for testing, serum IgM cannot be used as a diagnostic aid until the foal is older than 3 weeks. Previously, all suspected cases required confirmation by the necropsy finding of hypoplasia of the spleen, thymus, and lymph nodes with the absence of any normal lymphoid architecture. With the identification of the genetic defect causing SCID, the current standard for definitive diagnosis is demonstrating that the foal is homozygous for the defective SCID gene. This test depends on PCR amplification of a specific region of the DNA-PKcs gene, and evaluation of the amplicon in a Southern blot using probes specific for normal and mutant sequences.[7] This test is commercially available (VetGen, Ann Arbor, Mich.); requires whole blood or cheek swabs; and can identify homozygous affected, heterozygous carriers, and normal animals.

TREATMENT

Supportive care may prolong the course of disease, but affected foals die by 5 months. Immunologic reconstitution is currently impractical and an ethically questionable procedure.

CLIENT EDUCATION

Arabian mares and stallions intended for breeding should be tested for SCID carrier status. When two heterozygous carriers are bred, the progeny will include 25% SCID foals, 50% carriers, and 25% homozygous normal foals. Therefore prevention of SCID requires identification of carriers and either removing them from the breeding population or breeding them exclusively with homozygous normal animals and subsequent testing of progeny before their own breeding future is planned.

Anemia, Immunodeficiency, and Peripheral Ganglionopathy—Fell Pony Immunodeficiency Syndrome

In the late 1990s a new syndrome of anemia, immunodeficiency, and peripheral ganglionopathy was described in Fell pony foals.[73,74] Affected foals become ill within 2 to 3 weeks of birth and die by 3 months of age. Affected animals have been described in the United Kingdom, elsewhere in Europe,[75] and in the United States.[76]

CLINICAL SIGNS AND LABORATORY FINDINGS

Clinical signs include ill thrift, anemia, respiratory infection, glossal hyperkeratosis, and diarrhea. Anemia can be severe and is normochromic and normocytic to macrocytic, with small numbers of late erythroid precursors in bone marrow.[74,77] Some foals are affected by cryptosporidial enteritis and adenoviral bronchopneumonia and pancreatitis. Plasma proteins and blood lymphocyte counts can be normal or low. T cell subsets measured by flow cytometry are normal, although MHC II expression is low.[78] In vitro lymphoproliferative responses are normal.[78] On necropsy lymphoid organs can be small, and secondary lymphoid follicles and plasma cells are absent.[74] Neuronal changes are characterized by neuronal chromatolysis in the cranial mesenteric, dorsal root, and trigeminal ganglia.

ETIOLOGY AND PATHOGENESIS

There is preliminary evidence that this is a genetic disease inherited as an autosomal recessive trait, although the underlying defect is unknown.[79]

DIAGNOSIS

Previously, diagnosis depended on the antemortem presence of clinical signs in Fell pony foals and histologic confirmation of erythroid hypoplasia in the bone marrow, neuronal chromatolysis in peripheral nerve ganglia, absence of secondary lymphoid follicles, and low numbers of plasma cells in spleen and mesenteric lymph nodes. More recently, it has been shown that IgM levels measured after 4 weeks of age can assist in diagnosis, as can flow cytometric measurement of B lymphocytes.[80,81]

TREATMENT

Treatment of specific infections is of limited efficacy in affected foals, particularly those affected by severe anemia and diarrhea, and all die by 3 months of age.

CLIENT EDUCATION

While the underlying basis of this disease is unknown, it is difficult to give specific advice. If the condition is shown to be an autosomal recessive trait, then both the dam and sire of affected foals will be confirmed as carriers and breeding is discouraged.

Selective IgM Deficiency

Selective IgM deficiency is characterized by substantially reduced or absent serum IgM with normal or increased concentrations of other immunoglobulins and no other evidence of immunodeficiency.[1,82] Serum IgM concentrations are more than two standard deviations below the mean of age-matched control animals. All other immunologic parameters are normal, although in one case a lack of response to the B cell mitogen lipopolysaccharide was reported.[83] The syndrome has been most frequently described in Arabians and Quarter Horses, although the diagnosis has been made in other breeds.

CLINICAL SIGNS AND LABORATORY FINDINGS

Two clinical syndromes have been described. The first condition affects foals between 2 and 8 months of age, which develop severe pneumonia, arthritis, and enteritis with or without septicemia; many die before 10 months of age. Gram-negative bacterial infections are common (especially with *Klebsiella* species), and age at onset of signs is generally older than in foals with combined immunodeficiency. Some affected foals survive but have a history of repeated bacterial infections that respond temporarily to therapy but recur once antimicrobials are discontinued. These foals grow poorly and generally die within 2 years. Rarely, foals can recover from IgM deficiency, suggesting that such cases may actually be secondary rather than primary immunodeficiencies.[84]

The second presentation involves horses between 2 and 5 years of age, many of which have or ultimately develop lymphosarcoma. These individuals may have external or internal lymphadenopathy or both. Chronic weight loss, depression, and other nonspecific signs usually accompany lymphosarcoma. In cases associated with lymphosarcoma, the IgM deficiency is presumed to be a secondary rather than a primary immunodeficiency.

Routine laboratory findings are not diagnostically specific. Hematologic abnormalities consistent with chronic inflammatory disease, such as anemia, neutrophilia, and hyperfibrinogenemia, are commonly present. The total plasma protein and serum globulins are usually normal.

ETIOLOGY AND PATHOGENESIS

Although a genetic basis is suspected, the pathogenesis of selective IgM deficiency is unknown.[1] It seems likely that there are primary and secondary forms of this syndrome.

DIAGNOSIS

Definitive diagnosis of selective IgM deficiency is made by measuring the major serum immunoglobulins by RID and determining the absolute lymphocyte count. Horses with selective IgM deficiency have serum IgM concentrations persistently less than 2 standard deviations below that of age-matched controls (<15 mg/dl at 4 to 8 months old; <25 mg/dl at >8 months old) coupled with normal concentrations of IgG (≥400 mg/dl) and a normal lymphocyte count. Normal values for equine IgM concentrations have recently been reported.[85] Because seriously ill foals may have transiently depressed serum IgM concentration, suspected cases should be tested at least twice to document that IgM concentrations remain low. All other immunoglobulin concentrations are normal.

TREATMENT

Other than supportive care and antimicrobial therapy, there is no effective treatment for selective IgM deficiency. Because transfused plasma concentrations of IgM are low and the half life is quite short, any benefit would be only temporary.

CLIENT EDUCATION

The prognosis must be guarded; however, recovery has been reported.[84] If primary immunodeficiency is diagnosed or suspected, it is probably inadvisable to rebreed the sire and dam.

Other Primary Immunodeficiencies

Transient hypogammaglobulinemia and agammaglobulinemia are reported as established primary immunodeficiency syndromes in horses. However, these conditions have been infrequently reported and consequently remain poorly defined. Available information is presented later in this chapter. A further form of immunodeficiency affecting humoral immunity was described by Boy et al.[86] in a 10-month-old Arabian colt. The animal exhibited an absence of serum IgM, IgA, and IgG(T) and a normal concentration of IgG. In vitro testing of peripheral blood mononuclear cells (PBMCs) with T cell mitogens elicited normal responses, and responses to B cell mitogens were weak. On postmortem examination there was generalized lymphocyte depletion of lymphoid organs.

To increase our understanding of these and other currently unidentified immunodeficiency syndromes of horses, it is critical that every effort be made to identify such cases and thoroughly investigate them. Newly available immunologic resources may make it possible to define these diseases further and increase our diagnostic and prognostic resources, provided the case material can be identified.

COMMON VARIABLE IMMUNODEFICIENCY

Common variable immunodeficiency is the most common primary immunodeficiency in humans,[87] and sporadic cases have been reported in recent years in horses.[88-90] The disease is characterized by a deficiency of all immunoglobulin classes, accompanied by various defects in cellular function, but most consistently by a failure of B lymphocyte maturation. A pattern of recurrent infections and decreased serum immunoglobulin levels is seen. Medical management of these cases has been reported, with survival times of more than 1 year in some instances, even without the use of immunoglobulin replacement therapy.[88]

TRANSIENT HYPOGAMMAGLOBULINEMIA

Transient hypogammaglobulinemia has been reported in only two foals, an Arabian and a Thoroughbred, and is characterized by delayed onset of immunoglobulin synthesis.[84,91] Affected foals manifested signs consistent with bacterial and viral infections when passively acquired immunoglobulins are catabolized to nonprotective concentrations. For unknown reasons, the onset of autologous immunoglobulin production, which generally occurs at birth, is delayed until these foals are approximately 3 months of age. Hematologic studies may be suggestive of chronic infection, although total plasma protein is normal or reduced slightly. Diagnosis is based on the presence of low serum IgG (<200 mg/dl) and IgG(T) (<20 mg/dl) at 2 to 4 months of age, with low-normal serum IgM (>15 mg/dl) and IgA (>20 mg/dl). Lymphocyte counts are normal. Antimicrobial therapy and plasma transfusions are necessary to minimize infections. Affected foals usually survive if they have not concomitantly suffered failure of passive transfer and they receive appropriate support between 2 and 4 months of age. The fact that foals spontaneously recover from this condition raises the question of whether it may be a secondary immunodeficiency.

AGAMMAGLOBULINEMIA

Agammaglobulinemia is characterized by absence of B lymphocytes and failure to produce immunoglobulins in the presence of normal cell-mediated immunity.[1] The disease has been described in five colts of Thoroughbred, Standardbred, and Quarter Horse breeds.[84,92,93] Clinical signs commence between 2 and 6 months of age and result from bacterial infections such as pneumonia, enteritis, and arthritis. Multisystemic infections that respond poorly to therapy are common, and laboratory changes reflect chronic inflammatory disease. The fact that this syndrome has only been described in colts suggests an X-linked mode of inheritance, as occurs in a similar disease of humans. A maturation defect from stem cells to B cells has been suggested.[1] Affected foals have persistently subnormal serum concentrations of all immunoglobulin classes and normal lymphocyte counts. Serum IgM and IgA are generally absent at the time of evaluation and maternally derived IgG and IgG(T) decline with time. At 2 months of age, IgG is less than 300 mg/dl, which declines to less than 100 mg/dL by 6 months. There is no serologic response to immunization, and B lymphocytes, as determined by immunofluorescence, are absent. Tests of cell-mediated immune function such as intradermal PHA and in vitro blastogenesis are normal. Plasma and antimicrobial therapy result only in transient improvement. Affected horses die from disseminated infection between 1 and 2 years of age.

SECONDARY IMMUNODEFICIENCIES

Failure of Passive Transfer

Failure of passive transfer is the most common immunodeficiency disorder of horses and has recently been extensively reviewed.[2,94] It occurs in all breeds secondary to inadequate absorption of colostral antibodies. Failure of passive transfer is significantly correlated with increased susceptibility to infectious disease and death in neonatal foals.[95,96] The newborn foal is capable of mounting a normal immune response, as described earlier in this chapter. However, neonatal foals are immunologically naïve and thus have not yet developed memory responses or produced antigen-specific antibody and other forms of adaptive immunity. During the first 1 to 2 months of life, foals are dependent on passively transferred immunity for protection from infectious disease. The diffuse epitheliochorial nature of the equine placenta does not allow for in utero immunoglobulin transfer to foals. Although minor concentrations of some immunoglobulins can be detected at birth, the foal is born essentially agammaglobulinemic and acquires passive immunity by the ingestion and absorption of colostrum from the dam.[97,98] Colostrum is a specialized form of milk containing immunoglobulins, which are produced during the last 2 weeks of gestation under hormonal influences. Colostrum contains primarily IgGa, IgGb (IgGa plus IgGb is the equivalent of IgG) and IgG(T), with smaller quantities of IgA and IgM, all of which have been concentrated into mammary secretions from the mare's blood.[13,99] Colostrum is produced only one time each pregnancy and is replaced by milk that contains negligible immunoglobulins within 24 hours of the initiation of lactation.[13,97,99] Normal foals suckle within 1 to 3 hours of birth, and the absorptive capacity of the foal's gastrointestinal tract for immunoglobulins is greatest during the first 6 hours after birth, and then steadily declines until immunoglobulins can no longer be absorbed, when the foal is 24 hours old. The incidence of failure of passive transfer is highly variable among groups of horses and seems to depend primarily on management factors that ensure early colostral ingestion.[100] The reported prevalences of at least partial failure of passive transfer have ranged between 3% to 37%.[22,84,95,100]

CLINICAL SIGNS AND LABORATORY FINDINGS

Failure of passive transfer does not directly cause any clinical signs of disease. Failure of passive transfer is suspected when signs of generalized or localized bacterial infections such as septicemia, pneumonia, enteritis, and arthritis develop during the first 3 weeks of life. Routine laboratory findings may suggest sepsis, but the presence of infection in the neonatal period is not pathognomonic for failure of passive transfer. Common abnormalities include neutropenia or neutrophilia, hypoglycemia, and hyperfibrinogenemia. The total plasma protein may be low, normal, or elevated in foals with failure of passive transfer because of the wide variation in normal presuckle total plasma protein and the confounding effects of dehydration secondary to sepsis.

ETIOLOGY AND PATHOGENESIS

Causes for failure of passive transfer in foals include (1) failure of the foal to ingest an adequate volume of colostrum in the early postpartum period; (2) loss of colostrum via premature lactation; (3) inadequate immunoglobulin content of the colostrum; and (4) insufficient immunoglobulin absorption via the intestine.[2,101] There is a highly negative correlation between foal serum IgG concentration and the incidence of severe infections;[95] however, the minimum amount of IgG necessary for protection of a foal from infection varies with the amount and virulence of environmental pathogens, concomitant stress factors, and colostral antibody titer against specific pathogens. Although a serum IgG concentration of at least 400 mg/dl has been considered evidence of adequate passive transfer, most normal foals attain values more than twice this high[95,100] and serum IgG greater than 800 mg/dl may be required for adequate immunity.[96] Numerous other colostral factors may be important for the immune protection of foals. Colostrum has been variously shown to regulate cell-mediated immunity, activate granulocytes, promote intestinal absorption of macromolecules, decrease intestinal colonization by pathogens, and contain constituents of innate immunity (e.g., lactoferrin, complement) and leukocytes that have a local protective role in the neonatal digestive tract and may be systemically absorbed.[102,103] At this time the significance of these various phenomena for the health of neonates and their immunologic development is largely unknown. The one exception is the finding that colostral ingestion suppresses de novo antibody responses in foals in both a nonspecific and an antigen-specific manner.[97,104]

Neonatal weakness or lack of maternal cooperation (common in maiden mares) are common reasons for the foal to ingest an inadequate volume of colostrum. If colostral ingestion is delayed beyond 6 hours, the absorption of immunoglobulins is significantly reduced. Lactation before parturition is another common reason for failure of passive transfer because colostrum is produced only one time each gestation. The causative factors for premature lactation are unknown at this time, but foals from mares that "leak" milk hours to days before parturition are likely to suffer failure of passive transfer.[101]

Subnormal colostral immunoglobulin content (<3000 mg/dl) is rare in mares that do not prelactate,[100] but wide individual variation in colostral concentration of immunoglobulins does occur.[100,105-107] Poor-quality colostrum will undoubtedly cause failure of passive transfer. Colostral immunoglobulin content can be estimated by specific gravity or sugar (Brix) refractometry or quantitated by RID.[101]

Malabsorption is implicated as a cause of failure of passive transfer when foals are known to have ingested an adequate volume of good-quality colostrum within 12 hours of birth. Because glucocorticoids hasten the maturation of specialized enterocytes, stress-causing endogenous corticosteroid release may be a cause of reduced immunoglobulin absorption. However, obvious stress factors are often not found in foals with apparent impaired ability to absorb IgG.[6]

DIAGNOSIS

Subnormal serum IgG concentration 24 hours after birth is the basis for diagnosis of failure of passive transfer. Serum IgG of less than 200 mg/dl indicates complete failure of passive transfer, whereas 200 to 800 mg/dl should be considered partial failure of passive transfer. Many foals under good management conditions may remain healthy if the serum IgG concentration is at least 400 mg/dl, and consequently this cut point is measured by several rapid diagnostic tests. The most quantitatively accurate method to determine serum IgG is the SRID test (VMRD, Pullman, Wash.); however, this assay is time consuming and expensive, thus inappropriate for the diagnosis of failure of passive transfer when timely therapeutic intervention is paramount.[108] Numerous field screening procedures for IgG have been evaluated.[2,15,16,22,108-110] Criteria for selecting a screening test for equine failure of passive transfer must include accuracy, the time necessary to perform the test, ease of performance, and cost. Although the zinc sulfate turbidity, turbidimetric immunoassay, and glutaraldehyde coagulation tests are inexpensive and provide results within 1 hour, the ease and reported accuracy of membrane-based ELISA tests often makes them the test of choice in many practice situations. However, results of a recent study suggest that the choice of screening test is not so straightforward.[111] Although a variety of screening assays produced acceptable screening results, a membrane-based ELISA assay (SNAP test; Idexx, Westbrook, Me.) gave the greatest sensitivity, specificity, and accuracy at a cutoff of 400 mg/dl. However, at a cutoff of 800 mg/dl, this same test had a lower specificity that would have led to unnecessary treatment of some foals if that cutoff had been used. These data highlight the difficulty faced by equine clinicians in selecting a rapid diagnostic test for failure of passive transfer. Because failure to diagnose and treat the condition could result in the death of many foals, a sensitive test is required. However, specificity is also important, particularly given the cost of treatment (plasma transfusion) and the fact that treatment is not without its own inherent complications. Individual clinician judgment is therefore important in test selection, although at this time the relatively good performance of semiquantitative SNAP test, and its convenience, may continue to make it a popular choice.[112] Turbidimetric immunoassays offer a somewhat more complex but potentially more accurate assay that can be conducted at the point of care.[16,110] Generally, all screening tests are relatively accurate in identifying foals with complete failure of passive transfer; however, there is variation in their ability to detect marginally deficient foals.[2] In the future new technologies such as infrared spectroscopy have considerable promise for providing accurate and economical results.[17]

TREATMENT

If failure of passive transfer is anticipated because of premature lactation, neonatal weakness, dam death, or low-specific-gravity colostrum, an alternative colostral source can be given orally. A minimum of 2 L of equine colostrum given in 500-ml increments during the first 8 hours after birth is optimal. Bovine colostrum may be safely substituted if equine colostrum is not available;[61,113] however, foals given bovine colostrum may also require plasma transfusion because bovine immunoglobulins have a very short half life in foals and are not specifically directed against equine pathogens.

If the foal is more than 12 hours old when failure of passive transfer is suspected or diagnosed, an intravenous plasma transfusion is indicated. There are numerous commercial sources of equine plasma. Use of these products is convenient, saves time, and is safe because donors are free of alloantibodies and negative for infectious diseases. The only potential drawback to the use of commercial plasma is that antibodies specific for pathogens in the foal's environment may be lacking. Optimal plasma would be obtained from a local blood-typed donor, one that is known to lack serum alloantibodies and alloantigens Aa and Qa. The volume of plasma necessary to bring serum IgG into an acceptable range cannot be accurately predicted because it depends on the severity of failure of passive transfer, the immunoglobulin content of the plasma, and on concomitant diseases, which may hasten immunoglobulin catabolism. Generally, 1 L of plasma will increase the serum IgG concentration of a 50-kg foal by 200 to 300 mg/dl;[40] thus 2 to 4 L may be necessary to achieve serum IgG greater than 800 mg/dl. A therapeutic dose of plasma should be administered, and then foal serum IgG remeasured. If the desired concentration has not been attained, more plasma is necessary. Some foals with partial failure of passive transfer (IgG >400 and <800 mg/dl) may do well without plasma therapy if there are no preexisting infections and exposure to pathogens is minimized. These foals should be monitored closely for the development of infections.

CLIENT EDUCATION

The prognosis for foals with failure of passive transfer depends on the degree of failure, the environment to which the foal is exposed, the foal's age at the time of diagnosis, and the presence and severity of secondary infections. Management factors that ensure the ingestion of at least 2 L of high-quality colostrum within 6 hours of birth are paramount in failure of passive transfer prevention. Foaling should be witnessed so that any mispresentations can be corrected, and foals that do not readily nurse within 3 hours can be given colostrum via nasogastric tube. The evaluation of colostral specific gravity with a hydrometer (Lane Manufacturing, Denver, Colo.) or Brix 0-50% sugar refractometer may aid in prediction of failure of passive transfer.[101] A colostral specific gravity of 1.060 measured with a hydrometer corresponds to approximately 3000 mg/dl IgG, which is the minimum acceptable value. When dam colostral specific gravity is less than 1.060, some degree of failure of passive transfer should be suspected in the foal and corrected. A Brix % sugar reading of 20% to 30% correlates with adequate colostral quality and a reading of >30% indicates very good-quality colostrums. A commercial kit based on glutaraldehyde coagulation (Gamma-Check-C, Veterinary Dynamics, Inc., San Luis Obispo, Calif.) is also available for stallside screening of immunoglobulin concentrations in mare colostrums.

Routine screening of foal serum IgG at 24 to 48 hours after birth allows necessary plasma therapy before the onset of infections. This can be done with any of a variety of stallside or laboratory tests described earlier in this chapter. Ideally, foals should have an IgG concentration of >800 mg/dl at 24 to 36 hours of age.

Foals that are born prematurely, are weak, or from prelactating mares should be provided with an alternative colostral source within 6 hours of birth. A colostrum bank can be established by collecting and freezing (−20° C) 250 ml of colostrum from mares that have not prelactated within 6 hours of foaling, once their own foals have suckled. Ideally, banked colostrum should be screened for alloantibodies, although they are unlikely if the mare's own foal remains healthy. The immunoglobulins in banked frozen colostrum are stable for at least 1 year.

Exercise

Exercise, when conducted at a stressful level, can significantly affect equine immune function.[114] Strenuous exercise significantly suppresses lymphoproliferative responses, while increasing lymphokine activated killer cell activity.[53,115] In racehorses decreased lymphoproliferative responses can be demonstrated 12 to 16 hours after racing.[116] Protracted high-intensity training results in decreased phagocytosis and oxidative burst activity in neutrophils and lymphocytes, although pulmonary alveolar macrophage function was unaffected.[51] Other studies have demonstrated decreased neutrophil and pulmonary alveolar macrophage (PAM) function in response to single bouts of intense exercise[117,118] and prolonged suppression of innate immunity after exercise of long duration.[119] In unconditioned ponies strenuous exercise increases susceptibility to experimental infection with equine influenza virus.[120,121] In an influenza infection study in trained horses, moderate exercise led to increased signs of clinical disease, although duration of disease was unaffected.[121]

Overall, these various studies have demonstrated a clear immunomodulatory effect of exercise, with some specific evidence for increased susceptibility to infectious disease. Although this remains an active area of investigation with much to be learned, it is clear that the potentially immunosuppressive effect of high-intensity exercise, particularly of protracted duration or in unconditioned animals, needs to be recognized.

Age

There is a high incidence of *respiratory infections in foals and weanlings*, which frequently relapse on cessation of antibiotic treatment.[122] It is also possible that the normal level of immunocompetence in this age group leads to increased susceptibility to pyogenic respiratory infections, particularly under group housing conditions. Features of the foal's immune system that may predispose to such infections are discussed earlier in this chapter.

Old age has the potential to result in relative immunodeficiency, although there have been few equine studies to investigate this possibility. Older horses display decreased lymphoproliferation to mitogens,[123] and in an exercise study they demonstrated reduced immunologic response to exercise.[115] The implications of such phenomena for disease risk in older horses remains uncertain. The high incidence of pituitary pars intermedia dysfunction in older horses is a risk factor for infectious disease, as a consequence of high steroid levels.

Leukoproliferative Disease-associated Immunodeficiency

Lymphosarcoma is often associated with IgM deficiency[2,85] and can also be associated with decreased lymphocyte blastogenesis.[124,125] Affected horses were diagnosed with bacterial pneumonia in some instances, and in another report a horse suffering from myelomonocytic leukemia was found to be suffering from pulmonary aspergillosis.[126] These cases demonstrate the importance of considering leukoproliferative disease, and particularly lymphosarcoma, in cases of persistent infections that are refractory to treatment.

Drug-induced Immunodeficiency

The most common iatrogenic cause of immunosuppression is corticosteroid treatment, often given with the specific aim of treating a hypersensitivity disorder. The mode of action and the effects of corticosteroids are reviewed later in this chapter, but there is evidence for the capacity of corticosteroids to induce recrudescence of viral diseases such as equine infectious[127] anemia or EHV-1 infection[128] and to lead to development of life-threatening bacterial infection.[129] There is also evidence that corticosteroid treatment can bias adaptive immune responses to vaccination in horses, specifically suppressing IgGa and IgGb responses without affecting IgG(T) responses.[39] This phenomenon may be consistent with the capacity of corticosteroids to specifically suppress Th1 immune responses without affecting Th2 responses.[130,131]

Infectious Disease

Several infectious diseases have been associated with immunodeficiency in horses. The best-characterized example may be perinatal EHV-1 infection.[132] Foals that are infected late in gestation with EHV-1 are often born weak, with interstitial pneumonia, and develop a variety of bacterial diseases.[133] Affected foals have profound lymphopenia and generally die, despite therapy. The immunodeficiency is thought to be due to viral-induced lymphoid damage because necropsy reveals marked necrosis of lymphoid tissue in the thymus, spleen, and lymph nodes.

Undifferentiated Immunodeficiencies

A group of *foals with oral candidiasis and bacterial septicemia* between 2 weeks and 4 months of age had laboratory or histologic evidence of immunodeficiency that did not fulfill diagnostic criteria for any of the recognized primary immunodeficiencies.[134] Oral lesions ranged from focal white plaques on tongue margins to a generalized thick, white pseudomembrane covering the tongue and gingiva. Affected foals showed bruxism, ptyalism, fever, and depression in addition to pneumonia, arthritis, or diarrhea, singly or severally. The lymphocyte counts of the foals were usually normal. Several foals had IgM deficiency coupled with depressed blastogenesis, suggesting cellular immune dysfunction. Many of the foals had low or marginally reduced serum IgG in addition to IgM deficiency or reduced blastogenesis. It was not determined whether the immunologic defects were primary or secondary. All foals died despite extensive therapy with parenteral antimicrobials, topical antimycotics, and intravenous plasma. Localized or systemic candidiasis has also been described in neonatal foals receiving broad-spectrum intravenous antimicrobials for treatment of presumed bacterial sepsis. This may represent an opportunistic infection in foals with loss of normal bacterial flora secondary to antimicrobial use and exacerbated by immune suppression secondary to the underlying primary disease process.

Acquired immunodeficiency was identified in a 7-year-old Appaloosa gelding that had no history of previous illness.[135] Clinical signs included lethargy, anorexia, and dyspnea. Pneumonia and septicemia caused by *Rhodococcus equi* were confirmed by tracheal wash and blood culture, respectively. Immunologic evaluation revealed marked lymphopenia, subnormal serum IgG and IgA with marginally low IgG concentrations, failure to respond serologically to immunization, and reduced in vitro lymphocyte blastogenesis. Histologic examination of lymph nodes and spleen revealed lymphoid atrophy.[117,118]

IMMUNOMODULATORS

Clinicians frequently seek to increase normal, restore deficient, and temper over exuberant host immune responses. For these reasons modulation of the immune system, which provides critical defense against many types of disease, has become an area of intense interest in clinical medicine. Both immunostimulants and immunodepressants are considered immunomodulators. There are a variety of ways to classify immunomodulators beyond this distinction, but for practical purposes they may be best classified on the basis of their origin (i.e., physiologic products [actual normal components of the immune response], microbial products, and chemically defined agents). Immunomodulation can also result from modes of therapy not considered here, including bone marrow transplantation and irradiation.

Although a scientific rationale for the use of immunomodulators exists, a major limitation is the complexity of the immune response to be modulated. We are faced with several major problems in the rational clinical application of immunomodulators. Our current diagnostic methods do not allow us to precisely identify the in vivo defects, deficiencies, or excesses of substances or regulators present within the immunoregulatory network. Consequently, our attempts to intervene with immunomodulators are often relatively crude and nonspecific. Some of the information on which we base our use of immunomodulators has come from controlled, experimental studies, some performed in vitro and others in vivo. In clinical patients expectations based on these types of studies are frequently not realized. Reasons for this include the timing of the administration of the immunomodulator during the course of disease, and the fact that observation of a single immunologic phenomenon resulting from use of an immunomodulator, for example, an increase in lymphocyte count or lymphoproliferative responses, does not necessarily translate into improved clinical performance in the face of an infectious disease. Because of the complexity of the immune network, the rational use of immunomodulators can be considerably more difficult than the use of antimicrobial agents. An example of the importance of timing in immunomodulatory intervention is the relative success of immunosuppressive therapy in the context of organ allografts, compared with the frequent treatment failures experienced in treating autoimmune disease. In the former case, therapy is planned in advance of the introduction of the allograft, whereas in the case of autoimmunity the immune response and resulting disease are well established before they are detected and therapy is initiated.

Immunomodulators have been embraced by clinicians with great enthusiasm, and the concept of their use remains appealing. However, although the clinical value of immunosuppressive drugs such as corticosteroids and immunostimulant adjuvants in vaccines is clearly established, evidence for the clinical value of many immunostimulants is sparse. It is important to look critically at the immunomodulatory drugs on the market and objectively evaluate the effects of therapy. Many agents that have been discarded for use in humans are now being resurrected for veterinary use. Is it realistic to expect better results in veterinary patients?

This discussion will be limited to drugs currently marketed for use as immunomodulators or for which there is published evidence of activity. Advances in genetic engineering have made available recombinant forms of many cytokines with immunomodulatory potential, but only those with some established value will be discussed.

IMMUNOSUPPRESSORS

Corticosteroids

Corticosteroids are classic examples of immunosuppressive agents. Corticosteroids exhibit an extensive range of effects on elements of both the innate (inflammatory) and adaptive immune response. The mechanism of action of corticosteroids is illustrated in Figure 1-24. Corticosteroids, acting through their cytoplasmic steroid receptors, directly regulate as many as 1% of genes in the genome, usually resulting in induction of transcription.[1] The useful antiinflammatory effects of corticosteroids are summarized in Table 1-9. The effect on the adaptive immune response is complex.[2] For example, in cases of autoimmune disease such as autoimmune hemolytic anemia, corticosteroids may act by reducing phagocytosis of antibody-coated cells by the reticuloendothelial system rather than decreasing antibody production. Nevertheless, corticosteroids have been shown to have effects on antibody production, and in the horse they can suppress de novo antigen-specific IgGa and IgGb responses while sparing IgG(T) responses.[3] This may be consistent with the action of corticosteroids to suppress Th1 responses while sparing Th2 responses.[4-7] Cell migration is significantly affected by corticosteroids, and in the horse corticosteroids suppress neutrophil migration, together with phagocytic and bactericidal activity.[8] The mechanism whereby migration is decreased involves decreased expression of integrin molecules, including selectins and integrins.[9]

Although corticosteroids are powerful immunosuppressive agents, they may also predispose patients to life-threatening opportunistic infections[10] or recrudescence of viral infection.[11-13] Additional extensive undesirable side effects include fluid retention, decreased wound healing, and the concern that their use can be associated with the development of laminitis in some circumstances.[14-17] For this reason prolonged or high-dose corticosteroid therapy must be used judiciously.

Cytotoxic Drugs

The two commonly used immunosuppressive cytotoxic drugs, *azathioprine* and *cyclophosphamide,* interfere with DNA synthesis and act primarily on dividing cells.[1] This activity is useful for treatment of cancer and for suppression of dividing lymphocytes. Toxicity limits the use of these drugs, although at lower doses they can be used in combination with corticosteroids. Two case reports describe the use of these drugs in horses suffering from immune-mediated hemolytic anemia or thrombocytopenia when corticosteroid therapy alone had failed, with some success.[18,19]

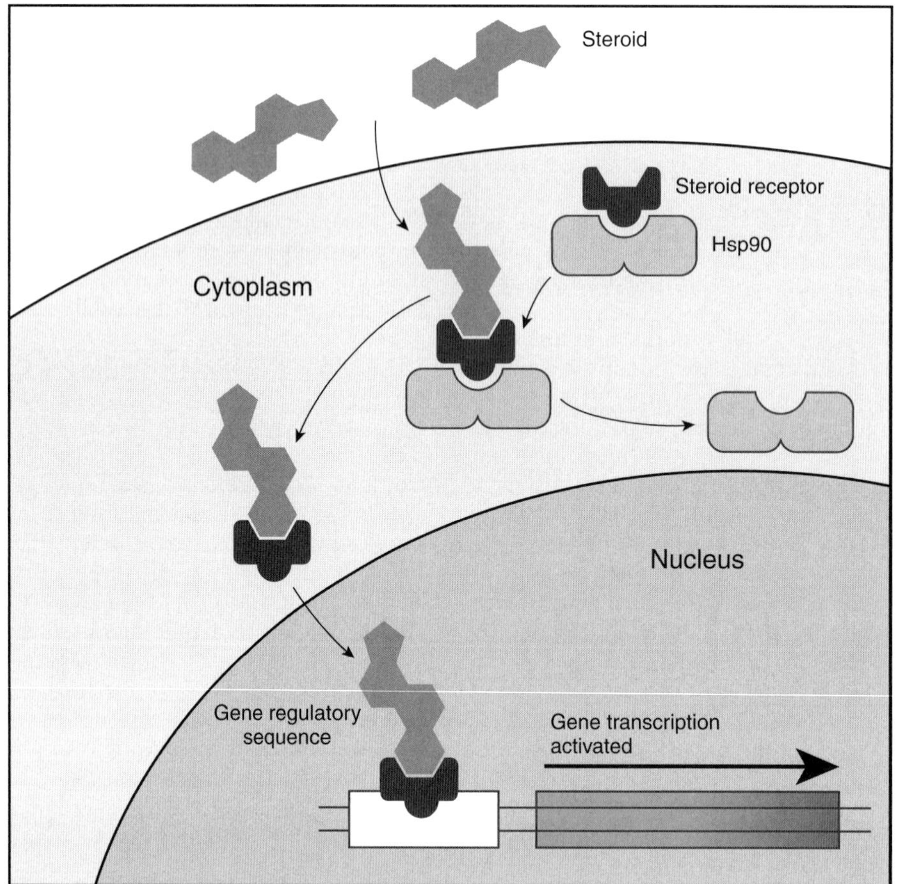

FIGURE 1-24 Lipid soluble corticosteroid molecules diffuse across the plasma membrane into the cytosol and bind to steroid receptors. This displaces a heat-shock protein (Hsp90) normally bound to the nascent steroid receptor, exposing a DNA binding region. The new complex enters the nucleus and binds to specific regulatory DNA sequences, resulting in modulation of transcription of a wide variety of genes.

TABLE 1-9

Antiinflammatory Effects of Corticosteroid Therapy Mediated by Regulation of Gene Transcription

ACTION OF CORTICOSTEROIDS	
Direct Effect	**Physiologic Effects**
↓ IL-1, TNF-a, GM-CSF, IL-3, IL-4, IL-5, IL-8	↓Inflammation caused by cytokines
↓NOS	↓NO
↓ Phospholipase A2, Cyclo-oxygenase type 2 ↑ Lipocortin-1	↓Protaglandins, Leukotrienes
↓Adhesion molecules	↓Emigration of leukocytes from vessels
↑Endonucleases	↑Apoptosis in lymphocytes and eosinophils

From Murphy KM, Travers P, Walport M: Janeway's Immunobiology, 7th ed. New York, 2007, Garland Science, New York, 2008, Garland Science.
IL, Interleukin; *TNF*, tumor necrosis factor; *GM-CSF*, granulocyte-macrophage colony-stimulating factor; *NOS*, nitric oxide synthase; *NO*, nitric oxide.

Bacterial and Fungal Derivatives

Bacterial and fungal derivatives are a class of drugs that includes relatively nontoxic alternatives to immunosuppressive cytotoxic drugs. *Cyclosporine* is a fungal derivative and has emerged as a major immunosuppressive agent for allograft survival; it selectively inhibits proliferation, cytotoxicity, and lymphokine production of T cells by binding to intracellular proteins known as immunophilins and interfering with signaling pathways that are important for clonal expansion of lymphocytes.[1] Cyclosporin is efficacious in suppressing specific immune responses with minimal nonspecific toxic effects on polymorphonuclear leukocytes, monocytes, and macrophages. Thus immunosuppressed patients suffer fewer severe secondary infections. The drug is not hazard free; in addition to suppressing lymphocyte responses in general, it is also toxic to the kidneys and other organs.

In horses the use of cyclosporin has been limited to topical therapy for ocular inflammatory disease, including keratitis[20] and uveitis.[21,22] In the treatment of uveitis, numbers of infiltrating T lymphocytes and IL2 and γ-IFN levels were suppressed by cyclosporin treatment.[23]

IMMUNOSTIMULANTS

Physiologic Products

IMMUNOGLOBULINS

The use of immunoglobulins for treatment of failure of passive transfer of immunity is discussed earlier in this chapter, and antigen-specific passive immunoglobulin therapy is discussed later. Other forms of immunoglobulin immunomodulation include the use of monoclonal or polyclonal sera directed against components of the immune system. This type of therapy has still found limited practical application in the 30 years since the advent of monoclonal antibody technology, largely as a result of the immunogenicity of the antibodies themselves. Although recombinant technology now has the prospect of resolving this problem, there are no current examples of clinical applicability in the horse.

Another mode of immunoglobulin therapy is polyclonal intravenous immunoglobulin (PIVIG) therapy using pools of immunoglobulin derived from several thousand donors.[24,25] It was serendipitously observed that PIVIG administration was useful for treatment of autoimmunity; [26,27] proposed mechanisms include idiotype-antiidiotype network regulation,[28] cytokine regulation, specific antibody interactions, Fc-receptor blockade, inhibition of activated complement deposition, and long-term selection of immune repertoires.[29] Although the exact mechanisms underlying the effects of PIVIG are uncertain, there are good examples of therapeutic success in patients with immunothrombocytopenic purpura.[30] However, diseases such as autoimmune diabetes mellitus are resistant to therapy.[31] There are no publications describing PIVIG therapy in horses, although this treatment modality remains an intriguing possibility in this species.

CYTOKINES

Given the central role of cytokines in immunoregulation, their potential as immunomodulators is obvious and a discussion of the possible use of cytokines as therapeutic agents in this regard would be extensive, although largely hypothetical. Therefore consideration will be limited to the two cytokines that have found clinical application in horses to date.

Interferon-α The clinical application of interferon-α in the horse has been extensively reviewed.[32,33] Interferon-α has antiviral and immunostimulant properties, and oral administration of interferon-α reduces inflammatory airway disease (IAD)[34] in racehorses.[35] The treatment employed was low-dose (50 to 150 IU) "natural" human interferon-α, and it resulted in decreased BAL cell counts and a noninflammatory cytologic profile.[36] Higher doses (450 IU) were less effective, consistent with results in other species.[33] The efficacy of oral therapy probably depends on effects mediated through oropharyngeal lymphoid tissue, as the agent is destroyed in the stomach.

Granulocyte-colony Stimulating Factor The clinical application of granulocyte colony-stimulating factor (G-CSF) in the horse has been extensively reviewed.[33] Treatment with G-CS Fin neonatal foals results in a sustained, dose-dependent increase in neutrophil count and a left shift[37,38] by increasing neutrophil production in the bone marrow and shortening the time to release into the circulation; half life remains unchanged at 8 hours. In horses, canine recombinant G-CSF (Amgen) has been used to treat sepsis and endotoxemia with some success.[33]

Bacterial, Viral, and Plant Products

A variety of bacterial and fungal microorganisms or microbial products have been identified that have an immunomodulating effect on the immune system. A common feature of many of these products is a nonspecific immunostimulant effect, purportedly due to macrophage activation and release of cytokines, including interferons, IL-1, TNF, or IL-6.[33,39] Consequently, mild fever and malaise may be associated with this form of treatment. In the horse these treatments are most commonly used in cases of respiratory infection or sarcoids. An extensive review of the use of these and other immunostimulants in the horse has been published.[33]

MYCOBACTERIAL PRODUCTS

A wide range of mycobacterial fractions have been identified with immunomodulating ability.[33,39] The minimal structure with immunologic (adjuvant) activity is muramyl dipeptide (MDP), which is a potent adjuvant.[40] Preparations commercially available for use in horses include BCG (bacille Calmette-Guérin), a modified live human tuberculosis vaccine, and protein-free mycobacterial cell wall extracts (Nomagen, Fort Dodge Laboratories, Inc., Fort Dodge, Iowa.; Equimune, Vetrepharm Inc., London, Ont.). Efficacy is claimed for treatment of equine respiratory disease. Adverse reactions have been reported after multiple intravenous treatments in horses, resulting in marked interstitial lung infiltration and progressive pulmonary fibrosis. As a result, caution should be exercised before selecting this treatment modality. In horses the major successful application of these products has been in the intralesional treatment of sarcoids, particularly periocular sarcoids, and this is discussed elsewhere in this text.

PROPIONIBACTERIUM ACNES (CORYNEBACTERIUM PARVUM)

Propionibacterium acnes is a gram-positive anaerobe, marketed for use in horses as a killed preparation under the tradename EqStim (Immunovet, Inc., Tampa, Fla.) for treatment of equine respiratory disease.[39] It is recommended for use prophylactically before weaning, transport stress or co-mingling, or for the therapy of chronic infectious respiratory disease. In a blind randomized clinical trial, *P. acnes* treatment resulted in early resolution of spontaneously occurring respiratory disease.[33] In healthy horses *P. acnes* resulted in increased CD4+ T lymphocyte numbers and LAK activity in peripheral blood and BAL fluid, increased nonopsonized phagocytosis in peripheral blood leukocytes, and decreased pulmonary cellularity.[41] Overall, this agent is one of the most popular immunostimulants currently marketed for horses, but substantive peer-reviewed evidence to confirm its value is lacking.

CpG DNA

In recent years an extensive literature has developed describing the immunomodulatory effects of certain bacterial DNA motifs.[42] The specific immunostimulatory DNA motifs are called *CpG sequences,* and appropriate sequences for immunostimulation of domestic species have been identified.[43] Much work has been done on examining the efficacy of CpG sequences as vaccine adjuvants,[44] immunomodulators for hyposensitization, or cancer therapy.[45] The value of CpGs in horses as both vaccine adjuvants[46] and as potential nonspecific immunomodulators[47] has been demonstrated, although commerical products are not yet available.

ACEMANNAN

Acemannan is an extract of the aloe vera plant mostly used for treatment of fibrosarcomas in dogs and cats.[33] It can also be used as a vaccine adjuvant and, in addition, has antiviral activity. Anecdotal reports describe efficacy for treatment of equine respiratory disease (intravenous) and sarcoids (intralesional), although both forms of treatment are associated with side effects, including syncope, tachycardia, tachypnea, and sweating. Controlled studies of efficacy in the horse are lacking.

PARAPOXVIRUS OVIS

Marketed under the trade name Baypamun (Bayer Animal Health, Del.), and currently in the United States as Zylexis (Pfizer Animal Health), inactivated parapoxvirus ovis has been used extensively in Europe for prophylaxis and treatment of infectious disease in companion animals (including horses) and pigs.[33] The immunostimulant properties depend on a component of the viral envelope and increase NK activity and macrophage activation. Efficacy has been demonstrated against viral and bacterial disease in several species,[33] and there is some evidence in horses that prophylactic administration before weaning reduces signs of respiratory disease after weaning.[48] In studies of treatment of sarcoid, there was no evidence of efficacy.[49] In a model of transport stress, treatment with Zylexis led to restoration of suppressed antibody responses to influenza virus infection in horses.[50]

ECHINACEA

Extracts of *Echinacea angustifolia* are reported to be immunostimulatory. One study in horses evaluated the effect of an experimental oral *Echinacea* sp. extract on neutrophil number and phagocytosis and lymphocyte count.[51] Findings provided only limited evidence of immunostimulation based on changes in cell count and behavior.

CHEMICALLY DEFINED AGENTS

Levamisole Levamisole is a synthetic anthelmintic used for treatment of nematode infections that has also been reported to restore impaired host immune defenses.[33] Levamisole appears to have little effect on the normal immune system, but it appears to stimulate a subnormal response and suppress hyperactive responses. The effects are dose related, and low doses are reported to enhance, whereas higher doses suppress, responses. In cattle levamisole enhances lymphoproliferative responses in vitro, although in vivo co-administration with a vaccine had no immunostimulant effect.[52] Similarly, levamisole did not prevent corticosteroid-mediated immunosuppression in cattle[53] or enhance postpartum lymphoproliferative responses in pigs.[52] Aside from anecdotal reports, there are no published controlled studies of its value in horses.

ANTIGEN-SPECIFIC IMMUNOMODULATION

VACCINATION AND ADJUVANTS

Vaccination is a critically important tool in preventing infectious disease in humans and animals, and both passive and active vaccination are extensively employed in the horse. Specific equine vaccination strategies are presented elsewhere in this book, and the scientific principles and practice of equine vaccination have been extensively reviewed.[54] Active vaccination induces an antigen-specific immune response in the vaccinated animal by administration of dead or live antigen or DNA capable of expressing protein antigens in vivo. Success of all these forms of vaccination often depends on the use of an effective adjuvant, a compound capable of amplifying and directing immune responses.[55] As such, adjuvants are one of the most important forms of immunomodulation agents in use in equine medicine.

Passive vaccination is accomplished by administering preformed antibodies either as a plasma transfusion or in a concentrated form, as in commercially available tetanus antitoxin. This strategy can be highly effective in diseases for which there is no available form of active vaccination (e.g., *Rhodococcus equi*) or in high-risk situations when there is inadequate time for protection to be generated by active vaccination. Generally, passive vaccination should be avoided when possible because of the risk of transmission of infection in serum-derived products. An example of this is the association of acute hepatic necrosis with a previous administration of tetanus antitoxin.[56]

HYPOSENSITIZATION

Because horses suffer from a number of hyposensitivity diseases, attempts have been made to perform antigen-specific immunosuppression. Examples include insect bite hypersensitivity (IBH) and recurrent airway obstruction (RAO).[57] The principle of this type of therapy is that the immune response to an allergen can be redirected in order to reduce hypersensitivity disease.[58] For example, Type 1 hypersensivity disease may depend on a Th2 immune response, and treatments that can change this to a Th1 immune response may eliminate or control the hypersensitivity disease by changing the immune response from one dominated by IgE to IgG.[1] Typically, hyposensitization treatments use injections of the allergen itself, starting with very small doses and gradually increasing the dose over time. This form of treatment depends on correct identification of the allergen against which the hypersensitivity disease is directed, and the difficulty in identifying these allergens using available intradermal testing methodologies[59,60] may provide an explanation for the mixed success of hyposensitization treatment in horses.[61] Prospects for hyposensitization therapy may be improved by new techniques to produce large numbers of recombinant allergens.[62,63] These allergens are far better defined than conventionally prepared allergen extracts, and in initial experimental studies of RAO they were found to be far superior in terms of specificity and sensitivity for detection of allergen-specific IgE. Such developments, together with the developments of DNA vaccination strategies incorporating CpG immunomodulation for hyposensitization,[64-66] and additional therapeutic vaccination strategies[67] targeting MHC II antigen presentation[68,69] and formation of Tregs,[70] mean that there is a good chance that new and effective therapies will be developed in the future.

CONCLUSION

The properties and efficacy of immunosuppressive agents are generally well documented, as are the effects of antigen-specific immunostimulant adjuvants. Of all the nonspecific equine immunostimulants described in the literature, only interferon-α and *P. acnes* are supported by well-designed and well-performed studies.[35,36,41] Given the interest in this modality of therapy, this is regrettable and evidence of the difficulty in designing studies to establish immunostimulant efficacy, possible lack of efficacy of such products in some instances, and the dire need for additional scientific research.

REFERENCES

Equine Immunity

1. Murphy K, Travers P, Walport M: *Janeway's immunobiology*, New York, 2008, Garland Science.
2. Abbas A, Lichtman A, Pillai S: *Cellular and molecular immunology*, Philadelphia, 2007, Saunders.
3. Paul WE, editor: *Fundamental immunology*, ed 6, Philadelphia, 2008, Lippincott-Raven.
4. Oikawa MA, Kamada M, Yoshihara T, et al: Clinicopathological analysis of foal diseases from 237 autopsy cases, *Kitasato Arch Exp Med* 64:149-156, 1991.
5. Coombs SL, Webbon PM: Tracheal mucus transport in the horse following equine influenza vaccination, *Vet Rec* 119:601-602, 1986.
6. Dixon PM: Respiratory mucociliary clearance in the horse in health and disease, and its pharmaceutical modification, *Vet Rec* 131:229-235, 1992.
7. Oikawa M, Takagi S, Anzai R, et al: Pathology of equine respiratory disease occurring in association with transport, *J Comp Pathol* 113:29-43, 1995.
8. Nordengrahn A, Rusvai M, Merza M, et al: Equine herpesvirus type 2 (EHV-2) as a predisposing factor for Rhodococcus equi pneumonia in foals: prevention of the bifactorial disease with EHV-2 immunostimulating complexes, *Vet Microbiol* 51:55-68, 1996.
9. MacKay RJ: Inflammation in horses, *Vet Clin North Am Equine Pract* 16:15-27, 2000.
10. Netea MG, van der Graaf C, Van der Meer JWM, et al: Toll-like receptors and the host defense against microbial pathogens: bringing specificity to the innate-immune system, *J Leukoc Biol* 75:749-755, 2004.
11. Petersen HH, Nielsen JP, Heegaard PM: Application of acute phase protein measurements in veterinary clinical chemistry, *Vet Res* 35:163-187, 2004.
12. Grondahl G, Sternberg S, Jensen-Waern M, et al: Opsonic capacity of foal serum for the two neonatal pathogens Escherichia coli and Actinobacillus equuli, *Equine Vet J* 33:670-675, 2001.
13. Camp CJ, Leid RW: Chemotaxis of radiolabeled equine neutrophils, *Am J Vet Res* 43:397-401, 1982.
14. Higgins AJ, Lees P: The acute inflammatory process, arachidonic acid metabolism and the mode of action of anti-inflammatory drugs, *Equine Vet J* 16:163-175, 1984.
15. Gibson KT, Hodge H, Whittem T: Inflammatory mediators in equine synovial fluid, *Aust Vet J* 73:148-151, 1996.
16. Verburg KM, Maziasz TJ, Weiner E, et al: Cox-2-specific inhibitors: definition of a new therapeutic concept, *Am J Ther* 8:49-64, 2001.
17. Morton AJ, Campbell NB, Gayle JM, et al: Preferential and non-selective cyclooxygenase inhibitors reduce inflammation during lipopolysaccharide-induced synovitis, *Res Vet Sci* 78:189-192, 2005.
18. Tilley SL, Coffman TM, Koller BH: Mixed messages: modulation of inflammation and immune responses by prostaglandins and thromboxanes, *J Clin Invest* 108:15-23, 2001.
19. Schror K, Mehta P, Mehta JL: Cardiovascular risk of selective cyclooxygenase-2 inhibitors, *J Cardiovasc Pharmacol Ther* 10:95-101, 2005.
20. Bertolini A, Ottani A, Sandrini M: Dual acting anti-inflammatory drugs: a reappraisal, *Pharmacol Res* 44:437-450, 2001.
21. Hardy J, Bertone AL, Weisbrode SE, et al: Cell trafficking, mediator release, and articular metabolism in acute inflammation of innervated or denervated isolated equine joints, *Am J Vet Res* 59:88-100, 1998.
22. Gangur V, Birmingham NP, Thanesvorakul S: Chemokines in health and disease, *Vet Immunol Immunopathol* 86:127-136, 2002.
23. Marr KA, Lees P, Cunningham FM: Agonist-induced adherence of equine neutrophils to fibronectin- and serum-coated plastic is CD18 dependent, *Vet Immunol Immunopathol* 71:77-88, 1999.
24. Smith CW: Endothelial adhesion molecules and their role in inflammation, *Can J Physiol Pharmacol* 71:76-87, 1993.
25. Stickle JE: The neutrophil. Function, disorders, and testing, *Vet Clin North Am Small Anim Pract* 26:1013-1021, 1996.
26. Jones SL, Sharief Y, Chilcoat CD: Signaling mechanism for equine neutrophil activation by immune complexes, *Vet Immunol Immunopathol* 82:87-100, 2001.
27. Foster AP, Cunningham FM: Differential superoxide anion generation by equine eosinophils and neutrophils, *Vet Immunol Immunopathol* 59:225-237, 1997.
28. Re F, Muzio M, De Rossi M, Polentarutti N, et al: The type II "receptor" as a decoy target for interleukin 1 in polymorphonuclear leukocytes: characterization of induction by dexamethasone and ligand binding properties of the released decoy receptor, *J Exp Med* 179:739-743, 1994.
29. Healy DP: New and emerging therapies for sepsis, *Ann Pharmacother* 36:648-654, 2002.
30. Lewis MJ, Wagner B, Woof JM: The different effector function capabilities of the seven equine IgG subclasses have implications for vaccine strategies, *Mol Immunol* 45:818-827, 2008.
31. Wagner B, Miller DC, Lear TL, Antczak DF: The complete map of the Ig heavy chain constant gene region reveals evidence for seven IgG isotypes and for IgD in the horse, *J Immunol* 173:3230-3242, 2004.
32. Lunn DP, Holmes MA, Antczak DF, et al: Report of the Second Equine Leucocyte Antigen Workshop, Squaw Valley, California, July 1995, *Vet Immunol Immunopathol* 62:101-143, 1998.
33. Gritzmacher CA: Molecular aspects of heavy-chain class switching, *Crit Rev Immunol* 9:173-200, 1989.
34. DeKruyff RH, Rizzo LV, Umetsu DT: Induction of immunoglobulin synthesis by CD4+ T cell clones, *Semin Immunol* 5:421-430, 1993.
35. Xu L, Rothman P: IFN-gamma represses epsilon germline transcription and subsequently down-regulates switch recombination to epsilon, *Int Immunol* 6:515-521, 1994.

36. Siebenkotten G, Esser C, Wabl M, Radbruch A: The murine IgG1/IgE class switch program, *Eur J Immunol* 22:1827-1834, 1992.
37. McIntyre TM, Kehry MR, Snapper CM: Novel in vitro model for high-rate IgA class switching, *J Immunol* 154:3156-3161, 1995.
38. Taussig MJ: Molecular genetics of immunoglobulins, *Immunol Suppl* 1:7-15, 1988.
39. Ford J, Home W, Gibson D: Light chain isotype regulation in the horse. Characterization of Ig kappa genes, *J Immunol.* 153:1099-1111, 1994.
40. Home W, Ford J, Gibson D: L chain isotype regulation in horse. I. Characterization of Ig lambda genes, *J Immunol.* 149:3927-3936, 1992.
41. Alcover A, Alarcon B: Internalization and intracellular fate of TCR-CD3 complexes, *Crit Rev Immunol* 20:325-346, 2000.
42. Chen CH, Six A, Kubota T, et al: T cell receptors and T cell development, *Curr Top Microbiol Immunol* 212:37-53, 1996.
43. Bromley SK, Burack WR, Johnson KG, et al: The immunological synapse, *Annu Rev Immunol* 19:375-396, 2001.
44. Kisielow P, Miazek A: Thymic selection and tolerance, *Transplant Proc* 28:3429-3430, 1996.
45. Antczak DF, Allen WR: Maternal immunological recognition of pregnancy in equids, *J Reprod Fertil Suppl* 37:69-78, 1989.
46. Maloy WL: Comparison of the primary structure of class I molecules, *Immunol Res* 6:11-29, 1987.
47. Tallmadge RL, Lear TL, Antczak DF: Genomic characterization of MHC class I genes of the horse, *Immunogenetics* 57:763-774, 2005.
48. Ansari HA, Hediger R, Fries R, et al: Chromosomal localization of the major histocompatibility complex of the horse (ELA) by in situ hybridization, *Immunogenetics* 28:362-364, 1988.
49. Donaldson WL, Crump AL, Zhang CH, et al: At least two loci encode polymorphic class I MHC antigens in the horse, *Anim Genet* 19:379-390, 1988.
50. Zinkernagel RM, Doherty PC: Immunological surveilance against altered self-components by sensitized T lymphocytes in lymphocytic choriomeningitis, *Nature* 251:547-548, 1974.
51. Bjorkman PJ, Saper MA, Samraoui B, et al: The foreign antigen binding site and T cell recognition regions of class I histocompatibility antigens, *Nature* 329:512-518, 1987.
52. Braciale TJ, Morrison LA, Sweetser MT, et al: Antigen presentation pathways to class I and class II MHC-restricted T lymphocytes, *Immunol Rev* 98:95-114, 1987.
53. Monaco JJ, Nandi D: The genetics of proteasomes and antigen processing, *Annu Rev Genet* 29:729-754, 1995.
54. Lechner F, Cuero AL, Kantzanou M, et al: Studies of human antiviral CD8+ lymphocytes using class I peptide tetramers, *Rev Med Virol* 11:11-22, 2001.
55. Mealey RH, Sharif A, Ellis SA, et al: Early detection of dominant Env-specific and subdominant Gag-specific CD8+ lymphocytes in equine infectious anemia virus-infected horses using major histocompatibility complex class I/peptide tetrameric complexes, *Virology* 339:110-126, 2005.
56. Cresswell P: Assembly, transport, and function of MHC class II molecules, *Annu Rev Immunol* 12:259-293, 1994.
57. Halaby DM, Mornon JP: The immunoglobulin superfamily: an insight on its tissular, species, and functional diversity, *J Mol Evol* 46:389-400, 1998.
58. Crepaldi T, Crump A, Newman M, et al: Equine T lymphocytes express MHC class II antigens, *J Immunogenet* 13:349-360, 1986.
59. Lunn DP, Holmes MA, Duffus WP: Equine T-lymphocyte MHC II expression: variation with age and subset, *Vet Immunol Immunopathol* 35:225-238, 1993.
60. Frayne J, Stokes CR: MHC Class II positive cells and T cells in the equine endometrium throughout the oestrous cycle, *Vet Immunol Immunopathol* 41:55-72, 1994.
61. Horohov DW, Siegel JP: Lymphokines: progress and promise, *Drugs* 33:4, 1987.
62. Mizel SB, Farrar JJ: Revised nomenclature for antigen-nonspecific T-cell proliferation and helper factors, *Cell Immunol* 48:433-436, 1979.
63. Hanlon AM, Jang S, Salgame P: Signaling from cytokine receptors that affect Th1 responses, *Front Biosci* 7:D1247-D1254, 2002.
64. Bowie A, O'Neill LA: The interleukin-1 receptor/Toll-like receptor superfamily: signal generators for pro-inflammatory interleukins and microbial products, *J Leukoc Biol* 67:508-514, 2000.
65. Imada K, Leonard WJ: The Jak-STAT pathway, *Mol Immunol* 37:1-11, 2000.
66. Leonard WJ, Lin JX: Cytokine receptor signaling pathways, *J Allergy Clin Immunol* 105:877-888, 2000.
67. Heyninck K, Beyaert R: Crosstalk between NF-kappaB-activating and apoptosis-inducing proteins of the TNF-receptor complex, *Mol Cell Biol Res Commun* 4:259-265, 2001.
68. Akgul C, Moulding DA, Edwards SW: Molecular control of neutrophil apoptosis, *FEBS Lett* 487:318-322, 2001.
69. Sampson AP: The role of eosinophils and neutrophils in inflammation, *Clin Exp Allergy* 30(Suppl 1):22-27, 2000.
70. Sandersen C, Bureau F, Turlej R, et al: Homodimer activity in distal airway cells determines lung dysfunction in equine heaves, *Vet Immunol Immunopathol* 80:315-326, 2001.
71. Horohov DW: Equine T-cell cytokines. Protection and pathology, *Vet Clin North Am Equine Pract* 16:1-14, 2000.
72. Aggarwal N, Holmes MA: Characterisation of equine T helper cells: demonstration of Th1- and Th2-like cells in long-term equine T-cell cultures, *Res Vet Sci* 66:277-279, 1999.
73. Kim CH: Trafficking of FoxP3+ regulatory T cells: myths and facts, *Arch Immunol Ther Exp (Warsz)* 55:151-159, 2007.
74. Cools N, Ponsaerts P, Van Tendeloo VF, Berneman ZN: Regulatory T cells and human disease, *Clin Dev Immunol* 2007:89195, 2007.
75. Tang Q, Krummel MF: Imaging the function of regulatory T cells in vivo, *Curr Opin Immunol* 18:496-502, 2006.
76. Gilger BC, Malok E, Cutter KV, et al: Characterization of T-lymphocytes in the anterior uvea of eyes with chronic equine recurrent uveitis, *Vet Immunol Immunopathol* 71:17-28, 1999.
77. Lavoie JP, Maghni K, Desnoyers M, et al: Neutrophilic airway inflammation in horses with heaves is characterized by a Th2-type cytokine profile, *Am J Respir Crit Care Med* 164:1410-1413, 2001.
78. McGorum BC, Dixon PM, Robinson NE, et al (eds): *Equine respiratory medicine and surgery*, Edinburgh, 2007, Saunders.
79. Ganusov VV, De Boer RJ: Tissue distribution of lymphocytes and plasma cells and the role of the gut: response to Pabst et al, *Trends Immunol* 29:209-210, 2008.
80. Pabst R, Russell MW, Brandtzaeg P: Tissue distribution of lymphocytes and plasma cells and the role of the gut, *Trends Immunol* 29:206-208, 2008.
81. Mazanec MB, Nedrud JG, Kaetzel CS, Lamm ME: A three-tiered view of the role of IgA in mucosal defense, *Immunol Today* 14:430-435, 1993.
82. Kumar P, Timoney JF, Sheoran AS: M cells and associated lymphoid tissue of the equine nasopharyngeal tonsil, *Equine Vet J* 33:224-230, 2001.
83. Breathnach CC, Yeargan MR, Timoney JF, et al: Detection of equine herpesvirus-specific effector and memory cytotoxic immunity in the equine upper respiratory tract, *Vet Immunol Immunopathol* 111:117-125, 2006.
84. Perryman LE, McGuire TC, Torbeck RL: Ontogeny of lymphocyte function in the equine fetus, *American Journal of Veterinary Research* 41:1197-1200, 1980.

85. Hannant D, Rossdale PD, McGladdery AJ, et al. Immune responses of the equine foetus to protein antigens. *Proceedings of the Sixth International Conference on Equine Infectious Diseases,* UK, 1991:86, Cambridge.
86. Martin BR, Larson KA: Immune response of the equine fetus to coliphage T2, *American Journal of Veterinary Research* 34:1363-1364, 1973.
87. Morgan DO, Bryans JT, Mock RE: Immunoglobulins produced by the antigenised equine foetus, *Journal of Reproduction and Fertility Supplement* 23:735-738, 1975.
88. Roitt IM, Brostoff J, Male DK, eds: *Immunology*, St. Louis, 1993: pp 11.1-11.16, Mosby.
89. Boyd RL, Tucek CL, Godfrey DI, et al: The thymic microenvironment, *Immunology Today* 14:445-459, 1993.
90. Godfrey DI, Zlotnik A: Control points in early T-cell development, *Immunology Today* 14:547-553, 1993.
91. Palmer DB, Hayday A, Owen MJ: Is TCR β expression an essential event in early thymocyte development? *Immunology Today* 14:460-462, 1993.
92. Blanchard-Channell M, Moore PF, Stott JL: Characterization of monoclonal antibodies specific for equine homologues of CD3 and CD5, *Immunology* 82:548-554, 1994.
93. Lunn DP, Holmes MA, Duffus WPH: Three monoclonal antibodies identifying antigens on all equine T-lymphocytes, and two mutually exclusive T-lymphocyte subsets, *Immunology* 74:251-257, 1991.
94. Giguere S, Polkes AC: Immunologic disorders in neonatal foals, *Vet Clin North Am Equine Pract* 21:241-272, v, 2005.
95. Wichtel MG, Anderson KL, Johnson TV, et al: Influence of age on neutrophil function in foals, *Equine Vet J* 23:466-469, 1991.
96. Morris DD, Gaulin G, Strzemienski PJ, Spencer P: Assessment of neutrophil migration, phagocytosis and bactericidal capacity in neonatal foals, *Vet Immunol Immunopathol* 16:173-184, 1987.
97. Hietala SK, Ardans AA: Neutrophil phagocytic and serum opsonic response of the foal to Corynebacterium equi, *Vet Immunol Immunopathol* 14:279-294, 1987.
98. Bernoco M, Liu IKM, West-Ehlert CJ, et al: Chemotactic and phagocytic function of peripheral blood polymorphonuclear leucocytes in newborn foals, *J Reprod Fertil Suppl* 35:599-605, 1987.
99. Demmers S, Johannisson A, Grondahl G, et al: Neutrophil functions and serum IgG in growing foals, *Equine Vet J* 33:676-680, 2001.
100. McTaggart C, Yovich JV, Penhale J, et al: A comparison of foal and adult horse neutrophil function using flow cytometric techniques, *Res Vet Sci* 71:73-79, 2001.
101. Liu IKM, Walsh EM, Bernoco M, et al: Bronchalveolar lavage in the newborn foal, *J Reprod Fertil Suppl* 35:587-592, 1987.
102. Bernoco MM, Liu IK, Willits NH: Hemolytic complement activity and concentrations of its third component during maturation of the immune response in colostrum-deprived foals, *American J Vet Res* 55:928-933, 1994.
103. Lavoie JP, Spensley MS, Smith BP, Bowling AT, Morse S: Complement activity and selected hematologic variables in newborn foals fed bovine colostrum, *Am J Vet Res* 50:1532-1536, 1989.
104. Smith III R, Chaffin MK, Cohen ND, Martens RJ: Age-related changes in lymphocyte subsets of quarter horse foals, *Am J Vet Res* 63:531-537, 2002.
105. Flaminio MJ, Rush BR, Shuman W: Peripheral blood lymphocyte subpopulations and immunoglobulin concentrations in healthy foals and foals with Rhodococcus equi pneumonia, *J Vet Int Med* 13:206-212, 1999.
106. Flaminio MJ, Rush BR, Davis EG, et al: Characterization of peripheral blood and pulmonary leukocyte function in healthy foals, *Vet Immunol Imunopathol* 73:267-285, 2000.
107. Sanada Y, Noda H, Nagahata H: Development of lymphocyte blastogenic response in the neonatal period of foals, *Zentralblatt Fur Veterinarmedizin Reihe A* 39:69-75, 1992.
108. Breathnach CC, Sturgill-Wright T, Stiltner JL, et al: Foals are interferon gamma-deficient at birth, *Vet Immunol Immunopathol* 112:199-209, 2006.
109. Jansen BC, Knoetze PC: The immune response of horses to tetanus toxoid, *Onderstepoort J Vet Res* 46:211-216, 1979.
110. Wilson WD: Vaccination of foals British Equine Veterinary Association Conference, Harrogate, 2001, R&W Publications.
111. Jeffcott LB: Studies on passive immunity in the foal. 1. Gamma-globulin and antibody variations associated with the maternal transfer of immunity and the onset of active immunity, *J Comp Pathol* 84:93-101, 1974.
112. Rouse BT: The immunoglobulins of adult equine and foal sera: a quantitative study, *Br Vet J* 127:45-51, 1971.
113. Sellon DC: Secondary immunodeficiencies of horses, *Vet Clin North Am Equine Pract* 16:117-130, 2000.
114. Rouse BT, Ingram DG: The total protein and immunoglobulin profile of equine colostrum and milk, *Immunology* 19:901-907, 1970.
115. Sheoran AS, Timoney JF, Holmes MA: Immunoglobulin isotypes in sera and nasal mucosal secretions and their neonatal transfer and distribution in horses, *Am J Vet Res* 61:1099-1105, 2000.
116. Jeffcott LB: Duration of permeability of the intestine to macromolecules in the newly-born foal, *Vet Rec* 88:340-341, 1971.
117. Holmes MA, Lunn DP: A study of bovine and equine immunoglobulin levels in pony foals fed bovine colostrum, *Equine Vet J* 23:116-118, 1991.
118. Lavoie JP, Spensley MS, Smith BP, Mihalyi J: Absorption of bovine colostral immunoglobulins G and M in newborn foals, *Am J Vet Res* 50:1598-1603, 1989.
119. Sheoran AS, Sponseller BT, Holmes MA, et al: Serum and mucosal antibody isotype responses to M-like protein (SeM) of Streptococcus equi in convalescent and vaccinated horses, *Vet Immunol Immunopathol* 59:239-251, 1997.
120. Nelson KM, Schram BR, McGregor MW, et al: Local and systemic isotype-specific antibody responses to equine influenza virus infection versus conventional vaccination, *Vaccine* 16:1306-1313, 1998.
121. Hoffman AM, Viel L, Juniper E, Prescott JF: Clinical and endoscopic study to estimate the incidence of distal respiratory tract infection in thoroughbred foals on Ontario breeding farms, *Am J Vet Res* 54:1602-1607, 1993.
122. Prescott JF: Rhodococcus equi: an animal and human pathogen, *Clin Microbiol Rev* 4:20-34, 1991.
123. Holznagel DL, Hussey S, Mihalyi JE, et al: Onset of immunoglobulin production in foals, *Equine Vet J* 35:620-622, 2003.
124. Wilson WD, Mihalyi JE, Hussey S, et al: Passive transfer of maternal immunoglobulin isotype antibodies against tetanus and influenza and their effect on the response of foals to vaccination, *Equine Vet J* 33:644-650, 2001.
125. Gibbs E, Wilson J, All B: Studies on passive immunity and the vaccination of foals against eastern equine encephalitis in florida. *Equine infectious disease V: Proceedings of the Fifth International Conference* 5:201–205, 1988.
126. Galan JE, Timoney JF, Lengemann FW: Passive transfer of mucosal antibody to Streptococcus equi in the foal, *Infect Immun* 54:202-206, 1986.
127. van Maanen C, Bruin G, de Boer Luijtze E, et al: Interference of maternal antibodies with the immune response of foals after vaccination against equine influenza, *Vet Q* 14:13-17, 1992.
128. Oirschot JT, Bruin G, Boer-Luytze E, et al: Maternal antibodies against equine influenza virus in foals and their interference with vaccination, *J Vet Med* 38:391-396, 1991.

129. Adkins B: T-cell function in newborn mice and humans, *Immunol Today* 20:330-335, 1999.
130. Ridge JP, Fuchs EJ, Matzinger P: Neonatal tolerance revisited: turning on newborn T cells with dendritic cells [see comments], *Science* 271:1723-1726, 1996.
131. Forsthuber T, Yip HC, Lehmann PV: Induction of TH1 and TH2 immunity in neonatal mice, *Science* 271:1728-1730, 1996.
132. Sarzotti M, Robbins DS, Hoffman PM: Induction of protective CTL responses in newborn mice by a murine retrovirus, *Science* 271:1726-1728, 1996.
133. Boyd NK, Cohen ND, Lim WS, et al: Temporal changes in cytokine expression of foals during the first month of life, *Vet Immunol Immunopathol* 92:75-85, 2003.

Hypersensitivity and Autoimmunity

1. Gell PGH, Coombs RRA, Lachman P, editors: *Clinical aspects of immunology*, Oxford, 1975, Blackwell, pp 761-781.
2. Murphy K, Travers P, Walport M: *Janeway's immunobiology*, New York, 2008, Garland Science.
3. Swiderski CE: Hypersensitivity disorders in horses, *Vet Clin North Am Equine Pract* 16:131-151, 2000.
4. McAleese SM, Halliwell RE, Miller HR: Cloning and sequencing of the horse and sheep high-affinity IgE receptor alpha chain cDNA, *Immunogenetics* 51:878-881, 2000.
5. Watson JL, Jackson KA, King DP, Stott JL: Molecular cloning and sequencing of the low-affinity IgE receptor (CD23) for horse and cattle, *Vet Immunol Immunopathol* 73:323-329, 2000.
6. Klei TR: Equine immunity to parasites, *Vet Clin North Am Equine Pract* 16:69-78, 2000:vi.
7. Forsthuber T, Yip HC, Lehmann PV: Induction of TH1 and TH2 immunity in neonatal mice, *Science* 271:1728-1730, 1996.
8. Blue JT, Dinsmore RP, Anderson KL: Immune-mediated hemolytic anemia induced by penicillin in horses, *Cornell Veterinarian* 77:263-276, 1987.
9. Suter M, Fey H: Further purification and characterization of horse IgE, *Vet Immunol Immunopathol* 4:545-553, 1983.
10. Matthews AG, Imlah P, McPherson EA: A reagin-like antibody in horse serum: 1. Occurrence and some biological properties, *Vet Res Commun* 6:13-23, 1983.
11. Wagner B, Siebenkotten G, Radbruch A, et al: Nucleotide sequence and restriction fragment length polymorphisms of the equine Cvarepsilon gene, *Vet Immunol Immunopathol* 82:193-202, 2001.
12. Navarro P, Barbis DP, Antczak D, et al: The complete cDNA and deduced amino acid sequence of equine IgE, *Mol Immunol* 32:1-8, 1995.
13. Marti E, Szalai G, Bucher K, et al: Partial sequence of the equine immunoglobulin epsilon heavy chain cDNA, *Vet Immunol Immunopathol* 47:363-367, 1995.
14. Halliwell RE, McGorum BC, Irving P, et al: Local and systemic antibody production in horses affected with chronic obstructive pulmonary disease, *Vet Immunol Immunopathol* 38:201-215, 1993.
15. Halliwell RE, Hines MT: Studies on equine recurrent uveitis. I: Levels of immunoglobulin and albumin in the aqueous humor of horses with and without intraocular disease, *Current Eye Res* 4:1023-1031, 1985.
16. Marti E, Peveri P, Griot-Wenk M, et al: Chicken antibodies to a recombinant fragment of the equine immunoglobulin epsilon heavy-chain recognising native horse IgE, *Vet Immunol Immunopathol* 59:253-270, 1997.
17. van der Haegen A, Griot-Wenk M, Welle M, et al: Immunoglobulin-E-bearing cells in skin biopsies of horses with insect bite hypersensitivity, *Equine Vet J* 33:699-706, 2001.
18. Wilson AD, Harwood LJ, Bjornsdottir S, et al: Detection of IgG and IgE serum antibodies to Culicoides salivary gland antigens in horses with insect dermal hypersensitivity (sweet itch), *Equine Vet J* 33:707-713, 2001.
19. Eder C, Curik I, Brem G, et al: Influence of environmental and genetic factors on allergen-specific immunoglobulin-E levels in sera from Lipizzan horses, *Equine Vet J* 33:714-720, 2001.
20. Eder C, Crameri R, Mayer C, et al: Allergen-specific IgE levels against crude mould and storage mite extracts and recombinant mould allergens in sera from horses affected with chronic bronchitis, *Vet Immunol Immunopathol* 73:241-253, 2000.
21. Wagner B, Radbruch A, Rohwer J, et al: Monoclonal anti-equine IgE antibodies with specificity for different epitopes on the immunoglobulin heavy chain of native IgE, *Vet Immunol Immunopathol* 92:45-60, 2003.
22. Wilson AD, Harwood L, Torsteinsdottir S, et al: Production of monoclonal antibodies specific for native equine IgE and their application to monitor total serum IgE responses in Icelandic and non-Icelandic horses with insect bite dermal hypersensitivity, *Vet Immunol Immunopathol* 112:156-170, 2006.
23. Wagner B, Flaminio JB, Hillegas J, et al: Occurrence of IgE in foals: evidence for transfer of maternal IgE by the colostrum and late onset of endogenous IgE production in the horse, *Vet Immunol Immunopathol* 110:269-278, 2006.
24. Hanna CJ, Eyre P, Wells PW, et al: Equine immunology 2: immunopharmacology–biochemical basis of hypersensitivity, *Equine Vet J* 14:16-24, 1982.
25. Nielsen IL, Jacobs KA, Huntington PJ, et al: Adverse reaction to procaine penicillin G in horses, *Aust Vet J* 65:181-185, 1988.
26. Kurotaki T, Narayama K, Oyamada T, et al: Immunopathological study on equine insect hypersensitivity ("kasen") in Japan, *J Comp Pathol* 110:145-152, 1994.
27. Wagner B, Miller WH, Morgan EE, et al: IgE and IgG antibodies in skin allergy of the horse, *Vet Res* 37:813-825, 2006.
28. Lazary S, Marti E, Szalai G, et al: Studies on the frequency and associations of equine leucocyte antigens in sarcoid and summer dermatitis, *Animal Genetics* 25(Suppl 1):75-80, 1994.
29. Marti E, Gerber H, Lazary S: On the genetic basis of equine allergic diseases: II. Insect bite dermal hypersensitivity, *Equine Vet J* 24:113-117, 1992.
30. Robinson NE, Derksen FJ, Olszewski MA, et al: The pathogenesis of chronic obstructive pulmonary disease of horses, *Br Vet J* 152:283-306, 1995.
31. Schmallenbach KH, Rahman I, Sasse HH, et al: Studies on pulmonary and systemic Aspergillus fumigatus-specific IgE and IgG antibodies in horses affected with chronic obstructive pulmonary disease (COPD), *Vet Immunol Immunopathol* 66:245-256, 1998.
32. Kunzle F, Gerber V, Van Der Haegen A, et al: IgE-bearing cells in bronchoalveolar lavage fluid and allergen-specific IgE levels in sera from RAO-affected horses, *J Vet Med A Physiol Pathol Clin Med* 54:40-47, 2007.
33. Cordeau M-E, Joubert P, Dewachi O, et al: IL-4, IL-5 and IFN-g mRNA expression in pulmonary lymphocytes in equine heaves, *Vet Immunol Immunopathol* 97:87-96, 2004.
34. Ainsworth DM, Grunig G, Matychak MB, et al: Recurrent airway obstruction (RAO) in horses is characterized by IFN-gamma and IL-8 production in bronchoalveolar lavage cells, *Vet Immunol Immunopathol* 96:83-91, 2003.
35. Berndt A, Derksen FJ, Venta PJ, et al: Elevated amount of Toll-like receptor 4 mRNA in bronchial epithelial cells is associated with airway inflammation in horses with recurrent airway obstruction, *Am J Physiol Lung Cell Mol Physiol* 292:L936-L943, 2007.
36. Horohov DW, Beadle RE, Mouch S, et al: Temporal regulation of cytokine mRNA expression in equine recurrent airway obstruction, *Vet Immunol Immunopathol* 108:237-245, 2005.
37. Traub-Dargatz JL, McClure JJ, Koch C, et al: Neonatal isoerythrolysis in mule foals, *J Am Vet Med Assoc* 206:67-70, 1995.
38. McClure JJ, Koch C, Traub-Dargatz J: Characterization of a red blood cell antigen in donkeys and mules associated with neonatal isoerythrolysis, *Anim Genet* 25:119-120, 1994.

39. Buechner-Maxwell V, Scott MA, Godber L, et al: Neonatal alloimmune thrombocytopenia in a quarter horse foal, *J Vet Int Med* 11:304-308, 1997.
40. Ramirez S, Gaunt SD, McClure JJ, et al: Detection and effects on platelet function of anti-platelet antibody in mule foals with experimentally induced neonatal alloimmune thrombocytopenia, *J Vet Int Med* 13:534-539, 1999.
41. Galan JE, Timoney JF: Immune complexes in purpura hemorrhagica of the horse contain IgA and M antigen of Streptococcus equi, *J Immunol* 135:3134-3137, 1985.
42. Divers TJ, Timoney JF, Lewis RM, et al: Equine glomerulonephritis and renal failure associated with complexes of group-C streptococcal antigen and IgG antibody, *Vet Immunol Immunopathol* 32:93-102, 1992.
43. Hines MT: Immunologically mediated ocular disease in the horse, *Vet Clin North Am Large Anim Pract* 6:501-512, 1984.
44. Deeg CA, Kaspers B, Gerhards H, et al: Immune responses to retinal autoantigens and peptides in equine recurrent uveitis, *Invest Ophthalmol Vis Sci* 42:393-398, 2001.
45. Davidson MG, Nasisse MP, Roberts SM: Immunodiagnosis of leptospiral uveitis in two horses, *Equine Vet J* 19:155-157, 1987.
46. Faber NA, Crawford M, LeFebvre RB, et al: Detection of Leptospira spp. in the aqueous humor of horses with naturally acquired recurrent uveitis, *J Clin Microbiol* 38:2731-2733, 2000.
47. Parma AE, Fernandez AS, Santisteban CG, et al: Tears and aqueous humor from horses inoculated with Leptospira contain antibodies which bind to cornea, *Vet Immunol Immunopathol* 14:181-185, 1987.
48. Gilger BC, Malok E, Cutter KV, et al: Characterization of T-lymphocytes in the anterior uvea of eyes with chronic equine recurrent uveitis, *Vet Immunol Immunopathol* 71:17-28, 1999.
49. McClure JJ: Equine autoimmunity, *Vet Clin North Am Equine Pract* 16:153-164, 2000.
50. Wilkerson MJ, Davis E, Shuman W, et al: Isotype-specific antibodies in horses and dogs with immune-mediated hemolytic anemia, *J Vet Int Med* 14:190-196, 2000.
51. Geor RJ, Clark EG, Haines DM, et al: Systemic lupus erythematosus in a filly, *J Am Vet Med Assoc* 197:1489-1492, 1990.
52. Pfeiffer CJ, Spurlock S, Ball M: Ultrastructural aspects of equine pemphigus foliaceus-like dermatitis. Report of cases, *J Submicrosc Cytol Pathol* 20:453-461, 1988.
53. Fordyce PS, Edington N, Bridges GC, et al: Use of an ELISA in the differential diagnosis of cauda equina neuritis and other equine neuropathies, *Equine Vet J* 19:55-59, 1987.
54. Wright JA, Fordyce P, Edington N: Neuritis of the cauda equina in the horse, *J Comp Pathol* 97:667-675, 1987.
55. Kadlubowski M, Ingram PL: Circulating antibodies to the neuritogenic myelin protein, P2, in neuritis of the cauda equina of the horse, *Nature* 293:299-300, 1981.
56. Piercy RJ, Swardson CJ, Hinchcliff KW: Erythroid hypoplasia and anemia following administration of recombinant human erythropoietin to two horses, *J Am Vet Med Assoc* 212:244-247, 1998.
57. Woods PR, Campbell G, Cowell RL: Nonregenerative anaemia associated with administration of recombinant human erythropoetin to a Thoroughbred racehores, *Equine Vet J* 29:326-328, 1997.

Immunodeficiency

1. Perryman LE: Primary immunodeficiencies of horses, *Vet Clin North Am Equine Pract* 16:105-116, vii, 2000.
2. Sellon DC: Secondary immunodeficiencies of horses, *Vet Clin North Am Equine Pract* 16:117-130, 2000.
3. Halliwell REW, Gorman NT, editors: *Veterinary clinical immunology*, Philadelphia, 1989, Saunders.
4. Clabough DL, Levine JF, Grant GL, Conboy HS: Factors associated with failure of passive transfer of colostral antibodies in Standardbred foals, *J Vet Intern Med* 5:335-340, 1991.
5. Stoneham SJ, Wingfield Digby NJ, Ricketts SW: Failure of passive transfer of colostral immunity in the foal: incidence, and the effect of stud management and plasma transfusions, *Vet Rec* 128:416-419, 1991.
6. Raidal SL: The incidence and consequences of failure of passive transfer of immunity on a thoroughbred breeding farm, *Aust Vet J* 73:201-206, 1996.
7. Shin EK, Perryman LE, Meek K: A kinase-negative mutation of DNA-PK(CS) in equine SCID results in defective coding and signal joint formation, *J Immunol* 158:3565-3569, 1997.
8. Prescott JF: Immunodeficiency and serious pneumonia in foals: the plot thickens, *Equine Vet J* 25:88-89, 1993.
9. Pastoret P-P, Griebel P, Bazin H, Govaerts A, editors: *Handbook of vertebrate immunology*, San Diego, 1998, Academic Press.
10. Riggs MW: Evaluation of foals for immune deficiency disorders, *Vet Clin North Am Equine Pract* 3:515-528, 1987.
11. Flaminio MJ, Rush BR, Shuman W: Peripheral blood lymphocyte subpopulations and immunoglobulin concentrations in healthy foals and foals with Rhodococcus equi pneumonia, *J Vet Int Med* 13:206-212, 1999.
12. McFarlane D, Sellon DC, Gibbs SA: Age-related quantitative alterations in lymphocyte subsets and immunoglobulin isotypes in healthy horses, *Am J Vet Med* 62:1413-1417, 2001.
13. Sheoran AS, Timoney JF, Homes MA, et al: Immunoglobulin isotypes in sera and nasal mucosal secretions and their neonatal transfer and distribution in horses, *Am J Vet Res* 62:1413-1417, 2001.
14. Koterba AM, Drummond WH, Kosch PC, eds: *Equine clinical neonatology*, Philadelphia, 1990, Lea and Febiger.
15. Clabough DL, Conboy HS, Roberts MC: Comparison of four screening techniques for the diagnosis of equine neonatal hypogammaglobulinemia, *J Am Vet Med Assoc* 194:1717-1720, 1989.
16. Davis DG, Schaefer DM, Hinchcliff KW, Wellman ML, Willet VE, Fletcher JM: Measurement of serum IgG in foals by radial immunodiffusion and automated turbidimetric immunoassay, *J Vet Intern Med* 19:93-96, 2005.
17. Riley CB, McClure JT, Low-Ying S, Shaw RA: Use of Fourier-transform infrared spectroscopy for the diagnosis of failure of transfer of passive immunity and measurement of immunoglobulin concentrations in horses, *J Vet Intern Med* 21:828-834, 2007.
18. Beetson SA, Hilbert BJ, Mills JN: The use of the glutaraldehyde coagulation test for the detection of hypogammaglobulinaemia in neonatal foals, *Aust Vet J* 62:279-281, 1986.
19. Perkins GA, Miller WH, Divers TJ, et al: Ulcerative dermatitis, thrombocytopenia, and neutropenia in neonatal foals, *J Vet Intern Med* 19:211-216, 2005.
20. McTaggart C, Penhale J, Raidala SL: Effect of plasma transfusion on neutrophil function in healthy and septic foals, *Aust Vet J* 83:499-505, 2005.
21. Davis EG, Rush B, Bain F, Clark-Price S, Wilkerson MJ: Neonatal neutropenia in an Arabian foal, *Equine Vet J* 35:517-520, 2003.
22. McClure JT, DeLuca JL, Miller J: *Comparison of five screening tests for detection of failure of passive transfer in foals, Journal of Veterinary Internal Medicine: ACVIM 20th Annual Veterinary Medical Forum Abstract Program* 16:336, 2002.
23. McGuire TC, Perryman LE, Davis WC: Analysis of serum and lymphocyte surface IgM of healthy and immunodeficient horses with monoclonal antibodies, *Am J Vet Res* 44:1284-1288, 1983.
24. Robinson NE, editor: *Current therapy in equine medicine*, ed 6, St. Louis, 2009, Saunders.
25. Lunn DP, Holmes MA, Antczak DF, et al: Report of the Second Equine Leucocyte Antigen Workshop, Squaw valley, California, July 1995, *Vet Immunol Immunopathol* 62:101-143, 1998.

26. Akens MK, Holznagel E, Franchini M, et al: Comparative analysis of equine lymphocyte subsets in whole blood and gradient-purified samples, *Vet Immunol Immunopathol* 58:231-237, 1997.
27. Kidd PG, Vogt RF: Report of the workshop on the evaluation of T-cell subsets during HIV infection and AIDS, *Clin Immunol Immunopathol* 52:3-9, 1989.
28. Stewart C: Clinical applications of flow cytometry, *Cancer* 69:1543-1552, 1992.
29. McClure JT, Fiste M, Sharkey L, et al: Immunphenotypic classification of leukemia in three horses, *J Vet Int Med* 15:144-152, 2001.
30. Lunn DP, Holmes MA, Gibson J, et al: Haematological changes and equine lymphocyte subpopulation kinetics during primary infection and attempted re-infection of specific pathogen free foals with EHV-1, *Equine Vet J* 1991; Supplement 12:35-41.
31. Kydd JH, Hannant D, Mumford JA: Residence and recruitment of leucocytes to the equine lung after EHV-1 infection, *Vet Immunol Immunopathol* 52:15-26, 1996.
32. Dascanio JJ, Zhang CH, Antczak DF, Blue JT, Simmons TR: Differentiation of chronic lymphocytic leukemia in the horse, *J Vet Int Med* 6:225-229, 1992.
33. Rendle DI, Durham AE, Thompson JC, Archer J, Mitchell M, Saunders K, Millere J, Paillot R, Smith KC, Kydd JH: Clinical, immunophenotypic and functional characterisation of T-cell leukaemia in six horses, *Equine Vet J* 39:522-528, 2007.
34. Flaminio MJ, Rush BR, Davis EG, et al: Characterization of peripheral blood and pulmonary leukocyte function in healthy foals, *Vet Immunol Immunopathol* 73:267-285, 2000.
35. Smith III R, Chaffin MK, Cohen ND, Martens RJ: Age-related changes in lymphocyte subsets of quarter horse foals, *Am J Vet Res* 63:531-537, 2002.
36. Patton EA, Soboll G, Coombs D, Lunn DP. Evaluation of T cell proliferatifve responses following EHV-1 infection Conference of Research Workers in Animal Diseases, St. Louis, 2001.
37. McClure JT, Lunn DP, McGuirk SM: Combined immunodeficiency in 3 foals, *Equine Vet Ed* 5:14-18, 1993.
38. Hutchison JM, Garry FB, Belknap EB, et al: Prospective characterization of the clinicopathologic and immunologic features of an immunodeficiency syndrome affecting juvenile llamas, *Vet Immunol Immunopathol* 49:209-227, 1995.
39. Slack JA, Risdahl JM, Valberg S, et al: Effects of corticosteroids on equine IgG sub-isotype responses to vaccination, *Am J Vet Res* 61:1530-1533, 1997.
40. Bernoco M, Liu IK, Wuest Ehlert CJ, et al: Chemotactic and phagocytic function of peripheral blood polymorphonuclear leucocytes in newborn foals, *J Reprod Fertil Suppl* 35:599-605, 1987.
41. Flaminio MJ, Rush BR, Shuman W: Immunologic function in horses after non-specific immunostimulant administration, *Vet Immunol Immunopathol* 63:303-315, 1998.
42. Morris DD, Gaulin G, Strzemienski PJ, et al: Assessment of neutrophil migration, phagocytosis and bactericidal capacity in neonatal foals, *Vet Immunol Immunopathol* 16:173-184, 1987.
43. Zink MC, Yager JA, Prescott JF, Wilkie BN: In vitro phagocytosis and killing of Corynebacterium equi by alveolar macrophages of foals, *Am J Vet Res* 46:2171-2174, 1985.
44. Foerster RJ, Wolf G: Phagocytosis of opsonized fluorescent microspheres by equine polymorphonuclear leukocytes, *Zentralbl Veterinarmed B* 37:481-490, 1990.
45. Johannisson A, Grondahl G, Demmers S, Jensen-Waern M: Flow-cytometric studies of the phagocytic capacities of equine neutrophils, *Acta Veterinaria Scandinavica* 36:553-562, 1995.
46. Raidal SL, Bailey GD, Love DN: The flow cytometric evaluation of phagocytosis by equine peripheral blood neutrophils and pulmonary alveolar macrophages, *Vet J* 156:107-116, 1998.
47. Raidal SL, Bailey GD, Love DN: Flow cytometric determination of oxidative burst activity of equine peripheral blood and bronchoalveolar lavage-derived leucocytes, *Vet J* 156:117-126, 1998.
48. Grondahl G, Sternberg S, Jensen-Waern M, et al: Opsonic capacity of foal serum for the two neonatal pathogens *Eschericia coli* and *Actinobacillus equuli*, *Equine Vet J* 33:670-675, 2001.
49. Demmers S, Johannisson A, Grondahl G, et al: Neutrophil functions and serum IgG in growing foals, *Equine Vet J* 33:676-680, 2001.
50. McTaggart C, Yovich JV, Penhale J, et al: A comparison of foal and adult horse neutrophil function using flow cytometric techniques, *Res Vet Sci* 71:73-79, 2001.
51. Raidal SL, Rose RJ, Love DN: Effects of training on resting peripheral blood and BAL-derived leucocyte function in horses, *Equine Vet J* 33:238-243, 2001.
52. Hormanski CE, Truax R, Pourciau SS, et al: Induction of lymphokine- activated killer cells of equine origin: specificity for equine target cells, *Vet Immunol Immunopathol* 32:25-36, 1992.
53. Horohov DW, Keadle TL, Pourciau SS, et al: Mechanism of exercise-induced augmentation of lymphokine activated killer (LAK) cell activity in the horse, *Vet Immunol Immunopathol* 53:221-233, 1996.
54. Nunokawa Y, Fujinaga T, Taira T, et al: Evaluation of serum amyloid A protein as an acute-phase reactive protein in horses, *J Vet Med Sci* 55:1011-1016, 1993.
55. Okumura M, Fujinaga T, Yamashita K, et al: Isolation, characterization, and quantitative analysis of ceruloplasmin from horses, *Am J Vet Res* 52:1979-1985, 1991.
56. Takiguchi M, Fujinaga T, Naiki M, Mizuno S, Otomo K: Isolation, characterization, and quantitative analysis of C-reactive protein from horses, *Am J Vet Res* 51:1215-1220, 1990.
57. Topper MJ, Prasse KW: Analysis of coagulation proteins as acute-phase reactants in horses with colic, *Am J Vet Res* 59:542-545, 1998.
58. Yamashita K, Fujinaga T, Okumura M, et al: Serum C-reactive protein (CRP) in horses: the effect of aging, sex, delivery and inflammations on its concentration, *J Vet Med Sci* 53:1019-1024, 1991.
59. Reis KJ: A hemolytic assay for the measurement of equine complement, *Vet Immunol Immunopathol* 23:129-137, 1989.
60. Grondahl G, Johannisson A, Jensen-Waern M, Nilsson Ekdahl K: Opsonization of yeast cells with equine iC3b, C3b, and IgG, *Vet Immunol Immunopathol* 80:209-223, 2001.
61. Lavoie JP, Spensley MS, Smith BP, et al: Complement activity and selected hematologic variables in newborn foals fed bovine colostrums, *Am J Vet Res* 50:1532-1536, 1989.
62. McGuire TC, Poppie MJ: Hypogammaglobulinemia and thymic hypoplasia in horses: a primary combined immunodeficiency disorder, *Infect Immun* 8:272-277, 1973.
63. McGuire TC, Poppie MJ, Banks KL: Combined (B- and T-lymphocyte) immunodeficiency: a fatal genetic disease in Arabian foals, *J Am Vet Med Assoc* 164:70-76, 1974.
64. Perryman LE: Molecular pathology of severe combined immunodeficiency in mice, horses, and dogs, *Vet Pathol* 41:95-100, 2004.
65. Wiler R, Leber R, Moore BB, et al: Equine severe combined immunodeficiency: a defect in V(D)J recombination and DNA-dependent protein kinase activity, *Proc Natl Acad Sci U S A* 92:11485-11489, 1995.
66. Poppie MJ, McGuire TC: Combined immunodeficiency in foals of Arabian breeding: evaluation of mode of inheritance and estimation of prevalence of affected foals and carrier mares and stallions, *J Am Vet Med Assoc* 170:31-33, 1977.

67. Bernoco D, Bailey E: Frequency of the SCID gene among Arabian horses in the USA, *Anim Genet* 29:41-42, 1998.
68. Ding Q, Bramble L, Yuzbasiyan-Gurkan V, Bell T, Meek K: DNA-PKcs mutations in dogs and horses: allele frequency and association with neoplasia, *Gene* 283:263-269, 2002.
69. Perryman LE, McGuire TC, Crawford TB: Maintenance of foals with combined immunodeficiency: causes and control of secondary infections, *Am J Vet Res* 39:1043-1047, 1978.
70. Bjorneby JM, Leach DR, Perryman LE: Persistent cryptosporidiosis in horses with severe combined immunodeficiency, *Infect Immun* 59:3823-3826, 1991.
71. Perryman LE, Bue CM, Magnuson NS, Mottironi VD, Ochs HS, Wyatt CR: Immunologic reconstitution of foals with combined immunodeficiency, *Vet Immunol Immunopathol* 17:495-508, 1987.
72. Perryman LE, McGuire TC, Torbeck RL: Ontogeny of lymphocyte function in the equine fetus, *Am J Vet Res* 41:1197-1200, 1980.
73. Holliman A, Scholes SP: Possible immune deficiency in Fell ponies, *Vet Rec* 137:176, 1995.
74. Scholes SF, Holliman A, May PD, Holmes MA: A syndrome of anaemia, immunodeficiency and peripheral ganglionopathy in Fell pony foals, *Vet Rec* 142:128-134, 1998.
75. Butler CM, Westermann CM, Koeman JP: Sloet van Oldruitenborgh-Oosterbaan MM. The Fell pony immunodeficiency syndrome also occurs in the Netherlands: a review and six cases, *Tijdschr Diergeneeskd* 131:114-118, 2006.
76. Gardner RB, Hart KA, Stokol T, Divers TJ, Flaminio MJ: Fell Pony syndrome in a pony in North America, *J Vet Intern Med* 20:198-203, 2006.
77. Richards AJ, Kelly DF, Knottenbelt DC, Cheeseman MT, Dixon JB: Anaemia, diarrhoea and opportunistic infections in Fell ponies, *Equine Vet J* 32:386-391, 2000.
78. Bell SC, Savidge C, Taylor P, Knottenbelt DC, Carter SD: An immunodeficiency in Fell ponies: a preliminary study into cellular responses, *Equine Vet J* 33:687-692, 2001.
79. M. Holmes, personal communication, 2002.
80. Thomas GW, Bell SC, Carter SD: Immunoglobulin and peripheral B-lymphocyte concentrations in Fell pony foal syndrome, *Equine Vet J* 37:48-52, 2005.
81. Thomas GW, Bell SC, Phythian C, et al: Aid to the antemortem diagnosis of Fell pony foal syndrome by the analysis of B lymphocytes, *Vet Rec* 152:618-621, 2003.
82. Perryman LE, McGuire TC, Hilbert BJ: Selective immunoglobulin M deficiency in foals, *J Am Vet Med Assoc* 170:212-215, 1977.
83. Weldon AD, Zhang C, Antczak DF, Rebhun WC: Selective IgM deficiency and abnormal B-cell response in a foal, *J Am Vet Med Assoc* 201:1396-1398, 1992.
84. Perryman LE, McGuire TC: Evaluation for immune system failures in horses and ponies, *J Am Vet Med Assoc* 176:1374-1377, 1980.
85. Perkins GA, Nydam DV, Flaminio MJ, Ainsworth DM: Serum IgM concentrations in normal, fit horses and horses with lymphoma or other medical conditions, *J Vet Intern Med* 17:337-342, 2003.
86. Boy MG, Zhang C, Antczak DF, Hamir AN, Whitlock RH: Unusual selective immunoglobulin deficiency in an arabian foal, *J Vet Int Med* 6:201-205, 1992.
87. Murphy K, Travers P, Walport M: *Janeway's immunobiology*, New York, 2008, Garland Science.
88. Pellegrini-Masini A, Bentz AI, Johns IC, et al: Common variable immunodeficiency in three horses with presumptive bacterial meningitis, *J Am Vet Med Assoc* 227:114-122, 87, 2005.
89. Franklin RP, Long MT, MacNeill A, et al: Proliferative interstitial pneumonia, Pneumocystis carinii infection, and immunodeficiency in an adult Paso Fino horse, *J Vet Int Med* 16:607-611, 2002.
90. Flaminio MJ, LaCombe V, Kohn CW, Antczak DF: Common variable immunodeficiency in a horse, *J Am Vet Med Assoc* 221:1296-1302, 2002.
91. McGuire TC, Poppie MJ, Banks KL: Hypogammaglobulinaemia predisposing to infection in foals, *J Am Vet Med Assoc* 166:71-75, 1975.
92. Deem DA, Traver DS, Thacker HL, Perryman LE: Agammaglobulinaemia in a horse, *J Am Vet Med Assoc* 175:469-472, 1979.
93. Banks KL, McGuire TC, Jerrells R: Absence of B lymphocytes in a horse with primary agammaglobulinaemia, *Clin Immunol Immunopathol* 5:282-290, 1976.
94. Giguere S, Polkes AC: Immunologic disorders in neonatal foals, *Vet Clin North Am Equine Pract* 21:241-272, 2005.
95. McGuire TC, Crawford TB, Hallowell AL, Macomber LE: Failure of colostral immunoglobulin transfer as an explanation for most infections and deaths of neonatal foals, *J Am Vet Med Assoc* 170:1302-1304, 1977.
96. Koterba AM, Brewer BD, Tarplee FA: Clinical and clinicopathological characteristics of the septicaemic neonatal foal: review of 38 cases, *Equine Vet J* 16:376-382, 1984.
97. Jeffcott LB: Studies on passive immunity ini the foal. 1. Gamma-globulin and antibody variations associated with the maternal transfer of immunity and the onset of active immunity, *J Comp Pathol* 84:93-101, 1974.
98. Rouse BT: The immunoglobulins of adult equine and foal sera: a quantitative study, *Br Vet J* 127:45-51, 1971.
99. Rouse BT, Ingram DG: The total protein and immunoglobulin profile of equine colostrums and milk, *Immunology* 19:901-907, 1970.
100. Morris DD, Meirs DA, Merryman GS: Passive transfer failure in horses: incidence and causative factors on a breeding farm, *Am J Vet Res* 46:2294-2299, 1985.
101. Leblanc MM, Tran T, Baldwin JL, Pritchard EL: Factors that influence passive transfer of immunoglobulins in foals, *J Am Vet Med Assoc* 200:179-183, 1992.
102. Le Jan C: Cellular components of mammary secretions and neonatal immunity: a review, *Vet Res* 27:403-417, 1996.
103. Xu RJ: Development of the newborn GI tract and its relation to colostrum/milk intake: a review, *Reprod Fertil Dev* 8:35-48, 1996.
104. Wilson WD, Mihalyi JE, Hussey S, et al: Passive transfer of maternal immunoglobulin isotype antibodies against tetanus and influenza and their effect on the response of foals to vaccination, *Equine Vet J* 33:644-650, 2001.
105. Pearson RC, Hallowell AL, Bayly WM, et al: Times of appearance and disappearance of colostral IgG in the mare, *Am J Vet Res* 45:186-190, 1984.
106. Townsend HG, Tabel H, Bristol FM: Induction of parturition in mares: effect on passive transfer of immunity to foals, *J Am Vet Med Assoc* 182:255-257, 1983.
107. Lavoie JP, Spensley MS, Smith BP, Mihalyi J: Colostral volume and immunoglobulin G and M determinations in mares, *Am J Vet Res* 50:466-470, 1989.
108. Rumbaugh GE, Ardans AA, Ginno D, Trommershausen Smith A: Measurement of neonatal equine immunoglobulins for assessment of colostral immunoglobulin transfer: comparison of single radial immunodiffusion with the zinc sulfate turbidity test, serum electrophoresis, refractometry for total serum protein, and the sodium sulfite precipitation test, *J Am Vet Med Assoc* 172:321-325, 1978.
109. Kent JE, Blackmore DJ: Measurement of IgG in equine blood by immunoturbidimetry and latex agglutination, *Equine Vet J* 17:125-129, 1985.
110. McCue PM: Evaluation of a turbidimetric immunoassay for measurement of plasma IgG concentration in foals, *Am J Vet Res* 68:1005-1009, 2007.
111. Davis R, Giguere S: Evaluation of five commercially available assays and measurement of serum total protein concentration via refractometry for the diagnosis of failure of passive transfer of immunity in foals, *J Am Vet Med Assoc* 227:1640-1645, 2005.

112. Pusterla N, Pusterla JB, Spier SJ, et al: Evaluation of the SNAP foal IgG test for the semiquantitative measurement of immunoglobulin G in foals, *Vet Rec* 151:258-260, 2002.
113. Holmes MA, Lunn DP: A study of bovine and equine immunoglobulin levels in pony foals fed bovine colostrums, *Equine Vet J* 23:116-118, 1991.
114. Hines MT, Schott HC, Bayly WM, Leroux AJ: Exercise and immunity: a review with emphasis on the horse, *J Vet Int Med* 10:280-289, 1996.
115. Horohov DW, Dimock A, Guirnalda P, et al: Effect of exercise on the immune response of young and old horses, *Am J Vet Res* 60:643-647, 1999.
116. Nesse LL, Johansen GI, Blom AK: Effects of racing on lymphocyte proliferation in horses, *Am J Vet Res* 63:528-530, 2002.
117. Wong CW, Smith SE, Thong YH, Opdebeeck JP, Thornton JR: Effects of exercise stress on various immune functions in horses, *Am J Vet Res* 53:1414-1417, 1992.
118. Wong CW, Thompson HL, Thong YH, Thornton JR: Effect of strenuous exercise stress on chemiluminescence response of equine alveolar macrophages, *Equine Vet J* 22:33-35, 1990.
119. Robson PJ, Alston TD, Myburgh KH: Prolonged suppression of the innate immune system in the horse following an 80 km endurance race, *Equine Vet J* 35:133-137, 2003.
120. Folsom RW, Littlefield-Chabaud MA, French DD, et al: Exercise alters the immune response to equine influenza virus and increases susceptibility to infection, *Equine Vet J* 33:664-669, 2001.
121. Gross DK, Hinchcliff KW, French PS, et al: Effect of moderate exercise on the severity of clinical signs associated with influenza virus infection in horses, *Equine Vet J* 30:489-497, 1998.
122. Hoffman AM, Viel L, Prescott JF: Microbiologic changes during antimicrobial treatment and rate of relapse of distal respiratory tract infections in foals, *Am J Vet Res* 54:1608-1614, 1993.
123. Horohov DW, Kydd JH, Hannant D: The effect of aging on T cell responses in the horse, *Dev Comp Immunol* 26:121-128, 2002.
124. Furr MO, Crisman MV, Robertson J, Barta O, Swecker WS Jr: Immunodeficiency associated with lymphosarcoma in a horse, *J Am Vet Med Assoc* 201:307-309, 1992.
125. Dopson LC, Reed SM, Roth JA, Perryman LE, Hitchcock P: Immunosuppression associated with lymphosarcoma in two horses, *J Am Vet Med Assoc* 182:1239-1241, 1983.
126. Buechner-Maxwell V, Zhang C, Robertson J, et al: Intravascular leukostasis and systemic aspergillosis in a horse with subleukemic acute myelomonocytic leukemia, *J Vet Int med* 8:258-263, 1994.
127. Tumas DB, Hines MT, Perryman LE, Davis WC, McGuire TC: Corticosteroid immunosuppression and monoclonal antibody-mediated CD5+ T lymphocyte depletion in normal and equine infectious anaemia virus-carrier horses, *J Gen Virol* 75:959-968, 1994.
128. Gibson JS, Slater JD, Field HJ: The pathogenicity of Ab4p, the sequenced strain of equine herpesvirus-1, in specific pathogen-free foals, *Virology* 189:317-319, 1992.
129. Mair TS: Bacterial pneumonia associated with corticosteroid therapy in three horses, *Vet Rec* 138:205-207, 1996.
130. DeKruyff RH, Fang Y, Umetsu DT: Corticosteroids enhance the capacity of macrophages to induce Th2 cytokine synthesis in CD4+ lymphocytes by inhibiting IL-12 production, *J Immunol* 160:2231-2237, 1998.
131. Ramierz F, Fowell DJ, Puklavec M, Simmonds S, Mason D: Glucocorticoids promote a TH2 cytokine response by CD4+ T cells in vitro, *J Immunol* 156:2406-2412, 1996.
132. Wernery U, Wade JF, Mumford JA, Kaaden O-R, eds. Equine infectious diseases VIII. Proceedings of the Eighth International Conference, Dubai 23rd-26th March, 1998. Newmarket, 1999:129–146, R & W Publications.
133. Bryans JT, Allen GP: Herpesviral diseases of the horse, In Wittmann G, editor: *Herpesvirus diseases of cattle, horses, and pigs*, Boston, 1989, Kluwer Academic Publishers, pp 176-229.
134. McClure JJ, Addison JD, Miller RI: Immunodeficiency manifested by oral candidiasis and bacterial septicemia in foals, *J Am Vet Med Assoc* 186:1195-1197, 1985.
135. Freestone JF, Hietala S, Moulton J, Vivrette S: Acquired immunodeficiency in a seven-year-old horse, *J Am Vet Med Assoc* 190:689-691, 1987.

Immunomodulators

1. Murphy K, Travers P, Walport M: *Janeway's immunobiology*, New York, 2008, Garland Science.
2. Wilckens T, De Rijk R: Glucocorticoids and immune function: unknown dimensions and new frontiers, *Immunol Today* 18:418-424, 1997.
3. Slack JA, Risdahl JM, Valberg S, et al: Effects of corticosterioids on equine IgG sub-isotype responses to vaccination, *Am J Vet Res* 61:1530-1533, 1997.
4. Blotta MH, DeKruyff RH, Umetsu DT: Corticosteroids inhibit IL-12 production in human monocytes and enhance their capacity to induce IL-4 synthesis in CD4+ lymphocytes, *J Immunol* 158:5589-5595, 1997.
5. Franchimont D, Louis E, Dewe W, et al: Effects of dexamethasone on the profile of cytokine secretion in human whole blood cell cultures, *Regul Pept* 73:59-65, 1998.
6. DeKruyff RH, Fang Y, Umetsu DT: Corticosteroids enhance the capacity of macrophages to induce Th2 cytokine synthesis in CD4+ lymphocytes by inhibiting IL-12 production, *J Immunol* 160:2231-2237, 1998.
7. Ramierz F, Fowell DJ, Puklavec M, et al: Glucocoricoids promote a TH2 cytokine response by CD4+ T cells in vitro, *J Immunol* 156:2406-2412, 1996.
8. Morris DD, Strzemienski PJ, Gaulin G, et al: The effects of corticosteroid administration on the migration, phagocytosis and bactericidal capacity of equine neutrophils, *Cornell Vet* 78:243-252, 1988.
9. Burton JL, Kehrli Jr ME, Kapil S, et al: Regulation of L-selectin and CD18 on bovine neutrophils by glucocorticoids: effects of cortisol and dexamethasone, *J Leukoc Biol* 57:317-325, 1995.
10. Mair TS: Bacterial pneumonia associated with corticosteroid therapy in three horses, *Vet Rec* 138:205-207, 1996.
11. Kono Y, Hirasawa K, Fukunaga Y, et al: Recrudescence of equine infectious anemia by treatment with immunosuppressive drugs, *Natl Inst Anim Health Q (Tokyo)* 16:8-15, 1976.
12. Tumas DB, Hines MT, Perryman LE, et al: Corticosteroid immunosuppression and monoclonal antibody-mediated CD5+ T lymphocyte depletion in normal and equine infectious anaemia virus-carrier horses, *J Gen Virol* 75:959-968, 1994.
13. Gibson JS, Slater JD, Awan AR, et al: Pathogenesis of equine herpesvirus-1 in specific pathogen-free foals: primary and secondary infections and reactivation, *Arch Virol* 123:351-366, 1992.
14. Bathe AP: The corticosteroid laminitis story: 3. The clinician's viewpoint, *Equine Vet J* 39:12-13, 2007.
15. Bailey SR, Elliott J: The corticosteroid laminitis story: 2. Science of if, when and how, *Equine Vet J* 39:7-11, 2007.
16. Dutton H: The corticosteroid laminitis story: 1. Duty of care, *Equine Vet J* 39:5-6, 2007.
17. Johnson PJ, Slight SH, Ganjam VK, et al: Glucocorticoids and laminitis in the horse, *Vet Clin North Am Equine Pract* 18:219-236, 2002.
18. Messer NTt, Arnold K: Immune-mediated hemolytic anemia in a horse, *J Am Vet Med Assoc* 198:1415-1416, 1991.
19. Humber KA, Beech J, Cudd TA, et al: Azathioprine for treatment of immune-mediated thrombocytopenia in two horses, *J Am Vet Med Assoc* 199:591-594, 1991.

20. Gratzek AT, Kaswan RL, Martin CL, et al: Ophthalmic cyclosporine in equine keratitis and keratouveitis: 11 cases, *Equine Vet J* 27:327-333, 1995.
21. Gilger BC, Wilkie DA, Davidson MG, et al: Use of an intravitreal sustained-release cyclosporine delivery device for treatment of equine recurrent uveitis, *Am J Vet Res* 62:1892-1896, 2001.
22. Gilger BC, Michau TM, Salmon JH: Immune-mediated keratitis in horses: 19 cases (1998-2004), *Vet Ophthalmol* 8:233-239, 2005.
23. Gilger BC, Malok E, Stewart T, et al: Effect of an intravitreal cyclosporine implant on experimental uveitis in horses, *Vet Immunol Immunopathol* 76:239-255, 2000.
24. Nimmerjahn F, Ravetch JV: The antiinflammatory activity of IgG: the intravenous IgG paradox, *J Exp Med* 204:11-15, 2007.
25. Anthony RM, Nimmerjahn F, Ashline DJ, et al: Recapitulation of IVIG anti-inflammatory activity with a recombinant IgG Fc, *Science* 320:373-376, 2008.
26. Dwyer JM: Immunoglobulins in autoimmunity: history and mechanisms of action, *Clin Exp Rheumatol* 14:S3-S7, 1996.
27. Dwyer JM: Manipulating the immune system with immune globulin, *N Engl J Med* 326:107-116, 1992.
28. Dietrich G, Kaveri SV, Kazatchkine MD: Modulation of autoimmunity by intravenous immune globulin through interaction with the function of the immune/idiotypic network, *Clin Immunol Immunopathol* 62:S73-S81, 1992.
29. Vassilev T, Kazatchkine MD: Mechanisms of immunomodulatory action of intravenous immunoglobulin in autoimmune and systemic inflammatory diseases, *Ther Apher* 1:38-41, 1997.
30. Imbach P, Akatsuka J, Blanchette V, et al: Immunthrombocytopenic purpura as a model for pathogenesis and treatment of autoimmunity, *Eur J Ped* 154:S60-S64, 1995.
31. Colagiuri S, Leong GM, Thayer Z, et al: Intravenous immunoglobulin therapy for autoimmune diabetes mellitus, *Clin Exp Rheumatol* 14:S93-S97, 1996.
32. Moore BR: Clinical application of interferons in large animal medicine, *J Am Vet Med Assoc* 208:1711-1715, 1996.
33. Rush BR, Flaminio MJ: Immunomodulation in horses, *Vet Clin North Am Equine Pract* 16:183-197, viii, 2000.
34. Moore BR, Krakowka S, Robertson JT, et al: Cytologic evaluation of bronchoalveolar lavage fluid obtained from standardbred racehorses with inflammatory airway disease, *Am J Vet Res* 56:562-567, 1995.
35. Moore BR, Krakowka S, Cummins JM, et al: Changes in airway inflammatory cell populations in standardbred racehorses after interferon-alpha administration, *Vet Immunol Immunopathol* 49:347-358, 1996.
36. Moore BR, Krakowka S, McVey DS, et al: Inflammatory markers in bronchoalveolar lavage fluid of standardbred racehorses with inflammatory airway disease: response to interferon-alpha, *Equine Vet J* 29:142-147, 1997.
37. Zinkl JG, Madigan JE, Fridmann DM, et al: Haematological, bone marrow and clinical chemical changes in neonatal foals given canine recombinant granulocyte-colony stimulating factor, *Equine Vet J* 26:313-318, 1994.
38. Madigan JE, Zinkl JG, Fridmann DM, et al: Preliminary studies of recombinant bovine granulocyte-colony stimulating factor on haematological values in normal neonatal foals, *Equine Vet J* 26:159-161, 1994.
39. Rush BR, Lunn DP: Immunomodulation in horses: indications and preparations Proceeding of the 50th Annual Convention of the American Association of Equine Practitioners, Denver, 2004, Colorado, 454–458.
40. Audibert FM, Lise LD: Adjuvants: current status, clinical perspectives and future prospects, *Trends Pharmacol Sci* 14:174-178, 1993.
41. Flaminio MJ, Rush BR, Shuman W: Immunologic function in horses after nonspecific immunostimulant administration, *Vet Immunol Immunopathol* 63:303-315, 1998.
42. Hacker G, Redecke V, Hacker H: Activation of the immune system by bacterial CpG-DNA, *Immunology* 105:245-251, 2002.
43. Rankin R, Pontarollo R, Ioannou X, et al: CpG motif identification for veterinary and laboratory species demonstrates that sequence recognition is highly conserved, *Antisense Nucleic Acid Drug Dev* 11:333-340, 2001.
44. Sato Y, Roman M, Tighe H, et al: Immunostimulatory DNA sequences necessary for effective intradermal gene immunization, *Science* 273:352-354, 1996.
45. Whitmore MM, Li S, Falo Jr L, Huang L: Systemic administration of LPD prepared with CpG oligonucleotides inhibits the growth of established pulmonary metastases by stimulating innate and acquired antitumor immune responses, *Cancer Immunol Immunother* 50:503-514, 2001.
46. Lopez AM, Hecker R, Mutwiri G, et al: Formulation with CpG ODN enhances antibody responses to an equine influenza virus vaccine, *Vet Immunol Immunopathol* 114:103-110, 2006.
47. Flaminio MJ, Borges AS, Nydam DV, et al: The effect of CpG-ODN on antigen presenting cells of the foal, *J Immune Based Ther Vaccines* 5:1, 2007.
48. Ziebell KL, Steinmann H, Kretzdorn D, et al: The use of Baypamun N in crowding associated infectious respiratory disease: efficacy of Baypamun N (freeze dried product) in 4-10 month old horses, *Zentralblatt Fuer Veterinaermedizin Reihe B* 44:529-536, 1997.
49. Studer U, Marti E, Stornetta D, et al: [The therapy of equine sarcoid with a non-specific immunostimulator–the epidemiology and spontaneous regression of sarcoids], *Schweizer Archiv fur Tierheilkunde|Sat, Schweizer Archiv fur Tierheilkunde* 139:385-391, 1997.
50. Lunn DP, Rush BR. Immunomodulation: Principles and Mechanisms Proceeding of the 50th Annual Convention of the American Association of Equine Practitioners. Denver, Colorado, 2004:447–453.
51. O'Neill W, McKee S, Clarke AF: Immunological and haematinic consequences of feeding a standardised Echinacea (*Echinacea angustifolia*) extract to healthy horses, *Equine Vet J* 34:222-227, 2002.
52. Babiuk LA, Misra V: Levamisole and bovine immunity: In vitro and in vivo effects on immune responses to herpesvirus immunization, *Can J Microbiol* 27:1312-1319, 1981.
53. Roth JA, Kaeberle ML: Effect of levamisole on lymphocyte blastogenesis and neutrophil function in dexamethasone-treated cattle, *Am J Vet Res* 45:1781-1784, 1984.
54. Lunn DP, Townsend HGG: Equine vaccination, *Vet Clin North Am Equine Pract* 16:199-226, 2000.
55. Macy DW: Vaccine adjuvants, *Semin Vet Med Surg (Small Anim)* 12:206-211, 1997.
56. Moore J, editor: *Equine medicine and surgery*, St. Louis, 1999, Mosby.
57. Marti E, Horohov DW, Antzak DF, Lazary S, Lunn DP: Advances in equine immunology: Havemeyer workshop reports from Santa Fe, New Mexico, and Hortobagy, Hungary, *Vet Immunol Immunopathol* 91:233-243, 2003.
58. Crameri R: Allergy vaccines: dreams and reality, *Expert Rev Vaccines* 6:991-999, 2007.
59. Jose-Cunilleras E, Kohn CW, Hillier A, Saville WJ, Lorch G: Intradermal testing in healthy horses and horses with chronic obstructive pulmonary disease, recurrent urticaria, or allergic dermatitis, *J Am Vet Med Assoc* 219:1115-1121, 2001.
60. DeBoer DJ: Survey of intradermal skin testing practices in North America, *J Am Vet Med Assoc* 195:1357-1363, 1989.
61. Barbet JL, Bevier D, Greiner EC: Specific immunotherapy in the treatment of Culicoides hypersensitive horses: a double-blind study, *Equine Vet J* 22:232-235, 1990.
62. Schmid-Grendelmeier P, Crameri R: Recombinant allergens for skin testing, *Int Arch Allergy Immunol* 125:96-111, 2001.
63. Crameri R: High throughput screening: a rapid way to recombinant allergens, *Allergy* 56:30-34, 2001.

64. Jahn-Schmid B, Wiedermann U, Bohle B, et al: Oligodeoxynucleotides containing CpG motifs modulate the allergic TH2 response of BALB/c mice to Bet v 1, the major birch pollen allergen, *J Allergy Clin Immunol* 104:1015-1023, 1999.
65. Broide D, Raz E: DNA-Based immunization for asthma, *Int Arch Allergy Immunol* 118:453-456, 1999.
66. Broide D, Schwarze J, Tighe H, et al: Immunostimulatory DNA sequences inhibit IL-5, eosinophilic inflammation, and airway hyperresponsiveness in mice, *J Immunol* 161:7054-7062, 1998.
67. Crameri R, Rhyner C: Novel vaccines and adjuvants for allergen-specific immunotherapy, *Curr Opin Immunol* 18:761-768, 2006.
68. Rhyner C, Kundig T, Akdis CA, Crameri R: Targeting the MHC II presentation pathway in allergy vaccine development, *Biochem Soc Trans* 35:833-834, 2007.
69. Crameri R, Fluckiger S, Daigle I, Kundig T, Rhyner C: Design, engineering and in vitro evaluation of MHC class-II targeting allergy vaccines, *Allergy* 62:197-206, 2007.
70. Mantel PY, Kuipers H, Boyman O, et al: GATA3-driven Th2 responses inhibit TGF-beta1-induced FOXP3 expression and the formation of regulatory T cells, *PLoS Biol* 5:e329, 2007.

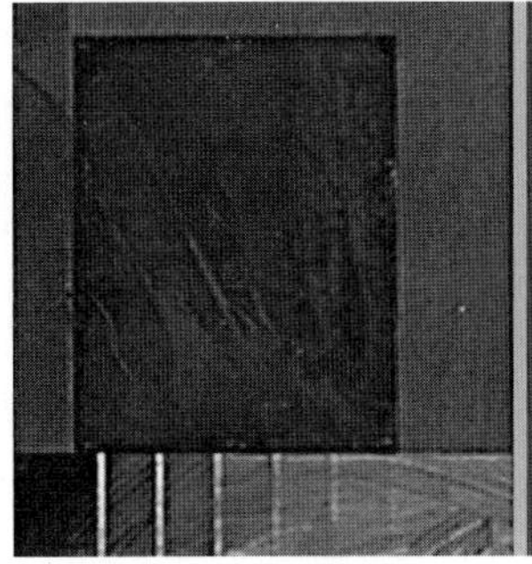

Mechanisms of Infectious Disease

CHAPTER 2

Maureen T. Long

MECHANISMS OF ESTABLISHMENT AND SPREAD OF BACTERIAL AND FUNGAL INFECTIONS

Maureen T. Long

NORMAL FLORA

Dermal and mucosal surfaces provide a life-preserving protective barrier composed of physical, chemical, and microbial defenses.[1] *Normal flora* is an essential component of this protective barrier against pathogens yet paradoxically provides a source for opportunistic invasion. *Commensal bacteria* are those living on or within a host in a way such that both derive mutual benefit and in which interruption of this association results in abnormal host development or overt disease.[1] A pathogen is any disease-producing organism; thus a commensal is potentially pathogenic. Colonization is infection without disease; colonization of skin, gastrointestinal, respiratory, and urogenital tracts occurs early in life and persists during the healthy lifetime of the host.

Skin Flora

The combination of normal flora and mucosal immunity provides an effective barrier against infectious colonization of nondisrupted skin surfaces. Specific bacteria are stratified by site, and certain bacteria multiply and colonize depending on associated adnexa.[2] Most bacteria and fungi on the surface of the skin are not associated with disease; however, yeast and bacteria associated with hair follicles are more likely to be related to a disease process.[3] Even though horses inhabit an environment heavily contaminated with fecal flora, normal dermal flora in the horse is surprisingly devoid of members of the Enterobacteriaceae.[4] Normal inhabitants include mixed populations of bacteria of species of *Acinetobacter, Aerococcus, Aeromonas, Bacillus, Corynebacterium, Flavobacterium, Micrococcus, Nocardia,* coagulase negative *Staphylococcus, Staphylococcus aureus, Streptomyces,* and nonhemolytic *Streptococcus* generae.[2] Certain *Staphylococcus* spp. have been associated with skin disease in the horse, and these include *S. aureus, S. intermedius,* and *S. hyicus,* whereas species such as *S. xylosus* and *S. sciuri* were more associated with normal skin.

More than 30 species of fungi can inhabit the skin and *Alternaria, Aspergillus, Candida, Fusarium, Rhizopus,* and *Trichophyton* spp. are commonly present.[2] Until recently the presence of *Malassezia* yeast species has been considered pathogenic. Recent fungal culturing of the skin of normal, healthy horses has confirmed colonization by a species of *Malassezia* yeast that is novel to the horse (tentatively named *M. equi*). Colonized sites include groin, axilla, and perineal regions.[5]

Oral, Pharyngeal, and Respiratory Flora

Oral and pharyngeal mucosal flora is associated with both health and disease of the upper and lower respiratory system. The oral and pharyngeal mucosa is richly populated with many bacteria, including obligate aerobes, anaerobes, and facultative anaerobes.[6] Gram positive and negative anaerobes are the predominant flora in the mouth and pharyngeal tonsils of the normal horse, with *B. fragilis* and *Bacteroides spp.* most commonly found. Genera consisting of *Fusobacterium* spp., *Eubacterium* spp., *Clostridium* spp., *Veillonella* spp., and *Megasphaera* spp. are also cultured. Aerobic and facultative anaerobic populations mostly comprise *S. zooepidemicus, Pasteurella* spp., *E. coli, Actinomyces* spp., and *Streptococcus* spp. Because these same genera are also consistently found in horses with lower respiratory infections, opportunistic colonization by pharyngeal flora is the likely mechanism of disease.[6] Contamination of the trachea of the horse is a frequent occurrence, as evidenced by the fact that trans-tracheal aspiration (TTA) yields positive bacterial cultures in approximately 30% of both normal adult horses and foals.[7] As with skin flora, normal horses have multiple fungal species inhabiting conjunctival, nasal, and oral mucosa.[8] Stabling increases the frequency of ocular fungi in normal horses.[8]

Intestinal Flora

In animal models and chronic human conditions, normal flora is considered important for intestinal maturity and containment of disease. Changes in cecal weight, villus:crypt ratio, and volatile fatty acid production and the development of gut IgA responses are all affected by suboptimal cecal colonization in germ-free animals.[9] A relationship between severity of mucosal disease and normal flora has also been demonstrated in models of inflammatory bowel disease of humans.[10]

Bacteria are present in all parts of the intestinal tract of the horse, and the microbial fauna increases in complexity and density aborally.[11] The stomach of the horse is not a sterile environment. A dense population of gram positive bacterial rods, primarily composed of *Lactobacillus* spp., colonizes the nonsquamous portion of the equine stomach. Substantial colonization of the duodenum is present with a large population of proteolytic bacteria, and this colonization increases by tenfold in the ileum.[12]

Microbial degradation and fermentation of plant material in the large intestine are important components of nutrient acquisition in the equid. The consumption of cellulose and starch results in the production of volatile fatty acids (VFAs).[13] The major cellulolytic bacterial strains in the horse produce arrays of fermentation products that differ from those of cattle.[14] The common bovine rumen bacteria *Ruminococcus flavefaciens* is one of the most predominant cellulolytic bacteria of the equine cecum based on standard microbiologic techniques.[15] Genetic techniques also demonstrate that the predominant flora are the low GC-content bacteria, which include *Cytophaga-Flexibacter-Bacteroides* and *Clostridium* bacteria; the actual species are completely novel.[15] Standard microbiologic techniques specifically demonstrate Enterobacteriaceae, *Butyrivibrio* spp., *Streptococci* spp., *Bacteroides* spp., *Lactobacilli* spp., *Selenomonas* spp., *Eubacterium* spp., *Propionibacterium* spp., and *Staphylococcus* spp. in residence.[16] In addition, there are completely different compositions of bacteria between the differing segments of the colon, especially between the ascending colon and cecum, indicating highly specialized digestive functions associated within the large intestine itself.[15] Yeasts and fungi of the order *Mucorales* have been identified in the cecum of normal horses and are capable of digesting cellulose and starch.[17]

Routine surveillance demonstrates a relative lack of intestinal pathogens in the flora of normal horses. In the largest study to date, fecal shedding of *Salmonella enteriditis* as detected by fecal culture in normal horses from farms without evidence of salmonellosis was 0.8% in resident horses.[18] Molecular diagnostics, once hoped to provide a tool for understanding the incidence of *Salmonella* spp. in the clinically normal horse, has provided inconsistent information, and polymerase chain reaction (PCR) is most useful for identification of subclinical shedders and environmental contamination during an outbreak.[19,20] On the basis of limited investigations, the carriage rates of *C. difficile* in normal horses and foals appear to be low (<1.5%).[21]

Intestinal flora in the horse is an important source for extraintestinal pathogens. In studies examining the carriage rate of *Rhodococcus equi*, all horses cultured carried the bacteria regardless of age.[22,23] Furthermore, if the farm had endemic *R. equi* and respiratory isolates contain the 90 kDa plasmid, which has been associated with disease, fecal isolates also contained this plasmid.

Urogenital Flora

By far, most of the work that characterizes equine normal flora has focused on urogenital flora to address infertility and fetal loss. Although vaginal and vestibular mucosa of mares should be colonized with normal mucosal flora, the uterus is considered sterile. However, typical culturing techniques result in frequent isolation of what could be considered pathogens, and cytology and bacterial counts are essential supplemental tests for detecting true uterine infection. Counts less than 10 colony-forming units and lack of inflammatory cells indicate uterine or technical contamination.[24]

Many bacteria inhabit the external genitalia of stallions, including bacteria considered to be associated with metritis in mares. The predominant aerobe isolated is coagulase-negative *Staphylococcus* spp., followed by *Corynebacterium* spp., α-hemolytic *Streptococcus* spp., and *Lactobacillus* spp. Pathogens such as β-hemolytic *Streptococcus* spp., *Pseudomonas aeruginosa*, and *Klebsiella* spp. can be frequently found in servicing stallions.[25,26] Pregnancy rates appear to be the same in mares bred to *P. aeruginosa* semen–infected stallions.[27]

Fungal Flora

Essentially the same principals apply regarding normal flora, host immunity, and specific virulence factors for the pathogenesis of fungal infection. Fungal infections can be divided into primary or opportunistic pathogens. True pathogens are less dependent on host status than opportunistic pathogens, although even a true pathogen may require some degree of alteration of normal flora or host immunity to become established. Long-term antibiotic use, immunosuppression, and compromised organ function (especially involving the pulmonary or endocrine system) are three primary host factors highly associated with establishment of opportunistic fungal infection. Fungi in particular can adapt to the mammalian environment over a relatively short course in order to become established. Establishment usually requires a change in thermal range, oxygen requirements, and resistance to host defenses.

POPULATION BIOLOGY OF BACTERIAL INFECTIONS

Inoculum size, virulence of the organism, and microbial resistance are three important determinants in the outcome of infectious challenge. Minimizing the size of bacterial challenge by controlling environmental contamination must be the primary goal for successful disease control in the natural environment and hospital settings.

Inoculum Size

Little dose-response work has been published that demonstrates a clear relationship between frequency or severity of disease and dose for many equine bacterial pathogens. In general, for systemic infections, inoculum size has been shown to be the most important determinant of disease in hematogenously disseminated infections such as meningitis and, in rodent models, osteomyelitis.[28] The equine literature emphasizes animal and environmental risk factors[29] as important determinants in survival for conditions such as neonatal osteomyelitis, but these factors ultimately control the degree of bacterial challenge at birth. For skin infections, colonization of experimentally induced wounds with *Staphylococcus* spp. is historically dependent on inoculum size. However, attainment of antibiotic resistance and new virulence factors are predominant factors in the development of human *S. aureus* colonization and disease.[30,31] The occurrence of diarrhea is dose dependent in salmonellosis in calves,[32] but little is known regarding challenge dose in the foal or the adult horse. Very small numbers of *Streptococcus equi* subsp. *equi* inoculated intranasally result in rapid colonization of the equine lingual and nasopharyngeal tonsils within hours.[33] Minimal inoculum size is required for certain pathogens that form toxins, such as *E. coli* O157H7and *Clostridium* spp. in humans.[34]

Virulence

Virulence is the relative ability of an organism to cause disease.[1] Virulence of an organism is frequently tested by inoculation of different strains or genetically modified organisms of a pathogen into groups of a rodent species (or cell culture), and lethality or invasiveness is evaluated. When this particular methodology is used, the severity of many diseases frequently is found to be strain dependent and virulence is commonly associated with certain phenotypic characteristics of a particular strain.

Antibiotic Resistance

Widespread use of antibiotics in both animal and human infection occurred after World War II.[35,36] Within 30 years resistance of gram positive organisms was already occurring in human pneumococcal infections.[37] From the 1960s to the 1980s, staphylococcal resistance progressed from initial methicillin-resistant organisms to vancomycin-resistant organisms.[36] Specific types and mechanisms of bacterial resistance are discussed in association with particular diseases. Briefly, there is intermediate resistance that occurs in geographically defined isolates in a step-wise fashion resulting from genetic changes under antibiotic pressure.[37,38] Thus proper dose and length of antibiotic exposure are important in preventing the development of these isolates.[37,38] In high-grade and multidrug-resistant (MDR) forms of antibiotic resistance, there is clonal expansion of small numbers of isolates.[39] In addition to selective antibiotic pressure, individual carrier animals and people are important for development and maintenance of high-grade and MDR resistance. Virulence and antibiotic resistance are not synonymous; commensal or relatively noninvasive pathogens have higher rates of resistance,[40] whereas more highly pathogenic or invasive organisms have less resistance. Because commensal organisms are ubiquitous, with a higher likelihood of contact with bacteria that have multiresistance genes, commensal organisms become a reservoir for resistance genes.[40]

DEVELOPMENT OF DISEASE AND THE ROLE OF NORMAL FLORA

Disruption of Normal Flora

The pathophysiology of certain types of equine colitis and pleuropneumonia is consistent with either disruption of normal flora and invasion by a pathogen or the conversion of a common commensal organism into a pathogen. Development of colitis in the horse has been associated with feed change, antibiotics, surgery, nonsteroidal inflammatory drugs, and transport, all events that disrupt flora.[41,42] Rapid change from a roughage diet to concentrate results in increased anaerobes, decreased cellulolytic bacteria, decreased cecal protozoa diversity, and decreased pH in the equine cecum.[41] Isolation of *Clostridium difficile* is more likely from horses treated with antibiotics, and clinical disease has been associated with ampicillin, erythromycin, penicillin, and potentiated sulfonamide administration in adult horses.[43,44] In ponies infected with *Salmonella* spp., transport and surgery reactivated infection and diarrhea, and antibiotics (oxytetracycline) prolonged shedding but did not induce recrudescence.[42] In a case control study, use of potentiated sulfonamides was not significantly associated with the development of diarrhea in hospitalized horses; however, overall antibiotic use was highly associated with the occurrence of diarrhea.[45]

There are several mechanisms by which antibiotics disrupt normal gastrointestinal flora and function.[46] The most important include (1) disruption of carbohydrate metabolism, (2) decreased metabolism of bile acids, (3) direct effects on intestinal motility, and (4) shortening of intestinal villi. Changes in carbohydrate metabolism are a large intestinal event secondary to reduced microbial reduction of carbohydrates to short-chain fatty acids (SCFAs). Because SCFA metabolism and absorption result in fluid and electrolyte absorption, a sudden decrease in SCFA leads to osmotic diarrhea with an intraluminal accumulation of organic acids, cations, and carbohydrates. In human studies, reduced SCFAs have been demonstrated with many antibiotics, including ampicillin, metronidazole, and erythromycin.[46] Bile acids, reduced in the colon by dehydroxylating bacteria, are potent colonic secretogues. Increases in fecal bile acids have been demonstrated in humans with the use of ampicillin and clindamycin.[46] Erythromycin and amoxicillin directly affect colonic motility.[46] Erythromycin is a motilin receptor agonist resting in contraction of antral and duodenal smooth muscles.[47] In the horse erythromycin results in a dose-dependent increase in ileocecal emptying.[48] Motility enhancing effects have also been observed in human patients treated with amoxicillin.[46]

Disease Caused by Colonization of Commensal Flora

Occurrence of infectious lower respiratory disease in adult horse is an example of how contamination of a normally sterile site with several commensal bacteria results in disease. Changes in upper respiratory mucosal flora and transportation are two important elements that contribute to the development of pleuropneumonia in the horses. The tonsillar mucosa of the oropharynx is heavily colonized with *S. equi* subsp. *zooepidemicus,* and necrosis of this tissue occurring during viral infection is associated with spread to the lower respiratory tract.[6] Transport of horses (especially for distances >500 miles) is a primary risk factor for pleuropneumonia as demonstrated in a large retrospective study.[49] Elevation of the head for an extended period of time is likely a contributing factor. Horses normally feed from the ground for most of the day, and this posture promotes effective tracheal clearance of inhaled debris and particulate matter. Under experimental conditions elevation of the head for prolonged periods of time results in an increase in the variety and multiplication of oral/pharyngeal commensal bacteria within the trachea. *Pasteurella, Actinobacillus,* and *Streptococcus* spp. are the most frequent and prolific colonizers of the trachea after prolonged head elevation.[50,51] In addition to prolonged head elevation imposed by extended transport periods, there is decreased phagocytosis of equine peripheral neutrophils in these horses.[51] As a result, common commensal bacteria of the nasal and oropharyngeal mucosa become opportunistic pathogens.

Nosocomial Infections

Nosocomial infection (health care–associated infections) is defined by the Centers for Disease Control and Prevention (CDC) as a localized/systemic condition resulting from an adverse reaction to the presence of an infectious agent or its toxin. There must be no evidence that the infection was present or incubating at the time of hospital admission.[52] Nosocomial infections are becoming a major problem for large animal veterinary teaching and private referral hospitals. Infections with *Serratia marcescens*, *Acinetobacter baumannii*, *S. aureus*, methicillin-resistant *Staphylococcus* spp., *Enterococcus* spp., and various *Salmonella enteritidis* serovars have all been reported in association with nosocomial infection in equine patients.[53,54] Surgical incision infection, joint sepsis, catheter phlebitis, wounds, and diarrhea represent the common clinical syndromes reported in horses.[53-55] When nosocomial infection involves the acquisition of isolates from the hospital environment, these isolates are more difficult to treat because they frequently undergo high-level antibiotic pressure and attain multiresistance. Nosocomially transmitted salmonellosis in equine hospital wards is increasingly reported, with *Salmonella enteritidis* serotypes Krefeld, Saint Paul, DT104, and Anatum all demonstrating attainment of MDR over the course of the outbreak.[56,57] Only one study of a nosocomially transmitted *Salmonella enteritidis* (serotype Heidelberg) did not demonstrate significant acquisition of multidrug resistance over time.[58]

PATHOGENESIS OF BACTERIAL INFECTIONS

The ability of bacteria to gain entry and cause disease results from a combination of factors possessed by the agent itself, environmental conditions, and status of host defenses. Bacteria either gain entry through a body surface by direct inoculation or colonize and damage a dermal or mucosal barrier to cause disease. Environmental or risk factors specific for individual diseases increase the probability of successful penetration or colonization and are discussed for specific diseases in various chapters. Innate immunity and specific immunity, which alter host susceptibility to disease, are also discussed elsewhere in this chapter. General mechanisms that are specific to bacteria and enhance disease are virulence factors that enhance the entry, spread, and damage to host tissues (Table 2-1). Virulence factors may either allow bacteria an advantage to gain entry and disseminate or directly cause damage to the host once entry has been gained. Major virulence factors are listed for specific equine pathogens.

FACTORS THAT ENHANCE ENTRY OF BACTERIA

Adhesion, Entry, and Secretion

Protein secretion systems (PSSs) are a structurally diverse complex of essential virulence factors for bacteria that allow specialized interactions between cells.[59] Classifications of associated pili are separated on the basis of their biogenesis by a particular PSS and their resulting final structure, which accounts for their wide diversity. These main systems function to translocate various sized molecules and are important in the formation of adhesins upon attachment to host cells.

TABLE 2-1

General Mechanisms of Bacterial Pathogenesis

Action	Mechanism	Examples
Entry of bacteria	Adhesion Entry	Fibrillar adhesins Nonfibrillar adhesins Curli fimbriae Lipoteichoic acid Biofilm adhesion proteins Membrane ruffling
Enhancement of spread	Immune resistance Host substrate utilization	Capsule Lipopolysaccharide Anticomplement Resistance to phagocytosis Phagolysosomal survival Iron acquisition
Damage to host membranes	Toxins	Exotoxin Endotoxin Apoptosis

Fibrillar adhesins (FAs) and nonfibrillar adhesins (NFAs) are the most important PSS subgroup not used for bacterial conjugation. They specifically target host cells and biofilms for enhancement of colonization and invasion.

Fibrillar Adhesions

There are multiple types of FAs in both gram positive and gram negative bacteria, with gram negative the most well characterized (Table 2-2).[60-62] Pili or fimbriae are rod-shaped structures composed of an orderly array of a single protein usually arranged in a helical fashion to form a cylinder. The tip of the fimbria mediates attachment to carbohydrate moieties on cell surfaces and is integral to bacterial invasion and colonization. Bacteria can also contain multiple types of pili. Both the bacterial pili themselves and the cellular pathways they use for secretion and formation of pili are targets for pharmacologic intervention, and there are multiple subclasses depending on their configuration.[60]

Type I fimbriae (Figure 2-1) are distributed in the periplasmic space and translocated to the cell surface by a chaperone-usher (C-U) pathway.[62-65] These pili are made up of multiple major pilin subunits compiling a rigid shaft with minor pili proteins composing the flexible tip. These require a C-U secretion system for biogenesis. The C-U prevents the pili from achieving their final figuration while in the periplasmic space located between the inner and outer membrane before assuming their position on the outer membrane. Although once considered Type I, the formation of the pili associated with enterotoxigenic *E. coli* (ETEC) is now considered an alternate C-U pathway, which functions to confer species-specific binding to intestinal epithelium and mediate agglutination of erythrocytes. In gastrointestinal and urinary tract infection, fimbriae are likely one of the most important virulent factors for successful invasion.[61] Although the importance of *E. coli* adhesive fimbriae is questionable in equine disease and

TABLE 2-2

Major Types of Bacterial Adhesins		
Adhesin	**Definition**	**Example**
Type 1 fimbriae	Cell surface structure primarily on gram (–) bacteria that bind to the terminal mannose of glycoproteins on cells	*Escherichia coli*
Type 4 pili	Cell surface structure primarily on gram (–) bacteria that function in adhesion, twitching, and DNA uptake, which bind on CD46 and other glycolipids	*Pseudomonas aeruginosa*
Curli fimbriae	Coiled aggregative fimbrial structures that bind to fibronectin, laminin, and plasminogen and function in adhesion, aggregation, and biofilm formation	Enterohemorrhagic *Escherichia coli* (EHEC) Salmonella
Fibrils and flexible rods	Short, thin rodlike adhesins that bind to fibronectin for adhesion to host tissues	*Streptococcus* species
(Lipo) Teichoic acid	Part of the peptidoglycan layer of cell walls	Gram positive bacteria
Biofilm	Exopolysaccharide produced by bacteria that allows matrix formation of embedded material	Gram positive and negative bacteria

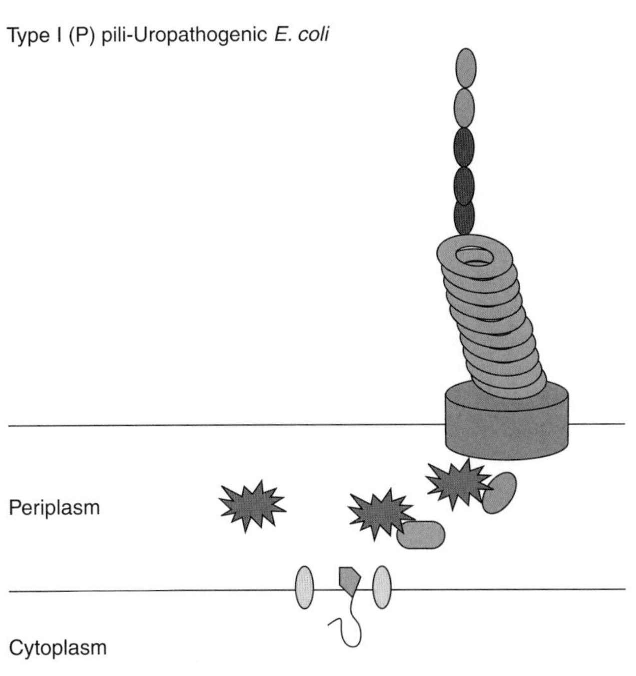

FIGURE 2-1 Idealization of Type 1 fimbrial adhesion where pilus subunits are ushered from the cytoplasm to the periplasmic space and secrete through the cell membrane.

specific receptors for these fimbriae have not been identified, their action provides the general framework of bacterial-host cell interaction. Once receptor-mediated attachment occurs, intracellular calcium increases in the host cell.[61] Proteins and protein kinases involved in the breakdown of actin are activated, resulting in the disruption of microvilli. There is a change in the cytoskeleton of the cells and permeability to ions and water. Ions are secreted, resulting in the classic secretory diarrhea.

Type IV pili (Figure 2-2) are located at the pole of the cell and assembled via the Type II secretion system that is called the *general assembly pathway*.[62,63] These pili are flexible fibers of variable length that can aggregate, are important in the formation of microcolonies, and are responsible for the twitching motion of bacteria. The proteins are secreted into the periplasmic space but remain anchored to the inner membrane. The protein is then assembled and passed through a pore formed in the outer membrane. Curli fimbriae are solid surface structures that use the extracellular nucleation-precipitation pathway.[63] This pilus is secreted as a soluble protein extracellularly with a second protein, the nucleator, for stability. These have been identified as important for binding to extracellular matrix proteins and biofilm formation.

Although discussed in greater detail later, the antiphagocytic M-protein of *Streptococcus* spp. is actually a fibrillar protein and also assists, but is not essential for, adhesion. In anaerobic bacteria, antibodies to flagella proteins can block *Clostridium difficile* adhesion.[66] These proteins are thought to mediate intestinal adherence and colonization.[66]

Afimbrial Adhesins

Afimbrial adhesins are cell proteins that enhance the binding of bacteria to host cells. They are also called *microbial surface components recognizing adhesive matrix molecules*.[67,68] Gram positive organisms possess afimbrial proteins on their surfaces that presumably aid in binding to host cells. The three most commonly studied afibrillar adhesins are those that bind salivary glycoprotein, bind fibronectin, or are composed of lipoteichoic acid (LTA).[68,69] Salivary binding proteins are commonly found in pathogens and commensals of the oral cavity. Both *Streptococcus* spp. and *Actinomyces* spp. possess these proteins. Fibronectin binding protein (FBP) is necessary for *S. aureus* invasion and binds both fibronectin and collagen to form a bridge between the FBP and the host cell integrin (integrin $\alpha_5\beta_1$).[70,71] The FBPs are essential for invasion of both epithelial and endothelial cells in *S. pyogenes*.[67-68] Heterologs of FBP have been demonstrated in *S. pneumoniae* of humans, *S. equi* subsp. *equi*, and *S. equi* subsp. *zooepidemicus*. Other potential equine pathogens that have FDPs on their surface include *Actinomyces* spp. *E. faecalis*, and *L. monocytogenes*.[69,72] Lipoteichoic acid (LTA), a common binding factor found in *Streptococcus* group A bacteria, is important in adhesion of bacteria to cells.[73] This

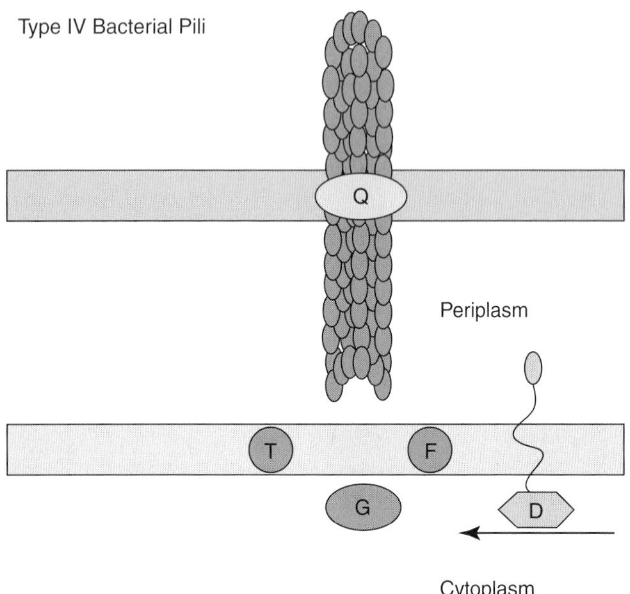

FIGURE 2-2 Idealization of Type IV fimbrial adhesion where pilus subunits are secreted through the membrane by an adenosine triphosphate–mediated process.

protein is also important in stimulation of cytokine secretion from the cells during infection and has been demonstrated in group B *Streptococcus*, including *S. equi* subsp. *equi*.[74] A less commonly described afibrillar adhesin is composed of surface polypeptide chains in *Corynebacterium* that binds to lectin.[75] Binding of these proteins can be abolished by trypsin treatment. Afibrillar adhesins are also present in gram negative organisms; the most commonly studied are conserved high molecular weight adhesion proteins of *Haemophilus influenzae* and *Bordetella pertussis*.[73]

Biofilm Ahesins

Bacterial ecology has emphasized the importance of biofilm for colonization of both biotic and abiotic surfaces of bacteria.[59] A requirement for biofilm formation is a tight interaction of bacterial adhesins with surface receptors that promote further bacterial aggregation. The most important family of biofilm adherence proteins (BAPs) is that of *Staphylococcus aureus*. These proteins have high molecular mass and repetitive structures whose size and number can be varied during the course of infection, possibly allowing for immune evasion.

Cytoskeletal Changes

Binding of bacteria frequently results in cytoskeleton changes within the host cell in order to enhance susceptibility to invasion. "Membrane ruffling" is a virulence factor that results in either internalization or breakdown of intracellular components to allow for invasion of tissues. Once bacteria attach, the change in the membrane itself (ruffling) aids in colonization of host surfaces or even uptake of the bacteria. The most common virulence proteins of both gram positive and gram negative are bacteria lectins.[63-76] Although attachment is thought to be the primary role of these proteins, attachment itself results in an intracellular change, including actin rearrangements, cell signaling regulation, or actual secretion of bacterial substances into the host cell. These proteins are highly conserved in bacteria and are important targets for immunoprophylaxis.

Membrane transformation for uptake of intracellular bacteria such as *Yersinia* spp., *Listeria monocytogenes*, *Salmonella* spp., and *Shigella flexneri* can be either zipperlike or triggerlike. Binding results in actin rearrangement and engulfment of these intracellular bacteria by both phagocytic and nonphagocytic cells. *Yersinia* and *Listeria* spp. form a zipperlike relationship wherein the tightly adhered bacteria result in actin polymerization and formation of a phagocytic cup through actin nucleation, polymerization, and depolamerization.[77] Alternatively, *Salmonella* and *Shigella* bacteria adhere and secrete proteins that are translocated into the host cell cytoplasm and trigger actin polymerization.[78] In addition to membrane ruffling, *Mycobacterium avium* and *Salmonella* spp. also rely on activation of intracellular GTPases, leading to phagocytosis.[79,80]

FACTORS THAT ENHANCE SPREAD OF BACTERIA

Once colonization occurs, multiplication and spread of bacteria are enhanced through virulence factors. These factors assist bacteria in survival in the hostile host environment and breakdown of tissue barriers. Many of these defenses overlap, but the result is avoidance of destruction by the host and sublimation of host tissues into a new bacterial niche.

Survival in Host Environment

CAPSULE

One of the most common and potent strategies for avoidance of phagocytosis is the presence of a capsule. Despite the remarkable diversity of bacteria, assembly and structure of capsule are remarkably similar across species.

It was observed as early as 1928 that engulfment and digestion of *S. pneumoniae* were associated with lack of capsule,[81] and by 1940 it was clear that this virulence factor was genetically encoded.[82] Early studies with *S. equi* subsp. *equi* demonstrated that resistance to phagocytosis was associated with an increase in capsule and M-protein,[83] and in a model of *S. equi* subsp. *zooepidemicus* infection in mice, enhancement of virulence was associated with increased amount of capsule, which increased resistance to phagocytosis.[84] Although colonization of the guttural pouch occurs with nonencapsulated *S. equi* subsp. *equi* strains, induction of lymphadenopathy is associated with capsular strains.[85] In more recent studies of *S. equi* subsp. *equi* infection, rapid colonization in the lingual and pharyngeal tonsil is dependent on genetically associated virulence factors that control colony morphology, with the mucoid strain having enhanced virulence.[33]

Escherichia coli capsule is the "prototype" capsule of gram negative bacteria.[86] Ultrastucturally, this capsule forms a fine fibrillar meshwork covering the bacteria surface.[87] The K antigen is one of the major antigens, is temperature dependent in its antigenic structure and amount, [88] and is highly associated with increased pathogenicity and resistance to phagocytosis.[89,90] The other major antigen for gram negative bacteria is the lipopolysaccharide (LPS) minus the lipid A component of the molecule. A third minor component, colanic acid, appears to exhibit antiphagocytic activity in some *E. coli*. Classically, the presence of capsule on *E. coli* prevents complement mediated phagocytosis.[91] The LPS itself activates complement, and the capsule prevents immune activation by concealing the LPS molecule.[92]

Capsules of anaerobic bacteria are unique, and these structures may directly account for the formation of abscesses within the host. The capsule of *B. fragilis* has two distinct polysaccharides composed of repeating subunits with oppositely charged groups (Zwitter ion).[93] This polysaccharide complex injected alone promotes the induction of abscess. Infection of rodents with the encapsulated form of *Bacteroides* and *Fusobacterium* spp. results in the formation of intraperitoneal abscesses, whereas nonencapsulated bacteria do not cause abscessation.[94-96] Synergism of capsular anaerobes with other bacteria occurs; nonencapsulated bacteria have enhanced survival in abscesses and produce capsule when cultured or inoculated with encapsulated bacteria.[95]

ANTICOMPLEMENT FACTORS

Similar to and overlapping with capsule are structural proteins that block complement. The O side chain of LPS on gram negative bacteria is an anticomplement factor.[97] The longer the side chain, the greater the distance between phagocytes and bacteria. The capsular component, sialic acid, interacts with O antigen to prevent the formation of C3 converatase.[98] Bacterial enzymes are formed by *Streptococcus* spp. and other organisms that damage the polymorph chemoattractant, C5a.[99,100] Production of a protein in *Salmonella* spp., encoded by the *rck* gene, prevents insertion of the C9 fragment of complement into the bacterial membrane.[9] The M protein of *S. equi* subps. *equi* appears to decrease deposition of complement on the surface of bacteria.

RESISTANCE TO PHAGOCYTOSIS

Recent studies of streptococci have shown that when M-protein content is kept constant, the amount of capsule is actually correlated with resistance to phagocytosis.[85] Resistance to in vitro phagocytosis can be abolished with treatment with hyaluronidase and induction of specific immunity against M-protein of *S. equi* subsp. *equi* and *S. equi* subsp. *zooepidemicus*.[101] The M proteins of *Streptococcus* spp. are also essential for resistance to phagocytosis blocking complement.[83,102-104] This mechanism for complement resistance appears to be through enhancement of binding of fibrinogen to the bacteria in the presence of M protein.[105-107]

PHAGOLYSOSOMAL SURVIVAL

The intracellular environment should be inhospitable for bacteria, yet many organisms are ingested by phagocytic cells and utilize this environment to multiply and disseminate. In normal phagolysomal fusion, the phagocytic vesicle first becomes fused with a host cell endosome. Shortly thereafter, fusion with the lysosome occurs. Several digestive proteins are released within the lysosome, and there is a decrease in pH, resulting in inactivation and digestion of a foreign protein or microorganism. Bacteria have devised ways to escape the phagosome or use the phagosome as a niche for extended survival. *Shigella* spp. and *Listeria monocytogenes* are bacteria that escape the phagocytic vesicle to multiply in the host cell cytoplasm.[108] Before escape from the phagosome, *Listeria* modulates maturation of the phagosome by delaying fusion with the lysosome.[109] Both *Mycobacterium* and *Legionella* spp. cause a change in the maturation of the phagosome leading to uninhibited replication within macrophages.[110,111] Engulfment of *Salmonella* spp. in the phagosome appears to induce formation of an actual phagolysosome, but the organism survives acidification and reactive oxygen intermediates (ROIs), likely through production of catalase and superoxide dismutase.[112,113] The acid tolerance response (ATR) is important primarily for intracellular bacteria that are able to withstand highly acidic environments, including *L. monocytogenes*, *R. equi*, and *Salmonella* spp.[114,115] Genes that control virulence in *Salmonella* are actually upregulated by an acidic environment. *Rhodococcus equi* suppresses acidification of the phagolysosome in addition to inhibiting phagolysosomal fusion.[116] Recently, homologous genes that regulate survival under high temperature and oxidative stress were also determined to be essential for phagolysomal survival in *R. equi*.[117] Although the mechanism by which *R. equi* inhibits phagolysosomal fusion is unknown, opsonization by an *R. equi*–specific antibody results in enhanced fusion and killing.[115,118] Resistance to phagolysosomal fusion and replication in the phagolysosome appears dependent on the presence of the 90 kDA virulence plasmid.[114] *Rickettsia*, *Neorickettsia* (formerly *Ehrlichia*), and *Rhodococcus* bacteria appear to inhibit phagolysosomal fusion.

HOST SUBSTRATE UTILIZATION

Nutrition of bacteria is intimately associated with cellular and tissue environments. The proper level of iron is important because iron is required for the production of reactive oxygen intermediates. The *fur* gene in *E. coli* was first identified as the major regulator of iron acquisition.[119] Homologs of this gene have been identified in many other bacteria, including *Salmonella* spp., *Vibrio* spp., *Pseudomonas aeruginosa*, *S. aureus*, and *B. fragilis*.[119,120] *Rhodococcus equi* has its own chromosomally encoded genes (iupABC) that allow survival in low iron environments.[121] In addition, bacteria possess siderophores, which are very potent chelators of iron.[122] These siderophores are secreted outside of the bacterial cell, uptake iron, and are taken back up by the cells through a receptor-mediated process. After internalization the iron is cleaved and utilized by the bacteria. Resistance to carbon, nitrogen starvation, and new substrate utilization are also important means by which bacteria survive inhospitable environments. The latter has been demonstrated as important for *R. equi* survival in the phagosome, where bacteria become more efficient at membrane fatty acid and cholesterol utilization under anaerobic conditions.[123]

Damage to Host Tissues

TOXINS

Exotoxins are virulence factors secreted by the host that frequently function to aid spread of infection (Figure 2-3). Both gram positive and gram negative organisms secrete an array of exotoxins. Classically, there are three types of exotoxins.[61] The first is the A-B form, in which there are two distinct parts to the toxin: one for binding and one for enzymatic action. The second does not appear to have distinct parts and forms pores within host membranes. The third is superantigen, which forms a bond between the major histocompatibility complex (MHC) class II receptor of macrophages, resulting in release of various T cell helper–mediated cytokine cascades. Several examples of common equine pathogens are discussed.

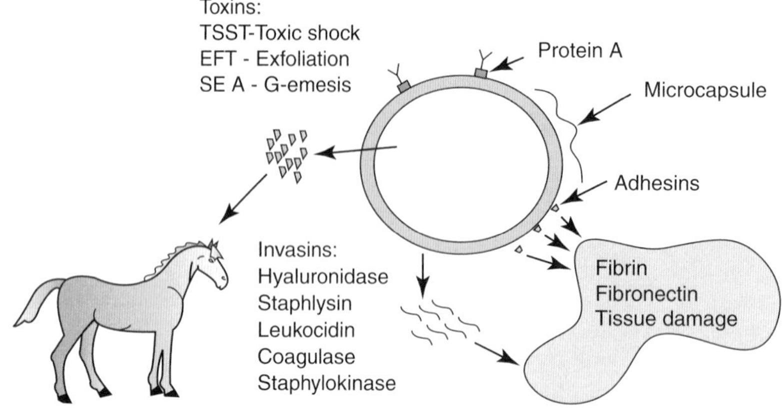

FIGURE 2-3 Mechanisms of virulence of *Staphylococcus aureus*. (Redrawn from Todar K: Todar's Online Textbook of Bacteriology, textbookofbacteriology.net, © Kenneth Todar Ph.D., University of Wisconsin-Madison.)

STAPHYLOCOCCUS AUREUS

Toxins of *Staphylococcus aureus* are well characterized, provide examples of several types of toxins produced by the same organism, and are directly associated with the pathogenesis of this disease (see Figure 2-3).[124] Although there are few overt syndromes recognized in the horse that are specifically caused by *S. aureus,* toxins that may be important for disease in the horse include the four hemolysins, toxic shock syndrome toxin-1 (TSST-1), exfoliative toxins, and leukocidin (Table 2-3). For example, cellulitis induced by *S. aureus* in the horse may be similar to wound-associated toxic shock in humans. Toxic shock syndrome is a disease of increased capillary permeability characterized by hypotension, hypoalbuminemia, and edema. The toxins of *S. aureus* work in concert to (1) induce massive release of cytokines, (2) increase sensitivity to cytokines, and (3) damage endothelial cells directly. The superantigen toxin of *S. aureus* forms a bridge between the MHC receptor on macrophages and the T cell receptor. This bridge results in a massive release of interleukin-2 with the downstream effect of T cell proliferation and induction of Type 1 cytokines that stimulate release of pro-inflammatory cytokines from macrophages. Exfoliative toxin, which induces T cell proliferation, and TSST-1 have been identified in equine *S. aureus* isolates associated with severe phlegmon and metritis.[125,126]

The enhanced virulence displayed by community-acquired methicillin resistant *Staphylococcus aureus* (CA-MRSA) has been associated with the cytotoxin Panton-Valentine leukocidin (PVL), which is a β-pore former that causes enhanced spread through skin necrosis.[127,128] PVL has been identified in almost all CA-MRSA strains, but a causal role in enhanced virulence is still subject to debate; recent work with this toxin was not proved in in vivo models.[129] Other toxins, such as arginine catabolic mobile elements (ACMEs) and phenol soluble modules (PSMs), are under intense scrutiny. Deletion of ACME from MRSA strains greatly decreased in vivo virulence, and acquisition of this genetic element likely confers a more robust ability to colonize over non-ACME strains, giving rise to an epidemic-prone bacterial clone.[128-130] The PSM-αprotein demonstrates enhanced destruction of white blood cells.[127]

CLOSTRIDIUM INFECTIONS

Clostridrium bacteria mediate clinical disease by producing exotoxins. The *Clostridium* bacteria causing botulism and tetanus excrete neurotoxins to which horses are highly susceptible. The main toxins of botulism (BNT) and tetanus (TNT) are remarkably similar even though both toxins exert effects that appear to be polar opposites, with botulism causing a flaccid paralysis and tetanus a spastic paralysis.[131] Both toxins share amino acid sequences of metalloproteinases that are most similar to zinc-requiring endopeptidases. With botulism there are six serologically different neurotoxins, with most reports in horses caused by type B toxin, although A, C, and D have also been identified.[131-135] There is only one tetanus neurotoxin that is responsible for the clinical signs of spastic paralysis.

Neurotoxin is secreted as a progenitor and must be cleaved by proteases (trypsin) to the derivative toxin to produce clinical signs. The active toxin consists of a light and heavy chain (A-B type toxin) that mediates paralysis by blockage of acetylcholine esterase in a three-step process.[61,136] The first step is the rapid step, which is involved in recognition by the neurotoxin of the receptor on the nerve and rapid binding. In the second, translocation occurs as the active site of the molecule is internalized into the nerve cell ending by endocytosis. The acidified vesicle induces a conformational change in the toxin so that it can be translocated to the cytosol. The third and final step is the slow step, wherein cell neuroproteins called *synaptopeptidases* are cleaved and acetylcholine release prevented. Neurotoxin cleaves the proteins synaptobrevin (SNAP), synaptosome associated membrane proteins (VAMP), and syntaxin, which are involved with neurotransmitter release, exocytosis of the neurotransmitter vesicle, and vesicle-cell membrane fusion, respectively. The inactivation of one or more of these proteins accounts for the prevention of release of synaptic vesicles. The different botulinum neurotoxins exhibit variable specificity to these proteins. Types B, D, F, and G are active against VAMP, whereas A, C, and E are active against SNAP, and C is the only form that cleaves syntaxin.

The difference in clinical signs noted between the *C. tetanus* and *C. botulinum* is a reflection of the binding and level of activity of the respective toxin. *Clostridium botulinum* binds to peripheral nerves and *C. tetanus* to cells within the CNS. Further, *C. botulinum* toxin binding results in prevention of downstream release of other neurotransmitters, such as γ-aminobutyric acid. Injection of *C. tetanus* toxin intravenously in low doses results in flaccid paralysis.

TABLE 2-3

Mechanisms of Virulence of *Staphylococcus aureus*

Factor	Mechanism of Action
Toxic shock syndrome toxin	Hemolysin
Exfoliative toxin	Hemolysin, T cell proliferation
Leukocidin	Hemolysin
Superantigen	Cross linking and activation of macrophages and T cells
Staphylokinase	Plasminogen activator (lysis of fibrin clots)
α toxin	Damage to erythrocytes, skin, nerve, lethal
	Edema formation: forms pores in cells, activation of arachidonic acid cascade and release of procoagulant factors.
β hemolysis (Sphingomyelinase C)	Toxic to erythrocytes
δ toxin	Erythrocytes, cellular
γ-hemolysin	Degranulation of leukocytes
Leukocidin	Degranulation of leukocytes
Panton-Valentine leukocidin	Pore former in white blood cells; skin necrosis
Arginine catabolic mobile elements	Increased colonization of community-acquired methicillin resistant *Staphylococcus aureus* (CA-MRSA)
PSM-alpha	Enhanced destruction of white blood cells in CA-MRSA

The main pathologic features of disease cause by *C. perfringens* are edema, necrosis, and death regardless of the site of action.[136] Toxins elaborated by these clostridia include both lethal and nonlethal toxins that cause necrosis and hemolysis and frequently contain lecithinases and lipases. *Clostridium perfringens* has four major lethal toxins, including an enterotoxin and three minor toxins. Thus far genetic characterization of equine isolates associated with diarrhea indicate that the majority are type A, the toxic effects of which are mediated in part by α-toxin.[137] The *cpe*-toxin or enterotoxin has been detected by enzyme-linked immunosorbent assay (ELISA) in approximately 16% to 19% of equine isolates, so disease has been linked to both enterotoxigenic type A and nonenterotoxigenic type A strains.[21,138] There are individual case reports of neonatal diarrhea associated with Type B (β and ε toxins), Type C (β toxin), and Type D (ε toxin) strains that also carry the α toxin.[139,140] Table 2-4 is a summary of the mechanisms of actions of the toxins of *Clostridium perfringens*.[136,141-145]

Clostridium difficile has five toxins, although disease causation is thought to rely on the production of toxins A and B.[146,147] The evidence to date indicates that both toxin A and B mediate the pathogenesis of *C. difficile* diarrhea.[147] Research suggests that the formation of the classic pathologic lesion, the pseudomembrane, is a result of the combined actions of toxin A, toxin B, and interleukin-8. Classically, toxin A is considered an enterotoxin and lethal, whereas toxin B is a virulent cytotoxin. Toxin A appears to be the primary mediator of fluid accumulation; injection of toxin A results in fluid accumulation, cell necrosis, and recruitment of inflammatory cells.[148,149] One mechanism of this fluid accumulation appears to be by interruption of actin filaments and destruction of tight junctions. Toxin A also results in neutrophil recruitment, and evidence suggests that this is mediated through the direct action of the toxin on macrophages to release interleukin-1, tumor necrosis factor α, and leukotrienes. In cell culture toxin A can cause interleukin-8 secretion (a potent recruiter of neutrophils), cell detachment, and apoptosis of separated cells. This direct activation of macrophages and secretion of IL-8 is through a calcium- and calmodulin-dependent mechanism that results in direct nuclear upregulation after nuclear translocation of transcription factors NF-κβ and AP-1.[148] Toxin B is more cytotoxic than toxin A, especially to human epithelial cells.

TABLE 2-4

Mechanisms of Virulence of *Clostridium perfringens* Toxins

Factor	Mechanism of Action
α	Zinc metalloproteinase: hemolysis, lethality through cardiovascular collapse and death, disruption of endothelium and erythrocytic cell membranes by *hydrolyzation* of lecithin and sphingomyelin, platelet aggregation. Stimulates the release of massive amounts of inflammatory cytokines. Activation of coagulation, aggregation of red blood cells, which occurs throughout body, including muscle cells, which results in myositic syndromes
β	Massive catecholamine release with drop in heart rate and blood pressure. Forms pores especially in neurons, resulting in neurotoxicity
ε	Pore former within neuronal cell membrane, resulting in irreversible cell membrane damage and death
Enterotoxin	Change in ion movements of enterocytes affecting cellular metabolism
β-2	Mechanism of action in dispute; associated with enteritis of large animals

CELL DEATH

Apoptosis is a distinctive morphologic process that results in cleavage of nuclear material and scavenging of unwarranted cells without immune activation.[150] Apoptosis or programmed cell death is an important pathway for complex organisms to deal with damaged and diseased tissue. Apoptosis avoids the release of the tissue-damaging enzymes and nonspecific elimination of tissue that occurs in cellular necrosis. Several bacteria have modulated the host apoptotic pathways for enhancement of survival.[151] *Shigella flexneri, S. typhimurium,* and toxins of *S. aureus, Pseudomonas* spp., and *C. diphtheriae* have demonstrated programmed cell death as a consequence of cellular infection or exposure.[150,152] The protein of *S. flexneri*, IpaB, induces apoptosis by binding to and activating the cellular enzyme caspase 1, which induces apoptosis of macrophages.[108] *Staphylococcus aureus* α toxin, which is similar to listeriolysin O (LLO) presumably escapes the macrophage after engulfment and induces host cell apoptosis.[124] The TSST toxin of *S. aureus* induces B cell apoptosis and blocks immunoglobulin production.

PATHOGENESIS OF FUNGAL INFECTIONS

Of the 250,000 species of fungi, fewer than 200 are true pathogens.[1] Superficial mycoses affect the hair shaft and the superficial epidermis. Cutaneous mycoses (dermatophytosis) infect the epidermis, dermis, hair, and nails of animals, and *Microsporum, Trichophyton,* and *Epidermophyton* spp. are the most commonly associated pathogenic genera. Subcutaneous tissues can become infected with *Sporothrix, Conidiobolus, Basidiobolus* spp., and members of the Dematiaceae fungi, including the *Chromoblastomycosis, Mycetoma,* and *Phaeohyphomycosis* spp. infections. Most of these infections are introduced by penetration through skin or opportunistic invasion of damaged skin surfaces. *Histoplasma capsulatum, Coccidioides immitis, Blastomyces dermatitidis,* and *Paracoccidioides brasiliensis* are the four most important fungal pathogens that can cause systemic infection. The most common opportunistic infections include *Candida albicans, Aspergillus* spp., *Cryptococcus neoformans, Mucor* spp., and *Pneumocystis carinii.*

FACTORS THAT ENHANCE ENTRY OF FUNGI

Adherence

Fungal virulence factors may be more complex than those of bacteria because of the higher degree of opportunism that occurs with a change in host status. There may be subtle factors that, combined with host status, result in a certain fungus attaining a virulent state. For instance, the typical fungal wall is composed of three major polysaccharides: mannose; β-1,3 and β-1,6 linked glucans; and chitin. Chitin mutants in *C. albicans* are less virulent when tested in rodent models than are wild-type fungi.[153] Further, a mutant *C. albicans* that cannot synthesize complex mannose oligosaccharides does not adhere to other yeast and epithelial cells and has lost virulence in a guinea pig model.[154] Both of these mutants can proliferate in vitro normally, and whether or not this is an actual virulence factor is unclear.

As with bacteria, cellular adherence is an important prerequisite for infection and colonization of the host. Adhesins have been identified in *C. albicans* and *B. dermatitidis*. Two genes have been associated with adhesion in *C. albicans*. The first is a glycoprotein that has sequences consistent with agglutinating activity. Transformation of this gene into other nonadherent fungal species results in adhesion of the transformed yeast to cells.[155] *Candida albicans* also has integrin-like proteins, the disruption of which results in diminished hyphal growth, adhesion to cells, and loss of virulence in mice[156,157] The *B. dermatitidis* adhesin mediates binding to human monocyte-macrophages through the CD14 receptor.[158]

FACTORS THAT ENHANCE SPREAD OF FUNGI

Evasion of Immune Defenses

CAPSULE

Many fungi have polysaccharide capsules that, like bacteria, help resist phagocytosis and immune activation. The capsule of *C. neoformans* inhibits leukocyte accumulation, cytokine secretion, and macrophage phagocytosis.[159] Mutants without capsule are highly infective and avirulent. As indicated earlier, many fungi are engulfed by macrophages, and intracellular survival is mediated by virulence factors. Macrophages are decimating cells for *C. albicans,*[160] *H. capsulatum,*[161] and *B. dematitidis. Histoplasma capsulatum* is primarily a yeast in vivo, and this form infects macrophages. Phagolysosomal fusion occurs at a normal rate,[162] but blockage of acidification of the phagolysosome occurs.[163]

Adaptation to Host Environment

MORPHOLOGY AND TEMPERATURE

Adaptability to the host environment is also a trait that enhances fungal virulence. Fungal dimorphism, which is the ability to adopt another morphologic state, is clearly tied to virulence. Mutants of *C. albicans* that cannot switch to the hyphal form are avirulent in certain in vivo models, although both forms likely contribute to pathogenesis.[164] A second adaptation is called phenotypic switching, in which colonies of fungi change during in vitro growth. *Candida albicans, C. neoformans,* and *H. capsulatum* all display phenotypic switching, and these different phenotypes are associated with degrees of virulence.[165,166] *Histoplasma capsulatum* spontaneously gives rise to mutants that have less capsule, are less virulent, and are not cytotoxic to macrophages.[167] The signal for dimorphic fungi to change form is usually temperature change. Many fungal species germinate within the host with increased temperature, allowing for dissemination within the host. Calcineurin is found in many yeast and mammalian cells, and in *C. neoformes* this protein mediates the ability of this fungus to grow at 37° C.[168] Temperature and heat shock are also mediated by the calcium-dependent protein cyclophilin B in *Aspergillus*.[169] Adaptation to mammalian pH is genetically controlled in *C. albicans*. Mutants display abnormal cell morphology at physiologic pH ranges.[170]

NUTRIENTS

Nutrient requirements that affect virulence include primarily melanin, iron, and calcium. Melanins are present in the wall of *C. neoformans,* and melanin can scavenge ROI intermediates, making the organism resistant to the oxidative burst of neutrophils.[171] Pathogenic fungi have siderophores and high affinity ferric iron reductase to acquire iron from low iron environments.[172,173] *Histoplasma capsulatum* secretes a calcium-binding protein that enhances calcium uptake from calcium-poor environments.[174,175] Without this protein *H. capsulatum* cannot form colonies and does not survive in cultured macrophages.

DAMAGE TO HOST TISSUES

Toxins

Exposure to both pathogenic and saprophytic fungi is an everyday occurrence. Respiratory contamination and infection are important for many pulmonary species, but skin penetration and dissemination from necrotic gut are important portals for large animals also. Dissemination after the initial infection is dependent on previous damage to host tissues, deeper mechanical penetration, or actual invasion of new tissues. *C. albicans* can actually grow through and replace cell membranes.[160] True molds invade blood vessels and grow along the intima of the vessels. Fungi secrete many degradative enzymes, including proteinases, phosphatases, and DNAses in order to surmount structural barriers.[176] A group of genes called *secreted aspartyl proteinase* (SAP) genes allow more persistent colonization of host surfaces and deeper penetration.[177]

When *C. immitis* invades the host, the fungi form endospores. These endospores secrete a proteinase and a urease that likely aid in the breakdown of pulmonary tissues.[178-180] The two proteinases of *A. fumigatus* break down elastin, a major component of lung tissues.[181,182] Phospholipase activity has been demonstrated in *C. albicans, C. neoformans,* and *A. fumigatus*.[183] Strains of *Candida* spp. with high amounts of this enzyme have higher virulence,[184] and abolishing this activity results in decreased adherence of the organism.[185] Host eicosanoids enhance fungal colonization. Recent evidence demonstrates production of eicosanoids by both dermatophytosis and systemic fungi.[186]

Apoptosis

Fungi induce apoptosis, which may be due either to the direct effect of a fungal toxin or secondary to host cell cytoskeleton rearrangements.[187] The gliotoxin of *A. fumigatus* can induce DNA fragmentation and apoptosis in macrophages.[188] This toxin also has many other immunosuppressive qualities, which include inhibition of the neutrophil respiratory burst and T cell activation.

MECHANISMS OF ESTABLISHMENT AND SPREAD OF VIRAL INFECTIONS

J. Lindsay Oaks

Viral infections are responsible for some of the most medically and economically important diseases of horses. A few notable examples include influenza, equine rhinopneumonitis and abortion (Herpesviridae), African horse sickness (Reoviridae), equine infectious anemia (Retroviridae), various encephalitis viruses (Alphaviridae), and most recently in the United States the West Nile virus (Flaviviridae). Specific therapy of viral infections remains a significant challenge because antiviral drugs are generally ineffective, impractical, or prohibitively expensive for the treatment of horses. Treatment of most viral infections focuses on supportive care of the affected organ systems and control of secondary complications such as bacterial infection. Currently control of most clinically significant viral diseases in horse populations relies on vaccination, quarantine, or even destruction of infected animals.

Despite the great significance of some viral infections, recognizing that many equine viruses are ubiquitous, weakly pathogenic, or not associated with any known disease under normal circumstances is also important. Some examples include equine adenovirus,[1] respiratory and enteric reoviruses[2] (the term *reo* is derived from the acronym for respiratory enteric orphan, indicating that these isolates have not been associated with disease), and equine herpesvirus (EHV) type 2.[3] Some host-virus relationships may be mutualistic in that virally derived genetic elements are theorized to benefit the host by facilitating genetic variability and evolution.[4] Thus many viruses are of no practical clinical significance, and no control efforts are warranted. For this reason, the veterinarian should never assume that the recovery of a virus from a clinical specimen is significant without proof that the virus can cause the disease in question.

Veterinary virology is a rapidly changing field. New diseases continue to emerge or be discovered; a dramatic example is the Hendra paramyxovirus that appeared in Australia in 1994, killing horses and human beings.[5] More recently, another paramyxovirus, the Salem virus, has been identified in the United States, although the clinical importance of this virus is unclear.[6] Less dramatic, but of more relevance to most equine veterinarians, is the association of bovine papillomavirus with sarcoids.[7,8] A number of equine diseases occur in which viral involvement has yet to be excluded, including Theiler's hepatitis[9] and lymphosarcoma.[10] Viral origins also likely will be discovered for diseases in which viruses were not suspected previously to play a role; in human beings and mice, viruses have been proposed to have a role in everything from diabetes to obesity.[11,12] However, the greatest advances in veterinary virology are in understanding the molecular biology of viral replication, virus-cell interactions, and virus-host interactions. Related advances in molecular biology techniques, such as PCR and immunohistochemistry, also are providing sensitive, specific, and rapid tools for the diagnosis of viral infections. In the realm of antiviral drugs, aggressive searches are ongoing for effective and economical drugs for treatment of human beings, and in the near future antiviral drugs likely will be a realistic therapeutic option for equine veterinarians.[13,14] Finally, significant advances in the design of vaccines likely will improve the efficacy of immunization.

This chapter outlines the general ways that viruses cause disease and describes the most important virus-cell and virus-host interactions that result in pathologic conditions. Although the focus is on equine viruses whenever possible, the principles described are generally not species dependent, and no attempt is made to limit the discussion to recognized equine viral pathogens or diseases. Discussion of a particular mechanism or virus also should not be taken to suggest that this mechanism or type of virus has been documented in horses. When possible, supporting references have been selected to include review articles or texts for additional information about key concepts.

VIRUSES AND VIRUS-CELL INTERACTIONS

An in-depth discussion of viral structure, taxonomy, and replication is beyond the scope of this chapter, and the reader is referred to textbooks of veterinary or human virology for more detailed information.[15,16] However, a brief overview is presented to emphasize those features that have clinical relevance.

Virus Structure, Taxonomy, and Replication

The fundamental structure of all viruses is a DNA or RNA genome enclosed by a coat of protein called the *capsid* (Figure 2-4). For viruses that are enveloped, the capsid is enclosed further by a host cell–derived lipid membrane into which viral proteins have been incorporated. In addition to protecting the viral genome, the capsid and other associated structural proteins (e.g., matrix proteins) are important for virus assembly, packaging the viral genome, releasing the genome into a target cell, and for nonenveloped viruses, providing receptors that bind to host cells. For enveloped viruses the receptors are incorporated into the lipid membrane. The primary clinical significance of these features is that enveloped viruses, because of their fragile lipid membrane, are highly susceptible to inactivation by heat, desiccation, or detergents, and transmission typically requires direct exchange of body fluids, short distance aerosols, or arthropod vectors.

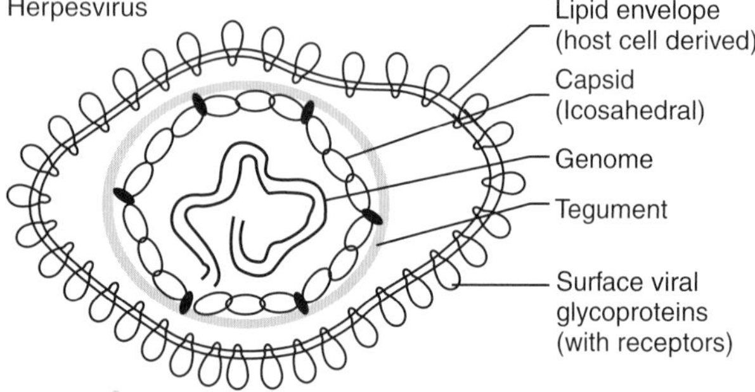

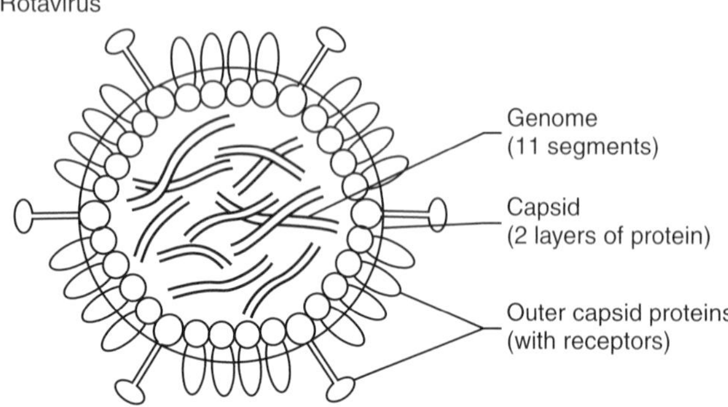

FIGURE 2-4 Schematic representations of basic viral structure. The basic structure of an enveloped virus is shown by the drawing of a herpesvirus. The basic structure of a nonenveloped virus is shown by the drawing of a rotavirus.

In contrast, nonenveloped viruses (e.g., equine rotavirus) are resistant to physical inactivation, and environmental contamination is more likely to be a significant factor in their transmission.

The composition of the viral genome is an important basis for virus classification (Figure 2-5). The type of viral genome also determines the strategies required to replicate the genome and transcribe messenger ribonucleic acid (mRNA; Figure 2-6). Viral genomes may be single-stranded RNA, double-stranded RNA, single-stranded deoxyribonucleic acid (DNA), or double-stranded DNA. The genomes of single-stranded RNA viruses may have positive polarity, in which the genome also serves directly as mRNA for translation of viral proteins. To replicate genomes, these viruses must first synthesize a strand of complementary RNA that can be used as a template to replicate genomes and transcribe new mRNA. Retroviruses are a subset of single-stranded, positive polarity RNA viruses that use their RNA genomes as templates to produce double-stranded DNA, which in turn is used for the transcription of mRNA and new viral genomes. Single-stranded RNA viruses may also have negative polarity, in which the genome is antisense to mRNA, and synthesis of a complementary RNA strand is required to serve as mRNA and as a template for new genomes. The clinical significance of these types of replication strategies is that they require polymerases and other enzymes not normally found in eukaryotic host cells. Eukaryotic cells, which exclusively use DNA as genetic material and as templates for mRNA transcription, use DNA-dependent DNA polymerases and DNA-dependent RNA polymerases for these functions, respectively. RNA viruses require RNA-dependent RNA polymerases to replicate or transcribe RNA, or RNA-dependent DNA polymerase (reverse transcriptase) to produce DNA from an RNA template. These unique viral enzymes are important targets for antiviral drugs because they can be used selectively to inhibit viral replication. The most common antiviral drugs currently available are nucleotide analogs that are used selectively by viral but not cellular enzymes and result in defective DNA or RNA.[17,18] Although most DNA viruses follow the eukaryotic pattern of replication and transcription, in many cases these viruses produce homologs of host cell enzymes that are sufficiently unique to make them selectively susceptible to nucleotide analogs. Additional targets for current and future antiviral agents are viral proteins used for translation and post-translational protein processing.[17]

Viral polymerases and the genetic organization of viruses are also important for rapid antigenic variation and immunologic evasion. Viral RNA polymerases are low fidelity and lack proofreading functions and thus randomly introduce errors into new RNA at an average rate of about one nucleotide mismatch per 10,000 bases copied.[19] Therefore in a population of viruses, virtually every individual virus differs slightly, and this population is referred to as a *quasi species*. Although many of these mutations are neutral or even deleterious, in the face of selective pressures such as the host immune response or antiviral drugs, this genetic plasticity allows rapid development of resistant virus populations.[20] Secondary structures or certain sequences in the viral genome may facilitate polymerase errors further at selected regions that are important for immune evasion, such as in sequences that code for neutralizing epitopes.[19] The genomes of some viruses, such as influenza, comprise separate segments, which allows reassortment of entire gene segments and sudden and dramatic changes in antigenicity.[21]

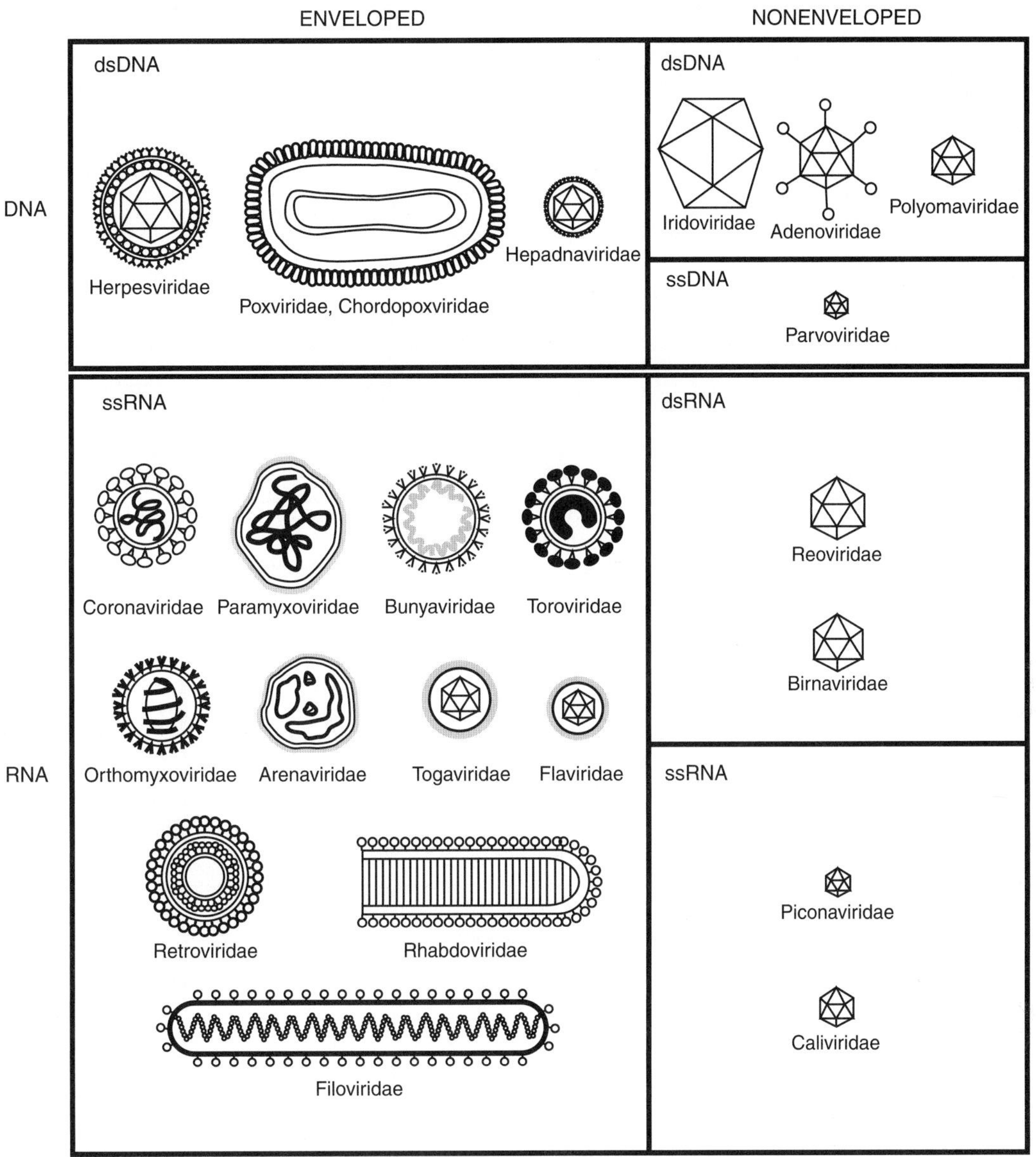

FIGURE 2-5 Virus family classification based on genome composition and presence of envelope or absence of envelope. The relative size of the viruses to each other is also shown.

Virus Life Cycle

All viruses are obligate intracellular parasites. Viral replication can occur only within living cells, and all viruses to some extent depend on the host cell synthetic machinery. The life cycle of all viruses includes the following steps: attachment to the target cell, entry into the cell, uncoating and release of the viral genome, transcription and translation of viral proteins, replication of the viral genome, assembly of new virions, and release of progeny virions[15,16] (Figure 2-7). Although the biochemistry of these steps is beyond the scope of this discussion, recognizing that they are all specific, energy-requiring interactions between the virus and the host cell is important. The inability of the virus to interact appropriately with a cell at any of these steps prevents replication in that cell type and defines the tropism of the virus. All of these steps are also important potential targets for antiviral drugs and host immune responses.

One of the most critical virus-cell interactions is attachment and entry. This initial step is one of the most important determinants of species susceptibility and host cell tropism and is an important target for antiviral antibodies that neutralize infectivity. Attachment and entry requires a specific interaction between a viral receptor and a cell-surface protein that acts as the host cell receptor. Many viruses also require interaction with additional cell surface molecules (co-receptors) for successful attachment and entry. Influenza provides a good example of this process. The influenza virus hemagglutinin molecule binds to sialic acid residues of cell-surface glycolipids or glycoproteins. Binding induces a conformational change in the hemagglutinin protein, exposing a cleavage site to a host cell protease. Cleavage of hemagglutinin induces fusion of the viral envelope to the host cell membrane and release of the capsid into the cytosol.[22,23] Equine influenza does not infect human beings because the hemagglutinin molecules do not recognize human sialic acid molecules.[24]

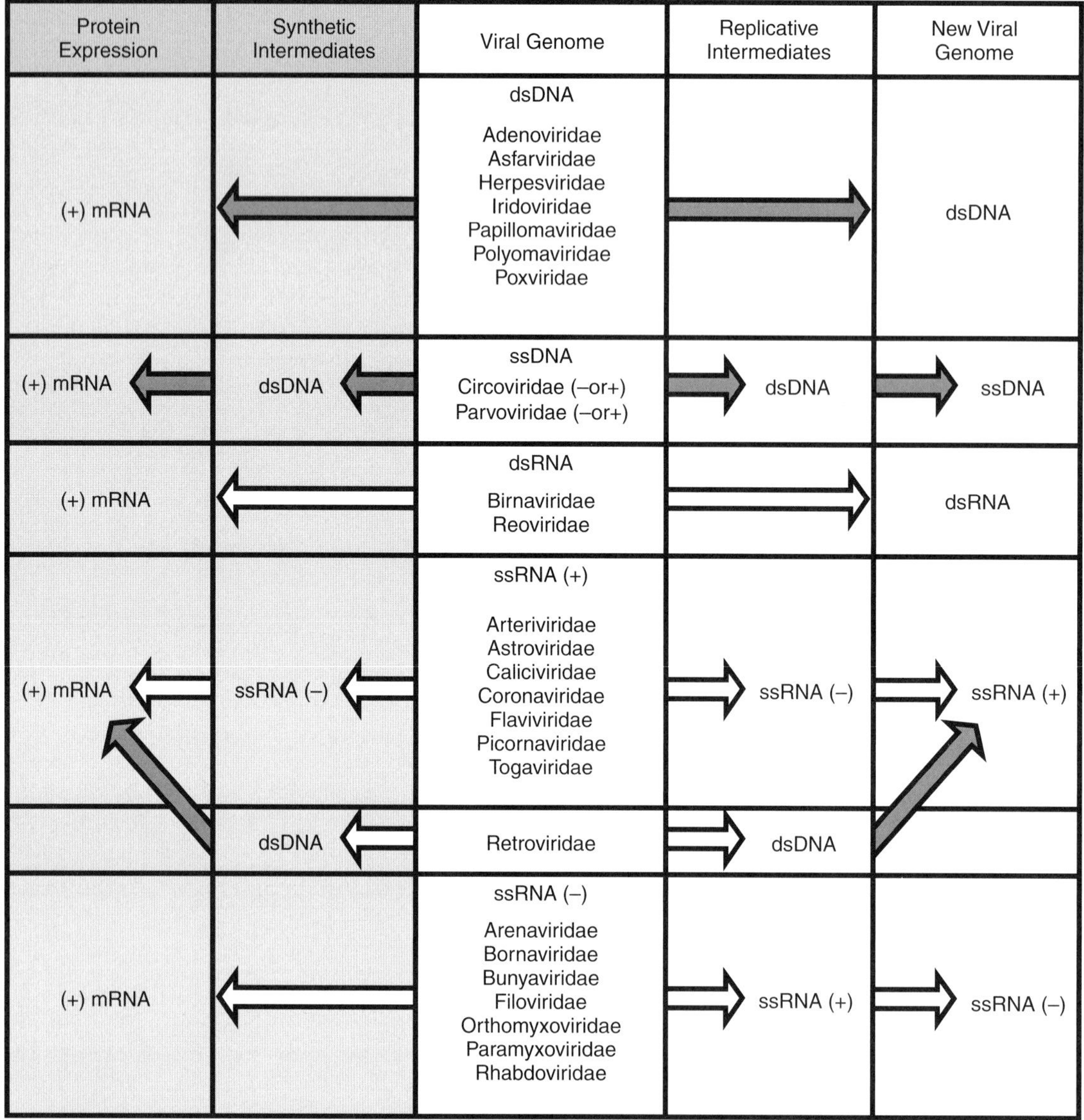

FIGURE 2-6 Summary of the main virus families that infect vertebrates and general strategies employed by these viruses to produce mRNA for protein expression and to replicate genomes. Required intermediate molecules are indicated. *White arrows* indicate the need for unique viral polymerases, including RNA-dependent RNA polymerase and RNA-dependent DNA polymerase (reverse transcriptase). *Dark arrows* indicate the use of cellular polymerases or viral homologs of cellular polymerases. *ds,* Double-stranded; *ss,* single-stranded; (+) for RNA = positive polarity, polarity of RNA used for protein translation; (+) for DNA = coding strand, sequence same as for (+) RNA; (– or +) DNA = contains single strands of DNA of both polarities. (Modified from Baltimore D: Expression of animal virus genomes, *Bacteriol Rev* 35:235-241, 1971.)

Within the horse equine influenza infection is restricted to respiratory epithelial cells by the distribution of the appropriate host cell protease.[22] Viruses may infect other cell types by using a different host cell receptor for attachment and entry. Highly pathogenic strains of avian influenza are able to spread systemically because of mutations in the hemagglutinin that allow cleavage by host cell proteases found on cells outside of the respiratory tract.[22] Other ways in which a virus can infect multiple cell types are using a host cell receptor that is present on different cell types or infecting a single cell type that is present in different tissues (e.g., macrophages and vascular endothelium). Host cell receptors also may be present in an age-dependent fashion, accounting for age-related differences in susceptibility to diseases such as polioencephalomyelitis and rotaviral enteritis.[25,26]

Once the viral nucleocapsid gains entry to the cytosol of the cell, the viral genome is released through the process of uncoating. After uncoating, depending on the genetic composition of the virus, the viral genome localizes to the appropriate regions of the cell for replication and mRNA transcription. DNA viruses typically replicate genomes and transcribe mRNA in the nucleus and then transport the mRNA to the cytoplasm for translation. RNA viruses typically replicate, transcribe mRNA, and translate viral proteins in the cytoplasm. These

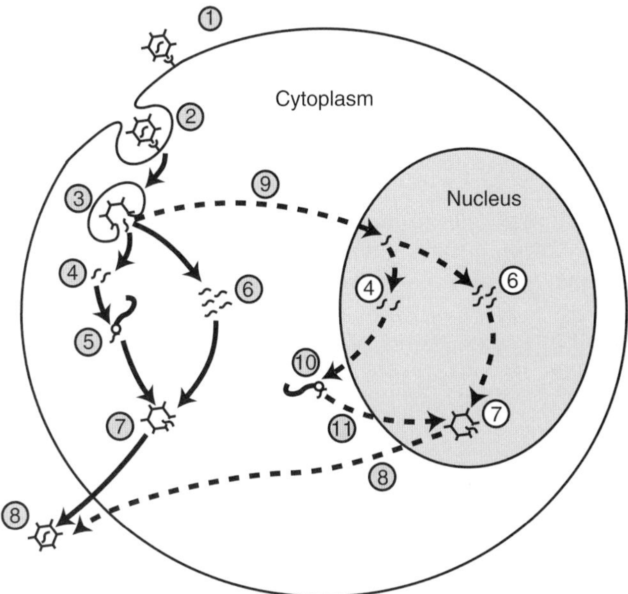

FIGURE 2-7 Schematic representation of the general virus life cycle. Both RNA and DNA viruses share the initial steps, including attachment (1); entry/fusion (2); and uncoating and release of viral genome into the cell (3). *Solid arrows* indicate remaining steps for RNA viruses, which all occur in the cytoplasm, including transcription of mRNA (4); translation of viral proteins (5); replication of the viral genome (6); assembly of new virions (7); and release of progeny virions (8). *Dashed arrows* indicate steps for a DNA virus. The life cycle is similar except that the DNA genome is translocated to the nucleus (9) for transcription (4) and replication of viral genomes (6). Viral mRNA is then translocated back to the cytoplasm for translation (10), and newly synthesized viral proteins are translocated back to the nucleus (11) for assembly (7); new virions are then released from both nuclear and cytoplasmic membranes (8).

sites of replication account, respectively, for the location of viral inclusion bodies that are diagnostically useful in histopathologic sections. In general, the first viral proteins expressed are regulatory factors, enzymes, and polymerases required for initiation of viral gene expression and diversion of host cell resources to viral replication. Subsequently, viral structural proteins are expressed and assembled with new viral genomes into virions. Enveloped viruses require the additional step of acquiring a lipid envelope by budding the nucleocapsid through areas of the nuclear or plasma membrane into which viral proteins have been incorporated. Viruses then are released, usually in association with death of the host cell, into the extracellular space and blood. Some viruses, such as herpesviruses and paramyxoviruses, also may transfer progeny virions directly into an adjacent cell by inducing fusion between the two cells, a strategy that allows the virus to avoid contact with neutralizing antibodies in the extracellular space.

Virus-Cell Interactions

After a cell is infected, the process of viral replication may have a number of effects on the host cell. Viruses have evolved a number of strategies and host cell interactions to facilitate their own replication and circumvent host responses that may eliminate the infected cell. In general, virally driven effects favor viral replication, transmission, and persistence and often result in death or dysfunction of the infected cell. Cellular or host responses generally favor control and elimination of the virus from the host. These responses may block viral replication, may initiate innate and specific host immune responses, and are frequently evident clinically as inflammation.

CELL CYCLE AND VIRAL REPLICATION

Viral replication requires that the host cell support high levels of nucleic acid replication, mRNA transcription, and protein translation. The growth and division phase of the cell cycle (S phase) is most suited for this purpose. However, many cells infected by viruses already are differentiated fully and in the resting phase (G_0 or G_1 phase). Some of the more complex viruses, such as herpesviruses, poxviruses, and adenoviruses, have virally encoded proteins that activate the cellular systems for growth and division, thus manipulating the cell to create an environment favorable for viral replication. This ability allows tropism for cells that otherwise might not be able to support viral replication. The "immediate early" genes expressed by herpesviruses, which initiate viral replication in differentiated cells, induce progression of the cell cycle from G_0 to the S phase.[27,28] Other viruses, particularly the genetically simpler viruses such as parvoviruses, lack the ability to activate resting cells.[27,29] Thus their tropism is restricted to cells that naturally go through a growth and division phase, such as intestinal crypt cells and hematopoietic cells. Consequently, parvoviral diseases such as feline panleukopenia typically involve replication in the rapidly dividing cells of the intestine (diarrhea) and bone marrow (pancytopenias). If infection occurs in utero during development of tissues such as the cerebellum, neurologic disease also may be observed.

CELL KILLING

Cells that replicate virus often are killed as a direct consequence of infection. One mechanism by which viruses kill cells is lysis, often associated with the release of progeny virions. Insertion of viral proteins into cell membranes, budding, direct toxicity of viral proteins, and diversion of normal host cell homeostatic processes to viral replication may result in death of the cell.[15,16,30] Viruses also may activate the cellular self-destruct mechanism of programmed cell death (apoptosis). Although cells may induce apoptosis in an attempt to prevent completion of the virus life cycle, viruses also may use this mechanism to kill the cell and facilitate release of virions.[31]

NEOPLASIA

Viral infection can cause neoplastic transformation of infected cells. The most common examples in horses include warts (equine papillomavirus) and sarcoids (bovine papillomavirus). Virally induced invasive neoplastic diseases such as leukemia or lymphosarcoma have not been recognized in the horse, unlike other species. However, these types of diseases may be identified. Viral proteins that activate the cell cycle into the growth and division phases may lead to neoplastic transformation if expressed in a cell that is not killed by the infection. Papillomavirus infections induce epithelial neoplasms (fibropapillomata) using a virally encoded protein (E5 oncoprotein) that induces proliferation of normally quiescent cells and that presumably is needed for viral replication.[8] The E1A oncoproteins and immediate early proteins of adenoviruses and herpesviruses, respectively, are highly oncogenic in cells that do not allow full virus expression.[32,33] Adenoviral and herpesviral infections in horses currently are not recognized as oncogenic. The lack of oncogenic transformation by these viruses is most likely because abortive infections may not occur in vivo, transformed cells are always removed by the immune system, or the requisite co-factors for transformation are not present. As an example of the role of co-factors, infection of human beings with human herpesvirus 4 (Epstein-Barr virus, the cause of infectious mononucleosis) is not associated commonly with neoplasia in North America or Europe, whereas infection with this virus in Africa is associated strongly with Burkitt's lymphoma and in China with nasopharyngeal carcinoma.[34]

Oncogenic retroviruses, including leukemia and sarcoma viruses, induce neoplastic transformation in several ways but in all cases do so by integration into the host cell genome and activation of cellular oncogenes.[35] Specifically, a retrovirus and its viral promoter sequences may insert upstream from and activate a normally quiescent cellular oncogene in the process of viral gene expression. Other retroviruses, such as the bovine leukemia virus, produce a virally encoded protein, tax, which transactivates and upregulates the expression of cellular oncogenes. These are believed to be the primary mechanisms of transformation by the leukemia viruses. Integration of the retroviral genome also may inactivate by insertion host cell repressors required to actively suppress the expression of cellular oncogenes. Some retroviral genomes, such as those of the rapidly transforming sarcoma viruses, may transform the cell by acquiring cellular oncogenes that are then co-expressed along with other viral gene products during replication.

INTERFERENCE WITH DIFFERENTIATED CELL FUNCTION

Although not described in horses and still poorly documented in other species, such as humans, some viral infections are theorized to play a role in chronic diseases such as diabetes and obesity. For example, the hepatitis C virus may infect the B cells of the pancreas and interfere with the production of insulin.[11] In experimental infections of rodents, canine distemper virus and Borna disease virus cause obesity, possibly by infection of the hypothalamus and downregulation of leptin receptors.[12] Although the role of viruses in these types of infections is still controversial, advances in the detection of viruses are likely to uncover unusual and previously unsuspected roles for viruses in chronic diseases, including those of horses.

INTERACTIONS WITH HOST IMMUNE RESPONSES

One of the main obstacles to successful viral replication in vivo is the host immune response. In response to infection, cells can react in a number of ways to block viral replication, initiate the expansion of specific antiviral immune responses, and target the infected cell for immunologic recognition and destruction. As a result, many viruses have developed counterstrategies to block cell signals that promote these host cell responses.

Interferons induce the expression of a number of cellular proteins that inhibit viral replication in the cell. Secreted interferons similarly impart resistance to viral replication in adjacent cells and are an important mechanism for controlling the local spread of infection. Some viruses, including paramyxoviruses, adenoviruses, and herpesviruses, produce proteins that interfere with the cell signaling mechanisms required for the expression of interferon-induced proteins.[36,37]

One of the most important systems for recognition of virally infected cells by cytotoxic lymphocytes is endocytic processing of viral proteins followed by expression of the resultant viral peptides on the cell surface complexed with MHC class I molecules. Viral products may interfere directly with the processing, transport, or cell surface expression of MHC I molecules or viral peptides, thereby preventing recognition by cytotoxic, $CD8^+$ T lymphocytes.[36,38] In antigen-presenting cells, cell surface expression of viral peptides with MHC II molecules to immune regulatory cells, mainly $CD4^+$ helper T lymphocytes and B cells, is required for initiation and upregulation of antibody- and cell-mediated antiviral immune responses. Similar interference with the processing, transport, or cell surface expression of MHC II molecules or viral peptides can interfere with antiviral immune responses.[36] Some herpesviruses also have been shown to interfere with recognition of virally infected cells by natural killer cells, an early, nonspecific cell-mediated immune response.[39]

An interesting and more recently recognized viral mechanism for interference with host immune responses is the use of virally encoded cytokine mimics. Cytokines are critical cell signaling molecules that coordinate and regulate the development of host immune responses. Some viruses, including poxviruses, herpesviruses, and adenoviruses, express cytokine homologs that mimic and interfere with the activity of interferons, interleukin-1, interleukin-8, interleukin-10, tumor necrosis factor, epidermal growth factor, and granulocyte-macrophage colony-stimulating factor.[36,40] Although the role of these homologs in natural disease is not clear, experimentally they can modulate immune responses and affect disease severity.[36]

VIROLOGIC LATENCY

At the host level viruses may use several mechanisms to establish persistent infections and avoid immune clearance. Some persistent infections are characterized by continual replication despite the presence of antiviral immune responses. If these types of persistent infections are subclinical, they often are described as clinically latent. However, the viral dynamics at the host level should be differentiated from events at the cellular level. In cells virologic latency is a specific type of cell interaction and an important mechanism of persistence for some viruses. *Virologic latency* is defined as the presence of a viral genome that is not producing infectious virus.[41] The genomes of latent viruses are transcriptionally suppressed and translationally silent so that no viral proteins are expressed that may identify the cell to the immune system as infected. The definition of *latency* also stipulates that on reactivation, viral gene expression and the production of infectious progeny virions can be resumed, differentiating latently infected cells from cells infected with defective viruses.

The classic latent infection is that of the herpesviruses. For the α herpesviruses, such as EHV1 and EHV4, latent infections are established in the nuclei of sensory neurons and can be maintained indefinitely, and infected animals serve as the reservoir of the virus.[42-44] The only detectable viral gene products in latently infected neurons are a small RNA message called *latency-associated transcripts,* which are required for maintenance of latency.[41] On reactivation viral nucleic acids are translocated across synapses to epithelial cells of the nasopharynx, which produce infectious virus. In adult horses the amount of viral replication in the nasopharynx is usually not sufficient to result in clinical disease.[44] The stimuli that induce reactivation are poorly defined, but reactivation can be induced by immunosuppression (e.g., corticosteroids) and presumably by other stressors, such as pregnancy, transport, and social stress.[44,45]

MECHANISMS OF DISEASE: VIRUS-HOST INTERACTIONS

Viral interactions with individual cells are the basis for viral pathogenesis. However, for the whole animal, the severity of disease, or whether infection even results in clinical disease at all, is a much more complex interaction between the classic triad of virus, host, and environment. More specifically, these factors include viral virulence, viral spread within the animal, the intensity of direct and immune-mediated pathologic response elicited by the virus, and the ability of the virus to avoid clearance by the host. Other than the virulence of the virus, which is strictly a property of the virus, the other virus-host interactions can be influenced by the age and genetics of the host and by environmental factors such as stress and nutrition. These factors account for the observation that considerable variation in disease signs can occur among a group of animals infected with the same viral strain.

Viral Virulence

Certain strains of a virus are well recognized as causing more severe disease. Although many host factors may influence the severity of clinical disease, virulence per se is strictly a property of the virus. The main properties of a virus that may affect virulence include host cell tropism and replication rate. A tropism change that leads to involvement of additional tissues or facilitates virus spread generally results in more severe disease. The systemic spread of highly pathogenic avian influenza strains described earlier is one example. Outbreaks of EHV1 abortion or neurologic disease strongly suggest that EHV1 strains exist that have a tropism for these tissues compared with EHV1 strains that cause respiratory disease. However, the appropriate studies have not been performed yet to determine the exact basis for this observation. Limited studies of EHV1 genetics and virulence in mouse models have not identified differences between the abortigenic, neurogenic, and respiratory strains.[46] However, the severity of EHV1 respiratory disease in experimentally infected foals can be decreased by deletion of genes that facilitate cell-to-cell spread.[47]

An increase in the viral replication rate is usually associated with an increase in virulence, presumably because of the greater number of infected cells and amount of tissue damage. The virulence of equine infectious anemia virus strains can be correlated directly to plasma virus titers and numbers of infected cells, without any changes in tropism.[48,49] The molecular basis for the increased replication rate is not clear but most likely is caused by variation in viral regulatory sequences and proteins.[50,51]

Spread of Infection in the Host

Viral infections generally are regarded as localized or systemic. Localized viral infections are those that are restricted to a single organ system, often at the site of entry. Because infection of the tissue is direct, the incubation period for localized viral infections is usually short, often only a few days. Many infections of the skin or mucosal surfaces are localized, and examples in the horse include infections with enteric rotavirus and influenza. For influenza, virus is inhaled into the nasopharynx and replicates in epithelial cells of the upper respiratory tract and trachea. Virus is not present in the blood or tissues outside of the respiratory tract. In general, viruses remain localized because they lack the receptors to infect cells of other tissues or circulating cells, such as monocytes or lymphocytes, that can disseminate the virus. Some viruses are temperature sensitive and remain localized because they are unable to replicate efficiently at core body temperatures. EHV3, the cause of coital exanthema, is restricted to the surface of the genitalia in horses because of its temperature sensitivity.[52] EHV1 and EHV4 are not temperature sensitive, however, and systemic infection may occur with these viruses. The feline respiratory herpesvirus is also temperature sensitive and normally is restricted to the cooler mucosal surfaces. However, hypothermia may lead to dissemination and multiorgan infections.[53] Temperature sensitivity is also a means by which some viruses, such as equine influenza and infectious bovine rhinotracheitis virus, may be attenuated for use as modified-live intranasal vaccines. Infection by the vaccine strain is limited to the cooler mucosal surfaces; the inability to spread systemically prevents sequelae such as abortion and pneumonia.[54,55]

Systemic infections are those in which virus is disseminated to multiple tissues by blood or lymph. This viremia may exist in the form of cell-free virions in the plasma or lymph or may be cell associated in circulating blood cells, usually monocytes or lymphocytes. The classic paradigm for a systemic infection is infection of mice with ectromelia virus[56] (Figure 2-8). Localized viral replication first occurs at the site of entry and in regional lymph nodes. Depending on the level of replication, clinical disease may be present. The virus then enters the blood or lymphatics and spreads to other tissues, such as spleen and liver, in which clinical disease may occur. Virus is amplified and then released again for a second, usually higher-titered, viremia that further disseminates the virus to other organs. Each viremic episode is associated with a febrile response and is the basis for the biphasic fever response associated with some viral infections. Because systemic infections require multiple steps, the incubation periods are longer than for localized infections, typically 1 to several weeks. Infections in the horse by eastern, western, or Venezuelan equine encephalitis virus closely follow this paradigm. Localized viral replication occurs at the site of entry (mosquito bite) followed by viremia and dissemination to the central nervous system.[57] For most horses, even nonvaccinated horses, dissemination is controlled before infection of the brain, and neurologic disease is a rare outcome of infection. A variation on the theme is infection of horses with EHV1. The most common clinical disease associated with EHV1 infection is rhinopneumonitis caused by a localized infection of the nasopharyngeal mucosa.[58] In almost all cases, a cell-associated viremia also occurs in lymphocytes, but in most infected horses this does not result in disease. However, in some cases, viremia is associated with infection of endothelial cells, and in the pregnant mare vascular damage to the uterus and placenta may lead to abortion.[58,59] Similarly, infection of the vascular endothelium in the central nervous system results in neurologic disease.[60]

Some viruses also may spread in the host through nerves. In the horse rabies is the best known infection that relies on neural spread. Following local replication in myocytes at the site of entry, usually a bite wound, rabies virus ascends peripheral nerves into the central nervous system, where it replicates in neurons, and then egresses by way of cranial nerves to the salivary gland.[61] EHV1 and EHV4 establish latency in the nuclei of sensory neurons that innervate the nasopharynx

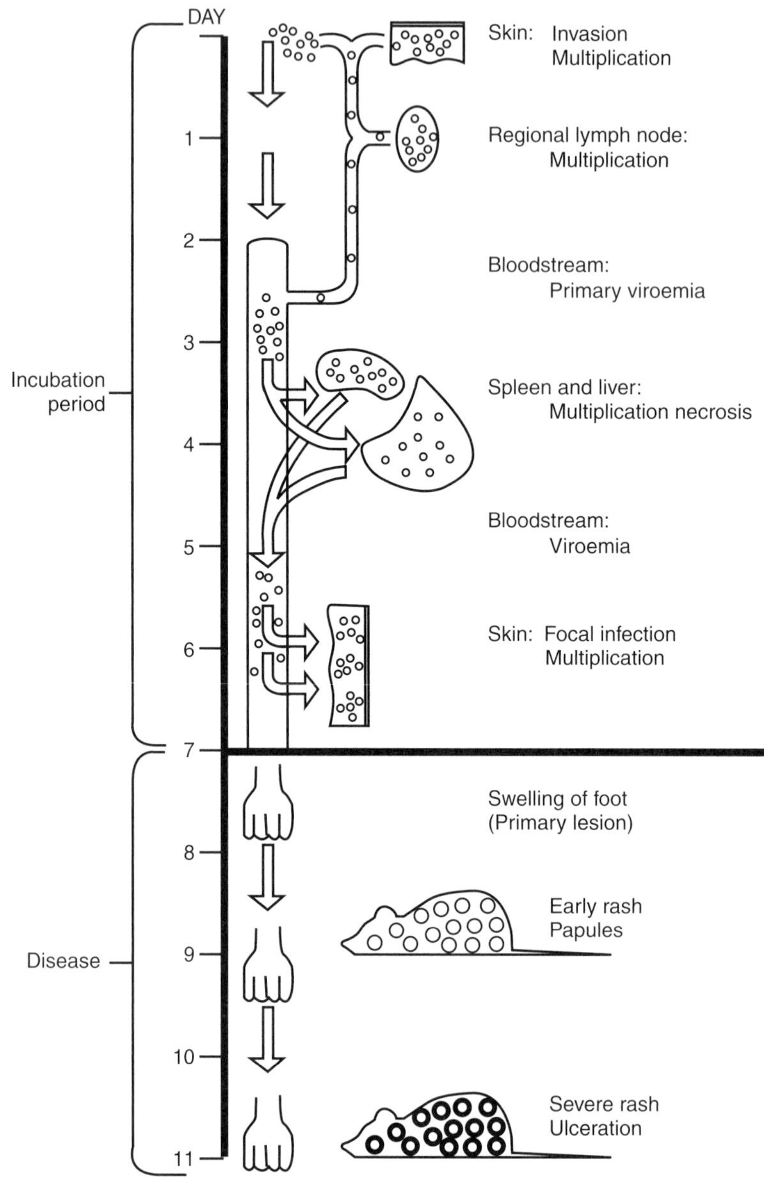

FIGURE 2-8 Schematic representation of the pathogenesis of mousepox (ectromelia), illustrating the classic paradigm for the events in a systemic infection. (From Fenner F: The pathogenesis of the acute exanthems, *Lancet* 255:915, 1948.)

and reach the nucleus by ascending nerve axons. Similarly, on reactivation these viruses egress back down the axon to infect epithelial cells.[43,62]

Viral Pathology

Once a virus reaches a target organ, virally mediated cell death is the fundamental source of pathologic response, disease, and clinical signs observed by the veterinarian. Despite the great complexity of virus-host interactions and the many factors that influence the expression of clinical disease, in actuality viruses have a limited number of ways by which to cause infection. Cells and tissues may be destroyed directly by cytolytic viral infections or by infections that affect the differentiated function of target cells (e.g., neoplasms and immunodeficiencies). Viral infections of organ systems with bacterial flora (e.g., intestinal and respiratory tracts) can disrupt the normal barrier functions of these organs and result in secondary bacterial infections and toxemia that may contribute significantly to the pathologic response. Cell death and pathologic response also may be caused by host immune responses specifically directed against virally infected cells or by indiscriminate inflammatory responses. Virally induced autoimmune diseases have not been described in horses but are another potential source of pathologic response that may be identified in the future.

For most of the clinically important viral diseases of horses, disease manifestation results from some combination of cytolytic infection and immune-mediated tissue destruction. The relative contribution of these mechanisms is primarily a function of viral virulence and host factors that influence the type and intensity of immune responses. The predominant mechanism of pathologic response also can vary with different stages of the same disease, as seen in acute versus chronic equine infectious anemia. In acute disease most of the disease manifestation is caused by direct viral damage and cytokines, whereas in chronic disease immune complex–mediated anemia and glomerulonephritis become more significant.

DIRECT VIRAL PATHOLOGY

The most straightforward cause of damage and disease in an organ system is for the virus directly to kill or cause dysfunction in the infected cells. As described previously, cell death may be caused by cytolysis resulting from viral replication and interference with normal cell homeostasis or by initiation of apoptosis. Cell dysfunction usually is observed as neoplastic transformation, although more vague effects on other differentiated cell functions, such as insulin secretion, remain possibilities.

The disease associated with a given viral infection is related to the affected organ system(s), the number of cells destroyed, and the sensitivity of the affected organ system to dysfunction. If the number of infected cells is not sufficient to lead to clinically significant organ dysfunction, then the result is a subclinical infection. Vaccination and naturally acquired immunity are important factors that limit the number of infected cells. However, epidemiologically these infections may still be important because these animals may still be infectious. When enough cells are infected to lead to overt organ dysfunction, then clinical disease becomes apparent. The threshold for clinically significant damage varies considerably between organs and the types of cells. EHV1 infections of the respiratory epithelium, which has a large number of cells with a high turnover rate, produce mild clinical disease even with a high rate of infection. On the other hand, much more significant clinical manifestations of EHV1 infection such as abortion and neurologic disease are caused by infection of a few endothelial cells because minimal vascular damage can lead to thrombosis, ischemic necrosis, and damage to large amounts of tissue. If viral infection results in neoplastic transformation of a cell type, then disease may progress according to the characteristics of the neoplasm, whether or not the virus remains associated with the tumor.

Of particular importance are infections of the respiratory and intestinal tracts that contain normal bacterial flora and have important barrier functions to prevent access of bacteria and toxins to deeper tissues. Consequently, complications of bacterial infection and toxemia are important secondary problems of viral infections.[63,64] For example, upper respiratory viral infections damage the ciliated epithelial cells that function to move mucus and other respiratory secretions outward and provide a barrier between the mucosal bacterial flora and the underlying subepithelial tissues. Damage to this barrier may lead to opportunistic bacterial pneumonias by normal bacterial flora such as *Streptococcus equi* subsp. *zooepidemicus* or *Mannheimia haemolytica* in horses or cattle, respectively.

IMMUNE-MEDIATED VIRAL PATHOLOGY

In most viral infections immune-mediated pathologic response contributes significantly to disease and in some cases may be the predominant cause of disease manifestation. This paradigm has been documented elegantly in classic experiments with lymphocytic choriomeningitis virus infections of mice in which immunodeficient mice develop persistent infections but do not develop disease and do develop disease if their immune systems are reconstituted.[65] Equine immune and inflammatory responses are covered in detail in Chapter 1 and are described in this section only in general terms and as they relate to viral infections.

The primary antiviral immune responses initiated in viral infections include natural killer cells, virus-specific cytotoxic ($CD8^+$) T lymphocytes, and to a lesser extent antibody-mediated lysis of infected cells (antibody-directed cellular cytotoxicity, complement fixation, and phagocytosis by macrophages and neutrophils). These immune responses detect and selectively kill virally infected cells and are a significant cause of cell death. Indiscriminate inflammatory responses also may kill uninfected cells in the vicinity of infected cells, primarily from activation of monocytes and granulocytes with release of a wide array of cytotoxic molecules (e.g., lysozyme, proteases, lipases, and oxygen radicals). Secondary bacterial infections greatly exacerbate indiscriminate tissue damage, not only from the direct effect of bacterial toxins but also because of extensive recruitment of neutrophils and complement, which are highly nonselective components of the antibacterial immune response.

Antibody-mediated immune complex hypersensitivity reactions also may play a major role in the genesis of viral disease. Antibodies bound to soluble viral antigens fix complement and opsonize neutrophils, again leading to indiscriminate cell and tissue destruction. Viral antigens may be on the surface of cells, such as erythrocytes or platelets, resulting in immune-mediated anemia and thrombocytopenia, respectively.[66] When viral antigen is in excess relative to antibody, circulating immune complexes are formed that can be deposited in the capillary beds of tissues such as joints and renal glomeruli. In chronic equine infectious anemia virus, with persistent viral replication and antigenemia in the presence of antiviral antibodies, these mechanisms are primarily responsible for the characteristic lesions of anemia, thrombocytopenia, and glomerulonephritis.[66,67] Non-neutralizing antiviral antibodies actually may serve to increase the number of infected cells and the severity of disease through the mechanism of antibody-dependent enhancement. This enhancement occurs when antibodies bind to the virus and facilitate attachment and entry into Fc receptor–bearing cells such as macrophages by serving as a form of alternative receptor.[68] Antibody-dependent enhancement has been shown to be involved in the pathogenesis of a number of diseases, including feline infectious peritonitis,[69] human respiratory syncytial virus,[70] and dengue hemorrhagic fever.[71]

Soluble inflammatory mediators released by infected cells and inflammatory cells in response to viral infections are also significant contributors to clinical signs and disease manifestation. These mediators include a wide array of cytokines, interleukins, and other pro-inflammatory molecules with potent systemic and local effects. The most evident of these is the febrile response caused by interleukin-1 released by macrophages in response to virally infected cells. Increased levels of other soluble factors, including interferons, interleukins, transforming growth factor, and tumor necrosis factor, are also present in many viral infections.[72,73] These cytokines are primarily proinflammatory and immunoregulatory and are generally important for the control of viral infections but also can be responsible for many of the nonspecific clinical signs of viral infection, such as depression; malaise; and, in chronic infections, cachexia. Soluble mediators also may have important local effects. Vasoactive factors such as prostaglandins and leukotrienes cause edema and swelling. In equine infectious anemia virus, tumor necrosis factor α, transforming growth factor β, and interferon-α have been shown to suppress hematopoiesis and contribute to the development of anemia and thrombocytopenia.[74]

AUTOIMMUNITY

Although not described in horses, viral infections in other species can induce immune-mediated responses to host cell antigens and autoimmune diseases. The best documented human autoimmune disease suspected to be initiated by viral infections is Guillain-Barré syndrome, in which infection with cytomegalovirus or Epstein-Barr herpesvirus elicits antinerve ganglioside immune responses and demyelinating disease.[75] Postinfluenza myocarditis is an occasional sequela in horses and human beings and is a potential autoimmune disease. Although no direct evidence supports this theory, influenza virus is not identified consistently in affected heart muscle and the pathogenesis is not known.[76]

Immune Avoidance

A key requirement for viruses to be maintained in nature is to persist successfully in a reservoir host (if the reservoir is an infected animal) and to be transmitted to another susceptible host. One of the most important obstacles to persistence and transmission is detection and elimination by the host immune system. Transmission to a new host also may require that the virus avoid preexisting immunity from prior natural exposures or vaccination. Within the host rapidly replicating viruses such as influenza may shed and transmit virus before the host can mount specific antiviral immune responses. Herpesviruses avoid detection during latency by not expressing any viral proteins. For persistent viral infections that continually replicate within a host, such as retroviruses, evasion of developing immune responses is necessary. Immunodeficiency viruses may cripple antiviral immune responses by directly infecting immunoregulatory $CD4^+$ T lymphocytes. As described previously, many other viruses can dysregulate host immune responses by expressing cytokine mimics.

One of the most important mechanisms of immunologic avoidance is antigenic variation in which neutralizing viral antigens are altered so that they are no longer recognized or accessible by host immune responses. The most important of these antigens includes viral proteins bound by neutralizing antibodies (e.g., virus receptors) and any peptides presented in the context of MHC I or II cell surface molecules for recognition by cytotoxic ($CD8^+$) T lymphocytes or helper ($CD4^+$) T lymphocytes, respectively. Antigenic variation is generated by nucleotide errors during transcription or replication, which result in amino acid substitutions in the relevant epitopes. This process is facilitated by viral polymerases that are inherently error prone and lack proofreading functions and by placing the sequences for the relevant epitopes adjacent to other genomic sequences or structures that further predispose to transcriptional errors.[19] Other mechanisms by which some viruses may modify their antigenicity is through intramolecular recombination/duplication or reassortment of segmented genomes (e.g., influenza and African horse sickness).[19,21] For reassortment, co-infection of a single cell with genetically different virions may result in a progeny virion with segments derived from both virions and a major change in antigenicity. In influenza these are called *antigenic shifts,* and the radical change in the antigenicity of the virus may render preexisting immunity in the host population ineffective at preventing outbreaks of disease with high morbidity and mortality.[21] Viruses also may facilitate the production of non-neutralizing antibodies that sterically interfere with the ability of neutralizing antibodies to bind. Although the mechanism of antigenic variation is primarily random, immunologic selection determines which variants successfully emerge and are capable of replicating within the host or the host population.

Host Genetics

Genetic differences in susceptibility to disease have been well documented. In an outbred population of animals, the considerable variation in the type or severity of clinical disease is well recognized, even when animals are infected with the same virus strain and have no recognizable differences in other factors such as age, challenge dose, nutrition, and general health status. Conversely, highly inbred populations may be more uniformly susceptible to a viral disease.[77] Thus inbreeding can pose problems for endangered species, such as Przewalski's horse, or other populations with limited genetic variability, which may incur high rates of morbidity or mortality if the animals are infected with a virulent virus.

Although in many virus-host interactions the basis for genetic resistance to disease is not well defined, host genetics have been shown to affect the tropism of the virus and influence the type and intensity of immune responses to a viral infection. In human immunodeficiency virus infections, genetically determined absence or presence of certain co-receptors has a significant effect on susceptibility to disease.[78,79] Immunologically, host genetics defines the repertoire of antigen-specific recognition molecules (antibodies and T cell receptors) and antigen-presenting molecules (MHC I and II). Consequently, genetically different animals respond to different subsets of viral antigens. The relative inability to react to a neutralizing epitope prevents or delays effective control of viral replication.[80] Different subsets of viral antigens may favor the development of a type 1 T helper cell (cell-mediated) or type 2 T helper cell (antibody-mediated) immune response, which has implications for the ability to control infection and for immune-mediated pathologic response.[81-83]

ADVANCES IN THE DIAGNOSIS OF VIRAL DISEASES

The diagnosis of viral infections traditionally has relied on the detection of antiviral antibodies by serologic tests and the direct demonstration of virus by isolation in cultures of living cells or in laboratory animals. Although these principles are still the foundation for the diagnosis of viral diseases, recent molecular biology advances have greatly improved the clinical use of viral diagnostics.

The sensitivity and specificity of antibody testing have been enhanced by the recombinant viral proteins or peptides for use as antigens in serologic tests. One example is the use of recombinant antigens in antibody tests for equine infectious anemia virus. The replacement of whole-virus antigen preparations with recombinant viral proteins has improved the sensitivity and specificity of the agar gel immunodiffusion (Coggins) and enzyme-linked immunosorbent assay tests.[84,85] The improvement in specificity is especially important when screening for a low-prevalence disease in which the predictive value of a positive result is low, as is the case for equine infectious anemia in the United States.

However, the greatest advances have been in the area of detection of virus in clinical specimens. The clinical utility of traditional methods of virus isolation in cell culture often is limited by the sensitivity, specificity, predictive value, or the length of time needed to perform this type of assay. Another significant limitation of virus isolation, particularly for the more labile enveloped viruses, is the requirement for viable virus, which may be compromised by autolysis or transport to the laboratory. In many diagnostic laboratories, virus isolation in cell culture has been replaced by immunohistochemistry and the PCR, both of which are sensitive and specific tests that can be completed in one or two days. Immunohistochemistry is a method that detects viral antigens in formalin-fixed tissue samples. Although immunohistochemistry technology has been available for many years, this assay has become more widely used because of improvements in the methods for antigen retrieval and the greater availability of antiviral monoclonal or polyclonal antibodies. The aldehydes in formalin cross-link proteins during the fixation process and prevent the recognition of epitopes by antibodies. For many viruses reliable protocols now have been established that use carefully controlled protease digestion of the tissue sections so that the availability of epitopes is restored.[86] The tissue sections then can be incubated with antiviral antibodies, and bound antibodies can be visualized with a variety of colorimetric systems. The specificity of immunohistochemistry depends highly on the antiviral antiserum and has been improved greatly by the availability of antiviral monoclonal antibodies and recombinant viral proteins that can be used to generate monospecific antisera.[87-89]

The PCR is a nucleic acid amplification method that detects viral DNA or RNA extracted from fresh or formalin-fixed tissue samples. Only a few years ago the techniques used to purify nucleic acids and perform the PCR reaction were limited by expense and practicality to the research laboratory. However, the simplification and commercialization of these procedures have made this type of test economical and clinically useful for diagnostic laboratories.[90,91] The PCR test uses oligonucleotide primers and a thermostable DNA polymerase (Taq polymerase) to amplify exponentially the viral nucleic acids. The basis for specific amplification in the PCR assay is the sequence of the oligonucleotide primers, which are produced synthetically to be complementary and thus bind to the viral nucleic acid sequences. To produce complementary primers, the sequence of the viral DNA or RNA must be known. Consequently, this assay is only useful for testing for viruses that have been sequenced, and in the past sequence data limited the ability to design PCR primers. However, because of advances in the technology for sequencing and database management, virtually all of the significant equine pathogens now have complete sequence data available. At the end of the PCR procedure, the amplified nucleic acids (i.e., a positive result) are visualized most commonly with agarose gel electrophoresis in which the amplicons in the gel are viewed with a fluorescent dye, and the product presumptively is confirmed as the correct one on the basis of its molecular size (Figure 2-9).

Immunohistochemistry and PCR are now routine tests that generally are sensitive, specific, and rapid. However, care must be taken not to make assumptions about the performance characteristics of new tests. For example, although PCR assays are often more sensitive than virus isolation, this is not automatically true. The sensitivity and specificity of any new test must be evaluated individually and with respect to the performance of the previous test. Also, the significance of any virus identified in a specimen still must be interpreted in the context of the pathogenicity of the virus and clinical disease, regardless of the method used to detect the virus.

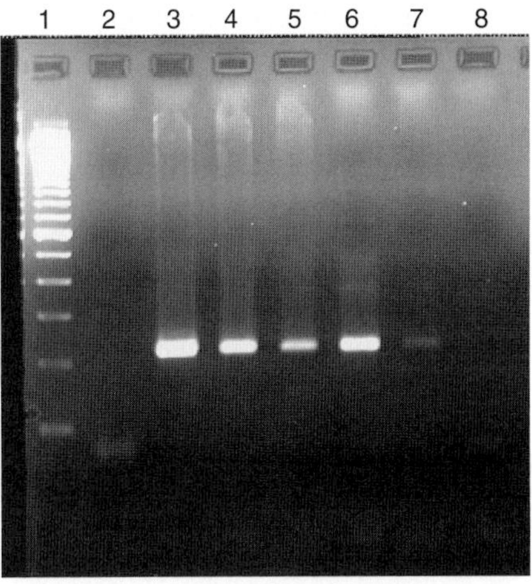

FIGURE 2-9 Analysis of polymerase chain reactions (PCRs) for equine infectious anemia virus. PCR products are electrophoresed in an agarose gel. DNA in the gel is stained with ethidium bromide and visualized with ultraviolet light that causes the DNA to fluoresce and appear as white bands in the gel. Lane 1 is a size standard to determine the size of the DNA amplicons. Lane 2 is a negative control, and lane 3 is a positive control. The samples in lanes 4, 5, 6, and 7 are positive; the sample in lane 8 is negative.

INTERNAL PARASITE INFECTIONS

Thomas R. Klei

Horses serve as hosts for numerous parasites, which induce a wide range of pathologic and immunologic responses.[1,2] Many of the latter are of a hypersensitive nature and also result in disease conditions. Immune responses leading to protective resistance against reinfection occur, but the level of this resistance is most often incomplete. Mechanisms associated with these responses have not been investigated extensively in the horse, but information is available from other host-parasite systems that may be relevant to the equine. The purpose of this section is to acquaint the reader with contemporary thoughts on host-parasite interactions. Because of their prevalence, major importance to equids, and information available, coverage is limited to helminth parasites that occur in most developed and nontropical countries.

PARASITE-INDUCED LESIONS

Infection with most metazoan parasites results in inflammation and structural and functional changes of the organs invaded. The outcome of these changes is an alteration of the host's physiologic state. The degree of alteration depends on the existing physiologic condition of the animal, which is dictated to a great degree by its age, nutritional status, and previous immunologic experience with the parasite. The numbers of parasites introduced and the specific parasite also affect the degree of physiologic change that occurs.

When these factors favor major alterations, the results are readily identifiable clinical signs of infection. Subclinical infections, although less apparent, are potentially important to the general health of the animal and continued transmission of the agent. The pathophysiologic effects of infection by ectoparasites, helminths, and microorganisms are in many cases similar.[3,4] Abnormalities in weight gain, skeletal growth, reproduction, and lactation may result from infections with any of these agents. These changes are often directly related to parasite-induced anorexia, disruption of metabolic processes, and anemia. An understanding of the morphologic and biochemical lesions produced by specific parasites clarifies the role of these agents in clinical and subclinical conditions associated with the infections. A majority of detailed studies on the pathophysiology of parasitic infections have been conducted in laboratory animal models and domestic animal species other than the horse.[3] However, the classical pathology of parasitic infections of the horse has been reviewed.[2,5] The following discussion outlines some recent observations on host-parasite interactions that may be of significance to equine medicine. Examples of host-parasite interactions responsible for alterations in host homeostasis are presented as they relate to the gastrointestinal tract, lungs, and skin.

Gastrointestinal Tract

Internal parasites are most important to equine health as mediators of gastrointestinal problems, including colic and diarrhea. Although almost all internal parasites have been inferentially implicated as causative agents of colic at some time, significant evidence-based experimental or field obsevations have emerged to support this contention for some parasites. The helminth parasites include large strongyles, principally *Strongylus vulgaris, Parascaris equorum, Anoplocephala perfoliata,* and as a group the cyathostomins.

STRONGYLUS VULGARIS

Details of the pathogenesis of colic associated with migration of *Strongylus vulgaris* through the mesenteric arteries and the resultant thrombosis, infarctions, and necrosis of the intestine have been described in detail elsewhere.[2,5] Large strongyles are easily controlled with currently available macrocyclic lactone anthelmintics and are rare in horses kept on well-managed farms in developed countries. Nonetheless, this parasite-host interaction has arguably been experimentally studied in more detail that other internal parasites of the horse and some points are particularly noteworthy. Histologic studies of experimentally infected parasite-free pony foals during the initial stages of infection indicate that the severity of lesions produced in the intestine cannot be attributed solely to mechanical disruption caused by larval migrations and that these larval stages induce some biologic amplification system within the mucosa, which results in the degree of inflammation observed.[6] Although the mechanisms involved in this response have not been investigated, the histologic nature of the lesion is characteristic of an Arthus reaction, suggesting an involvement of the immune response. Other experimental studies using the parasite-free pony–*S. vulgaris* system have implicated a role for the immune response in the mediation and regulation of the arterial lesions produced by this parasite. Passive transfer of immune serum but not normal serum reduced the severity of arteritis seen and clinical signs associated with experimental infections without reducing the numbers of parasites that develop in these ponies.[7] However, treatment with immune serum also induced an anamnestic eosinophilia and marked perivascular infiltration of eosinophils in the cecum. The reduction in intravascular lesions may have been associated with an inactivation of parasite-secreted inflammatory factors either by antibody or serum enzymes or circulating cytokines. This serum may also have contained nonspecific host-derived anti-inflammatory substances. The exacerbation of the eosinophil response may have been associated with the formation of immune complexes. Although the mechanisms are unknown, the results suggest that the immune response may simultaneously modulate and potentiate inflammation. It has been postulated that larvacidal treatment of *S. vulgaris*–infected horses and killing of intravascular larvae may release a bolus of antigenic factors from these larvae within the mesenteric vasculature, resulting in an exacerbation of arterial and intestinal lesions and colic. Experimental testing of this hypothesis indicates that this phenomenon does not occur and further that viable larvae are necessary to maintain the arteritis and eosinophilia seen.[8,9] Experimental studies using parasite-free ponies that were immunized with crude adult worm antigens and subsequently challenged with *S. vulgaris* larvae showed an exacerbation of the pathologic responses seen in the mesenteric vasculature and including an anamnestic eosinophilia, further suggesting a role for the immune response in the development of these lesions.[10]

PARASCARIS EQUORUM

Colic associated with *Parascaris equorum* infection in foals has been related to intestinal impaction and rupture and is not considered to be of major significance in adult horses.[11] These conditions in foals may become more important with the widespread identification of *P. equorum* resistance to ivermectin.[12] However, ascarid nematodes are particularly potent sources of allergens, and it is not inconceivable that the hypersensitized mature horse may respond to low-level infections with this parasite. Observations made in the author's laboratory are noteworthy in this regard. Two mature *Parascaris*-free adult horses were inoculated intradermally with less than 90 μg of saline-soluble somatic extract of adult *P. equorum* in order to test for immediate hypersensitivity to this antigen. Both horses experienced an immediate systemic response and colic. One of the horses died within 3 hours of intradermal inoculation. Necropsy results were consistent with the diagnosis of acute severe colitis. Because of the allergic potential of ascarid nematodes and the sensitivity of the equine gut to immediate hypersensitivity reactions, this potential is worthy of further characterization and consideration.

ANOPLOCEPHALA PERFOLIATA

Clinical observations have maintained an interest and concern over the pathogenic potential of *Anoplocephala perfoliata* infections. Earlier case reports have described cecal ruptures and intussusceptions of the cecum and colon associated with these infections.[13,14] However, detailed retrospective analyses of the concomitant occurrence of intussusception and colic with *A. perfoliata* infections have failed to consistently demonstrate any causal relationship between these conditions and tapeworm infections.[15] These parasites inhabit the region of the ileocecal junction and produce ulcerated lesions of the mucosa and submucosal inflammation. However, the parasites are not uncommon, and it is possible that the association of tapeworm infections and clinical signs attributed to them are caused by chance alone. Detailed experimental investigations of these infections have not been conducted, and thus specific details on the pathogenesis and relevance of these lesions are lacking. However, an association between tapeworm infections and colic of ileocecal origin has been suggested in a case control study of 231 horses.[16] The development of a test to measure IgG(T) levels to specific secreted *A. perfoliata* antigens was shown to correlate to parasite burdens. Use of this method in the United Kingdom has shown by a matched case control study that *A. perfoliata* is a significant risk factor for spasmodic colic and ileal impactions. The risk of spasmodic colic was also associated in these studies with increased numbers of parasites.[17]

CYATHOSTOMINS

Cyathostomins (cyathostomes or small strongyles) have not generally been considered to be of major importance, particularly as causative agents of colic. In this regard, field studies of Uhlinger are of particular importance.[18] In these controlled experiments different anthelmintic treatment regimens were used to test their efficacy in reducing the incidence of colic. The more efficacious treatment programs significantly reduced the incidence of colic by 2 to 13 times of that seen in the same herds before implementation of the more efficacious treatment. Because of the management programs used before the initiation of this study and the results of fecal cultures, it can be assumed that the primary parasites present in these horses were cyathostomes. These data strongly implicate a role for cyathostomins in a substantial proportion of colics observed under field conditions. The parasite or host factors involved in these colic cases are unknown but may be the dynamic turnover of parasites during the life cycle in the mucosa and the related inflammatory responses seen that they induce.

Cyathostomins have been implicated in numerous case reports with seasonal diarrhea in adult horses, which is a condition called *larval cyathostominiasis*. These cases are characterized by a sudden onset of diarrhea during the late winter or spring. Mature horses are usually affected, and these cases are often fatal. These are difficult to diagnose, and the only consistent signs are weight loss and diarrhea.[19] Large numbers of larval cyathostomes are found in the feces or in intestinal contents and within the mucosa of these horses. These symptoms are related to the synchronous emergence of fourth-stage larvae of these parasites from the mucosa. These larvae build to potentially large numbers within the mucosa owing to the arrested development of infective larvae. The seasonality of the occurrence of this condition at present does not appear to vary in different climatic regions as does the analogous bovine condition of type II ostertagiasis. Specific parasite or host factors associated with the regulation of the hypobiotic state of the larvae or the inflammatory response initiated at parasite emergence have not been described. Other clinical reports have suggested that cyathostome-related diarrhea and weight loss are not related to the seasonal presentation described previously.[20] This is supported by experimental studies demonstrating that pathophysiologic effects occur as large numbers of parasites enter the intestine as well as when they leave.[21]

In view of the paucity of specific mechanistic information on the pathophysiologic effects of equine gastrointestinal parasites, a synopsis of relevant information gathered from other model systems is warranted, particularly for nematodes.[3,22] Parasitic organisms may induce changes in gastrointestinal function directly by mechanical disruption of tissues and cells or by the release of factors that directly alter cell function. Induction of the immune response serves as an anamnestic amplification system. The result of these changes is an alteration in function of the smooth muscle and epithelium of the bowel.

A number of helminth parasites, including *P. equorum*, have been demonstrated to produce intestinal smooth muscle hyperplasia. Evidence suggests that this response may be induced by intestinal inflammation or stenosis associated with parasitism. Contractility of these muscles has also been demonstrated to be induced in a Schultz-Dale reaction by stimulation with parasite antigens. This response is mediated in rats by mast-cell–derived 5-hydroxytryptamine (5-HT) and in guinea pigs by histamine. A regulatory relationship of myenteric neurons to these antigen-induced changes has also been demonstrated in this model system. These latter experiments suggest that antigen-induced stimulation of smooth muscle contractility may be correspondingly blocked by γ-aminobutyric acid similarly stimulated by mast cell products. This complex system may be an adaptation by the host to maintain homeostasis in the face of continued antigenic stimulus. It is noteworthy that strongyle-induced alterations in myoelectric activity of the equine small intestine and colon have been demonstrated in vivo.[23,24] In some of these experiments, dead *S. vulgaris* larvae evoked an alteration of the smooth muscle response in previously exposed ponies, suggesting a role for the immune response in the stimulation of the hyperactivity.[25]

There is a rapidly growing literature on the host-parasite interactions of a number of mouse models of gastrointestinal nematode infections.[26-29] The mouse models include infections of *Trichinella spiralis, Nippostrongylus brasiliensis, Heligmosomoides polygyrus,* and *Trichuris muris*. Because of the use of the mouse the most contemporary of immunologic, genetic, molecular, and cell biologic techniques are available and may provide useful insights into potential explanations of immunologic and pathophysiologic responses of the horse to nematode parasites, particularly the cyathostomins. Although differences in specifics exist between these murine models, it is clear that these worms induce a type 2 T helper cell cytokine response consisting of IL-4, IL-5, IL-9, and IL-13. IL-4 and IL-13 induction of the Stat6 pathway is central to most of the resulting responses. There is a consistent mastocytosis and eosinophil infiltration of the intestine. The resulting responses also involve goblet cells, the enteric nervous system, epithelial cells, and alternately activated macrophages as effector cells. Cell junctions are disrupted, smooth muscle hypercontractility is stimulated and epithelial cell secretion increased, and goblet cell productions of mucus production stimulated. Although these mechanisms are used most often to explain expulsion of the nematodes in question, they could be equally important in the disruption of the homeostasis seen in the parasitized equine intestine.

RESPIRATORY SYSTEM

Several nematode parasites infect the equine lung. These include *S. westeri* and migrating stages of *P. equorum* en route to the small intestine. Migrating stages of aberrant parasites, such as *Habronema* sp., *Draschia megastoma* and *Strongylus* spp., which induce granulomatous foci in the lung parenchyma, and adults and larvae of the lungworm *Dictyocalus arnfieldi*, which inhabit the bronchi, also occur. Host responses to two of these are noted.

Parascaris equorum larval migrations in the lungs of yearling horses produce more severe clinical signs and inflammatory responses than in foals that are reared parasite free. These infections in yearlings are accompanied by focal accumulations of lymphoid tissue, indicating an induction of an active local immune response. It is suggested that this is an age-related phenomenon.[11] However, it is likely that more severe reactions could be the result of previous sensitization to *P. equorum* antigens. Increased responses of this nature have been described in the livers of pigs immunized with *Ascaris suum* antigens following challenge infections.

Dictyocalus arnfieldi infections of donkeys rarely produce clinical signs, and it has been suggested that these equids are the natural host for this parasite. Infections of horses produce a more severe and prolonged bronchial inflammatory response similar to *Dictyocalus* sp. infection in other hosts. The mechanisms associated with this differential response have not been defined but are not uncommon in unadapted host-parasite associations. It is possible that the more marked inflammatory reaction of the horse to these parasites is due to the absence of downregulatory mechanisms that are established in the more adapted natural host, the donkey.

Skin

Whereas *Onchocerca cervicalis* infections in horses are rare where macrocyclic lactone anthelmintics are regularly used, reactions to the filarial nematode illustrate variations seen in responses to chronic parasite infection. Focal, alopecic, depigmented, pruritic lesions are often seen in infected horses. Not all infected horses react to this infection, and the appearance of clinical signs is often seasonal. Detailed studies have not been conducted on the pathogenesis of these lesions in horses. However, similar conditions occur in human onchocerciasis,[30] and it is likely that the host-parasite responses active in humans are also present in the horse. Lesion development is associated with immune-mediated killing of microfilariae in the skin. Parasites appear to be killed in an antibody-dependent cell-mediated reaction. In this response antimicrofilarial surface IgG and IgE antibodies mediated adherence and degranulation of granulocytes, which are predominantly eosinophils. Major basic protein of eosinophils has been demonstrated in the tissues of patients with dermal lesions, and it has been suggested that eosinophil toxic enzymes and proteins are responsible for many of the changes seen. The reason for the absence of these lesions in most horses is unclear. Human onchocerciasis and filariasis are spectral diseases. In these diseases regulation of immune responses has been associated with the lack of pathologic responses to the parasites.[31,32] Immune regulatory mechanisms associated with these infections include immune tolerance, anergy, induction of immune regulation involving Treg cells or macrophages, and the production of IL-10 and TGF β-altering Th cell subsets and the production of specific cytokines during different phases of the infections. Recent studies have also focused on the role of an intracellular commensal microorganism, *Wolbachia,* which is a parasite of *Onchocerca* and other filarial nematodes. These bacteria have been shown to mediate type 1 inflammatory lesions in humans and mouse models.[32]

The presence of these types of parasite-associated immune regulatory events has yet to be critically studied in the horse. However, the seasonal variability in skin responses to the *Onchocerca microfilariae* by horses in some regions has been investigated. In this instance the onset of ventral-midline dermatitis during the summer may be related to a seasonal fluctuation in microfilarial burdens of the skin, which have been demonstrated to correspondingly peak at this time.[33] Not only do total numbers increase, but microfilariae are also found more commonly in the surface layers of the skin. Interestingly, this period of abundant microfilariae corresponds with the seasonal peak in numbers of the vector, *Culicoides varripennis*. Although speculative, correlations in the peak availability of microfilariae and vectors may be an evolutionary adaptation by these parasites to maximize transmission and survival of this parasite species.

PROTECTIVE RESISTANCE

Resistance to infection may be innate or acquired. In some instances innate resistance to equine parasites has been attributed to age, with older individuals being resistant. Most equine helminth parasites develop only in the horse, and conversely the horse exhibits an innate resistance to most nonequine parasites. Exceptions to this rule are parasites with a broader host range that occasionally infect horses, such as larvae of the tapeworm *Echinococcus granulosus* and the liver fluke *Fasciola hepatica*. *Trichostrongylus axei*, a parasite of ruminants, establishes readily in the equine stomach and produces significant lesions only when present in large numbers. In some cases parasites that develop in the horse induce more severe lesions and clinical signs than in their apparent normal host, as has been described for *D. arnfieldi*.

Age resistance to *P. equorum* and *S. vulgaris* has been described in horses by comparing susceptibility of young and old ponies reared under parasite-free conditions. It is apparent that the reaction of the lung to migrating *P. equorum* larvae is more marked in mature horses and suggests that an immune response occurs in this site.[13,14] Initial reports on age-acquired resistance to *S. vulgaris* infection[34] have not been substantiated, and experimental observations in our laboratory indicate that this does not occur.

The occurrence of acquired resistance to equine parasites can be inferred from the observation that older chronically exposed horses generally have lower burdens of parasites than do similarly exposed young horses. On the basis of these criteria, acquired resistance is apparent to infections of *S. westeri, P. equorum, Strongylus* spp., and cyathostome species. Extensive experiments are limited, however, to those on *S. vulgaris* and to some degree cyathostomins.

Although *S. vulgaris* has been largely eliminated from well-managed horse farms, examination of details of the immune response to it illustrates some equine immune mechanisms. Resistance that is acquired to *S.vulgaris* in most cases is partial and of a concomitant type; that is, some stages of the parasite, such as arterial larvae of *S. vulgaris*, may reside within the horse in the face of an active acquired resistance against newly acquired infective stages.

Resistance to infection with *S. westeri* adult parasites is inferred by the short duration of their life cycle within the small intestine and the failure of subsequent exposures to establish patent infections. Mares, however, remain infected with arrested third-stage larvae, which subsequent to foaling are transmitted to the foals in milk 4 days postpartum. Although not studied in horses, similar phenomena occur in swine strongyloidosis. In these infections there is apparent protective resistances against the migrating L_3, which is effective in preventing re-establishment of the intestinal infection but is ineffective against L_3, which are sesquestered in the abdominal fat of the sow.[35] Similar epidemiologic phenomena occur in *S. westeri* infection of horses, and it may be implied that similar immunologic mechanisms are also active.

Immunologic mechanisms associated with protective resistance are presented primarily as they relate to parasites that inhabit the lumen of the gastrointestinal tract and secondly as those that undergo extraintestinal tissue migration.

Gastrointestinal Parasites

Immune responses directed toward gastrointestinal nematodes vary significantly among hosts and against different parasite species within a given host. However, some generalities may serve as a background for understanding these responses in the horse. A phenomenon termed *self-cure* has been described in sheep, in which the ingestion of significant numbers of infective larvae induces the expulsion of existing adult parasites. This expulsion is initiated by a species-specific immediate-type hypersensitivity response that may cause the nonspecific expulsion of other nematode species. Although this phenomenon has not been examined in the horse, experimental infections of naturally parasitized ponies with large numbers of *S. vulgaris* L_3 induced a dramatic decrease in preexisting strongyle fecal egg counts, suggesting that a self-cure–like reaction may occur under some conditions.

More typically, establishment of primary infections results at some time in spontaneous expulsions of these worms as a result either of senility or, as demonstrated in laboratory animal model systems, of active acquired immune responses. This phenomenon occurs experimentally in the absence of reinfection and is thus separate from the self-cure phenomenon. A large number of immune effectors has been identified with this phenomenon in various model systems, and it is likely that some if not all are at some time active in the equine intestine. The mechanisms involved are T cell dependent. Antibodies may be involved but are not sufficient in themselves to induce expulsion. T cell–mediated mastocytosis, eosinophilia, and goblet cell hyperplasia have all been demonstrated to be related to expression of expulsion in some systems. These accessory cells are involved in the nonspecific efferent arm of this response. Mediators of inflammation, such as vasoactive amines, prostaglandins, and increased production of mucus, have been linked to immune elimination of primary infections in some but not all model systems. The increased secretion and hyperreactivity of intestinal smooth muscle associated with worm expulsion have been termed "weep and sweep" phenomena. It is likely that a number of specific immunologic events initiate several nonspecific effector mechanisms, resulting in this expulsion. These mechanisms vary with the species of parasite involved. The elimination of adult *S. westeri* and *P. equorum* from maturing horses and the hypothetical seasonal turnover in *Strongylus* spp. and cyathostome spp. may be mediated by such responses.

In addition to immune responses that occur during tissue migrations, protective resistance to reinfection by gastrointestinal nematodes occurs at the surface of the epithelium. This reaction, termed *rapid expulsion* or *immune exclusion,* is separate from self-cure or immune expulsion of primary infection. Infective larvae are expelled from the intestine in a matter of hours. Again, mechanisms of expulsion described vary between parasite and host species. However, anaphylactic reactions and mucus entrapment have been observed. Some experiments using the *T. spiralis*–rat system suggest that alterations in the epithelial cells in immune animals are directly involved in the exclusion of these parasites. Although immune-mediated damage of intestinal helminths such as decreased fecundity, reduced size, and morphologic alterations have been noted, infective larvae expelled by rapid expulsion mechanisms remain viable and undamaged. It may be speculated that reactions of this nature are responsible, in part, for resistance to reinfection of equines with cyathostomes.

Some specific observations have been made on the equine acquisition of resistance to reinfection with cyathostomins.[36] This resistance is acquired over time with continued exposure to pasture L3; is incomplete; and, like other parasitic helminth infections, appears to be genetically regulated in that parasite numbers are overdispersed within a given herd of adult animals. The limited number of experimental and field studies completed to date suggest that immunity may be directed toward all stages of the parasite life cycle. Challenge infections of previously exposed and naïve ponies with mixed strongyle infections indicate that a nonspecific self-cure–like phenomenon occurs, reducing numbers of adult and fourth stage larvae (L4) in the lumen as well as within the mucosa.[10] Fecal egg counts are significantly reduced in older animals when compared with yearlings even when adult parasite numbers are similar. These observations suggest that immune responses are directed at female fecundity or that the species of cyathostomins present in the older animals are inherently less fecund. Numbers of early L3 (EL3) are reduced following challenge infections of previously exposed adult ponies when compared with previously exposed young animals or age-matched naïve controls.[37] Other studies have suggested that acquired resistance is important in the induction of hypobiosis.[38,39] Resistance to acquisition of EL3 was not seen when numbers were compared in young previously exposed and age-matched ponies raised under parasite-free conditions. However, these previously exposed young animals demonstrated significantly fewer developing larvae (DL) in the mucosa, suggesting that once the EL3 began to develop, they were susceptible to immune attack.[37] This response is likely driven by cytokines produced by T cells of the Th2 lineage with demonstrated increases in IL-4 and IL-5.[40] This response mimics in some ways the results described in studies of murine nematodes.[29]

Tissue-migrating Parasites

A number of intestinal helminths as well as others migrate through extraintestinal tissues as part of their life cycle. These include parasites such as *P. equorum, S. westeri,* and *Strongylus* spp., all of which stimulate an acquired immune response in the horse. During this migration these larvae are vulnerable to attack by immune effectors that may either encapsulate them in an immune-mediated inflammatory response, disrupt their migrations by interfering with important metabolic or invasive processes, or inhibit molting from the L_3 to L_4 stages. The most studied phenomenon in this regard is antibody-mediated adherence of inflammatory cells, which may result in killing of the larvae. This phenomenon involves many cell types and immunoglobulin isotypes in different host-parasite systems.

In vitro studies of this nature have been conducted using *S. vulgaris* third-stage larvae and equine immune effectors.[41] In these experiments an antibody-dependent adherence of cells was demonstrated and shown to be parasite species-specific. In vitro killing was mediated by eosinophils and not by neutrophils or monocytes. Activated eosinophils were necessary to mediate this response, and *S. vulgaris* infections have been demonstrated to activate eosinophils and neutrophils in vivo.[42] Although it is not certain that eosinophils are essential in this protective immune response, an anamnestic eosinophilia is characteristic in immune ponies but not nonimmune ponies following experimental *S. vulgaris* challenge.[10] Because of its prominence and compelling in vitro and correlative in vivo data, the eosinophil is considered a major effector in immune-mediated helminth killing. However, recent studies in murine parasite model systems in which eosinophilia was blocked by anti-IL-5 treatment suggest that this type of cell is not essential for protective resistance in some systems.[43] Significant increases in equine IL-5 have been measured in ponies vaccinated against *S. vulgaris*. It is possible, in vivo, that a number of cells function as effectors and may overcome the absence of sufficient eosinophils under some circumstances. Antibody reactivity with parasite-secreted enzymes and molting fluids, factors important in parasite homeostasis, has been demonstrated in vitro; similar reactions may be important in vivo.

T-cell responses are essential for the induction of protective resistance to tissue-migrating helminths in most systems studied, including the experimental *S. vulgaris* pony model. This dependency is likely due to the T cell dependency of the antibody response and to the mediation of secondary effector cell responses. It is likely that antigenic substances secreted or excreted (ES) by migrating nematodes are important in the induction of these responses. It is probable that a combination of immune responses elicited by a combination of specific parasite antigens, including surface antigens and ES products, is necessary to induce an immune response sufficient to provide protective resistance.

PARASITE-INDUCED REGULATORY RESPONSES

Helminth parasites have evolved elaborate mechanisms to evade the host's immune responses, live in the face of an active specific host response, and yet establish chronic infections. These immune evasion strategies include the production and secretion of molecules such as proteases, protease inhibitors, antioxidants, prostaglandins, and phosphophrylcholin-antigens, which disrupt host effector responses.[44,45] Other molecules that mimic host immune regulatory factors, such as TGFβ and MIF, have also been identified in parasitic helminth genomes.[45] These mimics likely downregulate host-parasite–directed protective response and add to immune evasion.

Helminth parasites can induce a regulatory immune response, which promotes their survival but also has bystander effects on host responses to other infectious agents, vaccines, allergic responses, and autoimmune diseases. These observations have progressed to the point that helminth therapy is being developed for the treatment of human inflammatory bowel disease and ulcerative colitis.[46,47] In this situation infection with the swine whipworm *T. suis* impedes the regulation of type 1 inflammatory responses responsible for these conditions and reduces disease activity. The generally accepted and simple model that has emerged for this type of helminth-induced regulation is that parasite factors stimulate dendritic cells that activate regulatory T cells and alternately activated macrophages. These cells, through the production of TGF β and IL-10, may suppress both Th1- and Th2-mediated inflammatory responses.[48-50]

Detailed studies of the effects of equine helminths on the regulation of parasite-induced responses or to heterologous immunogens have not been reported. The effects of different levels of gastrointestinal helminth infection on the response of ponies to keyhole limpet hemocyanin immunization was measured.[51] Antibody levels determined by ELISA showed that animals with low levels of parasites had a trend toward increased KLH specific total immunoglobulin, IgG(T) and IgA compared with heavily parasitized ponies. Medium and heavily parasitized ponies demonstrated a trend toward reduced lymphoproliferative response to KLH that was not restored after the addition of IL-2. Cells from these ponies also produced significantly lower levels of IL-4 compared with lightly parasitized ponies. These data indicate that heavily parasitized animals have uniformly decreased cellular and humoral immune responses to soluble protein immunization. The mechanisms involved are unknown. The significance of these observations, particularly to vaccination against specific pathogens and the subsequent protective response to challenge infection, should be considered in the future.

REFERENCES

Mechanisms of Establishment and Spread of Bacterial and Fungal Infections

1. In Murray PR, Baron EJ, Jorgensen JH, et al, editors: *Manual of clinical microbiology*, ed 9, Washington DC, 2007, ASM Press.
2. Scott DW: *Large animal dermatology*, Philadelphia, 1988, Saunders.
3. Scott DW: Bacteria and yeast on the surface and within non-inflamed hair follicles of skin biopsies from dogs with non-neoplastic dermatoses, *Cornell Vet* 82:379-386, 1992.
4. Galuppo LD, Pascoe JR, Jang SS, Willits NHGSL: Evaluation of iodophor skin preparation techniques and factors influencing drainage from ventral midline incisions in horses, *J Am Vet Med Assoc* 215:963-969, 1999.
5. Nell A, James SA, Bond CJ, et al: Identification and distribution of a novel Malassezia species yeast on normal equine skin, *Vet Rec* 150:395-398, 2002.
6. Bailey GD, Love DN: Oral associated bacterial infection in horses; studies on the normal anaerobic flora from the pharyngeal tonsilar surface and its association with lower respiratory tract and paraoral infections, *Vet Microbiol* 15:367-379, 1991.
7. Crane SA, Ziemer EL, Sweeney CR: Cytologic and bacteriologic evaluation of tracheobronchial and aspirates from clinically normal foals, *Am J Vet Res* 50:2042-2048, 1989.
8. Moore CP, Heller N, Majors LJ, et al: Prevalence of ocular microorganisms in hospitalized and stabled horses, *Am J Vet Res* 49:773-777, 1988.
9. Koopman JP, Kennis HM, Millink JW, et al: Normalization of germ free mice with anaerobically cultured ceacal flora of normal mice, *Lab Anim* 18:188-194, 1984.
10. Blumberg RS, Saubermann LJ, Strober W: Animal models of inflammation and their relation to human inflammatory bowel disease, *Curr Opin Immunol* 11:648-656, 1999.
11. Makie RI, Wilkins CA: Enumeration of anearobic bacterial microflora of the equine gastrointestinal tract, *Appl Environ Microbiol* 54:2155-2160, 1988.
12. Yuki N, Shimazaki T, Kushiro A, et al: Colonization of the stratified squamous epithelium of the nonsecreting area of horse stomach by lactobacilli, *Appl Environ Microbiol* 66: 5030-5034, 2000.

13. Davies MK: Studies on the microbial flora of the large intestine of the horse by continuous culture in an artificial colon, *Vet Sci Commun* 3:39-44, 1979.
14. Jullinand V, de Vaux A, Millet L, Fonty G: Identification of *Ruminococcus flavefaciens* as the predominant cellulolytic bacteria species of the equine cecum, *Appl Environ Microbiol* 65:3738-3741, 1999.
15. Daly K, Stewart CS, Flint HJ, Shirazi-Beechey SP: Bacterial diversity within the equine large intestine as revealed by molecular analysis of cloned 16S rRNA genes 3, *Fems Microbiol Ecol* 38:141-151, 2001.
16. Maczulak AE, Dawson KABJP: Nitrogen utilization in bacterial isolates from the equine cecum, *Appl Environ Microbiol* 50:1439-1443, 1985.
17. Orpin CG: Isolation of cellulolytic phycomycete fungi from the caecum of the horse, *J Gen Microbiol* 123(Pt 2):287-296, 1981.
18. Traub-Dargatz JL, Garber LP, Fedorka-Cray PJ, et al: Fecal shedding of *Salmonella* spp by horses in the United States during 1998 and 1999 and detection of *Salmonella* spp in grain and concentrate sources on equine operations, *J Am Vet Med Assoc* 217:226-230, 2000.
19. Ward MP, Alinovi CA, Couetil LL, Wu CC: Evaluation of a PCR to detect Salmonella in fecal samples of horses admitted to a veterinary teaching hospital, *J Vet Diagn Invest* 17: 118-123, 2005.
20. Alinovi CA, Ward MP, Couetil LL, Wu CC: Detection of Salmonella organisms and assessment of a protocol for removal of contamination in horse stalls at a veterinary teaching hospital, *J Am Vet Med Assoc* 223:1640-1644, 2003.
21. Weese JS, Staempfli HR, Prescott JF: A prospective study of the roles of *Clostridium difficile* and enterotoxigenic *Clostridium perfingens* in equine diarrhoea, *Equine Vet J* 33:403-409, 2001.
22. Nakazawa M, Sugimoto C, Isayama Y: Quantitative culture of *Rhodococcus equi* from the feces of the horse, *Natl Instit Anim Health Q (Tokyo)* 23:67-68, 1983.
23. Woolcock JB, Mutimer MD, Farmer AM: Epidemiology of Corynebacterium in horses, *Res Vet Sci* 28:87-90, 1980.
24. Hinrichs K, Cummings MF, Sertrich PL, Kenney RM: Clinical significance of aerobic bacterial flora of the uterus, vagina, vestibule and clitoral fossa of clinically normal mares, *J Am Vet Med Assoc* 193:75, 1988.
25. Madsen M, Christensen P: Bacterial flora of semen collected from Danish warmblood stallions by artificial vagina, *Acta Vet Scand* 36:1-7, 1995.
26. Platt H, Atherton JG, Orskov L: *Klebsiella* and *Enterobacter* organisms isolated from horses, *J Hyg* 77:401-408, 1976.
27. Newcombe JR: Comparison of the bacterial flora of three sites in the genital tract of the mare, *Vet Rec* 102:160-170, 1978.
28. Giampaolo C, Scheld M, Boyd J, et al: Leukocyte and bacterial interrelationships in experimental meningitis, *Ann Neurol* 9:328-333, 1981.
29. Emslie KR, Ozanne NR, Nade SM: Acute haematogenous osteomyelitis: an experimental model, *J Pathol* 141:157-167, 1983.
30. Sanden G, Ljungh A, Wadstrom T, et al: Staphylococcal wound infection in the pig: part II. Inoculation, quantification of bacteria and reproducibility, *Ann Plas Surg* 23: 219-223, 1989.
31. Tenover FC, McDougal LK, Goering RV, et al: Characterization of a strain of community-associated methicillin-resistant Staphylococcus aureus widely disseminated in the United States, *J Clin Microbiol* 44:108-118, 2006.
32. Smith BP, Habasha F, Reina-Guerra M, Hardy AJ: Bovine salmonellosis: experimental production and characterization of the disease in calves, using oral challenge with *Salmonella typhoid, Am J Vet Res* 40:1510-1513, 1979.
33. Timoney JF, Kumar P: Early pathogenesis of equine Streptococcus equi infection (strangles), *Equine Vet J* 40:637-642, 2008.
34. Dorn R: *Escherichia coli* O157:H7, *J Am Vet Med Assoc* 206: 1583-1585, 1995.
35. Neu HC: The crisis in antibiotic resistance, *Science* 257: 1064-1073, 1992.
36. Finland M: Emergence of antibiotic resistance in hospitals, 1935-1975, *Rev Infect Dis* 1:4-22, 1979.
37. Amsden GW, Amankwa K: Pneumococcal resistance: the treatment challenge, *Ann Pharmacother* 35:480-488, 2001.
38. Charpentier E, Tuomanen E: Mechanisms of antibiotic resistance and tolerance in, *Streptococcus pneumoniae, Microbes Infect* 2:1855-1864, 2000.
39. Gillespie SH: Antibiotic resistance in the absence of selective pressure, *Int J Antimicrob Agents* 17:171-176, 2001.
40. Witte W: Antibiotic resistance in gram-positive bacteria: epidemiological aspects, *J Antimicrob Chemother* 44(Suppl A):1-9, 1999.
41. Goodson J, Tyznik WJ, Cline JH, Dehority BA: Effects of an abrupt diet change from hay to concentrate on microbial numbers and physical environment in the cecum of the pony, *Appl Environ Microbiol* 54:1946-1950, 1988.
42. Owen RS, Fullerton J, Barnum DA: Effects of transportation, surgery and antibiotic therapy in ponies infected with, *Salmonella, Am J Vet Res* 44:46-50, 1983.
43. Gustafsson A, Baverud V, Gunnarsson A, et al: The association of erythromycin ethylsuccinate with acute colitis in horses in Sweden, *Equine Vet J* 29:314-318, 1997.
44. Baverud V, Gustafsson A, Franklin A, et al: *Clostridium difficile* associated with acute colitis in mature horses treated with antibiotics, *Eq Vet J* 29:279-284, 1997.
45. Wilson DA, MacFadden KE, Green EM, et al: Case control and historical cohort study of diarrhea associated with administration of trimethoprim-potentiated sulphonamides to horses and ponies, *J Am Coll Vet Int Med* 10:258-264, 1996.
46. Hogenauer C, Hammer HF, Krejs GJ, Reisinger EC: Mechanisms and management of antibiotic-associated diarrhea, *Clin Infect Dis* 27:702-710, 1998.
47. Peeters TL, Matthijs G, Depoortere I, et al: Erythromycin is a motilin receptor agonist, *Am J Physiol* 257:G470-G474, 1989.
48. Lester GD, Merrit AM, Neuwirth L, et al: Effect of erythromycin lactobionate on myoelectric activity of ileum, cecum, and right ventral colon, and cecal emptying of radiolabeled markers in clinically normal ponies, *Am J Vet Res* 58:328-334, 1998.
49. Austin SM, Foreman JH, Hungerford LL: Case-control study of risk factors for development of pleuropneumonia in horses, *J Am Vet Med Assoc* 1995:325-328, 1995.
50. Raidal SL, Love DN, Bailey GD: Inflammation and increased numbers of bacteria in the lower respiratory tract of horses within 6 to 12 hours of confinement with the head elevated, *Austr Vet J* 72:45-50, 1995.
51. Raidal SL, Bailey GD, Love DN: Effect of transportation and lower respiratory tract contamination and peripheral blood neutrophil function, *Austr Vet J* 75:433-438, 1997.
52. Gaynes R, Richards C, Edwards J, et al: Feeding back surveillance date to prevent hospital-acquired infections, *Emerg Infect Dis* 7:295-298, 2001.
53. Boerlin P, Eugster S, Gaschen F, et al: Transmission of opportunistic pathogens in a veterinary teaching hospital, *Vet Microbiol* 82:347-359, 2001.
54. Colahan PT, Peyton LC, Connelly MR, Peterson R: *Serratia* spp. infection in 21 horses, *J Vet Med Sci* 185:209-211, 1984.
55. Weese JS, Baird JD, Poppe C, Archambault M: Emergence of *Salmonella typhimurium* definitive type 104 (DT 104) as an important cause of salmonellosis in horses in Ontario, *Can Vet J* 42:788-792, 2001.

56. Ikeda JS, Hirsh DC: Common plasmid encoding resistance to ampicillin, chloramphenical, gentamicin, and trimethroprim-sulfadiazine in two serotypes of *Salmonella* isolated during and outbreak of equine salmonellosis, *Am J Vet Res* 46:769-773, 1985.
57. Begg AP, Johnston KG, Hutchins DR, Edwards DJ: Some aspects of the epidemiology of equine salmonellosis, *Austr Vet J* 65:221-223, 1988.
58. Amavisit P, Markham PF, Lightfoot D, et al: Molecular epidemiology of *Salmonella* Heidelberg in an equine hospital, *Vet Microbiol* 80:85-98, 2001.
59. Gerlach RG, Hensel M: Protein secretion systems and adhesins: the molecular armory of Gram-negative pathogens, *Int J Med Microbiol* 297:401-415, 2007.
60. Fernandez LA, Berenguer J: Secretion and assembly of regular surface structures in Gram-negative bacteria, *FEMS Microbiol Rev* 24:21-44, 2000.
61. Salyers AA, Whitt DD: *Bacterial pathogenesis,* Washington, DC, 1994, ASM Press.
62. Wu H, Fives-Taylor PM: Molecular strategies for fimbrial expression and assembly 1, *Crit Rev Oral Biol Med* 12:101-115, 2001.
63. Hultgren SJ, Abraham S, Caparon M, et al: Pilus and non-pilus bacterial adhesins: assembly and function in cell recognition, *Cell* 73:887-901, 1993.
64. Proft T, Baker EN: Pili in Gram-negative and Gram-positive bacteria—structure, assembly and their role in disease, *Cell Mol Life Sci* 66:613-635, 2008.
65. Mandlik A, Swierczynski A, Das A, Ton-That H: Pili in Gram-positive bacteria: assembly, involvement in colonization and biofilm development, *Trends Microbiol* 16(1):33-40, 2008.
66. Tasteyr A, Barc MC, Collignon A, Boureau H, Karjalainen T: Role of FliC and FliD flagellar proteins of *Clostridium difficile* in adherence and gut colonization, *Infect Immun* 69: 7937-7940, 2001.
67. Wizemann TM, Moskovitz J, Pearce BJ, et al: Peptide methionine sulfoxide reductase contributes to the maintenance of adhesins in three major pathogens, *Proc Natl Acad Sci U S A* 93:7985-7990, 1996.
68. van der FM, Chhun N, Wizemann TM, et al: Adherence of *Streptococcus pneumoniae* to immobilized fibronectin, *Infect Immun* 63:4317-4322, 1995.
69. Gilot P, Andre P, Content J: *Listeria monocytogenes* possesses adhesins for fibronectin, *Infect Immun* 67:6698-6701, 1999.
70. Sinha B, Francois PP, Nusse O, et al: Fibronectin-binding protein acts as *Staphylococcus aureus* invasion via fibronectin bridging to integrin alpha5beta1, *Cell Microbiol* 1:101-117, 1999.
71. Sinha B, Francois P, Que YA, et al: Heterologously expressed *Staphylococcus aureus* fibronectin-binding proteins are sufficient for invasion of host cells, *Infect Immun* 68:6871-6878, 2000.
72. Rich RL, Kreikemeyer B, Owens RT, et al: Ace is a collagen-binding MSCRAMM from, *Enterococcus faecalis. J Biol Chem* 274:26939-26945, 1999.
73. Wizemann TM, Adamou JE, Langermann S: Adhesins as targets for vaccine development 2, *Emerg Infect Dis* 5:395-403, 1999.
74. Srivastava SK, Barnum DA: The role of lipoteichoic acids on the adherence of *Streptococcus equi* to epithelial cells, *Vet Microbiol* 8:485-492, 1983.
75. Colombo AV, Hirata R Jr, de Souza CM, et al: *Corynebacterium diphtheriae* surface proteins as adhesins to human erythrocytes, *FEMS Microbiol Lett* 197:235-239, 2001.
76. Smyth CJ, Marron MB, Twohig JMGJ, Smith SGJ: Fimbrial adhesins: similarities and variations in structure and biogenesis, *FEMS Immunol Med Microbiol* 16:127-139, 1996.
77. Bierne H, Gouin E, Roux P, et al: A role for cofilin and LIM kinase in *Listeria*-induced phagocytosis, *J Cell Biol* 55: 101-112, 2001.
78. Zhou D, Mooseker MS, Galan JE: An invasion-associated Salmonella protein modulates the actin-bundling activity of plastin, *Proc Natl Acad Sci USA* 96:10176-10181, 1999.
79. Reddy VM, Kumar B: Interaction of *Mycobacterium avium* complex with human respiratory epithelial cells, *J Infect Dis* 181:1189-1193, 2000.
80. Sangari FJ, Goodman J, Bermudez LE: *Mycobacterium avium* enters intestinal epithelial cells through the apical membrane, but not by the basolateral surface, activates small GTPase Rho and, once within epithelial cells, expresses an invasive phenotype, *Cell Microbiol* 2:561-568, 2000.
81. Griffith F: The significance of pnuemococcal types, *J Hyg* 47:89-115, 1928.
82. Avery OT, MacLoeon DM, McCarty M: Studies on the chemical nature of the substance inducing transformation of pneumococcal types. Induction of transformation by a deoxyribonucleic acid fraction isolated from pneumococcus type III, *J Exp Med* 79:137-158, 1944.
83. Srivastava SK, Barnum DA, Prescott JF: Production and biological properties of M-protein of, *Streptococcus equi, Res Vet Sci* 38:184-188, 1985.
84. Gilmour MI, Park PI, Selgrad MK: Ozone-enhanced pulmonary infection with *Streptococcus zooepidemicus* in mice. The role of alveolar macrophage function and capsular virulence factors, *Am Rev Respir Dis* 147:753-760, 1993.
85. Anzai T, Timoney JF, Kuwamoto Y, et al: In vivo pathogenicity and resistance to phagocytosis of *Streptococcus equi* strains with different levels of capsule expression, *Vet Microbiol* 67:277-286, 1999.
86. Whitfield C, Roberts IS: Structure, assembly and regulation of expression of capsules in, *Escherichia coli, Mol Microbiol* 31:1307-1319, 1999.
87. Amako K, Meno Y, Takade A: Fine structures of the capsules of *Klebsiella pneumoniae* and *Escherichia coli* K1, *J Bacteriol* 170:4960-4962, 1988.
88. Bortolussi R, Ferrieri P, Quie PG: Influence of growth temperature of Escherichia coli on K1 capsular antigen production and resistance to opsonization, *Infect Immun* 39:1136-1141, 1983.
89. Guze LB, Harwick HJ, Kalmanson GM: Klebsiella L-forms: effect of growth as L-form on virulence of reverted Klebsiella pneumoniae, *J Infect Dis* 133:245-252, 1976.
90. Takahashi M, Yoshida K: San Clemente CL: Relation of colonial morphologies in soft agar to morphological and biological properties of the K-9 strain of *Klebsiella pneumoniae* and its variants, *Can J Microbiol* 23:448-451, 1977.
91. Horwitz MA, Silverstein SC: Influence of the Escherichia coli capsule on complement fixation and on phagocytosis and killing by human phagocytes, *J Clin Invest* 65:82-94, 1980.
92. Wacharotayankun R, Arakawa Y, Ohta M, et al: Enhancement of extracapsular polysaccharide synthesis in Klebsiella pneumoniae by RmpA2, which shows homology to NtrC and FixJ, *Infect Immun* 61:3164-3174, 1993.
93. Tzianabos AO, Kasper DL, Onderdonk AB: Structure and function of *Bacteroides fragilis* capsular polysaccharides: relationship to induction and prevention of abscesses, *Clin Infect Dis* 20(Suppl 2):S132-S140, 1995.
94. Patrick S, Lutton DA, Crockard AD: Immune reactions to *Bacteroides fragilis* populations with three different types of capsule in a model of infection, *Microbiology* 141(Pt 8): 1969-1976, 1995.
95. Brook I: The role of encapsulated anaerobic bacteria in synergistic infections, *FEMS Microbiol Rev* 13:65-74, 1994.
96. Brook I: Encapsulated anaerobic bacteria in clinical infections, *Zentralbl Bakteriol* 279:443-446, 1993.
97. Tomas JM, Ciurana B, Benedi VJ, Juarez A: Role of lipopolysaccharide and complement in susceptibility of *Escherichia coli* and *Salmonella typhimurium* to non-immune serum, *J Gen Microbiol* 134(Pt 4):1009-1016, 1988.

98. Morrison DC, Brown DE, Vukajlovich SW, Ryan JL: Ganglioside modulation of lipopolysaccharide-initiated complement activation, *Mol Immunol* 22:1169-1176, 1985.
99. Jagels MA, Travis J, Potempa J, Pike R, Hugli TE: Proteolytic inactivation of the leukocyte C5a receptor by proteinases derived from, *Porphyromonas gingivalis, Infect Immun* 64: 1984-1991, 1996.
100. Hill HR, Bohnsack JF, Morris EZ, et al: Group B streptococci inhibit the chemotactic activity of the fifth component of complement, *J Immunol* 141:3551-3556, 1988.
101. Chanter N, Ward CL, Talbot NC, et al: Recombinant hyaluronate associated protein as a protective immunogen against *Streptococcus equi* and *Streptococcus zooepidemicus* challenge in mice, *Microb Pathog* 27:133-143, 1999.
102. Hoe NP, Kordari P, Cole R, et al: Human immune response to streptococcal inhibitor of complement, a serotype M1 group A *Streptococcus* extracellular protein involved in epidemics, *J Infect Dis* 182:1425-1436, 2000.
103. Johnsson E, Berggard K, Kotarsky H, et al: Role of the hypervariable region in streptococcal M proteins: binding of a human complement inhibitor, *J Immunol* 161:4894-4901, 1998.
104. Mitchell TJ: Virulence factors and the pathogenesis of disease caused by, *Streptococcus pneumoniae, Res Microbiol* 151: 413-419, 2000.
105. Timoney JF, Artiushin SC, Boschwitz JS: Comparison of the sequences and functions of *Streptococcus equi* M-like proteins SeM and SzPSe, *Infect Immun* 65:3600-3605, 1997.
106. Boschwitz JS, Timoney JF: Inhibition of C3 deposition on *Streptococcus equi* subsp. *equi* by M protein: a mechanism for survival in equine blood, *Infect Immun* 62:3515-3520, 1994.
107. Boschwitz JS, Timoney JF: Characterization of the antiphagocytic activity of equine fibrinogen for *Streptococcus equi* subsp, *equi, Microb Pathog* 17:121-129, 1994.
108. Goebel W, Chakraborty T, Domann E, et al: Studies on the pathogenicity of, *Listeria monocytogenes. Infection* 4 (Suppl 19):S195-S197, 1991.
109. Alvarez-Dominguez C, Roberts R, Stahl PD: Internalized *Listeria monocytogenes* modulates intracellular trafficking and delays maturation of the phagosome, *J Cell Sci* 110(Pt 6): 731-743, 1997.
110. Armstrong JA, Hart PD: Phagosome-lysosome interactions in cultured macrophages infected with virulent tubercle bacilli. Reversal of the usual nonfusion pattern and observations on bacterial survival, *J Exp Med* 142:1-16, 1975.
111. McDonough KA, Kress Y, Bloom BR: The interaction of *Mycobacterium tuberculosis* with macrophages: a study of phagolysosome fusion, *Infect Agents Dis* 2:232-235, 1993.
112. Oh YK, Alpuche-Aranda C, Berthiaume E, et al: Rapid and complete fusion of macrophage lysosomes with phagosomes containing Salmonella typhimurium, *Infect Immun* 64: 3877-3883, 1996.
113. Gallois A, Klein JR, Allen LA, et al: Salmonella pathogenicity island 2-encoded type III secretion system mediates exclusion of NADPH oxidase assembly from the phagosomal membrane, *J Immunol* 166:5741-5748, 2001.
114. Benoit S, Benachour A, Taouji S, et al: Induction of vap genes encoded by the virulence plasmid of *Rhodococcus equi* during acid tolerance response, *Res Microbiol* 152:439-449, 2001.
115. Zink MC, Yager JA, Prescott JF, Fernando MA: Electron microscopic investigation of intracellular events after ingestion of Rhodococcus equi by foal alveolar macrophages 3, *Vet Microbiol* 14:295-305, 1987.
116. Toyooka K, Takai S, Kirikae T: *Rhodococcus equi* can survive a phagolysosomal environment in macrophages by suppressing acidification of the phagolysosome 1, *J Med Microbiol* 54(Pt 11):1007-1015, 2005.
117. Pei Y, Nicholson V, Woods K, Prescott JF: Immunization by intrabronchial administration to 1-week-old foals of an unmarked double gene disruption strain of Rhodococcus equi strain 103+, *Vet Microbiol* 125:100-110, 2007.
118. Hietala SK, Ardans AA: Interaction of *Rhodococcus equi* with phagocytic cells from *R. equi*- exposed and non-exposed foals, *Vet Microbiol* 14:307-320, 1987.
119. Hantke K: Cloning of the repressor protein gene of iron-regulated systems in *Escherichia coli* K12, *Mol Gen Genet* 197:337-341, 1984.
120. Goldberg MB, Boyko SA, Calderwood SB: Positive transcriptional regulation of an iron-regulated virulence gene in Vibrio cholerae, *Proc Natl Acad Sci USA* 88:1125-1129, 1991.
121. Miranda-Casoluengo R, Duffy PS, O'Connell EP, et al: The iron-regulated iupABC operon is required for saprophytic growth of the intracellular pathogen Rhodococcus equi at low iron concentrations, *J Bacteriol* 187:3438-3444, 2005.
122. Neilands JB: Siderophores: structure and function of microbial iron transport compounds, *J Biol Chem* 270:26723-26726, 1995.
123. Wall DM, Duffy PS, Dupont C, et al: Isocitrate lyase activity is required for virulence of the intracellular pathogen, *Rhodococcus equi, Infect Immun* 73:6736-6741, 2005.
124. Dinges MM, Orwin PM, Schlievert PM: Exotoxins of Staphylococcus aureus, *Clin Microbiol Rev* 13:16-34, 2000.
125. Shimizu A, Kawano J, Ozaki J, et al: Characteristics of *Staphylococcus aureus* isolated from lesions of horses, *J Vet Med Sci* 53:601-606, 1991.
126. Sato H, Matsumori Y, Tanabe T, et al: A new type of staphylococcal exfoliative toxin from *Staphylococcus aureus* strain isolated from a horse with phlegmon, *Infect Immun* 62: 3780-3785, 1994.
127. Boyle-Vavra S, Daum RS: Community-acquired methicillin-resistant *Staphylococcus aureus*: the role of Panton-Valentine leukocidin, *Lab Invest* 87:3-9, 2007.
128. Diep BA, Palazzolo-Ballance AM, Tattevin P, et al: Contribution of Panton-Valentine leukocidin in community-associated methicillin-resistant Staphylococcus aureus pathogenesis, *PLoS ONE* 3(9):e3198, 2008.
129. Diep BA, Otto M: The role of virulence determinants in community-associated MRSA pathogenesis, *Trends Microbiol* 16:361-369, 2008.
130. Diep BA, Carleton HA, Chang RF, et al: Roles of 34 virulence genes in the evolution of hospital- and community-associated strains of methicillin-resistant Staphylococcus aureus, *J Infect Dis* 193:1495-1503, 2006.
131. Critchley EMR: A comparison of human and animal botulism: a review, *J R Soc Med* 84:295-298, 1991.
132. Ricketts SW, Greet TRC, Glyn PJ, et al: Thirteen cases of Botulism in horses fed big bale silage, *Equine Vet J* 16:515-516, 1984.
133. Kelley AP, Jones RT, Gillick JC, Sims LD: Outbreak of botulism in horses, *Equine Vet J* 16:519-521, 1984.
134. Swerczek TW: Toxicoinfectious botulism in foals and adult horses, *J Am Vet Med Assoc* 176:217-220, 1980.
135. Wichtel JJ, Whitlock RH: Botulism associated with feeding alfalfa hay to horses, *J Am Vet Med Assoc* 199:471-472, 1991.
136. Hathaway P: Toxigenic *Clostridia, Clin Microbiol Rev* 3:66-98, 1990.
137. Kaneo M, Inoue S, Abe T, et al: Isolation of *Clostridium perfingens* from foals, *Microbios* 64:153-158, 1990.
138. Donaldson MT, Palmer JE: Prevalence of *Clostridium perfingens* enterotoxin and *Clostridium difficile* toxin A in feces of horses with diarrhea and colic, *J Am Vet Med Assoc* 215: 358-361, 1999.
139. Howard-Martin M, Morton RJ, Qualls CW, MacAllister CG: *Clostridium perfingens* type C enterotoxemia in a newborn foal, *J Am Vet Med Assoc* 189:564-565, 1986.

140. Montgomery RF, Rowlands WT: Lamb dysentery" in a foal, *Vet Rec* 189:398-399, 1937.
141. Alape-Giron A, Flores-Diaz M, Guillouard I, et al: Identification of residues critical for toxicity of *Clostridium perfingens* phospholipase C, the key toxin in gas gangrene, *Eur J Biochem* 267:5191-5197, 2000.
142. Rood JI: Virulence genes of C. perfingens, *Annu Rev Microbiol* 52:330-360, 1998.
143. Tweten RK: *Clostridium perfingens* beta toxin and *Clostridium septicum* alpha toxin: their mechanisms and possible role in pathogenesis, *Vet Microbiol* 82:1-9, 2001.
144. Petit L, Maier E, Gilber M, et al: *Clostridium perfingens* epsilon toxin induces a rapid change of cell membrane permeability to ions and forms channels in artificial lipid bilayers, *J Biol Chem* 276:15736-15740, 2001.
145. Herholz C, Miserez R, Nocolet J, et al: Prevalence of beta2-toxigenic *Clostridium perfingens* in horses with intestinal disorders, *J Clin Microbiol* 37:358-361, 1999.
146. Pothoulakis C, Lamont JT: Microbes and microbial toxins: Paradigms for microbial-mucosal interactions II. The integrated response of the intestine to *Clostridium difficile* toxins, *Am J Physiol Gastrointest Liver Physiol* 2:G178-G183, 2001.
147. Borriello SP: Pathogenesis of *Clostridium difficile* infection, *J Antimicrob Chemother* 41(Supplement C):13-19, 1998.
148. Jefferson KK, Smith MF, Bobak DA: Roles of intracellular calcium and NF-kappa-Beta in the *Clostridium difficile* Toxin A-induced up-regulation and secretion of IL-8 from human monocytes, *J Immunol* 163:5183-5191, 1999.
149. Feltis BA, Wiesner SM, Kim AS, et al: *Clostridium difficile* toxins A and B can alter the epithelial permeability and promote bacterial paracellular migration through HT-29 enterocytes, *Shock* 14:629-634, 2000.
150. Gao LY, Kwaik YA: The modulation of host cell apoptosis by intracellular bacterial pathogens, *Trends Microbiol* 8:306-313, 2000.
151. Grassme H, Jendrossek V, Gulbins E: Molecular mechanisms of bacteria induced apoptosis, *Apoptosis* 6:441-445, 2001.
152. Yrlid U, Wick MJ: Salmonella-induced apoptosis of infected macrophages results in presentation of a bacteria-encoded antigen after uptake by bystander dendritic cells 4, *J Exp Med* 191:613-624, 2000.
153. Bulawa CE, Miller DW, Henry LK, Becker JM: Attenuated virulence of chitin-deficient mutants of, *Candida albicans, Proc Natl Acad Sci U S A* 92:10570-10574, 1995.
154. Buurman ET, Westwater C, Hube B, et al: Molecular analysis of CaMnt1p, a mannosyl transferase important for adhesion and virulence of *Candida albicans, Proc Natl Acad Sci U S A* 95:7670-7675, 1998.
155. Fu Y, Rieg G, Fonzi WA, et al: Expression of the *Candida albicans* gene ALS1 in *Saccharomyces cerevisiae* induces adherence to endothelial and epithelial cells, *Infect Immun* 66: 1783-1786, 1998.
156. Gale CA, Bendel CM, McClellan M, et al: Linkage of adhesion, filamentous growth, and virulence in *Candida albicans* to a single gene, INT1, *Science* 279(5355):1355-1358, 1998.
157. Kinneberg KM, Bendel CM, Jechorek RP, et al: Effect of INT1 gene on *Candida albicans* murine intestinal colonization, *J Surg Res* 87(2):245-251, 1999.
158. Newman SL, Chaturvedi S, Klein BS: The WI-1 antigen of *Blastomyces dermatitidis* yeasts mediates binding to human macrophage CD11b/CD18 (CR3) and CD14, *J Immunol* 154:753-761, 1995.
159. Fries BC, Taborda CP, Serfass E, Casadevall A: Phenotypic switching of *Cryptococcus neoformans* occurs in vivo and influences the outcome of infection, *J Clin Invest* 108: 1639-1648, 2001.
160. Rotrosen D, Edwards JE Jr, Gibson TR, Moore JC, Cohen AH, Green I: Adherence of *Candida* to cultured vascular endothelial cells: mechanisms of attachment and endothelial cell penetration, *J Infect Dis* 152:1264-1274, 1985.
161. Eissenberg LG, Goldman WE: *Histoplasma capsulatum* fails to trigger release of superoxide from macrophages, *Infect Immun* 55:29-34, 1987.
162. Eissenberg LG, Schlesinger PH, Goldman WE: Phagosome-lysosome fusion in P388D1 macrophages infected with Histoplasma capsulatum, *J Leukoc Biol* 43:483-491, 1988.
163. Eissenberg LG, Poirier S, Goldman WE: Phenotypic variation and persistence of *Histoplasma capsulatum* yeasts in host cells, *Infect Immun* 64:5310-5314, 1996.
164. Lo HJ, Kohler JR, DiDomenico B, Loebenberg D, Cacciapuoti A, Fink GR: Nonfilamentous *C. albicans* mutants are avirulent, *Cell* 90:939-949, 1997.
165. Kvaal C, Lachke SA, Srikantha T, Daniels K, McCoy J, Soll DR: Misexpression of the opaque-phase-specific gene PEP1 (SAP1) in the white phase of *Candida albicans* confers increased virulence in a mouse model of cutaneous infection, *Infect Immun* 67:6652-6662, 1999.
166. Fries BC, Goldman DL, Cherniak R, Ju R, Casadevall A: Phenotypic switching in *Cryptococcus neoformans* results in changes in cellular morphology and glucuronoxylomannan structure, *Infect Immun* 67:6076-6083, 1999.
167. Eissenberg LG, Moser SA, Goldman WE: Alterations to the cell wall of *Histoplasma capsulatum* yeasts during infection of macrophages or epithelial cells, *J Infect Dis* 175:1538-1544, 1997.
168. Cruz MC, Sia RA, Olson M, et al: Comparison of the roles of calcineurin in physiology and virulence in serotype D and serotype A strains of Cryptococcus neoformans, *Infect Immun* 68:982-985, 2000.
169. Joseph JD, Heitman J, Means AR: Molecular cloning and characterization of *Aspergillus nidulans* cyclophilin B, *Fungal Genet Biol* 27:55-66, 1999.
170. De Bernardis F, Muhlschlegel FA, Cassone A, Fonzi WA: The pH of the host niche controls gene expression in and virulence of, *Candida albicans, Infect Immun* 66:3317-3325, 1998.
171. Doering TL, Nosanchuk JD, Roberts WK, Casadevall A: Melanin as a potential cryptococcal defence against microbicidal proteins, *Med Mycol* 37:175-181, 1999.
172. Howard DH: Acquisition, transport, and storage of iron by pathogenic fungi, *Clin Microbiol Rev* 12:394-404, 1999.
173. Holzberg M, Artis WM: Hydroxamate siderophore production by opportunistic and systemic fungal pathogens, *Infect Immun* 40:1134-1139, 1983.
174. Woods JP, Heinecke EL, Luecke JW, et al: Pathogenesis of Histoplasma capsulatum, *Semin Respir Infect* 16:91-101, 2001.
175. Sebghati TS, Engle JT, Goldman WE: Intracellular parasitism by *Histoplasma capsulatum*: fungal virulence and calcium dependence, *Science* 290:1368-1372, 2000.
176. van Burik JA, Magee PT: Aspects of fungal pathogenesis in humans, *Annu Rev Microbiol* 55:743-772, 2001.
177. Hube B: *Candida albicans* secreted aspartyl proteinases, *Curr Top Med Mycol* 7:55-69, 1996.
178. Resnick S, Pappagianis D, McKerrow JH: Proteinase production by the parasitic cycle of the pathogenic fungus, *Coccidioides immitis, Infect Immun* 55:2807-2815, 1987.
179. Yuan L, Cole GT: Isolation and characterization of an extracellular proteinase of Coccidioides immitis, *Infect Immun* 55:1970-1978, 1987.
180. Yu JJ, Smithson SL, Thomas PW, et al: Isolation and characterization of the urease gene (URE) from the pathogenic fungus, *Coccidioides immitis, Gene* 198:387-391, 1997.
181. Iadarola P, Lungarella G, Martorana PA, et al: Lung injury and degradation of extracellular matrix components by *Aspergillus fumigatus* serine proteinase, *Exp Lung Res* 24: 233-251, 1998.

182. Rodriguez E, Boudard F, Mallie M, Bastide JM, Bastide M: Murine macrophage elastolytic activity induced by *Aspergillus fumigatus* strains in vitro: evidence of the expression of two macrophage-induced protease genes, *Can J Microbiol* 43:649-657, 1997.
183. Ghannoum MA: Potential role of phospholipases in virulence and fungal pathogenesis, *Clin Microbiol Rev* 13:122-143, 2000.
184. Mitrovic S, Kranjcic-Zec I, Arsic V, Dzamic A: In vitro proteinase and phospholipase activity and pathogenicity of *Candida* species, *J Chemother* 4(Suppl 7):43-45, 1995.
185. Prakobphol A, Leffler H, Hoover CI, Fisher SJ: Palmitoyl carnitine, a lysophospholipase-transacylase inhibitor, prevents *Candida* adherence in vitro, *FEMS Microbiol Lett* 151:89-94, 1997.
186. Noverr MC, Toews GB, Huffnagle GB: Production of prostaglandins and leukotrienes by pathogenic fungi, *Infect Immun* 70:400-402, 2002.
187. Mendes-Giannini MJ, Taylor ML, Bouchara JB, et al: Pathogenesis II: fungal responses to host responses: interaction of host cells with fungi, *Med Mycol* 38(Suppl 1):113-123, 2000.
188. Golden MC, Hahm SJ, Elessar RE, et al: DNA damage by gliotoxin from *Aspergillus fumigatus*. An occupational and environmental propagule: adduct detection as measured by 32P DNA radiolabelling and two-dimensional thin-layer chromatography, *Mycoses* 41:97-104, 1998.

Mechanisms of Establishment and Spread of Viral Infections

1. Castro AE, Heuschele WP, editors: *Veterinary diagnostic virology*, St Louis, 1992, Mosby.
2. Herbst W, Gorlich P, Danner K: Virologico-serologic studies in horses with respiratory tract diseases, *Berl Munch Tierarztl Wochenschr* 105:49, 1992.
3. Telford EAR, Studdert MJ, Agius CT, et al: Equine herpesviruses 2 and 5 are gamma-herpesviruses, *Virology* 195:492, 1993.
4. Bock M, Stoye JP: Endogenous retroviruses and the human germline, *Curr Opin Genet Dev* 10:651, 2000.
5. Selvey LA, Wells RM, McCormack JG, et al: Infection of humans and horses by a newly described morbillivirus, *Med J Aust* 162:642, 1995.
6. Renshaw RW, Glaser AL, Van Campen H, et al: Identification and phylogenetic comparison of Salem virus, a novel paramyxovirus of horses, *Virology* 270:417, 2000.
7. Carr EA, Theon AP, Madewell BR, et al: Bovine papillomavirus DNA in neoplastic and nonneoplastic tissues obtained from horses with and without sarcoids in the western United States, *Am J Vet Res* 62:741, 2001.
8. Carr EA, Theon AP, Madewell BR, et al: Expression of a transforming gene (E5) of bovine papillomavirus in sarcoids obtained from horses, *Am J Vet Res* 62:1212, 2001.
9. Tennant B: Acute hepatitis in horses: problems of differentiating toxic and infectious causes in the adult, *Proc Am Assoc Equine Pract* 24:465, 1978.
10. Tomlinson MJ, Doster AR, Wright ER: Lymphosarcoma with virus-like particles in a neonatal foal, *Vet Pathol* 16:629, 1979.
11. Mason A: Viral induction of type 2 diabetes and autoimmune liver disease, *J Nutr* 131:2805S, 2001.
12. Dhurandhar NV: Infectobesity: obesity of infectious origin, *J Nutr* 131:2794S, 2001.
13. Murray MJ, del Piero F, Jeffrey SC, et al: Neonatal equine herpesvirus type 1 infection on a thoroughbred breeding farm, *J Vet Intern Med* 12:36, 1998.
14. Rees WA, Harkins JD, Lu M, et al: Pharmacokinetics and therapeutic efficacy of rimantadine in horses experimentally infected with influenza virus A2, *Am J Vet Res* 60:888, 1999.
15. In Murphy FA, Gibbs EPJ, Horzinek MC, et al, editors: *Veterinary virology*, ed 3, San Diego, 1999, Academic Press.
16. Flint SJ, Enquist LW, Krug RM, et al: *Virology: molecular biology, pathogenesis, and control*, Washington DC, 2000, ASM Press.
17. De Clercq E: In search of a selective antiviral chemotherapy, *Clin Microbiol Rev* 10:674, 1997.
18. Bean B: Antiviral therapy: current concepts and practices, *Clin Microbiol Rev* 5:146, 1992.
19. Preston BD, Dougherty JP: Mechanisms of retroviral mutation, *Trends Microbiol* 4:16, 1996.
20. Domingo E, Baranowski E, Ruiz-Jarabo CM: Quasispecies structure and persistence of RNA viruses, *Emerg Infect Dis* 4:521, 1998.
21. Scholtissek C: Molecular epidemiology of influenza, *Arch Virol* 13(suppl):99, 1997.
22. Steinhauer DA: Role of hemagglutinin cleavage for the pathogenicity of influenza virus, *Virology* 258:1, 1999.
23. Skehel JJ, Wiley DC: Receptor binding and membrane fusion in virus entry: the influenza hemagglutinin, *Annu Rev Biochem* 69:531, 2000.
24. Ito T, Kawaoka Y: Host-range barrier of influenza A viruses, *Vet Microbiol* 74:71, 2000.
25. Kuhlenschmidt MS, Rolsma MD, Kuhlenschmidt TB, et al: Characterization of a porcine enterocyte receptor for group A rotavirus, *Adv Exp Med Biol* 412:135, 1997.
26. Weinstein L: Influence of age and sex on susceptibility and clinical manifestations in poliomyelitis, *N Engl J Med* 257:47, 1957.
27. De Beek O: Caillet-Fauquet: Viruses and the cell cycle, *Prog Cell Cycle Res* 3:1, 1997.
28. Sinclair J, Baille J, Bryant L, et al: Human cytomegalovirus mediates cell cycle progression through G(1) into early S phase in terminally differentiated cells, *J Gen Virol* 81:1553, 2000.
29. Berns KI: Parvovirus replication, *Microbiol Rev* 54:316, 1990.
30. Puvion-Dutilleul F, Besse S, Pichard E, et al: Release of viruses and viral DNA from nucleus to cytoplasm of HeLa cells at late stages of productive adenovirus infection as revealed by electron microscope in situ hybridization, *Biol Cell* 90:5, 1998.
31. Thomson BJ: Viruses and apoptosis, *Int J Exp Pathol* 82:65, 2001.
32. Moore M, Horikoshi N, Shenk T: Oncogenic potential of the adenovirus E4orf6 protein, *Proc Natl Acad Sci U S A* 93:11295, 1996.
33. Sullivan DC, Atherton SS, Caughman GB, et al: Oncogenic transformation of primary hamster embryo cells by equine herpesvirus type 3, *Virus Res* 5:201, 1986.
34. de The Gde: Epstein-Barr virus and associated diseases: course of medical virology, Institut Pasteur, 1995/1996, *Ann Med Interne (Paris)* 148:357, 1997.
35. Burmeister T: Oncogenic retroviruses in animals and humans, *Rev Med Virol* 11:369, 2001.
36. Haig DM: Subversion and piracy: DNA viruses and immune evasion, *Res Vet Sci* 70:205, 2001.
37. Young DF, Didcock L, Goodbourn S, et al: Paramyxoviridae use distinct virus-specific mechanisms to circumvent the interferon response, *Virology* 10:383, 2000.
38. Xiao-Ning X, Screaton GR, McMichael AJ: Virus infections: escape, resistance, and counterattack, *Immunity* 15:867, 2001.
39. Tomasec P, Braud VM, Richards C, et al: Surface expression of HLA-E, an inhibitor of natural killer cells, enhanced by human cytomegalovirus gpUL40, *Science* 287:1031, 2000.
40. Haig DM: Poxvirus interference with the host cytokine response, *Vet Immunol Immunopathol* 63:149, 1998.
41. Garcia-Blanco MA, Cullen BR: Molecular basis of latency in pathogenic human viruses, *Science* 254:815, 1991.
42. Welch HM, Bridges CG, Lyon AM, et al: Latent equid herpesviruses 1 and 4: detection and distinction using the polymerase chain reaction and co-cultivation from lymphoid tissues, *J Gen Virol* 73:261, 1992.
43. Borchers K, Wolfinger U, Lawrenz B, et al: Equine herpesvirus 4 DNA in trigeminal ganglia of naturally infected horses detected by direct in situ PCR, *J Gen Virol* 78:1109, 1997.

44. Edington N, Bridges CG: Experimental reactivation of equid herpesvirus 1 (EHV 1) following the administration of corticosteroids, *Equine Vet J* 17:369, 1985.
45. Padgett DA, Sheridan JF, Dorne J, et al: Social stress and the reactivation of latent herpes simplex virus type 1, *Proc Natl Acad Sci U S A* 95:7231, 1998.
46. Chowdhury SI, Kubin G, Ludwig H: Equine herpesvirus type 1 (EHV-1) induced abortions and paralysis in a Lippizaner stud: a contribution to the classification of equine herpesviruses, *Arch Virol* 90:273, 1986.
47. Matsumura T, Kondo T, Sugita S, et al: An equine herpesvirus type 1 recombinant with a deletion in the gE and gI genes is avirulent in young horses, *Virology* 242:68, 1998.
48. Crawford TB, Wardrop KJ, Tornquist SJ, et al: A primary production deficit in the thrombocytopenia of equine infectious anemia, *J Virol* 70:7842, 1996.
49. Oaks JL, McGuire TC, Ulibarri C, et al: Equine infectious anemia virus is found in tissue macrophages during subclinical infection, *J Virol* 72:7263, 1998.
50. Maury W, Perryman S, Oaks JL, et al: Localized sequence heterogeneity in the LTR of in vivo isolates of equine infectious anemia virus, *J Virol* 71:4929, 1997.
51. Belshan M, Baccam P, Oaks JL, et al: Genetic and biological variation in equine infectious anemia virus rev correlates with variable stages of clinical disease in an experimentally infected pony, *Virology* 279:185, 2001.
52. Jacob RJ, Price R, Bouchey D, et al: Temperature sensitivity of equine herpesvirus isolates: a brief review, *SAAS Bull Biochem Biotechnol* 3:124, 1990.
53. Gaskell R, Dawson S: Feline respiratory diseases. In Greene CE, editor: *Infectious diseases of the dog and cat*, Philadelphia, 1998, WB Saunders.
54. Younger JS, Whitaker-Dowling P, Chambers TM, et al: Derivation and characterization of a live attenuated equine influenza vaccine virus, *Am J Vet Res* 62:1290, 2001.
55. Cravens RL, Ellsworth MA, Sorensen CD, et al: Efficacy of a temperature-sensitive modified-live bovine herpesvirus type-1 vaccine against abortion and stillbirth in pregnant heifers, *J Am Vet Med Assoc 208*:2031, 1996.
56. Fenner F, Mousepox: (infectious ectromelia of mice): a review, *J Immunol* 63:341, 1949.
57. Calisher CH: Medically important arboviruses of the United States and Canada, *Clin Microbiol Rev* 7:89, 1994.
58. Walker C, Love DN, Whalley JM: Comparison of the pathogenesis of acute equine herpesvirus 1 (EHV-1) infection in the horse and the mouse model: a review, *Vet Microbiol* 68:3, 1999.
59. Edington N, Smyth B, Griffiths L: The role of endothelial cell infection in the endometrium, placenta and foetus of equid herpesvirus 1 (EHV-1) abortions, *J Comp Pathol* 104:379, 1991.
60. Whitwell KE, Blunden AS: Pathological findings in horses dying during an outbreak of the paralytic form of equid herpesvirus type 1 (EHV-1) infection, *Equine Vet J* 24:13, 1992.
61. Green SL: Rabies. Vet Clin North, *Am Equine Pract* 13:1, 1997.
62. Baxi MK, Efstathiou S, Lawrence G, et al: The detection of latency-associated transcripts of equine herpesvirus 1 in ganglionic neurons, *J Gen Virol* 76:3113, 1995.
63. Sutton GA, Viel L, Carman PS, et al: Pathogenesis and clinical signs of equine herpesvirus-1 in experimentally infected ponies in vivo, *Can J Vet Res* 62:49, 1998.
64. Yates WD: A review of infectious bovine rhinotracheitis, shipping fever pneumonia and viral-bacterial synergism in respiratory disease of cattle, *Can J Comp Med* 46:225, 1982.
65. Allan JE, Dixon JE, Doherty PC: Nature of the inflammatory process in the central nervous system of mice infected with lymphocytic choriomeningitis, *Curr Top Microbiol Immunol* 134:131, 1987.
66. Clabough DL, Gebhard D, Flaherty MT, et al: Immune-mediated thrombocytopenia in horses infected with equine infectious anemia virus, *J Virol* 65:6242, 1991.
67. Clabough DL: The immunopathogenesis and control of equine infectious anemia, *Equine Pract* 85:1020, 1990.
68. Sullivan NJ: Antibody-mediated enhancement of viral disease, *Curr Top Microbiol Immunol* 260:145, 2001.
69. Hohdatsu T, Yamada M, Tominaga R, et al: Antibody-dependent enhancement of feline infectious peritonitis virus infection in feline alveolar macrophages and human monocyte cell line U937 by serum of cats experimentally or naturally infected with feline coronavirus, *J Vet Med Sci* 60:49, 1998.
70. Openshaw PJ, Culley FJ, Olszewska W: Immunopathogenesis of vaccine-enhanced RSV disease, *Vaccine* 20(suppl 1):S27, 2001.
71. Mady BJ, Erbe DV, Kurane I, et al: Antibody-dependent enhancement of dengue virus infection mediated by bispecific antibodies against cell surface molecules other than Fc gamma receptors, *J Immunol* 147:3139, 1991.
72. Van Reeth K: Cytokines in the pathogenesis of influenza, *Vet Microbiol* 74:109, 2000.
73. Herbein G, O'Brien WA: Tumor necrosis factor (TNF)-alpha and TNF receptors in viral pathogenesis, *Proc Soc Exp Biol Med* 223:241, 2000.
74. Tornquist SJ, Oaks JL, Crawford TB: Elevation of cytokines associated with the thrombocytopenia of equine infectious anaemia, *J Gen Virol* 78:2541, 1997.
75. Winer JB: Guillain-Barré syndrome, *Mol Pathol* 54:381, 2001.
76. Nolte KB, Alakija P, Oty G, et al: Influenza A virus infection complicated by fatal myocarditis, *Am J Forensic Med Pathol* 21:375, 2000.
77. Evermann JF, Heeney JL, Roelke ME, et al: Biological and pathological consequences of feline infectious peritonitis virus infection in the cheetah, *Arch Virol* 102:155, 1988.
78. Murakami T, Yamamoto N: Roles of cytokines and chemokine receptors in HIV-1 infection, *Int J Hematol* 72:412, 2000.
79. Carrington M, Nelson G, O'Brien SJ: Considering genetic profiles in functional studies of immune responsiveness to HIV-1, *Immunol Lett* 79:131, 2001.
80. Crowe JE Jr, Suara RO, Brock S, et al: Genetic and structural determinants of virus neutralizing antibodies, *Immunol Res* 23:135, 2001.
81. Copeland KF, Heeney JL: T helper cell activation and human retroviral pathogenesis, *Microbiol Rev* 60:722, 1996.
82. Brown WC, Rice-Ficht AC, Estes DM: Bovine type 1 and type 2 responses, *Vet Immunol Immunopathol* 63:45, 1998.
83. Karupiah G, Type: 1 and type 2 cytokines in antiviral defense, *Vet Immunol Immunopathol* 63:105, 1998.
84. Kong XG, Pang H, Sugiura T, et al: Evaluation of equine infectious anemia virus core proteins produced in a baculovirus expression system in agar gel immunodiffusion test and enzyme-linked immunosorbent assay, *J Vet Med Sci* 60:1361, 1998.
85. Soutullo A, Verwimp V, Riveros M, et al: Design and validation of an ELISA for equine infectious anemia (EIA) diagnosis using synthetic peptides, *Vet Microbiol* 79:111, 2001.
86. Kanai K, Nunoya T, Shibuya K, et al: Variations in effectiveness of antigen retrieval pretreatments for diagnostic immunohistochemistry, *Res Vet Sci* 64:57, 1998.
87. Patteson JS, Maes RK, Mullaney TP, et al: Immunohistochemical diagnosis of eastern equine encephalomyelitis, *J Vet Diagn Invest* 8:156, 1996.
88. Del Piero F: Diagnosis of equine arteritis virus infection in two horses by using monoclonal antibody immunoperoxidase histochemistry on skin biopsies, *Vet Pathol* 37:486, 2000.
89. Hooper PT, Russell GM, Selleck PW, et al: Immunohistochemistry in the identification of a number of new diseases in Australia, *Vet Microbiol* 68:89, 1999.
90. Belak S, Thoren P: Molecular diagnosis of animal diseases: some experiences over the past decade, *Expert Rev Mol Diagn* 1:434, 2001.
91. Mackay IM, Arden KE, Nitsche A: Real-time PCR in virology, *Nucleic Acids Res* 30:1292, 2002.

Internal Parasite Infections

1. Jacobs DE: *A colour atlas of equine parasites*, Philadelphia, 1986, Lea & Febiger.
2. Slocombe JOD: Pathogenesis of helminths in equines, *Vet Parasitol* 18:139, 1985.
3. Symons LEA: *Pathophysiology of endoparasitic infection compared with ectoparasitic infestation and microbial infection*, San Diego, 1989, Academic Press.
4. Fox MT: Pathophysiology of infection with gastrointestinal nematodes in domestic ruminants: recent developments, *Vet Parasitol* 72:285-297, 1997.
5. Herd RP: *The Veterinary Clinics of North America Equine Practice*, Philadelphia, 1986, WB Saunders, vol 2: Parasitology.
6. McCraw BM, Slocombe JOD: *Early development of Strongylus vulgaris in pony foals (abstr), Proc Am Assoc Vet Parasitol* 57.
7. Klei TR: *Recent observations on the epidemiology, pathogenesis and immunology of equine helminth infections. Proceedings of the 6th International Conference on Equine Infectious Diseases*, Newmarket, 1991, R&W Publications, pp 129-136.
8. Klei TR, Turk MAM, McClure JR, et al: Effects of repeated experimental *Strongylus vulgaris* infections and subsequent ivermectin treatment on mesenteric arterial pathology in pony foals, *Am J Vet Res* 51:54, 1990.
9. Holmes RA, Klei TR, McClure JR, et al: Sequential mesenteric arteriography in pony foals during a course of repeated experimental *Strongylus vulgaris* infections and ivermectin treatments, *Am J Vet Res* 51:661, 1990.
10. Monahan CM, Taylor HW, Chapman MR, Klei TR: Experimental immunization of ponies with Strongylus vulgaris radiation-attenuated larvae or crude soluble somatic extracts from larval or adult stages, *J Parasitol* 80:911-923, 1994.
11. Clayton HM: Ascarids: Recent advances. In Herd RP, editor: *The veterinary clinics of North America equine practice parasitology*, Philadelphia, 1986, WB Saunders, pp 313.
12. Lyons ET, Tolliver SC, Ionita M, Collins SS: Evaluation of parasiticidal activity of fenbendazole, ivermectin, oxibendazole, and pyrantel pamoate in horse foals with emphasis on ascarids (Parascaris equorum) in field studies on five farms in Central Kentucky in 2007, *Parasitol Res* 103:287-291, 2008.
13. Beroza GA, Barclay WP, Phillips TN, et al: Cecal perforation and peritonitis associated with *Anoplocephala perfoliata* infection in three horses, *J Am Vet Med Assoc* 183:804, 1983.
14. Barclay WP, Phillips TN, Foerner JJ: Intussusception associated with, *Anoplocephala perfoliata, Vet Rec* 124:34, 1989.
15. Owen RR, Jagger DW, Quan-Taylor R: Cecal intussusceptions in horses and the significance of, *Anoplocephala perfoliata, Vet Rec* 124:34, 1989.
16. Proudman CJ, Edwards GB, Gareth B: Are tapeworms associated with equine colic? A case control study, *Equine Vet J* 25:224, 1993.
17. Proudman CJ, French NP, Trees AJ: Tapeworm infection is a significant risk factor for spasmodic colic and ileal impaction colic in the horse, *Equine Vet J* 30:194-199, 1998.
18. Uhlinger CA: Effects of three anthelmintic schedules on the incidence of colic, *Equine Vet J* 22:251, 1991.
19. Uhlinger CA: Equine small strongyles: epidemiology, pathology and control, *Compend Contin Educ Pract Vet* 13:863, 1991.
20. Love S, Murphy D, Mellor D: Pathogenicity of cyathostome infection, *Vet Parasitol* 85:113-121, 1999.
21. Murphy D, Love S: The pathogenic effects of experimental cyathostome infections in ponies, *Vet Parasitol* 70:99-110, 1997.
22. Castro GA: Immunophysiology of enteric parasitism, *Parasitol Today* 5:11, 1989.
23. Bueno L, Ruckenbusch Y, Dorchies PH: Disturbances of digestive motility in horses associated with strongyle infection, *Vet Parasitol* 5:253, 1979.
24. Lester GD, Bolton JR, Cambridge H, et al: The effect of *Strongylus vulgaris* larvae on the equine intestinal myoelectrical activity, *Equine Vet J Suppl* 7:8, 1989.
25. Berry CR, Merrit AM, Burrows CF, et al: Evaluation of the myoelectrical activity of the equine ileum infected with *Strongylus vulgaris* larvae, *Am J Vet Res* 87:27, 1986.
26. Artis D: New weapons in the war on worms: identification of putative mechanisms of immune-mediated expulsion of gastrointestinal nematodes, *Int J Parasitol* 31:723-733, 2006.
27. Finkelman FD, Shea-Donohue T, Goldhill J, et al: Cytokine regulation of host defense against parasitic gastrointestinal nematodes: lessons from studies with rodent models, *Annu Rev Immunol* 15:505-533, 1997.
28. Maizels RM, Yazdanbakhsh M: Immune regulation by helminth parasites: cellular and molecular mechanisms, *Nat Rev Immunol* 9:733-744, 2003.
29. Patel N, Kreider T, Urban JF Jr, Gause WC: Characterisation of effector mechanisms at the host:parasite interface during the immune response to tissue-dwelling intestinal nematode parasites, *Int J Parasitol* 39:13-21, 2009.
30. In Soulsby EJL, editor: *Immune responses in parasitic infections: immunology, immunopathology and immunoprophylaxis, Nematodes,* Boca Raton, Fla, 1987, CRC Press, vol. 1.
31. King CL, Nutman TB: Regulation of immune responses in lymphatic filariasis and onchocerciasis, *Immunol Today* 3:A54, 1991.
32. Allen JE, Adjei O, Bain O, et al: Of mice, cattle, and humans: the immunology and treatment of river blindness, *PLoS Negl Trop Dis* 30:e217, 2008.
33. Foil LD, Klei TR, Miller RI, et al: Seasonal changes in density and tissue distribution of *Onchocerca cervicalis* microfilariae in ponies and related changes in *Culicoides varnipennis* populations in Louisiana, *J Parasitol* 73:320, 1987.
34. Ogbourne CP, Duncan JR: *Strongylus vulgaris in the Horse: Its Biology and Veterinary Importance,* ed 2. Misc. Pub. No. 9. St. Albans, U.K., Commonwealth Institute of Parasitology.
35. Murrell KD: Induction of protective immunity to *Strongyloides ransomi* in pigs, *Am J Vet Res 42* :1981, 1915.
36. Klei TR, Chapman MR: Immunity in equine cyathostome infections, *Vet Parasitol* 199; 85: 123-133.
37. Monahan CM, Chapman MR, Taylor HW, et al: Experimental cyathostome challenge of ponies maintained with or without benefit of daily pyrantel tartrate feed additive: comparison of parasite burdens, immunity and colonic pathology, *Vet Parasitol* 31:229-241, 1998.
38. Murphy D, Love S: The pathogenic effects of experimental cyathostome infections in ponies, *Vet Parasitol* :99-110, 1997.
39. Chapman MR, French DD, Taylor HW, Klei TR: One season of pasture exposure fails to induce a protective resistance to cyathostomes but increases numbers of hypobiotic third-stage larvae, *J Parasitol* 88:678-683, 2002.
40. Klei TR, et al: Unpublished data
41. Klei TR, Chapman MR, Dennis VA: Role of the eosinophil in serum-mediated adherence of equine leukocytes to infective larvae of, *Strongylus vulgaris, J Parasitol* 78:477-484, 1992.
42. Dennis VA, Klei TR, Chapman MR, et al: In vivo activation of equine eosinophils and neutrophils by experimental *Strongylus vulgaris* infections, *Vet Immunol Immunopathol* 20:61, 1988.
43. Finkelman FD, Pearce EJ, Urban JF, et al: Regulation and biological function of helminth-induced cytokine responses, *Immunol Today* 12:A62, 1991.
44. Maizels RM, Bundy DA, Selkirk ME, et al: Immunological modulation and evasion by helminth parasites in human populations, *Nature* 365:797-805, 1993.
45. Maizels RM, Blaxter ML, Scott AL: Immunological genomics of *Brugia malayi*: filarial genes implicated in immune evasion and protective immunity, *Parasite Immunol* 23:327-344, 2001.

46. Elliott DE, Summers RW, Weinstock JV: Helminths and the modulation of mucosal inflammation, *Curr Opin Gastroenterol* 21:51-58, 2005.
47. Summers RW, Elliott DE, Weinstock JV: Is there a role for helminths in the therapy of inflammatory bowel disease? *Nat Clin Pract Gastroenterol Hepatol* 2:62-63, 2005.
48. Hoerauf A, Satoguina J, Saeftel M, Specht S: Immunomodulation by filarial nematodes, *Parasite Immunol* 27:417-429, 2005.
49. Van Riet E, Hartgers FC, Yazdanbakhsh M: Chronic helminth infections induce immunomodulation: consequences and mechanisms, *Immunobiology* 212:475-490, 2007.
50. Jackson JA, Friberg IM, Little S, Bradley JE: Review series on helminthes, immune modulation and the hygiene hypothesis: immunity against helminthes and immunological phenomena in modern human populations: coevolutionary legacies? *Immunology* 126:18-27, 2009.
51. Edmonds JD, Horohov DW, Chapman MR, Pourciau SS, Antoku K, Snedden K, Klei TR: Altered immune responses to a heterologous protein in ponies with heavy gastrointestinal parasite burdens, *Equine Vet J* 33:658-663, 2001.

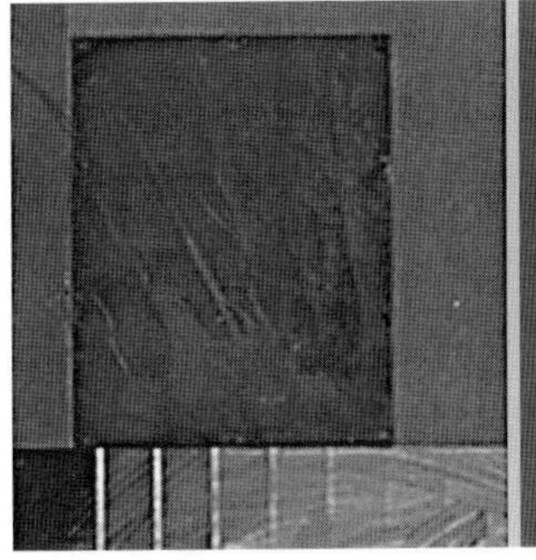

Clinical Approach to Commonly Encountered Problems

CHAPTER 3

Melissa T. Hines

CHANGES IN BODY TEMPERATURE

Melissa T. Hines

Assessment of body temperature is an essential part of every physical examination. As with all mammalian species, horses normally maintain their core body temperatures within a narrow range despite extremes in environmental conditions. The core temperatures may vary by approximately 1° C (2° F) between individuals. In adult horses the average normal body temperature is 38.0° C (100.5° F), whereas in neonatal foals the temperature tends to be slightly higher, ranging between 37.8° to 38.9° C (100.0° to 102.0° F). A diurnal variation of up to 1° C (2° F) may occur, with the low point typically in the morning and the peak in the late afternoon.

CONTROL OF BODY TEMPERATURE

The set-point is the crucial temperature that the body attempts to maintain, primarily via neuronal control operating through temperature centers in the hypothalamus.[1,2] Peripheral and central thermoreceptors sense changes in ambient and core body temperatures and activate feedback mechanisms that bring the temperature back to the set-point. Specifically, the anterior hypothalamic-preoptic area contains large numbers of heat-sensitive neurons and lower numbers of cold-sensitive neurons that function as temperature detectors. Peripheral receptors, which are generally most sensitive to low temperatures, are located in the skin and in some deep tissues, such as the spinal cord and abdominal viscera, and around certain great veins. The anterior hypothalamic-preoptic area and the peripheral receptors transmit signals into the posterior hypothalamic area, subsequently activating autonomic and behavioral effector responses to regulate body temperature.

When the body temperature is too high, heat loss increases and heat production diminishes. Increasing blood flow to the skin is an effective mechanism for heat transfer from the body core to the surface. In response to changes in core body temperature and environmental temperature, the sympathetic nervous system regulates the degree of vasoconstriction and thus the amount of blood flow. Heat is lost from body surfaces to the surroundings by several physical mechanisms, including radiation, conduction, and convection. Evaporation is also an important mechanism of heat loss in horses.[3] The rate of sweating controls to some extent the amount of evaporative heat loss. However, even when the animal is not sweating, water evaporates insensibly from the skin and lungs, causing continual heat loss. In horses evaporative heat loss, primarily through increased sweating but also through increased respiration, becomes more important as the ambient temperature rises and during exercise.[3,4] In addition to increased heat loss when the body temperature rises, the horse also decreases temperature further by inhibiting means of heat production, such as shivering, and by behavioral responses, such as seeking shade and wind currents and wading into water.

Mechanisms that increase body temperature come into play when the body temperature is too low.[2] Heat is conserved by stimulation of the posterior hypothalamic sympathetic centers, leading to cutaneous vasoconstriction and piloerection. Heat production also increases and may occur through increased muscle activity ranging from inapparent contractions to generalized shivering. Shivering may increase heat production by four to five times baseline. The primary motor center for shivering is in the posterior hypothalamus, which normally is stimulated by cold signals from the peripheral receptors and to some extent the anterior hypothalamic-preoptic area. Signals from heat-sensitive neurons in the anterior-hypothalamic-preoptic area inhibit the center. Digestion of food also contributes to total body heat. Sympathetic stimulation may increase the rate of cellular metabolism, increasing heat production by chemical thermogenesis. Cooling also increases the production of thyrotropin-releasing hormone, ultimately increasing thyroid hormones and cellular metabolism and further contributing to chemical thermogenesis. In addition to these physiologic adaptations, behavioral responses to conserve heat also occur, such as adopting a huddled stance, aggregating in groups, and seeking shelter.

CONDITIONS OF INCREASED BODY TEMPERATURE

Elevation of the body temperature above normal is one of the most common clinical problems encountered, and although classically associated with infection, a variety of disorders may cause increased body temperature. Veterinarians should distinguish between conditions of hyperthermia, in which the temperature set-point is unaltered, and true fever, in which the set-point actually increases.

HYPERTHERMIA

The body temperature may become elevated without an increase in the set-point when a loss of equilibrium occurs in the heat balance equation. Increased heat production or absorption of heat beyond the ability of the body to dissipate heat may occur. In some conditions impaired heat loss also may occur. Hyperthermic conditions include problems such as exercise-related hyperthermia, heat stroke, malignant hyperthermia, anhidrosis, central nervous system disorders, and reactions to certain toxins or drugs. In general, these conditions do not respond to treatment with antipyretic drugs.

EXERCISE-RELATED HYPERTHERMIA

During sustained or high-intensity exercise, increased heat production is associated with muscular activity.[3,4] The heat produced may exceed the ability of the body to lose heat, resulting in an increased core body temperature. Typically, the temperature returns to normal with rest as heat loss mechanisms remain activated. Elevated temperature also may occur with the intense muscle activity associated with generalized seizures.

HEAT STROKE

Heat stroke occurs when the body temperature rises above a critical temperature, leading to multisystemic problems. In horses signs of heat stroke may develop when the body temperature is above 41.5° C (107° F), which most often occurs in association with exercise in environmentally stressful conditions. Although horses can acclimatize to various weather conditions to some extent, the efficiency of evaporative heat loss may be compromised significantly in hot, humid weather.[4,5] Susceptibility to heat stroke may increase if sweating leads to dehydration and electrolyte imbalances. Once the body temperature reaches the critical point, the homeostatic mechanisms of thermoregulation fail, resulting in peripheral vasoconstriction, decreased cardiac output, and decreased blood pressure. Affected horses are lethargic, with weak, flaccid muscles. Prostration, circulatory shock, disseminated intravascular coagulation, multiple organ failure, and death may occur.

ANHIDROSIS

Especially in hot, humid climates, horses may develop anhidrosis, which is characterized by a partial or total loss of the ability to sweat.[6] Because of the resulting impaired heat loss, hyperthermia may develop. Clinical signs of poor performance, increased respiratory rate, and poor hair coat also are observable.

MALIGNANT HYPERTHERMIA

Malignant hyperthermia encompasses a group of inherited skeletal muscle disorders in which calcium metabolism is altered.[7] Although the condition is most common in human beings and pigs, it has been reported in several species, including horses.[8,9] The disorder is characterized by a hypermetabolic state of muscle that generally is induced by halogenated inhalation anesthetics, depolarizing skeletal muscle relaxants, and occasionally local anesthetics or stress. Clinical signs include a rapid increase in core body temperature, skeletal muscle rigidity, and tachycardia. Affected animals may develop significant acidosis and muscle necrosis and in some cases may die. In pigs, malignant hyperthermia has been linked to a single point mutation in the gene for the skeletal muscle ryanodine receptor, but a genetic basis has not yet been established in horses.[7]

CENTRAL NERVOUS SYSTEM DISORDERS

Any condition affecting those areas of the hypothalamus involved in thermoregulation may alter the body temperature, with hyperthermia being more common than hypothermia.[1,2] Thus central hyperthermia occurs in association with a variety of conditions, including hemorrhage, neoplasms or abscesses, infectious/inflammatory changes, and degenerative disorders. Central hyperthermia usually is characterized by a lack of any diurnal variation, absence of sweating, resistance to antipyretic drugs, and excessive response to external cooling.

CERTAIN TOXINS OR DRUGS

Occasionally, hyperthermia has been associated with toxins or drugs. Exposure to compounds that act to uncouple oxidative phosphorylation, such as the wood preservative pentachlorophenol, potentially could cause a significant rise in body temperature.[10] Foals treated with the antibiotic erythromycin and possibly other macrolides are at risk of developing hyperthermia.[11] Such predisposition has been attributed to a reaction to the erythromycin itself or to an alteration of the thermoregulatory system of the foal by mechanisms not yet described. Environmental conditions may exacerbate the development of hyperthermia, with foals exposed to high ambient temperatures and direct sunlight being at greatest risk.

PATHOGENESIS OF TRUE FEVER

In true fever the set-point for the desired core body temperature increases and then is maintained by the same mechanisms that maintain the normal body temperature. Although primarily associated with infectious diseases, fever is also a prominent component of many inflammatory, immunologic, and neoplastic conditions. Although the pathogenesis of the febrile response is complex, essentially all of these conditions initiate fever by stimulating the release of endogenous pyrogens (Figure 3-1).

Endogenous pyrogens are substances with the biologic property of fever induction.[12,13] Initially endogenous pyrogen was assumed to be a single molecule produced by leukocytes—thus the name *leukocytic* or *granulocytic pyrogen*. Now, multiple cytokines are known to act as pyrogens, and a variety of cell types produce them, with monocytes and macrophages predominating. Currently, the following cytokines are thought to be intrinsically pyrogenic in that they produce a rapid-onset fever via direct action on the hypothalamus without requiring formation of another cytokine: interleukin-1α (IL-1α) and IL-1β, tumor necrosis factors (TNF) α and β, interferon-α, and IL-6. IL-1α and IL-1β and TNF-α appear to be among the most potent pyrogens. Many endogenous pyrogens use the cell-signaling apparatus gp130. Cytokines that act through this receptor include IL-6, IL-11, oncostatin M, ciliary neurotrophic factor, cardiotropin-1, and leukemic inhibitory factor. From a clinical standpoint, several pyrogenic cytokines

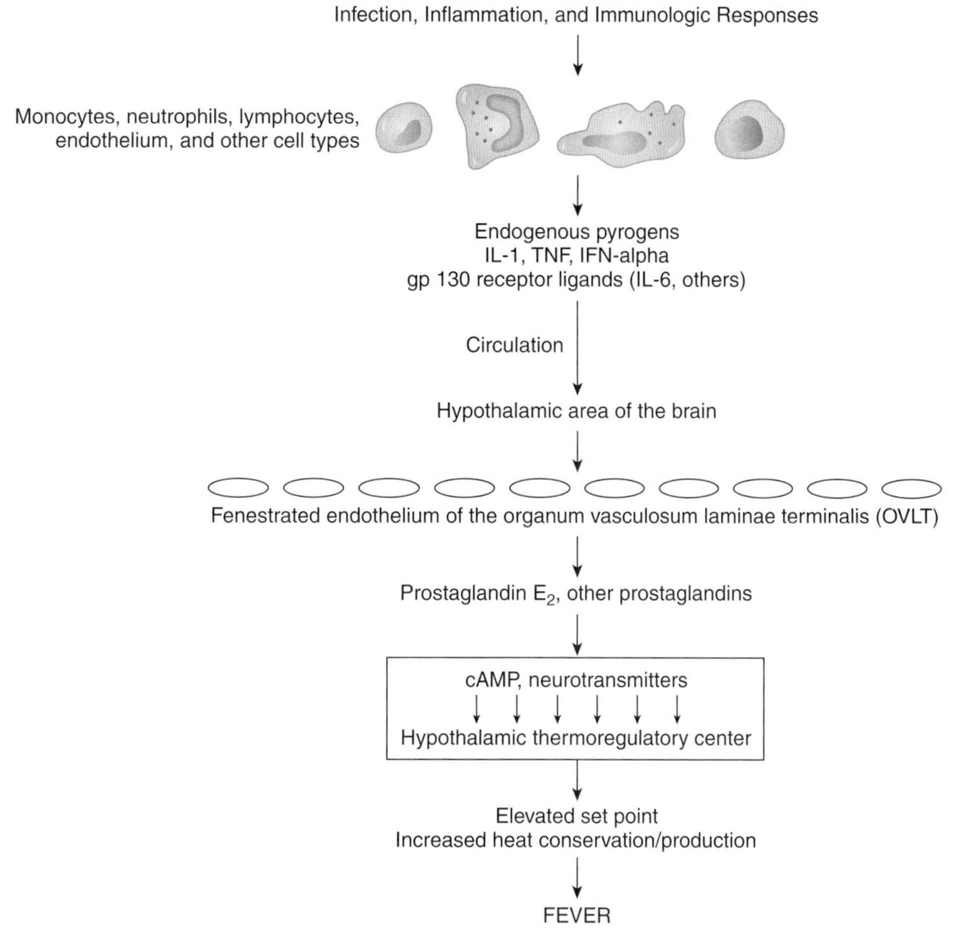

FIGURE 3-1 Schematic representation of the pathogenesis of fever. *cAMP,* Cyclic adenosine monophosphate; *IFN,* interferon; *IL,* interleukin; *TNF,* tumor necrosis factor.

are produced during most febrile diseases and contribute to the febrile response.

The precise mechanism of action of pyrogenic cytokines in the central nervous system is still unclear. Endogenous pyrogens probably act on the circumventricular organs or organum vasculosum laminae terminalis (OVLT), a rich vascular network associated with neurons of the preoptic anterior hypothalamus.[13-15] Ablation of the OVLT prevents fever after a peripheral injection of endogenous pyrogens but has no effect when endogenous pyrogens are injected directly into the brain tissue.[14] In the region of the OVLT the blood-brain barrier is minimal, and endothelial cells lining this region may allow direct movement of endogenous pyrogens into the brain or may release arachidonic acid metabolites in response to endogenous pyrogens, which then move into the brain. The production of arachidonic acid metabolites, particularly prostaglandin E_2 via the cyclooxygenase 2 (COX-2) pathway, is clearly important in the pathogenesis of fever because COX inhibitors, and specifically COX-2 inhibitors, effectively reduce the febrile response but have no effect on the normal body temperature. The prostaglandins do not act directly but initiate neuronal signaling by producing a cascade of changes in cyclic nucleotides, calcium, and monoamines leading to a higher set-point in the hypothalamic thermoregulatory center.

Physiologic mechanisms exist to control the febrile response and prevent extremes that are incompatible with life. Multiple feedback mechanisms limit the activity of the pyrogenic cytokines, and many endogenous cryogens or antipyretics have been identified.[16,17] For example, IL-10, which can be induced by pyrogenic cytokines, inhibits further production of IL-1 and TNF. Arginine vasopressin and α-melanocyte-stimulating hormone act within the brain to decrease fever.[16-19] When administered to human beings, α-melanocyte-stimulating hormone is a much more potent antipyretic than acetaminophen. Nitric oxide also has been shown to have an antipyretic role, mediated by cyclic guanosine monophosphate, in the anterior hypothalamic-preoptic region.[20]

The cytokines that act as endogenous pyrogens have a variety of biologic effects. Therefore the onset of fever is accompanied by several hematologic, immunologic, and metabolic changes referred to as the *acute phase response.* In particular, IL-6 and IL-11 induce the synthesis of acute phase proteins by hepatocytes, including fibrinogen, C-reactive protein, haptoglobin, and others. Similarly, hypoferremia, hypozincemia, and hypercupremia are cytokine mediated, as is the activation of lymphocytes, which in turn produce additional cytokines.

Pyrogenic cytokines, particularly IL-1 and TNF-α, cause membrane perturbation with an increase in phospholipases and the production of arachidonic acid.[12,13] The subsequent production of mediators depends on the metabolic pathways for arachidonic acid in the target tissue. Prostaglandins induced by endogenous pyrogens stimulate the muscle catabolism associated with fever and induce collagenase synthesis from synovial cells, contributing to the muscle and joint pain often seen with fever. Local tissue responses to IL-1β and TNF-α may stimulate afferent neural impulses that lead to behavioral responses associated with fever, such as lethargy and anorexia. As expected, treatment with COX inhibitors can diminish many of the signs of fever.

EFFECTS OF FEVER

Fever is a normal physiologic response with beneficial and adverse effects to the animal. With the exception of some viral infections, the elevation in temperature is generally not high enough to affect pathogens directly. However, studies on bacterial infections in several species have demonstrated an increase in survival with fever, which is thought to be caused primarily by enhanced host defenses.[21-23] In addition, the concentration of iron, which is required by many bacteria for multiplication, decreases during the acute phase response.[24-26] If the temperature becomes extremely high, many of the beneficial effects are reversed.[2,27,28] In rabbits the severity of bacterial infection increases when the body temperature is more than 3° C (5° F) above normal. The increased catabolism, variable anorexia, and increased metabolic rate can lead to muscle wasting and weakness when fever is prolonged. Although seizures induced by fever are uncommon in horses, they can be seen in neonates when the temperature is above 42° C (108° F).[29] In debilitated animals prolonged fever has been associated with cardiovascular failure.

APPROACH TO FEVER

Increased body temperature is a common clinical sign with diverse causes (Figure 3-2). Fortunately, in many cases the cause may be readily apparent on the basis of the signalment, history, and physical examination. Conditions of increased temperature, such as exercise-related hyperthermia and malignant hyperthermia, are often apparent from the history. Infectious diseases remain the most common cause of fever, and often localizing clinical signs such as nasal discharge or diarrhea aid in the diagnosis. In other cases an increased temperature may be one component of another obvious condition, such as neoplasm, immune-mediated disease, or a drug reaction.

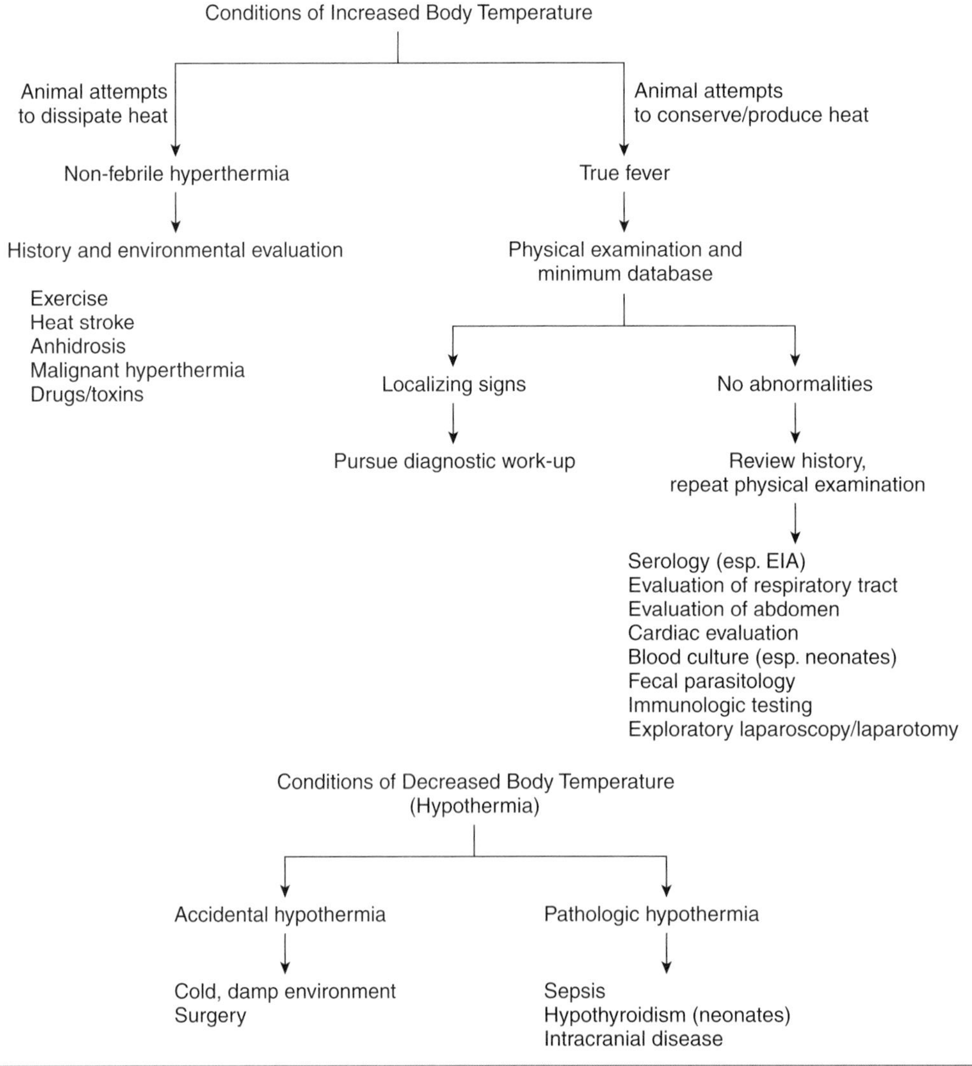

FIGURE 3-2 Approach to changes in body temperature.

FEVER OF UNKNOWN ORIGIN

Fever of unknown origin exists when fever is prolonged with no other specific signs. In many cases the cause is a common disease with an unusual presentation. The specific criteria used to define fever of unknown origin in the horse in a review of 63 cases included the following: (1) illness of at least 3 weeks' duration associated with nonspecific signs, (2) body temperature of at least 38.6° C (101.5° F) on several occasions, and (3) no clear diagnosis after an initial complete blood count and serum biochemical profile.[30] The most common cause was found to be infection, which was responsible for 43% of the cases. Other causes included neoplasms in 22% of cases; immune-mediated diseases in 6.5%; and miscellaneous diseases such as toxic hepatopathy, parasitism, and others in 19%. In 9.5% of cases no diagnosis was made. Therefore diagnosis of fever of unknown origin requires a systematic approach with emphasis on the evaluation of infectious disease.

The clinician can have the body temperature taken twice daily over a period of time to document fever and identify any pattern. Although some inconsistencies in the precise terminology used to define patterns of fever exist, intermittent fevers generally are characterized by recurring paroxysms of elevated temperature followed by periods of normal temperature, such as those fevers that demonstrate diurnal variation. Intermittent fevers most often are associated with infectious causes, particularly viral infections, although they may be seen with a variety of other conditions. In most cases of intermittent fever the temperature tends to peak in the late afternoon or evening, though this is not always the case. Remittent fevers are those in which diurnal variation is exaggerated without a return to normal body temperature or those with a cyclic pattern in which the temperature elevation lasts for several days, such as may be seen with equine infectious anemia virus. Biphasic fevers, in which an initial rise in body temperature precedes a period of normal temperature and then a second rise, are characteristic of certain diseases such as equine monocytic ehrlichiosis (Potomac horse fever). Sustained fevers are those in which the elevation of temperature is consistent.

A complete history is important when investigating fever of unknown origin. Any exposure to *Streptococcus equi* ssp. *equi* (strangles) may be significant because of the association of this organism with internal abscessation. Travel history may be relevant, especially regarding diseases with a geographic influence such as babesiosis and coccidioidomycosis.

The clinician always should perform a careful physical examination, including rectal palpation. Repeating the physical examination may yield new information. The clinician also should perform a complete neurologic examination because disorders of the central nervous system may cause aberrations in temperature through pyrogenic cytokines or in some cases through direct effects on thermoregulatory centers.

Ancillary diagnostic tests usually are required to diagnose fever of unknown origin. A database, including complete blood count, fibrinogen, biochemical profile with bile acids, and urinalysis, should be obtained. Hemoparasites occasionally may be seen on the blood smear, but the apparent absence of organisms does not rule out a parasitemia that is below readily detectable limits. Abnormalities consistent with chronic infection or inflammation, including anemia, hyperfibrinogenemia, and hyperglobulinemia, are common but nonspecific findings. If an elevation of serum protein occurs, further assessment by serum protein electrophoresis and specific immunoglobulin quantitation may be indicated. A monoclonal gammopathy is characteristic of plasma cell myeloma and other tumors of the reticuloendothelial system, both of which may initiate fever directly and increase susceptibility to bacterial infection. In general, immunodeficiencies may be associated with chronic infections. If the serum albumin is low, the veterinarian should investigate the causes of hypoalbuminemia, including decreased production because of significant hepatic disease, increased gastrointestinal or renal loss, or loss into a third space. The presence of hypercalcemia can be helpful in establishing a diagnosis because in horses hypercalcemia most often is linked with renal disease or neoplasms.

Infections of the respiratory tract and abdomen frequently are associated with fever of unknown origin in the horse, and therefore these systems should be thoroughly evaluated. Careful auscultation of the thorax using a rebreathing bag should be performed at rest and, if possible, after exercise. Endoscopy, including examination of the guttural pouches, can be useful. Diagnostic imaging of the thorax, including radiographs and ultrasound, often is indicated. The clinician also should include thoracocentesis in evaluation of the thorax because abnormalities occasionally are apparent even without increases in the volume of pleural fluid. Pleuroscopy, which allows direct visual examination of the pleural space and which may facilitate biopsy of any masses, can be helpful in establishing a diagnosis, especially when neoplasia is suspected.

Peritonitis and abdominal abscessation are common causes of fever of unknown origin, and the veterinarian should include abdominocentesis in the diagnostic plan. The peritoneal fluid should be evaluated for protein, cellularity, and cell morphology, and culture should be performed. The veterinarian should remember that although many neoplastic conditions involve the abdomen, neoplastic cells are not always observed in the peritoneal fluid. In cases of gastric squamous cell carcinoma, gastroscopy is helpful in establishing the diagnosis. Radiographs of the abdomen may be useful, especially in neonates, and ultrasound of the abdomen may help identify fluid for collection or abnormalities that indicate further evaluation, such as abdominal masses or pathologic liver conditions.

Gastrointestinal parasitism is a common clinical problem in the horse, although it is associated only occasionally with fever. However, feces should be examined for parasite ova in horses with fever of unknown origin. In cases of suspected gastrointestinal protein loss, diarrhea, or melena, one should consider diagnostic procedures such as fecal culture, polymerase chain reaction for *Salmonella,* rectal mucosal biopsy, or absorption tests.

Bacterial endocarditis can cause a fever of unknown origin, although the condition is not as common in horses as in some other species. In the study by Mair, Taylor, and Pinsent, the authors identified endocarditis in 3 of 63 cases of fever of unknown origin.[30] In each case a murmur they did not identify initially became apparent several weeks after the onset of illness. Therefore a thorough cardiac evaluation, including echocardiography, is indicated.

Blood cultures are generally most useful in neonates but can yield valuable information in adult horses with fever as well. Ideally, collect three to five samples at least 45 minutes apart when the horse is not on a regimen of antibiotic therapy. Sampling just before and during a temperature rise is most likely to yield a positive culture.

The clinician should consider equine infectious anemia as a differential diagnosis for horses with fever of unknown origin and should perform a serologic examination. Recently, a serologic test for detection of antibodies to the M protein of *Streptococcus equi* ssp. *equi* was developed as an aid in the diagnosis of internal abscessation.[31] Serologic tests for equine babesiosis, brucellosis, and coccidioidomycosis are also available.

Immune-mediated disorders such as immune-mediated hemolytic anemia, immune-mediated thrombocytopenia, systemic lupus erythematosis, vasculitides, and rheumatoid arthritis have been implicated as causes of fever of unknown origin, but more commonly in human beings and small animals than in horses. However, appropriate diagnostic tests, such as the Coombs' test, skin biopsy, and antinuclear antibody testing, may be useful in some cases.

Exploratory laparoscopy or laparotomy is indicated when abdominal involvement is evident or the animal is becoming progressively debilitated. Occasionally, bone marrow aspiration may be useful, particularly in those horses with persistent abnormalities in circulating cell populations. In cases in which a specific diagnosis has not been made, therapeutic trials with antimicrobials may help, and in cases of suspected immune-mediated disease, corticosteroids may help.

HYPOTHERMIA

Hypothermia occurs when the core body temperature drops below accepted normal values. In clinical cases hypothermia can be characterized as accidental or pathologic (see Figure 3-2). In accidental hypothermia a spontaneous decrease in the core body temperature occurs independent of actual disruption to the thermoregulatory system. These cases often can be identified from the history. Mild accidental hypothermia sometimes occurs with surgical procedures. Most often, accidental hypothermia is associated with exposure to cold or cold, damp environments, which can lead to severe hypothermia and death. Neonates are particularly susceptible to hypothermia, although central thermoregulation through the hypothalamus is normal.[29] Sick foals often decrease their activity and nutritional intake and have alterations in circulation. They also have a large ratio of surface area to body weight, enhancing heat loss. Geriatric and otherwise debilitated animals are also at increased risk of hypothermia.

One should consider pathologic causes of hypothermia when no clear reason for accidental hypothermia is evident. Pathologic hypothermia occurs in association with disorders that decrease metabolic activity or directly affect the thermoregulatory center and occurs with endocrine disorders, sepsis, and intracranial disease. In horses hypothyroidism is probably an uncommon clinical problem; however, impaired thermoregulation has been seen in foals with congenital hypothyroidism.[32] Lesions of the thyroid gland also have been associated with hypothermia in donkeys.[33] Hypothermia has been observed with septicemia and shock, especially in neonates, in which 24% of septic foals were found to have a decreased body temperature.[29]

The ability to generate heat through shivering is impaired or lost when the body temperature becomes too low. The animal experiences a decrease in the metabolic rate of most tissues. Heart rate, cardiac output, glomerular filtration, and blood pressure may decrease.

CHANGES IN BODY WEIGHT

Jonathan H. Foreman

An unwelcome or unexpected change in the body weight of a horse is a commonly encountered problem in equine practice. Although obesity may be a more common problem, weight loss often represents a more serious situation, with potentially severe consequences. Normal or acceptable body weight is also in the eye of the beholder because a horse with a given body weight might look overweight as an endurance horse, appropriate as a Thoroughbred racehorse, or too thin as a show hunter.

Whether dealing with a problem of weight loss or weight gain, the veterinarian always should investigate the feeding practices of the horse. Not uncommonly the owner reports that the horse is receiving 3 lb of grain twice daily when the actual measuring device (usually the everyday coffee can) differs in net grain weight once the volume of the measuring device and grain density are taken into account. Observing firsthand the feeding practices of the stable may be necessary to document that the horse actually is getting the reported amount of grain 2 or 3 times daily. Hay should be examined for type, quality (color, texture, leafiness, and steminess), mold, weeds, and potentially toxic plants. Hay analysis will help in the accurate assessment of the nutritional value of the hay. The horse in question should be observed eating hay and grain to ensure that it really does consume the amounts the owner or feeder reports.

The veterinarian also should observe nursing foals when they suckle. The udder should be examined before and after nursing to ensure that the mare actually is producing sufficient milk and that the foal actually is nursing the mare completely until her udder is empty. The milk itself should be examined from both halves of the udder to see that it appears grossly normal (no evidence of mastitis). The nostrils of the foal should be examined after nursing to determine the presence of milk reflux caused by dysphagia, esophageal obstruction, or gastric reflux associated with gastrointestinal ulcers.

DECREASED BODY WEIGHT

Losses in body weight are usually insidious and chronic but may be surprisingly rapid in the face of acute overwhelming systemic infections (Table 3-1). Causes have been classified variously as gastrointestinal, nutritional, infectious, or hypoproteinemic.[1,2] Differential mechanisms include decreased feed intake, decreased absorption of nutrients, decreased nutrient utilization, and increased loss of energy or protein leading to a catabolic "sink."[1-3]

Decreased feed intake may be caused by management factors, poor dentition, dysphagia, or esophageal obstruction. Management factors leading to weight loss may be multifactorial and include inadequate amounts of feed, inadequate quality of feed, or inability of the horse to eat the proper amounts of the feed given. A horse with severe lameness (e.g., chronic laminitis) may not be able to ambulate to the feed source. A horse low on the pecking order in a pasture hierarchy may be unable to eat because it cannot approach the feed without

TABLE 3-1

Mechanisms and Selected Differential Diagnoses for Decreased Body Weight

Mechanism	Differential Diagnoses
Lack of access to appropriate food	Unappetizing or inappropriate types of feed Poor-quality feed Insufficient quantity of feed Inability to access the available feed: *Lameness, other musculoskeletal abnormality* *Social factors within the herd ("pecking order")*
Lack of ingestion of available nutrients	Lack of appetite Inadequate prehension *Nigropallidal encephalomalacia* *Masseter myodegeneration* Abnormal mastication *Poor dentition* *Masseter myodegeneration* Abnormal swallowing *Dysphagia* Abnormal esophageal transit *Esophageal abnormalities*
Abnormal digestion, absorption, or metabolism of nutrients	Gastrointestinal dysfunction *Gastrointestinal ulceration* *Inflammatory bowel disorder* *Neoplasia* *Parasitism* Hepatic dysfunction Toxicities
Inadequate delivery of nutrients to peripheral tissues	Cardiovascular disease *Heart failure* Respiratory disease *Recurrent airway obstruction (chronic obstructive pulmonary disease)* Hepatic disease
Increased rate of protein and energy use or loss	Unusual levels of physical activity Late gestation, early lactation Adaptation to environmental conditions (e.g., cold) Neoplasia Infection, inflammation *Pneumonia* *Pleuritis* *Peritonitis* *Equine infectious anemia* Pain Heart failure Endocrine disorder *Pituitary pars intermedia dysfunction* Gastrointestinal disease Renal disease
Primary muscle wasting disorders	Neurogenic muscle atrophy Primary muscle disease *Equine motor neuron disease* *Immune-mediated myopathy* *Polysaccharide storage myopathy*

the other horses bullying it and fending it away. The feed must be palatable and digestible. Appropriate amounts and types of concentrates must be fed with consideration to the work schedule or pregnancy status of the horse. Proper investigation of stable feeding practices is described earlier.

Poor dentition may cause the horse not to eat some or all of its grain or hay. Parrot-mouthed horses or aged horses with receding incisor teeth (more than 25 years old) may have difficulty in tearing off grass when grazing. A horse with one or more oral sores from a poorly fitting bit or sharp cheek teeth may exhibit partial or complete inappetence because of pain associated with chewing. Sharp cheek teeth, wave mouth, or step mouth may lead to poor digestion and incomplete absorption of nutrients because of inadequate mastication of hay leading to poor fiber use during the hindgut (cecum) fermentation process.

Dysphagia has many causes, including abnormal prehension, chewing, or swallowing.[4] Abnormal prehension can be caused by tongue lacerations; dental, mandibular, or maxillary fractures; damage to nerves supplying the tongue or facial musculature (local trauma, equine protozoal myelitis, or polyneuritis equi); or central neurologic disease (equine protozoal myelitis). Basal ganglia lesions caused by poisoning by ingestion of yellow star thistle or Russian knapweed prevent normal prehension in the pharynx.[4] Swallowing abnormalities may be caused by neurologic (equine protozoal myelitis, viral encephalitis, or guttural pouch infection); muscular; or physical obstructions such as strangles, abscesses, or guttural pouch distention.[4] Muscular causes include hyperkalemic periodic paralysis in Quarter Horse foals, vitamin E or selenium deficiency in neonates, botulism in neonates and adults, and local trauma subsequent to laryngeal surgery (laryngoplasty).

Esophageal obstruction usually presents acutely because an apparently dysphagic horse regurgitates food from its nostrils while attempting to eat or drink. Chronic choke, or anorexia related to painful swallowing caused by partial esophageal obstruction, may lead to weight loss without the owner realizing that the horse is not eating adequately. Megaesophagus and esophageal diverticula may also result in dysphagia, intermittent obstruction, aspiration pneumonia, and chronic weight loss. The accurate diagnosis of some esophageal disorders may require esophageal endoscopy or contrast radiography.

If the horse with weight loss has been observed to fully ingest adequate amounts of good-quality hay and grain, then decreased feed absorption must be considered the reason for weight loss. Maldigestion and malabsorption are not easily confirmed diagnoses, but tests based on luminal absorption of simple sugars (xylose or glucose tolerance tests) have been used to document malabsorption syndromes.[3,5,6] These tests are described in greater detail in Chapter 15. Malabsorption may be caused by parasitism, diarrhea, and inflammatory or neoplastic intestinal disease.

Gastrointestinal parasitism results in weight loss because of several mechanisms.[2] Parasites may compete directly for nutrients within the lumen of the bowel. Malabsorption may result from a lack of mucosal integrity, a decrease in intestinal villi size and number (and subsequent decrease in mucosal absorptive surface area), and a decrease in digestive enzymes that originate in the mucosa. Competition of parasites for protein sources may result in decreased availability of amino acids for production of digestive enzymes or mucosal transport proteins. Increased mucosal permeability caused by leakiness in mucosal intercellular bridges may result in mucosal edema and increased transudation of intercellular fluid and its associated electrolytes, amino acids, and sugars into the lumen of the intestine.

Chronic diarrhea may result in partial or complete anorexia, which contributes directly to weight loss. More rapid (decreased) gastrointestinal transit time results in increased losses of incompletely digested dietary feedstuffs. Malabsorption may result from decreased transit time and from villus blunting caused by specific pathogens, such as in viral diarrhea (see Chapter 15). Bacterial pathogens may compete directly for luminal nutrients. Mucosal invasion by viral and bacterial pathogens may cause mild to severe degrees of mucosal sloughing (ulcers), which results in maldigestion, malabsorption, and increased mucosal losses of intercellular fluid (e.g., in parasitism).

Assuming that the horse has adequate feed intake and absorption, inappropriate hepatic use of amino acids and sugars must be considered as a differential diagnosis for weight loss. Chronic liver disease may result in weight loss because of inappetence, maldigestion (caused by inadequate bile acid production), and inadequate or improper processing of amino acids into normal plasma proteins in the liver. These abnormalities may result in lowered concentrations of serum albumin, liver-dependent clotting factors (factors II, VII, IX, and X), and total plasma or serum protein. Lowered circulating proteins (especially albumin) may result in decreased plasma colloid osmotic pressure and thus may manifest as peripheral dependent edema in the distal limbs, pectoral region, and ventral midline. This peripheral edema may mask further weight loss by making the torso of the horse appear to be heavier than it actually is. Decreases in clotting factors may result in bleeding diatheses. Hyperlipemia, hyperlipidemia, fatty liver syndrome, and ketosis may be seen in poorly fed ponies and in miniature horses with acute anorexia or overwhelming energy demands, such as pregnancy or lactation.[7]

Increased loss of protein or energy is a common cause of decreased body weight in horses. Luminal losses of fluid, electrolytes, and nutrients were described earlier for intestinal parasitism and diarrhea. Acute inflammatory protein losses may occur into major body cavities in overwhelming infections such as pleuritis or peritonitis. Chronic abscessing pneumonia, pleuritis, and peritonitis often result in increased, rather than acutely decreased, serum total protein because of increased γ-globulin production in response to chronic antigenic stimulation from the chronic infection. These chronic infections also usually have weight loss as an additional clinical sign because of the continuing catabolic processes associated with the infection itself. Equine infectious anemia is a type of persistent systemic infection that in its symptomatic form may result in chronic weight loss and varying levels of anemia.[8] Asymptomatic equine infectious anemia carriers may have no weight loss or other obvious clinical signs but can infect pasture mates via vector transmission.

Protein-losing enteropathy is not a definitive diagnosis but rather is a group of diseases, each of which results in luminal losses of fluid, electrolytes, plasma proteins, and nutrients. Mechanisms of protein and fluid loss were described earlier for intestinal parasitism and diarrhea. Gastrointestinal ulcers, especially in the right dorsal colon, have been reported to result in lowered serum total protein and weight loss.[9] One of the early indications of nonsteroidal anti-inflammatory drug toxicity is detection of a lowered serum total protein. Horses with such a condition also may manifest varying degrees of inappetence and colic, especially during the immediate postprandial period. Intestinal neoplasms (usually lymphosarcoma) often manifest as a protein-losing enteropathy with weight loss.[10]

Acute or chronic renal diseases, especially involving glomerulonephritis, can result in urinary protein loss and subsequent body weight loss.[2] Horses with this condition may have polyuria and polydipsia as associated clinical signs. Owners or handlers often report polyuria as increased wetness in stall bedding. The veterinarian should question owners thoroughly regarding the water intake of the horse. The veterinarian may need to observe stable watering habits, often including actually measuring the volume of the water buckets to establish definitively the presence of polydipsia. Turning off automatic water feeders in the stall or pasture and offering the horse measured volumes of water from additional buckets may be necessary to establish a diagnosis of polydipsia. Urine puddles in stalls or collected urine samples may foam excessively because of increased protein concentrations. Increased urinary protein concentrations can be diagnosed quickly on the farm with the proper interpretation of urine dipstick protein indicators.

Neoplasms or abscesses within the thorax or abdomen serve as catabolic energy and protein sinks, resulting in chronic weight loss.[2,10,11] Chronic pain, such as that associated with severe, unresponsive laminitis, results in increased catabolism and weight loss, probably because of chronically elevated systemic catecholamine levels. Increased circulating epinephrine and norepinephrine levels result in a whole-body catabolic state with increased breakdown of stored energy sources and ultimately result in chronic weight loss. Similar weight loss caused by systemic catabolism can result from chronically elevated serum cortisol associated with pituitary adenoma and secondary hyperadrenocorticism.

Heart murmurs and resultant heart failure can cause weight loss because of inefficiency of circulation of nutrients and oxygen to peripheral tissues. Chronic obstructive pulmonary disease or heaves may result in weight loss because of an increase in the work of breathing and poor oxygenation of peripheral tissues. Although ventral abdominal musculature may hypertrophy and result in a heave line, weight loss is manifested by increased depth between the ribs and decreased muscular thickness and definition along the dorsal midline. Suckling foals with severe pneumonia may manifest weight loss if they become inappetent because of decreased suckling related to their severe dyspnea.

Approach to the Diagnosis of Weight Loss

An appropriately taken history should document the type, amount, and quality of feed and hay being provided daily. Documentation of deworming products used and intervals of administration is critical. The history also may document the presence of anorexia, depression, polyuria, polydipsia, diarrhea, and other important historical signs that may point more quickly toward a specific cause of the weight loss.

The physical examination should reveal the presence of weight loss, a cardiac murmur, pneumonia or pleuropneumonia (increased lung sounds), chronic obstructive pulmonary disease (increased abnormal expiratory lung sounds), dental abnormalities, peripheral edema, urine staining on the hindlimbs, diarrhea, icterus, nasal discharge (dysphagia, pneumonia), fever, or hirsutism (secondary hyperadrenocorticism). The rectal examination may document the presence of intra-abdominal masses (abscesses or neoplasms), enlarged left kidney, thickened intestinal or rectal wall, colonic displacement, gritty peritoneal surfaces (peritonitis), gritty feces (sand impaction), or diarrhea.

Fecal flotation may serve as an adequate screening tool to determine whether any evidence of parasitism exists. In the event of a positive fecal flotation, Baermann sedimentation may be necessary to determine quantitatively the severity of the patent parasitic load in the horse with weight loss. Fecal occult blood may be positive with gastrointestinal ulceration or neoplasms, but parasites or a recent rectal examination also may result in positive results.

Routine hematologic testing (complete blood count and fibrinogen) should assist in diagnosing infectious conditions such as pleuritis or peritonitis. Decreased serum or plasma total protein and albumin concentrations are evidence of hypoproteinemia and make the following conditions more likely: severe malnutrition, protein-losing enteropathy (diarrhea, parasitism, ulceration, intestinal neoplasms, or inflammatory intestinal disease), glomerular disease, acute pleuritis or peritonitis, and chronic liver disease. Increased total protein concentrations, especially γ-globulins, make chronic closed-cavity infections such as abscesses, peritonitis, or pleuritis more likely. Increased γ-globulin fractions suggest the presence of parasitism.

Routine serum biochemistries should aid in diagnosing renal (renal azotemia, electrolyte abnormalities) and liver disease (increased γ-glutamyltransferase, aspartate aminotransferase, serum alkaline phosphatase, and lactate dehydrogenase). Urinalysis should reveal increased protein levels on dipstick or quantitative analysis in the event of glomerular protein losses. Metabolic alkalosis may be evident in the aftermath of salivary bicarbonate losses caused by dysphagia or esophageal obstruction.

Endoscopy may aid in diagnosing causes of dysphagia or esophageal obstruction. Lengthy endoscopes are necessary for examination of large adult horses for suspected gastrointestinal ulcers, but shorter endoscopes may suffice for foals or shorter-necked adults (e.g., Arabians and ponies).

Peritoneal fluid analysis documents the presence of a transudate (equivocal infection) or exudate (probable infection).[12,13] Aerobic and anaerobic peritoneal fluid cultures should be performed if intra-abdominal infection is suspected. Exfoliative cytologic examination rarely may document the presence of neoplastic cells from intra-abdominal neoplasms.[2,10-14]

Nonroutine tests should be performed only as indicated and should include oral absorption tests (see Chapter 15) and biopsies of the liver, kidney, or intestinal wall. Abdominal or thoracic ultrasonography should help in ruling out abnormalities of the liver or kidneys and may document the presence of abnormal fluid (peritonitis or pleuritis) or masses (abscesses or neoplasms). Cardiac ultrasound should be definitive in the event of a murmur and suspected heart failure. Radiography also may be helpful to document the presence of thoracic masses or chronic obstructive pulmonary disease, but increased pleural fluid obscures visualization of other intrathoracic structures.

INCREASED BODY WEIGHT

Overfeeding may be the most common cause of obesity in horses and also may be the easiest to correct. The veterinarian should investigate the feeding practices of the stable and feed and hay sources thoroughly. Novice horse owners, single-horse owners, and pony owners commonly overfeed their animals.

Ponies seem to be particularly susceptible to obesity, perhaps because their size renders them more easily overfed. However, at least one author has proposed that this tendency toward obesity in ponies receiving modern confinement diets may be because of their having evolved in the inhospitable ice age climates of northern Europe.[15] In that era the lack of readily available grazing feedstuffs might have placed greater selection pressure on survival of ponies with more efficient dentition and better nutrient and fluid absorption from the gastrointestinal tract. The author argues that those ponies that had greater feed conversion efficiency would have been stronger, had longer lives, and been more available for breeding. Current illustrations of this theory may lie in the Welsh and Connemara pony breeds that still thrive and flourish in the wild in the inhospitable north Atlantic climates of the western coasts of Wales and Ireland, respectively.

Obesity has also been associated with equine metabolic syndrome, also known as *peripheral Cushing's disease* or *prelaminitic metabolic syndrome*.[16-18] Affected horses are insulin resistant and at increased risk of developing laminitis. They may exhibit either generalized obesity or regional adiposity, typically manifested as a cresty neck or fat pads next to the tailhead. Although equine metabolic syndrome has been recognized in many breeds, some breeds, including ponies, Morgans, Paso Finos, and Norwegian Fjords, appear to be predisposed. Certain management practices, such as the provision of a starch-rich, high glycemic–index diet to horses that are relatively inactive, may contribute to the development of the syndrome. Previously, affected horses were sometimes assumed to suffer from hypothyroidism, but recent studies do not support a primary role for thyroid dysfunction in equine metabolic syndrome.

Horses with pituitary pars intermedia dysfunction (PPID; equine Cushing's syndrome) may also have insulin resistance and abnormal accumulation of fat.[19] Although horses with PPID often have loss of muscle mass or weight loss, some individuals will also have excess fat deposition, especially along the crest of the neck, over the tailhead, in the sheath or in the supraorbital fossa. The presence of additional clinical signs, such as hirsutism, as well as specific testing for PPID, will help to differentiate these horses from those with insulin resistance and fat accumulation resulting from metabolic syndrome.

Hypothyroidism has been reported to be associated with weight gain in horses and obesity and infertility in broodmares.[15,20] However, evidence for hypothyroid-associated weight gain and infertility was lacking in surgically created hypothyroid pony[21] and Quarter Horse[22] subjects. Also, a clinical study demonstrated that decreased thyroid function was uncommon in broodmares and was not a common cause of infertility.[23] In general, hypothyroidism remains a somewhat controversial disorder in adult horses, both because of difficulties in accurately diagnosing the condition and the numerous extrathyroidal factors that can affect thyroid function.[24-27] Because resting thyroid hormone concentrations can vary widely depending on a number of factors, documentation of hypothyroidism may require performance of a thyroid-stimulating hormone or thyroid-releasing hormone stimulation test or determination of thyroid-stimulating hormone concentrations.[25-27] The diagnosis and treatment of thyroid dysfunction is described in greater detail elsewhere in this text.

Pregnancy in mares is a normal physiologic event that leads to increased body weight. Surprisingly, many new owners of mares may not know that their new purchase is pregnant. For an earlier negative pregnancy diagnosis to have been in error is not uncommon. Any mare that is gaining weight in an unexpected manner should be examined rectally, and by ultrasonography if necessary, for a possible pregnancy.

Approach to the Diagnosis of Increased Body Weight

Major differential diagnoses for increased body weight include overfeeding; pregnancy; metabolic syndrome; and other conditions that result in abdominal distention, such as bloat, ascites, uroperitoneum, fetal hydrops, and rupture of the prepubic tendon or abdominal wall musculature. The latter conditions are described in greater detail in Chapter 18.

Feeding practices should be investigated and observed firsthand if necessary. A positive pregnancy status should be an easy historical and rectal diagnosis. Most hematologic and biochemical tests are normal in the pregnant or simply overweight horse. Horses should be evaluated for insulin resistance and PPID. Thyroid status should be assessed appropriately, not by simple resting thyroid hormone concentrations.[24-26]

Education of the client regarding feeding practices is important, especially if the overweight horse is determined simply to have been overfed by a novice owner. Dangerous consequences, including colic and laminitis, should be explained to the client.

CLINICAL ASSESSMENT OF POOR PERFORMANCE

Melissa T. Hines

Any decrease in performance may be critical to the equine athlete. Numerous factors influence performance, including genetics, training, desire, and overall health. Peak athletic performance requires optimal function of all body systems, particularly those involved in locomotion and oxygen transport.

APPROACH TO POOR PERFORMANCE

Determining the cause of poor performance in those horses without overt clinical disease often is challenging.[1-4] In a study by Martin, Reef, Parente, et al. of 348 cases of poor performance, a definitive diagnosis was established in 73.5% of cases after in-depth examination, which included the use of a high-speed treadmill.[3] Subtle abnormalities may be sufficient to impair performance, and in some cases problems may be evident only during exercise, contributing to the difficulty of making a diagnosis. Additionally, multiple problems may occur concurrently. In a study by Morris and Seeherman of 275 racehorses with a history of poor racing performance, 84% were found to have more than one abnormality.[2] Therefore determining the actual clinical significance of any given problem may be difficult.

Equine athletes presented for poor performance should undergo a comprehensive evaluation, the basic components of which include a history, detailed physical examination, and laboratory screening. The clinician should emphasize examination of the respiratory, musculoskeletal, and cardiovascular systems because these systems most often are linked to performance problems. In many cases standardized exercise testing, generally on a high-speed treadmill, is critical in identifying the problem. Endoscopic examination of the upper airways during exercise has proved particularly useful.

HISTORY

Obtaining a complete history is a fundamental part of evaluating poor performance. The clinician should establish the use of the horse, the time in training, and the specifics of the training program. Determining whether the horse has never performed as expected or has experienced a decline in the level of performance is crucial. If the horse has never performed as expected, the veterinarian should consider a lack of ability, congenital abnormalities, and training problems. A change in performance, either sudden or insidious, often is associated with an acquired problem. The clinician should characterize specifically the decline in performance, including the intensity of exercise at which signs are observed and whether performance is abnormal from the onset of exercise or declines during an exercise bout. In those cases in which performance drops off during exercise, the clinician should determine whether the decline is acute or gradual and whether any other signs, such as stridor, are associated with it.

Other elements of the history with particular relevance to athletic performance include any previous respiratory disease, respiratory noise, or respiratory distress associated with exercise. Any change in gait also may be significant. Establishing the feeding practices, changes in appetite or body condition, the type of tack used, and whether sweating is appropriate is important. The clinician should determine the response to any medications that have been used, such as phenylbutazone or furosemide. The information obtained in the history may help direct the investigation.

GENERAL PHYSICAL EXAMINATION AND LABORATORY SCREENING

The clinician should perform a complete physical examination in all cases. Hematologic testing and a biochemical profile are indicated, although in most horses presented for poor performance without obvious clinical abnormalities, routine evaluation of a single sample is within normal limits. Because exercise can induce some changes in laboratory parameters, such as an increase in the packed cell volume and neutrophil count, considering the time of sample collection relative to exercise is important.[5-7] Potentially significant findings include changes consistent with chronic inflammation, such as anemia, hyperglobulinemia, and possibly hyperfibrinogenemia. Subclinical infections may have only slight alterations in the leukocyte count and differential. Viral infections, especially in the early stages, may be associated with a leukopenia and neutropenia. A decrease in the neutrophil-to-lymphocyte ratio has been associated with overtraining, although this is not a reliable correlation.[7]

Horses at rest normally maintain a significant proportion of red blood cells and hemoglobin in the splenic reserve.[5,6,8] Thus although total body hemoglobin increases in response to training and may correlate with performance, this cannot be determined from a resting sample. Special techniques must be used to document total red cell mass or hemoglobin.[8,9] Anemia can decrease the oxygen-carrying capacity during exercise, resulting in suboptimal performance.

Signs of organ dysfunction in horses presented for poor performance are not common findings. Muscle enzymes may be elevated, although many cases of myopathy are subclinical and require evaluation of muscle enzymes after exercise.[10] Much attention has been paid to the importance of electrolytes and exercise; however, abnormalities seldom are found. In general, circulating electrolyte concentrations are regulated tightly and may not reflect closely the total body electrolyte status.[11] However, a concentration of potassium consistently below 3 mEq/L may suggest a potassium deficit. Chronic electrolyte deficiencies may be detected by performing renal fractional excretion of electrolytes.

EVALUATION OF THE RESPIRATORY SYSTEM

The clinician should give careful attention to examining the respiratory tract because abnormalities of this system frequently influence performance. The examination should include evaluation of air flow from the nares and percussion of the sinuses, as well as assessment of any cough or nasal discharge. Careful palpation of the larynx may reveal an increase in prominence of the muscular process of the left arytenoid cartilage resulting from a loss of mass of the left dorsal cricoarytenoid muscle associated with idiopathic hemiplegia. The clinician can use the laryngeal adductor response test, or slap test, to evaluate adduction of the arytenoid cartilages by slapping the withers during expiration and evaluating movement of the contralateral arytenoid by endoscopy or palpation. The clinician should perform a thorough auscultation of the trachea and lungs. Having the horse rebreathe from a plastic bag placed over the nostrils increases the respiratory rate and tidal volume, thus accentuating sounds. In addition to auscultation, the clinician should note the character and pattern of respiration, including the presence of any abdominal component, and the recovery time. Percussion of the thorax may be useful in establishing the lung border and any dull or hyperresonant areas, as well as in detecting pleural pain.

Dynamic obstruction of the airway is among the most common causes of poor performance in the equine athlete.[2,3,12-14] In the study by Morris and Seeherman of 275 racehorses evaluated for poor performance, 40% were found to have dynamic obstruction.[2] Similarly, in the study by Martin, Reef, Parente, et al. of 348 racehorses and show horses with poor performance, 148 (42.6%) had dynamic obstruction of the airways.[3] Of these 148 affected horses, 39 were found to have multiple airway abnormalities. An additional 22 horses had dynamic airway obstruction concurrently with a cardiac arrhythmia. In both studies of poor performance, the most common conditions causing airway obstruction were dorsal displacement of the soft palate and idiopathic left laryngeal hemiplegia with arytenoid collapse. Other conditions diagnosed included dynamic pharyngeal collapse, epiglottic entrapment, subepiglottic cyst, rostral displacement of the palatopharyngeal arch, and redundant alar folds. An important note is that many of the horses with airway obstruction did not have a history of abnormal respiratory noise and did not have abnormalities at rest. Also, not all abnormalities observed at rest caused obstruction. Therefore these studies emphasize the importance of treadmill videoendoscopy as a component of the evaluation of poor performance. In most cases the clinician should perform a treadmill videoendoscopy regardless of the history and physical examination findings.

Endoscopy also can be useful in identifying respiratory problems other than dynamic airway collapse. For example, the clinician can identify narrowing of the ventral nasal meatus associated with sinusitis, nasal masses, and pharyngitis. If the endoscope is sufficiently long, tracheal injury and secretions in the lower respiratory tract can be visualized. Sampling of airway secretions by bronchoalveolar lavage may aid in the diagnosis of low-grade respiratory infections, small airway inflammatory disease, or exercise-induced pulmonary hemorrhage. In some cases evidence of inflammation and retropharyngeal lymphadenopathy on endoscopic examination of the guttural pouches has been associated with dorsal displacement of the soft palate, which may result from neuropathy of the pharyngeal branch of the vagus nerve.[15]

Radiographs and ultrasound may be indicated on evaluation of the respiratory system of horses with poor performance, especially in those horses with evidence of lower respiratory tract disease. Radiographs also can be useful in assessing upper respiratory disorders, allowing for the evaluation of soft tissue masses or fluid accumulations. In addition, sometimes the clinician can identify abnormalities of the pharyngeal and laryngeal structures such as thickening of the soft palate or hypoplasia of the epiglottis.

EVALUATION OF THE CARDIOVASCULAR SYSTEM

Any decrease in cardiac output potentially can limit performance, making thorough evaluation of the cardiovascular system essential. On basic physical examination the clinician should evaluate the mucous membrane color, capillary refill time, and arterial and venous peripheral pulses, although finding abnormalities in these parameters in horses presented for decreased performance is uncommon. The clinician should perform careful auscultation of the heart on both sides of the thorax to evaluate the cardiac rhythm and murmurs. Many horses have murmurs that are of little clinical significance.[2,16] In the study by Martin, Reef, Parente, et al., 102 of the 348 horses were found to have murmurs, the most common being mitral regurgitation.[3] In all cases the murmur was determined to be clinically unimportant.

The clinician can use electrocardiography to evaluate the cardiac rhythm further and ideally should perform the procedure before, during, and after exercise using radiotelemetry. Cardiac arrhythmias were the only abnormality found in 33 of the 348 horses evaluated by Martin, Reef, Parente, et al. and were found in conjunction with dynamic airway obstruction in 22 horses.[3] However, in the study by Morris and Seeherman, arrhythmias were noted in just 2 of 275 horses.[2] The most frequent arrhythmias observed include atrial and ventricular premature depolarizations. Ventricular tachycardia and paroxysmal atrial fibrillation also have been noted. Changes in the T wave, once thought to be related to poor performance, and second-degree atrioventricular block have been found to have no effect on exercise capacity.[17]

Echocardiography before and after exercise helps to evaluate cardiac function. Martin, Reef, Parente, et al. found decreased fractional shortening indicating left ventricular dysfunction after exercise in 19 horses, only 8 of which had echocardiographic changes at rest.[3] Six of the 19 horses had clinically significant arrhythmias. Myocardial disease may contribute to left ventricular dysfunction and arrhythmias. Elevations in myocardial fractions of creatine kinase, lactate dehydrogenase, and troponin support myocardial disease but are not present in all cases.

EVALUATION OF THE MUSCULOSKELETAL SYSTEM

A surprising number of horses presented for poor performance are found to be lame, even when lameness is not part of the presenting complaint.[1,2,4] Therefore the clinician should perform a complete lameness examination in all cases. In some horses presented for poor performance, the gait asymmetry may be subtle and only discernible at high speed, making diagnosis by traditional methods difficult. In these cases gait analysis on the treadmill and advanced diagnostic techniques such as nuclear scintigraphy, thermography, and computed tomography or magnetic resonance imaging may be useful. The clinician also should perform a neurologic examination to identify any deficits that could contribute to poor performance.

Myopathy can lead to decreased performance. In many cases the condition is subclinical and requires an exercise challenge test to make the diagnosis.[3,10] The clinician should measure creatine kinase before exercise and ideally 4 to 6 hours after an exercise bout consisting of 15 to 30 minutes at the trot. In normal horses this light exercise rarely causes more than a threefold increase in creatine kinase. An increase of fivefold or more indicates exertional rhabdomyolysis. A muscle biopsy can help to define the myopathy. In the study by Martin, Reef, Parente, et al., 10 of 348 horses developed clinical exertional rhabdomyolysis after exercise, and an additional 53 demonstrated subclinical myopathy as demonstrated by increased creatine kinase levels after exercise.[3]

EXERCISE TESTING

Exercise testing provides a mechanism for evaluating a range of body systems under standard exercise conditions. In particular, measurements of cardiorespiratory and metabolic function taken during an exercise test provide information about the capacity and efficiency of key body systems involved in energy production. From a clinical standpoint exercise testing is generally most useful in assessing the effect on performance of abnormalities found on a physical examination. Testing also may help to establish the reason for reduced athletic capacity in horses that have no abnormalities on basic examinations. Exercise testing can be done in the field, which mimics the condition in which the horse actually performs. However, most testing is currently done on a treadmill, which provides more consistent conditions and an opportunity to perform a greater range of measurements. The specific protocol used for exercise testing may vary somewhat.[1,18,19] Occasionally a high-speed test is performed in which the horse is accelerated rapidly to maximal speed and run to fatigue. However, the most common type of test is an incremental test in which the speed increases every 1 to 2 minutes until the horse reaches fatigue, allowing for the generation of data during submaximal and maximal exercise. In most cases the test is performed with the treadmill at a slope of 10%. This slope is not so steep as to be completely unrepresentative of normal exercise, and yet it ensures that maximum-intensity exercise can be performed without reaching speeds that may be too fast for horse safety. Some parameters that can be assessed in an exercise test include heart rate, blood lactate level, arterial blood gases, total red cell volume, stride length, and oxygen uptake. Various spirometers, which are masks for measuring pulmonary ventilation, can be used to measure parameters such as air flow rates, tidal volume and the durations of phases of the respiratory cycle.[20] As previously discussed, treadmill videoendoscopy is often valuable.

Heart Rate During Exercise

Evaluation of the heart rate during exercise provides an indirect index of cardiovascular capacity and function. Several heart rate monitors are available.[21] Radiotelemetry also can be used to evaluate the heart rate and rhythm, particularly at the end of exercise. Because the stroke volume does not change greatly with increasing exercise speed, the heart rate provides a guide to changes in cardiac output. In general, a linear increase in heart rate occurs with increasing exercise speed up to the point at which the maximal heart rate is reached.[22-24] The maximal heart rate (HRmax) is identified when no further increase in heart rate occurs despite an increase in exercise speed. The HRmax does not change with training state, although the speed at which it is reached increases with increasing fitness.

One reference point for comparison of cardiovascular capacity is the treadmill speed at a heart rate of 200 beats/min (V_{200}). At a heart rate of 200 beats/min, most horses are close to the point of onset of blood lactate accumulation. The V_{200} can be calculated by linear regression analysis or plotted using measurements taken at three to four submaximal exercise speeds, without the horse reaching maximal exercise. The clinician should take care when using the V_{200} to assess exercise capacity because at a heart rate of 200, horses may be exercising at different proportions of their HRmax and therefore their maximal oxygen uptake (VO_{2max}). In general, however, horses with the highest cardiovascular and metabolic capacities have the highest V_{200} values; that is, the better horses reach a heart rate of 200 at higher speeds than those with a lower exercise capacity. The V_{200} increases with training and can be useful for monitoring changes in fitness. The better-quality Thoroughbreds have a V_{200} of 8 to 9 m/sec in an exercise test with the treadmill set at a 10% slope. Values less than 7 m/sec are abnormal and if found in a fit horse indicate decreased cardiac capacity.

Another measurement of cardiovascular capacity is the treadmill speed at which the horse reaches HRmax, known as V_{HRmax}. This value correlates with VO_{2max} and exercise capacity but requires the horse to exercise up to maximal speeds so that a plateau in heart rate can be identified.

Heart rate measurements are helpful in determining the actual significance of cardiac abnormalities such as murmurs and arrhythmias. In horses with functional cardiac disease, the reduced stroke volume necessitates higher heart rates to maintain adequate cardiac output. Also, studies in Standardbred racehorses have suggested that horses with musculoskeletal problems have an increased V_{200} and that monitoring the V_{200} may help to identify subclinical lameness.

Blood or Plasma Lactate Measurement

Exercising muscles produce lactate to some extent during all intensities of exercise, but production increases exponentially with the intensity of exercise.[24-26] As exercise becomes more intense, the aerobic energy contribution becomes insufficient to meet total energy requirements, and increased anaerobic metabolism results in increased lactate production. Lactate diffuses from muscle to blood, and therefore blood or plasma concentrations of lactate reflect muscle lactate. Some evidence suggests that whole blood concentrations most accurately measure lactate accumulation because red blood cells actively take up lactate.[26-29]

The rate of increase of lactate in the blood may be used as an indirect indicator of cardiovascular and metabolic capacity. Horses with the highest aerobic capacities because of a high maximal cardiac output tend to have lower lactate values at submaximal exercise intensities than those with lower aerobic capacities. Lactate values can be used to compare horses or to evaluate training in the same horse. The treadmill speed at which a plasma lactate of 4 mmol/L (V_{LA4}) is reached is one measure of lactate production, and a high value reflects good aerobic capacity. The V_{LA4} has been used to monitor changes in fitness. In fit Thoroughbred horses 3 years of age and older, values for V_{LA4} range from 8.0 to 9.5 m/sec. Horses that are not fit or that have respiratory disease have lower values. Another useful reference is the blood or plasma lactate at conclusion of the 10 m/sec exercise step of the incremental test, and highly fit, athletic horses usually have values below 5 mmol/L. High-quality sprint horses, which perform largely under anaerobic conditions and have a high anaerobic capacity, may have high peak lactate values.

Oxygen Uptake

The measurement of oxygen uptake (VO_2) is critical to assessing athletic performance.[22,23] The VO_{2max} has been used as a key indicator of exercise capacity in human athletes since the 1950s. As the VO_2 increases linearly with increasing treadmill speed, VO_{2max} can be identified when VO_2 reaches a plateau despite an increase in speed. The Thoroughbred horse has VO_{2max} values that are higher than those of many other mammalian species when expressed on a mass-specific basis. The major factor responsible for the high VO_{2max} in athletic horses is their high oxygen-carrying capacity, which arises from a high maximum stroke volume and to some extent a large arteriovenous oxygen content difference. The VO_{2max} is a good index of changes in fitness and a measurement of exercise capacity in performance horses.

Maximum Oxygen Pulse

The oxygen pulse is defined as the VO_2/heart rate and is expressed as ml/kg/beat. This value provides an indication of the maximum stroke volume, and in high-quality horses values range between 0.66 to 0.76 ml/kg/beat. Those horses with cardiac problems resulting in low cardiac outputs and individuals with low VO_{2max} values usually have values in the range of 0.5 to 0.56 ml/kg/beat. The maximum oxygen pulse also has been shown to correlate with treadmill total run time.

Arterial Blood Gas Analysis During Exercise

Arterial blood gas analysis during exercise may be indicated, especially in horses in which respiratory disorders are the suspected cause of poor performance. For an accurate blood gas analysis, the clinician should take into account the temperature of the blood because it may reach 42° C during maximal exercise. At exercise intensities above 65% VO_{2max}, athletic horses become hypoxemic, although the extent varies between individuals.[30-33] Horses with low VO_{2max} values do not necessarily have a significant decrease in arterial oxygen tension.

Hematocrit and Total Red Cell Volume During Exercise

The total volume of red cells is a major determinant of oxygen-carrying capacity, and therefore measurement of red cell volume can give some index of exercise capacity. A postexercise packed cell volume test is not a reliable indicator of total red cell volume primarily because of plasma volume variations, but it does provide a rough estimate of total circulating red cells.

The clinician can make an accurate determination of red cell volume by techniques that use dye dilution after mobilization of the splenic erythrocyte pool to measure the plasma volume. Although total red cell volume increases with training, some evidence indicates that Standardbred racehorses with overtraining syndrome may develop an abnormal red cell hypervolemia that contributes to poor performance.[9]

Peak Running Speed and Total Run Time

The peak treadmill running speed and the total run time may indicate exercise capacity. In some studies of human athletes, the peak treadmill running speed during an exercise test was shown to be a predictor of performance. Athletic Thoroughbred racehorses can complete 60 seconds at 13 m/sec during an incremental exercise test at a 10% slope.

Stride Length

Athletic horses are thought to have better stride characteristics.[4,34] Some studies have shown a correlation between maximum stride length and the treadmill run time. An accelerometric device has been used to provide quantitative information about locomotory variables that may be useful in evaluating performance.[34]

DYSPHAGIA

Laurie A. Beard

NORMAL EATING

Normal eating is complex and requires normal anatomic structures and neurologic function. The process of eating can be divided into prehension (uptake of food into the oral cavity) and deglutition (transport of food from the oral cavity to the stomach). Prehension requires the lips to grasp and the incisors to tear the food.[1] Motor innervation to the tongue, lips, and muscles of mastication is provided by the hypoglossal, facial, and trigeminal nerves. Sensory input is important for successful prehension and requires intact olfactory, optic, and trigeminal nerves, providing smell, sight, and sensation of the rostral oral mucosa and lips. Normal prehension depends on the central nervous system to coordinate movements of the tongue and lips.

Deglutition involves mastication, swallowing, and transport of food through the esophagus to the stomach. Mastication initiates mechanical digestion and insalivation. Mastication is specifically a function of the molars to grind feed and the tongue and buccal muscles to position the food. The facial nerve provides motor and sensory fibers to the tongue and pharynx. The glossopharyngeal nerve provides sensory fibers to the caudal third of the tongue. The trigeminal nerve is sensory to the teeth and provides the important parasympathetic fibers to the parotid salivary gland. Function of this gland is critical to help liquefy food and provides a small amount of digestive enzymes.

Swallowing is complex and is performed in a series of steps. Initially, food must be moved to the base of the tongue and formed into a bolus. This action requires coordinated movements of the tongue and pharynx. Second, the bolus is forced caudally. As this action takes place, the oropharynx relaxes and the soft palate elevates to seal the palatopharyngeal arch and nasopharynx.[1] Next, the bolus enters the oropharynx and the hyoid apparatus swings rostrodorsally, which draws the larynx and the common pharynx forward.[1,2] The epiglottis is tipped caudally and prevents the bolus from entering the larynx. Finally, the bolus is moved into the common pharynx with pharyngeal muscle contractions and enters the open cranial esophageal sphincter. The sphincter closes to prevent esophagopharyngeal reflux and aerophagia. Herbivores are unique in that breathing continues uninterrupted during swallowing, unlike as in other animals.[1] The glossopharyngeal, vagus, and spinal accessory nerves provide sensory and motor fibers to the pharynx, larynx, and soft palate.

The esophageal phase of eating involves the transport of the food bolus to the stomach, with primary peristaltic waves, which are generated by continuous contraction of the pharyngeal peristalsis. The bolus is transported to the caudal esophageal sphincter, which relaxes to allow the bolus to enter the stomach and then contracts to prevent gastroesophageal reflux. If reflux does occur, esophageal clearance is achieved by secondary peristaltic waves. Antiperistalsis is normal in ruminants during eructation and regurgitation but is not normal in horses.[1]

DYSPHAGIA

Dysphagia is defined as difficulty in swallowing but often is used to describe problems with eating.[2] Problems with eating may include problems with prehension, mastication, swallowing, and esophageal transport. In this section the term *dysphagia* is used in the broader sense to describe problems with eating. Dysphagia can result from a number of disorders affecting any part of the upper gastrointestinal system (i.e., oral cavity, pharynx, and esophagus). Clinical signs of dysphagia vary depending on the cause and the location of the problem but may include ptyalism (excessive salivation), gagging, dropping food, nasal discharge, and coughing. Dysphagia can result from morphologic or functional disorders. The causes of these diseases may be acquired or congenital. Morphologic causes of dysphagia include abnormal anatomy, obstruction of the upper gastrointestinal tract, inflammation, and pain. Examples of anatomic abnormalities include a cleft palate and subepiglottic cysts.[3,4] Obstruction of the upper gastrointestinal tract most commonly includes feed impactions of the esophagus but also can include pharyngeal obstructions secondary to retropharyngeal lymph node masses or severe guttural pouch tympany.[1,2,5-8] Inflammatory conditions resulting in pain and dysphagia include periodontal diseases, foreign bodies, pharyngitis, epiglottitis, and mandibular or maxillary fractures.[1,3]

Functional disorders resulting in dysphagia include neurologic, neuromuscular, and muscular diseases. Functional disorders frequently result in problems with swallowing but less commonly involve mastication and prehension and rarely occur with esophageal transport. Neurologic diseases resulting in dysphagia may be peripheral or central. Peripheral neurologic problems frequently result from abnormalities of the guttural pouch but also can include toxic peripheral neuropathies, such as lead toxicity. Problems of the guttural pouch include infection (tympany, empyema, or mycosis), iatrogenic problems (infusion of caustic substances), and trauma (rupture of the longus capitis muscle from the basisphenoid bone and hemorrhage into the guttural pouch).[2,9,10] Central neurologic diseases may result in problems in prehension, mastication, or swallowing. Specific examples include equine protozoal myelitis, viral encephalitis (rabies and eastern and western encephalitis), toxic neuropathies (leukoencephalomalacia and nigropallidal encephalomalacia), and cerebral trauma.[1,2,5,11,12] Neuromuscular problems resulting in dysphagia generally manifest as a systemic disease and include diseases such as botulism and organophosphate toxicity.[1,2,13] Muscular diseases resulting in dysphagia are rare but include nutritional muscular dystrophy (white muscle disease).[14] Although reported more frequently in foals, nutritional muscular dystrophy is also seen in adult horses, and in some cases signs are limited to dysphagia associated with myodegeneration of the masseter muscles or tongue.[15,16]

Basic Approach to Dysphagia

The initial evaluation of dysphagia focuses on determining whether morphologic or functional abnormalities exist. To answer these questions best, the signalment, history, physical examination (including observation of the horse eating), and additional tests (e.g., endoscopic examination and radiographs) should be considered. Some morphologic abnormalities, such as a cleft palate, will be apparent at an early age. There is some evidence that esophageal disorders may be more common in Friesian horses.[17] A history of an acute onset of dysphagia is often consistent with trauma, whereas a slow, progressive onset of clinical signs is more consistent with a neurologic problem such as guttural pouch mycosis, equine protozoal myelitis, or toxicities. The clinician should assess exposure of the horse to toxic substances or plants (lead or yellow star thistle). A history of treatment before the onset of dysphagia suggests trauma or injury to the pharynx. Use of a balling gun or flushing of guttural pouches may result in iatrogenic injury to the pharynx, esophagus, and guttural pouches. The clinician should determine concurrent problems in other horses (e.g., strangles or other bacterial infections of the submandibular lymph nodes).

In performing the physical examination, the clinician should pay close attention to the head and neck. Because rabies is a potential cause of dysphagia, protective measures should be taken while performing a careful and thorough physical examination. Ideally, all clinicians working on horses should have an adequate rabies antibody titer. An examination of the oral cavity is best accomplished with a mouth speculum; good light; and, if necessary, the administration of sedation. The teeth should be examined carefully for retained deciduous caps, sharp points or hooks, wave mouth or step mouth, dental fractures, and patent infundibula.[3] Foreign bodies may become wedged between the molars or under the tongue. The tongue should be examined for lacerations, foreign bodies, and evidence of neoplasia. The throat latch area and neck should be examined for heat or swelling, which might be caused by a ruptured esophagus. The lungs should be auscultated carefully to determine if the horse shows evidence of aspiration pneumonia resulting from dysphagia.

A valuable activity is to watch the horse eat. The distinction between dysphagia and anorexia is important. Dysphagic horses usually are hungry and will attempt to eat. Problems with prehension generally suggest a primary neurologic problem. Watching the horse try to graze and eat hay or grain may be necessary. Ingestion of yellow star thistle or Russian knapweed results in basal ganglia lesions (nigropallidal encephalomalacia). Horses with these lesions are unable to prehend food (with lack of coordination of the lips and tongue), but they can swallow.[2] Their ability to drink water should be evaluated carefully because some horses continue to drink despite swallowing difficulties. Horses that expel food while chewing may have problems with mastication. Coughing and nasal discharge indicate aspiration of food into the trachea. Problems with swallowing or regurgitation may cause aspiration. Esophageal obstruction results in regurgitation of food through the nares. Regurgitation often is observed during feeding but may occur shortly after or even hours after feeding. Ptyalism, without dysphagia, may result from ingestion of legume plants (especially second-cutting red clover) contaminated with *Rhizoctonia leguminicola.* This fungus produces a mycotoxin called *slaframine,* which has parasympathomimetic properties.[2] The excess salivation disappears once the animal stops feeding on the plant.

Morphologic Abnormalities

Morphologic abnormalities that cause dysphagia are more easily diagnosed than functional disorders. Morphologic problems of the oral cavity generally result in problems of prehension or mastication. An oral examination (as outlined earlier) is particularly useful. The passing of a nasogastric tube, endoscopic examination, and radiographs (if necessary) are other diagnostic tests that may help to identify the anatomic localization and cause of dysphagia. Complete obstruction of the esophagus can be excluded if a nasogastric tube is passed successfully into the stomach. Feed impactions of the esophagus are common in horses. Esophageal impactions of feed may occur because of poor mastication or esophageal strictures or diverticulum.[1,2,5] The most common sites for obstructions occur in the cranial esophagus, at the thoracic inlet, and at the base of the heart.[5] Other esophageal abnormalities include rupture, fistula, cyst, diverticula, megaesophagus, and neoplasms.[2,18] An endoscopic examination allows visualization of the nasal passageways, nasopharynx, guttural pouches, pharynx, larynx, and esophagus. Inflammation of the pharynx, larynx, or esophagus is assessed best by endoscopic examination. Partial obstructions of the pharynx often result in dyspnea, especially during exercise, and sometimes can cause dysphagia. Retropharyngeal masses, guttural pouch tympany, and rarely neoplasms may result in pharyngeal obstruction and collapse.[2,7,8] Depending on the length of the endoscope available, the clinician can evaluate all or part of the esophagus for inflammation or obstruction.

Although they are not required in all situations, radiographs can provide additional information about horses with morphologic causes of dysphagia. Radiographs of the skull can help demonstrate the presence of periodontal disease, fractures of the mandible or maxilla, lesions of the temporomandibular joint, or radiopaque foreign bodies.[3] Radiographs of the larynx or pharynx are indicated in cases of pharyngeal obstruction and are especially useful to evaluate retropharyngeal masses, neoplasms, or trauma.[6-8] Radiographs of esophageal perforations reveal subcutaneous air, which shows up as extraluminal radiolucencies.[1] Contrast studies of the esophagus, with the use of barium sulfate, may help differentiate cases of esophageal strictures, dilation, or diverticulum.[2] Radiographs of the thorax are indicated in horses with nasal discharge and abnormal thoracic auscultation because of the concerns of aspiration pneumonia.

Functional Abnormalities

Functional disorders that cause dysphagia are more difficult to diagnose and should be pursued after morphologic causes are not identified. The clinician also should consider a functional abnormality if the initial physical examination provides strong evidence of a neurologic, neuromuscular, or muscular problem. The initial step to evaluate functional causes of dysphagia is to perform a neurologic examination. The neurologic examination helps establish a neuroanatomic localization by (1) assessing brain, brainstem, and spinal cord functions; (2) determining if the problem is focal, multifocal, or diffuse; and (3) determining if the problem is a peripheral or central problem.

Cerebral disease usually manifests as seizures, head pressing, wandering, depression, and changes in mentation. Brainstem function can be assessed by cranial nerve examination. Evaluation of an abnormal response of the cranial nerves should establish the location of the problem within the brainstem. For example, the optic nerve can be assessed by the menace response (requiring the facial nerve) and by the pupillary light reflex (requiring the oculomotor nerve). Abnormalities of the oculomotor, trochlear, and abducens nerves manifest as strabismus or lack of a pupillary light reflex. Facial nerve paralysis (ear, eyelid, and muzzle droop) and vestibular disease (circling, nystagmus, and head tilt) often occur together because of the close proximity of these nerves as they exit the brainstem.[19] Endoscopic examination is a valuable tool to determine if pharyngeal or laryngeal paralysis is present. These problems may be caused by peripheral or central diseases. The dorsolateral wall of the medial compartment of the guttural pouch contains a plexus of nerves, including the glossopharyngeal nerve; branches of the vagus, spinal accessory, and hypoglossal nerves; and the cranial cervical ganglion. Mycotic plaques, empyema, and trauma (hematoma) of the guttural pouch can result in pharyngeal paralysis, dorsal displacement of the soft palate, laryngeal hemiplegia, and occasionally Horner's syndrome.[1,2,9,10,19] The clinician should obtain skull radiographs in many horses with dysphagia; these are especially helpful when traumatic injuries are suspected. Rupture of the longus capitis muscle results in ventral deviation of the dorsal pharynx and narrowing of the nasopharynx. Bony fragments may be evident ventral to the basisphenoid bones in these horses.[10] Otitis media and pathologic fracture of the petrous temporal bone frequently result in vestibular disease and facial nerve paralysis and occasionally in glossopharyngeal and vagus nerve involvement. An endoscopic examination of the guttural pouches is helpful with this problem because the distal stylohyoid bone is thickened and irregular. Ventrodorsal, lateral, and rostrolateral oblique radiographs also may reveal osseous changes of the stylohyoid bone, tympanic bulla, or petrous temporal bone.[19]

The clinical examination should include an evaluation of gait. Signs of ataxia, generalized weakness, and hypermetria along with cranial nerve signs may be observable with brainstem involvement. The clinician should evaluate the horse at the walk, the trot, down an incline, over a step, and backing and turning in tight circles. The clinician may wish to place the feet of the horse in abnormal positions and determine if the horse can reposition the leg correctly in a reasonable time. Generalized weakness (without ataxia) may manifest with a decrease in tail, eyelid, and tongue tone and muscle fasciculations. Weakness generally suggests a neuromuscular (botulism, organophosphate poisoning) or muscular problem.[2,13,14] Equine lower motor neuron disease results in generalized weakness and weight loss; however, affected horses are not dysphagic and do not exhibit cranial nerve abnormalities.[20] Ataxia or hypermetria along with dysphagia suggests a diffuse or multifocal disease that affects the spinal cord and brainstem. Examples of such diseases include equine protozoal myelitis, rabies, equine herpes myeloencephalopathy, polyneuritis equi, and a migrating parasite.[10,21,22] Further diagnostic tests are indicated in these cases, such as an evaluation of spinal fluid for cytologic abnormalities and chemistry and Western blot analysis for antibodies to *Sarcocystis neurona*.[23] Grass sickness, a disease found in Great Britain and other northern European countries, results in ileus and colic. Grass sickness can result in dysphagia, with problems in swallowing or esophageal transport.[24] Grass sickness is regarded as a fatal disease, resulting in ileus of the gastrointestinal tract, dysphagia, and weight loss, which most likely is caused by an unidentified neurotoxin. *Grass sickness* can be defined as a dysautonomia characterized by pathologic lesions in autonomic ganglia, enteric plexi, and specific nuclei in the central nervous system.[25] Additional information about the specific causes of dysphagia are covered elsewhere in this text.

ABDOMINAL DISTENTION

Jonathan H. Foreman

Increases in body weight because of overeating or pregnancy must be distinguished from increases in body girth caused by bloat, ascites, uroperitoneum, fetal hydrops, or ruptured prepubic tendon. In each of these conditions body weight actually may increase because of fetal growth or fluid accumulation. More important, however, a perceptible change in the shape of the abdomen of the horse occurs.

Bloat usually is associated with colic signs in horses and is caused by gaseous intestinal distention resulting from ileus or simple obstruction of the large intestinse or, rarely, the small intestine. Ileus caused by diarrhea, peritonitis, colic surgery, or parasympatholytic agents (e.g., atropine) can result in sufficient accumulation of intraluminal gas to be manifested as tympany, bloat, and mild to severe abdominal pain.[1] If optic topical atropine application is overly aggressive, secondary ileus and bloat may result. Rapid and severe gas production may follow grain overload; cecal and colonic fermentation of readily available carbohydrate sources results in rapid-onset colonic tympany and abdominal distention.[2] Exhaustion in endurance horses also is associated with intestinal shutdown and subsequent abdominal distention.[3] In any of these bloat conditions, abdominal auscultation in the flank area reveals decreased or absent intestinal motility sounds (borborygmi) and perhaps increased gaseous distention sounds (pinging). Decreased borborygmi in the right flank are specific for cecal ileus.

Simple colonic obstruction also results in tympany and bloat. Strangulating obstruction results in greater pain than usually is manifested in simple obstruction and bloat. Colonic displacements are more common in older postpartum mares.[4] These horses often initially show mild colic signs and progressively develop more dramatic pain and abdominal distention. Miniature horses with simple obstructions caused by fecaliths often have bloat as the initial clinical sign.[5] Such cases have the additional complication that rectal examination may be impossible for differentiation of the source of the bloat. Even in full-sized horses, rectal examination may reveal that the abdomen is so filled with distended colon that the examiner cannot push an arm into the rectum any farther than wrist-deep. Colonic or cecal bloat can be relieved by trocarization through the flank, but relief is merely palliative and is usually temporary because the cause of the obstruction still has not been resolved.

Ascites does not occur commonly in horses and usually is caused by peritonitis or abdominal neoplasms. Peritonitis is caused by septicemia, laparotomy, intestinal leakage, internal abscess, or a penetrating external wound resulting in inflammation and usually infection of the peritoneal lining of the abdomen. Such inflammation results in increased fluid production by the squamous abdominal epithelium. Initially, this increased abdominal fluid may be characterized as a transudate (low cell count and low total protein). If inflammation with infection persists, the character of the fluid may change to that of an exudate (increased cell count >5000 nucleated cells/μl, increased neutrophil count, increased degenerate neutrophils, microscopically visible bacteria, and increased total protein).[6,7] These increases in abdominal fluid volume can be substantive and can result in abdominal distention that eventually becomes clinically apparent. Fluid ballottement in the equine abdomen is not an easily performed diagnostic technique but may be easier in foals, ponies, or miniature horses than in full-sized horses.

Ascites also may result from abdominal neoplasms. Tumors reported to cause ascites and weight loss in horses include lymphosarcoma, squamous cell carcinoma, mammary adenocarcinoma, and mesothelioma.[8,9] Although rare, mesothelioma may cause the most fluid production because it is a tumor of the fluid-producing cells of the peritoneal lining. Mesothelioma may result in the production of large volumes of fluid (several liters) in a short time (24 hours) after a similarly large volume is drained from the same horse via abdominal catheterization or trocarization.

Ascites also may result from any condition that produces lowered serum total protein and albumin. With lowered intravascular colloid osmotic pressure, fluid diffuses or moves from the vasculature and results in dependent peripheral edema. Fluid also may accumulate within the major body cavities (i.e., the thorax and the abdomen).[7] The mechanisms for such low-protein conditions include poor protein intake, malabsorption, poor hepatic utilization, and increased rate of protein loss such as in glomerular renal disease, peritonitis/pleuritis, or gastrointestinal transudation (diarrhea or ulceration). Causes of peripheral edema are described elsewhere in this text.

Increased preload because of right ventricular heart failure also can result in a transudate fluid accumulation within the abdomen.[7] A horse with right ventricular heart failure usually has tricuspid insufficiency and manifests other signs of right ventricular heart failure, such as a murmur; exercise intolerance; jugular pulse; and edema of the ventral abdomen, pectoral muscles, and distal limbs. Severe mitral insufficiency also can result in right ventricular heart failure but only after the development of left ventricular heart failure and its associated pulmonary edema, which is manifested by exercise intolerance, coughing, epistaxis, and increased respiratory effort.

Uroperitoneum results from leakage of urine from some part of the urinary tract into the abdomen and most commonly is associated with a ruptured bladder in neonatal foals (usually male). Uroperitoneum also may result from a necrotic bladder caused by neonatal sepsis and urachal abscesses. Such foals often have pendulous, bloated abdomens that ballotte more easily than do the abdomens of adult horses with accumulation of fluid. Abdominal fluid actually may smell like urine, and peritoneal fluid creatinine concentrations will be high—often more than twice those of peripheral blood.[10-12] Because most classically described neonatal urinary bladder tears are dorsal near the trigone, the foal still may be able to produce a stream of urine despite having a leaking bladder. A ruptured urinary bladder abscess should be suspected in a foal with sepsis that initially responds to therapy for sepsis and then, several days later, exhibits acute-onset depression, anorexia, ileus, and abdominal distention. Adults horses rarely have uroperitoneum; however, uroperitoneum has been associated with ruptured urinary bladders during stressful parturition in mares that manifest mild postpartum abdominal pain and abdominal distention.[12,13]

Fetal hydrops results from an accumulation of excessive amounts of fluid within the amnion (hydrops amnion) or chorioallantois (hydrops allantois).[14] Hydrops results in a bilaterally pendulous abdomen in a late-term pregnant mare. A rapid accumulation of fluid over 10 to 14 days may make walking or perhaps even breathing difficult for the mare. A diagnosis may be made after taking history and performing a rectal examination, although palpating the fetus is usually difficult because the excess fluid causes the uterus to descend out of reach of the examiner. If necessary, a percutaneous ultrasonographic examination may be used to confirm the diagnosis by documenting the presence of increased intrauterine fluid within the fetal membranes.

A ruptured prepubic tendon results in a unilateral lowering of the abdominal margin and apparent distention of the abdomen only on the affected side. The condition is associated routinely with later-term pregnancy in mares and is thought to occur simply because of the increased weight of the pregnant uterus pressing downward on the abdominal wall. Rupture of the rectus, transverse, or oblique abdominal muscles also can result in ventral dropping or herniation of the abdomen late in gestation.[14] Ruptures may be more common in older or more sedentary mares, probably because of decreased abdominal wall strength and tone. Other than a focal abdominal wall hernia, a unilateral prepubic tendon rupture results in the only form of prominent unilateral abdominal distention in horses. Mares with ruptured prepubic tendons may have elicitable pain in the local abdominal wall and may be reluctant to walk. They may need assistance during parturition because they may have difficulty performing an effective abdominal press to aid in fetal expulsion.

APPROACH TO THE DIAGNOSIS OF ABDOMINAL DISTENTION

Pregnancy, diarrhea, colic signs, colic surgery, and the use of parasympatholytic agents should be evident from the history. The rate of onset of abdominal distention may help to distinguish more acute conditions (e.g., gastrointestinal bloat from grain overload) from more chronic conditions (e.g., ascites caused by heart or liver failure). Signalment and history may assist in indicating specific conditions. A depressed, 48- to 72-hour-old male foal with fluid abdominal distention may be a likely candidate to have a ruptured urinary bladder and uroperitoneum. Miniature horses with bloat and colic signs frequently have simple obstructions owing to fecaliths or enteroliths.

A complete physical examination reveals the presence of a murmur that may be associated with heart failure and ascites. Other signs of heart failure also may be evident on physical examination. An actual defect in the integrity of the abdominal wall may be palpable on external examination of the abdomen in a mare with a ruptured prepubic tendon or ruptured abdominal wall musculature.[14] The veterinarian should attempt ballottement to discern the presence of increased free abdominal fluid in suspected ascites or uroperitoneum. Fever may indicate the presence of an infectious peritonitis or umbilical abscess.

A rectal examination is a critical part of examining a horse with bloat or colic but may be difficult to accomplish if colonic distention is dramatic or if the patient is small (i.e., a foal, pony, or miniature horse). A rectal examination may document advanced pregnancy, resulting in mild bilateral abdominal distention (normal pregnancy), abnormal or severe bilateral distention (hydrops or bilateral ruptured prepubic tendon), or unilateral distention (unilateral ruptured prepubic tendon or focal abdominal wall hernia). A rectal examination also may reveal abnormalities of the urinary tract (enlarged kidney or ureter, abscess, or neoplasm), which may result in uroperitoneum in adults.

An ultrasonographic examination may be helpful and is sometimes necessary to examine the distended abdomen and fetus in a pregnant mare. Such an examination must be performed percutaneously in late gestation. Ultrasonography can determine the location of increased abdominal fluid (intrauterine or extrauterine) and the health status of the fetus. Percutaneous placement of base-apex electrocardiographic leads across the abdomen of the mare may help to document that the fetus is still viable if an ultrasound examination does not produce definitive evidence (heart movement or gross fetal movement).[15]

Cardiac ultrasonography may help to document the presence of a cardiac valvular defect that can be the cause of ascites in a horse with heart failure. Abdominal radiography may assist in the diagnosis of abdominal distention caused by intestinal obstruction in a foal or miniature horse. Percutaneous ultrasound examination also may assist in documenting the source of abdominal distention (e.g., intussusception) in smaller horses or foals [3,16] and in characterizing umbilical and urachal abnormalities.[3]

Complete blood counts and plasma fibrinogen concentrations assist in diagnosing inflammatory conditions such as infectious peritonitis. Urachal or urinary bladder abscesses also may be associated with inflammatory leukograms. Blood or peritoneal fluid cultures may assist in documenting the offending bacterial agent(s). Foals or adults with uroperitoneum have elevated serum urea nitrogen, creatinine, and potassium and decreased serum sodium, chloride, and bicarbonate concentrations.[10,11]

Abdominocentesis should be attempted to distinguish the cause of ascites. Care must be taken, however, when obtaining peritoneal fluid from late-term pregnant mares to avoid penetrating directly into the distended uterus. Analysis of peritoneal fluid reveals abdominal fluid to be a transudate (equivocal infection) or exudate (probable infection).[6,7] Fluid should be cultured aerobically and anaerobically when infectious peritonitis is suspected. Exfoliative cytologic examination rarely may document the presence of neoplastic cells.[8,9] Peritoneal fluid creatinine concentration approaches or often exceeds (more than twice) that of serum if uroperitoneum is present.[10,11] Serum and peritoneal urea nitrogen concentrations are less reliable for such a diagnosis because the peritoneal membrane does not differentially sequester urea nitrogen (but does creatinine) within the abdominal cavity.

COLIC

Siddra Hines

Colic is defined as the manifestation of abdominal pain. In horses colic is a serious medical and economic problem worldwide. In the United States the annual incidence of equine colic has been reported to be anywhere between 3.5% and 26%. A study performed by the National Animal Health Monitoring System in 1998 assessed the annual incidence to be 4.2%.[1] In this study only 1.4% of colic episodes resulted in surgery, but the overall fatality rate for all colic was 11%, making colic second only to old age as a leading cause of death in horses.[1] The estimated total cost of colic nationally in 1998 was $115 million.[1] These numbers illustrate the enormous impact that colic has on the equine population.

Colic encompasses a wide variety of conditions, and determining the specific cause of colic is a complex and sometimes impossible task. Because many cases resolve with minimal intervention, a specific diagnosis is often not made. Most cases of colic, often referred to as "true colics," are conditions of the gastrointestinal tract. However, disorders of other body systems, such as cholelithiasis and uterine torsion, may also manifest as colic. In addition, a number of other clinical problems may be confused with colic, including pleuritis, exertional rhabdomyolysis, laminitis, hyperkalemic periodic paralysis, renal disease, and even neurologic abnormalities.[2] A thorough physical examination and further diagnostic tests help ascertain whether or not a horse is exhibiting actual gastrointestinal pain.

Horses express clinical signs of colic in a variety of ways. Often, the first sign recognized by owners is inappetence, but other early signs include general restlessness and extended periods of lying down. More overt signs, such as kicking or biting at the abdomen, pawing, and stretching out as if to urinate, may also be observed. As the level of discomfort increases, horses may repeatedly get up and down and try to roll, sometimes violently.[3] The level of stoicism varies widely between individual horses, and the severity of signs does not always correlate to the severity of the lesion.

PATHOPHYSIOLOGY

The precise pathophysiologic mechanisms involved in cases of colic may vary because of the myriad causes for colic in the horse. True colic can be classified on the basis of small intestinal versus large intestinal disorders, physical versus functional disorders, obstructive versus nonobstructive lesions, and strangulating versus nonstrangulating lesions. In all of these colic classifications, the simplest basic etiologies for damage to the gastrointestinal tract are inflammation and ischemia. Gastrointestinal distention, ileus, and endotoxemia also play a role in the development of disease in many cases.

Ischemia of the intestine can result from a strangulating lesion or even from a simple obstruction. Strangulating lesions cause acute direct occlusion of vessels leading to rapid tissue hypoxia, ischemia, and ultimately necrosis. With obstructions significant pressure within the distended intestine may lead to venous collapse, which over time may result in ischemia as the intestinal vasculature becomes increasingly compromised.[3]

The mucosa is the layer most sensitive to hypoxia because of its high metabolic activity. Damage to the mucosa can be assessed on a scale of Grade I through Grade V, with Grade V being the most severe.[4] The villous tips are especially sensitive to ischemia and damage typically begins there. Crypt cells are affected later as the ischemia becomes more complete and longer in duration. In the equine colon complete ischemia leads to necrosis and detachment of surface epithelial cells and most likely to capillary thrombosis and occlusion.[4] Smooth muscle is less sensitive to hypoxia, and therefore it is destruction of the mucosa that is the main factor leading to the pathologic changes associated with colic.

Prolonged intestinal distention proximal to an obstructive lesion can eventually lead to tissue ischemia. Distention also results in edema and additional secretion of fluid into the lumen of the gut as venous collapse occurs.[4] As veins are occluded, hydrostatic pressure within the capillaries increases, causing increased filtration. Lymphatic drainage is also often impaired, and the resultant excess fluid becomes edema and secreted intestinal fluid. Distention is one of the main causes of pain associated with colic, as stretch pain receptors are triggered within the wall of the intestine.[4]

Inflammation plays a major role in almost every type of colic and often occurs secondary to ischemia. The inflammatory response is generally meant to protect the intestine against long-term damage. The pathophysiology of inflammation is complex and beyond the scope of this section, but the basic process in the gut is similar to that of other body systems. Almost all cells in the intestine can play a role in the development of inflammation by either cytokine production or cell activation. Some specific cell types involved in the initiation of intestinal inflammation include mucosal cells, endothelial cells, fibroblasts, neutrophils, macrophages, neurons, eosinophils, and mast cells.[5] Cytokines, growth factors, and adhesion molecules produced by these cells are important in the initiation of inflammation. Some important cytokines include interleukin-1, tumor necrosis factor (TNF) α, platelet activating factor, complement, interferon (IFN), and histamine.[5]

Endothelial cells are stimulated by ischemia or macrophage cytokines to attract neutrophils, which subsequently migrate to the affected tissue facilitated by adhesion molecules. Vascular permeability is also increased, resulting in the formation of edema and facilitating the migration of inflammatory cells. Neurons, fibroblasts, and muscle cells detect and release other cytokines, leading to the activation of many effector cell types.[5]

Eventually the intestinal barrier is compromised to the extent that endotoxin begins to leak into systemic circulation. Endotoxemia (discussed in detail in Chapter 15) is most common with colitis and to a lesser extent with strangulating lesions. The response to endotoxin is complex, involving a massive release of cytokines and mediators that results in systemic inflammation and fever. Classical endotoxemia has more recently been described as *systemic inflammatory response syndrome* (SIRS), because it appears to involve more than just endotoxin as an initiating factor.[5] The result is hemodynamic responses that include both vasodilation and vasoconstriction, platelet aggregation, and eventual development of a hypercoagulable state and consumptive coagulopathy.[4]

Finally, ileus should be addressed as an important component of the pathophysiology of colic. Ischemic bowel has decreased motility, although bowel more proximal to the lesion tends to have an increase in motility until it becomes so distended that it can no longer contract normally. Postoperative ileus appears to involve both dopaminergic and adrenergic stimulation. It has also been suggested that prostaglandins E_1 and E_2, as well as nitric oxide, play a role in disrupting intestinal motility patterns.[4]

APPROACH TO THE PATIENT WITH COLIC

Colic may be caused by a number of conditions. Fortunately, in most affected horses, such as those with gas or spasmodic colics, the problem can be resolved without extensive intervention. However, in some cases, a delay in surgical exploration can result in increased mortality. Thus the initial goal in the assessment of a horse with colic is often to determine whether the case is an uncomplicated one rather than one requiring either extensive medical management or surgical exploration. Signalment, history, physical examination, clinicopathologic data, and imaging findings may all contribute to the evaluation of a patient with colic.

The signalment of the horse can provide some information that may increase the degree of suspicion for a specific cause of colic. Weanling-age foals are more prone to ascarid impactions,[2,6] whereas younger foals are at higher risk for small intestinal volvulus or intussusception.[7] Older horses have a far greater likelihood of developing strangulating lipomas.[4,8] In general, Arabians are considered to be at higher risk for colic than other breeds and are specifically predisposed to ileal impaction, small colon impaction, and enterolith formation.[2] Miniature horses, especially younger horses, are prone to small colon impactions and fecaliths.[2,4] Standardbreds, Tennessee Walking Horses, and Warmblood stallions have a higher risk of developing inguinal hernias.[2,4]

With regard to sex, stallions are susceptible to testicular torsion in addition to inguinal hernias.[4] Postpartum mares are predisposed to torsion of the large colon,[2,4] whereas colic in a late-gestation mare may indicate normal parturition or dystocia. Pregnant mares also exhibit signs of colic with uterine torsion.[2,3] Nonpregnant mares can have mild transient signs of colic associated with ovarian activity.

The history of the patient can provide vital clues as to the severity and possible etiology of the colic. Previous history of colic, including colic surgery, history of other surgeries, recent management changes, geographic area, breeding history and pregnancy status, duration and severity of pain, recent defecation, appetite, previous treatment, and response to treatment are all important components in the medical history of a colicky horse. Additionally, specific details as to feed, deworming, dentistry, history of medications (e.g., nonsteroidal anti-inflammatory drugs [NSAIDS], antibiotics), and activity level may also provide valuable diagnostic information. Factors that tend to increase risk of colic include inadequate deworming or dentistry, use of NSAIDs, stall confinement, recent feed changes, feeding of Coastal Bermuda grass hay, feeding of excessive concentrate or infrequent large meals, and off-the-ground feeding.[2,9] A link has also been identified between cribbing and an increased likelihood of developing epiploic foramen entrapment.[10]

A thorough physical examination is essential to the evaluation of colic. It is possible that a horse will be so uncomfortable initially that sedation will be necesssary for safe completion of the examination. If possible, heart rate, respiratory rate, and auscultation of gut sounds should be evaluated before sedation because these can change significantly in response to sedation.[11,12] Because rectal temperature can also be significantly decreased after rectal palpation, it is advisable to obtain the body temperature before palpation.[3] A finding of pyrexia may increase suspicion of colitis, enteritis, peritonitis, or intra-abdominal abscessation in the patient, although previous administration of an NSAID may mask this clinical finding.[2,4] Tachycardia is considered to be an indicator of pain, hypovolemia, tachyarrhythmia, or endotoxemia and rates of >80 beats/min generally indicate serious disease.[2,4] During auscultation the patient should be evaluated for the presence of any cardiac abnormalities that would put the horse at increased risk under sedation. Respiratory rate may be increased in horses with colic as a response to some combination of pain, fever, and/or metabolic acidosis. Mucous membranes and capillary refill time (CRT) give a rough assessment of cardiovascular status and peripheral perfusion. Mucous membranes should be pink with a CRT <2 seconds. Prolonged CRT and either grayish or dark red mucous membranes indicate impaired cardiovascular status and poor perfusion. With poor perfusion, there may also be cool extremities and reduced jugular fill. Significant changes in mucous membrane color, often with a dark "toxic" line adjacent to the teeth, may accompany endotoxemia, which is common in gastrointestinal disease, particularly in those horses with colitis, proximal enteritis, and strangulating lesions. Icterus does not always indicate hepatobiliary disease because horses that have been off feed for more than 48 hours will also exhibit hyperbilirubinemia. Finally, tacky mucous membranes are generally observed with dehydration of at least 5% to 7%.[2]

Other important considerations include assessment of hydration status, attitude, abdominal distention, and the presence of injuries that indicate self-trauma. As previously mentioned, in stallions careful palpation of the inguinal region must be performed to identify an inguinal hernia or testicular torsion. Severe abdominal distention may markedly increase the respiratory effort and eventually lead to respiratory distress. During auscultation of gastrointestinal sounds, auscultation of the most ventral part of the abdomen should also be performed to assess for the presence of sand. Although not always present, a characteristic "waves on the beach" sound can sometimes be heard, indicating the presence of sand in the colon.[13] If feces can be collected from the horse, it is very useful to evaluate for the presence of sand. A simple way to do this is to mix a few fecal balls with warm water in a rectal sleeve and hang the sleeve with the fingers down. After about 5 minutes any sand in the feces should sediment into the ends of the glove fingers.[2]

Adequate restraint is essential for colic diagnostics such as rectal palpation, nasogastric intubation, and abdominocentesis. Not only is the veterinarian at increased risk of injury with an uncooperative horse, but the horse also is at increased risk of rectal tears, significant epistaxis, and abdominocentesis complications such as enterocentesis or contamination of the collection site. Depending on the case, restraint for further examination can be accomplished using sedation or application of a nose twitch. Care should be taken when determining appropriate restraint for an individual animal. The safety of the examiner and the horse must be considered; at the same time, it is important not to further compromise an unstable patient or dramatically affect assessment of the horse's level of pain. Use of xylazine hydrochloride IV at 0.2 to 0.5 mg/kg (typically 100 to 250 mg for a 500-kg horse) is often adequate, but butorphanol tartrate at 0.01 to 0.08 mg/kg IV can be added when necessary.[3] Use of detomidine is usually discouraged in the initial management of colic because of its long duration of action and heightened ability to mask more significant pain that may affect determination of the horse's treatment.[12] However, if indicated, detomidine can be administered at 0.01 to 0.04 mg/kg IV or IM.[3] It is most commonly used when a longer duration of sedation is required to keep a horse quiet during transport to a referral center.

Nasogastric intubation should be performed as a part of a complete colic examination. If a horse is exhibiting significant pain or has a heart rate greater than 60 beats/min on initial evaluation, nasogastric intubation should be performed before other diagnostic procedures because it may have both diagnostic and therapeutic value. It is important to note that if a horse has significant gastric distention, gastric decompression may help prevent gastric rupture and allow for a more thorough physical exam. The nasogastric tube can be left in place if a significant amount of net reflux is obtained to allow for repeated decompression. If no reflux is obtained and a simple colic is suspected, oral fluids with or without electrolytes or magnesium sulfate (Epsom salt) can be administered via the tube. Although mineral oil has long been considered a part of standard colic treatment, its use is controversial. Mineral oil may be valuable as a diagnostic tool, providing an estimate of gastrointestinal transit time. In a normal horse mineral oil can be observed in the feces and on perineum and tail in 12 to 24 hours.[14] The absence of mineral oil after this period indicates delayed gastrointestinal transit. However, mineral oil can sometimes pass around an impaction that is present, thereby falsely suggesting adequate gastrointestinal transit when in fact digesta is not moving normally.[14] In addition, if a horse ultimately requires abdominal surgery, the presence of mineral oil can complicate an enterotomy.[15]

Rectal palpation can be important in the assessment of colic. Even with the use of appropriate sedation, some horses remain resistant to rectal examination, placing them at increased risk for rectal tears. To facilitate palpation per rectum, application of lidocaine within the rectal lumen or intravenous administration of N-butylscopolammonium can help to decrease rectal pressure and peristalsis.[16] Although rectal palpation can provide valuable diagnostic information, the presence or absence of a particular lesion cannot always be definitively determined. For instance, although a pelvic flexure or cecal impaction may be palpable, if no impaction is palpated, it cannot be ruled out. Additionally, gas distention might be palpable in gas colic, but it may also reflect a more serious problem, such as a displacement or torsion. Rectal palpation therefore can provide evidence to support a diagnosis but is often not diagnostic in itself. Nephrosplenic entrapment may be suspected if the spleen is displaced medially or the gut is palpated between the spleen and kidney.[2] Another useful finding is the identification of distended small intestine. Although small intestinal distention may occasionally occur secondary to a large intestinal problem such as a displacement, it is most often an indication of small intestinal disease. Although rectal palpation cannot differentiate a surgical small intestinal problem such as a strangulating lesion from a medical problem such as proximal enteritis, small intestinal disease is almost always an indication for referral.[17] Therefore palpable loops of distended small intestine are a significant finding on rectal examination. Rectal palpation can also be useful for identifying masses in the abdomen, which may be a cause of chronic colic.

A packed cell volume (PCV) and total protein should ideally be evaluated to assist with a assesssment of hydration status and possible protein loss. These values can be affected by stress, which can increase the PCV, anemia, protein loss, or hyperproteinemia, confounding the effects of dehydration.[4] Therefore these values must be evaluated in the context of the history and physical examination of the patient as well as their relationship to each other. In general, the greatest negative indicator is a significantly increased PCV (i.e., >65%) coupled with a significantly low plasma protein concentration (i.e., <4 g/dl), especially if serial values are trending toward these extremes.[2,4]

Although further bloodwork usually is not performed on a standard simple colic, a complete blood count (CBC) and serum chemistry can provide valuable information if a colic goes beyond simple treatment and requires more advanced care. In acute colic, CBC values will typically be normal or reflect stress, but in more chronic conditions nonspecific signs of inflammation such as leukocytosis and hyperfibrinogenemia can develop as well as a possible normochromic normocytic anemia of chronic disease. If significant colon wall compromise occurs, leukopenia with neutropenia and a left shift with toxic changes can occur as a result of endotoxemia.[2,3] Thrombocytopenia may also be present with endotoxemia.

Electrolyte abnormalities, especially hypokalemia and hypocalcemia, are the most common abnormalities observed on a chemistry panel in horses with colic.[18] Anorexia, dehydration, diarrhea, and excessive nasogastric reflux can all contribute to derangement of electrolytes. In addition to calcium and potassium, sodium, chloride, magnesium, and bicarbonate can be lost with diarrhea or significant gastric reflux.[18] Leakage from damaged cells may result in elevated serum phosphate. Metabolic acidosis caused by elevation of lactate, loss of bicarbonate, or both may also be observed. Occasionally, hepatic enzyme activities are increased, especially γ-glutamyltransferase. This most commonly occurs with large colon displacement or proximal enteritis.[19,20] Dehydration often results in elevations in creatinine and serum urea nitrogen, and these parameters should be monitored, especially when NSAIDs or aminoglycoside antibiotics are used.

Abdominocentesis can be performed in the field as well as in a referral setting. Most often the procedure requires either an 18-g, 1.5-inch needle or a teat cannula for the collection of fluid. The typical location in which the procedure is performed is to the right of midline (to avoid splenocentesis) on the most ventral point of the abdomen at least several inches caudal to the xiphoid.[4] If severe gas distention or small intestinal distention is present, or if a sand enterocolitis is suspected, it may be advisable to forego abdominocentesis in order to avoid puncture of a distended compromised viscus or a heavy sand-filled viscus that is sitting flush with the ventral body wall.

Although a practitioner may not have access to a full fluid analysis and cytology, a basic assessment of abdominal fluid can be made by visual evaluation for color and clarity, and total protein can be evaluated with a refractometer. Normal fluid should be odorless, nonturbid, and a clear to pale yellow color.[4] Increased turbidity can indicate increased protein, increased total nucleated cell count, or both. Total protein should be less than 2.5 g/dL.[4,21] A normal cell count is typically less than 5000 cells/μl, although it may be normal up to 10,000/μl.[4,21] Serosanguinous fluid usually reflects a strangulating obstruction or significant compromise to the bowel wall. With a ruptured gastrointestinal structure, the fluid is generally dark and smells of ingesta. These results should be confirmed, however, because an accidental enterocentesis will appear the same.[4] If the spleen is accidentally punctured, the fluid will look like frank blood and will usually have a PCV equal to or greater than the peripheral PCV.[22]

Ultrasound examination of the abdomen may be useful in the evaluation of horses with colic. It is particularly valuable in the identification of small intestinal distention or nephrosplenic entrapment. With a nephrosplenic entrapment the spleen cannot be visualized against the body wall, or the kidney cannot be visualized on the left side because of the interference of large colon.[23] Small intestine can most reliably be found in the inguinal region or on the ventral abdomen, and it should normally be collapsed or have a very small diameter with frequent peristalsis.[21,24] Small intestine can be evaluated for dilation, motility, and thickening of the intestinal wall.[24] An intussusception may be identified as a target-shaped lesion on cross-sectional view.[25] Ultrasonographic assessment of peritoneal fluid volume and character may be useful in assessing the patient and in identifying pockets of representative fluid for abdominocentesis. The thickness of intestinal wall should be evaluated at numerous locations, especially the right dorsal colon, which may be extraordinarily thickened with right dorsal colitis.[24] Investigation for abdominal masses also is often undertaken using ultrasound, coupled with rectal palpation. Adequate transabdominal ultrasound examination is most easily performed with a 2.5 to 5 MHz curved linear transducer; however, an examination can also be performed using a transrectal probe, which is more likely to be available to the general practitioner.[24,26]

Radiographs of the abdomen are of limited usefulness but may be diagnostic for two problems associated with colic in the adult horse: sand accumulation and enterolithiasis. Sand is usually visualized best in the ventral large colon. It is important to keep in mind that some sand can be visualized in many normal horses, so the presence of sand in and of itself has no diagnostic relevance. Radiographs may, however, provide some information as to the volume of sand present.[27] Enteroliths represent the other main lesion identifiable by radiographs, although, depending on the location, they may be difficult to visualize.[21] In a study of 141 horses evaluated for enterolithiasis, abdominal radiography had a sensitivity of 76.9% and a specificity of 94.4%.[28] The abdomen can be more thoroughly assessed via radiography in a neonate as opposed to an adult horse, although results still cannot be considered conclusively diagnostic. Radiographs of a foal's abdomen can identify gas distention of the stomach, small intestine, or large colon, which are nonspecific but generally pathologic findings.[7] A radiographic pattern known as *pneumatosis intestinalis,* characterized by linear radiolucencies within the bowel wall, is typical for necrotizing enterocolitis.[7] Excessive peritoneal fluid and pneumoperitoneum can also be identified.

Referral to a secondary care center is indicated when there is a strong likelihood that the horse will require surgery or more extensive medical care is necessary. The most common basis for referral is severe or persistent pain with a lack of response to analgesics.[17] If a horse demonstrates intractable pain or requires repeated doses of analgesics to remain comfortable, referral is warranted. Referral is also indicated when a horse has not resolved the signs of colic in 24 to 48 hours after onset, or if a 1.1 mg/kg dose of flunixin meglumine does not maintain comfort for at least 8 to 12 hours.[17] A persistently elevated heart rate can be a good indicator of pain or endotoxemia and necessitates referral. Other indications of endotoxemia or impaired cardiovascular status include weak pulses, abnormal mucous membrane color (pale, hyperemic, injected, purple, or cyanotic), and delayed capillary refill time. Rectal palpation of a potentially surgical lesion or small intestinal distention, an abnormal abdominocentesis, net nasogastric reflux of >2 to 3 L, or significant depression are all findings that would also support referral.[17] In addition, significant dehydration may require extensive treatment with intravenousor oral fluids or both because dehydration has the potential to exacerbate even apparently simple colic problems and affects the patient's systemic health. Dehydration can result in worsening of an impaction that is already present or contribute to development of an impaction when coupled with ileus and an inciting primary colic problem such as colonic displacement.

DIARRHEA

Melissa T. Hines

Diarrhea, defined as an increase in the frequency, fluidity, or volume of bowel movements, is a commonly encountered clinical problem in the horse. Diarrhea may occur as a primary disease of the gastrointestinal tract or as a secondary response to another disease process, such as sepsis, endotoxemia, or hepatic disease.

The function of the equine gastrointestinal tract is complex and involves maintenance of normal fluid balance and digestion and absorption.[1-3] As a result of dietary intake and endogenous secretions, normally a large volume of fluid enters the gastrointestinal tract, most of which is reabsorbed. In the adult horse absorption occurs predominantly in the large bowel, where a volume of water approximately equal to the total extracellular fluid volume of the animal, or about 100 L, is recovered during the course of the day. Because the large colon is the primary site of water resorption, most significant diarrheal disease in the adult horse involves the colon. In young foals, however, small intestinal disorders such as rotaviral infection also may result in diarrhea.[4]

A second critical function of the large bowel is that of microbial digestion of carbohydrates and, to some extent, protein or nonprotein nitrogen.[1-3] Microbial fermentation of carbohydrates in the cecum and colon results primarily in the production of volatile fatty acids, which are absorbed readily, providing up to 75% of the energy requirement of the horse. Therefore maintaining a stable environment for the microbial population is important. In general, efficient function of the large bowel requires mechanisms that limit the rate of digesta passage, provide optimal conditions for microbial digestion, and allow for efficient transport of solutes and water.

The characteristics of normal equine feces vary somewhat with diet. Generally, equine feces are tan, brown, or greenish, and, although approximately 75% water, they are well formed. An adult horse on a diet of grass hay and approximately 3 lb of oats per day produces about 20 to 28 g of feces per kilogram of body mass per day, or about 11 to 13 kg of feces per day.[5] In cases of diarrhea the amount of feces may increase up to tenfold, with horses producing more than 200 g/kg/day, or more than 90 L of diarrhea. As a result, diarrhea can cause significant losses of electrolytes and water and significant systemic acid-base imbalances. However, despite large water losses, horses with chronic diarrhea seldom develop severe dehydration or electrolyte abnormalities because they compensate for increased fecal losses.

MECHANISMS OF DIARRHEA

Inflammation within the bowel plays a central role in the pathogenesis of diarrhea. Several basic mechanisms of diarrhea have been described, and in most diarrheal diseases more than one mechanism is involved. These mechanisms include the following:

1. *Malabsorption:* Malabsorption results from a decrease in the functional absorptive surface area of the gastrointestinal tract. Villus atrophy in the small intestine, seen with rotaviral enteritis and infiltrative bowel disease, can result in malabsorption because of the loss of functional epithelium and maldigestion caused by decreased production of digestive enzymes. A number of insults to the colon result in inflammation and disruption of absorptive cells and tight junctions, leading to decreased absorptive capacity and decreased ability to retain absorbed fluid (i.e., increased loss). Several inflammatory mediators, such as histamines and prostaglandins, contribute to the colonic inflammation. These mediators are produced primarily by inflammatory cells in the lamina propria and inhibit absorption through a variety of mechanisms.[6-10]
2. *Increased secretion:* The increased secretion of solutes and water by the inflamed colon can contribute significantly to the development of diarrhea. Although the precise mechanisms of secretion in the equine colon are not understood fully, active secretion and passive fluid loss occur.[6-12] Control of active secretion is complex, involving two primary pathways: first, the activation of adenyl cyclase, resulting in an increase of intracellular cyclic adenosine monophosphate concentrations, and second, the activation of calcium channels, leading to increased intracellular calcium concentrations.[11,12] Cyclic adenosine monophosphate and calcium stimulate specific secretory activities, primarily through chloride channels. In some cases of diarrhea, bacterial enterotoxins such as those produced by certain strains of *Escherichia coli* and *Salmonella* spp. stimulate adenyl cyclase activity, thus

increasing active secretion. This is true hypersecretory diarrhea. Also, a number of inflammatory mediators produced by the inflamed colon, particularly prostaglandin E, increase intracellular concentrations of cyclic adenosine monophosphate and to some extent calcium, thereby increasing active secretion by mucosal cells.[11-13] Inflammation also enhances passive fluid loss through a number of factors, such as changes in hydrostatic pressure in the colonic capillaries, mucosal damage, and loss of tight junctions. In horses with severe mucosal injury, the loss of protein can decrease vascular oncotic pressure and further potentiate fluid exchange across the endothelium.

3. *Decreased transit time (abnormal motility):* Progressive motility must be present for diarrhea to occur. Primary motility disorders causing diarrhea are not well recognized, although diarrhea associated with stress or excitement may represent this phenomenon. Inflammation is known to influence gastrointestinal motility, in addition to altering absorption and secretion. However, the precise significance of the altered motility in the pathogenesis of diarrhea is not clear. Sufficient retention time and thorough mixing are required for digestion and absorption of nutrients and fluid to occur, and decreased intestinal transit time has been recognized in association with many gastrointestinal diseases, including infectious diarrhea. Absorption of endotoxin and the release of inflammatory mediators, including prostaglandins, disrupts normal motility patterns.[14] In some cases of acute colitis, a period of ileus may occur without diarrhea. With diarrheal diseases, the elimination of gut contents is part of the normal host defense mechanism, and thus decreasing motility is not indicated in most cases.
4. *Osmotic overload:* Any increase in osmotically active particles within the intestinal lumen can result in diarrhea. The increase can be associated with the administration or ingestion of osmotically active substances such as magnesium sulfate. The increase also may be associated with overloading of the intestine with carbohydrates or occasionally lipids beyond the amount that can be digested and absorbed. Therefore sudden dietary changes that result in significant shifts in gut flora and changes in fermentation or gastrointestinal diseases that result in malabsorption or maldigestion also may result in an osmotic diarrhea. In foals the loss of villus epithelial cells in the small intestine associated with disorders such as rotavirus infection and clostridiosis may lead not only to malabsorption but also to maldigestion caused by the decreased production of lactase.[4,15] The resulting lactose intolerance allows excess lactose to enter the large intestine, increasing the osmotic load.
5. *Increased hydraulic pressure from the blood to the lumen:* This mechanism of diarrhea is more common in chronic conditions, such as congestive heart failure or inflammatory bowel disease. The condition may result from decreased oncotic pressure associated with hypoproteinemia, increased capillary hydrostatic pressure (as in heart failure), or decreased lymphatic drainage associated with inflammation of lymphatics and lymph nodes.

Understanding the mechanisms of diarrhea can be helpful in directing therapy. However, it is important to remember that most disorders that cause diarrhea, whether infectious or noninfectious, do so through inflammatory mechanisms resulting in multiple functional alterations.

DIAGNOSTIC APPROACH TO THE PATIENT WITH DIARRHEA

Diarrhea is a common, and sometimes fatal, clinical problem of adult horses and foals. A number of specific causes for acute and chronic diarrhea have been identified (Tables 3-2, 3-3, and 3-4). A comprehensive evaluation may help in establishing a diagnosis and developing a treatment plan (Box 3-1). However, even in severe cases a definitive diagnosis often is not made, making the problem particularly frustrating.[16,17]

HISTORY AND PHYSICAL EXAMINATION

The veterinarian should consider the signalment and history carefully when evaluating a patient with diarrhea. Age is particularly important because several disorders, such as foal heat diarrhea and rotavirus, are age related. The genetic background also may be significant because diarrhea has been associated with certain heritable immunodeficiencies, and granulomatous bowel disease has been identified in three sibling horses.[18-20] Establishing whether the diarrhea is acute or chronic is important. Other historical questions of particular relevance include dietary changes; deworming program; involvement of single versus multiple animals; exposure to sand; and the use of medications, especially antibiotics and NSAIDs.[21-23] Other concurrent diseases, stress, possible exposure to toxins, weight loss, water consumption, and salt availability also may be significant. The information obtained helps the veterinarian prioritize differential diagnoses and direct further testing.

TABLE 3-2

Differential Diagnoses for Acute Diarrhea in Adult Horses

Common Causes	Major Diagnostic Test(s)
Salmonellosis	Fecal culture or polymerase chain reaction (PCR), culture of rectal mucosal biopsy
Potomac horse fever *(Neorickettsia risticii)*	PCR (feces, peripheral blood), paired serologic tests
Clostridiosis *(Clostridium difficile, C. perfringens)*	Fecal culture, toxin analysis
Antibiotic-associated diarrhea	History
Nonsteroidal anti-inflammatory toxicity (primarily right dorsal colitis)	History and supportive clinicopathologic findings, ultrasonography, exploratory surgery with biopsy
Undiagnosed	Other conditions ruled out
Less Common	
Cantharidin toxicity	
Parasitism (strongylosis, cyathostomiasis, other)	
Aeromonas, Campylobacter spp.	
Sand	
Carbohydrate overload	
Arsenic toxicity, other toxicities	
Thromboembolic disease	
Anaphylaxis	

TABLE 3-3

Differential Diagnoses for Chronic Diarrhea in Adult Horses

Cause of Diarrhea	Major Diagnostic Test(s)
Chronic salmonellosis	Fecal culture or polymerase chain reaction, culture
Sand	Fecal sedimentation
Parasitism (strongylosis, cyathostomiasis)	Fecal egg count, empirical deworming
Nonsteroidal anti-inflammatory toxicity (primarily right dorsal colitis)	History and supportive clinicopathologic findings, ultrasonography, exploratory surgery with biopsy
Inflammatory or infiltrative disorders	Histopathologic exam, absorption tests (supportive but nonspecific)
Inflammatory bowel disease (granulomatous, lymphocytic-plasmacytic, or eosinophilic enterocolitis)	
Mucosal lymphosarcoma	
Amyloidosis	
Dietary: abnormal fermentation	History
Neoplasms: lymphosarcoma, squamous cell carcinoma	Histopathologic exam
Peritonitis, abdominal abscessation	Peritoneal fluid analysis, ultrasound, exploratory surgery
Nongastrointestinal causes (chronic liver disease, congestive heart failure, renal disease)	Physical exam, clinicopathologic findings

TABLE 3-4

Differential Diagnoses for Diarrhea in Foals

Cause of Diarrhea	Major Diagnostic Test(s)
Salmonellosis	Fecal culture or PCR
Clostridiosis *(Clostridium difficile, C. perfringens)*	Fecal culture, toxin analysis
Endotoxemia, gram negative septicemia	Blood culture, physical examination, complete blood count, sepsis score
Antibiotic-associated diarrhea	History
Foal heat diarrhea	History, physical examination
Viral: rotavirus; rarely coronavirus or adenovirus	Electron microscopy, enzyme immunoassay
Protozoan: cryptosporidiosis	Fecal analysis
Secondary lactose intolerance therapy	Oral lactose tolerance test, response to
Rhodococcus equi	Culture, PCR
Lawsonia intracellulare	Fecal PCR, serologic testing
Gastric ulcer disease syndrome	Gastric endoscopy
Strongyloides westeri	Fecal egg count
Sand	Fecal sedimentation

PCR, Polymerase chain reaction.

The clinician should perform a complete physical examination. The body condition of the horse and the presence of any edema should be noted. The presence of fever, dehydration, or signs of endotoxemia may help in assessing the severity of the disease and differentiating the cause because some causes of diarrhea are not associated typically with systemic signs of illness. Careful evaluation of the abdomen should be performed. Visible abdominal distention is often an indication of large intestinal distention, which may occur in association with acute colitis. However, distention also may be visible with extreme dilation of multiple loops of small intestine. Careful auscultation of the abdomen can be useful in assessing motility. Generally, progressive borborygmi heard about every 3 to 4 minutes on both sides of the abdomen suggest normal motility of the cecum and colon. Auscultation behind the xiphoid process may help identify the presence of sand or gravel if particles can be heard grinding together during contractions of the colon.[24] Particularly in foals, transabdominal palpation and ballottement may be useful to identify increased abdominal fluid or large masses near the body wall. Transrectal palpation can be helpful in assessing the size of intestinal segments, consistency of contents, and wall thickness as well as in identifying masses, enlarged lymph nodes, or mesenteric arteritis.

Clinical Pathology

Routine analysis of blood work rarely identifies a specific cause of diarrhea but can be important in directing appropriate supportive care and may help to establish whether diarrhea is caused by another condition, such as hepatic or renal disease. Some important parameters to evaluate include the presence of leukopenia, particularly neutropenia with a left shift and toxic changes in the white blood cells. These abnormalities suggest a systemic inflammatory response, which also may be associated with thrombocytopenia and coagulopathies. The clinician also should evaluate the concentration of protein, as well as the albumin:globulin ratio. Significant hypoproteinemia, especially hypoalbuminemia caused primarily by protein loss, may occur with acute and chronic diarrhea. Hyperglobulinemia may indicate a chronic inflammatory condition. Disturbances in acid-base balance, especially metabolic acidosis, and electrolyte abnormalities frequently occur in horses with acute

BOX 3-1

OUTLINE OF DIAGNOSTIC APPROACH TO DIARRHEA

I. Signalment, history, and physical examination
II. Clinical pathology
  1. Minimum database: complete blood count, fibrinogen, and serum chemistry profile
    a. Assess hydration, acid-base status, electrolyte abnormalities, and protein status.
    b. Assess renal and hepatic function.
    c. Assess endotoxemia.
  2. Serum protein electrophoresis and immunoglobulin quantitation
  3. Serologic testing: *Neorickettsia risticii* and *Lawsonia intracellulare*
  4. Peritoneal fluid analysis
III. Evaluation of feces
  1. Gross appearance: severity, hemorrhage, odor, and presence of sand
  2. Direct smear: evaluation of protozoan populations and presence of leukocytes and epithelial cells
  3. Parasite evaluation: including evaluation for *Cryptosporidium parvum,* especially in foals
  4. Evaluation of bacterial pathogens
    a. Gram stain and spore stain
    b. Aerobic and anaerobic culture (culture of multiple samples or rectal mucosal biopsy for *Salmonella* spp.)
    c. Clostridial toxin analysis
    d. Polymerase chain reaction: *Salmonella,* spp. *N. risticii,* and *L. intracellulare*
  5. Foals: evaluation of viral pathogens, primarily rotavirus (electron microscopy and enzyme immunoassay)
IV. Diagnostic imaging: radiography and ultrasonography
V. Endoscopic examination: stomach, rectum, and descending colon
VI. Absorption tests (glucose or xylose absorption): primarily for chronic protein-losing enteropathy
VII. Histopathologic examination
VIII. Toxin evaluation: cantharidin in urine or gastrointestinal contents, arsenic in liver, or other
IX. Response to therapy

diarrhea but are uncommon with chronic diarrhea. Because of the dehydration frequently seen with acute diarrhea, prerenal azotemia is common and is important to recognize because some therapies, especially NSAIDs, may worsen the condition. In a study of 122 horses with acute diarrhea, horses with azotemia and clinicopathologic findings consistent with hemoconcentration and hypoproteinemia were less likely to survive.[17]

The diagnostic and prognostic value of serum protein electrophoresis has been evaluated in horses with chronic diarrhea.[25] Significantly higher levels of β_1-globulin were found in horses with larval cyathostomiais than in other horses, and such values in conjunction with a decreased albumin were helpful in diagnosing intestinal parasitism. However, a normal β_1-globulin concentration was not a reliable indicator of the absence of the disease. Significantly lower albumin concentrations and significantly higher α_2-globulin concentrations were found in horses that did not survive, suggesting that these parameters are nonspecific indicators of the severity of inflammatory changes within the intestinal wall. Parasitic infections, particularly strongylosis, also may be associated with elevated serum concentrations of immunoglobulin G(T).[26]

Infrequently, immunodeficiencies are associated with diarrhea.[18,19] Therefore in some horses, further evaluation of immune status may be indicated and may include specific immunoglobulin quantitation, evaluation of specific lymphocyte subsets, or functional assays. The clinician should consider genetic testing for severe combined immunodeficiency in sick foals of Arabian breeding.

Analysis of peritoneal fluid may be useful in some horses with diarrhea. Abnormalities in the peritoneal fluid may reflect the severity of inflammation and in some cases may help to establish a specific diagnosis. Increases in protein and sometimes nucleated cell count may be seen in association with ulcerative colitis.[23] In horses with bacterial peritonitis, the veterinarian may find organisms on cytologic examination or culture. Occasionally, the veterinarian may identify neoplastic cells in the peritoneal fluid, although their absence does not rule out the presence of neoplasia.

Evaluation of Feces

Evaluation of the feces may yield important information in cases of diarrhea. Even the gross appearance of the feces can be helpful. For example, profuse, watery diarrhea is not generally consistent with a diagnosis of right dorsal colitis. Frank blood in the feces suggests bleeding into the distal colon from mucosal damage. Hemorrhagic, foul-smelling feces often are seen in association with clostridial diarrhea. The clinician also can assess the feces for the presence of occult blood, which indicates bleeding from any source. Although excess sand in the feces is readily apparent in some cases, other cases require mixing the feces in a rectal sleeve with water and allowing the sand to settle.

Microscopic examination of the feces for evidence of parasitism and evaluation of viable protozoal populations also may be useful. A direct smear of fresh feces allows for observation of the motility of ciliates and can be used as a screen for the presence of ova and oocysts, although more sensitive techniques, including fecal flotation and sedimentation, are recommended for evaluation of parasitism. Ideally, a quantitative method that allows for estimation of the number of eggs per gram of feces, such as McMaster's or Stolley's, is recommended. However, it is important to remember that fecal examination for parasites sometimes can be misleading, giving false-negative results. *Cryptosporidium parvum* infection can be difficult to diagnose, but oocysts can be detected in the feces by acid-fast staining or by immunofluorescence assay.[27]

Fecal samples also can be examined microscopically for leukocytes and epithelial cells. In general, the cellularity increases with the severity of diarrhea. Fecal leukocytes and epithelial cells are increased in salmonellosis but are not specific for this disorder.[28] More than 10 leukocytes per high-power field may indicate salmonellosis.

Evaluation of the feces for infectious agents is essential in the diagnostic evaluation of horses with diarrhea. *Salmonella* and *Clostridium* species are among the most common causes of bacterial diarrhea in horses. Other, less common bacterial agents include *Campylobacter* spp.; *Aeromonas* spp.; and, particularly in weanling age foals, *Lawsonia intracellulare*.[29,30] Although primarily a respiratory pathogen, *Rhodococcus equi* also can cause diarrhea, particularly in foals 2 to 4 months of age.[31] *Escherichia coli* is an uncommon cause of diarrhea in foals, unlike in calves and piglets. However, enterotoxigenic strains, characterized by the presence of virulence factors, have been identified in foals. Gram stain and spore stain of fecal smears can help to identify and quantitate the bacterial populations present, particularly clostridial species. However, although large numbers of gram positive rods or spores have been identified in foals with clostridial enterocolitis, the results of direct staining may be misleading.[32,33] In one study *Clostridium perfringens* was cultured from 59% of samples in which no gram positive rods were visible. Some clostridial strains also are likely part of the normal microflora.[34] Large numbers of yeast in the feces should alert the clinician to the possibility of candidiasis, especially in compromised neonatal foals.

Fecal culture is used commonly to establish a diagnosis in cases of bacterial diarrhea. When culturing feces, especially if an outside laboratory is used, the clinician must consider proper sample handling, particularly for anaerobic clostridia.[35] *Salmonella* spp. are one of the most significant bacterial pathogens in equine feces.[36] Although the number of *Salmonella* spp. organisms isolated from the feces of horses with clinical salmonellosis is generally greater than from horses with asymptomatic infections, the volume of feces in horses with profuse diarrhea may decrease the likelihood of positive culture. Culture of multiple fecal samples, typically five, is recommended to increase the sensitivity. Culture of a rectal mucosal biopsy or rectal scraping is an alternative to fecal cultures and may increase sensitivity because *Salmonella* spp. are intracellular organisms. Identifying clostridial species requires anaerobic culture. However, evaluating the presence of toxin in cases of suspected clostridial diarrhea also is critical because *Clostridium* spp., particularly *C. perfringens* type A, may be present in normal equine feces.[34] Depending on the clostridial species and the laboratory, toxin can be assessed by detecting preformed toxin in the feces, toxin being produced by the isolate in culture, or the toxin gene in the isolate.[32-35]

An increasing number of polymerase chain reaction (PCR) assays are available for detecting causative agents of equine diarrhea. In comparing a PCR with microbial culture for detection of salmonellae in equine feces and environmental samples, the PCR method was found to be more sensitive and more rapid and required submission of fewer samples.[37,38] Currently, PCR is also available for detection of *Neorickettsia risticii (Ehrlichia risticii)*, the causative agent of Potomac horse fever, in feces and peripheral blood.[39,40] Fecal PCR analysis also has been shown to be useful in documenting equine proliferative enteropathy caused by *Lawsonia intracellulare*.[30] Serologic methods, evaluating the presence of antibodies, are additional diagnostic tests used for diagnosis of Neorickettsia and Lawsonia.[30,40]

Rotaviral infection is associated with diarrhea in foals and is most common in foals from 1 to 4 weeks of age.[4,41] The veterinarian generally makes a diagnosis by detecting the virus through electron microscopy or the viral antigen by enzyme immunoassay (Rotazyme, Abbot Laboratories, North Chicago, Ill.), which is generally more sensitive than direct electron microscopy.[42] Coronavirus appears to have a low prevalence in foals but has been isolated from a horse with diarrhea.[43]

Less commonly used tests include evaluation of fecal osmolality and electrolyte concentrations (sodium and potassium). If the concentration of sodium plus potassium is much less than the osmolality, the result indicates the presence of osmotically active nonelectrolytes, confirming an osmotic diarrhea.

Diagnostic Imaging

Diagnostic imaging, although particularly useful in foals, also can be valuable in adult horses. In foals radiographs can detect gas distention in the lumen of the gastrointestinal tract, and the gas pattern may help to differentiate ileus from mechanical obstruction. Occasionally, gas may be seen within the bowel wall in severe cases of clostridial necrotizing enterocolitis. In adult horses abdominal radiography is limited somewhat by having the proper facilities and equipment to perform the procedure safely. However, radiographs can be effective in identifying radiodense material, such as enteroliths and sand. Ultrasonography can be used in horses of all ages to evaluate the amount and character of the peritoneal fluid, masses, intestinal distention, and wall thickness. In horses with of right dorsal colitis the diagnosis has been supported by ultrasonographic evidence of thickening of the right dorsal colon. Although isotope-labeled white blood cell scintigraphic scans also may help identify colonic ulcerations, the availability and sensitivity of the procedure are limited.

Other Diagnostics

Endoscopic examination of the stomach and proximal duodenum may reveal the presence of neoplasms or ulceration. Diarrhea and inappetence are common clinical signs in symptomatic foals with ulceration of the squamous gastric mucosa. Endoscopy also can be used for inspection of the mucosa of the rectum and descending colon, allowing for evaluation of mural masses or mucosal inflammation.

Absorption tests are used primarily in horses with chronic diarrhea or weight loss to evaluate the small intestinal absorptive capacity. Oral glucose and oral xylose absorption tests have been used.[44,45] Although the plasma concentration of glucose may reflect glucose metabolism as well as absorption from the gastrointestinal tract, the assay has been shown to be reliable in the diagnosis of significant malabsorptive conditions. Xylose is influenced less by the metabolic status of the horse, but the compound is more expensive than glucose, and the assay is not available in many laboratories. Results of both assays are nonspecific, but abnormal results support malabsorption and may indicate the necessity of biopsy.

Diagnosing neoplasms and chronic inflammatory or infiltrative disorders often requires histopathologic examination. A rectal mucosal biopsy is easy to collect and also can be cultured, but the area that can be reached for biopsy is limited. Laparoscopy allows for visualization of the abdomen and certain biopsies. The veterinarian can obtain full thickness intestinal biopsy during exploratory celiotomy.

Diarrhea is a component of the clinical syndrome associated with several toxins. Cantharidin (blister beetle toxin) can be detected in urine or gastrointestinal contents.[46,47] The veterinarian can measure lead in the blood and liver, selenium in the blood and liver, or arsenic in the liver if they are suspected.[47,48] He or she should consider oleander toxicity in horses with diarrhea, arrhythmias, and renal disease, especially if exposure is possible.[47] Oleandrin is detectable in urine and gastrointestinal contents.

Evaluation of Response to Therapy

Evaluating the response to empirical therapy may be helpful in some horses with undiagnosed diarrhea, especially in chronic cases. Dietary changes may decrease diarrhea in some cases, and often a diet of grass hay alone is recommended. In cases in which right dorsal colitis is suspected but cannot be confirmed, using pellet feed may be beneficial. Addition of psyllium mucilloid and corn oil to the diet also may be beneficial in right dorsal colitis. Psyllium mucilloid also has been used in cases in which sand was suspected as contributing to the diarrhea. Any medications that the horse has been receiving, especially NSAIDs or antibiotics, should be discontinued in case they are contributing to the diarrhea.

Transfaunation can be used in an attempt to restore normal flora. Fresh colonic or cecal contents are considered the best source of organisms, but feces can be used. Several commercial prebiotics and probiotics are available, and their efficacy is under investigation. The yeast *Sacchromyces boulardii* may decrease the severity and duration of clinical signs in horses with acute enterocolitis.[49]

A course of corticosteroids can be tried in cases of chronic diarrhea in which infectious causes have been ruled out. Treatment with a larvicidal anthelmintic may be beneficial in some cases and sometimes is used with corticosteroids. Some horses with chronic diarrhea have responded to iodochlorhydroxyquin (10 g/450 kg/day for 2 weeks). This drug sometimes has been used concurrently with trimethoprim-sulfa. Occasionally, transfusion with plasma seems to suppress diarrhea in young horses.

RESPIRATORY DISTRESS

Bonnie R. Rush

Respiratory distress is defined as labored breathing and is characterized by an inappropriate degree of effort to breathe based on rate, rhythm, and subjective evaluation of respiratory effort.[1] *Dyspnea* refers to the sensation of arduous, uncomfortable, or difficult breathing that occurs when the demand for ventilation exceeds the patient's ability to respond.[2] *Dyspnea* describes a symptom rather than a clinical sign, and although the term is used often, dyspnea is not technically applicable in veterinary medicine. The clinical signs of respiratory distress vary with the severity and origin of impaired gas exchange. Clinical signs commonly observed in horses with respiratory distress include flared nostrils, exercise intolerance, inactivity, exaggerated abdominal effort, abnormal respiratory noise (stridor), anxious expression, extended head and neck, cyanosis, and synchronous pumping of the anus with the respiratory cycle.[1] Horses with chronic respiratory distress may develop a heave line resulting from hypertrophy of the cutaneous trunci and abdominal muscles, which assist during forced expiration.[3] Respiratory distress usually results from inefficient exchange of oxygen and carbon dioxide caused by primary pulmonary disease, airway obstruction, or impairment of the muscles and supporting structures necessary for ventilation. In some cases ventilation increases in the absence of impaired gas exchange in response to pain, metabolic acidosis, or high environmental temperature. Familiarity with the mechanics of breathing and control of ventilation in healthy and diseased lungs facilitates the diagnosis and treatment of respiratory distress.[3,4]

CONTROL OF VENTILATION

The partial pressure of oxygen (Pa_{O_2}) and carbon dioxide (Pa_{CO_2}) in arterial blood are maintained within a narrow range through rigid control of gas exchange.[2] The central controller of respiration in the medulla alters the rate and depth of respiration via efferent signals to the muscles of respiration in response to afferent signals from chemoreceptors in the peripheral vasculature and central nervous system and mechanoreceptors in the upper and lower respiratory tract, diaphragm, and thoracic wall. The central controller therefore adjusts alveolar ventilation to the metabolic rate of the individual.[4]

Sensors

The chemoreceptors identify changes in metabolism and oxygen requirements and provide feedback to the central controller, thus allowing for modification of ventilation. Central chemoreceptors respond predominantly to hypercapnia, whereas peripheral chemoreceptors respond to hypoxia and hypercapnia. Central chemoreceptors, located in the ventral medulla, monitor alterations in the pH of intracerebral interstitial fluid and cerebrospinal fluid. The blood-brain barrier is impermeable to bicarbonate and hydrogen ions but is freely permeable to carbon dioxide. Therefore acidification of the intracerebral interstitial fluid and stimulation of the central chemoreceptors occur predominantly in response to hypercapnia. The severity of acidosis in the intracerebral interstitial fluid caused by hypercapnia is amplified by two features of the central nervous system: (1) hypercapnia produces cerebral vasodilation, increasing the delivery of CO_2 to the central nervous system, and (2) cerebrospinal fluid has poor buffering capacity because of low total protein concentrations.[2]

Peripheral chemoreceptors are located in the arterial circulation and respond to acidemia, hypercapnia, and hypoxemia. The carotid bodies are situated at the bifurcation of the common carotid artery, and the aortic bodies are located near the aortic arch. These receptors relay information to the central controller regarding arterial gas tensions via the glossopharyngeal and vagus nerves. Their responsiveness to alterations in Pa_{CO_2} is less consequential than the central chemoreceptors; however, the peripheral chemoreceptors are solely responsible for the hypoxic ventilatory drive. The peripheral chemoreceptors demonstrate a nonlinear response to low arterial oxygen tension. They are insensitive to alterations in Pa_{O_2} above 100 mm Hg, exhibit moderate response to arterial O_2 tensions between 50 and 100 mm Hg, and demonstrate a dramatic increase in responsiveness when the partial pressure of oxygen falls below 50 mm Hg in the arterial circulation.[2] The respiratory pattern elicited by hypoxia differs from that stimulated by hypercapnia.[5,6] Hypoxia evokes an increase in respiratory frequency, whereas hypercapnia triggers an elevation in tidal volume. In addition, hypoxia stimulates recruitment of the inspiratory muscles, whereas hypercapnia potentiates the activity of inspiratory and expiratory muscles.

The sensitivity of peripheral chemoreceptors should be considered in the treatment of patients with complex acid-base and blood-gas abnormalities. A patient suffering from impaired gas exchange caused by pulmonary disease and metabolic acidosis resulting from shock manifests respiratory distress in response to hypoxemia, hypercapnia, and acidosis. Oxygen supplementation likely will improve the patient's arterial oxygen tension. Such treatment, however, may abolish the hypoxic ventilatory drive and consequently slow the ventilatory rate. This decreased ventilation could exacerbate respiratory acidosis and may result in decompensation of the patient.[4] To prevent life-threatening acidemia, treatment of metabolic acidosis in addition to oxygen supplementation is indicated.

Receptors located in the upper and lower respiratory tract respond to mechanical and chemical stimuli and relay afferent information to the central controller of respiration via the vagus nerve.[1,2] Vagal blockade abolishes tachypnea in horses with pulmonary disease; therefore these receptors are likely to play an important role in development of respiratory distress associated with primary pulmonary disease.[7-9] Pulmonary stretch receptors, also called *slow-adapting stretch receptors,* are located within smooth muscle fibers in the walls of the trachea and bronchi.[1,2,4] These receptors are stimulated by pulmonary inflation and inhibit further inflation of the lung (Hering-Breuer reflex). Conversely, at end expiration these receptors stimulate inspiratory activity. These receptors are considered to be partially responsible for controlling the depth and rate of respiration.

Irritant receptors (rapid-adjusting stretch receptors) are believed to be located between epithelial cells of the conducting airways.[2] They are not likely to function in regulation of breathing in a normal resting horse.[4] Stimulation of these receptors by noxious stimuli triggers bronchoconstriction, cough, tachypnea, mucus production, and release of inflammatory mediators.[1,2] Irritant receptors can be triggered by exogenous stimuli (e.g., smoke, irritant gases, dust) or by endogenously produced inflammatory mediators, including histamine and prostaglandins. Production of histamine, prostaglandins, and other inflammatory mediators increases in horses with recurrent airway obstruction (RAO; chronic obstructive pulmonary disease [COPD]).[10-12] Stimulation of irritant receptors by these inflammatory mediators may be responsible in part for bronchoconstriction, mucus production, and tachypnea observed in horses with allergic airway disease. In addition to their role as chemoreceptors, irritant receptors also function as mechanoreceptors.[1] An abrupt change in end-expiratory lung volume, such as occurs with pneumothorax or pleural effusion, produces tachypnea attributed to stimulation of irritant receptors. Juxtacapillary receptors are believed to be located within the wall of the alveolus. Stimulation by increased interstitial fluid volume triggers the sensation of difficult breathing.[2] Nonmyelinated C fibers are located in the pulmonary parenchyma, conducting airways, and blood vessels. These receptors respond to pulmonary edema, congestion, and inflammatory mediators, and stimulation activates tachypnea. In addition, C fiber receptors may stimulate the release of pulmonary neuropeptides, which produce bronchoconstriction, vasodilation, protein extravasation, and cytokine production.[1] Increased negative pressure (upper airway obstruction) within the airway stimulates mechanoreceptors of the larynx and produces prolongation of inspiratory time and activation of upper airway dilator muscles.[13]

Central Control of Respiration

The central controller consists of a group of motor neurons in the pons and medulla that receive input from the peripheral and central receptors and initiate phasic activity of diaphragmatic, intercostal, and abdominal respiratory muscles.[2] The medullary respiratory center, which is located in the reticular formation, controls the rhythmic pattern of respiration. The dorsal respiratory group coordinates inspiratory activity by assimilating afferent information from the glossopharyngeal and vagus nerves and transmits efferent signals to the muscles of inspiration and neurons in the ventral respiratory group. The ventral respiratory group consists of inspiratory and expiratory motor neurons. This nucleus is relatively inactive at rest and has a more dominant role during exercise. The apneustic center, located in the pons, provides stimulatory input to inspiratory motor neurons. Damage to the apneustic center, from trauma or neonatal maladjustment syndrome, results in prolonged inspiratory gasps interrupted by transient expiratory efforts.[4] The pneumotaxic center, also located in the pons, inhibits the inspiratory centers and regulates the volume and rate of respiration. The pneumotaxic center is not required to maintain a normal respiratory rhythm; instead, this center functions to fine tune the respiratory rhythm,[2] receiving afferent input from the vagus nerve regarding Pa_{O_2}, Pa_{CO_2}, and pulmonary inflation.

Effectors of Respiration

The muscles required for ventilation include the diaphragm, the external and internal intercostal muscles, and the abdominal muscles. The single most important muscle required for the inspiratory phase of the respiratory cycle is the diaphragm. Contraction of the diaphragm forces the abdominal contents back, increasing the length of the thoracic cavity, and pulls the ribs abaxially, increasing the width of the abdominal cavity. In addition, the external intercostal muscles participate in inspiration by pulling the ribs abaxially to increase the width of the thoracic cavity. The net effect is an increase in the size of the thoracic cavity, producing subatmospheric intrathoracic pressure, to drive inspiration and pulmonary inflation. Expiration at rest is a passive process in most species and relies on elastic recoil of the lung to create positive intrathoracic pressure.[2] In horses the first portion of expiration relies on elastic recoil of the lung to the point of relaxation volume, whereby the tendency for pulmonary collapse equals the tendency for expansion by the thoracic wall. However, horses further decrease lung volume by active compression of the chest wall, through contraction of the internal intercostal muscles and muscles of the abdominal wall.[14] Conversely, the first part of inhalation is passive until the relaxation volume is reached, at which point the diaphragm and external intercostal muscles complete the inspiratory phase. Mechanical (abdominal distention, trauma to the thoracic wall) and neuromuscular (botulism, phrenic nerve damage, nutritional muscular dystrophy) dysfunction of the diaphragm and intercostal muscles prevents expansion of the thoracic wall and produces hypoventilation, hypoxemia, and respiratory distress.[4] Horses with torsion of the large colon develop significant abdominal distention and respiratory distress. Respiratory failure caused by impaired diaphragmatic function plays an important role in the pathophysiology and mortality associated with this intestinal accident.

The diameter of the conducting airways is an important determinant of the degree of pulmonary resistance and work of breathing and is controlled by the autonomic nervous system. Vagal-mediated parasympathetic stimulation causes airway narrowing and is one mechanism of bronchoconstriction associated with allergic airway disease. Administration of atropine results in rapid relief of bronchoconstriction in some horses with RAO, demonstrating the important role of parasympathetic bronchoconstriction in the pathogenesis of this disease.[3,4] β_2-Receptor stimulation produces smooth muscle relaxation and bronchodilation. β_2-Adrenergic receptors are abundant throughout the lung; however, sympathetic innervation is sparse, and β-receptors within the lung must rely on circulating catecholamines for stimulation.[4] Airways must be constricted for β_2-receptor stimulation or atropine blockade to produce increased airway caliber.[15,16] β-Adrenergic receptors are less abundant than β_2-receptors and play no important role in the regulation of airway diameter. However, β-receptors appear to be upregulated in horses with RAO and contribute to bronchoconstriction associated with this disease.[17]

Nonadrenergic-noncholinergic (NANC) innervation also contributes to large airway diameter. Smooth muscles of the trachea and bronchi relax in response to activation of the inhibitory NANC system. In RAO-affected horses with clinical signs of airway obstruction, inhibitory NANC function is absent.[18] Failure of the inhibitory NANC system may result from the inflammatory response during acute RAO or may be an inherent autonomic dysfunction of the conducting airways of RAO-affected horses.

HYPOXEMIA

Respiratory distress most often originates from inadequate pulmonary gas exchange to meet the metabolic demands of the individual, resulting in hypoxemia and hypercapnia. Hypoxemia results from one or more of five basic pathophysiologic mechanisms: hypoventilation, ventilation-perfusion mismatch, right-to-left shunting of blood, diffusion impairment, and reduced inspired oxygen concentration. The degree of hypercapnia and response to oxygen supplementation varies depending on the mechanism of impaired gas exchange. Determination of these two parameters is useful in identifying the pathophysiologic process predominantly responsible for the development of hypoxemia.[2]

Hypoventilation

The hallmark of hypoventilation is hypercapnia.[2] The elevation in $Paco_2$ is inversely proportional to the reduction in alveolar ventilation; halving alveolar ventilation doubles $Paco_2$.[2] The reduction in arterial oxygen tension is almost directly proportional to the increase in CO_2. For instance, if $Paco_2$ increases from 40 to 80 mm Hg, then the Pao_2 decreases from 100 to 60 mm Hg. Therefore hypoxemia resulting from hypoventilation is rarely life-threatening. In addition, oxygen supplementation easily abolishes hypoxemia caused by pure hypoventilation. Acidosis caused by hypercapnia is the most clinically significant feature of hypoventilation and may threaten the life of the patient.[2] Metabolic alkalosis or central nervous system depression (e.g., from head trauma, encephalitis, narcotic drugs) can produce hypoventilation; however, horses with these disorders may not demonstrate clinical signs of respiratory distress. The following disorders can cause alveolar hypoventilation, and affected patients usually demonstrate clinical signs of respiratory distress: mechanical (abdominal distention, trauma to the thoracic wall) and neuromuscular (botulism, phrenic nerve damage, nutritional muscular dystrophy) dysfunction of the diaphragm and intercostal muscles, restrictive pulmonary disease (silicosis, pulmonary fibrosis, pneumothorax, pleural effusion), and upper airway obstruction.[4]

Ventilation-Perfusion Mismatch

Ventilation-perfusion (V-Q) mismatch is the most common cause of hypoxemia and is characterized by unequal distribution of alveolar ventilation and blood flow.[4] Pulmonary regions that are overperfused in relation to ventilation (low V-Q ratio) contribute disproportionate amounts of blood with low arterial oxygen content to the systemic circulation.[2] Respiratory diseases characterized by low V-Q ratios include RAO, pulmonary atelectasis, and consolidation.[4] If ventilation exceeds perfusion (high V-Q ratio), the ventilated pulmonary units are inefficient for CO_2 elimination and O_2 uptake. Ventilation of poorly or nonperfused units is wasted ventilation, termed *alveolar dead space*.[2] Conditions associated with high V-Q ratios include pulmonary thromboembolism and shock (low pulmonary artery pressure). Patients with V-Q mismatch often have a normal arterial Pco_2. The ventilatory drive to maintain normal $Paco_2$ is powerful. Because the CO_2 dissociation curve is basically a straight line (direct relationship), increased ventilation efficiently decreases $Paco_2$ at high and low V-Q ratios. Because of the nearly flat shape of the O_2 dissociation curve, increasing ventilation is inefficient for proportionally increasing the arterial Po_2. Only pulmonary units with moderate to low V-Q ratios benefit from increased ventilation. Therefore the increased ventilatory effort to maintain normal $Paco_2$ is wasted and unnecessarily increases the work of breathing. Oxygen supplementation increases $Paco_2$ in patients with a V-Q mismatch. However, elevation in arterial O_2 is delayed compared with hypoventilation and in some cases may be incomplete.[2] Compensatory mechanisms are present to minimize unequal distribution of ventilation and perfusion in diseased lungs to prevent the development of hypoxemia until the pulmonary pathologic condition is severe.[23] Reflex pulmonary arterial constriction (hypoxic vasoconstriction) prevents perfusion of unventilated alveolar units and attempts to redirect blood flow to alveoli that are ventilated adequately. Airway hypocapnia causes bronchoconstriction of airways that conduct to unperfused alveolar units, redirecting air flow to better-perfused alveoli.

Shunt

Shunt is defined as blood that is not exposed to ventilated areas of the lung and is added to the arteries of the systemic circulation.[2] Shunting can occur as an extreme form of V-Q mismatch or with direct addition of unoxygenated blood to the arterial system. *Physiologic shunting* is defined as perfusion of nonventilated or collapsed regions of the lung and occurs with pulmonary consolidation, atelectasis, and edema. Congenital heart disease, such as tetralogy of Fallot and some cardiac septal defects, is an example of a direct right-to-left shunt wherein unoxygenated blood from the right side of the heart is added to oxygenated blood from the left side of the heart. In these conditions hypoxemia cannot be abolished by increasing the oxygen content of inspired air. The shunted blood is never exposed to the higher concentration of inspired oxygen in the alveolus, and the addition of a small amount of shunted blood with its low O_2 content greatly reduces the Po_2 of arterial blood. Compared with breathing room air, the decrement in Po_2 is much greater at Po_2 levels associated with the inhalation of O_2-enriched air because the O_2 dissociation curve is so flat at high Po_2 levels. Only hypoxemia caused by right-to-left shunting behaves in this manner when the patient is permitted to inspire high percentages of oxygen (70% to 100%). Shunts do not usually cause hypercapnia.[2] Chemoreceptors detect excess arterial CO_2, and ventilation increases to reduce the content of CO_2 in unshunted blood until arterial Pco_2 reaches the normal range. In some cases of shunt the arterial Pco_2 is below normal because of hyperventilation stimulated by the hypoxemic ventilatory drive.

Diffusion Impairment

Gas exchange between the alveolus and the capillary occurs by passive diffusion, which is driven by the property of molecules to move randomly from an area of high concentration to one of low concentration.[2] Factors that determine the rate of gas exchange include the concentration gradient between the alveolus and capillary blood, solubility of the gas, surface area available for diffusion, and the width of the air-blood barrier. Diseases characterized by pure diffusion impairment are rare in veterinary medicine.[4] Diffusion impairment can occur with pulmonary fibrosis, interstitial pneumonia, silicosis, or edema caused by increased width of the barrier or decreased surface area available for gas exchange. The clinician should recognize that the major component of hypoxemia for these conditions is a V-Q mismatch; however, diffusion impairment can contribute to the severity of hypoxemia. Supplemental oxygen therapy is effective in treating hypoxemia caused by diffusion impairment because it creates a more favorable concentration gradient and increases the driving pressure of oxygen to move from the alveolus into the blood. Transport of CO_2 is less affected by diseases of diffusion impairment because of its greater solubility compared with O_2.[2]

Reduction of Inspired Oxygen

Hypoxemia resulting from decreased inspired oxygen content is uncommon and occurs only under special circumstances. High altitude and iatrogenic ventilation with a low oxygen concentration are the most common circumstances in which hypoxemia is attributed to reduction of inspired oxygen content.[2]

Most pulmonary diseases in horses incorporate more than one of these pathophysiologic mechanisms for the development of hypoxemia. Horses with pleuropneumonia, for example, may develop hypoxemia caused by hypoventilation (extrapulmonary restriction by pleural effusion), V-Q mismatch (accumulation of exudate and edema within alveoli and conducting airways), and diffusion impairment (exudate and edema within the interstitial spaces).

OBSTRUCTIVE DISEASE

The location (intrathoracic or extrathoracic) and nature (fixed or dynamic) of airway obstruction determines whether impedance to air flow occurs during inspiration, expiration, or both.[3] The phase of the respiratory cycle affected by air flow obstruction is prolonged and may be associated with a respiratory noise (stridor or wheeze).[2,19]

The horse is an obligate nasal breather and can breathe efficiently only through the nares.[4] Therefore upper airway obstruction within the nasal passages cannot be bypassed by mouth breathing. In addition, approximately 80% of the total airway resistance to air flow is located in the upper airway.[19] A 50% decrease in the radius of an airway increases its resistance by 16-fold (Poiseuille's law).[2] Therefore small changes in the upper airway diameter dramatically affect the overall resistance to air flow and work of breathing for the horse. Extrathoracic airway pressures are subatmospheric during inspiration; therefore poorly supported structures in the upper airway narrow or collapse during inspiration (dynamic collapse). The most common cause of non–fixed upper airway obstruction in horses is laryngeal hemiplegia, which produces inspiratory stridor during exercise. Intraluminal masses and arytenoid chondritis cause fixed upper airway obstruction and produce inspiratory and expiratory respiratory distress.[3]

Of the total airway resistance 20% is attributable to the small airways.[19] Although the radius of individual bronchioles is small, many of them exist and the sum or collective radius is large, with the result that their overall contribution to pulmonary resistance is low.[2] Because the resistance of the bronchioles is low, advanced disease must be present for routine measurements of airway resistance to detect an abnormality, and obstruction of these airways must be extensive before a horse would suffer from respiratory distress. During pulmonary inflation intrathoracic pressures are subatmospheric. Small airways are pulled open by negative intrathoracic pressure and stretched parenchymal attachments at high lung volumes. Thus resistance to air flow in small airways is low during the inspiratory phase of respiration.[2] During exhalation intrathoracic pressure is positive and the diameter of small airways is decreased, and bronchioles may even close at low lung volumes. Therefore resistance to air flow in small airways is greatest during the expiratory phase. In horses with RAO the airway diameter is reduced by inflammatory exudate, edema, and bronchoconstriction.[3,4] As lung volume decreases during expiration, the narrowed bronchioles are compressed shut (dynamic airway collapse) and trap air distal to the site of closure.[4] This is an example of severe flow limitation, which may lead ultimately to the development of emphysema. Flow limitation forces horses with RAO to breathe at higher lung volumes and maintain a higher functional residual capacity to reduce or prevent dynamic airway collapse. Affected horses attempt to reduce the end-expiratory lung volume by recruiting abdominal muscles to increase the intrathoracic pressures during expiration. However, the greater the end-expiratory pressure, the greater is the likelihood of small airway compression and collapse. Hypertrophy of the cutaneous trunci and expiratory abdominal muscles, especially the external abdominal oblique, produces the characteristic "heave line" associated with RAO.[4] Because dynamic airway narrowing and collapse occur during exhalation, wheezes are typically loudest at end expiration in horses with RAO.[3,4]

RESTRICTIVE DISEASE

Restrictive disease is less common than obstructive pulmonary disease in horses.[4] By definition, restrictive disease inhibits pulmonary expansion and leads to inspiratory respiratory distress.[2]

The vital capacity and compliance (pulmonary or chest wall) decrease, expiratory flow rates and elastic recoil increase, and airway resistance is normal. The characteristic respiratory pattern in horses with restrictive pulmonary disease is rapid, shallow respiration at low lung volumes.[4] This strategy takes advantage of high pulmonary compliance at low lung volumes and decreases the work of breathing. This respiratory pattern has the disadvantage of increased ventilation of anatomic dead space.[2] Restrictive diseases may be classified as intrapulmonary (pulmonary fibrosis, silicosis,[20] and interstitial pneumonia[21,22]) and extrapulmonary (pleural effusion, pneumothorax, mediastinal mass, botulism, and nutritional muscular dystrophy).[4] Hypoxemia observed in horses with intrapulmonary restrictive disease is attributed to V-Q mismatch and diffusion impairment. Stimulation of juxtacapillary receptors may contribute to respiratory distress observed in these patients.[2] The pathophysiologic mechanism for hypoxemia in horses with extrapulmonary restriction is hypoventilation.[4] In horses with pleural effusion and pneumothorax, respiratory distress is likely to be exacerbated by thoracic pain.

NONPULMONARY RESPIRATORY DISTRESS

Respiratory distress does not always originate from dysfunction of the pulmonary system and its supporting structures. Nonpulmonary respiratory distress can occur because of inadequate oxygen-carrying capacity of the blood, compensation for metabolic acidosis, pain, and hyperthermia.

Impaired oxygen-carrying capacity of the blood may occur because of anemia (blood loss, hemolytic, or aplastic) or dysfunction of red blood cells (methemoglobinemia, carbon monoxide toxicity). In these cases the arterial Po_2 tension (quantity of dissolved oxygen) is normal; however, the total oxygen content of the blood is reduced greatly.[2] Tachypnea and respiratory distress occur in response to impaired oxygen delivery and tissue hypoxia.[3]

The respiratory system can compensate for metabolic acidosis by increasing ventilation to lower $Paco_2$ and attenuate acidemia.[2] The ventilatory drive increases in response to stimulation by peripheral chemoreceptors by circulating hydrogen ions. Hypocarbic compensation for mild to moderate metabolic acidosis is effective in returning blood pH to normal until renal compensatory mechanisms can be established.[2]

Pain and anxiety are physiologic causes of tachypnea and hyperpnea. Horses with musculoskeletal pain are unlikely to demonstrate significant respiratory distress; however, rhabdomyolysis and laminitis are painful musculoskeletal conditions that may produce tachypnea.[3] Marked respiratory distress is observed frequently in horses with abdominal pain; however, the respiratory distress is not caused solely by pain and is exacerbated by abdominal distention, shock, acidosis, and endotoxemia.

Hyperthermia caused by fever, high environmental temperature, exercise, and heat stress can produce respiratory distress in horses. Tachypnea and elevation in body temperature are the most prominent clinical signs in horses with anhydrosis.[23] Hyperpnea is an effective mechanism for heat dissipation in human beings, dogs, and ruminants.[3] Unfortunately, increased ventilation is an inefficient mechanism for heat dissipation in horses and appears to be wasted effort.[3,4]

CLINICAL EVALUATION OF RESPIRATORY DISTRESS

A thorough physical examination is essential to determine the origin of respiratory distress, identify concurrent disease, and direct further diagnostic testing. Prolonged inspiration is consistent with restrictive or extrathoracic, nonfixed, obstructive disease, whereas horses with intrathoracic airway obstruction exhibit expiratory difficulty.[2,3] Respiratory distress associated with inspiration and expiration may indicate an extrathoracic fixed obstruction. Stridor is an abnormal respiratory noise that usually is generated by obstruction of the upper airway and is audible most often during inspiration.[3] Horses with nonpulmonary respiratory distress demonstrate increased rate and depth of respiration without producing abnormal respiratory noise.

Thoracic auscultation identifies abnormal respiratory sounds (crackles and wheezes) or regions of decreased breath sounds caused by pleural effusion, pneumothorax, or pulmonary consolidation. Percussion of the thoracic wall generates a resonant and hollow sound when performed over regions of normal lung. Pleural effusion and pulmonary consolidation sound dull and flat during thoracic percussion, whereas pneumothorax produces a hyperresonant sound.[4]

Normal air flow occurs in laminar flow; therefore normal horses at rest do not generate easily audible sounds.[4] Respiratory sounds are generated from vibration in tissue and sudden changes in pressure of gas moving within the airway lumen. Airway narrowing and exudate generate audible sounds by creating disturbances in laminar flow, turbulence, and sudden changes in pressure of moving gas.[2] Crackles are intermittent or explosive sounds, generated by bubbling of air through secretions or by equilibration of airway pressures after sudden opening of collapsed small airways. The generation of crackles requires an air-fluid interface, and these abnormal lung sounds occur in horses with pneumonia, interstitial fibrosis, RAO, pulmonary edema, and atelectasis.[4] Wheezes are continuous, musical sounds that originate from oscillation of small airway walls before complete closing (expiratory wheeze) or opening (inspiratory wheeze).[2] Expiratory wheezes are the hallmark of obstructive pulmonary disease.[2]

Arterial blood gas determination provides a quantitative evaluation of pulmonary function, alveolar ventilation, and acid-base status and may identify the origin of respiratory distress (hypercapnia, hypoxemia, or acidemia).[2] The clinician may determine the pathophysiologic mechanism of hypoxemia by examining the $Paco_2$ level and by investigating the response of Pao_2 to supplemental oxygen therapy. In addition, serial blood gas monitoring can determine response to bronchodilator, parasympathomimetic, or anti-inflammatory therapy.

Additional diagnostic tests that may be indicated in horses with respiratory distress include thoracic radiography, thoracic ultrasonography, endoscopic examination of the upper airway, and atropine challenge. The findings during thoracic auscultation and percussion are valuable in determining whether ultrasonography rather than radiography is indicated. Pulmonary consolidation, abscessation, fibrosis, interstitial pneumonia, peribronchial infiltration, and mediastinal mass are differentiated and diagnosed readily via thoracic radiography. Thoracic ultrasonography is superior to radiography in detecting and characterizing pleural fluid and peripheral pulmonary abscessation and consolidation in horses. Air reflects the ultrasound beam; therefore ultrasonography does not image deep pulmonary lesions if the overlying lung is aerated.[24] An endoscopic examination of the upper airway is indicated in horses with inspiratory stridor and suspected upper airway obstruction.[4] Horses with extreme respiratory distress may resent endoscopic examination, and forced examination may precipitate a respiratory crisis. Atropine administration in horses with RAO may provide rapid relief of respiratory distress if the major component of airway obstruction is reversible bronchoconstriction. Horses that respond to an atropine challenge likely will respond favorably to bronchodilator therapy. Incomplete response to atropine in horses with RAO indicates that exudate or fibrosis is contributing to airway obstruction, and limited response to bronchodilator therapy is anticipated.[3,4]

COUGH

Catherine W. Kohn

Cough, a sudden explosive expulsion of air through the glottis, is a common sign of respiratory disease and a reflex pulmonary defense mechanism. Coughing facilitates the removal of noxious substances and excessive secretions from the airways by creating maximum expiratory airflow. A high-velocity airflow generates the shear forces required to separate mucus from the airway walls, enabling expulsion of exudate and debris from the airway.[1] An understanding of the cough reflex provides insight into the pathophysiology of diseases characterized by cough.

The cough reflex has been studied infrequently in horses. Descriptions of the cough cycle and the neural basis of cough presented in this section are based on data from other species. The author infers that similar events occur in horses. Because differences exist among species regarding the cough reflex,[2] studies on horses will be required to define the physiologic events of the cough reflex in this species.

COUGH CYCLE

The cough cycle has four phases: inspiration, compression, expression, and relaxation.[1] Deep inspiration, which immediately precedes cough, increases lung volume. As lung volume increases, the ability to generate maximum expiratory airflow increases because of the greater force of contraction achieved by the muscles of respiration when their precontraction length increases and because of the greater elastic recoil pressure of the lung at high lung value.[3] Thus precough expansion of lung volume maximizes the velocity of expiratory airflow. Achievement of maximum expiratory airflow rates requires a relatively gentle expiratory effort, and airflow maxima are therefore independent of effort.[2]

After deep inspiration the glottis closes. While the glottis remains closed, compression of the chest cavity occurs by contraction of the thoracic and abdominal musculature during an active expiratory effort. Compression of the chest results in an increase in pleural pressure from 50 to 100 mm Hg.[2] This increase in pleural pressure is transmitted to pressure in the intrathoracic airways and trachea. Intra-alveolar pressures actually exceed intrapleural pressures by an amount equal to the elastic recoil pressure of the lung.[4]

Expression occurs when the glottis opens abruptly, thus producing a gradient in airway pressure (atmospheric at the pharynx and high in the alveoli), and air is expired forcefully. The occurrence of dynamic airway compression in larger airways maximizes the velocity of airflow toward the mouth (Figure 3-3). The intra-airway pressures vary in the respiratory system according to the instantaneous transpulmonary pressure.[3] At the equal pressure point the airway pressure equals the pleural pressure. Toward the mouth from the equal pressure point (downstream), the pleural pressure is greater than intrathoracic airway pressure, and the intrathoracic airways therefore are compressed dynamically. Partial collapse of the airways downstream of the equal pressure point maximizes airflow velocities in these airways by decreasing their diameter. At high lung volumes the equal pressure point likely is in the larger airways and therefore only the intrathoracic trachea may be subject to dynamic compression and maximal airflow velocity.[4] Maximum airflow velocity produces high shearing forces that dislodge mucus and debris from airway walls, thus facilitating expectoration. Cough is therefore most effective as a defense mechanism for clearing the larger airways in healthy animals. Removal of noxious substances from the smaller peripheral airways depends on the presence of mucus in the airways, and irritants that stimulate cough also may stimulate mucus production.[5]

In diseases characterized by increased resistance in small peripheral airways caused by partial obstruction (e.g., RAO), maximal expiratory flow rates are reduced. When small airways are obstructed partially, the equal pressure point moves toward the periphery of the lung during coughing because

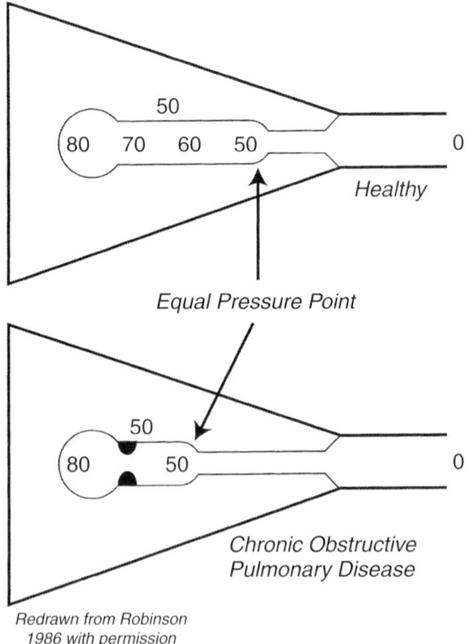

FIGURE 3-3 Dynamic airway compression during cough or maximum expiratory airflow. Lungs are represented at total lung capacity. When chronic obstructive pulmonary disease is present, the equal pressure point moves toward the alveoli. This peripheral migration of the equal pressure point results in dynamic compression in more peripheral airways during cough than would be found in a healthy individual. Redrawn from Robinson NE: Pathophysiology of coughing, Proceedings of the thirty-second convention of the American Association of Equine Practitioners, Nashville, 1986.

pressures in airways downstream of the partial obstruction are lower than are pressures in those airways in healthy lungs (see Figure 3-3). This shift in the equal pressure point subjects more peripheral airways to dynamic compression. Coughing is likely to be less effective as a clearance mechanism when obstructive diseases of the small airways are present. Bronchodilator therapy may increase the effectiveness of cough in such patients by increasing expiratory airflow rates.[4]

The sound of cough is generated by vibration of laryngeal and pharyngeal structures caused by the rapid expulsion of air immediately after opening of the glottis,[3] by narrowing and deformation of airways, and by vibration of surrounding lung tissue. Variations in the sound of cough most likely relate to the quantity and quality of mucus in the airway.[6]

At the end of cough relaxation occurs. Intrapleural pressure falls, and the muscles of expiration relax. Transient bronchodilation occurs.[1]

NEURAL BASIS OF THE COUGH REFLEX

The afferent input for the cough reflex is carried predominantly in the vagus nerves, and the cough reflex depends uniquely on vagal afferents in the species studied.[5,7,8] Sensory myelinated nerves in the larynx respond to mechanical and chemical irritation and mediate cough and changes in airway diameter.[7] The identity of receptors that initiate cough in the lower airways is subject to debate; however, all of the receptors described in this section likely contribute to the cough response.[8] Rapidly adapting receptors are located in the airway mucosa in the region of the carina and are stimulated primarily by mechanical deformation produced, for example, by inhaled particles, mucus, or cellular debris accumulating near the carina. Chemical irritants (e.g., ammonia fumes, ozone, and inflammatory mediators) evoke cough by stimulation of receptors located in the peripheral airways. Pulmonary C fibers may mediate a chemically evoked cough, although this issue is currently under debate. Chemical mediators known to stimulate pulmonary C fibers and cough when inhaled as aerosols by human beings include bronchodilator prostaglandins, bradykinin, and capsaicin.[8] Forced expiration during coughing may be facilitated by the modulating effects of information from these receptors on central respiratory neurons.

Bronchoconstriction is a constant component of cough,[3,6] and stimuli of cough also may cause bronchoconstriction; however, cough and bronchoconstriction are separate airway reflexes. Inhalation of dust and irritant gases causes reflex bronchoconstriction in the species studied. Reflex bronchoconstriction has a slow onset and is long lasting compared with the cough reflex.[2] Bronchoconstriction may increase the efficiency of cough by decreasing airway diameter and therefore increasing airflow velocity. In some cases bronchodilating drugs may suppress the cough reflex by desensitizing airway receptors that elicit cough.[6]

Sensory nerves mediating bronchoconstriction and cough are distributed unevenly along the airways.[7] Laryngeal receptors and sensory nerves in the extrapulmonary airways may be more sensitive to mechanical stimuli, whereas intrapulmonary receptors may respond preferentially to chemical mediators and irritants.

Little is known about the brainstem neuronal pathways of the cough reflex. In the cat the cough center is reported to be in the medulla at the level of the obex, alongside the solitary nucleus of the vagus and close to the expiratory neurons of the respiratory center. On the motor side of the cough reflex, the vagal, phrenic, intercostal, and lumbar nerves and motor portions of the trigeminal, facial, hypoglossal, and accessory nerves are distributed to the striated and smooth muscles of respiration, the vocal fold abductors and adductors, and glands of the respiratory tract.[3]

STIMULI OF COUGH

Cough may be stimulated by airway smooth muscle contraction (bronchoconstriction), excessive mucus production, presence of inhaled particles in the airways, release of inflammatory mediators (infectious diseases), exposure to cold or hot air, intramural or extramural pressure or tension on the airways (tumor, granuloma, abscess, or decreased pulmonary compliance caused by restrictive disease such as interstitial fibrosis or pleuritis), sloughing of airway epithelial cells, and enhanced epithelial permeability (pulmonary edema).[5] Epithelial sloughing and enhanced epithelial permeability theoretically increase the accessibility of cough receptors to the mechanical or chemical agents that stimulate them. Loss of the integrity of the epithelial lining of the respiratory tract is a common feature in many respiratory diseases associated with cough (infectious diseases); however, a cause-and-effect relationship between alterations in respiratory epithelium and cough has not been established.[5]

Diseases of the respiratory tract may alter the sensitivity of the cough reflex.[5] For example, viral diseases may increase the responsiveness of cough receptors to stimuli.

DELETERIOUS CONSEQUENCES OF COUGH

Although cough is an important defense mechanism of the respiratory system that promotes expectoration of inhaled noxious substances and voluminous airway secretions, cough may lose its original defensive function and may contribute to the morbidity and discomfort associated with bronchopulmonary disease.[8] This is especially true when the effort to cough is intense and when multiple coughs occur sequentially. Chronic coughing is exhausting and, especially in foals, may decrease food intake. Paroxysmal or persistent cough may impair respiration. Coughing may have profound effects on the cardiovascular system. During the deep inspiratory phase of cough, the rise in intra-abdominal pressure because of contraction of the diaphragm and the fall in intrathoracic pressure combine to aspirate blood from the vena cava to fill the right atrium and ventricle abruptly.[3] Because the pleural pressure decreases, the pulmonary artery pressure also decreases. During the expiratory phase of cough, an initial increase in systemic arterial blood pressure and a simultaneous and commensurate increase in cerebral venous and cerebrospinal fluid pressures occur. However, venous return to the heart soon decreases, and within a few heartbeats filling of the heart and stroke volume decrease.[2,3] Hypotension ensues. Falling arterial blood pressure in the face of high cerebral venous pressures reduces the effective perfusion pressure of the brain. Cerebral hypoperfusion and anoxia may occur. Cough-induced syncope has been reported in human beings[2] and in dogs.[9]

In chronic cough bronchial muscular hypertrophy may develop. Bronchial mucosal edema or emphysema may accompany chronic cough. During cough inspiration inflammatory debris may be aspirated into previously uncontaminated areas of the lung. Cough in dogs has been associated with pneumothorax (from rupture of preexisting pulmonary bullae) and lung lobe torsion.[10] Rib and vertebral fractures have been reported in human beings with powerful coughs but have not been reported in horses.[2,3]

CLINICAL APPROACH TO THE COUGHING HORSE

Cough is a common sign of respiratory disease in horses (Figure 3-4). Cough is an indication of mechanical or irritant stimulation of cough receptors for which the potential causes are diverse. Many clinical approaches exist for anatomic localization of the origin of the cough stimulus in respiratory disease and for discovery of the cause. All methods have in common a systematic and thorough evaluation of the history and physical examination of the patient. To aid the clinician in formulating a rational approach to diagnosis, diseases associated with cough may be grouped according to those characterized by fever (current or historical) and those characterized by lack of an elevated body temperature. The clinician should keep in mind that exceptions to generalizations always occur concerning disease processes, and the following discussion therefore serves only as a guide to develop a logical approach to differentiating diseases characterized by cough.

Cough with Fever

Horses with cough and fever should have a thorough physical examination (see Chapter 9 for a complete description of a physical examination for horses with respiratory disease). A minimal laboratory database for the coughing horse with fever should include the results of a hemogram and a fibrinogen determination. The clinician carefully should auscultate the thorax of the horse in a quiet room with the horse breathing quietly. If the horse is not dyspneic or hypoxemic, the clinician also should undertake auscultation during forced breathing. A plastic bag loosely held over the nostrils of the horse forces the horse to increase tidal volume and respiratory rate. This maneuver causes many horses with exudate in the airways to cough, and deep breathing may be frankly painful for some horses with pleuropneumonia. Auscultation during forced breathing is not necessary in horses with obviously abnormal lung sounds during quiet breathing and is not advisable in horses with pneumonia (especially aspiration pneumonia) or in horses with foreign material in the trachea. Crackles and wheezes heard repeatedly during the inspiratory and early expiratory phases of breathing suggest that pulmonary parenchymal disease is present.

Accentuated normal bronchovesicular sounds sometimes are present in horses with pulmonary consolidation because of referral of sounds from the aerated lung. Absence of lung sounds in dependent portions of the thorax indicates that pulmonary consolidation, atelectasis, or fluid in the pleural cavity may be present. Thoracic percussion and sonographic evaluation are particularly helpful in documenting the presence of fluid in the pleural cavity. Ultrasonography also may show pleural irregularities and superficial parenchymal abscessation, atelectasis, or consolidation. Thoracic radiographs are especially helpful in demonstrating deeper parenchymal disease. Many equine practitioners do not have access to thoracic radiography but can perform thoracic ultrasonography.

Abnormal lung sounds, percussion irregularities, and sonographic evidence of fluid or consolidation are indications for performing transtracheal aspiration (TTA) and bronchoalveolar lavage (BAL). When both procedures are to be performed on the same patient, the clinician should perform TTA first to obtain a sample for culture before the airway is contaminated by the BAL tube. Many practitioners prefer to obtain TTA samples transendoscopically to prevent percutaneous aspiration. Despite the development of guarded culture swabs for transendoscopic use, this technique does not always prevent contamination of lower airway fluid samples. One study demonstrated that *Pseudomonas* spp. and anaerobic bacteria in cultures of tracheal fluid obtained transendoscopically should be viewed as potential contaminants.[11]

Cytologic evaluation of the TTA/BAL, indicating an increase in polymorphonuclear leukocytes (PMNs), is consistent with parenchymal disease. Some PMNs may be degenerate. Although some clinicians believe that PMNs may be seen in the tracheal aspirates of normal horses, few PMNs are found in bronchoalveolar lavage fluids from healthy horses (4.4 ± 3.3 cells to 8.9 ± 1.2 cells/μl).[12] How well the results of cytologic evaluation of BAL fluids represent the environment of the lower airways is a matter of some debate. BAL fluids are harvested from a focal area of the lung. If parenchymal disease is not generalized, BAL may miss the diseased region. Results of BAL fluid analysis are normal in some horses with pneumonia and pleuropneumonia. Transtracheal wash fluid consists of secretions from both lungs, and TTA cytologic examination was abnormal in all horses with pneumonia and pleuropneumonia in one study.[13] The prevalence of PMNs in TTA fluid from horses without lower respiratory tract disease has not been determined.

The presence of degenerate PMNs and extracellular or intracellular bacteria in TTA/BAL fluid is consistent with the diagnosis of a septic process. The clinician should evaluate a Gram stain to guide the initial choice of antimicrobial agents while awaiting results of culture and sensitivity determinations. Growth of aerobic or anaerobic bacteria in a culture of TTA fluid confirms the presence of bacterial pneumonia if clinical and radiographic findings are also consistent with this disease process. Contamination of cultures of airway secretions obtained via TTA occasionally may occur. Lack of growth of bacterial pathogens from TTA fluid suggests that viral, interstitial, or fungal pneumonia might be present. These possibilities should be investigated by evaluating paired serum samples taken 10 to 14 days apart for influenza virus, equine herpesvirus 1 (EHV1), EHV4, rhinovirus, and equine viral arteritis. Identification of virus by DNA or antigen detection (PCR, immunoflourescence) or virus isolation may also be indicated. Serologic testing for histoplasmosis, blastomycosis, coccidioidomycosis (especially in the southwestern United States), and possibly mycobacteria should be evaluated. Fungal cultures of tracheal fluid should be evaluated when other, more common causes of pneumonia have been ruled out and if the clinical signs of the patient are consistent with this diagnosis. Negative results on serologic tests and fungal cultures in patients with a significant interstitial pattern on thoracic radiographs should prompt consideration of the diagnosis of interstitial pneumonia, a condition for which the inciting cause has not been established and for which the prognosis is grave.

Percussion, radiographic, or ultrasonic evidence of increased intrapleural fluid is an indication for thoracocentesis. Many horses with bacterial pleuropneumonia have elevated pleural fluid PMN concentrations, and PMNs may be

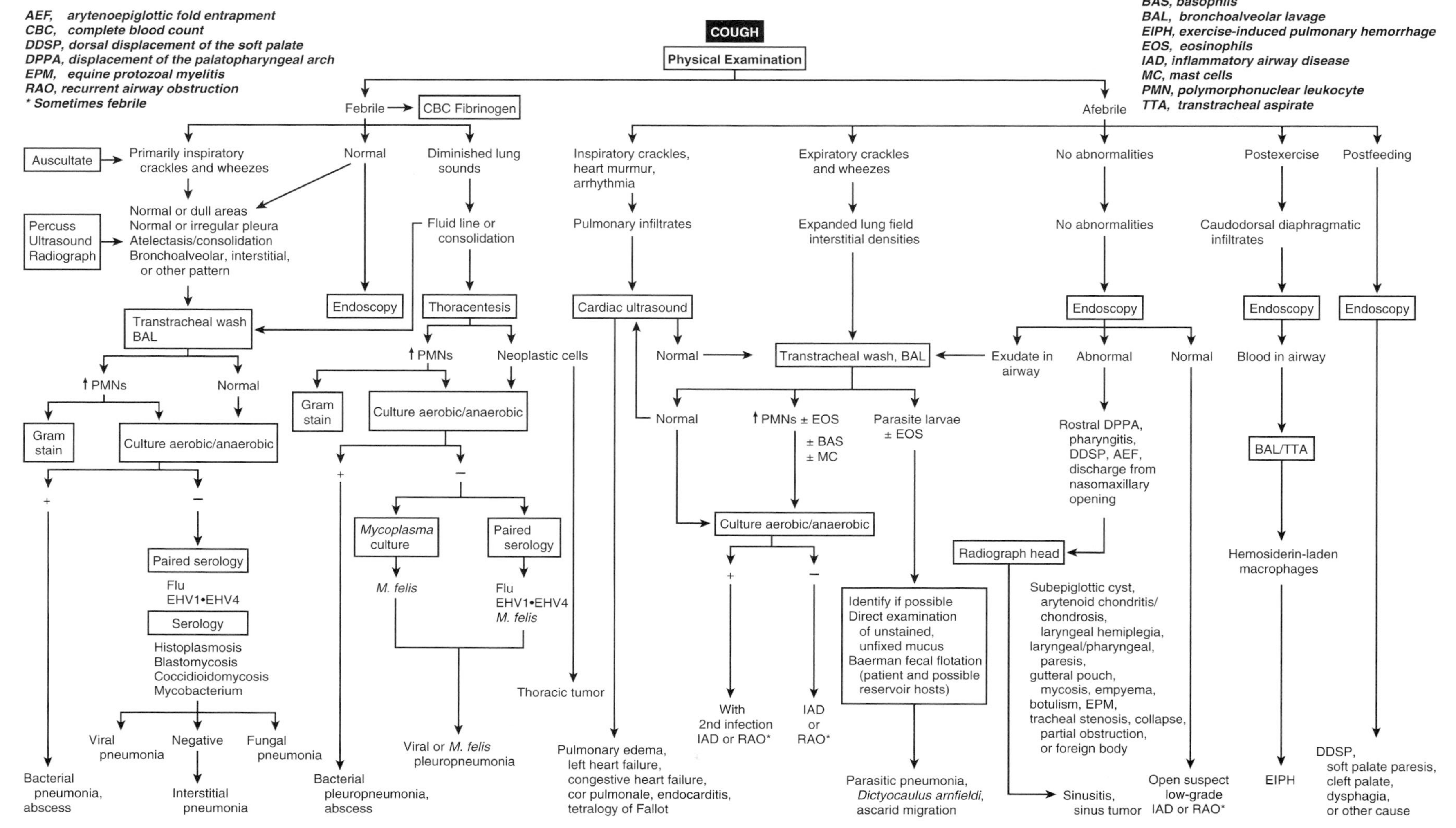

FIGURE 3-4 Approach to cough. *EHV1, 4,* Equine herpesvirus 1 or 4.

degenerate. Intracellular or extracellular bacteria may be seen on cytologic evaluation. Occasionally, frankly neoplastic cells may be identified in thoracic fluid (usually squamous cells or lymphocytes). Many cytologists are uncomfortable diagnosing thoracic neoplasia solely on the basis of an evaluation of pleural fluid. Thoracic fluid should be cultured aerobically and anaerobically. A positive culture identifies the cause of bacterial pleuritis; however, pleural fluid cultures often may be negative. Cultures of TTA fluid are more likely to be positive in horses with pleuropneumonia, and TTA cultures should be performed routinely for these patients. Primary viral pleuritis, although rare in the author's experience, has been reported in horses, and paired serologic examinations for influenza virus and EHV1/EHV4 may be helpful when cultures are negative. One case of pleuritis caused by *Mycoplasma felis* has been reported.[14] Culture of pleural fluid and paired serologic examinations for this organism should be performed in patients for which other tests have not proved diagnostic.

Intrathoracic neoplasms may cause cough with or without accompanying fever. Confirmation of a thoracic tumor may require an ultrasound-guided biopsy or an exploratory thoracotomy and a biopsy. Secondary bacterial pleuritis may complicate thoracic neoplasms, and aerobic and anaerobic cultures of thoracic fluid from patients suspected of having thoracic neoplasms should be performed.

Some febrile coughing horses have no abnormalities on auscultation, percussion, thoracic radiography, or ultrasound. In such patients occult pulmonary disease may be present and TTA/BAL and culture of TTA fluid are indicated. Alternatively, such horses may have upper airway disease (sinusitis, sinus tumor, guttural pouch empyema), and an endoscopic evaluation is also indicated.

Cough Without Fever

When auscultation of the thorax demonstrates primarily expiratory crackles and wheezes, thoracic percussion often reveals a caudoventral expansion of the lung borders. These findings suggest that RAO may be present. Thoracic radiographs usually show increased interstitial densities; radiographs are useful to rule out occult underlying pulmonary disease (such as a well walled-off abscess) but are not required for diagnosis in most cases. TTA and BAL are indicated. Horses with RAO usually have an increase in well-preserved PMNs, and sometimes eosinophils, in TTA and BAL fluids. Growth of pathogens in aerobic or anaerobic culture of TTA fluid identifies secondary bacterial infection. No growth in cultures of TTA fluid is also consistent with the diagnosis of RAO.

Inflammatory airway disease (IAD) is a syndrome most often associated with chronic intermittent cough, decreased performance and increased mucoid airway secretions.[15] However, the absence of a cough does not rule out IAD. Evaluation of BAL fluid reveals nonseptic inflammation. IAD and RAO share a number of clinical, cytologic, and functional characteristics. In general, IAD is not associated with the labored breathing and severe exercise intolerance seen with active cases of RAO. Also, in horses with IAD the BAL fluid tends to have less pronounced neutrophilic inflammation and is more likely to have increased mast cells, basophils, or eosinophils compared with BAL fluid from horses with RAO.

TTA/BAL fluids may occasionally contain parasite larvae or many eosinophils. If horses historically have been housed with donkeys or mules, the veterinarian should suspect *Dictyocaulus arnfieldi* infestation. Coughing horses younger than 18 months of age with eosinophilic TTA fluid may be experiencing migration of *Parascaris equorum* larvae. The clinician should attempt to identify the larvae, although this may be difficult. A direct cytologic evaluation of unfixed, unstained, or iodine-stained mucus may be helpful to identify larvae of *D. arnfieldi*. The clinician should perform a Baermann flotation on feces from the patient and potential reservoir hosts, but the test may not demonstrate ascarid larvae because pulmonary migration occurs early in the prepatent period.[16] The diagnosis of pulmonary ascarid migration is based on ruling out other causes of pneumonia.

When TTA/BAL fluids have no abnormal cells, cultures still should be assessed. For afebrile coughing horses with thoracic auscultation findings of inspiratory crackles and wheezes and cardiac murmur or arrhythmia, thoracic radiographs are appropriate. The presence of diffuse pulmonary infiltrates in a bronchoalveolar pattern suggests that pulmonary edema may be present. A complete ultrasonic evaluation of the heart is indicated.

Some coughing, afebrile horses have no abnormalities on auscultation or percussion, and endoscopy of the upper airway and trachea is indicated. Some horses have endoscopic evidence of exudate in the trachea and likely have low-grade RAO. The clinician should take thoracic radiographs of these horses if possible and perform TTA/BAL testing followed by culture of TTA fluid. A transtracheal aspirate should not be obtained immediately after tracheoscopy because bacteria on the endoscope may contaminate airway cultures.

In other patients, cough may be a symptom of upper airway obstructive disease (dorsal displacement of the soft palate; rostral displacement of the palatopharyngeal arch; arytenoepiglottic fold entrapment; subepiglottic cyst; arytenoid chondritis/chondrosis; laryngeal hemiplegia; or tracheal stenosis, collapse, or partial obstruction) or maxillary or frontal sinusitis with discharge into the nasal passages via the nasomaxillary opening or laryngeal/pharyngeal paresis. The latter may be a symptom of guttural pouch mycosis, empyema, or systemic disease (e.g., botulism or equine protozoal myelitis). Cough also may be a symptom of a tracheal foreign body (e.g., a twig or TTA catheter) in the airway. The veterinarian should suspect low-grade RAO or IAD in horses with cough but no abnormalities on endoscopic examination.

Cough after exercise or feeding also should prompt an endoscopic evaluation. Evidence of hemorrhage in the trachea after exercise indicates that exercise-induced pulmonary hemorrhage is likely. This diagnosis can be confirmed by finding hemosiderin-laden macrophages in BAL or TTA fluid. Thoracic radiographs may show interstitial densities and pleural thickening in the caudodorsal lung field. Postprandial cough may be associated with soft palate paresis, dorsal displacement of the soft palate, cleft palate (neonates and foals), or dysphagia of any cause. A detailed description of diagnostic and therapeutic strategies for diseases of the respiratory system can be found in Chapter 9.

POLYURIA AND POLYDIPSIA

Catherine W. Kohn, Bernard Hansen

The complaint of excessive urination and drinking may be heard with some frequency in equine practice. Before pursuing a lengthy diagnostic workup, the veterinarian should

TABLE 3-5

Voluntary Water Consumption in Healthy Horses

	WATER CONSUMPTION	
Ambient Temperature	**ml/kg/day**	**L/450 kg**
5° to 16°C (41° to 61° F)	44 to 61	19.8 to 27.5
25° C (77° F)	70	31.5

(Data from Tasker JB: Fluid and electrolyte studies in the horse, III. Intake and output of water, sodium, and potassium in normal horses, *Cornell Vet* 57: 649-657, 1967; Rose BD: *Clinical physiology of acid-base and electrolyte disorders,* New York, 1989, McGraw-Hill Information Services; and Groenedyk S, English PB, Abetz I: External balance of water and electrolytes in the horse, *Equine Vet J* 20: 189-193, 1988.)

confirm that 24-hour urine production and voluntary water consumption exceed reference ranges. Urine production in adult horses may range from 15 to 30 ml/kg/day, and values as high as 48 ml/kg/day have been reported.[1-4] Daily urine volume is affected by diet; more water is lost in the urine of horses fed pelleted diets and legume hays than in that of horses fed grass hay. The latter excrete more water in feces.[5,6] Generally, any component of the diet that increases renal solute load increases urine volume (e.g., high salt content in the diet). Voluntary water intake also is affected by the ambient temperature (Table 3-5). When temperatures are high and evaporative water losses increase to cool the horse, voluntary water intake also increases. Diet and climatic conditions therefore must be considered when interpreting water consumption and urine production data. Water requirements are proportional to metabolic body size rather than to body mass. Thus larger horses, particularly draft breeds, require less water per kilogram than do smaller horses, ponies, or miniature horses. In addition, fat is low in water content compared with lean body tissue, and fat animals require proportionately less water than do lean animals.[7]

Some owners may misinterpret pollakiuria (frequent urination usually of small volume) as polyuria. Quantitative collection of urine for a 24-hour period may be required to verify excessive urine production. Several simple collection apparatuses have been described.[8,9]

MAINTENANCE OF WATER BALANCE IN HEALTH

Maintenance of water homeostasis depends on establishing a balance between intake and excretion such that plasma osmolality remains constant (within approximately 2% of normal).[10] The primary determinant of renal water excretion is antidiuretic hormone (ADH).[11] ADH is a polypeptide synthesized in three nuclei in the hypothalamus (suprachiasmatic, paraventricular, and supraoptic nuclei)[12] and transported from the latter two nuclei in secretory granules down axons of the supraopticohypophyseal tract into the posterior lobe of the pituitary, where ADH is stored. Some ADH enters the cerebrospinal fluid or portal capillaries of the median eminence from the paraventricular nucleus.[11] In addition, neurons from the suprachiasmatic nucleus deposit ADH in other areas in the central nervous system.[12] In human beings lesions of the posterior pituitary or supraopticohypophyseal tract below the median eminence usually do not lead to permanent central diabetes insipidus because ADH still has access to systemic circulation in these cases.[11] The clinical importance of these anatomic relationships in horses is not known.

ADH increases renal water reabsorption and urine osmolality by augmenting water permeability of luminal membranes of cortical and medullary collecting tubules. ADH augments urea, and in some species NaCl, accumulation in the interstitium, therefore promoting medullary hypertonicity. The primary stimuli for ADH release are plasma hyperosmolality and depletion of the effective circulating blood volume. Osmoreceptors in the hypothalamus detect changes in plasma osmolality of as little as 1%.[11] Although the threshold for ADH release in the horse is not known, 24-hour water deprivation in healthy ponies resulted in approximately an 8 mOsm/kg increase in plasma osmolality (about 3%), from 287 ± 3 mOsm/kg to 295 ± 4 mOsm/kg, which was associated with an increase in plasma ADH concentration between 1.53 ± 0.36 pg/ml to 4.32 ± 1.12 pg/ml.[13] In another study of ponies water deprivation for 19 hours resulted in an increase in plasma osmolality from 297 ± 1 mOsm/L to 306 ± 2 mOsm/L.[14] In human beings plasma osmolalities of 280 to 290 mOsm/L stimulate ADH release. The organs that sense changes in effective circulating blood volume include arterial and left atrial baroreceptors. These stretch receptors function indirectly as volume sensors by responding to the reductions in intraluminal pressure that typically accompany loss of plasma volume. Reduced activation of these receptors by hypovolemia or heart failure is a potent cause of ADH release, even in the absence of increased plasma osmolality. ADH secretion also may be stimulated by stress (pain), nausea, hypoglycemia, and certain drugs (e.g., morphine, lithium).[11]

When the need for water in body fluids cannot be met by conservation via the renal/ADH axis, thirst is stimulated. Thirst is regulated primarily by plasma tonicity; however, in human beings the threshold for stimulation of thirst is approximately 2 to 5 mOsm/kg greater than that for stimulation of ADH release.[11] Thirst is controlled by osmosensitive neurons in close proximity in the hypothalamus to osmoreceptors that mediate ADH secretion.[12] Thirst is sensed peripherally by oropharyngeal mechanoreceptors as dryness of the mouth. Thirst also may be stimulated by volume depletion through an incompletely understood mechanism. Experimental ponies drank when their plasma osmolalities increased by 3% after water deprivation, when plasma Na concentrations increased by approximately 5%, and after induction of a plasma volume deficit of 6%.[14]

MECHANISM OF URINE CONCENTRATION

For the kidney to make concentrated urine, ADH must be produced, the renal collecting tubules must respond to ADH, and the renal medullary interstitium must be hypertonic. Generation of medullary hypertonicity is initiated in the thick ascending limb of the loop of Henle by active transport of NaCl out of the lumen. Because the thick ascending limb is impermeable to water, active resorption of NaCl results in hypotonicity of the fluid entering the distal tubule in the renal cortex (Figure 3-5, *A*). The distal tubules and cortical portions of the collecting ducts are permeable to water (see Figure 3-5, *B*), which is reabsorbed down its concentration gradient into the interstitium. Reabsorbed water is transported rapidly out of the interstitium by the extensive cortical capillary network, and interstitial hypertonicity is preserved. Urea remains in the lumen of the distal tubule and cortical collecting duct and is concentrated further. Luminal fluid flows into the medullary collecting duct, which is permeable to water and urea when under the influence of ADH (see Figure 3-5, *C*). Water is reabsorbed down its progressively steeper concentration gradient as luminal fluid moves through the medullary collecting ducts. Some urea also is reabsorbed into the interstitium. Reabsorbed water is removed efficiently by the vasa recta in the renal medulla. Because these blood vessels also are arranged in a hairpin loop, minimal loss of medullary interstitial solute occurs with water removal. Some reabsorbed urea enters the loop of Henle (see Figure 3-5, *D*) and thus is recycled, helping to maintain medullary hypertonicity. In the absence of ADH the collecting ducts are relatively impermeable to water and urea, resulting in water and urea loss in urine and reduction of medullary solute. Prolonged diuresis of any cause may result in the loss of medullary hypertonicity (medullary washout) with subsequent impairment of renal concentrating ability. Water is reabsorbed down its concentration gradient from the thin descending limb of the loop of Henle (see Figure 3-5, *E*) as a consequence of medullary hypertonicity. This segment of the nephron is impermeable to NaCl and urea; thus the osmolality of luminal fluid in the most distal portion of the loop approaches that of the interstitium. The thin ascending limb of the loop of Henle is permeable to NaCl, which diffuses down its concentration gradient into the interstitium (see Figure 3-5, *F*). As previously mentioned, this segment is also permeable to urea, and some interstitial urea enters the tubule lumen by diffusion down its concentration gradient. Luminal fluid entering the thick ascending limb of the loop of Henle is thus hypotonic to the interstitium.

When luminal fluid reaches the thick ascending limb of the loop of Henle, approximately 80% of the glomerular filtrate has been reabsorbed. Therefore only 20% of the glomerular filtrate is available for reabsorption via the action of ADH.[15,16]

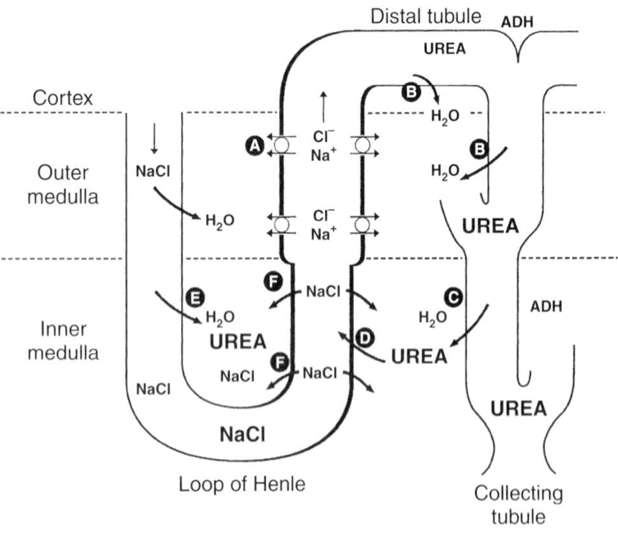

FIGURE 3-5 The countercurrent hypothesis identifies the roles of sodium chloride and urea transport in the generation of concentrated urine. From Fenner WR: *Quick reference to veterinary medicine,* ed 3, Philadelphia, Wiley-Blackwell, 2001. Originally adapted from Jamison RL, Maffly RH: The urinary concentration mechanism, *N Engl J Med* 295:1059-1067, 1976.

PRIMARY POLYDIPSIA

Excessive water intake may result in water diuresis. Primary polydipsia has been described in horses residing in the southern United States during months when ambient temperature and humidity are high. Apparent psychogenic polydipsia may result from boredom, especially in stalled young horses.[8] Psychogenic polydipsia also has been reported anecdotally in horses with chronic liver disease and central nervous system signs that had been treated with intravenous fluids.[17] Primary disorders of thirst are poorly understood in horses.

CAUSES OF POLYURIA WITH SECONDARY POLYDIPSIA

Increased urine flow may be induced by solute or water diuresis (Box 3-2). Solute diuresis results in increased urine flow because of excessive renal excretion of a nonreabsorbed solute such as glucose or sodium. During solute diuresis the urine osmolality is equal to or higher than the plasma osmolality. Primary renal insufficiency or failure (33% or fewer intact nephrons) result in solute diuresis, because each functional nephron must filter an increased amount of solute to maintain daily obligatory solute excretion. Fractional clearances of solutes such as Na, K, and Cl therefore appropriately increase. Solute diuresis caused by glucosuria occurs in hyperglycemic horses when the maximal renal reabsorptive capacity for glucose is exceeded (180 to 200 mg/dl).[18] Solute diuresis caused by glucosuria has been reported in horses with pituitary pars intermedia dysfunction (PPID pituitary adenoma) and in a hyperglycemic horse with bilateral granulosa cell tumors.[19,20] Primary diabetes mellitus, a common cause of hyperglycemia and glucosuria in other species, is uncommon in the horse, although type 2 diabetes mellitus was diagnosed in a 15-year-old Quarter Horse mare.[21] Primary renal tubular glucosuria caused by a defect in proximal tubular glucose reabsorption (as is seen in Basenji dogs with Fanconi-like syndrome)[15] has not been reported in horses. Psychogenic salt consumption also has been reported to cause solute diuresis in a horse.[22] Postobstructive solute diuresis is not diagnosed commonly in horses because nephrolithiasis and ureterolithiasis are uncommon; when they occur, the condition is often bilateral and associated with chronic renal failure, and treatment is usually unsuccessful.[23,24]

Decreased water resorption in the collecting tubules or inappropriately large voluntary water intake causes water diuresis. The osmolality of the urine during water diuresis is less than that of plasma. Water diuresis may be caused by insufficient ADH secretion, insensitivity of the receptors of the distal collecting duct and collecting tubules to the action of ADH, renal medullary solute washout, or apparent psychogenic polydipsia. Insufficient secretion of ADH (central diabetes insipidus) may be associated with PPID of horses but has never been documented[25] and with head trauma and potassium depletion in other species. A case of idiopathic central diabetes insipidus was reported in a Welsh pony.[26] Insensitivity of collecting duct receptors to ADH may occur during endotoxemia and hyperadrenocorticism (glucocorticoid excess associated with PPID). In other species potassium

BOX 3-2

CAUSES OF POLYURIA AND POLYDIPSIA

Solute Diuresis

Primary renal insufficiency or failure
Glucosuria (PPID)
Psychogenic salt consumption
Diabetes mellitus
Postobstructive diuresis

Water Diuresis

Insufficient antidiuretic hormone (central diabetes insipidus)
- PPID
- Head trauma
- (Potassium depletion)*

Insufficient response of collecting ducts to antidiuretic hormone
Acquired nephrogenic diabetes insipidus
- Hyperadrenocorticism (glucocorticoid excess with PPID)
- Endotoxemia
- (Drugs: gentamicin, lithium, methoxyflurane, amphotericin B, propoxyphene, etc.)
- (Congenital nephrogenic diabetes insipidus)

Renal medullary solute washout
- Chronic diuresis of any cause
- Inappropriate renal tubular sodium handling

Apparent psychogenic polydipsia
(Chronic liver disease)
(Polycythemia)
(Pyometra)
(Hypercalcemia)
(Potassium depletion)

Iatrogenic

Intravenous fluid therapy
Excess dietary salt
Drugs:
- Diuretics
- Glucocorticoids
- (Drugs causing acquired diabetes insipidus)

Modified from Fenner WR: *Quick reference to veterinary medicine,* ed 3, Philadelphia, Wiley-Blackwell, 2001
PPID, pituitary pars intermedia dysfunction
*Not reported in horses.

depletion, hypercalcemia, and the administration of certain drugs (e.g., gentamicin) have been reported to cause insensitivity of the collecting duct receptors to ADH.[15] Congenital diabetes insipidus also has been reported in other species.[26] True nephrogenic diabetes insipidus implies isolated dysfunction of response to ADH by collecting tubules that are not associated with other structural or metabolic lesions of the kidney. The occurrence of nephrogenic diabetes insipidus in two sibling Thoroughbred colts suggests that the condition might be heritable in some horses.[27] Renal medullary washout (loss of medullary Na, Cl, and urea) leading to water diuresis may result from chronic diuresis of any cause. Diuresis is associated with increased tubular flow rates and inability to resorb sodium and urea adequately from the tubular lumen. Enhanced medullary blood flow may deplete medullary solute further. Water diuresis also has been reported in association with pyometra, hypoadrenocorticism (chronic renal sodium loss), chronic liver disease (increased aldosterone concentration promotes sodium retention, smaller daily load of urea for excretion caused by decreased conversion of ammonia to urea), primary polycythemia, hypercalcemia, and potassium depletion in other species.[15]

APPROACH TO THE HORSE WITH POLYURIA AND POLYDIPSIA

Iatrogenic causes of polyuria and polydipsia (see Box 3-2) should be ruled out by careful assessment of the history and by documentation of return to normal urine volume and water intake after withdrawal of intravenous fluids, excess dietary salt, or drugs implicated in causing polyuria and polydipsia (Figure 3-6). Verification of 24-hour urine volume and water intake should be undertaken for horses suspected of having polyuria and polydipsia that do not display obvious polyuria (frequent large volume urination and wet stall) and polydipsia (water bucket always empty and overt thirst). Hemogram, serum biochemistries, and urinalysis should be assessed for all horses with polyuria and polydipsia. A hallmark finding in horses with polyuria and polydipsia is a decreased urine specific gravity (USG). Identification of other abnormalities on laboratory tests (e.g., increased blood urea nitrogen or creatinine concentrations, hyperglycemia, and hypokalemia) necessitates ruling out the presence of underlying diseases (e.g., renal insufficiency and PPID) using specialized laboratory tests.

The hydration status of horses then should be assessed carefully. Horses that are dehydrated should be rehydrated judiciously with intravenous fluids, with care taken not to overhydrate horses with renal insufficiency. After rehydration, when possible, creatinine clearance should be determined by using a urine collection apparatus to allow 24-hour volumetric urine collection. A creatinine clearance value below the reference range (1.46 to 3.68 ml/min/kg)[28] suggests that renal insufficiency with decreased glomerular filtration rate and solute diuresis are likely present. A creatinine clearance within the reference range indicates that central diabetes insipidus (CDI), nephrogenic diabetes insipidus (NDI), or apparent psychogenic polydypsia (APP) is present. To distinguish among these differential diagnoses, an exogenous ADH challenge test should be performed (see the subsequent discussion).

Horses with polyuria and polydipsia that are well hydrated and healthy according to physical examination and results of hemogram and serum biochemistry determinations should be subjected to a water deprivation test to assess renal ability to conserve water.[2,29,30] Water deprivation testing is contraindicated in a dehydrated horse with a low USG. Such horses have already undergone an endogenous water deprivation test (clinical dehydration is present) and have responded with an inappropriately low USG. The following guidelines for interpretation of water deprivation test results are based on practical experience and the limited data available. A positive response to water deprivation (USG >1.030) indicates that the horse has APP, whereas a negative response (USG <1.008) after 24 hours of water deprivation or greater than 5% weight loss[31] is consistent with a diagnosis of CDI, true NDI, insensitivity

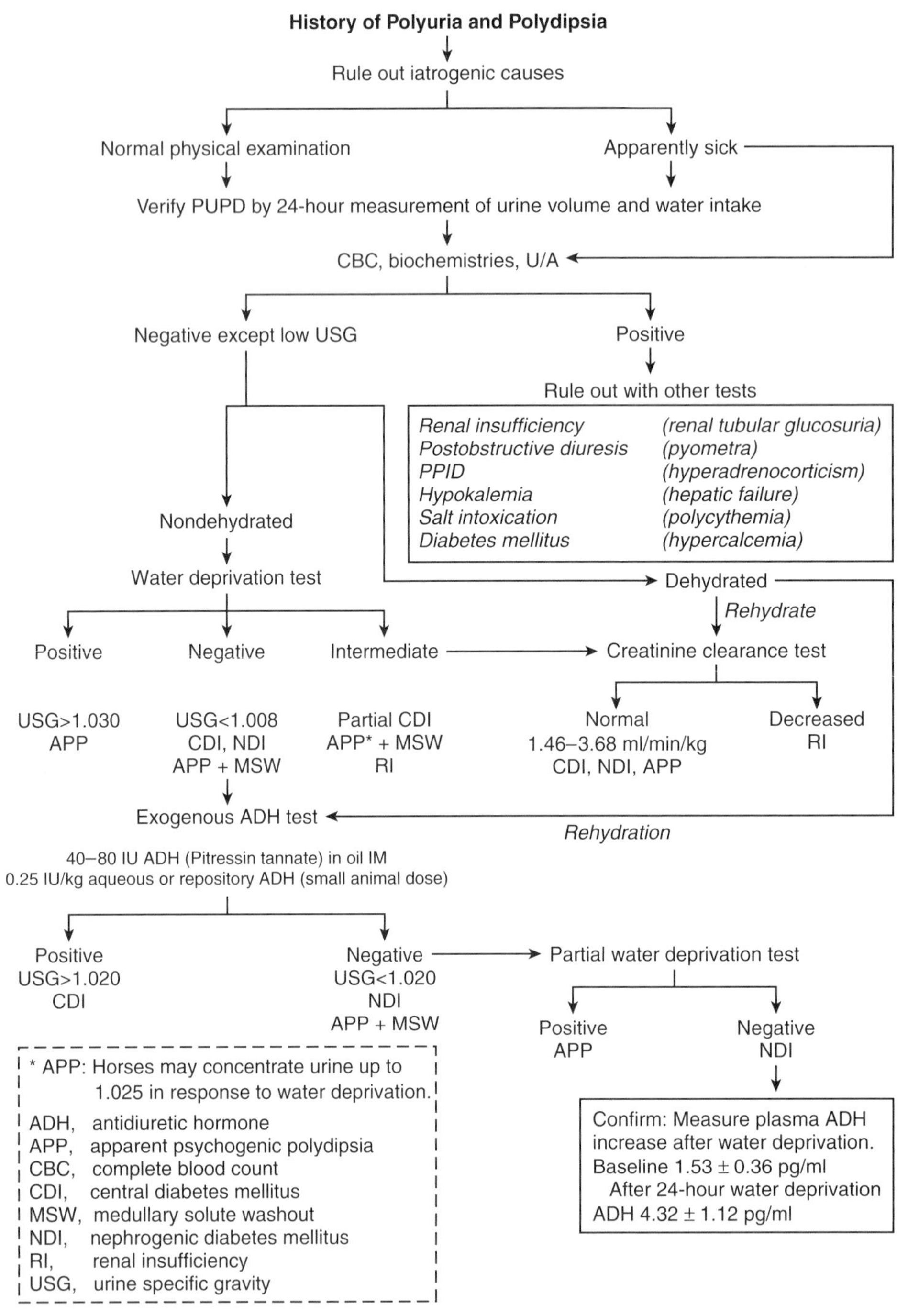

FIGURE 3-6 Approach to the polyuric patient. *PPID,* pituitary pars intermedia dysfunction; *PUPD,* Polyuria and polydipsia; *U/A,* Urinalysis. Modified from Fenner WR: *Quick reference to veterinary medicine,* ed 3, Philadelphia, Wiley-Blackwell, 2001.

of collecting duct receptors to ADH, or apparent psychogenic polydipsia and medullary solute washout (APP plus MSW). Horses with a negative response to water deprivation testing should undergo an exogenous ADH challenge. Some horses may have an intermediate response to water deprivation. An intermediate response is consistent with partial CDI or APP plus MSW or renal insufficiency, and assessment of creatinine clearance is indicated. Consult Chapter 19 for a more detailed discussion of water deprivation testing.

An evaluation of a response to the administration of exogenous ADH is indicated for horses that do not concentrate their urine adequately during water deprivation testing, for horses that require rehydration and subsequently demonstrate creatinine clearance values within reference ranges, and for rehydrated horses for which creatinine clearance determinations are impractical. Two regimens for exogenous ADH administration have been reported: 40 to 80 IU ADH as Pitressin tannate in oil intramuscularly[32] or 0.25 IU/kg aqueous or repository ADH intramuscularly. A few reports of responses of horses to exogenous ADH administration have been made, and the following recommendations are based on clinical experience. A positive response to exogenous ADH (USG < 1.020) confirms the diagnosis of CDI. A negative response (USG > 1.020) implies that NDI or APP plus MSW is present.[31]

MSW may result in a decreased USG despite the presence of adequate ADH. A partial water deprivation test should result in an increase in USG in horses with APP plus MSW but should have no effect on horses with true NDI or insensitivity of collecting duct receptors to ADH. The horse is allowed to consume its normal diet and water ad libitum. Voluntary water consumption is monitored closely for 3 to 4 days to establish a baseline. Water available to the horse then is decreased by 5% to 10% of the baseline voluntary intake. Water should be offered in aliquots several times a day to prevent the horse from consuming most of the water in a short time. Water intake should never be restricted below maintenance requirements (about 40 ml/kg/day). During water restriction the horse is allowed to eat its regular diet. The horse should be weighed daily if possible and observed carefully for signs of dehydration (prolonged capillary refill time, increasing heart rate, prolonged skin tenting, and hypernatremia). Moderate water restriction in the face of continued intake of dietary solutes facilitates re-establishment of the corticomedullary osmotic gradient.[15] Results of partial water deprivation tests in horses have been reported infrequently.

The diagnosis of true NDI or insensitivity of collecting duct receptors to ADH may be confirmed by measuring plasma ADH concentrations before and after partial water deprivation. ADH concentrations have been reported to increase from baseline values of 1.53 ± 0.36 pg/ml to 4.32 ± 1.12 pg/ml after 24 hours of water deprivation in ponies.[13]

Because CDI, NDI, and APP are uncommon in horses, the presenting complaint of polyuria and polydipsia usually signifies other underlying disease. The most likely underlying disease is renal insufficiency. PPID should be considered in horses with compatible clinical signs (hirsutism, weight loss, and laminitis) and supporting laboratory data (hyperglycemia and failure of suppression of cortisol production by dexamethasone).[33] Medullary washout may be a more common complication of primary diseases and their therapy in horses than has been reported to date. Potential causes of diuresis compatible with the case history and clinical signs should be investigated, and a partial water deprivation test should be considered when horses exhibit polyuria and polydipsia.

EDEMA

Kenneth W. Hinchcliff

Edema is defined as the excessive and abnormal accumulation of fluid in the interstitium. Interstitial fluid accumulates because of imbalances in the rates with which fluid enters and exits the interstitium. Factors that increase the rate of fluid flux from the capillary or impair lymph drainage sufficiently to overwhelm normal compensatory mechanisms result in accumulation of fluid and the development of edema.

PHYSIOLOGY

The volume of interstitial fluid and lymph fluid in the normal horse is 8% to 10% of body mass,[1] or 36 to 45 L in a 450-kg horse. Interstitial fluid consists of water, protein, and electrolytes. Compared with plasma, interstitial fluid has a slightly lower concentration of cationic electrolytes, a slightly higher concentration of chloride, and a much lower concentration of protein (1.2 versus 0.2 mOsm/L of water).[2] The amount and function of plasma proteins within the interstitial space are not inconsequential. A constant circulation of plasma proteins occurs between the vascular and interstitial spaces, with about half of the protein circulating every 24 hours in human beings. More than half of the plasma protein content of the body is contained within the interstitial space at any one time. Plasma proteins within the interstitial space are important in the transport of water-insoluble substances from the vascular space and in resistance to infection.[3]

Interstitial fluid is contained within the interstitium, the intercellular connective tissues that lie between the cellular elements of the vascular and cellular compartments of the body. The extracellular tissue of the interstitium, except in the case of bone, consists of a three-dimensional collagen fiber network embedded in a proteoglycan gel matrix.[4] Interstitial water exists as free water and as water within the proteoglycan gel. Normally, only a small proportion of interstitial fluid exists as free water, most of the water being contained in the interstitial gel. However, in edematous states, the proportion of fluid as free water within the interstitium increases.[2]

The source of interstitial fluid is the intravascular space. The volume of interstitial fluid is determined by the functional relationships of three major anatomic structures: the capillary, the interstitial space, and the lymphatics.[5] Functionally, the volume of fluid that accumulates in the interstitium is determined by the rate of ingress of fluid from the vascular space, the compliance of the interstitium, and the rate at which fluid is evacuated from the interstitium. The net rate of ingress of fluid from capillaries into the interstitium is determined by a number of factors acting across the capillary membrane, the effects of which are related by Starling's equation:

$$J = Kf[P_c - P_t) - \sigma(\pi_p - \pi_t)]$$

in which J equals the volume flow across the capillary wall; Kf equals the filtration coefficient of the capillary wall (volume flow per unit time per 100 g of tissue per unit pressure); P_c equals capillary hydrostatic pressure; P_t equals interstitial fluid hydrostatic pressure; σ equals the osmotic reflection coefficient; π_p equals the colloid osmotic (oncotic) pressure of the plasma; and π_t equals the colloid osmotic (oncotic) pressure of the interstitial fluid.[6] Although all these factors act in concert to determine the rate of net fluid efflux from the capillary, considering them individually is conceptually easier.

FILTRATION (KF) AND REFLECTION (σ)COEFFICIENTS

Together the filtration and reflection coefficients describe the properties of the capillary membrane that determine the ease with which water, protein, and other plasma constituents move from the vascular space to the interstitium. The filtration coefficient, which is the product of the hydraulic permeability and surface area of the capillary, is a measure of the ease with which water crosses the capillary membrane. The reflection coefficient is an indicator of the degree to which the capillary membrane resists the passage of a substance, such as protein. A reflection coefficient can be defined for each substance; a reflection coefficient of 0 indicates that the molecule crosses the membrane as readily as does water, whereas a value of

1 indicates that the membrane is impermeable to the substance. The reflection coefficient for a substance may vary with the anatomic site of the capillary[7,8]: capillaries in the liver are permeable to albumin, whereas capillaries in muscle are much less permeable and cerebral capillaries are among the least permeable to albumin.

The movement of fluid and protein across the vascular membrane is assumed to be passive, with plasma water and protein exiting the vascular space through pores in the capillary membrane. However, the rate with which various plasma constituents cross the capillary membrane varies considerably depending on the constituent and the tissue. For example, muscle capillary pores are permeable to water molecules (reflection coefficient of 0) but much less permeable to albumin (reflection coefficient of approximately 0.9).[2] Movement of solutes across the endothelium is not understood fully, being complex, but is affected by the concentration of the solutes on either side of the membrane, solute charge and interaction with other solutes, and capillary pore configuration.[9]

Together the filtration and reflection coefficients partially determine the rate of fluid flux across the capillary wall and the composition of the fluid. For a given hydrostatic and oncotic pressure difference, tissues with higher filtration coefficients (whether because of a larger capillary surface area or more porous capillaries) will have a greater fluid flux. Conversely, under the same circumstance, increases in the reflection coefficient of the capillary wall reduce fluid flux. The differential permeability of the capillary membrane to water and protein has important consequences in the maintenance of the oncotic pressure difference between plasma and interstitial fluid.

Aquaporins are a diverse family of membrane proteins that are expressed predominantly in tissues in which edema and fluid imbalances are of major concern.[10,11] While water movement across cell membranes is driven by osmotic and hydrostatic forces, the speed of this process can be influenced by the presence of specific aquaporin channels. These channels are primarily water channels, although some are also permeable to small solutes. The pharmacologic modulation of the expression and activity of various aquaporins potentially could provide novel treatments for a variety of disorders, including brain edema.

Hydrostatic and Colloid Osmotic Pressures

Transcapillary fluid flow results from an imbalance between the hydraulic forces favoring movement of water from the capillary into the interstitium and the forces favoring movement of water in the reverse direction. The forces contributing to fluid movement out of the capillary are the intracapillary hydrostatic pressure and the interstitial colloid osmotic pressure, whereas those forces favoring movement of fluid from the interstitium to the capillary are the interstitial hydrostatic pressure (if it is positive) and the plasma colloid osmotic pressure.[12]

The principal force favoring fluid efflux from the capillary is the hydrostatic pressure within the capillary. Capillary hydrostatic pressure varies among different tissues and decreases along the length of the capillary. Hydrostatic pressure within a capillary is determined by the arterial and venous pressures and by the precapillary and postcapillary resistances.[13] Specifically, capillary pressure is determined by the ratio of the postcapillary resistance (R_a) to the precapillary resistance (R_v), and the arterial (P_a) and venous (P_v) pressures:

Thus a small increase in venous pressure has a much greater effect on capillary pressure than does an increase in arterial pressure. For this reason the hydrostatic pressure is greater in capillaries below the heart (e.g., legs) than in those above the heart (e.g., head).

The colloid osmotic pressure of the plasma is the principal force minimizing fluid efflux from the capillary. The colloid osmotic pressure is generated because the plasma and interstitial fluid are separated by a semipermeable membrane—the endothelium—and vary slightly, but significantly, in composition. As noted previously, the interstitial fluid has a lower protein concentration than does plasma but has an essentially identical electrolyte concentration. The difference in protein concentration across the semipermeable endothelium generates an osmotic force that tends to draw water from the interstitium into the plasma.

In addition to the capillary hydrostatic pressure, the colloid osmotic pressure and negative hydrostatic pressure of the interstitial fluid favor fluid movement out of the capillary. Fluid flux across the capillary results from the summation of these forces (Table 3-6). These figures should be recognized as representing the forces at the midpoint of an idealized capillary; the forces are dynamic, changing between tissues and even along the length of the capillary. In fact, a large net flux of fluid from the capillary occurs at its arteriolar end, where capillary hydrostatic forces are greatest and plasma oncotic forces are least, and a net flux of fluid into the capillary toward its venous end, where capillary hydrostatic forces are least and plasma oncotic pressure is greatest.

The small imbalance in filtration forces results in a net efflux of fluid from the capillary into the interstitial tissue. This fluid does not accumulate in the interstitium; it is removed by the lymphatics.

Lymphatics

The lymphatics drain the interstitium of fluid and substances, notably proteins, that are not absorbed by the capillaries. The lymphatics represent the only means by which

TABLE 3-6

Mean Forces (mm Hg) Influencing Fluid Movement into or out of the Capillary

Type of Pressure	Mean Force
HYDROSTATIC PRESSURES	
Mean capillary pressure	17.0
Interstitial pressure	–5.3
Total hydrostatic pressure favoring filtration	22.3
COLLOID ONCOTIC PRESSURES	
Plasma oncotic pressure	28.0
Interstitial oncotic pressure	6.0
Total oncotic pressure opposing filtration	22.0
TOTAL PRESSURE FAVORING FILTRATION	0.3

Data from Guyton AC: *Textbook of medical physiology,* ed 11, Philadelphia, Saunders, 2005. #T3-6 interstitial protein is returned to the circulation. Interstitial fluid (and, with it, protein) moves down a pressure gradient into lymphatic capillaries through clefts between the lymphatic endothelial cells. Lymphatic endothelial cells are supported, and the lymphatic capillaries maintained patent, by anchoring filaments that attach the endothelial cells to surrounding connective tissue. Lymphatic fluid progresses centripetally through progressively larger vessels before draining into the great veins of the chest. Lymphatic valves prevent the retrograde flow of fluid from the lymphatics. Lymph is propelled by factors extrinsic to the lymphatics, including muscle activity, active and passive motion, posture, respiration, and blood vessel pulsation. Exercise causes a significant increase in lymph flow, at least in part because of the increase in tissue pressure that is associated with muscle contraction, although passive motion also increases lymph flow. Standing results in significant diminution or cessation of lymph flow from, and the prompt accumulation of interstitial fluid in, the lower extremities of human beings. In addition to the extrinsic factors affecting lymph flow, coordinated contractions of lymphatic vessels contribute substantially to the centripetal flow of lymph.[4]

BOX 3-3

PATHOGENESIS OF EDEMA

Increased Capillary Hydrostatic Pressure

Venous obstruction
- Thrombophlebitis
  - Compression (mass, tourniquet)

Venous congestion
- Posture (dependent limbs)
- Congestive heart failure

Arteriolar dilation
- Inflammation
- Increased body water

Decreased Plasma Oncotic Pressure

Panhypoproteinemia
Hypoalbuminemia

Increased Interstitial Oncotic Pressure

Increased capillary permeability

Decreased Lymph Flow

Lymphatic obstruction

MECHANISMS OF EDEMA FORMATION

Simply stated, accumulation of excessive fluid in the interstitial spaces—edema—results from an imbalance of the rates of fluid filtration from the capillaries and drainage by the lymphatics. Perturbations of one or more of the forces that affect filtration across the capillary alter the rate at which fluid enters the interstitium. Increases in capillary hydrostatic pressure, decreases in plasma oncotic pressure, and increases in interstitial oncotic pressure all favor increased fluid filtration. Conversely, increased interstitial hydrostatic pressure and decreased interstitial oncotic pressure act to inhibit fluid filtration.

Box 3-3 lists the fundamental mechanisms by which excessive interstitial fluid accumulates. Increases in capillary hydrostatic pressure, which occur with venous obstruction or arteriolar dilation, such as that associated with inflammation, increase net fluid efflux. The edema that occurs with congestive heart failure likely has an increase in capillary hydrostatic pressure as one of its causes, although the mechanism is complex.[4] Posture also affects capillary hydrostatic pressure; capillaries below the level of the heart have higher hydrostatic pressures than do capillaries above the level of the heart.

A decrease in the oncotic gradient across the capillary endothelium, which occurs with a decreased plasma oncotic pressure or an increased interstitial oncotic pressure, results in an increase in efflux of fluid from the capillary. A decrease in plasma oncotic pressure decreases the oncotic gradient that favors movement of fluid into the capillary. Consequently, the capillary hydrostatic pressure, which favors filtration, predominates and fluid accumulates in the interstitium. Plasma oncotic pressure decreases when plasma protein concentration declines. Albumin is the plasma protein that exerts the preponderance of the oncotic force[8]; therefore clinically, edema often is associated with hypoalbuminemia. An increase in the permeability of the capillary membrane greatly increases fluid and protein transport into the interstitium and decreases the ability of the membrane to maintain a difference in oncotic pressure between the plasma and the interstitium.[5] Capillary permeability increases when the endothelium is damaged, such as by vasculitis or inflammatory reactions.

Lymphatic obstruction prevents the removal of interstitial fluid and protein. Filtration of fluid and passage of small amounts of protein into the interstitial space continues in the presence of lymphatic obstruction. The interstitial fluid is reabsorbed by the capillaries; however, the protein is not. Consequently, the protein content of the interstitial fluid gradually increases, with a resultant increase in interstitial oncotic pressure that favors filtration of fluid. The increased interstitial oncotic pressure causes fluid to accumulate in the interstitium, thus exacerbating the edema.[2]

Alterations in the magnitude of one or more of Starling's forces may be offset by compensatory changes in lymph flow and other of Starling's forces. In concert Starling's forces and lymph flow act as "edema safety factors" to prevent the excess accumulation of interstitial fluid and development of frank edema. For example, lymph flow increases with the increased filtration associated with increased capillary hydrostatic pressure. Thus a larger volume of fluid enters and is removed from the interstitial space. The interstitial protein concentration decreases as increased fluid flow washes protein out of the interstitial space. Reduced interstitial space protein concentration increases the oncotic gradient, inhibiting fluid efflux from the capillary, and decreases the rate of movement of fluid from the capillary to the interstitial space.[6]

DIAGNOSTIC APPROACH TO THE PATIENT WITH EDEMA

Edema is not in itself a disease; rather, it is a sign of a disease process. Therefore the diagnostic approach to the patient with edema is based on an understanding of the pathogenesis of edema and knowledge of the diseases likely to be involved (Box 3-4). The diagnostic approach to an animal with edema should not be any different from that for any other sign of disease. A clinical examination, including history and physical examination, permits the development of a list of potential diagnoses and dictates the appropriate subsequent steps in confirming the diagnosis. The reader is referred to those sections of the text that deal with specific diseases for a description of the appropriate diagnostic aids.

When taking the history of a horse that has edema, the veterinarian should focus on acquiring facts that have the greatest diagnostic use in differentiating among those diseases that have edema as a sign. The veterinarian should consider the following aspects:

- Housing, season, and geographic region
- Vaccine and parasiticide administration
- Exposure to other horses and diseases present within the herd
- The duration of the edema, its distribution, and the presence of any other clinical signs

The veterinarian should investigate the remainder of the history depending on the responses to initial questions.

The physical examination should begin with a visual evaluation of the attitude and physical condition of the horse. The temperature, pulse, and respiration should be recorded. Although the physical examination should be complete, particular attention should be paid to those body systems that the preliminary examination indicates may be involved in the disease process. The physical examination reveals the distribution and severity of edema. Edema that is localized to one extremity or is not bilaterally symmetric is more likely to be caused by local factors (e.g., lymphangitis, venous obstruction) than by systemic disease. Conversely, edema that involves several areas of the body and has a symmetric distribution is likely to be associated with systemic disease (e.g., the ventral edema of congestive heart failure).

After the initial clinical examination, the clinician will have developed an ordered list of potential diagnoses. Confirmation or elimination of these diagnoses depends on subsequent diagnostic procedures, including the response to therapy. Sections of this text deal with the specific disease processes for appropriate diagnostic procedures.

BOX 3-4

COMMON CAUSES OF PERIPHERAL OR VENTRAL EDEMA IN HORSES

Congestive Heart Failure

Valvular disease
Myocarditis
Monensin toxicosis

Vasculitis

Equine viral arteritis
Equine ehrlichiosis
Purpura hemorrhagica
Equine infectious anemia

Venous Obstruction and Congestion

Catheter-related thrombophlebitis
Disseminated intravascular coagulation
Tight bandages
Tumors
Immobility

Cellulitis

Staphylococcal
Clostridial
Counterirritant application

Lymphatic Obstruction

Ulcerative lymphangitis
Lymphadenitis *(Streptococcus equi, Corynebacterium pseudotuberculosis)*
Lymphosarcoma
Tumors

Hypoalbuminemia

Parasitism
Pleural and peritoneal effusions
Protein loss (gastrointestinal, renal, or wounds)
Inadequate production (starvation)
Hemodilution (subsequent to hemorrhage)

Shock

Hemorrhagic
Endotoxic

Pleuritis

Late-term pregnancy
Prepubic tendon rupture
Starvation
  Inadequate intake
  Malabsorption

SPINAL ATAXIA

Kathy K. Seino

The complaint of incoordination or ataxia is a commonly encountered clinical problem in the horse. Horses might exhibit obvious gait deficits such as weaving of the feet at the walk ("walking like a drunken sailor"), a broad-based stance when stopped from a trot, truncal sway, crossing over when turning, or pivoting on the inside limb when spun. More challenging may be the horse that exhibits poor performance in which the degree of ataxia may be a subtle manifestation appreciated only under saddle by the rider when a higher degree of coordination is required, such as in dressage or jumping.[1] Common complaints may be that the horse "is not bending as well," "refusing fences," "stumbling," or "switching leads." Spinal ataxia is the most commonly reported manifestation of neurologic disease in the horse, and there are numerous causes (Table 3-7).[2,3]

Spinal ataxia or sensory ataxia is distinguished from vestibular and cerebellar ataxia in that it occurs secondary to damage of the ascending proprioceptive pathways (primarily the spinocerebellar tracts) as they originate in the white matter of the spinal cord and travel to the higher levels of brainstem and brain.[4] Ataxia associated with focal lesions in the proprioceptive pathways at the level of the brain (cranial to the red nucleus) varies in severity but is usually mild with proprioceptive deficits and some alteration of mentation. Cranial nerve deficits also may be present with brain and brainstem lesions. With ataxia caused by spinal cord lesions caudal to the

TABLE 3-7

Differential Diagnoses for Horses Presenting with Signs of Spinal Ataxia

Common Causes	Major Diagnostic Tests
Cervical compressive myelopathy	Cervical radiography, myelogram
Equine protozoal myeloencephalitis	Western Blot, IFAT
Equine herpesvirus-1 myeloencepahalopathy	PCR, titers, virus isolation
West Nile encephalitis	IgM capture ELISA, PRNT
Trauma	Radiography, nuclear scintigraphy, ultrasound, MRI, CT, CSF analysis
Equine degenerative myeloencephalopathy	Rule out other causes, serum Vitamin E levels
Neoplasia	CSF analysis, rule out other causes
Rabies	Rule out other causes
	Postmortem FA testing of brain
LESS COMMON CAUSES	
Eastern and Western Equine Encephalitis	ELISA, titers, virus isolation
Occipitoatlantoaxial malformation	Age, breed, radiographs
Vertebral osteomyelitis, diskospondylitis, spinal abscess	CSF analysis, culture, radiography, nuclear scintigraphy
Diskospondylosis	Radiography, nuclear scintigraphy
	Rule-out bacterial diskospondylitis
Cervical vertebral spinal hematoma	Radiographs, myelogram, CT, rule out other causes
Intervertebral disc disease	
Synovial cyst, arachnoid cyst	Radiographs, myelography, CT, MRI
Verminous meningoencephalitis	Rule out other causes
Stronglyus vulgaris	CSF (eosinophilic leukocytosis supportive)
Halicephalobus gingivalis	CBC (eosinophilia supportive)
Setaria spp.	
Draschia megastoma	
others	
Equine infectious anemia	Coggins test (agar gel immunodiffusion), ELISA
Aortic-iliac thrombosis	Rectal palpation
Cauda equina neuritis	Rule out other causes
Polyneuritis equi	
Toxic agents	
Stinging nettles	
Ivermectin, moxidectin	
Ionophores	
Moldy corn	
Locoism	
Sorghum, Rye grass, Dallis grass	
Heavy metals (lead, arsenic)	
Crotalaria	
Fluphenazine	
Propylene glycol	

IFAT, Indirect fluorescent antibody test; *PCR,* polymerase chain reaction; *IgM,* immunoglobulin M; *ELISA,* enzyme-linked immunosorbent assay; *PRNT,* plaque reduction neutralization test; *MRI,* magnetic resonance imaging; *CT,* computed tomography; *CSF,* cerebrospinal fluid; *FA,* fluorescent antibody; *CBC,* complete blood count.

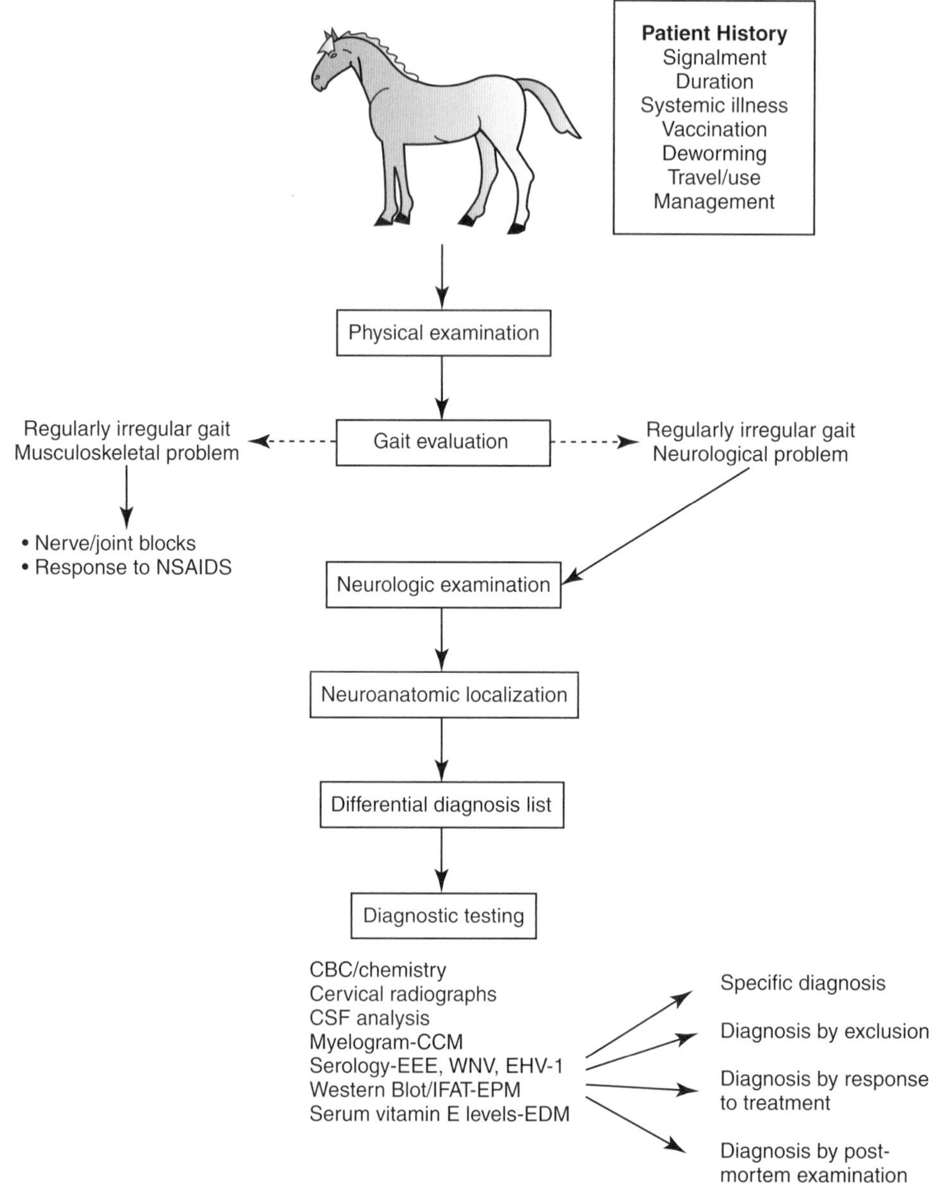

FIGURE 3-7 Diagnostic approach for a horse presenting with signs of spinal ataxia.

foramen magnum, mentation is normal. Spinal ataxia in the horse often manifests with a concomitant weakness or paresis as a result of simultaneous damage and involvement of the descending motor pathways.[4,5]

Accurate diagnosis of the cause of spinal ataxia in the horse requires a comprehensive evaluation of available historical information, a thorough physical examination, and a neurologic examination to localize the neuroanatomic lesion (Figure 3-7). These initial steps are critical in the development of a differential diagnosis list and the selection of appropriate ancillary tests to make a final diagnosis.

HISTORY AND SIGNALMENT

The signalment may offer important information for the clinician because breed, age, and gender predilections have been associated with certain causes of spinal ataxia in horses. For instance, occipitoatlantoaxial malformations (OAAMs) occur most frequently in Arabian foals, in which it is an inherited disorder.[6,7] Neuroaxonal dystrophy has been reported in Morgan Horses.[8] In retrospective studies, although cervical compressive myelopathy (CCM) has been reported in most light and draft breeds, Thoroughbreds were more likely to develop CCM, with a predisposition for males more than females (3:1).[2] Warmblood breeds and Tennessee Walking Horses also seem to have a predisposition for development of CCM.[5,9] A breed predilection for equine degenerative myeloencephalopathy (EDM) has been associated with Appaloosas, Quarter Horses, and Peruvian Pasos.[10,11]

Consideration of age in the manifestation of spinal ataxia may also be beneficial. Congenital abnormalities are likely to manifest at an early age. Foals with occipitoatlantoaxial malformations typically develop neurologic deficits between birth and 6 months of age.[7,12]

Spinal ataxia caused by EDM typically manifests before the horse is 2 to 3 years of age, with most affected horses exhibiting symptoms before 6 months of age.[13] However, the condition can be recognized in horses at any age. During halter breaking and handling, weanlings are at more risk for cranial and cervical trauma.[14] Young horses of training age presenting for ataxia without cranial nerve signs should be assessed for cervical compressive myelopathy. In horses older than 10 years with spinal ataxia and cervical neck pain, CCM should also be considered as these horses may have developed osteoarthritis of the caudal cervical vertebrae (C6 to T1) sufficient to cause spinal cord compression.[2] Horses older than 5 years of age are more likely to have lumbar fractures and sacroiliac subluxations and fractures.[15]

The onset of clinical signs (acute or chronic) and progression is an important part of the evaluation of the horse with spinal ataxia. Acute onset of clinical signs may suggest a traumatic event as the cause. However, the clinician must consider whether an underlying proprioceptive deficit may have contributed to the traumatic event (e.g., falling, stumbling) or whether trauma may have worsened a preexisting condition (e.g., CCM). Horses affected with CCM are reported to have a waxing and waning of clinical signs.[2] Equine protozoal myeloencephalitis (EPM) may present as a slow and insidious course of disease or in some horses as an acute manifestation of neurologic disease.[16] Infectious causes of spinal ataxia such as equine herpesvirus-1 (EHV-1) myeloencephalopathy (EHM) and West Nile virus (WNV) encephalitis (WNE) typically manifest in a rapid progression of clinical signs over a few days that then stabilize.[17,18] Eastern equine encephalitis (EEE) is also rapidly progressive, and the disease is often fatal. In most affected horses cerebral signs predominate, especially as the disease progresses.[19] Rabies, which should be considered in any horse with acute neurologic disease, can initially present as ataxia. The disease is generally rapidly progressive and fatal.

By skillfully questioning the client, the clinician can elicit other important historical information, including previous systemic illnesses, vaccinations, deworming protocol, medications, travel history, and general management practices (e.g., feed, environment). Any history of systemic illnesses should be noted in a horse that exhibits signs of spinal ataxia. In foals neonatal septicemia could result in the hematogenous spread of bacteria (*E.coli, Salmonella* spp., *Streptococcus* spp., and *Actinobacillus* spp.) and subsequent vertebral osteomyelitis, with acute onset of neurologic signs caused by spinal cord compression even after the foal recovers from septicemia. A recent history of tail docking or injections may be linked with an ascending infection and subsequent hindlimb ataxia. Similarly, vertebral osteomyelitis may be iatrogenic from contaminated vaccines or drugs injected near the spinal column.[20] Various anthelminthics and tranquilizers have been reported to cause central nervous system (CNS) disease, and the history of recent medications should be noted (see Table 3-7).[5] Conversely, verminous meningoencephalomyelitis should not be ruled out as a differential in a horse with spinal ataxia that has a history of deworming with anthelmintics.[20] Type of feed and forage should also be evaluated because ataxia has been linked with grazing various types of grasses (see Table 3-7).[21] EDM has been linked in some cases to diets with a lack of green forage and commercially heated pellets.

The vaccination status of the horse for the arboviruses (EEE and Western equine encephalitis [WEE] viruses, WNV) as well as for rabies and tetanus should be determined because these pathogens may cause neurologic disease. Specific information on the type of vaccine and when the vaccine was given is necessary to determine whether the horse was adequately protected. In particular, for the viral encephalomyelitides in endemic areas, the mosquito season may be prolonged; therefore it is recommended that horses receive multiple boosters when using a killed virus vaccine product.[22] Recent vaccination of a naïve horse should be noted because onset of protective immunity may not have been induced before the horse was infected, and recent vaccination history may also have a bearing on the interpretation of serologic tests.

Travel history may provide useful information to the clinician. Certain geographic distributions of several infectious CNS pathogens have been reported. EEE is endemic in the southeastern states, although it has been detected in all states east of the Mississippi River and a number of western states.[20] In areas of the geographic habitat of the definitive host *Didelphis viginiana* (opossum), approximately 50% of horses are exposed to *Sarcocystis neurona,* the causative agent for EPM, whereas in central Wyoming and Montana, the exposure rate in horses has been 6.5% and 0% respectively. A history of recent travel from a showing or racing venue, hospitalization in a veterinary facility, boarding at a riding school, and subsequent stress has been associated with horses that have developed EHM.[18,23]

Finally, whether the horse is seronegative for equine infectious anemia (EIA) virus (via Coggins test or one of the three other U.S. Department of Agriculture–approved ELISA tests) should be determined. Although rare, ataxia has been reported as the predominant clinical sign in horses with EIA.[24]

PHYSICAL EXAMINATION

A thorough physical examination is an integral part of the evaluation of a horse with spinal ataxia for many reasons. Evidence of underlying systemic infection may help to narrow down the cause of neurologic disease. Infectious diseases such as arboviral encephalomyelitides and EHV-1 may cause generalized clinical signs of fever, depression, and inappetence that may precede neurologic signs. In light of the highly contagious nature of the recent outbreaks of the neurotropic equine herpesvirus-1 myeloencephalopathy, it is recommended that a horse with acute neurologic signs should be isolated and tested to rule out infection with EHV-1. High-level biosecurity measures should be instituted when the clinician is faced with multiple febrile horses, with one or more showing concomitant neurologic disease, because these horses may be viremic and shedding high levels of EHV-1.[18,25]

Underlying metabolic disturbances (i.e., electrolyte abnormalities, hypoglycemia in foals, hypocalcemia), circulatory shock, hyperammonia, and hepatoencephalopathy may manifest with neurologic signs and should be ruled out. Some horses may manifest severe abdominal pain with stumbling and trembling rather than the typical signs of colic. In horses with hindlimb gait deficits, a rectal examination with evaluation of the internal iliac artery pulses should be performed to rule out an aortic-iliac thombosis. Palpation of large muscle masses for pain and firmness and palpation of the joints for distention should be done to help eliminate musculoskeletal problems. Assessment of digital pulses to rule out the possibility of laminitis as a non-neurologic cause of gait abnormality should be performed.

NEUROLOGIC EXAMINATION AND NEUROANATOMIC LOCALIZATION

Neuroanatomic localization of the lesion based on the neurological examination is critical in the formation of the differential list for a horse with spinal ataxia. The neurologic examination should confirm that the horse is exhibiting neurologic deficits and the absence of musculoskeletal disease. This differentiation may be difficult, but it is important to establish because a normal response during a neurologic examination requires a sound musculoskeletal system. A horse with lameness resulting from a musculoskeletal problem will have a gait that is consistent or regularly irregular, whereas a gait in a neurologic horse is irregularly irregular and varies from step to step.[5] A horse with a neurologic gait deficit will have an abnormality that is apparent in all phases of the examination. Further assessment with nerve blocks, joint anesthesia, or response to NSAIDs may be beneficial in differentiating between musculoskeletal or neurologic disease.[5]

Once the presence of neurologic abnormalities has been established, it should then be determined whether the signs are central or peripheral; are from a single lesion, multifocal sites, or diffuse inflammation; and are symmetric or asymmetric because answers to these questions narrow down the differential diagnoses. EPM, for instance, is the most common cause of multifocal and diffuse lesions and should be considered in a horse with spinal ataxia and cranial nerve deficits as presenting symptoms. Other differentials include verminous meningoencephalomyelitis, WNE, EHM, and polyneuritis equi. Focal single lesions are likely to be caused by compressive lesions (CCM, intervertebral disc protrusion, fractures). Causes for spinal ataxia that manifest most often as symmetric lesions include CCM, EDM, cauda equina syndrome, and neuroaxonal dystrophy. A common presentation of horses affected with EPM is asymmetric muscle atrophy of the gluteal or quadriceps muscles and other muscles (e.g., infraspinatus, triceps) being reported.[20] Other conditions with asymmetric manifestation include verminous meningioencephalomyelitis and neoplasia.

A comprehensive review of neurologic examination of the horse and the means for neuroanatomic localization is provided elsewhere in this text. Briefly, for horses with ataxia, normal mentation, and no cranial deficits, the lesions are expected to be caudal to the foramen magnum. Cervical lesions (spinal cord C1-C6) result in proprioceptive deficits, weakness, and ataxia of all four limbs, with deficits typically one grade worse in the rear limbs than the front limbs. Lesions in the brachial intumescence (C7-T2) will result in worse deficits in the front limbs than the rear limbs. Lesions in the thoracolumbar region (T3-L3) will result in normal front limbs but deficits in the hindlimbs. Horses will manifest urinary incontinence, difficulty defecating, abnormal tail tone, and perineal hypalgesia with lesions in the sacral region (S3-S5). Poor tail tone with normal front and rear limbs indicates that the lesion is in the coccygeal region.[5] Certain conditions have been associated with a predilection for affecting specific regions. For instance, CCM can result from compression anywhere from C1 through C7, with most lesions occurring at C3-C4 in young horses and at C5-C6 or C6-C7 in older horses.[21] In horses with spinal ataxia, urinary incontinence, and difficulty defecating, EHM should be considered as a differential. In EDM neuronal fiber degeneration often occurs most prominently in the midthoracic region, with horses manifesting more severe deficits in the rear limbs than the forelimbs.[26] Horses affected with cauda equina neuritis may manifest only anal and tail tone hyperalgesia or deficits with no gait abnormalities, and horses with true polyneuritis equi will often manifest cranial nerve abnormalities, head tilt, and gait abnormalities (ataxia and weakness) as well as sacral signs.[27]

DIAGNOSTIC TESTS

A list of potential differential diagnoses for spinal ataxia is made by synthesis of the history, physical examination, and neuroanatomic localization of the lesion or lesions. The causes of spinal ataxia in the horse are listed in Table 3-7. CCM is the most common cause of spinal ataxia in the horse. Complete evaluation of a horse with spinal ataxia often includes a complete blood count, serum biochemistry profile, radiographs of the cervical spine, and cerebrospinal fluid (CSF) evaluation. Clinical pathologic findings may help identify an inflammatory leukogram (elevated leukocyte count with elevated fibrinogen) suggestive of an underlying systemic infection or abscess, leukopenia (which may be present with the viral CNS pathogens), underlying electrolyte abnormalities, and metabolic derangements. CSF findings may be surprisingly normal (even with trauma or spinal abscesses), or there may be evidence consistent with trauma and hemorrhage (xanthochromia and erythroid pleocytosis).[21] There also might be evidence of inflammation or infection. In horses with viral and other encephalitides, abnormal CSF findings may include elevated total protein levels with a moderate mononuclear pleocytosis, and, in the case of EHV-1, xanthochromia may be present. In acute infection EEE is unique in that it typically causes a marked neutrophilic pleocytosis.[20] Further selection of specific diagnostic tests depends on differential diagnoses determined during the evaluation (see Table 3-7) and are described in detail in the succeeding chapters of this book.

With some conditions a final diagnosis can be made only after excluding other differentials. For instance, antemortem diagnosis of EDM in horses is difficult. Low serum vitamin E levels are only supportive of EDM and are not often found in young horses exhibiting clinical signs of progressive spinal ataxia.[13] Because of the high prevalence of horses with antibody to *S. neurona* and limitations of the antemortem diagnostic tests for EPM, a response to antiprotozoal therapy is considered by some the diagnostic test of choice for EPM after exclusion of other differential diagnoses.[20] Diagnosis of verminous meningoencephalitis is often based on postmortem findings, but this disorder should be considered as a differential diagnosis in a horse with cervical signs that has negative cervical radiographs and myelogram results, negative EPM test results, and negative response to antiprotozoal therapy.[20]

SYNCOPE AND WEAKNESS

Mark V. Crisman

Syncope is a clinical syndrome consisting of a generalized weakness, sudden collapse, and a transient cessation of consciousness. Syncopal episodes are uncommon in horses, and generally few or no premonitory warning or presyncopal (faintness) signs are evident to the rider or handler. The subsequent loss of consciousness and collapse may be potentially harmful or dangerous to the horse and the rider. Despite the infrequent reports of true syncopal episodes in horses, the clinical signs are sufficiently dramatic to cause great concern on the part of the owner. Syncope in horses has been virtually unstudied. Consequently, most of the following information has been drawn from studies of humans and other animal species.

Although presyncopal signs have been well described in human beings (i.e., dizziness, yawning, confusion, spots before the eyes), these signs are generally not evident in horses. Horses may stumble initially and go down or suddenly collapse. The depth and duration of unconsciousness may vary, but generally unconsciousness lasts a few minutes. Horses may be slightly unsteady or struggle during recovery. After a syncopal attack the horse will completely recover and appear normal.

PATHOPHYSIOLOGY

Syncope results from a sudden reduction in cerebral blood flow and subsequent cerebral ischemia. Cerebral blood flow is maintained primarily by arterial blood pressure and cerebrovascular resistance. In response to falling or rising systemic blood pressure, the cerebral blood flow autoregulatory mechanism automatically regulates cerebral vessels to constrict or dilate. This control phenomenon maintains a constant cerebral blood flow despite fluctuations in arterial blood pressure, whether or not these fluctuations are physiologic or pathologic. If perfusion pressure in human beings falls below 60 mm Hg, the cerebral blood flow autoregulatory mechanism may fail. Mean resting arterial pressure measured at the carotid artery in horses has been reported to be 97 ± 12 mm Hg at a heart rate of 42 ± 10 beats/min.[1] Systolic pressure in horses experiencing syncope has not been determined.

Disturbances in oxygen supply to the brain generally result from three primary causes: hypoxemia, anemia, and ischemia. Although a variety of conditions or diseases may cause these disturbances, all three potentially deprive the brain of its critical oxygen supply.[2] *Hypoxemia* generally is defined as insufficient oxygen reaching the blood so that arterial oxygen content and tension are low. This insufficiency results from an inability of oxygen to cross the alveolar membrane (e.g., pulmonary disease) or low oxygen tension in the environment (e.g., high altitude). In situations of mild hypoxemia the cerebral blood flow autoregulatory mechanism maintains oxygen delivery to the brain. When the hypoxemia is severe or the compensatory mechanism fails, cerebral hypoxia occurs and syncope may result.

Anemia is defined functionally as a decreased oxygen-carrying capacity of the blood. This may be characterized by several mechanisms, including a reduction in the amount of hemoglobin available to bind and transport oxygen or changes in hemoglobin that interfere with oxygen binding (e.g., methemoglobin). If the anemia is severe, the oxygen concentration drops below the metabolic requirements of the brain despite increased cerebral blood flow.

Finally, cerebral ischemia results when cerebral blood flow is insufficient to supply cerebral tissue. Any disease that greatly reduces cardiac output, such as myocardial infarction or an arrhythmia, ultimately may result in cerebral ischemia. If any of these aforementioned conditions occurs and cerebral blood flow is interrupted or stops with resultant cerebral underperfusion, consciousness is lost. If tissue oxygenation is restored immediately, consciousness generally returns quickly without sequelae.

Areas of the brain that maintain or control consciousness have been the subject of much debate and research. Generally, the level of activity of the brain (alertness) is maintained through sensory input to the ascending reticular activating system in the rostral brainstem, thalamus, and cerebral cortex. More specifically, the bulboreticular facilitatory area within the reticular substance of the middle and lateral pons and mesencephalon is considered to be the central driving component of the excitatory area of the brain. Recent studies have identified the role of the midbrain reticular formation and the thalamic intralaminar nuclei in maintaining consciousness and arousal in animals and human beings.[3] Syncope may result if regional cerebral blood flow to this area is disrupted for any reason.

In horses syncope may be cardiogenic or extracardiac (neurocardiogenic) in origin. The primary cause of syncope in horses is generally cardiovascular disease. Cardiogenic syncope may result from (1) myocardial disease, (2) cardiac dysrhythmias (i.e., atrial fibrillation and third-degree heart block), (3) congenital heart disease, (4) pulmonary hypertension or stenosis, and (5) pericardial disease. Although many of these conditions are uncommon in horses, atrial fibrillation has been associated with several reports of syncope.[4]

Cardiovascular disease, resulting in an inability to regulate heart rate or stroke volume, ultimately decreases cardiac output. Atrial fibrillation can lead to heart rates greater than 240 beats/min with submaximal exercise. The lack of effective atrial contraction prevents complete ventricular filling at the end of diastole, thus causing a great reduction in effective cardiac output. Complete heart block may be persistent or intermittent and also has been associated with syncopal episodes in horses. When the block is complete and the pacemaker below the block fails to function, syncope occurs. This situation has been reported in human beings and horses as Morgagni-Adams-Stokes syndrome. This syndrome is the most frequent arrhythmic cause of syncope in human beings.[5] Morgagni-Stokes-Adams attacks result from an advanced atrioventricular block and usually involve a momentary sense of weakness followed by an abrupt loss of consciousness. After cardiac standstill or prolonged periods of asystole, unconsciousness results from cerebral ischemia. These "cardiac faints" have been reported to occur several times a day in human beings. Additional, less common causes of cardiogenic syncope usually involve the distal conduction system (His-Purkinje system) and may be persistent or episodic. Heart block involving the atrioventricular node or proximal conduction system may be congenital or drug induced (e.g., digitalis). Sick sinus syndrome, a condition described in elderly human beings, involves impaired sinoatrial impulse formation or conduction and has been associated with cerebral anoxia. With any of these conditions, cardiac output does not increase sufficiently during skeletal muscle exercise to meet peripheral oxygen demands. Blood preferentially flows to exercising muscle, resulting in systemic arterial hypotension, which results in cerebral ischemia leading to weakness or syncope.

Extracardiac causes of syncope indirectly may involve the cardiovascular system and were referred to previously as *vasovagal* or *vasodepressor syncope*. The term *neurocardiogenic syncope* more accurately describes this phenomenon.

Neurocardiogenic syncope is the most common type of syncope reported in human beings and often is precipitated by stress or pain.[6] Although not specifically described in horses, a similar mechanism of collapse likely may exist. The critical cardiovascular features include hypotension and paradoxical sinus bradycardia, heart block, or sinus arrest after sympathetic excitation. Additionally, cardiac asystole may occur as an extreme manifestation of neurocardiogenic syncope. The mediating mechanisms of neurocardiogenic syncope are not well understood; however, several theories have been proposed. Hypercontractile states may cause excessive stimulation of the myocardial mechanoreceptors (C fibers) located in the left ventricle. The result is an exaggerated parasympathetic afferent signal carried by the vagus and glossopharyngeal nerves with a subsequent decrease in sympathetic tone. Inhibition of sympathetic vasoconstrictor activity results in vasodilation, which may be especially evident during periods of vigorous activity and increased heart rates and blood pressure. The excess vagal activity produces bradycardia and a decrease in cardiac output. This combination, along with a decrease in peripheral vascular resistance, ultimately leads to syncope.

Regardless of the specific cause, syncope results from a sudden fall in cerebral blood flow. The loss of consciousness is caused by a reduction of oxygenation to the parts of the brain that maintain consciousness. In horses syncope usually is caused by a fall in systemic blood pressure resulting from a decrease in cardiac output.

Additional, less common causes of syncope in horses may include neurologic disease from space-occupying lesions or increased intracranial pressure. Syncopal episodes have been reported in foals with severe respiratory or congenital heart disease.[7] After minimal exercise or restraint in these foals, hypoxemia and subsequently reduced cerebral blood flow may result in syncope. Certain drugs, specifically phenothiazine tranquilizers (acepromazine), have been reported to cause syncope in horses. These tranquilizers produce antiadrenergic effects primarily through α_1-blockade with resultant vasodilation and hypotension. If phenothiazine tranquilizers are administered to severely hypovolemic horses or to horses that have hemorrhaged, severe hypotension and syncope may result.

Several disorders often are confused with syncope and should be differentiated carefully by an accurate history and thorough physical examination. These disorders include (1) epilepsy, (2) hypoglycemia, (3) narcolepsy and cataplexy, (4) sleep deprivation, (5) cerebrovascular disease, and (6) hyperkalemic periodic paralysis.

Epileptic seizures generally differ from syncope in that they have immediate onset and involve loss of consciousness, tonic and clonic convulsive activity with opisthotonos, and changes in visceral function (urination and defecation). Seizures commonly last for several minutes and often are followed by a postictal phase in which the horse may pace, appear blind, and not recognize its surroundings.

Metabolic disturbances such as hypoglycemia frequently are observed in neonatal foals and may be associated with weakness or syncopal-like episodes. Typically affected foals are premature or are subject to perinatal stress with subsequent increased glucose use following hypoxia or sepsis. Serum glucose determination is necessary to evaluate hypoglycemia.

Narcolepsy, an abnormal sleep tendency, and cataplexy occasionally may be difficult to distinguish from syncope as a cause of unconsciousness. Attacks of narcolepsy or cataplexy may be preceded by signs of weakness (buckling at the knees) followed by total collapse and areflexia. Rapid eye movements may occur with an absence of spinal reflexes. No other neurologic abnormalities are observed between attacks, although animals may appear sleepy between episodes. Provocative testing with physostigmine (0.05 mg/kg) may induce narcoleptic attacks and might be helpful in differentiating syncope from narcolepsy or cataplexy. Recumbent sleep deprivation may also cause excessive drowsiness, often manifested by buckling and episodes of collapse.[8] Therefore potential physical and behavioral causes for a reluctance to lie down and sleep should be investigated.

Cerebrovascular disease associated with head trauma and subarachnoid hemorrhage may cause temporary unconsciousness in horses. Clinical signs resulting from brain trauma generally are associated with focal cerebral dysfunction and therefore are readily distinguishable from syncope.

Hyperkalemic periodic paralysis causes weakness and collapse without alterations in consciousness. This autosomal dominant disorder has been reported in certain lines of registered Quarter Horses, Paints, and Appaloosas. A reliable DNA-based test is available to diagnose hyperkalemic periodic paralysis in horses.

EVALUATION OF SYNCOPE

A thorough evaluation of syncope in the horse consists of the following:

1. *History*: Emphasis should be placed on obtaining a detailed history. The onset and the duration of the problem, along with performance history and possible reasons for recumbent sleep deprivation, should be determined.
2. *Physical examination*: After a thorough physical examination and determination of vital signs, a detailed cardiovascular and neurologic examination should be performed. In addition to heart rate at rest and pulse characteristics, a thorough cardiac auscultation should be performed in a quiet room to identify any murmurs or cardiac dysrhythmias. An electrocardiogram (ECG) and echocardiogram also provide valuable information. Because some arrhythmias may be paroxysmal, continuous ECG monitoring may be useful. A neurologic examination should evaluate reflexes and sensory and motor function carefully to identify any central or peripheral neuropathies.
3. *Complete blood count and biochemical profile*: To rule out other potential causes of syncope-like episodes (e.g., hypoglycemia and sepsis), a complete blood count and biochemical profile should be performed. Additionally, serum lactate dehydrogenase (isoenzymes 1 and 2), creatine kinase (CK-2), and cardiac troponin I concentration determinations may be helpful in identifying cardiac dysfunction.[9]
4. *Exercise/stress test:* A thorough cardiac evaluation should be performed following strenuous exercise, including auscultation and an electrocardiogram. If available, a high-speed treadmill may be helpful in this phase of the evaluation. If any cardiac abnormalities are detected on physical examination, exercise testing on a treadmill will allow a more thorough evaluation of the cardiovascular system, although care must be taken to ensure that such testing does not exacerbate the condition of the horse.

Diagnosis of the cause of syncope in horses is not always easy because the cause should be considered a sign complex rather than a primary disease. In addition to the infrequent reports of syncope, the history is often vague, and the neurologic and cardiovascular examinations may not lead to a specific cause. Even in the absence of apparently overt cardiovascular disease (e.g., atrial fibrillation), cardiac dysrhythmias cannot be excluded as the possible cause of syncope.

TREATMENT OF SYNCOPE

Options for treating syncope in horses are limited. The frequency of the syncopal attacks and the underlying cause (i.e., cardiogenic or neurocardiogenic) may determine if a course of treatment should be undertaken. Generally, treatment of syncope should be directed toward preventing or correcting the cause of the decreased cerebral perfusion. An accurate pathophysiologic diagnosis is essential for treating cardiogenic syncope. A few reports in the literature indicate successful treatment of syncope associated with atrial fibrillation in horses.[4] A horse with a complete heart block returned to work after implantation of a transvenous cardiac pacing system.[10]

REFERENCES

Changes in Body Temperature

1. Dinarello CA: Thermoregulation and the pathogenesis of fever *Infect Dis Clin North Am* 10:433-450, 1996.
2. Guyton AC, Hall JE: *Textbook of medical physiology*, ed 11, Philadelphia, 2006, Saunders.
3. Guthrie AJ, Lund RJ: Thermoregulation: base mechanisms and hyperthermia *Vet Clin North Am Equine Pract* 14:45-59, 1998.
4. Marlin DJ, Schroter RC, White SL et al: Recovery from transport and acclimatisation of competition horses in a hot humid environment, *Equine Vet J* 33:371-379, 2001.
5. Geor RJ, McCutcheon LJ, Ecker GL, et al: Heat storage in horses during submaximal exercise before and after humid heat acclimation, *J Appl Physiol* 89:2283-2293, 2000.
6. Mayhew IG, Ferguson HO: Clinical, clinicopathological, and epidemiological features of anhidrosis in central Florida thoroughbred horses, *J Vet Intern Med* 1:136-141, 1987.
7. Fujii J, Otsu K, Zorzato F, et al: Identification of a mutation in porcine ryanodine receptor associated with malignant hyperthermia, *Science* 253:448-451, 1991.
8. Manley SV, Kelly AB, Hodgson D: Malignant hyperthermia-like reactions in three anesthetized horses, *J Am Vet Med Assoc* 183:85-89, 1983.
9. Smyth GB: Spinal cord decompression and stabilization of a comminuted axis fracture complicated by intraoperative malignant hyperthermia-like reaction in a filly, *Aust Equine Vet* 10:133-136, 1992.
10. Exon JH: A review of chlorinated phenols, *Vet Hum Toxicol* 26:508-520, 1984.
11. Stratton-Phelps M, Wilson WD, Gardner IA: Risk of adverse effects in pneumonic foals treated with erythromycin versus other antibiotics: 143 cases (1986-1996), *J Am Vet Med Assoc* 217:68-73, 2000.
12. Dinarello CA: Cytokines as endogenous pyrogens, *J Infect Dis* 179(suppl 2):S294-S304, 1999.
13. Luheshi GN: Cytokines and fever: mechanisms and sites of action, *Ann N Y Acad Sci* 856:83-89, 1998.
14. Blatteis CM, Bealer SL, Hunter WS, et al: Suppression of fever after lesions of the anteroventral third ventricle in guinea pigs, *Brain Res Bull* 11:519-526, 1983.
15. Still JT: Evidence for the involvement of the organum vasculosum laminae terminalis in the febrile response of rabbits and rats, *J Physiol* 368:501-511, 1985.
16. Kozak W, Kluger MJ, Tesfaigzi J, et al: Molecular mechanisms of fever and endogenous antipyresis, *Ann N Y Acad Sci* 917: 121-134, 2000.
17. Tatro JB: Endogenous antipyretics, *Clin Infect Dis* 5(suppl): S190-S201, 2000.
18. Catania A, Lipton JM: Peptide modulation of fever and inflammation within the brain, *Ann N Y Acad Sci* 856:62-68, 1998.
19. Lipton JM, Catania A: Anti-inflammatory actions of the neuroimmunomodulator alpha-MSH, *Immunol Today* 18:140-145, 1997.
20. Steiner AA, Antunes-Rodrigues J, McCann SM, et al: Antipyretic role of the NP-cGMP pathway in the anteroventral preoptic region of the rat brain, *Am J Physiol Regul Integr Comp Physiol* 282:R584-R593, 2002.
21. Weinstein MP, Iannini PB, Stratton CW, et al: Spontaneous bacterial peritonitis: a review of 28 cases with emphasis on improved survival and factors influencing prognosis, *Am J Med* 64:592-598, 1978.
22. Banet M: Fever and survival in the rat: the effect of enhancing fever, *Pflugers Arch* 381:35-38, 1979.
23. Jiang Q, Cross AS, Singh IS, et al: Febrile core temperature is essential for optimal host defense in bacterial peritonitis, *Infect Immun* 68:1265-1270, 2000.
24. Grieger TA, Kluger MJ: Fever and survival: the role of serum iron, *J Physiol* 279:187-196, 1978.
25. Kluger MJ, Rothenburg BA: Fever and reduced iron: their interaction as a host defense response to bacterial infection, *Science* 203:374-376, 1979.
26. Ballantyne GH: Rapid drop in serum iron concentrations as a host defense mechanism: a review of experimental and clinical evidence, *Am Surg* 50:405-411, 1984.
27. Mackowiak PA, Plaisacne KI: Benefits and risks of antipyretic therapy, *Ann N Y Acad Sci* 856:214-223, 1998.
28. Plaisacne KI, Mackowiak PA: Antipyretic therapy: physiologic rationale, diagnostic implications and clinical consequences, *Arch Intern Med* 160:449-456, 2000.
29. Koterba AM, Drummond WH, Kosch PC, editors: *Equine clinical neonatology*, Philadelphia, 1990, Lea & Febiger.
30. Mair TS, Taylor FG, Pinsent PJ: Fever of unknown origin in the horse: a review of 63 cases, *Equine Vet J* 21:260-265, 1989.
31. Sheoran AS, Sponseller BT, Holmes N, et al: Serum and mucosal antibody isotype responses to M-like protein (SeM) of Streptococcus equi in convalescent and vaccinated horses, *Vet Immunol Immunopathol* 59:239-252, 1997.
32. Irvine CH: Hypothyroidism in the foal, *Equine Vet J* 16: 302-306, 1984.
33. Stephen JO, Baptiste KE, Townsend HG: Clinical and pathologic findings in donkeys with hypothermia: 10 cases (1988-1998), *J Am Vet Med Assoc* 216:725-729, 2000.

Changes in Body Weight

1. Ettinger SJ, Feldman EC, editors: *Textbook of veterinary internal medicine*, ed 6, St. Louis, 2005, Saunders.
2. Smith BP, editor: *Large animal internal medicine*, ed 4, St. Louis, 2009, Mosby.
3. Brown CM, editor: *Problems in equine medicine*, Philadelphia, 1989, Lea & Febiger.
4. Robinson NE, Sprayberry K, editors: *Current therapy in equine medicine*, ed 6, St. Louis, 2009, Saunders.
5. Roberts MC: Malabsorption syndromes in the horse, *Compend Cont Educ Pract Vet* 7:S637, 1985.
6. Jacobs KA, Bolton JR: Effect of diet on the oral D-xylose absorption test in the horse, *Am J Vet Res* 43:1856, 1982.
7. Moore BR, Abood AS, Hinchcliff KW: Hyperlipemia in 9 miniature horses and miniature donkeys, *J Vet Intern Med* 8:376, 1994.
8. Clabough DL: Equine infectious anemia: the clinical signs, transmission, and diagnostic procedures, *Vet Med* 85:1007, 1990.
9. Snow DH, Douglas TA, Thompson H, et al: Phenylbutazone toxicosis in Equidae: a biochemical and pathophysiologic study, *Am J Vet Res* 42:1754, 1981.

10. Traub JL, Bayly WM, Reed SM, et al: Intra-abdominal neoplasia as a cause of chronic weight loss in the horse, *Compend Cont Educ Pract Vet* 5:S526, 1983.
11. Rumbaugh GE, Smith BP, Carlson GP: Internal abdominal abscesses in the horse: a study of 25 cases, *J Am Vet Med Assoc* 172:304, 1978.
12. Nelson AW: Analysis of equine peritoneal fluid, *Vet Clin North Am Large Anim Pract* 1:267, 1979.
13. Duncan JR, Prasse KW: Cytology. In Duncan JR, Prasse KW, editors: *Veterinary laboratory medicine*, ed 2, Ames, 1986, Iowa State University Press.
14. Foreman JH, Weidner JP, Parry BA, et al: Pleural effusion secondary to thoracic metastatic mammary adenocarcinoma in a mare, *J Am Vet Med Assoc* 197:1193, 1990.
15. Schafer M: *An eye for a horse*, London, 1980, JA Allen.
16. Frank N: Insulin resistance in horses, *Proc Am Assoc Equine Pract* 52:51, 2006.
17. Johnson PJ: The equine metabolic syndrome peripheral Cushing's syndrome, *Vet Clin North Am Equine Pract* 18:271, 2002.
18. Treiber KH, Kronfeld DS, Hess TM, et al: Evaluation of genetic and metabolic predispositons and nutritional risk factors for pasture-associated laminitis in ponies, *J Am Vet Med Assoc* 228:1538, 2006.
19. Schott HC: Pituitary pars intermedia dysfunction: challenges of diagnosis and treatment, *Proc Am Assoc Equine Pract* 52:60, 2006.
20. McKinnon AO, Voss JL, editors: *Equine reproduction*, Philadelphia, 1993, Lea & Febiger.
21. Lowe JE, Kallfelz FA: Thyroidectomy and the T4 test to assess thyroid dysfunction in the horse and pony, *Proc Am Assoc Equine Pract* 16:135, 1970.
22. Vischer CM: *Hypothyroidism and exercise intolerance in the horse [thesis]*, Urbana-Champaign, 1996, University of Illinois.
23. Meredith TB, Dobrinski I: Thyroid function and pregnancy status in broodmares, *J Am Vet Med Assoc* 224:892, 2004.
24. Frank N, Sojka J, Messer NT: Equine thyroid dysfunction, *Vet Clin North Am Equine Pract* 18:305, 2002.
25. Breuhaus BA: Thyroid-stimulating hormone in adult euthyroid and hypothyroid horses, *J Vet Intern Med* 16:109, 2002.
26. Morris DD, Garcia M: Thyroid-stimulating hormone response test in healthy horses, and effect of phenylbutazone on equine thyroid hormones, *Am J Vet Res* 44:503, 1983.
27. Duckett WM, Manning JP, Weston PG: Thyroid hormone periodicity in healthy adult geldings, *Equine Vet J* 21:125, 1989.

Clinical Assessment of Poor Performance

1. Rose RJ: *Poor performance: a clinical and physiological perspective, Proceedings of the nineteenth American College of Veterinary Internal Medicine Forum*, Denver, Colo, 2001, pp 224-225.
2. Morris EA, Seeherman HJ: Clinical evaluation of poor performance in the racehorse: the results of 275 evaluations, *Equine Vet J* 23:169-174, 1991.
3. Martin BB, Reef VB, Parente EJ, et al: Causes of poor performance of horses during training, racing or showing: 348 cases (1992-1996), *J Am Vet Med Assoc* 216:554-558, 2000.
4. Seeherman HJ, Morris E, O'Callaghan MW: The use of sports medicine techniques in evaluating the problem equine athlete, *Vet Clin North Am Equine Pract* 7:259-269, 1991.
5. Rose RJ, Allen JR, Hodgson DR, et al: Response to submaximal treadmill exercise and training in the horse: changes in haematology, arterial blood gas and acid base measurements, plasma biochemical values and heart rate, *Vet Rec* 113: 612-618, 1983.
6. Rose RJ, Allen JR: Hematologic responses to exercise and training, *Vet Clin North Am Equine Pract* 1:461-476, 1985.
7. Tyler-McGowan CM, Golland LS, Evans DL, et al: Haematological and biochemical responses to training and overtraining, *Equine Exerc Physiol Suppl* 30:621-635, 1999.
8. McKeever KH, Hinchcliff KW, Reed SM, et al: Role of decreased plasma volume in hematocrit alterations during incremental treadmill exercise in horses, *Am J Physiol* 265:R404-R408, 1993.
9. Persson SGB, Osterberg I: Racing performance in red blood cell hypervolaemic Standardbred trotters, *Equine Vet J Suppl* 30:617-620, 1999.
10. Valberg SJ, MacLeay JM, Mickelson JR: Exertional rhabdomyolysis and polysaccharide storage myopathy in horses, *Compend Cont Educ Pract Vet* 19:1077-1085, 1997.
11. Rose RJ: Electrolytes: clinical applications, *Vet Clin North Am Equine Pract* 6:281-294, 1990.
12. Dart AJ, Dowling BA, Hodgson DR, et al: Evaluation of high-speed treadmill videoscopy for diagnosis of upper respiratory tract dysfunction in horses, *Aust Vet J* 79:109-112, 2001.
13. Christley RM, Hodgson DR, Evans DL, et al: Cardiorespiratory responses to exercise in horses with different grades of idiopathic laryngeal hemiplegia, *Equine Vet J* 29:6-10, 1997.
14. King CM, Evans DL, Rose RJ: Cardiorespiratory and metabolic responses to exercise in horses with various abnormalities of the upper respiratory tract, *Equine Vet J* 71:200-202, 1994.
15. Holcombe SJ, Derksen FJ, Stick JA, et al: Pathophysiology of dorsal displacement of the soft palate in horses, *Equine Vet J Suppl* 30:45-48, 1999.
16. Kriz NG, Hodgson DR, Rose RJ: Prevalence and clinical importance of heart murmurs in racehorses, *J Am Vet Med Assoc* 216:1441-1445, 2000.
17. King CM, Evans DL, Rose RJ: Significance for exercise capacity of some electrocardiographic findings in racehorses, *Aust Vet J* 71:200-202, 1994.
18. Seeherman HJ, Morris EA: Methodology and repeatability of a standardized treadmill exercise test for clinical evaluation of fitness in horses, *Equine Vet J Suppl* 9:20-25, 1990.
19. Seeherman HJ: Treadmill exercise testing: treadmill installation and training protocols used for clinical evaluations of equine athletes, *Vet Clin North Am Equine Pract* 7:259-269, 1991.
20. Evans DL: Physiology of equine performance and associated tests of function, *Equine Vet J* 39:373, 2007.
21. Evans DL, Rose RJ: Method of investigation of the accuracy of four digital-display heart rate meters suitable for use in the exercising horse, *Equine Vet J* 18:129-132, 1986.
22. Evans DL, Rose RJ: Cardiovascular and respiratory responses in thoroughbred horses during treadmill exercise, *J Exp Biol* 134:397-408, 1988.
23. Evans DL, Rose RJ: Determination and repeatability of maximum oxygen uptake and other cardiorespiratory measurements in the exercising horse, *Equine Vet J* 20:94-98, 1988.
24. Rose RJ, Hendrickson DK, Knight PK: Clinical exercise testing in the normal thoroughbred racehorse, *Aust Vet J* 67:345-348, 1990.
25. Evans DL, Harris RC, Snow DH: Correlation of racing performance with blood lactate and heart rate after exercise in thoroughbred horses, *Equine Vet J* 25:441-445, 1993.
26. Rasanen, Lampinen KF, Poso AR: Responses of blood and plasma lactate and plasma purine concentrations to maximal exercise and their relation to performance in standardbred trotters, *Am J Vet Res* 56:1651-1656, 1995.
27. Vaihkonen LK Hyyppa, Poso AR: Factors affecting accumulation of lactate in red blood cells, *Equine Vet J Suppl* 30:443-447, 1999.
28. Rainger JE, Evans DL, Hodgson DR, et al: Distribution of lactate in plasma and erythrocytes during and after exercise in horses, *Br Vet J* 151:299-310, 1995.
29. Poso AR, Lampinen KJ, Rasanen LA: Distribution of lactate between red blood cells and plasma after exercise, *Equine Vet J Suppl* 18:231-234, 1995.

30. Bayly WM, Shultz DA, Hodgson DR, et al: Ventilatory responses of the horse to exercise: effect of gas collection systems, *J Appl Physiol* 63:1210-1217, 1987.
31. Christley RM, Evans DL, Hodgson DR, et al: Blood gas changes during incremental and sprint exercise, *Equine Vet J Suppl* 30:24-26, 1999.
32. Bayly WM, Hodgson DR, Schulz DA, et al: Exercise-induced hypercapnia in the horse, *J Appl Physiol* 67:958-1966, 1989.
33. Christley RM, Hodgson DR, Evans DL, et al: Effects of training on the development of exercise-induced arterial hypoxemia in horses, *Am J Vet Res* 58:653-657, 1997.
34. Barrey E, Evans SE, Evans DL, et al: Locomotion evaluation for racing in thoroughbreds, *Equine Vet J Suppl* 33:99-103, 2001.

Dysphagia

1. Anderson NY, editor: *Veterinary gastroenterology*, ed 2, Malvern, Penn, 1992, Lea & Febiger.
2. Robinson NE, editor: *Current therapy in equine medicine*, ed 6, St. Louis, 2009, Saunders.
3. Baum KH, Modransky PD, Halpern NE, et al: Dysphagia in horses: the differential diagnosis, part I, *Compend Cont Educ Pract Vet* 10:1301-1307, 1988.
4. Stick JA, Boles C: Subepiglottic cyst in three foals, *J Am Vet Med Assoc* 177:62, 1980.
5. Baum GH, Halpern NE, Banish LD, et al: Dysphagia in horses: the differential diagnosis, part II, *Compend Cont Educ Pract Vet* 10:1405-1408, 1988.
6. McCue PM, Freeman DE, Donawick WJ: Guttural pouch tympany: 15 cases (1977-1986), *J Am Vet Med Assoc* 12:1761-1763, 1989.
7. Sweeny CR, Benson CE, Whitlock RH, et al: Streptococcus equi infection in horses, part I, *Compend Cont Educ Pract Vet* 9: 689-693, 1987.
8. Todhunter RJ, Brown CM, Stickle R: Retropharyngeal infections in five horses, *J Vet Med Assoc* 187:600-604, 1985.
9. Greet TRC: Outcome of treatment in 35 cases of guttural pouch mycosis, *Equine Vet J* 19:483-487, 1987.
10. Sweeny CR, Freeman DE, Sweeny RW, et al: Hemorrhage into the guttural pouch (auditory tube diverticulum) associated with rupture of the longus capitis muscle in three horses, *J Am Vet Med Assoc* 202:1129-1131, 1993.
11. MacKay RJ, Davis SW, Dubey JP: Equine protozoal myeloencephalitis, *Compend Cont Educ Pract Vet* 14:1359-1367, 1992.
12. Uhlinger C: Clinical and epidemiologic features of an epizootic of equine leukoencephalomalacia, *J Am Vet Med Assoc* 198:126-128, 1991.
13. Swerczek TW: Toxicoinfectious botulism in foals and adult horses, *J Am Vet Med Assoc* 176:217-220, 1980.
14. Moore RM, Kohn CW: Nutritional muscular dystrophy in foals, *Compend Cont Educ Pract Vet* 13:476-490, 1991.
15. Step DL, Divers TJ, Cooper B, et al: Severe masseter myonecrosis in a horse, *J Am Vet Med Assoc* 198:117, 1991.
16. Pearson EG, Snyder SP, Saulez MN: Masseter myodeneration as a cause of trismus or dysphagia in adult horses, *Vet Rec* 156:642, 2005.
17. Broekamn LE, Kuiper D: Megaesophagus in the horse. A short review of the literature and 18 own cases, *Vet Q* 24:199, 2002.
18. Green S, Green EM, Arson E: Squamous cell carcinoma: an unusual cause of choke in the horse, *Mod Vet Pract* 67:870-875, 1986.
19. Power HT, Watrous BJ, de Lahunta A: Facial and vestibulocochlear nerve disease in six horses, *Am J Vet Med Assoc* 183: 1076-1080, 1983.
20. Divers TJ, Mohammed HO, Cummings JR, et al: Equine lower motor neuron disease: findings in 28 horses and proposal of a pathophysiological mechanism, *Equine Vet J* 26:409-415, 1994.
21. Kohn CW, Fenner WR: Equine herpes myeloencephalopathy, *Vet Clin North Am Equine Pract* 3:405-419, 1987.
22. Yvorchuk-St. Jean K: Neuritis of the cauda equina, *Vet Clin North Am Equine Pract* 3:421-426, 1987.
23. Granstrom DE, Dubey JP, Davis SW, et al: Equine protozoal myeloencephalitis: antigen analysis of cultured Sarcocystis neurona merozoites, *J Vet Diagn Invest* 5:88-90, 1993.
24. Doxey DL, Milne EM, Gilmour JS, et al: Clinical and biochemical features of grass sickness (equine dysautonomia), *Equine Vet J* 23:360-364, 1991.
25. Griffiths IR, Kydriakides E, Smith S, et al: Immunocytochemical and lectin histochemical study of neuronal lesions in autonomic ganglia of horses with grass sickness, *Equine Vet J* 25:446-452, 1993.

Abdominal Distention

1. Ducharme NG, Fubini SL: Gastrointestinal complications associated with the use of atropine in horses, *J Am Vet Med Assoc* 182:229, 1983.
2. Dietz O, Wiesner F, editors: *Diseases of the horse*, New York, 1984, Karger.
3. Robinson NE, editor: *Current therapy in equine medicine*, ed 6, St. Louis, 2009, Saunders.
4. White NA, editor: *The equine acute abdomen*, Philadelphia, 1990, Lea & Febiger.
5. Ragle CA, Snyder JR, Meagher DM, et al: Surgical treatment of colic in American miniature horses: 15 cases (1980-1987), *J Am Vet Med Assoc* 201:329, 1992.
6. Nelson AW: Analysis of equine peritoneal fluid, *Vet Clin North Am Large Anim Pract* 1:267, 1979.
7. Latimer KS, Mahaffey EA, Prasse KW: *Duncan and Prasse's veterinary laboratory medicine*, ed 4, Philadelphia, 2003, Wiley-Blackwell.
8. Traub JL, Bayly WM, Reed SM, et al: Intra-abdominal neoplasia as a cause of chronic weight loss in the horse, *Compend Cont Educ Pract Vet* 5:S526, 1983.
9. Foreman JH, Weidner JP, Parry BA, et al: Pleural effusion secondary to thoracic metastatic mammary adenocarcinoma in a mare, *J Am Vet Med Assoc* 197:1193, 1990.
10. Behr MJ, Hackett RP, Bentinck-Smith J, et al: Metabolic abnormalities associated with rupture of the urinary bladder in neonatal foals, *J Am Vet Med Assoc* 178:263, 1981.
11. Richardson DW, Kohn CW: Uroperitoneum in the foal, *J Am Vet Med Assoc* 182:267, 1983.
12. Smith BP, editor: *Large animal internal medicine*, ed 4, St Louis, 2009, Mosby.
13. Nyrop KA, DeBowes RM, Cox JH, et al: Rupture of the urinary bladder in two post-partum mares, *Compend Cont Educ Pract Vet* 6:S510, 1984.
14. McKinnon AO, Voss JL, editors: *Equine reproduction*, Philadelphia, 1993, Lea & Febiger.
15. Colles CM, Parkes RD, May CJ: Foetal electrocardiography in the mare, *Equine Vet J* 10:32, 1978.
16. Bernard WV, Reef VB, Reimer JM, et al: Ultrasonographic diagnosis of small intestinal intussusception in three foals, *J Am Vet Med Assoc* 194:395, 1989.

Colic

1. USDA-APHIS: Incidence of colic in U.S. horses. Available at http://www.aphis.usda.gov/vs/ceah/ncahs/nahms/equine/equine98/colic.PDF Accessed 3/4/09.
2. Moore BR, Moore RM: Examination of the equine patient with gastrointestinal emergency, *Vet Clin N Am-Equine* 10:549, 1994.
3. Orsini JA, Divers TJ, editors: *Equine emergencies: treatment and procedures*, St. Louis, 2008, Saunders.
4. Mair T, Divers T, Ducharme N, editors: *Manual of equine gastroenterology*, St. Louis, 2002, Saunders.
5. White NA II: Intestinal response to injury, *Proc Ann Conv AAEP* 52:115, 2006.

6. Cribb NC, Cote NM, Boure LP, et al: Acute small intestinal obstruction associated with Parascaris equorum infection in young horses: 25 cases (1985-2004), *N Z Vet J* 54:338, 2006.
7. Chaffin MK, Cohen ND: Diagnostic assessment of foals with colic, *Proc Ann Conv AAEP* 45:235, 1999.
8. Proudman CJ: A two year, prospective survey of equine colic in general practice, *Equine Vet J* 24:90, 1992.
9. White NA II: Causes and risks for colic, *Proc Ann Conv AAEP* 52:115, 2006.
10. Archer DC, Pinchbeck GK, French NP, et al: Risk factors for epiploic foramen entrapment colic: an international study, *Equine Vet J* 40:224, 2008.
11. Wagner AE, Muir WW 3rd, Hinchcliff KW: Cardiovascular effects of xylazine and detomidine in horses, *Am J Vet Res* 52:651, 1991.
12. Daunt DA, Steffey EP: Alpha-2 adrenergic agonists as analgesics in horses, *Vet Clin N Am-Equine* 18:39, 2002.
13. Ragle CA, Meagher DM, Schrader JL, et al: Abdominal auscultation in the detection of experimentally induced gastrointestinal sand accumulation, *J Vet Intern Med* 3:12, 1989.
14. Tillotson K, Traub-Dargatz JL: Gastrointestinal protectants and cathartics, *Vet Clin N Am-Equine* 19:599, 2003.
15. White NA, editor: *The equine acute abdomen*, Malvern, 1990, Lea & Febiger.
16. Luo T, Bertone JJ, Greene HM, et al: A comparison of N-butylscopolammonium and lidocaine for control of rectal pressure in horses, *Vet Ther* 7:243, 2006.
17. White NA: Equine colic: how to make the decision for surgery. In AAEP Focus Proceedings 2005, Philadelphia.
18. Navarro M, Monreal L, Segura D, et al: A comparison of traditional ad quantitative analysis of acid-base and electrolyte imbalances in horses with gastrointestinal disorders, *J Vet Intern Med* 19:871, 2005.
19. Davis JL, Blikslager AT, Catto K, et al: A retrospective analysis of hepatic injury in horses with proximal enteritis (1984-2002), *J Vet Intern Med* 17:896, 2003.
20. Gardner RB, Nydam DV, Mohammed HO, et al: Serum gamma glutamyl transferase activity in horses with right or left dorsal discplacements of the large colon, *J Vet Intern Med* 19:761, 2005.
21. Fischer AT Jr.: Advances in diagnostic techniques for horses with colic, *Vet Clin N Am-Equine* 13:203, 1997.
22. Cowell RL, Tyler RD, editors: *Diagnostic cytology and hematology of the horse*, ed 2, St. Louis, 2007, Mosby.
23. Santschi EM, Slone DE, Frank WM: Use of ultrasound in horses for diagnosis of left dorsal displacement of the large colon and monitoring its nonsurgical correction, *Vet Surg* 22:281, 1993.
24. Freeman SL: Diagnostic ultrasonography of the mature equine abdomen, *Equine Vet Educ* 15:319, 2003.
25. Bernard WV, Reef VB, Reimer JM, et al: Ultrasonographic diagnosis of small-intestinal intussusception in three foals, *J Am Vet Med Assoc* 194:395, 1989.
26. Bradecamp EA: How to image the adult equine abdomen and thorax in ambulatory practice using a 5-mHz rectal probe, *Proc Ann Conv AAEP* 53:537, 2007.
27. Keppie NJ, Rosensein DS, Holcombe SJ, et al: Objective radiographic assessment of abdominal sand accumulation in horses, *Vet Radiol Ultrasound* 49:122, 2008.
28. Yarbrough TB, Langer DL, Snyder JL, et al: Abdominal radiography for diagnosis of enterolithiasis in horses: 141 cases (1990-1992), *J Am Vet Med Assoc* 205:592, 1994.

Diarrhea

1. Argenzio RA, Lowe JE, Pickard DW, et al: Digesta passage and water exchange in the equine large intestine, *Am J Physiol* 226:1035-1042, 1974.
2. Argenzio RA, Stevens CE: Cyclic changes in ionic composition of digesta in the equine intestinal tract, *Am J Physiol* 228: 1224-1230, 1975.
3. Argenzio RA: Functions of the large intestine and their interrelationship with disease, *Cornell Vet* 65:303-327, 1975.
4. Conner ME, Darlington RW: Rotavirus infection in foals, *Am J Vet Res* 41:1699-1703, 1980.
5. Holland JL, Kronfeld DS, Sklan D, et al: Calculation of fecal kinetics in horses fed hay or hay and concentrate, *J Anim Sci* 76:1934-1944, 1998.
6. O'Louglin EV, Scott RB, Gall DG: Pathophysiology of infectious diarrhea: changes in intestinal structure and function, *J Pediatr Gastroenterol Nutr* 12:5-20, 1991.
7. Rachmilewitz D: Prostaglandins and diarrhea, *Dig Dis Sci* 25: 897-899, 1980.
8. Hardcastle J, Hardcastle PT: Involvement of prostaglandin in histamine-induced fluid and electrolyte secretion by rat colon, *J Pharm Pharmacol* 40:106-110, 1988.
9. Wang YZ, Cooke, Su HC, et al: Histamine augments colonic secretion in guinea pig distal colon, *Am J Physiol* 258: G432-G439, 1990.
10. Clarke LL, Argenzio RA: NaCl transport across equine proximal colon and the effect of endogenous prostaglandins, *Am J Physiol* 259:G62-G69, 1990.
11. Halm DR, Rechkemmer GR, Schoumache RA, et al: Apical membrane chloride channels in a colonic cell line activated by secretory agonists, *Am J Physiol* 254:C505-C511, 1988.
12. Cliff WH, Frizzell RA: Separate Cl^- conductances activated by cAMP and Ca^2 in Cl(-)-secreting epithelial cells, *Proc Natl Acad Sci U S A* 87:4956-4960, 1990.
13. Ling BN, Kokko KE, Eaton DC: Prostaglandin E2 activates clusters of apical Cl^- channels in prinicipal cells via a cyclic adenosine monophosphate-dependent pathway, *J Clin Invest* 93:829-837, 1994.
14. King JN, Gerring EL: The action of low dose endotoxin on equine bowel motility, *Equine Vet J* 23:11-19, 1991.
15. Weese JS, Parsons DA, Staempfli HR: Association of Clostridium difficile with enterocolitis and lactose intolerance in a foal, *J Am Vet Med Assoc* 214:229-232, 1999.
16. Stewart MC, Hodgson JL, Kim H, et al: Acute febrile diarrhoea in horses: 86 cases (1986-1991), *Aust Vet J* 72:41-44, 1995.
17. Cohen ND, Woods AM: Characteristics and risk factors for failure of horses with acute diarrhea to survive: 122 cases (1990-1996), *J Am Vet Med Assoc* 214:382-390, 1999.
18. Mair TS, Taylor FG, Harbour DA, Pearson GR: Concurrent cryptosporidium and coronavirus infections in an Arabian foal with combined immunodeficiency syndrome, *Vet Rec* 126:127-130, 1990.
19. Richards AF, Kelly DF, Knottenbelt DC, et al: Anaemia, diarrhoea and opportunistic infections in Fell ponies, *Equine Vet J* 32:386-391, 2000.
20. Sweeney RW, Sweeney CR, Saik J, et al: Chronic granulomatous bowel disease in three sibling horses, *J Am Vet Med Assoc* 188:1192-1194, 1986.
21. Wilson DA, MacFadden KE, Green EM, et al: Case control and historical cohort study of diarrhea associated with administration of trimethoprim-potentiated sulphonamides to horses and ponies, *J Vet Intern Med* 10:258-264, 1996.
22. Stratton-Phelps M, Wilson WD, Gardner IA: Risk of adverse effects in pneumonic foals treated with erythromycin versus other antibiotics: 143 cases (1986-1996), *J Am Vet Med Assoc* 217:68-73, 2000.
23. Karcher LF, Dill SG, Anderson WI, et al: Right dorsal colitis, *J Vet Intern Med* 4:247-253, 1990.
24. Ragle CA, Meagher DM, Schrader JL, et al: Abdominal auscultation in the detection of experimentally induced gastrointestinal sand accumulation, *J Vet Intern Med* 3:12-14, 1989.
25. Mair TS, Cripps PJ, Ricketts SW: Diagnostic and prognostic value of serum protein electrophoresis in horses with chronic diarrhoea, *Equine Vet J* 25:324-326, 1993.

26. Patton S, Mock RE, Drudge JH, et al: Increase of immunoglobulin T concentrations in ponies as a response to experimental infection with the nematode Strongyles vulgaris, *Am J Vet Res* 39:19-22, 1978.
27. Cole DJ, Cohen ND, Snowden K, et al: Prevalence of and risk factors for fecal shedding of Cryptosporidium parvum oocysts in horses, *J Am Vet Med Assoc* 213:1296-1302, 1998.
28. Morris DD, Whitlock RH, Palmer JE: Fecal leukocytes and epithelial cells in horses with diarrhea, *Cornell Vet* 73:265-274, 1983.
29. Hathcock TL, Schumacher J, Wright JC, et al: The prevalence of Aeromonas species in feces of horses with diarrhea, *J Vet Intern Med* 13:357-360, 1999.
30. Lavoie JP, Drolet R, Parsons D, et al: Equine proliferative enteropathy: a cause of weight loss, colic, diarrhoea and hypoproteinemia in foals on three breeding farms in Canada, *Equine Vet J* 32:418-425, 2000.
31. Cimprich RE, Rooney JR: Corynebacterium equi enteritis in foals, *Vet Pathol* 14:95-102, 1977.
32. East LM, Savage CJ, Traub-Dargatz JL, et al: Enterocolitis associated with Clostridium perfringens infection in neonatal foals: 54 cases (1988-1997), *J Am Vet Med Assoc* 212:1751-1756, 1998.
33. Magdesian KG, Hirsh DC, Jang SS, et al: Characterization of Clostridium difficile isolates from foals with diarrhea: 28 cases (1993-1997), *J Am Vet Med Assoc* 220:67-73, 2002.
34. Tillotson K, Traub-Dargatz JL, Dickinson CE, et al: Population-based study of fecal shedding of Clostridium perfringens in broodmares and foals, *J Am Vet Med Assoc* 220:342-348, 2002.
35. Weese JS, Staemplfi HR, Prescott JF: Test selections and interpretation in the diagnosis of Clostridium difficile-associated colitis, *Proc Annu AAEP Conv* 45:50-52, 1999.
36. Smith BP: Salmonella infection in horses, *Compend Cont Educ Pract Vet* 3:S4-S17, 1981.
37. Cohen ND, Neibergs HL, Wallis DE, et al: Genus-specific detection of salmonellae in equine feces by use of the polymerase chain reaction, *Am J Vet Res* 55:1049-1054, 1994.
38. Cohen ND, Martin LJ, Simpson RB, et al: Comparison of polymerase chain reaction and microbiological culture for detection of salmonellae in equine feces and environmental samples, *Am J Vet Res* 57:780-786, 1996.
39. Barlough JE, Rikihisa Y, Madigan JE: Nested polymerase chain reaction for detection of Ehrlichia risticii genomic DNA in infected horses, *Vet Parasitol* 68:367-373, 1997.
40. Mott F, Rikihisa T, Zhang Y, et al: Comparison of PCR and culture to the indirect fluorescent-antibody test for diagnosis of Potomac horse fever, *J Clin Microbiol* 35:2215-2219, 1997.
41. Browning GF, Chalmers RM, Snodgrass DR, et al: The prevalence of enteric pathogens in diarrhoeic thoroughbred foals in Britain and Ireland, *Equine Vet J* 23:397-398, 1991.
42. Ellis GR, Daniels E: Comparison of direct electron microscopy and enzyme immunoassay for the detection of rotaviruses in calves, lambs, piglets and foals, *Aust Vet J* 65:133-135, 1988.
43. Guy JS, Breslin JJ, Breuhaus B, et al: Characterization of a coronavirus isolated from a diarrheic foal, *J Clin Microbiol* 38: 4523-4526, 2000.
44. Mair TS, Hillyer MH, Taylor FGR, et al: Small intestinal malabsorption in the horse: an assessment of the specificity of the oral glucose tolerance test, *Equine Vet J* 23:344-346, 1991.
45. Roberts MC, Norman P: A re-evaluation of the D (+) xylose absorption test in the horse, *Equine Vet J* 11:239-243, 1979.
46. Schmitz DG: Cantharidin toxicosis in horses, *J Vet Intern Med* 3:208-215, 1989.
47. Smith BP, editor: *Large animal internal medicine*, ed 4, St Louis, 2009, Mosby.
48. Pace LW, Turnquist SE, Casteel SW, et al: Acute arsenic toxicosis in five horses, *Vet Pathol* 34:160-164, 1997.
49. Desrochers AM, Dolente BA, Roy MF, et al: Efficacy of Sacchromyces boulardii for treatment of horses with acute enterocolitis, *J Am Vet Med Assoc* 227:954, 2005.

Respiratory Distress

1. Ainsworth DM, Davidow E: Respiratory distress in large animals, *Proc Forum ACVIM* 12:589, Veterinary 1994.
2. West JB, editor: *Respiratory physiology: the essentials*, Baltimore, 1990, Williams & Wilkins.
3. Smith BP, editor: *Large animal internal medicine*, ed 4, St Louis, 2009, Mosby.
4. Beech J, editor: *Equine respiratory disorders*, Philadelphia, 1991, Lea & Febiger.
5. Ainsworth DM, Ducharme NG, Hackett RP: Regulation of equine respiratory muscles during acute hypoxia and hypercapnia, *Am Rev Respir Dis* 147:A700, 1993.
6. Muir WW, Moore CA, Hamlin RL: Ventilatory alterations in normal horses in response to changes in inspired oxygen and carbon dioxide, *Am J Vet Res* 36:155-161, 1975.
7. Derksen FJ, Robinson NE, Slocombe RF: Ovalbumin induced allergic lung disease in thepony: role of vagal mechanisms, *J Appl Physiol* 53:719-724, 1982.
8. Derksen F, Robinson N, Slocombe R: 3-Methylindole-induced pulmonary toxicosis in ponies, *Am J Vet Res* 43:603-607, 1982.
9. Derksen FJ, Robinson NE, Stick JA: Technique for reversible vagal blockade in the standingconscious pony, *Am J Vet Res* 42:523-531, 1981.
10. McGorum BC: Quantification of histamine in plasma and pulmonary fluids from horses with chronic obstructive pulmonary disease, before and after "natural (hay and straw) challenges," *Vet Immunol Immunopathol* 36:223-237, 1993.
11. Watson E, Sweeney C, Steensma K: Arachidonate metabolites in bronchoalveolar lavage fluid from horses with and without COPD, *Equine Vet J* 24:379-381, 1992.
12. Grunig G, Hermann M, Winder C, et al: Procoagulant activity in respiratory tract secretions from horses with chronic pulmonary disease, *Am J Vet Res* 49:705-709, 1988.
13. Sant'Ambrogio G, Mathew OP, Fisher JT: Laryngeal receptors responding to transmural pressure, airflow, and local muscle activity, *J Appl Physiol* 65:317-330, 1983.
14. Koterba AM, Kosch PC, Beech J: The breathing strategy of the adult horse (Equus caballus) at rest, *J Appl Physiol* 64:337-343, 1988.
15. Derksen FJ, Scott JS, Slocombe RF, et al: Effect of clenbuterol on histamine-induced airway obstruction in ponies, *Am J Vet Res* 48:423-429, 1987.
16. Scott J, Broadstone R, Derksen F, et al: Beta adrenergic blockade in ponies with recurrent obstructive pulmonary disease, *J Appl Physiol* 64:2324-2328, 1988.
17. Scott JS, Garon HE, Broadstone RV, et al: Alpha 1 adrenergic induced airway obstruction in ponies with recurrent pulmonary disease, *J Appl Physiol* 65:686-791, 1988.
18. Robinson NE, Derksen FJ, Olszewski MA, et al: The pathogenesis of chronic obstructive pulmonary disease of horses, *Br Vet J* 152:283-306, 1996.
19. Macklem PT, Mead J: Resistance of central and peripheral airways measured by retrograde catheter, *J Appl Physiol* 22: 395-402, 1967.
20. Berry CR, O'Brien TR, Madigan JE, et al: Thoracic radiographic features of silicosis in 19 horses, *J Vet Intern Med* 5:248-256, 1991.
21. Buergelt CD, Hines SA, Cantor G, et al: A retrospective study of proliferative interstitial lung disease of horses in Florida, *Vet Pathol* 23:750-756, 1986.
22. Lakritz J, Wilson WD, Berry CR, et al: Bronchointerstitial pneumonia and respiratory distress in young horses: clinical, clinicopathologic, radiographic, and pathological findings in 23 cases (1984-1989), *J Vet Intern Med* 7:277-288, 1993.

23. Mayhew IG, Ferguson HO: Clinical, clinicopathologic, and epidemiologic features of anhidrosis in central Florida thoroughbred horses, *J Vet Intern Med* 1:136-141, 1987.
24. Reimer JM: Diagnostic ultrasonography of the equine thorax, *Compend Cont Educ Pract Vet* 12:1321-1327, 1990.

Cough

1. Crystal RG, West JB, editors: The lung: scientific foundation, New York, 1991, Raven Press.
2. Lenfant C, editor: *Lung biology in health and disease*, vol 5 New York, 1977, Marcel Dekker.
3. Korpas J, Tomori Z: Cough and other respiratory reflexes, *Prog Respir Res* 12:15-148, 1979.
4. Robinson NE: Pathophysiology of coughing, *Proceedings of the thirty-second convention of the American Association of Equine Practitioners,* Nashville, 1986, pp 291-297.
5. Karlsson JA, Sant'Ambrogio G, Widdicombe J: Afferent neuronal pathways in cough and reflex bronchoconstriction, *J Appl Physiol* 65:1007-1023, 1988.
6. Korpas J, Widdicombe JG: Aspects of the cough reflex, *Respir Med* 85(suppl A):3-5, 1991.
7. Karlsson J-A, Hansson L, Wollmer P, et al: Regional sensitivity of the respiratory tract to stimuli causing cough and reflex bronchoconstriction, *Respir Med* 85(suppl A):47-50, 1991.
8. Coleridge HM, Coleridge JCG: Pulmonary reflexes: neural mechanisms of pulmonarydefense, *Annu Rev Physiol* 56:69-91, 1994.
9. Nelson RW, Couto CG, editors: *Essentials of small animal internal medicine*, ed 2, St Louis, 1992, Mosby.
10. Sherding R: Personal communication, Ohio State University, June 1995.
11. Sweeney CR, Sweeney RW, Benson CE: Comparison of bacteria isolated from specimens obtained by use of endoscopic guarded tracheal swabbing and percutaneous tracheal aspiration in horses, *J Am Vet Med Assoc* 195:1225-1229, 1989.
12. Moore BR, Dradowka S, Robertson JT, et al: Cytologic evaluation of bronchoalveolar lavage fluid obtained from standardbred racehorses with inflammatory airway disease, *Am J Vet Res* 56:562-567, 1995.
13. Rossier Y, Sweeney CR, Ziemer EL: Bronchoalveolar lavage fluid cytologic findings in horses with pneumonia or pleuropneumonia, *J Am Vet Med Assoc* 198:1001-1004, 1991.
14. Ogilvie TH, Rosendal S, Blackwell TE, et al: Mycoplasma felis as a cause of pleuritis in horses, *J Am Vet Med Assoc* 192: 1374-1376, 1983.
15. Couetil LL, Hoffman AM, Hodgson J, et al: Inflammatory airway disease of horses, *J Am Vet Intern Med* 21:356, 2007.
16. Colahan PT, Mayhew IG, Merritt AM, et al, editors: *Equine medicine and surgery*, ed 5, St. Louis, 1999, Saunders.

Polyuria and Polydipsia

1. Tasker JB: Fluid and electrolyte studies in the horses. III. Intake and output of water, sodium and potassium in normal horses, *Cornell Vet* 57:649-657, 1967.
2. Rumbaugh GE, Carlson GP, Harrold D: Urinary production in the healthy horse and in horses deprived of feed and water, *Am J Vet Res* 43:735-737, 1982.
3. Morris DD, Divers TJ, Whitlock RH: Renal clearance and fractional excretion of electrolytes over a 24-hour period in horses, *Am J Vet Res* 45:2431-2435, 1984.
4. Kohn CW, Strasser SL: 24-hour renal clearance and excretion of endogenous substancesin the mare, *Am J Vet Res* 47:1332-1337, 1986.
5. Cymbaluk NF: Water balance of horses fed various diets, *Equine Pract* 11:19-24, 1989.
6. Rose RJ: Electrolytes: clinical application, *Vet Clin North Am Equine Pract* 6:281-294, 1990.
7. DiBartola SP: *Fluid, electrolyte, and acid-base disorders in small animal practice (fluid therapy in small animal practice)*, ed 3, St. Louis, 2005, Saunders.
8. Brown CM: *Problems in equine medicine*, Philadelphia, 1989, Lea & Febiger.
9. Harris P: Collection of urine, *Equine Vet J* 20:86-88, 1988.
10. LeFever Kee J, Paulanka BJ, *Polek C: Fluids and electrolytes with clinical applications*, Philadelphia, 2009, Delmar.
11. Rose BD: *Clinical physiology of acid-base and electrolyte disorders*, New York, 1989, McGraw-Hill Information Services.
12. Narins RG, editor: *Maxwell and Kleeman's clinical disorders of fluid and electrolyte metabolism*, New York, 1994, McGraw-Hill.
13. Houpt KA, Thornton SN, Allen WR: Vasopressin in dehydrated and rehydrated ponies, *Physiol Behav* 45:659-661, 1989.
14. Suffit E, Houpt KA, Sweeting M: Physiological stimuli of thirst and drinking patterns in ponies, *Equine Vet J* 17:12-16, 1985.
15. Fenner WR: *Quick reference to veterinary medicine*, ed 3, Philadelphia, 2001, Wiley-Blackwell.
16. Jamison RL, Maffly RH: The urinary concentrating mechanism, *N Engl J Med* 295:1059-1067, 1976.
17. Carlson GP: Discussion: practical clinical chemistry, *Proceedings of the 23rd AAEP Convention*, Golden, Colo, 1977, American Association of Equine Practitioners.
18. Stewart J, Holman HH: The "blood picture" of the horse, *Vet Rec* 52:157-165, 1940.
19. Corke MJ: Diabetes mellitus: the tip of the iceberg, *Equine Vet J* 18:87-88, 1986.
20. McCoy DJ: Diabetes mellitus associated with bilateral granulosa cell tumors in a mare, *J Am Vet Med Assoc* 188:733-734, 1986.
21. Ruoff WW, Baker DC, Morgan SJ: Type II diabetes mellitus in a horse, *Equine Vet J* 18:143-144, 1986.
22. Buntain BJ, Coffman JR: Polyuria and polydypsia in a horse induced by psychogenic salt consumption, *Equine Vet J* 13: 266-268, 1981.
23. Laverty S, Pascoe JR, Ling GV, et al: Urolithiasis in 68 horses, *Vet Surg* 21:56, 1992.
24. Ehnen SJ, Divers TJ, Gillette D, et al: Obstructive nephrolithiasis and ureterolithiasis associated with chronic renal failure in horses: eight cases (1981-1987), *J Am Vet Med Assoc* 197:249, 1990.
25. Baker JR, Ritchie HE: Diabetes mellitus in the horse: a case report and review of the literature, *Equine Vet J* 6:7-11, 1974.
26. Breukink HJ, Van Wegen P, Schotman AJH: Idiopathic diabetes insipidus in a Welsh pony, *Equine Vet J* 15:284-287, 1983.
27. Schott HC, Bayly WM, Reed SM, et al: Nephrogenic diabetes insipidus in sibling colts, *J Vet Intern Med* 7:68-72, 1993.
28. Kohn CW, Chew DJ: Laboratory diagnosis and characterization of renal disease in horses, *Vet Clin North Am Equine Pract* 3:585-615, 1987.
29. Brobst DF, Bayly WM: Responses of horses to a water deprivation test, *J Equine Vet Sci* 2:51-56, 1982.
30. Genetzky RM, Loparco FV, Ledet AE: Clinical pathologic alterations in horses during a water deprivation test, *Am J Vet Res* 48:1007-1011, 1987.
31. Ziemer EL: Water deprivation test and vasopressin challenge. In *Equine medicine and surgery,* Goleta, Calif, 1991, American Veterinary Publications.
32. Robinson NE, editor: *Current therapy in equine medicine*, ed 6, St. Louis, 2009, Saunders.
33. Smith BP, editor: *Large animal internal medicine*, ed 4, St Louis, 2009, Mosby.

Edema

1. Carlson GP: Blood chemistry, body fluids, and hematology, In Gillespie JR, Robinson NE, editors: *Equine exercise physiology*, ed 2, Davis, Calif, 1987, ICEEP Publications.
2. Guyton AC, Hall JE: *Textbook of medical physiology*, ed 11, Philadelphia, 2005, Saunders.

3. Renkin EM: Some consequences of capillary permeability to macromolecules: Starling's hypothesis revisited, *Am J Physiol* 250:H706-H710, 1986.
4. Staub NC, Taylor AE, editors: *Edema*, New York, 1984, Raven Press.
5. Demling RH: Effect of plasma and interstitial protein content on tissue edema formation, *Curr Stud Hematol Blood Transfus* 53:36-52, 1986.
6. Taylor AE: Capillary fluid filtration: Starling forces and lymph flow, *Circ Res* 49:557-575, 1981.
7. Renkin EM, Michel CC, editors: *Handbook of physiology*, New York, 1984, Oxford University Press.
8. Raj JU, Anderson J: Regional differences in interstitial fluid albumin concentration in edematous lamb lungs, *J Appl Physiol* 72:699-705, 1992.
9. Costanzo L, editor: *Physiology*, ed 3, St Louis, 2006, Saunders.
10. Verkman AS: Mammalian aquaporins: diverse physiological roles and potential clinical significance, *Expert Rev Mol Med* 10: e13, 2008.
11. Frigeri A, Nicchia GP, Svelto M: Aquaporins as targets for drug discovery, *Curr Pharm Des* 13:2421-2427, 2007.
12. Michel CC: Microvascular permeability, venous stasis and oedema, *Inter Angiol* 8:9-13, 1984.
13. Green JF: *Fundamental cardiovascular and pulmonary physiology*, Philadelphia, 1987, Lea & Febiger.

Spinal Ataxia

1. Whitwell K: Causes of ataxia in horses, *In Practice* 2:17-24, 1980.
2. Rush B, Grady JA: Cervical stenotic myelopathy, *Compendium Contin Educ Pract Vet Equine* 3:430-436.
3. Tyler CM, Davis RE, Begg AP, Hutchins DR, et al: A survey of neurological diseases in horses, *Aust Vet J* 70:445-449, 1993.
4. Lornez MD, Kornegay JE, editors: *Handbook of veterinary neurology*, ed 4, St. Louis, 2004, Saunders.
5. Furr M, Reed S, editors: *Equine neurology*, Philadelphia, 2008, Wiley-Blackwell.
6. Mackay RJ: Neurologic disorders of neonatal foals, *Vet Clin North Am-Equine Prac* 21:387, 2005.
7. Watson AG, Mayhew IG: Familial congenital occipitoatlantoaxial malformation (OAAM) in the Arabian horse, *Spine* 11:334-339, 1986.
8. Beech J, Haskins M: Genetic studies of neuraxonal dystrophy in the Morgan, *Am J Vet Res* 48:109-113, 1987.
9. Levine JM, Ngheim PP, Levine GJ et al: Associations of sex, breed, and age with cervical vertebral compressive myelopathy in horses: 811 cases (1974-2007), *J Am Vet Med Assoc* 233: 1453-1458, 2008.
10. Blythe LL, Hultgren BD, Craig AM, et al: Clinical, viral, and genetic evaluation of equine degenerative myeloencephalopathy in a family of Appaloosas, *J Am Vet Med Assoc* 198: 1005-1013, 1991.
11. Gandini G, Fatzer R, Mariscoli M, et al: Equine degenerative myeloencephalopathy in five Quarter Horses: clinical and neuropathological findings, *Equine Vet J* 36:83-85, 2004.
12. Mayhew IG, Watson AG, Heissan JA: Congenital occipitoatlantoaxial malformations in the horse, *Equine Vet J* 10: 103-113, 1978.
13. Miller MM, Collatos C: Equine degenerative myeloencephalopathy, *Vet Clin North Am Equine Pract* 13:43-52, 1997.
14. Vos NJ, Pollock PJ, Harty M, Brennan T, et al: Fractures of the cervical vertebral odontoid in four horses and one pony, *Vet Rec* 162:116-119, 2008.
15. Reed S, Bayly W, Traub JL: Ataxia and paresis in horses Part 1: Differential diagnosis, *Compend Contin Educ Pract, Vet Equine* :S88-S98, 1981.
16. Mackay RJ: Equine protozoal myeloencephalitis, *Vet Clin North Am Equine Pract* 13:79-96, 1997.
17. Porter MB, Long MT, Getman LM, et al: West Nile virus encephalomyelitis in horses: 46 cases (2001), *J Am Vet Med Assoc* 222:1241-1247, 2003.
18. Pusterla N, David WW, Madigan JE, et al: Equine herpesvirus-1 myeloencephalopathy: A review of recent developments, *Vet J* 180:279-289, 2009.
19. Del Piero F, Wilkins PA, Dubovi EJ, et al: Clinical, pathologic, immunohistochemical, and virologic findings of eastern equine encephalomyelitis in two horses, *Vet Pathol* 38: 451-456, 2001.
20. Sellon DC, Long MT, editors: *Equine infectious diseases*, St. Louis, 2007, Saunders.
21. Mayhew IGJ: Milne Lecture: the equine spinal cord in health and disease, *Proc Annu Conv AAEP* 45:67-84, 1999.
22. American Association of Equine Practitioners: *Guidelines for vaccination of horses,* 2008. Available at: http://www.aaep.org/vaccination_guidelines.htm. Accessed March 5, 2009.
23. Henninger RW, Reed SM, Saville WJ, et al: Outbreak of neurologic disease caused by equine herpesvirus-1 at a university equestrian center, *J Vet Intern Med* 21:157-165, 2007.
24. McClure JJ, Lindsay WA, Taylor W, et al: Ataxia in four horses with equine infectious anemia, *J Am Vet Med Assoc* 180: 279-283, 1982.
25. American Association of Equine Practitioners: *Equine infectious disease outbreak: AAEP control guidelines,* 2009. Available at: http://www.aaep.org/control_guidelines_nonmember.htm. Accessed March 5, 2009.
26. Mayhew IG, deLahunta A, Whitlock RH, et al: Equine degenerative myeloencephalopathy, *J Am Vet Med Assoc* 170:195-201, 1977.
27. Rousseaux CG, Futcher KG, Clark EG, et al: Cauda Equina Neuritis: A Chronic Idiopathic Polyneuritis in Two Horses, *Can Vet J* 25:214-218, 1984.

Syncope and Weakness

1. Physick-Shepard PW: Cardiovascular response to exercise and training in the horse, *Vet Clin North Am Equine Pract* 1:383, 1985.
2. Plum F, Posner JB, editors: *The diagnosis of stupor and coma*, ed 3, Philadelphia, FA, 1986, Davis.
3. Kinomura S, Larsson J, Gulyas B, et al: Activation by attention of the human reticular formation and thalamic intralaminar nuclei, *Science* 271:512-515, 1996.
4. Deegen E, Buntenkotter S: Behavior of the heart rate of horses with auricular fibrillation during exercise and after treatment, *Equine Vet J* 8:26-29, 1976.
5. Stein JH, Klippel JH, Reynolds HY, et al: *Internal medicine*, ed 5, St. Louis, 1998, Mosby.
6. Sra JS, Jazayeri MR, Avitall B, et al: Comparison of cardiac pacing with drug therapy in the treatment of neurocardiogenic (vasovagal) syncope with bradycardia or systole, *N Engl J Med* 328:1085-1090, 1993.
7. Vitamus A, Bayly WM: Pulmonary atresia with dextroposition of the aorta and ventricular septal defect in three Arabian foals, *Vet Pathol* 19:160-168, 1982.
8. Bertone JJ: Excessive drowsiness secondary to recumbent sleep deprivation in two horses, *Vet Clin North Am Equine Pract* 22:157-162, 2006.
9. Cornelisse CJ, Schott HC, Olivier NB, et al: Concentration of cardiac troponin I in horse with a ruptured aortic regurgitation jet lesion and ventricular tachycardia, *J Am Vet Med Assoc* 217:231-235, 2000.
10. Reef VB, Clark ES, Oliver JA, et al: Implantation of a permanent transvenous pacing catheter in a horse with a complete heart block and syncope, *J Am Vet Med Assoc* 189:449-452, 1986.

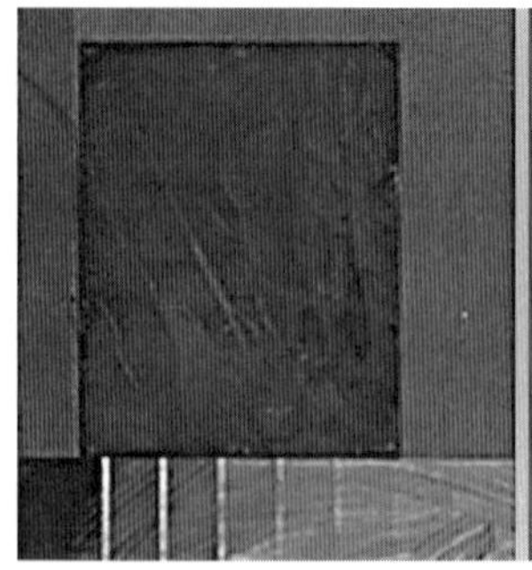

PHARMACOLOGIC PRINCIPLES

CHAPTER 4

INTRODUCTION TO CLINICAL PHARMACOLOGY

Patricia M. Dowling

Drug administration is a daily and income-generating activity in equine practice. Before a drug is administered, the veterinarian must select a safe and efficacious dosage regimen based on the individual horse's physiology and the nature and formulation of the drug. If the ultimate goal of drug therapy is to improve or cure a disease, then it is the veterinarian's responsibility to ensure that the selected drug is efficacious with minimal toxicity or adverse reactions in the patient. Individual animals of various ages and species vary widely in their handling of an administered drug. Given that most veterinary practitioners deal with a number of animal species and frequently administer more than one drug at time, it becomes obvious that there is a great potential for therapeutic error and adverse drug interactions. A basic understanding of pharmacokinetics and the effects of pathophysiology on drug disposition enables the clinician to optimize therapy while minimizing the risk of adverse drug effects.

PHARMACOKINETICS

Pharmacokinetics is the mathematics of drug dosage determination. It involves mathematical evaluation of the rates of drug absorption and distribution throughout the body, along with metabolism and ultimate excretion from the body. Basic pharmacokinetic studies are usually performed in healthy animals. Unfortunately, however, veterinarians do not often administer drugs to normal, healthy animals. Dosage regimens derived from studies in healthy animals may not be accurate for diseased animals. Clinical pharmacokinetics is the study of the effects of disease states or other variables (age, sex, pregnancy) on the pharmacokinetics of drugs. Clinical pharmacokinetics guides veterinarians in adjusting dosage regimens determined in healthy animals to optimize treatment of diseased animals.

PLASMA DRUG CONCENTRATIONS AS THERAPEUTIC GUIDELINES

Most pharmacokinetic information is derived from plasma drug concentrations, even though pharmacologic action depends on drug concentration at a particular effector site, which is often a specific drug receptor. In reality, measuring drug concentrations at the drug receptor site is not practical. Instead, plasma (or serum) drug concentrations are measured and assumed to represent drug concentrations in the target tissues. Most cells in the body are perfused with tissue fluids or plasma, and drug concentrations usually reach equilibrium between tissue fluids and the blood. Therefore for most drugs pharmacologic action correlates well with the plasma drug concentration.

VARIATION BETWEEN DRUG DOSE AND PLASMA DRUG CONCENTRATION

Drug dosages needed for a therapeutic effect differ widely among individuals. The "usual" dose has no effect in some individuals, causes serious toxicity in others, and produces an optimal effect in a few. The relationship between the dosage of a drug and its concentration in plasma is affected by its bioavailability, the animal's body size and fluid composition, variability in drug distribution within the body, and variability in rates of metabolism and excretion. These factors are all influenced by genetic differences in metabolism and excretion, environmental factors, disease alterations in system function, and concurrent administration of other drugs. Therefore the plasma concentration of a drug is not a perfect index of pharmacologic response. However, pharmacologic response is more closely related to plasma drug concentration than to drug dose. But therapeutic decisions should never be made on the basis of the plasma drug concentration alone. Knowledge of plasma drug concentration should always be used with careful medical observation and judgment to determine optimal therapy.

DEFINITIONS IN PHARMACOKINETICS

Pharmacokinetic information is used to determine drug dosage regimens in clinical patients. An understanding of the way in which drug dosage regimens are derived and how they can be adjusted for different disease states requires knowledge of some basic pharmacokinetic terms. Mathematical *models* provide equations to describe drug concentration as a function of time. With an *open model* the drug is eliminated from the body. An open model describes the fate of most drugs. With a *closed model* the drug is recirculated within the body (e.g., a drug that undergoes enterohepatic recirculation). In pharmacokinetic models the body is represented by a series of *compartments* that communicate reversibly with one another. A *compartment* is a tissue or group of tissues with similar blood flow and drug affinity. A drug is assumed to be uniformly distributed within a compartment and can move dynamically in and out of compartments. Rate constants represent the entry and exit of drugs from each compartment. The *central compartment* is made up of the highly perfused tissues that equilibrate rapidly with the drug. Overall drug elimination occurs mainly from the central compartment, because the kidneys and liver are well-perfused tissues. The *peripheral compartment* is made up of less-perfused tissues such as muscle and connective tissues. The *deep compartment* consists of slowly perfused tissues or depot tissues such as fat and bone. The presence of a deep compartment for drug distribution is important for toxins and drug residues. Most drugs in clinical use are described by one or two compartment models. Models with more than three compartments are usually not physiologically relevant. Describing drug disposition with compartment models creates differential equations that describe drug concentration changes in each compartment and provides a visual representation of the rate processes among compartments.

RATES AND ORDERS OF REACTIONS

The drug absorption or elimination rate is the speed with which it occurs. If the amount of drug in the body is decreasing over time, then the elimination rate is expressed as follows:

$$\Delta C / \Delta t$$

The absorption and elimination rate of a drug is determined experimentally by measuring the plasma drug concentration at given time intervals. *Rate constants* relate the observed rate of a kinetic process to the drug concentration that controls the process. The elimination rate constant (K) is equal to the rate of drug elimination divided by the amount of drug in the body. The absorption rate constant (Ka) describes the rate of drug absorption into the central compartment. *Reaction order* refers to the way that drug concentration influences reaction rate.

With a *zero order reaction* the amount of drug changes at a constant time interval, regardless of the drug concentration. The rate of drug elimination is as follows:

$$\Delta C / \Delta t = -K_0$$

where K_0 is the zero order rate constant in mg/ml min. A graph of drug concentration versus time on regular graph paper for a zero order reaction produces a straight line (Figure 4-1), described by the equation:

$$C = -K_0 t + C_0$$

where *C* is the drug concentration at any time *t*, and C_0 is the drug concentration at time zero. For most drugs zero order elimination occurs only when elimination mechanisms become saturated. Renal tubular secretion and bile secretion of drugs are examples of potentially saturable processes. The most well-known zero order reaction is the oxidation of ethanol in humans. The alcohol dehydrogenase system becomes saturated with very small amounts of ethanol. To achieve mild intoxication (1 mg/ml) throughout a 75-kg person, an intake of about 56 ml of absolute alcohol (or 4 oz of whiskey, vodka,

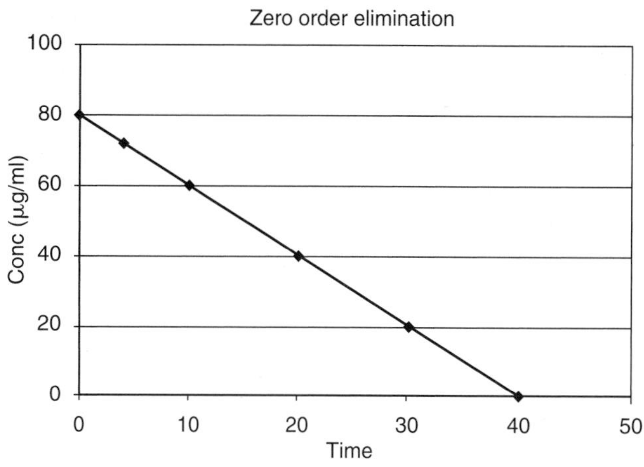

FIGURE 4-1 Drug concentration versus time for a zero order reaction produces a straight line on regular graph paper.

or gin) is required. The maximum amount of alcohol that can be eliminated is 10 ml per hour; therefore it takes 5 hours to totally eliminate the original 56 ml. Therefore to maintain a constant level of mild intoxication requires only 10 ml of ethanol or 25 ml of liquor per hour. In veterinary medicine, drugs with well-known zero order elimination include phenylbutazone in horses and deracoxibin dogs. Once elimination processes are saturated, increased dosages of such drugs result in wildly unpredictable plasma concentrations and easily result in toxicity.

With a first order reaction, the amount of drug changes at a rate proportional to the amount of drug remaining. The first order elimination rate is expressed as follows:

$$\Delta C / \Delta t = -KC$$

where *K* is the first order rate constant, is expressed in units of time^{-1} (min^{-1} or hr^{-1}), and defines the fraction of drug eliminated from the body per unit time; *C* is the plasma drug concentration at any time *t*. Although K remains constant, the rate (>C/>t) is always changing because *C* is always decreasing. A graph of drug concentration versus time for a first order reaction produces an exponential curve on regular graph paper but produces a straight line on semilogrithmic graph paper (Figure 4-2) and is described by the following equation:

$$C = C_0 e^{-Kt}$$

where *C* is drug concentration at any time *t*, *K* is the first order rate constant in minutes or hours, and C_0 is the drug concentration at time zero (the moment of injection). Most drugs are absorbed and eliminated by first order processes. Glomerular filtration by the kidney is a first order process.

CLINICAL APPLICATION OF COMPARTMENTAL MODELING, RATES, AND ORDERS OF REACTIONS

The aforementioned concepts can be combined to mathematically describe the changes in the drug concentration in the body over time. Drug disposition described by a one-compartment open model with intravenous (IV) injection and first order elimination (Figure 4-3) means that the body acts as one homogeneous compartment. A drug's concentration in one part of the body is assumed to be proportional to its concentration in any other part. Many drugs administered by routes other than IV, such as oral, subcutaneous, intramuscular, or intradermal, are described by a one-compartment open model with first order absorption (Ka) and elimination (K) (Figure 4-4). With a two-compartment open model with IV injection and first order elimination, the model assumes the body acts as two compartments: the central compartment (blood and highly vascularized tissues) and a peripheral compartment (less vascularized tissues). Most drugs administered in veterinary medicine are described by this model (Figure 4-5). Elimination is considered to occur only from the central compartment, because the liver and kidneys are highly vascularized tissues. The plasma concentration versus time graph does not produce a straight line on semilogrithmic paper but can be broken into two sections and described by the following biexponential equation:

$$C = Ae^{-\alpha t} + Be^{-\beta t}$$

Where C is the concentration at any time t, A is the y-intercept of the first portion of the curve extrapolated to zero, and α is the slope of the line; B is the y-intercept of the latter portion of the curve extrapolated to zero, and β is its slope. The movement of drug between the central and peripheral compartments is described by the rate constants K_{12} and K_{21}.

For some concentration versus time data, the line can be broken into three or more straight lines, and described mathematically with three or more exponential terms. Theoretically, drug distribution in the body can be described by as many compartments as there are different tissues, but for practical purposes more than three compartments models are not necessary. Drugs that are described by three compartment models usually have some tissue site where the drug is sequestered and slowly eliminated from the body, such as the aminoglycosides, which sequester in the renal tubular epithelial cells, and oxytetracycline, which sequesters in teeth and bone.

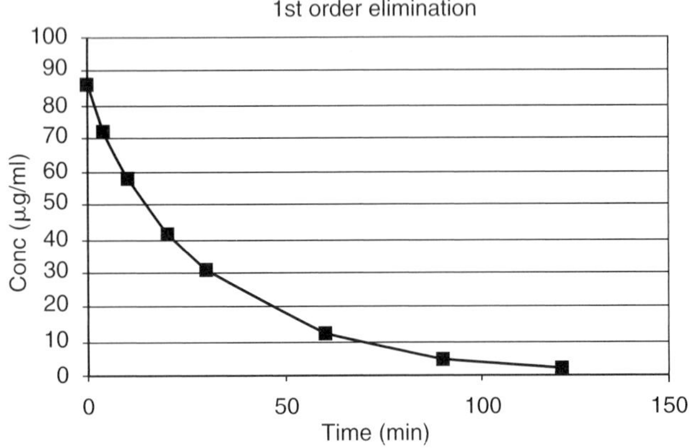

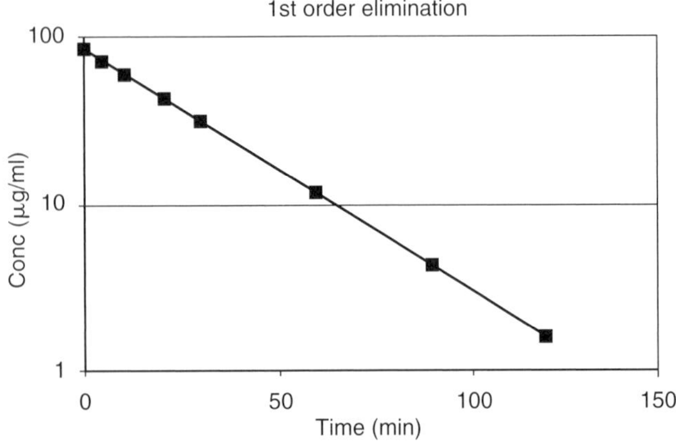

FIGURE 4-2 Drug concentration versus time for a first order reaction produces an exponential curve on regular graph paper but produces a straight line on semilogarithmic graph paper.

DISTRIBUTION OF DRUGS IN THE BODY

The volume of distribution (Vd) of a drug is the mathematical term used to describe the apparent volume of the body in which a drug is dissolved.[1] The Vd is the parameter used to assess the amount of drug in the body from the measurement of a "snapshot" plasma concentration. The numerical value of Vd can give some indication of the distribution of the drug in the body. A drug's distribution is determined by its ability to cross biologic membranes and reach tissues outside

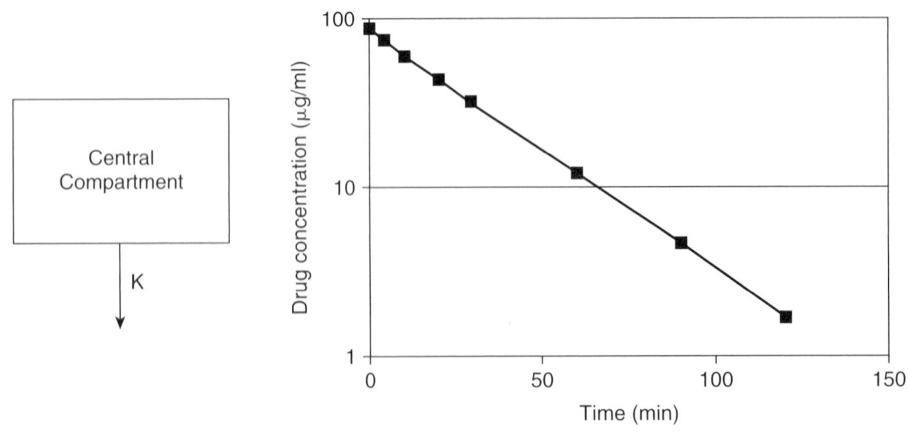

FIGURE 4-3 Graphic representation of a one-compartment open model with IV administration and first order elimination.

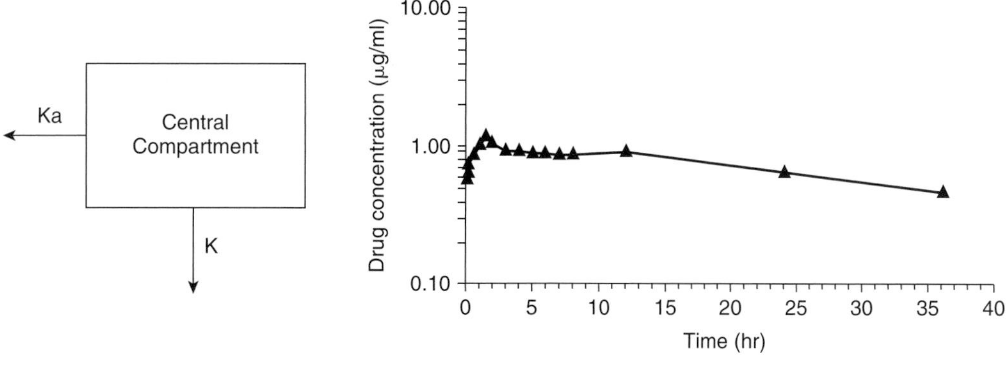

FIGURE 4-4 Plasma concentration versus time graph after intramuscular administration of long-acting OTC to a horse, demonstrating a one-compartment open model with first order absorption and elimination.

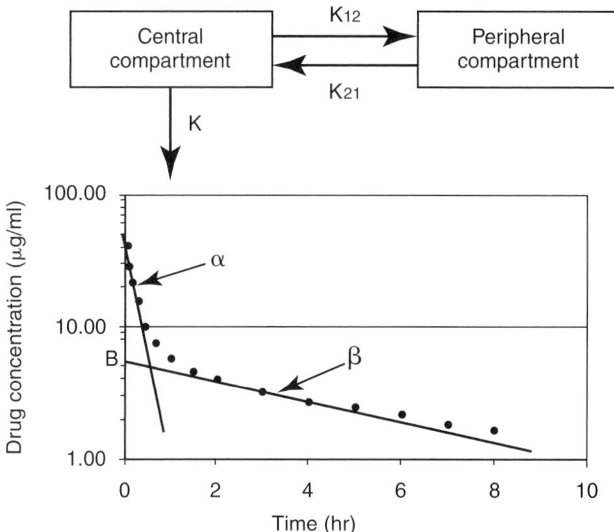

FIGURE 4-5 Plasma concentration versus time graph after IV administration of gentamicin to a horse, demonstrating a two-compartment open model with first order elimination from the central compartment. The equation of the line is biexponential, where $C = Ae^{-\alpha t} + Be^{-\beta t}$.

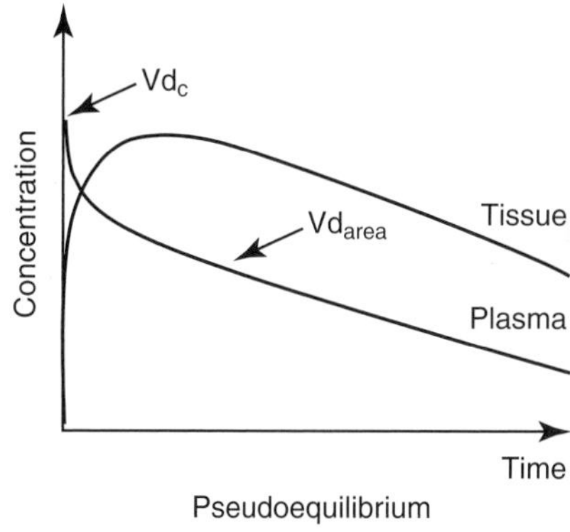

FIGURE 4-6 Graphical representation of the difference between the volume of the central compartment and the volume of distribution by area.

the vascular system. The physical characteristics of the drug molecule, such as ionization, lipid solubility, molecular size, and degree of protein binding, determine its ability to cross biologic membranes.

Three volumes of distribution (Vd) are reported in the veterinary literature: the volume of the central compartment, the steady-state volume of distribution, and the volume of distribution calculated by the area method. Conceptually, the easiest demonstration of the volume of distribution is with the volume of the central compartment (Vd_c). Just after an IV dose, plasma drug concentration is maximal (Figure 4-6). Assuming that the instant drug concentration (C_0) results from the drug mixing in the blood, the Vd_c is the apparent volume from which drug elimination occurs, because the kidneys and liver belong to the central compartment, and is calculated from the following equation:

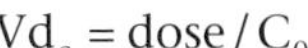

$$Vd_c = \text{dose} / C_0$$

where C_0 is the concentration at time zero, extrapolated from the plasma concentration versus time graph. To understand what the Vd_c for a drug represents, consider the body as a beaker filled with fluid (Figure 4-7). The fluid represents the plasma and other components of extracellular water. If a drug is administered intravenously, it rapidly distributes in the extracellular fluid. If the drug does not readily cross lipid membranes, it will be confined mainly to the extracellular fluid and a plasma sample therefore will have a high drug concentration. The higher the measured concentration in relation to the original dose, the lower the numerical value for Vd_c. Drugs such as the β-lactam and aminoglycoside antibiotics are poorly lipid soluble and therefore remain predominantly in the extracellular fluid and have low values for Vd. In contrast, some drugs readily cross lipid membranes and distribute into tissues. This is represented by the beaker on the right, where the stars at the bottom of the beaker represent drug molecules that have been taken up by tissues. A plasma sample will have a low drug concentration in proportion to the original dose and therefore will have a high numerical value for Vd_c. Given the limitations on measuring drug concentrations at "time zero" and using the aforementioned formula, the measured concentration of highly lipid-soluble drugs can be low enough to result in a value of Vd_c that is greater than 1 L/kg, so it is often referred to as an *apparent*

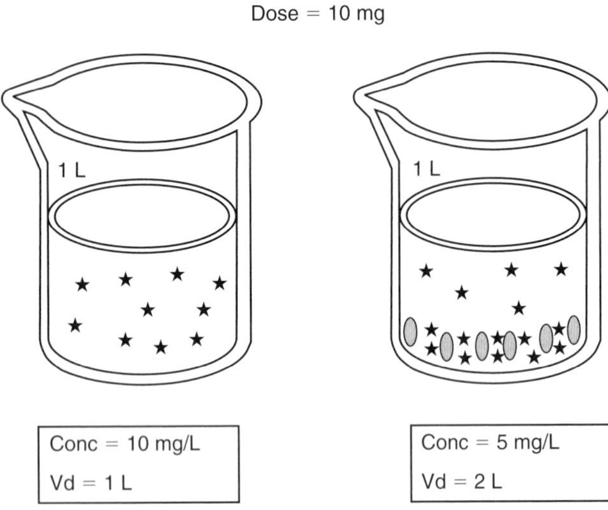

FIGURE 4-7 The beaker on the left represents a low Vd drug that is mainly distributed to the extracellular fluid. A sample from the fluid will contain a high concentration of drug and therefore will have a low value for Vd. The beaker on the right represents a high Vd drug that readily crosses membranes and moves out of the extracellular fluid into tissues. A sample from the fluid will contain a low concentration of drug and therefore will have a high value for Vd.

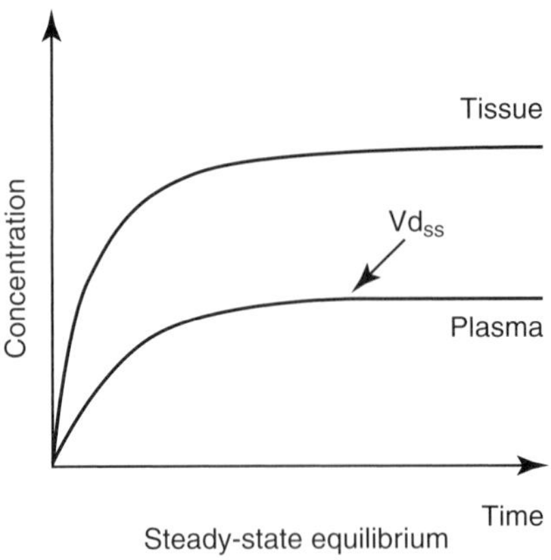

FIGURE 4-8 Graphical representation of the volume of distribution when plasma concentrations are measured at steady-state conditions.

volume of distribution. In the example on the right, the "apparent" Vd is 2 L/kg even though the beaker contains only 1 L of fluid.

For most drugs after a single IV dose, the drug is distributed and begins to be eliminated simultaneously. When concentrations are measured and the data graphed, there is a distribution phase, wherein the plasma drug concentration that is due to elimination and not distribution increases until it reaches an asymptotic value at which pseudoequilibrium is achieved (see Figure 4-6). When pseudoequilibrium is reached, the movement of drug between the peripheral and central compartments reaches equilibrium, and decreasing plasma concentrations are now due only to irreversible elimination (described by the elimination rate constant, β). The applicable Vd value in this situation is the volume of distribution by area (Vd_{area}),

$$Vd_{area} = Dose \div AUC^{0\text{-}\infty}/\beta$$

where $AUC^{0\text{-}\infty}$ is the area under the plasma concentration time curve from zero to infinity. To be calculated accurately, the amount of drug that enters the systemic circulation must be accurately known and the terminal phase must be a pure elimination phase. An inaccurate Vd_{area} is frequently published for "long-acting" intramuscular or subcutaneous administered drugs, where prolonged elimination is due to delayed absorption.

With an IV infusion or with a multiple dose regimen, the rate of drug entry into the body is equal to its elimination rate, and the body becomes a closed system with no clearance. In this situation the correct Vd to describe distribution is the Vd at steady-state (Vd_{ss}; Figure 4-8):

$$Vd_{SS} = \text{Drug in body at steady-state}/\text{Concentration in plasma}$$

Clinical Use of the Different Volume of Distribution Values

The Vd_c is used to predict the initial plasma drug concentration after an IV bolus of a drug when a loading dose is needed to rapidly achieve a therapeutic drug concentration. The Vd_{ss} is used to calculate a loading dose when it is clinically necessary to rapidly reach steady-state concentrations. The Vd_{area} is used to predict the amount of drug remaining in the body. For all drugs the value of Vd_{area} is greater than Vd_{ss}, but generally the difference is small and the values are used interchangeably. However, with the IV administration of drugs that are rapidly eliminated into urine (e.g, aminoglycosides), Vd_{area} can be much larger than Vd_{ss} because a large fraction of the drug is eliminated before pseudoequilibrium is reached.

It is useful to compare a drug's Vd to the distribution of water in the body in order to get an idea of its distribution. Drugs with a Vd value of less than 0.3 L/kg are predominantly confined to the ECF, whereas drugs with a Vd value of greater than 1 L/kg are highly lipid soluble and tend to distribute out of the extracellular fluid and into tissue compartments (Box 4-1). Although the value of Vd does not confirm penetration of a drug into specific tissues, in general the higher the value of the Vd, the more likely it is that the drug will reach sequestered sites such as the brain and cerebrospinal fluid, the prostate and other sex organs, the eye, and the mammary gland. Studies must be performed to confirm that therapeutic concentrations are achieved in such sites.

Conditions That Affect Volume of Distribution

The Vd is constant for any drug and will change only with physiologic or pathologic conditions that change the distribution of the drug. Drugs with high Vds are usually very lipid soluble and typically are not significantly affected by changes in body water status and do not require dosage adjustment. However, there are many medical conditions that affect the disposition of low Vd drugs in a patient

BOX 4-1

VOLUME OF DISTRIBUTION (Vd) OF VARIOUS DRUGS

Low Vd Drugs (<0.3 L/kg)

Penicillins
Cephalosporins
Aminoglycosides
Nonsteroidal anti-inflammatory drugs
Medium Vd Drugs (> 0.3 - < 1 L/kg)
Phenobarbital
Sulfonamides
Prednisolone
Rifampin

High Vd Drugs (>1 L/kg)

Macrolides
Tetracyclines
Fluoroquinolones
Chloramphenicol
Metronidazole
Trimethoprim
Dexamethasone
Furosemide
Ketamine
Diazepam
Firocoxib

(e.g., nonsteroidal anti-inflammatory drugs and aminoglycosides), and these drugs do require dosage adjustment because of their narrow therapeutic index. Many conditions in horses, such as colic, are characterized by volume contraction and dehydration and changes in acid-base balance, which affect the extracellular fluid volume. Neonatal foals have a higher percentage of body water than adult horses (80% versus 60% total body water), and the extra 20% is primarily confined to the extracellular fluid, so the Vd of drugs such as gentamicin are higher in neonatal foals than older foals or adult horses.[2] Therefore to achieve equivalent therapeutic plasma concentrations of gentamicin in a neonatal foal, the dose must be higher than that administered to the older foal or adult horse.

BIOAVAILABILITY

Bioavailability (F) is a measure of the systemic availability of a drug administered by a route other than IV.[3] Bioavailability is determined by comparing the area under the plasma drug concentration curve versus time (AUC) for the extravascular formulation to the AUC for the IV formulation. The AUC is calculated by computer or by the trapezoidal method, wherein the entire curve is divided into trapezoids, then the area of each trapezoid is calculated and summed to give the AUC. For an orally administered drug, use the following equation:

$$F = (AUC_{oral} \div AUC_{iv}) \times 100 = \%\ \text{bioavailable}$$

If *F* is significantly less than 100%, the drug dose must be increased to achieve systemic drug concentrations similar to the IV formulation:

$$\text{Adjusted dose} = \text{dose}_{iv}/F$$

If the oral formulation of a drug has a mean bioavailability of 50%, the drug dose must be doubled to achieve the same concentrations in plasma as achieved using the IV formulation. However, the variability of the bioavailability in the population is more clinically significant than the mean. To make sure that the horse with the poorest absorption is dosed appropriately, the dose must be increased according to the lowest bioavailability, not the mean. For example, if a drug has a mean F of 50% with a range of 20% to 70%, then to achieve an exposure of 100% for all the treated horses, the dose must be multiplied by 5, not just 2. However, if this is done, the horses with an F of 70% will be overdosed by a factor of 3.5. For a drug with a narrow therapeutic window and a poor bioavailability, there may be no dose that is ideal for all horses in the population. Low bioavailability of antimicrobials and anthelmintics is a major cause of subtherapeutic dosages that promote drug resistance. Poor oral bioavailability is a major limitation of many drugs administered to horses.[4]

LIPID SOLUBILITY AND DRUG IONIZATION (THE PH-PARTITION HYPOTHESIS)

The degree of lipid solubility determines how readily a drug will cross biologic membranes. Drugs are classified as lipid soluble (or nonpolar) versus water soluble (or polar). Highly lipophilic drugs diffuse easily across almost all tissue membranes. Most of the drugs used in equine practice exist as weak acids or weak bases. Their lipid solubility depends a great deal on their degree of ionization (charged state). An *ionized* drug is hydrophillic and poorly lipid soluble. A *nonionized* drug is lipophilic and can cross biologic membranes. The degree of ionization for a weak acid or weak base depends on the pKa of the drug and the pH of the surrounding fluid. At a given pH, there is an equilibrium between the ionized and nonionized proportions of drug. When the pH is equal to the pKa of the drug, then the drug will be 50% ionized and 50% nonionized (log 1 = 0). As the pH changes, the proportion of ionized to nonionized drug will change according to the *Henderson-Hasselbach* equations:

For a weak acid:

$$pH = pKa + \log\ (\text{ionized drug} / \text{nonionized drug})$$

For a weak base:

$$pH = pKa + \log\ (\text{ionized drug} / \text{nonionized drug})$$

Whereas the precise ratios of ionized versus nonionized drug can be calculated from the Henderson-Hasselbach equations, the relevance of the equations can be understood by simply remembering the sentence "like is nonionized in like." For example, a weak acid will be most nonionized in an acidic environment, so aspirin is most nonionized in the stomach and is readily absorbed. The fluid of most sequestered sites in the body (cerebrospinal fluid, accessory sex gland fluid, milk, abscesses) has a pH more acidic than plasma. In cattle with mastitis weak acid antibiotics are typically administered by intramammary infusion, whereas weak bases are administered parenterally. This makes sense according to the pH-partition concept. Weak bases in the plasma are highly nonionized and readily cross into the mammary gland. Then, as the equilibrium shifts, they become "ion-trapped" in the more acidic milk, but the fraction of nonionized drug in the mammary gland is available to cross the bacterial cell membrane for antimicrobial action. Weak acids such as penicillins and cephalosporins are highly ionized in plasma and therefore do not penetrate into the mammary gland very well, so these are most effective when administered by local infusion into the udder, where the extremely high local concentrations negate local pH effects.

Typically, drugs that are weak acids will have low Vd values and weak bases will have high values for Vd (Box 4-2). Amphoteric drugs such as the fluoroquinolones and tetracyclines have acidic and basic groups on their chemical structures. These drugs have a pH range where they are maximally nonionized. For example, enrofloxacin is most lipid soluble (nonionized) in the pH range of 6 to 8, so it is lipid soluble at most physiologic pHs. In acidic urine significant ionization occurs, which reduces enrofloxacin's antibacterial activity. But this reduction in activity is offset by the extremely high concentrations of enrofloxacin achieved in urine, so it is of no clinical importance. Despite being weak bases, the aminoglycosides are very large, hydrophilic molecules and have high pKa values, so they are highly ionized at physiologic pHs. Therefore parenterally administered aminoglycosides do not cross lipid membranes well and do not achieve therapeutic concentrations in milk, accessory sex gland fluids, abscesses, or cerebrospinal fluid.

Drug Protein Binding

Protein binding can involve plasma proteins, extracellular tissue proteins, or intracellular tissue proteins. Many drugs in circulation are bound to plasma proteins, and because bound drug is too large to pass through biologic membranes, only free drug is available for delivery to the tissues and to produce the desired pharmacologic action. Therefore the degree of protein binding can greatly affect the pharmacokinetics of drugs. Acidic drugs such as nonsteroidal anti-inflammatory drugs tend to bind predominantly to albumin.[5] Albumin is the most abundant plasma protein, and it is critical to maintaining the colloidal oncotic pressure in the vascular system. As a negative acute phase protein, albumin concentration decreases during inflammation. Hypoalbuminemia results from decreased production, seen with severe hepatic insufficiency, or by loss through increased rates of urinary excretion, such as in nephrotic syndrome or with mucosal damage, as with protein losing enteropathies. Basic drugs typically bind to α-1 acid glycoprotein, which is an acute phase protein, whose hepatic production increases significantly with inflammatory conditions.[6] Other proteins, including corticosteroid binding globulin, are important for binding of some specific drugs but are less important in overall drug-protein binding.[7] There is equilibrium between free and bound drug, however, just like the relationship of ionized and nonionized drug molecules. Protein binding is most clinically significant for antimicrobial therapy, where a high degree of protein binding serves as a drug "depot," allowing for increased duration of the time the drug concentration remains above the bacterial minimum inhibitory concentration, adding to antimicrobial efficacy.[8] For other drugs changes in plasma protein binding can influence individual pharmacokinetic parameters, but changes in plasma protein binding usually do not influence the clinical exposure of the patient to a drug. Changes in protein binding caused by drug interactions are assumed to instantaneously change free drug concentrations and have been frequently cited as a cause of adverse drug reactions. But the increase in free drug concentration is only transient, because drug distribution and drug elimination change to compensate. The often-cited example of the concurrent administration of phenylbutazone and warfarin leading to bleeding caused by increased free concentrations of warfarin is erroneous. The true interaction is from phenylbutazone-induced inhibition of the hepatic metabolism of warfarin, which results in increased plasma concentrations and increased anticoagulant effect.[7] Therefore adjustments in dosing regimens because of hypoproteinemia or concurrent administration of highly bound drugs are not necessary except in the rare case of a drug with a high hepatic extraction ratio and narrow therapeutic index that is given parenterally (e.g., IV dosing of lidocaine).[9]

BOX 4-2

DRUGS CLASSIFIED BY pH

Acidic Drugs
Penicillins
Cephalosporins
Sulfonamides
Nonsteroidal anti-inflammatory drugs

Basic Drugs
Macrolides
Trimethoprim
Chloramphenicol
Metronidazole
Aminoglycosides

Amphoteric Drugs
Fluoroquinonolones
Tetracyclines

DRUG ELIMINATION FROM THE BODY

Drug elimination refers to the irreversible removal of drug from the body by all routes of elimination. Elimination may be divided into two major components: excretion and biotransformation. Drug excretion is the removal of the intact drug. Most drugs are excreted by the kidney into the urine. Other pathways include the excretion of drug into bile, sweat, saliva, or milk. Biotransformation (drug metabolism) converts the drug in the body to a metabolite that is more readily excreted, usually by adding a chemical group to the molecule to make it more water soluble. Enzymes involved in biotransformation are mainly located in the liver. Other tissues, such as the kidney, lung, small intestine, and skin, contain biotransformation enzymes.

ELIMINATION RATE CONSTANT AND ELIMINATION HALF-LIFE

The rate of elimination for most drugs is a first order process. The elimination rate constant (K) represents the sum of drug elimination by excretion and metabolism. Drug elimination

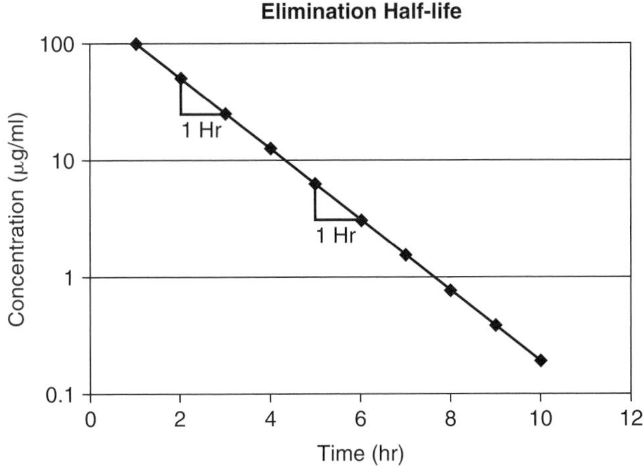

FIGURE 4-9 For a drug with first order elimination, the plasma concentration decreases by 50% every hour, so the elimination half-life is 1 hour.

TABLE 4-1

Half-Life of Elimination of a Drug

Number of Half-Lives	Fraction of Drug Remaining (%)
0	100
1	50
2	25
3	12.5
4	6.25
5	3.125
6	1.56
7	0.78
8	0.39
9	0.195
10	0.0975

is considered always to occur from the central compartment, because the liver and kidney are well-perfused tissues. The elimination rate constant is used to calculate the drug's half-life ($T_{1/2}$), or the time required for drug concentration to decrease by one half (Figure 4-9). For first order reactions, $T_{1/2}$ is constant across the plasma concentration versus time curve and is calculated from:

$$T_{1/2} = 0.693/K$$

where 0.693 = ln2 (the natural logarithm of 2). Mean residence time (MRT) is roughly the equivalent of $T_{1/2}$ when pharmacokinetics are calculated using statistical moment theory. The MRT is the time it takes for drug concentration to decrease by 63.2%, so the MRT value is typically slightly greater than $T_{1/2}$. The $T_{1/2}$ determines the drug dosage interval, how long a toxic or pharmacologic effect will persist, and drug withdrawal times for food animals or performance horses. Notice that it takes 10 $T_{1/2}$s to decrease the plasma concentration by 99.9% (Table 4-1). Knowing a drug's plasma $T_{1/2}$ can give the clinician some idea of the drug's withdrawal time for food or performance animals. However, for drugs that undergo hepatic metabolism (e.g., phenylbutazine) or drugs that sequester in specific tissues (e.g., aminoglycosides, isoxuprine), simply multiplying the $T_{1/2}$ by a factor of 10 for a withdrawal time may not be sufficient to prevent violative residues. Also note that doubling a drug dose does not double the withdrawal time; it merely adds one half-life to the time it takes to reach the acceptable threshold concentration (Figure 4-10).

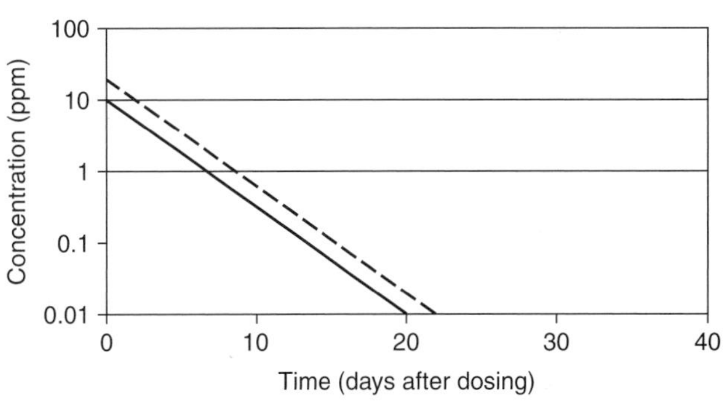

FIGURE 4-10 Doubling a drug dose adds only one half-life to its withdrawal time. For this drug with an elimination half-life of 24 hours, if the dose is doubled to reach a plasma concentration of 20 µg/ml, then it will take 21 days instead of 20 days to reach an acceptable threshold of 0.01 µg/ml.

Flip-Flop Kinetics

Long-acting drug formulations are often products whose carriers cause them to be slowly absorbed into the systemic circulation. Therefore the drug elimination rate is limited by the drug absorption rate. The value for *K* (the elimination rate constant) calculated from the plasma concentration versus time curve is actually the value for *Ka* (the absorption rate constant). The easiest way to identify "flip-flop" kinetics is to compare the plasma concentration versus time curve for the extravascular route of administration to the curve after the drug is given intravenously (Figure 4-11). If the elimination phases of the

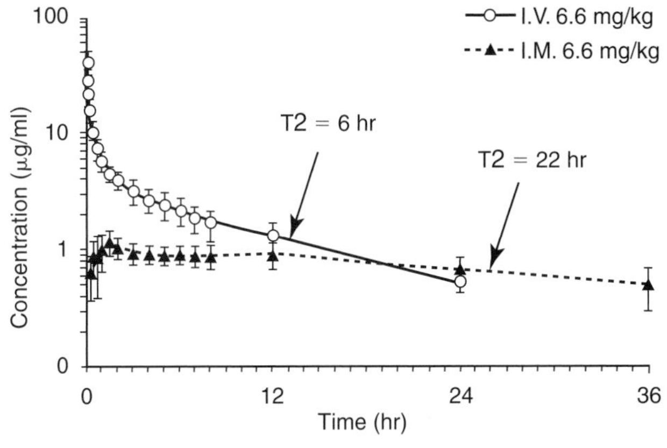

FIGURE 4-11 Plasma concentration versus time graph for long-acting oxytetracycline in horses, demonstrating "flip-flop" kinetics. The delayed absorption from the intramuscular injection results in the slow elimination and triples the elimination half-life value.

curves are not parallel, then delayed absorption is prolonging elimination and the flip-flop phenomenon has occurred.

For a two-compartment model, β (from the equation $C = Ae^{-\alpha t} + Be^{-\beta t}$) is the drug elimination rate constant from the entire body once the drug has reached equilibrium between the two compartments. Therefore β is used to calculate the elimination half-life:

$$T_{1/2} = 0.693/\beta$$

Clearance

Clearance is a measure of drug elimination from the body without reference to the mechanism of elimination. It is always reported in pharmacokinetic papers, but its significance is rarely explained in pharmacokinetic studies in horses. Clearance is the most important pharmacokinetic parameter because it is the only parameter that controls overall drug exposure and it is used to calculate the dosage required to maintain a specific average steady-state concentration.[10]

Clearance (Cl) is the total drug clearance and is the sum of renal clearance (Cl_R), hepatic clearance (Cl_H), and all other elimination mechanisms. By definition, Cl is the volume of fluid containing drug that is cleared of drug per unit of time (ml/kg/min). The most frequent technique for determining plasma Cl is to administer a single IV dose of a drug and then measure plasma concentrations over time. Then,

$$Cl = Dose/AUC$$

where *AUC* is the area under the plasma concentration time curve.

If the body is considered as the whole system clearing the drug, *Cl* can also be determined by the animal's cardiac output and the extraction ratio *(E)*, where *E* is a numerical value between 0 and 1 that is the percentage of the drug that is cleared by a single pass through the clearing organ:

$$Cl = \text{Cardiac output} \times E$$

For a drug with an extraction ratio of 1 (100% removal by the liver and kidney on the first pass), then the expected value of Cl is about 50% of the cardiac output, because blood flow to the liver and the kidneys represents about half of the cardiac output.

In contrast to Vd values, Cl values have to be interpreted according to the value of cardiac output for the species involved. Given that most drugs are extracted primarily by renal and hepatic mechanisms, the extraction ratio is considered high if E is greater than 0.7, medium if E equals 0.3, and low if E is less than 0.1. Because the liver and kidneys receive about 50% of cardiac output, then the overall E is high if it is greater than 0.35, medium if it is about 0.15, and low if it is less than 0.05. From this and the cardiac output of the species, breakpoint values can be determined to classify drugs as having high, medium, and low clearance. For the horse with a cardiac output of 55 ml/kg/min, a high Cl value is 19 ml/min/kg, medium Cl is 8.25 ml/min/kg, and low Cl is 3.6 ml/min/kg.

It is sometimes difficult to understand the difference between the elimination half-life and clearance. The relationship is as follows:

$$Cl = (Vd)(K) \text{ or}$$
$$C1 = (Vd)(0.693/T_{1/2})$$

Consider the values for clearance and $T_{1/2}$ values for four antimicrobial drugs (Table 4-2). Note that the plasma clearance values are similar, but the elimination half-lives are very different. Because the $T_{1/2}$ is influenced by the extent of drug distribution, the drugs have similar clearance, but oxytetracycline has the largest Vd and the longest $T_{1/2}$. Because $T_{1/2}$ is derived from rate constants and does not have a physiologic basis, it is influenced by the sensitivity of the analytical method and by many pharmacokinetic parameters, and it is a poor parameter alone to evaluate physiologic (e.g., age, sex) or pathologic (e.g., renal failure) changes that effect drug disposition.

Renal Clearance of Drugs

Renal excretion is the major route of elimination from the body for most drugs. Drug disposition by the kidneys includes glomerular filtration, active tubular secretion, and tubular reabsorption (Figure 4-12), such that renal drug clearance is defined by the following equation:

$$Cl_R = Cl_F + Cl_S - FR$$

where Cl_R = total renal clearance
Cl_F = clearance attributed to glomerular filtration
Cl_S = clearance attributed to active tubular secretion
FR = fraction reabsorbed from the tubule back to circulation

Glomerular filtration (Cl_F) occurs with small molecules (<300 molecular weight) of free drug (not bound to plasma proteins). Large molecules or protein-bound drugs do not get filtered at the glomerulus because of size and electrical hindrance. The kidneys receive approximately 25% of cardiac output, so the major driving force for glomerular filtration is the hydrostatic pressure within the glomerular capillaries. Glomerular filtration rate (GFR) is estimated by measuring a substance or drug that is eliminated only by glomerular filtration, such as creatinine or inulin.

If Cl_R is greater than Cl_F, then some tubular secretion is occurring. Active tubular secretion is a carrier-mediated transport system, located in the proximal renal tubule. It requires energy input because the drug is moved against a concentration gradient. Two active tubular secretion systems have been identified: anion secretion for acids and cation secretion for

TABLE 4-2

Comparison of Clearance to Elimination Half-life

	Penicillin	Gentamicin	Oxytetracycline	Tylosin
Cl (ml/min/kg)	3.5	3.1	4.0	2.2
T2 (min)	30	75	360	54

bases. Drugs with similar structures may compete with each other for the same transport system. For example, probenecid competes with penicillin or the fluoroquinolones for the same transport system, effectively decreasing Cl of these antimicrobials. In patients with reduced functional renal tissue, remaining transport systems become easily saturated and drug accumulation occurs.

If Cl_R is less than *GFR,* tubular reabsorption of drug is occurring. Tubular reabsorption is an active process for endogenous compounds (e.g., vitamins, electrolytes, glucose). It is a passive process for the majority of drugs. It occurs along the entire nephron but primarily in the distal renal tubule. Factors that affect reabsorption include the pKa of the drug, urine pH, lipid solubility, drug size, and urine flow. Drug reabsorption is highly dependent on ionization, which is determined by the drug's pKa and the pH of the urine. According to the Henderson-Hasselbach equation, a drug that is a weak base will be mainly nonionized in alkaline urine and a weak acid will be mainly ionized in alkaline urine. The nonionized form of the drug is more lipid soluble and has greater reabsorption (Table 4-3). The pKa of a drug is constant, but urinary pH is highly variable in animals and varies with the diet, drug intake, time of day, and systemic acidosis/alkalosis. Species differences have a major influence on the renal excretion of ionized drugs. Carnivores, with a urine pH of 5.5 to 7.0, will have a greater renal excretion of basic drugs than herbivores, with a urine pH of 7.0 to 8.0.

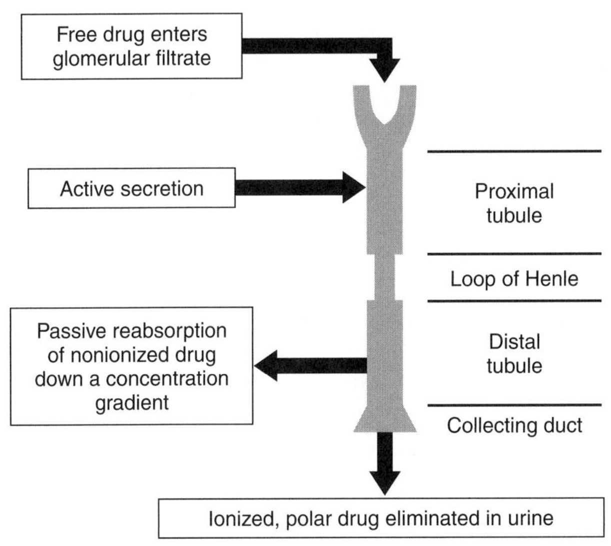

FIGURE 4-12 Movement of drugs in the renal tubule.

TABLE 4-3

Renal Clearance (ml/min/kg) at Different Urinary pHs

			URINE pH		
		pKa	**4.4**	**6.4**	**7.9**
Penicillin	Acid	2.4	0.001	0.1	3.0
Oxytetracycline	Base	10.4	1000	10	0.3

Hepatic Clearance of Drugs

Nonrenal drug elimination is assumed to be due primarily to biotransformation (hepatic metabolism) and biliary excretion. Clearance of a drug by the liver is determined by hepatic blood flow *(Q_H)* and the intrinsic ability of the liver to extract the drug *(extraction ratio,* or *ER_H)*:

$$Cl_H = (Q_H)(ER_H)$$

Drugs with a high extraction ratio (approaching 1) have Cl_H equal to the hepatic blood flow. These drugs are called *high clearance drugs.* Examples of drugs with high ER_H are lidocaine, propranolol, and isoproterenol. Clearance of drugs with high ER_H is highly influenced by changes in hepatic blood flow. Drugs that are administered orally and are absorbed across the intestinal mucosa must first pass through the liver via the portal circulation before being distributed to the rest of the body. Most of a drug with a high ER_H will be cleared in one pass through the liver; this is called the *first pass effect,* and it limits the oral administration of such drugs. Drugs that have a low hepatic extraction rate ($ER_H \le 0.2$) are not greatly affected by changes in hepatic blood flow. However, their clearance will be affected by changes in the hepatic microsomal enzyme systems and protein binding. A first pass effect does not interfere with the systemic availability of these drugs. Drugs with a low ER_H include chloramphenicol, phenylbutazone, phenobarbital, and digoxin.

Biotransformation (Hepatic Metabolism) of Drugs

Metabolism is necessary for removal of lipophilic drugs from the body (Figure 4-13). Biotransformation depends on the chemical composition of the liver, activity of major drug metabolism enzymes, hepatic volume (perfusion rate), drug accessibility to and extraction by hepatic metabolic sites, and physicochemical properties of the drug. Biotransformation of a parent drug results in metabolites that may be active or inactive themselves. A *prodrug* is a drug administered in an inactive form that must be biotransformed to its active form, such as prednisone to prednisolone. Drug metabolic pathways are divided into *phase I* and *phase II* reactions. Phase I reactions (oxidation, reduction, hydrolysis, hydration, dethioacetylation, isomerization) typically

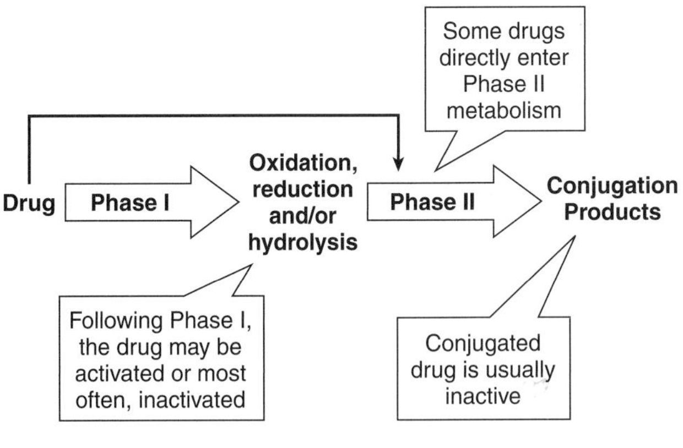

FIGURE 4-13 Hepatic metabolism increases the water solubility of drugs, facilitating excretion from the body.

add functional groups to the drug molecule necessary for phase II reactions. Phase II reactions (glucuronidation, glucosidation, sulfation, methylation, acetylation, amino acid conjugation, glutathione conjugation, and fatty acid conjugation) typically include conjugation reactions that increase the water solubility of the drug, facilitating excretion from the body.

Among the reactions catalyzed by drug metabolism enzymes, the cytochrome P450 mixed function oxidase system is the most intensively studied. This reaction catalyzes the hydroxylation of hundreds of structurally diverse drugs, whose only common characteristic is high lipid solubility. Species differences in drug metabolic rate are the primary source of variation in drug activity and toxicity. Cats have a poor ability to glucuronidate drugs, pigs are deficient in sulfate conjugation, and dogs are relatively poor acetylators.

Induction and Inhibition of Metabolism

Metabolism of drugs can be substantially affected by enzyme induction or inhibition by other drugs or chemicals (Box 4-3). In some cases the drug itself may alter its own metabolic fate by induction or inhibition. Many drugs are capable of inducing enzyme activity, thereby increasing the rate of metabolism and hepatic clearance of concurrently administered drugs, which typically results in a decreased pharmacologic effect. Enzyme induction typically occurs slowly, requiring several weeks to reach maximum effect. Induction is accompanied by increased hepatic ribonucleic acid (RNA) and protein synthesis and increased hepatic weight. Enzyme induction is important in the pathogenesis of hepatotoxicity and therapeutic failure of many drugs. Phenobarbital is a potent enzyme inducer known for hepatotoxicity and for inducing its own metabolism. Rifampin induces the metabolism of azole antifungals; concurrent administration with itraconazole results in subtherapeutic itraconazole concentrations.

BOX 4-3

DRUGS THAT AFFECT ENZYME FUNCTION

Enzyme Inducers

Chlorinated hydrocarbons
Griseofulvin
Omeprazole
Phenobarbital
Phenytoin
Rifampin

Enzyme Inhibitors

Chloramphenicol
Cimetidine
Dexamethasone
Erythromycin
Fluoroquinolones
Ketoconazole
Phenobarbital
Phenylbutazone
Prednisolone
Quinidine

Drug-induced enzyme inhibition also occurs and typically results in prolonged clearance of a concurrently administered drug. The potential for toxicity or an exaggerated pharmacologic response is increased. In contrast to induction, inhibition occurs rapidly. Erythromycin and enrofloxacin are known inhibitors of the metabolism of theophylline; concurrent administration can cause central nervous system toxicity and seizures.[11,12]

Kinetics of Drug Metabolism

The enzymes that catalyze drug metabolism typically obey Michaelis-Menten kinetics as a *first order reaction*:

$$V = \frac{V_{max}[C]}{K_m + [C]}$$

where V is the rate of drug metabolism, K_m is the Michaelis constant, and C is the drug concentration. In most clinical situations the drug concentration is much less than the Michaelis constant, so the equation reduces to the following:

$$V = \frac{V_{max}[C]}{K_m}$$

that is, the rate of drug metabolism is directly proportional to the concentration of free drug and first order kinetics are observed in that a constant fraction of drug is metabolized per unit of time. With a few drugs, such as phenylbutazone, ethanol, deracoxib, and phenytoin, or if very large doses of a drug are given, the drug concentrations achieved are much greater than K_m and the rate equation is as follows:

$$V = \frac{V_{max}[C]}{[C]} = V_{max}$$

The enzymes are saturated by the high free drug concentrations, and the rate of metabolism remains constant over time. This is *zero-order kinetics* or *nonlinear kinetics*, and a constant amount of drug is metabolized per unit of time.

DRUG ACCUMULATION

Drugs are often given in multiple-dosage regimens. To predict plasma drug concentrations, it is necessary to decide whether successive doses of a drug have any effect on the previous dose. The *principle of superposition* assumes that early doses of drug do not affect the pharmacokinetics of subsequent doses. For most drugs, as equal doses are given at a constant dosage interval, the plasma concentration-time curve plateaus and a *steady-state* is reached. At steady-state the plasma drug concentration fluctuates between a maximum concentration (Cmax, or peak) and minimum concentration (Cmin, or trough). Once steady-state is reached, Cmax and Cmin are constant and remain unchanged from dose to dose (Figure 4-14). The time to steady-state depends solely on the elimination half-life. It takes approximately six $T_{1/2}$s to reach 99% steady-state levels. The drug dose and dosage frequency influence the values of Cmax and Cmin at steady-state, while the dosage frequency and $T_{1/2}$ influence the fluctuation between Cmax and Cmin.

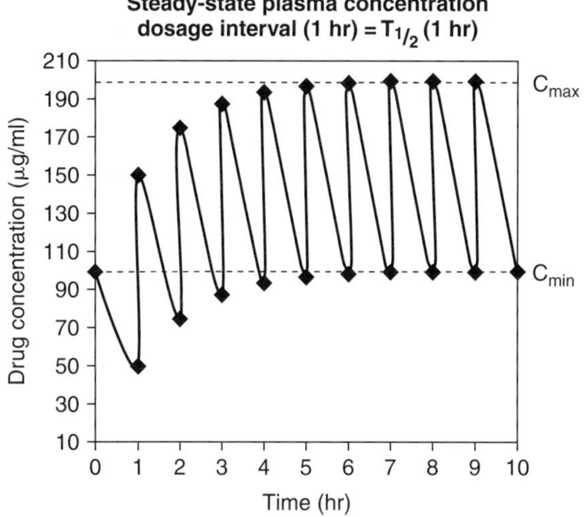

FIGURE 4-14 Plasma concentration versus time graph for an IV drug that produces a peak plasma concentration of 100 μg/ml after a single dose. After 6 hours (which equals 6 half-lives), the maximum and minimum drug concentrations become constant, further drug accumulation does not occur, and the drug is steady-state.

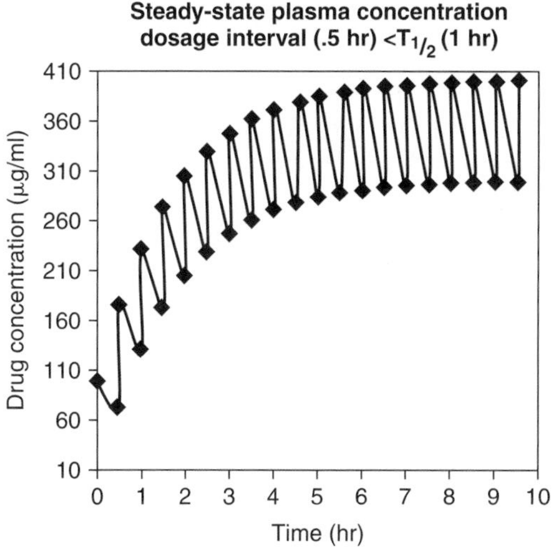

FIGURE 4-15 Plasma concentration versus time graph for a drug with a dosage interval (0.5 hour) less than the half-life (1 hour), demonstrating significant drug accumulation at steady-state.

Clinical Consequences of Dosage Intervals Less than the Half-Life

Drugs such as phenobarbital, potassium bromide, phenylbutazone, and digoxin are commonly given at dosage intervals much shorter than their $T_{1/2}$=s (Figure 4-15). This results in a Cmax at steady-state that is greater than the peak concentration after a single dose. There is minimal fluctuation between Cmax and Cmin, and missing a single dose will not affect plasma concentrations greatly. There is a lag time to reach the desired plasma concentrations at steady-state, and there will be a lag time for plasma concentrations to change in response to a dose change.

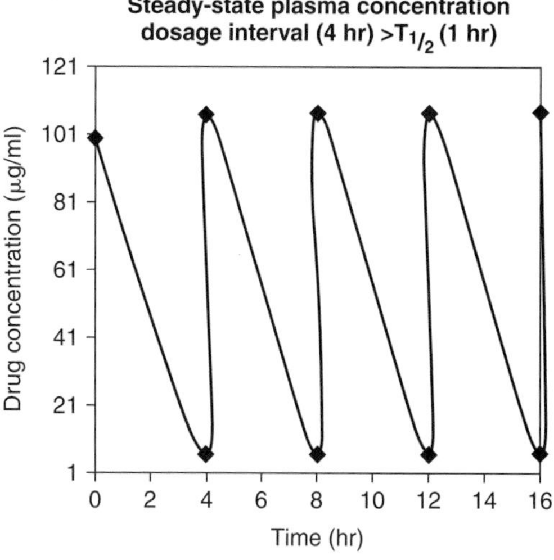

FIGURE 4-16 Plasma concentration versus time graph for a drug with a dosage interval (4 hours) greater than the half-life (1 hour), resulting in no significant drug accumlation at steady-state.

Clinical Consequences of Dosage Intervals Greater than the Half-Life

Drugs such as IV formulations of penicillin and cephalosporins are administered at dosage intervals that are greater than the $T_{1/2}$ (Figure 4-16). As the dosage interval increases, Cmax at steady-state is closer in value to the peak concentration after a single dose. If the dosage interval is greater than 10 $T_{1/2}$ s (the time required to eliminate 99.9% of the previous dose), drug accumulation essentially does not occur. There is marked fluctuation between Cmax and Cmin (peak and trough), and missing a dose will greatly affect plasma concentrations. However, there is minimal lag time to achieve the desired plasma concentration.

DESIGNING DRUG DOSAGE REGIMENS

The success of drug therapy is highly dependent on the dosage regimen design. Not all drugs require rigid individualization of the dosage regimen. In the case of antimicrobials with a broad safety range, such as the penicillins and cephalosporins, the dosage is not titrated precisely but rather determined on the basis of clinical judgment to maintain an effective plasma concentration above the minimum inhibitory concentration of the bacterial pathogen. For drugs with a narrow therapeutic margin, such as digoxin, the aminoglycosides, and theophylline, the individualization of the dosage regimen is very important. The objective of the dosage regimen for these drugs is to produce a safe plasma drug concentration that does not exceed the minimum toxic concentration or fall below a critical minimum concentration below which the drug is not effective. Factors that influence the concentration of drug attained at the drug's site of action include the dose administered, the route of administration, release and absorption of drug from dosage form, the extent of drug distribution, and the rate of drug elimination.

The horse's age may have a profound effect on drug disposition (Table 4-4).[13] The definition of *geriatric* varies between

TABLE 4-4

Age-Related Changes in Geriatric and Pediatric Patients

Body Part/Function Affected	Geriatric	Pediatric
Organ blood flow	Decreased	Increased
Total body water	Decreased	Greatly increased
Body fat	Increased	Decreased
Serum proteins	Decreased albumin	Decreased albumin
	Increased globulins	
Hepatic metabolism	Decreased	Greatly decreased

species, and in small animals it varies between breeds. Body composition and regional blood flow change in geriatric horses. Cardiac output decreases, so regional and organ blood flow also decrease. These changes have an impact on drug absorption, distribution, and elimination. Blood flow is preferably redistributed to the brain and heart, so there is an increase in risk of drug toxicity in these organs. Gastrointestinal motility and absorptive capacity are reduced. Hepatocyte number and function decrease along with hepatic and splanchnic blood flow. As renal blood flow decreases, GFR and active secretory capacity of the nephron decreases, resulting in decreased renal clearance of drugs. Lean body mass decreases while fatty tissues increase. The plasma concentrations of water-soluble (low volume of distribution) drugs tend to increase, whereas the plasma concentrations of lipid-soluble (high volume of distribution) drugs tend to decrease. Serum albumin decreases while gamma globulins increase, so total plasma protein concentrations essentially remain the same.

The definition of *neonate* also varies with species and age, but all the determinants of drug disposition are altered as the foal matures.[14] Blood flow to the heart and brain is greater and faster, making the foal more susceptible to drug-induced cardiotoxicity and neurotoxicity. Gastrointestinal absorption tends to be decreased as a result of decreased gastric emptying and decreased intestinal peristalsis. Absorption from intramuscular and subcutaneous sites changes as muscle mass and blood flow change. Neonates have less fat and greater total body water (primarily extracellular fluid) than adults. Therefore low Vd drugs (e.g., gentamicin, ketoprofen) distribute into a larger volume, making it necessary to increase the dose to avoid therapeutic failure. Because of low body fat stores, lipid-soluble drugs will have higher plasma concentrations in foals. For example, moxidectin is much more lipid soluble than ivermectin, so it is more easily overdosed in foals.[15] Drug elimination by both hepatic metabolism and renal excretion is limited in neonates, so drug dosing intervals need to be increased for many drugs, such as aminoglycosides and nonsteroidal anti-inflammatory drugs.

In addition, the sick horse usually has impaired drug detoxifying ability. Hepatic damage reduces drug metabolism and may increase drug action, whereas renal damage and impaired excretion decrease drug clearance. Alterations in gastrointestinal motility affect drug absorption, and are a concern in horses with postoperative ileus. Peripheral circulation is decreased in shock, resulting in decreased absorption of intramuscularly and subcutaneously administered drugs.

Pharmacokinetic-Based Dosage Regimens

A drug dose regimen is composed of a dose and a dosing frequency. Some drugs are given as single doses, so a specific plasma concentration will be targeted. When multiple doses of a drug are given, the dosage frequency and drug accumulation must be considered. There are simple calculations that can be used to design a patient-specific dose regimen.

SINGLE DOSE REGIMEN

A single drug dose has its duration of action determined by the size of the dose, its elimination rate, and the volume of distribution. To calculate a single dose of a drug, or when assuming a once-a-day dosing, only the Vd and the desired plasma concentration are needed:

$$\text{Dose} = (\text{Vd})(C_0)$$

For drugs administered other than intravenously, the dose must be corrected for bioavailability:

$$\text{Dose} = (\text{Vd})(C_0)/(F)$$

CONTINUOUS RATE INFUSION

When the desired response needs to be constant, the drug may be infused intravenously at a constant rate (R) following the initial IV dose:

$$R = (C)(\text{Vd})(K)$$

The infusion rate is essentially the rate of drug loss from the body (mg/min or mg/hr). Therefore to maintain the established concentration of drug in the body, it is necessary to infuse drug at the rate equal to its loss (K = elimination rate). For example, the vasopressive drugs dopamine and dobutamine have extremely short elimination half-lives, so they must be administered by constant infusion.

MULTIPLE DOSE REGIMEN

Continuous IV infusion offers the most precise control of drug levels in the body and is essential for precise control of drugs with a narrow safety margin or very rapid elimination. This method is not feasible for most drugs in veterinary medicine. It is possible to maintain an average desired plasma concentration by repeating doses at constant dosing intervals. Obviously, the highest plasma concentrations will occur soon after drug administration, and the lowest concentrations will be just before the next dose is administered. As long as the lowest concentration is acceptable for therapy and the highest concentration does not cause toxicity, these variations in plasma concentration are acceptable:

$$\text{Dose} = \frac{(C_{ave})(V_d)(\tau)}{(1.44)T_{1/2}}$$

where τ = dosage interval and 1.44 is a constant to correct for log scale.

LOADING DOSE FOLLOWED BY MAINTENANCE DOSE REGIMEN

Drugs that have long elimination half-lives, such as digoxin and the sulfonamides, have a long lag time to acceptable drug concentrations and therefore are usually given by a large loading dose ($Dose_L$) followed by maintenance doses ($Dose_M$).

$$Dose_L = \frac{Dose_M}{1 - e^{-K\tau}}$$

THERAPEUTIC DRUG MONITORING

Monitoring plasma drug concentrations is valuable if there is a relationship between the plasma drug concentration and the desired clinical effect or an adverse effect. It is particularly helpful in horses with gastrointestinal, cardiovascular, hepatic, or renal disease. It is also useful when many drugs are being administered at the same time and may be altering one another's metabolic effects. Therapeutic drug monitoring (TDM) is often valuable for regulating the dosage of drugs used chronically or prophylactically. For those drugs in which plasma concentration and clinical effect are not related, other pharmacodynamic parameters may be monitored. For example, clotting times may be measured in patients on anticoagulant therapy.

The drugs for which TDM is commonly used are characterized by serious toxicity (e.g., digoxin, phenobarbital, aminoglycosides); a steep dose-response curve, wherein a small increase in dose can cause a marked increase or decrease in response (e.g., theophylline); marked pharmacokinetic variability among individual patients, so dose is poorly predictive of plasma drug concentration (e.g., cyclosporine); easily saturated elimination mechanisms that lead to nonlinear kinetics; or when the cost of therapy justifies confirming a desired plasma drug concentration (Table 4-5).

Performing Therapeutic Drug Monitoring

Samples for TDM should not be submitted until plasma drug concentrations have reached steady-state in the patient (after approximately 6 elimination half-lives have passed). For conditions in which steady-state concentrations must be reached immediately, administer a loading dose. The risk of adverse drug reactions is obviously increased, so TDM can be used to proactively determine the proper maintenance dose. When a loading dose is being administered, TDM should be done after the loading dose to establish a baseline. The second TDM should be one drug half-life later to ensure that the maintenance dose is able to maintain the concentrations achieved by the loading dose. If the drug concentrations at the second sample do not match those of the first sample, the maintenance dose can be adjusted at this time rather than waiting for steady-state, with the risk of therapeutic failure or toxicity. The third time to do TDM is at steady-state to ensure an appropriate dosage regimen.

TABLE 4-5

Recommendations for Therapeutic Drug Monitoring

Drug	Therapeutic Range	Vd (L/kg)	T½	Time to Steady-State	Sample Collection
Amikacin	25 μg/ml peak <5 μg/ml trough	0.25	1-2 h	1 day	Peak: 0.5-1 hour after administration Trough: just before next dose or 8 hours after dosing if using once-daily administration; collect in plastic only
Bromide	Monotherapy: 2-3 μg/ml (20-30 mmol/L) W/phenobarb: 1-2 μg/ml (10-20 mmol/L)		24 d	4 months	Anytime
Digoxin	0.9-3.0 ng/ml	6.7	23 h	7 days	2-5 h post dose, collect in glass only
Gentamicin	10 μg/ml peak <2 μg/ml trough	0.3	1 h	1 day	Peak: 0.5-1 hour after administration Trough: just before next dose or 8 hours after dosing if using once-daily administration; collect in plastic only
Phenobarbital	14-45 μg/ml (70-170 mmol/L)	0.96	24 hours	6 days	Anytime
Theophylline	10-20 μg/ml	.8	13 hours	3 days	1-2 hours postdose

BOX 4-4

INTERPRETING THE RESULTS OF THERAPEUTIC DRUG MONITORING

Plasma Concentrations Lower Than Anticipated

Poor compliance with regimen
Error in dosage regimen
Wrong product (e.g., controlled release instead of immediate release)
Poor bioavailability
Rapid elimination
Increased apparent volume of distribution
Poor timing of blood sample

Plasma Concentrations Higher Than Anticipated

Poor compliance with regimen
Dose incorrect
Very rapid drug absorption
Decreased apparent volume of distribution
Slow elimination

Plasma Concentration Correct, but Poor Patient Response to Therapy

Diagnosis incorrect
Altered tissue receptor sensitivity (tolerance)
Drug interaction at receptor site

The number of samples collected for TDM depends on the drug, its $T_{1/2}$, and the reason for monitoring. To determine optimal aminoglycoside therapy, peak and trough samples are needed. To allow for the distribution phase, blood sampling for the peak concentration is done 0.5 to 1 hour after administration, and the trough sample is usually taken before the next dose. With very long elimination half-lives and twice-daily dosing, there are no statistically significant differences between Cmax and Cmin values for phenobarbital or potassium bromide. Therefore a single sample can be collected for TDM at any time during the dosing interval. However, Cmax and Cmin samples should be collected in any horse that is not responding as expected to therapy in order to determine if the horse has a shorter- or longer-than-normal elimination time for the drug (Box 4-4).

Adjustment of Dosage Regimens

Adjustment of the dosage regimen is frequently required when drugs are administered to diseased horses, whereas the dosage regimens have been established in relatively healthy, normal horses. Adjustment is indicated when drug elimination or the drug's distribution is significantly altered in the animal. In general, the following rules are true:

- If the volume of distribution changes, change the drug dose.
- If the elimination of the drug changes, change the dosing interval.

For drug dosage regimens determined by TDM, modifications are made on a percentage basis:

New Dose = Old Dose × (Target + Concentration ÷ Measured Concentration)

DOSAGE ADJUSTMENTS IN RENAL FAILURE

The ultimate route for drug elimination from the body is the kidney. Therefore it is not surprising that renal disease has a profound impact on the disposition of drugs administered to animals in renal failure. With reduced renal clearance, the parent drug, its metabolites, or both may accumulate in the patient and cause toxicity. Loss of proteins and electrolytes in urine and the alterations in acid-base balance associated with renal failure affect the pharmacokinetics and pharmacodynamics of drugs. Enhanced drug activity or toxicity can occur as a result of synergy with uremic complications. Altogether, these effects make it difficult to determine safe and effective drug dosages for veterinary patients in renal failure.

The goal of dosage adjustment is to provide a drug concentration-time profile in the horse with renal failure that is as similar as possible to that of a normal horse. The best approach to modifying drug therapy in horses with renal failure would be to carry out therapeutic drug monitoring and adjust the dosage for each patient. This is possible with some drugs, such as gentamicin and amikacin, but it is impractical and cost prohibitive for most drugs used in veterinary practice. The best approach for most drugs is to estimate a corrected dose from available renal function tests and then to monitor the patient closely for evidence of efficacy or toxicity. For drugs that are eliminated primarily by renal mechanisms, creatinine (Cr) clearance correlates well with drug clearance. Cr is an endogenous product of creatinine phosphate metabolism in muscle. It is removed by glomerular filtration, and serum concentrations are relatively constant in healthy people and animals. The elimination half-life of a drug that is eliminated in urine remains stable until Cr clearance is reduced to 30% to 40% of normal, which is why drug dosage regimens are typically not adjusted until two thirds of renal function has been lost.[16] In human patients Cr clearance is quantified by determining urinary Cr excretion over a 24-hour period. The measured Cr clearance is then used in formulas to make drug dosage adjustments. Unlike in human medicine, values for Cr clearance are not usually available for veterinary patients. When Cr clearance is not available, a single value of the patient's serum creatinine can be substituted in the formulas. However, the relationship between serum creatinine is not linear once serum creatinine is above 4 mg/dl, so the adjustment formulas are even less accurate for predicting an ideal dose adjustment.[16] These formulas do not account for changes in the volume of distribution, degree of protein binding, and nonrenal clearance mechanisms of the drug that may be caused by the renal dysfunction. Therefore these dosage adjustments must be regarded as preliminary estimations to be followed by adjustments based on observed clinical response.

Dose-Reduction Method

With the dose-reduction method the normal dosage regimen is adjusted by reducing the drug dose and maintaining the drug dosing interval.

Adjusted dose = Normal Dose × (Patient's Cr clearance ÷ Normal Cr clearance)

or

Adjusted dose = Normal Dose × (Normal Cr) Patient's Cr)

Interval-Extension Method

With the interval-extension method the drug dose is maintained and the drug dosing interval is extended.

Adjusted Interval = Normal Interval [1/(Patient's Cr clearance/Normal Cr clearance)]

or

Adjusted Interval = Normal Interval [1/(Normal Serum Cr/ Patient's Serum Cr)]

Both methods attempt to keep the average plasma drug concentrations constant. The interval-extension method produces Cmax and Cmin values similar to those seen in healthy patients (Figure 4-17), but it does produce substantial periods of time during which drug concentrations may be subtherapeutic. This is the preferred method with aminoglycosides, which have a long postantibiotic effect and in which a low trough concentration is desirable to reduce the risk of nephrotoxicity. Depending on the relationship of the elimination half-life to the dosage interval, significant drug accumulation may occur with the dose-reduction method (Figure 4-18), but at steady-state there are no periods of time during which concentrations are subtherapeutic. This is the preferred method for the penicillin and cephalosporin antibiotics, wherein maintaining the plasma concentration above the pathogen's minimum inhibitory concentration (MIC) correlates with efficacy and the drugs are relatively nontoxic even if accumulation occurs. To decide which method to use, the practitioner should determine if drug efficacy and toxicity are related to peak, trough, or average plasma concentrations and then select the method that best balances efficacy against potential toxicity. The interval-extension method is more convenient for the client because the normal recommended dose is simply administered less frequently. In addition, if the drugs are available only in fixed dosage forms (e.g., capsules, unbreakable tablets), it is easier to adjust the dosage interval.

Because the elimination half-life is prolonged in patients with renal disease and it always takes six elimination half-lives to reach 99% of steady-state concentrations, there is a delay in reaching steady-state in horses with renal failure compared with horses with normal renal function. Therefore it may be necessary to administer a loading dose to rapidly achieve therapeutic drug concentrations. If the dose-reduction method

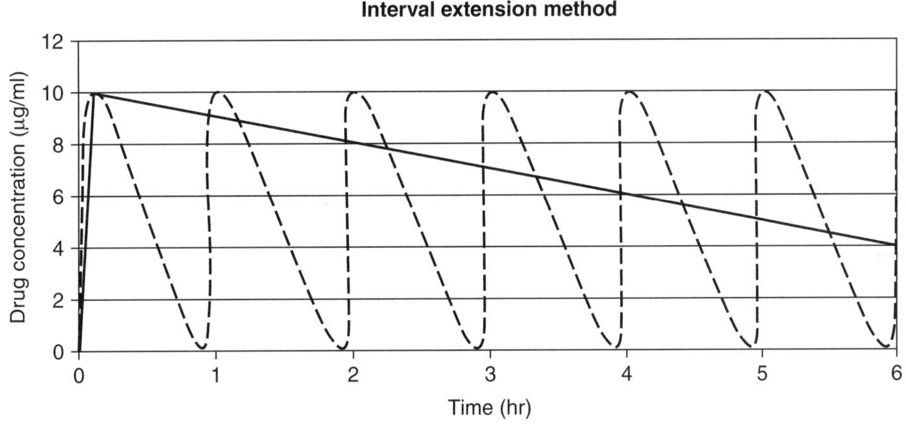

FIGURE 4-17 Comparison of an interval-extension dosage regimen *(solid line)* in a renal failure patient with a normal dosage regimen in a healthy patient *(dotted line).* Normal elimination half-life was 15 minutes; in the patient with renal failure, it increased to 8 hours.

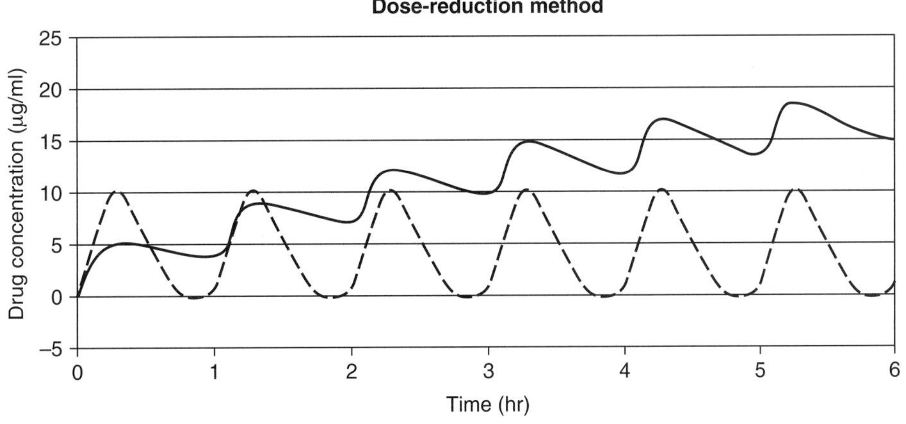

FIGURE 4-18 Comparison of a dose-reduction dosage regimen in a renal failure patient *(solid line)* compared with a normal dosage regimen in a healthy patient *(dotted line).* Normal elimination half-life was 15 minutes; in the renal failure patient, it increased to 8 hours.

is used, this is achieved by giving the usual dose initially, followed by the reduced dose at the next time. If the interval-extension method is used, this is accomplished by giving a double dose initially.

For renal failure patients in general, the practitioner must consider the following:

1. Avoid using any drugs at all, unless there are definite therapeutic indications. If a drug is absolutely necessary, try to select one that is hepatically metabolized and excreted in bile rather than eliminated by the kidneys (e.g., doxycycline).
2. If therapeutic drug monitoring is available, tailor the drug dosage regimen to that specific patient.
3. If therapeutic drug monitoring is unavailable, determine if there are clinically proven, adjusted dosage regimens for specific drugs. The package insert that accompanies pharmaceuticals intended for human use often gives guidelines for adjusting dosages.
4. If the drug has not been sufficiently studied to have dosage adjustment recommendations, determine if there is sufficient information about its kinetics to estimate the proper drug dose in renal failure.
5. Carefully monitor treated patients for signs of efficacy and toxicity.

ANTIMICROBIAL THERAPY

Patricia M. Dowling, Jennifer L. Davis

Successful antimicrobial therapy relies on administering sufficient doses so that pathogens at the site of infection are killed or suppressed to the extent that they can be eliminated by the host's immune system. There are complex pharmacokinetic (PK) and pharmacodynamic (PD) relationships among the host, the bacteria, and the antimicrobial. Pharmacokinetics is what the body does to a drug; the processes of absorption, distribution to the various organs and tissues, metabolism of lipid-soluble drugs into water-soluble metabolites, and finally renal excretion. Pharmacodynamics is what the antimicrobial does to the bacteria. It describes the drug action and responses of the bacteria. Pharmacokinetics and pharmacodynamics are interrelated in that PK effects determine the amount of drug that reaches the site of action, and the intensity of a PD effect is associated with the drug concentration at the site of action. New information on the PK/PD relationships of veterinary pathogens and antimicrobials is rapidly emerging and changing the way in which the dosage of antimicrobials is determined in equine practice.

RATIONAL USE OF ANTIMICROBIAL AGENTS

The following questions must be considered when developing an antimicrobial regimen:

1. *Does the diagnosis warrant antimicrobial therapy?* Using antimicrobials to treat minor infections or purely viral or inflammatory diseases is irrational, expensive, and potentially hazardous to the patient; it also encourages antimicrobial resistance. Clients have come to expect antimicrobials for trivial infections or in the event that an infection may develop. Equine practitioners must resist client pressure to use or prescribe unnecessary drugs.
2. *What organism(s) are likely to be involved?* For many infections the likely organism can be successfully predicted on the basis of the history and clinical signs.
3. *What is the in vitro antimicrobial susceptibility of the organism?* For many pathogens the *in vitro* susceptibility can be reliably predicted. For example, *Streptococcus* species are typically susceptible to penicillin. However, many gram negative bacteria have unpredictable susceptibilities, and susceptibility testing is essential for determining appropriate drug therapy.
4. *In what part of the body or tissue is the infection located? Will the antimicrobial penetrate to the infection?* Consideration of the pathophysiology of the infection will help the practitioner select an effective therapy. Treatment of sequestered infections such as mastitis or meningitis requires antimicrobials that readily cross membrane barriers. Antimicrobials characterized by low values for volume of distribution (Vd) are unlikely to reach therapeutic concentrations in such sites.
5. *Will the antimicrobial be effective in the local environment of the organism?* The local infection environment reduces the efficacy of some antimicrobials. Sulfonamides are ineffective in purulent debris because para-amino benzoic acid (PABA) released from decaying neutrophils serves as a PABA source for bacteria and reduces the competitive effect of the sulfonamide. Aminoglycosides are ineffective in an abscess because of the acidic, anaerobic environment along with the presence of nucleic acid material from decaying cells, which inactivates the aminoglycosides.
6. *What drug formulation and dose regimen will maintain the appropriate antimicrobial concentration for the proper duration of time?* Label doses apply only to label pathogens. For off-label uses the dosage regimen must be adjusted depending on the antimicrobial susceptibility of the specific pathogen.
7. *What adverse drug reactions or toxicities might be expected? Do the benefits outweigh the risks?* The risks of adverse reactions from antimicrobials are often underappreciated. A serious adverse reaction may complicate treatment of the original problem and even be fatal. Failure to communicate the risks of adverse drug reactions to clients is a common cause of litigation.
8. *Can you choose an approved product? If using an antimicrobial in an off-label manner, can you determine appropriate withdrawal times for food animals? Can you determine appropriate withdrawal times for performance horses?* The antimicrobials used in horses are not approved for horses intended for food, and information on appropriate withdrawal times is lacking. Also, competitive horses are subject to the rules of the sport's governing association regarding drugs, which vary according to the organization, state or province, and country. Understanding the principles of drug elimination allows the practitioner to determine appropriate withdrawal times for competitive or slaughter horses.

DOCUMENTING THE INFECTION

A diagnosis must be established before any therapy can be administered. It is not always necessary to culture samples from all patients with infectious diseases to identify the organism involved. Often the practitioner can base a diagnosis on clinical experience from similar cases. The signs of some infectious diseases are so obvious that the need for microbiological identification is minimal; however, for those infectious diseases of unknown cause or for those attributable to organisms with irregular antimicrobial susceptibility, there is no substitute for isolation and identification of the causative agent. For these organisms initial therapy while waiting for culture results must include an antimicrobial with a broad spectrum of activity. However, broad spectrum drugs are usually more toxic and more expensive than narrow spectrum drugs. The use of broad spectrum antimicrobials for relatively trivial infections encourages development of antimicrobial-resistant organisms. Without evidence of a susceptible pathogen, such use is irrational and exposes the patient to unnecessary risks.

Whenever possible, the veterinarian should obtain a representative sample of material from a clinical patient. Beware of sampling grossly contaminated sites such as purulent nasal discharges. An immediate Gram stain can be performed from a direct smear and will direct initial therapy. Samples are submitted for appropriate culture and identification. If the identified organism has unpredictable susceptibility patterns, the practitioner should request a susceptibility test, such as Kirby-Bauer, E test, or MIC method.

In some clinical cases identification of the pathogen may be made by serologic demonstration of antibodies (e.g., anaplasmosis, leptospirosis, brucellosis).

Antimicrobial Dosage Regimen Design

Successful antimicrobial therapy relies on administering sufficient doses so that pathogens at the site of infection are killed or suppressed to the extent that they can be eliminated by the host's immune system. The relationship among the host, the bacteria, and the drug may be very complex. High plasma antimicrobial concentrations are *assumed* to be advantageous in that a large concentration of drug will diffuse into various tissues and body fluids. Drug concentration at the infection site is assumed to be of major importance in determining drug efficacy. Drug movement from the plasma to extravascular tissues depends on molecular size, lipid solubility, drug pKa, local pH, specific cellular transport mechanisms, and degree of protein binding. The relationship between bacteria and drug in the laboratory is described by the following:

MIC: The lowest drug concentration that inhibits bacterial growth.

Minimum bactericidal concentration (MBC): The lowest drug concentration that kills 99.9% of bacteria.

The MICs are used to determine the drug dose, in an attempt to achieve blood and tissue concentrations that exceed the in vitro MIC for the pathogen.

Interpreting Minimum Inhibitory Concentrations

According to the Clinical Laboratory Standards Institute (CLSI, formerly known as *NCCLS)* definition, the MIC values are derived as serially doubled concentrations (in μg/ml). Susceptible (S), intermediate (I), and resistant (R) designations are derived from *breakpoints* assigned by laboratory-based PK and PD data, pathogen population MIC distribution, and clinical trial results.[1] A CLSI-approved breakpoint is specific for the animal species, disease, pathogen, antimicrobial, and dosage regimen. When a pathogen is reported as *susceptible*, it means that the recommended dosage of the antimicrobial will reach plasma or tissue concentrations that will inhibit bacterial growth in vivo. When a pathogen is reported as *resistant*, inhibitory antimicrobial concentrations are not safely attainable in the patient. If the pathogen is reported as *intermediate*, then administering the antimicrobial at higher-than-recommended doses may result in effective therapy.[2] Susceptibility testing results predict which bacteria have intrinsic or acquired resistance mechanisms to a particular antimicrobial. In vitro tests do this because bacterial susceptibility usually clusters around a small range of MICs. In Figure 4-19 the bacterial inhibition of *E. coli* by amoxicillin has a bimodal distribution. The large cluster of *Escherichia coli* inhibited by amoxicillin concentrations of 0.5 to 16 μg/ml are considered the *normal range* and 16 μg/ml is considered the breakpoint of susceptibility. *E. coli* requiring an amoxicillin concentration of 16 μg/ml to be inhibited are likely to have intrinsic or acquired resistance mechanisms, and amoxicillin is unlikely to be a successful treatment for patients infected with these isolates. In vitro susceptibility tests predict treatment outcome

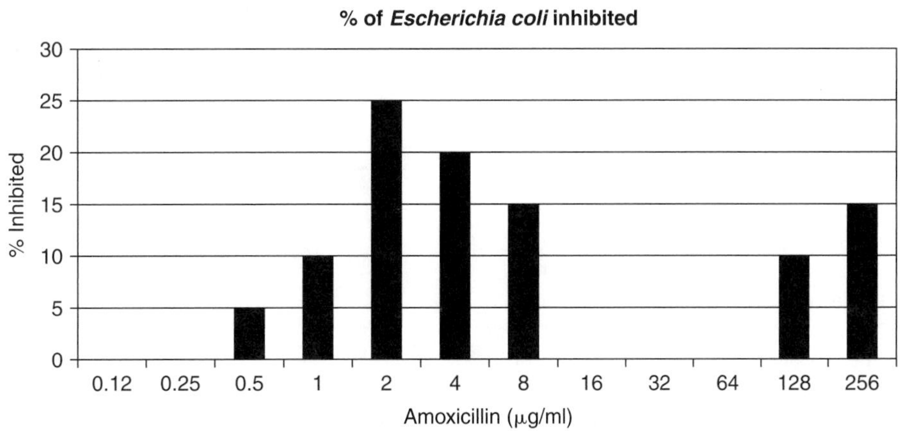

FIGURE 4-19 The percentage of *Escherichia coli* inhibited by increasing concentrations of amoxicillin has a bimodal distribution. *E. coli* requiring more than 16 μg/ml of amoxicillin to be inhibited are likely to have intrinsic or acquired resistance mechanisms. Amoxicillin therapy in patients with this pathogen is unlikely to be effective.

fairly well, considering that many variables in the host-pathogen relationship are not taken into account.[1] Antimicrobial susceptibility data may not account for the following:

1. *Host defenses*: The interaction between the host and the pathogen is complex and not predicted by in vitro tests. Antimicrobial drug action takes place in concert with host defenses such as humoral and cell-mediated immunity; complement components; and nonspecific antibacterial factors such as lactoferrin, lactoperoxidase, and lysozyme.[3]
2. *Drug distribution in the body:* The *S, I,* and *R* designations assigned by the microbiology laboratory are typically based on safely achievable plasma concentrations. This does not necessarily take into account extremely high concentrations of antimicrobials achieved in organs and fluids of excretion (kidney, urine, bile) or with local administration of high drug concentrations (e.g., ophthalmic ointments). Macrolide antimicrobials are characterized by negligible plasma concentrations despite very high lung concentrations.[4] Pathophysiology may alter drug distribution, and some antimicrobials, such as the tetracyclines, accumulate in pneumonic lung tissues.[5]
3. *Growth rates and size of inoculum:* The incubator of the microbiology laboratory is an ideal setting for bacterial growth. Conditions are managed to promote rapid growth, and rapidly dividing bacteria are more susceptible to antimicrobial drugs. Replication rates may be much slower at the infection site, and MICs are generally unreliable for slow-growing bacteria. Standardized inoculums used in the laboratory may over- or under-represent pathogen numbers in infected tissues.[3]
4. *Mixed infections*: Separate susceptibility testing of pathogens in a mixed infection does not account for the pathologic synergism between bacteria. The by-products of one bacterium may facilitate the establishment and growth of another.[6]
5. *Infection environment:* Many antimicrobials are inactive in purulent exudate, which is typically anaerobic, acidic, and hyperosmolar. Some antimicrobials have different activity in body fluids (e.g., plasma, milk, bile) than in nutrient-rich laboratory media. Deposition of fibrin may alter tissue penetration of antimicrobials. Many bacteria are capable of producing a polysaccharide slime capsule to protect them from host factors. Mastitis pathogens typically increase their replication rate when incubated in mastitic milk.[3]
7. *Topically administered antimicrobials are not tested:* Veterinary microbiology laboratories may not routinely do susceptibility testing for antimicrobials that are used only topically. Polymixin B is one of the most effective antimicrobials for superficial *Pseudomonas* infections,[7] but because it causes neurotoxicity and nephrotoxicity if administered systemically, it is rarely included in susceptibility testing. Bacitracin and mupirocin are other examples of topical antimicrobials rarely tested by diagnostic laboratories.
8. *In vivo synergism may occur with antimicrobial combinations:* Despite predictions of resistance from susceptibility testing, therapy may be successful because of synergistic combinations of antimicrobials. Synergism between penicillins and aminoglycosides has been recognized for streptococcal, enterococcal, and staphylococcal infections.[8] The synergism is attributed to increased cellular uptake of the aminoglycoside after cell wall damage from the penicillin.
9. *The CLSI breakpoints may be inappropriate:* The CLSI breakpoints were originally established with bacterial isolates from humans, using human PK data and clinical trials. A veterinary subcommittee was established in 1993 and has proposed veterinary-specific guidelines for susceptibility tests for a limited number of antimicrobials.[9] Currently, only ceftiofur, ampicillin, and gentamicin have CLSI-approved breakpoints for equine pathogens. Diagnostic laboratories use human-derived breakpoints for other bacteria-drug combinations.

Therefore the true relevance of any in vitro MIC in predicting the in vivo results of drug therapy is questionable. The MIC results are not a positive order to use a particular antimicrobial. Selection of the optimal antimicrobial must take into consideration other factors, such as the site of infection, pharmacokinetics of the drugs, and effect of underlying diseases. Considering all of these factors, most veterinarians determine a drug dosage regimen that uses a target plasma drug concentration based on a multiple of the in vitro MIC (usually 2 to 10).

Bactericidal Versus Bacteriostatic Antimicrobials

It is common to classify antimicrobials as *bactericidal* or *bacteriostatic* (Box 4-5). If the ratio of the MBC to MIC is small (<4 to 6), a drug is considered bactericidal, and it is possible to obtain drug concentrations that will kill 99.9% of the organisms exposed. If the ratio of MBC to MIC is large, it may not be possible to safely administer dosages of the drug to kill 99.9% of the bacteria, and the drug is considered bacteriostatic.

For many drugs the distinction between bactericidal and bacteriostatic is not exact and depends on the drug concentration attained in the target tissue and the pathogen involved. Specific situations in which a bactericidal drug is preferred over a bacteriostatic drug include immunocompromised patients such as neonates, life-threatening infections such as bacterial endocarditis and meningitis, and surgical prophylaxis.

Postantibiotic Effect

For some bacteria-antimicrobial interactions, bacterial growth remains suppressed for a period after drug concentration has decreased below the MIC.[10] This postantibiotic effect (PAE) may be the reason that dosage regimens that fail to maintain

BOX 4-5

CLASSIFICATION OF ANTIMICROBIALS

Bactericidal

Aminoglycosides
β-lactams
Fluoroquinolones
Trimethoprim/sulfonamides

Bacteriostatic

Chloramphenicol
Macrolides
Sulfonamides
Tetracyclines

TABLE 4-6

Length of Postantibiotic Effect for Selected Antimicrobials and Antibiotics

Microbe	Long PAE (>3 Hours)	Intermediate PAE	Short PAE (<1 Hour)
Gram positive	Fluoroquinolones	Aminoglycosides	—
	Macrolides	Penicillins	—
	Chloramphenicol	Cephalosporins	—
	Tetracycline	—	—
Gram negative	Fluoroquinolones	—	Penicillins
	Aminoglycosides	—	Cephalosporins
	—	—	Trimethoprim/sulfanomides
Anaerobes	Metronidazole	—	—

PAE, Postantibiotic effect.

drug concentration above the MIC are still efficacious. The PAE depends on the antimicrobial and the bacterial pathogen (Table 4-6).

Pharmacokinetic-Pharmacodynamic Relationships

The PK-PD relationship between an antimicrobial and a pathogen determines the way that the dosage regimen is calculated.[11] The PK parameters used in drug dosage design are the area under the plasma concentration versus time curve (AUC) from 0 to 24 hours, the maximum plasma concentration (Cmax), and the time the antimicrobial concentration exceeds a defined PD threshold (T). The most commonly used PD parameter is the MIC. In relating the PK and PD parameters to clinical efficacy, antimicrobial drug action is classified as either concentration dependent or time dependent (Box 4-6; Figures 4-20 and 4-21). For antimicrobials whose efficacy is concentration dependent, high plasma concentrations relative to the MIC of the pathogen (Cmax:MIC) and the area under the plasma concentration-time curve that is above the bacterial MIC during the dosage interval (area under the inhibitory curve, AUC_{0-24}:MIC) are the major determinants of clinical efficacy. These drugs also have prolonged PAEs, thereby allowing once-a-day dosing while maintaining maximum clinical efficacy. For fluoroquinolones (e.g., enrofloxacin, orbifloxacin, difloxacin, marbofloxacin), clinical efficacy is associated with achieving either an AUC_{0-24}:MIC greater than 125 or a Cmax:MIC greater than 10. For aminoglycosides (e.g., gentamicin, amikacin), achieving a Cmax:MIC greater than 10 is considered optimal for efficacy. Other antimicrobials that appear to have concentration-dependent activity include metronidazole (Cmax:MIC>10-25) and azithromycin AUC_{0-24}:MIC):MIC>25). For some pathogens with very high MIC values, such as *Pseudomonas aeruginosa*, achieving the optimum PK/PD ratios may be impossible with label or even higher-than-label dosages. In such cases underdosing is ineffective and merely contributes to antimicrobial resistance.

For antimicrobials whose efficacy is time dependent, the time during which the antimicrobial concentration exceeds the MIC of the pathogen determines clinical efficacy (T>MIC). How much above the MIC and for what percentage of the dosing interval concentrations should be above the MIC are still being debated and are likely specific for individual bacteria-drug combinations. Typically, exceeding the MIC by 1 to 5 multiples for between 40% and 100% of the dosage interval is appropriate for time-dependent killers. The T>MIC should be closer to 100% for bacteriostatic antimicrobials and for patients that are immunosuppressed. These drugs typically require frequent dosing or constant rate infusions for appropriate therapy. In sequestered infections penetration of the antimicrobial to the site of infection may require high plasma concentrations to achieve a sufficient concentration gradient. In such cases the AUC_{0-24} hr:MIC and/or Cmax:MIC may also be important in determining efficacy of otherwise time-dependent antimicrobials.

BOX 4-6

CLASSIFICATION OF ANTIMICROBIALS BASED ON MEANS OF EFFECT

Concentration-Dependent

Aminoglycosides
Fluoroquinolones
Metronidazole

Time-Dependent

Cephalosporins
Chloramphenicol
Macrolides
Penicillins
Sulfonamides
Tetracyclines

DESIGNING THE DRUG DOSAGE REGIMEN

When designing specific antimicrobial dosage regimens, the practitioner targets a specific plasma drug concentration. High plasma antimicrobial concentrations are *assumed* to be advantageous in that a large concentration of drug will diffuse into various tissues and body fluids. In light of the previous information, antimicrobial dosage regimens are designed in one of two ways: either to maximize plasma concentration or to

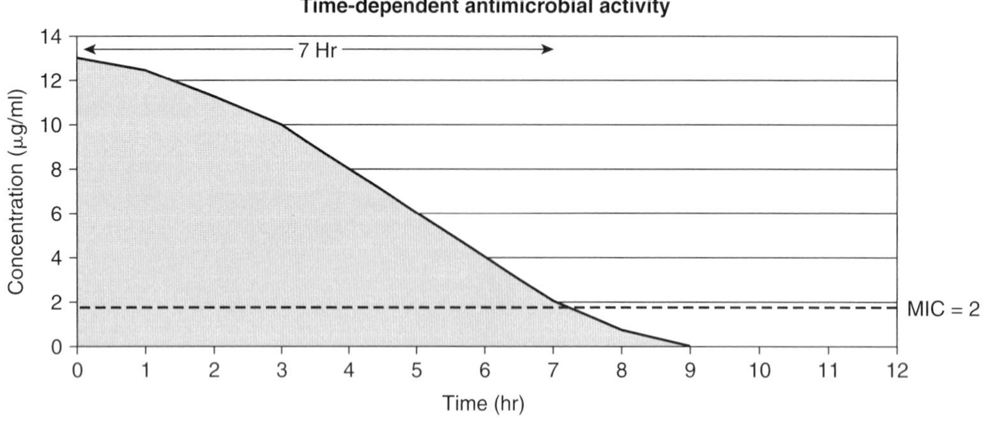

FIGURE 4-20 For time-dependent antimicrobials the time during which the antimicrobial concentration exceeds the minimum inhibitory concentration of the pathogen determines clinical efficacy.

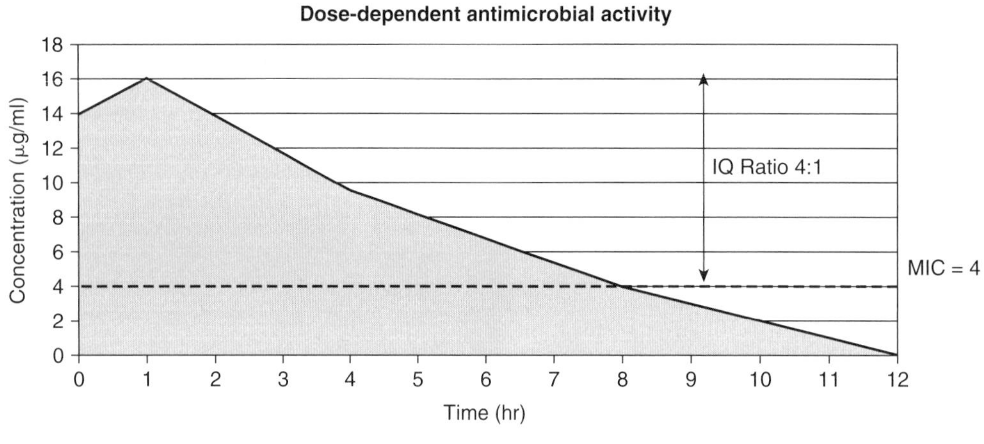

FIGURE 4-21 For concentration-dependent antimicrobials, the inhibitory quotient *(IQ)* and the area under the inhibitory curve are the major determinants of clinical efficacy.

provide a plasma concentration above the bacterial MIC for some percentage of the dosage interval.

For *concentration-dependent killers* with a prolonged PAE whose PK-PD relationship is to have an ideal Cmax:MIC, and if the volume of distribution (Vd) of the antimicrobial is known, a precise drug dosage regimen for the pathogen can be calculated from the following equation:

$$\text{Dose} = (V_d)\,(\text{desired plasma concentration})$$

where the desired plasma concentration is some multiple of the MIC (usually 8-10) and once-daily dosing is assumed.

For *concentration-dependent killers* whose PK-PD relationship is to have an ideal AUC_{0-24}:MIC, the following equation can be used to calculate a daily dose:

$$\text{Dose} = \frac{(AUC_{0-24}:\text{MIC})\,(\text{MIC})\,(\text{Cl})}{(\text{F})\,(24\ \text{hr})}$$

where AUC_{0-24}:MIC is ≥ 100, Cl is clearance (volume of blood cleared of drug per day in ml/kg/day), and F is bioavailability.

For *time-dependent killers* the objective is to keep the average plasma drug concentration above the pathogen's MIC for the duration of the dosage interval. Again, by using Vd and elimination half-life information, the practitioner can precisely calculate a dosing regimen:

$$\text{Dose} = \frac{(\text{desired avg plasma conc})\,(\text{Vd})(\text{dosage interval})}{1.44(t1/2)}$$

CONCURRENT USE OF ADDITIONAL ANTIMICROBIALS

Combination antimicrobial therapy is commonplace in veterinary medicine, but combination therapy has rarely been demonstrated as superior to single drug therapy through clinical trials. Use of multiple antimicrobial drugs should be limited to the following cases:

1. Known synergism against specific organisms[8]
2. Prevention of rapid development of bacterial resistance[12]
3. To extend antimicrobial spectrum of initial therapy of life-threatening conditions[13]
4. To treat known mixed bacterial infections[14]

Multiple antimicrobial therapy is implicated as a cause of diarrhea in horses, likely from the additive antibacterial effects against normal gastrointestinal flora.[15] Antagonistic combinations such as penicillin and tetracyclines should be avoided; penicillins require actively dividing bacteria to exert their bactericidal effects on the bacterial cell wall, and the bacteriostatic action of tetracyclines suppress cell wall formation.[2]

PROPHYLACTIC USE OF ANTIMICROBIALS

There are few reports examining the efficacy of prophylactic antimicrobials in veterinary medicine in general and in horses specifically.[16] Because of the lack of controlled veterinary studies, information on prophylaxis is largely extrapolated from human studies. The relative risk of infection must warrant the use of prophylactic antimicrobials. The risks of adverse effects from the prophylactic drug must be less than the risk of development of disease and its consequences. In veterinary medicine most of the risk of infection depends on the skill of the surgeon and handling practices in the hospital.[17] The organism or organisms that are likely to cause the infection and their antimicrobial susceptibility should be known or accurately predicted. The antimicrobial should be bactericidal and must be administered and distributed to the site of potential infection before the onset of infection. The veterinarian should consider drugs that can be given intravenously and have a high volume of distribution. Drugs used prophylactically should not be those that would be used therapeutically. The duration of antimicrobial prophylaxis should be as abbreviated as possible. Most of the time a single preoperative dose is sufficient and cost effective.[18]

β-LACTAMS: PENICILLINS AND CEPHALOSPORINS

The β-lactam antibiotics are among the most commonly used antibiotics. Their use and popularity are due to their safety, efficacy, flexibility in dosage forms, and relatively low expense. Both penicillins and cephalosporins have a four-member β-lactam ring. The β-lactam ring is unstable and is a major target for bacterial resistance mechanisms.

Mechanism of Action

β-lactam antibiotics act on enzymes called *penicillin-binding proteins (PBPs)* responsible for building the bacterial cell wall.[2] Therefore they are active only against rapidly multiplying organisms in which the binding of penicillin within the cell wall interferes with production of cell wall peptidoglycans and results in cell lysis in a hypo- or iso-osmotic environment. There may be anywhere between two to eight PBPs in a bacteria. When β-lactam antibiotics bind covalently and irreversibly to the PBPs, the bacterial cell wall is disrupted and lysis occurs. Differences in the spectrum and action of β-lactam antibiotics are due to their relative affinity for different PBPs. To bind to the PBPs, the β-lactam antibiotic must first diffuse through the bacterial cell wall. Gram negative organisms have an additional lipopolysaccharide layer that decreases antibiotic penetration. Therefore gram positive bacteria are usually more susceptible to the action of β-lactams than gram negative bacteria. Because the penicillins poorly penetrate mammalian cells, they are ineffective in the treatment of intracellular pathogens.

Resistance Mechanisms

Resistance mechanisms to the β-lactams include failure of the antibiotic to penetrate the outer bacterial cell layers and alteration of PBPs that decrease the affinity of the PBP for the antibiotic.[19-21] Alterations of the PBPs occur with methicillin-resistant staphylococci.[22] A third mechanism of resistance is from production of β-lactamase enzymes.[23,24] There may be as many as 50 β-lactamase enzymes (penicillinases, cephalosporinases) produced by bacteria. These enzymes hydrolyze the cyclic amide bond of the β-lactam ring and inactivate the antibiotic. Staphylococcal β-lactamases are produced by coagulase positive *Staphylococcus* spp. The synthesis of these enzymes is plasmid encoded, and the enzymes are exocellular. These enzymes typically do not inactivate cephalosporins and antistaphylococcal penicillins. Most of these β-lactamases can be inactivated by inhibitors such as clavulanic acid and sulbactam. The Gram negative β-lactamases are a diverse group of enzymes that can be chromosomal coded, plasmid coded, or both. *E. coli* lactamase is coded by plasmids and hydrolyzes both cephalosporins and penicillins. Chromosomal-mediated lactamases hydrolyze penicillin, cephalosporins, or both.

BENZYLPENICILLIN (PENICILLIN G)

Penicillin G was the first antibiotic developed and remains one of the most effective antibiotics available. It is still the initial drug of choice for many bacterial infections.

Spectrum of Activity

Aerobic bacteria susceptible to penicillin G include most β-hemolytic streptococci, β-lactamase-negative staphylococci, *Actinomyces* spp., some *Bacillus anthracis, Corynebacterium* spp., and *Erysipelothrix rhusiopathiae*.[25] Most species of anaerobes are susceptible, excluding β-lactamase–producing *Bacteroides* spp.[26] Penicillin G is easily inactivated by β-lactamases and has little efficacy against organisms that can produce these enzymes. In addition, penicillin G is ineffective against those bacteria that are resistant by other mechanisms, such as having a relatively impermeable cell wall. Therefore penicillin G has little activity against many staphylococci and most gram negative bacteria.[23]

Pharmacokinetics

ABSORPTION

Because penicillin is a weak acid with a pKa of 2.7, it is highly ionized in plasma. Gastric absorption of penicillin G is poor because it is rapidly hydrolyzed in the acid environment of the stomach. Phenoxymethyl penicillin (penicillin V) can be given orally to horses and has a half-life of absorption of 0.2 hours.[27] The sodium and potassium salts of penicillin G are the only dosage forms that are suitable for IV administration and are quickly absorbed from intramuscular or subcutaneous sites of administration.[28] Procaine penicillin G is more slowly absorbed from intramuscular administration than are the sodium or potassium salts and so produces lower but more sustained plasma concentrations. Benzathine penicillin G is the least soluble of the dosage forms; it is very slowly absorbed, producing sustained but subtherapeutic plasma concentrations of penicillin G.[28] The rate of absorption from intramuscular injections of procaine penicillin G varies depending on the injection site, with injections into the neck muscle producing more rapid absorption and higher plasma concentrations than with injections into the hindquarters.[29]

DISTRIBUTION

The Vd of sodium penicillin G is 0.7 L/kg,[30] and there is a moderate degree of protein binding (52%-54%).[31] After absorption penicillin is distributed mainly in extracellular fluid and may not reach therapeutic concentrations in sequestered infections.[32]

ELIMINATION

Elimination of penicillin is primarily renal, as unchanged drug by glomerular filtration and active renal tubular secretion. The elimination half-life of penicillin G is 1 hour,[31,32] and total clearance is 8.5 ± 1.33 mL/min/kg.[30] Oral penicillin V has an elimination half-life of 3.7 hours.[27]

Adverse Effects and Drug Interactions

IMMUNE-MEDIATED REACTIONS

Penicillin is associated with immune-mediated hemolytic anemia (Type II hypersensitivity),[33,34] and anaphylaxis (Type I hypersensitivity) in horses.[35] The immune-mediated anemia usually resolves with discontinuation of penicillin therapy. Anaphylaxis usually occurs after previous exposure to penicillin and can be fatal. IV epinephrine and oxygen administration and respiratory support are indicated. Although it is widely assumed that penicillin and cephalosporins are cross-reactive in sensitive individuals, the actual incidence in humans is extremely low.[36]

PROCAINE REACTIONS AND USE IN PERFORMANCE HORSES

When procaine penicillin G products are accidentally administered intravascularly, they cause extreme central nervous system stimulation.[37,38] Most horses will survive unless they fatally traumatize themselves during the reaction. Diazepam will attenuate the reaction if given before procaine administration but has no effect if given afterwards.[37] Veterinary formulations contain higher concentrations of procaine than human formulations, and high temperatures increase the solubility of procaine. Therefore penicillin procaine G should be kept refrigerated and administered by careful intramuscular injection. Even with careful intramuscular injection, adverse reactions are still reported in horses. Repeated injections increase the chance of intravascular administration and may increase the sensitivity to procaine as a result of neuronal sensitization (kindling). Once absorbed into the circulation, procaine is hydrolyzed by plasma esterases to the nontoxic metabolites PABA and diethylaminoethanol.[39] Horses that have had documented adverse reactions to intramuscular procaine penicillin G injections had significantly lower procaine hydrolyzing capacity compared with horses that did not have a history of adverse reactions.[40] Procaine is slowly eliminated in urine, is easily detectable by regulatory laboratories, and commonly causes violative residues in racehorses and performance horses given penicillin procaine G.[41]

ELECTROLYTE IMBALANCES

The sodium or potassium content of IV formulations can contribute to electrolyte imbalances associated with congestive heart failure and renal function impairment. A million units of potassium penicillin contain 1.7 mEq of potassium, so it should be administered by slow IV injection.

PHENYLBUTAZONE

Concurrent administration with phenylbutazone in horses increases plasma concentrations of penicillin G but lowers tissue concentrations. The effect is likely due to a lower peripheral distribution.[30]

Formulations

Na^+ and K^+ penicillin (also called *crystalline penicillin*) are water-soluble formulations and may be injected intravenously, intramuscularly, or subcutaneously. They achieve rapid plasma concentrations but have very short elimination half-lives and therefore must be administered frequently or by continuous rate infusion. Potassium penicillin is usually less expensive than sodium penicillin but must be administered more carefully because rapid IV administration can cause cardiac arrhythmias. Procaine penicillin G is a poorly soluble salt that is slowly absorbed after intramuscular injection. It is the most commonly used formulation of penicillin in horses. Benzathine penicillin G is a very insoluble salt that is used in long-acting penicillin preparations, which contain a 50:50 mixture of procaine penicillin G and benzathine penicillin G. Because the benzathine fraction is poorly absorbed and plasma concentrations are below the MICs of most pathogens, use of these products is not recommended in horses.[32]

Clinical Use

Penicillin is still the antimicrobial of choice for many diseases in horses, such as streptococcal and anaerobic infections. Traumatic wounds are frequently infected with *Streptococcus zooepidemicus*, which is routinely susceptible to penicillin.[13] However, iatrogenic wounds are frequently infected with penicillinase-producing *Staphylococcus aureus* or other staphylococci, so culture and susceptibility testing is necessary before initiating penicillin therapy.[13,42]

The IV formulations are used when high doses are necessary for adequate concentrations at the site of infection in life-threatening situations. The dosage of penicillin G varies greatly depending on the formulation, species, and disease being treated.

AMINOPENICILLINS

Spectrum of Activity

The aminopenicillins are able to penetrate the outer layer of gram negative bacteria better than penicillin G; therefore they have activity against many of the gram negative bacteria (*E. coli, Salmonella, Pasteurella* spp.) as well as gram positive bacteria.[2] However, resistance to the aminopenicillins is easily acquired by gram negative bacteria, so they are not usually effective against *Klebsiella, Proteus, Pseudomonas, and S. aureus*. Most anaerobes are sensitive, except β-lactamase producing strains of *Bacteroides*.[26] Amoxicillin penetrates the gram negative cell more easily than does ampicillin; therefore it has greater activity against gram negative bacteria.[25]

Pharmacokinetics

ABSORPTION

In horses ampicillin sodium is well absorbed after intramuscular or subcutaneous administration; however, oral dosage forms are poorly absorbed by adult horses.[43] The intramuscular administration of ampicillin trihydrate produces lower ampicillin blood concentrations that extend over a longer period of time than does intramuscular ampicillin sodium.[43] Oral absorption of amoxicillin is between 5.3% and 10.4% in adult horses[44,45] but between 36% and 42% in foals.[46] The ampicillin prodrugs are converted to ampicillin as they are absorbed from the gastrointestinal tract. Compared with the bioavailability of oral ampicillin (2%), the ampicillin esters have improved oral bioavailabilities in adult horses: pivampicillin (31%), bacampicillin (39%), and talampicillin (23%).[47] The low oral bioavailability of ampicillin esters is due to chemical hydrolysis in the high pH of equine ileal contents.

DISTRIBUTION

The aminopenicillins are rapidly and widely distributed into most body fluids; distribution into cerebrospinal fluid is low unless the meninges are inflamed. The Vd of amoxicillin in adult horses is 0.19[48] and 0.27 L/kg in neonatal foals.[46] The Vd of ampicillin in horses ranges between 0.18 to 0.7 L/kg.[49,50] Peak serum concentrations of ampicillin are 6.2 to 9.7 μg/ml 16 minutes after an intramuscular dose of 10 mg/kg of ampicillin sodium.[43] Penetration into synovial fluid is high,[43,51] and concentrations are increased and persist in infected joints.[52] In a subcutaneous tissue chamber model in ponies, concentrations of IV ampicillin sodium, oral pivampicillin, and intramuscular procaine penicillin G remained above the MIC of *Streptococcus zooepidemicus* for 8, 12, and 24 hours, respectively.[53] The protein binding of amoxicillin is moderate (37%-38%),[54] whereas it is low for ampicillin (6%-8%).[31]

ELIMINATION

Amoxicillin and ampicillin are primarily excreted unchanged in the urine. The elimination half-life of amoxicillin is approximately 1 hour in horses and foals.[45,46,52,54] The elimination half-life of ampicillin ranges between 0.5 hour to 2.3 hours.[43,49,50,55,56]

Adverse Effects and Drug Interactions

Amoxicillin and ampicillin have the same adverse effects as penicillin G. Their spectrum of action is greatly enhanced when combined with β-lactamase inhibitors such as clavulanic acid and sulbactam.

Formulations

Sodium ampicillin is available as a human aqueous formulation for IV, intramuscular, and subcutaneous injection. The reconstituted aqueous formulations are unstable after more than a few hours. Ampicillin trihydrate is a poorly soluble, slow-release aqueous suspension approved for use in large animals. Absorption is erratic, and it produces prolonged but low plasma concentrations.

Clinical Use

Indications for ampicillin or amoxicillin are few insofar as they offer little advantage over benzyl penicillins because of acquired resistance in gram negative bacteria. Based on a tissue cage inflammation model, an intramuscular dosage of 15 mg/kg of ampicillin sodium given every 6 hours would be required to treat ampicillin-susceptible bacteria.[50] Sodium ampicillin may be substituted for sodium or potassium penicillin as a choice for surgical prophylaxis.

ANTIPSEUDOMONAL PENICILLINS

Because of its strong antipseudomonal activity, ticarcillin is used to treat endometritis in mares.

Spectrum of Activity

Carbenicillin, ticarcillin, and piperacillin are the antipseudomonal penicillins.[2] This group of penicillins can penetrate the outer cell wall of *Pseudomonas* sp. and other gram negative bacteria. They are susceptible to β-lactamase inactivation by *Klebsiella* spp. This group has activity against gram negative bacteria at the expense of activity against gram positive bacteria. They retain activity against anaerobic bacteria and are synergistic when administered with aminoglycosides.

Pharmacokinetics

Absorption of intramuscular ticarcillin is 65%, and the elimination half-life is less than 1 hour in horses.[57,58] Peak endometrial concentrations after IV administration were 12.9 μg/g but were greater than 150 μg/g when 6 grams of ticarcillin were diluted in 250 ml of saline and infused into the uterus.[57]

β-LACTAMASE INHIBITORS

Spectrum of Activity

The β-lactamase inhibitors are a specific class of drugs that inhibit bacterial β-lactamase, so they are administered in combination with β-lactam antibiotics.[59] These drugs combine with β-lactamase enzymes produced by gram negative and some gram positive bacteria. An inactive enzyme complex is formed, and the co-administered antibiotic is then able to exert its effect. New evidence suggests that ß-lactamase inhibitors, once thought to have little antimicrobial activity of their own, bind to different PBPs, affecting autolysis and contributing to the activity of the concomitantly administered β-lactam antibiotic.[60] The primary drugs of this class are clavulanic acid and sulbactam. They extend the spectrum of amoxicillin and ampicillin to include β-lactamase–producing *E coli, Klebsiella, Proteus,* and *Staphylococcus* spp.[24] Most anaerobes, including *Bacteroides fragilis*, are susceptible.[26]

Pharmacokinetics

ABSORPTION

Absorption of ticarcillin and clavulanic acid in foals is age dependent; neonatal foals have a higher systemic bioavailability after IM administration than older foals (100% and 88% versus 100% and 27%, respectively).[61] When administered intramuscularly in combination with clavulanic acid, ticarcillin demonstrates "flip-flop" kinetics, wherein the elimination half-life is longer after intramuscular than IV injection as a result of slow absorption from the injection site.[62] Systemic absorption of both ticarcillin and clavulanic acid is poor after intrauterine administration.[63]

DISTRIBUTION

The Vd of ticarcillin in older foals was 0.24 L/kg, and the Vd of clavulanic acid was 0.48 L/kg. In neonatal foals the Vd of ticarcillin was higher at 0.69 L/kg, as would be expected for a low-Vd drug in a neonate, with its increased extracellular fluid volume.[61] In mares the Vd of ticarcillin was 0.13 L/kg, and the Vd of clavulanic acid was 0.18 L/kg.[63]

ELIMINATION

Ticarcillin demonstrates age-dependent elimination in foals. In neonatal foals the Vd and clearance of ticarcillin were approximately double those reported for older foals and mares.[61] The renal elimination mechanism of ticarcillin appears immature in a 3-day-old foal but near normal adult function by 28 days of age. In mares the elimination half-life of clavulanic acid is 0.4 hour.[63]

Adverse Effects and Drug Interactions

When ticarcillin is administered intramuscularly into the hindquarters at a concentration of 400 mg/ml with 13.2 mg/ml clavulanic acid, foals showed signs of significant local discomfort.[61] A lower concentration of drug did not cause signs of discomfort in neonatal foals. The penicillin β-lactam inhibitor drugs can be used in combination with aminoglycosides for a synergistic effect against the pathogens commonly encountered in septicemic foals.[64]

Formulations

Amoxicillin-clavulanic acid is available only as oral tablets or suspension for humans and small animals. Ampicillin-sulbactam was available as a trihydrate formulation labeled for cattle and used in Canada, but it is no longer marketed. Sodium ampicillin-sulbactam and ticarcillin disodium-clavulanic acid formulations are available for human use.

Clinical Use

IV ampicillin-sulbactam or ticarcillin-clavulanic acid are treatment options for gram negative bacterial infections in valuable foals. Clavulanic acid concentrations were too low when the combination was administered to mares through IV or intrauterine routes to be of value over straight ticarcillin in the treatment of endometritis.[63]

CEPHALOSPORINS

Spectrum of Activity

The widespread emergence of penicillin-resistant staphylococci in the 1950s provided the impetus for the development of the cephalosporin antibiotics. In human medicine cephalosporins are widely used; however, it is said that cephalosporins are drugs in search of diseases to treat—meaning that precise therapeutic indications for these drugs are difficult to define, and there is a tendency to use these drugs when older, cheaper drugs would suffice.[65] Their use in equine medicine is not widespread because of their relative expense and because equine clinical experience includes only a few specific agents. They were initially grouped into three "generations" primarily on the basis of their antibacterial activity, but some of the newer cephalosporins did not easily fit into this scheme, so an expanded classification was developed (Table 4-7).[2] By convention, cephalosporins discovered before 1975 are spelled with a *ph* and after 1975 with an *f*.

Cephalosporins are broad spectrum antibiotics with a wide range of antimicrobial activity.[2,66] They are usually active against β-hemolytic streptococci and against β-lactamase–producing staphylococci but not against methicillin- (oxacillin-) resistant *Staphylococcus aureus* (MRSA) or mycobacteria. Most enterococci are resistant. In the absence of acquired resistance, *E. coli* and *Salmonella* are usually susceptible, as are some *Proteus* and *Klebsiella* spp. Group 7 cephalosporins are effective against Enterobacteriaecae and other gram negative bacteria that are resistant to earlier generations of cephalosporins because of acquired β-lactamase resistance. Common gram negative aerobic respiratory pathogens such as *Haemophilus* and *Pasteurella*, including β-lactamase producers, are usually susceptible to cephalosporins. Although most corynebacteria are susceptible, *Rhodococcus equi* is usually resistant. Only antipseudomonal (group 6) and group 7 cephalosporins are effective against *Pseudomonas aeruginosa*. Activity against non–spore-forming anaerobic bacteria is variable and similar to that of the aminopenicillins. Cefoxitin is notably resistant to β-lactamase–producing anaerobes, including *Bacteroides fragilis*. Ceftiofur is active against respiratory pathogens such as streptococci, *Pasteurella* spp., and *Histophilus* spp. and most anaerobes but has less activity against *S. aureus* and Enterobacteriaceae than other group 4 drugs. *Bacteroides* spp. and *Pseudomonas* spp. are resistant to ceftiofur. When administered, ceftiofur is rapidly metabolized to the active metabolite desfuroylceftiofur. Desfuroylceftiofur is less active than ceftiofur against *S. aureus* and *Proteus* spp.[67] Diagnostic laboratories use a ceftiofur disc for susceptibility testing because of the instability of desfuroylceftiofur, so susceptibility testing results for staphylococci and *Proteus* spp. may not reliably predict the efficacy of ceftiofur therapy.

The broad spectrum antibacterial activity of the cephalosporins may cause overgrowth ("superinfection") by inherently resistant bacteria, including *Clostridium difficile*, which no longer have to compete with the normal microbial flora. Nosocomial infection with vancomycin-resistant enterococci (VRE) has become a serious problem in human hospitals. One of the highest risk factors for contracting a VRE infection in a human hospital is treatment with a cephalosporin.[68]

Pharmacokinetics

ABSORPTION, DISTRIBUTION, AND ELIMINATION

See Table 4-7 for the PK parameters for the cephalosporins in horses. Intramuscular and subcutaneous administration of cephalosporins results in rapid drug absorption, but the extent varies with the drug and the species. Oral bioavailability is acceptable in neonates but rapidly becomes too low to be practical for older foals or adults.[69,70] The values for Vd in horses for the cephalosporins are typically low (< 0.3 L/kg), indicating distribution primarily to extracellular

TABLE 4-7

Pharmacokinetics of Cephalosporins in Horses

CLASSIFICATION OF CEPHALOSPORINS

Group	Characteristics	Examples
1 (First generation)	Parenteral; resistant to staphylococcal β-lactamase; sensitive to enterobacterial β-lactamase	Cephacetrile, cephaloridine, cephalothin, cephapirin, cephazolin
2 (First generation)	Oral; resistant to staphylococcal β -lactamase; moderately resistant to some enterobacterial β-lactamase	Cefadroxil, cephadrine, cephalexin
3 (Second generation)	Parenteral and oral; resistant to many β-lactamases	Cefaclor, cefotetan, cefoxitin, cefuroxime, cefamandole
4 (Third generation)	Parenteral; resistant to many β-lactamases	Cefotaxime, ceftizoxime, ceftriaxone, ceftiofur, cevofecin, latamoxef
5 (Third generation)	Oral; resistant to many β-lactamases	Cefetamet, cefixime, cefpodoxime
6 (Third generation)	Parenteral; resistant to many β-lactamases; active against *Pseudomonas aeruginosa*	Cefoperazone, cefsulodin, ceftazidime
7 (Fourth generation); included with group 6 in some classifications	Parenteral; resistant to staphylococcal, enterobacterial and pseudomonal β-lactamases	Cefepime, cefquinome, cefpirome

RELATIVE ACTIVITY OF CEPHALOSPORINS AGAINST COMMON BACTERIA[a]

Drug	Group	*S. aureus*[b]	*E. coli, Klebsiella, Proteus*	*Enterobacter*	*Pseudomonas aeruginosa*	*Bacteroides*	*Other anaerobes*
Cephalothin	1	+++	++	-	-	-	+
Cefuroxime	3	++	+++	-	-	-	+
Cefoxitin	3	+	+++	+	-	++	++
Cefotaxime	4	++	+++	+	-	+	++
Ceftriaxone	4	+	+++	+	-	-	+
Ceftazidime	6	+	+++	++	+++	-	-
Cefepime	7	++	+++	+++	+++	-	+

a +++, highly active; ++, moderately active; +, limited activity; -, no clinical activity. Susceptibilities for individual isolates may vary.
b Methicillin-susceptible *Staphylococcus aureus*.

Drug	Vd (L/kg)	T½ or MRT (hr)	Protein Binding (%)	Clearance (ml/min/kg)	F (%)	Dose (mg/kg)
GROUP ONE (FIRST GENERATION)						
Cefazolin[60]	0.19	0.6-0.8	8	5.51		IV: 11
cephalothin[63]	0.15	0.25	18	13.6		IV: 11
cephapirin[64]	0.17	0.9		10	95	IV, IM: 20
GROUP TWO (FIRST GENERATION)						
cephradine[66]	0.4	1.6		6.7		IV, PO: 25
cefadroxil						
adults[62]	0.46	0.8		7		IV: 25
foals[61]	0.52	1.4			37-100	IV: 5, PO: 5-20
GROUP THREE (SECOND GENERATION)						
cefoxitin67	0.12	0.8		4.32	77	IV, IM: 20

Continued

TABLE 4-7—cont'd

Pharmacokinetics of Cephalosporins in Horses—cont'd

Drug	Vd (L/kg)	T½ or MRT (hr)	Protein Binding (%)	Clearance (ml/min/kg)	F (%)	Dose (mg/kg)
GROUP FOUR (THIRD GENERATION)						
ceftriaxone[69]	0.15	0.81		2.81		IV: 14
cefotaxime[70]	0.29	0.6		5.2		IV: 40
ceftiofur						
adults[76]	0.43	5.11	99		42	IM: 2.2
foals[78]	0.76			3		
GROUP SIX (THIRD GENERATION)						
cefoperazone[68]	0.68	IV: 0.77 IM: 1.52		12	42	IV, IM: 30
GROUP SEVEN (FOURTH GENERATION)						
cefepime						
adults[73]	0.23	2.1			100	IV, IM: 2.2
foals[72]	0.18	1.65		1.33		IV: 14

fluid. However, they have good distribution into the extracellular fluid of most tissues, including pleural, pericardial, and synovial fluid. Penetration into cortical and cancellous bone is usually adequate.[71] Cephalosporins penetrate poorly into the ocular humour and, except for some third-generation drugs, do not achieve therapeutic concentrations in the central nervous system.[2] In general the group 4-6 cephalosporins have an increased ability to penetrate the central nervous system.[72] Higher Vd values for foals reflect the increased extracellular fluid compartment of the neonate.[69,73] Most cephalosporins are rapidly eliminated as the unchanged drug in the urine. Cephalothin, cephapirin, cefotaxime, and ceftiofur are deacetylated by the liver, and their metabolites have significant antibacterial activity. For ceftiofur most of the antibacterial activity is attributed to its metabolite, desfuroylceftiofur.[74] Renal excretion of cephalosporins occurs through a combination of glomerular filtration and active tubular secretion. Therefore it may be necessary to modify the dosage regimen of most cephalosporins for patients in renal failure. For the cephalosporins that undergo hepatic metabolism, hepatic insufficiency may decrease metabolism and increase drug accumulation. Dose-dependent kinetics occurred in foals administered cefadroxil, as demonstrated by increasing mean residence time, which suggests saturation of immature renal tubular secretion at high doses.[69] For some cephalosporins delayed absorption from the intramuscular injection site results in flip-flop kinetics.[75]

ADVERSE EFFECTS AND DRUG INTERACTIONS

The adverse effects of the cephalosporins are similar to those reported for the penicillins. In general cephalosporins have a high therapeutic index. Bleeding disorders have been reported in humans but not in animals.[76] The reaction appears to be related to vitamin K antagonism. Ceftriaxone and cefepime cause gastrointestinal disturbances after administration to foals and horses.[77-79] Ceftiofur is associated with injection site inflammation and diarrhea caused by altered gastrointestinal flora in horses.[80,81] The currently available cephalosporins are considered to be potentially nephrotoxic by way of deposition of immune complexes in the glomerular basement membrane or from a direct toxic effect leading to acute tubular necrosis.[82] Like the penicillins, cephalosporins can be synergistic with aminoglycosides against many pathogens.[83] In human medicine it is recommended that cephalosporins not be used in conjunction with aminoglycosides; however, animal studies demonstrate a protective effect of the cephalosporins against nephrotoxicity.[84]

FORMULATIONS

Cefadroxil is available as veterinary formulated tablets or suspension for small animals. Cephalexin is available as human tablets and suspensions for oral administration. The parenteral formulations of cephalosporins are usually sodium salts (e.g., cefazolin, cefoxitin, ceftiofur). Cefepime (human) and ceftiofur (food animal "ready to use") are available as hydrochloride formulations. Cephapirin is available in the United States only in bovine mastitis and intrauterine formulations.

CLINICAL USE

Of the group 1 to 3 cephalosporins, cefazolin,[85,86] cephalothin,[87] cephapirin,[88-90] cefadroxil,[69,70] cephradine,[91] and cefoxitin[92] have been used in horses. In addition to ceftiofur, ceftriaxone[77] and cefotaxime [78,93] are group 4 drugs that have been used in horses and septic foals. Cefpodoxime is a group 5 drug that has been investigated for oral use in foals.[94] Cefoperazone,[75] a group 6 drug, and cefepime,[98,110] a group 7 drug, have been studied for use in horses and neonatal foals. Both drugs have strong resistance to β-lactamases, including those produced by *Pseudomonas*.

Ceftiofur is the only cephalosporin approved for equine use and the only one routinely used in equine practice, where it is a good alternative to penicillin or trimethoprim/sulfonamides for the treatment of streptococcal infections.[13,96-98] Other than ceftiofur, clinical use of group 3 to 7 cephalosporins is usually restricted to septic foals with bacterial infections caused by strains with multiple drug resistance. Ceftiofur or any of the parenteral cephalosporins are effectively used for local treatment of musculoskeletal infections.[99-101]

AMINOGLYCOSIDES

The aminoglycoside antibiotics include streptomycin, neomycin, gentamicin, amikacin, tobramycin, and kanamycin. They have a chemical structure of amino sugars joined by a glycoside linkage. The importance of this group in veterinary medicine is to treat serious infections caused by aerobic gram negative bacteria and staphylococci. Amikacin and tobramycin have excellent activity against *Pseudomonas aeruginosa.* However, the use of aminoglycosides has been eclipsed by the fluoroquinolones, which have stronger safety profiles and better distribution kinetics.[2] Nevertheless, the aminoglycosides remain important drugs in the treatment of severe gram negative sepsis, although their highly cationic, polar nature means that distribution across membranes is limited. Single daily dosing is now recommended for most dosage regimens because it maximizes efficacy and reduces toxicity.

Mechanism of Action

The aminoglycosides are large molecules with numerous amino acid groups, making them basic polycations that are highly ionized at physiologic pHs. Aminoglycosides must penetrate the bacteria to assert their effect. Susceptible, aerobic gram negative bacteria actively pump the aminoglycoside into the cell. This is initiated by an oxygen-dependent interaction between the antibiotic cations and the negatively charged ions of the bacterial membrane lipopolysaccharides. This interaction displaces divalent cations (Ca^{++}, Mg^{++}), which affects membrane permeability.[102] Once inside the bacterial cell, aminoglycosides bind to the 30S ribosomal subunit and cause a misreading of the genetic code, interrupting normal bacterial protein synthesis. This changes the cell membrane permeability, resulting in additional antibiotic uptake, further cell disruption, and ultimately cell death.

Aminoglycoside action is bactericidal and concentration dependent. For example, concentrations of gentamicin in the range of 0.5 to 5.0 μg/ml are bactericidal for gram positive and some gram negative bacteria. At 10 to 15 μg/ml, gentamicin is effective against the more resistant bacteria such as *Pseudomonas aeruginosa, Klebsiella pneumoniae,* and *Proteus mirabilis.*[103] The clinical implication is that high initial doses of aminoglycosides increase ionic bonding, enhancing the initial concentration-dependent phase of rapid antibiotic internalization, which leads to greater immediate bactericidal activity. Human clinical studies demonstrate that proper initial therapeutic doses of aminoglycosides are critical in reducing mortality from gram negative septicemia. For antimicrobials whose efficacy is concentration dependent, high plasma concentration levels relative to the MIC of the pathogen (Cmax:MIC ratio, also known as the *inhibitory quotient,* or *IQ)* and the area under the plasma concentration-time curve that is above the bacterial MIC during the dosage interval (area under the inhibitory curve, AUIC = AUC/MIC) are the major determinants of clinical efficacy. For the aminoglycosides a Cmax:MIC ratio of 10 is suggested to achieve optimal efficacy.[11]

The aminoglycosides have a significant PAE, the period of time during which antimicrobial concentrations are below the bacterial MIC but the antimicrobial-damaged bacteria are more susceptible to host defenses. The duration of the PAE tends to increase as the initial aminoglycoside concentration increases.[104]

Antimicrobial activity of aminoglycosides is enhanced in an alkaline environment (pH of 6-8). They bind to and are inactivated by the nucleic acid material released by decaying white blood cells. Therefore they are usually ineffective in the acidic, hyperosmolar, anaerobic environment of abscesses.

Spectrum of Activity

The aminoglycosides are effective against most aerobic gram negative bacteria, including *Pseudomonas.*[2] They are somewhat effective against staphylococci, although resistance can occur. They are often effective against enterococci, but therapy against streptococci is more effective when combined with a β-lactam antibiotic. *Salmonella* and *Brucella* spp. are intracellular pathogens and are often resistant. Some mycobacteria, spirochetes, and mycoplasma are susceptible. Aminoglycosides are ineffective against anaerobic bacteria because aminoglycoside penetration into the bacteria requires an oxygen-dependent transport mechanism. Amikacin was developed from kanamycin and has the broadest spectrum of activity of the aminoglycosides. It is effective against strains not susceptible to other aminoglycosides because it is more resistant to bacterial enzymatic inactivation and is considered the least nephrotoxic. However, it is poorly active against *Streptococcus zooepidemicus* compared with gentamicin, so amikacin should be reserved for pathogens known to be resistant to gentamicin.[13]

Resistance Mechanisms

Aminoglycoside resistance is primarily due to enzymes encoded by genes located on bacterial plasmids. These phosphotransferases, acetyltransferases, and adenyltransferases act internally to alter the aminoglycoside and prevent it from binding to ribosomes.[2] Amikacin is least susceptible to enzyme inactivation. Plasmid-mediated resistance to the aminoglycosides is transferable between bacteria. A single type of plasmid may confer cross-resistance to multiple aminoglycosides and to other unrelated antimicrobials. A single bacterial isolate may have any one of a variety of combinations of resistance to different antibiotics conferred by the particular plasmid it carries. As an example, an *E. coli* strain may be resistant to ampicillin, apramycin, chloramphenicol, gentamicin, kanamycin, sulfonamide, streptomycin, tetracycline, and trimethoprim.[105] The nature of resistance in organisms such as *E. coli* and *Salmonella* species has been a focus of international research because of concerns about potential transference of antimicrobial resistance from animal to human pathogens. Bacteria may also utilize other methods that reduce the efficacy of aminoglycosides. Some strains of bacteria are less permeable to aminoglycosides, requiring much higher concentrations of aminoglycosides to kill them, and therefore can be selected for during treatment. Resistance resulting from chromosomal resistance is minimal and develops slowly for most of the aminoglycosides, with the exception of streptomycin or dihydrostreptomycin; resistance to streptomycin can occur from a single-step mutation.

FIRST EXPOSURE ADAPTIVE RESISTANCE

Both subinhibitory and inhibitory aminoglycoside concentrations produce resistance in bacterial cells surviving the initial ionic binding.[106] This adaptive resistance is due to decreased aminoglycoside transport into the bacteria. Exposure to one dose of an aminoglycoside is sufficient to produce resistant variants of an organism with altered metabolism and impaired aminoglycoside uptake. In vitro animal and clinical studies show that the resistance occurs within 1 or 2 hours of the first dose. The duration of adaptive resistance relates directly to the elimination half-life of the aminoglycoside. With normal aminoglycoside pharmacokinetics, the resistance may be maximal for up to 16 hours after a single dose of aminoglycoside, followed by partial return of bacterial susceptibility at 24 hours and complete recovery at approximately 40 hours.[107] If the aminoglycoside is dosed multiple times a day or the drug concentration remains constant, as with a continuous infusion, adaptive resistance persists and increases. Adaptive resistance is likely to persist in peripheral compartments, which are often the site of infection because of the persistence of aminoglycosides at these sites. Dose administration at 24-hour intervals, or longer, may increase efficacy by allowing time for adaptive resistance to reverse.[106,108,109] Some clinicians have expressed reservations about once-daily dosing when intestinal damage allows continued exposure to bacteria that may replicate during the prolonged periods of subtherapeutic aminoglycoside concentrations, but this has not been documented clinically.

PHARMACOKINETICS

Absorption See Table 4-8 for the pharmacokinetics of gentamicin and amikacin in horses. Amikacin and gentamicin are rapidly and well absorbed from intramuscular and subcutaneous routes of administration but are not absorbed orally.[102]

Distribution The aminoglycosides are polar antibiotics; therefore distribution is limited to the extracellular fluid space. The Vd in most species ranges between 0.15 to 0.3 L/kg but is higher in neonates.[110,111] After parenteral administration, effective concentrations are obtained in synovial, perilymph, pleural, peritoneal, and pericardial fluid.[112] Therapeutic concentrations are not achieved in bile, cerebrospinal fluid, respiratory secretions, and prostatic and ocular fluids.[102,113] Gentamicin does not cross the placenta of late-term mares.[114] The predominant site of drug accumulation is the renal cortex in most species. The following general relative gentamicin concentrations are reached over time with repeated doses, from highest to lowest concentrations: renal cortex > renal medulla > liver/lung/spleen > skeletal muscle.[102] Gentamicin distributes into jejunal and colonic tissue, with a peak gentamicin concentration of 4.13 μg/ml in the large colon and 2.26 μg/ml in the jejunum.[115]

In endotoxemia gentamicin concentrations increase in serum as a result of a fever-induced decrease in the volume of the extracellular fluid compartment.[116] The administration of therapeutic fluids, similar to those that are used in the treatment of colic, does not significantly change the pharmacokinetics of concurrently administered gentamicin.[117] The pharmacokinetics of gentamicin are unchanged in horses undergoing colic surgery.[118] Peritoneal lavage had no effect on pharmacokinetics of gentamicin in healthy horses after abdominal surgery, in which localized nonseptic peritonitis was induced.[119]

Endometrial tissue concentrations of gentamicin were higher than plasma concentrations after 7 days of intramuscular therapy with a dose of 5 mg/kg every 8 hours.[120] Intrauterine administration of 2 grams of amikacin produced a peak of more than 40 μg/gram of endometrial tissue within 1 hour after infusion. Between 2 and 4 μg of amikacin per gram of endometrial tissue were still present 24 hours after infusion.[121] Intrauterine administration of 2.5 grams of gentamicin once daily for 5 days resulted in endometrial tissue concentrations of 41.65 μg/gram 24 hours after the last dose.[122]

Gentamicin distributed into synovial fluid in normal horses and reached a peak of 6.4 μg/ml at 2 hours with a single 4.4 mg/kg IV dose.[123] However, local inflammation may increase drug concentrations in the joint, and concentrations may also increase with repeated doses. Intra-articular administration of 150 mg of gentamicin resulted in a peak synovial concentration of 1828 μg/ml 15 minutes after injection, and synovial concentrations remain greater than 10 μg/ml for at least 24 hours.[124] Regional perfusion techniques are excellent methods to deliver aminoglycosides locally and prevent the adverse effects of systemic therapy.[125-130] When intraosseous perfusion was compared with IV perfusion, each technique produced mean peak concentrations of amikacin ranging between 5 to 50 times that of recommended peak serum concentrations for therapeutic efficacy.[131] Gentamicin-impregnated polymethylmethacrylate beads or collagen sponges may also be used to achieve extremely high local concentrations of drug, while avoiding systemic toxicity.[99,132-135]

ELIMINATION

The aminoglycosides are almost exclusively eliminated in urine by glomerular filtration.[102] The plasma elimination half-lives range between 1 to 3 hours in adult animals but are increased in neonates or animals with renal dysfunction.[111] Renal accumulation results in extended withdrawal times for food animals.

Adverse Effects and Drug Interactions

NEPHROTOXICITY

The aminoglycosides enter the renal tubule after filtration through the glomerulus (Figure 4-22). From the luminal fluid the cationic aminoglycoside molecules bind to anionic phospholipids on the proximal tubular cells.[136] The aminoglycoside is taken into the cell by way of carrier-mediated pinocytosis and translocated into cytoplasmic vacuoles, which fuse with lysosomes.[137] The drug is sequestered unchanged in the lysosomes. With additional pinocytosis drug continues to accumulate within the lysosomes. The accumulated aminoglycoside interferes with normal lysosomal function, and eventually the overloaded lysosomes swell and rupture. Lysosomal enzymes, phospholipids, and the aminoglycoside are released into the cytosol of the proximal tubular cell, disrupting other organelles and causing cell death.[138]

TABLE 4-8

Pharmacokinetics of Aminoglycosides in Horses

Drug	Volume of Distribution (L/kg)	Half-life or MRT (hour)	Clearance (ml/min/kg)	Dose (mg/kg)
AMIKACIN				
Foals, 3-day-old[2]	0.42	2.7	1.92	7
Foals, premature, hypoxic[188]	0.60	5.4	1.9	7
Neonatal, high sepsis score[111]	0.34	4.10	1.17	IV: 6.6
Horses[189]	0.14-0.2	1.14-1.57	1.28-1.49	IV: 4.4, 6.6, 11
Horses[190]	0.21	2.8	0.75	IV: 6
GENTAMICIN				
Foals, 1-day-old[110]	0.31	2.2	1.75	4
Foals, 1-month-old[220]	0.24	3.07	0.9	IV: 4
Mares, late pregnancy[114]	0.15	2.26	1.06	—
Horses[116]	0.17	1.66	1.41	IV: 3
Horses, endotoxic[116]	0.14	1.54	1.17	IV: 3
Horses[113]	0.12	0.78	—	IV: 6.6
Horses[112]	0.27	2.17	1.56	IV: 2.2
Horses[150]	0.14	3.0	—	IV, IM: 6.6
Ponies[120]	0.19	1.82	1.27	IV, IM: 5
Horses, intravenous fluids[117]	0.15	1.96	1.04	IV: 2.2
Horses, postoperative[118]	0.17	1.47	1.27	IV: 6.6

MRT, Mean residence time; *IV,* intravenous; *IM,* intramuscular.

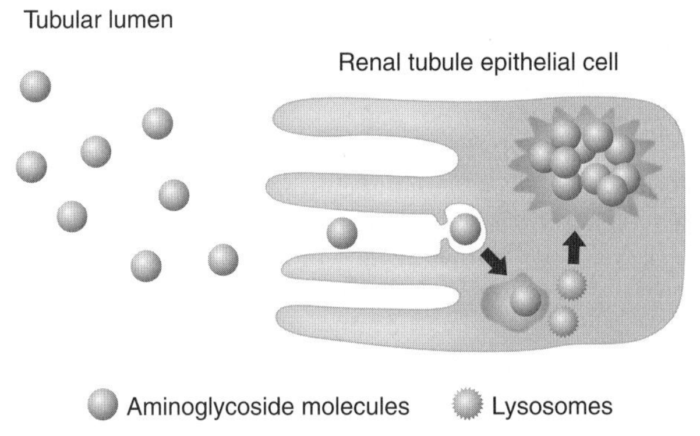

FIGURE 4-22 Neprotoxicity occurs from ionic binding of aminoglycoside molecules to polysaccharide cations on the proximal tubular epithelium, followed by pinocytosis and accumulation within lysosomes.

The risk factors for aminoglycoside toxicity include: prolonged therapy (>7 to 10 days), acidosis and electrolyte disturbances (hypokalemia, hyponatremia), volume depletion (shock, endotoxemia), concurrent nephrotoxic drug therapy, preexisting renal disease, and elevated plasma trough concentrations.[139-144] Calcium supplementation can reduce the risk of nephrotoxicity.[145] Administration of antioxidants such as silymarin and vitamin E may decrease aminoglycoside nephrotoxicity.[146] The risk of nephrotoxicity can also be decreased by feeding the patient a diet high in protein and calcium, such as alfalfa hay, because protein and calcium cations compete with aminoglycoside cations for binding to renal tubular epithelial cells.[147] High dietary protein also increases GFR and renal blood flow, reducing aminoglycoside accumulation.[148]

Uptake and accumulation of aminoglycosides into renal tubular epithelium demonstrates saturable kinetics. Because nephrotoxicity is related to aminoglycoside accumulation in the renal proximal tubular cells, it is logical that peak concentrations are not related to toxicity and that longer dose intervals results in less total drug exposure to the renal brush border membrane. High-dose, once-daily dosing of aminoglycosides has now become common in human and veterinary medicine; it takes advantage of the concentration-dependent killing and long PAE of these drugs and prevents first exposure adaptive resistance and toxicity.[113,118,149-151]

OTOTOXICITY

Aminoglycoside ototoxicity occurs from the same accumulation mechanisms as nephrotoxicity. In the inner ear aminoglycosides appear to generate free radicals that subsequently do permanent damage to sensory cells and neurons.[152-154] Gentamicin damages the cochlear division of the eighth cranial nerve, resulting in vertigo, and amikacin damages the auditory division of the eighth cranial nerve, resulting in permanent deafness. This drug-specific toxicity may be due to the distribution characteristics of each drug and concentration achieved in each sensory organ.[155,156]

THERAPEUTIC DRUG MONITORING

Individual horses can differ widely in the serum concentrations produced by the same aminoglycoside dosage regimen. When this relative unpredictability is combined with the often small difference between therapeutic and toxic serum concentrations, determining serum concentrations in a particular patient becomes very valuable. There is a tendency to underdose neonatal patients, especially those that are receiving aggressive fluid therapy.[157] To maximize efficacy and minimize toxicity, therapeutic drug monitoring of gentamicin or amikacin is recommended. Peak concentrations are targeted to achieve a peak plasma concentration:MIC ratio of 10.[11,102,107] Because the trough concentration is associated with nephrotoxicity, it is recommended that trough concentrations be less than 2 μg/ml for gentamicin and less than 5 μg/ml for amikacin before the next dose is administered.[102,107] To allow for the distribution phase, blood sampling for the peak concentration is performed 0.5 to 1 hour after IV administration, and the trough sample is usually taken before the next dose. The peak and trough concentrations can then be used to estimate the elimination half-life for the individual patient. An increase in the elimination half-life during therapy is a very sensitive indicator of early tubular insult.[158] If a once-daily regimen is used, a blood sample just before the next dose will be well below the recommended trough concentrations and may even be below the limit of detection of the assay. For these patients an 8-hour postdose sample will provide a more accurate estimate of the elimination half-life.

If therapeutic drug monitoring is unavailable, then once-daily high-dose therapy is recommended; the development of nephrotoxicity is detected by an increase in urine gamma glutamyl transferase (UGGT) enzyme and an increase in the urine GGT:urine creatinine (UCr) ratio. The UGGT:UCr may increase to two to three times baseline within 3 days of a nephrotoxic dose.[139,158,159] If these tests are not available, the development of proteinuria is the next best indicator of nephrotoxicity and is easily determined in a practice setting.[158,159] Elevations in serum urea nitrogen and Cr confirm nephrotoxicity but are not seen for 7 days after significant renal damage has occurred.[111] Elimination half-lives of 24 to 45 hours have been reported in horses with renal toxicity, further prolonging the toxic exposure to the drug.[142] While peritoneal dialysis is useful in lowering creatinine and serum urea nitrates, it may not be effective in significantly increasing the elimination of the accumulating aminoglycoside.[142] The horse's ability to recover most likely depends on the type of medication exposure and the amount of healthy renal tissue remaining to compensate.

NEUROMUSCULAR BLOCKADE

Neuromuscular blockade is a rare effect, related to blockade of acetylcholine at the nicotinic cholinergic receptor.[160] It is most often seen when anesthetic agents are administered concurrently with aminoglycosides.[161] Affected patients should be treated promptly with parenteral calcium chloride at 10 to 20 mg/kg intravenously or calcium gluconate at 30 to 60 mg/kg intravenously to reverse dyspnea from muscle response depression. IV edrophonium at 0.5 mg/kg will also reverse neuromuscular blocking effects.[160]

DRUG INTERACTIONS

Aminoglycosides are inactivated if combined in vitro with other drugs because of pH incompatibilities. The aminoglycosides are synergistic against streptococci, *Pseudomonas*, and other gram negative bacteria if combined with β-lactam antibiotics as a result of the bacterial cell wall being disrupted by the β-lactam antibiotic. Halothane anesthesia causes significant changes in the pharmacokinetics of gentamicin; total body clearance and volume of distribution decrease, and half-life of elimination increases.[162] A longer gentamicin dosing interval after anesthesia may help correct for the changes, but the practitioner should seriously consider selecting another antimicrobial. Neuromuscular blocking agents or drugs with neuromuscular blocking activity should not be used concurrently with aminoglycosides because they can increase the risk of neuromuscular blockade, particularly during anesthesia.[161] Other nephrotoxic drugs should be avoided when possible during aminoglycoside therapy. Concurrent administration of phenylbutazone with gentamicin decreases the elimination half-life of gentamicin by 23% and decreases the Vd by 26%; the pharmacokinetics of phenylbutazone are not affected.[163] Flunixin has no effect on the pharmacokinetics of gentamicin when administered concurrently to adult horses.[118]

Formulations

Gentamicin and amikacin are available as brand name and generic solutions for intrauterine infusion in mares. Although not labeled for other routes of administration, they are commonly administered by IV, intramuscular, subcutaneous, intra-articular, and intraosseous routes to horses. Gentamicin is also available in ophthalmic formulations for the treatment of gram negative keratitis.

Clinical Use

Gentamicin and amikacin are commonly used to treat serious gram negative infection in horses and septicemia in foals. Amikacin is used when antimicrobial resistance to gentamicin has developed in gram negative pathogens, but gentamicin has greater activity against streptococci than amikacin.[13] The aminoglycosides are usually administered concurrently with β-lactam antimicrobials for a possible synergistic effect. The use of aminoglycosides in horses has been limited because of toxicity concerns, but high-dose once-daily dosing greatly reduces the risks. Use of the aminoglycosides is also limited by their poor penetration of cellular membranes and inactivation in purulent environments.

CHLORAMPHENICOL AND FLORFENICOL

Chloramphenicol (CHPC) was isolated in 1947 from a soil actinomycete from Venezuela. Florfenicol (FLF) is a fluorinated derivative of CHPC.

Mechanism of Action

Both CHPC and FLF are bacteriostatic antibiotics that inhibit protein synthesis by binding to ribosomal subunits of susceptible bacteria, leading to the inhibition of peptidyl transferase and thereby preventing the transfer of amino acids to growing peptide chains and subsequent protein formation.[164] These antibiotics have a very wide spectrum of activity, including streptococci, staphylococci, anaerobes, *Haemophilus, Salmonella, Pasteurella, Mycoplasma,* and *Brucella* spp. FLF has activity against CHPC-resistant strains of *E. coli, Klebsiella, Proteus, Salmonella,* and *S. aureus*. Both are also active against rickettsia, chlamydia, and hemobartonella.[2]

Mechanisms of Resistance

Bacterial resistance to CHPC results from plasmid-mediated bacterial production of acetylase enzymes. Acetylation of hydroxyl groups prevents drug binding to the 50-S ribosomal subunit. FLF has a fluorine atom instead of the hydroxyl group located at C-3 in the structure of CHPC and thiamphenicol. Initially FLF was less susceptible to deactivation by bacteria with plasmid-transmissible resistance to CHPC. Recently, new resistances to CHPC and FLF have been identified in cattle pathogens.[165,166]

Pharmacokinetics

ABSORPTION

CHPC and FLF are rapidly absorbed after oral administration. The oral bioavailability of CHPC in foals is 83%,[167] but only 40% after a single administration in mares and bioavailability declines to 20% after five doses.[168] The oral bioavailability of FLF in horses is 81%.[169] The commercially available formulation of FLF is a long-acting injectible product for cattle and is characterized by delayed absorption and low plasma concentrations.[170]

DISTRIBUTION

Because of high lipid solubility and low protein binding, CHPC and FLF are widely distributed throughout the body. Highest drug levels are attained in the liver and kidney, but therapeutic drug concentrations are attained in most tissues and fluids, including ocular humor and synovial fluid.[2] CHPC may achieve cerebrospinal fluid concentrations of up to 50% of plasma concentrations when the meninges are normal, and more if inflammation is present.[171] FLF does not penetrate the blood-brain barrier as readily as CHPC.[172] The Vd of CHPC is 2.83 L/kg in horses[173] and 1.6 L/kg in neonatal foals.[167] The Vd of FLF is 0.72 L/kg in horses.[184] The degree of protein binding of CHPC in horses is 30%,[174] whereas FLF has a low degree of protein binding in cattle.[175]

ELIMINATION

In most species these drugs are eliminated by renal excretion of parent drug and by hepatic glucuronide conjugation and elimination in feces. The elimination half-life of CHPC in foals older than 7 days and adult horses is less than 1 hour.[167,173,174,176,177] In 1-day-old foals the elimination half-life is 5.3 hours, indicating the immaturity of the foal's hepatic metabolism capacity.[176] FLF has an elimination half-life of 1.8 hours in horses after IV administration.[169] The long-acting formulation for cattle is slowly eliminated on account of the prolonged absorption from the intramuscular injection site (flip-flop kinetics).[170]

Adverse Effects and Drug Interactions

Insofar as these drugs are protein synthesis inhibitors, dose-related anemia and pancytopenia are associated with chronic therapy (>14 days), causing a decrease in protein synthesis in the bone marrow. FLF is more likely than CHPC to cause reversible bone marrow suppression with chronic dosing[172] or overdose.[178] In humans an idiosyncratic aplastic anemia occurs with exposure to CHPC.[179] The reaction is rare (1 in 30,000), and not dose related. Toxic effects are related to the presence of the para-nitro group on the CHPC molecule. This reaction does not occur with FLF, insofar as it lacks the para-nitro group. CHPC is a hepatic microsomal enzyme inhibitor. It decreases the clearance of other drugs metabolized by the same cytochrome P450 enzymes, including phenytoin, phenobarbital, pentobarbital, phenylbutazone, xylazine, and cyclophosphamide.[180,181] Whether FLF affects the metabolism of other drugs is unknown.

Although CHPC is well-tolerated by horses, FLF alters fecal consistency with single doses administered intravenously, orally, or intramuscularly.[169] In a chronic dosing study with the cattle intramuscular formulation, all horses remained clinically normal but had dramatic alterations in enteric flora. *Salmonella* spp., *E. coli,* and *Clostridium perfringens* in these horses rapidly developed resistance to FLF.[170]

In general, CHPC or FLF should not be administered concurrently with penicillins, macrolides, aminoglycosides, or fluoroquinolones. CHPC or FLF may antagonize the activity of penicillins or aminoglycosides, and they act on the same ribosomal site as the macrolides.[182,183] Inhibition of protein synthesis by CHPC or FLF interferes with the production of autolysins necessary for cell lysis after fluoroquinolones interfere with DNA supercoiling.[184]

Formulations

CHPC sodium succinate is a water-soluble formulation for IV use and is hydrolyzed to CHPC in the liver. CHPC free base and CHPC-palmitate are available for oral administration. The CHPC-palmitate is hydrolyzed in the gastrointestinal tract to CHPC. Ophthalmic formulations of CHPC are also available. FLF is available only as a cattle product in three carriers (2-pyrrolidone, propylene glycol, and polyethylene glycol) to give it a long-acting effect.

Clinical Use

CHPC is banned for use in any type of food animal because it can lead to idiosyncratic aplastic anaemia in humans. It is used in small animals and horses for a variety of bacterial infections, especially when penetration into the central nervous system is desired, but appropriate precautions should be taken in handling the product to prevent human exposure. FLF should not be routinely used in horses because of its effects on gastrointestinal flora and the clinical limitations of the long-acting cattle formulation.

POTENTIATED SULFONAMIDES

The sulfonamides are a group of organic compounds with chemotherapeutic activity (hence they are antimicrobials, not antibiotics). They have a common chemical nucleus that is closely related to *p*-aminobenzoic acid, an essential component in the folic acid pathway of nucleic acid synthesis. Sulfonamides are combined with diaminopyrimidines such as trimethoprim (TMP) and pyrimethamine (PYM), which inhibit an essential step further along the folate pathway. Because the potentiated sulfonamides are remarkably synergistic and nontoxic, they are commonly used in equine medicine. Their use is complicated by differences in pharmacokinetics among TMP and PYM and the various sulfonamides used in the combinations.

Mechanism of Action

The sulfonamides inhibit the bacterial enzyme dihydropteroate synthetase (DPS) in the folic acid pathway, thereby blocking bacterial nucleic acid synthesis. Sulfonamides substitute for PABA, preventing its conversion to dihydrofolic acid. Alone, this action is considered bacteriostatic. Because the activity is by competitive substitution, the sulfonamide tissue concentration must be kept high enough to prevent bacterial access to PABA. Therefore the sulfonamides are ineffective in pus and necrotic tissue, which provide additional sources of PABA to the bacteria. The sulfonamides are nontoxic to mammalian cells because they use dietary folate for synthesis of dihydrofolic acid and do not require PABA. The addition of TMP or PYM to a sulfonamide creates a bactericidal combination. TMP inhibits bacterial folic acid synthesis at the next step in the folic acid sequence, inhibiting the conversion of dihydrofolic acid to tetrahydrofolic acid by inhibiting dihydrofolate reductase. This enzyme is present in both bacteria and mammalian cells, but the bacterial enzyme is inhibited at much lower concentrations than necessary to inhibit the mammalian enzyme.[185] The MICs against specific susceptible bacteria for each drug are generally lowered when the antimicrobials are administered in the potentiated sulfonamide combination. The resistance developed to the potentiated sulfonamides is lower than that to each individual drug; this is an important benefit because resistance to sulfonamides is very common and resistance develops rapidly to diaminopyrimidines when used alone.[186]

The potentiated sulfonamides have a broad spectrum of activity. The following bacteria are usually susceptible: *Streptococcus, Proteus, E. coli, Pasteurella, Haemophilus,* and *Salmonella* spp. Staphylococci, anaerobes, *Nocardia, Corynebacterium, Klebsiella,* and *Enterobacter* are susceptible but may become resistant. *Pseudomonas* spp., *Bacteriodes* spp., and enterococci are usually resistant.[13,42,187] Other significant organisms that are susceptible to potentiated sulfonamides include protozoa (*Toxoplasma gondii, Sarcocystis neurona*) and coccidia. PYM is more effective than TMP against protozoa.[186] The potentiated sulfonamides are formulated at a fixed ratio of 1:5 of TMP to sulfonamide. The optimum concentration for bactericidal action is 1:20.[185] When and where this optimum concentration is achieved are difficult to predict in vivo, but a 1:20 ratio is used in susceptibility testing.[188]

Mechanisms of Resistance

Bacterial resistance to the sulfonamides is common and may be from chromosomal mutations or mediated by plasmids. Chromosomal mutations can lead to bacterial hyperproduction of PABA, which overcomes the competitive substitution of the sulfonamides. Plasmid-encoded resistance results in a by-pass of the drug-sensitive step by production of altered forms of the DPS enzyme with a lower affinity for sulphonamides. Resistance to TMP usually occurs by plasmid-encoded production of TMP-resistant dihydrofolate reductase. Other resistance mechanisms include excessive bacterial production of dihydrofolate reductase (DHFR) and reduction in the ability of the drug to penetrate the bacterial cell wall. Cross-resistance among sulfonamides is considered complete and often occurs with pyrimidines.[185] Resistance to the TMP-sulfonamide combinations develops slowly but is now common among equine bacterial isolates.[13,189]

Pharmacokinetics

Pharmacokinetics of the potentiated sulfonamides are complicated by the distinct differences between disposition of TMP and PYM and the various sulfonamides. When sulfonamides and diaminopyrimidines are administered concurrently to horses, the pharmacokinetics of each drug appears to be unaffected by the presence of the other. Table 4-9 outlines the pharmacokinetics of specific potentiated sulfonamide combinations in horses. Although the potentiated sulfonamides are frequently used interchangeably, pharmacokinetics studies show that they are not bioequivalent in horses.

ABSORPTION

In general, potentiated sulfonamides are readily absorbed from the gastrointestinal tract of horses but may be affected by feeding.[190-192] For TMP and sulphachlorpyridazine, peak plasma concentrations and bioavailabilities are significantly reduced when the drug is mixed with concentrate compared with nasogastric administration.[193] Both drugs also demonstrate a biphasic absorption pattern, and it appears that this is due to a portion of the TMP and sulphachlorpyridazine dose binding to feed, with a second absorption phase occurring in the large intestine.[194] Bioavailability following intrauterine administration was 23% to 43% for TMP and 29% to 34% for sulfadoxine, and both were detected in the milk of lactating mares.[195] The oral bioavailability of PYM is 56% in horses.[196]

DISTRIBUTION

Because the sulfonamides are weak acids and relatively hydrophilic, they distribute well in extracellular and interstitial fluids and typically have values for Vd of 0.3 to 0.7 L/kg. Concentrations of sulfonamides in tissues are generally lower than those in plasma. The diaminopyrimidines are lipophilic weak bases and penetrate intracellularly better than sulfonamides, resulting in values for Vd of 1.5 to 2.7 L/kg and higher tissue concentrations than plasma concentrations.[185] Distribution of potentiated sulfonamides has been broadly investigated in the horse. Sulfadiazine and TMP and sulfamethoxazole and TMP are all well distributed into peritoneal fluid, cerebrospinal fluid, synovial fluid, and urine.[197-199] Inflammation in the meninges or synovium does not significantly affect distribution into the respective fluids. After repeated doses sulfamethoxazole, unlike TMP, accumulates in the cerebrospinal fluid.[197] Cerebrospinal fluid concentrations of PYR reach 25% to 50% of serum concentrations but do not appear to accumulate in horses with daily dosing.[200]

Sulfonamides can be highly bound to plasma proteins, but the extent of binding depends on species, drug, and concentration. In the horse the degree of protein binding varies between 33% for sulfaphenazole to 93% for sulfamethoxine.[185] Approximately 50% of TMP is protein bound, and binding is independent of plasma concentration.[201] Although only free drug is available for antimicrobial action, protein-bound drug serves as a reservoir and extends the duration of action of these drugs.

METABOLISM

Diaminopyrimidines and sulfonamides are metabolized by the liver, usually by acetylation, aromatic hydroxylation, and glucuronidation.[185] The acetylated, hydroxylated, and conjugated forms of the sulfonamides are significantly less microbiologically active than their parent compounds. The precise metabolic pathways for TMP or PYR have not been elucidated. Metabolites may compete with the parent drug for involvement in folic acid synthesis. They have little detrimental effect on bacteria, so their presence can decrease the activity of the remaining parent drug.[202,203]

TABLE 4-9

Pharmacokinetics of Trimethoprim, Pyrimethamine, and Sulfonamides in Horses

Drug	Volume of Distribution (L/kg)	Half-life or MRT (hour)	Protein Binding (%)	Clearance (ml/min/kg)	Dose† (mg/kg)
Trimethoprim	—	2.4	—	—	PO: 5
Sulfadiazine[191]		7.4			PO: 25
Trimethoprim	2.0	2.8	35	8.8	IV: 2.5
Sulfadiazine[213]	0.5	4.6	20	1.5	IV: 12.5
Trimethoprim	1.5	3	50	—	IV: 8
Sulfadoxine[201]	0.39	14	14-72		IV: 40
Trimethoprim	2.8	3.4	—	11	IV: 7.5
Sulfamethoxazole[222]	0.5	4.8	—	1.4	IV: 36.5
Trimethoprim	1.6	1.9	—	13	IV: 2.5
Sulfamethoxazole[197]	0.33	3.5	—	1.3	IV: 12.5
Trimethoprim	1.5	2.6	—	7.7	IV: 5
Sulfachlorpyridazine[193]	0.26	3.8	—	2.6	IV: 25
Pyrimethamine[196]	1.5	12	—	1.6	IV, PO: 1
Sulfadiazine[202]	0.4	3.8	43	2.3	IV: 20
Sulfamerazine[202]	0.49	3.2	44	1.8	IV: 20
Sulfamethazine[192]	0.63	11.4	—	0.8	IV: 160
Sulfamethazine[202]	0.33	5.4	69	0.9	IV: 20

MRT, Mean residence time; *PO,* oral; *IV,* intravenous.

ELIMINATION

Sulfonamides are primarily excreted in urine, but excretion in feces, bile, milk, sweat, and tears also occurs. Renal excretion of unchanged drug and metabolites occurs by glomerular filtration and active tubular secretion.[185] Reabsorption occurs in the distal tubule by passive diffusion. Because most sulfonamides are weak acids, alkaline urine increases their ionization and elimination. Renal excretion of TMP occurs by glomerular filtration, active tubular secretion, and reabsorption. In horses it appears that a large percentage of TMP is metabolized before elimination in urine (46%) and feces (52%). The clearance of the diaminopyrimidines is affected by urine pH, plasma concentration, and extent of diuresis. In contrast to the sulfonamides, alkaline urine increases the reabsorption of the basic TMP.[201]

Adverse Effects and Drug Interactions

The potentiated sulfonamides are noted for their widely varying adverse effects. Crystalluria, hematuria, and renal tubular obstruction can result from poorly soluble sulfonamides, especially in dehydrated patients with acidic urine.[185] However, the lower doses of sulfonamide used in the potentiated sulfonamide combinations make crystallization less likely than with sulfonamides administered alone. Local infusion of potentiated sulfonamides into the uterus of mares caused irritation of the endometrium and a decreased pregnancy rate.[195] Intramuscular administration is not recommended because of tissue irritation from the organic solvents, high concentration, and high pH of the formulations. IV administration must be done by slow and careful injection. Rapid administration is associated with thrombophlebitis and anaphylaxis.[185,204] The concurrent use of IV potentiated sulfonamides with detomidine is contraindicated because it appears that the potentiated sulfonamide sensitizes the myocardium and results in cardiac dysrhythmias and hypotension that may be fatal.[205,206] The procaine in procaine penicillin G is a PABA analog and may reduce efficacy if used concurrently with potentiated sulphonamides.[2]

FOLATE ANTAGONISM EFFECTS

The nonregenerative anemias seen in response to long-term administration of potentiated sulfonamides are believed to be related to folate reduction with long-term, high-dose administration, such as in the treatment of equine protozoal myeloencephalitis (EPM). Concurrent therapy with TMP and PYR does not increase the efficacy against protozoa and is suspected to increase the incidence of adverse effects caused by folate reduction. Supplementation with oral folic acid is often recommended for horses on long-term potentiated sulfonamide therapy.[207] The administration of oral folic acid to pregnant mares being treated for EPM may not protect the fetus from the effects of folate deficiency. Mares have delivered foals with congenital defects after oral administration of potentiated sulphonamides.[208] These mares had also been supplemented with oral folic acid and vitamin E during the period of antibiotic treatment. Each of three mares on this dosage regimen produced a foal with renal hypoplasia or nephrosis and bone marrow aplasia or hypoplasia. In both mares and foals, serum folate concentrations were below the laboratory reference range, and in two foals folate was less than 30% of the minimum reference range. The risk of congenital defects should be considered when treating pregnant mares with PYM and sulfonamide. Treatment with TMP-sulfamethoxazole and PYM does not affect semen quality, testicular volume, sperm production efficiency, erection, or libido of healthy stallions. However, treatment may induce changes in copulatory form and agility and alter the pattern and strength of ejaculation.[209] Stallions that develop neurologic signs during treatment should be bred with caution. TMP/sulfamethoxazole has been associated with immune-mediated hemolytic anemia in a horse.[210]

EFFECTS ON GASTROINTESTINAL FLORA

The effects of potentiated sulfonamides on normal gastrointestinal flora are controversial. In some studies potentiated sulfonamides alone or with concurrent penicillin therapy are associated with diarrhea in horses.[211,212] Other studies show little effect on fecal flora.[213,214] The likelihood of any antimicrobial therapy causing diarrhea in a horse depends on several factors, including the antibacterial spectrum of the drug and the drug concentrations achieved in the gastrointestinal tract. The presence or absence of potential pathogens in the composition of the individual horse's microflora and the presence of antimicrobial-resistant pathogens in the hospital or clinic environment are also important factors in the incidence of gastrointestinal disturbances.

FORMULATIONS

TMP/sulfadiazine is available as a 48% injectable solution for IV administration in horses. It is also available as oral paste and powder formulations for horses. Generic tablets of TMP/sulfamethoxazole available for human use are commonly administered to horses. A commercially available PYR/sulfadiazine formulation is marketed for the treatment of equine protozoal myelitis in horses.

CLINICAL USE

It is very difficult to apply pharmacokinetic principles to determine drug dosage regimens for the potentiated sulfonamides. Different pathogens have varying MIC values, and the optimal ratio of TMP or PYM to sulfonamide also varies among bacteria and protozoa. The most important component of the formulation for efficacy appears to be the diaminopyrimidine, and the choice of sulfonamide may not be nearly as important. Therefore there is considerable controversy regarding the dosage regimen of these combinations. The veterinary products are labeled for once-daily administration, but studies indicate that twice-daily dosing is better for attaining therapeutic plasma concentrations.[213,215] Despite frequent clinical use for equine streptococcal infections, even prophylactic administration failed to prevent abscessation caused by *Streptococcus equi* subsp. *zooepidemicus*.[216]

TETRACYCLINES

Tetracycline was discovered after a team of workers examined 100,000 soil samples from around the world. Tetracycline derivatives include *oxytetracycline, chlortetracycline, doxycyline*, and *minocycline*. Oxytetracycline (OTC) and doxycycline (DXC) are used in horses.

MECHANISM OF ACTION

The tetracyclines bind to the 30-S ribosomal subunit and interfere with bacterial protein synthesis. They are bacteriostatic at usual therapeutic concentrations but bactericidal at high concentrations. Drug entry into the bacteria is by an energy-dependent mechanism. Mammalian cells do not possess the tetracycline transport mechanism. Tetracyclines are most active at an acidic pH. The tetracyclines are broad-spectrum in activity; they are effective against gram positive and gram negative bacteria, as well as *Chlamydia, Mycoplasma*, and *Rickettsia* spp. and some protozoa (*Haemobartonella, Anaplasma* spp.). Their activity against staphylococci is limited, and they are not active against group D streptococci (enterococci). *Pseudomonas, E. coli, Klebsiella*, and *Proteus* are usually resistant. Most anaerobes are susceptible to DXC.[2] In vitro concentrations of OTC above 0.01 μg/ml effectively suppress growth of *Neorickettsia risticii*.[217] Tetracyclines are also effective against intracellular pathogens of foals, such as *Lawsonia intracellularis* and *Rhodococcus equi*.[218] Multiple other actions have been attributed to DXC, including anticollagenolytic activity through inhibition of matrix metalloproteinases (MMPs), anti-inflammatory activity, and ability to enhance corneal repair. [219]

MECHANISMS OF RESISTANCE

Widespread acquired resistance in many pathogens limits the clinical usefulness of the tetracyclines. Resistance occurs from plasmid-mediated failure in the active transport of the drug into the bacterial cell and increased efflux from the cell. Another major mechanism of resistance involves cytoplasmic production of a protein that protects the ribosome from tetracycline action.[2]

PHARMACOKINETICS

ABSORPTION

Oral absorption of OTC is erratic, and oral administration is not recommended in horses because its adverse effects on gastrointestinal flora.[214] At an oral dose of 10 mg/kg in fed horses, DXC produced serum, synovial fluid, peritoneal fluid, and endometrial tissue concentrations above 0.25 μg/ml, suggesting effective therapy for gram positive infections.[220] At an oral dose of 20 mg/kg in fasted horses DXC produced mean maximum plasma concentration of 0.91 μg/ml following a single dose and 1.74 μg/ml after multiple doses using a 12-hour dosing interval.[221] A precise bioavailability cannot be determined because IV administration of DXC causes cardiac toxicity.[222] However, using allometric scaling, the estimated systemic absorption for DXC after oral administration in horses is only 2.7%.[221] Oral absorption of DXC in foals is higher, with a single oral dose of 10 mg/kg producing mean maximum plasma concentrations of 2.54 μg/ml and 4.05 μg/mL after multiple doses using a 12-hour dosing interval.[223] The long-acting formulation of OTC in polyethylene glycol has a bioavailability of 83% after intramuscular injection in horses.[224]

DISTRIBUTION

The tetracyclines are well distributed to most tissues, except the central nervous system. Therapeutic levels may be achieved, however, when the meninges are inflamed. Tetracyclines readily diffuse into milk.[2] OTC reaches 50% of plasma concentrations in synovial fluid and peritoneal fluid. Urine OTC concentrations are relatively high, with peak concentrations above 1500 µg/ml.[225] The Vd of OTC in neonatal foals is 2 L/kg [226] and 0.34 to 0.95 L/kg in adult horses.[224,227] The apparent Vd of DXC in horses after oral absorption is 25 L/kg, indicating the high lipid solubility and tissue penetration of DXC. Synovial and peritoneal fluids achieve the same DXC concentrations as plasma, and endometrial tissue concentrations are more than twice plasma concentrations. DXC is not detectable in cerebrospinal fluid after oral administration.[220] DXC concentrates intracellularly, with mean maximum concentrations in polymorphonuclear cells approximately 17 times higher than concentrations found in plasma.[221] In foals peritoneal fluid, synovial fluid, and bronchoalveolar lavage cell activity of DXC were similar to plasma concentrations; however, activity in the cerebrospinal fluid was significantly lower, and activity in pulmonary epithelial lining fluid and urine was significantly higher.[223]

Ocular penetration of systemic DXC has been studied. Vitreal drug concentrations were 0.17 µg/mL after multiple doses of 10 mg/kg.[228] Aqueous humor concentrations were approximately 0.11 µg/mL after multiple doses of 20 mg/kg, which represented 7.5% of corresponding plasma concentrations.[221] DXC was also detectable in the preocular tear film of horses without ocular disease after once-daily administration of 20 mg/kg.[219]

OTC is 50% protein bound in horses.[229] Plasma protein binding of DXC is high (82%), which is similar to that of other species.[221] This impairs distribution of DXC into the extracellular fluid.

ELIMINATION

The tetracyclines are not known to be biotransformed to any significant extent before elimination. OTC is eliminated in urine unchanged primarily by glomerular filtration. Unmetabolized drug is also eliminated with bile into the gastrointestinal tract and may undergo enterohepatic recirculation, prolonging its effects.[2] DXC is primarily excreted into the feces by way of nonbiliary routes in an inactive form. Therefore DXC does not accumulate in patients with renal insufficiency.[230] The clearance of OTC in foals is 3.3 ml/min/kg[226] and 2.2 ml/min/kg in adult horses.[224] When administered intravenously, the elimination half-life is 7 hours in foals[226] and 6 hours in horses.[224] Because of flip-flop kinetics, the elimination half-life is 22 hours after intramuscular administration of OTC in polyethylene glycol.[224] DXC clearance cannot be accurately determined from oral dosing.[221]

Adverse Effects and Drug Interactions

GASTROINTESTINAL EFFECTS AND INTERACTIONS

Calcium-containing products (e.g., milk, antacids) or other divalent cations will chelate with tetracyclines and interfere with gastrointestinal absorption.[2] Because DXC is less likely than the older tetracyclines to form chelation complexes with divalent and trivalent metals, there is less interference with oral absorption by calcium or other substances.[230]

The clinical use of OTC in horses is controversial because of reports of adverse gastrointestinal effects. However, adverse effects were also associated with excessive dosage,[231] concomitant use of other antimicrobials, and stressors such as surgery and transport.[232-235] Anecdotally, OTC therapy has been used successfully in equine practice, and recognition of the equine rickettsial diseases has increased OTC use in horses.[236-238] In a chronic dosing study using a long-acting formulation of OTC, no deleterious effects on fecal flora were detected and treated horses remained clinically normal.[239] DXC is less likely to cause adverse gastrointestinal effects because it is bound in an inactive form in the intestines; however, at higher doses the risk of adverse effects may be increased. One study reported that doses of 20 mg/kg orally twice daily produced signs of abdominal discomfort in one horse and a severe enterocolitis in another. The other four horses in that study were unaffected.[221] DXC administered to foals at 10 mg/kg orally twice daily for 8 to 17 days for treatment of *Lawsonia intracellularis* infection did not produce any adverse effects.[218]

RENAL EFFECTS

Renal tubular necrosis caused by OTC is associated with high doses, outdated parenteral products, endotoxemia, dehydration and hypovolemia, and concurrent pigment nephropathy.[2,240] In normal foals high-dose IV OTC administration for the correction of flexural deformities does not cause renal toxicity.[241] Oliguric renal failure developed in a foal that had concurrent neonatal isoerythrolysis given 70 mg/kg of IV OTC for a flexural deformity.[240]

CARDIOVASCULAR EFFECTS

Rapid IV administration of OTC results in hypotension and collapse. This is attributed to intravascular chelation of calcium, decreased blood pressure from the drug vehicle (propylene glycol), or both. Pretreatment with IV calcium borogluconate prevents collapse.[242,243] Rapid IV administration of DXC to horses causes tachycardia, systemic arterial hypertension, collapse, and death.[222,244] It is suggested that this reaction is due to chelation of intracellular calcium, resulting in neuromuscular blockade of the myocardium. Plasma total and ionized calcium concentrations are not affected by IV DXC administration.

MUSCULOSKELETAL EFFECTS

Intramuscular injection of long-acting OTC formulations causes localized pain and swelling at the injection site.[2,239] OTC causes flexor tendon relaxation; this effect has been used to treat foals with flexural deformities.[245,246] OTC induces a dose-dependent inhibition of collagen gel contraction by equine myofibroblasts. Inhibition of normal collagen organization may provide the mechanistic explanation for the results seen after the pharmacologic treatment of flexural deformities by OTC administration.[247] Because of the neuromuscular blocking effects, tetracyclines are not recommended for the treatment of diseases affecting the neuromuscular junction, such as botulism.

Formulations

Injectable OTC products are formulated as short- or long-acting products. The short-acting solutions are in propylene glycol and have concentrations of 50 or 100 mg/ml. The long-acting solutions are in 2-pyrrolidone or polyethylene glycol and have a concentration of 200 mg/ml. The polyethylene glycol formulation is less irritating than the 2-pyrrolidone formulation. The long-acting formulations may be administered by slow IV injection, but the long-acting effect is lost.[194] DXC tablets are available in multiple generic and proprietary formulations.

Clinical Use

OTC is the drug of choice for treatment of Potomac horse fever *(Neorickettsia risticii)* and equine anaplasmosis *(Anaplasma phagocytophilum)*. It is also used to treat contracted flexor tendons in foals and calves. Its use for other microbial infections in horses is controversial because of concerns related to adverse gastrointestinal effects and widespread antimicrobial resistance. DXC is also indicated for rickettsial diseases in horses and may be a suitable oral alternative to OTC. Tetracyclines are commonly used for treatment of proliferative enteropathy caused by *Lawsonia intracellularis*. DXC is also used for the treatment of keratomalacic diseases in horses because it may decrease corneal proteinases such as MMP-2 and MMP-9.[219]

MACROLIDES AND AZALIDES

The macrolide antibiotics include *erythromycin, clarithromycin, tylosin, tilmicosin,* and *tiamulin. Azalides,* such as *azithromycin,* have a similar mechanism of action but have a methylated nitrogen in the macrocyclic ring. Triamilides, such as tulathromycin, are semisynthetic macrolides prepared by fermentation followed by organic synthesis. Because of their adverse gastrointestinal effects, these drugs are typically contraindicated in adult horses; however, erythromycin, clarithromycin, and azithromycin are commonly used in foals.

Mechanism of Action

The macrolides and their derivatives bind to the 50-S ribosomal subunit in a manner similar to that of CHPC and FLF, and they interfere with protein synthesis. They are usually considered bacteriostatic but may be bactericidal at high concentrations. Macrolides are not effective against gram negative bacteria, except some strains of *Pasteurella* and *Haemophilus* in cattle.[2] Azithromycin is more active than the macrolides against gram negative bacteria and anaerobes.[217,248] Susceptible bacteria include staphylococci, streptococci, *Campylobacter jejunii, Clostridium* spp., *Rhodococcus equi, Lawsonia intracellularis, Mycoplasma* spp., and *Chlamydia* spp.[249]Antimicrobial activity of these weak bases is optimum at an alkaline pH; therefore they have reduced activity in acidic environments (e.g., pus, abscesses) but may be clinically effective because of high concentrations due to ion-trapping. Erythromycin has nonantimicrobial effects on host cell metabolism, inflammatory mediators, and gastrointestinal motility.[250,251]

Mechanisms of Resistance

The routine use of the macrolides is limited because bacterial resistance develops quickly after repeated exposure.[252] Mechanisms of resistance include decreased drug entry into bacteria, inability to bind to the bacterial 50-S ribosomal subunit, and plasmid-mediated production of esterases.[2] Resistance to erythromycin has been reported in 13% of *R. equi* isolates.[253] Extensive cross-resistance occurs among the macrolides.[2]

Pharmacokinetics

ABSORPTION

Erythromycin is available for oral administration as enteric-coated erythromycin base, erythromycin esters (ethylsuccincate or estolate), and erythromycin salts (phosphate or stearate). Because of expense, many practitioners administer the drug as crushed enteric-coated tablets of erythromycin base. However, erythromycin base is degraded in the stomach by gastric acid. The esterified formulations are absorbed intact and must be hydrolyzed to the active erythromycin A. The erythromycin salts are absorbed unchanged.[250] The oral bioavailability of erythromycin base is 17% in fasted foals, with most of the drug being degraded and absorbed as the microbiologically inactive anhydroerythromycin A.[254] Microencapsulation of the base improves the oral bioavailability of erythromycin base to 26% in fasted foals, but it remains only 7.7% in fed foals.[255] The oral bioavailability of erythromycin estolate in fasted foals is 36% but only 16% for erythromycin phosphate.[256] The estolate formulation appears to have the best pharmacokinetic profile in foals. Because of injection site irritation, intramuscular administration of erythromycin is not recommended in horses. The reported oral bioavailability of azithromycin in foals ranges between 39% to 56%.[257,258] The oral bioavailability of clarithromycin in foals is similar (57%).[259] The bioavailability of tulathromycin has not been determined; however, after intramuscular administration the drug is rapidly detected in the plasma of foals, with maximum concentrations of 0.41 μg/ml 4 hours after administration.[260]

DISTRIBUTION

The macrolides are well distributed into most tissues. Erythromycin, clarithromycin, and azithromycin concentrate in leukocytes, making them very effective against intracellular pathogens such as *Rhodococcus equi*.[261] Concentrations of azithromycin and clarithromycin in bronchoalveolar lavage cells were significantly higher than erythromycin, and azithromycin had a significantly longer elimination half-life from the cells.[262] Bronchoalveolar cell and pulmonary epithelial lining fluid concentrations of azithromycin are 15- to 170-fold and 1- to 16-fold higher than concurrent serum concentrations, respectively, and did not decrease for up to 48 hours after administration.[257] Clarithromycin concentrations in bronchoalveolar cell and pulmonary epithelial lining fluid are 91- to 105-fold and 324- to 585-fold higher than concurrent serum concentrations, respectively; however, in contrast to azithromycin, clarithromycin concentrations significantly decreased within 12 hours of administration.[259] Tulathromycin concentrates in bronchoalveolar cells, and concentrations are detectable for at least 8 days after a single administration. Concentrations are higher 192 hours after administration than at 24 hours after administration, indicating ongoing accumulation within these cells.[260]

Because they are weak bases, macrolides are ion trapped in milk, cerebrospinal fluid, and gastric fluids. The Vd for erythromycin is 2.7 L/kg in foals.[254] Azithromycin is known for its high degree of lipid solubility, and the Vd of azithromycin in foals is 11.6 to 18.6 L/kg.[257,258] Clarithromycin also exhibits a large volume of distribution, with reported values of 10.4 L/kg [259] Peritoneal and synovial fluid concentrations of azithromycin and clarithromycin parallel serum concentrations.[259] The apparent Vd for tulathromycin after intramuscular administration is 15.2 L/kg.[260]

ELIMINATION

Erythromycin is extensively metabolized, with much of the parent drug and active metabolite excreted into the bile, resulting in an elimination half-life of 1 to 2 hours.[254-256,263] Erythromycin inhibits the metabolism of a number of other drugs by interfering with cytochrome P450 enzymes.[2] In addition, the degradation product anhydroerythromycin A is a potent inhibitor of cytochrome P450-mediated metabolism.[264] Erythromycin undergoes enterohepatic cycling.[2] Azithromycin is not highly metabolized and is primarily eliminated in bile. The elimination half-life is 16 to 20.3 hours in foals.[257,258] Clarithromycin is extensively metabolized in humans, and the active metabolite, 14-hydroxy-clarithromycin, is produced in foals, although the pharmacokinetics have not been quantitated.[259] The elimination half-life of clarithromycin in foals is intermediate between erythromycin and azithromycin at 5.4 hours.[259] Tulathromycin has the longest elimination half-life, reported at 117 hours in foals.[260]

Adverse Effects and Drug Interactions

The use of erythromycin in horses is associated with a number of adverse effects. Since erythromycin came into clinical use in the 1950s, it was apparent that therapy was frequently accompanied by adverse gastrointestinal effects. Macrolide antibiotics, including erythromycin and clarithromycin, are motilin receptor agonists. They also appear to stimulate motility via cholinergic and noncholinergic neuronal pathways. At microbially ineffective doses they stimulate migrating motility complexes and antegrade peristalsis in the gastrointestinal tract.[251,263,265,266] When used at antimicrobial doses, erythromycin is associated with potentially fatal colitis from *Clostridium* spp.[267-269]

Erythromycin is also associated with acute respiratory distress syndrome, hyperthermia, gastroenteritis, and hepatoxicity in foals.[264,270,271] The mechanism of hyperthermia in erythromycin-treated foals has not been elucidated but likely results from derangement of the hypothalamic temperature set-point.[270] Extreme care should be taken when administering erythromycin to foals with respiratory disease during periods of hot weather. Foals should not be left outside on hot, sunny days while on erythromycin therapy. Erythromycin also interferes with host cell metabolism and decreases inflammatory responses in airways, but the clinical significance of this has not been determined.[264]

Erythromycin is commonly administered in conjunction with rifampin to take advantage of antimicrobial synergism and reduce the chance of resistance development.[12] Erythromycin may interact with other drugs metabolized by the same cytochrome P450 enzyme system. Concurrent administration of erythromycin with theophylline results in a doubling of plasma theophylline concentrations and can result in seizures in foals.[2]

Azithromycin is associated with fewer adverse effects than erythromycin in human beings. No adverse reactions were detected during or after repeated intragastric administration of azithromycin or clarithromycin in foals.[257,259] Azithromycin has been used successfully in adult horses without adverse effects; however, there are anecdotal reports of antimicrobial-associated colitis in older weanlings.

In a study that evaluated the use of tulathromycin in foals with evidence of pulmonary abscessation, self-limiting diarrhea, fever, and injection site reactions were the only adverse effects noted. In one foal in that study, the injection site reaction was severe and resulted in temporary lameness and severe swelling.[272]

Formulations

Because the base of erythromycin is unstable in gastric acid, it is formulated as enteric-coated erythromycin tablets. Erythromycin stearate and erythromycin phosphate are insoluble salt formulations that disassociate in the intestine, allowing absorption of the free erythromycin base. Erythromycin ethylsuccinate and erythromycin estolate are ester formulations that are absorbed intact from the intestine, and then plasma esterases release active drug. Erythromycin is available in an intramuscular formulation approved for cattle. Because of its highly irritating nature, this formulation is not recommended for intramuscular use in horses and it can be fatal if injected intravenously. A human-labeled formulation of erythromycin lactobionate is available for IV use. Tablet formulations are available for azithromycin in 250-, 500-, and 600-mg strengths. Clarithromycin is available as an immediate and extended release tablet. The extended release formulations have not been studied in horses. Tulathromycin is available as a 100-mg/ml injectable solution for cattle and swine.

Clinical Use

On account of its association with potentially fatal adverse effects, erythromycin is usually limited to treatment of *Rhodococcus equi* infections in foals. It also has been shown to be an effective therapy for Potomac horse fever[273] and equine proliferative enteropathy caused by *Lawsonia intracellularis*.[274] Its motilin-like activity is exploited for use as a treatment for adynamic ileus in horses.[251] Azithromycin has become an attractive alternative to erythromycin for the treatment of *R. equi* infections in foals because of its pharmacokinetic profile, which allows once-daily or every-other-day dosing and an apparent reduced incidence of adverse effects.[275] However, in a retrospective study of 81 foals treated for naturally occurring *R. equi* infection, the combination of clarithromycin and rifampin was shown to be superior to combinations of azithromycin and rifampin and erythromycin and rifampin.[261] Tulathromycin may be an acceptable treatment for pulmonary abscesses in foals. Pharmacokinetic and efficacy studies suggest that a once-weekly dosing regimen at 2.5 mg/kg, administered intramuscularly, may be effective.[260,272] This provides a more affordable treatment alternative, although injection site reactions may limit the use of this drug in horses.

FLUOROQUINOLONES

The quinolones are a group of synthetic antimicrobials. The first was *nalidixic acid*, which was introduced in 1964. It had good activity against gram negative bacteria but had a low Vd and numerous adverse effects and was limited to treatment of urinary tract infections. Further chemical manipulation resulted in development of the fluorinated quinolones, which had extended antimicrobial activity with improved safety. Included in this group are *ciprofloxacin, enrofloxacin, danofloxacin, difloxacin, orbifloxacin, marbofloxacin, fleroxacin, moxifloxacin,* and *levofloxacin.* No fluoroquinolones are approved for use in horses, but because of their pharmacokinetics and antimicrobial activity, they are commonly used for serious gram negative infections.

Mechanism of Action

The fluoroquinolones have a unique mechanism of action for bacterial killing. The fluoroquinolones inhibit bacterial deoxyribonucleic acid (DNA) gyrase (also known as *topisomerase II).*

Bacteria have a single chromosome consisting of double-stranded DNA. Within the bacterial cell the chromosome is folded around an RNA core, and each fold is supercoiled. DNA gyrase, which has been found in every organism examined, is responsible for supercoiling the strand of bacterial DNA. The DNA gyrase structure has four subunits: two A monomers and two B monomers. The enzyme forms a heart-shaped molecule, with the A monomers forming the atria and the B monomers forming the ventricles. The bacterial DNA binds to the gyrase in the cleft between the A and B subunits. The DNA gyrase nicks double-stranded DNA, introduces negative supercoils, and seals the nicked DNA. The fluoroquinolones bind to the DNA-DNA gyrase complex and inhibit the DNA resealing, resulting in abnormal spatial DNA configuration, which leads to DNA degradation by exonucleases.[276]

Fluoroquinolone activity is concentration dependent, and clinical efficacy is most associated with achieving either a AUC_{0-24}:MIC greater than 125 or a Cmax:MIC greater than 10. These PK/PD relationships are related, insofar as increasing the dose to increase the peak plasma concentration will also increase the AUC value.[2]

All of the fluoroquinolones are bactericidal, although these drugs have an optimum concentration for bacterial killing. Higher or lower drug concentrations result in reduced bactericidal activity. It is thought that the DNA-DNA gyrase complex has two binding sites for fluoroquinolones. At low drug concentrations only one binding site is occupied, resulting in single-stranded nicks in the DNA. Reduced killing at high concentrations is thought to be due to dose-dependent inhibition of RNA or protein synthesis. RNA and protein synthesis are required for production of bacterial autolysins, which are responsible for the fluoroquinolone-induced cell lysis.[2,276]

The fluoroquinolones are broad spectrum in activity, with activity against most gram negative bacteria; some gram positive bacteria; and *Mycoplasma, Chlamydia,* and *Rickettsia* spp. They are particularly effective against the enteric gram negative pathogens, including some strains resistant to aminoglycosides and cephalosporins. Reported MICs are very low, and MBCs are one to two times the MIC for most pathogens. They are usually active against staphylococci but have variable activity against streptococci and enterococci. Most diagnostic laboratories use ciprofloxacin or enrofloxacin to determine pathogen susceptibility; however, MIC values vary among the fluoroquinolones. Ciprofloxacin has the greatest activity against *Pseudomonas* spp. Orbifloxacin has lower MIC values than enrofloxacin for the gram negative bacteria *Actinobacillus equuli, E. coli, Pasteurella* spp., and *Salmonella* spp. Enrofloxacin has lower MIC values for the gram positive bacteria and *Pseudomonas* spp.[2]

Most fluoroquinolones are not active against anaerobic bacteria.[277] This susceptibility pattern may be a therapeutic advantage in the treatment of enteric infections in horses, because gastrointestinal anaerobes rarely cause disease and usually are protective by competitively inhibiting colonization by pathogenic aerobic organisms.

The fluoroquinolones concentrate within phagocytic cells. Uptake occurs by simple diffusion, and intracellular concentrations may be several times greater than plasma concentrations. Intracellular drug is microbiologically active against intracellular pathogens such as *Brucella* spp., *Mycoplasma* spp., and *Mycobacterium* spp.[2] Exposure of gram negative bacteria to fluoroquinolones at concentrations several times the MIC for 1 to 2 hours results in a PAE with a recovery period of 1 to 6 hours. This effect suggests that fluoroquinolone dosage regimens can tolerate plasma concentrations below the pathogen's MIC for extended periods of time without a reduction in efficacy.[278]

Mechanisms of Resistance

Microbial resistance to the fluoroquinolones is primarily due to chromosomal mutations that alter bacterial DNA gyrase, decrease cell wall permeability, or increase fluoroquinolone efflux from the cell. Plasmid-mediated resistance has only recently been documented for the fluoroquinolones. Fluoroquinolone-resistance plasmids can be transmitted horizontally and provide low-level resistance that facilitates the emergence of higher-level resistance at therapeutic levels.[279] The fluoroquinolones must penetrate bacteria to reach the target DNA gyrase. The fluoroquinolones diffuse through porin channels in the outer membrane of gram negative bacteria. *Pseudomonas* spp. resistance is associated with alterations in a wide range of outer-membrane proteins. From these mutations the increase in the MICs of the fluoroquinolones is relatively low (2- to 32-fold). However, there is cross-resistance with unrelated antibiotics, most frequently TMP, tetracycline, CHPC, and cefoxitin.[280]

Since the fluoroquinolones have been used intensively in human medicine in the last 2 decades, high-level resistance has emerged in some pathogens. Chronic fluoroquinolone use encourages the development of chromosomally mediated resistance. In high-level resistant bacterial strains, one resistance mechanism alone is usually not responsible; rather, two or three mechanisms of resistance operate in conjunction. In resistant *S. aureus* increased efflux is often coupled with a gyrase mutation.[281] In resistant *E. coli* gyrase mutations are usually associated with changes in the outer membrane proteins.[282]

Pharmacokinetics

ABSORPTION

The fluoroquinolones are rapidly and well absorbed from the gastrointestinal tract of monogastrics and preruminant calves. Enrofloxacin is more lipid soluble than ciprofloxacin and has a higher oral bioavailability than ciprofloxacin in horses and small animals. The oral bioavailability of ciprofloxacin is only 6.8% in adult ponies.[283] The oral bioavailability of enrofloxacin is approximately 60% in adult horses and 42% in foals.[284-286] The moderate oral absorption of enrofloxacin has been determined to be due to hepatic first pass effect.[287] Oral absorption of enrofloxacin is not affected by feeding.[288] Antacids containing divalent cations (calcium, magnesium) chelate fluoroquinolones and reduce oral bioavailability.[2] Bioavailability from parenteral injection is nearly 100% for all fluoroquinolones, but intramuscular injections of enrofloxacin are irritating to tissues.[289] For economic reasons and client convenience, practitioners have attempted to administer the bovine injectable solution of enrofloxacin orally to horses. This results in a bioavailability of approximately 65% in horses when administered intragastrically.[290] Unfortunately, the injectable formulation is highly irritating to the oral mucosa and may cause ulceration with repeated use. A methylcellulose gel formulation has better oral absorption but may also cause oral ulceration.[291]

DISTRIBUTION

The fluoroquinolones are extremely lipid soluble and well distributed to most tissues. Tissue concentrations typically exceed plasma concentrations during therapy. Extremely high concentrations are achieved in the kidney, urine, liver, and bile. Therapeutic concentrations for gram negative bacteria may be achieved in cerebrospinal and ocular fluids.[283,285,292,293] Aqueous humor concentrations of enrofloxacin after IV administration of 3 daily doses of 7.5 mg/kg were 0.32 μg/ml.[294] Plasma protein binding of fluoroquinolones is low to moderate in most species. Protein binding data are available only for orbifloxacin and levofloxacon in the horse, which are reported to be 21%[295] and 28%,[296] respectively.

ELIMINATION

The fluoroquinolones are predominantly excreted in the urine by glomerular filtration and active tubular secretion.[2] For marbofloxacin approximately 40% is excreted unchanged in the urine, whereas with enrofloxacin only 3.4% is excreted unchanged in the urine.[287] Ciprofloxacin undergoes some sulfoxidation, and its metabolites also have antimicrobial activity. Enrofloxacin is metabolized (de-ethylated) to ciprofloxacin in horses, with serum ciprofloxacin concentrations reaching 20% to 35% of enrofloxacin concentrations.[289] Metabolism of enrofloxacin to ciprofloxacin is negligible in foals, and ciprofloxacin was not detected in the plasma of foals in which IV or oral enrofloxacin was administered.[284] The elimination half-life of ciprofloxacin in ponies is 2.5 hours and 5 hours in horses.[283] Enrofloxacin has an elimination half-life of 4.4 hours after IV administration and 10 hours after intramuscular administration, indicating flip-flop kinetics.[289] With oral administration the elimination half-life of enrofloxacin is 8 hours.[293]

Adverse Effects and Drug Interactions

Toxicity of fluoroquinolones is mild in most species, and gastrointestinal irritation is the most common side effect.[2] The only fluoroquinolone reported to cause gastrointestinal effects in experimental horses is moxifloxacin.[297] The effects of most clinical concern are arthropathies. Transient arthropathies occur when fluoroquinolones are used in the therapy of *Pseudomonas* pneumonia in children with cystic fibrosis, but their benefits are considered to outweigh the risks of use.[298] Chronic high-dose fluoroquinolone therapy causes articular cartilage lesions in juvenile dogs, particularly in weight-bearing joints.[299] No documented arthropathies have been reported for calves, swine, or poultry. An in vitro study using equine cartilage explants did not demonstrate cartilage damage from enrofloxacin, although proteoglycan synthesis was reduced at high doses.[300] Arthropathies have been documented in 2-week-old foals after receiving 10 mg/kg of enrofloxacin orally.[301] Damage was characterized by synovial joint effusion and lameness and erosion and cleft formation in articular cartilage. Arthropathies were not seen in adult horses that were given up to 25 mg/kg of IV enrofloxacin daily for 3 weeks or 15 mg/kg orally every 12 hours for 3 weeks.[292,302] Although they are not recommended for use in pregnant humans or animals, the fluoroquinolones appear to have little effect on the developing fetus.[303] Enrofloxacin was successfully used to treat chronic pleuritis in a pregnant mare with no apparent detrimental effects on the foal.[304]

Ciprofloxacin and enrofloxacin interfere with the cytochrome P450 system metabolism of methylxanthines such as theophylline. Serum theophylline concentrations may double and result in central nervous system and cardiac toxicity, so concentrations must be monitored during therapy.[305]

The fluoroquinolones may cause adverse central nervous system effects in humans and animals as a result of a γ-aminobutyric acid (GABA) receptor antagonism. This has been associated with an increase in the incidence of seizures in human beings and dogs. Administration of enrofloxacin to human beings results in hallucinations.[2] Rapid IV administration of high doses of enrofloxacin to horses causes transient neurologic signs, including excitability and seizurelike activity.[302] This can be prevented by slow injection or dilution of the dose. Dilution of the dose should be performed in sterile saline solution, because the cations found in other fluids, such as lactated Ringer's solution, may chelate and inactivate the drug. Photosensitivity reactions and Achilles tendon rupture have been associated with fluoroquinolone use in humans but have not been reported in animals.[276]

The fluoroquinolones have been used in combination with other antimicrobial agents to expand the therapeutic spectrum, suppress emergence of drug-resistant bacterial populations, or exploit inhibitory or bactericidal synergism against drug-resistant populations. Minimal synergy occurs between fluoroquinolones and β-lactams or aminoglycosides against gram negative enteric bacteria because of the already high susceptibility of these organisms. Combinations with aminoglycosides, β-lactams, or vancomycin are additive or indifferent against staphylococci. Antagonism between fluoroquinolones and CHPC or rifampin appears to be due to the inhibition of bacterial autolysin synthesis from concurrent administration of bacterial protein synthesis inhibitors.[2]

Formulations

Ciprofloxacin is available as human-labeled tablets, a diluted solution for IV administration, and a solution for ophthalmic use. Enrofloxacin is available as oral tablets and a 50 mg/ml injectable solution for intramuscular injection in dogs and as a 100 mg/ml injectable solution for the subcutaneous treatment of cattle. Both injectable solutions can be administered intravenously to horses. Orbifloxacin, marbofloxacin, and danofloxacin are available as oral tablets for small animals.

Clinical Use

The use of fluoroquinolones in horses has been limited because of the risk of arthropathies; however, enrofloxacin has been successfully used in clinical cases, and fluoroquinolones may be the only viable option for treating some infections.[304,306-308] Informed consent from the client should always be obtained before using fluoroquinolones in young horses. Because the fluoroquinolones are concentration-dependent killers with a long PAE, the ideal dosage regimen is once-daily high-dose therapy.

RIFAMPIN

Mechanism of Action

The rifamycins are antibiotics produced from *Streptomyces mediterranei*. Rifampin inhibits DNA-dependent RNA polymerase in susceptible organisms, suppressing RNA synthesis.

It has no effect on the mammalian enzyme. Its action is bacteriostatic or bactericidal depending on the susceptibility of the bacteria and the concentration of the drug. Rifampin is effective against a variety of mycobacterium species and *S. aureus, Haemophilus,* and *Rhodococcus equi*. Rifampin is considered especially active in the treatment of staphylococcal and rhodococcal infections and in the eradication of pathogens located in difficult-to-reach target areas, such as inside phagocytic cells. It is active at an acid pH, making it a rational choice for the treatment of septic foci and granulomatous infections. It has moderate activity against *Actinobacillus suis, Actinobacillus equuli, Bordetella bronchiseptica,* and *Pasteurella* spp. Equine isolates of *Pseudomonas aeruginosa, E. coli, Enterobacter cloacae, Klebsiella pneumoniae, Proteus* spp., and *Salmonella* spp. are resistant. The ability of rifampin to reach intracellular bacteria can make it difficult to predict in vivo therapy results on the basis of in vitro sensitivity tests.[309] Because bacterial resistance to rifampin develops rapidly, it is usually administered with another antimicrobial.[310] Although it is commonly combined with erythromycin for the treatment of *R. equi*,[12] resistance to the combination has been reported.[252,311] The combination is also effective for treatment of equine monocytic ehrlichiosis (Potomac horse fever).[273] Rifampin is also commonly administered with newer macrolide and macrolide derivative drugs, such as clarithromycin and azithromycin.[261]

Pharmacokinetics

ABSORPTION

The oral bioavailability of rifampin varies between 70% in fasted horses to 26% when administered with feed.[29,309,312] Because rifampin is usually administered with feed, recommended dosages compensate for the decreased bioavailability. Bioavailability after intramuscular injection is 60%.[313]

DISTRIBUTION

Rifampin is highly lipophilic and penetrates most tissues as well as milk, bone, abscesses, and the central nervous system. Feces, saliva, sweat, tears, and urine may be discolored red-orange by rifampin and its metabolites.[314] The Vd of rifampin in horses is 0.6 to 0.9 L/kg.[312,313] Rifampin is 78% bound to plasma proteins.[312]

ELIMINATION

In other species rifampin is deacetylated in the liver to a metabolite that also has antibacterial activity. Desacetylrifampin was not detected in equine serum samples after an IV dose of 10 mg/kg or oral doses of 10 mg/kg every 12 hours for seven doses.[312] Desacetylrifampin was measured in urine, but rifampin was much more predominant. However, only 6.82% of the total dose was recovered in the urine as either rifampin or desacetylrifampin. The elimination half-life of rifampin is 6 to 8 hours after IV administration and 12 to 13 hours after oral administration.[309,312] Because of immature hepatic metabolism, elimination of rifampin is delayed in very young foals.[315,316] Plasma clearance ranges between 1.14 to 1.34 ml/min/kg.[312,313] As a hepatic enzyme inducer, rifampin induces its own metabolism so that multiple oral dosing significantly decreases the elimination half-life. Enzyme induction is typically not been seen with fewer than 5 days of therapy, but once it occurs, the increase in enzyme activity may last for more than 2 weeks after discontinuation of treatment.[317]

Adverse Effects and Drug Interactions

Rifampin stains everything it touches red, and treated animals may produce red urine, tears, sweat, and saliva. There are no harmful consequences from this effect. Most horses object to the taste of rifampin, so care must be taken to deposit a dose quite far back on the tongue and rinse the horse's mouth afterward. Microsomal enzyme induction from rifampin may shorten the elimination half-life and decrease plasma drug concentrations of CHPC, corticosteroids, theophylline, itraconazole, ketoconazole, warfarin, and barbiturates.[314]

Formulations

Rifampin is available as human-labeled capsules or suspension for oral administration or as a diluted solution for IV use.

Clinical Use

Rifampin is primarily used in the treatment of pulmonary abscess caused by *R. equi* and *L. intracellularis* proliferative enteropathy in foals in combination with a macrolide or a macrolide derivative.

METRONIDAZOLE

Mechanism of Action

Metronidazole is rapidly taken up by bacteria, where it is metabolized by a reduction process to cytotoxic derivatives (short-lived free radical compounds). These cytotoxic compounds damage DNA and other critical intracellular macromolecules. Aerobic bacteria lack the reductive pathway necessary to produce the radical compounds.[318] Metronidazole is highly effective against anaerobic bacteria, including *Bacteroides fragilis* (penicillin resistant), *Fusobacterium,* and *Clostridium* spp. Metronidazole-resistant *Clostridium difficile* may cause diarrhea in foals.[319] Metronidazole has good activity against protozoa, including *Giardia* and *Trichomonas* spp.[320] Metronidazole has anti-inflammatory effects in human beings, particularly in the gastrointestinal tract, and has been used in them for the treatment of chronic inflammatory bowel diseases.[321]

Pharmacokinetics

ABSORPTION

Metronidazole is rapidly and well absorbed after oral administration in horses, with an oral bioavailability of 75% to 85%.[320,322] In horses with gastrointestinal ileus, metronidazole may be administered rectally and is rapidly absorbed; however, the bioavailability is only 30%.[323]

DISTRIBUTION

Metronidazole is lipophilic and widely distributed in tissues. It penetrates bone, abscesses, and the central nervous system. The Vd in mares is 0.7 to 1.7L/kg.[320,322]

ELIMINATION

Metronidazole is primarily metabolized in the liver. Both metabolites and unchanged drug are eliminated in urine and feces. Plasma clearance is 2.8 ml/min/kg, and elimination half-life is 3 to 4 hours in horses.[320,322-324]

Adverse Effects and Drug Interactions

With clinical use in horses, anorexia is the only adverse effect associated with the oral use of metronidazole.[325] Metronidazole produces mutations in bacteria, and carcinogenicity occurs in laboratory mice with prolonged exposure. Therefore metronidazole is banned from use in food animals. Because it has been implicated as a teratogen in laboratory animals, use in pregnant animals is not recommended.[2]

Because of its limited antimicrobial spectrum, metronidazole is merely additive to aminoglycosides and β-lactams in the treatment of polymicrobial infections.[2]

Formulations

Metronidazole is available only as human-labeled formulations. It is most commonly administered orally as tablets and capsules. Because it is poorly soluble, the IV formulation must be diluted in a large volume for administration, and it is cost prohibitive in adult horses.

Clinical Use

Metronidazole is used to treat anaerobic infections, especially pleuropneumonia and lung abscesses caused by penicillin-resistant *Bacteroides fragilis* and clostridial enterocolitis.[14,325-327] Although rectal absorption is inferior to oral absorption, it is a viable option for treatment when oral administration is not feasible. Metronidazole has also been used for the treatment of infiltrative bowel diseases in the horse.[328]

NONSTEROIDAL ANTI-INFLAMMATORY DRUGS

Patricia M. Dowling

The most commonly used drugs for treatment of pain and inflammation in horses are the nonsteroidal anti-inflammatory drugs (NSAIDs). The NSAIDs inhibit the enzyme cyclooxygenase (COX), which converts arachadonic acid to the prostaglandins thromboxane and prostacyclin (Figure 4-23). Blocking these ecosanoids results in anti-inflammatory, analgesic, antipyretic, antiendotoxic, and antithrombotic effects.[1]

MECHANISM OF ACTION

Cyclooxygenase Inhibition

Two different, distinct forms of COX have been identified. The constitutively expressed form was considered normal for homeostasis and is referred to as *COX-1,* whereas the inducible form produced in response to injury was considered detrimental and is referred to as *COX-2.*[2] COX-1 is found in platelets, the kidneys, and the gastrointestinal tract; COX-2 is identified in fibroblasts, chondrocytes, endothelial cells, macrophages, and mesangial cells. COX-2 is induced by exposure to various cytokines, mitogens, and endotoxin and is upregulated at sites of inflammation.[3] Unfortunately, this classification of "good" versus "bad" COX proved too simplistic to explain the roles of the different forms of COX.[4] COX-2 is produced constitutively in the brain, spinal cord, kidney, ovary, uterus, placenta, thymus, bone, cartilage, synovia, endothelia, prostate, and lung. COX-2 is involved in cellular processes such as gene expression, differentiation, mitogenesis, apoptosis, bone modeling, wound healing, and neoplasia[5] but can also be induced by hormones, nitric oxide, cytokines, and lipoxygenase products.

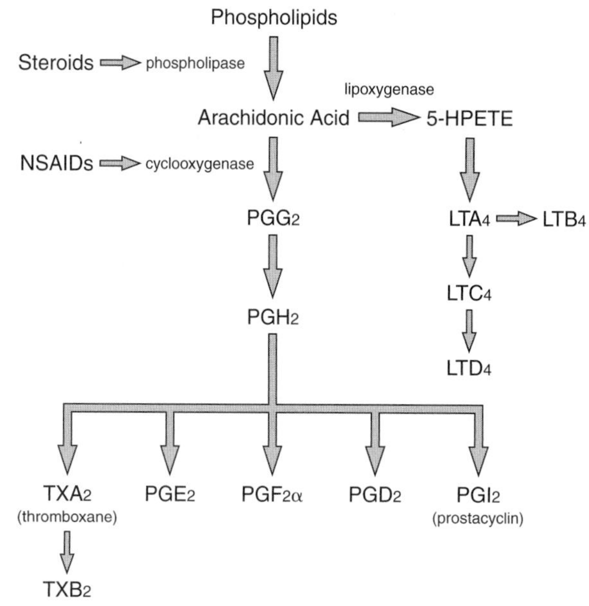

FIGURE 4-23 In the arachidonic acid cascade, cycloxygenase works on arachidonic acid to produce prostaglandins (*PG*), thromboxanes (*TX*), and prostacyclin, whereas lipoxygenase works on arachidonic acid to produce leukotrienes (*LT*). *NSAIDS,* Nonsteroidal anti-inflammatory drugs; *HPETE,* hydroperoxyeicosatetraenic acid.

The prostaglandins produced in the gastrointestinal tract and kidney that maintain mucosal integrity in the upper gastrointestinal tract and renal perfusion, respectively, originally appeared to be derived only from COX-1. It was suggested that COX-2–selective NSAIDs would suppress prostaglandin synthesis at sites of inflammation but would spare constitutive prostaglandin synthesis in the gastrointestinal tract and kidney.[6] Most of the currently available NSAIDs vary in their potency as inhibitors of COX-1, but are far more potent inhibitors of COX-2 than COX-1. The pharmaceutical companies raced to develop COX-2–selective NSAIDs, but this now appears to be an imperfect solution.[5] If COX-2 is primarily responsible for the prostaglandins that mediate pain, inflammation, and fever, then COX-2–selective drugs are not necessarily more therapeutically effective, because the nonselective NSAIDs are already very effective inhibitors of COX-2.[7] Moreover, COX-1–derived prostaglandins contribute to pain, inflammation and fever, so COX-2–selective NSAIDs may actually be less effective.[8] Studies are now published showing that some COX-2 "selective" drugs are therapeutically effective only at doses high enough to inhibit COX-1.[7] Because COX-2 also produces beneficial prostaglandins, the highly selective COX-2 inhibitors produced adverse reactions not seen with traditional NSAIDs.[9] Also, gastrointestinal ulceration is associated with significant mucosal inflammation and expression of COX-2, yet COX-2–derived prostaglandins are responsible for promoting healing.[10] It is now widely accepted that both COX-1 and COX-2 are involved in mucosal defense in the gastrointestinal tract.[11] Likewise, both COX-1 and COX-2 are involved in normal renal function, insofar as prostaglandins affect renal circulation through vasodilation, renin secretion, and sodium and water excretion. As in the gastrointestinal tract, it was thought that COX-1–derived prostaglandins were involved in regulating homeostatic functions and COX-2–derived prostaglandins were involved only in inflammation or tissue damage. However, constitutive expression has been demonstrated for both isoforms in the kidney. Traditional NSAIDs and COX-2–selective NSAIDs both reduce sodium excretion and may cause acute renal failure when maintenance of adequate renal perfusion is prostaglandin dependent.[12]

Anti-inflammatory Effects

The NSAIDs are primarily anti-inflammatory as a result of their inhibition of prostaglandin production. Therefore NSAIDs do not resolve inflammation but prevent its ongoing occurrence. Whereas prostaglandin production will rapidly diminish, any previously present prostaglandin must be removed before inflammation will subside. From tissue cage work, it has been shown that phenylbutazone, ketoprofen, and carprofen have delayed peak concentrations at the site of inflammation and persist in inflammatory exudates for long periods of time after plasma concentrations are negligible.[13-15] This explains the delayed onset and prolonged duration of anti-inflammatory action that does not correlate with plasma pharmacokinetics of the NSAIDs.

The NSAIDs are commonly used in horses to attenuate the prostaglandin-mediated effects of endotoxin.[16-18] Low-dose flunixin has anti-endotoxin effects without obscuring the signs of colic pain, but because it does not alter endotoxin-induced leukopenia, there is little benefit in using the low dose over the recommended dose.[19-25] Flunixin and phenylbutazone significantly inhibit movement of polymorphonuclear and mononuclear cells and antagonize the effects of endotoxin on bowel motility.[16,26]

Other Anti-inflammatory Effects

COX inhibition does not explain all of the anti-inflammatory activity of NSAIDs. NSAIDs are more lipophilic at a low pH, such as is found in inflamed tissues. Some anti-inflammatory action appears to be related to their ability to insert into the lipid bilayer of cells and disrupt normal signals and protein-protein interactions in cell membranes. In the cell membrane of neutrophils, NSAIDs inhibit neutrophil aggregation, decrease enzyme release and superoxide generation, and inhibit lipoxygenase.[27,28]

Analgesic Effects

The NSAIDs act as analgesics by inhibiting COX and preventing the production of prostaglandins that sensitize the afferent nociceptors at peripheral sites of inflammation. However, increasing evidence suggests that some NSAIDs have a central mechanism of action at the level of the spinal cord for analgesia unrelated to COX inhibition.[29] This action is synergistic with opioids and β_2-receptor--adrenergic drugs.[29,30] Work with the specific enantiomers of some NSAIDs has shown the S enantiomers to have good COX-inhibitory effects, whereas R forms can have weak activity against COX yet still produce analgesia.[31,32]

Clinical Implications for Treating Pain and Inflammation

For managing pain and inflammation in horses, NSAIDs are more effective as analgesics when inflammation is a part of the pain process and when they are given before the onset of the inflammatory process or insult. The time to onset and duration of analgesia of NSAIDs does not correlate well with their anti-inflammatory properties. Because the analgesic effect has a more rapid onset and shorter duration of action than the anti-inflammatory action, dosage regimens for effective analgesia may need to be different than those for anti-inflammatory effects.

CHIRALITY

Many of the NSAIDs are *stereoisomers*. Stereoisomers consist of enantiomers with the same molecular formula, but because of asymmetrically oriented chemical groups on a central carbon, they form three-dimensional, nonsuperimposable mirror images and are known as *chiral* compounds.[33] This means that they are like one's hands: superimposable palm to palm but not palm to back. For the NSAIDs it is common to use the *S (sinister)* and *R (rectus)* designations for each of a pair of enantiomers.[34] Although each member of a pair of enantiomers differs in three-dimensional orientation, their physical properties (e.g., melting and boiling points, refractive index, solubility) are identical. Biologic systems are highly chiral environments, and the pharmacokinetics and pharmacodynamic effects of each of a pair of enantiomers may be very different. Stereospecificity may occur in the pharmacokinetic processes of absorption, distribution, metabolism, and excretion, especially if the process involves a carrier protein.[35] If the fit of a drug molecule into the binding site on a protein, enzyme, or receptor involves the chiral center, then the affinity for attachment will be different for each of a pair of enantiomers. Therapeutic efficacy, toxicity, or both may be related specifically to one enantiomer. For the chiral NSAIDs the S enantiomer typically is associated with COX inhibition and the R enantiomer is associated with analgesic effects.[33] Most chiral drugs are formulated as racemic mixtures, containing equal amounts of each enantiomer, because pure enantiomeric compounds are difficult and expensive to manufacture. All of the propionic acid NSAIDs (i.e., ketoprofen, carprofen, vedoprofen, naproxen) are chiral compounds, and, except for naproxen, they are formulated as racemic mixtures. After administration some enantiomers undergo *chiral inversion*, as hepatic enzymes convert one form of the enantiomer to the other form. When chiral inversion of the propionic acid derivatives occurs, it is almost invariably unidirectional, from R to S.[33] The degree of chiral inversion varies among species and cannot be predicted from one species to another, making extrapolating dosages for NSAIDs extremely hazardous.

PHYSICAL PROPERTIES

Almost all NSAIDs are weak acids and highly bound to plasma proteins such as albumin.[1] Therefore they are well absorbed from the stomach, and most of the drug in the plasma is protein bound. Because of protein binding, they are predominantly distributed in the extracellular fluid and only low concentrations of NSAIDs are found in normal tissues and joint fluid. In damaged tissues and joints, however, NSAID concentrations increase to therapeutic levels because of increased blood flow, vascular permeability, and acute phase protein penetration into sites of inflammation. Most NSAIDs undergo hepatic metabolism either through oxidation or glucuronide conjugation before being eliminated in the urine.[1]

DRUG INTERACTIONS

The occurrence and potential hazards of drug interactions must be considered before initiating therapeutic use of the NSAIDs. In general, any two NSAIDs administered together will be additive in their effect.[36-39] Because most NSAIDs act by similar mechanisms of COX inhibition, a higher dose of a single NSAID should produce the same response. Antacids, mucoprotective agents, and adsorbent antidiarrheal drugs can interfere with the absorption of NSAIDs.[36] Concurrent use of corticosteroids is generally contraindicated because corticosteroids increase the secretion of gastric acid, pepsin, and trypsin; alter the structure of gastric mucin; and decrease mucosal cell proliferation. This action is synergistic with NSAID-induced gastrointestinal mucosal damage, but the specific risks of concurrent NSAID and steroid administration are unknown.[40] CHPC decreases the elimination rate, and rifampin significantly increases the elimination rate of phenylbutazone.[41] Concurrent administration of phenylbutazone and procaine penicillin G results in higher serum concentrations of penicillin because of decreased tissue distribution.[42] Concurrent administration of gentamicin and phenylbutazone results in increased distribution and delayed elimination of gentamicin.[43] Phenylbutazone decreases urinary excretion of furosemide and attenuates furosemide-induced increases in urinary excretion of sodium and chloride.[44,45]

ADVERSE EFFECTS OF NONSTEROIDAL ANTI-INFLAMMATORY DRUGS

The adverse effects of the NSAIDs are primarily related to COX inhibition in tissues where prostaglandins are beneficial and protective. NSAIDs classically inhibit platelet aggregation by preventing thromboxane production via the COX-1 pathway.[1] Recovery of platelet function is dependent on the pharmacokinetics of the NSAID and the mechanism of COX inhibition.[46-50] Aspirin permanently modifies COX, so platelet function is restored only by the production of new platelets.[46,50] Renal papillary necrosis (medullary crest necrosis), oral and gastrointestinal ulceration, and right dorsal colitis have been associated with NSAID use in the horse.[51-59] The NSAIDs have a higher incidence of toxicity in neonates because kidney and liver function is not fully developed.[58,60-62] When indicated in neonates, NSAIDs should be administered at the lowest possible doses and at extended dosing intervals. NSAIDs should be administered very cautiously to dehydrated animals.[53,55] Because they mostly distribute in extracellular water, plasma concentrations will be greater than normal in the dehydrated animal and more likely to cause toxicity.

Treatment of NSAID-induced gastrointestinal toxicity is intensive and mainly symptomatic.[51] The hypoproteinemia that results from loss of plasma proteins into the ulcerated gastrointestinal tract can be corrected with IV infusions of plasma. The fluid and electrolyte losses that accompany the diarrhea are managed with commercially available IV fluids. Broad-spectrum antimicrobials are indicated when bacterial septicemia appears to exist. Pain must be managed with opioid analgesics. Anti-ulcer medications may be beneficial and speed recovery. Surgical removal of damaged sections of stomach or colon may be necessary in some cases.[51] Recovery is usually slow, and in severe cases the prognosis is always guarded.

The renal toxicity of NSAIDs is a major concern, particularly in the perioperative period. NSAIDs typically have little effect on renal function in normal adult animals.[63] However, they decrease renal blood flow and GFR in patients with congestive heart failure, that are hypotensive or hypovolemic (especially during anesthesia and surgery), or that have chronic renal disease.[12] A more severe dose-dependent toxicity associated most commonly with phenylbutazone is renal papillary necrosis.[53,58,59] Although attributed to impaired renal blood flow, other mechanisms, such as direct nephrotoxicity of the drug or its metabolites, also may be involved.

The effects of NSAIDs on proteoglycan synthesis should be considered in their clinical use for equine joint disease. Many NSAIDs affect cartilage anabolism in addition to their anti-inflammatory actions.[64,65] A few NSAIDs, such as carprofen, increase proteoglycan synthesis.[64,66] Phenylbutazone does not affect proteoglycan synthesis or chondrocyte viability, but it is protective against chondrocyte-mediated catabolism.[65] The effects of NSAIDs on bone healing are currently controversial, with some laboratory animal studies showing detrimental effects and others showing little or no effect on bone healing.[67] Currently the only NSAID that has shown negative bone healing effects in horses is phenylbutazone.[68] Clinicians should consider the clear benefits of analgesia in equine patients against the potential adverse effects.

ASPIRIN

Aspirin (sodium salicylate) is available only in oral forms. Because it is a weak acid, it is best absorbed in the acidic environment of the upper gastrointestinal tract. During absorption aspirin is partially hydrolyzed to salicylic acid and distributed throughout the body. Highest concentrations are attained in the liver, heart, lungs, renal cortex, and plasma. Extent of protein binding is moderate (about 60%) and depends on species and drug and albumin concentrations.[1] Aspirin is hepatically metabolized by glycine and glucuronide conjugation. Salicylates and their metabolites are rapidly excreted in urine by way of glomerular filtration and active tubular excretion, with an elimination half-life in the horse of approximately 1 hour.[69] In the horse salicylic acid is the primary salicyl compound found in urine.[70] Significant tubular reabsorption occurs, which depends greatly on pH.[1]

Aspirin is the most effective NSAID for antiplatelet therapy.[46,71,72] Aspirin irreversibly acetylates the COX present in platelets, which inhibits the formation of thromboxane A_2, which is responsible for vasoconstriction and platelet aggregation.[46,71,72] Antiplatelet therapy may be beneficial in the management of equine laminitis, disseminated intravascular coagulation, and equine verminous arteritis. A precise antiplatelet dose has not been established, but a dose of 12 mg/kg prolongs bleeding time for 48 hours.[46]

CARPROFEN

Carprofen is a propionic acid derivative formulated as a racemic mixture. Currently available for use in horses in Europe, approval is being sought for North America. The Vd is 0.1 L/kg for the R enantiomer and 0.29 L/kg for the S enantiomer.[13] At the recommended dose of 0.7 mg/kg, carprofen has a longer elimination half-life in horses than most other NSAIDs. After IV administration, the plasma elimination half-life is 21 hours for the R enantiomer and 17 hours for the S enantiomer. The R enantiomer predominates in plasma and exudates because of the hepatic stereospecificity for glucuronidation of the S enantiomer, leading to its more rapid clearance.[73] Chiral inversion of carprofen does not occur in the horse.[73] Like other NSAIDs, carprofen accumulates in inflammatory exudate but produces only modest reductions in the concentrations of ecosanoids compared with flunixin or phenylbutazone.[31,74] Despite this, carprofen produces significant analgesia, probably owing to the central actions of the R enantiomer.[74]

DICLOFENAC

Diclofenac is available as a 1% liposomal suspension cream for topical application in horses. It is used to control pain and inflammation associated with osteoarthritis in the tarsal, carpal, metacarpophalangeal, metatarsophalangeal, and proximal interphalangeal joints in horses. A 5-inch ribbon of dicolfenac topical cream is applied twice daily over the affected joint for up to 10 days. Owners should wear rubber gloves to prevent absorption into the hands. A single topical application of diclofenac cream produced measurable concentrations of diclofenac in transudate within 6 hours and significantly attenuated carrageenan-induced local production of prostaglandin E_2.[75] However, in an amphotericin B acute synovitis model, there was no overall difference between the diclofenac treated group and the control group.[76] In a controlled field study in horses with osteoarthritis of the tarsal, carpal, metacarpophalangeal, metatarsophalangeal, and proximal interphalangeal joints, average lameness scores showed statistically significant improvement after treatment with diclofenac topical cream.[77] The limited systemic absorption of diclofenac makes it useful in the treatment of acute lameness in competitive horses.[78] However, as a result of central sensitization and windup, locally administered diclofenac will be less effective than systemically administered NSAIDs for therapy of chronic pain.

FIROCOXIB

Firocoxib is a COX-2–selective NSAID in an oral paste formulation for treatment of musculoskeletal pain in horses. Firocoxib is dosed at 0.1 mg/kg for up to 14 days. In horses firocoxib is well absorbed, with an oral bioavailability of 79%, and Vd values are approximately 2 L/kg. Firocoxib is slowly eliminated, with reported elimination half-lives as long as 2 days.[79,80] In horses renal clearance of firocoxib is less than total body clearance, which indicates that hepatic clearance through metabolism of firocoxib is the main pathway for elimination in horses.[80] In clinical trials of horses with naturally occurring osteoarthritis, overall clinical efficacy of firocoxib was comparable to that of a paste formulation of phenylbutazone.[81]

FLUNIXIN MEGLUMINE

Flunixin meglumine is a very potent inhibitor of COX that is approved for use in horses and is available in injectable and oral formulations. Flunixin is rapidly absorbed after oral administration, with a bioavailability of 86% and peak serum levels within 30 minutes.[82] Absorption is delayed by feeding.[83] The Vd is 0.1 to 0.3 L/kg in horses, and the plasma elimination half-life is 1 to 2 hours.[82-84] In newborn foals the elimination half-life is prolonged at 13.4 hours. The Vd is also increased in the newborn foal, as is expected with a low Vd drug in the neonate.[85] It is highly protein bound (86%) but appears to readily partition into tissues, hence the relatively high volume of distribution.[86,87] The elimination half-life in inflammatory exudate is 16 hours.[88] The onset of anti-inflammatory action is within 2 hours, peak response occurs between 12 and 16 hours, and duration of action is 36 hours. Analgesic effects have a more rapid onset and shorter duration. Only 14% of a dose is excreted in urine, but otherwise little is known about the metabolism of flunixin.[1]

Flunixin is used in horses for a variety of inflammatory and painful conditions, including colic, colitis, exertional rhabdomyolysis, endotoxic shock, respiratory disease, ocular disease, general surgery, and laminitis.[1] Flunixin is more effective than phenylbutazone in preventing the clinical signs of endotoxemia but appears equivalent to ketoprofen.[89] Flunixin may prevent abortion in endotoxic mares.[90] Flunixin is dosed at 1.1 mg/kg every 24 hours for musculoskeletal pain but may be administered more frequently (every 8 to 12 hours) for colic pain. Low-dose therapy at 0.25 mg/kg every 8 hours is used for anti-endotoxic effects but will not provide much analgesia at this dose. Extremely high doses of flunixin may mask signs of surgical colic pain and interfere with treatment decisions.

Flunixin has a good safety profile, but high doses or chronic dosing can cause anorexia, depression, and gastrointestinal ulcers.[56,91] In normal foals the label dose of flunixin administered for 5 days did not produce adverse effects, but 6 times the label dose resulted in gastrointestinal ulcers.[62] In another study foals were administered flunixin at the label dose for 30 days, and all treated foals developed gastric ulcers.[60] Intramuscular injections of flunixin are highly irritating to muscle and have been incriminated in cases of clostridial myonecrosis in horses; they should therefore be avoided when possible, despite the label directions.[92,93] If not treated promptly and aggressively, clostridial myonecrosis causes severe tissue damage and may be rapidly fatal. Flunixin treatment of horses with ischemic gastrointestinal disease may cause prolonged permeability defects in recovering mucosa.[94-96]

KETOPROFEN

Ketoprofen is a chiral propionic acid derivative approved for horses as a racemic solution for IV or intramuscular injection. Oral and rectal bioavailability is too poor for these routes to be used clinically.[15,97,98] Ketoprofen is 92.8% protein bound in horses.[99] Ketoprofen has a moderate Vd for both enantiomers of approximately 0.5 L/kg and short plasma elimination half-lives of 1 to 1.5 hours.[15,32,88,99,100] Ketoprofen is hepatically metabolized by conjugation reactions, with only 25% of a dose eliminated as unchanged drug in urine.[99] The S enantiomer is associated with antiprostaglandin activity and toxicity, whereas the R enantiomer is associated with analgesia and does not produce gastrointestinal ulceration.[15,101] Because of chiral inversion, the S enantiomer predominates in horses.[15] Ketoprofen accumulates in inflammatory exudates in the horse, where the elimination half-life of the S enantiomer is 23 hours and the R enantiomer is 20 hours. The maximum anti-inflammatory effects of ketoprofen occur at 4 hours after a dose and last for 24 hours, illustrating that the anti-inflammatory effects are not related to plasma concentrations.[88]

In studies of noninfectious arthritis, endotoxemia, and colic, ketoprofen is clinically similar to flunixin meglumine in efficacy.[88,89,101] In an experimentally induced synovitis model, phenylbutazone was more effective in reducing lameness and synovial fluid prostaglandin concentrations.[102] In horses with chronic laminitis, ketoprofen was more effective than phenylbutazone at relieving pain but only at a higher-than-label dose.[103] In a comparative toxicity study, ketoprofen at the label dose had less potential for toxicity than flunixin meglumine or phenylbutazone.[56] In drug tolerance studies using 25 times the label dose for 5 days, horses developed depression, icterus, nephritis, hepatitis, and hemorrhagic necrosis of the adrenal glands.[104]

PHENYLBUTAZONE

Phenylbutazone is the most widely used NSAID in the horse and is available in many generic IV and oral formulations. After oral administration, phenylbutazone is well absorbed, but time to peak concentration may be delayed by feeding.[105-107] The Vd is 0.15 L/kg, with highest concentrations in the liver, heart, kidney, lungs, and plasma.[108] The elimination half-life is 3.5 to 7 hours.[109] In neonatal foals the Vd is higher (0.27 L/kg) and the elimination half-life is longer (6.4 to 22.1 hours) than in adult horses.[110] Plasma protein binding in horses is greater than 99%.[109] Phenylbutazone is metabolized in the liver to oxyphenbutazone, an active metabolite that is eliminated more slowly from the body than phenylbutazone. Oxyphenbutazone inhibits the metabolism of phenylbutazone. Phenylbutazone and its metabolite cross the placenta and are excreted in milk. Less than 2% is excreted in the urine as unchanged drug. The capacity of the liver to metabolize phenylbutazone becomes overwhelmed at relatively low drug doses, resulting in dose-dependent kinetics.[111] The elimination half-life increases with increasing dose rates and increasing age.[111-113] The elimination half-life from exudate is 24 hours.[14] Therapeutic efficacy lasts for more than 24 hours as a result of the irreversible binding of phenylbutazone to COX, slow elimination from inflamed tissues, and long elimination half-life of oxyphenbutazone.[109] Therefore high or frequent doses of phenylbutazone result in disproportionately increasing plasma concentrations, which easily result in toxicity.

Phenylbutazone is used extensively in horses for a variety of musculoskeletal disorders. Although phenylbutazone also antagonizes the disruptive effects of endotoxin on bowel motility, flunixin meglumine is generally preferred for treatment of colic in horses.[16] Phenylbutazone appears to inhibit prostaglandin synthesis at low plasma concentrations in the horse (5-15 μg/ml), whereas much higher drug concentrations are needed in human beings (50-150 μg/ml).[109] This discrepancy is probably due to a species difference in the structure of COX. An initial dose of 4.4 mg/kg every 12 hours on the first day of therapy is followed by a decreased dose and increased dosing interval for subsequent therapy. Because of the accumulation from the long elimination half-life of phenylbutazone and oxyphenbutazone, chronic therapy should be every other day or only as needed to control pain.

Phenylbutazone has a narrow safety margin, especially in foals and ponies and dehydrated horses.[53,62] Phenylbutazone toxicity most commonly results in adverse gastrointestinal effects, including oral, esophageal, gastric, cecal, and right dorsal colonic ulcerations, and accompanying protein-losing enteropathy, hypoproteinemia, leukopenia, and anemia.[51-55,114] Renal papillary necrosis (renal medullary crest necrosis) results from inhibition of prostaglandins that maintain renal blood flow and direct toxicity of phenylbutazone and metabolites.[59] Because phenylbutazone can mask symptoms of lameness in horses for several days after therapy, it may be used to disguise lameness during soundness examinations or for competitive purposes.[109] Extravascular administration results in severe tissue necrosis. Phenylbutazone may have a negative effect on bone healing in horses.[68] Phenylbutazone significantly suppresses total T4 and free T4 concentrations in horses for 10 days.[115]

VEDAPROFEN

Vedaprofen is structurally related to ketoprofen and carprofen and also is formulated as a racemic mixture of S and R enantiomers. It is available in some countries as an IV injectable solution and as a palatable gel for oral administration with a loading dose of 2 mg/kg followed by 1 mg/kg every 12 hours. Oral bioavailability is approximately 100%, and it is highly protein bound (99%). Within 2 hours after IV administration, the mean R:S plasma concentration ratio is 95:5. This is due to marked distribution and elimination differences between the enantiomers, and not chiral inversion. The R enantiomer has an elimination half-life of 2.2 hours and a volume of distribution of 0.23 L/kg, and the S enantiomer has an elimination half-life of 0.76 hours and a volume of distribution of 0.5 L/kg.[116] Both enantiomers accumulate in inflammatory exudate and are more slowly cleared from exudate than from plasma. In an equine acute nonimmune inflammation model, vedaprofen produced significant inhibition of inflammatory swelling and partially inhibited leukocyte migration into the exudate. Inhibition of leukocyte migration was not seen in this model with other NSAIDs.[116]

REFERENCES

Introduction to Clinical Pharmacology

1. Toutain PL, Bousquet-Melou A: Volumes of distribution, *J Vet Pharmacol Ther* 27:441-453, 2004.
2. Baggot JD, Love DN, Stewart J, et al: Gentamicin dosage in foals aged one month and three months, *Equine Vet J* 18: 113-116, 1986.
3. Toutain PL, Bousquet-Melou A: Bioavailability and its assessment, *J Vet Pharmacol Ther* 27:455-466, 2004.
4. Baggot JD: Bioavailability and bioequivalence of veterinary drug dosage forms, with particular reference to horses: an overview, *J Vet Pharmacol Ther* 15:160-173, 1992.
5. Bertucci C, Domenici E: Reversible and covalent binding of drugs to human serum albumin: methodological approaches and physiological relevance, *Curr Med Chem* 9:1463-1481, 2002.
6. Bailey DN, Briggs JR: The binding of selected therapeutic drugs to human serum alpha-1 acid glycoprotein and to human serum albumin in vitro, *Ther Drug Monit* 26:40-43, 2004.
7. Toutain PL, Bousquet-Melou A: Free drug fraction vs free drug concentration: a matter of frequent confusion, *J Vet Pharmacol Ther* 25:460-463, 2002.

8. Craig WA, Ebert SC: Protein binding and its significance in antibacterial therapy, *Infect Dis Clin North Am* 3:407-414, 1989.
9. Benet LZ, Hoener BA: Changes in plasma protein binding have little clinical relevance, *Clin Pharmacol Ther* 71:115-121, 2002.
10. Toutain PL, Bousquet-Melou A: Plasma clearance, *J Vet Pharmacol Ther* 27:415-425, 2004.
11. Intorre L, Mengozzi G, Maccheroni M, et al: Enrofloxacin-theophylline interaction: influence of enrofloxacin on theophylline steady-state pharmacokinetics in the beagle dog, *J Vet Pharmacol Ther* 18:352-356, 1995.
12. von Rosensteil NA, Adam D: Macrolide antibacterials, *Drug interactions of clinical significance, Drug Saf* 13:105-122, 1995.
13. Boothe DM: *Drug disposition and extrapolation of dosing regimens*, St Louis, 2001, Saunders.
14. Baggot JD, Short CR: Drug disposition in the neonatal animal, with particular reference to the foal, *Equine Vet J* 16:364-367, 1984.
15. Johnson PJ, Mrad DR, Schwartz AJ, et al: Presumed moxidectin toxicosis in three foals, *J Am Vet Med Assoc* 214:678-680, 1999.
16. Riviere JE: *Comparative pharmacokinetics: principles, techniques and applications*, Hoboken, NJ, 2003, Wiley-Blackwell.

Antimicrobial Therapy

1. Lorian V, Burns L: Predictive value of susceptibility tests for the outcome of antibacterial therapy, *J Antimicrob Chemother* 25:175-181, 1990.
2. Giguere S, Prescott JF, Baggot JD, et al: *Antimicrobial Therapy in Veterinary Medicine*, 4th ed, Ames, 2006, Blackwell Publishing.
3. Sandholm M, Kaartinen L, Pyorala S: Bovine mastitis: why does antibiotic therapy not always work? An overview, *J Vet Pharmacol Ther* 13:248-260, 1990.
4. Clark C, Dowling PM, Ross S, et al: Pharmacokinetics of tilmicosin in equine tissues and plasma, *J Vet Pharmacol Ther* 31: 66-70, 2008.
5. Ames TR, Patterson EB: Oxytetracycline concentrations in plasma and lung of healthy and pneumonic calves, using two oxytetracycline preparations, *Am J Vet Res* 46:2471-2473, 1985.
6. Kuriyama T, Nakagawa K, Kawashiri S, et al: The virulence of mixed infection with Streptococcus constellatus and Fusobacterium nucleatum in a murine orofacial infection model, *Microbes Infect* 2:1425-1430, 2000.
7. Hariharan H, McPhee L, Heaney S, et al: Antimicrobial drug susceptibility of clinical isolates of Pseudomonas aeruginosa, *Can Vet J* 36:166-168, 1995.
8. Fantin B, Carbon C: In vivo antibiotic synergism: contribution of animal models, *Antimicrob Agents Chemother* 36:907-912, 1992.
9. Marshall SA, Jones RN, Wanger A, et al: Proposed MIC quality control guidelines for National Committee for Clinical Laboratory Standards susceptibility tests using seven veterinary antimicrobial agents: ceftiofur, enrofloxacin, florfenicol, penicillin G-novobiocin, pirlimycin, premafloxacin, and spectinomycin, *J Clin Microbiol* 34:2027-2029, 1996.
10. Vogelman BS, Craig WA: Postantibiotic effects, *J Antimicrob Chemother* 15:A37-46, 1985.
11. McKellar QA, Sanchez Bruni SF, Jones DG: Pharmacokinetic/pharmacodynamic relationships of antimicrobial drugs used in veterinary medicine, *J Vet Pharmacol Ther* 27:503-514, 2004.
12. Prescott JF, Nicholson VM: The effects of combinations of selected antibiotics on the growth of Corynebacterium equi, *J Vet Pharmacol Ther* 7:61-64, 1984.
13. Clark C, Greenwood S, Boison JO, et al: Bacterial isolates from equine infections in western Canada, *Can Vet J* 2008(49): 153-160, 1998-2003.
14. Sweeney CR, Holcombe SJ, Barningham SC, et al: Aerobic and anaerobic bacterial isolates from horses with pneumonia or pleuropneumonia and antimicrobial susceptibility patterns of the aerobes, *J Am Vet Med Assoc* 198:839-842, 1991.
15. Cohen ND, Woods AM: Characteristics and risk factors for failure of horses with acute diarrhea to survive: 122 cases (1990-1996), *J Am Vet Med Assoc* 214:382-390, 1999.
16. Raidal SL, Taplin RH, Bailey GD, et al: Antibiotic prophylaxis of lower respiratory tract contamination in horses confined with head elevation for 24 or 48 hours, *Aust Vet J* 75:126-131, 1997.
17. Whittem TL, Johnson AL, Smith CW, et al: Effect of perioperative prophylactic antimicrobial treatment in dogs undergoing elective orthopedic surgery, *J Am Vet Med Assoc* 215:212-216, 1999.
18. Haven ML, Wichtel JJ, Bristol DG, et al: Effects of antibiotic prophylaxis on postoperative complications after rumenotomy in cattle, *J Am Vet Med Assoc* 200:1332-1335, 1992.
19. Dever LA, Dermody TS: Mechanisms of bacterial resistance to antibiotics, *Arch Intern Med* 151:886, 1991.
20. Gold HS, Moellering RC: Antimicrobial-drug resistance, *N Engl J Med* 335:1445-1453, 1996.
21. Ayala J, Quesada A, Vadillo S, et al: Penicillin-binding proteins of Bacteroides fragilis and their role in the resistance to imipenem of clinical isolates, *J Med Microbiol* 54:1055-1064, 2005.
22. de Lencastre H, Oliveira D, Tomasz A: Antibiotic resistant Staphylococcus aureus: a paradigm of adaptive power, *Curr Opin Microbiol* 10:428-435, 2007.
23. Geddes AM, Klugman KP, Rolinson GN: Introduction: historical perspective and development of amoxicillin/clavulanate, *Int J Antimicrob Agents* 30(Suppl 2):S109-112, 2007.
24. Essack SY: The development of beta-lactam antibiotics in response to the evolution of beta-lactamases, *Pharm Res* 18:1391-1399, 2001.
25. Papich MG: The beta-lactam antibiotics: clinical pharmacology and recent developments, *Compend Contin Educ Pract Vet* 9:68-74, 1987.
26. Falagas ME, Siakavellas E: Bacteroides, Prevotella, and Porphyromonas species: a review of antibiotic resistance and therapeutic options, *Int J Antimicrob Agents* 15:1-9, 2000.
27. Schwark WS, Ducharme NG, Shin SJ, et al: Absorption and distribution patterns of oral phenoxymethyl penicillin (penicillin V) in the horse, *Cornell Vet* 73:314-322, 1983.
28. Schipper IA, Filipovs D, Ebeltoft H, et al: Blood serum concentrations of various benzyl penicillins after their intramuscular administration to cattle, *J Am Vet Med Assoc* 158:494-500, 1971.
29. Baggot JD: Bioavailability and bioequivalence of veterinary drug dosage forms, with particular reference to horses: an overview, *J Vet Pharmacol Ther* 15:160-173, 1992.
30. Firth EC, Nouws JF, Klein WR, et al: The effect of phenylbutazone on the plasma disposition of penicillin G in the horse, *J Vet Pharmacol Ther* 13:179-185, 1990.
31. Durr A: Comparison of the pharmacokinetics of penicillin G and ampicillin in the horse, *Res Vet Sci* 20:24-29, 1976.
32. Love DN, Rose RJ, Martin IC, et al: Serum concentrations of penicillin in the horse after administration of a variety of penicillin preparations, *Equine Vet J* 15:43-48, 1983.
33. McConnico RS, Roberts MC, Tompkins M: Penicillin-induced immune-mediated hemolytic anemia in a horse, *J Am Vet Med Assoc* 201:1402-1403, 1992.
34. Wilkerson MJ, Davis E, Shuman W, et al: Isotype-specific antibodies in horses and dogs with immune-mediated hemolytic anemia, *J Vet Intern Med* 14:190-196, 2000.
35. Nielsen IL, Jacobs KA, Huntington PJ, et al: Adverse reaction to procaine penicillin G in horses, *Aust Vet J* 65:181-185, 1988.

36. Romano A, Mayorga C, Torres MJ, et al: Immediate allergic reactions to cephalosporins: cross-reactivity and selective responses, *J Allergy Clin Immunol* 106:1177-1183, 2000.
37. Chapman CB, Courage P, Nielsen IL, et al: The role of procaine in adverse reactions to procaine penicillin in horses, *Aust Vet J* 69:129-133, 1992.
38. Tobin T, Blake JW: The pharmacology of procaine in the horse: relationships between plasma and urinary concentrations of procaine, *J Equine Med Surg* 1:188-194, 1977.
39. Tobin T, Blake JW, Sturma L, et al: Pharmacology of procaine in the horse: procaine esterase properties of equine plasma and synovial fluid, *Am J Vet Res* 37:1165-1170, 1976.
40. Olsen L, Ingvast-Larsson C, Brostrom H, et al: Clinical signs and etiology of adverse reactions to procaine benzylpenicillin and sodium/potassium benzylpenicillin in horses, *J Vet Pharmacol Ther* 30:201-207, 2007.
41. Stevenson AJ, Weber MP, Todi F, et al: Plasma elimination and urinary excretion of procaine after administration of different products to standardbred mares, *Equine Vet J* 24: 118-124, 1992.
42. Adamson PJ, Wilson WD, Hirsh DC, et al: Susceptibility of equine bacterial isolates to antimicrobial agents, *Am J Vet Res* 46:447-450, 1985.
43. Firth EC, Klein WR, Nouws JF, et al: Effect of induced synovial inflammation on pharmacokinetics and synovial concentration of sodium ampicillin and kanamycin sulfate after systemic administration in ponies, *J Vet Pharmacol Ther* 11:556-562, 1988.
44. Ensink JM, Moi A, Vulto AG, et al: Bioavailability of pivampicillin and ampicillin trihydrate administered as an oral paste in horses, *Vet Q* 18:2s117-120.
45. Wilson WD, Spensley MS, Baggot JD, et al: Pharmacokinetics and estimated bioavailability of amoxicillin in mares after intravenous, intramuscular, and oral administration, *Am J Vet Res* 49:1688-1694, 1988.
46. Baggot JD, Love DN, Stewart J, et al: Bioavailability and disposition kinetics of amoxicillin in neonatal foals, *Equine Vet J* 20:125-127, 1988.
47. Ensink JM, Vulto AG, van Miert AS, et al: Oral bioavailability and in vitro stability of pivampicillin, bacampicillin, talampicillin, and ampicillin in horses, *Am J Vet Res* 57:1021-1024, 1996.
48. Ensink JM, Klein WR, Mevius DJ, et al: Bioavailability of oral penicillins in the horse: a comparison of pivampicillin and amoxicillin, *J Vet Pharmacol Ther* 15:221-230, 1992.
49. Sarasola P, McKellar QA: Pharmacokinetics and applications of ampicillin sodium as an intravenous infusion in the horse, *J Vet Pharmacol Ther* 16:63-69, 1993.
50. van den Hoven R, Hierweck B, Dobretsberger M, et al: Intramuscular dosing strategy for ampicillin sodium in horses, based on its distribution into tissue chambers before and after induction of inflammation, *J Vet Pharmacol Ther* 26:405-411, 2003.
51. Bowman KF, Dix LP, Riond JL, et al: Prediction of pharmacokinetic profiles of ampicillin sodium, gentamicin sulphate, and combination ampicillin sodium-gentamicin sulphate in serum and synovia of healthy horses, *Am J Vet Res* 47: 1590-1596, 1986.
52. Errecalde JO, Carmely D, Marino EL, et al: Pharmacokinetics of amoxycillin in normal horses and horses with experimental arthritis, *J Vet Pharmacol Ther* 24:1-6, 2001.
53. Ensink JM, Klein WR, Barneveld A, et al: Distribution of penicillins into subcutaneous tissue chambers in ponies, *J Vet Pharmacol Ther* 19:439-444, 1996.
54. Montesissa C, Carli S, Sonzogni O, et al: Pharmacokinetics of sodium amoxicillin in horses, *Res Vet Sci* 44:233-236, 1988.
55. Beech J, Leitch M, Kohn CW, et al: Serum and synovial fluid levels of sodium ampicillin and ampicillin trihydrate in horses, *J Equine Med Surg* 3:3503-3504, 1979.
56. Traver DS, Riviere JE: Ampicillin in mares: a comparison of intramuscular sodium ampicillin or sodium ampicillin-ampicillin trihydrate injection, *Am J Vet Res* 43:402-404, 1982.
57. Spensley MS, Baggot JD, Wilson WD, et al: Pharmacokinetics and endometrial tissue concentrations of ticarcillin given to the horse by intravenous and intrauterine routes, *Am J Vet Res* 47:2587-2590, 1986.
58. Sweeney CR, Soma LR, Beech J, et al: Pharmacokinetics of ticarcillin in the horse after intravenous and intramuscular administration, *Am J Vet Res* 45:1000-1002, 1984.
59. Sandanayaka VP, Prashad AS: Resistance to beta-lactam antibiotics: structure and mechanism based design of beta-lactamase inhibitors, *Curr Med Chem* 9:1145-1165, 2002.
60. Finlay J, Miller L, Poupard JA: A review of the antimicrobial activity of clavulanate, *J Antimicrob Chemother* 52:18-23, 2003.
61. Wilson WD, Spensley MS, Baggot JD, et al: Pharmacokinetics and bioavailability of ticarcillin and clavulanate in foals after intravenous and intramuscular administration, *J Vet Pharmacol Ther* 14:78-89, 1991.
62. Sweeney RW, Beech J, Simmons RD, et al: Pharmacokinetics of ticarcillin and clavulanic acid given in combination to adult horses by intravenous and intramuscular routes, *J Vet Pharmacol Ther* 11:103-108, 1988.
63. Van Camp SD, Papich MG, Whitacre MD: Administration of ticarcillin in combination with clavulanic acid intravenously and intrauterinely to clinically normal oestrous mares, *J Vet Pharmacol Ther* 23:373-378, 2000.
64. Hoffman AM, Viel L, Muckle CA, et al: Evaluation of sulbactam plus ampicillin for treatment of experimentally induced Klebsiella pneumoniae lung infection in foals, *Am J Vet Res* 53:1059-1067, 1992.
65. Brogan JC: Sorting out the cephalosporins, *Postgrad Med* 91:301-304, 1992:307-308, 311-302 passim.
66. Hornish RE, Kotarski SF: Cephalosporins in veterinary medicine: ceftiofur use in food animals, *Curr Top Med Chem* 2:717-731, 2002.
67. Salmon SA, Watts JL, Yancey RJ: In vitro activity of ceftiofur and its primary metabolite, desfuroylceftiofur, against organisms of veterinary importance, *J Vet Diagn Invest* 8:332-336, 1996.
68. Rice LB: Emergence of vancomycin-resistant enterococci, *Emerg Infect Dis* 7:183-187, 2001.
69. Duffee NE, Christensen JM, Craig AM: The pharmacokinetics of cefadroxil in the foal, *J Vet Pharmacol Ther* 12:322-326, 1989.
70. Wilson WD, Baggot JD, Adamson PJ, et al: Cefadroxil in the horse: pharmacokinetics and in vitro antibacterial activity, *J Vet Pharmacol Ther* 8:246-253, 1985.
71. Lovering AM, Walsh TR, Bannister GC, et al: The penetration of ceftriaxone and cefamandole into bone, fat and haematoma and relevance of serum protein binding to their penetration into bone, *J Antimicrob Chemother* 47:483-486, 2001.
72. Cunha BA: Third-generation cephalosporins: a review, *Clin Ther* 14:616-652, 1992; discussion 615.
73. Meyer JC, Brown MP, Gronwall RR, et al: Pharmacokinetics of ceftiofur sodium in neonatal foals after intramuscular injection, *Equine Vet J* 24:485-486, 1992.
74. Jaglan PS, Roof RD, Yein FS, et al: Concentration of ceftiofur metabolites in the plasma and lungs of horses following intramuscular treatment, *J Vet Pharmacol Ther* 17:24-30, 1994.
75. Soraci AL, Mestorino ON, Errecalde JO: Pharmacokinetics of cefoperazone in horses, *J Vet Pharmacol Ther* 19:39-43, 1996.
76. Strom BL, Schinnar R, Gibson GA, et al: Risk of bleeding and hypoprothrombinaemia associated with NMTT side chain antibiotics: using cefoperazone as a test case, *Pharmacoepidemiol Drug Saf* 8:81-94, 1999.

77. Gardner SY, Aucoin DP: Pharmacokinetics of ceftriaxone in mares, *J Vet Pharmacol Ther* 17:155-156, 1994.
78. Gardner SY, Sweeney RW, Divers TJ: Pharmacokinetics of cefotaxime in neonatal pony foals, *Am J Vet Res* 54:576-579, 1993.
79. Guglick MA, MacAllister CG, Clarke CR, et al: Pharmacokinetics of cefepime and comparison with those of ceftiofur in horses, *Am J Vet Res* 59:458-463, 1998.
80. Foreman JH: *Does ceftiofur cause diarrhea? AAEP 44th Annual Convention Proceedings* :146-147, 1994.
81. Mahrt CR: Safety of ceftiofur sodium administered intramuscularly in horses, *Am J Vet Res* 53:2201-2205, 1992.
82. Fanos V, Cataldi L: Renal transport of antibiotics and nephrotoxicity: a review, *J Chemother* 13:461-472, 2001.
83. Miranda-Novales G, Leanos-Miranda BE, Vilchis-Perez M, et al: In vitro activity effects of combinations of cephalothin, dicloxacillin, imipenem, vancomycin and amikacin against methicillin-resistant Staphylococcus spp. strains, *Ann Clin Microbiol Antimicrob* 5:25, 2006.
84. Beauchamp D, Theriault G, Grenier L, et al: Ceftriaxone protects against tobramycin nephrotoxicity, *Antimicrob Agents Chemother* 38:750-756, 1994.
85. Donecker JM, Sams RA, Ashcraft SM: Pharmacokinetics of probenecid and the effect of oral probenecid administration on the pharmacokinetics of cefazolin in mares, *Am J Vet Res* 47:89-95, 1986.
86. Sams RA, Ruoff WW: Pharmacokinetics and bioavailability of cefazolin in horses, *Am J Vet Res* 46:348-352, 1985.
87. Ruoff WW, Sams RA: Pharmacokinetics and bioavailability of cephalothin in horse mares, *Am J Vet Res* 46:2085-2090, 1985.
88. Brown MP, Gronwall RR, Houston AE: Pharmacokinetics and body fluid and endometrial concentrations of cepharpirin in mares, *Am J Vet Res* 47:784-788, 1986.
89. Brown MP, Gronwall RR, Houston AE: Pharmacokinetics and serum concentrations of cepharpirin in neonatal foals, *Am J Vet Res* 48:805-807, 1987.
90. Juzwiak JS, Brown MP, Gronwall R, et al: Effect of probenecid administration on cephapirin pharmacokinetics and concentrations in mares, *Am J Vet Res* 50:1742-1747, 1989.
91. Henry MM, Morris DD, Lakritz J, et al: Pharmacokinetics of cephradine in neonatal foals after single oral dosing, *Equine Vet J* 24:242-243, 1992.
92. Brown MP, Gronwall RR, Houston AE: Pharmacokinetics and body fluid and endometrial concentrations of cefoxitin in mares, *Am J Vet Res* 47:1734-1738, 1986.
93. Morris DD, Rutkowski J, Lloyd KC: Therapy in two cases of neonatal foal septicaemia and meningitis with cefotaxime sodium, *Equine Vet J* 19:151-154, 1987.
94. Carrillo NA, Giguere S, Gronwall RR, et al: Disposition of orally administered cefpodoxime proxetil in foals and adult horses and minimum inhibitory concentration of the drug against common bacterial pathogens of horses, *Am J Vet Res* 66:30-35, 2005.
95. Gardner SY, Papich MG: Comparison of cefepime pharmacokinetics in neonatal foals and adult dogs, *J Vet Pharmacol Ther* 24:187-192, 2001.
96. Dyke TM, Hinchcliff KW: Treatment of respiratory infections in horses with ceftiofur sodium, *Equine Vet J* 25:197-198, 1993.
97. Folz SD, Hanson BJ, Griffin AK, et al: Treatment of respiratory infections in horses with ceftiofur sodium, *Equine Vet J* 24: 300-304, 1992.
98. Verheyen K, Newton JR, Talbot NC, et al: Elimination of guttural pouch infection and inflammation in asymptomatic carriers of Streptococcus equi, *Equine Vet J* 32:527-532, 2000.
99. Holcombe SJ, Schneider RK, Bramlage LR, et al: Use of antibiotic-impregnated polymethyl methacrylate in horses with open or infected fractures or joints: 19 cases (1987-1995), *J Am Vet Med Assoc* 211:889-893, 1997.
100. Pille F, De Baere S, Ceelen L, et al: Synovial fluid and plasma concentrations of ceftiofur after regional intravenous perfusion in the horse, *Vet Surg* 34:610-617, 2005.
101. Schneider RK, Andrea R, Barnes HG: Use of antibiotic-impregnated polymethyl methacrylate for treatment of an open radial fracture in a horse, *J Am Vet Med Assoc* 207:1454-1457, 1995.
102. Brown SA, Riviere JE: Comparative pharmacokinetics of aminoglycoside antibiotics, *J Vet Pharmacol Ther* 14:1-35, 1991.
103. Barclay ML, Begg EJ, Hickling KG: What is the evidence for once-daily aminoglycoside therapy? *Clin Pharmacokinet* 27:32-48, 1994.
104. Nestaas E, Bangstad HJ, Sandvik L, et al: Aminoglycoside extended interval dosing in neonates is safe and effective: a meta-analysis, *Arch Dis Child Fetal Neonatal Ed* 90:F294-300, 2005.
105. Pohl P, Glupczynski Y, Marin M, et al: Replicon typing characterization of plasmids encoding resistance to gentamicin and apramycin in Escherichia coli and Salmonella typhimurium isolated from human and animal sources in Belgium, *Epidemiol Infect* 111:229-238, 1993.
106. Barclay ML, Begg EJ: Aminoglycoside adaptive resistance: importance for effective dosage regimens, *Drugs* 61:713-721, 2001.
107. Barclay ML, Begg EJ: Aminoglycoside toxicity and relation to dose regimen, *Adverse Drug React Toxicol Rev* 13:207-234, 1994.
108. Daikos GL, Jackson GG, Lolans VT, et al: Adaptive resistance to aminoglycoside antibiotics from first-exposure downregulation, *J Infect Dis* 162:414-420, 1990.
109. Daikos GL, Lolans VT, Jackson GG: First-exposure adaptive resistance to aminoglycoside antibiotics in vivo with meaning for optimal clinical use, *Antimicrob Agents Chemother* 35:117-123, 1991.
110. Cummings LE, Guthrie AJ, Harkins JD, et al: Pharmacokinetics of gentamicin in newborn to 30-day-old foals, *Am J Vet Res* 51:1988-1992, 1990.
111. Wichtel MG, Breuhaus BA, Aucoin D: Relation between pharmacokinetics of amikacin sulfate and sepsis score in clinically normal and hospitalized neonatal foals, *J Am Vet Med Assoc* 200:1339-1343, 1992.
112. Anderson BH, Firth EC, Whittem T: The disposition of gentamicin in equine plasma, synovial fluid and lymph, *J Vet Pharmacol Ther* 18:124-131, 1995.
113. Godber LM, Walker RD, Stein GE, et al: Pharmacokinetics, nephrotoxicosis, and in vitro antibacterial activity associated with single versus multiple (three times) daily gentamicin treatments in horses, *Am J Vet Res* 56:613-618, 1995.
114. Santschi EM, Papich MG: Pharmacokinetics of gentamicin in mares in late pregnancy and early lactation, *J Vet Pharmacol Ther* 23:359-363, 2000.
115. Snyder JR, Pascoe JR, Hietala SK, et al: Gentamicin tissue concentrations in equine small intestine and large colon, *Am J Vet Res* 47:1092-1095, 1986.
116. Wilson RC, Moore JN, Eakle N: Gentamicin pharmacokinetics in horses given small doses of Escherichia coli endotoxin, *Am J Vet Res* 44:1746-1749, 1983.
117. Jones SL, Wilson WD, Milhalyi JE: Pharmacokinetics of gentamicin in healthy adult horses during intravenous fluid administration, *J Vet Pharmacol Ther* 21:247-249, 1998.
118. Tudor RA, Papich MG, Redding WR: Drug disposition and dosage determination of once daily administration of gentamicin sulfate in horses after abdominal surgery, *J Am Vet Med Assoc* 215:503-506, 1999.
119. Easter JL, Hague BA, Brumbaugh GW, et al: Effects of postoperative peritoneal lavage on pharmacokinetics of gentamicin in horses after celiotomy, *Am J Vet Res* 58:1166-1170, 1997.

120. Haddad NS, Pedersoli WM, Ravis WR, et al: Pharmacokinetics of gentamicin at steady-state in ponies: serum, urine, and endometrial concentrations, *Am J Vet Res* 46:1268-1271, 1985.
121. Orsini JA, Park MI, Spencer PA: Tissue and serum concentrations of amikacin after intramuscular and intrauterine administration to mares in estrus, *Can Vet J* 37:157-160, 1996.
122. Pedersoli WM, Fazeli MH, Haddad NS, et al: Endometrial and serum gentamicin concentrations in pony mares given repeated intrauterine infusions, *Am J Vet Res* 46:1025-1028, 1985.
123. Beech J, Kohn C, Leitch M, et al: Therapeutic use of gentamicin in horses: concentrations in serum, urine, and synovial fluid and evaluation of renal function, *Am J Vet Res* 38: 1085-1087, 1977.
124. Lloyd KC, Stover SM, Pascoe JR, et al: Effect of gentamicin sulfate and sodium bicarbonate on the synovium of clinically normal equine antebrachiocarpal joints, *Am J Vet Res* 49: 650-657, 1988.
125. Lescun TB, Adams SB, Wu CC, et al: Continuous infusion of gentamicin into the tarsocrural joint of horses, *Am J Vet Res* 61:407-412, 2000.
126. Murphey ED, Santschi EM, Papich MG: Regional intravenous perfusion of the distal limb of horses with amikacin sulfate, *J Vet Pharmacol Ther* 22:68-71, 1999.
127. Whitehair KJ, Blevins WE, Fessler JF, et al: Regional perfusion of the equine carpus for antibiotic delivery, *Vet Surg* 21: 279-285, 1992.
128. Whitehair KJ, Bowersock TL, Blevins WE, et al: Regional limb perfusion for antibiotic treatment of experimentally induced septic arthritis, *Vet Surg* 21:367-373, 1992.
129. Errico JA, Trumble TN, Bueno AC, et al: Comparison of two indirect techniques for local delivery of a high dose of an antimicrobial in the distal portion of forelimbs of horses, *Am J Vet Res* 69:334-342, 2008.
130. Parra-Sanchez A, Lugo J, Boothe DM, et al: Pharmacokinetics and pharmacodynamics of enrofloxacin and a low dose of amikacin administered via regional intravenous limb perfusion in standing horses, *Am J Vet Res* 67:1687-1695, 2006.
131. Butt TD, Bailey JV, Dowling PM, et al: Comparison of 2 techniques for regional antibiotic delivery to the equine forelimb: intraosseous perfusion vs. intravenous perfusion, *Can Vet J* 42:617-622, 2001.
132. Booth TM, Butson RJ, Clegg PD, et al: Treatment of sepsis in the small tarsal joints of 11 horses with gentamicin-impregnated polymethylmethacrylate beads, *Vet Rec* 148:376-380, 2001.
133. Butson RJ, Schramme MC, Garlick MH, et al: Treatment of intrasynovial infection with gentamicin-impregnated polymethylmethacrylate beads, *Vet Rec* 138:460-464, 1996.
134. Farnsworth KD, White NA 2nd, Robertson J: The effect of implanting gentamicin-impregnated polymethylmethacrylate beads in the tarsocrural joint of the horse, *Vet Surg* 30:126-131, 2001.
135. Ivester KM, Adams SB, Moore GE, et al: Gentamicin concentrations in synovial fluid obtained from the tarsocrural joints of horses after implantation of gentamicin-impregnated collagen sponges, *Am J Vet Res* 67:1519-1526, 2006.
136. Kaloyanides GJ: Antibiotic-related nephrotoxicity, *Nephrol Dial Transplant* 9:4130-4134, 1994.
137. Tulkens PM: Nephrotoxicity of aminoglycoside antibiotics, *Toxicol Lett* 46:107-123, 1989.
138. Kaloyanides GJ: Drug-phospholipid interactions: role in aminoglycoside nephrotoxicity, *Ren Fail* 14:351-357, 1992.
139. van der Harst MR, Bull S, Laffont CM, et al: Gentamicin nephrotoxicity-a comparison of in vitro findings with in vivo experiments in equines, *Vet Res Commun* 29:247-261, 2005.
140. Molitoris BA, Meyer C, Dahl R, et al: Mechanism of ischemia-enhanced aminoglycoside binding and uptake by proximal tubule cells, *Am J Physiol* 264:F907-916, 1993.
141. Riviere JE, Coppoc GL, Hinsman EJ, et al: Species dependent gentamicin pharmacokinetics and nephrotoxicity in the young horse, *Fundam Appl Toxicol* 3:448-457, 1983.
142. Sweeney RW, MacDonald M, Hall J, et al: Kinetics of gentamicin elimination in two horses with acute renal failure, *Equine Vet J* 20:182-184, 1988.
143. Matzke GR, Frye RF: Drug administration in patients with renal insufficiency. Minimising renal and extrarenal toxicity, *Drug Saf* 16:205-231, 1997.
144. Thatte L, Vaamonde CA: Drug-induced nephrotoxicity: the crucial role of risk factors, *Postgrad Med* 100:83-84, 1996.
145. Brashier MK, Geor RJ, Ames TR, et al: Effect of intravenous calcium administration on gentamicin-induced nephrotoxicosis in ponies, *Am J Vet Res* 59:1055-1062, 1998.
146. Varzi HN, Esmailzadeh S, Morovvati H, et al: Effect of silymarin and vitamin E on gentamicin-induced nephrotoxicity in dogs, *J Vet Pharmacol Ther* 30:477-481, 2007.
147. Schumacher J, Wilson RC, Spano JS, et al: Effect of diet on gentamicin-induced nephrotoxicosis in horses, *Am J Vet Res* 52:1274-1278, 1991.
148. Behrend EN, Grauer GF, Greco DS, et al: Effects of dietary protein conditioning on gentamicin pharmacokinetics in dogs, *J Vet Pharmacol Ther* 17:259-264, 1994.
149. Drusano GL, Ambrose PG, Bhavnani SM, et al: Back to the future: using aminoglycosides again and how to dose them optimally, *Clin Infect Dis* 45:753-760, 2007.
150. Magdesian KG, Hogan PM, Cohen ND, et al: Pharmacokinetics of a high dose of gentamicin administered intravenously or intramuscularly to horses, *J Am Vet Med Assoc* 213: 1007-1011, 1998.
151. Magdesian KG, Wilson WD, Mihalyi J: Pharmacokinetics of a high dose of amikacin administered at extended intervals to neonatal foals, *Am J Vet Res* 65:473-479, 2004.
152. Bates DE: Aminoglycoside ototoxicity, *Drugs Today (Barc)* 39:277-285, 2003.
153. Selimoglu E: Aminoglycoside-induced ototoxicity, *Curr Pharm Des* 13:119-126, 2007.
154. Wu WJ, Sha SH, Schacht J: Recent advances in understanding aminoglycoside ototoxicity and its prevention, *Audiol Neurootol* 7:171-174, 2002.
155. Selimoglu E, Kalkandelen S, Erdogan F: Comparative vestibulotoxicity of different aminoglycosides in the Guinea pigs, *Yonsei Med J* 44:517-522, 2003.
156. Kalkandelen S, Selimoglu E, Erdogan F, et al: Comparative cochlear toxicities of streptomycin, gentamicin, amikacin and netilmicin in guinea-pigs, *J Int Med Res* 30:406-412, 2002.
157. Green SL, Conlon PD, Mama K, et al: Effects of hypoxia and azotaemia on the pharmacokinetics of amikacin in neonatal foals, *Equine Vet J* 24:475-479, 1992.
158. Brown SA, Garry FB: Comparison of serum and renal gentamicin concentrations with fractional urinary excretion tests as indicators of nephrotoxicity, *J Vet Pharmacol Ther* 11: 330-337, 1988.
159. Whiting PH, Brown PA: The relationship between enzymuria and kidney enzyme activities in experimental gentamicin nephrotoxicity, *Ren Fail* 18:899-909, 1996.
160. Paradelis AG, Triantaphyllidis C, Giala MM: Neuromuscular blocking activity of aminoglycoside antibiotics, *Methods Find Exp Clin Pharmacol* 2:45-51, 1980.
161. Hildebrand SV, Hill T 3rd: Interaction of gentamycin and atracurium in anaesthetised horses, *Equine Vet J* 26:209-211, 1994.
162. Smith CM, Steffey EP, Baggot JD, et al: Effects of halothane anesthesia on the clearance of gentamicin sulfate in horses, *Am J Vet Res* 49:19-22, 1988.
163. Whittem T, Firth EC, Hodge H, et al: Pharmacokinetic interactions between repeated dose phenylbutazone and gentamicin in the horse, *J Vet Pharmacol Ther* 19:454-459, 1996.

164. Cannon M, Harford S, Davies J: A comparative study on the inhibitory actions of chloramphenicol, thiamphenicol and some fluorinated derivatives, *J Antimicrob Chemother* 26: 307-317, 1990.
165. Berge AC, Epperson WB, Pritchard RH: Assessing the effect of a single dose florfenicol treatment in feedlot cattle on the antimicrobial resistance patterns in faecal Escherichia coli, *Vet Res* 36:723-734, 2005.
166. Cloeckaert A, Baucheron S, Flaujac G, et al: Plasmid-mediated florfenicol resistance encoded by the floR gene in Escherichia coli isolated from cattle, *Antimicrob Agents Chemother* 44:2858-2860, 2000.
167. Brumbaugh GW, Martens RJ, Knight HD, et al: Pharmacokinetics of chloramphenicol in the neonatal horse, *J Vet Pharmacol Ther* 6:219-227, 1983.
168. Gronwall R, Brown MP, Merritt AM, et al: Body fluid concentrations and pharmacokinetics of chloramphenicol given to mares intravenously or by repeated gavage, *Am J Vet Res* 47:2591-2595, 1986.
169. McKellar QA, Varma KJ: Pharmacokinetics and tolerance of florfenicol in Equidae, *Equine Vet J* :209-213, 1996.
170. Dowling PM. Florfenicol in horses: pharmacokinetics and tolerance, 19th Annual ACVIM Forum 198-199, 2001.
171. Nau R, Sorgel F, Prange HW: Pharmacokinetic optimisation of the treatment of bacterial central nervous system infections, *Clin Pharmacokinet* 35:223-246, 1998.
172. de Craene BA, Deprez P, D'Haese E, et al: Pharmacokinetics of florfenicol in cerebrospinal fluid and plasma of calves, *Antimicrob Agents Chemother* 41:1991-1995, 1997.
173. Brown MP, Kelly RH, Gronwall RR, et al: Chloramphenicol sodium succinate in the horse: serum, synovial, peritoneal, and urine concentrations after single-dose intravenous administration, *Am J Vet Res* 45:578-580, 1984.
174. Sisodia CS, Kramer LL, Gupta VS, et al: A pharmacological study of chloramphenicol in horses, *Can J Comp Med* 39: 216-223, 1975.
175. Adams PE, Varma KJ, Powers TE, et al: Tissue concentrations and pharmacokinetics of florfenicol in male veal calves given repeated doses, *Am J Vet Res* 48:1725-1732, 1987.
176. Adamson PJ, Wilson WD, Baggot JD, et al: Influence of age on the disposition kinetics of chloramphenicol in equine neonates, *Am J Vet Res* 52:426-431, 1991.
177. Varma KJ, Powers TE, Powers JD: Single- and repeat-dose pharmacokinetic studies of chloramphenicol in horses: values and limitations of pharmacokinetic studies in predicting dosage regimens, *Am J Vet Res* 48:403-406, 1987.
178. Tuttle AD, Papich MG, Wolfe BA: Bone marrow hypoplasia secondary to florfenicol toxicity in a Thomson's gazelle (Gazella thomsonii), *J Vet Pharmacol Ther* 29:317-319, 2006.
179. Page SW: Chloramphenicol 1. Hazards of use and the current regulatory environment, *Aust Vet J* 68:1-2, 1991.
180. Burrows GE, MacAllister CG, Tripp P, et al: Interactions between chloramphenicol, acepromazine, phenylbutazone, rifampin and thiamylal in the horse, *Equine Vet J* 21:34-38, 1989.
181. Grubb TL, Muir WW, Bertone AL, et al: Use of yohimbine to reverse prolonged effects of xylazine hydrochloride in a horse being treated with chloramphenicol, *J Am Vet Med Assoc* 210:1771-1773, 1997.
182. Asmar BI, Prainito M, Dajani AS: Antagonistic effect of chloramphenicol in combination with cefotaxime or ceftriaxone, *Antimicrob Agents Chemother* 32:1375-1378, 1988.
183. Ruiz NM, Ramirez-Ronda CH: Tetracyclines, macrolides, lincosamides & chloramphenicol, *Bol Asoc Med P R* 82:8-17, 1990.
184. Neu HC: Synergy of fluoroquinolones with other antimicrobial agents, *Rev Infect Dis* 11(Suppl 5):S1025-1035, 1989.
185. Van Duijkeren E, Vulto AG, Van Miert AS: Trimethoprim/sulfonamide combinations in the horse: a review, *J Vet Pharmacol Ther* 17:64-73, 1994.
186. van Miert AS: The sulfonamide-diaminopyrimidine story, *J Vet Pharmacol Ther* 17:309-316, 1994.
187. van Duijkeren E, van Klingeren B, Vulto AG, et al: In vitro susceptibility of equine Salmonella strains to trimethoprim and sulfonamide alone or in combination, *Am J Vet Res* 55:1386-1390, 1994.
188. Grace ME, Bushby SR, Sigel CW: Diffusion of trimethoprim and sulfamethoxazole from susceptibility disks into agar medium, *Antimicrob Agents Chemother* 8:45-49, 1975.
189. Marsh PS, Palmer JE: Bacterial isolates from blood and their susceptibility patterns in critically ill foals: 543 cases (1991-1998), *J Am Vet Med Assoc* 218:1608-1610, 2001.
190. Bogan JA, Galbraith A, Baxter P, et al: Effect of feeding on the fate of orally administered phenylbutazone, trimethoprim and sulphadiazine in the horse, *Vet Rec* 115:599-600, 1984.
191. Sigel CW, Byars TD, Divers TJ, et al: Serum concentrations of trimethoprim and sulfadiazine following oral paste administration to the horse, *Am J Vet Res* 42:2002-2005, 1981.
192. Wilson RC, Hammond LS, Clark CH, et al: Bioavailability and pharmacokinetics of sulfamethazine in the pony, *J Vet Pharmacol Ther* 12:99-102, 1989.
193. van Duijkeren E, Vulto AG, Sloet van Oldruitenborgh-Oosterbaan MM, et al: Pharmacokinetics of trimethoprim/sulphachlorpyridazine in horses after oral, nasogastric and intravenous administration, *J Vet Pharmacol Ther* 18:47-53, 1995.
194. Van Duijkeren E, Kessels BG, Sloet van Oldruitenborgh-Oosterbaan MM, et al: In vitro and in vivo binding of trimethoprim and sulphachlorpyridazine to equine food and digesta and their stability in caecal contents, *J Vet Pharmacol Ther* 19:281-287, 1996.
195. Boyd EH, Allen WE: Absorption of two trimethoprim/sulphonamide combinations from the uterus of pony mares, *J Vet Pharmacol Ther* 12:438-443, 1989.
196. Clarke CR, Burrows GE, MacAllister CG, et al: Pharmacokinetics of intravenously and orally administered pyrimethamine in horses, *Am J Vet Res* 53:2292-2295, 1992.
197. Brown MP, Gronwall R, Castro L: Pharmacokinetics and body fluid and endometrial concentrations of trimethoprim-sulfamethoxazole in mares, *Am J Vet Res* 49:918-922, 1988.
198. Brown MP, Kelly RH, Stover SM, et al: Trimethoprim-sulfadiazine in the horse: serum, synovial, peritoneal, and urine concentrations after single-dose intravenous administration, *Am J Vet Res* 44:540-543, 1983.
199. Brown MP, McCartney JH, Gronwall R, et al: Pharmacokinetics of trimethoprim-sulphamethoxazole in two-day-old foals after a single intravenous injection, *Equine Vet J* 22:51-53, 1990.
200. Clarke CR, MacAllister CG, Burrows GE, et al: Pharmacokinetics, penetration into cerebrospinal fluid, and hematologic effects after multiple oral administrations of pyrimethamine to horses, *Am J Vet Res* 53:2296-2299, 1992.
201. Rasmussen F, Gelsa H, Nielsen P: Pharmacokinetics of sulphadoxine and trimethoprim in horses. Half-life and volume of distribution of sulphadoxine and trimethoprim and cumulative excretion of [14C]-trimethoprim, *J Vet Pharmacol Ther* 2:245-255, 1979.
202. Nouws JF, Firth EC, Vree TB, et al: Pharmacokinetics and renal clearance of sulfamethazine, sulfamerazine, and sulfadiazine and their N4-acetyl and hydroxy metabolites in horses, *Am J Vet Res* 48:392-402, 1987.
203. Nouws JF, Vree TB, Baakman M, et al: Disposition of sulfadimidine and its N4-acetyl and hydroxy metabolites in horse plasma, *J Vet Pharmacol Ther* 8:303-311, 1985.
204. Gray AK, Kidd AR, O'Brien J, et al: Suspected adverse reactions to medicines during 1988, *Vet Rec* 124:286-287, 1989.

205. Dick IG, White SK: Possible potentiated sulphonamide-associated fatality in an anaesthetised horse, *Vet Rec* 121:288, 1987.
206. Taylor PM, Rest RJ, Duckham TN, et al: Possible potentiated sulphonamide and detomidine interactions, *Vet Rec* 122:143, 1988.
207. Fenger CK, Granstrom DE, Langemeier JL, et al: Epizootic of equine protozoal myeloencephalitis on a farm, *J Am Vet Med Assoc* 210:923-927, 1997.
208. Toribio RE, Bain FT, Mrad DR, et al: Congenital defects in newborn foals of mares treated for equine protozoal myeloencephalitis during pregnancy, *J Am Vet Med Assoc* 212:697-701, 1998.
209. Bedford SJ, McDonnell SM: Measurements of reproductive function in stallions treated with trimethoprim-sulfamethoxazole and pyrimethamine, *J Am Vet Med Assoc* 215:1317-1319, 1999.
210. Thomas HL, Livesey MA: Immune-mediated hemolytic anemia associated with trimethoprim-sulphamethoxazole administration in a horse, *Can Vet J* 39:171-173, 1998.
211. Ensink JM, Klein WR, Barneveld A, et al: Side effects of oral antimicrobial agents in the horse: a comparison of pivampicillin and trimethoprim/sulphadiazine, *Vet Rec* 138:253-256, 1996.
212. Wilson DA, MacFadden KE, Green EM, et al: Case control and historical cohort study of diarrhea associated with administration of trimethoprim-potentiated sulphonamides to horses and ponies, *J Vet Intern Med* 10:258-264, 1996.
213. Gustafsson A, Baverud V, Franklin A, et al: Repeated administration of trimethoprim/sulfadiazine in the horse-pharmacokinetics, plasma protein binding and influence on the intestinal microflora, *J Vet Pharmacol Ther* 22:20-26, 1999.
214. White G, Prior SD: Comparative effects of oral administration of trimethoprim/sulphadiazine or oxytetracycline on the faecal flora of horses, *Vet Rec* 111:316-318, 1982.
215. Bertone AL, Jones RL, McIlwraith CW: Serum and synovial fluid steady-state concentrations of trimethoprim and sulfadiazine in horses with experimentally induced infectious arthritis, *Am J Vet Res* 49:1681-1687, 1988.
216. Ensink JM, Bosch G, van Duijkeren E: Clinical efficacy of prophylactic administration of trimethoprim/sulfadiazine in a Streptococcus equi subsp. zooepidemicus infection model in ponies, *J Vet Pharmacol Ther* 28:45-49, 2005.
217. Rikihisa Y, Jiang BM: In vitro susceptibilities of Ehrlichia risticii to eight antibiotics, *Antimicrob Agents Chemother* 32:986-991, 1988.
218. Sampieri F, Hinchcliff KW, Toribio RE: Tetracycline therapy of Lawsonia intracellularis enteropathy in foals, *Equine Vet J* 38:89-92, 2006.
219. Baker A, Plummer CE, Szabo NJ, et al: Doxycycline levels in preocular tear film of horses following oral administration, *Vet Ophthalmol* 11:381-385, 2008.
220. Bryant JE, Brown MP, Gronwall RR, et al: Study of intragastric administration of doxycycline: pharmacokinetics including body fluid, endometrial and minimum inhibitory concentrations, *Equine Vet J* 32:233-238, 2000.
221. Davis JL, Salmon JH, Papich MG: Pharmacokinetics and tissue distribution of doxycycline after oral administration of single and multiple doses in horses, *Am J Vet Res* 67:310-316, 2006.
222. Riond JL, Riviere JE, Duckett WM, et al: Cardiovascular effects and fatalities associated with intravenous administration of doxycycline to horses and ponies, *Equine Vet J* 24:41-45, 1992.
223. Womble A, Giguere S, Lee EA: Pharmacokinetics of oral doxycycline and concentrations in body fluids and bronchoalveolar cells of foals, *J Vet Pharmacol Ther* 30:187-193, 2007.
224. Dowling PM, Russell AM: Pharmacokinetics of a long-acting oxytetracycline-polyethylene glycol formulation in horses, *J Vet Pharmacol Ther* 23:107-110, 2000.
225. Brown MP, Stover SM, Kelly RH, et al: Oxytetracycline hydrochloride in the horse: serum, synovial, peritoneal and urine concentrations after single dose intravenous administration, *J Vet Pharmacol Ther* 4:7-10, 1981.
226. Papich MG, Wright AK, Petrie L, et al: Pharmacokinetics of oxytetracycline administered intravenously to 4- and 5-day-old foals, *J Vet Pharmacol Ther* 18:375-378, 1995.
227. Horspool LJ, McKellar QA: Disposition of oxytetracycline in horses, ponies and donkeys after intravenous administration, *Equine Vet J* 22:284-285, 1990.
228. Gilmour MA, Clarke CR, Macallister CG, et al: Ocular penetration of oral doxycycline in the horse, *Vet Ophthalmol* 8:331-335, 2005.
229. Pilloud M: Pharmacokinetics, plasma protein binding and dosage of oxytetracycline in cattle and horses, *Res Vet Sci* 15:224-230, 1973.
230. Shaw DH, Rubin SI: Pharmacologic activity of doxycycline, *J Am Vet Med Assoc* 189:808-810, 1986.
231. Andersson G, Ekman L, Mansson I, et al: Lethal complications following administration of oxytetracycline in the horse, *Nord Vet Med* 23:9-22, 1971.
232. Baker JR, Leyland A: Diarrhoea in the horse associated with stress and tetracycline therapy, *Vet Rec* 93:583-584, 1973.
233. Cook W: Diarrhoea in the horse associated with stress and tetracycline therapy, *Vet Rec* 93:15-17, 1973.
234. Owen R: Post stress diarrhoea in the horse, *Vet Rec* 96:267-270, 1975.
235. Owen RA, Fullerton J, Barnum DA: Effects of transportation, surgery, and antibiotic therapy in ponies infected with Salmonella, *Am J Vet Res* 44:46-50, 1983.
236. Palmer JE: Potomac horse fever, *Vet Clin North Am Equine Pract* 9:399-410, 1993.
237. Palmer JE, Benson CE, Whitlock RH: Effect of treatment with oxytetracycline during the acute stages of experimentally induced equine ehrlichial colitis in ponies, *Am J Vet Res* 53:2300-2304, 1992.
238. Palmer JE, Whitlock RH, Benson CE: Equine ehrlichial colitis: effect of oxytetracycline treatment during the incubation period of Ehrlichia risticii infection in ponies, *J Am Vet Med Assoc* 192:343-345, 1988.
239. Dowling PM: Long-acting oxytetracycline in horses, 17th Annual ACVIM Forum :217-219, 1999.
240. Vivrette S, Cowgill LD, Pascoe J, et al: Hemodialysis for treatment of oxytetracycline-induced acute renal failure in a neonatal foal, *J Am Vet Med Assoc* 203:105-107, 1993.
241. Wright AK, Petrie L, Papich MG, et al: Effect of high dose oxytetracycline on renal parameteres in neonatal foals, *American Association of Equine Practitioners* 297-298, 1992.
242. Gyrd-Hansen N, Rasmussen F Smith M: Cardiovascular effects of intravenous administration of tetracycline in cattle, *J Vet Pharmacol Ther* 4:15-25, 1981.
243. Smith M, Gyrd-Hansen N, Rasmussen F: Tetracycline intravenously to cattle: cardiovascular side-effects, *Nord Vet Med* 33:272-273, 1981.
244. Riond JL, Duckett WM, Riviere JE, et al: Concerned about intravenous use of doxycycline in horses, *J Am Vet Med Assoc* 195(846):848, 1989.
245. Kasper CA, Clayton HM, Wright AK, et al: Effects of high doses of oxytetracycline on metacarpophalangeal joint kinematics in neonatal foals, *J Am Vet Med Assoc* 207:71-73, 1995.
246. Madison JB, Garber JL, Rice B, et al: Effect of oxytetracycline on metacarpophalangeal and distal interphalangeal joint angles in newborn foals, *J Am Vet Med Assoc* 204:246-249, 1994.
247. Arnoczky SP, Lavagnino M, Gardner KL, et al: In vitro effects of oxytetracycline on matrix metalloproteinase-1 mRNA expression and on collagen gel contraction by cultured myofibroblasts obtained from the accessory ligament of foals, *Am J Vet Res* 65:491-496, 2004.

248. Neu HC: Clinical microbiology of azithromycin, *Am J Med* 91:12S-18S, 1991.
249. Jacks SS, Giguere S, Nguyen A: In vitro susceptibilities of Rhodococcus equi and other common equine pathogens to azithromycin, clarithromycin, and 20 other antimicrobials, *Antimicrob Agents Chemother* 47:1742-1745, 2003.
250. Lakritz J: Erythromycin: clinical uses, kinetics and mechanism of action, 15th Annual ACVIM Forum: 368-370, 1997.
251. Lester GD, Merritt AM, Neuwirth L, et al: Effect of erythromycin lactobionate on myoelectric activity of ileum, cecum, and right ventral colon, and cecal emptying of radiolabeled markers in clinically normal ponies, *Am J Vet Res* 59:328-334, 1998.
252. Kenney DG, Robbins SC, Prescott JF, et al: Development of reactive arthritis and resistance to erythromycin and rifampin in a foal during treatment for Rhodococcus equi pneumonia, *Equine Vet J* 26:246-248, 1994.
253. Giguere S, Prescott JF: Clinical manifestations, diagnosis, treatment, and prevention of Rhodococcus equi infections in foals, *Vet Microbiol* 56:313-334, 1997.
254. Lakritz J, Wilson WD, Mihalyi JE: Comparison of microbiologic and high-performance liquid chromatography assays to determine plasma concentrations, pharmacokinetics, and bioavailability of erythromycin base in plasma of foals after intravenous or intragastric administration, *Am J Vet Res* 60:414-419, 1999.
255. Lakritz J, Wilson WD, Marsh AE, et al: Effects of prior feeding on pharmacokinetics and estimated bioavailability after oral administration of a single dose of microencapsulated erythromycin base in healthy foals, *Am J Vet Res* 61:1011-1015, 2000.
256. Lakritz J, Wilson WD, Marsh AE, et al: Pharmacokinetics of erythromycin estolate and erythromycin phosphate after intragastric administration to healthy foals, *Am J Vet Res* 61:914-919, 2000.
257. Jacks S, Giguere S, Gronwall PR, et al: Pharmacokinetics of azithromycin and concentration in body fluids and bronchoalveolar cells in foals, *Am J Vet Res* 62:1870-1875, 2001.
258. Davis JL, Gardner SY, Jones SL, et al: Pharmacokinetics of azithromycin in foals after i.v. and oral dose and disposition into phagocytes, *J Vet Pharmacol Ther* 25:99-104, 2002.
259. Womble AY, Giguere S, Lee EA, et al: Pharmacokinetics of clarithromycin and concentrations in body fluids and bronchoalveolar cells of foals, *Am J Vet Res* 67:1681-1686, 2006.
260. Scheuch E, Spieker J, Venner M, et al: Quantitative determination of the macrolide antibiotic tulathromycin in plasma and broncho-alveolar cells of foals using tandem mass spectrometry, *J Chromatogr B Analyt Technol Biomed Life Sci* 850:464-470, 2007.
261. Giguere S, Jacks S, Roberts GD, et al: Retrospective comparison of azithromycin, clarithromycin, and erythromycin for the treatment of foals with Rhodococcus equi pneumonia, *J Vet Intern Med* 18:568-573, 2004.
262. Suarez-Mier G, Giguere S, Lee EA: Pulmonary disposition of erythromycin, azithromycin, and clarithromycin in foals, *J Vet Pharmacol Ther* 30:109-115, 2007.
263. Prescott JF, Hoover DJ, Dohoo IR: Pharmacokinetics of erythromycin in foals and in adult horses, *J Vet Pharmacol Ther* 6:67-73, 1983.
264. Lakritz J, Wilson WD, Watson JL, et al: Effect of treatment with erythromycin on bronchoalveolar lavage fluid cell populations in foals, *Am J Vet Res* 58:56-61, 1997.
265. Steiner A, Roussel AJ: Drugs coordinating and restoring gastrointestinal motility and their effect on selected hypodynamic gastrointestinal disorders in horses and cattle, *Zentralbl Veterinarmed A* 42:613-631, 1995.
266. Nieto JE, Rakestraw PC, Snyder JR, et al: In vitro effects of erythromycin, lidocaine, and metoclopramide on smooth muscle from the pyloric antrum, proximal portion of the duodenum, and middle portion of the jejunum of horses, *Am J Vet Res* 61:413-419, 2000.
267. Baverud V, Franklin A, Gunnarsson A, et al: Clostridium difficile associated with acute colitis in mares when their foals are treated with erythromycin and rifampicin for Rhodococcus equi pneumonia, *Equine Vet J* 30:482-488, 1998.
268. Gustafsson A, Baverud V, Gunnarsson A, et al: The association of erythromycin ethylsuccinate with acute colitis in horses in Sweden, *Equine Vet J* 29:314-318, 1997.
269. Larsen J, Dolvik NI, Teige J: Acute post-treatment enterocolitis in 13 horses treated in a Norwegian surgical ward, *Acta Vet Scand* 37:203-211, 1996.
270. Stratton-Phelps M, Wilson WD, Gardner IA: Risk of adverse effects in pneumonic foals treated with erythromycin versus other antibiotics: 143 cases (1986-1996), *J Am Vet Med Assoc* 217:68-73, 2000.
271. Traub-Dargatz J, Wilson WD, Conboy HS, et al: Hyperthermia in foals treated with erythromycin alone or in combination for respiratory disease during hot environmental conditions, *Am Assoc Equine Pract* :243-244, 1996.
272. Venner M, Kerth R, Klug E: Evaluation of tulathromycin in the treatment of pulmonary abscesses in foals, *Vet J* 174: 418-421, 2007.
273. Palmer JE, Benson CE: Effect of treatment with erythromycin and rifampin during the acute stages of experimentally induced equine ehrlichial colitis in ponies, *Am J Vet Res* 53:2071-2076, 1992.
274. Lavoie JP, Drolet R, Parsons D, et al: Equine proliferative enteropathy: a cause of weight loss, colic, diarrhoea and hypoproteinaemia in foals on three breeding farms in Canada, *Equine Vet J* 32:418-425, 2000.
275. Chaffin MK, Cohen ND, Martens RJ: Chemoprophylactic effects of azithromycin against Rhodococcus equi-induced pneumonia among foals at equine breeding farms with endemic infections, *J Am Vet Med Assoc* 232:1035-1047, 2008.
276. Brown SA: Fluoroquinolones in animal health, *J Vet Pharmacol Ther* 19:1-14, 1996.
277. Appelbaum PC: Quinolone activity against anaerobes, *Drugs* 58(Suppl 2):60-64, 1999.
278. Nicolau DP: Predicting antibacterial response from pharmacodynamic and pharmacokinetic profiles, *Infection* 29 (Suppl 2):11-15, 2001.
279. Robicsek A, Jacoby GA, Hooper DC: The worldwide emergence of plasmid-mediated quinolone resistance, *Lancet Infect Dis* 6:629-640, 2006.
280. Hooper DC: Mechanisms of fluoroquinolone resistance, *Drug Resist Updat* 2:38-55, 1999.
281. Schmitz FJ, Perdikouli M, Beeck A, et al: Molecular surveillance of macrolide, tetracycline and quinolone resistance mechanisms in 1191 clinical European Streptococcus pneumoniae isolates, *Int J Antimicrob Agents* 18:433-436, 2001.
282. Webber M, Piddock LJ: Quinolone resistance in Escherichia coli, *Vet Res* 32:275-284, 2001.
283. Dowling PM, Wilson RC, Tyler JW, et al: Pharmacokinetics of ciprofloxacin in ponies, *J Vet Pharmacol Ther* 18:7-12, 1995.
284. Bermingham EC, Papich MG, Vivrette SL: Pharmacokinetics of enrofloxacin administered intravenously and orally to foals, *Am J Vet Res* 61:706-709, 2000.
285. Giguere S, Belanger M: Concentration of enrofloxacin in equine tissues after long-term oral administration, *J Vet Pharmacol Ther* 20:402-404, 1997.
286. Giguere S, Sweeney RW, Belanger M: Pharmacokinetics of enrofloxacin in adult horses and concentration of the drug in serum, body fluids, and endometrial tissues after repeated intragastrically administered doses, *Am J Vet Res* 57: 1025-1030, 1996.
287. Peyrou M, Bousquet-Melou A, Laroute V, et al: Enrofloxacin and marbofloxacin in horses: comparison of pharmacokinetic parameters, use of urinary and metabolite data to estimate first-pass effect and absorbed fraction, *J Vet Pharmacol Ther* 29:337-344, 2006.

288. Steinman A, Britzi M, Levi O, et al: Lack of effect of diet on the pharmacokinetics of enrofloxacin in horses, *J Vet Pharmacol Ther* 29:67-70, 2006.
289. Kaartinen L, Panu S, Pyorala S: Pharmacokinetics of enrofloxacin in horses after single intravenous and intramuscular administration, *Equine Vet J* 29:378-381, 1997.
290. Boeckh CBC, Boeckh A, Wilkie S, Davis C, Buchanan T, Boothe D: Pharmacokinetics of the Bovine Formulation of Enrofloxacin (Baytril 100) in Horses, *Veterinary Therapeutics* 2:129-134, 2001.
291. Epstein K, Cohen N, Boothe D, et al: Pharmacokinetics, stability and retrospective analysis of use of an oral get formulation of the bovine injectable enrofloxacin in horses, *Vet Ther* 5:155-167, 2004.
292. Giguere S, Sweeney RW, Habecker PL, et al: Tolerability of orally administered enrofloxacin in adult horses: a pilot study, *J Vet Pharmacol Ther* 22:343-347, 1999.
293. Langston VC, Sedrish S, Boothe DM: Disposition of single-dose oral enrofloxacin in the horse, *J Vet Pharmacol Ther* 19:316-319, 1996.
294. Divers TJ, Irby NL, Mohammed HO, et al: Ocular penetration of intravenously administered enrofloxacin in the horse, *Equine Vet J* 40:167-170, 2008.
295. Davis JL, Papich MG, Weingarten A: The pharmacokinetics of orbifloxacin in the horse following oral and intravenous administration, *J Vet Pharmacol Ther* 29:191-197, 2006.
296. Goudah A, Abo El-Sooud K, Shim JH, et al: Characterization of the pharmacokinetic disposition of levofloxacin in stallions after intravenous and intramuscular administration, *J Vet Pharmacol Ther* 31:399-405, 2008.
297. Gardner SY, Davis JL, Jones SL, et al: Moxifloxacin pharmacokinetics in horses and disposition into phagocytes after oral dosing, *J Vet Pharmacol Ther* 27:57-60, 2004.
298. Alghasham AA, Nahata MC: Clinical use of fluoroquinolones in children, *Ann Pharmacother* 34:344-413, 2000:347-359; quiz.
299. Burkhardt JE, Hill MA, Turek JJ, et al: Ultrastructural changes in articular cartilages of immature beagle dogs dosed with difloxacin, a fluoroquinolone, *Vet Pathol* 29:230-238, 1992.
300. Beluche LA, Bertone AL, Anderson DE, et al: In vitro dose-dependent effects of enrofloxacin on equine articular cartilage, *Am J Vet Res* 60:577-582, 1999.
301. Vivrette SL, Bostian A, Bermingham EC, et al: *Quinolone-induced arthropathy in neonatal foals, 47th Annual American Association of Equine Practioners Convention* :376-377, 2001.
302. Bertone AL, Tremaine WH, Macoris DG, et al: Effect of long-term administration of an injectable enrofloxacin solution on physical and musculoskeletal variables in adult horses, *J Am Vet Med Assoc* 217:1514-1521, 2000.
303. Larsen H, Nielsen GL, Schonheyder HC, et al: Birth outcome following maternal use of fluoroquinolones, *Int J Antimicrob Agents* 18:259-262, 2001.
304. Heath SE: Chronic pleurits in a horse, *Can Vet J* 30:69, 1989.
305. Intorre L, Mengozzi G, Maccheroni M, et al: Enrofloxacin-theophylline interaction: influence of enrofloxacin on theophylline steady-state pharmacokinetics in the beagle dog, *J Vet Pharmacol Ther* 18:352-356, 1995.
306. Dechant J: Combination of medical and surgical therapy for pleuropneumonia in a horse, *Can Vet J* 38:499-501, 1997.
307. MacDonald DG, Bailey JV, Fowler JD: Arthrodesis of the scapulohumeral joint in a horse, *Can Vet J* 36:312-315, 1995.
308. Rodger LD, Carlson GP, Moran ME, et al: Resolution of a left ureteral stone using electrohydraulic lithotripsy in a thoroughbred colt, *J Vet Intern Med* 9:280-282, 1995.
309. Wilson WD, Spensley MS, Baggot JD, et al: Pharmacokinetics, bioavailability, and in vitro antibacterial activity of rifampin in the horse, *Am J Vet Res* 49:2041-2046, 1988.
310. Fines M, Pronost S, Maillard K, et al: Characterization of mutations in the rpoB gene associated with rifampin resistance in Rhodococcus equi isolated from foals, *J Clin Microbiol* 39:2784-2787, 2001.
311. Takai S, Takeda K, Nakano Y, et al: Emergence of rifampin-resistant Rhodococcus equi in an infected foal, *J Clin Microbiol* 35:1904-1908, 1997.
312. Kohn CW, Sams R, Kowalski JJ, et al: Pharmacokinetics of single intravenous and single and multiple dose oral administration of rifampin in mares, *J Vet Pharmacol Ther* 16:119-131, 1993.
313. Burrows GE, MacAllister CG, Beckstrom DA, et al: Rifampin in the horse: comparison of intravenous, intramuscular, and oral administrations, *Am J Vet Res* 46:442-446, 1985.
314. Frank LA: Clinical pharmacology of rifampin, *J Am Vet Med Assoc* 197:114-117, 1990.
315. Burrows GE, MacAllister CG, Ewing P, et al: Rifampin disposition in the horse: effects of age and method of oral administration, *J Vet Pharmacol Ther* 15:124-132, 1992.
316. Castro LA, Brown MP, Gronwall R, et al: Pharmacokinetics of rifampin given as a single oral dose in foals, *Am J Vet Res* 47:2584-2586, 1986.
317. Burrows GE, MacAllister CG, Ewing P, et al: Rifampin disposition in the horse: effects of repeated dosage of rifampin or phenylbutazone, *J Vet Pharmacol Ther* 15:305-308, 1992.
318. Baggot JD, Wilson WD, Hietala S: Clinical pharmacokinetics of metronidazole in horses, *J Vet Pharmacol Ther* 11:417-420, 1988.
319. Magdesian KG, Hirsh DC, Jang SS, et al: Characterization of Clostridium difficile isolates from foals with diarrhea: 28 cases (1993-1997), *J Am Vet Med Assoc* 220:67-73, 2002.
320. Sweeney RW, Sweeney CR, Soma LR, et al: Pharmacokinetics of metronidazole given to horses by intravenous and oral routes, *Am J Vet Res* 47:1726-1729, 1986.
321. Rubin DT, Kornblunth A: Role of antibiotics in the management of inflammatory bowel disease: a review, *Rev Gastroenterol Disord* 5(Suppl 3):S10-S15, 2005.
322. Steinman A, Gips M, Lavy E, et al: Pharmacokinetics of metronidazole in horses after intravenous, rectal and oral administration, *J Vet Pharmacol Ther* 23:353-357, 2000.
323. Garber JL, Brown MP, Gronwall RR, et al: Pharmacokinetics of metronidazole after rectal administration in horses, *Am J Vet Res* 54:2060-2063, 1993.
324. Specht TE, Brown MP, Gronwall RR, et al: Pharmacokinetics of metronidazole and its concentration in body fluids and endometrial tissues of mares, *Am J Vet Res* 53:1807-1812, 1992.
325. Sweeney RW, Sweeney CR, Weiher J: Clinical use of metronidazole in horses: 200 cases (1984-1989), *J Am Vet Med Assoc* 198:1045-1048, 1991.
326. Jones RL: Clostridial enterocolitis, *Vet Clin North Am Equine Pract* 16:471-485, 2000.
327. McGorum BC, Dixon PM, Smith DG: Use of metronidazole in equine acute idiopathic toxaemic colitis, *Vet Rec* 142: 635-638, 1998.
328. Barr BS: Infiltrative intestinal disease, *Vet Clin North Am Equine Pract* 22:e1-e7, 2006.

Nonsteroidal Anti-Inflammatory Drugs

1. Lees P, Higgins AJ: Clinical pharmacology and therapeutic uses of non-steroidal anti-inflammatory drugs in the horse, *Equine Vet J* 17:83-96, 1985.
2. Wallace JL: How do NSAIDs cause ulcer disease? *Baillieres Best Pract Res Clin Gastroenterol* 14:147-159, 2000.
3. Wallace JL: Distribution and expression of cyclooxygenase (COX) isoenzymes, their physiological roles, and the categorization of nonsteroidal anti-inflammatory drugs (NSAIDs), *Am J Med* 107:11S-16S, 1999; discussion 16S-17S.
4. Wallace JL, Ma L: Inflammatory mediators in gastrointestinal defense and injury, *Exp Biol Med (Maywood)* 226:1003-1015, 2001.

5. Wallace JL: Selective cyclooxygenase-2 inhibitors: after the smoke has cleared, *Dig Liver Dis* 34:89-94, 2002.
6. Wallace JL: NSAID gastroenteropathy: past, present and future, *Can J Gastroenterol* 10:451-459, 1996.
7. Wallace JL, Reuter BK, McKnight W, et al: Selective inhibitors of cyclooxygenase-2: are they really effective, selective, and GI-safe? *J Clin Gastroenterol* 27(Suppl 1):S28-S34, 1998.
8. Wallace JL, Bak A, McKnight W, et al: Cyclooxygenase 1 contributes to inflammatory responses in rats and mice: implications for gastrointestinal toxicity, *Gastroenterology* 115:101-109, 1998.
9. Wallace JL, Muscara MN: Selective cyclo-oxygenase-2 inhibitors: cardiovascular and gastrointestinal toxicity, *Dig Liver Dis* 33(Suppl 2):S21-S28, 2001.
10. Perini RF, Ma L, Wallace JL: Mucosal repair and COX-2 inhibition, *Curr Pharm Des* 9:2207-2211, 2003.
11. Wallace JL: Prostaglandins, NSAIDs, and gastric mucosal protection: why doesn't the stomach digest itself? *Physiol Rev* 88:1547-1565, 2008.
12. Giovanni G, Giovanni P: Do non-steroidal anti-inflammatory drugs and COX-2 selective inhibitors have different renal effects? *J Nephrol* 15:480-488, 2002.
13. Armstrong S, Tricklebank P, Lake A, et al: Pharmacokinetics of carprofen enantiomers in equine plasma and synovial fluid — a comparison with ketoprofen, *J Vet Pharmacol Ther* 22:196-201, 1999.
14. Higgins AJ, Lees P, Sedgwick AD: Development of equine models of inflammation. The Ciba-Geigy Prize for Research in Animal Health, *Vet Rec* 120:517-522, 1987.
15. Landoni MF, Lees P: Pharmacokinetics and pharmacodynamics of ketoprofen enantiomers in the horse, *J Vet Pharmacol Ther* 19:466-474, 1996.
16. King JN, Gerring EL: Antagonism of endotoxin-induced disruption of equine bowel motility by flunixin and phenylbutazone, *Equine Vet J Suppl* :38-42, 1989.
17. Moses VS, Hardy J, Bertone AL, et al: Effects of anti-inflammatory drugs on lipopolysaccharide-challenged and unchallenged equine synovial explants, *Am J Vet Res* 62:54-60, 2001.
18. Danek J: Effects of flunixin meglumine on selected clinicopathologic variables, and serum testosterone concentration in stallions after endotoxin administration, *J Vet Med A Physiol Pathol Clin Med* 53:357-363, 2006.
19. Dunkle NJ, Bottoms GD, Fessler JF, et al: Effects of flunixin meglumine on blood pressure and fluid compartment volume changes in ponies given endotoxin, *Am J Vet Res* 46:1540-1544, 1985.
20. Olson NC, Meyer RE, Anderson DL: Effects of flunixin meglumine on cardiopulmonary responses to endotoxin in ponies, *J Appl Physiol* 59:1464-1471, 1985.
21. Semrad SD: Comparison of flunixin, prednisolone, dimethyl sulfoxide, and a lazaroid (U74389F) for treating endotoxemic neonatal calves, *Am J Vet Res* 54:1517-1522, 1993.
22. Semrad SD, Hardee GE, Hardee MM, et al: Flunixin meglumine given in small doses: pharmacokinetics and prostaglandin inhibition in healthy horses, *Am J Vet Res* 46:2474-2479, 1985.
23. Semrad SD, Hardee GE, Hardee MM, et al: Low dose flunixin meglumine: effects on eicosanoid production and clinical signs induced by experimental endotoxaemia in horses, *Equine Vet J* 19:201-206, 1987.
24. Semrad SD, Moore JN: Effects of multiple low doses of flunixin meglumine on repeated endotoxin challenge in the horse, *Prostaglandins Leukot Med* 27:169-181, 1987.
25. Templeton CB, Bottoms GD, Fessler JF, et al: Endotoxin-induced hemodynamic and prostaglandin changes in ponies: effects of flunixin meglumine, dexamethasone, and prednisolone, *Circ Shock* 23:231-240, 1987.
26. Dawson J, Lees P, Sedgwick AD: Actions of non-steroidal anti-inflammatory drugs on equine leucocyte movement in vitro, *J Vet Pharmacol Ther* 10:150-159, 1987.
27. Pillinger MH, Capodici C, Rosenthal P, et al: Modes of action of aspirin-like drugs: salicylates inhibit erk activation and integrin-dependent neutrophil adhesion, *Proc Natl Acad Sci U S A* 95:14540-14545, 1998.
28. Weissmann G, Montesinos MC, Pillinger M, et al: Non-prostaglandin effects of aspirin III and salicylate: inhibition of integrin-dependent human neutrophil aggregation and inflammation in COX 2- and NF kappa B (P105)-knockout mice, *Adv Exp Med Biol* 507:571-577, 2002.
29. Chambers JP, Waterman AE, Livingston A: The effects of opioid and alpha 2 adrenergic blockade on non-steroidal anti-inflammatory drug analgesia in sheep, *J Vet Pharmacol Ther* 18:161-166, 1995.
30. Johnson CB, Taylor PM, Young SS, et al: Postoperative analgesia using phenylbutazone, flunixin or carprofen in horses, *Vet Rec* 133:336-338, 1993.
31. Armstrong S, Lees P: Effects of R and S enantiomers and a racemic mixture of carprofen on the production and release of proteoglycan and prostaglandin E2 from equine chondrocytes and cartilage explants, *Am J Vet Res* 60:98-104, 1999.
32. Verde CR, Simpson MI, Frigoli A, et al: Enantiospecific pharmacokinetics of ketoprofen in plasma and synovial fluid of horses with acute synovitis, *J Vet Pharmacol Ther* 24:179-185, 2001.
33. Landoni MF, Soraci AL, Delatour P, et al: Enantioselective behaviour of drugs used in domestic animals: a review, *J Vet Pharmacol Ther* 20:1-16, 1997.
34. Landoni MF, Lees P: Chirality: a major issue in veterinary pharmacology, *J Vet Pharmacol Ther* 19:82-84, 1996.
35. Lapicque F, Muller N, Payan E, et al: Protein binding and stereoselectivity of nonsteroidal anti-inflammatory drugs, *Clin Pharmacokinet* 25:115-123,1993.
36. Brouwers JR, de Smet PA: Pharmacokinetic-pharmacodynamic drug interactions with nonsteroidal anti-inflammatory drugs, *Clin Pharmacokinet* 27:462-485, 1994.
37. Semrad SD, Sams RA, Harris ON, et al: Effects of concurrent administration of phenylbutazone and flunixin meglumine on pharmacokinetic variables and in vitro generation of thromboxane B2 in mares, *Am J Vet Res* 54:1901-1905, 1993.
38. Keegan KG, Messer NT, Reed SK, et al: Effectiveness of administration of phenylbutazone alone or concurrent administration of phenylbutazone and flunixin meglumine to alleviate lameness in horses, *Am J Vet Res* 69:167-173, 2008.
39. Reed SK, Messer NT, Tessman RK, et al: Effects of phenylbutazone alone or in combination with flunixin meglumine on blood protein concentrations in horses, *Am J Vet Res* 67: 398-402, 2006.
40. Peng S, Duggan A: Gastrointestinal adverse effects of non-steroidal anti-inflammatory drugs, *Expert Opin Drug Saf* 4: 157-169, 2005.
41. Burrows GE, MacAllister CG, Tripp P, et al: Interactions between chloramphenicol, acepromazine, phenylbutazone, rifampin and thiamylal in the horse, *Equine Vet J* 21:34-38, 1989.
42. Firth EC, Nouws JF, Klein WR, et al: The effect of phenylbutazone on the plasma disposition of penicillin G in the horse, *J Vet Pharmacol Ther* 13:179-185, 1990.
43. Whittem T, Firth EC, Hodge H, et al: Pharmacokinetic interactions between repeated dose phenylbutazone and gentamicin in the horse, *J Vet Pharmacol Ther* 19:454-459, 1996.
44. Dyke TM, Hinchcliff KW, Sams RA: Attenuation by phenylbutazone of the renal effects and excretion of frusemide in horses, *Equine Vet J* 31:289-295, 1999.
45. Hinchcliff KW, McKeever KH, Muir WW 3rd, et al: Pharmacologic interaction of furosemide and phenylbutazone in horses, *Am J Vet Res* 56:1206-1212, 1995.

46. Cambridge H, Lees P, Hooke RE, et al: Antithrombotic actions of aspirin in the horse, *Equine Vet J* 23:123-127, 1991.
47. Hardee MM, Moore JN, Hardee GE: Effects of flunixin meglumine, phenylbutazone and a selective thromboxane synthetase inhibitor (UK-38,485) on thromboxane and prostacyclin production in healthy horses, *Res Vet Sci* 40:152-156, 1986.
48. Heath MF, Evans RJ, Poole AW, et al: The effects of aspirin and paracetamol on the aggregation of equine blood platelets, *J Vet Pharmacol Ther* 17:374-378, 1994.
49. Lees P, Ewins CP, Taylor JB, et al: Serum thromboxane in the horse and its inhibition by aspirin, phenylbutazone and flunixin, *Br Vet J* 143:462-476, 1987.
50. Baxter GM, Moore JN: Effect of aspirin on ex vivo generation of thromboxane in healthy horses, *Am J Vet Res* 48:13-16, 1987.
51. Cohen ND, Carter GK, Mealey RH, et al: Medical management of right dorsal colitis in 5 horses: a retrospective study, *J Vet Intern Med* 1995(9):272-276, 1987-1993.
52. Collins LG, Tyler DE: Experimentally induced phenylbutazone toxicosis in ponies: description of the syndrome and its prevention with synthetic prostaglandin E2, *Am J Vet Res* 46:1605-1615, 1985.
53. Gunson DE, Soma LR: Renal papillary necrosis in horses after phenylbutazone and water deprivation, *Vet Pathol* 20:603-610, 1983.
54. Hough ME, Steel CM, Bolton JR, et al: Ulceration and stricture of the right dorsal colon after phenylbutazone administration in four horses, *Aust Vet J* 77:785-788, 1999.
55. Karcher LF, Dill SG, Anderson WI, et al: Right dorsal colitis, *J Vet Intern Med* 4:247-253, 1990.
56. MacAllister CG, Morgan SJ, Borne AT, et al: Comparison of adverse effects of phenylbutazone, flunixin meglumine, and ketoprofen in horses, *J Am Vet Med Assoc* 202:71-77, 1993.
57. Meschter CL, Gilbert M, Krook L, et al: The effects of phenylbutazone on the morphology and prostaglandin concentrations of the pyloric mucosa of the equine stomach, *Vet Pathol* 27:244-253, 1990.
58. Leveille R, Miyabayashi T, Weisbrode SE, et al: Ultrasonographic renal changes associated with phenylbutazone administration in three foals, *Can Vet J* 37:235-236, 1996.
59. Read WK: Renal medullary crest necrosis associated with phenylbutazone therapy in horses, *Vet Pathol* 20:662-669, 1983.
60. Carrick JB, Papich MG, Middleton DM, et al: Clinical and pathological effects of flunixin meglumine administration to neonatal foals, *Can J Vet Res* 53:195-201, 1989.
61. Traub JL, Gallina AM, Grant BD, et al: Phenylbutazone toxicosis in the foal, *Am J Vet Res* 44:1410-1418, 1983.
62. Traub-Dargatz JL, Bertone JJ, Gould DH, et al: Chronic flunixin meglumine therapy in foals, *Am J Vet Res* 49:7-12, 1988.
63. Held JP, Daniel GB: Use of nonimaging nuclear medicine techniques to assess the effect of flunixin meglumine on effective renal plasma flow and effective renal blood flow in healthy horses, *Am J Vet Res* 52:1619-1621, 1991.
64. Frean SP, Cambridge H, Lees P: Effects of anti-arthritic drugs on proteoglycan synthesis by equine cartilage, *J Vet Pharmacol Ther* 25:289-298, 2002.
65. Jolly WT, Whittem T, Jolly AC, et al: The dose-related effects of phenylbutazone and a methylprednisolone acetate formulation (Depo-Medrol) on cultured explants of equine carpal articular cartilage, *J Vet Pharmacol Ther* 18:429-437, 1995.
66. Frean SP, Abraham LA, Lees P: In vitro stimulation of equine articular cartilage proteoglycan synthesis by hyaluronan and carprofen, *Res Vet Sci* 67:183-190, 1999.
67. Pountos I, Georgouli T, Blokhuis TJ, et al: Pharmacological agents and impairment of fracture healing: what is the evidence? *Injury* 39:384-394, 2008.
68. Rohde C, Anderson DE, Bertone AL, et al: Effects of phenylbutazone on bone activity and formation in horses, *Am J Vet Res* 61:537-543, 2000.
69. Broome TA, Brown MP, Gronwall RR, et al: Pharmacokinetics and plasma concentrations of acetylsalicylic acid after intravenous, rectal, and intragastric administration to horses, *Can J Vet Res* 67:297-302, 2003.
70. Murdick PW, Ray RS, Noonan JS: Salicylic acid concentration in plasma and urine of medicated and nonmedicated horses, *Am J Vet Res* 29:581-585, 1968.
71. Judson DG, Barton M: Effect of aspirin on haemostasis in the horse, *Res Vet Sci* 30:241-242, 1981.
72. Trujillo O, Rios A, Maldonado R, et al: Effect of oral administration of acetylsalicylic acid on haemostasis in the horse, *Equine Vet J* 13:205-206, 1981.
73. Soraci A, Benoit E, Jaussaud P, et al: Enantioselective glucuronidation and subsequent biliary excretion of carprofen in horses, *Am J Vet Res* 56:358-361, 1995.
74. Lees P, McKellar Q, May SA, et al: Pharmacodynamics and pharmacokinetics of carprofen in the horse, *Equine Vet J* 26:203-208, 1994.
75. Caldwell FJ, Mueller PO, Lynn RC, et al: Effect of topical application of diclofenac liposomal suspension on experimentally induced subcutaneous inflammation in horses, *Am J Vet Res* 65:271-276, 2004.
76. Schleining JA, McClure SR, Evans RB, et al: Liposome-based diclofenac for the treatment of inflammation in an acute synovitis model in horses, *J Vet Pharmacol Ther* 31:554-561, 2008.
77. Lynn RC, Hepler DI, Kelch WJ, et al: Double-blinded placebo-controlled clinical field trial to evaluate the safety and efficacy of topically applied 1% diclofenac liposomal cream for the relief of lameness in horses, *Vet Ther* 5:128-138, 2004.
78. Anderson D, Kollias-Baker C, Colahan P, et al: Urinary and serum concentrations of diclofenac after topical application to horses, *Vet Ther* 6:57-66, 2005.
79. Kvaternick V, Pollmeier M, Fischer J, et al: Pharmacokinetics and metabolism of orally administered firocoxib, a novel second generation coxib, in horses, *J Vet Pharmacol Ther* 30: 208-217, 2007.
80. Letendre LT, Tessman RK, McClure SR, et al: Pharmacokinetics of firocoxib after administration of multiple consecutive daily doses to horses, *Am J Vet Res* 69:1399-1405, 2008.
81. Doucet MY, Bertone AL, Hendrickson D, et al: Comparison of efficacy and safety of paste formulations of firocoxib and phenylbutazone in horses with naturally occurring osteoarthritis, *J Am Vet Med Assoc* 232:91-97, 2008.
82. Soma LR, Behrend E, Rudy J, et al: Disposition and excretion of flunixin meglumine in horses, *Am J Vet Res* 49:1894-1898, 1988.
83. Welsh JC, Lees P, Stodulski G, et al: Influence of feeding schedule on the absorption of orally administered flunixin in the horse, *Equine Vet J Suppl* :62-65, 1992.
84. Coakley M, Peck KE, Taylor TS, et al: Pharmacokinetics of flunixin meglumine in donkeys, mules, and horses, *Am J Vet Res* 60:1441-1444, 1999.
85. Crisman MV, Wilcke JR, Sams RA: Pharmacokinetics of flunixin meglumine in healthy foals less than twenty-four hours old, *Am J Vet Res* 57:1759-1761, 1996.
86. Galbraith EA, McKellar QA: Protein binding and in vitro serum thromboxane B2 inhibition by flunixin meglumine and meclofenamic acid in dog, goat and horse blood, *Res Vet Sci* 61:78-81, 1996.
87. Higgins AJ, Lees P, Sharma SC, et al: Measurement of flunixin in equine inflammatory exudate and plasma by high performance liquid chromatography, *Equine Vet J* 19:303-306, 1987.
88. Landoni MF, Lees P: Comparison of the anti-inflammatory actions of flunixin and ketoprofen in horses applying PK/PD modelling, *Equine Vet J* 27:247-256, 1995.
89. Jackman BR, Moore JN, Barton MH, et al: Comparison of the effects of ketoprofen and flunixin meglumine on the in vitro response of equine peripheral blood monocytes to bacterial endotoxin, *Can J Vet Res* 58:138-143, 1994.

90. Daels PF, Stabenfeldt GH, Hughes JP, et al: Effects of flunixin meglumine on endotoxin-induced prostaglandin F2 alpha secretion during early pregnancy in mares, *Am J Vet Res* 52:276-281, 1991.
91. MacAllister CG, Sangiah S: Effect of ranitidine on healing of experimentally induced gastric ulcers in ponies, *Am J Vet Res* 54:1103-1107, 1993.
92. Brehaus BA, Brown CM, Scott EA, et al: Clostridial muscle infections following intramuscular injections, *Equine Vet Science* 3:42-46, 1983.
93. Rebhun WC, Shin SJ, King JM, et al: Malignant edema in horses, *J Am Vet Med Assoc* 187:732-736, 1985.
94. Tomlinson JE, Blikslager AT: Effects of cyclooxygenase inhibitors flunixin and deracoxib on permeability of ischaemic-injured equine jejunum, *Equine Vet J* 37:75-80, 2005.
95. Tomlinson JE, Wilder BO, Young KM, et al: Effects of flunixin meglumine or etodolac treatment on mucosal recovery of equine jejunum after ischemia, *Am J Vet Res* 65:761-769, 2004.
96. Tomlinson JE, Blikslager AT: Effects of ischemia and the cyclooxygenase inhibitor flunixin on in vitro passage of lipopolysaccharide across equine jejunum, *Am J Vet Res* 65:1377-1383, 2004.
97. Corveleyn S, Deprez P, Van der Weken G, et al: Bioavailability of ketoprofen in horses after rectal administration, *J Vet Pharmacol Ther* 19:359-363, 1996.
98. Corveleyn S, Henrist D, Remon JP, et al: Bioavailability of racemic ketoprofen in healthy horses following rectal administration, *Res Vet Sci* 67:203-204, 1999.
99. Sams R, Gerken DF, Ashcraft SM: Pharmacokinetics of ketoprofen after multiple intravenous doses to mares, *J Vet Pharmacol Ther* 18:108-116, 1995.
100. Landoni MF, Lees P: Influence of formulation on the pharmacokinetics and bioavailability of racemic ketoprofen in horses, *J Vet Pharmacol Ther* 18:446-450, 1995.
101. Landoni MF, Foot R, Frean S, et al: Effects of flunixin, tolfenamic acid, R(-) and S(+) ketoprofen on the response of equine synoviocytes to lipopolysaccharide stimulation, *Equine Vet J* 28:468-475, 1996.
102. Owens JG, Kamerling SG, Stanton SR, et al: Effects of pretreatment with ketoprofen and phenylbutazone on experimentally induced synovitis in horses, *Am J Vet Res* 57:866-874, 1996.
103. Owens JG, Kamerling SG, Stanton SR, et al: Effects of ketoprofen and phenylbutazone on chronic hoof pain and lameness in the horse, *Equine Vet J* 27:296-300, 1995.
104. Ketofen: In Arrioja A, editor: *Compendium of Veterinary Products*, 10th ed, Hensall, ON, 2007, North American Compendiums Ltd, pp 1673.
105. Rose RJ, Kohnke JR, Baggot JD: Bioavailability of phenylbutazone preparations in the horse, *Equine Vet J* 14:234-237, 1982.
106. Smith PB, Caldwell J, Smith RL, et al: The bioavailability of phenylbutazone in the horse, *Xenobiotica* 17:435-443, 1987.
107. Sullivan M, Snow DH: Factors affecting absorption of non-steroidal anti-inflammatory agents in the horse, *Vet Rec* 110:554-558, 1982.
108. Soma LR, Gallis DE, Davis WL, et al: Phenylbutazone kinetics and metabolite concentrations in the horse after five days of administration, *Am J Vet Res* 44:2104-2109, 1983.
109. Tobin T, Chay S, Kamerling S, et al: Phenylbutazone in the horse: a review, *J Vet Pharmacol Ther* 9:1-25, 1986.
110. Wilcke JR, Crisman MV, Sams RA, et al: Pharmacokinetics of phenylbutazone in neonatal foals, *Am J Vet Res* 54:2064-2067, 1993.
111. Tobin T, Blake JW, Valentine R: Drug interactions in the horse: effects of chloramphenicol, quinidine, and oxyphenbutazone on phenylbutazone metabolism, *Am J Vet Res* 38:123-127, 1977.
112. Lees P, Maitho TE, Taylor JB: Pharmacokinetics of phenylbutazone in two age groups of ponies: a preliminary study, *Vet Rec* 116:229-232, 1985.
113. Piperno E, Ellis DJ, Getty SM, et al: Plasma and urine levels of phenylbutazone in the horse, *J Am Vet Med Assoc* 153:195-198, 1968.
114. Hunt JM, Lees P, Edwards GB: Suspected non-steroidal anti-inflammatory drug toxicity in a horse, *Vet Rec* 117:581-582, 1985.
115. Ramirez S, Wolfsheimer KJ, Moore RM, et al: Duration of effects of phenylbutazone on serum total thyroxine and free thyroxine concentrations in horses, *J Vet Intern Med* 11:371-374, 1997.
116. Lees P, May SA, Hoeijmakers M, et al: A pharmacodynamic and pharmacokinetic study with vedaprofen in an equine model of acute nonimmune inflammation, *J Vet Pharmacol Ther* 22:96-106, 1999.

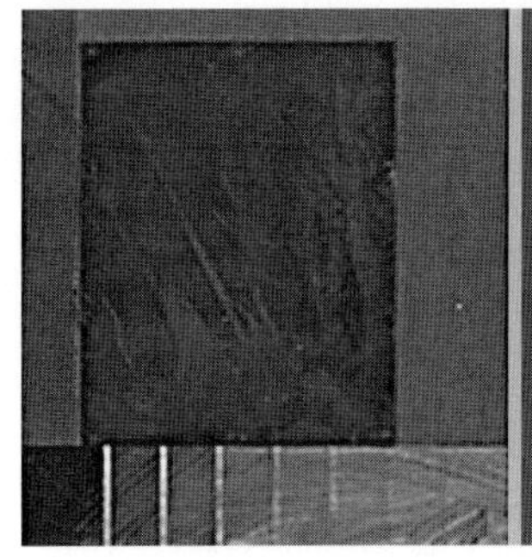

Aspects of Clinical Nutrition

CHAPTER 5

*Raymond J. Geor**

Veterinarians are a primary source of nutritional information and advice for horse owners. Therefore it is reasonable to expect equine practitioners to have some expertise in the clinical assessment of nutritional status and feeding programs so that they may assist horse owners in the selection of rations for an individual horse or group of horses. Additionally, because diet composition can contribute to the pathophysiology and clinical manifestations of certain chronic diseases (e.g., some forms of chronic exertional rhabdomyolysis), the veterinarian is often consulted to make recommendations for special diets. Special dietary considerations are also required for sick neonatal foals or adult horses. This chapter provides an overview of the principles of clinical assessment of nutritional status and feeding programs, reviews carbohydrate nutrition for horses (including the types of carbohydrates in horse feeds, terminology and methods for analysis of carbohydrates in feeds, and strategies for mitigation of gastrointestinal disturbances associated with carbohydrate nutrition), and summarizes current recommendations for the nutritional support of neonatal or adult horses with acute illness. Other topics are feeding management of thin and starved horses and dietary recommendations for the management of obesity, which is becoming a significant problem in equine medicine. The reader is referred to the most recent edition of the National Research Council's *Nutrient Requirements of Horses* for a complete discussion of equine nutrition.[1]

EVALUATION OF NUTRITIONAL STATUS AND FEEDING PROGRAMS

Clinical assessment of a feeding program for an individual or group of horses involves three basic elements: assessment of general health and dietary history, clinical examination, and evaluation of current diet and feeding method (i.e., types and amounts of feeds and how they are fed). The physiologic state and intended use of the horse (e.g., pregnant, lactating, in athletic work) affect its nutritional requirements and therefore are vital with respect to the evaluation of the feeding program and the making of any necessary adjustments. It also is useful to inspect housing and feeding facilities, including feed bins, hay storage, and the watering system. Commercial software programs are available to assist with ration evaluation in relation to nutrient requirements.[2] Figure 5-1 shows an example of a simple form that can be used to collect clinical data, including signalment, body weight and condition, and details regarding the horse's current and recommended ration. Box 5-1 provides explanations for a number of nutritional terms used to describe feed nutrients and fractions, the knowledge of which is relevant to the interpretation of feed analysis data.

Clinical Examination

Body condition scoring (BCS) and measurement of body weight are the cornerstones of the clinical assessment of nutritional status. In some situations laboratory analysis of blood or other tissue samples may be indicated as part of the nutritional evaluation (e.g., measurement of whole blood selenium concentration). It must be recognized that no single laboratory value is a reliable indicator of nutritional status in an individual animal. Nonetheless, blood or tissue measurements may be valuable for evaluation of herd problems, wherein samples should be obtained from a representative number of animals.

Body weight and BCS, which assesses subcutaneous fat deposition, are indicators of long-term energy balance: energy (calorie) intake relative to the horse's needs. In general, horses that receive inadequate dietary energy will lose body weight and condition, whereas weight gain and the development of overconditioning (high BCS) signify energy intake in excess of requirements. Although a number of systems have been used to determine BCS, the most widely applied method is that developed by Henneke.[3] The Henneke system uses a 1- to 9-point scale and requires the assessment of subcutaneous fat deposition in six areas: over the crest of the neck, withers, behind the shoulder, over the ribs, along the back, and around the tail-head. Considerable variation may exist in the pattern of fat deposition among horses; for example, some horses have little fat deposited over the ribs even when other areas of the body are well covered. In addition, fat deposits are sometimes asymmetrically distributed. Therefore it is important to evaluate all six areas of the body on both sides. A score between 1 and 9 is assigned, wherein 1 indicates severe emaciation and 9 indicates extreme fatness (Table 5-1). Body condition scores of 4 to 6 are regarded as ideal depending on use of the horse. Studies of weight gain and loss in moderately conditioned

*The editors acknowledge and appreciate the contribution of Debra K. Rooney, a former author of this chapter. Her original work has been incorporated into this edition.

NUTRITIONAL STATUS AND FEEDING PROGRAM EVALUATION FORM

HORSE INFORMATION Date ________

Owner ______________________________ Horse Name _________________________

Description ____

(e.g., age, gender, breed)

Use/physiological state ____

Housing/environment ____

Medical history____

____

PHYSICAL ASSESSMENT

Dentition _______ Normal _________ Poor

Hooves _______ Normal _________ Founder lines (laminitic)

Hair Coat _______ Normal _________ Long _________Other

Current Body Condition Score _________

(1 = very thin; 5 = moderate; 9 = very obese)

Notes:____

(e.g., abnormal fat deposits)

Optional: Neck Circumference (cm or inches)_____________

ESTIMATED ENERGY INTAKE ON CURRENT DIET

Forage Consumption

Excellent hay (1.1 Mcal/lb) × __________ lb/d = ________________ Mcal digestible energy (DE)

Very good hay (0.9 Mcal/lb) × __________ lb/d = ________________ Mcal

Average hay (0.8 Mcal/lb) × __________ lb/d = ________________ Mcal

Below-average hay (0.7 Mcal/lb) × __________ lb/d = ________________ Mcal

Concentrate Consumption

Oat grain (1.3 Mcal/lb) × _____________ lb/d = ________________ Mcal

Sweet feed (1.4 Mcal/lb) × __________ lb/d = ________________ Mcal

High-fat sweet feed (1.5 Mcal/lb) × ________ lb/d = ________________ Mcal

Other Feeds (e.g., protein supplements, beet pulp)

____________ (_____ Mcal/lb) × ________ lb/d = _________________ Mcal

____________ (_____ Mcal/lb) × ________ lb/d = _________________ Mcal

____________ (_____ Mcal/lb) × ________ lb/d = _________________ Mcal

Current Total Energy Intake __________________**Mcal/d**

(NOTE: Other nutrient intakes should also be checked for adequacy)

FIGURE 5-1 Worksheet for evaluation of nutritional status and feeding program (adapted from Dr. Laurie Lawrence, University of Kentucky).

ESTIMATING THE APPROPRIATE DAILY ENERGY INTAKE

Target Body Condition Score (BCS) ________________

Recommended Change in BCS ___________________
(+1, +2, -1,-2, etc.)

Current Horse Weight ____________ **Target Horse Weight** ____________

Guide: For an 1100- to 1200-lb horse, change in 1 BCS unit = 45 to 70 lb, but greater weight change may be necessary to alter BCS in very thin or very obese horses. Also, note that altering feed intake can have a rapid effect on body weight by increasing or decreasing gut fill. Thus, a change in gut fill can affect body weight by 10 to 20 lb, without a concomitant change in body condition score.

Recommended Energy Intake for Target Weight __________________**Mcal/d**
(see Box 2)

Suggested Adjustments for Weight Change (estimates)
- Increase BCS 1 unit in 60 days (add 6 to 7 Mcal/d)
- Increase BCS 2 units in 90 days (add 9 to 10 Mcal/d)
- Decrease BCS 1 unit in 60 days (subtract 6 to 7 Mcal/d)
- Decrease BCS 2 units in 120 days (subtract 6 to 7 Mcal/d)

Adjusted Recommended Daily Energy Intake _____________**Mcal/d**

RECOMMENDED DIET

Current Level of Dietary Energy
Adequate _______ Insufficient _________ Excessive __________

Current Diet Could Include Minor Modifications: _____________________

Current Diet Should Be Adjusted as Follows:

Suggestions:
- For weight loss: concentrate amounts should be reduced first
- For weight gain: hay intake and quality should be adjusted first

ENERGY INTAKE WITH SUGGESTED DIET

Forage Consumption
Excellent hay (1.1 Mcal/lb) × __________ lb/d = ________________ Mcal DE
Very good hay (0.9 Mcal/lb) × __________ lb/d = ________________ Mcal
Average hay (0.8 Mcal/lb) × __________ lb/d = ________________ Mcal
Below-average hay (0.7 Mcal/lb) × __________lb/d = _______________ Mcal

Concentrate Consumption
Oat grain (1.3 Mcal/lb) × _____________ lb/d = ________________ Mcal
Sweet feed (1.4 Mcal/lb) × ___________ lb/d = ________________ Mcal

FIGURE 5-1, cont'd

High-fat, sweet feed (1.5 Mcal/lb) × ________ lb/d = ________________ Mcal

Other Feeds (e.g., protein supplements, beet pulp)

___________ (_____ Mcal/lb) × ________ lb/d = ________________ Mcal

___________ (_____ Mcal/lb) × ________ lb/d = ________________ Mcal

___________ (_____ Mcal/lb) × ________ lb/d = ________________ Mcal

Total Energy Intake ________________ **Mcal/d**

FIGURE 5-1, cont'd

BOX 5-1

NUTRITIONAL TERMINOLOGY RELEVANT TO THE INTERPRETATION OF FEED COMPOSITION DATA

Moisture: % of feed that is water

Dry matter: 100% minus the water in feed
Most hays and concentrates are approximately 90% water.
Fresh pasture can contain 60%-80% water.
Feed compositions are usually compared on a *dry matter basis* (100% dry matter), but feeds with similar concentrations of dry matter can be compared on an *as-fed basis.*

Crude protein (CP): Also called *total protein;* this value is calculated by measuring total nitrogen.

Acid detergent fiber (ADF): A chemically determined fraction that contains cellulose and lignin. ADF is inversely related to digestibility and is used to estimate the digestible energy content of horse feeds.

Neutral detergent fiber (NDF): A chemically determined fraction that contains cellulose, lignin, and hemicellulose. NDF contains most of the structural carbohydrates in plants; as plants mature, they contain more stem (more structure), and therefore DF increases with maturity. The NDF fraction includes the ADF fraction. There is a general inverse relationship between NDF in forages and voluntary forage intake by horses—in other words, when two hays of similar variety are compared, the forage with lower NDF will be consumed in higher amounts by horses.

Nonfiber carbohydrates (NFCs): Not a measured fraction. NFC is determined by calculating the difference between total DM and the sum of NDF, crude fat, ash, and crude protein. Types of carbohydrates that are included in the NFC fraction are true nonfiber carbohydrates such as monosaccharides and starch, but it also includes some carbohydrates that are resistant to mammalian enzymatic digestion such as pectin (found in beet pulp and alfalfa hay) and fructan (found in some grasses).

Ethanol soluble carbohydrates (ESCs): Part of the nonstructural carbohydrate fraction. The ESC fraction contains mostly simple sugars, disaccharides. Some laboratories categorize this fraction as *sugars.*

Starch: Contains amylose and amylopectin. The starch analysis does not separate easily digested starch and starch resistant to small intestinal digestion.

Nonstructural carbohydrate (NSC): Previously, the NSC fraction included all carbohydrates not included in NDF, but today it is commonly defined as starch plus ESC. Therefore the NSC in a feed represents the carbohydrates that are expected to be digested and absorbed from the small intestine as glucose or other simple sugars.

Water-soluble carbohydrates (WSCs): This fraction includes the simple carbohydrates that appear in the ESC fraction as well as *some* longer chain carbohydrates, including fructans. Fructans are storage carbohydrates synthesized by some plants, especially cool season grasses. Some nutritionists calculate fructan as the difference between WSC and ESC, but this estimate has not been validated.

Digestible energy (DE): Not a measured value. DE is calculated from other analyzed fractions, including ADF and crude protein. The amount of fat in the feed affects the true DE value of a feed, but if crude fat was not a requested item on the feed analysis, the DE might be calculated using an average value for crude fat. For common forages (e.g., hay and pasture), the DE value calculated by a laboratory is a relatively accurate assessment of the true DE value. For concentrate feeds the calculated DE value may not represent the true DE value.

Adjusted Crude Protein, %TDN, NEL, NEM, NEG, relative feed value: Not relevant to horse diet analyses.

TABLE 5-1

Description of Body Condition Scores in Horses

Condition Score	General Condition	Neck	Shoulder	Withers	Ribs	Loin	Tailhead
1	Very Poor	Individual bone structure visible; feels very bony	Bone structure very visible and sharp to touch	Bones easily visible; no fat; razorlike	Ribs very visible and skin furrows between ribs	Spine bones visible; ends feel pointed	Tailhead and hips very visible
Animal extremely emaciated; no fatty tissue can be felt							
2	Very Thin	Bones just visible; animal emaciated	Possible to outline bone structure	Withers obvious, very minimal fat covering	Ribs prominent, slight depression between ribs	Slight fat covering other vertical and flat spin projections; ends feel rounded	Tailhead and hipbones obvious to the eye
3	Thin	Thin, flat muscle covering, no raised muscle or fat	Shoulder accentuated; some fat cover but thinner than is desirable	Withers thin and accentuated with some, although little, fat cover	Slight fat cover over ribs. Rib outline obvious to the eye	Fat buildup halfway on vertical spines, but easily visible; flat spinal bones not felt	Tailhead prominent; hip bones rounded but easily visible; pin bones covered
4	Moderately Thin	Neck with some fat; horse not obviously thin	Shoulder not obviously thin with some fat cover	Withers not obviously thin, smooth edges but prominent	Faint outline visible to the eye	Slight outward ridge along back	Fat palpable
5	Moderate	Neck blends smoothly into body with some fat cover	Shoulder blends smoothly into body	Withers smoothly rounded over top	Ribs cannot be seen but can be easily felt	Back level	Fat around tailhead beginning to feel spongy
6	Moderately Fleshy	Fat easily palpable	Fat layer palpable	Fat palpable	Fat over ribs feels spongy	May have slight inward crease	Fat around tailhead soft and palpable
7	Fleshy	Visible fat deposits or lumps along neck	Fat buildup behind shoulder	Fat covering withers is firm	Individual ribs still palpable	May have slight inward crease down back	Fat around tailhead soft and rounded off
8	Fat	Noticeable thickening of neck	Area behind shoulder filled in flush with body	Area along withers filled with fat	Difficult to feel ribs	Crease down back evident	Tailhead fat very soft and flabby
Fat deposited along inner buttocks							
9	Extremely Fat	Bulging fat	Bulging fat	Bulging fat	Patchy fat over ribs	Obvious deep crease down back	Building fat around tailhead
Fat along inner buttocks may rub together; flank filled in flush							

(BCS = 4-7) Thoroughbred, Quarter Horse, and Arabian horses indicate that one BCS unit represents approximately 25 to 35 kg of body weight.[4,5] The body weight associated with each unit of body condition may be higher in fat or thin horses.

The Henneke BCS system, originally developed for use in Quarter Horse broodmares,[3] is most appropriate for use in light breeds such as Thoroughbreds, Arabians, and Standardbreds. This system may not be suitable for ponies and larger-breed horses (e.g., drafts) that have a different pattern of fat distribution. A 9-point BCS system for Warmblood horses was developed to account for differences in conformation and patterns of fat deposition in this breed when compared with Quarter Horses.[6] For example, fat begins to cover the hip bones of Quarter Horses at a BCS of 4, whereas the hip bones of Warmblood horses remain prominent at a BCS of 6 (using the system developed for Warmbloods).

It also should be noted that the BCS system does not register differences in regional adiposity that may signify increased risk of disease. In humans visceral (abdominal) adiposity is more closely linked than generalized obesity to the risk for diabetes and cardiovascular disease, and measurement of waist circumference is a better indicator of abdominal fat accumulation than is body mass index.[7] In horses and ponies there may be a similar association between regional adiposity and disease risk. In studies of horses and ponies with a predisposition to pasture-associated laminitis, some affected animals are not obese on the basis of BCS (i.e., BCS <7) and have no external evidence of regional adiposity, but others have enlarged fat deposits on the neck ("cresty neck") and thoracic and tailhead regions; these fat deposits are sometimes asymmetrically distributed.[8,9] Neck crest adiposity, assessed by the ratio of mean neck circumference to height at the withers (NCHR), is negatively associated with insulin sensitivity in horses and ponies.[9,10] Although cutoff values for NCHR in relation to obesity and disease risk have not been defined, repeated measurement of mean neck circumference is useful for monitoring the effectiveness of a weight loss program.

Knowledge of a horse's body weight is needed for accurate calculation of nutrient and feed requirements. It is important to note that the body weight of an individual horse can vary between 5% to 15% depending on hydration and feeding status and on gastrointestinal fill. Accordingly, it is important to standardize the time of feeding relative to measurement of body weight. Body weight may be measured directly by use of a platform scale or, in mature horses, estimated from body measurements such as heart girth circumference and body length.[11,12] Heart girth is measured immediately behind the elbows, and body length is measured from the point of the shoulder to the tuber ischii:

$$\text{Body weight (kg)} = [\text{Heart girth (cm)}^2 \times \text{length (cm)}]/11{,}800$$

Body weight also can be estimated from measurement of heart girth circumference by use of a weight tape calibrated for horses. Measurements should be taken in a consistent manner, with the horse standing on a flat surface, and care must be taken not to pull the tape too tightly. Clinicians are advised to take the average of several (e.g., 3 or 4) measurements. Accuracy of these measurements is affected by a number of factors, including breed, conformation, level of fitness, thickness of hair coat, gastrointestinal fill, and pregnancy status.[12] Body weight based on heart girth is most accurate when this method is applied to mature horses with an average BCS (i.e., 5-7). Underestimation or overestimation of body weight may occur when weight tapes are used to estimate the body weight of horses with low or high condition scores.

Diet and Ration Evaluation

It is useful to first examine the physical characteristics of feeds (i.e., visual appearance [color, presence of foreign material such as mold and dust] and odor). Preserved forages (e.g., hay) should be evaluated for type (grass versus legume), leaf -to-stem ratio, and presence of seed heads. Hays with good nutritional value are characterized by a large proportion of leaf; when compared with stems, leaves have higher nonstructural carbohydrates (starches, sugars, fructans), lower structural carbohydrates (hemicellulose, cellulose, lignin), and higher protein.[1] Therefore second- and third-cutting hays, which often have a higher stem-to-leaf ratio, tend to provide higher nutritional value than first-cutting hay. The latter is usually harvested at a more mature stage. The presence of seed heads and a stemmy, coarse appearance are also indications of advanced maturity at cutting. Some studies have reported an inverse relationship between the neutral detergent fiber (NDF, the fraction that contains cellulose, hemicellulose, and lignin) and voluntary hay intake (i.e., the voluntary intake of stemmy hays with high NDF content will be lower compared with that of hays with high leaf-to-stem ratio).[1,13]

The next step in the evaluation is to estimate daily feed intake. Owners or stable managers should be questioned to determine the amounts of hay, concentrates, and supplements provided (and whether the horse regularly refuses any of these feedstuffs). All feeds, including several flakes or biscuits of hay, should be weighed to estimate the actual amounts of feed provided to the horse. Significant errors may occur when volume (e.g., "a coffee can full") rather than weight is used to estimate feed provision because grains, concentrates, and hays vary markedly in weight per unit volume. A handheld fish scale or similar scale works well for this task. It is difficult to measure actual feed intake, particularly when forage is fed on the ground, where wastage can be as high as 25%, or fed to groups of horses. The other challenge is estimation of pasture forage intake, which is generally taken as the difference between the mean intake of digestible energy (DE) for horses, with consideration given to their weight, age, and physiologic condition, minus actual daily intakes of hay and grains. As previously mentioned, regular assessment of body weight and BCS over time will provide the best guide to the adequacy of energy intake. Reported values for daily dry matter intake (DMI) by horses, ponies, and donkeys range between 0.8% to 5.2% of body weight.[1] Young and mature horses appear to have a maximal daily DMI of 3% to 3.2% of body weight, but intakes in the range of 2.0% to 2.5% of body weight are more typical (this includes horses maintained on an all-hay diet). Some evidence suggests that ponies may have higher daily DMI than horses.[1]

The clinician also should evaluate feeding management, particularly when a problem under investigation may be due to poor feeding practices (e.g., weight loss, colic). For example, what are the relative proportions of forage and grain/concentrate? Does the ration contain adequate high-quality forage? How many times a day is the horse fed? How frequently is the diet changed, and are these changes made gradually (ideally over 7 to 10 days) or suddenly? Several epidemiologic studies have reported that changes in diet (grain/concentrate or hay, even when switching to hay of the same type) significantly increase the risk of colic.[14-16] The risk of gastrointestinal problems also increases when horses are fed large quantities of starch-rich grain and concentrate feeds or inadequate long-stem roughage.[14,16] As a general guide, all horses should receive a *minimum* of 1.0% of body weight per day as hay or the equivalent; forage at 1.5% of body weight per day is preferred. For a 450- to 500-kg horse, grain or concentrate meals should be no more than 2.5 kg (approximately 5 lb) to reduce risk of hindgut disturbances associated with the cecal delivery of undigested starch. If the daily ration includes more than 5.0 kg of grain or concentrate, it should be provided in more than two feedings per day (see the section on carbohydrates in equine nutrition).[16]

Information on the nutrient content of the diet is needed to determine the adequacy of the ration. Several approaches can be used to estimate the nutrient contents of feeds. The feed tags on commercial feeds provide some nutritional information, including a list of ingredients and data on some nutrients. However, feed manufacturers are required to guarantee only that minimums were met and maximums were not exceeded; in other words, the actual content of listed nutrients is not provided. An alternative source of data on the nutrient content of feeds is published databases (e.g., National

Research Council [NRC] publications, feed company Web sites). Although the nutrient profiles available from these databases provide a useful guide, these data may not correspond exactly to the feedstuff provided to the horse under evaluation because of differences in geography, growing and harvesting conditions, and other factors. The ideal, although not always practical, approach is to submit samples of feed and forages (core hay samples, pasture clippings) for laboratory analysis of nutrient content. At least two samples (approximately 250 g each) of each grain or concentrate should be taken; these should be mixed thoroughly with the composite sample submitted for analysis. Approximately 10% of the hay store should be sampled by use of a hay probe. Again, these samples should be well mixed, with the composite sample shipped to the laboratory in a sealable plastic bag. Garden shears can be used to obtain pasture clippings, which should be sampled in a Z pattern and cut to grazing height. It may be necessary to sample clippings taken from several pastures to determine the range of nutrients on the farm. The basic nutrient profile from analysis includes dry matter (DM), DE, crude protein (CP), acid detergent fiber (ADF), NDF, fat (EE, ether extract), ash, calcium, magnesium, phosphorus, sodium, and potassium (see Box 5-1). Trace element and vitamin analyses are available depending on need and expense. Some laboratories will perform additional analyses and calculations to provide estimates of some of the carbohydrate fractions. For example, Equi-Analytical Inc. (Ithaca, NY; www.equi-analytical.com) analyzes starch and ethanol-soluble carbohydrates (which are mostly simple sugars). More information on dietary carbohydrates is presented later in this chapter.

With data on feed composition (and estimated intake of feeds), it is possible to formally evaluate the ration against published feeding standards (e.g., NRC 2007[1]). The NRC developed a simple Web-based program that calculates nutrient requirements derived from the 2007 *Nutrient Requirements of Horses* (http://nrc88.nas.edu/nrh/); this program can also be downloaded to a personal computer. The user is first required to enter basic information such as age, body weight, and physiologic state (e.g., stallion, lactating mare, working horse) and then data on the horse's ration—specifically, the amount and nutrient profile of each feed and supplement fed to the horse. The program uses these data to calculate nutrient requirements, dietary supply, and the difference between the two amounts. Unfortunately, only a limited number of nutrients are evaluated: DE, CP, lysine, Ca, P, Na, Cl, and K. The NRC recommendations are also based on minimum nutrient requirements, whereas many nutritionists favor feeding standards based on optimal ranges. Several nutrition companies have developed more comprehensive computer software programs. For example, Microsteed, developed by Kentucky Equine Research (KER), Inc., can evaluate the ration against both the NRC minimums and a set of optimums recommended by company nutritionists.[17]

The process outlined in the preceding paragraphs will facilitate decisions regarding the adequacy of the current ration. If gross deficiencies or excesses are identified, adjustments can be recommended and implemented. Another important aspect is the need for follow-up monitoring, particularly if a goal has been set for weight loss or gain. Figure 5-1 outlines a simple way to estimate energy needs and intake and calculate ration adjustments necessary to facilitate weight loss or gain. A more detailed discussion of dietary management of thin or obese horses is presented later in this chapter.

CARBOHYDRATES IN EQUINE NUTRITION

Carbohydrates are the primary source of energy in the diet of horses. As nonruminant herbivores, horses evolved to utilize forages high in structural carbohydrates, with bacterial fermentation and production of volatile fatty acids (VFAs) in a highly developed large intestine. However, modern horses, particularly those in athletic training, are often fed cereal grains or other starch-rich feeds to meet energy requirements. For example, some survey studies indicate that racehorses weighing 450 to 550 kg typically receive 3 to 6 kg of feed per day, with some horses receiving more than 8 kg per day.[18,19] Such high grain intakes by horses (or a low forage-to-grain ratio such as 30:70) have been implicated in the development of gastrointestinal problems, particularly colic associated with disturbances to hindgut function[20,21] and gastric ulcer disease.[22,23] Additionally, diets rich in starch and sugar contribute to the clinical expression of chronic muscle diseases (polysaccharide storage myopathy and recurrent exertional rhabdomyolysis) in genetically susceptible horses[24] and likely exacerbate insulin resistance and susceptibility to laminitis in horses and ponies with the metabolic syndrome phenotype.[25] Therefore equine veterinarians should have working knowledge of carbohydrate digestion and metabolism and methods for assessment of the carbohydrate fractions in feeds. This information can be used in the formulation of diets and feeding programs that control intake of certain carbohydrates and potentially mitigate risk of these conditions.

Classification and Nomenclature

Plant carbohydrates in equine feeds can be subdivided into the structural carbohydrates (SCs), which largely make up the fibrous portion of the diet and originate from the plant cell wall, and the nonstructural carbohydrates (NSCs), which originate from the cell content. Diets for horses, whether based on pasture, conserved forage, concentrates, or a combination of all three, contain both SCs and NSCs.[26]

All dietary carbohydrates contain similar amounts of gross energy. However, when utilized by the horse, they provide variable amounts of DE, metabolizable energy, and net energy.[27] Carbohydrates digested and absorbed as monosaccharides in the small intestine yield more energy than carbohydrates digested by microbial action (predominantly fermentation), and a glycemic response to the ingestion of such carbohydrates tends to occur.[28] The type of linkage between the monosaccharide residues in the carbohydrate also affects the site of digestion of these compounds and thus their nutritional value. Hydrolysis of the α1-6 and the α1-4 linkages of starch and maltose, for example, can occur in the equine small intestine, but horses do not produce the enzymes necessary to digest the β1-4 linkages found in cellulose or the mixed linkages found in hemicellulose.[28] Therefore digestion of cellulose and hemicellulose must occur as a result of microbial fermentation, which does not result in a pronounced glycemic response. Stachyose, raffinose, β-glucans, fructooligosaccharides (or fructans), and pectin are also thought to be resistant to enzymatic hydrolysis. Thus an understanding of the various carbohydrates fractions in plants (including means of digestion) is needed to determine the potential for a feed to result in a glycemic-insulinemic response.

SIMPLE SUGARS

This fraction comprises monosaccharides and disaccharides (i.e., glucose, fructose, and sucrose). The simple sugar content of these plants is low; the sugars produced by way of photosynthesis can be used immediately by the plant to supply energy for metabolism, protein synthesis, and growth, or they can be elaborated into more complex *oligosaccharides* (e.g., raffinose and stachyose) or the *structural polysaccharides* of the plant cell wall (e.g., cellulose, hemicellulose, and pectin). When sugar production exceeds the immediate requirements for metabolism, the excess sugars are polymerized to form "storage," or "reserve," carbohydrates. Storage carbohydrates mostly are in the form of starch or fructan. Starches, fructans, together with the simple sugars and the oligosaccharides, make up the NSC fraction of the diet.[26]

OLIGOSACCHARIDES

The raffinose family of oligosaccharides are α-galactosyl derivatives of sucrose. The most common are the trisaccharide, raffinose (composed of galactose, fructose, and glucose) and the tetrasaccharide, stachyose. These oligosaccharides are found in sugar beet molasses and whole grains. Soybean oligosaccharides make up approximately 5% of DM in whole beans and up to 8% of DM in soybean meal. Together raffinose and stachyose rank second only to sucrose in abundance as water-soluble carbohydrates. However, raffinose and stachyose cannot be directly digested by the horse because of the absence of the enzyme α-galactosidase.

STRUCTURAL POLYSACCHARIDES

This fraction includes dietary fiber that is composed of cellulose, pectin, and hemicelluloses, along with mannans, galactans, and xyloglucans.[26] Total nonstarch polysaccharides (NSPs) are the sum of the water-soluble and water-insoluble NSPs and include cellulosic and noncellulosic polysaccharides. Although some of the NSPs are water soluble, these are not digestible by mammalian enzymes, and digestion therefore can occur only through fermentation, which may occur proximal to the cecum.

STARCH

Starch is the main storage polysaccharide in most higher plants, including the forage legumes (e.g., clover, alfalfa). Starch is stored in both the vegetative tissues (i.e., nonreproductive tissues such as leaves and stems) and the reproductive tissues (i.e., flowers, seeds). The starch content of grass seed ranges from approximately 300 to 400 g starch/kg seed DM, whereas oats, barley, and corn contain approximately 400, 550, and 700 g starch/kg DM, respectively.[26] The amount of starch stored in the leaves of legumes rarely exceeds 75 g starch/kg DM.

Starch consists of polymers of glucose, which occur in two forms: amylose and amylopectin. Amylose is a linear α-(1-4) linked molecule, and amylopectin is a larger, highly branched molecule containing both α-(1-4) and α-(1-6) linkages. The ratio of amylose to amylopectin largely depends on the botanical origin of the starch. For example, in wheat flour amylose is around 30% of the total starch, whereas corn can contain up to 70% amylose. The extent to which starch is digested prececally depends on many factors, including the availability of the starch to mammalian enzymes (e.g., the extent to which any outer husk or hull has been broken down), the ratio of amylose to amylopectin within the starch granule, the effect of processing (thermal treatment, for example, improves the digestibility of corn and barley starch), and intestinal passage rate.[29] Glucose availability in the small intestine tends to be higher for starches with high amylopectin content. As discussed in more detail later, the ingestion of excessive levels of starch may exceed the relatively limited amylolytic capacity of the equine foregut. Any undigested starch (including resistant starch) that has not been fermented in the stomach and small intestine by resident microbes will pass into the large intestine, where it will be fermented, yielding less net energy than when it is absorbed as glucose.[29]

FRUCTAN

Fructan is the major storage carbohydrate of the vegetative tissues of temperate grasses. Depending on the number of fructose molecules, fructans can be described as oligosaccharides (<10 monosaccharide units) or polysaccharides (>10 units). High levels of fructan can accumulate in the vegetative tissues of pasture grasses, with implications for the development of pasture-associated laminitis.[26] In a 3-year northern European study of the water-soluble carbohydrate (WSC; sugar plus fructan) components in the vegetative structures of temperate grasses, fructan contents of up to 279 g/kg DM were recorded.[26] Fructan accumulation (unlike that for starch) can occur below the temperature threshold for plant growth (approximately 6° C).[30] Therefore cold, bright days that result in high rates of photosynthesis but minimal plant growth may lead to the production of large quantities of excess sucrose and, in turn, substantial fructan accumulation.

Evaluation of the Carbohydrate Content in Feeds

A number of analytical techniques and terms have been used to describe the carbohydrate fractions in feeds. It is important to understand what the different terms mean—and recognize the variation among laboratories with respect to analytical methods and definitions (see Box 5-1).

WATER-SOLUBLE CARBOHYDRATES

The WSC fraction includes the simple (glucose, sucrose, fructose) and more complex (oligosaccharides and fructans) sugars. Although not all of these components can be digested by mammalian enzymes, most can be rapidly fermented by gram positive bacteria, resulting in the production of lactic acid. However, it is important to note that starch, which also can be fermented in this way, is not included in this category. Some commercial laboratories measure WSC (i.e., free sugars plus oligosaccharides and fructans) but report it simply as sugar, whereas others use the term *sugar* to describe the free sugar fraction only.

ETHANOL SOLUBLE CARBOHYDRATES

The term *ethanol soluble carbohydrates* (ESCs) refers to the component of the WSC that is digestible by mammalian enzymes and elicits a glycemic response (i.e., simple sugars). The difference between the WSC and ESC fractions has been used to approximate the amount of fructan in a particular feedstuff, although the accuracy of this calculation has not been verified.

NONSTRUCTURAL CARBOHYDRATES

The NSC fraction includes the monosaccharides and disaccharides, oligosaccharides (including fructan), fructan polysaccharides, and starch. Several methods have been used to estimate the NSC content of feeds. The system developed by Van Soest[31] estimates NSC *by difference,* wherein the feed is partitioned into neutral detergent solubles and NDF. The NDF fraction contains cellulose, most of the hemicellulose, and lignin. Until recently, the NSC content of a feed was determined on the basis of feed analysis and the "by-difference method," according to the following equation:

$$NSC = 100 - (\text{crude protein }\% + \text{NDF }\% + \text{moisture }\% + \text{fat }\% + \text{ash }\%)$$

This estimate was taken to represent the combined sugar, starch, and fructan content of the feed. However, it also includes pectins, gums, and mucilages that, unlike starch, sugar, and fructan, are not subject to very rapid fermentation and therefore do not induce the marked changes in lactic acid concentrations and pH within the hindgut that can occur with excess intake of sugars, starch, or fructan. Therefore the NSC by-difference fraction is now referred to as *nonfiber carbohydrate,* or *NFC.* The quantitative difference between measured NSC and NFC is small for some feeds (e.g., cereal grains) but can be quite large for other feeds (e.g., feeds with substantial pectin, such as sugar beet pulp) (Table 5-2).

Most commercial feed analysis laboratories do not completely fractionate the carbohydrates that make up the NSC, but in most feeds the amount of NSC can be approximated by summing the amount of starch and WSC. The extent to which the sum of starch and WSC accounts for all NSC depends on the analytic procedures used to measure these fractions. This determination probably more accurately reflects the potential for a feed to be rapidly fermented to produce lactic acid.

Carbohydrate Nutrition and Colic

Colic is caused by many conditions, each of which may be related to specific risk factors, such as changes in diet, feeding practices, exercise patterns, and housing or inappropriate parasite control programs. An association between feeding practices and disturbances in gastrointestinal function has long been hypothesized,[32,33] but the mechanisms linking diet with the development of intestinal dysfunction are poorly understood. Indeed, the exact relationship between diet and colic is difficult to determine because of the variety of feeds and feeding practices used throughout the world as well as differences in study populations. Furthermore, it is often difficult to separate the effects of diet and feeding schedule from other management practices, which often depend on the horse's breed and use. Nonetheless, the results of recent epidemiologic studies support the proposition that diet composition and recent changes in diet are important risk factors for development of colic.[34-39] Tinker et al.[37] prospectively examined the risk for colic at 31 horse farms over a 1-year period. Both a change in concentrate feeding (odds ratio [OR] = 3.6 relative to no colic) and the feeding of high levels of concentrate (>2.5 kg/day dry matter, OR = 4.8, >5 kg/day dry matter, OR = 6.3, relative to feeding no concentrate) were identified as risk factors for colic. In addition, colic risk increased when processed feeds such as pellets were fed. Hudson et al.[36] reported that a recent (within 2 weeks) change in type of grain or concentrate fed (OR = 2.6), the feeding of more than 2.7 kg of oats per day (OR = 5.9), and a change in the batch of hay fed (OR = 4.9) were significant risk factors for an episode of colic. In another prospective case-control study, neither the amount nor type of concentrate fed was associated with the colic risk, although the researchers did conclude that horses at pasture may have a decreased risk of colic.[38] On the other hand, a recent (within 2 weeks) change in diet, in particular the type of hay fed (including hay from a different source or cutting of the same type of hay) was a significant risk factor for colic.[38] In this study feeding hay other than coastal/Bermuda or alfalfa significantly increased the colic risk, but this finding may have reflected hay quality and digestibility rather than type of hay per se. Changing to a poorer quality, less digestible hay or feeding wheat straw or cornstalks may predispose horses to large colon impaction.[38] In a practitioner-based colic study in the United Kingdom, a recent change in management was associated with at least 43% of the cases of spasmodic or mild undiagnosed colic. The most common management change was turnout onto lush pasture in the spring.[39] In reviewing the results of available epidemiologic studies, Cohen estimated that approximately one third of colic cases had a history of a recent change in diet.[40] The ingestion of high-concentrate and low-forage diets has also been implicated in the development of gastric ulcers, which in turn may result in signs of colic.[23]

These observations raise several questions regarding the effects of diet composition and dietary change on gastrointestinal function, including the capacity of the equine digestive tract for grain (starch) digestion, possible reasons for increased colic risk with high levels of grain feeding, and the effect of a sudden change in diet (grain or forage) on gastrointestinal function.

TABLE 5-2

Neutral Detergent Fiber, Nonfiber Carbohydrate, and Nonstructural Carbohydrate Composition of Selected Feedstuffs on a Dry Matter Basis*

Feedstuff	% NDF	% NFC†	% NSC‡
Alfalfa hay	43.1	22.0	12.5
Beet pulp	47.3	36.2	19.5
Corn gluten meal	7.0	17.3	12.0
Mixed, mostly grass hay	60.9	16.6	13.6
Soybean meal (48% CP)	9.6	34.4	17.2
Soyhulls	66.6	14.1	5.3

NDF, Neutral detergent fiber; *NFC,* nonfiber carbohydrate; *NSC,* nonstructural carbohydrate.
*The values shown here may vary from those shown elsewhere in this chapter. The values are provided to illustrate differences among feeds and carbohydrate categories. Actual values for individual feeds may vary by stage of maturity, variety, and source.
†%NFC = (100% - %CP-%EE-%Ash-%NDF); CP = crude protein, EE = ether extract.
‡%NSC determined by direct measurement.

Carbohydrate Digestion and Hindgut Function

From a digestive viewpoint carbohydrates in horse feedstuffs can be divided into three main fractions: (1) hydrolyzable carbohydrates (CHO-H), which can be digested in the small intestine by mammalian enzymes (or they can be fermented, both in the foregut and hindgut); (2) rapidly fermented carbohydrates (CHO-F_R), which cannot be broken down by mammalian digestive enzymes but are readily available for microbial fermentation; and (3) slowly fermentable carbohydrates (CHO-F_S). The hydrolyzable fraction includes hexoses, disaccharides, some oligosaccharides, and the nonresistant starches. Although some fermentation of these compounds may occur in the stomach, the primary products of digestion of these compounds are monosaccharides that can be absorbed in the small intestine, with a relatively high energy yield. The rapidly fermentable fraction included pectin, fructan, and some oligosaccharides not digested in the small intestine. Resistant starch and neutral detergent hemicellulose could also be included in the rapidly fermentable fraction. The slowly fermentable carbohydrate fraction includes cellulose, hemicellulose, and ligno-cellulose that result primarily in the production of acetate in the large intestine.

FOREGUT DIGESTION

Carbohydrate digestion begins in the stomach, which in the horse is relatively small and inelastic (capacity 9-15 L for a 500-kg horse). Bacterial fermentation of ingested feed is initiated in the cranial (squamous) portion of the stomach, with conversion of some of the available simple sugars or starches to lactic acid.[41] This microbial activity and starch/sugar degradation slows when the gastric contents pass to the fundic gland region and are mixed with gastric secretions containing pepsinogen. Horse saliva contains minimal amylase activity, and little enzymatic carbohydrate digestion occurs in the stomach.

The small and large intestines are the primary sites of carbohydrate digestion. Starch digestion in the small intestine first involves degradation by α-amylase into disaccharide (maltose), trisaccharide (maltotriose), and α-dextrin units. Subsequently, there is hydrolysis of maltose, maltotriose, and α-dextrin units by small intestine brush border glycanases, primarily amyloglucosidase (AMG), to form free glucose.[42] The disaccharidases sucrase, lactase, and maltase are expressed along the length of the small intestine.[43] D-glucose and D-galactose are transported across the equine intestinal brush border membrane by a Na^+/glucose co-transporter type 1 isoform (SGLT1),[43] and fructose is absorbed by way of an equine-specific GLUT-5 transporter.[15] The activity of both transport proteins is highest in the duodenum and lowest in the ileum.[15] Sugars taken up by enterocytes are transported down concentration gradients into the circulation by way of the GLUT-2 transporter. Preliminary studies have demonstrated upregulation of small intestinal SGLT1 expression with an increase in dietary starch content.[44]

It has been proposed that starch digestion in the small intestine is limited by amylolytic activity (e.g., the availability and activity of α-amylase). The activity of α-amylase in pancreatic tissue of horses is low relative to that of other species,[45] although the activities of brush border glycanases appear to be comparable to those observed in humans, pigs, and dogs.[46,47] The activity of α-amylase in pancreatic tissue of horses fed either hay or hay and concentrate for at least 8 weeks was unaffected by diet.[46] However, in a related study, the amylase activity of jejunal chyme was modestly higher in horses that received a diet with added corn, oats, or barley when compared with only hay.[47]

The extent of starch digestion in the small intestine is affected by the type and amount of starch digested (see the section on strategies for minimizing gastrointestinal disturbances).[48] At low levels of starch intake (<100 g/100 kg body weight from oats, barley, or corn as a single meal), approximately 80% of the starch was digested in the small intestine. When starch feeding was doubled (250 to 270 g/100 kg body weight), precedal starch digestibility decreased to between 50% and 55%.[49] Therefore most nutritionists recommend that an individual grain or concentrate meal contain no more than 2 g starch per kg body weight. For example, if a grain concentrate is 50% starch, no more than 4 g/kg bodyweight (Bwt) or approximately 2 kg for a 500-kg horse should be fed. At higher intakes in a single meal, particularly when unprocessed corn or barley is fed, there is the risk of substantial starch overflow into the hindgut, where it will undergo rapid fermentation.

HINDGUT DIGESTION

The equine large intestine (cecum and colon) is an enlarged fermentative chamber that contains an extremely abundant and highly complex community of microorganisms. Although some fermentation of feedstuffs occurs in the stomach and small intestine, most fermentation occurs in the hindgut. The microbial hydrolysis of dietary plant fiber within the large intestine leads to the release of soluble sugars that are subsequently fermented to the VFAs acetate, propionate, and butyrate, which are an important source of energy. In addition, the VFAs (particularly butyrate) regulate the expression of genes controlling proliferation, apoptosis, and differentiation of gut epithelial cells.[50]

The rate of fermentation and the microbial and biochemical contents of the large intestine are affected by diet composition and feeding pattern (i.e., continuous grazing, or small, frequent meals, versus large meals administered twice daily). A change from forage only to a forage and concentrate diet will result in an increased rate of fermentation and marked changes in the microbial population, luminal pH, and the contents of VFA and lactate.[51] The extent of these changes is likely dependent on the nature and abruptness of the dietary change. With a sudden increase in grain (i.e., starch) feeding, a portion of the ingested starch passes into the cecum undigested, where it undergoes rapid fermentation with increased production of lactate and gas and a decrease in cecal-colonic pH. Increasing proportions of grain result in decreased acetate and increased propionate and lactate contents of the cecum and colon.[51] Other biochemical changes with the rapid fermentation of starch (or other CHO-F_R, such as fructan) in the hindgut may include an increase in the production of vasoactive monoamines (e.g., tyramine, tryptamine), endotoxins, and exotoxins, all of which have been implicated in the pathogenesis of laminitis.[52]

After an increase in starch feeding, the numbers of lactobacilli and total anaerobic bacteria increase, whereas the numbers of xylanolytic and pectinolytic bacteria decrease.[53] Overall, there is an increase in amylolytic, lactic acid–producing bacteria and decreases in the proportions of acid-utilizing (particularly lactate) and cellulolytic (i.e., fiber-degrading) bacteria. Reduced efficiency of fiber utilization and decreased energy yield may result from the decline in cellulolytic bacteria with high grain feeding. In horses fed forage only, pH within the cecum and colon is in the range of 6.7 to 7.0. The feeding of increasing amounts of corn or barley starch is associated with proportionate decreases in cecal pH, with values approaching 6.0 when 3 to 4 g/kg Bwt is fed as a single meal.[51,54,55] A similar dose of oat starch was not associated with a significant decrease in pH, consistent with other data demonstrating higher precedal digestibility of oat starch versus barley and corn starch.[55] Some nutritionists have suggested that a cecal pH of 6.0 represents subclinical acidosis and that the risk of clinically apparent intestinal dysfunction (e.g., increased permeability) is substantially increased when hindgut pH is less than 6.0.[2,55] Similar disruptions to the hindgut environment probably occur with the delivery of other rapidly fermentable substrate, such as fructan, which can compose 5% to 40% of grass DM,[26] particularly temperate species such as perennial ryegrass and timothy. In vitro experiments have demonstrated that fructan induces a more rapid decrease in the pH of cecal contents compared with corn starch,[56] and one type of fructan (raftilose) has been used to induce carbohydrate overload and laminitis.[57]

These disturbances to the hindgut environment put the horse at greater risk for digestive disturbances such as colic, osmotic diarrhea, and laminitis.[32,33] Scenarios favoring the presentation of large loads of rapidly fermentable substrate to the hindgut include (1) a sudden introduction to grain feeding or an abrupt increase in the amount of grain concentrate; (2) the feeding of large grain meals that, even in horses adapted to such feeds, overwhelm the hydrolytic or absorptive capacity of the small intestine; and (3) the grazing of lush pasture or forage with high contents of rapidly fermentable substrate such as fructan and simple sugars. It is therefore apparent that feeding strategies designed to minimize hindgut disturbances must focus on reducing the flow of rapidly fermented substrate to the cecum and large colon.

Recommendations for Minimizing Digestive Disturbances

FEEDING FREQUENCY

Ideally, feeding strategies for horses kept under intensive conditions would mimic the pattern of a grazing animal—that is, an almost continuous feeding pattern that minimizes fluctuations in the rate of delivery of substrate to the large intestine and, when forage makes up the bulk of the diet, ensures some stability of the hindgut ecosystem. A more continuous feeding pattern also may minimize fluctuations in gastric acidity and therefore be of benefit in horses at risk for squamous mucosal ulcer disease. For stabled horses fed two large meals daily, foraging behavior should be encouraged by increasing the availability of hay (or even a variety of different forages) and pasture or dry lot turnout (with forage available). Provision of more frequent (e.g., thrice daily rather than twice daily), smaller concentrate meals throughout the day is also recommended to minimize delivery of undigested hydrolyzable carbohydrate to the hindgut. Extending eating time by diluting the energy density of the meal (e.g., chopped hay mixed with concentrates) or feeding forage before grain or concentrate may be helpful. For some greedy eaters placement of several large stones in the feeder trough may slow the rate of intake.

ADEQUATE FORAGE AND FIBER

For hard-working horses with high DE requirements, the provision of roughage is often restricted in favor of grain concentrates to ensure adequate DE intake within limits of typical dry matter consumption. However, there is considerable circumstantial evidence associating low-roughage diets with digestive disturbances (e.g., hindgut acidosis, colic, gastric ulcers) and behavioral problems. There also is evidence that the adverse effects of high starch intake on hindgut function are mitigated when the ration is at least 50% NDF.[58] Accordingly, there is rationale for feeding programs that promote higher roughage intake. An absolute fiber requirement has not been defined, but a minimum of 1.0 kg long-stem forage per 100 kg Bwt (i.e., 5.0 kg for a 500-kg horse, as fed basis) has been recommended. Some nutritionists have suggested that a rate of 1.5 kg per 100 kg Bwt is preferable. Alternatively, fiber intake can be increased by feeding other sources such as sugar beet pulp or soya hulls, both of which are highly digestible (i.e., the DE yield is higher compared with that of hay) and are now commonly added to energy supplements for horses. This approach also facilitates a decrease in reliance on grain or sweet feed for energy, thereby decreasing the risk of digestive disturbances associated with high starch intake.

Forage quality is another important consideration. The feeding of highly lignified fiber sources (e.g., straw), which are poorly degraded in the large intestine, may increase the risk of impaction colic. High intake of straw is possible when it is used for bedding, particularly when an inadequate amount of hay (or roughage with low palatability) is offered. An increase in the provision of palatable forage or a change in bedding can be helpful in these situations. Moldy forage should not be fed to equids.

LIMITING DELIVERY OF RAPIDLY FERMENTED SUBSTRATE TO THE HINDGUT

Size of Grain-concentrate Meals The feeding of large meals rich in starch and sugar can overwhelm the digestive capacity of the small intestine and destabilize the hindgut because of rapid fermentation of these substrates. No more than 2 g starch/kg Bwt should be fed in a single meal. For a grain or sweet feed mix that is 40% to 50% starch, this upper limit equates to approximately 2.0 kg per meal for a 500-kg horse.

Feed Starch Sources with High Prececal Digestibility Prececal starch digestibility varies with the type of grain and the nature of any mechanical or thermal processing. Whereas oat starch has a prececal digestibility of around 80% to 90%, approximately 35% of equivalent doses of barley or corn starch (from unprocessed grains) reaches the cecum undigested. The higher prececal digestibility of oat starch may relate to the small size of the starch granules when compared with other grains, providing a large surface area for exposure to intestinal amylase. Milling, grinding, and various heat treatments (e.g., steam flaking, micronization, extrusion) improves the prececal starch digestibility of oats, barley, and corn. In one study the pre-ileal digestibility of ground oats was 97% when compared with 83% for whole oats. Rolling or breaking did not improve the pre-ileal digestibility of oats. For corn and barley pre-ileal starch digestibility is substantially increased after heat (e.g., steam-flaked corn, micronized barley) but not mechanical treatment. Overall, oats appear to be the safest source of starch for horses, although barley and corn are acceptable *if* they are subjected to some form of heat treatment.

Use Alternative Sources of Energy The energy demands of growth, lactation, and performance can be readily met by provision of alternative energy sources such as vegetable oil (fat) and nonstarch carbohydrates (e.g., sugar beet pulp, soya hulls). Commercial concentrates made with these ingredients contain varying amounts of starch and sugar, but in general amounts are substantially lower compared with straight cereals or sweet feed mixes. Compared with more traditional fiber sources such as hay, soya hulls and beet pulp contain lower indigestible material (e.g., lignin) and higher amounts of nonstarch polysaccharides, pectins, and gums, which can be digested to a large extent within the time period that they remain within the gastrointestinal tract. This translates to a higher energy yield. A variety of vegetable oils (e.g., corn, soy, safflower, or flaxseed) and other sources of fat (e.g., stabilized rice bran; approximately 20% fat) are suitable for inclusion in equine diets. Corn oil tends to be the most palatable oil, but most types have acceptable palatability provided that they are fresh and not rancid. One recommendation is to feed up to 100 g oil/100 kg body weight daily. For reference purposes, 450 ml of oil (approximately 420 g) provides about 3.4 megacalories (Mcal) of DE. This daily amount should be divided into two or three meals and introduced gradually (e.g., starting at 50 ml/day). Vitamin E (100 to 200 IU/100 ml of oil) should be added to the ration if supplemental vegetable oil is provided.

Pasture Grazing An unresolved problem is management of the intake of rapidly fermentable substrate (e.g., fructan) by horses at pasture, particularly animals with a history of pasture-associated laminitis or those with recognized risk factors for this disease (i.e., obesity, insulin resistance). The most obvious avoidance strategy is to prevent access to pasture and feed preserved forage with low NSC content (e.g., <10% NSC). Alternative approaches are to restrict access to pasture at certain times of the day, avoiding peaks in forage NSC content that may increase risk of laminitis, or to apply a grazing muzzle that limits forage intake (but allows water intake). Several factors affect the accumulation of fructans and other forms of NSC in pasture plants, including plant growth rate, temperature, and light intensity. There also is marked diurnal variation, with peak concentrations in the afternoon and a nadir during the night and early morning, and it has been suggested that horses grazing in the afternoon may ingest twofold to fourfold quantities of NSC when compared with that ingested during night or early morning grazing. These observations are the basis for the recommendation to restrict grazing to late night and early morning, with removal of the horse or pony from pasture by midmorning.

GRADUAL DIETARY CHANGES

The increased risk of colic in the 2-week period after a change in hay or grain feeding suggests that all changes in diet and pattern of feeding should be gradual. Horses should receive a blend of old and new hays during the transition between hay batches (e.g., over a 7- to 10-day period, with a gradual increase in the proportion of the new forage) and a conservative introduction to concentrate feeding or changes in type of grain or concentrate. One suggestion is to start at about 0.5 kg/day (split into two feedings) for a 450- to 500-kg horse, with increasing increments of no more than 0.5 kg per day until attainment of the target feeding rate.

EFFICACY OF PROBIOTIC SUPPLEMENTS AND FEED ADDITIVES PURPORTED TO STABILIZE THE HINDGUT ENVIRONMENT

There is considerable interest in the use of feed additives such as live yeast culture, probiotics (bacterial species), and buffers (e.g., sodium bicarbonate) as a strategy to minimize the negative effects of cereal-based diets. Yeast cultures might be beneficial for stabilization of the hindgut environment in the face of high cereal feeding. In horses fed high starch meals (3.4 g/kg Bwt/meal, as barley), daily supplementation with 10 g of a live yeast *(Saccharomyces cerevisiae)* culture preparation attenuated postfeeding decreases in cecal and colonic pH and alterations in hindgut microbial populations.[59] Thus supplementation with live yeast culture may be beneficial in horses fed a high grain ration, but from a practical standpoint it may be more important to ensure adequate fiber in the diet, decrease the quantity of grain, and emphasize use of nonstarch energy sources that do not adversely affect the hindgut environment.

Probiotics have been defined as live microorganisms that, when ingested or administered orally, provide a beneficial effect beyond that of their nutritional value.[60] Many probiotics are marketed for use in horses, the primary rationale being the treatment or prevention of gastrointestinal diseases (e.g., as an adjunct therapy in the management of acute or chronic diarrhea) or prophylactic administration for prevention of colic associated with disturbances to gut microflora (e.g., for horses fed a high cereal ration). Anecdotal data suggest that the use of probiotics in horses is widespread; however, as with many nutritional supplements, there is a dearth of scientific data regarding safety and efficacy. An effective probiotic organism must be resistant to destruction by gastric acid, pancreatic secretions, and bile salts and be able to colonize the intestinal tract. Weese and Rousseau have screened equine intestinal microflora for organisms meeting these criteria and initially identified *Lactobacillus pentosus* (WE7) as a potential equine probiotic. However, in a randomized controlled clinical trial of 153 neonatal foals (24-48 hours old), the administration of freeze-dried *L. pentosus* WE7 for 7 days was significantly associated with the development of signs of depression, anorexia, and colic and more days with diarrhea compared with the placebo treatment.[60] On the other hand, supplementation with *Saccharomyces boulardii* reduced significantly the duration of diarrhea in horses with enerocolities.[61]

The feeding of a protected sodium bicarbonate product has been reported to moderate the decrease in fecal pH associated with grain feeding in horses,[62] perhaps as a result of the buffering of lactic acid produced in the cecum and colon. This approach may be useful for mitigation of hindgut disturbances associated with grain feeding or the grazing of lush pasture.

NUTRITIONAL SUPPORT OF SICK HORSES

There are little data on the effects of different feeding practices on short- and long-term outcomes of sick horses, and many recommendations regarding nutritional management are based on anecdotal evidence or clinician experience rather than the results of controlled studies. In human medicine nutritional status is an independent determinant of morbidity in hospital patients.[63,64] Nutrient deprivation is associated with immunosuppression and alterations in gastrointestinal function, including decreased motility, villus atrophy, and a decrease in gut barrier function resulting from an increase in intestinal permeability, particularly in patients with preexisting malnutrition.[65] Consequently, nutritional support is standard practice in the care of sick people.

Healthy adult horses can tolerate 2 to 3 days of feed withdrawal without ill effect. Starvation invokes neuroendocrine responses that lower metabolic rate, conserve lean tissues (i.e., skeletal muscle), and promote use of fat stores to meet energy demands.[66] This strategy prolongs life in the face of nutrient deprivation. The metabolic response to critical illness (e.g., sepsis) contrasts with that of simple starvation. Increased sympathetic nervous system activity, inflammatory cytokines (e.g. interleukin-1[IL-1], IL-2, IL-6, tumor necrosis factor α [TNF-α]), and catabolic hormones (catecholamines, cortisol, and glucagon) combine to increase metabolic rate and induce a state of hypercatabolism.[67] Stimulation of proteolytic pathways in skeletal muscle provides amino acids for hepatic gluconeogenesis and synthesis of acute phase proteins. Amino acids (from catabolism of lean tissues) rather than fatty acids are the primary source of energy substrate. There also is disruption of glucose regulation with development of marked insulin resistance. Unabated, this hypercatabolic state results in large nitrogen losses, severe muscle wasting, and compromise of immune function and tissue healing.[66-68]

Severe hyperlipidemia has been described in horses with colic, colitis, or both that had clinical and laboratory evidence of systemic inflammatory response syndrome (SIRS).[69] The increase in circulating lipids likely reflects both an increase in the mobilization of fat reserves (lipolysis) and a decrease in lipid clearance from blood, with both processes potentially modulated by SIRS, endotoxemia, or both. Studies in other species have demonstrated that the activity of endothelial lipoprotein lipase, the enzyme responsible for tissue uptake of circulating lipids, is decreased by TNF-α, whereas the activity of hormone-sensitive lipase is increased during endotoxemia.[68,70,71] In horses with severe hypertriglyceridemia, treatment with intravenous dextrose solution or partial parenteral nutrition resulted in a decrease in serum triglyceride concentrations to reference limits, and appetite improved coincident with the decrease in circulating lipids.[69]

Candidates for Nutritional Support

Several factors affect the decision to provide nutritional support to a sick horse, including the duration of inappetence or anorexia, the nutritional state before illness (e.g., poor versus good body condition), physiologic state (e.g., growing animals, last trimester of pregnancy, lactation), and the presence of clinical indicators of a hypercatabolic state (e.g., hyperlipidemia or lipemia).[72,73] As a general guide, horses that have not eaten for 48 to 72 hours are candidates for nutritional support. However, earlier intervention should be considered when there is evidence of compromised nutritional status, such as horses in thin body condition (BCS <3); those with a history of weight loss, poor feed intake, or both for more than 48 hours before examination; and those with evidence of sepsis, SIRS, or severe hyperlipidemia (e.g., triglycerides >500 mg/dl). Aggressive nutritional support also is indicated for obese (BCS >7) animals, particularly pony breeds, miniature horses, donkeys, and lactating mares, all of which are at high risk for development of hyperlipemia and hepatic lipidosis during periods of negative energy balance. Old horses or those with evidence of endocrine (pituitary pars intermedia dysfunction [PPID], equine Cushing's disease) and metabolic disease (equine metabolic syndrome) also are candidates for early nutritional intervention.

Estimating Nutrient and Feed Requirements

The nutritional requirements of sick horses have not been determined, so recommendations are largely based on data from healthy horses, with some extrapolation from data in other species. As for healthy animals, however, the first consideration is energy (calories). As discussed, negative energy balance caused by starvation or underfeeding can compromise immune function, delay wound healing, and result in a marked decrease in lean mass (e.g., skeletal muscle), the latter resulting from the breakdown of endogenous protein for use in energy-requiring processes. On the other hand, studies in humans and other species have shown that an oversupply of energy *(hyperalimentation)* is also detrimental, with complications such as hyperglycemia, hyperinsulinemia, hypertriglyceridemia, insulin resistance, and increased risk of septic complications.[74] A proposed mechanism of increased complications induced by hyperalimentation is an increase in the expression of TNF receptors associated with an increase in nuclear factor κB binding to the nucleus.[75] Furthermore, in septic animals high caloric intake results in an increase in mortality.[76,77] For these reasons, the current thinking in human medicine is to underfeed nonprotein calories (15 to 25 kilocalories [kcal]/kg daily or no more than 66% of calculated energy requirements) to minimize risk of septic complications.[74]

The sixth edition of *Nutrient Requirements of Horses*[1] reported that the DE needs of mature horses at maintenance ranges between 30.3 to 36.3 kcal/kg body weight daily. The lower end of this range is suitable for minimally active animals with a tendency to gain weight ("easy keepers"), and the high value should be applied to animals with a nervous temperament ("hard keepers"). For healthy horses confined to a stall, daily energy requirements are probably 25% to 40% lower than in horses kept at pasture or in similar circumstances that require it to engage in some voluntary activity. Pagan and Hintz[78] reported that the DE requirement of healthy horses kept in stalls was approximately 22 to 23 kcal/kg Bwt per day, or 30% lower than the DE required by horses kept at pasture. This *stall maintenance* caloric requirement can be estimated by the following equation: RER = [21 kcal × Bwt (kg)] + 975 kcal, where RER is resting energy requirement. Energy requirements are also affected by the level of feed intake. Thermogenesis associated with the digestion, fermentation, and metabolism of feed can account for 15% to 25% of daily energy expenditure. Because horses recovering from illness generally consume less feed, some reduction in the energy losses associated with digestion and nutrient processing is to be expected.

Another consideration in the estimation of energy requirements is the effect of disease or surgical intervention on metabolic rate. There is conflicting evidence from human studies regarding the effects of surgery, injury, or illness (e.g., sepsis) on metabolic rate and energy requirements. Some studies have demonstrated that abdominal surgery increases energy needs by as much as 30%, whereas others have reported minimal change in energy requirements after gastrointestinal surgery, perhaps a reflection of the decrease in physical activity during hospitalization.[79,80] On balance, it appears that energy needs are minimally altered by surgery or injury unless there are major complications such as generalized burns or sepsis, in which case energy requirements may increase by 40% to 100%.[80] The potential effects of underlying disease (e.g., endotoxemia or SIRS) on the energy requirements of horses are unknown. However, in sick neonatal foals resting metabolic rate and energy requirements were considerably lower compared with those of healthy foals of the same age,[81,82] and horses that underwent resection of the small intestine gained weight when fed at true maintenance (i.e., 32 to 33 kcal/kg/day) during the postoperative period.[83] This author recommends that the caloric requirements of sick horses initially be based on the RER or stall maintenance equation (i.e., 22 to 23 kcal/kg/day). Thereafter there should be a gradual increase in the ration, although true maintenance DE may not be required until the horse returns to normal management (e.g., field turnout). Practitioners should keep in mind that regular measurement of body weight or assessment of BCS should be undertaken during convalescence to judge the adequacy of energy provision and provide a basis for adjustments in feeding.

Protein serves an important role in tissue maintenance, immune function, wound healing, and the slowing of endogenous protein catabolism. Protein requirements must be considered in light of caloric intake and underlying disease process. When energy supply from carbohydrate and fat is limited, endogenous protein will be used for energy, contributing to a loss of lean body mass. Therefore the practitioner should, when developing a nutritional plan, first ensure that minimal energy needs are met and then calculate protein requirements. For humans suggested protein requirements range between 1.2 and 2.0 g protein/kg/day, with the higher end of this range recommended for patients undergoing major intestinal surgery.[84] The crude protein (CP) requirement of healthy adult horses at maintenance is approximately 1.25 g CP/kg body weight/day and this value is an appropriate starting point in the development of a nutritional plan for sick horses: As the efficiency of digestion for most dietary proteins in horse feeds is about 70%, this level of CP will provide approximately 0.9 g available protein/kg body weight. For parenteral feeding a slight lowering of protein feeding is reasonable given the higher metabolic availability of amino acids administered by the intravenous route. In recent reports of parenteral feeding of horses, 0.6 to 0.8 g protein/kg/day (1 g per 40 to 50 kcal) was administered (as a balanced amino acid solution).[83,85] There may be justification for higher levels of dietary protein (e.g., 2 g CP/kg/day), particularly for horses in poor body condition (BCS <3) or those with SIRS, hypoproteinemia, or hypoalbuminemia.

Modes of Nutritional Therapy

The mode of nutritional therapy will depend on the underlying disease, the horse's appetite, and complications that arise during convalescence. The popular phrase in human clinical nutrition "if the gut works, use it" is used when discussing the pros and cons of enteral nutrition (EN) versus parenteral nutritional (PN) support. Historically, PN has been associated with several complications, including intestinal atrophy, failure of gut barrier function, bacterial translocation, increased incidence of sepsis, and hyperglycemia. In rodent models intestinal villous atrophy develops within a few days of the start of PN, and withdrawal of enteral feeding has been associated with bacterial translocation, systemic inflammation, and sepsis.[86-88] Early human studies also suggested that complication rates (particularly sepsis) and mortality were higher in patients receiving PN compared with those who received EN. However, critical review of human studies has indicated that PN (i.e., complete bowel rest) is not associated with intestinal atrophy, whereas the incidence of bacterial translocation is the same in patients receiving PN and those receiving EN.[74] Although EN is preferable when the gastrointestinal tract is functional, the weight of evidence from human studies indicates that PN is an important alternative to EN when a risk of malnutrition is present and EN is not tolerated or not possible because of poor gastrointestinal function. These same principles can be applied when developing a plan for the nutritional management of sick horses. Parenteral nutrition should be considered for horses with ileus and other intestinal conditions that prevent voluntary or enteral feeding, particularly when the withholding of oral feeding is expected to exceed 48 hours.

ASSISTED ENTERAL FEEDING

Assisted enteral feeding (AEF) is accomplished by the infusion of a liquid diet through a nasogastric tube. Diet options for AEF include human-marketed enteral products, commercial pelleted horse feeds, and homemade recipes.[89,90] Formulations marketed for humans that have been administered to adult horses include Vital HN and Osmolyte HN (Ross Laboratories, Columbus, Ohio). Both formulations are devoid of fiber, which is an advantage because it facilitates administration through a small diameter nasogastric tube but also a disadvantage insofar as it may lead to the development of diarrhea when these products are fed to horses. There also have been anecdotal reports of laminitis in horses fed these diets. Risk of these complications may be mitigated by gradually introducing the liquid diet over a 3- to 4-day period, but diarrhea remains common, perhaps indicating the importance of dietary fiber for maintenance of normal hindgut function. It also should be recognized that the mix of energy substrates in these fiber-free enteral formulas for human use differs from that in typical equine rations. Osmolyte contains approximately 29% of calories from lipid and 54% of calories from hydrolyzable carbohydrate (mostly sugars), and Vital HN provides about 10% calories from lipid and 74% from carbohydrate. The high lipid content of Osmolyte may contribute to digestive disturbances in horses not adapted to fat-supplemented rations, and use of a high carbohydrate diet such as Vital HN may be contraindicated for horses with abnormal glucose metabolism (insulin resistance). Collectively, these considerations argue against the use in horses of fiber-free enteral products intended for human use. Diets containing a moderate amount of fiber (10% to 20% crude fiber [CF], DM basis) appear to be a more suitable choice for AEF in horses.

A simple approach is to use a commercially available pelleted feed that contains a source of fiber, such as Equine Senior (Land O' Lakes-Purina Feed, St. Louis, Mo.) or similar "complete feeds" that contain added fiber and can be fed without hay. These products contain about 14% to 25% CF and provide 2.6 to 3.1 Mcal DE/kg diet (as fed). Therefore 3.5 to 4.0 kg of diet would be needed to meet the stall energy requirements of a 500-kg horse. Vegetable oils (75 to 375 ml per day) can be added to increase the caloric density of the diet (Table 5-3). One standard cup (approximately 225 ml or 210 g) of oil provides about 1.7 Mcal of DE. Vitamin E (100 to 200 IU per 100 ml of oil) should be added to the ration if supplemental vegetable oil is provided. When providing supplemental fat to a sick horse (450 to 500 kg Bwt), 75 to 125 ml per day (¼ to ½ cup) should be given initially and then gradually increased if no adverse response is seen (e.g., diarrhea, steatorrhea, lipemia). Feeding vegetable oil may be contraindicated in horses and ponies with hypertriglyceridemia (triglyceride concentration >40 to 500 mg/dl) or hepatic lipidosis.

Variations on the alfalfa/dextrose/casein enteral formulation first described by Naylor et al.[90] also can be used for AEF (Table 5-4). The recipe designed by Naylor et al.[90] provides about 3 Mcal DE/kg diet and is 33% CP and 12% CF. The higher protein content, compared with that of typical equine diets, may be beneficial for debilitated or hypoproteinemic horses. In healthy horses this diet reportedly maintained body weight and serum biochemical parameters within reference limits. However, diarrhea and laminitis were occasional complications.

TABLE 5-3

Enteral Formulation Based on a Complete Pelleted Ration and Recommended Feeding Schedule for a 500-kg Horse*

Ingredient	Day 1 (¼ ration)	Day 2 (½ ration)	Day 3 (¾ ration)	Day 4 (Full ration)
Complete pelleted horse feed (g)†	885	1770	2650	3530
Vegetable oil (ml)	100	177	265	354
Water (L)	8	16	24	24
Digestible energy (Mcal)	3	6	9	12

*Energy requirements are at *stall maintenance* for a 500-kg horse (~12 Mcal DE/day). These allowances should be divided and administered into a minimum of four feedings daily.
†Equine Senior (Land 'O Lakes-Purina Feed, St. Louis, Mo.), 2.6 Mcal DE/kg (as fed).

TABLE 5-4

Alfalfa/Dextrose/Casein Enteral Formulation and Recommended Feeding Schedule for a 500-kg Horse*

	DAY						
Parameter	1	2	3	4	5	6	7
Electrolyte mixture (g)†	230	230	230	230	230	230	230
Water (L)	21	21	21	21	21	21	21
Dextrose (g)	300	400	500	600	800	800	900
Dehydrated cottage cheese or casein (g)	300	450	600	750	900	900	900
Dehydrated alfalfa meal (g)	2000	2000	2000	2000	2000	2000	2000
Digestible energy (Mcal)	7.4	8.4	9.4	10.4	11.8	11.8	12.2

Adapted from Naylor JM, Freeman DE, Kronfeld DS: Alimentation of hypophagic horses, *Compend Cont Educ Pract Vet* 6:S93-S99, 1984.
*These allowances should be divided and administered into three or four feedings daily. Stall maintenance requirements for a 500-kg horse are 12 Mcal DE/day.
†Composition of electrolyte mixture: sodium chloride (NaCl) 10 g; sodium bicarbonate ($NaHCO_3$) 15 g; potassium chloride (KCl) 75 g; potassium phosphate (dibasic anhydrous, K_2HPO_4) 60 g; calcium chloride ($CaCl_2 \cdot 2H_2O$) 45 g; magnesium oxide (MgO) 25 g.

Suggested feeding protocols for a complete pelleted feed with supplemental vegetable oil and for the alfalfa/dextrose/casein formulation are presented in Tables 5-3 and 5-4, respectively. The rate of diet administration should be gradually increased over a 3- to 5-day period. A suggested rate of introduction is to administer ¼ of the final target volume of feed on day 1, ½ total volume on day 2, ¾ total volume on day 3, and the total volume on day 4 or 5. Clinical signs of intolerance to enteral feeding will dictate a slower rate of introduction. In hospital settings the enteral diet should be administered in a minimum of four and preferably six feedings per day, with no more than 6 to 8 L per feeding for a 450- to 500-kg horse (including volume of water used to flush the tube). This volume should be administered over a 10- to 15-minute period. In field settings a more practical approach is to administer two treatments daily, although it will not be possible to meet stall maintenance nutritional requirements with this treatment regimen.

Pelleted feeds should be soaked in warm water to soften before mixing in a blender (ratio of 1 kg pelleted feed to 6 liters of water). A fresh batch of diet should be made before each feeding. A tube with a ½-inch (12-mm) inner diameter is suitable for most enteral diets that contain fiber. The end of the tube should be open ended, rather than fenestrated, to prevent the tube from becoming clogged. Intermittent nasogastric intubation or placement of an indwelling nasogastric tube can be used to facilitate feeding. In hospitalized horses feeding tubes can be left in place for up to 8 days, although nasopharyngeal irritation and mucoid nasal discharge are expected outcomes (when longer-term AEF is anticipated, placement of the tube through cervical esophagostomy is recommended). Softer silicon tubes are less irritating compared with tubes made of polyvinylchloride, do not tend to harden when left in place, and are generally recommended for horses requiring AEF for a number of days. Before placing the tube, the clinician should establish that the diet solution flows adequately through the tube. It may be necessary to add more water or to mix the feed in a blender a second time. The tube should be positioned in the stomach rather than the distal esophagus to minimize risk of reflux of feed around the tube. The tube should be secured to the halter; between feedings application of a muzzle may be necessary to prevent the horse from dislodging the tube. A marine bilge pump is recommended for infusion of fiber-containing diets. After administration of the diet, the tube should be flushed with approximately 1 L of water followed by a small volume of air to ensure that no feed material remains in the tube. The end of the tube should be capped with a syringe case between feedings.

Close clinical monitoring, particularly of gastrointestinal function, is imperative for horses receiving AEF. Repeated ultrasonographic examinations can be useful for evaluation of gastric distention and intestinal motility. The presence of residual gastric fluid should be assessed (i.e., by siphoning) before each feeding. Substantial gastric reflux (>1 to 2 L) is an indication to withhold enteral feeding for at least 1 to 2 hours, with re-evaluation before recommencement of diet administration. Persistent gastric reflux indicates intolerance to enteral feeding and the need for parenteral feeding. Similarly, signs of colic, ileus, abdominal distention, and increased digital pulses suggest an intolerance to enteral feeding and are an indication to discontinue therapy or decrease the volume and frequency of feedings. The passage of loose feces is not uncommon in horses receiving AEF and of minimal concern if not accompanied by clinical signs of depression, dehydration, ileus, or colic. It is important to measure the total volume of water administered through the nasogastric tube. Daily water requirements (approximately 50 ml/kg/day) can generally be met during AEF if the horse is fed four to five times daily. Frequent measurements of hematocrit and plasma total protein concentration also are useful for monitoring hydration status and the adequacy of water administration. Hypokalemia, ionized hypomagnesemia, and ionized hypocalcemia can occur in horses with gastrointestinal disease. Accordingly, frequent measurements of serum electrolytes and ionized calcium and magnesium are recommended during AEF in these patients. Supplementation with potassium, calcium, magnesium, or both may be necessary. Horses also should be monitored for development of complications associated with repeated or indwelling nasogastric intubation, including rhinitis, pharyngitis, and esophageal ulceration. Body weight should be measured daily to assess the adequacy of nutritional support, although changes in body weight may reflect alterations in fluid balance rather than the effect of feeding.

PARENTERAL NUTRITIONAL SUPPORT

Parenteral nutrition is indicated for horses with gastrointestinal tract dysfunction (e.g., ileus, gastric reflux) or conditions that mandate complete bowel rest (e.g., small intestinal resection, duodenitis-proximal jejunitis). Durham et al.[83,85] examined the effects of postoperative PN in 15 horses (versus 15 control horses) recovering from resection and anastomosis of strangulated small intestine and reported no beneficial effect of PN on time to first oral feeding, duration of hospitalization, costs of treatment, or short-term survival (up until 5 months after discharge), although the PN protocol did confer improved nutritional status, as reflected by lower serum concentrations of triglycerides and total bilirubin and higher concentrations of glucose. However, the duration and volume of postoperative gastric reflux were longer in the PN group than in the control horses, perhaps as a result of alterations in gastric or small intestinal motility, and there was an insignificant trend for catheter-site complications in the PN group.[83] The authors concluded that further study of a larger number of horses is necessary to determine the clinical benefits and possible harmful side effects of PN in horses recovering from small intestinal surgery. Studies of the effects of PN in human patients also have yielded equivocal findings. Several studies have demonstrated that perioperative PN is associated with reduced morbidity and mortality in malnourished patients.[91-93] In contrast, perioperative PN in well-nourished human patients has been associated with increased morbidity, particularly septic complications.[94,95] Nonetheless, as previously discussed, the current consensus in human clinical nutrition is that PN is an important component of overall case management, particularly in patients with evidence of malnourishment, gut failure, and increased nutritional requirements (e.g., pregnancy, lactation, growth).

The following paragraphs provide a brief overview of the composition of PN solutions, methods for delivery, and potential complications. As with EN support, the goal of PN is to administer calories and amino acids such that loss of body protein (and lean body mass) is minimized.[73] Carbohydrates, in the form of a 50% dextrose solution (3.4 kcal/g or 1.7 kcal/ml; osmolarity 2525 mOsm/L), and lipid, as a 10% to 20% emulsion (20% emulsion: 9 kcal/g or 2 kcal/ml; osmolarity 260 mOsm/L), are the primary sources of energy used in PN solutions, whereas an amino acid solution (e.g., Travasol 8.5% or 10%; Baxter Health Care Corporation) is used to meet protein requirements (e.g., protein synthesis, immune function). Commercial lipid emulsions (e.g., Intralipid 20%; Baxter Health Care Corporation, Deerfield, IL) consist of soybean oil, egg yolk phospholipid, and glycerin. These emulsions provide mainly unsaturated fatty acids (linoleic, 44% to 62%; oleic, 19% to 30%; linolenic, 4% to 11%; palmitic, 7% to 14%). PN solutions with and without lipid can be used (i.e., dextrose/amino acid or dextrose/lipid/amino acid mixtures). The addition of lipids to the PN formula results in a solution with lower osmolarity compared with a dextrose/amino acid mixture of similar caloric density. Hence the lipid-containing solution should be less irritating to peripheral veins. Lipid solutions must be included in the formula if target calorie provision approaches true maintenance (32 to 33 kcal/kg/day) because this level of calorie delivery from a dextrose/amino acid PN solution often results in marked hyperglycemia and glucosuria. However, when the target daily energy provision is 20 to 22 kcal/kg/day, dextrose/amino acid mixtures can be used. In human medicine this approach is referred to as a *partial parenteral nutrition* and is often employed in postoperative patients who require only a few days of intravenous nutritional support;[74] similarly, partial PN is recommended for horses requiring short-term (3 to 7 days) intravenous feeding. Lipid administration is not recommended for patients at high risk for severe hypertriglyceridemia or hyperlipemia (e.g., ponies, miniature horses, donkeys). Serum triglyceride concentrations should be monitored on a regular basis if lipid solutions are administered to these patients. As discussed previously, provision of amino acids (protein) at a rate of 0.6 to 0.8 g/kg body weight daily is one guideline for meeting protein requirements in adult horses, although some authors have recommended 1 to 1.5 g/kg/day, and provision of amino acids at 0.6 to 2 g/kg/day has been used in sick horses without apparent complications.

A suggested PN formula (Table 5-5) comprises 1 L of 50% dextrose (0.5 g/ml dextrose × 3.4 kcal/g × 1000 ml = 1700 kcal), 1 L of a 10% amino acid solution (0.1g/ml of amino acids × 4 kcal/g × 1000 ml = 400 kcal), and 500 ml of 20% lipid emulsion (0.2 g/ml lipid × 9 kcal/g × 500 ml = 900 kcal). These components are diluted with 4 L of isotonic fluid, yielding a final volume of 6.5 liters and a caloric density of approximately 0.45 kcal/ml. A multivitamin supplement may be added to this mixture. This solution can be prepared up to 24 hours before administration, with storage at 4° C until use. Administration of PN solutions should be through a dedicated intravenous catheter (i.e., do not administer other medications with

TABLE 5-5

Parenteral Nutrition Formula and Recommended Administration Rate for a 500-kg Horse*

Formula Variable	First 12 hours	Second 12 hours	Day 2
Dextrose 50%	1000 ml	1000 ml	1000 ml
Lipid 20%	500 ml	500 ml	500 ml
Amino acids 10%	1000 ml	1000 ml	1000 ml
Isotonic fluids	4000 ml	4000 ml	4000 ml
Total volume	6500 ml	6500 ml	6500 ml
Kcal per bag	3000	3000	3000
Kcal per hour	210	333	480
Rate (ml/hour)		470	740
1070			
Bags required	0.90 per 12 h	1.4 per 12 h	4.0 per 24 h
Kcals per day	—	—	11,500

Adapted from Robinson NE, Sprayberry K, editors: *Current therapy in equine medicine,* ed 6, St Louis, 2009, Saunders.
*For parenteral nutrition, daily energy needs are estimated at 23 kcal/kg/day (11.5 Mcal per day for a 500-kg horse).

this catheter), preferably one inserted into a large vein such as the jugular to minimize the risk of complications associated with the infusion of hyperosmotic solutions. Alternatively, a double-lumen catheter can be used, allowing the PN solution to be given through one port and medications and other fluids through the other port. To minimize the risk of thrombophlebitis, nonthrombogenic catheters such as those made from polyurethane are recommended. Meticulous attention to sterile technique is needed during catheter placement to further minimize the risk of thrombophlebitis and other septic complications. The fluid lines used for delivery of the PN solution should be changed every 24 hours. An infusion pump is required to ensure accurate delivery of the PN solution. The bag containing the PN solution should be covered with a brown bag during administration to protect it from light, which can degrade the amino acids within the solution.

Table 5-5 provides a recommended rate of parenteral feeding for a 500-kg horse. The initial rate of PN solution administration should be approximately 35% of target calorie provision, increasing to 60% to 65% after 12 hours and 100% (23 kcal/kg/day) at 24 hours, provided that there are no complications, such as the development of marked hyperglycemia, glucosuria, or hyperlipemia. Hyperglycemia and hyperlipemia were the most common complications of postoperative PN in horses after intestinal surgery. In one report hyperglycemia was observed in 52 of 79 horses receiving PN,[96] perhaps because of insulin resistance, an excessive rate of administration, or both. Blood glucose concentrations should be measured every 4 to 8 hours in horses receiving PN, and the rate of dextrose administration should be decreased if glucose concentrations exceed renal threshold (approximately 180 to 200 mg/dl). A constant-rate insulin infusion (e.g., regular insulin at a starting dose of 0.05 to 0.1 IU/kg/hr) can be instituted if the reduction in dextrose administration rate fails to correct the hyperglycemia. Blood glucose concentrations must be closely monitored (e.g., every 2 to 6 hours). Adjustments in insulin dose may be required to achieve glycemic control. Serum blood urea nitrogen (BUN), triglycerides, and electrolytes should be monitored at least daily. Hypokalemia, hypocalcemia, and hypomagnesemia have been reported in horses receiving PN, and it may be necessary to supplement these nutrients if parenteral feeding is used for more than 48 hours. Finally, body weight should be recorded daily or every other day.

TRANSITION TO VOLUNTARY FEEDING

A decrease in AEF or PN is indicated when appetite returns (or when voluntary oral feeding is no longer contraindicated). Initially, small amounts of palatable (e.g., fresh grass or leafy hay) feed should be offered. If these feedings are tolerated, the level of tube or parenteral feeding can be gradually reduced as the provision of feed for voluntary consumption is increased. Nutritional support can be withdrawn when voluntary feed intake provides at least 75% of stall maintenance DE and protein requirements. As with any feeding program, all changes in diet should be gradual. Hay should be the primary, if not sole, component of the convalescent diet, preferably leafy hay with a fresh aroma. Grain or commercial grain-concentrate feeds should be offered only if hay alone does not meet requirements. An alternative to grain is to feed 1 to 2 lb/day of a high-protein product (approximately 20% to 25% CP, usually with added minerals and vitamins) as a supplement to hay.

NUTRITIONAL MANAGEMENT OF THE ORPHANED OR SICK FOAL

Foal Metabolism and Nutrient Requirements

The foal's nutritional requirements and dietary composition change substantially during the gradual transition from neonate to weanling. At birth the foal must transition from a continuous supply of nutrients provided by the dam by way of the placenta to intermittent absorption of ingested nutrients. At the same time, the metabolism of the neonate is no longer able to depend on the maternal glucose concentration to maintain normoglycemia, and the pancreas assumes responsibility for regulating glucose homeostasis.[97] These dramatic alterations in energy metabolism may not always occur smoothly, and the neonatal foal possesses limited energy reserves in the form of glycogen and fat. The result is that hypoglycemia occurs frequently in even the normal neonatal foal, and the sick foal is at risk for profound hypoglycemia if deprived of energy intake for even a few hours.[97]

The neonatal foal has a high metabolic rate and requires frequent ingestion of high volumes of milk to meet its energy requirements for maintenance and growth. In light breeds the average rate of daily gain over the first month of life is 1 to 1.5 kg/day. During the first week of life, calorie needs are as follows: approximately 150 kcal/kg/day, with a gradual decrease to approximately 120 kcal/kg/day at 3 weeks of age, and then to 80 to 100 kcal/kg/day by 1 to 2 months of age.[81,82] Healthy neonatal foals (<7 days of age) have up to 7 nursing bouts per hour, most lasting for 1 to 2 minutes. Subsequently, there is a gradual decrease in the frequency of nursing but an increase in the duration of each nursing bout. During the first 24 hours of life, foals consume approximately 15% Bwt as milk (i.e., 8 L in a 50-kg foal), increasing to between 23% and 25% Bwt (15 L) by day 3 or day 4.[98] On a DM basis, mare's milk averages about 64%, 22%, and 13% sugar (as lactose), protein, and fat, respectively, as compared with cow's milk, which contains 38%, 26% and 30% sugar, protein, and fat, respectively. As a result, glucose (from lactose) is the primary source of energy for the foal.

Starting as early as the second day of life, foals begin ingesting small amounts of hay, grass, and grain while also ingesting maternal feces, which likely provides the initial microbial flora required to support digestion of these feedstuffs. It is unlikely that grain and roughage are well digested until at least several weeks of age, at which point the foal begins the gradual transition from a milk-based diet to a forage-based diet. The amount of milk produced by the mare peaks after approximately 2 months of lactation and then begins a steady decline, which continues until the time of weaning, when the foal must begin relying on solid feed for an increasing proportion of its nutritional requirements. Full maturation of hindgut function may occur by 3 to 4 months of age.

Nutritional Support of Orphan Foals

The primary options for management of orphan foals are to raise by hand or foster to a nurse mare.[98,99] Fostering is the best option for a foal younger than 6 to 8 weeks of age. Draft or Draft-cross mares that are mild in temperament make good nurse mares. Any disparity between the stage of lactation and age of the foal should be noted. A mare that is 4 to 6 weeks into lactation may not have the quality of milk needed to sustain a neonate; it may be necessary to provide the neonatal foal with a mineral supplement when fostered to a mid-to-late lactation mare.

Hand rearing has several disadvantages, including the need for high labor input, the expense of milk substitute, and a high incidence of behavioral problems. The risk of behavioral problems can be mitigated by ensuring that the foal is raised with an equine companion (e.g., a quiet horse or pony or even another orphan foal). Teaching a foal to drink from a bucket is preferable to bottle feeding because it is less labor intensive for the owner and allows the foal to drink milk on demand. Feeding from a bucket also helps prevent some of the behavioral problems that develop in foals that have bonded to people. Bottle feeding may be the only option in newborn foals, but a quick transition to bucket feeding is recommended. It is also important to ensure adequate colostral intake (and acquisition of passive immunity) in foals that are orphaned at birth.

Fortified cow's milk (by the addition of 20 g/L dextrose to 2% part skimmed milk); goat milk; and calf, lamb, and kid milk substitutes have been used to rear foals, but a high-quality mare-milk formula is preferred. On a DM basis foal milk replacers should contain approximately 15% fat and 22% CP, with a fiber content of less than 0.5%.[99] Milk replacers should be fed as a 10% to 15% solution when diluted with water. Milk replacers generally provide about 500 kcal/L when mixed according to the manufacturer's instructions. The volume of milk should be fed over a 7- to 10-day period. One recommendation is to start at 5% to 10% of Bwt, increasing to 20% to 25% Bwt by day 10. Intake of 20% to 25% Bwt/day as milk replacer will meet energy and nutrient requirements for growth. As a general guide, most light-breed foals need 14 to 17.5 L (4 to 5 gallons) of milk substitute each day during the first 2 to 3 weeks of life, and draft foals require 21 to 28 L (6 to 8 gallons). Foals may be fed as infrequently as two to four times daily, although more frequent feedings (six to nine daily) are recommended for young foals and during the initial phase of hand rearing to keep from overwhelming the digestive tract. Feeding buckets should be thoroughly cleaned on a daily basis. Similarly, strict hygiene is required during the preparation of the milk substitute. Fresh water should be available at all times.

Body weight or linear measures that predict weight and height gain[100] should be monitored on a regular (e.g., weekly) basis. Expected rates of growth and weight gain are available for some horse breeds. Studies of hand-reared foals have demonstrated growth rates similar to those observed in foal reared with their dams.[101] Solid feed should be introduced as early as 2 to 3 weeks of age (e.g., small amounts of high-quality hay, milk-based pellets, or both). Up to 1 kg of milk pellets/day can be fed with a concomitant reduction in liquid milk feeding. Orphan foals can be weaned from milk at 10 to 12 weeks of age, with a transition to a diet of forage and a balanced foal feed (16% to 18% CP).

Nutrition of the Sick Neonatal Foal

The energy (calorie) requirements of sick, recumbent foals are less than those of healthy foals, in part because of their lower physical activity and a temporary decrease in growth rate compared with healthy neonates. In one study the metabolic rate of healthy foals was 130 to 140 kcal/kg Bwt/day, whereas metabolic rate in immature foals and foals with perinatal asphyxia syndrome was approximately 62 to 69 kcal/kg Bwt/day.[81] It is possible that sepsis and endotoxemia increase metabolic rate, although studies in neonatal humans indicate that critical illness is not accompanied by a hypermetabolic state. Currently providing critically ill, recumbent foals approximately 45 to 50 kcal/kg Bwt/day is recommended.[98,102] This "hypocaloric" approach to nutritional support may prevent complications associated with overfeeding, such as hyperglycemia and glucosuria, particularly in foals with sepsis wherein the systemic inflammatory response contributes to insulin resistance and carbohydrate intolerance. Neonatal foals require approximately 1.5 g protein/kg Bwt/day.

The adage "if the gut works, use it" also applies to the nutritional support of sick neonatal foals. Milk contains trophic substances that promote growth and development of the gastrointestinal tract. Additionally, enteral feeding is believed to lower the risk of sepsis associated with bacterial translocation. However, parenteral feeding is required in foals with poor gastrointestinal tract function.

ENTERAL NUTRITION

Thorough assessment of gastrointestinal function is needed before institution of EN support, including abdominal auscultation and evaluation of abdominal distention and the presence of gastric reflux. Abdominal radiographs and ultrasonographic examination for evaluation of bowel dimensions and motility also may be indicated. Foals with evidence of gastrointestinal dysfunction such as gastric reflux, bowel distention, increased bowel wall thickness, and ileus are unlikely to tolerate enteral feeding. A conservative approach to enteral feeding is also indicated for premature or immature foals in which the gastrointestinal tract may not be completely developed. Foals with perinatal asphyxia syndrome or severe sepsis may be intolerant of enteral feeding as a result of intestinal ischemic injury.

Mare milk is the preferred substrate for enteral feeding; it is highly digestible and obviously provides the correct balance of nutrients for normal growth and development. Commercial mare milk replacers can be used, but practitioners should bear in mind that these products are bovine in origin and have lower digestibility compared with mare's milk. This may increase the risk of intestinal dysfunction associated with enteral feeding. Part skimmed (2% fat) cow's milk to which 20 g/L dextrose (corn sugar) is added can be used if mare's milk (or a mare's milk replacer) is unavailable. Foals that are unable to nurse the mare (or when no mare is available) may be fed through a bottle, bowl, or nasogastric feeding tube. Bottle feeding is recommended when the foal is expected to be transitioned to a mare within a short period of time. The practitioner should remember, however, that bottle feeding is very labor intensive and does carry some risk of milk aspiration if the milk flow rate from the bottle exceeds the foal's capacity to nurse properly. The risk of aspiration is lower with bowl feeding because the head is positioned with the nose down during drinking.

Many sick, recumbent foals have a weak or uncoordinated suck reflex and are at risk of milk aspiration and pneumonia. Milk should be administered to these patients through a feeding tube. Use of small-bore, indwelling nasogastric feeding tubes (e.g., NG1243-12fr × 108 cm [43 inches], MILA International, Erlanger, Kentucky) and feeding of small volumes at frequent intervals (e.g., every 20 minutes) is preferred over repeated passage of a nasogastric tube at 1- to 2-hour intervals. Large-bolus feedings may overwhelm digestive capacity, and repeated passage of a stomach tube is an unnecessary stress on the foal. Another advantage of the small-bore, indwelling tubes is that they do not interfere with the suckle response. Therefore the tube may be left in place as the foal is transitioned to feeding from the mare. The feeding tube should be inserted with the foal in sternal recumbency, and correct placement within the esophagus should be confirmed by radiography or endoscopy. The tube should be fastened to the external nares by sutures or may be retained using a circumferential elastic bandage around the muzzle. It is important to check at each feeding that the tube is still in place and there is no gastric reflux. The foal should be in sternal recumbency or standing when it is fed. Milk should be administered by gravity flow and followed by a small amount of clean water to flush the tube. The tube should be capped between feedings to prevent aspiration of air. Feeding tubes should be replaced every 1 or 2 days to reduce the risk of gastrointestinal tract infection.

A suggested initial rate of milk delivery is 2 to 3 ml/kg Bwt/hr or 100–150 ml/hr for a 50-kg foal, which will provide 2.4 to 3.6 L of milk to a 50-kg foal during the first 24 hours of enteral feeding (Table 5-6). Dextrose-containing fluids can be administered intravenously to provide additional calories during the transition to an adequate level of enteral feeding. The feeding rate can be gradually increased over the next 2 to 3 days (e.g., increase to 4 to 5 ml/kg/hr on day 2 and then to 6 to 8 ml/kg/hr on day 3), which represents a total daily intake of 10% to 15% Bwt. As the rate of enteral feeding increases, intravenous caloric support (dextrose) can be gradually withdrawn. This feeding level will likely meet the maintenance energy requirements of hospitalized foals. Depending on the rate of clinical improvement and the length of hospitalization, it may be possible to increase the volume of feeding to 22% to 23% Bwt/day, which approximates the milk intake of healthy neonatal foals. Clinical monitoring should include frequent assessments of gastrointestinal function, including gastric reflux, intestinal sounds, abdominal distention, and quantity and quality of feces. Gastric reflux, bloating, colic, diarrhea, or constipation can indicate intolerance to enteral feeding and the need for adjustments to the feeding program. Adjustments may involve a decrease in the volume or frequency of enteral feedings. Foals fed milk replacers appear to be more likely to develop loose feces than foals fed mare's milk. In some cases clinical improvement is observed after supplementation with 6000 units of lactase (Lactaid; McNeil Nutritionals, LLC, Ft. Washington, Pa.) per 50 kg foal every 3 to 8 hours, mixed into the milk replacer before feeding.[103]

PARENTERAL NUTRITION

Parenteral nutrition support is indicated for foals with poor gastrointestinal function and intolerance to enteral feeding. Short-term parenteral supplementation (less than 24 hours) does not require the use of a balanced PN solution that contains sources of carbohydrate, amino acids, and lipids. However, if PN is expected to be administered for a longer period, then a more complete formula should be used.

Short-term caloric supplementation can be accomplished by administrations of an intravenous fluid containing 5% dextrose (e.g., 5% dextrose in water [D_5W], Lactated Ringer's solution with 5% dextrose, 0.45% saline with 5% dextrose), and hypotonic maintenance electrolyte solutions containing 5% dextrose.[97] Fluids containing dextrose should not be used for initial large volume fluid resuscitation because this often results in profound hyperglycemia. After initial fluid resuscitation the solutions containing electrolytes as well as

TABLE 5-6

Feeding Recommendations for Neonatal and Growing Foals

Foal Age (days)	Energy Requirement	Volume of Mare's Milk or Milk Replacer	Percentage of Body Weight Fed
0-1	150 kcal/kg/day	2-3 ml/kg/hr	5%-7%
2-3	150 kcal/kg/day	4-5 ml/kg/hr	10%-12%
4-7	150 kcal/kg/day	6-8 ml/kg/hr	14%-20%
8-30	120 kcal/kg/day	9-10 ml/kg/hr	22%
30-weaning	80-100 kcal/kg/day	Gradually decreasing and replaced with solid feed	

dextrose may be used as the primary fluids for maintenance therapy in foals with minimal ongoing fluid losses. As a maintenance solution, D_5W is not a good choice because it lacks electrolytes; it is primarily useful in providing free water to patients suffering from hyperosmolar conditions. The caloric content of a 5% dextrose solution is 0.17 kcal/ml, so an infusion rate of 10 ml/kg/hr would be required to deliver approximately 40 kcal/kg/day (0.17 kcal/kg/hr × 24 hours/day = 41 kcal/kg/day). However, this rate of infusion is more than twice the maintenance fluid requirements of neonatal foals (4 to 5 ml/kg/hr). Therefore an infusion rate of 5 ml/kg/hr (providing approximately 20 kcal/kg/day) is a more appropriate target for partial caloric support using 5% dextrose solutions.[97] Caution is required when adjusting the infusion rate in response to changes in hydration state to prevent excessive dextrose administration, especially in premature or very sick foals that may be glucose intolerant.

An alternative approach involves the administration of a 50% dextrose solution by use of an infusion pump, provided that isotonic fluids are administered concurrently to minimize the risk of vascular endothelial injury caused by the hyperosmolar 50% dextrose solution. Use of 50% dextrose solution is not recommended unless an infusion pump is available. The caloric content of 50% dextrose solution is 1.7 kcal/ml; therefore an infusion rate of 1 ml/kg/hr will provide about 40 kcal/kg/day (1.7 kcal/kg/hr × 24 hours/day = 41 kcal/kg/day). At this low rate of infusion, the primary fluid needs of the patient can be met with a dextrose-free isotonic electrolyte-containing fluid, the infusion rate of which can be altered in response to changes in patient fluid status without concerns related to the requirements of the nutritional plan.[97]

Two approaches have been used for formulation of PN solutions for foals.[97,98,104] The first involves the exact determination of the anticipated metabolic needs of the patient, followed by the development of a formulation that will meet all of these needs using a mixture of dextrose, amino acids, and lipids. The second approach is simpler and more practical and uses one of two basic PN formulas (Table 5-7):

1. Solution I: a mix of equal volumes of 50% dextrose and 8.5% amino acid solutions, intended for short-term use (caloric density = 1.02 kcal/ml).
2. Solution II: a mix of 3 parts 50% dextrose, 4 parts 8.5% amino acid, and 1 part 20% lipid solutions. This solution is preferred for foals that are poorly tolerant of infused dextrose (caloric density = 1.08 kcal/ml).

As previously discussed, protein degradation in muscle tissue occurs during critical illnesses such as sepsis. Thus provision of adequate energy and amino acids to counter this catabolic response is an important goal of PN support. The recommended ratio for nonprotein calories to nitrogen is 100 to 200 nonprotein calories per gram of nitrogen.[105] In one report the amount of protein provided affected weight gain of neonatal foals, with a negative association between the nonprotein nitrogen calories: grams nitrogen ratio (NPC/g N) and the rate of weight gain.[106] Solution I provides 125 NPC/g N, and Solution II contains 131 NPC/g N.

The inclusion of lipids in the PN formulation allows for the provision of a larger number of calories per unit volume compared with solutions containing only dextrose. Another advantage of lipid emulsions is that they are isotonic, thereby moderating the hypertonicity of the PN formulation and potentially decreasing the risk of thrombophlebitis. In a recent report the use of lipid-containing PN solutions allowed for the provision of 40 to 92 kcal/kg/day (mean = 63 kcal/kg/day) to foals, compared with 25 to 66 kcal/kg/day (mean = 41 kcal/kg/day) with a dextrose-based solution.[104]

Methods for delivery of PN solutions have been discussed (see the section on nutritional support of sick horses). The catheter and catheter site should be monitored at least twice daily for heat, swelling, or exudation. Increased resistance to fluid flow in the catheter may be an indication of thrombosis deeper within the vasculature and will often necessitate the placement of a catheter in an alternative site, such as the opposite jugular vein, a cephalic vein, or a lateral thoracic vein. The rate of infusion (in ml/hr) is calculated on the basis of the desired kcal/kg/day to be administered. A reasonable initial goal is 40 to 50 kcal/kg/day; higher rates of energy administration often result in hyperglycemia and hyperlipidemia. The initial infusion rate of PN solutions should be 50% of the calculated final rate, and the rate should be gradually increased every 1 to 3 hours after monitoring of the blood glucose concentration to ensure that hyperglycemia (blood glucose >180 mg/dl) is not present.

Rectal temperature should be closely monitored during PN support because fever is a common early manifestation of systemic infection. Blood glucose concentrations should be closely monitored, the frequency of which depends on the stability of blood glucose concentrations. Blood glucose should be maintained between 90 and 180 mg/dl. Although the renal threshold for glucose is not well described in foals, glucosuria and diuresis will be observed in many when blood glucose levels exceed 180 mg/dl. Urine output should be monitored continuously, in combination with intermittent monitoring of urine glucose concentration, because of the risk of hyperglycemia-induced diuresis and glucosuria. Additional clinicopathologic monitoring should consist of daily complete blood counts and serum chemistry profiles in the critical case; these can be performed every 48 to 72 hours in more stable patients. Body weight should be assessed on a daily basis to ensure that the foal is at least maintaining body weight while on PN support.

Some critically ill foals are intolerant of even a conservative rate of dextrose administration because of insulin resistance.

TABLE 5-7

Formulation of Parenteral Nutrition Solutions for Neonatal Foals

Formulation	Composition	Caloric Density (kcal/ml)	Nonprotein calories/g nitrogen
Formula I	1500 ml 50% dextrose, 1500 ml 8.5% amino acids	1.02	125
Formula II	1500 ml 50% dextrose, 500 ml 20% lipids, 2000 ml 8.5% amino acids	1.08	131

The administration of insulin is needed to control hyperglycemia and allow attainment of the goal level of PN support.[97] Use of continuous rate infusion (CRI) for the administration of insulin is preferred to intermittent bolus dosing. An initial insulin infusion rate of 0.07 IU/kg/hr is generally well tolerated. If possible, simultaneous alterations in both the insulin and PN infusion rate should be avoided, because this can result in marked fluctuations in blood glucose concentrations. Blood glucose monitoring should be performed at least hourly for the first 2 to 3 hours after initiation of the insulin CRI, and if hyperglycemia (blood glucose >150 mg/dl) is persistent beyond the first 2 hours of insulin therapy, then the insulin infusion rate may be increased by 50%, followed by hourly blood glucose monitoring for an additional 2 or 3 hours. This procedure for increasing the insulin infusion rate may be repeated if hyperglycemia persists. Conversely, if hypoglycemia (blood glucose <60 mg/dl) is noted, then a bolus of 0.25 to 0.5 ml/kg of 50% dextrose solution should be administered intravenously over 3 to 5 minutes. The blood glucose level should then be reassessed every 30 minutes for at least 90 minutes. If hypoglycemia recurs, a second bolus of dextrose should be administered and the insulin infusion rate decreased by 50%. Close monitoring will then be required for an additional 60 to 90 minutes to assess the stability of blood glucose concentration. Further changes to the insulin infusion rate are not usually necessary once a steady state has been achieved, wherein the blood glucose level is stable and the desired rate of PN administration has been achieved.

When PN support is to be discontinued, it is recommended that the infusion rate be gradually reduced by 25% to 50% increments every 4 to 6 hours while gradually introducing enteral feeding. The monitoring of blood glucose must continue during this weaning process to prevent severe hypoglycemia.

MANAGEMENT OF OBESITY

Obesity is an emergent problem in companion animal equid populations. Obesity has been associated with insulin resistance in horses and ponies, and both obesity and insulin resistance have been associated with increased risk of laminitis, particularly the pasture-associated form of this disease.[8,9,107] There is no universal definition of obesity in horses and ponies. According to the Henneke system, horses with a BCS of 8 (fat) or 9 (extremely fat) can be defined as obese, and animals with a BCS of 7 might be considered overweight, if not obese. Few studies have examined the prevalence of obesity in horse and pony populations. The 1998 National Animal Health Monitoring System (NAHMS) study estimated that 4.5% of the horse population in the United States was overweight or obese.[108] However, the accuracy of this estimate may be questioned because it was based on owner reports, not the results of physical examination. Anecdotal observations by equine veterinarians suggest that the prevalence of obesity is far higher than the NAHMS estimate. In support of this contention, a recent cross-sectional, prospective study of 300 mature horses (ponies were excluded) in southwestern Virginia reported obesity (BCS of 8 or 9) in 57 animals (i.e. a prevalence of 19%).[109] In a study of 319 pleasure riding horses in Scotland, 32% were obese and a further 35% were considered fat.[110]

The cause of obesity in horses and ponies is likely multifactorial. However, overfeeding and lack of physical activity are likely contributing factors. Many horses are kept in confinement (e.g., stall, small pen) for much of the day, and even if used for riding activities 2 or 3 days per week, they may not require any more than maintenance energy intakes. Nevertheless, many of these horses are fed much more than the maintenance energy requirement, a problem that is compounded by the provision of grains, sweet feeds, and other feeds with high caloric density. Obesity also can be a problem in some horses and ponies given unrestricted access to pasture, particularly during the spring and fall, when pasture forage is actively growing, plentiful, and energy rich. In a study by Thatcher et al., more than 60% of the surveyed horses were maintained at pasture year round and were not used for any type of riding activity.[109]

Maintenance DE requirements for horses range between 30 and 36 kcal/kg Bwt (Table 5-8), with variation among horses resulting from differences in dietary composition, age, breed, environment, and body composition, among other factors.[1] Thus for a 500-kg (1100-lb) horse, minimum maintenance energy needs are 15.2 Mcal DE/day. This requirement can be met by about 7 kg (15 lb) of high-quality hay (i.e., no supplemental grain is required). To illustrate the impact of even moderate overfeeding on body weight, consider the effect of adding 1 kg of grain or sweet feed/day to this horse's ration for a 1-year period (i.e., an additional 3 Mcal/day or >1000 Mcal over the 1-year period); if it is assumed that 20 to 25 Mcal of DE *over maintenance* is required for 1 kg of weight gain, the horse in this example will gain upwards of 40 kg Bwt during this period (with a 1- to 1½-unit increase in BCS).

Genetics may be another factor in the predisposition to obesity. Horse owners and veterinarians often use the term *easy keeper* to describe a horse or pony that has a tendency to be overweight and appears to require fewer calories than most horses to maintain condition. Ponies and certain horse breeds (e.g., Morgans, Arabians, Paso Finos) appear to fit this description. One hypothesis is that certain lines of horses and ponies have inherited genetic traits that have facilitated survival on poor-quality forages or in the face of limited feed availability: the so-called thrifty genotype.[8,111] When these animals are supplied with abundant feed, particularly grains or pasture forage rich in NSC, weight gain and obesity result.

Obesity in horses and ponies is a risk factor for laminitis. Mechanical trauma caused by increased load on the feet is one possible reason that obesity is linked with laminitis. However, the increased risk of laminitis in obese equids is more likely related to the attendant insulin resistance. In one recent study of ponies, a phenotype characterized by generalized or regional adiposity (especially a cresty neck), hyperinsulinemia, and hypertriglyceridemia was associated with tenfold higher risk for development of pasture-associated laminitis. The clustering of these risk factors for laminitis is termed *prelaminitic syndrome*.[8] Similar associations between obesity, insulin resistance, and laminitis have been observed in horses, leading to the use of the term *equine metabolic syndrome*.[112] Obese ponies, donkeys, and miniature horses are prone to the development of hyperlipemia during times of stress or negative energy balance (e.g., concurrent disease, lactation). Other proposed effects of obesity include impaired thermoregulation in hot weather, reduced athletic performance, and increased risk of joint injuries, but evidence is lacking. In broodmares obesity and insulin resistance have been associated with prolonged luteal phase and lengthened interovulatory intervals,[112] but the impact of these alterations in the estrous cycle on reproductive performance has not been extensively studied.

TABLE 5-8

Recommended Digestible Energy Intake by Mature Horses (Mcal/day)*

Type of Horse	400 kg (880 lb)	Target Bodyweight 500 kg (1100 lb)	600 kg (1320 lb)
Adult sedentary†			
Minimum voluntary activity	12.1	15.2	18.2
Average voluntary activity	13.3	16.7	20.0
Elevated voluntary activity	14.5	18.2	21.8
Adult light exercise	16.0	20.3	24.0
Adult moderate exercise	18.6	23.3	28.0
Adult heavy exercise	21.3	26.6	32.0
Adult very heavy exercise	27.6	35.6	41.4
Pregnant—0-4 mo	13.3	16.7	20.0
Pregnant—5 mo	13.7	17.1	20.5
Pregnant—6 mo	13.9	17.4	20.9
Pregnant—7 mo	14.3	17.9	21.5
Pregnant—8 mo	14.8	18.5	22.2
Pregnant—9 mo	15.4	19.2	23.1
Pregnant—10 mo	16.2	20.2	24.2
Pregnant—11 mo	17.1	21.4	25.7
Lactating—1st mo	25.4	31.7	38.1
Lactating—2nd mo	25.3	31.7	38.0
Lactating—3rd mo	24.5	30.6	36.7
Lactating—4th mo	23.6	29.4	35.3
Lactating—5th mo	22.7	28.3	34.0
Lactating—6th mo	21.8	27.2	32.7

From Committee on Nutrient Requirements of Horses, National Research Council: *Nutrient requirements of horses*, ed 6, rev, Washington DC, 2007, National Academic Press.

*Recommended intakes for stallions and growing horses can be found in the NRC publication.

†Sedentary adults: Minimum = very inactive in stall/paddock, *easy keeper;* elevated = very active in stall/paddock, *hard keeper.* Light exercise: 1 to 3 hours/wk; walking, trotting. Moderate exercise: 3 to 5 hours/wk; walking, trotting, some canter; easy skills. Heavy exercise: 4 to 5 hours/wk; trotting, cantering; hard skills. Very heavy: racing; elite 3-day; endurance racing.

WEIGHT MANAGEMENT PROGRAMS

In horses, as in humans, eating less and exercising more are the key strategies to improve body weight and condition. Important steps in the development of a weight management program include the following:

- Owner/trainer recognition that the horse or pony is overweight or obese: As the old adage states, "Beauty is in the eye of the beholder," and different equestrian disciplines and breeds have adopted different standards to evaluate body condition. Nonetheless, the effectiveness of any weight loss program is critically dependent on the willingness of the owner or caregiver to comply with the plan.
- Evaluation of the current feeding program and housing: this includes a thorough evaluation of the type of feed that is being provided (including supplementary feed, hay, pasture quality, and time allowed for grazing) and in what quantities.
- Assessment of the weekly workload and soundness for exercise: Is the horse or pony engaged in structured physical activity (e.g., being ridden)? If so, how much? Many obese equids receive little structured exercise. Information on current activity level and soundness for exercise forms the basis for recommendations regarding physical activity.
- Set realistic goals for weight loss and regularly monitor progress: In this author's experience, there is wide variation in the response of obese horses and ponies to weight loss treatment programs. Some undergo a substantial loss of body weight and adiposity after 2 to 3 months of diet restriction and increased physical activity. In others, progress can be frustratingly slow, and further adjustments to diet and the level of physical activity may be needed for satisfactory improvement. As a guide, an effective weight loss regimen should result in the loss of approximately 25 to 30 kg over a 4- to 6-week period. This decrease in body weight may be accompanied by the loss of approximately 1 unit of BCS. However, initial weight loss may result from a decrease in abdominal fat or abdominal fat mass, and further weight loss may be required before noticeable changes in BCS occur. Body weight and body condition should be assessed regularly (e.g., every 2-4 weeks) during the *weight reduction* program so that progress can be monitored and the program adjusted accordingly.

- Make all dietary changes gradually, and avoid prolonged periods of feed withholding. Abrupt starvation in obese ponies, donkeys, and miniature horses carries the risk of hyperlipemia and hepatic and renal lipidosis.
- Develop an appropriate *weight maintenance* program once the target weight and body condition have been achieved. This includes monthly assessment of body weight and condition to ensure that the feeding program is appropriate to the current level of physical activity and other environmental influences on energy requirements (e.g., ambient conditions).

In obese people the combination of caloric restriction and regular physical activity can result in more substantial weight loss than either strategy alone. However, studies in human beings also have demonstrated that physical activity is beneficial even when weight loss does not occur, as demonstrated by improvements in insulin resistance, blood lipid profile, and markers of inflammation, all of which are risk factors for cardiovascular disease. Similarly, a study in a small number of obese mares demonstrated improvements in insulin sensitivity without a change in body weight after 7 days of round pen exercise (15 to 20 min/day).[113] Accordingly, a program of regular exercise is likely to be beneficial in the management of obese (but sound) horses and ponies. In the author's experience, weight reduction and subsequent control are improved when dietary restriction is combined with a program of riding or longeing. A suggested exercise regimen is to start with two or three exercise sessions per week (20-30 min/session), subsequently building to 4 or 5 times per week, with a gradual increase in the intensity and duration of exercise.

FEEDING OBESE HORSES

Caloric restriction is of paramount importance in the management of obese equids; creation of a state of negative energy balance is needed to achieve loss of body weight. Several different dietary strategies can be applied depending on the horse's present and desired body condition and other individual circumstances. A certain amount of trial and reassessment is invariably required to achieve the goal weight and condition in an individual animal. Key considerations are the quantity and composition of the ration. Removal from pasture (e.g., to a large dry lot) is necessary for adequate control of dietary intake. Some nutritionists and veterinarians have recommended restrictive grazing as a means to decrease caloric intake in overweight equids. However, a study in obese pony mares reported no change in body weight when ponies were allowed access to pasture for 12 hours daily (either during day or night),[114] perhaps because of increased forage consumption during the restricted grazing period. In another study it was estimated that ponies could consume 40% of their daily DM intake during 3 hours of pasture turnout.[115] Strategies that allow turnout while minimizing forage intake include application of grazing muzzles, strip grazing behind other horses, mowing the pasture and removing clippings before providing access, putting a deep layer of wood chips over a small paddock, and using dry lots or indoor arenas. It is important to ensure that horses wearing grazing muzzles are able to consume water. In some obese horses and ponies, a return to less restricted pasture access is possible after attainment of goal body weight and condition. Even then, however, reduced grazing may be justified during periods of rapid growth (i.e., spring and fall) given the likelihood for weight gain and exacerbation of insulin resistance, with attendant increased risk of laminitis.

In general, rations for overweight and obese horses should be high in fiber and low in NSC. Horses at maintenance require approximately 2% Bwt as forage or forage plus supplement to meet daily nutrient requirements. As a first step toward calorie restriction and weight loss, grain and other concentrated sources of calories (e.g., commercial sweet feeds, feeds containing added fats) should be reduced (for overweight animals) or totally removed (for obese animals) from the diet. Excessive feeding of other treats, such as carrots and apples, also should be curtailed. Forage (as hay or hay substitute such as chop, chaff, or haylage) should be the primary, if not sole, energy-providing component of the ration. In some areas forage-based, low-calorie feeds complete with vitamins and minerals are available commercially; this type of feed is convenient and may be used as a substitute for hay or fed as a component of the ration along with hay. In a study of obese ponies provided a free-choice forage (chaff) diet during winter and summer, voluntary intake (DM basis) was about 2% of body weight, and BCS was unchanged during the study period.[116] As a general guide, therefore, hay or hay substitute should initially be provided at no more than 1.5% of current body weight per day (clients should be instructed to weigh the ration), with subsequent further reductions in feed depending on the extent of weight loss (e.g., 1% of *target* body weight). It is preferable not to decrease forage provision below 1% of body weight; feeding smaller amounts of forage can increase the risk of hindgut dysfunction, stereotypical behaviors (e.g., wood chewing), ingestion of bedding, and coprophagy. The ration should be divided into three to four feedings per day.

Mature grass hay (i.e., with visible seedheads and a high stem-to-leaf ratio) has higher fiber and lower energy and NSC than immature hay and is suitable forage for the obese horse or pony. Alfalfa hay or other legumes, such as clover, are less preferred because, on average, these forages have higher energy and NSC content than grass hay. Ensiled forages generally have lower NSC contents than hay made from the same crop. However, despite the generally lower NSC content of haylage compared with hay, the high palatability of some haylages may result in higher total NSC intake. Ideally, the results of proximate nutrient analysis, including direct measurement of starch and ESC, should be reviewed before selection of the hay. An NSC content of less than 10% is recommended. Poorly digestible, highly silicated forages should be used with caution; according to anecdotal reports, this practice increases the risk of impaction colic in some animals.

Forage-only diets do not provide adequate protein, minerals, or vitamins. It is possible that the lack of protein over the long term could lead to the loss of muscle mass rather than fat. Therefore the forage diet should be supplemented with a low-calorie commercial ration balancer product that contains sources of high-quality protein and a mixture of vitamins and minerals to balance the low vitamin E, vitamin, copper, zinc, selenium, and other minerals typically found in mature grass hays. These products are often designed to be fed in small quantities (e.g., 0.5 to 1.0 kg/day); they can be mixed with chaff (hay chop) to increase the size of the meal and extend feeding time, which may alleviate boredom in animals provided a restricted diet.

Ponies, donkeys, and miniature horses must not be abruptly starved to reduce their body weight or prevented from eating for prolonged periods; these strategies have been associated with the development of hyperlipemia. This risk is increased at times of stress, such as during transportation, lactation, pregnancy, and management changes. As mentioned, the target duration for weight loss should be weeks to months rather than days.

Additional factors should be considered when planning a weight reduction program, including strategies to extend feeding time and relieve boredom in the face of limited feed provision, the need for individual rather than group feeding, the potential need for a change in the type of bedding, and the potential use of pharmacologic agents (e.g., levothyroxine) purported to enhance weight loss or mitigate co-morbidities such as insulin resistance. Recent studies have demonstrated that levothyroxine sodium (48 mg/day for an adult horse) can enhance weight loss in healthy horses.[117]

Use of hay nets with small openings or double hay nets can extend feeding time in some horses. The size of the meal and duration of feeding can be increased by mixing the feed with chaff or chopped straw. In group housing situations it may be necessary to separate the obese horse or pony to allow strict control of feed intake. For animals housed in stalls, dietary restriction can promote intake of bedding. Because some straws retain some of the cereal heads, ingestion of bedding can substantially increase daily caloric intake (and possibly the risk of colic). In this situation use of shavings, paper, or other nonstraw alternatives for bedding is recommended.

FEEDING THIN AND STARVED HORSES

Failure to meet a horse's energy (DE) requirements will result in weight loss. Prolonged nutritional restriction (energy and protein) will result in emaciation and, in severe cases, death. Chronically starved horses have low body condition (BCS of 2 or lower), with minimal subcutaneous fat and reduced muscle mass. The hair coat is often unthrifty in appearance, and muscle weakness may result in recumbency. Healthy horses starved of feed take approximately 60 to 90 days to become recumbent. After 36 to 48 hours of recumbency, horses are often in lateral recumbency, may not be able to raise their heads, and can display seizurelike activity. The prognosis for survival is very poor in horses recumbent for more than 72 hours, even when appropriate nutritional support and nursing care are instituted.[118]

Laboratory findings in chronically starved horses may include anemia, hypertriglyceridemia, hyperbilirubinemia (especially unconjugated bilirubin), high nonesterified fatty acid concentrations, lymphopenia, hypophosphatemia, and hypomagnesemia. Protein deficiency may result in hypoalbuminemia and low BUN concentration. When presented with a thin or emaciated horse, the clinician first must determine the cause (e.g., feed restriction versus medical problems such as intestinal parasites, malabsorption syndromes, poor dentition, and old age). Thorough clinical evaluation is therefore required to identify the cause of weight loss and emaciation. If the horse has been neglected, obtaining an accurate history of its diet and feeding program may be difficult. However, observation of the environment and other horses on the farm may indicate feed restriction as the cause of thin body condition or starvation. Herd mates also may be in poor body condition, pastures overgrazed, and hay quality poor or fed in quantities insufficient to meet the requirements of the individual or herd. Harsh environmental conditions (e.g., dry summer, cold winter) can contribute to feed restriction in horses kept at pasture.

Recommendations for feeding management of thin and emaciated horses vary depending on the severity and chronicity of starvation and appetite. Severely debilitated horses with poor appetite may require AEF with a slurry made from commercial complete feeds or PN support (as described earlier in this chapter). For horses in moderately poor body condition (BCS 3 or 4) with good appetite, a simple increase in energy intake will result in weight gain. The first step is to thoroughly evaluate the current ration, with particular reference to the adequacy of DE and protein intake (see Figure 5-1 and Table 5-8). Requirements for weight gain can then be estimated. The relationships among energy intake, change in body weight, and change in BCS have not been well described. However, in light-breed horses it appears that each unit of body condition increase requires at least 20 kg of weight gain. Some experts suggest that 16 to 24 Mcal of DE are required per kilogram of gain in mature horses of about 500 kg (1100 lb) Bwt.[1] Using an average value of 20 Mcal DE/kg weight gain, a 1-unit increase in BCS (20 kg gain) will require 400 Mcal of DE over maintenance requirements—or an additional 6 to 7 Mcal per day for the 500-kg horse over a 60-day period. Using similar assumptions, a 2-unit increase in BCS (approximately 40 kg) may be achieved over a 90-day period by feeding an additional 9 to 10 Mcal of DE per day (see Figure 5-1). Note that these estimates have been derived from limited data, and individual responses are likely to vary. Also bear in mind that the efficiency of conversion of DE to usable energy for tissue deposition (net energy) varies among energy sources; less DE may be needed per unit of gain if a high-fat feed is provided as compared with a high-fiber feed such as grass hay. The addition of 3 kg of good-quality hay (e.g., alfalfa, DE 2.4 Mcal/kg on dry matter [DM] basis) or sugar beet pulp (2.8 Mcal DE/kg DM) to the ration will provide the extra DE required for a 1-unit increase in BCS over a 60-day period. Alternatively, a smaller amount of additional hay or beet pulp may be combined with vegetable oil (1.7 Mcal DE per standard cup [225 ml]). The provision of 2 to 2.5 kg per day of a commercial fat-supplemented feed (8% to 10% fat; typical DE of 3 to 3.5 Mcal per kg) is another option.

A more conservative approach is indicated for the initial nutritional support of starved horses. In malnourished human patients aggressive refeeding can result in potentially fatal shifts in fluids and electrolytes as a result of hormonal and metabolic responses to rapid refeeding, whether enteral or parenteral; this problem has been named *refeeding syndrome*. The hallmark biochemical feature of refeeding syndrome is hypophosphatemia, but other electrolyte abnormalities may occur, including hypokalemia and hypomagnesemia.[119] Thiamine deficiency is another possible feature of refeeding syndrome. During prolonged starvation the intracellular concentrations of these substances become severely depleted, although serum concentrations may remain within reference limits. With refeeding, glycemia leads to an increase in circulating insulin, which stimulates glycogen, fat and protein synthesis. These processes require co-factors such as phosphate, magnesium, and thiamine. Insulin stimulates cellular uptake of potassium, and magnesium and phosphate also move into the cells. Water follows by osmosis. Consequently, there can be marked decreases in serum phosphate, magnesium, and potassium, with potential development of cardiac dysfunction (e.g., arrhythmias, cardiac arrest) and neuromuscular complications.

The incidence of refeeding syndrome in chronically starved horses is unknown. Anecdotally, however, metabolic and electrolyte derangements similar to those observed in humans with refeeding syndrome have been observed in starved horses provided a diet rich in starches and sugars (i.e., high NSC). Therefore some experts recommend restricting dietary NSC in the ration provided to chronically starved horses, specifically less than 20% NSC in the total diet.[73] One study evaluated the metabolic responses of chronically starved horses refed one of three diets: alfalfa hay, oat hay, or a diet of half oat hay and half an extruded (commercial) feed.[120] The diets were initially offered at 50% of estimated daily DE requirements and, over the subsequent 10-day period, gradually increased to 100% of daily needs. There were minimal differences among treatments with regard to metabolic responses (e.g., blood glucose, nonesterified fatty acid, and mineral concentrations), but serum insulin concentrations were higher in horses fed hay in addition to extruded feed. Weight gain over the 10-day period did not differ among treatments. Another study compared starved horses fed a diet of alfalfa alone and those fed alfalfa and corn oil.[121] Phosphorus intake was lower in horses fed the alfalfa and corn oil diet, which is associated with lower serum phosphorus concentrations.

In general, a diet consisting mostly of forage (e.g., hay) is recommended during the rehabilitation of chronically starved horses. Grass or legume hay (or a mixture of the two) should be fed. The NSC content of these forages is generally less than 15% DM. Alfalfa hay is a good choice for initial refeeding because it has a higher mineral content than grass hay. Grains (e.g., oats, corn, barley) and sweet feeds are not recommended because of their high NSC content. It is advisable to supplement the hay ration with a vitamin and mineral supplement or balancer pellet. The energy density of the ration may be increased by adding vegetable oil (e.g., ¼ to 1 cup per day, starting at the low end of this range) or providing a commercial fat-supplemented feed (8%-12% fat, as fed with NSC <20%). As previously mentioned, thiamine deficiency is thought to contribute to the pathophysiology of refeeding syndrome in humans. Accordingly, the administration of a B-vitamin preparation may be justified.

The DE (caloric) requirements should be calculated on the basis of *resting energy requirements* at the current body weight (22 to 23 kcal/kg/day) and the true maintenance requirements at the ideal body weight (30-36 kcal/kg/day; see Table 5-8). Starved, emaciated horses may have lost 25% to 30% of body weight; therefore maintenance DE needs for ideal body weight will be based on 125% to 130% of body weight measured at the time of first examination. A gradual increase in daily DE intake has been recommended,[73] starting at 25% to 50% of resting requirements at current body weight, building to 100% of resting requirements over the next 2 to 3 days, and followed by a gradual (over 7 to 10 days) transition to maintenance energy requirements for the ideal body weight. Energy provision should not exceed 100% of resting requirements if AEF is used for provision of the ration, with transition to true maintenance after the start of voluntary feed consumption. Regardless of feeding method (voluntary versus AEF), the ration should be divided into four to six feedings daily during the first 10 to 14 days of rehabilitation. Subsequently, the ration can be provided into two to three meals per day.

Regular (every 1 to 2 days) measurement of blood glucose, serum magnesium, phosphorus, and potassium is advised during the first 7 to 10 days of refeeding. Frequent assessment of hydration status and gastrointestinal function (e.g., borborygmi, quantity and character of feces) is also recommended. Administration of intravenous fluids, oral electrolyte-mineral preparations, or both may be necessary to correct electrolyte imbalances.

REFERENCES

1. National Research Council: *Nutrient requirements of horses*, ed 6, Washington, D.C, 2007, The National Academies Press.
2. Pagan JD, Geor RJ, editors: *Advances in equine nutrition II, Nottingham,* Untied Kingdom, 2001, Nottingham University Press.
3. Henneke DR, Potter GD, Kreider JL, et al: Relationship between condition score, physical measurements and body fat percentage in mares, *Equine Vet J* 15:371-372, 1983.
4. Pratt SE, Geor RJ, McCutcheon LJ: Effect of dietary energy source and physical conditioning on insulin sensitivity and glucose tolerance in standardbred horses, *Equine Vet J* (Suppl 36):579-584, 2006.
5. Suagee JK, Burk AO, Quinn JK, et al: Effects of diet and weight gain on body condition scoring in Thoroughbred geldings, *J Equine Vet Sci* 28:156-166, 2008.
6. Kienzle E, Schramme S: Body condition scoring and prediction of bodyweight in adult warm-blooded horses, *Pferdeheilkunde* 20:517-524, 2004.
7. Lee S, Bacha F, Gungor N, et al: Waist circumference is an independent predictor of insulin resistance in black and white youths, *J Pediatr* 148:188-194, 2006.
8. Treiber KH, Kronfeld DS, Hess TM, et al: Evaluation of genetic and metabolic predispositions and nutritional risk factors for pasture-associated laminitis in ponies, *J Am Vet Med Assoc* 228:1538-1545, 2006.
9. Carter RA, Treiber KH, Geor RJ, et al: Prediction of incipient pasture-associated laminitis from hyperinsulinemia, hyperleptinemia, and generalized and localized obesity in a cohort of ponies, *Equine Vet J* 41:171-178, 2009.
10. Frank N, Elliott SB, Brandt LE, et al: Physical characteristics, blood hormone concentrations, and plasma lipid concentrations in obese horses with insulin resistance, *J Am Vet Med Assoc* 228:1383-1390, 2006.
11. Caroll C, Huntington P: Body condition scoring and weight estimation of horses, *Equine Vet J* 20:41-45, 1988.
12. Ellis JM, Hollands T: Accuracy of different methods of estimating the weight of horses, *Vet Rec* 143:335-336, 1998.
13. St. Lawrence AC, Lawrence LM, Coleman R: Using an empirical equation to predict the voluntary intake of grass hays by mature equids. *Proceedings of the 17th Equine Nutrition and Physiological Society Sumposium* 99-100, 2001.
14. Archer DC, Proudman CJ: Epidemiological clues to preventing colic, *Vet J* 172:29-39, 2006.
15. Shirazi-Beechey SP: Molecular insights into dietary induced colic, *Equine Vet J* 40:414-421, 2008.
16. Geor RJ, Harris PA: How to minimize gastrointestinal disease associated with carbohydrate nutrition in horses. In: *Proceedings of the 53rd Annual Convention of the American Association of Equine Practitioners* 178-185, 2007.
17. Pagan JD, Jackson S, Duren S: Computing horse nutrition: how to properly conduct an equine nutrition evaluation using Microsteed equine ration evaluation software, *World Equine Vet Rev* 1:11-17, 1996.
18. Gallagher K, Leech J, Stowe H: Protein, energy and dry matter consumption by racing Thoroughbreds: a field study, *J Equine Vet Sci* 12:43-47, 1988.
19. Southwood LL, Evans DL, Bryden WL, et al: Nutrient intake of horses in Thoroughbred and Standardbred stables, *Aust Vet J* 70:164-168, 1993.
20. White NA: Equine colic. II. Causes and risk factors for colic. In: *Proceedings of the 52nd Annual Convention of the American Association of Equine Practitioners* 2006, pp. 115-119.

21. Richards N, Hinch GN, Rowe JB: The effect of current grain feeding practices on hindgut starch fermentation and acidosis in the Australian racing Thoroughbred, *Aust Vet J* 84: 402-407, 2006.
22. Nadeau JA, Andrews FM, Mathew AG, et al: Evaluation of diet as a cause of gastric ulcers in horses, *Am J Vet Res* 61:784-790, 2000.
23. Reese RE, Andrews FM: Nutrition and dietary management of equine gastric ulcer syndrome, *Vet Clin Nth Am Equine Pract* 25:79-92, 2009.
24. McKenzie EC, Valberg SJ, Godden SM, et al: Effect of dietary starch, fat and bicarbonate content on exercise responses and serum creatine kinase activity in equine recurrent exertional rhabdomyolysis, *J Vet Intern Med* 17:693-701, 2003.
25. Geor RJ: Metabolic predispositions to laminitis in horses and ponies: obesity, insulin resistance and metabolic syndromes, *J Equine Vet Sci* 28:753-759, 2008.
26. Longland AC: Starch, sugar and fructans, what are they and how important are they in diets for horses. In: *Proceedings of the 1st WALTHAM-RVC laminitis conference* 7-14, 2007.
27. Harris PA: Energy requirements of the exercising horse, *Ann Rev Nutr* 17:185-210, 1997.
28. Harris PA, Geor RJ: Primer on dietary carbohydrates and utility of the glycemic index in equine nutrition, *Vet Clin Nth Am Equine Pract* 25:23-37, 2009.
29. de Fombelle A, Veiga L, Drogoul C, et al: Effect of diet composition and feeding pattern on the prececal digestibility of starches from diverse botanical origins measured with the mobile nylon bag technique, *J Anim Sci* 82:3625-3634, 2004.
30. Pollock CJ, Lloyd EJ: The effect of low temperature upon starch, sucrose and fructan synthesis in leaves, *Ann Bot* 60:231-235, 1987.
31. Van Soest PJ: *Nutritional ecology of the ruminant*, ed 2, Ithaca, New York, 1995, Comstock Publishing.
32. Argenzio RA: Functions of the equine large intestine and their interrelationship in disease, *Cornell Vet* 65:303-330, 1979.
33. Clarke LL, Roberts MC, Argenzio RA: Feeding and digestive problems in horses. Physiologic responses to a concentrated meal, *Vet Clin North Am Equine Pract* 6:433-450, 1990.
34. Cohen ND, Gibbs PG: Dietary and other management factors associated with colic in horses, *J Am Vet Med Assoc* 215:53-60, 1999.
35. Hillyer MH, Taylor FGR, Proudman CJ, et al: Case control study to identify risk factors for simple colonic obstruction and distension colic in horses, *Equine Vet J* 34:55-463, 2002.
36. Hudson JM, Cohen ND, Gibbs PG, et al: Feeding practices associated with colic in horses, *J Am Vet Med Assoc* 219: 1419-1425, 2001.
37. Tinker MK, White NA, Lessard P, et al: Retrospective study of equine colic risk factors, *Equine Vet J* 29:454-458, 1997.
38. Cohen ND, Peloso JG: Risk factors for history of previous colic and for chronic, intermittent colic in a population of horses, *J Am Vet Med Assoc* 208:607-703, 1995.
39. Proudman CJ: A two year, prospective survey of equine colic in general practice, *Equine Vet J* 24:90-93, 1992.
40. Cohen ND: The John Hickman Memorial Lecture: Colic by numbers, *Equine Vet J* 35:343-349, 2003.
41. Varloud M, Goachet AG, de Fombelle A, et al: Effect of the diet on prececal digestibility of dietary starch measured in horses with acid insoluble ash as an internal marker. In: *Proceedings of the 18th Equine Nutrition and Physiological Society Sumposium*, East Lansing, Michigan, 117-118, 2003.
42. Cummings JH, Englyst HN: Gastrointestinal effects of food carbohydrate, *Am J Clin Nutr* (Suppl 61):S938-S945, 1995.
43. Dyer J, Fernandez-Castano E, Salmon KS, et al: Molecular characterisation of carbohydrate digestion and absorption in equine small intestine, *Equine Vet J* 34:349-358, 2002.
44. Dyer J, Al Rammahi M, Waterfall L, et al: Adaptive response of equine intestinal Na(+)/glucose co-transporter (SGLT1) to an increase in dietary soluble carbohydrate, *Pflugers Arch* 458:419-430, 2009.
45. Lorenzo-Figueras M, Morisset SM, Morriset J, et al: Digestive enzyme concentrations and activities in healthy pancreatic tissue, *Am J Vet Res* 68:1070-1072, 2007.
46. Kienzle E: Small intestinal digestion of starch in the horse, *Revue Med Vet* 145:199-204, 1993.
47. Kienzle E, Radicke S, Wilke W, et al: Activity of amylase in the gastrointestinal tract of the horse, *J Anim Physiol Am Nutr* 72:234-241, 1994.
48. Meyer H, Radicke S, Kienzle E, et al: Investigations on preileal digestion of oats, corn and barley starch in relation to grain processing, *Proceedings of the 13th Equine Nutrition and Physiological Society Symposium,* 92-97, 1993.
49. Potter GD, Arnold FF, Householder DD, et al: Digestion of starch in the small or large intestine of the equine, *Pferdeheilkunde* 1:107-111, 1992.
50. Bugaut M, Bentejec M: Biological effects of short chain fatty acids in nonruminant mammals, *Annu Rev Nutr* 13:217-241, 1993.
51. De Fombelle A, Julliand V, Drogoul C, et al: Feeding and microbial disorders in horses: part 1—effects of an abrupt incorporation of two levels of barley in a hay diet on microbial profile and activities, *J Equine Vet Sci* 21:439-445, 2001.
52. Bailey SR, Marr CM, Elliott J: Current research and theories on the pathogenesis of acute laminitis in the horse, *Vet J* 167:129-142, 2004.
53. Goodson J, Tyznik WJ, Cline JH, et al: Effects of an abrupt diet change from hay to concentrate on microbial numbers and physical environment in the cecum of the pony, *Appl Environ Microbiol* 54:1946-1950, 1988.
54. Willard JG, Willard JC, Wolfram SA, et al: Effect of diet on cecal pH and feeding behavior of horses, *J Anim Sci* 45:87-93, 1977.
55. Radicke S, Kienzle E, Meyer H: Preileal apparent digestibility of oat and corn starch and consequences for cecal metabolism, *Proceedings of the 13th Equine Nutrition and Physiological Society Symposium,* 43-48, 1991.
56. Bailey SR, Rycroft A, Elliott J: Production of amines in equine cecal contents in an *in vitro* model of carbohydrate overload, *J Anim Sci* 51:1930-1934, 2002.
57. French KR, Pollitt CC: Equine laminitis: loss of hemidesmosomes in hoof secondary epidermal lamellae correlates to dose in an oligofructose induction model: an ultrastructural study, *Equine Vet J* (Suppl 36):230-235, 2004.
58. Drogoul C, de Fombelle A, Julliand V: Feeding and microbial disorders in horses. 2: effect of three hay:grain ratios on digesta passage rate and digestibility in ponies, *J Equine Vet Sci* 21:487-490, 2001.
59. Medina B, Girard ID, Jacotot E, et al: Effect of preparation of *Saccharomyces cerevisiae* on microbial profiles and fermentation patterns in the large intestine of horses fed a high fiber or a high starch diet, *J Anim Sci* 80:2600-2609, 2002.
60. Weese JS, Rousseau J: Evaluation of *Lactobacillus pentosus* WE7 for prevention of diarrhea in neonatal foals, *J Am Vet Med Assoc* 226:2031-2034, 2005.
61. Desrochers AM, Dolente BA, Roy MF, et al: Efficacy of *Saccharomyces boulardii* for treatment of horses with acute enterocolitis, *J Am Vet Med Assoc* 227:954-959, 2005.
62. Pagan JD, Lawrence TJ, Lawrence LA: Feeding protected sodium bicarbonate attenuates hindgut acidosis in horses fed a high-grain ration, *Proceedings of the 54th Annual Convention of the American Association of Equine Practitioners,* 530-533, 2007.
63. Heyland DK: Nutritional support in the critically ill patient: a critical review of the evidence, *Critical Care Clinics* 14: 423-440, 1998.

64. Silk DBA, Gow NM: Postoperative starvation after gastrointestinal surgery: early feeding is beneficial, *Br Med J* 323: 761-766, 2001.
65. Shukla VK, Roy SK, Kumar J, Vaida MP: Correlation of immune and nutritional status with wound complications in patients undergoing abdominal surgery, *Ann Surg* 51:442-445, 1985.
66. Hasselgren PO, Fischer JE: Counter–regulatory hormones and mechanisms in amino acid metabolism with special reference to the catabolic response in skeletal muscle, *Curr Opin Clin Nutr Metab Care* 2:9-14, 1999.
67. Romijn JA: Substrate metabolism in the metabolic response to injury, *Proc Nutr Soc* 59:447-449, 2000.
68. Leverve X: Inter-organ substrate exchanges in the critically ill, *Curr Opin Clin Nutr Metab Care* 4:137-142, 2001.
69. Dunkel B, McKenzie HC: Severe hypertriglyceridemia in clinically ill horses: Diagnosis, treatment and outcome, *Equine Vet J* 35:590-595, 2003.
70. Gelfand RA, Mathews DE, Bier D, et al: Role of counterregulatory hormones in the catabolic response to stress, *J Clin invest* 74:2238-2248, 1984.
71. Langhans W: Peripheral mechanisms involved with catabolism, *Curr Opin Clin Nutr Metab Care* 5:419-426, 2002.
72. Magdesian KG: Nutrition for critical gastrointestinal illness: feeding horses with diarrhea or colic, *Vet Clin Equine* 19: 617-644, 2003.
73. Robinson NE, Sprayberry K, editors: *Current therapy in equine medicine*, ed 6, St Louis, 2009, Saunders.
74. Jeejeebhoy KN: Enteral and parenteral nutrition: evidence-based approach, *Proc Nutr Soc* 60:399-402, 2001.
75. Raina N, LaMarre J, Liew C-C, et al: Effect of nutrition on the expression of plasma soluble tumor necrosis factor (TNF) receptors, membrane TNF receptors and MRNA of TNF receptors in rats receiving oral and parenteral nutrition, *Am J Physiol* 277:E464-E473, 1999.
76. Yamazaki K, Maiz A, Moldaver LL, et al: Complications associated with overfeeding of infected animals, *J Surg Res* 40:152-158, 1986.
77. Matsui J, Cameron RG, Kurian R, et al: Nutritional, hepatic, and metabolic effects of cachetin/tumor necrosis factor in rats receiving parenteral nutrition, *Gastroenterology* 104:235-243, 1993.
78. Pagan JD, Hintz HF: Equine energetics. I. Relationship between body weight and energy requirements in horses, *J Anim Sci* 63:815-821, 1986.
79. Stapleton RD, Jones N, Heyland KD, et al: Feeding critically ill patients: what is the optimal amount of energy? *Crit Care Med* 35:S535-S540, 2007.
80. Jeejeebhoy KN: Permissive underfeeding of the critically ill patient, *Nutr Clin Pract* 19:477-480, 2004.
81. Ousey JC, Holdstock NB, Rossdale PD, et al: How much energy do sick neonatal foals require compared to healthy foals? *Pferdeheilkunde* 12:231-237, 1996.
82. Ousey JC, Prandi S, Zimmer J, et al: Effects of various feeding regimens on the energy balance of equine neonates, *Am J Vet Res* 58:1243-1251, 1997.
83. Durham AE, Phillips TJ, Walmsley JP, et al: Study of the clinical effects of postoperative parenteral nutrition in 15 horses, *Vet Rec* 153:493-498, 2003.
84. Adam S, Forrest S: ABC of intensive care, *Br Med J* 319: 175-178, 1999.
85. Durham AE, Phillips TJ, Walmsley JP, et al: Nutritional and clinicopathological effects of post operative parenteral nutrition following small intestinal resection and anastomosis in the mature horse, *Equine Vet J* 36:390-396, 2004.
86. Frost P, Bihari D: The role of nutritional support in the critically ill: physiological and economic considerations, *Nutrition* (Suppl 13):58-63, 1997.
87. Miura S, Tanaka S, Yoshioka M, et al: Changes in intestinal absorption of nutrients and brush border glycoproteins after total parenteral nutrition in rats, *Gut* 33:484-489, 1992.
88. Mosenthal AC, Xu D, Deitch EA: Elemental and intravenous total parenteral nutrition diet-induced gut barrier failure is intestinal site specific and can be prevented by feeding nonfermentable fiber, *Crit Care Med* 30:396-402, 2002.
89. Buechner-Maxwell VA, Elvinger F, Thatcher CD, et al: Physiologic response of normal adult horses to a low residue liquid diet, *J Equine Vet Sci* 23:310-317, 2003.
90. Naylor JM, Freeman DE, Kronfeld DS: Alimentation of hypophagic horses, *Comp Cont Educ Pract Vet* 6:S03-S99, 1984.
91. Detsky AS, Baker JP, O'Rouke K, Goel V: Perioperative parenteral nutrition: a meta-analysis, *Ann Intern Med* 107:195-203, 1987.
92. Silk DB, Green CJ: Perioperative nutrition: parenteral versus enteral, *Curr Opin Clin Nutr Metab Care* 1:21-27, 1998.
93. Bozzetti F, Gavazzi C, Miceli R, et al: Perioperative total parenteral nutrition in malnourished gastrointestinal cancer patients: a randomized, clinical trial, *J Parenter Enteral Nutr* 24:7-14, 2000.
94. Klein S, Kinney J, Jeejeebhoy K, et al: Nutrition support in clinical practice: review of published data and recommendations for future research directions, *J Parenter Enteral Nutr* 21:133-156, 1997.
95. Farinas-Alvarez C, Farinas MC, Fernandez-Mazarrasa C, et al: Analysis of risk factors for nosocomial sepsis in surgical patients, *Br J Surg* 87:1076-1081, 2000.
96. Lopes MA, White NA: Parenteral nutrition for horses with gastrointestinal disease: a retrospective study of 79 cases, *Equine Vet J* 34:250-257, 2002.
97. McKenzie HC III, Geor RJ: Feeding management of sick neonatal foals, *Vet Clin North Am Equine Pract* 25:109-119, 2009.
98. Stoneham S: How to feed the sick neonatal foal. In: *Proceedings of the 1st British Equine Veterinary Association and WALTHAM Nutrition Symposia, Equine Veterinary Journal Limited,* Suffolk, United Kingdom, 33-37, 2005.
99. Naylor JM, Bell R: Raising the orphan foal, *Vet Clin N Am Equine Pract* 1:169-178, 1985.
100. Staniar WB, Kronfeld DS, Hoffman RM, et al: Weight prediction from linear measures of growing thoroughbreds, *Equine Vet J* 36:149-154, 2004.
101. Cymbaluk NF, Smart ME, Bristol F, et al: Importance of milk replacer intake and composition in rearing orphan foals, *Can Vet J* 34:479-486, 1993.
102. Ousey JC: Feeding the newborn foal in health and disease, *Equine Vet Educ* 6:50-54, 2003.
103. Magdesian KG: Neonatal foal diarrhea, *Vet Clin N Am Equine Pract* 21:295-312, 2005.
104. Krause JB, McKenzie HC III: Parenteral nutrition in foals: a retrospective study of 45 cases, *Equine Vet J* 2007(39):74-78, 2000-2004.
105. Koterba AM, Drummond WH, Kosch PC, editors: *Equine clinical neonataology*, Philadelphia, 1990, Saunders.
106. Spurlock SL, Donaghue S: Weight gains in foals on parenteral nutrition, *Proceedings of the 2nd Conference of the International Society of Perinatology,* 61, 1990.
107. Geor R, Frank N: Metabolic syndrome: from human organ disease to laminar failure in equids, *Vet Immunol Immunopath* 129:151-154, 2009.
108. United States Department of Agriculture. NAHMS Equine '98. Part III. Management and Health of Horses (www.aphis.usda.gov/vs/ceah/cahm; accessed September 15, 2008).
109. Thatcher C, et al. Unpublished data, 2007.
110. Wyse CA, McNie KA, Tannahil VJ, et al: Prevalence of obesity in riding horses in Scotland, *Vet Rec* 162:590-591, 2008.
111. Treiber KH, Kronfeld DS, Geor RJ: Insulin resistance in Equids: possible role in laminitis, *J Nutr* 136:S2094-S2098, 2006.

112. Johnson PJ: The equine metabolic syndrome: peripheral Cushing's syndrome, *Vet Clin N Am Equine Pract* 18:271-293, 2002.
113. Powell DM, Reedy SE, Sessions DR, et al: Effect of short-term exercise training on insulin sensitivity in obese and lean mares, *Equine Vet J* (Suppl 34):81-84, 2002.
114. Buff PR, Johnson PJ, Wiedmeyer CE, et al: Modulation of leptin, insulin and growth hormone in obese pony mares under chronic nutritional restriction and supplementation with ractopamine hydrochloride, *Vet Ther* 7:64-72, 2007.
115. Ince JC, Longland AC, Moore-Colyer M, et al: A pilot study to estimate the intake of grass by ponies with restricted access to pasture. *Proceedings of the British Society of Animal Science* :109, 2005.
116. Dugdale AHA, Curtis GC, Knottenbelt DC, et al: Changes in body condition and fat deposition in ponies offered an *ad libitum* chaf-based diet, *Proceedings of the 12th Congress of the European Society of Veterinary Clinical Nutrition*, 39, 2008, [abstract].
117. Frank N, Elliott SB, Boston RC: Effects of long-term oral administration of levothyroxine sodium on glucose dynamics in healthy adult horses, *Am J Vet Res* 69:76-81, 2008.
118. Whiting TL, Salmon RH, Wruck GC: Chronically starved horses: predicting survival, economic, and ethical considerations, *Can Vet J* 46:320-324, 2005.
119. Stanga Z, Brunner A, Leuenberger M, et al: Nutrition in clinical practice: the refeeding syndrome: illustrative cases and guidelines for prevention and treatment, *Eur J Clin Nutr* 62:687-694, 2008.
120. Witham CL, Stull CL: Metabolic responses of chronically starved horses to refeeding with three isoenergetic diets, *J Am Vet Med Assoc* 212:691-696, 1998.
121. Stull CL: Nutrition for rehabilitating the starved horse, *J Equine Vet Sci* 23:456-459, 2003.

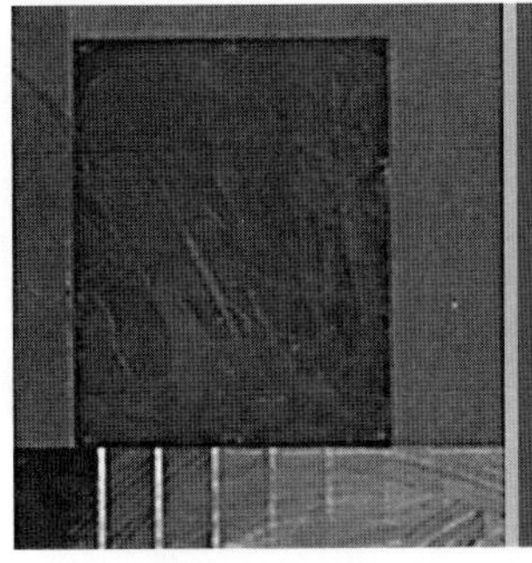

Recognizing and Treating Pain in Horses

CHAPTER 6

William Muir

Attitudes, opinions, and therapeutic approaches concerning the treatment of pain in horses continue to evolve.[1] Traditionally, pain was used as a diagnostic and prognostic tool that helped determine the source and severity of disease (e.g., articular damage, laminitis, abscess, colic), More recently, however, pain has become appreciated for its ability to produce profound behavioral, neuroendocrine, metabolic, and immunologic effects. Chronic pain, for example, can produce avoidance and protective behaviors, poor performance, inappetence, and weight loss and predisposes to infection, resulting in a generalized "sickness syndrome," which often contributes to the death or euthanasia of the horse.[2] Improved knowledge of the neuroanatomic and molecular mechanisms responsible for pain and the discovery that untreated pain induces changes in the central nervous system (CNS) that contribute to the development of chronic pain have focused attention on the development of more aggressive and effective analgesic protocols for horses.[3-5] Pain in horses should be considered an independent, rather than dependent, variable particularly when the cause of pain is uncertain (idiopathic pain), the pain is difficult to treat (e.g., myopathy or uveitis), or the cause of pain is impossible to eliminate (e.g., laminitis or osteoarthritis). Pain, like heart rate, respiratory rate, and temperature, should be considered a clinical sign that requires evaluation, documentation, and treatment. This approach will hasten the development of practical and clinically relevant diagnostic and evaluative methods that will aid in identifying the most efficacious therapies. This chapter presents an abbreviated review of the physiologic and pathophysiologic mechanisms responsible for pain and suggests clinically useful methods for evaluating and treating pain in horses.

PAIN

Pain is defined as "an unpleasant sensory and emotional experience associated with actual or potential tissue damage, or described in terms of such damage"[6] (Box 6-1). This definition encompasses those neurophysiologic processes that warn and protect the horse from actual or potential tissue damage, help prevent further injury, and promote healing. Clinically, pain results from two multifaceted components, nociception and perception.[4] Both facets are integrated to provide the immediate recognition and elimination (if possible) of the painful stimulus. Nociception is the detection of a noxious (mechanical, thermal, chemical) stimulus and by itself is not pain, because the transformation of noxious stimuli to electric impulses (transduction), their transfer to the spinal cord (transmission), and their eventual projection to the brain do not ensure that the electric impulses will be recognized (perceived; e.g., as during anesthesia; Figure 6-1). Perception is the recognition that nociception has occurred or continues to occur and triggers responses that protect the horse from further insult and help maintain homeostasis. Pain perception or the actual registration of a noxious stimulus depends on external (environmental) and internal (patient-related) issues and is responsible for the secondary behavioral (vigilance, immobilization, fear), metabolic (hyperglycemia), neuroendocrine (cortisol, catecholamines), and physiologic (heart rate, respiratory rate, pupillary) responses that are frequently used to evaluate the severity of pain, determine stress, and ultimately ascertain the horse's quality of life.

Physiologic and Pathologic Pain

Under normal circumstances pain is caused by the activation of high-threshold (high stimulus intensity) pain receptors (nociceptors) located at the distal ends of unmyelinated (C) or poorly myelinated (Aδ) nerve fibers[2,4] (see Figure 6-1). The free nerve endings of these peripheral afferent nerve fibers encode noxious stimuli depending on the modality, intensity, duration, and location of the stimulus. The intensity of the stimulus required to produce painful sensations is considerably more than that required to produce nonpainful sensations (touch) and is the most important factor determining the severity of pain.[2] Pain that is not associated with tissue damage is referred to as *physiologic* or *nociceptive pain* and serves to warn and protect the horse from potential tissue damage. Pain that occurs in association with tissue or nerve damage is considered pathologic and is frequently categorized as inflammatory or neuropathic, depending on the primary causative factor.[5] Pathologic pain is exaggerated by the development of peripheral and central sensitization. The temporal aspects of pathologic pain are dynamic and characterized by a reduction in the intensity of the stimulus required to initiate pain (hypersensitivity), the persistence of pain after removal of the noxious stimulus (hyperpathia), and the sensation of pain by stimuli that do not normally provoke pain (allodynia).[7] Inflammatory and neuropathic

BOX 6-1

TERMS USED TO DEFINE AND DESCRIBE PAIN

1. ***Pain:*** Unpleasant sensory or emotional experience associated with actual or potential tissue damage or described in terms of such damage.
2. ***Noxious stimulus:*** Stimulus (mechanical, chemical, thermal) of sufficient intensity to threaten or overtly cause tissue damage.
3. ***Nociception:*** Process of pain perception via pain receptors (nociceptors), transmission of noxious (painful) stimuli. Includes transduction, transmission, modulation, and perception.
4. ***Hyperalgesia:*** Increased response (hypersensitivity) to a noxious stimulus, either at the site of injury (primary) or in surrounding undamaged tissue (secondary).
5. ***Hyperesthesia:*** Increased sensitivity to *non*-noxious stimuli.
6. ***Hyperpathia:*** Greatly exaggerated pain sensation to nociceptive stimuli.
7. ***Allodynia:*** Pain produced by *non*-noxious stimuli.
8. ***Preemptive analgesia:*** Prevention or minimization of pain by the administration of analgesics before the production of pain or before the introduction of a noxious stimulus (surgery) if pain already exists. The goal of preemptive analgesia is to provide a therapeutic intervention in advance of pain to prevent or minimize the central nervous system response to a noxious stimulus.
9. ***Multimodal therapy:*** Administration of multiple drugs that act by different mechanisms of action to produce the desired (analgesic) effect.

pain are often characterized by an exaggerated response (hyperalgesia) when a noxious stimulus is applied to the injured area.

Peripheral Sensitization

Peripheral sensitization is caused by the production and activation of enzymatic and reparative processes initiated by tissue damage and inflammation at the site of injury. The production or dissemination of the by-products of damaged tissues, the infiltration and activation of inflammatory cells (lymphocytes, neutrophils, mast cells, macrophages), and increased sympathetic nerve activity excites and increases the sensitivity (lower activation threshold) of peripheral nociceptors (Figure 6-2).[4,8] Tissue damage results in the production of prostaglandins, bradykinin, and neurotrophic growth factors, the local release and spread of adenosine, adenosine triphosphate and ions (H^+, K^+), and an exaggerated pain response. Leukocytes and macrophages release cytokines (interleukin-1 [IL-1], IL-6, tumor necrosis factor). Primary afferent sensory nerve fibers release neuropeptides (substance P, calcitonin gene-related peptide) causing mast cells to degranulate, local vasodilation, and plasma extravasation, further amplifying the inflammatory response. Collectively, this "sensitizing soup" lowers nociceptor threshold and activates additional, so-called silent, nociceptors, thereby amplifying the pain response.[8] Peripheral sensitization is responsible for primary hyperalgesia or pain that is initiated by innocuous stimuli applied within the area of tissue injury.

Central Sensitization

Central sensitization results from the cumulative effects (temporal summation) of repetitive and sustained nociceptive inputs on the dorsal horn of the spinal cord.[4,7,8] Normally, temporary noxious stimuli generate fast but short-lived excitatory potentials within the CNS that indicate the onset, duration, intensity, and location of the painful stimulus. This fast excitatory transmission is transmitted by Aδ and C fibers and is mediated by glutamate acting on α-amino-3-hydroxy-5-isoxazole proprionic acid (AMPA) and kainite (KA) receptors within the dorsal horn of the spinal cord. Sustained input from damaged tissue or injured nerves, however, releases neuropeptides (substance P, neurokinin A) in addition to glutamate that activate *N*-methyl-D-aspartate (NMDA) and tachykinin receptors, resulting in a gradual "windup" of neurons in the dorsal horn of the spinal cord and central sensitization (see Figure 6-2). [8] Windup, central sensitization, and biochemical changes that occur in the CNS associated with their development represent a continuum of the pain process that is initiated by an acute painful process or untreated acute or chronic pain. Central sensitization can last for hours to days and is believed to be responsible for increases in the receptive field and hypersensitivity to noxious stimuli outside the area of primary tissue damage (secondary hyperalgesia).[8,9] Changes in spinal cord segmental inhibitory input also contribute to dorsal horn hyperexcitability, resulting in the perception of pain from otherwise innocuous stimuli carried by Aδ (touch) nerve fibers.[8] Central sensitization is fundamentally different from peripheral sensitization in that it enables low-intensity stimuli to produce pain because of changes in sensory processing in the spinal cord. The projection of electric impulses, initiated by a painful stimulus from the spinal cord to the brain, can modify memory and may be the reason that severe or untreated acute or chronic pain results in permanent behavioral changes.[10] The development of central sensitization has several clinically relevant implications, including a change in the therapeutic focus from peripheral (local anesthetics, nonsteroidal antiinflammatory drugs [NSAIDs]) to central sites (opioids, α_2-adrenoceptor agonists), the selection of potent centrally acting analgesic drugs, and the introduction of strategies that help limit or prevent the development of central sensitization (preemptive and multimodal).[5] Once hyperexcitability (central sensitization) is established, larger doses of analgesics are required for longer periods of time for therapy to be effective. In other words, pain should be treated as early as possible and preemptively when possible.

In summary, peripheral sensitization is caused by the local production, release, and accumulation of chemicals (prostaglandins, leukotrienes, neuropeptides, nerve growth factors) that sensitize peripheral nerve fibers and activate additional ("silent") pain receptors.[4,8] Some of the hypersensitivity at the site of injury and all of the hypersensitivity

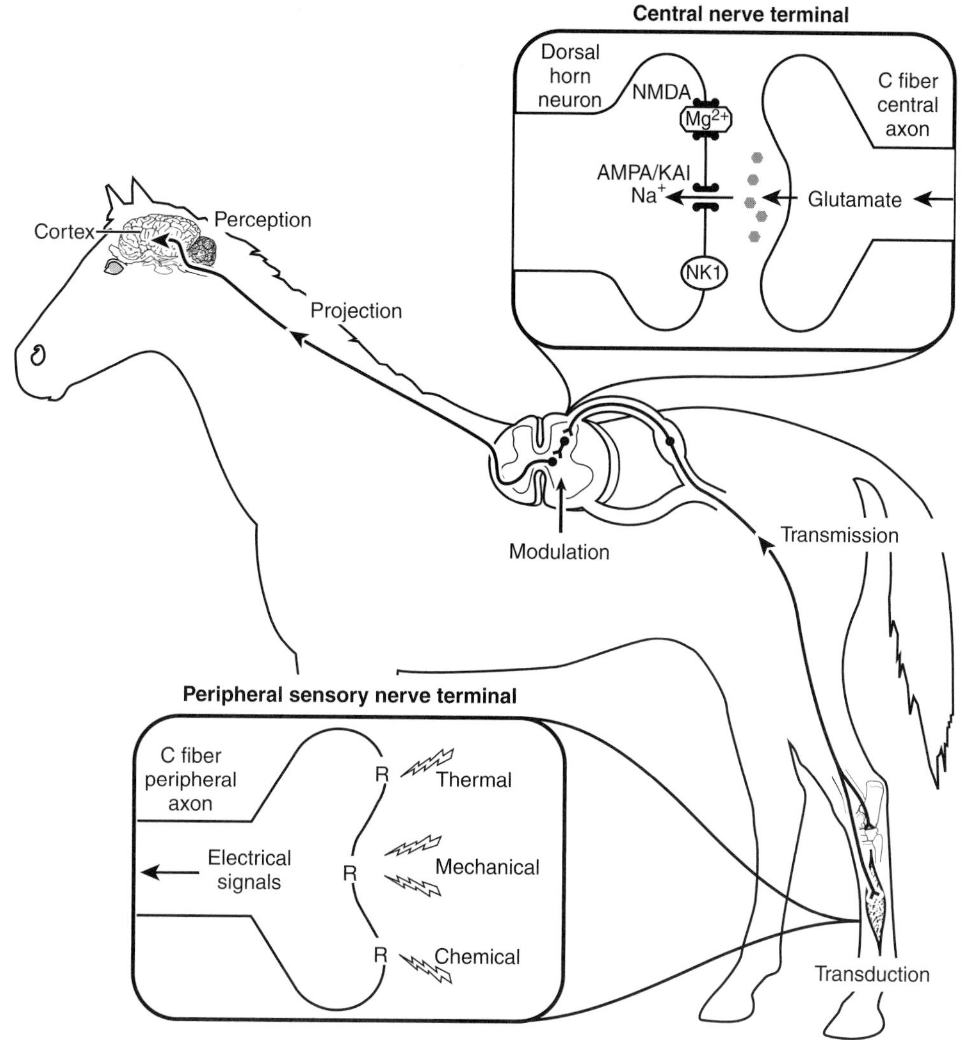

FIGURE 6-1 Pain nociception and perception. Painful thermal, mechanical, and chemical stimuli are tranduced to electric potentials (action potentials) that are transmitted to the spinal cord, where they are modulated and then projected to the brain (perception). The major excitatory neurotransmitter in the spine is glutamate, which normally activates α-amino-3-hydroxy-5-isoxazole proprionic acid (AMPA) and kainate (KAI) receptors. *NMDA,* N-methyl-D-aspartate; *NK1,* neurokinin.

outside the site of injury (secondary hyperalgsia) result from central sensitization.[7-11] The primary difference between peripheral and central sensitization is that the former activates and sensitizes nociceptors at the terminal ends of Aδ and C fibers, whereas the latter changes sensory processing in the spinal cord, resulting in pain from stimuli that activate low-threshold sensory (touch) receptors.[5,8] Visceral pain (e.g., pain from intestine, liver, spleen, kidney, or bladder), unlike somatic pain, is transmitted by parasympathetic (principally vagal) and sympathetic splanchnic afferent nerve fibers.[12,13] The autonomic fibers involved in transmitting noxious inputs from visceral organs, including the distal colon, rectum, and bladder, are diffuse and extensively overlap. These differences from somatic transmission (transmission by parasympathetic and sympathetic nerves and extensive overlap) result in a significant autonomic response (tachycardia, tachypnea, mydriasis) and difficulty in localization of the site of pain.[12] Generalized or diffuse inflammation, ischemia, and mesenteric stretching or intestinal dilation (e.g., of the stomach or cecum) can produce severe, unrelenting pain in horses.

STRESS AND DISTRESS

Pain associated with disease, accidental, or surgical trauma or originating from unknown causes can result in activation of the sympathetic nervous system, secretion of glucocorticoids (primarily cortisol), hypermetabolism, sodium and water retention, and altered carbohydrate and protein metabolism. The term given to this response is *stress,* which encompasses the biologic processes whereby the horse attempts to maintain homeostasis and cope with threats to its well-being.[14] Acute and chronic pain are capable of producing a significant stress response in horses, thereby reducing their quality of life. The stress response is an adaptive pattern of behavioral, neural, endocrine, immunologic, hematologic, and metabolic changes directed toward the restoration of homeostasis (Figure 6-3). During threatening circumstances the stress response prepares

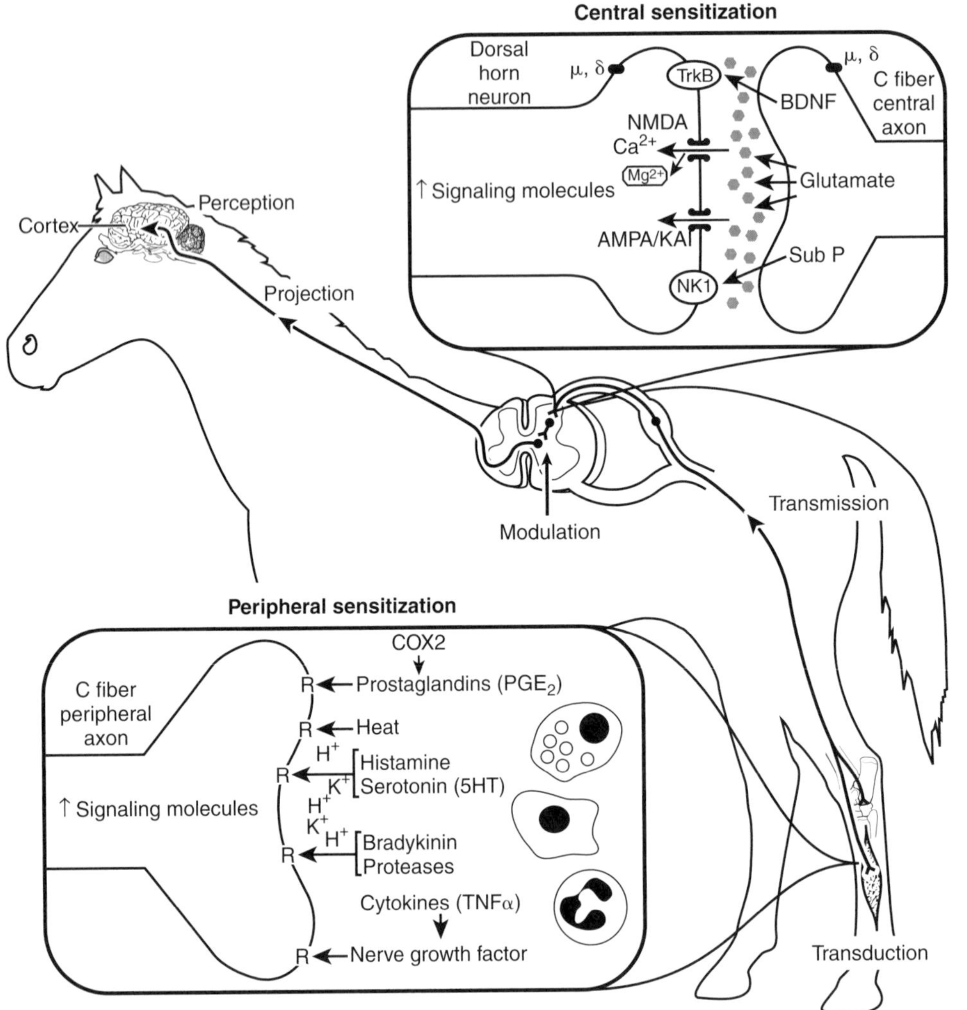

FIGURE 6-2 Peripheral and central sensitization. Peripheral sensitization caused by tissue or nerve injury lowers the threshold of nociceptors and activates "silent" nociceptors, leading to primary hyperalgesia. Central sensitization caused by the temporal summation of nociceptive input activates N-methyl-D-aspartate (NMDA) receptors in the spinal cord, resulting in secondary hyperalgesia. *TrkB,* Tyrosine kinase B; *AMPA,* α-amino-3-hydroxy-5-isoxazole proprionic acid; *KAI,* kainate; *NK1,* neurokinin; *Sub P,* substance P; *COX-2,* cyclooxygenase 2; *5-HT,* 5-hydroxytryptamine; *TNF-α,* tumor necrosis factor α.

the horse for an emergency reaction that fosters survival in the face of immediate threats (fight or flight). Most stress in horses is temporary because of the removal or short duration of exposure to the stressor. Surgery and anesthesia are common sources of stress in horses that can be modified by appropriate selection and use of preanesthetic and anesthetic drugs.[15] Suffering occurs when horses are forced to endure the infliction or imposition of physical pain or develop the feeling of impending harm (fear).[16] Severe or chronic stress can become maladaptive, producing distress and triggering self-sustaining cascades of neural and endocrine responses that upset physiologic homeostasis and negatively affect biologic functions critical to the well-being of the animal (Box 6-2). Stress and distress negatively affect the well-being of horses, produce immune incompetence, and can lead to gradual physical deterioration and death.[17] At a minimum, all animals should be granted the "five freedoms": freedom from hunger and malnutrition, freedom from discomfort, freedom from disease, freedom from injury, and freedom from pain.

Neuroendocrine and Autonomic Stress

The noxious stimuli that produce acute and chronic pain induce stress that activates the hypothalamus-pituitary-adrenal axis.[14] This afferent information stimulates the secretion of corticotropin-releasing factor, vasoactive intestinal peptide, and adrenocorticotropic hormone (ACTH). Corticotropin-releasing factor acts synergistically with vasopressin to stimulate the production of ACTH and β-endorphin, thereby enhancing cell survival and producing analgesic effects, respectively. Corticotropin-releasing factor also stimulates the adrenomedullary release of ACTH and catecholamines. Corticotropin-releasing factor is an excitatory neurotransmitter in the locus ceruleus that increases norepinephrine release and excitatory behaviors. Adrenocorticotropic hormone stimulates the adrenal cortex to secrete cortisol, corticosterone, and aldosterone and also stimulates increased glucocorticoid production and the adrenomedullary secretion of catecholamines. Cortisol stimulates gluconeogenesis, increases proteolysis

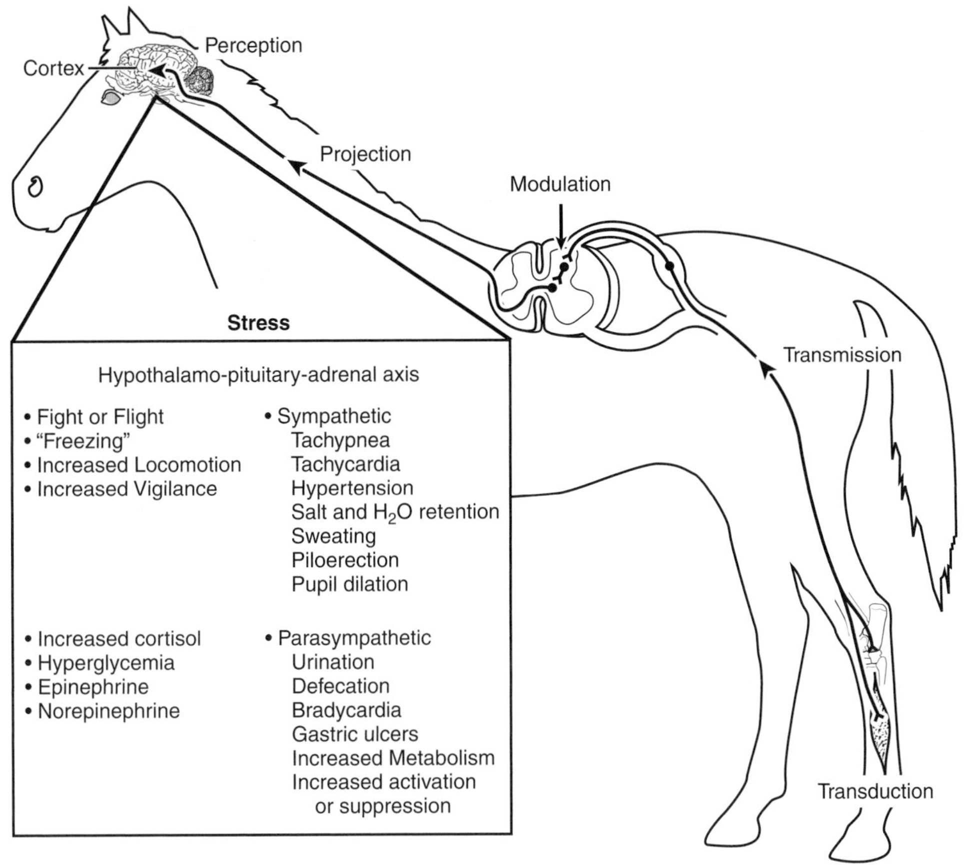

FIGURE 6-3 Pain produces stress that activates the hypothalamus-pituitary-adrenal axis, resulting in varied behavioral, neuroendocrine, metabolic, and immune responses.

BOX 6-2

INDICATORS OF PAIN, STRESS, AND WELL-BEING

- Attitude
- Activity
- Appearance
- Appetite
- Facial expression
- Behavior
- Posture
- Response to handling
- Willingness to perform work

and lipolysis, facilitates catecholamine effects, and produces antiinflammatory actions. It is important to note that many of these same factors (corticotropin-releasing factor, ACTH, and corticosterone) are significant modulators of learning and memory processes.[18] Increases in CNS sympathetic output increase respiratory rate, heart rate, and arterial blood pressure and produce sweating, piloerection, and pupillary dilation. Catecholamines are released from the adrenal medulla into the systemic circulation, amplifying these effects. Increased concentrations of circulating catecholamines augment glycogenolysis, increase gluconeogenesis, inhibit insulin release, and promote insulin resistance. Skeletal muscle blood flow generally increases out of proportion to increases in blood flow to other organ systems, preparing the animal for fight or flight. Epinephrine causes glycogenolysis and gluconeogenesis and inhibits insulin release while promoting peripheral insulin resistance and lipolysis. Thyroid hormones stimulate carbohydrate metabolism and heat production and increase and sensitize α-adrenergic receptors in the heart, thereby sensitizing it to the effects of circulating catecholamines.

Metabolism

The neurohumoral changes produced by stress increase the secretion of catabolic hormones, promoting the production of food substrates from the breakdown of carbohydrates, fats, and protein.[17] Hyperglycemia is produced and may persist because of the production of glucagon and relative lack and resistance to insulin, although insulin levels may periodically increase. Cortisol, catecholamines, and growth hormone stimulate lipolytic activity, resulting in an increase in circulating glycerol and free fatty acids. Protein catabolism is a common occurrence and a major concern after severe trauma or extensive surgical procedures. Cortisol increases protein catabolism, resulting in the release of amino acids.

Immune System

The immune system functions as a diffusely distributed sense organ that communicates injury-related information and the severity of stress to the brain. Pain therefore can modulate the immune response.[19] The key elements for determining the immune response to pain are its intensity and duration. The messengers of the immune system are cytokines (interleukin-1 [IL-1], IL-6, tumor necrosis factor α). IL-1 and IL-6 induce the release of acute phase (inflammatory) reactants, cause fever, and initiate prostaglandin production (PGE_2). Severe stress from any cause can trigger the acute phase response.[14] The main feature of the acute phase response is the release of proteins from the liver that act as inflammatory mediators and scavengers in tissue repair. These proteins include C-reactive protein, fibrinogen, macroglobulin, and antiproteinases. IL-1 and IL-6 can stimulate the secretion of ACTH from the pituitary gland and the subsequent release of cortisol. Tumor necrosis factor α produces signs of shock, including hypotension, hemoconcentration, hyperglycemia, hyperkalemia, and nonrespiratory acidosis, and activates the complement cascade. Excessive production of these proteins can contribute to systemic inflammatory response syndrome, as discussed in the chapter on gastrointestinal diseases in this text. The peripheral white blood cell count generally reflects a stress leukogram typified by an elevated number of immature polymorphonuclear leukocytes (left shift) and reduced numbers of lymphoctes. Chronic pain produces sustained increases in circulating concentrations of cortisol, epinephrine, norepinephrine, and glucagon and suppresses the humoral and cellular immune response.[17] The systemic release of endogenous opioids (endorphin and enkephalin) may contribute to immunosuppression.

Behavior and Morphology

Pain produces changes in behavior, attitude, performance, and memory. Pain activates the locus ceruleus, limbic regions (hypothalamus, hippocampus, amygdala), and cerebral cortex, which are involved in the adaptive responses to stress.[17] Pain-induced increases of corticotropin-releasing factor in the hypothalamus, amygdala, and locus ceruleus, for example, produce an increased startle response, anxiety, and fear. Corticotropin-releasing factor therefore serves as an excitatory neruotransmitter in the locus ceruleus, resulting in release of cortical norepinephrine, dopamine, and 5-hydroxytryptamine with resultant behavioral hyper-responsiveness, hyperarousal, vigilance, and agitation. Prolonged stress impairs the desire and ability of the horse to perform or learn. Chronic stress caused by pain can result in phenotypic changes that include a failure to thrive, poor hair coat, weight loss, and an acceleration of aging.

BOX 6-3

POTENTIAL BEHAVIORAL INDICATORS OF PAIN IN HORSES

- Considerable restlessness, agitation, and anxiety
- Rigid stance and reluctance to move
- Lowered head carriage
- Fixed stare and dilated nostrils, clenched jaw
- Aggression toward own foal
- Aggression toward handlers, horses, objects, and self
- Decreased interactions with handlers
- Vocalization (deep groaning, grunting)
- Rolling
- Kicking at abdomen
- Flank watching
- Stretching
- Dullness and depression
- Weight-shifting among limbs
- Limb guarding
- Abnormal weight distribution
- Pointing, hanging, and rotating limbs
- Abnormal movement
- Reluctance to move
- Arched back
- Head shaking
- Abnormal bit behavior
- Altered eating; anorexia, quidding, food pocketing

PAIN ASSESSMENT

Although truly rational therapeutic approaches cannot be developed until most, if not all, of the specific mechanisms responsible for the physiologic and pathologic causes of pain are known, the use of simple yet detailed pain-scoring systems can help categorize the intensity, duration, and location of pain, thereby suggesting potential treatments. Pain-scoring systems, however, are of little value in suggesting therapy until the evaluator has a general understanding of the behavioral changes and physiologic and pathophysiologic processes involved in the production of pain (Box 6-3; Figure 6-4).[7] This includes an understanding of the reasons for tissue hypersensitivity, peripheral sensitization, central sensitization, primary and secondary hyperalgesia, allodynia, spontaneous and referred pain, and the differences between somatic and visceral pain. All the aforementioned changes modify the gain of the pain system, leading to permanent alterations in the neurochemical regulation of the CNS and phenotypic (physical characteristics) changes.[8] One of the most challenging problems in the clinical study of pain in horses is the development of a universally accepted method of classification. The absence of a universally accepted, clinically relevant pain-scoring system has made it difficult to categorize patients, prescribe therapy, evaluate treatment, and compare research trials. Pain classification systems based on anatomy, etiology, body system, severity, duration, behavior, or cause are descriptive but do not identify the mechanisms responsible for pain and therefore do not provide the type of information required for determining effective therapy. One classification system proposes to diagnose pain on the basis of the relationship among clinical signs, tissue type, disease, and the patient's response to predefined neurobiologic criteria.[20] This approach suggests that pain should be classified as inflammatory, neuropathic, or both and that the presence of peripheral sensitization, central sensitization, allodynia, and hyposensitivity to pain be used to subcategorize patients further and guide therapeutic decisions. Application of this approach along with anatomic, etiologic, and time- and behavior-based schemes may lead to the development of more informative diagnostic methods.

DRUGS USED TO TREAT PAIN

A vast array of drug and complementary therapies are claimed to be efficacious in the treatment of pain in horses. Most evidence is anecdotal or reflects individual opinions and preferences.[1] Some therapies have been evaluated in experimental pain models (balloon colic, heat lamp, hoof nail) using otherwise normal horses, but few therapies have been subjected to blinded, randomized, controlled clinical trials, and fewer still have been evaluated in horses with spontaneous disease.[21-25, 26] Regardless, a great deal of anecdotal data suggests that many of the same drugs used to treat pain in humans, dogs, and cats should be effective for treating pain in horses. Similarly, alternative therapies such as acupuncture, chiropractic, and nutraceuticals may provide pain relief in horses when applied in the right circumstances.[2,27-31] Pharmacologic approaches for the treatment of pain in horses derive their greatest benefits when drugs are selected for specific purposes (inflammation, nerve injury), scaled to the severity of pain, and used in combination (multimodal therapy) or preemptively (Figure

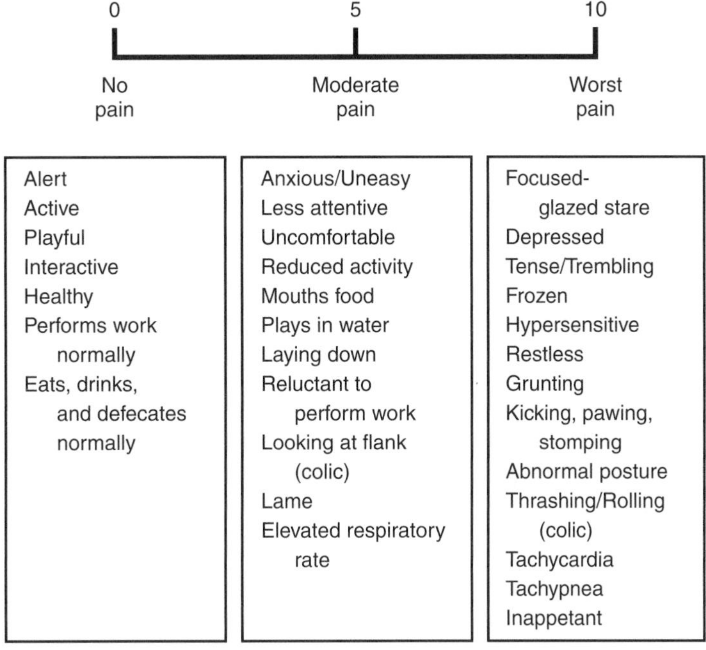

FIGURE 6-4 The visual analog scale is a simple, practical method for evaluating the severity of pain and the efficacy of therapy.

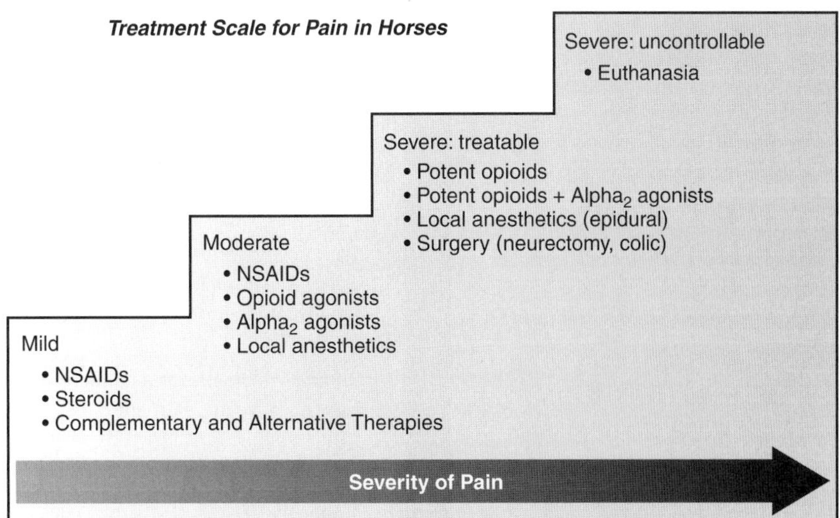

FIGURE 6-5 A drug treatment pain scale for horses. *NSAIDs,* Nonsteroidal antiinflammatory drugs.

6-5). Most drugs used to treat pain fall into one of five broad categories and include the steroidal antiinflammatory drugs, NSAIDs, opioids, α_2-adrenoceptor agonists, and local anesthetics. To this arsenal can be added an expanding list of adjunct medications that produce anticonvulsants (gabapentin, pregabalin), opioid (tramadol), or calming (acepromazine) effects[29] (Tables 6-1 to 6-3). It is important to remember that a multimodal approach to pain management is often most effective, although the potential for drug-related adverse effects may be increased (see Box 6-1).

Antiinflammatory Drugs

Antiinflammatory drugs are comparatively weak analgesics but are extremely effective for the treatment of acute inflammatory conditions.[32-38] Glucocorticosteroids produce antiinflammatory effects by inhibiting phospholipase A_2 and the breakdown of membrane phospholipids to arachadonic acid and subsequently to prostaglandins and leukotrienes (Figure 6-6).[33] Prostaglandins and leukotrienes exaggerate the inflammatory response and are key factors

TABLE 6-1

Commonly Used Analgesic Agents and Suggested Doses in Horses*

Drug	Route	Dose	Comments
ANTI-INFLAMMATORY DRUGS			
CORTICOSTEROIDS			
Dexamethosone isonicotinate	IV	0.015-0.050 mg/kg	
Hydrocortisone sodium succinate	IV	1.0-4.0 mg/kg	
Prednisolone	IV	0.25-1.0 mg/kg	
NON-STEROIDAL ANTI-INFLAMMATORY DRUGS			
Carprofen	IV	0.5 mg/kg q12-24hr	
Firocoxib	PO	0.1 mg/kg q24hr	Selective COX-2 inhibitor. Decreased risk of gastrointestinal adverse effects compared with nonselective NSAIDs. Maintain adequate hydration.
Flunixin meglumine	IV, PO	0.25 mg/kg q6hr 0.5 mg/kg q8hr 1.1 mg/kg q12hr	Adverse gastrointestinal and renal effects possible. Maintain adequate hydration. Avoid IM use if possible.
Ketoprofen	IV, IM	2.2-3.3 mg/kg q24hr	Adverse gastrointestinal and renal effects possible. Maintain adequate hydration.
Phenylbutazone	IV, PO	2.2-4.4 mg/kg q12hr	Adverse gastrointestinal and renal effects possible. Maintain adequate hydration.
OPIOIDS			
Buprenorphine	IV	0.01-0.04 mg/kg	Little information available regarding clinical use in horses.
Butorphanol	IV IM	0.01-0.05 mg/kg q4hr 0.04-0.1 mg/kg q4-6hr	Adverse effects may include increased locomotion in adult horses, sedation in foals. May increase appetite. High doses or prolonged use may decrease GI motility.
Meperidine	IV	0.2-1.0 mg/kg	
Methadone	PO	0.1-0.2 mg/kg	Used more commonly in Europe than in U.S.
Morphine	IV, IM	0.05-0.3 mg/kg	μ agonist. Adverse effects include decreased GI motility (constipation or impaction), excitation (especially when given intravenously). Combine with α2 agonists to lessen CNS effects.
α-2 AGONISTS			
Detomidine	IV, IM	0.005-0.03 mg/kg q6-12hr	Sedative; higher doses for IM use. See text for adverse effects.
Romifidine	IV	40-120 μg/kg	May provide insufficient analgesia for some procedures. See text for adverse effects.
Xylazine	IV, IM	0.2 – 1.1 mg/kg	Sedative; higher doses for IM use. See text for adverse effects.
MISCELLANEOUS AGENTS			
Gabapentin	PO	2.5-5 mg/kg q8-12hr	Originally marketed as an anticonvulsant agent. Probably most effective in treatment of neuropathic pain.
N-butylscopolamine	IV	0.3 mg/kg	Antispasmodic for GI tract disorders.

IV, Intravenous; *PO,* by mouth; *NSAIDs,* nonsteroidal anti-inflammatory drugs; *GI,* gastrointestinal; *CNS,* central nervous system.
*The dose and route of administration used for each patient must be determined on the basis of the clinical problems, systemic status of the horse, concurrent drug use, and other relevant medical factors.

in the production of peripheral sensitization. Prostaglandins (PGE_2, thromboxane A_2) activate prostaglandin receptors throughout the body, producing pain, inflammation, and fever. Prostaglandins also are responsible for producing a protective gastric barrier to intralumenal acidity, sustaining normal gastric secretory activity, and maintaining normal gut motility. Prostaglandins regulate renal blood flow and maintain normal renal tubular function. Cyclooxygenase (COX) metabolizes arachidonic acid to prostaglandins. At least two types of COX (COX-1, COX-2) exist. COX-1 is constitutive in most tissues and helps maintain normal cell and tissue function. COX-2 is constitutive in the CNS, kidney, eye, and reproductive organs and is highly inducible in inflamed tissues. COX-2 is produced by inflammatory cells and is upregulated following tissue injury. Most NSAIDs produce their antiinflammatory and analgesic effects by differentially inhibiting both COX-1 and COX-2.[33] These drugs are discussed in more detail in the pharmacology chapter of this text. Inhibition of COX-1 is believed to be responsible for mild analgesic effects and NSAID toxicity (gastrointestinal ulceration). The availability of newer NSAIDs that are more selective for COX-2 versus COX-1; (firocoxib [Equiox]) may provide COX-1–sparing effects, thereby minimizing toxic effects on the gut.[37] Future pharmacologic manipulation of NSAIDs may result in the development of drugs that effectively inhibit both the COX and lipoxygenase pathways for inflammation in horses (see Figure 6-6). It should be emphasized that all NSAIDs are nephrotoxic. Gastrointestinal, renal, or liver toxicity and the potential for delayed clotting are important issues that are more common with chronic drug administration.[36,39] NSAIDs alter platelet function and may produce blood dyscrasias in sick or hemorrhaging horses. Toxicity is more common in very young or old, dehydrated, or immunocompromised horses or in horses with preexisting cardiovascular, renal, or liver disease.

Opioids

Opioids vary widely in their analgesic potency, clinical efficacy, and adverse effects.[40-44] Opioid agonist-antagonists and partial agonists produce μ-receptor or morphinelike effects and are in general less toxic but less potent analgesics than morphine.[44] Opioid antagonists are relatively devoid of agonist activity and are used clinically to antagonize or reverse opioid effects. Morphine is considered the prototypic opioid to which all other opioids are compared.[45,46] Opioids produce their effects by activating opioid receptors (μ, κ, δ).[47] Most opioids produce beneficial (analgesic, euphoric) pharmacologic effects by activating central and peripheral μ-receptors, although evidence indicates that drugs with κ-receptor activity may be equally or more effective in treating gastrointestinal pain.[43,46] Butorphanol, an opioid agonist-antagonist with κ-receptor activity, for example, is excellent for the treatment of mild to moderate visceral pain.[40,44,48,49] The beneficial properties of opioids, however, are overshadowed by the requirement for special licensing and record keeping; the occasional development of ileus, constipation, and colic (morphine); and the potential for all opioids and especially μ-opioid agonists to produce excitement (increased locomotor activity), disorientation, and ataxia in horses. Opioids delay gastric emptying and prolong intestinal transit time.[43] Increases in intestinal smooth muscle tone are caused by centrally mediated increases in vagal tone and activation of opioid receptors throughout the gastrointestinal tract. These effects are followed by a decrease in propulsive peristaltic activity and absorption of water from the intestinal lumen, predisposing horses to constipation and colic from impaction of the colon, a condition that becomes more prominent when opioids are administered for several

TABLE 6-2

Neuroleptanolagesic Combinations for Intravenous Use in Horses

Drug	Dose
Acepromazine Butorphanol	0.05-1.0 mg/kg 0.05-0.1 mg/kg
Acepromazine Burpenorphine	0.05-1.0 mg/kg 0.005-0.01 mg/kg
Acepromazine Xylazine	0.05-1.0 mg/kg 0.2-0.5 mg/kg
Xylazine Butorphanol	0.5-1.0 mg/kg 0.01-0.05 mg/kg
Xylazine Morphine	0.5-1.0 mg/kg 0.1-0.5 mg/kg

TABLE 6-3

Drugs by Continuous Rate Infusion for Analgesia in Horses.

Drug	Route	Dose	Comments
Lidocaine	CRI	Bolus 1.3 mg/kg; then 0.05 mg/kg/min	Overdose may result in seizures, CNS excitation. May be used for several days.
Detomidine	CRI	Bolus 8.4 μg/kg; then 0.5 μg/kg/min for 15 min; then 0.3 μg/kg/min for 15 min; then 0.15 μg/kg min thereafter	Will cause sedation, ataxia. For sedation and analgesia of 1-4 hr; not for long-term (days) use.
Butorphanol	CRI	Bolus 17.8 μg/kg; then 10-15 μg/kg/hr	Tolerance may develop; usually used for 12-24 hr.
Ketamine	CRI	0.4-1.2 mg/kg/hr	Ataxia and sensitivity to sound possible at higher doses.

CRI, Constant rate infusion; *CNS,* central nervous system.

days. Large or repeated doses of opioids can inhibit the urinary voiding reflex and increase external urethral sphincter tone, resulting in urine retention. Urine retention can be an important postoperative consideration in horses that have received large volumes of fluids during surgery and results in discomfort, agitation, and premature attempts to stand in horses recovering from anesthesia. Recommended dosages of opioids can produce sympathetic activation (sweating, mydriasis), nervousness, increased locomotor activity, agitation, and dysphoria in some horses.[47,50] These latter effects (excitement, disorientation, ataxia) are particularly troublesome when repeated dosages of μ-opioid agonists are administered to young, untrained, or fractious horses. Opioids, especially morphine, produce profound analgesic effects when combined with α_2-agonists (xylazine, detomidine).[51] The combination of opioids and α_2-agonists (morphine, butorphanol, and xylazine, detomidine, romifidine) produces neuroleptanalgesia and has been administered preemptively to perform standing medical and surgical procedures that otherwise would require general anesthesia.[51-53] Fentanyl is a particularly potent μ-opioid agonist with a short duration of action, making its clinical use impractical unless administered by constant rate infusion to horses in pain (severe colic, laminitis).[54] Alternatively, a fentanyl transdermal drug-delivery system (patch) is available, but clinical experience is limited, adequate or effective blood plasma concentrations may not be attained, and adverse effects such as agitation and tachycardia may occur with higher doses. Furthermore, it may be necessary to replace the patches every 24 hours in horses to maintain analgesia.

As previously suggested, different opioids produce their pharmacologic effects on the basis of their ability to combine with and differentially activate opioid receptors. Very little is known about opioid receptor distribution, density, and selectivity in horses compared with other species. Furthermore, the potential for opioids to produce CNS agitation, increased locomotor acitivty, and inhibitory gastrointestinal effects when used alone or in combination with other sedatives or inhalant anesthesia may limit their potential usefulness as analgesics.[47,50,55] Finally, there are few comparative studies or large-scale randomized, controlled, and blinded multicenter clinical trials evaluating the efficacy of opioids in horses with naturally occurring disease, making their clinical use a trial-and-error process.[26,41,48]

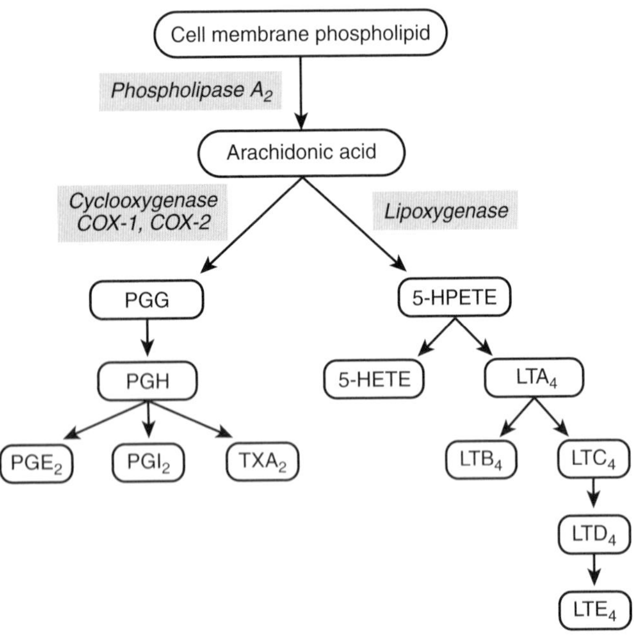

FIGURE 6-6 Tissue or nerve injury damages cell membranes, leading to the production of arachadonic acid, prostaglandins, and leukotrienes through the activity of phospholipase A_2, cylcooxygenase, or lipoxygenase enzymes, respectively. These enzymatic pathways are important for producing inflammation and pain. They can be inhibited by corticosteroids, nonsteroidal antiinflammatory drugs (NSAIDS), and lipoxygenase inhibitors.

α_2-Agonists

α_2-Agonists (xylazine, detomidine, medetomidine, romifidine) produce sedation, muscle relaxation, and analgesia by activating various α_2-receptors in the CNS and peripherally.[56] Sedation is attributed to activation of the CNS α_2- receptors in areas of the brain that are responsible for awareness, arousal, and vigilance. Activation of α_2-receptors in the brain and spinal cord decreases the release of excitatory neurotransmitters and interferes with sensory processing and transmission.[56] Individual drug effects vary according to chemical structure, α_2 versus α_1 selectivity, metabolism, and elimination. Xylazine is considered the prototypic α_2-agonist and demonstrates a comparatively low α_2-receptor selectivity and short half-life. Xylazine also produces local anesthetic effects, presumably because of its structural similarity to lidocaine. Analgesia is confounded, however, by mild to significant sedation that can result in stupor, ataxia, and reluctance to move. These effects may be beneficial but can mask clinical signs in horses suffering from colic.[34,48,57] Regardless, α_2-agonists are particularly effective therapy for the acute treatment of moderate to severe pain (colic) and can be administered by infusion to treat acute injuries or intraoperatively to reduce injectable or inhalant anesthetic requirements.[42,,56] α_2-Agonists are particularly effective when administered with opioids (butorphanol, morphine) or acepromazine.[51,53,58] The effects of α_2-agonists can be antagonized by the α_2-antagonists yohimbine, tolazoline, and atipamezole.

Clinically, the administration of α_2-agonists typically produces profound sedation, bradycardia, respiratory depression, and occasionally unexpected or aggressive behavior. Sinus bradycardia and bradyarrhythmias are common after the administration of α_2-agonists. Decreases in heart rate and atrioventricular block are caused by the combined effects of decreases in CNS sympathetic output and increases in vagal tone.[59] Atropine or glycopyrrolate can help prevent bradycardia and atrioventricular block but generally are not required. Arterial blood pressure initially increases and then decreases from baseline values. Arterial hypertension is initiated by stimulation of peripheral vascular α_1- and α_2-receptors and increases in baroreceptor activity. The subsequent decrease in arterial blood pressure is caused by a decrease in CNS sympathetic output and heart rate.[56,60] Cardiac output decreases almost immediately in conjunction with decreases in heart rate.[59] Respiratory rate and tidal volume decrease as the horse becomes sedate and may contribute to the development of respiratory acidosis and hypoxemia. Relaxation of the muscles of the nostrils, pharynx, and larynx can result in respiratory stridor, snoring, irregular breathing patterns, inspiratory dyspnea, and upper airway obstruction in some horses, particularly those with upper airway disease.

α_2-Agonists produce immediate and pronounced decreases in gastrointestinal tone and motility that can be pronounced and last for 8 to 10 hours.[61-63] Gastrointestinal stasis is caused by stimulation of α_2-receptors in the gut and increases in serum gastrin concentration. The decrease in gut motility is dose dependent but is believed to be responsible for postoperative ileus, gas accumulation, and the occasional development of colic in some horses and may require the administration of an α_2-antagonist (yohimbine).[64] α_2-Agonists promote diuresis in horses by increasing blood pressure and producing direct actions on the renal tubules to decrease renal tubular salt and water absorption. Labor can be delayed or prolonged because of sedative and muscle relaxant effects.[65]

Local Anesthetics

Local anesthetics (lidocaine, mepivacaine) are frequently used alone or in combination with other analgesic drugs to produce a loss of sensation. They are administered at specific sites (topical, local) or on nerves (regional). Analgesia results from blockade of sodium ion channels, thereby preventing the initiation and conduction of electric activity (action potentials) in small-diameter (C, Aδ) sensory nerve fibers. Larger (clinical) dosages of local anesthetics also block electric activity in large fibers (Aβ), thereby producing loss of motor function and temporary motor paralysis. Most local anesthetic drugs produce mild CNS depression with antiarrhythmic, antishock, and gastrointestinal promotility effects.[43,66-69] They can be administered epidurally and systemically to decrease the need for additional analgesics (Table 6-4).[43,66] The systemic infusion of lidocaine decreases the requirement for inhalant (isoflurane, sevoflurane) or injectable (ketamine, propofol) anesthetics (anesthetic sparing) and potentiates the analgesic actions of opioids or α_2-agonists.[65,67] Mild sedation occurs because of membrane-stabilizing effects, a generalized decrease in neuronal activity, and a centrally mediated decrease in sympathetic tone. Local anesthetics have the potential to produce a loss of motor function (paralysis) that can become problematic in some surgical patients (rectal-vaginal fistula repair), leading to untoward behavioral responses. Local anesthetics produce minimal cardiovascular or respiratory effects in otherwise normal, healthy horses but can decrease cardiac output, arterial blood pressure, and heart rate when administered intravenously because of decreases in CNS sympathetic output, myocardial contractile force, and venous return.[65,67] These effects are more prominent in stressed or sick animals that depend on sympathetic nervous system activity for maintaining homeostasis. Although local anesthetics are considered to have antiarrhythmic effects, they can produce sinus bradycardia and bradyarrhythmias and hypotension when administered rapidly and intravenously. Significant differences exist among the various local anesthetics regarding these effects and their metabolism, elimination, and potential to produce CNS toxicity (disorientation, ataxia, seizures).[69] Horses are comparatively sensitive to the neurotoxic side effects of local anesthetics, and bolus dosages exceeding 2 mg/kg usually produce CNS stimulation typified by nervousness, excitement, agitation, disorientation, nystagmus, and seizures. These effects can result in death from respiratory paralysis. Local anesthetic drugs can produce respiratory paralysis when administered by epidural or spinal (subarachnoidal) routes. The migration of the local anesthetic cranially to the sixth cervical nerve roots

TABLE 6-4

Drugs Used for Epidural Analgesia

Drug	Dose (mg/kg)	Duration of effect	Comments
CAUDAL EPIDURAL ANALGESIA (FIRST COCCYGEAL SPACE)			
Lidocaine		30-90 min	Ataxia or recumbency at higher doses.
Xylazine	0.03-0.35	3-5 hr	Perineal sweating is common.
Detomidine	0.06	2-3 hr	Sedation, ataxia, systemic effects.
Ketamine	0.1-2.0	30-90 min	
COMBINATIONS FOR CAUDAL EPIDURAL ANALGESIA (FIRST COCCYGEAL SPACE)			
Lidocaine Xylazine	0.22 0.17	5-6 hr	Ataxia or recumbency; perineal sweating.
Lidocaine Butorphanol	0.25 0.04	2.5 hr	Ataxia or recumbency.
LUMBOSACRAL EPIDURAL ANALGESIA (VIA CATHETER)			
Morphine	0.1-0.2 q8-18hr	8-24 hr	May cause skin wheals, pruritis.
Detomidine	0.03-0.06 q20-24hr	8-24 hr	May cause sedation, ataxia.
Ketamine	0.8		
COMBINATIONS FOR LUMBOSACRAL EPIDURAL ANALGESIA (VIA CATHETER)			
Morphine Detomidine	0.1 0.03 mg/kg	8-24 hr	Sedation, ataxia possible.
Ketamine Morphine	0.5 – 1.0 0.1	12-18 hr	Sedation, mild ataxia.
Ketamine Xylazine	0.5 – 1.0 0.2	>2 hr	Mild sedation, bradycardia.

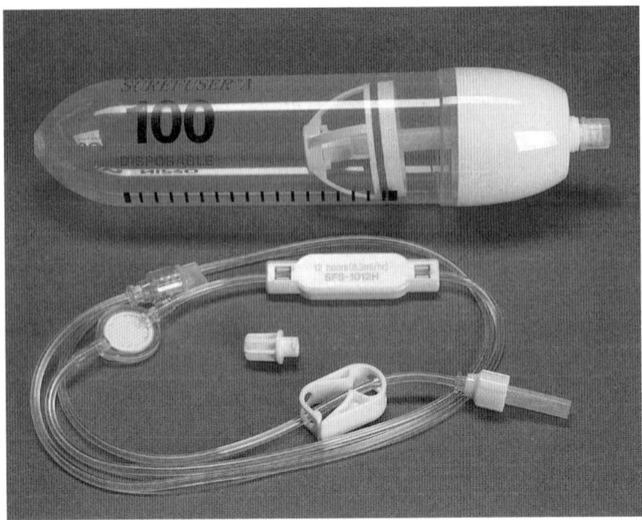

FIGURE 6-7 Photograph of a 100-ml balloon infuser and solution administration tubing with inline filter and fluid rate (8.3 ml/hr) controller (ReCathCo, LLC; Allison Park, PA: info@recathco.com).

can paralyze the diaphragm, resulting in hypoventilation and apnea.

Nontraditional Analgesics

New techniques (chiropractic) and drugs (gabapentin) are being evaluated for the treatment of acute and chronic pain in horses. New methods for continuous intravenous and, more important, peripheral site (local) drug administration are emerging (Figure 6-7). Anticonvlusants (gabapentin) and behavior-modifying drugs (chloripramine) have been administered to horses to produce adjunctive analgesic effects, but their efficacy and safety are unknown.[70-71] Alternative therapies such as acupuncture, chiropractic, and nutraceuticals are used to treat pain in horses as adjuncts to various drug regimens.[72] Several of these therapies are considered effective pain therapy by clinical experts, but most have not been evaluated carefully.[2,27-31]

REFERENCES

1. Price J, Marques JM, Welsh EM, et al: Pilot epidemiological study of attitudes towards pain in horses, *Vet Res* 151:570, 2002.
2. Gaynor GJ, Muir WW: *Handbook of veterinary pain management*, St Louis, 2002, Mosby.
3. Muir WW: Anaesthesia and pain management in horses, *Equine Vet Educ* 10:335, 1998.
4. Muir WW, Woolf CJ: Mechanisms of pain and their therapeutic implications, *J Am Vet Med Assoc* 219:1346, 2001.
5. Woolf CJ, Chong MS: Preemptive analgesia: treating postoperative pain by preventing the establishment of central sensitization, *Anesth Analg* 77:362, 1993.
6. Mersky R, Bogduk N: *Classification of chronic pain*, ed 2, Elsevier House, Brookville Plaza, East Park Co, Shannon Clare, Ireland, 1994, IASP Press.
7. Woolf CJ, Decosted I: Implications of recent advances in the understanding of pain pathophysiology for the assessment of pain in patients, *Pain Suppl* 6:S141, 1999.
8. Woolf CJ, Salter MW: Neuronal plasticity: increasing the gain in pain, *Science* 288:1765, 2000.
9. Dirls J, Moiniche S, Holsted KL, et al: Mechanisms of postoperative pain: clinical indications for a contribution of central neuronal sensitization, *Anesthesiol* 97:1591, 2002.
10. Coderre TJ, Katz J, Vaccarino AL, et al: Contribution of central neuroplasticity to pathological pain: review of clinical and experimental evidence, *Pain* 52:259, 1993.
11. Woolf CJ: A new strategy for the treatment of inflammatory pain: prevention or elimination of central sensitization, *Drugs* 47(suppl 5):1, 1994.
12. Blackshaw LA, Gabhart GF: The pharmacology of gastrointestinal nociceptive pathways, *Curr Opin Pharmacol* 2:642, 2002.
13. Bueno L, Fioramonti J, Delvaux M, et al: Mediators and pharmacology of visceral sensitivity: from basic to clinical investigations, *Gastroenterol* 112:1714, 1997.
14. Weissman C: The metabolic response to stress: an overview and update, *Anesthesiol* 73:308, 1999.
15. Taylor PM: Equine stress response to anaesthesia, *Br J Anaesth* 63:702, 1989.
16. Chapman CR, Garvin J: Suffering: the contributions of persistent pain, *Lancet* 353:2233, 1999.
17. Carstens E, Moberg GP: Recognizing pain and distress in laboratory animals, *ILAR J* 41:62, 2000.
18. Charney DS, Grillon C, Bremner JD: The neurobiological basis of anxiety and fear: circuits, mechanisms, and neurochemical interactions (part 1), *Neuroscientist* 4:35, 1998.
19. Chapman RC, Nakamura Y: A passion of the soul: an introduction to pain for consciousness researchers, *Conscious Cogn* 8:391, 1999.
20. Woolf CJ, Max MB: Mechanism-based pain diagnosis, *Anesthesiol* 95:241, 2001.
21. Higgins AJ, Lees P, Wright JA: Tissue-cage model for the collection of inflammatory exudate in ponies, *Res Vet Sci* 36:284, 1984.
22. Kamerling SG, Weckman TJ, Dequick DJ, et al: A method for studying cutaneous pain perception and analgesia in horses, *J Pharmacol Methods* 13:267, 1985.
23. Lowe JE, Hintz HF, Schryver HF: A new technique for long-term cecal fistulation in ponies, *Am J Vet Res* 31:1109, 1970.
24. Pippi NL, Lumb WV: Objective tests of analgesic drugs in ponies, *Am J Vet Res* 40:1082, 1979.
25. Chan WW, Chen KY, Liu H, et al: Acupuncture for general veterinary practice, *J Vet Med Sci* 63:1057, 2001.
26. Sullivan KA, Hill AE, Haussler KK: The effects of chiropractic, massage and phenylbutazone on spinal mechanical nociceptive thresholds in horses without clinical signs, *Equine Vet J* 40(1):14-20, 2008.
27. Haussler KK: Back problems: chiropractic evaluation and management, *Vet Clin N Am Equine Pract* 15:195, 1999.
28. Peck LS: Clarifying convention session on alternative therapies, *J Am Vet Med Assoc* 217:1458, 2000.
29. Skarda RT, Muir WW: Comparison of electroacupuncture and butorphanol on respiratory and cardiovascular effects and rectal pain threshold after controlled rectal distention in mares, *Am J Vet Res* 64:137, 2003.
30. Fleming P: Nontraditional approaches to pain management, *Vet Clin N Am Equine Pract* 18:83, 2002.
31. DeQuick D, Chay S, Kamerling S, et al: Pain perception in the horse and its control by medication: an overview. *Proceedings of the Fifth Annual International Conference on the Control of the Use of Drugs in Racehorses*, Toronto, 1983, Canada, p. 50.
32. Harkins JD, Carney JM, Tobin T: Clinical use and characteristics of the corticosteroids, *Vet Clin N Am Equine Pract* 9:543, 1993.
33. Hay WP, Moore JN: Management of pain in horses with colic, *Compendium* 19:987, 1997.
34. Kamerling S, DeQuick D, Crisman T, et al: Phenylbutazone: lack of effect on normal cutaneous pain perception in the horse. *Proceedings of the Fifth Annual International Conference on the Control of the Use of Drugs in Racehorses*, Toronto, 1983, Canada, p. 85.
35. Moore JN: Nonsteroidal anti-inflammatory drug therapy for endotoxemia: we're doing the right thing, aren't we?, *Compendium* 11:741, 1989.

36. Owens JG, Kamerling SG, Stanton SR, et al: Effects of ketoprofen and phenylbutazone on chronic hoof pain and lameness in the horse, *Equine Vet J* 27:296, 1995.
37. Doucet MY, Bertone AL, Hendrickson D, et al: Comparison of efficacy and safety of paste formulations of firocoxib and phenylbutazone in horses with naturally occurring osteoarthritis, *J Am Vet Med Assoc.* 1:232:91-97, 2008.
38. Masferrer JL, Isakson PC, Seibert K: Cyclooxygenase-2 inhibitors: a new class of anti-inflammatory agents that spare the gastrointestinal tract, *Gastroenterol Clin N Am* 25:363, 1996.
39. Van Hoogmoed LM, Snyder JR, Harmon FA: In vitro investigation of the effects of cyclooxygenase-2 inhibitors on contractile activity of the equine dorsal and ventral colon, *Am J Vet Res* 63:1496, 2002.
40. Kalpravidh M, Lumb WV, Wright M, et al: Analgesic effects of butorphanol in horses: dose-response studies, *Am J Vet Res* 45:211, 1984.
41. Kalpravidh M, Lumb WV, Wright M, et al: Effects of butorphanol, flunixin, levorphanol, morphine, and xylazine in ponies, *Am J Vet Res* 45:217, 1984.
42. Bennett RC, Steffey EP: Use of opioids for pain and anesthetic management in horses, *Vet Clin N Am Equine Pract* 18:47-60, 2002.
43. Robinson EP, Natalini CC: Epidural anesthesia and analgesia in horses, *Vet Clin N Am Equine Pract* 18:61-82, 2002.
44. Muir WW, Robertson JT: Visceral analgesia: effects of xylazine, butorphanol, meperidine and pentazocine in horses, *Am J Vet Res* 46:2081, 1985.
45. Combie J, Blake JW, Ramey BE, et al: Pharmacology of narcotic analgesics in the horse: quantitative detection of morphine in equine blood and urine and logit-log transformations of this data, *Am J Vet Res* 42:1523, 1981.
46. Combie J, Nugent TE, Tobin T: Pharmacokinetics and protein binding of morphine in horses, *Am J Vet Res* 44:870, 1983.
47. Combie J, Shults T, Nugent EC, et al: Pharmacology of narcotic analgesics in the horse: selective blockade of narcotic-induced locomotor activity, *Am J Vet Res* 42:716, 1981.
48. Jochle W, Moore JN, Brown J, et al: Comparison of detomidine, butorphanol, flunixin meglumine and xylazine in clinical cases of equine colic, *Equine Vet J Suppl* 7:111, 1989.
49. Sellon DC, Monroe VL, Roberts MC, et al: Pharmacokinetics and adverse effects of butorphanol administered by single intravenous injection or continuous intravenous infusion in horses, *Am J Vet Res* 62:183, 2001.
50. Nugent TE, Combie JD, Weld JM, et al: Effects of enkephalins versus opiates on locomotor activity of the horse, *Res Commun Chem Pathol Pharmacol* 35:405, 1982.
51. Robertson JT, Muir WW: A new analgesic drug combination in the horse, *Am J Vet Res* 44:1667, 1983.
52. Muir WW, Skarda RT, Sheehan W: Cardiopulmonary effects of narcotic agonists and a partial agonist in horses, *Am J Vet Res* 39:1632, 1978.
53. Muir WW, Skarda RT, Sheehan W: Hemodynamic and respiratory effects of xylazine-morphine sulfate in horses, *Am J Vet Res* 40:1417, 1979.
54. Kamerling SG, DeQuick DJ, Weckman TJ, et al: Dose-related effects of fentanyl on autonomic and behavioral responses in performance horses, *Gen Pharmacol* 16:253, 1985.
55. Steffey EP, Eisele JH, Baggot JD: Interactions of morphine and isoflurane in horses, *Am J Vet Res* 64:166, 2003.
56. England GCW, Clarke KW: Alpha$_2$ adrenoceptor agonists in the horse: a review, *Br Vet J* 152:641, 1996.
57. Lowe JE, Hilfiger J: Analgesic and sedative effects of detomidine compared to xylazine in a colic model using IV and IM routes of administration, *Acta Vet Scand* 82:85, 1986.
58. Muir WW, Skarda RT, Sheehan W: Hemodynamic and respiratory effects of a xylazine-acetylpromazine drug combination in horses, *Am J Vet Res* 40:1518, 1979.
59. Wagner AE, Muir WW, Hinchcliff KW: Cardiovascular effectsof xylazine and detomidine in horses, *Am J Vet Res* 52:651, 1991.
60. Kamerling SG, Cravens WMT, Bagwell CA: Dose-related effects of detomidine on autonomic responses in the horse, *J Auton Pharmacol* 8:241, 1988.
61. Lester GD, Merritt AM, Neuwirty L, et al: Effect of α2-adrenergic, cholinergic, and nonsteriodal anti-inflammatory drugs on myoelectric activity of ileum, cecum, and right ventral colon and on cecal emptying of radiolabeled markers in clinically normal ponies, *Am J Vet Res* 58:320, 1998.
62. Merritt AM, Burrows JA, Mstat H: Effect of xylazine, detomidine, and a combination of xylazine and butorphanol on equine duodenal motility, *Am J Vet Res* 59:619, 1998.
63. Sutton DG, Preston T, Christley RM, et al: The effects of xylazine, detomidine, acepromazine and butorphanol on equine solid phase gastric emptying rate, *Equine Vet J* 34:486, 2002.
64. Grubb TL, Muir WW, Bertone AL, et al: Use of yohimbine to reverse prolonged effects of xylazine hydrochloride in a horse being treated with chloramphenicol, *J Am Vet Med Assoc* 210:1771, 1997.
65. Nuñez E, Steffey EP, Ocampo L, Rodriguez A, Garcia AA: Effects of alpha$_2$-adrenergic receptor agonists on urine production in horses deprived of food and water, *Am J Vet Res* 65(10):1342-1346, 2004.
66. Doherty TJ, Frazier DL: Effect of intravenous lidocaine on halothane minimum alveolar concentration in ponies, *Equine Vet J* 30:300, 1998.
67. Robertson SA, Sanchez LC, Merritt AM, Doherty TJ: Effect of systemic lidocaine on visceral and somatic nociception in conscious horses, *Equine Vet J* 37:122-127, 2005.
68. Harkins JD, Mundy GD, Woods WE, et al: Lidocaine in the horse: its pharmacological effects and their relationship to analytical findings, *J Vet Pharmacol Ther* 21:462, 1998.
69. Harkins JD, Stanley S, Mundy GD, et al: A review of the pharmacology, pharmacokinetics, and regulatory control in the US of local anaesthetics in the horse, *J Vet Pharmacol Ther* 18:397, 1995.
70. Davis JL, Posner LP, Elce Y: Gabapentin for the treatment of neuropathic pain in a pregnant horse, *J Am Vet Med Assoc* 231:755-758, 2007.
71. Turner RM, McDonnell SM, Hawkins JF: Use of pharmacologically induced ejaculation to obtain semen from a stallion with a fractured radius, *J Am Vet Med Assoc.* 206:1906-1908, 1995.

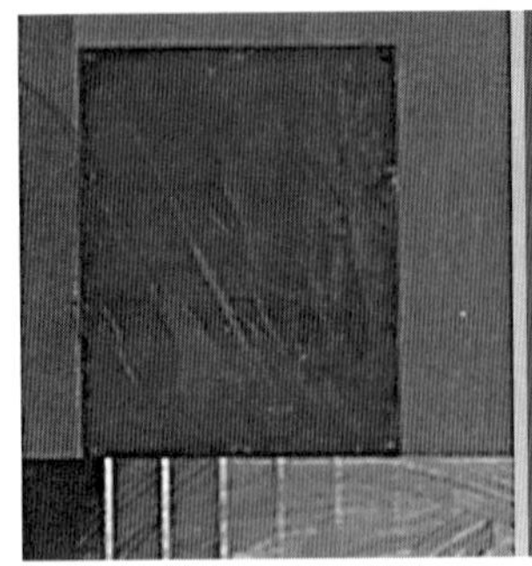

Critical Care

CHAPTER

7

APPROACH TO EQUINE CRITICAL CARE

Peggy S. Marsh

Critical care is provided in disease states of crisis or extreme complexity and involves thoughtful judgment and timely intervention. Typically, acute life-threatening conditions require this type of care. Because of the intricate, time-consuming, and often urgent nature of such situations, specially trained personnel are often best suited to deliver optimal care. This type of care is generally needed for days, rather than just a few minutes or hours, and therefore a team of health care providers is required. The provision of optimal diagnostic and monitoring alternatives is facilitated by access to a wide range of equipment. Segregating patients that need immediate as well as continuous attention in a particular area of a hospital or clinic, such as an intensive care unit (ICU), allows better use of resources. However, these are not absolute requirements for providing critical care. Adherence to a foundation principle that calls for serial evaluations of the entire patient, with particular attention to maintaining or restoring homeostasis for that individual, is at the heart of critical care medicine.

In equine practice there are no definitive universal guidelines to identify patients that would benefit from being treated in a centralized ICU by a team of specialized health care providers. In human medicine various studies have evaluated the potential benefits of such care. Most have shown increased efficiency, shorter duration of stay, and sometimes decreased cost when critical care patients are treated in a central hospital unit and managed by a specialized team of health care providers. The decision as to which equine patients would benefit from such care is based on a wide variety of criteria, including type of illness or trauma, degree of illness, availability of personnel and facilities, biosecurity measures, cost, and client preference. In veterinary medicine there is no clear evidence demonstrating when such care might improve outcome and efficiency or reduce cost.

*The editors acknowledge and appreciate the contributions of Joanne Hardy, a former editor of this chapter. Her original work has been incorporated into this edition.

Even with a wide range of inciting problems, there are some aspects of critical care medicine that are common in all critically ill individuals. Therapeutic goals for all patients include providing appropriate care for the primary problems, anticipating complications and initiating appropriate preventive therapy, and providing appropriate supportive care for all vital body systems.

The purpose of this chapter is to provide an outline of therapeutic guidelines for use in equine patients with life-threatening medical problems or patients with complex disease processes that simultaneously involve multiple body systems. Diagnosis and therapy of many specific critical care topics are covered in more detail in other chapters of this book, and the reader will be referred to the relevant chapters as appropriate. The goal for this chapter is to outline an approach to the entire patient and all body systems that will facilitate creation of an action plan to help restore systemic function in the critically ill equine patient.

EQUINE INTENSIVE CARE UNIT

Comprehensive care for critically ill horses can be provided anywhere, with some creativity and a large commitment of time; however, it can be argued that moving such patients to a hospital setting with experienced clinicians and a variety of diagnostic and therapeutic equipment allows for better use of resources and improved care. Equine ICUs are becoming increasingly prevalent in clinical practice. Common features include housing of patients according to type or severity of illness with appropriate biosecurity precautions; readily available equipment for diagnosing, monitoring, and treating the seriously compromised horse; and 24-hour staffing with professionals who have the knowledge and experience to treat these patients. The goals of these units are to pool resources, thereby increasing efficiency and reducing cost, and to improve patient outcomes.

The decision to offer ICU services should be based on the population needs and the economic environment of the hospital and community. Several recent studies describe the general case population and commonly performed procedures and treatments of patients admitted on an emergency basis to large university referral centers.[1,2] Because equine emergencies are relatively common among patients requiring critical care, such information provides an initial database for understanding population dynamics. In general, these studies revealed that although acute abdominal crisis is the most common type of case encountered, many cases will not require surgical intervention. Also, a variety of other problems presented as emergencies, and the required skills to deal with these included experience with dysfunction of most all body systems. Reviewing the anticipated distribution of cases within a given area, as well as the monthly distribution of cases, is important. Such reviews ensure an appropriate allocation of staff and equipment tailored to the needs of the population.

Human ICU treatment requires a multidisciplinary team that includes intensivists (i.e., physicians who specialize in critical illness care), nurses, respiratory care therapists, dieticians, pharmacists, and other consultants from a broad range of specialties, such as surgery, internal medicine, and anesthesiology. Compared with human medicine, the number of equine cases is limited and is handled without the same degree of clinician specialization. The most common advanced training programs in equine practice are anesthesia, internal medicine, and surgery. Individuals trained in these areas typically have experience with critically ill equine patients. More recently, specialty training in the area of equine emergency and critical care has been developed. Although the care of many extremely sick horses is performed in the general practice setting, it is useful to know that the number of veterinarians with extensive experience and specialty training in the area of critical care is growing.

Besides clinicians, intensive and continuous care usually is provided by licensed veterinary technicians. In general, good nursing care is pivotal to successful outcomes. The technical staff should be trained to identify subtle changes in patient status and feel comfortable using a range of equipment. The ability to perform common techniques and to recognize changes in condition early is essential.

The equipment used for the care of critically ill equine patients should be based on the anticipated case population and the maximal level of care required for that population. Purchasing a ventilator would be a poor economic decision if mechanical ventilation is performed rarely. Renting medical equipment that might be needed only occasionally or seasonally may be a more practical choice. Box 7-1 lists some equipment to consider when equipping an equine ICU. Regular review of equipment and training for all personnel on new equipment are essential.

Commonly performed procedures in equine critical care include monitoring, fluid administration, and pain control. Monitoring includes not only close, astute observation and serial physical examinations but also the use of appropriate equipment and laboratory support to monitor systemic health as appropriate for that patient. Fluid administration encompasses routine administration of a wide range of products, including crystalloids, synthetic colloids, blood, and blood substitutes. The selection of appropriate analgesia may vary widely depending on the origin of pain (e.g., musculoskeletal versus abdominal) and the possible adverse effects of different medications. All of these considerations should be based on the specific needs of the equine patient.

Emergency drugs should be readily available and mobile, possibly in a crash cart or box in the ICU. Table 7-1 lists several emergency drugs and dosages used in adult horses. Keeping a specific list such as this one readily available in the crash cart for easy reference is advisable. In addition, assembling packs for specific anticipated emergency situations, such as all the necessary items for delivering supplemental oxygen or supplies to perform an urgent tracheotomy, and placing these packs in key areas are recommended.

BOX 7-1

EQUIPMENT LIST FOR DIFFERENT LEVELS OF EQUINE INTENSIVE CARE UNITS

Basic
- Fluid administration system
- Electrocardiogram
- Centrifuge
- Refractometer
- Glucose strips
- Urinalysis strips
- Ultrasound
- Oxygen tank and regulator

Intermediate
- Blood pressure monitor
- Cytologic exam/Gram stain
- Glucometer
- Intravenous fluid pump delivery systems
- Sling and hoist for down horses

Advanced
- Blood gas/electrolyte analyzer
- Pulse oximeter
- Mechanical ventilator
- Colloid osmometer
- Capnograph
- Syringe infusion pumps

Monitoring equipment commonly used in an ICU includes an electrocardiogram, a blood pressure monitor, a stallside glucometer and a lactate analyzer, a stallside electrolyte and chemistry analyzer, an ultrasound unit, a centrifuge for hematocrit determination, a refractometer for determining total protein and urine specific gravity, and urine test strips for urinalysis. Other monitoring tools to consider are a microscope with 100× magnification, equipment for cytological examination (including Gram stains), and a blood gas and electrolyte monitoring unit. A colloid osmometer is useful for determining colloid oncotic pressure in sick horses. If mechanical ventilation is routine, further monitoring units, including capnographs and pulse oximeters, are useful. Standard operating protocol should be established for each piece of equipment, and regular maintenance should be performed.

Advanced imaging is becoming more common, and the use of ultrasound has become an essential component of diagnosing and monitoring critically ill patients. Ultrasound can be used for identifying and monitoring effusions, intestinal distention, and motility; identifying umbilical structures; monitoring pregnancy; and visualizing ocular structures, among other anatomic areas. To enable imaging of a wide variety of structures, access to a variety of transducers ranging from 2.5 to 10 MHz, as well as a rectal probe, is recommended.

Oxygen ports for supplementation through nasal insufflation or for mechanical ventilation should be available. When installing a new ICU, the practitioner should consider placements of ports for oxygen, vacuum, and air, as well as a remote gas source and a pipeline system to allow delivery of oxygen. Compressed gas cylinders can be used, but these must be stored

TABLE 7-1

Emergency Drug Chart for Adult Horses

Drug	Dose	Dose per 1000 lb	Route	Comment
Dobutamine (positive inotrope)	2-10 μg/kg/min (1vial [250 mg] in 1000 ml = 250 μg/ml)	900-4500 μg/min	IV	Use diluted solution within 24 hours. It is compatible with most IV fluids. Do not mix with alkaline solution calcium chloride/gluconate.
Doxapram (respiratory stimulant)	0.2 mg/kg	4.5 ml	IV or topical under tongue	Do not mix with alkaline drugs/fluid.
Epinephrine (for anaphylaxis or asystole)	0.01-0.02 mg/kg; 0.1-0.5 mg/kg	4.5-9 ml	IV/IM/SQ/Intratracheal	Do not give with bicarbonate, hypertonic saline, or aminophylline. It does not need to be diluted when given intravenously to adults.
Glycopyrrolate (for bronchodilation and bradycardia)	0.005-0.01 mg/kg	10-20 ml	IV/IM/SQ	Do not mix with alkaline drugs/fluids.
Lidocaine (treatment of ileus)	1.3 mg/kg loading slowly over 5 minutes 0.05 mg/kg/min infusion	Loading: 30 ml Infusion: 67 ml/hr	IV	Ensure that product does not contain epinephrine.
Lidocaine (treatment of arrhythmias)	Bolus: 0.25-0.5 mg/kg (slowly) Infusion: 20-50 μg/kg/min	Bolus: 5-10 ml Infusion: 30-60 ml/hr	IV	Ensure that product does not contain epinephrine.

IV, Intravenous; IM, intramuscula; *SQ*, subcutaneous

and handled appropriately to prevent injury. For each cylinder type, knowledge of the capacity of the cylinder and the flow rate enables calculation of the amount of time provided. The small portable E cylinders contain 655 L of oxygen when full and can provide oxygen for 260 minutes when set at a flow rate of 5 L/min. Adult horses may require flow rates of 10 to 15 L/min to have any significant effect on the fraction of oxygen inspired (FIO_2). Larger G or H cylinders containing 5290 or 6910 L, respectively, allow oxygen supplementation for longer periods.

The design of the ICU should accommodate the care of horses with a wide variety of problems. All stalls should have the equipment necessary for hanging large volume (e.g., 5 L) fluid bags. In addition, the design should include one or two stalls for easy unloading of down horses, and the structure must be able to withstand hoisting. If care of neonatal patients is expected to be routine, large foaling stalls should be available. These stalls may feature mobile separators to facilitate treatment of foals while allowing them access to their dams.

A central office facilitates oversight of the entire unit. For larger ICU facilities video monitoring of stalls from the central office is optimal. Sufficient storage space should be available to protect equipment that is not in use. A separate food preparation area should be available for preparation of enteral feeding. Staff members should pay attention to cleanliness in this area and particularly should refrain from washing their hands or contaminated material in the sink used for food preparation.

Although grouping critically ill patients in a single location allows for the greatest efficiency of personnel and equipment, maintaining biosecurity is essential. Grouping patients with similar disorders is therefore recommended. Strict disinfection and isolation protocols should be in place to prevent nosocomial infections and the spread of infectious disease. Thorough hand washing is an important component of most biosecurity protocols. Hand rubbing with an alcohol-based solution is more effective than hand washing with an antiseptic, probably because it does not require rinsing and drying of hands.[3] Adoption of this practice significantly reduces cross-contamination among patients.

Guidelines for the judicious use of antibiotic regimens are available for human ICUs, and some of these guidelines apply to equine ICUs. These guidelines usually include recommendations for initial empirical selection of effective antibiotic regimens based on history, disease process, possibility of nosocomial infection, and knowledge of specific isolates for the hospital. Once culture results are available, therapy can be modified. Other methods that have been proposed to minimize antibiotic resistance and superinfections include cycling of antibiotics and restricted use of potent, broad spectrum therapies.

Salmonella organisms also can be a cause of nosocomial infection in the equine hospital. *Salmonella* shedding is greater in horses with colic, and the use of common equipment such as stomach tubes and pumps may promote transmission. Careful attention to hospital design and disinfection practices can help minimize the risk of hospital outbreaks.

COMMON PHYSIOLOGIC FEATURES OF CRITICAL ILLNESS

Despite differing problems, the common denominator in the treatment of many critically ill patients is the need to maintain adequate delivery of oxygen to meet metabolic demand. Methods to return to a fully functional state include serial systemic evaluations, even when the problem appears focal; attention to minimize adverse affects of treatments; and restoration of homeostasis, in particular working toward adequate delivery of oxygen and nutrients to cells.

Often a disease affects a single organ, and therapy can be focused on a specific process in that organ. A simple bacterial bronchopneumonia is often resolved with a course of appropriate antimicrobial medication and possibly the use of a nonsteroidal agent to help control inflammation. However, it is not unusual for the infection to induce fevers. Fevers may cause generalized malaise as well as inappetence. In horses fevers may be associated with signs of colic and altered gastrointestinal function. Although this is an obvious and relatively simple example of how a focal lesion creates systemic effects, it elucidates the need for evaluation of the entire body, even in patients with an obvious primary problem. Severely ill patients require sequential, thorough, and systemic evaluations. These evaluations are fundamental in critical care medicine.

A more severe consequence of focal problems causing systemic effects can occur when the initial insult is recognized as foreign by the body, and the various components of the immune system become activated to eliminate the threat. Most of the time this process is appropriate, and the various inflammatory mediator or coagulation cascades are activated in an orderly fashion. However, sometimes the progression is not balanced, and activation of certain systems, such as those governing inflammation and coagulation, can lead to unchecked release of mediators and a generalized reaction. In sick horses the most commonly cited example of this is systemic inflammatory response syndrome (SIRS), which can occur as a consequence of endotoxemia. These aspects of equine medicine are discussed in detail in Chapter 15.

Therapeutic misadventures can occur. The adverse affects of some therapeutic modalities can inadvertently cause significant systemic issues. A common example of this problem may be seen with the use of antibiotics in sick horses. It is not unusual for critically ill patients that are being treated with appropriate antimicrobial agents to develop significant, potentially life-threatening colitis. Understanding the potential effects of prescribed medication, carefully monitoring the patient's clinical progression, and making adjustments to the treatment plan and management strategies may ameliorate some of these problems.

Many severe problems cause alteration of normal body function and lead to misdistribution of supplies needed to maintain cellular metabolism. When the delivery or utilization of oxygen is inadequate to the metabolic needs of tissue beds, the term *dysoxia* is used. Clinically, this syndrome is recognized as shock. If left untreated, such states may lead to metabolic acidosis, organ dysfunction, and death.

Shock usually results from oxygen delivery that is insufficient to meet tissue oxygen consumption. Oxygen delivery can be defined as cardiac output multiplied by arterial oxygen content ($DO_2 = CO \times CaO_2$). Cardiac output is measured as heart rate times stroke volume. Oxygen content is determined by both the amount of oxygen carried by hemoglobin in the red blood cells as well as the amount of oxygen dissolved within plasma. The formula for calculating arterial oxygen content is as follows:

$$[1.34 \times \text{Hb} \times (\text{saturation}/100)] + (0.003 \times P_aO_2)$$

It is important to note that the majority of oxygen that is delivered to tissues is carried in the red blood cells bound to hemoglobin and the commonly monitored partial pressure of oxygen (PaO_2; dissolved oxygen) represents only a small portion of total oxygen. This highlights the need to monitor anemia during critical illness.

The clinical condition of shock may be described or classified in several different ways, such as by stage of shock or by underlying etiology. The stages of shock include compensated, uncompensated, and irreversible. During the initial phase of compensated shock, vital organ function is maintained and blood pressure remains normal to increased. This is also called *warm shock*. During this time various compensatory mechanisms are activated, including baroreceptors and chemoreceptors, the renin-angiotensin system, humoral responses, and internal fluid shifts. When activation of these mechanisms fails to restore normal tissue oxygenation, microvascular perfusion becomes marginal and cellular function deteriorates. All of this leads to hypotension, the hallmark of shock. During this phase vasoconstriction predominates, and the term *cold shock* is used. When lack of perfusion becomes severe and is refractory to all attempts to correct it, organ dysfunction and failure occur. At this point the process is often irreversible despite all therapeutic attempts.

The categories of etiologies of shock include hypovolemia, cardiogenic, distributive, obstructive, and dissociative. It is important to consider these differential diagnoses of shock to help determine management strategies, but the goal for treatment of shock resulting from any cause is to improve perfusion. Attempting to restore normal physiology may be misguided in critically ill patients because such efforts can result in substantial iatrogenic risks; however, early goal-directed therapies have been shown to improve outcome.

BASIC STEPS

An understanding of the physiologic and pathologic processes that may be occurring in critically ill patients is key to a successful outcome. The goal is to evaluate the patient, recognize current problems, anticipate impending issues, and then create an action plan. Because critical illness is generally dynamic, the plan also must also be dynamic. In the often highly emotionally charged period of initial patient evaluation, a systematic, thorough approach to each patient is beneficial. A basic 12-step plan for assessing and treating a critically ill patient is outlined in Box 7-2.

BASIC PROCEDURES IN ADULT EQUINE CRITICAL CARE

Joanne Hardy

Critical care for adult horses varies depending on the underlying problem being addressed. Expertise in a variety of technical procedures is advisable to facilitate diagnostic and therapeutic efforts.

VASCULAR ACCESS AND ADMINISTRATION OF FLUIDS

Intravenous catheters are available in varying materials, constructions, lengths, and diameters (Table 7-2). In choosing a catheter, the practitioner should consider the desired fluid rate, fluid viscosity, the length of time the catheter will remain in the vein, the severity of the systemic illness, and the size of the animal. The rate of fluid flow is proportional to the diameter of the catheter and inversely proportional to the length of the catheter and the viscosity of the fluid.

BOX 7-2

TWELVE-STEP PLAN FOR CRITICAL CARE ASSESSMENT AND TREATMENT

1. Evaluate.
2. Provide respiratory stabilization if needed.
3. Obtain venous access.
4. Provide cardiovascular support, including developing a fluid plan that addresses hydration and metabolic needs.
5. Provide pain relief, which may include analgesic or sedative medications and/or directly addressing the cause of the pain.
6. Measure effectiveness of the above and continue with diagnostic procedures.
7. Develop a plan to prevent secondary infection, in particular to help preserve the gastrointestinal mucosal barrier.
8. Develop a nutritional plan.
9. Develop a plan for monitoring the patient.
10. Evaluate systemic response and adjust plan as needed.
11. Address special circumstances such as recumbency.
12. Assess effectiveness, re-evaluate patient, revise plan.

TABLE 7-2

List of Available Catheter Materials

Material	Example	Comment
Polypropylene	PE tubing, Medicut	Highly thrombogenic not recommended
Teflon	Angiocath	Less thrombogenic
Polyurethane	Mila	Much less thrombogenic
Silastic	Centrasil	Least thrombogenic

Standard adult horse catheter sizes are usually 14 gauge in diameter and 5.25 inches in length. For more rapid administration rates, larger-bore catheters, such as 12- or 10-gauge, could be used, with the caveat that these larger sizes may be more traumatic to the vascular endothelium, which increases the risk of thomobosis, Plasma, blood products, and synthetic colloids, because of their increased viscosity, flow more slowly; if the horse requires volume replacement, the practitioner can combine administration of these fluids with a balanced electrolyte solution.

Teflon catheters should be changed every 3 days, whereas polyurethane catheters may remain in the vein for up to 2 weeks. Regardless of the type of catheter, the site of vascular access should be closely monitored several times daily (discussed in more detail later in this chapter). Horses that are very ill (e.g., bacteremic, septicemic, endotoxic) are more likely to experience catheter problems and benefit from polyurethane or silicone catheters.

One also must consider the catheter construction (Table 7-3). Through-the-needle catheters are most common for standard-size adult horses. An over-the-wire catheter is best used in foals and miniature horses or when catheterizing the lateral thoracic vein. Short and long extension sets are available, as well as small- and large-bore diameters. Using an extension set that screws into the hub of the catheter is best, to prevent dislodgment. In horses with low central venous pressures (CVPs), disconnection of the line can result in significant aspiration of air and cardiovascular collapse. Double extensions are available for horses that require administration of other medication with the fluids.

Common sites for insertion of intravenous catheters in horses include the jugular, lateral thoracic, cephalic, and saphenous veins. The lateral thoracic vein makes an acute angle as it enters the chest at the fifth intercostal space; therefore an over-the-wire catheter is best to use when catheterizing this vein. Catheters placed in any location other than the jugular vein require more frequent flushings (every 4 hours) because they tend to clot more easily. Leg catheters usually are bandaged because they are more prone to dislodgment than jugular catheters.

In adult horses a catheter is usually not covered with a bandage so that potential problems can be quickly identified. The practitioner may need to apply bandages to foals if they are tampering with the catheter. A triple-antibiotic ointment may be applied at the insertion site to decrease infection. Catheters should be flushed with heparinized saline (10 IU/ml)

TABLE 7-3

List of Commercially Available Catheter Constructions

Type	Description	Advantage	Disadvantage
Butterfly	Needle attached to tubing	Ease of use	Laceration of vessel; vessel puncture and extravascular administration
Over-the-needle	Stylet inside catheter for venipuncture	Available in large diameter, ease of insertion	Limited length of catheter, not flexible, break at catheter and hub junction
Through-the-needle	Short needle inserted; catheter threaded through needle	All lengths available, flexible, peel-away needle	Technically more difficult to insert
Over-the-wire	Needle serving as guide to insert wire, which serves as guide for catheter	Flexible, long catheters available, ensures proper catheter placement	More technical expertise required to place catheter, expensive

four times per day if they are not used for fluid administration. When administering a medication, the clinician should wipe the injection cap with alcohol before inserting the needle and change the injection cap daily. The clinician should culture catheters if catheter site infection is suspected for identification of the causative organism and to facilitate early recognition of possible nosocomial infection.

Coil sets are used for stallside fluid administration for most adult horses. These are advantageous because they allow the horse to move around, lie down, and eat without restraint. An overhead pulley system with a rotating hook prevents fluid lines from becoming tangled.

Administration sets are used for short-term fluid or drug administration and are available at 10 drops/ml and 60 drops/ml. When using a calibrated fluid pump, one should take care to use the appropriate set calibrated for the brand of pump. Long coiled extension sets can then be used to connect fluids to the horse. Foal coil sets that deliver 15 drops/ml are also available.

Special foal fluid administration sets are available as pressurized bags that allow delivery of fluids at 250 ml/hr. These bags can be placed in a special harness on the foal's back, thereby preventing entanglement with the mare.

Calibrated pumps allow delivery at various rates. These pumps have alarms that signal air in the line, an empty fluid bag, or catheter problems. The maximal fluid rate that these pumps can deliver is 999 ml/hr, which is insufficient for most adult horses. The pumps are useful for recumbent foals or for combined drug infusions. For large volume fluid delivery, peristaltic pumps are available that can deliver up to 40 L/hr. One must supervise these pumps constantly when in use because they continue to run even if fluids run out. Large-bore catheters should be used to prevent trauma resulting from the jet effect on the endothelium of the vein.

BASIC FLUID THERAPY

Fluid administration for maintenance or replacement is one of the mainstays of equine critical care and should be readily available in any equine hospital. The availability of commercial materials and fluids for use in large animals makes fluid administration easy and cost-effective in most situations. This section provides a review of available materials and principles that should be followed when planning fluid administration.

DESIGNING A FLUID THERAPY REGIMEN

Fluids can be administered for maintenance or replacement purposes. Horses usually receive maintenance regimens orally, and electrolyte formulations are available for this purpose. Intravenous maintenance fluids are lower in sodium and higher in calcium, potassium, and magnesium than replacement fluids. Replacement regimens replace fluids lost through dehydration and ongoing losses. When designing a fluid therapy regimen, the clinician must consider the following questions:

- What volume of fluid must be given?
- What type of fluid will be given?
- What will be the rate of administration?

The volume of fluids to give equals the maintenance requirements plus the correction for dehydration and ongoing losses.

MAINTENANCE

In the adult horse maintenance fluid requirements have been estimated at 60 ml/kg/day. This figure probably overestimates the actual needs of a resting, fasted animal but appears to be safe in most situations. In horses with renal failure, in which elimination of excess fluids is problematic, monitoring of body weight and CVP is indicated. If weight gain, edema, or increased CVP is evident, the fluid administration rate should be decreased.

DEHYDRATION

Evaluation of dehydration is at best a subjective estimate, and the clinician must understand that this estimate must be adjusted on the basis of monitoring parameters. Table 7-4 lists useful parameters for evaluating acute, extracellular dehydration.

After obtaining an estimate of dehydration, the clinician can calculate the amount of fluids to be given as follows:

$$\text{Volume of fluid (L)} = \text{Estimate of dehydration (\%)} \times \text{body mass (kg)}$$

ONGOING LOSSES

Sometimes the clinician can measure and record ongoing losses (e.g., for nasogastric reflux), but ongoing losses usually must be estimated. The clinician monitors the patient to determine whether the calculated fluid volume is meeting the ongoing losses. Patients receiving fluids intravenously should be monitored at least twice a day, including assessment of heart rate and measurement of packed cell volume and total protein; the clinician should monitor patients more frequently (every 2, 4, or 6 hours) depending on the severity of cardiovascular compromise. The clinician should also monitor creatinine concentration once daily when initially elevated to ensure adequate return to normal. Additional means of monitoring

TABLE 7-4

Parameters Used for Estimation of Dehydration in the Horse

% Dehydration	Heart Rate (Beats per Minute)	CRT (Seconds)*	PCV/TP (%/g/L)*	Creatinine (mg/dl)
6	40-60	2	40/7	1.5-2
8	61-80	3	45/7.5	2-3
10	81-100	4	50/8	3-4
12	>100	>4	>50/>8	>4

*_CRT_, Capillary refill time; _PCV_, packed cell volume; _TP_, total protein

adequate fluid delivery may include measurement of CVP, arterial blood pressure, and urine output.

TYPE OF FLUID

The type of fluid to administer depends on evaluation of the chemistry profile and disease state. The first step is to decide on the baseline fluid (saline or balanced electrolyte solution), and the second step is to decide on the types of additives to add to the baseline fluid, which depends on specific deficits or excesses, such as hyponatremia or hypernatremia, hypokalemia or hyperkalemia, hypocalcemia or hypercalcemia, hypoglycemia, and acid-base disorders.

Two categories of fluids commonly are used for fluid replacement: 0.09% saline and balanced electrolyte solutions (BESs). Table 7-5 lists the composition of various commercially available fluids. In general, BESs are chosen when serum electrolytes are close to normal. All BESs contain some potassium. Saline is higher in sodium and much higher in chloride than serum concentrations and is used when sodium is lower than 125 mEq/L. Saline also is used in disease processes associated with high potassium levels, such as hyperkalemic periodic paralysis or renal failure, in which a potassium-free solution is preferable. In cases of long-term fluid maintenance therapy (greater than 4 to 5 days), if the oral route is not available, the practitioner should consider half-strength basic fluids to which potassium and calcium are added. Long-term fluid therapy with routine BESs results in hypernatremia, hypokalemia, hypomagnesemia, and hypocalcemia.

In horses routine fluid replacement includes calcium and potassium supplementation, in particular when the horse receives no oral intake because of gastrointestinal disease. Both electrolytes are important for smooth muscle function and vascular tone. Recently, magnesium supplementation also has received interest, particularly with fasting and ileus.[1,2]

Horses with metabolic acidosis also may require bicarbonate supplementation. Because the most common cause of nonrespiratory acidosis is lactic acidemia resulting from poor perfusion, providing fluid replacement should be the first and principal means of correcting this problem. Rules of thumb for bicarbonate supplementation in acute metabolic acidosis are as follows:

- Normal respiratory function: If the horse is unable to exhale the generated carbon dioxide (CO_2) because of a respiratory problem, the acidosis will worsen.
- pH lower than 7.2: In acute acidosis associated with dehydration, fluid replacement results in restoration of urine output, and renal compensation follows and usually is complete if the pH is greater than 7.2.
- Half of the calculated amount is rapidly administered, followed by the remainder over 12 to 24 hours.
- Intravenously administered bicarbonate and calcium-containing solutions are incompatible.

In chronic metabolic acidosis, particularly with ongoing losses of bicarbonate (e.g., diarrhea), the horse usually requires the full calculated amount, partly because the bicarbonate

TABLE 7-5

Crystalloid Solutions Available for Fluid Therapy

Product	Approximate pH	mOsm/L	Na (mEq/L)	K (mEq/L)	Ca (mEq/L)	Mg (mEq/L)	Cl (mEq/L)	Buffer (mEq/L)
Lactated Ringer's	6.5	273	130	4	3	—	109	Lactate 28
Lactated Ringer's and 5% dextrose	5	525	130	4	3	—	109	Lactate 28
PlasmaLyte A	7.4	294	140	5	—	3	98	Acetate 27 Gluconate 23
Plasmalyte 148	7.4	294	140	5	—	3	98	Acetate 27 Gluconate 23
Plasmalyte 148	5.5	294	140	5	—	3	98	Acetate 27 Gluconate 23
Plasmalyte 56 and 5% dextrose	5	362	40	13	—	3	40	Acetate 16
5% Dextrose	4	252	—	—	—	—	—	—
0.9% NaCl	5	308	154	—	—	—	154	—
7% NaCl	—	2400	1196	—	—	—	1196	—
5% Dextrose and 0.9% NaCl	4	560	154	—	—	—	154	—
5% Dextrose and 0.45% NaCl	4	280	77	—	—	—	77	—
5% $NaHCO_3$	8	1190	595	—	—	—	595	—
8.4% $NaHCO_3$	—	2000	1000	—	—	—	1000	—
1.3% $NaHCO_3$ (must be mixed)	—	308	154	—	—	—	1541	—

loss is distributed over all fluid compartments, not just the extracellular fluid. Orally administered bicarbonate is a good means of dealing with ongoing losses in horses with diarrhea.

Bicarbonate can be given orally as a powder, where

$$1 \text{ g } NaHCO_3 = 12 \text{ mEq of } HCO_3$$

RATE OF ADMINISTRATION

For patients in severe shock, the clinician should give a shock dose of fluids in the first hour (60 to 80 ml/kg), which can be done only with pressurized bags or a pump.

In other situations the rate of administration is based on 24-hour requirements and estimates as a volume per hour. Keeping tally of the fluids given is important to ensure that the correct amount is administered.

ORALLY ADMINISTERED FLUIDS

Oral fluid therapy should be administered using the fluid composition shown in Table 7-6. One should administer calcium separately because it causes precipitation of the solution. This electrolyte solution meets daily needs for an adult horse and can be given through a small, preplaced nasogastric feeding tube or by intermittent intubation.

Fluids Used to Expand Circulating Blood Volume

ISOTONIC CRYSTALLOIDS

Intravenous administration of isotonic crystalloids immediately reconstitutes circulating volume. However, because the fluids are crystalloids, they distribute to the entire extracellular compartment within a matter of minutes. Because the extracellular fluid compartment is three times the volume of blood, one must administer three times as much isotonic crystalloid to gain the desired amount of volume expansions. The dose is 60 to 90 ml/kg/hr, and the fluid types usually are BESs such as lactated Ringer's solution.

HYPERTONIC CRYSTALLOIDS (7.2% NACL)

Hypertonic crystalloids are approximately eight times the tonicity of plasma and extracellular fluid; their immediate effect is to expand the vascular volume by redistribution of fluid from the interstitial and intracellular spaces. However, this effect is short lived. As the electrolytes redistribute across the extracellular fluid, fluids shift again and the patient becomes hypovolemic again. Because the principal effect is fluid redistribution, a total body deficit still exists that must be replaced. The duration of effect of hypertonic solutions is directly proportional to the distribution constant, which is the indexed cardiac output. The dose is 4 ml/kg, administered as rapidly as possible, and the fluid is 5% or 7% saline. Because of its short duration of effect, one must follow hypertonic saline administration with isotonic volume replacement.

TABLE 7-6

Fluid Composition for Orally Administered Fluid Therapy

For Every L of Water, add:

FOR EVERY 21 L OF WATER	
Electrolyte	**Amount**
NaCl	10 g
$NaHCO_3$	15 g
KCl	75 g
K_2HPO_4	60 g

COLLOIDS

Colloids are fluids that contain a molecule that can exert oncotic pressure. These molecules do redistribute to the extracellular fluid but at a much slower rate than crystalloids, so that the duration of effect is prolonged compared with that of crystalloids. Table 7-7 describes the different colloids available.

A disadvantage of natural colloids (plasma or albumin) is that they are more antigenic and can cause allergic reactions. Synthetic colloids have a much lower antigenicity, but they can cause bleeding disorders because of their tendency to coat platelets or by causing a decrease in coagulation factor. In the horse Dextran 40 can cause anaphylactoid reactions. Hetastarch administration can cause a decrease in coagulation factors and prolong clotting times, particularly at high doses (20 ml/kg).[3] The dose is 10 ml/kg of 6% solutions.

Synthetic colloids do not register on a refractometer. Accurate evaluation of oncotic pressure requires use of a colloid osmometer. If one is not available, the clinician must use clinical evaluation (e.g., observing presence of edema and poor circulatory volume and pressure).

BLOOD SUBSTITUTES

Blood substitutes are hemoglobin solutions. Currently, only one commercial hemoglobin solution (oxyglobin, which is made from bovine hemoglobin) is available. The major advantage of oxyglobin is that it does not depend on 2,3-diphosphoglycerate for oxygen-carrying capacity, such that it can be stored and is immediately able to transport oxygen. The duration of effect is approximately 18 hours in horses, after which point another dose or a blood transfusion must be considered.[4,5] Unfortunately, cost limits the usefulness of oxyglobin in horses.

WHOLE BLOOD

Whole blood is the ideal fluid for blood loss or platelet loss, provided that it is fresh blood and has been crossmatched. It is important to remember that stored blood loses its oxygen-carrying capacity and that it can take several hours to restore it after administration.

Ideally, the ICU should maintain blood donors that are free of antigenic determinants, particularly Aa and Qa, and of isoantibodies. The practitioner can perform a major and minor crossmatch to select an appropriate donor, provided that complement is added to the test for hemolysin detection. Interpretation of the minor crossmatch may be difficult if autoagglutination is present. If crossmatch is unavailable, one can use a non-Thoroughbred gelding. A volume of 20 ml/kg can be safely collected every 3 weeks in adult horses,[3] and whole blood can be collected in sodium citrate using sterile technique. Commercial blood collection kits are also available. Complications of blood transfusion include acute anaphylactic reactions, allergic reactions, hemolysis, fever, tachypnea, and hypocalcemia caused by citrate chelation.

TABLE 7-7

Characteristics of Colloid Solutions Available for Fluid Therapy

Characteristics	5% Albumin	25% Albumin	Oxypolygelatin	Dextran 40	Dextran 70	Hetastarch
Molecular weight (d)						
Average	69,000	69,000	30,000	40,000	70,000	450,000
Number average	69,000	69,000	22,000-24,000	25,000	39,000	70,000
Range	—	—	5,600-100,000	10,000-80,000	15,000-160,000	10,000-3,400,000
Solvent	—	—	Balanced electrolyte solution	0.9% saline or 5% dextrose	0.9% saline or 5% dextrose	0.9% saline or balanced electrolyte solution
Maximum water binding (ml/g)	18	18	39	37	29	20
Concentration (%)	5	25	5.6	10	6	6
Half-life	14-16 days	14-16 days	2-4 hours	2.5 hours	6 hours	25 hours
Plasma percentage (after 24 hours)	—	—	12	18	29	38
Extravascular percentage (after 24 hours)	—	—	—	22	33	39
Overall survival in blood	—	—	168 hours	44 hours	4-6 weeks	17-26 weeks
Colloid oncotic pressure (mm Hg)	20	100	45-47	40	—	30

MONITORING ARTERIAL BLOOD PRESSURE

The practitioner can measure arterial blood pressure by direct catheterization of a peripheral artery or by indirect measurements that depend on a cuff placed over an artery and cuff inflation until blood flow is occluded. Measurement of arterial blood pressure is one of the indirect estimates of tissue perfusion, using the mean pressure as the driving pressure. Horses may have low mean arterial pressure (MAP) as a result of hypovolemia, SIRS, heart failure, or any of a wide variety of disorders.

Most monitoring equipment provides an estimation of systolic arterial pressure, diastolic pressure, and MAP. MAP is a calculated value determined by integrating the area under the pressure waveform and dividing this by the duration of the cardiac cycle.

Pulse pressure is the difference between systolic and diastolic pressure and is responsible for the palpable pulse. A bounding pulse pressure results from an increased systolic pressure, a decreased diastolic pressure, or both.

Ultimately, the clinician is interested in oxygen delivery to tissues, which depends on adequate perfusion of tissues, which in turn depends on functional capillary density and blood flow in capillaries. In the clinical arena measurement of tissue perfusion or of tissue blood flow is impractical. Therefore clinicians use blood pressure as an estimate of adequate blood flow and tissue perfusion. The problems with this assumption are as follows:

- Tissue blood flow is regulated locally; an adequate systemic blood pressure may not reflect local blood flow if vasoconstriction, shunting, poor capillary recruitment, edema, or thromboembolism exist. An example is the central redistribution of blood flow in shock, with preferential shunting of abdominal organs.
- Blood flow depends on pressure differential. If vasoconstriction is generalized, blood pressure may be normal but flow may be poor.
- Blood flow through a vessel depends on the viscosity of the fluid (blood) and the radius of the vessel. At high viscosity blood flow may be impaired. Severe vasoconstriction, although maintaining blood pressure, may impair flow.

DIRECT OR INVASIVE BLOOD PRESSURE MEASUREMENT

An over-the-needle catheter configuration is preferable for direct or invasive blood pressure measurement to prevent bleeding at the site of puncture. A small (20- or 22-gauge) catheter is preferable to minimize hematoma formation on catheter removal. The radial artery over-the-needle catheter (Arrow International, Reading, Pa.) with a wire guide is suitable for arterial catheterization of peripheral vessels in the horse. As an alternative, an over-the-wire catheter sheath that calls for a Seldinger technique for insertion (Seldinger technique transradial artery catheter, Arrow International) may be used. The catheter is connected to noncompliant tubing filled with heparinized saline, which is linked to a pressure transducer.

Suitable arteries for arterial catheterization in the horse include the transverse facial, facial, and greater metatarsal arteries. In the standing horse the transverse facial or the facial artery are most practical (Figure 7-1).

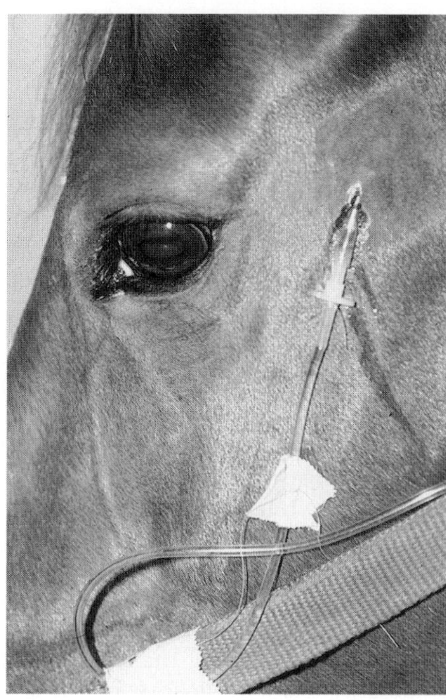

FIGURE 7-1 An adult horse with an arterial catheter in the tranverse facial artery for direct blood pressure monitoring.

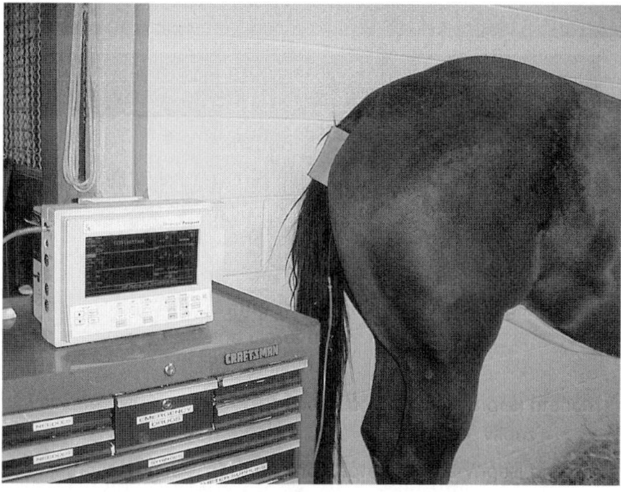

FIGURE 7-2 Indirect oscillometric blood pressure measurement in a horse using a cuff placed on the tail.

The reference unit for blood pressure is millimeters of mercury (mm Hg), meaning the force exerted by the blood against an area of the vessel wall to raise a column of mercury by a certain number of millimeters. Occasionally, centimeters of water (cm H_2O) is used. One mm Hg equals 1.36 cm H_2O. The mercury manometer is too slow, however, to record changes in blood pressure rapidly. Therefore a continuous method of pressure recording is preferable for clinical use. A transducer transforms the pressure signal to an electronic signal that can be displayed continuously. The transducer and flush device (Pressure Monitoring Kit with Truwave disposable pressure transducer; Edwards Lifescience, Irvine, Calif,) then can be used for continuous blood pressure measurement. One should place the transducer at the level of the heart base, as estimated by the point of the shoulder.

In addition to blood pressure measurement, invasive blood pressure measurement enables evaluation of the pressure waveform, which in turn can provide insight regarding the status of the stroke volume and peripheral vascular tone.

Indirect Measurement

Indirect blood pressure measurements depend on a cuff placed around the tail or the metatarsus. The diameter of the cuff influences the accuracy of the measurement, with cuffs that are too wide resulting in underestimation of the blood pressure. An ideal cuff width-to-circumference ratio of 0.25 to 0.35 has been recommended for use on the tail or limbs of horses. Cuff widths are available for neonate, pediatric, and adult horses. Once the cuff is in place, the practitioner measures blood pressure by recording the signal emitted by the changing blood frequency during the pulse wave. The following sections describe noninvasive blood pressure measurement methods.

DOPPLER

Doppler uses a small ultrasound probe placed on a peripheral artery, and a piezoelectric crystal within the probe converts the pulse wave into an audible signal. The probe must be placed over a shaved area (usually under the tail of the horse) after application of a coupling gel. Doppler allows measurement of only systolic pressure and is therefore not as useful as other methods.

OSCILLOMETRIC SPHYGMOMANOMETRY

Oscillometric sphygmomanometry relies on the recording of the change in oscillations generated by the change in blood flow during deflation of the cuff. Oscillations start as the cuff pressure reaches systolic pressure, are maximal at mean pressure, and disappear when the cuff reaches diastolic pressure. The meter records and displays systolic, diastolic, and mean pressures. When placing the meter on the tail, one can use tape or a bandage below the cuff to prevent its slipping, but should not restrain the cuff itself (Figure 7-2).

PHOTOPLETHYSMOGRAPHY

Photoplethysmography relies on the detection of arterial volume by attenuation of infrared radiation. Photoplethysmography originally was designed for use in human fingers and has been validated for use in small dogs and cats but has not been evaluated for use in horses.

TRANSESOPHAGEAL ULTRASOUND

Transesophageal ultrasound is a method of hemodynamic monitoring that uses a transesophageal probe with two ultrasound transducers (HemoSonic; Arrow International). An M-mode transducer continuously measures the aortic diameter, and a pulsed Doppler measures the flow velocity, providing hemodynamic measurements, including MAP. Although transesophageal Doppler echocardiography has been evaluated for determination of cardiac output in horses, the accuracy and repeatability of the combined probes for blood pressure determination have not been evaluated (Vingmed Sound, Horten, Norway).

Goals of Blood Pressure Measurement

The goal of blood pressure measurement is to identify hypotension and follow the response to therapy after interventions. Blood pressures of greater than 70 mm Hg are targeted in the adult, and greater than 60 mm Hg are targeted in neonates. In horses hypertension rarely is identified, other than after giving high doses of pressor agents such as phenylephrine.

Pitfalls

When using direct pressure monitoring, the clinician should ensure that a good waveform is visible on the oscilloscope. Dampening of the pressure waveform by an air bubble or improper catheter placement leads to flattening of the pressure waveform and falsely low pressure measurements. Alternatively, long connector tubing lengths (>4 feet) can lead to a resonant system that records a falsely elevated systolic pressure. The flush test can help determine whether the recording system is distorting the pressure waveform.

MONITORING CENTRAL VENOUS PRESSURE

Central venous pressure is the pressure in the central veins of the patient and is most often measured within the intrathoracic portion of the cranial vena cava. The CVP is affected by vascular volume, venous tone, and cardiac function. Monitoring CVP is most useful for patients in which the veterinarian is attempting to maintain adequate vascular volume without fluid overload. For example, assessment of CVP may be useful in horses with oliguric or anuric renal failure, horses with large volume gastric reflux, and horses predisposed to edema formation.

Central venous pressure is measured by using an intravenous catheter placed in the jugular vein and terminating in the intrathoracic portion of the cranial vena cava. The catheter is attached via an extension set to a water manometer positioned such that the pressure at the level of the base of the heart or point of the shoulder is zero.

TRACHEOSTOMY

Box 7-3 lists the materials needed for an emergency tracheostomy pack. If possible, the clinician should clip, prepare, and infiltrate with local anesthetic the planned incision site. In cases of acute respiratory distress, this may not be possible, however. The clinician makes an 8- to 10-cm longitudinal incision at the junction of the proximal and middle third of the neck, just above the V made by the junction of the sternothyrohyoideus muscles. It is important to stay on midline to favor drainage, separating the sternothyrohyoideus muscles on the midline and exposing the trachea. The clinician makes a transverse incision between two tracheal rings, taking care not to damage the tracheal cartilages. If the head of the horse is supported in elevation during the procedure, the clinician should make the tracheal incision distal in relationship to the skin incision to keep from covering the incision when the head is lowered. In emergency situations a J-type tracheostomy tube is used because of its ease of insertion. When the horse is calm, or if the situation is not critical, a self-retaining tube is preferable for maintenance because J-tubes tend to fall out. If the animal is to be ventilated, a silicone-cuffed tube is preferable to allow for closed-system ventilation.

BOX 7-3

MATERIALS NEEDED FOR AN EMERGENCY TRACHEOSTOMY PACK

- Local anesthetic
- Needle and syringe
- Sterile, disposable surgical blade
- Scissors
- Hemostats
- J-type tracheostomy tube

The tracheostomy tube should be cleaned daily and changed as needed. Petroleum gel applied around the incision prevents skin scalding. In general but particularly in foals, tracheostomy tubes should be removed as early as possible to avoid permanent tracheal deformity. To help decide when to remove the tube, the clinician can occlude the tube temporarily to see if the horse can breathe without it. After the tube is removed, the site should be cleaned of exudate twice daily and allowed to heal by second intention. The wound generally closes in 10 to 14 days and heals in 3 weeks.

THORACOCENTESIS

Thoracic drainage is an essential part of managing pleural effusion and can be lifesaving in cases of severe effusion. Pleural effusion is identified by typical increases in area of cardiac auscultation; dullness in the ventral area of auscultation; and, if unilateral, a discrepancy in auscultation between the two hemithoraxes. The clinician can use percussion, although ultrasound typically provides the best method of identifying fluid in the chest. Pleural fluid is drained through a cannula or by placement of a chest drain. The clinician clips, prepares, and infiltrates the site with a local anesthetic. An incision is made in the skin cranial to the proposed point of entry, and the trocar is inserted through the skin. The clinician moves the incision in a caudal direction to a point between two ribs and, using pressure, pushes the trocar into the chest. One hand serves as a stop to control depth of entry. After obtaining the fluid, the clinician places a Heimlich valve on the end of the tube and sutures the tube in place using a Chinese finger trap pattern.

Pneumothorax is classified as open (external wound) or closed. The pleural pressure equilibrates with atmospheric pressure, resulting in lung collapse. Tension pneumothorax develops when air continuously enters the chest without evacuation. The pleural pressure can reach supra-atmospheric levels and can be life threatening.

In open pneumothorax sealing of the chest must occur, followed by evacuation of air. The clinician can seal the chest with sheets of plastic wrapped around the site of entry or close the wound if possible. The chest is evacuated by placing a small trocar, or a 14-gauge catheter, in the dorsal twelfth intercostal space, and the trocar is removed once the air has been evacuated satisfactorily. In closed pneumothorax or tension pneumothorax, the catheter must be kept in place until the source of air entry can be sealed.

NASOGASTRIC INTUBATION

Nasogastric intubation is an essential and possibly lifesaving procedure performed in cases of equine colic. The horse should be adequately restrained, with a twitch and sedation if needed. The clinician should stand on the side of the horse, with the hand closest to the horse placed on the nose, and the thumb in the nostril. With the other hand, the clinician passes the tube in the ventral meatus, using the thumb to keep it directed correctly. If a hard structure is encountered, it is the ethmoidal area, and the tube should be redirected ventrally. On reaching the pharynx, the practitioner should feel a soft resistance. The tube can be turned 180 degrees to direct its curvature dorsally. The clinician stimulates the horse to swallow by gentle to-and-fro movement or by blowing in the tube. Keeping the head of the horse flexed at the poll is helpful. Once the horse swallows, the clinician pushes the tube into the esophagus. Blowing into the tube to dilate the esophagus facilitates insertion. If the horse coughs, the clinician withdraws the tube and repeats the procedure until the tube is positioned correctly. There are three ways to determine that the tube is placed correctly in the esophagus: gentle suction, which should elicit a negative pressure; shaking of the trachea, which should not elicit a rattle; and visual confirmation of correct placement. Direct observation is the safest method. The tube is advanced until it is in the stomach (fourteenth rib). If the clinician encounters difficulty in passing the cardia, 60 ml of mepivacaine may be injected into the tube. Once the tube is in place, the practitioner must force the horse to reflux if reflux is not spontaneous. Medication should never be administered by nasogastric tube to a horse with colic without checking first for reflux. To do this, one fills the tube with water using a pump and directs the end of the tube downward to verify the presence of gastric contents. Subtracting the amount pumped in from the amount obtained is useful to determine the net amount of reflux.

One removes the tube by first occluding it (putting a thumb on the end or folding it) to prevent its contents from spilling out in the pharynx and possibly the trachea as it is withdrawn. Gentle traction is then applied in a direction parallel to the nose. If bleeding occurs, a towel can be placed over the horse's nose. The bleeding, even if severe, is self-limiting.

Nasogastric reflux is not normal. Occasionally, a small amount of reflux (1 L or less) is obtained if a horse has had a tube in place for a long time. When reflux occurs, the clinician should note the amount, character, and timing in relation to the onset of colic. In addition, the clinician should note the response to gastric decompression. Reflux originating from the small intestine is alkaline, whereas reflux composed of gastric secretions is acidic. Typically, *reflux* refers to small intestinal ileus, functional or mechanical. Lesions of the proximal small intestine produce large amounts of reflux early in the onset of the colic. With lesions of the distal small intestine (ileum), one initially obtains no reflux, and as the condition persists, one obtains reflux but usually several hours after the onset of the colic. Occasionally, large colon disease can be associated with reflux if the colonic distention exerts pressure on the duodenum as it curves over the base of the cecum.

The clinician should note the amount of reflux obtained because this factors into ongoing losses, and the volume of fluids given intravenously must be adjusted accordingly. Horses with functional ileus need gastric decompression usually every 4 hours, although if the condition is severe, they may require decompression every 2 hours. The nasogastric tube should be left in place only as long as required because some horses develop pharyngeal and laryngeal irritation associated with its presence.[6] These horses then have pain when swallowing when they resume feeding.

ABDOMINOCENTESIS

Abdominocentesis is important for evaluating abdominal disease, whether it is colic, weight loss, or postoperative problems. Box 7-4 provides the materials needed to perform this procedure.

The clinician clips a 2×2–inch area approximately 3 cm caudal to the xyphoid and 1 to 2 cm to the right of midline. With sterile gloved hands, the clinician inserts an 18-gauge needle through the skin and gently advances it into the abdomen. If no fluid is obtained, another needle can be inserted next to the first one. If no fluid is obtained this time, a bitch catheter, cannula, or dialysis catheter may be tried. Obtaining fluid from very dehydrated horses is often difficult.

To insert a teat cannula, bitch catheter, or dialysis catheter, the clinician places a bleb of local anesthetic at the site, punctures the skin and abdominal wall with a 15-gauge scalpel blade using sterile technique, and then inserts the chosen device in the abdomen. Two points of resistance will be encountered: as the device goes through the abdominal wall and as it goes through the peritoneum. The clinician collects the fluid in ethylenediamine tetraacetic acid (EDTA; shaken out of the tube so that the amount in the sample is not excessive) and, if the fluid is cloudy, in a culture tube.

Normal values for abdominocentesis are as follows: total protein should be less than 2.5 g/dl, and white blood cells should be less than 5000 cells/μl. On cytologic examination neutrophils make up approximately 40% of cells, the rest being lymphocytes, macrophages, and peritoneal cells.

With intestinal strangulation, the protein increases first (in the first 1 to 2 hours) such that the fluid is clear but more yellow. After 3 to 4 hours of strangulation, red blood cells also leak, and the fluid is more orange. After 6 hours or more, white blood cells increase gradually, with the progression of intestinal necrosis.

Enterocentesis sometimes occurs and must be differentiated from intestinal rupture. With enterocentesis a cytologic examination reveals plant material, bacteria, and debris but no cells. The clinical condition of the horse is not consistent with rupture, although in early rupture clinical signs may not reflect rupture (2 to 4 hours are necessary for manifestation of signs). Cytologic examination of abdominal fluid with intestinal rupture shows neutrophils, bacteria, and bacteria that have been phagocytized by neutrophils.

BOX 7-4

MATERIALS NEEDED FOR ABDOMINOCENTESIS

- 18-gauge, 1 ½-inch needle
- Teat cannula
- Bitch catheter
- Dialysis catheter
- Sterile gloves
- EDTA and culture tubes
- Sterile, disposable scalpel blade

EDTA, Ethylenediaminetetraacetic acid.

Blood contamination can result from the procedure and must be differentiated from internal hemorrhage or severely devitalized bowel. Blood from skin vessels usually swirls in the sample and spins down when centrifuged, leaving the sample clear. If an abdominal vessel is punctured, blood also spins down. All fresh blood contamination shows platelets, which are not present with blood older than 12 hours. If the spleen is punctured accidentally, centrifugation reveals a packed cell volume higher than the peripheral packed cell volume. In internal hemorrhage blood is hemolyzed such that the supernatant is reddish after centrifugation; the sample has no platelets and shows erythrophagocytosis. Ultrasonography also reveals fluid swirling in the abdomen.

Excess EDTA in the sample falsely elevates the total protein. When performing an abdominocentesis, the clinician should shake out the EDTA from the tube to avoid this sampling error.

Abdominal surgery increases the total protein level and white blood cell count for some time after surgery. Typically, if no enterotomy occurred, the white blood cell count increases greatly for 4 to 7 days and returns to normal by 14 days. The total protein level may remain elevated for 3 to 4 weeks after surgery. Neutrophils appear to be nondegenerate. After an enterotomy or an anastomosis, degenerate neutrophils and occasional bacteria may be seen in the first 12 to 24 hours. Subsequently, the white blood cell count remains elevated for approximately 2 weeks, but on cytologic examination the neutrophils appear to be nondegenerate and no bacteria are apparent. The total protein level remains elevated for 1 month after surgery. If septic peritonitis is present, clinical signs are consistent with bacterial infection (i.e., fever, depression, anorexia, ileus, pain, endotoxemia). The white blood cell count and total protein level are elevated greatly. On cytologic examination greater than 90% of cells are neutrophils, and they appear to be degenerate. Free and phagocytized bacteria are visible.

TROCARIZATION OF THE LARGE COLON

Trocarization of the large colon is occasionally useful to decompress the abdomen for abdominal compartment syndrome (i.e., severe distention associated with pain and dyspnea). Box 7-5 lists the materials needed for this procedure.

Trocarization should be performed only for large colon distention and never to decompress the small intestine. Before deciding on trocarizatino, identifying the segment of intestine involved is important. In adult horses, such identification can be made by rectal palpation, and in foals or small horses, radiographs or ultrasound can be used. The distended segment of large colon also must be close to the body wall so that it can be reached safely.

The most common site for trocarization is the right upper flank area, just cranial to the greater trochanter at the location of the cecal base. The clinician clips, prepares, and infiltrates with a local anesthetic a 4 × 4-cm area of skin. With gloved hand, the clinician inserts a 14-g catheter with an extension tube perpendicular to the skin. The clinician places the end of the extension in water so that gas bubbles are visible when the tip of the catheter is positioned correctly. When gas is obtained, the trocar part of the catheter should be withdrawn slightly to keep from lacerating the bowel. It may be necessary to reposition the catheter several times when gas is not obtained. After decompression the clinician removes the trocar and infuses an antibiotic (e.g., gentamicin) while withdrawing the catheter.

BOX 7-5

MATERIALS NEEDED FOR TROCARIZATION

- 14-gauge, 5 ¼-inch catheter
- Local anesthetic
- Sterile gloves
- Extension tubing
- Small water container (syringe case works)

Peritonitis and local abscessation are the two most common problems encountered after trocarization. The horse should be observed for 24 hours for signs of peritonitis. If the practitioner suspects peritonitis, confirmation is with abdominocentesis, and systemic broad spectrum antibiotics should be administered to the horse until the condition resolves. If a local abscess develops, the practitioner can drain it externally.

URINARY CATHETERIZATION

Measurement of urine output in adult horses is an infrequent procedure, compared with foals, but it may be useful in horses with of oliguric renal failure or when 24-hour volumetric measurements are needed. Male horses with neurologic disorders that make them unable to express their bladder may require bladder decompression.

In the mare, urine is easily collected by placing a Foley catheter that is connected to collection tubing. One can make a closed system by using a solution administration set and empty fluid bag. In geldings one can insert a male urinary catheter and suture it in place using a Chinese finger trap pattern. If the horse is recumbent and thrashing, leaving as little as possible of the catheter protruding to keep it from being pulled out is important. Normal horses produce 1 to 2 ml/kg/hr of urine.

SUPPORT OF CARDIOVASCULAR FUNCTION*

Peter R. Morresey

REVIEW OF CARDIOVASCULAR PHYSIOLOGY

Cardiac output, the volume of blood pumped through the heart per minute, is calculated as the product of heart rate and stroke volume. Heart rate is determined by a number of neurologic, endocrinologic, and physical factors. Stroke volume is the

*The author wishes to acknowledge two excellent sources that were particularly helpful in the formulation of this manuscript: Magdesian's article on monitoring the critically ill equine patient published in *Veterinary Clinics of North America* in 2004,[47] and an article by Coley, Donaldson, and Durando on cardiac output technologies in the horse that was published in the *Journal of Veterinary Internal Medicine* in 2003.[56]

amount of blood expelled from the heart with each contraction (i.e., the difference between end-diastolic volume [maximal filling] and end-systolic volume within the ventricle [peak contraction]). The quantity of blood arriving as the arterial supply of a tissue depends on cardiac output.

Resistance to arterial blood flow varies among tissues. As a result, cardiac output is not evenly distributed throughout the body. Contraction of the smooth muscle of the arterioles largely determines that this resistance functions to maintain a pressure gradient across the tissue capillary beds, allowing flow from arterioles to venules. Systemic vascular resistance can be considered a measure of vasomotor tone and hence vascular capacity.

Delivery of oxygen to the tissues becomes inadequate when the cardiovascular system is dysfunctional, because the oxygen delivered is a product of blood flow through the tissue and arterial oxygen content. In patients with reduced blood flow and peripheral perfusion, fluid therapy is used to increase circulating volume. Increased venous return leads to an increased stroke volume, increasing cardiac output and therefore tissue blood flow. When fluid therapy fails to improve tissue perfusion as a sole therapeutic approach, the use of vasoactive drugs (e.g., vasopressors, inotropes) may be indicated.

CARDIOVASCULAR INSUFFICIENCY: SHOCK STATES

If the cardiovascular system fails to meet the demands of the animal for adequate oxygen delivery to tissues, a state of shock ensues. Shock is classified into four major types: hypovolemic shock, cardiogenic shock, obstructive shock, and distributive shock.[1] The first three of these categories of shock are associated with a decrease in cardiac output and uniform circulatory disturbances in the arterioles, venules, and capillaries. Anaerobic tissue metabolism ensues as a result of diminished oxygen delivery. The fourth type of shock, distributive or vasodilatory shock, is associated with a heterogenous disturbance of blood flow in the microcirculation and areas of shunting.[2]

Hypovolemic shock results from a loss of intravascular volume, whether by systemic dehydration with resultant hemoconcentration, loss of fluid into a third space, or by loss of whole blood through hemorrhage. Decreased circulating volume leads to diminished venous return, reducing cardiac preload. This reduction in preload decreases myocardial fiber length, with resultant decreased contractility and therefore cardiac output. Reduced tissue perfusion results.

Cardiogenic shock is the result of impaired ventricular function with resultant decreased cardiac output. Myocarditis, myocardial infarction, valvular pathology, or arrhythmias may be responsible.[3] Inflammatory cytokines, including tumor necrosis factor-α (TNF-α) and interleukin (IL)-2 and IL-6, decrease the contractility of cardiac myocytes, effects shown experimentally to be mediated by nitric oxide.[4]

Obstructive shock (of the heart, arteries, or large veins) results from a lack of blood flow. With respect to the heart, blood flow is decreased or prevented from entering the heart, culminating in circulatory failure and a cessation of blood pumping through the body.[5] This type of shock may be precipitated by conditions such as vascular thrombosis, pericardial constrictive diseases, and pneumothorax.[6]

Distributive (vasodilatory) shock, manifested as an abnormal distribution of microvascular blood flow, may be septic, anaphylactic, or neurogenic in origin.[5] Shunting of blood in the microcirculation occurs, resulting in tissue hypoxia and metabolic derangement. This may occur in the presence of normal or increased cardiac output.[2] Central to the pathogenesis of distributive shock is endothelial dysfunction, the result of neutrophil-generated cytokines, proteases, lipid mediators, and oxygen-derived free radicals. Neutrophil adherence to the endothelial surface, migration into underlying tissues, and tissue injury result.[7]

Regardless of the type of shock, if it is prolonged and severe, the terminal physiologic disturbance will manifest as distributive shock.[8] Successful management of shock depends on early recognition and aggressive intervention.[9]

THERAPEUTIC GOALS IN THE CARDIOVASCULAR PATIENT

Principles of Management

Treatment of patients with cardiovascular compromise centers on identification of the underlying cause followed by fluid resuscitation to restore an appropriate circulating volume and administration of vasoactive drugs (e.g., vasopressors, inotropic agents) to normalize cardiac output and restore adequate tissue perfusion (Table 7-8).[10] Fluid resuscitation, which optimizes cardiac preload and hence cardiac output, is the preferred first line of defense in the treatment of hypovolemia and hypotension. If the patient does not respond fully to fluid resuscitation, further improvement in cardiac output is achieved through augmentation of systemic vascular resistance and increasing cardiac contractility by administration of vasopressors and inotropes, respectively.[3]

Fluid Therapy for Resuscitation

The optimal fluid for resuscitation of the patient with shock combines the oxygen-carrying capacity of blood, the ability to provide volume expansion in the circulating pool, and constituents sufficient to replenish and maintain the composition and quantities of all body fluid compartments.[11] Because the ideal fluid has not yet been identified, fluid resuscitation is most commonly initiated with polyionic intravenous fluids.

Two basic types of intravenous fluids are available to correct dehydration and restore circulating volume: crystalloids and colloids. Crystalloids may be obtained as either replacement or maintenance fluids. *Replacement* fluids rapidly distribute to the compartments of the extracellular fluid (ECF). They are isotonic and should be used to replace deficits in hypovolemic and dehydrated animals. *Maintenance* fluids provide free water that distributes to both the intracellular fluid (ICF) and ECF. They should be used to maintain fluid balance after rehydration in horses that need ongoing intravenous support.

CRYSTALLOIDS: REPLACEMENT FLUIDS

Crystalloid replacement fluids are polyionic isotonic fluids formulated to have an electrolyte composition similar to that of plasma in healthy animals.[12] Examples include the following:

Lactated Ringer's Solution Lactated Ringer's solution (LRS) is useful in patients requiring rapid restoration of fluid volume. Sodium concentration is lower than in equine plasma, and Cl^- concentration is higher. Although K^+ concentration is relatively low (4 mEq/L), LRS should not be given to patients with hyperkalemia. Lactate in LRS is metabolized by

TABLE 7-8

Useful Drugs in Cardiovascular Critical Care

Type	Dose	Comments
Vasopressors		
Norepinephrine	0.05-1 μg/kg/min intravenously	
Epinephrine	0.02-0.05 mg/kg intravenously	
Dopamine	1-5 μg/kg/min intravenously	Renal dopaminergic receptors
	5-10 μg/kg/min intravenously	β_1-Adrenergic stimulation
	> 10 μg/kg/min intravenously	α-Adrenergic stimulation
Phenylephrine	3 μg/kg/min intravenously over 15 minutes	
Vasopressin	0.4-0.8 units/kg intravenously	
Inotropes		
Dobutamine	1-20 μg/kg/min intravenously	
Plasma volume expansion		
Crystalloids		
Isotonic	50-100 ml/kg intravenously	
Hypertonic saline	4-8 ml/kg intravenously	
Colloids		
Plasma	5-10 ml/kg intravenously	
Hetastarch	5-10 ml/kg intravenously	

Adapted from Orsini JA and Divers TJ: *Manual of equine emergencies,* ed 2, St Louis, 2003, Saunders.

the liver to glucose or CO_2 and water. In theory, lactate may accumulate and contribute to metabolic acidosis in patients with hepatic dysfunction. Calcium ions present in LRS may precipitate with citrate and bicarbonate additives.

Plasmalyte 148 and Normosol-R Plasmalyte 148 and Normosol-R are similar to LRS, but they contain magnesium rather than calcium and can therefore be used when precipitation with concurrently administered anticoagulants may occur. The alkalinizing agents in these fluids are acetate and gluconate, respectively. Relative to LRS, Na^+ concentration is increased and Cl^- concentration is decreased.

***Normal saline* (0.9% NaCl)** Normal saline is an isotonic fluid consisting solely of Na and Cl. Concentrations of both Na^+ and Cl^- (154 mEq/L of each) are higher than those of plasma. As a mildly acidifying solution, the use of normal saline in patients with hyperkalemia and metabolic alkalosis is indicated. Care should be taken when normal saline is used for treatment of hyponatremia because gradual correction of plasma Na^+ concentration is recommended to prevent the excessive osmotic draw of water from cells.

Hypertonic saline (7% NaCl) Hypertonic saline is a useful adjunct to other crystalloid fluids for use in the rapid restoration of intravascular fluid (IVF) volume. Administration of hypertonic saline causes a rapid but transient (30- to 60-minute duration) plasma volume expansion as a result of osmotic redistribution of fluid from the interstitial fluid (ISF) space. The rapid increase in vascular volume improves cardiac output and tissue perfusion with rapid administration of only a relatively small volume of fluid. However, to maintain tissue perfusion, concurrent or subsequent administration of isotonic replacement fluids is required for patients with hypovolemia. Iatrogenic hypernatremia and hypokalemia may occur after hypertonic saline is administered; therefore plasma electrolyte concentrations ideally should be evaluated in the patient before and after administration of hypertonic saline.

CRYSTALLOIDS: MAINTENANCE FLUIDS

Crystalloid maintenance fluids are polyionic isotonic or hypotonic fluids formulated for long-term use in patients needing chronic fluid support.[12] The high concentration of Na^+ and relatively low concentration of K^+ in replacement fluids may result in hypernatremia and hypokalemia in patients receiving high volumes of these fluids over several days' time. In contrast, maintenance fluids contain a lower Na^+ concentration and a higher K^+ concentration, maintaining isotonicity with the addition of dextrose. Maintenance fluids also contain increased concentrations of Ca^{++} and Mg^{++} compared with replacement fluids. Examples fluids include *Plasmalyte 56* and *Normosol-M. Half-strength dextrose and saline* (0.45% NaCl and 2.5% dextrose) is an isotonic fluid that provides free water as dextrose is metabolized. This fluid is useful for long-term management in patients with hyperkalemia.

COLLOIDS

Colloids are fluids that induce a more rapid expansion of IVF than occurs with the administration of similar volumes of crystalloid fluids. Colloid fluids contain large-molecular-weight particles that are unable to diffuse quickly across cellular barriers, thereby maintaining or increasing colloid oncotic pressure. This allows a more effective volume expansion that persists over a longer period of time than that possible with the administration of crystalloids alone. In emergency situations small-volume colloid infusion can draw fluid from the ECF, allowing rapid plasma volume expansion in the early stages of volume replacement. Colloids expand plasma volume without increasing interstitial water.[13] The utility of colloids for human fluid resuscitation is controversial; the mortality rate was either unchanged compared with that observed in patients receiving only crystalloids or even increased in some subgroups of trauma and nontrauma patients.[14]

Plasma *Plasma* is a colloid fluid that contains a variety of essential proteins as well as osmotically active albumin. However, albumin is effective as an osmole only if it remains within the intravascular space. Plasma administration can therefore worsen edema if albumin is rapidly lost from the vascular space, as might occur in patients with increased capillary permeability (vasculitis), gastrointestinal protein loss, or marked proteinuria or in patients with very low plasma oncotic pressure. Other important constituents of plasma include clotting factors, immunoglobulins, and antithrombin. Plasma proteins also provide carrier sites for exogenous (drugs) and endogenous (hormones) compounds. In addition to the relatively short duration of effect of plasma when administered for oncotic effect, disadvantages of plasma administration in horses include the potential for adverse reactions and the relatively high cost for large volume administration in adult horses.

Hetastarch *Hetastarch* (6% hydroxyethyl starch) is often a more cost-effective colloid replacement than plasma. The large starch molecules maintain their plasma oncotic effect for a relatively long time as the molecules are gradually removed from circulation through renal elimination. However, unlike plasma, there are no functional molecules present in hydroxyethyl starch solutions. Hetastarch can be given as a series of rapid bolus doses for plasma volume expansion, in contrast to plasma itself, which must be administered slowly. For this reason it offers an attractive way to rapidly ameliorate the effects of acute blood loss. However, one retrospective study suggests that intraoperative use of Hetastarch in human cardiac surgery may increase bleeding and subsequent blood transfusion requirements.[15] Levels of factor VIII and von Willebrand's factor were decreased in horses receiving Hetastarch.[16]

Blood Blood can be considered the ultimate colloid replacement fluid, providing replacement of lost circulating volume, oncotic activity in the form of plasma proteins, oxygen-carrying capacity, a vehicle for therapeutic drug transport, and replenishment of coagulation factors.[5] However, its use requires selection of an appropriate donor, with careful collection and administration technique.[17] In addition, use of citrate-based anticoagulants may lead to hypocalcemia in recipients after blood or plasma administration. Care must also be exercised in the choice of concurrently administered intravenous fluids because calcium chelation may occur in shared intravenous lines. The technique of donor selection and blood administration has been well reviewed by Slovis.[17]

PRACTICAL CONSIDERATIONS AND COMBINATION FLUID THERAPY

When time allows, the initial fluid selection will be made on the basis of the biochemical profile and the clinical appearance of the patient. The initial resuscitation is usually an isotonic crystalloid fluid such as LRS or an equivalent with a bicarbonate precursor. In patients with hyperkalemia (e.g., uroperitoneum, acute renal failure), 0.9% NaCl, a K-deficient fluid, is preferred. The use of hypertonic saline is beneficial for transient IVF expansion where ISF is still adequate.

Concurrent or sequential administration of both crystalloids and colloids is useful for restoring hydration and circulating volume. Crystalloids distribute to the ECF space, with approximately 75% distributing to the ISF space, allowing interstitial rehydration in patients where this fluid shift has occurred. Consideration should be given to the existing oncotic pressure because high volume crystalloid fluid administration to a patient with low plasma oncotic pressure may precipitate significant edema formation as a consequence of further decreases in colloid onocotic pressure.

After administration colloid fluids remain largely restricted to the intravascular space. Rapid expansion of IVF is therefore possible during hypovolemic shock. The administration of colloids increases oncotic pressure by allowing increased retention of crystalloid fluids within the IVF compartment. As suggested previously for hypertonic saline therapy, administration of isotonic crystalloids is usually recommended before or concurrently with colloid fluid administration to ensure adequate fluid volume redistribution to interstitial spaces.

The use of crystalloid versus colloid fluids in situations requiring rapid large volume fluid resuscitation is controversial. The decrease in oncotic pressure that may occur after administration of large volumes of crystalloid fluids is widely thought to promote pulmonary edema; however, some clinical evidence suggests that the lung is relatively resistant to edema because of the effects of hemodilution and decreased oncotic pressure.[18] Other studies of fluid resuscitation of hypovolemic shock patients with normal saline demonstrate increased pulmonary edema compared with patients who were resuscitated with colloid solutions.[19]

In patients with hemorrhagic shock, two scenarios are possible. With controlled hemorrhagic shock, the bleeding source has been occluded after hemorrhage. Uncontrolled hemorrhagic shock occurs where bleeding is ongoing. Hypertonic saline administration to patients with controlled hemorrhagic shock leads to a desirable increase in blood pressure and cardiac output; however, in patients with uncontrolled hemorrhage, hypertonic saline increases bleeding from injured blood vessels and increases the risk of death.[20]

VASOACTIVE DRUGS

Vasoactive drugs may be administered in an attempt to increase cardiac output if response to primary intravenous fluid resuscitation is inadequate. Desirable qualities of vasoactive drugs (e.g., vasopressors and inotropes) used to combat hypotension include a short onset of action and rapid metabolism, which enable these drugs to be administered as continuous-rate infusions in order to titrate their effects in response to rapid changes in patient condition.

Receptor Physiology

Vasopressors and inotropes can be divided into adrenergic and nonadrenergic agonists. Adrenergic receptors targeted by vasoactive therapy include α_1-, α_2-, β_1-, and β_2-adrenergic receptors and dopaminergic receptors. Nonadrenergic mechanisms include activation of vasopressin-specific receptors (chiefly V_1) and effects on phosphodiesterase activity.[3]

α_1-Adrenergic receptor stimulation results in vasoconstriction caused by contraction of smooth muscle surrounding blood vessels.[21,22] α_1 Activity is also associated with metabolic changes and increased cardiac contractility.[23] Postsynaptic α_2-receptor stimulation results in vasodilation.[24]

β_1-Adrenergic receptor stimulation results primarily in cardiac effects with increases in both heart rate (chronotropic effect) and contractility (inotropic effect). Chronotropic effects result from increased conductivity at the sinoatrial node and within the cardiac ventricular muscle. Inotropic effects increase stroke volume, thereby improving cardiac output. β_2-Receptor stimulation causes relaxation of smooth muscle with consequent vasodilation of the arteries of coronary vessels, visceral organs, and skeletal muscle. Slight chronotropic and inotropic improvement after β_2- stimulation is also seen.[25]

Dopaminergic receptors improve myocardial contractility and, at certain doses, increase heart rate.[26] Several types of dopaminergic receptors have been identified, and specific effects vary depending on receptor type. Other notable effects include renal stimulation, resulting in diuresis and naturesis (D_1 and D_2 receptors).[27]

Vasopressin receptors (V_1) are present throughout the vascular system, and their stimulation results in vasoconstriction, especially at peripheral arterioles.[28,29] After normal physiologic V_1 stimulation, resulting vasoconstriction leads to no net change in blood pressure as a result of modulation by reflex activation of the baroreceptors.[28,29] However, during hypovolemic shock, markedly increased levels of V_1 stimulation lead to significant increases in vascular resistance, an important mechanism for restoration of arterial blood pressure.[30]

Vasopressors

Vasopressors increase MAP, improving perfusion pressure and distribution of cardiac output. Decreased venous compliance increases venous return, which improves cardiac output.[21,22] Vasopressor use must be closely monitored because excessive vasoconstriction increases cardiac afterload, increasing cardiac workload while decreasing stroke volume and therefore cardiac output.

Adrenergic Vasopressors

NOREPINEPHRINE

Norepinephrine has predominantly α_1-adrenergic agonist activity. It is useful to improve organ perfusion pressure during distributive and vasodilatory shock, especially in patients nonresponsive to fluid resuscitation or inotrope administration. Systemic vascular resistance and MAP are increased, with greater arterial constriction (and therefore resistance increase) than occurs with epinephrine. Vasoconstriction increases cardiac afterload, potentially decreasing cardiac output; however, this effect is countered by the α_1- effects of norepinephrine, which facilitate increased stroke volume.[31]

EPINEPHRINE

Epinephrine is a strong α- and β-adrenergic agonist, making it a potent vasopressor. Splanchnic blood flow is decreased compared with norepinephrine.[32] Coronary and renal blood flow is also reduced. Myocardial irritability is increased, with resultant increased risk of arrhythmia. Postresuscitation myocardial depression and increased myocardial oxygen consumption are reported.[33]

Repetitive doses of epinephrine have not been shown to have significant additive pressor effect. High-dose epinephrine induces disproportionate increases in systolic and pulmonary vasculature pressure. Pulmonary edema may result.[24]

DOPAMINE

Dopamine is active at adrenergic (α-, β-) and dopaminergic receptors, with differing effects recognized depending on the dosage administered. High infusion rates of dopamine tend to result in a predominance of α-adrenergic effects and a vasopressor response. β-Adrenergic effects predominate at lower infusion rates with principally an inotropic response. Low infusion rates are purported to stimulate dopaminergic receptors, improving splanchnic perfusion with concurrent effects on the afferent renal vasculature.[35,36] Plasma concentrations of dopamine vary widely among individuals. As a result, the effect of any particular infusion rate may be highly variable.[34] Considerable controversy exists regarding the utility of dopamine administration, with variable experimental evidence of improved renal perfusion and meta-analysis data showing increased mortality in some subsets of patients.[5,37,38]

PHENYLEPHRINE

Phenylephrine is primarily an α-agonist. Systemic vascular resistance and MAP increase after administration, but cardiac output decreases as a result of a decreased heart rate with an unchanged stroke volume. When phenylephrine is used as a vasopressor, concurrent use of a β-agonist (e.g., norepinephrine, dobutamine) is often beneficial.

Nonadrenergic Vasopressors

VASOPRESSIN

Vasopressin, or antidiuretic hormone, is a peptide whose primary role is to regulate the body's retention of water. Released in response to dehydration, vasopressin acts at the kidneys, binding V_2 receptors promoting water conservation in the collecting tubule and thereby concentrating and reducing urine volume.

Vasopressin binds to peripheral V_1 receptors, causing vasoconstriction. Although catecholamines may be increased during sepsis, their vasoconstrictor effect can be reduced; this effect, however, can be restored by administration of vasopressin. Human research demonstrates beneficial effects of vasopressin when used concurrently with the catecholamines.[21,33]

Stimulation of V_1 receptors has been suggested to decrease blood flow in the gastrointestinal tract. Experimental studies have shown a detrimental effect in volume-deficient animals; however, in test subjects receiving aggressive fluid resuscitation, V_1 stimulation improved visceral circulation.[39] Therefore V_1 agonists may be unsuitable for use in horses that remain hypovolemic. It is vital to ensure adequate fluid resuscitation before administration of these drugs.[39] Current evidence suggests that vasopressin should be used in combination with a catecholamine vasopressor.[40,41] Reports of vasopressin use and physiology in the horse are few in number.[42-44]

Inotropes

The mode of action of inotropic drugs is to increase cardiac stroke volume. This is achieved by increased myocardial contractility, which increases ventricular emptying and decreases end-systolic volume. Cardiac workload and oxygen consumption are increased, which is of concern in hypoxemic patients. If response to fluid resuscitation is inadequate, inotropes provide another means to increase cardiac output and oxygen delivery.[3]

DOBUTAMINE

Dobutamine is a synthetic catecholamine that has primarily β_1-adrenergic receptor stimulating action with weak α and β_2 affinity. Dobutamine is useful in patients with diminished cardiac output or decreased central venous oxygen tension despite adequate fluid volume restoration. Beneficial effects include increased stroke volume and heart rate, with improved splanchnic perfusion and urine output. Blood pressure effects are variable.[3]

MONITORING CARDIOVASCULAR FUNCTION IN THE CRITICAL PATIENT

PHYSICAL EXAMINATION

Compromised cardiovascular function is suggested by poor peripheral pulse quality, discoloration of the mucous membranes with or without delayed refill time, cold extremities, and signs of generalized weakness. Heart rate and rhythm are likely disturbed, with cardiac auscultation revealing murmurs. Body weight may increase as a result of edema formation. In addition to these, other suggestive findings are discussed in the subsequent sections.

JUGULAR PULSATION

In the normal standing horse, jugular pulsation is restricted to the caudal one third of the neck. Increased jugular pulsation indicates tricuspid regurgitation or increased CVP.[45] The former can be distinguished by occlusion of the jugular vein proximally and stripping of blood down toward the heart. Should the jugular vein refill while occluded in this fashion, tricuspid regurgitation is likely.

VENTRAL OR PERIPHERAL EDEMA

Subcutaneous edema in dependent sites may form in patients with volume overload. Alternatively, increased capillary permeability or decreased colloid osmotic pressure (COP) may be responsible.[12]

URINE PRODUCTION

Urine production is considered a reflection of renal blood flow and hence cardiac output. This can be considered an indication of the adequacy of overall organ and tissue perfusion.[46] However, during vasopressor therapy urine output and glomerular filtration rate are unreliable indicators of human renal function.[36]

Specific gravity can vary widely, although when dehydration is present, urine should always be concentrated. In patients with renal compromise, isosthenuric urine is produced. In normal horses urine output is highly variable, depending on fluid intake and diet. Reported ranges in the horse are 0.6 to 1.25 ml/kg/hr.[47]

LABORATORY VALUES

Hematocrit, protein concentrations, and electrolyte concentrations (especially K^+, Mg^{++}, and Ca^{++}) should be monitored and normalized if possible in horses with cardiovascular compromise. Oxygen delivery to tissues, potential for edema formation, and cardiac rate and rhythm are dependent on appropriate values.

LACTATE

Lactate is the terminal product of anaerobic glycolysis. Increased blood lactate concentration results from inadequate delivery of oxygen to peripheral tissues. This may be the result of hypovolemia, hypoxemia, alterations in hemoglobin concentration, decreased perfusion pressure, or a combination of these factors. Increased tissue demands for oxygen may be secondary to sepsis or increased metabolic rate.[48] Tissue oxygen consumption may be impaired, leading to increased lactate production.[49] Therefore blood lactate concentration is an indication of the adequacy of peripheral perfusion and oxygen delivery to tissues. The need for and response to blood transfusion can be assessed by analysis of plasma lactate.[50]

Lactate measurement is useful clinically to monitor the response to fluid therapy and vasoactive drug treatments in patients with poor tissue perfusion. Decreases in plasma lactate concentration are considered to temporally follow improvements in cardiovascular performance; therefore the trend in changes in plasma lactate concentration is most clinically useful. In situations of appropriate volume restoration in which lactate concentration remains increased, unresolved inflammatory stimulus and uncontrolled sepsis should be suspected.

ARTERIAL BLOOD PRESSURE

Arterial blood pressure is the product of cardiac output (itself the product of heart rate and stroke volume) and systemic vascular resistance (vasomotor tone). Mean blood pressure, not systolic or diastolic blood pressure, is considered most important for organ and tissue perfusion (Table 7-9).[47]

Arterial blood pressure can be measured by direct (invasive) and indirect (noninvasive) means, as described earlier in this chapter. Trends in arterial blood pressure, as opposed to individual readings, should be used to guide therapy. Consideration of physical findings should also be given when altering therapy.

CENTRAL VENOUS PRESSURE

Central venous pressure is determined by central venous blood volume, muscular tone of the venous system, and the balance between venous return and cardiac output. The technique for

TABLE 7-9

Cardiovascular Parameters

Type of Blood Pressure	Blood Pressure Reading
Arterial pressure	
Mean arterial pressure	> 60 mmHg
Systolic (indirect)	111.8 ±13.3 mmHg
Diastolic (indirect)	67.7 ± 13.8 mmHg
Central venous pressure	mean 12 cmH_2O

Data from Cook VL, Bain FT: Volume (crystalloid) replacement in the ICU patient, *Clin Tech in Equine Pract* 2:122–129, 2003, and Magdesian KG: Monitoring the critically ill equine patient, *Vet Clin North Am Equine Pract* 20:11–39, 2004.

measuring CVP in horses is described earlier in this chapter. Central venous pressure is a measure of blood pressure within the intrathoracic cranial vena cava, estimating right atrial pressure and cardiac preload.

Central venous pressure can be used to guide fluid replacement therapy in patients with hypovolemia. The tendency to form edema in patients that are hypooncotic, have increased capillary permeability, or have diminished cardiac function can also be monitored. As with measurements of arterial blood pressure, the trend in CVP seen through repeated monitoring is most informative regarding restoration of fluid volume administration and attempts to manage cardiac failure.

Low CVP values are consistent with vasodilation or hypovolemia. Lack of an increase in CVP in response to a challenge fluid bolus is consistent with hypovolemia. Decreased CVP also occurs during inspiratory efforts that result in decreased intrathoracic pressure. Central venous pressure can be increased in patients with fluid overload (iatrogenic), increases in blood volume (renal failure, renin-angiotensin-aldosterone activation), systemic venoconstriction (sympathetic activation), and right-sided heart failure. Restrictions to cardiac filling, such as pericardial or pleural effusion, forced expiration, and positive pressure ventilation, may increase CVP. Increased CVP may falsely result from ventricular catheterization and air within the manometer or fluid lines.

COLLOID OSMOTIC PRESSURE

Colloid osmotic pressure, also referred to as *oncotic pressure,* results from the osmotic force caused by macromolecules within the intravascular compartment. This pressure is essential to retain appropriate intravascular volume. Proteins and colloid molecules retain water within the vasculature by virtue of their osmotic draw. They are sufficiently large in mass to limit their permeability across the vascular endothelium. In addition, the Gibbs-Donnan effect, wherein sodium cations are attracted to negative residues on protein (albumin), adds further to the intravascular osmotic draw.

Loss of plasma proteins resulting from increased capillary permeability can lead to a hypooncotic state. Severe loss of proteins leads to hypovolemia caused by simultaneous loss of plasma. Fluid resuscitation with crystalloids dilutes plasma proteins. In horses with hypoproteinemia, this further dilution leads to an increase in interstitial fluid volume and therefore to ventral and tissue edema with potential for reduced blood volume.[16,51]

Colloid osmotic pressure can be measured or calculated, with reasonable agreement in healthy but not hospitalized horses.[52] Because albumin is the major contributor to COP, alterations in the albumin-to-globulin ratio alter COP at any given total plasma protein concentration. Calculated COP in horses with hypoproteinemia (hypoalbuminemia) is therefore likely inaccurate.[51] Direct measurement of COP is necessary after synthetic colloid (hetastarch) administration because these starch molecules have considerable osmotic effect but are not measurable by refractometry.

VENOUS BLOOD GAS

Arterial blood gas values are required to assess pulmonary gas exchange, as described elsewhere in this chapter; however, in patients with cardiovascular compromise in which severe hypoperfusion may be present, tissue level hypercapnia and acidemia are more accurately represented in central venous blood.[53] Venous hypercapnia results from increased tissue CO_2 production and transference to blood in the capillaries of the hypoperfused peripheral tissues and a diminished CO_2 excretion because of pulmonary hypoperfusion.[54]

ELECTROCARDIOGRAM

Indications for electrocardiogram (ECG) monitoring of equine patients with cardiac compromise include dysrhythmias and marked electrolyte abnormalities (especially hyperkalemia); ECG is also useful to monitor response to vasoactive drug therapy. The base apex lead system is most commonly used in equine medicine. Telemetry units allow remote monitoring of horses free in stalls and are most convenient when seeking to diagnose an intermittent dysrhythmia.[45,47] A more complete review of the cardiovascular system and its monitoring is available in Chapter 10.

ECHOCARDIOGRAPHY

Echocardiography is extensively reviewed in Chapter 10. Visualization of the heart, pericardial space, and intrathoracic vessels gives invaluable insight into cardiac integrity and function.

Monitoring cardiac output in the horse is possible by Doppler echocardiography.[55] This technique allows determination of the velocity, turbulence, and direction of blood flow in the heart. Change in frequency between the emitted and the reflected ultrasound wave is used to calculate the velocity of the blood cells, and hence a measure of cardiac output can be made. Correct alignment of the waveform is essential for an accurate estimate of cardiac output, with the beam needing to be aligned as close to parallel to blood flow as possible.[56]

CARDIAC OUTPUT MEASUREMENTS

The use of advanced technologies such as lithium dilution, indicator dilution, bioimpedance, and pulse contour analysis for assessment of cardiac output has been extensively reviewed.[56] These techniques are impractical in the clinical setting or have not been validated for the horse.

Briefly, dilution techniques rely on injection of a known amount of an indicator dye into a vein upstream of the heart. The indicator is diluted by the blood passing through the heart. Once diluted, the concentration of indicator is measured in a peripheral artery; the volume of blood and therefore the cardiac output can be calculated as related to the area under the concentration-time curve of the indicator downstream of the heart.

Transthoracic electric bioimpedance is a noninvasive method of measuring cardiac output. Because blood has a relatively high electrical conductivity compared with solid tissues and air, alterations in arterial blood flow lead to changes in thoracic impedance. The amount of change relates to the amount of blood flowing (cardiac output). This change is measured as alterations in the conductivity of a small electric current applied to the thorax. Bioimpedance has not been used to measure cardiac output in horses.[56]

Pulse contour analysis calculates the cardiac output from arterial pressure waveforms, using the area under the arterial pressure tracing during systole to represent blood flow in the catheterized vessel. This is therefore a measure of cardiac output.[57]

SUPPORT OF RESPIRATORY FUNCTION

Bonnie Barr

A core skill in critical care medicine is rapid and thorough assessment of respiratory and cardiovascular function firmly grounded by the understanding of physiologic and pathophysiologic processes in each of these organ systems. The major function of the respiratory system is gas exchange and, in conjunction with the cardiovascular system, delivery of oxygen to tissues and elimination of CO_2 generated by tissue metabolism. Oxygen and CO_2 are exchanged between the inspired air and blood to maintain normal arterial partial pressure of oxygen (PaO_2) and CO_2 ($PaCO_2$). The respiratory control system maintains PaO_2 and $PaCO_2$ within a narrow homeostatic range despite the body's wide variety of demands. Adequate ventilation requires the complex interaction among central respiratory centers, spinal pathways, peripheral respiratory nerves, and primary respiratory muscles.[1] Under normal conditions the primary driving force of alveolar ventilation is changes in the $PaCO_2$, which are sensed by central chemoreceptors in the brainstem.[1] Changes in PaO_2, which are sensed by peripheral chemoreceptors in the carotid and aortic bodies, also have an impact on alveolar ventilation but typically only in states of marked hypoxemia.[1]

The basic components of the respiratory system are the upper airways, the respiratory passageways, and the alveolocapillary membrane. The upper airways and the respiratory passageways are not involved in gas exchange and therefore are referred to as *anatomic dead space*.[1] The alveolocapillary membrane is the primary area involved in gas exchange, although occasionally areas are ventilated but not perfused, resulting in physiologic dead space.[1] The alveolocapillary membranes are made up of the alveoli and the pulmonary capillaries, which form a dense network intertwined with the alveoli. This allows for maximum exchange of oxygen and CO_2. Factors that affect the rate of gas diffusion include thickness of the membranes, surface areas of the membrane, the diffusion coefficient of the gas, and the pressure difference between the two sides of the membrane.[1,2]

OXYGEN DELIVERY TO THE TISSUES

Oxygen is delivered to the alveoli, where it diffuses down a pressure gradient into the pulmonary capillary system and is delivered to the tissues. Under normal conditions approximately 97% of oxygen is transported in the blood bound to hemoglobin.[1,2] In the pulmonary capillaries the PaO_2 is high, and therefore oxygen binds with hemoglobin but when PaO_2 is low, in the tissues, oxygen is released. The oxygen-hemoglobin dissociation curve depicts the association between PaO_2 plotted on the x axis and percentage of oxygen saturation of hemoglobin plotted on the y axis. The resulting curve is sigmoid in shape, with the plateau portion at high PaO_2 values. At this point in the curve, a decrease in PaO_2 results in minimal changes in oxygen saturation within erythrocytes. In contrast, the steep part of the curve indicates that a relatively small decrease in PaO_2 in this range results in a very large decrease in the amount of oxygen bound to hemoglobin and resultant oxygen transfer to tissues at the level of the tissue capillary bed. Factors such as pH, temperature, and the concentration of 2,3-diphosphoglycerate can result in a shift of the curve increasing or decreasing oxygen affinity of hemoglobin.[1,2]

In its strictest definition *hypoxemia* refers to the condition of decreased oxygen content in the blood. Oxygen in the blood is present either combined with hemoglobin (Hb) in the erythrocyte or as dissolved oxygen (P_aO_2). Total oxygen content (CaO_2) is calculated as follows:

$$CaO_2 = (1.34 \times Hb \times SaO_2) + (P_aO_2 \times 0.003)$$

where 1.34 is the oxygen-binding capacity of hemoglobin, SaO_2 is the percentage of saturation of hemoglobin with oxygen, and 0.003 is the solubility constant for dissolved oxygen in plasma.[1,2] Disorders that affect the binding of oxygen to hemoglobin (e.g., carbon monoxide toxicity, methemoglobinemia) have a tremendous impact on oxygen delivery to the tissues. Relying solely on assessment of P_aO_2 can result in significant errors in clinical judgment. In spite of this important consideration, and because P_aO_2 is more easily and frequently referenced in most laboratory and clinical situations than is total oxygen content, *hypoxemia* is often used to refer to a condition of decreased dissolved oxygen in the blood (decreased P_aO_2), which is how that term will be used in the remainder of this discussion.

CAUSES OF HYPOXEMIA

Hypoxemia (low PaO_2) occurs for one of five reasons: decreased inspired oxygen content, diffusion impairment within the lungs, hypoventilation, right-to-left shunting of blood, or ventilation-perfusion mismatch. Horses breathing room air inspire sufficient quantities of oxygen to maintain adequate dissolved oxygen unless they are housed at extremely high altitudes. Occasionally, decreased inspired oxygen content may be a problem in horses under general anesthesia that are inhaling inadequate gas mixtures. However, for practical purposes decreased inspired oxygen is a very rare primary cause of hypoxemia.

Diffusion impairment occurs when the capillary-alveolar interface does not permit adequate gas exchange. This occurs with pulmonary diseases such as pulmonary fibrosis and consolidation that decrease the area or increase the thickness of the alveolocapillary membrane. Because CO_2 normally diffuses about 20 times more rapidly than O_2 across the alveolar-capillary interface, decreased diffusion results in hypoxemia before there is significant hypercapnia. However, oxygen is very diffusible, and under typical resting conditions in a normal horse, the partial pressure of O_2 in the blood is nearly identical to that of alveolar gas when the red cell is only one third of the way along the capillary. Pulmonary disease must be quite severe before diffusion will limit gas exchange in horses; therefore diffusion impairment as a primary cause of hypoxemia in resting horses is uncommon. However, in horses undergoing maximal exercise, oxygen transfer is likely to be diffusion limited because the extremely high cardiac output causes blood to pass through the pulmonary capillaries too quickly to permit complete oxygenation.

Hypoventilation occurs when there is a reduction in the amount of air entering and exiting the alveoli, resulting in decreased gas exchange. Alveolar ventilation is the amount of air that reaches the alveoli and participates in gas exchange. Because metabolic production of CO_2 is fairly constant under normal metabolic circumstances, the blood CO_2 level is primarily controlled by its rate of elimination through the lungs. A partial pressure gradient between the capillary venous blood and the alveoli of the lungs results in diffusion of CO_2 into the alveoli. Carbon dioxide is then removed from the alveoli by ventilatory exchange of atmospheric air with alveolar gases. Because CO_2 is highly diffusible, the partial pressure of CO_2 in alveolar gas and arterial blood are virtually identical and the $PaCO_2$ accurately reflects the current status of alveolar ventilation. In other words, hypoventilation always causes an increased alveolar, and therefore arterial, partial pressure of CO_2. Hypoventilation can also result in varying degrees of decreased PaO_2 and respiratory acidosis. Causes of hypoventilation include disorders of the central nervous system, resulting in depression of the respiratory center and disorders of the thoracic cavity, respiratory tract, and respiratory muscles.[1,2] Central nervous system depression can be due to the administration of certain medications, brain and spinal cord trauma, or space-occupying lesions in the brain. Impairment of respiration can result from upper airway obstruction, pleural space disease, neuromuscular disease, thoracic pain, and severe abdominal distention.

Hypoxemia caused by right-to-left shunt occurs when venous blood bypasses gas exchange areas of the lungs (alveoli) and mixes with oxygenated arterial blood, resulting in hypoxemia. Shunt can result from either right-to-left cardiac shunt (extrapulmonary; e.g., Tetralogy of Fallot) or atelectatic or consolidated lung lobes (intrapulmonary).[1,2] The latter mechanism is a result of severe ventilation-perfusion mismatch.

The most common cause of hypoxemia in the horse is ventilation-perfusion mismatch. This occurs when alveolar ventilation and blood flow are not closely matched, resulting in inefficient gas exchange. A high ventilation-perfusion mismatch occurs when regions of the lung are ventilated but not perfused, causing an increase in the physiologic dead space of the lung.[1,2] A low ventilation-perfusion mismatch occurs when regions of the lung are perfused but not ventilated. Ventilation-perfusion mismatch may result from all forms of pulmonary disease. For example, pulmonary thromboembolism can cause high ventilation-perfusion mismatch, whereas bronchopneumonia with consolidation results in a low ventilation-perfusion mismatch.[1,2] If ventilation-perfusion mismatch is severe, the functional result is a right-to-left intrapulmonary shunting of blood.[1,2]

CAUSES OF TISSUE HYPOXIA

Hypoxemia is only one of several possible causes of oxygen deficiency at the tissue level, a condition referred to as *hypoxia*. Tissue hypoxia may result from any condition that causes decreased oxygen delivery to the tissues. Horses with decreased cardiac output, such as that which occurs in any shock state; decreased blood oxygen-carrying capacity, such as that which occurs with anemia or in the presence of abnormal hemoglobin; peripheral arterial-venous shunting; histotoxic changes (e.g., inhibition of the cytochrome chain); increased peripheral oxygen consumption; hypermetabolic conditions (e.g., hyperthermia, seizures, sepsis); and localized obstruction of blood flow, may experience generalized or localized tissue hypoxia in the face of normal P_aO_2.[1,2]

ARTERIAL BLOOD GAS ANALYSIS

Arterial blood gas analysis is the most common method for assessment of pulmonary function and acid-base status in horses that are critically ill. In the adult horse the sample may be obtained from the facial artery or transverse facial artery (see Figure 7-1).[3] If continuous samples are to be obtained, an indwelling arterial catheter may be placed. Alternatively, a sample may be carefully obtained from the carotid artery in some horses.

Arterial blood gas analysis measures the amounts of oxygen and CO_2 in arterial blood, reflecting the functional efficiency of the lungs and response to oxygen therapy.[2,3] Correct interpretation of the arterial blood gas information allows one to assess the status of ventilation and oxygenation in the patient and determine whether an acid-base disorder is present. This can greatly facilitate appropriate diagnostic, therapeutic, and prognostic decision making for the patient.

Samples for blood gas analysis must be collected and handled appropriately to ensure accurate results. A small amount of heparin is used to coat the hub of the needle before aspiration of the sample. Excessive heparin dilutes the sample and may cause inaccurate results, including decreased pH, $PaCO_2$, and bicarbonate. After collection the sample should be stored anaerobically by removing the needle and placing a syringe cap over the tip of the syringe. Prolonged exposure to air bubbles can result in a decrease in $PaCO_2$ and an increase in PaO_2 as the sample equilibrates with room air in the bubble.[2,3] A sample stored at room temperature should be analyzed within 10 to 15 minutes.[4] In samples stored at 37° C, $PaCO_2$ will increase by approximately 0.1 mm Hg per minute and PaO_2 will increase at approximately 0.5 to 2.3 mm Hg per minute.[2,3] Delaying analysis for 1 hour will provide useful information only about acid-base status, not about oxygenation. If the sample is immediately stored on ice to decrease metabolic activity of cells, it should be analyzed within 2 hours. Exceeding these times may result in an increased P_{aCO2}, decreased pH, decreased glucose, and increased lactate as blood cells continue to metabolize nutrients.

BLOOD GAS ASSESSMENT OF RESPIRATORY FUNCTION

A systematic evaluation of blood gas values includes consideration of pH, P_aO_2, arterial oxygen saturation (usually a calculated value), P_aCO_2, and bicarbonate concentration. Normal blood gas measurements in the awake horse on room air are shown in Table 7-10.

The P_aO_2 is the partial pressure of oxygen dissolved in arterial blood and is a reflection of pulmonary oxygenating capability.[1-3] Hemoglobin or its binding state do not affect P_aO_2; once O_2 is bound to hemoglobin, it cannot exert any gas pressure. Causes of low P_aO_2 (hypoxemia) are discussed in preceding sections and include decreased inspired oxygen content, hypoventilation, diffusion impairment, right-to-left shunting of blood, and ventilation-perfusion mismatch. The P_aCO_2 is the partial pressure of CO_2 dissolved in the plasma of arterial blood and is a reflection of the balance between alveolar minute ventilation and metabolic CO_2 production.[1-3]

The first step in blood gas interpretation for evaluation of respiratory function is to assess ventilatory status. Increased P_aCO_2 indicates hypoventilation, and decreased P_aCO_2 indicates hyperventilation. Hypoventilation and hyperventilation are not clearly correlated with respiratory rate or effort and

TABLE 7-10

Normal Range of Arterial Blood Gas Values for Adult Horses

Variable	Normal Range
pH	7.4 ± 0.2
$PaCO_2$	40 ± 3 mmHg
PaO_2	94 ± 3 mmHg
Base excess	0 ± 1 mmHg
SpO_2	98-99%

From Aguilera-Tejero E, Estepa JC, Lopez I, et al: Arterial blood gases and acid-base balance in healthy young and old horses. *Equine Vet J* 30:352, 1998.

cannot be accurately assessed on the basis of physical examination. Hypoventilation may be caused by central apnea (central nervous system disease), obstructive apnea (upper respiratory tract disease), increased dead space ventilation (shunt, decreased cardiac output), reduced lung compliance (low lung volume), respiratory muscle weakness or fatigue, poor control when mechanical ventilation is employed, thoracic pain, or abdominal distention. Hyperventilation, with decreased P_aCO_2, may result from pain, hypoxemia of any cause, pulmonary disease, or neurologic disease.

Oxygenation status is determined by assessment of the P_aO_2 in light of the partial pressure of inspired oxygen, which is determined by the proportion of total volume of gas (fraction of inspired oxygen, or FiO_2) and the atmospheric pressure. Because most equine patients reside at elevations with reasonable atmospheric pressure, the most important variable to consider is FiO_2. P_aO_2 is typically four to five times the FiO_2. If the patient is breathing room air (FiO_2 = 21%), expected PaO_2 concentration is approximately 80 to 100 mm Hg; if the patient is breathing 100% oxygen (FiO_2 = 100%), expected P_aO_2 is approximately 400 to 500 mm Hg.

For many patients it is useful to calculate the alveolar-arteriolar oxygen difference (A-a difference) to determine whether the lungs are functioning properly with regard to gas exchange.[1,2] In the normal horse breathing room air, the P_aO_2 should be only slightly less than the alveolar oxygen concentration (P_AO_2) with an A-a difference of 5 to 20 mm Hg.

The formula for calculating the A-a difference is as follows:

$$[P_iO_2 - 1.2\,(P_aCO_2)] - P_aO_2$$

The alveolar oxygen concentration (P_A) in this equation is reflected as $[P_iO_2 - 1.2(P_aCO_2)]$, indicating that for any given PiO_2, as P_aCO_2 (ventilation) changes, there will be changes in P_AO_2. PiO_2 is the partial pressure of inspired oxygen as determined by the equation $FiO_2 \times (P_B - 47)$, where FiO_2 is the proportion of inspired oxygen (0.21 when breathing room air; 1 when breathing 100% oxygen), P_B is the barometric pressure, and 47 is the water vapor pressure. Barometric pressure may be approximated as average pressure for the altitude (approximately 760 mm Hg at sea level). These calculations can be simplified to approximate an A-a difference for an expected PiO_2 within most reasonable atmospheric pressures:

$$(150 - 1.2\ P_aCO_2) - P_aO_2$$

Calculating the A-a difference is particularly helpful in patients that are hypoventilating (increased P_aCO_2) to determine whether hypoxemia (decreased P_aO_2) is due solely to hypoventilation or whether there are concurrent pulmonary factors contributing to hypoxemia. If the A-a difference remains within normal limits in the face of hypoventilation, then the hypoxemia is likely attributable solely to hypoventilation. If the patient is hypoventilating (increased $PaCO_2$) and hypoxemic (decreased P_aO_2) with an increased A-a gradient, then the hypoxemia is due to hypoventilation in combination with ventilation-perfusion mismatching, right-to-left shunting, or diffusion impairment.

If decreased P_aCO_2 (hyperventilation) is present in combination with decreased P_aO_2, oxygen should be administered both as treatment and as a diagnostic aid. If the administration of oxygen fails to increase the PaO_2 about 100 mm Hg, right-to-left shunting should be suspected and appropriate diagnostic testing employed. Improvement of PaO_2 above 100 mmHg with oxygen administration suggests ventilation-perfusion mismatch or a diffusion disturbance, and additional diagnostic testing is employed. If hyperventilation is present and PaO_2 is normal, pH and bicarbonate should be carefully evaluated because the hyperventilation may be occurring in an attempt to maintain normal pH in the face of metabolic alkalosis, as discussed later in this chapter.

Arterial blood gas analysis will also provide a value for oxygen saturation (SaO_2) reported as a percentage. This value reflects the proportion of all heme-binding sites saturated with O_2. Its value is determined by P_aO_2 and other factors that alter the oxygen hemoglobin dissociation curve. Because total blood oxygen content (total of dissolved and hemoglobin-bound oxygen) depends largely on the total quantity of hemoglobin that is present, it is possible to have normal P_aO_2 and normal S_aO_2 despite profound deficiencies in total blood oxygen content (e.g., in the profoundly anemic patient). One should not assume that the total oxygen content is normal because the P_aO_2 and oxygen saturation are normal.

Venous blood gas analysis has limited usefulness for evaluation of respiratory tract disease. However, P_vO_2 may provide some information about tissue oxygenation in horses. If values fall between 28 and 35 mm Hg, there is likely limited oxygen reserve in the tissues. Values below 27 mm Hg often indicate the presence of anaerobic metabolism. A P_vO_2 value greater than 60 mm Hg in an animal breathing room air suggests the possibility of decreased oxygen delivery to tissues, which may occur in some patients with poor peripheral perfusion caused by shock or sepsis.

PULSE OXIMETRY

A useful adjunct to arterial blood gas analysis is pulse oximetry, a technique that relies on reflection of different wavelengths of light to detect and differentiate oxygenated and unoxygenated hemoglobin; the measurement is reported as SpO_2. Pulse oximeters provide an estimate of hemoglobin saturation with oxygen, which is related to the P_aO_2, as described by the oxygen-hemoglobin dissociation curve. Generally, oxygen saturation greater than 91% is considered indicative of an arterial oxygen level within physiologically normal limits.[2,5] When hemoglobin saturation exceeds 90%, the oxygen-hemoglobin dissociation curve is relatively flat, and large changes in PaO_2 are associated with small changes in hemoglobin saturation. Therefore pulse oximetry has a limited sensitivity for determining changes in pulmonary gas exchange at ranges above 90% hemoglobin saturation. As saturation falls below 91%, the curve sharply decreases, representing increasingly severe reductions in arterial oxygen levels.[2,5]

Pulse oximeters measure hemoglobin saturation by sensing the difference between light absorption at two different frequencies: red and infrared. The measurements are obtained by attaching a probe containing the light emitter and detector to a suitable site, such as a nasal septum, white lip, or vulva. Reports have indicated that below 90% oxygen saturation, pulse oximetry can either overestimate or underestimate SaO_2 in horses.[6] The accuracy is influenced by several factors, including dark-pigmented skin, hypoperfusion at the measurement site, anemia, hypothermia, and motion. These limitations become more problematic in a conscious, standing horse. Artificially increased results may result because the machine cannot differentiate oxyhemoglobin from carboxyhemoglobin and methemoglobin. Because of the limitations of pulse oximetry, response to treatment in a patient with critical hypoxemia is best monitored with arterial blood gas analysis.

ASSESSMENT OF ACID-BASE STATUS

An evaluation of blood gas results is not complete without assessment of the patient's acid-base status. The body must maintain blood pH within a fairly narrow range for metabolic processes to function smoothly. Because of this, the body has developed a variety of mechanisms to control the amount of acid present in the blood: (1) the chemical buffers system, the most important of which is bicarbonate; (2) respiratory elimination of CO_2 generated by cellular metabolism; and (3) renal excretion of excess acid or alkali.

The pH of blood is a logarithmic expression of hydrogen ion concentration that can be calculated using the Henderson-Hasselbalch equation:

$$pH = pK_a + \log [HCO_3^-/(PaCO_2 \times 0.03)]$$

This equation indicates that the pH of blood is determined by the ratio of bicarbonate to arterial CO_2. If the pH is to remain the same for any given change in bicarbonate, the P_aCO_2 needs to change in the same direction, and vice versa. This relationship between CO_2, water, and bicarbonate is reflected in the carbonic acid equilibrium equation:

$$CO_2 + H_2O \leftrightarrow H_2CO_3 \leftrightarrow H^+ + HCO_3^-$$

There are four primary acid-base disturbances that may occur in a patient: respiratory acidosis (hypoventilation or increased P_aCO_2), respiratory alkalosis (hyperventilation or decreased P_aCO_2), metabolic acidosis (decreased HCO_3^-), and metabolic alkalosis (increased HCO_3^-). These may exist as sole disorders or in combination (mixed disorders). In a simplified approach to blood gas analysis of acid-base status, the clinician first determines whether the blood pH is normal (approximately 7.40) or whether acidemia or alkalemia exist. If the blood pH is decreased (acidemia), the primary acid-base abnormality present in that patient is likely to be either respiratory acidosis or metabolic acidosis. If the blood pH is increased (alkalemia), the primary acid-base abnormality is probably respiratory alkalosis or metabolic alkalosis.

Differential diagnoses for primary hyperventilation and hypoventilation are discussed in preceding sections. It is clear that these disorders can significantly affect blood pH, and therapies to improve ventilation or treat underlying disorders will usually resolve these problems.

Metabolic acidosis is usually recognized as a decreased blood HCO_3^- concentration. It results from addition of a strong acid to body fluids (most frequently lactic acid) or from loss of bicarbonate through the kidneys or gastrointestinal tract. When this occurs, the body will often compensate by increasing ventilation to eliminate CO_2. The kidneys will also attempt to compensate by excreting excess acid and conserving HCO_3^-. It is important to note that lactic acid accumulation is the most common cause of metabolic acidosis in horses. This is often secondary to dehydration and decreased tissue perfusion. In most cases of mild to moderate metabolic acidosis, re-establishment of normal circulating blood volume will enhance clearance of lactic acid from the blood and decrease production of new lactic acid. Lactic acid is cleared from the blood by the liver. As the liver metabolizes lactate, it produces bicarbonate. As a result, metabolic acidosis secondary to lactic acidosis resulting from poor tissue perfusion will usually respond promptly to rehydration of the patient with replacement fluid therapy.

Metabolic alkalosis is associated with an increased blood HCO_3^- concentration and often a reciprocal decrease in plasma Cl^- concentration. The most common causes of metabolic alkalosis in horses are high volume nasogastric reflux, overzealous administration of chloride-wasting diuretics, or exhausted horse syndrome (with excessive Cl^- losses in sweat). These horses are treated with restoration of extracellular volume, including replacement of Cl^- and K^+ deficits.

APPROACH TO THE PATIENT WITH RESPIRATORY DISTRESS

Respiratory dysfunction may be the primary reason that a veterinarian is consulted, or it may occur while the horse is hospitalized for treatment of another problem. *Respiratory distress* is defined as an inappropriate degree of breathing effort, based on an assessment of respiratory rate, rhythm, and character. Causes of respiratory distress may be respiratory or nonrespiratory in origin, and the physiology of this condition is discussed in detail in Chapter 3.

Upper respiratory disorders that result in respiratory distress usually do so because of respiratory tract obstruction; Box 7-6 contains a partial list of differential diagnoses. Complete upper airway obstruction is a true emergency, insofar as the negative intrathoracic pressures resulting from inspiratory efforts against a closed airway lead to upper airway collapse and the inability to inspire or to pulmonary edema, which can be fatal even if the initial airway obstruction is resolved.[7] Diagnosis is usually based on physical examination and endoscopy of the upper airway. Most affected horses require an emergency tracheotomy. Additional therapies to consider are antimicrobial agents and antiinflammatory agents, including steroids.

Lower airway disease that may be associated with respiratory distress are shown in Box 7-7. Diagnosis is based on a thorough physical examination, thoracic ultrasound or radiographs, transtracheal aspirate, and arterial blood gas analysis. Treatment depends on the nature of the primary disorder and may include antimicrobial agents, antiinflammatory agents,

BOX 7-6

UPPER AIRWAY DISORDERS THAT MAY BE ASSOCIATED WITH RESPIRATORY DISTRESS IN ADULT HORSES

Nasal Disorders
Trauma, foreign body
Hemorrhage or hematoma
Neoplasia
Abscess

Pharyngeal Disorders
Neoplasia
Cyst
Dorsal displacement of soft palate
Trauma, foreign body
Abscess

Laryngeal Disorders
Laryngeal paralysis
Laryngeal hemiplegia
Trauma, foreign body
Edema
Arytenoid chondritis
Epiglottitis

Miscellaneous
Guttural pouch enlargement
Head edema

BOX 7-7

LOWER AIRWAY DISORDERS THAT MAY BE ASSOCIATED WITH RESPIRATORY DISTRESS IN ADULT HORSES

Pulmonary Disorders
- Pulmonary edema
- Diffuse interstitial pneumonia
- Aspiration pneumonia
- Abscessing or coalescing bronchopneumonia
- Acute respiratory distress syndrome
- Silicosis
- Smoke inhalation

Extrapulmonary Disorders
- Pleural effusion
- Intrathoracic hemorrhage
- Pneumothorax

and oxygen administration. Diseases involving the pleural space may respond to thoracic drainage or, in cases of a pnuemothorax, placement of a drain dorsally. Diagnosis and treatment of specific disorders are described in Chapter 9.

Nonpulmonary causes of respiratory distress include anemia, compensation for metabolic acidosis, pain, anxiety, and hyperthermia. Diagnosis of nonpulmonary causes of respiratory distress must start with a thorough history, physical examination, and bloodwork. After the initial evaluation, further diagnostic testing might include endoscopy, ultrasound, and radiographs.

OXYGEN THERAPY IN ADULT HORSES

Administration of oxygen by nasal cannula is the most common means of oxygen supplementation in adult horses. Initial studies of the efficacy of this form of oxygen administration in the adult horse produced equivocal results. However, a more recent study revealed that use of a nasal cannula to deliver oxygen increased both the fractional inspired oxygen concentration and P_aO_2 in control horses and horses with moderate to severe recurrent airway obstruction (RAO).[8] The nasal cannula is passed into the nasopharynx to the level of the medial canthus of the eye. At a flow rate of 30 L/min, P_aO_2 increased to 319 mm Hg in control horses and 264 mm Hg in RAO-affected horses.[8] This study indicated that flow rates of 10 to 20 L/min were well tolerated but higher rates produced irritation.[8] Thus if higher rates are needed, delivery should be through two cannulas. If a tracheotomy is present, oxygen can be delivered directly into the tracheotomy tube. With either method of administration, serial arterial blood gas measurements will determine the response to treatment.

INHALATION THERAPY

Inhalation therapy is an available method of treatment for horses with respiratory disorders, especially lower airway disease. Bronchodilators and corticosteroids administered with metered-dose inhalers are now common treatment modalities for horses with recurrent airway obstruction.[9] Horses with bacterial pneumonia or pleuropneumonia may benefit from aerosol administration of antimicrobial agents because the medication is delivered directly to the lungs. Additional advantages to aerosol administration include a rapid onset of action, decrease in the dose administered, and reduction in the incidence of adverse reactions. Proper administration requires an ultrasonic nebulizer. McKenzie and Murray reported that aerosol administration of gentamicin resulted in gentamicin levels in bronchial fluid that were higher than those observed after intravenous administration of the drug.[10] Thus inhalation therapy provides a good adjunctive therapy for the critical care patient.

SUPPORT OF GASTROINTESTINAL FUNCTION

Bonnie Barr

The gastrointestinal tract is the portal through which nutritive substances, vitamins, minerals, and fluids enter the body. Normal function of the gastrointestinal tract includes appropriate motility, absorption, and digestion so that food can be used for energy. Movement of the food through the gastrointestinal tract involves a complex interaction among the nervous system, the endocrine system, and the musculature of the gastrointestinal tract. The gastrointestinal tract has its own intrinsic enteric nervous system involved in motor control and intestinal secretions. In addition, the intestine receives extrinsic innervation from the autonomic nervous system. Digestion of food involves a large number of digestive enzymes that are found in glands throughout the gastrointestinal tract. The products of digestion are absorbed across the mucosa into the circulatory system or the lymphatic system.

The gastrointestinal mucosa forms a barrier between the body and a luminal environment, which not only contains nutrients but also is laden with potentially hostile microorganisms and toxins. Thus normal function also requires that nutrients be transported across the epithelium while excluding passage of harmful molecules and organisms.

Gastrointestinal complications are common in the critically ill horse and occasionally occur in postoperative elective patients. Those that are more at risk to develop gastrointestinal complications include horses that are septic or endotoxemic or suffer from poor perfusion. Many of the common complications have already been discussed, including ileus, endotoxemia, tympany, diarrhea, and gastric ulceration. Inappetence is probably the most common complication in the critical equine patient. Horses refuse to eat for many reasons, including physical factors such as pain, infection, and an inability to eat and psychological factors such as stress. The regulation of appetite is an immensely complex process involving the gastrointestinal tract, central and autonomic nervous systems, and many hormones. The hypothalamus is the main regulatory organ for appetite depending on the interaction between the feeding center and satiety center. Neurosubstances involved in regulation of appetite include neuropeptide Y, melanocyte-concentrating hormone, catecholamines, and leptin.[1] Gastrointestinal hormones involved in appetite regulation include glucagon, somatostatin, and cholecystokinin (CCK).[1] Loss of appetite can be caused by a variety of conditions and diseases. Some of the conditions are temporary and reversible, such as loss of appetite from the effects of medication. Some of the conditions are more serious, such as trauma to the head. Systemic mediators, such as TNF-α, IL-1 and IL-6, and corticotropin-releasing hormone have a negative influence on appetite. Many of these mediators are present in the critically ill patient because of inflammation, endotoxemia, and sepsis.

Methods used to recognize gastrointestinal dysfunction in the critically ill horse include changes in the physical examination, abdominal ultrasonography, and clinical pathologic evaluation. Serial physical examinations will identify changes in vital parameters, mentation, behavior, fecal production, and abdominal size. Some of the changes may not be specific for the gastrointestinal tract, but when combined with more specific changes, an abnormality of gastrointestinal function must be considered. An increase in heart rate can indicate pain, dehydration, endotoxemia, and decreased venous return. Increases in respiratory rate are not specific for gastrointestinal disease but do indicate that a systemic change has occurred in the horse. A decreasing temperature with rapid, weak pulse indicates the development of shock, which may be due to endotoxemia. An increase in temperature with additional signs of gastrointestinal dysfunction suggests colitis or acute peritonitis. Increased borborygmi may indicate a simple obstruction or hyperperistalsis associated with enterocolitis. A decrease or absence of borborygmi is associated with inflammation and ischemia, which may be due to postoperative ileus, peritonitis, or enterocolitis. Decreased or sudden changes in manure production or consistency indicate deterioration of the gastrointestinal motility or function. A normal 500-kg horse passes approximately 5 to 7 piles of manure per day, although one that is inappetent will pass less. Administering mineral oil and noting its presence in the feces can approximate transit time through the gastrointestinal tract. Urine output may be decreased if fluids are being sequestered to the gastrointestinal tract. Transabdominal ultrasound can be used to evaluate the anatomic location, contents, wall thickness, and motility of various regions of the intestine. In evaluating the small intestine, the clinician will see organized waves of motility when observing the intestinal walls and contents over a few seconds. Amotile bowel is observed with strangulating lesions, postoperative ileus, and enteritis. With mechanical lesions the small intestine is amotile with ingesta settled ventrally in the lumen of the intestine. The small intestinal wall may be thickened in patients that have enteritis, peritonitis, inflammatory bowel disease, and strangulating lesions. With colitis the large intestine may contain fluid ingesta, and the wall may be thickened. Gastrointestinal disorders may be accompanied by loss of integrity to the intestinal barrier, resulting in changes in the peritoneum and peritoneal cavity. The presence of peritoneal fluid, the echogenicity of the fluid, and the quantity of fluid can be assessed by transabdominal ultrasound. The presence of peritoneal fluid warrants abdominocentesis and fluid analysis to determine if the fluid is a transudate or exudate.

Hematologic alterations associated with gastrointestinal dysfunction are often nonspecific, reflecting systemic response to inflammation, endotoxemia, or sepsis. During the early stages of endotoxemia, an increase in the circulating concentrations of inflammatory mediators, epinephrine, and cortisol produces changes in the leukogram. The characteristic change includes leukopenia with neutropenia and a left shift, toxic changes in the neutrophilic cytoplasm, and lymphopenia. In later stages of disease a neutrophilia may be present because of enhanced myeloid proliferation of the bone marrow. Major fluid shifts occur when fluid accumulates in the small intestine, colon, or peritoneal cavity. These fluid shifts occur at the expense of the plasma volume, resulting in hemoconcentration and decreased circulating volume. Endotoxemia can cause redistribution of plasma volume into the splanchnic capillary beds and hypersecretion into the bowel lumen or peritoneal cavity. Increased capillary permeability leads to loss of albumin and water into the extravascular space, further depleting the plasma volume and intravascular oncotic pressure. Acute protein loss commonly results from damaged bowel in cases of enterocolitis and enteritis. Strangulating lesions can result in mucosal necrosis and leakage of plasma proteins into the lumen. Hypoproteinemia also occurs with inflammatory bowel disease because of inflammation of the bowel and the inability to absorb necessary protein owing to inappetence or inflammation of the bowel. Hyperfibrinogenemia occurs with generalized gastrointestinal inflammation or localized inflammation such as peritonitis or salmonellosis. Electrolyte imbalances are due to sequestration of sodium-rich fluids, anorexia, and changes in circulating volume. Serum biochemical changes result from dehydration, poor perfusion, and hypoxemia.

Severe illness or injury has been associated with hypermetabolism characterized by a pronounced catabolic state that is compounded by patients that are unable or unwilling to eat. Fatty acids are the primary source of energy in fully adaptive simple starvation, but in severe illness activation of a complex neurohormonal response results in utilization of body protein. This response is caused by inflammatory cytokines, such as TNF and ILs, which augment the effects of catecholamines and glucocorticoids associated with stress.[2,3] Inflammatory mediators increase the metabolic rate, contributing to the inefficient use of oxygen and calories, and may also directly dictate the body's normal response to starvation. The increased need for protein, specifically amino acids, as an alternative energy source compromises lean muscle mass and normal organ structure. Clinically and experimentally, the effects of negative energy balance have been well documented. Negative energy balance depletes the body of structural and functional protein, thereby impairing wound healing, immune function, and other normal organ functions. Negative energy balance leads to deficiencies in nonspecific and specific immune functions; gut mucosal atrophy; loss of visceral and muscular protein with consequent weakness and abnormal function; decreases in albumin, fibrinogen, complement proteins, and globulin; and poor wound healing. In addition, negative energy balance leads to depletion of glycogen stores; gastrointestinal ileus; disruption of the gastrointestinal barrier; and decreases in high turnover cell populations such as leukocytes, gastrointestinal mucosal cells, and fibroblasts. Inadequate nutrition sets the stage for serious complications resulting in sepsis, multiple organ failure, and death. In human critical care nutritional support has become a routine part of the care of the critically ill patient. Numerous reports in human-medicine literature document that nutritional support, especially early nutritional support, hastens recovery, diminishes some of the complications of the critically ill, and decreases length of stay.[2-4] The goal of aggressive early nutrition is to maintain host defenses by supporting the hypermetabolism and preserving lean body mass.

Assessment of the nutritional status of the critically ill equine patient at presentation and at regular intervals during hospitalization is necessary to identify patients that would benefit from early nutritional support. Horses with adequate nutritional status may not require nutritional support as early as underweight or obese horses. In addition, certain disease states, such as those associated with a severely compromised gastrointestinal tract and severe central nervous system disorders, may benefit from immediate nutritional support. Obese horses are prone to the development of hyperlipidemia when fasted after only a short period. Horses in poor body condition are especially vulnerable to impairment of immune function, poor tissue healing, and additional weight loss if deprived of nutrients for even a short period of time. Although horses in optimal body condition can tolerate periods of fasting, nutritional support may decrease complications and improve outcome.

In human critical care medicine, body composition is estimated and monitored by midarm circumference (i.e., muscle) and skin-fold thickness (i.e., fat); unfortunately, methods for monitoring nutritional status in the equine patient are not as sophisticated. The most practical methods in the equine are body weight measurement and body condition score. A body weight measurement, preferably on a walk-on scale, should be performed at admission and at regular intervals during hospitalization. If a walk-on scale is not available, a weight tape used to measure girth circumference can provide a reasonable estimate of body weight. Body condition score (BCS) is a subjective semiquantitative method of evaluating body fat and muscle mass by visual inspection and palpation of certain areas of the body. In 1983 Henneke developed the most commonly used BCS for horses. This score is positively correlated to body fat but not to weight or height. A total of nine scores are assigned: 1 is poor (extreme emaciation), and 9 is extremely fat.[5] An ideal BCS is 4 to 6.[5] The appropriate assessment and monitoring of nutritional status would include both the body weight and BCS.

The nutritional requirements of a critically ill horse have not been determined. Energy requirements can be calculated on the basis of size, age, condition, and metabolic stress. The daily energy expenditure is expressed as the basal energy requirement, which is the amount of energy used for maintenance of body function in a resting state in a thermoneutral environment. In small animal and human medicine, the basal energy requirement is often doubled for certain patients who have a higher caloric need, such as burn patients and multiple trauma patients. Maintenance requirements for healthy adult horses are estimated to be 35 to 40 kcal/kg/day.[6,7]

Enteral feeding is preferred if the gastrointestinal tract is completely or even partially functional. There are numerous advantages of enteral feeding, making it superior to parenteral feeding. Early enteral feeding is the current trend in human critical care patients because the nutrients are directly delivered to the gastric mucosa, preserving mucosal integrity and improving gastrointestinal function.[2-4] Enteral feeding is more physiologic, with nutrients being digested and absorbed by the gut and metabolized by the liver. Because enteral feeding stimulates insulin secretion, hyperglycemia is a less likely complication. Without local nutrients the gastrointestinal mucosa becomes leaky, and enterocytes are unable to maintain normal intercellular borders and immune function, thus creating a greater risk of secondary sepsis from translocation of bacteria and toxins. Enteral feeding also decreases the risk of intravenous catheter complications and reduces cost. In the horse voluntary intake is preferable to forced nasogastric feeding, but sometimes the actual caloric intake is difficult to estimate with voluntary intake. This problem can be overcome by weighing the feed and hay offered and the feed remaining in the stall, which allows for calculation of the calories ingested. If consumption is below 75% of the maintenance requirements for 48 hours or if the horse is anorexic or dysphagic, feeding by nasogastric tube is required.[7,8] The best enteral diet is a slurry of complete pelleted feed, which is inexpensive and well balanced for the horse and contains fiber to maintain gastrointestinal activity and growth. Vegetable oil can be added to increase the caloric density. (Chapter 5 contains appropriate enteral diet regimens). Complications of indwelling and repeated passage of nasogastric tubes include chronic irritation and trauma to the pharyngeal and esophageal region. An indwelling esophagostomy feeding tube is a good option if the horse is dysphagic and unable to swallow a nasogastric tube or if prolonged feeding is expected. Liquid diets designed for people have been fed to horses, although the efficacy of these diets is unknown. These diets offer the advantage of easy administration by a small-diameter nasogastric tube and administration of a known quantity of nutrients. Reported adverse effects of the commercial liquid diets include diarrhea and laminitis.[7,8] It is recommended that enteral feeding begin gradually, with a goal of reaching maintenance requirements over 5 to 7 days.[7,8] As with any diet, rapid changes may result in colic or diarrhea.

Parenteral nutrition is indicated for critical patients that cannot tolerate enteral feeding because of gastrointestinal dysfunction. Other candidates for parenteral nutrition include aged animals off their feed, pregnant or lactating mares off their feed, and horses with a body score off 3 or less.[9-11] The goal of parenteral nutrition is to provide a portion of daily nutritional requirements intravenously. Parenteral nutrition is a combination of nutrients designed to meet the energy requirements of the horses. Partial parenteral nutrition can be provided by supplementation with dextrose alone or with amino acids. Total parenteral nutrition includes dextrose, amino acids, and lipids. Carbohydrates and fats are used for energy requirements, and protein is used for protein synthesis and reduction of endogenous protein breakdown. Horses at risk for hyperlipidemia or those in poor body condition may benefit from the early addition of dextrose (2.5% to 5%) to crystalloid fluids. Dextrose supplementation may be beneficial even in healthy horses undergoing elective surgery that require prolonged withholding of feed.

Carbohydrates are the primary source of energy and are essential nutrients for certain tissues in healthy patients. Glucose is necessary for the body to oxidize free fatty acids by way of the citric acid cycle. In parenteral nutrition glucose is provided as a dextrose solution. Hyperglycemia is the most common complication reported in horses administered parenteral nutrition. A slow introduction of the fluid should allow an appropriate endogenous insulin response to occur, thus minimizing or eliminating the onset of hyperglycemia. Blood glucose levels should be monitored every 4 to 6 hours because if the renal threshold of glucose (180 to 220 mg/dl) is exceeded, glucosuria and osmotic diuresis can occur. A sudden onset of hyperglycemia in a patient that had been tolerating the parenteral nutrition can indicate the presence of complications, such as infection or sepsis. Protein is provided as an amino acid solution. Healthy adult horses require 0.7 to 1.5 g/kg/d of protein.[9,10] This amount is likely to increase in a critically ill horse, although the exact requirement is unknown. Supplementation of essential branched-chained amino acids (valine, leucine, and isoleucine) decreases trauma- and sepsis-induced muscle catabolism and improves nitrogen balance. Lipid emulsions are the most calorically dense nutrient and are a source of essential fatty acids. Fatty acids are required for several physiologic functions, including prostaglandin and leukotriene synthesis; surfactant production; wound healing; and the integrity of skin, hair, and nerves. Other components added to parenteral nutrition include vitamins (A, D, and E) and minerals. B-complex vitamins should be supplemented because they are required for carbohydrate metabolism. Macrominerals such as calcium and magnesium are best added to crystalloid fluids because divalent cations destabilize in lipids.

In choosing the amount of each component to be included in the solution, the practitioner must consider the energy requirement of the horse, the changes in nutrient utilization that accompany the specific disease, and the proper blend of nutrients to facilitate utilization. Dextrose, protein, and lipids can all be utilized as energy sources. The caloric density is as follows: dextrose provides 3.4 kcal/g, protein 4 kcal/g, and lipids 9 kcal/g. It is best to provide adequate nonprotein nitrogen as an energy source to permit efficient use of endogenous and exogenous proteins. A mixed-fuel system with 40% to 60% of the non-nitrogen calories as dextrose and 50% to 60% as lipid enables proteins to be utilized efficiently.[9-11] Chapter 5 contains a discussion of appropriate parenteral nutrition regimes.

Complications with parenteral nutrition include thrombophlebitis, hyperglycemia, hyperlipidemia, and hypokalemia. Patients with hyperlipidemia, hyperlipemia, and severe liver disease may not be able to tolerate lipids in the parenteral nutrition. Horses with severe endotoxemia or SIRS may also be lipid intolerant. Metabolic clearance of lipids involves the hydrolysis of triglycerides by lipoprotein lipase, an enzyme present in capillary endothelial cells. Bacterial endotoxins may induce inflammatory cells to release mediators that suppress lipoprotein lipase activity. In either of these cases, a diluted mixture of dextrose and amino acids (1:1) can be administered.[11] Hyperglycemia can be prevented by routine monitoring of blood glucose levels. In addition, slow and gradual introduction of parenteral nutrition might establish better tolerance in the patient. If hyperglycemia persists, endogenous insulin therapy should be considered. Electrolyte abnormalities, specifically hypokalemia, can result from decreased intake of food and the delivery of a high concentration of dextrose, which drives the potassium into the cell.

SUPPORT OF RENAL FUNCTION

Bryan Waldridge

Critical patients frequently are receiving multiple medications that may adversely affect renal function, such as nonsteroidal antiinflammatory drugs (NSAIDs), polymyxin B, and aminoglycosides. If the patient appears dehydrated, then renal function should be assessed before administration of potentially nephrotoxic drugs. Once the fluid deficit is corrected or clinicopathologic indices of renal function are within normal ranges, then treatment can proceed more safely. Patients that are at risk for dehydration or are receiving multiple drugs that can have adverse renal effects are probably best managed with at least maintenance rates (60 to 70 ml/kg/day) of intravenous fluids to prevent dehydration and support urine production. Specific treatment and diagnosis of acute renal failure is discussed in greater detail elsewhere in this text.

NONSTEROIDAL ANTIINFLAMMATORY DRUGS

The dehydrated horse depends on production of prostaglandins to maintain renal perfusion and glomerular filtration. Cyclooxygenase 1 (COX-1) is a constitutive enzyme that produces vasodilatory prostaglandins (PGE_2 and PGI_2) in response to decreased renal blood flow.[1] With the exception of firocoxib, other NSAIDs used in horses are not selective for COX-2, which is induced by inflammatory stimuli.[1] Therefore most NSAIDs inhibit activity of both enzymes to some degree, which blocks renal production of prostaglandins and prevents the compensatory increase in renal blood flow during dehydration. The mechanism of action and toxicity for NSAIDs is discussed in detail in Chapter 4.

AMINOGLYCOSIDE ANTIBIOTICS

Aminoglycoside antibiotics (e.g., gentamicin, amikacin, polymyxin B) are freely filtered at the glomerulus and excreted into the urine.[2] Renal proximal tubular cells actively take up aminoglycosides in the filtrate. Acute tubular necrosis and renal failure can occur with aminoglycoside therapy as a result of tubular cell organelle damage and blockage of tubules with necrotic debris.[2] These mechanisms of toxicity are discussed in Chapter 4.

PIGMENT NEPHROPATHY

Pigment nephropathy is relatively uncommon but can occur in horses with rhabdomyolysis (myoglobin) or intravascular hemolysis (hemoglobin). When either of these pigments is excreted into the urine, it may polymerize in the distal tubules and physically obstruct them. Additionally, myoglobin and hemoglobin induce renal vasoconstriction and are iron-containing pigments that may lead to hydroxyl radical production and further tubular damage.

METHODS TO RECOGNIZE RENAL PROBLEMS

Assessment of renal function is easily overlooked in critical care patients. It is advisable to measure serum blood urea nitrogen (BUN) and creatinine concentrations at least every 48 hours to assess glomerular filtration and renal function. Regular measurement of BUN and creatinine concentrations and assessment of results in light of physical examination findings (e.g., evidence of dehydration) and results of urinalysis are the most readily available methods to monitor renal function in equine critical care patients. Increases in serum creatinine concentration as small as 0.3 mg/dl can be significant.[3]

Dilute urine (specific gravity ≤ 1.012) concurrent with azotemia generally indicates decreased renal function. Urinary indicators of tubular damage include granular casts in urine, an increased urinary γ-glutamyltransferase-to-creatinine ratio (>25), and increased fractional excretion of electrolytes such as sodium and chloride.[3] Increased protein in urine (>1+ on dipstick test) can occur with glomerulonephritis; however, sulfosalicyclic acid precipitation is a more specific test for urinary protein. Laboratory assessment of renal function is discussed in detail in Chapter 19.

Monitoring for appropriate urination, especially in response to fluid therapy, is essential. Patients with anuria or oliguria after appropriate intravenous fluid volume replacement are at risk for pulmonary and peripheral edema. If fluid therapy to replace deficits and meet maintenance requirements does not stimulate urination, then the administration of diuretics or vasopressor agents should be considered, as outlined in Chapter 19.

TREATMENT GOALS AND MEASURING EFFECTIVENESS

Many cases of acute renal failure are reversible and will respond to fluid therapy and supportive care. Replacement of fluid deficits and administration of maintenance fluids should result in diuresis and gradual resolution of azotemia. Fluid rates can be increased to 1.5 to 2 times the maintenance rate to further stimulate diuresis and urination. At these fluid rates serum BUN and creatinine concentrations should generally decrease by approximately 50% within 24 hours.

If fluid therapy does not produce the expected increase in urine output, then diuretics (furosemide, 1 mg/kg, administered intravenously) can be administered. Urination should be expected within 30 minutes of furosemide administration. Diuretics may be most indicated in cases of pigmentary nephropathy to induce diuresis and physically clear clogged tubules of polymerized hemoglobin or myoglobin. However, it is imperative that adequate volume replacement occur before administration of diuretic agents; otherwise, the resultant diuresis will contribute to potentially severe dehydration and diminished peripheral perfusion and exacerbate renal damage.

Hypotension can be an unrecognized cause of decreased urine production. MAP should be maintained above 70 mm Hg to preserve tissue perfusion, glomerular filtration, and urine production.[4] Low-dose vasopressor therapy (dopamine at 2 to 5 μg/kg/min, constant-rate infusion; dobutamine up to 5 μg/kg/min, constant-rate infusion) will dilate renal capillaries without significant cardiac or systemic vascular effects.[3,4] Blood pressure should be measured in patients at risk for hypotension and those that fail to produce urine despite appropriate therapy. CVP may be monitored to assess the potential for fluid overload and edema formation in the horse with oliguric or anuric renal failure.

Aminoglycoside toxicity is best prevented by ensuring appropriate dosing regimens and limiting the use of aminoglycosides to hydrated animals without preexisting renal dysfunction.[4] Administering aminoglycoside antibiotics every 24 hours decreases the amount of time that renal tubular cells are exposed to higher concentrations of aminoglycosides. Therapeutic drug monitoring allows for detection of elevated trough (usually 24 hours after the previous dose) concentrations, which are more likely to cause toxicity than elevated peak concentrations. The dose of aminoglycoside may need to be reduced or the treatment interval prolonged if trough concentrations are elevated. High trough concentrations after an appropriate dose can indicate decreased glomerular filtration or glomerulonephritis.[2]

Once it appears that patients have responded well to therapy for acute renal failure, they can be gradually weaned from intravenous fluids and allowed to maintain hydration by voluntary water intake. A few days after discontinuing intravenous fluids, measurement of serum BUN and creatinine concentrations, urine specific gravity, and urinalysis can be repeated to determine if renal function has returned to normal. Some patients may have persistently elevated renal indices; however, this cannot be determined without repeated serum chemistry examinations.

SUPPORT OF NEUROLOGIC FUNCTION

Yvette S. Nout

Any horse with neurologic disease can present as an emergency. Neurologic disorders that have developed acutely warrant immediate veterinary attention, but deterioration of existing neurologic conditions may also require emergency veterinary attention. In particular, disorders that result in abnormal behavior or severe ataxia require emergency care. It is sometimes difficult to differentiate neurologic from nonneurologic disease because some conditions appear to be induced by a neurologic disorder when in fact they are not. Examples are recumbency caused by cardiovascular or respiratory diseases and gait abnormalities caused by musculoskeletal diseases such as bone fractures, rhabdomyolysis, or laminitis.

Emergency neurologic disease may arise from the central nervous system or peripheral nervous system, or they may be multifocal. The most commonly seen emergency neurologic conditions with a neuroanatomic location cranial to the foramen magnum are head injury, (myelo)encephalitis, and vestibular disease. Abnormal behavior caused by hepatic encephalopathy, seizure activity, neoplasia, abscessation, or toxicosis can also have an acute onset and therefore present as an emergency. Disorders that stem from the central nervous system distal to the foramen magnum include cervical vertebral stenotic myelopathy, equine degenerative myelopathy, trauma, and neoplasia. Except for spinal cord trauma, it is especially this group of disorders that typically would not manifest as emergencies because of the gradual onset of clinical signs. However, if onset is acute or clinical signs deteriorate, emergency care is required. Multifocal neurologic diseases such as equine protozoal myeloencephalitis, equine motor neuron disease, and botulism all can have acute severe onsets of clinical signs or progress to a degree that requires immediate veterinary attention. Peripheral nerve damage in horses is not uncommon and most often involves the suprascapular, radial, ulnar, femoral, and selected cranial nerves. Occasionally, the brachial plexus can be injured after a collision accident. Often, the cause of the nerve injury is traumatic, and horses should be examined carefully (e.g., for bone fractures).

Abnormal neurologic function can cause secondary excitement, agitation, and stress in the patient and worry for the owner or caretaker. When treating a neurologic emergency, the practitioner must first ensure protection and care of the people involved with the patient and limit further (self-inflicted) damage to the patient by protection and administration of drugs.

DIAGNOSTICS

Until a diagnosis is made, many emergency neurologic patients should be treated as rabies suspects. This requires that the number of people involved with the animal should be minimized and that all involved should be wearing protective clothing such as gloves and coveralls. Performing a thorough neurologic examination is critical. To come to a diagnosis, the practitioner performs a careful neurologic examination followed by appropriate ancillary diagnostics. Ancillary diagnostics used in emergency situations typically include hematology and serum chemistries, radiographs, and potentially cerebrospinal fluid analysis. When available, these patients may require further diagnostic tests such as computed tomography, magnetic resonance imaging, electrodiagnostics, or a combination thereof.

A neuroanatomic localization of the disease should be made after a thorough examination,[1,2] as described in Chapter 12. The neuroanatomical localization can be simplified by determining whether there is central nervous system, peripheral nerve, or multifocal nerve disease. In the case of central nervous system disease, it is helpful to determine whether the lesion is localized cranial or caudal to the foramen magnum (i.e., whether there is brain involvement). If there is brain involvement, it may be possible to further differentiate among cerebral, cerebellar, vestibular, or brainstem disease. If disease is localized caudal to the foramen magnum, the disease may be located in the cervical spinal cord or in the spinal cord caudal to T2.

Under emergency conditions the most important goal is stabilization of the patient before thorough neurologic evaluation. Figure 7-3 is a flowchart for management of the horse with an acute neurologic condition. Ideally, the practitioner examines the horse, diagnoses a disease, and treats the patient. Often, however, this is not so straightforward, and sedation or stabilization of the patient is required before continuing the evaluation. Also, it is likely that a final diagnosis cannot be reached on an emergency basis, which leaves the veterinarian to then select a treatment that benefits the horse and will not interfere too much with follow-up neurologic examinations. These empirical treatments will be based on differential diagnoses formed after the initial neurologic examination.

TREATMENT

During emergency situations, basic concepts of treatment and care should be followed. The ultimate goal is to optimize delivery of oxygen and nutrients to tissues. For the neurologic horse, sedation may be required to handle and examine the horse in a safe fashion or to treat seizure activity. Stabilization of hemorrhagic and hypovolemic conditions is necessary in trauma patients. Medical treatment of specific primary conditions is described in detail in Chapter 12. This section discusses select groups of drugs that are commonly used in horses with acute neurologic disease.

Sedatives and anesthetics are used to tranquilize the equine patient. Short-acting sedatives may be required for restraint during examination. Longer-term sedation or anesthesia is frequently required to avoid self-trauma in fractious horses. The use of tranquilizers or anesthetics may also be indicated to control abnormal behavior or seizure activity. Analgesic drugs are indicated if horses experience pain (e.g., in traumatic disease). NSAIDs are the mainstay drugs in equine medicine because of their antiinflammatory and analgesic properties. Opioids should be considered when additional analgesia is required or when analgesia is required in situations of suspected NSAID toxicity or when the risk of developing NSAID toxicity is high (e.g., dehydration). Opioids do not have specific antiinflammatory effects. The pharmacology and use of NSAIDs and opioids are described in detail in Chapters 4 and 6.

Corticosteroids, alone or in combination with other drugs, are still the classic drugs of choice for acute neurologic disease. Reported dosages of dexamethasone for horses range between 0.1 to 0.25 mg/kg, administered intravenously every 6 to 24 hours for 24 to 48 hours. A favorable response is expected within 4 to 8 hours after CS administration. Horses being given corticosteroid therapy should be monitored closely for the development of laminitis or secondary infection. If improvement in clinical signs is observed, the horse may be placed on oral prednisolone therapy (0.5 to 1.0 mg/kg daily tapered over 3 to 5 days) to decrease the chance of adverse effects. The neuroprotective effect of corticosteroids is thought

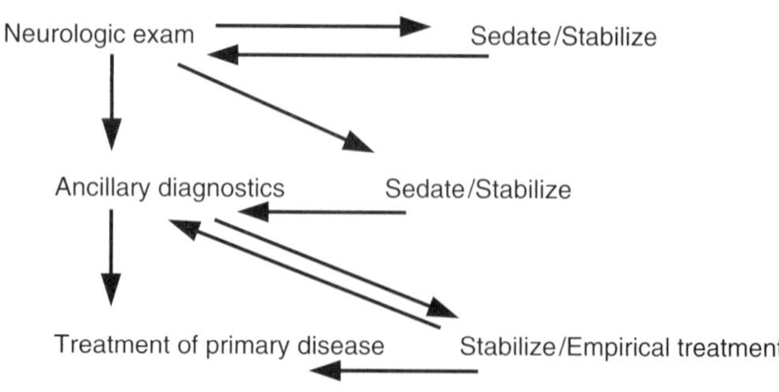

FIGURE 7-3 Flowchart for management of the acutely neurologic horse. Optimally, a neurologic examination is followed by ancillary diagnostics and treatment of the disease. However, in many acute neurologic horses, this is not so straightforward, and adjustment of this "optimal" path by using sedatives or therapeutic stabilization strategies is necessary before further assessment of the horse can continue.

primarily to be mediated by free radical scavenging.[3] Recently, it has been shown that, similar to methylprednisolone, dexamethasone decreases apoptosis-related cell death in rats that were subjected to traumatic spinal cord injury.[4] Other potential beneficial effects of corticosteroids include reduction in the spread of morphologic damage, prevention of the loss of axonal conduction and reflex activity, preservation of vascular membrane integrity, and stabilization of white matter neuronal cell membranes in the presence of central hemorrhagic lesions. Furthermore, their antiinflammatory properties may be useful in reducing edema and fibrin deposition, as well as their ability to reverse sodium and potassium imbalance caused by edema and necrosis. Methylprednisolone sodium succinate (MPSS) is a synthetic glucocorticoid with four times more antiinflammatory activity and 0.8 times less mineralocorticoid action compared with cortisol. Beneficial effects of MPSS on neural tissue include inhibition of lipid peroxidation, eicosanoid formation, and lipid hydrolysis, including arachidonic acid release, maintenance of tissue blood flow and aerobic energy metabolism, improved elimination of intracellular calcium accumulation, reduced neurofilament degradation, and improved neuronal excitability and synaptic transmission. Apparently, it is the cell membrane antilipid peroxidation effect of MPSS that is most beneficial. The dose of MPSS used in human trials (30 mg/kg) exceeds that necessary for activation of steroid receptors, which suggests that MPSS acts through mechanisms that are unrelated to steroid receptors. Investigators have concluded that high-dose MPSS treatment within 8 hours of spinal cord injury improved neurologic recovery.[5,6] However, controversy regarding the beneficial effects of MPSS remains.[7,8]

Osmotic diuretics such as 20% mannitol (0.25 to 2.0 mg/kg, administered intravenously over 20 minutes) and glycerol (0.5 to 2.0 mg/kg, administered intravenously every 6 to 12 hr for 24 hr) are effective in combating cerebral edema and increased intracranial pressure. These have a rapid onset of action (10 to 20 minutes) and work because of their hyperosmolar nature. Animals receiving osmotic diuretics should be adequately hydrated. Although mannitol administration is very effective in reducing intracranial pressure, there are technical limitations to the administration of this osmotic diuretic. Furthermore, the administration of multiple doses of mannitol can lead to intravascular dehydration, hypotension, reduction of cerebral blood flow (CBF), and elevation of spinal fluid osmolarity.[9,10] Therefore current research is focused on the use of hypertonic solutions that reduce intracranial pressure and support intravascular volume.[11] Hypertonic saline administered early in the treatment of shock associated with head trauma may enhance return of cerebral blood flow and cell membrane function. Effects of hypertonic saline are due to its ability to move water out of cells and decrease tissue pressure and cell size by osmotic plasma expansion. These effects result in a lowering of intracranial pressure and cerebral water content. Hypertonic saline may in fact be the maintenance fluid of choice in head injury. Hypertonic saline is associated with significant decreases in intracranial pressure and cerebral water content compared with isotonic fluid treatment. Another study comparing the effects of a hypertonic saline hydroxylethyl starch solution and mannitol on increased intracranial pressure found that the hypertonic saline hydroxylethyl starch reduced the intracranial pressure more effectively than mannitol.[12] Induction of prolonged hypernatremia using 3% hypertonic saline administered as a continuous infusion appears to be a promising therapy for control of cerebral edema.[13] Hypertonic saline may be given to head trauma horses in shock as a 5% or 7% sodium chloride solution in a 4- to 6-ml/kg bolus intravenous dose over 15 minutes.

Dimethyl sulfoxide (DMSO) 1 g/kg, administered intravenously as a 10% to 20% solution for 3 consecutive days followed by three treatments every other day, may be of benefit in acute neurologic disease. Reported benefits of DMSO include increased brain and spinal cord blood flow, decreased brain and spinal cord edema, increased vasodilating PGE_1, decreased platelet aggregation, decreased PGE_2 and PGF_2, protection of cell membranes, and trapping of hydroxyl radicals. The exact mechanism of DMSO remains unknown. This treatment remains controversial; some researchers have found no positive effects on neurologic outcome after the use of DMSO.[14] Although the antioxidants vitamin E and selenium have been shown to be beneficial in neurologic disease, they do not appear useful in acute injury because of the length of time required to achieve therapeutic concentrations in the central nervous system. Beneficial effects of vitamin E and selenium include reduced lipid peroxidation and free radical scavenging.[3]

Antimicrobial drugs may be required to treat the primary disease process (e.g., in bacterial meningitis); they may also be indicated for treatment of secondary complications, such as pneumonia and decubital sores in recumbent animals. The choice of antibiotic should be based on culture and sensitivity testing. Good empirical choices for broad spectrum coverage include trimethoprim-sulfamethoxazole at 30 mg/kg, administered orally or intravenously every 12 hours, or penicillin at 22,000 IU/kg, administered intramuscularly every 12 hours or intravenously every 6 hours in combination with gentamicin at 6.6 mg/kg, administered intramuscularly or intravenously every 24 hours. Appropriate monitoring for aminoglycoside toxicity should be undertaken with their use. In cases of meningitis caused by gram positive organisms, penicillin or ampicillin can be used. The use of penicillin is recommended only in cases of highly susceptible organisms because therapeutic cerebrospinal fluid concentrations are difficult to achieve. Third-generation cephalosporins are highly effective against gram negative cerebrospinal fluid pathogens. Fluoroquinolones also have adequate cerebrospinal fluid penetration. Sulfonamides are a cheaper alternative and have good cerebrospinal fluid penetration. Gentamicin and tetracyclines have poor cerebrospinal fluid penetration.

Treatment and prevention of decubital ulcers are critical in recumbent animals. The etiology of decubital ulcers, or pressure sores, is through prolonged or repeated unrelieved pressures to skin that result in damage and ischemia to underlying tissues and subsequent tissue ulceration. Prevention of decubital ulcers is aimed at protection of tissues and reduction of ischemic injury.[15-18] Microvascular thrombosis and ischemic necrosis occur and may result in secondary bacterial infection. Pressure ulcers usually occur over bony prominences. In horses the most common sites of decubital ulcers are the tuber coxae, the points of the shoulder, and the zygomaticotemporal protuberance. Futhermore, pressure sores can occur along the distal extremities. For horses preventive strategies include appropriate padding and bedding, frequent changes in body positioning (i.e., turning), efforts to improve mobility, frequent examination of skin, maintenance of a well-balanced diet, and skin that is kept dry. Pressure sores generally heal well once the horse is able to stand.

Surgical intervention may be required in, for example, head injury cases in which dislocation of bones has occurred. Indeed, a recent report described aggressive medical and surgical treatment of a horse with an open fracture of the calvarium. In this horse initial surgical débridement appeared successful; however, the horse succumbed to infection and necrosis of remaining brain matter.[19] The demand for and commitment of veterinarians and owners to advance our abilities in treating equine neurologic disease are growing. This will allow the field to move forward and continue with important basic and clinical research, with the goal of improving care of these horses.

CARE OF THE RECUMBENT HORSE

Examination, assessment, and subsequent management of a recumbent horse may be difficult and challenging. The horse is a "fight or flight" animal, and the combination of being debilitated and being in a strange environment surrounded by people may cause anxiety or fear, both of which can contribute to dangerous situations. Furthermore, the horse's primary disease can lead to an abnormal mentation and subsequent abnormal or dangerous behavior. The safety of all involved should be considered when working with a recumbent horse. If there is a risk of infectious or zoonotic disease, appropriate precautions should be taken, including wearing protective clothing and minimizing human exposure. Management of a recumbent horse requires a combination of intensive supportive care and specific treatment aimed at the underlying or complicating disease processes.[20,21] Supportive care is mainly directed at protection of the animal and maintenance of adequate hydration and nutritional status. Care of down horses is time consuming and more difficult if the horse is very large.

Prevention and care of muscle compartmental injury, peripheral nerve injury, and decubital ulcers are important aspects in the management of a down horse, insofar as these are frequent consequences of prolonged recumbency. Bedding should be absorbent, nonabrasive, and conformable. It may be necessary to adjust the type of bedding when the horse makes (successful) attempts to stand or is standing in the sling. Then it is very important that the bedding provide adequate footing. Deep bedding in those situations may hinder the horse's attempts to stand or ambulate, and straw may be slippery. The down horse should be turned regularly (every 2 to 6 hr) to provide adequate perfusion of the skin and musculature of the down side and improve perfusion and ventilation of the down lung. If the horse is able to maintain a sternal position, this should be encouraged and if necessary assisted with the placement of straw bales or other materials. Protection of the head is often required in recumbent horses, primarily to protect the eyes. Protection may be accomplished by use of adequate padding or of helmets or bandages. Damage to the eyes can occur directly by pressure to the eye or from bedding material. Furthermore, specific diseases may result in a horse's inability to blink (e.g., botulism, Horner's syndrome, facial nerve paralysis). The most common ophthalmic disorders seen in recumbent horses are corneal ulcers and keratitis. Eyes should be examined daily and assessed and treated carefully.

Unless horses can maintain themselves standing or in sternal recumbency long enough to drink, their water intake will not be sufficient to meet their maintenance requirement. Maintenance requirements for down horses may be slightly lower (50 ml/kg/day) than what is considered normal. Fluid therapy can be provided intragastrically by using a permanently placed small-bore feeding tube or by regular repeated nasogastric intubation, or fluids can be administered intravenously. Depending on the dietary protocol that is used, electrolytes and glucose may be added to the fluids. Recumbent animals lose body condition rapidly when no nutrition is provided. Dramatic changes are often noticeable within 1 week. Adequate nutrition is important in recumbent horses and may be beneficial for wound healing[22] and maintaining muscular strength and adequate immunity. Diets and routes of administration vary, depending on patient compliance, dietary tolerance, and budget. Dietary options can be divided into four categories.[21] Some horses are able to ingest a sufficient amount of roughage (±2% of bodyweight) with or without grain while they are in sternal recumbency or standing with sling assistance. The dietary intake and fecal output should be monitored closely, but in general no additional support is required. Many recumbent horses and horses that are dysphagic, however, are not able, or should not be allowed, to meet the required intake in this way. For these horses a soaked pellet gruel (30 cal/kg/day), liquid diet (Osmolite; Ross Products Division, Abbott Laboratories, Columbus, Ohio, or Critical Care Meals ™ MD's Choice Inc., Louisville, Tenn.), or parenteral nutrition may be used. Further discussion of nutritional support for sick horses is included in Chapter 5.

Down horses are prone to developing impactions of the cecum, large colon, or small colon. Reduced fecal output may be a preliminary sign of impaction, and the administration of laxatives such as magnesium or sodium sulfate solutions or mineral oil is indicated. Some horses may develop ileus, and this may have consequences for hydration and nutrition regulation. Urine and fecal retention may occur (e.g., in herpesvirus myeloencephalitis), and frequent emptying of rectum and bladder is then required. Alternatively, an indwelling urinary catheter can be placed.

Ensuring adequate ventilation, maintaining a clean stall environment, and preventing aspiration of food are important factors to reduce the chance of respiratory tract disease. A dysphagic horse should not be allowed to eat but should be offered an alternative source of nutrition. Antimicrobial drug therapy should be initiated when respiratory disease is present and may be indicated in a dysphagic horse. Regular turning of the horse may minimize development of lung disease. In addition to decubital ulcers, the development of aspiration pneumonia is the most common complication seen in horses with botulism.[23]

Physiotherapy is an important aspect of supportive care and the rehabilitative process of injured horses. Physiotherapy can be provided in the recumbent animal by manipulating limbs, depending on the horse's attitude, or assisting the horse to stand with a sling. Controlled exercise allows the unaffected parts of the nervous system to compensate for the affected parts by increasing strength and conscious proprioception. Exercise is especially helpful in improving weakness, ataxia, spasticity, and hypermetria.

A sling is an important tool in the assessment and management of a recumbent horse. When a horse is unable to rise, but otherwise appears to have a normal mentation (i.e., unaltered behavior), it may be very helpful in the examination to assist the horse to stand with a sling. The presence of lameness, weakness, and ataxia as well as the number of affected limbs are much more easily assessed when the horse is in an upright position. The horse may be able to stand freely and demonstrate clinical signs that may help in determining a diagnosis. Furthermore, using the sling to assist a horse to stand may provide valuable information for short-term management purposes. Deterioration or improvement of disease may be determined relatively easily by daily sling assistance in order to provide short-term recommendations and prognosis. For long-term management the sling can be useful, depending on the horse's primary disease and compliance. Horses may become used to using the sling and can be comfortably managed in the sling until they have regained sufficient control to ambulate freely. Periodic sessions of semistanding with sling assistance may function as a form of physiotherapy, and manipulation of limbs can occur during this time. Moreover, increasing the time that a horse can be maintained in an upright position decreases the detrimental effects of continuous pressure on skin and muscle. The time a horse is upright should also be used to clean and dry the horse and assess its food and water intake.

REFERENCES

Approach to Equine Critical Care

1. Hardy J, Burkhardt HA, Beard W: Equine emergency and intensive care: case survey and assessment of needs (1992-1994), *Proc Am Assoc Equine Pract* :182-183, 1996.
2. Dolente B, Lindberg S, Russell G, et al: Emergency case admissions at a large tertiary university referral hospital during a 12-month period, *J Vet Emerg Crit Care*, 18:298-305, 2008.
3. Girou E, Loyeau S, Legrand P, et al: Efficacy of handrubbing with alcohol based solution versus standard handwashing with antiseptic soap: randomized clinical trial, *Br Med J* 325:362, 2002.

Basic Procedures in Adult Equine Critical Care

1. Sevinga M, Barkema HW, Hesselink JW: Serum calcium and magnesium concentrations and the use of a calcium-magnesium-borogluconate solution in the treatment of Friesian mares with retained placenta, *Theriogenology* 57:941-947, 2002.
2. Garcia-Lopez JM, Provost PJ, Rush JE, et al: Prevalence and prognostic importance of hypomagnesemia and hypocalcemia in horses that have colic surgery, *Am J Vet Res* 62:7-12, 2001.
3. Jones PA, Tomasic M, Gentry PA: Oncotic, hemodilutional, and hemostatic effects of isotonic saline and hydroxyethyl starch solutions in clinically normal ponies, *Am J Vet Res* 58:541-548, 1997.
4. Belgrave RL, Hines MT, Keegan RD, et al: Effects of a polymerized ultrapurified bovine hemoglobin blood substituse administered to ponies with normovolemic anemia, *J Vet Intern Med* 16:396-403, 2002.
5. Maxson AD, Giger U, Sweeney CR, et al: Use of a bovine hemoglobin preparation in the treatment of cyclic ovarian hemorrhage in a miniature horse, *J Am Vet Med Assoc* 203:1308-1311, 1993.
6. Hardy J, Stewart RH, Beard WL, et al: Complications of nasogastric intubation in horses: nine cases (1987-1989), *J Am Vet Med Assoc* 201:483-486, 1992.

Support of Cardiovascular Function

1. Weil MH, Shubin H: Proposed reclassification of shock states with special reference to distributive defects, *Adv Exp Med Biol* 23:13-23, 1971.
2. Elbers PW, Ince C: Mechanisms of critical illness—classifying microcirculatory flow abnormalities in distributive shock, *Crit Care* 10:221, 2006.
3. Ellender TJ, Skinner JC: The use of vasopressors and inotropes in the emergency medical treatment of shock, *Emerg Med Clin North Am* 26:759-786, 2008.
4. Finkel MS, Oddis CV, Jacob TD, et al: Negative inotropic effects of cytokines on the heart mediated by nitric oxide, *Science* 257:387-389, 1992.
5. Spaniol JR, Knight AR, Zebley JL, et al: Fluid resuscitation therapy for hemorrhagic shock, *J Trauma Nurs* 14:152-160, 2007.
6. Rodgers KG: Cardiovascular shock, *Emerg Med Clin North Am* 13:793-810, 1995.
7. Lefer AM, Lefer DJ: Pharmacology of the endothelium in ischemia-reperfusion and circulatory shock, *Annu Rev Pharmacol Toxicol* 33:71-90, 1993.
8. Landry DW, Oliver JA: The pathogenesis of vasodilatory shock, *N Engl J Med* 345:588-595, 2001.
9. Tuite PK: Recognition and management of shock in the pediatric patient, *Crit Care Nurs Q* 20:52-61, 1997.
10. Mullner M, Urbanek B, Havel C, et al: Vasopressors for shock. Cochrane Database Syst Rev CD003709, 2004
11. Tremblay LN, Rizoli SB, Brenneman FD: Advances in fluid resuscitation of hemorrhagic shock, *Can J Surg* 44:172-179, 2001.
12. Cook VL, Bain FT: Volume(crystalloid) replacement in the ICU patient, *Clin Tech Equine Pract* 2:122-129, 2003.
13. Smiley LE: The use of hetastarch for plasma expansion, *Probl Vet Med* 4:652-667, 1992.
14. Velanovich V: Crystalloid versus colloid fluid resuscitation: a meta-analysis of mortality, *Surgery* 105:65-71, 1989.
15. Knutson JE, Deering JA, Hall FW, et al: Does intraoperative hetastarch administration increase blood loss and transfusion requirements after cardiac surgery? *Anesth Analg* 90:801-807, 2000.
16. Jones PA, Tomasic M, Gentry PA: Oncotic, hemodilutional, and hemostatic effects of isotonic saline and hydroxyethyl starch solutions in clinically normal ponies, *Am J Vet Res* 58:541-548, 1997.
17. Slovis N, Murray G: *How to approach whole blood transfusion in horses*, San Diego, Calif, 266-269, 2001.
18. Tranbaugh RF, Lewis FR: Crystalloid versus colloid for fluid resuscitation of hypovolemic patients, *Adv Shock Res* 9: 203-216, 1983.
19. Rackow EC, Falk JL, Fein IA, et al: Fluid resuscitation in circulatory shock: a comparison of the cardiorespiratory effects of albumin, hetastarch, and saline solutions in patients with hypovolemic and septic shock, *Crit Care Med* 11:839-850, 1983.
20. Krausz MM: Controversies in shock research: hypertonic resuscitation-pros and cons, *Shock* 3:69-72, 1995.
21. Holmes CL: Vasoactive drugs in the intensive care unit, *Curr Opin Crit Care* 11:413-417, 2005.
22. Ruffolo RR Jr, Nichols AJ, Stadel JM, et al: Pharmacologic and therapeutic applications of alpha 2-adrenoceptor subtypes, *Annu Rev Pharmacol Toxicol* 33:243-279, 1993.
23. Nagashima M, Hattori Y, Akaishi Y, et al: Alpha 1-adrenoceptor subtypes mediating inotropic and electrophysiological effects in mammalian myocardium, *Am J Physiol* 271: H1423-H1432, 1996.
24. Huang L, Tang W: Vasopressor agents: old and new components, *Curr Opin Crit Care* 10:183-187, 2004.
25. Steel A, Bihari D: Choice of catecholamine: does it matter? *Curr Opin Crit Care* 6:347-353, 2000.
26. Girault JA, Greengard P: The neurobiology of dopamine signaling, *Arch Neurol* 61:641-644, 2004.
27. Jose PA, Eisner GM, Felder RA: Regulation of blood pressure by dopamine receptors, *Nephron Physiol* 95:19-27, 2003.
28. Holmes CL, Landry DW, Granton JT: Science review: vasopressin and the cardiovascular system part 1: receptor physiology, *Crit Care* 7:427-434, 2003.
29. Vincent JL: Vasopressin in hypotensive and shock states, *Crit Care Clin* 22:187-197, 2006.
30. Holmes CL, Landry DW, Granton JT: Science review: vasopressin and the cardiovascular system part 2: clinical physiology, *Crit Care* 8:15-23, 2004.

31. Shepherd JT: Circulatory response to beta-adrenergic blockade at rest and during exercise, *Am J Cardiol* 55:87D-94D, 1985.
32. Woolsey CA, Coopersmith CM: Vasoactive drugs and the gut: is there anything new? *Curr Opin Crit Care* 12:155-159, 2006.
33. Zhong JQ, Dorian P: Epinephrine and vasopressin during cardiopulmonary resuscitation, *Resuscitation* 66:263-269, 2005.
34. MacGregor DA, Smith TE, Prielipp RC, et al: Pharmacokinetics of dopamine in healthy male subjects, *Anesthesiology* 92:338-346, 2000.
35. Schwartz LB, Gewertz BL: The renal response to low dose dopamine, *J Surg Res* 45:574-588, 1988.
36. Richer M, Robert S, Lebel M: Renal hemodynamics during norepinephrine and low-dose dopamine infusions in man, *Crit Care Med* 24:1150-1156, 1996.
37. Kellum JA, Pinsky MR: Use of vasopressor agents in critically ill patients, *Curr Opin Crit Care* 8:236-241, 2002.
38. Smit AJ: Dopamine in heart failure and critical care, *Clin Exp Hypertens* 22:269-276, 2000.
39. Asfar P, De Backer D, Meier-Hellmann A, et al: Clinical review: influence of vasoactive and other therapies on intestinal and hepatic circulations in patients with septic shock, *Crit Care* 8:170-179, 2004.
40. Patel BM, Chittock DR, Russell JA, et al: Beneficial effects of short-term vasopressin infusion during severe septic shock, *Anesthesiology* 96:576-582, 2002.
41. Malay MB, Ashton RC Jr, Landry DW, et al: Low-dose vasopressin in the treatment of vasodilatory septic shock, *J Trauma* 47:699-703, 1999.
42. Wong DM, Vo DT, Alcott CJ, et al: Plasma vasopressin concentrations in healthy foals from birth to 3 months of age, *J Vet Intern Med* 22:1259-1261, 2008.
43. Hurcombe SD, Toribio RE, Slovis N, et al: Blood arginine vasopressin, adrenocorticotropin hormone, and cortisol concentrations at admission in septic and critically ill foals and their association with survival, *J Vet Intern Med* 22:639-647, 2008.
44. Hollis AR, Boston RC, Corley KT: Plasma aldosterone, vasopressin and atrial natriuretic peptide in hypovolaemia: a preliminary comparative study of neonatal and mature horses, *Equine Vet J* 40:64-69, 2008.
45. Corley KTT, Marr CM: Cardiac monitoring in the ICU patient, *Clin Tech Equine Pract* 2:145-155, 2003.
46. Peitzman AB, Billiar TR, Harbrecht BG, et al: Hemorrhagic shock, *Curr Probl Surg* 32:925-1002, 1995.
47. Magdesian KG: Monitoring the critically ill equine patient, *Vet Clin North Am Equine Pract* 20:11-39, 2004.
48. Gutierrez G, Wulf ME: Lactic acidosis in sepsis: a commentary, *Intensive Care Med* 22:6-16, 1996.
49. Haupt MT, Gilbert EM, Carlson RW: Fluid loading increases oxygen consumption in septic patients with lactic acidosis, *Am Rev Respir Dis* 131:912-916, 1985.
50. Magdesian KG, Fielding CL, Rhodes DM, et al: Changes in central venous pressure and blood lactate concentration in response to acute blood loss in horses, *J Am Vet Med Assoc* 229:1458-1462, 2006.
51. Jones PA, Bain FT, Byars TD, et al: Effect of hydroxyethyl starch infusion on colloid oncotic pressure in hypoproteinemic horses, *J Am Vet Med Assoc* 218:1130-1135, 2001.
52. Brown SA, Dusza K, Boehmer J: Comparison of measured and calculated values for colloid osmotic pressure in hospitalized animals, *Am J Vet Res* 55:910-915, 1994.
53. Adrogue HJ, Rashad MN, Gorin AB, et al: Assessing acid-base status in circulatory failure. Differences between arterial and central venous blood, *N Engl J Med* 320:1312-1316, 1989.
54. Adrogue HJ, Rashad MN, Gorin AB, et al: Arteriovenous acid-base disparity in circulatory failure: studies on mechanism, *Am J Physiol* 257:F1087-F1093, 1989.
55. Marr CM: Equine echocardiography—sound advice at the heart of the matter, *Br Vet J* 150:527-545, 1994.
56. Corley KT, Donaldson LL, Durando MM, et al: Cardiac output technologies with special reference to the horse, *J Vet Intern Med* 17:262-272, 2003.
57. Berton C, Cholley B: Equipment review: new techniques for cardiac output measurement—oesophageal Doppler, Fick principle using carbon dioxide, and pulse contour analysis, *Crit Care* 6:216-221, 2002.

Support of Respiratory Function

1. West JB: *Respiratory physiology: the essentials*, ed 8, Baltimore, Lippincott, 2008, Williams & Wilkins.
2. Wingfield WE, Raffe MR, editors: *The veterinary ICU book*, Jackson Hole, Wyo, 2002, Teton New Media.
3. Aguilera-Tejero E, Estepa JC, Lopez I, et al: Arterial blood gases and acid-base balance in healthy young and old horses, *Equine Vet J* 30:352, 1998.
4. Picandet V, Jeanneret S: Jean-Pierre, L: Effects of syringe type and storage temperature on results of blood gas analysis in arterial blood of horses, *J Vet Intern Med* 21:476, 2007.
5. Matthews NS, Hartke S, Allen JC Jr: An evaluation of pulse oximeters in dogs, cats and horses, *Vet Anaesth Anal* 30:3, 2003.
6. Koenig J, McDonell W, Valverde A: Accuracy of pulse oximetry and capnography in healthy and compromised horses during spontaneous and controlled ventilation, *Can J Vet Res* 67:169, 2003.
7. Tute AS, Wilkins PA, Gleed RD, et al: Negative preesure pulmonary edema as a post-anesthetic complication associated with upper airway obstruction in a horse, *Vet Surg* 25:519, 1996.
8. Wilson DV, Schott HC, Robinson NE, et al: Response to nasopharyngeal oxygen administration in horses with lung disease, *Equine Vet J* 38:219, 2006.
9. Duvivier DH, Votion D, Roberts CA, et al: Inhalation therapy of equine respiratory disorders, *Equine Vet Educ* 11:124, 1999.
10. McKenzie HC, Murray MJ: Concentrations of gentamicin in serum and bronchial lavage fluid after intravenous and aerosol administration to horses, *Am J Vet Res* 61:1185, 2000.

Support Of Gastrointestinal Function

1. Ganong WG: *Review of medical physiology*, ed 19, Stamford, Connecticut, 1999, Appleton & Lange.
2. Souba WW: Nutritional support, *N Engl J Med* 336:41, 1997.
3. Weissman C: Nutrition in the intensive care unit, *Crit Care* 3:R67, 1999.
4. Heidegger CP, Darmon P, Pichard C: Enteral vs parenteral nutrition for the critically ill patient: a combined support should be preferred, *Curr Opin Crit Care* 14:408, 2008.
5. Henneke DR, Potter GD, Kreider JL, et al: Relationship between condition score, physical measurements and body fat percentages in mares, *Equine Vet J* 15:371, 1983.
6. National Research Council: *Nutrient requirements of horses*, Washington, DC, 2007, National Academies Press.
7. Robinson NE, editor: *Current therapy in equine medicine*, ed 6, St Louis, 2009, Saunders.
8. Dunkel BM, Wilkins PA: Nutrition and the critically ill horse, *Vet Clin North Am Equine Pract* 20:107, 204
9. Hansen TO, White NA, Kemp DT: Total parenteral nutrition in four healthy adult horses, *Am J Vet Res* 49:122, 1988.
10. Spurlock SL, Ward MV: Parenteral nutrition in equine patients: principles and theory, *Compend Cont Educ Pract Vet* 13:461, 1991.
11. Furr M: Intravenous nutrition in horses: clinical applications, *Proc Am Coll Vet Intern Med* 20:186, 2002.

Support of Renal Function

1. Doucet MY, Bertone AL, Hendrickson D, et al: Comparison of efficacy and safety of paste formulations of firocoxib and phenylbutazone in horses with naturally occurring osteoarthritis, *J Am Vet Med Assoc* 232:91-97, 2008.

2. Brashier MK, Geor RJ, Ames TR, et al. Effect of intravenous calcium administration on gentamicin-induced nephrotoxicosis in ponies, *Am J Vet Res* 59:1055-1062.
3. Divers TJ: Urine production, renal function, and drug monitoring in the equine intensive care unit, *Clin Tech Equine Pract* 2:188-192, 2003.
4. Corley KTT: Inotropes and vasopressors in adults and foals, *Vet Clin Equine* 20:77-106, 2004.

Support of Neurological Function

1. De Lahunta A, Glass EN: *Veterinary neuroanatomy and clinical neurology*, ed 3, St Louis, 2009, Saunders.
2. Matthews HK, Andrews FM: Performing a neurologic examination in a standing or recumbent horse, *Vet Med* November: 1229-1240, 1990.
3. Olby N: Current concepts in the management of acute spinal cord injury, *J Vet Intern Med* 13:399-407, 1999.
4. Zurita M, Vaquero J, Oya S, Morales C: Effects of dexamethasone on apoptosis-related cell death after spinal cord injury, *J Neurosurg* 96:83-89, 2002.
5. Bracken MB: Methylprednisolone in the management of acute spinal cord injuries, *Med J Austr* 153:368, 1990.
6. Bracken MB: Treatment of acute spinal cord injury with methylprednisolone: results of a multicenter, randomized clinical trial, *J Neurotrauma* 1(Suppl 8):S47-S50, 1991:discussion S51-S42.
7. Hugenholtz H: Methylprednisolone for acute spinal cord injury: not a standard of care, *CMAJ* 168:1145-1146, 2003.
8. Hugenholtz H, Cass DE, Dvorak MF, et al: High-dose methylprednisolone for acute closed spinal cord injury-only a treatment option, *Can J Neurol Sci* 29:227-235, 2002.
9. Arai T, Tsukahara I, Nitta K, Watanabe T: Effects of mannitol on cerebral circulation after transient complete cerebral ischemia in dogs, *Crit Care Med* 14:634-637, 1986.
10. Polderman KH, van de Kraats G, Dixon JM, et al: Increases in spinal fluid osmolarity induced by mannitol, *Crit Care Med* 31:584-590, 2003.
11. Qureshi AI, Suarez JI: Use of hypertonic saline solutions in treatment of cerebral edema and intracranial hypertension, *Crit Care Med* 28:3301-3313, 2000.
12. Schwarz S, Schwab S, Bertram M, et al: Effects of hypertonic saline hydroxyethyl starch solution and mannitol in patients with increased intracranial pressure after stroke, *Stroke* 29: 1550-1555, 1998.
13. Peterson B, Khanna S, Fisher B, Marshall L: Prolonged hypernatremia controls elevated intracranial pressure in head- injured pediatric patients, *Crit Care Med* 28:1136-1143, 2000.
14. Hoerlein BF, Redding RW, Hoff EJ, et al: Evaluation of dexamethasone, DMSO, mannitol and solcoseryl in acute spinal cord trauma, *J Am Anim Hosp Assoc* 19:216, 1983.
15. McDonald H: Preventing pressure ulcers, *Rehab Manag* 14: 40-46, 2001.
16. Thomas DR: Improving outcome of pressure ulcers with nutritional interventions: a review of the evidence, *Nutrition* 17:121-125, 2001.
17. Thomas DR: Issues and dilemmas in the prevention and treatment of pressure ulcers: a review, *J Gerontol A Biol Sci Med Sci* 56:M328-M340, 2001.
18. Thomas DR: Prevention and treatment of pressure ulcers: what works? what doesn't? *Cleve Clin J Med* 68:704-722, 2001.
19. Rayner SG: Traumatic cerebral partial lobotomy in a Thoroughbred stallion, *Austr Vet J* 83:674-677, 2005.
20. McConnico RS, Clem MF, DeBowes RM: Supportive medical care of recumbent horses, *Compend Cont Educ Pract Vet* 13:1287-1295, 1991.
21. Nout YS, Reed SM: Management and treatment of the recumbent horse, *Equine Vet Educ* 7:416-432, 2005.
22. Ferguson M, Cook A, Rimmasch H, et al: Pressure ulcer management: the importance of nutrition, *Medsurg Nurs* 9: 163-175, 2000:quiz 176-167.
23. Whitlock RH, Buckley C: *Botulism, Vet Clin North Am Equine Pract* 13:107-128, 1997.

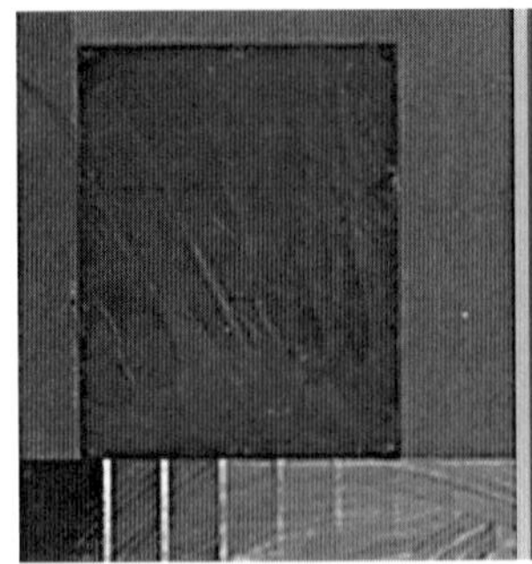

EPIDEMIOLOGY

CHAPTER 8

Noah Cohen

Like the field of equine medicine, the discipline of epidemiology is diverse. The previous edition of this textbook contains an excellent review of important epidemiologic concepts and principles relevant to equine medicine, including diagnostic testing, measures of disease association, causality, sample design and size, and basic statistical constructs. Those topics will not be revisited in this chapter, and readers interested in those aspects of epidemiology are directed to Chapter 21 in the previous edition. This chapter is devoted to the introduction of principles, techniques, and limitations of evidence-based medicine (EBM) and its essential and underlying role in epidemiology.

EVIDENCE-BASED MEDICINE

The concept of EBM was developed by clinical epidemiologists more than 20 years ago.[1] Since then, EBM has become very popular. Whereas a Medline search of EBM in 1993 yielded only six citations,[2] a search in early 2008 yielded more than 29,000 citations. The *Equine Veterinary Journal* currently dedicates a section to EBM, and the term *EBM* is increasingly used in presentations and publications. Recently, EBM has been described as "the integration of the best research evidence with our clinical expertise and our patient's unique values and circumstances."[3] The emphasis of EBM is on acquiring, assessing, and utilizing evidence to improve clinical decision making. A fundamental principle of EBM is that, whenever possible, evidence for clinical activities should be derived from well-designed studies of patients with spontaneous disease (i.e., epidemiologic studies).

The practice of equine medicine has traditionally been empiric and driven by the knowledge, wisdom, and experience of experts. The field has depended largely on combining an understanding of the pathogenesis and mechanisms of disease with authority, theory, logical deduction, and intuition. The human medical profession has moved away from these traditions toward a medical practice that is based on clinically relevant evidence.[2,3] The principle of EBM is to base all clinical decisions regarding prevention, diagnosis, treatment, and prognosis of disease on the use of the best existing evidence. It is difficult to dispute the value of this approach, which aims to discourage a reliance on authority ("I treat horses with equine protozoal myeloencepalitis [EPM] this way because that is what I was told" by a textbook or expert) and promote instead a reliance on the best available evidence ("Why do I treat EPM this way?" and "What is the most successful approach to treating EPM?"). Currently, *EBM* refers not only to this laudable principle but also to a methodology by which the principle is realized.

METHODOLOGY

The methodology of EBM consists of five steps: (1) defining, or asking, a clinical question; (2) searching for evidence to answer the question; (3) critically appraising the evidence gathered; (4) applying the results of answering the question; and (5) auditing the outcome of applying the results (i.e., how well did the EBM-derived answer work?).[2] Each of these steps is considered in turn. As will be discussed later, the state of development of the methodology is highly variable among steps.

STEP 1: ASKING THE QUESTION(S)

The first step in EBM is defining the question that pertains to the clinical circumstances of the patient. This is not always as simple as it might initially seem. A question that is too broad (e.g., "How do I treat pneumonia in horses?") may yield numerous citations that are not germane, whereas a question that is too focused (e.g., "How do I treat *Pneumocystis carinii* pneumonia in a foal with selective IgM deficiency?") may yield no results at all. Typically, veterinarians ask several questions about a given patient, including questions described as background and foreground varieties. Background questions are general knowledge questions, such as "How does cervical stenosis or instability develop in horses?" and "What causes abscessing pneumonia of foals?" Foreground questions are more specific to the particular case, such as "In a mare with congestive heart failure and atrial fibrillation that developed coincident with developing pleuropneumonia, what is the best approach for treating the arrhythmia?" Generally, veterinarians pose fewer background and more foreground questions as they gain experience with a particular condition.

Any clinical encounter will generate a number of questions pertaining to signalment and history (e.g., "Does the signalment suggest that certain disorders will be more common?" "Does the herd history help eliminate certain causes?"), clinical examination findings (e.g., "How do I interpret a head tilt and signs of facial nerve paralysis in this horse?"), etiology and differential diagnosis (e.g., "What might cause these signs?";

"What is the cause of these signs?"), diagnosis (e.g., "What tests are most meaningful in a patient with this clinical complaint?"), treatment (e.g., "What is the best way to treat temporohyoid osteoarthropathy?"), prognosis (e.g., "What is the probability that this horse will return to use?"), prevention (e.g., "What can be done to prevent recurrence?"), experiences and meanings (e.g., "Have I effectively communicated with the clients?"; "Does the client perceive that I empathize?"), and improvement (e.g., "Have I learned new information about managing this case from the experience?"; "Did my patient benefit?").

Attempting to answer all relevant questions simultaneously will be unrewarding for the clinician, client, and patient. Veterinarians must learn to prioritize their efforts. Often, first addressing certain questions of case management (i.e., history, physical examination and diagnosis) seems logical; however, the client's needs may also influence the order of the questions (e.g., matters of prognosis or experience and meaning). Moreover, veterinarians must consider which questions may feasibly be answered within the time and setting of the clinical encounter. The veterinarian should consider recording those questions that must be postponed so that they will not be forgotten.

The process of carefully considering questions to ask, prioritizing them, and saving unanswered ones to be answered later might seem like an inconvenience and a waste of time: Veterinarians do much of this already without needing to spend a lot of time formulating and recording their clinical inquiries. The principal advantage to the process is that it will help identify evidence-based solutions for the clinical problems that veterinarians face. With experience veterinarians become more proficient and expeditious in answering questions, and the process necessitates remaining current on new developments, such as new medical and surgical approaches to temporohyoid osteoarthropathy (and their evaluation) and new diagnostic tests for EPM.

Perhaps the most important principle of EBM is that veterinarians need to ask themselves what evidence exists for their clinical activities. Breaking away from the tradition of authority and empiricism in equine medicine will not be easy, and it will happen only if veterinarians are willing to question what they really know about their clinical decisions and interpretations.

STEP 2: SEARCHING FOR EVIDENCE

Once a question has been posed, it is important to find the best available evidence using a review of the literature that is as comprehensive as possible. Relying on book chapters or review articles will not suffice for at least two important reasons. First, new knowledge emerges more quickly than it can be incorporated into textbooks. Of course, well-written textbooks remain excellent resources for many background questions (e.g., pathophysiology of diseases, etiology of diseases with well-defined causes) and often will be fairly current in a field such as equine medicine, wherein the pace at which new information is generated is fairly slow. Unfortunately, it is often difficult to determine which information in these textbooks is current and which is outdated. Furthermore, authors of review articles have their own particular prejudices, beliefs, and perceptions, and these biases influence their interpretations and recommendations. Practitioners must guard against biases that may result in selecting reports that conform to their preexisting beliefs and perceptions, which is easier said than done.

In human medicine a hierarchy of *resources* for EBM has been proposed (note that this is a hierarchy of resources, not of evidence).[2] The highest tier of this hierarchy is a computerized decision support system (CDDS) in which clinical information from a patient's records is automatically linked to all relevant, important research findings pertaining to the patient's circumstances. The next highest-level resource is synopses of individual studies or reviews. These synopses are designed to be concise and precise distillations of the important facts needed by busy clinicians. The next level is syntheses of reports based on exhaustive searches for evidence, implementation of explicit scientific criteria for review, and systematic assembly of the evidence. Syntheses are epitomized by the Cochrane Reviews (www.Cochranelibrary.com/). At the bottom of this hierarchy are individual scientific reports.

Equine practitioners currently operate primarily at the level of individual reports. Although a veterinary CDDS will likely be developed in the future, it is not clear when. Synopses of numerous studies on a given topic are not likely to be available soon, primarily because numerous studies for a given topic do not yet exist. The same problem arises for systematic reviews: Although there are examples,[4] they are exceedingly rare. The advantage of relying on individual reports is that the information is generally current (whereas it can take many months or years to develop the evidence on which synopses and systematic reviews are based). The disadvantage is that the evidence is weaker from individual studies, and it puts the onus on the reader to critically appraise each study. Critical appraisal is discussed in greater detail in the next section, but first it is important to consider resources for finding information.

Those practitioners who are fortunate to work at institutions with appropriate licenses for digital publications will find that a great deal of information can be retrieved electronically with little effort, and librarians are generally available to assist. In settings without such licenses, it may still be possible to gain access to the necessary resources through colleges or universities. Regardless, veterinarians will find a considerable amount of high-quality information on the Internet through resources such as PubMed (http://wwwncbi.nlm.gov/PubMed/) and BioMed Central (http://www.biomedcentral.com). It is important to remember, however, that the Internet also offers much in the way of low-quality information. Relying on subscription journals is generally inefficient: There are simply too many journals with too many articles appearing each month that are relevant to the daily activities of equine specialists. Moreover, important articles are often published in journals to which few veterinarians subscribe. For example, not many veterinarians subscribe to the journal *Genomics,* but many would be interested in reading about the mutation that causes polysaccharide storage myopathy.[5]

STEP 3: CRITICAL APPRAISAL

Introduction Although the first two steps, formally stating questions and searching for the evidence, are fairly straightforward, the third step, critical appraisal, is more complex. It is also vitally important in equine EBM because the evidence for much of what equine practitioners do is sparse and primarily derived from observational (epidemiologic) studies or experiments (using horses or other animal species) from which practitioners must then extrapolate results to the clinical setting. These sources of evidence are not only low in terms of the hierarchy of resources for searching but also relatively low in the hierarchy of evidence that has been proposed for EBM.[6] Before further discussion of this hierarchy, it is necessary to briefly review these epidemiologic (patient- or population-based) study designs.

Study Designs EBM places a premium on information derived from patient-based epidemiologic studies. Epidemiologic study designs have been summarized in the previous edition, and a full discussion of all possible study designs and their strengths and limitations is beyond the scope of this chapter. Thus designs are reviewed briefly herein. Epidemiologic study designs can be defined as either experimental or observational (Box 8-1).

Experimental epidemiologic studies are ones in which the investigators control the exposure (e.g., a treatment group) to which patients are assigned. Assignment is most often at the level of the individual but may occasionally be at the level of population (e.g., fluoride added to the water of some communities but not others to evaluate effects on dental caries). Assignment of exposure should be randomized in an effort to render the treatment groups as similar as possible for both measured and unmeasured factors that may be independently associated with the outcome of interest. Randomization, however, does not ensure that there will not be significant differences among groups that occur by chance alone, and the chance of differences occurring is greater when the study population is small. In general, the randomized, controlled clinical trial (RCT) is considered the highest form of evidence from an individual study because of the extent to which biases are reduced through the processes of randomization, a priori specification of primary study outcomes, and so-called blinding of patients and clinicians assessing primary study outcomes. An example of an RCT is the report by Smith et al. regarding incisional complications after celiotomy.[7] It is worth noting that the term *RCT* is often used in equine medicine to refer to experimental studies involving research horses, rather than patients. At the time of this writing, a PubMed search for the term "randomized controlled trials and horses" yielded 518 results, of which fewer than a score were patient-based studies. The term *RCT* should be reserved for patient-based clinical studies to avoid imprecision in professional communications.

BOX 8-1

DESIGNS OF EPIDEMIOLOGIC STUDIES

Experimental Designs

Randomized, controlled trial
Population-based
N of 1 randomized, controlled trial

Observational Study Designs

Cohort study
- Prospective
- Retrospective/nonconcurrent
- Self-controlled case-series

Case-control study
- Case-control
- Case-crossover

Cross-sectional study
Reports of case series
Reports of individual cases or case series

A modification of the RCT is the N of 1 RCT design. The N of 1 RCT design is one in which individual patients are assigned to pairs of treatment periods: They receive a target treatment in one period and an alternative treatment (or placebo) during the other period. The approach continues until both patient and clinician are convinced that a given treatment (whose identity to which they may be blinded) is deemed to be effective for that patient.[2,6]

Unfortunately, experimental epidemiologic studies are exiguous in equine medicine, most likely because the resources to fund these generally expensive studies are often lacking. Thus the bulk of our evidence is derived from observational epidemiologic studies. Observational designs include cohort, case-control, and cross-sectional designs.

A cohort study is one in which investigators first define the exposure status of each group (cohort), and then the experiences of each cohort are followed over time for the occurrence of disease, such that disease incidence is determined. When more than one cohort is followed, comparisons can be made regarding the incidence of disease. The ratio of the risk in a cohort with an exposure of interest (e.g., a group of horses treated with omeprazole) relative to a reference cohort (e.g., a group of horses not treated with omeprazole) is termed the *relative risk* (RR), and it indicates how many times more likely the disease is to occur in the exposed cohort than in the unexposed cohort. The reader is encouraged to review the chapter on veterinary epidemiology in the second edition of this textbook for further discussion of the RR and other measures of risk in cohort studies.

Cohort studies may be prospective (concurrent), retrospective (nonconcurrent), or both. A prospective cohort study is one in which exposure status is determined during the present and horses are followed into the future for development of disease. A retrospective study is one in which exposure is determined in the past and individuals are monitored up to the present time for development of disease. A modification of the cohort study is the self-controlled case-series study in which the history of individual cases during defined periods of risk are studied; in this way each individual acts as its own control. For example, a practitioner might look at the association of colic with anthelmintic administration by identifying cases of colic, defining "at-risk periods" as the 3-day period after anthelmintic administration, and determine the incidence of colic during these risk periods for the individual horse.

In a case-control study disease status (whether a horse is a case of the disease of interest or is a member of the control group used for comparison) is first determined, and then the history of the exposure of interest. As a result of the selective sampling of cases, the incidence of disease (and thus the RR) generally cannot be determined in a case-control study. However, it is possible to determine the odds of exposure in cases relative to controls, which is equivalent to the odds of disease among exposed relative to unexposed, otherwise known as the *odds ratio* (OR). The OR will approximate the RR when the included cases are representative of all cases, controls reflect the reference population, and the disease is rare.

Case-control studies may be prospective, retrospective, or both. A prospective case-control study is one in which incident (new) cases of disease are compared with contemporaneously identified controls. Retrospective case-control studies are ones in which cases occurred before initiation of the study. The case-crossover design is a self-controlled equivalent of a case-control study. In this design exposures immediately preceding a disease event are compared with exposures occurring during earlier "control" periods when an event did not occur. The differences between the self-controlled case-series and the case-crossover studies may seem subtle, but they are technically important.

Cross-sectional studies are ones of a target population at a particular point in time: Exposure and disease status are determined simultaneously in cross-sectional studies. This design is best for descriptive studies and is considered particularly weak because, as a result of determining the outcome and exposure simultaneously, it is impossible to determine causality (because a cause must be demonstrated to precede its resultant effect).

Critical Appraisal: Identifying Bias Critical appraisal of studies entails trying to determine if the study results are valid and applicable to the clinical setting. Epidemiologic studies of patients generally contain estimates of a measure of association (e.g., the OR or RR) or other population parameter (e.g., the cumulative incidence of disease). Studies are considered valid when the observed or estimated parameter is the same as the true, or actual, value. The term *bias* refers to a systematic error in the study relating to its design, the means by which data were collected, or the way the study data were analyzed.[8] This type of systematic error is distinct from random error resulting from the imprecision of the device or devices (e.g., questionnaire, serum chemistry analyzer, blood pressure monitor) used for collecting data. Random error generally does not cause bias, and it can be reduced by increasing sample size. The fact that we never know the true value of the population parameter and cannot perform the infinite replicates needed for valid estimation means that we must use judgment and knowledge to identify potential biases in studies. Although a surfeit of biases have been identified, biases in epidemiologic or patient-based studies generally fall into one of three categories: selection bias, information bias, and confounding bias.[8]

Critical Appraisal Based on Study Design The study design can be used as a criterion for evaluating the quality of data. The ensuing discussion will proceed from designs with the weakest sources of information to those with the strongest. Because empiric observations can be misleading and experts can be wrong, anecdotes and recommendations should be considered as evidence of the weakest variety. It is important to remember, however, that many important clinical innovations have arisen because of an individual insight that proved valid, and experts also are often right.

Experimental research to describe biologic (e.g., physiologic, pathologic, pharmacologic) phenomena contributes significantly to our understanding of disease processes and potential interventions. Nevertheless, these studies are considered weak sources of evidence, particularly when they involve heterologous species of animals, for a number of reasons, including the disparities between experimental models of disease and spontaneous disease. In many instances, conclusions drawn from an experimental model that seem logical or plausible do not prove to be true when applied to patients. For example, although folate supplementation seemed logical (and was advocated by experts) in horses receiving folic-acid inhibitors to treat EPM, the practice appeared to pose a risk to fetuses of supplemented mares.[9] It is a basic tenet of EBM that, whenever possible, clinical decisions are based on evidence derived from patient-based studies, preferably those that are as similar as possible to the patients being treated.

Individual case reports are often important because they highlight new diseases, disease manifestations, potential therapies, and so forth. Because of their singularity, however, replication of their findings is important. In this way, case series are generally stronger evidence than individual case reports because they provide more information about variation among individuals with respect to clinical signs, diagnostic test results, and treatment responses. Case series can be very helpful in describing the clinical course and may represent the best available evidence for rare conditions. Nevertheless, bias may occur in the selection of cases and the subjective interpretation of findings. More important, these studies lack a comparison group for drawing inferences.

Although controlled studies are generally a preferred source of evidence, studies that use historical controls should be considered a very weak source of evidence because the controls and the group to which they are being compared are very likely different: Many factors change over time and can influence both exposure and disease. An exception is the circumstance in which mortality is essentially 100%. For example, it might be reasonable to compare a new treatment of rabies to the treatment of historical controls.

The case-control study design uses controls and is practical for studying rare diseases and identifying prognostic factors; however, this study design is subject to numerous biases. With respect to information bias, the historical nature of exposure data creates ample opportunities for error: Because data are not typically collected from patients for the purpose of future scientific study, data may be lacking in quality (e.g., incomplete dietary history among horses with colic) or absent (e.g., serum amyloid A concentrations in horses with various types of colic). With respect to selection bias, the representativeness of cases and controls can be problematic, particularly for the control group. Finally, confounding bias also can be a problem in case-control studies because the data regarding exposure to important confounding variables may be missing or of poor quality. Whenever possible, case-control studies should be designed to account for known risk factors to prevent confounding effects; when known variables associated with the disease of interest are not accounted for, study results should be interpreted with caution. Generally, the extent of the impact of ignoring confounders will be commensurate with the magnitude of the association of the confounder (e.g., activity level) and the outcome (e.g., colic). Consistency of the observed association also should be considered when readers attempt to assess the magnitude of the impact of ignored confounders: If a confounder has been repeatedly associated with an outcome, it may be particularly important to account for this confounder. Clearly, it is not always possible for investigators to collect data on all variables previously associated with the outcome of interest. Failure to account for a known confounder does not vitiate the value of a study, but readers should be aware that it will be necessary to substantiate the results of reports in which confounders are not accounted for because the magnitude and statistical significance of observed associations may be altered after accounting for confounding.

Cohort studies are superior to case-control studies in that the temporal association of exposure and disease tends to be better defined. Cohort studies are well-suited to identifying risk factors for disease, studying the outcome of an intervention, and examining the natural history of disease. Prospective cohort studies are generally superior to retrospective studies because of the problems associated with historical exposure data from the latter design. Other forms of information bias can occur but are much less likely when the study is well designed than in case-control studies. Given that the cohorts are chosen, some degree of selection bias should be expected in any cohort study. It is important to scrutinize the criteria for including and excluding cases to understand how representative the exposed and unexposed control groups are. Confounding biases also may occur, as discussed previously in reference to the case-control study design.

The RCT design is considered to be the superior design for patient-centered research because of its presumed ability to render study groups similar with respect to measured and unmeasured factors by way of randomization, thereby minimizing or eliminating confounding bias. Information biases may still occur in the RCT, but they are minimized or eliminated in well-designed studies. Selection biases also can occur, as discussed for cohort studies. As mentioned, RCTs are relatively rare in equine medicine because they are expensive as well as administratively and practically challenging to conduct. To reduce costs and complexity, the sample size of an RCT may be restricted. However, the favorable attributes of RCTs do not circumvent the problem of lack of power: RCTs of small sample sizes may lack sufficient power to detect clinically important differences among study groups.

Critical Appraisal Based on Clinical Activity The primary clinical activities of equine medicine are choosing and interpreting diagnostic tests, selecting treatments, and making prognoses. The types of evidence practitioners use varies to some extent by activity, and thus evidence can be considered for each activity.

Diagnostic Studies When appraising an article that relates to a diagnostic test, practitioners must evaluate three critical aspects: (1) the spectrum of disease patients represented in the population studied, (2) whether the reference standard (a.k.a. the "gold standard") was applied irrespective of the results of the diagnostic test, and (3) whether the reference standard was measured independently.[2]

It is not unusual for studies of diagnostic tests to assess the performance of the test to severe forms of disease (e.g., necropsy-confirmed cases of EPM) and horses free of signs of disease. Although the use of such case-control studies is useful for initial evaluation of tests, they are of limited clinical value. Useful evaluation of diagnostic tests will reflect the full spectrum of disease to which the test is to be applied, including patients with milder as well as florid forms of the disease, in early as well as late stages of disease, and among both treated and untreated patients. Thus case-control studies are generally weak sources of evidence for evaluating diagnostic tests. The best sources of evidence for diagnostic tests are prospectively designed studies of consecutive patients undergoing prespecified diagnostic testing criteria against a reference standard that is consistently applied (as described later in this chapter). Studies in which diagnostic testing criteria are developed in a consecutive series of patients should be considered as a valuable but lesser source of evidence. When patients are not consecutively evaluated, there is potential for bias in the selection of cases included; thus studies of nonconsecutive patients should be viewed as weaker evidence.

When a patient has a negative test, investigators are tempted to forego testing with the reference standard, especially when the latter is more invasive. For example, in a study evaluating the diagnostic sensitivity and specificity of thoracic ultrasound for detecting subclinical *Rhodococcus equi* pneumonia, it is probably not desirable to perform tracheobronchial aspiration to obtain a sample for microbiologic culture and cytologic evaluation in an apparently healthy foal from a farm with endemic *R. equi* pneumonia whose thoracic ultrasound findings were normal. However, failure to perform such testing introduces a bias that is an important limitation. One solution to this problem is conducting thorough follow-up: If the clinical outcome of interest is clinical signs of pneumonia, the foals not tested with the reference standard could be monitored throughout the period when signs are most likely to develop (e.g., until weaning or until the subject goes to the yearling sale); documenting the absence of clinical signs in foals that did not have tracheobronchial aspirates would minimize the limitation of differential ascertainment of the reference standard based on the results of the test being evaluated.

It is important that the diagnostic test and the reference standard be assessed independently. Caution is urged in evaluating results of studies in which the reference standard relies on expert opinion, such as the interpretation of biopsy results. It is best that the results of the diagnostic tests be unknown to those conducting the reference standard (and vice versa). Thus studies in which the same individuals are performing both tests should be regarded with suspicion. This is particularly important when either test has subjective levels for categorizing results (e.g., absent, mild, moderate, or severe; or negative, weak positive, moderate positive, strong positive).

It bears remembering that a good understanding of the principles of sensitivity, specificity, predictive values (positive and negative), and likelihood ratios (positive and negative) is essential in the interpretation of test results. If the study design is valid, it is necessary to ensure that the test can accurately distinguish patients with and without the disease. Although review of these topics is beyond the scope of this discussion, they are considered in the previous edition of this text and elsewhere.[3,10]

Therapeutic Studies From the standpoint of individual studies, the reference standard for treatment evaluation is the RCT.[1,3,6] However, just because a study is an RCT does not mean that the results of the study should be accepted as valid. As with other designs, RCTs are subject to biases. Individual RCTs should be evaluated for validity by answering each of the questions posed in Box 8-2. The importance of randomization has already been discussed. Ideally, the randomization

BOX 8-2

CRITERIA FOR EVALUATING RANDOMIZED CLINICAL TRIALS

1. Was treatment assignment randomized?
2. Was randomization concealed?
3. Were the groups similar at baseline?
4. Was follow-up adequate?
5. Were patients analyzed according to assigned treatment?
6. Were those involved in the study (e.g., patients, veterinarians, farm staff, hospital staff) kept blind with respect to treatment?
7. Apart from the treatment of interest, were the groups managed similarly?

procedure should be described in the materials and methods section of the report. When randomization has not been used for assignment, the trial should be interpreted with greater caution. If the effect of treatment in the nonrandomized trial is very large and compelling, results are unlikely to be invalid. When nonrandomized trials reveal absence of effect or harm, it also may be reasonable to accept the study conclusions, because false-negative results from nonrandomized studies are uncommon.

Ideally, allocation of treatment should be concealed from those managing and evaluating patients. Doing so makes it less possible that those assigning treatments might consciously or unconsciously distort the balance of treatment groups. The bias introduced by failing to conceal randomization cannot be predicted a priori: It may result in the treatment appearing more or less effective than it truly is. Although randomization should render treatment groups very similar at the onset of the study, it is possible that, due to chance alone, factors will be unequally distributed among groups. Thus it is important to examine the extent to which the study groups are similar at the time the study is initiated. If the groups differ for putative or known risk factors for the disease of interest, it will be important to ensure that efforts to account for confounding for these factors have been demonstrated.

Evaluation of the extent to which patients were followed is important. The proportion of patients lost to follow-up should be small because these patients may have had outcomes that would have influenced the results of the study. For example, if patients are withdrawn from the study preferentially from the group receiving the treatment of interest because that treatment caused adverse effects, the apparent efficacy of the treatment may be overstated. Although there is no magic number, studies in which more than 20% of patients are lost to follow-up should be viewed with caution. One approach to assessing the impact of losses to follow-up is to perform a sensitivity analysis in which each lost patient is assigned the worst possible outcome (e.g., developed the disease of interest); if the results of analysis are not significantly altered in magnitude or statistical significance of the association by this approach, the results are likely valid. When losses exceed 20%, results of the described type of sensitivity analysis to yield agreement cannot be expected to agree with the original results.

It is also important to assess that the duration of follow-up was adequately long for the disease process of interest. For example, a 4-week follow-up period may be inadequate for a study to evaluate the response to treatment for equine pleuropneumonia. It also is important to determine that follow-up is administered similarly to all patients regardless of treatment group and that all patients are monitored similarly irrespective of treatment group assignment. Failure to account for these factors can introduce information biases that may affect study results.

After random assignment events may occur unrelated to treatment that can affect the likelihood that a patient develops the disease of interest. Thus it is imperative that patients be considered in analysis according to the group to which they were assigned (even if it is known that the patient was inadvertently assigned another treatment or failed to take the assigned treatment). To many this approach seems overly conservative, if not illogical. The rationale for this process of analysis by assignment (intention to treat) is that patients that get crossed over to another treatment group or that do not take their treatments may possess characteristics such that the remaining members of their assigned group may no longer be comparable to the other group (or groups) as determined at the time of random assignment.

The term *blinding* refers to awareness of treatment assignment. To avoid biased interpreting and reporting, those administering treatment and monitoring patients must be unaware of which treatment is being given to each patient. This is particularly important when the outcome being assessed is subjective, such as a severity score or owner satisfaction. When blinding has not occurred among those administering the treatment, the study should be evaluated to determine if those assessing the outcome were blinded to treatment status (e.g., a farm-based study comparing two treatments for *R. equi* pneumonia wherein the farm staff administers the drugs and is aware of treatment status, but the veterinarian evaluating the foals for evidence of disease is kept blind to the treatment status). Jargon such as "double-blinding" should be avoided when describing studies because of its ambiguity; rather, the report should specify which individuals were specifically blind to treatment.[11]

Although it is important to know whether the groups were managed similarly apart from the treatment of interest, this information may not be collected or reported. If blinding is adequate, it is to be hoped that addition of treatments has not occurred.

In an effort to improve standards for documenting results of RCTs in human medicine, an international collaborative effort produced the Consolidated Standards for Reporting Clinical Trials (CONSORT). Interested readers may wish to review these standards (www.consort-statement.org) and the associated checklist and flow diagram because they are helpful in the assessment of strengths and weaknesses of reported trials.

If the results of a clinical trial seem valid, the reader should then ask whether the magnitude of treatment effect appears clinically important. Numerous measures of strengths of effect and association exist, as described previously. One useful measure that was not considered in the previous edition is the number needed to treat (NNT). The NNT is the number of patients that need to be treated during the period of the trial to prevent one additional case of disease.[3] The NNT is calculated by determining the inverse of the absolute value of the absolute risk difference. For example, in an RCT of azithromycin for prevention of *R. equi* pneumonia, the absolute risk difference through weaning between foals that received azithromycin and those that did not was 16%, such that the estimated NNT was 6.25 (1/0.16).[12] Thus it is estimated that at least six foals would need to be treated to prevent one new case of *R. equi* pneumonia from developing from birth to weaning. The NNT should always be reported in the context of a follow-up time. Moreover, it is important to recognize that NNTs are parameters estimated from data and should have confidence intervals calculated for them (as is done for RRs, ORs, and so on). For the *R. equi* chemoprophylaxis example, the 95% confidence interval for the estimated NNT was 4 to 12; thus we are 95% confident that the true NNT for the period from birth to weaning for azithromycin was between 4 and 12. It also merits noting that the NNT usually cannot be directly estimated from a case-control study because incidence is not measured using this design.

Given that all treatments have the potential for adverse effects, it is also possible to estimate the number needed to cause harm (NNH).[3] The NNH is calculated as the inverse of the absolute value of the absolute difference in risk of harm. For example, if the absolute risk difference of diarrhea in the aforementioned azithromycin trial is 1%, the NNT is estimated to be 100 (i.e., 100 foals would have to be treated for one foal to develop diarrhea from birth through weaning as a result of treatment).

Finally, if the study results seem valid and the observed effect appears important, it is still necessary to determine the extent to which the results of the trial are relevant to a given patient. The extent to which patients studied are representative of a given patient or patients in the veterinarian's practice must be assessed by carefully reviewing which patients were included and which were excluded and by applying clinical judgment. The patients in RCTs are not always representative of the full spectrum of patients with the condition of interest, let alone from the same environment or time period. Thus practitioners may have difficulty finding evidence that directly relates to their patients.

Unfortunately, valid RCTs are rarely available for most of the treatments used in equine medicine. Consequently, veterinarians rely heavily on weaker forms of evidence. In the absence of RCTs, veterinarians should try whenever possible to use evidence from well-designed cohort studies. Except for the absence of randomization, the principles of evaluating cohort studies for treatment should be the same as those for RCTs, including assessment of validity (summarized in Box 8-2), clinical importance of effects, and the extent to which the results apply to equine patients. Case-control studies should be viewed as weaker sources of evidence for evaluating therapies because they are more subject to biases. Equine practitioners should view case series and individual case reports as no more than preliminary and particularly prone to misinterpretation with respect to treatment effects.

Prognosis Practitioners must determine whether the results of a study for prognosis were valid, clinically important, and relevant to their patients. Cohort studies are considered the best design for assessing prognosis, although the case-control design may be useful for rare diseases or disorders for which follow-up must be very long.

The representativeness of patients selected for the cohort study depends on the criteria for inclusion and exclusion and the case definitions used. It is important that patients be included relatively early in the disease process to prevent missing out on more severely affected patients that might die before being included. The way in which individuals were identified for inclusion is critical for evaluating the potential for selection bias: Were all eligible horses with the disease included? Were the horses in some way selected? If so, was the selection process unbiased?

As for clinical trials, it is important for cohort studies that the follow-up procedures are consistent among groups, that losses to follow-up are not excessive, that events of interest are not missed, and that the length of the study period is appropriate for the disease of interest. Evidence that those lost to follow-up were compared with the baseline population and that the groups appeared similar enhances the validity of a cohort study. As for RCTs, the 20% guideline may be applied. Although assessing death is relatively objective, defining the cause of death or other outcomes for prognosis (e.g., failure to return to racing, infertility) may be more subjective and less accurately determined. Thus clear definitions for objective assessments of outcomes enhance the validity of prognostic studies.

If a prognostic cohort study is valid, it will need to be assessed for importance. Data pertaining to prognosis are generally of the time-to-event variety. Thus description of the timing of events may yield clear evidence of the importance of the findings. In general, graphic representation (e.g., Kaplan-Meier curves) of data is likely to be more informative than summary statistics (e.g., the median survival time or the proportion surviving for 1 year).[3] The precision of the estimated prognosis also must be provided so that confidence in the reported results can be properly assessed. Typically, this precision would be represented as a 95% confidence interval for estimated parameters or survival curves. Finally, it is important to consider the similarity of the patients studied to the patient being treated.

Grading Evidence In human medicine efforts have been made to develop grading systems for evidence.[2,3,6] Although similar systems may be developed for veterinary medicine, the need for application of these grading systems (e.g., formulating treatment policies or formal treatment guidelines) in equine medicine is unclear and likely premature.

STEP 4: APPLYING THE RESULTS

Ideally, the results of the first three steps would render the process of applying results relatively simple. Unfortunately, the framework of EBM becomes less stable with respect to application. Part of the problem with the application of results in equine medicine is the paucity of evidence derived from patient-centered studies on which to base treatment decisions; practitioners often must resort to weaker forms of evidence. The principal problem with this step, however, is that, although the basis for the first three steps (i.e., asking questions, finding information, and applying criteria to evaluate the evidence from clinical research studies) is well-defined and in many respects recursive, specifications for the proper application of results are not well-defined operationally. Inasmuch as equine practitioners must consider their clinical impressions and expertise as well as the preferences and particular circumstances of patients and clients, the process of how to apply results requires further development. Despite this limitation, awareness of the principles of clinical epidemiology and EBM will, it is to be hoped, lead to greater emphasis on the conduct of patient-centered studies in equine medicine and in the mentoring of trainees in the design, conduct, analysis, reporting, and interpretation of such studies. At the very least, principles of EBM will force equine practitioners to recognize the limitations of the evidence on which they act and accept these limitations with appropriate measures of skepticism and humility.

STEP 5: ASSESSING THE OUTCOMES

Clinicians often think of outcome assessment in terms of the patient: Did the horse survive? Did the disease resolve as a result of treatment? Did the horse return to use? Outcome assessments, however, should also include the perceptions of horse owners. Practitioners are sometimes irritated when owners ask them to implement certain treatments, particularly unfamiliar ones. However, in the absence of strong evidence for much of what equine practitioners do, it is important to recognize that clients' preferences may be as legitimate as those of veterinarians in terms of evidence. Moreover, clients' perceptions of their interactions with the veterinarian may influence their assessment of outcome as much as objective measurements of health or disease. All these types of outcome assessments (e.g., patient health, owner perceptions), when systematically evaluated, can help practitioners determine the extent to which their efforts benefit their patients and clients. Although there are some sophisticated outcome assessment studies of the impact of EBM on selected health disorders of human beings, such objective assessment is lacking in equine medicine. However, it is not unlikely that the success of EBM in human medicine will also hold true for horses.

Limitations of Evidence-based Medicine

Although the case for EBM is compelling, it has many limitations. Of those that will be mentioned, foremost is the lack of strong evidence in the form of well-designed, rigorously conducted clinical trials and observational studies on which to base clinical decisions. There are many explanations for the paucity of EBM resources. The roots of clinical veterinary medicine have been in the discipline of animal experimentation, and application of epidemiologic principles and methods for clinical investigation remains unfamiliar and troubling to many. The incentive for the pharmaceutical industry to develop a drug or biologic for horses is limited because of the small market share that horses represent relative to other companion animals or food-producing animals. The resources for conducting large clinical trials or observational studies are limited.

The definition of *EBM* remains vague, and it seems more intention based and motivational than stipulative or operational. It is easy to define the domain of a surgeon or a theriogenologist, but can we clearly identify an EBM practitioner?[13] A problem with ill-defined terms is that, no matter how noble the concept they represent, they can be inappropriately or inaccurately invoked to render credible or persuasive any particular point or effort.

The definition of *evidence* is also vague. It is wrong to think that EBM introduced evidence to medical practice. Clinicians have always used evidence in medicine, such as that derived from clinical experience, experimental research findings, and logical extrapolations or deductions of pathologic and physiologic knowledge. In general, the term *evidence* in the phrase *EBM* refers to clinical research findings, primarily those derived from patient-based studies. Some mistakenly interpret *evidence* in EBM to mean RCTs, others the most recent report pertaining to the topic, regardless of the design. The validity of EBM is largely determined by the extent to which *evidence* itself can be defined. Similarly, what is meant by "best," with respect to available evidence, is ill-defined. Just because there is a clinical trial germane to a research topic of interest does not mean that it is the best source of information: RCTs can have important deficiencies in terms of design and analysis (internal validity) or relevance to other populations of horses (external validity). Similarly, there can be sufficient evidence in the absence of clinical trials. A comical example was reported in the *British Medical Journal* in 2003: The authors identified the absence of RCTs to document the effectiveness of parachutes in preventing injuries during free fall from airplanes.[14] They concluded that RCTs of parachutes were needed to meet the criteria of some EBM adherents, and they proposed that these EBM proponents be recruited as participants for the trial. Although the report was intended to be humorous, the point that other sources of evidence than RCTs are valid bases for making clinical decisions is serious and important (and particularly relevant to equine medicine).[15]

Another limitation is that the process of EBM requires incorporating clinical experience and expertise, the expectations of clients, and the particular circumstances of each patient into the decision-making process.[13] However, no clear operational framework exists that explains how to accomplish this. EBM is compelling with respect to intent, but practitioners do not have much guidance in applying its findings.

Another limitation of EBM is that, although the principles are logical and commendable, it is impossible to know whether the approach will make any difference. Clinical trials comparing use of EBM with not using EBM for patient management are lacking. From the standpoint of outcome assessment, EBM is as much a system based on belief and credence as are other approaches that rely on credence of perceptions and authority of expert opinion.

CONCLUSION

The discipline of EBM developed as an extension of principles of clinical epidemiology during the early 1990s, and awareness of and interest in the application of EBM to equine medicine have grown in recent years. This chapter was intended to introduce the principles and techniques of EBM and to consider its limitations, with an emphasis on possible applications to equine medicine. The principal advantages of EBM for equine internal medicine appear to be twofold. First, the approach forces practitioners to question the basis for what they do at all steps in case management and thus to think more carefully about what they know or believe they know. Second, awareness of EBM has helped move practitioners away from the traditional approach of using their understanding of disease mechanisms in conjunction with their experiences, the opinions of experts, and logical deductions or extrapolations for basing their clinical decisions and toward an approach that relies more heavily on information derived from clinical research involving patients (but *not* experimental animals). Patient-based (epidemiologic) studies, even RCTs, are prone to biases. The paucity of systematic reviews and meta-analyses addressing most clinical questions in equine medicine means that our best evidence is primarily derived from individual studies, often ones that are observational in nature. Thus all who wish to apply EBM require the ability to critically appraise these studies. In this way, placing value on EBM should lead to better-informed, more careful evaluation of evidence.

Although the framework for the first three steps of EBM is well-established, EBM has some important limitations. The last two steps (application and assessment) are not well characterized from an operational standpoint, and the ambiguity of the definitions of the terms *EBM, evidence,* and *best evidence* may lead to confusion and imprecision.

There are good and bad aspects to EBM in its current state of development. The process of applying EBM to equine medicine is like the Neurathian predicament of trying to construct a ship while already at sea. The traditions of empiricism and authority are deep and their currents strong, whereas the resources for building equine EBM are thin and often tenuous. Despite these frailties, the principle of thinking critically about medical decisions and the evidence on which these decisions are based should benefit equine medicine.

REFERENCES

1. Evidence-based Medicine Working Group: Evidence-based medicine. A new approach to teaching the practice of medicine, *J Am Med Assoc* 268:2420-2425, 1992.
2. Fisher CG, Wood KB: Introduction to and techniques of evidence-based medicine, *Spine* 32:S66-S72, 2007.
3. Straus SE, Richardson WS, Glasziou P, Haynes RB: *Evidence-based medicine*, ed 3, Edinburgh, 2005, Churchill Livingstone.
4. Habacher G, Pittler MH, Ernst E: Effectiveness of acupuncture in veterinary medicine: systematic review, *J Vet Intern* 20: 480-488, 2006.
5. McCue ME, Valberg SJ, Miller MB, et al: Glycogen synthase (GYS1) mutation causes a novel skeletal muscle glycogenosis, *Genomics* 91:458-466, 2008.
6. Guyatt G, Rennie D: *User's guide to the medical literature. Essentials of evidence-based clinical practice*, Chicago, 2002, AMA Press.
7. Smith LJ, Mellor DJ, Marr CM, et al: Incisional complications following exploratory celiotomy: does an abdominal bandage reduce the risk? *Equine Vet J* 39:277-283, 2007.
8. Rothman KJ, Greenland S: Precision and validity in epidemiologic studies, In Rothman KJ, Greenland S, editors: *Modern epidemiology*, ed 2, Philadelphia, 1998, Lippincott-Raven.
9. Toribio RE, Bain FT, Mrad DR, et al: Congenital defects in newborn foals of mares treated for equine protozoal myeloencephalitis during pregnancy, *J Am Vet Med Assoc* 212:697-701, 1998.
10. Guyatt G, Sackett D, Hanes B: Evaluating diagnostic tests, In Haynes R, Sackett D, Guyatt G, et al., editors: *Clinical epidemiology: how to do clinical practice research,* ed 3, Philadelphia, 2005, Lippincott, Williams, and Wilkins.
11. Montori VM, Bhandari M, Devereaux PJ, et al: In the dark: the reporting of blinding status in randomized controlled trials, *J Clin Epidemiol* 55:787-790, 2002.
12. Chaffin MK, Cohen ND, Martens RJ: Chemoprophylactic effects of azithromycin against *Rhodococcus equi*-induced pneumonia among foals at equine breeding farms with endemic infections, *J Am Vet Med Assoc* 232:1035-1047, 2008.
13. Jenicek M: Evidence-based medicine: fifteen years later. Golem the good, the bad, and the ugly in need of review? *Med Sci Monit* 12:RA241-RA251, 2006.
14. Smith G, Pell JP: Parachute use to prevent death and major trauma related to gravitational challenge: systematic review of randomised, controlled trials, *Br Med J* 327:1459-1461, 2003.
15. Potts M, Prata N, Walsh J: Parachute approach to evidence based medicine, *Br Med J* 333:701-703, 2006.

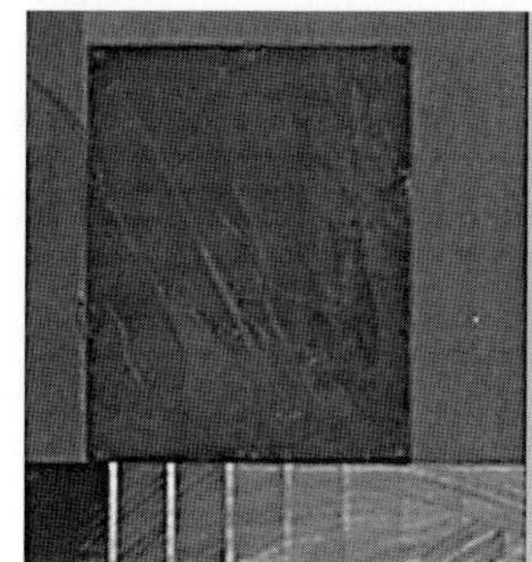

PART II

Disorders of Specific Body Systems

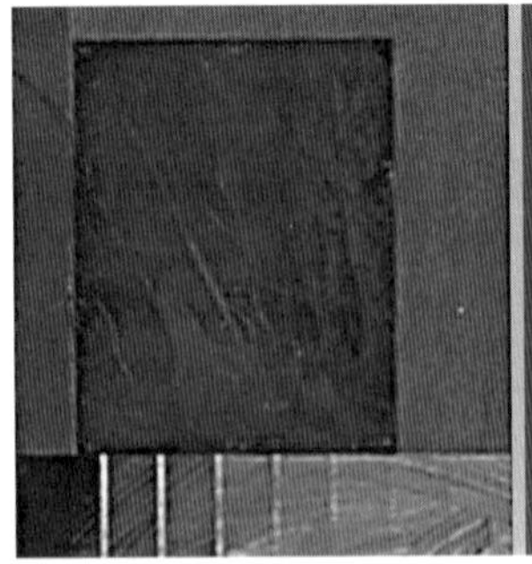

Disorders of the Respiratory System

CHAPTER 9

Dorothy M. Ainsworth, Jonathan Cheetham

Disorders of the respiratory system are second in importance only to those of the musculoskeletal system in limiting the athletic performance of the horse. Early detection and treatment of respiratory problems is essential to reduce economic losses and to prevent premature retirement of the horse from athletic performance.

DIAGNOSTIC APPROACH TO RESPIRATORY DISORDERS

History

The clinician should direct questions to the person most familiar with the performance and medical history of the horse. Accurately defining the problem, devoid of subjective impressions, can be the most difficult part of taking the history.

AGE AND BREED

The age of the animal exhibiting respiratory-related signs may provide clues as to the problem. Congenital defects (nasal septal deviations, choanal atresia, subepiglottic cysts, and hypoplastic lungs) are typically evident at birth, whereas other conditions, such as chronic bacterial pneumonia *(Rhodococcus equi),* may not be evident until the foal is 1 to 3 months of age. Viral and bacterial upper respiratory tract infections tend to occur in the weanling and yearling, whereas conditions such as inflammatory airway disease, pleuropneumonia, and exercise-induced epistaxis are found more commonly in performance horses 2 years or older. In contrast, recurrent airway disease (heaves) or neoplasia of the respiratory tract is diagnosed primarily in the middle-aged or older horse.

Breed considerations are also important in investigating respiratory disorders. For example, one should evaluate young Arabian foals with chronic infections for combined immunodeficiency syndrome, a heritable condition in which cell-mediated and humoral limbs of the immune system are deficient. In addition, solitary defects in the humoral immune system also predispose horses to develop chronic respiratory and enteric infections. Selective immunoglobulin M (IgM) deficiency tends to occur more frequently in Arabians and Quarter Horses than in other breeds, whereas agammaglobulinemia has been documented in Thoroughbreds and Standardbreds.[1,2]

ENVIRONMENT

One should ascertain the environment to which the horse was or presently is exposed. For example, is the horse stabled at a racetrack where population turnover is high and the potential for viral respiratory outbreaks is increased, or is the horse a sole inhabitant of a small pasture, seldom exposed to other horses? Does the farm have a history of endemic infections, as often occurs with *Streptococcus equi* subsp. *equi* outbreaks? Has the horse been exposed to pastures grazed by donkeys? This, along with information regarding the diet (hay, pelleted rations, or pasture), the nature of the bedding materials (straw, peat, or shavings), and the amount of time the horse is stabled are important considerations in establishing the risk factors for some respiratory disorders such as recurrent airway obstruction or lungworm infections. One should also obtain the deworming and vaccination schedules. Young horses are at risk for developing verminous pneumonia resulting from *Parascaris equorum* migration. Nematode eggs can survive for prolonged periods on a pasture. Thus establishing whether the foal was exposed to pastures grazed by yearlings or 2 year olds may help in establishing the diagnosis and treating the problems. If the horse is a performance animal and is at an increased risk for developing upper respiratory tract infections, one should determine how frequently equine influenza and equine herpesvirus type 1 (EHV1) and type 4 (EHV4) vaccinations are administered.

PRIOR MEDICAL PROBLEMS

Does the horse have a history of illness or trauma that might be related to the present complaint? Viral respiratory conditions often precede the development of bacterial pneumonia. Sequelae to *S. equi* subsp. *equi* infections include internal abscessation, guttural pouch empyema, retropharyngeal abscesses, and purpura hemorrhagica, which may ultimately affect the respiratory, cardiovascular, and gastrointestinal systems. Trauma may be implicated in the development of diaphragmatic herniae, pneumothorax, or tracheal injury and subsequent stricture formation.

PRESENT MEDICAL PROBLEM

Questions should be focused on defining the exact problem, establishing the chronicity of the disorder and the rapidity of its development. Is the problem insidious in onset or an acute disorder of less than 2 weeks' duration? Is the onset associated with a stressful event such as racing or a prolonged van ride? Does the farm have new arrivals that have not been quarantined? One should also determine the effect of the respiratory complaint on the expected athletic performance: Are clinical signs evident during eupneic (resting) breathing, or are they noticeable only during the hyperpnea of exercise? Has the horse received any medication, and did the clinical condition improve? Amelioration of signs during therapy suggests that the previous treatment protocols were not of sufficient duration or that an underlying immunodeficiency exists.

Physical Examination

Before physically examining the horse, it is helpful to simply step back and observe the demeanor and mental status (alert or depressed), posture, and manner of movement of the horse. Has the horse adopted a particular stance (extended head and neck), or is it reluctant to move because of pain (pleurodynia)? Are changes in the pattern of breathing from the normal eupneic state obvious (Box 9-1)? Is the breathing pattern rapid and shallow? Does nostril flaring accompany a pronounced expiratory effort? The normal respiratory rate of the adult horse varies from 8 to 15 breaths per minute, with a slightly noticeable abdominal component during expiration (an active process in the horse).

Abnormalities of the respiratory system are evident also by the production of unusual sounds associated with respiration; the presence of a cough; a nasal or ocular discharge; lymphadenopathy; epistaxis; facial, pharyngeal, or cervical swellings; and discolored mucous membranes. Ataxia or reluctance to move, the presence of ventral thoracic or limb edema, halitosis, and weight loss may occur with respiratory disorders.

During the physical examination, the clinician should assess the airflow from both nostrils to rule out potential masses that are obstructing the nasal cavity. This assessment is a very important and easily overlooked step of the physical examination. One can detect atheromata, which may restrict airflow during exercise, by palpating the false nostrils. Any peculiar breath odors are detectable at this time.

Percussion of the frontal and maxillary sinuses, performed by gently tapping over the sinuses while one holds the mouth of the horse slightly open, may reveal a dullness because of accumulations of fluid or inflammatory products. The absence of a percussible change does not rule out a sinus disorder. One also should assess evidence of swelling in the submandibular space (lymphadenopathy) or in the pharyngeal (guttural pouch or retropharyngeal disorders) and cervical areas (presence of accessory lungs).[3] Palpation of the laryngeal cartilages is important. Notably, the palpation of a more prominent muscular process of the arytenoid cartilage, caused by dorsal cricoarytenoid muscle atrophy, is subjective and may not be a good predictor of the presence of recurrent laryngeal neuropathy (RLN). A surgical scar can be detected by picking up and rolling the skin at the potential surgical site between the thumb and index finger. These sites include the dorsal lateral larynx (laryngoplasty), the intermandibular space in the midline and level with the vertical rami of the mandibles (laryngeal tie-forward) and cricothyroid notch (arytenoidectomy, vocal cordectomy). Any disparity in the angle of the lashes of the upper eyelids should also be noted. Vertical eyelashes and eyelid drooping in one eye (ptosis as a result of Horner's syndrome) suggest dysfunction of Müller muscle caused by damage of the vagosympathetic trunk.[4,5] Tracheal palpation is routine and should not elicit coughing episodes in the normal horse. The patency of the jugular veins should also be checked. Any evidence of perivascular injections that may contribute to upper respiratory tract obstructions by involving the recurrent laryngeal nerve or vagosympathetic trunks should be noted.

The clinician then should conduct a complete physical examination, paying attention to all organ systems (not simply focusing on the respiratory system). In respiratory emergencies, one conducts an abbreviated initial examination, making certain that a patent airway is established and that the patient is stabilized until such time when a more thorough physical examination can be conducted.

BOX 9-1

BREATHING PATTERNS

Eupnea. The normal quiet and seemingly effortless breathing pattern adopted by the healthy horse at rest. Inspiration and expiration in the horse are active processes.

Tachypnea. A breathing pattern characterized by rapid frequency and shallow depth or small tidal volume.

Hyperpnea. A breathing pattern characterized by an increase in the depth and rate of breathing, as might be found during exercise.

Apnea. A time period in which no discernible respiratory effort is made and airflow has ceased. Apnea may accompany sleep-related disorders or excessive ventilation (hypocapnia-induced apnea).

Hypoventilation. A pattern of breathing that alters gas exchange sufficiently to cause hypercapnia or elevations of arterial carbon dioxide tension.

Hyperventilation. A pattern of breathing that increases alveolar ventilation and results in arterial hypocapnia.

Respiratory Distress. A breathing pattern that appears to reflect difficulty in breathing. The animal appears to be distressed, and increased work of breathing is obvious.

AUSCULTATION OF THE LUNG FIELDS

Examine the horse during eupneic and hyperpneic (by use of a rebreathing bag) breathing. Normal breath sounds are those produced by turbulent air movement through the tracheobronchial tree and vary in intensity and quality depending on the portion of the lung field auscultated. The vesicular sounds, over the middle and diaphragmatic lung lobes, are the quietest sounds; the bronchial sounds, over the trachea and the base of the lung, are the loudest.[6-8] In the normal horse, one can hear breath sounds more easily on the right side than on the left. Considerable variation exists between normal patients in the intensity of the breath sounds. For example, vesicular sounds are often barely audible during eupneic (normal) breathing in the obese patient and are perceived as soft rustling sounds. However, one may hear breath sounds easily in the thin or young animal because of less attenuation of lung sounds by the chest wall. The intensity of breath sounds also increases with increased airflow. Thus breath sounds are accentuated in febrile or excited animals or in animals hyperpneic from a variety of causes (exercise, hypoxia, pain). However, auscultatory findings do not always correlate well with the degree of alveolar ventilation.[7] For example, in horses with lung consolidation, the transmission of breath sounds from adjacent areas gives the false impression that that region is well ventilated. Breath sounds also may become more difficult to hear in cases of (1) alveolar overinflation in which the aerated tissue of the lung is a poor conduction medium of sound or (2) pneumothorax and pleural effusions in which the sound is reflected at the pleural surface (acoustic impedance).[7]

Adventitious lung sounds are abnormal sounds superimposed on the normal breath sounds and have been described as crackles or wheezes. Crackles are short, explosive, discontinuous sounds that have been likened to the sound of salt thrown in a hot frying pan or the sound of cellophane being crumpled. They are usually of low intensity and are audible during the inspiratory phase of respiration. Their production has been attributed to the sudden equalization of pressure in two compartments after airways have reopened. Crackles are often audible in horses with pneumonia, pulmonary edema, or recurrent airway obstruction. Breathing 100% oxygen also may produce crackles because the nitrogen stent maintaining alveolar distention is eliminated.[9] Crackles are also audible in horses with subcutaneous emphysema. Wheezes are musical sounds thought to arise from the vibration of airway walls or tissue masses in close contact with the airway walls and may be audible during inspiration or expiration. Wheezes may be monophonic or polyphonic, the latter indicative of multiple sites of airway obstruction. Pleuritic friction rubs have been described as sandpaper-like sounds generated by the movement of the visceral and parietal pleurae across each other. One may detect them (infrequently) in the early stages of *dry* pleuritis, before the effusive stage.

PERCUSSION OF THE THORAX

Percussion of the thorax is accomplished by evaluating the type of sounds produced as one systematically taps the intercostal spaces of the thorax using a plexor and pleximeter (foals) or a large spoon and neurologic hammer (adults). Alternatively, an Azary pleximeter that is made of horn and a metal percussion hammer with a rubber tip may be used because of its improved sound quality.[10] Aerated tissues produce a resonant sound, whereas fluid-filled structures (bowel, heart, lung abscesses, consolidated lung) produce a dull sound. One should identify the transitional site where the sound quality changes during percussion (the site is marked with a piece of tape) and then compare with the normal limits in a healthy horse. The cranial limit is the shoulder musculature, the dorsal limit is the back musculature, and the caudoventral limits are the seventeenth intercostal space at the level of the tuber coxae, the sixteenth intercostal space at the level of the tuber ischii, the thirteenth intercostal space at the mid thorax, the eleventh intercostal space at the level of the scapulohumeral articulation, and the sixth intercostal space at the olecranon.[11] Defining the caudal lung borders of the lung field by thoracic percussion, at least in healthy horses, agrees well with the more routinely used method of ultrasonography.[10] Occasionally, the gas content of the large colon on the left side or of the cecum on the right side precludes detection of the caudal lung border in the sixteenth intercostal space in some horses.[10] Thoracic percussion should not be painful; resentment by the horse may indicate pleuritis or rib fractures. A ventral dullness suggests pleural effusion, pleural thickening, lung consolidation, masses, or pericardial effusion. Occasionally, caudal borders may be expanded, suggesting alveolar overinflation, which may accompany recurrent airway disease.

ENDOSCOPY

Fiberoptic endoscopy is an essential tool for assessing the equine respiratory tract. Endoscopy is helpful in establishing (1) the origin of respiratory noises that accompany laryngeal hemiplegia, dorsal displacement of the soft palate, epiglottic entrapment, rostral displacement of the palatopharyngeal arches, arytenoid chondritis, tracheal collapse or stenosis, and pharyngeal narrowing; (2) the existence of congenital defects such as subepiglottic cysts, cleft palate, or choanal atresia; and (3) the source of exudate or hemorrhage occurring with guttural pouch mycosis or empyema, ethmoidal hematoma, pulmonary epistaxis, retropharyngeal abscessation, and chronic pulmonary disease. Endoscopy also enables one to extract foreign bodies from the tracheobronchial tree and to obtain biopsies of tissues or masses in the respiratory tract. Endoscopic visualization of exudates within the pharynx or the trachea after exercise suggests the presence of inflammatory airway disease. Endoscopy is also used to obtain tracheobronchial aspirates (guarded swabs or catheters)[12] or to perform bronchoalveolar lavage (see later discussion). Several different fiberoptic endoscope models are available, but an 11-mm (outer diameter) endoscope is usually used in adult horses, and a smaller, 7.8-mm (outer diameter) pediatric scope is recommended for foals.

Videoendoscopic examination of the upper respiratory tract during maximal treadmill exercise (12 to 14 m/s) is a routine diagnostic modality at many referral centers, allowing visualization of dynamic collapse of the upper airway structures during exercise. Several studies have described the presence of multiple sources of airway collapse at high speed, including the aryepiglottic folds, vocal cords, and arytenoid cartilages.[13-15] Frequently, an abnormality in one structure produces narrowing of the airway, making inspiratory pressures more negative and leading to collapse of other structures. In one study, more than one abnormality was identified in 49% of the horses.[15] Accurate identification and appropriate treatment of these complex cases is not possible without a treadmill examination.

SINUSCOPY

Sinuscopy entails direct examination of the interior of the paranasal sinuses using an endoscope or an arthroscope that is introduced through a small trephine opening and is useful for diagnosing or treating sinus disease.[16,17] In selected cases, sinuscopy may be a diagnostic or therapeutic alternative to flap sinusotomy. The caudal maxillary sinus can be approached at a point 2 cm rostral to the midpoint of a perpendicular line drawn from the medial canthus of the eye to the facial crest. The rostral maxillary sinus can be accessed 2 cm caudal to the midpoint of a line drawn from the rostral end of the facial crest to the infraorbital foramen. The frontoconchal sinus is accessible through a portal placed 40% of the distance of a perpendicular line drawn from 0.5 cm caudal to the medial canthus from the midline. The site affords excellent visualization of the

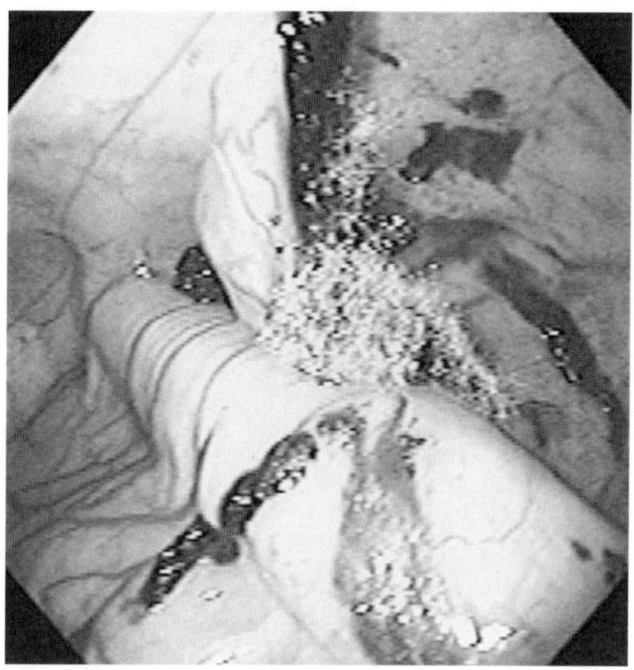

FIGURE 9-1 Sinuscopic view of the caudal maxillary sinus in 16-year-old Thoroughbred gelding with a history of epistaxis. A large fungal colony is on the infraorbital canal, and several small blood clots are visible. (Courtesy R. P. Hackett, Ithaca, N.Y., 2001.)

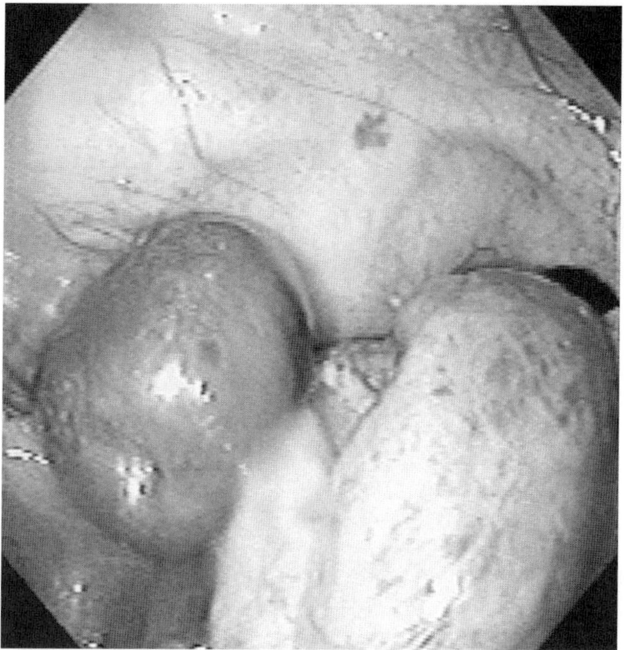

FIGURE 9-2 Sinuscopic view of small ethmoidal hematoma in 12-year-old Thoroughbred gelding. This lesion was injected with formalin transendoscopically. (Courtesy R. P. Hackett, Ithaca, N.Y., 2001.)

frontoconchal sinus and, via the large frontomaxillary opening, the caudal maxillary sinus. After sedation of the horse and surgical preparation and local anesthesia of the selected site, the clinician makes a small skin incision and opens the bone with either a 0.25-inch Steinmann pin (for a 4-mm diameter arthroscope) or a 10-mm trephine (for a 9-mm endoscope). The endoscope provides better illumination and a greater field of view. In addition to direct examination of the sinus interior for diagnosis (Figure 9-1), sinuscopy allows the examiner to biopsy tissues under direct visualization and to apply therapeutic procedures such as formalin injection of mass lesions (Figure 9-2), cyst removal, and removal of sequestered bone fragments. After the examination, the clinician may close the portal with cutaneous sutures or leave it open for therapeutic lavage.

COMPUTED TOMOGRAPHY

Interpretation of conventional radiographs of the equine head is notoriously difficult because of the complex anatomy and the spectrum of radiographic densities: air, soft tissue, bone, and tooth. Radiographs and clinical examination may not define accurately the location and extent of lesions in the head region, necessitating computed tomographic (CT) scans.[18] CT uses a rotating, highly columnated x-ray beam to generate digital cross-sectional images.[19,20] These cross-sectional images afford a much better evaluation of normal and pathologic anatomy than can be achieved through conventional radiographs (Figures 9-3 to 9-5). Additionally, the digital format enables three-dimensional reconstruction of structures and manipulation of images to optimize interpretation (see Figure 9-4). Constraints for this technique are its expense and limited availability and the need for general anesthesia of the horse.

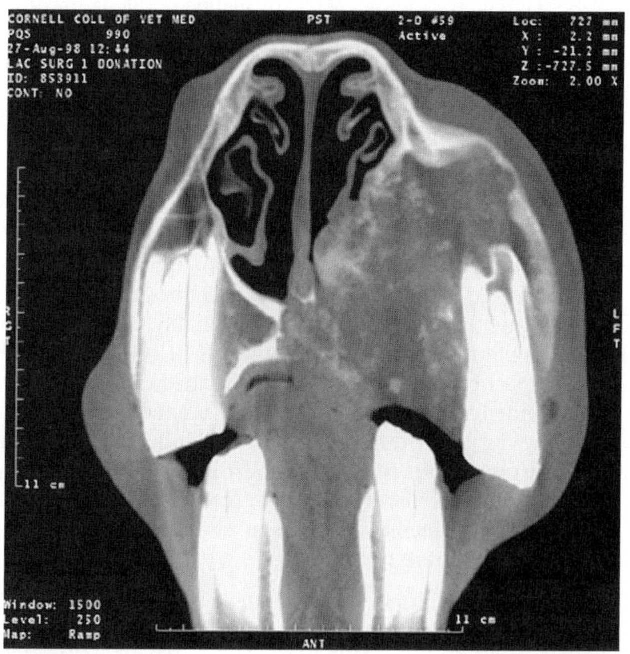

FIGURE 9-3 Cross-sectional image of an amelioblastoma involving the upper left premolars of a 4-year-old Warmblood gelding. A large soft tissue mass is encroaching on the nasal passages, and significant osseous destruction of the hard palate, ventral concha, and premaxilla is visible. (Courtesy R. P. Hackett, Ithaca, New York, 2001.)

Computed tomography has proved particularly useful for examining the anatomically complicated structures of nasal turbinates, paranasal sinuses, teeth, nasopharynx, and guttural pouches and for evaluating areas obscured by overlap of adjacent structures on conventional radiographs.[18,21-25] CT

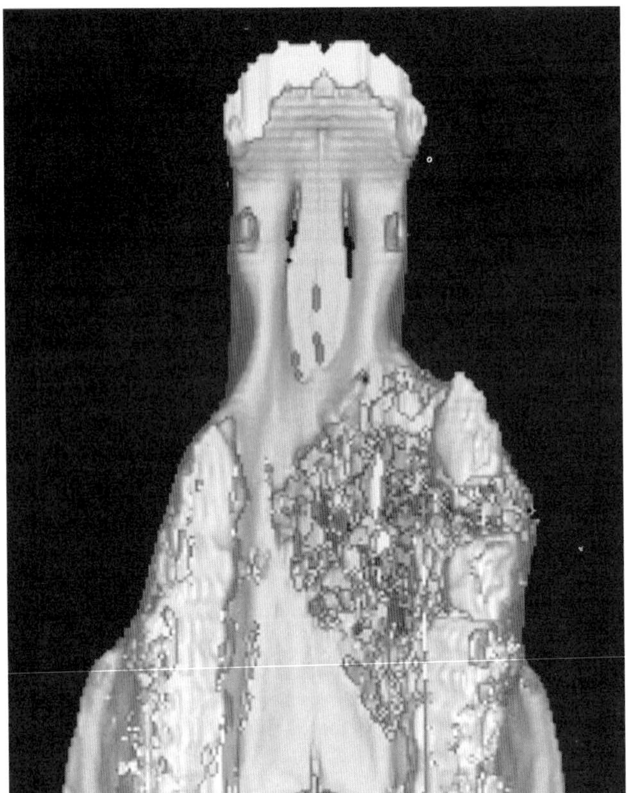

FIGURE 9-4 Three-dimensional reconstruction of the premaxilla in Figure 9-3. The extent of osseous destruction of the hard palate can be delineated clearly, as can separation of the second and third premolars. (Courtesy R. P. Hackett, Ithaca, N.Y., 2001.)

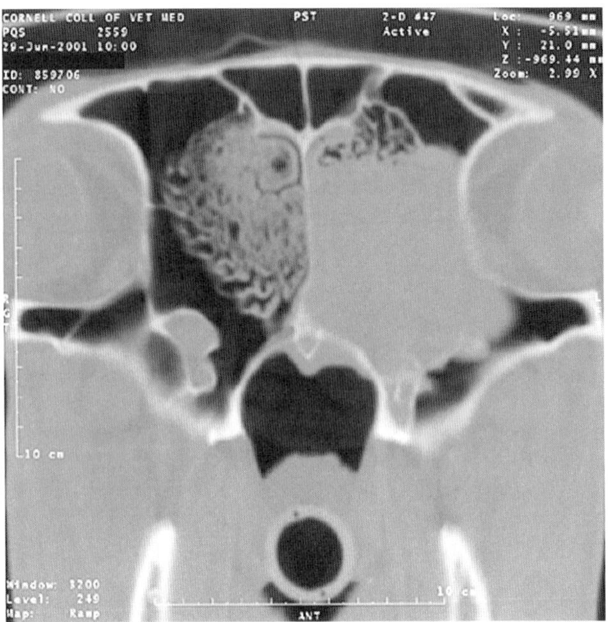

FIGURE 9-5 Cross-sectional image of an adenocarcinoma affecting the ethmoid turbinate in a 23-year-old hinny. (Courtesy R. P. Hackett, Ithaca, N.Y., 2001.)

is better than plain radiography for the diagnosis of dental disease caused by inherent avoidance of superimposition of the opposite dental arcade, excellent bone density characterization, and good spatial resolution.[26] Improved evaluation of these structures has enhanced considerably the clinician's ability to determine an accurate diagnosis, select optimal surgical approaches, and render an appropriate prognosis.

Computed tomography has been of limited usefulness in evaluating the lower respiratory tract in adult horses because of the size constraints of the gantry. However, CT is an excellent diagnostic modality for detecting and defining the extent of pulmonary or mediastinal masses in the thorax of foals, ponies, and miniature horses.[27]

MAGNETIC RESONANCE IMAGING

Magnetic resonance imaging (MRI) is another modality that can be used to investigate upper respiratory tract disorders. Magnetic resonance images represent a map of tissue protons that, under the influence of a magnetic field, are excited by brief pulses of radiofrequency waves.[19] As the magnetized excited protons relax back to their original magnetized state, a signal is emitted, the intensity of which is converted to a gray-scale image. MRI provides excellent cross-sectional evaluations of soft tissue structures, although it also provides useful information about bony structures. Contrast enhancement can be achieved by injecting an intravenous derivative of gadolinium during the T1-weighted scans.[19] Magnetic resonance images of the equine sinuses and nasal passages have been previously described,[28] although these images were obtained from cadaver heads. More recently, a detailed MRI study of horses with neurologic signs localized to the cerebrum, brainstem, or both was published demonstrating that equine skull structures can be imaged.[29] The authors note that compared with MRI in small animals, this imaging technique requires additional modifications with respect to the use of the contrast agent (gadolinium-diethylene triamine pentaacetic acid dose) and the scanning room, which must accommodate an anesthetized horse positioned on a nonmetallic support table. Because of equipment size constraints, MRI would likely be used only to evaluate thoracic structures in foals or miniature horses.

SAMPLING OF RESPIRATORY TRACT SECRETIONS

Centesis of the Paranasal Sinuses The clinician should perform centesis of the paranasal sinuses when radiographic or CT examination reveals fluid lines or soft tissue densities in the sinuses. In the sedated horse, the technique is performed aseptically using a Steinmann pin that has been advanced through a site that has been infiltrated with local anesthesia. One enters the rostral maxillary sinus at a site 2.5 cm dorsal to the facial crest and 2.5 cm caudal to the infraorbital foramen. One enters the caudal maxillary sinus, which communicates with the frontal sinus, at a site 2.5 cm dorsal to the facial crest and 2.5 cm rostral to the medial canthus. The clinician should submit aspirates for cytologic examination and bacterial culture.

Guttural Pouch Catheterization and Culture of the Exudate One performs guttural pouch catheterization in cases of empyema, chondroids, or distention of the pouches or in suspected cases of *S. equi* subsp. *equi* infections. With the horse sedated, the clinician passes a fiberoptic endoscope into the guttural pouch using the biopsy instrument or a Chambers catheter as a guide for the endoscope. One obtains a sample of the exudate with a triple-guarded catheter or protected swab. A technique for obtaining percutaneous aspirates of the guttural pouches recently has been described, but the authors prefer to use endoscopic visualization for sample collection.[30] Cytologic examination of guttural pouch aspirates from normal horses demonstrates the presence of mucus, a predominance of ciliated columnar epithelial cells, neutrophils, and a few (<1%) macrophages, lymphocytes, and eosinophils. Aspirates are not normally sterile; common bacterial isolates include β-hemolytic *Streptococcus, Staphylococcus,* and *Moraxella* species.[31] *S. equi* subsp. *equi* is not a normal inhabitant of the guttural pouch.

In horses suspected of having guttural pouch epistaxis, one should exercise caution regarding catheterization or endoscopic examination of the pouch. The procedure may dislodge a blood clot and cause fatal hemorrhage.

Sampling of Tracheobronchial Secretions Several techniques have been advocated for obtaining tracheobronchial samples. The choice of site for sample collection (tracheal versus bronchoalveolar) depends on the nature of the respiratory disorder. The appropriateness of using tracheal samples to evaluate chronic inflammatory disorders has been challenged because little correlation exists between tracheal and bronchoalveolar lavage cytologic findings or between tracheal and pulmonary histopathologic findings.[32,33] In contrast, a good correlation exists between bronchoalveolar lavage cytologic findings and pulmonary histopathologic findings.[34]

Tracheobronchial aspirates remain the method of choice for the investigation of infectious lower respiratory tract disorders. Collection of culture samples by fiberoptic endoscopy simplifies the procedure and eliminates some of the complications formerly associated with the transtracheal technique, such as cellulitis and pneumomediastinum. Guarded tracheal swabs[35] and the telescoping plugged catheter of Darien[12] are convenient techniques for obtaining representative samples. However, oropharyngeal contamination may still occur when one obtains tracheobronchial aspirates endoscopically using telescoping plugged catheters.[36,37] The authors prefer to obtain tracheobronchial aspirates percutaneously.

Characterization of the normal bacterial isolates from tracheobronchial aspirates in healthy horses has been well documented. When examining a horse with suspected respiratory disease, one must evaluate culture results in light of the cytologic findings and clinical examination. The tracheobronchial aspirates of approximately 8% of normal horses (pastured or stabled) were found to be culture positive for *Klebsiella,* β-hemolytic streptococci, *Pasteurella* species, and *Pseudomonas aeruginosa.* For a microorganism to be implicated in a lower airway disorder, one would expect (1) to obtain a moderate to heavy growth of the organism on culture ($\geq 1 \times 10^3$ colony-forming units), (2) to identify organisms within phagocytic cells, and (3) to have evidence of degenerative neutrophils. In contrast, anaerobes, which are a normal component of the oropharyngeal flora, are normally not isolated from aspirates of healthy horses, emphasizing their importance in disease processes when recovered from respiratory cases. Based on their studies, Sweeney, Beech, and Roby[38] also have described a group of transient bacterial flora of questionable pathogenicity such as *Enterobacter, Bacillus, Acinetobacter,* β-hemolytic streptococci (except for *Streptococcus pneumoniae* type 3), and *Staphylococcus epidermidis,* which may be isolated from tracheobronchial aspirates. In contrast, *S. pneumoniae* is now recognized as a pathogen of the respiratory tract in horses.[39-41] Fungal hyphae may be found free or engulfed within mononuclear cells in normal horses.

Bronchoalveolar Lavage This procedure is indicated in the investigation of chronic inflammatory diseases but may be performed with collection of transtracheal aspirates if one cannot dismiss an infectious process. Table 9-1 shows representative cytologic findings from bronchoalveolar lavage studies of normal horses. Before performing the bronchoalveolar lavage, the horse is sedated. Either a fiberoptic endoscope, which permits direct visualization of the lung segment to be lavaged, or a thick-walled flexible tube with a cuffed end, which is passed blindly into the distal airways, is wedged into the distal airway. Then, 20 to 35 ml of 2% lidocaine may be infused into the airways to desensitize the lung segment being sampled. Approximately 60 (foal) to 300 ml (adult horse) of physiologic saline solution is instilled and then aspirated. In *healthy* horses, nearly 75% of the fluid can be retrieved for cytologic examination. This volume is more difficult to obtain in horses with airway inflammation and mucus plugs.

Radiography

This technique may be helpful (1) in detecting soft tissue masses (abscesses, granulomata, neoplasms, hematomas, polyps) or fluid accumulations within the paranasal sinuses, the nasal cavity proper, the guttural pouches, and the retropharyngeal areas and (2) in evaluating orofacial deformations or

TABLE 9-1

Differential Counts in Bronchoalveolar Lavage Fluid*

Neutrophils	Macrophages	Lymphocytes	Eosinophils	Mast Cells	Epithelial Cells
8.9 ± 1.2	45.0 ± 2.8	43.0 ± 2.7	± 1.0	1.2 ± 0.3	3.5 ± 0.7
5.0 ± 4.0	72 ± 10	18 ± 3.0	2.0 ± 4.0	1.0 ± 1.4	—
6.2 ± 5.0	70.3 ± 15.2	7.6 ± 3.9	1.0 ± 1.4	0.6 ± 1.4	14.3 ± 13.4
6.2 ± 2.4	48.5 ± 2.5	35.3 ± 2.5	2.5 ± 0.9	5.2 ± 0.8	2.3 ± 1.4

Data from Derksen FJ, Brown CM, Sonea I, et al: Comparison of transtracheal aspirate and bronchoalveolar lavage cytology in 50 horses with chronic lung disease, *Equine Vet* J 21:23, 1989; Fogarty U: Evaluation of a bronchoalveolar lavage technique, *Equine Vet J* 22:174, 1990; Mair TS, Stokes, CR, Bourne FJ: Cellular content of secretions obtained by lavage from different levels of the equine respiratory tract, *Equine Vet J* 19:458, 1987; Deegan E, Beedle RE, editors: *Lung function and respiratory diseases in the horse,* Stuttgart, Germany, 1986, Hippiatrika.

*Percent of total white blood cell count plus-or-minus standard error or standard deviation.

fractures after trauma. Radiography also allows assessment of the anatomic dimensions of the pharyngeal and laryngeal structures (thickened soft palate, hypoplastic epiglottis, hyoid bone fractures). When nasal or sinus disorders are suspected, one should take lateral, dorsoventral, and oblique views. The clinician can usually achieve proper restraint of the horse for positioning of the cassette with xylazine, detomidine, or butorphanol sedation. In the horse that can be anesthetized safely, one may obtain a more thorough definition of the extent of nasal and upper respiratory tract diseases using CT scans.

Radiographic evaluation of the equine thorax remains preferable to ultrasonography for detecting diffuse parenchymal diseases such as interstitial pneumonia, pulmonary edema, and chronic airway disorders and for detecting deep parenchymal abscesses.[42] Imaging the thorax of the standing horse requires three to four overlapping lateral radiographs. However, compared with human or small animal medicine, in which correlations between the pulmonary disorders and the radiographic findings are well established, the radiographic changes in equine respiratory disorders tend to be rather nonspecific and lack predictive value in inflammatory airway diseases.[43] In addition, many pulmonary diseases such as inflammatory airway disease, exercise-induced pulmonary hemorrhage, lungworm infections, and recurrent airway obstruction may not have detectable radiographic abnormalities.[43]

Four types of radiographic patterns have been described: alveolar (airspace), interstitial, bronchial, and vascular. In the alveolar pattern, opaque areas coalesce and completely obliterate the vessels and bronchi. Air bronchograms may be notable. This pattern occurs with pneumonia, pulmonary edema, hemorrhage, or neoplastic infiltration. Interstitial patterns are found most commonly and are associated with a variety of conditions. This pattern causes a blurring of the edges of the pulmonary vessels, a diffuse increase in lung opacity, and variable reticular, linear, or nodular opacities.[43,44] A reticular pattern occurs with viral, bacterial, or parasitic pneumonia; pulmonary edema; interstitial pneumonia; and pulmonary fibrosis. An irregular linear pattern occurs with resolving bronchopneumonia, and a nodular pattern occurs with abscesses, granulomata, or neoplasms. Bronchial patterns alone are not found commonly but usually occur in association with interstitial patterns. Paired linear opacities or numerous small circular opacities represent thickening of the large- and medium-sized airways or of the septa around the lobules. This pattern occurs in cases of equine bronchitis. Bronchiolitis is generally not recognized radiographically.[45] Variations in the size, shape, and number of the pulmonary vessels cause a vascular pattern and may be visible in horses after exercise or in horses with left-to-right cardiac shunts.

Extraparenchymal disorders that are evident radiographically include the presence of free pleural fluid or of free gas (pneumothorax) represented by the separation of the right or left or both caudal lung lobes from the dorsal and dorsolateral body wall by a free-air density. Pleural fluid is characterized by an increased opacity in the ventral lung fields.

Ultrasonography

Thoracic ultrasonography is useful for diagnostic, therapeutic, and prognostic evaluation of peripheral parenchymal lung or pleural disorders. Unlike thoracic radiography, which requires technology limited to specialty practices or veterinary medical teaching hospitals, ultrasonography is a method readily available to the practicing veterinarian. Ultrasonography is considered to be superior to thoracic radiography for detecting pleural effusion, pulmonary consolidation, pulmonary or mediastinal abscesses, tumors, or granulomata[42] and should be performed when clinical examination or thoracic percussion reveals pain and areas of dullness within the thorax.

Normal lung tissue reflects the ultrasound beam, producing an echogenic pulmonary periphery (thin white line) and reverberation artifacts or concentric equidistant echoes. Normal pleural fluid appears as an anechoic (black) area separating the parietal pleura from the lung tissue, and one commonly detects a small amount of pleural fluid in the ventral thorax of racehorses.[46] In respiratory disorders, one may detect accentuated amounts of anechoic or hypoechoic (gray) pleural fluid. The clinician can determine the character of the pleural fluid, the presence of fibrin or gas, the degree of loculation, and the existence of pleural adhesions during the examination. Pulmonary abscesses appear on ultrasonography as encapsulated cavitated areas filled with fluid or echogenic (white) material, whereas areas of pulmonary consolidation appear as dense patterns of homogeneous internal echoes with a gray tone.[47] Depending on the degree of consolidation, one may visualize bronchial and vascular structures more easily on the sonogram, as well as mediastinal masses. Detection of caudal mediastinal masses improves when pleural effusion is concurrent, because the aerated caudal lungs impair examination. One may visualize masses located in the cranial mediastinum at the third right intercostal space in the absence of pleural effusions.

Diagnostically, certain limitations are inherent in ultrasonography. One may not detect a deep parenchymal lesion if the overlying aerated lung reflects the ultrasound beam. In addition, cases of pneumothorax may be difficult to identify because the free air in the dorsal thorax and the aerated ventral lung appear similar with ultrasound.[42] One also may use ultrasonography prognostically. The detection of free gas echoes (associated with anaerobic bacterial infections or bronchopleural fistulae), extensive fibrinous tags, or areas of loculations within the pleural fluid are associated with a poor prognosis, requiring a more extensive therapeutic regimen.[48]

Thoracocentesis

Sampling of the pleural fluid by means of thoracocentesis is beneficial for diagnostic, prognostic, and therapeutic purposes. Abnormal pleural fluid accompanies numerous respiratory disorders, including pulmonary abscessation (pleuropneumonia), chronic pneumonia, systemic mycoses, neoplasia, pulmonary granulomata, and equine infectious anemia. One may perform the technique easily at the sixth or seventh intercostal space approximately 10 cm dorsal to the olecranon by aseptically inserting a teat cannula through an anesthetized site in the intercostal space, just cranial to the border of the rib. To reduce the amount of air aspirated into the pleural cavity, one attaches a three-way stopcock to the cannula. The clinician should take samples from both sides of the thorax and submit the aspirate for cytologic and microbiologic examination. One may obtain up to 100 ml of pleural fluid, although smaller amounts (10 to 30 ml) are more routine.[49] Normal pleural aspirates contain less than 10,000 nucleated cells per μl (60% of which are neutrophils) and less than 2.5 g/dl of protein. Samples should be cultured aerobically and anaerobically. Fluid with a putrid odor is associated with anaerobic bacteria and carries a less-favorable prognosis for the horse.[50]

Nuclear Medicine Imaging

Scintigraphy, or nuclear medicine imaging, is a specialized technique available at some university and practice facilities. Using gamma-emitting radioisotopes such as krypton-81m or technetium-99m, the clinician can assess pulmonary ventilation and perfusion in the horse.[51,52] The horse, breathing through a closed circuit, inhales aerosolized technetium particles generated by a nebulizer. Aerosolized particles are of sufficiently small diameter to be deposited in the alveoli and small airways. Thus their distribution mirrors ventilation. A gamma camera records the sites of deposition within the lung fields. For the perfusion scan, one injects technetium-labeled macroaggregated albumin intravenously. The large protein particles lodge in the blood capillaries of the lung, enabling imaging of the pulmonary perfusion by the gamma camera. Hence lung scintigraphy permits evaluation of the ratio of regional ventilation to perfusion ($\dot{V}/\dot{Q}$) not possible by radiography or ultrasonography. Scintigraphic images may provide additional insights into the diagnosis and pathogenesis of such disorders as recurrent airway obstruction or exercise-induced pulmonary hemorrhage (EIPH) or in the evaluation of the horse with poor performance.[53,54] For example, horses with EIPH appear to have a perfusion deficit in the caudodorsal lung lobe that results in a high ($\dot{V}/\dot{Q}$) area.[53] Horses with recurrent airway obstruction may produce several patterns, including ($\dot{V}/\dot{Q}$) deficits in the costophrenic angle (caudoventral diaphragmatic margin), ventilation deficits in the mid dorsal lung area, or patterns similar to those seen in EIPH.[55]

In addition to assessment of pulmonary ventilation and perfusion, scintigraphy can show tracheal mucus transport after intratracheal injection of technetium. One performs the technique by timing the movement of the radioactive bolus over a given tracheal distance.[56,57] Normal values for the unsedated horse range between 16.6 to 20.7 mm/min. Further studies are needed to examine alterations in tracheal mucus transport during disease. For further information, the reader is referred to additional reviews.[56] Nuclear scintigraphy is not more useful than radiographs for the assessment of sinus disorders.[58]

Pulmonary Function Testing

Measurements of mechanical properties of the respiratory system, airway hyperreactivities, and arterial blood gas determinations have been used to assess the lower respiratory tract in horses and are generally available only at specialized pulmonary units associated with referral centers. The conventional techniques of pulmonary function testing require that (1) the horse wear a breathing apparatus to which an airflow meter has been attached and that (2) pleural pressure changes are measured by a catheter placed in the mid-esophagus, exteriorized through the nares, and attached to a pressure transducer. By integrating airflow relative to time, one obtains the inspiratory and expiratory volumes. Additional parameters obtained from measurements of airflow include inspiratory and expiratory times, breathing frequency, and peak airflows. In general, the simple measurement of tidal volume, breathing frequency, or minute volume (the product of tidal volume and breathing frequency) provides limited information regarding the functionality of the lung because these values tend to be maintained near normal limits until respiratory disease is advanced.[59]

Measures of lung distensibility (dynamic compliance) and airway obstruction (pulmonary resistance) provide meaningful information regarding pulmonary health. One measures dynamic compliance (C_{dyn}) by dividing the tidal volume by the change in pleural pressure occurring between the start and end of inhalation. One measures pulmonary resistance by several different techniques, depending on whether one measures the resistance at peak airflow or at specific ventilatory volumes (e.g., 50% tidal volume), and calculates it by dividing airflow by the change in pleural (esophageal) pressure. Alterations in these two values can provide information on the nature of the lung disorder. For example, in obstructive disorders of the tracheobronchial tree, dynamic compliance decreases and pulmonary resistance increases. A decrease in dynamic compliance in the absence of a change in pulmonary resistance suggests that the lung parenchyma has been stiffened by alveolar disease or by obstruction of the peripheral bronchioles. (Recall that peripheral bronchioles, because of their immense cross-sectional area, contribute little to the resistance of breathing until the disorder is well advanced.) Conversely, an increase in pulmonary resistance in the absence of a change in dynamic compliance suggests that the obstruction exists in the upper airway, trachea, or bronchus.[60]

An alternative and less-invasive technique for measuring pulmonary function uses the forced-oscillation method (or its modification, the impulse-oscillation method). While the horse wears an airtight facemask, an external test signal is imposed on the horse's breathing efforts that generate pressure-flow responses from the respiratory system. The mechanical properties derived from this technique over a wide range of frequencies (other than that of the horse's own breathing frequency) include total respiratory system impedance (Z_{rs}), respiratory system resistance (R_{rs}) and respiratory system reactance (X_{rs}).[61,62] The impedance represents the *impediment* that the system presents to oscillatory flow and consists of R_{rs} (resistive properties of the respiratory system) and X_{rs} (elastic and inertive properties of the respiratory system).

Measures of airway hyperreactivity are often obtained in conjunction with pulmonary function testing.[63-66] In this technique, one determines the dose of a nebulized bronchoconstrictor agent, such as histamine or methacholine, that causes a 35% increase in baseline R_{rs} or a 35% decrease in baseline lung compliance. As might be predicted, the dose to achieve this value in a horse with inflammatory airway disease or recurrent airway disease is much smaller than that needed to achieve a similar effect in a healthy horse. Measurement of airway hyperreactivity requires that the horse be sedated and outfitted with an airtight breathing mask. Laboratory assistants should wear protective masks to prevent inhalation of the bronchoconstrictor agent.

Pulmonary function testing of exercising horses and its use in assessing the poor performer is a new diagnostic approach offered at select referral centers. With the availability of high-speed treadmills and the ability to measure airflow during exercise,[67] analysis of tidal volume, breathing frequency, dynamic compliance, lung resistance, end-expiratory lung volume, and flow-volume and pressure-volume loops may provide additional insights into the cause of the poor performance, the recognition of expiratory flow limitation, and the documentation of EIPH on respiratory mechanics.

Lung Biopsy

A histopathologic diagnosis may prove useful in the therapeutic management of certain lung disorders. Percutaneous lung biopsy has been used to investigate (1) disorders characterized radiographically by a pulmonary miliary pattern and (2) disorders for which radiographic or ultrasonographic results are compatible with pulmonary neoplasia or granuloma.[68] Raphel and Gunson originally described the methods used,[69] which has since been modified because of the routine use of ultrasound during tissue sampling. The horse is sedated and biopsy locations are selected after ultrasonographic confirmation of landmarks (heart, diaphragm) and assessment of tissue accessibility. The biopsy instrument is aseptically advanced through the intercostal space (cranial to the rib) to the depth of the desired tissues, and samples are obtained for culture and for fixation in 10% formalin. In a study comparing biopsy instruments (manual Tru-cut versus automated biopsy needle), the investigators found airway bleeding developed in approximately one third of the cases sampled with the manual device and one tenth of the cases biopsied using the automated instrument.[70] The technique is not recommended in patients that are tachypneic, are in respiratory distress, exhibit uncontrollable coughing, or have bleeding disorders. The technique is not indicated in horses with pulmonary abscessation, pleuropneumonia, or pneumonia.[68] In a recent review of percutaneous lung biopsies performed in 66 horses, this technique yielded a definitive antemortem histologic diagnosis of pulmonary disease in 82% of cases.[71] In the same study, no complications were recognized in 91% of horses sampled.[71] The most common complications observed with lung biopsy are coughing, epistaxis, pulmonary hemorrhage, tachypnea, and respiratory distress. Hemothorax or accidental sampling of abdominal organs (liver, stomach) may occur.[70-72] When horses in respiratory distress are sampled using an automated instrument, epistaxis occurred in 13%, airway bleeding in 39%, and pneumothorax in 4% of patients.[70]

Thoracoscopy

Thoracoscopy or pleuroscopy is a diagnostic technique that is used in the standing sedated horse to visualize the intrathoracic structures that include the aorta, esophagus, intercostal vessels, sympathetic trunk, vagus nerves, lymph nodes, mainstem bronchi, pulmonary and azygous veins (right hemithorax), diaphragm, and dorsal and lateral surfaces of the lungs. The procedure is used to sample thoracic masses or nodules, to transect pleural adhesions, to place drains for the treatment of pleural abscesses, to repair diaphragmatic hernias, and to resect lung segments either for therapeutic or for diagnostic purposes.[73-77] Using thoracoscopy, one is able to obtain larger biopsy sizes and hence assess parenchymal and peripheral airway morphologic features better.[78]

Thoracoscopy is performed using aseptic procedures. An area in the eighth to twelfth intercostal space just ventral to the serratus dorsalis muscle is surgically scrubbed and infiltrated with local anesthetic to place an endoscopic portal.[79] Before insertion of the endoscopic portal (cannula), a pneumothorax is gradually created by inserting a teat cannula first through this intercostal space. The smaller cannula is replaced by a larger one through which a 10-mm (30-degree) rigid laparoscope connected to a video camera and light source can be advanced. Additional portals for biopsy or resection procedures are aseptically placed as needed. In most adult horses, the mediastinum is thought to be incomplete, thus a bilateral pneumothorax may ensue during this procedure. Hemodynamic effects of a unilateral thoracoscopy in healthy horses have been described.[79] In sedated healthy horses, thoracoscopy (and pneumothorax) produces a mild systemic hypertension and arterial hypoxemia. After completion of the examination or retrieval of samples or both, the pneumothorax is reduced, the lung is reinflated, and the skin is closed after removal of the laparoscope. Analgesic and antimicrobial agents should be administered to the horse after this procedure.

DISORDERS OF THE UPPER RESPIRATORY TRACT

A variety of disorders are encountered in the upper respiratory tract in horses. Presenting complaints for upper airway disorders include respiratory distress (especially during inspiration), nasal discharge, dysphagia, lymphadenopathy, swelling or pain in the throatlatch region, or decreased exercise tolerance. Endoscopic or radiographic examination of the head and upper airway facilitates a diagnosis of most upper respiratory disorders.

Sinus Disorders

SINUSITIS

Diagnosis and treatment of diseases of the paranasal sinuses are complicated by their large size, complex anatomy, difficult surgical access, and the advanced state of many diseases before a diagnosis is made.[80]

Anatomic Considerations Six pairs of sinuses communicate with the nasal cavity: dorsal, middle, and ventral conchal and maxillary, frontal, and sphenopalatine.[81] The frontal sinus has a large communication rostrally with the dorsal conchal sinus and thus forms the conchofrontal sinus. This drains through the frontomaxillary opening into the caudal maxillary sinus. The ventral conchal and rostral maxillary sinuses communicate over the infraorbital canal and drain through the nasomaxillary opening into the middle nasal meatus. The caudal maxillary sinus has a small opening medially into the middle conchal sinus. The sphenopalatine sinus drains over the infraorbital canal into the caudal maxillary sinus. In horses younger than 5 years, the last three cheek teeth—the first, second, and third molars (108-111 and 208-211)—occupy most of the maxillary sinus.[80] As the horse ages and the residual root decreases, the sinus cavity enlarges, and its rostral limit approaches the infraorbital foramen.

The sphenopalatine sinus has thin walls and a close relationship to the brain, pituitary gland, and cranial nerves II, III, IV, V, and VI.[82] The sinuses are lined by a respiratory epithelium—pseudostratified ciliated columnar—interspersed with goblet cells and underlying serous glands.[83] The nasomaxillary opening is a narrow slit that is easily occluded from inflammation of the mucosa, and this occlusion can lead to accumulation of exudate within the sinuses. Most clinically important conditions involve the maxillary or frontal sinuses.

Causes Primary sinusitis involves accumulation of exudate within the sinus cavities and is a sequela of viral or bacterial upper respiratory tract infections. Streptococcal (and rarely staphylococcal) organisms are the most frequent bacterial isolates. Secondary sinusitis is most commonly caused by dental disease or may be associated with sinus cyst, neoplasia, foreign body, or trauma.[17,84-87]

Dental sinusitis is associated with infection of the tooth root, fractured teeth, and patent infundibula.[85] The first molar is the most commonly involved tooth.[85,88,89] Sinus cysts act as a space-occupying lesion and have a variable wall that may be mineralized.[87,90,91] Neoplasia of the paranasal sinuses include squamous cell carcinoma (which, in some cases, can arise in the oral cavity and spread to the maxillary sinuses), adenocarcinoma, bone and dental tumors, fibrosarcoma, and hemangiosarcoma.[84,92] Although rare, fungal granulomata induced by *Cryptococcus neoformans* may cause secondary sinusitis.[80]

Clinical Signs Clinical signs depend on the inciting cause, location, and chronicity of the disorder. Clinical signs include nasal discharge that may be unilateral or bilateral, malodorous, or mucopurulent; reduced nasal airflow; epiphora; and facial swelling.[80,85] Sinus cysts and neoplasia are significantly more frequently associated with gross deformity of the nasal passages and facial bones than other disorders, which explains the high incidence of epiphora, reduced nasal airflow, and facial deformity in those conditions.[85] Dental sinusitis is strongly associated with malodorous nasal discharge.[80,85]

Diagnosis Diagnosis is based on the clinical history, age of the animal, and nature of the clinical signs. Percussion of the sinuses may reveal dullness. Culture and cytologic examination of the sinus fluid or biopsy of the tissue mass is helpful in the diagnosis, although differentiating between a neoplastic or dysplastic process and an inflammatory reaction may be difficult.

Endoscopic examination helps eliminate other potential causes of nasal discharge and demonstrates the presence of a discharge from the nasomaxillary opening, which confirms that the discharge originates from the sinus compartment. A thorough dental examination should be performed in all cases of suspected sinus disease. The presence of fractured or displaced teeth, receding gum lines, exudate around a specific tooth, or patent infundibula suggests that dental disease may be the cause of the disorder.

Lateral and lateral-oblique radiographs (30 to 45 degrees to the horizontal plane) are helpful in diagnosing sinusitis and may demonstrate single or multiple horizontal fluid-air interfaces, abnormalities of the teeth, lysis of alveolar bone, or any combination of these signs (Figures 9-6 and 9-7).[85,90] Dorsoventral radiographs are useful in selected cases (e.g., those with suspected empyema of the ventral conchal sinus). Strong diagnostic radiographic signs are present in approximately 57% of dental sinusitis cases.[85] In contrast, radiographs are strongly diagnostic of sinus cysts in only 35% of cases.[85] CT is the imaging diagnostic procedure of choice for diseases of the paranasal sinuses. The main advantage of CT is excellent cross-sectional imaging with no superimposition of structures.[93,94] Nuclear scintigraphy is not significantly more useful than radiographs for the assessment of sinus disorders.[58]

Treatment Treatment requires surgical removal of the primary cause (tooth, cyst, granulation tissue or neoplasia), the establishment of good drainage, and copious lavage. Nasofrontal surgical flaps provide good access to the majority of the paranasal sinuses[95,96] and can be performed in the standing horse. In the largest published case series, resolution of signs was obtained after surgery in 84% of primary sinusitis, 78% of dental sinusitis, and 93% of sinus cysts.[86] With neoplastic lesions, surgical resection or ablation achieves a low rate of success because of extensive infiltration of the neoplasm or recurrence of the tumor.[97,98]

PROGRESSIVE ETHMOIDAL HEMATOMA

Definition and Epidemiology Progressive ethmoidal hematoma (PEH) is characterized by encapsulated, expansive masses that usually arise from the submucosa of the ethmoidal labyrinth.[99,100] The mass is composed of blood and fibrous tissue, is encapsulated by respiratory epithelium,[101] and may extend into the paranasal sinuses.[99,101-103]

The condition occurs in 4% to 6% of horses with diseases of the nose and sinus.[85,100] The inciting factor in their development is not known, although they have been hypothesized to be associated with repeated episodes of submucosal

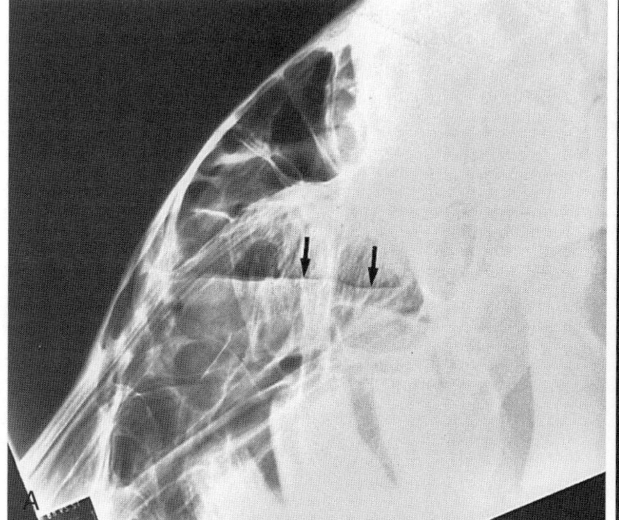

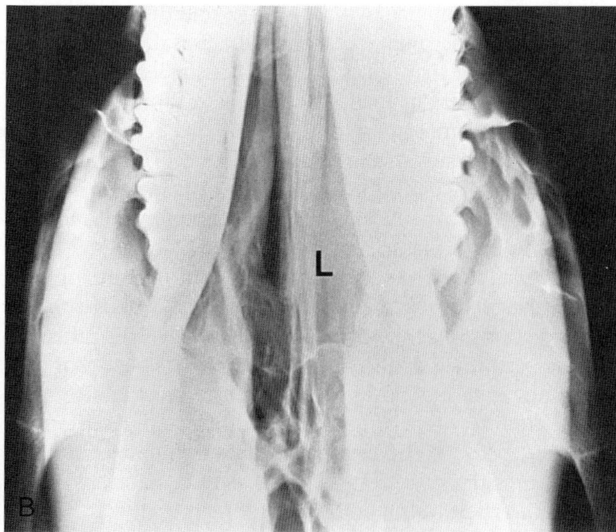

FIGURE 9-6 Five-year-old Thoroughbred with 7-month history of left-sided nasal discharge. **A,** Air-fluid interface *(arrows)* in the caudal maxillary sinus on the lateral radiograph is consistent with maxillary sinusitis resulting from dental disease. **B,** Increased soft tissue opacity in the left *(L)* maxillary sinus on the dorsoventral radiograph is notable. (Courtesy D. S. Biller, Manhattan, Kan., 1991.)

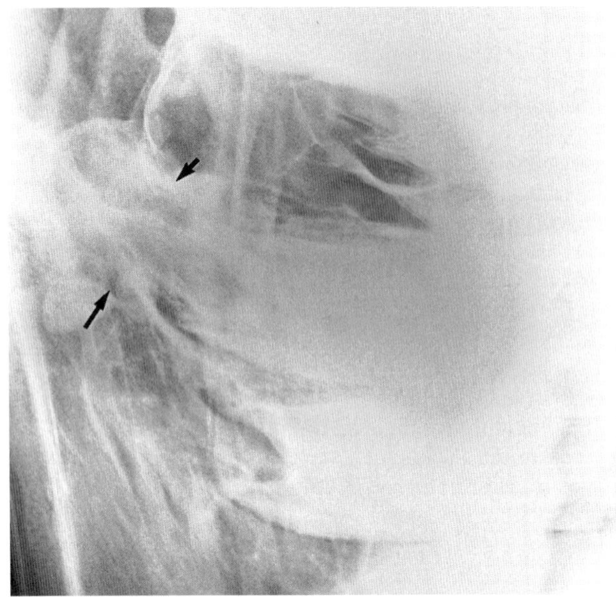

FIGURE 9-7 Lateral oblique radiograph of mid maxillary cheek teeth. The fourth cheek tooth had been removed previously. Sclerotic bony reaction *(arrows)* surrounds the root of the third cheek tooth. (Courtesy D. S. Biller, Manhattan, Kan., 1991.)

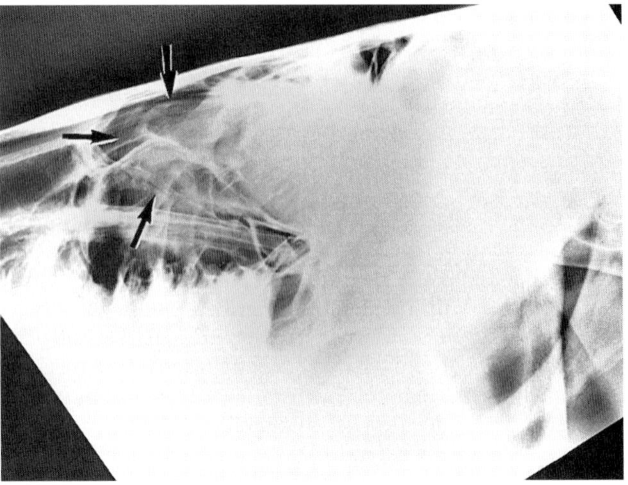

FIGURE 9-8 Ethmoidal hematoma. Focal increased soft issue opacity *(arrows)* adjacent to the ethmoids is notable. (Courtesy D. S. Biller, Manhattan, Kan., 1991.)

hemorrhage. PEH appear bilaterally in 50% of cases and are more prevalent in older horses.[103,104]

Clinical Signs The most common clinical sign caused by PEH is intermittent, serosanguineous discharge from the affected nasal passage.[101,103,105] Other clinical signs include facial swelling, halitosis, respiratory distress, and coughing.[101,103,105]

Diagnosis Diagnosis is based on the clinical signs, endoscopic examination, radiographic evaluation,[101-103,105] and, in some cases, CT findings to determine the extent of the lesion.[106] Endoscopy (see Figure 9-2) reveals a variably green-colored, smooth glistening mass originating from the ethmoid region. The mass may protrude beyond the nasal septum (and in such cases may cause a bilateral nasal discharge). Radiographs reveal a space-occupying soft tissue density with smooth margins and may demonstrate extension into the paranasal sinuses (Figure 9-8). Confirmation of the diagnosis is by histopathologic study of the removed tissue,[91,104] although the clinical appearance is highly suggestive.

Treatment Treatment options include formalin injection, surgical resection, and laser ablation. Smaller lesions (<10 cm in diameter) can be treated effectively by the intralesional injection of 4% to 10% formalin.[86,99,101,107] Most cases require multiple injections to achieve full resolution.[86,101] This procedure can be performed in the standing horse, has a low complication rate, and is associated with 60% resolution after a median of five injections.[101] Severe neurologic complications can, however, occur if the cribriform plate is fenestrated by the chronic pressure of a large PEH. CT may be indicated to determine the extent of the lesion before treatment.[107]

Surgical removal via a frontal sinus flap is associated with extensive hemorrhage and may require pre- or postoperative blood transfusions.[99,100,105] A preoperative crossmatch is warranted, and the horse may also require a postoperative tracheotomy if extensive packing of the nasal cavity is necessary to effect hemostasis. After surgical removal, approximately 20% to 50% of ethmoidal hematomas recur.[86,103-105] Postoperative complications may include facial incisional dehiscence, suture periostitis, facial bone sequestration, persistent nasal discharges, fungal sinus plaque formation, and encephalitis.[103,105] Laser excision has also been used to treat PEH, with a recurrence rate of 20% described in one report.[102] Recurrence is higher in bilateral PEH than other forms.

Guttural Pouch Disorders

ANATOMIC CONSIDERATIONS

The paired guttural pouches are diverticula of the external auditory tubes. Some investigators have suggested that the pouches play a role in cooling the arterial blood supply to the brain.[108] Each pouch has a capacity of 475 ml and is divided into medial and lateral compartments by the stylohyoid bone.[109] Each pouch fills on inspiration via the plica salpingopharyngeus. The mucosal lining of each pouch is secretory and covered by ciliated pseudostratified epithelium with goblet cells and glands.[110] The medial compartment is three times bigger than the lateral compartment and contains the internal carotid artery and a fold that encloses cranial nerves IX, XI, and XII. The pharyngeal branch of the vagus nerve (X) traverses the floor of the medial pouch, and the cranial sympathetic ganglia are also found within it. The rectus capitus ventralis and longus capitus muscle run just medially to the guttural pouch, and tearing of these muscles after a poll injury can be identified endoscopically as blood in the associated pouch. The lateral compartment of the guttural pouch contains the external carotid and maxillary artery. Branches of the facial nerve (VII), vestibulocochlear (VIII), and mandibular branch of the trigeminal nerve (V) run close to the wall of the lateral compartment.

TYMPANY

Definition Tympany is a nonpainful unilateral or bilateral distention of the guttural pouch by air that may produce an external swelling in the parotid region. Congenital tympany occurs in young foals (predominantly fillies), and acquired tympany uncommonly affects older horses.[111]

Causes The cause of congenital guttural pouch tympany is unknown. Tympany is more likely a functional defect rather than an anatomic defect because no abnormality is visible endoscopically or during surgical exploration. The condition may have a genetic component in Arabians.[112] Acquired tympany is typically associated with upper respiratory infection and is thought to be caused by swelling of tissues around the pharyngeal orifice, producing a unidirectional valve and trapping air or fluid within the pouch. This problem is transient, and rarely does pouch distention become severe.

Clinical Signs Clinical signs depend on the degree of pouch distention and hence the degree of compression of the nasopharynx. If distention is significant, the foal may exhibit stertorous breathing, respiratory distress, dysphagia, nasal discharge, or evidence of pneumonia caused by aspiration. Regurgitation of milk from the nostrils also may be evident.[113] Endoscopic examination may reveal significant compression of the nasopharyngeal area because of distention of the pouches.

Diagnosis Confirmation of the diagnosis is by the presence of tympanitic swelling in the area of Viborg's triangle. Radiographs reveal a large, air-filled guttural pouch with or without fluid accumulation (Figure 9-9). The distinction as to whether the problem is unilateral or bilateral can be difficult to make. Catheterization of one guttural pouch should correct the problem if a unilateral tympany exists. Dorsoventral radiographic views may help in diagnosing bilateral involvement.

Treatment Guttural pouch tympany can be relieved temporarily by percutaneous aspiration or placement of an indwelling catheter. Definitive treatment requires surgical correction. If percutaneous aspiration or indwelling catheter placement is unsuccessful, then surgical correction is required. For unilateral tympany, fenestration of the median septum, separating the two guttural pouches, by conventional or transendoscopic laser surgery allows movement of air into the normal pouch.[114] For bilateral tympany, a fistula can be made with a transendoscopic laser, just dorsal and caudal to the guttural pouch ostium, over a Chambers catheter placed in the pouch. A Foley catheter is then placed for 7 to 10 days. This technique is associated with complete resolution of clinical signs with one (70%) or two (30%) surgeries.[111] Prognosis for uncomplicated cases is good; however, the presence of aspiration pneumonia or dysphagia is associated with a guarded prognosis.

MYCOSIS

Definition Guttural pouch mycosis is characterized by development of fungal plaques on the mucosal walls of the guttural pouches. The majority of plaques are located on the roof of the medial compartment, associated with the internal carotid artery, and less frequently on the lateral wall of the lateral compartment of the pouch, associated with the external carotid or external maxillary artery.

Clinical Signs Many horses do not present until they experience significant spontaneous epistaxis caused by erosion of the fungal plaque through the arterial wall. Horses may also present with nasal discharge dysphagia, RLN, Horner's syndrome, abnormal head extension, swelling in the parotid region, facial paralysis, mycotic encephalitis, and atlantooccipital joint infections.[115-119] Although guttural pouch mycosis is uncommon in the young horse, it has been reported in foals younger than 6 months.[120] Repeated episodes of epistaxis can be fatal in approximately 48% of horses, and definitive surgical treatment should be sought urgently.[121]

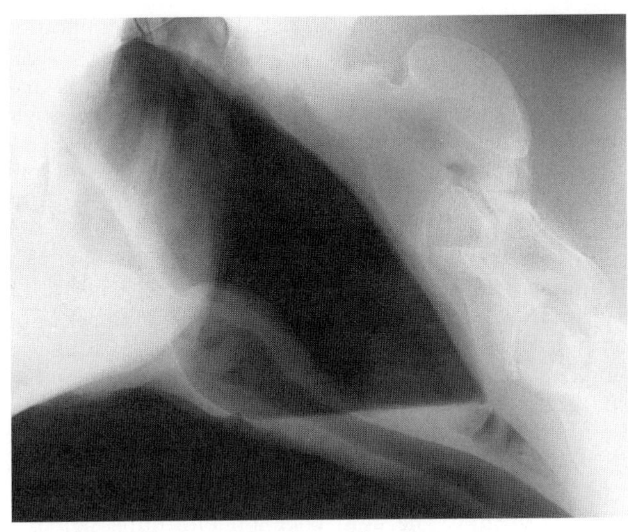

FIGURE 9-9 Guttural pouch tympany. Lateral radiograph of 5-month-old Arabian colt demonstrating a greatly distended gas-filled pouch. (Courtesy D. S. Biller, Manhattan, Kan., 1991.)

Pathogenesis The events leading to the formation of fungal plaques are not known. Some researchers have suggested that aneurysmal dilations of the vasculature, visualized radiographically, provide a suitable environment for fungal organisms to proliferate.[122] Fungal colonization leads to erosion of the underlying mucosa and vascular structures or injury to the adjacent nerves.

Diagnosis Confirmation of the diagnosis is by endoscopic observation of a fungal plaque in the guttural pouch. Shortly after an acute bout of epistaxis, endoscopic examination can confirm the presence of blood at the guttural pouch ostium, but attempts to visualize the interior of the pouch may be unsuccessful if blood obscures the visual field. Some risk exists of dislodging a blood clot during endoscopic examination of the pouch.[123] The presence of RLN or dysphagia should be documented at the initial examination because both are associated with a poor prognosis.[124] RLN is usually permanent, although some horses recover from dysphagia over 6 to 18 months. Horses may also recover from facial nerve paralysis and Horner's syndrome. Radiographs of the guttural pouch may show evidence of fluid accumulation or osteolytic changes in the stylohyoid bone or may suggest mycotic plaque formation.

Treatment Treatment depends on surgical occlusion of the affected vessel or vessels. In an emergency situation with acute epistaxis, ligation of the common carotid artery is contraindicated if the hemorrhage is from the internal carotid artery; flow in the internal carotid artery, from the circle of Willis, will be increased with ligation of the common carotid artery. Several different techniques have been advocated for occlusion.[124-129] Current therapies of choice use a coil or intravascular balloon to obliterate arterial flow proximal and distal to the fungal lesion.[117] The placement of transarterial coils, via an incision in the common carotid artery under fluoroscopic guidance, is associated with 84% survival and 71% return to performance.[124] If fluoroscopic guidance is not available, correct placement of the occluding balloon is essential to prevent postoperative complications, including blindness.[130,131] Correct placement can be difficult in the presence of aberrant vessels.[127,132] The fluoroscopic technique allows identification of such vessels before the occluding coils are placed.

Horses that have dysphagia, in which treatment is elected, may need enteral support via nasogastric intubation or esophagostomy. Medical treatment alone, with topical or parenteral antimycotic drugs, is not effective in eliminating the mycotic plaques.

EMPYEMA

Definition Empyema is an accumulation of exudate within the guttural pouches and is usually a sequela of upper respiratory tract infections (*Streptococcus* spp.). *Streptococcus equi* subsp. *equi* was isolated from 32% of cases evaluated for empyema in a large case series.[133] Empyema may also result from the rupture of abscessed retropharyngeal lymph nodes into the pouches or may accompany cases of guttural pouch tympany.[113] The condition may be unilateral or bilateral.

Clinical Signs The most common presenting sign is a nasal discharge that may be unilateral or bilateral.[133] Other clinical signs include lymphadenopathy, painful distention in the parotid region, stertorous breathing, dysphagia, and occasionally epistaxis.[113] Inspissation of the material may occur with chronic infections, forming masses called *chondroids* in approximately 20% of cases.[133]

Diagnosis Confirmation of the diagnosis is by radiographic examination or endoscopy. Radiographs demonstrate a fluid line or opacity in the pouch (Figure 9-10). Inspissated material also may be evident radiographically (Figure 9-11). Endoscopic examination may reveal a purulent material at the pharyngeal orifice of the auditory tubes and within the medial or lateral compartments of the guttural pouches. Distortion of the pharynx may occur if distention is significant.

Treatment Given that *S. equi* subsp. *equi* may be involved, the clinician should isolate affected horses and take precautions to prevent spread of the bacteria (see discussion on strangles). Treatment may entail medical and surgical modalities. In acute cases, daily irrigation with physiologic saline is usually effective.[133] The horse should be sedated to enhance lowering of its head and to improve drainage of flush materials. Administration of both topical and systemic benzylpenicillin improves treatment success. A gelatin-penicillin mixture can be instilled through a catheter inserted endoscopically into the guttural pouch.[134] A 50-ml mixture is prepared by first heat dissolving 2 grams of gelatin in 40 ml of sterile water and then cooling to 45° to 50° C. To this mixture is added 10 million units of sodium benzylpenicillin that have been reconstituted with 10 ml of sterile water. The mixture is dispensed in syringes and stored overnight at 4° C to set. For each treatment, 25 ml of the mixture is instilled.

One may attempt removal of chondroids with an endoscopic snare, preventing the complications or risk of surgery and minimizing the cost of treatment. However, this task is difficult if the chondroids are numerous.[134,135] Surgical removal of chondroids is effected via a modified Whitehouse approach or by using a transendoscopic laser to establish a permanent pharyngeal fistula into the guttural pouch.[136,137]

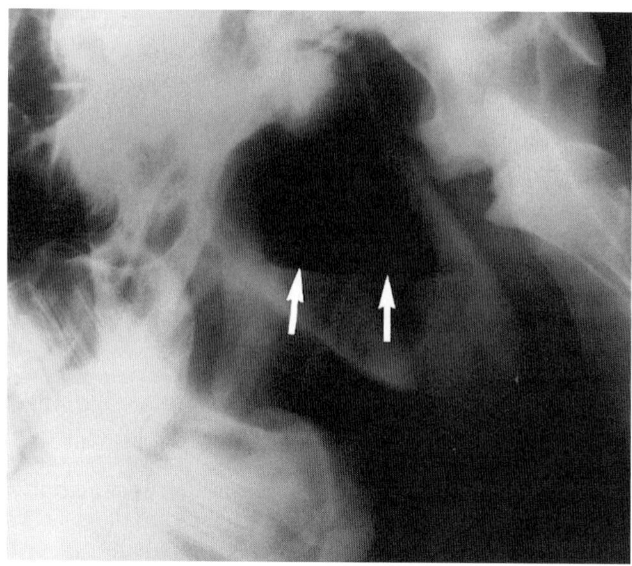

FIGURE 9-10 Guttural pouch empyema. Lateral radiograph shows a fluid line *(arrows)* or air-fluid interface within the guttural pouch. (Courtesy D. S. Biller, Manhattan, Kan., 1991.)

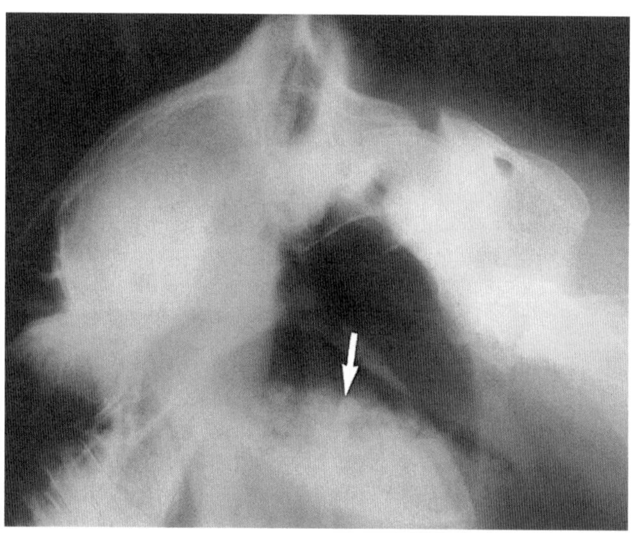

FIGURE 9-11 Guttural pouch chondroids. Lateral radiograph demonstrates irregular soft tissue opacities in the ventral guttural pouch outlined by gas *(arrow)*. (Courtesy D. S. Biller, Manhattan, Kan., 1991.)

Pharyngeal and Laryngeal Disorders

PHARYNGEAL LYMPHOID HYPERPLASIA

Causes The cause of chronic pharyngeal lymphoid hyperplasia (PLH) is not understood but is most likely multifactorial. The location of the nasopharynx exposes it to multiple allergens, irritants, and viral or bacterial agents. The local lymphoid tissue responds by stimulating mucus-producing cells and local immunoglobulins.

Epidemiology Pharyngeal lymphoid hyperplasia is predominantly a condition of young horses, and its prevalence decreases with age.[138-140] PLH is less severe if horses are housed on pasture rather than stabled.[141] PLH has been reproduced experimentally with inoculation of EHV2,[142,143] and although this virus can be isolated from young racehorses with PLH, its causality remains to be proven.[144]

Clinical Signs Some horses may show coughing, a nasal discharge, and mild mandibular lymphadenopathy.[145] PLH is diagnosed endoscopically by the appearance of raised hyperemic

BOX 9-2

GRADING SCHEME FOR LYMPHOID HYPERPLASIA

Grade I: A small number of inactive, white follicles scattered over the dorsal pharyngeal wall. The follicles are small and inactive, a normal finding in horses of all ages.

Grade II: Many small, white inactive follicles over the dorsal and lateral walls of the pharynx to the level of the guttural pouch. Numerous follicles that are larger, pink, and edematous are interspersed throughout.

Grade III: Many large pink follicles and some shrunken white follicles are distributed over the dorsal and lateral walls of the pharynx, in some cases extending onto the dorsal surface of the soft palate and into the pharyngeal diverticula.

Grade IV: More numerous pink and edematous follicles packed close together covering the entire pharynx, the dorsal surface of the soft palate and epiglottis, and the lining of the guttural pouches. Large accumulations appear as polyps.

(From Mansmann RA, McAllister ES, editors: *Equine medicine and surgery*, Santa Barbara, CA, 1982, Veterinary Publications.)

BOX 9-3

GRADING SCHEME FOR LARYNGEAL ANATOMY

Grade I: Synchronous full abduction and adduction of left and right arytenoid cartilages.

Grade II: Asynchronous movement such as hesitation, flutters, adductor weakness of the left arytenoid during inspiration or expiration or both, but full abduction induced by swallowing or nasal occlusion.

Grade III: Asynchronous movement of the left arytenoid during inspiration or expiration or both, but full abduction not induced and maintained by swallowing or nasal occlusion.

Grade IV: Significant asymmetry of the larynx at rest and lack of substantial movement of the left arytenoid.

(From Ducharme NG, Hackett RP: The value of surgical treatment of laryngeal hemiplegia in horses, *Compend Cont Educ Pract Vet* 13:472, 1991.)

and edematous follicles distributed throughout the nasopharyngeal walls (Box 9-2).[141,145,146] The condition, unless severe, has not been associated with poor performance per se,[138,139] although severe PLH has been proposed as a cause of dorsal displacement of the soft palate in young horses as a result of the proximity of the pharyngeal branch of the vagus nerve.[147]

Treatment Treatment options include rest, reducing the allergen content of the air through improved management, turnout to pasture, and throat spray (see section on chondritis).

TABLE 9-2

Function and Innervation of Muscles Controlling the Tone of the Equine Soft Palate

Muscle	Function	Innervation
Tensor veli palatini	Tenses the rostral aspect of the soft palate	Mandibular branch of the trigeminal nerve
Levator veli palatini	Elevates the palate during swallowing and closes the nasopharynx	Pharyngeal branch of the vagus
Palatinus	Shorten and depress the palate	Pharyngeal branch of the vagus
Palatopharyngeus	Shorten and depress the palate	Pharyngeal branch of the vagus

DORSAL DISPLACEMENT OF THE SOFT PALATE

Definition Dorsal displacement of the soft palate (DDSP) results in an upper airway expiratory obstruction at exercise. It is a common cause of poor performance in racehorses and has a prevalence of 10% to 20%.[14,15,148,149] Most affected horses make a loud, vibratory respiratory noise, known as *choking down*,[150,151] although a proportion are silent during displacement.[13,151] Endoscopic examination of the upper airway at rest is a poor predictor of DDSP.[152] A definitive diagnosis is made, during high speed treadmill examination, if the caudal border of the soft palate is seen dorsal to the epiglottis for more than 8 seconds.[153]

Anatomy The horse is an obligate intranasal breather, and the epiglottis is usually positioned dorsal to the caudal border of the soft palate. A common analogy is a *button through a buttonhole*.[154] The anatomy of this area is complex. The larynx is suspended from the pterous part of the temporal bone by a chain of paired hyoid bones, the stylohyoid, ceratohyoid, single basihyoid bone, and thyrohyoid, which articulates with the rostral aspect of the thyroid cartilage. The strap muscles (sternohyoid, sternothyroid, and omohyoid) contract during exercise and pull the larynx caudally. Similarly, the genioglossus, geniohyoid, and styloglossus muscles (through their direct or indirect attachments to the hyoid apparatus) pull the larynx rostrally.[155,156] The tone of the soft palate is determined by four pairs of muscles. The innervation and function of these muscles is shown in Table 9-2. The stylopharyngeus muscle is innervated by the glossopharyngeal nerve and tenses the dorsal wall of the nasopharynx.[157]

Etiology The etiologic factors of DDSP are not completely understood and can be divided into intrinsic and extrinsic causes. Intrinsic dysfunctions are seen with decreased tone in muscles of the palate. Dysfunction of the palatinus and palatopharyngeus muscles results in DDSP.[147] This cause is closely linked to PLH in young horses because the pharyngeal branch of the vagus nerve runs through the floor of the guttural pouch, which is also the roof of the pharynx. Transection of the tensor veli palatini tendon alone destabilizes the rostral aspect of the soft palate, leading to inspiratory airway obstruction but not DDSP.[158] Dysfunction of the caudal stylopharyngeus muscle destabilizes the nasopharynx but does not cause DDSP.[157]

Extrinsic causes are related to the musculature that controls the position of the larynx and hyoid apparatus. Transection of the paired thyrohyoid muscles produces DDSP[159] presumably because these muscles, innervated by the hypoglossal nerve, prevent caudal retraction of the larynx at exercise. Partial resection of the sternothyroid and sternohyoid tendons produces an inspiratory airway obstruction but not DDSP.[160]

Investigation targeting the role of the rostral hyoid muscles (geniohyoid, stylohyoid, and styloglossus) in horses are lacking, but, in humans at least, these muscles are critical to pharyngeal stability.[161,162] Indirectly, tongue-tie devices, which are designed to prevent caudal retraction of the hyoid apparatus at exercise, have been shown to prevent DDSP in some horses.[163]

In addition to these neuromuscular dysfunctions, structural abnormalities such as masses or granulomas associated with the epiglottic cartilage or the soft palate can induce DDSP.[148]

Treatment Surgical techniques aimed at preventing caudal retraction of the larynx, such as strap muscle resection and the Llewellyn procedure (transaction of the tendon of insertion of the sternothyroid muscle), are associated with success rates ranging between 58% to 73%.[151,164,165] Treatments aimed at intrinsic causes include staphylectomy[165] and soft tissue stiffening techniques such as rostral palatoplasty.[166] Conservative management of DDSP, incorporating rest, improvement of fitness, use of a tongue tie, or any combination, has also been reported, with a success rate of up to 61%.[163,167] A case-control study demonstrated that composite surgery including staphylectomy, sternothyrohyoideus myectomy, and ventriculocordectomy produced increased race earnings in 60% of horses compared with 40% in controls.[150]

Surgical advancement of the larynx (laryngeal tie-forward procedure) demonstrated a success rate of 80% to 82% in racehorses.[168] The proposed mechanism of this procedure is that it replaces the action of the thyrohyoid muscles and prevents ventral descent and caudal retraction of the larynx during exercise. This procedure is well described elsewhere.[168] Horses undergoing this procedure are as likely to race postoperatively as matched controls. The procedure restores race earnings to preoperative baseline levels and to those of matched controls.

In addition, an external device (Cornell Collar, Vet-Aire, Inc., Ithaca, NY) that applies forward and upward pressure to the hyoid apparatus and incorporates a figure-8 noseband also prevents experimentally induced DDSP during strenuous exercise.[169]

RECURRENT LARYNGEAL NEUROPATHY

Definition and Epidemiology Recurrent laryngeal neuropathy is a major cause of poor performance in racehorses and affects 1.6% to 8% of Thoroughbreds.[170-173] The prevalence in draft horses is nearly 42%,[174] and the risk of RLN increases with increasing height in Belgians and Percherons but not in Clydesdales.[174] Horses as young as 6 months may be affected.[175] The condition produces an inspiratory noise at exercise, which has been described as both *roaring* and *sawing*. The term *recurrent laryngeal neuropathy* is preferred to idiopathic laryngeal hemiplegia.[176]

Diagnosis A diagnosis can be made in most horses based on a resting endoscopic examination of the arytenoid cartilages. Some confusion has arisen from different grading systems used to diagnose the degree of arytenoid dysfunction present at this examination. A recent meeting of investigators reached consensus on a four-level grading system (Table 9-3), and this system should now be used.[176] This resting grading system is most useful in its ability to predict arytenoid function at high-speed exercise. Arytenoid position at exercise is shown in Table 9-4.[177]

TABLE 9-3

Grading System for Laryngeal Function Performed in the Standing Unsedated Horse[176]

Grade	Description
I	All arytenoid cartilage movements are synchronous and symmetrical, and full arytenoid abduction can be achieved and maintained.
II	Arytenoid cartilage movements are asynchronous at times, but full arytenoid abduction can be achieved and maintained.
III	Arytenoid cartilage movements are asynchronous or asymmetrical (or both). Full arytenoid cartilage abduction *cannot* be achieved and maintained.
IV	Immobility of the arytenoid cartilage and vocal fold is complete.

Grades II and III contain several subgrades. Readers are referred to the monograph for further information.

TABLE 9-4

Grading System for Laryngeal Function Performed During Treadmill Endoscopy[177]

Grade	Description
A	Full abduction of the arytenoid cartilages during inspiration
B	Partial abduction of the left arytenoid cartilage (between full abduction and the resting position)
C	Abduction less than resting position, including collapse into the contralateral half of the rima glottidis during inspiration

All grade 1 horses are normal (grade A) at exercise, and all grade 4 horses show dynamic collapse (grade C).[178] During exercise, 4% of grade 3 horses are normal (grade A), 19% are grade B, and 77% grade C.[179] For grade 2 horses, 4% are grade B or C at exercise.[178] Recently, a technique for examining the lateral cricoarytenoid muscle using ultrasound has been described, and this technique is a good predictor of arytenoid function at exercise.[180,181] It is especially useful if a high-speed treadmill examination cannot be performed.

Anatomy and Etiology The left recurrent laryngeal nerve curves medially around the aortic arch during development and is approximately 1 m long.[182] In contrast, the right recurrent laryngeal nerve courses around the right subclavian artery and is approximately 25% shorter.[182] The high prevalence of chronic demyelinating peripheral neuropathy in the left recurrent laryngeal nerve has been attributed to its length.[183,184] The myelin loss is most severe distally[185,186] and is associated with axonal loss.[187,188] RLN results in progressive atrophy of the left dorsal cricoarytenoid muscle and associated loss of arytenoid cartilage abduction.[183,185,188] The right recurrent laryngeal nerve is rarely affected, although direct trauma to the nerve can induce dysfunction.

During exercise, arytenoid dysfunction narrows the rima glottis and increases inspiratory impedance and noise.[189,190] This circumstance, in turn, results in airflow limitation and increased driving pressure during inhalation, leading to severe exercise-induced hypoxemia and decreased performance.[189,191-193]

Treatment The current gold standard for treatment of RLN in horses is prosthetic laryngoplasty, with or without vocal cordectomy or ventriculectomy.[194-197] This technique involves the placement of a nonabsorbable suture to create arytenoid abduction. One limitation of this technique is the frequent and significant loss of abduction of the arytenoid cartilage seen in the immediate postsurgical period.[197,198] This loss of abduction leads to a reduction in cross-sectional area of the rima glottidis and the return of exercise intolerance and abnormal respiratory noise.[197-199] Loss of abduction may also contribute to the modest postoperative success rate of 48% to 68% observed in racehorses.[194,195,200-203] A much higher success rate (73% to 91%) is reported in horses performing at submaximal exercise.[204]

In draft breeds, the degree of abduction required at laryngoplasty is lower than that for a racehorse, given that the goal is to prevent dynamic collapse of the arytenoid rather than to achieve a normal cross-sectional area of the rima glottidis. Some clinicians recommend vocal cordectomy alone for draft breeds. For racehorses and nonracehorses, the major complications are exercise intolerance, respiratory noise, and coughing.[195,196,203]

Restoration of physiologic function through reinnervation and nerve-muscle pedicle transplant techniques has also produced positive results,[205-207] although a delay of several months occurs before any improvement in arytenoid function is seen.

Partial arytenoidectomy is associated with a fair prognosis for the treatment of RLN in horses[200,208] and is not generally recommended as a first-line surgical option.

EPIGLOTTIC ENTRAPMENT

Definition and Epidemiology The aryepiglottic fold is the mucous membrane that extends from the lateral aspect of the arytenoid cartilages to the ventrolateral aspect of the epiglottis, where it blends with the subepiglottic mucosa and the glossoepiglottic fold. In epiglottic entrapment, this membrane envelopes the free border of the epiglottis.[209] Billowing of the entrapping membranes during respiration decreases the cross-sectional area of the pharynx and effectively obstructs the airflow, particularly during expiration.

The cause of epiglottic entrapment is not understood completely. In most cases, the epiglottic cartilage and associated soft tissues appear normal. In occasional cases, congenital epiglottic hypoplasia or inflammation of the upper respiratory tract structures appears to contribute to entrapment. Epiglottic entrapment is responsible for 1% to 3% of upper airway obstructive problems in horses.[15,173]

Clinical Signs Most horses exhibit exercise intolerance and respiratory stertor. Horses may occasionally cough during exercise or while eating.

Diagnosis Diagnosis is based on endoscopic examination. The membrane obscures the normal serrated margin of the epiglottis and its dorsal vasculature. In contrast to dorsal displacement of the soft palate, the shape of the epiglottis can still be seen. Ulceration of the free margin of the fold and erosion of the entrapped epiglottis may be apparent.[210]

Treatment Entrapment requires surgical correction. Several different approaches have been used and include transoral[209,211-213] or transnasal[214] axial division with a hooked bistoury and transendoscopic division with a laser.[215-217] The prognosis is good after surgery, although reentrapment and DDSP may occur after surgery.[209,213,217]

ARYTENOID CHONDRITIS

Definition and Epidemiology Arytenoid chondritis is a condition affecting the corniculate process of the arytenoid cartilage or its mucosal surface and may produce an abnormal enlargement of the arytenoid cartilages caused by chronic inflammation,[218,219] a mucosal ulceration of the vocal process,[220] and the formation of intralaryngeal granulation tissue.[221,222]

The condition is most commonly diagnosed in young racehorses between 2 and 4 years of age[223] and is more prevalent in North America, Australia, and New Zealand than in Europe.[208,218,220-224] Although the prevalence of the condition in North American horses has not been defined, its prevalence in Australian and New Zealand yearling Thoroughbreds (at sales) has been estimated at 0.21% to 0.6%.[220,223] In nonracehorses, arytenoid chondritis is more common in older animals.[221]

Cause The cause of arytenoid chondritis is not fully understood. The proposed etiologic factor is ascending infection and inflammation of the underlying cartilage after mucosal injury.[220,225] Affected arytenoid cartilage is thickened and laminated with fibrous connective tissue. Intraluminal granulation and sinus tracts are seen in some cases. The condition is typically unilateral, though often secondary contact damage (*kissing* lesion) occurs to the contralateral cartilage.

Diagnosis Diagnosis is made based on endoscopic examination. Mildly affected horses retain arytenoid mobility yet have ulcerations of the body of the affected cartilage or granulomata that project into the laryngeal lumen. In more advanced cases, the affected arytenoid cartilage is immobile and deviated medially. Laryngeal ultrasound may be useful for identifying concurrent abcessation.[180] Radiographs may reveal excessive mineralization of laryngeal cartilages.

Clinical Signs Clinical signs include exercise intolerance and inspiratory stridor during exercise. In severe bilateral cases, the reduction in rima glottidis cross-sectional area may be obstructive.

Treatment Mild cases of arytenoid chondritis may be treated with systemic antibiotics and application (20 ml every 12 hours) of a throat spray. The latter consists of 1 g nitrofurazone in 250 ml dimethyl sulfoxide, 500 ml water, 250 ml 99% glycerine, and 25 ml dexamethasone.

In moderate to severe cases, or if throat spray is not effective, a partial arytenoidectomy should be performed to remove the affected cartilage.[200,208] This procedure involves resection of the laryngeal ventricle, vocal fold, and arytenoid cartilage (excluding the muscular process) and the rostral strip of the corniculate cartilage and is associated with a fair prognosis for return to racing.[208] Intraluminal granulation tissue can be removed with a transendoscopic laser.[222] In severe bilateral cases, a tracheostomy may be required to create an effective airway.

ROSTRAL DISPLACEMENT OF THE PALATOPHARYNGEAL ARCH

In the horse, the soft palate terminates caudally by the confluence of the caudal pillars to form the palatopharyngeal arch that covers the esophageal orifice.[226] In rostral displacement of the palatopharyngeal arch, this fold of tissue appears to be displaced forward, overlying the apices of the arytenoid cartilages. The condition is uncommon, with a number of small case series and individual cases being reported.[14,227-230] The displacement of the palatopharyngeal arch may be associated with malformation of the laryngeal cartilages and the cricopharyngeal and cricothyroid muscles.[14] The condition may be present from birth. In most cases, abnormal respiratory noise and poor athletic performance are the presenting complaints. Abnormal pharyngeal conformation prevents normal deglutition, predisposing horses to develop aspiration pneumonia. In severe cases, horses may exhibit dysphagia, nasal discharge of food material, and persistent coughing.[229,231] The diagnosis is based on the clinical signs and history and confirmed with endoscopic examination. The rostrally displaced palatopharyngeal arch obscures the normal view of the apices of the arytenoid cartilages. Rostral displacement of the palatopharyngeal arch represents a major deformation of the laryngeal structures and is associated with a guarded prognosis. Resection of the arch by conventional surgery or laser surgery has not enabled successful athletic performance.[227]

NASOPHARYNGEAL CICATRIX

This condition is almost exclusively seen in horses on pasture in eastern and southern Texas, with occasional reports from Mississippi, Louisiana, and Florida.[210,232] The cause of the condition is unknown, but an environmental allergen may lead to nasopharyngeal inflammation with subsequent scarring and web formation and with reduction in the cross-sectional area of the rima glottidis[210,232] (Figure 9-12). Horses housed inside do not appear to be affected. Clinical signs include exercise intolerance and stridor. The arytenoid cartilages are involved in more than 70% of cases.[233] Horses should be removed from pasture and have antiinflammatory treatment initiated as soon as the diagnosis is made. If airway obstruction is present then a permanent tracheostomy should be performed.[233] This technique is associated with a high number of horses (89%) returning to their previous level of use.

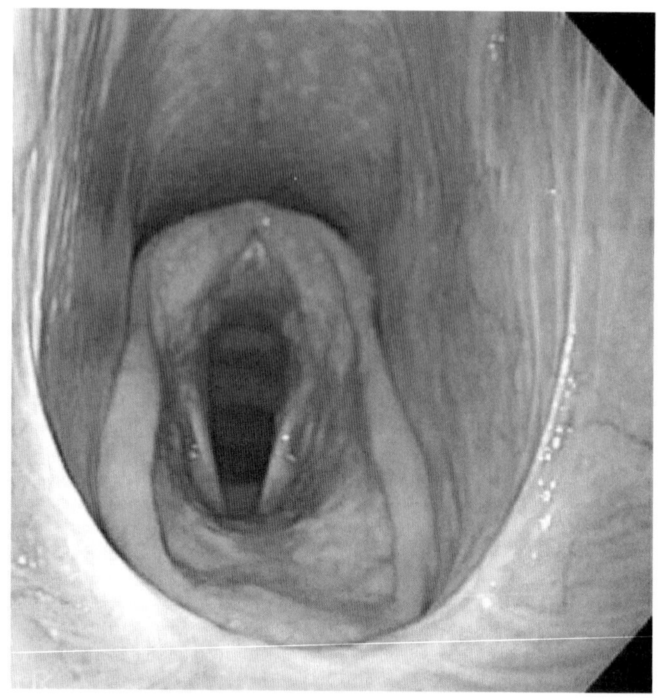

FIGURE 9-12 Nasopharyngeal cicatrix.

STREPTOCOCCUS EQUI SUBSP. *EQUI* INFECTIONS (STRANGLES)

Causes *Streptococcus equi* subsp. *equi*, a gram-positive β-hemolytic bacterium of the Lancefield group C, is the causative agent of strangles, a highly contagious disease of Equidae. The disease was recognized in the thirteenth century and occurs worldwide.[234] Multilocus enzyme electrophoresis studies have confirmed a close genetic relationship of *S. equi* subsp. *equi* and *S. equi* subsp. *zooepidemicus,* indicating that the former is a clone derived from the more genetically diverse *S. equi* subsp. *zooepidemicus*.[235] This finding has led to the recommendation that *S. equi* subsp. *equi* be reclassified as a biovar of *S. equi* subsp. *zooepidemicus*.[236] Although isolates of these two organisms show greater than 92% DNA homology, immunity is species specific; immunization with *S. equi* subsp. *zooepidemicus* does not protect against challenge by *S. equi* subsp. *equi*.

S. equi subsp. *equi* (hereafter termed *S. equi*) is not a normal inhabitant of the equine upper respiratory tract and does not require prior viral infections for successful colonization and infection.[237] Based on morphologic features of the bacterial colony, three strains of the organism occur that differ in virulence. The typical and highly virulent encapsulated *S. equi* strains produce golden, honey-colored mucoid colonies on blood agar. Atypical *S. equi* colonies exhibit a matte appearance within 24 hours of incubation. Nonencapsulated colonies are glossy, dry, and small.[238] Differences in the hyaluronic acid content of the capsule are responsible for the morphologically distinctive features of *S. equi* colonies.

Laboratory diagnosis of Lancefield group C streptococci (*S. equi, S. zooepidemicus, S. equisimilis*) is traditionally based on fermentation patterns of lactose, sorbitol, and trehalose. Typical *S. equi* isolates fail to ferment any of these sugars, whereas atypical *S. equi* isolates may ferment lactose or trehalose but not sorbitol.[239] In some laboratories, polymerase chain reaction (PCR) confirms the isolate to be *S. equi*.[240] Ideally, PCR should be performed using primers based on the nucleotide sequence of the gene encoding the *S. equi* M-like (SeM) protein.[241]

Epidemiology The infection occurs primarily in horses 1 to 5 years of age but is not restricted to this age group. Foals up to 3 months of age born from immune mares are known to be resistant to the development of strangles.[242] Thus infection in foals typically develops after weaning. In susceptible equine populations, morbidity is nearly 100%, whereas mortality is low (up to 10%).[243] Once having been infected, approximately 75% of the horses are immune to the organism for greater than 5 years.[244,245] However, 25% of these horses become susceptible to reinfection within months, which may represent a failure to produce or maintain an adequate level of the appropriate mucosal and systemic antibodies.[245] In one study of young horses that had been affected with clinical strangles as foals, researchers found that 83 were resistant to co-mingling exposure 6 months later.[246] Unfortunately, immunity is not lifelong. Epidemiologic studies report attack rates in horses greater than 3 years of age of 18%, 29%, and 35%.[243,247,248]

The organism is transmitted (1) via direct contact with nasal or ocular secretions or lymph node discharges from infected horses or (2) via exposure to fomites such as contaminated equipment, pails, halters, leads, brushes, clothing, horse vans, or stalls. Recent additions to a stable are most often the cause of a strangles outbreak because a recovering horse—one that is free of clinical signs—may shed the organism for several weeks. In closed herds, epidemics have been attributed to exposure of horses to asymptomatic chronic carriers of the organism. Such horses harbor the organism in the guttural pouches for periods as long as 39 months in the absence of clinical signs. Other sites of long-term carriage of *S. equi* include the paranasal sinuses.[249] The reason why the carrier state develops in certain horses is unknown. Waller (2007) suggested that incomplete drainage of the guttural pouches or sinuses (e.g., residual empyema or even chondroid formation) continuously stimulates an immune response that produces a modified humoral immunity profile that is distinct from that of a noncarrier. This hypothesis remains to be verified. Regardless of the mechanism, subclinical persistent carriage of *S. equi* is necessary for maintaining this infection between outbreaks.[250]

Controlled field studies that have documented the survivability of *S. equi* in the environment have not been conducted.[251] Although Jorm[252] found that *S. equi* survived for 63 days on wood at temperatures of 2° C and for 48 days on glass or wood at temperatures of 20° C, the effects of other competing bacteria (and their secreted bacteriocins) were not considered. The organism is susceptible to a 1:200 dilution of phenol and disinfectants such as povidone-iodine, chlorhexidine, and glutaraldehyde kill the organism within 90 minutes.

S. equi is traditionally thought to infect only Equidae. However, a fatal pneumonia attributed to the organism was reported in a dromedary camel.[253] In the literature on human beings, descriptions of *S. equi* bacteremia and meningitis exist, but infections in human beings are considered rare.[254]

Pathogenesis After infective droplets are inhaled or ingested, the organism adheres to the epithelial cells of the buccal and nasal mucosa of the horse. The mechanism or mechanisms involved in bacterial adherence is currently unknown[245] but may involve exposed bacterial surface proteins such as SzPSe, Se73.0, and Se51.9.[251] Within hours of adhesion, the organism has translocated below the mucosa and gained access to the local lymphatics and lymph nodes, where replication occurs extracellulary.[234] Complement-derived chemotactic factors generated after interaction of C1 with bacterial peptidoglycan attract large numbers of neutrophils that contribute to the lymphadenitis and abscess formation.[245] Spread of the organism to sites other than the upper respiratory tract lymphoid tissue may occur by hematogenous or lymphatic pathways. In experimental infections of *S. equi,* the organisms can be cultured from the blood 6 to 12 days after intranasal inoculation.[255]

Numerous virulence factors of *S. equi* contribute to its pathogenicity, a few of which include the hyaluronic acid capsule, the SeM protein, an antiphagocytic protein (Se18.9), a leukocidal toxin (streptolysin S-like [SLS] toxin), and cell membrane lipoproteins.[241,256-258] Synthesis of the hyaluronic acid capsule is controlled by the *has* operon, which consists of *hasA* (encodes hyaluronate synthase), *hasB* (encodes UDP-glucose dehydrogenase), and *hasC* (encodes UDP-glucose pyrophosphorylase). The capsule is antiphagocytic, ultimately reducing the number of bacteria that are subsequently ingested and killed. The capsule, by virtue of its negative charge and hydrophilicity, also produces a localized reducing environment that protects the activity of oxygen-labile proteases and toxins (SLS). Finally, the capsule is required for the activity of SeM. In nonencapsulated strains of *S. equi,* SeM aggregate and fail to achieve the three-dimensional structure required for their function.[245] Although nonencapsulated strains of *S. equi* are able to colonize the surface of the upper respiratory tract and stimulate production of serum antibody, they are unable to induce detectable pathologic changes in the retropharyngeal and mandibular lymph nodes.[259] The second virulence factor, the SeM protein, is a 58-kDa cell wall antigen that is also antiphagocytic. At its N-terminal end, SeM binds to fibrinogen, at its central region, to IgG. In doing so, it masks the C3b binding surface on the bacterial cell wall and inhibits the alternative C3 and classical C5 convertase.[245] Sequencing of the SeM gene between codons 38 and 143 from 142 *S. equi* strains has identified 43 alleles of SeM with each allele characteristic of a particular outbreak in a geographic location.[260] Thus SeM sequence analysis can be used to complement epidemiologic investigations of strangles outbreaks. The loss of SeM expression leads to a loss of virulence but not to a decrease in the infectivity of the organism. Another M-like protein of *S. equi,* SzPSe, exhibits antigenic cross reactivity with the M-like proteins of *S. zooepidemicus,* but its contribution to the virulence of *S. equi* is unknown.[235] Recently, a protein unique to *S. equi,* Se18.9, was found to also possess antiphagocytic properties.[258] The net effect of Se18.9 is to decrease deposition of C3 (and hence opsonic C3b) on the bacterial surface, reducing phagocytosis. SLS protein is thought to represent a fourth virulence factor by its cytotoxic properties. It damages host macrophages and neutrophils enabling immune evasion, as well as access to released essential nutrients.[241] A fifth virulence factor resides in the lipoprotein components of the *S. equi* cell membrane. When mutants of a specific lipoprotein are synthesized (PrtM) and the organisms are administered to susceptible ponies, clinical signs are markedly attenuated (0 of 5 infected ponies developed signs compared to controls). These data suggest that this lipoprotein is an important virulence factor and might become targeted for vaccine development.[257] Additional factors that contribute to the pathogenicity of *S. equi* include extracellular proteins or exotoxins that are mitogenic for peripheral blood mononuclear cells.[261] These mitogenic factors (SePE-H, SePE-I, SePE-K, and SePE-L) bind simultaneously to class II major histocompatibility complex (MHC) molecules on antigen presenting cells and to the T-cell receptor of T cells to induce nonspecific T cell stimulation, proliferation, and cytokine release. As a result, an acute phase response ensues characterized by release of interleukin-1 (IL-1), tumor necrosis factor α (TNF-α), and IL-6 from mononuclear cells that contribute to the production of fever, malaise, neutrophilia, and hyperfibrinogenemia.[245,261]

Humoral immune responses to many of these virulence factors are apparent in infected horses. During the initial stages of infection, serum IgGa to the SeM protein is induced, followed by the appearance of IgA and IgGb to SeM on the mucosal surfaces.[262] During convalescence, strong IgGb responses appear to SeM, as well as to other surface exposed proteins (Se44.2, Se46.8, Se45.5, Se42.0).[245]

Clinical Signs The incubation period ranges between 2 to 6 days. In typical cases, horses are febrile (103° F or higher), exhibit malaise, and develop a serous nasal discharge that becomes mucopurulent. Ocular and nasal mucosal membranes become hyperemic, and a mucopurulent ocular discharge may ensue. Mandibular and retropharyngeal lymph nodes are initially firm but become fluctuant before rupturing 7 to 10 days after the onset of signs. Retropharyngeal lymph nodes may rupture into the guttural pouches, causing neuropathy (dysphagia), empyema, and chondroid formation. Lymphadenopathy, one of the major signs of *S. equi* infections, may be asymmetrical and may become so severe that dysphagia, stridor, and respiratory distress ensue. Swelling of the throatlatch area or of Viborg's triangle may be apparent and palpation of this area may elicit pain. The affected horse may stand with its neck stretched out and be reluctant to swallow. A soft moist cough may be heard. The average course of the syndrome is 23 days.[237] In atypical *S. equi* infections, a mild inflammation of the upper respiratory tract occurs and is characterized by a slight nasal discharge, cough, and fever. Abscessation of the lymph nodes occurs only in a small number of the cases.[238,239,263] In the majority of horses, clinical signs resolve and bacterial shedding ceases by 4 to 6 weeks. In an estimated 10% of affected horses, continued intermittent shedding of *S. equi* may occur for several additional weeks.

Clinical Pathology A marked neutrophilic leukocytosis, hyperfibrinogenemia, hyperglobulinemia, and anemia of chronic infection are found in typical strangles cases. In cases complicated by concurrent pneumonia (aspiration), a left shift and the presence of neutrophils with toxic signs may be noted. In horses with purpura hemorrhagic, moderate to marked elevations in muscle enzymes occur.

Diagnosis The diagnosis is usually based on clinical signs and the isolation (culture) or detection (via PCR) of *S. equi* from a lymph node, a nasopharyngeal swab, nasal washings, or lavage fluid from the guttural pouches. Nasal shedding of *S. equi* occurs 2 to 3 days after the onset of fever and usually persists for several weeks. Thus culture of acutely affected horses may initially be negative.[251] Nasal washes appear to be more effective than nasopharyngeal swabs in detecting small numbers of *S. equi* because a greater surface area is inherently sampled. The wash is accomplished by instilling 50 ml of warm sterile saline into the nasal cavity via a 15-cm soft rubber tubing that has been inserted to the level of the medial canthus. Fluid is collected and centrifuged, and the pellet is cultured. Guttural pouch lavage is best performed endoscopically, allowing inspection of the medial and lateral compartments for evidence of lymphadenopathy, empyema, or (in more chronic infections) chondroid formation. For the lavage, 30 to 50 ml of sterile saline is instilled through the biopsy chamber and gently aspirated for culture or PCR or both. When endoscopy is not feasible, a guttural pouch lavage may yet be possible by advancing a Chambers catheter blindly into the guttural pouch of the sedated horse and lavaging the compartments. Finally, blood cultures may become positive for *S. equi* on days 6 to 12 after infection.[255] The PCR assay, based on the DNA sequence for SeM, is used in conjunction with bacterial culture in diagnostic workups. PCR is more sensitive than bacterial culture and can detect SeM DNA for weeks in guttural pouch lavages after the disappearance of live organisms.[264] It is useful in detecting asymptomatic carriers, in establishing *S. equi* infection status before or after transport or commingling, and in establishing success of treatment.[251]

Serologic diagnosis of *S. equi* infections entails measurement of SeM-specific antibody and can be helpful in detecting horses that have been exposed to *S. equi* or that have developed untoward sequelae as a result of infection. For example, a titer of more than 1:12,800 is highly supportive of a diagnosis of purpura hemorrhagica or of metastatic strangles.[251] Serologic testing can also be helpful in determining the need for vaccination or in identifying horses that may be hyperresponders and predisposed to the development of purpura hemorrhagica (SeM-specific antibodies > 1:1600). An enzyme-linked immunosorbent assay (ELISA) based on SeM-specific antibodies is commercially available (IDEXX Laboratories) but may not reliably detect subclinical carriers because of the overlap in the breakpoints between normal and convalescent horses.[250]

As previously stated, endoscopic examination of the guttural pouches for evidence of lymphadenopathy, empyema, or chondroids can be helpful in the diagnosis of *S. equi* infections. It can also aid in the identification of asymptomatic carriers, given that endoscopic abnormalities are often still present in these horses.[249] However, the absence of visible pathologic signs in one asymptomatic carrier emphasizes the need to still obtain samples for concurrent culture and PCR assay.[264,265]

Treatment Differences of opinion are marked as to whether or not to use antibiotics in horses with strangles.[251] Treatment is a function of the stage of the disease, and the general recommendations listed here are those included in the American College of Veterinary Internal Medicine (ACVIM) Consensus Statement developed by Sweeney, Timoney, Newton, et al.[251] The reader is referred to this excellent review. In treating horses with *S. equi,* penicillin is the drug of choice, although the organism is sensitive to oxytetracycline and the potentiated sulfonamides.[234,249]

The treatment plan is as follows:

1. For horses exhibiting early clinical signs of infection (fever, depression) in the absence of lymph node abscessation, penicillin G therapy for 3 to 5 days can arrest the progression of the disease. One should isolate the horses during their treatment protocol. Treated horses are likely to remain susceptible to infection because sufficient bacterial antigen to elicit a protective immune response may not have been produced as a result of treatment. No evidence has been found that the use of antibiotics during this stage will promote the development of metastatic strangles.[266]
2. For alert and otherwise healthy horses exhibiting lymph node abscessation, administration of penicillin slows the progression of lymph node abscessation and is generally contraindicated. Hot-packing the area or areas promotes maturation of the abscess. Once achieved, the clinician should lance the abscess and flush it with a 3% to 5% povidone-iodine solution and, if desirable, then institute antibiotic therapy. Horses may benefit from phenylbutazone or flunixin meglumine administration, which will reduce fever, lessen pharyngeal discomfort associated with the lymphadenitis, and improve their demeanor. The horses should be treated in isolation.
3. Horses that are systemically ill or that develop complications such as dysphagia, aspiration pneumonia, or respiratory distress require supportive care in addition to high levels of intravenous penicillin and other antimicrobials effective against gram negative organisms (aminoglycosides) or anaerobes (metronidazole). Horses may also require intravenous fluid therapy, a tracheostomy, nonsteroidal antiinflammatory drugs, and feeding via a nasogastric tube.

Sequelae The overall complication rate in horses with strangles is estimated to be 20%; most frequently, complications result from metastasis of the organism to other organ systems with the formation of purulent foci.[267] Complications include the following:

1. *Internal abscessation of the mesentery or of parenchymatous organs.* The causes of internal abscessation are not known,[268] and no evidence currently exists to suggest that the initiation of antimicrobial therapy predisposes the horse to the formation of internal abscessation.[266] Furthermore, internal abscesses have formed in the absence of prior antimicrobial treatment, making this risk factor unlikely.[269] The prevalence of metastatic abscessation is low, with estimates of 28% based on outbreaks on two farms.[269]

The horse with metastatic strangles may have a history of intermittent colic, periodic pyrexia, anorexia, depression, and weight loss. The clinician should direct diagnostic techniques, including rectal palpation, abdominocentesis, ultrasonography, CT (foal, miniature horse, or pony), and nuclear scintigraphy,[270] at determining the location of the abscess. In a review of 10 horses with internal abdominal abscesses caused by *S. equi,* abdominal ultrasonography (transabdominal or transrectal or both) was useful in detecting circular encapsulated hypoechoic masses of either homogenous or mixed echogenicity in seven of the horses.[271] Internal abscessation can be difficult to differentiate from abdominal neoplasms because both processes may induce similar abnormalities in the peritoneal fluid (leukocytosis and hyperproteinemia). Differentiation between the two processes may not be possible unless exfoliated neoplastic cells are identified.[272] Culture of the peritoneal fluid in horses with *S. equi* internal abdominal abscesses rarely yields positive (diagnostic) microbial isolates.[271]

Hematologic and serum biochemical abnormalities in horses with internal abscessation include (1) anemia, (2) neutrophilic and monocytic leukocytosis, (3) thrombocytosis, (4) hyperfibrinogenemia, (5) hyperglobulinemia and hypoalbuminemia, and (6) hypocalcemia.[268,271,272] However, these changes are not unique to internal abscessation and may be found in horses with intraabdominal neoplasms.[271,272] However, detecting an elevated SeM specific titer (>1:3200) is supportive evidence of metastatic strangles.[271] Once one confirms the diagnosis, long-term antimicrobial therapy is indicated and may be required for several months.

In the report of Pusterla et al. (2007), 7 of 10 horses with abdominal abscesses received a protracted course of antimicrobials (mean duration of 72 days) that initially consisted of a beta-lactam antimicrobial (ceftiofur, ampicillin) followed by chloramphenicol, trimethoprim sulfamethoxazole, or rifampin. Clinical signs, rectal palpation, repeated abdominocentesis, and multiple complete blood counts (CBCs) were used to monitor the progress of therapy. Nevertheless, survival rate was reported to be 40%.[271]

2. *Purpura hemorrhagica.* This aseptic necrotizing vasculitis may occur after reexposure to *S. equi* by natural infection or after vaccination. The prevalence of this disorder after natural outbreaks is not known. In a retrospective study of 53 horses diagnosed with purpura hemorrhagica at a university teaching hospital,[273] 17 horses had confirmed exposure or infection with *S. equi,* and 5 had been vaccinated with SeM protein. In horses with *S. equi*–associated purpura, IgA titers to the SeM and to nonspecific proteins in the *S. equi* culture supernatant (SC-P) are significantly greater than those titers found in horses with uncomplicated strangles.[274] The isolation of immune complexes consisting of IgA and M-like proteins in the sera of horses with purpura hemorrhagica has led to the suggestion that this isotype is involved in the development of purpura.[274,275] The immunologic basis for the increase in serum IgA levels is not known, but possible explanations include uncontrolled expansion of B cell populations that produce IgA against antigens of *S. equi;* failure of IgA removal mechanisms because of hepatic dysfunction; delayed, defective, or suppressed production of IgG or neutralization; or excess utilization of IgG. In the horse, purpura hemorrhagica has been likened to Henoch-Schönlein purpura, an immune complex–mediated disease of human beings.[275]

The clinical signs of purpura vary and range from a mild transient reaction to a severe and fatal form. Horses with purpura develop pitting edema of the limbs, head, and trunk and petechiation and ecchymoses of the mucous membranes. The vasculitis may cause skin sloughing or affect other sites, such as the gastrointestinal tract, lungs, and muscles. Death may ensue as a result of pneumonia, cardiac arrhythmias, renal failure, gastrointestinal disorders, or severe muscle infarcts.

Confirmation of the diagnosis is by skin biopsy specimen characterized as a leukocytoclastic vasculitis, isolation of the organism, or demonstration of elevated IgA titers to *S. equi* and IgG SeM titers of greater than 1:3200.

Treatment entails administration of intravenous penicillin (20,000 IU/kg four times daily), dexamethasone (0.1 mg/kg intravenously or intramuscularly), intravenous fluids, and antiinflammatory drugs. Treatment may be necessary for more than 7 days. Clinical recovery occurs as the source of the antigen is removed and as the immune response is suppressed. Coincidental with recovery is the production of IgG to *S. equi* antigens.[274]

3. *Guttural pouch empyema and chondroid formation* (see the previous discussion).
4. *Septicemia and the development of infectious arthritis and pneumonia.* These conditions warrant a poor prognosis.[276]
5. *Retropharyngeal abscessation.* This circumstance may cause the horse to develop respiratory distress or dysphagia (or both) and coughing. Endoscopy demonstrates collapse of the nasopharynx, deviation of the larynx, or drainage of purulent material into the nasopharynx when external pressure is applied to the parotid region.[277] Radiographs demonstrate a soft tissue density in the retropharyngeal area, thickening of the roof of the pharynx, reduction in the diameter of the pharyngeal airway, and distortion or compression of the guttural pouches, pharynx, and trachea.[278] Ultrasound of the region—caudal to the mandible, dorsal to the trachea, and between the linguofacial vein and maxillary vein—is used to determine the size and position of the retropharyngeal lymph nodes.[279] The retropharyngeal abscess may rupture into the pharynx and cause a secondary pneumonia (dysphagia) or may rupture dorsally into the guttural pouches.[267,277,278]

De Clercq and colleagues described an ultrasound-guided percutaneous technique for draining abscessed retropharyngeal lymph nodes that, when combined with local and systemic antimicrobial therapy, resolved clinical signs in four horses. When the purulent exudate was too viscous to be aspirated, surgical excision of the abscessed lymph node was performed.[279]

6. *Laryngeal hemiplegia.* This condition occurs when abscessed lymph nodes encroach on the recurrent laryngeal nerve.[280]
7. *Tracheal compression after abscessation of the cranial mediastinal lymph nodes has been reported.* The horse may show respiratory distress or exhibit stertorous breathing. Laryngeal hemiplegia may be an additional complication if the abscess compressing the trachea involves the recurrent laryngeal nerves.[280]
8. *Endocarditis, myocarditis, or cardiac conduction abnormalities.*
9. *Agalactia in periparturient mares.*
10. *Central nervous system abnormalities, including abscess formation and meningoencephalomyelitis.*[269,281,282] Clinical signs depend on the location of the abscess; but for those affecting the cerebrum, one may note circling, altered behavior, blindness, depression, and inappetence. In a report of four cases of brain abscesses, MRI localized the lesion, and a T2-weighted image revealed the abscess surrounded by a hyperintense rim. Additionally, the MRI demonstrated retropharyngeal lymphadenopathy and hyperintense areas within the sinuses.[269] Treatment was not attempted, and culture of the abscesses at postmortem confirmed *S. equi* as the etiologic agent. In a case of *S. equi* meningoencephalomyelitis in a foal, cerebral spinal fluid (CSF) analysis demonstrated an elevated total nucleated cell count and total protein concentration, as well as the presence of gram-positive cocci. *S. equi* infection was confirmed by PCR assay on the CSF.[282]
11. *Myopathies.* Several types of muscle disorders associated with *S. equi* infection have been described. One potentially fatal form is characterized by a vasculitis and infarction of skeletal muscles. In addition to muscle swelling and gait stiffness, horses may exhibit colic and unrelenting pain, necessitating euthanasia. Laboratory data often reveals neutrophilia with a left shift, hyperproteinemia, and hypoalbuminemia. Serum creatine kinase and aspartate transferase activities are markedly increased as a result of muscle inflammation and necrosis. Postmortem examination reveals muscle infarctions, as well as infarcts in the skin, gastrointestinal tract, pancreas, and lungs that are compatible with purpura hemorrhagica. Prognosis is guarded, and horses require treatment with intravenous fluids, antimicrobials, and corticosteroids.[283]

A second type of muscle disorder characterized by acute severe rhabdomyolysis without evidence of infarction or atrophy has been described in Quarter Horses exposed to *S. equi*.[284] Affected horses exhibit stiff gaits, muscle swelling, and recumbency. They also have elevations in neutrophils, fibrinogen, serum creatine kinase, and aspartate aminotransferase. However, on necropsy, pallor to the affected muscles (semimembranosus, semitendinosus, sublumbar, and gluteal muscles) is seen, with no evidence of infarction or muscle atrophy. *S. equi* can be isolated from affected muscles. Horses should be treated with penicillin and dexamethasone.[285]

Control Measures during an Outbreak The clinician should recommend that the following be implemented to reduce transmission of *S. equi* during an outbreak[251,286]:

1. Prevent spread of infection to horses on other premises and to new arrivals immediately by stopping all movement of horses on and off the premises.
2. Identify symptomatic and asymptomatic carriers by sampling nasopharyngeal or guttural pouch regions at weekly intervals and testing for *S. equi* by culture and PCR. Endoscopy of the guttural pouches to facilitate lavage and to inspect the compartments for evidence of abnormalities should be performed.
3. Isolate infectious horses from those screened negative for *S. equi*. Cordon off the isolation area, and have infectious horses looked after by a dedicated staff wearing protective clothing and footgear. Disinfect stalls, aisles, and equipment and water troughs (at least daily).
4. Once clinical signs have disappeared, perform at least three consecutive swabs or lavages for *S. equi* culture coupled with endoscopic examination of the guttural pouches to confirm that horses are noninfectious.
5. Manure and waste feed from infectious animals should be composted in an isolated location. Pastures used to hold infectious animals should be rested for 4 weeks.

Prevention Vaccines currently available include a protein-rich acid- and enzyme-extract product that is administered parenterally (e.g., Strepvax II) and attenuated live *S. equi* products that are administered intranasally (Pinnacle I.N.) or, in Europe, submucosally in the upper lip (Equilis StrepE). None of the vaccines guarantee prevention of strangles in vaccinated horses.

Parenteral (killed) vaccines induce strong serum bactericidal activity, but these antibodies are not necessarily protective because mucosal immunity plays a significant role in the resistance to infection.[287] For naïve horses and foals, two to three doses of the vaccine are administered at 2-week intervals and then boostered annually. Horses with high SeM titers should not be vaccinated.

In contrast to parenteral vaccination, mucosal immunization induces a combination of systemic and local responses that produce a greater variety of immunoglobulin isotypes and specificities that more closely mimic those induced by natural disease. Based on manufacturer's comments, approximately 40% of horses that have been vaccinated with the intranasal product before *S. equi* challenge develop clinical signs of the disease when challenged as compared with 60% of nonvaccinated controls that have been similarly challenged. Although intranasal vaccines are expected to produce fewer adverse reactions than parenteral vaccines, lethargy, inappetence, fever, lymphadenopathy, lymph node abscessation, purpura hemorrhagica, and intramuscular abscesses have occurred after vaccination.[245]

Submucosal vaccines have also been associated with the production of adverse reactions, including neck and mandibular lymph node abscesses.[288] In instances of suspected adverse vaccinal reactions, genetic typing of the isolate is required to confirm that coinfection of a wild type *S. equi* is not responsible for the problem. Attenuated live vaccines should be administered only to healthy afebrile animals free of nasal discharges. For the intranasal vaccine, it is recommended that two doses at 2-week intervals followed by an annual booster be administered. Foals may be vaccinated at 1 to 2 months of age, but vaccination may cause mandibular abscessation. For the submucosal vaccine that is available in Europe, two doses (0.2 ml) of the vaccine are injected at 4-week intervals in healthy horses older that 4 months. Because the duration of immunity by the submucosal vaccine is limited, it is recommended that high-risk horses receive a booster every 3 months, although boosting of horses vaccinated up to 6 month previously in the setting of an outbreak has been shown to improve clinical outcome and extends the usefulness of the vaccine.[250]

One should not administer intranasal (or submucosal) vaccines concurrently with other parenteral injections because of the risk of abscess formation at the site of the intramuscular injection. One should wash one's hands thoroughly after vaccination. Use of the vaccine during an outbreak remains controversial and should be restricted to select horses that are healthy and have not been exposed to horses infected with *S. equi*. Vaccination of horses with an SeM titer of more than 1:1600 may be associated with the development of purpura hemorrhagica. During vaccination, effective immune response still requires 7 to 10 days to develop. Thus protection may not be provided quickly enough during outbreaks. None of the vaccines provide cross-protection against *S. zooepidemicus* infections.

General Control Measures Whenever feasible, new additions to a farm should be isolated from the resident population for a minimum of 4 weeks. Horses should be monitored twice daily for evidence of fever spikes and examined for evidence of nasal discharge and lymph node enlargement. If possible, new additions to the herd while in isolation should be screened (via PCR) for *S. equi*. This assessment may require lavage of the guttural pouches to ensure that asymptomatic carriers have not been introduced to the facility. Measures should be implemented to prevent animal or personnel contact between the new additions and resident horses.

In a recent commentary, Prescott and Timoney (2007) suggested that strangles has all of the characteristics of an infection that should and could be eradicated.[289] These features include (1) infection limited to equids, (2) poor survival in the environment, (3) little to no antigenic variability, (4) availability of a PCR test to detect presence of organism, (5) low prevalence of a carrier state that could be eliminated by local treatment of the guttural pouches, and (6) existence of moderately effective vaccines that could be combined with eradication program. The envisioned eradication program entails making strangles a reportable disease (with agreed outbreak investigation procedures and published findings) and having each horse be issued a health passport that records exposure to strangles (or other infectious disease outbreaks) that could be used to institute movement controls and more rigorous import-export regulations, including providing results of a recent culture or PCR assay on the health passport.

Viral Infections

Viruses of known pathogenicity to the horse (or donkey) that are associated with respiratory tract disease include equine influenza virus (EIV), EHV1, EHV2, EHV4, EHV5, asinine herpesvirus 4 (AHV4), AHV5, equine arteritis virus (EAV), equine rhinitis viruses A (ERAV), equine rhinitis virus B1, 2, and 3 (ERBV1, ERBV2, ERBV3), equine adenoviruses 1 and 2, Hendra virus, and African horse sickness virus.

EQUINE INFLUENZA

Causes The influenza viruses are enveloped viruses with a segmented, single-strand RNA genome belonging to the family Orthomyxoviridae. Based on the internal nucleoproteins and matrix antigens, influenza viruses are classified as types A, B, or C. Types B and C infect only human beings, but type A infects many different species, including human beings, horses, swine, dogs, and fowl.[287] Type A is classified further into subtypes based on the surface antigens, the hemagglutinin (H, which is involved in binding of the virus to the host cell) and neuraminidase (N, which controls release of virus from infected host cells). Two subtypes of equine influenza are recognized as infectious for the horse: subtypes H7N7 and H3N8. Subtype H7N7 was first isolated in Prague in 1956 and has been called equine-1 influenza (A/equine/Prague/56). Subtype 1 is thought to have disappeared from horses worldwide because an isolate has not been confirmed since 1980. Subtype H3N8 was first isolated in Miami in 1963 (prototype) and was designated as equine-2 influenza (A/equine/Miami/63). Several variants of subtype 2 (antigenic drift) were identified and included A/equine/Fontainebleau/79, A/equine/Kentucky/81, A/equine/Saskatoon/90, and A/equine/Newmarket 2 (N2/93), among others.[290-292]

Recent studies of the H3N8 subtype have demonstrated that in the early 1990s, strains diverged into two distinct lineages designated as Eurasian and American (A/eq/Newmarket/1/93-like). In contrast, the oldest H3N8 strains circulating in the 1960s through the 1980s (Miami/63-like, A/eq/Fontainebleau/79-like) apparently became extinct.[293] Results from field observations indicate that the two lineages are sufficiently different that representatives of both lineages should be included in equine influenza vaccines.[294] Compared with the human influenza virus, EIV is relatively stable antigenically, not experiencing major antigenic shifts. This stability has been postulated to result from the shorter lifespan of horses relative to human beings and the lower mutation pressure placed on the EIVs because of low specific antibody titers.[295]

Epidemiology Equine influenza virus, as with the human influenza virus, is highly contagious and is transmitted through the air. It most commonly affects 2- and 3-year-old horses and may be the most common cause of respiratory illness in racehorses. Some racetrack facilities experience influenza outbreaks two to three times within a racing season.[291,292,296] This phenomenon may reflect poor ventilation systems (closed shedrows), lack of adequate immunization protocols, and rapid transmission of the virus from exercise ponies to racehorses.[291] Recent outbreaks in Japan and Australia during the summer of 2007 have raised questions about the failure of quarantine and vaccination to control the spread of disease, especially given the increased air transport of Thoroughbred stallions between the Northern and Southern hemispheres. Specifically, rapid air transport enables horses to arrive within 48 hours of departure, a time that is within the incubation period for influenza.

Although experimental infection of human beings with EIV (subtype 2) is possible, natural infections do not occur.[295] Interspecies transmission of influenza A2 was recently reported in Greyhound dogs, some of which eventually died of hemorrhagic pneumonia.[297] Interspecies transmission of viruses depends on several factors, one of which is ecology. It is unclear what association the dogs that developed influenza had with horses and whether infection resulted from aerosol transmission or from consumption of untreated meat (including lungs) from an infected horse.[298] A second factor that facilitates interspecies transmission is the presence of appropriate viral receptors (sialic acid linkages) in the host respiratory tract epithelium that are recognized by the viral hemagglutinin (H). When compared with equine influenza, canine isolates had undergone four amino acid modifications in the H antigen, and these changes are postulated to facilitate attachment of the virus to the canine epithelium.[297] Third, for successful interspecies transmission, the virus must be able to replicate efficiently within the cells of the new host for continued propagation and transmission. It is possible that recent equine H3N8 influenza strains have enhanced virulence and their transmission to dogs are now just being recognized.[298]

The reservoir of EIV between epizootics remains unknown. Some researchers speculate that the virus is maintained in the horse population itself and that asymptomatic carriers shed virus when stressed. Alternatively, the virus may be harbored in other species such as birds, which are asymptomatic but shed the virus in their feces.[295]

Pathogenesis The incubation period for equine influenza is 1 to 3 days. The virus infects and replicates primarily in respiratory epithelial cells of the upper respiratory tract with minimal pulmonary involvement. Healthy respiratory tract epithelium is ciliated and contains mucus that forms a protective layer over the cell surface. The mucus normally acts as a mechanical barrier between air and tissue and contains antibody and protein substances that deter the attachment of viral particles to the epithelium.[299] Neuraminidase activity of the viral particles alters the efficiency of the mucociliary apparatus, allowing the virions to attach via hemagglutinin antigens to the sialic acid moieties of the epithelial cells. The epithelial cell internalizes the bound virus and surrounds it with an endosome. However, in the mildly acidic conditions of the mature endosome, the H antigen protein becomes activated and promotes fusion of the viral and cellular membranes, leading to release of the nucleocapsid into the cytoplasm.[300] Release of replicated virions from the epithelial cell is controlled by the neuraminidase glycoproteins, enabling the cycle to continue.[301] Cell necrosis and patchy areas of desquamation follow viral replication within the respiratory tract epithelium. Exposure of irritant receptors causes hypersecretion of submucosal serous glands and further damage to the mucociliary apparatus. Inflammation leads to massive lymphocyte infiltration and edema. Recovery of the normal epithelial architecture can require more than 6 weeks.[302]

Humoral and cellular immunity are important in providing protection against viral disease, and the hemagglutinin and neuraminidase molecules are the main targets of the humoral immune responses against influenza. Thus small antigenic changes in the epitopes of these molecules enable the virus to evade the protective humoral immune responses of the host. IgA blocks viral penetration but is not cidal; certain IgG isotypes, IgGa and IgGb, opsonize the virus particles and enhance phagocytosis.[303] After natural infection, complete clinical and virologic immunity against reinfection with an homologous strain persists for at least 32 weeks, and partial protection is still evident after 1 year.[301] Exposure to the A2 subtype does not protect against infection with the A1 subtype, and vice versa.

Clinical Signs Clinical signs of influenza appear 3 to 5 days after exposure to the virus. Severity of signs is related to the strain of the virus and the immune status of the individual.[301] Horses exhibit a sudden onset of fever (103° to 105° F), which may be biphasic; a serous or mucopurulent nasal discharge (or both); anorexia; depression; and a dry, deep cough. Some horses exhibit myalgia, myositis, and limb edema and are thus reluctant to move.[295] A mild form of azoturia (myoglobinuria) occurs in some cases. One may find mandibular lymphadenopathy, as well as endoscopic evidence of pharyngitis and tracheitis. Bronchitis with minimal changes in lung sounds (wheezing) may occur. The severity of lower airway disease appears to be dependent on prior exposure (vaccination).[304] From experimental studies, inoculation with A/equine-1 produces a milder (subclinical) syndrome unless the animal is stressed before infection, whereas A/equine-2 usually generates the typical clinical signs. The course of the infection usually lasts 2 to 10 days in uncomplicated cases. Exercise exacerbates the clinical signs.[305] Secondary bacterial infections may occur, and donkeys and mules appear to have greater susceptibility to secondary infections than do horses.[306] Horses remain infectious for 3 to 6 days after the last signs of illness. In young foals and in donkeys or mules, influenza infections can be severe, producing signs of viral interstitial pneumonia and respiratory distress that may lead to death within 48 hours.[307,308] (See the later discussion on interstitial pneumonia.)

Clinical Pathology Horses may initially exhibit lymphopenia followed by monocytosis.

Diagnosis The clinician may diagnose equine influenza by the following methods:

1. *Detection of the virus.* Based on studies of influenza outbreaks, viral culture and isolation alone from nasopharyngeal swabs appears to be the least-sensitive method for diagnosing influenza,[291] probably because the chances of viral isolation are greatest when samples are collected within the first 24 hours.[296] A stall-side assay (Directigen Flu-A test, Becton Dickinson, Franklin Lakes, N.J.) allows rapid detection of influenza antigen and an immediate diagnosis.[302] PCR detection of viral nucleotides obtained from nasopharyngeal swabs enables a diagnosis of influenza infections within 48 hours of sample submission. In a natural outbreak of influenza in 11 horses at a riding school, a diagnosis was confirmed by viral isolation in five horses and by ELISA and by Directigen assay in five and seven horses, respectively, and by PCR in nine horses.[309] In testing horses for import quarantine, the Directigen or PCR should prove extremely useful in detecting impending or prior infections.
2. *Serologic testing.* Several diagnostic methods for detecting influenza virus antibodies in the horse are available and include complement fixation, hemagglutination inhibition, single radial hemolysis, viral neutralization, and enzyme immunoassay.[310] Acute and convalescent serum samples are needed to establish a definitive diagnosis, and although viral neutralizing antibodies may be detectable within a week of infection, up to 28 days may pass before a rise in hemagglutination titers is detected.[295] Serologic testing has been considered to be a sensitive method for diagnosing influenza outbreaks, although in one epidemic, approximately 24% of horses with clinical signs of influenza failed to seroconvert.[291]
3. *Pulmonary imaging.* In both experimental and clinical infections of influenza, pulmonary abnormalities can develop, although whether these infections result directly from the viral or from secondary bacterial infections is uncertain. The primary ultrasonographic alterations include mild lung consolidation and peripheral pulmonary irregularities and the absence of pleural effusion.[304,305] Thoracic radiographs, especially of foals with equine influenza, demonstrate an interstitial pattern. (See also the later discussion on interstitial pneumonia.)

Treatment Neuraminidase inhibitors such as oseltamivir phosphate and zanamivir have been used in human medicine for the treatment of influenza and have recently been investigated for use in equine medicine.[311,312] After oral administration, the phosphate salt of oseltamivir is absorbed and undergoes hepatic metabolism to the active drug oseltamivir carboxylate. When evaluated in vitro, both drugs (oseltamivir carboxylate and zanamir) inhibited the plaque-forming abilities of 12 equine influenza viral isolates tested.[311] In a small experimental challenge study, prophylactic treatment of horses with oseltamivir phosphate (2 mg/kg orally once daily) 24 hours before influenza challenge and continuing for 5 additional days, shortened the duration of pyrexia and viral shedding compared with the control group.[312] Administration of oseltamivir phosphate (2 mg/kg orally twice) approximately 2 days after influenza challenge (when horses were pyrexic) also reduced the magnitude of pyrexia and the duration of viral shedding relative to controls. Based on pharmacokinetic studies (2 mg/kg orally),[313] the investigators recommended that the dosing interval for oseltamivir should be less than 10 hours to maintain viricidal plasma levels of the drug. Because of its poor bioavailability, zanamivir is administered as an inhalant in human medicine. No studies have been conducted investigating the efficacy of inhaled zanamir in horses.

In the absence of a readily available and economically feasible source of neuraminidase inhibitors, treatment of affected horses is symptomatic with the primary objectives being to maintain adequate hydration and to prevent undue stresses. Nonsteroidal antiinflammatory drugs may be indicated to reduce the fever, eliminate the myalgia, and improve the appetite. The risk is that the owner will return the horse to strenuous exercise before the horse has rested a sufficient time. Horses that suffer severe infections may be unfit for competition for 50 to 100 days after infection. During the infection, frequent examinations of the respiratory tract are indicated to detect the development of secondary complications such as pneumonia, pleuropneumonia, and myocarditis.

Prevention Regular vaccination significantly reduces the population at risk. In fact, the suggestion has been made that at least 70% of the equine population (horses, ponies, and donkeys) should be vaccinated to prevent epidemics of influenza.[314] Dead and live vaccines are commercially available. The former include products containing killed whole virus (either A2 alone or with A1), subunit proteins (purified H or N proteins), and DNA plasmids. Inactivated whole influenza or subunit vaccines are typically administered intramuscularly (primary and secondary booster are required for naïve animals) and induce a humoral immune response characterized by serum antibodies that are able to neutralize the virus. However, the antibody response is short lived, and infection may occur in the case of low antibody concentrations or when a significant mismatch exists between the vaccine strain and the infecting strain of influenza.[301] In one study, the use of a killed vaccine reduced neither the rate of respiratory tract disease nor the severity of clinical scores compared with nonvaccinates.[315] The failure of vaccines to prevent infection is commonly known as *vaccine breakdown* and is most commonly reported in young racehorses. It has been attributed to variable vaccine potency, poor response to vaccination, antigenic drift, or a combination of these factors. This vaccine failure may also be a function of the number of boosters a horse receives before infection and of the strain of A2 contained within the vaccine. The transmission of influenza infection may be facilitated by vaccination that successfully attenuates the clinical signs but fails to prevent viral shedding.[316]

DNA vaccination is typically administered at mucosal sites or in the skin. However, based on experimental studies,[317,318] this approach requires multiple injections, reducing its field applicability; DNA vaccination can result in the in vivo expression of antigenic proteins that stimulate both humoral and cellular immune responses. A DNA vaccine for equine influenza is currently not commercially available.

The live influenza vaccines are products that contain the virus-based vector product or the temperature-sensitive (Ts) or cold-adapted virus. A live recombinant vaccine is commercially available in Europe (ProteqFlu, Merial Animal Health, Ltd). It contains a canarypox virus to express equine influenza hemagglutinin genes derived from both American (Kentucky/94) and Eurasian (Newmarket/2/93) strains. Thus far, the vaccine has shown promise in reducing clinical signs and nearly completely suppressing viral shedding in vaccinated ponies that were challenged with influenza. The vaccine induces both humoral and cellular immune responses.[294,319-321] The manufacturer's recommendation is to administer a series of three intramuscular injections beginning when the horse is 5 to 6 months of age, repeated 4 to 6 weeks later, and again 5 months after the first injection. Annual boosters are administered.

A second type of live commercially available influenza vaccine contains a cold-adapted, Ts virus that was derived from the wild-type A/eq/Kentucky/1/91 (H3N8) strain. After a single intranasal immunization, ponies were fully protected from clinical signs of disease when challenged with the parental influenza virus 5 weeks later.[301,322,323] Only 20% of vaccinates shed virus when challenged 5 weeks after the vaccination. Little data are available concerning the performance of the virus-based vector or modified-live vaccines during influenza outbreaks.

Vaccinating foals with killed, subunit, or attenuated virus vaccines may be ineffective because of interference by maternally derived antibodies.[301,324,325] Although the use of virus-based vectors for foals could circumvent the neutralizing effect of maternal antibody on vaccine efficacy, a complete understanding of the maturation of the foal's cell-mediated immune response is lacking. Thus most vaccination protocols are focused on enhancing maternal antibody production and providing secondary passive protection of the foal.

Some undesirable side effects of vaccination occur, including fever, depression, pain, swelling at the vaccination site, and muscular stiffness, but these adverse effects usually resolve within 1 or 2 days.[296]

Sequelae Secondary bacterial pneumonia and pleuropneumonia are potential complications that may follow viral respiratory diseases in horses that have not been rested adequately before being returned to training or that have undergone other potentially stressful events such as long trailer rides. Myocarditis, pericarditis, and cardiac arrhythmias are other possible sequelae to influenza infections. Interestingly, during an influenza outbreak in the United Kingdom in 2003, two unvaccinated Thoroughbred horses were purported to develop neurologic signs—ataxia, dog-sitting, and leaning. Postmortem examination attributed the neurologic deficits to an influenza-associated encephalopathy or encephalitis. However, this complication seems relatively rare.[326]

EQUINE HERPESVIRUSES

The Herpesviridae family of viruses contains a significant number of pathogens that have been grouped into alpha-, beta-, and gamma-herpesvirus subfamilies based on morphologic, biologic, and genomic characterizations.[327] The hallmark of these enveloped DNA viruses is their ability to establish lifelong infections achieved by a state of latency from which the virus may reactivate from time to time with recurrence of infections and transmission to other susceptible hosts.[328] In Equidae, several pathogenic herpesviruses in the alpha and gamma subfamilies have been identified.[329] In horses these include three alpha-herpesviruses, EHV1, EHV3, and EHV4, and two gamma-herpesviruses, EHV2 and EHV5. Note that EHV4, formerly called EHV1 subtype 2, serologically cross-reacts with EHV1 but is genetically distinct from that virus.[330] Similarly, EHV2 and EHV5 also cross-react with each other but are genetically distinct.

In donkeys, six herpesviruses have been identified thus far. AsHV1, an alpha-herpesvirus, was isolated from a donkey foal with vesicular lesions on its muzzle. The dam had similar lesions on the external genitalia and udder. This virus is related to, but genetically distinct from, EHV3. AsHV2 was isolated from the blood of a healthy donkey. Another herpesvirus, AsHV3, was isolated from donkeys after treatment with steroids. AsHV3 has the greatest genetic similarity to EHV1, suggesting that AsHV3 is a member of the alpha-herpesvirus subfamily. When experimentally inoculated with AsHV3, donkeys develop afebrile rhinitis. Three additional gamma-herpesviruses, AsHV4, AsHV5, and AsH6, have been detected in lung tissues of donkeys dying from acute interstitial pneumonia.[327,331] (See the later discussion on interstitial pneumonia.) However, to date, virus isolation of AsHV4, AsHV5, or AsHV6 has not been successful despite repeated inoculation attempts on a variety of primary and continuous cell lines.[332]

EQUINE HERPESVIRUS TYPES 1 AND 4

Causes Both viruses have a double-stranded DNA genome of 145 to 150 kbp that, based on sequence analysis, contains 76 unique genes for either virus.[333] The degree of DNA sequence homology between EHV1 and EHV4 varies between 55% and 84%; the degree of amino acid sequence identity varies between 55% and 96%.[334]

Although the host range of EHV1 was once considered to be restricted to the horse, EHV1 has been isolated from cattle, fallow deer, antelopes, alpacas, llamas, and camels.[335-337] In cattle at least, genomic analysis of the herpesvirus isolates failed to demonstrate any specific mutations that permitted interspecies transmission.[338] EHV1, in addition to causing respiratory disease, causes abortions, neonatal deaths, and myeloencephalitis. In horses that develop neurologic signs, the majority of the EHV1 isolates exhibit a single nucleotide polymorphism within the gene encoding the viral DNA polymerase (open reading frame 30).[339]

EHV4 is associated predominantly with respiratory disease in young horses, although the virus has been isolated from older horses exhibiting signs of acute febrile respiratory disease.[340] EHV4 only sporadically causes neurologic disease, abortion, or neonatal deaths.[341-344] In a study conducted by Van Maanen and colleagues (2000), 4% of 254 abortions were caused by EHV4.[345]

Epidemiology EHV1 and EHV4 may persist within a herd because of recrudescence of latent infections during periods of stress or immunosuppression. Dexamethasone or cyclophosphamide administration is a reliable reactivation stimulus for viral shedding in experimental studies.[346] For several years, the site of viral persistent was unknown. However, in a study of 40 abattoir horses, EHV1 and EHV4 were detectable by PCR methods in the bronchial lymph nodes of 88% of the horses examined. Of the trigeminal ganglia examined in nine of the horses, one was found to contain only EHV1, four had detectable EHV4 in the ganglia, and three had evidence of EHV1 and EHV4.[347] EHV2 also was isolated from all of the horses examined, leading some researchers to speculate that EHV2 activates the promoter gene of EHV1, although this has not been proven.[348] In addition to the clinical trials, experimental studies of EHV1 and EHV4 also have provided data supporting the fact that lymphoid and neural tissues are sites of viral latency.[346,348] Interestingly, in an investigation of a respiratory disease outbreak in young foals (7 to 17 months of age) attributed to EHV4, Pusterla, Leutenegger, Wilson, et al. (2005) were unable to demonstrate that EHV4 had established latency in the nasal mucosa or peripheral blood leukocytes within 28 days after developing of clinical signs.[349]

Some studies demonstrate that foals are infected during the first 5 weeks after birth and that horizontal spread continues up to and even after the time of weaning.[350-352] In a recent study of weanling foals with clinical signs of respiratory disease, EHV1 was not detected by PCR in the nasopharyngeal swabs from any of the foals, and EHV4 was identified in the nasopharyngeal swabs in two foals with respiratory disease.[353] Using diagnostic detection tools of seroconversion and viral isolation (nasopharyngeal swabs), Dynon, Black, Ficorilli, et al. (2007) investigated the prevalence of EHV1 and EHV4 in 20 Thoroughbred or Standardbred racehorses with acute febrile respiratory disease. In 3 of the 20 horses (ages 3, 4, and 6 years), EHV4 was diagnosed concurrently by viral isolation, PCR, and increasing antibody titers.[340] The fact that EHV4 was not detected in the other 17 clinically ill horses suggested to the investigators that EHV4 was not simply present in the nasal cavity as a consequence of a highly contaminated environment. For this same sample population, Dynon and colleagues found no evidence of EHV1 infection using either viral isolation techniques or serologic data. In another study, the prevalence of EHV1 was evaluated in a Thoroughbred breeding and racehorse training farm that historically had experienced abortions caused by EHV1. Despite numerous samplings of the asymptomatic horses (broodmares, foals, stallions, and racehorses) over the 9-month study period, EHV1 was detected only in the nasal secretions from 3 of 75 horses.[352] It was not detected (by PCR) in the whole blood samples from any of the horses.

Immunity to EHV1 or EHV4 is short lived (3 to 5 months); thus most horses are reinfected during their breeding or racing careers. Reexposure usually results in mild or inapparent infections, except in the case of broodmares in which reinfection may lead to abortion in the last trimester. Immunity after abortion is generally of longer duration, and in the field, repeat abortions rarely occur in the same mares. No clear relationship exists between gestational age or the level of virus-neutralizing antibody and the incidence of virus-induced abortion.[354] Perinatal disease characterized by weakness and respiratory distress is usually evident within 18 to 24 hours of birth, with foals dying within 24 to 72 hours.[355]

Pathogenesis Infection by EHV1 occurs via inhalation of the virus or contact with infected tissues (e.g., fetus, placenta). The virus is delicate and does not survive in the environment; thus close contact appears to be important for transmission.[355] Kydd, Smith, Hannant, et al.[356] have suggested that EHV1 enters the upper respiratory tract and, in the absence of mucosal antibody, immediately infects the epithelial lining of the nasopharynx and tonsils. Based on in vitro data, researchers thought that EHV1 attaches to the cell via the viral glycoproteins gB and gC.[357] After attachment, an interaction between a putative receptor enables fusion between the envelope of the virion and the cellular membrane. In vitro data also demonstrate that EHV1 can enter the cell by a second nonclassical endocytotic pathway. Both pathways require activation of an intracellular kinase, ROCK1, a potential site for therapeutic interventions. Once membrane fusion is completed, the capsid is released into the cytoplasm and transported to the nucleus. Subsequent events depend on whether EHV1 becomes a productive or limited infection. Productive infection results in the intercellular spread of EHV1 through susceptible cells (including leukocytes) in the stroma until the vascular or lymphatic endothelium becomes infected. Thereafter, infection spreads via leukocyte adhesion to the infected endothelium, leading to the development of cell-associated viremia. As a result of viremia and of inhalation of viral particles, the virus disseminates to the lower respiratory tract. In a limited infection, infected cells are phagocytized, and viral antigens are processed and presented to lymphocytes in mucosal lymphoid nodules or lymph nodes. The studies of Burrell[144] and Sutton, Viel, Carman, et al.[358] have demonstrated lower respiratory tract involvement in which hyperemia and mucous accumulations develop 2 to 12 weeks after the initial infection. EHV1 also has a tropism for lymphocytes and is reported to cause immunosuppression. Other clinical signs, such as abortion and neurologic disease, are a sequelae of the cell-associated viremia in which the virus is inaccessible to antibodies.[333]

Modes of transmission of EHV1 other than through the respiratory route have been investigated. Viral DNA has been isolated from semen collected from clinically normal stallions that were experimentally infected. However, venereal spread resulting in infection of susceptible mares has not yet been proven.[359] In another experimental investigation, 8-day-old equine embryos were inoculated for 24 hours with EHV1 before being washed 10 times according to guidelines established by the International Embryo Transfer Society. The investigators detected viral DNA (via PCR) and found evidence of cytopathic effects in 7 of the 10 embryos, suggesting a potential risk for transmission of EHV1 to recipient mares.[360]

The pathogenesis of EHV4 has not been investigated completely by experimental transmission studies but may be similar to that of EHV1. For example, EHV4 can multiply in the epithelia of the nasal cavities, pharynx, trachea, and bronchioli, with subsequent spread to the regional lymph nodes.[333] In contrast to EHV1, EHV4 generally does not cause viremia, and hence abortions and neurological disease are rare.[361]

Clinical Signs EVH1 and EHV4 produce similar respiratory-related signs, but for either virus, mild or subclinical infections are common. Clinical signs of rhinopneumonitis appear 1 to 3 days after infection and are indistinguishable from influenza. Horses are febrile and exhibit a cough and a serous nasal discharge, which may become mucopurulent with secondary bacterial infections. Horses develop rhinitis, pharyngitis, and tracheitis detectable endoscopically. A severe disseminated EHV1 infection that caused fever, depression, respiratory distress, and eventual death has been described in yearlings and 2-year-old horses.[362,363] This form is characterized by vasculitis, hemorrhage, and edema in the lung and has been attributed to a pulmonary vasculotropic form of EHV1. Perinatal disease characterized by weakness and respiratory distress is usually evident within 18 to 24 hours of birth, with foals dying within 24 to 72 hours.[355] With EHV4 infections, researchers believe that during the 6- to 8-month period after weaning, the majority of foals experience repeated infections with EHV4. The majority of such infections may go unnoticed.[345]

Clinical Pathology An epidemiologic survey by Mason, Watkins, McNie, et al.[364] during an outbreak of EHV1 infection on a racetrack in Hong Kong documented a monocytosis in infected horses (>500 cells/μl) during the first 5 days of clinically apparent infections. In experimental infections of EHV1, a decrease in neutrophils and monocytes occurs on day 3 after infection, but the absolute values of both cell types remain within normal limits.[358]

Diagnosis

1. *Viral isolation.* The virus has been recovered from peripheral blood mononuclear cells for up to 2 weeks after the infection or from nasopharyngeal swabs that have been collected in viral transport media. However, nasopharyngeal swabs should be obtained in the early febrile phase of the disease and transported to the laboratory as soon as possible in a sterile, cold-transport medium.[333] Viral isolation in cell culture is limited by time constraints and the need to confirm viral identity by immunostaining or PCR. In contrast, direct PCR on clinical materials is rapid and enables distinction between EHV1 and EHV4.[365] Recent work reveals poor sensitivity of a real-time PCR assay in detecting EHV1 DNA in buffy coat leukocytes.[366] A PCR assay of materials obtained from nasopharyngeal swabs is more sensitive.[352] However, because of the short duration of nasal shedding, viral DNA may not be detected, and thus diagnosis should also be supported by serologic assessment. A PCR has been developed that can distinguish between neuropathogenic and nonneuropathogenic strains of EHV1.[367]
2. *Serologic diagnosis* is via virus neutralization, immunoassay, complement fixation, or a radial immunodiffusion enzyme assay that detects antibodies against EHV1. A fourfold change in antibody titer is suggestive of infection.[368] A commercially available ELISA (Svanovir, Svanova Biotech AB, Uppsala, Sweden) based on the structural differences of the viral glycoprotein G of EHV1 and EHV4 distinguishes between antibodies against these two viruses.[352]
3. *Postmortem examination* of foals that died from EHV1 or EHV4 infection revealed interstitial pneumonia, pleural and peritoneal effusions, hypoplasia of the thymus and spleen, focal necrosis of the liver, and viral inclusion bodies within the hepatic parenchyma. Similar pathologic findings are observed in aborted fetuses. Immunohistochemistry, in situ hybridization, and PCR can be used on tissues to establish the diagnosis of EHV1.

Treatment Data available from experimental or clinical trials using antiviral drugs (nucleoside analogs) for the treatment of equine herpesvirus infections are limited. The key protein target for many of the antiviral compounds is the virus-encoded DNA polymerase. The activity of the second-generation nucleoside analogs such as acyclovir, valacyclovir (its prodrug), or ganciclovir is dependent on the drug being phosphorylated by the viral thymidine kinase. During latent infections, the virus does not express genes encoding for viral proteins (thymidine kinase, DNA polymerase), thus latent virus is unaffected by any of the conventional nucleoside analogs.[328] Nevertheless, in human medicine, routine use of these antivirals can suppress recurrent infections in patients for periods up to 10 years.

In a recent investigation, the in vitro activity of six nucleoside analogs in reducing plaque number or plaque size associated with EHV1-infected cells was examined.[369] The investigators used three different abortigenic and three neuropathic strains of EHV1. They found that the ED_{50} (defined as the 50% effective concentration for inhibition of plaque formation) of ganciclovir was less than that of acyclovir and that no differences in susceptibility of the six different EHV1 strains to these two drugs existed. Based on their studies, the researchers in the investigation suggested that an effective concentration for ganciclovir was 0.1 μg/ml and that of acyclovir was at least 2.0 μg/ml. Given that ganciclovir would be quite expensive to use clinically in the horse, it was more likely that acyclovir would be used. Indeed, during outbreaks of EHV1 involving neurologic disease or neonatal deaths, acyclovir has been administered at doses ranging between 8 to 16 mg/kg orally three times daily to 20 mg/kg orally three times daily.[370,371] The efficacy of acyclovir in treating respiratory diseases has not been demonstrated, and its poor bioavailability (3%) when given orally[372] may preclude it from achieving the requisite viricidal plasma levels (>2 μg/ml). Even when administered intravenously at 10 mg/kg,[373] the in vitro data suggest that the drug would have to be given either as a constant infusion or as a single treatment eight times a day to achieve plasma concentrations between 1.7 and 3.0 μg/ml.[369] In humans, the major reported adverse effect of parenteral administration of acyclovir is renal toxicity caused by precipitation of the acyclovir crystals in the renal tubules when maximal solubility is exceeded.[374]

Because of its improved bioavailability, interest in the acyclovir prodrug valacyclovir has prompted recent pharmacokinetic investigations. Garré, Shebany, Gryspeerdt, et al. (2007) reported that when valacyclovir was administered to horses at 20 mg/kg, its bioavailability was much improved, as compared with acyclovir (26%). However, plasma concentrations were maintained above the EC_{50} value for only 1.5 to 2.0 hours. Based on computer modeling, the investigators suggested dosing valacyclovir at 40 mg/kg orally three times daily in an effort (1) to maintain plasma concentrations greater than 1.7 μg/ml during the entire treatment interval and (2) to exceed plasma concentrations of 3.0 μg/ml during 30% of the treatment interval.[374] One potential drawback of acyclovir (or valacyclovir) is the development of viral resistance in strains lacking thymidine kinase, although this circumstance, to date, has not been realized.

Another antiviral drug, (s)-1-[(3-hydroxy-2-phosphonyl methoxyl)-propyl] cytosine (HPMPC), has been shown to be efficacious when given before EHV1 challenge in naïve foals but has not been used clinically in North America.[375]

Because evidence of immunosuppression during herpetic infections exists, the clinician may consider administering broad-spectrum antimicrobials for 7 to 10 days to affected horses. In addition, horses should be rested for 4 to 6 weeks before exercise training commences.

Management Recommendations during an Outbreak During an outbreak of EHV1, measures should be implemented to reduce the potential sequelae, such as abortion and neurologic disease. Affected animals should be isolated, and no horse should be permitted to leave the property or track until 3 weeks after recovering from the last clinical sign.[333] Stalls should be cleaned thoroughly of contaminated materials and then disinfected.

Prevention Commercially available vaccines include two single-component inactivated (killed) vaccines that are marketed for the prevention of EHV1-induced abortions in pregnant mares and respiratory infections (Pneumabort K, Fort Dodge Animal Health; Prodigy, Intervet Inc.). Three intramuscular doses are recommended for primary immunization followed by an annual booster. Multicomponent inactivated vaccines include products such as Prestige (Intervet Inc.) or Calvenza (Boehringer Ingelheim) that contain both EHV1 and EHV4 or Fluvac Innovator (Fort Dodge Animal Health) that contains influenza A1 and A2 with EHV1 and EHV4. A modified-live product (Rhinomune, Pfizer Animal Health) is also commercially available, although it is not recommended for use in pregnant mares. None of the products provides complete protection against clinical disease.

On the premises with confirmed clinical EHV1 infections, booster vaccination of horses that are likely to have been exposed to EHV1 is not recommended. Booster vaccinating nonexposed horses and horses that would come onto the premises is rational. This approach assumes that vaccination induces an anamnestic and not a primary response. The question of whether vaccination during an outbreak could induce nasal shedding (and thus preclude identification of clinically infected horses during an outbreak) was investigated. In a pilot study, 14 horses were vaccinated with either a killed product (Pneumabort K + 1b) or a modified-live product (Rhinomune). The investigators found that EHV1 DNA was not detected by PCR in nasopharyngeal swabs or in whole blood samples obtained from horses at 1-week intervals for 4 weeks after the vaccination.[376] These results suggested that in healthy unstressed horses, one should not detect vaccine DNA or reactivated latent EHV1 DNA after the vaccination.

A recent product that has been marketed to prevent EHV1 or EHV4 (or both) infections during disease outbreaks or during times in which the horse is stressed is Zylexis (Pfizer Animal Health), an inactivated *Parapox ovis* virus was purported to have immunomodulator activity. The manufacturer's recommendation are to administer the preparation to healthy horses 4 months of age or older via a series of three intramuscular injections given on days 0, 2, and 9. No scientific data establishing the efficacy of Zylexis have been published by independent groups.

EQUINE HERPESVIRUS 2

EHV2 is a slowly replicating virus, often known as *equine cytomegalovirus*. It is believed to establish latency in B-lymphocytes but can be found in lymphoid and neural tissue.[377]

Epidemiology EHV2 is endemic in horse populations tested worldwide with approximately 90% of horses tested being seropositive.[378,379] Because the prevalence of seropositivity and the magnitude of these titers are not different between healthy and diseased horses, opinions vary as to the true pathogenicity of EHV2.[142,380] In surveys of healthy adult horses, viral DNA can be recovered from the peripheral blood leukocytes in the majority of animals, with frequencies ranging between 68% to 71%[381] to 89%.[332] The virus has been isolated from nasopharyngeal swabs obtained in young racehorses with PLH, implicating EHV2 in the development of this condition.[144] The suggestion has been made that most foals are exposed to EHV2 at 2 to 3 months of age and shed the virus for 2 to 6 months until a humoral antibody response develops and eventually is associated with low viral recovery.[380] EHV2 has been isolated from 2- to 3-month-old foals during outbreaks of pneumonia in Hungary, Japan, Australia, New Zealand, and the United States.[380,382-385] In a longitudinal study of 27 foals in a Hungarian stable that experienced respiratory disease outbreaks, peripheral blood leukocytes and nasopharyngeal swabs were obtained from young foals until they reached 23 weeks of age.[381] By 6 weeks of age, 93% of the nasopharyngeal swabs were positive for EHV2 DNA, and by 8 weeks, 100% of the peripheral blood leukocytes were positive for EHV2 DNA. In some investigations of respiratory disease outbreaks in foals, EHV2 was the sole infectious agent isolated from the respiratory tract, whereas in other outbreaks, bacterial agents—*S. zooepidemicus* and *Rhodococcus equi*—complicated the pneumonitis.[384] This finding has led some researchers to speculate that if the foals are stressed or infected with a large dose of the virus during a period in which maternal antibodies are waning, then the virus may invade the cells of the immune system and cause further immunosuppression. Blakeslee, Olsen, McAllister, et al.[142] reported a dose-related immunosuppression after in vitro infection of lymphocytes with EHV2, and this effect has been documented in vivo using a rabbit model.

Pathogenesis After natural exposure, EHV2 is recoverable from nasal and nasopharyngeal swabs; from the kidney, bone marrow, spleen, mammary gland, salivary gland, vagina, tracheal mucus, neural tissue; and from the cornea and conjunctiva.[378,386] Leukocytes and lymph nodes draining the respiratory tract are major reservoirs of EHV2 DNA.[378]

Clinical Signs In foals that are experimentally infected with EHV2, pharyngitis and lymphoid hyperplasia develop, implicating the EHV2 as a causative agent of chronic lymphoid hyperplasia in young horses.[142] However, the role of EHV2 in the natural production of pharyngitis or lymphoid hyperplasia remains uncertain. The role of EHV2 in causing keratoconjunctivitis also remains equivocal, with clinical investigations both supporting[387] and refuting its involvement.[379]

Diagnosis EHV2 diagnosis depends on isolation of the virus, serologic evidence of an active viral infection, and the presence of clinical signs. EHV2 is highly cell associated but more slowly cytopathic than the equine alpha-herpesviruses. Its slow growth in culture may hinder its recognition if alpha-herpesviruses are present, increasing the time required for laboratory diagnosis.[353] Diagnosis is aided by PCR methods.

Treatment Treatment is symptomatic. Efficacy of antiviral agents has not been examined in EHV2 infections.

Prevention No commercial vaccine is available.

EQUINE HERPESVIRUS 5

Causes Originally classified as EHV2, examination of restriction endonuclease profiles of some slowly growing equine herpesviruses eventually led to its identification as a separate DNA virus in the gamma-herpesvirus subfamily.

Epidemiology The initial isolates of EHV5 were obtained from peripheral blood leukocytes and nasal swabs from Australian horses,[388] but the virus has been subsequently identified in horses in Switzerland, Germany, New Zealand, and the United States.[381,389,390] In a longitudinal study of mares and their foals that were monitored from birth to 6 months of age, latent EHV5 infections were detected in the peripheral blood mononuclear cells of 88% of the foals at 6 months of age. The presence of the virus was not associated with respiratory disease in that study.[390]

Pathogenesis Little is known about the natural course of disease in horses infected with EHV5. The initial isolates of EHV5 were from horses with upper respiratory tract disease and, similar to EHV2, has been implicated in the production of lymphadenopathy, immune suppression, malaise, and respiratory tract disease.[391]

Clinical Signs In a retrospective study of 24 horses with clinical signs and radiographic evidence of interstitial lung disease, EHV5 was detected by PCR in 79% of the paraffin-fixed lung samples obtained from these horses.[392] However, causality between EHV5 and multinodular interstitial lung disease remains to be established because EHV5 can be isolated from peripheral blood mononuclear cells (PBMCs) or nasal swabs of 24% to 33% of healthy horses.[381,389]

Diagnosis The diagnosis is confirmed by viral isolation and identification of the virus by PCR. Serologic tests are problematic because EHV2 and EHV5 share considerable cross-reactivity in ELISA and radioimmunoprecipitation because of common epitopes.[391]

Treatment Treatment is supportive if indicated. (See the later section on interstitial pneumonia.)

Prevention No vaccine is currently available.

EQUINE VIRAL ARTERITIS

Causes Equine arteritis virus (EAV), an enveloped single-stranded RNA virus, is a member of the family Arteriviridae (genus *Arterivirus*, order Nidovirales). EAV is genetically similar to corona viruses (also a member of Arteriviridae) but has a dissimilar viral structure and complement-fixing antigen.[393] The virus contains six envelope proteins (E, GP2b, GP3, GP4, GP5, and M) and a nucleocapsid protein (N). The major neutralization determinants of EAV are expressed by GP5, and although considerable variation in the sequence of this protein exists in field strains of the virus, only one serotype of EAV (the Bucyrus strain) has been found.[394] All strains of EAV evaluated thus far are neutralized by polyclonal antiserum raised against this highly virulent Bucyrus strain.[395] The virus, which has a worldwide distribution, may cause sporadic and sudden death in foals, abortion in mares, and mild or subclinical infections in adult horses.[393]

Epidemiology Before the 1984 epizootic of equine viral arteritis (EVA) in Kentucky, little attention was paid to this virus.[396] Most infections were assumed to be transmitted by inhalation until the important role of venereal transmission was demonstrated in those outbreaks. The virus is maintained in the equine population by long-term and short-term stallion carriers. The duration of the carrier status ranges between several weeks to years. Testosterone is essential for maintenance of persistence because long-term infections do not occur in colts exposed to the virus before the onset of peripubertal development or in mares.[396-398] During the carrier state, the virus is present solely in the reproductive tract, principally in the ampulla of the vas deferens. In the carrier stallion, genetic and antigenic variation (diversity of viral isolates) is generated in the course of persistence.[395] Primary exposure to the virus is presumed to be via the venereal route. Susceptible mares bred to carrier stallions almost always become infected with EAV. Viral shedding into the respiratory tract allows secondary horizontal transmission of the virus to occur. The latter type of transmission (aerosol or fomites) would be more typical of that occurring in young racehorses at training facilities. The mode of transmission to neonatal foals is not known and might entail both transplacental infection during late gestation or inhalation during or after the birth.[399,400]

In addition to the outbreak in Kentucky in 1984, several other outbreaks have been reported in North America, Europe,

Australia, New Zealand, and South Africa.[395] A significant difference in seropositivity to EAV exists not only between countries, but also among the horse breeds within a given country. Approximately 84% of Standardbreds and 93% of Austrian Warmblood stallions have circulating antibodies to EAV, whereas less than 5% of Thoroughbred and less than 1% of Quarter Horses are seropositive.[401] No evidence has been found of any breed-specific variation in susceptibility to EAV infection or in establishment of the carrier state, thus the number of actively shedding carrier stallions likely determines the prevalence of EAV infection in the individual horse breeds.[395] The virulence of the strains of EAV associated with individual horse breeds may not be constant, and those shed by carrier Standardbred stallions are often very highly attenuated and cause minimal if any disease in susceptible horses (regardless of breed).[395]

Pathogenesis After intranasal challenge (aerosolization), the virus invades the respiratory tract epithelium and the alveolar macrophages. By 72 hours after infection, replicating viruses are detectable in the bronchopulmonary lymph nodes, endothelium, and circulating macrophages. With venereal transmission (by natural cover or by artificial insemination), the virus can be isolated from swabs of the rectal and vaginal mucosa during the febrile periods. Dissemination of the virus by hematogenous routes allows infection of mesenteric lymph nodes; spleen; liver; kidneys; nasopharyngeal, pleural, and peritoneal fluid; and urine.[396] By 6 to 8 days after infection, the virus has localized within the endothelium and medial myocytes of blood vessels, where it causes a necrotizing arteritis, a panvasculitis.[393] Thus the clinical manifestations of EVA reflect vascular injury with increased permeability and leakage of fluid.[395] The vascular lesion may be caused by a direct cytopathic effect of the virus on the endothelium and medial myocytes, from the effects of anoxia or thrombosis induced by cell damage, or from virus-induced macrophage-derived vasoactive and inflammatory cytokines.[395] In neonatal foals, the virus, by virtue of its ability to cause lymphoid depletion in the spleen and lymph nodes, enhances the neonate's susceptibility to secondary bacterial infections.[400]

Clinical Signs The vast majority of EAV infections in equids (horses, donkeys, and mules) are inapparent or subclinical, but occasional outbreaks of EVA occur that are characterized by persistent infections in stallions, influenza-like illness in adult horses (with nasal and ocular discharge), abortion in pregnant mares, and fatal interstitial pneumonia and enteritis in neonatal foals.[395] The variation in clinical signs may be a function of host factors, such as age and immune status, and virus factors, including the virulence, the amount of infective virus, and the route of infection.[402] Thus very young, very old, debilitated, or immunosuppressed horses are predisposed to severe EVA. The incubation period ranges between 3 to 14 days (6 to 8 days if transmitted venereally). In the acute disease, horses are febrile (105° F) for 1 to 5 days, anorectic, depressed, and may cough. They may exhibit a serous nasal discharge, congestion of the nasal mucosa, mandibular lymphadenopathy, conjunctivitis, lacrimation, and, less frequently, corneal opacification. Edema of the sheath, scrotum, ventral midline, limbs, and eyelids occurs secondary to the vasculitis. Other signs may include respiratory distress, stiffness, soreness, diarrhea, icterus, skin rash on the neck, and papular eruptions on the inside of the upper lip. Most adult horses recover uneventfully; mortality rarely, if ever, occurs in natural outbreaks of EVA. Note that the highly virulent horse-adapted Bucyrus strain of EAV, which does cause high mortality in healthy adult horses, is not representative of field strains of the virus and is best regarded as a laboratory strain.[395]

Abortions occur between 10 to 34 days after exposure (during the third to tenth months of gestation), but the mechanism is not known. Abortion can occur with or without preceding clinical evidence of infection.[403] EVA has not been associated with teratologic abnormalities in fetuses or foals.

Neonates may die suddenly or develop severe respiratory distress followed by death.[396,399] In such cases, the dam of the affected foal may be completely asymptomatic.[393,400]

Clinical Pathology Infection causes leukopenia, lymphopenia, and thrombocytopenia.

Diagnosis In North America, EVA is a reportable disease. Although the virus may persist in the buffy coat for up to 36 days after infection, viral isolation can be difficult.[402] Samples to be submitted for viral isolation include citrated blood samples, nasopharyngeal and conjunctival swabs, vaginal swabs, and semen from an infected stallion.[404] PCR enhances viral detection and specificity, but the serum should also be submitted for detection of antibodies. Virus neutralization, complement fixation, immunodiffusion, and immunofluorescence are techniques used to demonstrate changes in antibody titers. A fourfold or greater rise in titer or a change in status from seronegative to seropositive may indicate a recent infection. Postmortem examinations of aborted fetuses demonstrate edema, excessive pleural fluid, and petechiation on the mucosal surfaces of the respiratory and gastrointestinal tracts, but focal necrosis of the liver or intranuclear inclusions are not features of the disease.[394] Foals that die acutely of EVA exhibit interstitial pneumonia characterized by a predominant macrophage infiltrate, hyaline membrane formation, and vasculitis of the small muscular arteries.[400] Infective virus particles or viral antigen can be identified by immunofluorescence in the small muscular arteries of the lung, kidney, spleen, thymus, and heart.

Treatment Treatment is symptomatic with the primary objectives being to keep the horse well hydrated and to provide analgesics (nonsteroidal antiinflammatory drugs) as needed. Fever in stallions can lead to sperm damage and temporary infertility; thus one should administer nonsteroidal antiinflammatory drugs. The horses should be isolated for 3 to 4 weeks to minimize the chances of transmission.

Prevention EAV infections are readily prevented through serologic and virologic screening of horses coupled with sound management practices that include appropriate quarantine and strategic vaccination.[395] Vaccination of seronegative stallions with a commercially available modified-live vaccine (ARVAC, Fort Dodge Animal Health) is credited with preventing the establishment of carrier states in the stallion or with further increases in the carrier state during the 1984 epizootic in Kentucky. (A modified-live vaccine is licensed for use in the United States and in Canada, whereas a killed vaccine [Artervac; Fort Dodge Animal Health] is available in the United Kingdom, Ireland, France, Denmark, and Hungary.[405]) For example, in the Kentucky outbreak, stallions were bred only to mares that were vaccinated or were seropositive from previous natural exposure to EVA. After vaccination, clinical immunity was found to develop rapidly and to last for 1 to 3 years.[396] Some vaccinates develop mild febrile reactions and transient lymphopenia, and the vaccine virus can be sporadically isolated from the buffy coat for 7 days (but occasionally up to 32 days). Thus mares should be vaccinated 3 to 4 weeks before breeding to an EAV carrier stallion and isolated.[403] Vaccinated stallions do not shed the virus in either semen or urine. Thus vaccination of prepubertal colts prevents them from becoming persistently infected carriers and is central to any effective control program. Vaccination is not recommended for pregnant mares or for foals younger than 6 weeks. Fetal infections have been documented after murine leukemia virus (MLV) vaccination of pregnant mares.[405] Passively derived antibodies to EAV decrease to undetectable amounts by 8 months postpartum for foals born to seropositive mares. Vaccination should be effective at this time if necessary.[406] Although the current MLV vaccine is effective, a recombinant subunit vaccine coexpressing the two major envelope proteins of EAV (GP5 and M) that experimentally has been shown to effectively induce neutralizing antibodies and protective immunization, may find commercial success.[405]

EQUINE RHINITIS VIRUSES

Causes Formerly termed *equine rhinoviruses,* at least four serotypes of equine rhinitis viruses have been identified to date. These viruses have been isolated from horses in the United Kingdom, mainland Europe, the United States, Australia, and Japan. Serotype 1, formerly called equine rhinovirus 1, has been renamed equine rhinitis A virus (ERAV) and is now reclassified as a member of the genus *Aphthovirus,* family Picornaviridae. The reclassification is based on (1) the homology of the nucleotide sequence of the ERAV genome with that of foot-and-mouth disease virus, (2) the physicochemical properties of ERAV, and (3) the production of viremia and persistent nasal, urine, and fecal shedding after ERAV infection.[407] Serotype 2, formerly called equine rhinovirus 2, has been renamed equine rhinitis B virus 1 (ERBV1) and has been reclassified to the genus *Erbovirus* (from **e**quine **r**hinitis **B v**irus), family Picornaviridae.[408] A third serotype, formerly designated P313/75 or equine rhinovirus 3 has also been assigned to the genus *Erbovirus*. It is now called equine rhinitis B virus 2 (ERBV2).[409] A fourth antigenically distinct, acid-stable equine picornavirus has also been assigned to the genus *Erbovirus* and is called equine rhinitis B virus 3 (ERBV3).[410,411] This virus had been originally classified with the ERBV1 isolates and exhibits weak serologic cross-reactivity with antibodies against ERBV1.[411]

Clinical Signs Infection of horses with ERAV causes acute fever, nasal discharge, coughing, anorexia, pharyngitis, laryngitis, and mandibular lymphadenitis.[412,413] Infection produces moderate increases in the neutrophil-to-lymphocyte ratios (from 50:49 in healthy horses to 57:43 in infected horses) and in plasma fibrinogen.[413] The importance of ERAV as a cause of respiratory disease has not been recognized previously because clinical signs may be mild and because viral isolation is difficult.[414] The incubation period is 3 to 8 days, with shedding of viral particles from pharyngeal secretions, urine, and feces being a feature of the infection. Young horses are infected more commonly than older horses. For example, the prevalence of serum neutralizing titers in 24-month-old Thoroughbreds just entering a training facility had increased from 18% to 63% when sampled 7 months later.[415] Other studies have found prevalence rates of neutralizing antibodies to ERAV to range between 73% to 90%.[413,416] ERAV has also been isolated from horses without clinical evidence of respiratory disease.[415] Equine rhinovirus A has a broad host range that includes rabbits, guinea pigs, monkeys, and human beings, although the virus does not seem to spread horizontally in each of these species. Intranasal inoculation of a human volunteer with ERAV resulted in severe pharyngitis, lymphadenitis, fever, and viremia.[412] Experimental and epidemiologic evidence of ERAV infection of human beings exists. High antibody titers were found in the sera of 3 of 12 stable workers, whereas no ERAV antibody was found in the sera of 159 non–stable workers.[417] In a serologic survey of 137 samples obtained from mixed-practice veterinarians, only 3% were seropositive for ERAV, suggesting that the risk of infection is low.[416] One can diagnose ERAV infections by serologic testing (fourfold changes in titers between acute and convalescent samples) or by PCR identification of the virus in nasopharyngeal swabs.[414]

Equine rhinitis viruses assigned to the genus *Erbovirus* are also respiratory tract pathogens. In a survey involving horses with acute respiratory disease, researchers isolated ERBV from 30% of the horses sampled. Of the 28 horses from which the virus was recovered, a serologic diagnosis was made in only 6 horses. Researchers attributed the low diagnostic rate to the difficulty of initially collecting samples during the acute phase: Antibody levels rise rapidly from day 6 after infection and peak between days 14 and 18.[418] Thus, in contrast to ERAV, viral isolation may be the more successful diagnostic method. In a survey involving Australian horses, serum neutralizing antibodies against ERBV1 were detected in 77% of the 2- to 3-year-old Thoroughbred horses in training and in nearly 94% of stable horses aged 10 to 22 years.[415] Interestingly, approximately 4% of mixed-animal veterinarians develop serum neutralizing antibodies against ERBV1, suggesting that, similar to ERAV, humans are at low risk for becoming infected with this virus.

The clinical significance of ERBV2 (formerly P313/75) is currently uncertain. ERBV2 has been isolated from one horse with a 6-day history of intermittent fever that began 4 days after an umbilical hernia operation and castration[419] and from another horse with signs of acute febrile respiratory disease and high titers against ERBV2.[340] In the epidemiologic survey conducted by Black, Wilcox, Stevenson, et al. (2007), 89% of 2- to 3-year-old Thoroughbreds at a training facility in Australia exhibited serum neutralizing antibodies to ERBV2. This prevalence rate contrasts with that found in older stable horses of 45%.[415]

The fourth rhinovirus, ERBV3 (originally classified as ERVA), was initially isolated from horses with acute respiratory disease. Additional studies are required to ascertain the severity of clinical disease that occurs with ERBV3 infections, as well as the seroprevalence in equine populations. No vaccine is currently available against ERAV or ERBV1, 2, or 3.

EQUINE ADENOVIRUSES

Two separate nonenveloped DNA viruses belonging to the family Adenoviridae have been isolated from horses and are recognized as equine adenovirus 1 (EADV1) and EADV2.[420]

EADV1 is endemic in most horse populations, and the belief is that most foals acquire the infection during the suckling period from the mares. Disease develops if maternal antibodies wane or if active immune responses are impaired. Susceptible foals include Arabian foals with combined immunodeficiency or Fell pony foals with an undefined immunodeficiency.[421] The virus replicates in the respiratory tract and can cause conjunctivitis, rhinitis, and bronchopneumonia. In one recent survey, EADV1 was detected by PCR in the nasal swabs of 40% of hospitalized foals and in 58% of healthy control foals.[422]

EADV2 has been isolated from the lymph nodes and feces of foals with upper respiratory tract disease and diarrhea.[423,424] For a more detailed description, the reader is referred to the section on foal pneumonia.

EQUINE HENDRA VIRUS

Cause Originally called equine morbillivirus but later renamed equine Hendra virus (HeV), this enveloped RNA virus is a prototype of a new genus, *Henipavirus,* within the subfamily Paramyxovirinae.[425] HeV is a pleomorphic (spherical or filamentous) structure, the genome of which exceeds 18 kbp. The latter encodes for eight different proteins, including the cell-attachment (G) and fusion (F) proteins that protrude from the viral envelop.[426]

Epidemiology The virus was first recognized as a causative agent of severe respiratory disease in Thoroughbred racehorses in a suburb of Brisbane, Australia, called Hendra.[427] During the 1995 outbreak in which 13 of 20 horses died or were euthanized, two humans also became infected, one fatally. However, in a retrospective analysis of postmortem tissues, it was later determined that in 1994, HeV was the cause of death of two other horses and a person assisting with their necropsy in Mackay, a city approximately 800 kilometers from the Brisbane area. Since that time, several additional outbreaks have occurred in Australia involving fewer numbers of horses or humans. In Australia, most equine cases have been documented to occur in the spring or summer and involve horses that were housed near food or the roost trees of flying foxes. Based on testing of wildlife, flying foxes (fruit bats, *Pteropus* spp.) were subsequently shown to be the source of infection of the horses. Despite the presence of antibody to HeV in fruit bats throughout their geographic range in Australia, suggesting that infection is quite common in that species,[428] HeV disease in horses in Australia has thus far been uncommon and sporadic.

Pathogenesis Natural and experimental infection in horses suggests an incubation period of 8 to 16 days or 4 to 10 days, respectively.[427,429] The means by which HeV infects horses is still unknown. The virus can be isolated from the oral cavity and urine of some infected horses but not from rectal or nasal swabs.[425] One hypothesized route of infection is via consumption of pasture or feed contaminated with bat urine, aborted bat fetuses, or reproductive fluids.[425] (The birthing season of the bats is consistent with the timing of the HeV cases that were recorded in horses between August and January.) In experimental infections, horses can be infected by eating material contaminated with the virus. Transmission to horses from exposure to infected cat urine is also possible. Horse-to-horse or horse-to-human transmission has been suggested to occur by direct contact with frothy nasal discharges, urine, blood, or pleural fluids of a viremic horse. No human-to-human transmission has been reported.

In experimental infections, horses kept in stalls adjacent to an infected horse fail to become infected, suggesting that the virus is not highly contagious and that aerosol transmission is inefficient. One additional hypothesis regarding transmission of the virus from bats to horses involves the Australian paralysis tick *Ixodes holocylus*. This tick is a blood feeder that feeds both on bats and horses (as well as other mammals, including humans).[430]

The mode of viral attachment and cell infectivity of HeV is different from that of other paramyxoviruses. It does not engage the sialic acid–containing receptors for attachment but rather depends on the viral G protein to interact with a cell-surface glycoprotein called ephrin-B2.[426] The ephrin-B2 receptors are highly concentrated on endothelial cells (hence the tropism of the virus for those cells), as well as neurons and smooth muscle cells. Fusion of the viral membrane is accomplished by the F glycoprotein. This process not only enables the virus to gain entrance into the cell but is also responsible for the formation of syncytial giant cells.[426] The virus replicates within the upper and lower respiratory tract epithelium and causes an interstitial pneumonia.

Clinical Signs Horses acutely develop signs of respiratory distress that are characterized by fever (>104° F), depression, tachycardia, tachypnea, sweating, poor capillary refill, and abnormal lung sounds (caused by pulmonary edema). Neurologic deficits such as ataxia, head pressing, and recumbency can also occur.[431] The time between the onset of signs until death is usually between 1 and 3 days.[425] Humans die as a result of respiratory and renal failure and relapsing encephalitic disease.[430]

Diagnosis Differential diagnoses to be considered in affected horses include heart failure, acute African horse sickness, highly virulent influenza, and plant intoxications.[431] Serologic testing (ELISA or virus neutralization tests) can be used to detect antibody titers in affected horses (or humans). Gross abnormalities in the lungs of affected horses are highly suggestive of but not pathognomonic for the disease. Histopathologic findings include alveolar edema, hemorrhage, lymphatic dilation, and vasculitis of pulmonary capillaries and arterioles. Within the walls of the blood vessels are the characteristic syncytial giant cells that contain cytoplasmic inclusion bodies.[425] From tissues, the virus can be isolated in cell culture, visualized by electron microscopy, and confirmed by indirect immunoperoxidase test, immunofluorescence test, or PCR.

Because of the susceptibility of humans, the high virulence of the virus, and the absence of therapeutic modalities and vaccines, HeV is classified as a biosecurity level 4 pathogen and requires the highest level of caution and preparedness when working with the tissues obtained from infected animals.[426] Such precautions include wearing effective eye, nose, and mouth protection from fomites and aerosols, complete covering of the body with plastic overalls, and double gloving with gloves tied by adhesive tape to the cuffs of the overalls.[431]

Treatment No antiviral agent exists that is effective against Hendra virus. The outbreak of the disease in Brisbane was controlled by a stamping-out program involving slaughter of all known infected horses, quarantine of premises, controls on the movement of horses within a defined disease control zone, and serologic surveillance to determine the extent of infection.[431]

Vaccination No vaccine is available.

Prevention In endemic areas, one should avoid confining horses to paddocks that contain roost trees for bats. The virus is susceptible to several different disinfectants, including 3% Lysol for 3 minutes at 20° C, 1% glutaraldehyde for 10 minutes at 20° C, irradiation, or formaldehyde fumigation.

AFRICAN HORSE SICKNESS VIRUS

Cause The African horse sickness virus (AHSV) is a double-stranded RNA nonenveloped member of the family Reoviridae (genus *Orbivirus*). It is morphologically similar to other orbiviruses, including bluetongue virus and equine encephalosis virus. Nine antigenically distinct serotypes of AHSV have been found: serotypes 1 to 8 are highly pathogenic for horses (90%-95% mortality rate), whereas infection with serotype

9 is associated with a mortality rate of 70%. Serotypes 1 to 8 are typically found only in restricted areas of sub-Saharan Africa, whereas type 9 is more widespread, being responsible for nearly all epidemics outside of Africa. The one exception to this report was in the 1987 to 1991 Spanish-Portuguese outbreaks resulting from infection with AHSV4.[432] The virus is transmitted by hematophagous arthropods, the most important being *Culicoides* spp. midges. Because of its severity and its ability to expand rapidly and without apparent warning out of its endemic areas, AHS is classified as a reportable disease by the World Organization for Animal Health, formerly known as the Office International des Epizooties (OIE).

Epidemiology Zebras are considered to be the natural vertebrate host and reservoir of the AHSV and thus play a role in its persistence in Africa. The single exception to this observation involves serotype 9, which is found in West Africa where zebras no longer occur.[432] Indeed, in the early and mid-1960s, serotype 9 spread across the Middle East (Saudi Arabia, Syria, Lebanon, Jordan, Iraq, Turkey, and Cyprus) and Central Asia (Iran, Afghanistan, Pakistan, and India) and later through North Africa into Spain. AHS was believed to have been effectively eradicated after its appearance in these regions. Then, in 1987, after the import of zebras from Namibia into Madrid, Spain again experienced an outbreak of AHS attributed to serotype 4. Unfortunately, because the climate was sufficiently moderate to permit overwintering of the virus or vector, outbreaks continued into 1991. *Culicoides imicola* is considered to be the most important field vector for AHSV, and although this biting midge is present in southern Europe (Spain, Portugal, Italy, Greece, and southern Switzerland), concern exists that with global warming and climatic change, the vector may extend its habitat to northern Europe.[433,434] Even more worrisome is that *Culicoides variipennis,* the North American vector of bluetongue virus, is an efficient laboratory vector of AHSV,[435] suggesting that should viremic equids gain entrance into North America, transmission of the virus could occur.

Although AHSV typically affects equids, dogs are experimentally susceptible to infection via ingestion of infected horse meat. This route is not considered to be an important means of transmission of the virus to susceptible equids.

Pathogenesis Once the virus gains entry into the host, it replicates in the regional lymph nodes before being spread hematogenously to most organs and tissues in the body. In the lungs, spleen, lymphoid tissues, and in certain endothelial cells, a secondary viral replication phase ensues. The incubation period from inoculation to secondary viremic phase is approximately 9 days.[432]

Clinical Signs Clinical signs arise as a result of increased capillary permeability and secondary circulatory impairment leading to serous effusion and hemorrhage in various tissues and organs. Four clinical syndromes of AHS infection have been identified (listed in order of decreasing severity): pulmonary or acute form, mixed form (cardiopulmonary), cardiac or subacute form, and the mild (horse sickness fever) form.[436] In the acute form, horses initially develop a fever (up to 107° F) and severe respiratory distress characterized by tachypnea, base-wide stance, extended neck, nostril flaring, and coughing. Frothy white and, occasionally, blood-tinged fluid may be evident at the nostrils. The course of the disease is usually 4 to 5 days. The mortality rate for this form is 95%. In the cardiac or subacute form, horses exhibit fever (104° F) and subcutaneous edema in the supraorbital fossa, head, neck, and chest regions. The conjunctiva may be congested, petechial hemorrhages may be evident, and the horse may develop signs of colic. Mortality rates may exceed 50%. The mixed form, the most common syndrome, represents a combination of the two syndromes, with death occurring within 3 to 6 days of fever. Mortality rates are 70% for this form. The AHS fever form typically affects mules, donkeys, zebras, and partially immune horses and is characterized by a mild to moderate fever and the development of edema in the supraorbital fossa. Affected animals recover.

Diagnosis Differential diagnoses include EVA, purpura hemorrhagica, equine infectious anemia, and babesiosis (early stages). Lesions are not pathognomonic for AHS, thus viral isolation or identification confirms the diagnosis. Samples of whole blood collected in an anticoagulant (preferably ethylenediaminetetraacetic acid) during the febrile phase or of pulmonary, lymphoid, or splenic tissues collected at postmortem enable viral isolation. AHSV can be detected in tissues by PCR or by ELISA.[432]

Treatment Specific therapy for this viral infection is not available, and treatment of individual affected horses is supportive and symptomatic. (See respiratory distress section later in this text.)

Prevention This noncontagious disease is spread by bites of infected midges, *Culicoides* spp. Control should be directed at restricting import of infected animals, slaughter of viremic animals to prevent them from serving as a source of the virus, reducing vector access to susceptible animals (by stabling), and implementing vector control by eliminating breeding sites of *Culicoides* and applying insecticides in and around stables and directly to equids.[432,437]

Polyvalent-attenuated vaccines (containing serotypes 1, 2, 4 and 2, 6, 7, 8) are available in Africa, where most animals are vaccinated twice in the first and second years of life and annually thereafter. A monovalent-attenuated vaccine containing serotype 9 is available for use in West Africa and outside of sub-Saharan Africa. The live vaccines are not recommended for use in pregnant mares.

TRACHEAL DISORDERS

Definition Tracheal disorders are not common in the horse. Tracheitis often accompanies viral upper respiratory tract diseases (see viral infections) and is characterized by areas of hyperemia and epithelial desquamation on endoscopy. Tracheitis may also develop after smoke inhalation or barn fires. Tracheal perforation or rupture can occur as a result of trauma. Tracheal compression may result from extraluminal masses such as streptococcal abscesses or neoplasms such as lymphosarcoma or lipoma. Intraluminal obstructions may follow fibrotic stricture formation secondary to trauma, tracheostomy, or pressure necrosis from inflated cuffs of endotracheal tubes or may be caused by granulomatous reactions within the trachea.[438] Foreign bodies, such as twigs, may be inhaled.[439] Tracheal collapse may occur as a congenital defect in miniature horses and ponies.[440]

Clinical Signs Clinical signs of tracheal disorders include subcutaneous emphysema and harsh tracheal sounds. Tracheal perforation can lead to pneumomediastinum and pneumothorax. Horses with viral infections or with tracheitis secondary to fires may have chronic and persistent coughing, bilateral nasal discharge, and a foul odor. Mild manipulation of the trachea may induce paroxysmal coughing.

Diagnosis A thorough physical examination or endoscopic evaluation of the trachea will identify these disorders.

Radiographs may aid in the visualization of foreign bodies, as well as in the detection of a concomitant pneumonia, pneumomediastinum, or pneumothorax.

Treatment Treatment is directed toward the primary cause. Primary inflammation after viral infection is not treated unless a persistent fever and a secondary bacterial tracheitis and pneumonia develop (see later discussion). In horses with tracheitis and pneumonitis secondary to smoke inhalation, a tracheostomy may be indicated to circumvent swollen soft tissues of the nasopharynx and to aid in the removal of casts and airway debris in the large airways. Foreign bodies may be retrieved by endoscopy snare but may require a tracheotomy to retrieve them if the endoscope is not long enough. In the adult horse, a 2-m endoscope is necessary to reach the level of the carina located at the fifth to sixth intercostal space. Extraluminal masses require careful drainage or excision, with the potential for spread of infection into the mediastinum. Minor tracheal tears usually resolve within 48 hours and may be managed conservatively. Large tears should be managed surgically with débridement and repair of the defect. If complete rupture occurs between tracheal rings or trauma is extensive, then tracheal resection and anastomosis is indicated.[441,442] Rupture of the trachea may require a temporary tracheotomy distal to the rupture to ensure patency of airflow. Broad-spectrum antimicrobial therapy may be indicated, especially if the mucociliary clearance mechanism is compromised. Complications such as subcutaneous emphysema, cellulitis, and pneumomediastinum usually resolve over 2 weeks. Horses with tracheal defects have a poor to guarded prognosis for return to athletic potential.

EMERGENCY TRACHEOSTOMY

An emergency tracheotomy may be necessary in horses with acute airway obstruction of any origin. Common indications include arytenoid chondritis, strangles, and anaphylactic reactions. The procedure is most readily performed in the standing horse. A site on the ventral midline at the junction of the proximal and middle third of the neck is selected and the trachea palpated between the paired sternothyrohyoid muscles. If time allows, the area is prepared for surgery, and the skin and subcutaneous tissues are infiltrated along the midline with local anesthetic. A 10-cm skin incision is made along the midline. The subcutaneous tissue and paired sternothyrohyoid muscles are separated bluntly until the trachea can be seen. A curved hemostat is placed on the midline and used to retract the musculature laterally to the left. A stab incision is made into the trachea between two tracheal rings and extended to the tracheal midline. This procedure is repeated on the right side so that the incisions connect. It is important to reflect the muscles and to avoid extending each incision beyond the midline to prevent inadvertent transaction of the common carotid artery or jugular vein. Removing a tracheal ring is not necessary for this emergency procedure.

A tracheostomy tube is placed in the incision to provide an airway. Two types of tubes are in common use. The older style metal tracheostomy tube is inserted in two pieces, locks, and is self-retaining. This tube has the advantage of not occluding the trachea if its lumen becomes blocked. The other type of tube is made of a synthetic material (commonly silicon) and has an inflatable cuff. The tube should be inserted with the lumen down (toward the lungs) and secured with umbilical tape to skin sutures and around the neck. The cuff should not be inflated because doing so will occupy the space around the tube and lead to airway obstruction should the tube's lumen become occluded with inflammatory exudate. Barrier cream should be placed below the surgical site to prevent serum scaling of the skin.

NORMAL LUNG

ANATOMY

The lungs of the horse differ from those of other domestic species in that they lack deep interlobar fissures and distinct lung lobes. Superficially, however, the left lung consists of a cranial and caudal lobe, whereas the right lung contains a cranial, an intermediate, and a caudal lobe.[443] The intrathoracic trachea bifurcates into the right and left mainstem bronchi at the level of the fifth or sixth intercostal space and enters the hilum of each lung. At its division from the trachea, the right bronchus assumes a straighter, more horizontal position relative to the left bronchus, a configuration that may predispose the horse to develop right-sided pulmonary disorders. Each bronchus divides into lobar, segmental, and subsegmental bronchi with the eventual formation of bronchioles. In the distal part of the bronchial tree, the terminal bronchioles lead into poorly developed respiratory bronchioles or open directly into alveolar ducts.[443,444] The tracheobronchial lining consists of tall columnar, pseudostratified epithelium interspersed with serous and goblet cells. The goblet cells and the underlying submucosal mucous glands function to produce mucus consisting of an outer gel and an inner sol layer.[445] Mucus serves to prevent epithelial dehydration, contains protective factors that guard against infectious agents, and is an integral part of the mucociliary apparatus. The rapid beating of the cilia moves mucus and any particulate matter to the pharynx to be swallowed. Approximately 90% of material deposited on the mucinous layer is cleared within 1 hour.

Ciliated cells decrease in frequency with successive divisions of the airways so that at the level of the bronchioles the epithelium is composed predominantly of low ciliated and taller nonciliated Clara cells.[446] Glands are also absent at this level. The bronchiolar epithelium becomes contiguous with that of the alveoli, which are characterized by two distinct cell types. Type I pneumocytes cover most of the alveolar surface with thin cytoplasmic extensions 0.2 to 0.5 μm thick.[445] Type II cells are considered to be stem cells, replacing the type I cells when damaged. Type II cells are cuboidal and contain the characteristic lamellar cytoplasmic inclusions thought to contain surfactant components. Surfactant is a complex mixture of phospholipids, surfactant-specific proteins (SP-A, -B, -C, and -D), and neutral lipids that functions to lower alveolar surface tension (SP-B, SP-C) and to enhance innate immune defenses (SP-A, SP-D). Age-related differences in the phospholipid components of surfactant exist. The concentrations of phosphatidylglycerol (a marker of lung maturity) are significantly lower in the bronchoalveolar lavage fluid (BALF) of term foals as compared with adult horses.[447]

Lymphocytes are scattered throughout the pulmonary epithelium, are associated with the bronchioles and bronchi, and occur in discrete nodules or patches.[448] These cells, along with alveolar macrophages, provide an integral component of the pulmonary immune surveillance system. Macrophages are derived from blood monocytes via the interstitium and are cleared continuously from the alveoli. They are the predominant cell type recovered from the bronchoalveolar lavage in normal horses (see Table 9-1). Pulmonary interstitial macrophages are able to ingest particles introduced within the pulmonary circulation rapidly.[449] The ability of these macrophages to localize antigenic particles within the pulmonary vasculature may predispose the equine lung to development of acute pulmonary inflammation (e.g., during endotoxemia).

Additional cells within the lung parenchyma include subepithelial and free mast cells. These cells bear IgE on their cell surface and release biogenic amines in response to specific antigen stimulation. They appear to be important in the pathogenesis of several equine pulmonary disorders, including anaphylaxis and lungworm infections.

Tracheobronchial secretions consist of substances secreted from mucous and serous glands, as well as serum transudates. The principal component of the secretions is water, with approximately equal amounts of protein, carbohydrate, lipid, and inorganic material. Contained within the protein fraction of the tracheobronchial secretions are albumin, IgA, IgG (the predominant immunoglobulin in the lower lung), lysozyme, lactoferrin, haptoglobulin, transferrin, and complement components.[445]

Vascular Supply

The lung has two sources of blood flow. The major source of blood is the pulmonary circulation, a low-pressure, low-resistance system that serves primarily to deliver blood to the alveoli for participation in gas exchange and secondarily to provide nutrients to the alveolar constituents. The distribution of the pulmonary arterial flow to the various lung regions depends largely on mechanical forces: gravity and pulmonary arterial, pulmonary venous, and alveolar pressures.[450] In the standing horse, a vertical perfusion gradient of the lung has been demonstrated,[451] the most dorsal part of the equine lung being less well perfused than the ventral dependent regions. The distribution of pulmonary blood flow is also influenced by vasoactive compounds such as catecholamines, histamine, and eicosanoids and by changes in alveolar oxygen and carbon dioxide. Alterations in pulmonary vascular resistance may help match ventilation with perfusion and optimize gas exchange.

The bronchial circulation, the second source of blood flow to the lungs, provides nutrient support to the lymphatics and vascular and airway components. Bronchial circulation provides arterial blood to the pleural surface and anastomotic connections with the alveolar capillary bed derived from the pulmonary circulation.[444] The magnitude of the anastomotic flow depends on the relative pressure in the bronchial and pulmonary microvasculature and on the alveolar pressure. Thus, in the dorsal part of the lung where pulmonary arterial flow is poor, blood flow from the bronchial circulation may be favored.[452] The degree of anastomotic bronchial blood flow through the alveolar capillaries increases with systemic arterial hypoxemia and alveolar hypoxia.[450] The bronchial circulation undergoes hypertrophy (angiogenesis) in response to inflammatory pulmonary diseases such as chronic bronchitis, bronchiolitis, and bronchiectasis.

Innervation

The autonomic nervous system supplies innervation to the pulmonary structures. This nervous system influences (1) airway smooth-muscle tone, (2) secretion of mucus from the submucosal glands, (3) transport of fluid across the airway epithelium, (4) permeability and blood flow in the bronchial circulation, and (5) release of mediators from mast cells and other inflammatory cells.[453] In the horse, the autonomic nervous system can be classified functionally into three categories: (1) parasympathetic, (2) sympathetic, and (3) nonadrenergic noncholinergic (NANC) pathways.[454] The vagus nerve is an integral component of the parasympathetic and NANC systems. The vagus nerve not only contains the efferent fibers of these pathways, which help alter airway resistance, lung volume, and compliance, but also contains the afferent fibers, the central input of which regulates the pattern of breathing. Stimulation of the parasympathetic fibers within the vagus nerve (i.e., the efferent limb) releases acetylcholine from the postganglionic fibers and combines with the muscarinic receptors of the airway smooth muscle to cause bronchoconstriction. Nonetheless, because atropinization (antagonism of muscarinic receptors) does not normally change airway resistance, the parasympathetic system appears to exert little influence on resting airway tone in the healthy horse.[455] However, vagal efferents are important in reflex bronchoconstriction during pulmonary disease.

As described previously, the vagus nerve also contains afferent nerve fibers that transmit information detected by three types of pulmonary mechanoreceptors: (1) the slowly adapting receptors, (2) the rapidly adapting receptors, and (3) the nonmyelinated C fibers. The receptors relay information to the central respiratory neurons located within the ventral medulla and pons. Changes in breathing depth and frequency occur in response to mechanical deformations or chemical stimulation of these receptors. Thus these receptors mediate the tachypneic breathing pattern that occurs in response to inhalation of irritant substances. Stimulation of these receptors also influences airway smooth-muscle tone,[456] inducing reflex bronchoconstriction in response to inhaled irritants.

In the lung, α- and β-adrenergic receptors mediate sympathomimetic effects. Postsynaptic fibers course from the sympathetic ganglion to airway smooth muscle where released norepinephrine interacts with α- and β-receptors. Postganglionic sympathetic fibers also innervate the parasympathetic ganglia. The released norepinephrine inhibits cholinergic neurotransmission.[454] However, numerous β_2-adrenergic receptors are distributed throughout the pulmonary parenchyma that lack innervation by the sympathetic fibers. Circulating catecholamines are probably important in activating these receptors and in causing subsequent bronchodilation. Interestingly, β_2-adrenergic stimulation does not alter airway diameter in the healthy horse[457] but does increase airway caliber in horses with recurrent airway disease. β-Agonists also promote ion transport and water secretion across human airway epithelium (in vitro) and may cause similar effects in vivo in the horse. This effect would benefit mucociliary clearance by increasing the sol component of the mucus. In addition, β-agonists stimulate surfactant secretion by type II pneumocytes, inhibit antigen-induced mast cell degranulation, and modulate cholinergic neural transmission.[453] Such effects remain to be demonstrated in the horse, however.

α-Adrenergic receptors also exist in the equine lung, but their stimulation induces bronchoconstriction only in horses with reactive airway obstruction and not in normal horses.[458] This finding suggests that, in health, these receptors are probably unimportant in the regulation of bronchomotor tone.

An additional autonomic pathway, the NANC inhibitory system, has been demonstrated in the equine lung, and its fibers course within the vagus nerve.[454] Although the mediators involved in neural transmission have not been identified definitively, some researchers speculate that vasoactive intestinal peptide or peptide histidine isoleucine or both may be the neurotransmitters.[459] Stimulation of this pathway causes a 50% reduction in smooth-muscle tone, thus exerting a vasodilating effect.[460] Interestingly, horses with recurrent airway disease appear to lack NANC innervation in the bronchioles, and this dysfunction may contribute to the airway hyperactivity observed.[454]

Lymph Drainage

Lymph drainage from the lung is accomplished by (1) the deep lymphatics, which begin at the level of the alveolar ducts and run with the conducting airway and arteries toward the hilar lymph nodes, and (2) the superficial lymphatics, which drain the visceral pleura through a plexus converging on the hilum.[445]

Pulmonary Physiology

The major function of the lung is gas exchange: diffusion of oxygen and elimination of carbon dioxide. During eupnea, an adult horse breathes at a frequency of approximately 12 breaths per minute and a tidal volume near 6.5 L, which represents a total minute ventilation of 77 L/min, or more than 100,000 L/day. During this same period, the resting horse consumes approximately 2.1 L/min of oxygen (3000 L/day) and produces approximately 1.7 L/min of carbon dioxide (2400 L/day).[67] Thus the lung provides an important means by which normal arterial oxygen and carbon dioxide tensions and arterial pH are maintained. In the absence of lung disease, pulmonary arterial oxygenation (Pao_2) depends on the inspired fraction of oxygen (normally 0.21) and the effective level of alveolar ventilation, which is approximated by a version of the alveolar gas equation:

$$PAo_2 = PIo_2 - (Paco_2/R)$$

where PAo_2 is the alveolar oxygen tension, PIo_2 is the inspired oxygen tension, $PAco_2$ is the alveolar carbon dioxide tension, and R is the respiratory exchange quotient (the ratio of carbon dioxide production to oxygen consumption). Because an admixture of venous blood with the pulmonary arterial circulation occurs, alveolar oxygen tension exceeds arterial oxygen tension by approximately 10 mm Hg.

In the absence of alterations in inspired oxygen tensions, arterial hypoxemia ($Pao_2 < 85$ mm Hg) may result from basically four processes, including (1) hypoventilation, (2) diffusion impairment, (3) $(\dot{V}/\dot{Q})$ inequality, and (4) right-to-left shunts.[461]

Alveolar and thus arterial carbon dioxide levels depend on the rate of carbon dioxide elimination relative to its production, given by the following equation:

$$PAco_2 = \dot{V}CO_2/\dot{V}A$$

where VCO_2 is the rate of CO_2 production and VA is alveolar ventilation. Hypoventilation is defined as inadequate CO_2 elimination relative to production, resulting in an elevated $Paco_2$ (hypercapnia, hypercarbia). Hypoventilation can result from a variety of abnormalities. A convenient diagnostic approach follows the control of breathing from (1) the respiratory center in the medulla, (2) the efferent nerves (phrenic), (3) the bellows (diaphragm and chest wall muscles), (4) the pleural space, and (5) the airways. Some situations in which hypoventilation may develop include (1) drug administration (barbiturates, diazepam, xylazine); (2) diseases of the brainstem after infection (encephalitis), trauma, hemorrhage, or neoplasia; (3) diseases of the respiratory muscles, including botulism, trauma, or fatigue; (4) pleuritis and space-occupying lesions; and (5) choke and upper airway obstruction.

In patients suffering from hypoventilation, arterial oxygenation improves with oxygen administration (by increasing inspired oxygen tension), but the most efficacious mode of correcting the hypercapnia and consequent hypoxemia is by mechanical ventilation. Diffusion impairment occurs when time is inadequate for equilibration of alveolar oxygen tensions with pulmonary capillary oxygen tensions. Under normal resting conditions, equilibration of oxygen tensions occurs within 0.25 seconds, approximately one third of the contact time of the blood in the pulmonary circulation.[461] Some evidence suggests that in the exercising horse, the arterial hypoxemia that normally develops at high exercise intensities is caused in part by the decrease in time available for oxygen diffusion.[462,463] During rest, diffusion impairment is unlikely to occur. Arterial hypoxemia caused by diffusion impairment can be corrected by administration of supplemental oxygen.

Inequalities are the primary cause of arterial hypoxemia and occur when alveolar ventilation and pulmonary blood flow are mismatched despite the existence of several reflexes that normally tend to prevent this problem. For example, a fall in the $(\dot{V}/\dot{Q})$ ratio causes alveolar hypoxia, which induces pulmonary vasoconstriction and decreases perfusion to that lung region. (However, this reflex also increases pulmonary vascular resistance and thus the work of the right side of the heart.) A second reflex is hypocapnic bronchoconstriction. When the $(\dot{V}/\dot{Q})$ ratio increases, regional ventilation of those lung units is reduced by smooth-muscle constriction. $(\dot{V}/\dot{Q})$ inequalities interfere with oxygen and carbon dioxide transfer such that hypoxemia and hypercapnia may ensue. Usually the consequent hypercapnia increases chemoreceptor drive and thus increases alveolar ventilation, which restores normocapnia. However, because of the shape of the oxyhemoglobin dissociation curve, the increase in oxygen tension in the normal alveoli caused by the hyperventilation does not significantly increase the oxygen content of the blood coming from these units. Several factors can exacerbate the hypoxemia of $(\dot{V}/\dot{Q})$ inequalities, including hypoventilation (sedation) and decrements in cardiac output (mechanical ventilation with positive end-expiratory pressure). $(\dot{V}/\dot{Q})$ inequalities respond to oxygen therapy, although this may lead to increases in arterial carbon dioxide tension by (1) a reduction of the chemoreceptor (hypoxic) drive, (2) an increase in $(\dot{V}/\dot{Q})$ inequalities, and (3) a shift in the carboxyhemoglobin dissociation curve to the right, decreasing its affinity for carbon dioxide.[464] Mechanical ventilation may be indicated in severe $(\dot{V}/\dot{Q})$ inequalities if hypercapnia is progressive.

Passage of blood through abnormal cardiovascular communications (atrial septal defects, ventricular septal defects, patent ductus arteriosus) or through pulmonary capillaries within the walls of atelectatic or fluid-filled alveoli causes shunts and consequent hypoxemia. Such defects may be considered as one extreme of ($\dot{V}/\dot{Q}$) inequality ($\dot{V}/\dot{Q}$ 0) and are resistant to correction by oxygen therapy.[464] In shunts caused by pulmonary disease, mechanical ventilation and positive end-expiratory pressure increase end-expiratory lung volume and thus the alveolar surface area available for gas exchange. The incremental increase in end-expiratory lung volume may also help redistribute the excessive extravascular lung water from the alveoli to the interstitium.

Metabolic Functions

The entire cardiac output passes through the pulmonary circulation, thus providing an ideal means by which hormones and drugs may be metabolized to inactive compounds. Indeed, relative to the hepatic blood flow (approximately 25% of the cardiac output), the contribution of the lungs to the total body clearance of drugs or xenobiotics may be significant. The lung contains hydrolytic enzymes that cleave peptides such as bradykinin and angiotensin I, thus serving to inactivate (bradykinin) or to bioactivate (angiotensin) compounds. The enzymatic activity responsible is concentrated within the caveolae of the pulmonary capillary endothelium or in pouchings in the plasma membranes of these cells.[465] Other pulmonary enzymes exist that are capable of cleaving phosphate groups from nucleotides (adenosine triphosphate, adenosine diphosphate, and adenosine monophosphate), of oxidizing steroid hormones (testosterone), of inactivating prostaglandins E and F, and of metabolizing biogenic amines such as 5-hydroxytryptamine, norepinephrine, and tyramine.[450,465,466]

Defense Against Infection

The sterile environment of the lung results from several mechanisms, including the mucociliary apparatus, which clears particulate debris from the lung at a rate of approximately 17 mm/min,[56] vagally mediated reflexes, which serve to initiate coughing and concomitant bronchoconstriction, and lung surfactant proteins, SP-A and SP-D, that act as collections against a large number of pathogens.[447,467] However, the predominant line of defense against noxious agents and bacteria are the alveolar macrophages and dendritic cells of the distal airways and alveoli. Recent investigations have shown depression in alveolar macrophage function after exercise or long transport.[468,469] Viral infections also depress macrophage function. Helping to maintain immunosurveillance and the sterile pulmonary environment are polymorphonuclear cells that respond to chemotactic stimuli and lymphocytes.

DISORDERS OF THE LOWER RESPIRATORY TRACT

Disorders of the lower respiratory tract are common in horses of all ages. Presenting signs and symptoms vary with these disorders and may include exercise intolerance, cough, nasal discharge, fever, respiratory distress, increased respiratory rate or effort, or generalized depression, inappetence, and weight loss. Careful clinical examination that includes auscultation while rebreathing often confirms the anatomic site of the problem. Ancillary diagnostic testing such as bronchoalveolar lavage, transtracheal wash, thoracic ultrasound, or thoracic radiography are often indicated to confirm a suspected diagnosis.

Bacterial Pneumonia

CAUSES

Normally the lungs contain only small numbers of bacteria (colony-forming units) that are considered to be transient contaminants in the process of being removed by clearance mechanisms.[470] When pulmonary defense mechanisms are overwhelmed, aspirated bacteria from the oropharynx may proliferate and cause pneumonia. The most common gram-positive bacteria involved are *Streptococcus equi* subsp. *zooepidemicus* (β-hemolytic), *Staphylococcus aureus,* and *S. pneumoniae* (α-hemolytic). The most frequent gram-negative isolates are *Pasteurella* and *Actinobacillus* spp., *Escherichia coli, Klebsiella pneumoniae,* and *Bordetella bronchiseptica.*[40,41,471-474] *Pseudomonas* sp. is rarely a cause of equine pneumonia, and its isolation from tracheobronchial aspirates suggests environmental contamination of equipment (endoscope). *Nocardia* organisms also have been isolated from horses with pulmonary infections, but these are rare and appear to require significant derangements of host defense mechanisms.[475] The anaerobic bacteria most commonly isolated are *Bacteroides fragilis, Peptostreptococcus anaerobius,* and *Fusobacterium* spp. Polymicrobic infections are not uncommon in cases of equine pneumonia and may represent a synergy between aerobic or facultatively anaerobic and anaerobic bacteria. Mechanisms of synergy may involve protection from phagocytosis and intracellular killing, production of essential growth factors, and lowering of local oxygen concentrations.[472]

PATHOGENESIS

Bacterial pneumonia may develop after viral infections, athletic events (races), trailer rides, and general anesthesia. It occurs in horses that are overcrowded, maintained on poor nutrition, or exposed to inclement weather. Laryngeal and pharyngeal dysfunction may predispose the horse to develop pneumonia by aspiration of oropharyngeal bacteria. Such predisposition occurs in horses (1) with primary neuropathies of the ninth and tenth cranial nerves (e.g., equine protozoal myeloencephalitis, botulism, *S. equi* infections, guttural pouch mycoses, neoplasia), (2) with primary myopathies of the pharyngeal, laryngeal, or esophageal musculature (e.g., vitamin E and selenium deficiency, megaesophagus), (3) after laryngeal surgery, or (4) with esophageal obstructions (choke). The pathogenic mechanisms described subsequently apply to the development of lung abscesses and pleuropneumonia.

Viral-induced modifications of respiratory tract defenses include (1) enhanced susceptibility to bacterial attachment and colonization after damage to the epithelial cells, (2) diminished mucociliary clearance and physical translocation of bacterial particles deposited on the bronchial ciliated epithelium, and (3) decreased surfactant levels and collapse of the airways because of viral destruction of alveolar type II cells.[476] The ensuing anaerobic environment predisposes the area to macrophage dysfunction. In addition, the alveolar exudate that accompanies viral pneumonitis may provide a nutrient medium for multiplication of aspirated bacteria.

During high-intensity exercise, the horse may aspirate track debris and oropharyngeal secretions. This, coupled with exercise-induced pulmonary hemorrhage, which provides a nutrient source, predisposes the horse to developing pneumonia.[477]

An exercise-associated increase in bacterial contaminants of the lower respiratory tract has been demonstrated experimentally. Strenuously exercised horses exhibit a tenfold and a 100-fold increase, respectively, in the number of aerobic and anaerobic bacteria isolated from transtracheal aspirates relative to preexercise samples.[478] The bacterial contamination, along with exercise-associated increases in bronchoalveolar cortisol concentrations, decreased pulmonary alveolar macrophage viability, and impaired phagocytic function, enables bacteria to proliferate and cause pneumonia.[468,469,477,479,480]

Transportation remains one of the most common causes of pneumonia and pleuropneumonia in the horse because physically restraining the head of the horse and preventing postural drainage enhances bacterial colonization of the lower respiratory tract.[477,481] Inflammation and increased numbers of bacteria are found in the transtracheal aspirates of horses within 6 to 12 hours of confinement with the head elevated.[482] Furthermore, although the stress response of horses during transport contributes to immunosuppression and enhanced susceptibility to pneumonia, the increase in serum cortisol levels are greater when horses are cross-tied compared with when left unrestricted in the box during transport.[483] Another hypothesis is that dehydration, associated with reduced fluid consumption before or during transportation, reduces mucociliary clearance and contributes to bacterial proliferation. Neither the prophylactic administration of antibiotics nor the intermittent release from the confined head posture reliably reduces tracheal bacterial numbers or prevents the accumulation of purulent tracheobronchial secretions in horses confined with their heads elevated.[481,482]

Horses undergoing general anesthesia may develop pneumonia when endotracheal intubation introduces oropharyngeal contaminants to the lower respiratory tract. Anesthesia may compromise mucociliary clearance and cause compression atelectasis and vascular congestion that results in regional ischemia and necrosis of lung regions. This circumstance provides local conditions suitable for bacterial multiplication.[477] In addition, excessive extension and flexion of the neck (e.g., during myelography) with secondary movement of the endotracheal tube may cause tracheal erosions that impair mucociliary clearance and predispose the horse to developing pleuropneumonia.[484]

CLINICAL SIGNS

In the early stages of bacterial pneumonia, clinical signs may not be obvious, being limited to a gurgling sound of exudates in the trachea, fever, or depression. As pneumonia progresses, horses may exhibit intermittent fever, tachypnea or respiratory distress, nasal discharge, coughing, inappetence, exercise intolerance, and weight loss. Nasal discharge is usually mucopurulent but may be hemorrhagic in some cases.[472] Epistaxis may be the result of bacterial hemolysin production *(Actinobacillus equuli)* or ischemic necrosis of lung tissue.[485] Auscultation of the thorax reveals increased harsh breath sounds dorsally, crackles, wheezes, and dullness of respiratory sounds ventrally. Manipulation of the trachea or larynx may induce a cough. Halitosis and a foul-smelling nasal discharge suggest an anaerobic infection. Mandibular lymphadenopathy may be apparent in aspiration pneumonia associated with strangles or with viral infections.

DIAGNOSIS

Clinical signs and history aid in the diagnosis. Clinical pathologic data consistent with bacterial pneumonia include leukocytosis caused by absolute neutrophilia with or without a left shift. Neutropenia may be evident if gram-negative organisms are involved. Hyperfibrinogenemia (>500 mg/dl), hyperglobulinemia, hypoalbuminemia, and anemia of chronic inflammation are compatible with the diagnosis of chronic bacterial pneumonia. Endoscopic evaluation of the upper respiratory tract may demonstrate a defect in laryngeal or pharyngeal function if this is the inciting cause. One may observe a mucopurulent exudate with or without traces of blood by endoscopy in the lower respiratory tract. Thoracic radiographs demonstrate a radiopacity in the anteroventral thorax and a loss of clarity in the lung fields caudal to the heart. Air bronchograms are occasionally found in the adult horse with bacterial pneumonia (Figure 9-13). Ultrasound may demonstrate consolidation of ventral lung lobes and extension of the pneumonia to the pleural surfaces as evident by the presence of comet tails. Tracheobronchial aspirates yield degenerative neutrophils, damaged epithelial cells, and microorganisms. The presence of squamous epithelial cells supports a diagnosis of aspiration pneumonia, provided that the tracheal catheter was not misplaced in the pharynx during sampling. The clinician should perform aerobic and anaerobic cultures on the tracheal aspirates.

TREATMENT

The clinician should direct treatment at the causative organism, but in the absence of culture and sensitivity results, one should administer broad-spectrum antimicrobials. Appropriate therapy might include intravenous aqueous sodium or potassium penicillin and an aminoglycoside or third-generation cephalosporin (Table 9-5). The aminoglycosides are efficacious against most gram-negative aerobes, but they lack efficacy against anaerobes. However, metronidazole is effective against most anaerobes, including the penicillin-resistant *B. fragilis* and is routinely included in the treatment protocol.

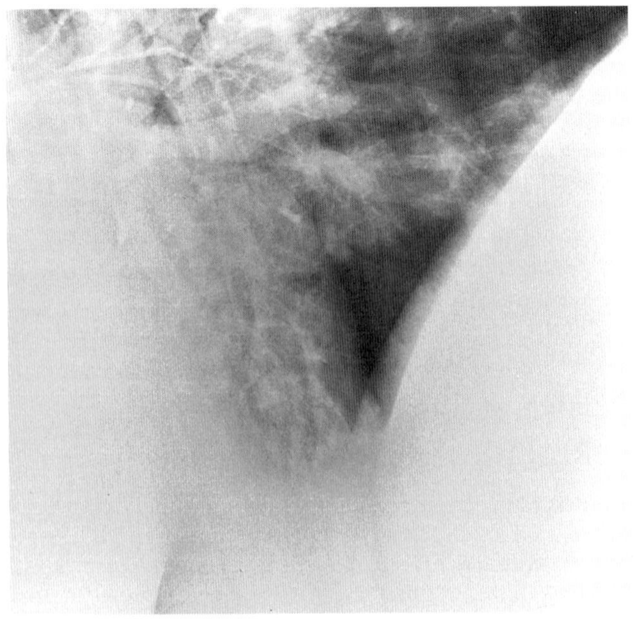

FIGURE 9-13 Two-year-old Thoroughbred with pneumonia. A patchy area of pulmonary consolidation is notable in the ventral dependent portion of the lung silhouetting the heart and diaphragm. (Courtesy D. S. Biller, Manhattan, Kan., 1991.)

TABLE 9-5

Antimicrobials and Other Drugs

Antimicrobial	Dose
Amikacin	16-18 mg/kg, IV, q 24 h
Ampicillin sodium	11-22 mg/kg, IV or IM, q 6-8 h
Ceftiofur	2.2 mg/kg, IV or IM, q 12 h
Chloramphenicol	50 mg/kg, PO, q 6 h
Doxycycline	10 mg/kg, PO, q 12 h
Enrofloxacin	7.5 mg/kg, PO or IV, q 24 h 5.0 mg/kg, PO or IV, q 12 h
Gentamicin	4.4-6.6 mg/kg, IV or IM, q 24 h
Metronidazole	15-25 mg/kg, PO, q 6-8 h
Oxytetracycline	6.6 mg/kg, IV, q 12-24 h
Potassium penicillin G	22,000 IU/kg, IV q 6 h
Procaine penicillin G	22,000 IU/kg, IM, q 12 h
Rifampin	5-10 mg/kg, PO, q 12 h
Sodium penicillin G	22,000 IU/kg, IV, q 6 h
Trimethoprim-sulfonamide	15-20 mg/kg, PO or IV, q 12 h
Other Agents Used	
Acetylcysteine	10-20 ml 20% solution (nebulized)
Albuterol	360-720 μg via inhalation
Clenbuterol	0.7-0.8 μg/kg, PO, q 12 h or nebulized
Fenoterol	1-2 mg via inhalation
Ipratropium bromide	2-3 μg/kg (nebulized)
Salmeterol	0.5-1 μg/kg via inhalation
Fluticasone	2-4 μg/kg via inhalation

IM, Intramuscularly; *IV,* intravenously; *PO,* orally; *q,* every.

Depending on the culture and sensitivity results, one may also administer potentiated sulfonamides. The clinician should use aminoglycosides judiciously in animals that have renal compromise or are dehydrated. (See the section on treatment for parapneumonic effusions.) Antimicrobial therapy may also be administered by nebulization. In general, one third of the calculated systemic dose of the antimicrobial (ceftiofur, gentamicin, marbofloxacin) is administered via an ultrasonic nebulizer two or three times daily.[486,487] With the nebulizate, one may also add 5 mg albuterol to enhance bronchodilation and 10 ml 20% acetylcysteine.

With gram negative infections and the potential for endotoxemia, small doses of flunixin meglumine (0.25 mg/kg three times daily) may be given to inhibit arachidonic acid metabolism. Other treatment modalities that have been advocated include prophylactic measures against laminitis. The goal of supportive care should be to minimize stress and ensure adequate ventilation and hydration. Ideally, horses should be bedded on paper or on other materials free of dusts or molds and should be fed forages of excellent quality. One should also direct attention to correcting the primary cause of the pneumonia. Depending on the chronicity of the pneumonia, one should note clinical improvement in 48 to 72 hours. The prognosis can be excellent if the pneumonia is treated aggressively, but the clinician should forewarn the owner of potential complications (see the following discussion). The clinician should administer treatment for 2 to 6 weeks, depending on the extent of the pneumonia and the underlying inciting cause. (See the section on treatment for parapneumonic effusions.)

Preventive measures that help deter the development of pneumonia include (1) adequate immunization protocols with vaccination against EIV, EHV1, and EHV4 every 4 to 6 months (in the performance horse); (2) the minimization of stressors such as long van rides in which the head is restrained constantly; and (3) the use of management or husbandry methods that minimize dust or noxious gas accumulations within the stall, prevent exposure to inclement weather, and provide adequate nutrition for the horse.

Lung Abscesses

CAUSES

In foals younger than 6 months, *R. equi* and *S. equi* subsp. *zooepidemicus* are the most common bacterial isolates recovered.[488] In adult horses, *Streptococcus* and *Actinobacillus* species are the most common gram-positive and gram-negative organisms implicated in the development of pulmonary abscesses.[488-490] This discussion addresses predominantly lung abscesses in the adult horse.

PATHOGENESIS

Lung abscesses may develop as a consequence of inhaling bacterial organisms resident to the oropharynx or contaminating the environment *(R. equi)*. The abscess may develop as a consequence of a focal pneumonia or may be a component of pleuropneumonia complex. (See discussion elsewhere in this chapter.) Racehorses may be at an increased risk for developing lung abscesses when bacteria proliferate in the blood in the airways and alveoli after episodes of EIPH. The regional location of lung abscesses in these cases supports this hypothesis.[490]

CLINICAL SIGNS

Clinical signs may vary, but most horses have periods of pyrexia, inappetence, lethargy, mild tachycardia, and respiratory-related signs ranging from tachypnea to distress.[489,490] Other signs that may be evident include cough, purulent nasal discharge, thoracic pain, epistaxis, and halitosis.

DIAGNOSIS

The adult horse may have a history of transport, strenuous exercise, surgery, prior pneumonia, or administration of medications. In most cases, evidence of an infection is found on the CBC and serum chemistry panel: mature neutrophilia, hyperfibrinogenemia, hyperglobulinemia, and anemia. Radiography and ultrasound are useful imaging modalities, and one may use them concurrently to detect lung abscesses (Figures 9-14 and 9-15). Pulmonary abscesses appear on ultrasonography as encapsulated cavitated areas filled with fluid or echogenic (white) material. Cardiac structures or an air-filled lung may overlie an abscess, obscuring its detection. In one study, two thirds of the abscesses were located in the caudodorsal lung field, whereas the remaining abscesses were located in the caudoventral region.[490]

Transtracheal aspirates or percutaneous aspirates of lung abscesses adhered to the body wall may help the clinician decide the choice of antimicrobials. One should culture isolates under aerobic and anaerobic conditions.

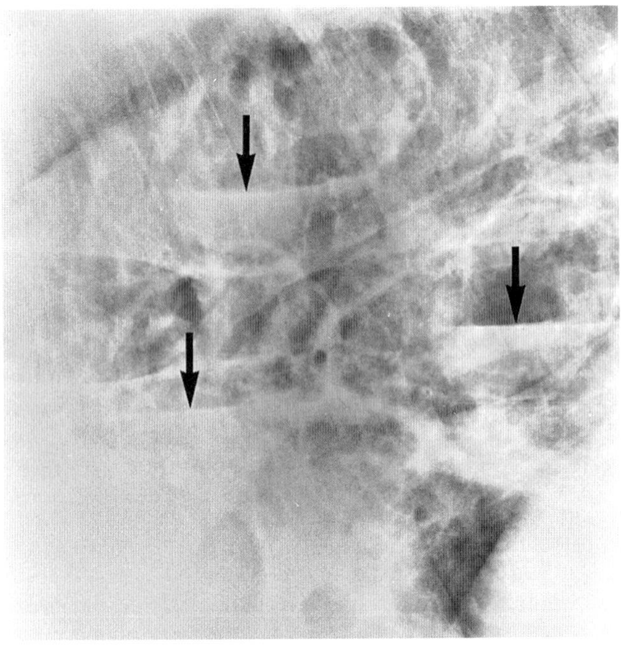

FIGURE 9-14 Nine-year-old saddle horse. Multiple cavitating pulmonary abscesses are present within the lungs. *Arrows* indicate air-fluid interfaces within the abscesses. (Courtesy D. S. Biller, Manhattan, Kan., 1991.)

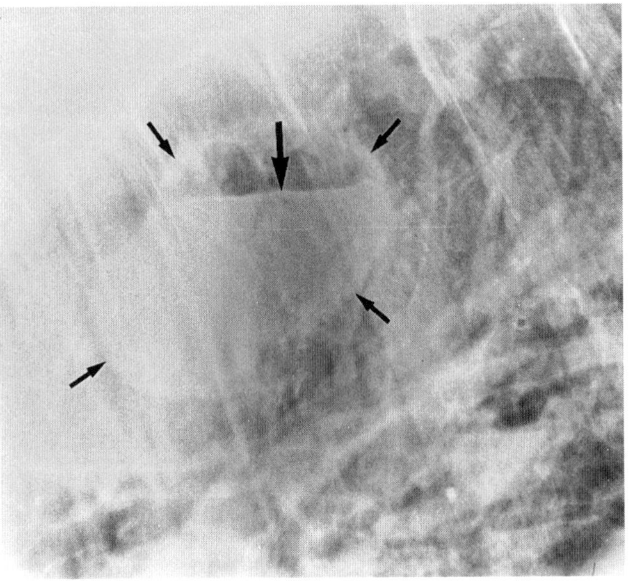

FIGURE 9-15 A large air-capped pulmonary abscess. *Small arrows* indicate an abscess; *large arrow* indicates the air-fluid interface. (Courtesy D. S. Biller, Manhattan, Kan., 1991.)

TREATMENT

Long-term antimicrobial therapy (8 to 10 weeks) along with prolonged periods of rest (5 to 6 months) before resuming strenuous exercise is recommended. (See the section on treatment for pneumonia and parapneumonic effusions for specific antimicrobial recommendations.) In human beings receiving antimicrobial treatment for pulmonary abscesses, an 80% reduction in the size of abscess cavities less than 3 cm in diameter usually occurs within 1 month of appropriate therapy.[491] Furthermore, 70% of cavitary lesions in human cases of lung abscessation resolve completely by 3 months.[492] For lung abscesses unresponsive to therapy, the clinician should consider drainage via a thoracotomy or thoracoscopy.[493]

The prognosis for resumption of athleticism is good if treatment is initiated early. In one study, 23 of 25 Standardbreds and 13 of 20 Thoroughbreds raced after the diagnosis and treatment of a lung abscess with no significant effect on race performance.[490]

Parapneumonic Effusions and Septic Pleuritis

CAUSES

Between two thirds and three quarters of cases of septic pleuritis arise as an extension of pneumonia or pulmonary abscessation.[494-496] Septic pleuritis also may occur in horses with thoracic trauma, esophageal rupture, or penetration of the esophagus or stomach by a foreign body.[477,497-499] The aerobic or facultatively anaerobic organisms most often isolated from horses with pleuropneumonia are bacterial species that normally reside in the oropharyngeal cavities: *Streptococcus* spp., *Pasteurella* and *Actinobacillus* spp., *E. coli,* and *Enterobacter* spp. Anaerobic organisms frequently isolated include *Bacteroides* spp., *Peptostreptococcus* spp., *Fusobacterium* spp., and *Clostridium* spp.[499-501]

EPIDEMIOLOGY

Risk factors for the development of pleuropneumonia are the same as those associated with pneumonia (see the previous discussion) and include long-distance transport, strenuous exercise, viral respiratory tract disease, surgery, dysphagia, general anesthesia, and systemic illness (enteritis). These conditions may enhance aspiration of oropharyngeal organisms or impair clearance of such organisms.[477,495,502]

PATHOGENESIS

The causative factors of equine pleuropneumonia are those that suppress the pulmonary defense mechanisms and allow bacterial contamination of the lower respiratory tract to progress to pneumonia or abscess formation. The subsequent extension of the infectious process into the pleural space causes pleuritis. The distribution of the pulmonary lesions—cranioventral with the right cranial and middle lung lobes more severely afflicted—is consistent with inhalation or aspiration of bacteria rather than infection from a hematogenous spread. Fluid accumulates within the pleural cavity as the parenchymal inflammation increases the permeability of the capillaries in the overlying visceral pleura, causing an outpouring of protein and cells. Bacteria may also invade the pleural fluid. (See previous discussion of pneumonia.)

CLINICAL SIGNS

Depending on the chronicity of disease, clinical signs may vary and may be confused with signs of colic or rhabdomyolysis. In the acute stages, horses are febrile and lethargic, have a slight nasal discharge, and exhibit a guarded cough, shallow breathing pattern, and painful, stilted gait.[501] The right hemithorax is affected more often than the left, presumably because of the more direct route of the right mainstem bronchus.[477] Thoracic auscultation may be abnormal, as evidenced by pleural friction rubs and ventral dullness. In severe acute cases, the horse may exhibit nostril flaring; tachycardia; jugular pulsations; toxic mucous membranes; a guarded soft, moist cough; and a serosanguineous fetid nasal discharge. In chronic cases of pleuropneumonia (duration longer than 2 weeks), horses may have bouts of intermittent fever and exhibit weight loss and substernal and limb edema.

DIAGNOSIS

The diagnosis is based on historical information, clinical examination, imaging results, and microbiologic and cytologic analysis of tracheal and pleural fluid aspirates. On auscultation of the thorax, one may hear vesicular sounds only dorsally, with an absence of lung sounds ventrally. One may hear bronchial or tracheal sounds if lung consolidation exists. Cardiac sounds radiate over a wider area of the lung field than normal, a finding distinct from clinical cases of pericarditis. On percussion of the chest, the clinician may elicit a painful response (pleurodynia) and detect an area of dullness or decreased resonance ventrally.

Laboratory assessment may reveal a normal or toxemic leukogram and chemistry findings in acute cases. In chronic cases, one may find anemia, neutrophilia, hyperfibrinogenemia, and hyperproteinemia.

Ultrasound is the diagnostic technique of choice in horses with suspected pleuropneumonia or pleural effusion. Using a 3.5- to 5-MHz transducer (sector scanner or linear probe), one can detect free or loculated fluid, pleural thickening, pulmonary and mediastinal abscesses, pulmonary consolidation, inundation of airways with fluid, fibrinous adhesions, and concurrent pericarditis. Pleural fluid may displace the lungs axially and dorsally. The fluid may appear anechoic or hypoechoic, depending on the relative cellularity.[501] Free gas echoes within the pleural fluid may reflect (1) the presence of anaerobic organisms,[48] (2) the presence of air introduced during a thoracocentesis, or (3) the presence of air introduced by a bronchopleural fistula. Ultrasonography enables accurate placement of the catheter during thoracocentesis and ensures productive yields during placement of a chest drain (Figures 9-16 to 9-18). Ultrasound examination fails to demonstrate deep parenchymal lesions if the overlying lung is normally aerated.

Thoracic radiography also remains a useful technique for evaluating horses with pleuropneumonia, permitting detection of a pneumothorax or an abscess located deep in aerated lung tissue. Pneumothorax may develop after transtracheal aspiration, thoracocentesis, thoracic drainage, or pleuroscopy. Pneumothorax may also develop as a sequela to gas-producing organisms in the pleural cavity or to air leaks from bronchopleural fistulae.[477] Although radiographs may detect pulmonary abscesses, they may fail to detect lesions obscured by the cardiac silhouette.

Thoracocentesis of both sides of the chest is indicated if one notes fluid bilaterally. Not only is thoracocentesis diagnostic and prognostic, it may also be a therapeutic life-saving procedure in horses with severe respiratory distress.[503] In healthy horses, the fenestrated caudal mediastinum allows communication of the fluid between the two sides of the chest. In horses with pleuropneumonia, fibrin may close mediastinal fenestrations, allowing for differences to develop in the pleural fluid of the two hemithoraces. The clinician should submit fluid for cytologic examination and for aerobic and anaerobic culture. Pleural fluid in healthy horses contains fewer than 10,000 cells/μl, approximately 60% of which are neutrophils, and has a total protein of less than 2.5 g/dl. In cases of pleuropneumonia, pleural fluid white blood cell counts and protein are elevated and glucose levels may be low (<40 mg/dl). The fluid may have a foul odor if anaerobes are contributing to the infection, but the absence of an odor should not preclude the possibility of an anaerobic component.

The clinician should always obtain a tracheobronchial aspirate to recover the inciting bacterial agents and to examine tracheobronchial secretions cytologically (Gram stain, cell types). One should submit aspirates for aerobic and anaerobic culture and Gram staining to provide guidance on

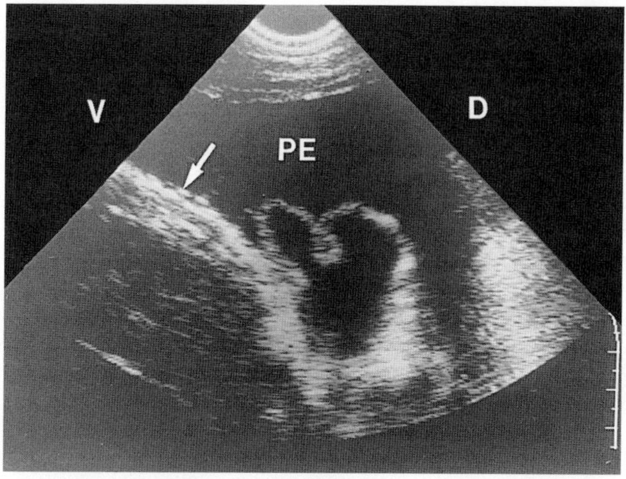

FIGURE 9-16 Ultrasound of pleural effusion. Anechoic (*black*) area represents pleural effusion (PE). The echogenic (*white*) tortuous fibrin strand is attached to the parietal pleura of the diaphragm. *V,* Ventral; *D,* dorsal; *arrow,* diaphragm. (Courtesy D. S. Biller, Manhattan, Kan., 1991.)

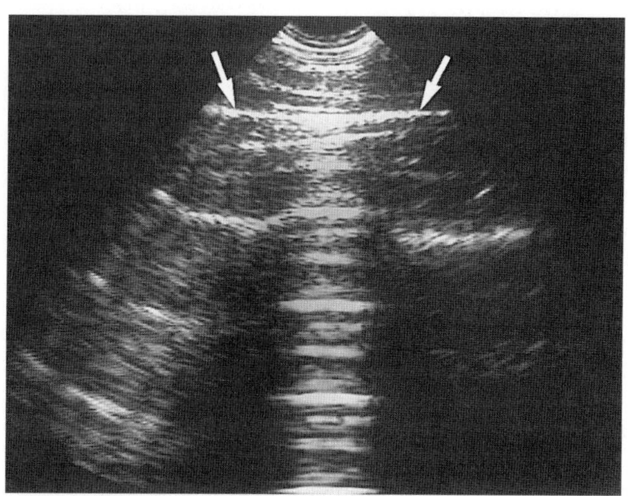

FIGURE 9-17 Normal thoracic ultrasound demonstrates a highly echogenic interface *(arrows)* between the chest wall and normal lung. A reverberation artifact is notable deep to the chest wall–lung interface. (Courtesy D. S. Biller, Manhattan, Kan., 1991.)

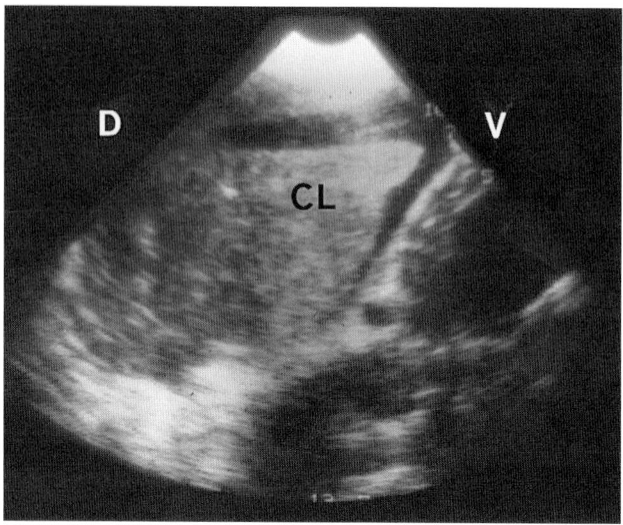

FIGURE 9-18 Ultrasound of ventrally consolidated lung *(CL)* surrounded by a small amount of pleural effusion. *V,* Ventral; *D,* dorsal. (Courtesy D. S. Biller, Manhattan, Kan., 1991.)

antimicrobial selection. During the course of the disease, one may obtain multiple tracheobronchial aspirates to identify new or resistant bacterial organisms.

One can use thoracoscopy, performed in standing sedated horses or in horses under general anesthesia, in acute and chronic cases of pleuropneumonia (1) for guided placement of drains into abscesses and loculated pleural effusions, (2) for assessment of the extent and progression of pleural disease, and (3) for the evaluation of therapeutic responses and the efficacy of pleural lavage or drainage.[75]

TREATMENT

For horses with pleuropneumonia, the aims of treatment are (1) to remove excessive pleural fluid, (2) to administer systemic antimicrobials to inhibit bacterial growth, (3) to provide antiinflammatory and analgesic drugs that deter the development of secondary complications, and (4) to provide supportive care.

Under ultrasound guidance, one can remove pleural fluid aseptically through the seventh or eighth intercostal spaces at a locale dorsal to the costochondral junction using a 24- to 32-Fr chest tube. One may remove as much as 30 to 50 L. If blood discoloration of the pleural fluid is caused by the underlying disease, the fluid remains blood-tinged throughout the drainage.[503]

The clinician should place indwelling chest tubes (1) if large volumes of foul-smelling fluid with microorganisms are obtained, (2) if the pleural fluid has a pH less than 7.2 or a glucose concentration less than 40 mg/dl, or (3) if the horse responds poorly to intermittent drainage.[496-503] To the end of the indwelling chest tube one should attach a Heimlich valve or a nonlubricated condom with its tip snipped off. Complications of chest tube placement include pneumothorax; lung laceration; hemothorax; cardiac arrhythmias; bowel, liver, or heart puncture; and localized swelling.[503]

Appropriate antimicrobial therapy is based on the results of the culture and sensitivity. Pending microbiologic test results, one should administer broad-spectrum intravenous antibiotics in most cases of pleuropneumonia because the infections are polymicrobic. Penicillin is one of the drugs of choice because it is efficacious against *Streptococcus* spp., *Staphylococcus* spp., and many anaerobes. Metronidazole is added routinely to the penicillin to broaden bactericidal activity against anaerobes, especially *B. fragilis*. Aminoglycosides lack efficacy against anaerobic bacteria and have poor penetration into respiratory tract secretions but still are administered with penicillin. Third-generation cephalosporins such as ceftiofur sodium, with activity against gram-negative aerobes and facultative anaerobes, showed excellent efficacy in the treatment of spontaneous clinical and posttransport pneumonia associated with *S. zooepidemicus, Actinobacillus* spp., and *Pasteurella* spp.[504]

Depending on the clinical response of the horse, 10 to 14 days after the onset of initial therapy, the clinician usually replaces parenteral antimicrobials with oral antibiotics. Chloramphenicol, a bacteriostatic drug, has excellent broad-spectrum activity against gram-negative, gram-positive, and anaerobic bacteria and can be given orally. (One must use caution when handling the drug.) Enrofloxacin, a fluoroquinolone, has excellent antibacterial action against aerobic gram-negative bacteria, many gram-positive bacteria, and mycoplasma bacteria but has limited activity against *Streptococcus* spp. and anaerobes.[505] Concentrations of the enrofloxacin in lung tissue are similar to those in serum.[506] Erythromycin and rifampin attain good concentrations in the lung and pleural fluid and within phagocytic cells, but rifampin is expensive and erythromycin may induce a fatal colitis, precluding their use in adult horses.[507] Antimicrobials may also be nebulized (see previous discussion on pneumonia).

Antimicrobial therapy should continue for 2 to 4 months until the horse is gaining weight, hematologic and serum chemistry values have normalized, and no evidence of respiratory tract disease exists. One should implement limited exercise (hand walking) and avoid stressing the horse. One should reevaluate refractory cases using the techniques of ultrasonography, thoracocentesis, or transtracheal aspiration to determine if drug resistance has developed, if additional pathogens are involved, or if untoward sequelae have occurred (see the following discussion).

In refractory cases, drainage of pulmonary or mediastinal abscesses or mechanical débridement of fibrinous material (decortication) may become necessary. One should consider initially attempting drainage using a large-bore chest tube (24 Fr) directed through the chest wall and then the capsular wall of the abscess followed by suction of the abscess contents. Lavage of the contents of the abscess may improve removal of the purulent material. One should take care to prevent spillage of the contents into the pleural cavity. For removal of fibrinopurulent material or necrotic lung segments, a standing thoracotomy may provide necessary access.[508] After removing accessible exudates and fibrin manually, one lavages the chest cavity with a warm 1% Betadine solution, packs it with a large lap sponge, and covers it with a self-adhering dressing and pad. One must lavage the pleural cavity daily. Fistulae formation is a common sequela in these clinical cases, but this does not preclude horses from returning to racing or breeding careers.

Nonsteroidal antiinflammatory drugs (flunixin meglumin, 0.25 to 0.50 mg/kg intravenously two to three times daily) provide analgesia, increase appetite, increase the comfort of the horse, and decrease the inflammatory response.

Many horses with pleuropneumonia benefit from the administration of intravenous fluids for the first 48 to 72 hours, until the horse is comfortable enough to resume drinking and the danger of endotoxemia has lessened. Nasal insufflation of oxygen (10 to 15 L/min) may be indicated if the horse is hypoxemic or in respiratory distress. One may achieve bronchodilation using inhaled or nebulized albuterol (600 to 720 μg three to four times daily). Because gram negative organisms are often involved in pleuropneumonia cases, one should implement prophylactic measures against laminitis.

PROGNOSIS

A favorable response most often relates to early identification and aggressive treatment of pleuropneumonia. Survival rates[495,509] of horses treated for acute pleuropneumonia range between 49% to 98%. The prognosis deteriorates with the increased duration of the illness because of involvement of anaerobic bacteria and the development of complicating factors such as pleural adhesions, pulmonary necrosis, cranial mediastinal abscesses, bronchopleural fistulae, constrictive pericarditis, and laminitis.[509,510] In a recent study, 61% of Thoroughbreds treated for pleuropneumonia raced after recovery, with 56% winning at least one race.[511]

COMPLICATIONS

Long-term medical treatment of pleuropneumonia may induce complications such as venous phlebitis or thrombosis (from intravenous catheter placement), cellulitis or pneumothorax after thoracocentesis, diarrhea resulting from antimicrobial and antiinflammatory therapy or endotoxemia, and laminitis. With minor changes in the therapeutic approaches, many of these complications resolve and do not impede the eventual return to health of the horse. The more complicated sequelae of infectious pleuropneumonia have been described in detail by Byars, Dainis, Seltzer, et al.[512] and Byars and Becht.[513] In a survey involving 153 horses brought to their veterinary hospital over a 4-year period with pleuropneumonia, the investigators detailed the development of cranial thoracic masses (7.2%), bronchopleural fistulae (6.5%), pericarditis (2.6%), and laminitis (1.3%).

One should suspect cranial thoracic masses when horses exhibit tachycardia, jugular distention, forelimb extension (pointing), and caudal displacement of the heart. One can confirm the presence of empyema, loculations, or encapsulated abscesses cranial to the heart by ultrasonography. In most cases, medical therapy is effective at reducing the abscess, and thus one should elect this conservative approach initially. Additional therapeutic modalities include the administration of a diuretic (furosemide) and a chronotropic agent (digitalis) to improve cardiac performance. However, refractory cases may require ultrasound-guided drainage of the abscess performed under short-term anesthesia (xylazine-ketamine combination).

Bronchopleural fistulae develop when necrotic pulmonary tissue sloughs, providing a direct communication of the airways with the pleural cavity. One confirms the diagnosis by visualization of the airways after pleuroscopy or by the intratracheal appearance of contrast media injected into the pleural cavity. Bronchopleural fistulae may close eventually as the pulmonary tissue adheres to the chest wall or as the airways close. In persistent cases, surgical removal of the affected tissue and closure of the airway may be indicated by thoracoscopy.

PLEURAL EFFUSION

CAUSES

Accumulation of fluid within the pleural space most often results from imbalances in Starling's law of fluid fluxes. As described previously, pleural effusions in the horse most commonly occur with bacterial pneumonia or lung abscesses.[514] (See the section on treatment for parapneumonic effusions.) Pleural effusions also may accompany a significant number of thoracic neoplasms such as fibrosarcoma, gastric or esophageal squamous cell carcinoma, hepatoblastoma, hemangiosarcoma, melanoma, mesothelioma, and metastatic mammary or ovarian adenocarcinoma, but they are most commonly associated with lymphoma.[515-524] Pleural effusion also develops in a significant number of other conditions, including thoracic trauma; pericarditis; peritonitis; viral, mycoplasmal, and fungal infections; congestive heart failure; liver disease; diaphragmatic herniation; hypoproteinemia; equine infectious anemia; pulmonary granulomata; and damage of the thoracic duct.[496,525-527]

PATHOGENESIS

Pleural fluid is the interstitial fluid of the parietal pleura. A pressure gradient driving its formation exists because the parietal pleura is supplied by the systemic circulation and because the pressure of the pleural space is more negative than that of the subpleural interstitium.[528] Pleural liquid and protein exit the pleural space via the parietal pleural stomata. Fluid production in the pleural space increases if any of the following occurs: (1) an elevation of the hydrostatic pressure gradient (congestive heart failure, portal hypertension); (2) a decrease in the colloid osmotic pressures (hypoproteinemia); (3) an increased permeability of the capillary vessels (infection, malignancy, inflammation); or (4) a decreased removal of fluid because of impaired lymphatic drainage or obstruction (neoplasia) or infiltration of the pleura or parenchyma (neoplasia).[529,530] Excessive amounts of peritoneal fluid may accumulate in the pleural cavity as the fluid moves through diaphragmatic defects or through diaphragmatic lymphatics.[528]

DIAGNOSIS

A physical and rectal examination, CBC and chemistry panel, cardiac evaluation, thoracic and abdominal ultrasound, and abdominocentesis may be helpful in determining the cause of the pleural effusion. When one suspects infectious agents, one should perform a transtracheal aspirate. One should also obtain a Coggins test and measure titers against *Coccidioides immitis, C. neoformans,* and *Mycoplasma felis,* depending on the nature of the effusion and the geographic location of the affected horse.

Cytologic and microbiologic evaluation of the pleural fluid (and pulmonary nodules or masses) may help identify neoplastic cells or fungal elements. Transudates, fluid with a total protein less than 2.5 g/dl, and few cells are usually associated with congestive heart failure, liver fibrosis, hypoalbuminemia, or early neoplastic processes. Modified transudates have low nucleated cell counts (<10,000 cells/μl) and moderate to high protein levels (>2.5 g/dl) and can be found in many disorders, including neoplasia. Exudates have nucleated cell counts exceeding 10,000 cells/μl and total protein levels greater than 3.0 g/dl and are found in infections and intraabdominal diseases.[514] One can distinguish septic effusions from nonseptic effusions by biochemical analysis of pleural fluid aspirates. For example, fluid that has a pH less than 7.2, a glucose concentration less than 40 mg/dl, and a lactate dehydrogenase concentration greater than 1000 IU/L has been suggested to indicate septic effusions. Chylous effusions, which are milky white to pale pink, have triglyceride concentrations exceeding that of simultaneously measured serum.[514]

TREATMENT

Treatment is aimed at the primary cause, but neoplastic conditions and pleural effusions associated with an end-stage organ failure carry a poor prognosis. Therapeutic thoracocentesis is indicated in malignant effusions when horses are experiencing breathing difficulties. Chest tube drainage and chemical pleurodesis, thoracoscopy with talc poudrage, or tunneled pleural catheters may be palliative approaches to reduce respiratory-related signs. The clinician should consider these procedures if (1) significant improvement in the status of the horse occurs with pleural fluid evacuation and (2) reexpansion of the lung is achieved once fluid is removed.

Pleurodesis is achieved by administering sclerosing agents that induce pleural inflammation, fibrosis, and, ultimately, a symphysis between parietal and visceral pleural surfaces. This action deters the accumulation of fluid (or air) in the pleural space.[531] Sclerosing agents such as talc (hydrated magnesium silicate) or tetracyclines are commonly used, although talc has been associated with the development of acute respiratory distress and hypoxemia.[532] These complications appear to be related to the talc particle size: Preparations that contain small-diameter particles (11 to 18 μm) are associated with a greater number of complications than are those preparations with particle diameters of 34 μ.[533] The belief is that the larger talc particles are disseminated through the lymphatic channels to a lesser degree and thus are less likely to induce systemic inflammation.[533]

Adapting protocols from human medicine[534] (given that successful management of malignant effusions in equine medicine has not been described) requires that the horse first be sedated. A chest tube is aseptically placed, and the effusion is drained. Before administering the sclerosing agent, physicians for humans will instill a local anesthetic to reduce patient discomfort. Patients also receive oral antiinflammatory drugs for analgesia. Then, one administers a sclerosing agent (e.g., in human medicine 500 mg doxycycline) in 100 to 500 ml of sterile solution through a chest tube and clamps the tube for 1 hour before reconnecting it to continuous suction.

Poudrage is the most widely used method of instilling talc into the pleural space and is usually performed under thoracoscopic guidance. Before spraying the talc over the visceral pleura, one should remove all pleural fluid; complete collapse aids in distributing the talc. In human medicine, one usually instills 5 g (8 to 12 ml) evenly over the pleural surface, places a chest tube, and applies progressive suction until the amount of fluid aspirated per day is less than 100 ml.[534] A slurry of talc can also be administered through a chest tube to induce pleurodesis if thoracoscopy is not an option.

Another option that is used in human medicine is the placement of a tunneled pleural catheter (TPC, Pleurx, Denver Biomedical, Denver, Colo.) that allows for continous home drainage of pleural effusions. The catheter, a 15.5-Fr silicone tubing, is 24 inches long and consists of a fenestrated distal end and a valve for draining purposes at the proximal end. The catheter is tunneled under the skin before entering the pleural space.[535] The drainage valve is accessed with a supplied adapter that can be attached to a plastic disposable vacuum bottle. In a randomized study comparing the efficacy of just TPC to doxycycline pleurodesis in the management of malignant pleural effusions, the degree of symptomatic improvement in dyspneic patients was comparable in both groups, but the late recurrence of pleural effusion was 13% in TPC patients compared with 21% in doxycycline-treated patients. Lastly, 46% of the TPC patients achieved spontaneous pleurodesis at a median of 27 days.[536]

FUNGAL PNEUMONIA

CAUSES AND PATHOGENESIS

The typical fungus exists in either a filamentous (mold) or a single-cell (yeast) form, although some fungi may exist in either form (hyphae in nature, yeast in tissue) and are termed *dimorphic*. Based on the mode of spore production and the morphologic characteristics of the colonies and constituent hyphae produced, fungi have been classified into five different phyla. In veterinary medicine, three of the most important phyla are Zygomycota *(Mucor, Absidia, Rhizopus)*, Ascomycota *(Aspergillus, Acremonium, Blastomyces, Coccidioides, Emmonsia, Histoplasma, Pneumocystis)*, and Basdiomycota *(Cryptococcus)*. Primary fungal pathogens causing respiratory disease in the horse include *Blastomyces dermatitidis, C. immitis, C. neoformans*, and *Histoplasma capsulatum*. Opportunistic fungi that cause respiratory disease include *Aspergillus* spp., *Pneumocystis carinii, Emmonsia crescens*, and *Acremonium strictum*.

Blastomyces dermatitidis is a thermally dimorphic fungus; it exists as a mold at room temperature and as a budding, round yeastlike cell when cultured at 37° C or when replicating in the host. As a soil saprophyte, *B. dermatitidis* can be found near decomposed vegetation or rotting wood.[537] In humans, inhalation of the fungi produces pulmonary infection that can disseminate to other organs and systems, including the central nervous system (CNS) and the reproductive and gastrointestinal tracts. Disease develops in both immunocompromised and immunocompetent individuals.[538] Although respiratory tract disease caused by this organism is rare in the horse, inhalation of the spores can cause a pyogranulomatous pneumonia.[539] No cases of animal (canine)-to-human transmission have been reported.

Coccidioides immitis, a soil saprophyte, is also dimorphic, existing as a mold on most culture media and as a nonbudding spherical form in the host tissue. Two variants, a California and non-California variant, exist, which are now classified as *C. immitis* and *C. posadasil*.[540] In humans, pulmonary infections ensue after inhalation of wind- or dust-borne arthroconidia. The infection is usually an acute and self-limiting respiratory disease in most hosts but can progress to chronic and sometimes fatal disseminated disease. Spontaneous healing can occur in 95% of healthy humans. Disease may also develop in immunocompromised individuals.[540] In horses, fungal pneumonia and pleuritis may occur after inhalation of arthrospores. Lymphohematogenous dissemination of the organisms may lead to the development of lesions in the bones, skin, and meninges, as well as cause abortion or mastitis.[541-543]

Cryptococcus neoformans is a yeastlike fungus that reproduces by budding, forming cells 4 to 7 μm in diameter. The organism has a predilection for the respiratory tract and for the CNS. The proposed route of infection is via inhalation with secondary hematogenous spread to the CNS. The virulence factors of the organism include an enzyme (phenol oxidase), a polysaccharide capsule, and the ability to grow at 37° C. The phenol oxidase enzyme aids in the production of melanin, which is thought to prevent formation of toxic hydroxyl radicals and to protect the fungal cell from oxidant stress and immune defenses.[544] The large polysaccharide capsule, which appears as a clear halo around the cell when organisms are stained with India ink, is antiphagocytic and immunosuppressive. Secreted capsular antigens bind opsonizing antibody before it reaches the organism.[545] Based on the capsular antigens, three variants of *C. neoformans* exist: *C. neoformans var. grubii* (serotype A), *C. neoformans var. gatti* (serotypes B and C), and *C. neoformans var. neoformans* (serotype D).[546]

Histoplasma capsulatum is a dimorphic fungus found in the soil and on decaying vegetation. Heavy concentrations of the organism accumulate in soils containing bat or bird feces. The organism is highly infectious as an airborne spore (microconidia) but is of low virulence when it converts to the yeast phase (2 to 4 μm) in the host.[546] In humans, acute benign pulmonary infection may become chronic pulmonary disease or progress to disseminated fatal systemic disease.[547] Systemic histoplasmosis is uncommon in proportion to the equine population exposed; the horse seems particularly resistant to infection.[548] The proposed route of infection is via inhalation or ingestion of the microconidia. Because the organism parasitizes mononuclear phagocytes and has an affinity for the reticuloendothelial system, it may disseminate to the liver, spleen, lymph nodes, and bone marrow.[549]

Opportunists such as *Aspergillus* spp., *P. carinii, E. crescens,* and *A. strictum* also cause pneumonia in horses that are immunosuppressed or have concurrent illnesses.[550-557] *Aspergillus* is a mold with septate hyphae 2 to 4 μm in diameter. The most prevalent pathogenic species is *A. fumigatus,* but *A. flavus, A. nidulans,* and *A. niger* also may cause disease.[558] These fungi are ubiquitous in the environment, growing on dead leaves, stored grain, compost piles, hay, and decaying vegetation.[545] In humans, *Aspergillus* spp. play a role in three clinical settings: (1) opportunistic infections; (2) allergic states; and (3) toxicoses (mycotoxins). Immunosuppression is the major factor leading to the development of opportunistic infections in humans.[559] In horses, aspergillosis has involved the guttural pouches, lungs, and mediastinum.[560,561] Inhalation of *Aspergillus* spores is suspected to be common, but disease is rare unless the horse is immunocompromised (neoplasia, steroid therapy), has been treated extensively with broad-spectrum antimicrobials, has a concurrent colitis (disruption of the mucosal barrier, allowing hematogenous spread), or has been stabled in an environment that contains high numbers of fungal organisms.[562] Infection is characterized by hyphal invasion of blood vessels, thrombosis, necrosis, and hemorrhagic infarction in pulmonary tissues. Because *Aspergillus* spp. occurs widely as an environmental contaminant, diagnosis may require repeated isolation or histologic demonstration. Dual mycotic pulmonary infections, although rare, have also been reported in horses involving *Aspergillus* spp. and fungal organisms in the order Mucorales *(Absidia corymbifera, Rhizopus stolonifer).*[560,562]

Pneumocystis carinii had been formerly considered a protozoan organism because of its morphologic features and its susceptibility to antiprotozoal agents.[563] However, the genes encoding the small subunit ribosomal RNA (16s) and the large subunit of mitochondrial rRNA demonstrate similarities to the genes encoding for the rRNA of several different fungal species.[564] As a result, *P. carinii* was reclassified as a fungus in 1988. Electron microscopy has revealed two parasite forms: trophozoite and cystic. The trophozoite is an ameboid form 2 to 5 μm in diameter with filopodia that attach to the surface of the type I epithelial cells. The trophozoite is visible with hematoxylin and eosin stains. The mature cyst is 4 to 6 μm in diameter and contains eight uninucleate intracystic bodies. The cyst stains with Gomori's or Grocott's methenamine silver stain and periodic acid–Schiff (PAS) stain. In keeping with the new taxonomic classification, some authors recommend replacing the terminology of the different parasite forms by the terms yeast cell (trophozoite), sporangia (cyst), and spores (intracystic bodies).[564] The infective stage or source of *P. carinii* is unknown, although several studies have reported discovery of *P. carinii* DNA in water and air samples, suggesting that these are environmental reservoirs.[565] It was long believed that *Pneumocystis* occurred only after reactivation of quiescent organisms (lung saprophytes) that had previously entered the lower respiratory tract of an immunocompetent host.[563] In rodent models, *P. carinii* can be transmitted from one animal to another via the airborne route, and evidence now exists that person-to-person transmission is the most likely mode of acquiring new pneumocystis infections.[566] *Pneumocystis* organisms have been identified in nearly every mammalian species, but the organisms have genetic characteristics that determine host specificity. For example, the *Pneumocystis* organism that infects humans (renamed as *P. jirovecii*) is unable to infect rodents.[567] In humans, pneumocystis pneumonia remains the most prevalent opportunistic infection in patients infected with human immunodeficiency virus (HIV) or in individuals receiving immunosuppressant medications.[568] In horses, it is a rare cause of pneumonia, affecting the younger foal as compared with the adult horse.

Other soil saprophytes that have been reported as rare causes of fungal pneumonia in the horse include *A. strictum* (a plant and insect pathogen)[569] and *E. crescens* (an opportunist pathogen of carnivores, insectivores, marsupials, lagomorphs, and rodents).[557] Both of these fungi are *cosmopolitan,* commonly isolated from soil and debris. In immunocompromised humans, *Acremonium* causes keratitis, endophthalmitis, endocarditis, meningitis, peritonitis, and osteomyelitis. Because *Acremonium* spp. can be an environmental contaminant, its isolation from respiratory tract secretions requires careful evaluation.[570] *Emmonsia* spp. are an occasional cause of animal and human infections, being endemic in the southwestern United States, Australia, and Eastern Europe. In rodents, an asymptomatic pulmonary infection develops after inhalation of the conidia. Rarely, in immunocompromised humans, disseminated infection may occur.[571]

EPIDEMIOLOGY

Fungal pneumonia in the horse as a primary entity is uncommon. Disease usually results when debilitating conditions that favor the penetration or growth of fungi exist. Contributory factors include (1) exposure to large numbers of mycotic organisms in the environment,[572] (2) stabling of horses within a moist or unhygienic environment,[573] (3) prolonged administration of antibiotics that upset the microfloral balance or interfere with vitamin synthesis, (4) existence of an immunosuppressive state primarily (combined immunodeficiency disorder) or secondarily because of the administration of drugs, development of an endocrinopathy, or neoplasia.[556,558]

For the pathogenic fungi, prevalence of the disease may be determined geographically. For example, *B. dermatitidis* is endemic to the Mississippi, Missouri, and Ohio River basins; the Canadian provinces of Quebec, Ontario, and Manitoba; the Great Lakes region; and the Eastern seaboard of the United States.[539] Although *H. capsulatum* is endemic to the Mississippi, Ohio, and St. Lawrence River valleys, it also is found in the southern United States.[549,574] *Coccidiodes immitis* is endemic to the arid and semiarid regions of North America, including the states of California, Texas, Arizona, New Mexico, Nevada, and Utah.[541,575] In contrast, *Cryptococcus neoformans* is widespread, being found in high concentrations in the soil and in avian manure *(C. neoformans var. neoformans)*. In Australia, an epizootiologic relationship of *C. neoformans var. gatti* exists with the eucalyptus tree *(Eucalyptus camaldulensis)*. Environmental dispersal of the fungus coincides with flowering of the eucalyptus tree in the spring, resulting in greater exposure and more cases of disease during that time.[576] A disproportionately large number of published equine cases have been recorded by Australian investigators, supporting the impression that this disease is more common in Australia than in North America or Europe.[577]

For the opportunistic fungus *P. carinii*, human clinical infections develop only in immunodepressed subjects, those individuals with low $CD4^+$ counts and with certain viral infections (cytomegalovirus, HIV), those in weakened nutritional states, or those receiving immunosuppressive therapy.[563,564] To date, most of the reported cases of equine pneumocystosis have occurred in foals 1.5 to 4 months of age. Predisposing factors include the existence of a combined immunodeficiency disorder,[554] *R. equi* or chronic bacterial pneumonia,[555,578] low $CD4^+$ counts,[579] and chronic debilitation or weight loss.[580,581] In two reports of equine pneumocystosis in foals, predisposing factors could not be identified.[582,583] The occurrence of pneumocystosis in young foals may reflect an age-dependent maturation of the immune system. Cell-mediated immune responses (in vitro) of foals younger than 2 months are reduced relative to those of adult horses, perhaps increasing the susceptibility of the foal to pneumocystosis.[584] If an adult horse becomes immunodeficient, it may be at risk for developing pneumocystis pneumonia as described in a 5-year-old Paso Fino mare.[163,585] This debilitated mare with respiratory distress had foaled 2 months previously. Immunologic testing of the mare at a tertiary referral center demonstrated an absence of serum IgM, low concentrations of serum IgG (800 mg/dl), and a low percentage of peripheral blood mononuclear cells expressing MHC class II molecules (28% compared with a normal range of 54% to 81%), suggesting immunocompromise.

CLINICAL SIGNS

Horses with primary fungal pneumonia (blastomycosis, histoplasmosis, cryptococcosis, and coccidioidomycosis) may have a chronic cough, anorexia, weight loss, exercise intolerance, and nasal discharge.[586-588] Tachypnea or respiratory distress may or may not be a clinical feature of the fungal pneumonia. Pleural effusion is found more commonly with coccidioidomycosis but has also been reported in cases of cryptococcosis and blastomycosis.[539,541,588]

In addition to causing pneumonia, these fungal organisms may cause disease in other body systems. *B. dermatitidis* causes weight loss, intraabdominal abscesses[539]; superficial abscesses around the anus, vulva, and udder[589,590]; and generalized cutaneous ulcerative skin lesions.[590] In a review of 15 cases of equine coccidioidomycosis, 43% of the cases had hepatic lesions, 29% had bone or periosteal involvement, 22% had lesions in the peritoneum, and 64% had pulmonary parenchymal disorders.[541] Other reports describe *Coccidioides immitis* lesions in the mammary gland,[543] the placenta and fetus,[542,591] and the skin.[592] *Cryptococcus neoformans* has been reported to cause granulomata in the skin, nasal cavity, paranasal sinuses, orbits, intestines, bones, meninges, placenta, and fetus.[576,593-597] In addition to pulmonary lesions (including abscessation),[598] *H. capsulatum* infections have been associated with abortions, disseminated histoplasmosis of foals, granulomatous colitis of adult horses, intraabdominal abscessation, and keratitis.[548,574,599-601]

A horse developing pneumonia caused by opportunistic fungi (aspergillosis, pneumocystosis) may have evidence of a debilitating or immunosuppressive problem such as colitis, peritonitis, septicemia, endotoxemia, an endocrinopathy, or chronic bacterial pneumonia. Young horses (foals) may be at an increased risk for developing opportunistic infections *(P. carinii)*.

In the majority of cases of pulmonary aspergillosis, pneumonia appears to be a sequela to mycotic invasion of the intestinal tract, the integrity of which has been compromised by severe acute enterocolitis.[550,551,553,572] Such horses also have typically received broad-spectrum antimicrobials and nonsteroidal anti-inflammatory drugs and are neutropenic—factors that may also predispose them to the development of systemic aspergillosis. Nevertheless, pulmonary aspergillosis also has been reported in horses with pleuropneumonia, myositis, renal failure, pituitary adenoma, and myelomonocytic leukemia.[553,556,558]

Horses with pulmonary aspergillosis may suddenly become febrile and tachypneic and may exhibit adventitious lung or pleural sounds and have a nasal discharge. Other horses with pulmonary aspergillosis may show only mild respiratory signs or fail to demonstrate any abnormalities of the respiratory tract.[553,599,602]

Pneumocystosis is a rare clinical entity. In the majority of cases, foals have evidence of chronic respiratory disease that has progressed to respiratory distress. Weight loss, dehydration, and inappetence also may be evident.[555,579-581,583] Similar signs were reported in a 5-year-old Paso Fino mare that developed pnuemocystosis.[585,603]

DIAGNOSIS

Tracheobronchial aspirates may reveal degenerated neutrophils, yeast cells, and bacteria. In the case of aspergillosis, the diagnosis may be difficult because one may recover fungal elements (*Aspergillus* spp., *Penicillium* spp., and *Mucor* spp.) from the tracheal washings of normal horses.[38] Definitive diagnosis may require repeated isolation of the *Aspergillus* organisms or histologic demonstration of hyphal elements in the pulmonary parenchyma. Transtracheal aspirates may be of limited usefulness in diagnosing pneumocystosis because the organism is rarely isolated by this method. For horses not in respiratory distress, isolation of the organism may be possible by bronchoalveolar lavage (BAL) or endobronchial brushings.[555,579-581] Cytocentrifugation of BAL samples followed by silver-staining of slides facilitates identification of *P. carinii*. Indeed, in human medicine, diagnostic sensitivity of cytology is considered to be 89% to 94% compared with sensitivity of histopathologic examination of lung biopsies of 73%.[585] A culture system has not been developed for diagnosis of *P. carinii*.

In horses with fungal pneumonia, radiographs may reveal circular masses with or without fluid lines and an accentuated interstitial pattern. In horses with cryptococcal pneumonia, the most common presentation is large cavitating granulomas (cryptococcomas) that tend to be located in the dorsocaudal lung lobes. Less commonly, miliary interstitial granulomas evenly distributed throughout the lung fields are evident.[577] Radiography or ultrasonography may detect pleural effusion. Ultrasonographic examination may reveal comet-tail signs, indicative of pleural roughening or inflammation, small areas of pulmonary consolidation, or masses of variable echogenicity delineated by hyperechoic capsules.[577,604] Ultrasound-guided aspirates of the masses may provide samples for culture and cytologic evaluation.

Serologic detection of an antibody response to *Coccidioides immitis, Cryptococcus neoformans,* and *H. capsulatum* has been useful in diagnosing fungal pneumonia because the organisms can be difficult to culture and tissue biopsies may lack evidence of the organisms. Repeated measurement of titers may be necessary. In a survey of immunoglobulin responses in healthy asymptomatic horses stabled in a *C. immitis* endemic areas, only 4% of the horses developed an IgG titer (all of which were ≤ 8). On resampling, the titer decreased or became negative within 2 to 6 months while horses remained disease free.[605] These data suggest that an elevated titer in a clinically ill animal strongly supports the diagnosis of *C. immitis* infection.[606] Interestingly, for *C. immitis* infections, the magnitude of the antibody response is associated with the clinical form. In comparing horses with miliary or interstitial pneumonia (sans thoracic effusion), with pneumonia and thoracic effusion (pleural or pericardial), and with pneumonia and disseminated disease, the geometric mean titers were 51, 225, and 104, respectively. Horses that had *C. immitis* abortions had titers less than 8. Similarly, in horses with cryptococcosis, serologic detection of capsular antigens (serum latex agglutination test) also has proved effective in the diagnosis.[588,593] In horses with histoplasmosis, an agar gel immunodiffusion (AGID) test has been used. There are two possible bands of precipitation in the test: an M-band that may indicate recent past infection (within 12 months) or active infection and an H-band. The simultaneous precipitation of both bands indicates current active infection.[548] The histoplasmin skin test is of little diagnostic value; in one endemic area, 73% of horses had a positive skin test.[607] Serologic diagnosis of pulmonary aspergillosis can be difficult because titers are detectable in healthy and diseased horses.[553] Nevertheless, Moore et al.[561] reported the existence of two precipitin bands against *Aspergillus* antigens in a horse confirmed to have an *Aspergillus* mediastinal granuloma. Precipitin bands were not evident in the eight control horses sampled. In a description of a horse with bronchial lymphadenitis caused by *Aspergillus,* precipitin bands against the fungus (titer of 1:8) were measured.[608] Recently, Guillot, Sarfati, DeBarros, et al.[609] reported the usefulness of an immunoblot analysis for the diagnosis of aspergillosis, detecting reactivity to low–molecular-mass antigens (22-26 kDa) in the sera of diseased horses that were not evident in clinically healthy horses. The investigators suggested that these antigens were released during mycelial growth in the tissues, a phase that would not develop in clinically healthy horses. However, until this experimental assay is commercially available, one should use the serologic diagnosis cautiously in suspected cases of pulmonary aspergillosis. One may confirm the diagnosis with lung biopsy and by the presence of other systemic alterations.

The immunocompetence status of the horse can be superficially evaluated by quantitation of immunoglobulin levels, by performing mitogen stimulation tests, and by immunophenotyping of peripheral blood leukocytes (granulocytes, monocytes, $CD5^+$, $CD4^+$, and $CD8^+$ T cells, B cells, and MHC I and II expression). Diagnostic investigations should rule out the existence of endocrinopathies and neoplasia.

TREATMENT

Treatment against the primary fungal pathogens requires long-term administration (weeks) of antifungal drugs and correction or elimination of the inciting cause of the fungal pneumonia. Many of the newer antifungal drugs have been designed to target differences in the cellular and biochemical properties of fungi compared with mammalian cells. Recall that fungi are eukaryotes that have DNA organized into chromosomes within the cell nucleus and endoplasmic reticulum, Golgi, mitochondria, and storage vacuoles within the cytoplasm. The fungal cell walls are rigid and consist of mannoproteins, β-glucans, and chitin. The fungal cell membrane is a lipid bilayer that contains ergosterol instead of cholesterol as the predominant sterol.

Four basic classes of antifungal drugs are commonly used in veterinary medicine. The polyenes are *cidal* compounds that are derived from *Streptomyces* species. Representatives of this class of drugs include amphotericin B, nystatin, and natamycin. The drugs work by combining irreversibly to the ergosterol in the fungal cytoplasmic membrane, causing depolarization, pore formation, and increased cell membrane permeability. Most bacteria are resistant to polyenes because they lack the necessary cell membrane binding sites. At high enough doses, the polyenes will bind with cholesterol and cause organ toxicity, most notably renal disease in mammalians.

A second class of drugs includes the azoles—miconazole, ketoconazole, itraconazole, fluconazole, and enilconazole (topical). These synthetic compounds reduce ergosterol production by inhibiting the P450 3A–dependent enzyme 14α-demethylase. As a result, aberrant sterols accumulate in the fungal cell membrane. This inhibition affects nutrient utilization and causes leaky cell membranes.[545] These compounds are considered to be either fungistatic or fungicidal. However, unlike the polyenes, some of these compounds have activity against gram-positive bacteria and protozoa. Because these drugs can inhibit the P450-dependent enzymes involved in cholesterol synthesis, hormone (cortisol, androgen, and testosterone) concentrations may be decreased.[610] Hepatotoxicities are also a potential side effect.

The allylamines are a third class of antifungals and include terbinafine and naftidine. These compounds also inhibit ergosterol synthesis in a site earlier than that of the azoles, specifically targeting the enzyme squalene epoxidase. Hepatotoxicities can also ensue.

A fourth class of antifungals includes the antimetabolites or substituted pyridimines that inhibit DNA and protein synthesis. An example is flucytosine, which is converted to 5-fluoruracil. Resistance develops when the active transport mechanism for flucytosine uptake is reduced.

Newer antifungal drugs are being marketed that target the synthesis of cell wall constituents by inhibiting the production of β-1,3 glucan (caspofungin, micafungin, and anidulafungin) or chitin (nikkomycin Z). However, because fungal pneumonia is relatively uncommon, the efficacy of various protocols has not been stringently assessed. Selection of the antifungal drug to use should also be guided by sensitivity patterns of the fungal isolates but more importantly on clinical response.

Amphotericin B has been used successfully to treat histoplasmosis,[549] pulmonary aspergillosis,[609] and pulmonary cryptococcosis.[577] The recommended dose is 0.1 to 0.6 mg/kg administered in a 5%-dextrose solution intravenously over 60 minutes, one to three times per week, although more frequent administration has been described.[577] Some clinicians have recommended starting at 0.35 mg/kg intravenously once daily for 3 days, then 0.4 mg/kg intravenously once daily for 3 days, and 0.5 mg/kg intravenously once daily for the remainder of the treatment course.[577] Possible adverse effects include anorexia, anemia, arrhythmias, hepatic and renal dysfunction, hypersensitivity reactions, tremors, and fever.[595] Pretreatment with flunixin meglumine has been suggested to ameliorate the adverse effects, although the risk of nephrotoxicity should be considered. Studies conducted in France have suggested that preheating amphotericin B to 60° to 70° C for 10 minutes before the administration increases the clinical efficacy and decreases nephrotoxicity by changing the physicochemical properties of the constituent colloidal dispersion.[577,611] Neither amphotericin B nor ketoconazole were found to be curative in a series of cases of coccidioidomycosis.[541] However, long-term administration of itraconazole (2.6 mg/kg orally twice daily) was effective in treating coccidioidomycosis vertebral osteomyelitis in a foal,[575] and long-term fluconazole (5 mg/kg orally once daily) proved efficacious for two horses with *C. immitis* interstitial pneumonia.[604] Higgins has found in horses with *C. immitis* pneumonia that the magnitude of the titer is associated with the severity of the infection and hence with prognosis.[606] Thus, when identified early in the course of their disease, horses with only miliary (interstitial) pneumonia have a better prognosis than horses with concurrent pleural effusion or disseminated disease. In the two horses with *C. immitis* interstitial pneumonia, clinical cure was achieved after a 4- to 6-month course of fluconazole (administered at a loading dose of 14 mg/kg orally followed by 5 mg/kg orally once daily).[604] Based on human medicine, clinicians should attempt to achieve peak plasma concentrations in the range of 4 to 8 μg/ml. Fluconazole therapy is terminated when clinical signs dissipate (weight gain is noted) and serum IgG titers decrease.

Too few cases of blastomycosis have, as yet, been described in the literature to recommend treatment protocols for this disorder. In the single case report of pneumonia caused by *Acremonia crescens,* fluconazole (loading dose of 14 mg/kg orally followed by 5 mg/kg orally once daily) for 30 days was efficacious. *P. carinii* infections require treatment with antiprotozoal drugs; Ewing et al.[581] has reported success using trimethoprim sulfamethoxazole (25 mg/kg orally twice daily) in combination with procaine penicillin G in foals with pneumocystosis. Furthermore, Flaminio et al.[579] supplemented trimethoprim sulfamethoxazole (30 mg/kg orally twice daily) with interferon-α (100 U orally once daily) and *Propionibacterium acnes* (EqStim) in an effort to increase $CD4^+$ and $CD8^+$ counts in a foal with pneumocystosis. The pneumonia eventually resolved and lymphocyte counts returned to normal. In another foal with pneumocystosis, dapsone, a dihydropterate synthase inhibitor, was administered at 3 mg/kg orally with a successful outcome.[612] In humans with acute respiratory distress caused by pneumocystosis and secondary hypoxemia, concurrent administration of glucocorticoids is recommended.[568]

Mycoplasmal Pneumonia

Several species of *Mycoplasma* may be isolated from the upper and lower respiratory tracts of healthy horses and from the nasal cavities of healthy foals soon after birth.[613] *M. felis* has been isolated from clinical and experimental cases of parapneumonic effusions[525,614,615] and from foals with pneumonia.[616] *M. felis, M. equirhinis,* and a non–*M. felis* glucose-fermenting mycoplasma (NFGM) species have been isolated, along with bacterial organisms, from the tracheobronchial aspirates of young athletic horses with inflammatory airway disease (IAD)[617,618] In a recent epidemiology survey of 800 young racehorses consisting of 632 controls and 170 with signs of IAD (cough at rest or exercise, mild pyrexia, abnormal mucous or serous nasal discharge), the isolation of *M. felis* but not *M. equirhinis* or NFGM mycoplasma was associated with an increased risk of IAD.[618] Furthermore, a recent Canadian survey documented serologic evidence of *M. felis* or *M. equirhinis* infection in 9% and 10%, respectively, of horses showing clinical signs of acute respiratory disease.[418]

The pathogenesis of the inflammatory or infectious airway disease (pneumonia) is generally believed to involve adherence of the organism to ciliated epithelium, causing loss of the cilia and subsequent death of the cell. This belief is supported by the finding of degenerative epithelial cells in the tracheobronchial aspirates of horses with mycoplasma infections.[617] Diagnosis of mycoplasmosis depends on isolation of the organism from tracheobronchial aspirates or from pleural fluid and on demonstration of seroconversion. The clinician should initiate treatment with broad-spectrum antibacterials (oxytetracycline) until antimicrobial culture and sensitivity reports are available given that bacterial coinfections are likely.

Interstitial Lung Disease

DEFINITION

Interstitial pneumonia describes an acute or chronic inflammatory process that involves primarily the alveolar walls (endothelium, basement membrane, and alveolar epithelium) and contiguous bronchiolar interstitium.[619,620] Horses that develop acute respiratory distress syndrome (discussed elsewhere in this chapter) may do so because of interstitial lung disease.

EPIDEMIOLOGY

Buergelt[621] has suggested that two types of equine interstitial disorders exist: one occurring in foals 6 days to 6 months of age[622,623] and one developing in adult horses older than 2 years. This discussion focuses on interstitial lung disorders in the adult horse.

CAUSES

Interestingly, in humans, interstitial lung disease is attributed to more than 200 different etiologic factors, including bacterial, fungal, viral, protozoal, and parasitic agents; collagen vascular disorders (systemic lupus erythematosus, rheumatoid arthritis, progressive systemic sclerosis, Sjögren syndrome); vasculitides; hypersensitivities; silica; asbestos; beryllium; and drugs.[624]

Most of the spontaneously occurring interstitial lung disorders in horses have been attributed to toxic or infectious (bacterial, viral, or parasitic agents) agents.[619] Toxic lung injury occurs after ingestion of Crofton weed (*Eupatorium adenophorum,* toxic agent unknown),[625,626] mist flower (*Eupatorium riparium,* toxic agent unidentified),[627] Crotalaria seeds (*Crotalaria juncea,* toxic agent is a pyrrolizidine alkaloid),[628] or exposure to Perilla mint (*Perilla frutescens,* toxic agent is a ketone).[629-631] Exogenous deposition of lipid (mineral oil) causes an interstitial pneumonia, often known as a lipoid pneumonia or lipid pneumonitis.[632-635] (Aspiration of mineral oil can occur after esophageal intubation if the oil is administered under pressure, in an incompletely emptied stomach, or after removal of the tube that still contains oil.[633])

Viral infections, particularly in foals or young horses,[304,308] also cause interstitial lung disease. Specific etiologic agents include equine influenza A2; EHV1 and 4; AHV4, 5, and 6; EVA; Hendra virus; and AHS virus.[327,636] In a recent retrospective study of 24 horses with clinical signs and radiographic evidence of interstitial lung disease, EHV5 was detected by PCR in 79% of the paraffin-fixed lung samples from these horses.[392] However, causality between EHV5 and this multinodular interstitial lung disease remains to be established as EHV5 can be isolated from PBMC or nasal swabs of 24% to 33% of healthy horses.[381,389]

Mycobacterial infections[637-639] are a rare cause of interstitial pneumonia in the horse. Etiologic agents include members of the *Mycobacterium tuberculosis* complex *(M. bovis, M. tuberculosis)* and of the *M. avium* complex (*M. avium* subsp. *avium, M. avium* subsp. *hominissuis, M. avium* subsp. *paratuberculosis).* In surveys of European abattoirs conducted in the mid-1950s, prevalence of mycobacterial infections was 0.3%, suggesting that horses were relatively resistant to infection.[640] Of the mycobacterial infections reported in that study, *M. avium* spp. *avium* was considered to be the most common cause of tuberculosis in the horse having been isolated from 91% of the affected horses. *M. bovis* was identified in 3% of the isolates.[641] Although airborne infections cannot be dismissed, the most common route of infection for equine tuberculosis is alimentary, with hematogenous dissemination to the liver, spleen, lung, lymph nodes, and bones.[638,640] Thus the clinical signs of tuberculosis will depend on which organ systems are affected. Fungal agents[569,603] also cause interstitial pneumonia. (See previous discussion on fungal pneumonia.)

Unfortunately, for many cases of interstitial pneumonia, a well-defined cause is lacking, and thus are known as *idiopathic interstitial* or *granulomatous disease*.[642-648] Idiopathic eosinophilic granulomatous pneumonia may occur as part of the syndrome of equine multisystemic eosinophilic epitheliotropic disease, or it may affect only the lungs, causing disseminated eosinophilic granulomas.[649]

PATHOPHYSIOLOGY

The inciting agent damages pulmonary epithelial or endothelial cells, causing coagulative necrosis of the alveoli. Pulmonary congestion, interstitial edema, erythrocyte extravasation, and alveolar flooding characterize the acute (exudative) phase of the disease. Fibrin, protein-rich fluid, cellular debris, and inflammatory cells (neutrophils and macrophages) form hyaline membranes. During the acute phase (1 to 5 days after the initial insult), the horse may exhibit respiratory distress. The exudative phase is followed by a proliferative stage in which the type II pneumocytes—the pulmonary stem cells—replace damaged type I pneumocytes. Interlobar septae widen because of the proliferation of fibroblasts and inflammatory cell infiltration by neutrophils and macrophages.[619] Chronic interstitial lung disease is characterized by fibrosis of the alveolar walls and accumulation of mononuclear cells in the interstitium. Granulomas and smooth muscle hyperplasia may form during the chronic phase, although this finding is not unequivocal in all cases of interstitial pneumonia.[620] For example, in an experimental model of interstitial lung disease (induced by intravenous administration of Perilla mint ketone), acute alveolar damage did not progress to interstitial fibrosis despite the enhanced collagen gene expression (COL1A1 and COL3A1).[631] It is possible that the changes of chronic interstitial lung disease require persistence of or repeated exposure to the causative agents—dusts, drugs, or infectious agents.[619]

The pathophysiologic stages of lipoid pneumonia have been described in humans. The first stage consists of hemorrhage and bronchopneumonia, which is followed by a severe macrophagic infiltrate that engulfs the oil droplets. The third and fourth stages entail fibroblastic proliferation and paraffinoma (fibrosis). Depending on the quantity of oil aspirated, the human patient can progress to stage 4 in a little as 3 to 4 weeks.[650]

CLINICAL SIGNS

Clinical signs of interstitial lung disease vary, depending on the stage of the disease and the causative agent involved. In the acute phase, horses may exhibit acute respiratory distress (tachypnea), adventitious lung sounds, and signs of hypoxemia caused by poor gas exchange (ataxia, altered mucous membrane color) with or without a fever.[630,651] In the later stages of the disease, horses also have clinical signs resembling those of heaves-affected horses—tachypnea, an accentuated expiratory effort, cough, and nasal discharge.[642-644] In chronic stages, horses may exhibit exercise intolerance,[643] weight loss, anorexia, and fever. Horses terminally affected by the pulmonary form of tuberculosis are febrile, exhibit respiratory distress, and have a cough. Occasionally, interstitial lung disease may produce pulmonary hypertension and cor pulmonale.[652] Interstitial lung disease also may be present in the absence of clinical signs.[643]

DIAGNOSIS

The diagnosis is based on the cumulative results of clinical examination, history, radiographic or ultrasonographic examination (or both), or isolation of a causative agent from respiratory secretions or tissue samples obtained from biopsy or postmortem examination. Clinical pathologic data are often nonspecific. Arterial hypoxemia may be evident on blood gas analysis. The CBC and serum chemistry panels may be normal or may demonstrate leukocytosis and hyperfibrinogenemia.[646,653] Confirmation of the horse's prior travel and area of residence may aid in the diagnosis. Silicosis develops in horses that have lived in arid or desert areas where soils are rich in silicates, as occurs, for example, in selected regions of California.[654] Other relevant historical information includes vaccination history (viral) and prior medications (e.g., lipid pneumonitis secondary to mineral oil administration).

Evaluation of tracheobronchial secretions or BALs may reveal the presence of a nonseptic inflammation characterized by neutrophilia with or without Curschmann's spirals.[646,648] Depending on the causative agent, analysis of respiratory secretions may also demonstrate pulmonary macrophages with (1) intracytoplasmic eosinophilic crystalline inclusions (silicosis),[655] (2) intracytoplasmic fungal organisms (fungal pneumonia),[569] or (3) acid fast–stained intracellular bacilli (tuberculosis).[639] In horses with lipid pneumonitis, the tracheal aspirates may be red to orange in color as a result of the presence of erythrocytes and contain a predominance of neutrophils. Sudan and Oil-Red-O stains of the aspirates confirm the presence of free lipid droplets, as well as lipid-laden macrophages.[633-635]

Radiographs demonstrate (1) an increase in the interstitial pattern of the lung (Figure 9-19) or (2) the presence of pulmonary infiltrates that form discrete and diffuse nodules. A reticulonodular radiographic pattern has been observed in horses

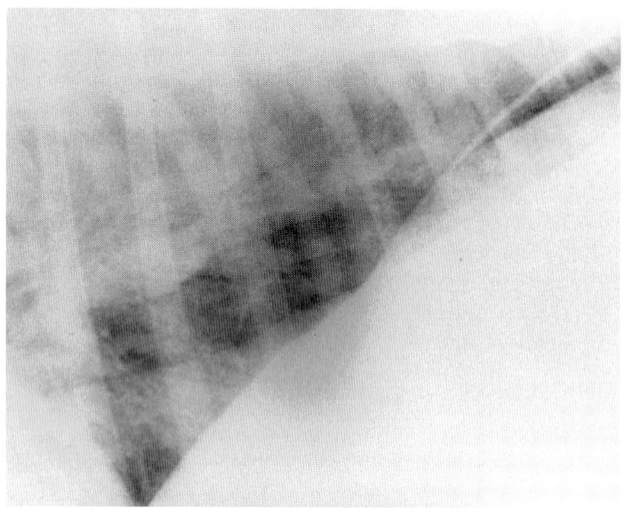

FIGURE 9-19 Overall increase in interstitial pulmonary opacity represents interstitial lung disease. (Courtesy D. S. Biller, Manhattan, Kan., 1991.)

with silicosis,[655] mycobacterial or fungal pneumonia, and EHV5 infections, as well as in idiopathic cases of interstitial lung disease. Radiographic changes do not allow one to distinguish these cases from those with neoplasia. Few descriptive studies of the ultrasonographic changes in interstitial lung disease exist. In general, the predominant changes in influenza consist of diffuse comet-tail signs with or without parenchymal defects consisting of consolidation,[304] or hypoechoic lesions in the caudal dorsal lung fields.[569,646]

Serology may be helpful in the diagnosis of viral infections[651] especially if acute and convalescent titers can be obtained for comparison. More rapid diagnostic approaches entail molecular techniques such as PCR (AHV4, AHV5, EHV5, EHV1, EIV, EHV).

Skin testing to diagnose mycobacterial infections are of low specificity and sensitivity,[641] given that up to 70% of clinically normal horses have a positive skin test.[656]

PATHOLOGIC SIGNS

The lung changes are a function of the stage and the causative agent. Histologic evaluation of lung biopsies confirms the diagnosis of interstitial pneumonia in the acute (exudative, proliferative) or chronic (fibrotic) stages. Postmortem examination may reveal diffuse pulmonary fibrosis, hypercellularity of the alveolar septa, and scarring of the interlobular septa and parts of the pleura. Severe chronic bronchitis and bronchiolitis also may be evident if concurrent airway disease exists, but this feature is atypical of interstitial pneumonia.[482] Multifocal granulomata may be detectable.[644,654] Microscopically, granulomas consist of epithelioid cells, giant cells, and lymphocytes. In horses with eosinophilic granulomatous pneumonia, the granulomas consist of central degenerated eosinophils surrounded by epithelioid macrophages, multinucleated giant cells, and collagenous fibrotic tissue.[649]

TREATMENT

Horses with acute interstitial pneumonia should receive supportive care, as outlined in the section Acute Respiratory Distress Syndrome. The following treatment recommendations pertain to horses with chronic interstitial lung disease. In human medicine, patients with chronic interstitial lung disease characterized by fibrosis (especially idiopathic pulmonary fibrosis) have received a variety of treatments, including corticosteroids, immunosuppressive or cytotoxic agents (azathioprine, cyclophosphamide), and antifibrotic agents (colchicine, D-penicillamine, *N*-acetylcysteine) alone or in combination.[657] Newer therapeutic approaches entail the administration of interferon-gamma, endothelin-1 receptor antagonists, and tyrosine kinase inhibitors,[658] although well-designed clinical trials for many of the drug treatments are lacking.

In equine medicine, the standard approach to the treatment of chronic interstitial lung disease, which lacks evidence of an active infection, has been corticosteroid administration singly or in combination with bronchodilators and broad-spectrum antimicrobials. Doxycycline, because of its anti-inflammatory effects, may also be indicated in the treatment of interstitial pneumonia. Well-controlled prospective studies are lacking, but the horse occasionally responds to treatment and is able to resume athletic ability.[646] For example, in one study of seven horses with idiopathic granulomatous interstitial pneumonia, only one of three horses that received a course of corticosteroid improved, although tachypnea remained.[648] Similarly, in a report of equine silicosis, of the eight horses that were treated with corticosteroids, 50% responded. Four of the eight had progressive radiographic pulmonary consolidation necessitating euthanasia within 12 months of initial diagnosis, whereas the remaining four showed no improvement in radiographic signs despite weight gains.[655] The prognosis for horses with lipoid pneumonia is poor, although Henninger, Hass, and Freshwater (2006) described the successful treatment of a 10-year-old Clydesdale stallion that had aspirated mineral oil administered by its owner for treatment of colic.[635] The treatment regimen consisted of antimicrobials (initially trimethoprim-sulfadiazine, later procaine penicillin, metronidazole and gentamicin before referral for 10 days) followed by a protracted course (weeks) of dexamethasone.

LUNGWORMS

CAUSES

Lungworm infections in the equine species are caused by *Dictyocaulus arnfieldi*. Infections in the donkey and mule are asymptomatic but provide a source of viable eggs for clinically apparent infections in the horse and pony.

EPIDEMIOLOGY

Lungworm infections have been diagnosed by recovery of larvae in live animals by bronchoscopic examination or at postmortem evaluation. Using this approach, the prevalence of lungworm infection is approximately 68% to 80% in donkeys, 29% in mules, and 2% to 11% in horses.[659,660]

PATHOGENESIS

Donkeys, mules, and asses are asymptomatic reservoirs of the parasite, but instances of lungworm infections have occurred in horses in which no contact with donkeys could be established, suggesting horse-to-horse transmission may be possible.[660] Experimental studies provide evidence that under field conditions, *Pilobolus* spp. fungi may facilitate the spread of lungworm infections in a manner similar to that which occurs in cattle lungworm infections.[661] The infective larvae ascend the coprophilous fungus as it grows on the manure and invade the sporangia. When the sporangia rupture, the infective larvae disperse with the fungal spores. After the infective larvae (0.4 mm) are ingested, they migrate through the gut wall and are carried to the lungs via the lymphatics. In hosts in which infections are patent, the larvae mature to egg-laying adults in the peripheral bronchioles. The prepatent period is approximately 2 to 3 months. Eggs are transported out of the lungs by the mucociliary apparatus, swallowed, and excreted in the feces where they become infective by 4 days.[662] First-stage larvae have survived for at least 49 days but do not survive over the winter.[663] In horses and ponies, larval development in the lungs is arrested (fifth stage), but airway inflammation still occurs.

CLINICAL SIGNS

Clinical signs can develop as early as 12 days after infection with a large number of larvae but are often delayed for several weeks in milder cases. Horses exhibit chronic coughing and an increased expiratory effort. Auscultation reveals crackles and wheezes, especially over the dorsal and caudal parts of the lung fields.[664] Signs are often indistinguishable from those associated with recurrent airway obstruction. Donkeys do not typically exhibit clinical signs of infection even when heavily parasitized.

DIAGNOSIS

Endoscopic examination may reveal a mild lymphoid follicular hyperplasia and copious amounts of exudate in the trachea and bronchioles. Tracheobronchial aspirates or BAL may contain a predominance of eosinophils, although isolated cases of probable lungworm infection have been reported in which eosinophils were absent in the lavage fluid. A peripheral eosinophilia is a variable finding in these horses. Definitive diagnosis is made by identification of *D. arnfieldi* larvae in the sediment of centrifuged mucus, although this process may be difficult.[663] One should examine stained and unstained cytologic preparations. In donkeys and in horses with patent infections, bronchoscopic identification of the lungworm, 16 cm in length, confirms the diagnosis. The Baermann technique is useful for diagnosing lungworms when the infections are patent. It is useful in testing the feces of potential in-contact reservoir hosts to help establish a diagnosis.

TREATMENT

Ivermectin (0.2 mg/kg) is effective against *D. arnfieldi* in controlled studies and field evaluations and did not cause any detrimental side effects.[665] Moxidectin (0.4 mg/kg) was found to be 99.9% effective in treating lungworm infections in donkeys.[666]

PREVENTION

Horses should not be pastured with donkeys or mules unless they are confirmed to be free of lungworms.

Acute Respiratory Distress Syndrome

CAUSES

Acute respiratory distress syndrome (ARDS) is a syndrome of lung injury characterized by alveolar damage, high-permeability pulmonary edema, and respiratory failure. Primary lung injury may result from aspiration (near drowning), improper administration of medications via nasogastric tubes, inhalation of smoke or noxious gases, oxygen toxicity, or pulmonary infection by viral, bacterial, mycoplasmal, or fungal agents. (See interstitial pneumonia.) Secondary lung injury may be a sequela of anaphylaxis, gram-negative sepsis or endotoxemia, trauma, embolism, and hypertransfusion.[510,632,667-670] Acute heart failure caused by rupture of the chordae tendinae, severe mitral valve regurgitation, or atrial fibrillation may increase left atrial and pulmonary capillary pressures, causing pulmonary edema.[671]

In human medicine, strict criteria have been established to define ARDS: impaired oxygenation (ratio of $Pa_{O_2}/FI_{O_2} \leq 200$ mm Hg, where FI_{O_2} is fractional inspired oxygen), detection of bilateral pulmonary infiltrates in chest radiographs, and a pulmonary artery wedge pressure less than 18 mm Hg or no clinical evidence of elevated left atrial pressures.[672,673] The milder form of ARDS is acute lung injury characterized by a Pa_{O_2}/FI_{O_2} ratio at or below 300 mm Hg. Similar criteria have been recommended for use in equine neonatal medicine. For example, in a retrospective study, Dunkel, Dolente, and Boston (2005) described acute lung injury or ARDS in 15 foals using radiographic, microbiologic, and gas exchange criteria. Unfortunately, unless the animal is mechanically ventilated, determining the fractional inspired oxygen level is difficult because it depends on the oxygen flow rate and the animal's ventilation.

PATHOGENESIS

Many different insults cause capillary permeability and alveolar damage leading to ARDS. This pathway may include complement and leukocyte activation with release of oxygen-free radicals and inflammatory mediators (IL-1, TNF) and secondary destruction of surfactant.[674] The net result is a deterioration of gas exchange and pulmonary mechanics. Whether horses that survive are more predisposed to the development of chronic interstitial lung disease with fibrosis has not been established (see the previous discussion of interstitial lung disease).

CLINICAL SIGNS

Horses with ARDS are tachypneic or in respiratory distress or both. A red-tinged or yellow frothy material, indicative of pulmonary edema, may be evident at the nares. Fever may be a component of the syndrome, depending on the primary cause. In cases of smoke inhalation, clinical signs may not become evident for several days after exposure to noxious gases.

DIAGNOSIS

Diagnosis depends on the physical findings and history. One may detect crackles on auscultation and may auscultate fluid within the trachea. Endoscopic examination, if performed without stressing the horse, may reveal the extent of airway edema, inflammation, mucosal necrosis, or sloughing and the presence of soot (smoke inhalation). Radiographs reveal an interstitial pattern, although an alveolar pattern caused by ventral consolidation of the lung fields may follow aspiration pneumonia. Arterial blood gases reveal hypoxemia and hypocapnia. In smoke inhalation, carboxyhemoglobin concentrations exceed 10%, indicating carbon monoxide toxicity.[670]

Echocardiographic evaluation of the heart should be performed to assess left ventricular function, chamber size, and valve patency. Serum troponin levels should be measured to ascertain cardiac injury.

TREATMENT

The clinician should direct treatment at the primary cause with the understanding that the prognosis is guarded. Lipid pneumonia resulting from aspiration of mineral oil is nearly always fatal.[632] (See interstitial pneumonia.) Cases of near drowning and smoke inhalation have been treated successfully, with return to athletic function in some cases.[667,668,675] Although in the latter, extensive lung injury and secondary necrosis of airways may eventually cause a fatal obstructive disease.

In horses with ARDS, one should administer intravenous fluid cautiously. Plasma may be needed if hypoproteinemia develops. Furosemide (1 mg/kg intravenously) helps mobilize lung extravascular water, and repetitive dosing at 2- to 4-hour intervals may be required. A continuous-rate infusion of furosemide may also be administered (0.12 mg/kg intravenous loading dose followed by 0.12 mg/kg/hr) in these cases.[676] Because of the reduced bioavailability, oral furosemide administration should be avoided.[677]

Humidified intranasal oxygen (10 to 15 L/min) or mechanical ventilation through a tracheotomy may be necessary. Although technically difficult to perform, adult horses in respiratory failure have been ventilated mechanically.[678] The clinician may perform tracheal suction to remove cell debris and other materials through the endoscope or through a tracheotomy. Surfactant, although expensive, may improve oxygenation and pulmonary mechanics when administered by intratracheal instillation. One may use bronchodilators to treat bronchospasm. β-Adrenergic agonists may be administered through an inhaler (see Table 9-5) or via nebulization. For example, one might nebulize a solution containing 0.9% saline (20 ml), 20% acetylcysteine (10 ml), and albuterol (5 mg). Antimicrobials can be added to the nebulizate. (See previous discussion on pneumonia.) Nonsteroidal antiinflammatory drugs and corticosteroids are also indicated for treating severe permeability edema. One should administer broad-spectrum antimicrobials, including metronidazole, in many of these cases but especially those involving aspiration pneumonia, bacterial and viral pneumonia, and smoke or noxious gas inhalation lung injury.

Recurrent Airway Obstruction

DEFINITION

Recurrent airway obstruction (RAO) is a naturally occurring respiratory disease characterized by periods of reversible airway obstruction caused by neutrophil accumulation, mucus production, and bronchospasm. The condition has been termed chronic obstructive pulmonary disease, chronic pulmonary disease, chronic airway reactivity, hyperactive airway disease, heaves, broken wind, and hay sickness. The consensus at the International Workshop of Equine Chronic Airway Disease was that the term chronic obstructive pulmonary disease not be used to describe this condition in horses because the pathophysiologic and morphologic aspects of the equine disease are quite different from those of human chronic obstructive pulmonary disease.[679]

Pulmonary function testing demonstrates a decrease in lung compliance, an increase in lung resistance, an increase in the work of breathing, and the development of arterial hypoxemia, usually in the absence of hypercapnia.[680,681] During airway obstruction, affected horses are hyperresponsive to nonspecific stimuli such as histamine, methacholine, and water.[682]

EPIDEMIOLOGY

The condition occurs worldwide, but the highest prevalence in the United States is in northeastern and midwestern horses that are fed hay and stabled. The condition is also found in horses stabled in the United Kingdom and in Europe. A similar condition, described in horses maintained on pasture in the southeastern United States, is termed summer pasture–associated obstructive disease (see later discussion). These horses improve when stabled.[683]

Recurrent airway obstruction affects middle-age or older horses, the median age of which is 12 years.[684] No breed predilection occurs, but a familial tendency has been found; a horse born to a dam and sire with RAO is at an increased risk for developing RAO.[685] Jost and colleagues investigated the genetics of RAO by focusing on the linkage association of the IL-4 receptor alpha chain gene (IL4RA), located on equine chromosome 13, to the severity of clinical signs of chronic airway disease.[686] They rationalized this approach because the IL-4 receptor is an integral component of a T helper cell type 2 (TH_2) (IL-4, IL-13)-mediated immune disorder (see the later discussion on etiopathogenesis) and because, in human asthmatics, linkages between the IL4RA gene (on human chromosome 16) and several distinct populations of asthmatics have been found.[687] Interestingly, Jost and colleagues found a significant haplotype association with clinical signs of airway disease (as assessed by surveys completed by owners) in the offspring of one sire but not that of another sire. This finding suggested the possible existence multiple genetic linkages to the severe chronic airway disease of the phenotype.

CAUSES

Much debate still occurs concerning the cause of RAO. Many investigators consider RAO to be a hypersensitivity reaction to organic dusts or molds commonly found in poorly cured hay or straw. Dust in horse stables contains more than 50 species of molds, large numbers of forage mites, endotoxins, and inorganic components—a variable mixture of agents, any one of which might induce pulmonary inflammation in a susceptible horse. The two most frequently implicated molds are *Aspergillus fumigatus* and *Faenia rectivirgula* (formerly *Micropolyspora faeni*, a thermophilic actinomycete).[688] Inhalation of aqueous extracts of *A. fumigatus, F. rectivirgula,* or *Thermoactinomyces vulgaris* partially but not fully induces RAO in susceptible horses.[682,689,690] Inhalation of endotoxin, a component of hay dust, induces airway neutrophilia but not all of the changes in pulmonary function that characterized RAO.[691,692] Full disease manifestation requires inhalation of hay dust either by natural challenge or by nebulization.

PATHOGENESIS

Recurrent airway obstruction is characterized by periods of reversible small airway obstruction caused by smooth-muscle contraction and accumulations of mucus and neutrophils. One hypothesis is that inhalation of the organic molds, dusts, and endotoxin induces a Th_2 response involving IgE-mediated degranulation of mast cells. This hypothesis is based on the following findings: (1) increased anti–*Micropolyspora faeni* and anti–*A. fumigatus* IgA and IgE concentrations in the BALF of asymptomatic and symptomatic RAO-affected horses,[693] (2) increased histamine levels in the BALF of RAO-affected horses 5 hours after natural challenge,[690] (3) increased serum IgE levels against recombinant *Aspergillus* antigens in RAO-affected horses,[694] and (4) increased numbers of BAL cells that are positive for IL-4 and IL-5 messenger RNA in RAO-affected horses.[695,696]

Data suggesting that RAO is not a Th_2 immune disorder include the following observations: (1) a poor correlation between antigen-specific IgE levels and expression of disease[694,697]; (2) the lack of a pulmonary eosinophilic response, as occurs in the Th_2 disorder of human asthma[698]; (3) the finding that the increased allergen-specific isotypes in the BALF of diseased horses are IgGa and IgGb (isotypes not compatible with a Th_2 response)[693]; (4) the lack of increase in IL-4 and IL-5 mRNA concentrations, as detected by quantitative PCR analysis of BAL lymphocytes[699-701]; (5) the lack of increase in IgE protein–positive cells in the lung tissue of RAO-affected horses as compared with controls[702]; and (6) the lack of up-regulation of GATA-3, a transcription factor required for IL-4 gene expression, in the bronchial epithelium of RAO-affected horses.[703]

In horses with RAO, IL-8 concentrations in the BALF are increased relative to levels found in healthy horses.[700,704] This cytokine may be derived from macrophages, neutrophils, or airway epithelial cells and is one of the primary chemoattractants for neutrophil migration into the airways. The gene expression of another neutrophil chemoattractant, IL-17, has also been found to be increased in the BALF cells of RAO-affected horses during the chronic but not acute stages of the disease and is thought to contribute to the persistent influx of neutrophils into the airways.[705,706] Furthermore, in horses chronically affected with RAO, pulmonary macrophages are not more hyperresponsive (ex vivo) to hay dust solutions than are cells isolated from controls.[707] This finding suggests again that the continued neutrophil influx in the chronic stages or RAO may be more dependent on the presence of neutrophil and bronchial-epithelial–derived chemokines than on macrophage activation.[706,707]

Other neutrophil- and macrophage-derived products such as reactive oxygen species and proteases also may contribute to the inflammatory process of RAO. Art, Kirschvink, Smith, et al.[708] suggested that an oxidative stress caused by the release of reactive oxygen species from granulocytes and macrophages develops in the airways of RAO-affected horses. Their conclusion is based on the finding that oxidized glutathione levels and glutathione redox ratios (the ratios of oxidized glutathione to total glutathione levels) are elevated in the pulmonary epithelial lining fluid of RAO-affected horses relative to controls. They further suggested that the oxidant stress does not incite but rather exacerbates the existing inflammation.

Interestingly, oxidative stress[709] has been found to activate NFκB, a transcription factor that regulates the expression of many proinflammatory cytokines and adhesion molecules, including tumor necrosis factor, IL-1β, IL-8, and intercellular adhesion molecule 1.[710] Recently, Bureau, Bonizzi, Kirschvink, et al.[711] demonstrated that levels of NFκB in the bronchial brushing cells of RAO-affected horses were increased many fold, the magnitude of which correlated with the severity of the clinical disease. Furthermore, the airway epithelial cell expression of intercellular adhesion molecule 1, a protein required for migration of neutrophils from the pulmonary vasculature into the lung parenchyma, paralleled the expression of NFκB, suggesting that this protein, along with IL-8, enhances the airway neutrophilia. Up-regulation of IL-8 in RAO-affected horses occurs at least 24 hours after hay dust exposure, suggesting that this epithelial chemokine is not responsible for early neutrophil influx into the airways.[706]

Proteases released from neutrophils and macrophages in the airways of RAO-affected horses may contribute further to inflammatory cell influx and possible tissue damage. The tracheal epithelial lining fluid of horses with RAO has increased concentrations of matrix metalloproteinases that exhibit collagenolytic, gelatinolytic, and elastinolytic activities.[712-714] The importance of these proteases, as well as other inflammatory mediators and arachidonic acid metabolites, to the initiation and development of bronchospasm, mucus secretion, and neutrophil influx remains to be determined.

CLINICAL SIGNS

Horses with RAO are usually afebrile and exhibit a chronic spontaneous cough, mucopurulent nasal discharge, and accentuated expiratory effort. Hypertrophy of the external oblique and rectus abdominis muscles caused by continued muscle recruitment is evident (heave line). Associated abdominal pressure changes may be large enough to cause the anus to protrude during expiration. The respiratory rate may be normal or increased. Exercise intolerance, weight loss, nostril flaring, reluctance to move, and cachexia may be evident in severe cases. Despite the development of pulmonary hypertension when horses are symptomatic,[715,716] RAO-affected horses rarely develop cor pulmonale—tachycardia, jugular distention, jugular pulsation, and ventral edema. Between episodes of severe RAO, cardiovascular alterations return to normal.[717] Nevertheless, a small percentage of horses do develop right ventricular hypertrophy and signs of right heart failure.[716]

DIAGNOSIS

The diagnosis is based on clinical signs, history of a seasonal disorder associated with husbandry alterations (e.g., being fed hay or being maintained in a dusty lot), and cytologic evidence of tracheobronchial aspirates supporting a nonseptic inflammation. Auscultation may reveal inspiratory or expiratory wheezes, crackles, or tracheal rattles, although it may require examination after a rebreathing bag to detect abnormal lung sounds in mildly affected horses. Percussion may be normal, or an expanded lung field may be detectable. A clinical scoring system has been developed to categorize the severity of RAO. Total clinical score is calculated as the sum of the score for nostril flaring (ranging between 1 to 4) and abdominal breathing effort (ranging between 1 to 4). Horses with a clinical score of 3 to 4, 5 to 6, or 7 to 8 are diagnosed as mild, moderate, or severe, respectively. However, for mildly affected horses, the physical examination findings underestimate the severity of changes in pulmonary function tests.[718]

Endoscopic examination reveals excessive mucopurulent exudate within the trachea. A bronchoalveolar lavage supports a nonseptic inflammatory reaction with increases in mucus and the percentage of intact neutrophils (>25% of the total nucleated cell count). In the BALF, the percentage of neutrophils may be as great as 90%, far exceeding the normal 5% to 15% found in healthy horses that are stabled and fed hay. In most affected horses, the percentages of eosinophils or mast cells are not increased. Albumin and immunoglobulin levels within the BAL may not increase.[719] Gram positive organisms may be retrieved by tracheobronchial aspirates if a concurrent septic inflammation exists, but this is rare. Pollen, fungal hyphae, and Curschmann's spirals (inspissated mucus plugs) also may be visible.

Thoracic radiography may demonstrate an increase in the interstitial and bronchial pattern throughout the lung fields. However, these changes may be difficult to interpret relative to the normal aging changes that occur. One may also detect exudate within the trachea by thoracic radiography (Figure 9-20). Radiographs are useful in ruling out thoracic neoplastic or infectious disorders in horses that have clinical signs

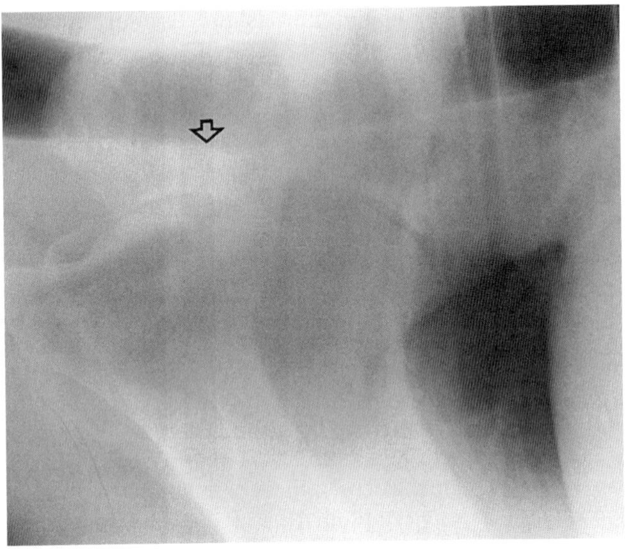

FIGURE 9-20 Tracheal fluid or exudate *(arrow)* is visible ventrally in the trachea at the level of the thoracic inlet. (Courtesy D. S. Biller, Manhattan, Kan., 1991.)

resembling RAO. In severely affected horses with RAO that repeatedly fail to respond to bronchodilators and glucocorticoids, radiographs should be obtained to rule out the existence of bronchiectasis (dilation or deformation of the bronchi or bronchioles).[720] This relatively uncommon complication of RAO causes irreversible airway obstruction as a result of collapse of the affected airways during expiration.

Ultrasound evaluation of RAO-affected horses confirms a shift of the caudal lung border caused by alveolar hyperinflation. However, gas in the large colon (left side) or in the cecum (right side) may preclude complete imaging of the most caudal extent of the lung fields at the sixteenth intercostal space. On ultrasound examination, small hypoechoic areas of irregularity on the lung surface may be detected, but, in general, this imaging modality does not detect airway inflammation.[721]

Echocardiographic findings of RAO-affected horses demonstrate an increase in the pulmonary artery diameter, an increase in the ratio of the diameters of the pulmonary artery to the aorta, and abnormalities in ventricular septal motion.[717] However, no changes in serum troponin I concentrations occur during experimentally induced RAO.[717]

Intradermal skin testing has been occasionally advocated for diagnosing RAO and for detecting sensitizing allergens. Theoretically, RAO-affected horses should react if sensitized to a given allergen, but the results supporting this theory have been inconclusive. For example, in some studies, clinically normal horses have positive skin test reactions to the allergens, whereas RAO-affected horses lack positive reactions.[722-724] In other studies, the percentage of RAO-affected horses exhibiting positive skin reactions (to any antigen) exceeds that of controls[725] or the response of RAO-prone horses to histamine challenge (measured at 0.5 hours after injection) or to *Aspergillus* spp. antigens (measured at 24 hours after injection) is enhanced.[726] Apparently, positive skin tests and serum precipitins to fungal and thermophilic actinomycete antigens are found in many normal and in RAO-affected horses and probably reflect a level of exposure of the horse rather than a susceptibility to RAO. In general, intradermal skin testing does not allow one to identify RAO-affected horses or the specific inhaled particulate that is inciting the inflammation.

A CBC and serum chemistry panel are of limited usefulness in diagnosing RAO because no abnormalities are detectable in the leukogram or in serum biochemistries.[684] These tests may be used to rule out the existence of a pneumonia or a neoplastic process. Arterial blood gas analyses are normal in approximately 25% of the horses with RAO, but in others, the development of arterial hypoxemia (Pa_{O_2} < 85 mm Hg) in the absence of arterial hypercapnia is noted.[727]

PATHOLOGIC SIGNS

Postmortem examination reveals a diffuse bronchiolitis with goblet cell metaplasia, airway smooth-muscle hypertrophy and hyperplasia, excess mucus, and inflammatory cells in the small airways.[728,729] Eosinophilic infiltration around the bronchioles is a variable finding present in approximately one third of affected horses. Varying degrees of alveolar overinflation and atelectases also are found, as well as evidence of fibrosis of the alveolar septa.[730] The larger airways—the bronchi and trachea—may show variable changes, including epithelial hyperplasia with loss of ciliated cells, goblet cell hyperplasia, and inflammatory cell infiltration.[731]

TREATMENT

Elimination of the source of mold or dust is not only the most beneficial step in the treatment regimen but also the most difficult management change to implement and achieve long term.[684] Horses should be switched to a diet consisting of pelleted feeds or hay cubes, making the dietary transition over 3 to 5 days. Some horses will tolerate hay that has been soaked in water, but this practice reduces the nutrient value of the hay and is often forsaken when the weather becomes cold. Unless pasture exacerbates the condition, the owner should keep horses outside, blanket them in the winter, and allow access to a three-walled shelter affording protection from the wind and rain. For chronically affected horses that have been turned out to pasture, clinical remission and normalization of conventional pulmonary function tests takes 4 to 8 weeks, depending on weather conditions. Recent data suggest that when RAO-susceptible horses are maintained in a low-dust environment (outside, no hay) for a prolonged period (years), they still exhibit a reduction in forced expiratory flow despite the absence of clinical signs. This finding suggests the existence of irreversible airway remodeling in affected animals.[732]

If the horse must be stabled, tall bedding should be shredded paper or shavings to reduce inhaled dusts and molds. Surrounding stalls should be bedded similarly. Although such stabling changes improve lung function somewhat, airway hyperreactivity still remains.[733,734] In a recent study of 12 RAO-affected horses that were stabled and fed a pelleted ration, pulmonary function tests and BALF neutrophil percentages improved within 4 weeks of implementing environmental changes. However, in four horses, pulmonary health (as assessed by BALF neutrophil percentages, maximal pleural pressure changes, and inflammatory cytokine profiles of the BALF cells) had not returned to normal by the conclusion of the study.[735]

Medical management is recommended in horses with clinical signs of RAO because environmental change alone takes several weeks to quiet the pulmonary inflammation. Corticosteroids are efficacious in reducing the inflammatory reaction in the lungs, whereas nonsteroidal antiinflammatory drugs provide no benefit. One potential regimen is to give oral prednisolone at

2.2 mg/kg once daily in the morning for 7 to 10 days, 1.1 mg/kg once daily for 7 to 10 days, 0.50 mg/kg once daily for 7 to 10 days, and 0.50 mg/lb every other day for 7 to 10 days. Alternatively, one may institute a course of parenteral or oral dexamethasone. For the 500-kg horse, the course is 40 to 50 mg intramuscularly once daily every other day for three treatments followed by 35 to 45 mg intramuscularly once daily every other day for three treatments, 30 to 40 mg intramuscularly once daily every other day for three treatments, and so forth until the horse is weaned off of the dexamethasone. A similar dosing schedule may be used when the parenteral dexamethasone formulation is given orally except that the initial dosage is 0.165 mg/kg for three treatments, followed by 0.084 mg/kg for three to four treatments, and 0.042 mg/kg for three to four treatments. In horses that remain stabled, are fed a pelleted feed, and receive oral dexamethasone protocol, a normalization of pulmonary function and a significant reduction in airway epithelial and luminal cell inflammatory gene expression (IL-8, IL-1β) is seen by 4 weeks after implementing the regimen.[735]

Other parenteral glucocorticoids that have been evaluated in RAO-affected horses maintained in dusty environments and fed hay include triamcinolone acetonide (0.09 mg/kg intramuscularly once) and isoflupredone (0.03 mg/kg intramuscularly once daily for several days).[736,737] The latter, because of its mineralocorticoid effects, can cause hypokalemia; therefore serum electrolytes should be supplemented and monitored. Corticosteroid use may be contraindicated in horses predisposed to laminitis or exhibiting endocrinopathies or those that have gastritis or gastric ulceration.

Inhaled steroids have been recommended to treat the pulmonary inflammation of RAO but may not provide a therapeutic benefit for 24 to 72 hours. For horses in respiratory distress, intravenous dexamethasone can provide an improvement within 4 to 6 hours. This application may be followed by treatment with inhaled steroids. A metered-dose inhaler containing fluticasone can be attached to a spacer on the Aeromask (Trudell Medical, London, Ontario, Canada) or to another drug delivery system (Equinehaler, Equine Health Care, Inc.) and administered to the horse during inspiration. The recommended dose is 2 mg twice daily. In RAO-affected horses that were still fed hay, fluticasone administration was associated with a marked improvement in pulmonary function, a normalization of BALF neutrophil counts, and a reduction in IL-8 copy numbers in BALF cells.[700]

Bronchodilators also are recommended for treating RAO. Three types of compounds are used to relax airway smooth muscle: β-adrenergics, methylxanthines, and anticholinergics. β_2-Adrenergic compounds include clenbuterol, albuterol, salmeterol, fenoterol, and trimetoquinol. Experimental investigations with clenbuterol suggest that when given at a dosage of 0.8 μg/kg once daily by mouth, the drug may be efficacious in alleviating some of the signs of RAO. In addition to a direct smooth-muscle effect, clenbuterol may stabilize mast cells, increase mucociliary clearance, improve airway secretions, and decrease inflammatory cytokine production.[738,739] If effects are not obtained at 0.8 μg/kg orally, then the dose may be increased step-wise by 25% increments. Adverse effects (tachycardia, tachypnea, sweating) are signs of toxicity. Albuterol is absorbed poorly from the gastrointestinal tract; thus inhalation is the recommended method of administration. Salmeterol is purported to be a long-acting β_2-agonist. However, in one study in RAO-affected horses, the investigators found that significant improvements in pulmonary function lasted for only 6 hours after its administration.[740] Aerosolized trimetoquinol (1000 μg administered via an ultrasonic nebulizer) significantly improved pulmonary function tests that lasted for 4 hours.[741] Some suggested doses of β_2-agonists that can be administered by metered-dose inhalers through the Aeromask are these: albuterol, 720 μg three to four times daily; fenoterol, 1 to 2 μg three to four times daily; and salmeterol, 210 μg three to four times daily. Administration of the β_2-agonist before corticosteroid dosing enhances the deposition of the latter in the smaller airways.[742] Long-term use of β_2-agonists has been associated with a down-regulation of β-receptors in humans, but whether this occurs in horses is unknown.

The methylxanthines include aminophylline (theophylline) and pentoxifylline, which dilate smooth muscle by increasing cyclic adenosine monophosphate levels intracellularly. Cyclic adenosine monophosphate also inhibits degranulation of mast cells and subsequent mediator release. One may give aminophylline at 4 to 6 mg/kg orally three times daily. However, in a recent study, aminophylline at 18 mg/kg intravenously provided clinical improvement in only 50% of horses.[743] Pentoxifylline, another methylxanthine derivative and phosphodiesterase inhibitor, is well absorbed orally and improves pulmonary function tests in RAO-affected horses when administered at 16 g twice daily by mouth.[744] It does not reduce BALF neutrophilia.

The third class of compounds used to affect smooth-muscle dilation is the anticholinergics, of which atropine, glycopyrrolate, and ipratropium are representatives. Atropine provides clinical improvement when administered intravenously at 0.02 mg/kg, but the duration of the effect is short lived (2 hours), and atropine may be associated with the development of ileus, abdominal pain, tachycardia, mydriasis, and thickening of airway secretions.[743] Atropine is generally used for emergency relief of airway obstruction. Glycopyrrolate is efficacious at a dose of 0.007 mg/kg, but it may also cause colic. One can also administer ipratropium bromide by inhalation at a dose of 180 to 360 mg three times daily with a low risk of inducing systemic side effects.[679] The powder form may be nebulized (dose of 2 to 3 μg/kg).

Disodium cromoglycate acts to stabilize mast cell degranulation and inhibit the vagal efferent component of histamine response. A suggested dose[688] is 80 mg once daily for 4 days administered by nebulization. Mucolytics (acetylcysteine, dembrexine) and mucokinetics (iodides, bromhexine) may provide some relief.[745] Antimicrobials are indicated if microorganisms are isolated on the tracheobronchial aspirate.

OTHER THERAPIES

In horses that develop respiratory distress caused by bronchospasm and airway inflammation, additional therapies are required. Administering nasal oxygen at flow rates as low as 5 L/min improves arterial oxygen tensions by as much as 30 mm Hg in some severely affected horses.[746] As the total nasal oxygen flow increases, so too will the mean arterial oxygen tension, although not to the same degree that occurs in healthy horses. Flow rates of 30 L/min (delivered by two nasal cannulae at 15 L/min) are associated with coughing and gagging in the horse. Nasal oxygen supplementation does not reduce breathing frequency, suggesting that stimulation of vagally mediated afferents—perhaps responding to inflammatory mediators—is responsible for the tachypnea.

Furosemide (1.0 mg/kg intravenously or nebulized) provides beneficial effects to RAO-affected horses within 20 minutes of its administration, decreasing total lung resistance

(R_L) and increasing C_{dyn} without affecting Pa_{O_2}.[747] Beneficial effects appear to be mediated by prostaglandin E_2, derived from either the renal or airway epithelium, that promotes smooth muscle relaxation. Prior treatment with the cyclooxygenase inhibitor flunixin meglumine prevents furosemide-induced bronchoconstriction.[748]

Therapies that are not efficacious in the treatment of RAO-affected horses include a single acupuncture treatment,[749] the oral administration of an herbal preparation containing thyme and Primula,[750] or the rapid intravenous administration of 30 L of isotonic saline.[751]

PROGNOSIS

RAO-prone horses are likely to develop acute exacerbations of the disease when husbandry practices lapse or when weather conditions become adverse. Horses do not *outgrow* the disorder, and, in fact, some clinicians believe that the inflammation becomes more difficult to manage as the horse ages. The basis for the lack of clinical response is unknown but might be the result of lung remodeling—development of fibromuscular hyperplasia in the alveolar septae,[716] excessive smooth-muscle hyperplasia,[729] bronchiectasis,[720] or potential down-regulation of the glucocorticoid receptor.

If proper environmental management changes are implemented, and if the appropriate therapy is initiated, clinical remission occurs in most cases. In a survey of RAO-affected horses that had been examined and treated at a referral center 2 to 4 years previously, 20% of the original cases (3 of 15) had been euthanized, 33% were still receiving bronchodilators on an as-needed basis, and athleticism had not decreased in 92% of the horses.[752] In a similar survey,[684] 13% of horses diagnosed with RAO 3 to 4 years earlier had been euthanized. However, more than 50% of the respondents in that survey stated that the athletic performance of the horse had been compromised by the disease. Perhaps this difference between the two surveys simply reflects a failure of the owners to comply with environmental management recommendations. When queried about the husbandry practices, 77% of the respondents still stabled the horse for part of the day, and 84% still fed dry hay. Because the effects of repetitive episodes on the development of irreversible changes in lung structure have yet to be determined, clients should be encouraged to implement effective husbandry changes that minimize the recurrences of RAO.

PREVENTION

Once the clinician has diagnosed RAO, the horse will always be susceptible to recurrences of disease. Husbandry changes should be implemented to decrease environmental dust and organic mold exposure. During periods of hot, humid, or dusty conditions, prophylactic administration of a steroid and bronchodilator via the metered-dose inhaler may be indicated. Routine immunizations against the viral respiratory pathogens and good management practices are logical suggestions.

Summer Pasture-Associated Obstructive Pulmonary Disease

DEFINITION

In the southeastern United States, a condition clinically similar to RAO, called summer pasture-associated obstructive pulmonary disease (SPAOPD), develops in mature horses that are maintained at pasture. Clinical signs typically show during late spring, summer, and early autumn.[683] This disorder has also been reported to occur in horses in the United Kingdom that are out on pasture.[753,754]

Horses with SPAOPD exhibit airway neutrophilia, excessive mucus production, and accentuated breathing efforts,[755] although the inciting environmental factors and the immunopathogenesis of this disorder have yet to be determined.

Because of its similarity to RAO, investigators have sought to determine if SPAOD reflects a TH_2 immune response to inhaled molds or antigens by examining BALF antibody isotypes and BAL cell cytokine profiles. Neither the total nor the antigen-specific IgE and IgG titers to *Aspergillus* spp., *Cladosporium herbarum*, *Penicillium* spp., *F. rectivirgula*, *Saccharomonospora viridis*, *Thermoactinomyces thalpophilus*, and the forage mite *Lepidoglyphus destructor* in tracheal lavage fluid are increased in SPAOD-affected horses relative to controls.[756] During the winter months, when horses are free of clinical signs, *A. fumigatus*–specific IgG titers in SPAOPD-affected horses exceed those of controls, but whether this increase reflects ongoing production or decreased consumption cannot be determined. Cytokine profiles of BALF cells isolated from SPAOPD-susceptible and -affected horses have also been examined. When horses are symptomatic, the mRNA copy numbers of *both* IL-4 and interferon-gamma in BALF cells are increased relative to controls.[757] This difference is not apparent when horses are asymptomatic, although the copy number of IL-4 in the SPAOPD-prone horses does not decrease during the asymptomatic periods either.

TREATMENT

Recommendations for treatment of RAO-affected horses include environmental management changes such as moving the horse from the pasture to a clean stable with wood shavings for bedding. Dusty and hot environments should be avoided because these conditions exacerbate SPAOD, although this task may be difficult to achieve in the southeastern United States.[758] As with RAO, corticosteroids and bronchodilators may be administered to reduce inflammation, airway hyperreactivity, and bronchoconstriction.

Inflammatory Airway Disease

DEFINITION

In a recent ACVIM Consensus Statement, the following criteria were listed to define the IAD phenotype: (1) poor performance, exercise intolerance or coughing, with or without excess tracheal mucus; (2) nonseptic inflammation detected by cytologic examination of BALF; and (3) pulmonary dysfunction based on evidence of lower airway obstruction, airway hyperresponsiveness, or impaired blood gas exchange at rest or during exercise.[759] Excluded from this group are horses with evidence of systemic infection (fever, depression, inappetence) and those with increased respiratory efforts at rest (RAO, SPAOPD). In defining the syndrome, the panel stated that airway inflammation should be determined by assessing inflammatory cell percentages in the BALF as opposed to tracheal washes.

EPIDEMIOLOGY

Although IAD is encountered predominantly in young performance horses,[65,144] those of any age may be affected.[760] A prevalence of 20% to 80% among racehorses in training has been reported.[144,761] The variation in prevalence may reflect differences in methods used. The amount of tracheal exudates detected endoscopically increases as a function of exercise intensity,[144] thus one may miss the diagnosis of IAD if one performs endoscopic examination in the resting horse.[762] A second factor contributing to the range in prevalence rates may be the age of the horse evaluated. In an epidemiologic survey of young racehorses in Britain, the prevalence rate of IAD decreased with age: In 4-year-old horses, it was 2% compared with 9% in the 2-year-old horses.[763] The relationship between IAD in young horses and RAO in mature horses is unknown. Current thinking holds that IAD progresses to RAO.[679] In non-racehorses or in sport horses, IAD is usually diagnosed at an older age than in racehorses.[764]

ETIOPATHOGENESIS

The definitive cause of lower airway inflammation observed in horses with IAD is currently unknown. It may be multifactorial, with the relative importance of a causative agent dependent on the age of the horse, its environment, and its athletic use. IAD may reflect the response of the lung to the presence of one or all of the following factors: (1) low-grade persistent bacterial or viral infections; (2) autologous blood from exercise-induced pulmonary hemorrhage; and (3) inhaled stable dusts, molds, endotoxin, particulate matter, or environmental pollutants such as hydrogen sulfide, ammonia, ozone, sulfur dioxide, nitrogen oxide, and carbon monoxide.

Studies in the United Kingdom and Australia suggest that bacterial agents may be involved in the pathogenesis of IAD.[144,765-770] Using an inflammatory score based on the amount of mucus, total nucleated cell count, and neutrophil percentages in endoscopically obtained tracheobronchial aspirates, investigators found that as the inflammatory score increased, the percentage of positive bacterial cultures also increased.[768] The most commonly isolated organisms were *S. equi* subsp. *zooepidemicus, S. pneumoniae, A. equuli,* and *Pasteurella* spp. *Mycoplasma* spp. were also isolated from some horses with IAD.[617,763] That the prevalence of IAD decreased with increasing age of the horse was attributed to the development of an effective immune response.

In studies in the United Kingdom and in Australia, no association between the onset of IAD and seroconversion to EHV1, ERAV, ERBV1, or equine influenza existed,[765,767,769] suggesting that IAD is not associated with viral infection. Nevertheless, a viral cause had been proposed for IAD based on the cytologic improvements in BALF constituents in horses treated with oral interferon-α. In a study of 32 Standardbred horses with a history of poor performance referable to the respiratory tract, the BALF total nucleated cell count and the percentages of BALF neutrophils, lymphocytes, and monocytes in horses with IAD were significantly increased as compared with control horses.[771-773] Lymphocytosis and monocytosis were consistent with a low-grade viral infection. A 5-day course of oral interferon-α (50 U/day) lowered total nucleated cell counts and converted the cell distribution to a noninflammatory profile for at least 15 days. The investigators did not describe whether the amelioration of pulmonary inflammation was associated with an improvement in athletic performance. They also did not evaluate horses endoscopically beyond 2 weeks to determine if cessation of interferon-α therapy was associated with a return of IAD.

Autologous blood, derived from rupture of pulmonary capillaries during intense exercise, has also been suggested as a cause of IAD. Instillation of blood causes a neutrophilic pulmonary inflammatory reaction in the lungs, suggesting that pulmonary hemorrhage may contribute to IAD.[774] Inoculation of blood into the bronchial tree of retired racehorses induced an inflammatory response 8 and 14 days later characterized by increased macrophage activity, alveolar septal thickness, and collagen content.[775] Similarly, in horses (2 to 4 years of age), a single intrabronchial instillate of autologous blood was associated with increased numbers of alveolar macrophages by 24 hours, 48 hours, and 7 days after blood inoculation. In contrast, by day 14, no evidence of alveolar fibrosis was found in lung tissues.[776]

Inhalation of stable dusts, environmental particulates, mites, endotoxin, and fungal wall components may also cause or contribute to IAD. The risk of IAD increases in horses that are stabled.[777,778] Episodes of IAD are shorter in horses bedded on shredded paper.[765] Environmental pollutants also have been suggested as a cause of IAD. Many racetracks and training facilities are located in metropolitan areas with significant accumulations of smog. No data exist verifying this agent as a cause of IAD, although Mills et al. (1996) found that when healthy horses were exposed to ozone, indices of oxidant stress in the pulmonary epithelial lining fluid increased (e.g., the amounts of reduced glutathione or glutathione disulfide, the glutathione redox ratio, the total iron concentrations), which were similar to those found in horses with poor performance. However, these changes can also occur in pulmonary disease not induced by ozone.

Another environmental factor that may contribute to development of IAD is the temperature of inspired air. In experimental studies of horses performing submaximal exercise, chilling of the inspired air to –5° C was associated with a modest increase in BALF neutrophil percentages (16% versus 11% in controls) measured 24 hours after the exercise cessation. Significant increases were found in the expression of IL-1, IL-5, IL-6, IL-8, and IL-10 in BALF relative to the control horses.[779]

Finally, Hare and Viel[63] have also suggested that a type I (IgE-mediated) hypersensitivity reaction to inhaled environmental allergens could be the cause of IAD. They studied young Standardbred racehorses with a history of poor performance and found evidence of peripheral blood and BALF eosinophilia (12% eosinophils). Normally, the percentage of eosinophils in BALF is less than 2%. Because they found no evidence of pulmonary or intestinal parasitism in this group of affected horses, the investigators attributed the eosinophilic IAD to an allergic reaction.

CLINICAL SIGNS

Inflammatory airway disease is frequently subclinical but in some cases may be associated with poor athletic performance, a chronic intermittent cough, and increased mucoid airway secretions. Serous to mucopurulent nasal discharge is commonly observed in young horses.[765] Thoracic auscultation is usually unremarkable. Affected horses may occasionally have increased respiratory rates and enhanced abdominal breathing. However, if maximal pleural pressure changes are measured, they are within the normal reference range (<10 cm H_2O).[65] Pyrexia is generally not a feature of the disorder. Horses may have evidence of concurrent EIPH.

DIAGNOSIS

With the exception of cases of IAD associated with pulmonary eosinophilia, CBC and chemistry profiles are usually within normal limits but are helpful in ruling out bacterial or viral pneumonia. The diagnosis of IAD is aided by endoscopic examination of the respiratory tract and the finding of exudate in the nasopharynx and in the trachea. Anecdotal reports that pulmonary inflammation is associated with thickening and blunting of the tracheal septum have recently been challenged.[780] Endoscopy permits one to obtain a sample of tracheobronchial aspirates for culture if so desired (using a guarded swab) and to perform a BAL. Cytologic analysis of the BALF demonstrates an increased total nucleated cell count, a mild neutrophilia, lymphocytosis, and monocytosis. In some young racehorses with IAD, the percentage of mast cells (>2%) and eosinophils (>1%) in the BALF are increased. Although it has been recommended that the diagnosis of IAD be based on BALF cytologic findings, a recent study demonstrated that this approach alone would miss the diagnosis of IAD in approximately one third of the affected horses.[781] These investigators suggested that the diagnosis of airway inflammation should be based on tracheal (>20% neutrophils) or BALF (>5% neutrophils) cytologic evaluations obtained 1 to 2 hours after the horse has performed a standardized treadmill exercise test. The exercise test is performed for two reasons: (1) the exercise hyperpnea enhances endoscopic and cytological evidence of IAD,[762,782] and (2) the exercise test eliminates (or identifies) other causes (musculoskeletal, cardiovascular) of poor performance. During the standardized treadmill exercise test, one should assess the upper respiratory tract with videoendoscopy; the cardiovascular system with electrocardiogram, postexercise echocardiogram, and pre- and postexercise serum troponin concentrations; and the musculoskeletal system with lameness examination and pre- and postexercise serum creatine kinase and aspartate transaminase concentrations. During the treadmill exercise testing, arterial blood gases should also be obtained for analysis. In exercising horses, the Pao_2 of select horses with IAD alone or in combination with EIPH was significantly less than in healthy control horses.[783]

Thoracic radiographs are a low-yield diagnostic modality in IAD cases because no correlation exists among radiographic score, BALF cytologic findings, lung function, and measures of airway hyperreactivity.[784] Thoracic radiographs can be used to exclude alternative diagnoses but not to confirm the diagnosis of IAD.

Specialized pulmonary function tests such as forced expiration and forced oscillation mechanics have been used to identify horses with IAD.[65,785,786] Measures of airway hyperreactivity, performed by determining dose-dependent alterations in respiratory mechanics after nebulization of methacholine or histamine, have demonstrated that some horses with IAD have hyperresponsive airways or airway narrowing or both.[63-65]

TREATMENT

Because the cause of IAD remains uncertain, most treatment recommendations aim at environmental alterations to decrease exposure to dust, molds, and allergens. Horses should have pasture turnout whenever possible. When stabled, horses should be maintained in a well-ventilated barn free of noxious gases. Horses with bacterial infections should receive a 7- to 10-day course of an antibiotic, the selection of which is based on culture and sensitivity results from the tracheobronchial aspirate. Horses may benefit from a 1-week period of rest coupled with a 5-day course of orally administered interferon-α (natural human interferon-α 50 U or recombinant human interferon-α 90 U). In a clinical trial of 34 young Standardbreds diagnosed with IAD, treatment with interferon-α was associated with recurrence of cough 4 weeks later in only 23% of the horses as compared with relapse in 75% of controls.[787] Interferon-α could reduce inflammation via elimination of persistent viral infections, modulation of an allergic response, or attenuation of proximal mediators of inflammation.[787]

One should also implement efforts to decrease the severity or frequency of EIPH by having horses train and race with furosemide. In the absence of an infectious cause, horses may also benefit from a 2- to 4-week course of corticosteroids: prednisolone at 2.2 mg/kg orally once daily for 7 to 10 days, followed by 1.0 mg/kg orally once daily for 7 to 10 days, and then 1.0 mg/kg orally once every other day for 7 to 10 days. As is the case with glucocorticoids, controlled studies examining the efficacy of bronchodilators in horses with IAD are lacking. Aerosolized albuterol (900 μg) administered to eight Standardbred horses (four of which exhibited airway hyperreactivity without clinical evidence of IAD) did not alter maximal oxygen consumption, maximal carbon dioxide production, or treadmill speed at which horses exhibited a heart rate of 200 beat/min.[788] Whether horses with overt signs of IAD benefit from treatment with bronchodilators remains to be determined.

EXERCISE-INDUCED PULMONARY HEMORRHAGE

CAUSES

Strenuous exercise is associated with hemorrhage from the pulmonary vasculature into the alveoli and airways, primarily in the caudal dorsal lung segments. Histologically, EIPH is characterized by the presence of edema, rupture of the pulmonary capillaries, and intraalveolar hemorrhage.

EPIDEMIOLOGY

Exercise-induced pulmonary hemorrhage has been detected in most breeds of horses undergoing strenuous exercise. The prevalence of EIPH is estimated to be between 44% and 75% in Thoroughbreds, 26% and 77% in Standardbreds, 62% in racing Quarter Horses, 50% in racing Appaloosas, 68% in steeplechasers, 67% in timber racing horses, 40% in 3-day event horses, 10% in pony club event horses, and 11% in polo ponies.[789-796] Indeed, EIPH probably occurs in any breed of horse that is strenuously exercised, but, apparently, the intensity of exercise rather than the duration of exercise is more important in its development. No clear correlation exists between EIPH and the location of stables, the condition of the track, or the track type.[797] In a recent study of Australian racing Thoroughbreds (ages 1 to 10 years) that were not permitted to receive furosemide prerace or to wear nasal dilator strips during the race,[798] EIPH was associated with the presence of excess tracheal mucus or tracheal dirt and with concentration of airborne particulates. EIPH was not associated with the age of the horse, gender, weight carried, and race distance, although previous studies have indicated a greater prevalence of EIPH in older horses.

PATHOGENESIS

Numerous mechanisms have been suggested to cause EIPH including ventilation inhomogeneities caused by inflammatory airway disease (IAD),[799,800] upper airway obstruction,[801,802] mechanical concussive forces associated with locomotion,[803,804] redistribution of blood flow in the lung,[805] and stress failure of the pulmonary capillaries.[806]

Robinson and Derksen[799] proposed that poor collateral ventilation in the horse coupled with small airway disease, and thus altered time constants for alveolar filling, caused underventilation of certain lung units. Extreme fluctuations in the alveolar pressure of these underventilated regions during exercise produced parenchymal tearing or alveolar capillary rupture. Small airway disease (IAD) has been detected in a large percentage of horses with EIPH.[800] However, its absence in the lungs of young racehorses that exhibit evidence of EIPH suggests that small airway disease, at least, is not an inciting cause of EIPH.[807] The role of small airway disease in propagating the cycle of EIPH cannot be dismissed.

Clarke[803] speculated that visceral constraint of the diaphragm caused greater mechanical forces or stresses to develop in the dorsal thorax. Thus, in the caudodorsal lung, these mechanical forces would be borne over a narrow area, leading to parenchymal tearing or rupture of capillaries during inspiration. However, evidence of widespread hemorrhage in the dorsal portions of the lung suggests that the distribution of extremely negative intrapleural pressures is more complex and not simply restricted to the region in close proximity to the caudal dorsal lung. An alternative mechanical theory has proposed that forelimb locomotory impact forces are transmitted through the chest wall, setting up waves converging caudodorsally in the lung parenchyma.[804] Although support for locomotory-impact forces as a cause of EIPH comes from the higher percentage of steeplechasers that bleed as compared with flatracers, the difference could simply reflect a greater exercise intensity and hence cardiac output and pulmonary artery pressures generated in the jumpers.[808] Furthermore, because horses still develop EIPH during swimming when concussive forces would be minimal, it seems less likely that mechanical forces alone cause EIPH.[809]

Currently, the most widely accepted hypothesis for the development of EIPH is stress failure of pulmonary capillaries.[806,810] Stress failure is thought to occur after development of high transmural pressures (the pressure difference between the pulmonary capillary bed and the adjacent alveoli) that disrupt capillary endothelial and alveolar epithelial tight junctions, leading to hemorrhage within the interstitium and alveoli. Elevated pulmonary capillary pressures, which may exceed 70 mm Hg in strenuously exercised horses, are a consequence of the high cardiac output, lack of sufficient pulmonary vascular vasodilation, and increased blood viscosity that occurs during exercise. The second component of transmural pressures is very negative intrapleural and alveolar pressures that are required to generate airflows exceeding 120 L/s through high resistance passages (nasal cavity, larynx).[811] More negative pressures would be generated when nasal, laryngeal, or pulmonary passages are narrowed from disease or if larger tidal volumes are generated, for example during exercise on an incline.[802,812] Evidence supportive of the stress failure theory is provided by electron micrographs prepared from lung segments taken from strenuously exercised horses. These micrographs demonstrate a breakdown of the endothelial and epithelial tight junctions and exudation of red blood cells into alveoli.[806] Although some investigators have found no correlation between pulmonary capillary pressures in exercising horses and the development of EIPH ascertained endoscopically,[813] others have found a correlation between mean pulmonary artery pressures in exercising horses and the number of erythrocytes in postexercise BALF samples.[814]

Thus the etiopathogenesis of EIPH may represent a complex interplay of many factors relating to the physiologic and pathologic features of pulmonary function and exercise.[815]

CLINICAL SIGNS

Physical examination of the resting horse that develops EIPH is unremarkable. In one study of 20 Standardbred racehorses, thoracic percussion, but not thoracic auscultation, identified abnormalities in the caudodorsal region of 50% (n = 5) of horses with EIPH.[816]

Epistaxis is an infrequent finding, occurring in less than 7% of Standardbreds, Thoroughbreds, or Quarter Horses after racing.[789-791,794,795] In one retrospective study of Japanese racehorses examined 30 minutes after racing either on the flat track or over hurdles, epistaxis was detected in 0.13% of the Thoroughbreds (>246,000 starts) and in 0.10% of the Anglo-Arabs (>4000 starts).[817] Similar prevalence rates were reported by Weideman et al. (2003) who found epistaxis in 0.17% of South African Thoroughbred racehorses (51,465 horses in 778,532 races). In the study by Takahashi et al.,[817] epistaxis occurred more frequently in horses that were older (0.04% in 2-year-olds versus 0.27% in horses > 5 years), raced over hurdles (0.11% flatracers versus 0.76% steeplechasers), and sprinted (0.13% in races < 1600 m long versus 0.11% in races 1601-2000 m long). They also found that the rate of recurrence of epistaxis was 13%. The lower frequency of epistaxis reported in this study by Takahashi et al.[817] may be because horses were examined 30 minutes after racing, and the horses were young (64% of horses were < 3 years of age). Sudden death attributed to EIPH is reported to occur in 82% to 87% of racehorses that die suddenly.[818,819]

Additional clinical signs that may be exhibited by some horses with EIPH after competition include difficult or labored breathing, coughing, or excessive swallowing.

Although long suspected to cause decreased athletic performance, it had been difficult to objectively ascertain because investigations had been confounded by any or all of the following: concurrent use of medications in horses (furosemide), statistical methods, and the numbers of horses evaluated. Nevertheless, owners or trainers often report that an affected horse does not perform up to expectations or that it exhibits a sudden loss of speed during competition.[809] In a prospective study of 744 Australian Thoroughbred racehorses (2396 starts) that competed without the benefit of furosemide or nasal dilator strips, an association between the presence and severity of tracheal blood and race performance was found.[798] Horses with a tracheal score at or above 2 (based on a scale of 0-4; see later discussion) had lower odds of winning or finishing in the first three positions and a lower likelihood of being in the 90th percentile or higher for race earnings. Although the exact pathophysiologic effect of EIPH on performance was not known, the investigators suggested that it may have reflected a deleterious effect of the bleeding on arterial oxygenation or on maximal oxygen consumption or both.[783,820]

DIAGNOSIS

Endoscopic detection of frank blood within the trachea is the usual method of diagnosis of EIPH. Optimal time for endoscopic examination is within 90 minutes of a race or a strenuous workout. An endoscopic scoring system for tracheal blood accumulation has been developed and achieves a high degree of concordance among evaluators.[798] The numeric scores range from 0 to 4, with a *0* assigned to cases for which no blood is detected in the pharynx, larynx, trachea, or mainstem bronchi and a *4* assigned to cases with multiple coalescing streams of blood covering more than 90% of the tracheal surface with blood pooling at the thoracic inlet. One limitation of the scoring system is that it does not provide a quantitative measure of the amount of hemorrhage.[798] Furthermore, confirmation of EIPH may require multiple endoscopic examinations of the same horse after exercise bouts of the same intensity. Whether, in a given horse, the tracheal blood score increases in severity over time is currently unknown.

Cytologic analysis of tracheobronchial or BAL constituents can aid one in the diagnosis of EIPH. Although total nucleated cell counts in BALF do not differ between racehorses and yearlings, the number of free erythrocytes and hemosiderophages in the BALF is greater in horses in training compared with horses not being trained.[821] Concern has surfaced that simple enumeration of erythrocytes recovered in the BALF to semiquantify the severity of EIPH may not be accurate and reproducible.[822] When EIPH positive and negative racehorses are compared, the total hemosiderin score (a reflection of cytoplasmic iron in alveolar macrophages) agrees well with EIPH status. Specifically, a total hemosiderin score above 75 has a sensitivity and specificity of 94% and 88%, respectively, in identifying EIPH-positive horses.[823] Hemosiderin scores should be interpreted cautiously because hemorrhage from prior episodes of pneumonia, pleuropneumonia, or abscessation will increase hemosiderin scores.

Pulmonary biopsy specimens obtained from the seventh or eighth intercostal space (10 cm above the level of the point of the elbow) from the lungs of EIPH-positive horses do not demonstrate histologic abnormalities that would distinguish affected horses from EIPH negative horse.[816] In contrast, histologic evaluation of lung samples obtained from the caudal dorsal lung regions (postmortem) of horses with EIPH reveals bronchiolitis, hemosiderophages, focal eosinophilic infiltration, and increased connective tissue.[800]

Radiographs are of limited usefulness in diagnosing horses with EIPH, given that the signs found in affected horses—an accentuated bronchial, bronchointerstitial, or interstitial pattern[824]—can also be observed in racehorses that do not exhibit evidence of pulmonary bleeding.[823] In severe cases of hemorrhage, a radiopaque region in the caudal dorsal lung lobe that obscures the pulmonary vasculature is detected[825,826] (Figure 9-21). Nuclear scintigraphy has not been useful in detecting areas of pulmonary hemorrhage after exercise.

Hemogram, serum biochemistry, and arterial blood gas values obtained from resting horses with EIPH are within normal limits. The mean platelet counts of EIPH-positive horses (128×10^9 cells/L) are significantly lower than those of EIPH negative horses (159×10^9 cells/L), although the total counts are within the normal range.[816]

TREATMENT

Drugs that reduce pulmonary capillary pressure during exercise have gained the most widespread use in the treatment and prevention of EIPH. Furosemide, 250 to 300 mg, is given intravenously 4 hours before the horse is strenuously worked or raced. Furosemide decreases plasma volume and decreases exercise-associated pulmonary artery and pulmonary capillary pressures.[827-829] Although furosemide administration has failed to prevent the development of EIPH in horses that were previously EIPH negative,[830,831] some evidence indicates

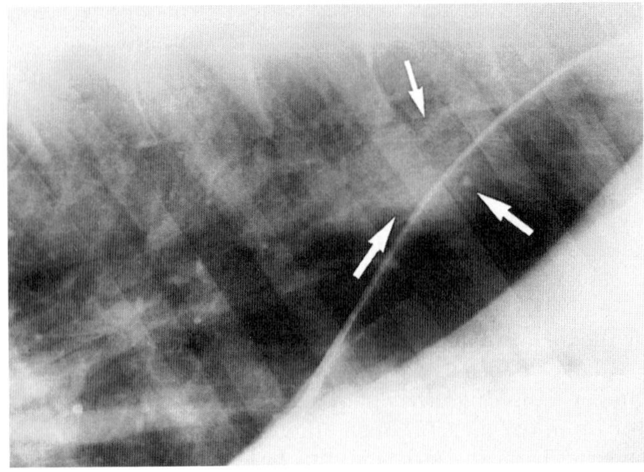

FIGURE 9-21 Focal area of increased interstitial pulmonary opacity *(arrows)* in the dorsal caudal lung field represents exercise-induced pulmonary hemorrhage. (Courtesy D. S. Biller, Manhattan, Kan., 1991.)

that it reduces the red blood cell counts in BALF or the EIPH endoscopic score.[832] Furosemide administration is also associated with improved performance in Thoroughbred racehorses.[833]

Nitric oxide, a potent vasodilator, has been administered to horses with EIPH. In one laboratory investigation of strenuously exercised horses, intravenous nitric oxide failed to reduce pulmonary artery or pulmonary capillary pressures and failed to prevent EIPH.[834] In another study, inhaled nitric oxide administered to horses maximally exercised on the treadmill reduced pulmonary arterial pressures but worsened erythrocyte counts in the BALF.[835]

Nasal dilators (Flair nasal strips) have been advocated as a treatment for horses with EIPH. These nasal dilators are adhesive strips containing springs that are applied externally 3 cm above the nostrils with the purpose of maintaining upper airway patency and reducing airway resistance during inspiration. In laboratory studies of exercising horses, the application of nasal strips failed to change arterial blood gases, pulmonary artery pressures, peak esophageal pressures, or tracheal blood accumulation compared with controls.[836,837] In one study, the nasal strips reduced erythrocyte counts in the BALF.[837]

The finding of concomitant small airway disease (IAD) in some horses suggests that one should attempt to minimize environmental dusts and molds. Corticosteroids and bronchodilators, inhaled or administered parenterally, have not been shown to reduce EIPH but may lessen the severity of small airway disease. In a laboratory study simulating airway responses in horses with EIPH (produced by intrapulmonary inoculation of 50 ml of autologous blood), each of three treatments consisting of oral prednisolone (1 mg/kg once daily), inhaled beclomethasone dipropionate (3.75 mg twice daily), or oral clenbuterol hydrochloride (0.8 μg/kg) decreased total erythrophage count in BALF compared to nontreated controls. This study suggested that the treatments suppressed numbers and possibly phagocytic function of macrophages.[838] In contrast, the antiinflammatory cromoglycate, which is believed to stabilize mast cell membranes, has not been efficacious in the treatment of EIPH.[839]

Other formulations that have been advocated for the treatment of EIPH include intratracheal immunoglobulin, oral herbal remedies (e.g., Yunnan paiyao, Single Immortal, Red Lung, and Red Lung Plus), intravenous aminocaproic acid, bioflavinoids, aspirin, and estrogens, but no scientific data exist that demonstrates their efficacy.[840]

Rest has been recommended, but pulmonary hemorrhage will likely recur once the horse resumes training. In severe cases of EIPH, a short course of broad-spectrum antimicrobials may be indicated to lessen the chance of secondary pneumonia or abscess formation.

PREVENTION

World wide, EIPH is of concern because of financial losses resulting from decreased performance, suspension of horses from racing, lost training days, and the cost of prerace mediation.[841] The efficacy of treatment regimens in the prevention of EIPH under race conditions has been difficult to determine even when speed handicapping methods are used. Variables such as the administration of drugs unknown to the investigators or the inability to diagnose or reproduce EIPH within a given horse on consecutive days make interpretation of these studies difficult.

Tumors of the Respiratory System

CAUSES

Based on postmortem surveys, the most frequently encountered tumors in the horse, regardless of the body system, are sarcoids, squamous cell carcinomas, fibromas, melanomas, papillomas, fibrosarcomas, and lymphomas.[653,842,843] Neoplastic involvement of the thoracic structures or pulmonary parenchyma per se is rare in horses and occurs at a prevalence rate of 0.15 to 0.62.[524,843] Tumors in the thoracic cavity arise as either primary neoplasms or from metastases and may involve extrapulmonary structures or the lung parenchyma. Examples of primary thoracic tumors are lymphomas and mesotheliomas.[524,761,844-847]

In addition to being the most common thoracic neoplasm, lymphoma is also the most common tumor of the equine hematopoietic system (see the discussion in the hematopoietic Chapter 14).[845,847] Lymphoma is classified according to its anatomic distribution as mediastinal, alimentary, cutaneous, multicentric, and generalized, although several forms may exist in the same horse. Horses affected with mediastinal lymphoma are young to middle-aged (mean age of 10 years) and exhibit weight loss, ventral edema, jugular distention caused by the presence of a mediastinal mass, tachypnea, or respiratory distress caused by pleural effusion secondary to compression of vessels.[845,848] Ultrasonography allows one to define the size and extent of the tumor, as well as to assess potential responses to treatment. Most mediastinal lymphomas are homogeneous hypoechoic masses greater than 4 × 4 cm in size, but some tumors exhibit focal hyperechoic areas.[849] As the size of the mass increases, the heart is displaced caudally causing it to be imaged in the sixth through the eighth intercostal spaces. Anechoic fluid surrounding the mass—indicative of pleural effusion—enhances the ultrasonographic image but may contribute to lung compression and breathing difficulties. Differential diagnoses for a cranial mediastinal mass include abscess, inflamed mediastinal lymph node, fatty tissue, and the thymus, which may be present in horses up to 4 years of age.[850] With the horse well sedated and its forelimb extended cranially, an ultrasound-guided biopsy specimen of the mass may be obtained aseptically through the third intercostal space.[850] Short-term intravenous anesthesia provides an alternative method of obtaining the ultrasound-guided biopsy if the horse will not remain stationary with sedation. In horses with concurrent pleural effusion, thoracocentesis may yield a modified transudate or nonseptic exudate, but neoplastic cells—lymphoblasts with mitotic figures—are not consistently found. After drainage of the pleural effusion, thoracic radiographs should be obtained to determine if the lung parenchyma is involved. Thoracoscopy may be another option to determine the extent of involvement of intrathoracic structures and possibly to obtain a biopsy, although the cranial and ventral position of the mass may preclude its clear visualization.[75,77,850,851] In affected horses, rectal examination and ultrasonographic evaluation of the abdomen should always be performed to detect involvement of abdominal organs or structures. The clinical course of the disease, from onset of signs until euthanasia, is often rapid and may be less than 8 weeks for most cases.[845] A recent report describes the successful treatment of a mixed-cell mediastinal lymphoma using cytarabine (170 mg/m^2 intramuscularly), cyclophosphamide (142 mg/m^2 intravenously), and prednisolone (86 mg/m^2 orally).[852]

Mesothelioma is the second most common primary thoracic tumor in the horse. This tumor arises from the serosal lining cells of the pleura and pericardium. In contrast to human disease, its development in horses has not been linked to asbestos exposure. Affected horses are often young to middle aged (2 to 13 years) and may exhibit respiratory distress caused by pleural effusion.[844,846,853-855] Thoracocentesis usually yields a dark to blood-tinged fluid of normal cellularity but with an increased total protein concentration. Cytologic examination of pleural fluid may reveal pleomorphic mesothelial cells with mitotic figures.[846] However, in other cases, distinguishing mesothelioma from other neoplasms or from reactive mesothelial cells may be impossible. Thoracoscopy may be used to confirm the presence of neoplastic nodules on the pleura, which should be biopsied for histologic examination and classification.[856] Malignant mesothelioma can be classified into three main histologic types: epithelioid, biphasic, and sarcomatoid. An immunohistochemical marker for epithelioid-type mesotheliomas that differentiates them from metastatic adenocarcinomas is calretinin, a protein that is related to the calcium-binding proteins and may be helpful in the diagnosis.[857] Treatment is not usually attempted in horses with mesothelioma. Whether pleurodesis would reduce the effusion and prolong the horse's life is unknown.

Primary equine lung tumors include granular cell tumors,[858-868] bronchial myxomas,[869] bronchial and pulmonary carcinomas,[653,870,871] bronchial and pulmonary adenocarcinomas,[872,873] bronchogenic squamous cell carinomas,[871] bronchioalveolar carinoma,[872] pulmonary chondrosarcomas,[874,875] and pulmonary leiomyosarcoma.[876] The prevalence rate of primary lung tumors (0.15%) is much less than that of metastatic pulmonary tumors. Of the primary lung tumors, the most common one is granular cell tumor (myoblastoma or Schwann cell tumor), and it is the only primary lung tumor that is mesenchymal rather than epithelial in origin. Based on a review of 26 reported cases,[651,858,860-866,868,877-880] the mean age of affected horses is 13 years; the majority of cases occur in mares (22 of 26 horses), and the tumor is often located in the right lung (16 of 26 horses). In a small number of horses, the tumor occurred in both lung lobes. In some horses, the tumor may be an incidental finding detected at necropsy; however, in most cases, clinical signs of chronic respiratory disease—coughing, increased respiratory rate or effort, and weight loss—develop. In the absence of an extensive workup, these signs may lead to a misdiagnosis of RAO. However, because the tumor or tumors protrude into the bronchus, airflow into that lung lobe may be reduced or completely lacking, making lung sounds difficult or impossible to detect. (This finding is in contrast to RAO in which adventitious lungs sounds may be heard over an expanded lung field.) Secondary bacterial infections may develop in the affected lung presumably because of impaired clearance of secretions caused by the tumor. In a few cases, hypertrophic osteopathy (Marie's disease) develops concurrently.[858,866,877,879] This condition is characterized by enlargement of the joints and the presence of bony swellings in the distal limbs caused by subperiosteal bony proliferation. As a result, affected horses exhibit generalized stiffness and shifting limb lameness. The diagnosis of granular cell tumor is based on imaging and endoscopic findings. On thoracic radiographs, single or multiple radioopaque nodules are evident. Endoscopic examination reveals mucosal-covered nodules protruding into the bronchi. A definitive diagnosis is obtained after histologic evaluation of endoscopically obtained biopsies. The cells are globoid or stellate and contain eosinophilic, PAS-positive cytoplasmic granules.[651,862] Immunohistochemical staining of the cells is positive for vimentin, an intermediate filament most commonly associated with cells of mesenchymal origin, and for S-100, a calcium-binding protein most commonly found in cells of neural crest origin.[865] Currently, no medical treatment has been developed for pulmonary granular cell tumors. In two cases, the tumor was resected successfully by transendoscopic electrosurgery[881] or via lung resection.[880] In general, the tumor does not usually metastasize to other sites, but bilateral lung involvement is a possibility.

The limited number of case reports in the literature describing clinical features of other primary lung tumors[653,869-876] precludes a detailed description of these tumors. In general, middle-aged to older horses are affected and exhibit weight loss, chronic cough, and tachypnea. In the absence of a thorough evaluation, the chronicity of the clinical signs may lead to a misdiagnosis of RAO, pneumonia, or even EIPH (epistaxis). Thoracic radiographs demonstrate the presence of pulmonary nodules that are confirmed to be neoplastic in lung biopsy obtained by ultrasound guidance. Cytologic examination of tracheal aspirates is not usually diagnostic. Treatment has not been attempted.

Thoracic tumors involving the pleural surfaces, lymph nodes, mediastinum, esophagus, diaphragm, or lungs may also arise from metastases from other neoplastic sites. Examples of metastatic tumors that affect the thoracic cavity include adenocarcinoma (primary sites of origin are in the kidney, uterus, ovary, mammary gland, and pancreas),[521,522,882-884] squamous cell carcinoma,[516,885-888] hepatoblastoma,[517] hymoma,[889] fibrosarcoma,[515] melanoma,[890] hemangiosarcoma,[518,524,891-903] and lymphoma.[524,845,904,905]

Hemangiosarcoma remains a rare tumor, occurring in 2 of 1322 horses in a study by Sundbery, Burnstein, Page, et al.[842] and in 1 of 4739 cases in a survey reported by Hargis and McElwain.[892] It is a malignant tumor of endothelial cells but does not appear to develop from a preexisting hemangioma.[895] A comprehensive review[896] provides a description of the clinical aspects of 35 cases of disseminated hemangiosarcoma, 21 of which were diagnosed at a participating veterinary hospital and 14 of which were previously reported in the literature.* The median age of horses was 12 years, and most clinical signs were referable to the respiratory or to the musculoskeletal systems. For example, respiratory distress and epistaxis were noted in 26% of cases, and muscular or subcutaneous swellings were noted in 24%. The majority of horses exhibited mucous membrane pallor either alone or in combination with icterus, reflecting prior hemorrhage. Ultrasonographic evaluation detected pleural effusion or hemothorax in four cases. Cytologic analysis of either the pleural or tracheobronchial aspirates (in horses that developed epistaxis) failed to demonstrate neoplastic cells. Antemortem diagnosis is difficult and may require thoracoscopy or pleuroscopy to visualize neoplasms and to obtain samples for histopathologic examination.[74,894] Microscopically, one may see vascular channels lined with plump, spindle-shaped cells. In some cases, well-differentiated channels are less conspicuous or are lacking, and cells have epithelioid morphologic appearance. When present, the tumor is classified as epithelioid (histiocytoid) hemangiosarcoma.[902] Immunohistochemical staining of tumor samples demonstrates cells that can be poorly reactive against factor VIII reactive antigen, positive for UEA-agglutinin I (a receptor of *Ulex europaeus I*) and negative for cytokeratin.[901,902] In affected horses, supportive care, including thoracocentesis, blood transfusions, and intravenous fluids, is generally unrewarding. Clinical deterioration is rapid, with death occurring, on average, 17 days from the onset of clinical signs. In a study of 11 young horses (younger than 4 years) with hemangiosarcoma, the investigators reported that the majority of cases had cutaneous masses or diffuse limb and joint swellings.[903] Although only one horse in this study developed disseminated hemangiosarcoma, the exact percentage of horses with cutaneous neoplasms that develop disseminated disease and over what time period is unknown.

In general, horses with metastatic thoracic neoplasia exhibit nonspecific clinical signs of depression, inappetence and weight loss, or clinical signs referable to the site of the primary neoplasm. In some cases, respiratory distress may occur if pleural effusion develops, or coughing may occur if the tumor compresses an airway.[847] Diagnostic examination, which requires a combination of imaging techniques including endoscopy, thoracic radiography, ultrasonography (and possibly thoracoscopy), and cytologic evaluation of respiratory secretions along with evaluation of the abdominal cavity and other body systems should be undertaken. Usually, hematologic and serum biochemical abnormalities are nonspecific and include anemia, leukocytosis, neutrophilia, and hyperfibrinogenemia.[846] The prognosis is poor for horses with neoplasms, and most patients are euthanized. In horses in which the tumor is localized and has a low metastatic potential, as exists with granular cell tumors, lung resection may be an option.[880] In cases with pleural effusion, the clinician may achieve temporary stabilization by thoracocentesis, but the therapeutic benefits of pleurodesis have not been established for equine patients (see the section on pleural effusion).

*References: 74, 518, 891, 893, 894, 897-900, and 906.

REFERENCES

1. Banks KL, McGuire TC, Jerrells TR: Absence of B lymphocytes in a horse with primary agammaglobulinemia, *Clin Immunol Immunopathol* 5:282, 1976.
2. Deem DA, Traver DS, Thacker HL, et al: Agammaglobulinemia in a horse, *J Am Vet Med Assoc* 175:469, 1979.
3. Davis DM, Honnas CM, Hedlund CS, et al: Resection of a cervical tracheal bronchus in a foal, *J Am Vet Med Assoc* 198:2097, 1991.
4. Bacon CL, Davidson HJ, Yvorchuk K, et al: Bilateral Horner's syndrome secondary to metastatic squamous cell carcinoma in a horse, *Equine Vet J* 28:500, 1996.
5. Simoens P, Lauwers H, De Muelenare C, et al: Horner's syndrome in the horse: a clinical, experimental and morphological study, *Equine Vet J* Suppl Sept(10):62, 1990.
6. Kotlikoff MI, Gillespie JR: Lung sounds in veterinary medicine I. Terminology and mechanisms of sound production, *Compend Contin Educ Pract Vet* 5:634, 1983.
7. Kotlikoff MI, Gillespie JR: Lung sounds in veterinary medicine part II. Deriving clinical information from lung sounds, *Compend Contin Educ Pract Vet* 6:462, 1984.
8. Viel L, Harris FW, Curtis RA: Terminology of lung sounds in large animal veterinary medicine. In Deegen E, Beadle RE, editors: *Lung Function and Respiratory Diseases*, Stuttgart, Germany, 1986, Hippiatrika.
9. Forgacs, P: *Lung Sounds,* Bailliere Tindall, London, 1978.
10. Bakos Z, Voros K: Thoracic percussion to determine the caudal lung border in healthy horses, *J Vet Intern Med* 21:504, 2007.
11. Roudebush P, Sweeney CR: Thoracic percussion, *J Am Vet Med Assoc* 197:714, 1990.
12. Darien BJ, Brown CM, Walker RD, et al: A tracheoscopic technique for obtaining uncontaminated lower airway secretions for bacterial culture in the horse, *Equine Vet J* 22:170, 1990.
13. Franklin SH, Naylor JR, Lane JG: Videoendoscopic evaluation of the upper respiratory tract in 93 sport horses during exercise testing on a high-speed treadmill, *Equine Vet J* Suppl (36):540, 2006.
14. Lane JG, Bladon B, Little DR, et al: Dynamic obstructions of the equine upper respiratory tract. Part 1: observations during high-speed treadmill endoscopy of 600 Thoroughbred racehorses, *Equine Vet J* 38:393, 2006.
15. Tan RH, Dowling BA, Dart AJ: High-speed treadmill videoendoscopic examination of the upper respiratory tract in the horse: the results of 291 clinical cases, *Vet J* 170:243, 2005.
16. Worster AA: Equine sinus endoscopy using a flexible endoscope: diagnosis and treatment of sinus disease in the standing sedated horse, *Proc Am Assoc Equine Pract* 45:128, 1999.
17. Ruggles AJ, Ross MW, Freeman DE: Endoscopic examination and treatment of paranasal sinus disease in 16 horses, *Vet Surg* 22:508, 1993.
18. Morrow KL, Park RD, Spurgeon TL, et al: Computed tomographic imaging of the equine head, *Vet Radiol Ultrasound* 41:491, 2000.
19. Kraft SL, Gavin PR: Physical principles and technical considerations for equine computed tomography and magnetic resonance imaging, *Vet Clin North Am Equine Pract* 17:115, 2001.
20. Tucker RL, Sande RD: Computed tomography and magnetic resonance imaging of the equine musculoskeletal conditions, *Vet Clin North Am Equine Pract* 17:145, 2001.
21. Smallwood JE, Wood BC, Taylor WE, et al: Anatomic reference for computed tomography of the head of the foal, *Vet Radiol Ultrasound* 43:99, 2002.
22. Chalmers HJ, Cheetham J, Dykes NL, et al: Computed tomographic diagnosis–stylohyoid fracture with pharyngeal abscess in a horse without temporohyoid disease, *Vet Radiol Ultrasound* 47:165, 2006.
23. Pease AP, van Biervliet J, Dykes NL, et al: Complication of partial stylohyoidectomy for treatment of temporohyoid osteoarthropathy and an alternative surgical technique in three cases, *Equine Vet J* 36:546, 2004.
24. Probst A, Henninger W, Willmann M: Communications of normal nasal and paranasal cavities in computed tomography of horses, *Vet Radiol Ultrasound* 46:44, 2005.
25. Walker AM, Sellon DC, Cornelisse CJ, et al: Temporohyoid osteoarthropathy in 33 horses (1993-2000), *J Vet Intern Med* 16:697, 2002.
26. O'Brien RT, Biller DS: Dental imaging, *Vet Clin North Am Equine Pract* 14:259, 1998.
27. Wion L, Perkins G, Ainsworth DM, et al: Use of computerised tomography to diagnose a Rhodococcus equi mediastinal abscess causing severe respiratory distress in a foal, *Equine Vet J* 33:523, 2001.
28. Arencibia A, Vazquez JM, Jaber R, et al: Magnetic resonance imaging and cross sectional anatomy of the normal equine sinuses and nasal passages, *Vet Radiol Ultrasound* 41:313, 2000.
29. Ferrell EA, Gavin PR, Tucker RL, et al: Magnetic resonance for evaluation of neurologic disease in 12 horses, *Vet Radiol Ultrasound* 43:510, 2002.
30. Chiesa OA, Vidal D, Domingo M, et al: Cytological and bacteriological findings in guttural pouch lavages of clinically normal horses, *Vet Rec* 144:346, 1999.
31. Chiesa OA, Garcia F, Domingo M, et al: Cytological and microbiological results from equine guttural pouch lavages obtained percutaneously: correlation with histopathological findings, *Vet Rec* 144:618, 1999.
32. Derksen FJ, Brown CM, Sonea I, et al: Comparison of transtracheal aspirate and bronchoalveolar lavage cytology in 50 horses with chronic lung disease, *Equine Vet J* 21:23, 1989.
33. Larson VL, Busch RH: Equine tracheobronchial lavage: comparison of lavage cytologic and pulmonary histopathologic findings, *Am J Vet Res* 46:144, 1985.
34. Fogarty U: Evaluation of a bronchoalveolar lavage technique, *Equine Vet J* 22:174, 1990.
35. Sweeney CR, Sweeney RW 3rd, Benson CE: Comparison of bacteria isolated from specimens obtained by use of endoscopic guarded tracheal swabbing and percutaneous tracheal aspiration in horses, *J Am Vet Med Assoc* 195:1225, 1989.
36. Racklyeft DJ: A tracheoscopic technique for obtaining uncontaminated lower airway secretions for bacterial culture in the horse, *Equine Vet J* 22(408):415, 1990.
37. Christley RM, Hodgson DR, Rose RJ, et al: Comparison of bacteriology and cytology of tracheal fluid samples collected by percutaneous transtracheal aspiration or via an endoscope using a plugged, guarded catheter, *Equine Vet J* 31:197, 1999.
38. Sweeney CR, Beech J, Roby KA: Bacterial isolates from tracheobronchial aspirates of healthy horses, *Am J Vet Res* 46:2562, 1985.
39. Burrell MH, Mackintosh ME, Taylor CE: Isolation of Streptococcus pneumoniae from the respiratory tract of horses, *Equine Vet J* 18:183, 1986.
40. ME Mackintosh, ST Grant and MH Burrell: Evidence of streptococcus pneumonia as a cause of respiratory disease in young thoroughbred horses in training. In DG Powell, editor: Equine Infectious Diseases V: *Proceedings of the Fifth International Conference, Lexington,* Kentucky, 1988, University of Kentucky Press.
41. Benson CE, Sweeney CR: Isolation of Streptococcus pneumoniae type 3 from equine species, *J Clin Microbiol* 20:1028, 1984.
42. Reimer JM: Diagnostic ultrasonography of the equine thorax, *Compend Contin Educ Pract Vet* 12:1321, 1990.
43. Lamb CR, O'Callaghan MW: Diagnostic imaging of equine pulmonary disease, *Compend Contin Educ Pract Vet* 11:1110, 1989.

44. King GK: Equine thoracic radiography II. Radiographic patterns of equine pulmonary and pleural diseases using air-gap rare-earth radiography, *Compend Contin Educ Pract Vet* 3:S283, 1981.
45. Farrow CS: Radiographic aspects of inflammatory lung disease in the horse, *Vet Radiol* 22:107, 1981.
46. Rantanen NW: Diseases of the thorax, *Vet Clin North Am Equine Pract* 2:49, 1986.
47. Reef VB, Boy MG, Reid CF, et al: Comparison between diagnostic ultrasonography and radiography in the evaluation of horses and cattle with thoracic disease: 56 cases (1984-1985), *J Am Vet Med Assoc* 198:2112, 1991.
48. Reimer JM, Reef VB, Spencer PA: Ultrasonography as a diagnostic aid in horses with anaerobic bacterial pleuropneumonia and/or pulmonary abscessation: 27 cases (1984-1986), *J Am Vet Med Assoc* 194:278, 1989.
49. Bennett DG: Evaluation of pleural fluid in the diagnosis of thoracic disease in the horse, *J Am Vet Med Assoc* 188:814, 1986.
50. Sweeney CR, Divers TJ, Benson CE: Anaerobic bacteria in 21 horses with pleuropneumonia, *J Am Vet Med Assoc* 187:721, 1985.
51. O'Callaghan MW, Hornof WJ, Fisher PE, et al: Ventilation imaging in the horse with 99mtechnetium-DTPA radioaerosol, *Equine Vet J* 19:19, 1987.
52. Attenburrow DP, Portergill MJ, Vennart W: Development of an equine nuclear medicine facility for gamma camera imaging, *Equine Vet J* 21:86, 1989.
53. O'Callaghan MW, Hornof WJ, Fisher PE, et al: Exercise-induced pulmonary haemorrhage in the horses: results of a detailed clinical, post mortem and imaging study. VII. Ventilation/perfusion scintigraphy in horses with EIPH, *Equine Vet J* 19:423, 1987.
54. O'Callaghan MW, Kinney LM: Pulmonary scintigraphy in horses with chronic obstructive pulmonary disease, *Comp Respir Soc* 8:78, 1989.
55. O'Callaghan MW: Scintigraphic imaging of lung disease. In Beech J, editor: *Equine respiratory disorders*, Philadelphia, PA, 1991, Lea & Febiger.
56. Nelson R, Hampe DW: Measurement of tracheal mucous transport rate in the horse, *Am J Vet Res* 44:1165, 1983.
57. Willoughby RA, Ecker G, Riddolls L: Mucociliary clearance in the nose and trachea of horses, *Comp Respir Soc* 8:36, 1989.
58. Barakzai S, Tremaine H, Dixon P: Use of scintigraphy for diagnosis of equine paranasal sinus disorders, *Vet Surg* 35:94, 2006.
59. Robinson NE: The physiologic basis of pulmonary function tests, *Proc Am Coll Vet Intern Med* 10:403, 1992.
60. Robinson NE: Tests of equine airway function, *Proc Am Coll Vet Intern Med* 10:284, 1992.
61. Young SS, Hall LW: A rapid, non-invasive method for measuring total respiratory impedance in the horse, *Equine Vet J* 21:99, 1989.
62. van Erck E, Votion D, Art T, et al: Measurement of respiratory function by impulse oscillometry in horses, *Equine Vet J* 36:21, 2004.
63. Hare JE, Viel L: Pulmonary eosinophilia associated with increased airway responsiveness in young racing horses, *J Vet Intern Med* 12:163, 1998.
64. Hoffman AM, Mazan MR, Ellenberg S: Association between bronchoalveolar lavage cytologic features and airway reactivity in horses with a history of exercise intolerance, *Am J Vet Res* 59:176, 1998.
65. Couëtil LL, Rosenthal FS, DeNicola DB, et al: Clinical signs, evaluation of bronchoalveolar lavage fluid, and assessment of pulmonary function in horses with inflammatory respiratory disease, *Am J Vet Res* 62:538, 2001.
66. Mazan MR, Hoffman AM, Manjerovic N: Comparison of forced oscillation with the conventional method for histamine bronchoprovocation testing in horses, *Am J Vet Res* 60:174, 1999.
67. Art T, Anderson L, Woakes AJ, et al: Mechanics of breathing during strenuous exercise in Thoroughbred horses, *Respir Physiol* 82:279, 1990.
68. Savage CJ, Traub-Dargatz JL, Mumford EL: Survey of the large animal diplomates of the American College of Veterinary Internal Medicine regarding percutaneous lung biopsy in the horse, *J Vet Intern Med* 12:456, 1998.
69. Raphel CF, Gunson DE: Percutaneous lung biopsy in the horse, *Cornell Vet* 71:439, 1981.
70. Venner M, Schmidbauer S, Drommer W, et al: Percutaneous lung biopsy in the horse: comparison of two instruments and repeated biopsy in horses with induced acute interstitial pneumopathy, *J Vet Intern Med* 20:968, 2006.
71. Pusterla N, Watson JL, Madigan JE, et al: Technique and diagnostic value of percutaneous lung biopsy in 66 horses with diffuse pulmonary diseases using an automated biopsy device, *Equine Vet Educ* 19:157, 2007.
72. Perkins G, Ainsworth DM, Yeager A: Hemothorax in 2 horses, *J Vet Intern Med* 13:375, 1999.
73. Mansmann RA, Bernardstrother S: Pleuroscopy in horses, *Mod Vet Pract* 66:9, 1985.
74. Rossier Y, Sweeney CR, Heyer G, et al: Pleuroscopic diagnosis of disseminated hemangiosarcoma in a horse, *J Am Vet Med Assoc* 196:1639, 1990.
75. Vachon AM, Fischer AT: Thoracoscopy in the horse: diagnostic and therapeutic indications in 28 cases, *Equine Vet J* 30:467, 1998.
76. Lugo J, Stick JA, Peroni J, et al: Safety and efficacy of a technique for thoracoscopically guided pulmonary wedge resection in horses, *Am J Vet Res* 63:1232, 2002.
77. Pollock PJ, Russell T: Standing thoracoscopy in the diagnosis of lymphosarcoma in a horse, *Vet Rec* 159:354, 2006.
78. Kirschvink N: The challenge of assessing inflammatory and structural changes in lower equine airways: a chance for thoracoscopic-guided pulmonary biopsy? *Vet J* 172:202, 2006.
79. Peroni JF, Robinson NE, Stick JA, et al: Pleuropulmonary and cardiovascular consequences of thoracoscopy performed in healthy standing horses, *Equine Vet J* 32:280, 2000.
80. Freeman DE: Sinus disease, *Vet Clin North Am Equine Pract* 19:209, 2003.
81. Hillman DJ: The skull. In Getty R, editor: *Sisson and Grossman's the anatomy of the domestic animals*, Philadelphia, 1975, WB Saunders.
82. McCann JL, Dixon PM, Mayhew IG: Clinical anatomy of the equine sphenopalatine sinus, *Equine Vet J* 36:466, 2004.
83. Pirie M, Pirie HM, Wright NG: A scanning electron microscopic study of the equine upper respiratory tract, *Equine Vet J* 22:333, 1990.
84. Head KW, Dixon PM: Equine nasal and paranasal sinus tumours. Part 1: review of the literature and tumour classification, *Vet J* 157:261, 1999.
85. Tremaine WH, Dixon PM: A long-term study of 277 cases of equine sinonasal disease. Part 1: details of horses, historical, clinical and ancillary diagnostic findings, *Equine Vet J* 33:274, 2001.
86. Tremaine WH, Dixon PM: A long-term study of 277 cases of equine sinonasal disease. Part 2: treatments and results of treatment, *Equine Vet J* 33:283, 2001.
87. Lane JG, Longstaffe JA, Gibbs C: Equine paranasal sinus cysts: a report of 15 cases, *Equine Vet J* 19:537, 1987.
88. Mason BJ: Empyema of the equine paranasal sinuses, *J Am Vet Med Assoc* 167:727, 1975.
89. Prichard MA, Hackett RP, Erb HN: Long-term outcome of tooth repulsion in horses. A retrospective study of 61 cases, *Vet Surg* 21:145, 1992.
90. Gibbs C, Lane JG: Radiographic examination of the facial, nasal and paranasal sinus regions of the horse. II. Radiological findings, *Equine Vet J* 19:474, 1987.

91. Tremaine WH, Clarke CJ, Dixon PM: Histopathological findings in equine sinonasal disorders, *Equine Vet J* 31:296, 1999.
92. Dixon PM, Head KW: Equine nasal and paranasal sinus tumours: part 2: a contribution of 28 case reports, *Vet J* 157:279, 1999.
93. Tucker RL, Farrell E: Computed tomography and magnetic resonance imaging of the equine head, *Vet Clin North Am Equine Pract* 17:131, 2001.
94. Henninger W, Frame EM, Willmann M, et al: CT features of alveolitis and sinusitis in horses, *Vet Radiol Ultrasound* 44:269, 2003.
95. Schumacher J, Dutton DM, Murphy DJ, et al: Paranasal sinus surgery through a frontonasal flap in sedated, standing horses, *Vet Surg* 29:173, 2000.
96. Freeman DE, Orsini PG, Ross MW, et al: A large frontonasal bone flap for sinus surgery in the horse, *Vet Surg* 19:122, 1990.
97. Boulton CH: Equine nasal cavity and paranasal sinus disease: a review of 85 cases, *J Equine Vet Sci* 5:268, 1985.
98. Hilbert BJ, Little CB, Klein K, et al: Tumours of the paranasal sinuses in 16 horses, *Aust Vet J* 65:86, 1988.
99. Marriott MR, Dart AJ, Hodgson DR: Treatment of progressive ethmoidal haematoma using intralesional injections of formalin in three horses, *Aust Vet J* 77:371, 1999.
100. Cook WR, Littlewort MC: Progressive haematoma of the ethmoid region in the horse, *Equine Vet J* 6:101, 1974.
101. Schumacher J, Yarbrough T, Pascoe J, et al: Transendoscopic chemical ablation of progressive ethmoidal hematomas in standing horses, *Vet Surg* 27:175, 1998.
102. Rothaug PG, Tulleners EP: Neodymium:yttrium-aluminum-garnet laser-assisted excision of progressive ethmoid hematomas in horses: 20 cases (1986-1996), *J Am Vet Med Assoc* 214:1037, 1999.
103. Greet TR: Outcome of treatment in 23 horses with progressive ethmoidal haematoma, *Equine Vet J* 24:468, 1992.
104. Laing JA, Hutchins DR: Progressive ethmoidal haematoma in horses, *Aust Vet J* 69:57, 1992.
105. Specht TE, Colahan PT, Nixon AJ, et al: Ethmoidal hematoma in nine horses, *J Am Vet Med Assoc* 197:613, 1990.
106. Colbourne CM, Rosenstein DS, Steficek BA, et al: Surgical treatment of progressive ethmoidal hematoma aided by computed tomography in a foal, *J Am Vet Med Assoc* 211:335, 1997.
107. Frees KE, Gaughan EM, Lillich JD, et al: Severe complication after administration of formalin for treatment of progressive ethmoidal hematoma in a horse, *J Am Vet Med Assoc* 219:950, 2001.
108. Baptiste KE, Naylor JM, Bailey J, et al: A function for guttural pouches in the horse, *Nature* 403:382, 2000.
109. Manglai D, Wada R, Endo H, et al: Macroscopic anatomy of the auditory tube diverticulum (guttural pouch) in the thoroughbred equine–a silicon mold approach, *Okajimas Folia Anat Jpn* 76:335, 2000.
110. Habel RE, editor: *Applied veterinary anatomy*, Ithaca, NY, 1975, WB Saunders.
111. Blazyczek I, Hamann H, Deegen E, et al: Retrospective analysis of 50 cases of guttural pouch tympany in foals, *Vet Rec* 154:261, 2004.
112. Blazyczek I, Hamann H, Ohnesorge B, et al: Inheritance of guttural pouch tympany in the arabian horse, *J Hered* 95:195, 2004.
113. Freeman DE: Diagnosis and treatment of diseases of the gutteral pouch (part 1), *Compend Contin Educ Pract Vet* 2:S3, 1980.
114. Tetens J, Tulleners EP, Ross MW, et al: Transendoscopic contact neodymium:yttrium aluminum garnet laser treatment of tympany of the auditory tube diverticulum in two foals, *J Am Vet Med Assoc* 204:1994, 1927.
115. Greet TR: Outcome of treatment in 35 cases of guttural pouch mycosis, *Equine Vet J* 19:483, 1987.
116. Cook WR, Campbell RS, Dawson C: The pathology and aetiology of guttural pouch mycosis in the horse, *Vet Rec* 83:422, 1968.
117. Freeman DE: Long-term follow-up on a large number of horses that underwent transarterial coil embolisation (TCE) for guttural pouch mycosis (GPM), *Equine Vet J* 38:271, 2006.
118. Walmsley JP: A case of atlanto-occipital arthropathy following guttural pouch mycosis in a horse. The use of radioisotope bone scanning as an aid to diagnosis, *Equine Vet J* 20:219, 1988.
119. Dixon PM, Rowlands AC: Atlanto-occipital joint infection associated with guttural pouch mycosis in a horse, *Equine Vet J* 13:260, 1981.
120. Millar H: Guttural pouch mycosis in a 6-month-old filly, *Can Vet J* 47:259, 2006.
121. Cook WR: The clinical features of guttural pouch mycosis in the horse, *Vet Rec* 83:336, 1968.
122. Colles CM, Cook WR: Carotid and cerebral angiography in the horse, *Vet Rec* 113:483, 1983.
123. Lane JG: The management of guttural pouch mycosis, *Equine Vet J* 21:321, 1989.
124. Lepage OM, Piccot-Crezollet C: Transarterial coil embolisation in 31 horses (1999-2002) with guttural pouch mycosis: a 2-year follow-up, *Equine Vet J* 37:430, 2005.
125. Leveille R, Hardy J, Robertson JT, et al: Transarterial coil embolization of the internal and external carotid and maxillary arteries for prevention of hemorrhage from guttural pouch mycosis in horses, *Vet Surg* 29:389, 2000.
126. Freeman DE, Ross MW, Donawick WJ, et al: Occlusion of the external carotid and maxillary arteries in the horse to prevent hemorrhage from guttural pouch mycosis, *Vet Surg* 18:39, 1989.
127. Freeman DE, Staller GS, Maxson AD, et al: Unusual internal carotid artery branching that prevented arterial occlusion with a balloon-tipped catheter in a horse, *Vet Surg* 22:531, 1993.
128. Freeman DE, Donawick WJ: Occlusion of internal carotid artery in the horse by means of a balloon-tipped catheter: clinical use of a method to prevent epistaxis caused by guttural pouch mycosis, *J Am Vet Med Assoc* 176:236, 1980.
129. Caron JP, Fretz PB, Bailey JV, et al: Balloon-tipped catheter arterial occlusion for prevention of hemorrhage caused by guttural pouch mycosis: 13 cases (1982-1985), *J Am Vet Med Assoc* 191:345, 1987.
130. Hardy J, Robertson JT, Wilkie DA: Ischemic optic neuropathy and blindness after arterial occlusion for treatment of guttural pouch mycosis in two horses, *J Am Vet Med Assoc* 196:1631, 1990.
131. Freeman DE, Ross MW, Donawick WJ: "Steal phenomenon" proposed as the cause of blindness after arterial occlusion for treatment of guttural pouch mycosis in horses, *J Am Vet Med Assoc* 197:811, 1990.
132. Bacon Miller C, Wilson DA, Martin DD, et al: Complications of balloon catheterization associated with aberrant cerebral arterial anatomy in a horse with guttural pouch mycosis, *Vet Surg* 27:450, 1998.
133. Judy CE, Chaffin MK, Cohen ND: Empyema of the guttural pouch (auditory tube diverticulum) in horses: 91 cases (1977-1997), *J Am Vet Med Assoc* 215:1666, 1999.
134. Verheyen K, Newton JR, Talbot NC, et al: Elimination of guttural pouch infection and inflammation in asymptomatic carriers of Streptococcus equi, *Equine Vet J* 32:527, 2000.
135. Seahorn TL, Schumacher J: Nonsurgical removal of chondroid masses from the guttural pouches of two horses, *J Am Vet Med Assoc* 199:368, 1991.
136. Gehlen H, Ohnesorge B: Laser fenestration of the mesial septum for treatment of guttural pouch chondroids in a pony, *Vet Surg* 34:383, 2005.

137. Hawkins JF, Frank N, Sojka JE, et al: Fistulation of the auditory tube diverticulum (guttural pouch) with a neodymium: yttrium-aluminum-garnet laser for treatment of chronic empyema in two horses, *J Am Vet Med Assoc* 218:405, 2001.
138. Hobo S, Matsuda Y, Yoshida K: Prevalence of upper respiratory tract disorders detected with a flexible videoendoscope in thoroughbred racehorses, *J Vet Med Sci* 57:409, 1995.
139. Holcombe SJ, Robinson NE, Derksen FJ, et al: Effect of tracheal mucus and tracheal cytology on racing performance in Thoroughbred racehorses, *Equine Vet J* 38:300, 2006.
140. Raker CW, Boles CL: Pharyngeal lymphoid hyperplasia in the horse, *J Equine Med Surg* 2:202, 1978.
141. Holcombe SJ, Jackson C, Gerber V, et al: Stabling is associated with airway inflammation in young Arabian horses, *Equine Vet J* 33:244, 2001.
142. Blakeslee JR, Jr, Olsen RG, McAllister ES, et al: Evidence of respiratory tract infection induced by equine herpesvirus, type 2, in the horse, *Can J Microbiol* 21:1975, 1940.
143. Prickett ME: The pathology of disease caused by equine herpesvirus-1. *Proceedings of the Second International Conference on Equine Infectious Diseases,* Princeton, NJ, 1969. Veterinary Publications.
144. Burrell MH: Endoscopic and virological observations on respiratory disease in a group of young Thoroughbred horses in training, *Equine Vet J* 17:99, 1985.
145. Christley RM, Hodgson DR, Rose RJ, et al: Coughing in thoroughbred racehorses: risk factors and tracheal endoscopic and cytological findings, *Vet Rec* 148:99, 2001.
146. Kannegieter NJ, Dore ML: Endoscopy of the upper respiratory tract during treadmill exercise: a clinical study of 100 horses, *Aust Vet J* 72:101, 1995.
147. Holcombe SJ, Derksen FJ, Stick JA, et al: Effect of bilateral blockade of the pharyngeal branch of the vagus nerve on soft palate function in horses, *Am J Vet Res* 59:504, 1998.
148. Ducharme NG: Pharynx. In Auer JA, Stick JA, editors: *Equine surgery*, St Louis, 2006, Elsevier Health Sciences.
149. Dart AJ, Dowling BA, Hodgson DR, et al: Evaluation of high-speed treadmill videoendoscopy for diagnosis of upper respiratory tract dysfunction in horses, *Aust Vet J* 79:109, 2001.
150. Barakzai SZ, Johnson VS, Baird DH, et al: Assessment of the efficacy of composite surgery for the treatment of dorsal displacement of the soft palate in a group of 53 racing Thoroughbreds (1990-1996), *Equine Vet J* 36:175, 2004.
151. Parente EJ, Martin BB, Tulleners EP, et al: Dorsal displacement of the soft palate in 92 horses during high-speed treadmill examination (1993-1998), *Vet Surg* 31:507, 2002.
152. Lane JG, Bladon B, Little DR, et al: Dynamic obstructions of the equine upper respiratory tract. Part 2: comparison of endoscopic findings at rest and during high-speed treadmill exercise of 600 Thoroughbred racehorses, *Equine Vet J* 38:401, 2006.
153. Rehder RS, Ducharme NG, Hackett RP, et al: Measurement of upper airway pressures in exercising horses with dorsal displacement of the soft palate, *Am J Vet Res* 56:269, 1995.
154. Cook WR: Some observations on form and function of the equine uppe airway in health and disease, I. The pharynx *Proc Am Assoc Eq Pract* 198:355, 1982.
155. Fogel RB, Trinder J, White DP, et al: The effect of sleep onset on upper airway muscle activity in patients with sleep apnoea versus controls, *J Physiol* 564:549, 2005.
156. Gumery PY, Roux-Buisson H, Meignen S, et al: An adaptive detector of genioglossus EMG reflex using Berkner transform for time latency measurement in OSA pathophysiological studies, *IEEE Trans Biomed Eng* 52:1382, 2005.
157. Tessier C, Holcombe SJ, Derksen FJ, et al: Effects of stylopharyngeus muscle dysfunction on the nasopharynx in exercising horses, *Equine Vet J* 36:318, 2004.
158. Holcombe SJ, Derksen FJ, Stick JA, et al: Effect of bilateral tenectomy of the tensor veli palatini muscle on soft palate function in horses, *Am J Vet Res* 58:317, 1997.
159. Ducharme NG, Hackett RP, Woodie JB, et al: Investigations into the role of the thyrohyoid muscles in the pathogenesis of dorsal displacement of the soft palate in horses, *Equine Vet J* 35:258, 2003.
160. Holcombe SJ, Beard WL, Hinchcliff KW, et al: Effect of sternothyrohyoid myectomy on upper airway mechanics in normal horses, *J Appl Physiol* 77:2812, 1994.
161. Malhotra A, Pillar G, Fogel RB, et al: Pharyngeal pressure and flow effects on genioglossus activation in normal subjects, *Am J Respir Crit Care Med* 165:71, 2002.
162. Brennick MJ, Gefter WB, Margulies SS: Mechanical effects of genioglossus muscle stimulation on the pharyngeal airway by MRI in cats, *Respir Physiol Neurobiol* 156:154, 2007.
163. Franklin SH, Naylor JR, Lane JG: The effect of a tongue-tie in horses with dorsal displacement of the soft palate, *Equine Vet J* Suppl (34):430, 2002.
164. Harrison IW, Raker CW: Sternothyrohyoideus myectomy in horses: 17 cases (1984-1985), *J Am Vet Med Assoc* 193:1299, 1988.
165. Anderson JD, Tulleners EP, Johnston JK, et al: Sternothyrohyoideus myectomy or staphylectomy for treatment of intermittent dorsal displacement of the soft palate in racehorses: 209 cases (1986-1991), *J Am Vet Med Assoc* 206:1909, 1995.
166. Ahren TJ: Oral palatopharyngoplasty: a survey of one hundred post-operative raced horses, *J Equine Vet Sci* 13:670, 1993.
167. Barakzai SZ, Dixon PM: Conservative treatment for thoroughbred racehorses with intermittent dorsal displacement of the soft palate, *Vet Rec* 157:337, 2005.
168. Woodie JB, Ducharme NG, Kanter P, et al: Surgical advancement of the larynx (laryngeal tie-forward) as a treatment for dorsal displacement of the soft palate in horses: a prospective study 2001-2004, *Equine Vet J* 37:418, 2005.
169. Woodie JB, Ducharme NG, Hackett RP, et al: Can an external device prevent dorsal displacement of the soft palate during strenuous exercise? *Equine Vet J* 37:425, 2005.
170. Goulden BE, Anderson LG: Equine laryngeal hemiplegia. Part III. Treatment by laryngoplasty, *N Z Vet J* 30:1, 1982.
171. Lane JG, Ellis DR, Greet TR: Observations on the examination of Thoroughbred yearlings for idiopathic laryngeal hemiplegia, *Equine Vet J* 19:531, 1987.
172. Dixon PM, McGorum BC, Railton DI, et al: Laryngeal paralysis: a study of 375 cases in a mixed-breed population of horses, *Equine Vet J* 33:452, 2001.
173. Brown JA, Hinchcliff KW, Jackson MA, et al: Prevalence of pharyngeal and laryngeal abnormalities in Thoroughbreds racing in Australia, and their association with performance, *Equine Vet J* 37:397, 2005.
174. Brakenhoff JE, Holcombe SJ, Hauptman JG, et al: The prevalence of laryngeal disease in a large population of competition draft horses, *Vet Surg* 35:579, 2006.
175. Harrison GD, Duncan ID, Clayton MK: Determination of the early age of onset of equine recurrent laryngeal neuropathy. 1. Muscle pathology, *Acta Neuropathol* 84:307, 1992.
176. Dixon P, Robinson E, Wade JF. 2003. Workshop summary. Proceedings of a Workshop on Equine Recurrent Laryngeal Neuropathy. Stratford-upon-Avon, United Kingdom, R & W Publications (Newmarket) Ltd.
177. Rakestraw PC, Hackett RP, Ducharme NG, et al: Arytenoid cartilage movement in resting and exercising horses, *Vet Surg* 20:122, 1991.
178. Ducharme N. 2003. 4-grade system of equine laryngeal function. Proceedings of a Workshop on Equine Recurrent Laryngeal Neuropathy. Stratford-upon-Avon, United KingdomR & W Publications (Newmarket) Ltd.
179. Hammer EJ, Tulleners EP, Parente EJ, et al: Videoendoscopic assessment of dynamic laryngeal function during exercise in horses with grade-III left laryngeal hemiparesis at rest: 26 cases (1992-1995), *J Am Vet Med Assoc* 212:399, 1998.

180. Chalmers HJ, Cheetham J, Yeager AE, et al: Ultrasonography of the equine larynx, *Vet Radiol Ultrasound* 47:476, 2006.
181. Chalmers HJ, Cheetham J, Mohammed HO, et al. Ultrasonography as an aid in the diagnosis of recurrent laryngeal neuropathy in horses. Proceedings 2006 ACVS Veterinary Symposium. 2006.
182. Quinlan TJ, Goulden BE, Barnes GR, et al: Innervation of the equine intrinsic laryngeal muscles, *N Z Vet J* 30:43, 1982.
183. Duncan ID, Griffths IR, McQueen A, et al: The pathology of equine laryngeal hemiplegia, *Acta Neuropathol* 27:337, 1974.
184. Gunn HM: Histochemical observations on laryngeal skeletal muscle fibres in 'normal' horses, *Equine Vet J* 4:144, 1972.
185. Cahill JI, Goulden BE: Equine laryngeal hemiplegia. Part I. A light microscopic study of peripheral nerves, *N Z Vet J* 34:161, 1986.
186. Dattilo DJ, Drooger SA: Outcome assessment of patients undergoing maxillofacial procedures for the treatment of sleep apnea: comparison of subjective and objective results, *J Oral Maxillofac Surg* 62:164, 2004.
187. Curtis RA, Hahn CN, Evans DL, et al: Thoracolaryngeal reflex latencies in Thoroughbred horses with recurrent laryngeal neuropathy, *Vet J* 170:67, 2005.
188. Cole CR: Changes in the equine larynx associated with laryngeal hemiplegia, *Am J Vet Res* 7:69, 1946.
189. Derksen FJ, Stick JA, Scott EA, et al: Effect of laryngeal hemiplegia and laryngoplasty on airway flow mechanics in exercising horses, *Am J Vet Res* 47:16, 1986.
190. Brown JA, Derksen FJ, Stick JA, et al: Laser vocal cordectomy fails to effectively reduce respiratory noise in horses with laryngeal hemiplegia, *Vet Surg* 34:247, 2005.
191. Shappell KK, Derksen FJ, Stick JA, et al: Effects of ventriculectomy, prosthetic laryngoplasty, and exercise on upper airway function in horses with induced left laryngeal hemiplegia, *Am J Vet Res* 49:1760, 1988.
192. Tetens J, Derksen FJ, Stick JA, et al: Efficacy of prosthetic laryngoplasty with and without bilateral ventriculocordectomy as treatments for laryngeal hemiplegia in horses, *Am J Vet Res* 57:1668, 1996.
193. Ehrlich PJ, Seeherman HJ, Morris E, et al: The effect of reversible left recurrent laryngeal neuropathy on the metabolic cost of locomotion and peak aerobic power in thoroughbred racehorses, *Vet Surg* 24:36, 1995.
194. Kidd JA, Slone DE: Treatment of laryngeal hemiplegia in horses by prosthetic laryngoplasty, ventriculectomy and vocal cordectomy, *Vet Rec* 150:481, 2002.
195. Hawkins JF, Tulleners EP, Ross MW, et al: Laryngoplasty with or without ventriculectomy for treatment of left laryngeal hemiplegia in 230 racehorses, *Vet Surg* 26:484, 1997.
196. Kraus BM, Parente EJ, Tulleners EP: Laryngoplasty with ventriculectomy or ventriculocordectomy in 104 draft horses (1992-2000), *Vet Surg* 32:530, 2003.
197. Dixon RM, McGorum BC, Railton DI, et al: Long-term survey of laryngoplasty and ventriculocordectomy in an older, mixed-breed population of 200 horses. Part 1: Maintenance of surgical arytenoid abduction and complications of surgery, *Equine Vet J* 35:389, 2003.
198. Brown JA, Derksen FJ, Stick JA, et al: Effect of laryngoplasty on respiratory noise reduction in horses with laryngeal hemiplegia, *Equine Vet J* 36:420, 2004.
199. Schumacher J, Wilson AM, Pardoe C, et al: In vitro evaluation of a novel prosthesis for laryngoplasty of horses with recurrent laryngeal neuropathy, *Equine Vet J* 32:43, 2000.
200. Radcliffe CH, Woodie JB, Hackett RP, et al: A comparison of laryngoplasty and modified partial arytenoidectomy as treatments for laryngeal hemiplegia in exercising horses, *Vet Surg* 35:643, 2006.
201. Davenport CL, Tulleners EP, Parente EJ: The effect of recurrent laryngeal neurectomy in conjunction with laryngoplasty and unilateral ventriculocordectomy in thoroughbred racehorses, *Vet Surg* 30:417, 2001.
202. Strand E, Martin GS, Haynes PF, et al: Career racing performance in Thoroughbreds treated with prosthetic laryngoplasty for laryngeal neuropathy: 52 cases (1981-1989), *J Am Vet Med Assoc* 217:1689, 2000.
203. Russell AP, Slone DE: Performance analysis after prosthetic laryngoplasty and bilateral ventriculectomy for laryngeal hemiplegia in horses: 70 cases (1986-1991), *J Am Vet Med Assoc* 204:1235, 1994.
204. Dixon PM, McGorum BC, Railton DI, et al: Long-term survey of laryngoplasty and ventriculocordectomy in an older, mixed-breed population of 200 horses. Part 2: Owners' assessment of the value of surgery, *Equine Vet J* 35:397, 2003.
205. Ducharme NG, Horney FD, Partlow GD, et al: Attempts to restore abduction of the paralyzed equine arytenoid cartilage. I. Nerve-muscle pedicle transplants, *Can J Vet Res* 53:202, 1989.
206. Fulton IC, Derksen FJ, Stick JA, et al: Treatment of left laryngeal hemiplegia in standardbreds, using a nerve muscle pedicle graft, *Am J Vet Res* 52:1461, 1991.
207. Fulton IC, Derksen FJ, Stick JA, et al: Histologic evaluation of nerve muscle pedicle graft used as a treatment for left laryngeal hemiplegia in standardbreds, *Am J Vet Res* 53:592, 1992.
208. Barnes AJ, Slone DE, Lynch TM: Performance after partial arytenoidectomy without mucosal closure in 27 Thoroughbred racehorses, *Vet Surg* 33:398, 2004.
209. Russell T, Wainscott M: Treatment in the field of 27 horses with epiglottic entrapment, *Vet Rec* 161:187, 2007.
210. McClure SR, Schumacher J, Snyder JR: Transnasal incision of restrictive nasopharyngeal cicatrix in three horses, *J Am Vet Med Assoc* 205:461, 1994.
211. Perkins JD, Hughes TK, Brain B: Endoscope-guided, transoral axial division of an entrapping epiglottic fold in fifteen standing horses, *Vet Surg* 36:800, 2007.
212. Lumsden JM, Stick JA, Caron JP, et al: Surgical treatment for epiglottic entrapment in horses: 51 cases (1981-1992), *J Am Vet Med Assoc* 205:729, 1994.
213. Ross MW, Gentile DG, Evans LE: Transoral axial division, under endoscopic guidance, for correction of epiglottic entrapment in horses, *J Am Vet Med Assoc* 203:416, 1993.
214. Greet TR: Experiences in treatment of epiglottal entrapment using a hook knife per nasum, *Equine Vet J* 27:122, 1995.
215. Tate LP, Sweeney CL, Bowman KF, et al: Transendoscopic Nd: YAG laser surgery for treatment of epiglottal entrapment and dorsal displacement of the soft palate in the horse, *Vet Surg* 19:356, 1990.
216. Tulleners EP: Correlation of performance with endoscopic and radiographic assessment of epiglottic hypoplasia in racehorses with epiglottic entrapment corrected by use of contact neodymium:yttrium aluminum garnet laser, *J Am Vet Med Assoc* 198:621, 1991.
217. Tulleners EP: Transendoscopic contact neodymium:yttrium aluminum garnet laser correction of epiglottic entrapment in standing horses, *J Am Vet Med Assoc* 196:1971, 1990.
218. Haynes PF, Snider TG, McClure JR, et al: Chronic chondritis of the equine arytenoid cartilage, *J Am Vet Med Assoc* 177:1135, 1980.
219. Behrens E, Pinero L: Laryngeal chondropathy in a group of broodmares, *J Equine Vet Sci* 10:113, 1990.
220. Kelly G, Lumsden JM, Dunkerly G, et al: Idiopathic mucosal lesions of the arytenoid cartilages of 21 Thoroughbred yearlings: 1997-2001, *Equine Vet J* 35:276, 2003.
221. Dean PW, Cohen ND: Arytenoidectomy for advanced unilateral chondropathy with accompanying lesions, *Vet Surg* 19:364, 1990.

222. Hay WP, Tulleners E: Excision of intralaryngeal granulation tissue in 25 horses using a neodymium:YAG laser (1986 to 1991), *Vet Surg* 22:129, 1993.
223. Smith RL, Perkins NR, Firth EC, et al: Arytenoid mucosal injury in young Thoroughbred horses: investigation of a proposed aetiology and clinical significance, *N Z Vet J* 54:173, 2006.
224. MacLean AA, Robertson-Smith RG: Chronic chondritis of the arytenoid cartilages in a pony mare, *Aust Vet J* 61:27, 1984.
225. Terry C, Shumpert K, Rashmir-Raven AM, et al: An unusual case of upper respiratory obstruction in a horse, *Vet Radiol Ultrasound* 43:43, 2002.
226. Haynes PF: Dorsal displacement of the soft palate and epiglottic entrapment: diagnosis, management and interrelationships, *Compend Contin Educ Pract Vet* 5:S379, 1983.
227. Blikslager AT, Tate LP, Tudor R: Transendoscopic laser treatment of rostral displacement of the palatopharyngeal arch in four horses, *J Clin Laser Med Surg* 17:49, 1999.
228. Klein HJ, Deegen E, Stockhofe N, et al: Rostral displacement of the palatopharyngeal arch in a seven-month-old Hanoverian colt, *Equine Vet J* 21:382, 1989.
229. Goulden BE, Anderson LJ, Davies AS, et al: Rostral displacement of the palatopharyngeal arch: a case report, *Equine Vet J* 8:95, 1976.
230. Crabill M, Schumacher J, Walker M: What is your diagnosis? Rostral displacement of the palatopharyngeal arch, *J Am Vet Med Assoc* 204:1347, 1994.
231. Cook WR: Some observations on diseases of the ear, nose and throat in the horse, and endoscopy using a flexible fibreoptic endoscope, *Vet Rec* 94:533, 1974.
232. Schumacher J, Hanselka DV: Nasopharyngeal cicatrices in horses: 47 cases (1972-1985), *J Am Vet Med Assoc* 191:239, 1987.
233. Chesen AB, Rakestraw PC: Indications for and short- and long-term outcome of permanent tracheostomy performed in standing horses: 82 cases (1995-2005), *J Am Vet Med Assoc* 232:1352, 2008.
234. Timoney JF: *Strangles, Vet Clin North Am Equine Pract* 9:365, 1993.
235. Timoney JF, Artiushin SC, Boschwitz JS: Comparison of the sequences and functions of Streptococcus equi M-like proteins SeM and SzPSe, *Infect Immun* 65:3600, 1997.
236. Jorm LR, Love DN, Bailey GD, et al: Genetic structure of populations of beta-haemolytic Lancefield group C streptococci from horses and their association with disease, *Res Vet Sci* 57:292, 1994.
237. Sweeney CR, Benson CE, Whitlock RH: Streptococcus equi infection in horses: Part I, *Compend Contin Educ Pract Vet* 9:689, 1987.
238. Prescott JF, Srivastava SK, deGannes R, et al: A mild form of strangles caused by an atypical Streptococcus equi, *J Am Vet Med Assoc* 180:293, 1982.
239. Grant ST, Efstratiou A, Chanter N: Laboratory diagnosis of strangles and the isolation of atypical Streptococcus equi, *Vet Rec* 133:215, 1993.
240. Artiushin S, Timoney JF: PCR for detection of Streptococcus equi, *Adv Exp Med Biol* 418:359-361, 1997.
241. Harrington DJ, Sutcliffe IC, Chanter N: The molecular basis of Streptococcus equi infection and disease, *Microbes Infect* 4:501, 2002.
242. Galan JE, Timoney JF, Lengemann FW: Passive transfer of mucosal antibody to Streptococcus equi in the foal, *Infect Immun* 54:202, 1986.
243. Sweeney CR, Benson CE, Whitlock RH, et al: Description of an epizootic and persistence of Streptococcus equi infections in horses, *J Am Vet Med Assoc* 194:1281, 1989.
244. Todd TG: Strangles, *J Comp Pathol Ther* 23:212, 1910.
245. Timoney JF: The pathogenic equine streptococci, *Vet Res* 35:397, 2004.
246. Hamlen HJ, Timoney JF, Bell RJ: Epidemiologic and immunologic characteristics of Streptococcus equi infection in foals, *J Am Vet Med Assoc* 204:768, 1994.
247. Piche CA: Clinical observations on an outbreak of strangles, *Can Vet J* 25:7, 1984.
248. George JL, Reif JS, Shideler RK, et al: Identification of carriers of Streptococcus equi in a naturally infected herd, *J Am Vet Med Assoc* 183:80, 1983.
249. Newton JR, Wood JL, Dunn KA, et al: Naturally occurring persistent and asymptomatic infection of the guttural pouches of horses with Streptococcus equi, *Vet Rec* 140:84, 1997.
250. Waller AS, Jolley KA: Getting a grip on strangles: recent progress towards improved diagnostics and vaccines, *Vet J* 173:492, 2007.
251. Sweeney CR, Timoney JF, Newton JR, et al: Streptococcus equi infections in horses: guidelines for treatment, control, and prevention of strangles, *J Vet Intern Med* 19:123, 2005.
252. Jorm LR. Factors affecting the survival of Streptococcus equi subsp equi. Sixth International Conference on Equine Infectious Disease. Newmarket, England, 1991.
253. Yigezu LM, Roger F, Kiredjian M, et al: Isolation of Streptococcus equi subspecies equi (strangles agent) from an Ethiopian camel, *Vet Rec* 140:608, 1997.
254. Breiman RF, Silverblatt FJ: Systemic *Streptococcus equi* infection in a horse handler: a case of human strangles, *West J Med* 145:385, 1986.
255. Evers WD: Effect of furaltadone on strangles in horses, *J Am Vet Med Assoc* 152:1394, 1968.
256. Muhktar MM, Timoney JF: Chemotactic response of equine polymorphonuclear leucocytes to Streptococcus equi, *Res Vet Sci* 45:225, 1988.
257. Hamilton A, Robinson C, Sutcliffe IC, et al: Mutation of the maturase lipoprotein attenuates the virulence of Streptococcus equi to a greater extent than does loss of general lipoprotein lipidation, *Infect Immun* 74:6907, 2006.
258. Tiwari R, Qin A, Artiushin S, et al: Se18.9, an anti-phagocytic factor H binding protein of Streptococcus equi, *Vet Microbiol* 121:105, 2007.
259. Anzai T, Timoney JF, Kuwamoto Y, et al: In vivo pathogenicity and resistance to phagocytosis of Streptococcus equi strains with different levels of capsule expression, *Vet Microbiol* 67:277, 1999.
260. Kelly C, Bugg M, Robinson C, et al: Sequence variation of the SeM gene of Streptococcus equi allows discrimination of the source of strangles outbreaks, *J Clin Microbiol* 44:480, 2006.
261. Anzai T, Sheoran AS, Kuwamoto Y, et al: Streptococcus equi but not Streptococcus zooepidemicus produces potent mitogenic responses from equine peripheral blood mononuclear cells, *Vet Immunol Immunopathol* 67:235, 1999.
262. Sheoran AS, Sponseller BT, Holmes MA, et al: Serum and mucosal antibody isotype responses to M-like protein (SeM) of Streptococcus equi in convalescent and vaccinated horses, *Vet Immunol Immunopathol* 59:239, 1997.
263. Timoney JF, Timoney PJ, Strickland KL: Lysogeny and the immunologically reactive proteins of Streptococcus equi, *Vet Rec* 115:148, 1984.
264. Newton JR, Verheyen K, Talbot NC, et al: Control of strangles outbreaks by isolation of guttural pouch carriers identified using PCR and culture of Streptococcus equi, *Equine Vet J* 32:515, 2000.
265. Sweeney CR: Strangles: Streptococcus equi infection in horses, *Equine Vet Educ* 8:317, 1996.
266. Ramey D: Does early antibiotic use in horses with 'strangles' cause metastatic Streptococcus equi bacterial infections? *Equine Vet Educ* 19:14, 2007.
267. Sweeney CR, Benson CE, Whitlock RH, et al: Streptococcus equi infection in horses. Part 2, *Compend Contin Educ Pract Vet* 9:845, 1987.

268. Rumbaugh GE, Smith BP, Carlson GP: Internal abdominal abscesses in the horse: a study of 25 cases, *J Am Vet Med Assoc* 172:304, 1978.
269. Spoormakers TJ, Ensink JM, Goehring LS, et al: Brain abscesses as a metastatic manifestation of strangles: symptomatology and the use of magnetic resonance imaging as a diagnostic aid, *Equine Vet J* 35:146, 2003.
270. Koblik PD, Lofstedt J, Jakowski RM, et al: Use of 111In-labeled autologous leukocytes to image an abdominal abscess in a horse, *J Am Vet Med Assoc* 186:1319, 1985.
271. Pusterla N, Whitcomb MB, Wilson WD: Internal abdominal abscesses caused by Streptococcus equi subspecies equi in 10 horses in California between 1989 and 2004, *Vet Rec* 160:589, 2007.
272. Zicker SC, Wilson WD, Medearis I: Differentiation between intra-abdominal neoplasms and abscesses in horses, using clinical and laboratory data: 40 cases (1973-1988), *J Am Vet Med Assoc* 196:1130, 1990.
273. Pusterla N, Watson JL, Affolter VK, et al: Purpura haemorrhagica in 53 horses, *Vet Rec* 153:118, 2003.
274. Heath SE, Geor RJ, Tabel H, et al: Unusual patterns of serum antibodies to Streptococcus equi in two horses with purpura hemorrhagica, *J Vet Intern Med* 5:263, 1991.
275. Galan JE, Timoney JF: Immune complexes in purpura hemorrhagica of the horse contain IgA and M antigen of Streptococcus equi, *J Immunol* 135:3134, 1985.
276. Yelle MT: Clinical aspects of Streptococcus equi infection, *Equine Vet J* 19:158, 1987.
277. Todhunter RJ, Brown CM, Stickle R: Retropharyngeal infections in five horses, *J Am Vet Med Assoc* 187:600, 1985.
278. Golland LC, Hodgson DR, Davis RE, et al: Retropharyngeal lymph node infection in horses: 46 cases (1977-1992), *Aust Vet J* 72:161, 1995.
279. De Clercq D, van Loon G, Nollet H, et al: Percutaneous puncture technique for treating persistent retropharyngeal lymph node infections in seven horses, *Vet Rec* 152:169, 2003.
280. Rigg DL, Ramey DW, Reinertson EL: Tracheal compression secondary to abscessation of cranial mediastinal lymph nodes in a horse, *J Am Vet Med Assoc* 186:283, 1985.
281. Bell RJ, Smart ME: An unusual complication of strangles in a pony, *Can Vet J* 33:400, 1992.
282. Finno C, Pusterla N, Aleman M, et al: Streptococcus equi meningoencephalomyelitis in a foal, *J Am Vet Med Assoc* 229:721, 2006.
283. Kaese HJ, Valberg SJ, Hayden DW, et al: Infarctive purpura hemorrhagica in five horses, *J Am Vet Med Assoc* 226:1893, 2005.
284. Sponseller BT, Valberg SJ, Tennent-Brown BS, et al: Severe acute rhabdomyolysis associated with Streptococcus equi infection in four horses, *J Am Vet Med Assoc* 227:1800, 1753.
285. Valaberg SJ, Bullock P, Hgetvedt W, et al. Muopathies associated with Streptococcus equi infections in horses. *Proceedings of the American Association of Equine Practitioners,* 1996.
286. Galan JE, Timoney JF: Mucosal nasopharyngeal immune responses of horses to protein antigens of Streptococcus equi, *Infect Immun* 47:623, 1985.
287. Wood JM: Antigenic variation of equine influenza: a stable virus, *Equine Vet J* 20:316, 1988.
288. Kemp-Symonds J, Kemble T, Waller A: Modified live Streptococcus equi ('strangles') vaccination followed by clinically adverse reactions associated with bacterial replication, *Equine Vet J* 39:284, 2007.
289. Prescott JF, Timoney JF: Could we eradicate strangles in equids? *J Am Vet Med Assoc* 231:377, 2007.
290. Newton R, Waller A, King A: Investigation of suspected adverse reactions following strangles vaccination in horses, *Vet Rec* 156:291, 2005.
291. Morley PS, Townsend HG, Bogdan JR, et al: Descriptive epidemiologic study of disease associated with influenza virus infections during three epidemics in horses, *J Am Vet Med Assoc* 216:535, 2000.
292. Newton JR, Verheyen K, Wood JL, et al: Equine influenza in the United Kingdom in 1998, *Vet Rec* 145:449, 1999.
293. Martella V, Elia G, Decaro N, et al: An outbreak of equine influenza virus in vaccinated horses in Italy is due to an H3N8 strain closely related to recent North American representatives of the Florida sub-lineage, *Vet Microbiol* 121:56, 2007.
294. Minke JM, Toulemonde CE, Coupier H, et al: Efficacy of a canarypox-vectored recombinant vaccine expressing the hemagglutinin gene of equine influenza H3N8 virus in the protection of ponies from viral challenge, *Am J Vet Res* 68:213, 2007.
295. Higgins WP, Gillespie JH, Holmes DR, et al: Surveys of equine influenze outbreaks during 1983 and 1984, *J Equine Vet Sci* 6:15, 1986.
296. Kemen MJ, Frank RA, Babish JB: An outbreak of equine influenza at a harness horse racetrack, *Cornell Vet* 75:277, 1985.
297. Crawford PC, Dubovi EJ, Castleman WL, et al: Transmission of equine influenza virus to dogs, *Science* 310:482, 2005.
298. Daly JM: Equine influenza in dogs: too late to bolt the stable door? *Vet J* 171:7, 2006.
299. McChesney AE: Viral respiratory infections of horses: structure and function of lungs in relation to viral infection, *J Am Vet Med Assoc* 166:76, 1975.
300. Carr CM, Kim PS: Flu virus invasion: halfway there, *Science* 266:234, 1994.
301. Paillot R, Hannant D, Kydd JH, et al: Vaccination against equine influenza: quid novi? *Vaccine* 24:4047, 2006.
302. Chambers TM, Holland RE, Lai A: Equine influenza: current veterinary perspectives, part 1, *Equine Pract* 17:19, 1995.
303. Nelson KM, Schram BR, McGregor MW, et al: Local and systemic isotype-specific antibody responses to equine influenza virus infection versus conventional vaccination, *Vaccine* 16:1306, 1998.
304. Gross DK, Morley PS, Hinchcliff KW, et al: Pulmonary ultrasonographic abnormalities associated with naturally occurring equine influenza virus infection in standardbred racehorses, *J Vet Intern Med* 18:718, 2004.
305. Gross DK, Hinchcliff KW, French PS, et al: Effect of moderate exercise on the severity of clinical signs associated with influenza virus infection in horses, *Equine Vet J* 30:489, 1998.
306. Chambers TM, Holland RE, Lai A: Equine influenza: current veterinary perspectives, Part 2, *Equine Pract* 27:26, 1995.
307. Britton AP, Robinson JH: Isolation of influenza A virus from a 7-day-old foal with bronchointerstitial pneumonia, *Can Vet J* 43:55, 2002.
308. Peek SF, Landolt G, Karasin AI, et al: Acute respiratory distress syndrome and fatal interstitial pneumonia associated with equine influenza in a neonatal foal, *J Vet Intern Med* 18:132, 2004.
309. van Maanen C, van Essen GJ, Minke J, et al: Diagnostic methods applied to analysis of an outbreak of equine influenza in a riding school in which vaccine failure occurred, *Vet Microbiol* 93:291, 2003.
310. Garin B, Plateau E, Gillet-Forin S: Serological diagnosis of influenza A infections in the horse by enzyme immunoassay. Comparison with the complement fixation test, *Vet Immunol Immunopathol* 13:357, 1986.
311. Yamanaka T, Tsujimura K, Kondo T, et al: In vitro efficacies of oseltamivir carboxylate and zanamivir against equine influenza A viruses, *J Vet Med Sci* 68:405, 2006.
312. Yamanaka T, Tsujimura K, Kondo T, et al: Efficacy of oseltamivir phosphate to horses inoculated with equine influenza A virus, *J Vet Med Sci* 68:923, 2006.

313. Yamanaka T, Yamada M, Tsujimura K, et al: Clinical pharmacokinetics of oseltamivir and its active metabolite oseltamivir carboxylate after oral administration in horses, *J Vet Med Sci* 69:293, 2007.
314. Baker DJ: Rationale for the use of influenza vaccines in horses and the importance of antigenic drift, *Equine Vet J* 18:93, 1986.
315. Morley PS, Townsend HG, Bogdan JR, et al: Efficacy of a commercial vaccine for preventing disease caused by influenza virus infection in horses, *J Am Vet Med Assoc* 215:61, 1999.
316. Newton JR, Daly JM, Spencer L, et al: Description of the outbreak of equine influenza (H3N8) in the United Kingdom in 2003, during which recently vaccinated horses in Newmarket developed respiratory disease, *Vet Rec* 158:185, 2006.
317. Soboll G, Horohov DW, Aldridge BM, et al: Regional antibody and cellular immune responses to equine influenza virus infection, and particle mediated DNA vaccination, *Vet Immunol Immunopathol* 94:47, 2003.
318. Lunn DP, Soboll G, Schram BR, et al: Antibody responses to DNA vaccination of horses using the influenza virus hemagglutinin gene, *Vaccine* 17:2245, 1999.
319. Edlund Toulemonde C, Daly J, Sindle T, et al: Efficacy of a recombinant equine influenza vaccine against challenge with an American lineage H3N8 influenza virus responsible for the 2003 outbreak in the United Kingdom, *Vet Rec* 156:367, 2005.
320. Paillot R, Kydd JH, Sindle T, et al: Antibody and IFN-gamma responses induced by a recombinant canarypox vaccine and challenge infection with equine influenza virus, *Vet Immunol Immunopathol* 112:225, 2006.
321. Paillot R, Kydd JH, MacRae S, et al: New assays to measure equine influenza virus-specific Type 1 immunity in horses, *Vaccine* 25:7385, 2007.
322. Chambers TM, Holland RE, Tudor LR, et al: A new modified live equine influenza virus vaccine: phenotypic stability, restricted spread and efficacy against heterologous virus challenge, *Equine Vet J* 33:630, 2001.
323. Lunn DP, Hussey S, Sebing R, et al: Safety, efficacy, and immunogenicity of a modified-live equine influenza virus vaccine in ponies after induction of exercise-induced immunosuppression, *J Am Vet Med Assoc* 218:900, 2001.
324. van Maanen C, Bruin G, de Boer-Luijtze E, et al: Interference of maternal antibodies with the immune response of foals after vaccination against equine influenza, *Vet Q* 14:13, 1992.
325. Wilson WD, Mihalyi JE, Hussey S, et al: Passive transfer of maternal immunoglobulin isotype antibodies against tetanus and influenza and their effect on the response of foals to vaccination, *Equine Vet J* 33:644, 2001.
326. Daly JM, Whitwell KE, Miller J, et al: Investigation of equine influenza cases exhibiting neurological disease: coincidence or association? *J Comp Pathol* 134:231, 2006.
327. Kleiboeker SB, Schommer SK, Johnson PJ, et al: Association of two newly recognized herpesviruses with interstitial pneumonia in donkeys (Equus asinus), *J Vet Diagn Invest* 14:273, 2002.
328. Field HJ, Biswas S, Mohammad IT: Herpesvirus latency and therapy—from a veterinary perspective, *Antiviral Res* 71:127, 2006.
329. Patel JR, Heldens J: Equine herpesviruses 1 (EHV-1) and 4 (EHV-4)—epidemiology, disease and immunoprophylaxis: a brief review, *Vet J* 170:14, 2005.
330. Blunden AS, Smith KC, Binns MM, et al: Replication of equid herpesvirus 4 in endothelial cells and synovia of a field case of viral pneumonia and synovitis in a foal, *J Comp Pathol* 112:133, 1995.
331. Browning GF, Ficorilli N, Studdert MJ: Asinine herpesvirus genomes: comparison with those of the equine herpesviruses, *Arch Virol* 101:183, 1988.
332. Kleiboeker SB, Turnquist SE, Johnson PJ, et al: Detection and nucleotide sequencing of a DNA-packaging protein gene of equine gammaherpesviruses, *J Vet Diagn Invest* 16:67, 2004.
333. van Maanen C: Equine herpesvirus 1 and 4 infections: an update, *Vet Q* 24:58, 2002.
334. Telford EA, Watson MS, Perry J, et al: The DNA sequence of equine herpesvirus-4, *J Gen Virol* 79:1197, 1998:Pt 5.
335. Kinyili JH, Thorsen J: Antigenic comparisons between herpesviruses isolated from fallow deer in Alberta and the viruses of infectious bovine rhinotracheitis, equine rhinopneumonitis and DN-599, a non-IBR bovine herpesvirus, *J Wildl Dis* 15:339, 1979.
336. Rebhun WC, Jenkins DH, Riis RC, et al: An epizootic of blindness and encephalitis associated with a herpesvirus indistinguishable from equine herpesvirus I in a herd of alpacas and llamas, *J Am Vet Med Assoc* 192:953, 1988.
337. Bildfell R, Yason C, Haines D, et al: Herpesvirus encephalitis in a camel (Camelus bactrianus), *J Zoo Wildlife Med* 27:409, 1996.
338. Pagamjav O, Yamada S, Ibrahim el-SM, et al: Molecular characterization of equine herpesvirus 1 (EHV-1) isolated from cattle indicating no specific mutations associated with the interspecies transmission, *Microbiol Immunol* 51:313, 2007.
339. Nugent J, Birch-Machin I, Smith KC, et al: Analysis of equid herpesvirus 1 strain variation reveals a point mutation of the DNA polymerase strongly associated with neuropathogenic versus nonneuropathogenic disease outbreaks, *J Virol* 80:4047, 2006.
340. Dynon K, Black WD, Ficorilli N, et al: Detection of viruses in nasal swab samples from horses with acute, febrile, respiratory disease using virus isolation, polymerase chain reaction and serology, *Aust Vet J* 85:46, 2007.
341. Bryans JT, Allen GP: Herpesviral disease of the horse. In Wittman G, editor: *Herpes virus disease of cattle, horses and pigs*, Boston, 1989, Kluvar.
342. O'Keefe JS, Alley MR, Jones D, et al: Neonatal mortality due to equid herpesvirus 4 (EHV-4) in a foal, *Aust Vet J* 72:353, 1995.
343. Thein P, Darai G, Janssen W, et al: Recent information about the etiopathogenesis of paretic-paralytic forms of herpesvirus infection in horses, *Tierarztl Prax* 21:445, 1993.
344. Verheyen K, Newton JR, Wood JL, et al: Possible case of EHV-4 ataxia in warmblood mare, *Vet Rec* 143:456, 1998.
345. van Maanen C, Vreeswijk J, Moonen P, et al: Differentiation and genomic and antigenic variation among fetal, respiratory, and neurological isolates from EHV1 and EHV4 infections in The Netherlands, *Vet Q* 22:88, 2000.
346. Slater JD, Borchers K, Thackray AM, et al: The trigeminal ganglion is a location for equine herpesvirus 1 latency and reactivation in the horse, *J Gen Virol* 75:2007, 1994:Pt 8.
347. Edington N, Welch HM, Griffiths L: The prevalence of latent Equid herpesviruses in the tissues of 40 abattoir horses, *Equine Vet J* 26:140, 1994.
348. Welch HM, Bridges CG, Lyon AM, et al: Latent equid herpesviruses 1 and 4: detection and distinction using the polymerase chain reaction and co-cultivation from lymphoid tissues, *J Gen Virol* 73:261, 1992:Pt 2.
349. Pusterla N, Leutenegger CM, Wilson WD, et al: Equine herpesvirus-4 kinetics in peripheral blood leukocytes and nasopharyngeal secretions in foals using quantitative real-time TaqMan PCR, *J Vet Diagn Invest* 17:578, 2005.
350. Foote CE, Love DN, Gilkerson JR, et al: Detection of EHV-1 and EHV-4 DNA in unweaned Thoroughbred foals from vaccinated mares on a large stud farm, *Equine Vet J* 36:341, 2004.
351. Foote CE, Love DN, Gilkerson JR, et al: EHV-1 and EHV-4 infection in vaccinated mares and their foals, *Vet Immunol Immunopathol* 111:41, 2006.

352. Brown JA, Mapes S, Ball BA, et al: Prevalence of equine herpesvirus-1 infection among Thoroughbreds residing on a farm on which the virus was endemic, *J Am Vet Med Assoc* 231:577, 2007.
353. Wang L, Raidal SL, Pizzirani A, et al: Detection of respiratory herpesviruses in foals and adult horses determined by nested multiplex PCR, *Vet Microbiol* 121:18, 2007.
354. Dolby CA, Hannant D, Mumford JA: Response of ponies to adjuvanted EHV-1 whole virus vaccine and challenge with virus of the homologous strain, *Br Vet J* 151:27, 1995.
355. Campbell TM, Studdert MJ: Equine herpesvirus type 1 (EHV1), *Vet Bull* 53:135, 1983.
356. Kydd JH, Smith KC, Hannant D, et al: Distribution of equid herpesvirus-1 (EHV-1) in respiratory tract associated lymphoid tissue: implications for cellular immunity, *Equine Vet J* 26:470, 1994.
357. Frampton AR Jr, Stolz DB, Uchida H, et al: Equine herpesvirus 1 enters cells by two different pathways, and infection requires the activation of the cellular kinase ROCK1, *J Virol* 81:108, 2007.
358. Sutton GA, Viel L, Carman PS, et al: Pathogenesis and clinical signs of equine herpesvirus-1 in experimentally infected ponies in vivo, *Can J Vet Res* 62:49, 1998.
359. Tearle JP, Smith KC, Boyle MS, et al: Replication of equid herpesvirus-1 (EHV-1) in the testes and epididymides of ponies and venereal shedding of infectious virus, *J Comp Pathol* 115:385, 1996.
360. Hebia I, Fiéni F, Duchamp G, et al: Potential risk of equine herpes virus 1 (EHV-1) transmission by equine embryo transfer, *Theriogenology* 67:1485, 2007.
361. Slater JD, Lunn DP, Horohov DW, et al: Report of the equine herpesvirus-1 Havermeyer Workshop, San Gimignano, Tuscany, June 2004, *Vet Immunol Immunopathol* 111:3, 2006.
362. Hamir AN, Vaala W, Heyer G, et al: Disseminated equine herpesvirus-1 infection in a two-year-old filly, *J Vet Diagn Invest* 6:493, 1994.
363. Del Piero F, Wilkins PA, Timoney PJ, et al: Fatal nonneurological EHV-1 infection in a yearling filly, *Vet Pathol* 37:672, 2000.
364. Mason DK, Watkins KL, McNie JT, et al: Haematological measurements as an aid to early diagnosis and prognosis of respiratory viral infections in thoroughbred horses, *Vet Rec* 126:359, 1990.
365. Sharma PC, Cullinane AA, Onions DE, et al: Diagnosis of equid herpesviruses-1 and -4 by polymerase chain reaction, *Equine Vet J* 24:20, 1992.
366. Hussey SB, Clark R, Lunn KF, et al: Detection and quantification of equine herpesvirus-1 viremia and nasal shedding by real-time polymerase chain reaction, *J Vet Diagn Invest* 18:335, 2006.
367. Allen GP: Development of a real-time polymerase chain reaction assay for rapid diagnosis of neuropathogenic strains of equine herpesvirus-1, *J Vet Diagn Invest* 19:69, 2007.
368. Gradil C, Joo HS: A radial immunodiffusion enzyme assay for detection of antibody to equine rhinopneumonitis virus (EHV-1) in horse serum, *Vet Microbiol* 17:315, 1988.
369. Garre B, van der Meulen K, Nugent J, et al: In vitro susceptibility of six isolates of equine herpesvirus 1 to acyclovir, ganciclovir, cidofovir, adefovir, PMEDAP and foscarnet, *Vet Microbiol* 122:43, 2007.
370. Murray MJ, del Piero F, Jeffrey SC, et al: Neonatal equine herpesvirus type 1 infection on a thoroughbred breeding farm, *J Vet Intern Med* 12:36, 1998.
371. Friday PA, Scarratt WK, Elvinger F, et al: Ataxia and paresis with equine herpesvirus type 1 infection in a herd of riding school horses, *J Vet Intern Med* 14:197, 2000.
372. Bentz BG, Maxwell LK, Erkert RS, et al: Pharmacokinetics of acyclovir after single intravenous and oral administration to adult horses, *J Vet Intern Med* 20:589, 2006.
373. Wilkins PA, Papich M, Sweeney RW: Pharmacokinetics of acyclovir in adult horses, *J Vet Emerg Crit Care* 15:174, 2005.
374. Garré B, Shebany K, Gryspeerdt A, et al: Pharmacokinetics of acyclovir after intravenous infusion of acyclovir and after oral administration of acyclovir and its prodrug valacyclovir in healthy adult horses, *Antimicrob Agents Chemother* 51:4308, 2007.
375. Gibson JS, Slater JD, Field HJ: The activity of (S)-1-[(3-hydroxy-2-phosphonyl methoxy) propyl] cytosine (HPMPC) against equine herpesvirus-1 (EHV-1) in cell cultures, mice and horses, *Antiviral Res* 19:219, 1992.
376. Pusterla N, Chaney KP, Maes R, et al: Investigation of the molecular detection of vaccine-derived equine herpesvirus type 1 in blood and nasal secretions from horses following intramuscular vaccination, *J Vet Diagn Invest* 19:290, 2007.
377. Drummer HE, Reubel GH, Studdert MJ: Equine gammaherpesvirus 2 (EHV2) is latent in B lymphocytes, *Arch Virol* 141:495, 1996.
378. Rizvi SM, Slater JD, Wolfinger U, et al: Detection and distribution of equine herpesvirus 2 DNA in the central and peripheral nervous systems of ponies, *J Gen Virol* 78:1115, 1997:Pt 5.
379. Borchers K, Ebert M, Fetsch A, et al: Prevalence of equine herpesvirus type 2 (EHV-2) DNA in ocular swabs and its cell tropism in equine conjunctiva, *Vet Microbiol* 118:260, 2006.
380. Fu ZF, Robinson AJ, Horner GW, et al: Respiratory disease in foals and the epizootiology of equine herpesvirus type 2 infection, *N Z Vet J* 34:152, 1986.
381. Nordengrahn A, Merza M, Ros C, et al: Prevalence of equine herpesvirus types 2 and 5 in horse populations by using type-specific PCR assays, *Vet Res* 33:251, 2002.
382. Pálfi V, Belák S, Molnár T: Isolation of equine herpesvirus type 2 from foals, showing respiratory symptoms, *Zentralbl Veterinarmed B* 25:165, 1978.
383. Sigiura T, Fukuzawa Y, Kamada M, et al: Isolation of equine herpesvirus type 2 from foals with pneumonitis, *Bull Equine Res Inst* 20:148, 1983.
384. Ames TR, O'Leary TP, Johnston GR: Isolation of equine herpesvirus type 2 from foals with respiratory disease, *Compend Contin Educ Pract Vet* 8:664, 1986.
385. Murray MJ, Eichorn ES, Dubovi EJ, et al: Equine herpesvirus type 2: prevalence and seroepidemiology in foals, *Equine Vet J* 28:432, 1996.
386. Borchers K, Wolfinger U, Ludwig H, et al: Virological and molecular biological investigations into equine herpes virus type 2 (EHV-2) experimental infections, *Virus Res* 55:101, 1998.
387. Kershaw O, von Oppen T, Glitz F, et al: Detection of equine herpesvirus type 2 (EHV-2) in horses with keratoconjunctivitis, *Virus Res* 80:93, 2001.
388. Browning GF, Studdert MJ: Genomic heterogeneity of equine betaherpesviruses, *J Gen Virol* 68:1441, 1987:Pt 5.
389. Dunowska M, Meers J, Wilks CR: *Isolation of equine herpesvirus type 5 in New Zealand, N Z Vet J* 47:44, 1999.
390. Bell SA, Balasuriya UB, Nordhausen RW, et al: Isolation of equine herpesvirus-5 from blood mononuclear cells of a gelding, *J Vet Diagn Invest* 18:472, 2006.
391. Holloway SA, Lindquester GJ, Studdert MJ, et al: Identification, sequence analysis and characterisation of equine herpesvirus 5 glycoprotein B., *Arch Virol* 144:287, 1999.
392. Williams KJ, Maes R, Del Piero F, et al: Equine multinodular pulmonary fibrosis: a newly recognized herpesvirus-associated fibrotic lung disease, *Vet Pathol* 44:849, 2007.
393. Del Piero F: Equine viral arteritis, *Vet Pathol* 37:287, 2000.
394. Mumford JA: Preparing for equine arteritis, *Equine Vet J* 17:6, 1985.
395. MacLachlan NJ, Balasuriya UB: Equine viral arteritis, *Adv Exp Med Biol* 581:429, 2006.

396. Timoney PJ, McCollum WH: Equine viral arteritis, *Can Vet J* 28:693, 1987.
397. Hedges JF, Balasuriya UB, Timoney PJ, et al: Genetic divergence with emergence of novel phenotypic variants of equine arteritis virus during persistent infection of stallions, *J Virol* 73:3672, 1999.
398. Holyoak GR, Little TV, McCollam WH, et al: Relationship between onset of puberty and establishment of persistent infection with equine arteritis virus in the experimentally infected colt, *J Comp Pathol* 109:29, 1993.
399. Del Piero F, Wilkins PA, Lopez JW, et al: Equine viral arteritis in newborn foals: clinical, pathological, serological, microbiological and immunohistochemical observations, *Equine Vet J* 29:178, 1997.
400. Szeredi L, Hornyak A, Denes B, et al: Equine viral arteritis in a newborn foal: parallel detection of the virus by immunohistochemistry, polymerase chain reaction and virus isolation, *J Vet Med B Infect Dis Vet Public Health* 50:270, 2003.
401. Hullinger PJ, Gardner IA, Hietala SK, et al: Seroprevalence of antibodies against equine arteritis virus in horses residing in the United States and imported horses, *J Am Vet Med Assoc* 219:946, 2001.
402. Traub-Dargatz JL, Ralston SL, Collins JK, et al: Equine viral arteritis, *Compend Contin Educ Pract Vet* 7:S490, 1985.
403. Timoney PJ, Klingeborn B, Lucas MH: A perspective on equine viral arteritis (infectious arteritis of horses), *Rev Sci Tech* 15:1203, 1996.
404. Chirnside ED: Equine arteritis virus: an overview, *Br Vet J* 148:181, 1992.
405. MacLachlan NJ, Balasuriya UB, Davis NL, et al: Experiences with new generation vaccines against equine viral arteritis, West Nile disease and African horse sickness, *Vaccine* 25:5577, 2007.
406. Hullinger PJ, Wilson WD, Rossitto PV, et al: Passive transfer, rate of decay, and protein specificity of antibodies against equine arteritis virus in horses from a Standardbred herd with high seroprevalence, *J Am Vet Med Assoc* 213:839, 1998.
407. Hartley CA, Ficorilli N, Dynon K, et al: Equine rhinitis A virus: structural proteins and immune response, *J Gen Virol* 82:1725, 2001.
408. King AMQ, Brown F, Christian P, et al: Family picornaviridae, In Fauquet CM, Mayo MA, Maniloff J, et al: *Virus Taxonomy: VIIIth Report of the International Committee on Taxonomy of Viruses*, Burlington, MA, 2005, Elsevier.
409. Huang JA, Ficorilli N, Hartley CA, et al: Equine rhinitis B virus: a new serotype, *J Gen Virol* 82:2641, 2001.
410. Black WD, Hartley CA, Ficorilli NP, et al: Sequence variation divides Equine rhinitis B virus into three distinct phylogenetic groups that correlate with serotype and acid stability, *J Gen Virol* 86:2323, 2005.
411. Black WD, Studdert MJ: Formerly unclassified, acid-stable equine picornaviruses are a third equine rhinitis B virus serotype in the genus Erbovirus, *J Gen Virol* 87:3023, 2006.
412. Plummer G, Kerry JB: Studies on an equine respiratory virus, *Vet Rec* 74:967, 1962.
413. Klaey M, Sanchez-Higgins M, Leadon DP, et al: Field case study of equine rhinovirus 1 infection: clinical signs and clinicopathology, *Equine Vet J* 30:267, 1998.
414. Li F, Drummer HE, Ficorilli N, et al: Identification of noncytopathic equine rhinovirus 1 as a cause of acute febrile respiratory disease in horses, *J Clin Microbiol* 35:937, 1997.
415. Black WD, Wilcox RS, Stevenson RA, et al: Prevalence of serum neutralising antibody to equine rhinitis A virus (ERAV), equine rhinitis B virus 1 (ERBV1) and ERBV2, *Vet Microbiol* 119:65, 2007.
416. Kriegshäuser G, Deutz A, Kuechler E, et al: Prevalence of neutralizing antibodies to Equine rhinitis A and B virus in horses and man, *Vet Microbiol* 106:293, 2005.
417. Feng L, Browning GF, Studdert MJ, et al: Equine rhinovirus 1 is more closely related to foot and mouth disease virus than to other picornaviruses, *Proc Nat Acad Sci USA* 93:990, 1996.
418. Carman S, Rosendal S, Huber L, et al: Infectious agents in acute respiratory disease in horses in Ontario, *J Vet Diagn Invest* 9:17, 1997.
419. Steck F, Hofer B, Schaeren B, et al: Equine rhinoviruses: new serotypes. In *Proceedings of the Fourth International Conference on Equine Infectious Disease*, Princeton, NJ, 1978, Veterinary Publications.
420. Studdert MJ: Equine adenovirus infections, In Studdert MJ, editor: *Virus Infections of Equines*, New York, 1996, Elsevier.
421. Richards AJ, Kelly DF, Knottenbelt DC, et al: Anaemia, diarrhoea and opportunistic infections in Fell ponies, *Equine Vet J* 32:386, 2000.
422. Bell SA, Leclere M, Gardner IA, et al: Equine adenovirus 1 infection of hospitalised and healthy foals and horses, *Equine Vet J* 38:379, 2006.
423. Horner GW, Hunter R: Isolation of two serotypes of equine adenovirus from horses in New Zealand, *N Z Vet J* 30:62, 1982.
424. Studdert MJ, Blackney MH: Isolation of an adenovirus antigenically distinct from equine adenovirus type 1 from diarrheic foal feces, *Am J Vet Res* 43:543, 1982.
425. Barclay AJ, Paton DJ: Hendra (equine morbillivirus), *Vet J* 160:165, 2000.
426. Eaton BT, Broder CC, Middleton D, et al: Hendra and Nipah viruses: different and dangerous, *Nat Rev Microbiol* 4:23, 2006.
427. Murray K, Selleck P, Hooper P, et al: A morbillivirus that caused fatal disease in horses and humans, *Science* 268:94, 1995.
428. Westbury H: Hendra virus: a highly lethal zoonotic agent, *Vet J* 160:165, 2000.
429. Baldock FC, Douglas IC, Halpin K, et al: Epidemiological investigations into the 1994 equine morbillivirus outbreaks in Queensland, Australia, *Sing Vet J* 20:1996.
430. Barker SC: The Australian paralysis tick may be the missing link in the transmission of Hendra virus from bats to horses to humans, *Med Hypotheses* 60:481, 2003.
431. Westbury HA: Hendra virus disease in horses, *Rev Sci Tech* 19:151, 2000.
432. Mellor PS, Hamblin C: African horse sickness, *Vet Res* 35:445, 2004.
433. Englund L, Pringle J: New diseases and increased risk of diseases in companion animals and horses due to transport, *Acta Vet Scand Suppl* 100:19, 2003.
434. Wittmann EJ, Baylis M: Climate change: effects on culicoides–transmitted viruses and implications for the UK, *Vet J* 160:107, 2000.
435. Boorman J, Mellor PS, Penn M, et al: The growth of African horse-sickness virus in embryonated hen eggs and the transmission of virus by Culicoides variipennis Coquillett (Diptera, Ceratopogonidae), *Arch Virol* 47:343, 1975.
436. Coetzer JAW, Erasmus BJ: In Coetzer JAW, Thommson GR, Tustin RC, editors: *Infections diseases of livestock with special reference to southern Africa, African horse sickness* Vol. 1. Cape Town, South Africa, 1994, Oxford University Press.
437. Sinclair M, Bührmann G, Gummow B: An epidemiological investigation of the African horsesickness outbreak in the Western Cape Province of South Africa in 2004 and its relevance to the current equine export protocol, *J S Afr Vet Assoc* 77:191, 2006.
438. Mair TS, Lane JG: Tracheal obstructions in two horses and a donkey, *Vet Rec* 126:303, 1990.
439. Urquhart KA, Gerring EL, Shepherd MP: Tracheobronchial foreign body in a pony, *Equine Vet J* 13:262, 1981.
440. Couetil LL, Gallatin LL, Blevins W, et al: Treatment of tracheal collapse with an intraluminal stent in a miniature horse, *J Am Vet Med Assoc* 225:1727, 2004.

441. Kirker-Head CA, Jakob TP: Surgical repair of ruptured trachea in a horse, *J Am Vet Med Assoc* 196:1635, 1990.
442. Tate LP Jr, Koch DB, Sembrat RF, et al: Tracheal reconstruction by resection and end-to-end anastomosis in the horse, *J Am Vet Med Assoc* 178:253, 1981.
443. Hare WCD: Equine respiratory system. In Getty R, editor: *Sisson and Grossman's the anatomy of the domestic animals*, Philadelphia, 1975, W.B. Saunders.
444. McLaughlin RF, Tyler WS, Canada RO: A study of the subgross pulmonary anatomy in various mammals, *Am J Anat* 108:149, 1961.
445. Breeze R, Turk M: Cellular structure, function and organization in the lower respiratory tract, *Environ Health Perspect* 55:3, 1984.
446. Pirie M, Pirie HM, Cranston S, et al: An ultrastructural study of the equine lower respiratory tract, *Equine Vet J* 22:338, 1990.
447. Christmann U, Livesey LC, Taintor JS, et al: Lung surfactant function and composition in neonatal foals and adult horses, *J Vet Intern Med* 20:1402, 2006.
448. Mair TS, Batten EH, Stokes CR, et al: The histological features of the immune system of the equine respiratory tract, *J Comp Pathol* 97:575, 1987.
449. Frevert CW, Warner AE, Adams ET, et al: Pulmonary intravascular macrophages are an important part of the mononuclear phagocyte system in the horse (Abstract), *J Vet Intern Med* 5:145, 1991.
450. Taylor AE, Rehder K, Hyatt RE, et al: *Clinical respiratory physiology*, Philadelphia, 1989, W.B. Saunders.
451. Amis TC, Pascoe JR, Hornof W: Topographic distribution of pulmonary ventilation and perfusion in the horse, *Am J Vet Res* 45:1597, 1984.
452. Robinson NE: Exercise induced pulmonary haemorrhage (EIPH): could Leonardo have got it right? *Equine Vet J* 19:370, 1987.
453. Barnes PJ: Neural control of human airways in health and disease, *Am Rev Respir Dis* 134:1289, 1986.
454. Derksen FJ, Broadstone RV. Bronchodilation therapy and the autonomic nervous system in horses with airway obstruction. Proceedings of the American College of Veterinary Internal Medicine, 1991.
455. Derksen FJ, Robinson NE, Slocombe RF: Ovalbumin-induced lung disease in the pony: role of vagal mechanisms, *J Appl Physiol* 53:719, 1982.
456. Sant'Ambrogio G: Nervous receptors of the tracheobronchial tree, *Annu Rev Physiol* 49:611, 1987.
457. Derksen FJ, Scott JS, Slocombe RF, et al: Effect of clenbuterol on histamine-induced airway obstruction in ponies, *Am J Vet Res* 48:423, 1987.
458. Scott JS, Garon H, Broadstone RV, et al: Alpha 1-adrenergic-induced airway obstruction in ponies with recurrent pulmonary disease, *J Appl Physiol* 65:687, 1988.
459. Sonea I, Bowker RM, Broadstone R, et al: Presence and distribution of vasoactive intestinal peptide-like and peptide histidine isoleucine-like immunoreactivity in the equine lung, *Am Rev Respir Dis* 143:A355, 1991:(Abstract).
460. Robinson NE, Wilson R: Airway obstruction in the horse, *J Equine Vet Sci* 9:155, 1989.
461. West JB: *Pulmonary pathophysiology*, Baltimore, 1982, Williams & Wilkins.
462. Bayly W, Grant BD, Breeze RG, et al: The effects of maximal exercise on acid-base balance and arterial blood gas tension in thoroughbred horses. In Snow DH, Persson SGN, Rose RJ, editors, *Equine exercise physiology*, Cambridge, England, 1983, Granta.
463. Wagner PD, Gillespie JR, Landgren GL, et al: Mechanism of exercise-induced hypoxemia in horses, *J Appl Physiol* 66:1227, 1989.
464. Dantzker DR: Physiology and pathophysiology of pulmonary gas exchange, *Hosp Pract (Off Ed)* 21:135, 1986.
465. Roth RA: Biochemistry, physiology and drug metabolism–implications regarding the role of the lungs in drug disposition, *Clin Physiol Biochem* 3:66, 1985.
466. Gillis CN, Pitt BR: The fate of circulating amines within the pulmonary circulation, *Annu Rev Physiol* 44:269, 1982.
467. Wright JR: Immunoregulatory functions of surfactant proteins, *Nat Rev Immunol* 5:58, 2005.
468. Wong CW, Thompson HL, Thong YH, et al: Effect of strenuous exercise stress on chemiluminescence response of equine alveolar macrophages, *Equine Vet J* 22:33, 1990.
469. Huston LH, Bayly WM, Liggitt HD, et al: Alveolar macrophage function in thoroughbreds after strenuous exercise. In Gillespie JR, Robinson NE, editors: *Equine exercise physiology*, Davis, CA, 1987, ICEEP Publications, Volume 2.
470. Blunden AS, Mackintosh ME: The microflora of the lower respiratory tract of the horse: an autopsy study, *Br Vet J* 147:238, 1991.
471. Spurlock SL, Spurlock GH, Donaldson LL: Consolidating pneumonia and pneumothorax in a horse, *J Am Vet Med Assoc* 192:1081, 1988.
472. Racklyeft DJ, Love DN: Bacterial infection of the lower respiratory tract in 34 horses, *Aust Vet J* 78:549, 2000.
473. Garcia-Cantu MC, Hartmann FA, Brown CM, et al: Bordetella bronchiseptica and equine respiratory infections: a review of 30 cases, *Equine Vet Educ* 12:45, 2000.
474. Anzai T, Walker JA, Blair MB, et al: Comparison of the phenotypes of Streptococcus zooepidemicus isolated from tonsils of healthy horses and specimens obtained from foals and donkeys with pneumonia, *Am J Vet Res* 61:162, 2000.
475. Biberstein EL, Jang SS, Hirsh DC: Nocardia asteroides infection in horses: a review, *J Am Vet Med Assoc* 186:273, 1985.
476. Jakab GJ: Viral-bacterial interactions in pulmonary infection, *Adv Vet Sci Comp Med* 26:155, 1982.
477. Raidal SL: Equine pleuropneumonia, *Br Vet J* 151:233, 1995.
478. Raidal SL, Love DN, Bailey GD: Effect of a single bout of high intensity exercise on lower respiratory tract contamination in the horse, *Aust Vet J* 75:293, 1997.
479. Bayly WM: Stress and equine respiratory immunity, *Proc Am Coll Vet Intern Med*, 1990 .
480. Raidal SL, Love DN, Bailey GD, et al: The effect of high intensity exercise on the functional capacity of equine pulmonary alveolar macrophages and BAL-derived lymphocytes, *Res Vet Sci* 68:249, 2000.
481. Raidal SL, Taplin RH, Bailey GD, et al: Antibiotic prophylaxis of lower respiratory tract contamination in horses confined with head elevation for 24 or 48 hours, *Aust Vet J* 75:126, 1997.
482. Raidal SL, Love DN, Bailey GD: Inflammation and increased numbers of bacteria in the lower respiratory tract of horses within 6 to 12 hours of confinement with the head elevated, *Aust Vet J* 72:45, 1995.
483. Stull CL, Rodiek AV: Effects of cross-tying horses during 24 h of road transport, *Equine Vet J* 34:550, 2002.
484. Rainger JE, Hughes KJ, Kessell A, et al: Pleuropneumonia as a sequela of myelography and general anaesthesia in a Thoroughbred colt, *Aust Vet J* 84:138, 2006.
485. Pusterla N, Jones ME, Mohr FC, et al: Fatal pulmonary hemorrhage associated with RTX toxin producing Actinobacillus equuli subspecies haemolyticus infection in an adult horse, *J Vet Diagn Invest* 20:118, 2008.
486. McKenzie HC: Characterization of antimicrobial aerosols for administration to horses, *Vet Ther* 4:110, 2003.
487. Art T, de Moffarts B, Bedoret D, et al: Pulmonary function and antimicrobial concentration after marbofloxacin inhalation in horses, *Vet Rec* 161:348, 2007.
488. Lavoie JP, Fiset L, Laverty S: Review of 40 cases of lung abscesses in foals and adult horses, *Equine Vet J* 26:348, 1994.
489. Mair TS, Lane JG: Pneumonia, lung abscesses and pleuritis in adult horses: a review of 51 cases, *Equine Vet J* 21:175, 1989.

490. Ainsworth DM, Erb HN, Eicker SW, et al: Effects of pulmonary abscesses on racing performance of horses treated at referral veterinary medical teaching hospitals: 45 cases (1985-1997), *J Am Vet Med Assoc* 216:1282, 2000.
491. Schachter EN: Suppurative lung disease: old problems revisited, *Clin Chest Med* 2:41, 1981.
492. Lubitz RM: Resolution of lung abscess due to Pseudomonas aeruginosa with oral ciprofloxacin: case report, *Rev Infect Dis* 12:757, 1990.
493. Colahan PT, Knight HD: Drainage of an intrathoracic abscess in a horse via thoracotomy, *J Am Vet Med Assoc* 174:1231, 1979.
494. Smith BP: Pleuritis and pleural effusion in the horse: a study of 37 cases, *J Am Vet Med Assoc* 170:208, 1977.
495. Raphel CF, Beech J: Pleuritis secondary to pneumonia or lung abscessation in 90 horses, *J Am Vet Med Assoc* 181:808, 1982.
496. Schott HC, Mansmann RA: Thoracic drainage in horses, *Compend Contin Educ Pract Vet* 12:251, 1990.
497. Fenno CH: Severe equine pleuritis due to wire penetration, *Vet Med Small Anim Clin* 70:458, 1975.
498. Tremaine WH, Dixon PM, McGorum BC, et al: Pleuropulmonary abscessation in a horse caused by a gastric foreign body, *Vet Rec* 136:637, 1995.
499. Collins MB, Hodgson DR, Hutchins DR: Pleural effusion associated with acute and chronic pleuropneumonia and pleuritis secondary to thoracic wounds in horses: 43 cases (1982-1992), *J Am Vet Med Assoc* 205:1753, 1994.
500. Hudson NPH, McClintock SA, Hodgson DR: Case of pleuro pneumonia with complications in a thoroughbred stallion, *Equine Vet Educ* 11:285, 1999.
501. Sprayberry KA, Byars TD: Equine pleuropneumonia, *Equine Vet Educ* 11:290, 1999.
502. Austin SM, Foreman JH, Hungerford LL: Case-control study of risk factors for development of pleuropneumonia in horses, *J Am Vet Med Assoc* 207:325, 1995.
503. Chaffin MK: Thoracocentesis and pleural drainage in horses, *Equine Vet Educ* 10:106, 1998.
504. Foreman JH: Equine respiratory pharmacology, *Vet Clin North Am Equine Pract* 15:665, 1999.
505. Orsini JA, Perkins S: The fluoroquinolones: clinical applications in veterinary medicine, *Compend Contin Educ Pract Vet* 14:1491, 1992.
506. Giguère S, Belanger M: Concentration of enrofloxacin in equine tissues after long-term oral administration, *J Vet Pharmacol Ther* 20:402, 1997.
507. Gustafsson A, Båverud V, Gunnarsson A, et al: The association of erythromycin ethylsuccinate with acute colitis in horses in Sweden, *Equine Vet J* 29:314, 1997.
508. Thoracotomy Grant B: *Proceedings of the 1997 Dubai International Equine Symposium*, Dubai, United Arab Emirates, 1997, Neyenesch Printers.
509. Byars TD: Pleuropneumonia: treatment and prognosis, The diagnosis and treatment of respiratory diseases. *Proceedings of the 1997 Dubai International Equine Symposium*. Dubai, United Arab Emirates, 1997, Neyenesch Printers.
510. Frevert CW, Warner AE: Respiratory distress resulting from acute lung injury in the veterinary patient, *J Vet Intern Med* 6:154, 1992.
511. Seltzer KL, Byars TD: Prognosis for return to racing after recovery from infectious pleuropneumonia in thoroughbred racehorses: 70 cases (1984-1989), *J Am Vet Med Assoc* 208:1300, 1996.
512. Byars TD, Dainis CM, Seltzer KL, et al: Cranial thoracic masses in the horse: a sequel to pleuropneumonia, *Equine Vet J* 23:22, 1991.
513. Byars TD, Becht JL: Pleuropneumonia, *Vet Clin North Am Equine Pract* 7:63, 1991.
514. Chaffin MK: Diagnostic assessment of pleural effusion in horses, *Compend Contin Educ Pract Vet* 16:1035, 1994.
515. Jorgensen JS, Geoly FJ, Berry CR, et al: Lameness and pleural effusion associated with an aggressive fibrosarcoma in a horse, *J Am Vet Med Assoc* 210:1328, 1997.
516. Wrigley RH, Gay CC, Lording P, et al: Pleural effusion associated with squamous cell carcinoma of the stomach of a horse, *Equine Vet J* 13:99, 1981.
517. Prater PE, Patton CS, Held JP: Pleural effusion resulting from malignant hepatoblastoma in a horse, *J Am Vet Med Assoc* 194:383, 1989.
518. Valentine BA, Ross CE, Bump JL, et al: Intramuscular hemangiosarcoma with pulmonary metastasis in a horse, *J Am Vet Med Assoc* 188:628, 1986.
519. Murray MJ, Cavey DM, Feldman BF, et al: Signs of sympathetic denervation associated with a thoracic melanoma in a horse, *J Vet Intern Med* 11:199, 1997.
520. Mair TS, Hillyer MH, Brown P: Mesothelioma of the pleural cavity in a horse: diagnostic features, *Equine Vet Educ* 4:59, 1992.
521. Foreman JH, Weidner JP, Parry BW, et al: Pleural effusion secondary to thoracic metastatic mammary adenocarcinoma in a mare, *J Am Vet Med Assoc* 197:1193, 1990.
522. Morris DD, Acland HM, Hodge TG: Pleural effusion secondary to metastasis of an ovarian adenocarcinoma in a horse, *J Am Vet Med Assoc* 187:272, 1985.
523. Thatcher CD, Roussel AJ, Chickering WR, et al: Pleural effusion with thoracic lymphosarcoma in a mare, *Compend Contin Educ Pract Vet* 7:S726, 1985.
524. Sweeney CR, Gillette DM: Thoracic neoplasia in equids: 35 cases (1967-1987), *J Am Vet Med Assoc* 195:374, 1989.
525. Ogilvie TH, Rosendal S, Blackwell TE, et al: Mycoplasma felis as a cause of pleuritis in horses, *J Am Vet Med Assoc* 182:1374, 1983.
526. Burbidge HM: Penetrating thoracic wound in a Hackney mare, *Equine Vet J* 14:94, 1982.
527. Mair TS, Pearson H, Waterman AE, et al: Chylothorax associated with a congenital diaphragmatic defect in a foal, *Equine Vet J* 20:304, 1988.
528. Sahn SA: The pathophysiology of pleural effusions, *Annu Rev Med* 41:7, 1990.
529. Tarn AC, Lapworth R: Biochemical analysis of pleural fluid: what should we measure? *Ann Clin Biochem* 38:311, 2001.
530. Das DK: Serous effusions in malignant lymphomas: a review, *Diagn Cytopathol* 34:335, 2006.
531. Yildirim E, Dural K, Yazkan R, et al: Rapid pleurodesis in symptomatic malignant pleural effusion, *Eur J Cardiothorac Surg* 27:19, 2005.
532. Kuzniar TJ, Blum MG, Kasibowska-Kuzniar K, et al: Predictors of acute lung injury and severe hypoxemia in patients undergoing operative talc pleurodesis, *Ann Thorac Surg* 82:1976, 2006.
533. Baron RD, Milton R, Thorpe JA: Pleurodesis using small talc particles results in an unacceptably high rate of acute lung injury and hypoxia, *Ann Thorac Surg* 84:2136, 2007.
534. Antony VB, Loddenkemper R, Astoul P, et al: Management of malignant pleural effusions, *Eur Respir J* 18:402, 2001.
535. Stather DR, Tremblay A: Use of tunneled pleural catheters for outpatient treatment of malignant pleural effusions, *Curr Opin Pulm Med* 13:328, 2007.
536. Putnam JB Jr, Light RW, Rodriguez RM, et al: A randomized comparison of indwelling pleural catheter and doxycycline pleurodesis in the management of malignant pleural effusions, *Cancer* 86:1992, 1999.
537. Carter GR, Changappa MM, Roberts AW: Systemic mycoses, In Carter GR, Changappa MM, Roberts AW, editors: *Essentials of Veterinary Mycology*, ed 5, Philadelphia, 1995, Lea & Febiger.
538. De Groote MA, Bjerke R, Smith H, et al: Expanding epidemiology of blastomycosis: clinical features and investigation of 2 cases in Colorado, *Clin Infect Dis* 30:582, 2000.

539. Toribio RE, Kohn CW, Lawrence AE, et al: Thoracic and abdominal blastomycosis in a horse, *J Am Vet Med Assoc* 214:1357, 1999.
540. Fisher MC, Koenig GL, White TJ, et al: Molecular and phenotypic description of *Coccidioides posadasil sp nov*, previously recognized as the non-California population of Coccidioides immitis, *Mycologia* 94:73, 2002.
541. Ziemer EL, Pappagianis D, Madigan JE, et al: Coccidioidomycosis in horses: 15 cases (1975-1984), *J Am Vet Med Assoc* 201:910, 1992.
542. Stoltz JH, Johnson BJ, Walker RL, et al: Coccidioides immitis abortion in an Arabian mare, *Vet Pathol* 31:258, 1994.
543. Walker RL, Johnson BJ, Jones KL, et al: Coccidioides immitis mastitis in a mare, *J Vet Diagn Invest* 5:446, 1993.
544. Casadevall A, Rosas AL, Nosanchuk JD: Melanin and virulence in Cryptococcus neoformans, *Curr Opin Microbiol* 3:354, 2000.
545. Carter GR, Changappa MM, Roberts AW: Mycoses caused by yeasts or yeast-like fungi. In Carter GR, Changappa MM, Roberts AW, editors: *Essentials of Veterinary Mycology*, ed 5, Philadelphia, 1995, Lea & Febiger.
546. Belay T, Cherniak R, O'Neill EB, et al: Serotyping of Cryptococcus neoformans by dot enzyme assay, *J Clin Microbiol* 34:466, 1996.
547. Sebghati TS, Engle JT, Goldman WE: Intracellular parasitism by Histoplasma capsulatum: fungal virulence and calcium dependence, *Science* 290:1368, 2000.
548. Rezabek GB, Donahue JM, Giles RC, et al: Histoplasmosis in horses, *J Comp Pathol* 109:47, 1993.
549. Cornick JL: Diagnosis and treatment of pulmonary histoplasmosis in a horse, *Cornell Vet* 80:97, 1990.
550. Slocombe RF, Slauson DO: Invasive pulmonary aspergillosis of horses: an association with acute enteritis, *Vet Pathol* 25:277, 1988.
551. Green SL, Hager DA, Mays MBC, et al: Acute diffuse mycotic pneumonia in a 7-month old colt, *Vet Radiol* 28:216, 1987.
552. Blomme E, Del Piero F, La Perle KMD, et al: Aspergillosis in horses: a review, *Equine Vet Educ* 10:86, 1998.
553. Sweeney CR, Habecker PL: Pulmonary aspergillosis in horses: 29 cases (1974-1997), *J Am Vet Med Assoc* 214:808, 1999.
554. Perryman LE, McGuire TC, Crawford TB: Maintenance of foals with combined immunodeficiency: causes and control of secondary infections, *Am J Vet Res* 39:1043, 1978.
555. Ainsworth DM, Weldon AD, Beck KA, et al: Recognition of Pneumocystis carinii in foals with respiratory distress, *Equine Vet J* 25:103, 1993.
556. Blue J, Perdrizet J, Brown E: Pulmonary aspergillosis in a horse with myelomonocytic leukemia, *J Am Vet Med Assoc* 190:1562, 1987.
557. Pusterla N, Pesavento PA, Leutenegger CM, et al: Disseminated pulmonary adiaspiromycosis caused by Emmonsia crescens in a horse, *Equine Vet J* 34:749, 2002.
558. Carrasco L, Mendez A, Jensen HE: Chronic bronchopulmonary aspergillosis in a horse with Cushing's syndrome, *Mycoses* 39:443, 1996.
559. Ho PL, Yuen KY: Aspergillosis in bone marrow transplant recipients, *Crit Rev Oncol Hematol* 34:55, 2000.
560. Thirion-Delalande C, Guillot J, Jensen HE, et al: Disseminated acute concomitant aspergillosis and mucormycosis in a pony, *J Vet Med A Physiol Pathol Clin Med* 52:121, 2005.
561. Moore BR, Reed SM, Kowalski JJ, et al: Aspergillosis granuloma in the mediastinum of a non-immunocompromised horse, *Cornell Vet* 83:97, 1993.
562. Carrasco L, Tarradas MC, Gómez-Villamandos JC, et al: Equine pulmonary mycosis due to Aspergillus niger and Rhizopus stolonifer, *J Comp Pathol* 117:191, 1997.
563. Santamauro JT, Stover DE: Pneumocystis carinii pneumonia, *Med Clin North Am* 81:299, 1997.
564. Ceré N, Polack B: Animal pneumocystosis: a model for man, *Vet Res* 30:1, 1999.
565. Morris AM, Swanson M, Ha H, et al: Geographic distribution of human immunodeficiency virus-associated Pneumocystis carinii pneumonia in San Francisco, *Am J Respir Crit Care Med* 162:1622, 2000.
566. Morris A, Beard CB, Huang L: Update on the epidemiology and transmission of Pneumocystis carinii, *Microbes Infect* 4:95, 2002.
567. Gigliotti F, Harmsen AG, Haidaris CG, et al: Pneumocystis carinii is not universally transmissible between mammalian species, *Infect Immun* 61:2886, 1993.
568. Thomas CF Jr, Limper AH: Pneumocystis pneumonia, *N Engl J Med* 350:2487, 2004.
569. Pusterla N, Holmberg TA, Lorenzo-Figueras M, et al: Acremonium strictum pulmonary infection in a horse, *Vet Clin Pathol* 34:413, 2005.
570. Fincher RM, Fisher JF, Lovell RD, et al: Infection due to the fungus Acremonium (cephalosporium), *Medicine (Baltimore)* 70:398, 1991.
571. England DM, Hochholzer L: Adiaspiromycosis: an unusual fungal infection of the lung. Report of 11 cases, *Am J Surg Pathol* 17:876, 1993.
572. Hattel AL, Drake TR, Anderholm BJ, et al: Pulmonary aspergillosis associated with acute enteritis in a horse, *J Am Vet Med Assoc* 199:589, 1991.
573. Long JR, Mitchell L: Pulmonary aspergillosis in a mare, *Can Vet J* 12:16, 1971.
574. Cooper VL, Kennedy GA, Kruckenberg SM, et al: Histoplasmosis in a miniature Sicilian burro, *J Vet Diagn Invest* 6:499, 1994.
575. Foley JP, Legendre AM: Treatment of coccidioidomycosis osteomyelitis with itraconazole in a horse. A brief report, *J Vet Intern Med* 6:333, 1992.
576. Petrites-Murphy MB, Robbins LA, Donahue JM, et al: Equine cryptococcal endometritis and placentitis with neonatal cryptococcal pneumonia, *J Vet Diagn Invest* 8:383, 1996.
577. Begg LM, Hughes KJ, Kessell A, et al: Successful treatment of cryptococcal pneumonia in a pony mare, *Aust Vet J* 82:686, 2004.
578. Shively JN, Dellers RW, Buergelt CD, et al: Pneumocystis carinii pneumonia in two foals, *J Am Vet Med Assoc* 162:648, 1973.
579. Flaminio MJ, Rush BR, Cox JH, et al: CD4+ and CD8+ T-lymphocytopenia in a filly with Pneumocystis carinii pneumonia, *Aust Vet J* 76:399, 1998.
580. Marrs GE: Pneumocystis carinii pneumonia in a Paso Fino colt, *Vet Med* 82:1172, 1987.
581. Ewing PJ, Cowell RL, Tyler RD, et al: Pneumocystis carinii pneumonia in foals, *J Am Vet Med Assoc* 204:929, 1994.
582. Whitwell K: Pneumocystis carinii infection in foals in the UK, *Vet Rec* 131:19, 1992.
583. Perron Lepage MF, Gerber V: Suter MM: A case of interstitial pneumonia associated with Pneumocystis carinii in a foal, *Vet Pathol* 36:621, 1999.
584. Prescott JF, Ogilvie TH, Markham RJ: Lymphocyte immunostimulation in the diagnosis of Corynebacterium equi pneumonia of foals, *Am J Vet Res* 41:2073, 1980.
585. MacNeill AL, Alleman AR, Franklin RP, et al: Pneumonia in a Paso-Fino mare, *Vet Clin Pathol* 32:73, 2003.
586. Pearson EG, Watrous BJ, Schmitz JA, et al: Cryptococcal pneumonia in a horse, *J Am Vet Med Assoc* 183:577, 1983.
587. Kramme PM, Ziemer EL: Disseminated coccidioidomycosis in a horse with osteomyelitis, *J Am Vet Med Assoc* 196:106, 1990.
588. Riley CB, Bolton JR, Mills JN, et al: Cryptococcosis in seven horses, *Aust Vet J* 69:135, 1992.
589. Benbrook EA, Bryant JB, Saunders LZ: A case of blastomycosis in the horse, *J Am Vet Med Assoc* 112:475, 1948.

590. Wilson JH, Olson EJ, Haugen EW, et al: Systemic blastomycosis in a horse, *J Vet Diagn Invest* 18:615, 2006.
591. Langham RF, Beneke ES, Whitenack DL: Abortion in a mare due to coccidioidomycosis, *J Am Vet Med Assoc* 170:178, 1977.
592. DeMartini JC, Riddle WE: Disseminated coccidioidomycosis in two horses and a pony, *J Am Vet Med Assoc* 155:149, 1969.
593. Cho DY, Pace W, Beadle RE: Cerebral cryptococcosis in a horse, *Vet Pathol* 23:207, 1986.
594. Welsh RD, Stair EL: Cryptococcal meningitis in a horse, *J Equine Vet Sci* 15:80, 1995.
595. Chandna VK, Morris E, Gliatto JM, et al: Localised subcutaneous cryptococcal granuloma in a horse, *Equine Vet J* 25:166, 1993.
596. Blanchard PC, Filkins M: Cryptococcal pneumonia and abortion in an equine fetus, *J Am Vet Med Assoc* 201:1591, 1992.
597. Lenard ZM, Lester NV, O'hara AJ, et al: Disseminated cryptococcosis including osteomyelitis in a horse, *Aust Vet J* 85:51, 2007.
598. Katayama Y, Kuwano A, Yoshihara T: Histoplasmosis in the lung of a race horse with yersiniosis, *J Vet Med Sci* 63:1229, 2001.
599. Johnson PJ, Moore LA, Mrad DR, et al: Sudden death of two horses associated with pulmonary aspergillosis, *Vet Rec* 145:16, 1999.
600. Nunes J, Mackie JT, Kiupel M: Equine histoplasmosis presenting as a tumor in the abdominal cavity, *J Vet Diagn Invest* 18:508, 2006.
601. Richter M, Hauser B, Kaps S, et al: Keratitis due to Histoplasma spp. in a horse, *Vet Ophthalmol* 6:99, 2003.
602. Pace LW, Wirth NR, Foss RR, et al: Endocarditis and pulmonary aspergillosis in a horse, *J Vet Diagn Invest* 6:504, 1994.
603. Franklin RP, Long MT, MacNeill A, et al: Proliferative interstitial pneumonia, Pneumocystis carinii infection, and immunodeficiency in an adult Paso Fino horse, *J Vet Intern Med* 16:607, 2002.
604. Higgins JC, Leith GS, Pappagianis D, et al: Treatment of Coccidioides immitis pneumonia in two horses with fluconazole, *Vet Rec* 159:349, 2006.
605. Higgins JC, Leith GS, Voss ED, et al: Seroprevalence of antibodies against Coccidioides immitis in healthy horses, *J Am Vet Med Assoc* 226:2005, 1888.
606. Higgins JC, Pusterla N, Pappagianis D: Comparison of Coccidioides immitis serological antibody titres between forms of clinical coccidioidomycosis in horses, *Vet J* 173:118, 2007.
607. Furcolow ML, Menges RW: Comparison of histoplasmin sensitivity rates among human beings and animals in Boone County, Missouri, *Am J Public Health Nations Health* 42:926, 1952.
608. Schar DL, Sage AM, Hayden DW, et al: What is your diagnosis? A large mass dorsal to the bifurcation of the trachea with tracheobronchial compression, *J Am Vet Med Assoc* 224:1757, 2004.
609. Guillot J, Sarfati J, de Barros M, et al: Comparative study of serological tests for the diagnosis of equine aspergillosis, *Vet Rec* 145:348, 1999.
610. deJaham C: Paradis M, Papich MG: Antifungal dermatologic agents: Azones and allylamines, *Comp Cont Educ Pract Vet* 22:548, 2000.
611. Gaboriau F, Chéron M, Petit C, et al: Heat-induced superaggregation of amphotericin B reduces its in vitro toxicity: a new way to improve its therapeutic index, *Antimicrob Agents Chemother* 41:2345, 1997.
612. Clark-Price SC, Cox JH, Bartoe JT, et al: Use of dapsone in the treatment of Pneumocystis carinii pneumonia in a foal, *J Am Vet Med Assoc* 224:407, 2004.
613. Antal T, Szabó I, Antal V, et al: Respiratory disease of horses associated with Mycoplasma infection, *Zentralbl Veterinarmed B* 35:264, 1988.
614. Rosendal S, Blackwell TE, Lumsden JH, et al: Detection of antibodies to Mycoplasma felis in horses, *J Am Vet Med Assoc* 188:292, 1986.
615. Hoffman AM, Baird JD, Kloeze HJ, et al: Mycoplasma felis pleuritis in two show-jumper horses, *Cornell Vet* 82:155, 1992.
616. Antal A, Szabó I, Vajda G, et al: Immunoglobulin concentration in the blood serum of foals suffering from pneumonia associated with mycoplasma infection, *Arch Exp Veterinarmed* 43:747, 1989.
617. Wood JL, Chanter N, Newton JR, et al: An outbreak of respiratory disease in horses associated with Mycoplasma felis infection, *Vet Rec* 140:388, 1997.
618. Newton JR, Wood JL, Chanter N: A case control study of factors and infections associated with clinically apparent respiratory disease in UK Thoroughbred racehorses, *Prev Vet Med* 60:107, 2003.
619. Dungworth DL: Interstitial pulmonary disease, *Adv Vet Sci Comp Med* 26:173, 1982.
620. Lopez A: Respiratory system, In McGavin MD, Zachary JF, editors: *Pathologic Basis of Veterinary Disease*, ed 4, St Louis, 2007, Mosby Elsevier.
621. Buergelt CD: Interstitial pneumonia in the horse: a fledgling morphological entity with mysterious causes, *Equine Vet J* 27:4, 1995.
622. Lakritz J, Wilson WD, Berry CR, et al: Bronchointerstitial pneumonia and respiratory distress in young horses: clinical, clinicopathologic, radiographic, and pathological findings in 23 cases (1984-1989), *J Vet Intern Med* 7:277, 1993.
623. Nout YS, Hinchcliff KW, Samii VF, et al: Chronic pulmonary disease with radiographic interstitial opacity (interstitial pneumonia) in foals, *Equine Vet J* 34:542, 2002.
624. Sharma OP: Interstitial lung disease, *Curr Opin Pulm Med* 1:345, 1995.
625. O'Sullivan BM: Crofton weed (Eupatorium adenophorum) toxicity in horses, *Aust Vet J* 55:19, 1979.
626. Oelrichs PB, Calanasan CA, MacLeod JK, et al: Isolation of a compound from Eupatorium adenophorum (Spreng.) [Ageratina adenophora (Spreng.)] causing hepatotoxicity in mice, *Nat Toxins* 3:350, 1995.
627. Gibson JA, O'Sullivan BM: Lung lesions in horses fed mist flower (Eupatorium riparium), *Aust Vet J* 61:271, 1984.
628. Nobre D, Dagli ML, Haraguchi M: Crotalaria juncea intoxication in horses, *Vet Hum Toxicol* 36:445, 1994.
629. Lindley WH: Acute pulmonary edema, *Mod Vet Pract* 59:64, 1978.
630. Breeze RG, Legreid WW, Bayly WM, et al: Perilla ketone toxicity: a chemical model for the study of equine restrictive lung disease, *Equine Vet J* 16:180, 1984.
631. Schmidbauer SM, Venner M, von Samson-Himmelstjerna G, et al: Compensated overexpression of procollagens alpha 1(I) and alpha 1(III) following perilla mint ketone-induced acute pulmonary damage in horses, *J Comp Pathol* 131:186, 2004.
632. Scarratt WK, Moon ML, Sponenberg DP, et al: Inappropriate administration of mineral oil resulting in lipoid pneumonia in three horses, *Equine Vet J* 30:85, 1998.
633. Davis JL, Ramirez S, Campbell N, et al: Acute and chronic mineral oil pneumonitis in two horses, *Eq Vet Educ* 13:230, 2001.
634. Bos M, de Bosschere H, Deprez P, et al: Chemical identification of the (causative) lipids in a case of exogenous lipoid pneumonia in a horse, *Equine Vet J* 34:744, 2002.
635. Henninger RW, Hass GF, Freshwater A: Corticosteroid management of lipoid pneumonia in a horse, *Eq Vet Educ* 18:205, 2006.
636. Field HE, Barratt PC, Hughes RJ, et al: A fatal case of Hendra virus infection in a horse in north Queensland: clinical and epidemiological features, *Aust Vet J* 78:279, 2000.
637. Mair TS, Taylor FG, Gibbs C, et al: Generalized avian tuberculosis in a horse, *Equine Vet J* 18:226, 1986.

638. Gunnes G, Nord K, Vatn S, et al: A case of generalised avian tuberculosis in a horse, *Vet Rec* 136:565, 1995.
639. Monreal L, Segura D, Segales J, et al: Diagnosis of Mycobacterium bovis infection in a mare, *Vet Rec* 149:712, 2001.
640. Pavlikel I, Jahn P, Dvorska L, et al: Mycobacterial infections in horses: a review of the literature, *Vet Med (Czech)* 49:427, 2004.
641. Muser R, Nassal J: Tuberculosis, tuberculin reaction any mycobacteria in horse, *Rindertuberkulose Brucell* 11:118, 1962.
642. Winder C, Ehrensperger F, Hermann M, et al: Interstitial pneumonia in the horse: two unusual cases, *Equine Vet J* 20:298, 1988.
643. Buergelt CD, Hines SA, Cantor G, et al: A retrospective study of proliferative interstitial lung disease of horses in Florida, *Vet Pathol* 23:750, 1986.
644. Derksen FJ, Slocombe RF, Brown CM, et al: Chronic restrictive pulmonary disease in a horse, *J Am Vet Med Assoc* 180:887, 1982.
645. Kelly DF, Newsholme SJ, Baker JR, et al: Diffuse alveolar damage in the horse, *Equine Vet J* 27:76, 1995.
646. Donaldson MT, Beech J, Ennulat D, et al: Interstitial pneumonia and pulmonary fibrosis in a horse, *Equine Vet J* 30:173, 1998.
647. Dixon PM, McGorum BC, Long KJ, et al: Acute eosinophilic interstitial pulmonary disease in a pony, *Vet Rec* 130:367, 1992.
648. Pusterla N, Pesavento PA, Smith P, et al: Idiopathic granulomatous pneumonia in seven horses, *Vet Rec* 153:653, 2003.
649. Uhlhorn M, Hurst M, Demmers S: Disseminated eosinophilic pulmonary granulomas in a pony, *Eq Vet Educ* 18:178, 2006.
650. Wright JL: Consequences of aspiration and bronchial obstruction. In Thurbeck WM, Churg AM, editors: *Pathology of the Lung*, ed 2, New York, 1995, Thieme Medical Publishing Co.
651. Turk JR, Brown CM, Johnson GC: Diffuse alveolar damage with fibrosing alveolitis in a horse, *Vet Pathol* 18:560, 1981.
652. Schwarzwald CC, Stewart AJ, Morrison CD, et al: Cor pulmonale in a horse with granulomatous pneumonia, *Equine Vet Educ* 18:182, 2006.
653. Bastianello SS: A survey on neoplasia in domestic species over a 40-year period from 1935 to 1974 in the Republic of South Africa. IV. Tumours occurring in Equidae, *Onderstepoort J Vet Res* 50:91, 1983.
654. Schwartz LW, Knight HD, Whittig LD, et al: Silicate pneumoconiosis and pulmonary fibrosis in horses from the Monterey-Carmel peninsula, *Chest* 80:82, 1981.
655. Berry CR, O'Brien TR, Madigan JE, et al: Thoracic radiographic features of silicosis in 19 horses, *J Vet Intern Med* 5:248, 1991.
656. Konyha LD, Kreier JP: The significance of tuberculin tests in the horse, *Am Rev Respir Dis* 103:91, 1971.
657. American Thoracic Society (ATS)the European Respiratory Society (ERS): Idiopathic pulmonary fibrosis: Diagnosis and treatment, *Am J Respir Crit Care Med* 161:646, 2000.
658. Raghu G: Idiopathic pulmonary fibrosis: treatment options in pursuit of evidence-based approaches, *Eur Respir J* 28:463, 2006.
659. Lyons ET, Tolliver SC, Drudge JH, et al: Parasites in lungs of dead equids in Kentucky: emphasis on Dictyocaulus arnfieldi, *Am J Vet Res* 46:924, 1985.
660. Lyons ET, Tolliver SC, Drudge JH, et al: Lungworms (Dictyocaulus arnfieldi): prevalence in live equids in Kentucky, *Am J Vet Res* 46:921, 1985.
661. Jorgensen RJ, Andersen S: Spread of equine lungworm (Dictyocaulus arnfieldi) larvae from faeces by Pilobolus fungi, *Nord Vet Med* 36:162, 1984.
662. Clayton HM: *Lung Parasites*, Philadelphia, 1983, W.B. Saunders.
663. George LW, Tanner ML, Roberson EL, et al: Chronic respiratory disease in a horse infected with Dictyocaulus arnfieldi, *J Am Vet Med Assoc* 179:820, 1981.
664. Clayton HM, Duncan JL: Natural infection with Dictyocaulus arnfieldi in pony and donkey foals, *Res Vet Sci* 31:278, 1981.
665. Lyons ET, Drudge JH, Tolliver SC: Ivermectin: treating for naturally occurring infections of lungworms and stomach worms in equids, *Vet Med* 80:58, 1985.
666. Coles GC, Hillyer MH, Taylor FG, et al: Activity of moxidectin against bots and lungworm in equids, *Vet Rec* 143:169, 1998.
667. Humber KA: Near drowning of a gelding, *J Am Vet Med Assoc* 192:377, 1988.
668. Austin SM, Foreman JH, Goetz TE: Aspiration pneumonia following near-drowning in a mare: a case report, *J Equine Vet Sci* 8:313, 1988.
669. Sembrat R, Di Stazio J, Reese J, et al: Acute pulmonary failure in the conscious pony with Escherichia coli septicemia, *Am J Vet Res* 39:1147, 1978.
670. Goer RJ, Ames TR: Smoke inhalation injury in horses, *Compend Contin Educ Pract Vet* 13:1162, 1991.
671. Davis JL, Gardner SY, Schwabenton B, et al: Congestive heart failure in horses: 14 cases (1984-2001), *J Am Vet Med Assoc* 220:1512, 2002.
672. Kollef MH, Schuster DP: The acute respiratory distress syndrome, *N Engl J Med* 332:27, 1995.
673. Ware LB, Matthay MA: The acute respiratory distress syndrome, *N Engl J Med* 342:1334, 2000.
674. Lewis JF, Jobe AH: Surfactant and the adult respiratory distress syndrome, *Am Rev Respir Dis* 147:218, 1993.
675. Kemper T, Spier S, Barratt-Boyes SM, et al: Treatment of smoke inhalation in five horses, *J Am Vet Med Assoc* 202:91, 1993.
676. Johansson AM, Gardner SY, Levine JF, et al: Furosemide continuous rate infusion in the horse: evaluation of enhanced efficacy and reduced side effects, *J Vet Intern Med* 17:887, 2003.
677. Johansson AM, Gardner SY, Levine JF, et al: Pharmacokinetics and pharmacodynamics of furosemide after oral administration to horses, *J Vet Intern Med* 18:739, 2004.
678. Mitten LA, Hinchcliff KW, Holcombe SJ, et al: Mechanical ventilation and management of botulism secondary to an injection abscess in an adult horse, *Equine Vet J* 26:420, 1994.
679. Robinson NE: International Workshop on Equine Chronic Airway Disease. Michigan State University 16-18 June 2000, *Equine Vet J* 33:5, 2001.
680. Muylle E, Oyaert W: Lung function tests in obstructive pulmonary disease in horses, *Equine Vet J* 5:37, 1973.
681. Derksen FJ, Scott D, Robinson NE, et al: Intravenous histamine administration in ponies with recurrent airway obstruction (heaves), *Am J Vet Res* 46:774, 1985.
682. Derksen FJ, Robinson NE, Scott JS, et al: Aerosolized Micropolyspora faeni antigen as a cause of pulmonary dysfunction in ponies with recurrent airway obstruction (heaves), *Am J Vet Res* 49:933, 1988.
683. Seahorn TL, Beadle RE: Summer pasture-associated obstructive pulmonary disease in horses: 21 cases (1983-1991), *J Am Vet Med Assoc* 202:779, 1993.
684. Aviza GA, Ainsworth DM, Eicker SW, et al: Outcome of horses diagnosed with and treated for heaves (recurrent airway obstruction), *Equine Vet Educ* 13:243, 2001.
685. Marti E, Gerber H, Essich G, et al: The genetic basis of equine allergic diseases. 1. Chronic hypersensitivity bronchitis, *Equine Vet J* 23:457, 1991.
686. Jost U, Klukowska- Rötzler J, Dolf G, et al: A region on equine chromosome 13 is linked to recurrent airway obstruction in horses, *Equine Vet J* 39:236, 2007.
687. Ewart SL, Robinson NE: Genes and respiratory disease: a first step on a long journey, *Equine Vet J* 39:270, 2007.
688. McPherson EA, Thomson JR: Chronic obstructive pulmonary disease in the horse. 1: Nature of the disease, *Equine Vet J* 15:203, 1983.

689. McPherson EA, Lawson GH, Murphy JR, et al: Chronic obstructive pulmonary disease (COPD) in horses: aetiological studies: responses to intradermal and inhalation antigenic challenge, *Equine Vet J* 11:159, 1979.
690. McGorum BC, Dixon PM, Halliwell RE: Phenotypic analysis of peripheral blood and bronchoalveolar lavage fluid lymphocytes in control and chronic obstructive pulmonary disease affected horses, before and after 'natural (hay and straw) challenges', *Vet Immunol Immunopathol* 36:207, 1993.
691. Pirie RS, Dixon PM, Collie DD, et al: Pulmonary and systemic effects of inhaled endotoxin in control and heaves horses, *Equine Vet J* 33:311, 2001.
692. Pirie RS, Collie DD, Dixon PM, et al: Inhaled endotoxin and organic dust particulates have synergistic proinflammatory effects in equine heaves (organic dust-induced asthma), *Clin Exp Allergy* 33:676, 2003.
693. Halliwell RE, McGorum BC, Irving P, et al: Local and systemic antibody production in horses affected with chronic obstructive pulmonary disease, *Vet Immunol Immunopathol* 38:201, 1993.
694. Eder C, Crameri R, Mayer C, et al: Allergen-specific IgE levels against crude mould and storage mite extracts and recombinant mould allergens in sera from horses affected with chronic bronchitis, *Vet Immunol Immunopathol* 73:241, 2000.
695. Lavoie JP, Maghni K, Desnoyers M, et al: Neutrophilic airway inflammation in horses with heaves is characterized by a Th2-type cytokine profile, *Am J Respir Crit Care Med* 164:1410, 2001.
696. Cordeau ME, Joubert P, Dewachi O, et al: IL-4, IL-5 and IFN-gamma mRNA expression in pulmonary lymphocytes in equine heaves, *Vet Immunol Immunopathol* 97:87, 2004.
697. Dixon PM, McGorum BC, Marley C, et al: Effects of equine influenza and tetanus vaccination on pulmonary function in normal and chronic obstructive pulmonary disease affected horses, *Equine Vet J* 28:157, 1996.
698. Corry DB, Kheradmand F: Induction and regulation of the IgE response, *Nature* 402:B18, 1999.
699. Ainsworth DM, Appleton JA, Antczak DF, et al: Immune responses in horses with recurrent airway obstruction, *Am J Respir Crit Care Med* 161:A842, 2000.
700. Giguère S, Viel L, Lee E, et al: Cytokine induction in pulmonary airways of horses with heaves and effect of therapy with inhaled fluticasone propionate, *Vet Immunol Immunopathol* 85:147, 2002.
701. Kleiber C, McGorum BC, Horohov DW, et al: Cytokine profiles of peripheral blood and airway CD4 and CD8 T lymphocytes in horses with recurrent airway obstruction, *Vet Immunol Immunopathol* 104:91, 2005.
702. van der Haegen A, Künzle F, Gerber V, et al: Mast cells and IgE-bearing cells in lungs of RAO-affected horses, *Vet Immunol Immunopathol* 108:325, 2005.
703. Couëtil LL, Art T, de Moffarts B, et al: DNA binding activity of transcription factors in bronchial cells of horses with recurrent airway obstruction, *Vet Immunol Immunopathol* 113:11, 2006.
704. Franchini M, Gilli U, Akens MK, et al: The role of neutrophil chemotactic cytokines in the pathogenesis of equine chronic obstructive pulmonary disease (COPD), *Vet Immunol Immunopathol* 66:53, 1998.
705. Debrue M, Hamilton E, Joubert P, et al: Chronic exacerbation of equine heaves is associated with an increased expression of interleukin-17 mRNA in bronchoalveolar lavage cells, *Vet Immunol Immunopathol* 105:25, 2005.
706. Ainsworth DM, Wagner B, Franchini M, et al: Time-dependent alterations in gene expression of interleukin-8 in the bronchial epithelium of horses with recurrent airway obstruction, *Am J Vet Res* 67:669, 2006.
707. Ainsworth DM, Wagner B, Erb HN, et al: Effects of in vitro exposure to hay dust on expression of interleukin-17, -23, -8, and -1beta and chemokine (C-X-C motif) ligand 2 by pulmonary mononuclear cells isolated from horses chronically affected with recurrent airway disease, *Am J Vet Res* 68:1361, 2007.
708. Art T, Kirschvink N, Smith N, et al: Indices of oxidative stress in blood and pulmonary epithelium lining fluid in horses suffering from recurrent airway obstruction, *Equine Vet J* 31:397, 1999.
709. Bowie A, O'Neill LA: Oxidative stress and nuclear factor-kappaB activation: a reassessment of the evidence in the light of recent discoveries, *Biochem Pharmacol* 59:13, 2000.
710. Barnes PJ, Karin M: Nuclear factor-kappaB: a pivotal transcription factor in chronic inflammatory diseases, *N Engl J Med* 336:1066, 1997.
711. Bureau F, Bonizzi G, Kirschvink N, et al: Correlation between nuclear factor-kappaB activity in bronchial brushing samples and lung dysfunction in an animal model of asthma, *Am J Respir Crit Care Med* 161:1314, 2000.
712. Koivunen AL, Maisi P, Konttinen YT, et al: Collagenolytic activity and its sensitivity to doxycycline inhibition in tracheal aspirates of horses with chronic obstructive pulmonary disease, *Acta Vet Scand* 38:9, 1997.
713. Raulo SM, Maisi P: Gelatinolytic activity in tracheal epithelial lining fluid and in blood from horses with chronic obstructive pulmonary disease, *Am J Vet Res* 59:818, 1998.
714. Raulo SM, Sorsa TA, Maisi PS: Concentrations of elastinolytic metalloproteinases in respiratory tract secretions of healthy horses and horses with chronic obstructive pulmonary disease, *Am J Vet Res* 61:1067, 2000.
715. Dixon PM: Pulmonary artery pressures in normal horses and in horses affected with chronic obstructive pulmonary disease, *Equine Vet J* 10:195, 1978.
716. Sage AM, Valberg S, Hayden DW, et al: Echocardiography in a horse with cor pulmonale from recurrent airway obstruction, *J Vet Intern Med* 20:694, 2006.
717. Johansson AM, Gardner SY, Atkins CE, et al: Cardiovascular effects of acute pulmonary obstruction in horses with recurrent airway obstruction, *J Vet Intern Med* 21:302, 2007.
718. Robinson NE, Olszewski MA, Boehler D, et al: Relationship between clinical signs and lung function in horses with recurrent airway obstruction (heaves) during a bronchodilator trial, *Equine Vet J* 32:393, 2000.
719. Derksen FJ, Scott JS, Miller DC, et al: Bronchoalveolar lavage in ponies with recurrent airway obstruction (heaves), *Am Rev Respir Dis* 132:1066, 1985.
720. Lavoie JP, Dalle S, Breton L, et al: Bronchiectasis in three adult horses with heaves, *J Vet Intern Med* 18:757, 2004.
721. Bakos Z, Vörös K, Kellokoski H, et al: Comparison of the caudal lung borders determined by percussion and ultrasonography in horses with recurrent airway obstruction, *Acta Vet Hung* 51:249, 2003.
722. Evans AG, Paradis MR, O'Callaghan M: Intradermal testing of horses with chronic obstructive pulmonary disease and recurrent urticaria, *Am J Vet Res* 53:203, 1992.
723. Lorch G, Hillier A, Kwochka KW, et al: Results of intradermal tests in horses without atopy and horses with chronic obstructive pulmonary disease, *Am J Vet Res* 62:389, 2001.
724. Lorch G, Hillier A, Kwochka KW, et al: Comparison of immediate intradermal test reactivity with serum IgE quantitation by use of a radioallergosorbent test and two ELISA in horses with and without atopy, *J Am Vet Med Assoc* 218:1314, 2001.
725. Jose-Cunilleras E, Kohn CW, Hillier A, et al: Intradermal testing in healthy horses and horses with chronic obstructive pulmonary disease, recurrent urticaria, or allergic dermatitis, *J Am Vet Med Assoc* 219:1115, 2001.

726. Wong DM, Buechner-Maxwell VA, Manning TO, et al: Comparison of results for intradermal testing between clinically normal horses and horses affected with recurrent airway obstruction, *Am J Vet Res* 66:1348, 2005.
727. Dixon PM, Railton DI, McGorum BC: Equine pulmonary disease: a case control study of 300 referred cases. Part 3: Ancillary diagnostic findings, *Equine Vet J* 27:428, 1995.
728. Slocombe R: Pathology of the airways. (In International Workshop on Equine Chronic Airway Disease, Michigan State University 16-18 June 2000.), *Equine Vet J* 33:6, 2001.
729. Herszberg B, Ramos-Barbón D, Tamaoka M, et al: Heaves, an asthma-like equine disease, involves airway smooth muscle remodeling, *J Allergy Clin Immunol* 118:382, 2006.
730. Kaup FJ, Drommer W, Damsch S, et al: Ultrastructural findings in horses with chronic obstructive pulmonary disease (COPD). II: Pathomorphological changes of the terminal airways and the alveolar region, *Equine Vet J* 22:349, 1990.
731. Kaup FJ, Drommer W, Deegen E: Ultrastructural findings in horses with chronic obstructive pulmonary disease (COPD). I: Alterations of the larger conducting airways, *Equine Vet J* 22:343, 1990.
732. Miskovic M, Couëtil LL, Thompson CA: Lung function and airway cytologic profiles in horses with recurrent airway obstruction maintained in low-dust environments, *J Vet Intern Med* 21:1060, 2007.
733. Jackson CA, Berney C, Jefcoat AM, et al: Environment and prednisone interactions in the treatment of recurrent airway obstruction (heaves), *Equine Vet J* 32:432, 2000.
734. Vandenput S, Votion D, Duvivier DH, et al: Effect of a set stabled environmental control on pulmonary function and airway reactivity of COPD affected horses, *Vet J* 155:189, 1998.
735. DeLuca L, Erb HN, Young JC, et al: The effect of adding oral dexamethasone to feed alterations on the airway cell inflammatory gene expression in stabled horses affected with recurrent airway obstruction (RAO), *J Vet Intern Med* 22:427, 2008.
736. Lapointe JM, Lavoie JP, Vrins AA: Effects of triamcinolone acetonide on pulmonary function and bronchoalveolar lavage cytologic features in horses with chronic obstructive pulmonary disease, *Am J Vet Res* 54:1310, 1993.
737. Picandet V, Léguillette R, Lavoie JP: Comparison of efficacy and tolerability of isoflupredone and dexamethasone in the treatment of horses affected with recurrent airway obstruction ('heaves'), *Equine Vet J* 35:419, 2003.
738. Genetzky RM, Loparco FV: Clinical efficacy of clenbuterol with COPD in horses, *J Equine Vet Sci* 5:320, 1985.
739. Laan TT, Bull S, Pirie RS, et al: The anti-inflammatory effects of IV administered clenbuterol in horses with recurrent airway obstruction, *Vet J* 171:429, 2006.
740. Henrikson SL, Rush BR: Efficacy of salmeterol xinafoate in horses with recurrent airway obstruction, *J Am Vet Med Assoc* 218:2001, 1961.
741. Camargo FC, Robinson NE, Berney C, et al: Trimetoquinol: bronchodilator effects in horses with heaves following aerosolised and oral administration, *Equine Vet J* 39:215, 2007.
742. Rush BR, Hoskinson JJ, Davis EG, et al: Pulmonary distribution of aerosolized technetium Tc 99m pentetate after administration of a single dose of aerosolized albuterol sulfate in horses with recurrent airway obstruction, *Am J Vet Res* 60:764, 1999.
743. Pearson EG, Riebold TW: Comparison of bronchodilators in alleviating clinical signs in horses with chronic obstructive pulmonary disease, *J Am Vet Med Assoc* 194:1287, 1989.
744. Léguillette R, Désévaux C, Lavoie JP: Effects of pentoxifylline on pulmonary function and results of cytologic examination of bronchoalveolar lavage fluid in horses with recurrent airway obstruction, *Am J Vet Res* 63:459, 2002.
745. Matthews AG, Hackett IJ, Lawton WA: The mucolytic effect of Sputolosin in horses with respiratory disease, *Vet Rec* 122:106, 1988.
746. Wilson DV, Schott HC 2nd, Robinson NE, et al: Response to nasopharyngeal oxygen administration in horses with lung disease, *Equine Vet J* 38:219, 2006.
747. Broadstone RV, Robinson NE, Gray PR, et al: Effects of furosemide on ponies with recurrent airway obstruction, *Pulm Pharmacol* 4:203, 1991.
748. Rubie S, Robinson NE, Stoll M, et al: Flunixin meglumine blocks frusemide-induced bronchodilation in horses with chronic obstructive pulmonary disease, *Equine Vet J* 25:138, 1993.
749. Wilson DV, Berney CE, Peroni DL, et al: The effects of a single acupuncture treatment in horses with severe recurrent airway obstruction, *Equine Vet J* 36:489, 2004.
750. van den Hoven R, Zappe H, Zitterl-Eglseer K, et al: Study of the effect of Bronchipret on the lung function of five Austrian saddle horses suffering recurrent airway obstruction (heaves), *Vet Rec* 152:555, 2003.
751. Jean D, Vrins A, Lavoie JP: Respiratory and metabolic effects of massive administration of isotonic saline solution in heaves-affected and control horses, *Equine Vet J* 36:628, 2004.
752. Naylor JM, Clark EG, Clayton HM: Chronic obstructive pulmonary disease: Usefulness of clinical signs, bronchoalveolar lavage, and lung biopsy as diagnostic and prognostic aids, *Can Vet J* 33:591, 1992.
753. Dixon PM, McGorum B: Pasture-associated seasonal respiratory disease in two horses, *Vet Rec* 126:9, 1990.
754. Mair TS: Obstructive pulmonary disease in 18 horses at summer pasture, *Vet Rec* 138:89, 1996.
755. Costa LR, Seahorn TL, Moore RM, et al: Correlation of clinical score, intrapleural pressure, cytologic findings of bronchoalveolar fluid, and histopathologic lesions of pulmonary tissue in horses with summer pasture-associated obstructive pulmonary disease, *Am J Vet Res* 61:167, 2000.
756. Seahorn TL, Beadle RE, McGorum BC, et al: Quantification of antigen-specific antibody concentrations in tracheal lavage fluid of horses with summer pasture-associated obstructive pulmonary disease, *Am J Vet Res* 58:1408, 1997.
757. Beadle RE, Horohov DW, Gaunt SD: Interleukin-4 and interferon-gamma gene expression in summer pasture-associated obstructive pulmonary disease affected horses, *Equine Vet J* 34:389, 2002.
758. McGorum BC, Dixon PM: Summer pasture associated obstructive pulmonary disease (SPAOD): an update, *Eq Vet Educ* 11:121, 1999.
759. Couëtil LL, Hoffman AM, Hodgson J, et al: Inflammatory airway disease of horses, *J Vet Intern Med* 21:356, 2007.
760. Robinson NE: Inflammatory airway disease: defining the syndrome. Conclusions of the Havemeyer Workshop, *Equine Vet Educ* 15:61, 2003.
761. Sweeney CR, Humber KA, Roby KA: Cytologic findings of tracheobronchial aspirates from 66 thoroughbred racehorses, *Am J Vet Res* 53:1172, 1992.
762. Martin BB Jr, Beech J, Parente EJ: Cytologic examination of specimens obtained by means of tracheal washes performed before and after high-speed treadmill exercise in horses with a history of poor performance, *J Am Vet Med Assoc* 214:673, 1999.
763. Wood JL, Newton JR, Chanter N, et al: Inflammatory airway disease, nasal discharge and respiratory infections in young British racehorses, *Equine Vet J* 37:236, 2005.
764. Allen KJ, Tremaine WH, Franklin SH: Prevalence of inflammatory airway disease in national hunt horses referred for investigation of poor athletic performance, *Equine Vet J* 529(36):Suppl, 2006.
765. Burrell MH, Wood JL, Whitwell KE, et al: Respiratory disease in thoroughbred horses in training: the relationships between disease and viruses, bacteria and environment, *Vet Rec* 139:308, 1996.

766. Wood JL, Burrell MH, Roberts CA, et al: Streptococci and Pasteurella spp. associated with disease of the equine lower respiratory tract, *Equine Vet J* 25:314, 1993.
767. Christley RM, Hodgson DR, Rose RJ, et al: A case-control study of respiratory disease in Thoroughbred racehorses in Sydney, Australia, *Equine Vet J* 33:256, 2001.
768. Chapman PS, Green C, Main JP, et al: Retrospective study of the relationships between age, inflammation and the isolation of bacteria from the lower respiratory tract of thoroughbred horses, *Vet Rec* 146:91, 2000.
769. Burrell MH, Whitwell KE, Wood JL, et al: Pyrexia associated with respiratory disease in young thoroughbred horses, *Vet Rec* 134:219, 1994.
770. Wood JL, Newton JR, Chanter N, et al: Association between respiratory disease and bacterial and viral infections in British racehorses, *J Clin Microbiol* 43:120, 2005.
771. Moore BR, Krakowka S, Robertson JT, et al: Cytologic evaluation of bronchoalveolar lavage fluid obtained from standardbred racehorses with inflammatory airway disease, *Am J Vet Res* 56:562, 1995.
772. Moore BR, Krakowka S, Cummins JM, et al: Changes in airway inflammatory cell populations in standardbred racehorses after interferon-alpha administration, *Vet Immunol Immunopathol* 49:347, 1996.
773. Moore BR, Krakowka S, Mcvey DS, et al: Inflammatory markers in bronchoalveolar lavage fluid of standardbred racehorses with inflammatory airway disease: response to interferon-alpha, *Equine Vet J* 29:142, 1997.
774. Tyler WS, Pascoe JR, Aguilera-Tejero E, et al: Morphological effects of autologous blood in airspaces of equine lungs. In *Proceedings of the 10th Veterinary Respiratory Symposium,* Michigan State University, September 22-24, 1991.
775. McKane SA, Slocombe RF: Alveolar fibrosis and changes in equine lung morphometry in response to intrapulmonary blood, *Equine Vet J* 451(34):Suppl, 2002.
776. Derksen FJ, Williams KJ, Uhal BD, et al: Pulmonary response to airway instillation of autologous blood in horses, *Equine Vet J* 39:334, 2007.
777. Tremblay GM, Ferland C, Lapointe JM, et al: Effect of stabling on bronchoalveolar cells obtained from normal and COPD horses, *Equine Vet J* 25:194, 1993.
778. Gerber V, Robinson NE, Luethi S, et al: Airway inflammation and mucus in two age groups of asymptomatic well-performing sport horses, *Equine Vet J* 35:491, 2003.
779. Davis MS, Williams CC, Meinkoth JH, et al: Influx of neutrophils and persistence of cytokine expression in airways of horses after performing exercise while breathing cold air, *Am J Vet Res* 68:185, 2007.
780. Koch C, Straub R, Ramseyer A, et al: Endoscopic scoring of the tracheal septum in horses and its clinical relevance for the evaluation of lower airway health in horses, *Equine Vet J* 39:107, 2007.
781. Hughes KJ, Malikides N, Hodgson DR, et al: Comparison of tracheal aspirates and bronchoalveolar lavage in racehorses. 1. Evaluation of cytological stains and the percentage of mast cells and eosinophils, *Aust Vet J* 81:681, 2003.
782. Malikides N, Hughes KJ, Hodgson JL: Comparison of tracheal aspirates before and after high-speed treadmill exercise in racehorses, *Aust Vet J* 85:414, 2007.
783. Sanchez A, Couëtil LL, Ward MP, et al: Effect of airway disease on blood gas exchange in racehorses, *J Vet Intern Med* 19:87, 2005.
784. Mazan MR, Vin R, Hoffman AM: Radiographic scoring lacks predictive value in inflammatory airway disease, *Equine Vet J* 37:541, 2005.
785. Hoffman A, Mazan M: Programme of lung function testing horses suspected with small airway disease, *Eqine Vet Educ* 11:322, 1999.
786. Pirrone F, Albertini M, Clement MG, et al: Respiratory mechanics in Standardbred horses with sub-clinical inflammatory airway disease and poor athletic performance, *Vet J* 173:144, 2007.
787. Moore I, Horney B, Day K, et al: Treatment of inflammatory airway disease in young standardbreds with interferon alpha, *Can Vet J* 45:594, 2004.
788. Mazan MR, Hoffman AM: Effects of aerosolized albuterol on physiologic responses to exercise in standardbreds, *Am J Vet Res* 62:2001, 1812.
789. Pascoe JR, Ferraro GL, Cannon JH, et al: Exercise-induced pulmonary hemorrhage in racing thoroughbreds: a preliminary study, *Am J Vet Res* 42:703, 1981.
790. Raphel CF, Soma LR: Exercise-induced pulmonary hemorrhage in Thoroughbreds after racing and breezing, *Am J Vet Res* 43:1123, 1982.
791. Speirs VC, van Veenendaal JC, Harrison IW, et al: Pulmonary haemorrhage in standardbred horses after racing, *Aust Vet J* 59:38, 1982.
792. MacNamara B, Bauer S, Iafe J: Endoscopic evaluation of exercise-induced pulmonary hemorrhage and chronic obstructive pulmonary disease in association with poor performance in racing Standardbreds, *J Am Vet Med Assoc* 196:443, 1990.
793. Lapointe JM, Vrins A, McCarvill E: A survey of exercise-induced pulmonary haemorrhage in Quebec standardbred racehorses, *Equine Vet J* 26:482, 1994.
794. Hillidge CJ, Lane TJ, Johnson EL, et al: Preliminary investigations of exercise-induced pulmonary hemorrhage in racing quarter horses, *J Equine Vet Sci* 4:21, 1984.
795. Hillidge CJ, Lane TJ, Whitlock TW: Exercise-induced pulmonary hemorrhage in the racing Appaloosa horse, *J Equine Vet Sci* 5:531, 1985.
796. Voynick BT, Sweeney CR: Exercised-induced pulmonary hemorrhage in polo and racing horses, *J Am Vet Med Assoc* 188:301, 1986.
797. Mason DK, Collins EA, Watkins KL: Exercise-induced pulmonary hemorrhage in horses. In Snow DH, Persson SGB, Rose RJ, editors: *Equine Exercise Physiology*, Cambridge, England, 1983, Burlington Press.
798. Hinchcliff KW, Jackson MA, Morley PS, et al: Association between exercise-induced pulmonary hemorrhage and performance in Thoroughbred racehorses, *J Am Vet Med Assoc* 227:768, 2005.
799. Robinson NE, Derksen FJ: Small airway obstruction as a cause of exercise-associated pulmonary hemorrhage: an hypothesis, *Am Assoc Equine Pract* 26:421, 1980.
800. O'Callaghan MW, Pascoe JR, Tyler WS, et al: Exercise-induced pulmonary haemorrhage in the horse: results of a detailed clinical, post mortem and imaging study. VIII. Conclusions and implications, *Equine Vet J* 19:428, 1987.
801. Cook WR, Williams RM, Kirker-Head CA, et al: Upper airway obstruction (paratial asphyxia) as the possible cause of exercise-induced pulmonary hemorrhage in the horse: an hypothesis, *J Equine Vet Sci* 8:11, 1988.
802. Ducharme NG, Hackett RP, Gleed RD, et al: Pulmonary capillary pressure in horses undergoing alteration of pleural pressure by imposition of various upper airway resistive loads, *Equine Vet J Suppl* 30:27, 1999.
803. Clarke AF: Review of exercise induced pulmonary haemorrhage and its possible relationship with mechanical stress, *Equine Vet J* 17:166, 1985.
804. Schroter RC, Marlin DJ, Denny E: Exercise-induced pulmonary haemorrhage (EIPH) in horses results from locomotory impact induced trauma–a novel, unifying concept, *Equine Vet J* 30:186, 1998.
805. Erickson HH, Bernard SL, Glenny RW, et al: Effect of furosemide on pulmonary blood flow distribution in resting and exercising horses, *J Appl Physiol* 86:2034, 1999.

806. West JB, Mathieu-Costello O, Jones JH, et al: Stress failure of pulmonary capillaries in racehorses with exercise-induced pulmonary hemorrhage, *J Appl Physiol* 75:1097, 1993.
807. Slocombe R: EIPH: the role of airways. *Proceedings of the World Equine Airway Symposium,* Edinburgh, Scotland, 2001.
808. Newton JR, Rogers K, Marlin DJ, et al: Risk factors for epistaxis on British racecourses: evidence for locomotory impact-induced trauma contributing to the aetiology of exercise-induced pulmonary haemorrhage, *Equine Vet J* 37:402, 2005.
809. Birks EK, Durando MM, McBride S: Exercise-induced pulmonary hemorrhage, *Vet Clin North Am Equine Pract* 19:87, 2003.
810. Birks EK, Mathieu-Costello O, Fu Z, et al: Very high pressures are required to cause stress failure of pulmonary capillaries in thoroughbred racehorses, *J Appl Physiol* 82:1584, 1997.
811. Poole DC, Epp TS, Erickson HH: Exercise-induced pulmonary haemorrhage (EIPH): mechanistic bases and therapeutic interventions, *Equine Vet J* 39:292, 2007.
812. Kindig CA, Ramsel C, McDonough P, et al: Inclined running increases pulmonary haemorrhage in the Thoroughbred horse, *Equine Vet J* 35:581, 2003.
813. Manohar M, Goetz TE: Pulmonary vascular pressures of exercising thoroughbred horses with and without endoscopic evidence of EIPH, *J Appl Physiol* 81:1589, 1996.
814. Meyer TS, Fedde MR, Gaughan EM, et al: Quantification of exercise-induced pulmonary haemorrhage with bronchoalveolar lavage, *Equine Vet J* 30:284, 1998.
815. Newton JR, Wood JL: Evidence of an association between inflammatory airway disease and EIPH in young Thoroughbreds during training, *Equine Vet J* 417(34):Suppl, 2002.
816. Doucet MY, Viel L: Clinical, radiographic, endoscopic, bronchoalveolar lavage and lung biopsy findings in horses with exercise-induced pulmonary hemorrhage, *Can Vet J* 43:195, 2002.
817. Takahashi T, Hiraga A, Ohmura H, et al: Frequency of and risk factors for epistaxis associated with exercise-induced pulmonary hemorrhage in horses: 251,609 race starts (1992-1997), *J Am Vet Med Assoc* 218:1462, 2001.
818. Gunson DE, Sweeney CR, Soma LR: Sudden death attributable to exercise-induced pulmonary hemorrhage in racehorses: nine cases (1981-1983), *J Am Vet Med Assoc* 193:102, 1988.
819. Boden LA, Charles JA, Slocombe RF, et al: Sudden death in racing Thoroughbreds in Victoria, Australia, *Equine Vet J* 37:269, 2005.
820. Art T, Tack S, Kirschvinck N, et al: Effect of instillation into lung of autologous blood on pulmonary function and tracheobronchial wash cytology, *Equine Vet J* 442(34):Suppl, 2002.
821. McKane SA, Canfield PJ, Rose RJ: Equine bronchoalveolar lavage cytology: survey of thoroughbred racehorses in training, *Aust Vet J* 70:401, 1993.
822. Hinchcliff KW: Counting red cells–is it an answer to EIPH? *Equine Vet J* 32:362, 2000.
823. Doucet MY, Viel L: Alveolar macrophage graded hemosiderin score from bronchoalveolar lavage in horses with exercise-induced pulmonary hemorrhage and controls, *J Vet Intern Med* 16:281, 2002.
824. Wisner ER, O'Brien TR, Lakritz J, et al: Radiographic and microscopic correlation of diffuse interstitial and bronchointerstitial pulmonary patterns in the caudodorsal lung of adult thoroughbred horses in race training, *Equine Vet J* 25:293, 1993.
825. Pascoe JR, O'Brien TR, Wheat JD, et al: Radiographic aspects of exercise-induced pulmonary hemorrhage in racing horses, *Vet Radiol* 24:85, 1983.
826. O'Callaghan MW, Goulden BE: Radiographic changes in the lungs of horses with exercise-induced epistaxis, *N Z Vet J* 30:117, 1982.
827. Manohar M, Hutchens E, Coney E: Furosemide attenuates the exercise-induced rise in pulmonary capillary blood pressure in horses, *Equine Vet J* 26:51, 1994.
828. Gleed RD, Ducharme NG, Hackett RP, et al: Effects of furosemide on pulmonary capillary pressure in horses exercising on a treadmill, *Equine Vet J* 30:102, 1999:Suppl, 1999.
829. Lester G, Clark C, Rice B, et al: Effect of timing and route of administration of furosemide on pulmonary hemorrhage and pulmonary arterial pressure in exercising thoroughbred racehorses, *Am J Vet Res* 60:22, 1999.
830. Sweeney CR, Soma LR: Exercise-induced pulmonary hemorrhage in thoroughbred horses: response to furosemide or hesperidin-citrus bioflavinoids, *J Am Vet Med Assoc* 185:195, 1984.
831. Sweeney CR, Soma LR, Maxson AD, et al: Effects of furosemide on the racing times of Thoroughbreds, *Am J Vet Res* 51:772, 1990.
832. Pascoe JR, McCabe AE, Franti CE, et al: Efficacy of furosemide in the treatment of exercise-induced pulmonary hemorrhage in Thoroughbred racehorses, *Am J Vet Res* 46:1985, 2000.
833. Gross DK, Morley PS, Hinchcliff KW, et al: Effect of furosemide on performance of Thoroughbreds racing in the United States and Canada, *J Am Vet Med Assoc* 215:670, 1999.
834. Manohar M, Goetz TE: Pulmonary vascular pressures of strenuously exercising Thoroughbreds during intravenous infusion of nitroglycerin, *Am J Vet Res* 60:1436, 1999.
835. Kindig CA, McDonough P, Finley MR, et al: NO inhalation reduces pulmonary arterial pressure but not hemorrhage in maximally exercising horses, *J Appl Physiol* 91:2674, 2001.
836. Goetz TE, Manohar M, Hassan AS, et al: Nasal strips do not affect pulmonary gas exchange, anaerobic metabolism, or EIPH in exercising Thoroughbreds, *J Appl Physiol* 90:2378, 2001.
837. Kindig CA, McDonough P, Fenton G, et al: Efficacy of nasal strip and furosemide in mitigating EIPH in Thoroughbred horses, *J Appl Physiol* 91:1396, 2001.
838. Walker HJ, Evans DL, Slocombe RF, et al: Effect of corticosteroid and bronchodilator therapy on bronchoalveolar lavage cytology following intrapulmonary blood inoculation, *Equine Vet J* 516(36):Suppl, 2006.
839. Hillidge CJ, Whitlock TW, Lane TJ: Failure of inhaled disodium cromoglycate aerosol to prevent exercise-induced pulmonary hemorrhage in racing quarter horses, *J Vet Pharmacol Ther* 10:257, 1987.
840. Erickson HH, Hidreth TS, Poole DC, et al: Management of exercise-induced pulmonary hemorrhage in nonracing performance horses, *Comp Cont Educ Pract Vet* 23:1090, 2001.
841. Weideman H, Schoeman SJ, Jordaan GF, et al: Epistaxis related to exercise-induced pulmonary haemorrhage in south African Thoroughbreds, *J S Afr Vet Assoc* 74:127, 2003.
842. Sundberg JP, Burnstein T, Page EH, et al: Neoplasms of Equidae, *J Am Vet Med Assoc* 170:150, 1977.
843. Cotchin E, Baker-Smith J: Correspondence: Tumours in horses encountered in an abattoir survey, *Vet Rec* 97:339, 1975.
844. Colbourne CM, Bolton JR, Mills JN, et al: Mesothelioma in horses, *Aust Vet J* 69:275, 1992.
845. Mair TS, Lane JG, Lucke VM: Clinicopathological features of lymphosarcoma involving the thoracic cavity in the horse, *Equine Vet J* 17:428, 1985.
846. Mair TS, Brown PJ: Clinical and pathological features of thoracic neoplasia in the horse, *Equine Vet J* 25:220, 1993.
847. Mair TS, Rush BR, Tucker RL: Clinical and diagnostic features of thoracic neoplasia in the horse, *Equine Vet Educ* 16:30, 2004.
848. Mair TS, Hillyer MH: Clinical features of lymphosarcoma in the horse: 77 cases, *Equine Vet Educ* 4:108, 1991.
849. Garber JL, Reef VB, Reimer JM: Sonographic findings in horses with mediastinal lymphosarcoma: 13 cases (1985-1992), *J Am Vet Med Assoc* 205:1432, 1994.

850. De Clercq D, van Loon G, Lefere L, et al: Ultrasound-guided biopsy as a diagnostic aid in three horses with a cranial mediastinal lymphosarcoma, *Vet Rec* 154:722, 2004.
851. Peroni JF, Horner NT, Robinson NE, et al: Equine thoracoscopy: normal anatomy and surgical technique, *Equine Vet J* 33:231, 2001.
852. Saulez MN, Schlipf JW Jr, Cebra CK, et al: Use of chemotherapy for treatment of a mixed-cell thoracic lymphoma in a horse, *J Am Vet Med Assoc* 224:733, 2004.
853. Kramer JW, Nickels FA, Bell T: Cytology of diffuse mesothelioma in the thorax of a horse, *Equine Vet J* 8:81, 1976.
854. Straub R, Tscharner C, Pauli B, et al: Mesothelioma of the pleura in a horse, *Schweiz Arch Tierheilkd* 116:207, 1974.
855. Kolbl VS: Pleural mesothelioma as a cause of death in a horse, *Wein tierarztl Mschr* 66:22, 1979.
856. Fry MM, Magdesian KG, Judy CE, et al: Antemortem diagnosis of equine mesothelioma by pleural biopsy, *Equine Vet J* 35:723, 2003.
857. Stoica G, Cohen N, Mendes O, et al: Use of immunohistochemical marker calretinin in the diagnosis of a diffuse malignant metastatic mesothelioma in an equine, *J Vet Diagn Invest* 16:240, 2004.
858. Nickels FA, Brown CM, Breeze RG: Myoblastoma. Equine granular cell tumor, *Mod Vet Pract* 61:593, 1980.
859. Turk MA, Breeze RG: Histochemical and ultrastructural features of an equine pulmonary granular cell tumour (myoblastoma), *J Comp Pathol* 91:471, 1981.
860. Misdorp W: Nauta-van Gelder HL: 'Granular-cell myoblastoma' in the horse. A report of 4 cases, *Pathol Vet* 5:385, 1968.
861. Parodi AL, Tassin P, Rigoulet J: Myoblastome a cellules granuleuses: Trois nouvelles observations a localisation pulmonair chez le cheval, *Rec Med Vet* 150:489, 1974.
862. Parker GA, Novilla NM, Brown AC, et al: Granular cell tumour (myoblastoma) in the lung of a horse, *J Comp Pathol* 89:421, 1979.
863. Inoue S, Okada N, Midoro K, et al: An equine case of granular cell tumor with chondroplasia, *Nippon Juigaku Zasshi* 49:581, 1987.
864. Kelly LC, Hill JE, Harner S, et al: Spontaneous equine pulmonary granular cell tumors: morphologic, histochemical, and immunohistochemical characterization, *Vet Pathol* 32:101, 1995.
865. Bouchard PR, Fortna CH, Rowland PH, et al: An immunohistochemical study of three equine pulmonary granular cell tumors, *Vet Pathol* 32:730, 1995.
866. Sutton RH, Coleman GT: A pulmonary granular cell tumour with associated hypertrophic osteopathy in a horse (abstract), *N Z Vet J* 43:123, 1995.
867. Kagawa Y, Hirayama K, Tagami M, et al: Immunohistochemical analysis of equine pulmonary granular cell tumours, *J Comp Pathol* 124:122, 2001.
868. Pusterla N, Norris AJ, Stacy BA, et al: Granular cell tumours in the lungs of three horses, *Vet Rec* 153:530, 2003.
869. Murphy JR, Breeze RG, McPherson EA: Myxoma of the equine respiratory tract, *Mod Vet Pract* 59:529, 1978.
870. Dill SG, Moise NS, Meschter CL: Cardiac failure in a stallion secondary to metastasis of an anaplastic pulmonary carcinoma, *Equine Vet J* 18:414, 1986.
871. Schultze AE, Sonea I, Bell TG: Primary malignant pulmonary neoplasia in two horses, *J Am Vet Med Assoc* 193:477, 1988.
872. Anderson JD, Leonard JM, Zeliff JA, et al: Primary pulmonary neoplasm in a horse, *J Am Vet Med Assoc* 201:1399, 1992.
873. Uphoff CS, Lyncoln JA: A primary pulmonary tumor in a horse, *Equine Pract* 9:19, 1987.
874. Sullivan DJ: Cartilaginous tumors (chondroma and chondrosarcoma) in animals, *Am J Vet Res* 21:531, 1960.
875. Clem MR, O'Brien TR, Feeney DA, et al: Pulmonary chondrosarcoma in a horse, *Compend Contin Educ Pract Vet* 8:S964, 1986.
876. Rossdale PD, Greet TRC, McGladdery AJ, et al: Pulmonary leiomyosarcoma in a 13 year-old Thoroughbred stallion presenting as a differential diagnosis to recurrent airway obstruction, *Equine Vet Educ* 16:21, 2004.
877. Godber LM, Brown CM, Mullaney TP: Polycystic hepatic disease, thoracic granular cell tumor and secondary hypertrophic osteopathy in a horse, *Cornell Vet* 83:227, 1993.
878. Heinola T, Heikkila M, Ruohoniemi M, et al: Hypertrophic pulmonary osteopathy associated with granular cell tumour in a mare, *Vet Rec* 149:307, 2001.
879. Alexander JE, Keown GH, Palotay JL: Granular cell myoblastoma with hypertrophic pulmonary osteoarthropathy in a mare, *J Am Vet Med Assoc* 146:703, 1965.
880. Facemire PR, Chilcoat CD, Sojka JE, et al: Treatment of granular cell tumor via complete right lung resection in a horse, *J Am Vet Med Assoc* 217:1522, 2000.
881. Ohnesorge B, Gehlen H, Wohlsein P: Transendoscopic electrosurgery of an equine pulmonary granular cell tumor, *Vet Surg* 31:375, 2002.
882. Rendle DI, Hewetson M, Barron R, et al: Tachypnoea and pleural effusion in a mare with metastatic pancreatic adenocarcinoma, *Vet Rec* 159:356, 2006.
883. Chaffin MK, Fuentealba IC, Schmitz DG, et al: Endometrial adenocarcinoma in a mare, *Cornell Vet* 80:65, 1990.
884. Gunson DE, Gillette DM, Beech J, et al: Endometrial adenocarcinoma in a mare, *Vet Pathol* 17:776, 1980.
885. Whiteley LO, Leininger JR, Wolf CB, et al: Malignant squamous cell thymoma in a horse, *Vet Pathol* 23:627, 1986.
886. Vaala WE: Pleuritis and pleural effusion in a mare secondary to disseminated squamous cell carcinoma, *Comp Cont Educ Pract Vet* 674, 1987.
887. Ford TS, Vaala WE, Sweeney CR, et al: Pleuroscopic diagnosis of gastroesophageal squamous cell carcinoma in a horse, *J Am Vet Med Assoc* 190:1556, 1987.
888. Hovda LR, Shaftoe S, Rose ML, et al: Mediastinal squamous cell carcinoma and thyroid carcinoma in an aged horse, *J Am Vet Med Assoc* 197:1187, 1990.
889. Furuoka H, Taniyama H, Matsui T, et al: Malignant thymoma with multiple metastases in a mare, *Nippon Juigaku Zasshi* 49:577, 1987.
890. Milne JC: Malignant melanomas causing Horner's syndrome in a horse, *Equine Vet J* 18:74, 1986.
891. Frye FL, Knight HD, Brown SI: Hemangiosarcoma in a horse, *J Am Vet Med Assoc* 182:287, 1983.
892. Hargis AM, McElwain TF: Vascular neoplasia in the skin of horses, *J Am Vet Med Assoc* 184:1121, 1984.
893. Freestone JF, Williams MM, Norwood G: Thoracic haemangiosarcoma in a 3-year-old horse, *Aust Vet J* 67:269, 1990.
894. Johnson JE, Beech J, Saik JE: Disseminated hemangiosarcoma in a horse, *J Am Vet Med Assoc* 193:1429, 1988.
895. Jean D, Lavoie JP, Nunez L, et al: Cutaneous hemangiosarcoma with pulmonary metastasis in a horse, *J Am Vet Med Assoc* 204:776, 1994.
896. Southwood LL, Schott HC 2nd, Henry CJ, et al: Disseminated hemangiosarcoma in the horse: 35 cases, *J Vet Intern Med* 14:105, 2000.
897. Collins MB, Hodgson DR, Hutchins DR, et al: Haemangiosarcoma in the horse: three cases, *Aust Vet J* 71:296, 1994.
898. Waller T, Rubarth S: Haemangioendothelioma in domestic animals, *Acta Vet Scand* 8:234, 1967.
899. Gruys E, Kok HA: Van Der Werff YD: Dyspnoea due to intrathoracic haemorrhage and haemangiosarcoma in a horse (author's transl), *Tijdschr Diergeneeskd* 101:310, 1976.
900. Reinacher VM: Hamangioenothelome in der skellettmuskulatur eines pferds, *Berl Munch Tierarztl Wochenschr* 91:121, 1978.
901. Katayama Y, Oikawa MA, Yoshihara T, et al: Clinical and immunohistochemicalobservationofhemangiosarcomainaracing thoroughbred, *Equine Pract* 18:24, 1996.

902. Warren AL, Summers BA: Epithelioid variant of hemangioma and hemangiosarcoma in the dog, horse, and cow, *Vet Pathol* 44:15, 2007.
903. Johns I, Stephen JO, Del Piero F, et al: Hemangiosarcoma in 11 young horses, *J Vet Intern Med* 19:564, 2005.
904. Rebhun WC, Bertone A: Equine lymphosarcoma, *J Am Vet Med Assoc* 184:720, 1984.
905. Keen JA, Swain JM, Rhind SM, et al: Lymphoproliferative disease resembling lymphomatoid granulomatosis in a thoroughbred mare, *J Vet Intern Med* 18:904, 2004.
906. Waugh SL, Long GG, Uriah L, et al: Metastatic hemangiosarcoma in the equine: report of two cases, *J Equine Med Surg* 1:311, 1977.

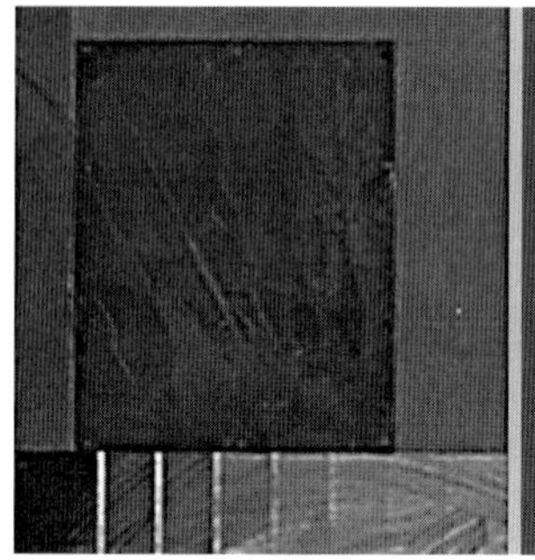

Cardiovascular Diseases

CHAPTER 10

John D. Bonagura, Virginia B. Reef, Colin C. Schwarzwald*

Cardiovascular (CV) system function is critical to exercise, thermoregulation, and the blood flow–dependent functions of the lungs, kidneys, gut, and reproductive system. Heart and vascular diseases are common in horses, but fortunately the underlying lesion is often minor and well tolerated. However, clinically significant CV disease can develop in horses with clinical signs that can include arrhythmia, exercise intolerance, congestive heart failure (CHF), weakness or collapse, systemic infection, or sudden death.

The clinical evaluation of the equine CV system is often perplexing. Horses are renowned for a variety of physiologic murmurs and arrhythmias. Furthermore, only when horses are undergoing exercise at the highest levels do they reach the limits of normal CV function. Clinical assessment is best served by an awareness of normal variation, the appreciation of relevant diseases, diagnostic studies and prognostic indicators, and an understanding of available management options. Communication of these issues constitutes the focus of this chapter.

Equine cardiology has advanced from a study of physiologic variation and speculation to one of accurate diagnosis and focused therapy, although many clinical issues remain unresolved. Much of the important groundwork in clinical equine cardiology was established by studies of normal CV physiology, cardiac catheterization, pathology, cardiac auscultation, electrocardiography, and echocardiography. These data, defining the normal anatomic and psychologic features of the equine CV system, constitute the backdrop of the clinical examination. Other examinations of importance to CV assessment include ambulatory electrocardiography, functional exercise testing, and biochemical tests of cardiac injury. Appropriate selection and interpretation of these tests allows the clinician to identify and quantify most diseases of the heart and circulation.

No recent comprehensive studies of CV *disease prevalence* are available. Holmes, Darke, and Else[33] observed that 2.5% of hospitalized horses were in atrial fibrillation (AF).[33] Else and Holmes[27-29] noted myocardial fibrosis in 14.3% of horses examined at necropsy and evidence of chronic valvular disease in approximately 25% of the hearts examined. Various CV lesions were considered important in 8.5% of 480 consecutive losses in a necropsy study conducted by Baker and Ellis.[52] CV diseases are probably the third most common cause of poor performance after musculoskeletal and respiratory diseases.[53-56] Occult heart disease, cardiac arrhythmias, and vascular lesions are considered important reasons for unexplained sudden death.[52,57-69] Certainly, most clinicians encounter manifestations of CV disease or dysfunction on a regular basis.

The assessment of CV disease in a horse is predicated on a competent clinical examination, the clinician's knowledge, and the ability to order and evaluate diagnostic studies. Incomplete information may impede an accurate diagnosis, foster miscommunication of risks to the client, or delay the proper course of management. Fundamentals of CV anatomy, physiology, and electrophysiology are reviewed elsewhere.[9,20,70-77] This chapter offers a framework for understanding the lesions, pathophysiology, diagnosis, and management of important congenital and acquired conditions of the heart and major vessels. Clinical aspects of circulatory shock are described in this volume, and the reader is referred elsewhere for the management of cardiopulmonary arrest.[78,79]

ANATOMIC CORRELATES OF CARDIOVASCULAR DISEASES

Most diagnostic techniques, including cardiac auscultation, electrocardiography, cardiac catheterization, and echocardiography, are predicated on an understanding of cardiac anatomy and physiology. The CV system is divided into two separate circulations: (1) systemic and (2) pulmonary. The systemic circulation has a greater venous capacitance, ventricular pumping pressure, arterial pressure, and vascular resistance.[73,75-77] Despite these differences, the functions of these two circulations are interdependent, as the following examples illustrate. Systemic and pulmonary circulations are arranged in series, therefore cardiac output (CO) from the left ventricle (LV) and the right ventricle (RV) must be equivalent. Accordingly, failure of either ventricle limits CO. Isolated LV failure, as with severe mitral regurgitation (MR), can cause right-sided failure; this is explained by the increased pulmonary venous pressure causing pulmonary hypertension and imparting a pressure load on the RV. A third example is the case of isolated RV failure with marked RV dilatation. Here the leftward bulging of the ventricular septum impairs filling of the LV. This last situation also can develop in chronic pericarditis. Arrhythmias also affect both sides of the

*When [DVD icon] appears, a corresponding video can be found on the DVD inside this book.

BOX 10-1

CARDIAC DIAGNOSES

Anatomic Diagnosis

Cardiac malformation
Valvular (endocardial) disease
Myocardial disease
Pericardial disease
Cor pulmonale (pulmonary disease leading to secondary heart disease)
Disorder of the impulse-forming or conduction system
Vascular disease

Physiologic Diagnosis

Systemic: pulmonary shunting
- Left to right
- Right to left

Valvular insufficiency
Valvular stenosis
Myocardial (systolic) dysfunction
Diastolic dysfunction
Cardiac rhythm disturbance
Cardiac-related syncope
Heart insufficiency or failure (limited cardiac output)
Congestive heart failure
Shock
Sudden cardiac death
Cardiopulmonary arrest

Etiologic Diagnosis

Malformation (genetic)
Degenerative disease
Metabolic or endocrine disease
Neoplasia
Nutritional disorder
Inflammatory disease
- Infective or parasitic
- Noninfective
  - Immune-mediated
  - Idiopathic

Ischemic injury
Idiopathic disorder
Iatrogenic disease
Toxic injury
Traumatic injury

heart so that the development of AF in the setting of structural heart disease can promote biventricular heart failure.

The heart consists of unique active and passive components,[75] and different diagnostic methods are needed to evaluate these structures and associated functions. Normal heart action requires coordination of electrical activity, muscular contraction and relaxation, and valve motion. When reviewing heart anatomy, and subsequently cardiac pathology, it is useful to consider the anatomic integrity of the pericardium, myocardium, endocardium, and valves, specialized impulse-forming and conduction systems, and blood vessels.[70] Using this approach, the causes of CV disease can be conveniently subdivided into anatomic, physiologic (functional), and causative diagnoses (Boxes 10-1 and 10-2).

Pericardial Disease

The pericardium limits cardiac dilatation, acts as a barrier against contiguous infection, and contributes to the diastolic properties of the heart. The pericardial space is formed by the reflection of the two major pericardial membranes—(1) the parietal pericardium and (2) the visceral pericardium (the epicardium)—and normally contains such a small amount of serous fluid that it cannot be seen by echocardiography. Pericardial effusion leading to cardiac compression (tamponade) impairs ventricular filling and diastolic function, typically causing right-sided CHF. Some cases of pericarditis progress to constrictive pericardial disease, which severely limits ventricular filling.

Pericardial effusion can develop as a primary disorder or secondary to pleuropneumonia. Infective pericarditis can produce an effusion sufficient to cause cardiac tamponade or eventual constriction of the heart.[55,80-97] Sterile, idiopathic pericardial effusion also has been reported in horses. The volume of effusion can be substantial and can lead to cardiac decompensation.[87] Cardiac mass lesions and intrapericardial tumors have been reported sporadically.[89,92,98,99] Cranial mediastinal tumors (lymphosarcoma) or abscesses secondary to pleuropneumonia also can compress the heart and mimic pericardial disease.[100] Clinical aspects of pericardial disease are discussed later in this chapter.

Myocardial Disease

The myocardium forms the bulk of the atrial and ventricular muscular walls. The right atrium (RA) communicates with the RV inlet through the right atrioventricular (AV) or tricuspid valve. The RV appears crescent shaped on cross-sectional echocardiographic examination and is functionally *U* shaped. The RV inlet is located in the right hemithorax and the outlet, pulmonary valve, and main pulmonary artery (PA) on the left side of the chest. The left atrium (LA) is caudal to the RA and separated by the atrial septum. The LA is dorsal to the LV through which it communicates across the left atrioventricular (mitral) valve. The LV is circular in cross-section when viewed by echocardiography and separated from the RV by the ventricular septum. The septum and free walls are thicker than the RV free wall (by approximately 2.5 to 3 times). Persistent embryologic openings in the cardiac septa are known as *septal defects,* with the ventricular septal defect (VSD) representing the most common cardiac anomaly in most equine practices (see Box 10-2). The LV is functionally *V* shaped with an inlet and outlet separated by the cranioventral (septal or "anterior") leaflet of the mitral valve (Figure 10-1). The aorta originates in the LV outlet, continuous with the ventricular septum cranially and in fibrous continuity with the septal mitral leaflet caudally. This great vessel exits from near the center of the heart and to the right of the main PA.

BOX 10-2

CAUSES OF CARDIOVASCULAR DISEASE

Congenital Cardiac Malformation

Simple systemic-to-pulmonary shunts (left to right)
- Atrial septal defect
- Ventricular septal defect
  - Paramembranous defect
  - Ventricular inlet defect
  - Subarterial (subpulmonic) defect
  - Muscular defect
- Patent ductus arteriosus

Patent foramen ovale (permitting right-to-left shunting)
Valvular dysplasia
- Mitral stenosis/atresia
- Pulmonic stenosis (bicuspid pulmonary valve)
- Pulmonary atresia (leading to a right-to-left shunt)
- Tricuspid stenosis/atresia (leading to a right-to-left shunt)
- Aortic stenosis/insufficiency (bicuspid or quadricuspid valve)

Subaortic rings with stenosis
Tetralogy of Fallot
Pulmonary atresia with ventricular septal defect (pseudotruncus arteriosus)
Double-outlet right ventricle
Subaortic stenosis
Hypoplastic left-side of the heart
Other complex malformations

Valvular Heart Disease Causing Valve Insufficiency or Stenosis

Congenital valve malformation
Semilunar valve fenestrations causing valve insufficiency
Degenerative (fibrosis) or myxomatous disease causing valve insufficiency
Vavular prolapse
Bacterial endocarditis causing valve insufficiency with or without stenosis
Rupture of a chorda tendinea causing mitral or tricuspid valve insufficiency
Rupture of a valve leaflet causing flail leaflet and valve insufficiency
Noninfective valvulitis
Valvular regurgitation following dilation of the heart or a great vessel
Papillary muscle dysfunction causing valvular insufficiency

Myocardial Disease

Idiopathic dilated cardiomyopathy: ventricular dilation and myocardial contractility failure
Myocarditis
Myocardial fibrosis
- Ischemic (embolic?) myocardial fibrosis
- Parasitic (Strongylus) embolization

Myocardial degeneration/necrosis
- Myocardial ischemia
- Myocardial infarction
- Toxic injury (e.g., monensin)
- Nutritional deficiencies (e.g., selenium deficiency)

Myocardial neoplasia
- Lymphosarcoma
- Melanoma
- Hemangioma/hemangiosarcoma
- Pulmonary carcinoma

Infiltrative myocardial disease (e.g., amyloidosis)

Pericardial Disease

Pericardial effusion with or without cardiac tamponade
- Infective: bacterial or viral
- Idiopathic pericardial effusion
- Constrictive pericardial disease
- Mass lesion (intrapericardial or extrapericardial) compressing the heart

Pulmonary Hypertension and Cor Pulmonale

Pulmonary hypertension following left-sided heart disease
Pulmonary vascular disease following left-to-right shunt
Immature pulmonary circulation
Primary bronchopulmonary or pulmonary vascular disease
Alveolar hypoxia with reactive pulmonary arterial vasoconstriction
Severe acidosis
Pulmonary thromboembolism

Cardiac Arrhythmias (see Box 10-9)

Atrial arrhythmias
Junctional (nodal) arrhythmias
Ventricular arrhythmias
Conduction disturbances

Vascular Diseases

Congenital vascular lesions
Rupture of the aorta, pulmonary artery, or systemic artery
Aneurysm of the aortic sinus of Valsalva
Aortic or aortoiliac degenerative disease
Arteritis
- Infective
- Immune-mediated

(Jugular) Venous thrombosis/thrombophlebitis
Pulmonary embolism
Mass lesion or tumor obstructing blood flow
Aorto-iliac thrombosis

The myocardium may dilate or hypertrophy in response to exercise,[101,102] increased work caused by structural cardiac disease, or as a consequence of a noncardiac disorder. Ventricular or atrial dilatation is recognized echocardiographically or at necropsy by distention and rounding of the affected chambers, including a "double-apex" sign when marked RV enlargement occurs. Lesions causing systolic pressure overload lead to concentric hypertrophy.[103] More common in horses

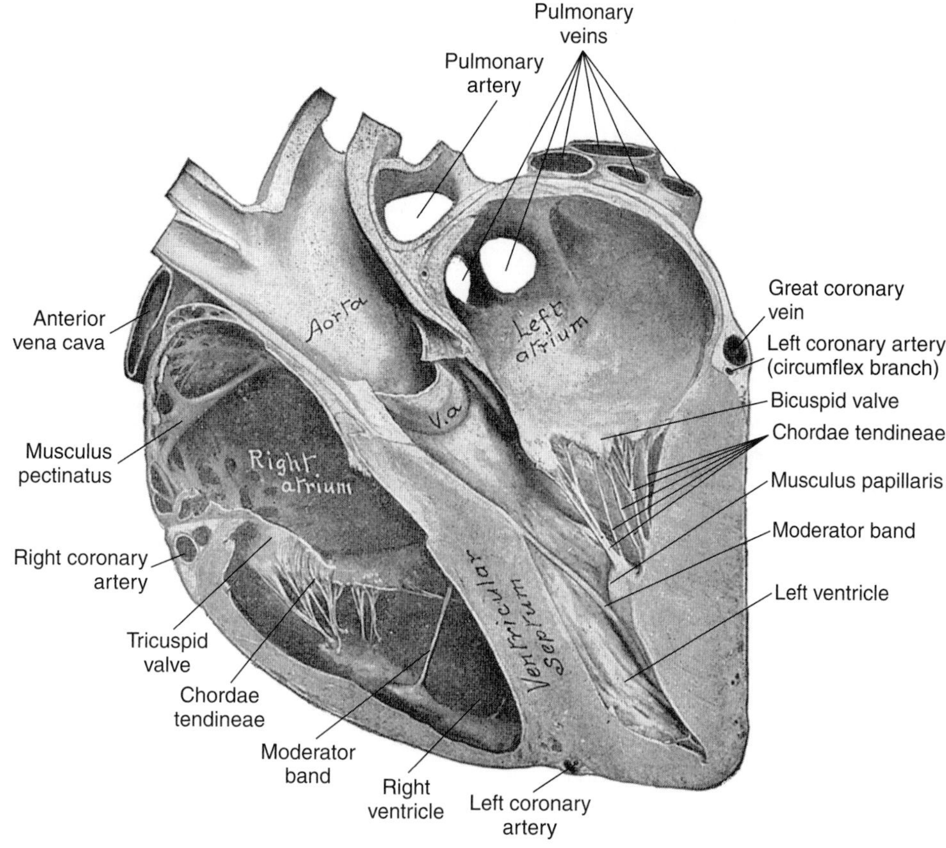

FIGURE 10-1 Sagittal view of the equine heart. The thicknesses of the ventricles, the position of the atria relative to the ventricles, and the relationship of the left ventricular (LV) inlet and outlet are evident. The bicuspid valve referred to in this figure is the mitral valve. The circular appearance of the left atrium (LA) and the relationship of the septal cusp of the mitral valve to the LV inlets and outlets are notable. These aspects are important when examining the heart by echocardiography. *v.a.,* Segment of aortic valve. (From Sisson S, Grossman JD: Anatomy of the domestic animals, ed 4, Philadelphia, 1953, WB Saunders.)

are lesions such as incompetent valves or shunts that cause ventricular volume overload with dilatation and eccentric ventricular hypertrophy. Increased cardiac work also occurs in response to exercise, severe anemia, and infections. In these situations, compensatory increases in CO, sympathetic activation, and peripheral vasodilation occur to maintain oxygen delivery to the tissues.[104,105]

The overall prevalence of myocardial disease is unknown; however, multifocal areas of fibrosis are commonly found at necropsy.[28,29,106-110] Whether these areas indicate prior inflammation, toxic injury, or ischemic necrosis caused by intramural coronary disease is uncertain. Cases of multifocal or diffuse myocarditis have been observed. Myocardial inflammation and myocardial failure can lead to cardiac arrhythmias and heart failure.[4,111,112] Idiopathic dilated cardiomyopathy develops sporadically and is recognized echocardiographically or by nuclear studies as a dilated, hypokinetic LV or RV.[90,113] Ingestion of monensin or other ionophores can cause mild to severe myocardial injury.[114-120] Neoplastic infiltration is considered rare.[59,98,99,121] Impaired myocardial function as a consequence of regional ischemia has been sought using stress echocardiography immediately after treadmill exercise or pharmacologic stress, but this diagnosis requires further definition.[122] Myocardial contraction is dictated by electrical activity of the myocardium; accordingly, cardiac arrhythmias—especially AF or ventricular tachycardia (VT)—can limit CO and cause exercise intolerance in performance animals (see later discussion). Clinical aspects of myocardial disease are discussed later in this chapter.

Valvular and Endocardial Diseases

The cardiac chambers are lined by the endocardium, which also covers the four cardiac valves and is continuous with the endothelium of the great vessels. Normal valves govern the one-way flow of blood through the heart by preventing significant regurgitation of blood from higher to lower pressure zones. The AV inlet valves—the tricuspid and the mitral—are anchored by the collagenous chordae tendineae and papillary muscles and are supported by a valve "annulus" and the caudal atrial walls (see Figures 10-1 and 10-2).[70] The mitral valve consists of two major cusps and several accessory cusps.[45] The tricuspid valve is the largest valve and consists of three well-defined leaflets. Lesions of any portion of the AV valve apparatus or dilatation of the ventricle can lead to valvular insufficiency (see Box 10-2). The aortic and pulmonary valves each consist of three semilunar leaflets that close during diastole to protect the ventricles from the higher arterial blood pressure (ABP). Aortic valvular tissue in horses is not simply passive and will contract in response to a number of adrenergic and vascular agonists, such as angiotensin II and

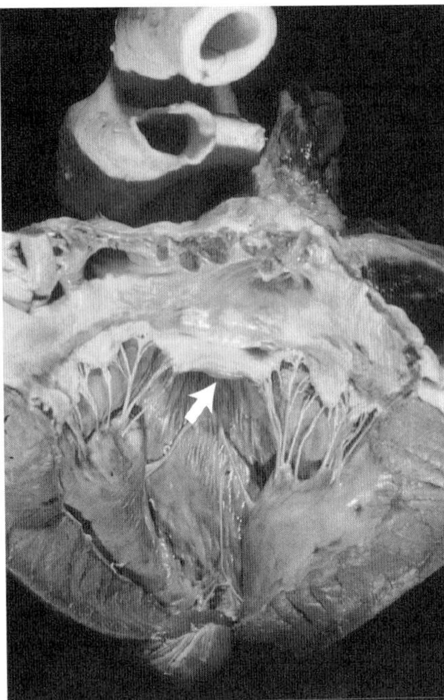

FIGURE 10-2 Anatomy of the left atrioventricular (mitral) valve. Opened left atrium (LA) and LV viewed from the caudal perspective. The large anterior (cranioventral or septal) leaflet in the center of the figure is notable. Chordae tendineae attach the valve to the papillary muscles. The ventricle has been cut so that the multiple cusps of the posterior (caudodorsal or mural) leaflet are visible to the left and the right of the anterior leaflet.

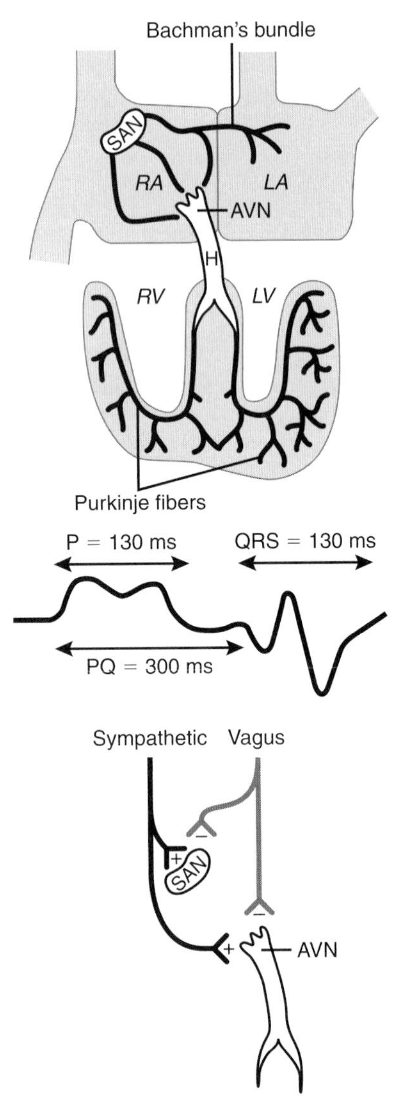

FIGURE 10-3 Impulse-forming and conduction systems of the heart. The impulse originates in the sinoatrial node (SAN) and is propagated across the right atrium (RA) and left atrium (LA), generating the P wave. Specialized internodal and interatrial (Bachmann's bundle) pathways facilitate impulse conduction. The impulse is delayed in the atrioventricular node (AVN) and rapidly conducted through the bundle of His (H), bundle branches, and Purkinje network *(top)*. Electrical activation of ventricular myocytes generates the QRS complex. The automaticity of the SA node and conduction across the AV node are modulated by the autonomic nervous system *(bottom)*. (Courtesy Dr. Robert L. Hamlin. From Schwarzwald CC, Bonagura JD, Muir WW: The cardiovascular system. In Muir WW, Hubbell JA, editors: Equine anesthesia: monitoring and emergency therapy, ed 2, St Louis, 2009, WB Saunders.)

endothelin.[123] The left and right main coronary arteries originate within the aortic valve sinuses (of Valsalva).

Valvular disorders in horses are common.* Congenital valve stenosis, dysplasia, or atresia are recognized sporadically in foals.[4,111,127,155-168] Degenerative diseases of the aortic, mitral, and tricuspid valves are very common in mature horses,[4,127,155-168] and endocarditis can develop on any cardiac valve† (see Box 10-2). Valvular lesions of obscure cause, including nonseptic valvulitis, have been recognized sporadically. Tricuspid and MR, of unspecified cause, is often detected in high performance animals, including Standardbred and National Hunt horses.[182-185] MR caused by rupture of a chorda tendineae is recognized in both foals and mature animals.[38,132,147,186] Clinical aspects of valvular heart disease are discussed later in this chapter.

Disease of the Impulse-Forming and Conduction Systems

The specialized cardiac tissues consist of the sinoatrial (SA) node, internodal pathways, AV node, bundle of His, bundle branches, fascicles, and Purkinje system (Figure 10-3). The SA node, a relatively large, crescent-shaped structure, is located subepicardially at the junction of the right auricle and cranial vena cava. Well-documented sinus node disease, although suggested,[187] is rare; in contrast, vagally induced sinus arrhythmias are common.[9,187-189] The equine atrial muscle mass is large and predisposes the horse to development of re-entrant rhythms and fibrillatory conduction.[190] The AV node, situated in the ventral atrial septum, and the bundle of His, which continues into the bundle branches, are sites for AV block, both physiologic (vagal), and infrequently, pathologic in nature. Conduction is slow across the normal AV node.[191-193] The His-Purkinje system in the ventricular septum and ventricular myocardium can act as substrates for junctional and ventricular ectopic

* References 5, 27, 28, 38, 45, 48, 56, 91, 109, 124-154.

†References 4, 31, 83, 84, 90, 91, 109, 111, 125, 139, 135, 144, 148, 169-181.

impulses and tachycardias. Because the horse has relatively complete penetration of Purkinje fibers in the ventricles—except for a small portion of the LV free wall—the substantial equine ventricles are electrically activated in a relatively short time (≈110 msec).[7]

The autonomic nervous system extensively innervates the heart and influences cardiac rhythms.[4,111,134,194-199] Interplay between the sympathetic and parasympathetic branches normally controls heart rate and rhythm in response to changes in ABP.[9,200] The vagus nerve innervates supraventricular tissues extensively and probably affects proximal ventricular tissues to a minor extent. Vagal influence generally depresses heart rate, AV conduction, excitability, and myocardial inotropic (contractile) state. However, because vagotonia also shortens the action potential and refractory period of atrial myocytes, high vagal activity is a predisposing factor in the development of AF.[201] Innervation of the stimulatory sympathetic nervous system is extensive throughout the heart and has effects generally opposite to those of the parasympathetic system. β_1-Adrenergic receptors dominate in the equine heart,[202] but presumably, other autonomic subtype receptors exist, including α-adrenergic receptors and small numbers of β_2-adrenoceptors.[76,203] The notable increase in heart rate that attends exercise is related to increased sympathetic efferent activity and withdrawal of parasympathetic tone.[9] Increases in heart rate to 220 to 240 beats/min are not uncommon with maximal exercise.[204-208] The exact role of dysautonomia in the genesis of cardiac arrhythmias has not been determined; however, infusion of autonomic receptor agonists and antagonists can be associated with direct or baroreceptor-induced changes in heart rate and rhythm.[209-212] Cardiac arrhythmias are discussed later in this chapter.

Vascular Diseases

There are three major subdivisions of the circulation: (1) systemic, (2) coronary, and (3) pulmonary. The arteries and veins consist of three layers: (1) adventitia, (2) media, and (3) intima. The overall structure and function of each layer varies with the vessel and location. Vascular receptors[20,73,75,76] and anatomic lesions influence vascular resistance and blood flow. α-Adrenoceptors dominate in the systemic vasculature, and blood pressure (BP) is generally raised by vasoconstriction after stimulation of postsynaptic α-adrenergic receptors by norepinephrine, epinephrine, or infused α-adrenergic receptor agonists like phenylephrine.[213,214] The presence of vasodilator β_2-adrenergic receptors is clinically relevant, insofar as infused β_2-agonists cause vasodilation in circulatory beds that contain high β-agonist adrenergic receptor density. Many vascular beds also dilate after the production of local vasodilator substances, such as nitric oxide, released during exercise, stress, or metabolic activity.[73,75] Dopaminergic receptors, when present in vascular walls, may be stimulated, causing vasodilation, provided vasoconstricting α-adrenergic activity does not dominate. Stimulation of histamine (H_1) receptors or serotonin (5-HT) receptors causes arteriolar dilatation, venular constriction, and increased capillary permeability.[75] Infusion of endothelin[215] or of calcium salts causes arterial vasoconstriction,[216] whereas administration of calcium channel antagonists (e.g., verapamil, diltiazem) causes vasodilation of vascular smooth muscle.[217]

Various vascular lesions have been reported in horses (see Box 10-2). Rupture of the aorta, PA, or middle uterine artery is devastating and often lethal.* The aorta may also rupture into the heart, creating an aortic to cardiac fistula.[220,221] Although parasitic arteritis may predispose to vascular injury, the cause of most vascular lesions, including aortic-iliac thrombosis, is unknown.[222-227] Causes of vasculitis include *Strongylus vulgaris* infestation of the cranial mesenteric artery, infective thrombophlebitis of the jugular veins, equine viral arteritis, and suspected immune-mediated disease.[106,108,228] Neoplasms can obstruct blood flow by external compression or through invasion, more often affecting the right side of the circulation. Examples include obstruction of the PA by a lung tumor and obstruction of venous return by neoplastic compression or invasion of the vena cava. Clinical features of vascular disease are discussed later in this chapter.

CLINICAL CARDIOVASCULAR PHYSIOLOGY

The clinician must appreciate elementary aspects of normal heart function to perform a clinical CV examination and understand the abnormalities associated with heart disease and CHF.[229] Central to this are the electrical-mechanical correlates of Wiggers cardiac cycle.

Cardiac Cycle

The association between electrical and mechanical events of the heart first described by Wiggers has been reviewed in standard physiology textbooks (Figure 10-4).[73,75-77] From a study of this cycle, it is evident that cardiac electrical activity precedes pressure and volume changes; therefore arrhythmias can exert deleterious hemodynamic effects, especially during exercise, illness, or anesthesia. Relevant aspects of this cycle are now considered.

The P wave of the electrocardiogram (ECG) stems from electrical activation of the atria, late in ventricular diastole and after the ventricles have been largely filled. During the ensuing atrial contraction, the *atrial sound* (fourth heart sound or S_4) is generated and the ventricle is filled to its end diastolic volume. The increase in atrial pressure, the atrial *a* wave, is reflected as a normal *jugular pulse* in the ventral cervical region. The magnitude of the atrial contribution to ventricular filling generally placed at 15% to 20% at rest, but increases dramatically during high heart rates. Therefore atrial tachyarrhythmias such as AF have the greatest effect on CO during exercise or tachycardia.

The QRS complex heralds ventricular systole. After depolarization of the ventricular myocytes, calcium enters the cell to trigger release of calcium stores in the sarcoplasmic reticulum. Increased cytosolic calcium interacts with the cardiac troponin complex on actin and myosin filaments to shorten the myofilaments and develop tension. These events are enhanced by sympathetic activity or drugs such as digoxin or dobutamine and depressed by anesthetics and drugs that impair calcium entry into cells. The abrupt increase in ventricular wall tension and chamber pressure closes the AV valves (coinciding with the vibrations of the *first heart sound,* S_1) and increases intraventricular pressure *(isovolumetric period)* until the semilunar valves open.[23,25] At this instant the ventricular walls move inward (Figure 10-5, *B* and *C*) and blood is ejected

*References 4, 34, 58, 111, 152, 218, 219.

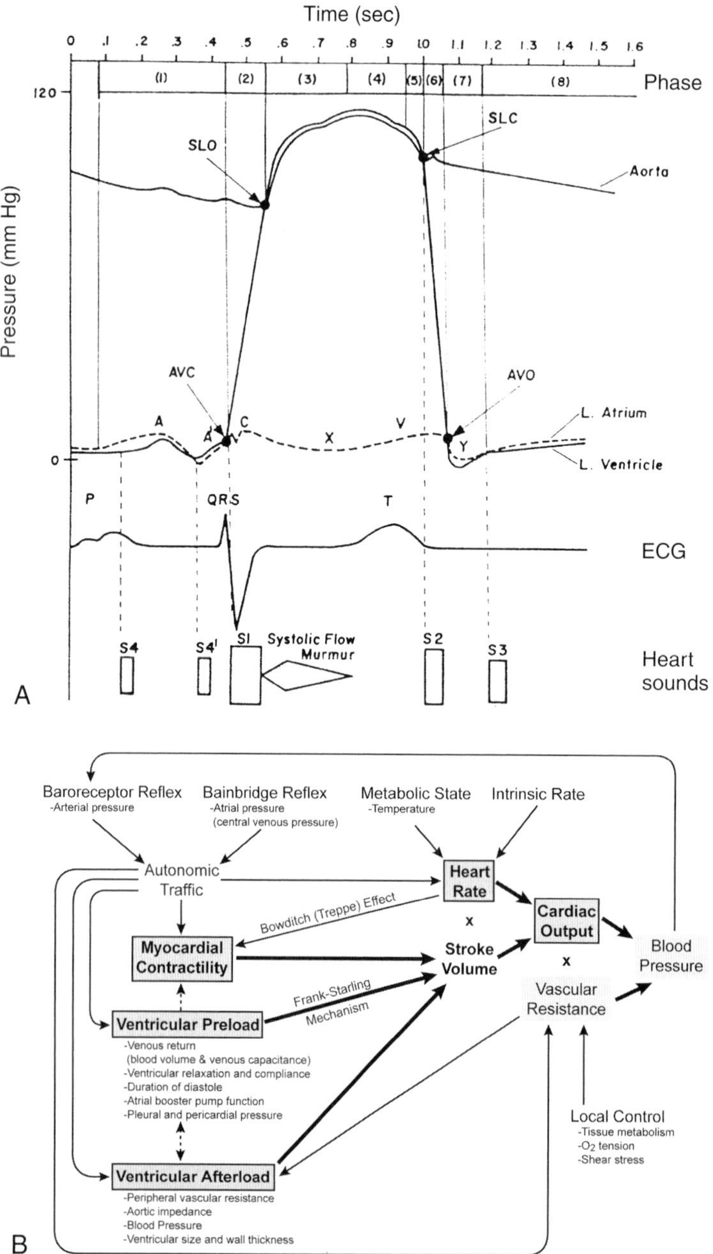

FIGURE 10-4 **A,** The cardiac (Wiggers) cycle of the horse. This drawing integrates the electric, pressure, mechanical, and flow events of diastole and systole and demonstrates the origins of the heart sounds. Electric activity precedes mechanical events. See the text for a full description. *AVC,* Closure of the mitral (atrioventricular) valve; *AVO,* opening of the mitral (atrioventricular) valve; *SLO,* opening of the aortic (semilunar) valve; *SLC,* closure of the aortic (semilunar) valve. **B,** Determinants of cardiac output (CO) and blood pressure (BP). (A, Modified from Detweiler DK, Patterson DF: The cardiovascular system. In Cattcott EJ, Smithcors JF, editors: Equine medicine and surgery, ed 2, Santa Barbara, CA, 1972, American Veterinary Publications. B, From Muir WW, Hubbell JA: Equine anesthesia, ed 2, St Louis, 2009, Saunders.)

into the great vessel as the ventricular pressure increases to peak value and creates a similar peak ABP (see Figures 10-5, *D,* and 10-6). The contracting heart twists during systole, and the LV strikes the chest wall caudal to the left olecranon causing the *cardiac impulse* or "apex beat." This early systolic movement, coincident with opening of the aortic valve, is a useful timing clue for cardiac auscultation and for identifying the mitral valve area for auscultation. The delay between the onset of the QRS and the opening of the semilunar valves, termed the *pre-ejection period,* can be measured by Doppler echocardiography and is an index of ventricular myocardial contractility such that positive inotropic drugs shorten the pre-ejection period.[46,230-237] Blood is ejected into the aorta and PA with an initial velocity that generally peaks near 1 ms/sec and can be measured by Doppler echocardiography.[149,230] The aortic ejection time usually exceeds 400 ms in a horse at rest, and reductions of either ejection velocity or ejection time are suggestive of reduced LV function. A *functional systolic ejection*

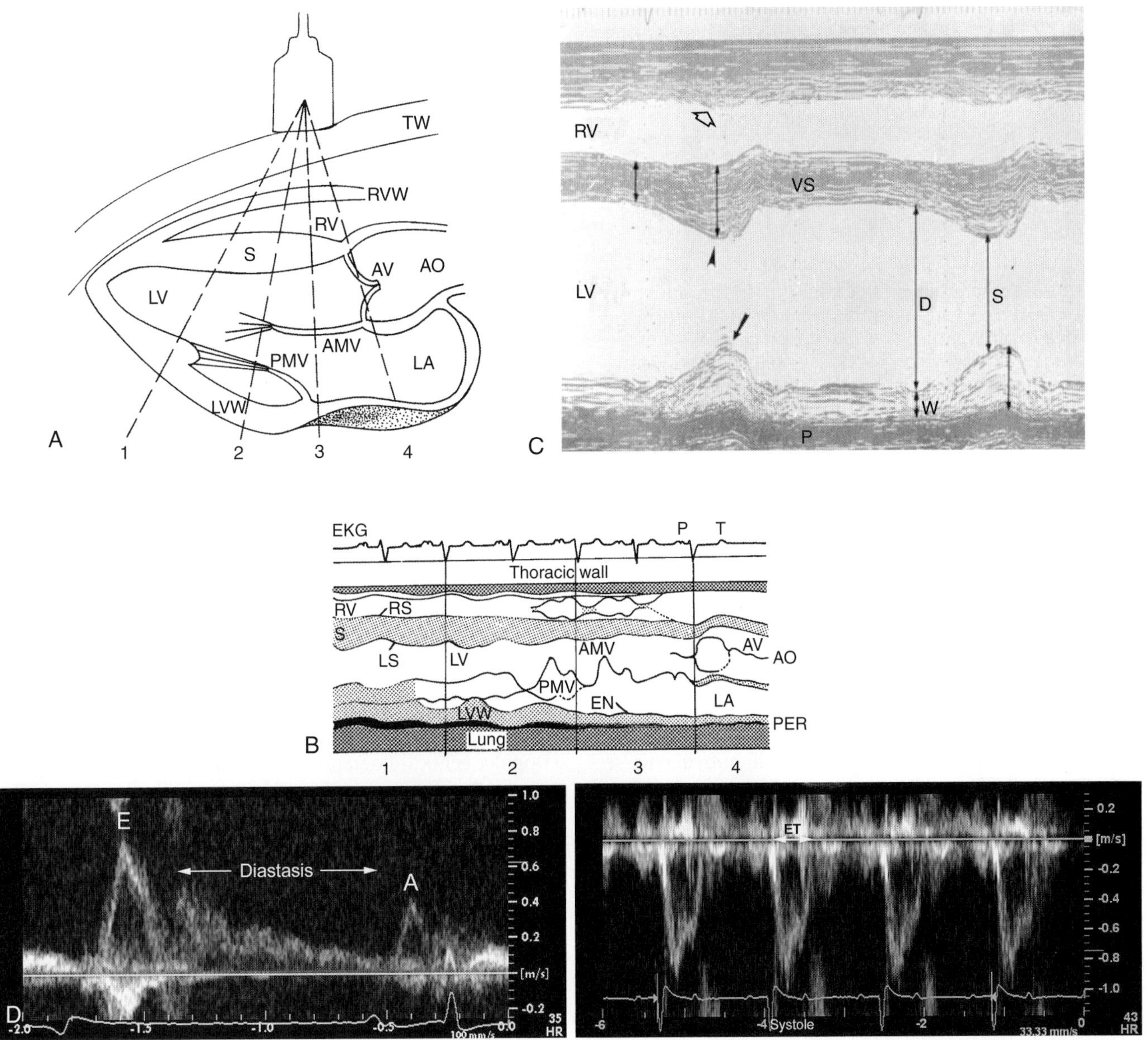

FIGURE 10-5 Ventricular function and echocardiography. **A,** Derivation of the M-mode echocardiogram. The lines demonstrate typical paths of M-mode recording planes (*1,* ventricular/papillary muscle; *2,* chordae tendineae; *3,* anterior mitral valve [AMV]; *4,* aortic root and left atrium [LA]/auricle; *TW,* thoracic wall; *RVW,* right ventricular wall; *RV,* right ventricle; *S,* septum; *LV,* left ventricle; *AV,* aortic valve; *AO,* aortic outflow tract; *LVW,* left ventricular wall; *PMV,* posterior mitral valve; *LA,* left atrium). **B,** The drawing demonstrates the appearance of the M-mode echocardiogram at each level (*PER,* pericardium; *RS, LS,* right and left sides of the ventricular septum; *EN,* endocardium). **C,** M-mode echocardiogram demonstrating the method of measuring left ventricular shortening fraction (LVSF), in which *D* is diastolic dimension and *S* is systolic dimension (LVSF = D – S/D). The prominent thickening of the walls during systole is notable. The end systolic excursion of the LV wall is visible (*arrow*). In practice, the systolic dimensions of the ventricular septum and the LV wall generally are measured along the same line as demonstrated for the LV lumen in systole (*S*) (*W,* LV wall; *VS,* ventricular septum). **D,** *Left:* Doppler echocardiographic recordings of LV filling (*left*) and ejection (*right*). Transmitral inflow is characterized by an early diastolic rapid-filling wave (*E*), low-velocity mid-diastolic filling (diastasis), and a presystolic atrial filling wave (*A*). *Right:* The velocity profile of aortic ejection is characterized by a roughly triangular appearance with rapid acceleration of blood flow into the ascending aorta in early to midsystole and termination of flow at the time of aortic valve closure. The area under the velocity spectrum curve (velocity-time-integral) correlates directly with ventricular stroke volume. The pre-ejection period (the time between the start of the QRS and beginning of ejection) and the ejection times (*ET, arrows*) are load-dependent indices of LV function.

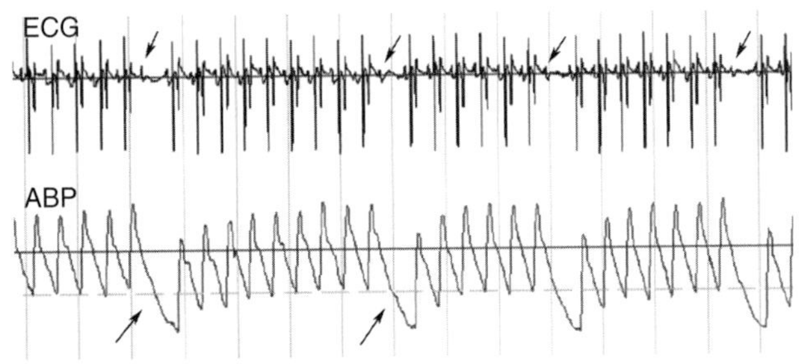

FIGURE 10-6 Compressed electrocardiogram (ECG) with simultaneous arterial blood pressure (ABP) recording in a horse with second-degree atrioventricular block. The progressive increase in ABP triggers a baroreceptor reflex leading to atrioventricular conduction block (*upper arrows*) and a corresponding fall in the ABP (*lower arrows*). Presumably this mechanism, along with sinus arrhythmia and sinus arrest, represents vagally induced mechanisms for controlling ABP in the standing horse.

murmur is often heard during ejection (see Figure 10-4, A). Such murmurs, by definition, must begin after the first sound and end before the second sound. The difference between the diastolic and systolic pressure (pulse pressure) and rate of rise of pressure contribute to a palpable *arterial pulse* during midsystole (see Figures 10-4, *A*, and 10-6). The precise timing of the pulse depends on the proximity of the palpation site relative to the heart. At the end of the *ejection period*, as ventricular pressures fall below those of the corresponding arteries, the semilunar valves close coincident with the high-frequency *second heart sound* (S2) or sounds and the incisura of the arterial pressure curves.[19,23,25] The pulmonary valve may close either after or before the aortic valve.[3,4,238] Asynchronous valve closure may lead to audible splitting of S_2, which is normal but can be extreme in some horses with lung disease. During the ejection period the ventricular volume curve graphs a marked reduction from the end diastolic volume: this volume ejected is defined as the *stroke volume*. The ratio of the stroke volume to the end diastolic volume is the *ejection fraction*, a commonly used index of systolic heart function and correlated to the often-used shortening fraction of the M (motion)-mode echocardiogram (see Figure 10-5). Contraction of the ventricles causes the atrial pressures to decline leading to the *x* descent of the atrial pressure curve and a brief systolic collapse of the jugular vein. Subsequent to atrial filling during ventricular systole, a positive pressure wave, the *v* wave, occurs in the atrial and venous pressure curves. Severe TR accentuates this wave and may lead to pathologic systolic pulsations extending up the jugular furrow. Finally, a decline in ventricular pressure (*isovolumetric relaxation*) occurs, related to off-loading of calcium from the troponin apparatus and resequestration into the sarcoplasmic reticulum. This active ventricular relaxation is associated initially with closure of the semilunar valves and eventually by opening of the AV valves. Relaxation in healthy hearts is enhanced by sympathetic activity. Conversely, myocardial ischemia can impair active relaxation, and it is likely that subendocardial ischemia combined with reduced diastolic filling time contribute to the marked elevations in LA pressures observed during galloping or other high-intensity exercise.[239,240]

Ventricular filling commences just as the AV valves open. As shown in Figure 10-5, *D*, ventricular diastole can be subdivided into three general phases: (1) rapid ventricular filling, (2) diastasis, and (3) atrial contraction.[73,75,76] These phases are readily observed using pulsed-wave Doppler echocardiography or Doppler tissue imaging.[241] Once the ventricles have relaxed and the atrial pressure exceeds the corresponding ventricular pressure, the AV valves open. At that instant, rapid filling ensues with a peak velocity of about 0.5 to 1 m/sec, but varying directly with the heart rate.[149] The ventricular pressures increase only slightly during this phase, whereas the ventricular volume curves change dramatically from the venous return. Rapid filling may be associated with a *functional protodiastolic murmur*, which is concluded by the *third heart sound* (S_3), the low-frequency vibrations occurring near the termination of rapid ventricular filling. The loss of atrial volume and corresponding decline in the atrial pressure (the y descent) is reflected in the jugular furrow as the vein collapses. After rapid filling, a period of greatly reduced low-velocity–filling diastasis ensues. This period may last for seconds during vagal arrhythmias such as sinus bradycardia, pronounced sinus arrhythmia, or second-degree AV block. With markedly exaggerated pauses, the jugular vein may begin to fill prominently. The last phase of diastole is the contribution to ventricular filling caused by the atrial contraction. A functional *presystolic murmur* has been associated with this period between the fourth and first heart sounds.

During the cardiac cycle the atrium functions as a reservoir for blood (ventricular systole), a conduit for venous return (early to mid-diastole), and as a pressure pump (atrial systole). Mechanical atrial function of the LA can be studied using two-dimensional (2D) echocardiography and advanced Doppler echocardiographic methods. Impaired electrical and mechanical function of the atria may predispose to recurrent atrial arrhythmias such as AF.[190,242-245]

ASSESSMENT OF VENTRICULAR FUNCTION

The ability of the ventricles to eject blood depends on both systolic and diastolic ventricular function, as well as heart rate and rhythm (Box 10-3). The most commonly used measurements of overall ventricular performance and circulatory function are invasively or noninvasively determined ABP, rate of ventricular pressure change (dp/dt), CO, stroke volume, ejection fraction, LV shortening fraction, systolic time intervals, central venous pressure, PA or wedge pressures, and arteriovenous oxygen difference (A-V DO_2).* CO, the amount of blood pumped by the left (or right) ventricle in 1 minute (L/min), is the product of ventricular stroke volume (ml/beat) multiplied by the heart rate (beats/min; see Figure 10-4, *B*). *Cardiac index* refers to the CO divided by (indexed to) the body surface area (or body mass). CO coupled to systemic vascular resistance determines the mean ABP: an increase in either variable raises mean arterial pressure. Values for CO vary widely with the size and activity of the horse and are often influenced by drug therapy or anesthesia.[210,260-275] A noninvasive estimate of CO can also be obtained using Doppler techniques.[233,234,257,276-285]

Ventricular stroke volume depends on myocardial contractility and loading conditions (preload and afterload; see Figure 10-4, *D*).[24,26] Although traditionally considered independent determinants of myocardial function, these variables are all interconnected and influence force, velocity, and duration of ventricular contraction.[76] Ultimately, the availability

*References 13, 24, 26, 46, 47, 246-259.

BOX 10-3

DETERMINANTS OF CARDIAC FUNCTION

Systolic Function: Determinants of Ventricular Stroke Volume

Preload [+]—ventricular end-diastolic volume
- Determinants of diastolic function (see below)
- Plasma volume
- Venous pressure/venous return

Myocardial inotropism [+]—contractility of the myocardium
- Sympathetic activity
- Myocardial disease
- Drugs (positive or negative inotropic agents)
- Myocardial perfusion

Ventricular afterload [–]—wall tension required to eject blood
- Aortic impedance
- Vascular resistance
- Ventricular volume (tension increases with dilation)
- Ventricular wall thickness (thin walls have higher tension)

Cardiac lesions increasing workload [–]
- Valvular regurgitation (common)
- Valvular stenosis (rare)
- Septal defects and shunts

Diastolic Function: Determinants of Ventricular Filling

Pleural/mediastinal factors (pressure, mass lesions)
Pericardial function (intrapericardial pressure, constriction)
Myocardial relaxation
Myocyte stiffness
Ventricular wall distensibility (chamber and myocyte compliance)
Venous pressure and venous return (must be matched with compliance)
Heart rate and ventricular filling time (shortened by tachycardia)
Myocardial perfusion (ischemia impairs relaxation)
Atrial contribution to filling (lost in atrial fibrillation)
Cardiac rhythm (arrhythmias can alter atrioventricular contraction sequencing)
Atrioventricular valve function

Cardiac Output

Cardiac output = Stroke volume [+] × heart rate [+]

Arterial Blood Pressure

Arterial blood pressure = Cardiac output [+] × vascular resistance [+]

of calcium to the sarcomere is modulated by the inotropic state, the initial myocardial stretch (preload), and the tension that must be generated to eject blood into the vascular system (afterload).

Myocardial *contractility* is increased by catecholamines, calcium, digitalis glycosides, and phosphodiesterase inhibitors.* Contractility is difficult to measure in the clinical setting but can be estimated noninvasively by observing directional changes in load-dependent pre-ejection or ejection phase indices of ventricular function. These include shortening and ejection fractions by M-mode and 2D echocardiography; pre-ejection period, ejection time, flow acceleration, velocity time integral of aortic or pulmonic ejection, and peak myocardial velocity by Doppler echocardiography; and myocardial deformation or strain by computerized analysis of 2D echocardiograms or tissue Doppler studies (see Figure 10-5).[49,50,51,237,303-306] Measured variables will be influenced by physiologic state, altered mildly by day-to-day variation[307,308] or sedatives,[231] and affected markedly by general anesthesia.

Ventricular fiber length or preload is a positive determinant of ventricular systolic function that depends on venous return and ventricular size and distensibility. The normal ventricle is highly preload dependent, such that increases in preload increase stroke volume. Dehydration, venous pooling, loss of atrial contribution to filling (AF), and recumbency all reduce ventricular filling and decrease stroke volume. When hypotension develops consequent to decreased ventricular filling, intravenous (IV) crystalloid or colloid is often administered initially to increase venous pressure and ventricular preload. Increased preload also can be observed in horses with heart disease as a consequence of impaired pump function, cardiac lesions, or fluid retention. Moderate to severe valvular insufficiency increases ventricular filling pressures and preload.[38,105,309-311] The increased ventricular diastolic dimension serves as a compensatory mechanism that maintains forward stroke volume in the setting of a failing ventricle or regurgitant heart valve.

Ventricular preload can be estimated by determining ventricular end diastolic volume or size, as measured by echocardiography, or by measuring venous filling pressures.[310] The measurement of venous filling pressures (central venous pressure, pulmonary diastolic or pulmonary capillary wedge pressure)[310-314] provides an accurate gauge of preload provided that heart rate and ventricular compliance (distensibility) are normal and ventilation is relatively stable. Myocardial ischemia, which impairs myocardial relaxation, and pericardial diseases, which constrict the ventricles, both reduce ventricular compliance; in such cases, the venous filling pressures may not accurately reflect chronic changes in ventricular preload.

Ventricular *afterload* is represented by the ventricular wall tension that must be developed to eject blood and relates to forces impeding this ejection. Peak wall tension occurs immediately before aortic valve opening. Vascular impedance

*References 209, 210, 213, 216, 234, 259, 264, 286-302.

during ejection also relates to the elastic, resistive, and dynamic properties of the connected great vessel and vascular tree. Increases in ventricular chamber size, arterial stiffness, or resistance, as well as marked increases in hematocrit, increase the impedance to ventricular ejection and reduce stroke volume. Afterload is difficult to measure clinically, and although BP is not identical to afterload, it may be used to estimate directional changes in afterload. LV failure, alveolar hypoxia-induced pulmonary vasoconstriction, atelectasis, and PA or venoocclusive diseases are important causes of increased RV afterload. Arterial vasodilators such as hydralazine and angiotensin converting enzyme (ACE) inhibitors decrease afterload.[268,315]

Ventricular synergy refers to the normal method of ventricular activation and contraction. Normal electrical activation causes a burst of activation of great mechanical advantage.[20] Cardiac arrhythmias, especially ventricular rhythm disturbances, can cause dyssynergy (dyssynchrony), with a resultant decrease in stroke volume. Coronary occlusions leading to ischemic myocardial necrosis also cause dyssynergy but are considered relatively rare.[57,108,316]

Structural and functional competency of the cardiac valves and the ventricular septa influence ventricular systolic function. Valvular insufficiency (or the rare stenosis) reduces ventricular stroke volume unless adequate compensation develops from ventricular dilatation and hypertrophy. Ventricular remodeling, combined with heart rate reserve, often allows small septal defects or mild to moderate valvular lesions to be well tolerated even during exercise. However, large defects or severe valvular lesions can create significant volume overload of the left heart, progressive myocardial dysfunction, and heart failure. Development of CHF is particularly likely when an arrhythmia such as AF is superimposed on a serious structural lesion.

Ventricular *diastolic function* determines ventricular filling and preload.[73,75,76,259] Factors that affect diastolic function are indicated in Box 10-3. When diastolic function is abnormal, often greater heart rate and higher venous pressure dependencies occur for maintenance of CO. A well-recognized cause of diastolic dysfunction is constriction or compression of the heart caused by pericardial disease. Marked ventricular chamber dilatation or hypertrophy also decreases ventricular compliance and requires higher ventricular distending pressures for filling. LV diastolic dysfunction as a consequence of severe RV dilatation or hypertrophy can be explained by bulging of the ventricular septum into the LV, which impedes left-sided filling. This influence of ventricular interdependence is observed clinically with chronic pericardial disease and severe pulmonary hypertension. Ventricular diastolic function also is affected by arrhythmias. Persistent tachycardia shortens diastole, cardiac filling time, and coronary perfusion. With AF, the atrial contribution to filling is lost. Junctional and ventricular arrhythmias lead to AV dissociation preventing normal AV sequencing and can also create marked dyssynchrony of ventricular contraction.

Objective measures of diastolic function are complicated, and no good clinical indicator of diastolic function is currently available for horses. However, diastolic dysfunction may be assumed when one of the aforementioned conditions is recognized. It is possible to measure transmitral and tricuspid inflow using Doppler techniques, but these methods are crude and depend on atrial pressure. Tissue Doppler imaging and rate of myocardial deformation also may provide insight into diastolic cardiac function but currently represent investigational techniques in horses.

Imbalance between *myocardial oxygen demand* and delivery can reduce both ventricular systolic and diastolic function and may affect cardiac rhythm as well. This relationship is also relevant when there is airway obstruction or bronchopulmonary disease, which can reduce arterial oxygenation.[317] Myocardial oxygen demand is augmented by increasing myocardial inotropic state, heart rate, and ventricular wall tension (related to preload and afterload).[76] Oxygen delivery depends on coronary anatomy and vasomotion (degree of vessel constriction), diastolic ABP, diastolic (coronary perfusion) time, and metabolic activity of the myocardium.[10,75,318-325] Normal coronary flow is highest to the LV myocardium in the ventricular septum and LV wall.[325] The immediate subendocardial layer of myocardium is probably most vulnerable to ischemic injury,[9,318] and altered ventricular depolarization may develop secondary to an imbalance in oxygen delivery. This probably accounts in part for the ST-T depression and changes in the T waves observed in hypotensive animals and in normal horses during sinus tachycardia. Coronary vasomotion is effective in augmenting coronary perfusion even at high heart rates (up to 200/min in ponies); however, coronary autoregulation is not as effective if diastolic perfusing pressure decreases in the aorta.[319,320,322]

The clinician may use the "double product" of ABP × heart rate as a general estimate of myocardial oxygen demand.[76] Persistent ST segment depression or elevation, especially at rest and normal heart rates, suggests deficient myocardial perfusion. However, ST segment and T wave changes are normal in horses examined during treadmill exercise and are therefore difficult to interpret.

CARDIOVASCULAR EXAMINATION OF THE HORSE

General Approach

A general approach to the recognition and diagnosis of heart disease and an assessment of its severity is summarized in Box 10-4. Undoubtedly, history and auscultation are the most important initial evaluation procedures in the CV examination of the horse. With the exception of abnormalities in ventricular function, normal cardiac auscultation in a horse with good exercise tolerance practically precludes significant heart disease. The initial CV physical examination should include a thorough auscultation of the heart at all valve areas, auscultation of both lung fields, palpation of the precordium, evaluation of the arterial pulses (head and limbs), inspection of the veins, and evaluation of the mucous membranes for pallor, refill time, and cyanosis, which may develop secondary to a right-to-left cardiac shunt or severe respiratory disease (see Box 10-4). An accurate resting heart rate and respiratory rate also should be recorded.

It is worth emphasizing that physical examination and a stethoscope can detect most serious cardiac disorders initially. Sustained or recurrent cardiac arrhythmias are easily discovered through cardiac auscultation and palpation of the arterial pulse, and diagnosis of the rhythm can be verified through electrocardiography. Pericarditis and cardiac tamponade are characterized by muffled heart sounds or pericardial friction rubs, jugular distension, and often RV failure.

BOX 10-4

CLINICAL EXAMINATION OF THE EQUINE CARDIOVASCULAR SYSTEM

History and Physical Examination

Work history and identification of possible hemodynamic dysfunction
Heart rate and rhythm
Examination of the arterial and venous pulses, refill, and pressure
Inspection of the mucous membranes
Evaluation for abnormal fluid accumulation: pulmonary, pleural, peritoneal, and subcutaneous
Auscultation of the heart and lungs
Measurement of arterial blood pressure (indirect method)

Electrocardiography

Heart rate, rhythm, and conduction sequence
P-QRS-T complexes: configuration, amplitude, duration, and axis (axis has limited value in horses)
Postexercise and exercise electrocardiography[†‡]
Holter (digitally recorded) electrocardiogram[†‡]

Echocardiography

M-mode echocardiography: cardiac dimensions and systolic ventricular function, cardiac anatomy and valve motion, and estimation of cardiac output
Two-dimensional echocardiography: cardiac anatomy and size, systolic ventricular function, identification of lesions, and estimation of cardiac output
Doppler echocardiography[‡]: identification of normal and abnormal flow, estimation of intracardiac pressures, estimation of cardiac output, and ventricular function
Postexercise echocardiography[‡]: identification of regional or global wall dysfunction or valve dysfunction exacerbated by exercise

Thoracic Radiography[‡]

Evaluation of pleural space, pulmonary parenchyma, and lung vascularity
Estimation of heart size (more beneficial in foals)

Clinical Laboratory Tests

Complete blood count and fibrinogen to identify anemia or inflammation
Serum biochemical tests, including electrolytes, renal function tests, and muscle enzymes: These studies may be useful for assessing arrhythmias, identifying low cardiac output (azotemia), and recognizing myocardial cell injury (cardiac isoenzymes of creatine kinase or lactic dehydrogenase)
Cardiac troponin-I concentration (cTnI): can be measured at rest and after exercise testing to identify myocardial damage
Serum protein to identify hypoalbuminemia and hyperglobulinemia
Arterial pH and blood gas analysis to evaluate pulmonary and renal function and to assess acid-base status
Urinalysis to identify renal injury from heart failure or endocarditis
Blood cultures for bacteremia and diagnosis of endocarditis
Serum/plasma assays for digoxin, quinidine, and other drugs

Radionuclide Studies[§]

Detection of abnormal blood flow or lung perfusion and assessment of ventricular function

Cardiac Catheterization and Angiocardiography[§]

Diagnosis of abnormal blood flow and identification of abnormal intracardiac and intravascular pressures

Modified from Bonagura JD: Clinical evaluation and management of heart disease, *Equine Vet Educ* 2:31–37, 1990.
*Most important part of the cardiac evaluation.
†May be needed to identify paroxysmal atrial fibrillation.
‡Generally done after referral.
§Not commonly performed.

Significant myocardial disease is usually associated with heart failure, arrhythmias, or a cardiac murmur, especially when ventricular dilatation or dysfunction causes insufficiency of the mitral or tricuspid valves. The presence of a cardiac murmur is the essential finding that leads one to consider degenerative or infective valvular disease or a congenital heart malformation.[111,156]

Laboratory studies, electrocardiography, and echocardiography are additional tests that are particularly useful in recognizing the underlying basis and severity of CV disease. Mild or subtle CV disease may require a detailed examination, including exercise testing before abnormalities can be objectively detected.[326-332]

History

Cardiovascular disease may be suspected from the history or a serendipitous finding during the course of a routine examination.* The horse with CHF may be presented for generalized venous distention, jugular pulsations, or edema. Conversely, other cardiac problems such as arrhythmia or murmur can be incidental findings, detected during a routine physical, prepurchase, or insurance examination. Once an abnormality has been found, a complete CV examination is aimed at

*References 32, 111, 112, 196, 256, 333-335.

BOX 10-5

CARDIOVASCULAR ASSOCIATION OF POOR PERFORMANCE

Arrhythmias

Atrial premature complexes
Ventricular premature complexes
Atrial fibrillation
Supraventricular tachycardia
Ventricular tachycardia
Advanced second-degree atrioventricular block
Complete third-degree atrioventricular block

Congenital, Valvular, or Myocardial Heart Diseases Associated with Murmurs

Ventricular septal defect
Mitral regurgitation
Tricuspid regurgitation
Aortic regurgitation
Cardiomyopathy with secondary atrioventricular valvular regurgitation

Occult Heart Disease

Pericardial disease
Cardiomyopathy or myocarditis
Ischemic myocardial disease (?)

Vascular Disorders

Aortic-iliac thrombosis
Jugular vein thrombosis/thrombophlebitis (bilateral)
Aortic root rupture (aorto-cardiac fistula)
Peripheral vein thrombosis/thrombophlebitis

BOX 10-6

CAUSES OF SUDDEN CARDIOVASCULAR DEATH

Electric Disorders of the Heart (Arrhythmias)

Ventricular tachycardia, flutter, or fibrillation
Complete atrioventricular block
Asystole

Toxic Injury to the Heart

Acute myocardial failure
Anesthetics
Drug- or toxin-induced arrhythmia
Toxic plants
Myocardial toxins
Systemic toxin secondarily affecting the heart

Cardiac Tamponade

Bacterial pericarditis
Idiopathic pericarditis
Viral pericarditis
Trauma

Hemorrhage

Rupture of the heart (with cardiac tamponade)
Rupture of the aorta or pulmonary artery (with or without cardiac tamponade)
Arterial rupture
  Middle uterine artery
  Mesenteric, omental, or other large arteries
Severe pulmonary hemorrhage
Rupture of the spleen or liver
Brain hemorrhage

Embolism

Carotid air embolism
Coronary embolism or thrombosis

Electrocution

Lightning
Alternating current electrocution

Cardiac Trauma

Cardiac catheterization or needle puncture of a ventricle leading to ventricular fibrillation
Penetrating thoracic wound

determining the lesion and the significance of disease in terms of safety, performance capabilities, and expected longevity.

The horse with clinically apparent CV disease may have subtle performance problems that are only apparent at peak performance levels. For example, slowing in the last quarter to three eighths of a race is a common historical complaint. In many cases, performance may deteriorate by only 2 to 3 seconds. In other horses, particularly in cases of AF, racing performance may decline greatly by 20 to 30 seconds or more. Horses with malignant VT may stop abruptly or even collapse. Horses with CV disease also may demonstrate excessively high heart and respiratory rates during and after exercise or may take a longer than normal time to return to a resting rate (or "cool out"). Coughing, either at rest or during exercise, tachypnea, and exercise-induced pulmonary hemorrhage are respiratory signs reported in some horses with heart disease. CV disease must always be considered along with musculoskeletal, respiratory, metabolic, and neurologic problems in the differential diagnosis of poor performance (Box 10-5).[54-56,122,317,336,337] Other performance-related problems with CV disease can include weakness, ataxia, collapse, and sudden death (Box 10-6).[52,57-68,219]

AUSCULTATION

CLINICAL METHOD

Cardiac auscultation is the systemic examination of the heart using a stethoscope. Auscultation is expedient and relatively sensitive for detection of serious heart disease when performed by a knowledgeable and experienced examiner. It provides information about heart rate, persistent arrhythmias, and presence or absence of congenital and acquired heart diseases. Pericardial diseases also may be recognized by auscultation. Auscultation should be conducted within the context of a medical history and general physical examination, which includes assessment of the precordium and pulses, auscultation of the thorax, and inspection for edema and abnormal ventilatory patterns.

Effective auscultation requires an understanding of anatomy, physiology, pathophysiology, and sound. Extensive clinical data regarding cardiac auscultation in the horse have been published* and experience with Doppler echocardiography has refined the clinician's understanding of heart sounds and murmurs.[130,145,354] Experience and training are also significant factors in effective cardiac auscultation,[355,356] and this examination method should be considered an acquired skill that can be constantly honed. The overall sensitivity of auscultation is high for identification of congenital heart diseases, *significant* valvular disease, and *persistent* cardiac arrhythmias. Sensitivity is lower for primary myocardial or pericardial diseases, unless obvious associated abnormalities exist (e.g., murmur, arrhythmia, prominent friction rub). The specificity of auscultation in the horse (e.g., the ability to distinguish a functional from a pathologic murmur or identify a specific flow disturbance) has not been sufficiently studied but most certainly depends on the clinician's knowledge and experience,[355] as well as one's opinion related to the physiologic versus pathologic nature of valvular regurgitation in some high-performance horses.

A prerequisite for auscultation is an appreciation of the normal heart sounds, the genesis of which has already been described (see Clinical Cardiovascular Physiology). The examiner must be familiar with the causes and clinical features of arrhythmias and murmurs (Tables 10-1, 10-2, and 10-3) and the areas for auscultation (Figure 10-8).† Auscultation is best carried out in a very quiet area because extraneous noise makes detection of soft to moderate murmurs quite difficult. The horse or foal should be sufficiently restrained so that the examiner can concentrate on listening. The venous pulse should be inspected and then the arterial pulse and the precordium palpated before commencing auscultation. Although uncommonly used today, practiced examiners can use percussion of the precordial area effectively to identify the region of cardiac dullness to identify heart size.[357]

The stethoscope examination generally commences on the left side. Both stethoscope chest pieces—the diaphragm (applied tightly) and the bell (applied lightly)—should be used. When using a single-piece tunable diaphragm, the pressure on the chest piece should be gradually increased to optimize the sounds of interest. All auscultatory areas should be examined. The locations of the cardiac valve areas can be identified using the following method:

- The left apical impulse located at the left thoracic wall is adjacent to or under the olecranon near the fifth intercostal space; this location identifies the ventral region of the LV inlet. The mitral valve is dorsal to the cardiac impulse, but mitral sounds and murmurs often project well to the apex while also radiating dorsally into the LA. The first heart sound (S_1) is best heard at this location, and the ventricular filling or third heart sound (S_3) is also heard well over this point.
- The aortic valve area is located one (or two) intercostal spaces cranially and is dorsal to the left apical impulse. The second sound (S_2) is loudest at this point, and aortic valve murmurs are heard best over this valve. The murmur of MR may also radiate dorsally and cranially to this area. Because of the central location of the aortic valve and the orientation of the ascending aorta to the right, aortic flow murmurs and the murmur of aortic regurgitation (AR) generally can be heard bilaterally, just medial to the triceps muscles.
- The pulmonic valve is located slightly cranioventral (generally one intercostal space) to the aortic valve, and the pulmonary component of S_2 is loudest at this point. This is also the location where splitting of the second sound is most obvious. The main PA extends dorsally from the pulmonic valve, high on the left cranial base. Murmurs that radiate into the PA are heard best at this location, including some functional murmurs and the murmur of patent ductus arteriosus (PDA). The murmur associated with an atrial septal defect (ASD) or a subarterial VSD, as well as the rare murmur of pulmonic stenosis, are typically loudest over the pulmonary valve and PA.
- The tricuspid valve area is located over a wide area on the right hemithorax, dorsal to the sternum and just cranial to the mitral valve; sounds and murmurs associated with tricuspid valve disease are usually heard best over the right hemithorax. Murmurs of paramembranous VSD are often detected ventral and slightly cranial to the tricuspid valve area, dorsal to the sternum.

It is worthwhile to concentrate first on the individual heart sounds when assessing the heart rhythm, because the generation of cardiac sounds depends on the underlying electrical rhythm and heart murmurs are timed relative to the heart sounds (Figure 10-9). The atrial sound (S_4) is heard after the P wave. The first and second heart sounds (S_1 and S_2) encompass systole, indicating the presence of a QRS complex. A murmur detected between the first and second sounds is termed *systolic*. In contrast, a murmur heard after S_2 is designated as *diastolic*. The distinctive atrial sound (S_4) is absent in AF. Normal variation in the P-R interval causes gradual changes in the S_4 to S_1 interval. Absence of a QRS complex, which occurs with second-degree AV block and with nonconducted atrial premature complexes (APCs), causes a pause in which the first and second heart sounds are absent. The heart sounds and precordial movements often can be palpated, especially over the left thoracic wall. Frequently the cardiac movements and low-frequency vibrations corresponding to the atrial contraction (S_4), onset of ventricular contraction (S_1), and closure of the semilunar valves (S_2) can be detected. With ventricular volume overloading or vigorous normal filling, an accentuated apex beat and third sound (S_3) will be palpable. Cardiac enlargement or displacement of the heart by an intrathoracic mass may lead to an abnormal location of the cardiac impulse. A loud cardiac murmur is often associated with a palpable vibration or *precordial thrill.*

HEART SOUNDS

Heart sounds should be readily heard on each side of the thorax, although some variability is found based on body type, and sounds are louder over the left thoracic wall. All four heart sounds can be detected in healthy horses, but all may not be present or evident at the same location (see Figures 10-9 and 10-10).[3,23,25] The ventricular filling sound (S_3) is most localized and variable, and may be difficult to detect unless the bell is placed lightly over the left apex. The intensity of the heart sounds should be consistent when the rhythm is regular, but variation of heart sound intensity occurs with arrhythmias (irregular cardiac filling). Muffled heart sounds are heard with pericardial effusions or pericardial abscesses (the muffling may only be on one side of the thorax) but also occur in some horses with large pleural

*References 3, 16, 19, 23, 25, 27, 32, 36, 48, 77, 111, 112, 134, 182, 196, 238, 256, 338-353.

†References 3, 19, 52, 57-65, 77, 219, 333-335, 340, 341, 343.

TABLE 10-1

Auscultation of Cardiac Arrhythmias

Rhythm	Heart Rate per Minute	Heart Sounds	Auscultation
SINUS MECHANISMS			
Sinus rhythm	Variable	S4-1-2 (3)*	Rate and rhythm dependent on autonomic tone
Sinus arrest/block	<26	S4-1-2 (3)	Irregular, long pauses
Sinus bradycardia	<26	S4-1-2 (3)	Generally regular unless escape rhythm develops
Sinus arrhythmia	25-50	S4-1-2 (3)	Irregular, cyclic change in heart rate; often interval varying between S4 and S1; often associated with second-degree atrioventricular block or sinus bradycardia
Sinus tachycardia	>50	S4-1-2-3	Typically regular, but second-degree atrioventricular block may develop if sympathetic tone decreases
SUSTAINED ATRIAL TACHYARRHYTHMIAS			
Atrial tachycardia and atrial flutter	>30	S1-2 (3)	Ventricular regularity and rate dependent on atrioventricular conduction sequence, sympathetic tone; consistent S_4 absent; variable-intensity S_1; may detect independent atrial sounds
Atrial fibrillation	>30	S1-2 (3)	Ventricular response irregular; rate related to sympathetic tone; heart rates consistently above 60 beats/min suggestive of significant underlying heart disease or heart failure; absence of consistent S_4
ECTOPIC RHYTHMS			
Junctional rhythm	26-200	S1-2 (3)	Heart rate usually regular idionodal rhythms or junctional tachycardia; heart rate dependent on the mechanism and sympathetic tone; inconsistent S_4; variable intensity sounds
Ventricular rhythm	26-200	S1-2 (3)	Heart rate possibly regular during monomorphic, unifocal ectopic rhythm or irregular during polymorphic or multifocal ectopic activity; heart rate dependent on the mechanism (e.g., escape rhythm versus ventricular tachycardia); variable intensity and split heart sounds possibly audible
Premature atrial and junctional beats	Varies	Early S1-S2	Intensity of S_1 may be louder or softer than normal; the sounds are not usually split; less than compensatory pause often follows premature beat; nonconducted atrial premature complexes result in pauses but not premature first heart sounds.
Premature ventricular beats	Varies	Early S1-S2	Intensity of S_1 often variable and ventricular beats possibly softer than normal; heart sounds possibly split from asynchronous ventricular activation heart sounds; compensatory pause typically following a premature beat
ATRIOVENTRICULAR BLOCKS			
Incomplete (first- and second-degree)	<50	S4-1-2 (3)	Heart rate variable; cyclic arrhythmia, variable S_4-S_1 interval; some variation in heart sounds
Complete (third-degree)	<26	S4-S1-2 (3)	Ventricular escape rhythm, usually regular; independent atrial (S_4) sounds; variable-intensity heart sounds

*Heart sounds in parentheses may be audible.

effusions and cranial mediastinal masses. Accentuation of all heart sounds, especially the third sound, may be detected with volume-loaded ventricles or with marked sympathetic activity. Projection of heart sounds over a wider area is sometimes evident in cases of pleuropneumonia with pulmonary consolidation.

The first heart sound varies with arrhythmias and often becomes louder (or sometimes softer) after prolonged diastolic periods. This in itself is not diagnostic of an abnormality. Splitting of the first heart sound, if pronounced, may indicate abnormal ventricular electrical activation or ventricular premature complexes.[238] Close splitting of the first sound may be more obvious when AF is present, and in the absence of an atrial sound, the split S_1 may be misinterpreted as a closely timed S_4 to S_1 complex.

The second sound is loudest normally over the aortic valve area and may be audibly split over the pulmonic valve area.[3,4,238] This sound can be very soft or absent after a premature beat, and it may be obscured by a holosystolic murmur. Audible splitting of S_2 occurs commonly in normal horses, varies with heart rate or respiration, and only infrequently is associated with pulmonary hypertension. The relative closure of the semilunar valves probably varies with the heart rate and PA pressure,[3,238] although the pulmonic component is most often detected after the aortic component in the healthy, resting horse. If the pulmonary component of the second sound develops a tympanic quality, becoming equal to or louder than the aortic component of S_2, then the clinician should consider pulmonary hypertension. Identification of a loud pulmonic S_2 is a useful clinical finding in cases of right-sided heart failure because it often indicates that a lesion on the *left* side of the heart has led to pulmonary hypertension and right-sided CHF.

Diastolic transient sounds are normal.[16,17,19,350] The atrial sound (S_4) should be detected in virtually all horses, and this sound may be quite loud in some cases. Isolated atrial sounds are commonly ausculted at slow resting heart rates caused by second-degree AV block; however, multiple isolated S_4 sounds indicate high-grade AV block. The ventricular sound (S_3) is normal and as a low-pitched sound may be difficult to hear. The sound often increases transiently in the setting of sinus tachycardia and enhanced rapid filling. This sound also achieves greater intensity when ventricular dilatation and elevated filling pressures develop, as with heart failure.

Other sounds may be detected with heart disease. Systolic clicks are uncommonly heard over the great vessels where they are thought to be benign. A systolic click loudest over the mitral area may be a marker for mitral valve disease or prolapse of the valve into the LA. Constrictive pericardial disease can create a loud early diastolic ventricular filling sound, a ventricular "knock," indicating abrupt termination of rapid filling under high venous pressures. In addition to muffling of sounds, pericarditis is often associated with a pericardial friction rub. These rubs are classically detected during three portions of the cardiac cycle (systole, early diastole, late diastole). These sounds must be distinguished from pleural friction rubs or respiratory mediated sounds, which are occasionally associated with the cardiac cycle. Pleural and pulmonary rubs tend to be heard only during one or two phases of the cardiac cycle and may not correlate closely.

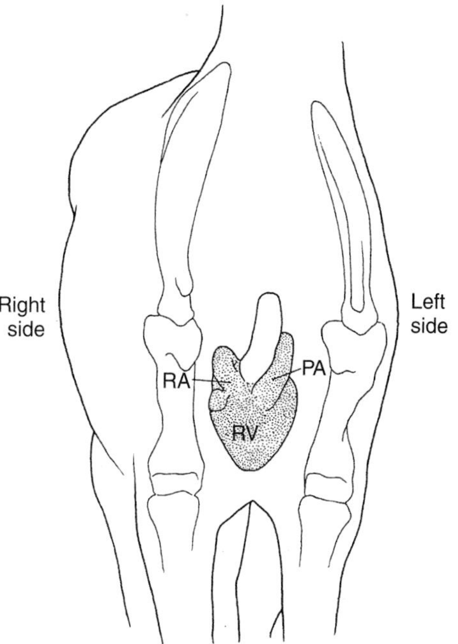

FIGURE 10-7 Cranial view of the heart demonstrating the U shape of the right ventricle *(RV)*. The tricuspid valve and the right ventricular inlet are located on the right side, whereas the outlet and pulmonary artery *(PA)* are on the left side. Murmurs of tricuspid regurgitation and perimembranous ventricular septal defects are typically loudest over the right hemithorax, whereas flow murmurs, and those caused by subaortic or subpulmonic septal defects are loudest over the left cardiac base. *RA,* Right atrium. (From Bonagura JD, Muir WW: The cardiovascular system. In Muir WW, Hubbell JAE, editors: *Equine anesthesia,* St. Louis, 1991, Mosby-Year Book.)

HEART RATE AND RHYTHM

Heart rate can change rapidly and dramatically, varying with autonomic efferent traffic and level of physical activity. Changes in the rate and rhythm are reflected in cardiac auscultation and palpation of the pulse (see Table 10-1).[344] The normal arterial pulse and cardiac rhythm is regular or cyclically irregular. Heart rate in mature horses varies between 28 and 44 beats/min, although slightly slower heart rates can be detected in some very fit racehorses and higher heart rates are often present in foals,[348] yearlings, draft horses,[358] and healthy but nervous horses. An elevated resting heart rate is commonly detected with late pregnancy, fever, pain, hypovolemia, severe anemia, infection, or shock. Persistent, otherwise unexplained tachycardia is also typical of heart failure wherein the standing heart rate usually exceeds 60 beats/min.

Physiologic arrhythmias associated with high resting vagal tone must be differentiated from pathologic arrhythmias. Vagal-induced arrhythmias are most often observed in healthy relaxed horses. The most common of these are sinus arrhythmia and second-degree AV block (see Figure 10-6), which is reported in 15% to 18% of normal horses at rest and has been detected in up to 44% of normal horses with 24-hour continuous electrocardiographic monitoring.[194,197,199,359,360] This arrhythmia is most common in fit racehorses or in other high-performance animals and disappears with stimulation of sympathetic nervous system activity. Sinus arrhythmia also occurs regularly in horses and is often associated with sinus bradycardia and resting heart rates between 24 to 28 beats/min. Sinus arrhythmia may wax and wane with respiration; however, synchronization with ventilation is not a consistent finding in the horse, and it is more likely related to changes in baroreceptor activity. SA block and SA arrest occur sporadically in fit horses. Because these physiologic arrhythmias are associated with high vagal tone, it is typical for the heart rate to range from a low-normal value to overt bradycardia. Maneuvers that reduce vagal activity and increase sympathetic tone can be undertaken to ensure that the rhythm becomes normal. Successful methods include leading the horse through three or four tight circles, jogging, or lunging. It should be recognized, however, that some horses redevelop physiologic AV block within 10 to 60 seconds after such maneuvers. If the arrhythmia persists after exercise, or if the auscultatory findings suggest another arrhythmia (see Table 10-1), then an ECG should be obtained.

The arrhythmias associated with heart disease occur most often with normal to increased heart rates, with the exception of advanced second-degree and complete (third-degree) AV block.* Atrial premature beats are characterized by a regular cardiac

*References 2, 4, 33, 111, 344, 361-363.

TABLE 10-2

Causes of Cardiac Murmurs

Cardiac Murmur	Lesion Identified by Echocardiography, Catheterization, or Necropsy
Functional murmurs*	No identifiable lesions
Congenital heart disease murmurs	Defect(s) in the atrial or ventricular septa; patent ductus arteriosus; atresia/stenosis of the tricuspid or pulmonic valve; valve stenosis; other malformations of the heart
Mitral regurgitation	High-level training; degenerative thickening of the valve; bacterial endocarditis; mitral valve prolapse into left atrium; rupture of a chorda tendinea; dilated-hypokinetic ventricle (dilated cardiomyopathy); papillary muscle lesion or dysfunction; valvulitis; malformation
Tricuspid regurgitation	High-level training†; same causes as for as mitral regurgitation; also pulmonary hypertension from severe left-sided heart failure or chronic respiratory disease
Aortic regurgitation	Degeneration of the aortic valve; congenital fenestration of the valve; bacterial endocarditis‡; aortic prolapse into a ventricular septal defect or the left ventricle; flail aortic valve leaflet; valvulitis; malformation; ruptured aorta or aortic sinus of Valsalva
Pulmonary insufficiency	Bacterial endocarditis‡; pulmonary hypertension; flail pulmonic valve leaflet; valvulitis; malformation; rupture of the pulmonary artery
Murmur associated with vegetative endocarditis	Insufficiency of the affected valve‡

Modified from Bonagura JD: Clinical evaluation and management of heart disease, *Equine Vet Educ* 2:31–37, 1990.

*Functional murmur may be innocent (unknown cause) or physiologic (suspected physiologic cause). Functional murmurs are common in foals and trained athletes (athletic murmur), associated with fever and high sympathetic nervous system activity (pain, stress, sepsis), and often are heard in anemic horses. Functional murmurs depend on the physiologic state and can be altered by changing the heart rate. Such dynamic auscultation is useful in detecting functional murmurs.

†Doppler echocardiography can identify "silent" regurgitation across a right-sided cardiac valve in some horses; this is probably a normal finding of no clinical significance.

‡Anatomic stenosis generally is caused by a large vegetation and also should be associated with a diastolic murmur of valvular insufficiency; increased flow across the valve, even in the absence of a true stenosis, may generate a murmur of "relative" valvular stenosis (e.g., with aortic regurgitation a systolic ejection murmur may occur because of an increased stroke volume).

rhythm, which is suddenly interrupted by earlier than normal beats. Because the sinus node is reset during an atrial premature beat, the following pause is usually incomplete or less than compensatory (provided the underlying sinus rhythm is regular). Premature atrial beats can also be blocked in the AV node, leading to a sudden pause in the rhythm without a premature first heart sound. A ventricular premature beat is often followed by a fully compensatory pause unless the extrasystole is interpolated between two normal sinus beats. Pulse deficits (more first sounds than arterial pulses) are common with premature beats.

Atrial fibrillation is characterized by an irregularly irregular pulse and ventricular rhythm, with some beats occurring sooner than expected, and with pauses in the rhythm demonstrating no consistent diastolic interval. The atrial contraction and hence the fourth sound are absent in AF. Infrequently, AF develops with recurring periodicity of cycle lengths that can cause difficulty in distinguishing this from second-degree AV block.[191,193,201] Another diagnostic pitfall can be the presence of a split first sound, because the clinician may mistake this for a closely timed S_4 to S_1 complex.

Conversely, atrial tachycardia can be conducted with patterns leading to a rapid but regular heart rhythm. However, most horses with atrial tachycardia develop irregular rhythms owing to frequent block of atrial impulses in the AV node, especially at rest. Heart rates are usually higher than normal at rest. Auscultation of the horse in a quiet area may reveal isolated audible fourth heart sounds associated with the second-degree AV block.

Junctional or nodal tachycardia and VT are usually manifested by a rapid regular rhythm, although some VTs cause an irregular rhythm. Owing to associated AV dissociation or abnormal ventricular activation, the heart sounds may sound split or variable in intensity.

CARDIAC MURMURS

Cardiac murmurs are prolonged audible vibrations developing in a usually quiet portion of the cardiac cycle. In general, murmurs are manifestations of either normal (functional) or abnormal (pathologic) blood flow in the heart and blood vessels. Although many heart murmurs are functional (physiologic, athletic, innocent), other murmurs provide evidence of heart disease and may require further investigation. Most *functional* cardiac murmurs are caused by vibrations that attend the *ejection* of blood from the heart during systole or the *rapid filling* of the ventricles during early diastole.* Causes of abnormal murmurs include incompetent cardiac valves, septal defects, vascular lesions, and (very rarely) valvular stenosis (see Tables 10-2 and 10-3). The continuous murmur of PDA is a normal finding in full-term foals for up to 3 days after parturition, but it occasionally persists for almost 1 week after foaling.[265,343,348,367]

One of the challenges of physical diagnosis is determination of the cause and clinical significance of a cardiac murmur. With knowledge and experience, the clinician can accurately determine the *likelihood* that a murmur is physiologic or pathologic in origin and efficiently select animals requiring additional

*References 18, 19, 32, 36, 134, 256, 333, 340, 343, 351, 364-366.

TABLE 10-3

Diagnostic Algorithm for Cardiac Auscultation in the Horse

Auscultation		Considerations		Further Observations		Probable Assessment		Other Tests
Irregular Rhythm	→	Vagally-mediated or Abnormal rhythm	⇒	Induce increased sympathetic tone[^] ⇓				
				↑ Rate & *regular* rhythm	→	Vagally-mediated (physiologic) rhythm[*]	→	None
				↑ Rate & *irregular* rhythm	→	Abnormal cardiac rhythm (see Table 10-1 for details)	→	ECG, ±Echo Electrolyes, Troponin-1
Regular tachycardia <90 beats/min[+]	→	Sympathetic activation [Pain, Volume depletion Infection, Anemia, Heart failure, etc.] or Ectopic cardiac rhythm	⇒	Manage underlying disorder ⇓				
				Appropriate HR reduction with normal heart sounds	→	Physiologic sinus tachycardia	→	None
				OR				
				Persistent Tachycardia abnormal heart sounds	→	Persistent sinus or ectopic tachycardia[$]	→	ECG, ±Echo Electrolyes, Troponin-1
Loud cardiac murmur with a precordial thrill	→	Organic heart disease	⇒	Determine timing & PMI (see below)	→	Congenital or acquired heart disease	→	Echo
Systolic murmur PMI: Left thorax	→	Functional or Organic	⇒	PMI: pulmonic or aortic valve Crescendo-decrescendo				
				Grade: 1 to 3/6[%]	→	Functional ejection murmur	→	None[#]
				Grade: 4 to 6/6	→	Congenital heart defect[&]	→	Echo
				PMI: mitral valve or left apex Any grade or configuration	→	Mitral regurgitation	→	Echo
Systolic murmur PMI: Right thorax	→	Organic Murmur	⇒	PMI: tricuspid valve Any grade or configuration	→	Tricuspid regurgitation	→	Echo[#]
				PMI: cranioventral thorax Holosystolic	→	Ventricular septal defect (VSD)	→	Echo
Diastolic murmur PMI: Left or right thorax	→	Functional or Organic	⇒	Brief (protodiastolic or presystolic) Soft or musical murmur	→	Functional murmur (or trivial AR)	→	None[#]
				PMI: aortic or pulmonic valve Holodiastolic	→	Aortic regurgitation (AR) or Pulmonic regurgitation with pulmonary hypertension	→ →	Echo[#] Echo[#]

Continued

TABLE 10-3

Diagnostic Algorithm for Cardiac Auscultation in the Horse—cont'd

Auscultation		Considerations		Further Observations		Probable Assessment		Other Tests
Continuous murmur PMI: Left or right thorax	→	Organic murmur	⇒	PMI: Pulmonary artery Foal or other signs of CHD	→	Patent ductus arteriosus (PDA) or a systemic to pulmonary shunt	→	Echo
				Mature horse	→	Aortic to cardiac fistula or Aortic to pulmonary artery fistula	→	Echo
Pericardia Friction Rub**	→	Organic murmur	⇒	Systolic or multi-phasic Distant (muffled) heart sounds Jugular venous distension	→	Pericarditis	→	Echo

Footnotes

^Endogenous sympathetic activity can be transiently increased by suddenly leading the horse in four or five tight circles or through trotting or lunging; the horse should be examined *immediately* after the activity has stopped.

*Vagally induced rhythms include sinus bradycardia, pause or arrest, sinoatrial block, sinus arrhythmia, and second-degree atrioventricular block.

+Resting tachycardia exceeding 90/minute should be evaluated with an ECG to qualify the rhythm; the cut-off rate is arbitrary but clinically useful.

$Ectopic rhythms include ectopic atrial tachycardia, junctional (nodal) tachycardia, and ventricular tachycardia.

%Functional murmurs due to ejection of blood into the great vessels often become transiently louder following an increase in sympathetic activity.

&Loud ejection murmurs over the semilunar valves and great vessels may indicate pulmonic stenosis or complex defects such as tetralogy of Fallot.

#Judgment should be exercised regarding the need for echocardiography. An echocardiogram might be indicated in the pre-purchase examination of any valuable foal or horse with a cardiac murmur; whereas, echocardiography may not be indicated in an older horse with a soft murmur of aortic regurgitation with normal arterial pulses or in a fit racehorse with a typical murmur of tricuspid regurgitation.

**Classic pericardial friction rubs are heard during systole, early diastole, and late diastole. Occasionally a functional pre-systolic murmur exhibits a frequency quality similar to a brief friction rub.

Abbreviations & Terminology:

- *Configuration* = the phonocardiographic 'shape' of a murmur, for example a plateau-shaped murmur that extends from the first sound through the second sound is termed holosystolic or pansystolic (e.g. MR or VSD); a 'diamond-shaped' murmur is crescendo-decrescendo in configuration (e.g., functional ejection); a "blowing" murmur that starts suddenly but dissipates gradually is decrescendo (e.g., aortic regurgitation), while a murmur that becomes progressively louder and then stops is crescendo in configuration (e.g., MR from mitral valve prolapse)
- *ECG* = perform an electrocardiogram to determine heart rhythm
- *Echo* = perform an echocardiogram to identify abnormal structure, cardiac size, or function; Doppler studies are added to assess normal and abnormal blood flow patterns and are optimal for evaluating horses with cardiac murmurs; Doppler studies must be interpreted relative to auscultatory findings.
- *Grade* = intensity of the murmur on a 1 through 6 scale; in most systems a grade 5 or 6 murmur is accompanied by a precordial thrill
- *HR* = heart rate
- *Organic* = related to a structural lesion in the heart or great vessels
- *PMI* = point of maximal murmur intensity
- *Precordial thrill* = the palpable thoracic vibration associated with a loud cardiac murmur
- *Troponin-I* = serum level of inhibitory cardiac troponin or cTn_I, a biomarker used to detect cardiomyocyte injury or necrosis
- *Valve* = refers to the general valve area of auscultation (see text for details)

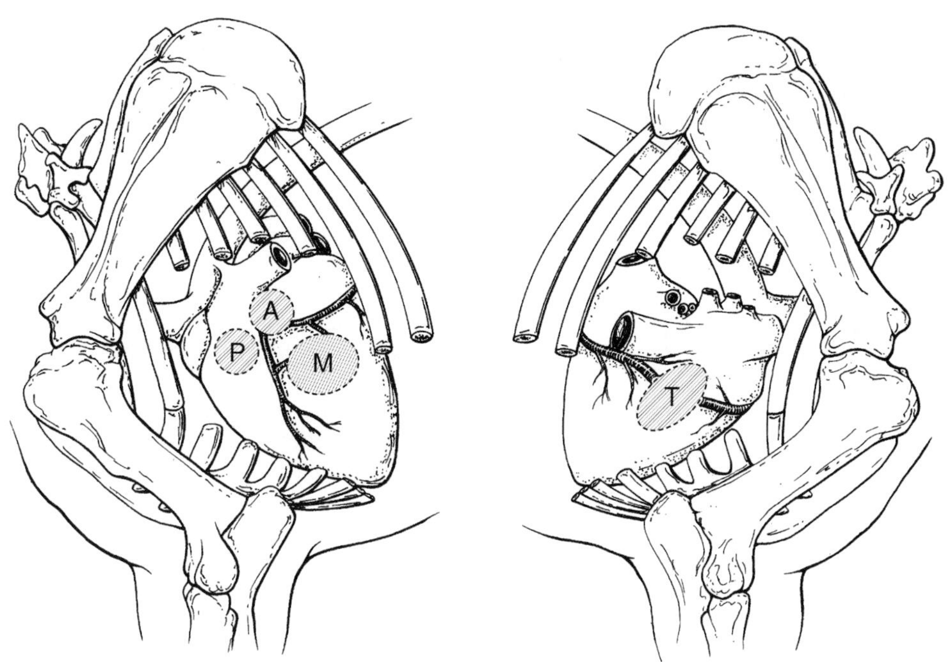

FIGURE 10-8 Cardiac auscultation areas in the horse from the left **(A)** and the right **(B)** side of the thorax. Note the size and anatomic position of the heart within the thorax. The cardiac apex (apical area) is usually located slightly above the level of the olecranon and can be identified by palpation of the apical beat. The cardiac base (basilar area) is located more cranially and at the level of the scapulohumeral joint. The shaded areas represent the respective valve areas (*P,* pulmonic; *A,* aortic; *M,* mitral; *T,* tricuspid). The right atrium (RA) (*above T*), tricuspid valve, and right ventricular (RV) inlet (inflow region, *below T*) are located on the right side of the thorax. Paramembranous ventricular septal defects (VSDs) that communicate with the RV inlet (below the tricuspid valve) are usually heard best along the lower right hemithorax (*below T*) and typically radiate from the right ventricle (RV) into the pulmonary artery (left hemithorax). Most (but not all) murmurs of tricuspid valve disease are heard best over the right chest wall, usually heard best more dorsally as they radiate into the RA (*above T*). The RV outlet projects to the left side of the thorax and continues into the pulmonary artery, which is located at the left dorsal cardiac base (*above P*). Thus murmurs originating in the RV outlet (e.g., murmurs from subpulmonic VSDs) systolic murmurs of relative pulmonic stenosis (from cardiac shunting), murmurs of pulmonic insufficiency (rare), and functional pulmonary arterial murmurs are heard best over the left chest wall *(P)*. The aortic valve is located centrally, and diastolic murmurs of aortic insufficiency may be heard at either hemithorax, although they are usually loudest on the left *(A)*. Functional murmurs generated in the ascending aorta are heard over the cranial basilar region of the heart. The systolic murmur of mitral regurgitation (MR) radiates to the left apex and is usually heard across the left ventricular (LV) inlet (area caudoventral of *M*). The regurgitant mitral jet can be directed craniodorsal or caudodorsal into the left atrium (LA) and can account for variability in murmur radiation. The functional protodiastolic murmurs associated with ventricular filling are usually evident over the ventricular inlets and may be heard on either side of the thorax. (From Reef VB: Cardiovascular system. In Orsini JA, Divers TJ, editors: Manual of equine emergencies: treatment and procedures, ed 2, Philadelphia, 2003, WB Saunders.)

studies. The clinician should describe the *timing, duration, quality or pitch, grade, point of maximal murmur intensity,* and *radiation* of a murmur, as well as the effect of changing heart rate on the sounds. Determination of timing is made relative to the heart sounds so that murmurs are designated as *systolic, diastolic,* or *continuous.* When the overall timing is not obvious, the clinician can either palpate the apical impulse, which occurs in early systole, or the systolic pulse in the brachial or median artery to identify the timing of the murmur. Skilled auscultators subdivide the timing of murmurs into proto-(early), meso-(middle), or tele-(late) systole or diastole, because the timing and duration of the murmur often correlate with specific flow disturbances. Shorter murmurs, especially those occurring in early systole or protodiastole, are more likely to be functional, although this is not always the case. Experience also teaches that relatively loud or long murmurs are more likely to be associated with cardiac pathology (see Figure 10-10 and Table 10-3), but again exceptions occur. The pitch or quality of the murmur provides additional insight. For example, mixed frequency (harsh or blowing) murmurs are typical of cardiac disease. A brief vibratory or musical murmur is typically functional; however, a prolonged musical murmur is suggestive of a valvular lesion. Applying the characteristics of murmurs to the clinical setting requires study, an organized scheme (see Table 10-3), and practice.

Functional, innocent, or physiologic heart murmurs are very common and are not attributed to cardiac pathology. Such murmurs may be related to the large size and tremendous inflow and outflow volumes of the equine heart.[364] Physiologic causes of functional murmurs include fever, high sympathetic activity (e.g., colic, exercise, pain), moderate to severe anemia, and peripheral vasodilation. These murmurs are typically soft (grades 1 to 3/6, of a possible 6), localized, relatively short, crescendo-decrescendo in timing, and labile. Increasing heart rate usually increases the intensity and duration of a functional murmur, although in some horses the murmur becomes less intense. Functional murmurs are neither holosystolic nor holodiastolic; therefore the heart sounds should still be evident.

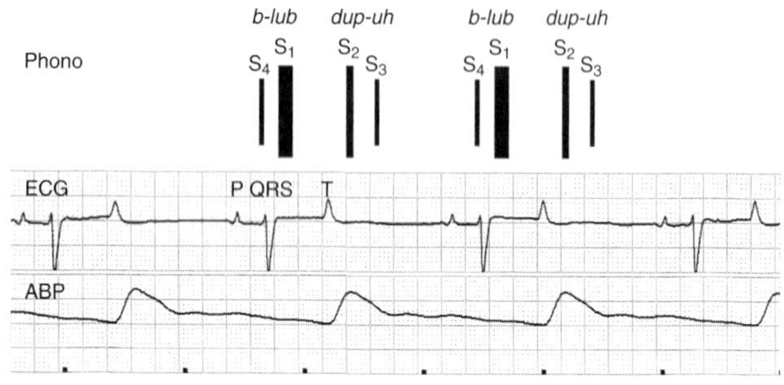

FIGURE 10-9 Schematic diagram of the normal heart sounds (Phono) in relation to a surface electrocardiogram (ECG) and an arterial blood pressure tracing (ABP) recorded from the transverse facial artery. *S1,* First (systolic) heart sound; *S2,* second (diastolic) heart sound; *S3,* third heart sound; *S4,* fourth (atrial) heart sound. *B-lub dup-uh* describes the sounds heard on auscultation. Note the timing of the heart sounds and the (peripheral) pulse pressure wave relative to the ECG. (From Schwarzwald CC, Bonagura JD, Muir WW: The cardiovascular system. In Muir WW, Hubbell JAE, editors: Equine anesthesia: monitoring and emergency therapy, ed 2, St Louis, 2009, WB Saunders.)

The most common functional murmur is the systolic ejection murmur heard over the aortic and pulmonic valves and projecting into their respective arteries at the left cardiac base (see Figure 10-8).[3] The functional ejection murmur is generated by flow into the great vessels, and by definition it must start after S_1 and end before S_2. Nonetheless, in some horses, the functional ejection murmur can achieve substantial intensity (rarely, a grade 4 or 5) and may seem holosystolic at higher heart rates. At times a remarkable change in functional murmur intensity is seen from day to day. An example of this is the varying murmurs identified in some horses with emergent colic. Because a loud functional murmur can radiate caudally, it may be confused with MR. In terms of diagnostic considerations, the clinician should not mistake a functional ejection murmur for that of aortic or pulmonic stenosis. Pulmonic stenosis is rare in the horse, and aortic stenosis even less common. Accordingly, these valvular malformations are rarely entertained in the differential diagnosis. The murmurs resulting from subpulmonic (subarterial) VSDs or the stenosis associated with tetralogy of Fallot may be loudest over the great vessels, but such murmurs are usually loud and prompt echocardiographic investigation.

Functional diastolic murmurs are also common, especially in young horses and in the Thoroughbred breed. These murmurs are generally soft and are detected over the LV or RV inlets—from the dorsal atrium to the ventricular apex. The functional protodiastolic murmur is an early diastolic murmur detected between S_2 and S_3. The murmur may be musical, vibratory, or "squeaky" and typically accentuates

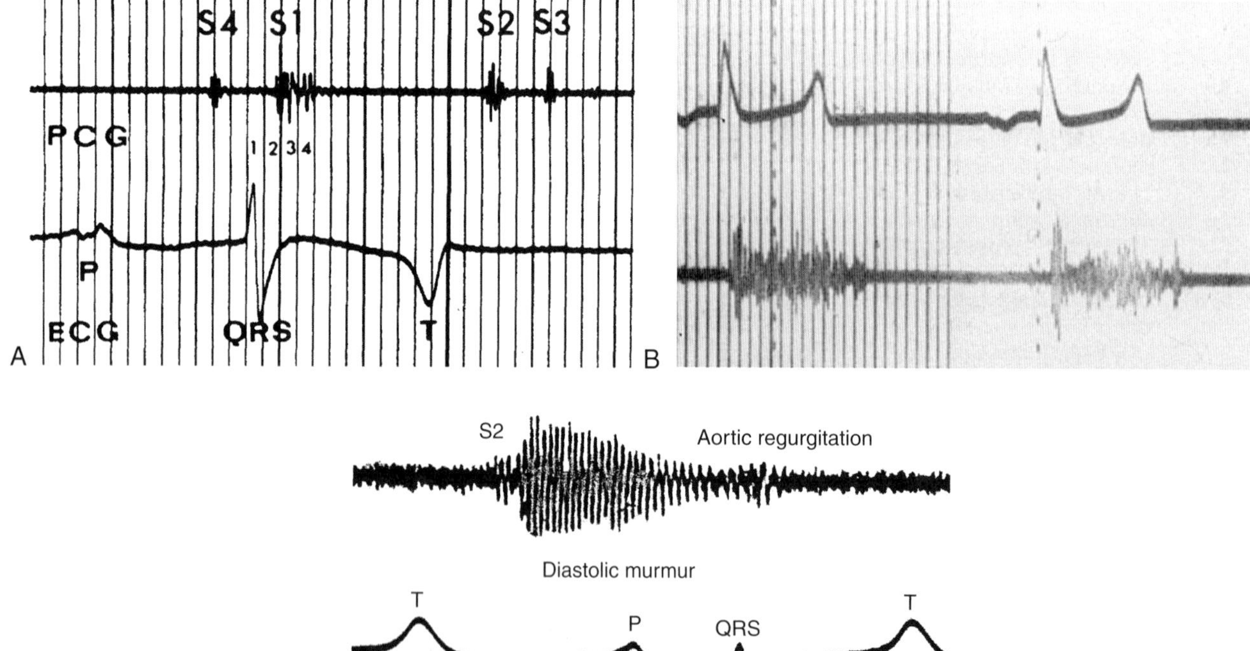

FIGURE 10-10 Phonocardiograms (PCG). **A,** The four normal heart sounds (S1 through S4) are evident in this recording. (The numbers *1* through *4* indicate the various components of the first heart sound; *ECG,* electrocardiogram.) **B,** Systolic murmur recorded from a yearling with a ventricular septal defect (VSD) (P waves on the ECG are negative in this tracing). **C,** Decrescendo, musical, holodiastolic murmur recorded from a horse with aortic regurgitation (AR). The murmur begins in early diastole (after the T wave) and ends at the QRS complex. (A recording courtesy of D. Smetzer, R.L. Hamlin, and C.R. Smith.)

with increased heart rate.[3] It most reasonably represents the rapid early filling of the ventricles. The presystolic functional murmur is heard between S_4 and S_1, and the vibrations may sound like a *rub* or long heart sound after the atrial contraction. It can be confused with an early systolic murmur or a friction rub.

The most commonly detected murmurs associated with structural or *organic heart disease* are those generated by tricuspid regurgitation (TR), MR, AR, and VSD. Typical causes and auscultatory features of these murmurs are indicated in Tables 10-2 and 10-3) and described in detail later in this chapter.

When a murmur is believed to represent underlying cardiac pathology, further investigation is required. The overall significance of the hemodynamic abnormality should include consideration of the work history, general physical examination, presence or absence of heart enlargement or cardiac failure, and results of ancillary tests such as echocardiography, electrocardiography, and exercise performance (or testing). Certainly, the history should be considered, because the horse with excellent performance and good exercise tolerance is less likely to have serious heart disease. Auscultation, however, is insufficient to distinguish trivial from significant heart disease in the poorly performing horse or in a horse with a cardiac arrhythmia. Echocardiography is helpful in these cases to quantify heart size and objectively assess ventricular function. Underlying lesions such as a valve vegetation, ruptured valve chorda tendineae, or dilated cardiomyopathy can be identified or discounted. Although there are no well-defined echocardiographic or Doppler correlates to functional heart murmurs, these studies can document abnormal blood flow and can pinpoint the cause of a pathologic murmur.

PULMONARY AUSCULTATION

Auscultation of the lungs should reveal normal breath sounds with the horse at rest, while ventilating into a rebreathing bag, and after exercise. Decreased or absent airway sounds or large airway sounds in the ventral portions of the thorax indicate a pleural effusion, a common finding in biventricular or right-sided heart failure. Moist or bubbling (fluid) sounds or crackles (i.e., rales) are uncommonly auscultated in the lungs of horses with pulmonary edema and left-sided heart failure. Instead, tachypnea associated with harsh bronchovesicular breath sounds is usually heard, because horses with chronic left-sided CHF seem to develop more interstitial than alveolar pulmonary edema. When alveolar edema does develop, respiratory distress may be severe, crackles may become evident, and free fluid may be auscultated in the trachea. On rare occasion, primarily with peracute left-sided heart failure, froth will be visible at the nares and the horse will cough and expel large quantities of pulmonary edema (Figure 10-11). Such horses demonstrate severe respiratory distress (marked tachypnea and dyspnea), anxiety, and agitation.

Examination of the Peripheral Vasculature

An evaluation of the peripheral vasculature is part of a CV workup and should include examination of the arteries and veins in the head, forelimbs, and hindlimbs. When important, ABP also should be measured. The genesis of the arterial and venous pulses has been described previously. The heart sounds should be correlated with both the jugular and the arterial pulses.

Normal-quality *arterial pulses* should be palpable in the facial, median, carotid, great metatarsal, coccygeal, and digital arteries. The arterial pulse represents the pulse pressure (i.e., the difference between peak systolic and diastolic pressures), the rate of rise of arterial pressure, and the physical characteristics of the artery and surrounding tissues. Palpating the facial artery pulse may identify heart rate and rhythm, as well as altered hemodynamic states. The arterial pulse can be described as *normal, hypokinetic (weak), hyperkinetic,* or *variable.* Irregularity often indicates a cardiac arrhythmia.

Thready or hypokinetic arterial pulses are associated with reduced stroke volume and peripheral vasoconstriction and therefore may be detected in CHF and in diseases associated with volume depletion or profuse hemorrhage. Thready arterial pulses may also be detected only in the hindlimbs with aortoiliac thrombosis. Bounding, hyperkinetic arterial pulses are palpable with clinically significant AR, PDA, and aortic to pulmonary or aortic to right-sided heart fistulas. The pulse in septic animals may be weak, owing to reduced pulse pressure, or normal to rapidly declining if peripheral vasodilation occurs. Marked variation in the intensity of the pulse usually occurs with arrhythmias, particularly AF and rapid or multiform VT. A pulse deficit (first heart sound without palpable pulse) occurs when developed LV pressure does not exceed aortic pressure. Deficits are likely to be palpated in association with pathologic arrhythmias, particularly premature beats, or after very short diastolic periods of tachyarrhythmias.

Palpation of the arterial pulse cannot quantify the actual ABP, which must be measured directly by arterial puncture or cannulation or indirectly using various auscultatory, Doppler, or oscillometric techniques.[71,253,269,368-393] Percutaneous placement of an arterial catheter in the facial or transverse tibial artery is frequently used to monitor pressure invasively in critically ill or anesthetized horses. Indirect methods have been used successfully to monitor pressure in the coccygeal artery; however, these methods are less sensitive in hypotensive animals and may lag in response during rapid changes in BP.[371,373,375] Attention must be directed to placement and

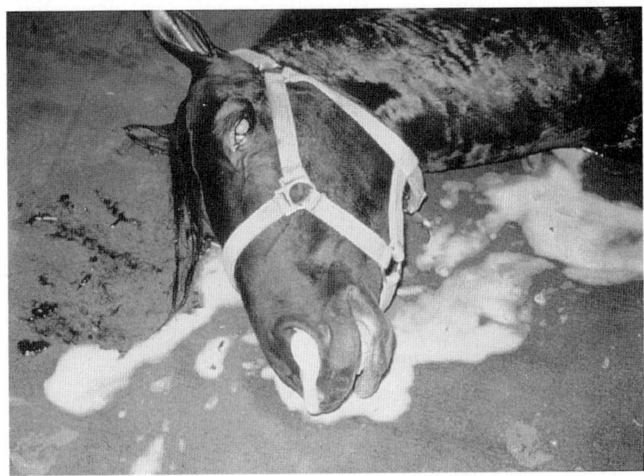

FIGURE 10-11 Peracute pulmonary edema in a horse with a ruptured chorda tendinea. The photo was taken immediately after euthanasia. An important note is that tracheal froth is often a postmortem artifact, particularly when observed hours after death.

diameter of the occluding cuff when indirect methods are used,[385] and the optimal width of the cuff (bladder) is between approximately one quarter to one fifth of the circumference of the tail when measuring pressure in the middle coccygeal artery.[379,384] The arterial pulse wave itself varies, depending on the site of measurement, and the distal arterial systolic pressure may be higher, and the diastolic pressure lower, than the corresponding central aortic pressures.

ABP monitoring includes determination of systolic, diastolic, and mean pressures. Arterial pressure is determined by the interplay between stroke volume, heart rate, and vascular resistance (see Box 10-3 and Figure 10-4, *B*). Marked increases in CO can lead to significant increases in ABP with systolic pressures exceeding 200 mm Hg.[246,390,394]

Normal reported values for indirect arterial pressure are 111.8 mm Hg systolic (ranging between 79 to 145 mm Hg) and 67.7 diastolic (ranging between 49 to 106 mm Hg).* BP is lowest in neonates and rises during the first month of life to the normal adult range.[253,373] Some variation is found among breeds. Draft breeds tend to have lower pressures than racehorses, and Standardbreds have lower pressures than Thoroughbreds.[389] Arterial pressures fluctuate slightly with ventilation and significantly under positive pressure ventilation or during cyclic changes in heart rate (see Figure 10-6). Posture imposes a significant influence on arterial pressure, because raising the head from the feeding position necessitates a higher aortic pressure to maintain cerebral perfusion. Obviously, when the head is lowered, the hydrostatic pressure imposed by an elevated head position is minimized. Mean arterial pressure measured in the middle coccygeal artery can vary approximately 20 mm Hg with the changing head position.[386] Abnormalities of arterial pressure and perfusion can result in changes in mucous membrane color and capillary refill time. Refill time is prolonged during hypotension or peripheral vasoconstriction; conversely, it may be shortened with vasodilation.

The systolic arterial pressure is generated by the LV and is consequently affected by the interplay between the stroke volume, heart rate, aortic compliance, and previous diastolic BP.[46] Arterial *pulse pressure* is highly dependent on stroke volume and the peripheral arteriolar resistance that determines the run off of diastolic pressure. Ventricular failure or reduced venous return reduces pulse pressure, creating a hypokinetic pulse; whereas abnormal diastolic run off (AR, generalized vasodilation) widens the pulse pressure, producing a stronger peripheral pulse. Diastolic and mean pressures are better estimates of perfusion pressure in anesthetized or critical equine patients; these variables are increased by arteriolar vasoconstriction or by higher CO. Mild variation in pulse pressure is normal across the respiratory cycle related to variation in ventricular filling. However, marked differences can be associated with cardiac tamponade, and the dramatic fall in pressure during inspiration is termed *pulsus paradoxus*.

The cutaneous veins should be examined for distensibility, refill, thrombosis, and estimated venous pressure. The jugular veins in normal horses are collapsed, but the veins of the limbs and torso are visible and somewhat filled. Venous pressure in the jugular vein is normally less than 10 cm of water above the phlebostatic point, and *jugular pulsations* are normally confined to the thoracic inlet and the ventral one third (10 cm) of the neck. These pulsations are reflections of the RA pressure changes that range from positive to subatmospheric over the cardiac cycle (discussed previously). Pulsations are normally visible along the entire length of the jugular vein when the head is lowered below the level of the heart and should not be misinterpreted. A pathologic jugular pulse also can be misdiagnosed if transmission of carotid arterial pressure into the jugular furrow occurs. Occluding the jugular vein ventrally can demonstrate if the pulses are actually originating within the RA or not, because venous pulse transmission, or prominent collapse, will be prevented by light digital pressure over the vein. Pronounced jugular pulsations are observed occasionally in excited but otherwise normal horses with high sympathetic tone. This might be caused by either vigorous RA contraction. Alternatively, an exaggerated venous collapse can create a "jugular pulse" that is simply a reflection of normal venous refilling during periods of positive RA pressure. When doubt persists, this finding can be verified by simple ultrasound imaging of the ventral portion of the vein.

Jugular abnormalities include abnormal pulses or elevated venous pressure. An abnormal jugular pulse is one that extends proximally up the jugular vein for more than 10 cm in systole (with the horse's head held in a normal position) or that demonstrates retrograde filling from the heart when the vein is occluded dorsally. Duplex Doppler studies of the jugular vein can distinguish a prominent pulse caused by retrograde flow from an apparent pulse caused by prominent collapse and normal filling. Abnormal jugular pulses are observed with arrhythmias causing AV dissociation (nonconducted atrial premature beats, junctional tachycardia, VT); with diseases of the tricuspid valve (moderate to severe TR or the rare case of tricuspid stenosis); and with RV failure from any cause including cardiac tamponade or constrictive pericardial disease. Elevated jugular venous pressure generally indicates right-sided CHF, pericardial disease, or hypervolemia. Generalized venous distention, particularly when accompanied by subcutaneous edema, is characteristic of CHF (Figures 10-12 and 10-13). Isolated distention of the veins cranial to the thoracic inlet is suggestive of a cranial mediastinal or pulmonary mass (or abscess) with obstruction of the cranial vena cava.[100] Prolonged refill of the saphenous vein indicates the possibility of aortoiliac thrombosis and decreased arterial supply to the affected limb.[222-227,396,397] A distended vein that is firm to palpation, and associated with marked distention of associated veins, indicates probable venous thrombus.[398] Pain or heat associated with venous swelling is suggestive of thrombophlebitis.

Congestive Heart Failure

Congestive heart failure in horses is relatively uncommon; however, the diagnosis often can be made from a thorough physical examination.[399] Clinical findings include persistent tachycardia (generally at 60/min or greater), jugular venous distention and pulsations, abnormal arterial pulses, fluid retention (ventral subcutaneous edema, pleural effusion, or pulmonary edema), and loss of body condition (see Figure 10-13). LV failure secondary to valvular or myocardial heart disease causes pulmonary venous congestion with pulmonary interstitial or, uncommonly, alveolar edema. Tachypnea or coughing associated with left-sided CHF can be misdiagnosed as pneumonia or chronic obstructive pulmonary disease. Exercise intolerance, lethargy, collapse (or syncope), anorexia, depression, and weight loss are other potential signs of heart

*References 371, 374, 375, 379, 380, 382-386, 389, 391, 395.

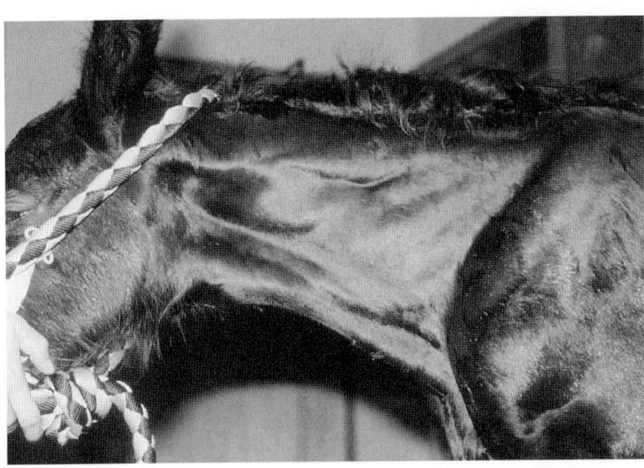

FIGURE 10-12 Jugular venous distention in a Shire foal with biventricular congestive heart failure (CHF) caused by congenital heart disease.

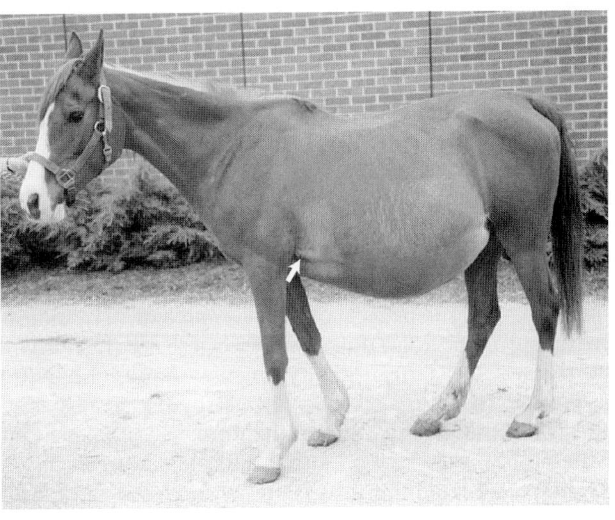

FIGURE 10-13 Ascites, ventral edema, and weight loss are evident in this mare with right-sided congestive heart failure (CHF). The distended lateral thoracic vein (*arrow*) is evident caudal to the triceps.

failure. This subject and management are discussed more fully later in this chapter.

DIAGNOSTIC AND LABORATORY STUDIES

Exercise Testing

Because most horses function as athletes, exercise testing represents an important method for identifying CV and other disorders in the underperforming horse. Additionally, some form of exercise testing should be included in the prepurchase CV examination, unless the animal is too young to perform or is to be used solely for breeding. Even in these situations, evaluation of a foal, weanling, or yearling after a period of free exercise is optimal. Furthermore, it should be determined that a stallion has sufficient stamina to perform in the breeding shed. For these reasons, it is recommended that CV system be evaluated at rest, immediately after exercise, and under the anticipated form of work required by the prospective owner. Having advanced this recommendation, it is also acknowledged that more data and information are needed to establish the reliability and predictive values of such studies relative to CV disease.

High-speed treadmill and other forms of exercise testing are increasingly used to detect subtle clinical abnormalities that limit peak performance.* The exercise examination provides valuable information about musculoskeletal diseases, airway diseases, and CV disorders. Treadmill exercise is also useful when evaluating the horse with a history of collapse or syncope, because the cardiac response to exercise can be evaluated without risk to a rider. A number of components to a standardized treadmill examination are available. Gait and lameness are evaluated and pre- and postexercise serum creatine kinase (CK) measured to identify subclinical myopathy. Videoendoscopy is used to identify laryngeal and other dynamic airway disorders. Arterial blood gases are often analyzed to assess pulmonary function. An exercise and postexercise ECG is recorded to identify heart rhythm disturbances. Pre- and postexercise echocardiography may be used to identify regional or global LV dysfunction. Doppler studies can be added to evaluate valvular insufficiency.[184]

Changes in heart rate with exercise have been well studied.[205,326-330,403,426] The normal horse develops sinus tachycardia, shortening of conduction intervals, and marked ST-T alterations associated with exercise. The maximal heart rate achieved depends on the level of exercise performed. At heart rates of less than 100 to 120 beats/min, SA node discharge is very labile and subject to psychologic influences. Once exercise has commenced, the heart rate should accelerate and then stabilize at a level appropriate for the work being performed. As a general guideline, heart rates of 70 to 120 beats/min are normal at the trot, 120 to 150 beats/min are normal at the canter, 150 to 180 beats/min are normal at the gallop, and more than 180 beats/min are normal when galloping at maximal exertion. The maximal heart rate for most horses is between 210 and 240 beats/min, although some develop higher rates. A linear relationship relates the heart rate and the velocity or work effort of exercise when the heart rate is between 120 and 210 beats/min. Heart rate usually recovers rapidly and falls to less than 100 beats/min within 2 to 5 minutes of cessation of exercise. The recovery of heart rate to the resting level is influenced by many factors, including the humidity, ambient temperature, training fitness, work performed, psychologic factors, and state of CV health. After maximal work, such as a race, 1 hour may pass before the heart rate completely recovers to the resting rate. An inappropriately high heart rate for a given level of exercise may simply denote a healthy, but unfit, horse; however, this finding can also indicate the presence of CV, pulmonary, or musculoskeletal disease. Information about the heart rate is particularly useful when a horse has the heart rate monitored routinely during exercise.

Exercise-induced arrhythmias may be observed during or after exercise. An exercising ECG obtained by radiotelemetry is necessary to determine if an arrhythmia is present during exercise. A heart rate monitor may provide some indication regarding arrhythmias during exercise; however, the detection

*References 122, 204, 273, 311, 313, 317, 327-330, 332, 337, 394, 400-425.

of erratic heart "blips" or "beeps" does not adequately characterize the rhythm disturbance. Exercise may induce supraventricular premature complexes, AF, ventricular extrasystoles, or VT. Exercise-induced (paroxysmal) AF should be included in the differential diagnosis of horses with poor performance during high-intensity exercise.[39,427,428] Exercise-induced ventricular arrhythmias are a particular concern because ventricular rhythm disturbances can lead to poor performance, sudden stopping, or even falling, and they have been suspected as one cause of sudden death.[60,62-65] Repetitive ventricular activity (paroxysmal VT) is particularly worrisome and may indicate preexisting myocardial disease or myocardial ischemia with altered cardiac electrical activity. In some horses, a maximal work effort is required to elicit heart rhythm disturbances. Thus when the history indicates performance problems only at the peak of exercise, or if other indicators of heart disease are present, a treadmill exercise test to exhaustion may be needed to reveal cardiac arrhythmias.

Horses demonstrate marked fluctuations in sympathetic and parasympathetic tone during the recovery period after exercise.[420,429,430] Arrhythmias are especially common during this time,[317,337] even if the resting and peak exercise heart rhythms were normal. Marked sinus arrhythmia, second-degree AV block, supraventricular ectopia, and ventricular premature complexes can be evident in the immediate postexercise period. With the exception of vagally mediated arrhythmias, postexercise arrhythmias should be considered suspicious. AF, ectopic supraventricular tachycardias, and VTs are considered abnormal at any point in the exercise test. However, the importance of single (isolated) ectopic complexes identified only in the immediate postexercise phase is less certain,[337] which is not surprising considering similar issues persist in assessing human athletes. In assessing these horses, attention also should be directed to the presence of coexisting respiratory disease, baseline auscultation and echocardiographic examinations, the heart rhythm during exercise, measurements of serum cardiac troponin I (cTn_I) before and after exercise, and the so-called stress echo immediately after work.

Echocardiography after the stress of exercise can be used in an attempt to identify global and regional myocardial dysfunction.[122,317,331,337] This examination must occur within 2 to 3 minutes after high-intensity exercise and with the heart rate in excess of 100 beats/min. However, the optimal heart rates and the influence of rapidly decreasing heart rates on echocardiographic measurements such as shortening fraction require better definition. Dynamic changes can be viewed from the short axis tomograms, and prominent thickening of the ventricular septum and LV free wall identified from long axis images. Persistent abnormalities in regional myocardial contraction are suggestive of vascular disease with ischemia, preexistent myocardial fibrosis, or a localized conduction disturbance. LV shortening fraction and LV fractional area change (two estimates of LV systolic function) are commonly measured during stress echocardiography. It is important to scrutinize multiple segments across the entire shortening area of the LV, because errors in cursor placement (e.g., too dorsal) or inconsistent orientation of the M-mode cursor placement between examinations can produce misleading results. Other methods used for stress echocardiographic assessment of LV function are the manual tracking of endocardial motion and subjective evaluation of regional wall motion. Newer echocardiographic modalities, including tissue Doppler imaging and 2D strain (2D speckle tracking) imaging, may have some advantages over conventional methods and could prove useful for quantitative assessment of regional and global LV function during stress echocardiography (CC Schwarzwald, unpublished observations), but more data and standardizations are needed before methods can be widely accepted.

Undoubtedly, CV disorders can be induced or worsened by the stress of exercise, and the likelihood of detecting disease is increased. However, the assessment is challenging because physiologic variability is also magnified. The immediate postexercise period involves rapidly changing autonomic traffic[420,429,430] that can result in confusing ECG and echocardiographic findings.[184,337] The presence of significant respiratory disease and associated arterial hypoxemia also creates the potential for secondary rhythm disturbances, unrelated to primary cardiac disease.[317] Thus the reliability and overall sensitivity, specificity, and predictive values of the exercise test (as it pertains to detection of arrhythmia and organic heart disease) are incompletely defined for a number of reasons. The "standardized" exercise test may not be identical across equine medical centers, so it may be difficult to compare results. The examiner's own reference for normal variation further qualifies the examination results. For example, the presence of isolated postexercise premature complexes may define the examination as *abnormal* for some[317] or *suspicious* or *uncertain* for others. Similarly, if the LV shortening fraction does not increase, but the LV fractional shortening area does, then one must ensure that the issue is not simply technical (i.e., cursor placement) as opposed to pathologic. Finally, the assessment of cardiac valve function after exercise or pharmacologic stress requires far better definition before any conclusions can be made.

Although the standardized treadmill examination is the most commonly used cardiac "stress test" at equine centers, some attention has been directed on performing *pharmacologic stress testing*. This examination involves increasing the heart rate and myocardial contractile force with dobutamine, either with or without atropine or glycopyrrolate, followed by echocardiographic assessment of ventricular contraction.[332,413,418,423,431] Pharmacologic stress echocardiography is used to identify regions of reduced myocardial perfusion or ischemic myocardial injury in human patients with coronary heart disease; the study is used in people who cannot perform physical exercise to stress the heart and increase myocardial oxygen demand.

Whether this form of stress testing should be used in horses is subject to debate. First, it must be emphasized that no compelling evidence from pathology studies indicates that horses develop significant coronary arterial disease. Admittedly, myocardial fibrosis is found in some horses at necropsy[29,432]; however, the pathogenesis or clinical relevance of these often-microscopic lesions is unresolved. In human patients, the diagnostic target is well-defined extramural coronary artery disease, and stress echocardiography generally predicts normal or abnormal findings at coronary arteriography. No evidence has been published at this time for a similar situation in horses, and this represents a major contextual issue when considering "stress echo" with either exercise- or pharmacologic-induced cardiac work. Furthermore, pharmacologic stress testing may not achieve the identical exercise endpoints in terms of heart rate or altered vascular resistances. The combination of dobutamine and atropine involves the use of proarrhythmic drugs,[413] making the heart rhythm assessment (a pivotal component of the exercise test) quite problematic. Pharmacologic stress testing does not provide an opportunity for dynamic assessment of the gait and airways.[417] Lastly, assessment of left heart valve function is complicated by changes in systemic ABP that may develop during drug-induced tachycardia (but have been poorly characterized in studies thus far.) Thus although pharmacologic stress testing carries the benefit of not requiring a treadmill, a number of outstanding issues must be addressed before this examination can be advocated for wider use.

Electrocardiography

NORMAL CARDIAC CELL ELECTRICAL ACTIVITY

Cardiomyocytes are excitable and capable of responding to electrical stimuli regardless of extrinsic innervation. Specialized cardiac tissues such as those in the SA node and the His-Purkinje system demonstrate spontaneous depolarization and can serve as pacemakers for the heart. The electrical processes responsible for the ECG are caused by ion fluxes across the cell membrane (Figure 10-14).[73,76,77] A general understanding of cellular activity, generation, and spread of the cardiac electrical impulse; effects of autonomic innervation; and electrocardiographic lead systems is required to interpret the equine ECG.

The partially selective nature of the cardiac cell membrane and the presence of various cell membrane pumps leads to an unequal partitioning of ions across the cell membrane.[73] This results in very high potassium and relatively low sodium concentrations intracellularly when compared with the extracellular fluid. Other ions including chloride and magnesium (but most notably calcium) are important to cellular electrical activity. Calcium also is essential for contraction of the cardiomyocytes. Sudden changes in cardiac cell membrane permeability or conductance to sodium, calcium, potassium, and chloride are responsible for the processes of depolarization, muscular contraction, and repolarization (see Figure 10-14). Serum electrolyte concentration, acid-base status, autonomic traffic, myocardial perfusion and oxygenation, heart disease, and drugs, in turn, affect these processes. The basic processes of cell depolarization, calcium influx, and cell repolarization form the basis for, respectively, the P and QRS complexes of the ECG, myocardial contraction, and the ST-T wave of the ECG.

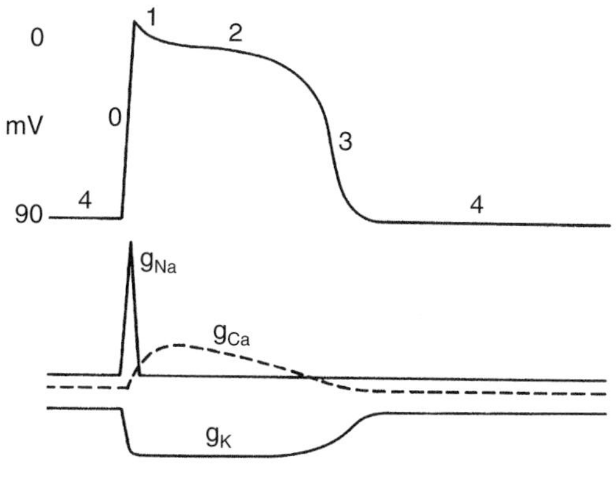

FIGURE 10-14 The cardiac action potential. The diagram demonstrates the phases of depolarization and repolarization, as well as membrane conductance (*g*) to important ions (see the text for details). (From Berne RM, Levy MN: Cardiovascular physiology, St Louis, 1986, CV Mosby.)

The resting membrane potential is determined primarily by the partitioning of potassium ions and proteins across the cell membrane and the relative impermeability of the membrane to sodium. *Depolarization* of atrial and ventricular myocytes and Purkinje fibers is caused by the rapid influx of extracellular sodium into the cell.[76,77] This current is represented by phase 0 of the cardiac cell action potential recording. Normal cardiac tissues depolarized in this manner conduct electrical impulses at high velocity. In contrast, the cells of the SA and AV nodes, as well as ischemic cells, demonstrate less negative diastolic membrane potentials. Nodal cells depend on a slow-inward current of depolarization that is carried mainly by calcium ions across the transient and long-lasting calcium channels. In ischemic cells, because of the less negative resting potential, some sodium channels remain in the inactivated state and thus are unavailable for activation and membrane depolarization during phase 0. Therefore cells in the SA node, AV node, and ischemic tissue conduct electrical impulses very slowly and can be involved in blocks, abnormal automatic mechanisms, or re-entrant pathways that promote cardiac arrhythmias. Antiarrhythmic drugs and calcium channel blockers act differently on tissues that are "fast" versus "slow" current dependent (see Cardiac Arrhythmias later in this chapter).

The influx of extracellular calcium into the cell during the *plateau phase* (phase 2) of the action potential triggers the release of intracellular calcium from the sarcoplasmic reticulum. Increases in cytosolic calcium cause myocardial contraction. Hypoxia, acidosis, anesthetics, and many other drugs can affect myocardial contractility by interfering with calcium entry into cells, with the release of calcium from the sarcoplasmic reticulum, or with the binding of calcium to contractile filaments.[73,76,104] Conversely, digitalis glycosides and dobutamine increase calcium influx and myocardial contractility.

Cellular *repolarization* is initiated by decreases in the cell membrane conductance to sodium and to calcium coincident with increased conductance to potassium. As intracellular potassium moves out of the cell, along its concentration gradient, phase 3 of the cardiac action potential occurs. Repolarization is complex, involves a number of ion currents,[433] and is affected by genetics and by drugs such as quinidine or amiodarone. Sympathetic stimulation may activate currents that facilitate repolarization at higher heart rates, explaining the shortening of the action potential under sympathetic drive. Paradoxically, vagotonia also enhances repolarization by opening potassium channels, an effect that is very prominent in the atria and may predispose to development of AF. Hypoxia and abnormalities in serum potassium or calcium also alter repolarization. Hyperkalemia accelerates repolarization and shortens the ST-T wave of the ECG. This occurs because hyperkalemia *increases* membrane permeability to potassium and the high intracellular potassium (exceeding 100 mmol/L) is more than adequate to drive potassium out of the cell (because extracellular potassium rarely exceeds 10 mmol/L).

Spontaneous depolarization or automaticity is a property of select cardiac tissues. Such activity is most prominent in the SA node but may also be encountered in cells around the AV node and in the His-Purkinje network. Normal automaticity is observed in these cells during phase 4 of the cardiac action potential. Spontaneous *pacemaker activity* is generated in normal pacemaker tissues by the background inward sodium current and a time-related decrease in membrane permeability to potassium ion efflux, as well as a transient inward calcium current.[76] Once membrane threshold is reached, ion flow across the

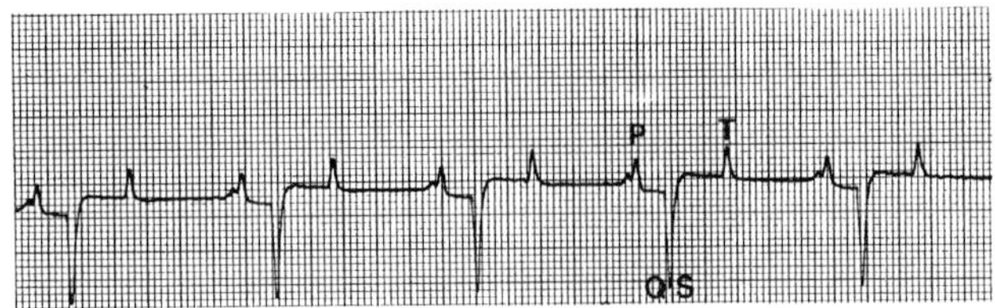

FIGURE 10-15 A normal equine base-apex lead electrocardiogram (ECG) (25 mm/sec; 1 cm = 1 mV). The waveforms are indicated. The normal P wave in this lead is positive and notched (bifid), and a depression occurs in the baseline after the P wave that indicates atrial repolarization (Ta wave). The QRS complex often lacks an R wave in this lead (QS complex). The T wave is labile and may be negative, biphasic, or positive. Increases in heart rate or sympathetic tone usually lead to positive T waves in this lead.

long-lasting calcium channels ("slow current") predominates and leads to cell depolarization (phase 0). Spontaneous depolarization is modified markedly by autonomic traffic. Vagal activity opens potassium channels and hyperpolarizes the membrane, depressing automaticity. With sympathetic stimulation or membrane hyperpolarization, the depolarizing funny current (I_F), becomes activated, enhancing pacemaker activity.

Autonomic innervation has profound effects on electrical activity[9,189,434] but is not distributed equally through the heart. The right and left vagus have preferential innervation to SA and AV nodes, and parasympathetic traffic is more extensive in supraventricular than ventricular myocardium. Sympathetic activity derived from paired ganglia is also not bilaterally symmetrical but does innervate both atria and ventricles extensively. Parasympathetic activity depresses SA nodal activity, enhances intra-atrial conduction by shortening atrial action potential duration, and slows AV nodal conduction. Conversely, sympathetic efferent traffic increases heart rate and shortens AV conduction time.[76] Sympathetic activity also increases cellular excitability, predisposes to some cardiac arrhythmias, and increases myocardial oxygen consumption by augmenting the heart rate, force of myocardial contraction, and myocardial wall tension. Parasympathetic efferent traffic dominates in the resting, standing horse and frequently fluctuates with changes in BP. The pronounced sinus arrhythmia, SA block, and second-degree AV block so often encountered in the normal horse is caused by changing vagal tone and serves to regulate ABP at rest (see Figure 10-6).[71]

Depression of normal SA automaticity or increased activity in other tissues in the atria, Purkinje system, or in cells around the AV node may lead to an abnormal or "ectopic" cardiac rhythm. This situation is often observed in healthy horses under general anesthesia. When the principal abnormality resides in depression of SA node function or blockage of the impulse in the AV node, the slow discharge of a subsidiary pacemaker is termed an *escape* mechanism. The purpose of these latent cardiac pacemakers is to rescue the heart from extreme bradycardia or asystole. However, drugs, inflammatory mediators, abnormal sympathetic activity, electrolyte disturbances, or ischemia also can enhance ectopic pacemakers abnormally, leading to *ectopic* rhythms that manifest as premature complexes or tachycardias. Additional abnormal electrophysiologic mechanisms, including abnormal automaticity in tissues other than nodal and conduction tissues (i.e., ischemic myocardium), after depolarizations, and re-entry account for the development of other arrhythmias.

GENESIS OF THE ELECTROCARDIOGRAM

The SA node is located near the right auricle; therefore initial cardiac muscle depolarization crosses the RA (see Figure 10-3). Activation waves spread through the atrial myocardial cells to the LA and also in the direction of the AV node. Specialized atrial muscle cells comprising internodal pathways and Bachman's bundle facilitate transmission of current across the atria.[8,435] These specialized pathways—as well as the SA node—are relatively resistant to high serum potassium concentrations and may function during hyperkalemia to cause a sinoventricular rhythm, even while normal atrial myocytes are inexcitable (atrial standstill).

Conduction continues across the AV tissues by first entering the AV node. Current transmission across the AV nodal cells is especially slow because this tissue depends on inward calcium currents and is subject to physiologic blockade from vagal efferent traffic.[192] Conduction proceeds at a greater velocity through the bundle of His and bundle branches. Propagation of the impulse through the ventricles is enhanced by a rapidly conducting Purkinje system that penetrates relatively completely through the ventricular myocardium.[6,7]

The ECG graphs the time-voltage activity of the heart. The average electrical potential generated by the heart muscle is recorded throughout the phases of the cardiac cycle with time displayed along the x-axis and electrical potential inscribed vertically (Figure 10-15). The normal waveforms are the P wave (atrial depolarization), the PR (or PQ) interval that is due mostly to slow AV nodal conduction, the QRS complex (ventricular depolarization), and the ST-T wave (ventricular repolarization). A prominent atrial repolarization wave (Ta wave) is often noted in the PR segment of the equine ECG, particularly at faster heart rates. The QT interval represents total electrical activation-repolarization time.

CLINICAL ELECTROCARDIOGRAPHY

The clinical application of electrocardiography to the horse has been studied extensively.* The principles of recording and interpreting the equine ECG are similar to those used for humans, dogs, and other species.[111,445] The lead systems used are identical, although some modified leads, such as the base to apex lead, are most useful for monitoring the cardiac rhythm. A number of semiorthogonal lead systems have been evaluated experimentally but are rarely used in clinical practice. The modified Einthoven's lead system, consisting of leads frontal planes I, II, III, $_a$VR, $_a$VL, and $_a$VF, and the precordial lead V_{10}, is quite applicable for ECG studies of horses (Box 10-7). The base-apex lead or chest leads are most often used for rhythm analysis.

The value of continuous, ambulatory (Holter) ECG monitoring is obvious for identification of infrequent rhythm disturbances, quantifying the severity of an arrhythmia, or objectively evaluating drug therapy (Figure 10-16). In one study it was observed that many horses that were historically and clinically without evidence of cardiac disease had supraventricular or (less often) ventricular arrhythmias on Holter ECG.[359] Ambulatory monitoring can be performed with contact electrodes using a bipolar lead system similar to that used for the equine heart rate monitors. Electrodes are

*References 1, 4, 6-8, 11, 30, 33, 35, 40, 43, 72, 77, 111, 188, 194, 195, 336, 344, 360, 436-470.

BOX 10-7

ELECTROCARDIOGRAPHIC LEADS

Frontal Plane Leads

Bipolar leads

Lead I = Left foreleg [+] – right foreleg [–]

Lead II = Left hindleg [+] – right foreleg [–]

Lead III = Left hindleg [+] – left foreleg [–]

Unipolar augmented limb leads

Lead aV_R = Right foreleg [+] – left foreleg and left hindleg [–]

Lead aV_L = Left foreleg [+] – right foreleg and left hindleg [–]

Lead aV_F = Left hindleg [+] – right foreleg and left foreleg [–]

Precordial Leads

Base-apex monitor lead

Positive electrode over the left apex compared with the negative electrode over the right jugular furrow

Precordial V leads

Positive electrode over the selected precordial site; -the lead is named based on the location of the exploring (V or C) electrode

Lead V_3: near the left apex

Lead V10: over the dorsal spinous processes (interscapular)

The most common method of obtaining the base-apex lead is to place the left foreleg electrode over the left apex, the right foreleg electrode over the jugular furrow (or at the top of the right scapular spine), and select lead I on the electrocardiograph. This lead is an excellent choice to monitor the cardiac rhythm. Precordial leads other than V10 (over the dorsal spine) are not commonly used.

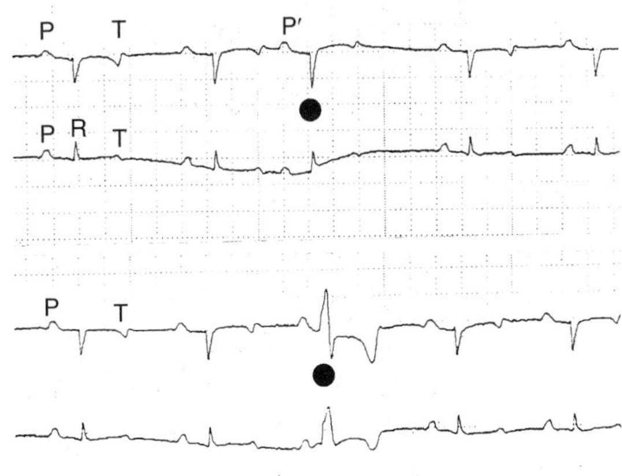

FIGURE 10-16 Examples of extrasystoles. Atrial (P′ at *top*) and ventricular (*bottom*) extrasystoles in a mare with heart failure, sinus tachycardia, and premature beats. The recordings are from a 24-hour tape-recorded (Holter) electrocardiogram (ECG). Two transthoracic leads recorded simultaneously. The waveforms are indicated. The dark circles indicate the premature complexes. The P-R interval of the APC is longer because of physiologic refractoriness in the atrioventricular node. The ventricular ectopic follows the sinus P wave (late diastolic) but discharges the ventricle before the sinus impulse can cause a normal QRS complex. The T wave of the ventricular extrasystole is abnormal (secondary T wave change). Paper speed is 25 mm/sec.

usually placed over the left saddle area and sternum and are kept moist and in contact with the horse using a surcingle and padding material. This type of continuous 24-hour rhythm monitor can be quite useful to evaluate the horse with a history of syncope or an arrhythmia, but in which an arrhythmia cannot be induced during resting, exercise, and postexercise ECG examinations. An alternative is an ECG event recorder that continuously records the rhythm and stores the ECG after an observed event, such as a sudden fall. These event recorders can be worn for longer periods of time.

Telemetry-based ECG recordings are commonly used in exercise testing (see Exercise Testing) and in monitoring of critical patients in hospital settings.[317,415] The lead systems used are often similar to those used for Holter ECG recordings; however, the degree of artifact that occurs during exercise is considerable. Those interested in consistent recordings must experiment with various electrode positions and lead systems.

The orientation, amplitude, and duration of the ECG waveforms depend on many factors, including the age of the horse,[348,464] the lead examined, the size of the cardiac chambers, the degree of training, and even the phase of ventilation.[439,440] The principal use of the ECG is to diagnose the heart rhythm, because in horses this examination is insensitive for detecting cardiomegaly, especially in horses with mild to moderate heart enlargement. A normal ECG does not exclude heart disease; moreover, the ECG is not a test of myocardial function. A systematic approach to ECG analysis should be undertaken and compared with reference values (Table 10-4).

Atrial depolarization generates the P wave. Normal activation proceeds from right-to-left and craniad to caudad, leading to positive P waves in left-right lead I and also in craniocaudal leads II and aVF.[8,11] The normal P wave is notched or bifid; however, single peaked, diphasic, and polyphasic P waves may be encountered in normal horses. A negative/positive P wave is often recorded if the focus of pacemaker activity shifts to the caudal RA near the coronary sinus (Figure 10-17). The initial peak of the common bifid P wave is reportedly caused by depolarization of the middle and caudal one third of the RA.[6] The second peak represents activation of the atrial septum and the medial surface of the LA. The P wave peaks can be subdivided with P_1 reported to be as high as 0.25 mV (mean of 0.14) and the second peak, P_2, reported to be as high as 0.5 mV (mean of 0.28).[445] Even subtle differences exist among breeds of horses. The P wave morphology can change cyclically with waxing and waning of vagal tone during sinus arrhythmia. During tachycardia, the P wave shortens, becomes more peaked, and is followed by a prominent atrial repolarization (T_a) wave that deviates the P-Q segment downwards. Such features make the diagnosis of atrial enlargement by electrocardiography very difficult.

The time required for conduction across the AV node and His-Purkinje system is estimated by measuring the P-R interval. Because physiologic AV block is so common, significant variation exists in the P-R interval, even within the same horse; thus normal maximal values for the P-R interval are difficult to state. Values that persistently exceed 0.5 seconds are probably abnormal. Variation in the P-R interval is not usually related to changes in ventilation[42] but is often correlated with changes in BP and baroreceptor activation.[71]

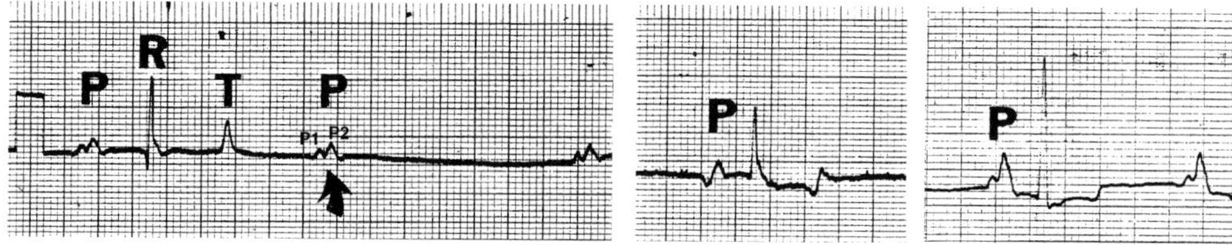

FIGURE 10-17 P waves of the horse are demonstrated. On the left is a normal, bifid P wave morphology with two distinct peaks (designated as *P1* and *P2*) and also a physiologic second-degree atrioventricular block (*arrow*). The center panel demonstrates a negative/positive P wave of coronary sinus origin. This is a normal variation. The right panel shows increased amplitude P waves recorded in a horse after conversion from atrial fibrillation (AF). The second peak is particularly large and may indicate atrial enlargement; however, such voltage criteria correlate poorly with cardiomegaly in horses. Echocardiography is a more accurate method for evaluating atrial size. Lead 2 paper speed is 25 mm/sec.

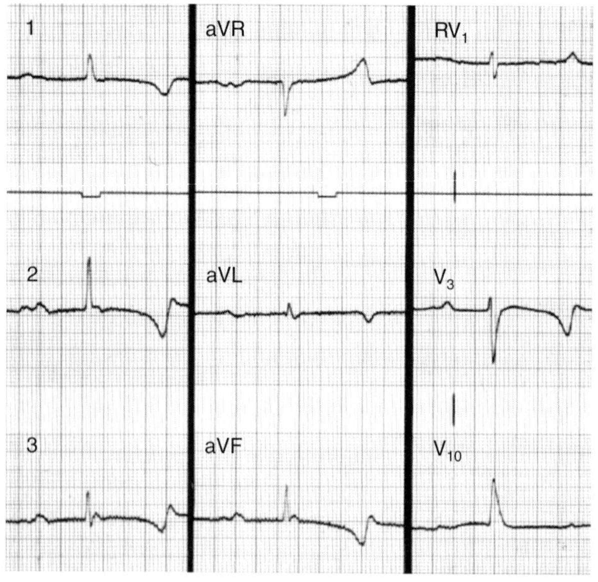

FIGURE 10-18 Multiple lead recordings in a normal horse. The varying configuration of the P-QRS-T complexes across the leads is notable.

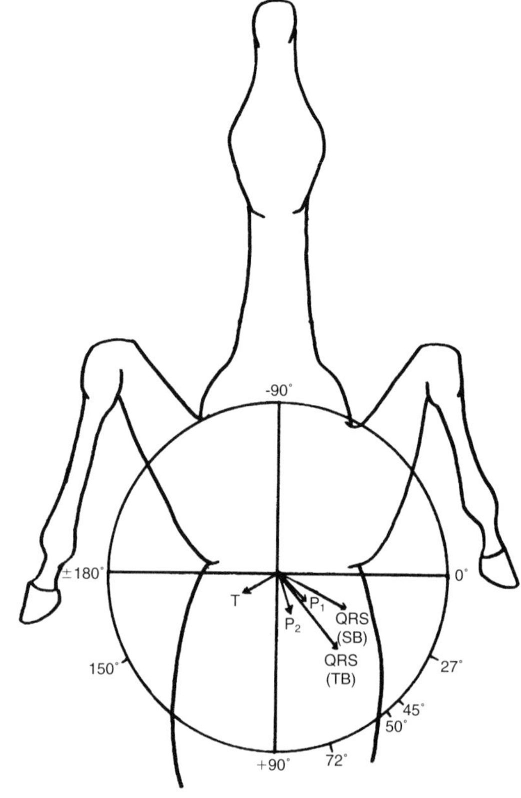

FIGURE 10-19 Diagram of the normal frontal plane lead axis. The predominant vectors for the QRS complex in Standardbred (SB) and Thoroughbred (TB) horses are indicated. The orientation of the two components of the normal P wave (P1 and P2; see Figure 10-17) differ slightly. (From Fregin GF: The cardiovascular system. In Mansmann RA, McAllister ES, Pratt PW, editors: Equine medicine and surgery, Santa Barbara, CA, 1982, American Veterinary Publications.)

The morphology of the QRS complex is variable. The relatively complete penetration of the conduction system into the free walls of the ventricle causes these chambers to be activated simultaneously with a burst of depolarization, which cancels much of the divergent electromotive forces.[6,7] Consequently, the normal electrical axis may vary and the amplitude of the QRS complex can be quite small in the frontal plane leads. A substantial dorsally oriented vector causes a prominent positive terminal deflection in lead V_{10}, while the (– electrode) right base to (+ electrode) left apex lead exhibits a prominent S wave (see Figures 10-15 and 10-18). The normal slur in the ST segment makes determination of QRS duration difficult in many horses.[35,471] The mean amplitude for the R wave in lead II for normal racehorses is about 0.8 to 1.1 mV.* Clinical experience suggests that R wave amplitudes exceeding 2.2 mV in lead II or 1.7 mV in lead I are often abnormal. However, occasionally the R wave amplitude in a normal horse exceeds even these limits.

The frontal plane leads can be inspected to estimate the mean electrical axis of depolarization, the "average" wave of depolarization (Figure 10-19). This determination is usually reported by direction, using a quadrant orientation (i.e., right or left, craniad or caudad), or is stated in degrees (e.g., lead I is 0 degrees, lead II is 60 degrees, lead aVF is 90 degrees, lead III is 120 degrees, lead aVR is minus 150 degrees, and lead aVL is minus 30 degrees). The general direction of the QRS axis can be quickly estimated by surveying the height

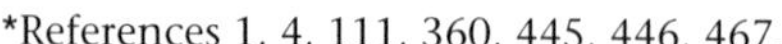

*References 1, 4, 111, 360, 445, 446, 467.

TABLE 10-4

Electrocardiography: Approximate Limits for Normal Frontal Plane Leads		
Variable	**Maximal Value**	**Comments**
Heart rate	44-50 beats/min	Resting mature horses; higher in foals, colts, and ponies
Cardiac rhythm	—	Sinus mechanisms, sinus arrhythmia, vagal-induced first- and second-degree atrioventricular block*
P wave	0.16 seconds	Atrial repolarization (Ta wave) possibly making measurement difficult
P-R interval	0.48 seconds	Varies; longer when vagal tone is high
QRS complex	0.14 seconds	May vary with the size of the heart (often longer in the base-apex lead)
QT interval	0.575 seconds	Inversely related to the heart rate
R wave lead I	0.85 mV	
R wave leads II, aV_F	2.3 mV	
Frontal axis	0-100 degrees	Axis variable in foals and yearlings

*When evaluating the electrocardiographic rhythm, one should consider the following points:
Technical aspects: paper speed, calibration, and lead(s)
Artifacts: electric, motion, twitching, and muscle tremor
Heart rate per minute: atrial and ventricular
Cardiac rhythm: atrial, atrioventricular conduction sequence, and ventricular conduction
Arrhythmias
Site or chamber of abnormal impulse formation, myocardial fibrillation, or conduction disturbance
Rate of abnormal impulse formation
Conduction of abnormal impulses
Patterns or repeating cycles
P wave: morphology, duration, amplitude, and variation
P-R interval: duration, variation, and conduction block (of P wave)
QRS: morphology, duration, and amplitude
Frontal plane mean electric axis
ST segment: depression or elevation
T wave: changes in morphology or size; QT interval
Miscellaneous: electrical alternans, synchronous diaphragmatic contraction

of the R waves in the frontal leads and selecting the lead with the greatest net-positive QRS complex. The axis in foals and yearlings is variable and frequently oriented craniad, whereas the frontal axis in most mature horses is directed left-caudad. Abnormal axis deviations have been observed with cardiomegaly, cor pulmonale, conduction disturbances, and electrolyte imbalance.[467]

After ventricular activation, repolarization of the ventricles is recorded. This period is measured from the end of the QRS complex (the "J point") and extends to the end of the T wave.[35,451,472] The T wave vector is most often directed toward the right caudal quadrant, resulting in a positive T wave in lead III and a negative or isoelectric T wave in lead I in resting horses.[445] Although some clinical surveys have suggested that abnormalities of the ST-T indicate cardiac dysfunction in performance animals, marked deviation of the ST segment and increased amplitude of the T wave are anticipated in healthy horses during exercise or even with excitement-induced tachycardia. No compelling evidence indicates that T wave abnormalities can be interpreted consistently. Progressive J point or ST segment deviation in the horse with hypovolemia or shock may indicate myocardial ischemia, whereas enlargement of the T wave may develop with myocardial hypoxia or hyperkalemia. Diagnosis and management of cardiac arrhythmias are discussed later in this chapter.

Thoracic Radiography

There are significant limitations to the use of thoracic radiography for evaluation of the equine heart related to the large size of the mature horse and the ability to obtain only a standing lateral thoracic radiograph in all except the smallest foals.[113] While recumbent lateral and, on occasion, ventrodorsal or dorsoventral projections can be obtained on neonatal foals, the stress of restraint or requirement for heavy sedation can make such positioning contraindicated. Thoracic radiographs may be useful to identify areas of pulmonary or pleural disease and assist in the differential diagnosis of respiratory problems.

Gross changes in cardiac size and shape may be detected in a lateral thoracic radiograph of a foal or horse with significant cardiomegaly.[113,342,473-475] A normal thoracic radiograph does not necessarily indicate that the heart is normal in size. Mild to moderate increases in the size of the cardiac chambers may go undetected, particularly in adult horses. Generalized enlargement of the cardiac silhouette is observed in cases of significant pericardial effusion or with CHF (Figure 10-20). Dorsal displacement of the trachea may be detected in some horses with LA and LV enlargement. In some horses with LA enlargement, the caudodorsal border of the cardiac silhouette bulges caudally. Increased contact between the ventral border

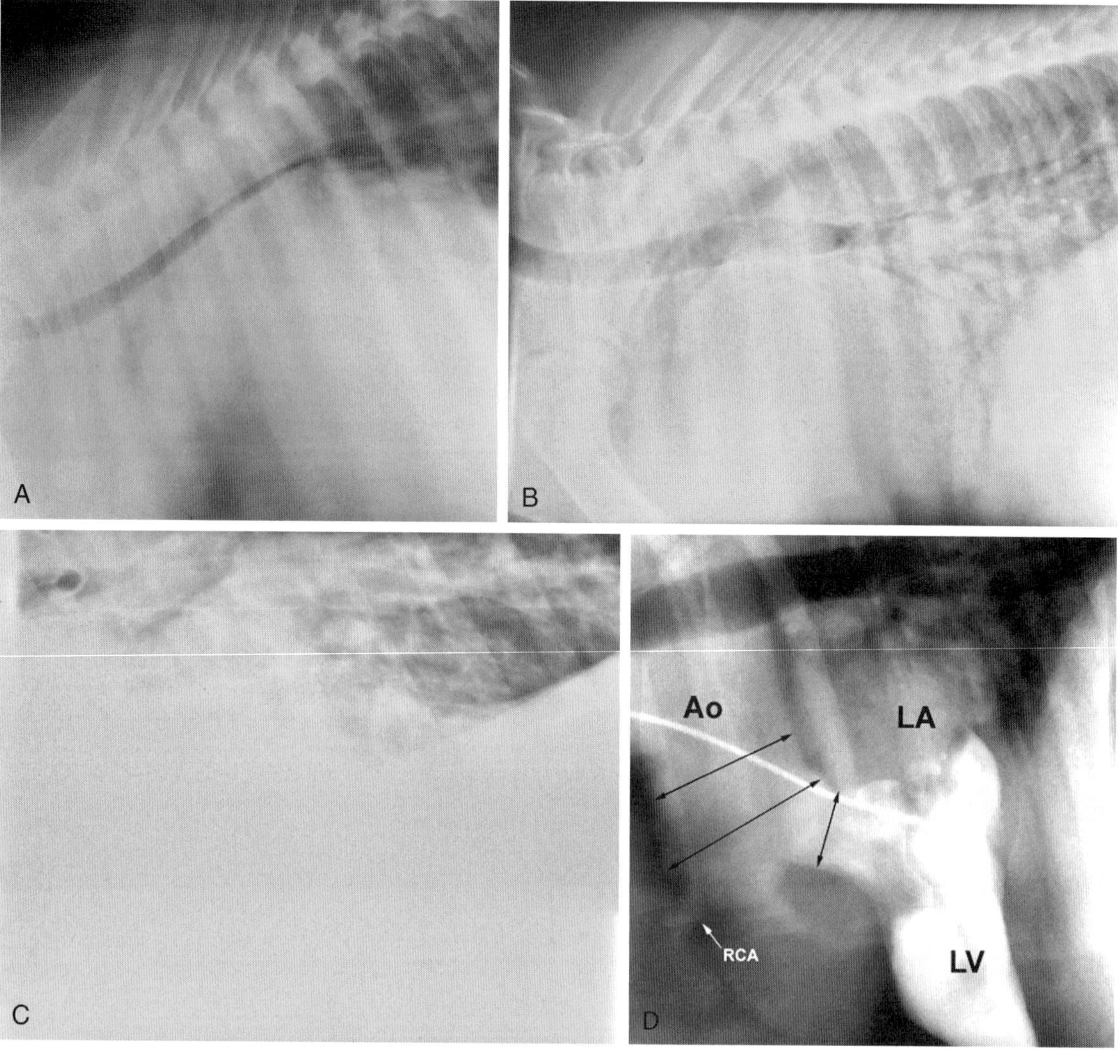

FIGURE 10-20 Thoracic radiography. **A,** Significant cardiomegaly in a Quarter Horse foal with complex congenital heart disease, including multiple ventricular septal defects (VSDs). **B,** Cardiomegaly and alveolar pulmonary edema in a filly with mitral regurgitation (MR) and left-sided congestive heart failure (CHF). **C,** Increased pulmonary density and pleural effusion in a Standardbred gelding with atrial fibrillation (AF), atrioventricular valvular regurgitation, myocardial failure, and biventricular CHF. **D,** Angiocardiogram obtained from an Arabian foal with pulmonary atresia and a large VSD (pseudotruncus arteriosus). Contrast medium was injected in the left ventricle (LV), and this medium opacifies a dilated, overriding aorta. Right-to-left shunting across the VSD results in dilution of contrast medium. The right arrow shows the subaortic LV outflow tract; the widened aorta is delineated by the arrows at the left. *Ao,* Aorta; *LA,* left atrium; *LV,* left ventricle; *RCA,* right coronary artery.

of the heart and the sternum may be detected with RV enlargement but is usually difficult to appreciate. A 50% decrease in the spinotracheal angle (the angle between the dorsal border of the trachea and the ventral border of the adjacent thoracic vertebrae) was demonstrated in young horses with cardiomegaly because of congenital cardiac disease.[113]

Evaluation of the pulmonary vasculature and pulmonary parenchyma is also difficult and very dependent on radiographic technique. Enlarged pulmonary vessels associated with pulmonary overcirculation can occasionally be observed in left-to-right shunts; the opposite is also true in congenital right-to-left shunts. Pulmonary edema causes generalized increased radiopacity, particularly in the hilar regions; the characteristic air bronchograms are more readily identified there when alveolar edema is present.

Angiocardiography is only practical in foals less than about 115 kg and usually requires general anesthesia, which may be contraindicated in the foal with a severely compromised CV system. Both selective and nonselective positive contrast angiocardiograms have been performed in foals and adult horses (see Figure 10-20, D),[156,473,476] but these techniques have been almost exclusively replaced by echocardiography and Doppler studies.

Nuclear medicine imaging has been developed in some equine referral institutions and has been used to assess cardiac function. First-pass nuclear angiocardiography permits the visualization of the cardiac chambers during sequential phases of the cardiac cycle.[113] Application of first-pass studies may be useful for identification of cardiac shunting, but again, this diagnosis is more simply attained by echocardiography.

Echocardiography

Ultrasound is the mechanical vibration of sound waves within a medium at frequencies greater than 20,000 c/s. These inaudible sound waves follow the laws of optics, can be transmitted through tissue, and can also be refracted and reflected. This last property permits the clinician to image the heart and other organs.[477] Echocardiography is the application of ultrasound diagnostics to the heart. When combined with Doppler studies,[478] transthoracic echocardiography has evolved to become the most important diagnostic study currently available for evaluation of the equine heart.* Transesophageal echocardiography (TEE) has been used in horses,[234,235,285] but (except in foals) it requires specially made endoscope-mounted transducers and is only practical in anesthetized or heavily sedated horses because of the fragile (and expensive) nature of the TEE probe.

Successful examination of the equine heart requires the use of crystals that vibrate at frequencies between 1.5 to 5.0 MHz, a detailed knowledge of ultrasound anatomy, thorough appreciation of equine cardiac diseases, and technical skills with imaging and instrumentation. Ultimately, a thorough echocardiographic examination yields information about the presence and nature of heart lesions, the size of the heart and great vessels, ventricular function, valvular function, blood flow, and the relevant hemodynamics of a cardiac lesion. Examination findings are relatively consistent when performed by experienced examiners, but day-to-day, subject, and examiner variation can be significant (>10%) for some variables and must be considered when performing serial examinations.[303,307,308,518]

The essential principle of echocardiography is straightforward: when ultrasound is directed into the chest and toward the heart, some of the sound energy reflects back to the transducer. This occurs because tissue interfaces with different acoustic impedance, such as muscle, collagen and blood, are encountered by the echobeam and ultrasound is reflected from these tissue interfaces. A hand-held transducer acts to both send and receive ultrasound.[486,520] The echocardiograph computer is capable of determining the spatial orientation and distance of the returning echoes, processing the signals, and displaying an image of the heart. The image is usually displayed, by convention, with that part of the heart closest to the transducer at the top of the display and adjacent to the transducer artifact. Two imaging modalities, the M-mode and 2D (B-mode or cross-sectional) formats, are in widespread use in equine practices. When Doppler studies or contrast echocardiography is added, blood flow can be detected relative to the 2D and M-mode images (Box 10-8; Figures 10-5 and 10-21 to 10-24).[149,303] M-mode, 2D, and Doppler studies can be used to quantify heart size and mass,[49,50,481] as well as estimate ventricular function. The influence of training on cardiac size can be assessed.[102,515,516] The technique also can be applied to assess the fetal heart.[521]

The M-mode echocardiogram is a single-crystal ice pick image of the heart (see Figures 10-5 and 10-22).[13,14,53,522] The movement of the cardiac structures (vertical axis) is displayed over time along the horizontal axis. The ECG can be recorded to provide a timing reference if desired, and the depth of the cardiac structures from the transducer (y-axis) is displayed in centimeters. Visualization of the characteristic movements of cardiac structures permits the experienced viewer to evaluate and quantify cardiac anatomy and function (see Figure 10-21). The high sampling rate of the M-mode study makes it excellent for visualizing rapidly vibrating structures, such as the oscillating mitral leaflet in AR.[138]

The 2D echocardiogram generates a cardiac field by mechanically or electrically sweeping one or more piezoelectric crystals across the heart.* In conventional transthoracic echocardiography, the operator hand-directs the imaging probe to achieve a suitable tomographic plane. The pie-shaped image obtained has both depth and breadth but has no significant thickness. Accordingly, different image planes must be used to interrogate the three-dimensional (3D) heart. These imaging planes are designated *long-axis* (sagittal), *short axis* (coronal), *apical* (when the transducer is near the left apex), and *angled* (hybrid) views. Apical images are difficult to obtain except in foals.

The 2D field is constantly updated to visualize cardiac motion in real time, and this is done at typical sampling rates of 20 to 40 frames/sec, with the update rate inversely related to penetration depth and angle of field. Fully digital echocardiographs can display much faster frame rates, often exceeding 60 frames/sec. In most cases the 2D study is watched in "real time" and also recorded digitally or on videotape for subsequent playback and analysis. Human interpretation is generally limited to 32 frames/sec so that recordings made at higher frame rates require slow-motion playback for detailed analysis. 2D echocardiography allows assessment of cardiac anatomy, detection of macroscopic structural lesions, subjective evaluation and measurement of chamber and vessel dimensions, and evaluation of LA and LV function.

Doppler echocardiography relies on the Doppler principle to measure the direction and velocity of red blood cells (RBCs) in the heart (see Figures 10-24 and 10-5).* In Doppler echocardiography, a portion of the ultrasound emitted by the transducer strikes moving RBCs. These targets cause ultrasound to be reflected back to the transducer. Because the RBCs constitute a moving "source" of (reflected) ultrasound, the returning sound waves attain a frequency that is slightly different from that originally transmitted (the "carrier frequency"). When the echocardiograph unit records the Doppler frequency shift, calculation of RBC velocity and direction relative to the transducer is possible. The information is displayed as a Doppler spectrum showing time along the horizontal axis, flow direction relative to the transducer as above (toward) or below (away from) a zero baseline, and calculated RBC velocity along the y-axis. Thus pulsed Doppler methods measure direction and velocity of RBCs within a discrete area of the heart or circulation. Disturbed flow, as might be recorded across a regurgitant orifice or VSD, results in a high-velocity and broadened-velocity spectrum.

Color-coded Doppler imaging is a more refined example of pulsed-wave technology, whereby flow toward the transducer is coded in red and flow away is represented in blue. Calculated velocity is displayed in relative shades of these colors,

*References 14, 41, 49, 51, 77, 83, 85, 90, 91, 94, 109, 122, 128-130, 137-139, 142, 143, 145, 149, 150, 163, 179, 183, 201, 220, 221, 230, 231, 233, 241, 257, 262, 276-280, 282, 283, 303-305, 342, 354, 251-254, 306-308, 479-519.

*References 50, 51, 90, 303, 403, 523, 524.

*References 149, 150, 233, 241, 257, 278, 354, 492.

BOX 10–8

INTERPRETATION OF ECHOCARDIOGRAPHIC AND DOPPLER STUDIES

General Principles of Interpretation

- Evaluate the electrocardiogram relative to cardiac motion and cardiac rhythm disturbances; arrhythmias can alter measures of ventricular function, cause aortic valvular regurgitation, and alter flow and pressure gradients.
- Remember that persistent tachyarrhythmias can lead to reversible form of dilated cardiomyopathy (tachycardia-induced cardiomyopathy).
- Determine the initial image planes needed for examination based on clinical examination and your standard operating procedures.
- Identify the general situs of the heart and cardiac structures; identify the atria, ventricles, cardiac septa, great vessels, and cardiac valves.
- Note any dilation, attenuation, or absence of the aorta or pulmonary artery and identify their origins and relationships to the atrioventricular valves and to the ventricles.
- Note the presence of unanticipated or lack of expected structures.
- Identify pleural effusion.
- Rule out extrapericardial mass lesions of the lung or thorax.

Pericardium and Pericardial Space

- Rule out pericardial effusion and pericardial mass lesion.
- Mixed echoic effusions or shaggy tags may indicate highly cellular or inflammatory effusate.
- In pericardial effusion: Identify diastolic collapse of the right atrium or right ventricle indicating cardiac tamponade or a large bilateral pleural effusion; protracted collapse or ventricular or atrial inversion are more reliable signs of tamponade. Exuberant swinging of heart may be seen.
- In pericardial effusion: Identify any heart-related lesions using multiple complementary planes.
- If there is concern about constrictive pericardial disease, evaluate the motion of the ventricular septum (for accentuated flutter or "septal bounce") and perform Doppler studies of the left and right ventricular inlets; large E-waves with abrupt termination of filling may be observed; evaluate the effects of ventilation because marked variation may be observed in E-waves; tissue Doppler may also be instructive in cases of constrictive disease.

Left Atrium, Pulmonary Veins, and Atrial Septum

- Identify pulmonary veins and pulmonary venous entry.
- Examine for attenuation or small size: Rule out volume depletion, right-to-left shunt, or low cardiac output.
- Examine for enlargement or rounding/turgid appearance: rule out left-to-right shunt, mitral valve disease, left ventricular systolic or diastolic failure, chronic arrhythmia (e.g., atrial fibrillation).
- Measure left atrial diameter and/or left atrial area by 2D imaging.
- Examine the atrial septum for abnormal bowing to the left or right atrium (high atrial pressure).
- Examine the atrial septum for septal defects or patent foramen ovale (perform Doppler and "bubble" contrast studies if necessary).
- Examine the blood pool for spontaneous contrast.
- Examine the atrioventricular groove for dilated vascular structure: Rule out dilated coronary sinus and left cranial vena cava.
- 2D Echocardiography and tissue Doppler can be used to evaluate atrial wall motion and function.

Mitral Valve

- Identify two valve leaflets and cusps in long and short axis planes; if evidence of mitral regurgitation, also examine mitral valve from left caudal imaging windows in two or more imaging planes.
- Observe motion during cardiac cycle by 2D and M-mode echocardiogram.
- Examine the support apparatus (chordae tendineae, papillary muscles).
- Increased valve echogenicity: Rule out degenerative thickening, valvulitis, vegetation (infective endocarditis), malformation (rare).
- Cleft or common septal leaflet: Rule out endocardial cushion defect/primum atrial septal defect (rare defects).
- M-mode: Reduced diastolic (E-F) slope: decreased transvalvular flow.
- Lack of diastolic separation or increased mitral E point to septal distance: Rule out aortic regurgitation (regurgitant jet impinging on the valve); left ventricular dilation with left ventricular failure (reduced transmitral flow), or mitral stenosis/tethering (rare defects or acquired from endocarditis).
- Prolapse of mitral leaflet into left atrium: Rule out degenerative disease, elongated or ruptured chordae tendineae, lesion of papillary muscle.
- Flail leaflet: Rule out ruptured chordae tendineae or avulsion of papillary muscle.
- Double line of mitral closure (mobile): Rule out ruptured chordae tendineae (flail leaflet).
- Diastolic mitral valve fluttering: Rule out aortic regurgitation.
- Systolic mitral fluttering: Rule out mitral regurgitation (musical).
- Chaotic valve motion: Rule out arrhythmia (atrial flutter, premature ventricular complexes); ruptured chordae tendineae.
- Premature (diastolic) closure: Rule out severe semilunar valve insufficiency, long P-R interval, or atrioventricular block.
- Delayed (systolic) closure (B-shoulder): rule out left ventricular failure and elevated atrial pressure.
- Systolic anterior motion of the mitral valve (systolic anterior motion, systolic mitral–septal contact): rule out dynamic left ventricular outflow tract obstruction due to valve malformation, subaortic stenosis, volume depletion, pulmonic stenosis, or hypertrophic or infiltrative cardiomyopathy (all very rare).

BOX 10-8

INTERPRETATION OF ECHOCARDIOGRAPHIC AND DOPPLER STUDIES—cont'd

- Doppler studies can be used to interrogate the mitral valve for regurgitation or abnormal flow; multiple planes should be obtained including short-axis images at the level of the left atrium immediately dorsal to the mitral valve.
- Mitral regurgitation is common. Eccentric jets are often observed. Do not confuse "backflow" color noise with true regurgitation. Horses can develop mid-to-late systolic mitral regurgitation (as with mitral prolapse). Multiple jets of mitral regurgitation are common.
- Always time flow events of mitral regurgitation (color M-mode and spectral Doppler); do not misdiagnose diastolic mitral regurgitation. Do not overemphasize receiving chamber color coding in mitral regurgitation because red blood cell entrainment and a "spray effect" can result in overestimation of mitral regurgitation severity, whereas wall-hugging jets underestimate severity of mitral regurgitation. Attempt to measure jet width at origin and correlate to left atrial and left ventricular chamber size.

Left Ventricle

- Evaluate from long and short axis tomograms; inspect contour and walls; dorsal septum is normally slightly thicker than left ventricle free wall.
- Echogenic smoke/contrast: Some spontaneous contrast may be normal; rule out low output states, bradycardia, systemic inflammation (?).
- Evaluate left ventricle dimensions (internal dimensions, thickness of interventricular septum and free wall) and left ventricle systolic function (fractional shortening, ejection fraction) using M-mode or 2D imaging.
- Left ventricle dilation: Rule out causes of volume overload or left ventricle failure: mitral or aortic valvular regurgitation, dilated cardiomyopathy, myocarditis, left-to-right shunt, persistent tachyarrhythmia.
- Left ventricle wall thinning: Rule out infarct, prior myocarditis, congenital aneurysm (rare).
- Left ventricle wall thickening: Consider "athletic heart"; rule out pseudohypertrophy from volume depletion, infiltrative cardiomyopathy (amyloid), myocarditis, chronic systemic hypertension, or left ventricle outflow obstruction (very rare).
- Hyperkinesis of left ventricle: Rule out mitral or aortic insufficiency, bradycardia, sympathetic stimulation.
- Hypokinesis or dyskinesis of the left ventricle: Rule out cardiomyopathy or other myocardial disease, ischemia, infarct, arrhythmia, regional wall infiltration, or myocarditis.
- Hyperechoic myocardium or subendocardium: Rule out recurrent ischemia, fibrosis, infiltration, infarction, myocarditis, amyloidosis.
- Tissue Doppler and 2D strain (2D speckle imaging) may be used to evaluate global and regional left ventricle function; transmitral flow can be obtained but is limited with respect to evaluation of left ventricle diastolic function

Left Ventricular Outlet, Aortic Valve, and Aorta

- Identify aortic valve leaflets and motion during cardiac cycle: Identify abnormal leaflet morphology (e.g., thickenings, fenestrations) or motion. Examine in both long-axis and short-axis image planes to see all leaflets.
- Thickened leaflets: diffuse or nodular: Rule out degeneration, endocarditis.
- Prolapse of aortic valve into the left ventricle: Rule out degenerative semilunar value disease (common), ventricular septal defect, or bacterial endocarditis with torn leaflet.
- Diastolic fluttering of the aortic valve: Rule out aortic insufficiency.
- Systolic fluttering or the aortic valve: normal or high flow state.
- Lack of systolic separation: Rule out low cardiac output, arrhythmia, stenosis (rare).
- Decreased aortic diameter: low cardiac output, hypotension.
- Aortic dilation: Rules out aortic regurgitation, tetralogy of Fallot, pulmonary artery atresia, truncus arteriosus, patent ductus arteriosus (rare).
- Aortic sinus of Valsalva aneurysm: focal dilation or ballooning of affected sinus: Evaluate for rupture into ventricular septum or right atrium.
- Doppler studies may be used to identify blood flow patterns in the left ventricle outflow tract, aortic regurgitation, paramembranous ventricular septal defect, and rare case of aortic stenosis. Doppler studies also can identify abnormal blood flow paths in rare cases of aortic sinus ruptured into the heart.

Ventricular Septum

- Septal hyperkinesis: as per the left ventricle.
- Septal hypokinesis: as per left ventricle; also rule out right ventricular pressure or volume overload.
- Paradoxical ventricular septal motion: rule out moderate to severe right ventricular volume overload such as atrial septal defect, severe tricuspid regurgitation, severe pulmonary hypertension with tricuspid regurgitation.
- Flat ventricular septum: rule out right ventricular volume overload (diastolic flattening) or right ventricular pressure overload (systolic flattening).
- Exaggerated and disparate ventricular filling rates with diastolic septal fluttering: Rule out constrictive pericardial disease.
- Examine for ventricular septal defects in both long-axis and short-axis image planes (perform Doppler studies if necessary).
- Echocardiogram drop-out or discontinuity of the ventricular septum: Rule out ventricular septal defect (peri/paramembranous adjacent to right/noncoronary cusps of the aortic valve and septal leaflet of tricuspid valve; inlet septal ventricular septal defect (ventral to tricuspid valve); muscular or trabecular ventricular

Continued

BOX 10–8

INTERPRETATION OF ECHOCARDIOGRAPHIC AND DOPPLER STUDIES—cont'd

septal defect; subpulmonic ventricular septal defect (also termed outlet, supracristal, subarterial, or doubly committed ventricular septal defect; directly underneath pulmonic and aortic valves); tetralogy of Fallot; pulmonary artery atresia; truncus arteriosus, or a false defect caused by angle of the ascending aorta or aortic dilation.

- Malalignment of the ventricular septum and anterior aortic root: examine for tetralogy of Fallot, malalignment type ventricular septal defect.
- Examine for dissection or "track" that may suggest rupture of the aorta into the ventricular septum with subsequent fistula.
- High-frequency fluttering of the ventricular septum: Rule out aortic regurgitation.
- Doppler studies, especially color Doppler, are useful for recognizing ventricular septal defects; continuous wave Doppler should be used to measure velocity across shunts to evaluate for "restrictive" versus unrestrictive septal defects. High velocity flow across a ventricular septal defect (>4.75 m/s) generally suggests a restrictive defect more likely to be well tolerated.

Right Atrium and Atrial Septum

- Examine for attenuation: If small, rule out volume depletion, external compression, or mass lesion impairing venous return.
- Examine for enlargement: If enlarged, rule out tricuspid regurgitation, tricuspid stenosis or atresia (rare), right heart failure, atrial septal defect, moderate to severe anemia or chronic arrhythmia.
- Examine the atrial septum for abnormal bowing into the left or right atrium (high atrial pressure).
- Examine the atrial septum for septal defects or patent foramen ovale (double mobile lines in foals).
- Doppler studies can be used to identify atrial septal defect, but streaming of normal flow patterns (i.e., caudal vena cava flow) is confusing.
- "Bubble studies" (by injecting agitated normal saline into the jugular vein) should be used to identify right-to-left shunting of blood. Caution: Similar to Doppler studies, streaming of normal blood from the caudal vena cava may produce negative contrast in the right atrium, falsely suggesting left-to-right shunting of blood.

Tricuspid Valve

- Identify valve leaflets and cusps in long- and short-axis image planes.
- Observe motion during cardiac cycle.
- Identify support apparatus (chordae tendineae, papillary muscles).
- Increased valve echogenicity: Rule out degenerative thickening, vegetation, malformation, thrombus on valve.
- Common septal leaflet: Rule out endocardial cushion defect/primum atrial septal defect (rare).
- Flail leaflet: Rule out ruptured chordae tendineae or avulsion of papillary muscle; rule out infective endocarditis.
- Chaotic valve motion: Rule out arrhythmia, ruptured chordae tendineae.
- Premature (diastolic) closure: Rule out severe pulmonic insufficiency, long P-R interval, or atrioventricular block.
- Doppler studies can interrogate the tricuspid valve for abnormal flow or regurgitation; most horses have some small jets of tricuspid regurgitation by color Doppler evaluation; use color M-mode and spectral Doppler to evaluate timing and peak velocity. High velocity tricuspid regurgitation (>3 m/s): Also rule out pulmonary hypertension, large ventricular septal defect, right ventricular outflow obstruction.

Right Ventricle

- Dilation: Rule out severe tricuspid insufficiency, chronic right ventricular pressure overload, biventricular congestive heart failure, atrial septal defect, large ventricular septal defect, severe pulmonary insufficiency, persistent tachyarrhythmia.
- Hypertrophy: Rule out large (unrestrictive) ventricular septal defect, pulmonary hypertension, pulmonic stenosis (rare), tetralogy of Fallot (rare), or complex congenital heart disease.
- Midventricular bands: Rule out double chambered right ventricle (examine for ventricular septal defect); remember that the right ventricular moderator band can be very prominent in horses.
- Hyperechoic tissue: Rule out myocardial fibrosis.

Right Ventricular Outlet, Pulmonary Valve, and Pulmonary Artery

- Identify valve leaflets and motion during cardiac cycle; if pulmonary valve lesion is suspected, also interrogate from a left cranial transducer position.
- Thick, fused, or hypoplastic leaflets: Rule out congenital stenosis or dysplasia (rare).
- Diastolic fluttering of pulmonic valve: Rule out valvular insufficiency.
- Systolic fluttering of pulmonic valve: normal or high flow state.
- Lack of systolic separation of the pulmonic valve: Rule out low cardiac output, arrhythmia, stenosis.
- Pulmonary artery, absence or attenuation: Rule out pulmonary atresia or pulmonary artery hypoplasia.
- Pulmonary artery, dilation of: Rule out pulmonary hypertension, left-to-right shunt, poststenotic dilation of pulmonic stenosis (rare); rupture of the aorta into the right heart or pulmonary artery (rare).
- Doppler studies can be used to identify abnormal flow in the pulmonary artery, including the rare pulmonic stenosis (high velocity), increased velocity flow from a left-to-right shunt, and patent ductus arteriosus in equine neonates. Pulmonary regurgitation is normal; high velocity pulmonary regurgitation indicates pulmonary hypertension.

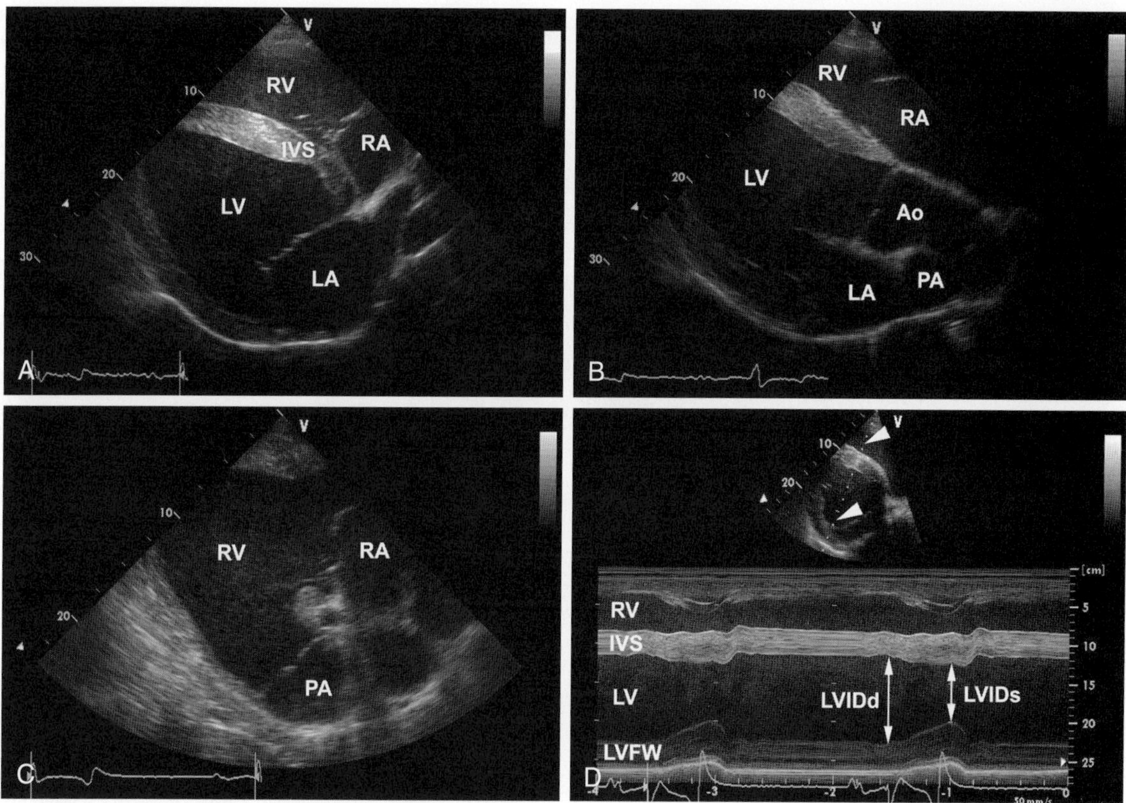

FIGURE 10-21 Two-dimensional (2D) echocardiograms obtained from the right side of the chest. An ECG is recorded simultaneously for timing. **A,** Four-chamber view. **B,** Left-ventricular outflow tract view. **C,** Right-ventricular inflow and outflow tract view. These images, recorded in a right-parasternal long-axis view, allow subjective assessment of cardiac structures and myocardial function and measurement of selected cardiac dimensions. **D,** M-mode echocardiogram of the normal left ventricle (LV) performed in a right-parasternal short-axis view at the level of the chordae tendineae. The myocardial wall motion (*y-axis*) along the cursor line (*arrowheads*) is displayed over time (*x-axis*). An ECG is recorded simultaneously for timing. This view allows subjective assessment of right- and left-ventricular dimensions and left-ventricular systolic function, measurement of the left-ventricular internal dimensions in systole and diastole, and calculation of the left-ventricular fractional shortening (percentage of change in the internal dimension; FS = [LVIDd – LVIDs]/LVIDd × 100). The latter provides an index of systolic left-ventricular function. *LV,* Left ventricle; *LA,* left atrium; *RV,* right ventricle; *RA,* right atrium; *IVS,* interventricular septum; *Ao,* aorta; *PA,* pulmonary artery; *LVFW,* left-ventricular free wall; *LVIDd,* left-ventricular internal diameter at end diastole; *LVIDs,* left-ventricular internal diameter at peak systole. (From Schwarzwald CC, Bonagura JD, Muir WW: The cardiovascular system. In Muir WW, Hubbell JAE, editors: Equine anesthesia: monitoring and emergency therapy, ed 2, St Louis, 2009, WB Saunders.)

and green or yellow are added to the flow mapping to identify "turbulence." Color-coding permits superimposition of flow information onto the 2D or M-mode image (see Figure 10-24). Although substantial technical challenges exist in terms of penetration and frame rate, color-Doppler imaging is useful in horses because a large area of the heart can be screened for flow disturbances. For example, it is much easier to find a jet of MR using color Doppler imaging than with other Doppler methods. A pivotal limitation of color Doppler regards temporal resolution. Depending on the system used, the frame rates of interrogation can be very slow (often <10/sec). Thus it is *mandatory to time flow events* using either spectral Doppler or by invoking the M-mode cursor and recording the event by color-M-mode echocardiography. In many cases, the color M-mode examination is simpler and provides excellent temporal resolution, reducing interpretation errors. This timing of blood flow prevents the clinician from misinterpreting normal "backflow" signals related to valve closure or diagnosing a diastolic flow event as systolic.

Pulsed-wave spectral and color Doppler techniques can provide accurate information about the location of flow disturbances but cannot measure high-velocity flow faithfully. High-velocity flow is encountered as RBCs are ejected from high- to lower-pressure zones across incompetent valves, stenotic valves, and intra- and extracardiac shunts (provided that there is a pressure difference across the defect). In general, once velocities exceed about 2.5 m/sec in either direction, part of the returning signal is displayed in the incorrect direction. This problem is called *signal aliasing*[257] (see Figure 10-24). To quantify high-velocity flow, a third modality must be invoked, either high pulse repetition frequency Doppler or continuous wave Doppler. Continuous wave Doppler has virtually unlimited ability to record very high velocity but does not provide the spatial discrimination found in pulsed-wave Doppler modalities.

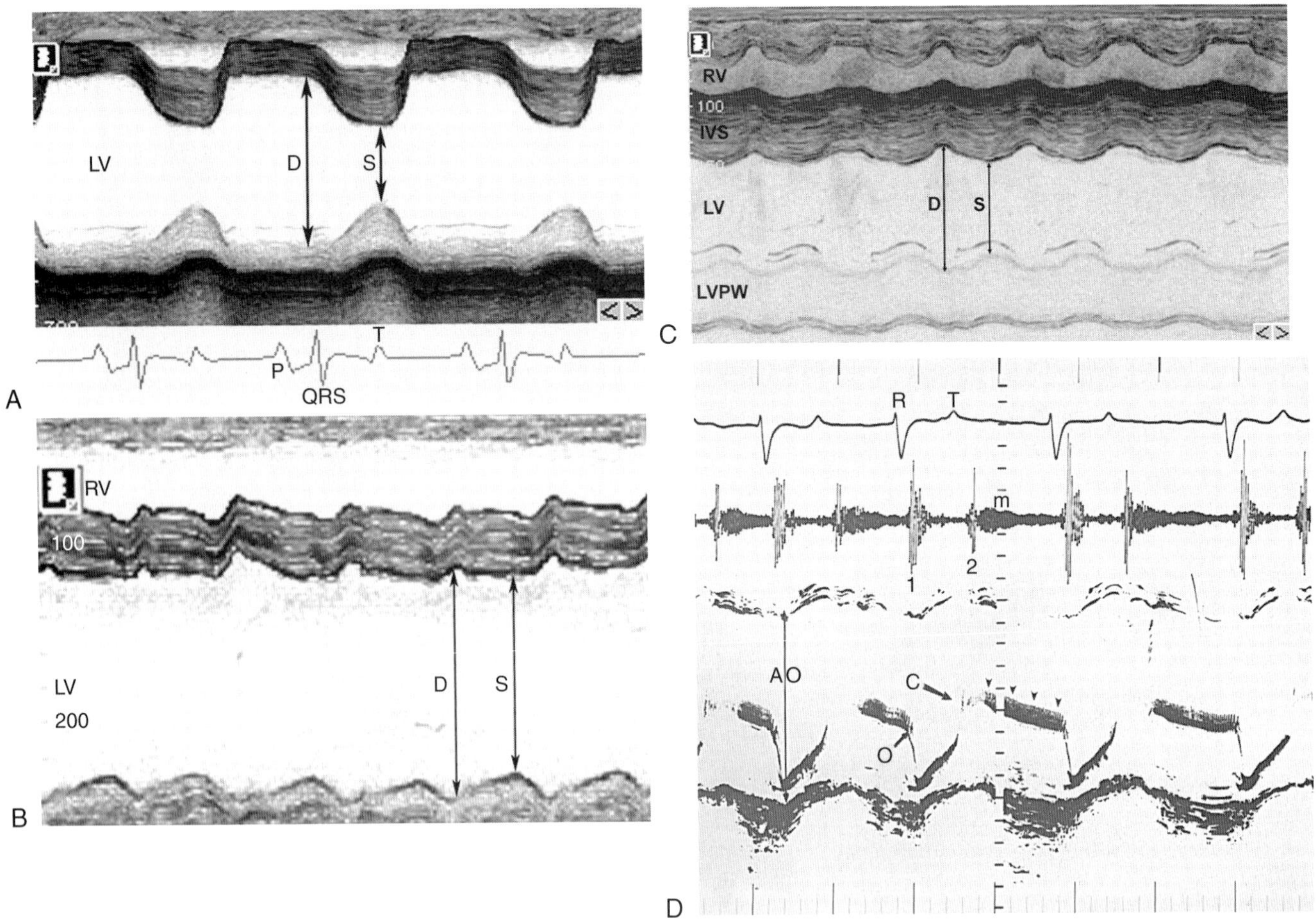

FIGURE 10-22 M-mode echocardiography. **A,** M-mode tracing demonstrating a hyperdynamic left ventricle (*LV*) in a horse with acute mitral regurgitation (MR). The significant change in LV dimensions from diastole (*D*) to systole (*S*) is notable and is typical of volume overloading with preserved ventricular function. Furthermore, the reduced resistance to ejection of blood into the left atrium (LA) enhances ventricular shortening. Depth calibration in millimeters is shown on the left. **B,** Recording through the ventricles demonstrating decreased contractility with a reduced LV shortening fraction. This pattern of contraction can be caused by myocarditis, myocardial injury (e.g., monensin), idiopathic dilated cardiomyopathy, chronic volume overload, protracted ventricular tachycardia (VT), or administration of negative inotropic drugs. Depth calibration in millimeters is shown on the left (*RV,* right ventricle). **C,** M-mode echocardiogram across the ventricles recorded from a horse with cardiac amyloidosis. Global LV systolic function is mildly reduced. The IVS and LVPW are thickened. The IVS also appears hyperechoic relative to the RV wall. The LVPW in the far field is less echogenic owing to attenuation of echoes in the far field. The right ventricle (RV) contained spontaneous echocontrast. Depth calibration in millimeters is shown on the left (*RV,* right ventricle; *IVS,* interventricular septum; *LV,* left ventricle; *LVPW,* left ventricular peripheral wall). **D,** Recording from a horse with aortic regurgitation (AR) and atrial fibrillation (AF), demonstrating fine diastolic fluttering of an aortic valve leaflet (*small arrows*). The aortic root (*AO*), valve opening (*O*), and valve closing (*C*) are indicated. The murmur (*m*) of AR is evident in the previous phonocardiogram. First (*1*) and second (*2*) heart sounds are labeled. Diastolic fluttering of the mitral valve (most common), aortic valve, ventricular septum, or walls of the aortic root may be observed in horses with this hemodynamic abnormality. The M-mode sampling rate (approximately 1000 pulses/sec) is ideal for detecting these high-frequency events.

Accurate recording of flow disturbances can provide qualitative and quantitative information about the severity of a lesion (see discussion later in this chapter). Furthermore, the pressure difference between the source and the sink of a high-velocity jet can be estimated by the modified Bernoulli equation, in which pressure drop in mm Hg equals $4V^2$ (where maximal velocity, V, is measured in m/sec by continuous wave Doppler). If, for example, a peak velocity of 4.8 m/sec is recorded across a VSD, and if the systolic systemic ABP is determined noninvasively to be 125 mm Hg, then the estimated RV systolic pressure would be calculated as follows:

$$\text{Pressure drop} = 4 \times 4.82^2 = 92 \text{ mm Hg}$$

$$\text{Estimated LV systolic pressure} = 125 \text{ mm Hg}$$

$$\text{Estimated RV systolic pressure} = 125 - 92 = 33 \text{ mm Hg}$$

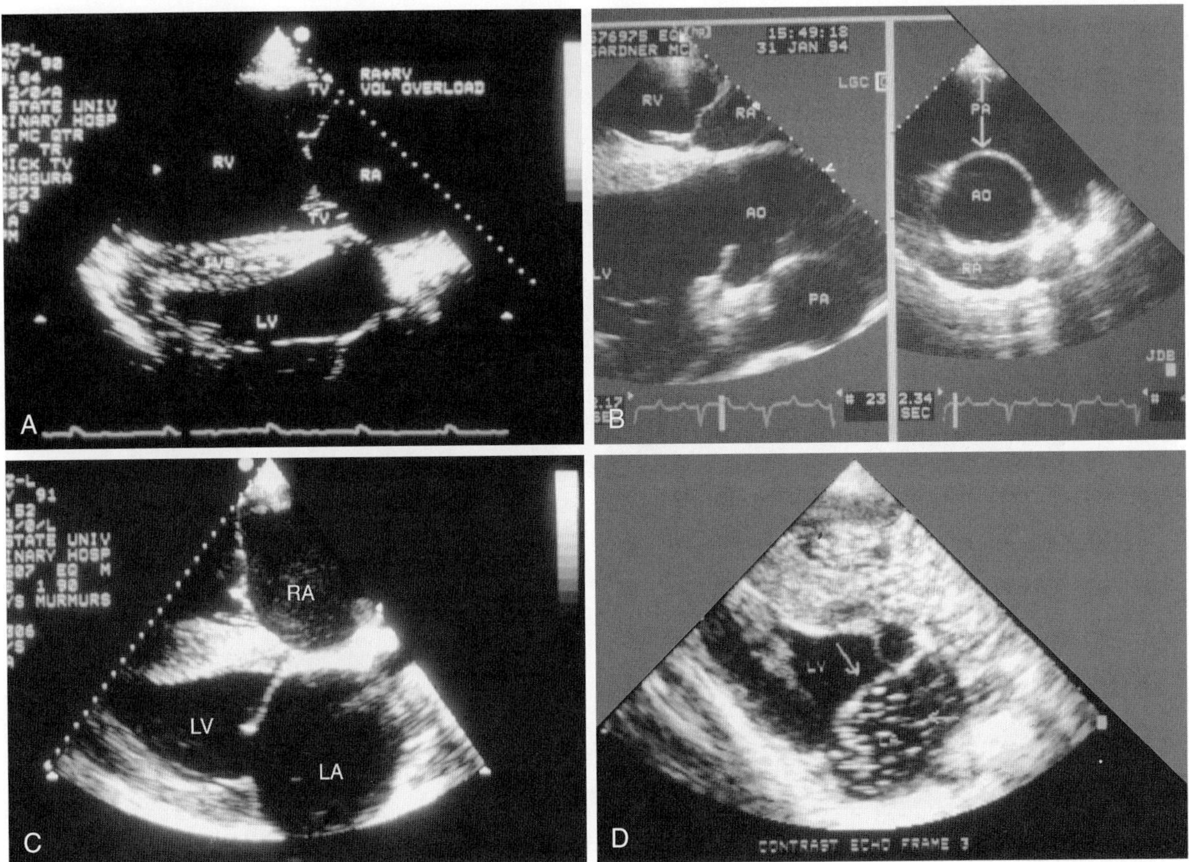

FIGURE 10-23 Two-dimensional (2D) echocardiograms. **A,** Long-axis image from the right thorax in a 12-year-old Quarter Horse gelding demonstrating significant right ventricular (RV) and right atrial (RA) dilation after tricuspid regurgitation (TR) and elevated pulmonary artery pressure. In this case a tumor that obstructed flow in the main pulmonary artery caused the pulmonary hypertension. The ventricular septum is flat and bulges slightly into the left ventricle (LV). **B,** Images of the ascending aorta and pulmonary artery obtained from the right hemithorax (*left panel*) and left cranial hemithorax. An evaluation of the pulmonary artery diameter relative to the aorta is useful when identifying pulmonary hypertension. **C,** Biatrial dilation in a Thoroughbred colt with mitral regurgitation (MR), pulmonary hypertension, atrial fibrillation (AF), and congestive heart failure (CHF). Both atria are rounded and appear turgid. The cause of mitral disease in this case was idiopathic lymphocytic-plasmacytic mitral valvulitis (*RA,* right atrium; *LV,* left ventricle; *LA,* left atrium). **D,** Contrast echocardiogram demonstrating right-to-left shunting at the level of the foramen ovale in a foal with severe respiratory disease. The saline generates echocontrast, opacifies the right atrium (RA) and right ventricle (RV), and visibly fills the left atrium (LA) (*arrows*), although the LV has not yet been opacified. This technique is easy and practical for demonstrating right-to-left shunts across the cardiac septa.

These findings indicate a restrictive septal defect, a lesion unlikely to cause difficulties for the horse except at highest levels of performance.

A similar quantitative approach is used to estimate the presence or absence of pulmonary hypertension when TR is identified in the absence of RV outflow tract obstruction (i.e., PA ejection velocity of <1.5 m/sec). Assuming the jet can be interrogated at nearly parallel to flow, peak regurgitant velocities exceeding 3.5 m/sec are suggestive of elevated PA systolic pressure. For this calculation, peak RA pressure must be estimated (around 10 mm Hg in horses without CHF). For example, a peak regurgitant velocity of 3.8 m/sec would result in calculated pressure drop from RV to RA of $(3.8)^2 \times 4$ or 58 mm Hg. When the RA pressure estimate (10 mm Hg) is added, estimated PA systolic pressure is 68 mm Hg. In cases of right-sided CHF, the RA pressure can be assumed to be at least 20 mm Hg or more or can be accurately measured by a catheter.

Advanced methods for assessing heart function by echocardiography includes measurement of various timing intervals of blood flow or tissue movements by Doppler methods. For example, systolic time intervals of aortic blood flow can be recorded from the aortic flow signal and may provide insight regarding LV function or changes related to valvular heart disease.[46,237] More advanced methods record longitudinal and radial tissue velocities by pulsed and color Doppler methods, or they assess of myocardial deformation (strain) by computer analysis of tissue movements (2D strain or 2D speckle tracking).[525,526] Strain and strain rate can be measured in longitudinal, radial, and circumferential planes and may provide more sensitive methods for assessing regional or global myocardial function. An additional application is measurement of atrial function using tissue velocities or time intervals.[244]

Echocardiography is most useful in the evaluation of congenital heart disease, heart murmurs, pericardial diseases,

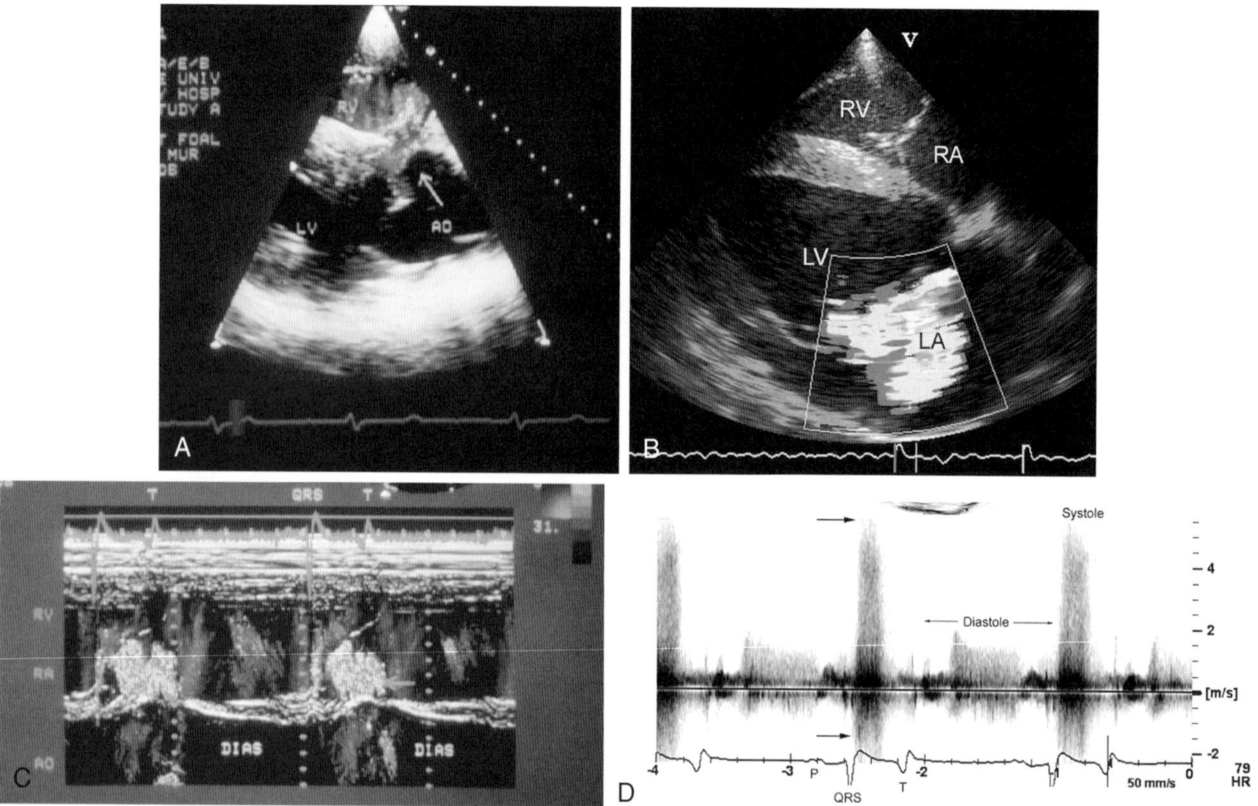

FIGURE 10-24 **A** to **C**, Black-and-white representations of color Doppler echocardiograms demonstrating mapping of blood through the heart. **A**, Perimembranous ventricular septal defect (VSD) in a foal (*arrow*). The flow pattern was coded red and aliased as the velocity increased across the defect. **B**, Wide spray of mitral regurgitation (MR) with flow moving from left ventricle (*LV*) into the left atrium (*LA*) in a horse with mitral valve prolapse (*RV*, right ventricle; *RA*, right atrium). **C**, Color M-mode study from a horse with tricuspid regurgitation (TR). The bright systolic flow pattern, following the QRS of the electrocardiogram (ECG), was mapped as turbulence in the color study. This is an excellent method for timing abnormal flow events. **D**, Example of continuous wave (*CW*) spectral Doppler echocardiogram obtained from a horse with a *VSD* and mild aortic regurgitation (AR). Time and the ECG waveforms are shown along the x-axis and velocity of flow along the y-axis with a meters per second scale (m/sec). Direction of flow relative to the transducer is also shown; flow toward the transducer is displayed as a positive signal (relative to the zero velocity baseline) and away from the transducer as a negative signal. A low-velocity flow pattern is evident in diastole related to diastolic shunting across the VSD, aortic regurgitant flow moving across the cursor line "off angle" (with parallel alignment, the AR velocity would be higher [i.e., >3.75 m/sec]), or contaminated transtricuspid flow. In systole a high positive velocity signal is recorded (>5 m/sec) compatible with a small (restrictive) left-to-right shunting VSD. However, the maximum velocity is not evident because the signal reaches the upper limit of the velocity scale (*arrow*). The negative signal (*lower arrow*) is either an aliased signal (if antialiasing filters are off) or VSD turbulence in the other direction. Moving the baseline down or increasing the velocity scale would have allowed for faithful recording of the peak velocity. (Note: For color images of color Doppler echocardiograms, see case examples included on the DVD.)

heart failure, and cardiac arrhythmias. Ultrasound can also identify other lesions of the lung, pleural space, or mediastinum that may masquerade as heart disease.[100,527] The source of a pathologic cardiac murmur, the size and function of the heart, and the overall influence of a cardiac lesion can be accurately determined by a complete echocardiographic and Doppler examination. A normal echocardiogram and Doppler study in a horse with a cardiac murmur is a favorable finding, suggesting a functional basis for the murmur. Conversely, identification of an abnormal flow pattern with associated cardiomegaly or abnormal ventricular function may indicate a high risk or limitation for work. As with all diagnostic studies, there can be ambiguous results, particularly regarding the tricuspid valve, because physiologic TR, silent to auscultation, is detectable by Doppler studies in many clinically normal horses. Contrast echocardiography,[528] whereby saline is used to delineate the path of blood flow, is especially useful for the detection of right-to-left shunts in foals, including patent foramen ovale (see Figure 10-23, *D*). Reference values for ventricular chamber size, wall thickness, and LV shortening fraction have been published,[51,231,252,303-305,502] and some representative data[252,303] are given in Table 10-5. Sedation can affect echocardiographic studies, mainly by altering sympathetic tone, ventricular loading, and subsequently LV size

TABLE 10-5

Reference Values for Equine Echocardiography in Adult Horses*

Measurement	Mode View	Normal Values Mean ± SD (Range) [Est. 95% range]	Population	N	Reference
LV STUDY – LINEAR MEASUREMENTS					
$LVID_s$ (cm)	M-mode	8.2 ± 0.6	Warmblood Dressage	15	1
Left ventricular internal diameter at peak systole	Right parasternal short-axis view—chordal level	8.6 ± 0.8	Warmblood Jumping	14	1
		8.2 ± 0.7	Warmblood Untrained	15	1
		7.4 ± 1.5 (5.9-8.9)	Warmblood Eventing	5	16
		7.4 ± 0.7 (6.1-8.7)	THB and THB cross	26	2
		7.3 ± 0.8 (5.9-9.1)	THB and THB cross	18	3
		7.5 ± 0.6 (5.8-8.8)	THB	37	4
		7.0 ± 1.0 (5.1-8.7)	THB (un-/trained)	8	7
		7.7 [7.0-8.3]	STB (untrained)	8	5
		7.5 ± 1.2 (5.4-8.8)	STB (untrained)	9	7
		7.5 ± 0.7 (6.9-8.7)	STB (trained)	7	7
$LVID_d$ (cm)		11.6 ± 0.7	Warmblood Dressage	15	1
Left ventricular internal diameter at end-diastole		12.1 ± 1.0	Warmblood Jumping	14	1
		11.5 ± 0.7	Warmblood Untrained	15	1
		11.6 ± 1.0 (10.3-12.5)	Warmblood Eventing	5	16
		11.9 ± 0.7 (10.5-13.4)	THB and THB cross	21	2
		11.3 ± 1.4 (8.0-14.0)	THB and THB cross	18	3
		11.9 ± 0.8 (9.7-13.1)	THB	37	4
		11.5 ± 0.7 (10.3-13.0)	THB (un-/trained)	8	7
		11.5 [10.7-12.3]	STB (untrained)	8	5
		10.9 ± 0.8 [9.4-12.4]	STB (untrained)	103	6
		12.2 ± 0.8 [10.6-13.8]	STB (trained)	103	6
		11.5 ± 1.1 (10.0-13.3)	STB (untrained)	9	7
		11.6 ± 0.5 (10.8-12.4)	STB (trained)	7	7
IVS_s (cm)		4.3 ± 0.7	Warmblood Dressage	15	1
Interventricular septal thickness at peak systole		4.0 ± 0.5	Warmblood Jumping	14	1
		4.0 ± 0.6	Warmblood Untrained	15	1
		4.5 ± 0.7 (3.5-5.2)	Warmblood Eventing	5	16
		4.6 ± 0.6 (3.3-5.6)	THB and THB cross	26	2
		4.7 ± 0.5 (3.9-5.7)	THB and THB cross	18	3
		4.2 ± 0.5 (3.2-5.2)	THB	38	4
		4.6 ± 0.3 (3.9-4.9)	THB (untrained)	8	7
		3.5 [3.2-3.8]	STB (untrained)	8	5
		4.3 ± 0.4 (3.5-4.9)	STB (untrained)	9	7
		4.4 ± 0.5 (3.4-5.0)	STB (trained)	7	7

Continued

TABLE 10-5

Reference Values for Equine Echocardiography in Adult Horses*—cont'd					
Measurement	Mode View	Normal Values Mean ± SD (Range) [Est. 95% range]	Population	N	Reference
LV STUDY – LINEAR MEASUREMENTS–CONT'D					
IVS_d (cm)		3.5 ± 0.4	Warmblood Dressage	15	1
Interventricular septal thickness at end-diastole		3.0 ± 0.3	Warmblood Jumping	14	1
		3.3 ± 0.5	Warmblood Untrained	15	1
		3.4 ± 0.3 (2.9-3.6)	Warmblood Eventing	5	16
		3.0 ± 0.4 (2.4-3.7)	THB and THB cross	26	2
		3.8 ± 0.3 (3.4-4.4)	THB and THB cross	18	3
		2.9 ± 0.3 (2.3-3.4)	THB	38	4
		3.3 ± 0.3 (2.9-3.6)	THB (untrained)	8	7
		2.6 [2.4-2.7]	STB (untrained)	8	5
		3.1 ± 0.3 (2.4-3.5)	STB (untrained)	9	7
		3.3 ± 0.5 (2.5-3.8)	STB (trained)	7	7
$LVPW_s$ (cm)		3.6 ± 0.5	Warmblood Dressage	15	1
Left ventricular free wall at peak systole		3.2 ± 0.5	Warmblood Jumping	14	1
		3.2 ± 0.6	Warmblood Untrained	15	1
		4.4 ± 0.3 (4.1-4.8)	Warmblood Eventing	5	16
		4.0 ± 0.6 (3.0-5.4)	THB and THB cross	9	2
		3.9 ± 0.4 (3.0-4.6)	THB	37	4
		4.4 ± 0.3 (3.9-4.8)	THB (untrained)	8	7
		3.5 [3.2-3.8]	STB (untrained)	8	5
		3.8 ± 0.4 (3.1-4.4)	STB (untrained)	9	7
		4.2 ± 0.4 (3.7-4.9)	STB (trained)	7	7
$LVPW_d$ (cm)		3.0 ± 0.3	Warmblood Dressage	15	1
Left ventricular free wall at end-diastole		2.6 ± 0.4	Warmblood Jumping	14	1
		2.7 ± 0.6	Warmblood Untrained	15	1
		2.7 ± 0.2 (2.4-2.8)	Warmblood Eventing	5	16
		2.3 ± 0.4 (1.7-3.4)	THB	37	4
		2.7 ± 0.3 (2.2-3.1)	THB (untrained)	8	7
		2.4 [2.2-2.6]	STB (untrained)	8	5
		2.3 ± 0.2 (2.0-2.5)	STB (untrained)	9	7
		2.8 ± 0.4 (2.2-3.2)	STB (trained)	7	7

TABLE 10-5

Reference Values for Equine Echocardiography in Adult Horses*—cont'd

Measurement	Mode View	Normal Values Mean ± SD (Range) [Est. 95% range]	Population	N	Reference
LV STUDY – LINEAR MEASUREMENTS–CONT'D					
LV-FS (%)		29 ± 5	Warmblood Dressage	15	1
LV fractional shortening		29 ± 5	Warmblood Jumping	14	1
$= (LVID_d - LVID_s)/LVID_d$		28 ± 5	Warmblood Untrained	15	1
		36 ± 9 (24.0-46.0)	Warmblood Eventing	5	16
		38.8 ± 4.6 (29.0-47.0)	THB and THB cross	21	2
		35.5 ± 3.9 (26.3-43.5)	THB and THB cross	18	3
		37.4 ± 3.9 (29.4-44.7)	THB	37	4
		40 ± 9	THB (untrained)	7	8
		31 ± 3	THB (trained)	7	8
		39.4 ± 5.6 (32.9-50.4)	THB (untrained)	8	7
		33	STB (untrained)	8	5
		34.1 ± 5.0 [24.1-44.2]	STB (untrained)	103	6
		30.9 ± 4.0 [22.9-38.9]	STB (trained)	103	6
		35.6 ± 5.9 (28.7-47.1)	STB (untrained)	9	7
		35.0 ± 4.1 (30.1-39.3)	STB (trained)	7	7
RWT		0.53 ± 0.05 (0.49-0.61)	Warmblood Eventing	5	16
Relative left ventricular wall thickness at end-diastole		0.36 – 0.38	TBH (trained, variable)	483	9
		0.4 ± 0.05	THB (untrained)	7	8
$= (LVPW_d + IVS_d)/ LVID_d$		0.45 ± 0.08	THB (trained)	7	8
		0.52 ± 0.05 (0.44-0.56)	THB (untrained)	8	7
		0.43	STB (untrained)	8	5
		0.40 ± 0.04 [0.32-0.48]	STB (untrained)	103	6
		0.40 ± 0.04 [0.32-0.48]	STB (trained)	103	6
		0.46 ± 0.02 (0.43-0.50)	STB (untrained)	9	7
		0.53 ± 0.07 (0.42-0.62)	STB (trained)	7	7
MWT		2.39-2.53 (range of means)	TBH (trained, variable)	483	9
Mean left ventricular wall thickness at end-diastole		2.4 ± 0.2	THB (untrained)	7	8
$= (LVPW_d + IVS_d)/2$		2.7 ± 0.1	THB (trained)	7	8
		2.98 ± 0.18 (2.70-3.22)	THB (untrained)	8	7
		2.19 ± 0.18 [1.83-2.55]	STB (untrained)	103	6
		2.43 ± 0.17 [2.09-2.77]	STB (trained)	103	6
		2.66 ± 0.20 (2.21-2.91)	STB (untrained)	9	7
		3.08 ± 0.43 (2.38-3.43)	STB (trained)	6	7
LV Mass (g)		4087 ± 727 (3175-4878)	Warmblood Eventing	5	16
Left ventricular mass		3358-4322 (range of means)	TBH (trained, variable)	483	9
$= 1.04 \times [(LVID_d+LVPW_d+IVS_d)^3 - LVID_d^3] - 13.6$		2866 ± 333	THB (untrained)	7	8
		3783 ± 240	THB (trained)	7	8
		2350 ± 383 [1584-3116]	STB (untrained)	103	6
		3263 ± 478 [2307-4219]	STB (trained)	103	6

Continued

TABLE 10-5

Reference Values for Equine Echocardiography in Adult Horses*—cont'd

Measurement	Mode View Timing	Normal Values Mean ± SD (Range) [Est. 95% range]	Population	N	Reference
LV SYSTOLIC TIME INTERVALS					
LVPEP (ms)	Ref 11, 15:	76 ± 18 [MM]	THB and THB cross	24	11
Pre-ejection period	M-mode	75 ± 110 (40-110) [PWD]	THB and THB cross	40	12
Ref 11: = time (R – O)	Right parasternal short-axis view – Aortic valve level	70 [PWD]	THB	7	13
Others: = time (Q – valve opening) or time (Q – onset flow)	Q: Onset Q wave	71 ± 10 (50-90) [MM]	THB and THB cross	112	14
	R: Peak R wave	68 ± 9 (58-88) [PWD]	THB and THB cross	112	14
	O: Point at which valve fully opened	46 ± 13/44 ± 13/41 ± 11 [MM]	STB	13	15
	C: Closure point	58 ± 21/61 ± 16/57 ± 15 [PWD]	STB	13	15
LVET (ms)	Ref 12, 13, 15:	407 ± 18 [MM]	THB and THB cross	24	11
Ejection time	PW-Doppler	467 ± 31 (410-550) [PWD]	THB and THB cross	40	12
Ref 11: = time (O – C)	Left parasternal long-axis view – Aortic outflow	480 [PWD]	THB	7	13
Others: = time (valve opening - closing) or time (onset – end of flow)		532 ± 97 (550-790) [MM]	THB and THB cross	112	14
	Ref 14:	527 ± 76 (400-700) [PWD]	THB and THB cross	112	14
	M-mode and PW-Doppler	452 ± 17/445 ± 16/447 ± 13 [MM]	STB	13	15
	Left-parasternal view	517 ± 28/507 ± 25/509 ± 23 [PWD]	STB	15	15
LVPEP/LVET		0.186 ± 0.04 [MM]	THB and THB cross	24	11
		0.138 ± 0.025 (0.09-0.24) [MM]	THB and THB cross	112	14
		0.131 ± 0.01 (0.092-0.31) [PWD]	THB and THB cross	112	14
		0.10 ± 0.03 [MM]	STB	13	15
		0.11 ± 0.04/0.12 ± 0.03 [PWD]	STB	13	15
LV STUDY – AREA MEASUREMENTS					
LV area$_s$ (cm^2)	2D	67.7 ± 10.1	THB and THB cross	18	3
LV internal area at peak systole	Right parasternal short-axis view—chordal level	40.8 ± 6.9 (29.3-57.2)	THB	37	4
LV area$_d$ (cm^2)		97.3-120 (range of means)	TBH (trained, variable)	483	9
LV internal area at end-diastole		100.9 ± 10.6 (81.2-124.0)	THB	37	4
LV myocardial area$_s$ (cm^2) LV myocardial area at peak systole		191.1 ± 16.8 (156.8-243.6)	THB	37	4
LV myocardial area$_d$ (cm^2) LV myocardial area at end-diastole		223.0 ± 15.2 (193-259.6)	THB	37	4
LV FAC (%) LV fractional area change = (LV Area$_d$ – LV Area$_s$)/LV Area$_d$		59.5 ± 5.0 (46.8-69.3)	THB	37	4

TABLE 10-5

Reference Values for Equine Echocardiography in Adult Horses*—cont'd

Measurement	Mode View Timing	Normal Values Mean ± SD (Range)	Population	N	Reference
LA STUDY					
LAD_{min} (cm)	2D	11.0 ± 0.8 (9.4-12.3)	THB and THB cross	18	3
Left atrial diameter at end-diastole	Left parasternal long-axis view	12.8 ± 0.8 (11.3-14.5)	THB	36	4
		max 13.5	THB and STB		10
	Mid-atrium min = end-diastole	max 14.0	Larger horses		10
LAD_{max} (cm)	max = end-systole	13.1 ± 0.5 (12.7-13.6)	Warmblood Eventing	5	16
Left atrial diameter at end-systole		12.6 ± 1.3 (10.8-15.7)	THB and THB cross	18	3
		12.9 ± 0.8 (11.2-14.5)	THB	28	4
LAD_{max} (cm)	2D	12.7 ± 0.9 (11.4-13.8)	Warmblood Eventing	5	16
Left atrial diameter at end-systole	Right parasternal long-axis view	12.6 ± 1.3 (10.9-14.6)	THB (untrained)	8	7
	(4-chamber view,	12.1 ± 0.9 (10.8-13.7)	STB (untrained, old)	9	7
	optimized for LA)	12.4 ± 1.4 (10.4-13.8)	STB (trained, young)	5	7
LAD_{max}/AAD	Mid-atrium	1.9 ± 0.2 (1.7-2.1)	Warmblood Eventing	5	16
LAD_{max} normalized to aortic annular diameter (see below)	max = end-systole (opening of mitral valve)	1.8 ± 0.2 (1.5-2.1)	THB (untrained)	8	7
	a = onset of atrial	1.9 ± 0.2 (1.7-2.1)	STB (untrained, old)	9	7
	contraction (P-wave)	1.9 ± 0.2 (1.6-2.1)	STB (trained, young)	5	7
LA $Area_{max}$ (cm^2)	min = end-diastole	103.5 ± 13.4 (82.1-117.6)	Warmblood Eventing	5	16
Left-atrial area at end-systole	(closure of mitral valve)	99.5 ± 11.3 (87.2-121.2)	THB (untrained)	8	7
		92.7 ± 9.1 (79.9-108.8)	STB (untrained, old)	9	7
		94.5 ± 12.6 (73.8-105.9)	STB (trained, young)	5	7
LA $Area_{max}$/AAD^2		2.6 ± 0.4 (2.1-3.1)	Warmblood Eventing	5	16
LA $Area_{max}$ normalized to the second power of aortic annular diameter		2.0 ± 0.3 (1.6-2.5)	THB (untrained)	8	7
		2.3 ± 0.4 (1.8-3.0)	STB (untrained, old)	9	7
		2.2 ± 0.3 (1.9-2.5)	STB (trained, young)	5	7
Passive LA FAC (%)		23.6 ± 4.9 (18.0-30.0)	Warmblood Eventing	5	16
Passive left atrial fractional area change		23.6 ± 4.3 (16.6-29.2)	THB (untrained)	7	7
= (LA $Area_{max}$ – LA $Area_a$)/ LA $Area_{max}$		26.7 ± 5.4 (17.1-31.8)	STB (untrained, old)	9	7
		19.8 ± 5.2 (11.4-24.2)	STB (trained, young)	5	7
Active LA FAC (%)		15.4 ± 5.3 (9.0-21.0)	Warmblood Eventing	5	16
Active left atrial fractional area change		18.7 ± 3.4 (13.6-23.2)	THB (untrained)	7	7
		19.7 ± 5.3 (11.4-27.6)	STB (untrained, old)	9	7
= (LA $Area_a$ – LA $Area_{min}$)/ LA $Area_a$		14.4 ± 6.2 (8.2-22.2)	STB (trained, young)	5	7

Continued

TABLE 10-5

Reference Values for Equine Echocardiography in Adult Horses*—cont'd

Measurement	Mode View Timing	Normal Values Mean ± SD (Range)	Population	N	Reference
LA STUDY—CON'D					
Total LA FAC (%) Total left atrial fractional area change $= (\text{LA Area}_{max} - \text{LA Area}_{min}) / \text{LA Area}_{max}$		35.2 ± 4.7 (29.0-42.0)	Warmblood Eventing	5	16
		38.0 ± 2.7 (34.9-43.0)	THB (untrained)	7	7
		41.3 ± 4.0 (35.3-48.8)	STB (untrained, old)	9	7
		31.6 ± 1.7 (30.4-34.7)	STB (trained, young)	5	7
Active: total LA AC Ratio of active to total LV area change		0.33 ± 0.11 (0.17-0.48)	Warmblood Eventing	5	16
		0.38 ± 0.08 (0.27-0.53)	THB (untrained)	7	7
		0.35 ± 0.12 (0.19-0.54)	STB (untrained, old)	9	7
		0.37 ± 0.18 (0.20-0.64)	STB (trained, young)	5	7
LA RI (Area) (%) Area-based left atrial reservoir index $= (\text{LA Area}_{max} - \text{LA Area}_{min}) / \text{LA Area}_{min}$		54.8± 11.4 (40.0-72.0)	Warmblood Eventing	5	16
		62.7 ± 7.3 (53.5-75.7)	THB (untrained)	7	7
		71.9 ± 12.2 (54.6-95.5)	STB (untrained, old)	9	7
		46.6 ± 3.7 (43.8-53.1)	STB (trained, young)	5	7
$\text{LA}_{sx}\text{Area}_{max}$ (cm^2) Left-atrial area at end-systole	2D Right parasternal short-axis view—aortic level max = End-systole	113.4 ± 18.1 (95.0-138.8)	Warmblood Eventing	5	16
		118.4 ± 10.4 (99.3-131.7)	THB (untrained)	8	7
		106.2 ± 17.5 (65.5-125.0)	STB (untrained, old)	9	7
		110.2 ± 8.8 (97.4-118.1)	STB (trained, young)	5	7
$\text{LA}_{sx}\text{Area}_{max}/\text{Ao}_{sx}\text{Area}$ $\text{LA}_{sx}\text{Area}_{max}$ normalized to aortic area		2.3 ± 0.3 (2.1-2.7)	Warmblood Eventing	5	16
		2.3 ± 0.3 (1.9-2.7)	THB (untrained)	8	7
		2.6 ± 0.5 (2.0-3.7)	STB (untrained, old)	9	7
		2.4 ± 0.2 (2.1-2.6)	STB (trained, young)	5	7
AORTA AND PULMONARY ARTERY					
AAD (cm) Aortic annular diameter	2D Right parasternal long-axis view Peak systole	6.7 ± 0.6 (6.0-7.6)	Warmblood Eventing	5	16
		7.0 ± 0.5 (6.4-7.8)	THB (untrained)	8	7
		6.4 ± 0.5 (5.4-6.9)	STB (untrained)	9	7
		6.5 ± 0.2 (6.2-6.8)	STB (trained)	5	7
AoD (cm) Diameter of the aortic sinus (sinus Valsalva)	2D Right parasternal long-axis view End-diastole	7.8 ± 0.7 (7.2-9.0)	Warmblood Eventing	5	16
		8.7 ± 0.5 (7.84-9.9)	THB	37	4
		8.2 ± 0.7 (7.3-9.5)	THB (untrained)	8	7
		7.4 ± 0.7 (6.2-8.4)	STB (untrained)	9	7
		7.5 ± 0.6 (7.2-8.5)	STB (trained)	5	7

TABLE 10-5

Reference Values for Equine Echocardiography in Adult Horses*—cont'd

Measurement	Mode View Timing	Normal Values Mean ± SD (Range)	Population	N	Reference
AORTA AND PULMONARY ARTERY—CONT'D					
PAD (cm)	2D	6.6 ± 0.6 (5.9-7.4)	Warmblood Eventing	5	16
Diameter of the pulmonary sinus	Right parasternal long-axis view	6.1 ± 0.5 (5.2-6.9)	THB	37	4
		6.4 ± 0.4 (5.5-6.8)	THB (untrained)	8	7
	End-diastole	6.1 ± 0.4 (5.6-6.8)	STB (untrained)	9	7
		6.5 ± 0.5 (5.9-6.9)	STB (trained)	5	7
PAD_{ann} (cm)	2D	5.5	STB (untrained)	8	5
Annular diameter of the pulmonary artery (at insertion of the PV)	Right parasternal long-axis view				
	Late-systole				
AoD/PAD	2D	1.2 ± 0.1 (1.0-1.3)	Warmblood Eventing	5	16
	Right parasternal long-axis view	1.3 ± 0.1 (1.1-1.6)	THB (untrained)	8	7
		1.2 ± 0.1 (1.0-1.5)	STB (untrained)	9	7
	End-diastole	1.2 ± 0.1 (1.1-1.4)	STB (trained)	5	7

This summary is intended to serve as a general guide for assessment of some of the most commonly used echocardiographic indices of cardiac dimensions and cardiac function in horses. Individual measurements may differ depending on echocardiographic techniques and breed, age, and athletic condition of the animal.

SD, Standard deviation; *THB,* Thoroughbred; *STB,* Standardbred; *N,* number of horses; *MM,* M-mode; *PWD,* Pulsed-wave Doppler.

References for Table

[1]Stadler P. et al: M-mode echocardiography in dressage- and show-jumping horses of class „S" and in untrained horses, *J Vet Med Assoc;* 40: 292-306, 1993.
[2]Long KJ et al: Standardized imaging technique for guided M-mode and Doppler echocardiography in the horse, *Equine Vet J* 24: 226–235, 1992.
[3]Voros K et al: Measurement of cardiac dimensions with two dimensional echocardiography in the living horse, *Equine Vet J* 23: 461-465, 1991.
[4]Patteson MW et al: Echocardiographic measurements of cardiac dimensions and indices of cardiac function in normal adult Thoroughbred horses, *Equine Vet J Suppl* 19: 18–27, 1995.
[5]Buhl R, Ersboll AK, Eriksen L, et al.: Sources and magnitude of variation of echocardiographic measurements in normal standardbred horses, *Vet Radiol Ultrasound* 45:505–512, 2004.
[6]Buhl R, Ersboll AK, Eriksen L, et al.: Changes over time in echocardiographic measurements in young Standardbred racehorses undergoing training and racing and association with racing performance, *J Am Vet Med Assoc* 226:1881–1887, 2005.
[7]Schwarzwald CC. Unpublished data. 2006. Techniques see: Schwarzwald CC, Schober KE, Bonagura JD. Methods and reliability of echocardiographic assessment of left atrial size and mechanical function in horses, *Am J Vet Res* 68:735–747, 2007.
[8]Young LE. Cardiac responses to training in 2-year-old thoroughbreds: an echocardiographic study. *Equine Vet J Suppl* 30:195–198, 1999.
[9]Young LE, Rogers K, Wood JL: Left ventricular size and systolic function in Thoroughbred racehorses and their relationships to race performance, *J Appl Physiol* 99:1278–1285, 2005.
[10]Reef VB. Cardiovascular ultrasonography. In Reef VB, editor: *Equine diagnostic ultrasound,* ed 1, Philadelphia, 1998, Saunders, 215–272.
[11]Patteson MW, Gibbs C, Wotton PR, et al: Effects of sedation with detomidine hydrochloride on echocardiographic measurements of cardiac dimensions and indices of cardiac function in horses, *Equine Vet J Suppl* 5:33–37, 1995.
[12]Blissitt KJ, Bonagura JD. Pulsed wave Doppler echocardiography in normal horses, *Equine Vet J Suppl* 5:38–46, 1995.
[13]Young LE, Scott GR: Measurement of cardiac function by transthoracic echocardiography: day to day variability and repeatability in normal Thoroughbred horses. *Equine Vet J* 30:117–122, 1998.
[14]Lightowler C, Piccione G, Fazio F, et al: Systolic time intervals assessed by 2-D echocardiography and spectral Doppler in the horse, *Anim Sci J* 74:505–510, 2003.
[15]Kriz NG, Rose RJ. Repeatability of standard transthoracic echocardiographic measurements in horses, *Aust Vet J* 80:362–370, 2002.
[16]Schwarzwald CC et al: The use of 2D speckle imaging in stress echocardiography in athletic horses. Unpublished data, 2008.

and function.[529] Clinical applications of echocardiography are illustrated later in this chapter.

Intravascular Pressures and Cardiac Catheterization

A large body of literature is derived from catheterization studies of the healthy standing, exercising, and anesthetized horse and pony along with limited catheterization data derived from horses with heart disease.* Normal published data relate in part to population and study methods; accordingly, reference ranges vary considerably and have been summarized recently.[77] Normal values also depend on the head and body positions of the horse, the influence of administered tranquilizers, sedatives, or anesthetic agents, and the size of the animal. Hemodynamic variables that can be measured or calculated by catheterization techniques include systolic, diastolic, and mean BP in the systemic and pulmonary circulations; PA occlusion (or pulmonary capillary wedge) pressure; central venous pressure; intracardiac pressures; CO; systemic and pulmonary vascular resistances; and arteriovenous oxygen difference.

Cardiac catheterization in the clinical setting has largely been replaced by Doppler echocardiography. However, indications for right heart catheterization persist, especially when accurate measurement of PA pressure is needed, the origin of pulmonary hypertension cannot be determined, or the diagnosis of occult constrictive pericardial disease is entertained. Knowledge of the general principles of hemodynamics and catheterization data in health and disease creates a useful framework for understanding clinical assessment of the CV system.

Pressures on the left side of the circulation include systemic arterial, LV, and LA pressures. Measurement of ABP has been described previously. Systemic arterial pressure is related in a directly positive manner to LV systolic function, impedance to blood flow in the aorta, systemic vascular resistance, and heart rate. Systolic pressures in the aorta and LV in the standing horse generally peak at approximately 110 to 130 mm Hg (with individual variation). Diastolic aortic pressure is usually near 75 mm Hg. An increase in heart rate as small as 10 beats/min can increase systemic BP by 20 mm Hg (or grater than these values). A peak systolic pressure gradient between the LV and central aorta indicates an obstruction to LV outflow, a very rare condition in horses. LV diastolic pressure reflects diastolic ventricular function and filling pressures, as well as ventricular emptying during systole. The diastolic pressure most often reported is the end diastolic pressure (typically 12 to 24 mm Hg in standing animals), which is higher than the early (often subatmospheric) minimal diastolic LV pressure. Horses and ponies have higher ventricular end diastolic pressures than do either human beings or dogs.[21,24,246,540] Exercise increases both LA and ventricular end diastolic pressures.* Pathologic elevation of resting LV end diastolic pressure indicates either reduced myocardial contractility, ventricular failure, LV volume overload (large VSD, MR, or AR), myocardial infiltration (lymphoma, amyloid), pericardial constraint, or increased ventricular wall stiffness. LA pressure is rarely measured directly, but can be estimated by a pulmonary capillary wedge pressure as described follows.

*References 37, 42, 46, 47, 71, 214, 258, 260, 261, 269, 270, 276, 280, 282, 284, 288, 309, 321, 368, 372, 376, 377, 381, 386, 393, 406, 498, 265-267, 277-279, 318-320, 530-552.

*References 239, 240, 321, 406, 530-533, 553.

A right heart catheterization is easily performed in most horses using a percutaneous technique involving placement of an 8-French introducer sheath and a 7-French balloon-tipped (Swan-Ganz) catheter of 110 to 120 cm in length. Pressures within the RA, RV, and PA can be obtained by advancing the catheter slowly from the jugular vein into a lobar branch of the PA. This is typically guided by pressure measurements and often with 2D ultrasound imaging. It may be possible to inflate the balloon tip briefly to occlude PA flow and "wedge" the distal catheter tip. This pulmonary capillary wedge pressure can be used to estimate the LV filling pressures of the pulmonary veins and LA.*

Mean RA and central venous pressures estimate the pressures filling the RV and are influenced by plasma volume, venomotor tone, body position, and heart function. Central venous pressure is typically about 5 to 10 mm Hg but increases significantly in recumbent horses, especially during general anesthesia. Values frequently double from the standing preanesthetic measurement, and central venous pressure determinations of 20 mm Hg are not uncommon.[538,554] A single measurement of the central venous pressure or of pressure in the RA is difficult to interpret unless the value is severely elevated. Trends are most important in assessment of plasma volume status and cardiac function. Markedly elevated RA pressures are observed with cardiac tamponade, constrictive pericardial disease (along with an abrupt y descent; see Figure 10-4, A), and in right-sided CHF. The *x* descent of the RA pressure waveform may be replaced by a positive c-v wave in the setting of severe TR; this pressure wave corresponds to a prominent jugular pulsation observed during inspection of the neck.

The peak RV systolic pressure is lower than that of the LV and is usually around 40 mm Hg (to up to 60 mm Hg) in standing horses. A small gradient (usually 10 to 15 mm Hg) may be measured between the ventricular apex and proximal pulmonary artery during systole in normal animals and relates in part to gravitational influences. RV end diastolic pressure is usually between 10 and 14 mm Hg, but values as high as 20 to 28 mm Hg have been reported. Hydrostatic effects can influence the RA and the RV end diastolic pressure if the horse's head is raised or lowered.[385] As with the LV, depression of contractility reduces the rate of systolic pressure development (dp/dt).[309] Elevated RV systolic pressure is recorded in pulmonary hypertension from any cause, with a large VSD, and with RV outflow obstruction as with pulmonic stenosis, tetralogy of Fallot, or obstructive pulmonary valve vegetation.[135] Pathologic elevations in RV diastolic pressure are encountered with pericardial disease, pulmonary hypertension, severe right-sided valvular disease, and CHF (Figure 10-25).

Pulmonary artery pressures in standing mature horses are considerably lower than values recorded from the aorta because of the lower resistance encountered in the pulmonary vascular tree. Mean PA pressure is higher in the newborn foal and decreases significantly during the first 2 weeks of life as pulmonary arteriolar resistance falls.[265] Average PA pressure in healthy horses and ponies is approximately 35 to 45 mm Hg in systole (but can be higher or lower depending on CO). Diastolic PA pressures are lower, approximately 20 to 30 mm Hg, but again showing some variation. Pulmonary pressures

*References 265, 312, 406, 497, 536, 553.

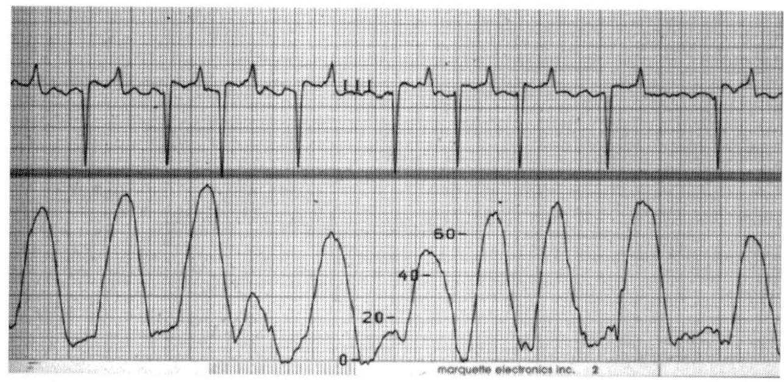

FIGURE 10-25 Recording of intravascular pressure during cardiac catheterization. Right ventricular (RV) pressure recordings from a Thoroughbred yearling with atrial fibrillation (AF), pulmonary hypertension, and biventricular congestive heart failure (CHF). The pressure waveforms vary because of ventilation and the arrhythmia. Peak pressures exceed 70 mm Hg. In the absence of pulmonic stenosis or a large ventricular septal defect (VSD), this indicates pulmonary hypertension. The ventricular end diastolic pressure also is elevated and is compatible with heart failure.

increase dramatically with increased CO as encountered during sinus tachycardia or with exercise.[390,406,532,536,553] The pressure that must be developed in the PA depends not only on pulmonary arteriolar resistance but also (unlike the systemic circulation) on the pulmonary capillary resistance and on the compliance and pressure in the LA. Pulmonary disease can influence these variables; for example, alveolar hypoxia and acidosis can induce reactive vasoconstriction, raising PA pressures.[555] This reaction may be particularly important in newborn foals where vascular resistance is already high.[265]

LV function also directly influences PA pressure because elevation of LA and pulmonary venous pressure places a direct burden on the PA and RV.[246] LV failure generally leads to secondary pulmonary hypertension that can be very severe, with systolic pressures exceeding 100 mm Hg. Presumably, other factors such as reactive vasoconstriction or anatomic changes in the pulmonary vascular tree must develop as a consequence of elevated LA pressures to sustain such high pressures at rest. In other cases the cause of pulmonary hypertension may not be evident.[556] Accordingly, elevated PA pressures must be assessed in light of heart rate, pulmonary wedge, LA or LV end diastolic pressure,[309,310] and CO. When PA pressure is increased, RV systolic pressure is also elevated to meet the pressure load. If pulmonary hypertension is chronic, then right-sided cardiac enlargement, TR, and right-sided heart failure can ensue.

The origin of pulmonary hypertension generally can be determined by conducting a thorough cardiorespiratory examination that includes echocardiographic and Doppler assessment of the left and right sides of the hearts. However, catheterization of the PA under sedation and local anesthesia can be instructive in confusing cases, especially if left-sided heart failure cannot be excluded. The pulmonary occlusion or wedge pressure estimates LV filling pressure and should approximate LV end diastolic pressure, provided that no obstructions are noted in the pulmonary veins or across the mitral valve. The PA diastolic pressure also can estimate PA wedge pressure provided that heart rate is normal and pulmonary vascular resistance is not increased. Increases in pulmonary capillary wedge pressure (or pulmonary diastolic pressure) are measured during exercise as LA pressure increases,[239,312,553] in left-sided CHF,[310,497] with severe MR,[311] and in some horses with AF.[313] Overinfusion of crystalloid solutions or marked depression of LV function are other causes of elevated pulmonary capillary wedge pressure; conversely, the wedge pressure is reduced in hypovolemia. When pulmonary hypertension is not caused by left heart failure, a near-normal wedge pressure is recorded in the setting of elevated PA diastolic pressure. This indicates increased vascular resistance across the small arteries because of pulmonary vasoconstriction or pulmonary vascular lesions. One caveat is that a pressure gradient between the PA diastolic and pulmonary capillary wedge pressures may be observed in normal horses in the setting of resting tachycardia.

CO is the volume of blood pumped by the left (or right) ventricle in 1 minute. This can be divided by body weight or surface area to calculate the cardiac index. The CO can be measured by thermodilution techniques, lithium dilution, arteriovenous oxygen difference (Fick methodology), 2D echocardiographic and Doppler studies, and other methods.* Determination of CO is most often done clinically when monitoring the effects of anesthetic agents or during fluid and drug therapy of the circulation in critical care situations wherein CO relates to tissue oxygen delivery. Reported values for cardiac index in standing horses or ponies are approximately 72 to 88 ml/min/kg. Noninvasive estimation of CO can be achieved using transthoracic 2D and Doppler echocardiographic methods, but (at least in adult horses) these estimates of CO are neither accurate nor reliable. In one study of foals, volumetric measurements by 2D echocardiography provided better estimates of CO than Doppler echocardiography.[275] The mixed venous (pulmonary artery) oxygen content (ml oxygen/dl blood) can be used as an indirect estimate of CO. As CO increases, the tissues extract less oxygen from each aliquot of blood; consequently, the venous oxygen content increases.[267] As CO decreases, the tissue extraction of oxygen increases, the oxygen content decreases, and the systemic-venous oxygen difference widens. Mixed venous samples obtained from PA catheters are probably superior to venous samples obtained from either the jugular or peripheral veins.[462]

Systemic and pulmonary vascular resistances strongly influence the mean pressures in their respective vascular systems. Vasoconstriction increases ABP. However, resistances cannot be measured directly in the intact animal and are generally calculated using a variation of Poiseuille's or Ohm's laws. The general formula for calculation of static vascular resistance is as follows:

Vascular resistance = (mean arterial pressure − mean atrial pressure)/CO

where CO is measured in liters per minute. The pressures used are mean aortic pressure and mean RA pressure for calculation of systemic vascular resistance and mean PA pressure and mean pulmonary wedge pressure for calculation of pulmonary vascular resistance. Correction values may be added to convert resistance to centimeter-gram-second (cgs) units.[561] Normal systemic vascular resistance in horses averages about 265 dynes·s·cm^{-5}.[5,77] Pulmonary vascular resistance should be about one fifth of the systemic value, but reported values vary more widely. Inasmuch as mean arterial pressure is similar between horses of different sizes, calculated vascular resistance is normally higher in smaller horses and ponies. Mechanisms

*References 260, 261, 265-267, 272-280, 282, 284, 285, 532, 534, 535, 551, 557-560.

that increase systemic vascular resistance include sympathetic activation, activation of the renin-angiotensin system, and the release of other vasoactive hormones into the blood, including arginine vasopressin (antidiuretic hormone) and epinephrine.[73] The pulmonary vascular resistance is tied to pulmonary vascular anatomy, age, total lung capillary resistance, LA pressure, and degree of pulmonary vascular constriction. The latter is controlled by the tension of alveolar oxygen and local mediators, including nitric oxide and endothelin.

Laboratory Studies

CV disorders may develop as a consequence of systemic or metabolic diseases such as electrolyte disturbances or septicemia. Conversely, circulatory failure or CV infections may alter routine laboratory tests. Prerenal azotemia and electrolyte disturbances (hyponatremia, hypokalemia, hypomagnesemia) may be detected in the horse with CHF, especially after diuretic therapy. Myocardial enzymes or troponins may be released in the circulation from primary or secondary cardiac muscle injury,[562] as might occur with hypotension, ischemia, or myocardial infarction. Increased cTn_I is often used as a biomarker for recent myocardial injury,[563,564] and this test can be obtained from most commercial laboratories. Elevated concentrations in a horse with an arrhythmia may indicate ongoing myocardial injury or myocarditis. Increased serum cTn_I also can be identified in horses after endurance races but does not necessarily indicate underlying structural heart disease.[563] Natriuretic peptides are released in the blood in response to a variety of stimuli, including myocardial stretch because of volume overload and increases in intracardiac pressures. Plasma atrial natriuretic peptide (ANP) concentrations may be elevated in horses with cardiac disease, particularly in the presence of LA enlargement or LA dysfunction (Schwarzwald CC, unpublished observations). To date, the use of ANP as a cardiac biomarker is limited to experimental settings, and more work is to be done to elucidate its clinical value in horses with heart disease.

An overview of the laboratory studies useful in assessment and management of CV diseases is found in Box 10-4. A complete blood count (CBC) and fibrinogen, biochemical profile, and urinalysis are indicated in horses with arrhythmias, heart failure, or when clinical evidence suggests endocarditis, pericarditis, vasculitis, or pleural effusion. Additional studies including blood cultures, blood gas tensions, oxygen saturation, other electrolytes (e.g., magnesium), cytology and culture of pericardial effusates, and myocardial isoenzymes of CK are indicated in selected cases. Monitoring of serum or plasma drug concentrations, especially quinidine and digoxin, are appropriate when these drugs are administered. Further application of these studies is discussed under specific diseases.

CONGESTIVE HEART FAILURE

Causes of Heart Failure

Heart failure is a clinical syndrome characterized by cardiac disease, limited CO in the setting of normal to high venous pressures, increased neurohormonal activity, renal sodium retention, accumulation of edema in tissues, and transudation of fluid into serous body cavities. The neurohormonal and renal abnormalities that characterize heart failure have not been extensively studied in horses but are probably similar to those reported in other species.[76,105] The most sensitive sign of heart failure is impaired

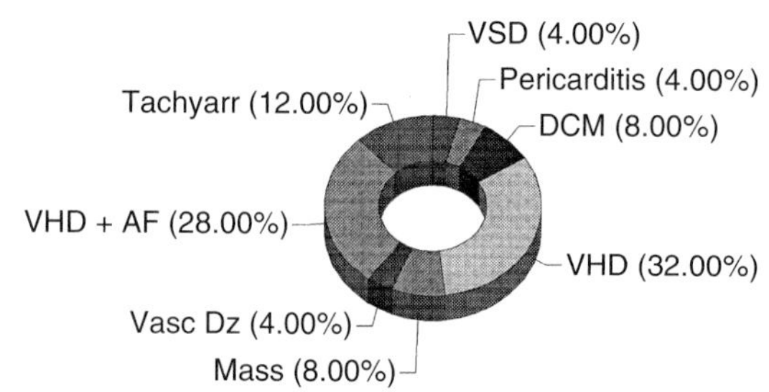

FIGURE 10-26 Graph demonstrating the overall causes of congestive heart failure (CHF) in 25 horses at a referral teaching hospital as a percentage of the total number of cases of equine CHF. *Tachyarr,* Tachyarrhythmia; *VSD,* ventricular septal defect; *DCM,* dilated cardiomyopathy; *VHD,* valvular heart disease; *Mass,* mass lesion; *Vasc Dz,* vascular disease; *VHD + AF,* valvular heart disease and atrial fibrillation. (Data from Ohio State University Veterinary Hospital.)

exercise capacity, but this is hardly specific in horses. The most characteristic clinical features of heart failure are increased venous pressures and fluid accumulation. The typical horse with cardiac failure is recognized in the overtly congested phase termed *CHF.*

Most cardiac lesions in horses are insufficient to cause CHF, and this syndrome is not common in equine practice. Nevertheless, CHF does develop in foals and mature horses as a consequence of diverse disorders, including congenital malformation, severe degenerative valvular disease, valvulitis, bacterial endocarditis, dilated cardiomyopathy, myocarditis, myocardial necrosis, pericardial disease, vascular rupture, pulmonary hypertension, artery obstruction, or persistent tachyarrhythmia.[112,564,565] The most common cause of CHF in horses is valvular heart disease—often complicated by AF (Figure 10-26). In addition to structural lesions of the heart and blood vessels, primary electrical disturbances, particularly sustained AV dissociation caused by intractable junctional or VT, can reduce myocardial function, decrease CO, and lead to CHF.[566] This is especially likely when the heart rate exceeds 100 beats/min for many days. Resolution of CHF in such cases may be possible if antiarrhythmic therapy is successful.

Clinical Recognition of Heart Failure

Congestive heart failure may develop suddenly or gradually. Peracute heart failure can occur after rupture of mitral valve chordae tendineae or consequent to acute endocarditis of a heart valve. Rapid multiform ventricular tachycardia can also result in the sudden development of congestive heart failure. Heart failure may progress rapidly in a foal with a large VSD as the pulmonary vascular resistance falls in the weeks after birth. Chronic valvular regurgitation can, after many years, lead to CHF; although only a small number of horses with degenerative valvular disease develop CHF.[567] Some lesions, which might otherwise be well tolerated, can cause heart failure if increased demands for CO develop. Examples include strenuous work, severe anemia, or persistent fever. Pregnancy is another example: the volume expansion and increased demands for CO in the latter stages of gestation may precipitate CHF in a mare with previously compensated heart disease. Development of AF in a horse with underlying structural disease, such as severe mitral or AR, can precipitate CHF.[568,569] Such cases are distinguished from the more typical case of AF by the presence of persistent, resting tachycardia and identification of structural lesions and cardiomegaly during echocardiography.

The clinical features of CHF are easily recognized,[399] but determination of the underlying cause of heart disease may be more difficult. The cause can be established if careful auscultation is combined with echocardiography, ECG, laboratory tests, and ultrasound examination of other body cavities.* Presenting clinical signs can vary but often include exercise intolerance, poor recovery after exercise, weight loss, coughing, tachypnea, ventral edema, and often colic-like signs.

The clinical features of right-sided CHF include resting tachycardia and prominent third (ventricular) sound along with generalized ventral, preputial, pectoral, and limb edema. Isolated limb edema, which is so common in hospitalized horses, is not a sign of CHF. Nor does ventral edema in the absence of generalized venous distention suggest a diagnosis of CHF. This finding should prompt consideration of other disorders including hypoproteinemia, vasculitis or severe pleural or abdominal effusion, or causes of generalized fluid retention. Scrutiny of the jugular and other superficial veins generally makes the recognition of right-sided CHF straightforward, because affected horses demonstrate elevated venous pressure and pathologic jugular pulses and filling (see Figures 10-12 and 10-13). The most common causes of "isolated" right-sided CHF are tricuspid or pulmonic valve lesions as with valvular endocarditis, diffuse pulmonary vascular disease, and pericardial disease. In most cases a prominent murmur of TR will be evident over the right thorax. When pulmonary hypertension underlies right-sided failure, the tricuspid murmur may be especially loud and the pulmonic component of the second heart sound tympanic. Because right-sided heart failure often develops consequent to pulmonary hypertension caused by left heart failure, left-sided murmurs are not uncommon. Another common association of right-sided CHF is persistent cardiac arrhythmia, such as AF, superimposed on structural heart disease of any form. Horses with long-standing uniform ventricular tachycardia can also present with right-sided heart failure. Cranial mediastinal lymphosarcoma and cranial thoracic masses including large pulmonary abscesses must be distinguished from RV failure.[100,581] Differential diagnosis is facilitated by examination with 2D echocardiography and thoracic ultrasonography.

The recognition of isolated left-sided heart failure, which causes pulmonary venous congestion and pulmonary edema, is more difficult in horses. In these cases, heart sounds and murmurs may be difficult to identify owing to loud airway sounds or even pulmonary crackles. If a cardiac murmur is present but missed, then an erroneous diagnosis of pneumonia may be entertained. Again, resting tachycardia and loud third heart sound are typical in these cases, and echocardiographic examination of the horse will be particularly useful. Typical findings in acute left-sided CHF are dilatation and rounding of the LA and ventricle, dilation of pulmonary veins, and often dilatation of the PA caused by pulmonary hypertension. A small aortic root may be evident, associated with low cardiac output. Careful examination may demonstrate anatomic lesions of the aortic root, ventricular septum, left heart valves, or chordae tendineae. Fulminant left-sided CHF can lead to coughing and expectoration of edema—a grave sign in most horses.

Biventricular CHF is most commonly observed when severe left sided disease results in chronic CHF and is complicated by AF. The clinical signs of advanced biventricular heart failure include resting tachycardia (usually >60 beats/min), loud ventricular filling sound, subcutaneous edema, tachypnea (from pulmonary edema or pleural effusion), varying amounts of ascites and pleural effusion, a small pericardial effusion, jugular distention, and abnormal jugular pulsations. Chronic biventricular CHF is frequently characterized by lethargy and also by loss of body condition. In most cases there will be one or more cardiac murmurs on the left typical of mitral or aortic valvular regurgitation and a murmur of TR on the right. Infrequently biventricular CHF is the result of congenital heart disease such as a VSD.

It is important to understand that *chronic* left-sided CHF in the horse is likely to cause interstitial lung edema and pulmonary hypertension. The magnitude of pulmonary hypertension is often impressive, with systolic PA pressures exceeding 80 mm Hg in many cases. The mechanisms by which the lung accommodates such severe and chronic elevations in pulmonary venous pressures without development of alveolar edema is speculative. It is likely that pulmonary arterial resistance increases, possibly related to remodeling in pulmonary arteries from chronic elevation of LA pressure. Chronic pulmonary hypertension also leads to RV dilatation and TR, which limits CO and predisposes to right-sided CHF. Furthermore, generalized fluid retention is a characteristic of chronic CHF in most species, and this retained fluid is generally pooled in the skin, pleural space, and peritoneal cavity.

Thus the clinician should anticipate signs of right-sided CHF even when the primary cardiac lesion is located on the left side of the heart. Clinical findings of severe pulmonary hypertension caused by left-sided CHF include a loud, tympanic, pulmonary component of the second heart sound (heard cranioventral to the aortic valve area), a systolic murmur and jugular pulse of tricuspid insufficiency, and dilatation of the PA, which can be identified by 2D echocardiography. Thoracic radiographs may demonstrate increased pulmonary vascularity, pulmonary infiltration near the hilus, pleural effusion, and rounding or enlargement of the cardiac silhouette. Further scrutiny of the echocardiogram identifies LA dilatation and lesions affecting the LV and usually the mitral valve, aortic valve, or the aorta. Doppler echocardiography can document abnormal flow patterns such as valvular regurgitation and predict PA pressures (using the Bernoulli relationship discussed previously). An ECG is needed to evaluate cardiac arrhythmias.

Therapy for Congestive Heart Failure

Therapy for CHF is realistic for potentially reversible disorders such as pericarditis or sustained ventricular tachyarrhythmia. It may also be feasible for valuable breeding stallions and mares, mares that develop CHF during gestation, or horses and ponies kept as pets.[146,399,582] Before therapy can commence, an accurate diagnosis is needed. For example, pericardiocentesis (not cardiac drugs) would be appropriate initial management of cardiac tamponade; thereafter, surgical drainage of the effusion (using drainage tubes) or a pericardiectomy could be considered.[86,87,94,583,584] Antibiotics would be essential in the treatment of bacterial endocarditis or infective pericarditis. Sustained junctional and ventricular tachyarrhythmias may lead to low CO and a potentially reversible dilated cardiomyopathy. Antiarrhythmic therapy with quinidine, magnesium sulfate solution, lidocaine, procainamide, propafenone, or amiodarone may be effective for treatment of some of these arrhythmias, and with resumption of normal rhythm, CHF may be reversed.

Furosemide[294,572,585-587] is administered to horses with CHF not associated with cardiac tamponade. The dosage initially

*References 87, 88, 105, 109, 112, 137, 146-148, 152, 186, 294, 299, 300, 309, 342, 504, 556, 565, 568-569, 570-580.

should be directed to mobilize edema and prevent its recurrence, and 1 to 2 mg/kg IV boluses are given to effect, whereby the higher or more frequent doses may be required when renal function is impaired.[588] Bolus administration may be followed by constant-rate infusion when profound diuresis is needed (Table 10-6). Respiratory effort should improve when pulmonary edema is evident. Short-term therapy with nasal oxygen, if available, also may be useful for horses with respiratory distress. Volume depletion, azotemia, and electrolyte imbalances are the most common adverse effects. Renal function should be followed and the dosage controlled to minimize prerenal azotemia. Diuretic therapy may eventually be discontinued in some horses, but others will require once- or twice-daily administration on the farm to prevent fluid retention.

Digoxin therapy is indicated for CHF not associated with pericardial disease or serious ventricular ectopy and is particularly beneficial when concurrent AF is superimposed on structural valvular heart disease. Treatment is initiated by the IV route, with most (450 to 550 kg) horses receiving a total dose of about 1 mg IV (see Table 10-6). The reported elimination half-life of digoxin has not been consistent (7.2 to 28 hours) and probably relates to the clinical state of the animals studied.* Long-term digoxin therapy involves once or twice daily oral administration, usually mixed with molasses and some grain. As expected, oral doses of digoxin are relatively higher because of lower bioavailability (20%).[300] Chronic digoxin therapy is monitored by measuring the serum digoxin concentration (drawn between 8 to 12 hours after the previous dose). Target therapeutic values range between 0.8 to 1.5 ng/ml (1-1.5 nmol/L), depending on the time of the blood sample, and drug therapy achieving these levels is usually well tolerated in terms of appetite and heart rhythm. Periodic cardiac examinations, measurements of serum biochemistries (creatinine, electrolytes), and recordings of ECG rhythm strips are be warranted during any long-term course of therapy.

Limited published experience is available regarding use of vasodilators and ACE inhibitors in horses with CHF. Hydralazine[268] might be considered in the initial management of severe MR caused by ruptured chordae tendineae or endocarditis, because systemic arterial dilatation can reduce the mitral regurgitant fraction. ACE inhibitors decrease renal sodium and water reabsorption, reduce volume overload, blunt the mechanisms leading to diuretic resistance, cause vasodilation, decrease in myocardial oxygen demand, and are considered cardioprotective by decreasing myocardial remodeling and fibrosis. In humans, ACE inhibitors have been shown to reduce mortality in heart failure. However, the benefits of ACE inhibitors have not been well studied in equine heart failure. Limited data are available in horses regarding enalapril,[315,591,592] ramipril,[593] and quinapril.[594] Although effective intravenously, oral enalapril did not significantly reduce ACE activity after oral administration. Ramipril administered at 200 μg/kg orally (PO) daily reduced indirect BP in healthy horses in an uncontrolled study, and this drug also has been used to treat CHF.[595] An open-label clinical study of quinapril in horses with MR but without CHF showed some evidence for increased stroke volume and reduced regurgitation fraction.[594] Most ACE inhibitors are contraindicated in humans during pregnancy. Therefore until appropriately studied, all ACE inhibitors should be considered as contraindicated in pregnant mares because of potential ill effects on the fetus.

*References 146, 286, 287, 289, 290, 294, 295, 297, 299, 363, 573, 582, 589, 590.

For horses with cardiomyopathy or valvular disease, or in pregnant mares with CHF, the development of AF may precipitate CHF. Furosemide and digoxin can effectively control CHF in many of these cases. All ACE inhibitors should be considered as contraindicated in pregnant mares because of potential ill effects on the fetus. Quinidine is also generally contraindicated in such cases, although horses may sometimes convert to sinus rhythm after the resolution of CHF by medical therapy. Reasonable long-term control of CHF may be achieved in some of chronic CHF, thus permitting a comfortable existence for the horse and—in the case of breeding animals—continued reproductive service.

Prognosis in CHF is at best guarded when irreversible structural heart disease is the cause of failure; thus the long-term outcome for life is poor. Of course, the horse with CHF requires rest to reduce demands on the heart and should never be worked or ridden owing to the risk of PA rupture, syncope, or fatal arrhythmia. Valuable horses may be used for breeding with great caution, but the stallion in CHF poses some risks for the handler, and pregnant mares are likely to be difficult to control in the later stages of gestation related to the volume expansion that accompanies the latter stages of pregnancy. Embryo transfer and freezing of semen are alternative approaches for valuable animals in CHF.

CONGENITAL HEART DISEASE

The prevalence of congenital heart disease in the overall equine population is unknown. In one survey of causes for neonatal death or euthanasia in 608 cases, the prevalence of congenital heart disease was 3.5%.[160] Congenital heart disease is often considered when a foal, weanling, or immature horse is identified with a prominent cardiac murmur, cyanosis, or signs of CHF.[365] A wide variety of cardiac malformations have been identified.* Theoretically, a great number of cardiac malformations could occur, including anomalies of (1) venous drainage, (2) atrial situs or septation, (3) atrioventricular connection, (4) atrial or ventricular development (including formation of the two atrioventricular valves), (5) ventricular outflow tracts, (6) semilunar valves, and (7) great vessels.[623,624] Furthermore, abnormal segmental connections might occur leading to "discordance" in the path of systemic or pulmonary venous return relative to the pulmonary artery or aorta. These abnormalities include transposition of the great vessels and double-outlet ventricle, wherein both great vessels exit the RV or LV cavity. However, practically speaking, the most common cardiac malformations in horses involve shunting of blood at the atrial or ventricular levels.

Although some defects are lethal to the neonate, other malformations are compatible with life but limit performance or reproductive value. Most cardiac malformations involve shunting of blood, with the VSD most often recognized (Figures 10-27 to 10-29). Isolated malformations leading to valvular stenosis or incompetency are uncommon. Rare lesions such as double-outlet RV,[598] transposition of the great vessels,[157,165,625] aorticopulmonary septal defect,[626] bicuspid pulmonary valve, pulmonary stenosis,[168] persistent fetal circulation,[627] hypoplastic left heart syndrome,[158,159] subaortic stenosis,[607] mitral valve malformation,[510,628]

*References 4, 14, 27, 28, 61, 90, 111, 112, 126, 127, 131, 134, 145, 151, 155-168, 171, 178, 265, 319, 334, 342, 367, 473, 479, 480, 482, 487, 504, 513, 528, 571, 575, 576, 578, 595-622.

TABLE 10-6

Drug Therapy of Heart Disease			
Drug	**Dose Recommendations**	**Comments–Therapeutic Drug Monitoring–Adverse/Toxic Effects**	**Indications (I) Contraindications (CI)**
ANTIARRHYTHMICS			
SODIUM CHANNEL BLOCKER (CLASS I_A)			
Quinidine sulfate (PO) or gluconate (IV)	22 mg/kg quinidine sulfate PO by NGT q2h for 4 (-6) doses until converted, adverse or toxic effects, or plasma quinidine concentration > 4 μg/ml. Do not exceed 6 doses PO q2h. Continue q6h until converted, adverse or toxic effects, or total dose of 180 mg/kg. 1-2.2 mg/kg quinidine gluconate IV q10min or 0.1-0.22 mg/kg/min CRI up to 12 (-24*) mg/kg total dose (*Caution: Can result in severe adverse effects!)	IV administration for AF of recent onset (< 2 weeks) without underlying structural heart disease or AF occurring during anesthesia. PO administration preferred for long-standing AF (> 2-4 weeks). Therapeutic drug monitoring: Therapeutic range: 2-5 μg/ml [6.2-15.4 μmol/L] 1-2 h after PO administration. Adverse effects: Commonly depression, diarrhea, colic, nasal mucosal swelling, and ataxia; rarely: paraphimosis, urticaria, and laminitis. Cardiovascular effects include acceleration of AV conduction and tachycardia (most common), prolonged QRS and QT interval, VT or torsades de pointes, hypotension, negative inotropism, exacerbation of heart failure, cardiovascular collapse, sudden death.	I: AF, SVT (ventricular arrhythmias) CI: Ventricular tachyarrhythmias, torsades de pointes, untreated heart failure, preexisting prolonged QRS or QT interval, complete AV block, digitalis intoxication. Use with caution in patients with uncorrected hypokalemia, hypomagnesemia, hypoxia, or acid-base disorders.
Procainamide	25-35 mg/kg PO q8h 1 mg/kg/min IV, up to 20 mg/kg total dose	Adverse effects: Hypotension, QRS and QT prolongation, negative inotropism, arrhythmias, GI and neurologic disorders. Similar but generally less severe than with quinidine.	I: Ventricular and supraventricular arrhythmias CI: See quinidine
SODIUM CHANNEL BLOCKER (CLASS I_B)			
Lidocaine	0.25-0.5 mg/kg slow IV, repeat in 5-10 min to effect, up to 1.5 mg/kg total dose; followed by 0.03-0.05 mg/kg/min CRI	Adverse effects: Low incidence at therapeutic doses. Occasionally depression and muscle fasciculations. Overdoses may lead to ataxia, CNS excitement, seizures, hypotension, VT, collapse, and sudden death.	I: Ventricular arrhythmias, (potentially vagally sustained AF) CI: SA, AV, or intraventricular block, bradycardia. Caution with hypovolemia, liver disease, shock, and heart failure.
Phenytoin	20 mg/kg PO q12h for 3-4 doses or until signs of sedation, followed by 10-15 mg/kg PO q12 maintenance dose 5-10 mg/kg IV, followed by 1-5 mg/kg IM q12h or 10-15 mg/kg PO q12h	Maintenance dose varies considerably. Therapeutic drug monitoring: Therapeutic range 5-10 μg/ml [19.8-39.6 μmol/L]. Adverse effects: Sedation, lip and facial twitching, gait deficits, excitation seizures, arrhythmias. Hepatotoxicity with chronic therapy. Hypotension and respiratory depression at high doses.	I: Digoxin-induced arrhythmias, other ventricular arrhythmias CI: SA or AV block, sinus bradycardia

Continued

TABLE 10-6

Drug Therapy of Heart Disease—cont'd

Drug	Dose Recommendations	Comments–Therapeutic Drug Monitoring–Adverse/Toxic Effects	Indications (I) Contraindications (CI)
SODIUM CHANNEL BLOCKER (CLASS I_C)			
Flecainide	1-2 mg/kg IV, infused at a rate of 0.2 mg/kg/min 4 mg/kg PO q2h for 4-6 doses, followed by 4 mg/kg PO q4h; adjust dose intervals if signs of toxicity occur.	Use with caution. Not generally recommended for treatment of AF. May not be effective for chronic AF. Adverse effects: Depression, colic, neurologic signs, negative inotropism, QRS and QT prolongation, severe ventricular arrhythmias, sudden death	I: Acute AF, supraventricular and ventricular arrhythmias resistant to other treatments CI: Structural heart disease, heart failure, SA or AV node dysfunction
Propafenone	0.5-2.0 mg/kg in 5% dextrose slowly IV over 10-15 min 2 mg/kg PO q8h	Can be used for IV or PO control of serious ventricular arrhythmias. IV formulation not available in U.S.A. Adverse effects: GI and neurologic disorders, bronchospasm, negative inotropism, exacerbation of heart failure, AV block, QRS and QT prolongation, arrhythmias	I: Supraventricular and ventricular arrhythmias resistant to other treatments CI: Structural heart disease, heart failure, SA or AV node dysfunction
β-ADRENOCEPTOR BLOCKER (CLASS II)			
Propranolol	0.03-0.16 mg/kg slow IV q12h 0.38-0.78 mg/kg PO q8h	Unspecific β_1/β_2-blocker. Variable oral bioavailability. Dosage should be individually adjusted. Adverse effects: Depression, lethargy, weakness, bradycardia, AV block, hypotension, negative inotropism, exacerbation of heart failure, bronchoconstriction (aggravation of recurrent airway obstruction)	I: SVT and AF (rate control, often in combination with digoxin), catecholamine-induced arrhythmias, unresponsive supraventricular and ventricular arrhythmias CI: Bradycardia, high-degree AV block, untreated heart failure, bronchopulmonary disease
POTASSIUM CHANNEL BLOCKER (CLASS III)			
Amiodarone	5 mg/kg/h IV for 1 h, followed by 0.83 mg/kg/h for 23h, and subsequently 1.9 mg/kg/h for 30h or to effect	Also class I, II, and IV effects. Poor and variable oral bioavailability, long half-life (16 days). Adverse reactions: Hindlimb weakness, weight shifting, torsades de pointes (supposedly low incidence), SA and AV nodal inhibition, bradycardia, hypotension. Prolonged treatment may affect lungs, liver, heart, thyroid gland, GI tract, eyes, skin, and nerves.	I: AF, ventricular arrhythmias (not investigated) CI: Sinus node dysfunction, bradycardia, AV block, cardiogenic shock
Bretylium tosylate	3-5 mg/kg IV, repeat up to 10 mg/kg	Also indirect anti-adrenergic effects Adverse effects: Excitement, GI disorders, hypotension, tachycardia, arrhythmias	I: Refractory, life-threatening ventricular tachycardia, ventricular fibrillation
CALCIUM CHANNEL BLOCKER (CLASS IV)			
Diltiazem	0.125 mg/kg over 2 min IV, repeated every 10 minutes to effect, up to 1.25 mg/kg total dose	Titrate to effect. Use diltiazem doses > 0.5-1.0 mg/kg with caution. Adverse effects of class IV drugs: Hypotension, tachycardia, sinus arrhythmia, bradycardia, sinus arrest, high-grade AV block, negative inotropism, exacerbation of heart failure (unless secondary to SVT or AF with rapid ventricular response rate)	I: Supraventricular arrhythmias (ventricular rate control in AF and interruption of SA/AV nodal-dependent SVT) CI: Hypotension, bradycardia, SA or AV block, ventricular systolic dysfunction, severe heart failure, cardiogenic shock, β-blocker
Verapamil	0.025-0.05 mg/kg IV q30min, up to 0.2 mg/kg total dose		

TABLE 10-6

Drug Therapy of Heart Disease—cont'd

Drug	Dose Recommendations	Comments–Therapeutic Drug Monitoring–Adverse/Toxic Effects	Indications (I) Contraindications (CI)
PHYSIOLOGIC CALCIUM CHANNEL BLOCKER, ACTIVATOR OF MEMBRANE NA⁺/K⁺-ATPASE			
Magnesium sulfate	2-6 mg/kg/min IV to effect, up 55 (-100) mg/kg total dose	Adverse effects: Overdoses (rare) may lead to CNS depressant effects, weakness, trembling, bradycardia, hypotension. Very high doses lead to neuromuscular blockade with respiratory depression and cardiac arrest.	I: Ventricular arrhythmias (especially for quinine induced and other causes of torsades de pointes and refractory VT), hypomagnesemia associated with cardiovascular disease CI: Bradycardia, SA and AV block, renal failure
DIGITALIS GLYCOSIDES			
Digoxin	IV loading dose: 0.0022 mg/kg IV q12h, for 2 doses IV maintenance dose: 0.0022 mg/kg IV q24h PO maintenance dose: 0.011 mg/kg PO q12h	Therapeutic drug monitoring: Peak (1-2h) and trough (12h) concentrations at steady state should fall within 0.8-1.2 (2.0) ng/ml [1-1.5 (2.6) nmol/L]. Adverse effects: Depression, anorexia, colic, diarrhea, sinus bradycardia, AV block, supraventricular and ventricular arrhythmias (bigeminy)	I: Heart failure, ventricular rate control in SVT or AF CI: AV block, diastolic ventricular dysfunction, preexisting digitalis toxicity, myocarditis, ventricular arrhythmias
ADRENERGIC (SYMPATHOMIMETIC) AGENTS			
INOTROPES			
Dopamine	1-5 μg/kg/min CRI, titrate to effect or adverse reactions	β_1-Adrenergic, also dose-dependent dopaminergic and α_1-adrenergic Adverse reactions: Tachycardia, ventricular arrhythmias, vasoconstriction and hypertension can occur at doses > 4-5 μg/kg/min	I: Hypotension, acute heart failure, cardiogenic shock, noncardiogenic shock (after adequate fluid loading), sinus arrest, bradycardia, high-grade or complete AV block, vagally induced bradyarrhythmias
Dobutamine	1-5 μg/kg/min CRI, titrate to effect or adverse reactions	β_1-Adrenergic, also β_2- and α_1-adrenergic. Preferred over dopamine. Adverse reactions: Tachycardia, ventricular arrhythmias, vasoconstriction	CI: Ventricular arrhythmias, tachycardia, atrial fibrillation (risk of severe tachycardia because of accelerated AV conduction)
Epinephrine	0.01-0.05 mg/kg IV 0.1-0.5 mg/kg IT Note different concentrations: *1:1,000 = 1 mg/ml* *1:10,000 = 0.1 mg/ml*	β-Adrenergic, α_1-adrenergic at higher doses Adverse effects: Tremor, excitability, arrhythmias, ventricular fibrillation. Overdoses can lead to hypertension, arrhythmias, renal failure, pulmonary edema, cerebral hemorrhage.	I: Ventricular asystole, cardiopulmonary resuscitation CI: Nonanaphylactic shock, arrhythmias, hypertension
VASOPRESSORS			
Norepinephrine	0.05-1 μg/kg/min CRI, titrate to effect	α_1-adrenergic. Norepinephrine also exerts some β_1-adrenergic effects.	I: Hypotension and shock associated with excessive peripheral vasodilation (i.e., septic or endotoxemic shock, quinidine toxicity; after adequate volume loading)
Phenylephrine	0.1-1 μg/kg/min CRI, titrate to effect	Usually administered in conjunction with fluid therapy and dobutamine. Adverse effects of vasopressors: Hypertension, reflex bradycardia, reduction in cardiac output because of increased afterload, CNS effects (excitement, restlessness), rarely arrhythmias. Overdosage can lead to seizures, ventricular arrhythmias, cerebral hemorrhage	CI: Hypertension, bradycardia, poor cardiac output, cardiac disease, ventricular tachycardia

Continued

TABLE 10-6

Drug Therapy of Heart Disease—cont'd

Drug	Dose Recommendations	Comments–Therapeutic Drug Monitoring–Adverse/Toxic Effects	Indications (I) Contraindications (CI)
ANTICHOLINERGIC (VAGOLYTIC) AGENTS			
Atropine Glycopyrrolate	0.01-0.02 mg/kg IV, IM 0.005-0.01 mg/kg IV	Adverse effects: Constipation, ileus, colic, bradycardia (initially or at very low doses), tachycardia, arrhythmias, CNS effects (stimulation, drowsiness, ataxia, seizures, respiratory depression). Glycopyrrolate is slightly less arrhythmogenic and rarely results in CNS effects	I: Vagally induced bradyarrhythmias, sinus bradycardia, sinus arrest, high-grade or complete AV block CI: Tachycardia, tachyarrhythmias, heart failure, GI disease, colic
ANGIOTENSIN-CONVERTING-ENZYME (ACE) INHIBITORS			
Enalapril Quinapril Ramipril	0.5 mg/kg PO q12h 0.25 mg/kg PO q24h 0.05-0.2 mg/kg PO q24h	Optimal doses and efficacy unknown Adverse effects: Cough, impairment of renal function, hypotension, hyperkalemia	I: Cardiovascular protection in cases with AR or MR, treatment of heart failure CI: Severe renal failure, hyperkalemia, hypotension
VASODILATORS AND INODILATORS			
Nitroglycerine	5-20 μg/kg/min CRI, titrate to effect	Venous vasodilator (preload reducer). Tolerance with long-term treatment (12-24h). Adverse effects: Severe hypotension, reflex tachycardia, weakness	I: Acute management of CHF CI: Hypotension, hypovolemia
Hydralazine	0.5-1.5 mg/kg PO q12h 0.5 mg/kg IV	Arterial vasodilator (afterload reducer) Adverse effects: Transient weakness, lethargy, hypotension, tachycardia, sodium/water retention (unless given with diuretics)	I: CHF, mitral regurgitation CI: Hypotension, hypovolemia, severe renal disease
Milrinone	0.2 μg/kg IV bolus, followed by 10 μg/kg/min CRI 0.5-1.0 mg/kg PO q12h	Phosphodiesterase inhibitor (inodilator) Adverse effects: Arrhythmias, hypotension, tachycardia, accelerated AV conduction	I: Acute management of CHF CI: Normal or low filling pressures, severe renal failure
DIURETICS			
Furosemide	Initial dose for CHF: 1.0-3.0 mg/kg IV or IM q8-12h as needed to produce diuretic effect Alternatively: 0.12 mg/kg IV bolus, followed by 0.12 mg/kg/h CRI Maintenance dose: 1 mg/kg IV or IM q12h	Start at higher/more frequent doses and reduce to minimal effective dose. Oral administration may be ineffective due to inconsistent bioavailability. Adverse effects: At high doses risk of hypovolemia, renal failure, electrolyte and acid-base imbalances	I: Congestive heart failure, edema CI: Dehydration, severe electrolyte disturbances

AF, Atrial flutter/fibrillation; *AR*, aortic regurgitation; *AV*, atrioventricular; *CHF*, congestive heart failure; *CNS*, central nervous system; *CRI*, constant-rate infusion; *GI*, gastrointestinal; *HF*, heart failure; *IM*, intramuscular; *IT*, intratracheal; *IV*, intravenous; *MR*, mitral regurgitation; *NGT*, nasogastric tube; *PO*, oral; *RAAS*, renin-angiotensin-aldosterone system; *SA*, sinoatrial; *SVT*, supraventricular tachycardia; *VT*, ventricular tachycardia.

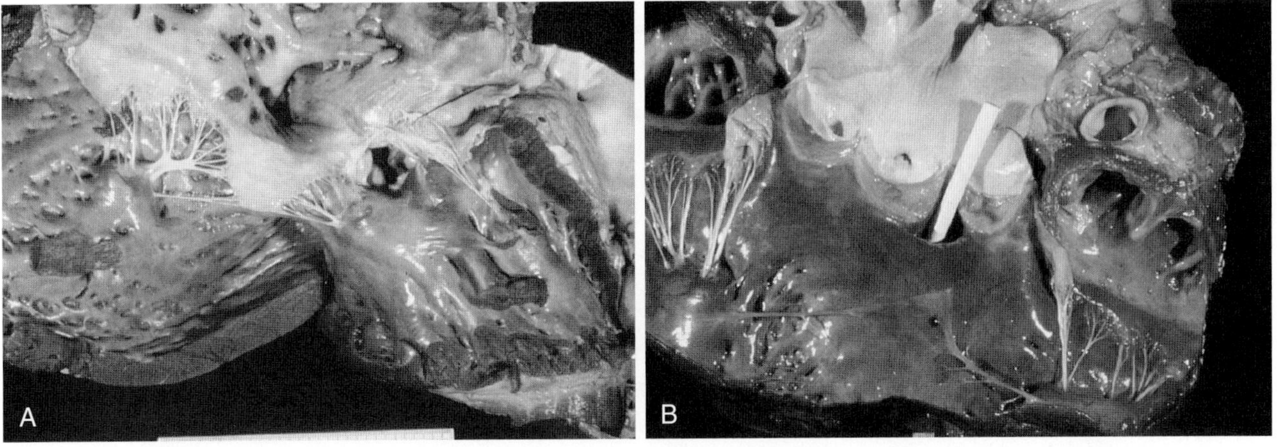

FIGURE 10-27 Pathologic evaluation of ventricular septal defects (VSDs). **A,** Opened right ventricle (RV) from a mare demonstrating a perimembranous septal defect opening just beneath the septal leaflet of the tricuspid valve. Aortic valve cusps are visible through the defect. Congestive heart failure (CHF) occurred late in life, after the development of atrial fibrillation (AF). **B,** A large VSD in a horse. A probe runs through the defect. The dorsal location immediately beneath the right and the noncoronary cusps of the aortic valve are notable. Ostia of both coronary arteries are also evident.

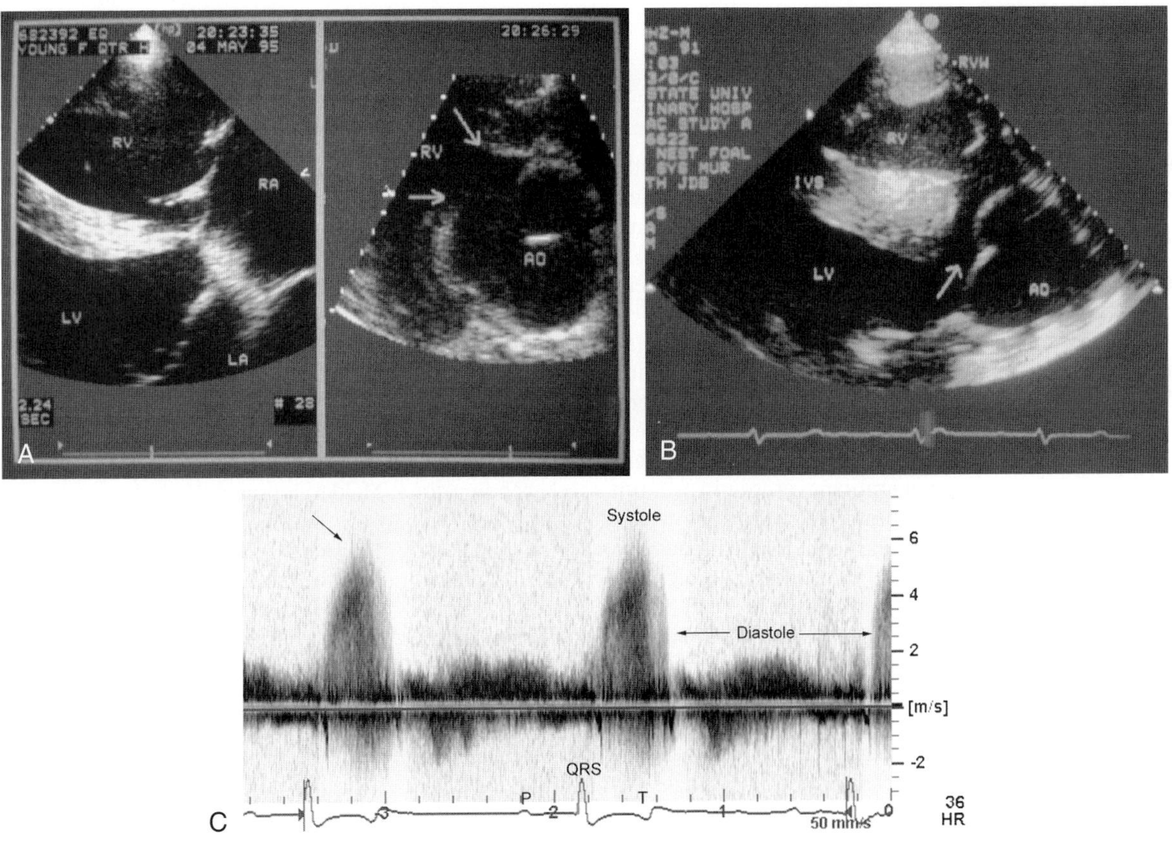

FIGURE 10-28 Echocardiograms demonstrating ventricular septal defects (VSDs). **A,** This subaortic VSD is not evident from the long-axis image (*left panel*) but is visible in the short-axis tomogram (*arrows*). This Quarter Horse gelding also had pulmonic stenosis. The elevated right ventricular (RV) pressures have led to significant RV enlargement with bulging of the septum toward the left ventricle (LV). **B,** Malalignment and a perimembranous septal defect associated with prolapse of an aortic valve leaflet across the defect (*arrow*) (*RVW,* Right ventricular wall). **C,** Continuous wave Doppler study recorded from a foal with a small, restrictive VSD. The maximal velocity of nearly 6 m/sec (*arrow*) predicts a pressure difference of up to 144 mm Hg between left and right ventricles.

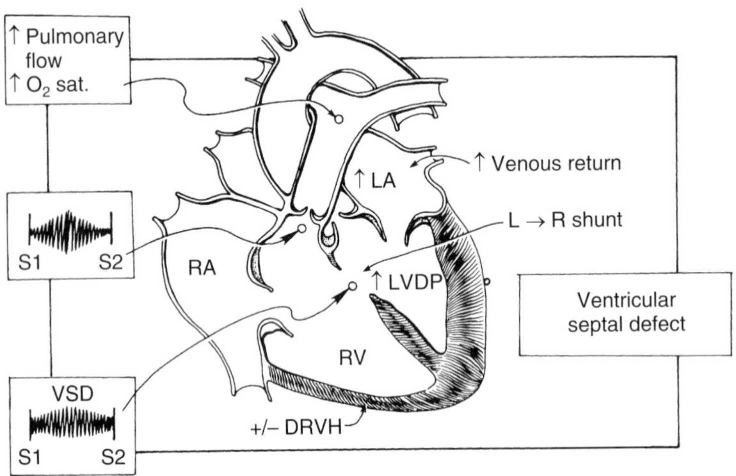

FIGURE 10-29 Pathophysiology of ventricular septal defects (VSDs). See text for details. *LA,* Left atrium; *RA,* right atrium; *LVDP,* left ventricular diastolic pressure; *RV,* right ventricle; *RVH,* right ventricular hypertrophy. (From Bonagura JD: Congenital heart disease. In Bonagura JD, editor: Cardiology, New York, 1987, Churchill Livingstone.)

endocardial fibroelastosis,[61,629] total anomalous pulmonary venous return,[630] and aortic origin of the pulmonary artery have been reported but will not be discussed further. Some of the more frequently recognized defects[342] are described following.

Pathogenesis of Congenital Heart Disease

The underlying genetic or other causative factors responsible for cardiac malformations in horses have not been studied. Potential but unproven causes include drugs, viral infection, environmental toxins, and nutritional disorders. Cardiac morphogenesis is complicated, but it is helpful to understand elementary aspects of cardiac development, especially as these pertain to CHD.[631] Among the fundamentals are septation of the atria, the anatomic components forming the ventricular septum, separation of the great vessels, and the normal fetal circulation.

The right and left atria are separated by incorporation of the right horn of the sinus venosus and through development and fusion of two prominent membranes: septum primum and septum secundum. The endocardial cushions close the gap between the atrial and ventricular septa. These tissues also contribute to the atrioventricular septum, the septal segment spanning the point of mitral valve septal insertion on the left to the tricuspid valve insertion on the right. The foramen ovale, a normal atrial structure, is located approximately in the middle of the atrial septum, continues almost directly from the entry of the caudal vena cava, and creates a passageway for blood to flow from RA to LA in the normal fetus. The equine foramen ovale resembles a fenestrated finger cot and can be observed echocardiographically as a mobile septal membrane even in healthy, full-term foals. This interatrial path may persist in foals with pulmonary hypertension and elevated RA pressures. Failure of normal development can lead to an ASD, which is typically designated by the location of the defective membrane (Figure 10-30).

The ventricular septum is a complicated partition that includes a small membranous portion located opposite the aortic root and craniodorsal to the tricuspid valve, an inlet septum immediately below the septal tricuspid leaflet, an apically located muscular or trabecular septum, and a dorsal outflow segment that separates the subaortic and the subpulmonic infundibulum. The ventral atrial septum connects to the dorsal ventricular septum by growth and differentiation of endocardial cushions. These swellings also form major parts of the atrioventricular valves. Insufficient development of any of these embryonic components can lead to a VSD, the most common cardiac malformation in horses. Defective differentiation of the endocardial cushions causes various combinations of an ostium primum (ventral) ASD, an inlet VSD, malformation of the atrioventricular valves, or common atrium with a single atrioventricular valve.

The aorta and pulmonary artery begin as a single vessel in the conus arteriosus. This common trunk or truncus arteriosus is eventually partitioned by migration of the conus and development of the conotruncal and spiral septa. Twisting of the spiral septum produces appropriate alignment (concordance) of the great vessels with their respective ventricular chambers. The descending aorta and pulmonary artery are connected by the ductus arteriosus, which carries fetal blood from pulmonary artery to descending aorta. Maldevelopment of conotruncal or spiral septal tissues leads to complicated congenital heart defects in the horse, including persistent truncus arteriosus,[632] double-outlet RV,[598] transposition of the great vessels,[157,165,625] and aorticopulmonary septal defect.[626] Persistence of the right aortic arch[633,634] and persistent PDA are both rare in horses (Figure 10-31).

There are two fetal circulations: one serving the embryo and the other communicating with the placenta. Functionally, two right-to-left shunts are present: one across the foramen ovale and the other across the ductus arteriosus. The fetal lungs are collapsed, pulmonary vascular resistance is high, and pulmonary blood flow is minimal. Desaturated blood returning from the fetal tissues is collected in the cardinal venous system and enters the sinus venosus and RA. This blood is largely earmarked for the RV and pulmonary artery. Most pulmonary arterial flow is diverted through the ductus arteriosus to the descending aorta and placenta where it is oxygenated. Well-saturated blood returning across the umbilical veins is delivered by the caudal vena cava to the RA, where it preferentially crosses the foramen ovale to enter the LA, LV, and ascending aorta. These patterns change dramatically with foaling. As the

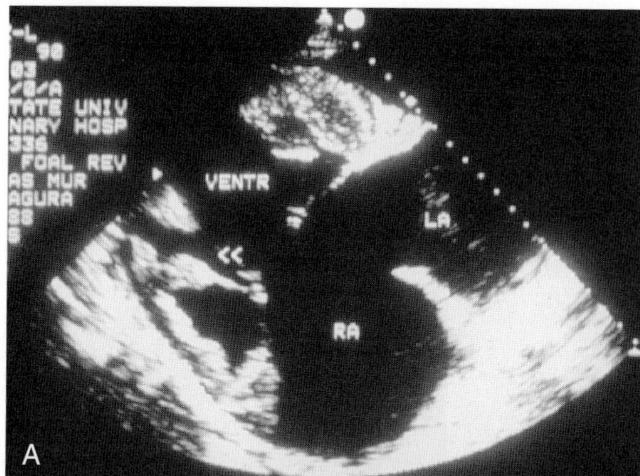

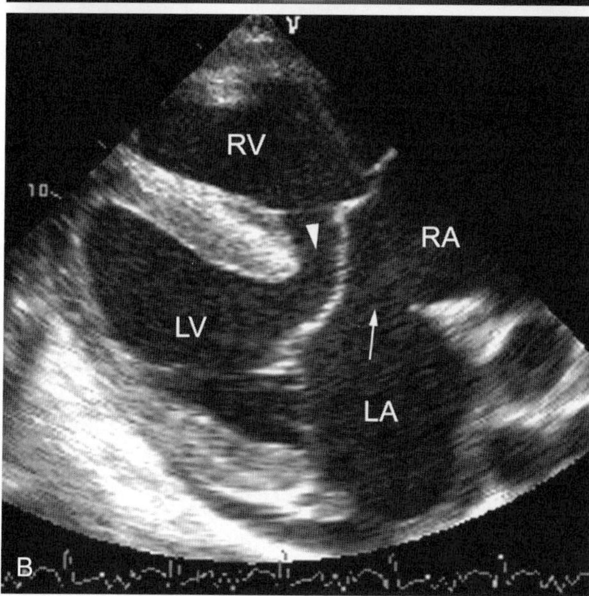

FIGURE 10-30 A, Echocardiogram demonstrating a primum atrial septal defect (ASD) in a foal with complex congenital heart disease that included a common (*left*) ventricle, rudimentary (*right*) ventricle, and double-outlet ventricle. The septal defect is evident between the four cardiac chambers. The dorsal secundum septum (*right*) is present, as well as the apical ventricular septum (*left*). **B,** Long axis image from a foal with a complete endocardial cushion defect. The primum ASD is evident in the ventral atrial septum (*arrow*), and an inlet ventricular septal defect (VSD) component (*arrowhead*) is observed below the closed common (or straddling) atrioventricular valve. Normal mitral and tricuspid septal leaflets would insert into the septum at slightly different levels (with tricuspid septal leaflet inserting more ventrally than the mitral septal leaflet).

lungs expand, pulmonary vascular resistance falls, and pulmonary blood flow increases. The resultant increase in LA pressure functionally closes the foramen ovale within the first 24 to 48 hours of life. Similarly, inhibition of local prostaglandins leads to functional closure of the ductus arteriosus within 72 hours in most full-term foals. Persistence of the right-to-left shunts, especially at the level of the foramen ovale, can occur in premature foals or those suffering from severe pulmonary disease with associated pulmonary hypertension. In these cases, shunting across the foramen ovale represents an additional mechanism for arterial desaturation and tissue hypoxia.

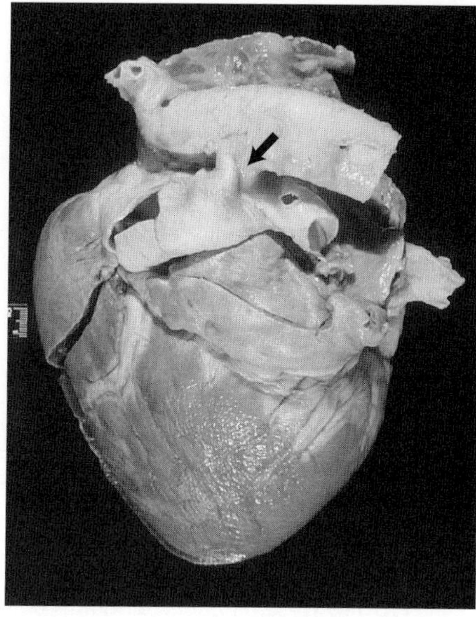

FIGURE 10-31 A postmortem demonstration of the ductus arteriosus (*arrow*) between the descending aorta and the pulmonary artery in a foal with complex congenital heart disease.

Clinical Pathophysiology of Shunts

Fundamental to understanding of cardiac malformations is an appreciation of shunt physiology and the responses of the heart and circulation to a shunt.[596] Shunting can be defined as an abnormal deviation of blood flow between systemic (left) and pulmonary (right) circulations. Shunting can be left-to-right, right-to-left, and bidirectional. Systemic to pulmonary (left-to-right) shunting is the expected consequence of an ASD, VSD, PDA, so long as systemic pressures and resistances exceed those on the right side and no stenosis limits PA flow. Even in cases of abnormal ventricular-arterial development, as with persistent truncus arteriosus, double-outlet RV, or univentricular heart, the clinical findings of a left-to-right shunt may predominate unless obstruction to blood flow or elevated pulmonary vascular resistance is seen.

The actual shunt volume carried to the lungs depends on the caliber (or "restrictive" nature) of the lesion orifice and the relative vascular resistances between systemic and pulmonary circulations. Shunting may not be significant for some weeks after foaling because pulmonary vascular resistance is relatively high and systemic arterial and LV pressures are relatively low. Eventually left-to-right shunts increase pulmonary arterial flow and augment pulmonary venous return. Small shunts are easily handled at the expense of mild left-sided dilation and hypertrophy. When the pulmonary to systemic flow ratio (Qp:Qs) exceeds about 1.8:1, the shunt is usually considered clinically significant and the consequences are obvious volume overload of the LA and LV. The greater the shunt volume, the higher is the potential for left-sided or biventricular CHF from ventricular dysfunction. Pulmonary hypertension can occur in the setting of left-to-right shunting from combinations of increased PA flow, lesions in the small pulmonary arteries, and LV failure. Thus consequences of significant left-to-right shunting may include any of the following: exercise intolerance, tachypnea, pulmonary edema, respiratory distress, pulmonary hypertension, AF, pleural effusion, jugular venous distension, or ventral edema. The foal may be smaller than

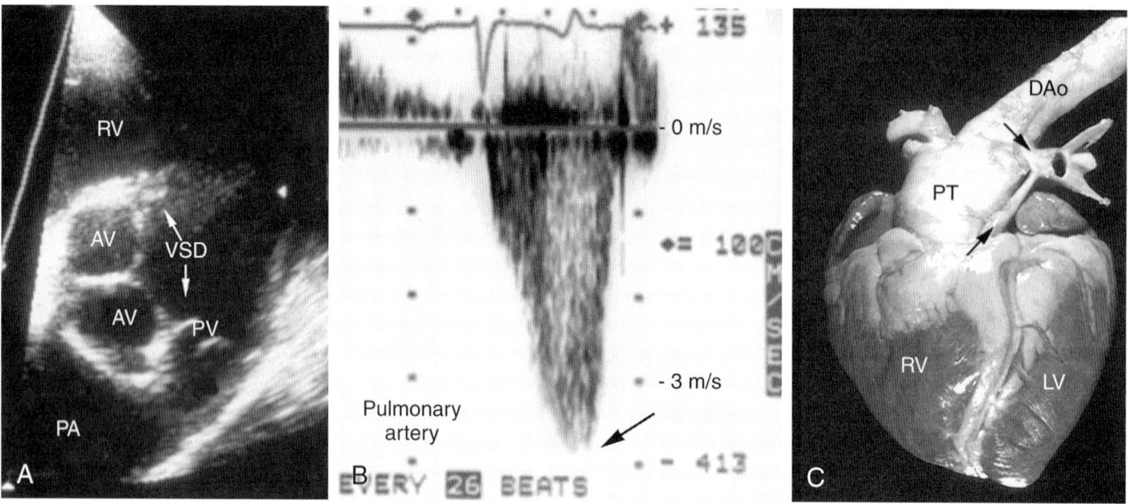

FIGURE 10-32 Phonocardiograms of cardiac murmurs caused by valvular heart disease. **A,** A holosystolic murmur of mitral regurgitation in a horse with chronic valvular degeneration. **B,** A variable, late systolic murmur of mitral regurgitation related to mitral valve prolapse. The murmur has a crescendo and peaks at end systole (*arrow*). Heart sounds are indicated. The murmur obscures the second sound. **C,** A holodiastolic, vibratory murmur of aortic regurgitation with presystolic accentuation. The accentuation probably is related to atrial contraction, altered ventricular volume and pressure, and an incremental increase in regurgitant volume. (From Bonagura JD: Congenital heart disease. In Robinson N, editor: Current therapy in equine practice, ed 5, Philadelphia, WB Saunders.)

expected and may have a history of antibiotic therapy for presumed bouts of "pneumonia."

Right-to-left shunting produces a different clinical presentation. When a shunt is complicated by a right-sided obstruction downstream from the defect, right-to-left shunting will develop once right-sided pressures exceed those on the left. This can occur in a foal with tricuspid valve atresia and ASD or with pulmonary valve atresia and VSD. Conversely, elevated right-sided resistance can develop more chronically from pulmonary vascular disease. For example, a large left-to-right shunt can induce medial hypertrophy and intimal thickening of small pulmonary arteries that elevates pulmonary vascular resistance. Though very uncommon, the resultant pulmonary hypertension may become severe and reverse the shunt to right-to-left (Eisenmenger's physiology). In these cases the left heart chambers are small and RV is hypertrophied to generate systemic BP.

The entrance of desaturated blood into the left side of the circulation causes arterial hypoxemia with potential consequences of tissue hypoxia, cyanosis, exercise intolerance, mild to moderate polycythemia, hyperviscosity of blood, and stunting of growth. CHF is rare, but sudden death can occur, presumably from arrhythmia. The degrees of hypoxemia and cyanosis in a right-to-left shunt depend on overall pulmonary blood flow and the degree of blood mixing between the circulations. Thus if pulmonary flow is markedly diminished, as with tricuspid atresia, then severe cyanosis is likely. However, effects of right-to-left shunting can be mitigated by overall increases in pulmonary blood flow as with truncus arteriosus or double-outlet RV without pulmonary obstruction. These lesions cause less hypoxemia because the volume of oxygenated blood reaching the LV is increased. The location or "commitment" of a VSD relative to the subaortic or subpulmonic region also influences clinical signs because oxygenated blood from the LV can actually stream preferentially through a VSD into the aorta. In these situations, cyanosis related to any mixing of blood in the RV may be negligible and the clinical condition predominated by left-sided or biventricular CHF. If the increased pulmonary flow is sufficient to minimize arterial hypoxemia but not create heart failure, then survival even beyond 5 years of age is possible.

Ventricular Septal Defects

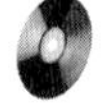

Ventricular septal defect is the most important CHD of horses.* A genetic basis is likely in the Arabian breed, and Welsh Mountain ponies also appear to be predisposed to VSD. In the authors' experience, VSD is also encountered regularly in Standardbred horses and in Quarterhorses. The VSD often accompanies more complicated heart malformations.

The location of a VSD depends on the embryogenesis of the lesion and influences the designation and even the clinical manifestations of the defect. The nomenclature of VSDs is confusing but can be remembered by considering the main components of the normal ventricular septum (see Figures 10-27 to 10-29). In most cases, a VSD is located dorsally ("high") on the ventricular septum, below the right and noncoronary cusp of the aortic valve on the left side, craniodorsal to the septal tricuspid leaflet on the right, and encompassing or contiguous with the fibrous part of the ventricular septum.[504] Such defects are generally termed *perimembranous, membranous,* or perhaps more correctly, *paramembranous.* Most of these holes are also "subcristal" because the VSD is located caudoventral to the supraventricular crest separating the RV inlet from the outlet. However, a very large paramembranous defect also can extend under the tricuspid valve toward the inlet septum or advance across the supraventricular crest toward the outlet septum. The (conotruncal-) septal defects associated with tetralogy of Fallot (Figure 10-32) and with pulmonary atresia are usually very large, and they fall into the latter appellation. Sometimes the aortic

*References 131, 145, 151, 157, 162, 165, 479, 482, 504, 513, 528, 576, 596, 602, 608, 614-617.

root is displaced ventrocranially and straddles the defect, creating a "malalignment" VSD. This is characteristic of the tetralogy of Fallot, but it also can be seen with large, isolated paramembranous defects. Malalignment is clinically significant because the right or noncoronary cusp of the aortic valve is likely to prolapse into the defect leading to AR (see Figure 10-28, B). A less common location for a VSD is immediately ventral to the septal tricuspid valve within the muscular septum. Such "inlet" VSDs are typical of a complete endocardial cushion defect and commonly related to a primum ASD, common atrioventricular valve leaflet, or persistent atrioventricular canal, which creates a gap between all four cardiac chambers (see Figure 10-30, B).[635] A subaortic VSD that communicates with the outlet portion of the ventricular septum directly below the pulmonary valve is variably termed a *subarterial, outlet, supracristal, subpulmonic,* or *doubly committed* VSD. This lesion also places the aortic valve at risk for prolapse. Finally, apical muscular (trabecular) defects or multiple VSDs are rare, but they have been observed in horses. Some of these are small, whereas others have been enormous.

Many VSDs close spontaneously in people, but whether or not this is common in horses is unknown. However, the flow across a VSD can be diminished by imposition of a cardiac valve. For example the rim, or even a major portion of a VSD, may be occluded by fibrotic tissue that ensnares the septal tricuspid leaflet, rendering the defect functionally smaller and possibly creating a hyperechoic aneurysm on the right septal surface. Large defects associated with malalignment of the ascending aorta to the upper border of the remaining septum are often associated with prolapse of an aortic valve leaflet (or of the aortic root) into the defect. Aortic prolapse can effectively close even a large VSD but at the risk of permitting chronic aortic valve insufficiency over time.[504]

The pathophysiology of the uncomplicated VSD is that of a left-to-right shunt as described previously (see Figure 10-29). Much of the shunt volume pumped by the LV is ejected immediately into the PA. As pulmonary flow increases, increased venous return to the LA and LV is noted, causing LV dilation and hypertrophy that can be recognized by echocardiography. Thus the left (not the right) ventricle performs most of the extra volume work. This is made more severe if aortic valve prolapse with AR is seen or if MR develops owing to LV enlargement. If the shunt is large and pulmonary arteriolar resistance does not increase significantly, then LV failure can develop. This is most likely to occur early in life, as the high fetal pulmonary vascular resistance declines, but late cases of CHF (with AF) also have been observed. The degree of RV hypertrophy and enlargement varies, depending on the location and size of the septal defect and pulmonary vascular resistance. Large nonrestrictive defects create a functional common chamber, allowing ventricular pressures to equilibrate and leading to marked RV hypertrophy, as well as pulmonary hypertension.

The clinical features of VSD are variable.[504,596] Clinical signs may be absent and the defect identified as an incidental finding. A mature horse may be presented for poor performance or with AF. Foals may be symptomatic for pulmonary edema or biventricular heart failure. Most commonly, a murmur is detected incidentally during the physical examination for another problem or during a prepurchase examination (see Figure 10-10, B). Because most defects communicate near the tricuspid valve, the most consistent physical examination finding is a harsh, holo- or pansystolic murmur that is loudest just below the tricuspid valve region and above the right sternal border. A slightly less intense ejection murmur because of increased flow across the RV outlet is usually evident over the left base. The second heart sound may be split more widely than normal, owing to disparate ventricular ejection times; the pulmonic component of S_2 will be tympanic if pulmonary hypertension is noted. In contrast the murmur of a subarterial (subpulmonic or supracristal) VSD is loudest over the left cranial base as the high velocity flow enters the main PA. When VSD is associated with complex cardiac malformation, the murmur is likely to be loud over each side of the thorax. The severity of the defect cannot be judged based on murmur intensity. In some cases, a small defect may be quite loud; whereas, a large, less restrictive defect may cause a murmur related entirely to the increased flow (relative pulmonic stenosis). A holodiastolic murmur of AR indicates prolapse of an aortic cusp and the likelihood that the lesion is relatively large. Substantial AR is associated with a hyperdynamic arterial pulse. If significant LV volume overload occurs, then the mitral valve may become incompetent and a holosystolic murmur of MR may be evident over the left apex. The rare trabecular (muscular) VSD may also create a systolic murmur over the left or right apex. The VSD associated with pulmonary atresia or persistent truncus arteriosus may not create a substantial murmur, but the increased flow through the dilated single vessel usually generates a loud ejection murmur over each side of the chest. If significant cardiomegaly develops, then atrial and ventricular premature complexes, or even AF, may be recognized.

Diagnostic studies are needed to confirm the lesion and determine the severity. The performance history is a useful overall indicator of effect, and the horse with an excellent work history is unlikely to have a large defect. The ECG is unreliable for diagnosing cardiomegaly in horses but is indicated in the setting of an arrhythmia. Thoracic radiography can be useful in foals to demonstrate cardiomegaly (see Figure 10-20, A), the pulmonary circulation, the lungs, and the pleural space; 2D echocardiography and color Doppler imaging establish the diagnosis.[478] M-mode studies and spectral Doppler examinations are useful for assessing the hemodynamic burden of the defect.

The VSD is delineated successfully using 2D echocardiography in almost every case, provided sufficient imaging planes are obtained (see Figures 10-24 and 10-28). It is important to collect long axis images of the LV outflow tract and aortic valve, as well as a short axis images at the level of the LV outflow tract, at and just ventral to the aortic leaflets. The typical paramembranous defect appears under the aortic valve and adjacent to the septal leaflet of the tricuspid valve. A true defect is characterized by a relatively echogenic tissue interface; whereas, an area of false echo dropout tends to be gradual. Most defects can be imaged in orthogonal (long axis/short axis) planes. The ostium of the right coronary artery of the horse is relatively large and may be confused with a subarterial (supracristal) VSD in short axis image planes. It also should be noted that a true inlet VSD of an endocardial cushion defect located immediately ventral to the septal tricuspid valve might not be easily seen in standard planes. Tipped or oblique views that show both atrioventricular valves may be required. Similarly, finding a muscular, apical, or small subarterial defect requires more imaging experience and is greatly assisted by color Doppler studies.

Attempts should be made to identify the largest diameter of the defect in complementary planes and compare this with the size of the aortic root, because orifice size is an important prognostic factor. While there are limitations to 2D sizing of the VSD, a defect exceeding 2.5 cm in diameter or a VSD/aortic root diameter of greater than 0.4 identifies a large defect with greater likelihood of clinical signs. Furthermore, 2D or M-mode evidence of left-sided cardiac dilatation, RV enlargement, or marked dilation of the main PA suggests a hemodynamically significant VSD and one more likely to affect performance or survival.

Identification of shunting across a VSD is confirmed using color Doppler studies. There will typically be high-velocity, turbulent flow entering the RV during systole with low velocity, uniform color shunting noted during diastole. Color Doppler imaging is extremely helpful for identifying a very small VSD or one with an atypical location. AR is identified in some horses, and the regurgitant flow is often directed into the VSD resulting in high-velocity diastolic shunting. Continuous wave Doppler is used to estimate the pressure difference between the two ventricles, because velocity (in m/sec) is proportional to the instantaneous pressure difference across the ventricles (by the modified Bernoulli equation: $\Delta P = 4V^2$; see Figures 10-24, *D,* and 10-28, *C*). A relatively small VSD is "restrictive" to flow, and the peak shunt velocity will generally exceed 4.5 m/sec, assuming proper alignment to shunt flow. In the setting of pulmonary hypertension, pulmonic stenosis, or systemic hypotension, the velocity of left-to-right shunting will be lower; when pulmonary hypertension is present, a TR jet of greater than 3.5 m/sec may be identified.

Potential outcomes of the isolated VSD include the following: (1) tolerance of the lesion; (2) partial or complete closure of a VSD by adherence of the septal tricuspid leaflet, fibrous tissue, RV hypertrophy, or aortic valve prolapse; (3) progressive AR, (4) AF; (5) left-sided or biventricular CHF, (6) pulmonary hypertension (with left-to-right shunting); or (7) reversal of the shunt with development of arterial hypoxemia and cyanosis. The last situation would be caused by either severe pulmonary vascular disease (Eisenmenger's physiology) or fibromuscular obstruction in the RV outlet leading to subpulmonic stenosis. The horse with a relatively small-diameter paramembranous defect, high-velocity left-to-right shunt, mild cardiomegaly, relatively normal RV cavity, and normal heart rhythm probably has a restrictive VSD that will be well tolerated. Most of these animals can perform sufficiently in the show ring, as hunter-jumpers, or even as endurance horses or racehorses. Large defects that are associated with echocardiographic evidence of moderate to severe cardiomegaly, RV hypertrophy, aortic root prolapse, or Doppler evidence of pulmonary hypertension are prone to complications and carry a less favorable prognosis for performance or life regardless of current clinical signs.

Definitive therapy for VSD involves cardiopulmonary bypass surgery and is impractical. Surgical banding of the PA elevates RV pressures and reduces left-to-right shunting; however, this procedure also limits CO and is not advised. New "hybrid" procedures involving catheter devices delivered by a transventricular approach and guided by epicardial echocardiography are now possible, although perhaps not practical. Medical management of CHF or of arrhythmias associated with CHD can be considered. However, even if the response to treatment is good, then the horse should not be used. In the authors' view, breeding of affected animals generally should be discouraged, especially in Arabian horses.

Atrial Septal Defects

Atrial septal defects, including endocardial cushion defects, are quite uncommon in foals.* As indicated earlier, an ASD may involve different portions of the atrial septum and is more likely

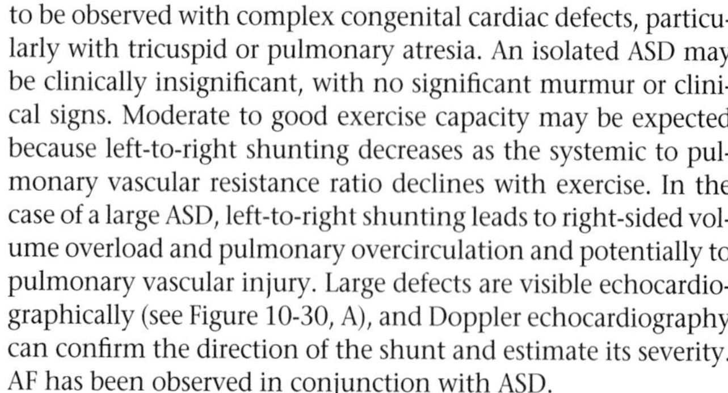

to be observed with complex congenital cardiac defects, particularly with tricuspid or pulmonary atresia. An isolated ASD may be clinically insignificant, with no significant murmur or clinical signs. Moderate to good exercise capacity may be expected because left-to-right shunting decreases as the systemic to pulmonary vascular resistance ratio declines with exercise. In the case of a large ASD, left-to-right shunting leads to right-sided volume overload and pulmonary overcirculation and potentially to pulmonary vascular injury. Large defects are visible echocardiographically (see Figure 10-30, A), and Doppler echocardiography can confirm the direction of the shunt and estimate its severity. AF has been observed in conjunction with ASD.

Complete endocardial cushion defects are rarely seen but are serious, usually leading to CHF or AF at an early age. Components of this defect typically include a large ASD involving the primum and the atrioventricular septa, a common atrioventricular valve leaflet, and often an inlet VSD (see Figure 10-30, B). The ventricles may be partitioned normally, unequally with one rudimentary ventricular chamber, or not at all, creating a single ventricle. In the most severe cases, there is a common atrioventricular canal, a single common atrioventricular valve, and a single ventricle from which both great vessels exit. The clinical signs of a complete endocardial cushion defect are variable. The foal with two ventricles and an unobstructed outlet to the pulmonary arteries will be hemodynamically similar to one with a large VSD. When a common ventricle is present, varying degrees of cyanosis may be observed. A systolic murmur is typical and may reflect flow across the VSD, ventricular outflow, or atrioventricular valve regurgitation. A 2D echocardiogram can reveal the lesions, and Doppler echocardiography can reveal the intracardiac shunts and AV valvular regurgitation. CHF may supervene, and the prognosis is poor.

Patent Ductus Arteriosus

Patent ductus arteriosus is rare as an isolated congenital cardiac defect in foals and is detected most frequently in combination with other, more complex malformations (see Figure 10-31).* The ductus arteriosus is a fetal vessel, derived from the left sixth aortic arch, which permits shunting from the PA to the descending aorta in the fetus. At birth the ductus arteriosus normally constricts, in response to increased local oxygen tension and inhibition of prostaglandins. It is functionally closed 72 hours after birth in the vast majority of foals. If the ductus arteriosus does not close, then a left-to-right shunt from the aorta to PA occurs. Although there may be some hereditary predisposition to PDA in other species, this lesion is so rare as an isolated congenital defect that this is not a significant concern. Premature foals, foals with persistent pulmonary hypertension, and foals whose dams have been given prostaglandin inhibitors may be more susceptible to the development of a PDA.

The clinical signs depend on the magnitude of the shunting through the PDA, which is determined by ductal diameter and vascular resistance in the pulmonary circulation. Physical examination findings (with a left-to-right PDA) include a continuous machinery murmur and thrill, usually loudest over the main PA (craniodorsal to the aortic valve area), and bounding arterial pulses. Differential diagnosis includes other systemic to pulmonary shunts in association with complex congenital heart disease.

*References 131, 159, 161, 163, 513, 528, 578.

*References 156, 159, 165, 168, 265, 367, 575, 597, 601.

Echocardiography will reveal volume overload of the PA, LA, and LV. The severity of these findings depends on the magnitude of the shunt. Direct visualization of the PDA is not always possible by 2D echocardiography, because overlying lung may obscure the ductus arteriosus. Ductal flow is best identified from the left cranial thorax by Doppler echocardiographic examination of the main PA that reveals continuous, high-velocity, turbulent flow directed toward the pulmonary valve. Cardiac enlargement and increased pulmonary vascularity may be detected in neonatal foals with a PDA, as well as radiographic evidence of pulmonary edema if the foal has developed CHF. Cardiac catheterization reveals elevated PA and capillary wedge pressures and increased PA oxygen saturation. The heart should be evaluated carefully for other congenital cardiac defects before surgical or catheter-based intervention is considered, because complex cardiac malformations are likely in a foal with PDA. Late complications of this lesion include rupture of the PA.

Tetralogy of Fallot

The tetralogy of Fallot is one of the more common congenital cardiac anomalies in foals responsible for right-to-left shunting, arterial desaturation, and cyanosis.[156,162,167,528] The four lesions are large paramembranous outlet VSD, RV outflow tract obstruction, cranial and rightward (dextro-) positioning of the aorta with overriding of the septal defect, and RV hypertrophy. Outflow obstruction can be the result of subvalvular fibromuscular obstruction, valvular pulmonic stenosis, or hypoplasia of the PA. Ventricular hypertrophy is caused by RV outflow obstruction and the large, unrestrictive, VSD that functionally creates a "common ventricle." Blood leaves the heart along the path of least resistance such that pulmonary flow depends on the severity of RV outflow tract stenosis. As previously discussed, the degree of cyanosis and severity of clinical signs depends on the volume of blood traversing the lungs. In some horses, a PDA is also present (pentalogy of Fallot), and this defect reduces signs by increasing pulmonary flow, left heart filling, and systemic arterial hemoglobin saturation.

Affected foals are usually smaller than normal, lethargic, and intolerant of exercise. Cyanosis is most evident after activity and is variably present at rest. Arterial blood gas analysis demonstrates hypoxemia with normal or reduced partial pressure of carbon dioxide (Pa_{CO_2}). Auscultation is typically characterized by a loud systolic murmur over the pulmonic valve area on the left side caused by (sub-) pulmonic stenosis. The second heart sound is usually unremarkable. Although polycythemia can be significant, it is usually mild, even when arterial oxygen tensions fall to 50 to 70 mm Hg.

Echocardiographic evaluation is diagnostic and reveals a large, unrestrictive VSD, RV outflow tract obstruction, malalignment and overriding of the aortic root, and RV hypertrophy (see Figure 10-32). Shunting can be identified by color Doppler or saline contrast echocardiography initiated by injection of agitated saline into the jugular vein. Both studies will demonstrate a right-to-left or bidirectional shunt. Conventional spectral Doppler studies can be used to delineate the shunt (typically bidirectional, low-velocity flow of <2 m/sec) and RV outflow obstruction (high-velocity flow exceeding 4 m/sec).

Although it is possible for horses to live for a number of years with tetralogy of Fallot, most affected animals are humanely destroyed because of the poor prognosis for life. Affected horses should not be used or bred if they survive to maturity. Tetralogy of Fallot must be distinguished from other causes of cyanotic heart conditions, including tricuspid atresia, pulmonary atresia with VSD, D-transposition of the great vessels, and double-outlet RV with pulmonary stenosis.

Pulmonary Atresia with Ventricular Septal Defect

Pulmonary atresia with VSD is rare, having been observed most often in Arabian foals (see Figure 10-32, C).[156,616,621,636] This malformation represents the exaggerated form of tetralogy of Fallot, with these findings: (1) the RV outlet does not connect into the pulmonary artery, (2) the RV hypertrophied, (3) a large malalignment VSD is present (in most cases), and (4) the fetal truncus arteriosus has been partitioned so unequally that the aorta is markedly dilated and the pulmonary trunk atretic or severely hypoplastic. Without careful ultrasound studies (or necropsy dissection) of the pulmonary circulation, the dilated aorta can be mistaken for a persistent truncus arteriosus, hence the moniker *pseudotruncus arteriosus*. Owing to the atretic pulmonary valve, pulmonary blood flow must be derived either from a PDA or the aorta. In the latter instance, the systemic collaterals are usually from bronchial arteries. Pulmonary atresia with intact ventricular septum has been diagnosed rarely.[622]

The diagnosis of pulmonary atresia is usually stimulated by clinical findings of cyanosis, cardiac murmur, and stunting in a foal or weanling. Diagnosis is confirmed by echocardiography. Careful imaging can identify the main lesions outlined previously. Of diagnostic importance is the inability to identify the pulmonary valve in the rudimentary RV outflow tract (though a small pouch may be seen). Careful ultrasound examination of the ascending aorta and aortic arch from the right and left sides of the thorax will fail to reveal a normal origin for the pulmonary trunk or an origin of the PA directly from a truncus arteriosus. The bifurcation of the PA may be found from a cranial imaging position, and continuous flow into that vessel documented by Doppler echocardiography suggests that pulmonary blood flow is derived from the ductus arteriosus or a collateral systemic artery.

Truncus Arteriosus

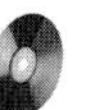

The failure of the fetal truncus arteriosus to partition into the aorta and PA represents a rare anomaly of the equine heart.[164,615] In this condition the fetal truncus never partitions and both ventricles continue to develop, communicating with the truncus arteriosus across a large malalignment type VSD. Systemic, coronary, and PA flows each arise from the truncus, which is guarded by a truncal valve (that can be incompetent or stenotic). Pulmonary blood flow originates from one or more pulmonary arteries connected directly to the truncus arteriosus (types I, II, III truncus) or indirectly from systemic to pulmonary collateral vessels (type IV truncus in older nomenclatures).

The pathophysiology and clinical findings of this malformation depend largely on the magnitude of pulmonary blood flow. If the PA origins are not stenotic and if pulmonary vascular resistance remains relatively low, then the clinical condition resembles a left-to-right shunt, except for right-to-left mixing of blood across the VSD. However, the degree of arterial hypoxemia may not be severe and cyanosis may not be obvious. Conversely, high pulmonary vascular resistance or obstruction to flow at the truncal origin of the PA is associated with arterial desaturation and findings similar to pulmonary atresia.

Clinical examination usually indicates a systolic cardiac murmur. The mucous membranes may be pink or cyanotic. If marked left-to-right shunting is noted, then CHF may occur. With careful ultrasound examination, the truncus and origin of the pulmonary arteries may be identified, allowing the condition to be distinguished from pulmonary atresia with VSD. Furthermore in some cases an abnormal truncal valve (with four leaflets) may be evident, further supporting the diagnosis. Management is best accomplished by consultation with a cardiac specialist.

Tricuspid Atresia

Another differential diagnosis for cyanotic heart disease is atresia of the tricuspid valve.[151,156,163, 165,636-638] This malformation dictates right-to-left shunting of systemic venous blood at the atrial level. The atrial shunt may be across a true ASD or a patent foramen ovale. Because all venous return must mix in the LA, this malformation generally causes marked hypoxemia with cyanosis. Affected foals rarely survive to weanling age unless there is a left-to-right shunting VSD into a functional RV outflow tract that provides good pulmonary flow. Otherwise, pulmonary flow must come from a ductus arteriosus or systemic collaterals (e.g., bronchial arteries). Most foals are stunted, nurse poorly, and exhibit severe exercise intolerance and cyanosis at rest. Arterial oxygen tension can be very low (40 to 60 mm Hg). Echocardiography reveals a markedly dilated RA and coronary sinus, atretic tricuspid valve, and rudimentary RV (larger if a functional left-to-right shunting VSD exists). Atrial shunting that allows systemic venous return to empty into the LA must be observed. Abnormal flow patterns can be verified by contrast or color Doppler echocardiography. Prognosis is grave.

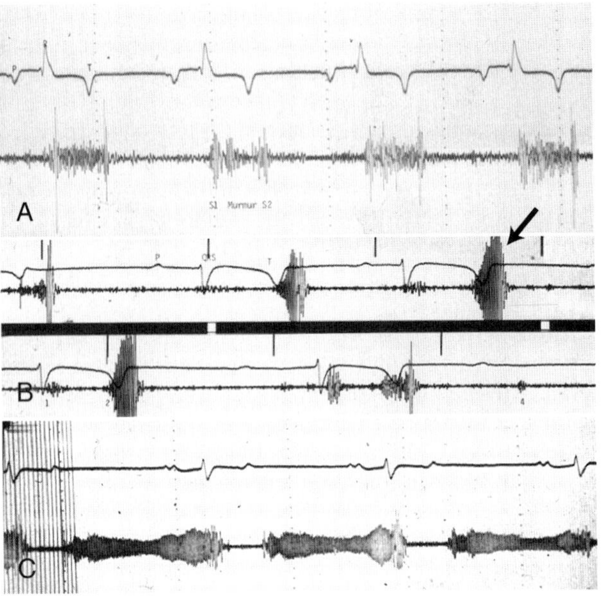

FIGURE 10-33 Phonocardiograms of cardiac murmurs caused by valvular heart disease. **A,** A holosystolic murmur of mitral regurgitation (MR) in a horse with chronic valvular degeneration. **B,** A variable, late systolic murmur of MR related to mitral valve prolapse. The murmur has a crescendo and peaks at end systole (*arrow*). Heart sounds are indicated. The murmur obscures the second sound. **C,** A holodiastolic, vibratory murmur of aortic regurgitation (AR) with presystolic accentuation. The accentuation probably is related to atrial contraction, altered ventricular volume and pressure, and an incremental increase in regurgitant volume.

ACQUIRED VALVULAR HEART DISEASE

Healthy cardiac valves maintain normal antegrade flow in the heart and prevent significant regurgitation of blood. Diseased cardiac valves, which can be stenotic or incompetent, limit CO and place an increased workload on the heart. Stenotic valvular lesions in horses are typically congenital in nature and are extremely rare.[126,156,157,168] However, acquired valvular regurgitation (also called *valvular insufficiency* or *valvular incompetency*) is very common.* The majority of valvular diseases in horses are degenerative in nature or related to high-level training.† Infective (bacterial) endocarditis, ruptured chordae tendineae, and inflammatory valvulitis are infrequent causes of valvular disease. Box 10-2 summarizes important causes of valvular dysfunction. Degenerative valvular disease and infective endocarditis are the valvular problems most often encountered by the equine practitioner (and the focus of this section).

The clinical significance of a valvular lesion depends largely on the severity of regurgitation across the valve. It is clear that many horses adapt to trivial or mild valvular regurgitation with no apparent consequence on performance.[643] The severity of valvular regurgitation is related to the dynamic cross-sectional area of the regurgitant orifice, the pressure gradient driving blood across the valve, and the time allowed for regurgitation, because not all incompetent valves leak throughout systole or diastole. Regardless of the volume, the movement of blood from a high to low pressure chamber is associated with a high-velocity jet that is proportional to the pressure drop between source and sink. The production of high-velocity jets leads to disturbed flow (with turbulence) and in many cases an audible cardiac murmur, the hallmark clinical feature of valvular heart disease (see Figures 10-10 and 10-22, *D*; Figure 10-33).

Valvular incompetency may be diagnosed by auscultation or with Doppler echocardiography.[129,354,509] Doppler studies are highly sensitive for identification of valvular incompetency and represent the gold standard for identification of valvular dysfunction. However, many horses with normal auscultation findings also demonstrate valvular regurgitation by Doppler examination. Most cardiologists consider these "silent" valvular leaks as normal,[354] especially when observed on the right side of the heart. Even on the left side, silent regurgitation is often observed by color Doppler examination.

Some of these flow signals are brief, representing "backflow" or valve closure signals; these are easily misinterpreted unless carefully timed by spectral Doppler or color M-mode examinations. Certainly some cases of silent regurgitation represent the earliest signs of degenerative valvular disease. However, there is no clinical benefit to screening horses by Doppler, and the approach is neither practical nor predictive of future outcome. Thus cardiac auscultation remains the most clinically important method for identifying *significant* valvular disease. Echocardiography including Doppler studies is used to verify the source of a pathologic murmur, identify heart lesions responsible, assess ventricular function, and quantify the degree of cardiac remodeling that has developed in response to the

*References 5, 18, 19, 38, 45, 48, 124, 127, 128, 130, 132, 136, 141, 149, 182, 183, 186, 366, 483, 496, 614, 639-641.

†References 31, 90, 91, 109, 125, 135, 138, 139, 142-144, 147, 148, 169, 170, 172-178, 185, 509, 642.

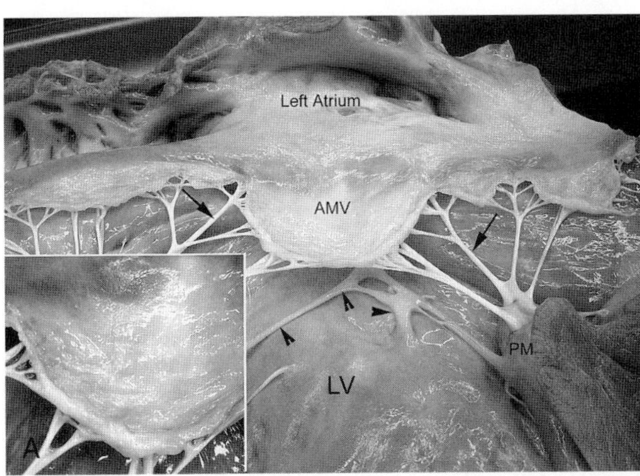

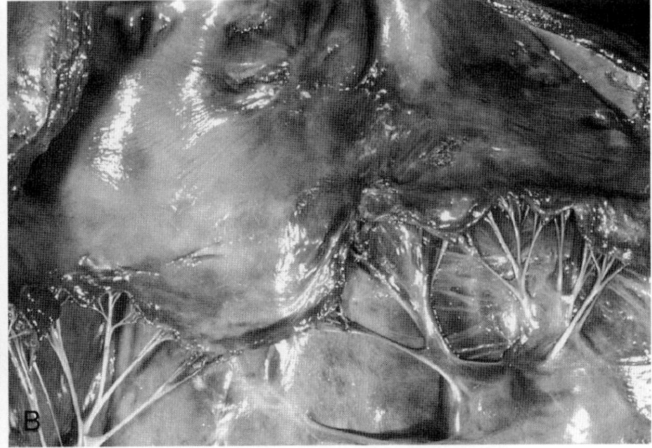

FIGURE 10-34 **A,** Postmortem images from a horse with mitral regurgitation (MR) and congestive heart failure (CHF) caused by severe degenerative valvular disease. The left ventricle (*LV*) is opened and the septal or anterior mitral valve leaflet (*AMV*) is shown. The free edges of the valve or cusps are slightly thickened for an equine valve. The body of the valve is very irregular and thick, changes most evident when viewed in close-up (see inset at lower left). The cut surface of a papillary muscle (*PM*) and intact chordal attachments to the valves are evident (*arrows*). The arrowheads *(left)* point to the LV moderator band or trabeculae septomarginalis, part of electrical conduction system. Myxomatous degeneration of the valve was evident on histopathology. The cause was unknown. **B,** Chronic suppurative valvulitis caused by chronic endocarditis has led to scarring, thickening, and distortion of the mitral valve. This horse developed severe left-sided CHF. Noninfective valvulitis also is recognized sporadically in horses, particularly in younger animals.

lesion. It is also emphasized that there is no echocardiographic or Doppler correlate to the functional ejection murmur.

Although examiners usually discount "silent" regurgitation, the clinical significance of *audible* valvular regurgitation also must be placed in context. For example, examination of high-performance athletes will demonstrate murmurs of tricuspid, mitral, or aortic valvular insufficiency in many of these horses. These findings are readily verifiable by Doppler imaging. In one study of 2-year-olds,[509] the prevalence of tricuspid and mitral regurgitant murmurs increased significantly over a 9-month training period to an incidence of 25.5% and 21.8%, respectively. The causes of these changes and the interpretation of these findings are problematic, especially when referenced to the clinical benchmark of "normal." It is possible that high-level training induces changes in ventricular geometry or in valvular thickness related to CV work, elevations of BP during training, or other factors. Nevertheless, whether these murmurs are actually "normal" or not, it is clear that the *clinical importance* of a regurgitant murmur in a horse must be interpreted with caution and certainly with the perspective of clinical and imaging findings.

The most practical evaluations for assessing the significance of a heart murmur are the work history, physical examination findings, and echocardiography. Other studies such as electrocardiography and exercise testing provide further information by which to judge the importance of a murmur. As a general rule, significant regurgitant murmurs tend to be loud and long. However, the intensity of an insufficiency murmur is related not only to the regurgitant volume but also to the driving pressures of blood and the physical characteristics of the thorax. Therefore although the examiner can grade the intensity of a heart murmur (see earlier in this chapter), it is not possible to grade the severity of regurgitation by auscultation alone. Relatively loud murmurs may be associated with regurgitant volumes that are inconsequential to an individual horse, especially when the murmur is high-pitched, vibratory, or musical in quality. Thus although clinically significant valvular heart disease is best *identified* by auscultation (see Tables 10-2 and 10-3), the *clinical relevance* of a valvular regurgitation must be assessed in other ways.* This approach is emphasized as follows.

Mitral Regurgitation

Mitral regurgitation is one of the more common murmurs detected in horses. The etiopathologic basis of mitral valve incompetency may involve any of the following: high-level training, degenerative thickening, idiopathic disease, prolapse of the valve, ruptured chordae tendineae, bacterial endocarditis, noninfective valvulitis, primary or ischemic myocardial disease, and congenital malformation of the valve (Figures 10-34 and 10-35).† Degenerative, fibrotic thickening of the mitral valve has been observed at necropsy in mature horses and is probably the basis for most cases of mild to moderate MR, including those with "normal" 2D echocardiographic imaging. The basis of mitral valve prolapse is uncertain but could involve connective tissue disease of the leaflets, stretched chorda tendineae, minor chordal ruptures, or injury to a papillary muscle. Ruptured mitral valve chordae tendineae with flail mitral leaflet can occur in animals of any age, including foals. Chordal ruptures, which often involve the accessory mitral cusps, may lead to severe MR with fulminant CHF. Necropsy findings in these cases often show degenerative thickening of the ruptured strand; rarely endocarditis is involved. Although uncommon, infective endocarditis can lead to ulceration, vegetation, or chordal injury and substantial MR (see later). The authors have observed MR because of severe mitral

*References 129, 130, 145, 278, 346, 354, 509.

†References 4, 38, 45, 48, 77, 109, 111, 124, 125, 128, 130, 132, 136, 138, 139, 141, 143, 144, 147, 148, 186, 366, 483.

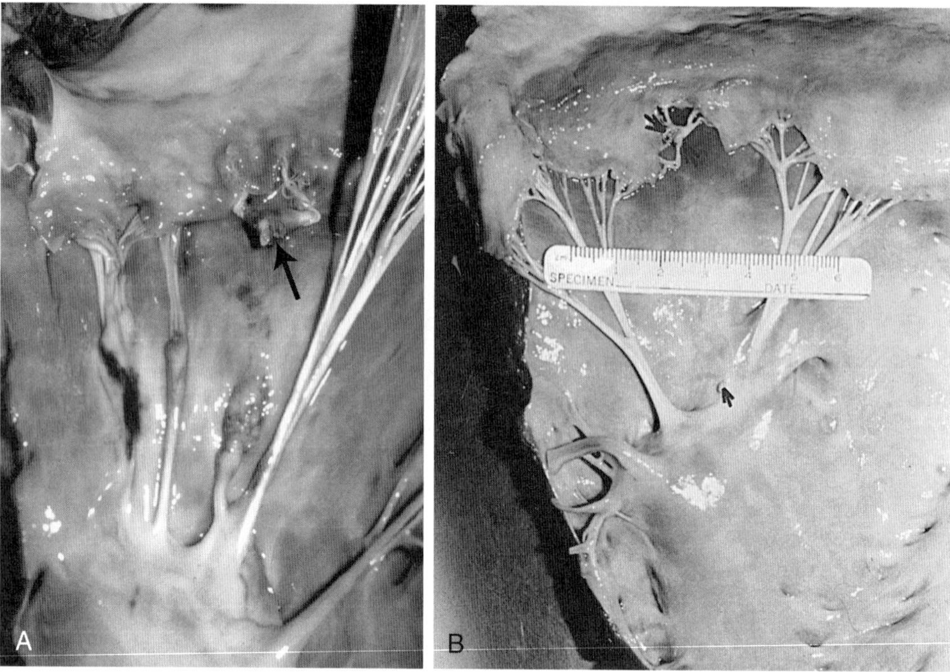

FIGURE 10-35 Rupture of the mitral valve chordae tendineae. **A,** Acute rupture of a chorda tendinea in a horse with lymphocytic plasmacytic valvulitis. The flail mitral cusp actually has twisted because of loss of support (*arrow*). The ventral portion of the tear is obvious adjacent to intact chords. **B,** Chronic rupture of a chorda tendinea in a horse. The contraction of the scarred segments (*arrow*) is notable.

scarring and thickening in young and mature horses. The cause of these lesions is unknown, but the nonsuppurative valvulitis identified might be related to an immune-mediated process. Cardiomyopathy, myocarditis, or myocardial infarction can lead to valvular insufficiency through dilatation of the mitral annulus or loss of papillary muscle support.

The *clinical presentation* of the horse with MR varies. MR is often an incidental finding detected during a routine examination. In other situations MR may be identified in a horse with suboptimal performance or overt clinical signs of heart failure. As indicated previously, relatively soft murmurs of MR are very common in high-performance horses.[509] When MR is only mild to moderate, significant LA dilatation and LV volume overload are not evident, LA pressure (as estimated by pulmonary capillary wedge pressures) increases little compared with healthy controls,[311] and the horse often performs satisfactorily. Two recent retrospective studies also suggest a good long-term prognosis for cases of mild MR in sport and pleasure horses[567] and in middle-aged to older horses and ponies[643] with left-sided valvular regurgitation. With moderate to severe MR, clinical signs are more likely, including poor performance, exercise-induced pulmonary hemorrhage, or overt CHF. Tolerance of the lesion depends largely on whether the horse is used for vigorous work. Some horses with MR also develop AF, which can further impair CO. When a murmur of MR is identified within the setting of fever, weight loss, polyarthritis, or systemic inflammation, infective endocarditis should be considered. MR related to chordal rupture is a rare but well-recognized cause of CHF, including peracute disease with fulminating pulmonary edema (see Figure 10-11). Chronic, hemodynamically significant MR from any cause can lead to pulmonary hypertension, AF, and biventricular CHF, with clinical signs of right-sided CHF dominating the clinical presentation (see earlier in this chapter).[48,109]

The *physical examination* of the horse with MR typically reveals a grade 2 to 5 (of a possible 6) holosystolic or pansystolic murmur. The murmur is detected most intensely at or dorsal to the palpable left apical impulse and over the mitral valve area (see Figure 10-8). Quite often the murmur is loud at the aortic valve, probably related to the proximity of the septal mitral leaflet to the aortic valve or to cranial projection of the regurgitant jet. Loud MR murmurs often project quite dorsally and to the right. The typical murmur of MR is long (holosystolic or pansystolic), extending into the second sound.[38] This timing may cause the listener to misinterpret the third sound as the second, thus preventing a full appreciation of the significance of the murmur. When the third sound is very loud, the clinician should consider significant volume overload or increased LV diastolic pressure. Because many horses with MR also have concomitant TR, echocardiographic examination and Doppler studies may be needed to differentiate bilateral AV valve insufficiency from isolated MR with radiation to the right. Finally, AF or premature beats can modify the murmur of MR.

Two variants of holosystolic MR murmur are the protomesosystolic decrescendo murmur and the mid-to-late systolic crescendo murmur. A decrescendo murmur may be detected with mild MR because coaptation of the leaflets can occur as the ventricular volume decreases during late systole. This type of murmur can be easily confused with a functional ejection murmur, unless the point of maximal murmur intensity is centered near the left apex. Conversely, severe MR with CHF could conceivably cause a decrescendo murmur because atrial and ventricular pressures may equilibrate in late systole. However, this is not a common finding and would be associated with CHF. The other variant of MR is the mid-to-late systolic crescendo murmur (see Figure 10-33, *B*). Presumably this murmur is caused by mitral valve prolapse as it starts *after* the LV

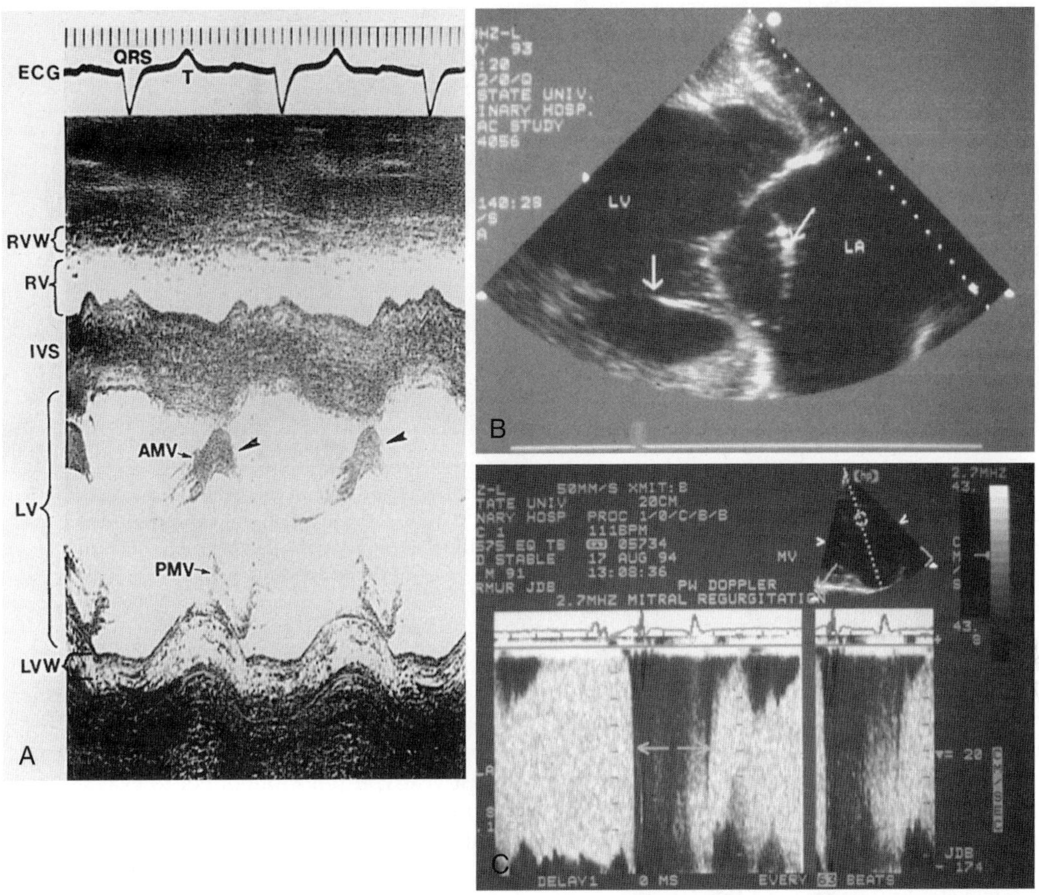

FIGURE 10-36 Echocardiograms recorded from horses with mitral regurgitation (MR). **A,** M-mode study demonstrating significant thickening of the anterior mitral valve (*AMV*) leaflet (*arrows*). This would be compatible with endocarditis or severe valvulitis (*RVW,* right ventricular wall; *RV,* right ventricle; *IVS,* intraventricular septum; *LV,* left ventricle; *LVW,* left ventricular wall). **B,** Flail mitral leaflet (*right arrow*) in a horse with multiple chordae ruptures. The prolapsed portion of the mitral valve forms a curved echodense line in the dilated left atrium (LA), whereas the other valve portions are to the left of this echocardiogram. A normal chord is evident (*left arrow*). **C,** Pulsed-wave Doppler study recorded from the LA demonstrating a turbulent, high-velocity, aliased systolic jet of MR in a Thoroughbred horse. The duration of the event is shown (*arrows*).

has begun ejection. Decreasing LV volume predisposes to leaflet prolapse and initiates midsystolic regurgitation that builds through the second heart sound. The resultant murmur can be harsh or musical, and the novice often confuses this flow event with an early diastolic murmur.

Both *echocardiography* and *Doppler examinations* play a pivotal role in the assessment of the horse with MR* (Figure 10-36); they are indicated to examine the valve anatomy; estimate the severity of MR; measure the size of the atria, ventricles, and great vessels; and quantify LV systolic function. The underlying cause of MR may be obvious from the echocardiographic examination. Mild to moderate valvular thickening, although admittedly subjective, is compatible with degeneration or nonbacterial valvulitis. Prolapse of the mitral valve cusps has been observed in horses with MR, but the limits of "normal" prolapse require further definition. Lesions caused by vegetative endocarditis cause the valves to appear irregularly thickened or shortened. In cases of acute endocarditis, evidence of valve thrombus can be seen; a high frame rate, real-time examination may show oscillation of this tissue. Small, focal lesions are more commonly observed on the atrial surface of the valve (see Figure 10-43, B). In chronic endocarditis, the valve may be more echodense or even appear calcified. Chordal rupture is recognized by observing chaotic flutter of a mitral structure (a flail leaflet), prolapse of a large portion of the valve into the atrium, or the contracted chordal remnant flipping into the atrium during systole (see Figure 10-36). High-frequency systolic vibrations of the mitral valve may be seen on the M-mode study in horses with a musical murmur of MR. Pulsed or continuous wave or color-Doppler studies can identify the mitral regurgitant jet (see Figure 10-36). The Doppler examination should be performed from both right- and the left-sided thoracic windows. High-velocity or turbulent jets may be difficult to find without a complete and thorough examination of the mitral valve that involves multiple image planes. When color-flow Doppler demonstrates both a wide *origin* of the regurgitant jet and a pattern of diffuse distribution of turbulence deep into the LA, the likelihood of hemodynamically significant MR is greater. Quantitation of cardiac size is instrumental in assessing

*References 129, 130, 354, 505, 509, 510.

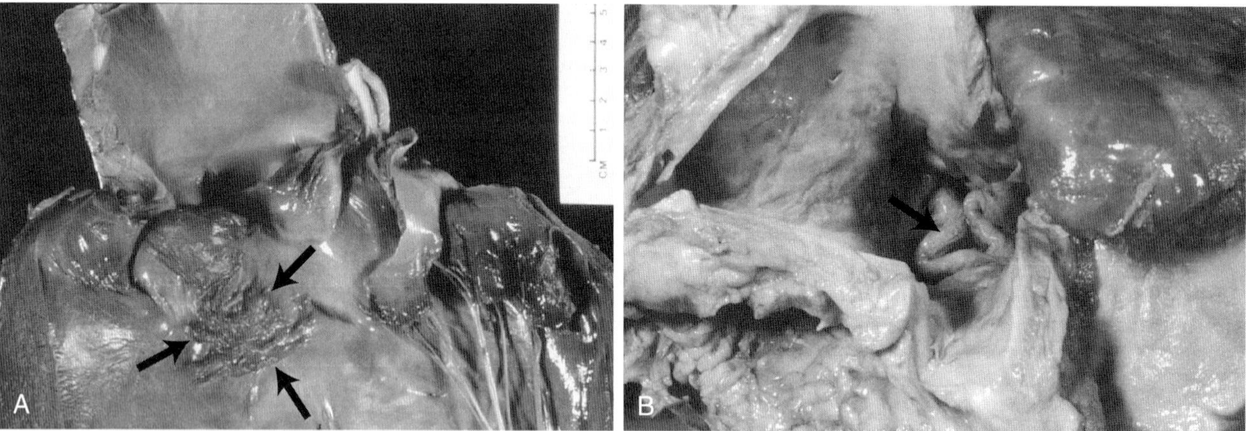

FIGURE 10-37 Postmortem lesions of aortic regurgitation (AR; see also Figure 10-41, *B*). **A,** A segment of the left ventricular (LV) outflow tract and the ascending aorta. Linear bands are evident on the two valves shown, and a large jet lesion also is visible below the valves *(between the arrows)*. The lesion is typical in aged horses. **B,** The aortic valve *(arrow)* viewed from the ascending aorta. Noninfective valvulitis and scarring have caused severe thickening.

severity. With severe MR and LV volume overload, rounding of the LV apex and increased end diastolic dimension will occur. Global LV function may appear normal to exuberant because ventricular preload is increased and afterload decreased in severe MR. However, when MR is both severe and chronic, or if the underlying basis for MR is cardiomyopathy, then the ventricular shortening fraction is normal to decreased. The LA often assumes a more circular, almost turgid, appearance when MR is hemodynamically importance, and the 2D echocardiographic measure of internal atrial dimension often exceeds 13.5 to 14.5 cm. With acute or chronic MR, the lobar and main PA may be dilated as a consequence of pulmonary hypertension, presumably related to increased LA pressure, interstitial lung edema, vascular remodeling, or other factors.

The prognosis for horses with MR is variable and, as discussed earlier, is related to clinical findings, work history, and results of echocardiographic studies. Abnormalities observed during echocardiography, including lesions of the mitral valve leaflets, the degree of LA and LV volume overloading, global LV function, and Doppler findings, should be considered when formulating the prognosis. Certainly, when MR is associated with CHF, AF, endocarditis, chordal rupture, marked cardiomegaly, severe valvular thickening, dilated cardiomyopathy, or pulmonary hypertension, the prognosis for life and performance is poor. The detection of PA dilatation indicates significant pulmonary hypertension and the low but concrete possibility of PA rupture associated with exercise. Fortunately, the vast majority of horses with MR appear to perform very well, indicating that MR in most cases is not clinically important.[567] Whether progressive exercise intolerance will develop in a particular case depends on the horse's use and on the progression of the underlying lesion. Generally, when MR is caused by valve degeneration and the heart size is normal, the progression is gradual, the prognosis for life is favorable, and performance is maintained. When MR is detected in an untrained colt or filly, the prognosis is less encouraging. The presence of even mild to moderate cardiac dilatation in a case of MR recommends a more guarded prognosis, although this assessment is best made by serial examinations. The significance of trivial to mild MR in the high performance horse or racehorse is uncertain. In some animals, treadmill exercise is normal, whereas others may demonstrate a higher heart rate for a given level of work than might otherwise be expected. The latter finding may be suggestive of a cardiac limitation to performance.

Regardless of cause or the severity of the condition, the horse diagnosed with MR merits follow-up examinations at least yearly, if not more often, to evaluate progression of the hemodynamic burden and to detect the development of CHF, pulmonary hypertension, or cardiac arrhythmias. Treatment of MR involves management of complications such as heart failure, endocarditis, or arrhythmias. These topics are covered elsewhere in this chapter.

Aortic Regurgitation

Aortic regurgitation is a common valvular insufficiency. Degeneration of the aortic valve is by far the most common reason for AR.* The degenerative nodular lesions and fibrous bands responsible for AR in older horses have been well described by Bishop, Cole, and Smetzer[5] (Figure 10-37, *A*). Prolapse of the aortic valve is a common echocardiographic finding and probably represents another manifestation of connective tissue degeneration affecting the valve. Small fenestrations of the valve also have been identified at necropsy but have uncertain clinical significance. Other potential causes of AR in horses include infective endocarditis, congenital valvular disease, VSD (see earlier in this chapter), noninfective valvulitis, and ruptured aortic sinus aneurysm.

In most cases, AR is an incidental finding encountered during a routine physical, prepurchase, or insurance examination. Most horses with this murmur are older than 10 years of age, and the murmur is especially common in aged horses, a testament to the degenerative nature of the lesion. Careful auscultation in a quiet area may identify a very soft diastolic murmur in a younger horse. Silent AR may also be considered physiologic or trivial, and it is not uncommon to identify a trivial jet of AR by Doppler studies in horses with no identifiable diastolic murmur.[354] When a loud murmur of AR is identified in a younger animal, a complete echocardiographic

*References 4, 18, 77, 111, 125, 127, 130, 136, 138, 139, 141, 142, 366, 496, 614, 640.

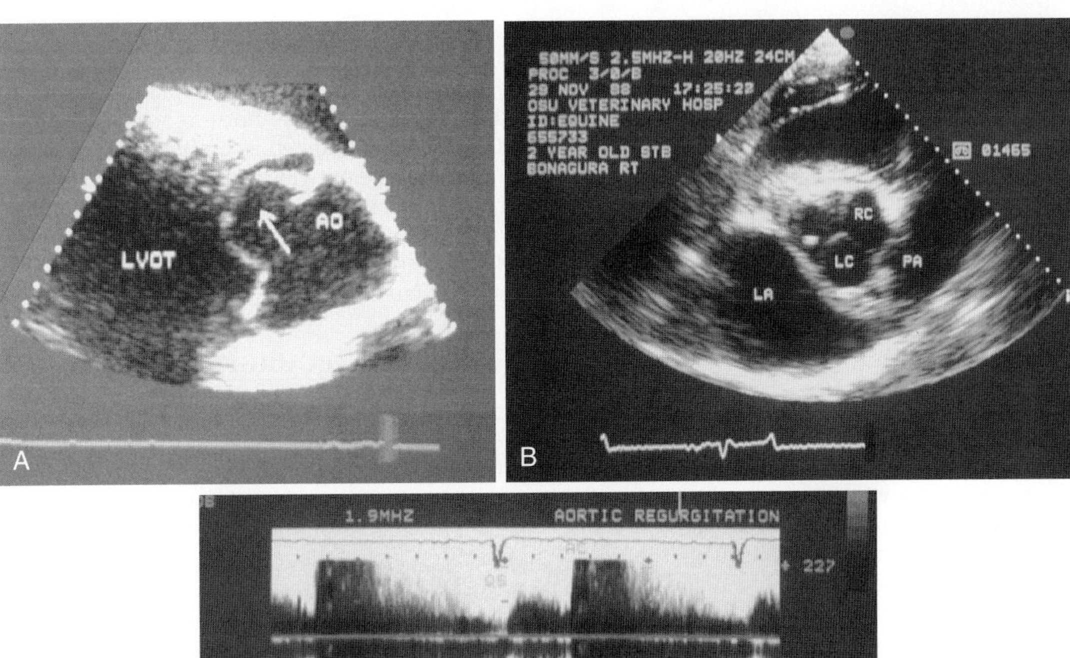

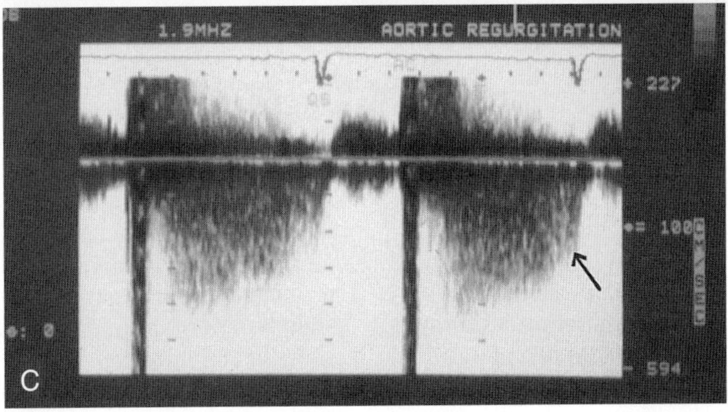

FIGURE 10-38 Echocardiograms recorded from horses with aortic regurgitation (AR; see also Figure 10-22, *D*). **A,** Aortic valve prolapse (*arrow*) in a 12-year-old Standardbred gelding. **B,** A well-circumscribed, echodense "bead" on the noncoronary cusp of the aortic valve in a 2-year-old Standardbred colt may represent a congenital or acquired lesion. This short-axis image plane is recorded across the base of the heart. **C,** Continuous wave Doppler recording from the same horse as in **A** demonstrates a turbulent diastolic signal that ends at the QRS complex (*arrow*). *LC/RC,* Left/right coronary cusps of the aortic valve in short axis; *PA,* pulmonary artery; *LA,* left atrium.

examination is warranted. Poor performance is an infrequent presenting complaint in horses with AR, because most will continue at their prior performance level, provided that no other clinical or cardiac abnormalities are present. Intermittent fevers, weight loss, or lameness should prompt consideration of endocarditis. CHF is infrequently observed in conjunction with isolated AR but may develop in the horses when AR occurs in combination with MR or AF.

Clinically important AR is identified by cardiac auscultation, which reveals a holodiastolic murmur, with the point of maximal intensity over the aortic valve area, and strong radiation to the right and toward the left cardiac apex in many instances. The murmur may vary greatly in intensity and character. The quality is typically harsh and decrescendo with a blowing nature (see Figure 10-10, *C*), but presystolic accentuation may be noted (see Figure 10-33, *C*). The character can be vibratory, musical, cooing, buzzing, or "dive bomber" in quality. A precordial thrill is palpable over the aortic valve area when the murmur is loud. A variant of the typical AR murmur is that associated with rupture of an aortic sinus into the RA, ventricular septum, or pulmonary artery. An aortic-cardiac fistula leads to a holodiastolic or continuous murmur that is louder over the right side of the thorax. However, in the majority of horses with an aortic-cardiac fistula, a continuous machinery type of murmur is detected. The quality of the arterial pulses is a good indicator of the severity of the isolated AR.[138] Bounding arterial pulses indicate significant LV volume overload and moderate to severe AR. A systolic ejection murmur is often present (particularly when the regurgitant volume is large) and is explained by ejection of a large stroke volume across the aortic valve. It should be emphasized that no evidence for anatomic stenosis as the result of degenerative aortic valve disease has been published.

A complete echocardiographic examination including Doppler echocardiography is useful for further evaluation of horses with AR, particularly when the arterial pulse is abnormal or cardiac-related clinical signs are suspected.* The most common abnormality observed by 2D echocardiography is mild valvular thickening in association with prolapse of one or more aortic leaflets (Figure 10-38). These findings are compatible with degenerative valvular disease. The aortic valve may flutter or vibrate. The 2D examination also assists with the differential diagnosis. In cases of endocarditis, the leaflets may appear thickened, irregular, and more highly echogenic. The valve may appear to oscillate if fresh thrombus is noted

*References 84, 130, 136, 138, 139, 141, 142, 152, 496, 501, 504.

within the vegetation. Other rare 2D echocardiographic findings related to AR include fenestrations of the aortic valve leaflets, flail aortic leaflet, aortic sinus aneurysm, and aortic root prolapse into a VSD. Dilatation of the aortic root (exceeding 10 cm) may be observed in some horses with AR.

The traditional M-mode examination in horses with AR is still useful. LV volume overload that develops with AR increases ventricular internal diameter at end diastole, increases shortening fraction, and decreased free wall thickness. An exaggerated or swinging septal motion on 2D or M-mode examination represents another subjective observation of volume overload. If myocardial failure develops, then the end systolic dimension may be increased, despite normal shortening fraction. Inspection of the mitral valve often reveals high-frequency diastolic vibrations of the anterior (septal) leaflet related to an eccentric high-velocity AR jet directed across the LV outflow tract to the left and caudally. Similar vibrations may also be detected on the intraventricular septum when the regurgitant jet is oriented in a right or cranial direction. High-frequency fluttering of the aortic valve leaflets or aortic walls is more common in horses with musical or vibratory murmurs. Increased mitral valve E-point septal separation can indicate the regurgitant jet is impinging on the valve or herald LV dilatation and failure. In the latter case, other markers of severe insufficiency will be evident, including ventricular dilatation, rounding of the LV apex, and a wide origin jet of AR on Doppler studies. Premature (presystolic) mitral closure is an uncommon but ominous finding of severe AR with elevated ventricular end diastolic pressure.

The flow disturbance of AR is confirmed by Doppler studies. The Doppler examination shows one or more central or eccentric diastolic jets of AR. The timing of the flow disturbance should be verified by spectral Doppler or color M-mode studies. Assessing the severity of AR by Doppler studies is rife with pitfalls, and the examiner should use multiple 2D, M-mode, and Doppler findings to assess severity. Importantly, a wide jet area in the LV outflow tract does not always indicate severe AR. The finding of a small, central perivalvular jet, with a small cross-sectional area, suggests trivial AR. Often these leaks are confined to mid-to-late diastole. Conversely, a strong spectral signal, holodiastolic timing, and wide-origin color Doppler signal suggests more significant regurgitation. Examination of the short axis jet area in cross-sectional studies of the aortic root is especially instructive because a wide ventricular spray is often associated with a small origin jet (this suggests mild AR). The CW Doppler spectrum can be assessed for a short pressure half-time (steep AR slope), which indicates LV diastolic pressure is rapidly increasing and that AR is severe. However, the examiner must be certain the ultrasound beam has remained in good alignment with the regurgitant jet before this assessment can be made.

The clinical significance and prognosis of AR is most accurately based on the history, physical examination, and echocardiogram. Because most cases of AR are associated with a slow degeneration of the aortic valve leaflets, and this occurs in older horses without other cardiac problems, the prognosis for life and performance is usually good. Such animals typically have minimal echocardiographic abnormalities or only mild echocardiographic signs of volume overload. Epidemiologic studies suggest that in general AR is mild in most cases and not an independent predictor of survival[643]; however, the occasional case is encountered with moderate to severe AR. The findings of flail aortic valve leaflet, endocarditis, or echo markers of moderate to severe volume overload or myocardial failure indicate a poor prognosis for life and performance. Ventricular dilatation can predispose to ventricular arrhythmias. Therefore an exercising ECG and exercise test should be obtained in performance horses with significant AR to determine if the horse remains safe to ride. A Holter ECG can be considered as a potential test in older, valuable animals to rule out ventricular ectopy. Follow-up clinical and echocardiographic examinations are indicated for the horse with moderate to severe AR. The development of secondary MR, AF, ventricular arrhythmias, CHF or sudden death should be anticipated in horses with severe volume overload.

Tricuspid Regurgitation

Tricuspid regurgitation might be the most frequently detected flow disturbance and murmur in the horse,* although little information confirms the etiopathogenesis of this condition aside from speculation that it might be related to recurrent physiologic pulmonary hypertension of high-intensity exercise. The prevalence and color of Doppler severity of TR increases with age, training, and subtle increases in RV size.[185] The anatomic basis of tricuspid valve incompetency can be any of the following lesions: idiopathic, degenerative thickening, prolapse, noninfective tricuspid valvulitis, bacterial endocarditis, pulmonary hypertension (including left-sided failure), ruptured chordae tendineae, myocardial disease with secondary cardiomegaly, chronic tachyarrhythmia, and congenital malformation of the valve. TR is common in horses of racing age[509]; however, the anatomic correlate to this incompetency is uncertain. Degenerative, fibrotic thickening of the tricuspid valve in mature horses may lead to mild to moderate TR. When compared with the mitral condition, ruptured tricuspid valve chordae tendineae are uncommon[639] and better tolerated unless associated with endocarditis. The tricuspid valve can be infected by bacteria, and in some cases is secondary to an injudicious or septic jugular venipunctures or catheterization. Pulmonary hypertension, cardiomyopathy, and myocarditis can lead to secondary dilatation of the tricuspid annulus or alteration of papillary muscle support, permitting valvular insufficiency. Tricuspid malformation does occur but seems more commonly associated with stenosis or atresia of the valve† (see earlier discussion in this chapter).

A soft, grade 2 to 3 systolic murmur of TR is most often an incidental finding detected during a routine examination. The murmur becomes more problematic when it is loud, or is identified in a horse that is performing poorly. Many horses with TR race well; therefore the clinician should first exclude other likely reasons for poor performance before incriminating the tricuspid valve. Of course, if chronic hemodynamically significant TR has developed, then peak work effort will suffer and even right-sided CHF may develop. The latter situation is very uncommon unless the TR is severe, related to pulmonary hypertension or infective endocarditis, or complicated by AF. Prominent jugular pulses (giant c-v waves) are typical of horses with TR associated with CHF.

Auscultation of the horse with TR typically reveals a grade 2 to 5 holosystolic murmur with the point of maximal intensity over the right hemithorax at the tricuspid valve area. The murmur can be holosystolic, decrescendo, or mid-to-late systolic.

*References 4, 77, 111, 125, 130, 149, 179, 180, 182, 184, 230, 354, 639, 644.

†References 151, 156, 161-163, 165, 366, 637, 638.

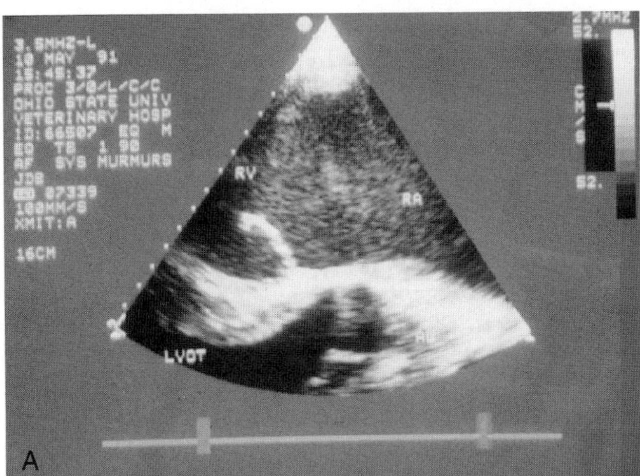

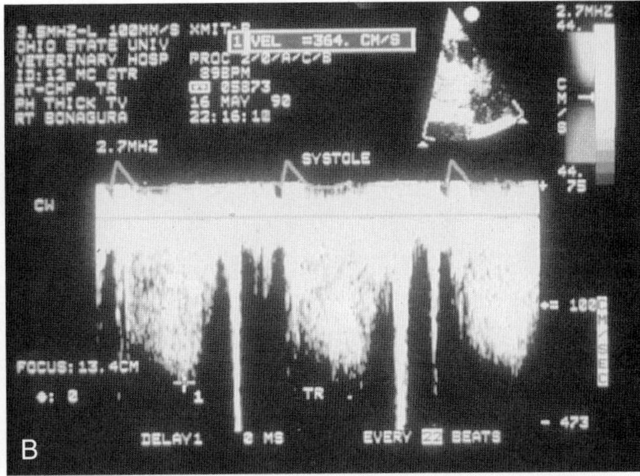

FIGURE 10-39 Echocardiograms from horses with tricuspid regurgitation (TR; see also Figure 10-24, *C*). **A,** Two-dimensional (2D) echocardiogram demonstrating probable valve thickening, significant right atrial (RA) distention, and spontaneous RA contrast in a horse with severe TR, atrial fibrillation (AF), and congestive heart failure (CHF) (1-cm calibrations at the left of the sector; *LVOT,* left ventricular outflow tract). **B,** Continuous wave Doppler recording of a high-velocity TR jet from a horse with TR caused by pulmonary artery obstruction as the result of a mass lesion. The high velocity of regurgitation (>3.6 m/sec) indicates that elevated right ventricular (RV) pressure is driving the regurgitant jet. In this case the high pressure is caused by supravalvular pulmonary stenosis resulting from the tumor. TR jets associated with normal RV pressures are typically less than 3.0 m/sec.

Although the timing and intensity may at times remind the examiner of a functional murmur, the location of greatest murmur intensity argues against that possibility. The murmur usually radiates dorsally and, if loud, to the extreme left cranioventral thorax. The intensity of the TR murmur in many cases does correlate well to the regurgitant volume, but loudness also depends on PA and RV systolic pressures. In general, a grade 4 or louder murmur is anticipated when there is moderate to severe TR or when TR is related to pulmonary hypertension. AF or atrial premature beats are present in some horses with TR, particularly when the RA is dilated or the regurgitant jet is large.

Echocardiographic examinations of the tricuspid valve (Figure 10-39) are typically performed from the right side of the thorax, because the tricuspid valve and RV inlet are closer to the right thoracic wall. However, an extreme left cranial transducer location with caudal angulation also can also be successful for examining the tricuspid valve. Because a number of potential reasons for tricuspid incompetency must be considered, careful attention must be directed to the valve and its support apparatus, the size of the PA, and the left side of the heart. In the vast majority of cases, a clear-cut lesion of the tricuspid valve leaflet is not evident. Valve thickening, prolapse, vegetations, chordal rupture, regurgitation secondary to RV dilatation, and pulmonary hypertension usually can be diagnosed or excluded with careful imaging. As with MR, moderate to severe TR leads to RA and RV volume overload; however, it is more difficult to quantify these chamber volumes owing to their complex geometry.[185]

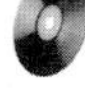

Doppler studies can identify the tricuspid regurgitant jet. In trivial or "silent" TR, this jet is typically very narrow at the origin and directed at the aorta. However, when the jet is wide at its origin, or projects centrally or laterally into the RA, cardiomegaly is more likely to be present and the heart should be examined carefully. The RV (and PA) systolic pressure can be estimated by faithfully recording the peak jet velocity. This requires the examiner to align the continuous wave Doppler cursor parallel to regurgitant flow and may demand a ventral or dorsal placement of the transducer with steep beam angulation. When the jet velocity is less than 2.5 m/sec, pulmonary hypertension is not present. Jets exceeding 3.2 to 3.4 m/sec are indicative of pulmonary hypertension—provided that no RV outflow obstruction or VSD are identified (see Figure 10-39, *B*). The identification of pulmonary hypertension should prompt careful examination of the left heart, because the main cardiac lesion may be centered over the mitral valve, aortic valve, or LV cavity and the right heart changes simply a secondary consequence.

The prognosis for horses with TR is generally very favorable. A soft murmur of TR in a trained athlete is disregarded as clinically insignificant; although, defining such a disturbance as "functional" would be imprecise in the opinion of the authors. The presence of TR is more likely to cause concern if right-sided cardiomegaly, pulmonary hypertension, or AF is evident. Visualization of a vegetation or chordal rupture would indicate a poor prognosis for performance and a guarded prognosis for life. The width of the regurgitant jet at its origin, recent performance history, and results of exercise testing are useful in developing a prognosis for life and future work. The affect of exercise and the associated pulmonary hypertension on the volume of TR may become better understood with the increased use of exercise testing and postexercise echocardiography.[184] When TR is judged to be moderate or severe, periodic re-examinations are indicated to follow the progression of the lesion and to detect cardiomegaly or cardiac arrhythmias if they develop.

Pulmonary Insufficiency

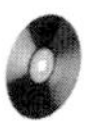

Trivial and clinically silent, physiologic pulmonic insufficiency can often be detected by Doppler studies; however, this is a normal finding.[130,149,230,354] Clinically significant pulmonic insufficiency is rare and occurs most frequently

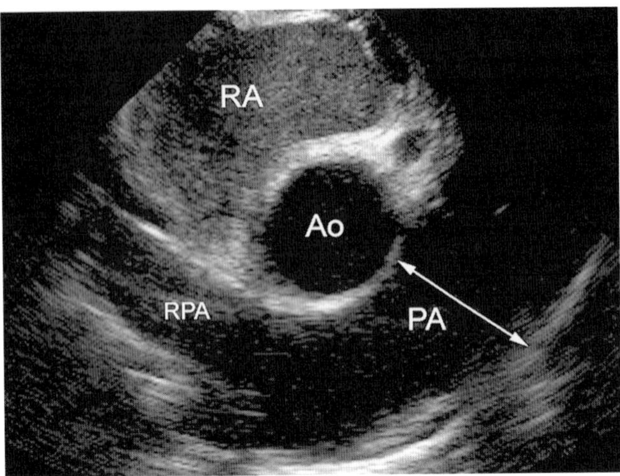

FIGURE 10-40 Right cranial echocardiogram with the aorta (*Ao*) in short axis demonstrating a dilated pulmonary artery (*PA*). The cause was pulmonary hypertension after left-sided congestive heart failure (CHF). *RA,* Right atrium (with spontaneous contrast in cavity); *RPA,* right branch of the pulmonary artery.

with pulmonary hypertension associated with left-sided heart failure. Infective endocarditis, congenital abnormalities of the valve leaflets (bicuspid or quadricuspid valve), and rupture of the pulmonary valve are rare causes of pulmonic insufficiency.[135,137] Murmurs of pulmonic regurgitation are usually undetectable unless the regurgitant volume is large or is driven by pulmonary hypertension; however, the regurgitant flow can be easily identified using pulsed-wave and color-flow Doppler echocardiography. Dilatation of the PA may be detected echocardiographically when pulmonic insufficiency is caused by pulmonary hypertension (Figure 10-40).

When severe pulmonic regurgitation does develop, it is generally a consequence of left-sided heart failure with pulmonary hypertension and accompanied by clinical signs of biventricular failure. Signs of right-sided CHF typically stem from the combination of pulmonary hypertension, pulmonic regurgitation, RV volume overload, and TR. If a murmur of pulmonic regurgitation is detected, then it is usually holodiastolic and a decrescendo murmur, with the point of maximal intensity at the pulmonic valve area, radiating toward the right cardiac apex. The prognosis for life and performance is usually poor in these cases.

Infective Endocarditis

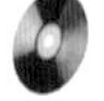

Infective (bacterial) endocarditis is caused by invasion of the heart valves or endocardium by bacteria. Endocarditis is not common in horses but occurs sporadically in most populations.*

Horses of any age can be affected, although the pathogenesis may differ in younger animals or in those that are immunosuppressed. In one report, the mean age of affected horses was 2.1 years.[179] Numerous bacteria have been associated with bacterial endocarditis. The offending microorganism likely depends on the environment, portal of entry (e.g., gastrointestinal tract, skin, lung, oral cavity, joint, surgical wound, or IV catheter), and the effects of prior antimicrobial therapy that may select for resistant strains. *Streptococcus* spp., *Actinobacillus equuli,* and *Pasteurella* spp. have been isolated most frequently. *Rhodococcus equi, Candida parapsilosis, Erysipelothrix rhusiopathiae,* meningococci, *Staphylococcus aureus,* and other organisms (e.g., aspergillosis) have also been isolated.

The pathogenesis involves bacterial invasion from the bloodstream and colonization of the heart valve or endocardial surfaces. Bacteremia is a prerequisite for development of this condition. Direct invasion of a previously normal valve by virulent bacteria, or in the context of overwhelming sepsis, represents the most likely pathogenic mechanism involved in foals with infective endocarditis. Disruption of the endocardial surface by jet lesions associated with congenital intracardiac shunts may also predispose to endocarditis, although this mechanism is not well established in horses. Preexisting valvular heart disease with endocardial changes or high-velocity jets may represent risk factors for bacterial colonization in older horses, but again this is completely unproven.

The most common sites of infective endocarditis are the aortic and mitral valves, although endocarditis lesions have been reported on all cardiac valves. Mural and chordal endocarditis lesions have also been reported but occur much less frequently. The combination of bacterial injury, exposure of valve collagen, thrombosis, and host leukocyte response contributes to development of the vegetation (Figure 10-41), which consists microscopically of bacteria, platelets, fibrin, leukocytes, and varying degrees of granulation or fibrosis. Bacteria may not be evident at necropsy, especially if antimicrobial therapy has sterilized the vegetation.

The pathophysiology of endocarditis in horses is probably similar to that in other species. A host response, as well as the primary cardiac lesions, contributes to the morbidity of this disease. Cardiac manifestations include valvular injury leading to regurgitation, chordal rupture, or rarely to stenosis; secondary cardiomegaly; myocarditis from extension of the infection or through coronary embolization; myocardial infarction if emboli are shed to the coronary arteries; arrhythmias from cardiomegaly, myocarditis, or infarction; and myocardial depression from bacteremia. Recurrent or chronic bacteremia, and hence fever, is characteristic of endocarditis. Metastatic infection, distant thrombosis and infarction, and immune-mediated host responses can occur. Distant infection or immune complex disease can lead to multisystemic clinical signs, including polyarthritis, osteomyelitis, vasculitis, or nephritis. Right-sided thrombi can lead to pulmonary thrombi, abscessation of the lungs, or both (see Figure 10-41).[135,169]

Clinical features of endocarditis are variable.[179] Affected horses usually have a history of intermittent fever, weight loss, depression, anorexia, lethargy, and often intermittent lameness (Figure 10-42). Synovial distension may be noted. A predisposing condition or a concurrent infection may be evident, including jugular vein thrombophlebitis, strangles, septic joint, or an abscess. In most horses no history of previous illness or evidence of concurrent infection is identified. The physical examination often reveals fever, and some horses may be tachypneic. The fever is often intermittent. Murmurs of mitral or aortic valvular insufficiency are most commonly detected; those of TR are less common. Systolic murmurs caused by valve destruction must be differentiated from the physiologic flow murmurs that are heard so often in febrile horses. Murmurs of valvular stenosis may also be detected with

*References 4, 31, 77, 90, 109, 111, 125, 135, 138, 139, 142-144, 147, 148, 169, 170, 172-180.

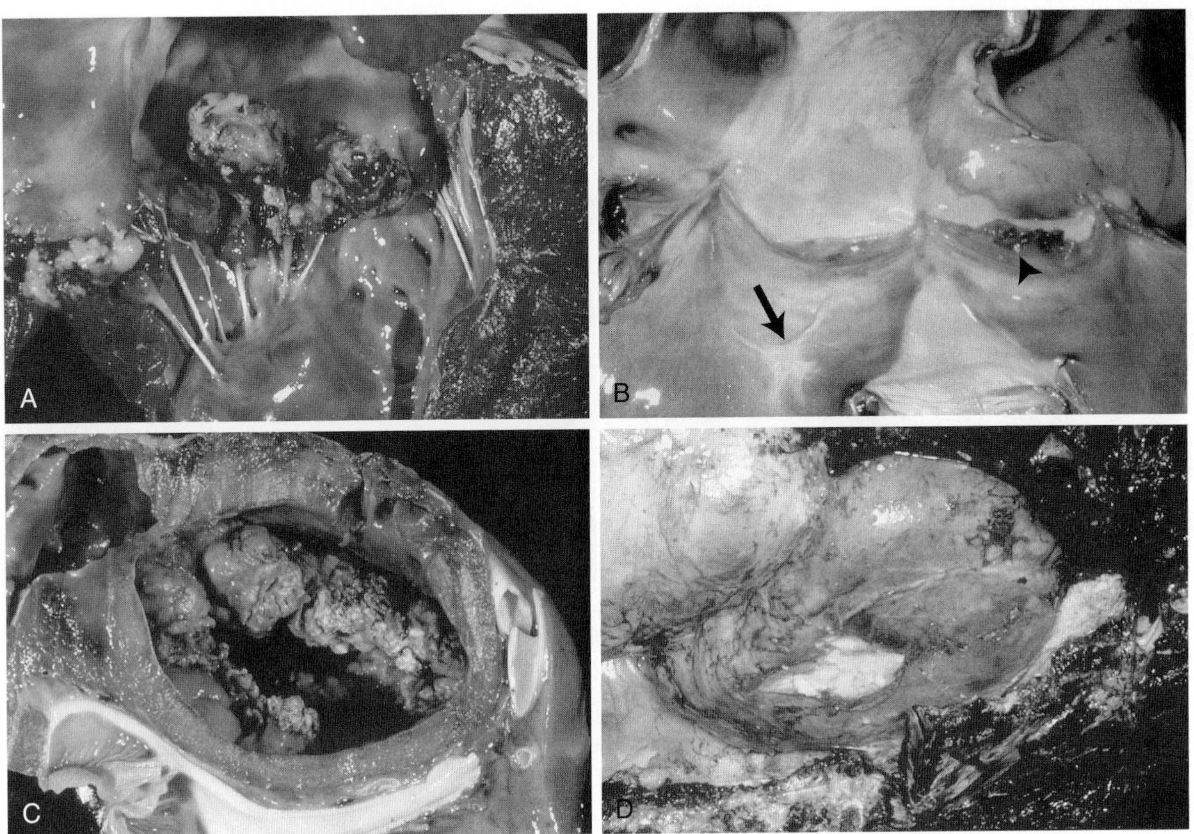

FIGURE 10-41 Bacterial endocarditis: postmortem lesions. **A,** Severe mitral valve endocarditis in a yearling. **B,** Focal aortic valve endocarditis is evident in this view of the left ventricular (LV) outlet and the ascending aorta. The septal mitral leaflet is at the lower right, and a jet lesion (*arrow*) is visible in the LV outflow tract. Above the mitral leaflet, in the center of the left coronary cusp, is a raised, irregular vegetation *(arrowhead)* that caused aortic regurgitation (AR). **C,** Tricuspid valve vegetation in a weanling. Although less common than mitral or aortic vegetations, right-sided endocarditis is a definite risk in horses, particularly in animals subjected to repeated jugular venous catheterization. **D,** A lung abscess in a horse after pulmonary valve endocarditis. The center of the abscess is incised and reveals caseous exudate. Systemic embolization and metastatic infection are recognized complications of valvular infections.

bacterial endocarditis but occur rarely.[135] Some horses with bacterial endocarditis have no auscultable murmur initially. The quality or intensity of the murmur may change over a number of days. AF, atrial or ventricular premature depolarizations, and VT have been observed with endocarditis.[109,174]

Laboratory studies obtained from horses with infective endocarditis may reveal anemia (of chronic inflammatory disease), hyperproteinemia (hyperglobulinemia with hypoalbuminemia), elevated fibrinogen, and leukocytosis with a mature neutrophilia.[179] Multiple blood cultures should be performed when bacterial endocarditis is suspected. The result of blood cultures may be negative, however, particularly after antimicrobial therapy. A positive blood culture may be more likely if multiple samples are drawn at different times of the day during or near febrile episodes. Antibiotic removal system media might also be of value when culturing blood from horses that have received antibiotics recently, and it can be helpful to consult with a clinical microbiologist regarding optimal broth media used for blood culturing.

Diagnosis of infective endocarditis may be definitive in the setting of a compatible clinical history with positive blood

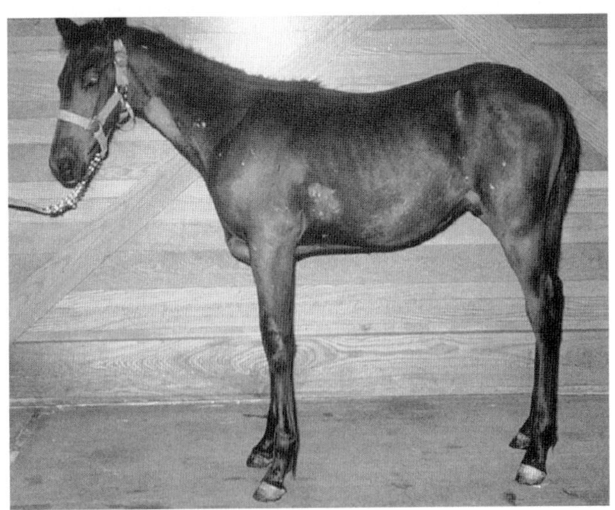

FIGURE 10-42 Weight loss, loss of condition, and ventral edema in this weanling with endocarditis and right-sided congestive heart failure (CHF; see also Figure 10-41, *C*).

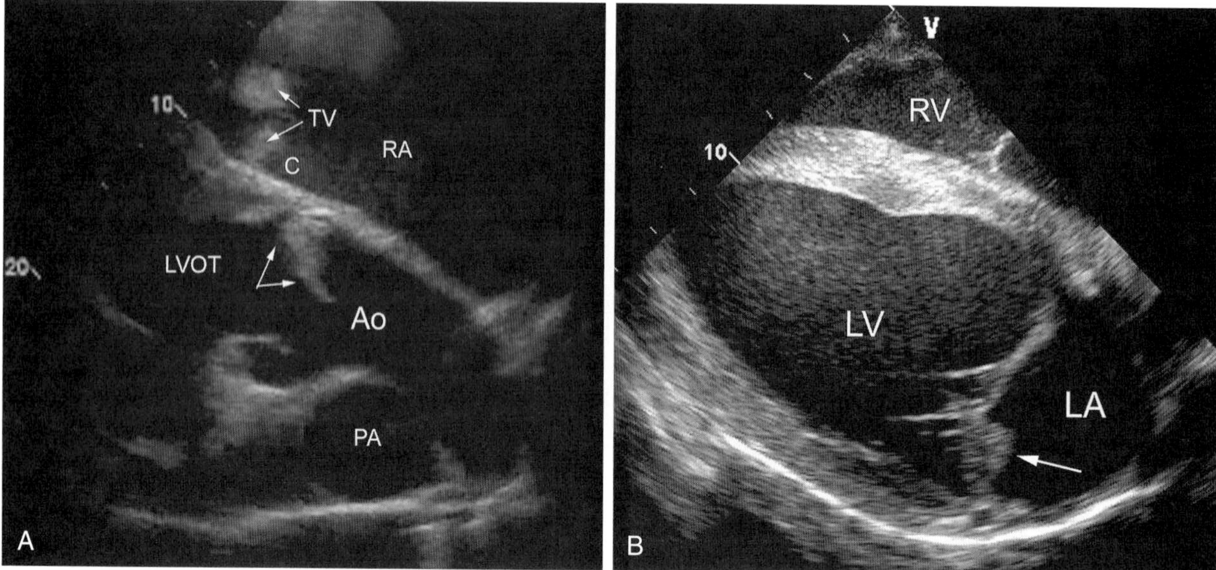

FIGURE 10-43 **A,** Right parasternal long axis two-dimensional (2D) image from a horse with infective endocarditis affecting multiple valves. Marked thickening of the tricuspid valve (*TV*) is evident, with spontaneous contrast (*C*) surrounding the valve. The right leaflet of the aortic valve is markedly thickened (*arrows*) between the left ventricular outflow tract (*LVOT*) and ascending aorta (*Ao*). Pulmonary artery (*PA*) and right atrium (*RA*) are seen in the far and near fields. **B,** Focal vegetation (*arrow*) is observed on a closed mitral valve in a long-axis image from the right thorax (*RV,* right ventricle; *LA,* left atrium; *LV,* left ventricle).

cultures or clear echocardiographic demonstration of a vegetation. In the absence of these, the relative likelihood of endocarditis is based on combinations of clinical findings and laboratory tests. Major and minor diagnostic criteria (Duke criteria) have been used for assessment of human patients,[645] and these principles are probably applicable to horses. Endocarditis should be considered in any horse that presents with a fever of unknown origin and one or more of the aforementioned clinical signs, particularly in association with synovial distension and lameness. Endocarditis becomes more likely when the cause of fever cannot be isolated to another body system and concurrent cardiac disease is identified. The diagnosis is confirmed with positive blood cultures in the setting of compatible clinical findings or by echocardiographic detection of vegetative lesions on the valve leaflets or endocardial surface (Figure 10-43).

Vegetative lesions usually appear echocardiographically as thickened, echogenic to hyperechoic masses with irregular or "shaggy" edges. The valve leaflet often demonstrates diffuse thickening as well. Discrete lesions are generally on the valve surface facing the normal path of blood flow. The typical endocarditis lesion adheres to the valvular endocardium (and therefore moves with the valve). When a fresh thrombus is attached to the vegetation, an oscillatory appearance may be evident with high frame rate, real-time imaging. Chronic lesions may contract, calcify, or develop a smooth contour. Rupture of the chordae tendineae or avulsion of a valve leaflet may also be detected echocardiographically, and this complication is not uncommon in mitral or tricuspid valve endocarditis. Pulsed-wave and color-flow Doppler echocardiography can be used to confirm that the valve is incompetent or (rarely) stenotic. Valvular regurgitation often progresses because of continued damage to the valve leaflets associated with ongoing bacterial infection or subsequent to fibrosis or calcification associated with a bacteriologic cure.

Early diagnosis and aggressive, prolonged treatment are important for successful treatment of infective endocarditis. Treatment should consist of high levels of bactericidal antibiotics, ideally based on culture and sensitivity patterns of blood culture isolates. Initial therapy should be broad spectrum, until the results of the blood culture are known or when a positive blood culture cannot be obtained. IV therapy is preferred in the initial stages of treatment. Drugs that penetrate fibrin well, particularly potassium penicillin (22,000 to 44,000 IU/kg, IV every 6 hours), are reasonable initial choices because bacteria may be sequestered in fibrin and may be unavailable to leukocytes. To extend the antimicrobial spectrum, penicillin is usually combined with gentamicin sulfate (6.6 mg/kg, IV every 24 hours) or amikacin sulfate (10 mg/kg, IV every 24 hours for adults; 25 mg/kg, IV every 24 hours for foals). Erythromycin estolate (25 mg/kg, PO every 6 to 12 hours) combined with rifampin (5 to 10 mg/kg, PO every 12 hours) may be useful in some cases. Nonsteroidal anti-inflammatory drugs (NSAIDs) (flunixin meglumine 1.1 mg/kg, IV every 12 hours) may be beneficial to reduce systemic and local inflammatory reactions. Aspirin (10 mg/kg, PO every 24 to 48 hours) and heparin (sodium heparin 40 IU/kg, SC every 8-12 hours; Fragmin 50 IU/kg, SC every 24 hours; or enoxaparin 40 IU/kg, SC every 24 hours) are used by some clinicians to prevent platelet adhesion, diminish growth of the vegetation, and reduce the risk of thrombotic complications, although the benefits of antithrombotic therapy are uncertain.

With effective antimicrobial therapy, the fever should resolve within 5 to 7 days. Response to treatment should be assessed by repeated examinations, including clinical assessment, laboratory analyses, and serial echocardiograms. Therapy should extend to at least 4 to 8 weeks or until body temperature, plasma fibrinogen concentration, and leukocyte counts have been normal for at least 2 weeks. The duration and type of long-term therapy depend on various factors, and the bacterial isolate, clinical response, cost, and potential toxicosis of the antimicrobial therapy must all be weighed in these decisions.

The expectation for long-term survival is poor in most cases of infective endocarditis causing severe valvular injury. Even in the absence of significant valvular regurgitation, difficulty may occur in achieving a bacteriologic cure, or valvular damage may progress as the vegetation heals and scars the valve. Although some horses have been treated successfully for endocarditis,[31,172,174] the prognosis for long-term use relative to athletic performance or breeding is low. The absence of an obvious echocardiographic lesion or signs of systemic inflammatory response creates a more favorable situation, provided that a bacteriologic cure can be obtained. Progressive cardiomegaly, CHF, rupture of the PA, development of AF, and sudden death have been reported in horses affected with endocarditis. Accordingly, periodic follow-up examination, including echocardiograms, should be performed in successfully treated cases.

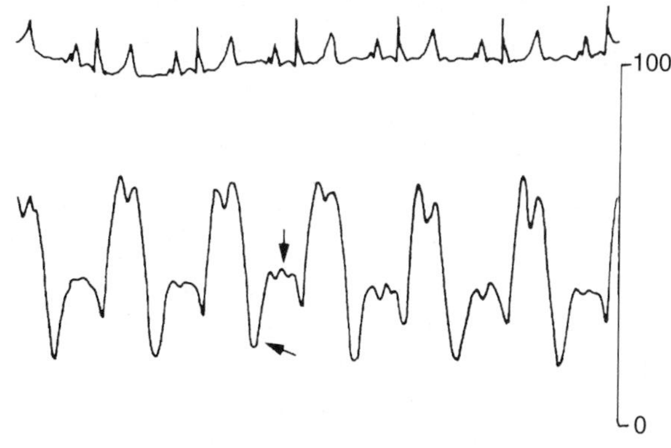

FIGURE 10-44 Pressure tracing demonstrating elevated right ventricular (RV) end diastolic pressure in a horse with constrictive pericarditis and heart failure. A quick rise occurs from the nadir of pressure (*lower arrow*) to a plateau (*upper arrow*), which is typical of constrictive disease and ventricular filling that is limited to early diastole.

PERICARDIAL DISEASE

Pericardial diseases occur uncommonly and are usually associated with pericardial effusion and fibrinous pericarditis.*

Pericarditis and pericardial effusion may be idiopathic, bacterial, viral, fungal, or traumatic in origin or associated with cardiac or pericardial neoplasia. Mesothelioma and lymphosarcoma are the most common neoplasms affecting the pericardium in horses. Pericardial hernias have also been seen but are rare. Not all cases of pericarditis are septic, but an infectious cause should be assumed until proven otherwise. *Streptococcus* spp. have most frequently been reported with pericarditis, but *Actinobacillus equi, Pseudomonas aeruginosa, Pasteurella* spp., *Corynebacterium* spp., *Mycoplasma* spp., and other microorganisms have been isolated.[87,94,96,652,654] Equine influenza and equine viral arteritis have been associated with fibrinous pericarditis (as well as abortion). Sterile inflammatory and eosinophilic effusates have been recognized, and an outbreak of pericarditis centered in Kentucky was attributed to a caterpillar vector[97] (see Figure 10-45, A). However, *Actinobacillus* spp. were the principal isolates obtained from necropsy and clinical cases.[95] External thoracic trauma or penetration by a gastric foreign body may lead to bacterial inoculation of the pericardial space.[646,649,650] The pathogenesis of noninfective pericarditis is unknown but might be immune mediated in some situations.[94]

The pathophysiology of pericardial disease in most cases is ascribed to impaired cardiac filling caused by either external compression (cardiac tamponade) or pericardial constriction. Typically, marked elevation is seen in the venous, atrial, and ventricular end diastolic pressures (Figure 10-44). Occasionally a mass lesion compresses the heart or obstructs venous drainage or ventricular outflow and mimics findings of pericardial disease. Other clinical signs may be referable to the underlying cause as with infection or neoplasia.

Reduced cardiac filling despite increases in ventricular filling pressures characterizes the clinical syndrome of pericardial effusion with tamponade. In acute cases, reduced ABP may be noted; chronically, BP is normal but signs of right-sided CHF are evident. The history usually includes systemic signs of illness, such as fever, lethargy, depression, anorexia, tachypnea, ventral edema, colic, and weight loss. A recent history of an upper or lower respiratory tract infection is not uncommon. Physical examination abnormalities include various combinations of tachycardia, fever, pericardial friction rub, muffled heart sounds, tachypnea, pleural effusion, jugular and generalized venous distention, ventral edema, thready pulses, and ascites. ABP may be decreased in cardiac tamponade and a pronounced inspiratory fall in BP (pulsus paradoxicus) may be identified by palpation of the pulse or through careful measurement of ABP. In chronic disease BP is normal, owing to fluid retention, elevated venous pressures, vasoconstriction, and tachycardia.

Laboratory studies are contributory to the diagnosis. Clinical laboratory abnormalities are not specific, but the most frequently detected abnormalities include anemia, hyperproteinemia, hyperfibrinogenemia, and a neutrophilic leukocytosis. Other hematologic abnormalities may be observed related to inflammation, CHF, or organ hypoperfusion. Thoracic radiographs usually reveal a globoid cardiac silhouette or pleural effusion and may reveal interstitial pulmonary infiltrates and enlarged pulmonary vessels. The ECG usually demonstrates decreased amplitude of the QRS complexes. If the effusion is large and the heart is swinging, then electrical alternans may be observed. Pericarditis may elevate the ST segment in multiple leads, but this change may occur simply as a result of tachycardia. Sinus tachycardia is typical, but ventricular or APCs may be detected.

The echocardiographic examination is diagnostic, demonstrating an anechoic or hypoechoic fluid space between the pericardium and epicardial surface of the heart (Figure 10-45, *B*), while excluding an extracardiac mass lesion, which can mimic pericardial disease.[100] Fibrin tags frequently are evident on the parietal and visceral pericardial surfaces. Findings of protracted diastolic collapse of the RV or systolic collapse of the RA are compatible with a clinical diagnosis of cardiac tamponade. Inflammatory processes may eventually lead to adhesions between the parietal and visceral pericardial layers, causing constrictive pericarditis with minimal or no obvious effusion. Associated pleural effusion is a

*References 4, 80-84, 86-95, 100, 125, 583, 584, 646-653.

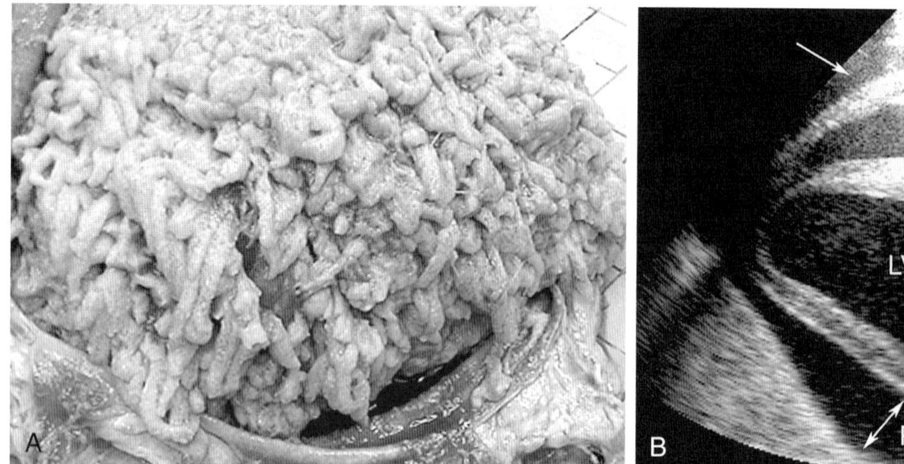

FIGURE 10-45 **A,** Considerably proliferative epicardial reaction in a horse with idiopathic, fibrinopurulent pericarditis. The heart is covered by a layer of organizing fibrin and inflammatory debris creating a shaggy appearance typical of inflammatory pericarditis. **B,** Two-dimensional (2D) long-axis echocardiogram from another horse demonstrating a moderate pericardial effusion. The effusion (*PE*) appears more prominent behind the left ventricle (*LV*) but is also evident (*arrow*) cranial to the right ventricle (RV) (*OT,* left ventricular outflow tract).

common ultrasound finding. Echocardiographic diagnosis of constrictive disease without effusion is more challenging, but typically reveals thickened pericardium, atrial dilatation, systemic venous dilation, exuberant movement of the ventricular septum, and exaggerated inspiratory filling of the heart as documented by pulsed-wave Doppler studies. In some cases right-sided heart catheterization is needed to establish the diagnosis. Typical findings are increased central venous pressure, elevated RV diastolic pressure, and possibly by a diastolic dip and plateau appearance to the RV waveform (see Figure 10-44).[86]

Cytologic evaluation of the pericardial effusion is essential to distinguish septic, aseptic, or neoplastic pericardial effusion. Fluid can be obtained in the course of needle pericardiocentesis or during the placement of an indwelling tube for pericardial lavage and drainage. Bacterial culture and sensitivity of the aspirated fluid should be performed so that antimicrobial therapy can be guided in cases of septic pericarditis.

The treatment of pericardial diseases varies, depending on the cause and clinical situation. Even when signs of right-sided CHF dominate the clinical picture, the use of furosemide is generally contraindicated, because aggressive diuresis results in lowered filling pressures, reduced ventricular filling, decreased CO, and possibly syncope. Instead, pericardiocentesis or catheter drainage should be considered as first-line therapeutic procedure in all cases of pericardial effusion with cardiac tamponade. Because the development of cardiac tamponade depends not only on the volume of pericardial fluid but also on the rate at which it accumulates, the clinician's urgency should be guided by BP, clinical signs, magnitude of pleural effusion, and echocardiographic evidence of cardiac tamponade. Tamponade is an indication for immediate drainage of the pericardial sac. Echocardiography can be used to localize a site for pericardiocentesis and choose an appropriate length of needle, catheter, or drainage tube. Pericardiocentesis should be performed after locally anesthetizing the intercostal muscles and pleura, and inserting an intravenous catheter to provide intravenous access should it be necessary. Electrocardiographic monitoring should be performed continuously during the procedure to monitor for cardiac puncture or in case ventricular arrhythmias develop. Pericardiocentesis is usually performed within the left fifth intercostal space, above the level of the lateral thoracic vein, although it can also be performed at the right hemithorax. Drainage is achieved using a large-bore catheter, teat cannula, or chest tube; the latter is recommended for repeated drainage and lavage of the pericardial sac and is most successful for aggressive management of septic or idiopathic fibrinous pericarditis. After insertion of an indwelling catheter, local therapy is administered that includes pericardial lavage and direct instillation of antimicrobials and possibly anticoagulants such as heparin. Combined with systemic antimicrobials, this therapy has been effective in the treatment of septic pericarditis.[583] Pericardial lavage should be continued for several days, until little accumulation of pericardial fluid (<1 L over 12 hours) is seen, clinical signs have improved, and the cytologic character of the fluid becomes less inflammatory. Initially, broad spectrum antibiotics should be used; the antibiotic regimen should then be adapted according to the results of bacterial cultures and antibiotic sensitivity patterns. NSAIDs are indicated to fight inflammation and to reduce the risk of constrictive pericarditis. If the cytologic analysis and culture are negative for bacteria, then anti-inflammatory doses of dexamethasone may be used for treatment of idiopathic, nonseptic, effusive pericarditis.[87,94] Exudative pericarditis may not respond in all cases to conservative treatment or even to drainage. Surgery is a rarely used option for treatment of pericardial disease but would be most appropriate for constrictive or constrictive-effusive pericarditis.[86] Presumably, introduction of minimally invasive thoracoscopic surgical techniques to management of pericardial diseases in horses might prove useful.

The prognosis for survival and maintenance of performance in horses affected by pericardial disease is guarded. The prognosis for cardiac or pericardial neoplasia is quite poor. Caution also must be expressed regarding inflammatory

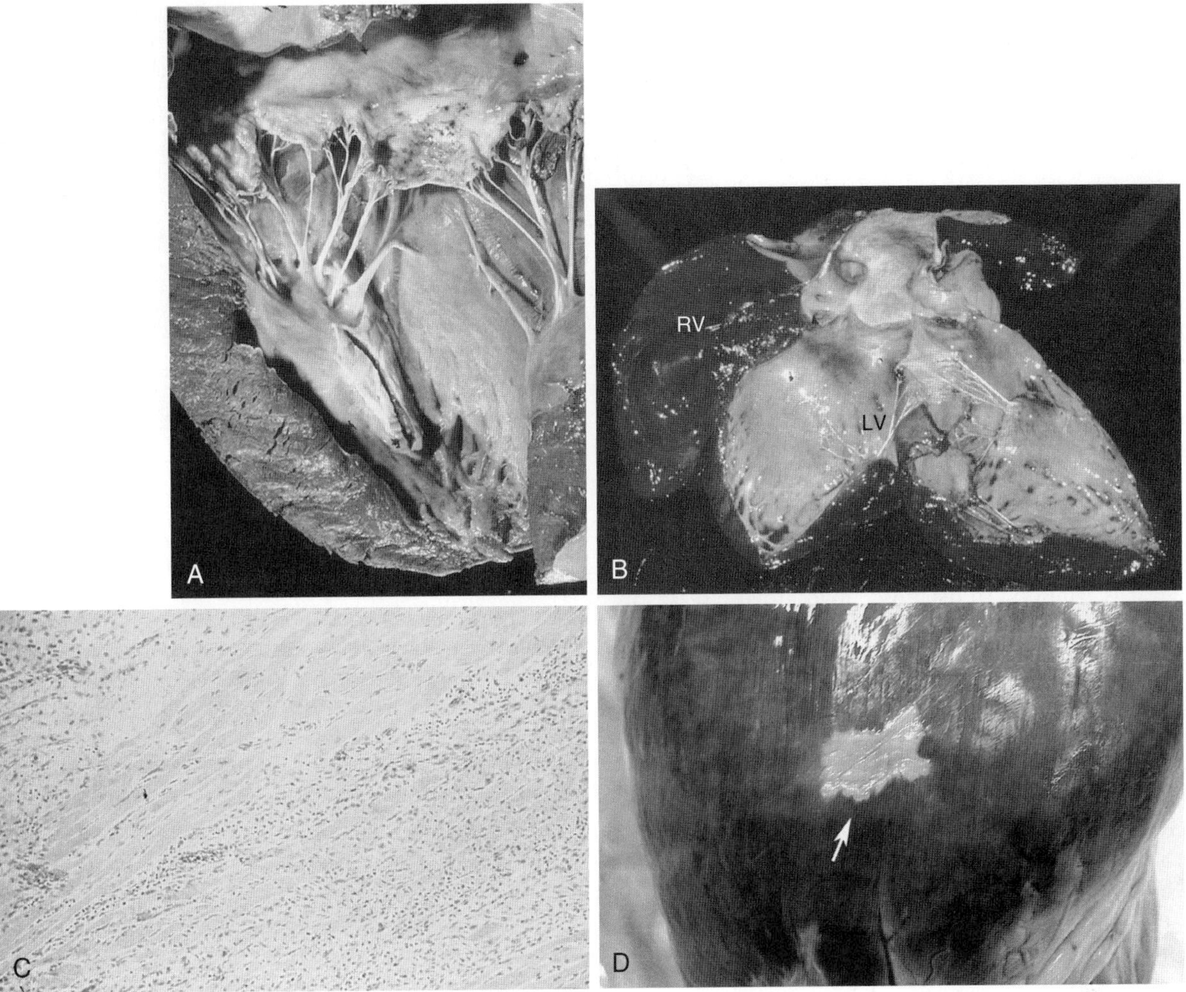

FIGURE 10-46 Myocardial diseases. **A,** An opened left ventricle (LV) revealing a (incised) large, oval area of subendocardial and myocardial fibrosis in a mare. No causative agent was found. **B,** Significant LV dilation and subendocardial fibrosis in a horse with idiopathic dilated cardiomyopathy. The white discoloration of the LV and left atrium (LA) may result from chronic distention or represent fibrosis after another injury. The opened right ventricle (RV) (to the left) is dilated but is not discolored. **C,** Myocardial lymphosarcoma. A substantial myocardial infiltration is evident in this photomicrograph. **D,** Close-up of the LV, subepicardial myocardial infarct (*arrow*) of undetermined cause.

pericarditis because the condition may become chronic, but very good results have been obtained in some reports.[94] The potential of eventual constrictive or fibrotic pericardial disease is also greatest with inflammatory pericardial conditions so that early success may be tempered by later complications of the disease.[87] The best prognosis of horses with fibrinous pericarditis is when treatment includes repeated drainage and lavage. Treated horses should be followed and re-evaluated by echocardiography.

MYOCARDIAL DISEASE

Myocardial diseases are probably under-recognized in clinical practice, and few published reports regarding these disorders are available.*

*References 4, 28, 29, 77, 98, 106-108, 110, 111, 114, 115, 121, 125, 432, 604, 655-664.

Certainly a potential exists for myocardial injury related to drugs, toxins (ionophore antibiotics, poisonous plants), ischemia, hypoxia, infective agents, parasite migration, heavy metals, trauma, relentless tachyarrhythmia, metabolic disease, or nutritional imbalance. Myocardial injury also can derive from extension of a preexisting infection (pericarditis, pericardial abscess, or endocarditis) or related to sepsis.[665] Infiltrative cardiomyopathies can occur consequent to neoplasia (melanoma, lipoma, lymphosarcoma, hemangiosarcoma, mesothelioma)[666] or the very rare amyloidosis[667] (Figure 10-46; see Box 10-2). Idiopathic, dilated cardiomyopathy also has been recognized in the horse. Tachyarrhythmias such as VT developing at a high rate (>160) can impair ventricular function and resolution of the rhythm disturbance may lead immediately to more normal LV function. A potentially reversible cardiomyopathy may accompany relentless ventricular or supraventricular tachycardia that has been present for days. Myocardial function in affected horses can only be assessed a number of days after conversion to sinus rhythm.

Clinical Features of Myocardial Diseases

The general manifestations of myocardial disease, regardless of the underlying injury, can be attributed to the following *pathophysiologic processes*: (1) reduced myocardial contractility and ventricular ejection fraction; (2) diastolic dysfunction with impaired ventricular filling; (3) mitral or tricuspid valve incompetency caused by cardiac dilatation or papillary muscle dysfunction; or (4) the development of arrhythmias. The overall cardiac disability engendered by myocardial disease varies greatly. Some horses have no detectable clinical signs; whereas, others demonstrate exercise intolerance, life-threatening arrhythmias, low-output CHF, or sudden death.

Persistent ventricular premature depolarizations or VT can be observed in horses with myocardial disease.[562] Atrial premature depolarizations, atrial tachycardia, or AF are more often primary electrical disturbances; although, these arrhythmias also can develop in horses with cardiomyopathies. Although it is tempting to diagnose "myocardial disease" in the setting of any cardiac rhythm disturbance, it should be appreciated that many rhythm abnormalities are "functional," without a gross anatomic substrate. This point is especially germane to horses suffering from electrolyte or other metabolic imbalances, high sympathetic tone, sepsis or toxemia, hypoxemia, or ischemia. In horses examined for sudden death at a racetrack, gross or microscopic myocardial lesions were relatively uncommon finding as compared with pulmonary hemorrhage.[69]

The onset of clinical signs may lag behind the initial myocardial insult, especially in cases of myocarditis or chronic myocardial injury. For example, a horse that has apparently recovered from an illness may develop problems once rigorous training is begun. The trainer may complain that the horse is unable to achieve faster speeds or may stop or suddenly slow during hard training. The affected horse may take a long time to "cool out" after a workout. In more severe cases, marked exercise intolerance, weakness, ataxia, or even collapse may occur. Respiratory distress, pulmonary edema, cyanotic mucous membranes, prolonged capillary refill time, and a rapid thready pulse may be detected after exercise. In case of severe myocardial injury, signs such as fever, persistent tachycardia, arrhythmia, murmur, pulmonary or ventral edema, or respiratory distress may be observed. Sudden death may occur without premonitory signs.

Results of the *clinical examination* in horses with myocardial disease are inconsistent. Resting physical examination findings can be normal, or signs of heart disease may be evident. These can include persistent tachycardia, tachypnea, frequent premature beats, sustained arrhythmias, systolic murmurs of AV valvular insufficiency, or CHF. A postexercise examination often detects an abnormally rapid heart rate, which remains persistently high after exercise is discontinued. The ECG may demonstrate atrial or ventricular arrhythmias, and an exercise ECG typically records an inappropriately high heart rate for the level of work undertaken. Resting echocardiography usually reveals a low normal or unambiguously reduced ventricular shortening fraction. Depending on the type of myocardial disease, the (relative) LV wall thickness can be increased (i.e., infiltrative cardiomyopathy) or decreased (i.e., dilated cardiomyopathy; see Figure 10-22). Postexercise echocardiography may demonstrate a paradoxic reduction

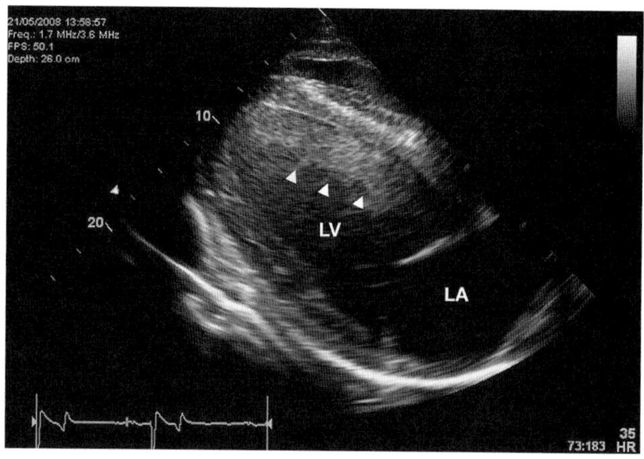

FIGURE 10-47 Spontaneous echo contrast (*SEC*), shown by arrowheads in the left ventricle (*LV*) of a 10-year-old Warmblood gelding with myocardial dysfunction. One can compare the LV density with the density within the left atrium (*LA*). A small amount of SEC is considered normal in horses, but marked increases in spontaneous contrast may be observed with very poor myocardial function. Bradycardia, low cardiac output (CO), rouleaux formation, systemic inflammation, and coagulation disorders are thought to contribute to this finding.

of LV shortening fraction or regional dysfunction characterized by LV wall motion abnormalities. Marked increases in LV or LA spontaneous contrast may be observed with very poor myocardial function, although this is not a specific finding (Figure 10-47). Abnormal areas of myocardial echogenicity have been observed; however, myocardial tissue characterization by echocardiography is not well established in horses, and gray scale also depends on technical factors.

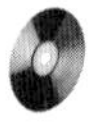

Clinical laboratory tests can be useful in the identification of myocardial damage but may not necessarily distinguish myocarditis from myocardial cell injury induced by a toxin or by ischemia. Elevated plasma or serum myocardial fractions of CK (i.e., creatine kinase *MB fraction* [CK-MB]) or of lactate dehydrogenase (LDH; both LDH_1 and LDH_2) suggest myocardial injury.[309] A more specific marker of myocardial is elevation of serum cTn_I or troponin T.[562,668-672] Although normal values or mild elevations do not exclude cardiomyopathy or myocardial infiltration, elevated values point to recent cardiac muscle damage.

Diagnosis of myocardial disease requires clinical suspicion and integration of findings from clinical and laboratory examinations. Because of the extreme variability of findings, the presumptive diagnosis of myocardial disease can be made only after reviewing the history, physical examination, echocardiogram, ECG, and clinical laboratory tests. Definitive diagnosis of myocarditis requires transvenous endomyocardial biopsy, but this test is largely impractical and may not identify piecemeal inflammation, degeneration, infiltration, or necrosis.

Treatment of horses affected by myocardial disease is primarily supportive. Prognosis depends on the cause and severity of myocardial injury and the hemodynamic consequences of myocardial disease. All horses should be rested, preferably in a stall, until myocardiasl function, ECG, and serum troponin return to normal or at least remain stable for several weeks. A minimum rest of 1 month (and usually more) should be instituted before a horse is returned to work. Supplementation with vitamin E and selenium may be beneficial, particularly in cases with suspected nutritional deficiencies. Antiarrhythmic therapy is administered when indicated for potentially life-threatening arrhythmias (see later in this chapter). Theoretically, an ACE inhibitor will reduce myocardial remodeling and unload the ventricle, assuming the drug can be sufficiently absorbed and biotransformed to an active state. When CHF has developed, digoxin and furosemide are prescribed as previously discussed in the section on CHF. Digitalization should be undertaken with caution in horses with ventricular extrasystoles because the arrhythmia may be aggravated, and it is not indicated in monensin toxicosis (see following discussion). If noninfective myocarditis is believed to be the cause of the arrhythmia or clinical signs, then corticosteroid therapy may be indicated, although its value is unsubstantiated. When the principal manifestation of myocardial disease is electrical (arrhythmias with otherwise normal myocardial function), the prognosis is fair to good for resolution of the arrhythmias. Horses with decreased myocardial function by echocardiography or those with CHF must be given a guarded prognosis for life and a poor prognosis for future performance. It is notable, however, that some horses with acute onset of CHF have recovered completely and returned to their prior performance levels. Such horses most likely suffered from acute myocarditis that resolved spontaneously or after anti-inflammatory therapy. Other horses may achieve a less spectacular recovery but still serve successfully as breeding animals

Myocarditis

Myocardial inflammation, or myocarditis, is difficult to diagnose. The diagnosis is often entertained in horses with cardiac arrhythmias or abnormal myocardial function, particularly when cardiac signs occur after another illness and are associated with elevated cardiac isoenzymes and serum troponin I concentrations. Often the prior disorder is a viral, influenza type of condition or an infection caused by *Streptococcus* spp. It is logical that immune-mediated myocarditis is operative in these cases, but definitive cause-and-effect proof is lacking. Myocarditis may also follow parasitic migration, pericarditis, or infective endocarditis. Hematogenous spread to the heart may be another mechanism for myocarditis. Severe necrotizing myocarditis can lead to arrhythmias or to signs of myocardial dysfunction as discussed earlier. The signs, prognosis, and treatment of myocarditis are similar to that described in the preceding section.

Toxic Injury of the Myocardium

A number of chemicals and plant toxins are potentially injurious to the myocardium. Ionophore antibiotics are among the most notorious causes of myocardial necrosis in horses.[114-120] Toxic myocardial injury also can occur after ingestion of white snakeroot *(Eupatorium)*, glycoside-containing Japanese yew plants (*Taxus* spp.), or cut oleander,[673,674] or also may occur from eating feed contaminated by *Epicauta* spp. (blister beetles), which contain the toxic element cantharidin.[658,660,675] Myocardial necrosis has also been observed after endotoxemia, particularly with clostridial infection, salmonellosis, and torsion of the large colon. Rattlesnake venom has been associated with cardiac injury and arrhythmias.[676]

Horses are uniquely sensitive to ionophore antibiotics, which are used as a coccidiostat in poultry production and as a growth promoter in cattle. Monensin toxicosis (>2 to 3 mg/kg) has occurred most frequently, but salinomycin (0.6 mg/kg or higher) and lasalocid (21.5 mg/kg or higher) also have caused myocardial injury and death in horses.[677] Ionophores react with polar cations to form lipid-soluble complexes, leading to cation transport across myocardial cell membranes. Various ionophores demonstrate particular affinities for different cations, although lasalocid may complex with a variety of ions. Exposure of horses to the ionophore antibiotics usually stems from accidental contamination of equine feedstuffs at the mill or through accidental delivery of poultry or cattle feed to horses. In most outbreaks, a recently acquired ration was fed.

Clinical signs of horses with ionophore toxicity vary with the specific type, quantity, and concentration of ionophore ingested and the preexisting health and body condition of the exposed horses. A wide range of clinical signs has been observed by one of the authors in exposed horses ranging from none to clinical signs involving almost all body systems. Weakness, lethargy, depression, anorexia, ataxia, colic, diarrhea, profuse sweating, and recumbency have been seen. The cardiac findings are similar to those previously described for myocardial diseases. If sudden death occurs, it is usually within 12 to 36 hours of ingestion of the contaminated feed. A single dose may lead to death from cardiac arrhythmias before the development of myocardial necrosis.

A recent report indicates that sublethal toxicosis may be well tolerated by some but not all horses, and echocardiography and exercise testing may help to identify horses affected more severely.[120] Polyuria and hematuria are other signs that have been reported in ponies after ionophore exposure.

A diagnosis of ionophore toxicity is based on the detection of the ionophore in the feed or stomach contents of exposed horses. Various clinicopathologic abnormalities are observed with monensin toxicity, including decreased serum calcium, potassium, magnesium, and phosphorus, as well as increases in serum urea, creatinine, unconjugated bilirubin, aspartate aminotransferase (AST), and muscle enzymes. Elevated concentrations of serum cardiac troponin cTn_I and isoenzyme patterns of CK and LDH have indicated cardiac, skeletal, and RBC damage. Elevated packed cell volume (PCV) and total solids have been associated with dehydration. Echocardiographic evaluation of affected horses has revealed marked decreases in shortening fraction with segmental wall motion abnormalities that range from mild to severe.

Prognostically, horses that exhibit decreased shortening fraction and dyskinesis shortly after exposure to monensin generally are unlikely to survive. Horses with mild decreases in shortening fraction survive and may be useful breeding animals, but most do not return to previous performance levels. Horses with normal echocardiograms typically survive and return to work at their previous levels. Postmortem findings range from no visible lesions to myocardial pallor and signs of CHF. Severe myocardial necrosis and fibrosis has been observed in horses with decreased shortening fraction or ventricular dyskinesis on echocardiography.

Treatment for affected horses is largely symptomatic (see previous discussion), unless very recent exposure is known. Vitamin E has been suggested to have a protective effect in other species and may be beneficial in affected horses. Digoxin and calcium channel blockers are contraindicated in acutely affected horses. If ingestion of the contaminated feedstuff is recent, then treatment with activated charcoal or mineral oil is indicated to reduce absorption of the ionophore. IV fluid and electrolyte replacement therapy may be indicated, as well as antiarrhythmic drugs, for any life-threatening arrhythmias. Stall rest in a quiet environment for up to 8 weeks after exposure is most important, because echocardiograms recorded after trivial exercise or excitement can reveal residual disease characterized by marked decreases in fractional shortening and myocardial dyskinesis.

Dilated Cardiomyopathy

Idiopathic dilated cardiomyopathy is a disorder of the myocardium characterized by global reduction of LV systolic function that cannot be explained by valvular, vascular, coronary, or congenital heart disease. The inciting cause of dilated cardiomyopathy is generally undetermined, although myocarditis or prior toxic injury is often suspected. Relentless junctional or VT also can lead to a dilated cardiomyopathic state that is reversible with control of the tachyarrhythmia. The clinical signs of cardiomyopathy are similar to those described earlier for myocardial diseases. Echocardiography is diagnostic, revealing cardiomegaly with biatrial and biventricular dilatation and depressed shortening fraction (see Figure 10-22, B). Symptomatic therapy with digoxin and diuretics may temporarily stabilize CHF and lead to transient improvement, but most horses deteriorate in the 3 to 12 months after diagnosis and are humanely destroyed. Neither the history nor the postmortem examination reveals the cause, and generally only diffuse or multifocal myocardial degeneration, necrosis, and fibrosis are observed.

A form of dilated cardiomyopathy also can be caused by vitamin E and selenium deficiency and is observed primarily in fast-growing foals from mares with a marginal or deficient selenium status raised in selenium-deficient areas. Affected foals are usually younger than 6 months of age and experience an acute onset of weakness, recumbency, respiratory distress, pulmonary edema, tachycardia, murmurs, and arrhythmias. The prognosis for foals affected with the myocardial manifestations of white muscle disease is poor, and most die within 24 to 48 hours after the onset of clinical signs. Laboratory abnormalities in affected foals include marked elevations of CK (including the MB fraction in foals with myocardial involvement), AST, and LDH, as well as hyperkalemia, hyponatremia, and hypochloremia. Myoglobinuria may occur. Echocardiography demonstrates the severity of myocardial involvement. Whole blood selenium, RBC glutathione peroxidase, and vitamin-E levels may be helpful in the diagnosis; however, tissue samples provide a more accurate indication of selenium stores. Treatment with vitamin E and selenium might be successful, but typically the myocardial necrosis is extensive and incompatible with life. Postmortem findings reveal pale streaking of the myocardium with intramuscular edema, myodegeneration, myocardial necrosis, and fibrosis or calcification. Prevention of white muscle disease is important in selenium-deficient areas. Supplementation of pregnant mares should occur during gestation based on individual blood and tissue selenium levels and should be continued during lactation, because more selenium is passed to the foal through the milk than across the placenta.

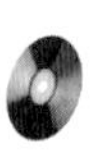

VASCULAR DISEASES

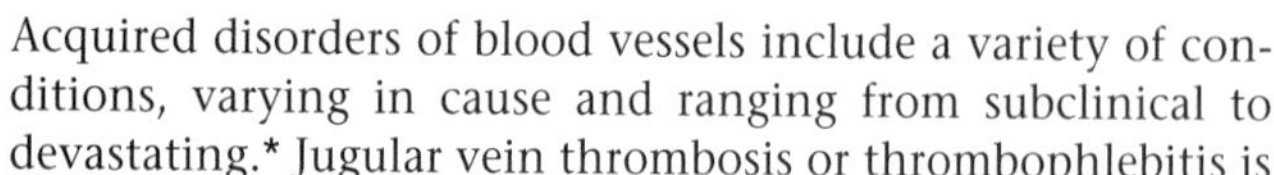

Acquired disorders of blood vessels include a variety of conditions, varying in cause and ranging from subclinical to devastating.* Jugular vein thrombosis or thrombophlebitis is probably the most common vascular problem encountered in clinical practice (Figure 10-48). Catheter embolization is observed periodically and has been amenable to surgical and percutaneous catheter retrieval.[699,700] Venous aneurysms,[680] vascular and lymphatic malformations, and angiomatous lesions are rare.[612] Rupture of the aorta or PA is usually a life-threatening event or leads to severe sequelae. Rupture of aortic sinus aneurysm into the ventricular septum or right heart chambers (Figures 10-49 and 10-50), aortic rupture into the pericardium, aortic aneurysms, and acquired aortic-pulmonary fistula have been reported.[34,58,219,221,698] Degenerative lesions (see Figure 10-50, *A*) including calcification may be observed in the aorta or PA.[701] Degenerative and calcific lesions affecting the bifurcation of the right and left pulmonary arteries also have been reported,[702,703] although the clinical importance of these is not well defined. Arteriosclerosis and arterial thrombosis may be caused by parasite migration in the mesenteric arteries[704] and possibly at the terminal aortic quadrifurcation (Figures 10-51 and 10-52). Aortic inflammation of unknown cause has been observed.[508,513] Rupture of the PA is a potential consequence of longstanding pulmonary hypertension and left heart failure. Arteriovenous communications occur rarely and may develop after vascular rupture or subsequent to growth of vascular tumors. Pulmonary vascular disease and associated hypertension may place a load on the RV, a condition called *cor pulmonale*. Although both acute and chronic airway obstruction can negatively affect right heart and overall cardiac function,[555,705] there is no compelling evidence to incriminate cor pulmonale as a common cause of clinically important heart disease in horses. Idiopathic pulmonary hypertension has been reported as a cause of AF in horses; however, left heart dysfunction was not completely excluded in the reported cases.[62] Tumors of the great arteries and veins are rare,[612] but neoplasms can compress or invade arteries and veins, including the PA and venae cavae. Mycotic disease within the guttural pouch is a well-recognized cause of arteritis and rupture of the affected arteries.

The echocardiographic observation of intravascular, spontaneous contrast within blood vessels and cardiac chambers has been suggested to indicate CV or rheologic disease,[490,706] as well as a normal phenomenon caused by rouleaux formation or platelet aggregates. This observation is common during ultrasound examinations and contrast may be observed in a variety of vessels, as well as in the heart (see Figure 10-47). Pronounced spontaneous echo contrast is especially likely when low flow rates exist as a result of bradycardia, arrhythmia, or myocardial failure, as well as when actual obstruction to blood flow in vessels is noted. Contrast is often prominent in valvular endocarditis. Lesions, thrombosis, or even venipuncture of the jugular vein can lead to spontaneous echo contrast in systemic veins and in blood flow entering the right side of the heart, often becoming more obvious if venous return suddenly increases. The identification of spontaneous contrast is also dependent on the operator with respect to transducer, gain, and gray-scale contrast settings. The clinical significance of isolated intravascular contrast cannot be stated with certainty; it has been observed in healthy horses, as well as those with CV disease.

Serious vascular disease often can be suspected from the clinical examination, although it may not be obvious until a catastrophic vessel rupture or fatal hemorrhage occurs. In general, significant *arterial* disease reduces perfusion to the

*References 4, 34, 52, 55-58, 62, 64, 66, 103, 106-108, 111, 125, 137, 152, 171, 207, 218, 219, 221-228, 316, 364, 368, 396-398, 476, 489, 501, 506, 549, 597, 600, 612, 678, 679, 698.

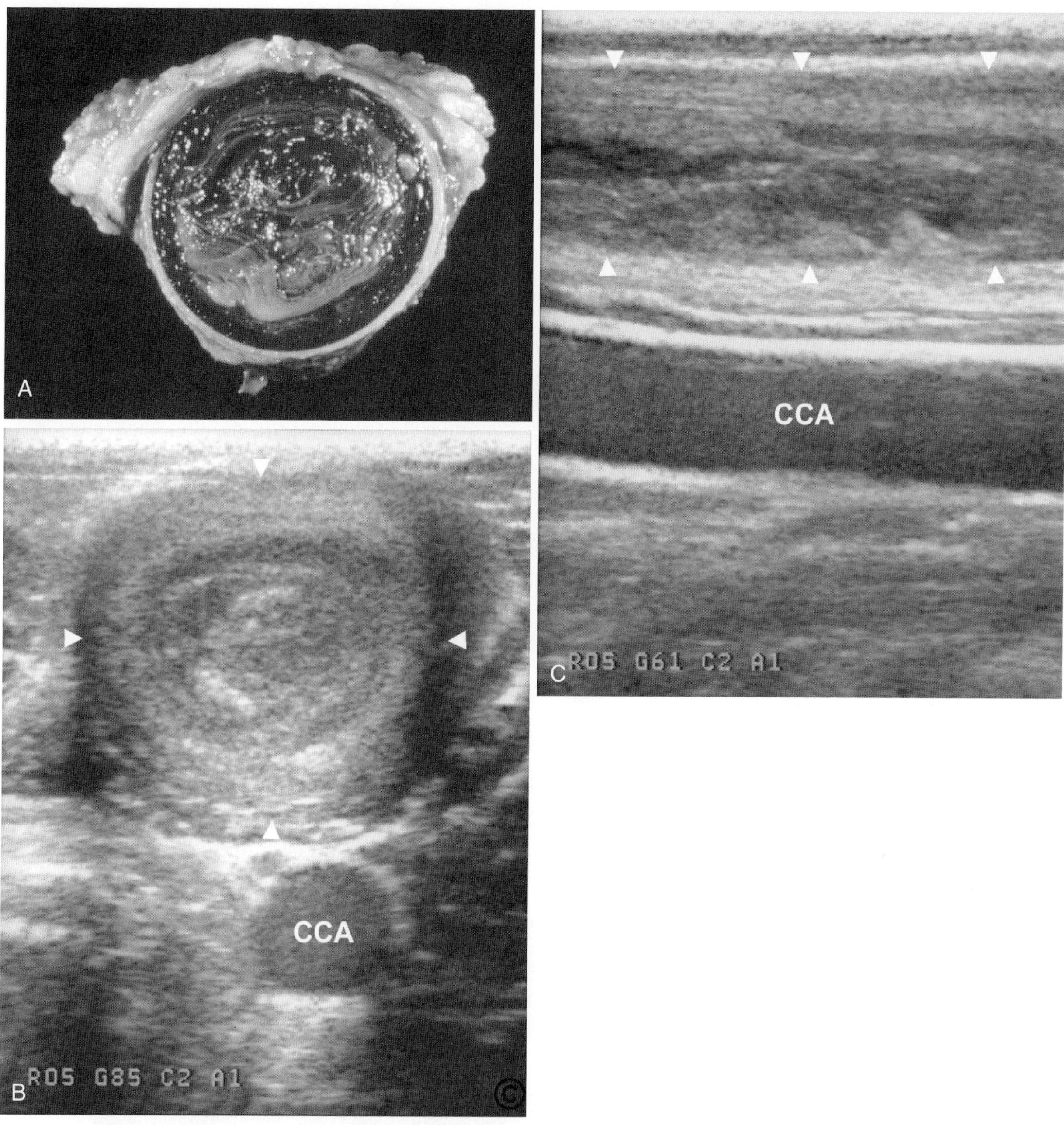

FIGURE 10-48 **A,** Postmortem specimen of a thrombosed jugular vein in cross-section. **B** and **C,** Ultrasonographic images obtained form a horse with jugular vein thrombosis in a cross-sectional **(B)** and a longitudinal **(C)** plane. The images show a mixed echogenic thrombus within the jugular vein (*arrowheads*). The common carotid artery (CCA) is displayed adjacent to the jugular vein. Residual blood flow through the affected area can be evaluated using duplex Doppler ultrasonography or newer vascular imaging technologies that directly visualize blood reflectors (e.g., red blood cells [RBCs]) in a gray-scale display (see DVD).

affected vascular bed, impairing tissue metabolism and function. If severe or complete, then ischemia may lead to tissue necrosis (infarction) and even perforation of a hollow organ. A bruit (auscultatory evidence of vascular narrowing or rupture) may be noted over the affected artery (or obvious hemorrhage if a superficial the vessel has ruptured). Ultrasound and Doppler examination can demonstrate serious arterial disease provided an acoustic window for examination is available. Rarely angiography or nuclear scintigraphy is required to demonstrate arterial thrombosis or disruption. In major *venous* disease, the typical sign is swelling of soft tissues drained by the affected vessel. Palpable evidence of local inflammation and thrombosis may be found in superficial venous disease. Right-sided endocarditis, embolic pneumonia, and pulmonary embolism are potential consequences of systemic venous disease.

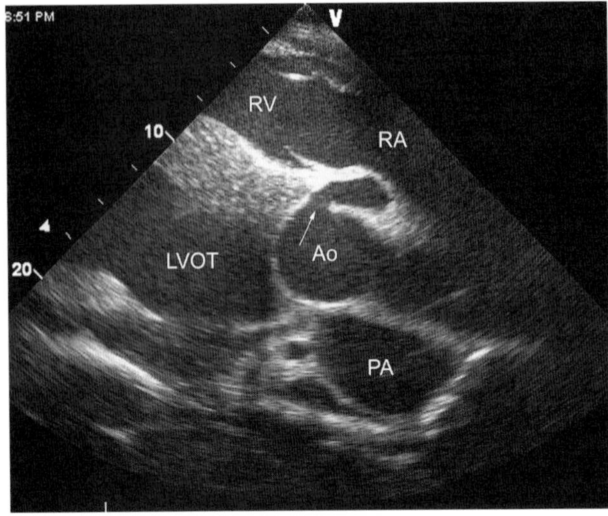

FIGURE 10-49 Aortic to cardiac fistula. Off-angle long-axis image of the proximal aorta (Ao) shows the origin *(arrow)* of a ruptured sinus of Valsalva aneurysm. This channel communicated with the right atrium (RA) in another plane. The right ventricle (RV) and pulmonary artery (PA) are slightly dilated because of left-to-right shunting.

Thrombophlebitis

Thrombophlebitis, the inflammation and thrombosis of a vein, is most commonly caused by IV catheterization or IV injection (see Figure 10-48).[398,689] The jugular veins are most often affected. Thrombosis can develop in the absence of preexisting vessel trauma subsequent to coagulation disorders. Clinical signs of phlebitis are straightforward, including swelling over the affected vein and pain on palpation of the involved tissues. Thrombotic occlusion results in distention of the veins and possibly subcutaneous edema adjacent to the affected area. Marked swelling, heat, and pain on palpation, combined with fever, hyperfibrinogenemia, or a neutrophilic leukocytosis, indicate infection of the thrombus.

The diagnosis and assessment of thrombophlebitis is based on the detection of the previously described clinical signs and examination by duplex Doppler ultrasonography (see Figures 10-48, *B* and *C*). Imaging of the affected vein reveals filling of the lumen with an anechoic, hypoechoic, hyperechoic (if gas filled), or mixed echogenic material that partially or completely occludes the vessel. Ultrasonographic evaluation may also reveal thickening of the vessel wall, perivascular swelling, tracts extending from the vein to the subcutaneous tissues or

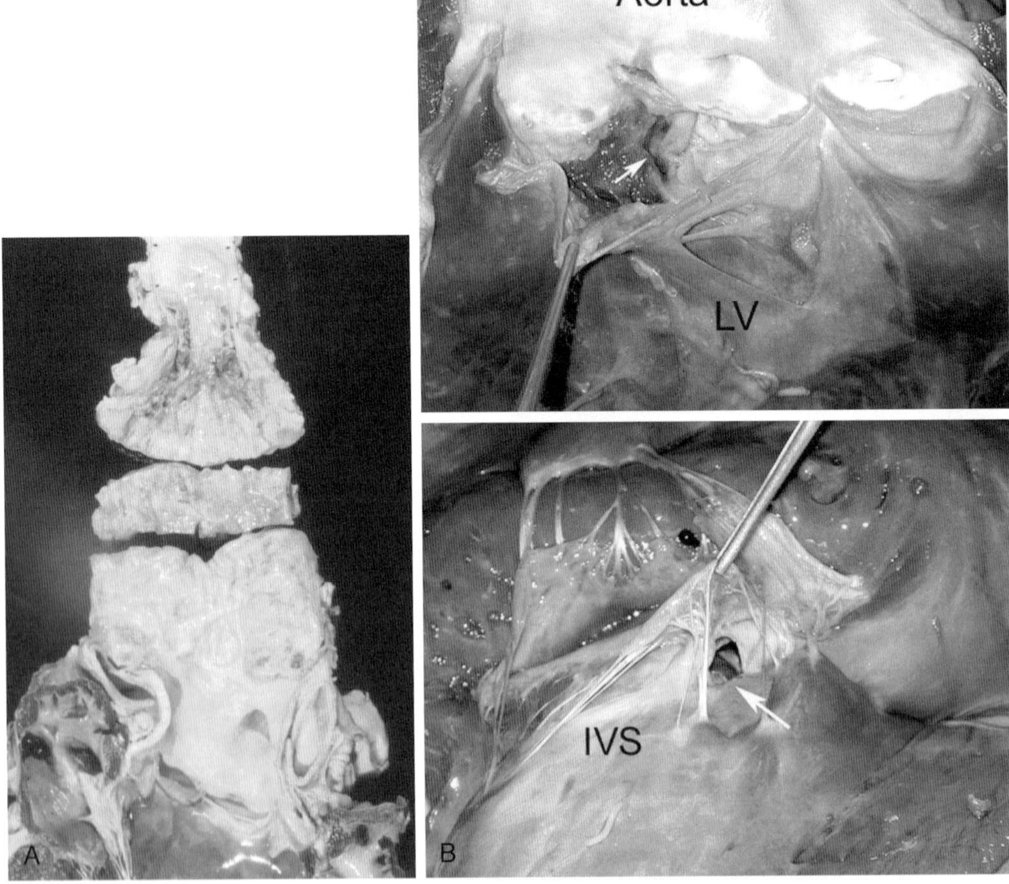

FIGURE 10-50 Aortic disease. **A,** Severe atheromatous change with secondary *Streptococcus* spp. infection of the proximal aorta. The intimal and subintimal change begins just distal to the coronary ostia. Representative sections of the ascending aorta are shown. *Strongylus vulgaris* was not found. The most distal segment was necrotic and severely narrowed flow across the region. **B,** Dissecting lesion communicating the root of the aorta *(top panel, arrow)* to the right side of the heart across the intraventricular septum (IVS). The distorted tricuspid valve is retracted to demonstrate the lesion on the right *(arrow).*

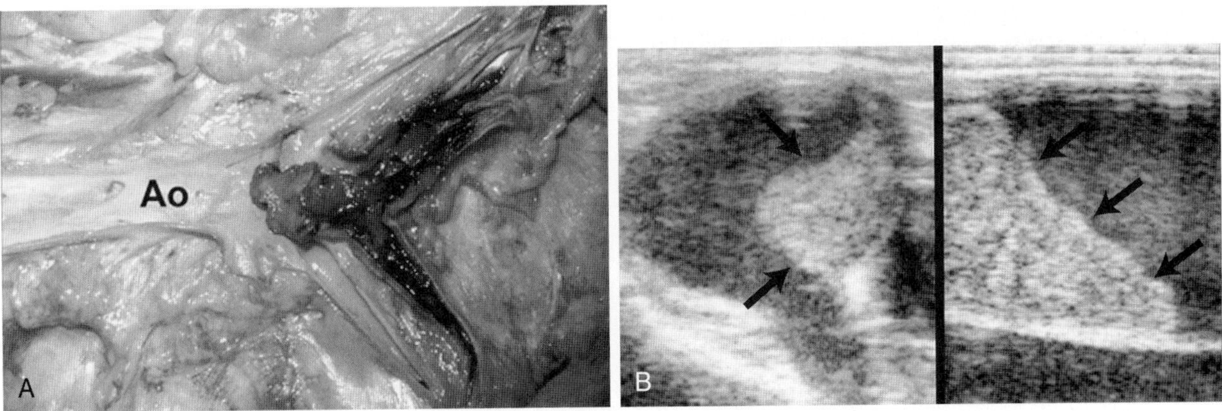

FIGURE 10-51 Aorto-iliac thrombosis. **A,** Postmortem image showing the thrombus in the terminal aorta (Ao) and the iliac arteries. **B,** Images obtained by rectal ultrasonographic examination in cross-sectional *(left)* and longitudinal *(right)* direction. The thrombus is evident as hyperechoic mass within the vessel *(arrows)*.

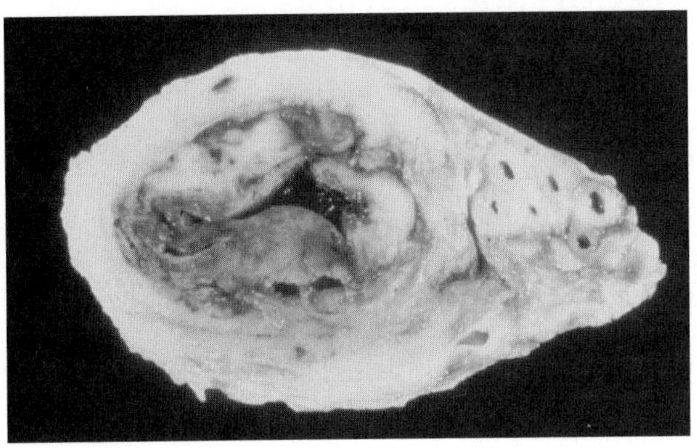

FIGURE 10-52 Verminous arteritis and thrombosis in the cranial mesenteric artery caused by *Strongylus vulgaris.*

skin, or subcutaneous abscesses. Cavitation in the center of a thrombus is suggestive of infection and represents a target for aspiration and bacterial culture. Stagnant or turbulent flow may be manifested by increased spontaneous venous contrast. Flow across the affected zone may be evaluated by contrast venography using agitated saline as a contrast agent, with pulsed-wave or color-coded Doppler studies, or with newer vascular imaging technologies that directly visualize blood reflectors (e.g., RBCs) in a gray-scale display. Venous drainage proximal and distal to the area of thrombosis also should be assessed, because collateral circulation may still enter the vein distally. A careful evaluation of the communicating large veins and of the heart should be performed in horses with infective thrombophlebitis. Bacterial endocarditis may develop secondary to embolization of infective thrombus or bacteremia.

Infections with multiple organisms should be anticipated in cases of infective thrombophlebitis, and high doses of broad spectrum antimicrobials should be administered until culture and sensitivity results of the aspirate are obtained. Metronidazole (15 mg/kg, PO every 6 hours, or 25 mg/kg, PO every 12 hours) should be considered if anaerobic infection is suspected. Flunixin meglumine (1 mg/kg every 12 hours) may be added to reduce inflammation. Local therapy including hot compresses and topical ichthammol (ammonium bituminosulfonate), NSAIDs (diclofenac sodium), heparinoids (chondroitin polysulfate), or dimethyl sulfoxide may be helpful in the treatment of thrombophlebitis. If antimicrobial therapy is unsuccessful, then surgical resection of the affected tissue may be indicated. Recanalization of an affected vein often occurs and can be documented by Doppler or contrast ultrasound studies demonstrating blood flow between the vessel wall and the thrombus. Occasionally, loculation may be detected within the ends of the thrombus. Such loculation may result in persistent fibrous webs within the vein that restrict venous return. Venous stricture also may occur because of longstanding thrombophlebitis. Complete fibrous occlusion of the jugular vein may impede venous return from the head such that if adequate collateral circulation does not develop, impaired venous drainage of the head and neck may limit performance. Vascular surgery may be required to regain venous drainage. Alternatively, an expert in interventional radiology or medicine can be consulted regarding other options, such as intravascular stenting.

Aortoiliac Thrombosis

Aortoiliac thrombosis is an uncommon, but potentially serious, disorder. The gross appearance, histologic features, and clinical findings of this vaso-occlusive disorder have been reviewed extensively, and the interested reader is directed to these and other related reports.*

The terminal aorta and the iliac arteries, including their proximal branches, are the focus of involvement in this disease. Vessels become partially to completely occluded by multifocal ingrowths of fibrous tissue, laminated thrombi, or fibrous plaques.[222] Histologic lesions include organized, fibrous connective tissue, hemosiderin-laden macrophages, irregular vascular channels, and disruption of the intima and internal elastic lamina. The lesions are generally devoid of fat. Arteriosclerotic and atherosclerotic aortic lesions have also been observed at other sites as well (see Figure 10-50, *A*). Suggested causes of these arterial disorders include *Strongylus vulgaris* infection, systemic infections, embolization, and vasculitis. No convincing evidence indicates that aortoiliac thrombosis is consistently caused by *Strongylus* spp. infection, and Azzie[224,226] has refuted this contention.

*References 56, 222-227, 396, 397, 683, 690, 707-713.

Although aortoiliac thrombosis is uncommon, it can be associated with severe performance problems, including reproductive failure.[690] The typical features include exercise-associated, typically unilateral, hindlimb lameness, ataxia, or collapse.[222,224,226,227] Aortoiliac thrombosis has also been diagnosed as a cause of breeding failure in stallions.[224,226,227] Physical examination of an affected horse at rest may reveal weak metatarsal arterial pulses or delayed saphenous refill in the affected limb. The temperature of the limb in the resting animal is usually normal, unless complete arterial occlusion has occurred, in which case the limb is cold and painful and may become edematous. Exercise in affected animals results in an exercise-associated gait abnormality (lameness, ataxia, or weakness), with a decreased or absent metatarsal and digital pulse and delayed or absent saphenous refill. Claudication may cause the horse to become very uncomfortable and reluctant to bear weight on the affected limb. Marked hyperpnea, other signs of distress, and profuse, generalized sweating are often present with trembling of the affected limb. A rectal examination may reveal fremitus, a weak or absent pulse, or aneurysmal dilatation of the affected artery or arteries. These abnormalities may be more evident after exercise and may help to confirm the diagnosis.

The diagnosis can be confirmed by ultrasonographic evaluation of the terminal aorta and iliac arteries (see Figure 10-51), using a high-frequency (5 or 10 MHz) rectal transducer,[223,225,397] or by nuclear techniques.[711,714] Doppler studies may indicate abnormal blood flow in the femoral arteries.[715] Essential abnormalities include a hypoechoic to echogenic mass protruding into the arterial lumen. An estimation of the degree of obstruction can be made based on the percentage of the artery occluded. Many cases are longstanding, and hyperechoic areas, even tissues sufficiently echo-dense to cast acoustic shadows, may be imaged within the aortic or iliac thrombus (these findings suggest mature scar tissue and calcification).

The prognosis for this disorder is guarded. No controlled studies have evaluated therapy for this condition. A case survey[709] suggests no treatment consistently improves outcome, but potential benefit of surgical or catheter-based thrombectomy or anticoagulation should be considered. Various medical treatments have been reported including IV sodium gluconate, larvicidal dewormings, phenylbutazone, low molecular weight dextran, anticoagulants,[713] and a controlled exercise program. Ultrasound-guided balloon thrombectomy[712] has been successful in some cases but is probably most useful in cases of active thrombosis in which the obstruction can be partially relieved. Early diagnosis is essential if therapy is to be beneficial. Treatment is aimed at improving collateral circulation and preventing additional thrombus formation.

Parasitic Infection

The migrating larval forms, particularly L_4, of *Strongylus vulgaris,* are known causes of arterial disease, particularly involving the aorta and the cranial mesenteric artery and its branches (see Figure 10-52). Lesions have been described as far forward as the bulbous aorta and the aortic sinuses in infected horses. Rounded fibrous plaques and mural thrombi have been reported in the thoracic and cranial abdominal aorta in 9.4% of horses examined immediately after death by Cranley and McCullagh.[106] These investigators reported a statistical association between the occurrence of proximal aortic *S. vulgaris* lesions and the presence of focal ischemic lesions in the myocardium. They hypothesized that these lesions were consequent to microembolism from parasitic lesions. With the advent of ivermectin and other new anthelmintics, as well as aggressive deworming programs currently recommended by practicing veterinarians, heavy *S. vulgaris* larval migration damage occurs much less frequently. However, migration of *S. vulgaris* L_4 larvae must be considered in horses with poor deworming histories, high potential of exposure, high fecal egg counts, and palpable abnormalities on rectal examination, as well as when fremitus or aneurysmal dilatation of the aorta is found, particularly in the region of the cranial mesenteric artery or iliac system. An ultrasonographic evaluation of the cranial mesenteric artery is possible and can be used to confirm the diagnosis of thrombosis in these vessels.[687,709] Treatment should consist of larvicidal deworming, combined with a rigorous individual and environmental parasite control program.

Arteriovenous Fistulas

Arteriovenous fistulas occur uncommonly and are most often detected with large vascular tumors (hemangiomas, hemangiosarcomas) or as a rare congenital defect or post-traumatic sequelae.[686,716] Classic features include a continuous thrill and murmur over the affected area, localized edema, slowing of the heart rate after occlusion of the shunt, and signs of increased CO if the shunt flow is great. Clinically important fistulas are more likely to develop where large arteries and veins run in parallel, as with the jugular vein and carotid artery. A diagnosis can be made with Doppler ultrasound, including pulsed-wave and color-flow Doppler to demonstrate continuous and pulsatile flow from the artery, through the associated communication, into the distended veins. A complete CV examination should be performed because a large arteriovenous communication could lead to cardiac failure. Treatment depends on the underlying cause, and an experienced surgeon should be consulted. No treatment may be indicated with small, uncomplicated arteriovenous communications. Large vascular neoplasms are usually inoperable at the time when they are diagnosed or complicated by the possibility of metastasis.

Arterial Rupture

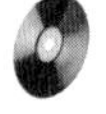

Rupture of the aorta or its branches or of the PA is reported sporadically. Rupture of the aortic root has been commonly reported in older breeding stallions but may also occur in older mares or in younger horses.[58] Rupture typically involves the right aortic sinus of Valsalva (see Figures 10-49 and 10-50, B). The aortic root can rupture into the RA, RV, intraventricular septum, or pericardial space.[58,152,220,221] Dystrophic changes in the media of the aorta have been reported, and the hypertension associated with breeding has been implicated as a cause of aortic root rupture. Aneurysms of the right sinus of Valsalva have also been reported and are related to congenital defects in the media of the aorta near the right aortic sinus. Rupture of the middle uterine artery can lead to fatal peripartum hemorrhage.[218] Ruptures of the extrapericardial aorta or other blood vessels leading to fatal hemorrhage or a systemic to pulmonary shunt have been reported.[52,57-60,62,64-68]

Rupture of an artery is often a catastrophic event, and most diagnoses are made at the necropsy floor. Antemortem diagnosis of an aortic sinus of Valsalva aneurysm is possible by echocardiography. Aside from breeding, horses with diagnosed aortic aneurysms or aortocardiac fistulas should not be used for athletic endeavor, because rupture of the aneurysm could occur at any time. When aortic root rupture or rupture of a sinus of Valsalva aneurysm communicates with the RA or RV, right-sided heart failure can occur. Rupture of the more distal aorta into the pulmonary artery also can occur.[34] These types of fistulas typically cause a continuous heart murmur. Cardiac arrhythmias (usually VT) may also develop, especially if dissection progresses into the intraventricular septum.[220] The prognosis for life in these horses is generally guarded, depending on the site and size of the communication. Some horses survive, and others may require supportive treatment for CHF.

Pulmonary artery rupture is most often caused by chronic pulmonary hypertension and PA dilatation. This is most commonly detected in conjunction with severe MR and pulmonary hypertension. The potential for PA rupture should be considered whenever a large dilated main PA or left and right PA is detected echocardiographically. Affected horses should be considered unsafe for riding or driving and should not be used, except for breeding, because of the possibility of sudden death. Focal medial calcification of the PA is not uncommon at necropsy[506,703] but is of uncertain clinical significance.

CARDIAC ARRHYTHMIAS

Cardiac arrhythmias are disturbances in heart rate, rhythm, or conduction and can be classified based on atrial and ventricular rate, anatomic origin of the impulse, method of impulse formation, and conduction sequence. A wide variety of cardiac arrhythmias have been recognized.[566,717] Of principal concern to the clinician are the hemodynamic consequences of arrhythmias (reduced pressure, flow, perfusion) and the potential for further electrical instability (myocardial fibrillation, sudden death).

The electrophysiologic basis of cardiac arrhythmias is not discussed in this section; however, other sections of the chapter provide information regarding abnormal automaticity, re-entry, and other mechanisms of arrhythmogenesis. Cardiac arrhythmias are classified based on the anatomic origin of the manifest ECG mechanism (Box 10-9). The reader should be aware that some arrhythmias, especially those originating in the AV junction, may mimic either atrial rhythm disturbances or "high" ventricular rhythms. For purposes of this discussion, the authors have elected to distinguish *atrial* from *junctional*; however, the term *supraventricular* may also be applied to these rhythm disturbances.

The clinical evaluation of the horse with an arrhythmia is reviewed in Box 10-10. Routine electrocardiography, clinical chemistry, hematology, echocardiography, exercising electrocardiography, postexercise electrocardiography, and continuous 24-hour electrocardiographic (Holter) monitoring can all play a role in the complete evaluation of a horse suspected of having intermittent cardiac arrhythmias. These points are discussed further following.

Sinus Rhythms

A number of physiologic sinus rhythms are recognized. These can be explained by the effects of autonomic nervous system traffic on the SA node (Figure 10-53). Normal horses at rest demonstrate vagal-mediated sinus bradycardia, sinus arrhythmia, sinus block, and sinus arrest; however, fear or a sudden stimulus may provoke sympathetically driven sinus tachycardia. Exercise leads to pronounced sinus tachycardia, with heart rates often exceeding 200 beats/min. AV conduction, as a general rule, tends to follow sinus activity. During sinus tachycardia, the P-R interval shortens, whereas during periods of progressive sinus node slowing, the P-R interval generally prolongs. Mobitz type I second-degree AV block (Wenckebach periodicity) often follows a progressive prolongation of the P-R interval. Sinus rate and AV conduction usually change in parallel; however, some horses appear to control BP during high sinus tachycardia by blocking impulses in the AV node. Second-degree AV block is more likely in a standing horse, in a horse that has suddenly stopped submaximal exercise, or after a brief surge of sinus tachycardia in an anxious animal.

Sinus rate and rhythm should be carefully monitored in the critically ill or anesthetized horse because heart rate is a major determinant of CO and ABP (see Figure 10-4, *B*). Sedative drugs and anesthetics can cause sinus bradycardia or sinus

BOX 10-9

CARDIAC RHYTHMS OF THE HORSE

Sinus Mechanisms*

Normal sinus rhythm
Sinus arrhythmia
Sinoatrial block or arrest
Sinus bradycardia
Sinus tachycardia

Atrial Rhythm Disturbances

Atrial escape complexes†
Atrial premature complexes
Atrial tachycardia: nonsustained and sustained
Atrial flutter
Atrial fibrillation
Reentrant supraventricular tachycardia

Junctional Rhythm Disturbances

Junctional escape complexes†
Junctional escape rhythm† (idionodal rhythm)
Junctional premature complexes
Junctional ("nodal") tachycardia
Re-entrant supraventricular tachycardia

Ventricular Rhythm Disturbances

Ventricular escape complexes†
Ventricular escape rhythm† (idioventricular rhythm)
Ventricular premature complexes
Accelerated ventricular rhythm (idioventricular tachycardia)
Ventricular tachycardia
Ventricular flutter
Ventricular fibrillation

Conduction Disturbances

Sinoatrial block*
Atrial standstill (hyperkalemia)
Atrioventricular blocks: first degree,* second degree,* third degree (complete)
Ventricular pre-excitation

*Generally physiologic.
†Escape complexes develop following another rhythm disturbance.

BOX 10-10

EVALUATION OF THE HORSE WITH A CARDIAC ARRHYTHMIA

- General medical history, past illnesses, past and current medications
- Work history and exercise tolerance
- General physical examination
- Physical examination: evidence of congestive heart failure
  - Subcutaneous edema
  - Jugular venous distention and pulsations
  - Pulmonary edema
  - Pleural and peritoneal effusion
  - Weight loss, poor condition
- Auscultation of the heart
  - Assessment of heart sounds (rhythm, third heart sound)
  - Assessment of heart murmurs
- Resting electrocardiogram
  - Heart rate and cardiac rhythm
  - Analysis of P-QRS-T waveforms
- Postexercise electrocardiogram
- Exercise (or treadmill) electrocardiogram
- Clinical laboratory studies
  - Complete blood count (rule out anemia, infection)
  - Blood culture (in cases of suspected endocarditis)
  - Serum electrolytes (particularly potassium and possibly magnesium)
  - Serum biochemical tests (especially renal function)
  - Skeletal muscle enzymes (cardiac isoenzymes)
  - Serum troponin concentration
  - Red blood cell potassium
  - Fractional excretion of potassium
- Echocardiogram/Doppler echocardiogram
  - Examine for cardiomegaly or reduced myocardial function
  - Identify predisposing cardiac lesions and abnormal flow
- Serum/plasma concentrations of cardioactive drugs
  - Serum digoxin concentration
  - Plasma quinidine concentration
- Response to medications

(Modified from Bonagura JD: Clinical evaluation and management of heart disease, *Equine Vet Educ* 2:31–37, 1990.)

arrest. Anesthetic drugs, hypoxia, traction on an abdominal viscus, ocular manipulation, hypothermia, increased intracranial pressure, and hypertension can depress sinus node function. Concurrent depression of the sinus node with stimulation of latent pacemakers in the coronary sinus or AV junction can lead to ectopic rhythms in the anesthetized horse. Conversely, an increasing sinus rate may indicate inadequate depth of anesthesia, pain, hypotension, hypovolemia, hypercarbia and hypoxemia, anemia, endotoxemia or sepsis, pyrexia, systemic inflammatory response syndrome (SIRS), anaphylaxis, or excessive catecholamine administration. Specific therapy for sinus tachycardia is rarely required because it represents a physiologic response to stress. However, when sinus tachycardia is identified, the cause must be sought and treated as appropriate.

Sinus bradycardia is generally a benign rhythm in standing horses; however, when encountered during sedation or anesthesia, this rhythm can lead to hypotension. Treatment of symptomatic sinus bradycardia can include the infusion of catecholamines (dobutamine, dopamine, epinephrine) or the administration of anticholinergic drugs (atropine, glycopyrrolate). Dopamine or dobutamine can be infused to increase heart rate, contractility, and ABP; however, reflex AV block may develop in some horses.[209,213,236,294] Excessive administration of catecholamines causes sinus tachycardia and ectopic beats. Anticholinergic drugs may not be effective in the setting of anesthetic-induced depression of SA function, particularly if vagal efferent traffic is low. Gastrointestinal complications including ileus and colic may develop after anticholinergic drug therapy; thus it should not be chosen for trivial rate problems.

Atrial Arrhythmias

Rhythms originating in the atria are common. These disturbances often develop as functional disorders with no overt structural cardiac lesion. Autonomic imbalance (including high sympathetic activity or high vagal tone), hypokalemia, drugs (catecholamines, anesthetics), infections, fever, anemia, hypoxia, and colic can be associated with APCs. Atrial rhythm disturbances are also very common in the setting of structural lesions of the heart valves, myocardium, and pericardium. Cardiac conditions known to predispose to atrial arrhythmias include mitral or tricuspid insufficiency, endocarditis, myocarditis, cardiac (atrial) enlargement, myocardial fibrosis, and myocardial ischemia. APCs can precipitate sustained atrial arrhythmias, including atrial tachycardia, atrial flutter, and AF. The large size of the equine atria and the frequent presence of microscopic atrial fibrotic lesions likely predispose the horse to these sustained arrhythmias. The high resting vagal tone present in most horses serves to shorten the duration of the action potential of atrial myocytes and also facilitates development of sustained atrial tachyarrhythmias, which probably depend on re-entry.

Atrial arrhythmias are the most common abnormal rhythms detected in horses (Figures 10-54 and 10-55).* APCs are the least complex of these rhythm disturbances; these can be clinically insignificant or associated with exercise intolerance or other signs of cardiac disease. In contrast, atrial tachycardia, atrial flutter, and AF are more likely to become clinically important. The overall importance of APCs is often difficult to ascertain. Routine ECG rhythm strips recorded from over 950 horses and interpreted by one of the authors indicated that atrial arrhythmias, overall, were present in less than 3% of the horses studied. However, when clinically normal horses were examined by Holter monitor, APCs were recorded in 28% of the horses. Thus it appears that the incidence of atrial arrhythmias depends not only on the population examined but also on the methods used for identification. These rhythm disturbances should be assessed in light of other clinical findings.

ATRIAL PREMATURE COMPLEXES

Atrial premature complexes are detected by auscultation and are documented by an ECG. Auscultation usually reveals a regular sinus rhythm that is interrupted by an obviously

*References 2, 33, 39, 42, 46, 55, 109, 134, 140, 174, 190, 191, 193, 195, 201, 293, 363, 469, 495, 546, 556, 568, 574, 576, 578, 718-731.

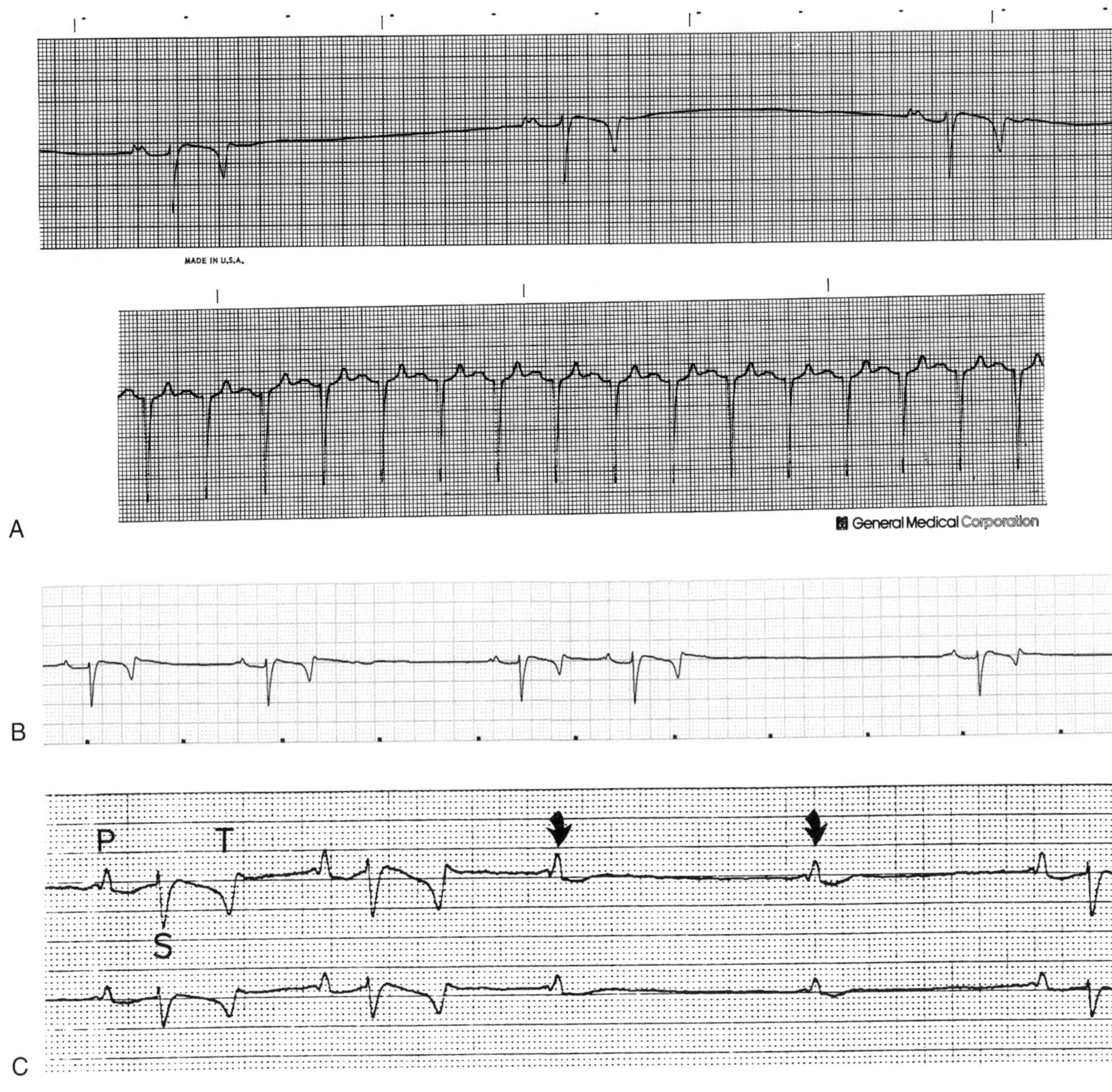

FIGURE 10-53 Sinus rhythms. **A,** Sinus bradycardia *(top)* and tachycardia *(bottom).* Base-apex lead recorded at 25 mm/sec. Whereas two consecutively blocked P-waves are considered normal on a 24-hour ECG, these phenomenon are observed infrequently (in approximately 1% of normal horses). **B,** Sinus arrhythmia with sinus arrest/sinus block recorded at 25 mm/sec paper speed. **C,** Sinus arrhythmia with second-degree atrioventricular block *(arrows).* An ambulatory electrocardiogram (ECG) is shown; transthoracic leads recorded at 25 mm/sec. Whereas two consecutively blocked P-waves are considered normal on a 24-hour ECG, these phenomena are observed infrequently (in approximately 1% of normal horses).

premature beat or—in case of a blocked APC—by an abnormal pause. Premature atrial contractions may be fully interpolated (continuation of the regular sinus rhythm after the premature atrial contraction is noted), or a pause may occur (if the sinus node is reset or the premature complex is nonconducted). The ECG is characterized by a premature (usually narrow) QRS complex, which is preceded by an abnormal, premature P wave (P′ [P prime wave]) that is often buried within the preceding T wave. If the impulse arrives in the AV node before complete repolarization, then the P-R interval is longer than normal (physiologic first-degree AV block). If the ectopic P′ wave is nonconducted (physiologic second-degree AV block), then a pause will be evident in the ventricular rhythm (see Figure 10-54). Premature atrial impulses can also be conducted aberrantly through the ventricle as a result of incomplete repolarization or persistent refractoriness of ventricular conducting tissues; this causes the QRS-T complex to be wider than normal or atypical in configuration. Care must be taken not to overdiagnose APCs. Sinus arrhythmia and sinus bradycardia often lead to variations in the P-P intervals, and often a "wandering atrial pacemaker" gradually alters the P wave morphology. Exercise or excitement will abolish such physiologic rhythms.

APCs, as a general rule, are more likely to be clinically significant in the following circumstances: When they (1) are frequent at rest, (2) associated with runs of atrial tachycardia, (3) related to poor performance (if other causes are excluded), (4) precipitate paroxysmal atrial flutter or fibrillation, or (5) develop in conjunction with structural cardiac disease.

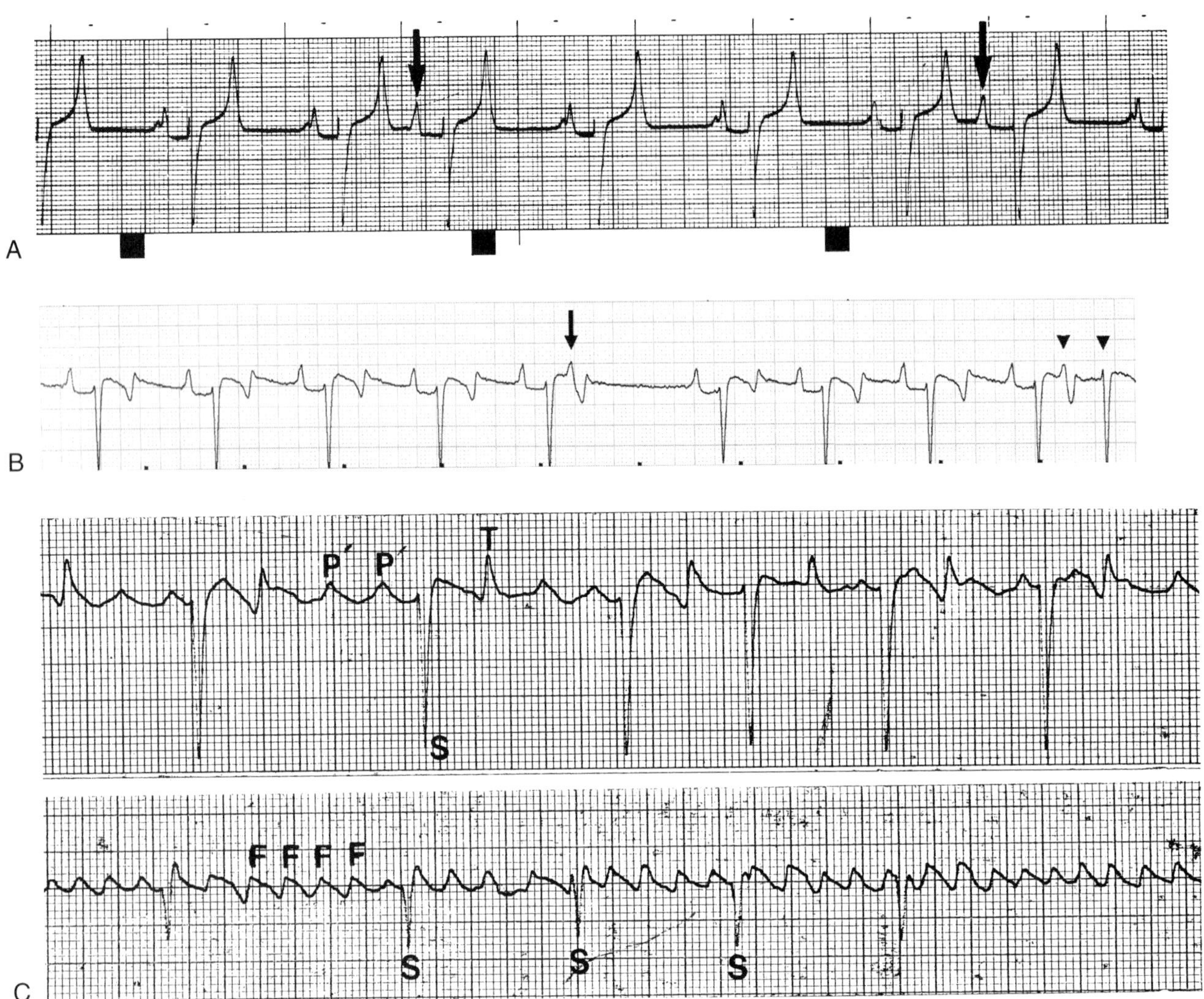

FIGURE 10-54 Electrocardiograms (ECGs) with atrial rhythm disturbances (recorded at 25mm/sec). **A,** Premature atrial complexes *(arrows)*. The premature P waves of different morphology, the slightly prolonged P-R interval indicating atrioventricular nodal refractoriness, and the normal-appearing QRS complex indicating a supraventricular origin are notable. A slight conduction aberrancy is evident in the second premature QRS complex (see also Figure 10-16). **B,** Premature atrial complexes occurring during the QT interval of the preceding complexes. The first premature complex is nonconducted (*arrow*), the second premature complex is conducted with first-degree AV block (*arrowheads*). **C,** Sustained atrial tachyarrhythmias. The top picture shows atrial tachycardia with rapid, regular P waves (*P′*) and a variable ventricular rate response to conducted P waves. The base-apex lead recorded at 25 mm/sec. The lower trace shows atrial flutter (*F*) with variable ventricular response (*S*). Lead 3 recorded at 25 mm/sec.

Documentation of atrial arrhythmias *during* exercise may be critical for determining if paroxysmal atrial tachycardia or fibrillation is likely to be the cause of poor performance.[428] Clinical judgment must be used; however, because supraventricular premature complexes are most likely to occur in the immediate postexercise period, probably associated with autonomic imbalance. If these postexercise arrhythmias are not associated with clinical signs and are not detected during exercise, then they are unlikely to be clinically significant. Cardiac rhythm monitoring during exercise may be necessary to be certain.

Isolated APCs generally are not treated. The hemodynamic consequences of these rhythm disturbances are minor, unless sustained abnormal activity develops. Consideration of antiarrhythmic therapy might be appropriate if frequent atrial extrasystoles are documented to precipitate AF. Unfortunately, neither quinidine nor procainamide are practical for chronic use, and the effectiveness of other antiarrhythmics including digoxin has not been established for this indication. Maintenance of normal serum potassium and magnesium may be important in suppressing atrial ectopic activity. In cases of suspected myocarditis, anti-inflammatory doses of dexamethasone might be considered as empiric therapy with consideration of adverse effects of such treatment.

ATRIAL TACHYCARDIA

Atrial tachycardia can be defined as a series of ectopic APCs. Atrial tachycardia may be sustained or nonsustained (paroxysmal) and is generally precipitated by a single APC. The atrial rate is rapid and regular; however, because ectopic P′ waves can be blocked physiologically in the AV node, an irregular ventricular rate response often results (see Figure 10-54, C). Atrial rates of 120 to 300 beats/min are typical in horses with sustained atrial tachycardia. At lower atrial rates, 2:1 AV conduction may yield a regular, relentless heart rate. At the higher atrial rates, the rhythm may be indistinguishable from atrial flutter. Differentiation of atrial tachycardia from flutter may not be critical because both arrhythmias seem to carry the same clinical significance and are treated in the same general way. Sustained atrial tachycardia is most often recognized during treatment of horses with quinidine sulfate. Before conversion of AF to sinus rhythm, atrial tachycardia may be observed (see Figure 10-55, A); thus in this setting, rhythm indicates a partial therapeutic effect of quinidine on the atrial myocardium. When this atrial tachycardia occurs as an isolated finding, structural or underlying myocardial disease should be suspected and the horse should be considered predisposed to the development or recurrence of AF. Treatment is the same as that described for AF. If the ventricular response rate is especially rapid (>120 beats/min), then consideration can be given to administration of either digoxin to block AV nodal conduction or possibly to diltiazem if digoxin is ineffective (see Table 10-6). ABP should be monitored carefully if diltiazem is administered.[243,732,733]

ATRIAL FLUTTER

Isolated atrial flutter is probably less common than atrial tachycardia and represents a form of atrial circuit movement or macroreentry. The clinical circumstances and assessment of this rhythm disturbance are identical to those of atrial tachycardia. The ECG in atrial flutter is characterized by a very rapid, abnormal, but regular atrial activity that is usually manifested as a "saw-toothed" ECG baseline. The atrial frequency often exceeds 300 beats/min. The RR intervals are usually irregular because of variable AV conduction, and fewer QRS and T complexes than flutter waves exist (see Figure 10-54, C). The ventricular rate depends on the refractory period of the AV node and on the strength of the atrial stimulus. Atrial flutter often alternates with AF in horses, creating so-called flutter-fibrillation. Treatment is similar to that for AF.

Atrial Fibrillation

Atrial fibrillation is the most common atrial arrhythmia associated with poor performance and exercise intolerance.* AF is most common in adult horses and has been reported infrequently in foals, weanlings, yearlings, or ponies. Several reports indicate a higher incidence in Standardbreds, draft horses, and Warmblood horses compared with the general hospital population.

CO at rest is normal in most horses with AF[546]; however, maximal CO during exercise is limited because the atrial contribution to filling is most important at higher heart rates. As expected, exercise intolerance is most common in high-performance horses (e.g., racehorses, advanced combined training horses, polo ponies, and some Grand Prix jumpers) and less common in show hunters and in pleasure, dressage, and endurance horses. The high LA pressures present in heavily exercising horses[240,553] is further exacerbated by the loss of active atrial transport function[313] and may contribute to exercise intolerance or other associated signs. Exercise-induced pulmonary hemorrhage, respiratory distress, CHF, ataxia or collapse, and myopathy have all been reported with AF; conversely, the arrhythmia is often detected as an incidental finding in horses with no overt signs.[363]

AF can be acute or chronic, and it can be paroxysmal, persistent, or permanent. Paroxysmal AF is often associated with a single episode of poor performance, with the horse often decelerating suddenly during a race. The arrhythmia usually disappears spontaneously within 24 to 48 hours. Paroxysmal AF may be associated with transient potassium depletion, particularly in horses treated with furosemide or bicarbonate solutions, and it is most often unrelated to other clinical or echocardiographic abnormalities of cardiac disease (lone AF). Although less common than paroxysmal AF, both persistent and permanent AF are easier to diagnose (persistent AF terminates after treatment, whereas permanent AF is sustained and resistant to therapy). Many horses with sustained AF have no other evidence of significant underlying cardiac disease when examined by physical examination and echocardiography. However, ultrastructural and functional myocardial pathology may be present, predisposing to AF. Furthermore, AF can induce atrial electrical, structural, and functional remodeling that may be responsible for the self-perpetuating, progressive, and recurrent nature of AF.[242,244,740] These remodeling changes are more likely to be reversible if AF is treated promptly. Recurrent episodes of AF are not uncommon and are more likely in the presence of concurrent structural or functional cardiac disease.

Horses with AF generally have a normal resting heart rate, although the rate decreases (and stroke volume tends to increase) after successful conversion of AF to normal sinus rhythm.[741] The presence of resting tachycardia in a horse with AF should give the clinician pause to consider intercurrent cardiac lesions or a disorder that increases sympathetic tone such as pain, anemia, fever, or infection. A number of factors interact in the prognosis of a horse with AF. Of these, the presence of CHF represents the overall worst prognostic indicator and is invariably associated with resting tachycardia. Severe structural heart disease, recurrent bouts of AF, long-standing AF, and failure to convert with therapeutic serum concentrations of quinidine represent negative prognostic factors inasmuch as affected horses can be more difficult to convert to sinus rhythm or more likely to revert back to AF even when therapy is successful.

The diagnosis of AF is initiated by recognition of an irregularly irregular heart rhythm, variable intensity heart sounds, and an absent fourth heart sound during cardiac auscultation. Arterial pulses vary in intensity, and pulse deficits may be present, especially when the ventricular rate is high (see Figure 10-55, *D*). The ECG is characterized by an absence of P waves; instead, fibrillation or *f* waves are seen in the baseline. These *f* waves may be coarse (large) or fine (small), and the number of atrial impulses per minute cannot be easily counted but usually exceeds 500 per minute. The QRS-T complexes are normal in morphology and duration, but ventricular rate response is quite irregular, although periodicity may be observed infrequently.[191] As for all atrial tachyarrhythmias, the ultimate ventricular rate response (and examination heart rate) depends on the refractory period of the AV node and the frequency and strength of the atrial stimuli. In the otherwise healthy horse in AF, vagal tone will be high and sympathetic tone

*References 2, 33, 39, 42, 46, 55, 109, 134, 140, 146, 174, 190, 191, 193, 201, 293, 361-363, 427, 428, 469, 495, 546, 556, 568, 574, 576, 578, 580, 718, 719, 721-731, 734-739.

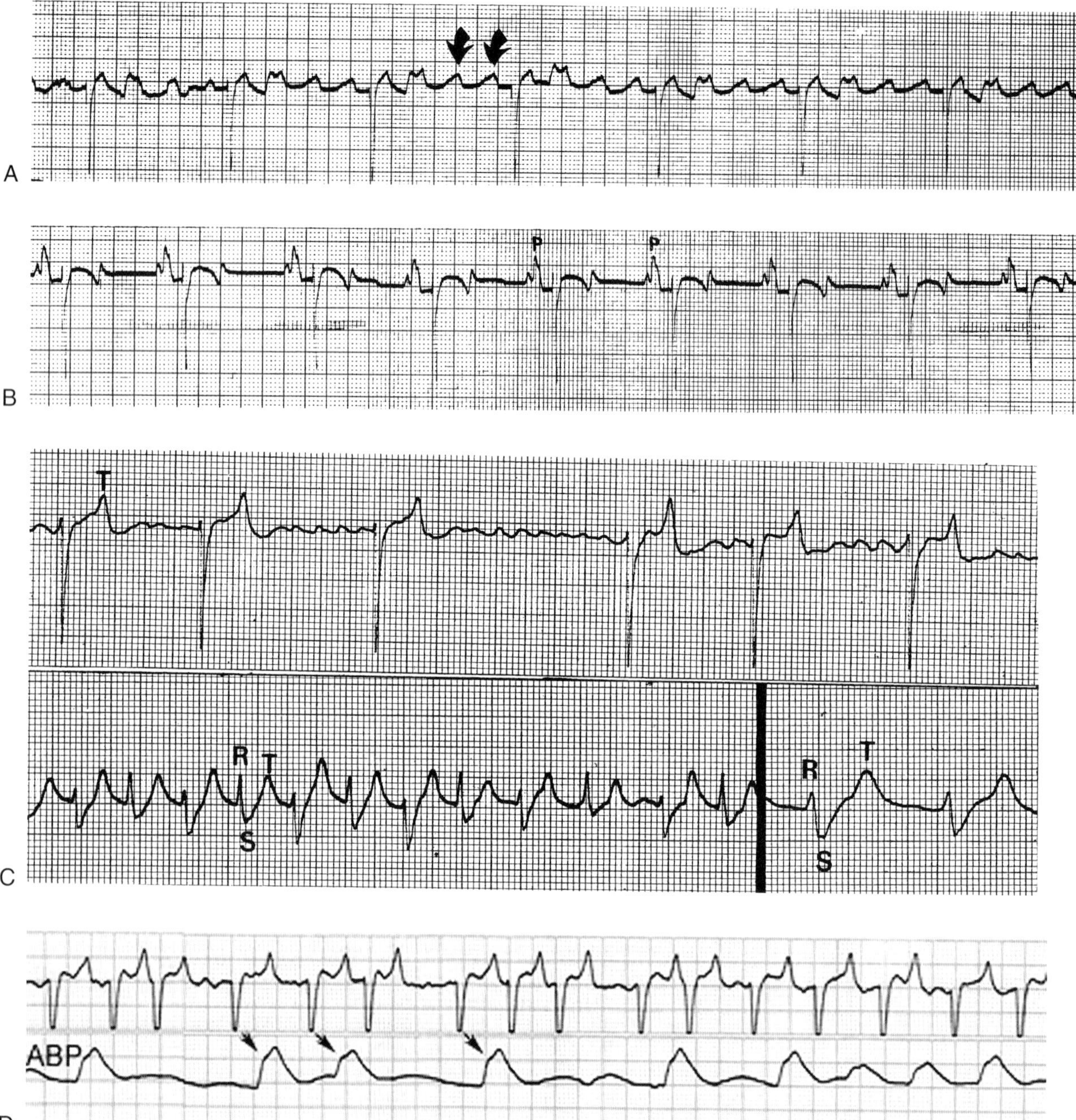

FIGURE 10-55 Atrial arrhythmias. **A** and **B,** Successful conversion of atrial fibrillation (AF) using a combination of digoxin and quinidine (see text for details). **A,** Incomplete conversion of AF to atrial tachycardia with rapid, regular atrial activity (*arrows*). **B,** Conversion to normal sinus rhythm during combination therapy. Notice the high amplitude of the second part of the P wave, indicating possible atrial enlargement. **C,** Quinidine toxicosis can be manifested as abnormalities on the electrocardiogram (ECG). In this horse, AF (*top;* base-apex lead recorded at 25 mm/sec) was not converted. The lower recording shows persistent AF with a rapid atrioventricular conduction response, electrical alternans, and widening of the QRS complex (lead 2 recorded at 25 mm/sec; *right panel,* at 50 mm/sec). The rapid rate response is related to the vagolytic effect of quinidine. The electrical alternans is common with regular supraventricular tachycardias with rapid ventricular response rates; this finding indicates varying conduction into the ventricle. The widened QRS is a sign of quinidine toxicosis. An idiosyncratic reaction leading to polymorphous ventricular tachycardia (VT) also has been recognized (see Figure 10-59). **D,** Hemodynamic consequences of increasing ventricular response rate in AF. The short QRS-QRS intervals do not generate effective arterial pulsations recorded in the arterial blood pressure (*ABP*) tracing, which is related to inadequate ventricular filling time during short cycles. Pulse deficits are detectable by physical examination.

low when standing; consequently, the ventricular rate will be close to normal or slightly increased. If sympathetic activity is increased for any reason, or if vagal activity is blocked (as occurs with quinidine sulfate therapy), then the ventricular rate response will increase as the AV nodal refractory period shortens. This explains the clinician's simple, but very useful, dependence on measuring pretreatment, resting heart rate in horses with AF.[363,574] Because the horse with structural heart disease will be more likely to require sympathetic support to maintain CO and ABP, persistent resting tachycardia, higher than 60 to 70 beats/min, indicates underlying cardiac disease and is associated with a poorer prognosis.

Laboratory studies in horses with AF are usually normal. Infrequently, a horse is found to have low serum potassium, fractional excretion of potassium, or RBC potassium. Chest radiographs are usually normal unless there is concurrent pulmonary disease. Thoracic radiography is not a high-yield procedure in horses without signs of lung disease or structural heart disease. The echocardiogram is usually normal, unless concurrent valvular or ventricular myocardial disease is noted. It is not uncommon for an otherwise normal horse to demonstrate a slightly reduced LV shortening fraction (usually in the 24% to 32% range), which returns to normal once the horse has been converted to sinus rhythm.[495,731] This decrease in fractional shortening is probably multifactorial in origin, probably related in part to decreased preload from loss of the atrial contribution to ventricular filling and irregular cardiac cycle. Doppler studies are useful in evaluating horses with concurrent valvular disease.

The most common treatment for AF involves conversion to normal sinus rhythm, unless concurrent CHF is noted or the horse is aged and therapy is deemed of little benefit. Conversion of AF to sinus rhythm can be accomplished using a number of drugs or through electrocardioversion, generally delivered by intracardiac catheters.[628,742-748] No prospective study has compared the two methods, and both quinidine and electrocardioversion are generally safe and effective treatments. Quinidine sulfate is the standard drug against which other drug treatments should be compared, although this agent is becoming more difficult to obtain in some countries. Quinidine cardioversion of AF is successful in many horses, and a number of different treatment plans can be followed (see Table 10-6).[319,717,739] The use of other drugs including flecainide,[738,749-753] propafenone,[754] and amiodarone[755-758] may be considered in unresponsive cases or when quinidine cannot be tolerated or obtained (see following). As a general principle, when AF occurs in the setting of CHF, the treatments should be aimed at controlling CHF and resting heart rate with furosemide, digoxin, and possibly an ACE inhibitor, as opposed to conversion back to sinus rhythm.

Based on the work of Reef, Levitan, and Spencer,[574] an excellent prognosis for quinidine conversion (>95% conversion rate) may be given for horses with heart rates of less than or equal to 60 beats/min, murmurs less than or equal to grade 3/6, and AF lasting less than 4 months. Recurrences affect approximately 25% of these horses. Quinidine conversion to sinus rhythm represents the standard therapy for most equine practices and has been used for the longest period of time. In general the use of other drugs (e.g., flecainide, amiodarone) is considered mainly for cases of resistant or recurrent AF or in situations in which quinidine or electrocardioversion are unavailable. In a study of electrocardioversion, the results were also very positive with a greater than 98% conversion rate (71 of 72 episodes in 63 horses).[747] Horses with longer duration of AF or significant structural cardiac disease may be more difficult to convert to sinus rhythm using quinidine or electrocardioversion, and they are more likely to have a higher recurrence rate independent of the treatment modality.

QUINIDINE THERAPY OF ATRIAL FIBRILLATION

Quinidine is typically administered by nasogastric tube because of its irrigating effects on the mucous membranes (see Table 10-6). Intravenous quinidine gluconate can be successful in conversion of horses with AF of recent onset or when nasogastric delivery is not feasible,[727] but failure to respond does not predict the response to oral treatment. Many successful approaches have been used to convert AF in horses, and the clinician should appreciate that the mean quinidine elimination half-life after an oral 10-g dose is about 6.7 hours.[294,759] One treatment approach for AF involves administration of a loading dose of 22 mg/kg quinidine sulfate by nasogastric tube every 2 hours for two to four doses, followed by every 6 hours dosing until the horse converts or develops initial signs of toxicosis. Aggressive every-2-hours dosing exceeding 88 to 132 mg/kg is especially likely to induce adverse effects. Therapeutic plasma quinidine concentrations for conversion from AF to sinus rhythm are 2 to 5 μg/ml (6.2 to 15.4 μmol/L) and should be measured if a horse fails to convert after an appropriate dosing regimen. If conversion to sinus rhythm has not occurred after 24 hours of therapy, then digoxin at 0.0055 to 0.011 mg/kg orally twice a day may be added to the treatment regimen for 24 to 48 hours. As in other species, a digoxin-quinidine interaction occurs that can effectively double the serum concentration of digoxin.[760] Thus combination therapy beyond 24 hours should be continued only with drug level monitoring of the serum digoxin (see Table 10-6) and consideration of using the lower end of the digoxin dosage range. Even horses that do not convert on the "standard" administration regimen may convert after the combined use of quinidine with digoxin. The value of using such a treatment plan every 6 hours is that steady-state levels are reached, sufficient time elapses to attain myocardial concentrations, and quinidine toxicity is less frequent when compared with the every-2-hour regimen. When prolonged treatment over more than 12 to 24 hours is necessary, adequate hydration and electrolyte balance (particularly potassium and magnesium) must be ensured by oral or IV administration of crystalloid solutions, because most horses undergoing oral quinidine treatment will become depressed and inappetent, will show reduced water intake, and may develop mild diarrhea.

Careful clinical and continuous electrocardiographic monitoring should be performed on horses with AF during conversion to sinus rhythm. The QRS duration should be monitored and compared with the pretreatment QRS duration before each additional treatment is administered. Prolongation of the QRS duration to greater than 25% of the pretreatment value is an indication of quinidine toxicity and should prompt discontinuation of therapy. The simplest ECG change is an acceleration of AV nodal conduction related to the vagolytic effect of quinidine (see Figure 10-55, C). Rapid supraventricular tachycardias with ventricular rate responses of up to 300 beats/min have been seen in several horses receiving quinidine sulfate. These horses have been treated with IV digoxin at 0.002 mg/kg to slow the ventricular response rate, IV replacement fluids to improve perfusion, IV sodium bicarbonate at 1 mEq/kg to reverse the sodium channel blocking effects of quinidine (probably by a combined effect of increasing extracellular sodium concentration and alkalinization,

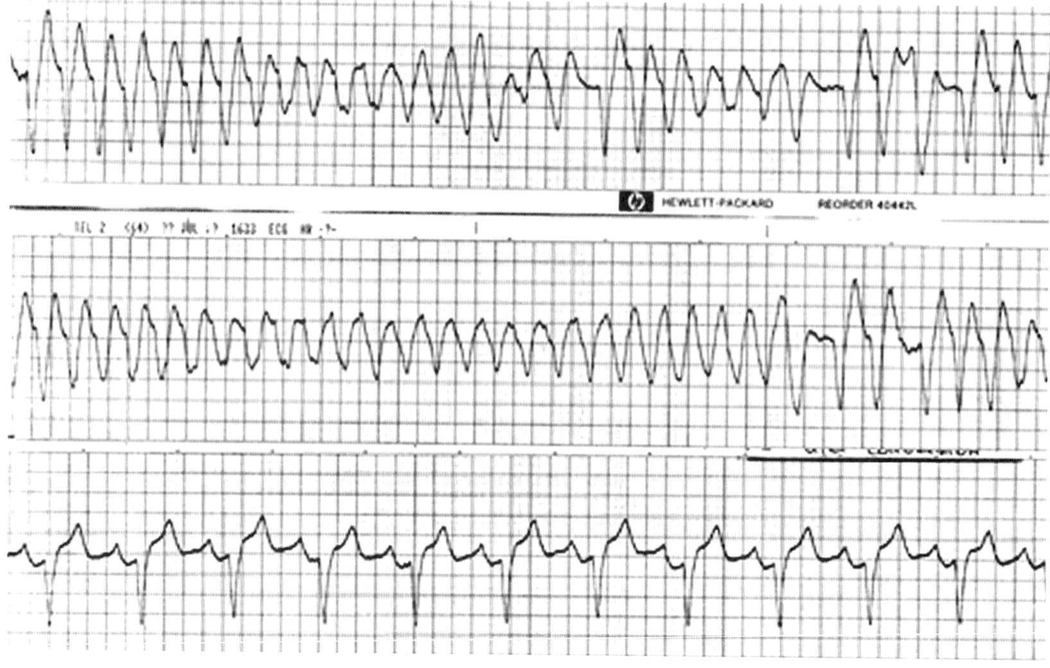

FIGURE 10-56 Polymorphous ventricular tachycardia (VT) after administration of quinidine sulfate for attempted conversion of atrial fibrillation (AF). In this case, normal sinus rhythm was established (*lower tracing*) after treatment with lidocaine, bicarbonate (to reverse sodium channel–blocking effects of quinidine), and phenylephrine (administered to maintain arterial blood pressure [ABP]).

leading to increased protein binding of quinidine and decreased extracellular concentrations of ionized calcium), and if needed, a phenylephrine drip to restore BP if critical hypotension develops. Ventricular arrhythmias (torsades de pointes, multiform VT, and ventricular premature complexes) have also been detected with quinidine toxicosis (Figure 10-56). Intravenous sodium bicarbonate is also indicated in these horses to bind free-circulating quinidine, whereas IV magnesium sulfate (up to 25 g in a 450- to 500-kg horse) is the treatment of choice for quinidine-induced ventricular arrhythmias (see Table 10-6). Lidocaine HCl may also be used if needed, starting with an IV bolus of 0.5 to 1.5 mg/kg, IV slowly. Conversely, administration of digoxin is contraindicated in horses with ventricular arrhythmias induced by quinidine.

Clinical markers of quinidine toxicosis include ataxia, colic, and nasal edema causing upper respiratory tract stridor. Most toxic reactions to quinidine sulfate are associated with higher plasma concentrations of the drug (>5 μg/ml) and can be avoided with careful clinical and electrocardiographic monitoring. Some of the adverse effects of quinidine administration, particularly polymorphic VT, are likely an idiosyncratic reaction. These adverse effects should prompt discontinuation of therapy or altering treatment intervals. Depression and paraphimosis occur in most horses treated with quinidine but disappear with the discontinuation of the drug. Diarrhea often develops with the administration of higher doses of quinidine, but this sign also disappears with discontinuation of the drug. Convulsions, hypotension because of vasodilation, CHF, laminitis, urticaria, and sudden death have rarely been reported with quinidine sulfate administration. A ventricular rate response in excess of 100 beats/min is an adverse reaction that may be more common in nervous horses or those prone to the vagolytic effects of quinidine. These horses may benefit from administration of digoxin to blunt the ventricular rate response, particularly if no other signs of quinidine toxicosis or elevated plasma concentration are present. If an increased ventricular response rate is anticipated, then one may even consider pretreatment with digoxin before initiation of quinidine therapy. Alternatively, diltiazem could be used for ventricular rate control, provided that BP can be closely monitored (see Table 10-6). However, the clinical experience with the use of diltiazem is limited, and doses should be carefully titrated to effect.

OTHER DRUGS FOR ATRIAL FIBRILLATION

Other drugs have been studied recently for treatment of AF in horses. Amiodarone administered as a constant-rate infusion has been used successfully for treating experimentally induced and natural AF in horses, but it cannot be recommended as a first-line therapy at this time.[755,757,758] Flecainide, a class Ic antiarrhythmic drug, may become more widely used if quinidine becomes unavailable. Although IV administration was generally ineffective at a dose of 2 to 3 mg/kg,[753] oral administration has demonstrated some success. Pharmacokinetics of flecainide have been studied in horses, and it has been successfully administered for treatment of AF, including recurrent AF.[738,749-753] The drug can be dissolved in water and delivered orally or by nasogastric tube. The approximate dosage is 4 to 6 mg/kg PO at intervals of 2 to 4 hours. Like quinidine, flecainide can prolong the QRS complex and become proarrhythmic, so the ECG must be carefully monitored from the first dose. Appreciation of the overall adverse effect profile of the drug in horses will require more clinical experience. IV propafenone also has been suggested for conversion of chronic AF,[754,761] but it has recently been shown to be ineffective at a dose of 2 mg/kg IV in horses with naturally occurring (and with pacing-induced) AF. Therefore the current knowledge does not support the use of this class Ic antiarrhythmic drug for treatment of AF.

ELECTROCARDIOVERSION OF ATRIAL FIBRILLATION

Electrical cardioversion of AF to sinus rhythm has been used at a number of referral centers as either the primary method of treatment or for management of horses that respond adversely or inadequately to quinidine therapy. As stated previously, electrocardioversion is very effective therapy, especially for AF of recent onset, but it requires special equipment and trained personnel. The procedure involves percutaneous placement of two specialized electrode catheters transvenously, with one catheter tip located within the left PA and the other within the RA cavity. Catheter placement is done under sedation and local anesthesia. The catheters are guided by pressure monitoring through the catheter lumen and 2D echocardiographic imaging (Figure 10-57). Radiography is used to verify the placement of the catheters either before or preferably after induction of general anesthesia. Although the catheters can be placed under local anesthesia, electrical cardioversion is very painful and must be performed under general anesthesia with the horse well padded because the shock results in a sudden jolt of the body and limbs.

The specific procedure used for cardioversion is beyond the scope of this textbook but has been well described in several studies.[743-747] In these reports, cardioversion was achieved with a mean energy level of 160 J. Experience indicates that some horses require higher energy doses, sometimes exceeding 300 J, and as with quinidine, not all cases result in conversion. The complications associated with electrocardioversion appear to be quite low but are finite related to general anesthesia or electrical shock. A case of transient complete AV block has been reported.[762]

FOLLOW-UP CARE

Horses can usually be returned to training within 24 to 48 hours after conversion. However, persistent sinus tachycardia, recurrent APCs (as detected by follow-up 24-hour Holter ECG), or persistent LV or LA dysfunction (as detected by follow-up echocardiography)[740] observed after successful conversion of AF to normal sinus rhythm may indicate subtle myocardial disease or AF-induced atrial remodeling. In addition, it may potentially indicate a higher risk of recurrent AF (although this contention has not been proven so far). These horses should probably be given more time to recover if possible (i.e., 1 to 2 weeks). Conversion of horses with AF generally results in a return to their previous performance level.[363,574] The exception is the horse with persistent LV dysfunction whose functional status will be improved following conversion to sinus rhythm, but whose performance will be less than its previous best. Horses with repeated episodes of AF are often converted numerous times with quinidine sulfate or electrocardioversion. Most horses that experience a recurrence of AF do so within 1 year of initial conversion, but much longer intervals have occurred between episodes of AF in some horses. If the duration of sinus rhythm becomes shorter, then repeated treatments may no longer be practical and a career change may be indicated. Some horses eventually become refractory to drug or electrical cardioversion, probably because of progressive atrial fibrosis or underlying myocardial disease. However, in the absence of significant, detectable cardiac disease, horses with persistent or permanent AF may still be used at lower levels of exercise (as long as the expected level of performance can be achieved), or they can be kept as breeding animals or pasture horses.

JUNCTIONAL AND VENTRICULAR ARRHYTHMIAS

Cardiac arrhythmias that originate within the AV conducting tissues, the ventricular specialized conducting tissues, or myocardium are classified as *junctional* (AV nodal or bundle of His) or *ventricular* in origin. Unlike sinus or atrial arrhythmias, these arrhythmias are not preceded by a conducted P wave. When sustained, junctional and ventricular rhythms often lead to dissociation between the SA (P wave) activity and that of the ventricle (QRS-T), resulting in AV dissociation.[447] In these cases an independent atrial rhythm is superimposed on the ectopic rhythm (see Figure 10-58, *C* and *D*). AV dissociation in these cases develops because the premature AV junctional or ventricular depolarization causes interference to the conduction of normal SA impulses. It is important to note that escape rhythms (see following) also cause AV dissociation. Therefore *AV dissociation* is a purely descriptive term of an ECG finding and neither characterizes the type and pathophysiologic mechanism of the arrhythmia nor determines the therapeutic approach.

With sustained junctional or VTs, P waves may be identified that are not conducted and therefore not consistently associated with a QRS complex (see Figure 10-58). Some of these P waves may be buried in the ectopic QRS-T complexes (especially at higher rates of ventricular activation), making their identification difficult. The use of ECG calipers helps determining the P-P interval and can greatly facilitate the identification of P waves. Occasionally, atrial impulses may be normally conducted, leading to capture beats or fusion beats. *Capture beats* are characterized by a normal P-QRS-T configuration, resulting from normal ventricular activation occurring before the ectopic focus discharges (see Figure 10-58, *D*). *Fusion beats* are seen when both the conducted impulse and an ectopic impulse cause simultaneous ventricular activation. The QRS-T morphology of a fusion beat represents the summation of a normal and an ectopic beat (see Figure 10-58, *C*).

It may be difficult to distinguish between junctional and ventricular arrhythmias and to determine the exact location of the abnormal impulse formation. The differentiation of junctional and ventricular rhythms can sometimes be made by inspection of the QRS complex. Junctional impulses are more likely to result in a narrow, relatively normal-appearing QRS complex with normal initial activation and electrical axis, because they originate above the ventricular myocardium. Complexes of ventricular origin, by contrast, are conducted abnormally and more slowly, resulting in a widened QRS, an abnormal QRS orientation, and abnormal T waves. However, junctional tachycardias also may be conducted aberrantly, resulting in a bizarre and wide QRS complex. When sustained, both types of rhythms cause AV dissociation with an independent atrial rhythm superimposed on the ectopic ventricular rhythm. Advanced echocardiographic methods that identify the sequence of ventricular activation may be of some value in distinguishing ventricular origin complexes from those starting above the ventricle and using the normal conduction system. The former are more likely to demonstrate ventricular dyssynchrony, characterized by wider dispersion of activation of different parts of the ventricles. Advanced electrophysiologic studies might also be applied to this differentiation.

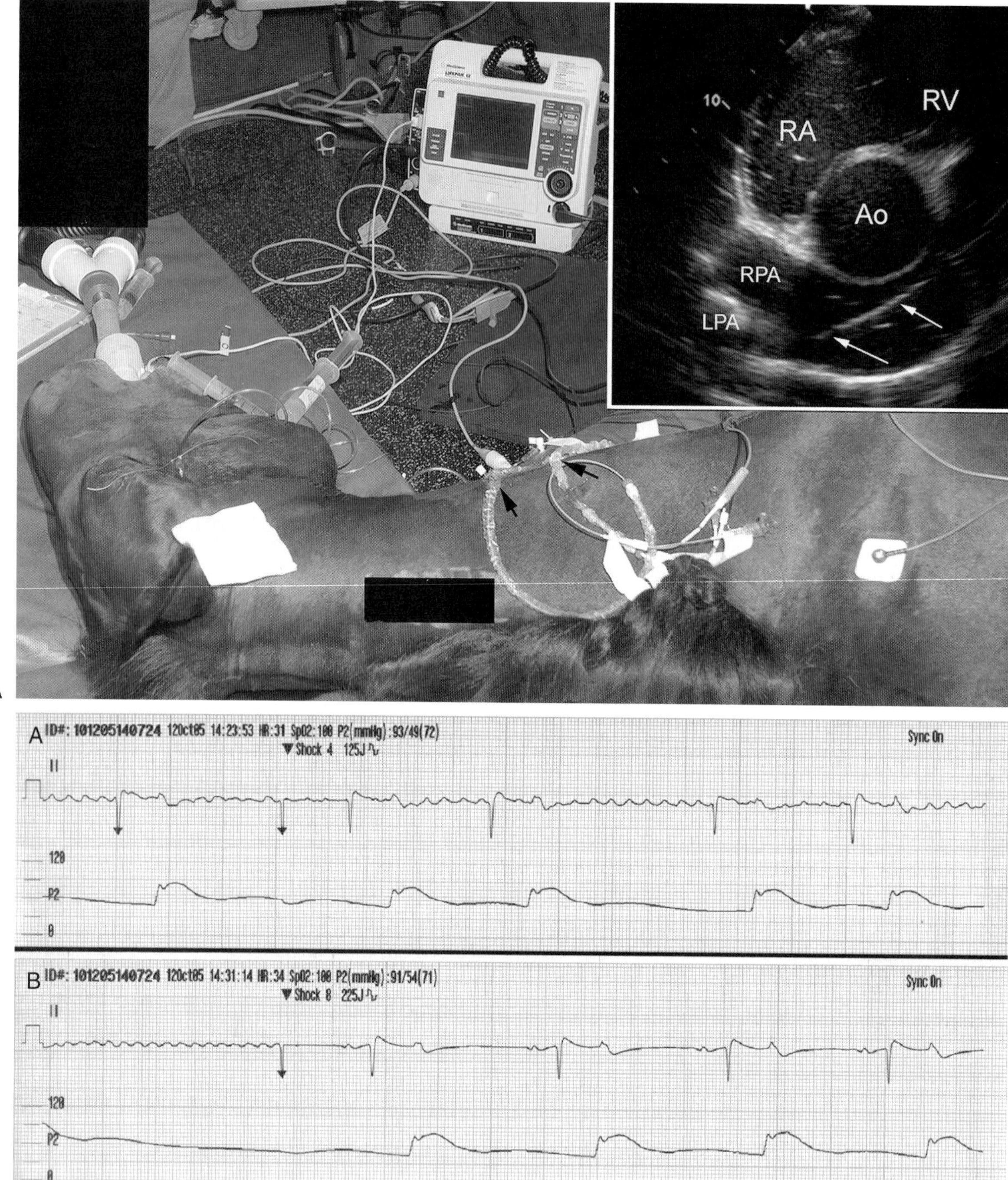

FIGURE 10-57 **A,** Electrocardioversion procedure in a Thoroughbred horse. The horse is under general anesthesia. Two specialized electrode catheters *(arrows)* were previously placed percutaneosly under local anesthesia into the right atrium (RA) and left pulmonary artery under guidance from two-dimensional (2D) echocardiography and intravascular pressure monitoring. The biphasic cardioverter (*top,* center of image) is connected to the catheters and is used to deliver the synchronized cardioversion shock, as well as monitor electrocardiogram (ECG) rhythm, invasive blood pressure (BP), and pulse oximetry. *Inset:* 2D image showing short axis image at base of heart. The catheter inserted into the left pulmonary artery (LPA) is indicated *(arrows)* (*RA,* right atrium; *RV,* right ventricle; *Ao,* aorta; *RPA,* right pulmonary artery). **B,** Transvenous electrical cardioversion for treatment of atrial fibrillation (AF) in an 2-year-old Standardbred racehorse under general anesthesia. A surface ECG (25 mm/sec) and an arterial blood pressure (ABP) tracing are displayed. The QRS complexes are automatically detected by the defibrillator unit and marked by small triangles. Biphasic electrical shocks (*larger triangles on top*) are applied at increasing energy levels. Delivery of the shocks is synchronized to the QRS complex to avoid the vulnerable period (T wave) and prevent induction of ventricular arrhythmias. **(A)** Unsuccessful attempt at an energy level of 125J. **(B)** Successful cardioversion at an energy level of 225J. Immediately after the shock, the baseline flattens and normal sinus rhythm resumes. No further treatment is required at this point. (From Schwarzwald CC, Bonagura JD, Muir WW: The cardiovascular system. In Muir WW, Hubbell JAE, editors: Equine anesthesia: monitoring and emergency therapy, ed 2, St Louis, 2009, WB Saunders.)

JUNCTIONAL ARRHYTHMIAS

Junctional complexes that arise early relative to the normal cardiac cycle are designated as *premature junctional complexes*. These complexes may occur as single or repetitive events and can resemble ectopic rhythms that might originate in the atria. Repetitive ectopic complexes that occur in short bursts or runs are termed *nonsustained* or *paroxysmal junctional tachycardias. Sustained junctional tachycardias* may also occur and can lead to CHF.

The clinical significance of an occasional junctional premature complex is difficult to ascertain. Persistent or repetitive junctional or ventricular rhythms are indicative of heart disease, systemic disease, or a drug-induced abnormality of cardiac rhythm. The best management choice is uncertain inasmuch as some junctional rhythms behave more like atrial tachyarrhythmias, whereas others cause AV dissociation and appear to act like ventricular ectopic impulses. Because the mechanism responsible for junctional tachycardias can be either abnormal automaticity or re-entry (circuit) movement using the AV node, empiric therapy is usually required to control sustained arrhythmias. If obvious AV dissociation is noted, then lidocaine, quinidine, or procainamide would seem reasonable choices (see Table 10-6). If the mechanism is uncertain but is clearly supraventricular, then IV digoxin or IV diltiazem may either silence the rhythm or slow the rate.

ESCAPE RHYTHMS

The normal heart contains potential cardiac pacemakers within the AV junctional and ventricular specialized tissues. These potential pacemakers may become manifest during periods of sinus bradycardia or AV block, creating *escape complexes* or *escape rhythms* (see Figure 10-60, *B*). Escape rhythms are characterized by slow ventricular rates, often in the realm of 15 to 25 beats/min. Specific antiarrhythmic drug suppression of escape rhythms is generally not necessary and is contraindicated because these rhythms serve as rescue mechanisms for the heart. Instead, management of escape rhythms should be aimed at resolving the underlying cause of sinus bradycardia or AV block.

ACCELERATED IDIONODAL (IDIOVENTRICULAR) RHYTHMS

Occasionally, the subsidiary nodal or ventricular pacemakers may be enhanced and discharge at a rate that is equal to or slightly above the SA rate (usually between 60 and 80 beats/min). The resulting rhythm is commonly referred to as *accelerated idionodal (idioventricular) rhythm* or *slow VT* (see Figure 10-58, *C*). Conditions that favor the development of these rhythms include gastrointestinal disease (possibly because of a combination of endotoxemia, autonomic imbalance, acid-base disturbances, and electrolyte abnormalities)[450] and administration of anesthetics or catecholamines. When the independent atrial and ventricular pacemaker foci discharge at similar rates, the P waves may appear to "march in and out" of the QRS complex. This phenomenon is called *isorhythmic AV dissociation* and is occasionally observed in adult horses during inhalation anesthesia. Accelerated idioventricular rhythms are often quite regular and may be misdiagnosed as sinus tachycardia on auscultation or palpation of peripheral pulses. Persistent, unexplained mild to moderate tachycardia should therefore prompt an electrocardiographic examination to ascertain a correct rhythm diagnosis. However, accelerated idioventricular rhythms generally are of little clinical (electrophysiologic and hemodynamic) significance and resolve spontaneously with appropriate treatment of potential underlying conditions and reduction of anesthetic dosages. Electrolyte supplementation (potassium, magnesium) and correction of fluid deficits and acid-base disturbances may be beneficial. Lidocaine (see Table 10-6) is sometimes administered as an intraoperative adjunct to general anesthesia, or it is used as an analgesic and prokinetic drug in the management of postoperative ileus. In these situations, its antiarrhythmic effects may provide some additional preventive or therapeutic benefits.

VENTRICULAR ARRHYTHMIAS

Ventricular arrhythmias are less common than atrial arrhythmias but are more likely to be associated with underlying structural cardiac disease, lesions of the myocardium, or a multisystemic disorder, including infections.* Ventricular arrhythmias may be observed with severe toxemia or sepsis or primary gastrointestinal disorders including proximal enteritis and large bowel disorders. Potassium, magnesium, and calcium activities can affect myocardial electrophysiology,[771] and electrolyte disorders can induce ventricular ectopy. Other potential causes of ventricular arrhythmias include metabolic disorders, ischemia, hypoxia, drugs, ionophores, and systemic inflammation. Primary heart diseases including severe valvular regurgitation, cardiomyopathy, myocarditis, endocarditis, and pericarditis can induce ventricular arrhythmias. Thus the approach to the horse with ventricular arrhythmias should emphasize ruling out the noncardiac causes, correcting them (if possible), and then following if necessary with a complete CV examination, including electrocardiography and echocardiography. Serum troponin should be measured to identify cardiac injury, although it may be problematic to separate primary from secondary causes of cardiac troponin elevations. Ventricular ectopic rhythms are classified as indicated in Box 10-9.

VENTRICULAR PREMATURE COMPLEXES

Ventricular premature complexes are characterized by premature, widened complexes, often followed by compensatory pauses. The pause occurs because the next sinus impulse is blocked by the refractory AV conduction system. If the sinus rate is slow or the ventricular premature complex is closely coupled to the preceding normal sinus beat, then it may be interpolated between two normal beats. Ventricular ectopic impulses are characterized by QRS and T waves that are wide and often bizarre in appearance (see Figures 10-58 and 10-59). The premature QRS bears no relationship to any preceding P waves, although the induction of ventricular ectopics may be dependent on underlying cardiac cycle length or heart rate. The morphology of the ventricular premature complexes may be uniform (monomorphic) or multiform (polymorphic) as shown in Figure 10-58, E. The relationship of a ventricular extrasystole to the preceding sinus QRS-T is expressed by the "coupling interval" between them. Often the coupling interval is fixed, although it may vary minimally[769] or markedly in horses. A very short coupling interval may place the ectopic QRS on the preceding T wave, a phenomenon called *R on T* and related experimentally to increased ventricular vulnerability for fibrillation.

Ventricular premature complexes are generally considered abnormal, except for possibly those occurring immediately after exercise.[337] However, ventricular ectopy was identified in

*References 110, 199, 359, 432, 447, 469, 489, 668, 672, 763-770.

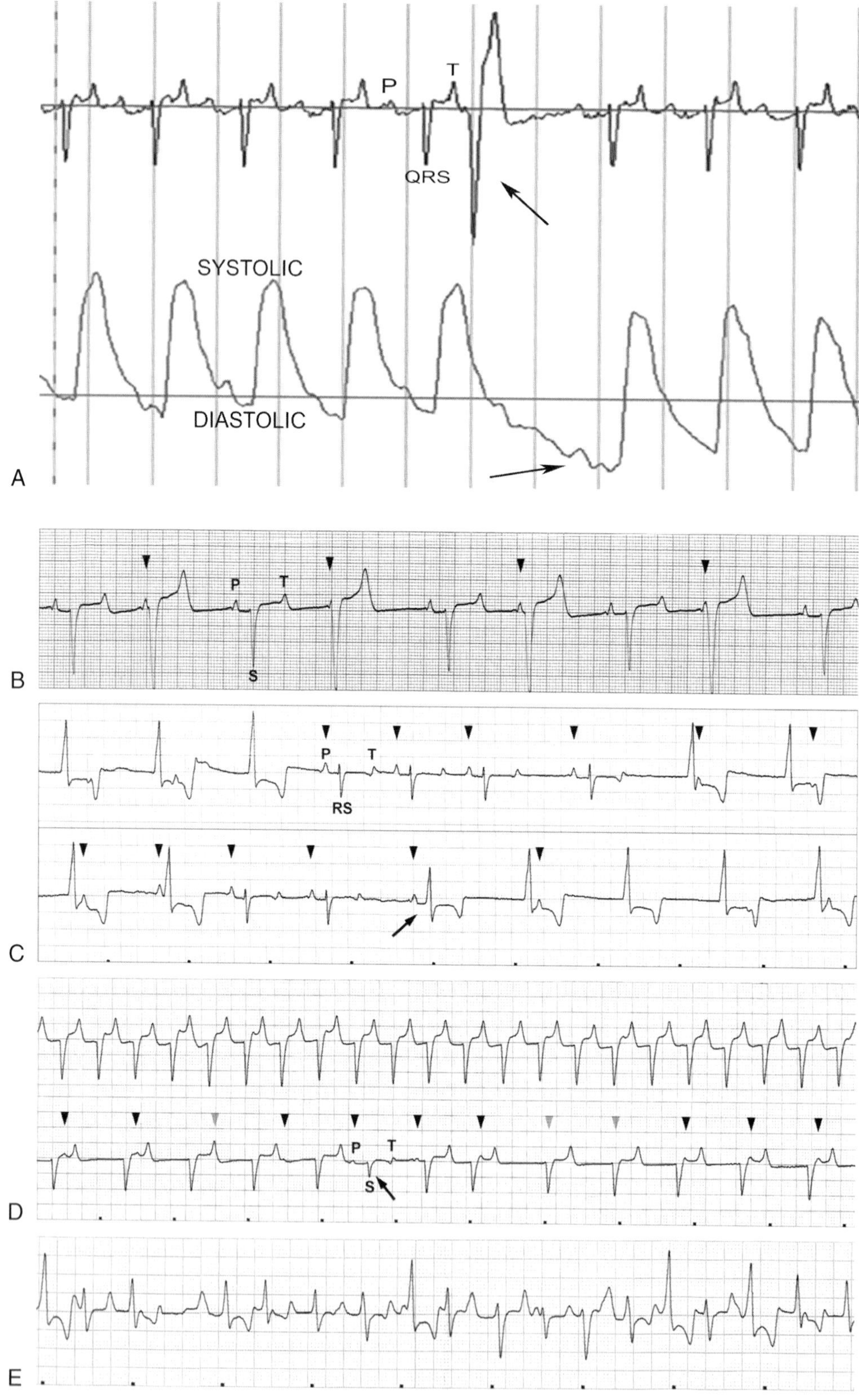

FIGURE 10-58 Ventricular arrhythmias. **A,** The ectopic complex *(arrow)* is premature and abnormal in morphology. A compensatory pause follows the extrasystole because the next sinus P wave is blocked in the atrioventricular node. The effect of the premature complex on arterial blood pressure (ABP) in the lower tracing *(arrow)* is noticeable. **B,** Base-apex lead electrocardiogram (ECG) recorded from a 15-year-old Arab mare with ventricular bigeminy. Normal sinus beats alternate with slightly larger and wider ventricular ectopic beats. SA node discharge is not affected by the ectopic beats, as indicated by the presence of nonconducted P waves immediately before the ectopic beats *(arrowheads)* (paper speed 25 mm/sec).

Figure 10-58, cont'd C, Base-apex lead ECG recorded from an 18-year-old Arab mare recovering from acute diarrhea and endotoxemia. The ECG shows an intermittent accelerated idioventricular rhythm at a rate of 50 beats/min. P wave intervals are indicated (*arrowheads*). The recording demonstrates that the ectopic focus is suppressed at higher rates of SA node discharge. The ventricular rhythm only becomes manifest when the sinoatrial (SA) rate drops below the rate of the ventricular pacemaker. SA node discharge is not affected by the ectopic rhythm, resulting in AV dissociation. A fusion beat is present (*arrow*), resulting from summation of a conducted sinus impulse with an ectopic ventricular beat (paper speed 25 mm/sec, voltage calibration 0.5 cm/mV). **D,** Base-apex lead ECG recorded from a 3-year-old Clydesdale gelding. The top recording shows a regular tachycardia at a rate of 120 beats/min. The appearance of the QRS-T complexes does not allow conclusive distinction between a supraventricular rhythm with rapid ventricular response and a ventricular rhythm. However, as the rate slows down (*bottom strip*), AV dissociation because of a ventricular tachycardia (VT) becomes apparent. P waves (*arrowheads*) and a capture beat (*arrow*) are indicated (paper speed 25 mm/sec, voltage calibration 0.25 cm/mV). **E,** Base-apex ECG recorded from a 5-year-old Clydesdale stallion with acute myocardial necrosis of unknown cause. The serum cardiac troponin I concentrations were severely elevated (404 ng/ml; normal <0.15 ng/ml). The ECG shows multiform VT at a rate of 120 beats/min (paper speed 25 mm/sec, voltage calibration 0.5 cm/mV). (B to E from Schwarzwald CC, Bonagura JD, Muir WW: The cardiovascular system. In Muir WW, Hubbell JAE, editors: Equine anesthesia: monitoring and emergency therapy, ed 2, St Louis, 2009, WB Saunders.)

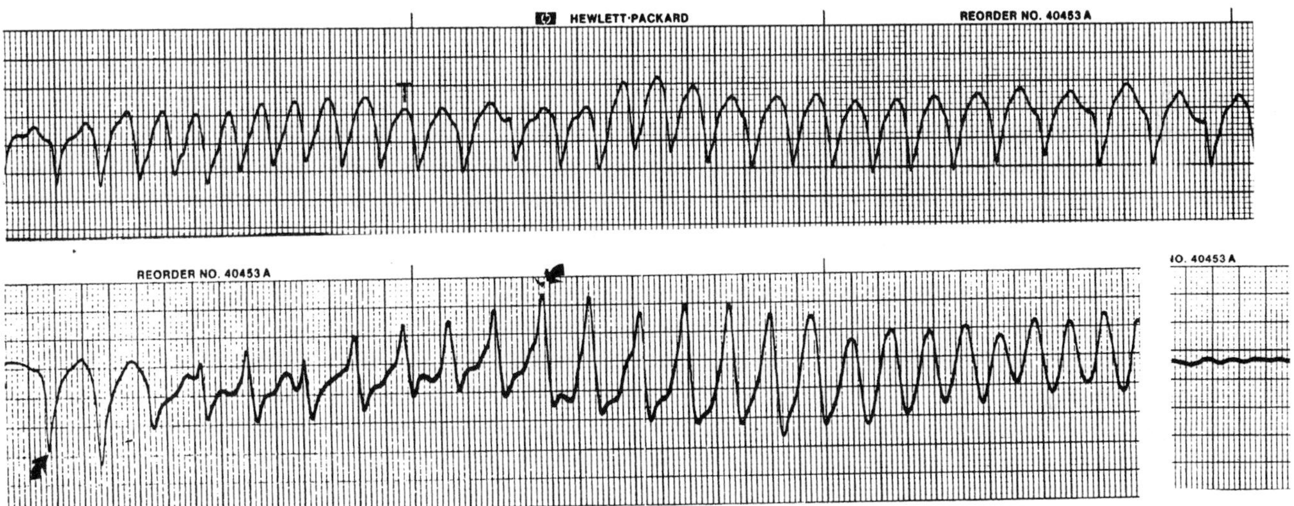

FIGURE 10-59 Sustained, rapid ventricular tachycardia (VT) (*top*) of varying rate that develops into a polymorphic ventricular rhythm with varying morphology complexes (torsades de pointes). The horse died of cardiac arrest (*lower right panel*). The arrows indicate QRS complexes of varying polarity (25 mm/sec).

14% of clinically normal horses during routine 24-hour continuous electrocardiographic monitoring.[359] The distributional pattern of ventricular ectopics may include haphazard distribution of single complexes, bigeminy (sinus beats followed, at a fixed coupling interval, by premature ventricular beats; Figure 10-58, *B*), couplets (pairs of ventricular premature complexes), triplets, or runs (four or more) of ventricular ectopics. Runs of accelerated ventricular rhythm, usually developing at relatively slow heart rates, are not uncommon. Runs of ventricular ectopics at a rapid rate—VT—are more likely to be hemodynamically and electrically unstable, particularly when they develop at rates higher than 100 per minute (see Ventricular Tachycardia below).

When premature ventricular beats are identified by auscultation, an ECG should be obtained, and a workup similar to that outlined in Box 10-4 should be undertaken. Occasional premature ventricular complexes, as with occasional supraventricular premature complexes, may be clinically insignificant and not require treatment. Rest is highly recommended for horses with frequent ventricular premature complexes. In the majority of horses with premature ventricular complexes occurring in the absence of significant structural heart disease, the arrhythmia seems to resolve spontaneously after 4 to 8 weeks of rest. The horse may then be able to return successfully to its prior performance level. Antiarrhythmic therapy is usually successful in abolishing ventricular premature complexes, but most return when the antiarrhythmic agent is discontinued, unless the underlying problem has been resolved and chronic administration is not practical. Dexamethasone and other anti-inflammatory drugs have been used to treat ventricular arrhythmias, but their use is controversial and they should certainly not be administered to horses with a recent or current infection.

VENTRICULAR TACHYCARDIA

Ventricular tachycardia is an ectopic ventricular rhythm characterized by either a regular or irregular ventricular rate (see Figures 10-58 and 10-59). *Torsades de pointes* represent a specific form of polymorphic VT, characterized by progressive changes in QRS direction leading to a steady undulation in the QRS axis (see Figure 10-59). VT is recognized clinically by an increased heart rate, often exceeding 100 beats/min. Arterial pulses are typically weak or variable in intensity. Multiform VT is characterized by an irregular rhythm (see Figure 10-58, E). With multiform VT, heart sounds are more likely to vary in intensity and arterial pulses are likely to be abnormal. Jugular pulsations may be detected because of AV dissociation. Syncope is associated with higher rates of VT (180 beats/min or higher). Respiratory distress and pulmonary edema may develop from impaired ventricular function. Protracted junctional tachycardias or VTs (>120 beats/min) may lead to CHF because of reversible myocardial failure (tachycardia-induced cardiomyopathy).[110] VTs can also progress to *ventricular flutter* and *ventricular fibrillation*, characterized by chaotic ventricular activation patterns leading to uncoordinated undulations of the electrical baseline. These rhythms often represent terminal rhythms and usually result in cardiac arrest (see Figure 10-59).

VT may be life threatening if R on T complexes are detected, if the arrhythmia is rapid (>180-200 beats/min), if multiform VT is detected, or if polymorphic tachycardia (torsades de pointes) is evident. Immediate treatment of CV collapse may be required.[717] IV therapies for VT include lidocaine, procainamide, quinidine magnesium salts, amiodarone, and propafenone (for refractory VT). Administration of antiarrhythmic drugs (see Table 10-6) can be associated with side effects, including proarrhythmia, seizures, and sudden death. Lidocaine causes central nervous system (CNS) excitation; however, boluses and infusions can be well tolerated in horses, and the drug causes minimal hemodynamic or electrophysiologic alterations at nontoxic doses.[623,624,772] Quinidine may be used for treatment of ventricular arrhythmias but is a myocardial depressant and vagolytic drug. Procainamide[773] has been studied to a limited degree, but it is generally well tolerated when given in graded doses. It has similar electrophysiologic effects to quinidine, but seems less vagolytic and possibly has less gastrointestinal side effects. Cumulative doses of up to 10 mg/kg are generally well tolerated; additional dosing should be guided by ECG, QRS duration, and ABP. Magnesium sulfate is an alternative antiarrhythmic that can be effective in both normomagnesemic and hypomagnesemic horses and is generally well tolerated at therapeutic doses. Amiodarone has been evaluated in a small number of horses[756,757] and can be considered as a second-line drug for serious, drug-resistant VT. Other antiarrhythmics, including IV propafenone[761] or phenytoin, may be tried in refractory ventricular arrhythmias.

A period of rest (4 to 8 weeks) followed by electrocardiographic and echocardiographic re-evaluation (including an exercising ECG) is indicated for follow-up of horses that have developed sustained VT. A substantial number of these horses can be successfully returned to performance after treatment with antiarrhythmics and rest, so long as significant and untreatable structural heart disease is not evident. The use of anti-inflammatory drugs in horses with VT is empiric.

Conduction Disturbances

Once a cardiac electrical impulse is formed, it is conducted rapidly throughout the heart. The sequence of cardiac electric activation is usually dictated by the specialized conducting tissues in the atria, the AV node, the bundle of His, the bundle branches, and the Purkinje fiber system. This conduction system permits orderly activation of atrial and ventricular muscle and facilitates effective mechanical activity of the heart. A variety of conduction disorders are recognized, including SA nodal exit block, atrial standstill (usually because of hyperkalemia), AV block, bundle branch block, and ill-defined ventricular conduction disturbances (Figures 10-60 and 10-61).*

Rarely, accelerated conduction occurs in the heart, which involves a pathway around the normally slow-conducting AV node and results in early excitation of the ventricles.[775] These syndromes are termed *pre-excitation* and have various associated labels related to similar human disorders (e.g., Wolff-Parkinson-White syndrome). A shortened P-R interval is typically found.

ATRIOVENTRICULAR CONDUCTION BLOCK

Delays in AV conduction are the most common conduction blocks. These delays are classified as *first-*, *second-*, and *third-degree* (or *complete*). *First-degree AV block* occurs when the PR (or PQ) interval exceeds a certain value (approximately 500 ms in large-breed horses and 320 ms in small breeds and ponies) while the atrial impulse still transmits through the AV conduction system and activates the ventricle, causing a QRS complex. Some P waves are not conducted to the ventricles during *second-degree AV block,* which results in occasional P waves not followed by a QRS-T complex (see Figure 10-60, *A*). Second-degree AV block after progressive prolongation of the PQ interval is classified as *Mobitz type I (Wenckebach)* block. Conversely, the AV block is termed *Mobitz type II* if the PQ interval is constant. Occurrence of two or more consecutive second-degree AV blocks in presence of a normal or slow sino atrial rate is called *high-grade (advanced) AV block,* although this can be a normal (vagally induced) finding in approximately 1% of healthy horses, based on 24-hour ECG findings of one of the authors (VBR). *Third-degree* or *complete AV block* is characterized by an absence of atrial to ventricular conduction. P waves are not followed by or related to QRS complexes, and to prevent ventricular asystole, a junctional or ventricular escape rhythm must develop below the level of the AV block (see Figure 10-60, *B*).

First- and second-degree AV block are considered normal variations.[764] These rhythms are most often associated with high vagal tone and may be seen with sinus bradycardia or sinus arrhythmia. Second-degree AV block can usually be abolished with exercise, stress, or vagolytic drugs such as atropine or glycopyrrolate (although drugs are rarely needed). Complete AV block is indicative of organic heart disease, severe drug toxicity, or abnormally high vagal activity. Generally speaking, third-degree AV block caused by vagal-efferent traffic is short-lived. Sudden development of high-grade or complete AV block may require the administration of atropine or a catecholamine, or it may require rapid transvenous insertion of a pacing wire into the RV. Chronic third-degree AV block requires treatment with a pacemaker;[507,776-779] and pacemakers have been successfully placed epicardially and transvenously in several horses and in a number of Miniature Donkeys with possible congenital complete AV block (see Figures 10-60, *C*, and 10-62).

INTRAVENTRICULAR CONDUCTION BLOCKS

Intraventricular conduction blocks, such as bundle branch block, are less common and more difficult to diagnose. Widening of the QRS complex and axis deviation are typical features. These abnormalities may also be found after APCs, from overdose with quinidine sulfate, from severe hyperkalemia, or secondary to supraventricular tachycardias with rapid ventricular response.

*References 173, 192, 198, 344, 470, 764, 774.

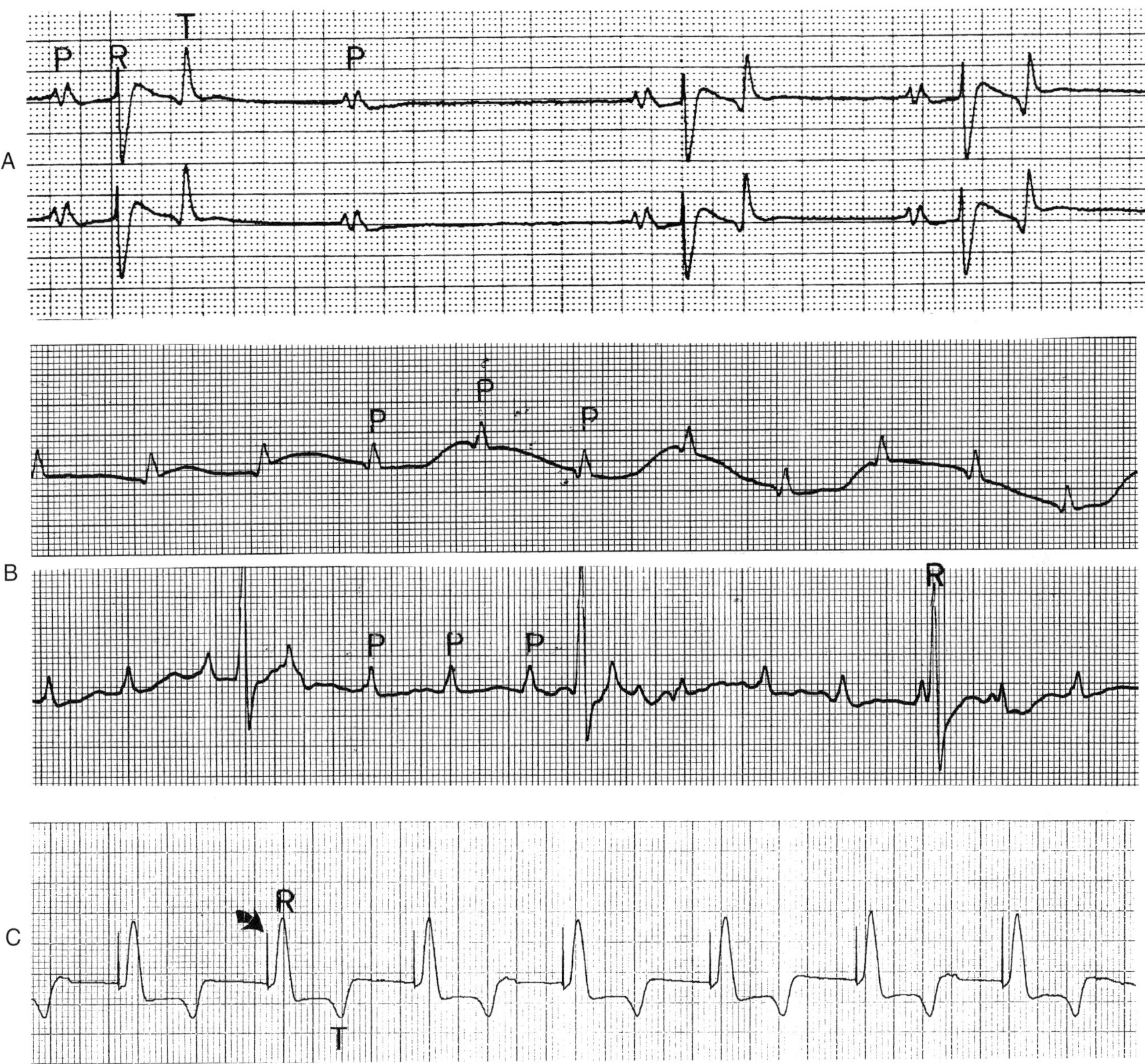

FIGURE 10-60 Conduction disturbances. **A,** Second-degree atrioventricular block. Nonconducted P waves and varying P-R intervals are evident (base-apex lead recorded at 25 mm/sec). **B,** The tracings are from a horse with third-degree atrioventricular block. The upper strip demonstrates multiple blocked P waves. The lower tracing shows nonconducted P waves and ventricular escape complexes (base-apex lead recorded at 25 mm/sec). **C,** Permanent transvenous ventricular pacing in a Miniature Donkey with a complete atrioventricular block. A pacemaker spike (*arrow*) precedes each paced ventricular complex.

PRE-EXCITATION

Pre-excitation, or accelerated AV conduction, has been reported sporadically,[775] but the clinical significance of this electrocardiographic abnormality has yet to be determined in this species. Ventricular pre-excitation in humans and in dogs is often due to an anomalous conducting pathway around the AV node, which serves as a path for re-entrant supraventricular tachycardias. These rhythm disturbances may cause hypotension and syncope. Whether pre-excitation syndromes are important has yet to be determined. Nevertheless, ECG traces occasionally show evidence of ventricular pre-excitation and are characterized by a P-QRS-T relationship but with an extremely short PR interval, early excitation of the ventricle characterized by a slurring of the initial QRS complex (a delta wave), and an overall widening of the QRS complex (see Figure 10-61, *A*).

HYPERKALEMIA

Hyperkalemia can cause significant depression of atrial, AV, and ventricular conduction and can shorten ventricular repolarization. Serum potassium is most likely to be markedly elevated after renal failure and oliguria, during shock, with severe metabolic acidosis, in foals with ruptured bladder or ureter and uroperitoneum, or after excessive IV potassium replacement. Hyperkalemia also occurs in Quarter Horses with hyperkalemic periodic paralysis.

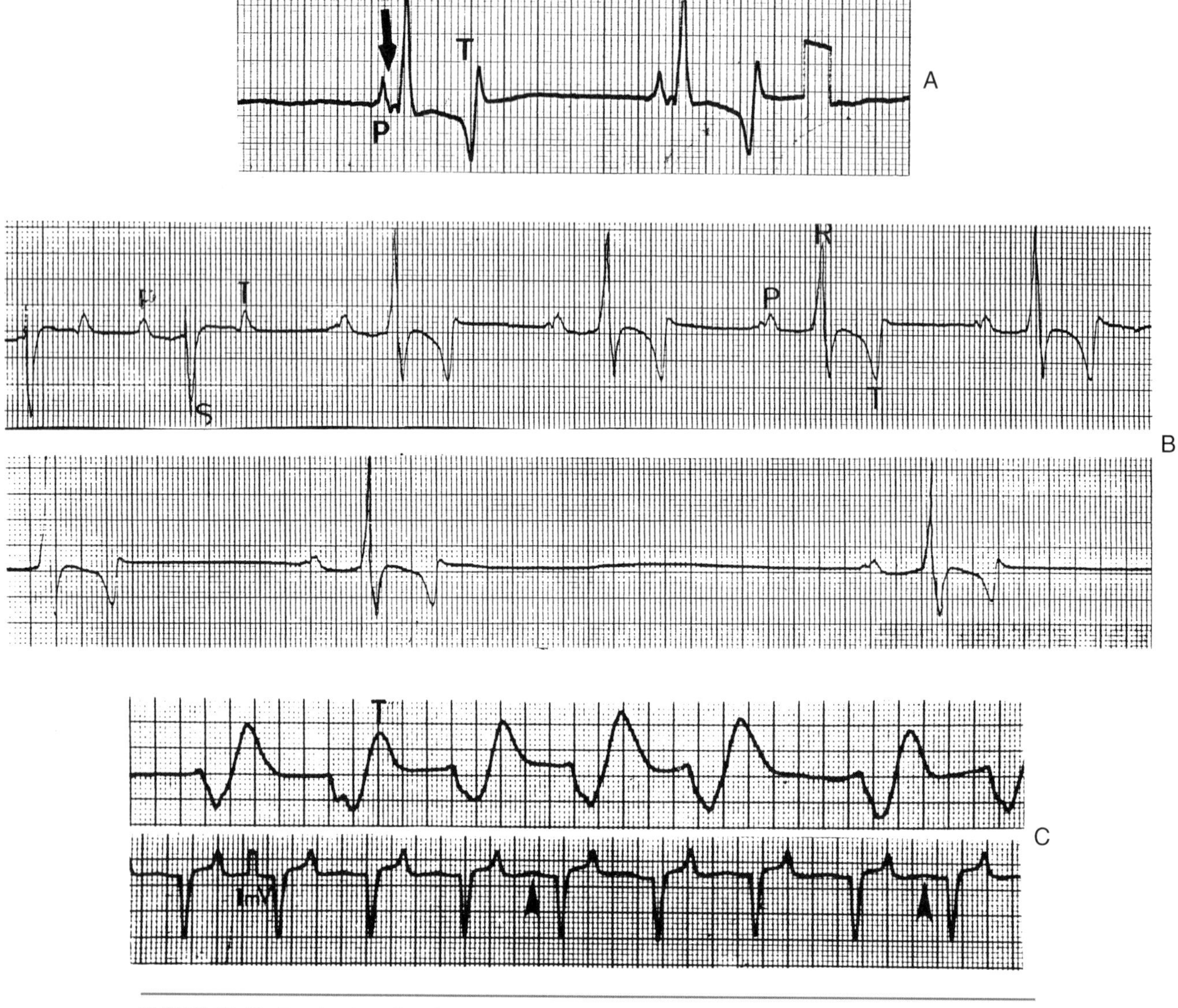

FIGURE 10-61 Conduction disturbances. **A,** Ventricular pre-excitation. The short P-R interval (*arrow*) and small deflection in the P-R segment (delta wave) indicate an accessory pathway around the atrioventricular node with premature activation of a portion of the ventricle (delta wave and initial portion of the QRS). The large QRS and secondary T wave changes can be explained by the loss of normal cancellation of ventricular electrical forces. **B,** A sinus arrhythmia and intraventricular conduction disturbance. The sudden change and widening of the ventricular conduction pattern are notable, despite the consistent P-R interval and probably represent a bundle branch block, although this diagnosis is difficult to make in horses (base-apex lead recorded at 25 mm/sec). **C,** Hyperkalemia in a foal with a ruptured bladder. The top strip demonstrates atrial standstill (no P waves), significant widening of the QRS complexes, and large T waves with a shortened ST segment. The lower tracing shows the effects after initial medical therapy for hyperkalemia, which included treatment with saline and sodium bicarbonate. The normalization of the QRS complexes and the appearance of low-amplitude P waves (*arrows*) are notable. (Tracing courtesy of Ron Hilwig, DVM, PhD.)

Changes in the ECG are usually evident at potassium serum concentrations greater than 6 mEq/L, with severe changes evident when serum concentrations are between 8 and 10 mEq/L.[198,780-782] Broadening and flattening of the P wave are the most consistently observed change. Prolongation of the PQ interval and bradycardia develop, excitability decreases, and atrial standstill (sinoventricular rhythm)—characterized by complete absence of P waves—may be observed. Either inversion or enlargement (tenting) of the T waves is also likely. Marked widening of the QRS complex may be noted as near-lethal concentrations of potassium are approached. Ventricular asystole or fibrillation can develop. The QT interval is not a reliable indicator of induced hyperkalemia, and other electrolyte and acid-base alterations, including serum calcium and sodium, influence the effect of hyperkalemia on the heart.

Therapy for hyperkalemia includes correction of the underlying problem, infusion of isotonic crystalloid solutions and dextrose, and administration of calcium salts and sodium bicarbonate. Lactated Ringer's solution (LRS) can be used in patients with hyperkalemia; the small amount

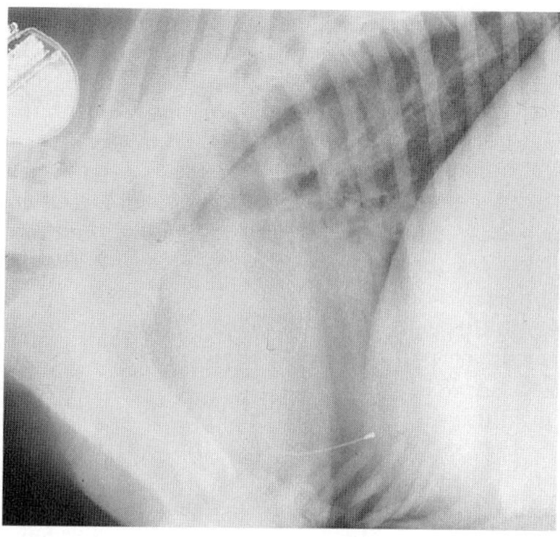

FIGURE 10-62 A lateral radiograph of a permanent transvenous pacing system in a Miniature Donkey. The pacemaker is evident at the upper left of the radiograph. The thin transvenous pacing wire extends from the device through the jugular vein and vena cava and into the right ventricular (RV) apex.

of potassium contained in LRS is generally not considered problematic, because the beneficial effects of volume replacement and treatment of metabolic acidosis largely overweigh the potential negative effects of additional potassium supply. Alternatively, sodium chloride (NaCl) or NaCl/dextrose solutions may be used, but maintenance solutions should not be used because of their relatively high potassium content. Dextrose (or glucose) can be administered as a bolus of 0.25 to 0.5 g/kg, IV over 15 minutes. The administration of regular insulin (0.1 IU/kg) in conjunction with dextrose infusion (0.5 to 1.0 g/kg, IV over 15 minutes) may be considered in cases of life-threatening hyperkalemia. Sodium bicarbonate may be used in cases of severe metabolic acidosis (provided that ventilation is adequate) at a dose of 1 to 2 mEq/kg, IV over 15 minutes (or depending on the base excess obtained by blood gas analyses [mEq sodium bicarbonate = 0.3 (−0.5) × BE × kg BWT]). In cases of severe arrhythmias, 1 ml/kg calcium gluconate 23% can be administered over a 10-minute period to effect.

REFERENCES

1. Detweiler DK: Electrocardiogram of the horse, *Fed Proc* 11:34, 1952.
2. Detweiler DK: Auricular fibrillation in horses, *J Am Vet Med Assoc* 126:47, 1955.
3. Patterson DF, Detweiler DK, Glendinning SA: Heart sounds and murmurs of the normal horse, *Ann N Y Acad Sci* 127:242, 1965.
4. Detweiler DK, Patterson DF: The cardiovascular system, In Catcott EJ, Smithcors JF, editors: *Equine medicine and surgery*, ed 2, Santa Barbara, CA, 1972, American Veterinary Publications, pp 277-347.
5. Bishop SP, Cole CR, Smetzer DL: Functional and morphologic pathology of equine aortic insufficiency, *Vet Pathol* 3:137, 1966.
6. Hamlin RL, Smetzer DL, Smith CR: Analysis of QRS complex recorded through a semiorthogonal lead system in the horse, *Am J Physiol* 207:325, 1964.
7. Hamlin RL, Smith CR: Categorization of common domestic mammals based on their ventricular activation process, *Ann N Y Acad Sci* 127:195, 1965.
8. Hamlin RL, Smetzer DL, Senta T, et al: Atrial activation paths and P waves in horses, *Am J Physiol* 219:306, 1970.
9. Hamlin RL, Klepinger WL, Gilpin KW, et al: Autonomic control of heart rate in the horse, *Am J Physiol* 222:976, 1972.
10. Hamlin RL, Levesque MJ, Kittleson MD: Intramyocardial pressure and distribution of coronary blood flow during systole and diastole in the horse, *Cardiovasc Res* 16:256, 1982.
11. Illera JC, Illera M, Hamlin RL: Unipolar thoracic electrocardiography that induces QRS complexes of relative uniformity from male horses, *Am J Vet Res* 48:1700, 1987.
12. McKeever KH, Hinchcliff KW, Reed SM, et al: Splenectomy alters blood pressure response to incremental treadmill exercise in horses, *Am J Physiol* 265:R409, 1993.
13. Pipers FS, Hamlin RL: Echocardiography in the horse, *J Am Vet Med Assoc* 170:815, 1977.
14. Pipers FS, Hamlin RL, Reef VB: Echocardiographic detection of cardiovascular lesions in the horse, *J Equine Med Surg* 3:68, 1979.
15. Senta T, Smetzer DL, Smith CR: Effects of exercise on certain electrocardiographic parameters, *Cornell Vet* 60:552, 1970.
16. Smetzer DL, Smith CR, Hamlin RL: The fourth heart sound in the equine, *Ann N Y Acad Sci* 127:306, 1965.
17. Smetzer DL, Smith CR: Diastolic heart sounds of horses, *J Am Vet Med Assoc* 146:937, 1965.
18. Smetzer DL, Bishop SP, Smith CR: Diastolic murmur of equine aortic insufficiency, *Am Heart J* 72:489, 1966.
19. Smetzer DL, Hamlin RL, Smith CR: Cardiovascular sounds, In Swenson MJ, editor: *Dukes' physiology of domestic animals*, ed 8, Ithaca, NY, 1970, Comstock Publishing Company Inc, pp 159-168.
20. Smith CR, Hamlin RL: Regulation of the heart and blood vessels, In Swenson MJ, editor: *Dukes' physiology of domestic animals*, ed 8, Ithaca, NY, 1970, Comstock Publishing Company Inc, pp 169-195.
21. Brown CM, Holmes JR: Haemodynamics in the horse. II. Intracardiac, pulmonary arterial, and aortic pressures, *Equine Vet J* 10:207, 1978.
22. Brown CM, Holmes JR: Haemodynamics in the horse. I. Pressure pulse contours, *Equine Vet J* 10:188, 1978.
23. Brown CM, Holmes JR: Phonocardiography in the horse. I. The intracardiac phonocardiogram, *Equine Vet J* 11:11, 1979.
24. Brown CM, Holmes JR: Assessment of myocardial function in the horse. II. Experimental findings in resting horses, *Equine Vet J* 11:248, 1979.
25. Brown CM, Holmes JR: Phonocardiography in the horse. II. The relationship of the external phonocardiogram to intracardiac pressure and sound, *Equine Vet J* 11:183, 1979.
26. Brown CM, Holmes JR: Assessment of myocardial function in the horse. I. Theoretical and technical considerations, *Equine Vet J* 11:244, 1979.
27. Else RW, Holmes JR: Cardiac pathology in the horse. III. Clinical correlations, *Equine Vet J* 4:195, 1972.
28. Else RW, Holmes JR: Cardiac pathology in the horse. I. Gross pathology, *Equine Vet J* 4:1, 1972.
29. Else RW, Holmes JR: Cardiac pathology in the horse. II. Microscopic pathology, *Equine Vet J* 4:57, 1972.
30. Gattland L, Holmes JR: ECG recording at rest and during exercise in the horse, *Equine Vet Educ* 2:28, 1990.
31. Hillyer MH, Mair TS, Holmes JR: Treatment of bacterial endocarditis in a Shire mare, *Equine Vet Educ* 2:5, 1990.
32. Holmes JR: The equine heart: problems and difficulties in assessing cardiac function on clinical examination, *Equine Vet J* 1:10, 1968.
33. Holmes JR, Darke PGG, Else RW: Atrial fibrillation in the horse, *Equine Vet J* 1:212, 1969.
34. Holmes JR, Rezakhani A, Else RW: Rupture of a dissecting aortic aneurysm into the left pulmonary artery in a horse, *Equine Vet J* 5:65, 1973.

35. Holmes JR, Rezakhani A: Observations on the T wave of the equine electrocardiogram, *Equine Vet J* 7:55, 1975.
36. Holmes JR: Prognosis of equine cardiac conditions, *Equine Vet J* 9:181, 1977.
37. Holmes JR: Sir Frederick Smith Memorial Lecture. A superb transport system—the circulation, *Equine Vet J* 14:267, 1982.
38. Holmes JR, Miller PJ: Three cases of ruptured mitral valve chordae in the horse, *Equine Vet J* 16:125, 1984.
39. Holmes JR, Henigan M, Williams RB, et al: Paroxysmal atrial fibrillation in racehorses, *Equine Vet J* 18:37, 1986.
40. Holmes JR: Electrocardiography in the diagnosis of common cardiac arrythmias in the horse, *Equine Vet Educ* 2:24, 1990.
41. Holmes JR: The development of clinical cardiology, *Equine Vet J* (Suppl 19) 2, September 1995.
42. Miller PJ, Holmes JR: Effect of cardiac arrhythmia on left ventricular and aortic blood pressure parameters in the horse, *Res Vet Sci* 35:190, 1983.
43. Miller PJ, Holmes JR: Beat-to-beat variability in QRS potentials recorded with an orthogonal lead system in horses with second-degree partial A-V block, *Res Vet Sci* 37:334, 1984.
44. Miller PJ, Holmes JR: Interrelationship of some electrocardiogram amplitudes, time intervals and respiration in the horse, *Res Vet Sci* 36:370, 1984.
45. Miller PJ, Holmes JR: Observations on structure and function of the equine mitral valve, *Equine Vet J* 16:457, 1984.
46. Miller PJ, Holmes JR: Relationships of left side systolic time intervals to beat-by-beat heart rate and blood pressure variables in some cardiac arrhythmias of the horse, *Res Vet Sci* 37:18, 1984.
47. Miller PJ, Holmes JR: Computer processing of transaortic valve blood pressures in the horse using the first derivative of the left ventricular pressure trace, *Equine Vet J* 16:210, 1984.
48. Miller PJ, Holmes JR: Observations on seven cases of mitral insufficiency in the horse, *Equine Vet J* 17:181, 1985.
49. Voros K, Holmes JR, Gibbs C: Left ventricular volume determination in the horse by two-dimensional echocardiography: an in vitro study, *Equine Vet J* 22:398, 1990.
50. Voros K, Holmes JR, Gibbs C: Anatomical validation of two-dimensional echocardiography in the horse, *Equine Vet J* 22:392, 1990.
51. Voros K, Holmes JR, Gibbs C: Measurement of cardiac dimensions with two-dimensional echocardiography in the living horse, *Equine Vet J* 23:461, 1991.
52. Baker JR, Ellis CE: A survey of post-mortem findings in 480 horses 1958 to 1980. I. Causes of death, *Equine Vet J* 13:43, 1981.
53. Pipers FS: Applications of diagnostic ultrasound in veterinary medicine, *Equine Vet J* 14:341, 1982.
54. Morris EA, Seeherman HJ: Clinical evaluation of poor performance in the racehorse: the results of 275 evaluations, *Equine Vet J* 23:169, 1991.
55. Mitten LA: Cardiovascular causes of exercise intolerance, *Vet Clin North Am Equine Pract* 12:473, 1996.
56. Reef VB: Clinical approach to poor performance in horses, *Proc Am Coll Vet Internal Med San Diego*:566, 1989.
57. Cronin MTL, Leader GH: Coronary occlusion in a Thoroughbred colt, *Vet Rec* 64:8, 1952.
58. Rooney JR, Prickett ME, Crowe MW: Aortic ring rupture in stallions, *Vet Pathol* 4:268, 1967.
59. Pascoe RR, O'Sullivan BM: Sudden death in a Thoroughbred stallion, *Equine Vet J* 12:211, 1980.
60. Platt H: Sudden and unexpected deaths in horses: a review of 69 cases, *Br Vet J* 138:417, 1982.
61. Hughes PE, Howard EB: Endocardial fibroelastosis as a cause of sudden death in the horse, *Vet Clin North Am Equine Pract* 6:23, 1984.
62. Gelberg HB, Zachary JF, Everitt JI, et al: Sudden death in training and racing Thoroughbred horses, *J Am Vet Med Assoc* 187:1354, 1985.
63. Kiryu I, Nakamura T, Kaneko M, et al: Cardiopathology of sudden death in the racehorse, *Heart Vessels Suppl* 2:40, 1987.
64. Lucke VM: Sudden death, *Equine Vet J* 19:85, 1987.
65. Brown CM, Kaneene JB, Taylor RF: Sudden and unexpected death in horses and ponies: an analysis of 200 cases, *Equine Vet J* 20:99, 1988.
66. Allen JR, Heidel JR, Hodgson DR, et al: Spontaneous rupture of the great coronary vein in a pony, *Equine Vet J* 19:145, 1987.
67. Leblond A, Villard I, Leblond L, et al: A retrospective evaluation of the causes of death of 448 insured French horses in 1995, *Vet Res Commun* 24:85, 2000.
68. Schiff P, Knottenbelt DC: Sudden death in a 11-year-old Thoroughbred stallion, *Equine Vet Educ* 2:8, 1990.
69. Boden LA, Charles JA, Slocombe RF, et al: Sudden death in racing Thoroughbreds in Victoria, Australia, *Equine Vet J* 37:269, 2005.
70. Sisson S, Grossman JD: *Anatomy of the domestic animals,* Philadelphia, 1953, WB Saunders.
71. Geddes LA, Hoff HE, McCrady JD: Some aspects of the cardiovascular physiology of the horse, *Cardiovasc Res Cent Bull* 3:80, 1965.
72. Miller MS, Bonagura JD: Genesis of the equine electrocardiogram and indications for electrocardiography in clinical practice, *J Equine Vet Sci* 5:23, 1985.
73. Guyton AC: *The circulation textbook of medical physiology*, ed 7, Philadelphia, 1986, WB Saunders, pp 205-346.
74. Jones WE: *Equine sports medicine,* Philadelphia, 1988, Lea & Febiger.
75. Shepherd JT, Vanhoutte PM: *The human cardiovascular system*, 1992, Lippincott, Williams, and Wilkins.
76. Opie LH: *Heart physiology: from cell to circulation* , Philadelphia, 2004.
77. Schwarzwald CC, Bonagura JD, Muir WW 3rd: The cardiovascular system, In Muir WW 3rd, Hubbell JAE, editors: *Equine anesthesia: monitoring and emergency therapy*, ed 2, St Louis, 2009, WB Saunders, pp 37-100.
78. Muir WW 3rd: Cardiopulmonary resuscitation and the prevention of hypotensive emergencies in horses, *Proc Am Assoc Equine Pract* 30:117, 1984.
79. Muir WW: 3rd: Anesthetic complications and cardiopulmonary resuscitation in the horse. In Muir WW, Hubbell JAE, editors: *Equine anesthesia*, St Louis, 1992, Mosby Year Book, pp 461-484.
80. Rainey JW: A specific arthritis with pericarditis affecting young horses in Tasmania, *Aust Vet J* 20:204, 1944.
81. Ryan AF, Rainey JW: A specific arthritis with pericarditis affecting horses in Tasmania, *Aust Vet J* 21:146, 1945.
82. Wagner P, Miller R, Merritt F, et al: Constrictive pericarditis in the horse, *J Equine Med Surg* 1:242, 1977.
83. Reef VB: Advances in echocardiography, *Vet Clin North Am Equine Pract* 7:435, 1991.
84. Rantanen NW: Diseases of the heart, *Vet Clin North Am Equine Pract* 2:33, 1986.
85. Marr CM: Equine echocardiography—sound advice at the heart of the matter, *Br Vet J* 150:527, 1994.
86. Hardy J, Robertson JT, Reed SM: Constrictive pericarditis in a mare: attempted treatment by partial pericardiectomy, *Equine Vet J* 24:151, 1992.
87. Freestone JF, Thomas WP, Carlson GP, et al: Idiopathic effusive pericarditis with tamponade in the horse, *Equine Vet J* 19:38, 1987.
88. Dill SG, Simoncini DC, Bolton GR, et al: Fibrinous pericarditis in the horse, *J Am Vet Med Assoc* 180:266, 1982.
89. Carnine BL, Schneider G, Cook JE, et al: Pericardial mesothelioma in a horse, *Vet Pathol* 14:513, 1977.

90. Bonagura JD, Herring DS, Welker F: Echocardiography, *Vet Clin North Am Equine Pract* 1:311, 1985.
91. Bonagura JD, Blissitt KJ: Echocardiography, *Equine Vet J* (Suppl 1)19:5, 1995.
92. Birks EK, Hultgren BD: Pericardial haemangiosarcoma in a horse, *J Comp Pathol* 99:105, 1988.
93. Wijnberg ID, Vink-Nooteboom M: Sloet van Oldruitenborgh-Oosterbaan MM: Idiopathic pericardial effusion with tamponade in a Friesian gelding, *Tijdschr Diergeneeskd* 122:216, 1997.
94. Worth LT, Reef VB: Pericarditis in horses: 18 cases (1986-1995), *J Am Vet Med Assoc* 212:248, 1998.
95. Bolin DC, Donahue JM, Vickers ML, et al: Microbiologic and pathologic findings in an epidemic of equine pericarditis, *J Vet Diagn Invest* 17:38, 2005.
96. Perkins SL, Magdesian KG, Thomas WP, et al: Pericarditis and pleuritis caused by *Corynebacterium* pseudotuberculosis in a horse, *J Am Vet Med Assoc* 224:1133, 2004.
97. Seahorn JL, Slovis NM, Reimer JM, et al: Case-control study of factors associated with fibrinous pericarditis among horses in central Kentucky during spring 2001, *J Am Vet Med Assoc* 223:832, 2003.
98. Baker D, Kreeger J: Infiltrative lipoma in the heart of a horse, *Cornell Vet* 77:258, 1987.
99. Dill SG, Moise NS, Meschter CL: Cardiac failure in a stallion secondary to metastasis of an anaplastic pulmonary carcinoma, *Equine Vet J* 18:414, 1986.
100. Byars TD, Dainis CM, Seltzer KL, et al: Cranial thoracic masses in the horse: a sequel to pleuropneumonia, *Equine Vet J* 23:22, 1991.
101. Evans DL: Cardiac responses to exercise and training. In Marr CM, editor: *Cardiology of the horse*, London, 1999, WB Saunders, pp 32-46.
102. Buhl R, Ersboll AK, Eriksen L, et al: Changes over time in echocardiographic measurements in young Standardbred racehorses undergoing training and racing and association with racing performance, *J Am Vet Med Assoc* 226:1881, 2005.
103. Rugh KS, Garner HE, Sprouse RF, et al: Left ventricular hypertrophy in chronically hypertensive ponies, *Lab Anim Sci* 37:335, 1987.
104. Braunwald E, Sonnenblick EH, Ross J Jr: Mechanisms of cardiac contraction and relaxation. In Libby P, Bonow R, Zipes D, et al: *Braunwald's heart disease: a textbook of cardiovascular medicine*, ed 8, Philadelphia, 2008, WB Saunders.
105. Braunwald E: Pathophysiology of heart failure. In Libby P, Bonow R, Zipes D, et al: *Braunwald's heart disease: a textbook of cardiovascular medicine*, ed 8, Philadelphia, 2008, WB Saunders.
106. Cranley JJ, McCullagh KG: Ischaemic myocardial fibrosis and aortic strongylosis in the horse, *Equine Vet J* 13:35, 1981.
107. Dudan F, Rossi GL, Luginbuhl H: Cardiovascular study of the horse: relationships between vascular and tissue lesions in the myocardium. II, *Schweiz Arch Tierheilkd* 126:527, 1984.
108. Dudan F, Rossi GL, Luginbuhl H: Cardiovascular study in the horse: relationship between vascular and myocardial lesions. III, *Schweiz Arch Tierheilkd* 127:319, 1985.
109. Reef VB, Bain FT, Spencer PA: Severe mitral regurgitation in horses: clinical, echocardiographic and pathological findings, *Equine Vet J* 30:18, 1998.
110. Traub-Dargatz JL, Schlipf JW Jr, Boon JA, et al: Ventricular tachycardia and myocardial dysfunction in a horse, *J Am Vet Med Assoc* 205:1569, 1994.
111. Fregin GF: The cardiovascular system. In Mansmann RA, McCallister ES, Pratt PW, editors: *Equine medicine and surgery*, ed 3, Santa Barbara, CA, 1982, American Veterinary Publications Inc.
112. Bonagura JD: Equine heart disease. An overview, *Vet Clin North Am Equine Pract* 1:267, 1985.
113. Koblik PD, Hornof WJ: Diagnostic radiology and nuclear cardiology. Their use in assessment of equine cardiovascular disease, *Vet Clin North Am Equine Pract* 1:289, 1985.
114. Doonan GR, Brown CM, Mullaney TP, et al: Monensin poisoning in horses—an international incident, *Can Vet J* 30:165, 1989.
115. Mollenhauer HH, Rowe LD, Witzel DA: Effect of monensin on the morphology of mitochondria in rodent and equine striated muscle, *Vet Hum Toxicol* 26:15, 1984.
116. Amend JF, Mallon FM, Wren WB, et al: Equine monensin toxicosis: some experimental clinicopathologic observations, *Compend Cont Educ Pract Vet* 2:S172, 1980.
117. Amend JF, Nichelson RL, Freeland LR, et al: Clinical toxicology of an antibiotic ionophore (monensin) in ponies and horses: diagnostic markers and therapeutic considerations, *Comparative veterinary pharmacology, toxicology and therapy*, Lancaster, UK, 1986, MTP Press Ltd, pp 381-389.
118. Bezerra PS, Driemeier D, Loretti AP, et al: Monensin poisoning in Brazilian horses, *Vet Hum Toxicol* 41:383, 1999.
119. Bila CG, Perreira CL, Gruys E: Accidental monensin toxicosis in horses in Mozambique, *J S Afr Vet Assoc* 72:163, 2001.
120. Hughes KJ, Hoffmann KL, Hodgson DR: Long-term assessment of horses and ponies post exposure to monensin sodium in commercial feed, *Equine Vet J* 41:47, 2009.
121. Sweeney RW, Hamir AN, Fisher RR: Lymphosarcoma with urinary bladder infiltration in a horse, *J Am Vet Med Assoc* 199:1177, 1991.
122. Reef VB: Stress echocardiography and its role in performance assessment, *Vet Clin North Am Equine Pract* 17:179, 2001.
123. Bowen IM, Marr CM, Chester AH, et al: In-vitro contraction of the equine aortic valve, *J Heart Valve Dis* 13:593, 2004.
124. Deprez P, Sustronck B, Vanroy M, et al: A case of mitral-valve insufficiency due to a ruptured chorda tendinea in a horse, *Vlaams Diergeneesk Tijdschr* 62:180, 1993.
125. Brown CM: Acquired cardiovascular disease, *Vet Clin North Am Equine Pract* 1:371, 1985.
126. Critchley KL: An interventricular septal defect, pulmonary stenosis and bucuspid pulmonary valve in a Welsh pony foal, *Equine Vet J* 8:176, 1976.
127. Clark ES, Reef VB, Sweeney C, et al: Aortic valve insufficiency in a one-year-old colt, *J Am Vet Med Assoc* 191:841, 1987.
128. Stadler P, Weinberger T, Kinkel N, et al: B-mode-, M-mode- and Dopplersonographic findings in mitral valve insufficiency (MVI) in horses, *Am J Vet Med* 39:704, 1992.
129. Blissitt KJ, Bonagura JD: Colour flow Doppler echocardiography in normal horses, *Equine Vet J (Suppl 1)* 19:5, 1995.
130. Blissitt KJ, Bonagura JD: Colour flow Doppler echocardiography in horses with cardiac murmurs, *Equine Vet J Suppl* 82, 1995.
131. Ecke P, Malik R, Kannegieter NJ: Common atrioventricular canal in a foal, *N Z Vet J* 39:97, 1991.
132. Marr CM, Love S, Pirie HM, et al: Confirmation by Doppler echocardiography of valvular regurgitation in a horse with a ruptured chorda tendinea of the mitral valve, *Vet Rec* 127:376, 1990.
133. Amada A: Diagnosis and treatment of valvular disease of the heart in the horse, *Advances in Animal Cardiology* 20:7, 1987.
134. Mill J, Hanak J: Diagnosis of heart valve defects, arrhythmia and functional disorders of cardiac conduction in competition horses and racehorses, *Arch Exp Veterinarmed* 39:319, 1985.
135. Nilsfors L, Lombard CW, Weckner D, et al: Diagnosis of pulmonary valve endocarditis in a horse, *Equine Vet J* 23:479, 1991.
136. Yamaga Y, Too K: Diagnostic ultrasound imaging in domestic animals: two-dimensional and M-mode echocardiography, *Nippon Juigaku Zasshi* 46:493, 1984.

137. Reimer JM, Reef VB, Sommer M: Echocardiographic detection of pulmonic valve rupture in a horse with right-sided heart failure, *J Am Vet Med Assoc* 198:880, 1991.
138. Reef VB, Spencer PA: Echocardiographic evaluation of equine aortic insufficiency, *Am J Vet Res* 48:904, 1987.
139. Bonagura JD, Pipers FS: Echocardiographic features of aortic valve endocarditis in a dog, a cow, and a horse, *J Am Vet Med Assoc* 182:595, 1983.
140. Wingfield WE, Miller CW, Voss JL, et al: Echocardiography in assessing mitral valve motion in 3 horses with atrial fibrillation, *Equine Vet J* 12:181, 1980.
141. Stadler P, Deegen E: Echocardiography in horses, *I. Mitral valve insufficiency. II. Aortic valve insufficiency.* Wiesbaden Proceedings, 1990, p. 11.
142. Stadler P, Hoch M, Fruhauf B, et al: Echocardiography in horses with and without heart murmurs in aortic regurgitation, *Pferdeheilkunde* 11:373, 1995.
143. Stadler P, Hoch M, Radu I: Echocardiography in the horse with special regard to color-flow Doppler technique, *Prakt Tierarzt* 76:1015, 1995.
144. Buergelt CD, Cooley AJ, Hines SA, et al: Endocarditis in six horses, *Vet Pathol* 22:333, 1985.
145. Reef VB: Heart murmurs in horses: determining their significance with echocardiography, *Equine Vet J* (Suppl) 19: 71, 1995.
146. Brumbaugh GW, Thomas WP, Hodge TG: Medical management of congestive heart failure in a horse, *J Am Vet Med Assoc* 180:878, 1982.
147. Reef VB: Mitral valvular insufficiency associated with ruptured chordae tendineae in three foals, *J Am Vet Med Assoc* 191:329, 1987.
148. Travers CW, van den Berg JS: *Pseudomonas* spp. associated vegetative endocarditis in two horses, *J S Afr Vet Assoc* 66:172, 1995.
149. Reef VB, Lalezari K, deBoo J, et al: Pulsed-wave Doppler evaluation of intracardiac blood flow in 30 clinically normal Standardbred horses, *Am J Vet Res* 50:75, 1989.
150. Stadler P, Weinberger T, Deegen E: Pulsed Doppler-echocardiography in healthy warm-blooded horses, *J Vet Med A Physiol Pathol Clin Med* 40:757, 1993.
151. Wilson RB, Haffner JC: Right atrioventricular atresia and ventricular septal defect in a foal, *Cornell Vet* 77:187, 1987.
152. Roby KAW, Reef VB, Shaw DP, et al: Rupture of an aortic sinus aneurysm in a 15-year-old broodmare, *J Am Vet Med Assoc* 189:305, 1986.
153. Habermehl KH, Schmack KH: The topography of the heart valves in horses, cattle and dogs, *Anat Histol Embryol* 15:240, 1986.
154. Lescure F, Tamzali Y: TM echocardiography in the horse. II. Acquired valvular heart disease. L'echocardiographie TM chez le cheval. II. Les cardiopathies orificielles acquises, *Point Veterinaire* 15:9, 1983.
155. Rooney JR, Franks WC: Congenital cardiac anomalies in horses, *Vet Pathol* 1:454, 1964.
156. Bayly WM, Reed SM, Leathers CW, et al: Multiple congenital heart anomalies in five Arabian foals, *J Am Vet Med Assoc* 181:684, 1982.
157. McClure JJ, Gaber CE, Watters JW, et al: Complete transposition of the great arteries with ventricular septal defect and pulmonary stenosis in a Thoroughbred foal, *Equine Vet J* 15:377, 1983.
158. Tadmor A, Fischel R, Tov AS: A condition resembling hypoplastic left heart syndrome in a foal, *Equine Vet J* 15:175, 1983.
159. Musselman EE, LoGuidice RJ: Hypoplastic left ventricular syndrome in a foal, *J Am Vet Med Assoc* 185:542, 1984.
160. Crowe MW, Swerczek TW: Equine congenital defects, *Am J Vet Res* 46:353, 1985.
161. Physick-Sheard PW, Maxie MG, Palmer NC, et al: Atrial septal defect of the persistent ostium primum type with hypoplastic right ventricle in a Welsh pony foal, *Can J Comp Med* 49:429, 1985.
162. Reef VB: Cardiovascular disease in the equine neonate, *Vet Clin North Am Equine Pract* 1:117, 1985.
163. Reef VB, Mann P: Echocardiographic diagnosis of tricuspid atresia in 2 foals, *J Am Vet Med Assoc* 191:225, 1987.
164. Sojka JE: Persistent truncus arteriosus in a foal, *Vet Clin North Am Equine Pract* 9:19, 1987.
165. Zamora CS, Vitums A, Nyrop KA, et al: Atresia of the right atrioventricular orifice with complete transposition of the great arteries in a horse, *Anat Histol Embryol* 18:177, 1989.
166. Leipold HW, Saperstein G, Woollen NE: Congenital defects in foals. In Smith BP, editor: *Large animal internal medicine*, St Louis, 1990, CV Mosby, pp 137-146.
167. Cargile J, Lombard CW, Wilson JH, et al: Tetralogy of Fallot and segmental uterine aplasia in a three-year-old Morgan filly, *Cornell Vet* 81:411, 1991.
168. Hinchcliff KW, Adams WM: Critical pulmonary stenosis in a newborn foal, *Equine Vet J* 23:318, 1991.
169. Innes JM, Berger J, Francis J: Subacute bacterial endocarditis with pulmonary embolism in a horse, *Br Vet J* 106:245, 1950.
170. McCormick BS, Peet RL, Downes K: *Erysipelothrix rhusiopathiae* vegetative endocarditis in a horse, *Aust Vet J* 62:392, 1985.
171. Wagenaar G, Kroneman J, Breukink H: Endocardtis in the horse. *Blue Book Vet Prof* 12:38, 1985.
172. Dedrick P, Reef VB, Sweeney RW, et al: Treatment of bacterial endocarditis in a horse, *J Am Vet Med Assoc* 193:339, 1988.
173. Hamir AN, Reef VB: Complications of a permanent transvenous pacing catheter in a horse, *J Comp Pathol* 101:317, 1989.
174. Collatos C, Clark ES, Reef VB, et al: Septicemia, atrial fibrillation, cardiomegaly, left atrial mass, and *Rhodococcus equi* septic osteoarthritis in a foal, *J Am Vet Med Assoc* 197:1039, 1990.
175. Ewart S, Brown C, Derksen FJ, et al: *Serratia marcescens* endocarditis in a horse, *J Am Vet Med Assoc* 200:961, 1992.
176. Ball MA, Weldon AD: Vegetative endocarditis in an Appaloosa gelding, *Cornell Vet* 82:301, 1992.
177. Pace LW, Wirth NR, Foss RR, et al: Endocarditis and pulmonary aspergillosis in a horse, *J Vet Diagn Invest* 6:504, 1994.
178. deGroot J, Sloet van Oldruitenborgh-Oosterbaan MM, van der Linde Sipman JS, et al: Heart diseases in foals. A literature review exemplified by 2 case reports, *Tijdschrift voor Diergeneeskunde* 121:382, 1996.
179. Maxson AD, Reef VB: Bacterial endocarditis in horses: ten cases, *Equine Vet J* 29(394):1997, 1984-1995.
180. Church S, Harrigan KE, Irving AE, et al: Endocarditis caused by *Pasteurella caballi* in a horse, *Aust Vet J* 76:528, 1998.
181. Little D, Keene BW, Bruton C, et al: Percutaneous retrieval of a jugular catheter fragment from the pulmonary artery of a foal, *J Am Vet Med Assoc* 220:212, 2002.
182. Patteson MW, Cripps PJ: A survey of cardiac auscultatory findings in horses, *Equine Vet J* 25:409, 1993.
183. Patteson MW, Blissitt KJ: Evaluation of cardiac murmurs in horses. I. Clinical examination, *In Pract* 18:367, 1996.
184. Buhl R, Ersboll AK: Effect of light exercise on valvular regurgitation in Standardbred trotters, *Equine Vet J* (Suppl) 36:178, 2006.
185. Lightfoot G, Jose-Cunilleras E, Rogers K, et al: An echocardiographic and auscultation study of right heart responses to training in young national hunt thoroughbred horses, *Equine Vet J* (Suppl 36):153-158, August 2006.
186. Brown CM, Bell TG, Paradis MR, et al: Rupture of mitral chordae tendineae in two horses, *J Am Vet Med Assoc* 182:281, 1983.
187. Kiryu K, Kaneko M, Kanemaru T, et al: Cardiopathology of sinoatrial block in horses, *Nippon Juigaku Zasshi* 47:45, 1985.

188. Matsui K, Sugano S, Amada A: Heart rate and ECG response to twitching in Thoroughbred foals and mares, *Nippon Juigaku Zasshi* 48:305, 1986.
189. Matsui K, Sugano S: Relation of intrinsic heart rate and autonomic nervous tone to resting heart rate in the young and the adult of various domestic animals, *Nippon Juigaku Zasshi* 51:29, 1989.
190. Moore EN, Spear JF: Electrophysiological studies on atrial fibrillation, *Heart Vessels* (Suppl 2:32), 1987.
191. Meijler FL, Kroneman J, van der Tweel I, et al: Nonrandom ventricular rhythm in horses with atrial fibrillation and its significance for patients, *J Am Coll Cardiol* 4:316, 1984.
192. Meijler FL: Atrioventricular conduction versus heart size from mouse to whale, *J Am Coll Cardiol* 5:363, 1985.
193. Meijler FL, van der Tweel I: Comparative study of atrial fibrillation and AV conduction in mammals, *Heart Vessels* (Suppl 2:24), 1987.
194. Raekallio M: Long-term ECG recording with Holter monitoring in clinically healthy horses, *Acta Vet Scand* 33:71, 1992.
195. Tschudi P: Electrocardiography in the horse. II. Disorders of impulse formation and impulse conduction, *Tierarztl Prax* 13:529, 1985.
196. Littlewort MCG: The equine heart in health and disease. In Hickman J (ed): *Equine Surgery and Medicine*. London, 1986, Academic Press.
197. Reef VB: Heart murmurs irregularities and other cardiac abnormalities. In Brown C, editor: *Problems in equine medicine*, New York, 1992, Lea & Febiger.
198. Bonagura JD, Miller MS: Common conduction disturbances [ECG in the horse], *J Equine Vet Sci* 6:23, 1986.
199. Reef VB: Twenty-four hour rhythm monitoring. In Mayhew I, editor: *Equine medicine and surgery IV*, ed 4, Santa Barbara, CA, 1991, American Veterinary Publications, pp 213-214.
200. Slinker BK, Campbell KB, Alexander JE, et al: Arterial baroreflex control of heart rate in the horse, pig, *calf, Am J Vet Res* 43:1982, 1926.
201. Meijler FL: Atrial fibrillation: a new look at an old arrhythmia, *J Am Coll Cardiol* 2:391, 1983.
202. Horn J, Bailey S, Berhane Y, et al: Density and binding characteristics of beta-adrenoceptors in the normal and failing equine myocardium, *Equine Vet J* 34:411, 2002.
203. Badino P, Odore R, Re G: Are so many adrenergic receptor subtypes really present in domestic animal tissues? A pharmacological perspective, *Vet J* 170:163, 2005.
204. Evans DL, Rose RJ: Determination and repeatability of maximum oxygen uptake and other cardiorespiratory measurements in the exercising horse, *Equine Vet J* 20:94, 1988.
205. Evans DL, Rose RJ: Cardiovascular and respiratory responses in Thoroughbred horses during treadmill exercise, *J Exp Biol* 134:397, 1988.
206. Landgren GL, Gillespie JR, Fedde MR, et al: o_2 transport in the horse during rest and exercise, *Adv Exp Med Biol* 227:333, 1988.
207. Littlejohn A, Snow DH: Circulatory, respiratory and metabolic responses in Thoroughbred horses during the first 400 meters of exercise, *Eur J Appl Physiol* 58:307, 1988.
208. Marsland WP: Heart rate response to submaximal exercise in the Standardbred horse, *J Appl Physiol* 24:98, 1968.
209. Donaldson LL: Retrospective assessment of dobutamine therapy for hypotension in anesthetized horses, *Vet Surg* 17:53, 1988.
210. Swanson CR, Muir WW 3rd, Bednarski RM, et al: Hemodynamic responses in halothane-anesthetized horses given infusions of dopamine or dobutamine, *Am J Vet Res* 46:365, 1985.
211. Trim CM, Moore JN, White NA: Cardiopulmonary effects of dopamine hydrochloride in anaesthetized horses, *Equine Vet J* 17:41, 1985.
212. Whitton DL, Trim CM: Use of dopamine hydrochloride during general anesthesia in the treatment of advanced atrioventricular heart block in four foals, *J Am Vet Med Assoc* 187:1357, 1985.
213. Hinchcliff KW, McKeever KH, Muir WW 3rd: Hemodynamic effects of atropine, dobutamine, nitroprusside, phenylephrine, and propranolol in conscious horses, *J Vet Intern Med* 5:80, 1991.
214. Hardy J, Bednarski RM, Biller DS: Effect of phenylephrine on hemodynamics and splenic dimensions in horses, *Am J Vet Res* 55:1570, 1994.
215. Benamou AE, Marlin DJ, Lekeux P: Equine pulmonary and systemic haemodynamic responses to endothelin-1 and a selective ET(A) receptor antagonist, *Equine Vet J* 33:337, 2001.
216. Gasthuys F, deMoor A, Parmentier D: Cardiovascular effects of low dose calcium chloride infusions during halothane anaesthesia in dorsally recumbent ventilated ponies, *Zentralbl Veterinarmed A* 38:728, 1991.
217. Schwarzwald CC, Bonagura JD, Luis-Fuentes V: Effects of diltiazem on hemodynamic variables and ventricular function in healthy horses, *J Vet Intern Med* 19:703, 2005.
218. Rooney JR: Internal hemorrhage related to gestation in the mare, *Cornell Vet* 54:11, 1964.
219. van der Linde Sipman JS, Kroneman J, Meulenaar H, et al: Necrosis and rupture of the aorta and pulmonary trunk in four horses, *Vet Pathol* 22:51, 1985.
220. Marr CM, Reef VB, Brazil TJ, et al: Aorto-cardiac fistulas in seven horses, *Vet Radiol Ultrasound* 39:22, 1998.
221. Sleeper MM, Durando MM, Miller M, et al: Aortic root disease in four horses, *J Am Vet Med Assoc* 219:491, 2001.
222. Maxie MG, Physick-Sheard PW: Aortic-iliac thrombosis in horses, *Vet Pathol* 22:238, 1985.
223. Reef VB, Roby KAW, Richardson DW: Use of ultrasonography for the detection of aortic-iliac thrombosis in horses, *J Am Vet Med Assoc* 190:286, 1987.
224. Azzie MAJ: Clinical diagnosis of equine aortic iliac thrombosis and its histopathology as compared with that of the strongyle aneurysm, *Proc Am Assoc Equine Pract San Francisco*, 1972, p 43.
225. Edwards GB, Allen WE: Aorto-iliac thrombosis in two horses: clinical course of the disease and use of real-time ultrasonography to confirm diagnosis, *Equine Vet J* 384:1988, 1988.
226. Azzie MAJ: Aortic/iliac thrombosis of Thoroughbred horses, *Equine Vet J* 1:113, 1969.
227. Physick-Sheard PW, Maxie MG: Aortoiliofemoral arteriosclerosis. In Robinson NE, editor: *Current therapy in equine medicine*, ed 1, Phildelphia, 1983, WB Saunders, pp 153-155.
228. Reef VB: Vasculitis in Robinson NE, *Current Therapy in Equine Medicine II*, Philadelphia, 1992, WB Saunders 1987, pp 312-314.
229. Elliott J: Control of Cardiovascular Function: Physiology and Pharmacology. In Marr CM, editor: *Cardiology of the Horse*, London, 1999, WB Saunders, pp 15-31.
230. Blissitt KJ, Bonagura JD: Pulsed wave Doppler echocardiography in normal horses, *Equine Vet J* (Suppl 19):18, 1995.
231. Patteson MW, Gibbs C, Wotton PR, et al: Effects of sedation with detomidine hydrochloride on echocardiographic measurements of cardiac dimensions and indices of cardiac function in horses, *Equine Vet J Suppl* 33, 1995.
232. Raisis AL, Young LE, Blissitt KJ, et al: A comparison of the haemodynamic effects of isoflurane and halothane anaesthesia in horses, *Equine Vet J* 32:318, 2000.
233. Young LE, Blissitt KJ, Clutton RE, et al: Feasibility of transoesophageal echocardiography for evaluation of left ventricular performance in anaesthetised horses, *Equine Vet J* (Suppl 19):225, 1992.
234. Young LE, Blissitt KJ, Clutton RE, et al: Temporal effects of an infusion of dopexamine hydrochloride in horses anesthetized with halothane, *Am J Vet Res* 58:516, 1997.

235. Young LE, Blissitt KJ, Clutton RE, et al: Temporal effects of an infusion of dobutamine hydrochloride in horses anesthetized with halothane, *Am J Vet Res* 59:1027, 1998.
236. Young LE, Blissitt KJ, Clutton RE, et al: Haemodynamic effects of a sixty minute infusion of dopamine hydrochloride in horses anaesthetised with halothane, *Equine Vet J* 30:310, 1998.
237. Lightowler C, Piccione G, Fazio F, et al: Systolic time intervals assessed by 2-D echocardiography and spectral Doppler in the horse, *Anim Sci J* 74:505, 2003.
238. Welker FH, Muir WW 3rd: An investigation of the second heart sound in the normal horse, *Equine Vet J* 22:403, 1990.
239. Smith BL, Jones JH, Pascoe JR, et al: Why are left atrial pressures high in exercising horses? *Physiologist*, 1992.
240. Jones JH, Smith BL, Birks EK, et al: Left atrial and pulmonary arterial pressures in exercising horses, *Physiologist* 35:225, 1992.
241. Long KJ: Doppler echocardiography in the horse, *Equine Vet Educ* 2:15, 1990.
242. DeClercq D, VanLoon G, Tavernier R, et al: Atrial and ventricular electrical and contractile remodeling and reverse remodeling owing to short-term pacing-induced atrial fibrillation in horses, *J Vet Intern Med* 22:1353, 2008.
243. Schwarzwald CC, Hamlin RL, Bonagura JD, et al: Atrial, SA nodal, and AV nodal electrophysiology in standing horses: normal findngs and electrophysiologic effects of quinidine and diltiazem, *J Vet Intern Med* 21:166, 2007.
244. Schwarzwald CC, Schober KE, Bonagura JD: Methods and reliability of echocardiographic assessment of left atrial size and mechanical function in horses, *Am J Vet Res* 68:735, 2007.
245. Schwarzwald CC, Schober KE, Bonagura JD: Echocardiographic evidence of left atrial mechanical dysfunction after conversion of atrial fibrillation to sinus rhythm in 5 horses, *J Vet Intern Med* 21:820, 2007.
246. Rugh KS, Garner HE, Miramonti JR, et al: Left ventricular function and haemodynamics in ponies during exercise and recovery, *Equine Vet J* 21:39, 1989.
247. Beglinger R, Becker M: Comparative study of the contractility measurement max. dp/dt in the horse, cow, swine, dog, cat and man, *Schweiz Arch Tierheilkd* 126:265, 1984.
248. Hillidge CJ, Lees P: Left ventricular systole in conscious and anesthetized horses, *Am J Vet Res* 38:675, 1977.
249. Koblik PD, Hornof WJ, Rhode EA, et al: Left ventricular ejection fraction in the normal horse determined by first-pass nuclear angiocardiography, *Vet Radiol Ultrasound* 26:53, 1985.
250. Hillidge CJ, Lees P: Studies of left ventricular isotonic function in conscious and anaesthetised horse, *Br Vet J* 133:446, 1977.
251. Robine FJ: Morphological and functional measurements on the equine heart by means of two-dimensional echocardiography, Dissertation, *Teirarztliche Hochscule*, Hanover, Germany, 1991.
252. Lescure F, Tamzali Y: Reference values for echocardiography applied to sport horses (English Thoroughbreds and French riding horses), *Rev Med Vet (Toulouse)* 135:405, 1984.
253. Lombard CW, Evans M, Martin L, et al: Blood pressure, electrocardiogram and echocardiogram measurements in the growing pony foal, *Equine Vet J* 16:342, 1984.
254. Stewart JH, Rose RJ, Barko AM: Echocardiography in foals from birth to three months old, *Equine Vet J* 16:332, 1984.
255. Van-Aarde MN, Littlejohn A, Van der Walt JJ: The ratio of cardiopulmonary blood volume to stroke volume as an index of cardiac function in horses, *Vet Res Commun* 8:293, 1984.
256. Reef VB: Evaluation of the equine cardiovascular system, *Vet Clin North Am Equine Pract* 1:275, 1985.
257. Goldberg SJ, Allen HD, Marx GR, et al: *Doppler echocardiography*, 2nd edition, Philadelphia, 1988, Lea & Febiger.
258. Wetmore LA, Derksen FJ, Blaze CA, et al: Mixed venous oxygen tension as an estimate of cardiac output in anesthetized horses, *Am J Vet Res* 48:971, 1987.
259. Bright JM: Ventricular function. In Marr CM, editor: *Cardiology of the horse*, London, 1999, WB Saunders, pp 3-14.
260. Hillidge CJ, Lees P: Cardiac output in the conscious and anaesthetised horse, *Equine Vet J* 7:16, 1975.
261. Muir WW 3rd, Skarda R, Milne D: Estimation of cardiac output in the horse by thermodilution techniques, *Am J Vet Res* 37:697, 1976.
262. Thomas DP, Fregin GF, Gerber NH, et al: Effects of training on cardiorespiratory function in the horse, *Am J Physiol* 245:R160, 1983.
263. Evans DL: Cardiovascular adaptations to exercise and training, *Vet Clin North Am Equine Pract* 1:513, 1985.
264. Swanson CR, Muir WW 3rd: Dobutamine-induced augmentation of cardiac output does not enhance respiratory gas exchange in anesthetized recumbent healthy horses, *Am J Vet Res* 47:1573, 1986.
265. Thomas WP, Madigan JE, Backus KQ, et al: Systemic and pulmonary haemodynamics in normal neonatal foals, *J Reprod Fertil Suppl* 35:623, 1987.
266. Ward DS, Fessler JF, Bottoms GD: In vitro calibration and surgical implantation of electromagnetic blood flow transducers for measurement of left coronary blood flow and cardiac output in the pony, *Am J Vet Res* 48:1120, 1987.
267. Weber JM, Dobson GP, Parkhouse WS, et al: Cardiac output and oxygen consumption in exercising Thoroughbred horses, *Am J Physiol* 253:R890, 1987.
268. Bertone JJ: Cardiovascular effects of hydralazine HCl administration in horses, *Am J Vet Res* 49:618, 1988.
269. Gasthuys F, deMoor A, Parmentier D: Haemodynamic changes during sedation in ponies, *Vet Res Commun* 14:309, 1990.
270. Hinchcliff KW, McKeever KH, Schmall LM, et al: Renal and systemic hemodynamic responses to sustained submaximal exertion in horses, *Am J Physiol* 258:R1177, 1990.
271. Schmall LM, Muir WW 3rd, Robertson JT: Haemodynamic effects of small volume hypertonic saline in experimentally induced haemorrhagic shock, *Equine Vet J* 22:273, 1990.
272. Lepiz ML, Keegan RD, Bayly WM, et al: Comparison of Fick and thermodilution cardiac output determinations in standing horses, *Res Vet Sci* 85:307, 2008.
273. Durando MM, Corley KT, Boston RC, et al: Cardiac output determination by use of lithium dilution during exercise in horses, *Am J Vet Res* 69:1054, 2008.
274. Valverde A, Giguere S, Morey TE, et al: Comparison of noninvasive cardiac output measured by use of partial carbon dioxide rebreathing or the lithium dilution method in anesthetized foals, *Am J Vet Res* 68:141, 2007.
275. Giguere S, Bucki E, Adin DB, et al: Cardiac output measurement by partial carbon dioxide rebreathing, 2-dimensional echocardiography, and lithium-dilution method in anesthetized neonatal foals, *J Vet Intern Med* 19:737, 2005.
276. Long KJ, Young LE, Utting JE et al: Determination of cardiac output in the standing horse by Doppler echocardiography and thermodilution, *Proc 30th British Equine Vet Assoc Congress* 30, 1991.
277. Mizuno Y, Aida H, Hara H, et al: Comparison of methods of cardiac-output measurements determined by dye dilution, pulsed Doppler-echocardiography and thermodilution in horses, *J Vet Med Sci* 56:1, 1994.
278. Stadler P, Kinkel N, Deegen E: Evaluation of systolic heart function of the horse with PW-Doppler-echocardiography compared with thermodilution, *Dtsch Tierarztl Wochenschr* 101:312, 1994.
279. Aida H, Hara H, Fujinaga T, et al: Comparison of methods of cardiac output measurements determined by dye dilution, pulsed Doppler echocardiography and thermodilution in horses, *J Vet Med Sci* 56:1, 1994.

280. Young LE, Blissitt KJ, Bartram DH, et al: Measurement of cardiac output by transoesophageal Doppler echocardiography in anaesthetized horses: comparison with thermodilution, *Br J Anaesth* 77:773, 1996.
281. Cipone M, Pietra M, Gandini G, et al: Pulsed wave-Doppler ultrasonographic evaluation of the common carotid artery in the resting horse: physiologic data, *Vet Radiol Ultrasound* 38:200, 1997.
282. Blissitt KJ, Young LE, Jones RS, et al: Measurement of cardiac output in standing horses by Doppler echocardiography and thermodilution, *Equine Vet J* 29:18, 1997.
283. Gratopp M: Estimation of cardiac output by Doppler echocardiography in healthy horses and horses with heart disease, Dissertation, Hanover, Tierarztl Hochsch, Hanover, Germany, 1996.
284. Kinkel N: Determination of cardiac minute volume in horses by Doppler ultrasonography in comparison with conventional methods, 1993, 169 pp 169 pp:1998.
285. Linton RA, Young LE, Marlin DJ, et al: Cardiac output measured by lithium dilution, thermodilution, and transesophageal Doppler echocardiography in anesthetized horses, *Am J Vet Res* 61:731, 2000.
286. Brumbaugh GW, Thomas WP, Enos LR, et al: A pharmacokinetic study of digoxin in the horse, *J Vet Pharmacol Ther* 6:163, 1983.
287. Button C, Gross DR, Johnston JT, et al: Digoxin pharmacokinetics, bioavailability, efficacy, and dosage regimens in the horse, *Am J Vet Res* 41:1388, 1980.
288. Dyson DH, Pascoe PJ: Influence of preinduction methoxamine, lactated Ringer solution, or hypertonic saline solution infusion or postinduction dobutamine infusion on anesthetic-induced hypotension in horses, *Am J Vet Res* 51:17, 1990.
289. Francfort P, Schatzmann HJ: Pharmacological experiments as a basis for the administration of digoxin in the horse, *Res Vet Sci* 20:84, 1976.
290. Gasthuys F, deMoor A, Parmentier D: Influence of digoxin followed by dopamine on the cardiovascular depression during a standard halothane anaesthesia in dorsally recumbent, ventilated ponies, *Zentralbl Veterinarmed A* 38:585, 1991.
291. Grubb TL, Foreman JH, Benson GJ, et al: Hemodynamic effects of calcium gluconate administered to conscious horses, *J Vet Intern Med* 10:401, 1996.
292. Keen P: The use of drugs in the treatment of cardiac disease in the horse, *Equine Vet Educ* 2:81, 1990.
293. Meijler FL, van der Tweel I: Digitalis and atrial fibrillation in 1985, *Ned Tijdschr Geneeskd* 129:729, 1985.
294. Muir WW 3rd, McGuirk SM: Pharmacology and pharmacokinetics of drugs used to treat cardiac disease in horses, *Vet Clin North Am Equine Pract* 1:335, 1985.
295. Muir WW 3rd, McGuirk S: Cardiovascular drugs. Their pharmacology and use in horses, *Vet Clin North Am Equine Pract* 3:37, 1987.
296. Muir WW 3rd: Cardiovascular effects of dopexamine HCl in conscious and halothane-anaesthetised horses, *Equine Vet J* 24:24, 1992.
297. Pedersoli WM Belmonte AA, Purohit RC, et al: Pharmacokinetics of digoxin in the horse, *J Equine Med Surg* 2:384, 1978.
298. Pedersoli WM, Ravis WR, Belmonte AA, et al: Pharmacokinetics of a single, orally administered dose of digoxin in horses, *Am J Vet Res* 42:1412, 1981.
299. Staudacher G: Individual glycoside treatment by means of serum concentration determination in cardiac insufficiency in horses, *Berl Munch Tierarztl Wochenschr* 102:1, 1989.
300. Sweeney RW, Reef VB, Reimer JM: Pharmacokinetics of digoxin administered to horses with congestive heart failure, *Am J Vet Res* 54:1108, 1993.
301. Trim CM: Inotropic agents and vasopressors in equine anesthesia, *Compend Cont Educ Pract Vet* 13:118, 1991.
302. Muir WW 3rd: The haemodynamic effects of milrinone HCl in halothane anaesthetised horses, *Equine Vet J* (Suppl) 9:108, 1995.
303. Long-Blissitt KJ, Bonagura JD, Darke PGG: Standardized imaging technique for guided M-mode and Doppler echocardiography in the horse, *Equine Vet J* 24:226, 1992.
304. Patteson MW, Gibbs C, Wotton PR, et al: Echocardiographic measurements of cardiac dimensions and indices of cardiac function in normal adult Thoroughbred horses, *Equine Vet J* (Suppl 19):18-27, September 1995.
305. Slater JD, Herrtage ME: Echocardiographic measurements of cardiac dimensions in normal ponies and horses, *Equine Vet J* (Suppl 19):28-32, September 1995.
306. Bakos Z, Voros K, Jarvinen T, et al: Two-dimensional and M-mode echocardiographic measurements of cardiac dimensions in healthy standardbred trotters, *Acta Vet Hung* 50:273, 2002.
307. Kriz NG, Rose RJ: Repeatability of standard transthoracic echocardiographic measurements in horses, *Aust Vet J* 80:362, 2002.
308. Gehlen H, Marnette S, Rohn K, et al: Precision-controlled echocardiographic left ventricular function parameters by repeated measurement on three consecutive days in trained and untrained Warmblood horses, *Dtsch Tierarztl Wochenschr* 112:48, 2005.
309. Nuytten J, Deprez P, Picavet T, et al: Heart failure in horses: hemodynamic monitoring and determination of LDH1 concentration, *J Equine Vet Sci* 8:214, 1988.
310. Fruhauf B, Stadler P, Deegen E: Evaluation of pulmonary wedge pressure in horses with and without left-heart abnormalities detected by echocardiography, *Pferdeheilkunde* 12:544, 1996.
311. Gehlen H, Bubeck K, Stadler P: Pulmonary artery wedge pressure measurement in healthy Warmblood horses and in Warmblood horses with mitral valve insufficiencies of various degrees during standardized treadmill exercise, *Res Vet Sci* 77:257, 2004.
312. Milne DW, Muir WW 3rd, Skarda RT: Pulmonary artery wedge pressure blood gas tensions and pH in the resting horse, *Am J Vet Res* 36:1431, 1975.
313. Gehlen H, Bubeck K, Rohn K, et al: Pulmonary artery wedge pressure during treadmill exercise in Warmblood horses with atrial fibrillation, *Res Vet Sci* 81:134, 2006.
314. Gehlen H, Groner U, Rohn K, et al: Day-to-day variability of cardiac pressure values in horses measured with right heart catheterization on 3 consecutive days, *Berl Munch Tierarztl Wochenschr* 119:400, 2006.
315. Muir WW 3rd, Sams RA, Hubbell JAE, et al: Effects of enalaprilat on cardiorespiratory, hemodynamic, and hematologic variables in exercising horses, *Am J Vet Res* 62:1008, 2001.
316. Rugh KS, Garner HE, Hatfield DG, et al: Ischemia induced development of functional coronary collateral circulation in ponies, *Cardiovasc Res* 21:730, 1987.
317. Martin BB Jr, Reef VB, Parente EJ, et al: Causes of poor performance of horses during training, racing, or showing: 348 cases (1992-1996), *J Am Vet Med Assoc* 216:554, 2000.
318. Parks CM, Manohar M: Distribution of blood flow during moderate and strenuous exercise in ponies (*Equus caballus*), *Am J Vet Res* 44:1983, 1861.
319. Parks C, Manohar M, Lundeen G: Regional myocardial blood flow and coronary vascular reserve in unanesthetized ponies during pacing-induced ventricular tachycardia, *J Surg Res* 35:119, 1983.
320. Parks CM, Manohar M: Transmural coronary vasodilator reserve and flow distribution during severe exercise in ponies, *J Appl Physiol* 54:1641, 1983.

321. Manohar M: Transmural coronary vasodilator reserve and flow distribution during maximal exercise in normal and splenectomized ponies, *J Physiol Lond* 387:425, 1987.
322. Manohar M, Parks C: Transmural coronary vasodilator reserve in ponies at rest and during maximal exercise, *J Appl Physiol* 54:1641, 1983.
323. Parks CM, Manohar M: Transmural distribution of myocardial blood flow during graded treadmill exercise in ponies, In Persson SGB, Rose RJ, editors: *Equine exercise physiology*, Cambridge, England, 1983, Granta, pp 105-120.
324. Parks CM, Manohar M: Regional blood flow changes in response to near maximal exercise in ponies: a review, *Equine Vet J* 17:311, 1985.
325. Reddy VK, Kammula RG, Graham TC, et al: Regional coronary blood flow in ponies, *Am J Vet Res* 37:1261, 1976.
326. Thornton JR: Exercise testing, *Vet Clin North Am Equine Pract* 1:573, 1985.
327. Evans DL, Rose RJ: Dynamics of cardiorespiratory function in Standardbred horses during different intensities of constant-load exercise, *J Comp Physiol* 157:791, 1988.
328. Foreman JH, Bayly WM, Grant BD, et al: Standardized exercise test and daily heart rate responses of Thoroughbreds undergoing conventional race training and detraining, *Am J Vet Res* 51:914, 1990.
329. Rose RJ, Hendrickson DK, Knight PK: Clinical exercise testing in the normal thoroughbred racehorse, *Aust Vet J* 67:345, 1990.
330. Seeherman HJ, Morris EA: Comparison of yearling, two-year-old and adult Thoroughbreds using a standardised exercise test, *Equine Vet J* 23:175, 1991.
331. Reef VB: Ambulatory and exercise electrocardiography and post-exercise echocardiography. In Marr CM, editor: *Cardiology of the horse*, London, 1999, WB Saunders, pp 150-160.
332. Durando MM, Slack J, Reef VB, et al: Right ventricular pressure dynamics and stress echocardiography in pharmacological and exercise stress testing, *Equine Vet J* (Suppl 36):183-192, August 2006.
333. Glendinning SA: The clinician's approach to equine cardiology, *Equine Vet J* 9:176, 1977.
334. King JM: Anomalous epicardial lymphatics, *Vet Med* 88:512, 1993.
335. Glazier B: Clinical aspects of equine cardiology, *Pract* 9:98, 1987.
336. Fregin GF: Medical evaluation of the cardiovascular system, *Vet Clin North Am Equine Pract* 8:329, 1992.
337. Jose-Cunilleras E, Young LE, Newton JR, et al: Cardiac arrhythmias during and after treadmill exercise in poorly performing Thoroughbred racehorses, *Equine Vet J* (Suppl 36):163-170, August 2006.
338. Gerring EL: Auscultation of the equine heart, *Equine Vet Educ* 2:22, 1990.
339. Kammerer H: Auscultation of the horse's heart, using a new stethoscope, *Dtsch Tierarztl Wochenschr* 90:521, 1983.
340. Littlejohn A, Button C: When is a murmur not a murmur? *J S Afr Vet Assoc* 53:130, 1982.
341. Littlewort MCG: The clinical auscultation of the equine heart, *Vet Rec* 74:1247, 1962.
342. Lombard CW: Cardiovascular diseases. In Koterba A, editor: *Equine clinical neonatology*, pp. 240-261; Philadelphia, 1990.
343. Machida N, Yasuda J, Too K: Auscultatory and phonocardiographic studies on the cardiovascular system of the newborn Thoroughbred foal, *Jpn J Vet Res* 35:235, 1987.
344. McGuirk SM, Muir WW 3rd: Diagnosis and treatment of cardiac arrhythmias, *Vet Clin North Am Equine Pract* 1:353, 1985.
345. Moore BR: Lower respiratory-tract disease, *Vet Clin North Am Equine Pract* 12:457, 1996.
346. Reef VB: The significance of cardiac auscultatory findings in horses—insight into the age-old dilemma, *Equine Vet J* 25:393, 1993.
347. Reimer JM: Performing cardiac auscultation on horses, *Vet Med* 88:660, 1993.
348. Rossdale PD: Clinical studies on the newborn Thoroughbred foal. II. Heart rate, *Br Vet J* 123:521, 1967.
349. Savage CJ: Evaluation of the equine respiratory system using physical examination and endoscopy, *Vet Clin North Am Equine Pract* 13(3):443-462, 1997.
350. Vanselow B, McCarthy M, Gay CC: A phonocardiographic study of equine heart sounds, *Aust Vet J* 54:161, 1978.
351. Blissitt KJ: Auscultation. In Marr CM, editor: *Cardiology of the horse*, London, 1999, WB Saunders, pp 73-92.
352. Young LE, Helwegen MM, Rogers K, et al: Associations between exercise-induced pulmonary haemorrhage, right ventricular dimensions and atrioventricular valve regurgitation in conditioned national hunt racehorses, *Equine Vet J* (Suppl 36):193-197, August 2006.
353. Naylor JM, Wolker RE, Pharr JW: An assessment of the terminology used by diplomates and students to describe the character of equine mitral and aortic valve regurgitant murmurs: correlations with the physical properties of the sounds, *J Vet Intern Med* 17:332, 2003.
354. Marr CM, Reef VB: Physiological valvular regurgitation in clinically normal young racehorses: prevalence and two-dimensional colour flow Doppler echocardiographic characteristics, *Equine Vet J* (Suppl 19):56-62, September 1995.
355. Naylor JM, Yadernuk LM, Pharr JW, et al: An assessment of the ability of diplomates, practitioners, and students to describe and interpret recordings of heart murmurs and arrhythmia, *J Vet Intern Med* 15:507, 2001.
356. Abbott J: Auscultation: what type of practice makes perfect? *J Vet Intern Med* 15:505, 2001.
357. Bakos Z, Voros K: Comparative examination of percussional and echocardiographic determination of the cardiac dullness area in healthy horses, *Acta Vet Hung* 55:277, 2007.
358. Hintz HF, Collyer C, Brant T: Resting heart rates in draft horses, *Vet Clin North Am Equine Pract* 11:7, 1989.
359. Reef VB: Frequency of cardiac arrhythmias and their significance in normal horses. In *Proceedings of the American College of Veterinary Internal Medicine*, 1989, San Diego, p 506.
360. Bonagura JD, Miller MS: Electrocardiography, In Jones WE, editor: *Equine sports medicine*, Philadelphia, 1985, Lea & Febiger, pp 89-106.
361. Bertone JJ: Atrial fibrillation in the horse: diagnosis; prognosis, treatment, *Vet Clin North Am Equine Pract* 6:6, 1984.
362. Bertone JJ, Wingfield WE: Atrial fibrillation in horses, *Compend Cont Educ Pract Vet* 9:763, 1987.
363. Deem DA, Fregin GF: Atrial fibrillation in horses, *J Am Vet Med Assoc* 180:261, 1982.
364. Li JK: Laminar and turbulent flow in the mammalian aorta: Reynolds number, *J Theor Biol* 135:409, 1988.
365. Marr CM: Cardiac murmurs: congenital heart disease. In Marr CM, editor: *Cardiology of the horse*, London, 1999, WB Saunders, pp 210-232.
366. Marr CM: Cardiac murmurs: acquired valvular disease. In Marr CM, editor: *Cardiology of the horse*, London, 1999, WB Saunders, pp 231-255.
367. Machida N, Yasuda J, Too K, et al: A morphological study on the obliteration processes of the ductus arteriosus in the horse, *Equine Vet J* 20:249, 1988.
368. Andersson B, Augustinsson O, Bademo E, et al: Systemic and centrally mediated angiotensin II effects in the horse, *Acta Physiol Scand* 129:143, 1987.
369. Bailey JE, Dunlop CI, Chapman PL, et al: Indirect Doppler ultrasonic measurement of arterial blood-pressure results in a large measurement error in dorsally recumbent anesthetized horses, *Equine Vet J* 26:70, 1994.

370. Branson KR: A clinical-evaluation of an oscillometric blood-pressure monitor on anesthetized horses, *J Equine Vet Sci* 17:537, 1997.
371. Ellis PM: The indirect measurement of arterial blood pressure in the horse, *Equine Vet J* 7:22, 1975.
372. Erickson BK, Erickson HH, Coffman JR: Pulmonary artery, aortic and oesophageal pressure changes during high intensity treadmill exercise in the horse: a possible relation to exercise-induced pulmonary haemorrhage, *Equine Vet J* (Suppl 9): 47-52, June 1990.
373. Franco RM, Ousey JC, Cash RS, et al: Study of arterial blood pressure in newborn foals using an electronic sphygmomanometer, *Equine Vet J* 18:475, 1986.
374. Fritsch R, Bosler K: Monitoring circulation in the horse during sedation and anesthesia by indirect blood pressure measurement, *Berl Munch Tierarztl Wochenschr* 98:166, 1985.
375. Fritsch R, Hausmann R: Indirect blood pressure determination in the horse with the Dinamap 1255 research monitor, *Tierarztl Prax* 16:373, 1988.
376. Gasthuys F, Muylle E, deMoor A, et al: Influence of premedication and body position during halothane anaesthesia on intracardial pressures in the horse, *Zentralbl Veterinarmed A* 35:729, 1988.
377. Will JA, Bisgard GE: Cardiac catheterization of unanesthetized large domestic animals, *J Appl Physiol* 33:400, 1972.
378. Gay CC, McCarthy M, Reynolds WT, et al: A method for indirect measurement of arterial blood pressure in the horse, *Aust Vet J* 53:163, 1977.
379. Geddes LA, Chaffee V, Whistler SJ, et al: Indirect mean blood pressure in the anesthetized pony, *Am J Vet Res* 38:2055, 1977.
380. Glen JB: Indirect blood pressure measurement in anesthetized animals, *Vet Rec* 87:349, 1970.
381. Hall LW: Cardiovascular and pulmonary effects of recumbency in two conscious ponies, *Equine Vet J* 16:89, 1984.
382. Johnson JH, Garner HE, Hutcheson DP: Ultrasonic measurement of arterial blood pressure in conditioned Thoroughbreds, *Equine Vet J* 8:55, 1976.
383. Kvart C: An ultrasonic method for indirect blood pressure measurement in the horse, *J Equine Med Surg* 3:16, 1979.
384. Latshaw H, Fessler JF, Whistler SJ, et al: Indirect measurement of mean blood pressure in the normotensive and hypotensive horses, *Equine Vet J* 11:191, 1979.
385. Parry BW, McCarthy MA, Anderson GA, et al: Correct occlusive bladder width for indirect blood pressure measurement in horses, *Am J Vet Res* 43:50, 1982.
386. Parry BW, Gay CC, McCarthy MA: Influence of head height on arterial blood pressure in standing horses, *Am J Vet Res* 41:1626, 1980.
387. Parry BW: Resting blood pressure values in various equine clinical cases, *J Equine Vet Sci* 4:49, 1984.
388. Parry BW, Anderson GA: Importance of uniform cuff application for equine blood pressure measurement, *Equine Vet J* 16:529, 1984.
389. Parry BW, McCarthy MA, Anderson GA: Survey of resting blood pressure values in clinically normal horses, *Equine Vet J* 16:53, 1984.
390. Physick-Sheard PW: Cardiovascular response to exercise and training in the horse, *Vet Clin North Am Equine Pract* 1:383, 1985.
391. Taylor PM: Techniques and clinical application of arterial blood pressure, *Equine Vet J* 13:271, 1981.
392. Wagner AE, Brodbelt DC: Arterial blood-pressure monitoring in anesthetized animals, *J Am Vet Med Assoc* 210:1279, 1997.
393. Wens HM: Catheterization of the heart by J.B.A. Chauveau in 1861, *Tierarztliche Umschau* 44:90, 1989.
394. Bayly WM, Gabel AA, Barr SA: Cardiovascular effects of submaximal aerobic training on a treadmill in Standardbred horses, using a standardized exercise test, *Am J Vet Res* 44:544, 1983.
395. Muir WW 3rd, Wade A, Grospitch B: Automatic noninvasive sphygmomanometry in horses, *J Am Vet Med Assoc* 182:1230, 1983.
396. Tillotson PJ, Kooper PH: Treatment of aortic thrombus in a horse, *J Am Vet Med Assoc* 149:766, 1966.
397. Tithof PK, Rebhun WC, Dietze AE: Ultrasonographic diagnosis of aorto-iliac thrombosis, *Cornell Vet* 75:540, 1985.
398. Dickson LR, Badcoe LM, Burbidge H, et al: Jugular thrombophlebitis resulting from an anesthetic induction technique in the horse, *Equine Vet J* 22:177, 1990.
399. Marr CM: Heart failure. In Marr CM, editor: *Cardiology of the horse*, London, 1999, WB Saunders, pp 289-311.
400. Hall MC, Steel JD, Stewart GA: Cardiac monitoring during exercise tests in the horse. II. Heart rate responses to exercise, *Aust Vet J* 52:1, 1976.
401. Maier-Bock H, Ehrlein HJ: Heart rate during a defined exercise test in horses with heart and lung diseases, *Equine Vet J* 10:235, 1978.
402. Rose RJ, Allen JR, Hodgson DR, et al: Responses to submaximal treadmill exercise and training in the horse: changes in haematology, arterial blood gas and acid base measurements, plasma biochemical values and heart rate, *Vet Rec* 113:612, 1983.
403. Rose RJ, Lovell DK: Symposium on exercise physiology, *Vet Clin North Am Equine Pract* 1:437, 1985.
404. Evans DL, Rose RJ: Method of investigation of the accuracy of four digitally displaying heart rate meters suitable for use in the exercising horse, *Equine Vet J* 18:129, 1986.
405. Evans DL, Rose RJ: Cardiovascular and respiratory responses to submaximal exercise training in the Thoroughbred horse, *Pflugers Arch* 411:316, 1988.
406. Erickson BK, Erickson HH, Coffman JR: Pulmonary artery and aortic pressure changes during high intensity treadmill exercise in the horse: effect of furosemide and phentolamine, *Equine Vet J* 24:215, 1992.
407. Evans DL, Harris RC, Snow DH: Correlation of racing performance with blood lactate and heart rate after exercise in Thoroughbred horses, *Equine Vet J* 25:441, 1993.
408. Christley RM, Hodgson DR, Evans DL, et al: Cardiorespiratory responses to exercise in horses with different grades of idiopathic laryngeal hemiplegia, *Equine Vet J* 29:6, 1997.
409. Hackett RP, Ducharme NG, Gleed RD, et al: Oral nitroglycerin paste did not lower pulmonary capillary pressure during treadmill exercise, *Equine Vet J Suppl* 30:153, 1999.
410. Betros CL, McKeever KH, Kearns CF, et al: Effects of ageing and training on maximal heart rate and VO2max, *Equine Vet J* (Suppl 34):100-105, September 2002.
411. Durando MM, Reef VB, Birks EK: Right ventricular pressure dynamics during exercise: relationship to stress echocardiography, *Equine Vet J* (Suppl 34):472-477, 2002.
412. Ohmura H, Hiraga A, Matsui A, et al: Physiological responses of young Thoroughbreds during their first year of race training, *Equine Vet J* (Suppl 34):140-146, September 2002.
413. Frye MA, Bright JM, Dargatz DA, et al: A comparison of dobutamine infusion to exercise as a cardiac stress test in healthy horses, *J Vet Intern Med* 17:58, 2003.
414. Gehlen H, Bubeck K, Stadler P: Pulmonary wedge pressure and heart frequency measurements during standardized treadmill exercise for extension of left atrial function diagnosis in warmblood horses, *Dtsch Tierarztl Wochenschr* 110:280, 2003.
415. Zucca E, Ferrucci F, Di FV, et al: The use of electrocardiographic recording with Holter monitoring during treadmill exercise to evaluate cardiac arrhythmias in racehorses, *Vet Res Commun* 27(Suppl 1):811, 2003.

416. Meyer C, Gerber R, Guthrie AJ: The use of the standard exercise test to establish the clinical significance of mild echocardiographic changes in a Thoroughbred poor performer, *J S Afr Vet Assoc* 75:100, 2004.
417. Durando M: Diagnosing cardiac disease in equine athletes: the role of stress testing, *Equine Vet J* 37:101, 2005.
418. Gehlen H, Marnette S, Rohn K, et al: Stress echocardiography in Warmblood horses: comparison of dobutamine/atropine with treadmill exercise as cardiac stressors, *J Vet Intern Med* 20:562, 2006.
419. Gramkow HL, Evans DL: Correlation of race earnings with velocity at maximal heart rate during a field exercise test in Thoroughbred racehorses, *Equine Vet J* (Suppl 36):118-122, August 2006.
420. Hada T, Ohmura H, Mukai K, et al: Utilization of the time constant calculated from heart rate recovery after exercise for evaluation of autonomic activity in horses, *Equine Vet J* (Suppl) 36:141, 2006.
421. Mukai K, Ohmura H, Hiraga A, et al: Effect of detraining on cardiorespiratory variables in young thoroughbred horses, *Equine Vet J* (Suppl) 36: 210, 2006.
422. Nankervis KJ, Williams RJ: Heart rate responses during acclimation of horses to water treadmill exercise, *Equine Vet J* (Suppl 36):110-112, August 2006.
423. Sandersen C, Detilleux J, Art T, et al: Exercise and pharmacological stress echocardiography in healthy horses, *Equine Vet J* (Suppl 36):159-162, August 2006.
424. Sandersen CF, Detilleux J, de Moffarts B, et al: Effect of atropine-dobutamine stress test on left ventricular echocardiographic parameters in untrained Warmblood horses, *J Vet Intern Med* 20:575, 2006.
425. Vincen TL, Newton JR, Deaton CM, et al: Retrospective study of predictive variables for maximal heart rate (HRmax) in horses undergoing strenuous treadmill exercise, *Equine Vet J* (Suppl 36):146-152, August 2006.
426. Poggenpoel DG: Measurements of heart rate and riding speed on a horse during a training program for endurance rides, *Equine Vet J* 20:224, 1988.
427. Amada A, Kurita H: Five cases of paroxysmal atrial fibrillation in the racehorse, *Exp Rep Equine Hlth Lab* 12:89, 1975.
428. Hiraga A, Kubo K: Two cases of paroxysmal atrial fibrillation during exercise in horses, *Equine Vet Educ* 11:6, 1999.
429. Physick-Sheard PW, Marlin DJ, Thornhill R, et al: Frequency domain analysis of heart rate variability in horses at rest and during exercise, *Equine Vet J* 32:253, 2000.
430. Thayer JF, Hahn AW, Pearson MA, et al: Heart rate variability during exercise in the horse, *Biomed Sci Instrum* 34:246, 1997.
431. Sandersen CF, Detilleux J, Delguste C, et al: Atropine reduces dobutamine-induced side effects in ponies undergoing a pharmacological stress protocol, *Equine Vet J* 37:128, 2005.
432. Coudry V, Jean D, Desbois C, et al: Myocardial fibrosis in a horse with polymorphic ventricular tachycardia observed during general anesthesia, *Can Vet J* 48:623, 2007.
433. Finley MR, Li Y, Hua F, et al: Expression and coassociation of ERG1, KCNQ1, and KCNE1 potassium channel proteins in horse heart, *Am J Physiol Heart Circ Physiol* 283:H126, 2002.
434. Kuwahara M, Hiraga A, Kai M, et al: Influence of training on autonomic nervous function in horses: evaluation by power spectral analysis of heart rate variability, *Equine Vet J Suppl* 30:178, 1999.
435. Glomset DJ, Glomset ATA: A morphologic study of the cardiac conduction system in ungulates, dog, and man. Part I: The sinoatrial node, *Am Heart J* 20:389, 1940.
436. Gross DR: Practical electrocardiography in the equine subject, *J Am Vet Med Assoc* 159:1335, 1971.
437. Grauerholz H, Jaeschke G: Construction of main and reference vectors from limb leads in the ECG of the horse, *Berl Munch Tierarztl Wochenschr* 101:376, 1988.
438. Grauerholz H, Jaeschke G: Training-induced changes of reference vectors in the QRS complex of the EKG of young trotting horses, *Berl Munch Tierarztl Wochenschr* 103:329, 1990.
439. Grauerholz H: Influence of respiration on the QRS complex of the ECG in clinically healthy horses and in horses with respiratory problems, *Berl Munch Tierarztl Wochenschr* 103:293, 1990.
440. Grauerholz H, Jaeschke G: Alterations induced by training in reference vectors of the electrocardiographic QRS complex of young trotting horses, *Berl Munch Tierarztl Wochenschr* 103:329, 1990.
441. Hartley JW, Hahn AW, DeLorey M, et al: Digital processing of equine exercise electrocardiograms, *Biomed Sci Instrum* 26:11, 1990.
442. Hilwig RW: Cardiac arrhythmias in the horse, *J Am Vet Med Assoc* 170:153, 1977.
443. Hanak J, Zert Z: Some ECG characters in Thoroughbred horses, common to parents and their offspring, *Vet Med (Praha)* 27:87, 1982.
444. Hanak J, Jagos P: Electrocardiographic lead system and its vector verification, *Acta Vet Brno* 52:67, 1983.
445. Fregin GF: The equine electrocardiogram with standardized body and limb positions, *Cornell Vet* 72:304, 1982.
446. Fregin GF: Electrocardiography, *Vet Clin North Am Equine Pract* 1:419, 1985.
447. Bonagura JD, Miller MS: Electrocardiography. What is your diagnosis? Junctional and ventricular arrhythmias, *J Equine Vet Sci* 5:347, 1985.
448. Amory H, Rollin F, Genicot B, et al: Bovine vectocardiography: a comparative study relative to the validity of four tridimensional lead systems, *J Vet Med* 39:453, 1992.
449. Clark DR, McCrady JD: Clinical use of the electrocardiogram in animals. I. Fundamentals of ECG examination, *Vet Med Small Anim Clin* 61:751, 1966.
450. Cornick JL, Seahorn TL: Cardiac arrhythmias identified in horses with duodenitis/proximal jejunitis: six cases (1985-1988), *J Am Vet Med Assoc* 197:1054, 1990.
451. Costa G, Illera M, Garcia-Sacristan A: Electrocardiographical values in non-trained horses, *Zentralbl Veterinarmed A* 32:196, 1985.
452. Illera JC, Illera M: Physiological electrocardiograms as the basis for diagnosis of heart diseases in horses, *Arch Med Vet* 3:239, 1986.
453. Illera JC, Illera M: Electrocardiography and heart score of horses competing in an endurance ride, *Aust Vet J* 64:88, 1987.
454. Illera JC, Illera M: Precordial heart score, *Aust Vet J* 65:355, 1988.
455. Irie T: A study of arrhythmias in Thoroughbred newborn foals immediately after birth, *Jpn J Vet Res* 38:57, 1990.
456. Kuwahara M, Hashimoto S, Ishii K, et al: Assessment of autonomic nervous function by power spectral analysis of heart rate variability in the horse, *J Auton Nerv Syst* 60:43, 1996.
457. Landgren S, Rutqvist L: Electrocardiogram of normal cold blooded horses after work, *Nord Vet Med* 5:905, 1953.
458. Lannek N, Rutqvist L: Normal area of variation for the electrocardiogram of horses, *Nord Vet Med* 3:1094, 1951.
459. Matsui K: Fetal and maternal heart rates in a case of twin pregnancy of the Thoroughbred horse, *Nippon Juigaku Zasshi* 47:817, 1985.
460. Polglaze K, Evans DL: The relationship between racing performance and electrocardiographic findings in the Standardbred racehorse, *Austr Equine Vet* 10:88, 1992.
461. Rose RJ, Davis PE: The use of electrocardiography in the diagnosis of poor racing performance in the horse, *Aust Vet J* 54:51, 1978.

462. Stewart JH, Rose RJ, Davis PE, et al: A comparison of electrocardiographic findings in racehorses presented either for routine examination or poor racing performance. In Persson SGB, Rose RJ, editors: *Equine exercise physiology*, Cambridge, England, 1983, Granta, pp 135-143.
463. Studzinski T, Czarnecki A: Relationship between the QRS duration (heart score) and ventricular weight in horses, *Ann Univ Mariae Curie Sklodowska Med*, 1980:35/36:33-43.
464. Tovar P, Escabias MI, Santisteban R: Evolution of the ECG from Spanish bred foals during the post natal stage, *Res Vet Sci* 46:358, 1989.
465. Tschudi P: Electrocardiography in the horse (1). Principles and normal picture, *Tierarztl Prax* 13:181, 1985.
466. Tschudi P: Electrocardiography in the horse. (3), *Tierarztl Prax* 14:365, 1986.
467. White NA, Rhode EA: Correlation of electrocardiographic findings to clinical disease in the horse, *J Am Vet Med Assoc* 164:46, 1974.
468. Yamamoto K, Yasuda J, Too K: Electrocardiographic findings during parturition and blood gas tensions immediately after birth in Thoroughbred foals, *Jpn J Vet Res* 39:143, 1991.
469. Yamamoto K, Yasuda J, Too K: Arrhythmias in newborn Thoroughbred foals, *Equine Vet J* 24:169, 1992.
470. Yamaya Y, Kubo K, Amada A, et al: Intrinsic atrioventricular conductive function in horses with a 2nd-degree atrioventricular block, *J Vet Med Sci* 59:149, 1997.
471. Persson SGB, Forssbergy P: Exercise tolerance in Standardbred trotters with T-wave abnormalities. In Gillespie JR, Robinson NE, editors: *Equine exercise physiology*, Davis, CA, 1987, ICEEP Publications, pp 772-780.
472. Matsui K, Sugano S: Species differences in the changes in heart rate and T-wave amplitude after autonomic blockade in Thoroughbred horses, ponies, cows, pigs, goats and chickens, *Nippon Juigaku Zasshi* 49:637, 1987.
473. Carlsten J, Kvart C, Jeffcott LB: Method of selective and nonselective angiocardiography for the horse, *Equine Vet J* 16:47, 1984.
474. Marr CM: Ancillary diagnostic aids in equine cardiology, *Equine Vet Educ* 2:18, 1990.
475. O'Brien RT, Biller DS: Field imaging of the respiratory tract radiology and ultrasonography, *Vet Clin North Am Equine Pract* 13:487, 1997.
476. Scott EA, Chaffee A, Eyster GE, et al: Interruption of aortic arch in two foals, *J Am Vet Med Assoc* 172:347, 1978.
477. Patteson MW: Two-dimensional and M-mode echocardiography. In Marr CM, editor: *Cardiology of the horse*, London, 1999, WB Saunders, pp 93-116.
478. Marr CM: Doppler echocardiography. In Marr CM, editor: *Cardiology of the horse*, London, 1999, WB Saunders, pp 117-134.
479. Lombard CW, Scarratt WK, Buergelt CD: Ventricular septal defects in the horse, *J Am Vet Med Assoc* 183:562, 1983.
480. Gerlis LM, Wright HM, Wilson N, et al: Left ventricular bands. A normal anatomical feature, *Br Heart J* 52:641, 1984.
481. O'Callaghan MW: Comparison of echocardiographic and autopsy measurements of cardiac dimensions in the horse, *Equine Vet J* 17:361, 1985.
482. Pipers FS, Reef VB, Wilson J: Echocardiographic detection of ventricular septal defects in large animals, *J Am Vet Med Assoc* 187:810, 1985.
483. Yamaga Y, Shibui I, Yasuda J, et al: Echocardiographic and ultrasonographic observations in a horse with mitral regurgitation and "intrahepatic cholangiocellular fibroadenomatosis," *Advances in Animal Cardiology* 18:65-75, 1985.
484. Bertone JJ, Paull KS, Wingfield WE, et al: M-mode echocardiographs of endurance horses in the recovery phase of long-distance competition, *Am J Vet Res* 48:1708, 1987.
485. Reef VB, Klumpp S, Maxson AD, et al: Echocardiographic detection of an intact aneurysm in a horse, *J Am Vet Med Assoc* 197:752, 1990.
486. Reef VB: Echocardiographic examination in the horse: the basics, *Compend Cont Educ Pract Vet* 12:1312, 1990.
487. Reef VB: Echocardiographic findings in horses with congenital cardiac disease, *Compend Cont Educ Pract Vet* 1:109, 1991.
488. Weinberger T: *Doppler echocardiography in horses*, Hannover, 1991, Germany, Tierarztliche Hochsc, p 237.
489. Lester GD, Lombard CW, Ackerman N: Echocardiographic detection of a dissecting aortic root aneurysm in a Thoroughbred stallion, *Vet Radiol Ultrasound* 33:202, 1992.
490. Mahony C, Rantanen NW, DeMichael JA, et al: Spontaneous echocardiographic contrast in the Thoroughbred: high prevalence in racehorses and a characteristic abnormality in bleeders, *Equine Vet J* 24:129, 1992.
491. Long KJ: Echocardiographic studies of valvular and ventricular function in horses, Dissertation, University of Edinburgh, Scotland, 1993.
492. Long KJ: Doppler echocardiography—clinical applications, *Equine Vet Educ* 5:161, 1993.
493. Young LE, Long KJ, Clutton RE, et al: The use of two dimensional and Doppler echocardiography for haemodynamic monitoring during general anaesthesia: preliminary findings in halothane-anaesthetised horses, *Vet Anaesth Analg* 20:42, 1993.
494. Bonagura JD: Echocardiography, *J Am Vet Med Assoc* 204:516, 1994.
495. Stadler P, Deegen E, Kroker K: Echocardiography and therapy of atrial-fibrillation in horses, *Dtsch Tierarztl Wochenschr* 101:190, 1994.
496. Cipone M, Pietra M, Guglielmini C, et al: Insufficienca aortica nel cavallo. Rilievi elettrofonocardiografici, ecocardiograficied eco-Doppler carotidei in due casi [Aortic insufficiency in horses. Results of electrophonocardiography, ultrasonic cardiography and carotid pulsed-wave Doppler echocardiography in two cases], *Obiettivi e Documenti Veterinari* 16:37, 1995.
497. Stadler P, Fruhauf B, Deegen E: Echocardiographic determination of diastolic heart function and measurement of pulmonary wedge pressure in horses, *Pferdeheilkunde* 11:109, 1995.
498. Tucker RL, Wickler SJ, London C, et al: Echocardiographic and right-sided cardiac pressure comparison of the mule and horse, *J Equine Vet Sci* 15:404, 1995.
499. Blissitt KJ, Marr CM, Rossdale PD, et al: Equine cardiovascular medicine, *Equine Vet J* (Suppl), 1996.
500. Darke PGG, Bonagura JD, Kelly DF: *Colour Atlas of Veterinary Cardiology*, London, 1996, Mosby.
501. Stadler P, Wohlsein P, Gratopp M, et al: Echocardiographic and radiographic imaging of aortic root and aortic arch aneurysm in the horse, *Pferdeheilkunde* 12:91, 1996.
502. Stadler P, Robine FJ: B-mode echocardiographic measurement of heart dimensions in warm-blooded horses without heart disease, *Pferdeheilkunde* 12:35, 1996.
503. Hoch M: Colour-coded Doppler echocardiography in horses. Dissertation, University of Hanover, Germany, 1998.
504. Reef VB: Evaluation of ventricular septal defects in horses using two-dimensional and Doppler echocardiography, *Equine Vet J Suppl* 86, 1995.
505. Reef VB: Heart murmurs in horses: determining their significance with echocardiography, *Equine Vet J* (Suppl 19):71-80, September 1995.
506. Cranley JJ: Focal medial calcification of the pulmonary artery: a survey of 1066 horses, *Equine Vet J* 15:278, 1983.
507. van Loon G, Fonteyne W, Rottiers H, et al: Dual-chamber pacemaker implantation via the cephalic vein in healthy equids, *J Vet Intern Med* 15:564, 2001.
508. Diaz OS, Sleeper MM, Reef VB, et al: Aortitis in a Paint gelding, *Equine Vet J* 32:354, 2000.

509. Young LE, Wood JL: Effect of age and training on murmurs of atrioventricular valvular regurgitation in young Thoroughbreds, *Equine Vet J* 32:195, 2000.
510. Schober KE, Kaufhold J, Kipar A: Mitral valve dysplasia in a foal, *Equine Vet J* 32:170, 2000.
511. Karlstam E, Ho SY, Shokrai A, et al: Anomalous aortic origin of the left coronary artery in a horse, *Equine Vet J* 31:350, 1999.
512. Southwood LL, Tobias AH, Schott HC, et al: Cyanosis and intense murmur in a neonatal foal, *J Am Vet Med Assoc* 208:835, 1996.
513. Reppas GP, Canfield PJ, Hartley WJ, et al: Multiple congenital cardiac anomalies and idiopathic thoracic aortitis in a horse, *Vet Rec* 138:14, 1996.
514. Lord PF, Croft MA: Accuracy of formulae for calculating left ventricular volumes of the equine heart, *Equine Vet J Suppl* 9:53-56, 1990.
515. Hoffmann KL, Wood AK, Kirby AC: Use of Doppler ultrasonography to evaluate renal arterial blood flow in horses, *Am J Vet Res* 58:697, 1997.
516. Rivas LJ, Hinchcliff KW: Effect of furosemide and subsequent intravenous fluid administration on right atrial pressure of splenectomized horses, *Am J Vet Res* 58:632, 1997.
517. Young L: Transoesophageal echocardiography. In Marr CM, editor: *Cardiology of the horse*, London, 1999, WB Saunders, pp 135-149.
518. Buhl R, Ersboll AK, Eriksen L, et al: Sources and magnitude of variation of echocardiographic measurements in normal Standardbred horses, *Vet Radiol Ultrasound* 45:505, 2004.
519. Zucca E, Ferrucci F, Croci C, et al: Echocardiographic measurements of cardiac dimensions in normal Standardbred racehorses, *J Vet Cardiol* 10:45, 2008.
520. Reimer JM: Cardiac evaluation of the horse using ultrasonography, *Vet Med* 88:748, 1993.
521. Adams Brendemuehl C, Pipers FS: Antepartum evaluations of the equine fetus, *J Reprod Fertil* (Suppl 35):565, 1987.
522. Stadler P, Rewel A, Deegen E: M-mode echocardiography in dressage horses, class S jumping horses and untrained horses, *Zentralbl Veterinarmed A* 40:292, 1993.
523. Carlsten JC: Two-dimensional, real-time echocardiography in the horse, *Vet Radiol Ultrasound* 28:76, 1987.
524. Stadler P, D'Agostino U, Deegen E: Real-time, two-dimensional echocardiography in horses, *Pferdeheilkunde* 4:161, 1988.
525. Schwarzwald CC, Bonagura JD: Methods and reliability of tissue Doppler imaging for assessment of left ventricular radial wall motion in horses, *J Vet Intern Med* , 2009:in press.
526. Schwarzwald CC, Schober KE, Berli ASJ, et al: Left ventricular radial and circumferential wall motion analysis in horses using strain, strain rate, and displacement by 2D speckle tracking, *J Vet Intern Med* 23:890, 2009.
527. Rantanen NW: Diseases of the thorax, *Vet Clin North Am Equine Pract* 2:49, 1986.
528. Bonagura JD, Pipers FS: Diagnosis of cardiac lesions by contrast echocardiography, *J Am Vet Med Assoc* 182:396, 1983.
529. Buhl R, Ersboll AK, Larsen NH, et al: The effects of detomidine, romifidine or acepromazine on echocardiographic measurements and cardiac function in normal horses, *Vet Anaesth Analg* 34:1, 2007.
530. Amend JF, Garner H, Rosborough JP, et al: Hemodynamic studies in conscious domestic ponies, *J Surg Res* 19:107, 1975.
531. Bove AA: Effects of strenuous exercise on myocardial blood flow, *Med Sci Sports Exerc* 17:517, 1985.
532. Davis JL, Manohar M: Effect of splenectomy on exercise-induced pulmonary and systemic hypertension in ponies, *Am J Vet Res* 49:1169, 1988.
533. Drummond WH, Sanchez IR, Kosch PC, et al: Pulmonary vascular reactivity of the newborn pony foal, *Equine Vet J* 21:181, 1989.
534. Dunlop CI, Hodgson DS, Chapman PL, et al: Thermodilution estimation of cardiac output at high flows in anesthetized horses, *Am J Vet Res* 52:1991, 1893.
535. Fisher EW, Dalton RG: Determination of cardiac output of cattle and horses by the injection, *Br Vet J* 117:141, 1961.
536. Goetz TE, Manohar M: Pressures in the right side of the heart and esophagus (pleura) in ponies during exercise before and after furosemide administration, *Am J Vet Res* 47:270, 1986.
537. Grossman W, Barry WH: Cardiac catheterization. In Braunwald E, editor: *Heart disease: a textbook of cardiovascular medicine*, ed 4, Philadelphia, 1992, WB Saunders, pp 180-203.
538. Hall LW, Nigam JM: Measurement of central venous pressure in horses, *Vet Rec* 97:66, 1975.
539. Hellyer PW, Dodam JR, Light GS: Dynamic baroreflex sensitivity in anesthetized horses, maintained at 1.25 to 1.3 minimal alveolar concentration of halothane, *Am J Vet Res* 52:1672, 1991.
540. Hillidge CJ, Lees P: Influence of general anaesthesia on peripheral resistance in the horse, *Br Vet J* 133:225, 1977.
541. Hlastala MP, Bernard SL, Erickson HH, et al: Pulmonary blood-flow distribution in standing horses is not dominated by gravity, *J Appl Physiol* 81:1051, 1996.
542. Manohar M: Right heart pressures and blood-gas tensions in ponies during exercise and laryngeal hemiplegia, *Am J Physiol* 251:H121, 1986.
543. Manohar M, Goetz TE, Hutchens E, et al: Atrial and ventricular myocardial blood flows in horses at rest and during exercise, *Am J Vet Res* 55:1464, 1994.
544. Manohar M: Pulmonary vascular pressures of strenuously exercising Thoroughbreds after administration of flunixin meglumine and furosemide, *Am J Vet Res* 55:1308, 1994.
545. Manohar M, Goetz TE, Hutchens E, et al: Effects of graded-exercise on pulmonary and systemic hemodynamics in horses, *Vet Clin North Am Equine Pract* 17:17, 1995.
546. Muir WW 3rd, McGuirk SM: Hemodynamics before and after conversion of atrial fibrillation to normal sinus rhythm in horses, *J Am Vet Med Assoc* 184:965, 1984.
547. Schatzmann U, Battier B: Factors influencing central venous pressure in horses, *Dtsch Tierarztl Wochenschr* 94:147, 1987.
548. Sheridan V, Deegen E, Zeller R: Central venous pressure (CVP) measurements during halothane anaesthesia, *Vet Rec* 90:149, 1972.
549. Sinha AK, Gleed RD, Hakim TS, et al: Pulmonary capillary pressure during exercise in horses, *J Appl Physiol* 80:1792, 1996.
550. Sporri H, Denac M: The ventricular pressure increase velocity as a parameter of myocardial strength development, *Schweiz Arch Tierheilkd* 111:239, 1969.
551. Staddon GE, Weaver BMG, Webb AI: Distribution of cardiac output in anaesthetized horses, *Res Vet Sci* 27:38, 1979.
552. West JB, Mathieu-Costello O: Stress failure of pulmonary capillaries as a mechanism for exercise-induced pulmonary hemorrhage in the horse, *Equine Vet J* 26:441, 1994.
553. Manohar M: Pulmonary artery wedge pressure increases with high-intensity exercise in horses, *Am J Vet Res* 54:142, 1993.
554. Klein L, Sherman J: Effects of preanesthetic medication, anesthesia, and position of recumbency on central venous pressure in horses, *J Am Vet Med Assoc* 170:216, 1977.
555. Bisgard GE, Orr JA, Will JA: Hypoxic pulmonary hypertension in the pony, *Am J Vet Res* 36:49, 1975.
556. Gelberg HB, Smetzer DL, Foreman JH: Pulmonary hypertension as a cause of atrial fibrillation in young horses: four cases (1980-1989), *J Am Vet Med Assoc* 198:679, 1991.
557. Corley KT, Donaldson LL, Furr MO: Comparison of lithium dilution and thermodilution cardiac output measurements in anaesthetized neonatal foals, *Equine Vet J* 34:598, 2002.
558. Corley KT, Donaldson LL, Durando MM, et al: Cardiac output technologies with special reference to the horse, *J Vet Intern Med* 17:262, 2003.

559. Wilkins PA, Boston RC, Gleed RD, et al: Comparison of thermal dilution and electrical impedance dilution methods for measurement of cardiac output in standing and exercising horses, *Am J Vet Res* 66:878, 2005.
560. Hallowell GD, Corley KT: Use of lithium dilution and pulse contour analysis cardiac output determination in anaesthetized horses: a clinical evaluation, *Vet Anaesth Analg* 32:201, 2005.
561. Orr JA, Bisgard GE, Forster HV, et al: Cardiopulmonary measurements in nonanesthetized resting normal ponies, *Am J Vet Res* 36:1667, 1975.
562. Schwarzwald CC, Hardy J, Buccellato M: High cardiac troponin I serum concentration in a horse with multiform ventricular tachycardia and myocardial necrosis, *J Vet Intern Med* 17:364, 2003.
563. Holbrook TC, Birks EK, Sleeper MM, et al: Endurance exercise is associated with increased plasma cardiac troponin I in horses, *Equine Vet J* (Suppl 36):27-31, August 2006.
564. Divers TJ, Krans MS, Jesty SA, et al: Clinical Findings and serum cardiac troponin I concentrations in horses after intragastric administration of sodium monensin, *J Vet Diagn Invest* 21:338, 2009.
565. Davis JL, Gardner SY, Schwabenton B, et al: Congestive heart failure in horses: 14 cases (1984-2001), *J Am Vet Med Assoc* 220:1512, 2002.
566. Bonagura JD: Diagnosis of cardiac arrhythmias. In Robinson NE, editor: *Current therapy in equine medicine*, ed 6, St Louis, 2009, WB Saunders.
567. Imhasly A, Tschudi PR, Lombard CW, et al: Clinical and echocardiographic features of mild mitral valve regurgitation in 108 horses, *Vet J*, March 7, 2009:[Epub ahead of print].
568. Belgrave JOS: A case of atrial fibrillation with congestive heart failure, *Equine Vet Educ* 2:2, 1990.
569. Bonagura JD: Clinical evaluation and management of heart disease, *Equine Vet Educ* 2:31, 1990.
570. Divers TJ, Whitlock RH, Byars TD, et al: Acute renal failure in six horses resulting from haemodynamic causes, *Equine Vet J* 19:178, 1987.
571. Glazier DB: Congestive heart failure and congenital cardiac defects in horses, *Vet Clin North Am Equine Pract* 8:20, 1986.
572. Hinchcliff KW, Muir WW 3rd: Pharmacology of furosemide in the horse: a review, *J Vet Intern Med* 5:211, 1991.
573. Marr CM: Treatment of cardiac arrhythmias and cardiac failure. In Robinson NE, editor: *Current therapy in equine medicine*, ed 6, St Louis, 2009, WB Saunders.
574. Reef VB, Levitan CW, Spencer PA: Factors affecting prognosis and conversion in equine atrial fibrillation, *J Vet Intern Med* 2:1, 1988.
575. Reimer JM, Marr CM, Reef VB, et al: Aortic origin of the right pulmonary artery and patent ductus arteriosus in a pony foal with pulmonary hypertension and right-sided heart failure, *Equine Vet J* 25:466, 1993.
576. Seahorn TL, Hormanski CE: Ventricular septal defect and atrial fibrillation in an adult horse—a case report, *J Equine Vet Sci* 13:36, 1993.
577. Smith HJ, Nuttall A: Experimental models of heart failure, *Cardiovasc Res* 19:181, 1985.
578. Taylor FG, Wotton PR, Hillyer MH, et al: Atrial septal defect and atrial fibrillation in a foal, *Vet Rec* 128:80, 1991.
579. Mogg TD: Equine cardiac disease. Clinical pharmacology and therapeutics, *Vet Clin North Am Equine Pract* 15:523, 1999.
580. Wijnberg ID, van der Kolk JH, van Garderen E, et al: Atrial fibrillation associated with central nervous symptoms and colic in a horse: a case of equine cardiomyopathy, *Vet Q* 20:73, 1998.
581. Garber JL, Reef VB, Reimer JM: Sonographic findings in horses with mediastinal lymphosarcoma—13 cases (1985-1992), *J Am Vet Med Assoc* 205:1432, 1994.
582. Southwood LL, Schott HC, Henry CJ, et al: Disseminated hemangiosarcoma in the horse: 35 cases, *J Vet Intern Med* 14:105, 2000.
583. Reef VB, Freeman D, Gentile D: Successful treatment of pericarditis in a horse, *J Am Vet Med Assoc* 185:94, 1984.
584. Bernard W, Reef VB, Clark ES, et al: Pericarditis in horses: six cases (1982-1986), *J Am Vet Med Assoc* 196:468, 1990.
585. Harkins JD, Hackett RP, Ducharme NG: Effect of furosemide on physiological variables in exercising horses, *Am J Vet Res* 54:2104, 1993.
586. Manohar M, Hutchens E, Coney E: Frusemide attenuates the exercise-induced rise in pulmonary capillary blood pressure in horses, *Equine Vet J* 26:51, 1994.
587. Johansson AM, Gardner SY, Levine JF, et al: Pharmacokinetics and pharmacodynamics of furosemide after oral administration to horses, *J Vet Intern Med* 18:739, 2004.
588. Johansson AM, Gardner SY, Levine JF, et al: Furosemide continuous rate infusion in the horse: evaluation of enhanced efficacy and reduced side effects, *J Vet Intern Med* 17:887, 2003.
589. Baggot JD: The pharmacological basis of cardiac drug selection for use in horses, *Equine Vet J* (Suppl 19):97-100, September 1995.
590. Pearson EG, Ayers JW, Wood GL, et al: Digoxin toxicity in a horse, *Compend Cont Educ Pract Vet* 9:958, 1987.
591. Gardner SY, Atkins CE, Sams RA, et al: Characterization of the pharmacokinetic and pharmacodynamic properties of the angiotensin-converting enzyme inhibitor, enalapril, in horses, *J Vet Intern Med* 18:231, 2004.
592. Sleeper MM, McDonnell SM, Ely JJ, et al: Chronic oral therapy with enalapril in normal ponies, *J Vet Cardiol* 10:111, 2008.
593. Luciani A, Civitella C, Santori D, et al: Haemodynamic effects in healthy horses treated with an ACE-inhibitor (ramipril), *Vet Res Commun* 31(Suppl1):297, 2007.
594. Gehlen H, Vieht JC, Stadler P: Effects of the ACE inhibitor quinapril on echocardiographic variables in horses with mitral valve insufficiency, *J Vet Med A Physiol Pathol Clin Med* 50:460, 2003.
595. Guglielmini C, Giuliani A, Testoni S, et al: Use of an ACE inhibitor (ramipril) in a horse with congestive heart failure, *Equine Vet Educ* 14:297, 2002.
596. Bonagura JD: Congenital heart disease. In Robinson NE, editor: *Current therapy in equine medicine*, ed 6, St Louis, 2009, WB Saunders.
597. Buergelt CD, Carmichael JA, Tashjian RJ, et al: Spontaneous rupture of the left pulmonary artery in a horse with patent ductus arteriosus, *J Am Vet Med Assoc* 157:313, 1970.
598. Chaffin MK, Miller MW, Morris EL: Double outlet right ventricle and other associated congenital cardiac anomalies in an American Miniature horse foal, *Equine Vet J* 24:402, 1992.
599. Cottrill CM, Rossdale PD: A comparison of congenital heart disease in horses and man, *Equine Vet J* 24:338, 1992.
600. Cox VS, Weber AF, Lima A, et al: Left cranial vena cava in a horse, *Anat Histol Embryol* 20:37, 1991.
601. Glazier DB, Farrelly BT, Neylon JF: Patent ductus arteriosus in an eight-month-old foal, *Ir Vet J* 28:12, 1974.
602. Glazier DB, Farrelly BT, O'Connor J: Ventricular septal defect in a 7-year-old gelding, *J Am Vet Med Assoc* 167:49, 1975.
603. Greene HJ, Wray DD, Greenway GA: Two equine congenital cardiac anomalies, *Ir Vet J* 29:115, 1975.
604. Guarda F, Rattazzi C, Appina S: Pathology of cardiac aneurysms in horses, *Pferdeheilkunde* 8:241, 1992.
605. Huston R, Saperstein G, Leipold HW: Congenital defects in foals, *J Equine Med Surg* 1:146, 1977.
606. Johnson JW, DeBowes RM, Cox JH, et al: Diaphragmatic hernia with a concurrent cardiac defect in an Arabian foal, *J Equine Vet Sci* 4:225, 1984.
607. King JM, Flint TJ, Anderson WI: Incomplete subaortic stenotic rings in domestic animals—a newly described congenital anomaly, *Cornell Vet* 78:263, 1988.

608. Koblik PD, Hornof WJ: Use of first-pass nuclear angiocardiography to detect left-to- right cardiac shunts in the horse, *Vet Radiol Ultrasound* 28:177, 1987.
609. Koterba AM, Drummond WH, Kosch PCE: *Equine clinical neonatology*, Philadelphia, Lea & Febiger, 1990.
610. Kvart C, Carlsten J, Jeffcott LB, et al: Diagnostic value of contrast echocardiography in the horse, *Equine Vet J* 17:357, 1985.
611. Lescure R, Tamzali Y: L'echocardiographie TM chez le cheval. III. Cardiopathie congenitale et troubles du rythme [TM echocardiography in the horse. III. Congenital heart disease and arrhythmias], *Point Veterinaire* 15:373, 1983.
612. Platt H: Vascular malformations and angiomatous lesions in horses: a review of 10 cases, *Equine Vet J* 19:500, 1987.
613. Reef VB: Equine pediatric ultrasonography, *Compend Cont Educ Pract Vet* 13:1277, 1991.
614. Staller GS, Reef VB: Aortic insufficiency associated with ventricular septal defect in a, *J Am Vet Med Assoc*, 1992:(submitted for publication).
615. Steyn PF, Holland P, Hoffman J: The angiocardiographic diagnosis of a persistent truncus arteriosus in a foal, *J S Afr Vet Assoc* 60:106, 1989.
616. Vitums A, Bayly WM: Pulmonary atresia with dextroposition of the aorta and ventricular septal defect in three Arabian foals, *Vet Pathol* 19:160, 1982.
617. Zamora CS, Vitums A, Foreman JH, et al: Common ventricle with separate pulmonary outflow chamber in a horse, *J Am Vet Med Assoc* 186:1210, 1985.
618. Zamora CS, Vitums A, Sande RD, et al: Multiple cardiac malformation in a horse, *Anat Histol Embryol* 17:95, 1988.
619. Patterson-Kane JC, Harrison LR: Giant right atrial diverticulum in a foal, *J Vet Diagn Invest* 14:335, 2002.
620. Gehlen H, Bubeck K, Stadler P: Valvular pulmonic stenosis with normal aortic root and intact ventricular and atrial septa in an Arabian horse, *Equine Vet Educ* 13:286, 2001.
621. Anderson RH: The pathological spectrum of pulmonary atresia, *Equine Vet Educ* 9:128, 1997.
622. Young LE, Blunden AS, Bartram DH, et al: Pulmonary atresia with an intact ventricular septum in a thoroughbred foal, *Equine Vet Educ* 9:123, 1997.
623. Anderson R: Nomenclature and classification: sequential segmental analysis. In Moller JH, Hoffman HJ, editors: *Pediatric cardiovascular medicine*, New York, 2003, Churchill Livingstone.
624. Van Praagh R: Nomenclature and classification: morphologic and segmental approach to diagnosis. In Moller JH HJ, editor: *Pediatric cardiovascular medicine*, New York, 2003, Churchill Livingstone.
625. Sleeper MM, Palmer JE: Echocardiographic diagnosis of transposition of the great arteries in a neonatal foal, *Vet Radiol Ultrasound* 46:259, 2005.
626. Valdes-Martinez A, Eades SC, Strickland KN, et al: Echocardiographic evidence of an aortico-pulmonary septal defect in a 4-day-old thoroughbred foal, *Vet Radiol Ultrasound* 47:87, 2006.
627. Cottrill CM, O'Connor WN, Cudd T, Rantanen NW: Persistence of foetal circulatory pathways in a newborn foal, *Equine Vet J* 19:252, 1987.
628. McGurrin MK, Physick-Sheard PW, Southorn E: Parachute left atrioventricular valve causing stenosis and regurgitation in a Thoroughbred foal, *J Vet Intern Med* 17:579, 2003.
629. Coumbe KM: Cardiac disease: endocardial fibroelastosis, *Equine Vet Educ* 14:81, 2002.
630. Seco DO, Desrochers A, Hoffmann V, et al: Total anomalous pulmonary venous connection in a foal, *Vet Radiol Ultrasound* 46:83, 2005.
631. Cottrill CM, Ho SY, O'Connor WN: Embryological development of the equine heart, *Equine Vet J* (Suppl 24):14-18, June 1997.
632. Stephen JO, Abbott J, Middleton DM, et al: Persistent truncus arteriosus in a Bashkir Curly foal, *Equine Vet Educ* 12:251, 2000.
633. Petrick SW, Roos CJ, van NJ: Persistent right aortic arch in a horse, *J S Afr Vet Assoc* 49:355, 1978.
634. van der Linde-Sipman JS, Goedegebuure SA, Kroneman J: Persistent right aortic arch associated with a persistent left ductus arteriosus and an interventricular septal defect in a horse, *Tijdschr Diergeneeskd* 104(Suppl 4):189-194, 1979.
635. Kutasi O, Voros K, Biksi I, et al: Common atrioventricular canal in a newborn foal—case report and review of the literature, *Acta Vet Hung* 55:51, 2007.
636. Meurs KM, Miller MW, Hanson C, et al: Tricuspid valve atresia with main pulmonary artery atresia in an Arabian foal, *Equine Vet J* 29:160, 1997.
637. Button C, Gross DR, Allert JA, et al: Tricuspid atresia in a foal, *J Am Vet Med Assoc* 172:825, 1978.
638. Honnas CM, Puckett MJ, Schumacher J: Tricuspid atresia in a Quarter Horse foal, *Southwestern Vet* 38:17, 1987.
639. Rooney JR, Robertson JL: Equine Pathology, Ames, Iowa, Iowa State University Press, 1996, p 15.
640. Littlewort MCG: Cardiological problems in equine medicine, *Equine Vet J* 9:173, 1977.
641. Buergelt CD: Equine cardiovascular pathology: an overview, *Anim Health Res Rev* 4:109, 2003.
642. Buhl R, Ersboll AK, Eriksen L, et al: Use of color Doppler echocardiography to assess the development of valvular regurgitation in Standardbred trotters, *J Am Vet Med Assoc* 227:1630, 2005.
643. Stevens KB, Marr CM, Horn JN, et al: Effect of left-sided valvular regurgitation on mortality and causes of death among a population of middle-aged and older horses, *Vet Rec* 164:6, 2009.
644. Kriz NG, Hodgson DR, Rose RJ: Prevalence and clinical importance of heart murmurs in racehorses, *J Am Vet Med Assoc* 216:1441, 2000.
645. Haldar SM, O'Gara PT: Infective endocarditis: diagnosis and management, *Nat Clin Pract Cardiovasc Med* 3:310, 2006.
646. Bertone JJ, Dill SG: Traumatic gastropericarditis in a horse, *J Am Vet Med Assoc* 187:742, 1985.
647. Wagner PC: Pericarditis. In Robinson NE, editor: *Current therapy in equine medicine*, ed 1, Philadelphia, 1983, WB Saunders, pp 149-151.
648. Robinson JA, Marr CM, Reef VB, et al: Idiopathic, aseptic, effusive, fibrinous, nonconstrictive pericarditis with tamponade in a Standardbred filly, *J Am Vet Med Assoc* 201:1593, 1992.
649. Bradfield T: Traumatic pericarditis in a horse, *Southwestern Vet* 23:145, 1970.
650. Voros K, Felkai C, Szilagyi Z, et al: Two-dimensional echocardiographically guided pericardiocentesis in a horse with traumatic pericarditis, *J Am Vet Med Assoc 198* :1991, 1953.
651. Buergelt CD, Wilson JH, Lombard CW: Pericarditis in horses, *Compend Cont Educ Pract Vet* 12:872, 1990.
652. Morley PS, Chirinotrejo M, Petrie L, et al: Pericarditis and pleuritis caused by *Mycoplasma felis* in a horse, *Equine Vet J* 28:237, 1996.
653. Wilson JH, Olson EJ, Haugen EW, et al: Systemic blastomycosis in a horse, *J Vet Diagn Invest* 18:615, 2006.
654. May KA, Cheramie HS, Howard RD, et al: Purulent pericarditis as a sequela to clostridial myositis in a horse, *Equine Vet J* 34:636, 2002.
655. Marcus LC, Ross JN: Microscopic lesions in the hearts of aged horses and mules, *Vet Pathol* 4:162, 1967.
656. King JM, Roth L, Haschek WM: Myocardial necrosis secondary to neural lesions in domestic animals, *J Am Vet Med Assoc* 180:144, 1982.
657. Fujii Y, Watanabe H, Yamamoto T, et al: Serum creatine kinase and lactate dehydrogenase isoenzymes in skeletal and cardiac muscle damage in the horse, *Bull Equine Res Institute* 20:87-96, 1983.

658. Shawley RV, Rolf LLJ: Experimental cantharidiasis in the horse, *Am J Vet Res* 45:2261, 1984.
659. Hulland TJ: Leptomeric fibrils in the myocardial fibers of a foal, *Vet Pathol* 25:175, 1988.
660. Schmitz DG: Cantharidin toxicosis in horses, *J Vet Intern Med* 3:208, 1989.
661. Freestone JF, Williams MM, Norwood G: Thoracic haemangiosarcoma in a 3-year-old horse, *Aust Vet J* 67:269, 1990.
662. Reef VB: Myocardial disease. In Robinson NE, editor: *Current therapy in equine medicine*, ed 3, Philadelphia, 1992, WB Saunders, pp 393-395.
663. Weldon AD, Step DL, Moise NS: Lymphosarcoma with myocardial infiltration in a mare, *Vet Med* 87:595, 1992.
664. Perkins JD, Bowen IM, Else RW, et al: Functional and histopathological evidence of cardiac parasympathetic dysautonomia in equine grass sickness, *Vet Rec* 146:246, 2000.
665. Slack JA, McGuirk SM, Erb HN, et al: Biochemical markers of cardiac injury in normal, surviving septic, or nonsurviving septic neonatal foals, *J Vet Intern Med* 19:577, 2005.
666. Delesalle C, VanLoon G, Nollet H, et al: Tumor-induced ventricular arrhythmia in a horse, *J Vet Intern Med* 16:612, 2002.
667. Nout YS, Hinchcliff KW, Bonagura JD, et al: Cardiac amyloidosis in a horse, *J Vet Intern Med* 17:588, 2003.
668. Cornelisse CJ, Schott HC, Olivier NB, et al: Concentration of cardiac troponin I in a horse with a ruptured aortic regurgitation jet lesion and ventricular tachycardia, *J Am Vet Med Assoc* 217:231, 2000.
669. O'Brien PJ, Landt Y, Ladenson JH: Differential reactivity of cardiac and skeletal muscle from various species in a cardiac troponin I immunoassay, *Clin Chem* 43:2333, 1997.
670. Smith GW, Constable PD, Foreman JH, et al: Cardiovascular changes associated with intravenous administration of fumonisin B1 in horses, *Am J Vet Res* 63:538, 2002.
671. Phillips W, Giguere S, Franklin RP, et al: Cardiac troponin I in pastured and race-training Thoroughbred horses, *J Vet Intern Med* 17:597, 2003.
672. Diana A, Guglielmini C, Candini D, et al: Cardiac arrhythmias associated with piroplasmosis in the horse: a case report, *Vet J* 174:193, 2007.
673. Galey FD, Holstege DM, Plumlee KH, et al: Diagnosis of oleander poisoning in livestock, *J Vet Diagn Invest* 8:358, 1996.
674. Tiwary AK, Puschner B, Kinde H, et al: Diagnosis of *Taxus* (yew) poisoning in a horse, *J Vet Diagn Invest* 17:252, 2005.
675. Beasley VR, Wolf GA, Fischer DC, et al: Cantharidin toxicosis in horses, *J Am Vet Med Assoc* 182:283, 1983.
676. Dickinson CE, Traub-Dargatz JL, Dargatz DA, et al: Rattlesnake venom poisoning in horses: 32 cases (1973-1993), *J Am Vet Med Assoc* 208:1866, 1996.
677. Aleman M, Magdesian KG, Peterson TS, et al: Salinomycin toxicosis in horses, *J Am Vet Med Assoc* 230:1822, 2007.
678. Vitums A: Origin of the aorta and pulmonary trunk from the right ventricle in a horse, *Vet Pathol* 7:482, 1970.
679. Vitums A, Grant BD, Stone EC, et al: Transposition of the aorta and atresia of the pulmonary trunk in a horse, *Cornell Vet* 63:41, 1973.
680. Hilbert BJ, Rendano VT: Venous aneurysm in a horse, *J Am Vet Med Assoc* 167:394, 1975.
681. Harrington DD, Page EH: Acute vitamin D_3 toxicosis in horses: case reports and experimental studies of the comparative toxicity of vitamins D_2 and D_3, *J Am Vet Med Assoc* 182:1358, 1983.
682. Lombardo de Barros CS: Aortic body adenoma in a horse, *Aust Vet J* 60:61, 1983.
683. Knezevic PF, Fessl L: Thrombectomy of the descending aorta in the horse, *Tierarztl Prax* (Suppl 1:94), 1985.
684. Spier S: Arterial thrombosis as the cause of lameness in a foal, *J Am Vet Med Assoc* 187:164, 1985.
685. Laging C, Grabner A: Malignant haemangioendothelioma in a horse, *Pferdeheilkunde* 4:273, 1988.
686. Parks AH, Guy BL, Rawlings CA, et al: Lameness in a mare with signs of arteriovenous fistula, *J Am Vet Med Assoc* 194:379, 1989.
687. Wallace KD, Selcer BA, Tyler DE, et al: In vitro ultrasonographic appearance of the normal and verminous equine aorta, cranial mesenteric artery, and its branches, *Am J Vet Res* 50:1774, 1989.
688. Johnson B, Baldwin C, Timoney P, et al: Arteritis in equine fetuses aborted due to equine viral arteritis, *Vet Pathol* 28:248, 1991.
689. Gardner S, Reef VB: Ultrasonographic evaluation of jugular vein thrombophlebitis in horses. 1992.
690. McDonnell SM, Love CC, Martin BB, et al: Ejaculatory failure associated with aortic-iliac thrombosis in two stallions, *J Am Vet Med Assoc* 200:954, 1992.
691. Welch RD, Dean PW, Miller MW: Pulsed spectral Doppler evaluation of a peripheral arteriovenous fistula in a horse, *J Am Vet Med Assoc* 200:1360, 1992.
692. Markey BKJ, Carter ME, Quinn PJ: Notes on equine viral arteritis—recent outbreaks in Britain, *Ir Vet J* 46:104, 1993.
693. Timoney PJ, McCollum WH: Equine viral arteritis, *Vet Clin North Am Equine Pract* 9:295, 1993.
694. West JB, Mathieu-Costello O, Jones JH, et al: Stress failure of pulmonary capillaries in racehorses with exercise-induced pulmonary hemorrhage, *J Appl Physiol* 75:1097, 1993.
695. Yanai T, Masegi T, Ishikawa K, et al: Spontaneous vascular mineralization in the brain of horses, *J Vet Med Sci* 58:35, 1996.
696. Birks EK, Mathieu-Costello O, Fu Z, et al: Very high pressures are required to cause stress failure of pulmonary capillaries in Thoroughbred racehorses, *J Appl Physiol* 82:1584, 1997.
697. Carr EA, Carlson GP, Wilson WD, et al: Acute hemorrhagic pulmonary infarction and necrotizing pneumonia in horses—21 cases (1967-1993), *J Am Vet Med Assoc* 210:1774, 1997.
698. Shirai W, Momotani E, Sato T, et al: Dissecting aortic aneurysm in a horse, *J Comp Pathol* 120:307, 1999.
699. Hoskinson JJ, Wooten P, Evans R: Nonsurgical removal of a catheter embolus from the heart of a foal, *J Am Vet Med Assoc* 199:233, 1991.
700. Lees MJ, Read RA, Klein KT, et al: Surgical retrieval of a broken jugular catheter from the right ventricle of a foal, *Equine Vet J* 21:384, 1989.
701. Fales-Williams A, Sponseller B, Flaherty H: Idiopathic arterial medial calcification of the thoracic arteries in an adult horse, *J Vet Diagn Invest* 20:692, 2008.
702. Imaizumi K, Nakamura T, Kiryu K, et al: Morphological changes of the aorta and pulmonary artery in Thoroughbred racehorses, *J Comp Pathol* 101:1, 1989.
703. Arroyo LG, Hayes MA, DeLay J, et al: Arterial calcification in race horses, *Vet Pathol* 45:617, 2008.
704. Guglick MA, MacAllister CG, Ewing PJ, et al: Thrombosis resulting in rectal perforation in a horse, *J Am Vet Med Assoc* 209:1125, 1996.
705. Johansson AM, Gardner SY, Atkins CE, et al: Cardiovascular effects of acute pulmonary obstruction in horses with recurrent airway obstruction, *J Vet Intern Med* 21:302, 2007.
706. Rantanen NW, Byars TD, Hauser ML, et al: Spontaneous contrast and mass lesions in the hearts of racehorses: ultrasound diagnosis—preliminary data, *J Equine Vet Sci* 4:220, 1984.
707. Barrelet A: Aorto-iliac thrombosis in a breeding stallion and an eventer mare, *Equine Vet Educ* 5:86, 1993.
708. Mouchot E, Desbrosse F: Aorto-iliac thrombosis in a horse. Clinical examination and use of ultrasonography as a diagnostic aid, *Pratique Vétérinaire Équine* 26:147, 1994.
709. Dyson SJ, Worth L: Aortoiliacofemoral thrombosis. In Robinson NE, editor: *Current therapy in equine medicine*, ed 4, Philadelphia, 1997, WB Saunders, pp 267-268.

710. Moore LA, Johnson PJ, Bailey KL: Aorto-iliac thrombosis in a foal, *Vet Rec* 142:459, 1998.
711. Duggan VE, Holbrook TC, Dechant JE, et al: Diagnosis of aorto-iliac thrombosis in a quarter horse foal using Doppler ultrasound and nuclear scintigraphy, *J Vet Intern Med* 18:753, 2004.
712. Hilton H, Aleman M, Textor J, et al: Ultrasound-guided balloon thrombectomy for treatment of aorto-iliac-femoral thrombosis in a horse, *J Vet Intern Med* 22:679, 2008.
713. Trachsel D, Cohausz O, Scharf G, et al: Aorto-iliac thrombosis in a gelding treated with the anticoagulant phenprocoumon (Marcoumar), *Schweiz Arch Tierheilkd* 150:613, 2008.
714. Ross MW, Maxson AD, Stacy VS, et al: First-pass radionuclide angiography in the diagnosis of aortoiliac thromboembolism in a horse, *Vet Radiol Ultrasound* 38:226, 1997.
715. Warmerdam EP: Ultrasonography of the femoral artery in six normal horses and three horses with thrombosis, *Vet Radiol Ultrasound* 39:137, 1998.
716. Guglielmini C, Bernardini D: Echo-Doppler findings of a carotid-jugular fistula in a foal, *Vet Radiol Ultrasound* 44:310, 2003.
717. Reef VB: Arrhythmias. In Marr CM, editor: *Cardiology of the horse*, London, 1999, WB Saunders, pp 179-209.
718. Glazier DB, Nicholson JA, Kelly WR: Atrial fibrillation in the horse, *Ir Vet J* 13:47, 1959.
719. Glendinning SA: The use of quinidine sulfate for the treatment of atrial fibrillation in horses, *Vet Rec* 77:951, 1965.
720. Glendinning SA: Significance of clinical abnormalities of the heart in soundness, *Equine Vet J* 4:21, 1972.
721. Rose RJ, Davis PE: Treatment of atrial fibrillation in three racehorses, *Equine Vet J* 9:68, 1977.
722. Oka Y: Studies on uses of quinidine sulfate for treatment of atrial fibrillation in heavy horses, *Jpn J Vet Res* 33:89, 1985.
723. Cipone M, Venturoli M: Atrial fibrillation in five horses. Changes in the ECG during quinidine therapy, *Summa Phytopathol* 3:53, 1986.
724. Petch MC: Atrial fibrillation: bad news for man and horse? *Equine Vet J* 18:3, 1986.
725. Shaftoe S, McGuirk SM: Valvular insufficiency in a horse with atrial fibrillation, *Compend Cont Educ Pract Vet* 9:203-208, 1987.
726. Machida N, Yasuda J, Too K: Three cases of paroxysmal atrial fibrillation in the Thoroughbred newborn foal, *Equine Vet J* 21:66, 1989.
727. Muir WW: 3rd, Reed SM, McGuirk SM: Treatment of atrial fibrillation in horses by intravenous administration of quinidine, *J Am Vet Med Assoc* 197:1607, 1990.
728. Stewart GA, Fulton LJ, McKellar CD: Idiopathic atrial fibrillation in a champion Standardbred racehorse, *Aust Vet J* 67:187, 1990.
729. Matsuda H: Treatment of atrial fibrillation in horses, *Jpn J Vet Res* 40:44, 1992.
730. Marr CM, Reef VB, Reimer JM, et al: An echocardiographic study of atrial fibrillation in horses: before and after conversion to sinus rhythm, *J Vet Intern Med* 9:336, 1995.
731. Reef VB, Reimer JM, Spencer PA: Treatment of atrial fibrillation in horses—new perspectives, *J Vet Intern Med* 9:57, 1995.
732. Schwarzwald CC, Sams RA: Determination of plasma protein binding of diltiazem in horses by ultrafiltration, *J Vet Pharmacol Ther* 29:579, 2006.
733. Schwarzwald CC, Sams RA, Bonagura JD: Pharmacokinetics of the calcium-channel blocker diltiazem after a single intravenous dose in horses, *J Vet Pharmacol Ther* 29:165, 2006.
734. Amada A, Kiryu K: Atrial fibrillation in the race horse, *Heart Vessels Suppl* 2:2, 1987.
735. Bertone JJ, Traub-Dargatz JL, Wingfield WE: Atrial fibrillation in a pregnant mare: treatment with quinidine sulfate, *J Am Vet Med Assoc* 190:1565, 1987.
736. Blissitt KJ: Diagnosis and treatment of atrial fibrillation, *Equine Vet Educ* 11:11, 1999.
737. Kuwahara M, Hiraga A, Nishimura T, et al: Power spectral analysis of heart rate variability in a horse with atrial fibrillation, *J Vet Med Sci* 60:111, 1998.
738. Ohmura H, Hiraga A, Aida H, et al: Determination of oral dosage and pharmacokinetic analysis of flecainide in horses, *J Vet Med Sci* 63:511, 2001.
739. van Loon G, Jordaens L, Muylle E, et al: Intracardiac overdrive pacing as a treatment of atrial flutter in a horse, *Vet Rec* 142:301, 1998.
740. Schwarzwald CC, Schober KE, Bonagura JD: Echocardiographic evidence of left atrial mechanical dysfunction after conversion of atrial fibrillation to sinus rhythm in 5 horses, *J Vet Intern Med* 21:820, 2007.
741. Gehlen H, Stadler P: Comparison of systolic cardiac function before and after treatment of atrial fibrillation in horses with and without additional cardiac valve insufficiencies, *Vet Res Commun* 28:317, 2004.
742. Frye MA, Selders CG, Mama KR, et al: Use of biphasic electrical cardioversion for treatment of idiopathic atrial fibrillation in two horses, *J Am Vet Med Assoc* 220:1039, 2002.
743. McGurrin MK, Physick-Sheard PW, Kenney DG, et al: Transvenous electrical cardioversion in equine atrial fibrillation: technique and successful treatment of 3 horses, *J Vet Intern Med* 17:715, 2003.
744. McGurrin MK, Physick-Sheard PW, Kenney DG: How to perform transvenous electrical cardioversion in horses with atrial fibrillation, *J Vet Cardiol* 7:109, 2005.
745. McGurrin MK, Physick-Sheard PW, Kenney DG, et al: Transvenous electrical cardioversion of equine atrial fibrillation: technical considerations, *J Vet Intern Med* 19:695, 2005.
746. Bellei MH, Kerr C, McGurrin MK, et al: Management and complications of anesthesia for transvenous electrical cardioversion of atrial fibrillation in horses: 62 cases (2002-2006), *J Am Vet Med Assoc* 231:1225, 2007.
747. McGurrin MK, Physick-Sheard PW, Kenney DG: Transvenous electrical cardioversion of equine atrial fibrillation: patient factors and clinical results in 72 treatment episodes, *J Vet Intern Med* 22:609, 2008.
748. DeClercq D, VanLoon G, Schauvliege S, et al: Transvenous electrical cardioversion of atrial fibrillation in six horses using custom made cardioversion catheters, *Vet J* 177:198, 2008.
749. Birettoni F, Porciello F, Rishniw M, et al: Treatment of chronic atrial fibrillation in the horse with flecainide: personal observation, *Vet Res Commun* 31(Suppl 1):273, 2007.
750. Ohmura H, Nukada T, Mizuno Y, et al: Safe and efficacious dosage of flecainide acetate for treating equine atrial fibrillation, *J Vet Med Sci* 62:711, 2000.
751. Ohmura H, Hiraga A, Aida H, et al: Influence of quinidine and flecainide on autonomic nervous activity in Thoroughbred horses, *Vet Rec* 152:114, 2003.
752. Risberg AI, McGuirk SM: Successful conversion of equine atrial fibrillation using oral flecainide, *J Vet Intern Med* 20:207, 2006.
753. VanLoon G, Blissitt KJ, Keen JA, et al: Use of intravenous flecainide in horses with naturally occurring atrial fibrillation, *Equine Vet J* 36:609, 2004.
754. DeClercq D, VanLoon G, Tavernier R, et al: Use of propafenone for conversion of chronic atrial fibrillation in horses, *Am J Vet Res* 70:223, 2009.
755. DeClercq D, VanLoon G, Baert K, et al: Intravenous amiodarone treatment in horses with chronic atrial fibrillation, *Vet J* 172:129, 2006.
756. DeClercq D, VanLoon G, Baert K, et al: Treatment with amiodarone of refractory ventricular tachycardia in a horse, *J Vet Intern Med* 21:878, 2007.

757. DeClercq D, VanLoon G, Baert K, et al: Effects of an adapted intravenous amiodarone treatment protocol in horses with atrial fibrillation, *Equine Vet J* 39:344, 2007.
758. Trachsel D, Tschudi P, Portier CJ, et al: Pharmacokinetics and pharmacodynamic effects of amiodarone in plasma of ponies after single intravenous administration, *Toxicol Appl Pharmacol* 195:113, 2004.
759. McGuirk SM, Muir WW 3rd, Sams RA: Pharmacokinetic analysis of intravenously and orally administered quinidine in horses, *Am J Vet Res* 42:938, 1981.
760. Parraga ME, Kittleson MD, Drake CM: Quinidine administration increases steady state serum digoxin concentration in horses, *Equine Vet J* (Suppl 19):114-119, September 1995.
761. Puigdemont A, Riu JL, Guitart R, et al: Propafenone kinetics in the horse. Comparative analysis of compartmental and noncompartmental models, *J Pharmacol Methods* 23:79, 1990.
762. VanLoon G, DeClercq D, Tavernier R, et al: Transient complete atrioventricular block following transvenous electrical cardioversion of atrial fibrillation in a horse, *Vet J* 170:124, 2005.
763. Cornick JL, Hartsfield SM, Miller M: ECG of the month. Premature ventricular complexes in an anesthetized colt, *J Am Vet Med Assoc* 196:420, 1990.
764. Gabriel F, Lekeux P: Cardiac arrhythmias encountered in 159 Belgian riding horses, *Ann Med Vet* 130:205, 1986.
765. Kiryu K, Machida N, Kashida Y, et al: Pathologic and electrocardiographic findings in sudden cardiac death in racehorses, *J Vet Med Sci* 61:921, 1999.
766. Marr CM, Reef VB: ECG of the month [Multifocal ventricular tachycardia in a horse], *J Am Vet Med Assoc* 198:1533, 1991.
767. Miller PJ, Rose RJ, Hoffman K, et al: Idioventricular tachycardia in a horse, *Aust Vet J* 64:55, 1987.
768. Nielsen IL: Ventricular tachycardia in a Thoroughbred racehorse, *Aust Vet J* 67:140, 1990.
769. Reimer JM, Reef VB, Sweeney RW: Ventricular arrhythmias in horses: 21 cases (1984-1989), *J Am Vet Med Assoc* 201:1237, 1992.
770. Vrins A, Doucet M, DeRoth L: Paroxysmal ventricular tachycardia in a horse, *Medecin Veterinaire du Quebec* 19:79, 1989.
771. Garcia-Lopez JM, Provost PJ, Rush JE, et al: Prevalence and prognostic importance of hypomagnesemia and hypocalcemia in horses that have colic surgery, *Am J Vet Res* 62:7, 2001.
772. Meyer GA, Lin HC, Hanson RR, et al: Effects of intravenous lidocaine overdose on cardiac electrical activity and blood pressure in the horse, *Equine Vet J* 33:434, 2001.
773. Ellis EJ, Ravis WR, Malloy M, et al: The pharmacokinetics and pharmacodynamics of procainamide in horses after intravenous administration, *J Vet Pharmacol Ther* 17:265, 1994.
774. Gasthuys F, Parmentier D, Goossens L, et al: A preliminary study on the effects of atropine sulphate on bradycardia and heart blocks during romifidine sedation in the horse, *Vet Res Commun* 14:489, 1990.
775. Muir WW 3rd, McGuirk SM: Ventricular preexcitation in two horses, *J Am Vet Med Assoc* 183:573, 1983.
776. Nihouannen JC, Sevestre J, Dorso Y, et al: Implantation of a cardiac pacemaker into horses. I. Equipment and techniques, *Rev Med Vet (Toulouse)* 135:91, 1984.
777. Nihouannen JC, Sevestre J, Dorso Y, et al: Implantation of a cardiac pacemaker into horses. II. Postoperative monitoring of a pacemaker with epicardial and myocardial electrodes in a pony, *Rev Med Vet (Toulouse)* 135:165, 1984.
778. Reef VB, Clark ES, Oliver JA, et al: Implantation of a permanent transvenous pacing catheter in a horse with complete heart block and syncope, *J Am Vet Med Assoc* 189:449, 1986.
779. van Loon G, Laevens H, Deprez P: Temporary transvenous atrial pacing in horses: threshold determination, *Equine Vet J* 33:290, 2001.
780. Castex AM, Bertone JJ: ECG of the month. Sinus tachycardia and hyperkalemia in a horse, *J Am Vet Med Assoc* 194:654, 1989.
781. Epstein V: Relationship between potassium administration, hyperkalaemia and the electrocardiogram: an experimental study, *Equine Vet J* 16:453, 1984.
782. Hardy J: ECG of the month. Hyperkalemia in a mare, *J Am Vet Med Assoc* 194:356, 1989.

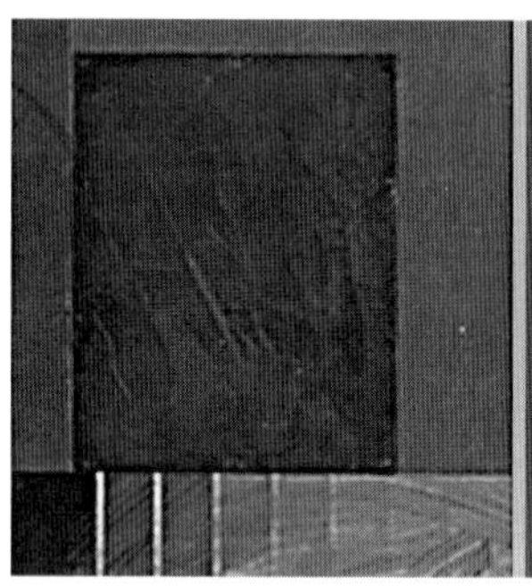

Disorders of the Musculoskeletal System

CHAPTER 11

Jennifer M. MacLeay

FUNDAMENTALS OF THE MUSCULOSKELETAL SYSTEM, DIAGNOSTIC TECHNIQUES, AND CLASSIFICATION OF MYOPATHIES

Jennifer M. MacLeay

The innate ability of the horse to learn and trust is a special attribute that allows human beings to take advantage of their extraordinary strength and agility. Horses have contributed to human life by assisting in agriculture, business, travel, and recreation. Although effective locomotion depends on the coordination of many body systems, movement ultimately depends on skeletal muscle. This chapter endeavors to review the many disorders that affect the muscular system of the horse.

STRUCTURE

Mammalian skeletal muscle consists of approximately 75% water, 18% to 22% protein, 1% carbohydrate, and 1% mineral, with variable lipid content. Depending on the breed and type of horse, between 44% and 53% of the live weight of a mature 500-kg horse has been estimated to be muscle.[1] The myofiber, or individual muscle cell, is the fundamental building block of muscle, and each is a fusiform, multinucleated cell. Combined, myofibers constitute 75% to 90% of the volume of muscle. The myofibers are arranged in parallel along the length of the muscle such that the force of contraction is additive. The rest of the muscle tissue is made up of fibroblasts, capillaries, adipose cells, nerves, and connective tissue fibers. The composition of any muscle varies depending on the muscle surveyed and the overall fitness level, age, and breed of the horse. Muscles begin and end with tendons of various sizes, which attach the muscle to bone. Golgi tendon organs act as end organs of muscle sense and are found in the major tendinous origins and insertions. The nerve and blood vessels that supply an individual muscle typically enter near the midpoint of the muscle belly at a region called the neurovascular hilum. The nerve bundle splits off into individual nerves once it enters the muscle. A single nerve contacts several myofibers such that they contract in unison when stimulated (motor unit). A single nerve innervates each myofiber at a single point known as the motor end plate.

Each myofiber is bounded by a complex membrane called the sarcolemma, which invaginates into the muscle fiber at numerous points to form the T, or transverse, tubules. The T tubules terminate within each muscle cell in proximity to the sarcoplasmic reticulum of the cell, contacting the myofibrils between the A and I band twice within each sarcomere. The T tubule lies between two terminal cisterns of the sarcoplasmic reticulum. Together these three structures form the triad.

A basement membrane surrounds the sarcolemma and attaches closely to a layer of connective tissue called the *endomysium*. The endomysium is continuous with the perimysium, which surrounds groups or bundles of muscle fibers. The perimysium, in turn, is continuous with the epimysium, which surrounds the entire muscle. Satellite cells, which consist of a simple cell membrane around a nucleus with a minimal amount of cytoplasm and few mitochondria, lie in shallow indentations on the myofiber surface between the sarcolemma and the basement membrane. Satellite cells give rise to new myofibers after rhabdomyolysis (dissolution of muscle fibers). The nuclei of the satellite cells and mature myofibers are oriented to the long axis of the muscle fiber. The muscle fiber nuclei lie at the periphery of the cells just within the sarcolemma.

Within each myofiber are parallel arrays of myofibrils, the basic contractile units of muscle. Myofibrils are composed of end-to-end stacks of rodlike structures or contractile units called *sarcomeres*. Each stack of sarcomeres forms a long filament, and arrays of filaments form the myofibrils. Sarcomeres are composed of the contractile proteins actin, myosin, tropomyosin, and troponin. Troponin is a complex of troponin T, troponin I, and troponin C, whereas myosin is made of heavy and light chains and a globular head that contains the myosin adenosine triphosphatase (ATPase). Figure 11-1 shows an electron micrograph of several myofibrils. The alternating bands of light and dark are notable. The dark A band is composed of the thick myosin filaments and is transected by a darker line called the M line. Each myosin filament is surrounded by, and interdigitates with, six thin filaments composed of actin, tropomyosin, and troponin. Areas where the thin filaments are

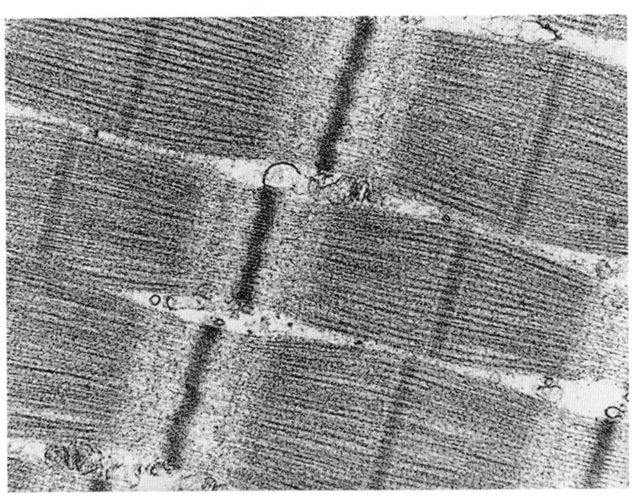

FIGURE 11-1 Electron micrograph of several muscle myofibrils (×45,000.)

not overlapping with myosin form the lighter I band. The dark line running across the I band is called the *Z line*. A sarcomere is defined as the region between each Z line. At the Z lines the protein α-actinin anchors actin. Because of the differing way these structures absorb light, the regular alternation of A bands and I bands in adjacent myofibrils produces the striated appearance characteristic of skeletal muscle fibers as viewed with light microscopy. Mitochondria fit into the small spaces around the myofibrils and produce the adenosine triphosphate (ATP) necessary for the contraction-relaxation cycle. The number, size, and shape of mitochondria vary depending on the fitness of the individual and the muscle fiber type predominant within the muscle sampled.[1-3]

MUSCLE CONTRACTION

To understand the pathophysiologic features of many muscle disorders, defining the sequential steps that lead to contraction is valuable. This process is known as *excitation-contraction coupling*.

Excitation

Excitation begins with the origination of a nerve impulse within the central nervous system. The impulse exits the spinal cord, travels along a motor neuron, and arrives at the motor end plate of an individual myofiber. Motor end plates are located in deep primary clefts or folds of the sarcolemma. The nerve impulse arrives at the motor end plate, releasing acetylcholine, which traverses the synaptic cleft and binds to nicotinic receptors. The binding of acetylcholine produces a conformational change in the nicotinic receptor, which results in the opening of ion channels, producing increased sodium and potassium conductance in the end plate membrane and causing depolarization and generation of an end plate action potential. The T tubule system propagates the action potential across the sarcolemma in all directions and carries it deep into the muscle fiber. Diffusion of acetylcholine from the receptors or hydrolysis by acetylcholine esterase causes depolarization to cease.

Excitation-Contraction Coupling

Coupling of excitation with contraction begins with the arrival of the action potential at the triad region, which causes opening of sodium channels embedded in the T tubule membrane and rapid influx of sodium into the cell. The rapid influx through the sodium channel results in a change of polarity across the membrane that we associate with depolarization. As a result the inside of the sarcolemma becomes more positive relative to the outside of the membrane. Depolarization of the T tubule membrane triggers a voltage-gated calcium channel known as the dihydropyridine receptor, which is also located within the T tubule membrane. Activation of the dihydropyridine receptor triggers the closely related ryanodine receptor in the terminal cisternae of the sarcoplasmic reticulum, causing it to release calcium into the sarcoplasm.

Contraction

Calcium released into the sarcoplasm binds to troponin C, resulting in a conformational change of the tropomyosin molecule and unmasking part of the actin filament responsible for binding to myosin: the G-actin monomer. With binding of myosin to the G-actin monomers, a 90-degree cross-bridge forms. As soon as the cross-bridge forms, myosin ATPase cleaves ATP to form adenosine diphosphate (ADP) and adenosine monophosphate (AMP), resulting in another conformational change converting the 90-degree angle to a 45-degree angle. The contractural force is generated by the movement of the cross-bridge myosin head from a 90-degree to a 45-degree angle with a coincident sliding of the myofilaments relative to one another toward the center of the sarcomere. The hydrolytic products of ATP then detach from the myosin head enabling the cycle to recommence. The addition of new ATP to the myosin molecule results in the rapid dissociation of the actin and myosin filaments.[4,5] Sustained contraction occurs with the rapid repetition of this mechanicochemical cycle.[5]

Each sarcomere shortens in unison in successive ratchetlike movements composed of multiple acts of relaxation and reengagement depending on the degree of shortening demanded by the nervous system. With input from the central nervous system to relax opposing muscles, the process of excitation-contraction coupling produces smooth coordinated movement.

Relaxation

For the cell to relax and return to baseline polarity, the sarcoplasmic reticulum and the plasmalemma must reaccumulate calcium, thereby lowering the concentration of calcium in the sarcoplasm and the T tubule while sarcolemmal membranes begin to repolarize. Sarcoplasmic calcium concentrations decrease when calcium-magnesium ATPase pumps return calcium to the sarcoplasmic reticulum and sodium-potassium ATPase pumps move sodium extracellularly and potassium intracellularly. Energy-dependent reaccumulation of calcium by the sarcoplasmic reticulum results in the release of calcium from troponin C, restoration of the resting configuration of the troponin-tropomyosin complexes, and ultimately disruption of the linkage between the myosin and actin filaments. Further details on muscle structure and contraction are available.[4-7]

TABLE 11-1

Energy Sources in Muscle*

	Creatine Phosphatase	Anaerobic Glycolysis	Aerobic Glycolysis	Fatty Acid Oxidation
Rate of ATP synthesis	73 mmol/s	40 mmol/s	17 mmol/s	7 mmol/s
Relative rate	100	55	23	10
Duration	4 s	2-3 min	1-2 h	Many hours

*Exact measurements vary somewhat by species; numbers are approximate.
ATP, Adenosine triphosphate.

An important note is that all of the processes necessary for relaxation are active, meaning they require energy in the form of ATP for them to occur. In the absence of ATP, actin and myosin remain engaged, and the muscle remains in the shortened or contracted position known as rigor.

Several terms are frequently used when referring to the shortening of muscle in veterinary medicine. *Contraction* implies a shortening or tightening of the muscle that is initiated by the central nervous system. This electrical activity is recorded readily using electromyography. A *contracture* is considered to be the shortening of a muscle because of abnormal activity within the muscle cell or cells. A contracture originates within the muscle fiber itself and is therefore electrically silent on electromyography. Contractures occur in disorders characterized by muscle cramping such as polysaccharide storage myopathy or recurrent exertional rhabdomyolysis in which muscle shortening is typically electrically silent. The term *spasm* is more generic and may refer to a transient or sustained contraction or contracture. If a spasm is painful, the term *cramp* is often used. Fibrous tissue within a muscle may prevent complete stretching and shortening of a muscle, thereby limiting the range of motion of a limb or joint. This process occurs in fibrotic myopathy as described in a subsequent section.

Source of Energy for Contraction

Understanding the sources of energy for contraction is important because most metabolic myopathies arise from derangements in these processes. ATP stores in muscle are very minimal and are quickly exhausted. Thereafter, ATP must be generated to sustain muscle function. In short, ATP is generated by either aerobic (oxidative) or anaerobic mechanisms. The primary substrates for aerobic metabolism include circulating nonesterified fatty acids and glucose or intramuscular stores (or both) of glycogen and triglycerides.

When the phosphate bond of ATP is cleaved, the resulting by-products include ADP, inorganic phosphate, and energy. At the onset of muscle activity, cleavage of the phosphate bonds of creatine phosphate (or phosphorylcreatine) in the presence of ADP by the enzyme creatine kinase produces creatine and ATP. This anaerobic pathway is quickly supplanted by other pathways to produce energy (Table 11-1).

Numerous different processes within the muscle fiber generate ATP after creatine phosphate and include glycogenolysis, glycolysis, Krebs cycle, β-oxidation of free fatty acids, and purine nucleotide deamination. Which pathways are most active depends on factors that include the underlying muscle fiber composition, the number of motor units recruited, capillarization of the muscle, the underlying oxidative and glycolytic capacities of the muscle fibers, and the delivery of oxygen and other energy substrates to the muscle. In turn, the breed and age of the horse, the length or stage of exercise, the intensity of exercise, and the fitness level of the horse influence these factors.

For specifics on glycolysis and generation of ATP via the Embden-Meyerhof pathway or the hexose monophosphate shunt, the reader is directed to a physiology text. Glycolysis or the breakdown of glucose (a 6-carbon molecule) to carbon dioxide and water in the presence of oxygen liberates 38 moles of ATP per mole of glucose. Whereas the fatty acid oxidation of a similar 6 carbon fatty acid yields 44 moles of ATP.

The primary sources of glucose include circulating glucose in the blood, small quantities of free glucose within the sarcoplasm, and stored glycogen within the muscle cell. Glycogen is a branched polymer of individual glucose molecules consisting of 1:4α and 1:6α linkages. Breakdown of glycogen, or glycogenolysis, results in the liberation of 37 moles of ATP per mole of glycogen. A large, extramuscular storage site of glycogen is the liver. With exercise, the liver begins to liberate free glucose into the blood. Muscle cells take up glucose by glucose transporters located in the cell membrane. Athletes who have exercised frequently over time develop a denser network of capillaries about each muscle cell to facilitate the delivery of oxygen, free fatty acids, and glucose to the cell and the removal of by-products.

Glycogen is made through the action of glycogen synthase and glycogen branching enzyme. The breakdown of glycogen's 1:4α linkages is mediated by phosphorylase, whereas the breakdown at the 1:6α linkages is mediated by glycogen debranching enzyme. To prevent a futile cycle of formation and degradation, these sets of enzymes are reciprocally regulated. Glycogen synthase is stimulated when glucose-6-phosphate is plentiful, whereas the presence of glucose-6-phosphate and ATP inhibit phosphorylase. Phosphorylase is activated when levels of AMP are elevated. Hormones may also activate phosphorylase. Epinephrine stimulates phosphorylase in both the liver and skeletal muscle, leading to elevations in blood lactate and glucose. Glucagon acts only on liver phosphorylase, resulting in elevations in blood glucose and not lactate.

Glycolysis and glycogenolysis are rapid processes and produce adequate energy for aerobic exercise. When exercise intensity increases and oxygen demand cannot be met, glucose is metabolized anaerobically. Anaerobic glycolysis of glycogen yields 3 moles of ATP and lactic acid as a by-product. The accumulation of lactic acid within the cell lowers the pH of the sarcoplasm, inhibits the function of many intracellular enzymes, and contributes to fatigue.

After a period of light aerobic exercise (this varies between individuals but in many is after approximately 15 to 20 minutes), the muscle begins to rely more on the β-oxidation of free fatty acids than on glycolysis for the production of ATP. Small stores of fat are located within the muscle. However, most of the free fatty acids are liberated from body fat stores or the liver and are taken up by the muscle cell during exercise. The longer the aerobic exercise, the more energy is derived from metabolism of free fatty acids. More intensive aerobic exercise uses a combination of carbohydrate and fatty acids as energy sources. The amount of energy derived from fatty acid metabolism appears also to be partially influenced by diet. The higher the intake of fat, the more muscle appears to rely on free fatty acids for energy. The optimal ratio of fat in the diet of the horse has yet to be determined.

The onset of fatigue during aerobic exercise is different from that during anaerobic exercise. During aerobic exercise, glycogen depletion, hyperthermia, and electrolyte depletion appear to be major factors, whereas during anaerobic exercise, lactic acidosis and depletion of creatine phosphate and ATP appear to be important factors initiating fatigue. Accumulation of lactic acid within the muscle cell leads to decreased intracellular pH and inhibition of the enzymes important in glycolysis. A low intracellular pH also inhibits excitation-contraction coupling. In aerobic and anaerobic forms of exercise, eventual onset of myalgia and decreased motivation appear to be additional factors in fatigue.

When most forms of energy within the muscle are exhausted the last source of energy within the cell is the formation of ATP from two molecules of ADP in a process known as the myokinase reaction. A by-product of this reaction is ammonia. Increasing ammonia concentrations in the circulation are well correlated with depletion of ATP. Depleted fibers may develop a painful, electrically silent contracture that is similar to rigor, and severely affected fibers may die. The death of muscle cells related to exercise is known as exertional rhabdomyolysis. Rhabdomyolysis is often assessed by the measurement of enzymes such as creatine kinase or lactate dehydrogenase that are released into the blood when muscle cells are severely stressed (the cell membranes become permeable) or the cells lyse.

FIBER TYPE

DIFFERENTIATION

Under light microscopy using simple staining techniques, skeletal muscle appears to be a homogeneous tissue. However, muscle is composed of many fibers with differing characteristics. Myofibers may be grouped into two categories: type 1 and type 2. Table 11-2 gives a summary of the characteristics of different fiber types. The type 1 and 2 classification is broad, and a spectrum of fibers has characteristics of both categories. The differences between fibers arise from variability in the proteins that comprise the contractile elements. Several different isoforms have been identified for the myosin heavy and light chains, tropomyosin, troponin I, troponin T, and troponin C. The greatest variability is in the isoform of the myosin heavy chain. In addition, the calcium pumping capacity of the sarcoplasmic reticulum may vary from cell to cell.

All types of fibers are found in most skeletal muscles. Type 1 fibers are high in oxidative capacity and therefore rely on glucose, free fatty acids, and a high amount of oxygen to supply energy for contraction. Their sarcoplasmic reticula have a moderately slow reuptake of calcium capacity. Therefore type 1 fibers are best suited to moderate contraction speeds and sustained contractions over long periods. As expected, these fibers predominate in muscles involved in posture. Type 2 fibers have a fast myosin ATPase rate and a rapid capacity to reuptake calcium into the sarcoplasmic reticulum. They are large-diameter fibers compared with type 1 fibers and have a higher glycolytic capacity, making them suited to powerful

TABLE 11-2

Fiber Type Characteristics

	TYPE 1	TYPE 2*	
		A	B
PHYSIOLOGIC CHARACTERISTICS			
Speed of contraction/twitch	Slow	Fast	Fast
Fatigability	Low	Intermediate	Rapid
Maximal tension developed	Low	High	High
HISTOCHEMICAL PROPERTIES			
Myofibrillar ATPase stain pH 9.4	Light	Dark	Dark
Preincubation at a pH of:			
≈4.5	Dark	Light	Medium
≈4.3	Dark	Light	Light
Oxidative capacity	High	Intermediate high	Low
Enzymes for glucose breakdown	Intermediate	High	High
Enzymes for free fatty acid breakdown	High	Intermediate	Low
No. of capillaries	High	Intermediate	Low
Glycogen content	Low	High	High

ATPase, Adenosine triphosphatase.
*Type 2C fibers have been described after acid preincubation with staining intensities between the light type 2A and medium type 2B fibers.

fast contractions. These fibers predominate in the skeletal muscles involved in locomotion and rapid fine-motor movements such as around the eye. Type 2 fibers that have activities closer to type 1 fibers are called type 2A, whereas those that exhibit high anaerobic capacity are characterized as type 2B. Because of the high oxidative capacity of type 1 fibers, these muscles often appear to have a deeper red color than fibers high in type 2A and 2B fibers.

Histologically, differentiation of muscle fiber types relies on the measurement of myofibrillar ATPase activity (the enzyme responsible for the breakdown of ATP at the actin-myosin cross-bridges). Staining for this enzyme distinguishes two distinct fiber types at pH 9.4. The slow-twitch type 1 fibers have a low activity at this pH and so appear lighter in color than the fast-twitch type 2 fibers. The type 2 fibers can be divided further by preincubation at a more acidic pH into types 2A, 2B, and even 2C (the pH values required for this differentiation vary with the laboratory but are around 4.5 and 4.3).

The varying capacities of muscle fiber types is largely the result of variations in myosin heavy-chain isoforms. These isoforms are identified through antibody and electrophoresis techniques. In mammals, at least nine have been identified. Two are developmental (embryonic and neonatal), two are found in cardiac muscle (alpha and beta), three are common in skeletal muscle (2a, 2b, and 2x), and two are rare with greatest expression in jaw, extraocular, and laryngeal muscles. Beta is also found in skeletal muscle and is an isoform with properties of slow twitch, high oxidative capacity, low glycolytic capacity, and low ATPase activity similar to the histologically identified type 1 myofibers. Type 2a myosin heavy-chain isoforms are typically found in fibers exhibiting fast twitch, high glycolytic, high ATPase activity, and high oxidative capacity and as such resist fatigue. Type 2b and 2x isoforms are found in muscles that are fast twitch, produce strong contractions, have high glycolytic and ATPase activity but have low oxidative capacity and, as such, fatigue faster than type 2a rich myofibers.[8-11]

Innervation

A neuron and all of its innervated myofibers constitute a motor unit. Each motor neuron may innervate a few or several hundred myofibers, and all of those myofibers exhibit similar contraction characteristics. Each myofiber, however, is innervated only by a branch of one motor neuron. Two types of motor nerve fiber are found, slow and fast. The type and pattern of electrical activity on a muscle cell is related to the type of myosin isoforms expressed: The large phasic motor nerve fibers innervate the type 2 myofibers, whereas the small tonic fibers innervate the type 1 fibers.[11]

Muscle spindles are a bundle of specialized muscle fibers that run parallel to nonsensory muscle fibers and which contact sensory axon endings. Muscle spindle cells are important in telling the nervous system about the tone and length of the muscle. They are also important in maintaining posture. Discharges are relayed directly to the ipsilateral spinal motor neurons that innervate the muscle in which the spindle is located, resulting in a reflex arc. Two types of sensory neurons innervate each spindle: the primary endings are from the large-diameter group 1A afferent axons, whereas the less elaborate secondary endings are from the smaller group 2 afferent axons. The spindle cell fibers also receive motor neuron innervation from small γ-motor neurons, which helps keep the spindle taut when the muscle contracts, which, in turn, enables the sensory endings to respond to a wide range of muscle lengths.

Muscle spindle cells are different from the muscle Golgi tendon organ. Golgi tendon organs are found at the ends of the muscle fibers at the musculotendinous junction and are formed from a common tendon to which several muscle fibers are attached. A sensory nerve ending wraps around each Golgi tendon organ. The sensory nerve innervating the Golgi tendon organ responds to tension generated by the contraction of any of these muscle fibers, and the discharge is relayed to the ipsilateral α-motor neurons, where it is inhibitory. This action forms another reflex arc responding to muscle tension and helps ensure that muscles of flexion and extension do not contract simultaneously.

Fiber Recruitment

Under neural control, an orderly selection of fibers occurs with increasing demands. When just maintaining posture or walking the horse uses only the nerves supplying the slow-twitch type 1 and possibly a few of the intermediate type fast-twitch high-oxidative type 2A fibers. As the speed or intensity of work increases, more and more fibers are recruited. Thus, at a medium trot, approximately 50% of the muscle cells within a muscle belly are contracting, whereas at a gallop, most or all fibers are involved. The fibers are recruited in a set order: type 1, type 2A, and then type 2B. The gradation in response of a muscle is known as the recruitment of motor units. A motor unit consists of a motor nerve and the cells it innervates. The smoothness of a muscular contraction occurs because of the asynchronous contraction of the various motor units.

Distribution

The proportions of fiber types present within a muscle vary according to individual traits of the horse, the muscle location, the breed, and the age of the horse.[1,8,10,12-15] In some muscles (in particular the middle gluteal muscle, which is sampled most commonly) the distribution also depends on the sampling site or depth because the distribution of fiber types is nonhomogeneous.[1,10,15,16] The suggestion has been made, however, that within a specific muscle of an individual, the variation in fiber types is small if samples are taken from the same site or an identical contralateral site under controlled conditions.[15,17] This arrangement is why it is generally recommended to biopsy specific muscles to diagnose certain disorders. It provides a relatively homogeneous baseline from which to evaluate a muscle. The exception is when a specific muscle is affected (e.g., exhibits atrophy) wherein it should be biopsied.

GROWTH, TRAINING, AND PERFORMANCE

Fiber type predominance does affect performance. However, with growth and training muscle cells adapt and may change fiber type over time.[1,7,18-22] Training results in (1) an increase in the ability of a fiber to use oxygen by increasing the number of mitochondria within the sarcoplasm, (2) a decrease in the use of muscle glycogen and blood glucose with a greater reliance on fat oxidation to supply ATP, and (3) a decrease in the amount of lactate produced per given intensity of exercise. Variable results have been reported on the effects of exercise on fiber size and capillarization. The extent and nature of the changes appear to depend on the duration, intensity, and type of exercise involved, as well as the age of the animal. Over the last decades, much information has been gained in the field of equine exercise physiology, and multiple texts are available on the subject both in print and online that extend beyond the scope of this chapter.[23-26]

PATHOLOGIC CHANGES

General Response of Muscle to Injury

Muscle responds to injury or damage in a limited number of ways. A growing body of evidence indicates that myopathic conditions share a similar final pathway of muscle fiber degeneration, although the number and type of fibers affected and the degree of damage varies.[27] The final common pathway involves failure to sequester calcium ions from the sarcoplasm. Prolonged calcium accumulation within the sarcoplasm leads to activation of cellular enzymes and prolonged activation of myofilaments. This process is visible histologically as hypercontraction. Consequently, mitochondria take up excess calcium in an attempt to prevent cellular damage. Accumulation of calcium within the mitochondria leads to failure of energy production (i.e., ATP) within the cell and eventually failure of all intracellular energy-dependent mechanisms, which leads to failure of membrane pumps and ultimately cell swelling and lysis.[27,28]

The exact nature of these calcium-activated degenerative pathways is still unknown. A key step may be calcium-induced membrane phospholipid hydrolysis via the activation of phospholipase enzymes, resulting in the production of tissue-damaging metabolites. Other processes, however, involving nonenzymatic lipid peroxidation also may be activated. During exercise the flow of oxygen increases. At the same time an overall depletion of ATP sources occurs. The resultant metabolic stress leads to a greatly increased rate of oxygen free radical production that may exceed the scavenger and antioxidant defense systems of the cell, leading to a loss of cell viability and damage. The increase in free radical activity can lead to a failure of calcium homeostasis and consequent muscle damage, or, alternatively, calcium overloading may lead to an activation of free radical–mediated processes.[29] Multiple initiators likely lead to this final common pathway, depending on the type of exercise, fitness level, presence or absence of underlying genetic defects in muscle metabolism, and nutritional status of the horse. Free radical–induced skeletal muscle damage may be especially important if reperfusion follows a period of ischemia.[30]

Atrophy and Hypertrophy

Atrophy may be defined as a decrease in muscle fiber diameter or cross-sectional area. Atrophy can occur in a variety of circumstances, including denervation, disuse, and cachexia, in many muscle diseases, after circulatory disturbances, and after extensive myolysis. Within 2 or 3 weeks after peripheral denervation, up to two thirds of the original muscle mass may be lost, although this may not always be obvious clinically because of the presence of superficial and intramuscular fat deposits. Histologic changes reflect the affected nerve and the muscle fiber supplied. In disuse (e.g., atrophy resulting from a tenotomy) a preferential atrophy of type 1 fibers is apparent, often with hypertrophy of type 2 fibers. In contrast, with cachexia and malnutrition, type 2 fibers are preferentially affected, especially in the postural muscles. Not all muscles show the same degree of atrophy, even within one disease process. In cachexia, the back and thigh muscles tend to be the first affected, and the loss of muscle is usually symmetric, with a concurrent loss of fat deposits. A localized asymmetric atrophy is associated with paralysis, immobilization, and denervation.[31]

As indicated previously, hypertrophy may occur through training. A compensatory hypertrophy may also occur in the fibers surrounding an area where fibers have been lost or have decreased greatly in size. Often, large fibers are visible histologically in such conditions, with evidence of incomplete longitudinal division.[31]

Repair after Denervation

Denervation results in atrophy, as remarked previously, but also leads to abnormal muscle excitability. Muscle becomes more sensitive to circulating acetylcholine. The result is the presence of fine, irregular contractions or fibrillations detectable using electromyography. Fibrillations are not visible clinically and should not be confused with fasciculations that appear grossly as jerky muscle contractions in response to pathologic spinal motor neuron discharges.[11] With reinnervation the fibrillations cease. Reinnervation can occur in two ways. Damage without severing the nerve is called axonotmesis. The axon is damaged but the Schwann cell and endoneural fibrous sheaths remain. Axons from the proximal part of the damaged nerve may reestablish connections within the empty residual Schwann cell sheath to the distal portion of the original nerve. Initially, atrophy of scattered muscle fibers is visible, but after reinnervation a proportion of the muscle fibers are restored to their normal size and function. Even if the affected muscle is not fully restored, other surrounding unaffected muscles may be able to compensate so that overall function is maintained, although slight gait abnormalities may remain.

The second type of reinnervation occurs when some nerve fascicles are severed completely or when the nerve lesion is located a great distance from the muscle, for example, when lesions involve the motor neuron cell bodies or nerve roots or both. In this case, collateral reinnervation from adjacent, unaffected axons can occur. Given that the nerve type characterizes the muscle type, this action results in regrouping of muscle fibers so that clusters of fibers of the same histochemical type are found rather than the normal checkerboard pattern. This phenomenon is known as fiber type grouping.

Repair after Injury

Regeneration where a break in the continuity of the muscle fiber has occurred differs considerably from neurologic damage. In such cases, repair involves multiplication of nuclei and formation of new internal structures and organelles followed by fusion and alignment into a new multinuclear myofiber. Regeneration can be swift when parts of the affected fiber remain intact. In this case, regeneration occurs at the healthy end of the severed fiber (continuous or budding regeneration). When damage is more severe, regeneration occurs by fusion of mononuclear myoblasts to form a myotube, which develops in a similar way to fetal fibers (discontinuous or embryonic regeneration). The origin of myoblasts is primarily satellite cells, and their origins and function have been well reviewed.[32,33] If the scaffolding, basement membrane, and supporting tissues remain intact, and if the initiating disease process subsides, new fibers tend to orient in a way similar to the original fibers. This type of regeneration usually occurs with segmental necrosis in which necrosis of the whole diameter of the fiber has occurred involving several sarcomeres. Fibroblastic and vascular reactions are minimal in this type of regeneration. Therefore full function of the muscle is restored without residual dysfunction.

Massive trauma, hemorrhage, infection, or infarction can result in damage to the basement membrane and other supporting structures resulting in complete disorientation of the regenerating fibers with significant proliferation of fibroblasts and vessels. In such cases, regeneration may result in significant deformation of the muscle with disruption of its normal function. Regenerated cells often have centrally located nuclei and larger diameters than older myofibers.

DIAGNOSIS OF SKELETAL MUSCLE DISORDERS

Because damage to muscle tissue often occurs along similar pathways, recognizing that muscle disorders can only rarely be diagnosed based on muscle histopathology alone is important. A thorough history that includes genetic background, exercise, nutrition, patient signalment, and clinical description of the muscular disorder is mandatory.

Skeletal muscle disorders broadly fall into two categories: acquired or inborn. Acquired myopathies include those of traumatic or infectious origin and ones arising secondarily from endocrine or nutritional disease or electrolyte imbalances (acquired metabolic myopathies).[34] Inborn errors of metabolism that manifest as metabolic myopathies originate primarily from defects in muscle energy metabolism. As such, they can be grouped as errors in carbohydrate, lipid, or purine metabolism; as mitochondrial defects; or as primary disorders of ion channels (channelopathies).

Acute trauma typically produces obvious clinical signs such as an open wound, severe lameness, heat, pain, swelling, or any combination. Healed traumatic injuries may be evident by abnormal gait or scar tissue, or both, within the muscle as primary complaints. Infectious myositis may also cause heat, pain, swelling, or crepitus, in addition to systemic signs of colic, endotoxemia, and shock if the infection is severe and widespread. In general the metabolic myopathies reveal a more chronic history involving some of the following client complaints: episodic weakness or muscle cramping, progressive weakness, atrophy, muscle wasting, reluctance to move, rapid muscle fatigue with exercise, intermittent or consistent gait abnormalities, muscle fasciculations, or discolored urine.

Modalities used to diagnose equine myopathies may include a thorough history (including use, diet, genetic background, signalment, and client complaint), physical examination, serum chemistry profile, complete blood count, urinalysis (including analysis for myoglobin and fractional excretions of sodium, potassium, phosphorus, and chloride), muscle biopsy (histology, histochemistry, electron microscopy), electromyography (EMG), thermography, genetic testing, nuclear scintigraphy, or any combination. In horses with suspected metabolic myopathies, diagnostics may be strategically put together as part of an exercise challenge test that includes the history, observation of the horse at work, pre- and postexercise measurement of serum muscle enzyme activity and lactate, urinalysis with fractional excretions of electrolytes, genetic testing, and muscle biopsy.

Plasma and Serum Enzyme Activities

The enzymes that are most useful in evaluating the equine muscular system are creatine kinase (CK), aspartate transferase (AST), and lactate dehydrogenase (LDH). A change in the plasma activity of any enzyme can occur for a variety of reasons, including alteration in the permeability of the enclosing cell membrane, cell necrosis, impaired removal or clearance of the enzyme, and increased or impaired synthesis. Decreases in plasma enzyme activities are not usually clinically significant. Often, no one specific organ of elimination is responsible, although most elimination occurs via the liver, kidneys, and lungs. Therefore, under most circumstances, the elimination rate of an enzyme from the plasma remains fairly constant, and the rate of influx to the plasma is the crucial factor.

Increases most commonly occur because of a defect in the integrity of the membrane containing the enzyme-rich sarcoplasm.[6,35] The defect results from complete disruption of the cell or a transient change in the permeability of the membrane without cell death. A complete explanation for the pattern of release of intracellular constituents from diseased muscles cannot be given here. Most of the enzymes that are detectable in increased concentrations in the blood with the various muscle disorders are the major soluble (sarcoplasmic) enzymes, although one can also detect the mitochondrial form of AST with severe injury.

The degree of muscle damage does not correlate with the magnitude of increase in serum muscle enzyme activity; a small amount of severely damaged muscle may release a similar amount of enzyme as a larger quantity of mildly damaged muscle. Under general circumstances, the rate of efflux of an enzyme most likely depends not only on its molecular weight and intracellular localization but also on its binding to various intracellular structures and relative intracellular and extracellular concentration. No explanation for the significant differences in half-lives of the various plasma muscle enzymes reported for human beings and horses has been given.

Creatine Kinase

Creatine kinase is the enzyme responsible for breaking down creatine phosphate to creatine and phosphate, releasing energy for muscular contraction. This reaction is the sole source of energy in muscle at the initiation of exercise. Thereafter, energy is supplied by oxidation of glucose and free fatty acids as described previously. Because this enzyme is responsible for the breakdown of creatine phosphate, it is often called creatine phosphokinase. This term, however, is inappropriate, and one should use creatine kinase. In the horse, CK is found mainly in skeletal muscle, the myocardium, and the brain.[36] Little or no exchange of CK between the cerebrospinal fluid and plasma appears to occur. A significant increase in total plasma CK activity therefore is caused by cardiac or skeletal muscle damage. CK (molecular weight, 80,000 daltons [Da]) does not enter the bloodstream directly after its release from the muscle cell but transits through the lymph via the interstitial fluid. The total quantity of circulating CK in the horse under normal conditions is estimated to be equivalent to the quantity of CK in approximately 1 g of muscle; a threefold to fivefold increase in plasma CK activity corresponds to the apparent myolysis of approximately 20 g of muscle.[37] However, as described previously, making assumptions as to the amount of muscle damaged based on serum CK activity is difficult because muscle cells appear to be able to release significant quantities of CK without necessarily being lysed.

In human beings, two monomers of CK are known and are designated M and B. The enzyme is dimeric, and three possible primary forms exist: MM, MB, and BB. In simplified terms, MM is found mainly in skeletal muscle, BB in the brain and epithelial tissues, and MB in the myocardium. In the horse, some confusion over CK isoenzymes exists, with workers reporting different electrophoretic bands and tissue activities, perhaps because of the different techniques used.[38-41] In one study the heart and skeletal muscle were found to contain predominantly the MM dimer; the brain, pancreas, and kidney, mainly the BB dimer; and the intestine, the MB and BB dimers.[39] This work suggests that in the horse, CK isoenzymes on their own could not be used to differentiate between skeletal and cardiac muscle damage. This problem is alleviated largely by the current availability of tests for cardiac troponin I. Unfortunately, commercial tests for skeletal troponin I are not available. In the absence of clinical cardiac disease, elevations in CK primarily can be attributed to skeletal muscle. The plasma half-life of CK in the horse is short (108 minutes, 123 ± 28 min with a plasma clearance of 0.36 ± 0.1 ml/kg/min)[37,42] in contrast to reports of 12 hours in human beings.[43]

Aspartate Aminotransferase

AST is found mainly in skeletal muscle, liver, and heart, although lower activities are present in several other tissues. Therefore AST is not tissue specific.[36,44,45] Two isoenzymes have been identified by electrophoresis: MAST (found exclusively in the mitochondria) and CAST (originating from the cytoplasm or sarcoplasm). The ratio of cytosolic to mitochondrial enzyme in horse serum is significantly greater than that found in human beings and many other mammals.[46] In the horse, the ratio of these two forms varies between tissues, and no tissue specificity is apparent for either isoenzyme. The plasma half-life of AST in the horse is 7 to 10 days,[42] far longer than the 11.8 hours in human beings.[43]

Lactate Dehydrogenase

Lactate dehydrogenase is a tetrapeptide that occurs in five different isozymic forms produced by combinations of two kinds of subunits (H [heart] and M [muscle]) in groups of four to produce the functional tetrameric molecule. The five isoenzymes are labeled as LDH_1 to LDH_5, or H_4, MH_3, M_2H_2, M_3H, and M_4, respectively. Similar to AST, LDH is found in most tissues and is therefore not organ specific. However, tissues contain various amounts of the LDH isoenzymes, and the isoenzyme profile obtained by electrophoretic separation has been used to identify specific tissue damage.[47] For the most part, LDH_5 (plus some LDH_4) is found in the locomotor muscles, the liver contains mainly LDH_3 (with some LDH_4 and LDH_5), the heart contains mainly LDH_1 (with LDH_2 and LDH_3), and all types have been found in certain nonlocomotor muscles.[38,41] Training has been shown to increase the percentage of LDH_1 to LDH_4 and decrease that of LDH_5 in skeletal muscle.[48] The practitioner should use nonhemolyzed samples for LDH determinations because red blood cells contain large amounts of LDH. In general, though, assays for CK and AST are most commonly used to evaluate skeletal muscle.

Urinalysis: Myoglobinuria

Myoglobin (molecular weight 16,500 Da) is essential for the transport of oxygen into and within muscle cells. Most mammalian muscles contain approximately 1 mg myoglobin per gram of fresh tissue, and the suggestion has been made that acute destruction of at least 200 g of muscle must occur before serum myoglobin levels rise sufficiently for detection in the urine.[49] Serum myoglobin has a short half-life, and therefore measuring serum myoglobin is of limited diagnostic value. In human beings, myoglobinuria occurs in a variety of conditions, including myocardial infarction, crush and burn injuries, malignant hyperthermia, idiopathic and exertional rhabdomyolysis, and certain genetic metabolic abnormalities.[6,49-52] In the horse, myoglobinuria has been seen in equine exercise or trauma-induced rhabdomyolysis,[53,54] white muscle disease in foals,[55] and postanesthetic myositis.[56]

Pigmenturia or dark urine may be caused by increased myoglobin, hemoglobin, or whole blood in the urine. Low levels of myoglobin, hemoglobin, or whole blood may occur in the urine and can be detected by urine dipstick or laboratory test before visible changes in the color of urine. Therefore considerable amounts of myoglobin, hemoglobin, or whole blood must be present for visible pigmenturia to occur. Many causes of hemolysis in the horse can result in hemoglobinuria, including oxidative damage to erythrocytes,[57] neonatal isoerythrolysis, hepatic disease, and renal disease.[59]

Unfortunately, stored urine, concentrated urine, and urine containing myoglobin, hemoglobin, or other porphyrins can appear similar in color[57,59,60] (Figure 11-2). Therefore myoglobinuria cannot be distinguished by color alone. The orthotoluidine-impregnated strips commonly used by veterinary clinicians (urine dipstick tests such as BM-Test-8, Boehringer Ingelheim Pharmaceuticals, Ridgefield, Conn.) are insensitive to the presence of myoglobin and hemoglobin.[54,61] The differential salting out of hemoglobin with ammonium sulfate gives false results in human beings[49,50,59,62] and the horse but is used commonly in many laboratories.[49,50,59,61,62] Visual inspection of the serum or plasma may indicate the cause of the pigmenturia. The low affinity of myoglobin for haptoglobin means that myoglobin is excreted at plasma concentrations around 0.2 g/L, whereas hemoglobin only appears in the urine at plasma concentrations greater than 1.0 g/L. At this concentration a pink discoloration of the plasma occurs, indicating that hemoglobin is present.[9,49,50,63]

On electrophoretic separation on cellulose acetate, myoglobin migrates as a β_2-globulin and hemoglobin as an α_2-globulin. This method can distinguish the two proteins in urine containing high concentrations (>125 μg/ml) of either protein, provided no other proteins, apart from albumin, are present. Immunoassays are the most sensitive and specific tests and can be used for detecting small amounts of myoglobin in blood and urine.[61,64,65] Sequelae of acute tubular necrosis and acute renal failure are associated with myoglobinuria in human beings[66] and horses.[44,63] Renal disease associated with myoglobinemia in the horse seems to be associated most with

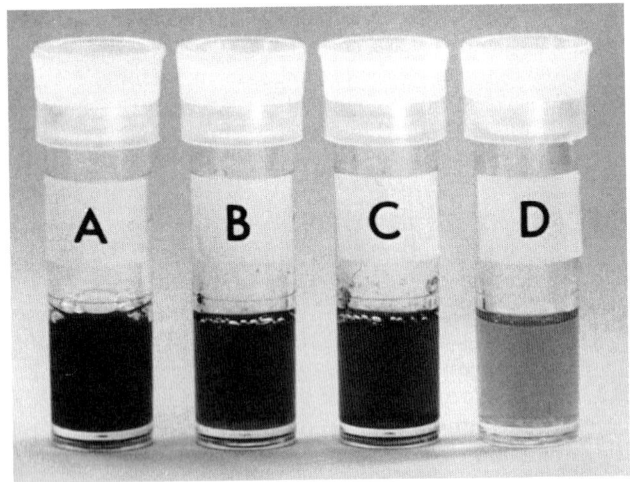

FIGURE 11-2 Four urine samples. **A,** With 3 mg/ml hemoglobin. **B,** With 3 mg/ml myoglobin. **C,** Normal stored for 1 month at 18° C. **D,** Control (fresh urine).

horses that are highly stressed (causing decreased renal blood flow), dehydrated, or have lactic acidosis associated with rhabdomyolysis. Therefore horses suffering from "capture" myopathy (e.g., cast in a stall or trailer accident and struggling for a prolonged period) and endurance horses are most at risk.

Muscle Biopsy

The practitioner can obtain muscle biopsy samples by surgical excision under general or local anesthesia[63] or by percutaneous needle biopsy from the standing horse.[9,14,67] Because of the variation in fiber composition in muscles, which muscle is chosen, as well as the position and depth of sampling, is important. Good specimen preparation for frozen sections is vital to prevent artifacts such as ice crystals.[6,9,68] For laboratories that prefer examination of frozen sections, specimens are typically shipped chilled overnight so that the laboratory may freeze the sample to minimize artifacts. Other laboratories prefer formalin-fixed specimens. The practitioner should discuss sample procurement, preparation, and shipment procedures with the laboratory before biopsy.

Muscle biopsy allows the morphologic, biochemical, and physiologic properties of the myofibers to be examined with the animal still alive and causes little morbidity. Typical sites used for percutaneous biopsy with a 6-mm modified Bergstrom needle in cases of generalized muscle disease or for research purposes include the semimembranosus, the biceps femoris, and most commonly the middle gluteal muscle. Although convenient, the necessity to have a modified Bergstrom needle means that most practitioners opt for open biopsy of the semimembranosus muscle over percutaneous middle gluteal muscle biopsy. Instructions on how to obtain a muscle biopsy are available online.[69]

To biopsy the semimembranosus a 6- to 10-cm^2 area is clipped and surgically prepared slightly lateral to and below the anus. At this location, if a scar occurs after the procedure the tail will hide it. An inverted L lidocaine block of the skin and subcutaneous tissues is performed. Local anesthetic is not injected into the muscle itself, which may induce artifact into the biopsy. The muscle belly is innervated poorly for pain, and reaction to transection of a small piece of muscle is minimal. A piece of muscle measuring approximately 1 × 1 × 2 cm is dissected free, and sutures are used to close the subcutaneous layer and skin. Buried skin sutures that do not need to be removed or skin staples appear to be preferable because they are less likely to cause skin irritation and therefore are less likely to be rubbed out by the patient. Should the horse open the biopsy site, the wound typically heals well by second intention with general wound care. This procedure rarely has complications; however, the horse should be current on tetanus prophylaxis as a general precaution. The biopsy is wrapped loosely in saline-dampened gauze and placed in a sealed container for shipment on icepacks to a laboratory skilled in muscle biopsy assessment.

Histochemical staining of frozen muscle sections aids in the detection of glycolytic enzyme deficiencies and storage of various atypical metabolic compounds.[6,70-72] Pathologic changes that can be found in muscle include presence of degenerate or regenerate myofibers, abnormal cytoplasmic inclusions, accumulations of polysaccharide, changes in fiber volume, number, shape, malformation, degeneration or proliferation of organelles, and disruption of the basic architecture of the fiber. Aggregates of inflammatory cells, reactive changes in vessel walls, occlusion of blood vessels, and increased amounts of fibrous tissue are other possible pathologic findings. In some conditions, such as tetanus or botulism, no significant changes may be seen. Further information on the types of changes that occur is available.[6,31]

Various histologic stains have been developed to highlight the different morphologic changes and inclusions that occur. The most important of these is the periodic acid–Schiff stain that highlights glycogen stores within a cell and membrane structures containing mucopolysaccharide, glycoproteins, mucoproteins, glycolipids, or phospholipids. Large aggregates of abnormal polysaccharide occur in Quarter Horses and Draft-breed horses with polysaccharide storage myopathy. Histochemical staining for fiber type enables the pathologic changes to be recognized as affecting all fibers or those of one type only. In cases of reinnervation, large groups of a single fiber type are visible as opposed to the more interspersed pattern typically observed.

Immunocytochemical studies have been used to investigate neuromuscular disorders in human beings and to diagnose autoimmune streptococcal-associated myositis in the horse.[73,74] Specialized staining techniques help to localize specific enzymes and intracellular and extracellular muscle components such as the various collagen and myosin types, complement, and fibronectin. Electron microscopic studies enable investigation into the ultrastructure of muscle fibers.

Electromyography

Needle EMG is the study of the electrical activity of muscles. EMG may be useful in horses with unusual gait or muscle changes and can be used to discriminate between neurogenic and myogenic causes and more specifically to identify areas or regions of an abnormality.[75] A recording needle electrode is placed into the muscle, and the electrical activity is amplified, recorded on an oscilloscope, and projected audibly into a loudspeaker. The electrical status of muscle membranes depends on the integrity of the whole motor unit. Thus an EMG evaluates the function of the ventral motor horn cell, its axon, axon terminals, and neuromuscular junctions, as well as the muscle fibers it innervates.

Investigations are usually carried out in two phases. First the practitioner assesses the electrical potentials associated with the physical disruption of the sarcolemma resulting from insertion of the needle. These insertional potentials, if relayed through a loudspeaker, tend to emit a sound similar to short bursts of loud static. They vary among muscles, probably because of differences in the size and number of motor units present.

The second phase involves assessment of electrical potentials when the needle electrode is at rest in the muscle. Normally, electrical silence occurs with cessation of needle movement, unless the needle is located in proximity to a nerve branch or the end plate zone when miniature end plate potentials are recorded continuously; these sound similar to low-intensity static.

In relaxed, diseased muscles, different types of abnormal electrical activity have been recognized. In cases of denervation, insertional activity may persist after needle movement has stopped because of increased excitability of the muscle fiber membranes. Positive, sharp waves are slow monophasic waves, rapid in onset, with a slow decay to the baseline, which occur repeatedly with variable amplitude (100 μV to 20 mV). Their cause is uncertain, they often occur with denervation, and they may represent a nonpropagated depolarization region in the muscle fibers near to the tip of the electrode. When occurring in trains, these positive sharp waves sound similar to a waning brrrr. Fibrillation potentials are electric signals generated by a single muscle fiber. Long, random volleys of mono- or biphasic (occasionally triphasic) potentials of short duration (0.5 to 5.0 ms), with amplitudes of usually less than 200 μV, commonly occur in denervation (depending on the stage). Constant and repetitive fibrillation potentials, which sound similar to rain on a tin roof or the sizzling of frying eggs, can be found especially in the early stages of denervation. Fibrillation potentials can also be seen in myopathic disorders in which segmental muscle necrosis may have caused, for example, the separation of a muscle fiber and its nerve supply.

Myotonic discharges—high-frequency (up to 1000 Hz) repetitive discharges with waxing and waning of potentials is seen and heard with a characteristic, musical, dive-bomber, or more precisely, revving motorcycle–like sound—are found in the myotonias (myotonia congenita, myotonia dystrophica, and hyperkalemic periodic paralysis) if the practitioner moves the exploring EMG electrode or percusses the muscle externally. Bizarre, high-frequency discharges (often called *pseudomyotonia*) may produce a dive bomber–like sound. No true waxing and waning occurs, although the amplitude and frequency of the potentials may change abruptly to mimic a revving motorcycle–like sound. The discharges are often in couplets or triplets and are likely to terminate abruptly. These, or similar discharges, occur in long-standing denervations, ventral horn cell disease, polymyositis, and certain myopathies. Unlike the myotonic discharges, pseudomyotonic discharges may be abolished by curare and therefore are believed to originate presynaptically.

Fasciculations, visible muscle twitching, are caused by the spontaneous contraction of some or all of the constituent fibers of a motor unit. They can be local or generalized and occur primarily with any cause of muscular weakness (myasthenia), especially in neurogenic disorders such as tetanus and certain debilitating and metabolic disorders. In addition, one can assess the electric activity induced by electric stimulation of nerves or associated with voluntary or induced muscle contraction. Further information on EMG is available.[76]

Thermography

An infrared thermographic scanner converts the radiated thermal energy of the skin to electric signals that can be amplified and displayed on a video screen. By using isotherm colors of known temperature, the examiner can obtain two-dimensional, graphic, and quantitative information regarding the precise temperature of the skin surface. The practitioner can use this technique noninvasively as a means of detecting changes in skin temperature resulting primarily from changes in peripheral blood flow. Inflammation, atrophy, neoplasia, and neurologic lesions, particularly of the autonomic supply to the skin, can alter local blood flow.

Abnormalities have been found in exercise-exacerbated focal thoracolumbar gait abnormalities, as well as disuse atrophy.[77] The technique has been useful in documenting hindlimb muscle strain as a cause of lameness in horses.

Scintigraphy

Bone-seeking radiopharmaceuticals have been used to detect and localize skeletal muscle involvement, especially in poor performance cases, but are of limited routine value in the field. Accumulation in damaged muscle may be related to the deposition of calcium in damaged fibers, binding by tissue hormones or enzyme receptors, tagging to denatured proteins, or altered capillary permeability. Uptake of labeled phosphates appears to occur only when muscle damage is ongoing and does not occur in areas of repair. Three main types of muscle uptake were identified in one study of horses with skeletal muscle damage: a diffuse, severe, and generalized uptake; bilateral symmetric uptake involving muscle groups that perform synergistic functions; and asymmetric radioisotope uptake in one or more muscle groups on one side of the animal.[78] The reasons for the various patterns have not been elucidated fully. Scintigraphy can be used as part of a series of tests to identify atypical or difficult-to-pinpoint lamenesses in horses that may have primary muscle lesions among other problems.[79,80]

Exercise Tests

Certain physiologic changes can result in a transient alteration in cell membrane permeability. Hypoxia, catecholamines, hypoglycemia, changes in pH, and altered ionic concentrations have been reported as causing such a change in membrane permeability.[45,81,82] Many of these changes are believed to act by decreasing the amount of ATP available for the maintenance of cell integrity, which becomes especially important during exercise.[83]

Measuring the CK and AST activities before and after a controlled period of exercise has been suggested as an aid to diagnosing certain muscle disorders. A major difficulty has been to establish exactly the normal enzyme response to exercise. Much confusion exists in the literature regarding this parameter, partly because of the differences in the intensity and duration of the exercise undertaken, the varying sampling intervals used in the reports, and the possible inclusion of individuals with muscular problems. The majority of workers have suggested that an increase in CK activities occurs with hard exercise,[83-85] whereas with slower work, others have shown no significant increase. This difference suggests that intensity could be an important factor.[86,87] Such a conclusion is supported by work in dogs, which shows that CK activities correlate with the intensity of muscular activity.[85] Another study in the horse,[88] however, suggested that CK elevations did not vary according to the intensity of the work, and one researcher[89] proposed that the duration of exercise was the more important factor. Another study suggested that when the duration of exercise was kept constant, the intensity of the exercise in fact did have an effect on the extent of CK activity increase.[90]

Although no significant increase in CK activity was found after trotting exercise in conditioned animals by one worker, others recorded significant increases when horses performed the same exercise after 1 or more days of rest.[87] Increases in AST activities of 35% have been reported after a 1500-m canter[91] and of 50% after strenuous exercise in previously rested animals.[84] Most other workers have found little increase in AST after different types of exercise.[42,46,89,92]

Therefore the effects of exercise on plasma muscle enzyme activities may depend on the fitness of the animal and the intensity and duration of the exercise, as well as on the environment.[38,63,89] However, concurrent lameness does not appear to alter postexercise CK activity significantly in healthy horses without myopathy.[93] In horses, as in human beings, large intersubject variability may occur in the postexercise rise in CK activities that must be taken into account.[37] Plasma volume changes may affect the activities recorded, especially if measured immediately after exercise.

As discussed previously, the physiologic increase in CK activity after exercise is believed to be caused by a change in cell membrane permeability, possibly caused by hypoxia, although other factors are likely involved. Hypoxia may occur at lower workloads in unconditioned horses, and these horses may be expected to show higher postexercise activities than a fit horse given the same work. The suggestion has been made that the magnitude of the exercise-induced increase in enzymes lessens with training.[42,88,89] Some workers have found no significant changes in the AST and CK responses to exercise during a training program,[92] whereas others have found that after an endurance ride the fittest animals (indicated by the speed of heart rate recovery after an endurance ride) had lower increases in CK activities.[86] The magnitude of exercise-induced changes in CK activities increases with detraining. This study concluded that increases of more than 100% in AST activity after exercise likely are abnormal, regardless of the intensity of the exercise or the fitness of the animal. Also, if a short, submaximal exercise test is carried out the serum CK and AST activities at 2 hours after exercise should not rise to more than 250% and 50% of the pre-exercise values, respectively, regardless of fitness.[90]

The point has been stressed that, although exercise might result in statistically significant changes in CK and AST activity, these may not always be of biologic or clinical significance.[94,95] The practitioner must always take into consideration the clinical history and clinical presentation when interpreting enzyme values. For example, a young racehorse given its first gallop often has activity changes greater than those described (e.g., from a pre-exercise level of 40 U/L to a 2-hour postexercise level of 350 U/L), although this is unlikely to be clinically significant. However, in cases of recurrent exertional rhabdomyolysis (RER) or polysaccharide storage myopathy (PSSM), similar changes may indicate ongoing subclinical muscular dysfunction. For example, in the author's experience, horses with RER or PSSM may have 4-hour postexercise serum CK activities of 10,000 to 15,000 U/L without outward clinical signs of rhabdomyolysis.

Currently the author recommends a standardized submaximal exercise test wherein the practitioner can interpret the results in the light of the horse's history and presentation. Box 11-1 shows the work up for a horse with chronic exertional rhabdomyolysis, and Box 11-2 illustrates a normal response to a standardized submaximal exercise test. Horses that have recently ridden in a trailer a long distance for evaluation may require 24 hours of hospitalization to ensure a normal CK value before the examination.

BOX 11-1

WORKUP FOR A HORSE WITH CHRONIC EXERTIONAL RHABDOMYOLYSIS

1. History: genetic background, diet, use, description of previous episodes, housing conditions
2. Physical examination
3. Collection of urine for fractional excretions (Na^+, K^+, Cl_-, and PO_4, if desired)
4. Collection of blood for baseline CK, AST, electrolytes, and lactate (if desired)
   a. A full profile is recommended in horses without a recent one performed.
   b. A complete blood count may be performed if inflammatory disease is suspected.
5. Exercise at a trot for 30 minutes either under saddle or on a lunge line; after 15 minutes, stop every 5 minutes for 1 minute to observe if stiffness or gait abnormalities are developing. If so, stop exercising the horse.
6. Postexercise CK analysis 4 to 6 hours after exercise. A 24-hour postexercise AST may be examined if desired.
7. Muscle biopsy. Middle gluteal, semimembranosus or other muscle if indicated.

AST, Aspartate transferase; *CK*, creatine kinase; *Cl*, chloride; *K^+*, potassium; *Na^+*, sodium; *P*, phosphorus.

Other Factors Affecting Activities of Aspartate Aminotransferase and Creatine Kinase

GENDER AND AGE

A group of Thoroughbreds was sampled over a 9-month period, and the 2-year-old fillies showed more significant fluctuations in AST and CK activities than the 3-year-old fillies and colts. Unfortunately, no 2-year-old colts were studied.[96] In a later study of 66 2- and 3-year-old Thoroughbred racehorses in training the fillies were more likely to have high CK and AST activities than colts, and 2-year-olds were more likely to have increased AST activity than 3-year-olds. The effect of age on the incidence of increased muscle enzyme activities

BOX 11-2

CRITERIA FOR A NORMAL RESPONSE TO A SUBMAXIMAL EXERCISE TEST DESIGNED FOR A GIVEN HORSE

1. Pre-exercise:
   CK activity <470 IU/L (laboratory resting reference range, 100 to 470 IU/L)
   AST activity <375 IU/L (laboratory resting reference range, 185 to 375 IU/L)
2. Not more than a doubling of the resting CK activity at 2 to 4 hours after exercise
3. Return to baseline CK activities at 24 hours after exercise
4. Not more than a 50% increase in AST activity
5. No clinical signs of stiffness

AST, Aspartate aminotransferase; *CK,* creatine kinase.

was thought not to have been caused by the natural loss of 2-year-olds from training with high enzyme activities, especially because several of these raced and won.[97] Certain animals may have physiologically higher plasma activities, or their muscle enzymes may be removed more slowly from the circulation. Alternatively, they may be more sensitive to the various insults that cause permeability changes in muscle fiber membranes. Age or training or both could have a dampening effect on muscle membrane changes. In dogs a significant decrease in CK activities has been reported with age, but no difference was found between males and females.[98] In one study, no correlation was found between plasma progesterone concentrations and the fluctuations in CK and AST activities.[99] However, a later study showed that when fillies with high median AST activities were removed from the study group, a highly significant relationship was found between progesterone and AST but not CK activities, and estradiol showed a significant effect on CK but not on AST activities. In rats, CK release after exercise or in vitro electric stimulation is greater in males than in females. Estradiol has been suggested to have a protective effect and to attenuate CK influx.[99,100] However, further work on the role of such hormones in CK and AST activities in the horse is necessary before conclusions can be drawn. In addition, all studies in large groups of horses must be examined with some scrutiny when one considers that the incidence of some underlying myopathies can be high within a population. Considering that AST and CK tend to rise exponentially with muscle damage, a few outliers in a study may skew results significantly. The incidence of RER in Thoroughbred horses may be as high as 5% of the population,[101] which may account for some of the increases in CK and AST activities observed in the studies cited.

TIME OF YEAR AND TRAINING

Several workers have suggested that AST plasma activities increase in the early stages of training and then decrease as training progresses.[102,103] Time of year does not have a significant effect on the number of animals with normal or with high AST and CK activities.[97] However, researchers observed an increase in mean activities peaking in April and May followed by a decrease to a low in September in a group of Thoroughbred racehorses in the Northern Hemisphere.[97] The high mean activities in April, May, and June were accompanied by high standard deviations, which made definitive conclusions difficult. Researchers also found large standard deviations in another study of Thoroughbreds in training.[9] On an individual basis a change in AST activities does not always seem to occur with training.[104] Therefore decreases or increases in the serum levels of AST activity are probably not good indicators of peak fitness or overtraining.[105]

In a study of AST activities in a small number of barren and pregnant Standardbred mares, researchers apparently found evidence for a diurnal rhythm, with the lowest activities occurring in the early morning (4 to 6 AM) and the highest activities at night (10 to 12 PM). The mean activities increased from September to November until March. Circannual cyclicity was found, but the pattern differed between the two groups. In barren mares the arcophase appeared to occur in the second half of January, whereas for pregnant animals it occurred in September (approximately month 5 of pregnancy). The standard error, however, was broad.[106]

RELATIONSHIP TO PERFORMANCE

Elevated CK and AST activities have been suggested to decrease the chance of a horse winning.[107] However, a group of 500 Standardbred trotters with a recent history of equine rhabdomyolysis and increased plasma muscle enzyme activities had a significantly better racing record compared with a large group of apparently unaffected horses.[1] Another study found that 50% of the horses with high median AST activities raced and won at least once.[97] However, determining whether these horses would have given better performances or won in better classes if they had not had such increased muscle enzyme activities obviously is not possible.

CLASSIFICATION OF MYOPATHIES

As the body of knowledge concerning equine myopathies grows the ability to classify them becomes more similar to that used in humans.[34] Broadly, equine myopathies may be inborn or acquired. Inborn errors of metabolism or primary myopathies may include disorders of carbohydrate, lipid or purine metabolism, mitochondrial myopathies, or disorders of ion movement across the cellular membranes (channelopathies). Secondary or acquired myopathies occur as a result of endocrine disorders (equine Cushing's syndrome), nutritional deficiencies (vitamin E, selenium), trauma (cast in a stall or other similar accident, overexertion under saddle, etc.), infection, and electrolyte imbalances. Manifestation of the aforementioned disorders may occur with or without recent exercise and may be obvious at birth or not until adulthood.

Practitioners may find approaching horses with muscle disorders from a problem-based approach most helpful. In this approach, horses are categorized into five categories: (1) those having muscle cramping with exercise, (2) those with permanent gait alterations, (3) those with muscle weakness, (4) those with muscle wasting, and (5) those with acute, severe rhabdomyolysis with or without recumbency or death. These clinically based classifications are not mutually exclusive, and some disorders fall into more than one category. However, the author believes that this approach is the most comprehensive, considering the current volume of knowledge relating to muscle disorders in the horse.

Box 11-3 shows how the various equine skeletal disorders might be classified under the pathophysiologic system using current information. Box 11-4 demonstrates a problem-based classification of the most common muscular disorders in the horse. The practitioner should note how many equine myopathies share common clinical presentations. Therefore a thorough history including genetic background, environment, and athletic history in conjunction with physical examination and laboratory workup are necessary to determine the most probable underlying cause in each case. Before discussing the specific muscle diseases the next section covers some general concepts and traditional thoughts concerning exertional rhabdomyolysis.

Exertional Rhabdomyolysis

Exertional rhabdomyolysis refers to the syndrome of muscle cramping that occurs during physical exertion or exercise. Differential diagnoses for exertional rhabdomyolysis are extensive (Box 11-5). Terms used to describe the disorder include

BOX 11-3

CLASSIFICATION OF EQUINE MYOPATHIES ACCORDING TO CAUSE

I. Neurogenic: may be hereditary or environmental in origin, acquired, or congenital
    A. Disorders of anterior horn cells
    B. Disorders of motor nerve roots
    C. Peripheral neuropathies
    D. Disorders of neuromuscular transmission
        1. Botulism
        2. Tetanus
        3. Tick paralysis
II. Myogenic
    A. Inborn errors of metabolism—genetic
        1. Disorders of carbohydrate metabolism
            a. Polysaccharide storage myopathy in Quarter Horses
            b. Polysaccharide storage myopathy in Draft Horses
            c. Polysaccharide storage myopathy in Warmblood Horses
            d. Glycogen branching enzyme deficiency
        2. Disorders of lipid metabolism
            a. Multiple acyl-CoA dehydrogenase deficiency (MADD)
        3. Disorders of purine metabolism—no known disorders in the horse
        4. Mitochondrial enzyme deficiencies
            a Complex I: NADH CoQ reductase deficiency
        5. Channelopathies, aberrations of ion and electrolyte flux
            a. Paramyotonias and myotonias
            a. Hyperkalemic periodic paralysis (paramyotonia)
            b. Myotonia congenita (myotonia)
            c. Myotonia dystrophica (myotonia)
            b. Recurrent exertional rhabdomyolysis in Thoroughbreds
            c. Idiopathic chronic exertional rhabdomyolysis (may be reclassified as additional diseases are identified)
    B. Acquired
        1. Traumatic
            a. Fibrotic myopathy
            b. Gastrocnemius muscle rupture
            c. Serratus ventralis muscle rupture
        2. Inflammatory
            a. Sore or pulled muscles
        3. Infectious
            a. Bacterial
                i. Clostridial myonecrosis
                ii. *Streptococcus* spp.
                    (1). Abscessation
                    (2). Autoimmune
                    (3). Purpura hemorrhagica
                    (4). Immunoglobulin G mediated
                    (5). Immunoglobulin A mediated (Henoch-Schönlein purpura)
                iii. *Staphylococcus* spp.
                iv. *Corynebacterium pseudotuberculosis*
            b. Viral
            c. Parasitic
                i. *Sarcocystis* spp.
                ii. *Trichinella spiralis*
        4. Circulatory
            b. Postanesthetic myositis
            c. Aortic-iliac thrombosis
        5. Nutritional
            a. Vitamin E deficiency; equine motor neuron disease, equine degenerative myelopathy
            b. Nutritional myodegeneration (white muscle disease); vitamin E with and without selenium deficiency
            c. Malnutrition
            d. Electrolyte deficiency
        6. Cachectic atrophy after chronic disease
        7. Exercise-related, overexertion, and the exhausted horse syndrome
        8. Toxic
            a. *Cassia occidentalis*
            b. White snakeroot
            c. Ionophores
        9. Endocrine
            a. Equine Cushing's syndrome
            b. Hypothyroidism (unsubstantiated)
        10. Disuse atrophy
        11. Malignancy: muscle tumors
        12. Miscellaneous or idiopathic
        13. Atypical myoglobinuria/pasture associated myopathy
        14. Postanesthetic myasthenia

NADH, Nicotinamide adenine dinucleotide.

BOX 11-4

PROBLEM-BASED APPROACH TO HORSES WITH MUSCLE DISEASE

Disorders are grouped according to similar clinical appearance. (No category is mutually exclusive. Disorders are grouped by most common clinical presentation. The reader is directed to the text for more extensive discussion for each disorder or disease.)

- I. Profound muscle cramping with exercise, tying-up syndrome, increased plasma/serum creatine kinase (CK) activity after exercise
  - A. Horses with inborn myopathy (inborn error of metabolism)
    1. Recurrent exertional rhabdomyolysis in Thoroughbreds
    2. Polysaccharide storage myopathy in Quarter Horses and Draft Horses
    3. Idiopathic chronic exertional rhabdomyolysis
    5. Mitochondrial myopathy (also has lactic acidosis)
  - B. Horses without inborn myopathy
    1. Overexertion
    2. Vitamin E or selenium deficiency
    3. Electrolyte depletion
- II. Horses with altered gait but without inborn myopathy and without muscle cramping; with or without elevated CK
  - A. Acute: muscle strain, sprain, tear
  - B. Chronic: fibrotic myopathy
- III. Muscle weakness
  - A. Hyperkalemic periodic paralysis (intermittent)
  - B. Myotonia congenita and myotonia dystrophica (worsens with exercise)
  - C. Equine motor neuron disease (worsens when standing still)
  - D. Equine polysaccharide storage myopathy in Draft Horses (can be progressive over time; rule out shivers as a differential diagnosis)
- IV. Muscle wasting
  - A. Generalized, may be accompanied by mild elevations in CK activity
    1. Equine motor neuron disease
    2. Streptococcal immune-mediated myositis: mediated by IgG
    3. Cachectic atrophy
    4. Disuse atrophy
    5. Endocrine; equine Cushing's syndrome
  - B. Segmental
    1. Neurogenic
    2. Disuse atrophy
    3. Fibrotic myopathy
    4. Posthealing of severe trauma
- V. Acute rhabdomyolysis, swollen painful musculature, with or without recumbency, with or without death
  - A. Severe, acute exercise-related rhabdomyolysis as from I.A. and I.B. above
  - B. Malignant hyperthermia/postanesthetic myopathy
  - C. Clostridial myonecrosis
  - D. *Sarcocystis* spp.
  - E. Streptococcal immune-mediated myositis; Henoch-Schönlein purpura
  - F. Aortic-iliac thrombosis
  - G. Toxic plants
    1. *Cassia occidentalis*
    2. White snakeroot
  - H. Ionophore toxicity (may also present as chronic heart failure without a history of acute rhabdomyolysis)
- VI. Disorders of the neonate
  - A. White muscle disease/nutritional myodegeneration
  - B. Foal rhabdomyolysis
  - C. Glycogen branching enzyme deficiency
  - D. Arthrogryposis
- VII. Miscellaneous disorders
  - A. Atypical myoglobinuria
  - B. Postanesthetic myasthenia
  - C. Polymyopathy
  - D. Abscesses
  - E. Tumors

Ig, Immunoglobulin.

chronic exertional rhabdomyolysis, equine rhabdomyolysis syndrome, azoturia, Monday morning disease, tying-up, myositis, setfast, and chronic intermittent rhabdomyolysis.[53,105,108-110] Broadly, horses experience exertional rhabdomyolysis for two main reasons: the horse has an underlying myopathy (chronic exertional rhabdomyolysis), or the horse has been overexerted physically (sporadic exertional rhabdomyolysis). Horses with underlying myopathies generally experience repeated episodes of rhabdomyolysis after short bouts of exercise; therefore the condition may be characterized as chronic. However, horses that are overexerted may experience only a single episode in their lifetime because the bout of rhabdomyolysis is caused by physical and environmental circumstances as opposed to an underlying pathologic condition of the muscle.

Identifying horses with underlying myopathies that are characterized by chronic exertional rhabdomyolysis is a rapidly developing field of veterinary medicine. To date, two major syndromes have been described: RER in Thoroughbred horses and PSSM in Quarter Horses and Draft-breed horses. Several less-common inborn errors of metabolism have also been described. Horses that have chronic exertional rhabdomyolysis but that cannot be diagnosed with any of the aforementioned disorders may be assumed to have a new or previously undescribed equine myopathy, provided no physical or environmental cause can be determined. Until more is known, horses with multiple bouts of rhabdomyolysis associated with minimal exercise that do not appear to fit into the categories of RER or PSSM are grouped and classified as having idiopathic chronic exertional rhabdomyolysis. One

BOX 11-5

DIFFERENTIAL DIAGNOSIS OF EQUINE RHABDOMYOLYSIS

Acorn poisoning
Anthrax
Arthritis (joint pain)
Back problems
Botulism
Castration sequelae
Colic
Cystitis
Hernia
Iliac thrombosis
Inguinal/popliteal lymphadenitis
Laminitis
Nephritis
Pleuritis
Postexhaustion syndrome
Proximal limb lameness
Spinal cord disease
Tetanus
Tick paralysis

should not assume that all Thoroughbreds, Quarter Horses, and Draft-breed horses demonstrating chronic or sporadic exertional rhabdomyolysis have RER or PSSM, respectively, simply because of their breed.

In the past, exertional rhabdomyolysis in the horse was described in the literature under diseases of the liver, kidney, blood, or muscle. Exertional rhabdomyolysis has also been attributed to infection, cold weather, intoxication, nervous irritation, calcium deficiency, excess of glycogen, lactic acid poisoning, an increase in red blood cells, and an unbalanced alkali reserve.[111] Most theories have not undergone thorough scientific scrutiny to rule them in or out as an inciting cause, contributing factor, or primary cause.

Exercise is the common triggering factor in horses with exertional rhabdomyolysis. However, in horses with underlying myopathies the amount of exercise necessary to trigger muscle cramping is often minimal in contrast to healthy horses exhibiting a sporadic episode of rhabdomyolysis because of overexertion. Similarly, horses with underlying myopathies suffer from repeated episodes, whereas overexerted but otherwise healthy horses do not, provided they are not pushed repeatedly beyond their level of fitness.

CLASSIC THEORIES FOR EXERTIONAL RHABDOMYOLYSIS

For centuries, horses were believed to tie up for a single as yet undetermined reason. The most popular reason was inactivity (i.e., stall rest) accompanied by a full ration of grain. This scenario was most likely to occur in Draft Horses rested on Sunday and worked on Monday, hence the name Monday morning disease. Currently the influence of diet, specifically carbohydrates, on exertional rhabdomyolysis is an area of active research. Diet plays a role in horses that are predisposed to exertional rhabdomyolysis from several different underlying myopathies (see specific disorders in the following sections), but how diet may influence muscle function in normal, healthy horses is still largely unknown.[112-114]

Lactic Acidosis From 1914 to 1915, history records that when oats were scarce and raw sugar was fed to horses as a substitute the incidence of metabolic diseases, especially azoturia, increased.[115] In two papers that are much quoted in the literature, excessive glycogen buildup was postulated to result in an overproduction of lactic acid during exercise.[116,117] These studies reproduced the condition by feeding horses 3 kg of molasses daily and then exercising the horses after a rest period. However, in these studies the levels of lactate measured in horses experiencing rhabdomyolysis were similar or lower than the values concurrently measured in normal, healthy horses exercising anaerobically. Therefore lactate alone is unlikely to trigger exertional rhabdomyolysis in healthy horses.[118] The role of lactic acid in horses with underlying myopathy has been investigated only in Thoroughbred horses with RER. That study found no correlation between lactate levels and CK activity measured 4 hours after exercise.[112] In investigations of other breeds of horses with chronic exertional rhabdomyolysis the relationships between rhabdomyolysis and lactate are less clear.[27,110,119,120]

Hypothyroidism Muscular problems are a common symptom of hypothyroidism in human beings.[121,122] In mild human cases, fatigue may be the only presenting symptom, although more severe cases may be accompanied by overt muscle cell damage, increased resting plasma CK activities, and sometimes increased myoglobin levels.[123] Poor racing performance and certain myopathies have been related to mild secondary hypothyroidism,[124] although this conclusion has been challenged.[125] Oral thyroxine supplementation may improve performance or decrease the incidence of myopathies in documented cases of hypothyroidism.[63,124] However, considerable debate still exists as to whether hypothyroidism is important in the pathogenesis of exertional myopathies in the horse.[53]

Resting thyroxine concentrations did not differ significantly between animals believed to be suffering from chronic rhabdomyolysis and those suffering from a variety of other conditions. However, some rhabdomyolysis sufferers may have a lowered response to thyrotropin-releasing hormone,[90] which may reflect a decreased thyroid reserve, but too few cases have been investigated to date. A study examined exercise in thyroidectomized horses and documented exercise intolerance but not increases in CK activity.[126] Conversely, in the author's experience, oversupplementation with thyroxine may lead to iatrogenic hyperthyroidism and symptoms of mildly increased CK activity and muscle wasting.

VIRAL CAUSES

Muscle pain or myalgia is a common symptom in the acute phase of influenza and other viral illnesses in human beings, although few reports of severe muscular problems are available.[51,127,128] Myalgia and myoglobinuria have been observed with herpesvirus infections.[51] Some horses are stiff and unwilling to work during or after an attack of the virus.[129] Viral infection has been reported as being one of the predisposing factors to equine rhabdomyolysis.[130]

A clinical investigation of an outbreak of muscle stiffness and poor performance in a flat-racing stable of Thoroughbreds revealed that more than one third of the horses demonstrated signs of muscular stiffness over 2 months, and 64% at one or more of the sampling times had increased CK and AST activities.[131] Serologic tests were highly suggestive of an equine herpesvirus type 1 infection. The possibility of a viral cause, at least in outbreaks of stiffness in racing yards, needs more in-depth evaluation. The virus could affect muscle directly, resulting in an increased susceptibility to exercise-induced damage. Alternatively, the increase in blood viscosity observed after infection could result in an impaired blood flow and decreased oxygen delivery to the peripheral tissues.[1] A study of horses exercised after experimental infection with equine influenza virus failed to demonstrate significant effects on muscle function or CK activity or evidence of muscle stiffness.[132]

Treatment of Rhabdomyolysis

Treatment of rhabdomyolysis depends on the underlying cause. For example, horses experiencing muscle damage because of sepsis or trauma require different approaches than horses experiencing rhabdomyolysis caused by underlying, heritable myopathies. Horses with rhabdomyolysis are often treated for colic or nonspecific signs of pain. Other differential diagnoses include disorders that are frequently associated with depression or a reluctance to move and include but are not limited to anthrax infection, postcastration abscesses, colic, cystitis, neurologic disorders, lymphadenitis, laminitis, nephritis, peritonitis, pleuritis, tetanus, and skeletal injury or infection.

The practitioner should perform a thorough physical examination and obtain a detailed history. The initial workup of a horse suspected of having rhabdomyolysis should include a complete blood count, chemistry profile, and urine collection. Treatment should follow the observations made on physical examination and changes observed in the blood count and chemistry profile. The practitioner should rehydrate horses with significant dehydration with fluids that reflect electrolyte deficiencies identified on a chemistry profile and should treat horses in significant discomfort with nonsteroidal antiinflammatory drugs (NSAIDs), provided renal perfusion and function are supported. The practitioner should not treat horses experiencing rhabdomyolysis in the face of extreme exhaustion and dehydration with nephrotoxic medications (aminoglycosides or NSAIDs) until ascertaining renal function. Horses that typically fall into this category include those with capture myopathies (e.g., horses that are trapped and struggle in trailer accidents, get wrapped up in ropes or fences, are being taught to tie to a fixed object, or get cast in a stall) and endurance horses. Treatment for horses with mild cases of rhabdomyolysis includes keeping them warm, minimizing movement, and providing stall rest and NSAIDs as appropriate. Muscle enzyme activity and the physical response of the horse to being asked to move and exercise can guide the practitioner as to when returning the horse to normal physical activity is appropriate. Therapies specific to each type of rhabdomyolysis are discussed in their respective sections.

Neurogenic Myopathy

Neurologic diseases are discussed in detail in Chapter 12, Disorders of the Neurologic System.

INBORN ERRORS OF METABOLISM

Jennifer M. MacLeay

DISORDERS OF CARBOHYDRATE METABOLISM

Polysaccharide Storage Myopathy

Polysaccharide storage myopathy is a disease characterized by repeated episodes of exertional rhabdomyolysis that may be induced with little exercise. Increased CK activity in the plasma or serum accompanies episodes of rhabdomyolysis. The most distinctive characteristic of the disease is a mild to severe accumulation of abnormal polysaccharide within the sarcoplasm. Based on a histologic diagnosis of abnormal polysaccharide, PSSM has been described in Quarter Horses, Warmbloods, Draft breeds (Belgians, Percherons, Clydesdales, Shires, Haflinger, Norwegian Fjord, Suffolk, Irish Draft, Draft crosses, and a Draft mule), and rarely in Thoroughbreds and Arabians. A mutation in the glycogen synthase enzyme gene (GYS1) is highly associated with the presence of abnormal polysaccharide in muscle biopsies.[1] The metabolic defect resulting from this mutation leads to the classic or type 1 form of PSSM that accounts for more than 90% of PSSM in some breeds of horses. A modifying genetic mutation in the RYR1 gene is associated with a more severe clinical phenotype of PSSM in Quarter Horses and related breeds than that observed in horses with the GYS1 mutation alone.[2] This RYR1 mutation is associated with malignant hyperthermia. Genetic tests for the PSSM and MH mutations are now commercially available through the University of Minnesota Veterinary Diagnostic Laboratory.

Based on the glycogen synthase mutation, PSSM has been diagnosed in Quarter Horses, Belgians, Percherons and their crosses, Paints, Appaloosas, Morgans, Mustangs, Tennessee Walkers, Rocky Mountain Spotted Horses, and some Warmbloods among others.[1] Among biopsies submitted to the University of Minnesota Neuromuscular Diagnostic Laboratory for horses with a suspicion of muscle disease, the overall prevalence of a diagnosis of PSSM was 22%. Quarter Horses were most likely to be diagnosed, followed by Draft and Warmblood horses. In a broader survey of Quarter Horses the overall prevalence of PSSM in American Quarter Horses at large was estimated to be between 6% and 12%.[3] Draft and Warmblood horses are more likely to have a client complaint of gait abnormality than Quarter Horses with PSSM. Among horses at necropsy, 86% of Draft horses had evidence of abnormal polysaccharide.[4] In a survey of 103 Belgian horses the incidence of PSSM was 36%, and the incidence of shivers, which can be mistaken for PSSM, was 18%, and 6% of horses had both.[5] This survey indicates that both diseases are common among Belgian horses but are not likely associated with one another. Of horses suspected of having a muscular problem and having muscle biopsies submitted for analysis, the incidence of PSSM among Draft horses was 54%.[6] In an epidemiologic study of Warmblood horses that had muscle biopsies submitted for analysis, 55% had a diagnosis of PSSM.[7] A general study concerning the overall incidence of PSSM among Warmblood horses has not been performed.

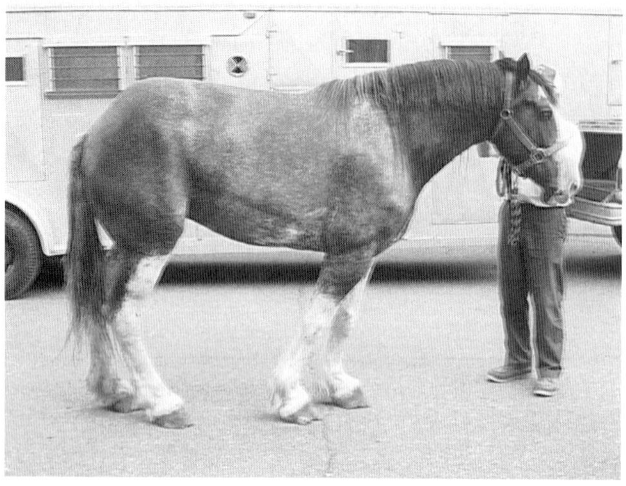

FIGURE 11-3 Draft Horse with equine polysaccharide storage myopathy standing with a base-narrow, weak stance.

CLINICAL SIGNS AND LABORATORY FINDINGS

Horses with PSSM have frequent episodes of muscle cramping and rhabdomyolysis that typically occur within the first 30 minutes of exercise. Clinical signs and laboratory changes (increased muscle enzymes, myoglobinuria) associated with an episode of PSSM rhabdomyolysis appear similar to other causes of rhabdomyolysis. Mild episodes are characterized by a stiff gait, anxiety, and a stretched-out stance. More severe episodes are characterized by anxiety, painful behavior, sweating, and reluctance to move or recumbency. Horses appear to vary in the severity or expression of the disorder. Some horses also appear to tolerate exercise better than others despite similar changes in CK activity after exercise. This finding may reflect a tolerance of the individual horse to muscular discomfort associated with exercise. Episodes are especially prevalent when exercise intensity increases. A complaint of a consistently abnormal gait or weakness is more common in Draft- and Warmblood-bred horses than Quarter Horses. Some Draft horses may exhibit progressive poor performance, shivers or a shiverslike gait, progressive muscle wasting, muscle weakness, recumbency, and death (Figure 11-3).

Horses that experience frequent episodes of rhabdomyolysis and have considerable accumulations of abnormal polysaccharide storage within the muscle fibers may have persistent elevations in serum or plasma CK activity even when stall confined. Whether this accumulation represents ongoing subclinical rhabdomyolysis or an alteration in the permeability of the muscle cell membrane is unknown. Muscle biopsy or genetic testing of horses with a history of chronic exertional rhabdomyolysis is indicated. Horses with PSSM have subsarcolemmal accumulations of an abnormal polysaccharide that is visible with a periodic acid–Schiff stain and is characteristically amylase resistant.

CAUSES AND PATHOPHYSIOLOGY

A glycogen synthase enzyme deficiency inherited as an autosomal recessive trait has been identified.[1] In addition the accumulations of abnormal polysaccharide observed in periodic acid Schiff–stained muscle sections appears to increase with age and therefore may be a secondary feature of the disease. Significant accumulations of abnormal polysaccharide may not be visible until 3 years of age in some horses, despite documented intermittent exercise-associated increases in serum and plasma CK activities at a younger age. Affected horses show great variability in expression of the disorder, as reflected in the amount of abnormal polysaccharide observed in muscle sections, desire and ability to exercise, frequency and severity of episodes of rhabdomyolysis, and degree of elevations in CK activity.

Studies have shown PSSM to be a disorder in which enhanced insulin sensitivity and elevated glucose excursion leads to increased synthesis of muscle glycogen, which appears to be independent of augmented glucose transport protein (GLUT4) or insulin receptor quantity.[8] Overall, affected horses demonstrate greater total muscle glycogen content compared with control horses. In addition, when fasted, horses with PSSM have consistently lower blood glucose concentrations than healthy controls. When given intravenous or oral glucose, horses with PSSM clear glucose from the blood stream at a faster rate than healthy controls. When administered insulin, horses with PSSM became severely hypoglycemic and remained so longer than healthy control horses. Why horses with PSSM have an increased sensitivity to insulin is unknown. However, this increased sensitivity results in increased uptake of glucose into the muscle cell. When the muscle cell takes up glucose from the blood, glycogen synthase is typically stimulated. However, the mutation affects the function of this enzyme. Horses with PSSM can break down the abnormal glycogen for energy albeit inefficiently. Horses with PSSM have glycogen branching enzyme with apparently normal activity.

Exercise influences glucose uptake into muscle cells. The physiologic changes associated with exercise result in changes in the number and activity of glucose transporters within the muscle cell membrane. Horses with PSSM have glucose tolerance curves more similar to healthy controls when they are exercised regularly,[9,10] which may explain why regular exercise and maintaining a certain level of fitness appears to help affected horses. Diets high in fat also appear to help these horses and may be related to a less severe postprandial glycemic response and decreased uptake of glucose by muscle cells.

DIAGNOSIS

A genetic test is now available and may be augmented by documenting the presence of abnormal polysaccharide on a periodic acid Schiff–stained muscle biopsy. Because the accumulation of abnormal polysaccharide appears to be a secondary feature of the disease, accurately diagnosing affected horses until 3 years of age or more may not be possible without genetic testing. Some anecdotal evidence supports the theory that mildly affected horses fed diets low in carbohydrates may accumulate polysaccharide in smaller amounts or more slowly than other affected horses.

An exercise tolerance test can be a useful diagnostic tool in horses with PSSM. Affected horses commonly experience a doubling or more of baseline CK activity after 15 to 30 minutes of trotting. The practitioner draws blood before and 4 to 6 hours after the exercise. The practitioner also should have fractional excretions of electrolytes (Figure 11-4), measurements of serum selenium (or GSHPx activity), and vitamin E concentration determined on horses with PSSM. The practitioner should supplement dietary electrolytes and selenium and vitamin E intake if these are abnormal.

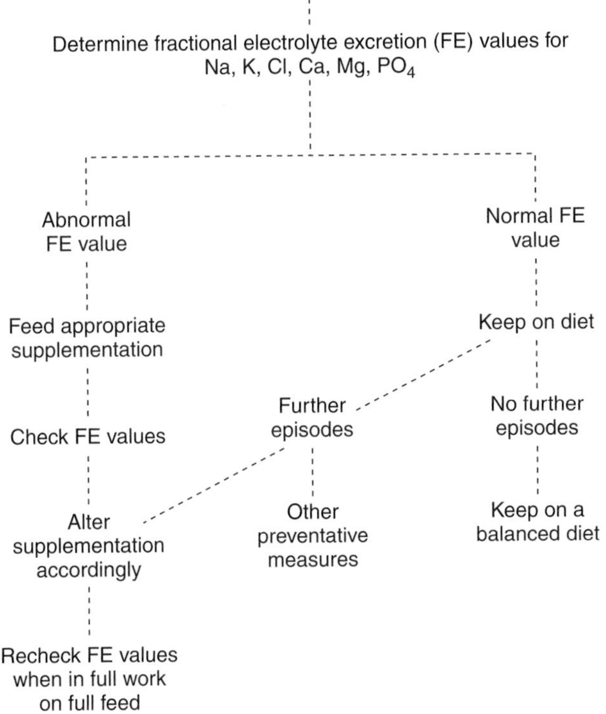

FIGURE 11-4 Protocol for using the fractional electrolyte excretion test in clinical cases of the equine rhabdomyolysis syndrome. The electrolyte status should not be evaluated without also evaluating vitamin E and selenium status.

TREATMENT

Horses with PSSM have a heritable myopathy that, in many horses, can be managed readily. Because of the nature of the disorder the practitioner should counsel owners, trainers, and riders of affected horses that the horse may not be able to perform at elite levels of competition if the condition is severe. However, many horses do perform well and have only occasional episodes of rhabdomyolysis. Horses should be exercised regularly because a good level of basal fitness appears to protect against episodes; however, increases in exercise intensity should be made gradually. Horses may live in stalls, but living outside where the horse may move around readily appears to lessen the frequency of episodes of rhabdomyolysis. A diet with less than 5% digestible energy as starch and more than 12% digestible energy as fat can reduce signs of exertional rhabdomyolysis potentially by increasing availability of free fatty acids for muscle metabolism.[11] Many horses can do well consuming only a grass or alfalfa hay and a simple vitamin and mineral supplement. If additional calories are necessary, they can be supplied as fats. Many different fat sources are available and include corn or vegetable oils, linseed oil, or rice bran. Commercial grain mixes that are high-fat, low-carbohydrate feeds are available and may be a good source of fat for the horse without the concern associated with other sources of fat. Oils can spoil, and larger quantities of oils or rice bran may not be palatable for some horses. Routine daily exercise helps with the metabolism of glucose in affected horses. Overall, owners that implement dietary changes with regular exercise have the greatest success in limiting the incidence of future episodes of rhabdomyolysis.[7,12]

Glycogen Branching Enzyme Deficiency

Glycogen branching enzyme deficiency was likely first identified in 1999 as amylopectinosis by Render et al.[13] It is a heritable disorder in human beings and cats.[14-16] Affected foals may be aborted, still born, or born weak, similar in appearance to foals with hypoxic ischemic encephalopathy or sepsis. Live foals have been presented to referral hospitals for sepsis, prematurity, and failure of passive transfer.[17] At presentation, foals often have concurrent sepsis, which necessitates treatment. These foals typically have elevated liver enzymes and persistent problems with hypoglycemia during hospitalization. Increases in serum CK activity may be present. Foals may die acutely during hospitalization or respond well to therapy and be discharged. Shortly after discharge the foal is discovered dead.

Muscle biopsy from affected horses shows a complete lack of normal glycogen staining. Normal glycogen is lacking in skeletal muscle, heart muscle, and liver. The disorder has been diagnosed only in Quarter Horses and Paint Horses and is inherited as a recessive trait. To date, all affected animals identified have been homozygous for a mutation (tyrosine to a stop codon) in the glycogen branching enzyme gene, and, where investigated, both parents have been heterozygous for this missense mutation.[18-20] A genetic test is available to identify affected offspring or carrier animals through the University of California Veterinary Genetics Laboratory, Davis, Calif.

DISORDERS OF LIPID METABOLISM

Multiple acyl-CoA dehydrogenase (MADD) deficiency was recently diagnosed in two Warmblood bred horses in Europe.[21] They exhibited clinical signs of a stiff gait and myoglobinuria progressing to recumbency. Both had elevations in AST, LDH, and CK; hyperglycemia and lactic acidemia; and impaired renal function. Urine and plasma had increased organic acids and acylcarnitines and free carnitine. Muscle biochemical analysis revealed deficiencies of short- and medium-chain acyl-CoA dehydrogenase and isovaleryl-CoA dehydrogenase. The disorder may be acquired as opposed to inherited. Further work is necessary to determine if MADD is more widespread and to determine the origin of the disorder.

Mitochondrial Enzyme Deficiencies

A small family of horses has been described with a syndrome of severe exercise intolerance. In this family, one mare was found to have a deficiency of complex I respiratory chain enzyme. She had severe exercise intolerance and muscle stiffness with extreme lactic acidosis in relationship to the degree of exercise but without rhabdomyolysis. Muscle biopsy demonstrated large accumulations of mitochondria with bizarre cristae formations. Biochemical analysis revealed low activity of nicotinamide adenine dinucleotide coenzyme Q reductase, the first enzyme complex of the mitochondrial respiratory chain, which resulted in impaired oxidative capacity for exercise and heavy reliance on anaerobic metabolism for muscular energy.[22] Examination of related horses provided evidence that the condition was likely familial.

CHANNELOPATHIES: ABERRATIONS OF ION AND ELECTROLYTE FLUX

Disorders discussed in this section have in common a defect in ion or electrolyte flow either across the sarcolemma or involving the sarcoplasmic reticulum. Hyperkalemic periodic paralysis, myotonia congenita, and myotonia dystrophica are characterized by an alteration in electric conduction across the outer muscle cell membrane. Equine motor neuron disease results from chronic vitamin E deficiency and consequential long-term oxidative stress, and although it results in altered membrane function, it is discussed under the acquired muscle disease section. The exact abnormality resulting in RER in Thoroughbreds is unknown. However, alteration in calcium homeostasis within the cell is the most likely candidate. Therefore it is included under this heading.

Hyperkalemic Periodic Paralysis

In human beings, three types of periodic paralysis are described: hypokalemic, hyperkalemic, and normokalemic. These disorders are caused by abnormalities in membrane permeability or a defective cation pump, resulting in an altered electrochemical gradient across the sarcolemma. The alteration, in turn, results in a change in resting membrane potential and threshold potential, resulting in a muscle fiber that is more or less excitable.[23] Together these disorders are classified as paramyotonias.

CLINICAL SIGNS AND LABORATORY FINDINGS

In horses, hyperkalemic periodic paralysis (HYPP) occurs in Quarter Horses, Paint Horses, Appaloosas, and other horses carrying bloodlines that trace back to the sire Impressive. Affected horses tend to be well muscled. Because of this phenotype the defect has been postulated to confer or be linked closely with other genes that are associated with a heavily muscled phenotype. Between episodes, horses appear to be clinically normal and can be highly successful show horses.[24] In fact, many breeders believe that being a heterozygote greatly enhances the physique of horses and is therefore necessary to compete in the show ring. Scientific research confirming or refuting this has not been performed.

Prolapse of the membrana nictitans may be the initial sign at the onset of an episode of HYPP with or without facial muscle spasm and generalized muscle tension. One may observe sustained contraction of the muscles of the muzzle and drooling. Heart rate and respiratory rate are often normal or only slightly increased. Whole-body sweating has been reported. Muscle fasciculations are common, especially in the shoulders, flanks, and neck area. One may observe myotonia (sustained muscle contraction in response to percussion).[24-26] Although the horse may remain standing, it may not be able to lift its head and may show intermittent buckling at the knees and hocks. In mild cases, however, the only signs observed may be mild muscle fasciculations or twitching similar to signs of shivering. Recumbency may occur in some horses with diminished tendon reflexes, although affected animals tend to remain conscious and alert and may eat if offered food. Duration of episodes is usually short (20 minutes to 4 hours, typically 30 minutes to 1 hour). Death can occur during an episode, usually from cardiac arrest, respiratory failure, or asphyxiation caused by upper airway obstruction (secondary to muscle flaccidity at the pharynx).

Some horses demonstrate altered vocalization and audible respiratory stridor, which may indicate laryngeal spasm or paralysis.[27] In a survey of 69 homozygous horses, more than 90% were reported to suffer some degree of abnormal airway noise, often between episodes, which tended to be an inspiratory stridor and was continuous in 21% of those evaluated. Exercise, excitement, and stress were possible triggering factors. Upper airway endoscopy of 24 horses revealed 9 with pharyngeal collapse, 10 with laryngeal spasm, 9 with pharyngeal edema, and 6 with a displaced soft palate. Clinically, homozygous affected animals tend to show exercise intolerance, whereas heterozygous animals may tolerate exercise well.[28]

In affected horses, one usually observes clinical episodes before 3 years of age.[29] However, a wide variation in clinical expression of the condition occurs (incomplete penetrance of the gene), with some affected animals showing minimal clinical signs. The variability in clinical signs may result from higher expression of mutant channels in the muscle of horses with symptoms than in those that are asymptomatic. Although variability in the severity of disease occurs between horses, in general, homozygous animals tend to have more severe clinical signs compared with heterozygotes. Muscle fiber diameter or fiber type is related to clinical expression. Management factors such as diet (high versus low potassium intake) and environmental stress may be more influential in the expression of the disorder.[28]

Between episodes, serum potassium concentration is usually within normal limits but may be increased slightly. During an episode, serum potassium concentration usually is increased (5.0 to 11.7 mmol/L),[28] although episodes without associated hyperkalemia have been reported.[30,31] Therefore the absence of hyperkalemia during an episode does not preclude a diagnosis of HYPP. Sodium and calcium concentrations may be decreased and hemoconcentration also may be observed during an episode. Serum CK and AST activities may be normal or mildly increased.[24,26,32] Recovery from an episode is associated with a decrease in serum potassium concentration.

Acute death from hyperkalemia-induced cardiac standstill may occur and is more likely in horses that are homozygous or poorly managed. Poor management may include feeding of diets high in potassium and irregular feeding, traveling, or strenuous exercise schedules.

CAUSES AND PATHOPHYSIOLOGY

Hyperkalemic periodic paralysis in human beings is inherited as an autosomal dominant trait and has been studied extensively, as has paramyotonia congenita. To date, only HYPP has been diagnosed in horses, and the disorder also appears to be inherited as an autosomal dominant trait.[28,33,34] In human beings and horses, HYPP is characterized by intermittent attacks of weakness or paralysis, which are precipitated by several factors, including potassium intake, fasting, cold, heavy sedation, anesthesia, and rest after exercise. Paramyotonia congenita is typically associated with a cold-induced myotonia. Both conditions have been linked to the human adult skeletal muscle sodium gene on chromosome 17q. The genetic mutation responsible for HYPP in human beings affects a gene at the SCN4A locus that encodes the α-subunit of the adult human skeletal muscle voltage-dependent sodium channel.[35] In the horse the mutation is a phenylalanine to leucine mutation in the transmembrane domain IVS3 of the α-subunit of the sodium channel.[36,37] In affected individuals an increase in membrane sodium conductance occurs because of the defective subpopulation of the voltage-dependent sodium channels failing to inactivate and remaining open or repeatedly opening. A small rise in the serum potassium concentration because of clinical variation, ingestion of potassium, or muscular activity may trigger a further increase in membrane sodium conductance, depolarization of the muscle membrane, and movement of potassium out of the muscle cells. As the membrane depolarization develops, the membrane initially becomes hyperexcitable and shows myotonic behavior. With further depolarization of the muscle the muscle cell membrane becomes unexcitable and paralysis occurs.[35,38] In Quarter Horses, all affected horses can trace their lineage to a stallion named Impressive.[36,37] For this reason the disorder is occasionally called Impressive disease. Whether the mutation in Impressive was a spontaneous mutation or was inherited is unknown. The mutation has become common in the Quarter Horse population because of the success of Impressive and his offspring in the show arena and the consequential extensive and long breeding career of Impressive. Of the more than 20,000 samples collected between 1992 and 1995, approximately 63% were homozygous normal (N/N), 36% were heterozygous affected (N/H), and 1% were homozygous affected (H/H).[28] These data translate to a gene-positive frequency of 4.4% of the Quarter Horse population. Because of the prevalence of the mutation the American Quarter Horse Association made genetic testing mandatory in 1998 and has not allowed homozygous affected horses to be registered since 2007.[33]

Plasma potassium concentrations of normal horses undergoing intensive exercise may reach the levels recorded during an episode of HYPP without any associated clinical signs,[39] which suggests that increased plasma potassium concentration alone is not responsible for all the clinical signs typically observed.[40]

HISTOLOGIC AND MUSCULAR CHARACTERISTICS

In human beings, periodic paralysis conditions are sometimes called vacuolar myopathies. The vacuoles, visible on light microscopy, arise from coalescence of dilated components of sarcoplasmic reticulum, fusion of T-system networks, or focal fiber destruction.[41] In the horse, no abnormalities are found on light microscopy.[26,34]

Affected animals have a lower intracellular potassium concentration and a higher intracellular water volume than normal horses. Using whole-fiber intercostal muscle biopsies, the mean resting membrane potential of five affected horses was significantly closer to the threshold potential compared with unaffected horses.[34] This finding may indicate a defect in membrane transport.

No difference is apparent between muscle fiber type distribution and fiber diameter between horses with HYPP and those without. However, the genetic defect may alter other less-measurable muscle traits such as tone, which is why it appears that breeders and judges prefer affected horses to unaffected ones.

ELECTROMYOGRAPHY

Numerous EMG abnormalities are apparent in HYPP horses at rest and during an episode.[30,31,34] Complex repetitive discharges are the most consistent abnormal finding, although one may observe myotonic potentials, fibrillation potentials, and positive sharp waves as well. The amount of abnormal spontaneous EMG activity can fluctuate substantially on repeated examinations.

DIAGNOSIS

The most accurate way to confirm a diagnosis of HYPP is a genetic test using DNA extracted from equine hair or whole blood samples. The American Quarter Horse Association recognizes results of HYPP genetic tests that are performed through a licensed laboratory. Tests are reported as homozygous normal (N/N), heterozygous (N/H), and homozygous affected (H/H). Before the development of the genetic test, a potassium challenge test was recommended to identify affected horses. This test has potential adverse affects and is no longer recommended. If a Quarter Horse dies acutely and HYPP is suspected, one may collect hair samples at postmortem for DNA testing. Increased potassium concentrations in aqueous humor samples support a diagnosis of hyperkalemia at the time of death.

Differential diagnoses for HYPP include other causes of collapse such as syncope, narcolepsy or cataplexy, and seizures, as well as other electrolyte disorders, neurologic dysfunction, and vitamin E–responsive and selenium-responsive myopathy.[32]

TREATMENT

Recommended treatment for horses with acute episodes of HYPP varies depending on the severity of clinical signs. Mildly affected horses (i.e., nonrecumbent but with muscle fasciculations) may be exercised lightly. Caution is advised because collapse is a potential risk in these horses. One may feed the horse a readily absorbable source of carbohydrate (oats or light Karo syrup) to promote insulin-induced cellular reuptake of potassium. Acetazolamide at 3 mg/kg orally also may be beneficial. Such procedures are often undertaken routinely by responsible and experienced owners of affected animals.

During more severe episodes, especially when recumbency occurs, one may administer 5% dextrose with sodium bicarbonate (with or without insulin) to decrease serum potassium concentration. Slow intravenous administration of 23% calcium gluconate at 0.2 to 0.4 ml/kg diluted in 1 to 2 L of 5% dextrose (5% dextrose at 4.4 to 6.6 ml/kg) or bicarbonate at 1 to 2 mEq/kg have been recommended for treatment of acute, severe episodes of HYPP.[24,26,34,41] Administration of calcium lowers the depolarization threshold and should make muscle cell membranes less likely to depolarize. If required, one may administer potassium-free isotonic fluids. Glucocorticoids may be contraindicated in susceptible horses because they induce episodes in human beings with similar disorders.[24] Inhalation of β-adrenergic agents has aborted acute attacks in human beings, but the use of such drugs has not been reported in HYPP-affected horses.[41,42]

PROGNOSIS

In humans with HYPP, the prognosis for normal activity is considered good, although a permanent myopathy and weakness may occur, which also seems to be the case in the horse. In at least one horse the condition progressed, necessitating euthanasia.[24] A recent report suggested that "the chances of a paralytic episode occurring while the horse is being ridden appear unlikely. However, because episodes of paralysis are unpredictable, we recommend that only persons experienced with the symptomatology handle and ride affected horses and to use caution if any abnormal clinical signs are observed."[28] Thousands of carrier horses are handled, ridden, and shown daily throughout the United States and elsewhere with little to no apparent danger to human beings.

PREVENTION

In horses, acetazolamide has been recommended as a daily medication to decrease the frequency and severity of HYPP episodes. The recommended dose is 2 to 3 mg/kg orally every 8 to 12 hours for maintenance.[24,28,33] Hydrochlorothiazide also has been used.[26] One should feed affected horses oats or timothy hay rather than alfalfa to decrease total potassium intake to less than 1.1% of the total ration as potassium. Feedstuffs generally low in potassium include fescue, Bermuda, Kentucky blue grass, oat or timothy hay, rice bran, fats and oils, beet pulp, corn, oats or barley, pasture grass, wheat, wheat bran, or soy hulls. Hays should be tested for potassium concentration because the amount of potassium varies with soil conditions and time of year harvested. Feeding grain two or more times a day, providing access to white salt (without potassium chloride added), and regular mild exercise also may be beneficial. One should establish a regular feeding and exercise schedule and should avoid rapid changes in diet, fasting, and water deprivation. Turnout to pasture or paddock may be beneficial.

In human beings, preventive therapy consists of frequent meals with high carbohydrate content, avoidance of fasting or of exposure to cold or overexertion, and the use of diuretics such as acetazolamide or chlorothiazide, which promote potassium wasting in the urine. Small doses of albuterol, a β-adrenergic agent, also have been recommended in human beings.[42] Albuterol is believed to work by stimulating sodium and potassium ion pumps, enhancing potassium transport across the muscle cell membrane. Tocainide, a frequency-dependent antiarrhythmic drug, may prevent the weakness caused by the myotonia.[41]

Myotonia Congenita and Dystrophica

Similar to HYPP, myotonia congenita and myotonia dystrophica are characterized by abnormal electric conduction across the muscle cell membrane.[41,43] Myotonia is defined as the "delayed relaxation of skeletal muscle after a voluntary contraction or a contraction induced by an electric or mechanical stimulus."[41] Two forms of myotonia congenita are described in human beings, Thomsen's disease and Becker myotonia. Both forms result from chloride channel mutations. Thomsen's disease is inherited as an autosomal dominant trait; Becker myotonia is inherited as a recessive trait.[41]

In the horse, no membrane chloride defect has been identified. As in human beings, at least one form of the condition in horses persists in the face of neuromuscular blockade.[41,44] Only a few horses with myotonia have been described. Affected foals have a severely abnormal gait at birth and are usually euthanized. Because of the small number of affected horses described, whether myotonia in this species is heritable or results from spontaneous point mutations is unknown. To date a complete description of clinical, histopathologic, and electrophysiologic findings in horses with myotonia congenita or myotonia dystrophica is not available.

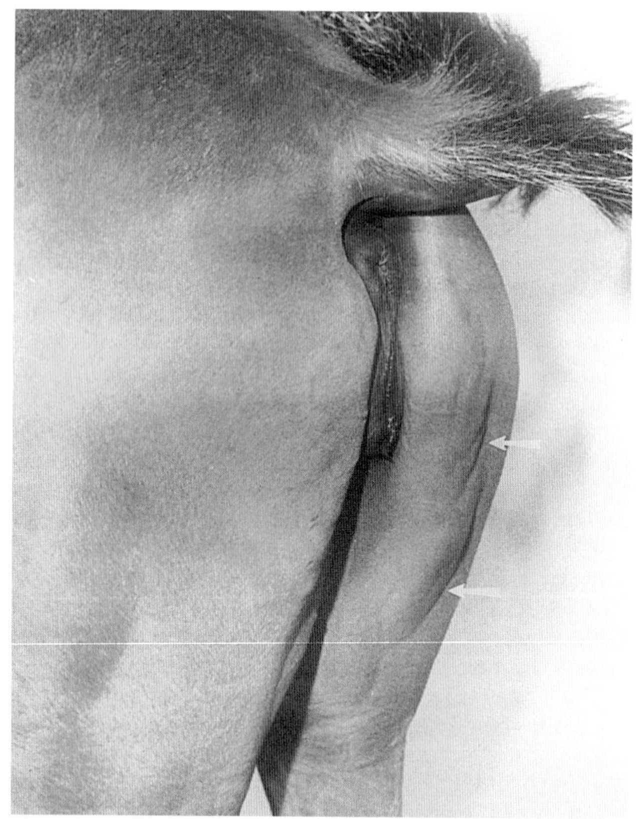

FIGURE 11-5 Prominent muscle groups of the hindquarters and a knot of sustained muscular contraction after mechanical stimulation in a foal suffering from clinical myotonia.

CLINICAL SIGNS AND LABORATORY FINDINGS

Stiffness of gait and prolonged contraction of affected muscle after local mechanical stimulation (finger flick) are the hallmarks of clinical myotonia (Figures 11-5 to 11-7). Clinical presentation of horses with myotonia varies.[32,45-50] One horse exhibited the presence of myotonic discharges on EMG with no overt primary muscular problems.

A second myotonic syndrome in horses is characterized by early onset of progressive deterioration in muscle function. Signs are usually apparent within the first 6 months of life. Initially, lameness associated with stiffness and hypertrophy of the affected muscles may occur. The lack of fluid, smooth movement is most pronounced after rest and diminishes with exercise. In most affected horses the abnormality is confined to the hindquarters, although all four limbs may be involved.[48,51] No other body systems are affected. In many cases the horses become progressively weaker, although the clinical course may vary. Based on clinical, electrophysiologic, and pathologic findings[46] this form of myotonia in horses has been suggested most to resemble human myotonia congenita or an undefined myotonia.[52]

A third, severe, and progressive form of myotonia reported in young horses is characterized by onset of clinical signs as early as 1 month of age.[48] Initially, horses exhibit generalized myotonia with hypertonicity of the larger proximal limb muscles, progressing rapidly to muscle stiffness, atrophy, and weakness. In one report the authors also observed testicular hypoplasia, early cataract formation, and mild glucose

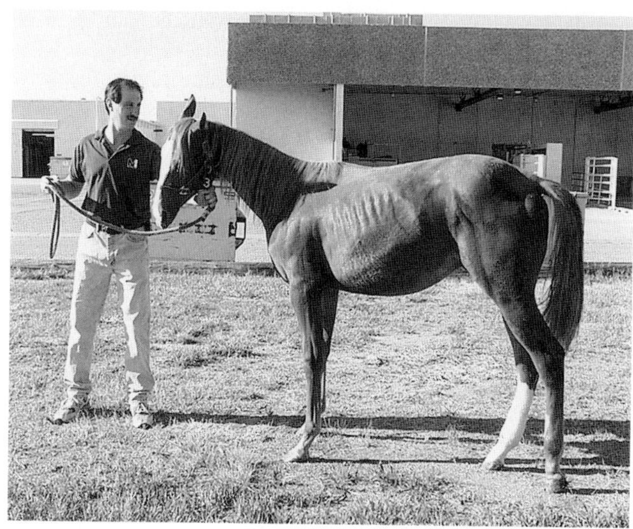

FIGURE 11-6 A young horse with myotonia. The heavy muscling of the hindquarters with atrophy of the distal limb and neck musculature are notable.

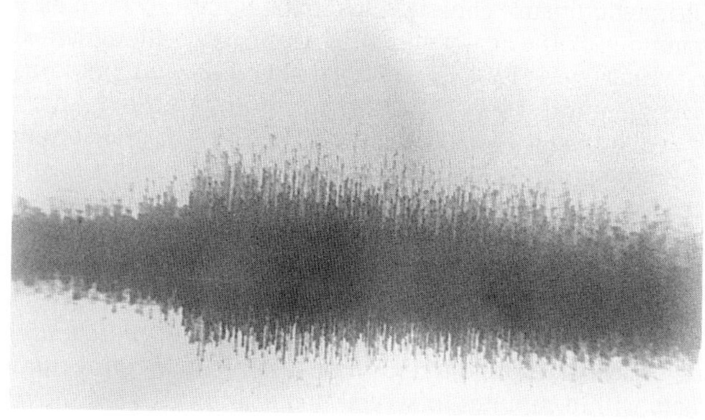

FIGURE 11-7 Prolonged myotonic discharges present on needle electromyographic examination. These high-frequency discharges emit a sound similar to a revving motorcycle but with no true waxing and waning. Instead the amplitude and frequency of the discharges change suddenly (as shown), altering the tone heard. Under general anesthesia, suxamethonium or tubocurarine does not abolish these discharges.

intolerance, suggesting multisystemic involvement. This myotonic dystrophy–like disorder is associated with specific histologic changes.[48,52]

Serum CK and AST activities may be elevated in horses with myotonia, but these increases are often not sustained throughout the course of the disease and tend to be unpredictable.

Not all muscles that exhibit classic myotonic discharges (see the diagnosis section) show histologic changes. Fiber size variation, changes in number and size of the individual fiber types, increased numbers of central nuclei, and clustering together of fiber types with signs of necrosis and degeneration have been reported.[23,46,53] Differences in the histologic findings may reflect different forms of the condition.[46] Dystrophic changes and a normal distribution of fibers would be more likely in a diagnosis of myotonia dystrophica. In a muscle biopsy from a yearling horse with a likely diagnosis of myotonia congenita, histopathologic examination of the muscle revealed small anguloid atrophy of type 2A and 2B fibers. In addition, the muscle fibers in the biopsy were almost exclusively type 2B with fewer type 1 and 2A fibers. No evidence of central nuclei, muscle necrosis, or macrophage infiltration was apparent.

DIAGNOSIS

The diagnosis of myotonia congenita or myotonia dystrophica is based on clinical signs, appropriate histopathologic changes in muscle, and the classic waning (dive bomber) or waxing and waning (revving motorcycle) sounds of the EMG trains of high-frequency discharges (see Figure 11-7). These waveforms are visible on insertion of the EMG electrode and on voluntary, mechanical, or chemical stimulation of the affected muscle. After percussion or stimulation, positive sharp waves and fibrillation potentials may be visible. These abnormal discharges ultimately subside when the muscle has been at complete rest for some time, although they can be initiated readily after the patient is given neuromuscular blockade (e.g., curarization).

TREATMENT

In human beings, quinine, procainamide, taurine, and phenytoin (diphenylhydantoin) have been recommended for treatment of myotonia. Most of these drugs decrease muscle excitability by blocking sodium movement.[38] The duration of EMG relaxation time after maximal voluntary effort is the only reliable indicator of muscle excitation and response to therapy in human beings[41] and is impractical in the horse.

Acepromazine, xylazine, thiopentone, pancuronium bromide, quinidine, and phenytoin have been used to treat horses with myotonia; however, significant improvement in clinical signs has not been observed.[54,55] Prolonged times to 90% muscle relaxation in vitro were observed in two horses with myotonia; these relaxation times were normalized by the administration of phenytoin to the affected horses. However, no obvious clinical improvement or significant effect on EMG was observed with the short duration of therapy.[45] The long-term effects of phenytoin on the clinical signs or progression of myotonia is unknown. The prognosis for horses with any type of myotonia is poor; most affected horses are euthanized because of their inability to function as athletes.

Recurrent Exertional Rhabdomyolysis

Racing Thoroughbreds share a high degree of relatedness. As much as 80% of the genome of the modern Thoroughbred directly traces to 31 animals.[56] This extensive amount of linebreeding makes associating diseases with a particular ancestor difficult because so many horses, healthy or not, may be related to a particular individual. The suggestion has been made that many Thoroughbred horses share a similar genetic trait that leads to RER.[57,58] Epidemiologic surveys of racing Thoroughbreds support that exertional rhabdomyolysis is common. A U.S. survey found approximately 5% of racing Thoroughbreds were affected, and a study in the United Kingdom found 6.7%.[59]

CLINICAL SIGNS AND LABORATORY FINDINGS

Thoroughbred horses with RER may have mild to moderate signs of muscle cramping. Clinical signs of RER are similar to those of other horses exhibiting exertional rhabdomyolysis.

The predominant clinical signs are mild to severe muscle cramping of the major muscle groups of the hindquarters, including the gluteal, semimembranosus, semitendinosus, biceps femoris, and quadriceps femoris muscles. Involvement of these muscle groups is not exclusive, and muscle cramping of the forelimb musculature may occur. Cramping is associated with mild to severe pain demonstrated by anxiety, profuse sweating, refusal to move, and increased heart and respiratory rates. Affected muscles are firm and painful on palpation. The practitioner can palpate generalized or focal areas of flocculation that may be associated with focal areas of muscle tearing or edema. In mild to moderate cases, muscle contractures abate within minutes to several hours, and the horse moves about more comfortably. In severe cases, rhabdomyolysis may lead to recumbency, necessitating a prolonged convalescence, which, in turn, may lead to further complications. Recovery is related to the severity of muscle fiber necrosis and may take days to weeks in mild and moderate cases and months in horses with severe rhabdomyolysis. In most cases, horses readily return to athletic function.

Damaged muscle fibers release myoglobin and the intracellular enzymes LDH, AST, and CK into the circulation. Myoglobin is filtered by the kidneys and is excreted in the urine. With moderate to severe muscle necrosis, myoglobin causes the urine to be orange to brown. In horses with systemic acidosis and dehydration that suffer significant muscle damage, myoglobin may cause tubular nephrosis with acute or delayed renal damage or failure.[60] In Thoroughbreds with RER, onset of rhabdomyolysis most commonly occurs soon after the onset of aerobic exercise, and for this reason accompanying systemic acidosis or dehydration does not occur and renal damage is rare.

After an episode of rhabdomyolysis, CK levels increase exponentially from the reference range to levels at or above 100,000 U/L. CK is a sensitive indicator of muscle damage, with activity peaking 4 to 6 hours after insult. If muscle necrosis is not ongoing, CK levels decrease rapidly over the next 24 to 48 hours because of the relatively short half-life (108 minutes). Serum AST activity takes 12 to 24 hours to peak, and activity may remain elevated for 7 to 14 days after insult.[61]

In Thoroughbred horses with RER, CK activity appears to peak 4 to 6 hours after activity, and affected horses have intermittent elevations in CK activity that are not associated with clinical signs of muscle cramping (subclinical exertional rhabdomyolysis).[62] Subclinical exertional rhabdomyolysis is common in Thoroughbred horses with RER, and CK activity may be at or above 10,000 U/L. Normal healthy horses participating in race training also may have occasional increases in CK activity but do not appear to have them as frequently as horses with RER.

ETIOLOGY

A group of Thoroughbreds with a history of chronic exertional rhabdomyolysis were studied and found to have similar abnormalities.[58,63-65] Muscle biopsies of the middle gluteal muscle did not identify any abnormal accumulations of polysaccharide, but an increased number of centrally located nuclei were found in mature muscle fibers. In vitro contracture studies demonstrated increased sensitivity to caffeine and halothane and faster times to peak contraction and 50% and 90% relaxation compared with healthy Thoroughbred horses or Quarter Horses with PSSM.[64] The in vitro contracture study is considered the gold standard for diagnosing RER in the Thoroughbred horse but requires a specialized laboratory. Therefore diagnosis is generally based on history, breed, and muscle biopsy results.

The muscle contracture results are similar to pigs with malignant hyperthermia.[66] However, further testing has demonstrated that the cellular defect in Thoroughbreds with RER and pigs with malignant hyperthermia is different. Therefore RER represents a disorder similar but not identical to malignant hyperthermia in swine.[67,68] Of interest is that occasional incidences of malignant hyperthermia in Thoroughbred horses with chronic exertional rhabdomyolysis have been reported.[25,69-73] This scenario may indicate that Thoroughbred horses with RER may be more susceptible to episodes of malignant hyperthermia while under general anesthesia, but the incidence is far less common than in swine. The exact cellular mechanism that leads to RER in Thoroughbred horses has yet to be elucidated, and genetic studies are currently under way.

PATHOPHYSIOLOGY

Recurrent exertional rhabdomyolysis affects as much as 5% of the racing Thoroughbred population and likely is inherited as an autosomal dominant trait.[57,74,75] However, expression of the disorder is multifactorial and depends on the fitness level and exercise schedule of the horse, diet, age, gender, temperament, and the presence of any skeletal lameness.[57] Expression of RER in Thoroughbred horses has been postulated to be related to the physicochemical changes experienced by the body during a high level of stress or anxiety. Such a trigger would be similar to that seen in swine with malignant hyperthermia. One study has ruled out the sarcoplasmic reticulum calcium release channel (RYR1) gene, the sarcoplasmic reticulum calcium ATPase (ATP2A1) gene, and the transverse tubule dihydropyridine receptor-voltage sensor (CACNA1S) gene.[67] Therefore the exact mechanism of how anxiety may trigger exertional rhabdomyolysis in susceptible horses remains unknown.

Many of the factors listed previously may influence the mental and physical state of the horse. For example, the typical Thoroughbred horse with RER has long been described as a 2- or 3-year-old filly with a nervous temperament.[57,59,76-78] A recent epidemiologic survey carried out in the United Kingdom showed that females are more likely than males to suffer from this condition, particularly in the birth to 2-year-old and 5- to 6-year-old age groups.[40,79] However, an equal sex ratio was reported in another study.[80] Genetic studies support that RER likely is inherited as an autosomal dominant trait.[74] The increased expression of RER in female Thoroughbreds and in younger horses might be because of temperament. Fillies are more likely to be described as having a nervous temperament by their trainers, and young horses may find the racetrack environment stressful.[57]

Diet also influences expression of RER, and affected horses often consume quantities of grain in excess of 10 lb (4.5 kg) per day. Higher CK activity has been documented in horses with RER compared with control horses when both groups were fed diets high in carbohydrates. In addition, dietary studies have shown that feeding horses diets high in carbohydrates at levels at which the caloric intake exceeds body demands may accentuate nervousness. This effect has been observed in Thoroughbreds with RER and in normal healthy horses.[62] Conversely, horses with RER that are fed diets higher in fat demonstrated a decrease in CK activity, and horses with RER and healthy horses consuming diets high in fat are often regarded as being more calm and less fearful.[81] Several high-fat, low-carbohydrate commercial grain mixes are now available for the horse owner, and anecdotal reports support laboratory findings that the number of incidences of rhabdomyolysis in horses with RER consuming these diets are reduced. Whether the influence of diet on the expression of RER is caused by temperament alone, another factor, or a combination of factors has yet to be determined.

Racehorses with RER are more likely to have an episode of rhabdomyolysis when exercised at a medium gallop as opposed to walking, trotting, breezing, or racing. Horses with RER that are exercised at the trot were more likely to have increased CK activity than when galloping at high intensity. The influence of temperament also may be a factor. Thoroughbreds at the race track are often trotted against traffic as a warm-up and then are turned around to gallop back home at a controlled rate of speed. This training scenario was the most frequent form of exercise associated with episodes of rhabdomyolysis and may result from excitement or anxiety that triggers the episode of rhabdomyolysis in susceptible horses. Horses that are fit for racing may find this training scenario especially exciting because they often pull and try to run faster. When racehorses were allowed to gallop full out, as in breezing or racing, episodes of rhabdomyolysis were infrequent.[57]

Horses with an underlying lameness are predisposed to episodes of exertional rhabdomyolysis. Whether changes in gait may be related to muscle pain or soreness or whether underlying skeletal disorders may alter a horse's way of going, precipitating an episode of rhabdomyolysis, or whether running in pain from a skeletal disorder may trigger an episode of rhabdomyolysis is unclear. Inclement weather has often been cited as causing an increase in the incidence of RER, as has the time of year.[82,83] In a 2-year survey in the United Kingdom, significantly more episodes of rhabdomyolysis were reported from November to February than during other times of the year.[40,79]

At the race track, large groups of horses are fed, exercised, and housed under similar conditions. Yet some horses are particularly predisposed to chronic exertional rhabdomyolysis, which underscores the likelihood of a genetic basis for the disorder. One is tempted to assume that all affected Thoroughbreds at the racetrack have RER. However, the practitioner must be wary about diagnosing all Thoroughbreds with chronic exertional rhabdomyolysis as having RER until the genetic fault is identified and a genetic test is available.

DIAGNOSIS

Currently the gold standard for diagnosing RER is the caffeine or halothane muscle contracture test.[65] However, this test requires a biopsy sample from intercostal muscle and is not readily available. Therefore diagnosis of RER is based on history, laboratory documentation of rhabdomyolysis, and histopathologic examination of muscle. Horses with RER should be Thoroughbreds or Thoroughbred crosses because of the likelihood that the disorder is inherited as an autosomal dominant trait. The horse should have experienced multiple bouts of muscle cramping after nonintensive exercise accompanied by documented elevations in CK activity. Muscle biopsy reveals recent rhabdomyolysis, regeneration, an increased number of central nuclei, and absence of abnormal polysaccharide.

TREATMENT

Treatment of horses with RER aims at managing the frequency of the clinical episodes of rhabdomyolysis, considering that the disorder is likely a primary myopathy. Environmental and dietary factors appear to influence the expression of RER. Such factors include dietary fat and carbohydrate content, dietary electrolytes, exercise regimens, housing and turnout conditions, and underlying skeletal lameness. The practitioner must pay particular attention to the temperament of the individual horse. The most successful trainers modify the affected workout schedule of the horse to minimize stress. For example, horses that prefer to work alone or with company should do so. If a horse is calmer to work when the track is empty, the trainer should exercise it early in the day; others may benefit from a long, slow warm-up to minimize stress. One should make similar stress-reducing modifications for affected horses used in other disciplines.

The diet should be modified to provide adequate but not excessive amounts of calories for the level of work being performed such that a greater proportion is supplied from fats as opposed to carbohydrates. High-calorie diets composed primarily of fat are effective in decreasing postexercise CK activities in affected horses.[84] The optimal fat source and percentage of fat in the diet have yet to be determined, but several commercially available feeds on the market have been found to be useful. The exact mechanism by which increased dietary fats lower CK activity in horses with RER has yet to be determined.

Dantrolene has been used in human medicine to treat and help prevent malignant hyperthermia. In this condition an abnormal release of calcium from the sarcoplasmic reticulum appears to occur, resulting in prolonged contracture, hyperthermia, metabolic and respiratory acidosis, and muscle damage. Dantrolene is thought to decrease the rate of calcium release from the sarcoplasmic reticulum and to affect charge movement in the T tubule system. Dantrolene has been used in human beings to treat chronic exertional rhabdomyolysis.[85] In one study, dantrolene (800 mg) given orally 1 hour before exercise in Thoroughbreds that had experienced a day of rest before exercise has been shown to be effective.[86]

Although dantrolene sodium has been suggested for treating equine rhabdomyolysis, the drug is used more commonly in prevention. Giving 2 mg/kg/day diluted in normal saline by a stomach tube for 3 to 5 days and then every third day for a month has been recommended.[76,87] A lower daily dose (300 mg) may be equally beneficial[87] and perhaps preferable because the drug is hepatotoxic.[76] Another recommendation is 500 mg orally for 3 to 5 days and then 300 mg every third day for a time. The time period depends on the circumstances and the effect on the liver, but prolonged treatment is not recommended. Monitoring of hepatic status and function is recommended because the effects on the liver seem to be individually variable. Up to 1 g of dantrolene, given with a small feed 1.5 to 2 hours before exercise for 3 to 5 days has been used with apparent success in racehorses, but in some cases the horses may have been suffering from overexertion rather than RER. Researchers have suggested that lower doses are unlikely to reach therapeutic levels. The drug appears not to be as bioavailable in the horse as in human beings and is cleared more quickly.[69]

Idiopathic Chronic Exertional Rhabdomyolysis

Horses of many breeds and types other than Thoroughbreds, Draft Horses, and Quarter Horses may experience recurrent episodes of exertional rhabdomyolysis. Of special note are

Standardbred and Arabian horses. These breeds share some common genetic heritage with Thoroughbred horses, and individuals with chronic exertional rhabdomyolysis may have muscle biopsy findings consistent with RER. These individual horses may respond favorably to management changes (high-fat diet and regular exercise) recommended for Thoroughbreds with RER. However, muscle contracture testing of affected Standardbred and Arabian horses has not been performed to confirm similar muscle pathophysiology.

Some horses with idiopathic exertional rhabdomyolysis do not respond to management and dietary recommendations described previously. Practitioners should counsel owners of horses that suffer from repeated episodes of rhabdomyolysis despite multiple management changes to decrease the exercise intensity the horse is performing or retire the horse from regular work.

ACQUIRED MYOPATHIES

Jennifer M. MacLeay

TRAUMATIC MUSCLE INJURY

Chronic Muscle Injury: Fibrotic Myopathy

Fibrotic myopathy tends to be a chronic, progressive disorder and may occur after excessive exercise over a long period that has resulted in the repeated tearing and stretching of muscle fibers.[1] Fibrotic myopathy has also been observed in Quarter Horses and stock horses after maneuvers such as sliding stops, in which the large thigh muscles are contracting while the stifle and hock are extending,[2,3] and in horses tied by a halter and shank that pull back and fight strongly. Fibrotic myopathy has also been described as congenital, perhaps caused by periparturient trauma,[4] and after intramuscular injection.[5] The semitendinosus muscle is most frequently affected, but adhesions to the semimembranosus and biceps femoris are common. Myopathy also may involve the gracilis or biceps brachii muscles.

The altered gait seen in horses with fibrotic myopathy of the hamstring muscles is characteristic. The horse walks with a shortened anterior phase of stride and then snaps the foot to the ground with a slap. The pathophysiologic process appears to involve trauma (external or work related) followed by inflammation, muscle fiber atrophy, and replacement by fibrous tissue. Occasionally, mineral deposits form in the affected tissues, in which case the condition has been labeled as an ossifying myopathy.[5] The characteristic gait likely results from a combination of scar tissue preventing normal extension and contraction of the muscle belly and possibly an altered γ-efferent loop with an abnormal setting of the muscle spindle trigger, which may allow the early unchecked contraction of caudal thigh muscles during the late swing phase of the stride.[6]

CLINICAL SIGNS

Fibrotic myopathy has been described as a nonpainful mechanical lameness associated with a distinct gait abnormality (Figure 11-8). The condition can be unilateral or bilateral,

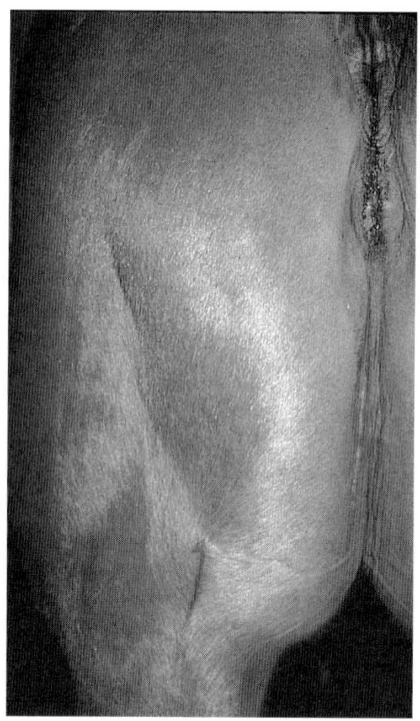

FIGURE 11-8 A horse with abnormal muscle contour secondary to fibrotic myopathy. (Courtesy Dr. Gary Baxter.)

and the horse pulls the affected limb or limbs back and down before the end of the protraction phase so that the foot slams down, resulting in a louder sound on impact than that of an unaffected limb and in a shortened cranial or swing phase and a lengthened weight-bearing phase,[4] which has been called a *goose-stepping gait*. The condition tends to be most obvious at the walk. If the condition involves the biceps brachii muscle the horse shows a shortened cranial phase of the thoracic limb with a tendency for the foot to land at the toe in a way similar to those animals affected by navicular syndrome. Occasionally, one can identify the area of muscle damage because of a dimpling or depression in the skin overlying the muscle. In cases in which significant fibrous tissue or calcification of the muscle occurs, the site is readily palpable. The lameness tends to be unresponsive to routine anti-inflammatory therapy.

DIAGNOSIS

The diagnosis of fibrotic myopathy is based on clinical signs and history. In one report, two horses with congenital fibrotic myopathy did not have palpable thickening of the muscle or tendon and had no evidence of scar formation.[7] Histologically, one may observe a band of dense collagenous connective tissue or irregular, jagged pieces of mineral. Diagnostic ultrasound has been useful in some cases to confirm the diagnosis and to determine whether mineralization is present in addition to the fibrosis.

Fibrotic myopathy may be distinguished from stringhalt by closely observing the gait. In horses with stringhalt the rear limb hyperflexes during the cranial or swing phase, and a stepwise caudal jerking movement does not occur just before the foot hits the ground.[3]

TREATMENT AND PROGNOSIS

Surgical treatments described for fibrotic myopathy include resection of the fibrotic band, semitendinosus myotenectomy, and simplified semitendinosus tenotomy.[5,7,8] Some improvement in gait may occur in some horses after surgery, but complete resolution of lameness is an unlikely result. Long-term prognosis is poor because the condition tends to recur after surgery. Postoperative problems with wound healing are common.[5] Transection of the semitendinosus tendon insertion on the tibia distal to the myotendinous junction has been said to result in much less postoperative trauma, which may help to decrease the potential for recurrence,[7] and full recovery has been reported anecdotally in a few cases. Performing a less-radical excision and combining this with passive postoperative flexion-and-extension physiotherapy therefore may be preferable. Surgery is unlikely to be of value if the biceps brachii is involved.[5]

Gastrocnemius Muscle Rupture

Rupture of the gastrocnemius muscle occurs in horses attempting to get up after a long period of recumbency (e.g., after anesthesia or postpartum paralysis). Rupture also occurs in animals that rear and fall over backward and occurs occasionally after overextension. In foals, ruptures have been reported after the first attempt of the foal to rise, especially if the foal has poor muscle tone or coordination. The condition also occurs in foals after an assisted delivery (dystocia) and in foals after manual attempts to straighten a fixed tibiotarsal joint. A rupture occurring in the tendon of insertion may result in avulsion of a portion of the tuber calcanei. If rupture occurs in the muscle belly, a hematoma may form and may calcify. The condition can occur unilaterally or bilaterally; however, the animal will be unable to stand if rupture is bilateral or if complete Achilles tendon rupture occurs. The affected hock or hocks may be flexed excessively because of the loss of the extensor influence of the gastrocnemius, giving the horse a squatting appearance. Heat, swelling, and pain are normally evident in the initial stages. The plasma muscle enzyme activities also tend to be elevated, at least initially.[9,10] Treatment involving support in a sling with the affected limb immobilized in an extended position has been recommended,[10] but the prognosis is guarded for a return to normal function.

Serratus Ventralis Rupture

Rupture of the serratus ventralis is rare and occurs as a consequence of dorsal impact trauma over the withers and neck region or after jumping a high fence or jumping off a raised platform. Animals are usually affected bilaterally. The thorax drops between the paired scapulae so that the dorsal borders are above the thoracic spinous processes. The croup is often higher than the withers. The condition is painful, and radiographs are needed to eliminate the possibility of dorsal spinous process fracture. The prognosis is poor. Recommended treatment is a prolonged period in a sling if the horse is suited temperamentally to such a restriction.[2]

Sore and Pulled Muscles

Pulled muscles (i.e., muscle tears or strains resulting in some disruption of muscle architecture and occasionally the formation of a hematoma) are often exhibited immediately after exercise. Depending on the extent of the trauma and the muscle groups involved, obvious swelling and apparent pain on palpation may or may not be present. Plasma CK and AST activities may or may not be elevated significantly. Definitive diagnosis may be difficult, especially in chronic cases. Faradic stimulation, scintigraphy, thermography, and diagnostic ultrasound are some of the more common techniques used to diagnose a pulled muscle. Treatment tends to be a combination of rest and physiotherapy (e.g., manipulation, faradism, ultrasound). Perhaps one should differentiate pulled muscles from the overexerted or sore muscle in which the associated damage tends to be at the cellular level involving structural damage of the contractile elements. Delayed-onset muscular soreness (DOMS) is a commonly recognized condition in human beings. The soreness tends to increase in intensity over the initial 24 hours after exercise and peaks around 24 to 72 hours, hence its name. Whether DOMS occurs in the horse is not certain, although the diagnosis has been suggested when a stiff gait, palpable soreness, and a reluctance to move, as well as increased hydroxyproline concentrations, are observed 24 hours after exercise. Free radicals may be involved in the pathophysiologic features of acute and delayed-onset postexercise muscular soreness. Treatment of DOMS in human beings varies from rest to light exercise with or without analgesia and the external application of heat. In the horse, continued exercise may be contraindicated if the horse has experienced significant exertional rhabdomyolysis as diagnosed by moderate to high CK activity and in horses with an obvious muscle tear as indicated by the presence of heat, pain, swelling, and abnormal gait. In human beings the best prevention for DOMS is moderate daily increases in the degree of training.

Infectious Myositis

Infectious agents (bacteria, viruses, and parasites) can affect skeletal muscles. Some agents produce inflammatory reactions (myositis), whereas others give rise to mild degenerative changes (i.e., myopathy). The differentiation can be difficult, especially in subacute and chronic cases, because an inflammatory reaction often induces secondary degenerative changes and vice versa.

CLOSTRIDIAL MYONECROSIS

Gas gangrene, malignant edema, and clostridial myonecrosis are terms used to describe infection of skeletal muscles with any of several *Clostridium* organisms (*C. septicum, C. perfringens, C. novyi,* C. *sordelli,* and *C. chauvoei*). Germination of spores and vegetative growth occur when suitable local anaerobic conditions (e.g., alkaline pH, low oxidative reduction potential) exist after castration, parturition injuries, puncture wounds, and, in particular, intramuscular injections.[11] Toxin production results in the destruction of the cellular defense mechanisms and significant tissue necrosis.

Affected animals may be found recumbent or dead. In less acute cases, mild to severe lameness, colic, or obtunded mentation may be the presenting complaint. Painful muscular swellings may be present, and one may feel flocculation or gas crepitation. The overlying skin may initially feel hot and then progressively becomes cool, tough, firm, and insensitive. Affected animals are often extremely obtunded with systemic signs of profound toxemia. The prognosis is poor without treatment because the condition often progresses rapidly with ataxia, recumbency, coma, and death.

Diagnosis usually is made from the clinical signs and history. The finding of a nonclotting, malodorous fluid on needle aspiration (with or without gas) can be indicative of clostridial infection. Anaerobic culture, cytologic examination, and fluorescent antibody identification of the organism in tissue specimens has been recommended for definitive diagnosis.[12]

Clinicopathologic changes tend to be nonspecific and similar to those seen in other septic-toxic conditions. Although increased serum muscle enzyme activities may be observed, they often do not appear to be in proportion to the degree of muscle damage.[13] In gas gangrene, extensive disintegration of muscle tissue occurs, with serosanguineous exudate and bubbles of gas. Malignant edema is characterized by a cellulitis with sparing of muscle fibers, although this may progress to gangrene.[12,14]

Treatment must be aggressive and typically includes initial administration of high doses of potassium penicillin G (44,000 IU/kg intravenously every 6 to 8 hours) and surgical débridement. One may administer penicillin with metronidazole (20 to 25 mg/kg orally every 8 hours or 20 mg/kg intravenously every 8 to 12 hours). Surgical débridement, fenestration, or both are essential to remove necrotic tissue and disrupt the anaerobic environment.[12] Long-term antibiotic and nursing care of the resulting wound usually is required. Antibiotic therapy should be continued until infection has resolved and for a minimum of 7 days thereafter. In many instances, diffuse cellulitis extending down fascial planes occurs, necessitating therapy for at least several weeks. Supportive fluid therapy and analgesics are often necessary in the initial stages while signs of systemic toxemia are evident. Corticosteroids should be used with caution, although initial short-term therapy may be beneficial in horses with evidence of shock. Prognosis in most horses is guarded.[11] Survival appears to be most frequent with *C. perfringens* infections, although extensive skin and muscle sloughing may occur, which, in turn, may necessitate euthanasia.

Immune-mediated hemolysis has been described in several horses with *C. perfringens* myositis.[15,16] The anemia may be characterized by regeneration, autoagglutination, and a positive Coombs' test. Type 3 echinocytes, spheroechinocytes, and reticulocytes may be observed. In such cases, immunosuppressive therapy must be judiciously implemented to treat the anemia without allowing the infection to go unchecked. Treatment of horses with penicillin has also resulted in immune-mediated hemolytic anemia.[17,18] In such cases, use of oxytetracycline and metronidazole should be considered.

Streptococcal Immune-Mediated Myositis

Purpura hemorrhagica is an immune-mediated vasculitis associated with sensitization and cross-reactivity to proteins in the cell wall of *Streptococcus equi* subsp. *equi*. Purpura hemorrhagica in its most common form may be associated with mild muscular lesions secondary to vasculitis.[19] Skeletal muscle necrosis with fragmentation and swelling of muscle fibers and a cellular infiltration may be visible histologically. Classically, the lesions are believed to be caused by a type III hypersensitivity vasculitis.

Some bacteria may share similar immunodeterminants with muscle so that antibodies produced against the bacteria also affect the muscle directly, causing necrosis.[20] This type of purpura has myositis as its primary clinical sign rather than vasculitis. Two forms of immune-mediated myositis have been described in horses in association with *S. equi* subsp. *equi:* immunoglobulin (Ig) G and IgA mediated. Both are less common complications of *S. equi* subsp. *equi* infection than purpura hemorrhagica.[21,22]

IgG-mediated myositis in horses is characterized by rapid onset of muscle wasting (2 to 14 days; Figure 11-9). The amount of muscle mass lost is often astounding considering the time frame. Horses typically have a history of clinical *S. equi* subsp. *equi* infection or live on farms where infection is endemic. Muscle biopsy reveals inflammatory cell infiltration of the muscle and muscle cell atrophy. Horses are otherwise bright and alert and have a normal appetite. Blood and serum profiles are within normal limits with the exception of increased CK and AST activity. Globulin fractions may increase slightly. Horses respond favorably to a 4- to 8-week course of corticosteroid therapy (dexamethasone or prednisolone, or both). In horses in which the practitioner suspects an internal nidus of infection (abscess) as the cause of long-term exposure to the antigen, concurrent antibiotic therapy should be instituted.

The IgA-mediated form of poststreptococcal myositis of horses is similar to Henoch-Schönlein purpura of humans and is a significantly more malignant form of myositis. Horses do not exhibit loss of muscle mass but may have residual loss of muscle mass should they survive. Affected horses have severe obtundation, muscle pain, stiff gait, thrombosis, and colic and may have areas of flocculent serosanguineous fluid several centimeters in diameter over the major muscle groups. Signs are progressive over the first 24 hours. In the first hours, blood analysis may show only a stress or endotoxic leukogram and high CK and AST activities. Physical examination and blood analysis progresses to support early disseminated intravascular coagulopathy and CK activities of greater than 100,000 U/L. Postmortem examination of these horses shows large areas of hemorrhagic necrosis within the large muscle groups (Figure 11-10). Histologic examination demonstrates myositis. Early, aggressive cardiovascular support combined with large doses of dexamethasone is essential in an attempt to treat these horses because mortality rates are high. If major vital organs are infarcted the horse will not likely survive. However, with aggressive support and long-term steroid therapy (1 to 2 weeks

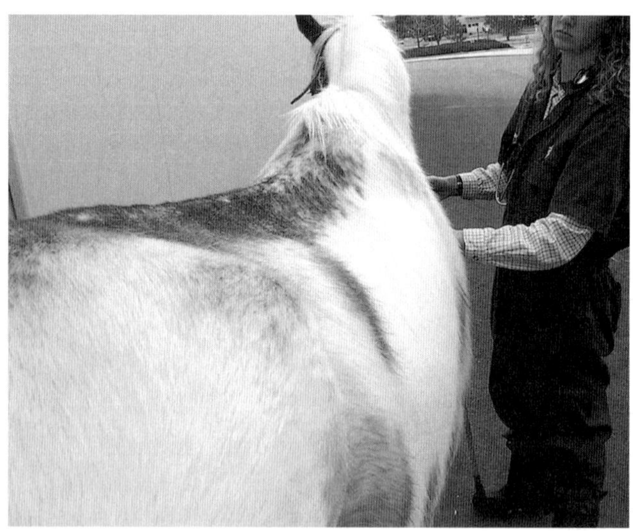

FIGURE 11-9 A horse with immunoglobulin G–mediated *Streptococcus equi* subsp *equi* myositis. The profound atrophy of the lumbar muscles is notable. The horse responded well to a course of prednisolone therapy.

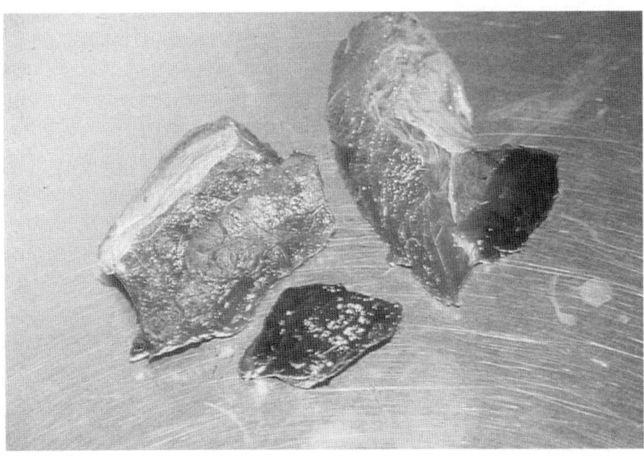

FIGURE 11-10 Muscle taken postmortem from a horse with immunoglobulin A–mediated *Streptococcus equi* subsp *equi* myositis. The sharp demarcation between normal and infarcted muscle is notable.

at high doses, followed by a longer-term, declining dose regimen) the horse may survive. These horses often have pockets of *S. equi* subsp. *equi* infection internally that may have been the nidus initiating the immune mediated reaction. Areas to be examined include the guttural pouches and thoracic and abdominal cavities. Because these horses may have a nidus of infection, treatment also should include aggressive antibiotic therapy.

Suppurative Myositis: Abscessation

Suppurative myositis may be hematogenous in origin or result from penetrating wounds, intramuscular injections, or an extension of an infective focus in an adjacent or distant structure. Almost any bacteria may be isolated from such abscesses, but two are particularly common in horses: *S equi* subsp. *equi* and *Corynebacterium pseudotuberculosis*. *S. equi* subsp. *equi* may occur secondary to (1) hematogenous spread, (2) misinjection of intranasal vaccines intramuscularly, or (3) skin contamination from aerosolized *S. equi* subsp. *equi* and subsequent intramuscular injection after administration of intranasal or intramucosal strangles vaccines.[23] Injections of a variety of intramuscular vaccinations can also lead to abscessation. Affected horses initially have an ill-defined cellulitis, which may heal, progress to a classic organized abscess, or in the case of certain staphylococci, may extend, resulting in extensive muscle damage. Abscesses may heal slowly, expand, or fistulate to the surface. Once fistulated, abscesses may collapse and heal, usually with scar tissue, or persist as chronic granulomata (especially *Staphylococcus aureus* in the neck and pectoral region).[14]

CORYNEBACTERIUM PSEUDOTUBERCULOSIS

Corynebacterium pseudotuberculosis is a gram-positive, pleomorphic, rod-shaped, intracellular, facultative anaerobe with worldwide distribution that may be isolated from large abscesses in various muscles, in particular, the pectorals. A significant geographic variation appears in the clinical presentation of *C. pseudotuberculosis* infection. Worldwide, ulcerative lymphangitis—usually with sores, abscesses, fever, lameness, anorexia, and lethargy, which may progress to chronic lameness and weight loss—is the most common condition associated with this infection. However, in the United States, especially in more arid regions, the organism tends to be associated with ventral midline, inguinal, and pectoral abscesses, although internal abscesses may occur. The condition has been called *pigeon fever* (after the swollen pectorals giving the appearance of a pigeon breast), dry land distemper, or Colorado strangles (after its geographic distribution).

Suppurative myositis can occur at any time of the year but is more common in late summer, fall, and early winter. One or more horses within a group may be affected. Outbreaks in a significant number of horses at a single establishment have been reported. *C. pseudotuberculosis* can survive in the soil and enter the body via lesions in the skin or mucous membranes and spread via the lymphatics. Insect vectors may be involved. Clinical signs vary with the stage of the condition and the site of the abscess or abscesses.[24,25] The affected horse may be pyrexic and anorectic during the maturation phase of the abscess. Ventral pitting edema, lameness, weight loss, and depression may also occur. If the abscesses are located in the axillary or inguinal regions the affected animal can be very lame and is more likely to be intermittently febrile. Such cases can be difficult to diagnose because the abscesses may take weeks or even months to develop fully. Increased white blood cell counts and plasma fibrinogen concentration may be observed, although, in the more chronic stages, few clinicopathologic changes are seen. Abscesses typically form deep in muscles and can be large with thick capsular walls filled with a nonodorous, light tan pus. The differential diagnosis includes seromata, tumors, and other bacterial abscesses. One can confirm the diagnosis by ultrasound or culture of any aspirated fluid. Abscesses in the axillary region in particular can be difficult to locate, even with ultrasound. A synergistic hemolysis inhibition test detects antibodies to the organism, but the intensity of the antibody response depends on several factors, including thickness of the capsule surrounding the abscess and chronicity of the infection. For example, horses with chronic thick-walled abscesses that have been lanced recently may have low or undetectable circulating antibody concentrations, perhaps because antibodies have been consumed during the massive toxin release. The test can be helpful in determining whether one should include internal *C. pseudotuberculosis* abscessation in the differential diagnosis.

Recommended treatments include encouraging the maturation process via hot poultices, lancing, flushing, and draining. In some cases, surgical intervention may be required to expose the abscess adequately. Some controversy exists over the use of antibiotics, especially respecting the timing of administration, which may depend on the stage of abscessation. Antibiotics commonly recommended include procaine penicillin G at 20,000 U/kg intramuscularly every 12 hours or potassium penicillin G at 40,000 U/kg intravenously every 6 hours, sulfadiazine (or sulfamethoxazole)-trimethoprim, or erythromycin. Rifampin (2.5 to 5.0 mg/kg) given orally every 12 hours is often recommended in combination with penicillin or sulfas. Antibiotic therapy should ideally continue for several weeks.

The prognosis is guarded; some abscesses do not resolve completely with treatment. Some recur when antibiotic therapy is discontinued; others may recur months later. In a few horses, internal abscesses may develop, resulting in chronic weight loss and sometimes ventral edema, ascites, dyspnea, recurrent colic, exercise intolerance, and recurrent pyrexia, among other conditions. Abortion can also be a sequela.[25] Avoiding contamination of paddocks from a draining lesion and dealing with contaminated bedding appropriately have been recommended. Good fly control can also be beneficial.

Parasitic Myositis

SARCOCYSTIS

Sarcocystis spp. are protozoal parasites that have an obligatory two-host life cycle. *Sarcocystis* spp. are found in horse muscle as part of the intermediate host infection. The horse consumes sporocysts with herbage that has been contaminated by carnivore feces. Sporozoites are released and migrate to various sites. Second- or third-generation schizonts develop within muscle fibers as thin-walled cysts. Entry into muscle fibers can result in extensive fiber degeneration and significant enzyme release if a heavy infestation occurs. Enlargement of the cysts over the next 100 days or so can result in further muscle damage and lameness. Four *Sarcocystis* species (*S. bertrami, S. equicanis, S. neurona,* and *S. fayeri*) have been recognized in horses, although some controversy exists as to whether they are all distinct species.[14,26] A high postmortem prevalence of sarcocysts in muscle sections (especially the tongue), occasional presence of sarcocysts in other skeletal muscle biopsies, and evidence of transplacental infection have been reported,[27,28] suggesting that inapparent infection is probably common. A light and electron microscope study of sarcocysts in the horse has been described.[29]

Some dispute exists as to how heavy an infestation is necessary to cause clinical muscle disease in the horse. Twelve of 91 horses with a history of chronic muscle problems were positive for sarcocysts on muscle biopsy.[28] Separating the group of animals with sarcocysts from others based on laboratory findings, history, or clinical signs was not possible. Weight loss, lethargy, difficulty in chewing and swallowing, generalized muscle weakness, and fasciculations have been reported in one horse with widely distributed sarcocysts, and clinical signs were attributed to the sarcocyst infestation.[30] Chronic illness in an experimentally infected pony also has been reported.[31] A heavy infestation is likely necessary to cause clinical disease.[32]

TRICHINELLA SPIRALIS

The nematode *Trichinella spiralis* can be found as an encysted larva in a bulging glassy segment of a muscle fiber in horses given feed containing contaminated porcine muscle tissue. Trichinosis is therefore rare. Interestingly, a survey in Serbia found that feeding meat to horses as food refuse was relatively common and may be practiced elsewhere in Europe as well. This observation lead the investigators to conclude that surveillance for *Trichinella,* a meat-born parasite, should continue in Europe.[33] Usually, one cyst per fiber is present, and the larva may be up to 100 μm long. Degeneration (plus regeneration) may occur in neighboring muscle fibers. The larva can live for many years, but if the parasitized segment degenerates, the larva is exposed and soon dies; this in turn results in an acute, predominantly eosinophilic inflammation.[14,34] The parasitic infection appears to be asymptomatic but may present a human health hazard in countries where consumption of horse meat is common.

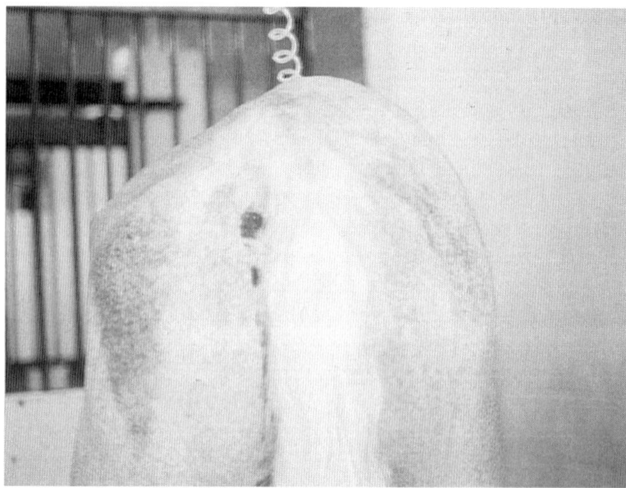

FIGURE 11-11 A horse with postanesthetic myositis of the right gluteal muscles. The severe swelling is notable. The horse recovered fully with supportive care.

CIRCULATORY PROBLEMS RESULTING IN MYOSITIS

Postanesthetic Myositis

Postanesthetic muscle damage may occur in 6% of anesthetized horses.[35] Postanesthetic myopathy may be divided into two forms: localized (the more common form) and generalized.

PATHOPHYSIOLOGIC CHARACTERISTICS OF LOCALIZED POSTANESTHETIC MYOSITIS

The localized form of postanesthetic myositis is likely a consequence of undergoing anesthesia combined with positioning of the horse during anesthesia with minimal padding (Figure 11-11). Recumbency results in direct pressure damage to the nerves or muscles (or both) or perfusion disturbances resulting in increased pressure within the osteofascial compartments, and local ischemia. In this context, compartment is defined as a muscle or group of muscles enclosed within a low-compliance envelope of fascia and sometimes periosteum.[36] This definition is comparable to compartmental syndrome described in human beings and down cattle. Venous occlusion tends to result in a greater inflammatory response and more extensive fibrous tissue repair than arterial occlusion. Sufficiently high intramuscular pressures have been reported during anesthesia of horses to compromise capillary blood flow and possibly affect neural transmission.[36-40] Postanesthetic compartmental syndrome per se has been reported only rarely in the horse, perhaps because compartmental pressures decrease rapidly when a horse stands.[41]

An increase in the lactate concentration of blood draining from dependent muscle, a significant postischemic hyperemia in dependent muscles, and increases in the plasma concentrations of thromboxane and prostaglandin E_2 have been reported in anesthetized horses. Damage may result from reperfusion of ischemic muscles rather than the ischemia itself. Reperfusion generates strong oxidants, possibly initiating membrane lipid peroxidation and muscle damage.[38]

Risk factors associated with postanesthetic myositis include the weight and fitness of the horse, positioning, padding, duration of anesthesia, hypoxemia, blood pressure, and the type of drugs or anesthetic used.

Postanesthetic myositis has been reported in the upper limb, as well as the dependent limb. Therefore support for the upper limb should be provided in addition to adequate padding. However, even when protective padding is used, hypotension and hypoxemia resulting may predispose horses to postanesthetic myositis.[36,38,42-44] No increase in the incidence of problems is apparent when repeated episodes of normotensive anesthesia are undertaken, even with halothane use.[42] Usually, the practitioner observes clinical signs in the limb that is down (compressed) when in lateral recumbency. In the forelimbs, the triceps, deltoids, and occasionally the brachiocephalic and cranial pectoral muscles tend to be affected. In the hind limbs the biceps and vastus lateralis are usually affected. The flank muscles and masseter muscles may also be involved. Occasionally the upper limb may be affected if its circulation is compromised. The position that appears to provide adequate surgical access to the lower limb with low compartmental and venous pressures in the upper limb is the flexed horizontal forward position (i.e., leg parallel to the floor, fully flexed at the carpus, and pushed gently forward).

When a horse is anesthetized in dorsal recumbency, the gluteal and occasionally the longissimus dorsi muscles tend to be affected. In one study, the adductor, pectineus, and gracilis muscles were involved, a finding attributed to arterial hypotension coupled with partial occlusion of the artery supplying these muscles (the medial circumflex femoral artery), perhaps because of the hind limbs being flexed passively.[45]

CLINICAL SIGNS

Clinical signs of postanesthetic myositis are normally seen during the initial recovery period but may occasionally be delayed for 1 hour or more. One may first suspect the condition if recovery is prolonged or the horse has repeated unsuccessful attempts to stand. Signs attributable to damage to one muscle group, one peripheral nerve, or mixtures of muscle groups and peripheral nerve or nerves may be visible. Affected muscle groups tend to be hot and swollen. The horse resents palpation and is usually reluctant to bear weight on the affected limb. One may observe signs of severe pain with sweating. Classically, with forelimb muscle involvement, the affected animal stands as if the radial nerve has been paralyzed but can use the extensor muscles. If hind limbs are involved, knuckling of the fetlock may occur; if the quadriceps femoris is involved, the stifle and hock may buckle, and the animal may not be able to rise, especially if both hind limbs are affected. Signs may persist for several days, even in uncomplicated cases.

Raised painful plaques of edematous muscle with or without fore or hind limb dysfunction may be seen. These swellings usually occur over the table contact areas (hip, rib, or facial area) and may be caused by inadequate padding, trauma from positioning devices, or the weight of the patient.[44] Serum CK and AST activities increase in affected individuals, and one may observe myoglobinuria with significant muscle damage.

On occasion, after recovery from general anesthesia, a horse demonstrates considerable discomfort with continued treading of the feet, sweating, holding its limbs (usually the hind limbs) in abnormal positions, and kicking out. The syndromes appear nonresponsive even to large doses of opiate or other analgesics, serum CK activities are not increased within the subsequent 48 to 96 hours, and no myoglobinuria is observable. These syndromes are assumed to be a form of paresthesia (pins and needles) caused by sensory neuropraxis, and a strong clinical similarity to the condition of postanesthetic neuromyopathy is suggested.

PATHOPHYSIOLOGIC CHARACTERISTICS OF GENERALIZED POSTANESTHETIC MYOSITIS

The generalized form of postanesthetic myositis may be caused by a condition similar to malignant hyperthermia in human beings and swine. Signs may appear during recovery, with many muscle groups affected independent of positioning. The cause of generalized postanesthetic myositis in horses is uncertain but has been suggested to result from local ischemia that becomes more generalized because of hypotension, sensitivity of muscle cells to anesthetic drugs, depolarizing muscle relaxants (suxamethonium), or a combination of these factors. In two studies that looked at the effect of hypotensive anesthesia, cases of generalized myositis occurred during recovery.[42,44] In vitro examination of muscle using an adapted human contracture test (used for the identification of malignant hyperthermia susceptibility) has shown increased sensitivity to caffeine and halothane in samples taken from certain susceptible Equidae.[46] Given that some of these studies are older, horses with inherited myopathies may have unwittingly been included.

Whether horses with inherited myopathies are more or less prone to malignant hyperthermic events or postanesthetic rhabdomyolysis compared with the general horse population is unknown. Certainly, given the common nature of these disorders, one can be confident in saying that not every horse anesthetized that has an underlying myopathy has a malignant hyperthermic or postanesthetic rhabdomyolytic event. However, in human beings, many different muscle disorders have been associated with an increased chance of malignant hyperthermic event when under general anesthesia. Therefore the potential exists, and inquiring whether a horse has a history of exertional rhabdomyolysis before performing general anesthesia is prudent. If a horse is believed to be at risk, premedicating that horse with dantrolene may be of benefit.

Generalized myositis may occur at any time during anesthesia. The temperature, heart rate, and respiratory rate increase, and muscles may fasciculate and contract. The horse may resist assisted ventilation and appear rigid. Death can occur. Postoperative cases also tend to occur regardless of the length of the anesthesia and positioning. Signs of extreme pain are apparent, and the affected animal is unable to rise. The muscles may be rigid, and excessive sweating usually occurs. Signs of colic with myoglobinuria may be present, as well as fluid disturbances.

One may need to differentiate the condition from postanesthetic myelopathy, in which signs can range from difficulty in standing to paraplegia with flaccid paralysis and analgesia involving the pelvic limbs. In addition, loss of sensation and spinal reflexes over several contiguous segments may occur.

LABORATORY FINDINGS

Plasma and serum CK, AST, and LDH activities usually increase in both forms of postanesthetic myositis of horses. Increased plasma muscle enzyme activities may help differentiate those animals with overt muscle damage from those with conditions similar to paresthesia (possibly caused by a reduced blood supply to sensory nerve endings). Fluid and electrolyte disturbances may also be present. Hypocalcemia, hypomagnesemia, hyperphosphatemia, metabolic acidosis, hyperkalemia, and hyperglycemia have been reported and should be treated if present. Myoglobinuria may occur, and renal function may be compromised, necessitating treatment with intravenous fluids, furosemide, and dopamine. Muscle biopsy histologic examination is consistent with rhabdomyolysis.

TREATMENT

The aims of treatment are to relieve pain, prevent further damage, correct fluid and electrolyte disturbances, and maintain renal function. The added clinical manifestation in some cases is malignant hyperthermia in which muscle contractures cause a rapid increase in body temperature. The treatment usually recommended is similar to that for exertional rhabdomyolysis. If a metabolic acidosis is present, the horse may require intravenous sodium bicarbonate. If the signs are recognized while the horse is anesthetized, one should stop using the anesthetic, whenever possible, and use alternative intravenous agents. If hyperthermia is present the horse should be cooled rapidly, and one should consider administration of fluids and dantrolene intravenously. Initial fluid infusion rates of up to 10 to 20 ml/kg/hour have been recommended, slowing to 4 to 5 ml/kg/hour. Analgesics that have been used include the NSAIDs and opioids. The effect of intravenously administered lidocaine in this scenario has not been evaluated. Diazepam and glyceryl guaiacolate to reduce muscle spasm may be of value, but one should use them with caution because of possible ataxia and therefore increased problems with standing. The horse may require sedation if it is awake and anxious because of the pain. The α_2-agonists (xylazine, detomidine, romifidine) may provide good sedation and analgesia, but may exacerbate ataxia; promote sweating, hypoinsulinemia, and hyperglycemia; and increase urine output, which may further exacerbate fluid loss. The vasoconstrictive effect of these agents together with their effect on cardiac output may compromise tissue blood flow further. Their use in the more violent cases may be warranted however. Acetylpromazine in combination with opioids may provide good sedation with minimal ataxia, and the vasodilatory effect may help improve tissue flow, provided circulatory volume is maintained and hypovolemia does not occur.

Intravenously and then orally administered dantrolene sodium has been suggested to be beneficial.[47] Dantrolene at 1 mg/kg body mass orally has been used successfully to treat postoperative cases. However, recent work on the pharmacokinetics of dantrolene[46] has suggested that higher doses are likely to be needed to establish and maintain effective blood levels. An intragastric dose of 2.5 mg/kg every hour after a loading dose of 10 mg/kg has been recommended.[48] Alternatively, an intravenous loading dose of 1.9 mg/kg has been suggested to achieve a more immediate therapeutic effect.[46] Dantrolene is not licensed for use in horses, is expensive, and is potentially hepatotoxic. Transient weakness and ataxia have been associated with intravenous administration.

PREVENTION

Correct positioning to prevent restriction of venous drainage or arterial input and the use of appropriate padding are recommended. Foam padding, for example, has been reported to be inferior to air mattresses or waterbeds.[43] Positioning is important, and various recommendations have been made. For example, the practitioner should elevate the upper limb and reduce pressure on the lower triceps by pulling the leg forward in a bent position.[40] In lateral recumbency the hind legs should be kept parallel or above parallel to the table and sufficiently separated to promote venous drainage. In dorsally recumbent horses, rather than letting the hind limbs position themselves passively, one should provide support for them in slight extension by a hoist. Problems with hind limb adductor myopathies do not always develop with passive positioning. The practitioner should avoid pulling back the hind limbs. If the hind limbs must be drawn back in full extension, for example, for certain arthroscopic examinations, one should keep the surgical time to a minimum to reduce the risk of quadriceps myopathy. The flexed horizontal forward position, with the uppermost (noncompressed) forelimb parallel to the floor, fully flexed at the carpus, and pushed gently forward, is preferable when the surgeon needs access to the medial aspect of the lower carpus and distal radius.[49]

Withholding grain feed for 48 to 72 hours before general anesthesia may be beneficial. Heavily muscled, Draft-breed, and more athletically fit horses may be at an increased risk for postanesthetic myositis, in particular those with athletic-induced sports injuries. The practitioner should maintain blood pressure at more than 80 mm Hg (mean arterial blood pressure) to maintain muscle perfusion, should minimize halothane use, and may find intraoperative fluids and inotropes valuable.

Prophylactically administered dantrolene has been recommended, especially if the horse has a history of exercise-induced rhabdomyolysis or muscle problems after previous episodes of general anesthesia or in Draft breeds. Various doses have been used. In the United Kingdom, intragastric administration at 2 to 4 mg/kg has been recommended, whereas higher doses (10 mg/kg) have been used in the United States.[50] However, no objective data exist to confirm the efficacy of prophylactic dantrolene administration for prevention of postanesthetic myositis in horses.

PROGNOSIS

Prognosis depends partially on the extent of the muscle damage, the treatment instituted, and the temperament of the individual. Affected horses often recover completely, especially if the condition is localized to one muscle group. Occasionally the horse may be left with residual muscle atrophy, fibrosis, and scarring. Death can occur with massive areas of ischemic myonecrosis and intrafascicular nerve fiber degeneration postmortem. Euthanasia may be required on humane grounds in horses that remain recumbent, have severe rhabdomyolysis, or that have uncontrollable pain.

Aortic-Iliac Thrombosis

PATHOPHYSIOLOGY

Predisposing factors and causes of aortic-iliac thrombosis remain unclear but can occur in adult athletes as well as foals.[51-53] Thrombi may result from damage to the vessel intima by migrating *Strongylus vulgaris* larvae or in hypercoagulable states associated with septicemia. Hormonal, nutritional, and mechanical factors, as well as prior infection with *S. equi* subsp. *equi* or equine influenza virus, have also been proposed as predisposing factors to thrombus formation.[52,54-56] The internal iliac arteries are bound more closely to fascia than many other arteries. This, coupled with the large forces generated during movement, could increase the risk of injury to these vessels.

CLINICAL SIGNS AND LABORATORY FINDINGS

Weakness of the hind limbs at rest or after exercise, lameness, ataxia, collapse and in one case failure to ejaculate have been reported.[52] After exercise in affected animals, ischemia of the muscle usually occurs because of circulatory interference. The ischemia is usually reversible because the blood flow may be adequate when at rest or at light work. The clinical signs vary in severity according to the degree of vascular occlusion, the vessels affected, and the extent of collateral circulation. The lameness tends to become more severe as exercise continues. Mild cases may be missed, however, because the horse appears normal when pulled up after a disappointing performance. Clinical signs may include poor performance, intermittent hind limb lameness, transient lameness or weakness with exercise, a tendency to drag the toe and occasionally knuckling over, and gradual shortening of the stride leading to a transient inability to move. A peracute condition with paraplegia, shock, and death also has been recognized.

Hind limbs may be affected, although usually one more than the other. After exercise the superficial veins on the more affected limb may appear collapsed (because of delayed filling) compared with the distended vessels on the more normal limb. The superficial veins of the affected limb or limbs may take up to 90 seconds to fill after intense exercise compared with approximately 10 seconds in normal horses. The affected limb often feels cooler than expected, especially around the gaskin, and may not sweat. One may feel a reduced digital pulse. The animal may sweat profusely on the body, head, and neck and sometimes cow-kicks or shakes the affected limb (perhaps because of paraesthesias following reduced blood supply to sensory nerve endings). Full recovery tends to occur within 20 to 30 minutes. On palpation of the peripheral pulses at rest, one may detect abnormalities, including a flattened, weak, and prolonged contour to the pulse distal to the site of obstruction, whereas proximally the pulse may be normal or increased in strength. Alternatively, certain pulses may be absent.

Aortic-iliac thrombosis has been reported in males and females, although a greater incidence of clinical problems has been reported in males. One of the reasons for this difference in incidence may be a more efficient collateral circulation in females. The mean age of affected animals was 5.2 years in one study. Plasma and serum muscle enzyme activities are usually within normal limits before and after exercise. In severe cases with significant muscle damage, however, increases in CK have been reported.[52]

On postmortem examination, affected vessels tend to be enlarged, and a large thrombotic mass is usually present at the aortic quadrification (Figure 11-12) that may be attached to, and therefore possibly originate from, organized masses in the internal and external iliac arteries. These may extend to the bifurcation of the popliteal artery, but rarely do they extend far into the tibial arteries or the muscular branches of the femoral artery. Histologically, affected muscles show signs of ischemia. Damaged fibers and supporting structures tend to be remodeled with little sign of inflammation or fibrosis.[51]

DIAGNOSIS

Diagnosis of aortic-iliac thrombosis is based on clinical signs and palpation of the thrombus per rectum or ultrasonic demonstration of the thrombus. Nuclear scintigraphy may also be used.[53] Abnormalities such as decreased arterial pulse or an unusual firmness of a vessel may easily be missed during rectal examination. The obstruction may be peripheral resulting in an increase in pulse quality proximally. Ultrasonography is therefore the definitive method for diagnosis. A linear array ultrasound probe with a frequency of 5.0 or 7.5 MHz has been recommended.[56,57] Differential diagnoses include exertional rhabdomyolysis, cervical vertebral malformation, and degenerative joint disease of the sacroiliac, lumbosacral, or coxofemoral or distal limb joints.

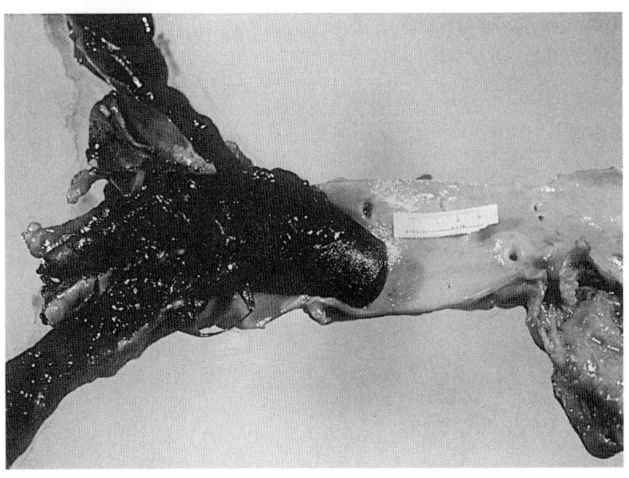

FIGURE 11-12 Aortic-iliac thrombosis.

TREATMENT

Diagnosis of aortic-iliac thrombosis rarely occurs before more than 75% of arterial flow has been compromised. As a result, therapy is difficult and often aimed at salvage rather than return to athletic function. Thrombolytics including sodium gluconate and recombinant tissue plasminogen activator have been used. Sodium gluconate at 450 mg/kg body mass by slow intravenous infusion has been recommended to treat horses with aortic-iliac thrombosis,[58] but no evidence exists that the drug has any effect on a mature thrombus.[52] Prednisolone sodium succinate (100 mg 30 minutes before administration of sodium gluconate) may help eliminate the systemic reactions frequently associated with this drug.[51,52] Aspirin (60 grains orally daily or every other day) is often recommended because of its antiplatelet actions that may prevent thrombus propagation. Heparin and low–molecular-weight dextran have been recommended for similar reasons. Other suggested protocols include monthly administration of ivermectin (Eqvalan, MSD-AGVET) and twice-daily oral doses of phenylbutazone at 2.2 mg/kg body mass for 3 months.[56] Improvement observed in some treated horses may be the result of the development of effective collateral circulation over time. Prognosis for severely affected horses is poor, and a hereditary predisposition has been suggested,[51] although little supporting evidence exists.

In humans, direct infusion of fibrinolytic agents into the body of the thrombus via an indwelling arterial catheter has been efficacious. The relative maturity and chronicity of thrombi frequently identified in affected horses suggests that mechanical clot removal may be more likely to be successful than this type of antifibrinolytic therapy. One horse was successfully treated with balloon catheter thrombectomy. The combination of surgical and medical therapy in this horse resulted in significant improvement, although a thrombus obstructing approximately 20% of the diameter of the arterial lumen remained present in the left external iliac artery when the horse was reexamined 8 weeks after surgery.[59]

NUTRITIONAL PROBLEMS ASSOCIATED WITH MUSCULOSKELETAL DISORDERS

VITAMIN E, SELENIUM, AND EXERTIONAL RHABDOMYOLYSIS

Vitamin E and selenium are powerful antioxidants that are essential for normal muscle function and deficiencies associated with neuropathy and myopathy. Historical studies examining vitamin E or selenium (or both) may be confounded by inclusion of animals with inherited myopathies. Although deficiencies in vitamin E have been described and will be summarized here, notably the optimal level of vitamin E for horses has not been determined, and toxicity has not been described, which may explain why some studies have found a benefit to supplementation while others have not.[60-69] A complex interaction likely exists between low or marginal vitamin E, selenium, electrolyte balance, and optimal muscle function (affected by glycogen concentration and fitness). Further, horses with heritable errors in muscle function may have altered basal needs for vitamin E, selenium, or electrolytes.

Disorders that have been attributed to dietary deficiencies of vitamin E and selenium include equine motor neuron disease, equine degenerative myelopathy, nutritional myodegeneration (white muscle disease), neonatal rhabdomyolysis, a predisposition to postanesthetic myopathy, and adult cases of exertional rhabdomyolysis. Severe masseter myonecrosis and tongue myopathy have also been attributed to selenium and vitamin E deficiency.[68]

Supplemental vitamin E may be beneficial in horses with underlying myopathies or healthy horses as an additional source of antioxidants in the diet. In fact, horses in heavy work do appear to need more vitamin E in their diet than many commercial feeds provide.[69] However, how chronic low vitamin E or selenium intake may affect performance in horses predisposed to rhabdomyolysis or in healthy horses is unknown. In horses with measured low levels of vitamin E or selenium, supplementation should always occur, and other causes for myopathy should be ruled in or out. In addition, it can be argued to increase vitamin E intake in horses with chronic exertional rhabdomyolysis and healthy horses performing hard work, even though the scientific work to uphold this recommendation has not been performed. Supplementation with selenium without serum measurements is not recommended because of the risk of toxicity.

ROLE OF VITAMIN E AND SELENIUM IN MUSCLE FUNCTION

GSHPx, a selenium-containing enzyme, and vitamin E help protect cells against free radicals,[70] which are formed by the reduction of molecular oxygen during normal oxidative processes. A free radical (or reactive oxygen species) is any chemical substance that has an unpaired electron in its outer orbit. The presence of this electron makes the free radical inherently unstable. Superoxide radicals, for example, in solution form hydrogen peroxide by dismutation. The superoxide radical can also react with hydrogen peroxide and hydrogen ions to produce the potent hydroxyl radical ($HO^\bullet$). The hydroxyl radicals can, in turn, react with almost any organic molecule to produce other organic radicals via chain reactions.

Free radical reactions are responsible for a significant number of key biochemical events, including mitochondrial electron transport, prostaglandin synthesis, phagocytosis, and degradation of catecholamines. Under controlled circumstances, free radicals are therefore necessary for life, but when uncontrolled, they may result in several degenerative disease processes. For example, free radicals can cause irreversible denaturation of essential cellular proteins and lipid peroxidation of exposed polyunsaturated fatty acids within the phospholipid structure of cellular membranes, resulting in structural damage and the formation of further hydroperoxides. The cellular membrane damage may, in turn, result in the release of liposomal enzymes and further damage. The free radicals can also cause damage to hyaluronic acid and collagen, resulting in enhanced prostaglandin production, and can uncouple oxidative phosphorylation and inactivate certain enzymes.

A system of natural antioxidant defenses is present within the body to counteract such free radical induced damage, including GSHPx and vitamin E. GSHPx acts to reduce the production of hydroxyl radicals by reducing hydroperoxides to alcohols as part of a cyclic system re-forming glutathione. Within red blood cells the enzyme acts as an integral part of the system, protecting against the conversion of hemoglobin to methemoglobin by hydroperoxides. Vitamin E acts as a scavenger of free radicals, and vitamin C may assist by reducing the tocopheroxyl radicals formed by this scavenging. In addition, vitamin E helps block lipid peroxidation and may also form an important part of the membrane structure because of its interaction with membrane phospholipids. Other naturally occurring antioxidant defenses include chelators that bind to and decrease the concentrations of transition metals (e.g., iron).

Vitamin E and selenium deficiencies have been implicated in muscular problems in several species, especially sheep, cattle and pigs.[34,71,72] In the horse, myopathy or white muscle disease attributed to vitamin E and selenium deficiency has been reported in foals from birth to 9 months of age.[73] In older animals, maxillary myositis, polymyositis, and dystrophic myodegeneration have also been attributed to such deficiencies.[74] In foals the syndrome apparently has been well documented in geographic areas of known selenium deficiency and inadequate vitamin E intake,[75] although many foals raised in such areas may have decreased GSHPx activities and low blood selenium concentrations without being affected.[76]

Two common sources of free radicals during exercise are increased activity of xanthine oxidase during anaerobic degradation of purine nucleotides and the partial reduction of oxygen during oxidative phosphorylation within mitochondria. The precise mechanisms leading to muscle damage and fatigue during exercise are uncertain, although free radicals or reactive oxygen species possibly play an important role. After strenuous exercise, especially under conditions of high heat and humidity, free radical production may exceed the capacity of the natural defense mechanisms of the cells, leading to muscle cell damage.[77]

Vitamin E has an apparent protective effect on experimental damage to rat skeletal muscle and may act via a non–antioxidant mechanism, with the hydrocarbon chain being an important mediator of the effects seen.[78] An apparent protective effect occurs from supranormal extracellular vitamin E concentrations on normal rat muscle, and exacerbation of exercise-induced damage to skeletal muscle by vitamin E deficiency has been reported. Nutritional modification of skeletal muscle, perhaps by reduction of the unsaturation of skeletal muscle membranes or enhancement of the antioxidant status of muscles, or a combination of both, may help prevent or reduce calcium-induced skeletal muscle damage.[79] Artificial methods to reduce oxidant damage during exercise include the administration of exogenous sources of naturally occurring antioxidant defenses (e.g., vitamin E) and limiting the formation of free radicals by minimizing the formation of inosine monophosphate from purine degradation during exercise.

Type 1 and type 2A fibers are most likely to participate in excess free radical formation because they are the most oxidative fibers and contain the most intracellular lipid stores. Selective type 1 fiber degeneration is found in nutritional myopathies of horses, sheep, and pigs that are responsive to vitamin E and selenium.[80]

Some differences in the pathologic processes exist between the equine conditions associated with vitamin E and selenium deficiencies and those in other species. Vitamin E deficiencies in calves and chicks show mitochondrial alterations early in the condition. In vitamin E–deficient and selenium-deficient lambs and chickens, early changes occur in small vessels, connective tissue, and neuromuscular elements. In the horse the changes appear to affect the myofibrils first. Morphologic changes in mitochondria and the sarcoplasmic reticulum seem to occur only in fibers with advanced lesions.[67,81]

Factors that may predispose horses to vitamin E and selenium deficiency include rancid feed, the addition of fish or plant oil to feed, prolonged storage of grain (e.g., dry grain loses tocopherol activities far more slowly than moist grain), poor-quality hay or hay stored for prolonged periods, and lush pastures.[2] Pastures associated with acid, poorly aerated soils, soils with a high sulfur content, or volcanic rock are more likely to be selenium deficient. Cases of deficiency are more likely to occur in areas with low (<0.05 ppm) plant selenium content. Dietary levels of selenium may be misleading, however, not only because other factors are likely to be involved in the pathogenesis of the condition but also because the biologic availability of the various types of selenium have not been determined. In addition, high but nontoxic levels of copper, silver, tellurium, and zinc can interfere with selenium availability and therefore induce typical lesions in animals on diets containing amounts of selenium usually considered to be adequate.

Other factors such as stress (including management and environment) and increased physical activity may be important for expression of clinical signs in the face of a deficiency or near deficiency and may explain why two similar groups of animals receiving the same dietary intake can show different clinical responses to similar dietary amounts of vitamin E or selenium or both. Acute selenium toxicity in the adult horse may also be associated with myodegeneration plus pulmonary edema, gastroenteritis, hepatic degeneration, and necrosis.[2,67]

Equine Motor Neuron Disease

Equine motor neuron disease is a disorder in horses characterized by neurologic and muscular dysfunction and muscle wasting. Initially the disorder was thought to have an inherited component or a specific geographic distribution.[82,83] Equine motor neuron disease is now accepted as being caused by chronic (6 to 24 months or more) vitamin E deficiency and has been reproduced experimentally.[84,85] Chronic vitamin E deficiency leads to chronic oxidative stress and resulting death of motor neurons and myopathy. Some horses exhibit equine motor neuron disease as a primarily neurogenic disorder, and others have pathologic conditions of the muscles and nerves. The disorder is also discussed in the chapter on neurologic diseases.

Clinically, affected horses exhibit various signs depending on the stage of the disease. Early complaints include weight loss and muscle atrophy (Figure 11-13). As the disease progresses, gait abnormalities become evident. The muscles of posture are primarily affected. The horse stands with a base-narrow stance, frequently shifts weight between legs, and may stand with the tail elevated, which progresses to tremors when the horse stands still. At the walk or trot, the gait initially appears normal despite the return of tremors when the horse stands still. Some horses stand with the head low, apparently too weak to hold it in an elevated position. The penis may be partially prolapsed. Affected horses may progress to recumbency or may stabilize without further progression. Ocular manifestations include a characteristic fundic abnormality with a mosaic pattern of dark brown to yellow brown pigment deposited in the tapetal zone and a horizontal band of pigment at the junction of the tapetum and nontapetum. This abnormal pigmentation is associated with chronic oxidative injury resulting in lipid peroxidation of the retina.[82]

Horses with equine motor neuron disease may have mild elevations in CK and AST activity. Complete blood counts are usually normal. Cerebrospinal fluid may have mild increases in protein and CK activity. Muscle biopsy may reveal neurogenic and myogenic atrophy.[86] Biopsy of the ventral branch of the accessory nerve reveals degeneration of the myelinated axon of the nerve and is present in acute and arrested cases. Muscle and nerve biopsies may yield important information. Vitamin E levels in affected horses are significantly decreased (too low to read to 100 μg/dl; normal 400 μg/dl). Often, multiple animals housed under identical conditions have similarly low vitamin E levels, but only one or a small number of horses may be demonstrating clinical signs. All horses should receive oral supplementation of vitamin E at 2000 to 5000+ IU/day. Horses eating a vitamin E–deficient diet for many months have consistently low serum vitamin E concentrations that

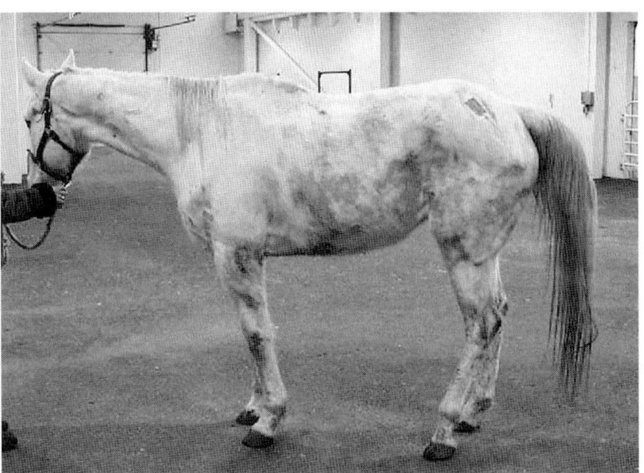

FIGURE 11-13 A horse with equine motor neuron disease. The generalized loss of muscle mass, the base-narrow stance, and raised tail head are notable.

may take weeks to months to return to the normal range even with supplementation of the grass hay diet with commercial grains. Horses displaying clinical signs at the time of diagnosis are unlikely to regain normal function. Once serum vitamin E levels are normal, aggressive vitamin E supplementation is no longer necessary. However, one should optimize daily intake to prevent future deficiency.

Low vitamin E intake is most common in horses eating hay and living without access to green pasture. Hay stored for long periods has less vitamin E than freshly cut hay. Many grain supplements have minimal quantities of vitamin E. Horses fed a grass hay diet without fresh pasture should have their vitamin E levels monitored and supplementation altered appropriately.

Nutritional Myodegeneration/White Muscle Disease

Vitamin E or selenium deficiency and the resulting muscle disorder are often described in the literature as a muscular dystrophy. The term is inappropriate considering that muscular dystrophy is defined in human medicine as a group of progressive genetically determined primary myopathies. They are usually not present at birth, and neural and vascular components are not involved initially. Regeneration of muscle cells is absent or inadequate, and replacement of muscle cells with fat and fibrous tissue occurs, which differs from the nutritionally associated disease in horses, and the term nutritional myodegeneration should be used.

CLINICAL SIGNS AND LABORATORY FINDINGS

Clinical signs and laboratory findings in horses with nutritional myodegeneration (NMD) vary depending on distribution of the muscular lesions and the extent of damage. Signs are seen most commonly in animals less than 2 months of age but may occur in any age horse. Differentials for NMD include atypical myoglobinuria, botulism, cerebellar disease, rhabdomyolysis, muscular dystrophy, spinal cord disease, meningitis, tetanus, dysphagia caused by cleft palate, HYPP, and cardiac defects leading to respiratory failure (Box 11-6). In severe cases, death may occur peracutely from a fatal arrhythmia, diaphragmatic failure, or after a few hours from exhaustion and circulatory collapse. The myocardium, diaphragm, and respiratory muscles are usually involved, leading to heart failure, dyspnea, and pulmonary edema.[87]

In less severe cases, clinical signs can include dysphagia, weakness, stiffness, and lethargy. Body temperature can vary from subnormal to supernormal. Affected horses may become recumbent and unable to rise and hind limb muscles may be sore upon palpation. Dysphagia may be the first sign noted because of involvement of the tongue and pharyngeal and sometimes masticatory muscles, and development of aspiration pneumonia may occur. Regurgitation, starvation, and ptyalism are other possible complications. If the heart is involved, tachycardia, arrhythmias, systolic murmurs, and respiratory distress are noted. Myoglobinuria has been reported in several cases. A swollen tongue and tachypnea are unusual presenting signs. A 10-month-old aborted fetus with histologic lesions typical of this condition has been reported.[76] No gender or breed predilection has been found. Recovery can occur within days or weeks of the presenting signs.[76] Signs may occur in an individual animal or several animals within a group.

BOX 11-6

DIFFERENTIAL DIAGNOSIS OF NUTRITIONALLY RELATED MYODEGENERATION

Atypical myoglobinuria
Botulism
Cerebellar diseases
Colic
Equine motor neuron disease
Equine rhabdomyolysis syndrome
Medullary diseases, such as herpesvirus type 1 and myelitis
Muscular dystrophy
Purpura hemorrhagica
Rabies
Septic polyarthritis
Spinal cord diseases
Suppurative meningitis
Tetanus
Tick paralysis
Trauma
Various causes of dysphagia (e.g., cleft palate, ulcers, and peripheral damage to certain cranial nerves)
Various causes of dyspnea (e.g., pneumonia and cardiac disease)

In the acute form, AST and CK activities are elevated. In the recovery stages the values may be increased only slightly or may be within the normal range. Increased CK and AST activities have also been found in approximately 25% of the mares of affected foals and in 20% of clinically normal foals in the same stable suggesting the existence of subclinical lesions.[88] Because selenium is incorporated into erythrocytes during erythropoiesis, the GSHPx activity of red blood cells may be a better indicator of long-term selenium status than serum selenium values. Low GSHPx, selenium, or vitamin E values have been reported in affected animals. In the author's laboratory, for example, GSHPx values of greater than 30 IU/ml of red blood cells would be expected in stabled animals fed a balanced diet. Values greater than 25 IU/ml may be expected in grazing animals with adequate intake and values less than 20 IU/ml are associated with deficient intake. Serum vitamin E concentrations of at least 400 μg/dl are considered normal. Concentrations between 200 and 400 μg/dl are considered marginal, and below 200 μg/dl suggests deficiency. Reference values vary according to the laboratory. One should take care with collection of samples, especially for vitamin E determination, because contact with rubber may interfere with analysis and heat may decrease values. Daily recommendations for vitamin E in foals are at minimum 2 to 6 IU/kg body weight and may be increased in a foal that appears to have NMD. Single-serum sample assays cannot be used as an indicator of vitamin E status in individual horses because of the high variability in values between animals and within the same animal.[89] Normal vitamin E concentrations have been reported in some affected foals, possibly reflecting recent ingestion of colostrum. Many of the dams of these foals had low serum vitamin E concentrations (<200 μg/dl), and possibly the selenium levels of affected foals were low before suckling. Mares should be supplemented with 1 mg of selenium orally per day in deficient areas.[66]

In foals with evidence of nutritional myodegeneration a full hematologic and clinical chemistry profile with a urinalysis is advisable. Laboratory analyses may reflect concurrent diseases such as failure of passive transfer, sepsis, pneumonia, or rhabdomyolysis. Electrolyte disturbances associated with rhabdomyolysis can include hyperkalemia, hyponatremia, hypocalcemia, and hypochloremia. Such findings may be associated with a poorer prognosis.

Some horses with NMD exhibit acute or chronic masseter myonecrosis or myodegeneration.[90] Acutely, horses show severely swollen and painful masseter muscles and difficulty eating or opening their mouths. Chronic cases are identified most often in young horses that exhibit rapid weight loss after weaning. On physical examination the masseter muscles are atrophied bilaterally, and it is impossible to open the mouth because of chronic fibrosis of the muscles. Serum activity of muscle enzymes is usually increased in affected horses. Whole blood selenium and glutathione peroxidase activity are usually below normal limits.

POSTMORTEM FINDINGS

Postmortem examination of neonatal foals with peracute white muscle disease reveals few macroscopic lesions. In acute cases, muscle may appear pale and streaks may be present, representing areas of coagulative necrosis next to less affected tissue. All muscle groups of the pelvic and thoracic limbs are commonly affected. The muscles of mastication, diaphragm, tongue, pharynx, and cervical musculature are commonly involved. Distribution of lesions is usually bilateral and symmetric. In subacute cases, one may observe yellow-white streaks in the heart and muscle, representing calcification.[13] Steatitis, yellow fat deposits, and fat necrosis have also been described in some but not all cases.[76] Typical histologic findings observed at various stages of NMD have been described. During the first few days, extensive floccular, granular, and severe hyaline degeneration of myofibers occurs. After approximately 1 week, phagocytosis of necrotic tissue occurs with endomysial thickening caused by edema, mononuclear infiltration, and proliferation of fibroblasts. By 2 weeks, epimyseal connective tissue has proliferated. Early regenerating fibers may coexist with signs of myodegeneration. Histologic lesions in horses with masseter myodegeneration may range from acute to subacute degeneration, with regenerative changes accompanying ongoing degeneration, to chronic degeneration with fibrotic replacement of muscle tissues. Affected horses may have lesions in skeletal and cardiac muscle as well.[90]

DIAGNOSIS AND TREATMENT

Diagnosis is made based on clinical signs, AST and CK activities, decreased blood selenium, GSHPx or vitamin E values (or both), or response to treatment. Reduction of physical activity and prompt administration of vitamin E and selenium usually are recommended. Ideally, mares are tested for vitamin E and selenium, and only supplemented as necessary to avoid toxicity. If needed, 1 mg of selenium per day or 600 to 2000 IU of vitamin E (or both) for a 500 kg horse is recommended for mares during gestation. In affected foals, selenium can be given by deep intramuscular injection at a dose of 0.06 mg/kg body weight (2 to 3 mg/45 kg of body weight).[91] The pectoral muscles are recommended to avoid making the neck sore, which would discourage the foal from nursing. Vitamin E concentration in many commercial, injectable preparations is too low to be used therapeutically. Therefore higher-concentration (300 IU/ml) preparations or oral therapy is recommended at 2 to 10 IU/kg daily. Aggressive daily oral supplementation of vitamin E coupled with a single intramuscular injection of selenium may be the best route of therapy when it is unknown whether low vitamin E or selenium is the cause of NMD in a particular case. Nasogastric feeding or feeding from a low bowl is preferable in dysphagic, anorectic, or recumbent foals. Other concurrent disorders such as pneumonia and sepsis should be treated appropriately. Prognosis for foals with NMD is guarded, especially if treatment has been delayed, signs are severe, or if complications are present. Prognosis also seems to be less favorable in animals with acid-base and electrolyte disturbances.

PREVENTION

Fresh pasture is typically associated with adequate vitamin E intake, although low vitamin E has been documented in horses on pasture in Europe.[92] Selenium status appears to be more dependent on access to pasture and geographic locale. Only limited amounts of selenium cross the placenta, which may explain why clinical cases may occur in offspring of supplemented mares.[13,93] The milk from mares that have been supplemented appears to contain more selenium than milk from unsupplemented animals, but the amount present is small because selenium is not concentrated in milk. Organic selenium supplementation appears to be more beneficial than inorganic. Therefore, although many authorities recommend, especially in deficient areas, that mares be supplemented from late gestation through lactation, others prefer to supplement the foals at birth, 2 weeks, and 6 weeks later.[76,93] This supplement action may not prevent the cases seen at birth or in the first few days of life. Other researchers recommend that, in problem areas, a selenium injection be given at birth and then every 2 to 3 months during the first 6 months of life.[2] In pigs, selenium may be teratogenic. Teratogenesis has not been observed in mares, but one recommendation is that selenium injections not be given early in a pregnancy. One must take special care with selenium administration because toxicity can occur. The single minimal lethal dose of oral sodium selenite is 3.3 mg/kg in the adult horse and results in a variety of clinical signs, including severe dyspnea, incoordination, diarrhea, recumbency, and death within a few hours. One should not expect increases in GSHPx activity in the blood until 2 to 3 weeks after selenium supplementation. GSHPx values tend to plateau before toxic levels of selenium are reached, and several months may pass before levels decrease after cessation of supplementation.

Electrolyte Depletion

Alterations in the intracellular or extracellular concentrations of electrolytes can occur in response to dietary deficiency and sweat losses or as a normal response to high-intensity exercise. The best way to assess the total-body level of electrolytes is to use fractional urinary excretions.[61,94,95] Table 11-3 lists recommendations for correcting abnormal dietary electrolytes. A table of fractional excretions for potassium, chloride, phosphorus, and calcium is provided in the chapter on Disorders of the Urinary System. For example, in endurance exercise, horses may lose significant amounts of sodium, potassium, and chloride in sweat, which may contribute to fatigue,

TABLE 11-3

Examples of Supplementation Given to 400- to 500-kg Horses Based on Fractional Electrolyte Excretion Test Results

FE Values	Supplementation
Low Na^+	2 oz (56 g)/day NaCl
Low Na^+ and K^+	2 oz (56 g) NaCl plus 10 oz (28 g) KCl/day for 2 weeks, then 2 oz (56 g) NaCl/day
High PO_4	Decrease bran intake if horse is fed, plus 2 oz (56 g) $CaCO_3$/day or alternative source(s) of calcium
High Na^+	Lower Na^+ intake (e.g., change source of hay if grown near the coast)

Data from Harris P, Colles C: The use of creatine clearance ratios in the prevention of equine rhabdomyolysis: a report of four cases, *Equine Vet J* 20:459, 1988.

FE, Fractional electrolyte; *CaCO3*, Calcium carbonate; *K+*, potassium; *KCl*, potassium chloride; *Na+*, sodium; *NaCl*, sodium chloride; *PO4*, phosphate.

Normal values: FE_{Na+} = 0.04-0.8; FE_{K+} = 35-80; FE_{PO4} = 0-0.2

exertional rhabdomyolysis, and synchronous diaphragmatic flutter. During anaerobic exercise, cellular acidosis occurs because of incomplete oxidation of pyruvate and the resulting accumulation of lactate. Volume depletion and poor circulation to muscle exacerbate acidosis. Systemic acidosis increases the serum fraction of ionized calcium and induces extrusion of potassium from muscle cells,[96] which may lead to changes in the action potential across the sarcolemma.

Aside from its role intracellularly in calcium-magnesium ATPase, extracellular magnesium influences muscle cell function. Extracellular magnesium concentration is inversely proportional to acetylcholine concentration at the neuromuscular junction; therefore small changes in the serum concentration of magnesium reflect proportionately large shifts in whole-body magnesium levels. Low blood levels of magnesium lead to increased membrane irritability and dysfunction of many enzymes necessary for protein, carbohydrate, and lipid metabolism. The most dramatic example of hypomagnesemia is grass tetany, which occurs in cattle grazing magnesium-deficient pasture.[97] Whole-body calcium balance is also important in muscular function, and hypocalcemia can be life threatening in most species. In horses, hypocalcemic tetany may be associated with blister beetle toxicosis, heavy lactation, intestinal disorders, endurance exercise, and malnutrition.[96]

Sodium, chloride, potassium, calcium, and magnesium play key roles in muscle fiber contractility and irritability. Therefore small imbalances may lead to muscle dysfunction and possibly exertional rhabdomyolysis. Diagnosis of whole-body electrolyte deficits can be difficult to confirm because of the rigorous homeostatic mechanisms in place that serve to maintain serum concentrations. Therefore a lack of correlation exists between intracellular ion concentrations and serum ion concentrations. In addition, electrolyte balance may shift in the body as a direct response to disease processes. For example, a whole-body deficit of potassium may exist, but plasma potassium may be normal because of efflux of potassium from damaged or acidotic muscle.[98]

Kinslow, Harris, Gray, et al.[99] performed one study examining the role of total body electrolyte balance and its effect on exertional rhabdomyolysis in 1995. The authors followed four mature Thoroughbred mares through their estrous cycles. Group mean percentage fractional excretion of electrolytes in urine showed cyclical trends that appeared to fluctuate in relation to the stage of the estrous cycle. They saw large increases in the urinary excretion of sodium, calcium, and magnesium in samples collected during the period from 2 days before to 4 days after estrus. The authors found significant correlations in individual animals between low progesterone concentrations and 24-hour fractional excretions of sodium, potassium, chloride, calcium, and phosphorus and between serum estradiol 17β and calcium, magnesium, and chloride. These results suggest that ovarian steroid hormones may exert an influence on urinary excretion of electrolytes in mares. Therefore estrous cycle–induced losses of sodium, calcium, and magnesium in mares consuming a diet marginal or deficient in electrolytes could predispose them to exertional rhabdomyolysis.

To examine the effect of total-body potassium on exertional rhabdomyolysis, Bain and Merritt[100] measured potassium concentrations within red blood cells and plasma in Thoroughbred horses with and without exertional rhabdomyolysis. The authors found that in fillies with exertional rhabdomyolysis, potassium concentration within red blood cells was lower than that of controls within 48 hours after an episode of exertional rhabdomyolysis. Whether decreased red blood cell potassium is an inciting cause of exertional rhabdomyolysis or results from exertional rhabdomyolysis is unknown. Beech and Lindborg[101] did not repeat these findings; they found no difference in red blood cell potassium concentration in horses with and without exertional rhabdomyolysis. However, the authors did find a significantly lower concentration of muscle potassium on a dry weight basis in horses with exertional rhabdomyolysis. Unfortunately, lower concentrations of muscle potassium did not correlate with the histologic appearance of the muscle. The authors concluded that low red blood cell potassium concentration may not be a valid indicator of reduced muscle potassium, and they did not associate potassium concentration with a predisposition for exertional rhabdomyolysis.

A study using potassium-depleted horses further clouds the role of potassium in exertional rhabdomyolysis.[102] In this study the authors depleted healthy horses of potassium by withdrawing feed and by administering sodium bicarbonate and furosemide. The result was decreased plasma potassium (2.9 ± 0.3 mEq/L, treatment group; 3.3 ± 0.5 mEq/L, control), chloride, calcium, and magnesium compared with control horses. Red blood cell potassium concentration remained unchanged. A significant increase in CK activity occurred in the potassium-depleted horses compared with controls 240 minutes after exercise (296 ± 211 U/L, potassium depleted; 86 ± 20 U/L, control). After exercise, three of the six horses developed diaphragmatic flutter, and two horses had CK activity beyond the normal range (685 U/L and 1374 U/L), and one horse was reported to walk with a stilted gait after exercise. The authors postulated that potassium depletion may play a role in exercise-induced muscle damage but could not conclude that it was the sole cause of increased serum CK activity. Unfortunately a similar study has not been performed in horses with underlying myopathies such as RER or PSSM to determine if potassium depletion influences rhabdomyolysis in a susceptible population.

Harris and Snow[64] also investigated the role of electrolyte imbalance in the pathophysiologic features of exertional rhabdomyolysis in 1991. The authors found that 100 of 144 Thoroughbred horses with exertional rhabdomyolysis had fractional excretions of electrolytes outside the normal range. Of those horses with abnormal fractional excretions, 72 of 100 responded favorably to additional electrolytes in their diet. However, the normal ranges for fractional excretions used in this study were narrower than other published normal ranges, and other investigators have not duplicated the authors' results.[97] The intermittent nature of exertional rhabdomyolysis in racehorses also makes the verification of a real response to therapy difficult to confirm.

One must consider the relative concentration of electrolytes in the diet when examining their influence on exertional rhabdomyolysis. Poorly balanced electrolyte supplements may exacerbate dietary deficiencies of other ions. For example, high concentrations of serum potassium may aggravate the effects of low serum calcium, resulting in muscular hyperactivity.[103] Such increased levels of serum potassium are found during normal exercise. In 1998, Harris and Colles[104] described a case study that may support this theory. In this study, low dietary calcium and increased phosphate excretion were found in two of four horses experiencing exertional rhabdomyolysis. Urinary clearance ratios were low for potassium in one case and low for sodium in another. All horses were reported to improve with dietary changes, according to the investigators.

Electrolyte balance within the body and interactions between the major electrolytes play important roles in normal muscular function. In healthy horses, imbalances and deficiencies may occasionally cause muscular dysfunction. The fractional electrolyte test is the best test available to assess electrolyte state but must be applied and interpreted with care,[105] and the different feeding practices among countries may mean that electrolyte supplementation based on the fractional electrolyte test may have more or less relevance. In horses predisposed to exertional rhabdomyolysis, identical imbalances or deficiencies may lead to more severe rhabdomyolysis because of preexisting abnormalities in muscular function.

Muscle Wasting with Malignant Disease/Cachectic Atrophy

Because of a combination of cachexia, malnutrition, disuse, infection, and old age, muscle weakness and occasionally muscle necrosis may develop with malignancies involving other body systems.

Overexertion

Overexertion may be defined as physical exertion to a state of abnormal exhaustion. Many horses willingly work to a point at which they are too exhausted to go on. If a horse is worked to a point of exhaustion, especially in an environment of heat and high humidity, multiple organ failure may result. Rhabdomyolysis is a frequent component of overexertion. Rhabdomyolysis may be precipitated from glycogen depletion and electrolyte depletion. Because horse sweat is hypertonic, profound and prolonged exercise leads to significant electrolyte depletion. Lactic acidosis induced by dehydration and anaerobic glycolysis further complicates electrolyte depletion. Laboratory tests typically reveal muscle enzymes 10 to 1000 times greater than normal; depletion of sodium, potassium, and chloride; dehydration; and azotemia. Muscle biopsy demonstrates acute rhabdomyolysis without evidence of previous rhabdomyolysis. Horses require emergency resuscitative therapy, including intravenous fluids and restoration of electrolytes. Horses in anuric or oliguric renal failure may respond favorably to furosemide or dopamine therapy.

The exhausted horse syndrome tends to occur when horses have been pushed past their performance limits. The syndrome is believed to have a complex cause involving a combination of fluid and electrolyte losses, depletion of energy stores, and extremes of environmental conditions. The syndrome therefore usually occurs in association with Three-Day Events, endurance contests, and long-distance rides.[3,106] A brief summary of some of the possible contributing factors follows. More detailed information is available.[60,96,107,108] The amount of sweat produced by an exercising horse depends on the environmental conditions, the nature of the work, and the fitness of the animal. Under favorable climatic conditions, sweat loss can be on the order of 5 to 8 L/hr on long-distance rides. In hot, humid conditions, where sweating is partially ineffective, sweat production can be as high as 10 to 15 L/hr. An endurance horse can lose at least 25 to 30 L or more if conditions are unfavorable, which far exceeds the 1 to 5 L lost by a racehorse performing a sprint at top speed. Early on in exercise and when the sweat losses are low, much of the water loss can be made up by absorption of water from the large intestine. However, if water losses via sweat are between 5% and 10% of body weight a decrease in circulatory volume occurs. The decrease tends to occur after approximately 3 hours of exercise with moderate sweating but occurs much sooner during exercise in high heat and humidity.

Sweat contains low concentrations of calcium and phosphate but is hypertonic to plasma with respect to sodium, potassium, and chloride. During exercise, the horse appears to be able to maintain, initially at least, its plasma electrolyte concentrations at the expense of other body compartments. This is especially true for sodium, for which the contents of the gastrointestinal tract are believed to provide an important reservoir. Decreases in plasma sodium of up to 6 mmol/L occur during endurance rides in hot weather. The decreases are likely to result from significant sodium and water losses followed by partial replacement of the water deficit by drinking. Sodium concentrations may in fact increase in those animals that are not allowed to drink or that refuse to drink.

Potassium losses in sweat are also significant during prolonged exercise. Potassium is lost in sweat and is exchanged for sodium and lost into the gastrointestinal tract. During heavy exercise and sweating, muscle tissue is the major source of potassium replacement. Hypochloremia is observed commonly after endurance rides, reflecting chloride losses in sweat. Chloride is the major anion absorbed in the kidney, and in its absence, bicarbonate is resorbed.

The most consistent acid-base alteration associated with endurance in hot environments is metabolic alkalosis, probably related to hypochloremia and hypokalemia caused by heavy sweating, and therefore may not be seen in cooler conditions. Hypocalcemia has sometimes been observed in endurance horses and might result from calcium losses in sweat or from disturbances of calcium homeostasis. These disturbances have been suggested to include energy deficiency, alkalosis, or competition with sodium and potassium exchange in the skeleton.

Even with frequent access to water, many endurance horses may develop clinical signs of slight to moderate dehydration during the course of a ride, as well as signs caused by some disturbance in electrolyte status. The combination of dehydration and sodium depletion results in a decreased plasma volume as determined by raised packed cell volume, total protein, and blood viscosity and may, in turn, result in inadequate tissue perfusion and inefficient oxygen and substrate transport, which can result in impaired renal function. Alterations in acid-base balance plus calcium, magnesium, and potassium depletion may contribute to the development of gastrointestinal tract stasis or ileus, as well as muscle cramps, synchronous diaphragmatic flutter, and rhabdomyolysis. If severe losses of water and electrolytes occur, then sweat production may decrease, resulting in even less effective thermoregulation.

Severe cases of dehydration coupled with electrolyte depletion may result in decreased renal perfusion and oliguria or anuria. Rhabdomyolysis may result from a combination of electrolyte depletion, poor perfusion, and resulting membrane instability. Myoglobinemia in human beings with decreased renal perfusion leads to kidney failure. Myoglobinemia leading to renal failure is less common in the horse, possibly because metabolic alkalosis occurs more commonly than metabolic acidosis in heavily exercised horses. If volume depletion is severe enough, metabolic acidosis may occur in the horse because of anaerobic glycosis and may contribute to kidney failure in some cases.

BOX 11-7

CLINICAL SIGNS AND LABORATORY FINDINGS IN THE EXHAUSTED HORSE

Clinical signs (not all are present in all cases):
Depression
Dehydration, anorexia, decreased thirst
Elevated respiratory rate
Elevated heart rate
Hypo or hyperthermia
Decreased pulse pressure
Decreased intestinal sounds
Laminitis
Muscle cramping
Poor sweating response
Poor jugular distention, increased capillary refill
Recumbency
Refusal to move
Synchronous diaphragmatic flutter
Laboratory findings:
Metabolic alkalosis
Paradoxical aciduria
Hypokalemia, hyponatremia, hypochloremia
Increased CK, AST, LDH activities
Proteinuria
Azotemia
Lipidosis
Signs of hepatic failure

AST, Aspartate aminotransferase; *CK,* creatine kinase; LDH, lactate dehydrogenase.

CLINICAL SIGNS AND LABORATORY FINDINGS

Box 11-7 shows some of the signs seen in exhausted horses and the associated laboratory findings. Signs may last for several days. Various guidelines have been given in the literature to help distinguish the exhausted horse from the nonexhausted, tired horse. The heart and respiratory rates may be similar in both cases at the end of an endurance ride, but in the nonexhausted horse the rates tend to return to normal far quicker, for example, to a heart rate of less than 60 to 70 beats per minute with a respiratory rate of less than 40 per minute within 25 to 30 minutes, unless the ambient temperature is high. In the exhausted horse the heart rate tends to remain greater than the respiratory rate, for example, greater than 70 beats per minute 30 minutes after exercise, with a persistently elevated rectal temperature.[2,3,96]

TREATMENT

Horses that appear depressed with persistently elevated heart and respiratory rates may respond to rest, cooling out, and access to salt, feed, and water. If no improvement is seen within 30 minutes the horse often needs fluid therapy. In the more severe case of a horse that refuses to eat or drink the horse needs prompt and vigorous fluid therapy. Fluids restore circulating blood volume, correct electrolyte deficits, and provide a source of readily metabolizable energy. Fluids may be administered orally or intravenously. The practitioner can give 5 to 8 L orally every 30 minutes to 1 hour, if required, but this should be stopped if any discomfort or gastric reflux becomes apparent. Oral hypertonic solutions should be avoided. In severely affected animals, up to 10 to 20 L/hr of fluids can be given intravenously; in addition, inserting a stomach tube may be necessary. One can use saline or lactated Ringer's solution with potassium chloride added to provide approximately 10 mEq/L. After the horse starts eating hay, potassium supplementation may be discontinued. The practitioner can administer glucose as 5% dextrose in saline or add 50% dextrose to Ringer's solution to deliver between 50 and 100 g/hr (concurrent insulin administration has been recommended). Slow administration of calcium also may be of value. Sodium bicarbonate administration is not indicated, because acidosis, if present, resolves with fluid volume expansion and is contraindicated if the horse is in a state of metabolic alkalosis. The horse may require other therapeutic agents to control pain and anxiety, although one should use the NSAIDs and phenothiazine derivatives with extreme caution in the face of dehydration (low blood pressure) and possible renal dysfunction. Avoiding corticosteroid administration has been recommended unless absolutely necessary.

The practitioner can use cold water body sprays and alcohol baths, particularly over the head and neck region, to cool the patient. A common myth is that ice water bathing may lead to muscle cramping. However, whole-body ice water bathing and cold water spray fans have been used successfully in major international events under hot and humid conditions without adverse effects. In recumbent, hyperthermic patients, one should give cold water enemas delivered via a handheld gravity-feed rectal tube. Further information concerning exercise physiology under environmental conditions of high heat and humidity is available.[60,96,106-108]

PREVENTION

Many endurance competitors train their endurance horses to drink electrolyte-rich water, which may help to restore electrolyte concentrations in addition to water during a race. However, plain water should always be available as an alternative. The proper amount of water intake during competition is unknown because the maximal absorption of water from the gastrointestinal tract is unknown, considering that exercise draws circulation away from the intestine. The amount of water contained in the intestinal tract depends on the amount of fiber contained therein. Research is ongoing to determine the optimal combination and time of feeding of grains, forage, electrolyte supplements, and water before and during long-distance competition. These findings also vary depending on the type of competition (endurance versus Three-Day Event) and length of course (10, 50, or 100 miles).

Various suggestions have been made as to the optimal nature of any electrolyte supplement. Supplements containing from one to four times more sodium than potassium have been recommended. Sodium bicarbonate has often been suggested as part of an electrolyte mix, but because most endurance horses tend to become alkalotic, this suggestion may in fact be counterproductive and is not recommended. Additional sodium and potassium chloride supplementation for a few days after competition may also be helpful in replenishing body stores but is often unnecessary if the basic diet is acceptable.[60,96,108]

Many workers have reported beneficial effects from oral or parenteral administration of vitamin E and selenium.[62,109] The beneficial effects of these compounds have been noted as being difficult to assess because they are often given in addition to changes in diet and exercise.[96] Benefit would presumably be the result of limiting or preventing free radical–induced muscle damage. Oral administration is preferable to intermittent injection.

TOXICOSES

Only a few available and palatable toxic compounds cause muscle fiber degeneration in the horse. White snakeroot *(Eupatorium rugosum)* and coffeeweed *(Cassia occidentalis)* are the most common plants that may cause rhabdomyolysis. Ionophore contamination of feed may also lead to life-threatening rhabdomyolysis. For additional information, see Chapter 22, Toxicologic Problems.

WHITE SNAKEROOT

White snakeroot is a common plant in the central midwestern and northeastern United States. White snakeroot is a shade-loving plant growing well in damp, wooded areas, shaded river banks, and in steep canyons.[110] The toxic principle is tremetol, a fat-soluble high–molecular-weight alcohol, and plants may be toxic in fresh and dried forms. Clinical signs of white snakeroot ingestion include progressive muscle tremors, weakness, choke, constipation, recumbency, arrhythmias, and death. Serum muscle enzyme activities increase significantly. At postmortem, one observes skeletal muscle necrosis and subepicardial and myocardial hemorrhages with grayish streaks in the myocardium.[111]

CASSIA OCCIDENTALIS

Cassia occidentalis (coffeeweed, senna) is toxic to horses and may cause ataxia, incoordination, recumbency, and death with liver and muscle damage. However, natural ingestion of this plant is uncommon.[112]

MISCELLANEOUS TOXICOSES

Selenium, iron, thallium, and perhaps sulfur and cobalt may cause muscle disease when fed at toxic levels. Metals such as iron may act by affecting vitamin E and selenium status or lipid peroxidation.[14] If ingested, bracken *(Pteridium aquilinum),* horsetail *(Equisetum arvense),* and rock fern *(Cheilanthes sieberi)* may induce thiamine deficiency with signs of anorexia, gait disturbances, staggering, lack of coordination, lethargy, a weak and irregular pulse, and muscular tremors.[113]

IONOPHORE TOXICITY

PATHOPHYSIOLOGY

Monensin, rumensin, lasalocid, and salinomycin are ionophores commonly fed as coccidiostats in food animals. Monensin is a carboxylic ionophorous antibiotic fermentation product derived from *Streptomyces cinnamonensis* and is used as a coccidiostat for poultry and as a feed additive for cattle because it increases feed utilization by altering rumen fermentation. Access to ruminant feed or accidental contamination of horse feed in a mill producing poultry, cattle, and horse feed are the most common causes for intoxication. Much is known about monensin toxicosis, and as such it will be used as the model for this discussion.

The lipid-soluble monensin-sodium complex releases sodium in exchange for a proton after it crosses the cell membrane. The protonated monensin leaves the cell to pick up more sodium, and the cycle repeats. The increase in intracellular sodium concentration stimulates the sodium-potassium ATPase pump and indirectly results in an increase in calcium. This increase in intracellular calcium may then result in the release of certain factors such as catecholamines, which, in turn, may be responsible for some of the clinical signs seen, especially in relation to the heart. When mitochondria become saturated with calcium, the process of oxidative phosphorylation is disturbed and supplies of ATP decrease. Swelling and disruption of mitochondria follows, resulting in release of stored calcium, which may potentiate or precipitate catecholamine-induced cardiac arrhythmias. Increased intracellular calcium concentrations may also result in a brief period of extreme contraction of muscle (because of effects on actin-myosin binding), as well as release of various cellular lytic enzymes. The rapid onset of cardiac or skeletal muscle necrosis may result from energy deficiency resulting from these lytic processes. Small concentrations of monensin also may result in an increase in intracellular potassium concentration; large concentrations of monensin tend to decrease intracellular potassium concentration. Other tissues less dependent on ATP may not show such severe signs.[34,114,115] In muscle, swelling and disintegration of mitochondria are the first visible lesions, although monensin does not cause mitochondrial structural defects in cultured muscle cells.[116] Further work is needed to determine if other substances or metabolites of monensin are involved in pathophysiologic features of toxicity in vivo.[114]

CLINICAL SIGNS

Horses are sensitive to monensin. Signs of toxicity may be apparent after ingestion of 2 to 3 mg/kg body mass of crystalline monensin (compared with 20 to 34 mg/kg for cattle). (The median lethal dose for mycelial monensin is estimated to be 1.38 ± 0.19 mg/kg body mass.) The increased susceptibility of horses to monensin toxicity may be because horses do not clear monensin from the bloodstream as rapidly as cattle. In addition, equine heart muscle is sensitive to the effects of catecholamines.[114] After ingestion of a single toxic dose, signs of lethargy, muscular weakness, and stiffness, often with recumbency, occur within 24 hours. In the early stages, progressive hypokalemia resulting in cardiac conduction disturbances occurs.[115] Cardiovascular signs may include tachycardia with possible arrhythmias, prominent jugular pulse, congested or pale mucous membranes, cold extremities, weak pulse, and profuse sweating. Tachypnea, hyperpnea, or dyspnea may be apparent. Early on, affected animals may show signs of colic, including sweating, increased heart rate, and increased or absent borborygmus. Amounts of feces may be reduced, or no feces may be passed. Animals may be anorectic. Myoglobinuria and muscle tremor also may be apparent, together with progressive ataxia and signs of central nervous system malfunction. Depending on the dose ingested (and the individual), death may occur within 24 hours. Hind limb muscles tend to be involved most severely.[14,34,114] Progressive cardiac insufficiency, weight loss, and sometimes renal failure are more common with chronic toxicity in the weeks after a single, lower dose exposure. In such cases, clinical signs related to skeletal muscle involvement may disappear, although poor performance and muscular weakness may be apparent if the horse is asked to perform. Signs of chronic toxicity may not be noticed for weeks after ingestion of the compound has stopped.[117] Monensin-containing feeds are often unpalatable, and owners may recollect a "bad" bag or shipment of feed that some horses refused to eat in the recent past.

LABORATORY FINDINGS

In peracute cases, in which the horse dies within 24 hours, a progressive hemoconcentration associated with increased urine output and decreased urine specific gravity, together with increased blood urea nitrogen and creatinine concentrations is typically observed.[115]

Serum CK and AST activities may be elevated moderately to significantly, primarily because of skeletal muscle damage. The increase in total LDH activity appears (at least initially) to be caused by LDH_1 and LDH_2 isoenzymes and may be related to increased erythrocyte fragility and hemolysis. Increases in alkaline phosphatase activity have also been observed, apparently from an increase in the bone isoenzyme.[115] Hemoglobinuria, myoglobinuria, or both may occur.

Sodium concentrations do not change greatly. Serum calcium concentration tends to decrease initially, within the first 12 to 24 hours, by approximately 10% to 15% and then recovers. Hypokalemia tends to occur in the first 24 hours with a decrease of 1 to 2 mmol/L followed by a return to normal by 36 hours. In chronic toxicity, clinical findings are often nonspecific and reflect the various organs involved. In one study of 32 horses with a history of unthriftiness and poor performance after prior ingestion of monensin-contaminated feed the authors observed decreased serum bilirubin concentration and increased alkaline phosphatase activity. In four horses, they also observed increased LDH_5 activity.[117]

In horses that die peracutely, one may not observe gross lesions and may rely on feed analysis for diagnosis. In less acute cases the gross changes are not pathognomonic for monensin toxicosis and can include edema, hydropericardium, hydrothorax, ascites, hemorrhages, and pale areas in the heart or diaphragm.[114,116,117]

DIAGNOSIS

Differentiating this condition histologically from vitamin E and selenium deficiency, atypical myoglobinuria (pasture myopathy), or exertional rhabdomyolysis may be difficult.[14] However, history of feed problems, signs in multiple horses, and evidence of heart failure in chronic cases aid in the diagnosis. The finding of high monensin concentrations in feed and stomach contents may confirm the diagnosis. The ingestion of blister beetles (*Epicauta* spp.) can cause cardiomyopathy, and one should exclude this from the differential diagnosis along with white snakeroot toxicosis.

TREATMENT AND PROGNOSIS

In acute monensin toxicosis, intensive isotonic polyionic fluid therapy with additional potassium has been recommended for treatment. Although this therapy may support the horse during the initial crisis, the prognosis is guarded because longer-term actions of monensin, particularly on the heart, still may cause death.[115,117] Activated charcoal or mineral oil administered orally may help to decrease further monensin absorption. The practitioner should avoid purgatives that act by stimulating the vagal system because of the risk of causing arrhythmias in an already damaged heart. Similarly, intravenously administered calcium may not be advisable. One should avoid cardiac glycosides because they may work synergistically with monensin, resulting in extensive cardiac muscle damage. Horses that have clinical signs of heart failure after previous exposure have a poor prognosis for long-term survival.

Muscle Tumors

Primary tumors of skeletal muscle are rare, malignant tumors being twice as frequent as benign ones. Rhabdomyosarcomata of the limbs, head, or neck appear as hard, spherical masses deep in the muscle. A significant proportion appears to occur in sites of earlier muscle fiber destruction and repair. Frequently, animals younger than 2 years are affected. Other benign and malignant primary tumors, including lipomata, liposarcomata, fibromata, fibrosarcomata, myxomata, and hemangiosarcomata, can occur in muscles. Metastatic spread to the muscles, especially of malignant melanomas, angiosarcomata, and tumors of the lymphoreticular system, also may occur.[14]

Atypical Myoglobinuria

Sudden death from exertional rhabdomyolysis is rare and usually occurs in an animal that has undergone some degree of exertion before the attack. Severe and often fatal attacks of a condition with similarities to exertional rhabdomyolysis have been reported in the United Kingdom and elsewhere in Europe in groups of animals out at pasture with no history of sudden exertion.[118-120] The condition has been called *atypical myoglobinuria* or *pasture myopathy*. A similar syndrome has been reported in the United States.[121] Clinical signs are consistent with rhabdomyolysis, and prolonged recumbency may be seen with weakness and tremors. Muscle enzymes are significantly elevated. Some horses may have signs consistent with cardiomyopathy as well.

PATHOPHYSIOLOGY

Factors common to many atypical myoglobinuria cases include adverse climatic conditions before the outbreak and the availability of tree bark, often on dead wood. This atypical syndrome characteristically affects a group of horses over a short period, and therefore the possible predisposing trigger or etiologic factor is thought to be environmental or toxic. No consistent abnormality in selenium or GSHPx values has been seen. Low vitamin E concentrations are inconsistently seen and have not been implicated.[119-121] In some but not all cases, *Trichoderma* spp. fungi were isolated from grass and wood taken from the fields grazed by the affected horses. Mycotoxins have therefore been suggested as being of possible significance.

No access to toxins such as monensin or salinomycin was demonstrated in any case. Oak trees with acorns were not always present, and gastrointestinal signs associated with acorn poisoning were not observed.[122] Spraying with an atrazine herbicide occurred before one outbreak.[123] Simazine residues were not thought to be at toxic levels and clinical signs were not those seen with triazene herbicide toxicity (i.e., severe colic, cessation of eating and drinking, and a dog-sitting posture).[120]

The cause of atypical myoglobinuria therefore has not been identified. In some cases the death may be inappropriately attributed to white snakeroot toxicity. In a case series in which white snakeroot was thought probable, retrospective analysis failed to identify tremetone.[121] In horses that died the precise cause of death was uncertain, but damage to the heart and diaphragm in association with biochemical alterations such as hypocalcemia may have been important. Renal failure may be a contributory cause but is unlikely to be the primary cause of death.

CLINICAL SIGNS

Atypical myoglobinuria occurs most frequently in horses and ponies grazing pasture of low quality. One or more animals in a group may be affected. A sudden onset of stiffness unrelated to exertion occurs, soon followed by severe myoglobinuria. Temperature, heart rate, and respiratory rate are generally within the normal range. No age, sex, or breed predilection has been observed, but few cases have been investigated. Of cases that have been well documented, progression of clinical signs is rapid and mortality is high. Serum CK activities are greatly increased, and advanced myodegeneration of all muscles, including the heart, may be present.[119-121]

Myodegeneration affecting mostly type 1 fibers with Zenker degeneration and necrosis has been described.[118] Large hyperchromatic hepatocyte nuclei were observed in some liver sections together with patchy vacuolation and infiltration of neutrophils into the portal areas. Pink proteinaceous granular material tended to be present in the kidney tubules and within Bowman's capsule.[120] Skeletal abnormalities may not be obvious on gross postmortem examination.

High CK activity (as much as 900,000 U/l) caused by myodegeneration is observable. AST activity also tends to be increased greatly. High sorbitol dehydrogenase values (up to 28.8 IU/dl; laboratory reference range, 4 to 15 IU/dl) were found in several cases in one investigation. Hypocalcemia may occur, especially in the terminal stages. Myoglobin is usually present in a sufficiently high concentration in the urine to be detectable by electrophoresis on cellulose acetate.

TREATMENT

Because the cause of the condition is unknown, symptomatic treatment is recommended, including intensive fluid therapy, which should be based on biochemical monitoring. The calcium status in particular should be monitored because horses may become hypocalcemic. Feeding a readily available source of calcium may be of benefit in some cases. In one study, horses were treated with supportive care and antioxidants, including polyionic fluids, vitamin E and selenium, vitamin C, dimethyl sulfoxide (DMSO), and flunixin meglumine.[121]

Postanesthetic Myasthenia

Postanesthetic myasthenia has been reported in three horses.[8] The condition could be a form of botulism or a drug-induced myasthenia. The characteristic signs were a difficult recovery from anesthesia, lack of any facial expression, flaccid tongue, mydriasis, an inability to raise the head, and dysphagia. All three patients recovered totally with supportive care.

PATHOPHYSIOLOGY AND TREATMENT OF ACUTE LAMINITIS

Ashley M. Stokes, Susan C. Eades, Rustin M. Moore

Acute laminitis (founder) is a severely debilitating, excruciatingly painful, and potentially career-ending and life-threatening disease of the soft tissues (sensitive and insensitive laminae) of the equine digit, affecting adult horses and ponies of any breed or use. Laminitis is frustrating for veterinarians because current knowledge and understanding of the pathophysiologic nature of the disease is incomplete, limiting efforts at prevention and treatment. Laminitis causes profound emotional stress and economic loss to horse owners and trainers because of the agonizing pain experienced by affected horses. Laminitis often leads to poor body condition and prolonged periods of recumbency with secondary pressure sores. Many affected horses rise only for short periods and demonstrate a characteristic stance of rocking or shifting their weight onto their rear feet, which is accompanied by anxiety, muscle fasciculations, and sweating.

PREDISPOSING CONDITIONS

Fifteen percent of horses in the United States are estimated to be afflicted with laminitis over the course of their lifetime. From an economic perspective the diagnosis and treatment of laminitis costs horse owners millions of dollars annually. Numerous primary diseases are known to be associated with the development of laminitis, such as colic, diarrhea, pneumonia, metritis, endocrine and metabolic disorders, and musculoskeletal injuries resulting in altered loading of a supporting limb.[1-3] A recent study examined records for horses that developed laminitis during hospitalization for illness or injury and found that endotoxemia was the condition with the greatest significant correlation to laminitis development. The diseases found most associated with endotoxemia in this study were acute diarrhea, surgically managed colic, interstitial pneumonia and bronchopneumonia, and retained placenta and metritis in postpartum mares.[2] Another study found that gastrointestinal disease occurred in 53% of horses that developed laminitis.[4] Of horses admitted for duodenitis or proximal jejunitis, the prevalence of laminitis was 28%, and a study of horses with acute diarrhea admitted to a referral hospital over a 7-year period found that 11.5% of those cases developed laminitis.[5,6]

A considerable amount of recent focus in laminitis research is in regard to the link between metabolic and endocrine abnormalities of horses and laminitis pathogenesis. Feeding of starch-rich (a diet with a high glycemic index) and fat-supplemented rations, combined with relative inactivity, can lead to metabolic syndrome and obesity in adult horses.[1] A review of equine insulin resistance found a significant relationship between this condition and laminitis.[7] In support of these concepts a recent study found that a definite interrelationship exists among obesity, inflammatory cytokines, and insulin sensitivity in the horse,[8] and other researchers have linked these metabolic abnormalities with laminitis.[9] Another study confirmed the prevalence and clinical features of horses with laminitis and the relationship with the endocrine disease pituitary pars intermedia dysfunction.[10] All of these studies point to the importance of the predisposition of laminitis development or progression in association with metabolic and endocrine abnormalities. More information is needed to understand fully the effects of these metabolic and endocrine conditions on laminitis in this particular group of horses.

Scientific investigations have identified some important pathophysiologic events involved with laminitis and have determined some pathways common to all initiating diseases. However, additional studies are needed to unravel the remaining mysteries regarding the initiation and propagation of laminitis. Currently, numerous and varied therapies are used to prevent and treat laminitis; however, clinicians' preferences and impressions regarding the most effective treatments are based on an incomplete understanding of the initiating events in this disease. Because of the gaps in knowledge of the pathophysiologic features of laminitis, the effectiveness of the currently used treatments is inconsistent at best. Therefore developing a more thorough understanding of the cascade of events involved with the onset and propagation of acute laminitis should help veterinarians develop more effective and cost-efficient therapies to prevent and treat a disease with profound humane, emotional, and economic effects on horses, horse owners, trainers, and veterinarians. This section provides a comprehensive review of the current knowledge of the pathophysiologic features of acute laminitis and presents experimental findings that should contribute to a better understanding of this pathogenic cascade and may ultimately help improve the prevention and treatment of laminitis in horses.

ANATOMY AND PHYSIOLOGY OF THE DIGIT

The normal laminar tissue and its vasculature are unique in numerous aspects. The ability of the horse to walk depends on the integrity of the interdigitating primary and secondary laminae, which structurally unite the hoof wall, distal phalanx, and the sole of the foot into a single unit.[11] The bulk of the hoof is composed of the stratum medium, which is composed of avascular, highly keratinized stratified squamous epithelium. This layer blends with the stratum internum, which comprises the primary and secondary epidermal laminae. Approximately 600 primary laminae form longitudinal grooves for interdigitation with the vascular laminae of the laminar dermis (corium). The laminar corium unites with the subcutis and periosteum of the distal phalanx.[12]

The bones of the digit are the proximal, middle, and distal phalanx and the distal sesamoid bone (navicular bone; Figure 11-14). The primary joint of the digit is the distal

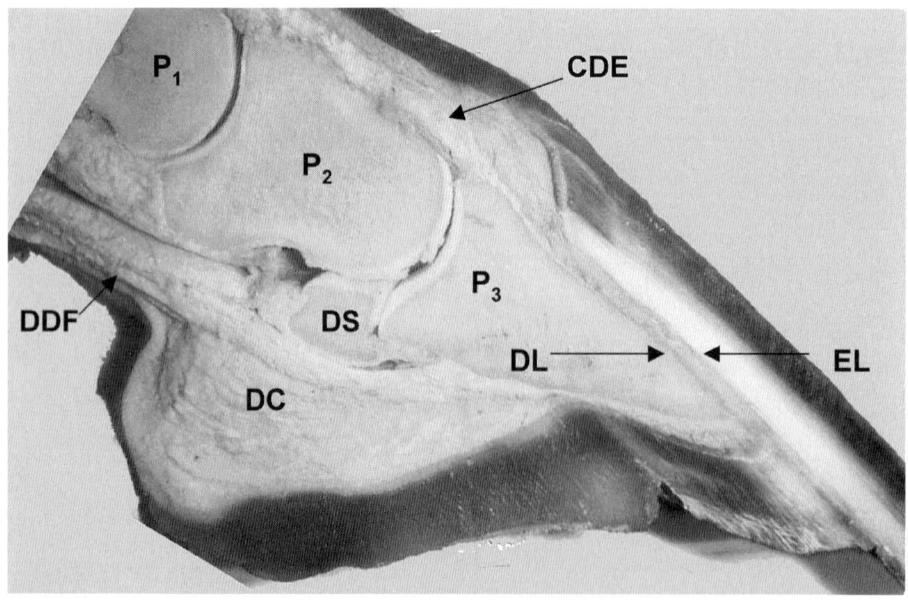

FIGURE 11-14 Cross-section of the equine digit. *CDE,* Common digital extensor tendon; *DC,* digital cushion; *DDF,* deep digital flexor tendon; *DL,* dermal laminae; *DS,* distal sesamoid bone; *EL,* epidermal laminae; P_1, proximal phalanx; P_2, middle phalanx; P_3, distal phalanx.

interphalangeal joint composed of the middle and distal phalanx and the distal sesamoid bone. The short collateral ligaments join the distal end of the middle phalanx and the proximal edges of the distal phalanx. The collateral sesamoidean ligaments extend from the distal aspect of the proximal phalanx and insert on the edges of the distal sesamoid bone. A branch of this ligament also inserts on the palmar process of the distal phalanx. The distal sesamoid impar ligament arises from the distal aspect of the distal sesamoid bone and extends to the palmar surface of the distal phalanx. A fibrous connection between the palmar surface of the middle phalanx and the deep digital flexor tendon forms a T-ligament. The deep digital flexor tendon inserts on the palmar aspect of the distal phalanx, and the common digital extensor tendon inserts on the extensor process of the distal phalanx.[12,13]

The distal interphalangeal joint capsule joins with the common digital extensor tendon, the collateral ligaments of the distal interphalangeal joint, the distal sesamoid impar ligament, and the T-ligament. The joint capsule has two main pouches, the dorsal pouch and the palmar pouch, and the palmar pouch is divided further into proximal and distal pouches. The digital cushion is a large soft-tissue structure located between the base of the cartilages, structures located palmar to the collateral ligaments composed of hyaline cartilage that progress to become predominantly fibrocartilage. The digital cushion is composed of fibroelastic tissue, adipose tissue, and a small percentage of fibrocartilage. A venous plexus is also located within the digital cushion.[12]

The nutrients to maintain the integrity of the corium come from the laminar arteries branching from the circumflex artery as it curves around the toe. These laminar arteries course in a distal to proximal direction. The laminar veins that course distally into the circumflex vein remove metabolic wastes and drain into the bulbar vein and digital veins. Arteriovenous shunts between the circumflex artery and vein have been demonstrated in acute laminitis.[12] These shunts provide a path of rapid flow from the laminar arteries to the veins, thus bypassing the laminar capillaries, and have the potential to rob the laminae of nutrient flow via its capillary bed. An example of the potential significance of this is that recent work using 15 micrometer microspheres injected into the arterial circulation of the digit has demonstrated that increased weight-bearing on a forelimb results in decreased laminar perfusion in that foot. Blood flow at the level of the fetlock was unaltered during this study, pointing to involvement of arteriovenous shunts in redirecting blood flow away from the laminae in the face of altered weight bearing.[14] There may be significant involvement of arteriovenous shunts in other aspects of laminitis pathogenesis that is currently unknown.

The conduction vasculature (digital arteries and veins) supplying the hoof has unique characteristics unlike other vascular beds. The digital veins are highly muscular compared with veins in other tissues and other species.[15] This muscular wall is probably needed to withstand the high vascular pressures exerted in these dependent tissues. The highly muscular wall is likely responsible for the low compliance of the veins.[16] In exercising horses the pressure in the venous circulation may reach 200 mm Hg.[17] The equine digital arteries and veins are highly sensitive to vasoconstrictive substances, most notably norepinephrine and endothelin.[18] Furthermore, the digital veins are most sensitive in vitro to vasoconstrictive substances.[19] For example, contraction induced by angiotensin, thromboxane, norepinephrine, serotonin, and endothelin is twice as strong in veins as arteries.[18-20] Recent studies have examined the nutrient vasculature (laminar arteries and veins) and have found similar patterns in their vascular reactivity.[21]

The culminating effects of low compliance and high sensitivity to vasoconstrictive substances predispose the equine digit to high venous pressures, thereby increasing hydrostatic pressure and thus the likelihood of edema formation. The microcirculation of the equine foot is adapted poorly to handling edema. In normal tissues, three safety factors counteract edema formation, including capillary permeability, pre- to postcapillary resistance, and lymphatic drainage. An impermeability of the capillary endothelium serves as a barrier to fluid and protein transudation, which results in a higher gradient between the capillary and tissue oncotic pressure, favoring movement of fluid into the capillary lumen. Paradoxically, the equine digital capillary bed is highly permeable to fluid and macromolecules and is more permeable than the vasculature of the dog and rat paw.[16] This permeability results in a higher concentration of interstitial protein, favoring edema formation. A high precapillary (arteriolar) resistance and low postcapillary (venous) resistance reduce the capillary pressure, thereby reducing the hydrostatic pressure for transcapillary fluid filtration. The precapillary-to-postcapillary resistance ratio in healthy horses is comparable to that in other musculoskeletal beds in other species. However, during the prodromal stages of experimentally induced laminitis (either the black walnut extract [BWE] or the carbohydrate overload [CHO] models) the contribution by the postcapillary portion increases, thus favoring edema formation. Lymphatic drainage provides the third edema safety factor. The small diameter and number of metacarpal lymphatics and the hydrostatic gradient to lymph flow reduce the likelihood that lymphatic circulation can effectively protect the foot against edema when the hydrostatic forces in the capillary favor edema formation.[22]

Clinical Signs and Diagnosis

Laminitis is a disease that can affect all four feet; however, laminitis most commonly affects the forelimbs because they bear approximately 60% of the mass of the horse.[11] The increased load of the forelimbs compared with the hind limbs is thought to account for the increased occurrence of laminitis in the forelimbs. To define better the severity of clinical signs exhibited by horses, Obel established a grading system in 1948. Grade 1 is the least severe and states that the horse alternately and incessantly lifts the feet and that lameness is not evident at a walk but is evident at a trot as a short, stilted gait. Horses that walk with a stilted gait but are still willing to have a foot lifted are classified as grade 2. Horses with grade 3 laminitis move reluctantly and vigorously resist lifting of a foot. The most severe classification is grade 4, noted by the horse refusing to move unless forced.[23] Other clinical signs characteristic of laminitis are heat present over the dorsal surface of the hoof wall, bounding of the digital pulse (increase in the difference between the systolic and diastolic digital arterial pressure), sensitivity to hoof testers, swelling of the coronary band, and alteration of stance to redistribute weight to the hind limbs (sawhorse stance or rocking of weight to the hind limbs) if laminitis is principally affecting the front limbs (Figure 11-15). More severe signs are a dropped sole or palpation of a depression located at the level of the coronary band, both indications of rotation or distal displacement (sinking) of the distal phalanx within the hoof wall.[13,24] Lateral radiographs of the digit are indicated for detection of rotation and distal displacement of the distal phalanx within the hoof capsule (Figures 11-16, *A* and *B*). The placement of a radiopaque marker 1 cm below the coronary band is helpful when determining the presence of distal displacement of the distal phalanx.

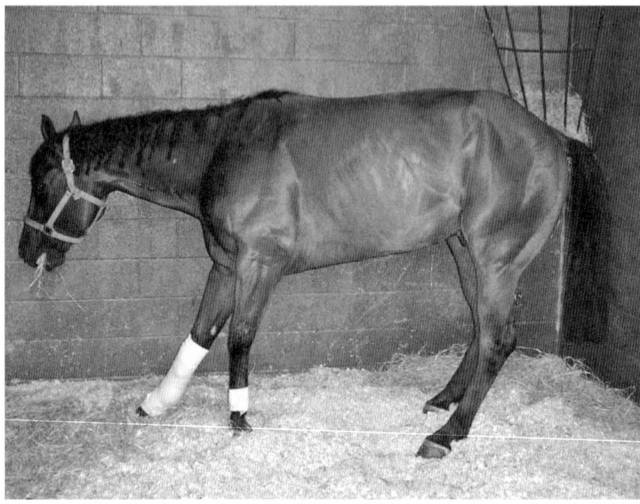

FIGURE 11-15 A few of the clinical signs commonly associated with laminitis include weight redistribution, pressure sores, and poor body condition, as demonstrated in this horse with forelimb laminitis.

The presence of a linear radiopaque marker in the block on which the horse stands is helpful to assess the angle and degree of rotation.

Histopathologic Findings

Histologic study of laminar changes during laminitis has been performed 48 to 96 hours after induction of laminitis with cornstarch or wheat flour gruel. Lameness begins approximately 30 hours after administration of the induction ration.[22] Evaluation of a progression of lesions by these studies is difficult because the onset and severity of lameness varies substantially from horse to horse. Studies using these models are confounded further by the fact that approximately 10% of horses appear to be resistant to the ration.

After the onset of lameness, the initial histologic alteration occurs in the digital vasculature, including swelling of the endothelial cells and mild edema formation.[25] Laminar capillaries become obstructed with erythrocytes within 8 hours. Within 6 to 12 hours, a perivascular leukocyte infiltration occurs that then dissipates as the inflammatory cells migrate into the epidermal layer. Arteriolar endothelial cells become deformed because of cytoplasmic processes that extend into the lumen. Microvascular thrombi and accompanying severe edema formation occur within 24 hours, and hemorrhage occurs within the primary dermal laminae by 72 hours.

Primary histologic alterations of the laminae occur within 8 hours after lameness develops.[25] Initially, thinning and lengthening of the lamellar structures is accompanied by reduction, flattening, and displacement of epithelial cells.

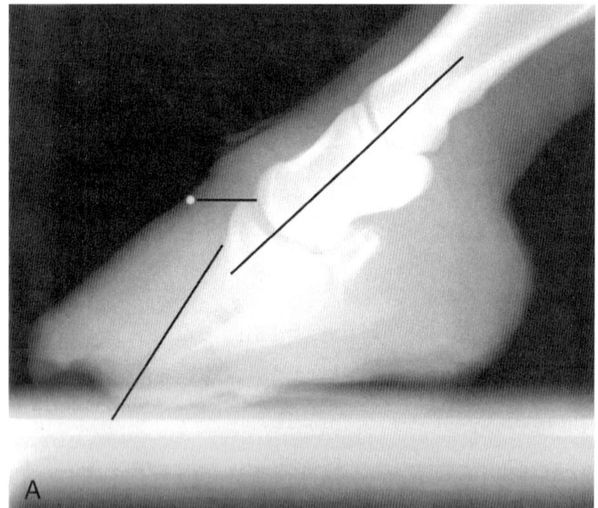

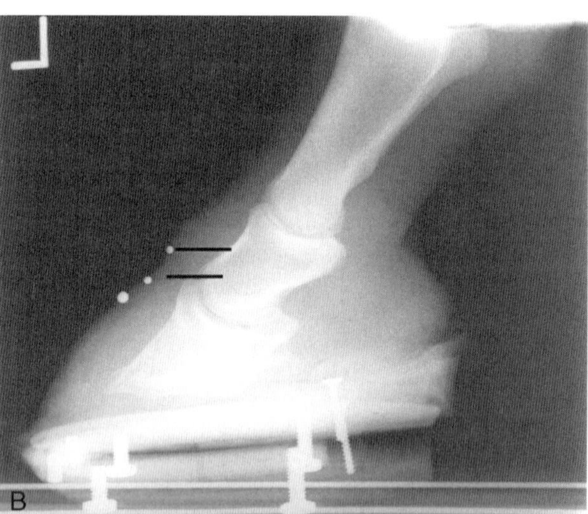

FIGURE 11-16 A, Lateral radiograph of the equine digit demonstrating rotation of the distal phalanx within the hoof capsule. Note the black line drawn parallel to the dorsal surface of the phalanx and the angle this forms with the radiopaque marker in the block, which is used to aid in the assessment of the magnitude of rotation. The line drawn axially through the proximal and distal interphalangeal joints should be approximately parallel to the dorsal surface of the distal phalanx in the normal horse, and deviation from this angle represents distal phalanx rotation. Also, note the placement of the round radiopaque marker in the dorsal hoof wall 1-cm distal to the coronary band, which is used to evaluate distal displacement of the phalanx. This marker should be approximately at the level of the extensor process in normal horses. The vertical distance between this line and the line drawn at the level of the extensor process represents the degree of displacement. **B,** Lateral radiograph of the digit demonstrating marked distal displacement of the phalanx. Note the three radiopaque markers that were used for serial radiographic evaluation. These can also be helpful in assessing dorsal hoof wall growth. (Courtesy Dr. Ralph E. Beadle.)

The secondary laminae become redirected such that laminae nearer the base of the dermal lamina are directed toward the coffin bone and those nearer the laminar tips are directed toward the hoof wall. Morphologic alterations after epithelial cell damage include swelling, vacuolization, nuclear swelling and pyknosis, and leukocytic infiltration of the secondary epidermal lamina, which is observable as early as 24 hours after the onset of lameness.

Pathogenesis

The mechanisms involved in the pathogenesis of laminitis are most likely numerous and interrelated. Inflammation (systemic inflammatory response syndrome [SIRS]), insulin resistance and endothelial dysfunction, enzyme activation, and excessive weight bearing and trauma are factors at the forefront of current investigations.

Systemic sequelae to inflammation (SIRS) commonly precede laminitis in horses with gastrointestinal disease, including pleuropneumonia, colitis, enteritis, peritonitis, and endometritis. Although researchers once questioned whether the disease should be called *laminar degeneration* because of the minimal neutrophilic infiltration present histologically, application of more sensitive research tools has produced abundant evidence of inflammatory changes during laminitis. In carbohydrate overload laminitis, neutrophils become aggregated to platelets in the early prodromal stage and at the onset of lameness.[26,27] During BWE laminitis, significant emigration of neutrophils and monocytes from the dermal capillaries[28] occurs along with emigration of activated leukocytes from the systemic circulation, which produce reactive oxygen species[29]; furthermore, expression of interleukin (IL)-1 and IL-10 in dermal tissues is increased.[30] Horses treated with BWE have increased concentrations of measured osmolality in plasma, laminar tissue, and skin, providing convincing evidence for systemic activation of neutrophils, neutrophil emigration into the integument and laminae, and neutrophil degranulation.[31,32] Calprotectin, a leucocyte marker and amplifier of the inflammatory state, was identified in myeloid cells and keratinocytes of horses with BWE-induced laminitis.[33] Significantly increased lamellar mRNA expression of cytokines important in the innate immune response are present at the developmental stage of the BWE model, and at the onset of acute lameness in both the BWE model and oligofructose model.[30,34] Cyclooxygenase (COX)-2 expression is also substantially increased in the early stages of laminitis.

Evidence also suggests endothelial cell dysfunction during equine laminitis. Substantial increases in digital venous resistance follow intense venous vasoconstriction and facilitate laminar edema formation in the early stages of carbohydrate overload and BWE-induced laminitis as also demonstrated by decreased endothelial-dependant vasodilator responses in vitro, suggesting decreased endothelial production of nitric oxide during these two diseases.[19,22,35-37] Although measurement of digital venous blood nitric oxide concentrations failed to confirm reduced nitric oxide synthase activity, researchers have found increased endothelial synthesis of endothelin (ET)-1 and restoration of digital hemodynamic changes after administration of ET-1 antagonists.[18,38,39] Concurrent with increased ET-1 concentrations are increased digital blood glucose, insulin, and platelet–neutrophil aggregates suggesting that endothelial dysfunction occurs during equine carbohydrate overload laminitis.[39] Laminar concentrations of IL-1beta, IL-6, IL-8, COX-2, intercellular adhesion molecule (ICAM)-1, and E-selectin mRNA increase in the first few hours after laminitis induction before the onset of lameness, suggesting early endothelial changes.[40]

Endothelial dysfunction can be caused by hyperglycemia, hyperinsulinemia, or insulin resistance. Insulin resistance and elevated plasma insulin concentrations often occur in obese horses with laminitis and in horses with pars intermedia dysfunction. Ponies predisposed to laminitis had higher plasma insulin concentrations that ponies not developing laminitis. Increased insulin concentrations in response to feeding inulin and fructan were greatest in horses predisposed to laminitis.[41] In addition, horses with carbohydrate overload laminitis develop elevations of plasma insulin concentration. Insulin resistance may be associated with development of laminitis by three mechanisms: (1) glucose uptake impairment, (2) insulin causes endothelial dysfunction, and (3) and insulin has proinflammatory effects.

Insulin stimulates glucose uptake into tissues via GLUT4 proteins, particularly in muscle and adipose tissue. Insulin resistance impairs GLUT4 function, potentially leading to glucose deprivation of tissues, starving them and causing cell death or damage. In support of this finding is the research that has shown that healthy hoof tissue has an absolute requirement for glucose such that when hoof explants are incubated in the absence of glucose, or in the presence of a glucose uptake inhibitor, the secondary epidermal laminae separate rapidly from their basement membrane, as they do when laminitis occurs.[42]

Insulin signal transduction pathways during insulin resistance in human patients and laboratory models have been recently reviewed.[43] Of interest to the pathogenesis of laminitis is the insulin pathway–specific impairment of the phosphatidylinositol (PI)-3-kinase–dependent signaling pathway that interferes with GLUT4-mediated glucose uptake in skeletal muscle reduces nitric oxide production in vascular endothelium. In contrast, insulin-stimulated secretion of ET-1 is mediated by mitogen-activated protein (MAP)-kinase signaling that is unimpeded during insulin resistance. That is, a key feature of insulin resistance is that it is characterized by specific impairment of PI-3-kinase–dependent signaling pathways, but the rennin-angiotensins system and MAP-kinase–dependent pathways are unaffected. Therefore hyperinsulinemia will promote secretion of ET-1 despite decreased production of nitric oxide. In addition, hyperinsulinemia activates the rennin-angiotensin system, thereby increasing generation of reactive oxygen species and adhesion molecules that accelerate cellular activation.[43] Evidence of oxidant stress during equine laminitis has been documented.[44] The end result of insulin resistance and hyperinsulinemia in people is endothelial dysfunction and an inflammatory state. Similar mechanisms in horses could contribute to epithelial damage and laminar separation. The importance of hyperinsulinemia in the pathogenesis of laminitis has been highlighted by a study inducing laminitis by infusing insulin intravenously causing hyperinsulinemia for 72 hours.[45]

Laminin and type IV and type VII collagen are components of the laminar basement membrane. The enzymes metalloproteinase-2 and metalloproteinase-9 are believed to dissolve these substances, and under normal physiologic states, controlled dissolution allows the movement of epidermal laminae past the dermal laminae as growth occurs.[46-48] Excessive activation of these enzymes leads to uncontrolled dissolution of the basement membrane components, resulting in separation of the epidermal laminae from the dermal laminae. Laminar samples from horses 48 hours after induction of laminitis using the CHO model demonstrated loss of basement membrane attachments.[49,50] In horses with naturally acquired acute and chronic laminitis, zymography of laminar connective tissues found increased activation of extracellular metalloproteinases compared with nonlaminitic horses.[51] Activation of the metalloproteinases is hypothesized to be induced by one or more exotoxins from *Streptococcus* species, especially *S. bovis,* a gram-positive bacteria found in the normal cecal flora.[46,52,53] Using the CHO model, researchers have identified changes in the bacterial population of the cecum with fermentation of the CHO, resulting in excessive lactate production, rapid decline in intracecal pH, and death of cecal bacteria including *Streptococcus* species.[52,54] In addition, activated neutrophils generate matrix metalloproteinase-9 capable of degrading the laminar basement membrane leading to laminar separation.[55] Thus evidence for the neutrophil's role in generating devastating tissue damage during equine inflammatory disease states is mounting.

The mechanical or traumatic theory is based on causes of laminitis resulting from direct trauma to the digit and not a primary systemic disease leading to the development of laminitis.[24] Common examples of traumatically linked laminitis are road founder, laminitis after unilateral lameness of the opposite foot (support limb laminitis), and development of laminitis after long trailer rides.[3,24] The exact mechanisms that lead to structural failure of the laminae are unknown, but several hypotheses have been suggested. Excessive force applied to the dermal and epidermal laminar interdigitations may initiate an inflammatory response with vasospasm, thereby increasing capillary hydrostatic pressure, leading to edema formation and ultimately resulting in a compartment-like syndrome similar to that of the ischemic-vascular theory. Another hypothesis is that application of excessive force results in tearing of the dermal and epidermal laminar interdigitations; the inflammatory response or vasospasm or both then ensue, leading to ischemic damage of the laminar interdigitations.[24]

Obviously, numerous mediators are present in acutely laminitic horses; therefore the authors believe that a single unifying mechanism is unlikely to cause the laminar damage. Most likely, vascular derangement and direct mediator damage coincide.

CURRENT TREATMENT

Treatment of laminitis remains empiric and is often based on the experience and preference of the clinician. Effective treatment of laminitis requires aggressive and appropriate treatment of the primary disease process. Additionally, the cornerstones of treatment of horses with acute laminitis are directed at different components of the pathophysiologic process. The practitioner should consider acute laminitis a medical emergency and should institute treatment immediately after clinical signs develop or, preferably, before the onset of clinical signs. The authors believe the goals of treatment are to eliminate or minimize any predisposing factors, reduce pain, reduce or prevent the magnitude of permanent laminar damage, and prevent further movement of the distal phalanx within the hoof capsule. Considerable controversy exists regarding the treatment of laminitis because of the lack of understanding of the pathophysiologic nature of this disease.

To institute preventive treatment for laminitis, one must identify those horses at risk. Many of the primary diseases thought to predispose horses to develop laminitis are associated with circulating endotoxin. One of the most important preventive measures is combating the effects of endotoxemia and sepsis effectively by decreasing the severity of the primary illness. Recommended treatments include administration of mineral oil (if the horse engorged on grain), intravenous fluids, parenteral antibiotics, NSAIDs, and hyperimmune serum or plasma. Corrective hoof trimming, placement of the horse in a deeply bedded stall, and frog support are vitally important preventative measures.

Because of the anatomy of the normal lamina and hoof and the microvascular alterations that develop with the onset of laminitis, horses are predisposed to developing significant laminar edema, which leads to compression of the nutrient capillaries, resulting in laminar ischemia, reduction of metabolic waste removal, and ultimately laminar necrosis and degeneration. Therefore steps should be taken to minimize laminar edema formation. The best approach is to ensure that the plasma oncotic pressure is sufficient by supplementation with plasma or another colloidal solution such as hydroxyethyl starch or plasma. Additionally, one should take care when administering intravenous fluid therapy to horses with acute laminitis or those predisposed to develop it because excessive intravascular volume caused by overzealous fluid administration could perpetuate development of laminar edema in horses with abnormal digital hemodynamics (i.e., increased capillary hydrostatic pressure). Therefore the authors suggest that fluid therapy be monitored carefully so as to avoid administering fluids in excess of the volume needed to maintain normal hydration. Although venous vasoconstriction is one of the events involved in the pathogenesis of laminitis, drugs currently available do not appear to be effective at blocking this vaso-constrictive response. Acepromazine (0.03 to 0.06 mg/kg intramuscularly or intravenously every 6 to 8 hours) must be administered at low doses to prevent hypotension and sedation. Glyceryl trinitrate applied topically (2 or 4 mg/hr patches) does not increase digital blood flow. Isoxsuprine hydrochloride (1.2 mg/kg orally every 12 hours) appears safe, but no evidence of efficacy has been found.

Continuous cooling of the limbs (up to the carpus and tarsus) reduces the severity of laminitis in experimental models. Expression of mRNA for matrix metallopeptidase (MMP)-2 and histologic lesions were reduced by continuous bathing of the limbs in water kept at 0° C.[56] Reduced blood flow, inflammation, and enzymatic activation are all possible sequelae to this intense cooling. The clinical efficacy of this practice is less than that reported experimentally. Maintaining constant immersion of limbs of compromised patients in these cold baths and initiating cryotherapy in the earliest stages of naturally occurring disease are very difficult.

Antiinflammatory medications are indicated to decrease inflammation, edema, and pain associated with laminitis. Phenylbutazone appears to have the best anti-inflammatory and analgesic effect of any of the NSAIDs commonly used in horses. The practitioner can administer a dose of 2.2 to 4.4 mg/kg of phenylbutazone intravenously or orally every 12 hours. Alternatively, flunixin meglumine can be administered at 0.5 to 1.1 mg/kg intravenously or orally every 8 to 12 hours. A dose of 0.25 mg/kg flunixin meglumine administered intravenously every 8 hours interrupts eicosanoid production associated with endotoxemia but provides little analgesic effect at that dose. Ketoprofen and firocoxib are also available for use in horses. DMSO is an antiinflammatory drug that scavenges hydroxyl radicals, decreases edema, and therefore is used to counteract the effects of ischemia-reperfusion injury. Although the involvement of oxygen free radicals generated by ischemia-reperfusion is questionable, oxygen free radical generation caused by insulin resistance is potentially an important event in the pathogenesis in some horses. DMSO can be administered at 0.1 to 1.0 g/kg intravenously diluted in a polyionic fluid with dextrose to a concentration of 10% to 20% every 8 to 12 hours. Some clinicians prefer to place DMSO topically on the coronary bands.

Pentoxifylline is a phosphodiesterase inhibitor that improves blood flow in people through actions on the red cell membrane. Pentoxifylline does improve red blood cell deformability in horses but does not increase digital blood flow in healthy horses when administered orally at relatively low doses.[57,58] Although pentoxifylline has not been evaluated in the treatment of equine laminitis, numerous in vivo and in vitro studies performed in horses document anti-inflammatory activities.[59-63] Recent data suggest intravenous (8.5 mg/kg) and oral (10 mg/kg) delivery yields plasma drug concentrations similar to those used for the treatment of intermittent claudication in people. The efficacy of these plasma concentrations in equine disease is not known.[64]

Doxycycline has recently been approved for use as an MMP inhibitor in human patients. Extrapolation has led to use of doxycycline in equine laminitis to inhibit MMP-mediated destruction of laminar connections. In contrast, results of recent studies in horses with endotoxemia reveal that doxycycline is a very weak inhibitor of MMPs in horses.[65] The alteration of microbial flora that may occur with oral administration of doxycycline may be contraindicated in horses with alimentary-associated laminitis.

Because microthrombi and platelet-platelet or platelet-neutrophil aggregates have been shown to form during laminitis, some clinicians prefer to administer heparin or aspirin to horses as a preventive or therapeutic agent. One can administer heparin using several regimens, but administration is often subcutaneous at a dose of approximately 20,000 to 40,000 units for a 450-kg horse. Heparin leads to microagglutination and a subsequent decrease in packed cell volume. No evidence indicates that administration of heparin prevents the onset of laminitis. Aspirin is often administered at a dose of 10 to 20 mg/kg orally once every 48 hours. Aspirin irreversibly inhibits platelet cyclooxygenase and therefore production of thromboxane, which should decrease platelet aggregation and vasoconstriction.

Efforts to reduce mechanical forces and stabilize the distal phalanx are imperative to effective treatment of acute laminitis. Horses should not be exercised during the acute stages because it can lead to increased mechanical forces that could lead to shearing of laminae. Owners should bed the stall deeply with sand or other material that provides support to the frog and provides some cushion if the horse spends long periods recumbent. Providing early and effective mechanical support of the distal phalanx can spare weakened, separating lamellae and improve the outcome. Ideally, mechanical support should be instituted before or at the onset of foot pain. Frog support is one of the more effective methods of providing support to the distal phalanx and can be achieved by using roll gauze taped to the frog in the shape of a triangle. One also can use a commercially available triangular, rubber frog pad. Using a moldable material such as dental putty or a thermoplastic material, a frog support can be conformed to the shape and sulci of the frog and sole, allowing for a more effective distribution of the mechanical support to the frog and subsequently the distal phalanx. The practitioner must take care to support the frog fully but not allow excessive pressure on the sole because this added pressure may increase pain.

Another method to decrease mechanical forces on the distal phalanx is to transect the deep digital flexor tendon to reduce caudal pull on the coffin bone. A deep digital flexor tenotomy has been performed in several horses in acute and chronic stages of laminitis to prevent or reduce coffin bone rotation. Although the short-term outcome was promising, the long-term survival and soundness proved to be less successful. The most appropriate use of a deep digital flexor tenotomy may be to perform it in association with corrective trimming and shoeing during the chronic stages of laminitis to help reverse the amount of rotation.

Each clinician will undoubtedly develop a therapeutic plan based on current literature and on past experiences with the effectiveness of these treatments. The information presented here simply represents some of the currently used methods. Obviously, other methods have not been discussed that may also have merit. The effectiveness of preventive and therapeutic measures needs to improve significantly to help manage this devastating disease. Improvement will become a reality only as researchers collectively work to unravel the remaining mysteries of the pathophysiologic events leading to acute laminitis.

Prognosis

Many horses that demonstrate clinical signs of acute laminitis that receive prompt, appropriate medical treatment and mechanical foot support may recover completely. However, horses, even with mild laminitis, should be withheld from exercise until all signs have subsided and only cautiously returned to athletic function. The primary disease that initiates the onset of laminitis also plays an important role in the prognosis and outcome. Management of the primary disease (i.e., strict dietary management and structured exercise in the case of obesity) is critical to slowing or stopping the progression of laminitis. If radiographs demonstrate signs of coffin bone rotation the prognosis for soundness and even survival must be more guarded. In general the greater the degree of coffin bone rotation, the worse the prognosis. Horses with greater than 15 degrees of rotation accompanied by distal displacement into the hoof capsule within 4 to 6 weeks of the onset of laminitis have a poor prognosis. Prolapse of the distal phalanx through the sole is often accompanied by subsolar abscessation. These horses often require extensive, long-term treatment, and the prognosis is grave because of the recurrent, crippling pain and recumbency, and they often require euthanasia for humane reasons. In one study of horses with acute laminitis admitted to a university veterinary hospital, 75% did not return to athletic function, and most were destroyed humanely within 1 year because of a lack of response to therapy or development of severe complications.[4]

Summary

Laminitis is very complex in its pathogenesis, and researchers and clinicians will need to dedicate substantial resources to continue studies of the various predisposing conditions, converging pathways, and effective treatments to decrease ultimately the numbers of horses with and the severity of laminitis.

REFERENCES

Fundamentals of the Musculoskeletal System, Diagnosis Techniques, and Classification of Myopathies

1. Gillespie J and Robinson N, eds, *Equine Exercise Physiology,* vol. 2, Davis, CA: ICEEP, 1987.
2. Kayar S, Hoppeler H, Essen-Gustavsson B: The similarity of mitochondrial distribution in equine skeletal muscles of differing oxidative capacity, *J Exp Biol* 137:253, 1988.
3. Kayar S, Hoppeler H, Mermod L: Mitochondrial size and shape in equine skeletal muscle. A three dimensional reconstruction study, *Anat Rec* 222:233, 1988.
4. Andrews T: *Biochemical Aspects of Human Diseases,* Oxford, 1983, Blackwell.
5. Kaneko JJ, Harvey JW, Bruss ML: *Clinical Biochemistry of Domestic Animals,* San Diego, 2009, Academic Press, 6.
6. Karpati G, Hilton-Jones D, Griggs RC: *Disorders of Voluntary Muscle, ed 7,* New York, 2009, Cambridge University Press.
7. Bechtel P, Lawrence L: *Equine Sports Medicine,* Philadelphia, 1989, Lea & Febiger.
8. Andrews F, Spurgeon T: Histochemical staining characteristics of normal horse skeletal muscle, *Am J Vet Res* 47:1843, 1986.
9. Snow DH: Equine Exercise Physiology, *Granta, Es.* vol. 1, England, 1983, Cambridge.
10. van den Hoven R, Wensing T, Breukink H: Variation of fiber types in the triceps brachii, longissimus dorsi, gluteus medius and biceps femoris of horses, *Am J Vet Res* 46:939, 1985.
11. Ganong W, editor: *Review of Medical Physiology,* New York, 2005, Lange Medical Books/McGraw Hill.
12. Lopez-Rivero J, Aguera E, Vivo J: Histochemical and morphological study of the middle gluteal muscle in Arabian horses, *J Equine Vet Sci* 10:144, 1990.
13. Raub R, Bechtel P, Lawrence L: Variation in the distribution of muscle fiber types in equine skeletal muscles, *J Equine Vet Sci* 5:34, 1985.
14. Snow D, Guy P: Percutaneous needle muscle biopsy in the horse, *Equine Vet J* 8:150, 1976.
15. Snow D, Guy P: Muscle fiber type composition of a number of limb muscles in different types of horse, *Res Vet Sci* 28:137, 1980.
16. Kline K, Bechtel P: Changes in the metabolic profile of the equine gluteus medius as a function of sampling depth (abstract), *Comp Biochem Physiol* 91A:815, 1988.
17. Hodgson D, Rose R: Effects of a nine month endurance programme on muscle composition in the horse, *Vet Rec* 121:271, 1987.
18. Hodgson D: Muscular adaptations to exercise training, *Vet Clin North Am Equine Pract* 1:533, 1985.
19. Hodgson D, Rose R, DiMauro J, et al: Effects of training on muscle composition in horses, *Am J Vet Res* 47:12, 1986.
20. McMiken D: Muscle fiber types and horse performance, *Equine Prac* 8:6, 1986.
21. Snow D, Guy P: *Biochemistry of Exercise IVB,* Baltimore, 1981, University Park Press.
22. Wood C, Ross T, Armstrong J: Variations in muscle fiber composition between successfully and unsuccessfully raced quarter horses, *J Equine Vet Sci* 8:217, 1988.
23. Committee I. International Conference on Equine Exercise Physiology, 2008
24. Essen-Gustavsson B, Lekeux P, Marlin D: *7th International Conference on Equine Exercise Physiology,* Suffolk: Equine Veterinary Journal, 2006
25. Hinchcliff K, Geor R, Pagan J: *6th International Conference on Equine Exercise Physiology,* Suffolk: Equine Veterinary Journal, 2002.
26. Jeffcott L: *5th International Conference on Equine Exercise Physiology,* Suffolk: Equine Veterinary Journal, 1999.
27. McEwen S, Hulland T: Histochemical and morphometric evaluation of skeletal muscle from horses with exertional rhabdomyolysis (tying-up), *Vet Pathol* 23:400, 1986.
28. Wrogemann K, Pena S: Mitochondrial calcium overload: A general mechanism for cell necrosis in muscle disease, *Lancet* 1:672, 1976.
29. Jackson M: Intracellular calcium, cell injury and relationships to free radicals and fatty acid metabolism, *Proc Nutr Soc* 49: 77-81, 1990.
30. Oredsson S, Plate G, Qwvarfordt P: Allopurinol-a free radical scavenger reduces reperfusion injury in skeletal muscle, *European J Vasc Surg* 5:47, 1991.
31. Hulland T: *Pathology of domestic animals,* ed 3, Orlando, FL, 1985, Academic Press.
32. Charge S, Rudnicki M: Cellular Regulation of Molecular Muscle Regeneration, *Physiol Rev* 84:209-234, 2004.
33. Grefte S, Kuijpers-Jagtman A, Torensma R, et al: Skeletal muscle development and regeneration, *Stem Cells Dev* 16:857-868, 2007.
34. Westermann C, Dorland J, Wijnberg I, et al: Equine metabolic myopathies with emphasis on the diagnostic approach Comparison with human myopathies, *Vet Q* 29:42-59, 2007.
35. Boyd J: The mechanisms relating to increases in plasma enzymes and isoenzymes in diseases of animals, *Vet Clin Pathol* 12:9, 1985.
36. Gerber H: The clinical significance of serum enzyme activities with particular reference to myoglobinuria, *Proc Am Assoc Equine Pract* 14:81, 1968.
37. Volfinger L, Lassourd V, Michaux J: Kinetic evaluation of muscle damage during exercise by calculation of amount of creatine kinase released, *Am J Physiol* 266:R434-R441, 1994.
38. Anderson M: The effect of exercise on the lactic dehydrogenase and creatine kinase isoenzyme composition of horse serum, *Res Vet Sci* 20:191, 1976.
39. Argiroudis S, Kent J, Blackmore D: Observations on the isoenzymes of creatine kinase in equine serum and tissues, *Equine Vet J* 14:317, 1982.
40. Fujii Y, Ikeda S, Watanabe H: Analysis of creatine kinase osoenzyme in racehorse serum and tissues, *Bull Equine Res Inst* 17:21, 1980.
41. Sighieri C, Longa A, Mariani A: Preliminary observations on the creatine kinase isoenzyme in equine blood serum by polyacrylamide-gel isoelectrofocusing. Influence of physical exercise, *Arch Vet Ital* 36:45, 1985.
42. Cardinet G, Littrell J, Freedland R: Comparative investigations of serum creatine phosphokinase and glutamic-oxaloacetic transaminase activities in equine paralytic myoglobinuria, *Res Vet Sci* 8:219, 1967.
43. Posen S: Turnover of circulating enzymes, *Clin Chem* 16:71, 1970.
44. Arighi M, Baird J, Hulland T: Equine exertional rhabdomyolysis, *Compend Continuing Educ Pract Vet* 6:5726, 1984.
45. Cornelius C, Burnham L, Hill H: Serum transaminase activities of equine thoroughbred horses in training, *J Am Vet Med Assoc* 142:639, 1963.
46. Rej U, Rudofsky R, Magro A: Effects of exercise on serum aminotransferase activity and pyridoxal phosphate saturation in Thoroughbred racehorses, *Equine Vet J* 22:205, 1990.
47. Littlejohn A, Blackmore D: Blood and tissue content of the iso-enzymes of lactate dehydrogenase in the thoroughbred, *Res Vet Sci* 25:118, 1987.
48. Guy P, Snow P: The effect of training and detraining on lactate dehydrogenase isoenzymes in the horse, *Biochem Biophys Res Commun* 75:863, 1977.
49. Rowland L, Penn A: Myoglobinuria. *Med Clin North Am* 56:1233, 1972.

50. Boulton F, Huntsman R: The detection of myoglobin in urine and its distinction from normal and variant hemoglobins, *J Clin Pathol* 24:816, 1971.
51. Dubowitz V: *Muscle Biopsy: A Practical Approach*, ed 2, London, 1985, Bailliere Tindall.
52. Schiff H, MacSearraigh E, Kallmeyer J: Myoglobin, rhabdomyolysis and marathon running, *Q J Med* 47:463, 1978.
53. Hodgson D: Myopathies in the athletic horse, *Compendium Continuing Educ Pract Vet* 7:551, 1985.
54. McLean J: Equine paralytic myoglobinuria A review, *Aust Vet J* 49:41, 1973:("azoturia").
55. Wilson T, Morrison H, Palmer N: Myodegeneration and suspected selenium/vitamin E deficiency in horses, *J Am Vet Med Assoc* 169:213, 1976.
56. Klein L: A review of 50 cases of post operative myopathy in the horse-Intrinsic and management factors affecting risk, *Proc Am Assoc Equine Pract* 24:89, 1978.
57. Anderson G, Mount M, Vrins A: Fatal acorn poisoning in a horse. Pathologic findings and diagnostic considerations, *J Am Vet Med Assoc* 24:1105, 1983.
58. Coffman J: Testing for Renal disease, *Vet Med Small Anim Clin* 75:1039, 1980.
59. Carlson G, Harrold D, Ocen P: Field laboratory evaluation of the effects of heat and work stress in horses, *Proc Am Assoc Equine Pract* 21:314, 1975.
60. Coffman J: *Equine Clinical Chemistry and Pathophysiology*, Kansas City, KS, 1981, Veterinary Medicine Pub Co.
61. Blackmore DJ, Eckersall PD, Evans GO, et al: *Animal Clinical Biochemistry*, Cambridge, England, 1988, Cambridge University Press.
62. Kelner M, Alexander N: Rapid separation and identification of myoglobin and hemoglobin in urine by centrifugation through a microconcentrator membrane, *Clin Chem* 31:112, 1985.
63. Colahan PT, Merritt AM, Moore JN: *Equine Medicine and Surgery*, St. Louis, 1999, Mosby, 5.
64. Valberg S, Holmgren N, Jonsson L, et al: Plasma AST, CK and myoglobin responses to exercise in rhabdomyolysis susceptible horses (abstract), *Can J Sport Sci* 13:34, 1988.
65. Watanabe M, Ireda S, Kameya T: Evaluation of myoglobin determination for the diagnosis of tying-up syndrome in racehorces in Japan, *Exp Rep Equine Health Lab* 15:79, 1978.
66. Knochel J: Rhabdomyolysis and Myoglobinuria, *Annu Rev Med* 33:435, 1982.
67. Lindholm A, Piehl K: Fibre composition enzyme activity and concentrations of metabolites and electrolytes in muscles of standardbred horses, *Acta Vet Scand* 15:287, 1974.
68. Mermod L, Hoppeler H, Rayer S: Variability of fiber size, capillary density and capillary length related to horse muscle fixation procedures, *Acta Anat* 133:89, 1988.
69. Valberg S: *Obtaining and submitting a muscle biopsy*, St. Paul, Minn, 2008, University of Minnesota.
70. Vd Hoven: *Some histochemical and biochemical aspects of equine muscles withspecial respect to equine exertional myopathy*, Netherlands, 1987, University of Utrecht.
71. Valberg S. Exertional rhabdomyolysis and polysaccharide storage myopathy in Quarter horses. In *Proceedings of the Forty-First Annual Convention of the American Association of Equine Practitioners* 1995;228-230.
73. van den Hoven R, Meijer A, Wensing T, et al: Enzyme histochemical features of equine gluteus muscle fibers, *Am J Vet Res* 46:1755, 1985.
73. Kaese H, Valberg S, Hayden D, et al: Infarctive purpura hemorrhagica in five horses, *J Am Vet Med Assoc* 226:1893-1898, 2005:1845.
74. Sponseller B, Valberg S, Tennent-Brown B, et al: Severe acute rhabdomyolysis associated with Streptococcus equi infection in four horses, *J Am Vet Med Assoc* 227:1800-1807, 2005: 1753-1754.
75. Wijnberg I, Back W, de Jong M, et al: The role of electromyography in clinical diagnosis of neuromuscular locomotor problems in the horse, *Equine Vet J* 36:718-722, 2004.
76. Wijnberg I, van der Kolk J, Franssen H, et al: Needle electromyography in the horse compared with its principles in man: a review, *Equine Vet J* 35:9-17, 2003.
77. Mayhew M: *Large Animal Neurology*, ed 2, Philadelphia, 2009, Wiley-Blackwell.
78. Morris E, Seeherman H, O'Callaghan M. Scintigraphic identification of rhabdomyolysis in horses. In *Proceedings of the Thirty-Seventh Annual Convention of the American Association of Equine Practitioners* 1991;315-324.
79. Archer D, Cotton J, Boswell J: Non-skeletal scintigraphy of the horse: indications and validity, *Vet J* 173:45-56, 2007.
80. Morris E, Seeherman H: Clinical Evaluation of poor performance in the racehorse: the results of 275 evaluations, *Equine Vet J* 23:169-174, 1991.
81. Cerny F, Haralambie G: *Biochemistry of exercise*, Champaign, Ill, 1983, Human Kinetics.
82. Raven P, Conners T, Evonuk E: Effects of exercise on plasma lactate dehydrogenase isoenzymes and catecholamines, *J Appl Physiol* 29:374, 1970.
83. Hambleton P, Slade L, Hamar D: Dietary fat and exercise conditioning effect on metabolic conditioning reduced exercise-induced increases in parameters in the horse, *J Anim Sci* 51:1330, 1980.
84. Milne D: Blood gases, acid-based balance and electrolyte enzyme changes in exercising horses, 1974 horses, *J S Afr Vet Assoc* 45:345, 1974.
85. Poso A, Soveri T, Oksanen H: The effect of exercise on blood parameters in standardbred and Finnish bred horses, *Acta Vet Scand* 24:170, 1983.
86. Milne D, Skarda R, Gabel A: Effects of training on biochemical values in standardbred horses, *Am J Vet Res* 37:285, 1976.
87. Shelle J, Van Huss W, Rook J. Blood parameters as a result of conditioning horses through short strenuous exercise bouts. Proceedings of the ninth equine Nutritional Physiology Symposium. 1985;206.
88. Aitken M, Anderson M, Mackenzie G: Correlations between physiological and biochemical parameters used to assess fitness in the horse, *J S Afr Vet Assoc* 45:361, 1974.
89. Anderson M: The influence of exercise on serum enzyme levels in the horse, *Equine Vet J* 7:160, 1975.
90. Harris P: *Aspects of the equine Rhabdomyolysis Syndrome*, 1988, Cambridge University.
91. Codazza D, Maffeo G, Redaelli G: Serum enzyme changes and haemato-chemical levels in thoroughbreds after transport and exercise, *J S Afr Vet Assoc* 45:331, 1974.
92. Rose R, Purdue R, Hensley W: Plasma biochemistry alterations in horses during an endurance ride, *Equine Vet J* 9:122, 1977.
93. Chaney K, MacLeay J, Enns R, et al: Effects of induced lameness via carpal osteochondral fragmentation on plasma creatine kinase activity in horses, *J Equine Vet Sci* 24:531-534, 2004.
94. Fayolle P, Lefebre H, Braun J: Effects of incorrect venepuncture on plasma creatine kinase activity in dogs and horses, *Br Vet J* 148:161-162, 1992.
95. Freestone J, Kamerling S, Church G: Exercise induced changes in creatine kinase and aspartate aminotransferase activities in the horse: effects conditioning, exercise tests and cepromazine, *J Equine Vet Sci* 9:275, 1989.
96. Frauenfelder H, Rossdale P, Ricketts S: Changes in serum muscle enzyme levels associated with training schedules and stage of the oestrous cycle in thoroughbred racehorses, *Equine Vet J* 18:371, 1986.
97. Harris P, Greet T, Snow D: Some factors influencing plasma AST/CK activities in thoroughbred racehorces, *Equine Vet J* 9(suppl):66, 1990.

98. Aktas M, Auguste D, Concorddet D: Creatine kinase in dog plasma: Preanalytical factors of variation, reference values and diagnostic significance, *Res Vet Sci* 56:30-36, 1994.
99. Serrantoni M, Harris P, Allen W: Muscle enzyme activities in the plasma of thoroughbred fillies in relation to exercise and stage of oestrous cycle, *Submitted for publication* 1996.
100. Amelink G, Koot R, Erich W: Sex linked variation in creatine kinase release and its dependence on oestradiol can be demonstrated in an in-vitro rat skeletal muscle preparation, *Acta Physiol Scand* 138:115-124, 1990.
101. MacLeay J, Sorum S, Valberg S, et al: Epidemiological factors influencing recurrent exertional rhabdomyolysis in Thoroughbred racehorses, *Am J Vet Res* 60:1560-1563, 1999.
102. Cardinet G 3rd, Fowler M, Tyler W: The effects of training, exercise and tying-up on serum transaminase activities in the horse, *Am J Vet Res* 24:980, 1963.
103. Mullen P, Hopes R, Sewell J: The biochemistry, nutrition and racing performance of two year old thoroughbreds throughout their training and racing season, *Vet Rec* 104:90, 1979.
104. Snow D, Harris P: Enzymes as markers for the evaluation of physical fitness and training of racing horses, *Adv Clin Enzymol* :6, 1988.
105. Rej U, Rudofsky R, Magro A, Prendergast J: Effects of exercise on serum aminotransferase activity and pyridoxal phosphate saturation in thoroughbred racehorces, *Equine Vet J* 22:205, 1990.
106. Flisińska-Bojanowska A, Komosa M, Gill J: Influence of pregnancy on diurnal and seasonal changes in glucose level and activity of FDPA, AlATand AspAT in mares (abstract), *Comp Biochem Physiol* 98A:32, 1991.
107. Sommer H: Blood profile testing in racehorses, *Equine Pract* 5:21, 1983.
108. Myositis Meginnis P: (tying-up) in race horses, *J Am Vet Med Assoc* 130:237, 1957.
109. Brennan B, Marshak R, Keown G: The tying up syndrome-a panel discussion, *Proc Am Assoc Equine Pract* 5:157, 1959.
110. Lindholm A, Johannson H, Kjaersgaard P: Acute rhabdomyolysis (tying-up) in standardbred horses. A morphological and biochemical study, *Acta Vet Scand* 15:325, 1974.
111. Udall D: *The Practice of Veterinary Medicine*, ed 3, Ithaca, NY, 1939, Udall.
112. MacLeay J, Valberg S, Pagan J: Effect of diet on Thoroughbred horses with recurrent exertional rhabdomyolysis performing a standardised exercise test, *Eq Vet J Suppl* 30:458, 1999.
113. Stashak T, editor: *Adam's lameness in horses*, ed, Philadelphia, 2002, Wiley-Blackwell, 5.
114. Valberg S, Mickelson J, Gallant E, et al: Exertional rhabdomyolysis in Quarter horses and Thoroughbreds: one syndrome, multiple etiologies, *Equine Vet J Suppl* 30:533-538, 1999.
115. Ursachen Hertha K: Verhu tung und Behandlung der Ha moglobina mie des pferdes, *Cornell Vet* 14:165, 1924.
116. Carlstrom B: U ber die Atiologie und Pathogenese der Kreuzlahmuns des Pferdes (Ha mglobina mia paralytica), *Skand Arch Physiol* 61:161, 1931.
117. Carlstrom B: U ber die Atiologie und Pathogenese der Kreuzlahmung des Pferdes (Ha moglobina mia paralytica), *Skand Arch Physiol* 63:164, 1932.
118. Snow D, Harris R, Gash S: Metabolic response of equine muscle to intermittent maximal exercise, *J Appl Physiol* 58:1689, 1985.
119. Harris P, Snow D: Tying up the loose ends of equine rhabdomyolysis (editorial), *Equine Vet J* 18:346, 1986.
120. Koterba A, Carlson G: Acid base and electrolyte alterations in horses with exertional rhabdomyolysis, *J Am Vet Med Assoc* 180:303, 1982.
121. DeGroot L, Larsen P, Refetoff S, editor: The thyroid and its diseases, In Chichester England, 1984, Wiley, 5.
122. Evered D, Ormston B, Smith P: Grades of hypothyroidism, *Br Med J* 1:657, 1973.
123. Docherty I, Harrop J, Hine K: Myoglobin concentration creatine kinase activity and creatine kinase B subunit concentrations in serum during thyroid disease, *Clin Chem* 30:42, 1984.
124. Waldron-Mease E: Hypothyroidism and myopathy in racing thoroughbreds and standardbreds, *J Equine Med Surg* 3:124, 1979.
125. Morris D, Garcia M: Thyroid-stimulating hormone response test in healthy horses and effect of phenylbutazone on equine thyroid hormones, *Am J Vet Res* 44:503, 1983.
126. Vischer CM, Foreman JH, Benson GJ, et al: Hypothyroidism and exercise intolerance in horses, *Proc 14th ACVM Forum* 1996.
127. Dietzman D, Shaller J, Ray C: Acute myositis associated with influenza B infection, *Pediatrics* 57:255, 1976.
128. Savage D, Forbes M, Pearce G: Idiopathic rhabdomyolysis, *Arch Dis Child* 46:594, 1971.
129. McQueen J, Davenport F, Keeran R, et al: Studies of equine influenza in Michigan 1963, *Am J Epidemiol* 83:280, 1966.
130. Carlson G: Medical problems associated with protracted heat and work stress in horses, *Compend Contin Educ Pract Vet* 5:542, 1985.
131. Harris P: Outbreak of the equine rhabdomyolysis syndrome in a racing yard, *Vet Rec* 127:468, 1990.
132. Gross D, Hinchcliff K, French P: Effect of moderate exercise on the severity of clinical signs associated with influenza virus infection in horses, *Equine Vet J* 30:489, 1998.

Inborn Errors of Metabolism

1. McCue M, Valberg S, Lucio M, et al: Glycogen Synthase 1 (GYS1) mutation in diverse breeds with polysaccharide storage myopathy, *J Am Vet Med Assoc* 91:458-466, 2008.
2. McCue ME, Valberg SJ, Jackson M, et al: Polysaccharide storage myopathy phenotype in quarter horse-related breeds is modified by the presence of an RYR1 mutation, *Neuromuscul Disord* 19(1):37-43, 2009:Epub 2008 Dec 3.
3. McCue M, Valberg S: Estimated prevalence of polysaccharide storage myopathy among overtly healthy Quarter Horses in the United States, *J Am Vet Med Assoc* 231:746-750, 2007.
4. Valentine B, Cooper B: Incidence of polysaccharide storage myopathy: necropsy study of 225 horses, *Vet Pathol* 42: 823-827, 2005.
5. Firshman A, Baird JD, Valberg S: Prevalences and clinical signs of polysaccharide storage myopathy and shivers in Belgian draft horses, *J Am Vet Med Assoc* 227:1958-1964, 2005.
6. McCue M, Ribeiro W, Valberg S: Prevalence of polysaccharide storage myopathy in horses with neuromuscular disorders, *Equine Vet J Suppl* 36:340-344, 2006.
7. Hunt L, Valberg S, Stepffenhagen K, et al: An epidemiological study of myopathies in warmblood horses, *Equine Vet J* 2007.
8. Annandale E, Valberg S, Mickelson J, et al: Insulin sensitivity and skeletal muscle glucose transport in horses with equine polysaccharide storage myopathy, *Neuromuscul Disord* 14:666, 2004.
9. De La Corte F, Valberg S, MacLeay J, et al: Developmental onset of polysaccharide storage myopathy in 4 Quarter Horse foals, *J Vet Int Med* 16:581-587, 2002.
10. De La Corte F, Valberg S, Mickelson J, et al: Blood glucose clearance after feeding and exercise in polysaccharide storage myopathy, *Equine Vet J Suppl* 30:324-328, 1999.
11. Ribeiro W, Valberg S, Pagan J, et al: The effect of varying dietary starch and fat content on serum creatine kinase activity and substrate availability in equine polysaccharide storage myopathy, *J Vet Int Med* 18:887-894, 2004.
12. Firshman A, Valberg S, Bender J, et al: Epidemiologic characteristics and management of polysaccharide storage myopathy in Quarter Horses, *Am J Vet Res* 64:1319-1327, 2003.
13. Render J, Commons R, Kennedy F, et al: Amylopectinosis in fetal and neonatal Quarter Horses, *Vet Pathol* 36:157-160, 1999.

14. Bao Y, Kishnani P, Wu J, et al: Hepatic and neuromuscular forms of glycogen storage disease type IV caused by mutations in the same glycogen-branching enzyme gene, *Am Soc Clin Invest* 97:941-948, 1996.
15. Fyfe J, Giger U, Van Winkle T, et al: Glycogen storage disease type IV: inherited deficiency of branching enzyme activity in cats, *Pediatr Res* 32:719-725, 1992.
16. Thon V, Khalil M, Cannon J: Isolation of human glycogen branching enzyme cDNAs by screening complementation in yeast, *J Biol Chem* 268:7509-7513, 1993.
17. Valberg S, Ward T, Rush B, et al: Glycogen branching enzyme deficiency in Quarter horse foals, *J Vet Int Med* 15:572-580, 2001.
18. Wagner M, Valberg S, Ames E, et al: Allele frequency and likely impact of the glycogen branching enzyme deficiency gene in Quarter Horse and Paint Horse populations, *J Vet Int Med* 20:1207-1211, 2006.
19. Ward T, Valberg S, Adelson D, et al: Glycogen branching enzyme (GBE1) mutation causing equine glycogen storage disease IV, *Mamm Genome* 15:570-577, 2004.
20. Ward T, Valberg S, Lear T, et al: Genetic mapping of GBE1 and its association with glycogen storage disease IV in American Quarter Horses, *Cytogenet Genome Res* 102:201-206, 2003.
21. Westermann C, de Sain-van der Velden M, Van der Kolk J, et al: Equine biochemical multiple acyl-CoA dehydrogenase deficiency (MADD) as a cause of rhabdomyolysis, *Mol Genet Metab* 91:362-369, 2007.
22. Valberg S, Carlson G, Cardinet G, et al: Skeletal muscle mitochondrial myopathy as a cause of exercise intolerance in a horse, *Muscle Nerve* 17:305-312, 1994.
23. Andrews T: *Biochemical aspects of human diseases*, Oxford, 1983, Blackwell.
24. Cox J: An episodic weakness in four horses associated with intermittent serum hyperkalemia and the similarity of the disease to hyperkalemic periodic paralysis in man, *Proc Am Assoc Equine Pract* 31:383, 1985.
25. Gillespie J, Robinson N: *Equine Exercise Physiology* vol. 2:Davis, Calif: ICEEP.
26. Steiss J, Naylor J: Episodic muscle tremors in a quarter horse. Resemblance to hyperkalemic periodic paralysis, *Can Vet J* 27:332, 1986.
27. Traub-Dargatz J, Ingram J, Stashak T, et al: Respiratory stridor associated with polymyopathy suspected to be hyperkalemic periodic paralysis in four quarter horse foals, *J Am Vet Med Assoc* 201:85-89, 1992.
28. Spier S, Valberg S, Carr E, et al. Update on hyperkalemic periodic paralysis, *AAEP Proceedings* 1995;231-233.
29. Naylor J, Jones V, Berry S: Clinical syndrome and diagnosis of hyperkalaemic paralysis in Quarter horses, *Equine Vet J* 25: 227-232, 1993.
30. Robinson J, Naylor J, Crichlow E: Use of electromyography for the diagnosis of equine hyperkalaemic periodic paresis, *Can J Vet Res* 54:495-500, 1990.
31. Stewart R, Bertone J, Yvorchuk-St Jean K: Possible normokalaemic variant of hyperkalemic periodic paralysis in two horses, *J Am Vet Med Assoc* 203:421-424, 1993.
32. Beech J. Myopathies in horses, *Proceedings from Equine Seminar* 1988 1988;101.
33. Spier S. Hyperkalemic periodic paralysis: 14 years later. Annual Convention of the AAEP 2006;347-350
34. Spier S, Carlson G, Pickar J: Hyperkalemic periodic paralysis in horses: Genetic and electrophysiologic studies, *Proc Am Assoc Equine Pract* 35:399, 1989.
35. McClatchey A, Trofatter J, McKenna-Yasek D: Dinucleotide repeat polymorphisms at the SCN4A locus suggest allelic heterogenity of hyperkalemic paralysis and paramyotonia congenita, *Am J Hum Genet* 10:896-901, 1992.
36. Rudolph J, Spier S, Bryns G, et al: Periodic paralysis in Quarter horses: A sodium channel mutation disseminated by selective breeding, *Nat Genet* 2:144-147, 1992.
37. Rudolph J, Spier S, Bryns G, et al: Linkage of hyperkalaemic periodic paralysis in Quarter horses to the horse adult skeletal muscle sodium channel gene, *Anim Genet* 23:241-250, 1992.
38. Peachey C, editor: *Handbook of Physiology*, Bethesda, 1983, Md, American Physiology Society.
39. Frauenfelder H, Rossdale P, Ricketts S: Changes in serum muscle enzyme levels associated with training schedules and stage of the oestrous cycle in thoroughbred racehorses, *Equine Vet J* 18:371, 1986.
40. Harris P: *Aspects of the equine rhabdomyolysis syndrome*, Cambridge, 1988, Cambridge University.
41. Karpati G, Hilton-Jones D, Griggs RC: *Disorders of voluntary muscle*, ed 7, New York, 2009, Cambridge University Press.
42. Bendheim P, Reale E, Berg B: Adrenergic treatment of hyperkalemic periodic paralysis, *Neurology* 35:746, 1985.
43. Griggs R: *Advances in neurology*, New York, 1977, Raven Press.
44. Colahan PT, Merritt AM, Moore JN: *Equine medicine and surgery*, St. Louis, 1999, Mosby, 5.
45. Beech J, Fletcher J, Lizzo F, et al: Effect of phenytoin on the clinical signs and in vitro muscle twitch characteristics in horses with chronic intermittent rhabdomyolysis and myotonia, *Am J Vet Res* 49:2130, 1988.
46. Hegreberg G, Reed S: Skeletal muscle changes associated with equine myotonic dystrophy, *Acta Neuropathol* 80:426, 1990.
47. Ptacek LJ, Johnson KJ, Griggs R: Genetics and physiology of the myotonic muscle disorders, *N Eng J Med* 328:482-488, 1993.
48. Reed S, Hegreberg G, Warwick M, et al: Progressive myotonia in foals resembling human dystrophia myotonica, *Muscle Nerve* 2:291-296, 1988.
49. Steinberg H, Botelho S: Myotonia in a horse, *Science* 137: 979-980, 1962.
50. Schooley E, MacLeay J, Cuddon P, et al: Myotonia congenita in a foal, *J Equine Vet Sci* 24:483-486, 2004.
51. Jamison J, Baird J, Smith-Maxie L, et al: A congenital form of myotonia with dystrophic changes in a Quarterhorse, *Equine Vet J* 19:353-358, 1987.
52. Beech J, Lindborg S, Braund KG: Potassium concentrations in muscle, plasma and erythrocytes and urinary fractional excretion in normal horses and those with chronic intermittent exercise-associated rhabdomyolysis, *Res Vet Sci* 55:43-51, 1993.
53. Hammel E, Marks H. Fifth International Congress on Neuromuscular Disease, 1982
54. Hegreberg G, Reed S: Muscle changes in a progressive equine myotonic dystrophy, *Fed Proc* 46:728, 1987.
55. Roneus B, Lindholm A, Jonsson L: Myotoni hos hast, *Svensk Vet Tidn* 35:217, 1983.
56. Cunningham P: The genetics of Thoroughbred horses, *Sci Am* 5:92, 1991.
57. MacLeay J, Sorum S, Valberg S, et al: Epidemiological factors influencing recurrent exertional rhabdomyolysis in Thoroughbred racehorses, *Am J Vet Res* 60:1560-1563, 1999.
58. Valberg S, Mickelson J, Gallant E, et al: Exertional rhabdomyolysis in Quarter horses and Thoroughbreds: one syndrome, multiple etiologies, *Equine Vet J Suppl* 30:533-538, 1999.
59. McGowan C, Fordham T, Christley R: Incidence and risk factors for exertional rhabdomyolysis in Thoroughbred racehorses in the United Kingdom, *Vet Rec* 23:623-626, 2002.
60. Andrews F: Acute Rhabdomyolysis, *Vet Clin North Am Equine Pract* 10:567-573, 1994.
61. Uehara N, Sawazaki H, Mochizuki K: Changes in the skeletal muscles volume in horses with growth, *Nippon Juigaku Zasshi* 47:161, 1985.
62. MacLeay J, Valberg S, Pagan J: Effect of ration and exercise on plasma creatine kinase activity and lactate concentration in Thoroughbred horses with recurrent exertional rhabdomyolysis, *Am J Vet Res* 61:1390-1395, 2000.

63. Lentz L, Valberg S, Herold L, et al: Myoplasmic calcium regulation in myotubes from horses with recurrent exertional rhabdomyolysis, *Am J Vet Res* 63:1724-1731, 2002.
64. Lentz LR, Valberg SJ, Balog EM, et al: Abnormal regulation of muscle contraction in horses with recurrent exertional rhabdomyolysis, *Am J Vet Res* 60:992-999, 1999.
65. Lentz LR, Valberg SJ, Mickelson JR, et al: In vitro contractile responses and contracture testing of skeletal muscle from Quarter Horses with exertional rhabdomyolysis, *Am J Vet Res* 60:684-688, 1999.
66. Mickelson JR: Malignant hyperthermia: excitation-contraction coupling, Ca2+ release channel and cell Ca2+ regulation defects, *Physiolog Rev* 76:2-56, 1996.
67. Dranchak P, Valberg S, Onan G, et al: Exclusion of linkage of the RYR1, CACNA1S, and ATP2A1 genes to recurrent exertional rhabdomyolysis in Thoroughbreds, *Am J Vet Res* 67:1395-1400, 2006.
68. Ward T, Valberg S, Gallant E, et al: Calcium regulation by skeletal muscle membranes of horses with recurrent exertional rhabdomyolysis, *Am J Vet Res* 61:242-247, 2000.
69. Court M, Engelking L, Dodman N: Pharmacokinetics of dantrolene sodium in horses, *J Vet Pharmacol Ther* 10:218, 1987.
70. Gronert G: Malignant hyperthermia, *Anesthesiology* 53:395, 1980.
71. Hildebrand S, Arpin D, Howitt G: Muscle biopsy to differentiate normal from malignant hyperthermia suspect horses and ponies, *Vet Surg* 17:172, 1988.
72. Manley S, Kelly A, Hodgson D: Malignant hyperthermia-like reactions in three anesthetized horses, *J Am Vet Med Assoc* 183:85, 1983.
73. Waldron-Mease E: Correlation of post-operative and exercise-induced equine myopathy with the defect malignant hyperthermia, *Proc Am Assoc Equine Pract* 24:95, 1978.
74. MacLeay JM, Valberg SJ, Sorum SA, et al: Heritability of recurrent exertional rhabdomyolysis in Thoroughbred racehorses, *Am J Vet Res* 60:250-256, 1999.
75. Dranchak P, Valberg S, Onan G, et al: Inheritance of recurrent exertional rhabdomyolysis in Thoroughbreds, *J Am Vet Med Assoc* 227:762-767, 2005.
76. Hodgson D: Myopathies in the athletic horse, *Compend Contin Educ Pract Vet* 7:551, 1985.
77. McLean J: Equine paralytic myoglobinuria ("azoturia"): a review, *Aust Vet J* 49:41, 1973.
78. Williams W: *The principles and practice of veterinary medicine*, ed 2, New York, 1879, William Wood 1879.
79. Harris P: Equine rhabdomyolysis syndrome, *Equine Pract* 11:3, 1989.
80. Beech J: Chronic exertional rhabdomyolysis, *Vet Clin North Am* 13:145, 1997.
81. MacLeay J, Valberg S, Pagan J: Effect of diet on Thoroughbred horses with recurrent exertional rhabdomyolysis performing a standardised exercise test, *Eq Vet J Suppl* 30:458, 1999.
82. Myositis Meginnis P: (tying-up) in race horses, *J Am Vet Med Assoc* 130:237, 1957.
83. Udall D: *The practice of veterinary medicine*, ed 3, Ithaca, NY, 1939, Udall.
84. McKenzie E, Valberg S, Godden S, et al: Plasma and urine electrolyte and mineral concentrations in Thoroughbred horses with recurrent exertional rhabdomyolysis after consumption of diets varying in cation-anion balance, *Am J Vet Res* 63: 1053-1060, 2002.
85. Haverkort-Poels P, Joosten E, Ruitenbeek W: Prevention of recurrent external rhabdomyolysis by dantrolene sodium, *Muscle Nerve* 10:45, 1987.
86. Edwards J, Newtont J, Ramzan P, et al: The efficacy of dantrolene sodium in controlling exertional rhabdomyolysis in the Thoroughbred racehorse, *Equine Vet J* 35:707-711, 2003.
87. Waldron-Mease E: Update on prophylaxis of tying-up using dantrolene, *Proc Am Assoc Equine Pract* 25:379, 1979.

Acquired Myopathies

1. Oliver J, Hoerlein B, Mayhew I: *Veterinary neurology*, Philadelphia, 1987, WB Saunders.
2. Stashak T, editor: *Adam's lameness in horses*, ed 5, Philadelphia, 2002, Wiley-Blackwell.
3. Beech J: Chronic exertional rhabdomyolysis, *Vet Clin North Am* 13:145, 1997.
4. Clayton H: Cinematographic analysis of the gait of lame horses. V: Fibrotic myopathy, *J Equine Vet Sci* 8:297, 1988.
5. Turner A, Trotter G: Fibrotic myopathy in the horse, *J Am Vet Med Assoc* 184:335, 1984.
6. Mayhew M: *Large animal neurology*, ed 2, Philadelphia, 2009, Wiley-Blackwell.
7. Bramlage L, Reed S, Embertson R: Semitendinosus tenotomy for treatment of fibrotic myopathy in the horse, *J Am Vet Med Assoc* 186:565, 1985.
8. Colahan PT, Merritt AM, Moore JN: *Equine medicine and surgery*, ed 5, St. Louis, 1999, Mosby.
9. Schneider J, Guffy M, Leipold H: Ruptured flexor muscles in a neonatal foal, *Equine Prac* 8:11, 1986.
10. Sprinkle F, Swerczek T, Crowe MW: Gastrocnemius muscle rupture and hemorrhage in foals, *Equine Prac* 7:10, 1985.
11. Valberg S, McKinnon A: Clostridial cellulitis in the horse: a report of five cases, *Can Vet J* 25:67, 1984.
12. Rebhun W, Shin S, King J, et al: Malignant edema in horses, *J Am Vet Med Assoc* 187:732-736, 1985.
13. Ronéus B: Glutathione peroxidase and selenium in the blood of healthy horses and foals affected by muscular dystrophy, *Nord Vet Med* 31:350, 1982.
14. Hulland T: *Pathology of domestic animals*, ed 3, Orlando, Fla, 1985, Academic Press.
15. Reef V: Clostridium perfringens cellulitis and immune-mediated hemolytic anemia in a horse, *J Am Vet Med Assoc* 182:251-254, 1983.
16. Weiss D, Moritz A: Equine immune-mediated hemolytic anemia associated with Clostridium perfringens infection, *Vet Clin Pathol* 32:22-26, 2003.
17. McConnico R, Roberts M, Tompkins M: Penicillin-induced immune mediated hemolytic anemia in a horse, *J Am Vet Med Assoc* 201:1402-1403, 1992.
18. Robbins R, Wallace S, Brunner C, et al: Immune-mediated haemolytic disease after penicillin therapy in a horse, *Equine Vet J* 25:462-465, 1993.
19. King A: Studies on equine purpura hemorrhagica: 3. Morbid anatomy and histology, *Br Vet J* 105:35, 1949.
20. Krisher K, Cunningham M: Myosin: A link between streptococci and heart, *Science* 227:413, 1985.
21. Sponseller B, Valberg S, Tennent-Brown B, et al: Severe acute rhabdomyolysis associated with Streptococcus equi infection in four horses, *J Am Vet Med Assoc* 227:1800-1807, 2005: 1753-1754.
22. Kaese H, Valberg S, Hayden D, et al: Infarctive purpura hemorrhagica in five horses, *J Am Vet Med Assoc* 226:1893-1898, 2005:1845.
23. Kemp-Symonds J, Kemble T, Waller A: Modified live *Streptococcus equi* (Strangles) vaccination followed by clinically adverse reactions associated with bacterial replication, *Equine Vet J* 39:284-286, 2007.
24. Aleman M, Spier S, Wilson W. Retrospective study of Corynebacterium pseudotuberculosis infection in horses: 538 cases (1982-1993). In *Proceedings of the Fortieth Annual Convention of the American Association of Equine Practitioners* 1994;117.
25. Miers K, Ley W: Corynebacterium pseudotuberculosis infection in the horse: Study of 117 clinical cases and consideration of etiopathogenesis, *J Am Vet Med Assoc* 177:250, 1980.
26. Mullaney T, Murphy A, Kiupel M, et al: Evidence to support horses as natural intermediate hosts for Sarcocystis neurona, *Vet Parasitol* 133:27-36, 2005.

27. Edwards G: Prevalence of equine sarcocysts in British horses and a comparison of two detection methods, *Vet Rec* :115, 1984.
28. Fransen JL, Degryse AD, Van Mol KA, et al: [Sarcocystis and chronic myopathies in horses], *Berl Munch Tierarztliche Wochenschr* 100:229, 1987.
29. Tinling S, Cardinet G, Blythe L: A light and electron microscopic study of sarcocysts in a horse, *J Parasitol* 66:458, 1980.
30. Freestone J, Carlson G: Muscle disorders in the horse: A retrospective study, *Equine Vet J* 23:86-90, 1991.
31. Fayer R, Hounsel C, Giles R: Chronic illness in a sarcocystis infected pony, *Vet Rec* 113:216, 1983.
32. Traub-Dargatz J, Schlipf JJ, Granstrom D, et al: Multifocal myositis associated with Sarcocystis sp in a horse, *J Am Vet Med Assoc* 205:1574-1576, 1994.
33. Murrell K, Djordjevic M, Cuperlovic K, et al: Epidemiology of Trichinella infection in the horse: the risk from animal product feeding practices, *Vet Parasitol* 123:223-233, 2004.
34. Goedegbuure S: Spontaneous primary myopathies in domestic animals: A summary of muscle biopsies from 159 cases, *Ann N Y Acad Sci* 317:290, 1987.
35. Richey M, Holland M, McGrath C: Equine postanesthetic lameness: a retrospective study, *Vet Surg* 19:392, 1990.
36. Lindsay W, McDonell W, Bignell W: Equine post-anesthetic forelimb lameness: Intracompartmental muscle pressure changes and biochemical patterns, *Am J Vet Res* 41:1919, 1980.
37. Serteyn D, Coppens P, Mottart E: Myopathie postanesthesique equine: Mesure de parame" tres respiratoires et hemodynamiques, *Ann Med Vet* 131:123, 1987.
38. Serteyn D, Mothart E, Deby C: Equine postanesthetic myositis: A possible role for free radical generation and membrane lipoperoxidation, *Res Vet Sci* 48:42, 1990.
39. White N: Post anesthetic recumbency myopathy in horses, *Compend Contin Educ Pract Vet* 4:S44, 1982.
40. White N, Suarez M: Changes in triceps muscle intracompartmental pressure with repositioning and padding of the lowermost thoracic limb of the horse, *Am J Vet Res* 47:2257, 1986.
41. Norman W, Williams R, Dodman N, et al: Postanesthetic compartmental syndrome in a horse, *J Am Vet Med Assoc* 195:502, 1989.
42. Grandy J, Steffy E, Hodgson D: Arterial hypotension and the development of post anesthetic myopathy in halothane-anesthetized horses, *Am J Vet Res* 48:192, 1987.
43. Lindsay W, Pascoe P, McDonnell W: Effect of protective padding on forelimb intracompartmental muscle pressures in anesthetized horses, *Am J Vet Res* 46:688, 1985.
44. Lindsay W, Robinson G, Brunson P, et al: Induction of equine postanesthetic myositis after halothane-induced hypotension, *Am J Vet Res* 50:404, 1989.
45. Dodman N, Williams R, Court M, et al: Postanesthetic hind limb adductor myopathy in five horses, *J Am Vet Med Assoc* 193:83, 1988.
46. Hildebrand S, Arpin D, Howitt G, et al: Muscle biopsy to differentiate normal from malignant hyperthermia suspect horses and ponies, *Vet Surg* 17:172, 1988.
47. Griggs R: *Advances in neurology*, New York, 1977, Raven Press.
48. Court M, Engelking L, Dodman N: Pharmacokinetics of dantrolene sodium in horses, *J Vet Pharmacol Ther* 10:218, 1987.
49. Taylor P, Young S: The effect of limb position on venous and compartmental pressure in the forelimb of ponies, *J Assoc Vet Anesth* 17:35, 1990.
50. Court MH, Engelking LR, Dodman NH, et al: Pharmacokinetics of dantrolene sodium in horses, *J Vet Pharmacol Ther* 10: 218-226, 1987.
51. Azzie M: Aortic iliac thrombosis of thoroughbred horses, *Equine Vet J* 1:113, 1969.
52. Maxie M, Physick-Sheard P: Aortic-iliac thrombosis in horses, *Vet Pathol* 22:238, 1985.
53. Duggan V, Holbrook T, Dechant J, et al: Diagnosis of aorto-iliac thrombosis in a quarter horse foal using Doppler ultrasound and nuclear scintigraphy, *J Vet Int Med* 18:753-756, 2004.
54. Mayhew I, Kryger M: Aortic-iliac-femoral thrombosis in a horse, *Vet Med Small Anim Clin* 70:1281, 1975.
55. Merillat L: Thrombosis of the iliac arteries in horses, *J Am Vet Med Assoc* 104:218, 1944.
56. Tithof P, Rebhun W, Dietze A: Ultrasonographic diagnosis of aorto-iliac thrombosis, *Cornell Vet* 75:540, 1985.
57. Reef V, Roby K, Richardson D: Use of ultrasonography for the detection of aortic-iliac thrombosis in horses, *J Am Vet Med Assoc* 190:286, 1987.
58. Branscomb B: Treatment of arterial thrombosis in a horse with sodium gluconate, *J Am Vet Med Assoc* 152:1643, 1968.
59. Hilton H, Aleman M, Textor J, et al: Ultrasound-guided balloon thrombectomy for treatment of aorto-iliac-femoral thrombosis in a horse, *J Vet Intern Med* 22:679-683, 2008.
60. Gillespie J, Robinson N: *Equine Exercise Physiology* vol. 2:Davis, Calif: ICEEP 1987.
61. Harris P: *Aspects of the equine Rhabdomyolysis Syndrome*, Cambridge, 1988, Cambridge University.
62. Hill H: Selenium-vitamin E treatment of tying-up in horses, *Mod Vet Pract* 43:66, 1962.
63. Lindholm A: Glutathione peroxidase, selenium and vitamin E in blood and in relation to muscular dystrophy and tying-up in the horse. 12th Linderstrom-Lang Conference, *IVB Symposium No.* 110:62, 1982.
64. Petersson K, Hintz H, Schryver H: *Equine Exercise Physiology* vol. 3:Davis, CA.: ICEEP.
65. Ronéus B, Hakkarainen R: Vitamin E in serum and skeletal muscle tissue and blood glutathione peroxidase activity from horses with azoturia-tying up syndrome, *Acta Vet Scand* 26:425, 1985.
66. Ronéus B, Hakkarainen R, Lindholm C: Vitamin E requirements of adult standardbred horses evaluated by tissue depletion and repletion, *Equine Vet J* 18:50, 1986.
67. Ronéus B, Jonsson L: Muscular dystrophy in foals, *Zentralbl Veterinarmed [A]* 31:441, 1984.
68. Step D, Divers T, Cooper B, et al: Severe masseter myonecrosis in a horse, *JAVMA* 198:117-119, 1991.
69. Siciliano P, Perker A, Lawrence L, . J Anim Sci: *Effect of dietary vitamin E supplementation on the integrity of skeletal muscle in exercised horses* 75:1553-1560, 1997.
70. Hitt M: Oxygen-derived free radicals: Pathophysiology and implications, *Compend Contin Edu Pract Vet* 10:939, 1988.
71. Rederstorff M, Krol A, Lescure A: Understanding the importance of selenium and selenoproteins in muscle function, *Cell Mol Life Sci* 63:52-59, 2006.
72. Blood D, Henderson J, Radostits O: *Veterinary Medicine. A Textbook of the diseases of cattle, sheep, pigs and horses*, Philadelphia, 1979, Lea & Febiger.
73. Hamir A: White muscle disease in a foal, *Aust Vet J* 59:57, 1982.
74. Owen L, Moore J, Hopkins J, et al: Dystrophic myodegeneration in adult horses, *J Am Vet Med Assoc* 17:343, 1977.
75. Hegreberg G, Reed S: Muscle changes in a progressive equine myotonic dystrophy, *Acta Neuropathol* 80(4):426-431, 1990.
76. Dill S, Rebhun W: White muscle disease in foals, *Compend Contin Educ Pract Vet* 7:S627, 1985.
77. Mills P, Smith NC, Cases I, et al: Effects of exercise intensity and environmental stress on indices of oxidative stress and iron homeostasis during exercise in the horse, *Eur J Appl Physiol* 74:60, 1996.
78. Phoenix J, Edwards R, Jackson M: The effect of vitamin E analogues and long carbon chain compounds on calcium-induced muscle damage. A novel role for alpha-tocopherol, *Biochem Biophys Acta* 1097:212, 1991.

79. Jackson M: Intracellular calcium, cell injury and relationships to free radicals and fatty acid metabolism, *Proc Nutr Soc* 49: 77-81, 1990.
80. McEwen S, Hulland T: Histochemical and morphometric evaluation of skeletal muscle from horses with exertional rhabdomyolysis (tying-up), *Vet Pathol* 23:400, 1986.
81. Ronéus B, Essén-Gustavsson B: Muscle fiber types and enzyme activities in healthy foals and foals affected by muscular dystrophy, *Zentralbl Veterinarmed A* 33:1, 1986.
82. de la Rúa-Domènech R, Mohammed H, Atwill E, et al: Epidemiologic evidence for clustering of equine motor neuron disease in the United States, *Am J Vet Res* 56:1433-1439, 1995.
83. Mohammed H, Cummings J, Divers T, et al: Epidemiology of equine motor neuron disease, *Vet Res* 25:275-278, 1994.
84. Jackson C, Riis R, Rebhun W, et al: Ocular manifestations of equine motor neuron disease, *Am Assoc Equine Pract* : 225-226, 1995.
85. Weber Polack E, King J, Cummings J: Quantitative assessment of motor neuron loss in equine motor neuron disease (EMND), *Eq Vet J* 30:256, 1998.
86. Jackson C, De La Hunta A, Cummings J, et al: Spinal accessory nerve biopsy as an ante mortem diagnostic test for equine motor neuron disease, *Equine Vet J* 28:215-219, 1996.
87. Beech J. Myopathies in horses. In *Proceedings from Equine Seminar,* 1988;101.
88. Higuchi T, Ichijo S, Osame S, et al: Studies on serum and tocopherol in white muscle disease of foals, *Nippon Juigaku Zasshi* 51:52-59, 1989.
89. Craig A, Blythe L, Lassen E: Variations of serum vitamin E, cholesterol, and total serum lipid concentrations in horses during a 72-hr period, *Am J Vet Res* 50:1527, 1989.
90. Pearson EG, Snyder SP, Saulez MN: Masseter myodegeneration as a cause of trismus or dysphagia in adult horses, *Vet Rec* 156:642-646, 2005.
91. Valberg S: A review of the diagnosis and treatment of rhabdomyolysis in foals, *Annual Convention of the American Association of Equine Practitioners* :117-121, 2002.
92. McGorum B, Mayhew I, Amory H, et al: Horses on pasture may be affected by equine motor neuron disease, *Equine Vet J* 38:47-51, 2006.
93. Maylin G, Rubin D, Lein D: Selenium and vitamin E in horses, *Cornell Vet* 70:272, 1980.
94. Coffman J, Amend J, Garner H: A conceptual approach to pathophysiologic evaluation of neuromuscular disorders in the horse, *J Equine Med Surg* 2:85, 1978.
95. Genetzky R, Loparco F, Ledet A: Clinical pathologic alterations in horses during water deprivation test, *Am J Vet Res* 48:1007, 1987.
96. Robinson N, editor: *Current Veterinary Therapy in Equine Medicine*, ed 6, St. Louis, 2009, Saunders.
97. Smith B, editor: *Large Animal Internal Medicine,* ed 4, St. Louis, 2009, Mosby.
98. Hodgson D: Myopathies in the athletic horse, *Compend Contin Educ Pract Vet* 7:551, 1985.
99. Kinslow P, Harris P, Gray, et al: Influence of the oestrous cycle on electrolyte excretion in the mare, *Equine Vet J Suppl* 18: 388-391, 1995.
100. Bain F, Merritt A: Decreased erythrocyte potassium concentration associated with exercise-related myopathy in horses, *J Am Vet Med Assoc* 196:1259, 1990.
101. Beech J, Lindborg S, Braund KG: Potassium concentrations in muscle, plasma and erythrocytes and urinary fractional excretion in normal horses and those with chronic intermittent exercise-associated rhabdomyolysis, *Res Vet Sci* 55:43-51, 1993.
102. Freestone J, Gossett K, Carlson G, et al: Exercise induced alterations in the serum muscle enzymes, erythrocyte potassium and plasma constituents following feed withdrawal or furosemide and sodium bicarbonate administration in the horse, *J Vet Int Med* 5:40-46, 1991.
103. Halperin ML, Goldstein MB: *Fluid, Electrolyte, and Acid-base Physiology*, ed 3, St. Louis, 1999, Saunders.
104. Harris P, Colles C: The use of creatinine clearance ratios in the prevention of equine rhabdomyolysis: A report of four cases, *Equine Vet J* 20:459, 1988.
105. Harris P, Gray J: The use of the urinary fractional electrolyte excretion test to assess electrolyte status in the horse, *Equine Vet Educ* 4(4):162-166, 1992.
106. Carlson G: Medical problems associated with protracted heat and work stress in horses, *Compend Contin Educ Pract Vet* 5:542, 1985.
107. Fowler M: Veterinary problems during endurance trail rides, *Proc Am Assoc Equine Pract* 25:460, 1979.
108. Smith C, Wagner P: Electrolyte imbalances and metabolic disturbances in endurance, *Compend Contin Educ Pract Vet* 7:S575.
109. Mansmann R, Podkonjak K, Jackson P: Panel report: Tying-up in horses, *Mod Vet Pract* 63:919, 1982.
110. Beier RC, Norman JO: The toxic factor in white snakeroot: identity, analysis and prevention, *Vet Hum Toxicol* 32(81):85, 1990.
111. Thompson LJ: Depression and choke in a horse: Probable white snakeroot toxicosis, *Vet Hum Toxicol* 31:321-322, 1989.
112. Martin B, Terry M, Bridges C, et al: Toxicity of Cassia occidentalis in the horse, *Vet Hum Toxicol* 23:416, 1981.
113. Hintz H: Bracken fern, *Equine Prac* 12:6, 1990.
114. Adams HR: *Veterinary Pharmacology and Therapeutics, ed 8*, Philadelphia, 2001, Wiley-Blackwell.
115. Whitlock R: Feed additives and contaminants as a cause of equine disease, *Vet Clin North Am* 6:467, 1990.
116. Mollenhauer H, Rowe L, Witzel D: Effect of monensin on the morphology of mitochondria in rodent and equine striated muscle, *Vet Hum Toxicol* 26:15, 1984.
117. Muylle E, Vandenhende C, Oyaert W, et al: Delayed monensin sodium toxicity in horses, *Equine Vet J* 13:107, 1981.
118. Cassart D, Baise E, Cherel Y, et al: Morphological alterations in oxidative muscles and mitochondrial structure associated with equine atypical myopathy, *Eq Vet J* 39:26-32, 2007.
119. Votion D, Linden A, Saegerman C, et al: History and clinical features of atypical myopathy in horses in Belgium, *J Vet Int Med* 2007(21):1380-1391, 2000-2005.
120. Whitwell K, Harris P, Farrington P: An outbreak of atypical myoglobinuria, *Equine Vet J* 20:357, 1988.
121. Finno C, Valberg S, Wunschmann A, et al: Seasonal pasture myopathy in horses in the midwestern United States: 14 cases, *J Am Vet Med Assoc* 2006(229):1134-1141, 1998-2005.
122. Coffman J: Testing for Renal disease, *Vet Med Small Anim Clin* 75:1039, 1980.
123. Egyed M, Nathan A, Eilat A: Poisoning in sheep and horses caused by the ingestion of weeds sprayed with simazine and aminotriazole, *Refuah Vet* 32:59, 1975.

Pathophysiology and Treatment of Acute Laminitis

1. Johnson PJ: The equine metabolic syndrome peripheral Cushing's syndrome, *Vet Clin North Am Equine Pract* 18:271-293, 2002.
2. Parsons CS, Orsini JA, Krafty R, Capewell L, Boston R: Risk factors for development of acute laminitis in horses during hospitalization: 73 cases (1997-2004), *J Am Vet Med Assoc* 230:885-889, 2007.
3. Peloso JG, Cohen ND, Walker MA, Watkins JP, Gayle JM, Moyer W: Case-control study of risk factors for the development of laminitis in the contralateral limb in Equidae with unilateral lameness, *J Am Vet Med Assoc* 209:1746-1749, 1996.
4. Slater MR, Hood DM, Carter GK: Descriptive epidemiological study of equine laminitis, *Equine Vet J* 27:364-367, 1995.
5. Cohen ND, Parson EM, Seahorn TL, Carter GK: Prevalence and factors associated with development of laminitis in horses with duodenitis/proximal jejunitis: 33 cases (1985-1991), *J Am Vet Med Assoc* 204:250-254, 1994.

6. Cohen ND, Woods AM: Characteristics and risk factors for failure of horses with acute diarrhea to survive: 122 cases (1990-1996), *J Am Vet Med Assoc* 214:382-390, 1999.
7. Firshman AM, Valberg SJ: Factors affecting clinical assessment of insulin sensitivity in horses, *Equine Vet J* 39:567-575, 2007.
8. Vick MM, Adams AA, Murphy BA, et al: Relationships among inflammatory cytokines, obesity, and insulin sensitivity in the horse, *J Anim Sci* 85:1144-1155, 2007.
9. Geor R, Frank N: Metabolic syndrome-From human organ disease to laminar failure in equids, *Vet Immunol Immunopathol* 129(3-4):151-154, 2008.
10. Donaldson MT, Jorgensen AJ, Beech J: Evaluation of suspected pituitary pars intermedia dysfunction in horses with laminitis, *J Am Vet Med Assoc* 224:1123-1127, 2004.
11. Hood DM: The mechanisms and consequences of structural failure of the foot, *Vet Clin North Am Equine Pract* 15:437-461, 1999.
12. Kainer RA: Clinical anatomy of the equine foot, *Vet Clin North Am Equine Pract* 5:1-27, 1989.
13. Riegel RJ, Hakola SE: *Illustrated atlas of clinical equine anatomy and common disorders of the horse*, Marysville, Ohio, 1997, Equistar Publications.
14. Stokes AM, Keowen ML, Eades SC, Moore RM: *Load and thermal effects on equine digital hemodynamics measured using microspheres, ACVS Veterinary Symposium*. Chicago, 2007, Ill.
15. Allen D Jr, Korthuis RJ, Clark S: Evaluation of Starling forces in the equine digit, *J Appl Physiol* 64:1580-1583, 1988.
16. Allen D Jr, Korthuis RJ, Clark ES: Capillary permeability to endogenous macromolecules in the equine digit, *Am J Vet Res* 49:1609-1612, 1988.
17. Ratzlaff MH, Shindell RM, DeBowes RM: Changes in digital venous pressures of horses moving at the walk and trot, *Am J Vet Res* 46:1545-1549, 1985.
18. Stokes AM: *Role of endothelin in the pathogenesis of acute laminitis in horses, Dissertation*. Baton Rouge, 2003, Louisiana State University.
19. Baxter GM, Laskey RE, Tackett RL, Moore JN, Allen D: In vitro reactivity of digital arteries and veins to vasoconstrictive mediators in healthy horses and in horses with early laminitis, *Am J Vet Res* 50:508-517, 1989.
20. Baxter GM: Alterations of endothelium-dependent digital vascular responses in horses given low-dose endotoxin, *Vet Surg* 24:87-96, 1995.
21. Peroni JF, Moore JN, Noschka E, Grafton ME, Aceves-Avila M, Lewis SJ, Robertson TP: Predisposition for Venoconstriction in the Equine Laminar Dermis: Implications in Equine Laminitis, *J Appl Physiol* 100:759-763, 2006.
22. Allen D Jr, Clark ES, Moore JN, Prasse KW: Evaluation of equine digital Starling forces and hemodynamics during early laminitis, *Am J Vet Res* 51:1930-1934, 1990.
23. Obel N: *Studies on the histopathology of acute laminitis, Almquist and Wiskells*. Uppsala, 1948, Sweden.
24. Hood DM: The pathophysiology of developmental and acute laminitis, *Vet Clin North Am Equine Pract* 15:321-343, 1999.
25. Hood DM, Grosenbaugh DA, Mostafa MB, et al: The role of vascular mechanisms in the development of acute equine laminitis, *J Vet Intern Med* 7:228-234, 1993.
26. Weiss DJ, Evanson OA, McClenahan D, et al: Effect of a competitive inhibitor of platelet aggregation on experimentally induced laminitis in ponies, *Am J Vet Res* 59:814-817, 1998.
27. Weiss DJ, Evanson OA, McClenahan D, Fagliari JJ, Jenkins K: Evaluation of platelet activation and platelet-neutrophil aggregates in ponies with alimentary laminitis, *Am J Vet Res* 58:1376-1380, 1997.
28. Black SJ, Lunn DP, Yin C, Hwang M, Lenz SD, Belknap JK: Leukocyte emigration in the early stages of laminitis, *Vet Immunol Immunopathol* 109:161-166, 2006.
29. Hurley DJ, Parks RJ, Reber AJ, Donovan DC, Okinaga T, Vandenplas ML, Peroni JF, Moore JN: *Dynamic changes in circulating leukocytes during the induction of equine laminitis with black walnut extract, 8th International Equine colic research symposium*. Quebec City, 2005, Canada, pp 167-168.
30. Belknap JK, Giguere S, Pettigrew A, et al: Lamellar pro-inflammatory cytokine expression patterns in laminitis at the developmental stage and at the onset of lameness: innate vs. adaptive immune response, *Equine Vet J* 39:42-47, 2007.
31. Loftus JP, Belknap JK, Stankiewicz KM, Black SJ: Laminar xanthine oxidase, superoxide dismutase and catalase activities in the prodromal stage of black-walnut induced equine laminitis, *Equine Vet J* 39:48-53, 2007.
32. Riggs LM, Franck T, Moore JN, et al: Neutrophil myeloperoxidase measurements in plasma, laminar tissue, and skin of horses given black walnut extract, *Am J Vet Res* 68:81-86, 2007.
33. Faleiros RR, Nuovo GJ, Belknap JK: Calprotectin in myeloid and epithelial cells of laminae from horses with black walnut extract-induced laminitis, *J Vet Intern Med* 23:174-181, 2009.
34. Stokes AM, Chirgwin SR, Hanly BK, Cardinale JP, Savois DM, Liford J, Eades SC, Moore RM: *Altered laminar gene expression indicative of vascular, inflammatory and metabolic events in horses with acute laminitis, Experimental biology*. San Francisco, 2006, Calif, p 267.
35. Eaton SA, Allen D, Eades SC, Schneider DA: Digital Starling forces and hemodynamics during early laminitis induced by an aqueous extract of black walnut (*Juglans nigra*) in horses, *Am J Vet Res* 56:1338-1344, 1995.
36. Peroni JF, Harrison WE, Moore JN, et al: Black walnut extract-induced laminitis in horses is associated with heterogeneous dysfunction of the laminar microvasculature, *Equine Vet J* 37:546-551, 2005.
37. Schneider DA, Parks AH, Eades SC, Tackett RL: Palmar digital vessel relaxation in healthy horses and in horses given carbohydrate, *Am J Vet Res* 60:233-239, 1999.
38. Eades SC, Stokes AM, Johnson PJ, et al: Serial alterations in digital hemodynamics and endothelin-1 immunoreactivity, platelet-neutrophil aggregation, and concentrations of nitric oxide, insulin, and glucose in blood obtained from horses following carbohydrate overload, *Am J Vet Res* 68:87-94, 2007.
39. Eades SC, Stokes AM, Moore RM: Effects of an endothelin receptor antagonist and nitroglycerin on digital vascular function in horses during the prodromal stages of carbohydrate overload-induced laminitis, *Am J Vet Res* 67:1204-1211, 2006.
40. Loftus JP, Black SJ, Pettigrew A, et al: Early laminar events involving endothelial activation in horses with black walnut-induced laminitis, *Am J Vet Res* 68:1205-1211, 2007.
41. Bailey SR, Menzies-Gow NJ, Harris PA, et al: Effect of dietary fructans and dexamethasone administration on the insulin response of ponies predisposed to laminitis, *J Am Vet Med Assoc* 231:1365-1373, 2007.
42. Pass MA, Pollitt S, Pollitt CC: Decreased glucose metabolism causes separation of hoof lamellae in vitro: a trigger for laminitis? *Equine Vet J Suppl* :133-138, 1998.
43. Kim JA, Montagnani M, Koh KK, Quon MJ: Reciprocal relationships between insulin resistance and endothelial dysfunction: molecular and pathophysiological mechanisms, *Circulation* 113:1888-1904, 2006.
44. Yin C, Pettigrew A, Loftus JP, et al: Tissue concentrations of 4-HNE in the black walnut extract model of laminitis: Indication of oxidant stress in affected laminae, *Vet Immunol Immunopathol* 129(3-4):211-215, 2008.
45. Asplin KE, Sillence MN, Pollitt CC, McGowan CM: Induction of laminitis by prolonged hyperinsulinaemia in clinically normal ponies, *Vet J* 174:530-535, 2007.
46. Pollitt CC: Equine laminitis: a revised pathophysiology, *Proceedings Am. Assoc. Equine Pract* 45:188-192, 1999.

47. Pollitt CC, Daradka M: Equine laminitis basement membrane pathology: loss of type IV collagen, type VII collagen and laminin immunostaining, *Equine Vet J, Suppl* 26:139-144, 1998.
48. Pollitt CC, Davies CT: its development coincides with increased sublamellar blood flow, *Equine Vet J Suppl* :125-132, 1998:Equine laminitis.
49. Kyaw-Tanner MT, Wattle O, van Eps AW, Pollitt CC: Equine laminitis: membrane type matrix metalloproteinase-1 (MMP-14) is involved in acute phase onset, *Equine Vet J* 40:482-487, 2008.
50. Pollitt CC: Basement membrane pathology: a feature of acute equine laminitis, *Equine Vet J* 28:38-46, 1996.
51. Johnson PJ, Tyagi SC, Katwa LC, Ganjam VK, et al: Activation of extracellular matrix metalloproteinases in equine laminitis, *Vet Rec* 142:392-396, 1998.
52. Garner HE, Moore JN, Johnson JH, et al: Changes in the caecal flora associated with the onset of laminitis, *Equine Vet J* 10:249-252, 1978.
53. Mungall BA, Kyaw-Tanner M, Pollitt CC: In vitro evidence for a bacterial pathogenesis of equine laminitis, *Vet Microbiol* 79:209-223, 2001.
54. Garner HE, Hutcheson DP, Coffman JR, et al: Lactic acidosis: a factor associated with equine laminitis, *J Anim Sci* 45: 1037-1041, 1977.
55. Loftus JP, Belknap JK, Black SJ: Matrix metalloproteinase-9 in laminae of black walnut extract treated horses correlates with neutrophil abundance, *Vet Immunol Immunopathol* 113: 267-276, 2006.
56. van Eps AW, Pollitt CC: Equine laminitis: cryotherapy reduces the severity of the acute lesion, *Equine Vet J* 36:255-260, 2004.
57. Ingle-Fehr JE, Baxter GM: The effect of oral isoxsuprine and pentoxifylline on digital and laminar blood flow in healthy horses, *Vet Surg* 28:154-160, 1999.
58. Weiss DJ, Geor RJ, Burger K: Effects of pentoxifylline on hemorheologic alterations induced by incremental treadmill exercise in thoroughbreds, *Am J Vet Res* 57:1364-1368, 1996.
59. Barton MH, Ferguson D, Davis PJ, Moore JN: The effects of pentoxifylline infusion on plasma 6-keto-prostaglandin F1 alpha and ex vivo endotoxin-induced tumour necrosis factor activity in horses, *J Vet Pharmacol Ther* 20:487-492, 1997.
60. Barton MH, Moore JN: Pentoxifylline inhibits mediator synthesis in an equine in vitro whole blood model of endotoxemia, *Circ Shock* 44:216-220, 1994.
61. Barton MH, Moore JN, Norton N: Effects of pentoxifylline infusion on response of horses to in vivo challenge exposure with endotoxin, *Am J Vet Res* 58:1300-1307, 1997.
62. Baskett A, Barton MH, Norton N, et al: Effect of pentoxifylline, flunixin meglumine, and their combination on a model of endotoxemia in horses, *Am J Vet Res* 58:1291-1299, 1997.
63. Chilcoat CD, Rowlingson KA, Jones SL: The effects of cAMP modulation upon the adhesion and respiratory burst activity of immune complex-stimulated equine neutrophils, *Vet Immunol Immunopathol* 88:65-77, 2002.
64. Liska DA, Akucewich LH, Marsella R, et al: Pharmacokinetics of pentoxifylline and its 5-hydroxyhexyl metabolite after oral and intravenous administration of pentoxifylline to healthy adult horses, *Am J Vet Res* 67:1621-1627, 2006.
65. Fugler LA: *Matrix metalloproteinases in the equine systemic inflammatory response: implications for equine laminitis. Electronic thesis and dissertation collection*, Baton Rouge, La, 2009, Louisiana State University.

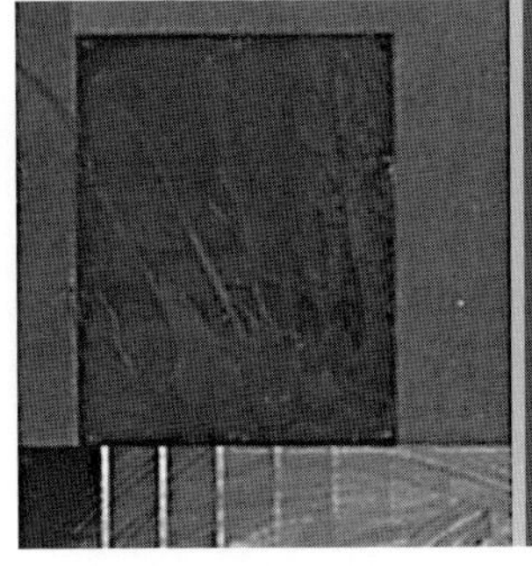

Disorders of the Neurologic System

CHAPTER 12

Stephen M. Reed, Frank M. Andrews

NEUROLOGIC EXAMINATION

Stephen M. Reed

Assessment of the central nervous system (CNS) in horses may seem a difficult task; however, with careful examination using a craniocaudal approach, assessment is not difficult. A craniocaudal approach is the most logical and efficient. The examination focuses on the neuroanatomic localization of the lesion or lesions and should be completed as part of the physical examination. Subtle neurologic deficits may be hidden by musculoskeletal disease or missed because of lack of knowledge or understanding of these disorders. To accomplish a complete and accurate neurologic examination, the veterinarian must feel comfortable with the format chosen for evaluating the nervous system and must have knowledge of which musculoskeletal disorders commonly are associated with neurologic disease. Problems such as osteochondrosis of the stifle, hock, and shoulder joints often occur concurrently in horses with cervical vertebral stenotic myelopathy.

Examples of typical histories in horses presented for neurologic examination, especially for signs of spinal ataxia, include previous medial patellar desmotomy, bilateral bog spavin in early life, osteochondrosis of the distal tibia or femur, and contracted tendons. All of these problems associated with developmental orthopedic diseases are examples of conditions that may occur simultaneously. Bilateral bog spavin often is associated with osteochondrosis of the distal tibia or other sites in the tibiotarsal joint. Patellar desmotomy to correct upward fixation of the patella may be necessary because of a conformational problem of the stifle joint or as a result of abnormal joint proprioception or quadriceps weakness after neurologic disease. The foregoing problem is more commonly associated with neurologic disease than many veterinarians realize, and the gait deficits caused by these lamenesses often mimic neurologic disease. Horses with bilateral osteochondritis dissecans (OCD) lesions of the stifle joints will often "bunny-hop" while running, which may be interpreted as a sign of neurologic disease rather than as a result of an underlying musculoskeletal disease.

The goals of a neurologic examination are to establish whether a neurologic problem is present and to determine the anatomic localization of the problem. Being able to account for all clinical signs with a single lesion is ideal; however, if this is not possible, then one should consider the possibility of multifocal disease or multiple diseases. In addition to anatomic localization of a lesion, it is important to record the findings of the examination as a baseline for comparison of future evaluations. After anatomic localization, one must decide what additional testing is necessary to determine the underlying cause of the clinical signs. Cervical radiography, cerebrospinal fluid (CSF) analysis, and electrodiagnostic testing may be useful in locating and determining the cause of the lesions.

The neurologic examination should be considered part of the physical examination. The author prefers to begin the examination at the head and proceed caudally to the tail. The examiner should proceed in a consistent fashion and should record findings in an orderly manner to avoid any part of the examination being omitted. Figure 12-1 shows a sample format. One may use the craniocaudal approach for all animals, whether ambulatory or recumbent.

The equine neurologic examination procedure has been described in detail elsewhere.[1-13] The author follows the format developed by Mayhew,[1] which divides the examination into five categories: (1) the head and mental status, (2) gait and posture, (3) neck and forelimbs, (4) trunk and hindlimbs, and (5) tail and anus. The functional divisions of the nervous system include the sensory, integration, and motor systems.

Before starting the examination, one should know the age, gender, breed, and use of the horse, although these are not essential. This information is useful because horses of various breeds behave differently. One should ask the owner about any unusual behavior the horse has exhibited and the date of onset of the behavior. Age is helpful because problems such as cervical vertebral stenotic myelopathy and cerebellar abiotrophy begin at a young age, usually less than 1 year. These problems occur more often in certain breeds. For example, cervical vertebral stenotic myelopathy is most common in Thoroughbreds, and cerebellar abiotrophy most often is observed in Arabians.

EXAMINATION

The evaluation of the head should include observation of the horse at rest and during motion; palpation, postural reactions, cranial nerve function, and cervicofacial reflexes; and evaluation of sensation. At the start of the examination the horse should be observed for alertness, mentation, attitude, and behavior (remembering that the animal's environment may influence its degree of excitement). Evaluation of the head includes observation of the behavior and mental status of the horse. One can complete this portion of the examination by careful observation even before handling the horse. A close and careful examination is necessary to evaluate the head and neck posture and coordination and to identify abnormalities of the cranial nerves. Initial consideration includes the environmental awareness of the horse. A normal horse appears bright and alert and responds appropriately to external stimuli. While the horse is being caught, the examiner can look for unusual behaviors such as yawning, abnormal or aimless wandering, seizures, or circling or head tilt and can begin to assess the vision and hearing of the horse. This is also a good time to observe how the horse is

NEUROLOGIC EXAMINATION

Date: ______
Sire ______
Dam ______
Dam's sire ______

History ______

General observations ______

CRANIAL NERVE EXAMINATION:

Menace (2, 7)	______	Facial symmetry:	______
Pupil size (2, 3, sym.)	______	Temporal/masseter (5)	______
Pupil symmetry (3, sym.)	______	Expressive muscles (7)	______
PLR (2, 3)	______	Palpebral reflex (5, 7)	______
Doll's eye (8, 3, 4, 6)	______	Retractor oculi (5, 6)	______
Ocular position (8, 3, 4, 6)	______	Gag reflex (9, 10)	______
Pathologic nystagmus	______	Tongue (12)	______

Symmetry of neck/body (muscle mass, scoliosis, etc.) ______

Manipulation of the neck L/R ______
up/down ______

Spontaneous involuntary movements (tremor, myoclonus, myotonia, etc.) ______

Description of gait (at walk and trot) ______

Circling	large L	______		
	R	______		
	small L	______		
	R	______		
Backing		______		
Up/down an incline		______		
Elevation of head		______		
Proprioception	LF	______	RF	______
	LR	______	RR	______
Sway reaction	fore	______		
	rear	______		
	tail pull	______		

Grading System—write in grading according to deLahunta
0 = No gait deficits
1 = Deficits barely perceptible—worsened with head elevation
2 = Deficits noted at a walk
3 = Deficits noted at rest, walking; nearly falls with head elevation
4 = Falls or nearly falls at normal gaits
5 = Recumbent patient

FIGURE 12-1 Example of a neurologic examination form. *PLR,* Pupillary light response.

Gait and posture (graded 0 to +4)

	Motor		Sensory
	Weakness	Spasticity	Ataxia
LF			
RF			
LR			
RR			

Reflexes Anal ______
Patellar ______
Triceps ______
Other ______

Nociceptive (withdrawal) ______

Tail tone ______

Autonomic Urinary ______
Rectal ______
Sweating ______

Cutaneous sensation ______

Assessment/comments ______

Lesion localization ______

Tentative DX ______

CSF	Cells	Protein	Culture	Cytology
L/S				
A/O				

Radiographs ______

Myelogram ______

Comments ______

FIGURE 12-1, cont'd.

standing and whether it has the limbs positioned appropriately under its body. The veterinarian should note any behavioral abnormalities, such as head pressing (a clear sign of cerebral disease) and aggressiveness (noted in animals that are not feeling well, as well as animals with CNS disease). If the examiner suspects rabies, then the examiner should take precautions to avoid unnecessary and potentially dangerous exposure.

Lesions of the reticular activating system or the cerebral hemispheres could result in coma or obtundation of consciousness. Horses demonstrating compulsive walking may have a diffuse cerebral disease, whereas a horse walking in large circles may have an asymmetrical forebrain lesion. Horses that have a serious systemic illness also may appear depressed or stuporous. One records the level of consciousness as *alert, depressed, stuporous, semicomatose,* or *comatose.* An animal that is depressed may react to its environment in an inappropriate or unresponsive fashion. Stuporous horses may appear to be asleep unless stimulated with pain, light, or noise and often demonstrate impaired reactivity.

Head posture and coordination are controlled by the cerebellar and vestibular regions of the brain and brainstem in response to sensory input from receptors in the head, limbs, and body. Examining the head and neck posture with the horse at rest, while eating, and while moving is helpful. In horses with normal head carriage, the head should be held straight and upright when viewed from the front. Head posture and coordination are controlled by the vestibular and cerebellar systems in response to sensory input from the head, neck, limbs, and trunk. Careful examination of the vestibular region is important because many horses develop a head tilt resulting from head trauma, temporohyoid osteoarthropathy (THO), or a guttural pouch infection. A head tilt is characterized by the poll deviated about the muzzle and must be distinguished from abnormal or unusual turning of the head or lateral deviation of the head as may occur with damage to the forebrain or injury to the cervical vertebrae. Additional signs that may accompany vestibular disease or injury include nystagmus, ipsilateral weakness, and facial nerve paralysis.

Postural abnormalities of the head and neck sometimes can be difficult to distinguish from head tilt. Horses with torticollis of the head and neck may have a congenital abnormality of the vertebrae or may have injured the muscles of the neck region. Damage to the dorsal gray columns can result in abnormal head and neck posture (acquired scoliosis) that has been described as a result of parasitic migration such as *Parelaphostrongylus tenuis*.[4] Careful examination, including palpation, should help identify fractures of the cervical vertebrae or painful muscles caused by trauma or an injection reaction. Neck pain may manifest as a reluctance to move the head and neck through a full range of motion. In the absence of pain or mechanical limitations to movement, normal horses should be able to turn their head to retrieve feed offered at the lateral thorax on each side, elevated to a level above the withers, or lowered to a point between the front legs just beneath the pectoral muscles. In some horses, radiographs of the cervical vertebrae may be useful to confirm a fracture or osteomyelitis. Blindness sometimes can lead to an abnormal head or neck posture.

The cerebellum helps regulate rate and range of motion. With damage to this area a horse often shows fine resting tremors of the head that worsen with intentional movements.[3] One may normally observe this tremorous movement of the head and neck in the newborn or young foal, but it is not normal in older foals and adult horses. In young Arabians and a few other breeds, a condition of cerebellar abiotrophy has been reported.[1-3] Horses with this condition show a hyper metric gait, failure to blink when exposed to bright light, and absence of a menace response.

After evaluating the alertness, mental attitude, head and neck posture, and coordination of the horse, the examiner should examine the cranial nerves closely. Systematic examination of the first to twelfth cranial nerves helps to ensure that a subtle lesion along the brainstem is less likely to be missed, although in fact the examiner assesses many of the cranial nerves simultaneously on approach to the horse. The examiner evaluates facial symmetry, facial sensation (including sensation inside the nares), head posture, eyes, nose, mouth, jaw tone, pharynx, and larynx. To determine if an animal can detect scent is usually not as important, but determining if it can see, hear, breathe, and swallow is critical.

Examination of the eyes should include evaluation of the blink or menace response, the ability of the horse to negotiate in a strange environment, pupillary light response, and in some cases a funduscopic examination. If a horse has a lesion of the eye or optic nerve, then the lesion will result in complete or partial ipsilateral blindness. To develop contralateral blindness, the horse would have to have a lesion in the optic tract or the lateral geniculate nucleus.[1]

Examination of the face should include evaluation of pupil size and symmetry, which are under control of the autonomic nervous system and are affected by environmental light and level of fear or excitement. To test the pupillary response, one should direct a light in each eye and note the constriction of the pupil. Identifying a consensual response in the horse is often difficult when one works alone. A swinging light test has been described.[1] In the performance of this test, the light is shone alternately into each eye and the more powerful direct pupillary light response is observed. A unilateral lesion affecting the afferent tracts in the eye, optic nerve, optic chiasm, or optic tract to the level of the midbrain will result in ipsilateral dilation when the light reaches the affected eye. Moving the light from side to side takes advantage of the ipsilateral light response being stronger than the consensual response. The examiner can perform this procedure alone. These reflexes are in the brainstem and are not affected by lesions in the visual cortex.

One possible cause of asymmetrical pupils in a horse is Horner's syndrome. Horner's syndrome is the collection of clinical signs associated with dysfunction of the sympathetic nerve supply to the head and neck. The sympathetic nerve supply to the head includes upper motor neurons in the caudal hypothalamus, parts of the midbrain and pons, as well as parts of the medulla oblongata. Axons from these centers descend in the cervical spinal cord to the preganglionic neurons in the cranial thoracic spinal cord. From here, preganglionic axons leave the cord and join the paravertebral sympathetic trunk, where they ascend up the neck to synapse in the cranial cervical ganglion in the guttural pouch.[4] This syndrome includes ptosis of the upper eyelid, miosis of the pupil, and protrusion of the third eyelid (nictitating membrane). In addition, the horse has unilateral facial sweating, increased facial temperature, and hyperemia of the nasal and conjunctival membranes. These signs should alert the examiner to the possibility of a previous perivascular injection, a guttural pouch infection, or damage to the sympathetic nerves in the vagosympathetic trunk, which courses from the cranial thoracic spinal cord through the thoracic inlet and upward to the orbit.[5] Loss of sympathetic innervation to the head results in the triad of clinical signs described, with the most prominent initial sign being increased sweating, which is not what one would expect and the exact cause of which is not well understood.[6,7]

Loss of symmetrical positioning of the eyes or the presence of abnormal deviation (i.e., strabismus) occurs when a horse has injured the third (oculomotor), fourth (trochlear), or sixth (abducens) cranial nerve or the connections between the eighth (vestibulocochlear) cranial nerve and these nuclei in the brainstem along the medial longitudinal fasciculus. Deviations of the eyes may occur with head trauma or midbrain lesions or can be normal variations in newborn foals. When the head is elevated dorsally, the eyes should move ventrally to maintain a normal horizontal gaze. When the head is moved from side to side, the eyes should move slowly opposite to the direction of the head movement, then move quickly in the direction of the head movement; this is referred to as *normal vestibular nystagmus*. Spontaneous or positional nystagmus is always abnormal.

The nuclei along the fifth (trigeminal) cranial nerve are among the largest nuclei along the brainstem of the horse. The fifth cranial nerve contains motor and sensory branches that supply innervation to the muscles of mastication and sensation to the skin and mucous membranes of the head. Injury to this nerve leads to dropped jaw and ipsilateral loss of, or decreased sensation to, the side of the face and the inside of the nares.

Damage to the seventh (facial) and eighth cranial nerves is common in horses. Injury to the seventh cranial nerve results in unilateral facial paralysis. This nerve contains branches that supply the ears, eyelids, and nares, and so injury to this nerve may affect all or only part of these structures. The most easily recognized sign is deviation of the nares toward the unaffected side coupled with drooping of the eyelid and ear on the affected side. Because this nerve also innervates the salivary and lacrimal glands, loss of or damage to this nerve may cause dry eye and decreased salivation.

Eighth cranial nerve deficits are easy to recognize, because unilateral injury to this nerve results in a head tilt toward the affected side. The eighth cranial nerve is important to hearing and control of balance. Projections from this nerve pass to the medulla and cerebellum. A horse that has damage to this nerve often appears disoriented and has a head tilt toward the side of the lesion along with abnormal position of the limbs and body and horizontal nystagmus. If the lesion involves the peripheral portion of the vestibular system, then the fast phase of the nystagmus is directed away from the side of the lesion. If the lesion involves the central portion of the vestibular system, then the nystagmus may appear vertical, rotary, or horizontal and may not always appear the same, depending on head position.

Horses that have peripheral damage to the vestibular system usually compensate for the deficits in a short time by use of visual and proprioceptive input. Therefore avoiding the use of a blindfold in cases of suspected vestibular disease is judicious. Using a blindfold hampers the ability of the horse to compensate, and the horse may become dangerous. However, blindfolding a horse with a suspected vestibular disease, but no longer showing an obvious head tilt, may be helpful to localize the lesion.

Within the medial compartment of the guttural pouch, along the caudodorsal and lateral walls, are the ninth (glossopharyngeal) cranial nerve and a branch of the vagus nerve. When a horse develops a guttural pouch infection, these nerves may be damaged, resulting in loss of innervation to the pharyngeal muscles. The clinical signs include dysphagia on the same side as the damaged nerve. If the infection is severe enough to involve the internal carotid nerve, which contains postganglionic sympathetic fibers to the structures of the head and eye, then Horner's syndrome results. As mentioned previously, the signs include ptosis of the upper eyelid, enophthalmos resulting in prolapse of the third eyelid, miosis of the pupil, and sweating along the side of the face.

Other diseases one should consider when Horner's syndrome is evident during a neurologic examination include injury or infarction to the cranial thoracic spinal cord, avulsion of the brachial plexus, a hematoma, or tumor invading the sympathetic trunk in the region of the caudal, cervical, or cranial thoracic sympathetic trunk. Mycosis of the guttural pouch can cause damage to the internal carotid nerve or the cranial cervical ganglion along the caudodorsal wall of the guttural pouch. Finally, an injury to or neoplasia of the structures within or just behind the orbit also may cause Horner's syndrome.

Focal sweating in a horse indicates involvement of the peripheral pre- or postganglionic sympathetic neurons. Identification of this problem also can aid in the anatomic localization of a neurologic lesion.[1]

Intact innervation to the larynx and pharynx is important, especially if the horse is to be used as an athlete. The easiest means to evaluate this region is by endoscopic examination of the pharyngeal and laryngeal regions. One can perform throat latch palpation and a laryngeal adductory slap test. Endoscopic examination is helpful and important to a complete evaluation. The innervation of the pharynx and larynx is via the ninth, tenth (vagus), and eleventh (accessory) cranial nerves and the connections of these nerves in the caudal medulla oblongata.

The twelfth cranial nerve, the hypoglossal nerve, has cell bodies in the hypoglossal nucleus of the caudal medulla oblongata and provides motor innervations to the muscle of the tongue. Normal horses provide a strong resistance to withdrawing the tongue from the mouth; horses with unilateral cranial nerve XII dysfunction have unilateral atrophy with weak retraction. Bilateral dysfunction interferes with prehension and swallowing, the tongue often protrudes from the mouth, and the horse has difficulty or is unable to withdraw the tongue. Severe cerebral leseions may also interfere with tongue retraction because of interference with voluntary control pathways.

After careful examination of the mental status and behavior of the horse and of the head, neck, and cranial nerves, the examiner should look for asymmetry of the muscles of the trunk, pelvic region, tail, and anus. Identification of focal sweating, focal muscle atrophy, or increased or decreased pain responses is helpful in localizing signs. In addition, the horse has two cervical reflexes. The cervicofacial reflexes result in a local twitch and drawing back of the lips (smile reflex) when one pricks the skin along the side of the neck down to the region of the second cervical vertebra. Below the region of the second cervical vertebra one should observe a local response.[14]

To evaluate the tail and anus, one should begin by observing the tail carriage at rest and with the horse in motion. The normal tail carriage is straight down but with free movement in all directions. Some normal horses allow the tail to be lifted, giving little resistance, whereas other horses strongly resist and clamp the tail. The usual response to anal stimulation is to clamp the tail and squat down, although with prolonged stimulation the horse may relax and eventually raise its tail.

Evaluation of Gait

Evaluation of the gait of the horse should include examination of postural reactions and may include evaluation of spinal reflexes in young or small horses. Although they may appear weak and ataxic, foals are ambulatory within hours after birth, making it possible to evaluate gait. Because postural reactions are sometimes difficult to interpret in horses, using gait abnormalities to help localize a lesion is essential. The author nearly always places the feet and limbs in an unusual position to observe the response of the horse. Gait abnormalities that are observed commonly in horses with neurologic disease include ataxia, spasticity, and weakness or paresis.[1-3,4,15,16]

Evaluation of gait is critical because subtle neurologic gait deficits often go unrecognized or sometimes, incorrectly, may be considered insignificant. One should conduct the examination to observe the horse at a walk and trot in a straight line and while turning. In some horses, observing the horse negotiate over small obstacles such as a curb is helpful. When possible, the examiner should observe the horse turned free and walking up and down an incline. Elevation of the head and walking on a slope may exaggerate a subtle deficit and make it more noticeable.

One should include in the examination observation of the horse at rest to observe its posture while standing, walking, trotting when possible, and sometimes while the horse is being ridden. The examiner should pay attention to which limbs show abnormal posture or abnormal movements and must be able to determine whether the horse has a painful or mechanical musculoskeletal problem or a neurologic gait deficit. The examiner must identify the presence of weakness, ataxia, and spasticity in each limb.

The important centers for posture and coordination in the brainstem and spinal cord are located in the regions of the sixth cervical to second thoracic (T2) and fourth lumbar to second sacral (S2) vertebrae in the spinal cord, along with coordination centers in the brainstem. Horses that demonstrate a wide base stance at rest often have a lesion of the cerebellum or vestibular system or may have conscious proprioceptive abnormalities.

To evaluate the gait of an animal, one begins by observing the horse at a walk and trot. At a walk the examiner can walk alongside, in step with first the pelvic limbs and then the thoracic limbs. This allows the examiner to more easily determine the stride length and foot placement. A weak limb often has a low arc and longer stride length.

One also should observe the horse walking in a circle, on a slope, and with its head elevated. These procedures provide a degree of "challenge" to the horse and may help to demonstrate if the horse is showing persistent irregular movements with its limbs. Horses with a musculoskeletal problem have been described as being a regularly irregular gait, whereas a horse with neurologic gait deficits shows less consistency placing its limbs (an irregularly irregular gait). Although observing the horse running free in a paddock or round pen and while being ridden can sometimes be helpful, this is not always possible. One must consider safety for the horse and rider, as well as certain legal ramifications before asking a person to ride a horse during the examination.

Additional tests that may be helpful during a neurologic examination include blindfolding the horse, walking it over a curb or other obstacle, and walking it with its head and neck extended. One can evaluate the strength and ability of the horse to correct body positions by performing a sway test by applying lateral pressure at the shoulder, hip, and tail while the horse is standing and walking. One should apply pressure several times while the horse is walking to catch the limb in various stages of weight bearing. Observing a horse during the backing process is important. When a normal horse is backing, it should lift each leg and place it in a coordinated and appropriate location. Horses with neurologic abnormalities often place the limbs in wide-based positions or lean back and are reluctant or refuse to move. The horse also may step on the feet of a pelvic limb with the front feet.

The horse should be observed closely while being turned in a tight circle to identify abnormal wide outward excursions of the pelvic limb (circumduction). Additional tests to assess proprioceptive function include a standing sway test in which one applies pressure to the shoulder. The horse initially should press into the examiner and then lean away, and finally it should step away with the offside limb. The author also crosses the limbs over the opposite thoracic or pelvic limb to determine if the horse recognizes and tolerates these unusual limb positions. After this, the examiner might lift one thoracic limb and force the horse to hop on the opposite limb in a modified postural reaction.

The examiner should observe the movements of each limb carefully to determine if a deficit is present and should assign a grade to the deficit. The author uses a system modified from the grades described by deLahunta[3] and Mayhew.[1] The severity is graded between 0 and 5. Grade 0 means no gait deficits. A grade 1 deficit requires careful observation to be certain the gait abnormality is caused by a neurologic dysfunction. Grade 2 deficits are mild to moderate but obvious to most observers as soon as the horse begins to move. Grade 3 deficits are obvious and are exaggerated during the negotiation of a slope or with head elevation. Grade 4 gait deficits may cause a horse to fall or nearly fall. When attempting to walk, an animal with these severe deficits often displays abnormal positioning while standing in its stall. Grade 5 horses are recumbent.

Weakness or paresis is a deficiency of voluntary movement as a result of loss of muscle power because of either damage to upper motor neurons, lower motor neurons, or the muscle. It can be described as knuckling, stumbling, or buckling and sometimes can be characterized by toe-dragging while walking. Weakness may be associated with an upper motor neuron or lower motor neuron lesion. In the case of a lower motor neuron or peripheral nerve injury or illness, the horse shows muscle atrophy and sensory loss. A spastic movement of the limbs often accompanies the weakness that results from loss of upper motor neurons. Ataxia is typified by abnormal foot placement and wide swaying of the foot and limb, especially while turning. Ataxia appears as a lack of coordination of motor movements. It can arise from damage to the vestibular, cerebellar, or sensory portions of the nervous system. Ataxia in horses is most often a result of loss of sensory input through injury, damage, or disease in the spinal cord blocking normal input to the cerebellum. Cerebellar ataxia is seen most often in young horses, typically Arabians with a condition known as *cerebellar abiotrophy*. Vestibular ataxia is often accompanied by a head tilt and other cranial nerve deficits.

Horses may also demonstrate dysmetria, which is characterized as exaggerated hypermetric or hypometric movements of the limbs. Horses with hypometric gaits often appear to have a straight leg or "tin soldier" way of moving (sometimes referred to as *spasticity*). A spastic gait is the result of increased muscle tone and is generally associated with upper motor neuron disease resulting from reduced inhibition of extensor motor neurons.

The gait abnormalities, along with the findings from other parts of the neurologic examination, allow the examiner to determine the neuroanatomic site of the problem. The severity of the clinical signs also helps one evaluate the extent or severity of the problem.

One should reexamine horses with an obscure or unusual gait that might be the result of lameners after the use of local anesthetics (to block selected peripheral nerves) or intra-articular medications. The use of nonsteroidal anti-inflammatory drugs (NSAIDs) for a period of 1 to 2 days also may alleviate pain and help one distinguish between lameness and a neurologic gait deficit.

One must realize that many horses that have minimal (grade 1 or mild grade 2) deficits often can race or perform other athletic activities.[13] The examining veterinarian has the responsibility of separating a neurologic from a musculoskeletal gait deficit and helping the owner determine the usefulness of the horse. For example, a horse with gait deficits up to grade 3 may be useful as a broodmare or breeding stallion (if the horse is handled by careful, knowledgeable persons who understand the risks and have the facilities to accommodate a horse in need of special management). Stallions with this degree of impairment may require assistance when mounting and dismounting mares. If the breed association allows artificial insemination, then the stallion may be easier to manage.

Localization of the Lesion

At the conclusion of the examination, the veterinarian needs to determine if a neurologic abnormality exists and where it is located. If the horse showed no evidence of abnormal behavior, seizures, or abnormal mental status and showed no cranial nerve deficits, then the lesion is most likely caudal to the foramen magnum.

The most difficult lesions to localize are in the brainstem, unless the signs include cranial nerve deficits or depression. Horses with brainstem lesions often show signs of weakness and ataxia similar to horses with a lesion in the cervical spinal cord. Two of the most common brainstem lesions in horses involve the seventh and eighth cranial nerves. Vestibular disease or injury may be a sequela of head trauma or an inner ear infection. Facial nerve paralysis may result from trauma to the nerve root origin in the brainstem or where the nerves course along the neck and face to the ears, eyelids, and nares.

Specific cranial nerve involvement, such as head tilt, facial nerve paralysis, or loss of facial sensation, can result from trauma, guttural pouch infection, THO, or equine protozoal encephalomyelitis. In addition, cranial nerve deficits may occur with polyneuritis equi and equine motor neuron disease (EMND).

Cerebellar lesions are characterized by a failure to blink to bright light, lack of a menace response, and a head tremor that worsens with intentional movements. The most common form of cerebellar disease in horses is abiotrophy, which occurs most frequently in Arabian horses.

Cervical spinal cord disease includes gait and proprioceptive deficits in all four limbs with no signs of brain, brainstem, or cranial nerve deficits. One should note that horses with cervical vertebral stenotic myelopathy might have mild pelvic limb deficits with minimal or barely detectable signs in the thoracic limbs.[16]

Horses with signs of neurologic gait deficits confined to the pelvic limbs have a neuroanatomic localization caudal to T2. When examining a horse with a lesion caudal to T2, carefully checking the tail and anus for involvement of the peripheral nerves or spinal cord segments in this region is important.

Horses that have peripheral nerve injury (Table 12-1), EMND, or polyneuritis equi show evidence of weakness, muscle atrophy, and in some cases selected areas of sensory loss. Primary muscle diseases such as exertional rhabdomyolysis, myotonia (congenita or dystrophica), and hyperkalemic periodic paralysis are covered elsewhere in this book (see Chapter 11). These conditions sometimes can mimic a neurologic problem.

Description of Normal Gaits

A walk is a natural four-beat gait in the horse. At this gait the normal horse has three feet on the ground at all times. Therefore the walk is a stable gait. Overtracking and interference may occur if the conformation of the horse is abnormal (e.g., with long limbs and a short body) and not as a result of neurologic disease.[11] The trot is a two-beat symmetrical gait in which the diagonal limbs are in contact with the ground at the same time. If one examines the horse on hard pavement, then the trot is the most helpful gait to distinguish lameness from a neurologic gait deficit. The pace is a two-beat symmetrical gait in which the legs on the same side of the body strike the ground simultaneously, resulting in significant truncal sway. In horses that have neurologic disease, identifying ataxia with truncal sway, which is often accompanied by pacing, is common. In horses with subtle ataxia, one observes pacing when horses walk with the head held in an extended position. Whenever one observes a horse pacing, the pacing may indicate an underlying neurologic disorder.

The gallop is a high-speed four-beat gait that often seems to be easier to perform than walking in a tight circle or moving at a slow trot. Therefore some horses with a neurologic gait deficit may perform better at high speed. As the horse accelerates or slows down, one may detect abnormalities, and one must observe the horse carefully at this time when an ataxic horse is most unsafe.

Abnormal gaits associated with stringhalt, upward fixation of the patella, and fibrotic myopathy deserve careful attention. Horses that show these gait abnormalities have a mechanical lameness, although the exact cause is unknown and may sometimes be associated with underlying neurologic disease.

Stringhalt often begins as an abrupt onset of excessive flexion of one or both rear limbs. In some horses the condition may worsen and result in frequent episodes of the foot hitting the abdomen. The condition has been reported for a long time and in some areas of the world may occur as an outbreak.[17] The clinical syndrome is similar to the movement of a horse with a tibial neurectomy with unopposed flexion of the hock and extension of the digit. In the case of Australian stringhalt, the forelimbs and neck muscles may be involved. Stringhalt deserves mention in this chapter because when the examiner observes this gait, the examiner should be certain no other signs of neurologic gait deficits exist. The primary condition usually can be corrected by a tenectomy of the lateral digital extensor tendon, including a portion of the muscle belly. The underlying cause of the disease may be a sensory neuropathy, a myopathy, or primary spinal cord disease. The defect likely affects the neuromuscular spindle, as well as the efferent and afferent pathways controlling muscle tone.[10]

Fibrotic myopathy results from scar tissue formation after injury to the semitendinosus and semimembranosus muscles. One may confuse the characteristic foot placement coupled with the abrupt rearward movement of the affected limb with a spastic gait caused by spinal cord injury (SCI) or disease. With careful examination, a horse suffering from fibrotic myopathy likely will not go undiagnosed.

Upward fixation of the patella in horses with neurologic disease may result from weakness in the quadriceps muscle group. This weakness is thought to occur because of a lack of use of these muscles or may be caused by abnormal transmission of proprioceptive information to and from the muscles and joint capsule because of damage to the spinal cord.

Horses with profound ataxia may pace when they walk, which often is accompanied by circumduction of the outside rear limb while turning. These signs suggest general proprioceptive deficits. If the horse has these deficits while walking, then the examiner should observe the horse walking with its

TABLE 12-1

Localization of peripheral nerve injuries in horses

Nerve	Clinical Signs	Common Causes of Injury
Suprascapular	Injury is termed sweeney. Eventual atrophy of supraspinatus and infraspinatus muscles. Lateral subluxation (popping) of the shoulder upon weight bearing. This may be caused by lack of lateral collateral support (suprascapular muscles) or by additional involvement of the pectoral nerve, subscapular nerve, caudal cervical nerve roots, or other muscular and tendinous supporting structures of the shoulder.	Collision of shoulder with objects.
Radial	Unable to bear weight on affected limb because of a lack of elbow extension. The shoulder is rested in an extended position and the limb rests with the dorsum of the pastern on the ground. The limb may be moved forward by the action of the pectoral girdle muscles while the horse walks.	Often damaged in conjunction with humeral fracture; Occasionally observed after recovery from general anesthesia.
Brachial plexus	Signs of radial nerve paralysis often predominate. Evidence of suprascapular involvement not uncommon. Involvement of other nerves and nerve roots may be confirmed with EMG. Possible long-term atrophy of triceps. May have diffuse hypalgesia of lower limb.	Compression of the brachial plexus and radial nerve roots between the scapula and the ribs.
Musculocutaneous	Paralysis not common. Gait not markedly altered. Elbow may be overextended. Hypalgesia of medial forearm. Ultimately biceps and brachial muscles atrophy.	Uncommon.
Median and ulnar	Stiff, goose-stepping gait with hyperextension of the carpal, fetlock, and pastern joints.	Uncommon.
Femoral	Unable to support weight as a result of lack of stifle extension. At a walk, the limb is advanced only with difficulty and the stride is markedly shortened. The limb buckles due to stifle, hock, and fetlock flexion if the horse attempts to bear weight. Quadriceps muscle will atrophy after 10-14 days. Patellar reflex is absent.	External blow to the limb; occasionally observed after recovery from general anesthesia.
Sciatic	Poor limb flexion with stifle and hock extended and fetlock flexed when the horse is not bearing weight. Weight can be supported if the foot is extended; otherwise weight is supported on the dorsal surface of the foot. Limb hypalgesia from stifle downward with the exception of the medial surface between stifle and hock.	Variety of injuries may be causal. Occasionally occurs secondary to intramuscular injections, especially in foals; occasionally observed after recovery from general anesthesia.
Tibial	Hypermetric or stringhalt-like gait with flexion of the hock (dropped hock) at rest. Hypalgesia of areas of caudal limb distal to the hock including most of the caudal and medial coronary band area.	Uncommon.
Peroneal	Frequently a component of sciatic nerve injury. Inability to flex the hock and extend the digits. Acutely there is hyperextension of the hock and hyperflexion of the fetlock and interphalangeal joints causing the horse to drag the fetlock along the ground. Short protraction phase to the stride. If the foot is placed in a normal position, the limb may bear weight. Hypalgesia of the craniolateral portion of the limb from the level of the hock to the fetlock.	Accessible to injury as it passes across the lateral surface of the tibia. Injury seen in horses after recovery from general anesthesia or secondary to a kick or blow to the lateral side of the pelvic limb.

head elevated and on a slope (these maneuvers often exaggerate a subtle problem).

If the horse shows signs only in the trunk and pelvic limbs, the neuroanatomic localization of the lesion is between T2 and S2 or involves the nerves and muscles of the pelvic limbs. However, horses with cervical spinal cord lesions often demonstrate signs in the pelvic limbs that are one grade worse than those observed in the thoracic limbs. Therefore a mild cervical spinal cord or brainstem lesion could show minimal or no thoracic limb signs with grade 1 or subtle signs in the pelvic limbs.

Palpating the horse over its back, rump, and muscles of the rear limbs while being careful to detect any muscle atrophy is helpful. The author routinely stimulates the horse over the side of its body and observes for any twitching of the cutaneous trunci muscles. Such twitching usually is accompanied by a cerebral response and requires a fairly severe lesion to detect areas of analgesia.

A sway reaction performed while the horse is standing and walking is also necessary to assess the pelvic limb strength and proprioceptive functions. In addition, one may evaluate strength by slow but deliberate and forceful pressure along the back and sacral muscles. A normal horse should reflexively arch its back upward, whereas a horse with rear limb weakness may be unable to withstand this pressure and its rear limbs may even buckle.

To complete the neurologic examination, one must examine the tail and anus to determine whether damage has occurred to the sacrococcygeal nerve and muscle segments. A normal perineal reflex results in contraction of the anus and clamping of the tail in response to light stimulation of the skin in this region. Cauda equina neuritis or polyneuritis equi, trauma, and iatrogenic injury resulting from an alcohol tail block are some disorders that may affect this area.

The evaluation of the major peripheral nerves in the horse is also an important part of the neurologic examination (Table 12-1). The important points to remember are that damage to a peripheral nerve can result in sensory and motor deficits in the area supplied by the nerve and that focal muscle atrophy follows within a short time after damage to one of these nerves. The examiner is referred to other portions of this book for a more detailed anatomic description of these nerves in the horse; however, a dropped elbow joint with radial nerve paralysis, inability to fix the stifle with femoral nerve paralysis, and atrophy of the supraspinatus and infraspinatus muscles (sweeney) with damage to the suprascapular nerve are classic examples of what to expect with peripheral nerve injuries.[1-3]

CONCLUSION

For a horse to be a good athlete, it must gather information from muscles, tendons, and nerves; process this information in the brain, brainstem, and spinal cord; and relay this information to the musculoskeletal system. The horse must accomplish all of this in a short time to perform complex maneuvers at a high rate of speed. When performing in a setting involving many other horses or when a rider or driver is involved, the horse needs to be able to control these movements in a coordinated fashion to protect itself, other horses, and especially those persons handling, riding, or driving the horse.

Beyond this, veterinarians must recognize which musculoskeletal and neurologic conditions occur together in order to assist prospective buyers with horse-purchasing decisions. Recognizing and understanding these things helps the veterinarian determine whether a particular horse with subtle neurologic gait deficits caused by trauma, infection, or compression may still be a safe and useful athlete.

CEREBROSPINAL FLUID EVALUATION

Frank M. Andrews

Cerebrospinal fluid evaluation has diagnostic importance regarding neurologic disease in horses. Collection and analysis of CSF is indicated to make or confirm a diagnosis of neurologic disease, but this is not without limitations. CSF values may be normal in an animal with severe neurologic deficits because the lesion is extradural, collection occurred early or late in the course of disease, collection occurred too far from the lesion, or the ventral roots and peripheral nerve have been affected by the disease. Even with its limitations, CSF provides valuable information about the CNS. However, one must emphasize that CSF evaluation is another piece of the diagnostic puzzle and together with the history, physical examination, neurologic examination, and other ancillary procedures may help in the diagnosis and prognosis of neurologic disease in horses.

FORMATION, FLOW, AND FUNCTION OF CEREBROSPINAL FLUID

CSF is an actively transported ultrafiltrate of plasma that bathes the CNS.[1] The CSF is located in the ventricles of the brain and subarachnoid space of the spinal canal (Figure 12-2) and originates from the choroid plexus and ependymal lining of the ventricles.[2] CSF flows from the ventricular system up and over the cerebral hemispheres and through the subarachnoid space surrounding the spinal cord.[1] Pulsation of blood in the choroid plexuses forces the CSF in a caudal direction. The rate of CSF production varies between 0.017 ml/min in cats to 0.5 ml/min in human beings[3] and is independent of the blood hydrostatic pressure. The rate of CSF production for horses has not been determined. Osmotic and hypertonic solutions such as mannitol and dimethyl sulfoxide (DMSO), when added to blood, decrease CSF production and decrease CSF pressure and edema.[1]

Collections of arachnoid villi (arachnoid granulations) are located in the venous sinus or the cerebral vein and absorb CSF. CSF absorption is related directly to the pressure gradient between the CSF and venous sinus. When CSF pressure exceeds venous pressure, these villi act as one-way ball valves, forcing CSF flow to the venous sinus.[4]

CSF functions to suspend the brain and spinal cord for protection, regulate intracranial pressure, and maintain the proper ionic and acid-base balance.[1]

COLLECTION OF CEREBROSPINAL FLUID

Techniques for collecting CSF in horses have been described in detail elsewhere.[1-5] One may collect CSF from the lumbosacral site in a standing horse sedated with an intravenous injection of 0.2 to 0.5 mg/kg xylazine or 0.01 to 0.02 mg/kg butorphanol (or a combination of both drugs). Alternatively, one can collect CSF from the atlantooccipital site of an anesthetized horse. In foals and recumbent adult horses, one can collect CSF while the animal is restrained and heavily sedated with 1.0 mg/kg xylazine and 0.2 mg/kg butorphanol, both administered intravenously. If the lesion is localized to an area above the foramen magnum (at least cranial to the second cervical vertebra), then CSF collected from the atlantooccipital site will be more diagnostic. If the lesion is localized to an area below the foramen magnum (caudal to the second cervical vertebra), then CSF collected from the lumbosacral site will be more diagnostic. These differences result from the craniocaudal circulation of CSF. Collecting CSF from both sites at the same time and comparing the findings may be helpful in cases in which neuroanatomic localization of the lesion is difficult.[5]

EXAMINATION OF CEREBROSPINAL FLUID

Reference values for CSF in horses have been reported,[6-11] but each laboratory should determine its own reference ranges. CSF determinations that are helpful in evaluating horses with

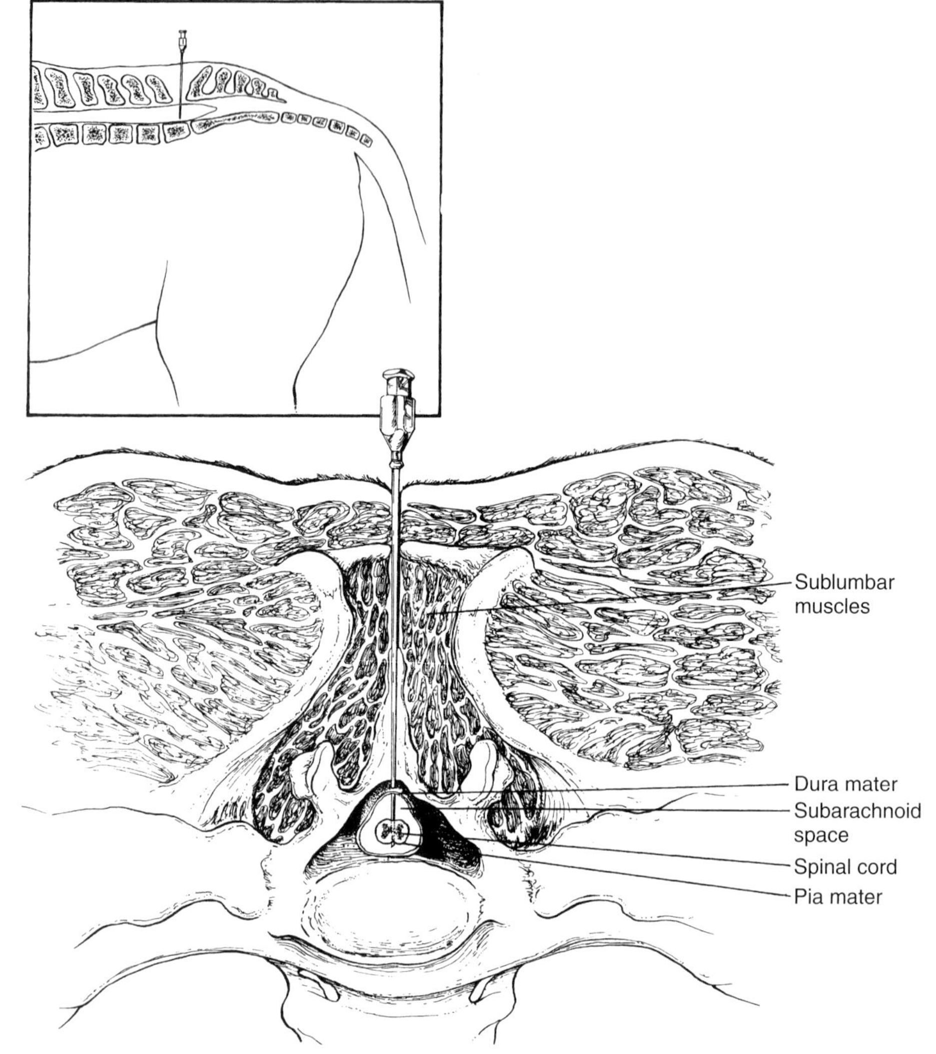

FIGURE 12-2 Lumbosacral spinal fluid collection from a horse showing the various tissue layers that the spinal needle must pass through to obtain a sample. The spinal fluid is collected ventral to the spinal cord in the subarachnoid space. *Inset,* Lateral view of spinal needle placement in the lumbosacral space for collection of cerebrospinal fluid (CSF). (From deLahunta A, Glass EN: Veterinary neuroanatomy and clinical neurology, ed 3, St Louis, 2009, WB Saunders.)

neurologic diseases include pressure, appearance, cellular content, protein concentration (total protein, albumin, immunoglobulin G [IgG]), enzyme activity (creatine kinase [CK], aspartate aminotransferase [AST], lactate dehydrogenase), and lactic acid concentration.

Pressure

One can measure opening CSF pressure before withdrawal of CSF by attaching a manometer tube with a three-way stopcock to a properly placed spinal needle, allowing the CSF to rise within it.[12] Because the cranial and vertebral cavities are enclosed in a rigid bony compartment, changes in blood pressure or volume can cause a concomitant increase in CSF pressure. Thus increased CSF pressure may occur from venous compression or jugular occlusion. Venous compression causes increased blood volume in the cranial cavity and compression of the CSF space, leading to increased CSF pressure. One can use jugular occlusion clinically to increase CSF pressure and facilitate collection of CSF fluid.[13] The jugular compression maneuver, or Queckenstedt's phenomenon, can help one diagnose compressive lesions, neoplastic lesions, or an abscess along the spinal cord. With compression and obliteration of the subarachnoid space by a compressive lesion in the cervical or thoracic spinal cord, jugular vein compression does not cause a CSF pressure increase in the lumbosacral site.[1]

Increased CSF pressure may occur after injury, after systemic changes in blood pressure, and in the presence of an intracranial space-occupying mass such as a tumor, abscess, hemorrhage, or edema. One must provide an adequate airway after injury and during surgery to prevent hypoxia-mediated cytotoxic cerebral edema and vasogenic cerebral edema.[14] Cytotoxic edema is caused by inadequate cerebral oxygenation and leads to neuronal, glial, and endothelial cell swelling. Such reactions are especially important during long surgical procedures or recumbency in which respiratory hypoxia and poor alveolar ventilation (hypercapnia) may occur. Hypercapnia increases cerebral blood flow in the cranial cavity and CSF pressure and may worsen existing cerebral edema.[1]

Increased CSF volume may occur in hydrocephalus, which is defined as an increased volume of CSF and can be classified as *compensatory* or *obstructive*.[15] Compensatory hydrocephalus is an accumulation of CSF in areas in which brain tissue has been destroyed and may occur from brain injury or inflammation. Hydranencephaly is destruction of brain tissue from a viral or other infectious agent and results in severe accumulation of CSF.[15] CSF pressure in compensatory hydrocephalus usually does not increase.[1]

Obstructive hydrocephalus is an accumulation of CSF in the ventricles from an obstruction to CSF outflow or absorption. Cerebral aqueduct malformation may lead to obstruction of ventricular CSF outflow. Inflammatory lesions, especially of the arachnoid villi, result in decreased absorption of CSF and increased CSF pressure. The white matter is affected more severely than the gray matter in obstructive hydrocephalus, but the cerebral cortex usually is spared.[1] CSF pressure in obstructive hydrocephalus usually increases. The presence of an abnormally high opening pressure that drops by 25% to 50% after removing 1 to 2 ml of fluid suggests a space-occupying intracranial mass or spinal cord compression cranial to the site of collection. The removal of more fluid would risk causing tentorial herniation.[12]

Appearance

One can evaluate the appearance of CSF immediately after collection. Normal CSF is clear and colorless and does not clot, and newsprint is visible through it.[16] CSF may be red tinged from blood contamination after a traumatic tap or from preexisting trauma to the CNS. In the case of a traumatic tap, the CSF usually will clear if allowed to flow for several seconds (about 0.5 to 1.0 ml). With preexisting trauma and secondary hemorrhage, the supernatant of CSF after centrifugation is xanthochromic.

Other causes of CSF xanthochromia include increased protein concentration (150 mg/dl)[16] and direct bilirubin leakage from serum in horses with high serum bilirubin concentration. In addition, indirect bilirubin may leak across a damaged blood-brain barrier. Clots in the CSF are abnormal and may be caused by increased amounts of fibrinogen resulting from inflammation.[1]

Turbid CSF may indicate an increased number of white blood cells (>200/μl), an increased number of red blood cells (RBCs) (>400/μl), epidural fat, bacteria, fungal elements, or amebic organisms.[1] Cytologic evaluation and cultures can help differentiate causes of turbidity.

Cytologic Evaluation

One can use a standard hemocytometer to obtain a complete blood count (CBC). In addition, a sedimentation chamber requiring 0.5 to 1.0 ml of CSF is a rapid method for cytologic evaluation.[17] One must perform cell counts and cytologic evaluation within 30 minutes to avoid degeneration. If cell counts or cytologic evaluation cannot be performed immediately, then one can mix a portion of the sample with an equal volume of 50% ethanol to preserve cellular characteristics.[12] CSF from normal horses and foals usually contains fewer than 10 white blood cells per microliter. However, much variation occurs in CSF white blood cell counts in horses.[9,10]

Most studies show no differences in white blood cell counts in normal CSF samples obtained from the atlantooccipital space as compared with samples obtained from the lumbosacral space.[10] However, one study did show a slightly higher total white blood cell count in CSF obtained from the lumbosacral site, but white blood cell counts in all of those horses were less than 10 per microliter.[6]

Small mononuclear cells (70% to 90%) and large mononuclear cells (10% to 30%) predominate in equine CSF. Rarely, one may see neutrophils in horse CSF. Increased CSF large mononuclear phagocytes are visible in horse CSF in diseases of axonal degeneration.[9] One may see increased CSF neutrophil numbers in encephalomyelitis, bacterial meningitis, parasitism, and diseases with extensive inflammation. Occasionally, in severe inflammatory diseases of the neurologic system or parasitism, eosinophils may be visible.[9,17,18] In some cases, cytologic evaluation of CSF may reveal specific agents causing neurologic disease such as fungal organisms,[16] bacteria, or tumor cells. Although CSF cytologic examination may support a diagnosis of neurologic disease, it may not yield a specific causative diagnosis.

Protein Concentration and Composition

Normal total protein values range between 20 to 124 mg/dl, depending on the measuring method used[1,6-10] (Table 12-2). Total protein concentration is higher in lumbosacral CSF compared with atlantooccipital CSF.[6] A difference of 25 mg/dl of protein between the atlantooccipital and lumbosacral spaces may suggest a lesion closer to the space with greater spinal fluid protein.[10] Proteins in the CSF are derived from the peripheral blood and include albumin, IgG, and possibly other globulins. Increased CSF albumin and IgG concentrations may occur with damage to the blood-brain barrier or increased intrathecal production of IgG. One can determine CSF albumin and IgG concentrations by electrophoresis and radial immunodiffusion, respectively, and can compare these with serum concentrations.[6] Special low-level radial immunodiffusion plates (VMRD Inc, Pullman, WA) are available to quantify CSF IgG concentration. One can calculate the albumin quotient (AQ) ([Albc]/[Albs] × 100) and IgG index ([IgGc]/[IgGs] × [Albs]/[Albc]) to determine blood-brain barrier permeability and intrathecal IgG production.[6] Increased intrathecal IgG production (increased IgG index) may occur in inflammatory spinal cord disease such as equine protozoal myeloencephalitis (EPM), bacterial meningitis, some tumors, and EMND. Increased blood-brain barrier permeability (increased AQ) may occur in equine herpesvirus-1 (EHV-1) after necrotizing vasculitis.[7] Determining blood-brain barrier integrity is also important in planning therapy. If the blood-brain barrier is damaged, then pharmacologic agents such as penicillin that do not normally penetrate the blood-brain barrier will penetrate a disrupted blood-brain barrier and attain bactericidal CSF concentration.

Enzyme Determination

CSF enzyme activity may be increased in neurologic disease. CK and AST activity may be increased in diseases with myelin degeneration and neuronal cell damage such as EPM, polyneuritis equi, equine degenerative myelopathy, and EMND. Increased CK activity also may occur in conditions that alter blood-brain barrier permeability, such as EHV-1. In diseases in which the blood-brain barrier is damaged, serum CK can leak

TABLE 12-2

Cerebrospinal Fluid Values from Atlantooccipital and Lumbosacral Spaces of Normal Healthy Adult Horses*

	Atlantooccipital Space (Mean ± SD [Range])	Lumbosacral Space (Mean ± SD [Range])
Red blood cell (RBC) count (per μl)	51.0 ± 160 (0-558)	36.8 ± 59.7 (0-167)
White blood cell count (per μl)	0.33 ± 0.49 (0-1)	0.83 ± 1.11 (0-3)
Total protein (mg/dl)*	87.0 ±± 17.0 (53 ± 11.6) (59-118) (35-74)	93.0 ± 16.0 (58.0 ± 11.0) (65-124) (39-78)
Albumin (mg/dl)	35.8 ± 9.7 (24-51)	37.8 ± 11.2 (24-56)
Albumin quotient (AQ)	1.4 ± 0.4 (1.0-2.0)	1.5 ± 0.4 (1.0-2.0)
Immunoglobulin G (IgG) (mg/dl)	5.6 ± 1.4 (3-8)	6.0 ± 2.1 (3-10)
IgG index	0.19 ± 0.046 (0.12-0.27)	0.19 ± 0.5 (0.12-0.26)
Creatine kinase (CK) (IU/L)	0-8	0-8
Lactate dehydrogenase (IU/L)	0-8	0-8
Aspartate aminotransferase (AST) (IU/L)	4-16	0-16
Glucose (mg/dl)	35%-70% of blood glucose	
Lactate (mg/dl)	1.92 ± 0.12	2.30 ± 0.21
Sodium (mEq/L)	140-150	140-150
Potassium (mEq/L)	2.5-3.5	2.5-3.5

*Total protein concentration next to the mean ± SD in parentheses is the value expected using a total protein standard.

into the CSF and increase CSF CK activity. This increased CK activity is not associated with damaged myelin.

Increased CK activity also may suggest other diseases of the CNS. In one study, CK activity (>1 IU/L) most often was associated with EPM in horses and may be helpful in differentiating compressive spinal cord disease from EPM. Furthermore, persistently increased CSF CK activity may be associated with a poor prognosis in horses with EPM.[19] Lactate dehydrogenase activity may be increased in spinal lymphosarcoma.

Lactic Acid Concentration

CSF lactic acid concentration may be an indicator of neurologic disease (see Table 12-2). CSF lactic acid concentration increases in eastern equine encephalomyelitis (4.10 ± 0.6 mg/dl), head trauma (5.40 ± 0.9 mg/dl), and brain abscess (4.53 mg/dl). Lactic acid concentration may be the only CSF parameter increased in horses with brain abscess.[20]

SUMMARY

Normal CSF findings do not always rule out the presence of neurologic disease. CSF values may be normal with lesions outside the CNS that are not bathed in the CSF, such as extradural, ventral root, and peripheral nerve lesions. Normal CSF values also may occur early or late in the disease process and in CSF samples obtained from a site distant from the lesion. Acute neurologic disease, especially if multifocal, may not have sufficient time to cause significant damage to the blood-brain barrier and alter CSF constituents, whereas in chronic CNS disease the blood-brain barrier may be repaired and functional but with nervous tissue replaced by fibrous tissue. Fibrosis of nervous tissue may result in significant neurologic gait deficits and normal CSF constituents. CSF taken away from the site of the lesion shows normal findings despite significant neurologic gait deficits. For example, CSF in a horse with a cervical spinal cord abscess may show a suppurative inflammation in the lumbosacral CSF and a normal atlantooccipital CSF. This discrepancy is caused by the caudad flow of CSF.

CSF may be helpful in supporting the diagnosis of neurologic disease in horses and is part of the diagnostic workup. Because CSF evaluation is an ancillary diagnostic test, one should use it with, and not as a substitute for, a thorough history, physical examination, neurologic examination, and other diagnostic tests.

ELECTRODIAGNOSTIC AIDS AND SELECTED NEUROLOGIC DISEASES

Frank M. Andrews, V.A. Lacombe

Localizing lesions to and within the nervous system can be difficult in some horses using only clinical and neurologic examinations. Generally, neurologic disease is characterized by changes in cell electric activity; because electric activity has amplitude and frequency, one can measure it by electronic equipment. The observed electric activity may be helpful in defining and localizing lesions of the nervous system.

Electromyography (EMG), auditory brainstem response (ABR) testing, and electroencephalography (EEG) are electrodiagnostic aids that may be helpful in the localization, diagnosis, and prognosis of neurologic disease in horses. Needle EMG and nerve conduction studies are helpful in localizing and defining diseases of the lower motor neuron or motor unit. ABR testing is helpful in localizing lesions to cranial nerve VIII and auditory pathways along the brainstem. EEG is helpful in diagnosing focal and diffuse intracranial lesions. Use of these diagnostic aids as an extension of the neurologic examination, separately or collectively, can provide valuable information about nervous system function and help in diagnosing neurologic disease. These techniques are noninvasive and in many cases can be done on the awake horse with mild sedation. Even when these techniques do not provide the information necessary to arrive at a diagnosis, they may provide a more complete understanding of the disease process.

ELECTROMYOGRAPHY

Needle EMG is the graphic recording of muscle cell electric activity during contraction or at rest from a recording electrode placed in the muscle. Electric activity is recorded by means of an amplifier on an oscilloscope.[1-3] Nerve conduction studies consist of stimulating a peripheral nerve with electric current and recording the resultant physiologic electric activity from other segments of the nerve or from the muscles innervated by those nerves.[4] Together, EMG and nerve conduction studies may help in the localization, diagnosis, and prognosis of diseases of the lower motor unit. The motor unit consists of the ventral horn cell bodies (located in the ventral horn of the spinal cord), its axon, the peripheral nerve, the myoneural junction, and the muscle fibers it innervates (Figure 12-3).

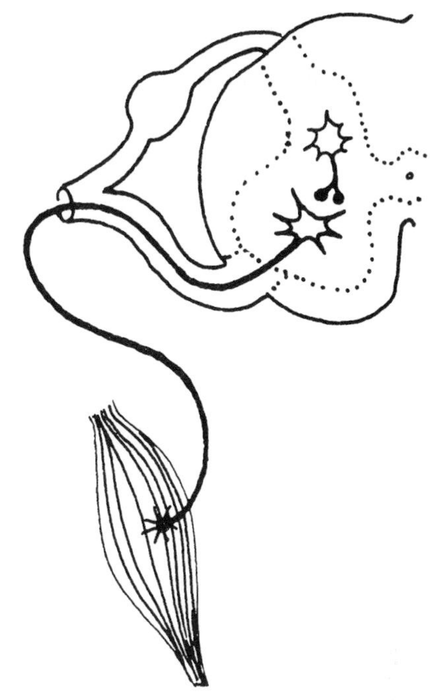

FIGURE 12-3 Illustration of the motor unit, including the ventral horn cell in the spinal cord, ventral root, peripheral nerve, neuromuscular junction, and muscle.

Electromyographic Examination

A history and physical and neurologic examination always should precede the EMG examination; these aid in localizing the lesion, shortening the examination time, and minimizing trauma to the horse. Initially, one examines the standing horse that is under mild sedation. One can tranquilize the horse with 0.2 to 0.5 mg/kg xylazine administered intravenously or 0.2 to 0.5 mg/kg xylazine and 2 to 10 mg butorphanol administered intravenously. Examination of the awake horse aids in evaluating individual motor unit action potentials (MUAPs), summated MUAPs, and interference pattern. One can evaluate normal and abnormal MUAPs and measure their amplitudes. Unfortunately, in the awake horse an interference pattern (many MUAPs) sometimes can obscure abnormal low-amplitude EMG potentials. In this case, further examination may require general anesthesia.

In the needle EMG examination, one should thrust the exploring electrode briskly into the muscle and hold it until the animal completely relaxes. To enable relaxation, one can force the animal to bear weight on the opposite limb. Once relaxation has occurred, one can evaluate the resting activity or any postinsertional activity of the muscle. One should evaluate at least four areas and depths of smaller skeletal muscles and six to eight areas and depths of larger skeletal muscles when possible. One should examine the horse systematically so as not to miss a lesion. Needle EMGs can also be performed in many of the major extrinsic muscles of the horse (Table 12-3). In addition, they can be performed on facial, laryngeal, esophageal, pectoral, and external anal sphincter muscles when indicated by neurologic examination. One may perform nerve conduction studies and collect muscle biopsy specimens to define suspected lesions further or confirm a diagnosis.

Nerve Conduction Studies

The evaluation of nerve conduction velocities requires knowledge of the topographic anatomy of nerves and muscles, plus a stimulator capable of delivering up to 150 V at durations of 0.1 to 3.0 ms at variable frequencies, up to 100 Hz. Most standard EMGs have built-in stimulators with adequate parameters to do nerve conduction studies. The peripheral nerve to be assessed can be located by palpation or by anatomic landmarks and then can be stimulated. One can palpate or observe the resultant muscle contraction and can view the evoked muscle action potential, which has a thumping sound, on the oscilloscope.

Nerve conduction studies are difficult to do in horses and therefore are not done routinely. However, the technique for radial and median nerve conduction studies in the horse has been reported.[5,6] One must perform nerve conduction studies with the horse under general anesthesia and may use them to evaluate the speed of conduction of large myelinated motor nerves. To do this, the horse should be placed in lateral recumbency, with the affected side up. One stimulates the appropriate motor nerve by monopolar needle electrodes inserted at or near the nerve and records an evoked MUAP from an innervated muscle (Figures 12-4 and 12-5). The examiner may see or palpate the contraction of appropriate muscles and insert needle electrodes until a repeatable response is obtained. The unaffected limb can be used as a control.

In horses, one can obtain radial nerve recordings from the extensor carpi radialis and abductor digiti longus (extensor carpi obliquus) muscles (see Figure 12-4) and can obtain median nerve recordings from the humeral and radial heads of the deep digital flexor tendon[5,6] (see Figure 12-5). Facial nerve recordings can be obtained from the levator nasolabialis muscle by stimulating the buccal branch of the facial nerve

TABLE 12-3

Muscles, Nerves, and Nerve Roots Evaluated during Routine Electromyographic Examination of Horses

Muscles	Peripheral Nerve	Spinal Nerve Root
REAR LIMB		
Long digital extensor	Peroneal nerve	L6-S1
Gastrocnemius	Tibial nerve	S1-S2
Deep digital flexor	Tibial nerve	S1-S2
Semimembranosus	Ischiatic nerve	L5-S2
Vastus lateralis	Femoral nerve	L3-L5
Biceps femoris	Caudal gluteal, ischiatic, and peroneal nerves	L6-S2
Middle gluteal	Cranial and caudal gluteal nerves	L5-S2
PARAVERTEBRAL		
Paravertebral muscles (segmentally)	Dorsal branches of ventral spinal nerves (L6-C1)	L6-C1
THORACIC LIMB		
Subclavius	Pectoral nerve	C6-C7, T1
Supraspinatus	Suprascapular nerve	C6-C8
Infraspinatus		
Deltoideus	Axillary nerve	C6-C8
Biceps brachii	Musculocutaneous nerve	C6-C8
Triceps	Radial nerve	C7-T1
Extensor carpi radials	Radial nerve	C7-T1
Superficial digital flexor	Ulnar nerve	C8-T2
Deep digital flexor	Ulnar and median nerve	C7-T1, T2

just ventral to the facial crest.[7] Often a supramaximal stimulus can be obtained at 70 to 90 V for 0.1-ms duration. Nerve conduction studies are helpful in diagnosing radial nerve, median nerve, and possibly facial nerve injury.

NORMAL ELECTROMYOGRAPHIC POTENTIALS

Normally occurring EMG potentials and nerve stimulation studies are described next. One can examine the muscle at rest, under submaximal contraction, under maximal contraction, and after direct nerve stimulation.

Insertional Activity

Insertional activity consists of short bursts of high-amplitude, moderate- to high-frequency (<200 Hz) electric activity after insertion or movement of the exploring electrode in the muscle (Figures 12-6 and 12-7). In normal skeletal muscle this activity stops a few milliseconds after cessation of needle movement. Insertional activity may be caused by mechanical stimulation, muscle fiber injury,[3,8,9] or depolarization of muscle fibers directly adjacent to the EMG needle.[1] Positive sharp waves and fibrillation potentials observed during (or associated with) needle insertion that stop after cessation of needle movement are considered normal. Damage to muscle fibers by needle insertion is probably the source of these potentials. However, positive sharp waves and fibrillation potentials persisting after needle insertion are considered abnormal and may suggest early muscle denervation.[3]

Resting Activity (Postinsertional Baseline)

Resting activity is observed in relaxed muscle and is characterized by electric silence. A flat line appears on the oscilloscope. When the needle comes to rest near a nerve twig or end plate, the needle may irritate small intramuscular nerve terminals, which results in the production of two characteristic potentials: (1) end plate noise and (2) end plate spikes. End plate noise produces a rippling of the baseline and a low-pitched continuous noise (Figure 12-8). End plate spikes, on the other hand, are high-amplitude intermittent spikes and make a popping sound. End plate noise and spikes can occur alone or together. The origin of end plate noise is thought to be extracellularly recorded miniature end plate potentials,[10,11] whereas end plate spikes are thought to be single muscle fiber contractions after needle electrode irritation of the nerve terminals.[11] In human beings, these potentials are associated with dull pain[3]; repositioning the needle often eliminates their activity.

Motor Unit Action Potentials

Motor unit action potentials (MUAPs) are voluntary or reflex muscle contractions observed after insertion of the needle electrode. They represent the sum of a number of single muscle fiber potentials belonging to the same motor unit. MUAPs are usually monophasic, biphasic, and triphasic. Because individual muscle fibers fire nearly synchronously, the prefixes refer to the number of phases above and below the baseline (see Figure 12-7). A few polyphasic potentials

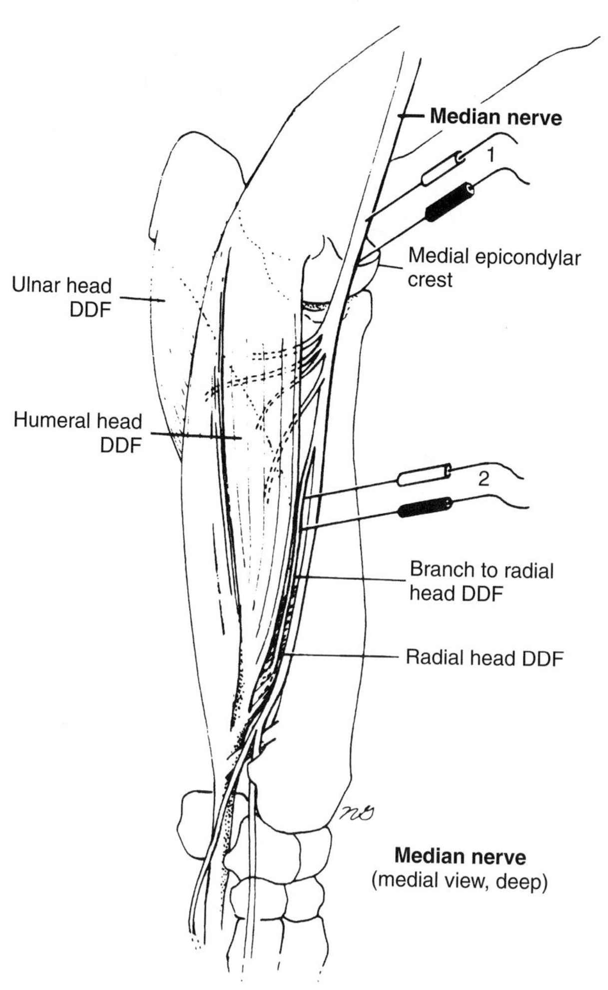

FIGURE 12-4 Illustration of anatomy and electrode placement used in median nerve conduction velocities. *DDF,* Deep digital flexor. (From Henry RW, Diesem CD, Wiechers MD: Evaluation of equine radial and median nerve conduction velocities, Am J Vet Res 40:1406–1410, 1979.)

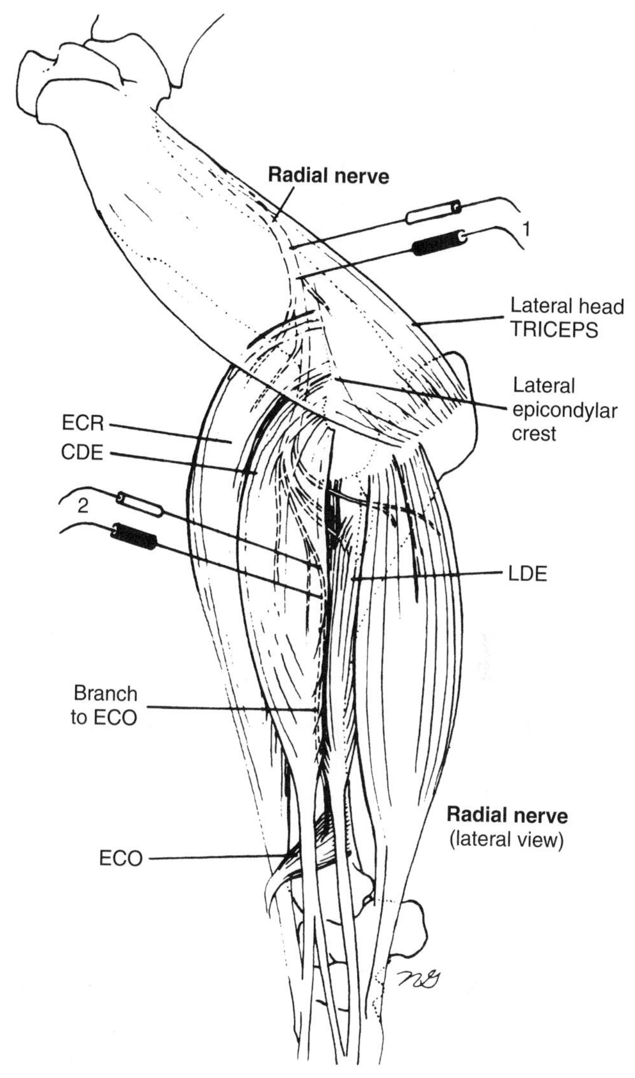

FIGURE 12-5 Illustration of anatomy and electrode placement used in radial nerve conduction velocities. *ECR,* Extensor carpi radialis; *CDE,* common digital extensor; *LDE,* long digital extensor; *ECO,* extensor carpi obliquus. (From Henry RW, Diesem CD, Wiechers MD: Evaluation of equine radial and median nerve conduction velocities, Am J Vet Res 40:1406–1410, 1979.)

(greater than four phases) may occur in normal muscle but usually do not exceed 5% to 15% of the population of MUAPs observed.[3] MUAPs have an amplitude ranging between 500 to 3000 μV and a duration ranging between 1 to 15 ms. Examination of the conscious horse enhances the evaluation of the amplitude and number of phases of MUAPs in the muscle.

One may see these MUAPs when one forces the animal to bear weight on or retract a limb, resulting in contraction of that explored muscle. In lightly stimulated muscle, one may see single MUAPs, because single motor units are recruited (see Figure 12-7). As muscle contraction becomes more intense, more motor units are recruited and the greater frequency of MUAPs appears on the oscilloscope. Once MUAPs fill the screen, one observes an interference pattern. Clinically, the number of phases and the duration of MUAPs are of greater importance than amplitude, because amplitude may be influenced by species, the muscle explored, the age of the horse, and electrode position.[9] Furthermore, MUAP duration has been shown to increase with age in human beings.[12]

EVOKED MUSCLE POTENTIALS

Stimulation of a mixed motor and sensory nerve results in two observed potentials: (1) the direct evoked muscle action potential (M wave) and (2) the reflex evoked muscle action potential (H wave). The M wave is the direct muscle action potential resulting from orthodromic conduction of direct nerve stimulation (Figure 12-9). The M wave is the most commonly used potential in veterinary medicine. This wave is usually biphasic or triphasic and is larger than the H wave. The amplitude of these evoked potentials depends on the number of motor units activated and on the size of the muscle, predominant fiber type, and type of recording electrode used.[4] With monopolar electrodes, amplitudes observed in the horse range between 5 to 60 mV for a 2- to 10-ms duration. Normal amplitudes and durations have been reported for several muscles in the horse. The time required for the potential to travel down the motor nerve, cross the neuromuscular

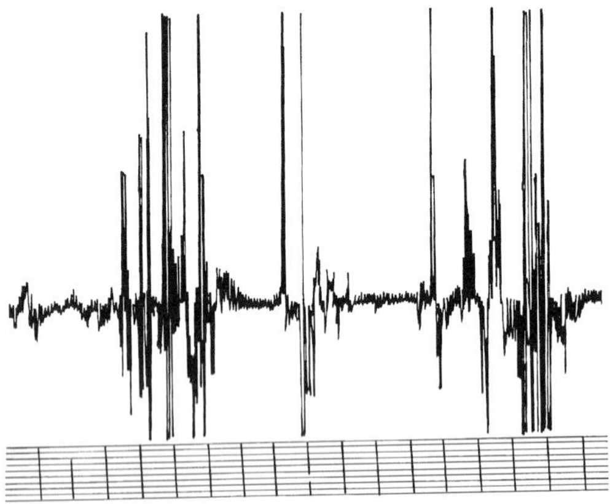

FIGURE 12-6 Normal insertional activity in the infraspinatus muscle. Gain: 0.500 mV/division; time: 10 ms/division.

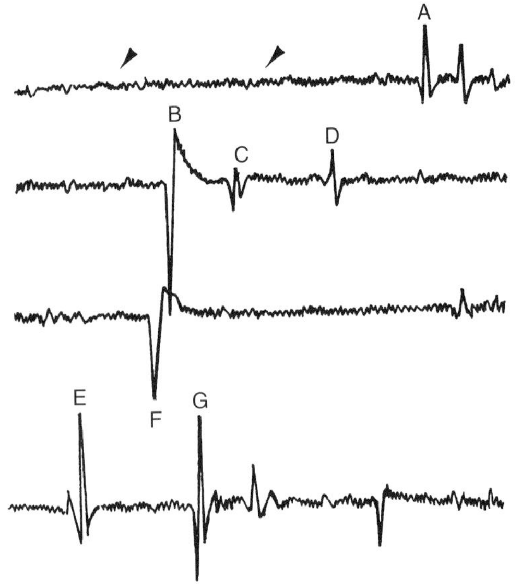

FIGURE 12-7 Electromyograph of the middle gluteal muscle showing normal resting activity *(arrowheads)*, fasciculation potentials (**A, E, G**), fibrillation potentials (**C**), positive sharp waves (**B, F**), and a small motor and action potential (**D**).

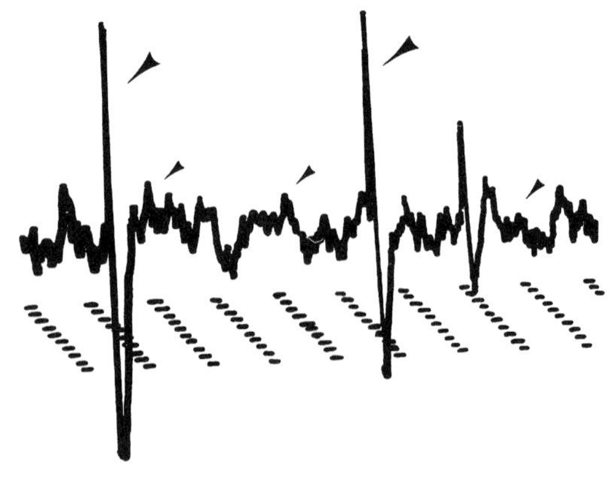

FIGURE 12-8 Electromyograph from triceps brachii muscle showing end plate spikes *(large arrowheads)* and end plate noise *(small arrowheads)*. Gain: 0.500 mV/stair step; time: 10 ms/division.

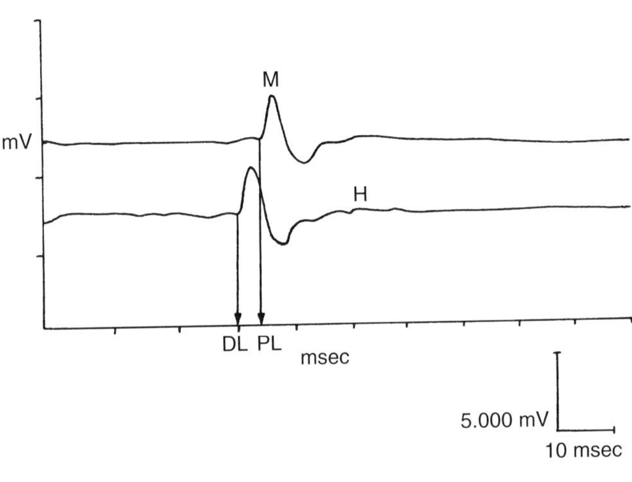

FIGURE 12-9 Evoked muscle action potentials from the levator nasolabialis muscle after direct stimulation of the buccal branch of the facial nerve illustrating the M wave and H wave. Nerve conduction velocity: 66.0 m/sec. *DL,* Distal latency; *PL,* proximal latency.

junction, travel down the muscle membrane, and stimulate a response in the muscle is called the *latency*. When two points along the motor nerve are stimulated, one can measure the distance between the stimulating electrodes (in millimeters) and divide it by the difference in latencies (in milliseconds). Normal median and radial nerve conduction velocities are 60 to 80 m/sec.[5,6] Normal facial nerve conduction velocities are 55 to 70 m/sec.[7]

ABNORMAL ELECTROMYOGRAPHIC POTENTIALS

Spontaneous activity in a relaxed muscle after cessation of needle movement may be clinically significant. Diseases affecting the motor unit can lead to altered muscle electric activity, such as prolonged or decreased insertional activity, postinsertional activity, altered waveforms, and complex repetitive discharges. Some abnormal EMG potentials are described next.

Prolonged or Decreased Insertional Activity

Prolonged electric activity continuing 1 to 10 ms after needle insertion and placement in the muscle is considered abnormal and probably is caused by hyperirritability and instability of the muscle fiber membrane.[9] This activity is most prominent 4 to 5 days after denervation in dogs.[13] Increased or prolonged insertional activity usually precedes the onset of other denervation potentials (fibrillation potentials and positive sharp waves) and may suggest early denervation atrophy.[9] However, one also may see prolonged insertional activity in myotonic disorders and myositis.[13]

Decreased insertional activity (decreased amplitude, duration, or both) may be associated with a decreased number of functioning muscle fibers and may suggest a long-standing neuropathy or myopathy. Infiltration of connective tissue and fat in the muscle can lead to a decreased number of muscle fibers, which can decrease insertional activity. Complete fibrosis of the muscle may result in loss of insertional activity. Insertional activity also may be absent when muscle fibers are functionally inexcitable, as occurs during attacks of familial periodic paralysis,[3,14] if one uses a faulty needle electrode, or if the EMG needle comes to rest in a normal muscle.[3]

Polyphasic Motor Unit Action Potentials

Polyphasic MUAPs (myopathic potentials) have increased frequency (greater than four phases) and decreased amplitude and duration (Figure 12-10), which one observes during submaximal muscle contraction and which result from an increased number of action potentials for a given strength of contraction. Myopathic potentials result from a diffuse loss of muscle fibers[15] and indicate the need for extra motor units to perform the work normally done by fewer motor units.[16] Myopathic potentials are polyphasic and most often occur in primary myopathies such as myotonia-like syndromes, periodic paralysis, myositis, botulism, and myasthenia gravis–like syndromes. These potentials also have been reported in steroid-induced myopathies, pars intermedia pituitary dysfunction, and membrane defect myopathies.[9]

Neuropathic Motor Unit Action Potentials

Neuropathic potentials are MUAPs of decreased frequency and longer duration than myopathic potentials and may occur during minimal and maximal muscle contraction (see Figure 12-10). Thus one observes fewer MUAPs of increased amplitude than expected for the strength of contraction, which is more noticeable during maximal contraction and produces a sputtering or motorboat sound. Neuropathic potentials probably are caused by a decreased number of functioning axons firing during maximal muscle contraction. These potentials are most often present in primary neuropathies in which collateral reinnervation has occurred.[16]

Fibrillation Potentials

Fibrillation potentials are the most commonly observed abnormal spontaneous electropotential in EMG (see Figure 12-7). These spontaneous discharges sound like frying eggs, crinkling cellophane, or frying bacon and have an initial positive deflection of 100 to 300 μV in amplitude and 2 to 4 ms in duration. They are diphasic or triphasic in waveform. Fibrillation potentials strongly suggest denervation but have been observed in polymyositis, muscular dystrophy, and botulism. Their origin is uncertain, but fibrillation potentials are thought to be spontaneous discharges from acetylcholine-hypersensitive denervated muscle fibers[1,17] or may result from muscle necrosis,[18] muscle inflammation, and focal muscle degeneration. A few fibrillation potentials have been observed in normal healthy muscle, but they are usually not reproducible in other areas of the muscle.

The onset of fibrillation potentials after denervation depends on the size of the animal. The larger the animal, the later the onset of fibrillation potentials[19]; they have been reported between days 5 and 16 postdenervation in dogs[20] and human beings.[18] The author has observed fibrillation potentials 4 to 10 days after nerve injury in horses. Fibrillation potentials often occurred along with positive sharp waves; they increase and then decrease in amplitude as the muscle atrophies, with activity ceasing on complete muscle atrophy. Fibrillation potentials occurring alone denote a more severe disease process than the presence of positive sharp wave potentials alone.[17] Fibrillation potentials are helpful in evaluating

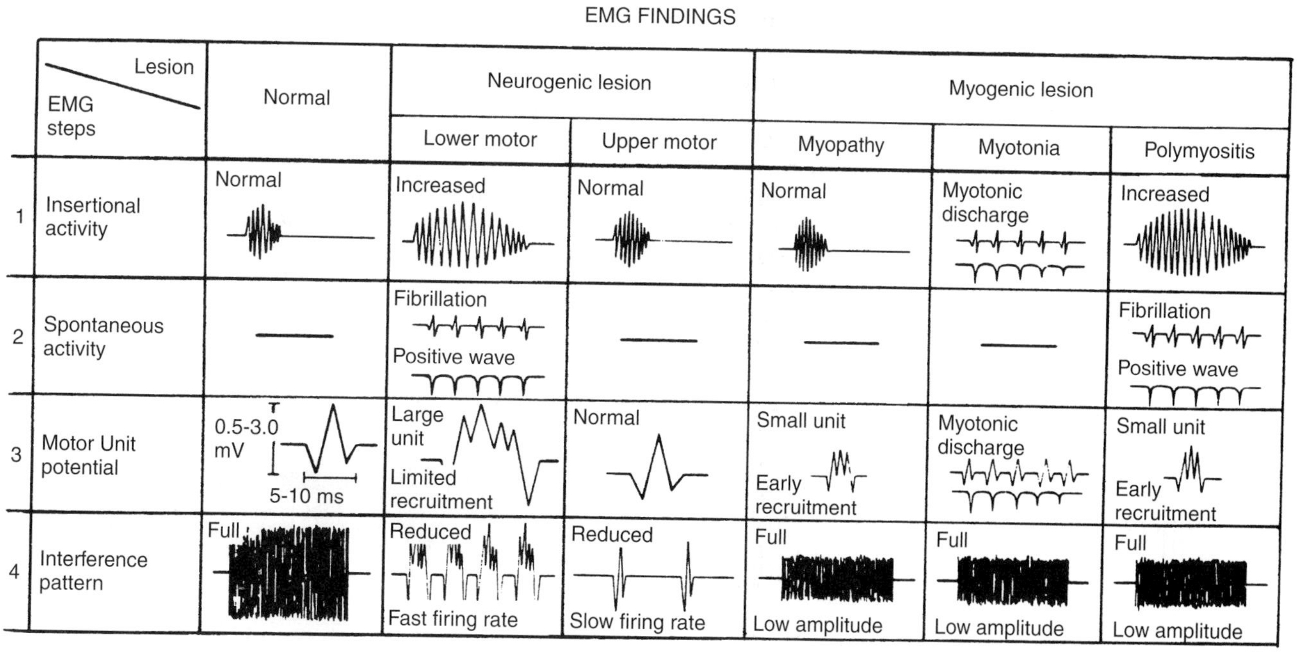

EMG FINDINGS

	EMG steps \ Lesion	Normal	Neurogenic lesion		Myogenic lesion		
			Lower motor	Upper motor	Myopathy	Myotonia	Polymyositis
1	Insertional activity	Normal	Increased	Normal	Normal	Myotonic discharge	Increased
2	Spontaneous activity	—	Fibrillation Positive wave	—	—	—	Fibrillation Positive wave
3	Motor Unit potential	0.5-3.0 mV 5-10 ms	Large unit Limited recruitment	Normal	Small unit Early recruitment	Myotonic discharge	Small unit Early recruitment
4	Interference pattern	Full	Reduced Fast firing rate	Reduced Slow firing rate	Full Low amplitude	Full Low amplitude	Full Low amplitude

FIGURE 12-10 Differential electromyographic findings in neurogenic and myogenic conditions. (Modified from Kimura J: Electrodiagnosis in diseases of nerve and muscle: principles and practice, Philadelphia, 1984, FA Davis.)

the length of time muscle denervation has been present and are important in diagnosing denervation before clinical muscle atrophy. One also can use fibrillation potentials as a prognostic indicator (by monitoring fibrillation frequency and amplitude changes with serial examinations, one can assess the extent and progress of denervation). In addition, a decrease in fibrillation potentials followed by the recording of MUAPs may indicate reinnervation and may suggest a favorable prognosis.[18]

Positive Sharp Waves

Positive sharp waves are potentials in which the primary deflection is downward, followed by a lower-amplitude, longer-duration negative deflection (see Figure 12-7). This waveform has been described as *resembling a sawtooth*.[3] Positive sharp waves occur with muscle denervation and muscular diseases such as myositis, exertional rhabdomyolysis (tying-up syndrome),[21] and spinal shock.[16] Sometimes one observes positive sharp waves in association with or shortly after insertional activity that persist after electrode placement. More than two positive sharp waves occurring after insertional activity may indicate early denervation. Positive sharp waves may occur in denervated muscle after chronic exertional rhabdomyolysis, myotonia,[21] EPM, laryngeal hemiplegia,[22] suprascapular nerve injury (sweeney),[23] and compressive myelopathies. Positive sharp waves often precede or appear along with fibrillation potentials in denervated muscle. One can observe these potentials singly or in trains (Figure 12-11), and they may sound like a machine gun. The origin of positive sharp waves is uncertain but may be associated with hyperexcitable muscle cell membranes.[17]

Fasciculation Potentials

Fasciculation potentials are spontaneous discharges from a group of muscle fibers representing the whole or part of a motor unit[3,17] (see Figure 12-7). The source of fasciculation potentials has not been determined yet, but evidence suggests they originate from neural discharges in the spinal cord or along the peripheral nerve.[24,25] Fasciculation potentials occur in diseases of anterior horn cells and irritative-type lesions of root or peripheral nerve, such as radiculopathies and nerve entrapments in human beings.[13] Little significance is placed on isolated fasciculation potentials in horses. However, fasciculation potentials in the presence of fibrillation potentials or positive sharp waves may indicate lower motor neuron disease and may occur in suprascapular nerve entrapment (sweeney) in horses.

Complex Repetitive Discharges versus Myotonic Potentials

Complex repetitive discharges (bizarre high-frequency potentials) and myotonic potentials occur less frequently in horses. Both of these potentials are repetitive MUAPs induced by insertion of the needle electrode or percussion of muscle. Bizarre high-frequency potentials tend to be shorter in duration and end abruptly compared with myotonic discharges. Bizarre high-frequency potentials sound like a machine gun. However, myotonic potentials often wax and wane in amplitude, last 4 to 5 seconds,[2,3,9] and sound like a dive-bomber, hence the nickname *dive-bomber potential*[1,9] (Figure 12-12). Myotonic and bizarre high-frequency potentials are thought to be associated with hyperexcitability of the muscle cell membrane.[1] Bizarre high-frequency potentials may occur in diseases of the lower motor unit such as muscular dystrophy,[1,9,21] steroid-induced myopathy,[9] polymyositis, chronic denervation,[26] and hyperkalemic periodic paralysis.[14] Myotonic potentials may occur in myotonia congenita and myotonia dystrophica[21] and may occur in hyperkalemic periodic paralysis in human beings, which may reflect abnormal muscle chloride or potassium conductance.[3] Myotonic potentials also have been observed in horses with hyperkalemic periodic paralysis, but some were obscured by concurrent complex repetitive discharges.[14]

DISEASES AFFECTING THE MOTOR UNIT AND PERIPHERAL NERVES

Diseases of the motor unit and peripheral nerves can lead to changes in skeletal muscle electric activity or nerve conduction velocity (or changes in both). In these diseases, EMG may be a useful diagnostic aid in localizing the lesion.

Focal and Multifocal Myelopathies

Compressive cervical myelopathies, cervical stenotic myelopathy (wobbler syndrome), and EPM are common causes of neurologic signs in the horse. These conditions are characterized by damage to the sensory pathways and in some instances damage to the ventral horn cells of the spinal cord, a component of the motor unit. Physical examination may reveal muscle atrophy and sweating over affected muscles. Needle EMG of the cervical axial musculature in horses with truncal, forelimb, and hindlimb ataxia, without cranial nerve deficits, may

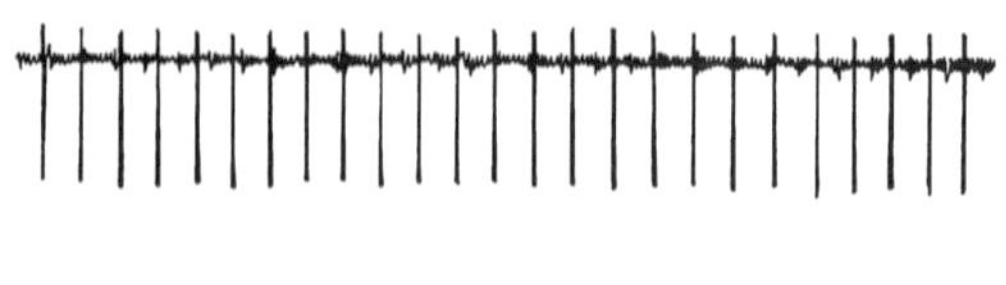

FIGURE 12-11 Electromyograph showing trains of positive sharp waves. Gain: 500 V/stair step.

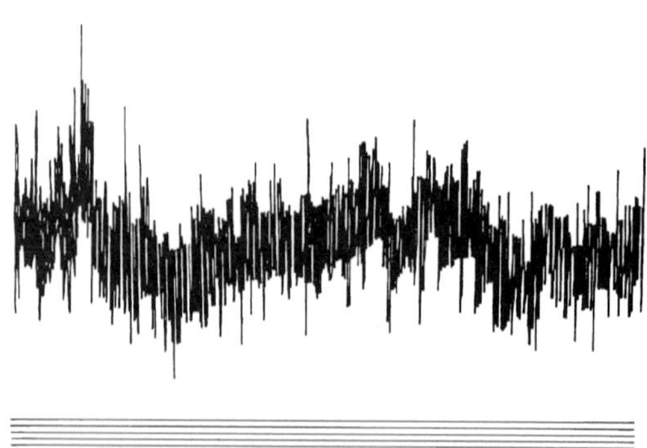

FIGURE 12-12 Electromyograph showing waxing and waning myotonic potentials. Gain: 500 V/stair step.

reveal increased insertional activity, fibrillation potentials, and positive sharp waves indicating compression of the ventral horn cells or ventral roots.[27] Abnormal postinsertional activity at the level of the spinal cord compression may allow the clinician to focus the radiographic examination.

In cases of EPM, needle EMG may reveal fibrillation potentials, positive sharp waves, and abnormal insertional activity in affected limb muscles in horses presented for obscure lameness. One also can examine horses with muscle asymmetry (Figure 12-13) via needle EMG to determine the extent of muscle involvement. The examination may lead to early diagnosis of EPM so that treatment can be prescribed. Serial needle EMG examination also may be helpful in monitoring the response to treatment and prognosis.

Radial and Suprascapular Nerve Injury

Damage to the peripheral nerves leads to muscle atrophy of the innervated muscle. Damage to the radial and suprascapular nerves can occur with trauma to the cranial aspect of the shoulder. Needle EMG and nerve conduction studies are helpful in evaluating the extent of damage to these and other peripheral nerves. Needle EMG and nerve conduction studies also may be able to differentiate lost or reduced limb function caused by nerve damage from painful conditions. Muscle groups that have atrophied because of disuse (disuse atrophy) caused by a painful condition show no postinsertional activity on needle EMG examination.

Positive sharp waves and fibrillation potentials in the triceps brachii and extensor carpi radialis muscles may suggest radial nerve injury. Positive sharp waves and fibrillation potentials in the supraspinatus and infraspinatus muscles may suggest suprascapular nerve injury (Figure 12-14). Postinsertional activity in these muscle groups and the lateral head of the triceps suggests damage to the brachial plexus (Figure 12-15). Thus needle EMG may be helpful in differentiating suprascapular nerve injury from brachial plexus injury. Visible evidence of muscle atrophy may not be present until several weeks after injury. To confirm a radial nerve injury, one can calculate the radial nerve conduction velocity (Figure 12-16). If the nerve conduction velocity is less than 60 m/sec or significantly less than the opposite limb, then one may suspect radial nerve injury. Radial nerve injury also may lead

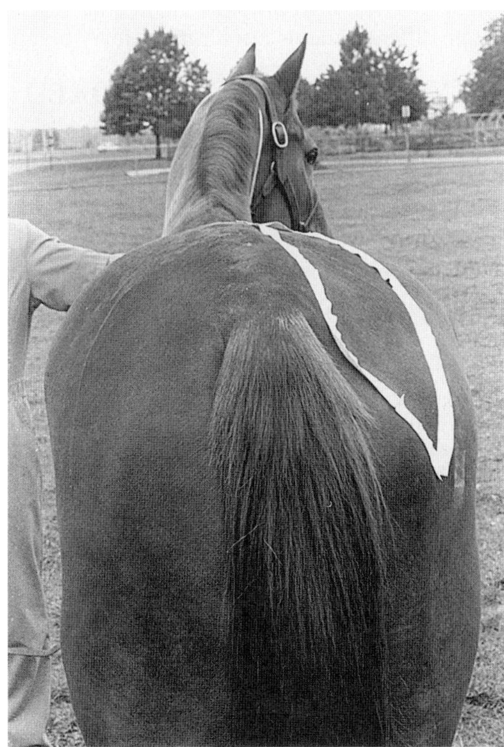

FIGURE 12-13 Horse with gluteal muscle atrophy due to EPM showing distribution of abnormal electro myographic potentials.

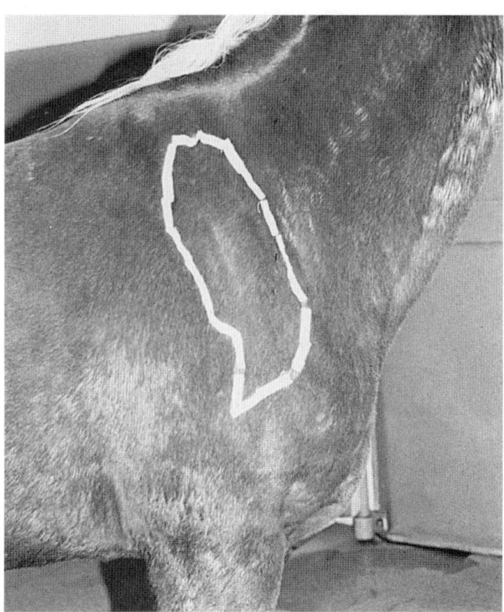

FIGURE 12-14 Horse with suprascapular nerve injury with characteristic electromyographic distribution of fibrillation potentials and positive sharp waves in supraspinatus and infraspinatus muscles.

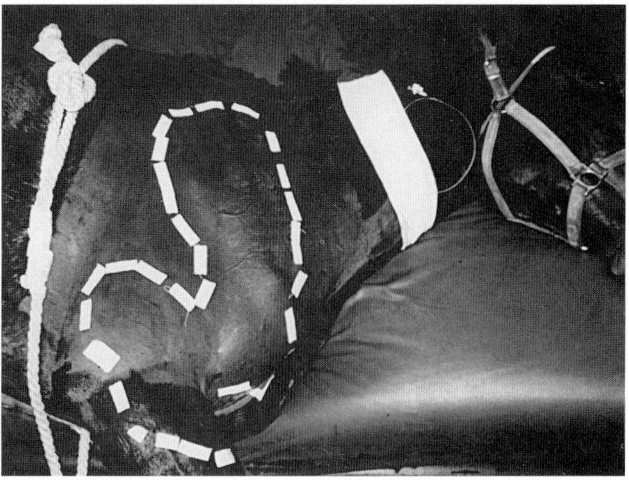

FIGURE 12-15 Horse with brachial plexus injury showing characteristic distribution of electromyographic charges, including fibrillations and positive sharp waves. The involvement of the supraspinatus, infraspinatus, triceps brachii, extensor carpi radialis, and pectoral muscles is notable.

to a decreased amplitude and duration of the evoked muscle action potential.

Needle EMG and nerve conduction studies may also be helpful in determining success of nerve decompression surgery. Once the nerve is decompressed surgically, serial needle EMG examinations may be helpful in determining if permanent nerve damage has occurred and the extent of return of nerve function.

Laryngeal Hemiplegia

Laryngeal hemiplegia has been described extensively in the literature as denervation of the intrinsic laryngeal musculature, specifically the recurrent laryngeal nerve.[5] One difficulty with this condition is that current diagnostic techniques (endoscopy, inspiratory stridor with exercise) are limited to recognizing laryngeal hemiplegia after onset of clinical signs.[28] However, fibrillation potentials and positive sharp waves in the dorsal cricoarytenoid muscle on needle EMG examination may appear before clinical signs. Thus needle EMG may be useful in the early detection of laryngeal hemiplegia in horses. Spontaneous EMG activity, including fibrillation potentials, positive sharp waves, or bizarre high-frequency discharges, have been reported in the dorsal cricoarytenoid muscle of horses affected with laryngeal hemiplegia. Fibrillation potentials and positive sharp waves are the most common abnormal electric potential observed in horses with laryngeal hemiplegia. Decreased insertional activity and bizarre high-frequency discharges were reported at a lesser frequency.[22]

Myopathies, Myositis, and Myotonia

Needle EMG may be helpful in evaluating horses with signs of primary muscle disease, such as muscle tremors, muscle fasciculations, muscle stiffness, weakness, and percussion dimpling. Myopathies generally are classified into *inflammatory* or *degenerative* types.[29] Degenerative myopathies are characterized by an intact motor unit but a loss of viable muscle fibers, which results in an increased number of polyphasic MUAPs with decreased duration (see Figure 12-10). Inflammatory myopathies (myositis) are characterized by a subacute or acute degeneration of muscle fibers with active infiltrates of inflammatory cells. The characteristic potentials are increased insertional activity, brief low-voltage MUAPs, fibrillation potentials, and positive sharp waves. Needle EMG is a valuable aid in the diagnosis and localization of focal and diffuse myopathies. Primary myopathies such as exertional rhabdomyolysis and myositis can be differentiated from myotonia and myotonia-like syndromes by needle EMG examination.[21] Furthermore, fibrillation potentials and positive sharp waves have been observed on EMG examination in horses with chronic myositis, exertional rhabdomyolysis, shivers, and hyperkalemic periodic paralysis.[14,21] After completing the needle EMG examination, one may evaluate muscles with postinsertional activity further by muscle biopsy and microscopic evaluation.[21,30]

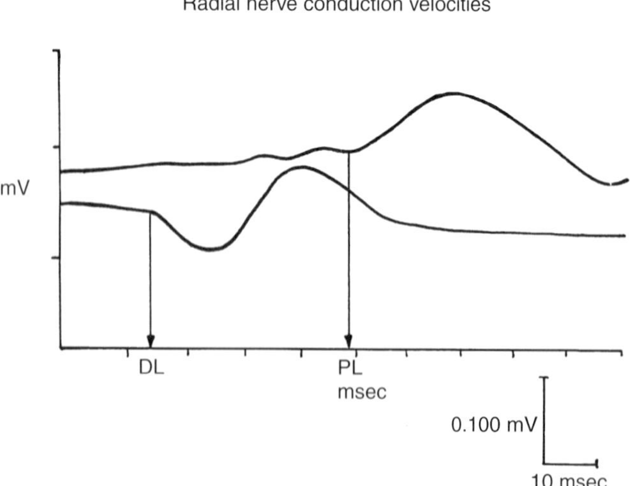

FIGURE 12-16 Evoked muscle action potential from the extensor carpi radialis muscle showing decreased amplitude and decreased nerve conduction velocity, suggesting radial nerve injury. *DL,* Distal latency; *PL,* proximal latency.

Myotonia

Myotonia is a disease characterized by an electrolyte conductance deficit in the skeletal muscle membrane.[3] One may observe fibrillation potentials, positive sharp waves, a train of positive sharp waves, and myotonic potentials on EMG examination in horses with myotonia congenita[21] and myotonia dystrophica.[31] Characteristic electrophysiologic findings include waxing-and-waning, high-frequency, spontaneous, and induced myotonic discharges (dive-bomber potentials) in many muscle groups, including the middle gluteal and semitendinosus muscles[21,31] (see Figure 12-12). One may use needle EMG to confirm the diagnosis of myotonia, to distinguish this condition from pseudomyotonia, and to localize areas for muscle biopsy (see Figure 12-10). Myotonia and myotonia-like syndromes also may present as tremors or even seizure activity. EMG along with a thorough physical and neurologic examination can help differentiate seizures from primary myopathy.

BRAINSTEM AUDITORY EVOKED RESPONSE TESTING

Brainstem auditory evoked response (BAER) testing is a method of recording potentials arising from the eighth cranial nerve and its projections in response to acoustic stimulation via surface or subcutaneously placed electrodes. The BAER is those evoked potentials, or waves, arising within the first 10 ms after delivery of an acoustic stimulus (clicks; Figure 12-17). In human beings, BAER is recognized as consisting of from five to seven waves, generally designated *I* through *VII*. Of these, waves I through V are the most common. In dogs and cats, fewer waves are observed.[32,33] In human beings and animals, a correspondence exists between these waves and certain anatomic generator sites[33-39]:

1. Wave I is generated by bipolar neurons of the eighth cranial nerve.
2. Wave II also may be generated partly by the eighth cranial nerve.
3. Waves II through V probably reflect more generalized activity in the auditory system in the medulla and pons and may represent neural activity ipsilateral and contralateral to the stimulated ear.

A wide range of clinical applications of BAER in human beings has been well described.[19,34,37,39-46] However, its use in the horse has been limited.[47-53]

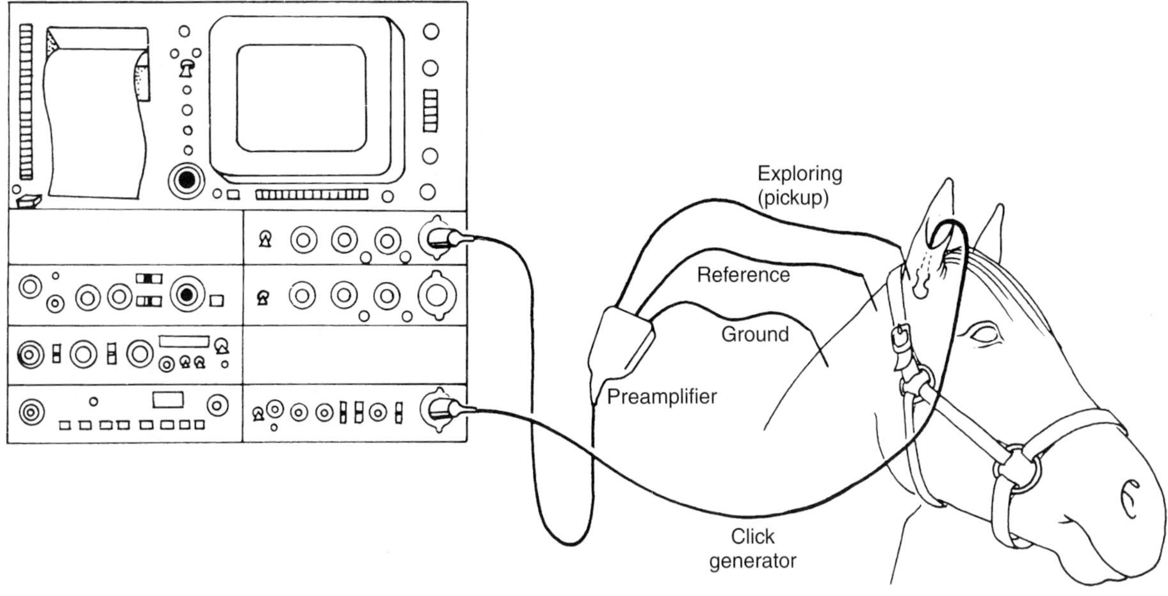

FIGURE 12-17 System used for auditory brainstem response (ABR) testing in the horse. (From Rolf SL, Reed SM, Melnick W et al: Auditory brainstem response testing in anesthetized horses, Am J Vet Res 48:910–914, 1987.)

ABR testing is a method of assessing not only auditory function but also a variety of neurologic disorders involving the brainstem. ABR testing is unaffected by the state of arousal of the test subject, and responses are not degraded by sedation or general anesthesia.[37,45]

One can examine horses awake, with or without mild sedation, or anesthetized (see Electromyography). If a conscious awake horse is tested, then one stimulates each ear and records the resultant waveforms independently. If the patient is anesthetized, then one examines the uppermost ear first, turns the horse, and examines the lower ear.

One commonly observes five peaks, and these are considered analogous to waves I through V in human beings (Figure 12-18).* Mean latencies have been reported previously in horses under general anesthesia.[55] As has been observed in dogs and cats,[32,33] latencies of the waves decrease as stimulus intensity increases. One can use the ABR clinically in horses with head tilts (Figure 12-19, A) to verify the presence of hearing loss (Figure 12-19, B), middle or inner ear infections, and stylohyoid osteomyelitis. ABR testing also may be helpful in the diagnosis and prognosis of traumatic, infectious, or inflammatory brainstem lesions such as vascular infarcts or anomalies, ischemic fibrocartilaginous emboli, basisphenoid bone fracture, and protozoal encephalomyelitis. One can assess the quantitative and qualitative characteristics of the ABR-generated waveforms. Persistent prolonged latencies suggest retrocochlear or conductive abnormalities.[37] Interaural latency differences of wave V may suggest unilateral brainstem disease, except when cochlear disease is present. Qualitative ABR changes are of greater use in equine medicine because quantitative measures of normal and abnormal horses are limited. In human beings, qualitative changes such as peak presence, waveform morphologic characteristics, and response stability are of greater use in the diagnosis of central disorders, particularly acoustic neuromata and demyelinating diseases.[37] The limitations of ABR include a dependence on cochlear function; susceptibility to extraneous noise, which may affect waveform morphology; and the limits of the machinery in excluding 60-cycle interference.

ELECTROENCEPHALOGRAPHY

Electroencephalography is the graphic recording of electric activity arising from the cerebral cortex. The origin of this electric activity is not known but is thought to arise from pyramidal cell dendrites located within a 2-mm depth of the cerebral cortex. This electric activity may be modified by deeper structures such as the brainstem, reticular activating system, and thalamus. EEG is an extension of the neurologic examination and is a valuable tool for determining the presence of a cerebral disease, localizing it, determining its extent (focal or diffuse), differentiating between inflammatory and degenerative changes, and establishing a prognosis.

EEG has been used and reviewed extensively in human beings[56,57] and small animals,[8,17] but little work has been done in the horse.[58-69] This discussion presents a brief description of the use, interpretation, and limitations of EEG so that one may gain a better understanding regarding its use.

NORMAL PATTERNS

One should evaluate the EEG for symmetry, waveform, morphology, frequency, and amplitude. The bipolar montage allows comparison of cortex to cortex. One can compare the potentials generated by the left occipital region with those of the right occipital cortex, the potentials generated by the left frontal cortex region with those of the right frontal area, and the potentials generated by the left side (left frontal-left occipital) with those of the right side (right frontal-right occipital; Figure 12-20). Normal EEG potentials in the horse consist of a dominant waveform in the awake alert

*References 4, 17, 35, 37, 39-44, 54.

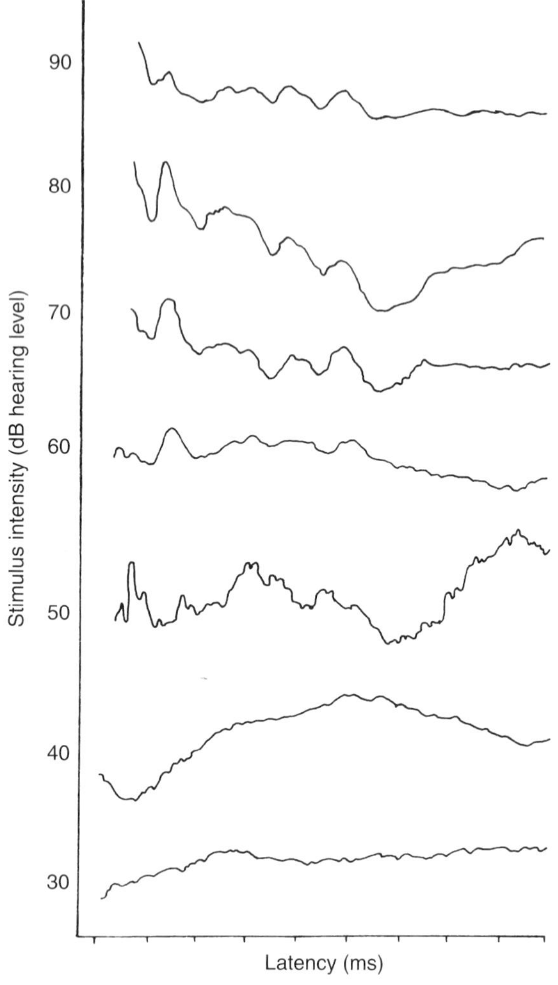

FIGURE 12-18 Mean latency waves at 136 dB, sound pressure level (SPL) through 87 dB SPL. Five waves are present, except at 40 of 80 dB SPL. (From Rolf SL, Reed SM, Melnick W et al: Auditory brainstem response testing in anesthetized horses, Am J Vet Res 48:910–914, 1987.)

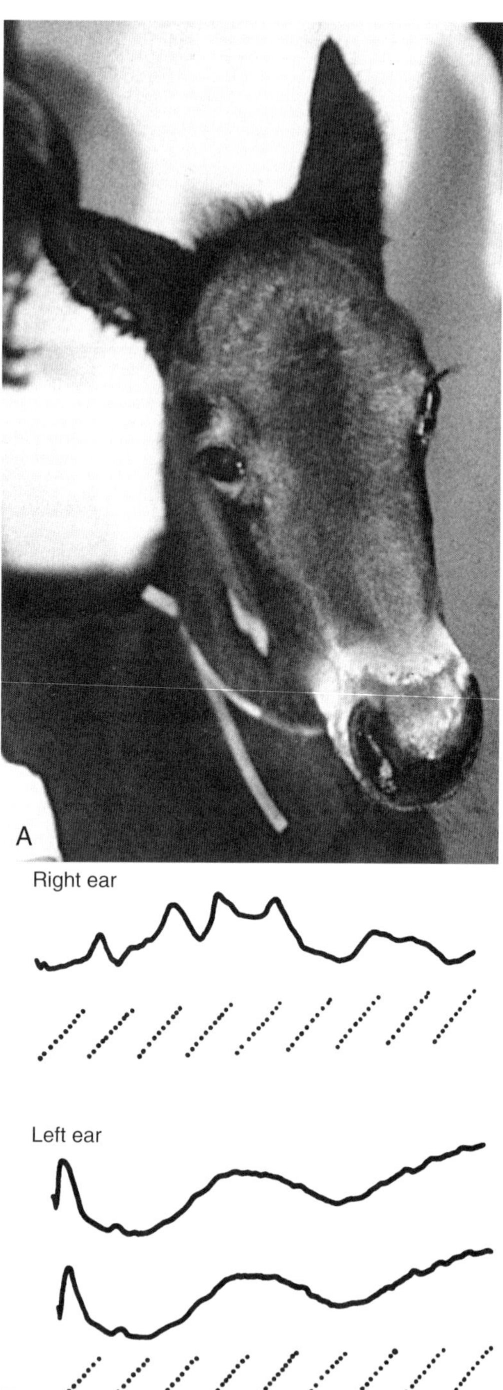

FIGURE 12-19 A, Photograph of foal with a right head tilt and drooping of the right ear. B, Auditory brainstem response (ABR) (see Figure 12-20) shows a hearing loss in the left ear, the presumed cause of the head tilt. The right ear was normal.

horse of low voltage (8 to 15 μV) and fast activity (18 to 30 Hz) (Table 12-4). Usually this activity is superimposed over a low- to medium-voltage (10 to 40 μV) and slow activity (5 to 10 Hz). Muscle artifact occasionally interrupts the baseline, when the animal shakes its head, moves its eyes, or twitches the facial muscles.

Abnormal Patterns

Diseases of the cerebral cortex can alter frequency, amplitude, and symmetry of EEG patterns. Low-voltage, fast activity, and spikes may occur with ongoing irritative processes such as seizures or inflammation (Figure 12-21). High-voltage, slow activity indicates death of neurons in diseases such as brain abscess (Figure 12-22) and neoplasia. However, low-voltage, fast activity and high-voltage, slow activity are not pathognomonic for any disease process but suggest the various disease states previously discussed. Localized EEG changes indicate focal cortical disease such as infarcts, hemorrhage, early tumor, or abscessation (see Figure 12-22), whereas generalized EEG changes may indicate a diffuse cortical or subcortical disease such as infection (see Figure 12-21), trauma, space-occupying lesions (hydrocephalus, tumor), idiopathic epilepsy, or a systemic metabolic illness (hepatic encephalopathy). Serial recordings may be helpful in following therapy and the progress of disease. Generally, artifacts such as ocular movement and facial muscle twitches produce asymmetrical and symmetrical low-voltage, slow activity, whereas hypothyroidism may produce symmetrical low-voltage, medium-to-slow

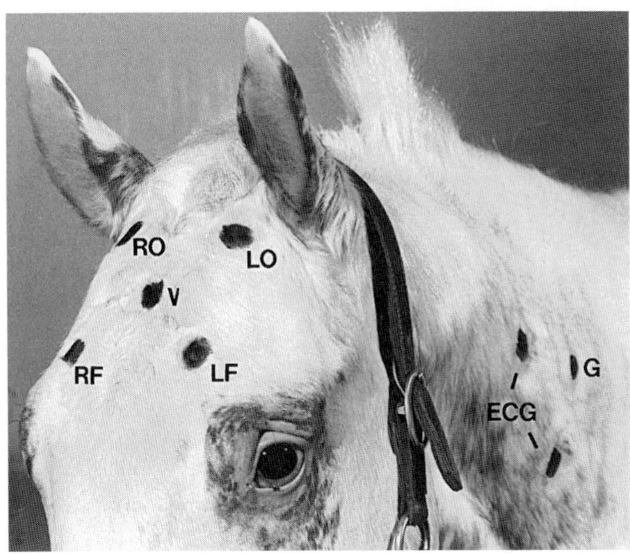

FIGURE 12-20 Photograph of horse illustrating bipolar montage for electroencephalography (EEG). *RO,* Right occipital; *LO,* left occipital; *RF,* right frontal; *LF,* left frontal; *V,* vertex; *G,* ground; *ECG,* electrocardiogram position.

TABLE 12-4

Amplitudes and Frequencies Observed in Normal Electroencephalographic Patterns from Awake and Sedated Adult Horses

		NORMAL PATTERNS	
		Voltage (μV)	Frequency (Hz)
Awake	Primary pattern	8-15	18-30
	Secondary pattern	10-40	5-10
Sedated with xylazine	Dominant	10-70	1-3
		10-80	10-15
		10-90	0.5-4
		5-30	25-40
Sedated with acetylpromazine	Primary pattern	5-40	25-40
	Secondary pattern	5-10	1-4

From Reed SM, Furr M, editor: Equine neurology, Oxford, 2008, Blackwell; Data from Purohit RC, Mysinger PW, Redding RW: Effects of xylazine and ketamine hydrochloride on the electroencephalogram and the electrocardiogram in the horse, Am J Vet Res 42:615–619, 1981; and Mysinger PW, Redding RW, Vaughan JT, et al: Electroencephalographic patterns of clinically normal, sedated, and tranquilized newborn foals and adult horses, Am J Vet Res 46:36–41, 1985.

activity.[54] The difficulty in EEG in the horse is differentiating artifact (muscle movement, eye movement, head shaking, EEG artifact) from true EEG changes. For reemphasis, EEG alone is only one part of the diagnostic workup. One always should interpret the EEG examination along with the history, clinical signs, and neurologic examination.

MAGNETIC RESONANCE IMAGING

Katherine S. Garrett

Although magnetic resonance imaging (MRI) has been used for diagnosis of neurologic disease in human beings for decades, it has only come into clinical use for horses within the past 10 years. Imaging of the brain and spinal cord is essentially impossible without MRI or computed tomography, so this represents an exciting new imaging modality to aid in the diagnosis of neurologic disease in horses.

PRINCIPLES

Magnetic field strength is measured in Tesla (T). The strength of the magnetic field varies between types of magnets, but is typically between 0.25 T and 1.5 T for most magnets currently in routine equine clinical use, although 3.0 T magnets will likely become more widely available in the near future.

Most MRI applications use hydrogen nuclei (protons) as the molecule of interest, but other nuclei can be used. Application of the strong magnetic field causes the magnetic moments of the protons within tissues to orient themselves parallel to the main magnetic field. A radiofrequency pulse at a specific frequency is then applied, which causes a change in the cumulative magnetic moment of the protons and synchronizes the phase of the protons' precessions (rotation about an axis). After the radiofrequency pulse is discontinued, the protons will return to the resting state governed by the main magnetic field alone and the precessional phase synchrony will degrade. Different tissues return to the resting state at different times and in different ways. In a basic sense, the time for the magnetic moment of a tissue to return to the direction of the main magnetic field is a description of the T1 time of the tissue and the time for the phase coherence to degrade is a description of the T2 time of the tissue. These are inherent properties, and the differences between tissues form the basis of MRI.

Different pulse sequences produce different types of contrast, based on each tissue's hydrogen content and its response. Proton density sequences have contrast determined by the proton content of each tissue. Cortical bone, tendons, ligaments, and air have low proton density, so they appear hypointense (dark) on all sequences, as well as on proton density–weighted sequences. T1-weighted sequences have contrast dominated by the T1 relaxation times of the tissues. Fat is hyperintense (bright) and fluid is hypointense. T2-weighted sequences have contrast dominated by the T2 relaxation time of the tissues. Fat is hypointense and fluid is hyperintense. Fluid attenuation inversion recovery (FLAIR) sequences have the signal from CSF specifically nulled using an inversion pulse. This allows abnormal fluid within the brain or spinal cord parenchyma to be more apparent. Intravenous contrast can also be used in MRI. Gadolinium compounds are typically used, which allow assessment of abnormal patterns of blood flow or delineation of anatomic structures, similar to the use of contrast in computed tomographic (CT) imaging.

Two major families of pulse sequences exist. Spin echo sequences use multiple radiofrequency pulses to generate a signal. Turbo or fast spin echo sequences are a subset of spin echo sequences that are faster than traditional spin echo sequences. Image contrast can be altered slightly; for example,

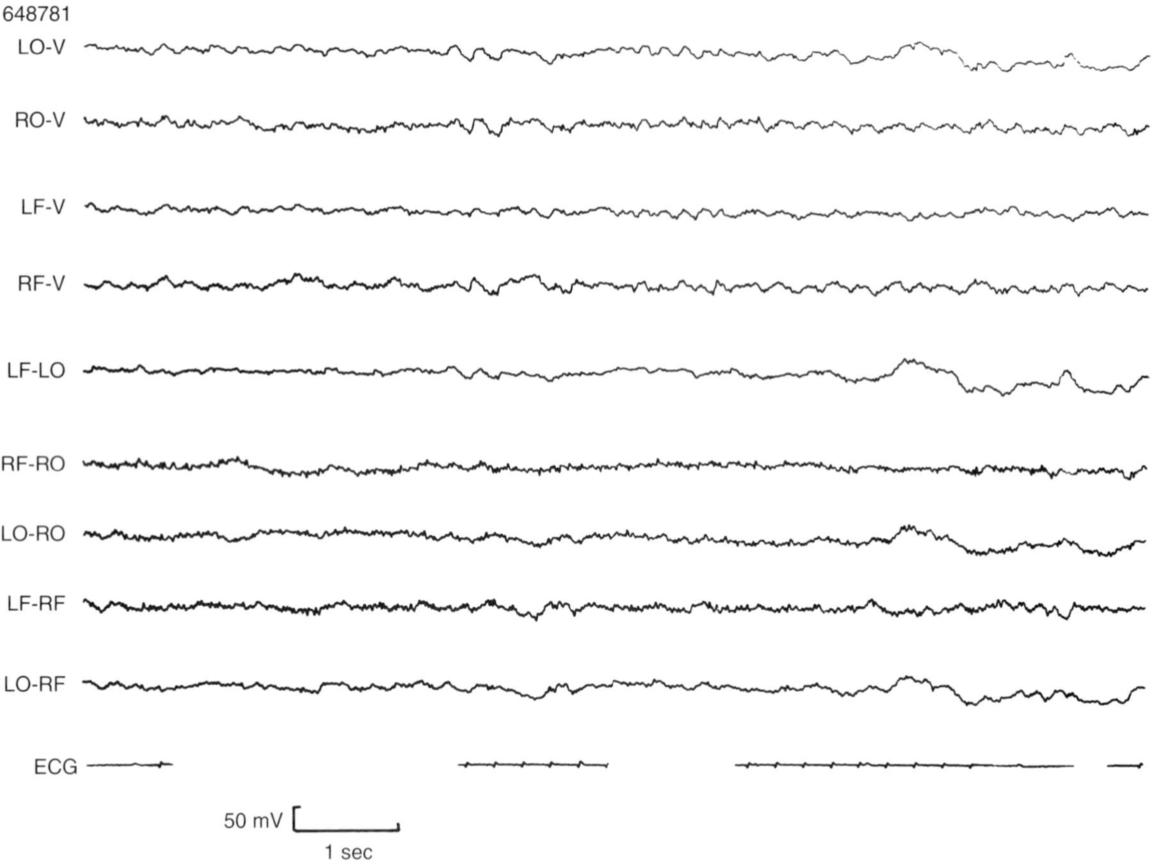

FIGURE 12-21 Electroencephalograph from a horse with cryptococcal meningitis showing generalized low-voltage, high-frequency activity and frequent spikes. *RO,* Right occipital; *LO,* left occipital; *RF,* right frontal; *LF,* left frontal; *V,* vertex; *G,* ground; *ECG,* electrocardiogram position.

fat on T2-weighted turbo spin echo sequences is hyperintense instead of hypointense. Gradient echo sequences use a changing magnetic field gradient to generate a signal. Gradient echo sequences can be acquired more quickly than spin echo sequences but are more susceptible to magnetic field inhomogeneities.

For each series of slices, the operator must choose the orientation of the slices, as well as the type of pulse sequence used. A typical MRI examination will consist of many series, each with a different combination of orientation and pulse sequence. Unlike CT imaging, the orientation of the images obtained during each pulse sequence can be selected by the operator. These are typically 1- to 5-mm thick slices. A complete examination produces hundreds of individual images to be reviewed and usually takes between 1 and 2 hours to complete the acquisition of images. Some series are acquired in a way that permits reconstruction in multiple planes or in three dimensions.

EQUIPMENT

The main magnetic field can be generated in a variety of ways. Permanent magnets are used in lower field systems (<0.4 T). These magnetic fields are generated by using ferromagnetic materials of the same type as in everyday magnets. Stronger magnetic fields are produced using superconducting electromagnets. These magnets use liquid helium to cool the electromagnetic coils and reduce the resistance, allowing much stronger magnetic fields to be generated. Liquid helium is expensive and requires periodic replenishment, but it is necessary to efficiently generate the stronger magnetic fields in clinical use. Regardless of the type of magnet, the room must be shielded to prevent any external radiofrequency pulses (e.g., radio signals, cellular phone transmission) from entering the room and introducing artifacts.

Two types of MRI systems are used for horses. One type consists of systems designed for use in human beings. These tend to be high field magnets with strengths ≥1.0 T of closed bore construction and require the horse to be under general anesthesia. The horse is positioned either in lateral or dorsal recumbency on a nonferromagnetic padded table with the body part of interest positioned into the bore. Foals can be imaged using the human patient table in any recumbency.

The other group consists of magnets that have been specifically designed for veterinary use. These magnets are generally low field magnets with a strength in the 0.25-T range. Many have an open bore design and can be positioned about a body part; some require general anesthesia and some only sedation. The images produced with these weaker magnets require longer scan times to obtain and are of lower resolution. Motion artifact in studies obtained on standing horses can significantly reduce image quality.

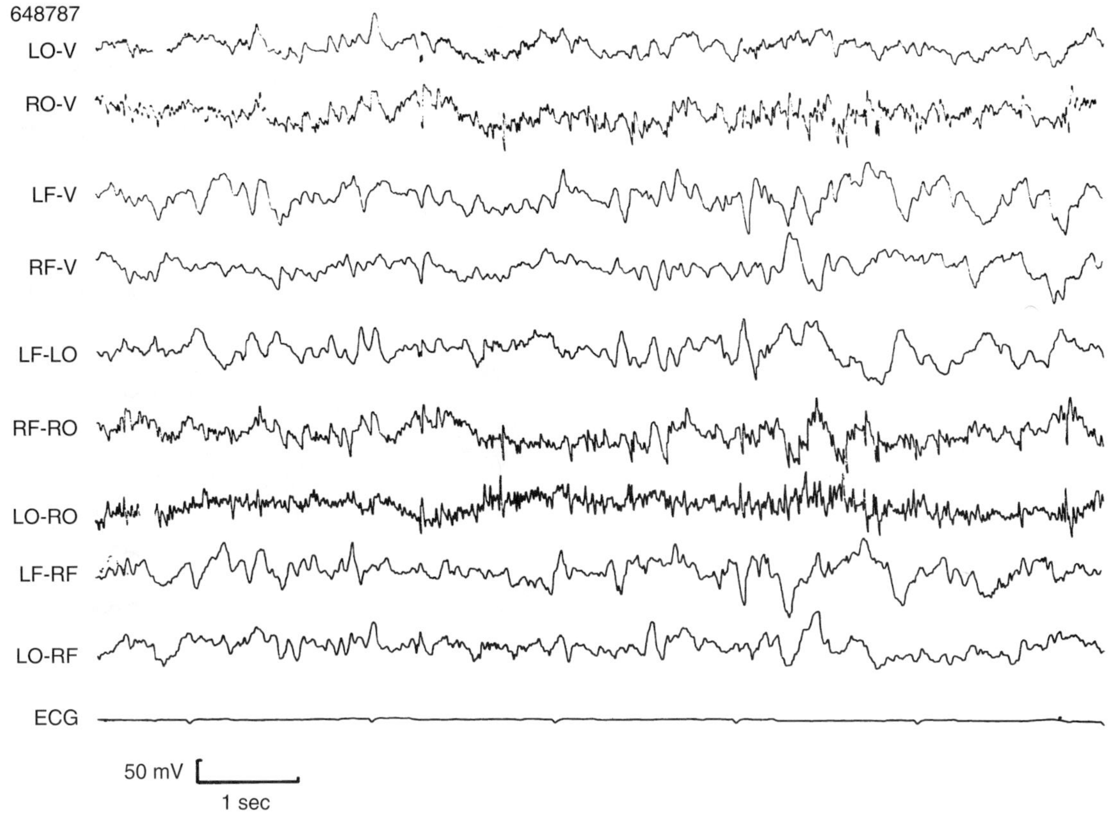

FIGURE 12-22 Electroencephalograph from a horse with a space-occupying mass in the left frontal area of the brain. The generalized high-voltage, low-frequency wave and asymmetry of left cortex are notable. *RO,* Right occipital; *LO,* left occipital; *RF,* right frontal; *LF,* left frontal; *V,* vertex; *G,* ground; *ECG,* electrocardiogram position.

Examinations are limited to regions that can fit into the bore of the magnet to be positioned at or near the isocenter (center of the magnetic field). Depending on the type of magnet, this requires that either the horse be pushed into the center of the magnet bore or that the magnet be positioned around the region of interest. These limits will vary between magnets based on their construction.

SAFETY

Most safety hazards associated with MRI are related to the introduction of ferromagnetic objects into a strong magnetic field, as opposed to the existence of the magnetic field itself. No known adverse effects have been reported for MRI at field strengths currently used in equine clinical imaging. Any object that is magnetic (scissors, oxygen tanks, scalpel blades) will be attracted to the magnet; thus all the equipment in the room must be nonmagnetic or MRI compatible, including the anesthesia equipment. The strength of the magnetic field increases exponentially as the distance to the magnet decreases. In practical terms, this means that the pull of the magnet on any ferromagnetic object becomes quickly stronger as the object approaches the magnet (to prevent injury this is especially important to bear in mind when considering stronger magnets).

The strong magnetic field can also affect internal implants and is especially dangerous for people with cardiac pacemakers, who should not enter a MRI room under any circumstances because of the potential for serious cardiac arrhythmias resulting from the effect of the magnetic field on the pacemaker. Metal shards in the cornea can also be affected by the magnet and can move within the cornea, causing ocular damage. The changing of the magnetic gradients can be quite loud. Any personnel who remain in the scan room during the examination should wear protective equipment to prevent hearing damage.

PATIENT PREPARATION

Horseshoes should be removed before the examination to eliminate the risk of potential magnetic attraction. Appropriate preparations should be carried out for images requiring general anesthesia. After induction to anesthesia but before entering the scan room, any metal objects (e.g., halters) should be removed from the horse. A specialized, nonferromagnetic table must be used to support the horse during the examination. After the horse is positioned in the bore of the magnet, it must remain completely motionless during image acquisition to prevent blurring of the image. Because MRI examinations typically take between 1 and 2 hours, urinary catheterization or some other means of urine collection is recommended to protect the equipment from contamination with fluid.

Because an MRI examination can be lengthy, it is extremely important that the primary region of interest be localized as specifically as possible. MRI has proven particularly useful in areas that are not amenable to examination using other diagnostic imaging modalities.

USE OF MAGNETIC RESONANCE IMAGING IN EQUINE NEUROLOGIC DISEASE

In adult horses, examination is limited to the brain and cranial cervical spine because of limitations of current magnet design. However, the trunk of foals up to approximately 500 lb may fit inside the bore of some magnets, enabling imaging of any part of the spinal column.

Few reports exist of clinical use of MRI in neurologic disease. Investigators at Washington State University described a case series of 12 horses with neurologic signs localized rostral to the foramen magnum imaged with MRI. Abnormal findings were seen in eight of these horses, and diagnoses included nigropallidal encephalomalacia, head trauma, cerebral abscess, stylohyoid bone fracture, pituitary mass, congenital hydrocephalus, and otitis media.[1] Additional case reports have described findings in cases of brain abscess,[2,3] cholesterol granuloma,[4] and EPM.[5] Diagnoses of equine protozoal myelitis, neoplasia, inflammatory disease, encephalomyelitis, meningitis, otitis media, hydrocephalus, and ischemic injury have been made at the author's clinic. In addition, substantial information has been gained regarding the extent of damage after traumatic injury. Although this clinic's experience with MRI of the nervous system is limited, the possibilities of this technique are exciting.

Pituitary Adenoma

A 13-year-old Thoroughbred mare had decreased mentation, poor appetite, weight loss, and absence of normal estrous cycles. The decreased mentation had progressed to prolonged periods of somnolence, slow circling behavior, and an apparent decrease in vision. The mare had decreased menace and pupillary light responses and demonstrated slight weakness on a tail pull test. An anatomic diagnosis of a CNS lesion rostral to the foramen magnum was made. Endogenous adrenocorticotropic hormone, triiodothyronine (T3), and thyroxine (T4) levels were normal. A MRI examination was undertaken in an attempt to find the cause of the neurologic signs and to further investigate a possible pituitary lesion.

A mass was found on the median plane ventral to the diencephalon, with the ventral aspect of the mass within the sella turcica (Figure 12-23). A portion of the pituitary distinct from the mass can be identified in part of the sella turcica. The mass compresses the thalamus, hypothalamus, and optic chiasm. Portions of the mass appear hemorrhagic and regions of the thalamus, and hypothalamus surrounding the mass are edematous.

This horse was treated with pergolide and cyproheptadine in an attempt to ameliorate the signs of pituitary pars intermedia dysfunction (PPID), and improvement was seen for a brief period of time. Its condition then deteriorated after 6 weeks with progressive anorexia, weight loss, and depression despite aggressive supportive care. The mare was euthanized, and necropsy results showed a large pituitary mass with histologic features consistent with a pituitary macroadenoma of the pars intermedia.

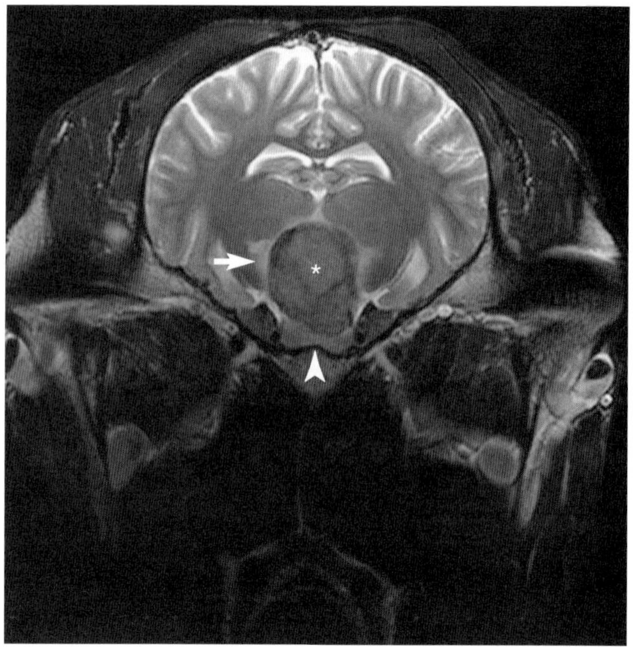

FIGURE 12-23 Transverse T2-weighted fast spin echo image of the brain at the level of the sella turcica. The asterisk indicates a large mass of heterogeneous signal intensity displacing the diencephalon laterally. The arrowhead indicates normal pituitary tissue compressed by the mass. The arrow indicates high T2 signal (edema) within the diencephalon adjacent to the mass.

Equine Protozoal Myeloencephalitis

An 18-year-old Thoroughbred gelding became ataxic 9 months before presentation. Two months before presentation, the horse started to exhibit weight loss, dysphagia, and facial muscle wasting. The animal had been treated for equine protozoal myelitis twice before presentation and exhibited grade 3/4 ataxia in all limbs. In addition, the horse had atrophy of the left facial muscles, as well as the left temporalis and masseter muscles, muzzle deviation to the right side, and difficulty moving food to the pharynx with normal tongue tone, prehension, and ability to swallow. These neurologic signs suggested multifocal disease with involvement of cranial nerves V, VII, IX, and X, as well as the cervical spinal cord and brainstem. Equine protozoal myelitis Western blot was weakly positive on the CSF and positive on serum.

MRI findings consistent with inflammation and edema were seen throughout the right side of the medulla and caudal pons in areas including the nuclei of cranial nerves V, VII, VIII, and XII (Figure 12-24). These findings are consistent with those seen in a previously reported case of EPM.[5]

Nitazoxanide (NTZ), vitamin E, and flunixin meglumine were administered. Supportive care, including intravenous fluid therapy and enteral feeding via nasogastric tube, was also performed. The horse became progressively more depressed and developed pleuropneumonia 1 week after admission, likely secondary to aspiration because of dysphagia. The next day, the horse became acutely more ataxic, was unable to rise, and died. On postmortem examination, neuronal degeneration, inflammation, and protozoal organisms consistent with *Sarcocystis neurona* were identified in the nuclei and nerves of cranial nerves V, VII, and VIII.

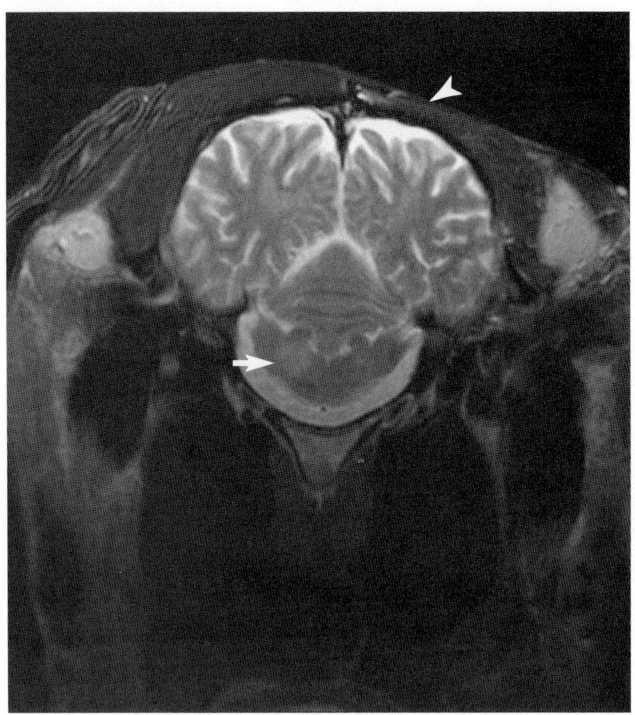

FIGURE 12-24 Transverse T2-weighted fast spin echo image of the brain at the level of the pons. The arrow indicates an area of T2 hyperintensity in the region of the nuclei of the seventh and eighth cranial nerves. The arrowhead indicates temporalis muscle atrophy.

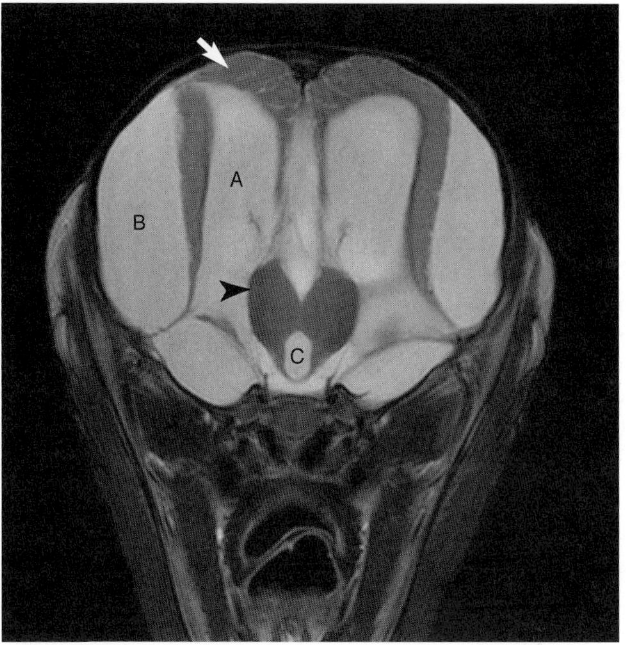

FIGURE 12-25 Transverse T2-weighted turbo spin echo image of the brain at the level of the thalamus. The lateral **(A)** and third **(C)** ventricles are massively dilated with cerebrospinal fluid (CSF) present outside of the brain **(B)**. The arrow indicates the cerebral cortex and the arrowhead indicates the thalamus.

Hydrocephalus

A 1-month-old Quarter Horse filly was noticed by the owners to have a dome-shaped head, blindness, and obtundation. A congenital brain lesion was suspected.

MRI images showed severe communicating hydrocephalus with a specific location of obstruction not identified (Figure 12-25). The ventricles were enlarged and filled with CSF. The parenchyma of the cerebral hemispheres was thinned, and the cerebellum was compressed and herniated through the foramen magnum. A meningocele and an open fontanelle were noted at the junction of the left and right frontal and parietal bones.

Treatment was not pursued, although the possibility of placement of a ventriculoperitoneal shunt was discussed with the owners. The foal remained alive and was weaned successfully.

Spinal Cord Compression

A 4-month-old Thoroughbred colt had a 2-day history of pyrexia and "knuckling over" of the left hind fetlock. Ultrasound examination of the lumbar, sacral, and gluteal regions showed an abscess within the musculature. The extent of the abscess could not be determined but was suspected to involve the pelvis, so MRI examination was undertaken.

Severe compression and inflammation of the spinal cord in the sacral region was seen on MRI (Figure 12-26). The left side of the sacrum had heterogeneous signal intensity suggestive of osteomyelitis.

The foal was treated with anti-inflammatory and antimicrobial medication and establishment of drainage of the

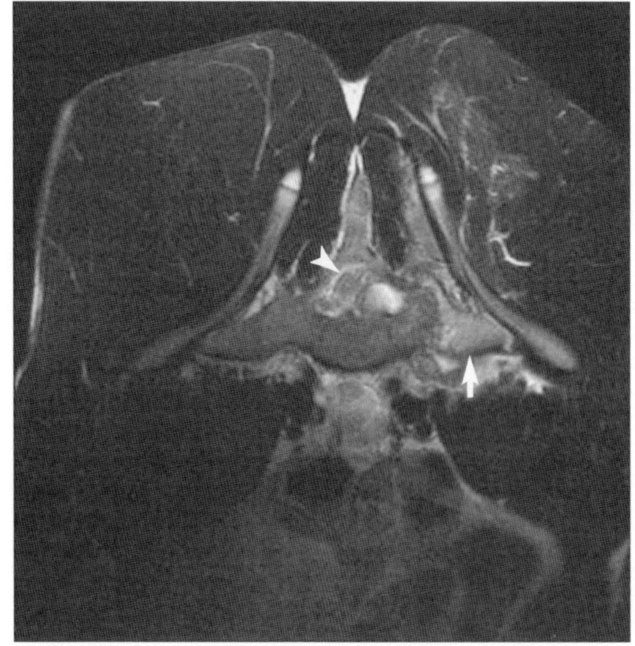

FIGURE 12-26 Transverse T2-weighted turbo spin echo image of the spinal canal at the level of the sacroiliac joint. The arrowhead indicates the laterally compressed spinal cord and the arrow indicates a region of edema and proteinaceous fluid accumulation within and around the sacrum (osteomyelitis).

intramuscular portion of the abscess. The foal's condition improved and it was discharged on long-term antimicrobial therapy. During follow-up MRI examination 2 months later, the compression of the spinal cord had been relieved and the intramuscular abscess had decreased in size. The heterogeneous signal intensity within the sacrum had improved but not resolved completely.

CONCLUSION

Although MRI of equine neurologic disease remains in its infancy, veterinarians are increasingly able to use this technology to make more specific and timely diagnoses. As the knowledge base regarding MRI progresses, practitioners will be able to advance their care and treatment of equine patients to new levels.

SEIZURES, NARCOLEPSY, AND CATAPLEXY*

Stephen M. Reed

SEIZURES

Seizures are clinical manifestations of rapid excessive electric discharges from the cerebral cortex that result in involuntary alterations of motor activity, consciousness, autonomic functions, or sensation and can be very difficult to diagnose and manage.[1-4] Seizures may be referred to as *fits, attacks, strokes, convulsions,* or *epilepsy*. A true seizure, however, refers to a specific clinical event regardless of cause or morphology. *Epilepsy* refers to reoccurring seizures with nonprogressive intracranial alterations, which may be genetic or acquired. True inherited epilepsy probably does not occur in horses.[2] *Convulsions,* however, refer to seizures accompanied by tonic-clonic muscle activity and loss of consciousness. Convulsions may include a generalized seizure.

Seizures in horses can be classified into three broad forms based on clinical signs: (1) partial seizure, (2) generalized seizure, and (3) status epilepticus. A partial seizure involves a discrete area of the cerebral cortex and results in localized clinical signs, such as facial or limb twitching, compulsive running in a circle, or self-mutilation. One may observe a partial seizure after a procedure such as collection of CSF, cervical myelography, anesthesia, or cranial trauma that may spread throughout the cerebral cortex and produce a secondary generalized seizure. A generalized seizure involves the entire cerebral cortex and results in generalized tonic-clonic muscle activity over the whole body, with loss of consciousness. Generalized seizures are the most common form of seizures observed in adult horses and foals.[2,3] Status epilepticus is characterized by generalized seizures occurring in rapid succession and is uncommon in horses.[2] In many cases the presence of a seizure might be suspected after recognition of unexplained trauma to the head or legs of a horse along with disruption of the stall or outside paddock. This is particularly important when signs such as this are recognized repeatedly. At other times the owner or caretaker may identify a change in attitude or behavior of the horse such as restlessness or a "far-off" appearance that might be a prodromal sign (aura) of an impending seizure.

PATHOGENESIS

Adult horses have a high seizure threshold. In most cases severe damage must occur to the brain before adult horses have seizures. Foals, however, have a lower seizure threshold and are more susceptible to conditions causing seizures.[5] Intracranial or extracranial factors may cause seizures[2] (Tables 12-5 and 12-6). The most common causes of seizures in foals under 2 weeks of age are hypoxic-ischemic encephalopathy, trauma, and bacterial meningitis.[5] The most common causes of seizures in foals less than 1 year of age are trauma and idiopathic epilepsy in Arabian foals.[2,3] The most common causes of seizures in adult horses older than 1 year of age are brain trauma, hepatoencephalopathy, and toxicity.[2] Tumors or pituitary enlargement secondary to pituitary pars intermedia dysfunction may cause seizures and blindness in horses older than 7 years.[2]

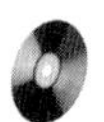

The pathophysiologic mechanisms of seizures are incompletely understood. Current research has focused on intracellular neuronal and synaptic events that initiate excessive and prolonged neuronal depolarization, known as *paroxysmal depolarization shift*. Several mechanisms are thought to cause paroxysmal depolarization shifts and seizures and include increased excitatory neural transmitters, decreased inhibitory neural transmitters (gamma-aminobutyric acid [GABA]), alteration in neural transmitter receptor sites, or a derangement in the internal cellular metabolism of the neuron.[6,7] The most widely held hypothesis for seizure initiation is development of excitatory postsynaptic potentials. Seizures may develop because of a summation of synchronous excitatory postsynaptic potentials in large groups of neurons that may be precipitated by an increase in excitatory neurons, a decrease in inhibitory neurons, a decrease in inhibitory neurotransmitters, or any combination of these.[6,8] Once a "critical mass" of neurons has fired, an uncontrolled spread of electric activity may occur over the cerebral cortex and precipitate a generalized seizure. Head trauma and decreased cerebral blood supply have been implicated in creating seizure foci. Head trauma may result in cerebral cortical hypoxia, which in turn may lead to necrosis of inhibitory neurons. Because cerebral inhibitory neurons are more sensitive to hypoxia than excitatory neurons, a loss of inhibitory neurons allows the spread of these excitatory postsynaptic potentials and seizure development.[9]

Inhibitory neurons surround excitatory neuron groups and check areas of intense stimulation. Decreased inhibitory neurotransmitters in these areas, such as GABA, have been implicated in seizure formation in animals. Application of penicillin directly to the brain of laboratory animals suppresses GABA and induces seizures.[10] These seizures can be blocked by use of other agents that potentiate inhibitory neurotransmitters. Phenobarbital and pentobarbital potentiate inhibitory neural transmitters, such as GABA, and block seizure foci caused by penicillin and hypoxia.

Alterations in the neuronal cell microenvironment may lead to seizure generation. Systemic and local neuronal electrolyte abnormalities may disturb excitatory neuron homeostasis and lead to spontaneous and excessive action potentials.[6]

*The authors wish to acknowledge Frank M. Andrews and Hilary K. Matthews, whose original work has been incorporated into this section.

TABLE 12-5

Known and Suspected Causes of Seizures in Horses Less than 1 Year of Age

DIFFERENTIAL DIAGNOSIS

Classification	Extracranial	Intracranial	Diagnostic Aids
Anomalies (congenital)		Hydrocephalus	
		Hydranencephaly	1-6, 8
		Benign epilepsy	11
Metabolic	Hypoxia, hyponatremia, hypoglycemia, hyperkalemia		2-4, 8, 11
Toxic	Organophosphates	Moldy corn	2-6
	Strychnine	Locoweed	9-11
	Metaldehyde		
Traumatic		Brain trauma	2-4
		Lightning	5, 6, 8, 10, 11
Vascular		Neonatal maladjustment syndrome (vascular accidents)	2-6
Infectious	Septicemia	Bacterial meningitis	2-4
	Endotoxemia	Cerebral abscesses	5-9
	Fever	Rabies	11
	Tetanus	Viral encephalitis	
	Botulism		

1, Breed; *2*, onset; *3*, clinical course; *4*, physical examination; *5*, neurological examination; *6*, clinical pathology: cerebrospinal fluid analysis; *7*, serologic testing; *8*, radiology (computed tomography scan, ultrasound, radiographs); *9*, toxicologic testing; *10*, electrodiagnostics (electroencephalography, electromyelography); *11*, pathologic examination.

Intracellular potassium released during neuronal activity may reach sufficient concentration to move the resting membrane potential toward the threshold and generate a seizure focus.[11] Spontaneous action potentials generated by alteration in intracellular potassium concentration may spread to other parts of the cerebral cortex, causing a generalized seizure.

Furthermore, alterations in one intracellular neuronal electrolyte may alter the homeostasis of other intracellular electrolytes. This alteration is supported by the observation of increased intracellular potassium concentration, together with decreased intracellular calcium, magnesium, and chloride concentrations, in the long-duration changes in excitability known to occur during interictal epileptogenesis and the transition from interictal to ictal activities.[12,13]

Alterations in sodium conductance also have been implicated in causing seizures. Rapid influxes of sodium into the neuron may lead to hyperexcitability of the neuron and rapid firing. Phenytoin, a hydantoin derivative, blocks these rapid influxes of sodium into neurons and suppresses repetitive firing by hyperexcitable neurons.[14] Thus a complex interaction may occur between these electrolytes and the internal cell homeostasis that precipitates seizure formation.

Clinical Signs and Diagnosis

Seizure activity is manifested clinically in a variety of ways, depending on the area and the extent of the cerebral cortex involved. In partial seizures, asymmetrical twitching of a limb, facial twitching, excessive chewing, compulsive running, or self-mutilation may occur.[2] A localized seizure may develop into a generalized seizure.

In a generalized seizure, one may observe three distinct clinical periods. Just before the seizure (aura), horses may exhibit signs of anxiety and uneasiness. During the seizure (ictus), horses may become recumbent, unconscious, and have symmetrical clonic muscle contractions (contractions and relaxations of muscles occurring in rapid succession), followed by symmetrical tonic muscle contractions (continuous unremitting muscle contractions).[2,3] Horses also may show deviation of eyeballs, dilated pupils, ptyalism, trismus or jaw clamping, opisthotonos, lordosis or kyphosis, violent paddling movements of the limbs, uncontrolled urination and defecation, and excessive sweating. A generalized seizure may last between 5 to 60 seconds.[2] After the seizure (postictus), horses may show depression and blindness for hours to days.[2,3]

Diagnosis of seizure is based on history, clinical signs, and ancillary diagnostic tests to determine an underlying cause, whenever possible (see Tables 12-5 and 12-6). In all paroxysmal, involuntary neurologic events, one should consider seizures first unless the cause is proved otherwise. Careful questioning of the owner can reveal information about the event, the time of day, relationship to feeding, date, unusual environmental circumstances (stimuli such as thunderstorms, fireworks, changes in housing), recent trauma, febrile episodes, exposure to drugs or toxins, recent behavioral changes, and the seizure history of the dam, sire, and other siblings. One must rule out other conditions that mimic seizures,

TABLE 12-6

Known and Suspected Causes of Seizures in Horses More than 1 Year of Age

	DIFFERENTIAL DIAGNOSIS		
Classification	**Extracranial**	**Intracranial**	**Diagnostic Aids**
Metabolic	Hepatoencephalopathy, hypomagnesemia, hypocalcemia, uremia, hyperlipidemia		2-6, 11
Toxic	Organophosphates	Moldy corn	2-6
	Strychnine	Locoweed	9-11
	Metaldehyde	Bracken fern	
		Lead, arsenic, mercury	
		Rye grass	
Traumatic		Brain trauma	8, 10, 11
Vascular		*Strongylus vulgaris*	2-4
		Cerebral thromboembolism	5, 6, 11
		Intracarotid injection	
Tumor		Neoplasia	2-5
		Hemarthroma	6, 8, 10, 11
		Cholesterol granuloma	
Infectious		Cerebral abscess	1, 3-6
		Rabies	7, 8, 12, 13
		Tetanus	
		Arbovirus encephalitides	
		Mycotic cryptococcosis	
		Protozoal encephalomyelitis	

1, Breed; *2,* onset; *3,* clinical course; *4,* physical examination; *5,* neurologic examination; *6,* clinical pathology: cerebrospinal fluid analysis; *7,* serologic testing; *8,* radiology (computed tomography scan, ultrasound, radiographs); *9,* toxicologic testing; *10,* electrodiagnostics (electroencephalography [EEG], electromyelography [EMG]); *11,* pathologic examination.

including painful conditions (colic, limb fractures, exertional myopathy), hyperkalemic periodic paralysis, and syncope. In these conditions horses do not lose consciousness but remain bright and alert. Horses with hyperkalemic periodic paralysis may show prolapse of the nictitating membranes of the eye and muscle fasciculations but remain anxious, alert, and have normal pain perception. This condition occurs in Quarter Horse and Quarter Horse crosses 2 to 3 years of age. Serum potassium concentration in these horses ranges between 5.5 to 9.0 mEq/L during or shortly before collapse.[15,16]

One can confuse narcolepsy and cataplexy with seizures. Most narcoleptic horses (except for some ponies) remain standing with the head hanging close to the ground. If recumbency occurs, then loss of muscle tone and rapid eye movement (REM) sleep may follow.[17] Cardiac arrhythmias or severe murmurs may precipitate syncopal episodes. Auscultation of the heart may help determine the presence of severe murmurs, and electrocardiography may help determine the presence of arrhythmias. Icteric mucous membranes may be apparent in horses with hepatoencephalopathy, and diarrhea may be evident in horses after toxin ingestion.

One should perform a complete neurologic examination to determine the presence of other neurologic signs. One should perform the neurologic examination during the interictal period, because an immediate postictal examination may reveal depression, weakness, blindness, and crossed extensor reflex and may lead to false anatomic localization of lesions.[1-3]

CSF from the cisterna magna may be helpful in determining the cause of seizures. Increased CSF protein, RBC count, white blood cell count, and abnormal differential white blood cell count may be helpful in determining the cause of the seizure.[1-3] Increased CSF lactic acid concentration may be evident in horses with cerebral abscess.[18]

Skull radiographs may help determine the presence of traumatic skull fractures. Bone scan may reveal nondisplaced skull fractures. A fundic examination may reveal papillary edema, detached retina, or active inflammation that may suggest trauma or an infectious cause. EEG and a CT scan may be helpful in localizing and determining the cause of a seizure.[19-21] If one cannot find an underlying cause, then a diagnosis of idiopathic epilepsy can be made.[2,3]

TREATMENT

The goals of treatment for horses or foals with a seizure disorder are to stop any ongoing seizure, to correct any underlying disease that is recognized, and to maintain the animal seizure free. One must base treatment of horses having seizures on medical considerations, client considerations, owner preference and compliance, and the long-term expense of medication. Starting anticonvulsant therapy should be based on the frequency and severity of the seizures of the horse. One may extrapolate guidelines for anticonvulsant therapy from treatment guidelines used in human beings and small animals. Generally, anticonvulsant therapy is indicated in status epilepticus (which occurs rarely in adult horses and uncommonly in foals): one seizure occurring every 2 months; clusters of seizures more than three or four times per year; or several multiple seizures occurring over 1 to 3 days.[22] Foals with idiopathic epilepsy that have several seizures over 1 to 3 days also may require short-term (1 to 3 months) anticonvulsant therapy.[2,3] The chronic use of anticonvulsants in horses is rare. Table 12-7 lists therapy guidelines.[2,3] One should decrease maintenance therapy slowly to determine if continued therapy is needed. The goals of anticonvulsant therapy are to reduce the frequency, duration, and severity of seizures without intolerable side effects. The complete elimination of a seizure may not be possible. The best initial treatment for seizures in horses is diazepam, a benzodiazepine anticonvulsant, and phenobarbital sodium, used for both immediate treatment, as well as for long-term management. Benzodiazepines act to hyperpolarize neuronal cells by binding to the GABA receptors, resulting in change of the chloride conductance pathways and making the cells resistant to depolarization.[23] Although quite effective, the half-life of diazepam is short, 10 to 15 minutes, making repeated doses sometimes necessary. Midazolam is another benzodiazepine that can be used in foals at 0.05 to 1.0 mg/kg intravenously or intramuscularly, as a continuous rate infusion.[24]

One must treat each horse as an individual and tailor the treatment dosages to fit the individual. The owners of horses with seizure disorders need to be made aware that therapy for the control of seizures, particularly in adult horses is often long term, sometimes for years. In addition, the initation of treatment does not guarantee complete elimination of seizures in that horse. A determination of when to begin therapy is based on the frequency and severity of the seizure episodes. Rarely is a horse identified in status epilepticus, meaning continuous seizure activity for more than 30 minutes; however, if present this would be a definite indication for treatment. If a horse has a recognized intracranial disease with seizures, then immediate initiation of treatment is indicated. When no definitive diagnosis exists for the cause of the seizures, then a decision to place the horse on long-term maintenance therapy for seizures is based on recognition of either a cluster of seizures, a frequency of two seizures per month, or occurrence of severe generalized seizures that results in risk of injury to the horse or to human beings in the environment, regardless of seizure frequency.

Adult horses and foals in seizure also may benefit from 1 g/kg DMSO given intravenously as a 10% solution with lactated Ringer's solution or 5% dextrose. DMSO scavenges free oxygen radicals released in damaged tissue and helps maintain cerebral blood flow by reducing thromboxane production, which may result in vasoconstriction and platelet aggregation.[25]

Corticosteroids may be effective initially as an anticonvulsant therapy. One should give a single dose of 0.1 to 0.2 mg/kg dexamethasone intravenously initially and should re-evaluate the horse the next day.[26] Corticosteroids may stabilize neuronal membranes and decrease seizure foci. Corticosteroids and DMSO may be synergistic.

Several drugs are contraindicated in seizures, and they include acetylpromazine, xylazine, and ketamine. Although acetylpromazine has been used to control seizures in foals, the drug is risky because of its ability to lower the seizure threshold.[2,3] Xylazine decreases cerebral blood flow and increases intracranial pressure, which may exacerbate cerebral hypoxia and worsen seizures. However, giving xylazine may be necessary in an emergency situation until a more appropriate drug becomes available. Ketamine increases cerebral blood flow, oxygen consumption, and intracranial pressure and

TABLE 12-7

Anticonvulsant Drugs Used to Treat Seizure Disorders in Horses

Regimen	Drug	50-kg Foal	450-kg Horse
Initial therapy (including status epilepticus)	Diazepam	5-20 mg IV	25-100 mg IV
	Pentobarbital	150-1000 mg IV	To effect
	Phenobarbital	250-1000 mg IV	2-5 g IV
	Phenytoin	50-250 mg IV or PO q4h	–
	Primidone	1-2 g PO	–
	Chloral hydrate (± magnesium sulfate, barbiturate)	3-10 g IV	15-60 g IV
	Xylazine*	25-100 mg IV or IM	300-1000 mg IV or IM
	Guaifenesin (± barbiturate)	To effect	40-60 g
	Carbamazine	250-500 mg	
	Triazolam	1 g	
Maintenance therapy	Phenobarbital	100-500 mg PO b.i.d.	1-5 g PO b.i.d.
	Phenytoin	50-250 mg PO b.i.d.	500-1000 mg PO t.i.d. (low therapeutic index)
	Primidone	1 g PO s.i.d. or b.i.d.	

IV, Intravenously; *IM,* intramuscularly; *PO,* by mouth.
*Should be used only in an emergency situation until an appropriate anticonvulsant agent can be started.

may exacerbate seizures. However, ketamine also antagonizes *N*-methyl-D-aspartate (NMDA) receptors, which are sometimes important in seizures of infants and foals. Use of ketamine in a rodent model, as well as on clinical cases of seizures in neonatal foals appears helpful.

Anticonvulsant medications for maintanence include phenobarbital, phenytoin, bromide, and primidone. In most horses with seizure disorders, phenobarbital is the medication of choice for long-term maintanence. This drug is well-absorbed after oral administration and is metabolized in the liver. After long-term oral administration of phenobarbital, the drug induces hepatic cytochrome P-450 enzyme complex, resulting in an increased rate of metabolism; therefore adjustment of the dose over time may be required. To achieve a steady-state concentration of anti-epileptic medication usually takes about five elimination half-lives, which is approximately 14 to 24 hours for phenobarbital. Therefore monitoring of trough levels 4 to 5 days after the initiation of treatment is important, aiming to achieve a plasma drug concentration of 15 to 45 μg/ml. Monitoring should be done at the time of establishment of initial seizure control, any time the dose of medication is adjusted, or whenever seizure control is inadequate. For most horses, monitoring plasma phenobarbital concentrations approximately every 60 days is adequate after seizure activity is controlled. In adult horses a once-daily oral phenobarbital dose of 10 to 12 mg/kg is usually adequate. In foals a loading dose of 20 mg/kg intravenously followed by repeated intravenous doses every 8 to 12 hours is often necessary.

Bromide is also used for long-term seizure control in adult horses. Bromide appears to compete with chloride to stabilize neuronal membranes. The elimination half-life of this drug in horses is 3 to 5 days. Steady-state concentrations can be expected after five elimination half-lives or after approximately 15 to 25 days of continuous therapy. A loading dose of 120 mg/kg daily for 5 days, followed by a daily oral dose of 40 mg/kg, achieved a serum level of 1 mg/ml, which has been reported to be therapeutic in horses and other species.[27]

NARCOLEPSY

True narcolepsy is an incurable nonprogressive sleep disorder of the CNS characterized by excessive daytime sleepiness with pathologic manifestations of REM sleep. These manifestations also include uncontrolled episodes of loss of muscle tone (cataplexy), although narcolepsy may also occur without cataplexy.[1-3,28] Narcolepsy has been recognized in human beings and in a variety of domestic animals, affecting 0.02% of adults worldwide and over 17 breeds of dogs.[28,29] Although its prevalence is not known in horses, narcolepsy cataplexy appears to be rare and is breed specific. As in human beings and dogs, both familial and sporadic cases of narcolepsy have been observed in horses. The disease has been reported in Suffolk and Shetland foals (the fainting disease),[30] Welsh ponies, Miniature Horses, as well as in Thoroughbred, Quarter Horse, Morgan, Appaloosa, and Standardbred.[1,3,4,31] A familial occurrence is thought to exist in affected Suffolk and Shetland pony foals, and in American Miniature Horses.[3,32] In general, narcolepsy is identified in two distinct groups: (1) in foals (for which the onset occurs at approximately 6 months of age) and (2) in adult horses.

A condition of excessive daytime sleepiness with episodes of collapse or near collapse is described in horses that have been deprived of recumbent sleep for a period of time.[33,34] This may be the result of medical conditions inhibiting recumbency, housing and environmental factors, or social and behavioral factors. Although this problem closely resembles narcolepsy in its clinical presentation, it is a result of sleep deprivation rather than the biochemical abnormalities suspected in horses with true narcolepsy.[35]

Pathophysiology

Four components of narcolepsy are apparent in human beings: (1) excessive daytime sleepiness associated with short periods of REM sleep, (2) cataplexy, (3) hypnagogic hallucinations, and (4) sleep paralysis.[2,36] Cataplexy or sudden collapse with complete inhibition of skeletal muscle tone occurs in horses with narcolepsy.[1,3,4] Respiratory and cardiac muscles are spared.[1]

The normal sleep cycle consists of two stages. Slow-wave sleep (non-REM sleep), mediated by serotonin, occurs first and originates from the midline raphe of the pons. Slow-wave sleep is followed by fast-wave (REM) sleep, which is mediated by norepinephrine. These centers are located in the locus caeruleus of the pons.[1,37] Slow- and fast-wave sleep act through the ascending and descending activation system of the reticular formation.[1] In fast-wave sleep, when REM occurs, the locus caeruleus activates the medial reticular formation nucleus, the axons of which descend the spinal cord to inhibit the lower motor neurons of the somatic efferent system. This inhibition produces atonia.[1,38,39] EEG recording during slow-wave sleep is characterized by synchronized high-voltage (100 μV) and slow-wave activities (2 to 4 Hz) in normal adult horses; in contrast, fast-wave sleep is characterized by desynchronized low-voltage and fast activity, which resembles the patterns of alert wakefulness.[40] Electromyographic recordings during fast-wave sleep show no recordable muscle tone.[1]

With narcolepsy and cataplexy, a biochemical abnormality of the brainstem or sleep-wake center may be responsible for the disease. In human beings, evidence suggests that narcolepsy with cataplexy begins in childhood and is related to an underlying deficiency in the hypothalamic orexin-hypocretin system.[41] Although their physiologic roles are not fully understood, hypocretins are hypothalamic-specific neuropeptides, which are involved in various functions such as sleep, feeding, energy homeostasis, and neuroendocrine and autonomic nerve functions. A mutation in the hypocretin receptor 2 gene has been identified in Dobermans and Labrador retrievers, with secondary impairment in postsynaptic hypocretin neurotransmission. In addition, in acquired canine narcolepsy, the concentration of hypocretin-1 in the brain and CSF was undetectably low, suggesting a loss of production of hypocretin peptides, similar to the pathophysiologic mechanisms reported in human beings.[29] Indeed, an autoimmune process on hypocretin-producing neurons has been suggested in human beings, although future research on this major issue is still required.[28] Although the role of hypocretins in equine narcolepsy is unknown, horses with pituitary pars intermedia dysfunction and with narcolepsy-like episodes also had low concentrations of hypocretin-1 in the CSF.[42]

Clinical Signs

Cataplectic episodes are triggered by strong emotions (usually positive), such as laughing or anger in human beings, and excitement associated with play or the presentation of food in dogs. In horses, the initiation of eating or drinking, petting

or stroking of the head and neck, hosing with cold water after exercise, and leading out of a stall may precipitate a cataplectic episode.[2] The episodes have also been reported during riding. However, one may observe narcolepsy in horses being in a stall or at pasture, without any obvious precipitating events. Tight whole-body restraint may induce a cataplectic state in neonatal foals. This response is thought to be an inherent in utero mechanism that prevents violent movements, especially during parturition.

Clinical signs of narcolepsy vary between mild muscle weakness to complete collapse. Adult horses may drop their heads, buckle at the knees, and stumble.[1-3] If forced to walk, then the horse may be ataxic. Pony breeds are more likely to become recumbent.[2] Horses and ponies that collapse may show absent spinal reflexes and REM sleep. Occasional sudden contraction of a limb or trunk muscle can occur, resulting in a spasmodic motion. Episodes may last between a few seconds to 10 minutes.[1-3] The horse maintains eye and facial responses, normal cardiovascular function, and normal respiratory function during the attack. Horses can be aroused from the attack with varying degrees of difficulty, and most recover and rise quietly without incident.[3] A predictable pattern of duration and frequency of attacks is set within the first 1 to 2 weeks after the onset of disease.[1] Affected horses are neurologically normal between attacks.[1,2]

Diagnosis

Diagnosis of narcolepsy is based on history, clinical signs, pharmacologic testing, and the absence of other diseases. Careful questioning of the caretaker should be performed to determine any event (or events) associated with the episode and video documentation of the episode (or episodes) is optimal. Physical examination may reveal the presence of superficial trauma, particularly over the dorsal aspect of the fetlocks and carpi in most, but not all, cases. A CBC and serum biochemical profile are normal in affected horses and may help to exclude underlying systemic and metabolic abnormalities. CSF is normal in affected horses.[2] EEG and needle EMG during an attack may reveal fast waves of REM sleep and the absence of postinsertional activity of resting muscle.[1]

A provocative test may be useful in diagnosing true narcolepsy or cataplexy in horses. Physostigmine salicylate, an anticholinesterase drug given at 0.05 to 0.1 mg/kg slowly intravenously, precipitates a cataplectic attack within 3 to 10 minutes after administration in affected horses.[2,3,31] This compound crosses the blood-brain barrier.[4] Careful monitoring of the horse after physostigmine administration is necessary because of untoward effects such as colic and cholinergic stimulation. In addition, lack of positive response to physostigmine does not rule out a diagnosis of narcolepsy because individual response to the drug is quite variable and some affected horses failed to respond to this provocative testing.[43]

Atropine sulfate, a muscarinic blocker, given at 0.04 to 0.08 mg/kg intravenously, reduces the severity of cataplectic attacks minutes after administration and can prevent their reoccurrence for 12 to 30 hours after administration.[2,3] Response to atropine sulfate supports a possible cholinergic mechanism for causing cataplexy. One must monitor horses given atropine sulfate for ileus and colic.

Neostigmine, a cholinesterase inhibitor given at 0.005 mg/kg intravenously, does not cross the blood-brain barrier and therefore has no effect on cataplectic attacks. However, neostigmine may help rule out conditions causing muscle weakness such as myasthenia-like syndromes and botulism. Horses with muscle weakness show increased muscle tone and a favorable response to neostigmine.

Differential Diagnosis

Cataplexy, which is specific to narcolepsy, is the best diagnostic marker of this disease and should be distinguished from other causes of episodic weakness. One should also consider other causes of acute collapse in the horse. Ruling out collapse secondary to prolonged sleep deprivation is important because it may be common in horses. This disorder may be caused by chronic pain, environmental factors, or social-behavioral factors. In these cases, administrating NSAIDs in animals with chronic pain, providing the horse with a comfortable environment (to encourage the horse to lay down), or both will improve the clinical signs.[44] Acute collapse without premonitory signs is characteristic of cardiovascular collapse or syncope, and unlike narcolepsy, it is not preceded by gradual lowering of the head and drowsiness. Atrial fibrillation, ruptured chordae tendineae, myocardial infarction, myocardial fibrosis, aortic endocarditis, and pericarditis have been associated with syncope in horses. Cerebral hypoxia may occur in these conditions and may lead to coma, with or without signs of cardiac failure. One should differentiate seizures from narcolepsy and cataplexy. One should also consider botulism (shaker foal syndrome, forage poisoning), myasthenia-like syndrome, postanesthetic neuromyopathy, exertional rhabdomyolysis, and metabolic causes such as hyperthermia, shock, hypoglycemia, hypocalcemia, hypokalemia or hyperkalemia, endotoxemia, anaphylaxis, and snakebite. Horses with hyperkalemic periodic paralysis also may have attacks similar to those in horses with narcolepsy. These horses typically have muscle tremors and may become recumbent with hyporeflexia but are alert and anxious. Attacks in horses with hyperkalemic periodic paralysis may last up to 15 minutes, and the horse usually stands without incident. Diagnosis of this condition is based on clinical signs, serum potassium concentration, potassium chloride provocation, and electromyographic findings.[45,46]

Treatment and Prognosis

In general, drugs that stimulate monoamine systems (e.g., dopamine) in the brain are effective suppressors of narcolepsy, whereas drugs that stimulate cholinergic activity in the brain exacerbate narcolepsy.[47] Imipramine, a tricyclic antidepressant drug, has been recommended to control narcolepsy and cataplexy.[1-3] The drug blocks the uptake of serotonin and norepinephrine and decreases REM sleep.[2] Oral administration (250 to 750 mg orally) produces inconsistent results.[2] Potentially serious adverse effects including muscle fasciculations, tachycardia, hyperresponsiveness to sound, and hemolysis may be seen in horses receiving intravenous doses of imipramine that exceed 2 mg/kg.[47] Adverse effects are not seen when the drug is administered orally, but that is likely because of very poor bioavailabilty. Anecdotally, tyrosine, which may increase dopamine concentration, may improve clinical signs of narcolepsy in some horses.[43]

As mentioned previously, atropine sulfate can provide relief from acute attacks for up to 30 hours, but one must weigh its use against the adverse gastrointestinal side effects it causes.

The prognosis for narcolepsy or cataplexy varies. Some newborn Thoroughbreds and Miniature Horses may have severe attacks but recover fully.[3] In Shetland and Suffolk ponies the disease may persist throughout life, as is true with the adult-onset form.[1-3] In horses 1 to 3 years of age, several episodes may occur but are without permanent consequence.[3]

CENTRAL NERVOUS SYSTEM TRAUMA

*Yvette S. Nout**

Trauma to the CNS is the most common cause of neurologic disease in horses. A recent study from Europe reported CNS trauma to account for 22% of neurologic disorders,[1] which is consistent with the findings from an older report out of Australia that indicated CNS trauma to account for 24% of neurologic cases.[2] Both studies reported trauma to the spinal cord to be more prevalent than brain injury. Feige et al.[1] reported a diagnosis of traumatic brain injury (TBI) in 5 out of 22 (23%) horses that were presented for traumatic neurologic disease, whereas 17 of the 22 (77%) were diagnosed with SCI. Tyler et al.[2] reported 47 cases of TBI and cranial nerve disease in 107 (44%) horses examined, whereas 60 horses in this group had SCI (56%). One study examining head fractures in 21 horses demonstrated that 24% had neurologic deficits secondary to their injuries.[3] Although mechanisms of CNS cell damage, to a certain degree, are similar after TBI and SCI, a few different processes exist with regards to cause and pathophysiology. Clinical syndromes as a result of traumatic injury to the CNS can vary tremendously, but the most common are coma; vestibular disease; tetraparesis, paraparesis, or tetraplegia; and cauda equina syndrome. Treatment regimens for CNS injury are aimed toward reducing inflammation and swelling, halting secondary injury mechanisms, and promoting regeneration and recovery of function. Prognosis depends primarily on severity of primary injury and on the extent and neuroanatomic location of CNS damage.

TRAUMATIC BRAIN INJURY

PATHOPHYSIOLOGY

Head trauma is typically caused by incidents such as collision with an immovable object such as a fencepost or another horse, falling down, flipping over backward, being kicked by another horse, and, although rare, impact by a projectile (e.g., gunshot). A recent study involving 34 horses with TBI showed that the most common cause (44%) of injury was rearing and falling backwards resulting in poll injury.[4] Another type of head injury that may lead to CNS damage is fracture of the petrous temporal bone associated with THO.[5,6]

Although traumatic injury to the head is reported to be common in horses, subsequent TBI occurs only in 25% to 50% of cases.[3,7] The remaining horses typically present for fractures of the orbit, periorbital rim, and zygomatic, mandibular, or maxillary bones.[3,7,8] TBI may occur with or without fracture of the calvarium; however, some of the most severe injuries to the brain occur when the injury is contained within the closed calvarium (i.e., no skull fractures).[9] Within the closed calvarium, the sum of the intracranial volumes of the brain, blood, and CSF are constant; volume or pressure changes within one of these compartments will affect volume (anatomy) or pressure of the other compartments.

Consequences of impact sustained to the poll in horses that flip over backward, include fracture of the bones on the side and base of the calvarium such as the petrous temporal, squamous temporal, and parietal bones. However, more commonly these bones remain intact and more serious injury occurs to the basilar bones as a result of strong traction forces from the rectus capitis ventralis muscles (Figure 12-27).[6,10,11] In addition, adjacent large vessels are lacerated, and hemorrhage into the retropharyngeal spaces or guttural pouches can occur. In severe cases, transverse fracture of the basilar bones at the level of the basioccipital-basisphenoidal suture can occur. Young horses may be more susceptible to this type of injury because the joint between the basilar bones fuses by 5 years of age.[11] In most cases the fracture site is stable and minimal displacement occurs. The cerebellum is seldom severely damaged after poll impact,[6] but the cerebral parenchyma is more commonly injured after being subjected to rapid acceleration-deceleration forces. Moreover, optic nerves and other attachments may be torn from the cerebral hemispheres.[12] Impact to the dorsal surface of the head may result in damage to the frontal or parietal bones, with subsequent cerebral cortical injury or, more commonly, damage to the cervical vertebrae with subsequent SCI.[6] In addition, cranial nerve XII may be injured as it exits the hypoglossal foramen. Furthermore, occipital cortical injury may occur and, as described for poll impact injuries, with frontal injuries the optic nerves may be stretched.

After trauma, most severe damage generally takes place at the place of impact (coup), opposite to the side of impact (contrecoup), or in both locations. Additionally, the brain is subjected to other forces after trauma, such as rotational and shock wave forces. TBI is a result of both direct, immediate mechanical disruption of brain tissue (primary injury) and indirect, delayed (secondary) injury mechanisms. The primary damage is a result of the biomechanical effects of the injury and is characterized by immediate and often irreversible damage to neuronal cell bodies, dendritic arborizations, axons, glial cells, and brain vasculature. This initial brain injury may be focal, multifocal, or diffuse.[13] Secondary injury is a complex cascade of molecular, cellular, and biochemical events that can occur for days to months after the initial insult, resulting in delayed tissue damage. In addition, systemic alterations further contribute to the tissue damage. Hypoxia, ischemia, brain swelling, alterations in intracranial pressure, hydrocephalus, infection, breakdown of blood-brain barrier, impaired energy metabolism, altered ionic homeostasis, changes in gene expression, inflammation, and activation and release of autodestructive molecules occur and exacerbate the initial injury.

Principles of raised intracranial pressure are described in the Monro-Kellie doctrine, which states that once the fontanelles and sutures of the skull are closed, the brain is enclosed in a nonexpandable case of bone, the brain parenchyma is nearly incompressible, the blood volume in the cranial cavity is therefore nearly constant, and a continuous outflow of venous blood from the cranial cavity is required to make

*The authors wish to acknowledge Hilary K. Matthews, whose original work has been incorporated into this section.

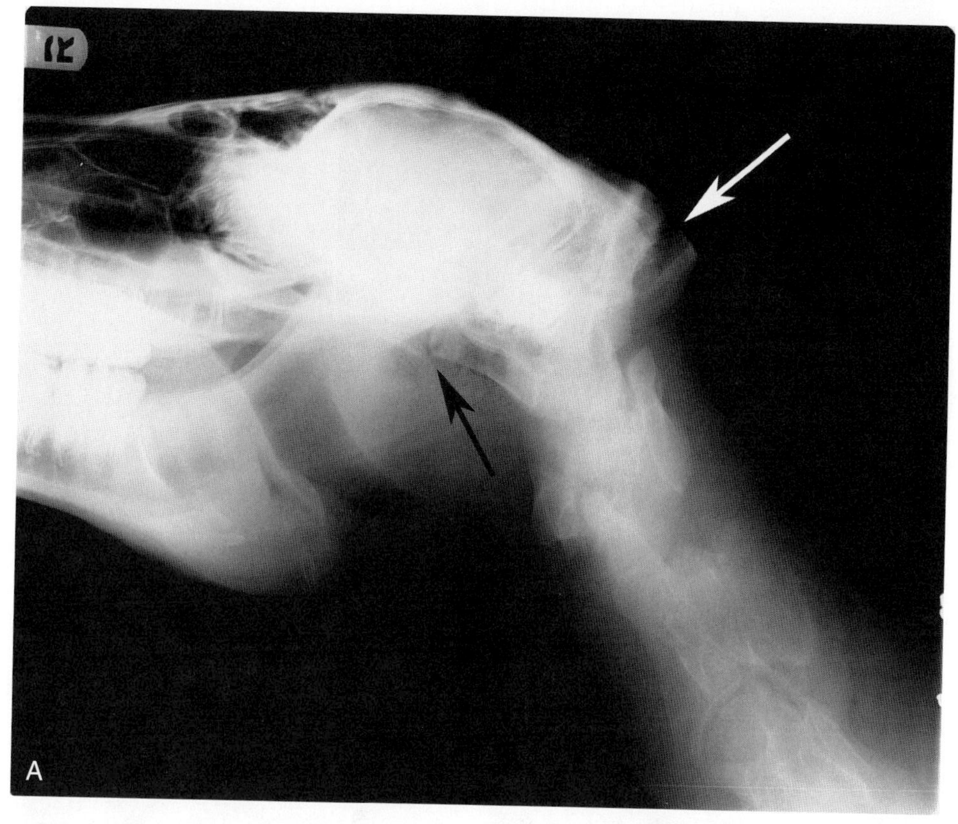

FIGURE 12-27, A, Radiographs taken from a foal that suffered head trauma. The black arrow is pointed at a fracture site at the level of the junction of the basisphenoid and basihyoid bones. A step is visible off the basisphenoid bone. The white arrow is pointed at a defect in the poll. The avulsed fragment of the caudal occipital bone is visible directly caudal to the fracture site.

Continued

room for continuous incoming arterial blood.[14] Blood flow to the brain is controlled by changes in diameter of resistance blood vessels, and cerebral blood flow is controlled by autoregulation whereby the perfusion pressure is maintained within a range of approximately 50 to 150 mm Hg.[15] Beyond these limits, cerebral blood flow decreases at pressures below the lower limit and increases at pressures above the higher limit. Cerebral perfusion pressure (mean arterial blood pressure minus intracranial pressure) is the stimulus to which the autoregulatory response of the vasculature occurs. Cerebral autoregulation is altered unpredictably after TBI, and it appears that the minimum acceptable cerebral perfusion pressure is higher than normal after trauma. Increased intracranial pressure leads to a decreased cerebral perfusion pressure and subsequently reduces cerebral blood flow. Reduced cerebral blood flow results in areas of ischemia and subsequent restriction of delivery of substrates such as oxygen and glucose to the brain. Reduced cerebral blood flow has been associated with an unfavorable neurologic outcome in human beings and has been implicated in increased susceptibility of the brain to secondary injury.[16,17] Brain swelling after TBI because of edema formation and hematoma formation within the skull are the most common causes of increased intracranial pressure. Vascular damage that occurs after head injury can occur epidural (between dura mater and the skull), subdural (between the dura mater and arachnoid mater), subarachnoid (between arachnoid mater and pia mater), superficial (vessels immediately under the pia mater), intraparenchymal, and intraventricular. Subarachnoid hemorrhage, or hemorrhage into the CSF, occurs commonly in horses.[8]

The cascade of secondary injury that results in necrotic and apoptotic cell death is described in more detail in the section on pathophysiology of SCI. Uncontrolled glutamate release and failure of energy systems in neuronal and supporting tissues lead to elevated intracellular calcium concentrations and subsequent cell death. Hemorrhage, ischemia, and the primary tissue damage lead to sequestration of vasoactive and inflammatory mediators at the injury site and are thus involved in the secondary injury cascade. Inflammation and endothelial damage cause derangements in normal cerebrovascular reactivity and contribute to a mismatch of oxygen delivery to tissue demand, resulting in local or diffuse ischemia.

A major consequence of ischemia is reduced delivery of oxygen and glucose. Blood flow interruption is responsible for disruption in ion homeostasis (especially calcium, sodium, and potassium), and a switch to anaerobic glycolysis resulting in lactic acid production and acidosis. Cell membrane lipid peroxidation with subsequent prostaglandin and thromboxane synthesis, formation of reactive oxygen species (ROS), nitric oxide, and energy failure also ensue. Because of the high metabolic rate and oxygen demand of the brain, disruption of blood flow rapidly compromises the energy-supplying processes and leads to impaired nerve cell function and even cell death. Impaired mitochondrial function with subsequent energy depletion leads to a loss in maintenance of membrane potentials resulting in depolarization of neurons and glia.[18]

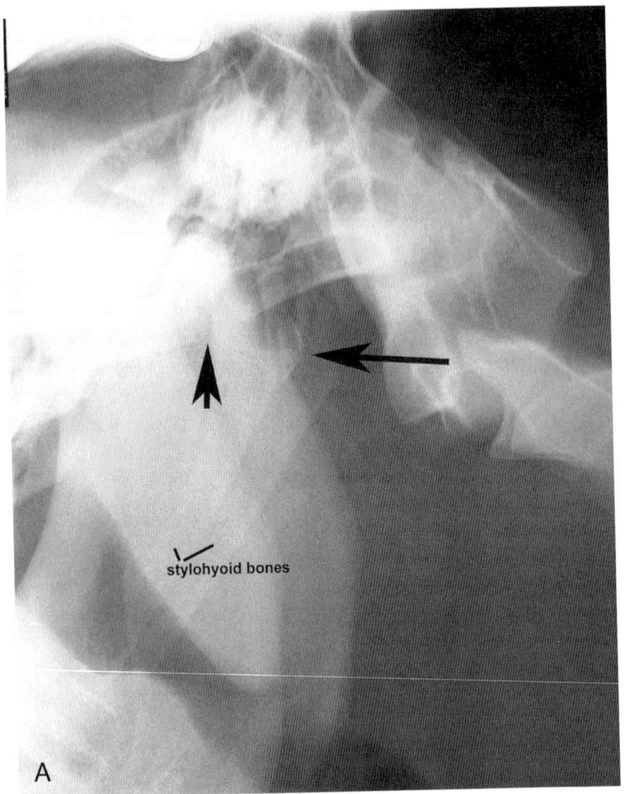

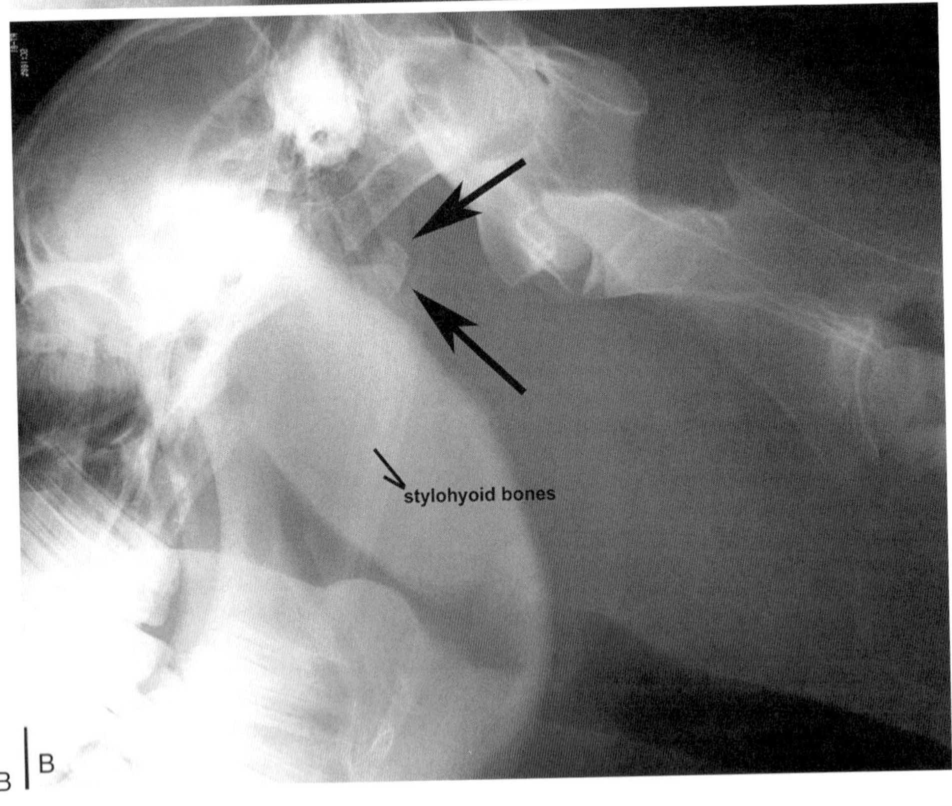

FIGURE 12-27, cont'd B, Radiographs taken from a horse that suffered trauma to the head that resulted in a fracture of the basisphenoid bone with avulsion of a fragment into the guttural pouch. The small arrow in (**A**) indicates the defect of the basisphenoid bone and the larger arrow the site of the avulsed bone. In (**B**) the avulsed bone is clearly visible between the two stylohyoid bones.

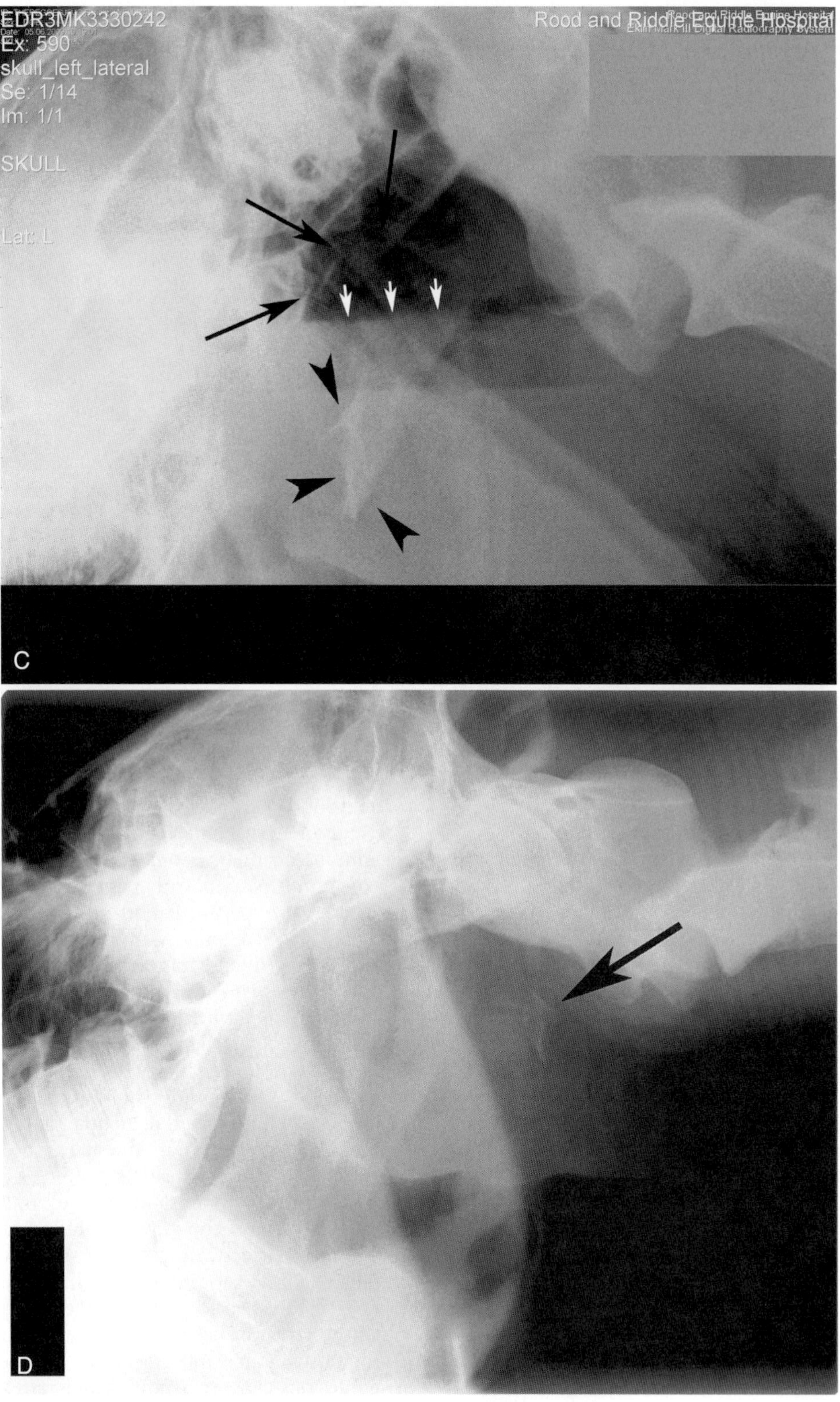

FIGURE 12-27, cont'd C, Radiograph from a 3-year-old thoroughbred colt that flipped while playing on the end of the lead shank. The horse hit its head on a small board along the side of the walkway and was unconscious for 3 to 5 minutes. The horse had blood coming from the nostrils, paralysis of the right eyelid, a corneal ulcer on the right eye, and weakness in all four limbs. The radiograph shows a fluid line in the guttural pouch *(small white arrows)*, a basisphenoid fracture *(large black arrows)* with a large fragment *(arrowheads)* visible in the guttural pouch area. **D,** This is a radiograph taken from a horse after head injury and subsequent rupture of the longus capitis muscle and an avulsion fracture from the basisphenoid bone. The arrow is pointed at the avulsed bone located behind the guttural pouch. Image from The Ohio State University. (A and C courtesy of Stephen Reed, DVM, Rood and Riddle Equine Hospital; B and D courtesy of The Ohio State University.)

Cytotoxic edema develops through the failure of the sodium-potassium ATPase-dependent pump in the presence of hypoxia and the subsequent influx of water that passively follows sodium and chloride. This type of edema occurs in gray and white matter and decreases the extracellular fluid volume.[19] If capillary endothelial cells are edematous, then the capillary lumen size will diminish, creating an increased resistance to arterial flow. Capillary permeability is usually not directly affected in cytotoxic edema. Major decreases in cerebral function occur with cytotoxic edema, with stupor and coma being common signs.[19] In addition to cytotoxic edema, vasogenic edema develops as a result of disruption of the blood-brain barrier, which includes damage of endothelial cells, degeneration of pericytes, and loss of astrocytes. Extravasation of blood components and water occurs resulting in increased extracellular fluid accumulation. This is referred to as *vasogenic edema*.[19] Understanding the complex pathophysiologic events that take place after TBI is important for development of effective monitoring and treatment strategies.

Neurologic Evaluation

Clinical signs associated with TBI range from inapparent to recumbency with unconsciousness or death (Figure 12-28). A complete physical examination is very important in head trauma cases, because fractures and other concurrent injuries are not uncommon and require identification and treatment. Physical examination findings as a result of head trauma can include fractures; hemorrhage from the nostrils, mouth, and ears; CSF draining from the ear (Figure 12-29); respiratory distress; cardiac arrhythmias; and hypo- or hypertension.[6,8,10]

Hemorrhage from the nose typically presents as dark-colored (venous) blood and originates from a paranasal sinus, ethmoid turbinates, or nasal cavity. Occasionally, blood is bright red and then usually originates from larger vessels in the guttural pouches.[6,20] Respiratory distress can occur associated with significant throat swelling after profuse hemorrhage into the guttural pouches. Furthermore, neurogenic pulmonary edema has been reported to occur. Acute elevation of intracranial pressure may result in the Cushing's reflex, which is a hypothalamic response to brain ischemia and is characterized by hypertension and secondary baroreceptor-mediated bradycardia. Continued elevation of intracranial pressure and reduction of cerebral blood flow results in increased sympathetic discharge (catecholamines), with subsequent myocardial ischemia and development of cardiac arrhythmias. This is referred to as the *brain-heart syndrome*.

Life-threatening injuries should be attended to first, and then a complete neurologic examination should be performed. Horses may be recumbent, intractable, or both after a traumatic incident; examination and management of these horses can be difficult and dangerous (see Figure 12-28).[21] Signs of focal brain injury are listed in Table 12-8. Sedation may be necessary for examination. Although α_2-agonists may transiently cause hypertension, which may potentiate intracranial hemorrhage,[22] xylazine has been found to cause a minor decrease in cerebrospinal pressure in normal, conscious horses.[23] Xylazine is probably a safe sedative to use in horses with head trauma, if the horse's head is not allowed to drop to such a low position that postural effects could lead to physiologic increases of intracranial pressure.[7]

The complete neurologic examination should include an assessment of the horse's mentation, cranial nerve function, posture, and ability to coordinate movements, as well as its ability to regulate rate and range of motion. In addition, reflex and nociceptive testing should be performed to investigate any concurrent SCI. Serial neurologic examinations, particularly during the first hours, are important for diagnostic purposes and to allow prediction of a more accurate prognosis. Furthermore, serial examinations are important to assess response to therapy.[7,21] Pupil size, symmetry, and response to light should be assessed in all horses and followed carefully, particularly in recumbent horses. A change from bilateral pupillary constriction to bilateral dilation with no response to light is a poor prognostic indicator.[7]

The most common neurologic syndromes after head trauma are a result of hemorrhage into the middle and inner ear cavities. Signs are those of central or peripheral vestibular disease and facial nerve damage and include recumbency, head tilt, neck turn, body lean, and circling, all toward the side of the lesion. The ipsilateral eye may be rotated ventrally and laterally, and there may be horizontal or rotary nystagmus with the fast phase away from the lesion.[6,22] Facial paralysis on the same side as the lesion is seen with cranial nerve VII damage. Central vestibular disease is suspected when signs of brainstem disease or other cranial nerve deficits are present. Central vestibular lesions can result in a paradoxical vestibular syndrome,, in which the lesion is located on the side opposite to that which is expected from the clinical signs.[6] More serious trauma can lead to alterations of mentation, behavior, or both.

The level of consciousness is affected by the degree of damage to the cerebrum and reticular activating system in the brainstem. Immediately after cerebral injury, a period of concussion occurs, with unconsciousness for various periods of time, or even coma. Usually a horse recovers from this in minutes to hours. Comatose horses may have an irregular breathing pattern with periods of either Cheyne-Stokes breathing or hyperventilation. In some horses, seizures can occur after initial concussion; these are typically generalized seizures. Level of mentation and responsiveness to reflexes should be assessed and recorded. Injury to the occipital cortex can result in impairment of vision and menace response of the eye contralateral to the lesion. Pupillary light reflex, however, should remain intact. Injury to the parietal cortex can result in decreased facial sensation on the contralateral side. Another sign of cerebral damage is dementia, or altered behavior, such as walking in circles (toward the side of the lesion), head pressing, hyperexcitability, or aggression.[6,7,22]

Severe rostral brainstem injuries (mesencephalon) can be associated with coma and depression because of damage to the reticular activating system. Strabismus, asymmetrical pupil size, and loss of pupillary light response can be present because of damage to cranial nerve III. Apneustic or erratic breathing reflects a poor prognosis, and bilaterally dilated and unresponsive pupils indicate an irreversible brainstem lesion. These lesions can occur immediately after injury, secondary to herniation of components of the cerebrum or cerebellum, or after hemorrhage. Severe brainstem injuries may result in a decorticate posture, characterized by rigid extension of neck, back, and limbs.[6] Injury to caudal parts of the brainstem (pons and medulla) result in dysfunction of multiple cranial nerves in addition to depression and limb ataxia and weakness. To make a distinction between a cranial cervical spinal cord and caudal brainstem lesion, careful assessment of the horse's mentation and function of cranial nerves X and XII is important.[6,7]

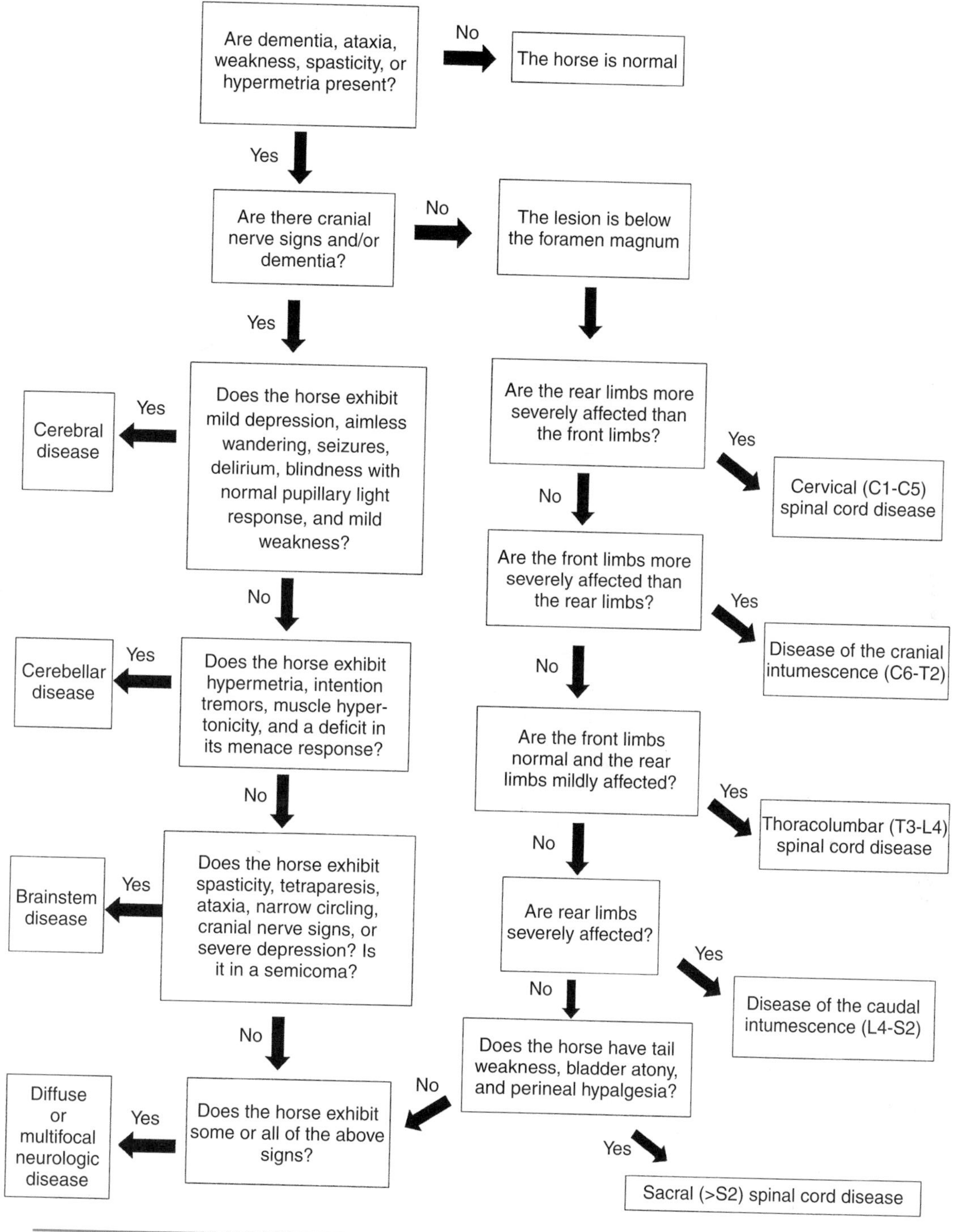

FIGURE 12-28 Flow chart for localizing a lesion in the nervous system in a recumbent horse.

Signs of cerebellar injury occur infrequently and include intention tremor, broad-based stance, spastic limb movements, and absent menace response with normal vision. If multiple areas of the brain are damaged, then this will be reflected in the different clinical signs. Multifocal damage or progression of disease through hemorrhage, secondary injury mechanisms, or both is suggested when clinical signs become more widespread.

Diagnostic tools that are helpful in further defining cranial trauma include radiography, computed tomography, MRI, endoscopy, electrodiagnostics, and CSF analysis. Radiographs are used to determine the presence and severity of fractures, hemorrhage in cavities, or thickening of stylohyoid bone or bulla (or both). A recent study determined that of the horses with bony fractures of the calvarium (22), only 50% were confirmed radiographically.[4] Computed tomography is very sensitive for detection of bony abnormalities and also provides some information on soft tissues and brain matter.[24-26] Soft tissue changes seen after TBI, for example, are change in the size, shape, and position of the ventricles, deviation of the falx cerebri, and focal changes in brain opacity.[6] In human beings, CT findings may include midline shift and obliteration of sulci and cisterns, for which a grading system exists that can be used in combination with other diagnostics for prognostication purposes.[27] Enhancement of areas of injury or hemorrhage is possible with iodinated contrast agents. MRI offers a higher sensitivity for examination of soft tissue structures and has the ability to acquire images in all planes. However, the use of MRI is not yet possible for all equine clinicians.

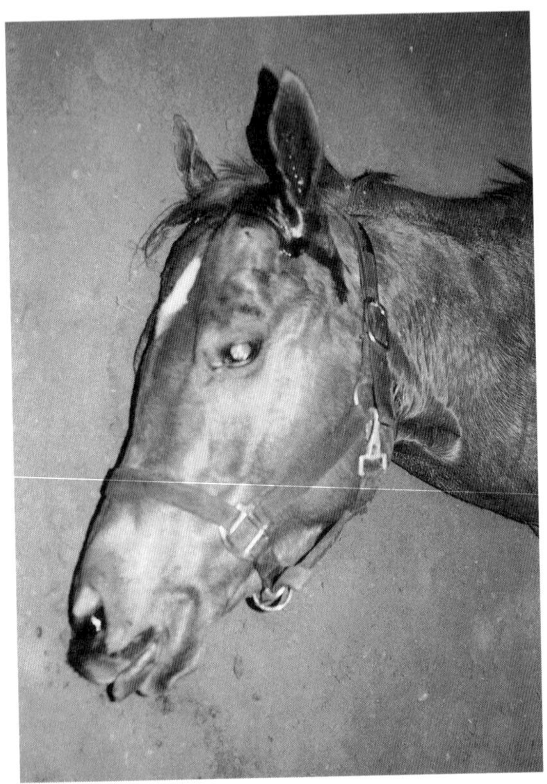

FIGURE 12-29 Blood and cerebrospinal fluid (CSF) draining from the ear after a basilar skull fracture.

Upper respiratory endoscopy is an important diagnostic procedure for evaluation of cranial nerve function, stylohyoid bones, retropharyngeal area, and appearance of guttural pouches. Use of electrodiagnostics is typically not indicated immediately after TBI; however, after stabilization or during recovery these techniques will provide information about certain levels of (dys)function. For example, electroencephalograms are used for assessment of seizure activity, BAER is used for examination of vestibular function, and visual function is examined with visual-evoked potential in combination with electroretinography. CSF analysis may not always be indicated after acute trauma, but it may be useful for excluding other diseases. Cisternal CSF collection is contraindicated if increased intracranial pressure is suspected because of the possibility of brain herniation through the foramen magnum. Lumbosacral collection is a safer alternative but can be normal despite a traumatic episode, especially in the acute phase, and because the sample is not obtained closest to the lesion, it may not reflect the changes that have occurred. CSF lactate concentrations are increased after trauma in horses.[28]

More invasive diagnostic and monitoring modalities are available. Methods to measure and monitor intracranial and cerebral perfusion pressures have been described for use in foals[29] and adult horses.[30,31] However, these techniques have thus far not been scientifically evaluated in clinical cases. In human medicine, development of advanced bedside neuromonitoring devices has been an important focus in neurocritical care. The four most important parameters to be determined are (1) intracranial pressure, (2) cerebral blood flow, (3) information on brain metabolism, and (4) functional outcome. In human beings, catheters may be placed into the brain tissue to determine glucose, glycerol, and glutamate concentrations, indicators of secondary ischemia,[32,33] by microdialysis. In addition, probes may be placed to determine brain tissue oxygen tension. It appears that use of multimodality monitoring techniques, in which complementary regional neuromonitoring

TABLE 12-8

Signs Characteristic of Focal Brain Injury

Levels	Consciousness	Motor Function	Pupils	Other Sign
Cerebrum	Behavior change, depression, coma	Circling	Normal	Blindness
Cerebellum		Ataxia and hypermetria, intention tremor		Menace response deficit without blindness
Diencephalon (thalamus)	Depression to stupor	Normal to mild tetraparesis, "aversive syndrome"*	Bilateral, nonreactive pupils with visual deficit	None
Midbrain	Stupor to coma	Hemiparesis, tetraparesis or tetraplegia	Nonreactive pupils, mydriasis, anisocoria	Ventrolateral strabismus
Pons	Depression	Ataxia and tetraparesis, tetraplegia	Normal	Head tilt, abnormal nystagmus, facial paralysis, medial strabismus
Rostral medulla oblongata (including inner ear)	Depression	Ataxia or hemiparesis to tetraplegia	Normal	Same
Caudal medulla oblongata	Depression	Ataxia, hemiparesis to tetraparesis, abnormal respiratory patterns	Normal	Dysphagia, flaccid tongue

From Robinson NE, editor: Current therapy in equine medicine, ed 6, St Louis, 2009, WB Saunders.
*Deviation of the head and eyes with circling toward the side of a unilateral lesion.

tools may measure tissue pH, cerebral blood flow, or biochemical metabolites would be part of an optimal overall strategy.[34]

Treatment and Prognosis

Based on the pathophysiology of events that occur after TBI, it is likely that single drug intervention would not be effective. Treatment of TBI is aimed at optimizing delivery of oxygen and substrates to brain tissue to salvage brain tissue that is undamaged or reversibly damaged. This requires optimizing cerebral blood flow (i.e., optimizing mean arterial blood pressure and hemoglobin concentration; ensuring intracranial pressure is not elevated). Emergency surgical treatment (although not commonly performed) is warranted in open cranial fractures and in the face of deterioration despite medical therapy. A recent report describes the surgical and medical treatment of a horse with severe and unfortunately fatal TBI.[35] In Figure 12-30 a flow chart is shown that can serve as a guide to the management of cranial trauma in horses. Evaluation of potential treatment strategies affecting secondary injury pathways has recently been reviewed.[36]

Methods to reduce intracranial pressure include hyperventilation, CSF drainage, treatment with hyperosmolar agents or barbiturates, head elevation, and decompressive surgery. Hyperventilation reduces the partial pressure of carbon dioxide in blood and subsequently leads to cerebral vasoconstriction. Reduced cerebral blood volume reduces intracranial pressure. However, cerebral vasoconstriction may lead to reduction of cerebral blood flow to ischemic levels. Hyperventilation could be considered in cases of increased intracranial pressure in horses. Proper hyperventilation requires monitoring of arterial blood gases and may require use of neuromuscular blockers if the horse is not comatose and is resisting the ventilator. CSF drainage is commonly used in people to reduce intracranial pressure; however, it is therapeutic only if CSF outflow obstruction is noted. If these methods are ineffective, then repeat imaging is pursued to investigate the presence of mass lesions before medical treatments are commenced such as administration of hyperosmolar substances and induction of barbiturate coma. Hyperosmolar treatment is commonly used in horses with neurologic signs attributable to TBI. This is discussed later in this section.

Mean arterial blood pressure should be maintained within normal limits. Blood transfusion may be indicated in cases of severe hemorrhage. Crystalloid fluids are recommended as fluid therapy of choice, particularly in light of findings of the serum versus albumin fluid evaluation (SAFE) study[37] that determined no difference between outcomes between administering albumin versus normal saline in the intensive care unit (and in which subgroup analysis demonstrated an increased mortality in TBI patients that were treated with albumin). However, isotonic crystalloid fluids administered in typical shock doses of 40 to 90 ml/kg/hr may produce worsening of cerebral edema and increased intracranial pressure.[38] Comparison of isotonic crystalloid fluids with hypertonic saline solutions has shown hypertonic saline to be the fluid of choice for fluid support of head trauma patients in shock.[39] Hypertonic saline is associated with significant decreases in intracranial pressure and cerebral water content compared with isotonic fluid treatment. Furthermore, hypertonic saline has positive effects on cerebral blood flow, oxygen consumption, and inflammatory response at a cellular level.[40] Hypertonic saline can be administered intravenously to head trauma horses in shock as 5% or 7% sodium chloride (NaCl) solutions (4 to 6 ml/kg) over 15 minutes. Isotonic fluids can then be used for maintenance if needed. Contraindications to the use of hypertonic saline include dehydration, ongoing intracerebral hemorrhage, hypernatremia, renal failure, hyperkalemic periodic paralysis, and hypothermia. Systemic side effects include coagulopathies, excessive intravascular volume, and electrolyte abnormalities. Monitoring central venous pressure and maintaining it within normal limits (5-7 cm H_2O) is therefore important, as well as monitoring serum sodium and potassium concentrations if hypertonic saline is used frequently.[39]

The use of carbohydrate-containing intravenous solutions should be avoided early in the treatment of head trauma patients. Glucose suppresses ketogenesis and may increase lactic acid production by the traumatized brain, limiting the availability of nonglycolytic energy substrates.[41] Furthermore, carbon dioxide liberated from glucose metabolism could cause vasodilation and worsening of cerebral edema. It has been well established that maintaining blood glucose concentrations at 80 to 110 mg/dl through intensive insulin therapy reduces morbidity and mortality in human critical care patients.[42] However, neurointensivists have shown that intensive insulin therapy increases markers of cellular distress in the brain and suggest that systemic glucose concentrations of 80 to 110 mg/dl is too low in TBI and may lead to cerebral hypoglycemia.[43] Recommendations now are to maintain blood glucose concentrations at 120 to 140 mg/dl in TBI.

Treatment with anti-inflammatories is likely the most commonly used treatment in equine TBI. Indications for use of anti-inflammatory treatment are to combat the inflammatory pathways of secondary injury mechanisms (cytokine release, free radicals), improve comfort level, and reduce fever. Fever is extremely common after TBI, and it has been well documented in animal models and in human beings to negatively affect outcome after TBI (e.g., by augmenting secondary injury mechanisms).[44,45] Researchers have proposed that a proactive approach should be taken toward reducing fever. In fact, hypothermia has been shown to be neuroprotective. Hypothermia results in decreased cellular metabolism and has been proven efficacious as a treatment for TBI in experimental and clinical settings.[46] The neuroprotective effects include reduced release of excitotoxins, reduction of free radical and inflammatory mediator formation, and reduction of blood-brain barrier disruption. However, long-term benefits and improved functional outcome has not been adequately demonstrated.[47,48] Therapeutics with anti-inflammatory properties that are common to equine practice include corticosteroids, NSAIDs, DMSO, and vitamin E. These drugs are discussed in more detail in the section pertaining to SCI.

Controlling seizure activity is very important after TBI, because seizure activity increases cerebral metabolic rate and is detrimental to secondary injury. It is not unusual for horses sustaining cranial trauma to develop seizures. Diazepam, midazolam, phenobarbital, or pentobarbital are drugs that can be used to control seizures. Intractable seizures may necessitate general anesthesia. Agents useful for general anesthesia include guaifenesin, chloral hydrate, barbiturates, and gas anesthesia. Ketamine is not recommended as part of a balanced anesthesia regimen because it increases cerebral blood flow and intracranial pressure.

Barbiturate treatment or coma may decrease cerebral metabolism, thereby providing a protective effect against cerebral ischemia. Barbiturates may also limit lipid peroxidation.

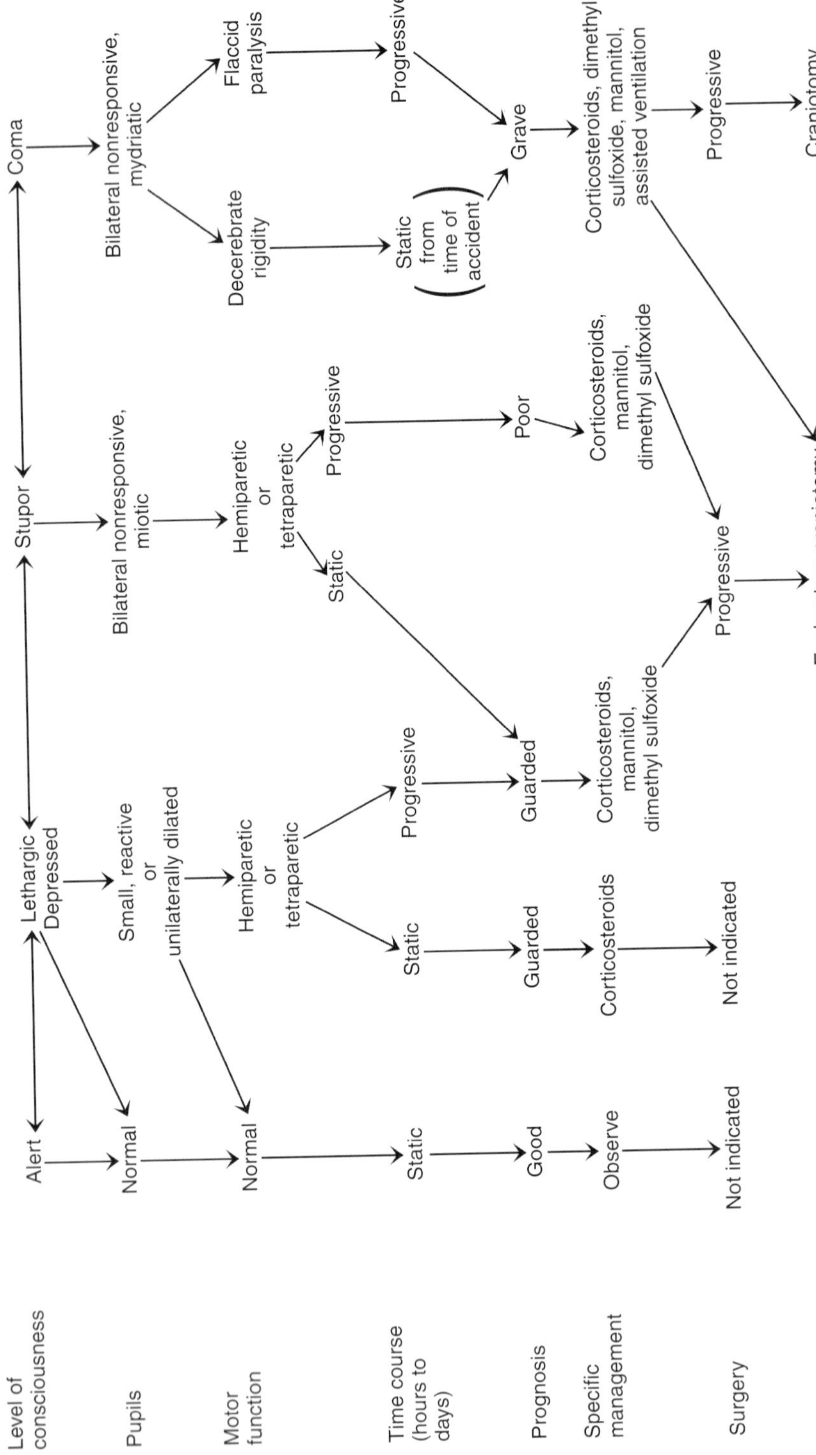

FIGURE 12-30 Flow chart for management of cranial trauma. (From Robinson NE, editor: Current therapy in equine medicine, ed 6, St Louis, 2009, WB Saunders; modified from Kirk KW, editor: Current veterinary therapy VII, Philadelphia, 1980, WB Saunders.)

However, the actual benefits of barbiturate use on the neurologic outcome remain controversial. The effects of barbiturates on lowering intracranial pressure are enhanced by concurrent hyperventilation. An exact dosage regimen for barbiturate treatment in horses has not been investigated, but 5 to 10 mg/kg intravenous to effect is reported to be useful. The major adverse effect of barbiturates is hypotension, especially if mannitol and furosemide have been administered, so they must be used with caution and adequate blood pressure monitoring. Barbiturates should be reserved for those cases in which elevated intracranial pressure is refractory to other treatments. Other methods to lower intracranial pressure include elevation of the head by 30 degrees if no cervical fractures are present[49] and decompressive craniectomy. Rationale for use of the latter is comparison of the effect of a durotomy for compartment syndrome of the brain to that of a fasciotomy in muscle compartment syndrome.[50,51] This technique has been used in normal dogs and was effective at reducing intracranial pressure.[52]

Furosemide has experimentally been found effective in decreasing intracranial pressure.[53] A 1 mg/kg bolus intravenous dose was administered at 5-hour intervals and a 0.5 mg/kg/hr dose was administered intravenously as a continuous rate infusion for 4 hours, 1 hour after the initial bolus. Normal hydration status is required before furosemide is administered. Furosemide may also be used concurrently with mannitol to increase the duration of intracranial pressure reduction provided by mannitol, and to diminish the potential for rebound intracranial pressure elevation. Hyperosmolar therapy forms the mainstay of treatment for elevated intracranial pressure.

Mannitol has been the primary osmotherapeutic drug for the last four decades. Mannitol induces changes in blood rheology and increases cardiac output, leading to improved cerebral perfusion pressure and cerebral oxygenation. Improved cerebral oxygenation induces cerebral artery vasoconstriction and subsequent reduction in cerebral blood volume and intracranial pressure. Mild dehydration after osmotherapy is desirable and may improve cerebral edema; however, severe dehydration can lead to hyperosmolality and renal failure. Mannitol also decreases CSF production by up to 50%, which can lead to prolonged intracranial pressure decrease.[39] In horses, 20% mannitol can be administered at 0.25 to 2.0 mg/kg intravenously over 20 minutes. Horses receiving osmotic diuretics should be adequately hydrated. The use of osmotic substances is warranted in any horse with worsening mental status, abnormal pupillary size or inequality indicating transtentorial herniation, or development of paresis. Although mannitol administration is very effective in reducing intracranial pressure, several limitations to its use exist. Hyperosmolality can be associated with renal and CNS effects. Furthermore, administration of multiple doses of mannitol may lead to intravascular dehydration, hypotension, and reduction of cerebral blood flow. Therefore current research is focused on the use of substitutes for mannitol, of which the most promising is hypertonic saline.

Hypertonic saline has a number of beneficial effects in TBI. The permeability of the blood-brain barrier to sodium is low. Hypertonic saline produces an osmotic gradient between the intravascular and the interstitial-intracellular compartments, leading to shrinkage of brain tissue and subsequent reduction of intracranial pressure. The reflection coefficient of NaCl is more than that of mannitol, making it potentially a more effective osmotic drug. As described previously, hypertonic saline augments volume resuscitation and increases circulating blood volume, mean arterial blood pressure, and cerebral perfusion pressure. Other beneficial effects include restoration of neuronal membrane potential, maintenance of the blood-brain barrier integrity, and modulation of the inflammatory response by reducing adhesion of leukocytes to endothelium.[39,54] Hypertonic saline typically is used as 3.0%, 5.0%, or 7.5% solutions, but a recent study showed beneficial effects of using small-volume 23.4% hypertonic saline to reduce intracranial pressure.[55]

Antibiotic treatment is usually warranted in cases of head trauma, especially when fractures are involved. The presence of hemorrhage increases the possibility of septic meningitis. Antibiotic choice should be based on culture and sensitivity testing. Good empiric choices for broad spectrum coverage include trimethoprim-sulfamethoxazole and penicillin in combination with gentamicin. Appropriate monitoring for aminoglycoside toxicity should be undertaken with their use. Owing to disruption of the blood-brain barrier, other antimicrobials probably penetrate into the CNS, and therefore their use may also be efficacious.

Nutritional support plays a role in the outcome after neurologic injury. In human beings, neurologic recovery from head injury occurs faster in patients receiving early adequate nutritional support.[56] If the horse is able to eat and the gastrointestinal tract is functioning normally, then water and good-quality hay should be available at all times. Small amounts of grain should be fed three to four times a day to boost caloric intake. The amount of grain fed should be based on the horse's condition and ability to tolerate grain feeding. Horses with a poor appetite or those unable to swallow may have to be tube fed using a gruel of alfalfa and complete feed pellets.[21] Horses in which enteral feeding is not possible are candidates for total parenteral nutrition. Thiamine may be of benefit in treating head injuries because thiamine aids in metabolism of lactic acid and is a necessary coenzyme in brain energy pathways.

The prognosis for cranial trauma is dependent on severity of insult and early treatment, and it is gauged by response to treatment. An early prognosis based on initial findings is important to establish for owners and thus can influence clinical decisions. However, in a study performed in human TBI patients, even with sophisticated clinical and radiologic technologies, it was not possible to predict outcome on the first day after the accident with sufficient accuracy to guide early management.[57] Here again, it is important to highlight the value of repeated neurologic evaluations. In general, basilar fractures and severe brainstem injuries carry a grave prognosis.[4,10] Recumbency, tetraparesis, and severe dementia carry a poor-to-grave prognosis.[8] A recent retrospective confirmed that recumbency of more than 4-hours duration after the initial onset of trauma and the presence of basilar skull fractures were associated with nonsurvival having odds ratios of 18 and 7.5, respectively.[4] Time, good nursing care, and adequate nutritional support, especially in the recumbent horse, are vital for a positive outcome.

SPINAL CORD AND VERTEBRAL INJURY

PATHOPHYSIOLOGY

Trauma to the vertebral column is typically caused by incidents, such as collision with an immovable object or falling down. Injury to the vertebral column can occur at all sites, but trauma to or fractures of the cervical vertebrae are the most common.[1,2,9,22] Foals appear to be more susceptible to vertebral trauma than adults and frequently suffer injury to the cranial cervical (C1-3), and caudal thoracic (T15-18) regions.[9] Fractures elsewhere along the vertebral column occur as well.[58] Vertebral fracture with subsequent SCI, not as a result of trauma but secondary to osteomyelitis, has been reported.[59] Predilection sites for vertebral trauma in adult horses are the occipital-atlanto-axial region, the caudal cervical region (C5-T1), and the caudal thoracic region.[9,22] Reports also exist of injuries at the sacral[60,61] and coccygeal[62,63] regions.

Typically, the more severe the insult is, the more damage occurs to the vertebral column (and the more severe clinical signs are due to soft tissue damage and osseous fragments compressing the spinal cord; Table 12-9). With very severe injury, soft tissue structures supporting the vertebral column may be disrupted, resulting in dislocation of vertebrae. Both subluxation and luxation of vertebrae have been reported in horses.[64] An increased incidence of luxations, subluxations, and epiphyseal separations is seen in young horses, which is likely because cervical vertebral growth plate closure does not occur until 4 to 5 years of age.[9] Compression injuries are associated with shortening of the vertebral body and result from a head-on collision with an immovable object.

SCI secondary to trauma is a dynamic process of which the severity is related to the velocity, degree, and duration of the impact. Cord concussion with transient neurologic deficits is a result of local axonal depolarization and transient dysfunction, whereas permanent paralysis is a result of primary tissue injury followed by spreading of secondary damage that expands from the injury epicenter.

Primary injury is the initial mechanical damage to the components of the spinal cord that follows acute insult. Blood vessels are broken, axons are disrupted, and neuron and glial cell membranes are damaged. Ensuing pathophysiologic processes involving ischemia, release of chemicals from injured cells, and electrolyte shifts alter the metabolic milieu at the level of the lesion and trigger a secondary injury cascade that substantially compounds initial mechanical damage. These secondary injury processes do not necessarily coincide with the clinical picture, because pathologic changes may progress in severity for weeks to months, even in the face of clinical improvement.

Secondary injury involves both necrotic and programmed cell death, and although mechanisms involved in this are not fully understood, some aspects of this process are well described. Disruption of cellular and subcellular membranes of glia, neurons, and vascular endothelial cells is believed to be the initiator of this autodestructive cascade of events, and it is likely that multiple mechanisms are involved such as ischemia, inflammation, free radical–induced cell death, excitotoxicity, cytoskeletal degradation, and induction of apoptotic pathways. The consequence of secondary injury is enlargement of the area of cell death. The phase of secondary injury is widely studied because this process progresses from minutes to months after injury and is thus considered to be a target for therapeutic interventions. Minimizing secondary injury through protection of neural elements that initially survived the mechanical injury would increase the quantity of spared tissue and could lead to reduced functional impairment.

Acute injury results in immediate hemorrhage and cell destruction within the central gray matter. Loss of microcirculation and cord swelling within minutes of injury occurs mainly because of hemorrhage and development of edema. The initial hemorrhage, edema, and hypoperfusion of the gray matter extends centripetally within minutes to hours of injury and results in central necrosis, white matter edema, and eventually, demyelination of axons through secondary injury processes. Spinal cord ischemia develops over several hours after injury and is considered one of the most important contributors to secondary injury.[65,66] Mechanical disruption of the microvasculature, vasospasm of intact vessels, and edema together lead to profound local hypoperfusion and ischemia. Cord swelling that exceeds venous blood pressure results in

TABLE 12-9

Common Types of Vertebral Trauma

Level of Injury	Age	Type of Vertebral Trauma	Common Traumatic Injury	Syndrome
Cervical	Foal to yearling	Fracture of dens, luxation C1-C2	Hyperflexion (e.g., somersault)	Tetraparesis, respiratory depression, death
Cervical	Young adult	Epiphyseal fracture	Hyperextension	Tetraparesis to tetraplegia
Cervical	Adult	Compression fracture	Head-on collision	Tetraparesis to tetraplegia
Cranial thoracic	Usually young	Fracture of dorsal spinous process	Flipping over backward	Often none
T2-S1	Any	Transverse fracture of vertebral arch, with dislocation	Somersaulting or falls	Paraparesis
Sacroiliac subluxation	Adult	Subluxation	Falls or slipping on ice	None
Sacral fracture	Any	Compression	Fall over backward or dog sitting when backed	Urinary and fecal incontinence with or without posterior paresis, paralysis of the tail and anus

From Robinson NE, editor: Current therapy in equine medicine, ed 6, St Louis, 2009, WB Saunders.

secondary ischemia, and ischemia is further exacerbated by cessation of autoregulation of spinal cord blood flow and systemic hypotension.

During the ischemic hypoxic state, cell metabolism is altered such that a shift occurs from aerobic to anaerobic metabolism, which is a less efficient method of energy production. Anaerobic metabolism results in lactic acid accumulation, causing acidosis in nervous tissue, thus decreasing glucose and oxygen consumption. Furthermore, lactic acid stimulates prostaglandin production, adenosine diphosphate release, platelet aggregation, thromboxane A_2 release, vasospasm, vasoconstriction, and the inhibition of neurotransmitter release. In addition, in hypoxic states, the sodium-potassium ATPase-dependent cell pump is inhibited or damaged, resulting in the cell's inability to maintain its electric polarity. Damage to this pump allows for accumulation of potassium extracellularly and sodium intracellularly, which contributes to the development of edema.[67]

Free radicals can cause progressive oxidation of fatty acids in cellular membranes (lipid peroxidation) through reactions with their unpaired electrons. Furthermore, oxidative stress can disable key mitochondrial respiratory chain enzymes, alter DNA/RNA and their associated proteins, and inhibit sodium-potassium ATPase. These changes can induce metabolic collapse and necrotic or apoptotic cell death and are considered important during the initial period of hypoperfusion (and perhaps even more important during the period of reperfusion). In addition to oxidative stress and membrane damage, nitric oxide production and excitatory amino acid–induced calcium entry are considered important mediators of necrotic and apoptotic cell death.[68]

Excitotoxicity refers to the deleterious cellular effects of excess glutamate and aspartate stimulation of ionotropic and metabotropic receptors. Extracellular concentrations of both of these excitatory amino acids are increased after acute SCI, which occurs through release from damaged neurons, decreased uptake by damaged astrocytes, and through depolarization-induced release. Ionotropic receptors include the NMDA and alpha-amino-3-hydroxy-5-methyl-4-isoxazole propionic acid (AMPA)/kainite receptors through which extracellular calcium and sodium can pass down a massive concentration gradient into the cell or, when activated, can result in release of calcium from intracellular stores. Metabotropic glutamate receptors are coupled to G proteins that act as secondary intracellular messengers to mediate a wide spectrum of cellular functions. Furthermore, elevation of intracellular calcium concentration can occur through direct membrane damage and voltage-gated calcium channels triggered by membrane depolarization. Elevated intracellular calcium concentrations can trigger a multitude of calcium-dependent processes that can lethally alter cellular metabolism, such as activation of lytic enzymes (calpains, phospholipase A_2, proteases, and lipoxygenase), generation of free radicals, impairment of mitochondrial function, spasm of vascular smooth muscle, and binding of phosphates with subsequent depletion of cell energy sources. Sodium dysregulation is thought to be important in the pathophysiology of damage to axonal and glial components in the white matter through similar mechanisms that lead to elevated intracellular calcium concentrations.

Controversy exists surrounding the role of inflammation in acute SCI, mainly because the effects of inflammatory cells can be both cytotoxic and protective. After SCI, the injury site is rapidly infiltrated by blood-borne neutrophils, which can secrete lytic enzymes and cytokines. Later, blood-borne macrophages and monocytes are recruited, as well as locally activated resident microglia, both of which subsequently invade to phagocytose the injured tissue. These and other reactive cells produce cytokines, such as tumor necrosis factor α (TNF-α), interleukins (ILs), and interferons, that mediate the inflammatory response and can further damage local tissue and recruit other inflammatory cells. Among the cytokines involved in secondary SCI, TNF-α is perhaps the most extensively studied. It is produced by a range of different cell populations, including neutrophils, macrophages and microglia, astrocytes, and T cells and has been shown to accumulate quickly at the site of SCI. It has been suggested that the early inflammatory phases are deleterious in nature, whereas the later inflammatory events appear to be protective.[65]

Currently much research is being performed on the role of apoptosis, or programmed cell death, in secondary injury. This slowly spreading form of cell death is induced by the injury and is characterized by apoptotic neurons at the lesion margins and, even later, apoptosis of oligodendrocytes in areas with degenerating axons that were injured at the original lesion site.[68,69] Apoptosis can thus occur at quite remote distances from the point of impact. Oligodendrocytes appear vulnerable to apoptosis, and death of these cells can result in demyelination of otherwise spared axons, thus contributing to the loss of distal neurologic function.

Neurologic Evaluation

Clinical signs seen as a result of SCI reflect the extent and location of the injury. Neurologic signs are usually observed immediately after the accident but may occur weeks to months after the initial insult because of delayed damage to the spinal cord caused by instability, arthritis, or bony callus formation at the site of impact. Clinical signs depend on the neuroanatomic location of injury and range between inapparent to severe incapacitating tetraparesis or tetraplegia (see Figure 12-28). Lesions causing recumbency are mostly found in the caudal cervical or thoracic spinal cord, whereas lesions of nonrecumbent horses are mostly found further cranial in the cervical spinal cord or in the lumbosacral cord.[1]

Initial evaluation of the patient should be directed toward stabilization and correction of any life-threatening problems such as airway obstruction, hemorrhage, cardiovascular collapse, and pneumothorax. In addition, major long-bone fractures must be identified, because these may be the limiting factor for survival of the horse. All affected horses may be nervous or agitated as a result of pain and the inability to stand. A systematic neurologic evaluation should then be performed to localize the site of injury.[9,21,70] In recumbent horses the use of a sling to assist standing may be a valuable diagnostic tool for localizing the site of injury and for assessing progression of disease and prognosis.[21,70]

In animals, SCI usually occurs as a solitary lesion and the level of the lesion can be diagnosed by neurologic examination.[71] Depression or loss of a segmental spinal reflex implies damage to either the afferent, efferent, or connecting pathways of the reflex arc. However, after acute SCI a phase of spinal shock can occur in which profound depression is noted in segmental spinal reflexes caudal to the level of the lesion, even though reflex arcs are physically intact.[71-73] Spinal shock occurs in all species; however, it appears to be of much shorter duration in dogs, cats, and rabbits when compared with primates.[71,74] Another syndrome that occurs infrequently and is short-lived in the horse is Schiff-Sherrington syndrome, in which extensor hypertonus is present in otherwise normal thoracic limbs in patients with severe cranial thoracic lesions.[74]

Cord injury typically results in damage that is worse in the large myelinated motor and proprioceptive fibers compared with the smaller or nonmyelinated nociceptive fibers. Therefore ataxia and loss of proprioception and motor function will occur before the loss of deep pain.[9] Flaccid paralysis with hypo- or areflexia, muscular hypotonia, and neurogenic muscle atrophy are characteristic of a lower motor neuron lesion. Signs resulting from an upper motor neuron spinal cord lesion include loss of voluntary motor function, whereas muscle tone may be increased and spinal reflexes may be normal to hyperactive.

In horses, lesions in the C1 to T2 region are most common and result in varying degrees of dysfunction ranging from tetraparesis to recumbency. Thoracolumbar SCI can result in paraparesis to recumbency and horses may dog sit. Sacral cord damage can result in fecal and urinary incontinence, loss of use of tail and anus, muscle atrophy, and mild deficits of pelvic limb function. Sacrococcygeal cord injury can produce hypalgesia; hypotonia and hyporeflexia of the perineum, tail, and anus; or total analgesia and paralysis of those structures. In addition to these clinical signs, loss of sensation can occur distal to the level of SCI. Furthermore, diffuse sweating can be seen as a result of loss of supraspinal input to the preganglionic cell bodies of the sympathetic system in the thoracolumbar intermediate gray matter. Patchy sweating can be seen with damage to specific preganglionic or postganglionic nerve fibers.[9,74]

Ancillary diagnostics that may aid in diagnosing or localizing SCI include radiography, myelography, computed tomography, MRI, nuclear scintigraphy, CSF analysis, nerve conduction velocities, EMG, and transcranial magnetic stimulation. Radiography may demonstrate fractures, luxations, subluxations, and vertebral compression. As presented previously, computed tomography or radiography are the diagnostic aids of choice to evaluate skeletal injury, whereas MRI is more sensitive for evaluation of soft tissue structures such as the spinal cord and ligaments. With respect to imaging the vertebral column with computed tomography and MRI devices, however, the size of the horse, the size of the equipment aperture, and the cost of the equipment aperture limit its use to investigations of the cervical and cranial thoracic spinal cord. Myelography may be required to confirm spinal cord compression and can be used at the level of the cervical, cranial thoracic, and sacral-coccygeal spinal cord. Nuclear scintigraphy can be useful in diagnosing nondisplaced or occult fractures and soft tissue lesions. Common CSF abnormalities after SCI include xanthochromia and mild-to-moderate increased total protein concentrations.[9] CSF analysis may be normal, especially in very acute or chronic cases. Nerve conduction velocity and electromyographic studies evaluate the lower motor neuron and aid in lesion localization. Electromyographic changes, however, may not develop until 4 to 5 days after nerve damage.[75] Transcranial magnetic stimulation allows detection of functional lesions in descending motor tracts through recording of magnetic motor-evoked potentials. This method has been validated and used to distinguish motor tract disorders from other causes of recumbency in clinical cases.[76-78]

Treatment and Prognosis

Treatment to reverse primary SCI does not currently exist, and it is the assortment of pathophysiologic processes that occur during the period of secondary injury that are considered the target for pharmaceutical intervention. The period of secondary injury can be divided into three therapeutic windows.[79] The first 48 hours after acute SCI are dominated by the vascular and biochemical changes that occur within the spinal cord. The second period is a result of the effects of inflammatory cells and occurs within hours of injury, peaking around 4 days after injury. The third period occurs approximately 1 week after injury and is characterized by axonal regeneration and lesion repair. The goals of treatment are to stop the cascade of cellular events initiated by the traumatic insult, to protect spared neural tissue, and to promote regeneration. Surgical intervention is warranted when the need exists for stabilization or fracture repair, as well as when a compressive lesion is evident; however, this is not routine practice. The use of medical treatment to stabilize the patient should always be instituted before surgery is performed.

Acute SCI often results in impaired cardiopulmonary function such as impaired ventilation, bradycardia, and hypotension. This is particularly the case in lesions cranial to C5 (respiratory center affected) and cranial to T2 (origin of sympathetic outflow = thoracolumbar spinal cord). Systemic hypotension may exacerbate spinal cord hypoperfusion and ischemia, and maintaining systemic blood pressure has been shown to improve spinal cord perfusion. Volume resuscitation is clearly indicated in shock and for restitution of tissue perfusion. The current recommendation is to maintain euvolemic normotension; because of sympathetic outflow disruption after cranial SCI, pressor therapy is commonly indicated in the treatment regimen. Maintaining normal mean arterial blood pressure is also important to consider during stabilization of the acutely injured horse, and it is particularly important when horses are placed under general anesthesia for various diagnostic and therapeutic procedures.

Similar to TBI, SCI has a complex multifactorial pathophysiology and likely requires a combinational treatment intervention for successful outcome. Many agents, which could target different aspects of the secondary injury mechanisms, have been investigated for use in SCI and have been reviewed.[65,80,81] Until now only methylprednisolone sodium succinate (MPSS) was shown to be efficacious in both animal models and human beings[82-87]; however, based on conflicting reports and small neurologic improvements, a number of reviews of the data have been published expressing concern with regards to the true beneficial effect of MPSS in acute SCI.[88-91] MPSS is a synthetic glucocorticoid with four times more anti-inflammatory activity and 0.8 times less mineralocorticoid action compared with cortisol.[92] Beneficial effects of MPSS on neural tissue include inhibition of lipid peroxidation, eicosanoid formation, and lipid hydrolysis, including arachidonic acid release, maintenance of tissue blood flow and aerobic energy metabolism, improved elimination of intracellular calcium accumulation, reduced neurofilament degradation, and improved neuronal excitability and synaptic transmission. MPSS was selected for human clinical trials rather than dexamethasone because the succinate radical has been shown to cross cell membranes more rapidly than other radicals.[85]

In 1984 the first National Acute Spinal Cord Injury Study (NASCIS I) was performed, and subsequent studies led to the conclusion that high-dose (30 mg/kg bolus followed by infusion at 5.4 mg/kg/hr for 23 hours) MPSS treatment within 8 hours of SCI improved neurologic recovery, and the use of naloxone in SCI was not recommended.[85,93,94] The dose of MPSS used exceeds that necessary for activation of steroid receptors, suggesting that MPSS acts through mechanisms that are unrelated to steroid receptors and apparently it is the cell membrane antilipid peroxidation effect of MPSS that is most beneficial.[85,94] In a fifth trial of MPSS (NASCIS III), using essentially the same protocol for drug administration and neurologic assessment as NASCIS II, no significant benefit was found when the NASCIS II regimen of 24-hour therapy was extended to 48 hours.[87,93] In addition, the NASCIS II and III studies have received intense criticism on several important methodological, scientific, and statistical issues that have been reviewed elsewhere.[91] Moreover, others have not been able to reproduce results obtained with NASCIS II and III.[91] Although there has been no report on increased incidence of adverse effects after MPSS treatment in human beings, a recent report in animals has shown that MPSS administration according to the doses recommended in the NASCIS II and III studies resulted in lymphocytopenia, intestinal necrosis, and eosinophilic pulmonary infiltrates.[95] Experts have suggested that a multinational study should be undertaken to review the current recommendation of MPSS administration.[91] The usefulness of high-dose MPSS treatment for spinal cord trauma in the horse remains to be investigated.

In horses, corticosteroids, alone or in combination with other drugs, are likely the most commonly used drugs for acute CNS trauma. Reported dosages of dexamethasone for horses range between 0.1 to 0.25 mg/kg intravenously every 6 to 24 hours for 24 to 48 hours. A favorable response is expected within 4 to 8 hours after administration. Horses on corticosteroid therapy should be monitored closely for the development of laminitis or *Aspergillus* spp. pneumonia. If improvement in clinical signs is observed, then the horse may be placed on oral prednisolone therapy (0.5 to 1.0 mg/kg tapered over 3 to 5 days) to decrease the chance of laminitis. The neuroprotective effect of corticosteroids is thought primarily to be mediated by free radical scavenging but may include decreased catecholamines and glutamate, as well as decreased apoptosis-related cell death.[96] Other potential beneficial effects of corticosteroids include reduction in the spread of morphologic damage, prevention of the loss of axonal conduction and reflex activity, preservation of vascular membrane integrity, and stabilization of white matter neuronal cell membranes in the presence of central hemorrhagic lesions.[67] Furthermore, their anti-inflammatory properties may be useful in reducing edema and fibrin deposition, as well as their ability to reverse sodium and potassium imbalance because of edema and necrosis. Another beneficial effect of corticosteroids is maintenance of normal blood glucose concentrations while maintaining electrolyte balance.[67]

As mentioned for TBI, the use of NSAIDs such as flunixin meglumine and phenylbutazone may decrease the inflammation associated with a traumatic episode. In addition, they may be beneficial in maintaining a normal rectal temperature. These compounds work by inhibiting cyclooxygenase, which converts arachidonic acid to inflammatory mediators (endoperoxides). In addition, the potential beneficial properties of DMSO, 1 g/kg intravenously as a 10% solution for 3 consecutive days followed by three treatments every other day, likely warrant inclusion of this drug in the treatment of CNS trauma.[7,8] Pharmacokinetic evaluation of DMSO in horses indicates that twice-daily dosing is necessary to maintain adequate blood levels.[97] Reported benefits of DMSO include increased brain and spinal cord blood flow, decreased brain and spinal cord edema, increased vasodilating prostaglandin E_1 (PGE_1), decreased platelet aggregation, decreased prostaglandin E_2 (PGE_2) and prostaglandin F_2 (PGF_2), protection of cell membranes, and trapping of hydroxyl radicals.[67] The exact mechanism of DMSO remains unknown, and this treatment remains controversial because some researchers have found no positive effects on neurologic outcome from the use of DMSO.[98] Although the free radical scavengers vitamin E and selenium have been shown to be beneficial in SCI, these antioxidants do not appear useful in the acute management because of the length of time required to achieve therapeutic concentrations in the CNS.[79]

Similar as is stated for TBI, antibiotics are not always necessary in the treatment of vertebral or spinal cord trauma; however, they are indicated in treating open fractures and secondary complications associated with a recumbent horse, such as pneumonia and decubital sores.

Physical therapy is important in the rehabilitative process in spine-injured horses. Controlled exercise allows the unaffected parts of the nervous system to compensate for the affected parts by increasing strength and conscious proprioception. Exercise is especially helpful in improving weakness, ataxia, spasticity, and hypermetria. In recumbent horses, massage, therapeutic ultrasound, and hydrotherapy of affected muscle groups for 10 to 15 minutes at least twice a day is important. These measures help combat necrosis and muscle atrophy of the horse's dependent muscle groups. Passive flexion and extension of all limbs is helpful in maintaining full range of motion in recumbent horses. Furthermore, experimental studies have shown that exercise enhances functional recovery after SCI.[99]

Prognosis is based on response to therapy and is directly related to the time from injury to the institution of treatment. Horses that show rapid neurologic improvement have a fair-to-good prognosis. Recumbent horses or horses suffering from fractures or luxations have a guarded-to-poor prognosis. Horses that have lost deep pain sensation have a functional or anatomic spinal cord transection and have a grave prognosis. The longer the time from loss of deep pain to treatment, the poorer the prognosis. Partial or complete recovery of horses with spinal cord trauma may take weeks to months, so time and nursing care are required.

VESTIBULAR DISEASE

Bonnie R. Rush

The vestibular system is a special proprioceptive system responsible for maintenance of balance and reflex orientation to gravitational forces. This system functions to maintain appropriate eye, trunk, and limb position in reference to movements and positioning of the head.[1,2]

VESTIBULAR APPARATUS

The afferent unit of the vestibular system comprises the receptor organ within the inner ear and the vestibulocochlear nerve (the eighth cranial nerve). The vestibulocochlear nerve processes auditory and vestibular input through a common physiologic mechanism. Acoustic stimuli and acceleration forces result in mechanical deformation of hair cells in the cochlea and vestibular receptor organs, which transform physical forces into electric impulses.[3] The inner ear is located in the petrous temporal bone and consists of the bony and membranous labyrinth. The membranous labyrinth is suspended within the bony labyrinth by perilymph, fluid similar to and likely derived from CSF.[2] The membranous labyrinth comprises the cochlea, the saccule, the utricle, and the three semicircular canals.[4] The cochlea is responsible for auditory functions and has no input to the vestibular system.[5] Endolymph fills the membranous labyrinth and is derived from blood vessels along one side of the cochlea.[2]

The three semicircular canals are oriented at right angles to one another, which allows for detection of rotation in any plane at any angle. At one end of each semicircular canal is a dilation of the canal called the *ampulla*. A ridge of connective tissue called the *crista* is located on one side of the ampulla. The internal surface of the crista is lined with hair cells (neuroreceptor cells) and sustentacular cells (support cells) that are oriented perpendicular to the flow of endolymph.[2,6] These cells are covered with a gelatinous protein-polysaccharide material called the *cupula,* which extends across the lumen of the ampulla.[5] Rotation of the head in any plane causes endolymph to flow in one or more of the semicircular ducts. Each hair cell has 40 to 80 stereocilia and a single modified kinocilium. Movement of endolymph causes the cupula to move across the stereocilia. Deformation of the stereocilia by the flow of endolymph toward the kinocilia results in increased neuronal activity of the vestibular nerve. Inhibition of vestibular neurons occurs with deviation of stereocilia away from kinocilia.[5] The semicircular canals are responsible for dynamic equilibrium and respond only to changing forces such as acceleration and deceleration but not to constant velocity or stationary positioning.[2] The semicircular canals can detect changing forces at a rate of 1 degree/sec.[2,5]

A similar receptor organ called the *macula* is located in the wall of the saccule and the utricle. The organ consists of a 2-mm oval plaque of dense connective tissue lined by neuroepithelial cells and covered with a gelatinous substance, termed the *otolithic membrane.* Calcium carbonate crystals called *statoconia (otoliths)* lie on the otolithic membrane, and their movement initiates stimulation of the vestibular neurons.[7] The macula sacculi is oriented vertically, and the macula utriculi is oriented horizontally. Gravitational forces continuously affect the position of otoliths in at least one of the maculae, supplying constant information regarding the static position of the head.[8] These receptor organs can detect changes in head position of one-half degree from the stationary plane.[5] The maculae of the saccule and utricle also detect linear acceleration and deceleration and are responsible for maintenance of static equilibrium.[8]

The hair cells of the crista ampullaris and maculae synapse with sensory neurons of the vestibular nerve. The cell bodies of these bipolar neurons are located within the petrous temporal bone and constitute the vestibular ganglion.[5] Axons leave the petrous temporal bone through the internal acoustic meatus adjacent to the cochlear portion of the eighth cranial nerve. Fibers course to the lateral aspect of the rostral medulla and penetrate the brainstem between the caudal cerebellar peduncle and the spinal tract of the trigeminal nerve. The majority of fibers of the eighth cranial nerve terminate in the four vestibular nuclei (rostral, medial, lateral, and caudal) located in the lateral wall of the fourth ventricle of the rostral medulla oblongata.[1] Some of these fibers form the vestibulocerebellar tract and directly enter the caudal cerebellar peduncle to terminate in the fastigial nucleus and flocculonodular lobes of the cerebellum. The afferent supply to the vestibular nucleus is primarily from the maculae, the crista ampullaris, and the cerebellum. These sensory fibers synapse with second-order neurons in the vestibular nuclei that extend fibers to the motor neurons of the spinal cord, the nuclei of the cranial nerves that control eye position, the cerebellum, the autonomic nervous system, the reticular formation, and the cerebral cortex.[2,5]

The vestibulospinal tract courses in the ipsilateral ventral funiculus and terminates in interneurons of the ventral gray column. Stimulation of the vestibulospinal tract is facilitatory to α- and γ-motor neurons of the ipsilateral extensor muscles, inhibitory to the α-motor neurons of the ipsilateral flexor muscles, and inhibitory to contralateral extensor muscles.[2] The net result is ipsilateral extensor tonus and contralateral flexor tonus that act as an adaptive mechanism against gravity by catching the body and preventing a fall in the direction of vestibular stimulation.[6]

Axons from the medial vestibular nucleus project through the medial longitudinal fasciculus. The ascending portions of the medial longitudinal fasciculus course to the motor nuclei of the third, fourth, and sixth cranial nerves (oculomotor, trochlear, and abducens).[4,9] These fibers coordinate conjugate eye movement with changes in head position. This pathway, along with cerebellar input, controls physiologic (vestibular) nystagmus.[2] Physiologic nystagmus is a normal reflex that allows the eyes to remain fixed on a stationary object while the head moves.[5] Nystagmus is characterized by involuntary, conjugate, rhythmic eyeball oscillations with a fast and slow phase. The direction of nystagmus is defined by the direction of the fast phase and is induced by rapid movements of the head. Rapid dorsiflexion of the neck results in vertical nystagmus, whereas side-to-side movement of the head induces horizontal nystagmus. Turning the head to the left results in a horizontal nystagmus with the fast phase to the left. The accompanying slow phase is in a direction opposite to body motion and allows the eyes to fix on a stationary image. The fast phase is initiated when the eyeball reaches the lateral limit of ocular movement and allows the eyeballs to jump forward and focus on a new image.[5,6] The slow phase is controlled by vestibular input, and the fast phase is a function of the brainstem.[2] Physiologic nystagmus induced by rapid manipulation of the head is called the *oculocephalic reflex*. This reflex occurs independent of vision.[10] Descending portions of the medial longitudinal fasciculus travel in the ventral funiculus of the cervical and cranial thoracic spinal cord segments and control the position and activity of the limbs and trunk in coordination with head position.[2,5]

Fibers from the vestibular nuclei that project to the reticular formation provide afferent nerves to the vomit center, which is the pathway for the development of motion sickness. Reticulospinal tracts also aid in the maintenance of extensor tone to support the body against gravity.[2,5]

Vestibular impulses enter the cerebellum via the caudal cerebellar peduncles. Fibers of the vestibulocerebellar tracts terminate primarily in the flocculonodular lobe and fastigial nucleus.[2] The flocculonodular lobe appears to be linked closely to the semicircular canals in the control of dynamic equilibrium.[5] The cerebellum functions to coordinate protagonistic, antagonistic, and synergistic muscle groups for controlled responses to gravity. The vestibular apparatus provides information to the cerebellum, dictating the relative degree of contraction necessary to maintain equilibrium.[5]

Vestibular signals travel through to the contralateral medial geniculate nuclei of the thalamus to the cerebral cortex. In addition to proprioceptive information from other parts of the body, the cerebral cortex facilitates conscious perception of orientation.[2]

The vestibular system is capable only of detecting movement and orientation of the head in relationship to the rest of the body. Afferent pathways from the neck allow the head to be cognizant of the orientation of the rest of the body.[5,8] Proprioceptive receptors in the joints of the neck that transmit signals to the reticular formation are essential to the righting reflex.[7,8] Exteroceptor receptors of the skin and proprioceptive receptors in other joints also are integrated in the cerebellum and reticular formation to aid in the maintenance of equilibrium. These signals allow the vestibular system to know if the body remains in an appropriate position with respect to gravity while the head is bent. Visual images can help to maintain balance by visual detection of the upright stance. In addition, slight linear or angular movement of the head shifts the image on the retina, which relays directional information to equilibrium centers. Visual compensation may be capable of maintaining balance in the face of complete vestibular destruction, if the eyes are open and motions are performed slowly.[5]

The seventh cranial nerve (the facial nerve) emerges from the lateral medulla ventral to the vestibulocochlear nerve at the level of the trapezoid body. The two nerves are associated closely with the petrous temporal bone and enter the internal auditory meatus together.[11] Within the internal auditory meatus, the facial nerve separates from the vestibular nerve and courses through the facial canal of the petrosal bone. The facial nerve exits the cranium from the stylomastoid foramen located immediately caudal to the external auditory meatus. Because of the proximity of the facial and vestibular nerves, a single disease process commonly affects both nerves simultaneously.[12]

Sympathetic innervation to the eye also is associated anatomically with the petrous temporal bone. Damage to this nerve (Horner's syndrome), along with vestibular and facial nerve deficits, frequently occurs with petrous temporal bone trauma and otitis media in small animals.[10] The association of Horner's syndrome, facial nerve paralysis, and vestibular disease rarely is documented in the horse.[2]

CLINICAL SIGNS

Knowledge of the anatomy and function of structures related to the peripheral and central vestibular system aids in neuroanatomic localization of the lesion.[10] Differentiation of central versus peripheral vestibular disease is important for establishing a list of differential diagnoses, initiating therapy, and formulating a prognosis. A thorough physical and neurologic examination of a horse with vestibular disease may identify nonvestibular neurologic signs, lending significant insight into the location of the lesion. Historical information, including duration of condition, rate of onset, and disease progression, also may aid in differentiation of central from peripheral vestibular disease.

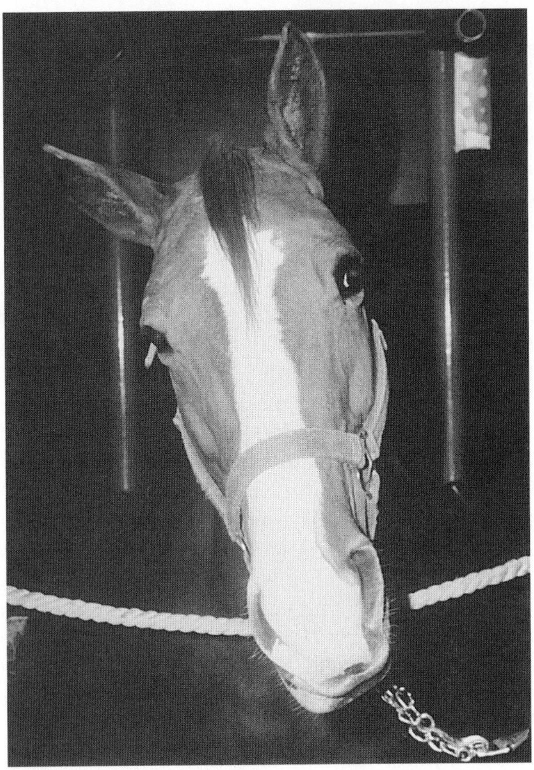

FIGURE 12-31 Thoroughbred with right-sided peripheral vestibular disease caused by a temporohyoid osteoarthropathy (THO) and acute fracture. The head tilt, dropped pinna, and eyelid droop occur on the affected side, whereas the muzzle is pulled toward the contralateral side.

Signs of acute peripheral vestibular system dysfunction include head tilt, nystagmus, falling, circling, reluctance to move, and asymmetrical ataxia with preservation of strength.* Horses affected with peracute vestibular disease are often violent because of disorientation.[1] A true head tilt is a consistent sign of vestibular disease and is characterized by ventral deviation of the poll of the head toward the affected side[4,14] (Figure 12-31). The horse prefers to lie on the side of the lesion and may lean on the wall toward the affected side when standing. When forced to move, the horse takes short, uncoordinated steps in a circle toward the direction of the lesion. The body may be flexed laterally with a concavity toward the lesion.[4,6] Extensor hypotonia ipsilateral to the lesion, and mild hypertonia and hyperreflexia of the extensor muscles of the contralateral side result in asymmetrical ataxia.[15] Extensor hypotonia occurs from loss of facilitatory neurons of the vestibulospinal tract to ipsilateral extensor muscles.

Contralateral extensor hypertonia occurs from loss of inhibitory neurons and unopposed extensor tone of the contralateral vestibulospinal tract.[2,6,14] Central vestibular disease has similar clinical signs, but general proprioceptive deficits, weakness, and multiple cranial nerve deficits also may be present, resulting from damage to the surrounding neurologic structures. The onset of vestibular signs in a horse with an expanding space-occupying central lesion is not as dramatic as peripheral nerve damage; adjustments by compensatory

*References 2, 4, 8, 10, 12, 13.

mechanisms occur during slow development of the lesion. These lesions, however, are not likely to show significant clinical improvement after the onset of clinical signs, as may occur with peripheral vestibular lesions.

Pathologic nystagmus is involuntary, rhythmic oscillations of the eyes occurring while the head is in a normal position and indicates a lesion in the vestibular system or cerebellum.[12] As in physiologic nystagmus, one can identify a fast and a slow phase. The direction of nystagmus is defined by the direction of the fast phase.[2,5,12] Pathologic nystagmus may be spontaneous, occurring with the head in the resting position, or positional, which is induced by elevation or lateral flexion of the head.[2] Nystagmus usually appears with the onset of other peripheral vestibular signs but may last only 2 to 3 days because of central compensation.[4,15] Concomitant blinking of the eyelid may hinder detection of nystagmus.[2]

Peripheral vestibular dysfunction may result in horizontal or rotary nystagmus. The fast phase of nystagmus is directed away from the lesion and does not change with changing head position.[2,3,6] The direction of rotary nystagmus is defined by the direction the limbus moves from the 12 o'clock position during the fast phase.[2] Horizontal, rotary, or vertical nystagmus can result from a central vestibular lesion. In addition, the type of nystagmus observed may change with changing head position in a patient with central vestibular disease.[1,12,14] Often the fast phase is directed away from the central lesion, but this is not a consistent finding.[2]

In the healthy animal a constant stream of electric stimulation arises in each vestibular end organ and transmits signals that control ocular position via the medial longitudinal fasciculus. These signals normally drive the eyes toward the opposite direction. The eyes are maintained centrally, however, because vestibuloocular pathways are opposed in an equal and opposite manner. Unilateral vestibular disease upsets this balance, resulting in slow deviation of both eyes toward the lesion. REM returns the eyes to midposition. Individuals that are blind at birth or have been blind for an extended time may exhibit irregular eyeball oscillation with no slow or fast component.[16]

Ataxia and dysmetria are often severe with peripheral ves tibular disease; however, strength is maintained. Postural reactions remain normal with the exception of the righting reflex. The motor system is unable to accurately control movement and identify the location of different parts of the body at a given time. Therefore the horse makes an exaggerated response toward the side of the lesion as it attempts to stand.[2]

Loss of hearing is a common finding with peripheral vestibular disease because of the proximity of the cochlea to the vestibular receptor organs. In the CNS, diffuse pathways control auditory signals and extensive central disease would be necessary to cause hearing loss.[14]

If vestibular signs are accompanied by depression, weakness, or conscious proprioceptive deficits, a central vestibular system lesion is likely. With a central lesion, abnormal conscious proprioception occurs because of damage within the brainstem of the descending upper motor neuron tracts to the limbs.[2] Damage to the spinocerebellar tracts or caudal cerebellar peduncles results in abnormal unconscious proprioception and hypermetria.[1] The nuclei of the trigeminal (fifth cranial nerve) and the abducens nerves (sixth cranial nerve) are in anatomic proximity to the vestibular nuclei and are damaged readily in a common disease process. Trigeminal nerve paralysis creates a loss of sensation to the head and atrophy of the muscles of mastication. Trochlear nerve damage results in medial strabismus.[10]

Destructive space-occupying lesions in the cerebellopontine angle or flocculonodular lobe may result in paradoxical central vestibular disease.[1,17] This syndrome is manifested by vestibular ataxia and a head tilt contralateral to the side demonstrating general proprioceptive ataxia and postural reaction deficits. When this unusual combination of neurologic signs is present, the side of general proprioceptive deficits defines localization of the lesion.[2,10]

Central or peripheral vestibular disease may produce strabismus. One observes ventrolateral strabismus ipsilateral to the vestibular lesion with elevation of the head and extension of the neck.[2,10] One observes mild ventral deviation of the eyes in normal horses when the head is elevated, but the finding is symmetric. Ventrolateral strabismus of vestibular disease is not a sign of a cranial nerve deficit of the extraocular muscles[2] but is a reflection of abnormal upper motor neuron influences on the oculomotor nucleus from the ipsilateral vestibular nucleus via the medial longitudinal fasciculus. If the strabismus is purely vestibular in origin, then normal ocular mobility is visible with manipulation of the head.[14]

Signs of vestibular disease may improve rapidly 2 to 3 weeks after onset because of visual and central accommodation.[2,13] Central vestibular lesions are slower to compensate than peripheral vestibular lesions; signs may even progress if the central lesion is an expanding space-occupying mass.[14] Human beings compensate satisfactorily for unilateral disease but are not required to be coordinated athletes performing at high speed.[4] Blindfolding a horse with compensated disease results in ataxia and a head tilt (Romberg's test). Blindfolding eliminates visual and limb proprioceptive orientation; the body is forced to rely on the impaired vestibular system for equilibrium.[2,10,11] This test is unreliable for localizing the side of the lesion.[3] Horses may decompensate dramatically when the blindfold is placed over the eyes, resulting in anxiety, disorientation, and falling.[2] One should perform the test with caution on a padded surface with good footing.

Horses affected with bilateral peripheral disease demonstrate no head tilt, circling, or pathologic nystagmus, and one cannot induce physiologic nystagmus by rapid manipulation of the head (the oculocephalic reflex) or by caloric testing. The head may sway with wide excursions from side to side.[4] As with all peripheral vestibular disease, strength is preserved.[2] Clinically, horses affected with bilateral vestibular disease exhibit more symmetrical ataxia similar to generalized cerebellar disease.[1]

Facial nerve (seventh cranial nerve) paralysis frequently occurs concurrently with peripheral vestibular disease because of its proximity to the vestibular nerve within the petrous temporal bone. Facial nerve paralysis worsens the long-term prognosis and complicates the management of vestibular disease patients. The facial nerve innervates the muscles of facial expression, and damage to this nerve results in muzzle deviation away from the affected side, lack of menace and palpebral response, ear droop, decreased nostril flare impeding air flow, and buccal impaction of feed.[4,11,12] Keratitis and corneal ulceration are common because of the inability to blink and decreased tear production.[4,18] Decreased tear production results from damage to parasympathetic fibers to the lacrimal gland. Preganglionic fibers travel with the facial nerve through the internal auditory meatus and separate in the facial canal proximal to the geniculate nucleus.[12] The fibers split from the facial nerve to join the superior petrosal nerve, which carries fibers to the sphenopalatine ganglion. Postganglionic fibers join the sympathetic fibers to the eye and travel with the vasculature to the lacrimal gland.[2,12] Corneal ulcerations occur in the inferior portion of the cornea and are slow to heal because of ongoing exposure.[11] Lack of tear production aids in localization of the lesion, indicating the damage is within the petrous temporal bone, proximal to the geniculate nucleus.[2,12] Clinical signs of facial nerve paralysis may not appear for several days after the onset of vestibular disease, because damage to the nerve may result from hematoma, callus, or an extension of inflammation and secondary neuritis.[4] Because of the proximity of the nuclei of the facial and vestibular nerves, extensive lesions of the medulla may involve both nerves. If no improvement of facial nerve deficits occurs within 3 to 4 months after the onset of disease, then the prognosis is poor for recovery. If one notes even mild improvement in the first 4 months, then facial nerve function may return.[4] Horses may learn to retract the globe, allowing the eyelid and nictitating membrane to slide across the surface of the cornea, distributing lubrication and protecting the eye from trauma.[11] Careful observation is necessary to differentiate this adaptation from improvement of lid function.

PERIPHERAL VESTIBULAR DISEASE

Acute onset of peripheral vestibular disease and facial nerve paralysis is not a rare occurrence in the horse.[15,19] Damage to the temporal bone is the most likely anatomic location when these nerves are affected concurrently. THO and traumatic skull fractures are the most common causes of these signs in large animals.[1] THO is the most common cause of peripheral vestibular disease in horses and should be the number one rule out for horses with acute onset of vestibular dysfunction, especially if accompanied by facial nerve palsy.

Temporohyoid Osteoarthropathy

Temporohyoid osteoarthropathy is one of the most common causes of acute onset peripheral vestibular disease, facial nerve paralysis, or both in horses.[4,11,20-22] Varying causes for the disorder have been suggested, including extension of inflammation and infection from otitis media-interna or guttural pouch infection, repetitive trauma, and nonseptic osteoarthritis. Much of the older veterinary literature refers to this disorder as *otitis media-interna,* whereas newer references use the designation *THO* because of the uncertaintly concerning underlying cause in most horses.* The earlier presumption of underlying otitis media-interna hypothesized that rather than rupturing the tympanic membrane, the inflammatory process might extend ventrally to involve the bones of the tympanic bulla and temporohyoid joint. However, this theory remains speculative, and relatively few horses with THO have evidence of otitis or guttural pouch infection at the time of diagnosis or historically. Some or all cases of THO are quite likely the result of primary degenerative joint disease rather than an extension of a bacterial ear or guttural pouch infection.

*References 4, 11, 15, 18, 23, 24.

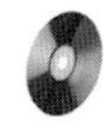

Regardless of initial cause, inflammation induces bony proliferation at the articulation of the stylohyoid bone with the petrous temporal bone, resulting in loss of the joint space and fusion of the temporohyoid joint. The hyoid apparatus is attached to the tongue and larynx; fusion of the temporohyoid joint results in impaired flexibility of the unit. A stress fracture of the petrous temporal bone, the stylohyoid bone, or both may result from eating, vocalization, or any activity associated with normal tongue movement.[6,15] Occasionally, fracture and acute onset of severe neurologic signs (collapse and seizure) may be associated with passage of a nasogastric tube or other veterinary procedure.[20] The fracture line may extend into the cranial vault at the level of the internal auditory meatus, resulting in direct neural tissue trauma and hemorrhage into the middle and inner ear.[1,15]

Neurologic signs are rarely apparent during the formation of proliferative osteitis and temporohyoid joint fusion. The onset of neurologic signs corresponds with the occurrence of the stress fracture. Early signs, before fracture, might include head shaking, resistance to the bit, ear rubbing, resentment of manipulation of the head or ears, or pain on pressure at the base of the ear. Occasionally more overt signs of otitis externa or otitis media-interna may be present, including evidence of exudate from the external ear canal.

Most horses exhibit acute onset of cranial nerve VII or VIII abnormalities (or both) at the time of fracture. Fractures can tear or stretch the facial or vestibulocochlear nerves as they exit the skull or within the skull, respectively. Some fractures extend into the cranial vault with resultant seizures, bacterial meningitis, or death.[15,20,23] Vestibular signs can vary between mild head tilt to circling with severe loss of balance and horizontal nystagmus or recumbency. Auditory abnormalities are evident in most affected horses when assessed by brainstem auditory-evoked responses.[25] If the facial nerve is damaged, then ptosis, muzzle deviation away from the side of the lesion, a drooping lower lip and ear on the side of the lesion, and accumulation of feed within the cheek occurs. Preganglionic parasympathetic fibers in the facial nerve that innervate the lacrimal gland may also be damaged with resultant keratoconjunctivitis sicca. Many affected horses have corneal ulceration varying between mild to severe. Corneal disease is secondary to decreased tear production and facial nerve dysfunction that diminishes the horse's ability to effectively close the eyelids and spread the tear film across the eye. Rarely, horses may have intermittent acute episodes of vestibular disease with intervening periods of apparent normal neurologic function. Occasionally, the fracture extends to the foramen lacerum, caudal to the petrous temporal bone, where the glossopharyngeal and vagus nerves exit the skull. Trauma to these nerves may result in dysphagia.[11]

A diagnosis of THO may be confirmed by imaging of the stylohyoid bone or petrous temporal bone by endoscopy, radiography, nuclear scintigraphy, computed tomography, or MRI.[20-22] Although most affected horses have acute onset of unilateral neurologic signs, it is not uncommon for imaging to identify bilateral THO and bony proliferation.

Endoscopy of the pharynx and guttural pouch is one of the most sensitive diagnostic tests for THO in horses.[20] One should perform this noninvasive procedure on every horse suspected of having proliferative osteitis, because one often can identify bony proliferation of the proximal stylohyoid bone within the guttural pouch[1,24] (Figure 12-32). Many horses also have evidence of hyperemia, bruising, or hematoma formation in

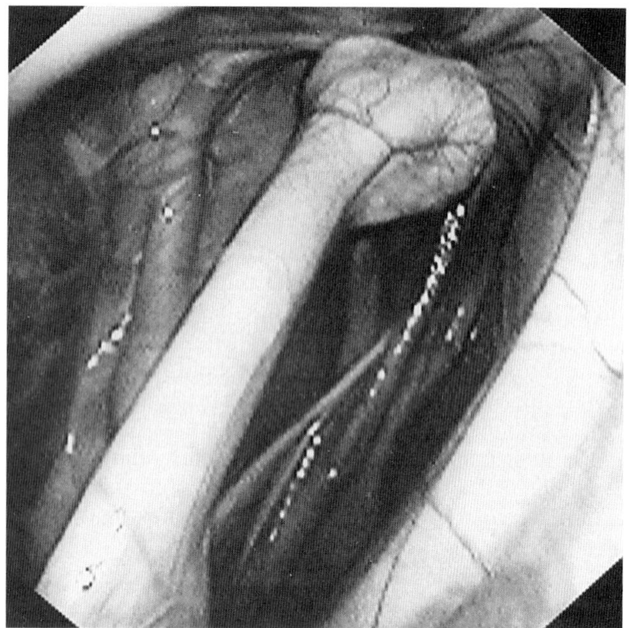

FIGURE 12-32 Endoscopic view of the right guttural pouch of a horse with acute onset of right-sided vestibular disease and facial nerve paralysis. Bony proliferation of the proximal stylohyoid bone is consistent with chronic THO.

the dorsal mucosa of the guttural pouch, near the head of the stylohyoid bone.

Dorsoventral radiographs of the caudal skull should reveal the characteristic periosteal proliferation and sclerosis of the stylohyoid bone and petrous temporal bone[4,11,18] (Figure 12-33). The fracture line is often difficult to identify because of minimal displacement of the fracture fragments. Lateral oblique radiographs obtained at varying angles may aid in localization of a fracture of the basisphenoid, occipital, or petrous temporal bones. Moderate bony proliferation may not occur for several weeks and must be present to diagnose the condition radiographically.[18]

Bone scintigraphy is a noninvasive technique that may allow for an immediate identification of early lesions of the petrous temporal bone. Radiography can identify only structural abnormalities of bone. Bone scintigraphy is capable of detecting dynamic characteristics of bone. Increased metabolic activity and blood supply to the bone, caused by infection or fracture, results in increased uptake of the radiolabeled compound (technetium-99m-labeled phosphate) before radiographic evidence of bony proliferation.[26-28]

When available, computed tomography and MRI are extremely sensitive diagnostic tests for identification of inflammation, bony proliferation, and fracture.[20-22] However, CT and MRI of the skull of horses requires general anesthesia. The risks associated with recovery from general anesthesia, when a horse has compromised neurologic function and possible skull fracture, should be considered seriously before recommendation of these procedures.

One may consider analysis of CSF in affected horses.[1,2] Cytologic evaluation, culture, and sensitivity may help to reveal the presence of secondary bacterial meningitis and can be used to direct the selection of an appropriate antimicrobial treatment plan.[15]

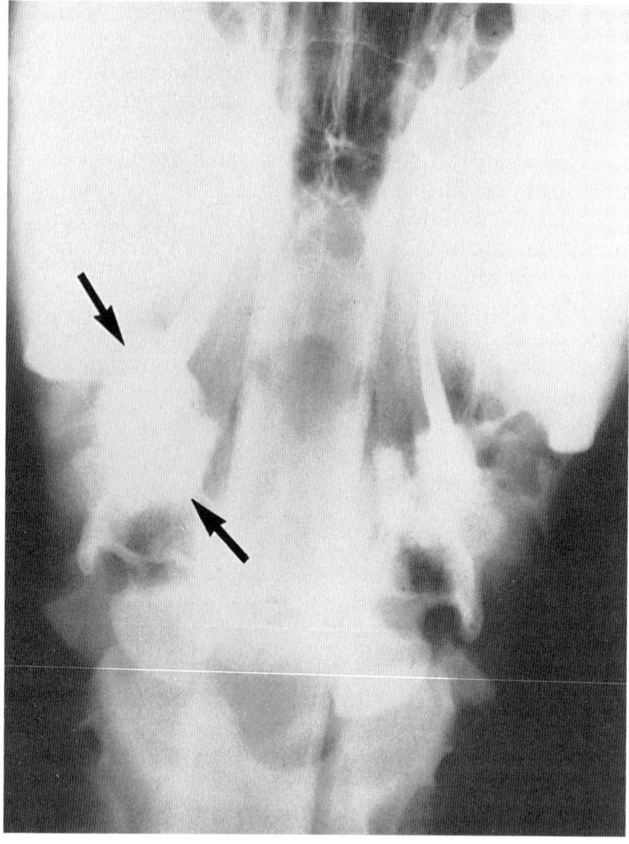

FIGURE 12-33 Ventrodorsal skull radiograph demonstrating bony proliferation of the proximal left stylohyoid and petrous temporal bones *(arrows)* associated with THO.

Treatment of horses with acute onset of neurologic dysfunction secondary to THO should focus on four areas[22]:

1. Stabilization of the horse and decreasing inflammation near the fracture site
2. Treatment with broad spectrum antimicrobials for either extension of a possible otitis interna-media or secondary infection in the hemorrhage that follows the fracture
3. Treatment of exposure keratitis and keratoconjunctivitis sicca
4. Surgical procedures to remove pressure on the temporohyoid articulation to decrease pain and to decrease the likelihood of repeated petrous temporal bone fracture

Medical therapy usually includes anti-inflammatory medications as described elsewhere in this text for treatment of acute head trauma. Trimethoprim-sulfonamide antimicrobials for 30 days are often recommended to treat potential bacterial infection. If culture and sensitivity of CSF or other diagnostic sample are available, then those results may direct alternative antimicrobial choices. Treatment of corneal ulceration and keratoconjunctivitis sicca is described elsewhere in this text.

Surgical treatment of THO may take the form of either a partial stylohyoid ostectomy or a ceratohyoidectomy.[22,29,30] Surgical removal of a 2- to 3-cm segment of the midbody of the stylohyoid bone results in a fibrous nonunion of the stylohyoid bone that should interrupt the transmission of hyoid forces to the temporohyoid joint. Reported complications include transection of the lingual artery, injury to the hypoglossal or facial nerve, and regrowth of the stylohyoid ostectomy site.[29,30] The goal of ceratohyoidectomy is also to remove mechanical stress on the fused temporohyoid joint, but the surgery is technically easier to accomplish without the risk of many of the more serious complications that may be seen with partial stylohyoidectomy.[30]

Diagnosis of THO before the acute onset of neurologic signs is difficult because most horses exhibit few, if any, clinical signs before fracture. Some horses may demonstrate ear rubbing, head tossing or shaking, chomping movements, and sensitivity or pain on palpation at the base of the ear.

Prognosis for life in horses with THO is fair to good if the horse survives the immediate fracture episode.[20] However, it may take up to 2 years for maximum neurologic improvement after fracture and the majority of affected horses have long-term, probably permanent, deficits. Some degree of facial nerve paralysis is common and persistent or recurrent corneal ulceration may result. However, many horses eventually learn to retract the globe to assist in eyelid closure to spread the tear film across the eye, lessening the severity and frequency of corneal ulceration. Many horses return to some level of athletic function after THO.[20] However, owners of horses with THO should be cautioned regarding the potential for acute onset of severe neurologic signs with no warning as a result of refracture. Therefore affected horses pose a risk to human beings in the environment and recognition of this risk is important. Surgical treatment may possibly diminish the risk for subsequent fracture; however, currently no long-term follow-up studies of large numbers of affected horses exist to quantify or compare risk with or without surgery.

Head Trauma

Traumatic fractures of the petrous temporal bone result in damage to the vestibular and facial nerves. Profuse aural hemorrhage or loss of CSF from the external ear canal frequently is observed. Bleeding from the nose occurs if the fracture extends to the cribriform plate.[4] Clinical signs usually appear immediately after trauma and include vestibular disease, facial nerve paralysis, recumbency, or coma. Damage to nervous tissue may be caused by hematoma, callus formation, or displacement of fracture fragments resulting in delayed onset of clinical signs. Signs from brainstem contusion or concussion may be more severe than vestibular dysfunction. If blindness is present, then the prognosis worsens because of the loss of visual compensation of vestibular disease in the future. If one cannot elicit the oculocephalic reflex (physiologic nystagmus), then the examiner should suspect damage to the medial longitudinal fasciculus, indicating extensive brainstem damage; a poor prognosis is indicated.[2] One may recall that bilateral peripheral vestibular disease also results in loss of the oculocephalic reflex; however, this is an unlikely scenario for trauma.

Fractures of the basioccipital and basisphenoid bones occur most frequently in horses that rear over backward and strike the poll of the head. This fracture does not result from referred impact from the poll but is thought to be an avulsion fracture from the pull of the powerful ventral straight muscle of the neck (rectus capitis ventralis) on its insertion on the basioccipital bone.[31] Basioccipital fractures result in neurologic signs associated with damage to the brainstem; signs of vestibular disease are common.

Petrous temporal bone fractures are difficult to identify radiographically; tympanosclerosis appears as early as 20 days after trauma and obscures the fracture line.[4] One often can identify basioccipital fractures easily but can confuse them with the suture lines in the base of the skull.[31] Treatment of vestibular signs after head trauma is similar to that of any acute head trauma as described previously in this chapter.

Drug Toxicities

Drug toxicities can result in unilateral or bilateral peripheral vestibular disease and deafness. Degeneration of the hair cells within the peripheral receptor organs of the auditory and vestibular system occurs with prolonged administration of aminoglycoside antibiotics. Severely affected animals also develop neural degeneration.[3] A more common manifestation of aminoglycoside toxicity is renal failure. As renal clearance of the aminoglycoside decreases, the ototoxic effects of the antibiotics are potentiated.[1,10,23] Clinical signs of vestibular disease appear before deafness. Early vestibular disease may be reversible or centrally compensated, but loss of auditory function is permanent.[2,10,23] Streptomycin preferentially affects the vestibular system, whereas dihydrostreptomycin, kanamycin, gentamicin, neomycin, and vancomycin are more toxic to the auditory system.[2,15] Vincristine, a vinca alkaloid, can cause bilateral cochlear nerve damage in human beings. Auditory function improves several months after discontinuation of the drug.[3] This antimitotic drug is a common component of multiagent chemotherapy protocols in the treatment of lymphosarcoma in the horse.[32] Vincristine also is used for immunosuppression and stimulation of platelet function in refractory cases of immune-mediated thrombocytopenia.[33] One should carefully monitor auditory function when using this drug.

Sudden loud noises can result in degeneration and necrosis of the sensory hair cells of the inner ear.[23] A lightning strike, although usually fatal, is reported to cause acute onset of unilateral vestibular disease in the horse. Facial nerve paralysis may or may not accompany the vestibular signs. Documentation of histopathologic findings in one case revealed hemorrhage and necrosis of the temporal bone, vestibular nerve, and adjacent tissue. Whether the mechanism of damage is electrocution or noise trauma is unknown.[1]

CENTRAL VESTIBULAR DISEASE

Any inflammatory disease or space-occupying mass of the CNS may damage the vestibular nuclei and related tracts. Clinical signs vary with the type and extent of the disease process. One should suspect a CNS disease if abnormal mentation, seizures, blindness, or multiple cranial nerve abnormalities are seen with general proprioceptive deficits. One should perform an electroencephalogram to detect the location and extent of the CNS lesion. The electroencephalogram can detect only cerebral damage and cannot identify lesions of the brainstem. Inflammatory, parasitic, and neoplastic diseases have been implicated in central vestibular disease of the horse.

Inflammatory disease affecting the CNS includes bacterial abscess, equine protozoal myelitis, polyneuritis equi, and viral encephalitis. One should perform CSF analysis to identify the inflammatory process. In the case of brain abscessation, a culture of the CSF may identify the causative organism; *Streptococcus equi* subsp. *equi* is a common causative agent.[34,35] EPM is a common neurologic disease in the United States and Canada and should be suspected if multifocal disease is present.[1] For polyneuritis equi to occur with vestibular dysfunction is common, but the signs of cauda equina neuritis predominate.[2]

Rabies may present as an encephalitis or spinal cord disease and should be considered in the differential diagnosis of any horse with neurologic disease. Spinal ataxia is the primary neurologic deficit observed in horses affected with equine herpesvirus (EHV) myelitis, but the presence of concurrent vestibular disease is reported.[36] The major clinical signs observed with a togavirus (eastern, western, and Venezuelan encephalitis) infection are depression and seizure, although cranial nerve deficits are observed.[6,35] Horses with West Nile virus (WNV) infection may display cranial nerve signs, including vestibular disease. Concurrent behavioral and mentation changes, ataxia, fever, and muscle fasciculations are common.

Aberrant parasite migration of the CNS in horses results in acute onset of neurologic signs. Clinical signs vary, but progression of clinical signs occurs in most instances. Neurologic signs are generally asymmetrical because of the random nature of migration. Neurologic disease secondary to parasite migration is discussed in detail later in this chapter. Fungal granulomata caused by *Aspergillus* spp. and *Cryptococcus neoformans* have been reported as space-occupying masses within the cranium of a horse.[1,37] Cholesteatoma (cholesterol granuloma) could involve the vestibular system by extending from the choroid plexus of the fourth ventricle of the brain.[1] Neoplastic diseases of the CNS are rare in the horse. Any tumor affecting the cerebellomedullary angle could result in vestibular signs.[2] Lymphosarcoma, ependymoma, meningeal melanoma, and melanotic hamartoma have been reported to affect the CNS of the horse.[2,38]

ANCILLARY DIAGNOSTIC TESTS

Caloric Testing

The caloric test is a diagnostic aid that may be helpful in differentiating central from peripheral vestibular disease. The test is able to assess each peripheral vestibular sensory organ separately. In the normal animal, irrigation of ice-cold water (12° C) into the external auditory canal for 3 to 5 minutes induces a horizontal nystagmus with the fast phase away from the tested labyrinth.[2,3,5,6] The water cools endolymph closest to the tympanic membrane, increasing its density. A density gradient is created within the semicircular canal and the cooled endolymph sinks, causing displacement of the hair cells. Warm water (45° C) irrigation of the external auditory canal results in horizontal nystagmus with a fast phase toward the tested labyrinth. The warm-water test is less reliable.[10,16] The test does not induce nystagmus in a nonfunctional labyrinth. Animals may resist the procedure, making the test difficult to interpret, and in some animals, one cannot induce nystagmus. If an asymmetrical response is obtained, then the depressed reaction indicates the abnormal labyrinth.[2] The test is difficult to perform and not entirely reliable, although it may be a helpful diagnostic aid in the anesthetized or comatose horse.[6]

Brainstem Auditory Evoked Response

The cochlea is damaged by trauma or inflammation of the peripheral vestibular receptor organs, and detection of hearing loss may help to differentiate central from peripheral vestibular disease. Unilateral hearing loss is difficult to assess subjectively in the horse. BAER is a method of objective assessment of auditory function in the horse. This noninvasive, electrodiagnostic test stimulates the auditory system with a series of clicks. Far-field potentials of the brainstem auditory components are recorded via cutaneous electrodes and a signal-averaging system.[6,39] The response is a series of evoked potentials occurring within 10 ms after the stimulus. In the horse the evoked potentials appear on the oscilloscope as a series of five waveforms.[40] In human beings, five to seven waveforms are present, and each corresponds to a specific neurologic structure.[39,40] Abnormalities of the specific waveforms can identify a lesion of the corresponding neurologic structure. In the horse, functional loss of the cochlea or eighth cranial nerve results in the loss of the entire waveform on the side of injury, and the presence or absence of the waveform can differentiate a central from a peripheral vestibular lesion. General anesthesia is not necessary to perform the test, but sedation is recommended.[39]

DISEASES OF THE CEREBELLUM

Barbara A. Byrne

Cerebellar abnormalities reported in horses consist primarily of neurodegenerative disorders confined primarily to a small number of breeds including Arabians and Gotland pony foals. The cerebellum is essential for the coordination of movement. Afferent information arises from the general and special (vestibular) proprioceptive systems and the special somatic (auditory and visual) systems. The cerebellum is responsible for regulation of the rate, range, and strength of movement, as well as integration and coordination for balance and posture. Cerebellar abnormalities in horses are unusual; however, when present, they can have a profound effect on gait and posture.

STRUCTURE AND FUNCTION

Knowledge of the structure and development of the cerebellum is important for understanding cerebellar function in health and disease. The cerebellum is located in the metencephalon dorsal to the pons and is attached to the pons via three cerebellar peduncles (Figure 12-34). The caudal peduncle is composed primarily of afferent fibers arising from the medulla, the vestibular nuclei via the vestibulocerebellar tracts, and the spinal cord via the spinocerebellar tracts. The middle cerebellar peduncle contains only afferent fibers to the cerebellum that arise from the transverse fibers of the pons. The rostral cerebellar peduncle is the primary connection to the mesencephalon and carries the majority of cerebellar efferent fibers, although a few afferent fibers arise from the spinocerebellar tracts. The cerebellum consists of two hemispheres and a central region known as the *vermis*.[1] The extensive convolutions of the cerebellar cortex are termed *folia*. The cortex covers the surface of the cerebellum. On cut section, the cerebellar medulla is a central region of white matter with multiple projections called *arbor vitae*. These branches extend to the cerebellar cortex and form the white matter portion adjacent to the cerebellar cortex.

The cerebellar medulla has three nuclei: (1) the fastigial, (2) the interpositional, and (3) the lateral nuclei from medial to lateral on each side of the cerebellum. The cerebellum also can be divided into three bilateral longitudinal regions in association with these nuclei.[1,2] The medial zone, containing the

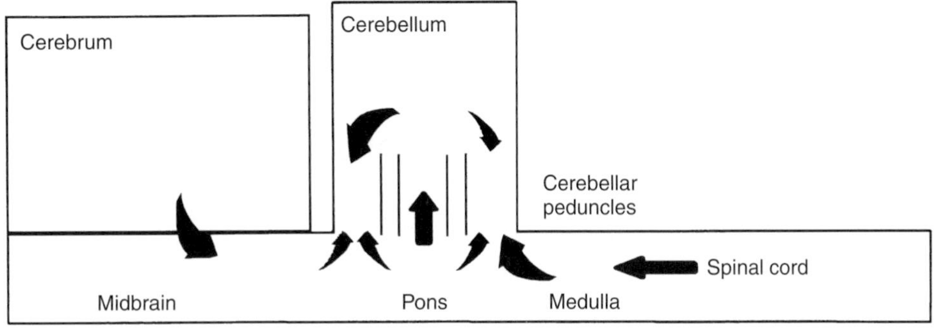

FIGURE 12-34 Schematic diagram of cerebellar efferent and afferent information pathways via the cerebellar peduncles. The arrow size reflects the relative contribution of each pathway (see text for details).

vermis and the fastigial nucleus, primarily regulates the tone, posture, and equilibrium of the body in general. The intermediate zones contain the interpositional nucleus and cortex adjacent to the vermis and adjust the orientation of limbs in space, maintaining balance, posture, and muscle tone during complex movements. The lateral zones, consisting of the lateral nuclei and lateral portions of the cerebral hemispheres, have a similar function but do not influence posture or muscle tone directly.[2]

The cerebellum arises from the alar plate region of the metencephalon and originates initially as a proliferation of cells in the rhombic lip that extend dorsally and medially to form the dorsal portion of the metencephalon. Germinal cells proliferating in the rhombic lip eventually migrate into the cerebellum and differentiate to form the specialized neurons of the cerebellar cortex. The cerebellar cortex has three layers: (1) the outer molecular layer, (2) the middle Purkinje layer, and (3) the inner granular layer (Figure 12-35). The molecular layer is acellular and consists primarily of the dendritic zones of the Purkinje cells and axons of the granular cells.[1] The Purkinje layer is only one cell thick and consists of Purkinje neurons. The granular layer is densely cellular with granular neurons. All layers must be present and aligned in proper orientation for normal function.

Organization of the specialized structure of the cerebellar cortex allows integration and coordination of movement. The cerebellum primarily provides regulation of skeletal movement, allowing coordinated movement; it does not initiate muscular activity. Afferent information regarding movement and balance arising from the mesencephalon, the brainstem, and the spinal cord enters the cerebellum via the cerebellar peduncles, and regulation of movement is coordinated by the inhibitory influence of Purkinje neurons on the cerebellar nuclei. Information enters the cerebellum via the cerebellar peduncles and is carried on two major afferent nerves termed *mossy fibers* and *climbing fibers*.[1] Mossy fibers originate from the brainstem and spinal cord. Mossy fibers send collateral fibers to synapse with the cerebellar nuclei; they terminate by synapsing with granule neurons in the cerebellar cortex. These fibers are facilitory at these synapses. The axons that granule neurons send to the molecular layer course transversely through this layer to synapse with the dendritic zone of multiple Purkinje cells and also provide facilitory influence at these synapses. Climbing fibers originate in the olivary nucleus, which provides most of the extrapyramidal projections to the cerebellum. Similar to mossy fibers, climbing fibers send collaterals to synapse on neurons in the cerebellar nuclei; however, the axon continues through the cerebellar cortex to synapse with the dendritic zone of the Purkinje neurons in the molecular layer. As with mossy fibers, climbing fibers provide a facilitative influence at the synapses.

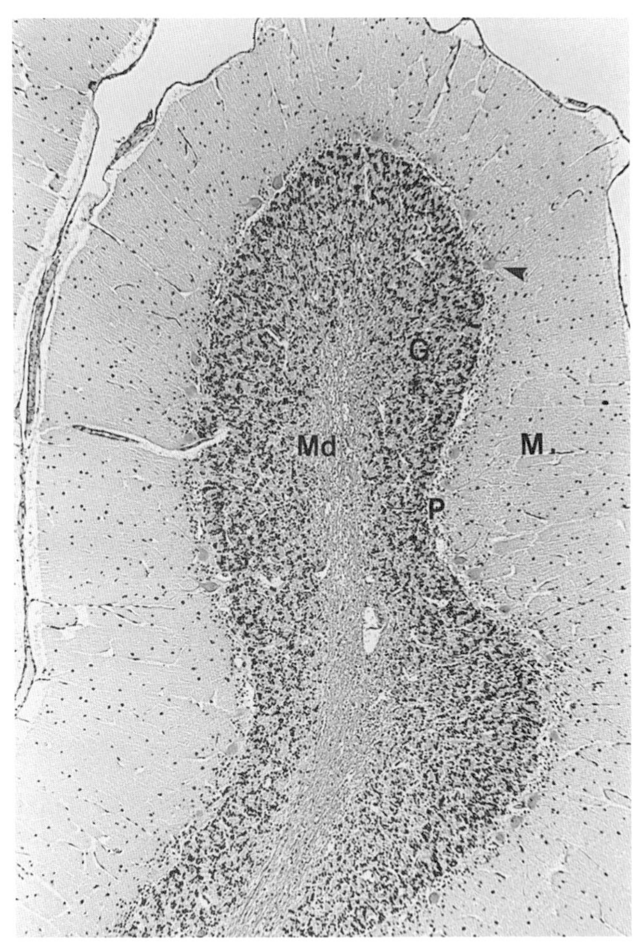

FIGURE 12-35 Photomicrograph of a normal cerebellum. *M,* Molecular layer; *P,* Purkinje layer; *G,* granular layer; *Md,* medulla; *arrowhead,* a Purkinje neuron. (Hematoxylin-eosin stain; ×55.) (Courtesy the Washington Animal Disease Diagnostic Laboratory, Pullman, WA.)

Purkinje neurons provide the sole efferent fibers from the cerebellar cortex. The majority of Purkinje cell axons terminate on neurons in the cerebellar nuclei, although direct projections from these neurons to the vestibular nuclei occur via the caudal cerebellar peduncle. Purkinje neurons are inhibitory and use the neurotransmitter GABA.[1] Efferent nerves from the cerebellum are primarily from the cerebellar nuclei that facilitate activity of upper motor neurons originating in the brainstem.

Thus much of the influence of the cerebellum on skeletal muscle activity is to modulate the upper motor neuron. Information regarding movement and balance enters the cerebellar cortex via the cerebellar peduncles. This afferent activity stimulates inhibitory Purkinje neurons by climbing or mossy fibers. Purkinje neurons in turn modulate the activity of the cerebellar nuclei to regulate movement and muscular tone. Purkinje neurons also provide direct inhibitory input to the vestibular nuclei.

CLINICAL SIGNS

Clinical signs associated with cerebellar disease generally reflect the loss of coordination. Mentation is normal in horses with cerebellar disease, provided that other regions of the brain are unaffected and metabolic disturbances such as septicemia or endotoxemia are not present. Cerebellar disturbances result in ataxia and inability to regulate the rate, range, and force of movement.[1] *Dysmetria* refers to alterations in the range of gait. *Hypermetria* is an exaggerated range of movement. When moving, the limb has a higher or longer flight compared with normal. Hypometria is a diminished movement; for example, the arc of flight of a limb in motion may be lower. Horses showing hypometria tend to hit objects with the limb when stepping over them and may fail to extend the limb far enough to set the foot down on a step. Initiation of movement may be jerky and awkward, and the trunk may sway from side to side when the horse moves. Spasticity is caused by hypertonia and results in a jerky stiff gait. Paresis is not a feature of cerebellar disease because the cerebellum does not initiate voluntary motion, although a horse that is unable to regulate rate and range of motion sometimes may appear weak and drag its toes. Diffuse cerebellar disease results in bilateral signs. In general, unilateral lesions result in signs ipsilateral to the lesion.

Intention tremor is another prominent sign of diffuse severe cerebellar disease. Tremor is most obvious as vertical or horizontal head motions and can be observed readily as a horse approaches feed or attempts to nurse. The tremor is present only when a movement is initiated and tends to become more exaggerated as the horse approaches an object.

Cerebellar disease also may cause loss of the blink reflex and vestibular abnormalities. The horse may fail to blink in response to an ocular menace. The exact mechanism for this deficiency is unknown; however, a portion of the visual pathway from the visual cortex to the facial nucleus (which initiates the blink) likely travels through the cerebellum. Disruption of the flocculonodular lobe, located in the ventral cerebellum, or the fastigial nucleus may result in vestibular signs characterized by disequilibrium; a variable nystagmus, which may be positional; and positioning difficulties.[1] Unilateral lesions may result in a head and body tilt toward the side of the lesion and nystagmus with the fast phase away from the lesion. Paradoxical vestibular syndrome, characterized by a head tilt away from the lesion and nystagmus with the fast phase toward the lesion, is apparent with unilateral lesions involving the cerebellar peduncle.[1,2]

DISEASES OF THE CEREBELLUM

Cerebellar Abiotrophy and Degeneration

Cerebellar abiotrophy is the most commonly reported cerebellar disease in horses.[3-10] *Abiotrophy in the nervous system* refers to premature degeneration of neurons caused by some intrinsic abnormality in their structure or metabolism.[11] Cerebellar abiotrophy has been reported in Arabian, Gotland pony, and Oldenburg horse breeds. Degenerative cerebellar lesions have been observed in one Thoroughbred and two Paso Fino newborn foals.[12] Arabian and part-Arabian horses in North America are affected most frequently and the disorder is believed to be inherited as an autosomal recessive trait in this breed.[3-6,8-10] The incidence in some Arabian horse herds has been reported to be as high as 8%. In one report, colts were affected more frequently than fillies, although subsequent reports have not substantiated this finding.[5] The cerebellar abiotrophy that occurs in Oldenburg horses is progressive and fatal, with atypical histologic lesions compared with the syndrome that occurs in Arabian foals, in which the degeneration is characterized by apoptosis of Purkinje cells.[13] Cerebellar abiotrophy generally affects foals less than 1 year of age and occurs most frequently in 1- to 6-month-old foals. Adult-onset cerebellar abiotrophy has been reported in other species such as the dog and has been observed in two horses.[1] Many foals are born with no abnormalities and later develop disease; however, occasionally they are affected at or shortly after birth.[5,6,9]

Clinical signs associated with cerebellar abiotrophy include intention tremors of the head, ataxia, wide-based stance and gait, dysmetria, and spasticity.[3-10] The most frequently reported initial signs noted by owners are an intention tremor of the head, vertical or horizontal, or a hypermetric forelimb gait.[3,9] The neurologic examination reveals no change in mentation. One almost never observes nystagmus, which has been reported in only one case of abiotrophy in a Gotland pony.[7] A menace reflex frequently is absent or diminished.[6,9] One must interpret this finding with caution because normal foals may lack or have a depressed menace reflex until at least 2 weeks of age.[14]

Stance and gait abnormalities seen with cerebellar abiotrophy generally consist of a wide-based stance or gait and ataxia.[6,8,9] The foal may move stiffly and have a high goose-stepping gait. The horse may protract the limb when walking, resulting in slamming of the foot to the ground. Movement may be spastic with circumduction. Walking on an incline, asking the foal to step over obstacles, and blindfolding the foal exacerbate gait abnormalities. Generally, gait abnormalities are symmetric, although in a Welsh Cob and Arabian cross foal the initial signs were characterized by a stiff motion in the left front limb. Signs in this foal progressed to severe ataxia.[4] Foals affected at birth may have difficulty rising.[5-7] Despite this finding, weakness is not a feature of the clinical signs associated with cerebellar abiotrophy. Spinal reflexes are usually normal. Some affected animals fall when startled or when raising their heads. Signs are generally progressive for several months after diagnosis. Once the animal has reached maturity, the condition becomes static, although mild improvement has been observed.[10]

Ancillary testing is of limited value in diagnosing cerebellar abiotrophy but can be helpful to rule out other causes of ataxia. The CBC and serum biochemistry profile are normal in affected foals. Abnormalities in CSF are detectable. In one study, three of four foals had an elevated CSF CK activity. Values in affected foals ranged between 6.6 to 62 IU/μl (normal range, 0 to 8 IU/μl).[9] CSF CK elevations generally are associated with neural necrosis or degeneration, although they are not associated specifically with a particular disease.[15-17]

In addition, CSF total protein may be elevated. In the study cited previously, three foals had elevated total protein with an average of 226 mg/dl (normal, 0 to 100 mg/dl) in all foals with cerebellar abiotrophy. As with CK, total protein elevations are not specific for abiotrophy and may occur with disruption of the blood-brain barrier or with CNS inflammation or degeneration. Many foals with cerebellar abiotrophy have normal CSF analysis. Electroencephalographic abnormalities, including increased synchrony and increased number of abrupt frequency changes, also may be detectable in affected foals.[9] In this study, these abnormalities were not observed in normal foals anesthetized under similar conditions. Skull and cervical radiographs are unremarkable. However, because mentation is normal in foals with cerebellar abiotrophy, electroencephalographic examination is not necessary to make a diagnosis and is primarily useful to exclude seizure disorders as a cause of the tremors observed.

Antemortem diagnosis of cerebellar abiotrophy is based on a typical history and the clinical signs of intention tremor, lack of menace, failure to blink to bright light, and ataxia in Arabian, part-Arabian, or Gotland pony foals. The differential diagnoses for cerebellar abiotrophy include cranial malformations; congenital spinal malformations, including atlanto-axial malformations and stenotic myelopathy; inflammation or infection of the cerebellum; and trauma. One can rule out these conditions based on the neurologic examination, CSF analysis, and radiography. The signs of characteristic ataxia and head tremor without weakness in the appropriate breed is nearly pathognomonic.

Postmortem examination provides a definitive diagnosis of this disorder. Generally, no gross abnormalities are notable; however, careful examination of the cerebellum may reveal an increased lobular pattern with prominent folia. In the Gotland pony, the weight ratio of the cerebellum to the cerebrum is reduced significantly in foals with cerebellar abiotrophy.[7] Normal foals had a 13% ratio, and affected foals had a 10% ratio. In the degenerative cerebellar condition in the Paso Fino and Thoroughbred foals, a decrease in the cerebellar-to-whole brain weight ratio was evident.[12] This ratio in normal foals was 8% and in affected foals was 6%.

Histologic abnormalities are consistent in cases of cerebellar abiotrophy. The most prominent finding is the widespread loss of Purkinje neurons[3-10] (Figure 12-36). Degenerative changes, such as shrunken and angular neurons with hyperchromasia and dispersion of Nissl's substance, are apparent. One may observe occasional "baskets" or clear spaces where the Purkinje neuron is lost. Thinning of the molecular layer occurs with gliosis. The granular layer is also thin with a loss of cellularity. Similar histologic findings were found in Thoroughbred and Paso Fino foals with vacuolation and proliferation of Bergmann's glia in the Purkinje cell layer.[12]

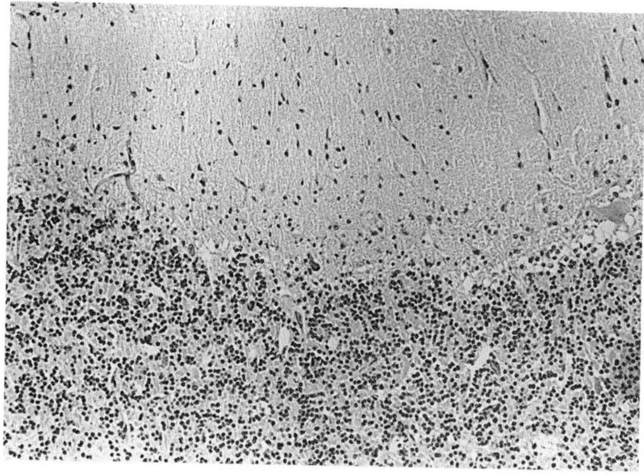

FIGURE 12-36 Photomicrograph of the cerebellum from a 9-month-old foal with cerebellar abiotrophy. The decreased number of Purkinje neurons is notable. (Hematoxylin-eosin stain; ×139.) (Courtesy the Washington Animal Disease Diagnostic Laboratory, Pullman, WA.)

The pathogenesis of cerebellar abiotrophy is unknown. Viral, toxic, and genetic causes have been investigated.[3,5,6,9] To date no evidence has been found to support an infectious cause. No virus has been isolated from the CSF or brain of affected foals, and no viral inclusions have been observed on histologic examination. No toxin has been associated consistently with cerebellar abiotrophy of Arabian foals. Experimental breedings of Arabian horses indicate an autosomal recessive mode of inheritance but an exact genetic basis for disease has not been determined. A pedigree analysis of Gotland ponies similarly suggests an autosomal recessive mode of inheritance[7]; however, a high degree of inbreeding was noted, making definitive conclusions difficult. Attempts to breed affected individuals in this study were unsuccessful.

No treatment exists for cerebellar abiotrophy. As noted previously, signs may be progressive until the foal reaches maturity. Signs may stabilize or improve slightly with time.

Gomen Disease

Gomen disease is a degenerative cerebellar condition recognized in the northwest part of New Caledonia.[18] Gomen disease is a progressive cerebellar disease that causes mild to severe ataxia. Horses that are indigenous or are introduced to the region may be affected. The disease occurs only in horses that are allowed to roam free, and signs may take 1 to 2 years to develop once a horse is introduced into an endemic area. Horses that are confined generally are unaffected. Clinical signs consist of ataxia, which is most prominent in the hindlimbs; toe dragging; and a wide-based stance. As the disease progresses, weakness becomes prominent and horses may have difficulty rising. The signs are primarily referable to involvement of the cerebellum; however, weakness likely is caused by brainstem or spinal cord involvement. Nystagmus is not observed. Ataxia is progressive over 3 to 4 years until the horse dies or is euthanized.

Mild cerebellar atrophy may be apparent on gross examination of the brain. Histologically, severe depletion of Purkinje neurons is evident throughout the cerebellum.[19] Purkinje neurons may contain lipofuscin pigment and vacuoles. One horse examined had moderate loss of granule cells. Moderate to severe lipofuscin pigmentation of neuron cell bodies occurs throughout the brain and spinal cord. Although lipofuscin accumulation may be considered a normal variation of aging, the degree of pigment accumulation is far more severe than that in horses of similar age.

The pathogenesis of this disease is unknown. Pedigree analysis has not revealed any genetic component for susceptibility to development of disease.[18] A condition of neuronal lipofuscinosis in dogs has some similarities to this disease.[19] The accumulation of lipofuscin pigment and association with free-ranging horses suggests a metabolic disorder, perhaps resulting from toxicity.[18,19]

Developmental Abnormalities

Dandy-Walker syndrome is characterized by a midline defect of the cerebellum and cystic dilation of the fourth ventricle, which separates the cerebral hemispheres.[20] Frequently, all or portions of the cerebellar vermis fail to form, and the corpus callosum may be absent. The condition is rare in horses and has been observed in Thoroughbred and Arabian foals.[21,22] Foals with this syndrome may be abnormal neurologically from birth, with difficulty rising, seizures, and absence of the suckle reflex.[21] The forehead may be domed excessively. Ataxia, nystagmus, aggression, and difficulty in training may persist as the foal ages.[21,22] Diagnosis generally is made at postmortem examination; however, one case was diagnosed antemortem using computed tomography.[21]

Several individual cases of equine developmental cerebellar abnormalities have been described. Cerebellar hypoplasia has been described in a Thoroughbred foal that had difficulty rising and developed seizures shortly after birth.[23] This report did not describe the histologic findings of cerebellar hypoplasia in detail; thus the relationship between this finding and cerebellar abiotrophy or degeneration in Arabian foals is unknown. Bilateral focal cerebellar cortical hypoplasia has been reported in a 6-year-old Thoroughbred gelding.[24] No gait abnormalities were detected in this horse, although it had fallen over repeatedly before euthanasia. The relationship between falling and the cerebellar abnormality is unclear. Possibly the abnormality in this adult horse resulted from a secondary problem, such as vascular injury, rather than a developmental defect.[13]

A single case of cerebellar dysplasia has been described in a 4-year-old Thoroughbred horse.[25] This horse had a 7-month history of circling and collapsing to the left side. In this case the horse had hyperplasia of the right side of the cerebellum with no associated central white matter. Histologically, the granule layer was thinning, with increased thickness of the molecular layer and cavitation of the white matter.

Additional reported developmental disorders include cerebellar hypoplasia with internal hydrocephalus and cerebellar aplasia with hydranencephaly in two fetuses from Haflinger mares with hydrops allantois.[26] Mild cerebellar degenerative changes consisting of Purkinje neuron granularity has been noted in a Standardbred filly with a chromosomal abnormality.[27] This abnormality was accompanied by mild spongiotic degeneration of the cerebrum. Abnormal neurologic signs in this filly included difficulty standing at birth, mental dullness, and a head tilt. Growth retardation, small inactive ovaries, and a consistently wrinkled muzzle accompanied these signs.

Infectious Conditions

Unlike in many other large animals, no infectious agents have the cerebellum as their primary target; however, a number of agents may affect the cerebellum. Any agent that targets the CNS, especially those that have a multifocal distribution, also may involve the cerebellum.

Equine protozoal myelitis is a protozoal disease caused by *Sarcocystis neurona*. This agent causes multifocal inflammation and necrosis of the CNS. The most common signs associated with *S. neurona* infection are spinal ataxia, weakness, and muscle atrophy, although this agent also can affect the cerebellum. Clinical signs associated with cerebellar involvement may reflect diffuse or focal involvement. A head tilt or asymmetrical ataxia without weakness or lower motor neuron signs may be associated with focal disease. Diagnosis is based on multifocal neurologic disease and the presence of antibody to *S. neurona* in the CSF. Additional information regarding this disease is found elsewhere in this chapter.

EHV-1 causes multifocal meningoencephalitis resulting from vasculitis, vascular thrombosis, and ischemia of nervous tissue. Although the primary signs associated with this agent include spinal ataxia, cranial nerve abnormalities, and signs associated with involvement of the cauda equina, this agent also may affect the cerebellum. As with equine protozoal myelitis, involvement may be focal, multifocal, or diffuse.

Occasionally, disseminated *Streptococcus equi* subsp. *equi* infection (bastard strangles) may result in a cerebellar abscess.[28] Neurologic abnormalities in one reported case included proprioceptive deficits in the right forelimb, nystagmus, and a head tilt. Meningitis contributed to other CNS signs such as depression, blindness, and recumbency. Diagnosis of this condition can be based on a history of previous *S. equi* subsp. *equi* infection, evidence of severe suppurative inflammation in the CSF, and culture of *S. equi* subsp. *equi* from the CSF. Treatment consists of penicillin. The prognosis is guarded; however, successful surgical drainage of a cerebral *S. equi* subsp. *equi* abscess has been reported.[29]

Focal involvement of the cerebellum has been associated with aberrant parasite migration in the horse.[4,30] In a 6-year-old pony, infection with *Halicephalobus deletrix* resulted in severe ataxia.[30] Histologic study showed lesions scattered throughout the cerebellum, brainstem, thalamus, and pituitary gland, and nematodes were observed throughout the lesions. A second case involving a 1-year-old Thoroughbred colt had a sudden onset of severe ataxia.[4] Multifocal malacia with numerous eosinophils was observed throughout the cerebellar white matter. No nematode was detected, although parasitic involvement was suspected based on the eosinophilic inflammation.

Miscellaneous Conditions

A familial neurologic condition in newborn Thoroughbred foals has been reported.[31] This syndrome affected three of five foals of a Thoroughbred mare. The foals were normal at birth and developed signs of severe incoordination, a wide-based stance, and recumbency at 2 to 5 days of age. The condition appeared more severe when the foals became excited or struggled; consequently, they were treated symptomatically with diazepam. The signs would improve with this treatment and return as the sedation diminished. These foals improved with stall rest over 7 to 10 days. The cause of the clinical signs in these foals is unknown; however, the authors suggested possible viral or toxic causes.

Cerebellar ataxia in two Thoroughbred fillies has been associated with hematoma in the fourth ventricle.[32] These two horses demonstrated fever, dysmetria, spasticity, and weakness. Clinical signs most likely resulted from compression of the adjacent cerebellum. CSF analyses in these cases revealed xanthochromia, elevated RBC and white blood cell counts, and elevated total protein concentrations. The cause of the hematomas was not identified; damage to regional small vessels and a vascular anomaly were suspected.

Chronic methylmercurial poisoning in horses can cause a number of clinical abnormalities, including cerebellar ataxia.[33] Severe poisoning can result in incoordination, dysmetria, and gross head nodding in the experimental setting. Associated clinical signs include lethargy, anorexia, exudative dermatitis, and laminitis. Lesions in the cerebellum consisted of focal atrophy and cellular depletion in the granular layer with little to no involvement of Purkinje cells. Additional abnormalities included neuronal necrosis and gliosis in the cerebrum, lymphocytic perivascular cuffing, and swollen axons in the spinal cord. Preferential accumulation of inorganic mercury in the brain and resulting cell injury most likely led to the neurologic signs observed. Diagnosis of methylmercurial poisoning can be based on clinical signs and measurement of mercury in the liver and kidney (see Chapter 22).

CERVICAL VERTEBRAL MALFORMATION

*Caroline N. Hahn**

Cervical vertebral malformation (CVM) is the most common cause of ataxia in horses in Europe and Australia and is an important differential diagnosis in regions affected by inflammatory diseases such as EPM and WNV. Differentiating CVM from other conditions that cause ataxia is important because some horses with vertebral malformation may be amenable to surgery.[1]

CVM resulting in spinal cord compression stems from bone and joint malformations and is seen as two broad categories. Younger lightbreed and warmblood horses and foals are predisposed to deformation of the vertebral bodies with malarticulation on flexion secondary to developmental bone disease (type 1 CVM). In older horses, spinal cord compression more commonly occurs secondary to vertebral malformation because of osteoarthritis of caudal cervical articular process joints (type 2 CVM),[2] although there is some overlap in this classification. Spinal cord compression has traditionally been separated into two further categories: (1) dynamic vertebral compressions, whereby the spinal cord compression is intermittent and occurs when the cervical vertebrae are flexed (more cranial vertebral) or extended (more caudal vertebrae), and (2) static compressions, in which spinal cord compression is continuous regardless of cervical position. Both syndromes are likely to occur in individual cases, and differentiating the two is probably not clinically important other than to remind clinicians of the risks associated with extreme neck manipulation under myelography.

CLINICAL SIGNS

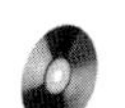

Cervical vertebral malformation is characterized by symmetrical ataxia, upper motor neuron paresis, and dysmetria, which are usually worse in the pelvic limbs than thoracic limbs.[3] Physical examination sometimes reveals palpable cranial cervical vertebral flexion-fixation, and affected horses tend to be large for their age and breed. Male animals appear to be more frequently affected. Often a history of increased clumsiness occurs, and mild to moderately affected horses show symmetrical ataxia with circumduction of the pelvic limbs, especially when the animal is made to walk in small circles. Proprioceptive deficits, toe dragging (flexor paresis), and varying degrees of upper motor neuron extensor paresis (assessed by pulling on the horse's tail at a walk) are also present. Thoracic limbs often have a hypometric, stiff (spastic) component to the strides, especially while walking the horse down a slope and with the head elevated. Thoracic limb deficits are usually less severe than pelvic limb deficits because of the more superficial location of pelvic limb spinocerebellar proprioceptive tracts in the spinal cord. Horses with chronic disease tend to show less paresis than those with recent onset clinical signs.[4] Neck pain or stiffness may be present in some older horses. An accident or injury to the neck is sometimes in the history, and clinical signs may have an abrupt onset or indeed the horse may be tetraplegic, especially if external trauma plays a major role. The ataxia, however, was likely present before the traumatic incident.

Clinical signs of concurrent developmental orthopedic disease of the appendicular skeleton, such as physeal enlargement of the long bones, joint effusion after osteochondrosis, and flexural limb deformities, are often present in young horses with CVM.[3] It is worth remembering that sometimes horses affected with CVM may have another concurrent neurologic disease such as equine protozoal encephalomyelitis.

PATHOGENESIS

Neurologic signs result from progressive spinal cord compression secondary to structural changes to vertebral and surrounding tissues. Pathologic changes of the cervical vertebrae leading to spinal cord compression consist of vertebral malformation with stenosis of the vertebral canal, abnormal formation of, and alterations to, the articular processes associated with osteochondrosis, angular deformity of vertebrae and cranioventral or, more commonly, caudal extension of the dorsal aspect of the vertebral arch (Figure 12-37).[3,4] Histopathologic examination of the spinal cord reveals wallerian-like degeneration, loss of axons and fibrosis at the sites of spinal cord compression, and axon loss in the ascending and descending white matter tracts within adjacent segments of the spinal cord cranial and caudal to the site of spinal cord compression.[3,5]

Type 1 CVM is as disease seen in young horses and may be a form of a developmental orthopedic disease (i.e., related to rapid skeletal growth in genetically predisposed horses). Cervical vertebrae in affected horses have lesions of osteochondrosis and epiphysitis similar to those seen in the limbs, found most commonly in more cranial cervical vertebrae, particularly C3, C4, and C5. A high dietary energy intake is almost certainly

*The authors wish to acknowledge Randolph H. Stewart and Bonnie R. Rush, whose original work has been incorporated into this section.

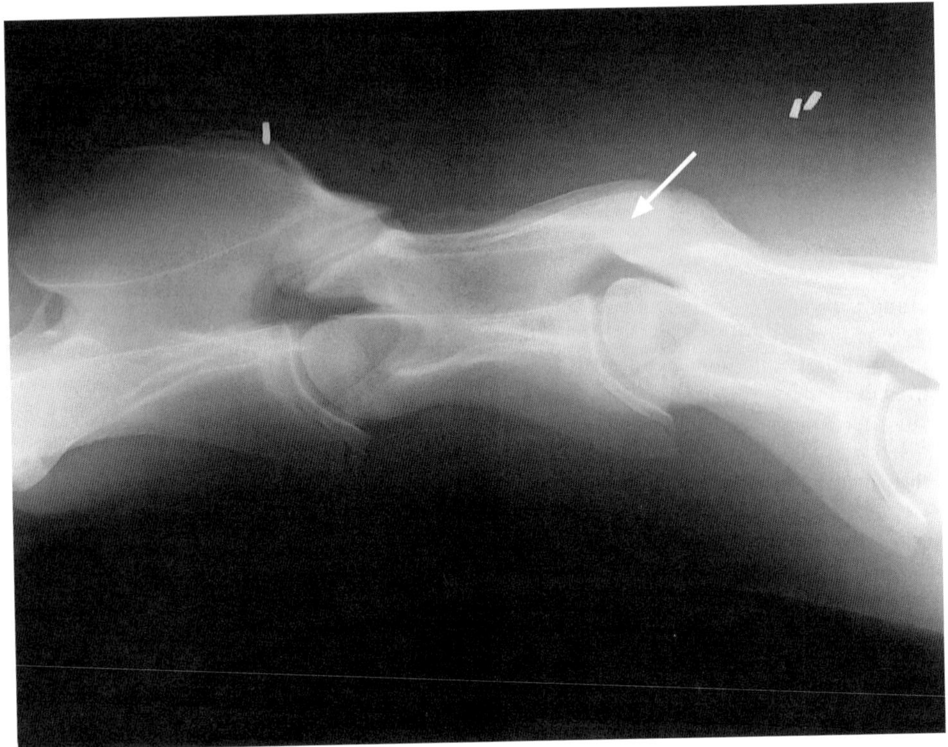

FIGURE 12-37 Cervical vertebrae 2, 3, and 4 of a horse with cervical vertebral malformation (CVM) showing stenosis of the vertebral canal subjectively obvious at C3-4, intervertebral malalignment of C3 and C4, and caudal extension of the dorsal aspect of the vertebral arch of C3 *(arrow)*.

necessary for expression of the disease and trauma to the neck probably plays a role as young, large, fast-growing animals (often male animals) are most commonly affected. Type 1 CVM almost certainly has a genetic basis; however, a breeding trial using horses with CVM that had had corrective surgery resulted in offspring that did not have CVM but did have a higher frequency of developmental orthopedic diseases than expected.[6]

Type 2 CVM more commonly occurs in older horses without evidence of developmental orthopedic disease but with arthritis of the caudal (C6-T1) cervical vertebrae. External injury is likely to play a part in the onset of the disease. Compression of the spinal cord is due to vertebral malformation at C5, C6, and C7, resulting in cone-shaped caudal cervical vertebrae with a reduction in a cross-sectional area of the vertebral canal and resultant impingement on the spinal cord by proliferating articular and periarticular soft tissues. There may be concurrent formation of epidural and periarticular cysts, which can result in sudden onset of symmetrical or asymmetrical signs without a contemporaneous episode of external injury. Bleeding into one of these cysts has been observed and adds to the compression. Occasionally these cause acute onset severe clinical signs that can abate within a few hours only to reappear later.

DIAGNOSIS

Fortuitously, the narrowing of the cervical vertebral canal and associated spinal cord compressive lesions in horses are most commonly in a dorsoventral in orientation, allowing the diagnosis to be made with good-quality, standing plain lateral radiographs of C1 to T1 vertebrae. However, it should be remembered that the lack of dorsoventral radiographic projections effectively makes this an incomplete diagnostic series. The horse should be sedated and the head pulled forward manually, thus straightening each vertebra along the median plain giving the best alignment of vertebral bodies. The assessment of qualitative features of vertebral malformation, including physitis of the caudal vertebral body, caudal extension of the dorsal arch of the vertebral body, intervertebral malalignment, and arthropathy of the articular processes, is useful; however, alone these findings offer poor positive and negative predictive values.[7]

The most important factor in the diagnosis of CVM in adult horses and foals is the identification of a decrease in the diameter of the vertebral canal, be it within a vertebra or, more commonly, between two vertebrae.[8] Corrected intravertebral and particularly intervertebral sagittal ratios (SRs) from C2-C7 calculated from lateral standing cervical radiographs can be used to accurately diagnose CVM in horses.[9] The intra- and intervertebral sagittal diameter of the vertebral canal are measured at the narrowest points and corrected for radiographic magnification and size of horse by being expressed as a ratio of the maximal height of the cranial vertebral physis (Figure 12-38). The minimum intravertebral diameter is measured at the point along the vertebral canal where the diameter is at a minimum, whereas the minimum intervertebral sagittal diameter ratio is made from the caudal aspect of the dorsal lamina of the vertebral arch of the more cranial vertebra to the dorsocranial aspect of the body of the more caudal vertebra, or from the caudal vertebral body of the more cranial vertebra to the cranial dorsal lamina of the vertebral arch of the more caudal vertebra, whichever was smaller. For vertebrae C2-C3 to C5-C6, the minimum diameter is invariably found to be the former measurement (see Figure 12-38).

Reference figures for intra- and intervertebral SR in a limited number of horses are shown in Tables 12-10 and 12-11. A specific site can be considered very likely to be compressed if it is more than two standard deviations smaller than the reference values. As a general rule of thumb, horses with signs of cervical spinal cord disease that have SR values at any inter- or intravertebral site that are less than 50% of reference values have a greatly increased risk of having cervical vertebral canal stenosis.

In horses with type II CVM, spinal cord compression is most often the result of coning of affected caudal cervical vertebrae. The measurements can be difficult to perform on caudal cervical vertebrae, particularly if the radiographs in large horses are underexposed. In addition, these horses have enlarged and remodeled intervertebral joints of the caudal cervical vertebrae. Many horses without neurologic signs have degrees of cervical vertebral osteoarthritis and considerable arthritic enlargement of articular processes that can occur well lateral and dorsal to the vertebral canal with no spinal cord compression.[4] Cervical scintigraphic examinations similarly cannot determine if active arthritis is actually causing spinal cord compression. Spinal magnetic motor evoked responses[10-14] may be used more in the future to objectively grade the degree of electric conductivity across a spinal lesion site.

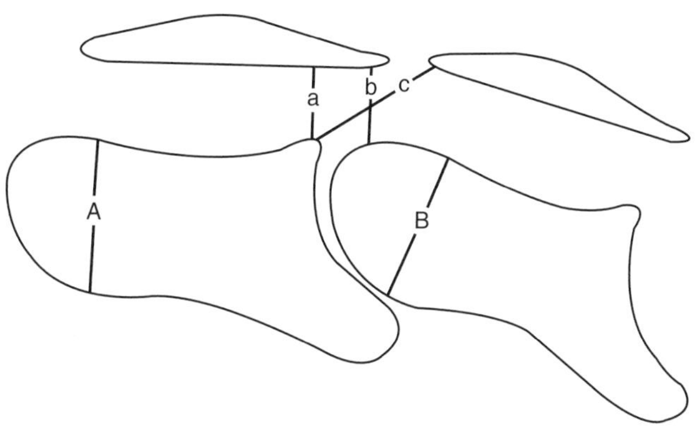

FIGURE 12-38 Two cervical vertebra showing sites for measuring the intra- and intervertebral sagittal diameter and the width of the vertebral body (**A**) (**B**). For a particular vertebra, the minimum intravertebral diameter could be anywhere along the vertebral canal (**a**), and the minimum intervertebral sagittal diameter is the smallest of the two measurements (**b**) or (**c**) compared with the diameter of the more caudal vertebral diameter (**B**).

Before deciding on surgical decompression or vertebral fusion, positive contrast myelographic evidence of spinal cord compression is mandatory. It should be remembered, however, that myelography under general anesthesia is not an innocuous procedure in the horse.[15,16] Myelography has traditionally been considered the gold standard antemortem diagnostic test; however, sagittal diameter ratio analysis may be more sensitive and specific than myelography, at least if the 50% or 2-mm reduction of the dorsal contrast medium myelographic rules are used.[17] Myelography can result in acceptable sensitivity and specificity for detecting sites of compression by using a 20% reduction of the total dural diameter reduction on a neutral myelographic view for the midcervical sites, and a 20% reduction of the same measurement at C6-7 with the neck in either neutral or flexed position.[18] In some horses with CVM, particularly those with caudal cervical arthropathy, spinal cord compression may occasionally occur in a lateral or transverse plane with no dorsoventral compression. In these cases, more subjective assessments, such as observing a blanching of the contrast column or split dorsal margins, may be the only myelographic abnormalities.

TREATMENT

Stall rest, glucocorticoids, DMSO, and other anti-inflammatory drugs may provide transient improvement in clinical signs in horses with CVM, especially if acute exacerbation of disease

TABLE 12-10

Summary Data for Sagittal Diameter Ratio by Vertebral Site in Eighteen Horses without Cervical Vertebral Malformation

	INTRAVERTEBRAL						INTERVERTEBRAL				
Site	**C2**	**C3**	**C4**	**C5**	**C6**	**C7**	**C2-3**	**C3-4**	**C4-5**	**C5-6**	**C6-7**
Mean	7.2	6.1	5.9	6.1	6.0	6.2	9.1	7.1	7.4	8.0	7.1
Standard Deviation	0.79	0.56	0.54	0.54	0.62	0.52	1.17	0.93	1.11	0.95	0.88

TABLE 12-11

Summary Data for Sagittal Diameter Ratio by Vertebral Site in Eight Horses with Cervical Vertebral Malformation

	INTRAVERTEBRAL						INTERVERTEBRAL				
Site	**C2**	**C3**	**C4**	**C5**	**C6**	**C7**	**C2-3**	**C3-4**	**C4-5**	**C5-6**	**C6-7**
Mean	6.3	4.8	4.8	4.9	4.8	4.8	7.0	5.5	5.7	5.8	5.9
Standard Deviation	1.19	0.33	0.37	0.26	0.44	0.17	1.93	1.28	0.59	1.14	0.68

secondary to trauma is seen. However, continued compression of the spinal cord is inevitable, and clinical signs will persist. In a controlled field study, in which growing foals with CVM were fed a diet restricted in protein and energy (65% to 75% of National Research Council recommendations), clinical signs and radiographic lesions resolved in some foals and significantly improved in others.[19] For most horses for which surgical treatment is not an option or with multiple intervertebral site involvement and severe, chronic clinical signs, the prognosis is poor to grave and humane destruction is advised.

Young patients with mild clinical signs of short duration and with only one site of cervical spinal cord compression have a good prognosis for return to athletic function with surgery. No controlled trials have been performed; however, it is estimated that more than 60% of such horses return to athletic function.[20-23] Ventral intervertebral fusion using a stainless steel fenestrated basket or threaded cylinder can allow expansion of the vertebral canal, atrophy of articular enlargements, and resolution of some or all the clinical signs in selected cases.[24] This procedure has been most successful in horses with acute clinical signs resulting from spinal cord compression at only one intervertebral site between C2 and C6 and in horses with absolute stenosis and enlarged articular processes of the caudal cervical vertebrae. Horses with persistent neck pain associated with cervical osteoarthritis but no evidence of fractures to the bodies of the vertebrae are also well suited to cervical intervertebral fusion surgery.

EQUINE DEGENERATIVE MYELOENCEPHALOPATHY

*Yvette S. Nout**

Equine degenerative myeloencephalopathy (EDM) is a noncompressive, diffuse, symmetrical, degenerative neurologic disease characterized by ataxia, weakness, and spasticity (hypometria) in young horses of many breeds and both genders. Mayhew first described the disease in 1976, and it has been subsequently diagnosed in many other breeds of horses.[1-3] In addition, identical syndromes have been observed in Mongolian wild horses *(Equus przewalskii)*[4] and Grant's zebras.[5] The pathogenesis of the disease is likely to be multifactorial. Currently it is thought that the combination of dietary vitamin E deficiency and genetic predisposition are the most important contributors to disease development.[5-8] A familial tendency to develop EDM has been suggested in the Arabian,[2] Thoroughbred,[8] and wild horses,[4] and it has been demonstrated in Morgans,[6] Appaloosas,[9] Strandardbreds, and Paso Finos.[8] Although a familial occurrence is suggestive of a genetic cause, this is so far unproven.

Neuroaxonal dystrophies (NADs) are a group of neurodegenerative diseases described in human beings and animals that are characterized by the formation of dystrophic axons. NAD can be considered a specific form of EDM and is clinically indistinguishable from EDM.[10] The disease has been described in Morgan horses.[6,11] Histologic lesions in NAD are confined to the cuneate and gracilis nuclei of the caudal myeloencephalon; in horses with EDM, lesions are found throughout the spinal cord and brainstem.

Equine degenerative myelopathy was one of the most prevalent causes of spinal cord disease in horses in the United States during an approximate 15-year span after it was first recognized. Although no recent epidemiologic surveys exist, the prevalence of EDM appears to have declined since about 1990.[12] In Europe the disease has been reported only sporadically, and just one recent report describes a cluster of five horses on one farm that were diagnosed with EDM.[13]

CLINICAL SIGNS

The age of onset of clinical signs varies between less than 1 month to several years, with most horses manifesting signs within the first year of life. However, in one study of 128 horses with EDM, age of onset ranged between 1 month to 20 years, with 16% of the horses showing signs at older than 28 months of age.[6]

Onset of signs may be abrupt but is usually insidious.[2] Signs are referable to upper motor neuron and general proprioceptive deficits and include symmetrical ataxia, weakness, and spasticity of all four limbs, often worse in the pelvic limbs.[2,12] Signs may begin in the pelvic limbs and progress to the thoracic limbs. Postural placing reactions may show conscious proprioceptive deficits. The gait is characterized by dysmetria and stabbing of the ground with the limbs. Horses may walk with a two-beat lateral gait, referred to as *pacing,* as also sometimes seen in horses with any spinal cord disease.[12] Often, hindlimb interference and dragging or scuffing of the toes are present. When walking backward, the horse may resist or rock back on the pelvic limbs and dog sit. When circling, affected horses often pivot on the inside hindlimb and circumduct the outside limb. Affected horses may have trouble stopping, and it is not unusual for them to fall while running in the pasture or being worked. Cranial nerve involvement, muscle atrophy, or changes in skin sensation or tail tone are absent in EDM.[2] Lower motor neuron signs such as hyporeflexia over the neck and trunk with diminished-to-absent cervical, cervicofacial, cutaneous trunci, and laryngeal adductor reflexes may be found, especially in severe and long-standing cases.[8,9]

Neuroaxonal dystrophy in Morgan horses has similar clinical signs; however, even in very severely affected horses, only pelvic limb deficits may be seen. Pelvic limb dysmetria, asynchrony, and ataxia are generally less severe than in EDM.[9]

PATHOLOGY

Gross necropsy findings in EDM are unremarkable.[2,3] Classic histologic changes are evident in the caudal brainstem nuclei (medulla oblongata) and especially the spinal cord and include diffuse neuronal fiber degeneration (dystrophy) of the white matter.[2,3] Generally, the lateral and medial cuneate nuclei, gracile nucleus, lateral cervical and thoracic nuclei, and lumbosacral and cervical intermediate gray columns are affected.[2,3] Astrocytosis, astrogliosis, vacuolization, myelin loss, spheroid formation (axonal swelling), and lipofuscin-like pigment accumulation are present in these areas.[2,3] With chronicity, the dorsal and ventral spinocerebellar tracts and the medial part of the ventral funiculi of the thoracic segments are more severely affected.[2,3] Neurochemical studies of the spinal

*The authors wish to acknowledge Hilary K. Matthews, whose original work has been incorporated into this section.

cord show a significant loss of myelin and component lipids.[3] Demyelination occurs to a greater extent than axon loss.[3]

Histologic changes in NAD of Morgan horses lack the diffuse nature of the changes seen in EDM. In NAD, histologic changes may be confined to the accessory cuneate nuclei.[6]

PATHOPHYSIOLOGY

The pathogenesis of EDM is unknown. However, it is most likely because of a complex interaction of many factors. Degenerative myelopathy in other species, which bears clinical and histopathologic similarities to EDM, has been linked to vitamin E and copper deficiencies, hereditary factors, and toxic insults.[14] Three risk factors associated with the development of EDM were identified in a study involving 56 affected and 179 control horses: (1) use of insecticides, (2) exposure to wood preservatives, and (3) spending frequent time on a dirt lot.[15] Spending time on green pastures was found to be a protective factor. Additionally, a foal was 25 times more likely to develop EDM if its dam had any other foals diagnosed with EDM.[15] These factors alone probably do not cause EDM but may interact with other factors to produce disease. In addition, these factors should be considered in preventing or minimizing the risk of developing EDM.

A hypothesis for the pathophysiology of EDM is exposure of genetically predisposed young foals to environmental oxidants and lack of antioxidants, including vitamin E. Oxidative stress is caused by the imbalance between production of prooxidants and the antioxidant defenses. ROS (e.g., superoxide anion, hydrogen peroxide, hydroxyl radical) are formed during the reduction of oxygen to water in normal cellular metabolism (Figure 12-39, *A*). Aerobic cells have antioxidant defense mechanisms that protect them from oxidative stress (Figure 12-39, *B*). The brain's high consumption of oxygen, high metabolic activity, and high concentration of polyunsaturated fatty acids, which can easily be oxidized to ROS, makes the CNS extremely vulnerable to oxidative attack by ROS.[14,16,17] Another source of ROS is through the metabolism of excitatory amino acids and neurotransmitters such as glutamate and aspartate. When present in excess, excitatory amino acids can trigger a series of events including an increase in intracellular calcium, which can lead to the production of free radicals and subsequent neuronal damage and death. Other sources of free radicals that arise from brain metabolism include cytochrome P-450 electron transport, monoamine oxidase activity, and endogenous guanidine compounds. Lipid peroxidation of cellular membranes and the direct oxidation of amino acids leading to inactivation of enzymes, receptors, and structural proteins are the main consequences of oxidative injury (Figure 12-40, A). Increased evidence exists for a role of redox signaling by oxygen radicals that targets mitochondrial cytochrome *c* release, DNA repair enzymes, and transcriptional factor nuclear factor-*k*B. Neuronal damage occurs once these physiologic systems are disrupted.[18]

The main endogenous antioxidants are superoxide dismutase, catalase, glutathione peroxidase (that contains selenium), α-tocopherol (vitamin E), and ascorbic acid (vitamin C) (see Figure 12-39, B; Figure 12-40, B).[16,17] Another protective mechanism is the existence of iron-binding proteins that keep iron in a less reactive form and prevent iron from catalyzing free radical reactions. Vitamin E reacts directly with OH^- and prevents oxidant injury to polyunsaturated fatty acids and thiol-rich proteins in cellular membranes (see Figure 12-40, B).

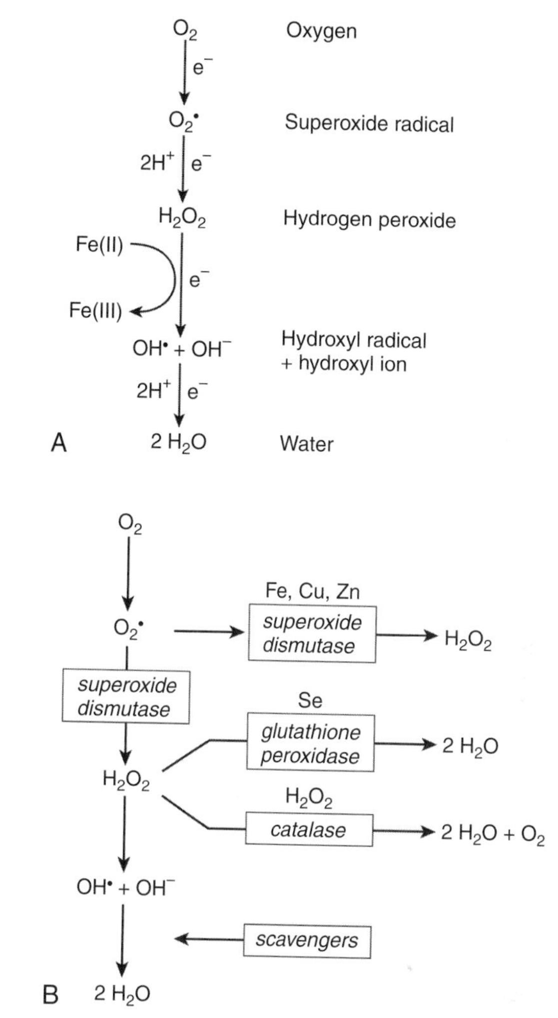

FIGURE 12-39 A, Physiologic metabolism of molecular oxygen to water. **B,** The mechanisms of action of four antioxidant systems. Superoxide dismutase may act as a pro-oxidant by increasing the formation of hydrogen peroxide and as an antioxidant by decreasing the superoxide radical concentration. Co-factors for superoxide dismutase are iron, zinc, and copper. The co-factor for glutathione peroxidase is selenium.

Vitamin E deficiency has received much attention as a possible cause of EDM. This association is based on the similarities between EDM and vitamin E deficiency in human beings and other animals, the reduced incidence of EDM seen after prophylactic treatment with vitamin E,[8] and the response to treatment with vitamin E in affected horses.[9] One study reported a high incidence of EDM on two breeding farms in which low serum vitamin E concentrations were found. Vitamin E supplementation decreased the incidence from 40% to less than 10%. However, affected and unaffected horses on both farms were found to be vitamin E deficient.[8] Another study found no significant differences in serum vitamin E and blood glutathione peroxidase concentrations between EDM affected horses and control horses.[19] A third study documented significantly lower vitamin E concentrations and clinical signs compatible with EDM in eight of nine foals sired by an EDM-affected stallion. Age-matched control foals raised in the same environment had normal serum vitamin E concentrations and no signs of EDM. Oral vitamin E absorption tests were performed

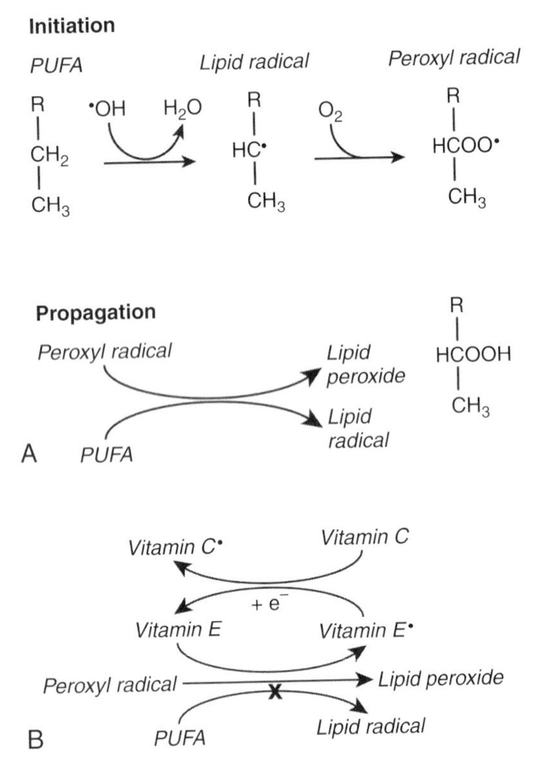

FIGURE 12-40 **A,** Mechanism of peroxidation of polyunsaturated fatty acids in cell membranes. **B,** Antioxidant mechanisms of α-tocopherol (vitamin E) and ascorbic acid (vitamin C). Polyunsaturated fatty acids are spared from oxidation because vitamin E is oxidized to a free radical instead. This prevents the propagation of lipid peroxidation in cell membranes and is referred to as *the chain-breaking action of vitamin E.* Vitamin C is a reducing agent that donates electrons to free radicals.

on both groups, and no significant differences were found between the groups.[20] Thus an inability to absorb vitamin E from the gastrointestinal tract does not appear to be a factor in the low serum vitamin E concentrations in EDM-affected horses.[20] Two other trials involving three[21] and nine[22] horses, respectively, support a role for vitamin E in the pathogenesis of EDM. Three foals developed neurologic disease and had low serum vitamin E concentrations after being housed on a dry lot. Two were examined post mortem at 6 months of age and had prominent neuroaxonal dystrophy. The third foal was put onto grass pasture and recovered.[21] Nine horses with a presumptive diagnosis of EDM improved after treatment with vitamin E at 6000 IU/day.[22] The role of vitamin E or glutathione peroxidase in the development of EDM remains unclear. The role of copper in the development of EDM is unclear. Although histologic changes and clinical signs consistent with degenerative myeloencephalopathy have been observed in copper-deficient animals, such as sheep, goats, calves, guinea pigs, pigs, and rats, no significant differences in plasma and liver copper concentrations between horses with confirmed EDM and age-matched control animals were found.[23]

Hereditary factors must also be considered in the pathogenesis of EDM and NAD in horses, as the diseases have been observed in familial clusters.[6,8,9] However, the mode of inheritance has so far not been identified in EDM- or NAD-affected horses. Toxic compounds such as organophosphates, diethyldithiocarbamate, and cycad palm have been reported to cause histologic changes and clinical signs similar to NAD in horses or other animals.[3] Their effect is due to the neurotoxic properties of the compounds. No direct association of toxic compounds with EDM or NAD in horses has been shown.

Recent research has shown that disruption of axonal transport plays a role in the pathogenesis of dystrophic axons in EDM.[24] Similar to what has been shown in canine NAD,[25] abnormal accumulation of synaptic proteins within dystrophic axons was demonstrated in horses with EDM in addition to altered presynaptic terminal attachment to swollen neurons. Furthermore, enhanced immunoreactivity to ubiquitin was demonstrated, implying activation of the ubiquitin system. Activation of this system would cause lysis of altered proteins within swollen neurons and finally result in dystrophic axons.

DIAGNOSIS

Definitive diagnosis of EDM can be made only with histopathologic examination of the spinal cord and brainstem. Antemortem diagnosis is based on clinical signs and ruling out other neurologic diseases (especially CVM and EPM). In EDM, CSF analysis and cervical spinal radiographs are usually within normal limits, although increased CSF creatine kinase (CK) levels have been found in horses affected with EDM.[3]

Measuring serum vitamin E concentrations may be unreliable when the animal is examined after the critical deficient period. Moreover, it should be noted that a single serum vitamin E sample may not adequately reflect the true vitamin E status of the horse, because up to 12% variation in concentrations can occur normally.[26] However, a low serum-plasma vitamin E concentration (<1.5 mg/ml) is supportive of the diagnosis.

TREATMENT AND PREVENTION

No specific treatment exists for EDM in horses. Affected horses may benefit from oral vitamin E supplementation coupled with monitoring of serum vitamin E concentrations. The earlier vitamin E treatment is instituted, the better the chance for a response. Horses with clinical signs of EDM may benefit from large doses of vitamin E (6000 to 10,000 IU/day) for an extended period of time.[27] Horses with very low serum vitamin E concentration may also benefit from 1000 (foals and yearlings) to 2000 (adults) IU of vitamin E in oil given intramuscularly every 10 days.[27] Dietary vitamin E levels should be maintained at 500 to 1000 IU/kg dry weight. Heat-treated pellets, stored oats, and sun-baked forages have marginal vitamin E concentrations (0 to 5 IU/kg dry weight).[8] Horses fed a diet of these should have frequent access to fresh green forage or vitamin E supplementation at 600 to 1800 mg or tocopheryl acetate 1.5 to 4.4 mg/kg/day to meet their reported needs.[28] To date, vitamin E toxicity associated with supplementation has not been reported. In addition, farms with a high incidence of EDM may benefit from prophylactic vitamin E supplementation.[8,13]

PROGNOSIS

EDM is generally progressive, necessitating euthanasia. Once clinical signs are evident, no improvement or remission occurs. However, signs may plateau.[8] Generally, horses with EDM do not progress to a state of recumbency.[3,8] Severely affected horses usually have an earlier age of onset and rapid disease progression, whereas mildly affected horses usually have a later age of onset, and the disease has a less rapid course.[29]

EQUINE PROTOZOAL MYELOENCEPHALITIS

*Martin Furr**

Equine protozoal myeloencephalitis is a commonly diagnosed condition of the horse, which J. Rooney originally described in 1964 and termed *segmental myelitis*. Later descriptions used the terminology *focal myelitis encephalitis*, recognizing that lesions within the brain occurred.[1] Eventually, an organism that resembled toxoplasma was seen in histologic sections, and the term *toxoplasma-like encephalitis* was coined.[2-4]

In 1976, Dubey first suggested that EPM was caused by a member of the genus *Sarcocystis*.[5] A *Sarcocystis* organism was eventually cultured from the spinal cord of an affected horse and named *Sarcocystis neurona* because it often develops within neurons.[6] Since that time, *S. neurona* or *S. neurona*-like organisms have been cultured from several ataxic horses, as well as numerous other animals including the zebra,[7] domestic cat,[8] Canadian lynx,[9] sea otter,[10,11] straw-necked ibis,[12] mink, raccoon, and skunk.[13-15]

Recently, another protozoan parasite *(Neospora hughesi)* has also been shown to be a cause of EPM in the horse; however, its role likely is limited.[16-21]

EPIDEMIOLOGY

EPM is one of the most commonly diagnosed neurologic diseases of the horse in the Western Hemisphere. It was reported that 25% of all equine neurologic disease submissions to the New York State Veterinary College were caused by EPM.[22] Similarly, EPM was diagnosed in 25% of all horses presented to the Ohio State University Veterinary Teaching Hospital with spinal ataxia in the early 1990s.[23] Given the complexity of clinical diagnosis, and the difficulty of finding conclusive lesions in the CNS, the true incidence is difficult to state conclusively. Based on a recent national study conducted by the United States Department of Agriculture (USDA), the average incidence of EPM was 14 + 6 cases per 10,000 horses per year. The lowest incidence was in farm and ranch horses (1 + 1 cases/10,000 horses), with 6 + 5 cases/10,000 horses for pleasure horses. A much higher incidence of 51 + 39 and 38 + 16 cases/10,000 horses was seen for competition and racing horses, respectively. An intermediate incidence of 17 + 12 cases was reported for breeding animals.[24] This is similar to the findings of other studies showing racing and showing animals to have a higher risk than breeding and pleasure horses.[25]

EPM is a disease of the Western Hemisphere, with cases reported from many states within the United States, as well as Canada, Mexico, Panama, Argentina, and Brazil. Most horses with a diagnosis of EPM outside this region appear to have spent some time in the endemic area. EPM has been reported in England among horses imported from the Eastern United States and in an 8-month-old Arabian horse in South Africa that had been imported from the United States approximately 5 months before the onset of signs.[26] The most recent report was a horse from California that developed clinical signs of EPM after 10 months in Hong Kong.[27] These cases demonstrate the probability of persistent, subclinical, latent infections.

However, a few reports exist of neurologic horses with consistent clinical signs, positive immunoblot test results, and no history of travel in the American continent.[28,29] The nature of the infection in these horses is unclear and may be because of cross-reacting antigens. Epidemiologic data of 364 horses with histologically confirmed EPM taken from across the United States and Canada revealed that Thoroughbreds, Standardbreds, and Quarter Horses were most commonly affected, although many other breeds were represented.[30] Standardbreds and Thoroughbred horses have also been reported to be over-represented in some studies[24,31,32]; however, this is not consistent and may reflect selection bias. Alternatively, this may reflect management, environment, or use of these breeds rather than an innate breed characteristic.[32] For example, neurologic disease would be difficult to discern in an animal not used for riding or strenuous athletic activity, unless the signs were severe.

All horses are susceptible to the development of EPM, but epidemiologic surveys have suggested that the average age of affected horses is 4.4 years in one study[31] and 3.6 years in another report.[32] More than 60% of cases were less than 4 years old. This bias toward younger animals being affected has been reported by other investigators[25,30,32]; however, one study also found an increased risk in horses older than 13 years of age.[33] It is unclear if the young age of most affected individuals reflects some specific physiologic effect or is rather a reflection of the animals use, because they are more likely to be involved in strenuous physical activity. The age range of reported cases is from 2 months[34] to 24 years[35]; no gender predilection exists. Most cases appear to be individual cases, and "outbreaks" of EPM appear to be very rare.[36] A report from Ohio, however, did find that previous diagnosis of the disease on the farm increased a horse's risk of subsequently developing EPM (>2.5 times higher).[25] This finding suggests clustering of cases may occur when all the risk factors for EPM are present. One author has described an epizootic of EPM on a single farm.[37]

After the development of the immunoblot test for *S. neurona*, numerous seroprevalence studies were performed, casting light on the distribution of the infection and life cycle of the organism.

Horses in the United States have a variable but generally high seropositive incidence to *S. neurona*, ranging between 10% among wild mustangs in Utah, 22% in the arid regions of Oregon, 45% in Pennsylvania, 53% in Ohio, and 60% in Michigan.[38-42] The Ohio study demonstrated increasing prevalence with increasing age, as well as differences from Southern to Northern Ohio. The authors concluded that this difference was the result of differences in the number of days of freezing temperature within the different regions, affecting parasite viability.[25] These results were confirmed by a different study in Colorado, showing increased incidence with increasing age and also associated with temperature (seroprevalence lowest in the colder months).[43]

Additional risk factors for EPM have been described. Risk increased if opossums were seen on the farm or if woods were

*The authors wish to acknowledge William J. Saville and David E. Granstrom, whose original work has been incorporated into this section.

present on the farm. The risk decreased if a creek or river was present on the farm and if the feed was kept protected from wildlife access.[25] Additional risk factors included an increased risk with increased numbers of horses, purchased versus home-grown grain, use of wood chips or shavings as bedding, presence of rats and mice on the premises, and increased human population density. A protective effect was apparent when woods were within 5 miles of the premises and where surface water was the primary drinking source. The National Animal Health Monitoring System (NAHMS) study also found the highest risk for disease was in the fall of the year.[24]

The seroprevalence for *Neospora hughesi*, in contrast to that for *Sarcocystis neurona*, is generally low and varies with the method of assay. Using an indirect immunofluorescence assay and a titer of 1:100 as the cutoff for a positive test, a seroprevalence of 37% in California, 20% in Montana, and 5% in New Zealand is noted.[44] In another study of horses in California, the *N. hughesi* seropositive rate was 1.7%/year of age.[45] A seroprevalence of 23.3% was found in an abattoir survey in the United States; the incidence was 0% in Argentina and Brazil.[46-48]

LIFE CYCLE

Sarcocystis spp. belongs to the phylum Apicomplexa, which includes several genera of coccidia that use an obligatory predator-prey or scavenger-carrion life cycle.[49,50] *Sarcocystis* spp. produce sporulated oocysts by sexual reproduction (gametogony) in the gut wall of the appropriate predator or definitive host. Infective sporocysts are introduced into the food and water supply of the prey animal or intermediate host by fecal contamination from the predator. In the *S. neurona* life cycle, the definitive host is the opossum, whereas the intermediate hosts are skunks, raccoons, and armadillos, among others. Once ingested by the intermediate host, sporocysts excyst, releasing four sporozoites that penetrate the gut and enter arterial endothelial cells in various organs. Meronts develop rapidly and eventually rupture the host cell, releasing merozoites into the bloodstream, which usually is followed by a second round of merogony in capillary endothelial cells throughout the body. Second-generation merozoites are released into the bloodstream and usually enter skeletal muscle cells, where they develop into specialized meronts known as *sarcocysts*. Mature sarcocysts contain bradyzoites, which are able to complete the life cycle only when ingested by the appropriate predator or scavenger.

S. neurona has been cultured from CNS lesions of several horses from different geographic locations within the United States and Central America.[6,51-55] Preliminary morphologic, immunologic, and DNA comparisons detected only minor differences among isolates[53,54]; however, more recent studies have demonstrated differences among isolates in the expression of surface receptors, which has substantial implications for immunodiagnosis.[56-58]

S. neurona may infect a large number of intermediate hosts aberrantly, unlike most *Sarcocystis* spp. Several species of animals and birds have been reported to exhibit signs similar to those in horses with EPM. This feature made the experimental elucidation of the *S. neurona* life cycle quite challenging. At the present time, domestic cats *(Felis domesticus)*, nine-banded armadillos (*Dasypus novemcinctus*), striped skunks *(Mephitis mephitis)*, raccoons *(Procyon lotor)*, and sea otters *(Enhydra lutris nereis)*[59-62] are considered to be viable intermediate hosts. Feeding studies, as well as epidemiologic and seroprevalence data, have determined this. Initially the domestic cat was thought to be only a laboratory intermediate host; however, several epidemiologic studies have now incriminated domestic cats as natural intermediate hosts.[63-65] The life cycle of *S. neurona* has been completed in a laboratory setting.[61] The horse has traditionally been considered an aberrant, dead-end host, in that sarcocysts have never been reported.[50] One report, however, describes mature sarcocysts that were well characterized as *S. neurona* and found in the tongue of a horse suffering from EPM.[66] This suggests that horses can be intermediate hosts but requires further confirmation.

Some evidence suggests that the organism may be transmitted by methods other than direct contact with opossum feces. It has been suggested that birds may mechanically disseminate sporocysts[67] and secondary transmission via "pass-through" of infective sporocysts in the feces of budgerigars, canaries, mice, and chickens fed opossum feces has occurred. At least some organisms appeared to retain viability and infectivity after transit through the digestive tract.[68] This is most likely to be a laboratory phenomenon; its importance in nature is unknown but likely to be small.

The life cycle of *Neospora hughesi* in horses is understood poorly. The definitive host of *N. caninum* has been demonstrated to be the dog,[69] but whether the dog is the definitive host of *N. hughesi* is not known. Tachyzoites, as well as tissue cysts, have been found in other horse tissues in two of the horses reported to have EPM caused by *Neospora* spp.[70] In one case of neosporosis, a foal was determined to have been infected congenitally, whereas congenital infections have not been demonstrated in horses infected with *Sarcocystis neurona* up to the present time.

PATHOGENESIS

Despite the often high rate of exposure to the organism, only a small percentage (perhaps <1%) of horses develop clinical illness.[24] This suggests that immune clearance of the parasite is very effective but that unknown factors must exist in certain cases to allow clinical disease to be expressed. Parasite dose is likely to be a factor, and in fact this has been experimentally demonstrated.[71] Strain-related variance in virulence may also be involved, although this has not been examined critically. Other factors that have been considered to have a role in the induction of EPM include physiologic stress associated with shipping, training, showing, and pregnancy that may make animals more susceptible to EPM.[25] Indeed, one reliable model of inducing EPM incorporates long-range shipping as a stressor, performed immediately before infection.[72] Other attempts to induce EPM using the oral infection route and that do not incorporate stressors such as shipping have lead to inconsistent and only mild illness.[73] The assumption is that these stressors lead to some degree of immune suppression, which is a commonly implicated factor in protozoan parasite infections. However, treatment of horses with immunosuppressive doses of steroids associated with oral infection with *S. neurona* did not result in significantly worse histopathologic changes in the CNS, although clinical signs were slightly more severe than in non–steroid-treated horses.[73] Additional evidence for the role of physiologic stress is found in the observation that stressed horses develop more severe clinical signs than naturally infected (nonstressed) horses.[74] It thus appears likely that stress has a role in the development of EPM; however, the interaction is complex and not fully understood at this time.

After infective sporocysts of *S. neurona* are passed from the definitive host and subsequently ingested by a horse, infection proceeds. Clinical disease results from the inflammation and neuronal necrosis associated with infection of the CNS with live organisms.

The mechanism (or mechanisms) by which *S. neurona* transits the blood-brain barrier and enters the CNS is unclear. One hypothesis is that *S. neurona* organisms that have been phagocytosed by leukocytes in the periphery are transported across the blood-brain barrier in the process of normal immune surveillance. Once within the CNS, the organisms proliferate. This "Trojan horse" hypothesis of CNS infection is attractive and has support from experimental work in which clinical disease can be induced by administering horses autologous lymphocytes, which have been infected with *S. neurona*.[75] When Arabian foals with severe combined immunodeficiency, lacking B and T lymphocytes, are infected with *S. neurona* they develop significant widespread parasite replication in visceral tissues, but parasites cannot be found within the CNS.[76] Alternatively, organisms enter the CNS by hematogenous dissemination, or directly through the cytoplasm of endothelial cells. Hematogenous dissemination is supported by the observation of a transient parasitemia in immunocompetent horses that have been experimentally challenged with *S. neurona*.[77]

There does not appear to be "targeting" of the CNS by the organism; rather the organism is not cleared from the CNS tissue while it is cleared elsewhere. Once organisms enter the CNS, it is likely that the immunosuppressive environment of the CNS plays a role by diminishing clearance of the organism in this immune-privileged tissue. The parasite itself may also induce some immunosuppresion.[78] Placental transmission with subsequent infection of the fetus is not believed to occur.

Resistance to *Sarcocystis neurona* is presumed to be the result of the combined effects of humoral and cellular immunity. After infection, a relatively rapid production of antibodies occurs. In horses challenged with live *S. neurona* organisms orally, all horses seroconverted within 32 days,[73] whereas in another study, horses challenged with a larger number of organisms seroconverted by day 13 after infection (if stressed by transport) and by day 30 if unstressed.[72]

It has been demonstrated with various apicomplexan parasites that antibody is at least partially protective. Research with *S. neurona* has demonstrated that antibodies to the Sn14 and 16 surface proteins block target cell penetration, while blocking the Sn30 surface protein had no effect.[79]

Although the effects of circulating antibody are likely to be very important, cell-mediated immunity is necessary for the elimination of intracellular forms of most organisms. Mouse studies have confirmed the importance of CD8+ T cells in protection against *S. neurona* encephalopathy in that species; it is presumed to be similar in horses. Endothelitis and meningoencephalitis developed in CD8 knockout mice after challenge with *S. neurona*, highlighting the importance of this cell subset in protection against *S. neurona*,[80] at least in the mouse. The CD8+ T cell is one important source of interferon gamma (IFN-γ), which is critical for protection against *S. neurona* induced neurologic disease in mice.[81] Infection of IFN-γ knockout mice leads to fulminant neurologic disease. These findings support the critical importance of IFN-γ in protection against *S. neurona*.

PATHOLOGY

Sarcocystis neurona probably causes few pathologic changes in immunocompetent intermediate hosts. However, CNS lesions in the horse are often extensive.[2-4,22] Multifocal areas of hemorrhage to light discoloration of the brain or spinal cord may be visible on gross examination. Lesions may be microscopic to several centimeters wide. The brainstem and spinal cord are affected most often; however, lesions have been seen in peripheral nerves. Microscopically, lesions are characterized by focal to diffuse areas of nonsuppurative inflammation and necrosis with perivascular infiltration of mononuclear cells, including lymphocytes, macrophages, and plasma cells. Giant cells, eosinophils, and gitter cells also are present in inflammatory infiltrates. Gray or white matter (or both) is affected. Organisms have been found in neurons, leukocytes, and vascular endothelium, although they tend to develop most often in neurons.

CLINICAL SIGNS

The clinical signs associated with *S. neurona* infection are variable and exclusively related to neurologic dysfunction. This variability reflects the random distribution of the lesions that may occur within the nervous system. Usually the physical examination is within normal limits, and the horse appears bright and alert, although one may observe focal muscle atrophy. A typical history is a slowly progressive ataxia, which may initially have been identified as a musculoskeletal disorder. Occasional acute and rapidly progressive disease is seen; empirically this presentation seems more commonly associated with brainstem disease, although this has not been formally evaluated. Neurogenic gait deficits seen with EPM are characteristically asymmetrical and may involve a single limb or multiple limbs. The presence of ataxia, asymmetry, and atrophy (the "three *A*'s of EPM") suggests multifocal or diffuse disease, which is characteristic of, although not pathognomonic for, EPM. Less commonly observed are diseases of the cerebrum, cerebellum, or brainstem resulting in a variety of cranial nerve deficits including dysphagia, head tilt, tongue or master paralysis, or masseter atrophy.

At least three horses have been observed with seizures as the only clinical signs of EPM.[82] Visual deficits and behavioral abnormalities have been reported in some horses with EPM.[83] A recent case series reported head shaking in three horses diagnosed with EPM that resolved after treatment for EPM.[84] The clinician needs to recognize that all of the clinical signs listed previously may be caused by conditions other than EPM, all of which should be considered in the differential diagnosis

DIAGNOSIS

An important point to remember is that EPM is an easy diagnosis to make but difficult to substantiate and confirm in a live patient. Experts recommend that at least three criteria be met before a diagnosis of EPM is rendered. First, the horse must have clinical signs arising from disease of the nervous system and that are consistent with EPM as described previously. Second one must confirm exposure to the causative agent by immunodiagnostic testing. Third, other conditions that could give rise to the clinical signs observed should be ruled out to the degree possible.

Ruling out other diseases may require radiographs of the cervical spine or head, nuclear scintigraphy, CSF evaluation, or testing for EHV, for example. These tests will be determined based on a careful physical and neurologic examination, as well as a consideration of the horse's history and progression, risk factors, and related information. The third component of the diagnostic triad is confirmation of exposure to the organism.

At the present time a number of tests are available to confirm exposure to the causative agents of EPM. An important consideration is that all currently available tests are intended to determine if antibodies to the causative agent are present, even though the test platforms may differ. Hence it is likely that the results obtained from such tests will be similar.

The first test developed to aid in the diagnosis of EPM was immunoblot analysis (Western blot) of serum and CSF to provide antemortem information regarding exposure to *Sarcocystis neurona*.[85] The test uses cultured merozoites to detect antibodies directed against proteins considered unique to *S. neurona*. Antibodies produced to proteins shared with *S. fayeri* or other organisms found in North America can be differentiated with this test.

Immunoblot testing of CSF samples has demonstrated greater than 90% specificity and sensitivity among approximately 100 horses with neurologic disease that received postmortem examination.[86] Approximately one half of the cases were histologically confirmed as EPM. Positive serum (specific antibody present) indicates exposure only; however, greater than 90% of histologically confirmed cases have tested seropositive. Given the widespread seroprevalence of this disease, however, this is not unexpected.

It was commonly believed for many years that the blood-brain barrier was impermeable to antibodies; hence it was thought that antibodies present in CSF confirmed that parasites had crossed the blood-brain barrier, entered the CNS parenchyma, and stimulated a local immune response. This has been shown not to be true. In fact, passive movement of antibodies into the CSF is readily demonstrated (the magnitude of the antibody in the CSF is directly related to serum concentrations of the same antibody).[87] When infection of the CNS occurs, the antibody titer is much higher because of local production of antigen-specific antibodies, however. Many of the false-positive CSF immunoblot tests probably arise from passive movement of antigen-specific antibody across the blood-brain barrier. In these cases, however, the immunoblot test is usually quite weakly reacting. Alternatively, blood contamination of the CSF sample at collection can lead to false-positive tests. Bleeding within the CNS, after trauma or infection, for example, will also lead to a false positive. In an effort to differentiate false-positive CSF antibody tests, a number of techniques have been described. The AQ is a measure of blood-brain barrier permeability and has been evaluated in horses as an aid in interpretation of the CSF immunoblot result. The normal AQ is 1.5 ± 0.4 in CSF of adult horses from the lumbosacral space and 1.86 ± 0.28 in CSF collected from the atlantooccipital space of neonatal foals.[88,89] Values greater than this suggest damage to the blood-brain barrier. Clinical experience and empiric evaluation of the value of the AQ has demonstrated a very low sensitivity for this test, however, and its use is no longer recommended as an aid in the diagnosis of EPM.[90] Determination of the IgG index was proposed as a method to differentiate intrathecal production versus passively acquired CSF antibodies. The range for IgG index in the CSF collected from the atlantooccipital space of normal horses is <0.27; values greater than this suggest intrathecal antibody production, consistent with CNS infection.[88] In one study the IgG index was found to be increased at the beginning of treatment and to drop slightly after treatment for EPM.[91] Unfortunately, the sensitivity of this test appears to be too low, and the use of the IgG index is no longer recommended as a diagnostic aid for EPM.[90]

False-negative results have been rare but may occur. The possible causes of false-negative responses are important to consider so that one does not misdiagnose affected horses. Some horses simply may fail to respond to the *Sarcocystis neurona*–specific proteins identified by the immunoblot. Horses that initially tested positive have become negative after several weeks of treatment and apparently have recovered. A chronically affected horse may test negative and still be infected, or the horse still may exhibit neurologic signs. Persistent neurologic damage (i.e., scarring) may be present in some cases, resulting in permanent neurologic damage in the absence of active infection. One should retest acute cases that initially test negative in 2 to 3 weeks. However, the incubation period appears to be sufficiently long to allow production of detectable amounts of IgG before the onset of clinical signs in most cases.

The original, conventional Western blot test has been modified at one testing laboratory (Michigan State) by blocking the 30-kD band with pooled serum with a high anti-*Sarcocystis cruzi* antibody titer.[91] This is considered by them to be a cross-reacting antigen. This modified Western blot was reported to have a sensitivity and specificity approaching 100%.[91] However, this study was performed on only a small number of EPM positive horses (6), and subsequent evaluation of the test by other investigators has found a much lower sensitivity and specificity of 89% and 69%, respectively.[92] A further modification of the Western blot has been proposed by another testing laboratory (Neogen Inc), in which the intensity of the staining reaction of the 17-kD band is reported as a unitless number referred to as the *relative quotient* (RQ). This number ranges between 0 to 100, with a higher value implying a more robust antibody response. The use of the RQ has not been found to improve diagnostic efficiency, although in one study the RQ did decrease slightly during treatment.[91]

A whole organism indirect fluorescent antibody test (IFAT), has been developed and is currently available from the University of California Diagnostic Laboratory.[93] Diagnostic performance of the IFAT was tested and compared with the Western blot tests and was reported to have a (slightly) better diagnostic efficiency than either test.[92] Serum titers of greater than 1:100 and CSF titers of greater than 1:5 were considered positive and diagnostic of active infection. This test is considered to be robust in the presence of blood contamination of the CSF sample. However, previous attempts using an indirect fluorescent test were disappointing, and the IFA was unable to distinguish between related *Sarcocystis* organisms.[94] This finding was further supported using the California IFAT, when it was demonstrated that the test was unable to differentiate between *S. neurona* and *S. fayeri* (a nonpathogenic *Sarcocystis*) infections.[95] Therefore the superiority of the IFAT as a diagnostic for EPM is not clearly established and awaits further evaluation.

Another diagnostic test described for EPM is an enzyme-linked immunosorbent assay (ELISA) for antibodies to the snSAG-1 protein. This test (currently commercially available from Antech Inc) provides a titer, and values greater than 1:100 in serum are considered to indicate active infection.[96] Use of this test is not without concern, however. The test has not been rigorously evaluated for sensitivity and specificity, and the cutoff values for a positive diagnosis appear to be arbitrary. Further, it has been clearly demonstrated that not all *S. neurona* isolates produce the SAG-1 protein[58]; hence false-negative results are possible with this test.

A stall-side ELISA test that uses the snSAG-1 protein is also available (Endocrine Technologies, Newark, CA); however, it has not been evaluated for accuracy. It does not appear at this time that any of these tests are clearly superior; the final diagnosis should not hinge on the results of the immunodiagnostic test alone.

Immunodiagnostic testing for *Neospora hughesi* (IFAT) is also available from the University of California. The accuracy of this test has not been rigorously evaluated in a large number of clinical patients, but in a small challenge study (14 total animals) demonstrated perfect assignment of infected and control horses when a serum IFAT cutoff of >1:640 was used.[97]

As previously noted, most horses with EPM do not show constitutional signs of illness, such as fever, depression, or anorexia. Changes in the CBC are not recognized, and changes in serum biochemistry analysis are not noted, unless the severity of the neurologic signs is such that the horse falls or is recumbent, or it is dysphagic and cannot drink or eat. In these horses, secondary changes in the serum biochemistry panel may be seen.

Collection and analysis of CSF is a common component of the neurologic evaluation and should not be ignored in evaluating the EPM suspect. The observation that CSF false-positive tests can occur has led some to question the value of analyzing CSF in horses being evaluated for EPM. An important point to remember is that the CSF is not collected for the sole purpose of doing an EPM test; additional information is obtained from the sample. Although it is true that some false-positive tests occur using CSF, this should not preclude the use of this diagnostic test. Horses exposed to *Sarcocystis neurona* will not necessarily and invariably develop a false-positive test on CSF. This appears to be associated with a high serum titer and is often transient. A negative CSF test has great value in eliminating EPM in most cases. A weak or suspect positive reaction in CSF is not compelling evidence for a diagnosis of EPM, whereas a stronger test reaction on immunoblot (or a titer exceeding the reference laboratory's high cutoff) is strong support for the diagnosis.

A key part of the diagnosis of EPM is ruling out other conditions that may be present; evaluation of CSF is necessary for this process. The author has identified conditions such as intrathecal hemorrhage, neoplasia, meningitis, and verminous encephalitis when evaluating EPM suspects (and would have been missed had the CSF analysis not been done). Hence the author considers CSF analysis a key part of the full diagnostic evaluation of horses with CNS disease.

Most horses with EPM have normal CSF. Early work identified the occasional increase in RBC count; however, in more recent times this finding has been considered to be spurious and a result of unrecognized blood contamination from the collection. The severe and fulminant case may have a mildly increased total protein or white blood cell count, but these situations are rare.

DIFFERENTIAL DIAGNOSIS

Given the variety of clinical abnormalities that may be expressed in horses with EPM, the differential diagnosis includes virtually all diseases of the equine CNS. However, the results of a careful history, physical examination, and neuroanatomic localization help to limit the number of rule outs and guide further diagnostic efforts. The most common and likely rule out is probably cervical compression. In contrast to EPM, cervical compression usually results in symmetrical gait deficits, which are worse in the pelvic limbs and are characterized by spasticity and hypermetria, with good retention of strength and no muscle wasting.

Infectious diseases such as WNV encephalitis, equine encephalitis (eastern equine encephalitis [EEE] and western equine encephalitis [WEE]), and equine herpesvirus-1 (EHV-1) may all cause neurologic disease that could resemble EPM. Horses affected with these conditions are typically systemically ill, demonstrating fevers and alterations in the leukogram. The neurologic deficits of EHV-1 are fairly characteristic in that dysuria is a common component that is not often seen in horses with EPM. CSF is abnormal in most such cases (e.g., WNV, EEE, EHV-1), in contrast to EPM, and a variety of specific diagnostic tests exist for each of these conditions, such as IgM capture ELISA for WNV and PCR testing for EHV-1.

Polyneuritis equi and equine degenerative encephalomyelitis may also be confused with EPM and can have signs of multifocal disease, ataxia, and muscle atrophy. Less common conditions, such as verminous encephalitis, bacterial meningitis or CNS abscessation, can be seen, but alterations in the leukogram and the CSF are usually present, distinguishing these cases from EPM.

TREATMENT

The cornerstone of treatment for horses with EPM is antiprotozoal medication. At the present time the Food and Drug Administration (FDA) has approved a number of compounds for the treatment of EPM. The first compounds used for the treatment of EPM were the sulfonamide drugs combined with pyrimethamine to achieve a synergistic effect. Clinical efficacy studies have been performed using sulfadiazine (20 mg/kg) and pyrimethamine (1 mg/kg) orally once per day, marketed as Re-Balance. Using this dose in well-characterized cases of EPM, the overall success rate (e.g., improvement by one clinical grade) was 61.5%. The duration of treatment varied between 90 to 270 days.[98] Complications of this drug regimen have been reported as anemia (22%), leukopenia (19%), and neutropenia (5%).[98] These signs are usually self-limiting and resolve with cessation of treatment. Folic acid supplementation has been advised by some authors to limit the degree of anemia; however, no support for this practice exists, and research has demonstrated increased toxicity when folic acid supplementation is provided. Hence its use is discouraged. Use of sulfadiazine in breeding animals is controversial, although one study has shown no effect on pregnancy rates or early embryonic death. Mild signs of ataxia associated with mounting and ejaculation were noted in a group of pony stallions treated with sulfamethoxazole and pyrimethamine.[99] At the time of this writing, Re-Balance was no longer commercially available.

The first FDA-approved drug for the treatment of EPM was ponazuril (Marquis, Bayer Animal Health). Ponazuril is well absorbed orally, and within 3 days achieves a therapeutic, steady-state concentration in the CSF of horses treated with 5 mg/kg body weight.[100]

A field efficacy study of 101 horses with well-characterized EPM and treated with ponazuril demonstrated successful treatment in 60% of treated animals, success defined as improvement by at least one neurologic grade. A 90-day relapse rate of 8% after the termination of treatment was found.[91] Animals typically responded within 10 days and often continued to improve even after treatment stopped at 28 days.

Safety studies have found ponazuril to be very safe, with no systemic toxicity, even at high doses (30 mg/kg body weight) for up to 56 days.[101] Treatment of breeding stallions with 10 mg/kg body weight ponazuril did not affect androgenic hormone production nor spermatogenesis.[102] Ponazuril has been used without obvious problems in pregnant mares, but the use of ponazuril in pregnant animals is off label, and owners should be made aware of this fact. Feeding 2 oz of corn oil immediately before the ponazuril is given results in blood concentrations that are 25% higher than if no corn oil is given.[103]

Diclazuril is chemically similar to ponazuril and has been investigated for the treatment of horses with EPM. In one study, treatment of EPM-affected horses with diclazuril resulted in improvement in 58% of the treated animals, when given for 28 days. Diclazuril is administered orally, once per day, at the rate of 5 mg/kg for 28 days.[98] At the time of this writing, diclazuril has been approved by the FDA to be administered as a top-dress pellet; however, the drug has not become commercially available. Diclazuril, like ponazuril, appears to be very safe. No adverse events attributable to the drug were reported during the efficacy study, but a specific target animal safety study has not been reported.

NTZ (Navigator, Idexx Pharmaceuticals) is a member of the 5-nitrothiazol class of antimicrobials and is currently approved for the treatment of EPM. NTZ also demonstrated a success rate of about 60% in horses in a well-controlled clinical field trial, which was scrutinized by the FDA and that was comparable in design to the ponazuril study.[98] A second study (open, uncontrolled field trial) reported a success rate of 81%. The standards for diagnosis, case inclusion, and definition of case success were very different from the FDA-regulated studies, however. The results of this study cannot logically be compared with the results of the FDA-controlled studies.

In safety testing, horses became very ill at two times the dose (and some deaths occurred at three times the dose after only a few doses).[98] Modification of the dosing schedule has reduced the apparent adverse effects; however, some diarrhea, depression, and laminitis has been seen. Results of the two reported efficacy studies for NTZ also demonstrate that only 51% to 59% of enrolled horses completed the study.[98] Although not confirmatory, this poor completion rate and study compliance raises the question of unreported toxicity. This is particularly noticeable in comparison with a completion rate of 68% for diclazuril and 90% for the ponazuril studies. To minimize toxicity, horses are given one half the dose each day for 1 week, then the dose is increased for the final 21 days of treatment. NTZ must be carefully dosed to minimize toxicity, which may occur even at the standard dosage. If toxic signs are observed, then withdrawal of the compound usually results in resolution of toxicity-related clinical signs. As of the writing of this chapter, NTZ is no longer available commercially in the United States.

Regardless of the drug used, the duration of treatment necessary and when to stop treatment is a consideration in all EPM cases. Definitive treatment durations are hard to define. Even successfully treated cases will remain immunoblot positive for long periods, so attempting to treat until the horse is seronegative is not a logical goal. The triazine-based drugs (Ponazuril [PNZ], Diclazuril [DCZ]) and NTZ are licensed to be given for only 28 days. Longer duration of treatment of clinical cases is often necessary; the need for this being determined by repeat examination after the first month of treatment. No response at all suggests misdiagnosis, and the case should be re-evaluated and further tested. If there has been a clinical response, yet the horse remains abnormal, then a second month of treatment is recommended. If finances are limited, then treatment can stop after 28 days, but the horse should be re-examined in 1 month to ensure that no deterioration occurs.

Relapses are a concern, and relapse rates of up to 25% have been suggested by one author when horses are treated with sulfadiazine and pyrimethamine; this was an empiric estimate, however.[104] The occurrence of a relapse is probably dependent on a number of factors, including the exact drug and dose used and the duration of treatment. Extended dosing may reduce the occurrence of relapse.[98] The relapse rate for horses treated for 28 days with ponazuril was 8%, when examined 90 days after cessation of therapy.[91] Relapse rates for the other drugs are not reported.

Relapse implies that the horse responded well to the initial drug treatment; hence horses that relapse can be treated with the same drug that was initially used but for a longer period. The author typically recommends 2 months of ponazuril, followed by a minimum 90-day course of sulfadiazine-pyrimethamine. Failure with a longer course of ponazuril usually prompts a change to a different medication from within a different chemical class. Other authors have recommended an immediate switch in drug class or indefinite intermittent therapy with sulfadiazine-pyrimethamine, 2 days per week at the standard dose.[98] The value of these strategies is currently unproven and purely anecdotal.

No studies have been conducted to determine the effectiveness of the currently approved antiprotozoal medications against *N. hughesi*. In vitro reports suggest effectiveness of NTZ against *N. caninum*,[105] yet treatment of one horse with culture positive *N. hughesi*–induced EPM did not result in improvement.[106] Ponazuril has also demonstrated in vitro effectiveness against *N. caninum*.[107,108] Ponazuril (5 mg/kg body weight, once per day for 28 days) was used in three horses with *N. hughesi* EPM. All three horses showed clinical improvement, and one showed complete resolution.[109]

In addition to specific antiprotozoal medication, ancillary treatment modalities are sometimes useful. In horses that are severely affected, the use of NSAIDs is recommended at standard dosages. Some practitioners routinely give NSAIDs during the first 1 to 2 weeks of treatment because of a concern that clinical signs might worsen as the parasite is killed and inflammation worsens transiently. This "treatment crisis" is occasionally observed but is only rarely of clinical significance; however, a modest course of NSAIDs is unlikely to be harmful. Intravenous DMSO (0.5-1.0 g/kg IV as a 10% solution) is widely recommended. Although specific studies showing effectiveness of this drug in horses is lacking, a substantial body of evidence in laboratory animals indicates that it lowers CSF pressure; clinical experience also indicates improvement in neurologic status after treatment. This treatment is usually reserved for more severely affected horses and is not necessary in the majority of cases.

The use of anti-inflammatory corticosteroids in horses with EPM is debated, with no universal agreement. Concern about immunosuppression and the observation that stress may be a risk factor for development of EPM has led some to conclude that steroids should be scrupulously avoided because they may make the condition worse. There seems little support for this position, however. In experimental models, large doses of steroids have not appeared to substantially increase the severity of the illness and, in fact, in some cases appear to lessen it. A critical aspect of the illness is the degree of neuroinflammation that occurs. Hence in severely affected horses that are in danger of becoming recumbent, a short course (2-5 days) of dexamethasone (0.05 mg/kg q12h) may be useful in stabilizing the patient until the antiprotozoal medications can take effect. Long-term use of corticosteroids should probably be avoided.

Immunomodulators have been recommended in an effort to "boost" the immune response in EPM-affected horses. No empiric research has been done in this area, and the clinical impression is that most nonspecific "immune enhancers" have no obvious effect. Levamisole (1 mg/kg PO q24h) has been recommended because it influences T cell–mediated immunity and enhances phagocytosis. More recently a parapox ovis virus (PPOV) immunomodulator (Zylexis, Pfizer Animal Health, Kalamazoo, Mich) has become available. This product is intended for use in the aid of treatment of horses with EHV-1 and EHV-4. PPOV has been demonstrated in a number of species (although not horses) to upregulate the secretion of numerous cytokines,[110] specifically IFN-γ, which is believed to be critical for clearance of *S. neurona*. For this reason, inclusion of PPOV vaccine in the treatment protocol for horses with EPM is logical, although unproven. It is possible, although unlikely, that immunomodulators or immunostimulants may enhance the immunopathologic effects associated with CNS infection.

Some clinicians recommend the use of additional supplements such as vitamin E and thiamine that may facilitate healing of nervous tissue when treating horses with EPM. Clinical trials have not been performed to establish the efficacy of this supplementation and it is unlikely to have significant effect, yet it is unlikely to be harmful.

In very ataxic animals, it is important to provide a stall with deep bedding and good footing. The best footing is a grassy field, and if the area is level with no obstacles, then turnout in such an area may be advisable. Turnout with other horses should be done carefully, because the ataxic horse cannot protect itself and may slip and fall when trying to get away from aggressive herd mates. Recumbent animals, or animals in slings, require additional care.

The prognosis for horses diagnosed with EPM appears to be similar regardless of the treatment used, because most reports suggest an approximate improvement rate of 60% to 75% with the standard therapy.[98]

PREVENTION

The widespread distribution of the parasite and the variety of intermediate hosts make control of EPM complicated. A vaccine was available; however, it has been removed from the market because of failure to demonstrate efficacy.

Monitoring high-risk age groups such as young and old horses closely for evidence of neurologic disease may help detect EPM early. That EPM may be the cause of the clinical signs when horses are presented for treatment of neurologic disease in the warmer months should raise the index of suspicion. Because many major horse competitions take place in the fall of the year, monitoring of horses before transport and competition may be helpful. Wildlife such as opossums and pests should be denied access to feed by using rodent-proof containers to help limit the contamination of feed with the infectious organism. One also should protect forages from wildlife access by storage in enclosed facilities. Close monitoring of broodmares close to foaling and horses that develop a major illness or injury is important, because it may help early diagnosis of EPM cases.

Prophylactic treatment with ponazuril has reduced the incidence and severity of clinical signs in one study.[111] Although unlikely to be financially viable in most situations, this suggests that treatment of horses with ponazuril before and during persistently stressful events such as long-distance shipping or a heavy travel and showing period, may reduce the risk of clinical illness. Alternatively, interval treatment with ponazuril (20 mg/kg PO every 7 days) significantly reduced *S. neurona* antibody in the CSF of challenged horses. This may also be a reasonable option for some specific circumstances.[107] Products have been marketed that are top-dressed on feed in an effort to kill the infective stage of the organism before ingestion. No empiric evaluation of these products exists, and they are highly unlikely to have any effect.

EQUINE HERPESVIRUS-1 MYELOENCEPHALOPATHY

W. David Wilson, Nicola Pusterla

EHV-1 is an economically important pathogen of horses and exerts its major effect by inducing abortion storms or sporadic abortions in pregnant mares, early neonatal death in foals, and respiratory disease in young horses.[1-8] Myeloencephalopathy is an uncommon manifestation of EHV-1 infection but can cause devastating losses during outbreaks on individual farms, racetracks, veterinary hospitals, or boarding stables.[9-11] Although EHV-4 rarely causes clinical manifestations of disease in organs other than the respiratory tract, isolated cases of myeloencephalopathy and sporadic abortions have been reported in EHV-4 infections.[1-3,12,13] Clinical signs of neurologic disease reflect a diffuse multifocal myeloencephalopathy after vasculitis, hemorrhage, thrombosis, and ischemic neuronal injury. Sudden onset and early stabilization of signs including ataxia, paresis, and urinary incontinence; involvement of multiple horses on the premises; and a recent history of fever, abortion, or viral respiratory disease in the affected horse or herd mates are typical features, although considerable variation exists between outbreaks concerning epidemiologic and clinical findings.[14] Prevention is difficult because many horses are latently infected with EHV-1, allowing the virus to circulate silently in horse populations, and current vaccines do not confer protection against neurologic manifestations of infection.[8,15] The distribution of lesions that can result after infection with neurotropic EHV-1 results in the need to include many conditions on the differential diagnosis list, including EPM, cervical vertebral instability, cervical stenotic myelopathy, vertebral or CNS trauma, polyneuritis equi, fibrocartilaginous emboli, aberrant parasite migration, degenerative myelopathy, togaviral encephalitis, rabies, botulism, toxins, and other disorders.

VIROLOGIC FINDINGS

Of the five distinct herpesviruses that are known to infect horses, three are typical α-herpesviruses with a double-stranded DNA genome and are designated EHV-1 (equine abortion virus, formerly known as *EHV-1, subtype 1*), EHV-4 (equine rhinopneumonitis virus, formerly known as *EHV-1, subtype 2*), and EHV-3 (equine coital exanthema virus), and two are γ-herpesviruses, designated *EHV-2* (formerly called *equine cytomegalovirus*) and *EHV-5* (which has recently been associated with interstitial pulmonary disease).[2,3,16-18] In addition, three asinine α-herpesviruses (AHV1, AHV2, and AHV3) have been isolated from donkeys. Of these, AHV3 has been shown by many criteria to be related closely to EHV-1. Indeed, EHV-1 and AHV3 are related more closely to each other than either is to EHV-4.[2,18-20] Phylogenetic analysis and epidemiologic evidence suggest that EHV-1 recently has been derived from AHV3 and that donkeys may remain an alternate host for EHV-1, serving as a reservoir to infect horses.[16,18]

EHV-1 and EHV-4 are distinguishable from EHV-2, EHV-3, and EHV-5 by biologic properties and virus neutralization tests (and distinguishable from each other by restriction endonuclease fingerprinting of DNA, DNA sequences, and several immunologic tests based on monoclonal antibodies to each virus).[1-3,16,17,21] EHV-1 and EHV-4 produce eosinophilic intranuclear inclusion bodies in infected cells in vivo and in vitro. Several strains have been identified within EHV-4 and EHV-1, although the epidemiologic, immunologic, and pathogenic significance of this finding is not known. The 1-p and 1-b subtypes of EHV-1 likely are capable of inducing neurologic disease. Apart from differences in endotheliotropism, genetic and antigenic fingerprinting and experiments in baby mice have not yielded clear markers distinguishing EHV-1 strains that induce neurologic disease or abortion (or both).[16,22-26] However, a recent analysis of EHV-1 isolates from neurologic and non-neurologic disease outbreaks revealed a point mutation within the DNA polymerase gene that was strongly associated with neuropathogenic disease.[27,28] Recently, a hamster model has been described showing some potential for discrimination between abortigenic and neuropathogenic EHV-1 strains.[29]

EPIDEMIOLOGY AND IMMUNITY

EHV-1 and EHV-4 are enzootic in most horse populations, and the majority of horses show serologic evidence of exposure to these viruses. Most horses become infected via the respiratory tract with EHV-1 or EHV-4 (or both) during the first year of life. After an incubation period of 2 to 10 days, clinical signs of respiratory disease of variable severity develop and resolve within 1 to 2 weeks in uncomplicated cases.[1-3] Resolution of clinical signs is coincident with development of virus-specific neutralizing antibody directed primarily against surface viral glycoproteins. The development of cell-mediated responses is probably critical for recovery.[30] Resistance to reinfection with homologous virus is demonstrable after recovery but generally persists for only 3 to 4 months. Subsequent infections typically induce milder clinical signs or subclinical infection, although virus shedding from the nasopharynx occurs.[1,2] The immune response frequently is not successful in clearing herpesviral infection, and the majority of clinically recovered horses remain latently (asymptomatically) infected with EHV-1 or EHV-4 (or both) for life.[1,2,31,32] Recently, EHV-1 has been shown to evade the host immune system in part by downregulating major histocompatibility complex class I expression at the cell surface. This process may be a prerequisite to the establishment of latency.[33]

Recrudescence of latent infection is important in the epidemiology of EHV-1 and EHV-4 and explains why these diseases can occur in closed populations without the introduction of new horses.[1,2,32,34] Signs of EHV-1 infection may occur in the horse in which stress-associated recrudescence of infection has occurred, or the horse may remain asymptomatic but shed infectious virus in nasal secretions to infect other horses. Natural infection with EHV-1 occurs by inhalation or ingestion of aerosolized infective virus or by direct contact with virus shed in the products of abortion or in the nasal and ocular discharges and saliva of horses with overt clinical disease, subclinically infected horses, or shedding carrier horses.[1,2,21] Infectious EHV-1 virus was detected in the feces of experimentally infected foals that developed diarrhea, suggesting that fecal spread is a possibility.[35] Virus may be shed by clinically affected and inapparently infected horses for 3 weeks or more, and EHV-1 may remain infective in the environment for up to 14 days and on horse hair for 35 to 42 days.[2,36,37]

The first definitive association between EHV-1 and myeloencephalopathy was made in 1966 in Norway with the isolation of the virus from the brain and spinal cord of a horse that showed signs of severe neurologic dysfunction.[38] The myeloencephalopathic form of EHV-1 infection now is considered to have a worldwide distribution, having been recognized in Denmark, The Netherlands, Germany, Sweden, Austria, Britain, Ireland, Australia, India, the United States, and Canada.[9,10,14,25,39,61] In view of the ubiquitous occurrence of EHV-1 infection in horse populations, outbreaks of EHV-1 myeloencephalopathy are rare. In many instances, cases of neurologic EHV-1 infection occur in association with outbreaks of abortion or respiratory disease, although some outbreaks occur in the absence of other manifestations of EHV-1 infection and without the introduction of new horses into the group.[21,34,62,63]

The myeloencephalopathic form of EHV-1 infection may occur as sporadic individual cases or, more often, as outbreaks involving multiple individuals over a period of several weeks on one or more premises within a limited geographic region.* Secondary or tertiary waves of clinical disease may occur as previously unexposed horses become infected from a common source over a short period.[10,21,44,60] Recently there has been an increased reporting of occurrences of EHV-1 myeloencephalopathy[65] in congregations of horses around the United States. Most of these outbreaks have been associated with a mutant strain of herpesvirus, which appears to replicate rapidly, leading to a very high level of viremia and an apparent increased incidence of neurologic manifestations of this disease.[27,28,66] Morbidity rates ranging between less than 1% to almost 90% of exposed individuals and mortality rates ranging between

*References 9, 10, 25, 38, 45, 49, 52, 54, 61, 64.

0.5% to 40% of in-contact horses have been reported.† Neurologic EHV-1 infection can occur at any time of year, but the highest incidence is in the late winter, spring, and early summer, perhaps reflecting the seasonal occurrence of abortigenic EHV-1 infections during the same months.[52]

The neurologic form of EHV-1 infection has been observed in pregnant mares, barren mares, geldings, stallions, and foals, although foals frequently do not show neurologic manifestations of infection during outbreaks that involve severe neurologic disease in adult horses.[9,44] The disease also appears to less commonly affect pony breeds. Pregnant mares and mares nursing foals appear be at increased risk for developing neurologic manifestations of EHV-1 infection, and the stage of gestation may be important in determining the outcome of infection in pregnant mares.[9,43,44,50,51] Mares infected during the first 2 trimesters of gestation appear to be more likely to develop neurologic signs without abortion, whereas mares infected during the last trimester are more likely to abort without showing neurologic signs.[21,41,43,51,58]

All breeds of horses are susceptible to the neurologic form of EHV-1 infection, and other Equidae also may be affected. EHV-1 was the suspected cause of myeloencephalopathy that developed in a zebra 1 week after an in-contact onager *(Equus hemionus onager)* aborted an EHV-1 infected fetus.[68] The authors are unaware of reports of neurologic EHV-1 affecting donkeys and mules, although donkeys and mules have shown seroconversion indicating infection with EHV-1 while in contact with affected horses during outbreaks.[56,57,64] Indeed, donkeys and mules returning from a show were thought to be responsible for dissemination of EHV-1 and propagation of multiple outbreaks of neurologic EHV-1 infection in Southern California in 1984 (and in several subsequent years), suggesting that a donkey-adapted variant of EHV-1 with an increased neuropathogenicity for horses may have been involved.[64]

A modified live EHV-1 vaccine of monkey cell line origin was associated with neurologic disease in 486 of 60,000 recipients, prompting its withdrawal from the U.S. market in 1977.[33] No reports of EHV-1 myeloencephalopathy have been associated with use of the modified live vaccine currently approved for use in horses in the United States.

PATHOGENICITY AND PATHOGENESIS

Natural infection with EHV-1 occurs by inhalation or ingestion, after which the virus attaches to and rapidly replicates in cells of the nasopharyngeal epithelium and associated lymphoreticular tissues, causing necrosis, exudation, and infiltration of phagocytic cells. Bronchial and pulmonary tissues also become infected, particularly in foals, thus predisposing them to secondary bacterial pneumonia.[1,2,21,30,69] Migration of virus-infected phagocytes into the circulation results in viremia associated with mononuclear cells (primarily T lymphocytes) of the buffy coat.[1,2,21,70] The immunologically privileged intracellular location of the virus appears to protect it from inactivation by circulating antibody and permits dissemination to other tissues, including the CNS, even in the presence of high levels of antibody.[71] EHV-1 is capable of spreading directly from one infected cell to contiguous cells without an extracellular phase.[21] Vascular endothelium is the initial site of infection in the CNS and appears to be the predilection site for replication of EHV-1 after transfer of the virus from circulating leukocytes.[51,72,73] Viremia, which may be of prolonged duration, can occur during primary and all successive infections with EHV-1, even when no clinical signs are apparent; thus all EHV-1 infections pose a threat of inducing neurologic disease or abortion.[1,9]

The acute onset of clinical signs of EHV-1 myeloencephalopathy appears to result from vasculitis and thrombosis of arterioles in the brain and especially the spinal cord. This causes functional impairment of blood flow and metabolic exchange and, in severe cases, hypoxic degeneration and necrosis (malacia) with hemorrhage into adjacent neural tissues of the white and, to a lesser extent, gray matter.* This proposed pathogenesis, based primarily on interpretation of the prominent vasculitis seen histopathologically in infected horses and the lack of definitive evidence of viral multiplication in neural tissues, contrasts greatly with the well-established pathogenesis of encephalitis caused by herpesviruses in other species.[16] The propensity of certain EHV-1 isolates to induce myeloencephalopathy does not appear to reflect specific neurotropism but rather a significant endotheliotropism.† The finding of chorioretinopathy and neural lesions in experimentally infected specific pathogen-free ponies, however, suggests that at least some strains of EHV-1 may exhibit neurotropism.[75] Furthermore, strong evidence indicates that in addition to circulating T lymphocytes, epithelial cells of the respiratory tract, and lymphoid tissues draining the respiratory tract, trigeminal ganglia are important sites for establishing and maintaining the lifelong state of latency that occurs in most, if not all, horses during primary infection with EHV-1 and EHV-4.[75-78] The ubiquitous EHV-2 has been proposed to play an important role in promoting reactivation of EHV-1 and EHV-4 from these sites in latently infected horses.[31]

No satisfactory explanation exists as to why some outbreaks of EHV-1 infection are associated with a high incidence of neurologic disease, whereas others are not, or why different horses show different clinical manifestations of EHV-1 infection during outbreaks.[9,10,45,60] A genetic strain of EHV-1 with an adenine-to-guanine mutation at the open reading frame 30, causing a mutation in the DNA polymerase, is associated with replicative aggressiveness and a greater potential for causing neurologic disease.[66] The nature and extent of lesions resulting from EHV-1 infection appear to be influenced by the age, gender, reproductive status (including stage of pregnancy), and immune status of the horse; the magnitude of challenge; strain variations; and perhaps the route of infection.[9,45,48] In one carefully monitored outbreak of EHV-1 infection on a stud farm in England, less than 17% of infected horses developed neurologic manifestations of infection, even though almost 60% of the horses on the farm were confirmed to have been infected.[9] Endothelial cell infection and perivascular cuffing within the CNS appeared to be at least as pronounced in foals that died during this outbreak without showing neurologic signs as in profoundly paretic mares with severe CNS lesions; however, parenchymal neural lesions were minimal in the foals.[9,45] A notable finding during this outbreak was that mares and stallions that developed neurologic signs had considerable antibody responses, whereas the majority of foals did not, despite experiencing a prolonged period of viremia.[9]

†References 9, 10, 25, 38, 45, 49, 52, 54, 61, 64, 67.

*References 9, 50, 51, 54, 58, 62, 74.

†References 26, 35, 45, 50, 51, 72, 73.

The majority of EHV-1 infections that cause neurologic signs probably represent reinfection rather than a new infection.[39,42,80] Infection occurs in horses with significant preexisting serum EHV-1 antibody titers. Affected horses frequently have high titers at the onset of neurologic signs, and those horses that develop the most severe clinical signs are frequently the ones that show the most rapid increase in antibody titer after infection.[9,50,51] In addition, the characteristic vascular lesions in neural tissues of affected horses are typical of type III (Arthus) hypersensitivity reactions, and circulating immune complexes have been demonstrated at the onset of neurologic signs, suggesting that they may result from an immune-complex vasculitis.* An immune-mediated mechanism is supported further by the difficulty experienced in isolating the virus from neural tissues of affected horses.[45,61,62] In addition, assessment of risk factors during outbreaks of neurologic EHV-1 infection in Southern California in 1984 revealed that horses vaccinated with killed or modified live EHV-1 vaccine within the previous year were significantly (9 to 14 times) more likely to develop neurologic manifestations of infection than were nonvaccinated horses.[64]

The finding of circulating antibodies to the myelin protein P2 in the serum of horses that died from EHV-1 myeloencephalopathy (but not in horses that recovered) has led to the suggestion that an alternate immune-mediated mechanism may play a role in the pathogenesis of neurologic EHV-1.[81] The presence of this antibody, however, may represent a response to leakage of the protein after damage induced by another mechanism.

Despite the foregoing observations, evidence for an immune-mediated pathogenesis for EHV-1 myeloencephalopathy is by no means conclusive. In experimental EHV-1 infections in which the onset of neurologic signs 8 to 9 days after infection correlated with a peak in the level of circulating immune complexes, vasculitis was not present in vessels in which endothelial cells did not support viral replication or in organs such as the kidney that one would expect to trap circulating immune complexes.[72] The finding of greatly depressed platelet counts several days before the onset of clinical signs, presumably the result of consumption in thrombi after endothelial damage, suggests that the neuropathologic changes are initiated before circulating immune complexes peak and that the action of immune complexes may be secondary and localized. Failure to isolate the virus from the CNS may be attributable to high levels of circulating antibody and to the endotheliotropism of the virus.[72]

CLINICAL SIGNS

In natural and experimental infections, neurologic signs appear 6 to 10 days after infection by the intranasal route.† The onset of neurologic signs may be preceded or accompanied by signs of upper respiratory disease, fever, inappetence, or hindlimb edema within the previous 2 weeks, although in many instances no antecedent signs are notable unless one routinely monitors rectal temperature. However, frequently one finds a herd or stable history of current or recent cases of respiratory tract infection, fever, inappetence, distal limb edema, abortion, neonatal death, foal diarrhea, or neurologic disease, and for one to encounter different signs of EHV-1 infection in different groups of horses on a particular farm is not unusual.[9]

Affected horses are occasionally febrile at the onset of neurologic disease, although most are normothermic and some are hypothermic. Neurologic signs are generally of acute or peracute onset, after which they tend to stabilize rapidly and generally do not progress after the first 1 or 2 days.[39,43,44,52,82] Clinical signs vary depending on the location and severity of lesions, but in most horses, signs reflect predominant involvement of the spinal white matter.[52] Ataxia and paresis of the limbs are the most common signs, with hypotonia of the tail and anus, tail elevation, and urinary incontinence being common but not invariable findings.* Clinical signs are usually bilaterally symmetrical or only mildly asymmetric, although hemiparesis or sudden onset of unilateral hind- or forelimb lameness progressing to unilateral or more generalized ataxia, paresis, and recumbency have been reported.[52,54,55,74,84] Lesions in peripheral nerves and spinal cord were observed in some of these cases.[54] The hindlimbs generally are affected more severely and earlier in the disease course than the forelimbs. In mildly affected horses, transient ataxia and stiffness of the pelvic limbs or dribbling of urine after overflow from a distended atonic bladder may be the only signs noted.[43,52] One may note conscious proprioceptive deficits in these cases as reluctance to move, clumsiness, toe dragging, knuckling, stumbling, pivoting, and circumduction in one or more limbs on circling, with spasticity evident in some cases.[44,52,85] These signs are often subtle and may go unnoticed. More severely affected horses show profound limb weakness and swaying of the hindquarters, and a small proportion show complete paralysis of affected limbs, manifested as paraplegia and sitting like a dog, complete recumbency, or tetraplegia.[9,21,52,85]

Distention of the urinary bladder is common and may cause signs of colic or dribbling of urine, which frequently results in scalding of the perineum, legs, and other areas.[57] Cystitis is a frequent complication, particularly when repeated catheterization is necessary to relieve bladder distention.[82] Affected stallions and geldings may develop penile flaccidity and paraphimosis or repeated erections, whereas mare may develop vulvar flaccidity.† In addition, stallions may experience reduced libido and swelling of the testes.[9,45] Scrotal edema may accompany hindlimb edema at the onset of neurologic signs in some cases.[9,43-45,58] Sensory deficits are uncommon, but perineal hypalgia or analgesia has been noted, and analgesia of the caudal half of the body was observed in one affected horse.[39,43,52,85] Consistent with predominant involvement of the white matter of the spinal cord, flexor reflexes are normal and perineal reflexes are preserved. In recumbent horses, spinal tendon reflexes can be tested and may be increased. Atrophy is rarely seen, even in the later stages of the disease.[52]Affected horses usually remain alert and have good appetites, even when recumbent, although some show modest depression and inappetence.[44,83] Severe depression, when it occurs, is more often caused by secondary complications than by brain involvement.[83] Unequivocal signs of brain disease are rare, although infarction of the brainstem may cause depressed sensorium, altered behavior, and cranial nerve damage leading to vestibular signs and to lingual, mandibular, and pharyngeal

*References 21, 42, 50, 51, 63, 73, 81.
†References 10, 35, 50, 51, 55, 60, 73.

*References 10, 39, 43, 52, 60, 83.
†References 9, 21, 39, 44, 83, 85.

paresis, which may manifest as dysphagia.[41,59,83,84,86] Strabismus, nystagmus, circling, and head tilt have been observed on occasion.[14,41,52,85]

Affected horses show variable progression of clinical signs. Those horses that are affected mildly frequently stabilize rapidly over a period of hours to a few days as edema and hemorrhage resolve; generally they recover completely over a period of days to several weeks.[9,10,39,44,60] If recumbency occurs, then it generally does so during the first 24 hours, with some horses showing such complete motor paralysis that they are unable to lift their heads.[54] Severely affected horses may show progression of signs during the first few days and may die in coma or convulsion or be euthanatized because of secondary complications.[9]

LABORATORY FINDINGS

CSF analysis typically, although by no means always, reveals xanthochromia, an increased protein concentration (100 to 500 mg/dl), and increased AQ (ratio of CSF to serum albumin concentration), reflecting vasculitis and protein leakage into CSF. The white blood cell count in CSF is usually normal (0 to 5 cells/μl) but occasionally is increased.* Abnormalities in CSF are not present at the onset of clinical signs in some horses, and changes resolve rather quickly; thus the CSF may be normal within 2 weeks of onset of clinical signs.[51,52,82]

The presence of antibodies to EHV-1 in the CSF of affected horses strongly suggests a diagnosis of EHV-1 myeloencephalopathy, although such antibodies are absent in many cases.[14,41,51,52,89] One should take into account the albumin concentration, IgG concentration, and EHV-1 antibody titer in serum and CSF when interpreting positive antibody titers in CSF.[87] Because the AQ usually is elevated in affected horses and the IgG index is normal, the presence of EHV-1 antibodies in CSF reflects leakage of protein across a damaged blood-brain or blood-CSF barrier after vasculitis rather than intrathecal antibody production.[81,87,89] Antibodies therefore are more likely to be present in the CSF of affected horses with concomitantly high serum titers.[51,52,81,87,89] Blood contamination during collection of CSF and other diseases that cause an increase in the permeability of the blood-brain barrier or bleeding into the subarachnoid space may elevate CSF antibody titers falsely if serum titers are also high. Isolation of EHV-1 from the CSF of affected horses would confirm a diagnosis but is rarely successful.[52,57]

Virus isolation and identification of EHV-1 from nasopharyngeal swabs or buffy coat samples strongly supports a diagnosis of EHV-1 myeloencephalopathy in a horse with compatible clinical signs and should be attempted by submission of nasopharyngeal swabs in viral transport medium and an uncoagulated blood sample (citrated or heparinized).† Diagnosis may be achieved more rapidly using real-time PCR for identification of EHV DNA from nasopharyngeal swabs or buffy coat samples. The likelihood of isolating EHV-1 during outbreaks of neurologic disease increases by monitoring in-contact horses and collecting nasal swab and buffy coat samples during the prodromal febrile phase before neurologic signs develop.[44] Even so, interpretation of positive results can be confusing because EHV-1 and EHV-4 have been isolated from the respiratory tract of normal horses.[36] Application of new diagnostic methods such as polymerase chain reaction (PCR), in situ hybridization, antigen-capture ELISA, and dot immunobinding to nasal swabs or scrapings, buffy coat samples, or pathologic specimens have improved the speed and specificity greatly with which one can diagnose EHV-1 infection.[91-99] Many conventional PCR protocols targeting specific genes of EHV-1 have been published in recent years for molecular detection of EHV-1 in nasopharyngeal swabs or buffy coat samples.[32,94-98] Although considerable progress has been made in developing PCR protocols for clinical use, quality control of nucleic acid amplification techniques remains an ongoing challenge because of lack of protocol standardization between laboratories.[100] Furthermore, the majority of PCR assays targeting genomic EHV-1 DNA are unable to differentiate between a lytic and latent infection. Novel technologies such as real-time PCR that allow quantitation of viral DNA and detection at the level of gene expression likely will feature prominently as molecular diagnostic approaches to EHV-1 infection are refined further in the future.

Serologic testing that demonstrates a fourfold or greater increase in serum antibody titer using serum-neutralizing or complement fixation tests on acute and convalescent samples collected 7 to 21 days apart provides presumptive evidence of infection.* Many horses with EHV-1 myeloencephalopathy, however, do not show a fourfold rise in serum-neutralizing titer, and some actually show a decline.[57] This may be explained by the finding that when antibody titers rise, they do so rapidly within 6 to 10 days of infection and already may have peaked by the time neurologic signs appear.† Although serologic testing has limitations in confirming a diagnosis of EHV-1 myeloencephalopathy in an individual horse, testing of paired serum samples from in-contact horses is recommended because a significant proportion of affected and unaffected in-contact horses seroconvert, providing indirect evidence that EHV-1 is the causative agent.‡ Interpretation of the results of serologic tests is complicated by the fact that the serum-neutralizing, complement-fixation, and ELISA tests in use at most diagnostic laboratories do not distinguish between antibodies to EHV-1 and EHV-4 because of cross-reaction between these viruses. A specific ELISA test based on the C-terminal portion of glycoprotein G of both viruses has been developed and should prove valuable in the investigation and management of disease outbreaks in the future.[102-104]

DIAGNOSIS

The multifocal distribution of lesions results in variability of clinical presentation, which necessitates inclusion of a number of conditions in the differential diagnosis. These conditions include EPM, cervical stenotic myelopathy, and cervical vertebral instability (wobbler syndrome), cervical vertebral fracture or other CNS trauma, neuritis of the cauda equina, fibrocartilaginous infarction, aberrant parasite migration, degenerative myelopathy, other viral encephalitides (flaviviruses and alphaviruses), rabies, botulism, CNS abscess, and a variety of plant and chemical intoxications.[14,52] Sudden onset

*References 50-52, 74, 82, 84, 87, 88.
†References 1, 2, 9, 14, 52, 90.

*References 9, 10, 14, 21, 39, 56, 59, 60, 83, 90.
†References 9, 10, 50, 51, 56, 60, 90, 101.
‡References 9, 10, 14, 56, 57, 59, 60.

and early stabilization of neurologic signs including ataxia, paresis, and urinary incontinence; involvement of multiple horses on the premises; and a recent history of fever (most consistently reported clinical sign before onset of ataxia), abortion, or viral respiratory disease in the affected horse or herd mates is sufficient to make a tentative diagnosis of EHV-1 myeloencephalopathy.[14] Antemortem diagnosis is supported by ruling out other conditions; demonstrating xanthochromia and elevated protein concentration in CSF; identifying EHV-1 in or isolating EHV-1 from the respiratory tract, buffy coat, or CSF; and demonstrating a fourfold increase in antibodies using serum-neutralizing, complement fixation, or ELISA tests performed on acute and convalescent serum samples collected from affected or in-contact horses 7 to 21 days apart.[10,60,105] Antemortem confirmation of a diagnosis of EHV-1 myeloencephalopathy is frequently not possible, however, particularly when an individual horse is affected, because the foregoing tests do not yield consistent results in all cases. Hematologic abnormalities with EHM are inconsistent but may include mild anemia and lymphopenia, followed by increased plasma concentration of fibrinogen.

TREATMENT AND PROGNOSIS

Because EHV-1 is a contagious and potentially devastating infection, horses suspected of being affected should be isolated promptly and strictly until EHV-1 is ruled out by confirmation of an alternate diagnosis.[83] No specific treatment is available; thus management of horses with EHV-1 myeloencephalopathy aims toward supportive nursing and nutritional care and reduction of CNS inflammation.[14] One should encourage horses that are not recumbent to remain standing and should protect them from self-inflicted trauma by the provision of good footing, such as a grass paddock, by placement of food and water in an accessible location at a convenient height above ground level, and by other measures, including the use of padded hoods and elimination of obstacles. Patients that become recumbent should be maintained in a sternal position on a thick cushion of dry absorbent bedding and should be rolled frequently (at least every 2 to 4 hours) to reduce the risk of myonecrosis and decubital ulcers. Whenever possible, one should lift and support the horse in the standing position using an appropriately fitting sling.[10] Slings are most beneficial for moderately affected horses that are too weak to rise but are able to maintain a standing position with minimal assistance.

Affected horses usually maintain a good appetite, even when recumbent, although hand feeding may be necessary to encourage some horses to eat. Maintenance of hydration is important, and provision of a laxative diet or the administration of laxatives such as bran mashes, mineral oil, or psyllium may be necessary to reduce intestinal impaction. One usually can meet the caloric and water needs of anorectic patients by feeding gruels of alfalfa-based or similar pelleted feeds in water or balanced electrolyte solution via nasogastric tube. If oral intake is insufficient to meet the daily water needs of 60 to 80 ml/kg of body mass per day, then one can maintain hydration by intravenous administration of balanced electrolyte solutions.[52] Partial or total parenteral nutrition can also be used to meet the caloric needs of anorectic, recumbent horses.

If affected horses are unable to stand and posture to urinate or if bladder function is impaired significantly, manual evacuation of the bladder by application of pressure per the rectum may be necessary. If these measures are unsuccessful, then judicious urinary catheterization is indicated and should be performed aseptically with the collection tubing attached to a sterile closed bag to minimize the risk of inducing urinary tract infection.[14,83,85] Cystitis is, however, a frequent complication, particularly in recumbent horses, and can lead to bladder wall necrosis, bladder rupture, and systemic sepsis. Urine scalding can become a major problem, particularly in mares that dribble urine. Prevention involves regular washing of the perineum, tail, and hind legs with water, application of water-repellent ointments, and braiding or wrapping the tail to simplify cleaning.[14] Administration of enemata or manual emptying of the rectum also may be necessary to promote defecation and improve patient comfort.[14]

Because vasculitis, hemorrhage, and edema are prominent early lesions and may have an immune basis, treatment with corticosteroids early in the disease course is recommended by some clinicians, although no objective data are available to document the efficacy of these or other anti-inflammatory drugs.[44,52,83] A short course of treatment with prednisolone acetate (1 to 2 mg/kg/day) or dexamethasone (0.05 to 0.25 mg/kg parenterally twice daily) for 2 to 3 days with decreasing doses over another 1 to 3 days may be beneficial.[14,52,85] Flunixin meglumine (1.1 mg/kg body mass every 12 hours) is indicated to treat CNS vasculitis. DMSO at a dose of 0.5 to 1.0 g/kg administered intravenously as a 10% to 20% solution in normal saline or 5% dextrose once daily for up to 3 days commonly is used to treat horses with suspected CNS trauma or inflammatory disease, such as EHV-1.[11,14] Although the efficacy of DMSO for treating herpesvirus myeloencephalopathy has not been evaluated, its reported ability to inhibit platelet aggregation and scavenge free radicals support its continued use. Because of the high risk of development of cystitis and other secondary bacterial infections, administering broad spectrum antibiotics such as potentiated sulfonamides (trimethoprim-sulfamethoxazole 30 mg/kg body mass orally every 12 hours) or ceftiofur (2.2 mg/kg body mass intramuscularly or intravenously every 12 hours) is advisable, particularly when corticosteroid treatment is used.[10,14,52] One should base the choice of antibiotics for treating established secondary bacterial infections of the urinary tract, respiratory tract, or other areas on the results of culture and susceptibility testing.

Acyclovir, a synthetic purine nucleoside analog with inhibitory activity against several human herpesviruses, has been shown to exert an inhibitory effect on EHV-1 in vitro.[106] Apparent efficacy of acyclovir was suggested by a successful treatment outcome in occasional outbreak situations.[60,107] Although these anecdotal reports seemed promising, data describing the pharmacokinetics, bioavailability, and safety of acyclovir in horses do not support claims of efficacy, especially after oral administration. Bioavailability of acyclovir after oral administration to horses is extremely low; in contrast, bioavailability of valacyclovir, a prodrug for acyclovir, is much higher.[108,109] Clearly, additional studies are needed to define the appropriate dose for valacyclovir in horses and to document its efficacy for the treatment of EHV-1 myeloencephalopathy. Another nucleoside analog, penciclovir, has been shown to have excellent activity against EHV-1 in tissue culture and in a mouse model of EHV-1 infection.[110]

Affected horses that remain standing have a good prognosis for recovery, and improvement generally is apparent within a few days, although a period of several weeks to more than a year may be required before horses with severe deficits show complete recovery.* In these instances, control of urination frequently returns before gait abnormalities resolve completely.[83] Some horses may be left with permanent residual neurologic deficits, including urinary incontinence and ataxia, that may necessitate euthanasia many months beyond onset of neurologic signs.[10,52,56,57] Horses that become recumbent have a greatly increased likelihood of developing complications such as myonecrosis, urinary tract infection, decubital ulcers, respiratory tract infection, gastrointestinal obstruction and ulceration, injuries, and complications of dehydration and malnutrition. Their prognosis for recovery is therefore poor, particularly if they remain recumbent for more than 24 hours and they are unable to stand after being lifted with a sling.[9,10] One should not elect euthanasia prematurely in valuable horses, however, because reports document horses standing again and recovering completely to race successfully after being recumbent for several days to 3 weeks.[44,54,58] Most mildly affected mares return to breeding soundness in the same season, whereas fertility is likely to be compromised in more severely affected mares that experience urinary retention.[9] Recurrence or exacerbation of neurologic signs in horses that have recovered completely has not been documented, even though the majority likely remain latently infected.[21,34,52,83]

PATHOLOGIC FINDINGS

When horses with suspected EHV-1 myeloencephalopathy die or are euthanized, one should submit the whole carcass or at least the head, spine, spleen, thyroid, and lung for postmortem examination because lesions frequently are not confined to the CNS of horses with EHV-1 myeloencephalopathy.* Gross pathologic lesions in the CNS frequently are not found, but small (2 to 6 mm) focal areas of hemorrhage distributed randomly throughout the meninges and parenchyma of the brain and spinal cord may be observed.† More diffuse dural hemorrhage is notable in some cases and may extend to spinal nerve roots and the cauda equina.[50,51,62] Small plum-colored areas of degeneration and hemorrhage are sometimes grossly visible in fresh tissue at various levels of the spinal cord (white matter), and malacic foci may be visible macroscopically in the gray and white matter in sliced fixed sections of brain.[50,51,58,59,62]

The gross and histologic lesions in the CNS reflect vasculitis, congestion, and secondary ischemic degeneration of nervous tissue.‡ Although vasculitis is a consistent finding, degeneration of nervous tissue is evident chiefly in those horses with clinical signs of severe neurologic disease.[45,50,51] The vasculitis is often severe and has a widespread, random, multifocal distribution, with the most severe lesions usually in the brainstem and spinal cord. In the brain the meningeal and penetrating or radiating vessels in gray matter are the major sites of vascular involvement. Thus foci of axonal swelling and malacia develop in the gray and white matter, particularly adjacent to the meningeal surface and in the deep cortex adjacent to the white matter.[50,51,62] In the spinal cord a similar orientation to meningeal vessels results in degeneration of white matter within ovoid, linear, or wedge-shaped foci, affecting predominantly the lateral and the ventral white columns.[51]

*References 10, 39, 44, 56, 60, 82, 84, 85.

*References 9, 21, 36, 45, 50, 51, 62.

†References 21, 45, 51, 58, 59, 62.

‡References 45, 50, 51, 58, 59, 62.

In some instances, sheaths of nerve roots and nerves and capsules of ganglia also are involved.[45,50,51,52] Trigeminal ganglionitis may be present but usually is not manifest clinically.[54]

Ocular lesions, including uveal vasculitis with perivascular mononuclear cell cuffing in the ciliary body and optic nerve or extensive retinal degeneration, have been observed in foals showing signs of bilateral hypopyon and iritis or severe visual impairment and chorioretinopathy without anterior segment involvement during field and experimental EHV-1 infections.[9,45,51,62,75] In some foals, EHV-1 appears to induce ocular and neural damage in the absence of gross signs of neurologic or visual impairment.[75] During paralytic infections, secondary viral replication occurs in blood vessels of the testis and epididymis in addition to CNS and may be responsible for reported signs of scrotal edema and loss of libido in affected stallions.[9,111]

EHV-1 infrequently is isolated from the CNS of affected horses that show typical lesions.* Thus one should attempt to isolate the virus from other sites to support the diagnosis. Those sites most likely to yield virus or to contain viral antigen include the turbinates and nasal passages, as well as lymph nodes draining the upper respiratory tract, lung, thyroid, spleen, and endometrium, in addition to the brain.[45,52,101] Immunofluorescent antibody testing of brain and spinal cord sections is considered to be more sensitive than virus isolation, but false-negative results have been observed.[45,52,61] An indirect immunoperoxidase method using orthodox light microscopy was highly sensitive for identifying individual antigen-containing cells in the CNS and other areas of the body, even at sites containing few or no lesions or inclusion bodies and in which virus could not be detected by immunofluorescent antibody testing or virus isolation.[45] Similarly, the PCR technique is more sensitive than virus isolation for detecting viral antigen in nasopharyngeal swabs collected from horses with respiratory tract disease caused by EHV-1 or EHV-4.[94] Both of these techniques—as well as antigen-capture ELISA tests, dot immunobinding, and in situ DNA hybridization, which are sensitive and readily differentiate between EHV-1 and EHV-4—show great promise for routine application to samples collected antemortem or at necropsy from affected horses.[45,73,92,95,99]

CONTROL AND PREVENTION

Control measures during outbreaks of EHV-1 infection aim at reducing spread by infectious aerosols, direct contact, and fomites, as well as at reducing stress-induced recrudescence of latent EHV-1 infection.[1,2,21] If neurologic signs or other clinical signs suggestive of EHV-1 infection occur, then one should isolate affected animals promptly and completely in a well-ventilated airspace separate from the remainder of the herd. In-contact horses should be isolated in their current location in small groups for at least 1 month; pregnant mares should be isolated preferably until they foal.[1-3,9,21,44,86] On breeding farms, one should suspend covering.[9] Aborted fetuses and fetal membranes are rich sources of infectious virus; therefore they should be collected and placed in leak-proof containers (e.g., heavy-gauge plastic bags) for submission for diagnostic evaluation or disposal by burning.[1,2] Similarly, bedding and dirt contaminated with fetal fluids should be disposed of or

*References 41, 45, 48, 52, 55, 58, 59, 72, 101, 112.

burned, and stalls or other areas occupied by infected horses should be cleaned thoroughly, disinfected with an iodophor or a phenolic product, and left empty for several weeks.[21] Equipment used to handle, groom, feed, water, muck out, or transport affected horses also should be cleaned and disinfected or disposed of properly. Thereafter separate equipment and personnel should be used for affected and unaffected horses, or at least caretakers should handle affected horses last and wear disposable gloves, surgical masks, and protective clothing that can be changed or disinfected between groups.[21] Although control measures are frequently successful in stopping further spread of infection during outbreaks, one should note that transmission of infection before control measures are implemented may result in a secondary waves of disease 1 to 2 weeks later.[9,21,44]

Traffic of horses and human beings on the premises should be minimized, and movement of horses onto and off of the infected premises should be suspended until at least 3 weeks after resolution of acute signs in the last clinical case or until tests show that virus transmission is no longer occurring.[1-3,14,21] Collection of nasal swabs and uncoagulated blood (buffy coat) samples from clinically affected and exposed horses within each group and demonstration of stable or declining antibody titers in serum samples proved to be helpful in determining patterns of exposure and spread and in establishing when virus transmission had ceased in one reported outbreak. Protracted viremia lasting several weeks or months occurs in some horses and extends the period during which movement of horses should be restricted.[9]

If horses must enter the farm, they should be current on EHV-1 vaccination and should be isolated away from the resident population. Although giving booster vaccinations to exposed pregnant mares during outbreaks of abortigenic EHV-1 infection is common practice,[1,2,21] vaccination of exposed horses during outbreaks of EHV-1 myeloencephalopathy has not been investigated and cannot be recommended at this time because of the possibility of an immune-mediated pathogenesis. Administering booster doses of inactivated EHV-1 vaccine to all unexposed horses that have not been vaccinated within the previous month is common practice, however.

Preventive measures should include routine management practices aimed at reducing the chances of introducing and disseminating infection.[3,21,74,113] New arrivals should be isolated for at least 3 weeks before joining the herd, distinct herd groups should be maintained based on the age and use of horses, and care should be taken to minimize or eliminate commingling of resident horses with visiting or transient horses. In particular, pregnant broodmares should be maintained in groups separate from the remaining farm population. In addition, minimizing stress associated with overcrowding and handling procedures is prudent in an attempt to reduce recrudescence of latent EHV-1 infection.[21,34,74,113]

No method is known that reliably prevents the neurologic form of EHV-1 infection. None of the EHV-1 or EHV-4 vaccines currently available carry a claim that they prevent EHV-1 myeloencephalopathy, and the disease has been observed in horses vaccinated regularly at 3- to 5-month intervals with inactivated or modified live vaccines.[14,52,57,59,60] Repetitive administration of currently available EHV-1 and EHV-4 vaccines appears to induce some immunity to respiratory disease and reduce the incidence of abortion but does not block infection and induction of viremia or eliminate the possibility of clinical disease and establishment of the carrier state.[1,2,21,59,113-118] Although the protection induced by inactivated EHV-1 vaccines is incomplete and of short duration, the vaccine reduces virus excretion in horses that do become infected.[115,118] To maintain appropriate vaccination procedures in an attempt to reduce the incidence of other manifestations of EHV-1 infection and reduce the magnitude of challenge experienced by in-contact horses is logical. This indirectly may help prevent EHV-1 myeloencephalopathy.[52] An attenuated live virus vaccine based on the temperature-sensitive and host range mutant clone 147 of EHV-1 has been evaluated recently. The novelty of this vaccine lies in the fact that a low dose administered intranasally replicated in conventional target species and conferred exceptional efficacy against respiratory disease, virus shedding, viremia, and abortion caused by a severe EHV-1 challenge.[119-121] Intranasal vaccine also claims to protect against less common manifestations of EHV-1 infection such as paresis and jaundice.[8]

POLYNEURITIS EQUI

William J. Saville

Polyneuritis equi is an uncommon neurologic disease of all equine species that is characterized by tail and anal sphincter paralysis, often accompanied by cranial and peripheral nerve damage.[1-13] Previous reports referred to the disease as *neuritis of the cauda equina* because of the susceptibility of this region, but frequent involvement of the cranial and peripheral nerves led to the term *polyneuritis equi*.[2] Although the disease has been recognized more readily in Europe, where Dexler first reported it in 1897, cases have now been reported in Great Britain, Canada, and the United States.[3,4,6,14] The disease does not appear to have a breed, gender, or age predilection, but the youngest horse affected was 17 months of age.[2,5,6,13-15]

The cause of this disease is unknown. Primary immune reaction and viral inflammatory disease have been suggested, although possibly one may be a consequence of the other.[2] Several infectious agents have been suggested, such as EHV-1, equine adenovirus, and streptococcal and *Campylobacter* spp. bacteria.[10,12,16] The pathologic lesions resemble those of Guillain-Barré syndrome in human beings, and the disease is similar to experimental allergic neuritis in rats.[10,13] Evidence suggests that the immune system is involved because horses with polyneuritis equi have circulating antibodies to P2 myelin protein, which is present in rats with experimental allergic neuritis.[10,17] Inflammatory lesions contain both T and B lymphocytes, suggesting the possibility of an immune-mediated reaction to myelin.[18]

CLINICAL SIGNS

Although the disease manifests itself in two forms, signs are generally slow and progressive: (1) the acute or early signs include hyperesthesia of the perineal or head regions (or both), and (2) in the chronic form, horses show paralysis of the tail, anus, rectum, and bladder. Paralysis often is accompanied by fecal and urinary retention, urinary scalding of the pelvic limbs, and penile paralysis in male horses.*

*References 1-3, 6, 8, 9, 12, 13, 15.

The pelvic limb signs are often symmetrical, whereas the signs involving the head and cranial nerves are often asymmetrical.[6,13,15] Muscle atrophy in the gluteal region is sometimes present along with mild degrees of ataxia.[2,3,5,6,9] Muscle atrophy associated with cranial nerve involvement may occur in the head region. Damage to peripheral motor nerves may result in gait deficits and abnormal use of thoracic or pelvic limbs.[1,12,13,15]

Although cranial nerve involvement is reported primarily to affect cranial nerves V, VII, and VIII, any of cranial nerves II, III, IV, VI, IX, X, and XII also may be involved.[2,4,5,8,13] As a result of damage to the cranial nerves, horses may have trouble with mastication and swallowing.[12] A head tilt, ear droop, lip droop, and ptosis are common signs.[8,12,13] One report describes a horse with brachial neuritis along with involvement of cranial nerves V, VII, and XII. The horse in that report also exhibited mild ataxia and weakness in all limbs. The horse performed the hopping test poorly on the right thoracic limb, and the horse resented palpation in the right caudal cervical and prescapular region.[2]

Colic caused by fecal retention may be the primary sign when one initially examines horses with polyneuritis equi. Fecal retention leads to an impaction caused by the flaccid anal sphincter, often accompanied by an atonic, distended bladder.[1] If the clinician sees these signs in the acute or hyperesthetic form, then they usually progress to the chronic form of hypalgesia or anesthesia. An area of hyperesthesia may surround the area of anesthesia.[1,2,8]

DIAGNOSIS

The definitive diagnostic test is a postmortem examination. The peripheral white blood cell count usually reveals a mature neutrophilia with hyperfibrinogenemia, mild to moderate anemia, and an increased total protein—all indications of a chronic inflammatory process.[3,5,13,15] Examination of the CSF may reveal an elevated protein (70 to 300 mg/dl), along with an elevated white blood cell count, which indicates a mononuclear inflammatory reaction, although cytologic examination of CSF may be normal, particularly in the acute stage of the disease.*

Radiography may be helpful to rule out trauma to the tailhead or cranial nerve involvement, such as a fractured petrous temporal or other bones of the skull.[2,8]

Some horses with clinical signs exhibit circulating serum antibodies to P2 myelin.[10,17] However, the presence of this antibody is only weakly supportive of the diagnosis, because the same antibody has been detected in horses with EHV-1 and equine adenovirus infections.†

Classically, the primary pathologic lesions involve the extradural nerve roots but also may involve the intradural nerve roots.[2,3,5,12,13] The lesions are granulomatous with various degrees of inflammation and infiltration of lymphocytes, eosinophils, macrophages, giant cells, and plasma cells. This inflammation leads to myelin degeneration, subsequent axonal degeneration, and thickening of the epineurium, endoneurium, and perineurium with proliferation, which causes obliteration of the neural architecture by the fibrous tissue.[1,2,9,13] The most severe lesions are in the cauda equina, but swelling, edema, and hemorrhage of cranial nerves may occur. The fibrous tissue formation may lead to adhesions between the meninges and the periosteum of the vertebral bodies.[13] Reports describe involvement of the autonomic nervous system, but no changes in clinical signs have been reported (post mortem only).[2,4]

The polyneuritis lesions are similar to those observed with Guillain-Barré syndrome in human beings, experimental allergic neuritis in rats, and coonhound paralysis in dogs.[2,5,11-13] This similarity may indicate a combination of inflammatory and immune-mediated mechanisms in the pathogenesis of polyneuritis equi.

*References 2, 3, 5, 6, 8, 11, 13.
†References 1, 2, 10, 13, 16, 19.

DIFFERENTIAL DIAGNOSIS

The most important differential diagnosis is trauma to the sacrococcygeal area of the spinal canal, which can be differentiated by radiography of the area looking for fractures or displacements.[2,6,8] EPM is the second most common disease in the differential diagnosis of polyneuritis equi. The usual signs of EPM include asymmetrical damage in the limbs and brain and brainstem lesions causing cranial nerve deficits with alterations in attitude, whereas the cranial nerve deficits of polyneuritis equi are peripheral, with no change in attitude.[6] This disease may be differentiated from polyneuritis equi by Western blot analysis of the CSF.[20] EPM is discussed in detail elsewhere in this text.

EHV-1 myeloencephalitis may be preceded by an episode of fever, cough, and nasal discharge or one or more abortions on a farm. This condition frequently affects more than one horse on a farm. Herpesvirus has a rapid onset and often results in severe hindlimb weakness and ataxia along with bladder dysfunction. Urinary dribbling sometimes may occur. The ataxia and weakness is usually symmetrical and may result in recumbency. Occasionally, affected horses sit like a dog because of profound pelvic limb weakness. Cranial nerve involvement is not common but may occur between 10% to 15% of affected horses.[21-24]

One should consider verminous myeloencephalitis as a differential diagnosis for polyneuritis equi. The signs vary and depend on the migratory pathway of the parasite. Diffuse or multifocal brain and spinal cord lesions have been reported. The onset is usually sudden with rapid deterioration and death. The incidence of this disease is low, perhaps because of more intense parasite control.[25-27]

One should consider EMND in the differential diagnosis. Horses with motor neuron disease have symmetrical muscle wasting or atrophy and weight loss with significant weakness, sweating, and muscle fasciculations. However, these horses are not ataxic and their unique clinical feature is that they walk better than they stand. This disease is a denervation atrophy of type 1 muscle fibers only and may be diagnosed by a spinal accessory nerve biopsy or sacrodorsalis caudalis muscle biopsy.[28]

TREATMENT

The primary therapy is palliative. No treatment for the disease is known. Removing feces from the rectum and evacuating the bladder are usually necessary. If cystitis caused by bladder distention occurs, then systemic antibiotics may be indicated. Some attempts have been made at treating the inflammation with corticosteroids, but the effects have been short lived. The prognosis is usually poor, but the progression of the disease is slow. Some animals may be maintained for many months.*

*References 2, 4-6, 8, 12, 13, 15.

VIRAL ENCEPHALITIS

Joseph J. Bertone

A wide variety of viruses can affect the CNS of horses, resulting in encephalitis or meningoencephalitis. Rabies, caused by a member of the Rhabdoviridae family, and WNV, a member of the Flaviviridae family, are discussed in detail elsewhere in this chapter. This section describes disease resulting from infections with members of the Togaviridae family of viruses (eastern, western, and Venezuelan encephalitis) and CNS infections caused by viruses from miscellaneous viral families.

TOGAVIRAL ENCEPHALITIS

Togaviridae are small, lipid- and protein-enveloped RNA viruses. Those that cause disease are insect-borne viruses (arboviruses) of the genus *Alphavirus*. The structure of the viruses and associated clinical presentations are similar among the viruses, but the epizootiology and antigenicity are distinct. In general, birds, rodents, and reptiles act as reservoirs. Mosquitoes often play a role in transmitting the disease among these species. Mosquitoes and, less commonly, other insects feed on sylvatic hosts and subsequently transmit the disease to horses and human beings.

Alphavirus Encephalitides: Eastern, Western, and Venezuelan Equine Encephalomyelitis

EEE, WEE, and Venezuelan (VEE) equine encephalitis viruses are the most frequently isolated alphaviruses from epidemics of encephalitis in horses and human beings in the Western Hemisphere (Table 12-12). The first recorded epidemic of EEE in North America likely occurred in Massachusetts in 1831.[1]

CAUSE

The alphaviruses are single-stranded, linear, positive-sense RNA viruses that measure between 60 to 70 nm in diameter. EEE and WEE are specific and discrete togaviral species; North and South American antigenic variants of EEE exist.[2] WEE is a recombinant between an EEE-like virus and a Sindbis-like virus.[3] Two antigenic subtypes of WEE virus exist: (1) WEE and (2) Highlands J viruses. The Highlands J virus causes most infections that occur east of the Mississippi River. The various strains have equivocal differences in antigenic properties and biologic behavior, and extensive geographic overlap occurs.[2] The molecular basis for the antigenic variation between EEE and WEE has been described.[4] VEE virus has six distinct subtypes designated by Roman numerals I through VI. Subtypes IAB, IC, and IE are responsible for large outbreaks of encephalitis in horses in the Western Hemisphere in the past 20 years. The so-called endemic types of VEE virus are considered to be of low pathogenicity for horses under most circumstances. These include ID and IF variants from Central America and Brazil, respectively; type II (Everglades) virus found in Florida; and types II, IV, V, and VI viruses.[5-8]

EPIZOOTIOLOGY

Encephalitis similar to the viral encephalitides has been reported in the United States for many years with high morbidity and mortality rates.[9-11] Evidence that an eastern and western virus exist and are antigenically distinct was first reported in 1933.[12] Horses immunized with strains of virus isolated from infected horses from the east or west were protected differentially when vaccinated with attenuated virus from one location and exposed to virus from the other.[12-15]

Distribution In general, disease associated with EEE, WEE, and VEE is restricted to the Western Hemisphere and ranges from temperate to desert climates. Each virus and incidence of associated equine disease has a characteristic distribution. The range of positive serologic tests for the viruses is often far greater than the range of clinical disease[15-41] (Figure 12-41).

EEE virus is found as far north as eastern Canada, south throughout the Caribbean, and in parts of Central and South America. Disease in the United States is primarily seen in the Southeastern United States but has been detected in all states east of the Mississippi River and some Western states. Outside the Western Hemisphere, EEE has been identified in the Philippines,[42] and some indications point to its presence in Europe.[43]

The WEE virus is recognized in reservoir avian hosts in the western United States; however, clinical disease rarely has been identified there in the last 20 years. Historically large outbreaks of WEE have been described in horses in California and other Western states. The reason for the dramatic decrease in incidence of clinical disease from WEE is largely unexplained to date. Geographic variation in virulence may be an explanation. Equine disease associated with WEE is rare on the Eastern seaboard of the United States but is recognized.[44]

Venezuelan equine encephalitis is a very important human and veterinary pathogen in the Western hemisphere that can cause large outbreaks of disease in human beings and horses

TABLE 12-12

A Summary of the Major Togaviral Equine Encephalitides*

Virus	Major Disease Vector	Zoonotic Potential	Amplification from Horses	Disease Spread	Viremia	Equine Mortality
EEE	*Aedes* spp.	Unlikely	Unlikely	Vector	Low	75%-100%
WEE	*Culex tarsalis*	Unlikely	Unlikely	Vector ± secretions	Low	20%-50%
VEE	*Culex melanconium, Aedes* spp. *Phosphora* spp.	Occurs	Occurs	Vector ± secretions	High	40%-80%

EEE, eastern equine encephalitis virus; *WEE*, western equine encephalitis virus; *VEE*, Venezuelan equine encephalitis virus.
*The statements made are generalizations, and some degree of variation occurs.

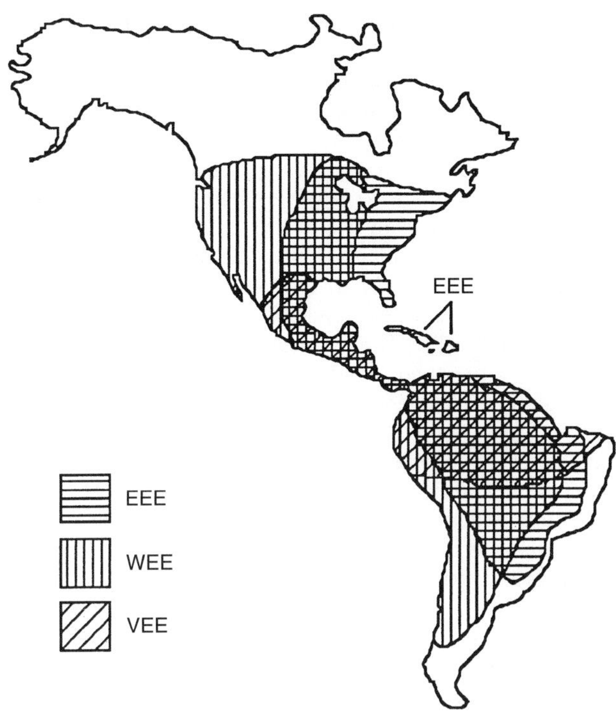

FIGURE 12-41 Predominant distribution of *Alphavirus* spp.–associated equine encephalitis in the Western Hemisphere. This figure represents the disease distribution. Positive serologic results for the diseases are more widespread. *EEE,* Eastern equine encephalitis virus; *WEE,* western equine encephalitis virus; *VEE,* Venezuelan equine encephalitis virus.

over large geographic areas. Outbreaks have occurred in Mexico, Venezuela, and Colombia in recent years. The virus has also been recently isolated in Trinidad, French Guiana, Peru, and Brazil.

Epidemic Several requirements must be met for epidemics associated with alphavirus encephalitis to develop. Long lapses can occur between outbreaks if all of these conditions are not met. These prerequisites include adequate and adjacent numbers of reservoir animals, sufficient quantities of virulent viruses, infected intermediate hosts, insect vectors, and susceptible horse and human populations.[45,46] Prediction of outbreaks has been attempted but without success,[1,38,47] which indicates that other, unknown factors may exist.

Reservoirs With minor exceptions, Togaviridae persist by asymptomatically infecting wild animals (sylvatic hosts) such as birds, small mammals, and reptiles by unknown mechanisms.[48] The viruses survive during the winter or nonvector season in sylvatic populations.[47,49]

Vectors Specificity of the viruses for particular vectors occurs. Vector distribution explains viral distribution to a large degree. The vectors for EEE include *Culiseta melanura* and *Aedes* spp.[15,31,50,51] *C. melanura* for the most part is confined to freshwater swamps, feeds primarily on swamp birds, and rarely is found in areas of increased horse populations.[15] In general, *C. melanura* serves as the vector for the enzootic cycle, which involves swamp birds. *Aedes* spp. appear to be more important in epizootics and epidemics.

Culex tarsalis is the primary vector that maintains WEE virus in an enzootic cycle with passerine birds. *Dermacentor andersoni* ticks,[52,53] *Triatoma sanguisuga* (assassin bug),[54,55] and the cliff swallow bug *(Oeciacus vicarius)* may also be involved as vectors or overwintering reservoirs for WEE.[52,56] Several species of mosquitoes from at least 11 genera have been determined to be naturally infected with epidemic strains of VEE virus, including *Culex melanconium*, and *Mansonia*, *Aedes*, and *Psorophora* spp.[18,19,25,26] Ticks may also be capable of virus transmission.

Vector Ecology Vector transmission is the most important way infection spreads for any of the alphavirus encephalitides. WEE and VEE may spread by nasal secretions, but this is less likely.[18,19,55,57] Vectors transmit viral particles between sylvatic hosts when taking a blood meal. If the virus is able to penetrate the gut of the vector, then it may pass through the hemolymph to oral glands, multiply, and subsequently be shed in saliva and other oral secretions. If the blood meal contains adequate numbers of viral particles, then multiplication may not be required for transmission. In most instances and judiciously assumed, the mosquito remains infected for life.[51,58]

Seasonal Incidence In most instances the diseases occur during the height of the vector season. In temperate climates the highest number of cases occurs between June and November. In warm climates, where the vector season is longer, the disease problem lasts longer. Some of these attributes have contributed to disease outbreaks in colder climates where the disease has been less usual.[59] We are likely to see more cold-climate outbreaks with the increase in global temperatures.

Zoonology Clinical infection in human beings usually involves old or young persons. Signs and morbidity and mortality rates are virus specific.[60] Circulating virus concentrations are usually insufficient for transmission of EEE from infected horses to human beings, mosquitoes, and other animals. Human disease most likely is associated with insect vector contact and often coincides temporally with or is preceded by equine epizootics.[1] In the acute stages of equine disease, a transient, substantial viremia occurs. Therefore if vector density increases, then an acutely infected horse could be a transient amplifier of EEE. Spread from horse to horse is possible.[50] Clinical signs in human beings include acute fulminant encephalitis, headache, altered consciousness, and seizures. The mortality rate in human patients is between 50% to 75%.[60]

Human beings and horses are terminal hosts for WEE. Human cases of WEE occur, but fatality and incomplete recovery are rare. These cases are associated with vector contact. Environmental conditions that decrease exposure to insects decrease the incidence of disease.[61] Increased numbers of animals with clinical equine disease are an indication of heavy sylvatic concentrations of virus and are not a potential source of infection for human beings. Generally, increased numbers of horse cases precede cases in human beings by 2 to 5 weeks.[62] Thus horses are sentinels for human beings in a given area. Clinical signs in human beings include fever, headache, confusion, stupor, and seizures, with a 5% to 15% mortality rate.[60]

Horses with VEE have sufficient circulating viral concentrations that act as amplifiers of disease.[25,63] Ocular and nasal secretions from infected horses contain high concentrations of VEE.[18,19] Infection via entry through the respiratory tract may occur by direct contact with infected animals. Equine and human survivors of VEE infection and clinical disease may develop chronic relapsing viremias and serve as chronic disease amplifiers.[63] Clinical signs in human beings include fever, headache, myalgia, and pharyngitis. The mortality rate in human beings is 1%.[60]

With any of the alphaviral equine encephalitides, sufficient viral particles for infection may be present in CNS and other tissues, and one should take precautions when performing a necropsy examination on suspect cases. Strict mosquito control and vaccination can prevent human and equine cases, and all equine cases should be reported to state health officials.[1,63] A recent study demonstrated that EEE has poor ability to replicate in lymphoid tissues, whereas VEE does so very efficiently. EEE can therefore avoid IFN-α and IFN-β induction in vivo, which may allow EEE to evade the host's innate immune responses and thereby enhance neurovirulence. Inhibition of genome translation restricts EEE infectivity for myeloid but not mesenchymal cells. This factor likely contributes to the observed differences in disease cause and presentation.[64]

Other Domestic Species Outbreaks of disease because of EEE have been described in emus, ostriches, and swine, with isolated cases in cattle, sheep, and nondomestic ungulates.[65-68] Pigs may also be affected by VEE.[68] The signs of disease in these species are similar but are milder than disease in horses for the respective viruses. Burros and mules may contract all three diseases, and the disease is as severe as that identified in horses.[69]

PATHOGENESIS

After viruses are inoculated, they multiply in muscle, enter the lymphatic circulation, and localize in lymph nodes. Viruses replicate in macrophages and neutrophils and subsequently are shed in small numbers. Many of the viral particles are cleared at this time. If clearance mechanisms are successful, then no further clinical signs develop. Neutralizing antibodies still will be produced. Several mechanisms of viral immunologic avoidance exist and include erythrocyte and leukocyte absorption. If viral elimination is not complete, then the remaining viruses infect endothelial cells and concentrate in highly vascular organs such as the liver and spleen. Viral replication in these tissues subsequently is associated with circulating virus. The second viremic period often is associated with early clinical signs of disease. Infection of the CNS occurs within 3 to 5 days.[7,19,70,71]

CLINICAL SIGNS

Clinical signs are more profound in unvaccinated animals.[62,72] Acute clinical signs of EEE and WEE are nonspecific and include mild fever to severe pyrexia, anorexia, and stiffness. Viremia occurs during this period. A 1- to 3-week incubation period exists after experimental infection with EEE or WEE. The incubation period is often shorter with EEE than WEE. Early signs of the diseases include fever and mild depression. This stage is transient and, presumably, often undetected because of lack of overt clinical signs. The acute signs may last for up to 5 days after they first manifest. Many cases of WEE do not progress beyond this point. With EEE, progression is more common. Once nervous signs develop, the viremia is past, and animals are unlikely to be able to amplify the disease. In progressive cases the fever may rise and fall sporadically. Cerebral signs may develop at any time but often occur a few days after infection. Acute signs often range from propulsive walking, depression, and somnolence to hyperesthesia, aggression, and excitability. Some horses may become frenzied after any sensory stimulation. Conscious proprioceptive deficits often are evident in the early stages. With progression, signs become less disparate and more consistent between EEE and WEE. The later signs are evidence of the dynamic nature of these conditions and increased severity of cerebral cortical and cranial nerve dysfunction. These signs include head pressing, propulsive walking, blindness, circling, head tilt, and facial and appendicular muscle fasciculations. Paralysis of the pharynx, larynx, and tongue is common. Death often is preceded by recumbency for 1 to 7 days. Comatose animals rarely survive. If animals are to survive, then they show gradual improvement of function over weeks to months.[72-75]

VEE may have similar or different clinical presentations compared with WEE and EEE, which is most likely because of the difference in strain pathogenicity and persistent high titer viremia with VEE.[18,71] The pyrexia in cases of VEE peaks early and remains increased through the course of the disease. In experimental disease, endemic strains are associated with mild fever and leukopenia. Epidemic strains are associated with severe pyrexia and leukopenia.[7,71] Diarrhea, severe depression, recumbency, and death may be prominent before neurologic deficits are evident. Neurologic signs occur at approximately 4 days after infection. Other associated signs include abortion, oral ulceration, pulmonary hemorrhage, and epistaxis.[18,19]

DIAGNOSIS

The presumptive diagnosis is based on findings at clinical presentation and the presence of associated epidemiologic features. Serologic and necropsy evaluation provide a definitive determination.

Clinical Immunology and Virology One usually identifies viral infections by complement fixation, hemagglutination inhibition, and cross-serum neutralization assays. A combination of these techniques increases the likelihood of a positive diagnosis.[76] A fourfold increase in antibody titer in convalescent sera commonly is recommended for diagnosis. However, one possibly may not detect a rise in titer. Viral antibodies are commonly present within 24 hours after the initial viremia, and their presence often precedes clinical encephalitis.[43] The concentration of antibodies increases rapidly and then decreases over 6 months.[77] An initial sample often is taken when encephalitic signs are present, which may be after titers have peaked. Therefore a second sample possibly may have a decreased titer compared with the initial sample. If increased titers exist for hemagglutination inhibition, complement fixation, and neutralizing antibody, then one can make a presumptive diagnosis on a single sample.[76] In the case of suspected VEE, an ELISA can detect viral-specific immunoglobulin M (IgM) antibodies to surface glycoprotein by 3 days after the onset of clinical signs. These antibodies are not produced in response to vaccine. The antibodies disappear by 21 days after infection.[77] The assay for confirming acute VEE infection should be used when one cannot collect convalescent serum samples. Viral cultures are unlikely to be fruitful, except in the case of acute VEE. One may isolate the virus from CSF of horses with acute infections.[19] The usefulness of CSF viral titers in light of a negative viral isolation is questionable. Fluorescent antibody, ELISA, and viral isolation are useful in identifying virus in brain tissue.[78,79]

Colostral antibodies may interfere with diagnosis in foals. The antibody titers to VEE, WEE, and EEE viruses in the sera of 2- to 8-day-old foals are similar to those of dams. The serum half-life of maternal antibodies in foals is approximately 20 days.[80]

Clinical Pathology The CSF changes associated with togaviral infections are similar to those of other viral encephalitides and include increased cellularity (50-400 mononuclear cells per microliter) and protein concentration (100 to 200 mg/dl).

Necropsy Findings For animals that die or are euthanatized, one should perform necropsy and gross and histologic examinations with special reference to the CNS. With any of the alphaviral equine encephalitides, sufficient viral particles for infection may be present in CNS and other tissues, and one should take precautions when performing a necropsy examination on suspect cases. The brain and spinal cord often have a normal gross appearance. In some cases vascular congestion and discoloration of the CNS is evident. Histologic findings include nonseptic mononuclear cell and neutrophilic inflammation of the entire brain.[18,81-83] Severe lesions are evident in the cerebral cortex, thalamus, and hypothalamus. Specific lesions include significant perivascular cuffing with mononuclear and neutrophil cell infiltration, gliosis, neuronal degeneration, and mononuclear cell meningeal inflammation. With VEE, liquefactive necrosis and hemorrhage of the cerebral cortex, atrophy of the pancreatic acinar cells, and hyperplasia of the pancreatic duct cells commonly occur.[82] Immunohistochemistry can be diagnostic on necropsy samples.[84,85]

Differential Diagnosis The differential diagnosis for EEE, WEE, and VEE should include other conditions associated with diffuse or multifocal neurologic deficits such as other togaviral encephalitides, trauma, hepatoencephalopathy, rabies, leukoencephalomalacia, bacterial meningoencephalitis, EPM, verminous encephalitis, and WNV. Plant and other toxins should also be considered.

TREATMENT

No known effective, specific treatment of the viral encephalitides exists. Treatment is primarily supportive. NSAIDs (phenylbutazone, 4 mg/kg every 12 hours; flunixin meglumine, 1 mg/kg every 12 to 24 hours) control pyrexia, inflammation, and discomfort. DMSO given at 1 g/kg intravenously in a 20% solution may be useful in controlling inflammation and provides some analgesia and mild sedation. The use of corticosteroids is controversial because beneficial effects are short term and the risk of developing secondary bacterial infections increases. One may control convulsions with pentobarbital, 0.05 to 2.2 mg/kg diazepam administered intravenously, 2 mg/kg phenobarbital given orally, or 0.2 to 1.0 mg/kg phenytoin administered intravenously. If horses develop secondary bacterial infections, then one should use appropriate antibiotic therapy. One should monitor hydration and administer balanced fluid solutions orally or intravenously as needed. Other supportive care should include dietary supplementation and administration of laxatives to minimize the risk of gastrointestinal impaction. If anorexia persists for more than 48 hours, then enteral or parenteral supplementation should be used; one can use commercial formulations. For the short term, pelleted feeds may be put into suspension for oral administration. Protection from self-induced trauma may require protective leg wraps and head protection. If the horse is recumbent, then one should attempt to provide support in a sling, and all animals should be bedded heavily.

PROGNOSIS

Complete recoveries from the neurologic deficits associated with these viruses are reported, but they are rare.[84] Animals that have recovered from EEE often have residual neurologic deficits that commonly include ataxia, depression, and abnormal behavior. Neurologic sequelae are similar but less common in horses that recover from WEE. For horses that develop neurologic disease, the mortality rate for EEE is between 75% to 100%; for WEE, 20% to 50%; and for VEE, 40% to 80%.[18,43] If horses recover from any of the diseases, then they seem to be protected variably for up to 2 years after infection. One would wisely assume that infection affords no protection.

PREVENTION

Prevention of alphavirus encphalitis should aim at reducing the concentration of insect vectors and implementing vaccination programs.[35-37,86-90] Most vaccines are killed (formalin inactivated) viruses of chick tissue culture origin. Significant increases in antibody titer occur at 3 days after vaccination.[18,19,89-92] One should vaccinate susceptible horse populations with monovalent, divalent, or trivalent vaccines containing EEE, WEE, or VEE. Administration of trivalent vaccines increases specific antibody production to all viruses. Some cross-protection exists between EEE and WEE and between EEE and VEE, but none exists between WEE and VEE.[80,93,94] If one is to give VEE vaccine, then simultaneous administration of all three vaccines is recommended.[95-97] The response to VEE vaccination alone is poorer in horses previously vaccinated against WEE and EEE.[91,92,96,97] VEE vaccination does not seem to interfere with responses to EEE or WEE vaccination.[98] One should complete annual vaccinations in late spring or several months before the beginning of the encephalitis season. Adequate titers appear to last for 6 to 8 months. In areas in which the mosquito problem is prolonged or continuous, biannual or triannual vaccination is suggested. Vaccination of susceptible horses in the face of an outbreak is recommended. If vaccinated horses develop disease, then the affected individuals are often young or old. Vaccination of mares 1 month before foaling enhances colostral antibody concentrations. Antibody concentrations in foals born to immunized mares appear by 3 hours after colostrum is fed and persist for 6 to 7 months.[80] Vaccination may begin at any age, but if they are vaccinated early, one should revaccinate foals at 6 months and 1 year to ensure adequate protection. Foals respond to vaccination with VEE in utero.[99] A prospective study to determine the serologic response of previously vaccinated horses to revaccination against EEE and WEE identified that horses responded variably to each antigen, and some horses had low or undetectable antibodies 6 months after vaccination. Some horses did not develop increasing titers to EEE or WEE despite recent vaccination. Geometric mean titers peaked 2 weeks after revaccination and were significantly increased from before revaccination.[100]

Owners should use insecticides and repellents when possible and practical, should eliminate standing water, and in endemic areas or during an outbreak should implement environmental insecticide application and should screen stalls. Horses with VEE can be persistently viremic and should be quarantined for 3 weeks after complete recovery. Cases of VEE must be reported to regulatory authorities in the United States. Public health officials may institute other measures of disease control.

MISCELLANEOUS VIRAL ENCEPHALITIDES

California encephalitis is a mosquito-borne disease caused by a group of closely related viruses belonging to the *Orthobunyavirus* genus of the Bunyaviridae family. Snowshoe hare and Jamestown Canyon viruses have been isolated in Canada and California. Snowshoe hare virus is the most widely occurring arbovirus in Canada and is maintained in an amplification cycle involving small mammals and mosquitoes primarily of the *Aedes* genus. Seroconversion without clinical disease is widespread.* One report exists of acute encephalitis with complete recovery in a horse that seroconverted to the snowshoe hare serotype of California encephalitis viruses.[116] Jamestown Canyon virus has been isolated from vesicular lesions in a horse.[117,118]

Main Drain virus, a member of the *Orthobunyavirus* genus of the Bunyaviridae family that is not part of the California encephalitis serogroup, was isolated from the brain of a horse with encephalitis in Sacramento County, California. Signs included incoordination, ataxia, stiffness of the neck, head pressing, dysphagia, fever, and tachycardia. The major vector is *Culicoides variipennis*, which transmits the virus from infected rabbits and rodents.[107] The Cache Valley virus, a member of the *Bunyamweravirus* genus of the Bunyaviridae family, has been isolated from a clinically normal horse; a high seroprevalence exists for this virus among horses in some geographic areas.[115]

St. Louis encephalitis virus is a member of the Flaviviridae family that is associated most commonly with encephalitis in human beings and may rarely be involved in equine disease. Experimental inoculation in horses produces viremia but no clinical signs. Neutralizing antibody is often present. *Culex pipiens* and *C. tarsalis* are the major vectors. Wild birds seem to be the primary reservoir.[29,108-109]

Powassan virus is also a member of the Flaviviridae family and has been associated with nonsuppurative, focal necrotizing meningoencephalitis in horses.[110] Antibodies for Powassan virus commonly are identified in Ontario and the Eastern United States. *Ixodes cookei*, *I. marxi*, and *Dermacentor andersoni* appear to be important vectors, with snowshoe hares and striped skunks as major reservoirs. Zoonoses occur after bites by infected ticks. Approximately 13% of horses sampled across Ontario in 1983 were serologically positive for the virus.[110] Experimental infection with Powassan virus strain M794 in horses was associated with neurologic deficits within 8 days. A nonsuppurative encephalomyelitis, neuronal necrosis, and focal parenchymal necrosis occur. Signs include tremors of the head and neck, ptyalism, myalgia, ataxia, and recumbency. No clinical signs were identified in inoculated rabbits, but widespread encephalitis characterized by lymphoid perivascular cuffing, lymphocytic meningitis, and lymphocytic choroiditis occurred.[45,110]

Experimental infection with Murray Valley virus, a member of the *Flavivirus* genus of the Flaviviridae family, results in transient pyrexia, myalgia, and ataxia. Horses are unlikely to be efficient amplifiers of this virus.[111-113] In Australia, the virus is more commonly a disease of human beings. An epidemic in human beings was associated with significant titers in horses. Some horses with clinical signs, significant titers, and histologic evidence of viral encephalitis were identified.[113,114]

Nipah virus, a member of the *Henipavirus* genus of the Paramyxoviridae family, causes encephalitis in human beings and pigs in Southeast Asia. It is transmitted from bats to pigs, and then spreads horizontally to other pigs and human beings. One anecdotal report exists of dilated meningeal vessels in a horse from which Nipah virus was isolated.[119]

*References 46, 62, 95, 101-106, 115.

Equine encephalosis virus, a member of the *Orbivirus* genus of the Reoviridae family, is an insect borne virus transmitted by a variety of *Culicoides* spp.[120,121] Horses, donkeys, and zebra in Southern Africa are frequently seropositive. The clinical importance of equine encephalosis virus as a cause of neurologic disease in equids appears to be limited despite the fact that it was originally isolated from a horse with clinical neurologic disease. Clinical signs that have been attributed to equine encephalosis virus include fever, depression, edema of the lips, acute neurologic signs, enteritis, and abortion.[122]

Borna disease virus is a member of the *Bornavirus* genus of the Bornaviridae family, a group of enveloped viruses with a nonsegmented, negative sense, single-stranded RNA genome. It is the cause of a naturally occurring, infectious, usually fatal, progressive meningopolioencephalitis that affects horses and sheep most commonly.[122] Less often the virus affects other equids, cattle, goats, rabbits, and possibly human beings. The disease is recognized to date in Germany, Switzerland, Liechtenstein, and Austria. Antibody-positive horses are present in the Middle East, Asia, Australia, and the United States. The route of transmission is unclear but may occur through virus shed in body secretions, gaining entrance to a new host through exposed nerve endings in the nasal and pharyngeal mucosa.[123] Borna disease is caused by a virus-induced immunopathologic reaction.[124] Natural infection in horses results in peracute, acute, or subacute meningoencephalitis leading to death in 1 to 4 weeks in 80% of affected animals. Specific neurologic signs are variable but may include slow-motion eating, chewing motions of the mouth, head pressing, somnolence and stupor, hyperexcitability, fearfulness, aggressiveness, hypokinesia, abnormal posture, hyporeflexia, head tilt, neurogenic torticollis, and inability to swallow. Disease is confirmed serologically by detection of specific antibodies.

Other viruses, identified in areas around the world, that have been implicated in equine encephalitis or that are associated with encephalitis in other species and for which significant titers have been identified in horses include the louping ill,[125,126] Maguari,[29,103,127] Aura,[28,127] Una,[28,127,128] Highlands J,[49,129] Semliki forest,[130] and Getah viruses.[131]

FLAVIVIRUS ENCEPHALITIS

Maureen T. Long

Emergence of new diseases or new outbreaks of previously described diseases are largely the product of globalization and global climate change. This has created an interface of exotic disease and new contacts with people, pests, and animals traveling over unprecedented distances as a result of modern transportation. Before 1999, the U.S. equine practitioner had little familiarity with flaviviruses and horse owners, for the most part, did not even know these diseases existed. After WNV was first identified in the United States, the widespread outbreak in human beings and horses residing in Middle and Northern latitudes of the North American continent was not predicted.[1-3]

This section is adapted from Sellon D and Long MT: Equine Infectious Diseases, St Louis, 2007, WB Saunders.

ETIOLOGY

The family Flaviviridae consists of a pathologically active group of viruses composed of three genera that are found worldwide.[4] The genus *Flavivirus* contains many viruses (approximately 70) that are usually transmitted by either ticks or mosquitoes (some are through direct contact or the vector is unknown) and organized into groups according to cross-neutralization with polyclonal hyperimmune mouse ascites. A quarter of these viruses are of veterinary importance. The other two genera have viruses of veterinary and human importance with the genus *Pestivirus* containing the ubiquitous bovine diarrhea virus (BVD) and *Hepacivirus* containing the human pathogen, hepatitis C virus (HCV). At least half of the members of Flaviviridae are zoonotic.

The members of the Japanese encephalitis (JE) serogroup that are most likely to cause overt disease in horses are JE virus, WNV, and Kunjin virus (KV) (an Australian flavivirus, now considered a variant of WNV).[5] Disease in horses caused by Murray Valley Fever (MVF) is geographically restricted to the South Pacific, and disease in horses is sporadic.[6-8] Other members of this group and those belonging to the other major groups of flaviviruses have been detected serologically in horses with limited reports of clinical disease. The following discussion will emphasize WNV and JE.

All Flaviviridae are positive sense single-stranded RNA viruses measuring approximately 50 nm.[9] The virions are spherical and enveloped with the C protein, making up a nucleocapsid of about 25 nm. Electron microscopy reveals an icosahedral symmetry of the envelope and capsid of these viruses. An approximately 11-kb genome contains a single open reading frame that is translated in its entirety and cleaved into 10 viral proteins by both cell and viral proteases.[10,11] Three structural and seven nonstructural proteins exist; the structural proteins include the capsid (C), premembrane (prM) and membrane (M), and envelop (E) proteins. The nonstructural (NS) proteins, numbered 1 through 5, are cleaved after translation and are required for viral replication and assembly.

The final M protein and the E protein are important for virulence.[12-17] The M protein is formed from a precursor protein (prM protein) that is modified as immature virions are secreted through the Golgi network of the cell. The E protein is only secreted in its native conformation through association with the prM protein. The E protein is the immunodominant viral protein and is important in receptor ligand binding and fusion to host cells.

EPIDEMIOLOGY

LIFE CYCLE

Japanese encephalitis serogroup viruses are vector-borne diseases with transmission occurring to avian and mammalian hosts from blood meal–seeking mosquitoes.[18] Virus is either maintained or cycled between vectors, and biological amplification occurs within the vector species. Vertical transmission within vectors must occur for maintenance of virus within a geographic area.[19] The primary nonarthropod reservoir hosts for these viruses (in which the virus is amplified and transmitted to vectors) are birds. Horses and human beings are dead-end hosts and do not amplify the virus in quantities sufficient to infect mosquitoes. In JE, swine are considered important amplifying hosts. Additional modes of transmission have been identified in the recent North American WNV outbreak. Transmission through oral ingestion in both avian and mammalian hosts has been proven, and oral and cloacal shedding has been demonstrated in birds.[20-24] West Nile virus may also be transmitted through contaminated blood transfusion or organ transplantation if donors are viremic.[25-29] Vertical transmission though placenta and milk has been demonstrated in people.[27,30,31]

RECENT EPIZOOTOLOGY

The largest documented outbreak of equine neurologic disease caused by a flavivirus began in 1999, with WNV encroachment into the United States. WNV was first detected in 1999 in New York City.[32] Since that time, more than 25,000 cases of equine West Nile encephalomyelitis (WNE), with an estimated 30% to 40% case fatality rate have been reported in horses in the United States. Overt clinical disease is still common in most states, with 1338 human cases (43 fatalities) and 218 veterinary cases reported during 2008.

By 2005, WNV had been identified in all of the 48 continental U.S. states.[33] Canadian provinces reporting disease include Quebec, Ontario, Manitoba, Saskatchewan, and Alberta, with New Brunswick and Nova Scotia reporting evidence of WNV–positive birds.[34] Serologic evidence of WNV has been reported in the Latin American countries of the Dominican Republic, Mexico, Guadeloupe, El Salvatore, Puerto Rico, Cayman Islands, Jamaica, Belize, and Cuba.[24,35-40] The incidence of equine and human disease appears low for Central and South America and the Caribbean compared with the United States.[41]

JE virus causes between 30,000 to 50,000 human encephalitis cases annually worldwide, with endemic areas including China, the southeast region of the Russian Federation, South and Southeast Asia, and Australia. Exact numbers of horses with clinical JE are difficult to ascertain; however, reports exist of JE isolation from horses in Taiwan, China, Pakistan, and Australia in the literature since the 1980s. Outbreaks in horses have also been reported in India, Nepal, the Philippines, Sri Lanka, and Northern Thailand. Seroconversion of young horses over their first year of exposure in Hong Kong is as high as 63% in some locales.

The spread and yearly incidence of JE serogroup viruses coincides with the availability of vectors and reservoir hosts with transmission potential. Thus outbreaks are seasonal and reflect mosquito activity. *Culex* spp. of mosquitoes are considered the primary mosquito vector for the JE serogroup.[24,42-45] WNV has been detected in approximately 60 species of North American mosquito, but the overall vector efficiency (moderate to high) and wide range of feeding activity of the *Culex* spp. indicates that the North American WNV outbreak is propelled mainly by this genera.[46] In the Northeastern United States, more than half of the WNV–positive mosquito pools are *Cx. pipiens*.[47-51] In the West, populations of the highly efficient *Cx. tarsalis* constitute the majority of positive pools with *Cx. pipiens* the next most commonly found *Culex* spp.[52-54] In the Southeast, *Cx. quinquefasciatus* and *Cx. nigripalpus* have the highest WNV infection rates.[55-59] In the Southwest, epidemics are most commonly associated with positive mosquito pools of *Cx. quinquefasciatus, Cx. tarsalis,* and *Cx. pipiens*.[60-64]

A reservoir host is one in which a pathogen is amplified in vivo so that it can be transmitted to a vector species.[49] A blood meal taken from a mammal containing 10^5 to 10^7 plaque-forming units (PFU) per millimeter (PFU/ml) of WNV results in infection of 30% to 100% of feeding mosquitoes, respectively. Human beings (voluntarily infected with the Egyptian strain of WNV) developed virus titers of 10^3 to 10^5 PFU/ml. In horses, the maximal titer after infection with this strain was similar.[65] Horses and human beings are considered dead-end (nonreservoir) hosts for WNV.

Viral titers capable of transmitting JE are similar to WNV. Swine are a notable reservoir host for JE (with little indication that the same is true for WNV here in the United States). The primary clinical manifestation of JE infection in swine is abortion. Affected litters contain weak pigs (which die soon after birth), dead fresh term fetuses, or mummies. Semen from infected boars contains infectious virus, and the semen has decreased sperm count and motility.

To date, more than 300 species of birds have been reported WNV-positive in the United States with 16 new species identified during the recent 2005 season.[66] High levels of viral amplification occur in many birds species (118), especially Passeriformes (e.g., songbirds) and Charadriiformes (e.g., shorebirds); the house sparrow and the American robin are considered two of the most important amplifying hosts for WNV. Although the crow is one of the most competent vectors, sparrows and robins have a lower mortality and hence longer days of infectious viremia. Strigiformes (owls) and Falconiformes (e.g., falcons) develop a viremia of shorter duration (but sufficient to infect mosquitoes). Psittaciformes (e.g., parrots) and Galliformes (e.g., game birds) develop the lowest viremias. By contrast, Anseriformes (e.g., waterfowl) are considered the most efficient avian reservoirs of JE and are essential for the spread of this virus through avian flyways.

Because transmission of JE serogroup viruses is via vectors, disease because of JE and WNV in horses and human beings is seasonal in temperate regions and year-round in subtropical regions. Intense virus activity in the United States begins in July, with a peak incidence in September and October.[67-70] A drop in ambient temperature with soft frost usually results in a rapid decrease in reporting activity.[71,72]

Older people appear more susceptible to neuroinvasive disease from both JE and WNV. This age bias in reporting appears true, at least for WNV, in horses.[24,73-77] Although men are more frequently affected with neuroinvasive disease, there appears to be no breed or gender predilection in horses. In one study of horses with WNV encephalomyelitis, female horses were 2.9 times more likely to die than male horses with neurologic signs.[78-80]

The remarkably explosive North American outbreak of WNV has introduced new potential hosts for the virus. Seropositive, free-ranging mammals include the big brown bat, little brown bat, eastern chipmunk, eastern gray squirrel, eastern striped skunk, white-tailed deer, and the brown bear.[24,49,66,81] Neurologic disease has been confirmed as WNV in gray squirrels and fox squirrels.[82,83] Alligators can have an extremely high titer of viremia and may be an important reservoir for WNV in the Southeast.[84] Reports exist of both farmed and free-ranging alligators with neurologic signs from which WNV has been isolated. In farm-raised alligators, cloacal shedding of virus has been demonstrated with oral infection likely.

Serologic evidence of natural infection has been demonstrated in domestic dogs and cats.[21] Experimental infection of cats resulted in a mild transient fever in some cats and a short-term viremia high enough to possibly transmit to mosquitoes. Oral transmission to cats has also been documented. New world camelids develop neurologic disease with natural exposure to WNV.[85,86]

PATHOGENESIS

Mammalian disease because of infection with the JE serogroup viruses uniformly demonstrates predilection of these viruses for nervous tissues. Neurologic disease in the horse consists of changes in mentation, signs consistent with spinal cord abnormalities, and defects in cranial nerves of the hindbrain.[87-97] The change in behavior is likely the result of viral infection and pathology induced in the neurons of the thalamus, medulla, and pons, with limited viral load in the cerebrum.[89,90,98] Although the thalamus integrates all sensory input to higher centers, lesions within the midbrain and rostral pons may affect the reticular formation, which has an important role in regulation of consciousness.[97,99] The reticular formation projects to the thalamus, which in turn sends diffuse projections to the entire cortex.[97] This formation also travels directly to the base of the forebrain, which is the source of cholinergic stimulation to the entire cerebral cortex. Disturbances of the reticular formation and the midbrain may induce behavioral changes ranging from severe aggression to somnolence and even coma.

WNV-induced motor deficits are multifocal, asymmetrical, and primarily characterized by weakness and ataxia.[89-91,98,100-102] These two clinical signs are likely a reflection of brain and spinal cord disease through direct infection of the spinal cord, interruption of motor tracts in the hindbrain, and loss of fine motor control through infection of the large nuclei of the thalamus and the basal ganglia. Ataxia can be attributable to interruption of general proprioception. Although ataxia is commonly detected and could be profound, many horses have difficulty standing primarily because of profound weakness. These clinical signs are attributable to infection of the gray matter within the midbrain and hindbrain. In some reports there appears to be with increasing severity in spinal cord lesions proceeding caudally.[101] Lower motor neuron disease characterized by weakness would be a common clinical sign associated with these spinal cord lesions.

Involuntary skin and muscle fasciculations, tremors, and hyperesthesia, extremely common in this disease, likely results from loss of fine motor control, which is regulated mainly by the basal ganglia.[103,104] Movement disorders are detected with flavivirus infection in a long-term Parkinson-like syndrome in rats and experimental infection in monkeys.[104] Infection in the pons and medulla oblongata can explain clinical deficits of CN VII, XII, and IX.[105]

In mammalian hosts, the actual virus load in neuronal tissues is low, indicating the possibility of another mechanism for severe neurologic clinical signs. Although cell lysis occurs with viral replication, WNV also induces apoptosis in neurons as demonstrated in cell culture and in vivo.[106] This apoptosis can be induced by the capsid protein through the caspase-9 pathway in the mitochondria. Another mediator of neuronal injury is the host immune response. Although CD8 T cells may be important in long-term protective immune responses, lesions in brains of mice with fatal WNV are predominantly composed of CD8+ T cells.[107,108]

CLINICAL FINDINGS

JE and WNV produce similar clinical signs, except that fatal JE infection in horses commonly results in blindness, coma, and death, whereas these signs are relatively limited in WNV horses.[109,110] For both these viruses, evidence exists of widespread subclinical infection in both people and horses. Horses develop clinical signs when infected with the neurally invasive lineage type I WNV, whereas infection with the African lineage type II viruses is universally subclinical in nature.[111,112] Infection with JE virus may result in severe clinical disease in naïve horses, but a great deal of variation is seen in virulence in JE viruses.

When clinically apparent disease occurs, both systemic and neurologic abnormalities are observed in horses with WNV. A mild to moderate increase in rectal temperature (38.6° to 39.4° C), anorexia and depression are the most common initial systemic signs.[87] Abdominal pain is not an uncommon initial presenting complaint.[87,90,113,114] Gait abnormalities, including overt lameness or dragging of a limb before development of an obvious neurologic syndrome, have also been reported. Both spinal cord disease and moderate mental aberrations occur. Onset of neurologic signs is frequently sudden and progressive, and the exact course of disease in any one animal is unpredictable.

The major hallmarks of equine WNV encephalomyelitis are muscle fasciculations and changes in personality. Many horses have periods of hyperexcitability and apprehension, sometimes to the point of aggression. Frequently a quiet horse will become hyperexcitable, and an abnormally aggressive horse will become compliant. Interspersed during periods of hyperexcitability, some horses appear to have abnormalities of sudden sleeplike activity resembling narcolepsy. This can occur to the point of cataplexy, and horses may partially or completely collapse for a short period of time. In some horses a change of mentation is persistent and a state of nonresponsiveness, resembling coma, results.

Fine and coarse fasciculations of the muscles of the face and neck are very common. Fasciculations can be quite severe and involve all four limbs and trunk, affecting normal activities such as walking, eating, and interactions with handlers and other horses. The fasciculations are most notable at the muzzle and eyelids. Eyelid activity during this period is enhanced with light and at times it appears that horses are quite photophobic.

One of the initial signs of motor abnormality is a short, slow, stilted gait described by observers as *lameness* (laminitis being a frequent differential diagnosis at this stage). However, in human patients, bradykinesia or slow, deliberate movement is frequently described, and this may be the equine corollary.[115] Spinal abnormalities are characterized by ataxia and paresis that can be highly asymmetrical or involve only one or two of the front limbs or hindlimbs. This may be of short duration, or horses may become suddenly recumbent and either die or require prolonged treatment. Horses that become recumbent often need aggressive supportive care.

Cranial nerves are frequently abnormal for short periods of time; weakness of the tongue, muzzle deviation, and head tilt are the most common abnormalities reported. Dysphagia has been reported with choke as a sequelae. A cauda equine syndrome consisting of stranguria and rectal impaction is infrequently reported.

Overall, the combination, severity, and duration of clinical signs can be highly variable. After initial signs abate, about 30% of clinical horses experience a recrudescence in clinical signs within the first 7 to 10 days of apparent recovery. Irrespective of recrudescence, about 30% of affected horses progress to complete paralysis of one or more limbs overall. Most of these horses are euthanized for humane reasons or die spontaneously.

Many horses will improve within 3 to 7 days of displaying clinical signs. If the horse demonstrates significant improvement, then full recovery within 1 to 6 months can be expected in 90% of patients. Residual weakness and ataxia appear are common with long-term loss of the use of one or more limbs infrequently described. Mild to moderate persistent fatigue on exercise has been observed.

DIAGNOSIS OF WEST NILE VIRUS

Ancillary diagnostic testing for horses with suspected WNV infection should include CBC, serum biochemistry analysis, and CSF analysis.[116,117] CBC and serum biochemistry profiles of West Nile virus–infected horses are usually normal. Horses may have a mild absolute lymphopenia. Horses can have elevated muscle enzymes secondary to trauma and prolonged periods of recumbency. A frequent finding is hyponatremia, which has also been described in human beings with encephalitis, potentially caused by inappropriate release of antidiuretic hormone.[118,119] CSF cell counts and protein concentration may be elevated. Differential cell counts in CSF of West Nile virus–infected horses are consistently increased, primarily because of increased mononuclear cell populations; in contrast, the most numerous cells in the CSF of horses with EEE are neutrophils, especially during the initial stages of disease.[117]

No pathognomic signs distinguish WNV infection in horses from other CNS diseases and a full diagnostic evaluation should be pursued. Infectious CNS diseases that should be considered as differential diagnoses include alphavirus encephalitis, rabies, EPM, EHV-1, botulism, and verminous meningoencephalomyelitis (e.g., *Halicephalobus gingivalis*, *Setaria* spp., *Strongylus vulgaris*). Noninfectious causes to consider include hypocalcemia, tremorgenic toxicities, hepatoencephalopathy, and leukoencephalomalacia. In alphavirus encephalitis and rabies, signs of cerebral involvement are characterized by behavioral alterations, depression, seizure, and coma. The appearance of seizure and coma is rare in WNV horses. Motor function is frequently abnormal in EEE and WEE. In WNV suspects, circling and propulsive walking may occur, but head pressing is rare. Cranial nerve signs common in EEE and WEE are common in WNV and include head tilt, pharyngeal and laryngeal dysfunction, and paresis of the tongue. Other clinical signs of alphavirus encephalitis that are observed with WNV infection are muscle fasciculations, hyperesthesia, excitability, blindness, somnolence, weakness of the tongue, and progression to recumbency. Differentiation of WNV from rabies is quite problematic, because clinical signs in horses with rabies frequently include ataxia, weakness, or gait abnormalities. Alphaviruses, rabies, *H. gingivalis* infection, hepatoencephalopathy, and leukoencephalomalacia are rapidly progressive with cortical signs. Although periods of somnolence, blindness, and some cranial nerve deficits occur, WNV horses appear to become rapidly recumbent or stabilize over several days. Spinal disease caused by EPM is a more difficult differential diagnosis if horses with WNV are not febrile and do not exhibit excessive muscle fasciculations. Both diseases demonstrate hindbrain disease with diffuse spinal cord abnormalities.

Confirmation of WNV infection with encephalitis in horses begins with assessment of whether or not a horse meets the case definition based on clinical signs, as well as whether or not the horse resides in an area in which WNV has been confirmed in the current calendar year in mosquitoes, birds, human beings, or horses.[100] Serologic testing developed by the National Veterinary Services Laboratory (NVSL) is based on detection of the IgM antibody response that uniformly occurs in acutely infected horses. The preferred test is an IgM capture ELISA (MAC-ELISA).[120] Horses develop a very intense IgM response on exposure to WNV that lasts approximately 6 weeks. This immunologic reaction is much more reliable than in human infection in which a more persistent IgM response is common. Most diagnostic laboratories use the WNV IgM capture ELISA (MAC) for actual confirmation of disease (increases in IgM rarely occur after vaccination). The sensitivity and specificity of this test is 81% and 100%, respectively.

In the nonvaccinated horse, a fourfold change in paired neutralizing antibody titers is confirmatory of a diagnosis of WNV infection. The most common neutralizing antibody test formats are the classic plaque reduction neutralizing antibody response (PRNT) and a more recently developed microwell format.[88,100,120,121] Vaccination induces formation of neutralizing antibody that likely confounds interpretation of the PRNT. Since 2001 reliance on the PRNT for serologic confirmatory diagnosis of WNV in horses has diminished because of widespread vaccination.

Other methods for confirmation of a diagnosis of WNV include postmortem detection of WNV by PCR, culture, and immunohistochemistry in tissues of the CNS. Nested PCR targeting the E protein has demonstrated sensitivity for relatively low viral load in equine tissues.[122,123] Real-time PCR methodology has been used to detect WNV in equine tissues.[123] The E-protein target appears less sensitive; however, the NS5 target has detected WNV nucleic acids in CNS tissues, heart, and intestine of clinically affected horses.

DIAGNOSIS OF JAPANESE ENCEPHALITIS

JE should be suspected in horses with compatible clinical signs that reside in an area of virus activity. Diagnostic confirmatory tests include serologic assays such as neutralizing, complement fixation, hemagglutination inhibition, and ELISA tests.[124-126] All single sera testing, including IgM assays, must be interpreted with caution in horses from areas with other endemic flaviviruses. In fatal JE cases, viral isolation, PCR assays, and immunohistochemistry for detection of virus in CNS tissues is confirmatory.

PATHOLOGIC FINDINGS

Gross pathologic findings are limited in WNV infection in the horse. The meninges may be congested. Small- to moderate-sized foci of hemorrhagic discoloration may be observed in the brain, spinal cord, or both. These areas occur most commonly in the basal ganglia, rostral colliculus, pons, medulla, and lumbar spinal cord. Edema and softening of tissues are also common findings.

Flaviviruses cause polioencephalomyelitis (inflammation of the gray matter) with lesions that increase in number from the diencephalon through the hindbrain and frequently increase in severity caudally through the spinal cord.* By contrast, these lesions are limited in the cortex and cerebellum. The basal ganglia, thalamus, pons, and medulla have the highest numbers of lesions with two to several cell layers of mononuclear perivascular cuffing. Most of the horses that are euthanatized with WNV have histological lesions that predominate in the gray matter with inflammatory foci within the midbrain and hindbrain and increasing severity caudally through the spinal cord. Neuronal damage includes chromatolytic neurons and neuronophagia. In long-standing disease, areas of neuronal dropout may exist. In the spinal cord, perivascular cuffing, gliosis, and damaged neurons may be seen. The inflammation associated with the neuropil is confined primarily to the gray matter.

*References 89, 91, 92, 95, 96, 127-131.

THERAPY

No known antiviral medications are marketed that demonstrate reliable activity against flaviviruses, thus treatment of disease is supportive.[87,90,132,133,134] In horses, the survival rate for WNV encephalitis is high compared with other infectious encephalitides. In most cases horses appear to begin recovery between 3 and 5 days after onset of signs. This fact makes it difficult to accurately assess the effect of any pharmacologic intervention when a feature of analysis is resolving clinical disease. Flunixin meglumine (1.1 mg/kg IV q12h) early in the course of the disease appears to decrease the severity of muscle tremors and fasciculations within a few hours of administration.

To date, much of the mortality in WNV horses results from euthanasia of recumbent horses for humane reasons. Recumbent horses are mentally alert and frequently thrash, sustaining many self-inflicted wounds and posing risk to personnel. Therapy of recumbent horses is generally more aggressive and may include dexamethasone sodium (0.05 to 0.1 mg/kg IV every 24 hours) and mannitol (0.25 to 2.0 gm/kg IV every 24 hours). Controversy remains as to whether corticosteroids enhance peripheral and CNS viral load.[135-138] Detomidine hydrochloride (0.02 to 0.04 mg/kg IV or IM) is effective for prolonged tranquilization. Low doses of acepromazine (0.02 mg/kg IV or 0.05 mg/kg IM) provide excellent relief from anxiety in both recumbent and standing horses. Until EPM is ruled out or WNV is confirmed, prophylactic therapy with antiprotozoal medications is recommended for horses in geographic areas where *Sarcocystis neurona* infection is prevalent. Other supportive measures may include oral and intravenous fluids and antibiotics for treatment of infections that frequently occur in recumbent horses (wounds, cellulitis, and pneumonia).

A variety of treatments has been recommended for horses with WNV; however, limited evidence exists to support their efficacy at this time.[1,139-143] The recommendation for interferon alpha (IFN-α) therapy is based on anecdotal reports in the human and veterinary literature. Limited information regarding efficacy in the horse is available. In a blinded study in which children with encephalitis because of JE were treated with IFN-α, survival was not enhanced. In fact, length of hospitalization was increased in the IFN-α treated group.

Therapy with intravenous WNV-specific immunoglobulin (Ig) has also been recommended. In a blinded placebo-controlled trial with low numbers of animals, the risk for development of recumbency was less in horses receiving plasma from horses immunized against WNV.[144] However, plasma treatment did not change outcome and severity of WNV disease. In human patients, high-dose glutamate therapy has been suggested to prevent neuronal cell death. Another experimental therapy in mice is administration of β-lactam inhibitors that stimulate GLT1, a chemical that activates glutamate.

PREVENTION

Epidemiological, experimental, and anecdotal evidence exists regarding the effectiveness of vaccination against flaviviruses.[145] Initial epidemiologic studies performed in 2000 established a point source for infection of WNV, demonstrating that outbreaks in horses may best be controlled by vaccination.[146-148] This finding was consistent with prior experience with JE, in which vaccines were advocated for horses before the WNV epizootic. Presently, four vaccines are licensed for prevention of WNV viremia in the United States. As of 2005 at least three vaccines are available for vaccination of horses against JE.[149-153] Vaccination before the mosquito season is critical. Manufacturer's labeling instructions must be followed for induction of immunity with initial immunization. All available vaccines are labeled for administration every 12 months after the initial series; however, only the modified live chimera vaccine has published 12-month efficacy data.[154] More frequent vaccination in areas with year-round mosquito seasons is recommended for most vaccines because it is not expected that the initial vaccine series will provide long-term protection, especially with killed virus vaccines with which antibody levels rapidly decrease after 4 to 6 months. Where these viruses are endemic, vaccination schedules should be maintained even when a decrease in the incidence of overt disease exists. This is evidenced by the persistence of reports of JE disease in naïve horses after introduction into endemic areas. Horses that have recovered from clinical disease have long-term immunity and should not require annual boosters.

PUBLIC HEALTH CONSIDERATIONS

West Nile virus is considered a zoonotic disease. A bird reservoir maintains the virus in an endemic life cycle in the environment, allowing for transmission by mosquitoes to human beings. Little risk exists of disease by direct contact with an infected horse, except during postmortem examination with inappropriate handling of infected tissues. The ecology of horse pastures and stables with standing water, a high degree of biological debris, and "bridge" vectors that feed on mammalian populations likely increase the risk of exposure in that environment. The same types of management tactics for prevention of disease in horses are important for human beings, except that no vaccine is available. Personal mosquito protection with a DEET-based product is recommended in areas with endemic disease.

The North American epidemic of WNV has demonstrated new modes of transmission including blood-borne and occupational risks. Blood-borne transmission can occur between viremic hosts. In addition, occupational infection has occurred through necropsy of avian hosts. Veterinarians and horse owners should institute personal protection with appropriate clothing, gloves, and eye protection when coming into contact with animal tissues during the arbovirus season.

RABIES

Carla S. Sommardahl

EPIDEMIOLOGY AND PATHOGENESIS

Rabies is an uncommon disease in equids, but because of its zoonotic potential, one should consider it in the differential diagnosis for horses showing neurologic signs lasting less than 10 days. In the United States during 2006, 547 cases of rabies were reported in domestic animals, with 53 of these being in horses and mules.[1]

The rabies virus is a large, cylindric, bullet-shaped neurotropic rhabdovirus (genus *Lyssavirus,* family Rhabdoviridae).[2] Rhabdoviruses are enveloped with single-stranded RNA. They are heat-labile and are susceptible to degradation by radiation, strong acids, alkalis, most disinfectants, lipid solvents, and anionic solvents.[2,3] Rabies virus is transmitted by saliva-contaminated wounds. In the horse the most common method of infection is a bite wound from a wild carnivore or insectivorous bat carrying the virus.[4] The most common reservoir hosts in the United States are skunks, raccoons, and the red fox.[2] However, domestic dogs, cats, and other horses may transmit rabies to horses by bite wounds. Furthermore, rabies virus can be transmitted by droplet inhalation, orally, or transplacentally. Droplet transmission has been reported to have occurred in foxes, coyotes, opossums, and raccoons in a bat cave in Texas. In that report the virus was isolated from the air in the cave.[5] Aerosolization of the virus also caused an outbreak of rabies in a laboratory. Transplacental transmission of the virus has occurred in naturally infected cattle and experimentally infected mice and bats.[2]

Rabies virus infects and replicates in myocytes at the inoculation site and may remain undetectable for weeks or months before moving centrally. The virus infects peripheral nerves by traversing neuromuscular and neurotendinous spindles. Progression along the nerve is thought to occur in the tissue spaces of the nerve fasciculus.[5] After progressing centripetally up the peripheral nerve by axoplasmic flow, the virus replicates in spinal and dorsal root ganglia of the corresponding peripheral nerve. Once the virus reaches the CNS, spread occurs rapidly through multiplication in neurons of the brain, spinal cord, sympathetic trunk, and glial cells. Spread of rabies virus also can occur through passive transport within CSF or blood.[2-4] Finally, the virus reaches tissues outside the CNS via centrifugal movement of the virus along nerve axons.[2,3]

The incubation period for rabies varies between 9 days to 1 year in horses. The incubation period can be affected by the virus strain, host species, inoculum size, and proximity of the inoculation site to the CNS.[2,4] Retention of virus in myocytes at the inoculation site may be a mechanism for variation in the incubation period. A shorter incubation period also may be explained by the virus entering peripheral nerves soon after exposure and rapidly migrating centripetally to the CNS without replication in nonneural tissue.[2]

CLINICAL SIGNS

No signs are pathognomonic for rabies infection in horses. Clinical signs on presentation vary and range from lameness to sudden death.[6-9] Hyperesthesia, ataxia, behavior change, 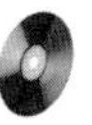

anorexia, paralysis or paresis, and colic have been reported as initial clinical signs.[6-11] One rarely finds a bite wound, and the horse may or may not be febrile. The site of inoculation and its proximity to the CNS influence what clinical signs one observes.[2,7,8] The neurologic signs exhibited in rabies-infected horses can be classified into three forms, depending on the neuroanatomic location in the CNS infected by the virus. First, in the cerebral or furious form, one may see aggressive behavior, photophobia, hydrophobia, hyperesthesia, straining, muscular tremors, and convulsions.[12] Second, in the brainstem or dumb form, one commonly sees depression, anorexia, head tilt, circling, ataxia, dementia, excess salivation, facial and pharyngeal paralysis, blindness, flaccid tail and anus, urinary incontinence, and self-mutilation.[10,12,13] Finally, in the paralytic or spinal form, one sees progressing ascending paralysis, ataxia, or shifting lameness with hyperesthesia, and self-mutilation of an extremity.[11-14] Most affected animals with the paralytic form become recumbent in 3 to 5 days, with normal eating and drinking often remaining.[13] The neurologic signs may vary as the virus spreads to other portions of the CNS. Thus horses may have clinical signs of two or all forms of rabies. Disease progresses rapidly, and death is usually inevitable regardless of the clinical manifestation. Anti-inflammatory therapy can delay virus progression,[12] but death usually occurs within 5 to 10 days after onset of clinical signs.[9,13]

DIAGNOSIS

Antemortem diagnosis of rabies is difficult, but one should consider the disease in horses showing rapidly progressing or diffuse neurologic signs. Other diseases that one should consider include hepatoencephalopathy, togaviral encephalitis, protozoal encephalomyelitis, nigropallidal encephalomalacia, botulism, lead poisoning, cauda equina neuritis, meningitis, space-occupying mass, trauma to the brain or spinal cord, and esophageal obstruction.[3,5,13] Clinical laboratory data of body fluids are nonspecific. CSF may be within normal reference range or may show a moderate increase in total protein concentration (60 to 200 mg/dl) and a pleocytosis (5 to 200 mg/dl).[3,5,13] Fluorescent antibody testing of tactile hair follicles of facial skin taken on biopsy or corneal epithelium may help diagnose rabies ante mortem. The fluorescent antibody technique detects the rabies virus antigen in these tissues. Unfortunately, a negative test does not exclude rabies as a differential diagnosis.[9] One can achieve definitive postmortem diagnosis by submitting half the brain in 10% formaldehyde for histologic examination and the other half frozen to a public health diagnostic laboratory for immunofluorescent antibody tests, mouse inoculation, and monoclonal antibody techniques. The whole brain may be shipped unfrozen on ice for further rabies evaluation and testing. One should examine the rest of the carcass only with careful precautions against transmission of the virus, if present, by wearing gloves, caps, and masks until a negative rabies diagnosis is made.

Common histopathologic changes are a mild, nonsuppurative encephalomyelitis; perivascular cuffing by mononuclear cells; gliosis; glial nodules; and neuronal degeneration.[3,13] These lesions occur most commonly in the hippocampus, brainstem, cerebellum, and gray matter of the spinal cord. Large intracytoplasmic eosinophilic inclusions within neurons and ganglion cells, known as *Negri bodies,* are pathognomonic for rabies.[2,3,13] However, in 15% to 30% of confirmed rabies cases, Negri bodies are not present in histopathologic sections, especially if the animal died or was euthanized early in the disease process.[2] The most commonly used and fastest diagnostic test for rabies is the fluorescent antibody test. This technique may identify 98% of infected brain specimens. The mouse inoculation test is the most accurate method for diagnosing rabies virus infection but requires 5 to 6 days to complete. The mouse inoculation test involves the injection of suspect brain or salivary gland tissue homogenates intracerebrally in mice and observation of clinical and neurologic signs or death.[2,3] The monoclonal antibody test has been used most recently for rabies diagnosis in horses. The test can differentiate specific street, fixed, or vaccinal strains of rabies virus by their glycoprotein or nucleocapsid antigens.[2] This is important in postexposure vaccination of human beings and animals when using the specific strain of virus.

TREATMENT AND PREVENTION

No specific treatment exists for rabies in horses. Symptomatic treatment and supportive care may help prolong the disease course to complete diagnostics and to rule out other diseases with similar signs. Prolonging the course, however, creates a risk of exposure to handlers and other animals. Therefore one should isolate any animal suspected of having rabies and should handle it as little as possible. Horses that are known to have been exposed to rabies should have all wounds cleaned and lavaged with iodine or quaternary ammonium disinfectant (and rabies antiserum, if available, infiltrated around the bite wound).[3,13] No postexposure protocol exists for unvaccinated or vaccinated horses. However, exposed horses should be quarantined for 6 months and observed for the occurrence of neurologic signs. Unvaccinated horses should not receive postexposure prophylaxis until after the 6 months of quarantine. Currently, the American Association of Equine Practitioners recommends that all horses in the United States be vaccinated against rabies. Available vaccines are inactivated tissue culture–derived products with an adjuvant. Foals from vaccinated mares should be vaccinated no earlier than 6 months of age. The second dose of vaccine should be given 4 to 6 weeks after the first. A third dose should be given at 10 to 12 months of age. The first dose of vaccine should be given to foals from unvaccinated mares at 3 to 4 months of age. A second dose should be given at 10 to 12 months of age. Adult horses should receive annual revaccination. Pregnant mares may be vaccinated annually before breeding or 4 to 6 weeks before foaling.

EQUINE MOTOR NEURON DISEASE

Yvette S. Nout

Equine motor neuron disease is an acquired neurodegenerative disease of adult horses that has been reported in North and South America, Japan, and Europe.[1-9] Lower motor neuron disease was recognized in 1988 based on histologic changes in skeletal muscle,[10] and EMND was first described in 1990.[1] In the 1990s, EMND was recognized worldwide in an apparently increasing frequency[3,11]; however, recently the number of EMND cases appears to be decreasing.[9] The decrease may be the result of preventive management measures taken for horses at risk of developing the disease.

The disease affects primarily the motor neurons in the spinal cord ventral horn cells and brainstem and leads to characteristic clinical signs, including generalized neuromuscular weakness and neurogenic muscle atrophy.[1,2,5,12] EMND closely resembles human motor neuron disease, which is known as *amyotrophic lateral sclerosis (ALS)* or Lou Gehrig disease.[1,13] However, EMND only affects the lower motor neurons, which is not the case in ALS. A chronic lack of antioxidants is implicated in the pathogenesis of this disease.

CLINICAL SIGNS

EMND occurs in adult horses with a mean age of onset of clinical signs of 9 years (range of 2 to 23 years).[14] The risk for EMND increases with age, peaking at around 15 years.[15] Quarter Horses appear at increased risk for developing EMND; however, this may reflect management factors.[2,15] No gender predilection is apparent.

Clinical signs vary depending on the stage or duration of the disease. Currently, a subacute and a chronic form are recognized.[9]

SUBACUTE FORM

During the early phase of EMND, trembling, muscle fasciculations, base-narrow stance, shifting of weight in the rear limbs, abnormal sweating, excessive recumbency, muscle atrophy, and weight loss despite a normal or even ravenous appetite are the most characteristic clinical signs (Figure 12-42).[1,2,6,8,9] Ataxia is not a clinical sign of EMND. A horse with EMND moves better than it stands.[2,8] Muscle wasting is most noticeable in the quadriceps, triceps, and gluteal areas. In more than 50% of cases, horses may display a lower than normal head carriage with muscle wasting of the cervical musculature (hangdog appearance).[8] Onset of muscle wasting may occur for approximately 1 month before the acute onset of clinical signs.

CHRONIC FORM

Owners may present horses for poor performance, gait abnormalities (stringhalt-like movement), and failure to gain weight. Trembling and muscle fasciculations are not pronounced in the chronic form of EMND. Horses with the chronic form of EMND are often horses that have stabilized from the subacute form; however, some horses develop the chronic form without experiencing the subacute form. Muscle atrophy varies from mild to severe, and some horses may appear emaciated.[1,8,9]

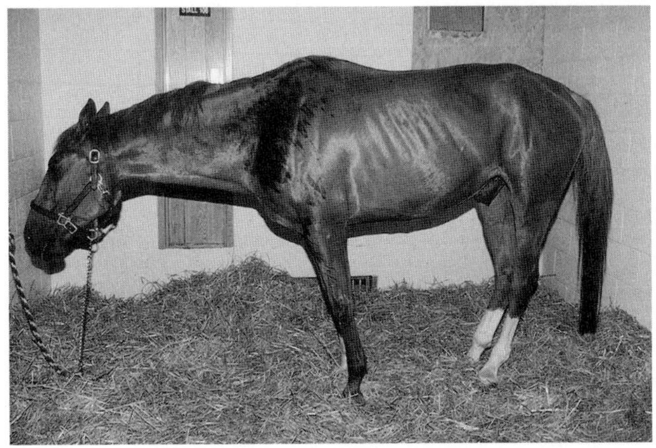

FIGURE 12-42 Characteristic appearance of a horse with equine motor neuron disease (EMND), including muscle wasting, sweating, base-narrow stance, low head carriage (hangdog appearance), and tailhead elevation.

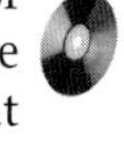

SUBCLINICAL FORM

Experimental evidence indicates that horses may develop a subclinical form of EMND, which may affect performance and safety.[8,9] In the subacute and chronic forms of EMND, the tailhead often is elevated because of denervation atrophy and fibrotic contracture of the sacrococcygeus dorsalis medialis muscle.[6,8,9] In approximately 30% of cases, ophthalmoscopic examination may reveal a distinctive retinopathy with a mosaic pattern of brown pigment deposition in the fundus. These horses are not necessarily visually impaired.[16,17]

PATHOLOGIC FINDINGS

Gross necropsy findings in EMND include diffuse muscle atrophy and pallor (especially of the intermediate vastus and medial head of the triceps muscles). The CNS and peripheral nerves are grossly normal. Histologically, one may detect noninflammatory neuronal degeneration and neuronal loss at all levels of the spinal cord, but such loss is most obvious in the cervical and lumbar intumescence. One finds the lesions in the ventral horn cells (lower motor neurons) of the spinal cord gray matter; the nuclei of cranial nerves V, VII, and XII in the brainstem; and the nucleus ambiguus. Secondary axonal degeneration with loss of myelinated fibers because of dysfunction or death of these motor neurons is present in the ventral spinal roots; spinal nerves; cranial nerves V, VII, IX (sometimes), and XII; and peripheral motor nerves.[1,12] Peripheral motor nerve degeneration also may be evident on antemortem muscle biopsy.[18]

Skeletal muscle changes include nonspecific myopathic changes such as excessive fiber size variation, internal nuclei, and cytoarchitectural alterations. Scattered fiber degeneration and necrosis is a consistent finding in EMND. Atrophy of type I and type II muscle fibers occurs in severely affected muscles in EMND and is pathognomonic of denervation atrophy.[1,12,13] EMND predominantly affects type I fibers, in contrast to denervating diseases in other species, and has not been reported in ALS. Motor neurons supplying the type I fibers have a higher oxidative activity and thus may be more susceptible to oxidative injury.[12] Similar to ALS, in which at least 30% of motor axons must be destroyed before clinical evidence of atrophy occurs, in horses with muscle wasting caused by EMND, a mean motor neuron loss of 31% was recorded.[19]

A pigment retinopathy may be visible, as well as deposition of lipopigment in the endothelial capillaries of the spinal cord. These findings have been reported in other animals with vitamin-E deficiency.[16,17] Besides the abnormalities in the neuromuscular system, no other pathologic findings have been found consistently in horses with EMND.

PATHOGENESIS

The clinical signs of neuromuscular weakness result from the generalized denervation muscle atrophy found in horses with EMND. The pathogenesis of the neuron damage and death in EMND is not understood fully but is thought to result from free radical damage. EMND occurs sporadically and affects horses of all ages and breeds. Therefore infectious agents or environmental toxins are less likely to be a cause of the disease.[2]

A chronic vitamin E deficiency is thought to be the most important factor in the development of EMND based on the fact that affected horses consistently have low plasma vitamin E concentrations and have not had access to pasture or green forages for a prolonged time.[2,11,15,20] Vitamin E concentrations in the CNS, peripheral nerves, muscle, liver, and adipose tissue have been found to be correlated to blood concentrations.[9] Horses generally have been on the same premises for more than 2 years before developing clinical signs.[15] The type I muscle fiber atrophy and the lipopigment deposition in the capillaries of the spinal cord are pathologic findings suggesting an oxidative type of injury as a cause of the neuronal death.[13] The pigment retinopathy found in approximately 30% of cases, and the lipopigment deposition in the vasculature of the spinal cord occurs in other species and is related to a vitamin E deficiency.[8,16]

EDM, another neurodegenerative disease in horses, also is associated with a vitamin E deficiency; however, the CNS lesions in EDM are different from those in EMND. Vitamin E–deficient adult horses have been suggested to develop EMND after a transitory period of triggering events such as exposure to neurotoxins or excessive amounts of pro-oxidants.[2,9] So far a neurotoxin has not been identified. The presence of pro-oxidants such as copper and iron in spinal cord, liver, and plasma has been investigated but has not been confirmed to play a role in the development of EMND.[9,21]

Although EMND is the only naturally occurring model for ALS[13] and oxidative injury is implicated in the cause of both diseases, some important differences exist between the two.[6,12,13] In contrast to EMND, in which the disease process is limited to the lower motor neurons, ALS affects upper and lower motor neurons. Only mild degeneration of the pyramidal tracts is present in horses with EMND, but the pyramidal tracts in horses are less extensive and poorly developed compared with human beings. ALS is familial in approximately 10% of cases, and 20% of patients with familial ALS carry a mutation of the Cu/Zn superoxide dismutase 1 gene.[22] This metalloenzyme is one of the principal oxygen-derived free radical scavengers and protectants against oxidant injury to the nervous system. The mutation of this gene leads to an altered form of the enzyme that is actively toxic to cells.[23] In these patients the quantity of oxidants is increased, whereas in horses with EMND, a lack of antioxidants is the presumed cause of neuronal degeneration and death.[2,24] Mutations in the Cu/Zn superoxide dismutase 1 gene have not been found in EMND.[25] The cause of spontaneously occurring ALS is unknown; however, the similarities between familial ALS and spontaneous ALS suggest a common pathway for neuronal death.[13] The question of why the disease affects motor neurons so selectively has not been answered thus far. Motor neurons are particularly susceptible to oxidative injury by having high energy requirements associated with the maintenance of long axons. The high concentration of polyunsaturated fatty acids in neuronal cell membranes make these cells particularly susceptible to lipid peroxidation.[26] A recent investigation has shown that chronic or episodic deficits in oxygen and glucose, through an altered function of vascular endothelial cell growth factor, result in a failure of the motor neurons to meet their metabolic requirements. This altered function of vascular endothelial cell growth factor resulted in ALS-like symptoms and neuropathy.[27] If a relationship between superoxide dismutase 1 and altered vascular endothelial cell growth factor function exists, then it remains to be investigated.

DIAGNOSIS

Clinical signs and a history of other EMND cases in the stable and absence of pasture or green hay may lead to a tentative diagnosis of EMND. Ophthalmoscopic examination may reveal fundic lesions in approximately 30% of cases. Serum enzyme activities of AST and CK are generally mildly to moderately increased. The plasma vitamin E concentration is consistently low (less than 1 μg/ml). CSF analysis has been performed in horses with EMND and demonstrated elevated IgG concentrations in approximately 50% of cases. Intrathecal production of IgG also occurs in ALS; however, in both diseases this is considered a secondary effect of the disease process rather than a cause. The AQ was normal in most horses examined, indicative of normal blood-brain barrier function.[2]

EMG of cervical, facial, triceps, rear limb, and tailhead muscles may be useful in acute cases.[1,28] To eliminate motion artifacts, one can sedate horses or place them under general or caudal epidural anesthesia.[28] However, the electromyographic changes, which include positive sharp waves and fibrillation potentials, may be difficult to evaluate because they are expected in any peripheral nerve disease, myopathy, or myositis.[1,6,28]

In some horses with EMND, the glucose absorption test has been found to be abnormal; however, histopathologic examination of the small intestine has failed to identify lesions. The plasma glucose concentration increases only by 40% after 1 g/kg of 20% glucose administered orally, but relatively normal peak concentrations occur after 0.5 g/kg xylose administration (18-25 mg/dl). An abnormality in intestinal glucose transport has been identified in vitro.[6,8,9] The clinical significance of this finding is unknown.

More invasive diagnostic tests to confirm the tentative antemortem diagnosis of EMND are the examination of muscle and nerve biopsies. A biopsy of the sacrocaudalis dorsalis muscle is easy to obtain in a standing horse, and microscopic examination of this muscle may reveal changes consistent with denervation muscle atrophy and scattered muscle necrosis. This test has a sensitivity of approximately 90%. One should place the muscle biopsy sample on a tongue depressor in 10% formalin to prevent contracture artifact.[18] Examination of a biopsy of the ventral branch of the spinal accessory nerve may be more sensitive in chronic cases. Horses generally need to be anesthetized for one to obtain a biopsy from this nerve. As with muscle biopsies, nerve biopsies must be placed on a tongue depressor and in 10% formalin or another fixative suitable for electron microscopy. An experienced neuropathologist should examine nerve biopsies carefully; samples may reveal only evidence of smaller Bungner's bands (columns of proliferated Schwann cells).[12,29]

The definitive diagnosis is based on postmortem examination of spinal cord, brainstem, nucleus ambiguus, and skeletal muscle. The most important differential diagnoses that one should consider are laminitis, rhabdomyolysis, and colic. Other diseases that may cause similar signs are botulism, EPM, polysaccharide storage myopathy, iliac thrombosis, equine grass sickness (EGS), and lead toxicosis.[8,9,30]

TREATMENT AND PREVENTION

Currently, no treatment for EMND has been proved efficacious. In acute cases an anti-inflammatory dose of corticosteroids or nonspecific antioxidant treatment with DMSO may be beneficial. The only recommended treatment is based on the idea that this disorder is caused by oxidative injury and on the fact that horses with EMND consistently have low plasma vitamin-E concentrations.

Treatment with vitamin E (5000 to 7000 IU/horse/day) results in an increase of plasma vitamin-E concentrations to 2.0 μg/ml or greater after 4 to 6 weeks.[9] This treatment may be beneficial; however, full recovery is unlikely because neuronal death is irreversible.[6,8,9] Treatment with vitamin E has been associated with improvement of clinical signs; however, no published studies examining the effect of treatment exist at this time. Response to treatment is thought to depend on the number of neurons that are damaged versus those that are dead. Currently, no diagnostic modality exists to examine this in live horses.

One should give vitamin E supplements to horses that have limited or no access to green grass or hay for prolonged periods. The recommended dose for supplementation is 2000 IU/day of dl-α-tocopherol acetate. Not all commercial feeds or supplements contain required amounts of vitamin E for deficient horses. Periodic monitoring of plasma vitamin E concentrations is recommended in horses that are at risk for developing EMND.[8,9]

PROGNOSIS

The prognosis is poor for return to performance and guarded for life. Although no published investigations exist regarding the survival rate and follow-up of horses with EMND, horses with EMND generally have been shown to follow one of three possible clinical courses.[8,9] Approximately 20% of horses continue to deteriorate, and the severe weakness and excessive recumbency necessitate euthanasia. In approximately 40% of horses, clinical signs appear to stabilize; however, these horses do not regain muscle mass and may develop severe gait abnormalities. Continued clinical abnormalities frequently lead to euthanasia within 1 year of onset of clinical signs. The third group of horses (approximately 40%) show dramatic improvement after treatment with vitamin E, and many may regain a normal muscle mass. These horses may remain stabilized, that is, appear normal, for 1 to 6 years or more; however, many relapse, resulting in euthanasia. In a small number of human beings with ALS, a similar scenario occurs when clinical signs stabilize without progression for years.[13] In horses with EMND, the relapse appears associated with return to exercise and may be caused by exercise-induced premature death of remaining neurons.[8,9]

TETANUS

Peter R. Morresey

Tetanus is an infectious disease of all domestic animals and human beings. Although tetanus has long been recognized, it is only recently that the nature of the toxins of *Clostridium tetani* and their mechanisms of action have been described.

Tetanus has been recognized since ancient times, including mention in the writings of Hippocrates. Tetanus (from the Greek *tetanos,* to contract) was first identified as a neurologic disease more than 20 centuries ago by Greek physicians.[1] A causative infectious agent was first hypothesized in the 1860s. Transfer of tetanus by injection of infected material from a human wound into a rabbit was demonstrated in 1884. Inoculation of soil into small mammals caused classical symptoms of tetanus.[2] Reinforcing the transmissible nature of an infectious agent, smears of wounds from infected patients showed a bacillus-like organism under microscopy. Pure culture of the toxigenic organism was obtained in 1889, and it was subsequently shown that animals immunized with modified tetanus toxin generated neutralizing serum antibodies.[2] In 1986 the amino acid sequence of tetanus toxin was revealed,[3] with the mechanism of action elucidated in 1992.[4]

BIOLOGY OF CLOSTRIDIUM TETANI

Clostridium tetani is a common soil inhabitant found throughout the world. It can be readily isolated from the intestinal tract and feces of a wide range of animals, with fecal surveys in North America, Brazil, and Canada revealing between 30% and 42% positive samples.[2]

C. tetani is a strict anaerobe and thus requires anaerobic conditions to grow. Organisms are highly motile by means of flagellae uniformly distributed over the entire bacterial surface allowing them to swarm over a culture plate. Optimal growth occurs at 37° C. Colonies have irregular margins, are flat, translucent, and gray with a matte surface on blood agar. Colonies are 4 to 6 mm in diameter with a narrow zone of clear (β-type) hemolysis. Microscopically, the bacilli often possess terminal endospores giving them a "drumstick" appearance.[2]

In adverse environmental conditions, *C. tetani* produces round terminal spores able to survive in the environment for a prolonged period (years) in the absence of direct sunlight. Spores are resistant to boiling water and many standard disinfection techniques. The vegetative form is susceptible to heat and numerous disinfectants.

TOXINS

As is common with all clostridial bacteria, *C. tetani* produces a number of toxins. Two of importance to pathogenesis of disease have been identified.

Tetanospasmin

The classical tetanus toxin (tetanospasmin) is produced in the bacterial cell as a single polypeptide chain of 1315 amino acids,[3] with a molecular mass of approximately 150 kd.[5] The amino acid sequence of tetanus toxin shares marked similarities to the amino acid sequences of botulinum toxins A, B, and E, suggesting that although neurotoxins from *Clostridium tetani* and *C. botulinum* have different clinical effects, they are derived from a common ancestral gene.[3]

After release from the cell, the molecule is cleaved into two polypeptide fragments by proteases produced by the organism—a heavy chain of about 100 kd and a light chain of about 50 kd that remain joined by a disulfide bond.[6] Toxin spreads from the infected site by diffusing into the adjacent tissues and is subsequently transported by the lymphatic system, allowing entrance to the bloodstream.[2] Toxin is also transported by retrograde movement centrally along the nerve axons.[2] Tetanospasmin is poorly absorbed across mucous membranes, is destroyed by gastric juices, and is unable to cross the placenta as result of its high molecular weight.

Tetanospasmin travels centripetally along the α motoneurons via membrane associated endoplasmic reticulum.[7] Once at the synaptic cleft, the toxin crosses to affect the presynaptic inhibitory interneurons (Renshaw cells). Tetanospasmin causes blockage of the inhibitory synapses of spinal cord motor neurons by inhibiting neurotransmitter release (glycine and gamma-amino butyric acid [GABA]), thereby inducing the characteristic spastic paralysis.

Three main steps exist at the level of the cell that result in action of this toxin: (1) binding to the neuronal cell membrane, (2) internalization by endocytosis, and (3) the intracellular blockade of neurotransmitter release.[8] Binding to receptors on the nerve endings is the initial step in the paralytic process. Membrane receptors for these toxins consist of membrane gangliosides and a receptor protein. Tetanus neurotoxin acts mainly at CNS synapses.[9]

Once toxin is bound, it is internalized by endocytosis. The light chain, where it displays its zinc-endopeptidase activity specific for protein components of the neuroexocytosis apparatus, is translocated into the cytosol where it can exert its effect.[9,10] This process of internalization makes toxin unavailable to be bound and neutralized by circulating antibodies.

The target of tetanus toxin is vesicle-associated membrane protein (VAMP), also known as *synaptobrevin,* an integral membrane protein of the synaptic vesicles of nerve cell terminals crucial for normal vesicle physiology.[8,11] Synaptobrevin is one of three proteins present in every cell, these being conserved from yeast to human beings. They are essential for a variety of vesicle docking and fusion events.[9] Mutant studies have shown that any alteration in synaptobrevin leads to disturbed vesicle function.[11] Two copies of a nine-residue motif situated in tandem, each with three negatively charged residues, appear to be responsible for toxin specificity.[11] Cleavage of synaptobrevin by proteolytic action of the zinc-dependent endopeptidase of tetanospasmin light chain is the mechanism of toxicity, incapacitating cellular exocytotic machinery and blocking neurotransmitter release.[1]

Recent findings show that both binding and internalization are mediated only by the heavy chain of the toxin, whereas the intracellular blockade of neurotransmitter release involves the light chain alone.[8]

TETANOLYSIN

Tetanolysin facilitates the spread of infection by increasing the amount of local tissue necrosis. The mechanism of action is to cause permeability changes in liposomes and biologic membranes resulting in cell lysis.[12] Tetanolysin is an oxygen-sensitive hemolysin similar to streptolysin and can affect a variety of cells including erythrocytes, neutrophils, macrophages, fibroblasts, and platelets. Tetanolysin has an affinity for cholesterol and related sterols that inhibit its lytic and lethal actions. The amount of tetanolysin produced by the organism in vivo is unknown.[2]

RISK FACTORS FOR DISEASE

Entry of organisms to the animal is usually by inoculation into a deep wound. Complicating diagnosis, the wound that served as the initial site of introduction of *Clostridium tetani* may involve unbroken skin or be healed by the time clinical signs are observed. Other potential sites of entry include lacerations, surgical sites, the umbilicus of the neonatal foal, and the postfoaling reproductive tract. Once traumatized or devitalized tissue has become contaminated with spores, the spores can remain dormant until necrosis of the tissue provides the strict anaerobic environment necessary for germination to the vegetative, toxin-producing form.

CLINICAL SIGNS AND COURSE OF DISEASE

Tetanus is manifest as hypertonia of the striated muscles, with clonic paroxysmal muscular spasms superimposed. Muscular activity may be increased to the point that rectal temperature becomes markedly elevated. It may be generalized or localized.

Localized tetanus involves muscular rigidity and spasms in the vicinity of the infected wound. With time, this usually progresses to a more generalized tetanus affecting the entire body; however, the initial manifestation of tetanus is most often generalized rather than localized.[2]

With generalized tetanus, a characteristic "sawhorse" stance, with an extended, rigid tail, may be present, and the gait is stiff if the horse remains ambulatory (Figure 12-43). Difficulty in standing or laying down is due to extensor muscle rigidity that is exacerbated by external stimuli. As a result of hyperesthesia, painful reflex muscle spasms progressing to generalized tonic contractions with opisthotonus may be the result of even mild stimulation. Progression of the disease makes voluntary movement impossible because of marked extensor rigidity of all four limbs, often leading to recumbency.

Tetanospasmin affects both the sympathetic and parasympathetic nervous systems. Sympathetic hyperactivity associated with adrenergic stimulation may lead to tachycardia, cardiac arrhythmias, and peripheral vasoconstriction. Parasympathetic hyperactivity increases vagal tone that may result in bradyarrhythmias, arterioventricular block, and sinus arrest.

Intracranial signs, when present, are due to the action of tetanospasmin on cranial motor nuclei. Trismus is due to contraction of the masticatory muscles, with sustained facial muscle contracture and lip retraction resulting in risus sardonicus (a sardonic grin). Dorsomedial retraction of the ears and excessive wrinkling of the skin of the forehead can be seen. Prolapse of the nictitating membrane and enophthalmos is due to retraction of the globe by the hypertonic extraocular muscles (Figure 12-44). Miosis, dysphagia, ptyalism, and laryngeal spasm may also occur.

Complications from tetanus include decubital ulcers after periods of recumbency, regurgitation because of dysphagia, dysuria because of a hypertonic urethral sphincter, and constipation with gaseous distention because of a hypertonic anal sphincter and lack of exercise.

Death may result from respiratory failure secondary to the spasm of respiratory muscles or central respiratory arrest from medullary intoxication. Aspiration pneumonia secondary to dysphagia or increased airway secretions may also be fatal. No characteristic necropsy lesions can be ascribed to the tetanus toxins themselves.

Various factors were found to influence survival in one study. Younger horses were significantly less likely to survive

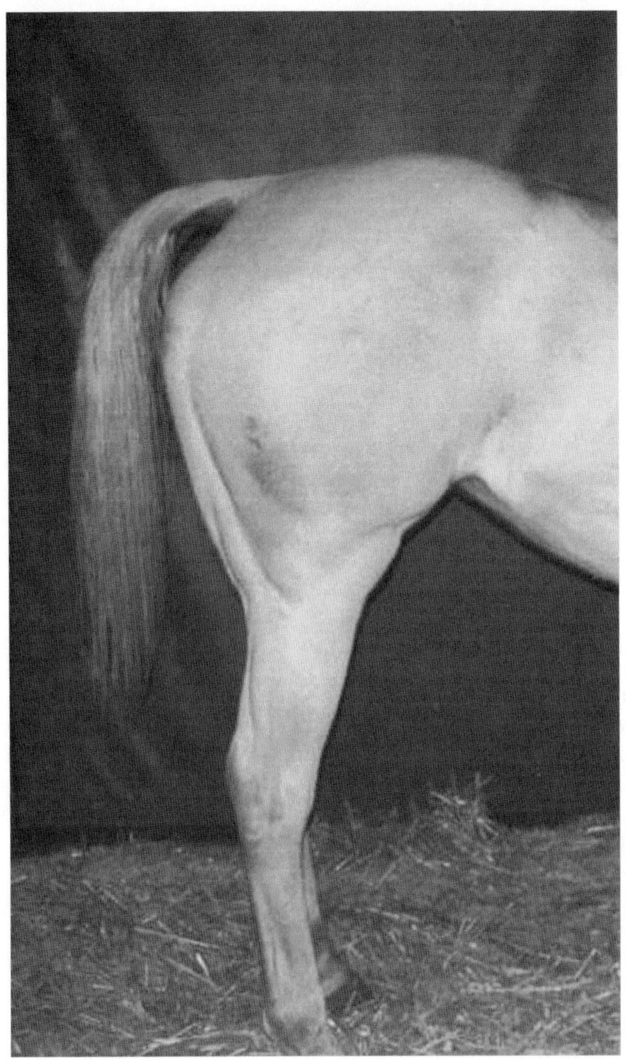

FIGURE 12-43 The extended, rigid tail seen in this horse is characteristic of generalized tetanus.

than older horses.[13] Dyspnea, dysphagia, and recumbency were significantly more common in nonsurvivors than survivors and can be considered indicators of a poor prognosis.[13] Of interest, a significant relationship has also been found in dogs between younger age and the development of more severe clinical signs, with more severe disease also decreasing survival.[14]

DIAGNOSIS

A presumptive diagnosis of tetanus is based on history, clinical signs, and response to treatment. Confirmation is difficult. On physical examination, a recent or healed wound may be found; however, absence of a detectable wound at the time of clinical onset is not uncommon. Devitalization of deep tissue undetectable externally may be the site of toxin production.

Gram staining of samples from the wound is of limited diagnostic value. Sporulated and vegetative forms of *Clostridium tetani* appear similar to other anaerobic bacteria. Furthermore, *C. tetani* may be present as a wound contaminant, with some strains of *C. tetani* nontoxigenic because they lack the 75-kilobase plasmid containing the toxin gene.[3,15]

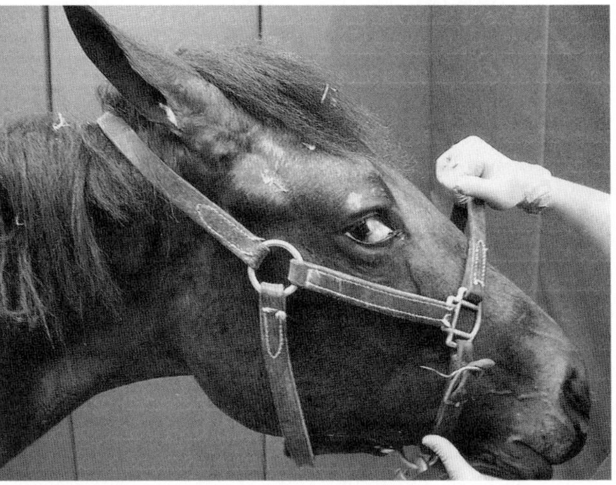

FIGURE 12-44 This horse exhibits enaphthalmus, prolapsed nictitors, and rigidity of facial muscles, typical of generalized tetanus.

Bacteriologic confirmation of tetanus is not often attempted but would be obtained by isolating *C. tetani* from the infected wound. However, isolation of *C. tetani* can be difficult and often fails because of low concentration of organisms present in the wound and strict anaerobic conditions required for culture.

Hematology, serum chemistry, and CSF analysis are usually unremarkable. If a wound or aspiration pneumonia is present, then neutrophilic leukocytosis with a left shift may be observed. Muscle enzymes may be elevated (CK and AST) because of muscle trauma from sustained contracture and prolonged recumbency.

TREATMENT

The binding of tetanospasmin to the α-motor neuron is extremely difficult to combat. Recovery is slow and does not occur until new interneuronal synapses develop to replace those that were inactivated by toxin. Therapeutic management of clinical cases of tetanus is centered on five goals discussed following.

Interruption of Toxin Production

Local and parenteral antibiotic therapy is initiated to prevent further production of tetanospasmin by eradication of the vegetative form of *Clostridium tetani* at the site of infection. Penicillin is the drug of choice for eliminating the vegetative form and is recommended to be administered at high dosages. Other antimicrobials that may be effective include the tetracyclines, macrolides (to be avoided in adults), and metronidazole. Metronidazole is indicated for deep and contaminated wounds because it is able to penetrate necrotic tissues without losing efficacy.

Neutralizing Unbound Toxin

Neutralizing any toxin that is not already bound to the CNS is of primary importance. Tetanus antitoxin (TAT) is produced from the sera of hyperimmunized horses. Once administered to the affected horse, the passively acquired antibodies neutralize unbound toxin both circulating in the blood and present in the wound. Injection of TAT, both around and proximal to the wound site, has been suggested to be beneficial in neutralizing unbound toxin.

It is vitally important to realize that once the toxin is internalized it can no longer be neutralized by antitoxin. Therefore the disease will likely continue to progress after the administration of TAT.

Control of Muscular Spasms

Sedatives can be used to control muscle spasms and rigidity. Phenothiazines work at the level of the brainstem, depressing descending excitatory input on the lower motor neurons within the spinal cord. Although these medications have been reported to lower the seizure threshold, their effectiveness in the management of clinical cases strongly supports the use of these drugs. Phenothiazines potentiate barbiturates, which are also useful because of their ability to depress the motor areas of the brain and abolish spontaneous spinal cord activity.

Muscle relaxants such as the benzodiazepines, which act as GABA agonists, indirectly antagonize tetanospasmin. Methocarbamol, as a central acting muscle relaxant, would also be considered a rational and useful therapeutic agent.

Supportive Care

Supportive care is of utmost importance in the successful treatment of tetanus. Patients should be placed in a dark, quiet environment, with minimal stimulation and handling. If recumbent, then deep soft bedding and regular turning (every 4 hours) to minimize decubital ulcers and pulmonary congestion is essential. Urinary catheterization, enemas, and manual rectal evacuation of feces may be required because of hypertonic urethral and anal sphincters and lack of an effective abdominal press. If dysphagic, then an esophagostomy or gastrostomy tube may be required for feeding. Tracheostomy may be required should laryngeal spasm and respiratory obstruction occur. Generalized muscle contraction can result in hyperthermia that must be managed.

Generation of Active Immunity to Tetanus Toxins

Unfortunately, the concentration of tetanus toxin required to cause overt neurologic disease is insufficient to generate a protective immunologic response. Therefore at the initiation of treatment for tetanus, all horses should be immunized with tetanus toxoid to initiate a protective antibody response. Experimentally, horses were resistant to challenge 8 days after receiving a single dose of toxoid.[16] To ensure optimal antibody production, affected horses should receive a second dose 1 to 2 months later.

PROGNOSIS

Prognosis depends on the incubation period, duration of onset, severity of clinical signs, and presence of any secondary complications. Therefore a short incubation period, short duration of onset, and rapid progression of signs results in a poor prognosis. When attempting to treat clinical cases, it must be realized that the required supportive care is prolonged, labor intensive, and costly.

PREVENTION

Where possible, management of contaminated or necrotic wounds should include thorough débridement, large volume flushing, and comprehensive cleansing. After this, rational antibiotic therapy should be instituted. Together these procedures, in conjunction with the following, should greatly minimize the occurrence of tetanus.

Tetanus Toxoid

Low concentrations of tetanospasmin are capable of inducing clinical signs. As a result, neither exposure to tetanospasmin nor recovery from clinical disease induces the development of immunity. Prophylactic antibody formation and generation of immunity is stimulated by vaccination with tetanus toxoid, derived from inactivation of tetanospasmin with formaldehyde. Significant differences were found in antibody response (IgG titers) between commercially available multivalent vaccines.[17] It was suggested that differences were the result of variations in antigenic mass.

Vaccination with tetanus toxoid markedly reduces the occurrence of clinical disease, with annual vaccination of all horses recommended. However, no vaccination is absolute,[18] with protection being dependent on proper administration and subject to breakdown in the face of overwhelming challenge. Experts recommend that tetanus toxoid be administered to horses with susceptible wounds if longer than 6 months since vaccination.

Tetanus Antitoxin

TAT is produced by hyperimmunization of horses with tetanus toxoid. Administration of 1500 U of antitoxin to unvaccinated horses provides immediate passive protection lasting approximately 3 weeks.[19] Higher doses result in longer duration of protection.

In one study monitoring antitoxin levels as a measure of protection, combined active-passive immunization (tetanus toxoid concurrently with TAT) was effective at providing rapid and prolonged protection for previously unvaccinated horses.[20] Administration in separate, remotely located sites on the horse was recommended.

Subclinical and clinical hepatic disease after TAT administration has been reported.[21-23] Known as *idiopathic acute hepatic disease,* this condition has also been called *Theiler's disease*, serum hepatitis, serum sickness, and postvaccinal hepatitis. Signs vary from hepatic enzyme elevation to hepatic encephalopathy in severe cases. Occurrence of this disease is rare and sporadic, but prognosis is poor in most affected horses.

Foal Vaccination

Tetanus-specific IgG antibodies inhibiting the foal's response to tetanus toxoid are passively transferred via colostrum. High titres of IgGa, IgGb, and IgG(T) subisotypes were detected in postsuckling serum samples collected from foals born to mares that had received booster doses of multicomponent vaccines during the last 2 months of gestation. Because these maternal antibodies exert a significant inhibitory effect on the response of foals to tetanus toxoid, it is recommended that primary immunization of foals born to vaccinated mares should not commence before age 6 months.[24] In addition, antibody response to vaccination of younger foals was shown to be poor,[19] necessitating multiple doses of toxoid. Vaccination for foals born to unvaccinated mares should begin at a younger age (3 months).

BOTULISM

Stephen M. Reed

Botulism is a severe neuroparalytic disease caused by toxins produced by *Clostridium botulinum,* a gram-positive, spore-forming, obligate anaerobic bacterium.[1-5] The bacteria are distributed widely in nature and can be found in soil, agricultural products, and marine environments. Organisms produce several types of antigenically distinct toxins designated as *A, B, C1, C2, D, E, F,* and *G.* Bacteria-producing toxin types A, B, E, F, and G are found in the environment, whereas types C and D are found within the intestinal tract of animals and birds.[3,5,6] Human disease is caused by types A, B, E, and rarely F.[1] The molecular weight of botulinum toxins is approximately 150 kd.[3]

In general, type B botulinum spores are most frequently isolated from the soil of the Northeastern and Appalachian regions of the United States. As a result, type B botulism is most often seen in the Mid-Atlantic states and Kentucky. In contrast, *C. botulinum* type C is most common in Florida, and type A occurs predominantly in the Western United States. Most reported cases (>85%) of botulism in horses in the United States result from type B botulism.[2,3,5,6,8-11] Less frequently, cases of type C and A botulism have been recognized. Type D botulism in horses has been suspected in the United States, but no cases have been confirmed at this time.

Botulinum toxins act presynaptically at the peripheral cholinergic neuromuscular junction. The toxin first binds to polysialogangliosides on the nerve terminal and is then internalized into the nerve terminus via a specific receptor.[7] The toxin then binds to SNARE (soluble *N*-ethylmaleimide-sensitive factor attachment *protein* receptor) proteins, preventing fusion of synaptic vesicles with the plasma membrane at the neuromuscular junction.[7] By attacking the SNARE proteins, the toxin prevents the synaptic vesicle from releasing acetylcholine, thus resulting in flaccid paralysis. Once the toxin is bound, improvement in clinical signs is achieved only by the regeneration of new motor end plates, explaining the delay of 4 to 10 days before noticeable clinical improvement even after treatment with antitoxin.

Clinical botulism in horses may occur by any of three mechanisms. Forage poisoning typically occurs in adult horses after ingestion of preformed toxin in feed material that has been contaminated by bacteria. Contaminated feed material may be spoiled grain, haylage, silage, or hay. In most cases, feed material contains decaying vegetable matter with bacterial proliferation and toxin production; however, occasionally feed is contaminated with decomposing animal carcasses.[5] In horses that had disease resulting from type C toxin, the cause was the ingestion of decomposing tissue of animals that contained the bacteria within the lumen of the intestinal tract.[8] A report describes type C1 and C2 toxins resulting in signs of neurotoxicity in one horse.[8,9] The same feed given to horses and cattle has been shown to result in disease in the horses, although not affecting the cattle, suggesting a species difference in susceptibility to these toxins.[6,8] Whenever more than one horse on a premise demonstrates clinical signs compatible with botulism, quick analysis of the entire ration and the feeding methodology to determine if contamination has occurred is recommended. This aggressive approach may prevent additional horses or other animals on the farm from becoming infected. Beginning the investigation with the feed, especially ensilage, is always best, because this is the most common source of toxin. Conditions may be optimal for proliferation of botulism spores and toxin production in improperly prepared hay or hay stored in plastic bags.[8]

Wound botulism occurs when wounds become contaminated with *C. botulinum,* producing toxin in vivo.[2] Published reports have described this type of infection after castration, an injection abscess, an infected umbilicus, and other contaminated wounds.[2,4,5,10] This problem is unique to horses, although a few cases have been described in other species (e.g., in human beings after sharing of needles during illicit drug use).

In foals a syndrome referred to as *toxicoinfectious botulism,* or *shaker foal syndrome,* occurs.[5,6,11] The disease appears to be a sporadic condition affecting foals from a few days to several months of life[10] and most commonly is associated with type B toxin. A high percentage (94%) of soil samples collected from farms that previously have had affected foals contained type B neurotoxin gene.[12] The foals on these farms are suspected to have ingested contaminated soils, and this may have led to the proliferation of spores within the intestinal tract, toxin production and absorption from the intestinal tract, and disease. A similar condition has been described in human infants fed honey or other food contaminated with botulism spores. In adult horses the intestinal flora appears to have a protective effect against the proliferation and absorption of spores and toxin.

CLINICAL SIGNS

The clinical signs of botulism in horses are similar, regardless of the source of contamination or the type of toxin.[5,6,10,11] The time of onset of clinical signs after ingestion of contaminated feed may vary from as short as 12 hours to as long as several days, but it usually occurs within 24 hours of exposure.[1] The incubation period may be associated with inoculum size, which suggests that the shorter the incubation, the more severe the disease. The disease usually affects motor nerves with high efferent traffic, resulting in weakness, dysphagia, and poor muscle tone. One can detect the lack of normal muscle clinically by evaluating eyelid tone, which often is weak. Affected horses appear to maintain coordination and therefore appear weak but not ataxic. Early in some cases the owners will note prolongation of the time the horse takes to eat its grain, or they will note abdominal discomfort and colic. The time to ingest a small quantity (usually a cup) of grain can be useful as a predictor of whether the horse has botulism. Some horses may have colic, decreased salivation, and occasionally urinary retention resulting from involvement of the cholinergic autonomic nervous system.

Over time affected horses demonstrate muscle fasciculations, often first in the triceps region, that eventually progress to the entire body and result in recumbency. At first the horse appears to gain strength after lying down for a short time and may return to standing spontaneously or with coaxing. Eventually the horse is unable to rise. Clinical evaluation should include careful examination of the tongue, eyelid and tail tone, and the pupillary light response, which appears sluggish. One will note ptosis of the eyelids. In horses affected for a longer time, an abnormal pattern of respiration may be noted. Death often results from respiratory failure.[5,6,9]

DIFFERENTIAL DIAGNOSIS

The differential diagnosis for horses affected with botulism can be any cause of weakness and dysphagia in horses and should include protozoal myeloencephalitis; EMND; EHV-1 myeloencephalopathy; WNV; rabies; several toxins such as lead, yew, and yellow star thistle; low blood calcium; and hyperkalemic periodic paralysis.[5,6,11] One also should consider less common clinical diseases such as tick paralysis, vascular accident, or even unusual examples of exercise intolerance.

The diagnosis of botulism is difficult and frequently is based on compatible clinical signs of acute onset of flaccid paralysis, weak or poor eyelid tone, poor tail tone, slow or difficult eating, and dysphagia, as well as a compatible history of possible exposure to toxin. To confirm the diagnosis, one must detect the toxin in feed, serum, gastrointestinal contents, feces, or debris collected from a wound.[4,5,11-14] The toxin is stable in frozen tissues or plasma and can be stored at −20° C for several weeks. The presence of botulism spores in intestinal contents or feed or the presence of an antibody response to *C. botulinum* in a recovered patient are also useful to confirm the diagnosis of botulism in horses.

Methods for detecting botulinum toxin include mouse bioassay, ELISA, PCR test, and use of an optical-based biosensor.[4,9,12-14] The mouse bioassay is sensitive but requires several days to complete and uses many mice. If serum has been collected from a horse in the acute stage of infection, then this assay is most accurate. One of the problems associated with this test in serum of horses is that because these animals are so sensitive to botulinum toxin, clinical signs may appear before the toxin reaches threshold levels required for detection. One must add specific antiserum to the test to detect the exact toxin type. Other tests are available, although these are less sensitive than mouse inoculation. The ELISA may be less specific because of cross-reactivity with other clostridial toxins, but it does have a turnaround time of 24 hours. The PCR test was used to identify an outbreak in Australia caused by type B botulism.[12] The fastest but least sensitive is the optical fiber–based biosensor.[13] The detection of botulism spores from the feces of infected horses has been useful in some outbreaks.[5,9] Compared with normal horses, the detection of spores in the feces is a rare occurrence (16 out of 507 samples). The use of ELISA for the detection of antibody in the serum of horses has been helpful to detect type C and D toxin in horses and cattle.[5]

EMG of horses with botulism will often identify a decremental response after repetitive stimulation. Although this test has been helpful in human beings, it is rarely helpful in horses.

TREATMENT

Treatment of horses with botulism is expensive, time consuming, and often unrewarding. The first therapeutic objective is prompt administration of specific or multivalent antitoxin to bind circulating toxin. Additional therapy includes appropriate nursing care, tube feeding, sedation to reduce muscle activity, antimicrobial agents, and laxatives. In severely affected foals or adults with respiratory failure, mechanical ventilation is indicated.[2,5,6,9,11]

Prognosis for horses with untreated botulism is poor; however, for horses that remain standing and that have been given antitoxin, the survival may approach 70%.[4] The shorter the time is that the horse is recumbent and the more rapidly it regains the ability to swallow, the better is the prognosis. In horses that do survive, recovery is complete but it can take months for the horse to regain full strength. Type B botulism is preventable by vaccination using type B toxoid, which was initially developed to prevent disease in newborn foals. The recommended vaccination schedule includes an initial three doses at 1-month intervals followed by an annual booster. For pregnant mares it is best to administer the annual booster 4 to 6 weeks before foaling.[5,6,11] Additional preventative measures involve good husbandry and proper processing and storage of feed material.

EQUINE GRASS SICKNESS (EQUINE DYSAUTONOMIA)

Yvette S. Nout

Equine grass sickness is an acquired degenerative polyneuropathy that predominantly affects the neurons of the autonomic and enteric nervous system. The disease was recognized first in Scotland in 1909.[1] Since then it has been reported in other parts of England, continental Europe, and Australia.[2,3] A clinically and histopathologically similar disease, mal seco, occurs in Argentina, southern Chile, and the Falkland Islands.[4] So far the disease has not been recognized in North America.

The disease affects postganglionic parasympathetic and sympathetic neurons and is characterized as a dysautonomia. Clinical signs vary, and the severity of EGS is suggested to be related to the extent of neuronal damage. The disease occurs sporadically and is often fatal. Although EGS has been studied extensively, the cause of the disease remains unknown.

CLINICAL SIGNS

EGS has been reported in other equids such as the Przewalski's Horse, zebra, donkey, and pony, but it occurs primarily in young, mature horses that have access to pasture. Horses with EGS are generally between 2 and 12 years of age, and horses between the ages of 3 and 5 years are at greatest risk for developing the disease. No breed or gender predilection to the disease is apparent.[3]

Acute, subacute, and chronic forms of EGS are recognized, of which clinical signs overlap from one form to the other.[5,6] Most horses are depressed and dysphagic. The dysphagia is caused by cranial nerve involvement and is recognized by drooling of saliva, feed material in the nares, impacted feed material in the buccal pouches, and difficulty drinking.

Acute Form

Clinical signs are related to acute onset of gastrointestinal ileus. The course of disease is generally less than 48 hours. Signs of abdominal pain may be severe and are caused by gastric and small intestinal distention. Affected horses are hypovolemic, and the reduced circulating volume may cause death from cardiac failure. Other clinical signs are generalized or patchy sweating, fine muscular fasciculations, pyrexia, severe dysphagia, and bilateral ptosis. Examination per rectum reveals small intestinal distention and often a mild secondary impaction of the large colon. One can obtain a large quantity of reflux after nasogastric intubation.

Subacute Form

The course of disease is 3 to 7 days, and clinical signs are less severe than in acute EGS. Horses with subacute EGS do not develop gastric or small intestinal distention but develop large colon impactions. These horses have a characteristic "tucked up" stance. Clinical signs include intermittent colic and patchy sweating. These horses often have rhinitis sicca.

Chronic Form

The course of the disease is weeks to months. Cachexia is the most prominent clinical abnormality in horses with chronic EGS. The entire gastrointestinal tract is empty in these horses, and they usually have rhinitis sicca characterized by accumulation of mucopurulent material in the nasal passages. Other clinical signs in animals with chronic EGS are sweating, muscle tremors, gait abnormalities (short strided), leaning against walls, base-narrow stance, snoring, pica, and penile prolapse. In a later stage, one may observe coat abnormalities such as areas of piloerection, growth of a long coat, and pallor of the coat.

PATHOLOGIC FINDINGS

Gross necropsy findings in acute EGS are consistent with gastrointestinal ileus. A large fluid-filled stomach and distended small intestine are present. Secondary impacted ingesta is often present in the large colon and cecum. Splenomegaly and erosions of the esophageal mucosa are other findings in acute EGS. Gross necropsy findings in subacute EGS are less severe and include colonic impaction.[2,5] One may find inspissated mucus in the lumen of the small colon and rectum and evidence of intraluminal hemorrhage such as inspissated blood or black feces. In horses with subacute and chronic EGS, one may find rhinitis sicca.

Neuronal lesions are most severe in the autonomic ganglia (cranial cervical, stellate, celiacomesenteric) and enteric nerves. One finds less severe lesions in some brainstem nuclei and parts of the spinal cord.[2,5-7] Changes detected in affected neurons are degenerative and include chromatolysis, loss of Nissl's substance, loss of the nucleus, spheroid formation, neuronal swelling, and an increase in the number of lysosomes and mitochondria.[2,5,6] Loss of a recognizable Golgi apparatus appears to be an early neuropathologic event in EGS.[5]

A recent study has demonstrated a reduction of neuropeptide expression in nasal mucosal innervation in horses with EGS.[8] This is suggested to underlie the presentation of rhinitis sicca seen in this disorder.

Similarly to other neurodegenerative diseases, one finds a specific anatomic distribution of neuropathologic conditions in EGS, which supports the hypothesis of a common factor sensitizing the neurons to specific insults. As in EGS, multiple system involvement is a common feature in human neurodegenerative disorders. The central pathologic condition in EGS appears to be specific and repeatable, consistent with findings in primary dysautonomias in other species. However, in EGS, one does not see the increasing severity of pathologic findings and severity of clinical signs with increased duration of disease consistently as is seen in classical neurodegenerative diseases. Moreover, the decrease in severity of pathologic conditions of the brain with increased duration of disease may suggest a healing process from the initial insult. The association between central neuronal pathologic findings and severity of clinical disease is unclear. In one study, increased neuronal pathologic findings were observed in milder clinical cases (chronic EGS),[7] which contrasts to another study that demonstrated increased neuronal pathologic findings in acute cases of EGS.[9]

PATHOGENESIS

Clinical signs are related to the damage of the autonomic nervous system. The most severe lesions are found in the myenteric and submucosal plexuses of the ileum and less severe changes occur in the celiacomesenteric ganglion. The altered autonomic activity results in cessation or decrease of intestinal peristalsis and subsequently leads to the development of ileus and colonic impaction. The dysphagia in most cases of EGS is caused by cranial nerve or brainstem involvement.[5] Based on epidemiologic and pathologic findings in horses with EGS, an unidentified neurotoxin is implicated as the causative agent of the disease; however, because of the complexity of the disease, multiple factors are suspected to be involved in the pathogenesis of EGS.[2,3,5]

Multiple experimental studies have failed to identify the causative agent or agents of EGS. Risk factors for developing the disease have been identified, however. Young horses between 3 and 5 years of age are at greatest risk for developing EGS.[3] Older horses have been suggested to be resistant to EGS, perhaps after nonfatal exposure to the causative agent. Moreover, horses that had been in contact with cases of EGS were 10 times less likely to develop the disease.[10] Similarly, transfer of maternal antibodies against this causative agent may explain the fact that EGS has not been reported in horses younger than 6 months. Horses that are kept solely at pasture are at increased risk of developing EGS; however, the disease has been reported in stabled horses and in horses that had no access to grass at all. The type of pasture or the type of supplementary feeds do not appear to be associated with the development of EGS. Horses that have been on the premises for less than 2 months and horses that have been moved recently to a different pasture are at increased risk of developing EGS. Horses are more likely to be affected with EGS when they are housed on premises that have experienced the disease previously. Although cases of EGS can occur throughout the year, the incidence of EGS consistently has been found to be greatest during the spring months, particularly if a period of warm weather is followed by a period of wet weather.

Paravertebral ganglionic damage exceeds and occurs earlier than prevertebral ganglionic damage. The putative neurotoxin is suggested to be ingested and initiates damage in the enteric plexuses, which leads to immediate functional deficits seen in the acute form of EGS.[5] Functional lesions precede structural lesions caused by secondary retrograde axonal degeneration. In chronic EGS, less initial enteric nerve damage occurs, and subsequently fewer secondary prevertebral ganglionic lesions occur. Consequently, the body has more time to develop functional and structural compensatory mechanisms. The less severe damage to the celiacomesenteric ganglion compared with the damage in the paravertebral ganglia is suggested to be caused by hematogenous spread of an ingested neurotoxin.

Currently, toxicoinfection with *Clostridium botulinum* type C is being investigated as a cause of the disease.[11-13] This organism grows and produces toxin in the gastrointestinal tract. The role of this organism in the cause of EGS is supported by the fact that type C botulinum neurotoxin has been detected in the gastrointestinal tract of 67% of horses with acute and 74% of horses with chronic EGS compared with 10% of control horses.[14] Moreover, horses with EGS were found to have lower IgG concentrations to the surface antigens of *C. botulinum* type C and to type C botulinum neurotoxin. An association between antibody concentration and form of EGS was not demonstrated, but horses that had been exposed to other horses with EGS or that had been grazing on pasture where the disease had occurred previously had significantly higher antibody concentrations to these antigens.[11] These findings may indicate the development of a protective immune response against the putative neurotoxin. More recently it has been demonstrated that fresh grass may contain botulinum neurotoxin, and this supports the hypothesis that EGS may be a form of soil-borne botulism in horses.[12] The suggestion is that natural-occurring biofilms may protect bacteria and improve their chance of survival; however, further research in the areas of cause, pathogenesis, treatment, and prevention of EGS is necessary.

The sulfur amino acid depletion in horses with EGS has been suggested to contribute to the pathogenesis of this disease through the increase of oxidative neuronal death; however, this has not been proven.[15] A further study found no evidence of systemic macromolecular oxidative damage in horses with EGS.[16] Mycotoxin toxicity also has been implicated as a cause for EGS,[13] and low sulfur amino acid concentrations may enhance the toxicity of mycotoxins.

DIAGNOSIS

No noninvasive definitive test exists to obtain an antemortem diagnosis of EGS. Serum biochemical and hematologic examinations do not reveal specific changes in horses with EGS. Plasma amino acid analysis in horses with acute EGS demonstrated a significant increase in plasma taurine concentration and a significant decrease in plasma cysteine, arginine, citrulline, histidine, isoleucine, leucine, methionine, threonine, tyrosine, and valine concentrations. In horses with subacute and chronic EGS, these changes were less significant (and the plasma amino acid profile normalized). Although one cannot use the amino acid analysis as a definitive test for EGS because of overlap in individual amino acid concentrations for control horses, horses with EGS, and horses grazed with EGS-affected horses, the test may have value as an additional diagnostic aid, because adequate plasma cysteine concentrations (>17 μmol/L) may exclude EGS.[15] Most horses with EGS and healthy co-grazed horses had significantly decreased plasma sulfur amino acid (cysteine and methionine) concentrations compared with healthy control animals.

When watching a horse eat, one may notice signs of abnormal esophageal function such as esophageal spasm and reverse peristalsis. Contrast radiography and endoscopy of the esophagus may reveal abnormalities such as megaesophagus and esophageal erosions.[6]

Examination of an ileal biopsy, collected via laparotomy, is the only method to confirm EGS ante mortem.[17,18] Neuronal degeneration is present in the enteric plexuses from the esophagus to the rectum, but the most severe changes are present in the terminal ileum. Examination of a rectal mucosal biopsy is specific but not sensitive for EGS.

The most important differential diagnoses for acute EGS are a small intestinal strangulating lesion and duodenitis-proximal jejunitis. Clinical signs and neuronal lesions in chronic EMND and chronic EGS may be similar, and these similarities have led to the speculation that these two diseases are related.[19] Further examination, however, reveals important differences such as the fact that EMND occurs in older horses that have not had access to pasture, and EGS occurs in young horses with access to pasture. EGS sometimes occurs along with EMND.[2,19]

TREATMENT AND PREVENTION

No effective cure exists for EGS. Horses with acute EGS may respond initially to gastric decompression and intravenous fluid therapy. Management of horses with chronic EGS includes nursing care and the use of the prokinetic drug cisapride and the appetite stimulant diazepam.[6]

PROGNOSIS

EGS is usually fatal. The case fatality rate for acute and subacute cases is 100%. If horses with acute EGS are not euthanized within 48 hours, then they die from circulatory failure or gastric rupture. Horses with subacute grass sickness usually are euthanized within 7 days.[7] Horses with chronic EGS often are euthanized because of weakness and emaciation; however, when given appropriate care at a referral hospital, approximately 50% of horses may survive.[6] Survivors may return to work, but some display residual abnormalities such as mild dysphagia, sweating, and coat changes.

LYME DISEASE IN HORSES

Stephen M. Reed, Ramiro E. Toribio

Lyme disease is the most common vector-borne infectious disease in human beings in the United States. Initially recognized in the mid-1970s in Lyme, Connecticut, as the cause of unexplained rheumatoid arthritis in children, the causative agent of Lyme disease was discovered to be a spirochete, *Borrelia burgdorferi (sensu lato)*. In addition to human beings, Lyme disease affects domestic animals such as dogs, cats, cattle, and horses.[1-7]

Human beings and animals acquire Lyme disease by transmission of *B. burgdorferi* through the bite of infected hard ticks (*Ixodes* spp.). In the Eastern and Midwestern United States the vector is the blacklegged tick or deer tick, *Ixodes scapularis* (formerly *I. dammini*), whereas in the Western United States the vector is the western blacklegged tick, *I. pacificus*. In Europe the sheep tick, *I. ricinus* is the vector of Lyme borreliosis.

Not all ticks are infected with the spirochete, and infection varies by tick species and geographic region. These ticks have a 2-year, three-stage life cycle and feed once during each stage.[8,9] The larvae hatch in the spring and summer and are usually noninfective because transovarial transmission is rare.[10] The tick may become infected at any stage of the life cycle by feeding on small mammalian hosts, typically the white-footed mouse *(Peromyscus leucopus)*, which is a natural host for the spirochete. The nymphal stage emerges the next spring and is most likely to transmit the disease because it is small, difficult to see, and engorges faster; engorgement is necessary to transmit *B. burgdorferi*. The white-tailed deer *(Odocoileus virginianus)* is the host for adult ticks. The life cycle of *I. ricinus* in Europe involves birds and mammals because immature stages feed on birds and reptiles. Nymphal *I. scapularis* are the main vectors of *B. burgdorferi* in human beings. These ticks are more active from May to July. Once the tick has engorged, *B. burgdorferi* is transmitted to the host via lymphatics or blood. Although larval and nymph stages are responsible for *B. burgdorferi* transmission to other mammals, the stage responsible for transmitting Lyme disease in horses is unknown.

EPIDEMIOLOGY

In endemic areas of the Northeast and Midwestern United States, approximately 20% of nymphal stages and 30% to 40% of adult stages of *Ixodes scapularis* are infected with *Borrelia burgdorferi*. In contrast, *I. pacificus* often feeds on lizards that are poor reservoirs for *B. burgdorferi*, and only 1% to 3% of these ticks, including the nymphal stages, are infected with the spirochete.[10] This difference in the number of infected ticks may explain the difference in the prevalence of Lyme borreliosis between the Eastern and Western United States. Equine seroprevalence is high in the Northeastern United States, but limited information is available for other parts of the country.[2,6] In Europe, clinical cases and equine serorologic surveys have documented Lyme borreliosis as a cause of equine disease in Poland, Germany, Scandinavia, and England.[5,11,12]

The apparent increasing incidence of disease in human beings and animals may result from an increased deer population, increased number of ixodid ticks, expansion of human and horse populations into previously rural woodland areas, or increased recognition of the disease manifestations.

The disease has a seasonal prevalence and is most common in spring, summer, and fall, with a peak incidence in June and July. In some climates such as California, ticks may be active throughout the year. The organism is maintained in a complex life cycle of small wild mammals and immature stages of the blacklegged tick. Larval and nymphal stages of the tick acquire the infection when they feed on infected mice. The white-tailed deer *(Odocoileus virginianus)* is not a reservoir for Lyme disease but rather the host for the adult stages of the tick. This is relevant to tick and Lyme disease control programs, because regional reductions in the number of *I. scapularis* has only been possible when the deer population has been decreased.[8]

CLINICAL SIGNS

Clinical signs associated with *Borrelia burgdorferi* in horses, as in human beings, are often nonspecific and involve multiple body systems. In human beings, clinical signs frequently include annular rash, erythema migrans, myalgia, aseptic meningitis, arthritis, and seventh cranial nerve palsy.[10] The disease usually begins as a skin rash and often progresses to involve joints and the nervous and cardiac systems but may involve other body systems as well. In human beings the skin rash may be slowly progressive and sometimes may take up to 1 month before becoming apparent.

In horses, reported clinical signs of Lyme borreliosis include chronic weight loss, sporadic lameness, laminitis, low-grade fever, swollen joints, muscle tenderness, anterior uveitis, encephalitis, and abortion.[3,4,13] Some horses may demonstrate clinical illness and depression and may go off feed in a short time. The bacteria may enter the CNS within a short time after exposure. Chronic arthritis may develop as a result of autoimmune mechanisms, although this is not fully understood. *Ixodid* spp. ticks are often co-infected with *Borrelia burgdorferi* and *Anaplasma phagocytophila*; however, dual infections remain to be documented in the horse. An important consideration is that limb swelling and response to tetracycline treatment, indicating Lyme borreliosis could be the result of *A. phagocytophila* infection.

DIAGNOSIS

The diagnosis of Lyme disease is often difficult. History of tick exposure or living in a Lyme disease endemic area is helpful; when combined with the identification of clinical signs and the elimination of other diseases, this information allows the clinician to make a presumptive diagnosis. Examination of blood work for other diseases may be more beneficial than a positive blood test for Lyme, although one should complete such a test as well. In human beings an early increase in serum IgM often occurs. Response to therapy also helps to support a presumptive diagnosis of Lyme disease. Diagnosis of Lyme disease in horses is difficult,[14] and in many cases one bases a presumptive diagnosis on history, clinical signs, and response to antibiotic therapy in an animal with probable cause to be infected (i.e., possible exposure). In human beings the skin lesions are obvious. Blood tests are of limited value; however, ELISA, kinetic ELISA, Western blot testing, and PCR on blood samples and synovial fluid from suspect animals have been evaluated.[2,5-7,14,15] One may test samples of joint fluid, CSF, and tissues from affected patients for presence of organisms. Several pathologic conditions should be considered in the differential diagnosis of equine borreliosis, including *Anaplasma phagocytophila* infection, chronic diseases, vasculitis, and immune-mediated arthritis if limb or periarticular swelling are present, as well as causes of neurologic disease.

PATHOGENESIS

Borrelia burgdorferi organisms are capable of nonspecifically activating monocytes, macrophages, and synovial lining cells, as well as natural killer cells, B cells, and complement, leading to production of host proinflammatory mediators. These proinflammatory mediators seem to localize in joints, leading to chronic arthritis and lameness. *B. burgdorferi* has developed strategies to interact with the mammalian host, including adhesion to host cells and components of the extracellular matrix such as fibronectin, β_3 integrins, and glycosaminoglycans. The current thinking in the development of arthritis is that outer-surface proteins (Osps) of *B. burgdorferi* trigger an autoimmune reaction because antibodies to OspA and OspB have been detected in 50% to 80% of human patients with arthritis.[16,17] Natural killer cells also play a central role in joint inflammation by producing excessive amounts of TNF-α and IL-8.[16]

TREATMENT AND PREVENTION

Many horses are treated annually for a presumptive diagnosis of Lyme disease. Recommended treatment includes oxytetracycline (6.6 mg/kg IV every 24 hours) or doxycycline (10 mg/

kg PO every 12 hours).[18] Treatment can be started with tetracycline for 1 week followed with doxycycline for 3 to 4 weeks. Ceftiofur (2.2 to 4.4 mg/kg IV every 12 hours) has also been evaluated.[18] In animals infected with *B. burgdorferi,* a rapid clinical response (2 to 4 days) is expected with tetracyclines. In some horses the clinical signs may show an initial worsening as a response to toxins released after death of the organisms. Currently, no licensed vaccine is available to prevent Lyme disease in horses, although vaccines are available for dogs and human beings. A recombinant OspA vaccine was evaluated in horses with promising results.[19]

Aids to prevention include daily grooming with removal of ticks, along with the use of tick repellents that contain permethrin. One should apply tick repellents to the head, neck, legs, abdomen, and under the tail. Keeping pastures mowed and removing brush and woodpiles makes the environment less hospitable for rodents, which in turn decreases the tick population. Regional programs to control Lyme disease are based on reducing the deer population.

HEAD SHAKING

Robert H. Mealey

CLINICAL SIGNS

Head shaking is a widely recognized disorder characterized by persistent or intermittent, spontaneous, and frequently repetitive vertical, horizontal, or rotary movements of the head and neck.[1] The affected horse shakes, jerks, or flicks its head uncontrollably in the absence of obvious physical stimuli, and the condition can be severe enough to render the horse unusable and dangerous.[2-5] Head shaking often is accompanied by snorting and sneezing, and many horses rub their noses on stationary objects or on the ground while moving. In addition to shaking the head up and down, flipping the upper lip, or shaking the head side to side, horses also may act as if a bee has flown up the nostril or may strike at the face with the forelimbs.[2,6,7] Head-shaking horses also may exhibit avoidance behavior, with low head carriage, corner seeking, and nostril clamping.[1,8] To characterize the severity of clinical signs, a grading system of 1 to 5 has been described, with grade 1 being a rideable horse with intermittent and mild signs (facial muscle twitching) and grade 5 being an unrideable, uncontrollable, dangerous horse with bizarre behavior patterns.[1] Clinical signs are usually worse during exercise; however, head shaking can affect horses at rest.[1-5,7] Mean age of onset is typically 7 to 9 years, and Thoroughbreds and geldings appear to be over-represented in some studies.[2,3,6] Head shaking can be seasonal or nonseasonal. Early literature suggested an increased incidence of head shaking during the warmer months of the year,[5] and a later study indicated that the peak periods of onset were spring and early summer.[3] Recent studies have found that 64%[6] and 59%[2] of head-shaking horses are affected seasonally, with the majority developing signs in the spring or early summer.

PATHOGENESIS

Early work suggested 58 possible causes for head shaking, including two that have received considerable attention recently: (1) photophobia and (2) trigeminal neuralgia.[9] Other reported and suggested causes include behavioral resentment to rider-induced head and neck flexion, exercise-induced hypoxia, ear mites, cranial nerve dysfunction, otitis media or otitis interna, cervical injury, ocular disease, guttural pouch mycosis, dental periapical osteitis, vasomotor rhinitis, allergic rhinitis, *Trombicula autumnalis* (harvest mite) larval infestation, maxillary osteoma, and EPM.[3,4,9-14] A study of 100 head-shaking horses revealed a potential specific cause in only 11 horses, and elimination of the abnormality resulted in resolution of the head shaking in only two of them.[3] Idiopathic head shaking has been used to describe the majority of cases in which no specific underlying cause is found, and necropsy results in these horses reveal no lesions.

The clinical signs exhibited by most head-shaking horses now generally are thought to result from sharp, electric-like, burning pain involving the trigeminal nerve.[1,2] Trigeminal nerve involvement is supported by the observations that some horses improve after blocking the infraorbital nerve (part of the maxillary branch),[15,16] and that most horses improve after blocking the posterior ethmoidal nerve (part of the ophthalmic branch).[1] Horses that head shake in response to light stimulation have been described as *photic head shakers*.[8] Most of these horses are affected seasonally (spring and summer), improve at night or when brought indoors, and improve when blindfolded or when gray lenses are placed over their eyes. Photic head shaking is hypothesized to be caused by optic-trigeminal summation (stimulation of the optic nerve that results in referred sensation to parts of the nose innervated by the trigeminal nerve), a mechanism similar to that proposed for photic sneezing in human beings.[2,8] Many features of head shaking in the horse are similar to trigeminal neuralgia in human beings—a severe chronic pain syndrome characterized by dramatic, brief stabbing or electric shocklike pain paroxysms felt in one or more divisions of the trigeminal distribution, spontaneously or on gentle tactile stimulation of a trigger point on the face or oral cavity. The disease is associated with microvascular compression and pathologic changes in the trigeminal root and trigeminal ganglion.[17] The basic underlying cause of head shaking in the horse may be trigeminal neuralgia,[1] and recent work suggests a degenerative disorder of the brainstem nucleus of the trigeminal nerve (D.C. Knottenbelt, personal communication). The trigeminal nerve is postulated to be hypersensitive and to fire in response to a variety of trigger factors including wind, airway turbulence, increased blood flow, pollen, dust, warmth, cold, insects, allergies, or other irritations. These trigger factors appear to act intranasally in many horses but could act in any trigeminal sensory region.[1]

DIAGNOSIS AND TREATMENT

One should perform a complete physical examination, including neurologic, dental, ophthalmic, and otoscopic examinations to rule out potential underlying causes. Other diagnostics could include endoscopy of the nasal passages, pharynx, and guttural pouches; radiography of the skull and cervical spine; CBC; and serum biochemistry profile. These examinations reveal no abnormalities in most cases. A recent survey suggests that one should consider idiopathic head shaking if two of the following three clinical signs are present: (1) vertical flipping of the head, (2) acting as if an insect has flown up the nostril, or (3) rubbing the muzzle on objects.[2] For photic head-shaking horses, clinical signs should improve after blindfolding or after placement of a mask shielding the eyes from the sun.

Cyproheptadine, an antihistamine (histamine$_1$) and serotonin antagonist with anticholinergic effects, has been used (0.3 mg/kg orally b.i.d.) to treat head-shaking horses, resulting in improvement in 5 of 7 horses in one study[8] and 43 of 61 horses in another.[2] Horses that respond do so within 1 week, and some may respond within 24 hours. Although the mechanism for efficacy of cyproheptadine in these cases is unknown, blocking of serotonin-mediated pain sensation could be involved.[8] Other investigators have found cyproheptadine alone to be ineffective, but the addition of carbamazepine (4 to 8 mg/kg PO q6-8h) resulted in 80% to 100% improvement in seven of nine cases, with horses responding within 3 to 4 days.[1] Carbamazepine is a sodium channel–blocking antiepileptic drug and is the drug of choice for treating trigeminal neuralgia in human beings.[18] Carbamazepine alone was reported to be effective in head shaking horses, but results were unpredictable.[1] The elimination half-life of carbamazepine in the horse is less than 2 hours, making sustaining therapeutic concentrations difficult; the drug is therefore of more benefit diagnostically than therapeutically in head-shaking horses (D.C. Knottenbelt, personal communication). Other medications and therapies including NSAIDs, corticosteroids, antihistamines, acupuncture, chiropractic manipulation, homeopathy, and feed supplements are generally ineffective in most horses.[2,19]

Diagnostic blockade of trigeminal nerve branches can be useful for identifying trigger points in head-shaking horses. Blockade of the infraorbital nerve may improve some horses and might identify candidates for infraorbital neurectomy.[15,16] However, results of infraorbital blockade and infraorbital neurectomy do not correlate, and because of neuroma formation, self-trauma, and low success rate, infraorbital neurectomy is not a recommended procedure.[15] A high percentage of horses improve after blockade of the posterior ethmoidal nerve, and sclerosis of this nerve results in temporary improvement in some horses.[1]

Therapies aimed at decreasing the response to trigger factors can be effective and include tinted contact lenses; face masks or hoods that block sunlight, wind, insects, and dust, with mesh or dark eye cups; and nose nets.[1,2,8,19,20] A recent owner survey found that nose nets that cover the nostrils with mesh and include a drawstring or elastic band that applies pressure to the upper lip resulted in some improvement in 70% of head-shaking horses, and that 70% or more improvement occurred in about 30% of the horses.[20] Finally, permanent tracheostomy is effective in some horses,[1,4] presumably because airflow then bypasses the nasal cavity where the majority of trigger factors are thought to act.[1]

VERMINOUS ENCEPHALOMYELITIS

Eduard Jose-Cunilleras

Aberrant migration of helminth and fly larvae through the CNS of horses and donkeys is a rare but important cause of severe neurologic disease. Parasites that have been reported to affect the brain and spinal cord of equids include rhabditid nematodes *(Halicephalobus* [*Micronema*] *deletrix* [syn. *H. gingivalis*]), strongyloid nematodes *(Strongylus vulgaris, S. equinus,* and *Angiostrongylus cantonensis)*, protostrongyloid nematodes *(Parelaphostrongylus tenuis)*, spiruroid nematodes *(Draschia megastoma)*, filarid nematodes (*Setaria digitata* and other *Setaria* spp.), and warble fly larvae (*Hypoderma* spp.).

Antemortem diagnosis is often impossible; however, a high index of suspicion may be warranted for certain clinical signs (acute onset or rapidly progressive asymmetric, focal, or multifocal brain or spinal cord signs) and changes in CSF analysis, in which case the treatment regimen should include specific antiparasitic drugs (e.g., fenbendazole) in addition to the more routinely used symptomatic and anti-inflammatory treatments (e.g., NSAIDs, DMSO, corticosteroids, antiprotozoal drugs).

CAUSES

Halicephalobus (Micronema) Deletrix (Halicephalobus Gingivalis)

Halicephalobus deletrix is synonymous with *H. gingivalis*, the latter being the most recent terminology.[1] The parasite was referred to as *Micronema deletrix* until 1970s and 1980s with use of the new nomenclature beginning in 1990.

The life cycle of *Halicephalobus* spp. nematodes is unknown. This small roundworm generally is considered a saprophytic organism that occasionally acts as a facultative parasite in horses and human beings. The likely route of entry is through nasal and oral mucosa, followed by possible hematogenous spread to organs with high vascularization such as the brain, spinal cord, and kidneys. *H. deletrix* recently has been shown to be transmitted from a mare to her foal because of mammary infestation.[2]

Organs affected by migration of *Halicephalobus* spp. include the brain, spinal cord, nasal and oral cavities, pituitary gland, and kidneys and less commonly the lymph nodes, heart, lungs, stomach, liver, and bones.[3,4] Organisms affecting the CNS have been reported to have a predilection for the basilar, pituitary region of the brainstem.[5] Characteristic histopathologic lesions in the CNS include malacia, granulomatous and lymphohistiocytic inflammatory infiltration, meningitis, and vasculitis in addition to identification of the nematodes. Other clinical signs include oral and nasal granulomata, renal involvement (*H. deletrix* is visible in the urine), granulomatous osteomyelitis,[6] and granulomatous chorioretinitis.[7]

Most of the cases of *Halicephalobus* encephalomyelitis in adult horses reported in the literature during the last 30 years describe simultaneous renal granulomatous lesions encapsulating the nematodes (Table 12-13). Granulomata within or adjacent to the renal parenchyma were observed on postmortem examination in 13 of 16 horses with neurologic disease; of the other three horses, in one case lesions were confined to the sacral spinal cord and cauda equine, and in another case only the skull and brain were examined at postmortem examination. In contrast, all three cases reported to date in foals showed no renal involvement but did show pulmonary granulomata.[2,5]

Strongylus Vulgaris, Strongylus Equinus, and Angiostrongylus Cantonensis

Aberrant strongyle larval migration is a much less common cause of neurologic signs because of routine broad spectrum antiparasitic treatment with ivermectin and moxidectin. The

TABLE 12-13

Signalment, Organism Identified, Clinical Signs, and Organs Affected in Cases of Verminous Encephalomyelitis

Signalment	Organism	Clinical Signs	Organs Affected	Affected Areas in Central Nervous System (CNS)	Reference
19-year-old Saddlebred gelding	*Halicephalobus*	Stranguria Ataxia Blindness Fever Recumbency	Kidneys Brain	Cerebrum Thalamus Hypothalamus	8
12-year-old pony gelding	*Halicephalobus*	Incoordination Voracious appetite Fever Recumbency	Kidneys Brain	Cerebrum Cerebellum	9
6-year-old pony gelding	*Halicephalobus*	Ataxia Recumbency	Kidneys Brain	Thalamus Cerebellum Pons and medulla	3
8-year-old Arabian female horse	*Halicephalobus*	Ataxia Mandibular swelling	Mandible Brain	Thalamus Midbrain	10
18-year-old Quarter Horse	*Halicephalobus*	Ataxia Recumbency	Kidneys Brain	—	11
4-year-old Appaloosa gelding	*Halicephalobus*	Mandibular mass	Mandible	—	12
13-year-old Paso Fino male horse	*Halicephalobus*	Ataxia Head pressing Recumbency	Kidneys Brain	Cerebellum Hippocampus	13
19-year-old Tennessee gelding	*Halicephalobus*	Ataxia Head pressing Decreased PLR Nystagmus	Kidneys Brain	Thalamus Midbrain Meninges	13
12-year-old female horse	*Halicephalobus*	Ataxia Recumbency	Brain	Meninges	14
14-year-old Paint gelding	*Halicephalobus*	Ataxia Urinary incontinence Cauda equina syndrome Recumbency	Caudaequina Sacral spinal cord and sacral rootlets Sacral rootlets	Cauda equina	15
23-year-old Saddlebred gelding	*Halicephalobus*	Fever Ataxia Blindness	Brain Eye	Cerebrum Cerebellum Brainstem Optic nerve and retina	16
6-year-old female Quarter Horse	*Halicephalobus*	Ataxia Recumbency	Brain	Midbrain Cerebrum Cerebellum	17
16-year-old male Holsteiner	*Halicephalobus*	Renal disease Blindness in right eye Seizures Comatose	Kidneys Eye Brain	Optic nerve Cerebellum Hippocampus	4
5-year-old male Miniature Horse	*Halicephalobus*	Ataxia Uveitis Testicular enlargement	Kidneys Brain Testicles	Cerebral cortex	4

TABLE 12-13

Signalment, Organism Identified, Clinical Signs, and Organs Affected in Cases of Verminous Encephalomyelitis—cont'd

Signalment	Organism	Clinical Signs	Organs Affected	Affected Areas in Central Nervous System (CNS)	Reference
17-year-old male Tennessee Walking Horse	*Halicephalobus*	Ataxia Hyperesthesia Opisthotonus Nystagmus	Brain	Cerebrum Cerebellum Brainstem Cervical spinal cord	18
10-year-old Thoroughbred gelding	*Halicephalobus*	Uveitis Head pressing Aggressive behavior	Eyes Brain Kidneys	Hypothalamus Thalamus Brainstem	7
12-year-old male Thoroughbred	*Halicephalobus*	Weakness Ataxia	Kidneys Brain	Brainstem Cerebellum Meninges	19
13-year-old Quarter Horse gelding	*Halicephalobus*	Draining tract in right side of mandible Ataxia Fever	Mandible Kidneys Brain	–	6
18-day-old male horse	*Halicephalobus*	Weakness, inability to stand	Lungs Brain	Neurohypophysis Hypothalamus	5
7-week-old male horse	*Halicephalobus*	Ataxia Convulsions Blindness	Lungs Brain	Cerebellum Cerebellar peduncles Meninges	5
3-week-old male Thoroughbred	*Halicephalobus*	Seizures Fever Ataxia	Lungs Brain	Cerebellum	2
12-year-old female Quarter Horse	*Setaria*	Ataxia Recumbency Urinary incontinence Decreased tail tone	Brain	C1 spinal cord	20
Group of eight ponies	*Strongylus*	Visual deficits Incoordination Convulsions	Brain	Cerebral cortex Thalamus Mesencephalon	21
2-year-old male donkey	*Strongylus*	Paraparesis Tetraparesis	Lumbar spinal cord	—	22
10-year-old male Paint	*Draschia*	Circling to left Tetraparesis Blindness in left eye Facial nerve paralysis	Brain	Midbrain Pons Temporal cortex Globus pallidus	23
9-month-old Appaloosa gelding	*Angiostrongylus*	Tetraparesis	Brainstem Spinal cord	—	24
4-month-old male Thoroughbred	*Angiostrongylus*	Tetraparesis	Spinal cord	—	24
14-year-old Quarter Horse gelding	*Hypoderma*	Ataxia Circling Right facial nerve paralysis Blindness in right eye	Brain	Midbrain Pons	25
	Hypoderma	—	Brain	Left corpus striatum	26
	Hypoderma	—	Brain	Brainstem	27

PLR, pupillary light response.

pathogenic mechanisms described for strongyle encephalomyelitis include aberrantly migrating fourth- and fifth-stage larvae in the intima of the aorta or left ventricle, which causes endothelial damage, stimulates the clotting cascade, and results in formation of a thrombus that often contains the parasitic larva.[21] Lesions are generally asymmetrical because of random migration in the brain, although migration along the spinal cord has been reported in a donkey.[22]

Parelaphostrongylus tenuis

The meningeal worm *Parelaphostrongylus tenuis* causes neurologic disease in cervids, ovids, bovids, and camelids. Recently, there have been multiple reports of similar disease in horses ranging in age between 6 months to 9 years.[28-30] Affected horses have a history of sudden onset of scoliosis with no history or evidence of trauma.

Draschia megastoma

Adult *Draschia megastoma* worms are found in the stomach of equids where they cause mucosal granulomatous masses and mild chronic gastritis. The life cycle of *Draschia* is indirect because the organism uses flies as the intermediate host. Eggs and larvae are released into the gastric lumen, and the first larval stage passes in the feces and is ingested by fly larvae of the genus *Musca* in which *Draschia* spp. organisms develop to infective larvae. Finally, horses become infected when the third larval stage is deposited on the host by adult flies. Infective larvae that are ingested and reach the stomach develop into adults and complete the life cycle. Larvae deposited in damaged skin result in local inflammation and development of extensive granulation tissue, which is the typical lesion of cutaneous habronemiasis.

Stray *D. megastoma* larvae may be found anywhere throughout the body, and a case has been reported of *D. megastoma* migration in the brainstem of a horse in Southern United States, resulting in asymmetrical brainstem disease.[23]

Setaria Species

Infestation with the filarial nematode *Setaria* is common in the abdominal cavity of ungulates where the organism does not cause significant clinical effects. *S. labiatopapillosa* is found in cattle, and *S. equina* is found in horses. Microfilariae gain access to peripheral circulation and then are transmitted to other potential hosts via mosquitoes. In a postmortem examination study of 305 horses in Japan, *S. equina* was recovered from 66 of those horses (≈22%).

The cattle parasite *S. digitata* occurs only in Asia, and infestation in unnatural hosts (horses, sheep, goats, camel, and human beings) has been associated with cerebrospinal nematodiasis. This condition can be enzootic in India, Burma, and Sri Lanka, is called *Kumri* (weak back), and has a seasonal occurrence, usually during the fly season (late summer and fall).[31]

Two cases of aberrant *S. digitata* CNS migration have been reported in Japanese racehorses, and one case of *Setaria* spp. larval migration in the brainstem and cervical spinal cord has been reported in a 12-year-old Quarter Horse mare in the Midwestern United States.[20,32]

Angiostrongylus cantonensis

Adult parasites are found in the right ventricle and pulmonary artery of rats. The pulmonary circulation carries eggs released by adult worms to the alveoli, where the first larval stage develops and migrates up the trachea, is swallowed, and passes in feces. Snails and slugs are intermediate hosts, and ingestion of the snail results in ingestion of the infective larvae that migrate through CNS, and finally, the larvae reach the heart via the circulation.

Aberrant CNS migration of *Angiostrongylus cantonensis* larvae has been reported in two foals with tetraparesis in Australia,[24] and aberrant migration is a recognized cause of eosinophilic meningoencephalitis in human beings and dogs.[33]

Hypoderma Species

Cattle are normal hosts of *Hypoderma* spp., but horses are accidental hosts of warble fly larvae. In cattle, *Hypoderma* larvae penetrate the skin after hatching from eggs attached to hair in the rump and lower legs. These larvae migrate through connective tissues to reach the esophagus, in the case of *H. lineatum*, or to the vertebral canal around epidural fat, in the case of *H. bovis*. Finally, the larvae migrate back to the skin over the back where they create a breathing hole. Cutaneous myiasis is uncommon in horses, and warble fly larvae occasionally may migrate aberrantly into the brain. Tissue damage causing necrosis and hemorrhage is extensive because of the big size of the instars.[25] Instars can enter through large natural foramina such as the foramen magnum, optic foramen, and occasionally intervertebral foramina.

CLINICAL SIGNS

Severity and duration of clinical signs vary from mild, transient, and insidious to severe and fatal. In some cases, clinical signs progress over 2 to 4 months, with periods of improvement or stabilization.[4,8,23] Variability of clinical signs depends on the number of parasites (thromboembolic shower of *Strongylus vulgaris*), on the size of the migrating organism (*Hypoderma* spp. larvae are large and cause severe necrosis and hemorrhage as they migrate in the CNS parenchyma), and neuroanatomic localization of the lesions. Horses suffering from larval migrations in the brain *(S. vulgaris, Halicephalobus deletrix, Draschia megastoma*, and *Hypoderma* spp.*)* may display head tilt, circling, recumbency, blindness, hyperesthesia, stiff neck, ataxia, head pressing, recumbency, seizures, and coma. In those cases in which larvae cause lesions in the spinal cord *(S. vulgaris, H. deletrix, Setaria* spp., *Angiostrongylus cantonensis)*, clinical signs may include focal or multifocal asymmetrical ataxia, weakness, dog-sitting posture caused by paraparesis, increased patellar reflexes, atonic bladder, poor tail tone, and poor rectal tone with impaction of feces (see Table 12-12). Recently, a case of cauda equine neuritis has been reported that was caused by *H. gingivalis* migration in the sacral spinal cord and cauda equina nerves.[15]

Clinical signs of *Parelaphostrongylus tenuis* infection are quite characteristic and include acute onset of scoliosis (observed in 90% of reported cases), with progressive gait deficits. Scoliosis is most common in the cervical area.[28-30] The affected area of the vertebral column is usually C shaped, with flaccid muscles and decreased cutaneous sensation on the convex side of the curve. Tetraparesis and ataxia is mild to moderate and predominantly ipsilateral to the convex side of the curve. If bilateral gait deficits are observed, then they are worse on the convex side. The proposed pathogenesis for clinical signs involves unilateral weakness of the paraspinal epaxial muscles on the convex side of the curve.[30] A linear lesion that extends for several segments, most likely in the dorsal gray column, is most likely to cause the observed signs.

DIFFERENTIAL DIAGNOSIS

One should consider verminous encephalomyelitis in all cases of acute or progressive asymmetrical disease of the spinal cord, cerebrum, cerebellum, or brainstem. If brain involvement is evident without other localizing signs, then the differential diagnosis list may include equine togaviral encephalomyelitis, rabies, equine protozoal myelitis (EPM), trauma, cerebral abscess or basilar epidural empyema, bacterial meningitis, hepatic encephalopathy, neoplasia, and leukoencephalomalacia. If the neurologic signs are limited to spinal cord involvement, then other diseases to include in the differential diagnosis list may be cervical stenotic myelopathy, EPM, EHV-1 myeloencephalopathy, trauma, WNV meningoencephalitis, EDM, trauma, spinal osteomyelitis or discospondylitis, vertebral fracture, and neoplasia. If the only signs present are related to cauda equina syndrome, then other conditions to consider are polyneuritis equi, sacral or coccygeal fracture, EPM, EHV-1 myeloencephalopathy, sorghum or Sudan grass toxicity, epidural abscess from tail blocking, and neoplasia.

Initial diagnostics should include CBC, serum chemistry profile, urinalysis, and CSF collection for cytologic evaluation. In addition, serologic examination and viral isolation and CSF Western blot for EPM may help eliminate several more common viral and protozoal myeloencephalitides. Radiographs of the cervical or lumbosacral spine and myelography may be required to rule out more common causes of spinal cord disease (cervical stenotic myelopathy, trauma, fractures). Although only routinely available at referral hospitals, advanced imaging techniques (e.g., computerized axial tomography, MRI) may be useful in diagnosing parasitic encephalomyelitis or other conditions with similar clinical signs.

CSF analysis in cases of parasitic encephalomyelitis can be normal; however, CSF changes are common and include xanthochromia, increased protein, and neutrophilic and mononuclear pleocytosis, but eosinophils rarely occur (Table 12-14). Only in a case of *Angiostrongylus cantonensis* were eosinophils the predominant cell type on CSF cytologic examination. In addition, *Halicephalobus deletrix* eggs are visible on microscopic examination of a CSF sample subjected to cytocentrifugation.[5] Similarly, *H. deletrix* larvae may be visible on microscopic examination of urine sediment or semen in cases of renal and testicular involvement.[4] Analysis of CSF obtained from horses with *Parelaphostrongylus tenuis* neurologic disease has been within normal limits.[30]

TABLE 12-14

Cerebrospinal Fluid Analysis in Verminous Encephalomyelitis

Organism	White Blood Cells in CSF	Protein in CSF	Cells in CSF	Larvae Present in Urine	Reference
Halicephalobus	2030 cells/μl	89 mg/dl	Mostly PMNs	—	10
Halicephalobus	25 cells/μl	69 mg/dl	15% N, 56% L, 22% M, 5% E, 2% B	—	13
Halicephalobus	81 cells/μl	114 mg/dl	9% N, 41% L, 50% M	—	13
Halicephalobus	60 cells/μl	710 mg/dl	-	—	14
Halicephalobus	495 cells/μl	112 mg/dl	34% N, 37% L, 29% M	No	15
Halicephalobus	—	—	—	Yes	4
Halicephalobus	—	—	—	No	19
Halicephalobus	179 cells/μl	71 mg/dl	Predominantly N; few L, M, and E	No	6
Halicephalobus	35 cells/μl	100 mg/dl	25% N, 58% M, 17% E, 2% L	No	5
Halicephalobus	16 cells/μl	76 mg/dl	31% N, 22% L, 47% M	—	2
Setaria	Increased	Increased	—	—	20
Strongylus	Two of eight ponies had increased white blood cell counts: 42 cells/μl and 1080 cells/μl	One of eight ponies had high protein at 175 mg/dl.	—	20	
Strongylus	9988 cells/μl	550 mg/dl	72% N, 14% L, 12% M, 2% E	—	22
Draschia	Normal	Normal	—	—	23
Angiostrongylus	1560 cells/μl	—	1% N, 8% L, 14% M, 77% E	No	24

CSF, cerebrospinal fluid; *PMN,* polymorphonuclear neutrophil leukocytes; *N,* neutrophils; *L,* small lymphocytes; *M,* large mononuclear cells; *E,* eosinophils; *B,* basophils.

Antemortem diagnosis may be possible in those cases in which renal or bony involvement is detected and nematodes are identified in biopsies of the affected tissues.[6] As described previously, renal involvement with granulomatous lesions encapsulating *Halicephalobus deletrix* worms is observed in most cases of *H. deletrix* encephalomyelitis. Therefore transabdominal renal ultrasound examination and ultrasound-guided biopsy (in those cases with renal lesions present), as well as microscopic examination of urine sediment, may prove useful in cases of acute onset progressive asymmetrical neurologic disease, especially if one suspects cerebrospinal nematodiasis caused by *H. deletrix*.

Additionally, a PCR–based diagnostic test has been developed for confirmation of *Setaria* encephalomyelitis in goats, sheep, and horses.[34] This test is based on specific amplification of *Setaria* spp. filarial DNA from a blood sample from the host.

PATHOLOGIC FINDINGS

The gross and histopathologic lesions depend on the parasite involved. Thorough postmortem examination with sectioning and histopathologic examination of all areas of the CNS relevant to the antemortem clinical signs are important to identify migrating parasites. *Strongylus vulgaris* and *Hypoderma* spp. larvae are easy to see, but other nematodes are only visible on microscopic examination. Some reports describe how one may recover and examine whole, fixed nematodes for distinctive morphologic features by centrifugation of formalin solution in which the brain had been fixed.[9,18] Gross examination of other tissues for evidence of *S. vulgaris* thrombi or presence of *Halicephalobus deletrix* granulomatous lesions may help establish a postmortem diagnosis.

On histopathologic examination, one generally sees extensive tissue necrosis with mixed inflammatory response. *H. deletrix* migration in the CNS typically results in histiolymphocytic infiltrates, malacia, glial proliferation, and perivascular lymphocytic cuffing. Migrations of warble fly and *S. vulgaris* larvae result in severe hemorrhage, large malacic tracts, and edema caused by their relative larger size.

TREATMENT

Treatment of verminous encephalomyelitis in horses is often unrewarding. None of the cases reported in the literature have responded favorably to anti-inflammatory drugs and antihelmintics. Only in one case of *Halicephalobus deletrix* granuloma limited to the prepuce, therapy with ivermectin and diethylcarbamazine was successful.[35] However, numerous cases of cerebrospinal nematodiasis likely respond favorably to anti-inflammatory drugs and antihelmintics, but one never reaches a definitive diagnosis because diagnosis requires a postmortem examination.

Therapeutic recommendations depend on the severity, progression, and localization of neurologic signs, as well as on consideration of possible contraindications (e.g., if one suspects bacterial or viral cause, then one should avoid using corticosteroids). In cases of acute neurologic disease use of the following anti-inflammatory drugs may be warranted: NSAIDs such as phenylbutazone (2.2 mg/kg b.i.d.), flunixin meglumine (1 mg/kg b.i.d.), or ketoprofen (2 mg/kg b.i.d.); intravenously administered DMSO (1 g/kg as a 10% solution once daily for 3 to 5 days); and corticosteroids (dexamethasone at 0.1 to 0.25 mg/kg once daily or prednisolone at 0.2 to 4.4 mg/kg once daily). If cerebral signs are observed, then one may administer mannitol (0.25 to 2 g/kg as a 20% solution once daily), or hypertonic saline may be warranted in an attempt to minimize cerebral edema. In countries in which EPM is known to occur, antiprotozoal treatment is recommended.

Specific antiparasitics suggested for treating verminous encephalomyelitis include benzimidazole compounds (oxfendazole, thiabendazole, fenbendazole, and mebendazole), diethylcarbamazine and ivermectin for the treatment of nematodes, and organophosphates (trichlorfon and dichlorvos) for the treatment of warble fly larvae. Although ivermectin is effective against most equine parasites, it may not be the best choice because of its delayed method of killing, which may take as long as 10 to 14 days. Some authors have suggested administration of fenbendazole at 50 mg/kg by mouth once daily for 3 days[36,37]; however, specific data on the efficacy of antihelmintics in treating nematode or warble fly larvae migration through the CNS are not available.

MISCELLANEOUS NEUROLOGIC DISORDERS

Debra C. Sellon

In addition to the numerous neurologic problems discussed in detail earlier in this chapter, horses can develop a wide variety of acute or chronic neurologic disorders with clinical signs related to brain, spinal cord, or peripheral nerve dysfunction. Clinical signs can occur because of primary disease or dysfunction of the CNS or secondary to a variety of metabolic disorders or disorders of other body systems. This section will mention the most important of the miscellaneous CNS disorders and refer the reader to relevant chapters for more detailed information.

NEUROLOGIC NEOPLASIA

Many types of neoplastic lesions have been identified in the brain and spinal cord of horses. A comprehensive review of the clinical and pathologic aspects of equine CNS neoplasia, however, is lacking in the peer-reviewed veterinary literature. Available case reports and summaries of pathologic studies suggest that CNS neoplasia is quite uncommon in horses. In one Australian survey of 450 horses with neurologic disease, the prevalence of neurologic disease secondary to neoplasia was less than 2%.[1] This percentage is likely to be much lower in horses in the United States because of the much higher incidence of encephalitic disorders and EPM.

Tumors of the nervous system can be classified on the basis of their cellular origin as tumors of nerve cells, neuroepithelium, glia, peripheral nerves and nerve sheaths, mesodermal structures, and endocrine organs. Neoplasms of nerve cell origin appear to be extremely uncommon in horses with only a few reports of ganglioneuromas, complex tumors arising in peripheral ganglia and composed of well-differentiated neurons, nerve processes, Schwann cells, and glial cells.[2,3] These tumors may cause intestinal obstruction and signs of colic in affected horses.

Tumors of neuroepithelial origin in horses include ependymoma, choroid plexus papilloma, neuroepithelial tumor of the optic nerve, malignant medulloepithelioma, ocular medulloepithelioma, and pineoblastoma.[4-19] Glial cell tumors include optic disc astrocytoma, retinoblastoma, and microglioma.[13,19,20] Neoplasms of peripheral nerves and nerve sheaths appear to be more common than CNS neoplasia and include neurofibromas and neurofibrosarcomas.[21-26] The most common sites for neurofibromas are in the cutaneous tissues of the pectoral region, abdomen, neck, and face but gastrointestinal tract lesions have also been described.[21] There are also reports of intracranial and mediastinal schwannomas in horses.[27,28]

The most common mesodermal neoplasm in horses appears to be meningioma.[5,18,29] Neoplastic reticulosis, lipoma in the mesencephalic aqueduct, angioma in the cervical spinal cord, primary meningeal lymphoma, and melanoblastoma of the cerebellar meninges have also been described.[30-32]

Older texts often refer to pituitary pars intermedia dysfunction (PPID) of older horses as a neoplastic lesion. This disorder is most likely a manifestation of oxidative damage to dopamine-producing neurons in the central nervous system with subsequent dysregulation of hormone production within the pars intermedia of the pituitary gland. PPID is discussed in detail in the Endocrinology chapter of this text.

Cholesterol granulomas (cholesteatomas, cholesterinic granulomas) are likewise not neoplastic lesions, though they may have been described as such in the past.[33-41] These lesions are found in the choroid plexus of up to 20% of older horses.[42] Although more common in the choroid plexus of the fourth ventricle, lesions in the lateral ventricles may be more likely to result in clinical signs. Lesions may represent a chronic granulomatous reaction to deposition of cholesterol crystals associated with chronic choroid plexus leakage. Grossly the granulomas are circumscribed, firm, granular, and yellow-brown with a glistening cut surface. They are most often recognized as incidental findings at necropsy of horses without noticeable clinical signs. If they are large enough, however, they might cause CNS signs as a result of direct pressure on cerebral tissues or obstructive hydrocephalus. In affected horses, reported clinical signs have included altered behavior, depression, somnolence, seizures, ataxia, weakness, and coma. CSF from affected horses may have an elevated protein and appear xanthochromic.[33-35]

Secondary neoplastic conditions affecting the CNS may penetrate the cranial vault or vertebrae, extend through osseous foramina, or metastasize via the vascular system. Clinical signs vary depending on the type, site, and extent of the lesion. Lymphosarcoma is probably the most common secondary neoplasm of the CNS in horses.[32,43-48] Lesions may cause forebrain signs if present in the cranial vault or ataxia and paresis if causing compression of the spinal cord.

Melanoma of the spinal cord, meninges, and brain may occur with metastasis of primary cutaneous lesions.[49-51] Alternatively, clinical signs may represent spread from affected sublumbar lymph nodes.[32,52] Melanoma of the CNS is most common in gray horses.

Hemangiosarcoma and undifferentiated sarcoma have been reported to affect the CNS of horses[32,53-55] There are numerous descriptions of adenocarcinomas and carcinomas (including squamous cell carcinoma) affecting the CNS of horses by direct spread from a primary site in the head or by metastasis from a distant site.[32,56-62] Tumors of the bone or bone marrow may involve the skull or vertebrae resulting in compression of the brain or spinal cord, respectively.[32,63-65]

Malformation tumors, including epidermoids, dermoids, teratomas, and teratoids, may also affect the CNS.[32] They are often incidental findings at necropsy but may occasionally be clinically significant.

Supportive evidence for the presence of CNS neoplasia can be obtained with advanced imaging (i.e., computed tomography, magnetic resonance imaging) of the brain or spinal cord in select equine patients. Definitive diagnosis of primary CNS neoplasia in horses requires cytologic or histopathologic identification of neoplastic cells or tissues. This diagnosis necessitates biopsy, cytologic evaluation of an aspirate from a suspect lesion, or identification of neoplastic cells in cerebrospinal fluid (CSF). Analysis of CSF is rarely diagnostic of neoplasia in horses because of the rarity of the presence of neoplastic cells in the fluid. Given the practical difficulties inherent in obtaining biopsy samples from the brain or spinal cord, definitive diagnosis of primary CNS neoplasia in horses rarely occurs antemortem. Definitive diagnosis is more likely in horses with secondary CNS neoplasia in which a diagnosis is made by biopsy or cytologic evaluation of primary lesions identified external to the CNS.

TOXIC DISORDERS

A wide variety of toxic substances can affect the CNS of horses. Most of these are discussed in detail in the Toxicology chapter of this text. Three toxic neurologic conditions merit mention in this chapter because of their common occurrence in some geographic areas and their distinctive clinical appearance as demonstrated in the referenced video segments on the DVD accompanying this text.

LEUKOENCEPHALOMALACIA

Equine leukoencephalomalacia is a seasonal disorder of horses, ponies, donkeys, and mules, occurring most commonly in late fall through early spring. Most outbreaks are associated with a dry growing period followed by a wet period. The disorder is caused by ingestion of the mycotoxin fumonisin B1, a metabolite of *Fusarium moniliforme*.[66-88] Two clinical syndromes are associated with fumonisin B1 intoxication. The more common is a neurologic syndrome characterized initially by incoordination, aimless walking, intermittent anorexia, lethargy, depression, blindness, and head pressing. These signs may be followed by hyperexcitablity, belligerence, extreme agitation, profuse sweating, and delirium. Recumbency and clonic-tetanic seizures may occur before death. Less commonly, horses develop a hepatotoxic syndrome with swelling of the lips and nose, somnolence, severe icterus and petechiation of mucous membranes, abdominal breathing, and cyanosis. Gross lesions include liquefactive necrosis and degeneration of the cerebral hemispheres; changes may also occur in the brainstem, cerebellum, and spinal cord.

NIGROPALLIDAL ENCEPHALOMALACIA

Yellow star thistle and Russian knapweed grow over much of the western United States in nonirrigated pastures during dry seasons of summer and fall. Ingestion of these plants result in unilateral or more commonly bilateral softening and necrosis in areas of the globus pallidus and substantia nigra.[89-98] Lesions are often sharply defined and may be cavitary. Although the plants are generally considered unpalatable by most horses, some horses may develop a craving for the plants and selectively seek them out. The exact toxic principle in these plants has not been determined. Affected horses demonstrate variable degrees of impairment of eating and drinking with lack of coordination of movements of prehension, mastication, and deglutition. Most horses appear to be able to swallow if food or water is placed in the posterior pharynx. Severely affected horses might attempt to drink by immersing their muzzle deeply into the water in an apparent attempt to force water into the posterior pharynx. Hypertonicity of facial muscles is common with the horse often holding the mouth partially open with the lips retracted. The tongue may protrude from the mouth and many horses display constant chewing movements.

Fluphenazine Toxicity

Fluphenazine administration to horses may result in characteristic clinical signs of toxicity.[99-103] Fluphenazine is a highly potent phenothiazine neuroleptic that is widely used in human medicine for a variety of psychological disturbances. In horses, fluphenazine decanoate has been used to provide a persistent sedative effect. It binds avidly to dopamine D_2 receptors in the brain. The very slow dissociation of fluphenazine from these receptors is associated with a greater risk of adverse extrapyramidal signs than is observed with newer atypical antipsychotic medications.[99] Its administration to some horses can result in severe extrapyramidal effects and Parkinsonism with clinical signs including agitation, profuse sweating, hypermetria, aimless circling, intense pawing and striking with the thoracic limbs, and rhythmic swinging of the head and neck alternating with periods of severe stupor. There are no published reports of the pharmacokinetics of fluphenazine in horses. A long-acting depot formulation for IM administration is available and appears to be most commonly used. One published report suggests a dosage of 0.05 to 0.08 mg/kg IM every 2 weeks with a warning to beware of idiosyncratic reactions.[104] Horses have exhibited signs of extrapyramidal effects of fluphenazine decanoate after receiving doses as low as 40 mg IM.[99] Given that recommended doses for adult humans range between 25 to 50 mg, it is reasonable to assume that at least some horses are much more susceptible than humans to the adverse effects of fluphenazine decanoate. The severity of clinical signs observed in some affected horses is sufficient to pose considerable safety risks for veterinarians and handlers treating these horses. This author is aware of at least one horse that was euthanized because of the extreme danger of clinical signs after administration of fluphenazine; other authors have indicated similar adverse outcomes.[99] Treatment consists of discontinuation of drug administration and enhancing cholinergic function by administering anticholinergic medications. Diphenhydramine chloride results in significant improvement in some, but not all, affected horses.[99,101] Benztropine mesylate (0.018 mg/kg IV every 8 hours) has also been helpful for treatment of some affected horses.[99] Other horses apparently benefited from sodium pentobarbital (2 mg/kg IV followed by a constant rate infusion at 2.5 mg/kg/h) in an attempt to control maniacal behavior without inducing recumbency or anesthesia.[99]

METABOLIC DISORDERS

A wide variety of metabolic disorders can cause clinical signs indicative of central nervous system dysfunction. These signs include hepatic dysfunction, hypoglycemia, hypoxemia and ischemia, and severe abnormalities in plasma electrolyte concentrations.

Hepatoencephalopathy

An excellent review of the etiology, pathogenesis, clinical signs, diagnosis, and treatment of liver disease is included elsewhere in this text. A normally functioning liver is necessary to maintain normal brain neuron and astrocyte function. With acute liver disease hepatoencephalopathy is most often a result of astrocyte swelling, acute cytotoxic cerebral edema and intracranial hypertension. In chronic hepatic disease astrocytes are swollen but also show evidence of Alzheimer type II changes. Horses with hepatoencephalopathy show signs of cerebral cortex dysfunction. The earliest recognizable clinical signs in horses are often depression, lethargy, mild ataxia, and various forms of inappropriate behavior. These signs can progress to head pressing, circling, somnolence, and diminished responsiveness to external stimuli. Eventually affected horses become recumbent and comatose. Seizures may occasionally be observed but they are not common. The type and severity of clinical signs do not correlate with type or reversibility of the underlying hepatic disease.

Hypoglycemia, Hypoxemia, and Ischemia

Severe hypoglycemia is not common in adult horses but is common in neonates, often as a complication of sepsis, prematurity, hypoxic ischemic encephalopathy, or hypothermia. When hypoglycemia does occur it may result in weakness, depression, ataxia, and eventually loss of consciousness. Seizure activity is not common in adult horses but may occasionally be observed in affected foals. Iatrogenic hypoglycemia can occur in horses treated with insulin or with abrupt cessation of intravenous glucose therapy. Clinical signs are rapidly reversed with intravenous administration of glucose-containing solutions. Guidelines for intravenous glucose therapy are included in the chapter on foal diseases elsewhere in this text (Chapter 21).

Because of the brain's high and continuous demand for oxygen, the CNS is extremely susceptible to hypoxic or ischemic damage. This is most apparent in the neonate with hypoxic ischemic encephalopathy, discussed in detail in the chapter on foal diseases. As nervous tissue switches to anaerobic glycolysis to meet its energy needs brain glucose is depleted and localized lactic acidosis occurs. Neurons swell and cytotoxic edema exacerbates ischemia. The end result is irreversible cell damage and neuronal death. Clinical signs depend on what areas of the brain are affected. Localized hypoxia may occur with thromboembolic disorders or intracarotid injections. Deprivation of oxygen to the entire CNS results in more dramatic clinical signs of impaired cerebral function ultimately leading to seizures, coma, and death. This type of generalized severe tissue hypoxia may result from decreased inspired oxygen, ventilation/perfusion abnormalities, right to left shunting of blood, impairment of gas diffusion within the lungs, hypoventilation, severe anemia, impaired oxygen utilization by tissues, or profound hypotension secondary to sepsis, hemorrhage, anaphylaxis, or cardiac failure. These disorders are discussed in detail in the appropriate chapters elsewhere in this text.

Electrolyte Abnormalities

Severe hyponatremia or hypernatremia can result in CNS dysfunction. Hyponatremia most often results from water intoxication because of excessive IV or oral administration or consumption of hypotonic solutions. A common clinical scenario resulting in hyponatremia is oral consumption of large quantities of water by a patient with a disorder that results in significant concurrent electrolyte loss (e.g., diarrhea, excessive sweating, polyuric renal failure). Clinical signs are most common in horses with a serum sodium concentration of <110 mEq/L. Profound hypernatremia may result in clinical signs of spasticity, myoclonus, and depression. Therapy of foals affected with profound hyponatremia or hypernatremia is discussed in the chapter on foal disorders.

REFERENCES

Neurologic Examination

1. Mayhew J: *Large animal neurology*, Philadelphia, 2009, Wiley-Blackwell.
2. Blythe LL: Neurologic examination of the horse, *Vet Clin North Am Equine Pract* 3:255-281, 1987.
3. deLahunta A, Glass EN: *Veterinary neuroanatomy and clinical neurology*, ed 3, St Louis, 2009, WB Saunders.
4. Van Biervliet J, de Lahunta A, Divers TJ: Sporadic conditions affecting the spinal cord: parasitic migration and neoplastic disease, *Clin Tech Equine Pract* 5:49-53, 2006.
5. Matthews HK, Andrews F: Performing a neurologic examination in a standing or recumbent horse, *Vet Med* 85:1229-1240, 1990.
6. Firth E: Horner's syndrome in the horse: experimental induction and a case report, *Equine Vet J* 10:9-13, 1978.
7. Mayhew IG: Horner's syndrome and lesions involving the sympathetic nervous system, *Vet Clin North Am Equine Pract* 2:44-47, 1980.
8. Hahn CN: Miscellaneous disorders of the equine nervous system: Horner's syndrome and polyneuritis equi, *Clin Tech Equine Pract* 5:43-48, 2006.
9. Andrews FM, Matthews HK: Localizing the source of neurologic problems in horses, *Vet Med* 85:1107-1120, 1990.
10. Mayhew IG: Equine neurologic examination, *Prog Vet Neurol* 1:40-47, 1981.
11. Mayhew IG: Neurological and neuropathological observations on the equine neonate, *Equine Vet J Suppl* 5:28-33, 1999.
12. Woods JR: Neurological examination of the horse, *OVMA* 24:13-18, 1972.
13. Mayhew IG: Neurologic examination of the horse with a discussion of common diseases and syndromes. In *Proceedings of the twenty-fourth annual convention of the American Association of Equine Practitioners,* St Louis,1978, AEEP.
14. Rooney JR: Two cervical reflexes in the horse, *J Am Vet Med Assoc* 162:162, 1973.
15. Jones WE, editor: *Equine sports medicine*, Philadelphia, 1989, Lea & Febiger.
16. Yeager MJ, Middleton DL, Render JA: Identification of spinal cord lesions through the use of Zenker's fixation and radiography, *J Vet Diagn Invest* 1:264-266, 1989.
17. Robertson-Smith RG, Jeffcott LB, Friend SCE, et al: An unusual incidence of neurological disease affecting horses during a drought, *Aust Vet J* 62(1):6-12, 1985.

Cerebrospinal Fluid Evaluation

1. deLahunta A, Glass EN: *Veterinary neuroanatomy and clinical neurology*, ed 3, St Louis, 2009, WB Saunders.
2. Milhort TH: The choroid plexus and cerebrospinal fluid production, *Science* 166:1514, 1969.
3. Blood DC, Henderson JA, Radostits O: *Veterinary medicine*, ed 5, Philadelphia, 1979, Lea & Febiger.
4. Tripathi R: Tracing the bulk outflow of cerebrospinal fluid by transmission and scanning electron microscopy, *Brain Res* 80:503, 1974.
5. Mayhew J: *Large animal neurology*, Philadelphia, 2009, Wiley-Blackwell.
6. Andrews FM, Maddux JM, Faulk DS: Total protein, albumin quotient, IgG, and IgG index determinations in horse cerebrospinal fluid, *Prog Vet Neurol* 1:197-204, 1990.
7. Blythe LL, Mattson DE, Lassen ED, et al: Antibodies against equine herpesvirus 1 in the cerebrospinal fluid of horses, *Can Vet J* 26:218, 1985.
8. Wilson JW: Clinical application of cerebrospinal fluid creatine phosphokinase determination, *J Am Vet Med Assoc* 171:1977, 2000.
9. Beech J: Cytology of equine cerebrospinal fluid, *Vet Pathol* 20:553-562, 1983.
10. Mayhew IG, Whitlock RH, Tasker JB: Equine cerebrospinal fluid: reference values of normal horses, *Am J Vet Res* 38:1271, 1977.
11. Rossdale PD, Falk M, Jeffcott LB, et al: A preliminary investigation of cerebrospinal fluid in the newborn foal as an aid to the study of cerebral damage, *J Reprod Fertil Suppl* 27:593, 1979.
12. Hayes TE: Examination of cerebrospinal fluid in the horse, *Vet Clin North Am Equine Pract* 3:283-291, 1987.
13. Smith BP, editor: *Large animal internal medicine*, ed 4, St Louis, 2009, Mosby.
14. Fishman RA: Brain edema, *N Engl J Med* 293:706, 1975.
15. Greene HJ, Leipold HW, Vestwebor J: Bovine congenital defects: variations of internal hydrocephalus, *Cornell Vet* 64:596, 1974.
16. Andrews FM, Matthews HK, Reed SM: The ancillary techniques and tests for diagnosing equine neurologic disease, *Vet Med* 85:1325-1330, 1990.
17. Jamison JM, Prescott JF: Bacterial meningitis in large animals, part 1, *Compend Contin Educ Pract Vet* 9:399-406, 1987.
18. Darian BJ, Belknap J, Niefield J: Cerebrospinal fluid changes in two horses with central nervous system nematodiasis (Micronema deletrix), *J Vet Intern Med* 2:201-205, 1988.
19. Furr MO, Tyler RA: Cerebrospinal fluid creatine kinase activity in horses with central nervous system disease: 69 cases (1984-1989), *J Am Vet Med Assoc* 197:245-248, 1990.
20. Green EM, Green S: Cerebrospinal fluid lactic acid concentration: reference values and diagnostic implications of abnormal concentrations in adult horses. In McGuirk SM, editor: *Proceedings of the American College of Veterinary Internal Medicine,* Blacksburg, VA, 1990, ACVIM.

Electrodiagnostic Aids and Selected Neurologic Diseases

1. Chrisman DC, Burt JK, Wood PK, et al: Electromyography in small animal neurology, *J Am Vet Med Assoc* 160:311-318, 1972.
2. deLahunta A, Glass EN: *Veterinary neuroanatomy and clinical neurology*, ed 3, St Louis, 2009, WB Saunders.
3. Kimura J: *Electrodiagnosis in diseases of nerve and muscle: principles and practice*, Philadelphia, 1984, FA Davis.
4. Sims MH: Electrodiagnostic techniques in the evaluation of diseases affecting skeletal muscle, *Vet Clin North Am Small Anim Pract* 13:145-162, 1983.
5. Henry RW, Diesem CD, Wiechers MD: Evaluation of equine radial and median nerve conduction velocities, *Am J Vet Res* 40:1406-1410, 1979.
6. Henry RW, Diesem CD: Proximal equine radial and median motor nerve conduction velocity, *Am J Vet Res* 42:1819-1822, 1981.
7. Andrews FM: Facial nerve conduction velocities in the horse, 1989-2001.
8. Klemm WR: *Animal electroencephalography*, New York, 1969, Academic Press.

9. Klemm WR: *Applied electronics for veterinary medicine and small animal physiology*, Springfield, IL, 1976, Charles C Thomas.
10. Buchthal F, Rosenfalck P: Spontaneous electrical activity of human muscle, *Electroencephalogr Clin Neurophysiol* 20:321, 1966.
11. Weiderholt WC: End plate noise in electromyography, *Neurology* 20:214, 1970.
12. Buchthal F: *An introduction to electromyography*, Copenhagen, 1957, Scandinavia University Books.
13. Kugelberg E, Petersen I: Insertion activity in electromyography with notes on denervated muscle response to constant current, *J Neurol Neurosurg Psychiatry* 12:268-273, 1949.
14. Spier SJ, Carlson GP, Holiday TA, et al: Hyperkalemic periodic paralysis in horses, *J Am Vet Med Assoc* 197:1009-1017, 1990.
15. Warmolts JR, Engel WK: A critique of the "myopathic" electromyogram, *Trans Am Neurol Assoc* 95:173-177, 1970.
16. Buchthal F, Guild C, Rosenfalck D: Multielectrode study of the territory of a motor unit, *Acta Physiol Scand* 39:83-104, 1957.
17. Ettinger S, editor: *Textbook of veterinary internal medicine*, ed 6, St Louis, 2005, WB Saunders.
18. Feinstein B, Pattle RE, Weddell G: Metabolic factors affecting fibrillation in denervated muscle, *J Neurol Neurosurg Psychiatry* 8:1-11, 1945.
19. Thompson DS, Woodward JB, Ringel SP, et al: Evoked potential abnormalities in myasthenic dystrophy, *Electroencephalogr Clin Neurophysiol* 56:453-456, 1983.
20. Inada S, Sugaro S, Ibaraki T: Electromyographic study on denervated muscles in the dog, *Nippon Juigaku Zasshi* 25: 327-336, 1963.
21. Andrews FM, Spurgeon TL, Reed SM: Histochemical changes in skeletal muscles of four male horses with neuromuscular disease, *Am J Vet Res* 47:2078-2083, 1986.
22. Moore MP, Andrews FM, Reed SM, et al: Electromyographic evaluation of horses with laryngeal hemiplegia, *J Equine Vet Sci* 8:424-427, 1988.
23. Andrews FM: Indication and use of electrodiagnostic aids in neurologic disease, *Vet Clin North Am Equine Pract* 3:293-322, 1987.
24. Denny-Brown D, Pennybacker JB: Fibrillation and fasciculation in voluntary muscle, *Brain* 61:311, 1938.
25. Wettstein A: The origin of fasciculations in motor neuron disease, *Ann Neurol* 5:295, 1979.
26. Farnbach GC: Clinical electrophysiology in veterinary neurology. I. Electromyography, *Compend Contin Educ Pract Vet* 11:791-797, 1980.
27. Mayhew IG, deLahunta A, Whitlock RH: Spinal cord disease in the horse, *Cornell Vet* 68(Suppl):44-70, 1978.
28. Cook WR: The diagnosis of respiratory unsoundness in the horse, *Vet Rec* 77:516, 1965.
29. Kornegay JN, Gorageaz EJ, Dawe DL, et al: Polymyositis in dogs, *J Am Vet Med Assoc* 176:431, 1980.
30. Andrews FM, Reed SM, Johnson G: Indications and techniques for muscle biopsy in the horse, *Proc Am Assoc Equine Pract* 35:357-366, 1989.
31. Reed SM, Hegreberg GA, Bayly WM, et al: Progressive myotonia in foals resembling human dystrophia myotonia, *Muscle Nerve* 2:291-296, 1988.
32. Achor LJ, Starr A: Auditory brainstem response in the cat. I. Intracranial and extracranial responses, *Electroencephalogr Clin Neurophysiol* 48:155-173, 1980.
33. Marshall AE: Brainstem auditory-evoked response of the nonanesthetized dog, *Am J Vet Res* 46:966-973, 1985.
34. Fria TJ: The auditory brainstem response: background and clinical applications, *Monogr Contemp Audiol* 2:1-5, 1980.
35. Glattke TJ, Runge CA: Comments on the origin of short latency auditory potentials. In Beasley DS, editor: *Audition in childhood: method of study*, San Diego, 1984, College Hill Press.
36. Hashimoto I, Ishiyama Y, Yoshimoto T, et al: Brainstem auditory evoked potentials recorded directly from human brainstem and thalamus, *Brain* 103:841-859, 1981.
37. Hosford-Dunn H: Auditory brainstem response audiometry: applications in central disorders, *Otolaryngol Clin North Am* 18:257-284, 1985.
38. Jewett DL, Williston JS: Auditory evoked potential for far fields averaged from the scalp of human beings, *Brain* 94: 681-696, 1971.
39. Keranishvili ZS: Sources of the human brainstem auditory evoked potential, *Scand Audiol* 9:75-82, 1980.
40. Anziska BJ, Cracco RQ: Short latency somatosensory evoked potentials in brain-dead patients, *Arch Neurol* 37:222-225, 1980.
41. Cushman MZ, Rossman RN: Diagnostic features of the auditory brainstem response in identifying cerebellopontine angle tumors, *Scand Audiol* 12:35-41, 1983.
42. Greenberg RP, Becker DP, Miller JD, et al: Evaluation of brain function in severe human head trauma with multimodality evoked potentials. II. Localization of brain dysfunction and correlation with post-traumatic neurological conditions, *J Neurosurg* 47:761-768, 1975.
43. Jabbari B, Schwartz DM, MacNeil B, et al: Early abnormalities of brainstem auditory evoked potentials in Friedreich's ataxia: evidence of primary brainstem dysfunction, *Neurology* 33:1071-1074, 1983.
44. Jay WM, Hoyd CS: Abnormal brainstem auditory-evoked potentials in Stelling-Turk-Duane retraction syndrome, *Am J Ophthalmol* 89:814-818, 1980.
45. Robinson D, Rudge P: The use of the auditory evoked potential in the diagnosis of multiple sclerosis, *J Neurol Sci* 45: 235-244, 1980.
46. Starr A, Achor J: Auditory brainstem response in neurological disease, *Arch Neurol* 32:761-768, 1975.
47. Marshall AE, Byars TD, Whitlock RH, et al: Brainstem auditory evoked response in the diagnosis of inner ear injury in the horse, *J Am Vet Med Assoc* 178:282-286, 1978.
48. Marshall AE: Brainstem auditory-evoked response in the nonanesthetized horse and pony, *Am J Vet Res* 46:1445-1450, 1985.
49. Harland MM, Stewart AJ, Marshall AE, et al: Diagnosis of deafness in a horse by brainstem auditory evoked potential, *Can Vet J* 47:151-154, 2006.
50. Steiss JE, Brendemuehl JP, Wright JC, et al: Nerve conduction velocities and brain stem auditory evoked responses in normal neonatal foals, compared to foals exposed to endophyte-fescue, *Progr Neurol Psychiatry* 2:252-260, 1991.
51. Mayhew IG, Washbourne JR: Brainstem auditory evoked potentials in horses and ponies, *Vet J* 153:107-113, 1997.
52. Mayhew IG: The clinical utility of brainstem auditory evoked response testing in horses, *Equine Vet Educ* 15:27-33, 2003.
53. Mayhew IG, Washbourne JR: Short latency auditory evoked potentials recorded from non-anesthestized thoroughbred horses, *Br Vet J* 148:315-327, 1992.
54. Stockard JE, Stockard JJ, Westmoreland BF, et al: Brainstem auditory-evoked responses: normal variation as a function of stimulus and subject characteristics, *Arch Neurol* 36:823-831, 1979.
55. Rolf SL, Reed SM, Melnick W, et al: Auditory brainstem response testing in anesthetized horses, *Am J Vet Res* 48: 910-914, 1987.
56. Elul R: Specific site of generation of brain waves, *Physiologist* 7:125, 1964.
57. Gibbs FA, Gibe EL: *Atlas of electroencephalography*, vols. 1-3, Reading, Mass, 1958, 1959, 1964, Addison Wesley.
58. Mysinger PW, Redding RW, Vaughan JT, et al: Electroencephalographic patterns of clinically normal sedated and tranquilized newborn foals and adult horses, *Am J Vet Res* 46:3641, 1985.

59. Williams DC, Aleman M, Holliday TA, et al: Qualitative and quantitative characteristics of the electroencephalogram in normal horses during spontaneous drowsiness and sleep, *J Vet Intern Med* 22:630-638, 2008.
60. Aleman M, Gray LC, Williams DC, et al: Juvenile idiopathic epilepsy in Egyptian Arabian foals (1985-2005), *J Vet Intern Med* 20:1443-1449, 2006.
61. Lacombe VA, Podell M, Furr M, et al: Diagnostic validity of electroencephalography in equine intracranial disorders, *J Vet Intern Med* 15:385-393, 2001.
62. Otto KA, Voight S, Piepenbrock S, et al: Differences in quantitated electroencephalographic variables during surgical stimulation of horses anesthetized with isoflurane, *Vet Surg* 25:249-255, 1996.
63. Haga HA, Dolvik NI: Electroencephalographic and cardiovascular variables as nociceptive indicators in isoflurane-anaesthetized horses, *Vet Anaesth Analg* 32:128-135, 2005.
64. Robinson C, Lacombe VA, Reed S, et al: Predicting factors for abnormal computed tomography of the head in 58 horses affected by neurologic disorders, *J Am Vet Med Assoc*, 235(2):176–183, 2009.
65. Williams DC, Aleman M, Holliday TA, et al: Qualitative and quantitative characteristics of the electroencephalogram in normal horses during spontaneous drowsiness and sleep, *J Vet Intern Med* 22(3):630-638, 2008.
66. Ernst Niedermeyer: *Fernando Lopes da Silva: Electroencephalography: basic principles, clinical applications, and related fields*, ed 5, Philadelphia, 2005, Lippincott Williams & Wilkins.
67. Hepburn RJ, Furr MO: Sinonasal adenocarcinoma causing central nervous system disease in a horse, *J Vet Intern Med* 18(1):125-131, 2004.
68. Johnson CB, Bloomfield M, Taylor PM: Effects of midazolam and sarmazenil on the equine electroencephalogram during anaesthesia with halothane in oxygen, *J Vet Pharmacol Ther* 26(2):105-112, 2003.
69. Murrell JC, White KL, Johnson, et al: Investigation of the EEG effects of intravenous lidocaine during halothane anaesthesia in ponies, *Vet Anaesth Analg* 32(4):212-221, 2005.

Magnetic Resonance Imaging

1. Ferrell EA, Gavin PR, Tucker RL, et al: Magnetic resonance for evaluation of neurologic disease in 12 horses, *Vet Radiol Ultrasound* 43:510-516, 2002.
2. Audigie F, Tapprest J, George C, et al: Magnetic resonance imaging of a brain abscess in a 10-month-old filly, *Vet Radiol Ultrasound* 45:210-215, 2004.
3. Spoormakers TJ, Ensink JM, Goehring LS, et al: Brain abscesses as a metastatic manifestation of strangles: symptomatology and the use of magnetic resonance imaging as a diagnostic aid, *Equine Vet J* 35:146-151, 2003.
4. Maulet BEB, Bestbier M, Jose-Cunilleras E, et al: Magnetic resonance imaging of a cholesterol granuloma and hydrocephalus in a horse, *Equine Vet Educ* 20:74-79, 2008.
5. Javsicas LH, Watson E, MacKay RJ: What is your neurologic diagnosis? Equine protozoal myeloencephalitis, *J Am Vet Med Assoc* 232:201-204, 2008.

Seizures, Narcolepsy, and Cataplexy

1. deLahunta A: *Glass EN: Veterinary neuroanatomy and clinical neurology*, ed 3, St Louis, 2009, WB Saunders.
2. Robinson NE, editor: *Current therapy in equine medicine*, ed 6, St Louis, 2009, WB Saunders.
3. Mayhew J: *Large animal neurology*, Philadelphia, 2009, Wiley-Blackwell.
4. Lane SB, Bunch SE: Medical management of recurrent seizures in dogs and cats, *J Vet Intern Med* 4:26-39, 1990.
5. Podell M: Seizures in dogs, *Vet Clin North Am Small Anim Pract* 26:779-809, 1996.
6. Aleman M, Gray LC, Williams DC, et al: Juvenile idiopathic epilepsy in Egyptian Arabian foals: 22 cases (1985-2005), *Vet Intern Med* 20:1443-1449, 2006.
7. Working group on status epilepticus: Treatment of convulsive status epilepticus: recommendations of the epilepsy foundation of Americas working group on status epilepticus, *J Am Med Assoc* 270:854-859, 1993.
8. Robinson C, Lacombe VA, Reed S, et al: Predicting factors for abnormal computed tomography of the head in 58 horses affected by neurologic disorders, *J Am Vet Med Assoc*, 2009: (in press).
9. Berendt M, Gram L: Epilepsy and seizure classification in 63 dogs: a reappraisal of veterinary epilepsy terminology, *J Vet Intern Med* 13:14-20, 1999.
10. Furr M: Perinatal asphyxia in foals, *Compend Contin Educ Pract Vet* 18:1342-1351, 1996.
11. Collatos C: Seizures in foals: pathophysiology, evaluation, and treatment, *Compend Contin Educ Pract Vet* 12:393-400, 1990.
12. Berendt M: Epilepsy. In Vite CH, editor: *Braund's clinical neurology in small animals: localization, diagnosis and treatment*, Ithaca, NY, 2004, International Veterinary Information Service.
13. Prince D: Neurophysiology of epilepsy, *Annu Rev Neurosci* 1:395-415, 1978.
14. Delgado-Escueta AV, Ward AA, Woodbury DM, et al: New wave of research in the epilepsies, *Adv Neurol* 44:3-55, 1986.
15. Podell ML: Antiepileptic drug therapy, *Clin Tech Small Anim Pract* 13:185-192, 1998.
16. Trommer BL, Pasternak JF: NMDA receptor antagonists inhibit kindling epileptogenesis and seizure expression in developing rats, *Brain Res Dev Brain Res* 53:248-252, 1990.
17. Platt SR: The role of glutamate in neurologic diseases. In *Proceedings of the American College of Veterinary Internal Medicine*, Denver, 2001, ACVIM.
18. Slovis NM: Perinatal asphyxia syndrome (hypoxic ischemic encephalopathy). In *Proceedings of the American College of Veterinary Internal Medicine*, Charlotte, NC, 2003, ACVIM.
19. Jasper HH, Ward AA Jr, Pope A, editors: *Basic mechanisms of the epilepsies*, Boston, 1969, Little, Brown.
20. Russo ME: The pathophysiology of epilepsy, *Cornell Vet* 71:221-247, 1981.
21. Ayala GF, Dichter M, Gumnit RJ, et al: Genesis of epileptic interictal spikes: new knowledge of cortical feedback systems suggests neurophysiological explanation of brief paroxysms, *Brain Res* 52:1-17, 1973.
22. Fertiziger AP, Ranck JB: Potassium accumulation in interstitial space during epileptiform seizures, *Exp Neurol* 26:571-585, 1970.
23. Bertone JJ, Horspool LJI: *Equine clinical pharmacology*, St Louis, 2004, WB Saunders.
24. Higgins AJ, Snyder JR: *The equine manual*, ed 2, St Louis, 2006, WB Saunders.
25. Prince DA: Cortical cellular activities during cyclically occurring interictal epileptiform discharges, *Electroencephalogr Clin Neurophysiol* 31:469-484, 1971.
26. Heinemann U, Lux HD, Gutnick MJ: Extracellular free calcium and potassium during paroxysmal activity in the cerebral cortex of the cat, *Exp Brain Res* 27:237-243, 1977.
27. Radial SL, Edwards S: Pharmacokinetics of potassium bromide in adult horses, *Aust Vet J* 83:425-430, 2005.
28. Dauvilliers Y, Arnulf I, Mignot E: Narcolepsy with cataplexy, *Lancet* 369:499-511, 2007.
29. Tonokura M, Fujita K, Nishino S: Review of pathophysiology and clinical management of narcolepsy in dogs, *Vet Rec* 161:375-380, 2007.
30. Sheather AL: Fainting in foals, *J Comp Pathol Ther* 37:106-113, 1924.
31. Sweeney CR, Hendricks JC, Beech J, et al: Narcolepsy in a horse, *J Am Vet Med Assoc* 183:126-128, 1983.

32. Lunn DP, Cuddon PA, Shftoe S, et al: Familial occurrence of narcolepsy in Miniature Horses, *Equine Vet J* 25:476-477, 1993.
33. Bertone JJ: Excessive drowsiness secondary to recumbent sleep deprivation in two horses, *Vet Clin North Am Equine Pract* 22:157-162, 2006.
34. Aleman M, Williams DC, Holliday T: Sleep and sleep disorders in horses, *Proc Am Assoc Equine Pract* 64:180-185, 2008.
35. Bertone JJ: Sleep deprivation—not narcolepsy—in horses, *Proceedings of the North American Veterinary Conference* vol. 21, 2007, Orlando, FL, pp 91-93..
36. Katherman AE: A comparative review of canine and human narcolepsy, *Compend Contin Educ Pract Vet* 11:818, 1980.
37. Henley K, Morrison AR: A reevaluation of the effects of lesions of the pontine tegmentum and locus coeruleus on phenomena of paradoxical sleep in the cat, *Acta Neurobiol Exp (Wars)* 34:215, 1974.
38. Sakai K, Sastre JP, Salvert D, et al: Tegmentoreticular projections with special reference to the muscular atonia during paradoxical sleep in the cat: an HRP study, *Brain Res* 176:233, 1979.
39. Jones BF: Elimination of paradoxical sleep by lesions of the pontine gigantocellular tegmental field in the cat, *Neurosci Lett* 13:385, 1979.
40. Ruckebush Y, Barbey P, Guillemot P: Les états de sommeil chez le cheval, *C R Seances Soc Biol Fil* 164:638-665, 1970.
41. Kothare SV, Kaleyias J: Narcolepsy and other hypersomnias in children, *Curr Opin Pediatr* 20:666-675, 2008.
42. McFarlane D, Maidment NT, Lam H et al: Cerebrospinal fluid concentration of hypocretin-1 in horses with equine pituitary pars intermedia disease and its relationship to oxidative stress. In *Proceedings of the twenty-fifth annual meeting of the American College of Veterinary Internal Medicine, ****, 2007, ACVIM, p 791.
43. Hines MT: Narcolepsy: more common than you think?, *Proceedings of the North American Veterinary Conference: Large Animal* vol. 19, 2005, Orlando, FL, pp 189-190.
44. Mayhew IGJ: Sleep attacks, *Proceedings of the North American Veterinary Conference: Large Animal*, 2003, Orlando, FL, pp 174-175.
45. Cox JH: An episodic weakness in four horses associated with intermittent serum hyperkalemia and the similarity of the disease to hyperkalemic periodic paralysis in man, *Proc Am Assoc Equine Pract* 31:383-391, 1985.
46. Spier S, Carlson GP, Pikar J, et al: Hyperkalemic periodic paralysis in horses: genetic and electrophysiologic studies, *Proc Am Assoc Equine Pract* 35:399-402, 1989.
47. Peck KE, Hines MT, Mealey KL, et al: Pharmacokinetics of imipramine in narcoleptic horses, *Am J Vet Res* 62:783-786, 2001.

Central Nervous System Trauma

1. Feige K, Fürst A, Kaser-Hotz B, et al: Traumatic injury to the central nervous system in horses: occurrence, diagnosis and outcome, *Equine Vet Educ* 12:220-224, 2000.
2. Tyler CM, Begg AP, Hutchins DR, et al: A survey of neurological diseases in horses, *Aust Vet J* 70:445-449, 1993.
3. Little CB, Hilbert BJ, McGill CA: A retrospective study of head fractures in 21 horses, *Aust Vet J* 62:89-91, 1985.
4. Feary DJ, Magdesian KG, Aleman MA, et al: Traumatic brain injury in horses: 34 cases (1994-2004), *J Am Vet Med Assoc* 231:259-266, 2007.
5. Johnson PJ, Kellam LL: The vestibular system. II. Differential diagnosis, *Equine Vet Educ* June :185-194, 2001.
6. MacKay RJ: Brain injury after head trauma: pathophysiology, diagnosis, and treatment, *Vet Clin North Am Equine Pract* 20:199-216, 2004.
7. Reed SM: Management of head trauma in horses, *Comp Contin Educ Pract Vet* 15:270-273, 1993.
8. Robinson NE, editor: *Current therapy in equine medicine*, ed 6, St Louis, 2009, WB Saunders.
9. Reed SM: Medical and surgical emergencies of the nervous system of horses: diagnosis, treatment, and sequelae, *Vet Clin North Am Equine Pract* 10:703-715, 1994.
10. Stick JA, Wilson J, Kunze D: Basilar skull fractures in three horses, *J Am Vet Med Assoc* 176:228, 1980.
11. Ramirez O 3rd, Jorgensen JS, Thrall DE: Imaging basilar skull fractures in the horse: a review, *Vet Radiol Ultrasound* 39: 391-395, 1998.
12. Martin L, Kaswan R, Chapman W: Four cases of traumatic optic nerve blindness in the horse, *Equine Vet J* 18:133-137, 1986.
13. Nout YS: Central nervous system trauma. In Reed SM, Furr MO, editors: *Equine neurology*, Ames, IA, 2007, Blackwell Publishing.
14. Andrews PJ, Citerio G: Intracranial pressure. Part one: historical overview and basic concepts, *Intensive Care Med* 30: 1730-1733, 2004.
15. Steiner LA, Andrews PJ: Monitoring the injured brain: ICP and CBF, *Br J Anaesth* 97:26-38, 2006.
16. Narayan RK, Greenberg RP, Miller JD, et al: Improved confidence of outcome prediction in severe head injury. A comparative analysis of the clinical examination, multimodality evoked potentials, CT scanning, and intracranial pressure, *J Neurosurg* 54:751-762, 1981.
17. Golding EM: Sequelae following traumatic brain injury. The cerebrovascular perspective, *Brain Res Brain Res Rev* 38: 377-388, 2002.
18. Verweij BH, Muizelaar JP, Vinas FC, et al: Impaired cerebral mitochondrial function after traumatic brain injury in humans, *J Neurosurg* 93:815-820, 2000.
19. Fishman RA: Brain edema, *N Engl J Med* 293:706-711, 1975.
20. Sweeney CR, Freeman DE, Sweeney RW, et al: Hemorrhage into the guttural pouch (auditory tube diverticulum) associated with rupture of the longus capitis muscle in three horses, *J Am Vet Med Assoc* 202:1129-1131, 1993.
21. Nout YS, Reed SM: Management and treatment of the recumbent horse, *Equine Vet Educ* 7:416-432, 2005.
22. Mayhew IG: Equine neurology and nutrition, *Glenelg, Australia* , 1996:AEVA Bain-Fallon Memorial Lectures.
23. Moore RM, Trim C: Effect of Xylazine on cerebrospinal fluid pressure in conscious horses, *Am J Vet Res* 53:1558-1561, 1992.
24. Tietje S, Becker M, Bockenhoff G: Computed tomographic evaluation of head diseases in the horse: 15 cases, *Equine Vet J* 28:98-105, 1996.
25. Barbee DD, Allen JR: Computed tomography in the horse: general principles and clinical applications. In *Proceedings of the American Association of Equine Practitioners*, AEEP, Lexington, KY; 1986, pp 483-493.
26. Tucker RL, Farrell E: Computed tomography and magnetic resonance imaging of the equine head, *Vet Clin North Am Equine Pract* 17(vii):131-144, 2001.
27. Marshall LF, Marshall SB, Klauber MR, et al: The diagnosis of head injury requires a classification based on computed axial tomography, *J Neurotrauma* 1(Suppl 9):S287-292, 1992.
28. Green EM, Green S: Cerebrospinal fluid lactic acid concentration: reference values and diagnostic implications of abnormal concentrations in adult horses. In *Proceedings of the American College of Veterinary Internal Medicine*, Blacksburg, VA, 1990, ACVIM, pp 495-499.
29. Kortz GD, Madigan JE, Goetzman BW, et al: Intracranial pressure and cerebral perfusion pressure in clinically normal equine neonates, *Am J Vet Res* 56:1351-1355, 1995.

30. Brosnan RJ, Esteller-Vico A, Steffey EP, et al: Effects of head-down positioning on regional central nervous system perfusion in isoflurane-anesthetized horses, *Am J Vet Res* 69:737-743, 2008.
31. Brosnan RJ, LeCouteur RA, Steffey EP, et al: Direct measurement of intracranial pressure in adult horses, *Am J Vet Res* 63:1252-1256, 2002.
32. Hillered L, Persson L, Nilsson P, et al: Continuous monitoring of cerebral metabolism in traumatic brain injury: a focus on cerebral microdialysis, *Curr Opin Crit Care* 12:112-118, 2006.
33. Bellander BM, Cantais E, Enblad P, et al: Consensus meeting on microdialysis in neurointensive care, *Intensive Care Med* 30:2166-2169, 2004.
34. Rose JC, Neill TA, Hemphill JC 3rd: Continuous monitoring of the microcirculation in neurocritical care: an update on brain tissue oxygenation, *Curr Opin Crit Care* 12:97-102, 2006.
35. Rayner SG: Traumatic cerebral partial lobotomy in a Thoroughbred stallion, *Aust Vet J* 83:674-677, 2005.
36. Marklund N, Bakshi A, Castelbuono DJ, et al: Evaluation of pharmacological treatment strategies in traumatic brain injury, *Curr Pharm Des* 12:1645-1680, 2006.
37. Finfer S, Bellomo R, Boyce N, et al: A comparison of albumin and saline for fluid resuscitation in the intensive care unit, *N Engl J Med* 350:2247-2256, 2004.
38. Gunnar W, Jonasson O, Merlotti G, et al: Head injury and hemorrhagic shock: studies of the blood brain barrier and intracranial pressure after resuscitation with normal saline solution, 3% saline solution, and dextran-40, *Surgery* 103:398-407, 1988.
39. White H, Cook D, Venkatesh B: The use of hypertonic saline for treating intracranial hypertension after traumatic brain injury, *Anesth Analg* 102:1836-1846, 2006.
40. Kempski O: Cerebral edema, *Semin Nephrol* 21:303-307, 2001.
41. Robertson CS, Goodman JC, Narayan RK, et al: The effect of glucose administration on carbohydrate metabolism after head injury, *J Neurosurg* 74:43-50, 1991.
42. Van den Berghe G, Wouters P, Weekers F, et al: Intensive insulin therapy in the critically ill patients, *N Engl J Med* 345:1359-1367, 2001.
43. Vespa P, Boonyaputthikul R, McArthur DL, et al: Intensive insulin therapy reduces microdialysis glucose values without altering glucose utilization or improving the lactate/pyruvate ratio after traumatic brain injury, *Crit Care Med* 34:850-856, 2006.
44. Busto R, Dietrich WD, Globus MY, et al: Small differences in intraischemic brain temperature critically determine the extent of ischemic neuronal injury, *J Cereb Blood Flow Metab* 7:729-738, 1987.
45. Dietrich WD: The importance of brain temperature in cerebral injury, *J Neurotrauma* 2(Suppl 9):S475-485, 1992.
46. Clifton GL, Jiang JY, Lyeth BG, et al: Marked protection by moderate hypothermia after experimental traumatic brain injury, *J Cereb Blood Flow Metab* 11:114-121, 1991.
47. Clifton GL, Miller ER, Choi SC, et al: Lack of effect of induction of hypothermia after acute brain injury, *N Engl J Med* 344:556-563, 2001.
48. Robertson CL, Clark RS, Dixon CE, et al: No long-term benefit from hypothermia after severe traumatic brain injury with secondary insult in rats, *Crit Care Med* 28:3218-3223, 2000.
49. Feldman Z, Kanter MJ, Robertson CS, et al: Effect of head elevation on intracranial pressure, cerebral perfusion pressure, and cerebral blood flow in head-injured patients, *J Neurosurg* 76:207-211, 1992.
50. Hutchinson PJ, Corteen E, Czosnyka M, et al: Decompressive craniectomy in traumatic brain injury: the randomized multicenter RESCUEicp study (www.RESCUEicp.com), *Acta Neurochir Suppl* 96:17-20, 2006.
51. Timofeev I, Kirkpatrick PJ, Corteen E, et al: Decompressive craniectomy in traumatic brain injury: outcome following protocol-driven therapy, *Acta Neurochir Suppl* 96:11-16, 2006.
52. Bagley RS, Harrington ML, Pluhar GE, et al: Effect of craniectomy/durotomy alone and in combination with hyperventilation, diuretics, and corticosteroids on intracranial pressure in clinically normal dogs, *Am J Vet Res* 57:116-119, 1996.
53. Albright AL, Latchaw RE, Robinson AG: Intracranial and systemic effects of osmotic and oncotic therapy in experimental cerebral edema, *J Neurosurg* 60:481-489, 1984.
54. Soustiel JF, Vlodavsky E, Zaaroor M: Relative effects of mannitol and hypertonic saline on calpain activity, apoptosis and polymorphonuclear infiltration in traumatic focal brain injury, *Brain Res* 1101:136-144, 2006.
55. Ware ML, Nemani VM, Meeker M, et al: Effects of 23.4% sodium chloride solution in reducing intracranial pressure in patients with traumatic brain injury: a preliminary study, *Neurosurgery* 57:727-736 discussion 727-736, 2005.
56. Young B, Ott L, Twyman D, et al: The effect of nutritional support on outcome from severe head injury, *J Neurosurg* 67: 668-676, 1987.
57. Kaufmann MA, Buchmann B, Scheidegger D, et al: Severe head injury: should expected outcome influence resuscitation and first-day decisions? *Resuscitation* 23:199-206, 1992.
58. Pinchbeck G, Murphy D: Cervical vertebral fracture in three foals, *Equine Vet Educ February*:24-28, 2001.
59. Rashmir-Raven A, DeBowes RM, Hudson L, et al: Vertebral fracture and paraplegia in a foal, *Prog Vet Neurol* 2:197-202, 1991.
60. Collatos C, Allen D, Chambers J, et al: Surgical treatment of sacral fracture in a horse, *J Am Vet Med Assoc* 198:877-879, 1991.
61. Haussler KK, Stover SM: Stress fractures of the vertebral lamina and pelvis in Thoroughbred racehorses, *Equine Vet J* 30: 374-381, 1998.
62. Tutko JM, Sellon DC, Burns GA, et al: Cranial coccygeal vertebral fractures in horses: 12 cases, *Equine Vet Educ August*: 250-254, 2002.
63. Wagner PC, Long GG, Chatburn CC, et al: Traumatic injury of the cauda equina in the horse: a case report, *Equine Med Surg* 1:282-285, 1977.
64. Jeffcott LB: Disorders of the thoracolumbar spine of the horse—a survey of 443 cases, *Vet J* 12:197, 1980.
65. Kwon BK, Tetzlaff W, Grauer JN, et al: Pathophysiology and pharmacologic treatment of acute spinal cord injury, *Spine J* 4:451-464, 2004.
66. Tator CH, Fehlings MG: Review of the secondary injury theory of acute spinal cord trauma with emphasis on vascular mechanisms, *J Neurosurg* 75:15-26, 1991.
67. de la Torre JC: Spinal cord injury. Review of basic and applied research, *Spine* 6:315-335, 1981.
68. Beattie MS: Inflammation and apoptosis: linked therapeutic targets in spinal cord injury, *Trends Mol Med* 10:580-583, 2004.
69. Beattie MS, Farooqui AA, Bresnahan JC: Review of current evidence for apoptosis after spinal cord injury, *J Neurotrauma* 17:915-925, 2000.
70. Matthews HK, Andrews FM: Performing a neurologic examination in a standing or recumbent horse, *Vet Med November*: 1229-1240, 1990.
71. Smith PM, Jeffery ND: Spinal shock—comparative aspects and clinical relevance, *J Vet Intern Med* 19:788-793, 2005.
72. Sherrington CS: Croonian lecture (1897): the mammalian spinal cord as an organ of reflex action, *Philos Trans R Soc Lond* 190B:128-138, 1898.
73. Ditunno JF, Little JW, Tessler A, et al: Spinal shock revisited: a four-phase model, *Spinal Cord* 42(7):383-395, 2004.
74. deLahunta A: *Glass EN: Veterinary neuroanatomy and clinical neurology*, ed 3, St Louis, 2009, WB Saunders.
75. van Wessum R, Sloet van Oldruitenborgh-Oosterbaan MM, Clayton HM: Electromyography in the horse in veterinary medicine and in veterinary research—a review, *Vet Q* 21:3-7, 1999.

76. Nollet H, Deprez P, van Ham L, et al: Transcranial magnetic stimulation: normal values of magnetic motor evoked potentials in 84 normal horses and influence of height, weight, age and sex, *Equine Vet J* 36:51-57, 2004.
77. Nollet H, Van Ham L, Deprez P, et al: Transcranial magnetic stimulation: review of the technique, basic principles and applications, *Vet J* 166:28-42, 2003.
78. Nollet H, Vanschandevijl K, Van Ham L, et al: Role of transcranial magnetic stimulation in differentiating motor nervous tract disorders from other causes of recumbency in four horses and one donkey, *Vet Rec* 157:656-658, 2005.
79. Olby N: Current concepts in the management of acute spinal cord injury, *J Vet Intern Med* 13:399-407, 1999.
80. Thuret S, Moon LD, Gage FH: Therapeutic interventions after spinal cord injury, *Nat Rev Neurosci* 7:628-643, 2006.
81. Baptiste DC, Fehlings MG: Pharmacological approaches to repair the injured spinal cord, *J Neurotrauma* 23:318-334, 2006.
82. Hall ED, Wolf DL, Braughler JM: Effects of a single large dose of methylprednisolone sodium succinate on experimental posttraumatic spinal cord ischemia. Dose-response and time-action analysis, *J Neurosurg* 61:124-130, 1984.
83. Behrmann DL, Bresnahan JC, Beattie MS: Modeling of acute spinal cord injury in the rat: neuroprotection and enhanced recovery with methylprednisolone, U-74006F and YM-14673, *Exp Neurol* 126:61-75, 1994.
84. Bracken MB, Shepard MJ, Holford TR, et al: Administration of methylprednisolone for 24 or 48 hours or tirilazad mesylate for 48 hours in the treatment of acute spinal cord injury. Results of the Third National Acute Spinal Cord Injury Randomized Controlled Trial. National Acute Spinal Cord Injury Study, *JAMA* 277:1597-1604, 1997.
85. Bracken MB, Shepard MJ, Collins WF Jr, et al: Methylprednisolone or naloxone treatment after acute spinal cord injury: 1-year follow-up data. Results of the Second National Acute Spinal Cord Injury Study, *J Neurosurg* 76:23-31, 1992.
86. Bracken MB, Holford TR: Effects of timing of methylprednisolone or naloxone administration on recovery of segmental and long-tract neurological function in NASCIS 2, *J Neurosurg* 79:500-507, 1993.
87. Bracken MB, Shepard MJ, Holford TR, et al: Methylprednisolone or tirilazad mesylate administration after acute spinal cord injury: 1-year follow up. Results of the Third National Acute Spinal Cord Injury Randomized Controlled Trial, *J Neurosurg* 89:699-706, 1998.
88. Hurlbert RJ: The role of steroids in acute spinal cord injury: an evidence-based analysis, *Spine* 26:S39-46, 2001.
89. Short DJ, El Masry WS, Jones PW: High dose methylprednisolone in the management of acute spinal cord injury—a systematic review from a clinical perspective, *Spinal Cord* 38:273-286, 2000.
90. Coleman WP, Benzel D, Cahill DW, et al: A critical appraisal of the reporting of the National Acute Spinal Cord Injury Studies (II and III) of methylprednisolone in acute spinal cord injury, *J Spinal Disord* 13:185-199, 2000.
91. Sayer FT, Kronvall E, Nilsson OG: Methylprednisolone treatment in acute spinal cord injury: the myth challenged through a structured analysis of published literature, *Spine J* 6:335-343, 2006.
92. Hall ED: The neuroprotective pharmacology of methylprednisolone, *J Neurosurg* 76:13-22, 1992.
93. Bracken MB, Shepard MJ, Hellenbrand KG, et al: Methylprednisolone and neurological function 1 year after spinal cord injury. Results of the National Acute Spinal Cord Injury Study, *J Neurosurg* 63:704-713, 1985.
94. Bracken MB, Shepard MJ, Collins WF, et al: A randomized, controlled trial of methylprednisolone or naloxone in the treatment of acute spinal-cord injury. Results of the Second National Acute Spinal Cord Injury Study, *N Engl J Med* 322:1405-1411, 1990.
95. Kubeck JP, Merola A, Mathur S, et al: End organ effects of high-dose human equivalent methylprednisolone in a spinal cord injury rat model, *Spine* 31:257-261, 2006.
96. Zurita M, Vaquero J, Oya S, et al: Effects of dexamethasone on apoptosis-related cell death after spinal cord injury, *J Neurosurg* 96:83-89, 2002.
97. Blythe LL, Craig AM, Christensen JM, et al: Pharmacokinetic disposition of dimethyl sulfoxide administered intravenously to horses, *Am J Vet Res* 47:1739-1743, 1986.
98. Hoerlein BF, Redding RW, Hoff EJ, et al: Evaluation of dexamethasone, DMSO, mannitol and solcoseryl in acute spinal cord trauma, *J Am Anim Hosp Assoc* 19:216, 1983.
99. Van Meeteren NL, Eggers R, Lankhorst AJ, et al: Locomotor recovery after spinal cord contusion injury in rats is improved by spontaneous exercise, *J Neurotrauma* 20:1029-1037, 2003.

Vestibular Disease

1. Mayhew J: *Large animal neurology*, Philadelphia, 2009, Wiley-Blackwell.
2. deLahunta A, Glass EN: *Veterinary neuroanatomy and clinical neurology*, ed 3, St Louis, 2009, WB Saunders.
3. Dyke P, Thomas P, Lambert E, editors: *Peripheral neuropathy*, Philadelphia, 1975, WB Saunders.
4. Firth E: Vestibular disease and its relationship to facial paralysis in the horse: a clinical study of 7 cases, *Aust Vet J* 53:560, 1977.
5. Guyton A, editor: *Organ physiology: structure and function of the nervous system*, Philadelphia, 1976, WB Saunders.
6. Watrous B: Head tilt in horses, *Vet Clin North Am Equine Pract* 3:353, 1987.
7. Ganong W: Control of posture and movement. In Ganong W, editor: *The nervous system*, Los Altos, CA, 1979, Lange.
8. Kuffler S, Nicholls J, Martin A, editors: *From neuron to brain*, Sunderland, MASS, 1984, Sinauer Associates.
9. Swenson MJ, Reece WO, editors: *Duke's physiology of domestic animals*, ed 11, Ithaca, NY, 1993, Comstock.
10. Chrisman C: Disorders of the vestibular system, *Compend Contin Educ Pract Vet* 1:744, 1979.
11. Power H, Watrous B, deLahunta A: Facial and vestibulocochlear nerve disease in six horses, *J Am Vet Med Assoc* 183:1076, 1983.
12. Geiser D, Henton J, Held J: Tympanic bulla, petrous temporal bone, and hyoid apparatus disease in horses, *Compend Contin Educ Pract Vet* 10:740, 1988.
13. Palmer A: Pathogenesis and pathology of the cerebello-vestibular syndrome, *J Small Anim Pract* 11:167, 1970.
14. Ettinger S, editor: *Textbook of veterinary internal medicine*, ed 6, St Louis, 2005, WB Saunders.
15. Blythe L, Watrous B, Schmitz J, et al: Vestibular syndrome associated with temporohyoid joint fusion and temporal bone fracture in three horses, *J Am Vet Med Assoc* 185:775, 1984.
16. Palmer A: Nystagmus and its focal causes. In Palmer A, editor: *Introduction to animal neurology*, Blackwell, 1976, Oxford.
17. Raphel C: Brain abscess in three horses, *J Am Vet Med Assoc* 180:874, 1982.
18. Pidgeon G, editor: *Proceedings of the seventh American College of Veterinary Internal Medicine Forum*, Madison, WI, 1989, OmniPress.
19. Montgomery T: Otitis media in a thoroughbred, *Vet Med Small Anim Clin* 76:722, 1981.
20. Walker AM, Sellon DC, Cornelisse CJ, et al: Temporohyoid osteoarthropathy in 33 horses (1993-2000), *J Vet Intern Med* 16:697-703, 2002.
21. Hilton H, Puchalski SM, Aleman M: The computed tomographic appearance of equine temporohyoid osteoarthropathy, *Vet Radiol Ultrasound* 50:151-156, 2009.
22. Divers TJ, Ducharme NG, deLahunta A, et al: Temporohyoid osteoarthropathy, *Clin Tech Equine Pract* 5:17-23, 2006.

23. Jubb K, Kennedy P, Palmer N, editors: *Pathology of domestic animals*, Orlando, FL, 1985, Academic Press.
24. Grunsell O, editor: *The veterinary annual*, Bristol, England, 1971, John Wright & Sons.
25. Aleman M, Puchalski SM, Williams DC, et al: Brainstem auditory-evoked responses in horses with temporohyoid osteoarthropathy, *J Vet Intern Med* 22:1196-1202, 2008.
26. Ueltschi G: Bone and joint imaging with 99mTc labeled phosphates as a new diagnostic aid in veterinary orthopedics, *Vet Radiol Ultrasound* 18:80, 1977.
27. Lamb C, Koblik P: Scintigraphic evaluation of skeletal disease and its application to the horse, *Vet Radiol Ultrasound* 29:16, 1988.
28. Devous M, Twardock R: Techniques and applications of nuclear medicine in the diagnosis of equine lameness, *J Am Vet Med Assoc* 3:318, 1984.
29. Blythe LL, Watrous BJ, Shires GMH, et al: Prophylactic partial stylohyoidectomy for horses with osteoarthropathy of the temporohyoid joint, *J Equine Vet Sci* 14:32-37, 1994.
30. Pease AP, Van Biervliet J, Dykes NL, et al: Complication of partial stylohyoidectomy for treatment of temporohyoid osteoarthropathy and an alternative surgical technique in three cases, *Equine Vet J* 36:546-550, 2004.
31. Cook W: Skeletal radiology of the equine head, *Vet Radiol Ultrasound* 11:35, 1970.
32. Couto G: Personal communication, 1992.
33. Robinson E, editor: *Current therapy in equine medicine*, ed 6, St Louis, 2009, WB Saunders.
34. Ford J, Lokai M: Complications of *Streptococcus equi* infections, *Vet Clin North Am Equine Pract* 2:41, 1980.
35. Mittel L: Seizures in the horse, *Vet Clin North Am Equine Pract* 3:323, 1987.
36. Kohn CW: Equine herpes myeloencephalitis, *Vet Clin North Am Equine Pract* 3:405, 1987.
37. Teuscher E, Vrins A, Lemaire T: A vestibular syndrome associated with *Cryptococcus neoformans* in a horse, *Zentralbl Veterinarmed A* 31:132, 1984.
38. Mair T, Pearson G: Melanotic hamartoma of the hind brain in a riding horse, *J Comp Pathol* 102:239, 1990.
39. Marshall A, Byars T, Whitlock R, et al: Brainstem auditory evoked response in the diagnosis of inner ear injury in the horse, *J Am Vet Med Assoc* 178:282, 1981.
40. Rolf S, Reed S, Melnick W, et al: Auditory brainstem response testing in anesthetized horses, *Am J Vet Res* 48:910, 1987.

Diseases of the Cerebellum

1. deLahunta A, Glass EN: *Veterinary neuroanatomy and clinical neurology*, ed 3, St Louis, 2009, WB Saunders.
2. Holliday TA: Clinical signs of acute and chronic experimental lesions of the cerebellum, *Vet Sci Commun* 3:259, 1979.
3. Dungworth DL, Fowler ME: Cerebellar hypoplasia and degeneration in a foal, *Cornell Vet* 55:17, 1966.
4. Fraser H: Two dissimilar types of cerebellar disorder in the horse, *Vet Rec* 78:608, 1966.
5. Sponseller ML: Equine cerebellar hypoplasia and degeneration, *Proc Am Assoc Equine Pract* 13:123, 1967.
6. Palmer AC, Blakemore WF, Cook WR, et al: Cerebellar hypoplasia and degeneration in the young Arab horse: clinical and neuropathological features, *Vet Rec* 93:62, 1973.
7. Bjork G, Everz KE, Hansen HJ, et al: Congenital cerebellar ataxia in the Gotland pony breed, *Zentralbl Veterinarmed A* 20:341, 1973.
8. Baird JD, MacKenzie CD: Cerebellar hypoplasia and degeneration in part-Arab horses, *Aust Vet J* 50:25-28, 1974.
9. Turner-Beatty MT, Leipold HW, Cash W, et al: Cerebellar disease in Arabian horses, *Proc Am Assoc Equine Pract* 31:241, 1985.
10. DeBowes RM, Leipold HW, Turner-Beatty M: Cerebellar abiotrophy, *Vet Clin North Am Equine Pract* 3:345, 1987.
11. deLahunta A: Abiotrophy in domestic animals: a review, *Can J Vet Res* 54:65, 1990.
12. Mayhew IG: Neurological and neuropathological observations on the equine neonate, *Equine Vet J Suppl* 5:28, 1988.
13. Blanco A, Moyano R, Vivo J: Purkinje cell apoptosis in Arabian horses with cerebellar abiotrophy, *J Vet Med A Physiol Pathol Clin Med* 53:286-287, 2006.
14. Adams R, Mayhew IG: Neurological examination of newborn foals, *Equine Vet J* 16:306, 1984.
15. Sherwin AL, Norris JW, Bulcke JA: Spinal fluid creatine kinase in neurologic disease, *Neurology* 19:993, 1969.
16. Furr MO, Tyler RD: Cerebrospinal fluid creatine kinase activity in horses with central nervous system disease: 69 cases (1984-1989), *J Am Vet Med Assoc* 197:245, 1990.
17. Culebras-Fernandez A, Richards NG: Glutamic oxaloacetic transaminase, lactic dehydrogenase, and creatine phosphokinase content in cerebrospinal fluid, *Cleve Clin Q* 38:113, 1971.
18. LeGonidec G, Kuberski T, Daynes P, et al: A neurologic disease of horses in New Caledonia, *Aust Vet J* 57:194, 1981.
19. Hartley WJ, Kuberski T, LeGonidec G, et al: The pathology of Gomen disease: a cerebellar disorder of horses in New Caledonia, *Vet Pathol* 19:399, 1982.
20. Jubb KVF, Kennedy P, Palmer N: *Pathology of domestic animals*, San Diego, 1993, Academic Press.
21. Cudd TA, Mayhew IG, Cottrill CM: Agenesis of the corpus callosum with cerebellar vermian hypoplasia in a foal resembling the Dandy-Walker syndrome: pre-mortem diagnosis by clinical evaluation and CT scanning, *Equine Vet J* 21:378, 1989.
22. Oaks GL: Personal communication, 1994.
23. Oliver RE: Cerebellar hypoplasia in a thoroughbred foal, *N Z Vet J* 23:15, 1975.
24. Wheat JD, Kennedy PC: Cerebellar hypoplasia and its sequela in a horse, *J Am Vet Med Assoc* 131:291, 1957.
25. Poss M, Young S: Dysplastic disease of the cerebellum of an adult horse, *Acta Neuropathol* 75:209, 1987.
26. Waelchli RO, Ehrensperger F: Two related cases of cerebellar abnormality in equine fetuses associated with hydrops of fetal membranes, *Vet Rec* 123:513, 1988.
27. Makela O, Gustavsson I, Hollmen T: A 64, X, i(Xq) karyotype in a Standardbred filly, *Equine Vet J* 26:251, 1994.
28. Bell RJ, Smart ME: An unusual complication of strangles in a pony, *Can Vet J* 33:400, 1992.
29. Allen JR, Barbee DD, Boulten CR, et al: Brain abscess in a horse: diagnosis by computed tomography and successful surgical treatment, *Equine Vet J* 19:552, 1987.
30. Blunden AS, Khalil LF, Webbon PM: *Halicephalobus deletrix* infection in a horse, *Equine Vet J* 19:255, 1987.
31. Mayhew IG, Schneiders DH: An unusual familial neurological syndrome in newborn thoroughbred foals, *Vet Rec* 133:447, 1993.
32. Miller LM, Reed SM, Gallina AM, et al: Ataxia and weakness associated with fourth ventricle vascular anomalies in two horses, *J Am Vet Med Assoc* 186:601, 1985.
33. Seawright AA, Costigan P: Chronic methylmercurialism in a horse, *Vet Hum Toxicol* 20:6, 1978.

Cervical Vertebral Malformation

1. Moore BR, Reed SM, Robertson JT: Surgical treatment of cervical stenotic myelopathy in horses: 73 cases (1983-1992), *J Am Vet Med Assoc* 203:108-112, 1993.
2. Nout YS, Reed SM: Cervical vertebral stenotic myelopathy, *Equine Vet Educ* 15:212-223, 2003.
3. Mayhew IG, deLahunta A, Whitlock RH, et al: Spinal cord disease in the horse, *Cornell Vet* 68(Suppl 8):110-120, 1978.
4. Mayhew J: *Large animal neurology*, Philadelphia, 2009, Wiley-Blackwell.
5. Summers BA, Cummings JF, deLahunta A: *Veterinary neuropathology*, St Louis, 1995, Mosby.

6. Wagner PC, Grant BD, Watrous BJ, et al: A study of the heritability of cervical vertebral malformation in horses. In *Proceedings of the thirty-first Annual Convention of the American Association of Equine Practitioners,* AEEP, Lexington, KY, 1985.
7. Mayhew IG, Green SL: *Accuracy of diagnosing CVM from radiographs,* San Antonio AEEP, Lexington, KY, 2000, British Equine Veterinary Association.
8. Mayhew IG, Green SL: *Radiographic diagnosis of equine cervical vertebral malformation,* Denver, 2002, ACVIM.
9. Hahn CN, Handel I, Green SL, et al: Assessment of the utility of using intra- and intervertebral minimum sagittal diameter ratios in the diagnosis of cervical vertebral malformation in horses, *Vet Radiol Ultrasound* 49:1-6, 2008.
10. Mayhew IG, Washbourne JR: Magnetic motor evoked potentials in ponies, *J Vet Intern Med* 10:326-329, 1996.
11. Nollet H, Van Ham L, Gasthuys F, et al: Influence of detomidine and buprenorphine on motor-evoked potentials in horses, *Vet Rec* 152:534-537, 2003.
12. Nollet H, Van Ham L, Dewulf J, et al: Standardization of transcranial magnetic stimulation in the horse, *Vet J* 166:244-250, 2003.
13. Nollet H, Van Ham L, Deprez P, et al: Transcranial magnetic stimulation: review of the technique, basic principles and applications, *Vet J* 166:28-42, 2003.
14. Nollet H, Deprez P, van Ham L, et al: Transcranial magnetic stimulation: normal values of magnetic motor evoked potentials in 84 normal horses and influence of height, weight, age and sex, *Equine Vet J* 36:51-57, 2004.
15. Nyland TG, Blythe LL, Pool RR, et al: Metrizamide myelography in the horse: clinical, radiographic, and pathologic changes, *Am J Vet Res* 41:204-211, 1980.
16. Beech J: Metrizamide myelography in the horse, *J Am Vet Rad Soc* 20:22-31, 1979.
17. Van Biervliet J, Mayhew IG, de Lahunta A: Cervical vertebral compressive myelopathy: diagnosis, *Clin Tech Equine Pract* 5:54-59, 2006.
18. Van Biervliet J: Value of contrast radiography in the assessment of cervical spinal lesions, *Brit Eq Vet Assoc Congress,* 2004.
19. Donawick WJ, Mayhew IG, Galligan DT, et al: Results of a low-protein, low-energy diet and confinement on young horses with wobbles. In *Proceedings of the thirty-ninth Annual Convention of the American Association of Equine Practitioners,* AEEP, Lexington, KY, 1993.
20. Walmsley JP: Surgical treatment of cervical spinal cord compression in horses: a European experience, *Equine Vet Educ* 17:39-43, 2005.
21. Nixon AJ, Stashak TS: Surgical therapy for spinal cord disease in the horse. In *Proceedings of the thirty-first Annual Convention of the American Association of Equine Practitioners,* Lexington, KY, 1985.
22. Grant BD, Barbee DD, Wagner PC et al: Long term results of surgery for cervical vertebral malformation. In *Proceedings of the thirty-first Annual Convention of the American Association of Equine Practitioners,* AEEP, Lexington, KY, 1985.
23. Grant BD, Hoskinson JJ, Barbee DD et al: Ventral stabilization for decompression of caudal cervical spinal cord compression in the horse. In *Proceedings of the thirty-first Annual Convention of the American Association of Equine Practitioners,* AEEP, Lexington, KY, 1985.
24. Furr M, Reed SM: *Equine neurology,* Philadelphia, 2007, Blackwell Publishing.

Equine Degenerative Myeloencephalopathy

1. Mayhew IG, deLahunta A, Whitlock RH: Equine degenerative myeloencephalopathy, *American Association Equine Practitioners*:103-105, 1976.
2. Mayhew IG, deLahunta A, Whitlock RH, et al: Equine degenerative myeloencephalopathy, *J Am Vet Med Assoc* 170:195-201, 1977.
3. Mayhew IG, deLahunta A, Whitlock RH, et al: Spinal cord disease in the horse, *Cornell Vet* 68(Suppl 6):1-207, 1978.
4. Liu SK, Dolensek EP, Adams CR, et al: Myelopathy and vitamin E deficiency in six Mongolian wild horses, *J Am Vet Med Assoc* 183:1266-1268, 1983.
5. Montali RJ, Bush M, Sauer RM, et al: Spinal ataxia in zebras. Comparison with the wobbler syndrome of horses, *Vet Pathol* 11:68-78, 1974.
6. Beech J, Haskins M: Genetic studies of neuraxonal dystrophy in the Morgan, *Am J Vet Res* 48:109-113, 1987.
7. Blythe LL, Craig AM, Lassen ED, et al: Vitamin-E-deficiency as a causative factor in equine degenerative myeloencephalopathy, *Ann N Y Acad Sci* 570:415-416, 1989.
8. Mayhew IG, Brown CM, Stowe HD, et al: Equine degenerative myeloencephalopathy: a vitamin E deficiency that may be familial, *J Vet Intern Med* 1:45-50, 1987.
9. Blythe LL, Hultgren BD, Craig AM, et al: Clinical, viral, and genetic evaluation of equine degenerative myeloencephalopathy in a family of appaloosas, *J Am Vet Med Assoc* 198:1005-1013, 1991.
10. Miller MM, Collatos C: Equine degenerative myeloencephalopathy, *Vet Clin North Am Equine Pract* 13:43-47, 1997.
11. Beech J: Neuroaxonal dystrophy of the accessory cuneate nucleus in horses, *Vet Pathol* 21:384-393, 1984.
12. Furr M, Reed SM, editors: *Equine Neurology,* Ames, IA, 2008, Blackwell Publishing.
13. Gandini G, Fatzer R, Mariscoli M, et al: Equine degenerative myeloencephalopathy in five Quarter Horses: clinical and neuropathological findings, *Equine Vet J* 36:83-85, 2004.
14. Toenniessen JG, Morin DE: Degenerative myelopathy—a comparative review, *Compend Contin Educ Pract Vet* 17:271-277, 1995.
15. Dill SG, Correa MT, Erb HN, et al: Factors associated with the development of equine degenerative myeloencephalopathy, *Am J Vet Res* 51:1300-1305, 1990.
16. Facchinetti F, Dawson VL, Dawson TM: Free radicals as mediators of neuronal injury, *Cell Mol Neurobiol* 18:667-682, 1998.
17. Bains JS, Shaw CA: Neurodegenerative disorders in humans: the role of glutathione in oxidative stress-mediated neuronal death, *Brain Res Brain Res Rev* 25:335-358, 1997.
18. Chan PH: Reactive oxygen radicals in signaling and damage in the ischemic brain, *J Cereb Blood Flow Metab* 21:2-14, 2001.
19. Dill SG, Kallfelz FA, deLahunta A, et al: Serum vitamin E and blood glutathione peroxidase values of horses with degenerative myeloencephalopathy, *Am J Vet Res* 50:166-168, 1989.
20. Blythe LL, Craig AM, Lassen ED, et al: Serially determined plasma alpha-tocopherol concentrations and results of the oral vitamin-E absorption test in clinically normal horses and in horses with degenerative myeloencephalopathy, *Am J Vet Res* 52:908-911, 1991.
21. Mayhew IG: Equine degenerative myeloencephalopathy (EDM): clinical findings and suspected aetiology. In *Proceedings of the International Equine Neurology Conference,* Ithaca, NY, 1997, pp 18-29.
22. Blythe LL: Equine degenerative myeloencephalopathy—genetics and treatment. In *Proceedings of the International Equine Neurology Conference,* Dallas, 1997.
23. Dill SG, Hintz HF, deLahunta A, et al: Plasma and liver copper values in horses with equine degenerative myeloencephalopathy, *Can J Vet Res* 53:29-32, 1989.
24. Siso S, Ferrer I, Pumarola M: Abnormal synaptic protein expression in two Arabian horses with equine degenerative myeloencephalopathy, *Vet J* 166:238-243, 2003.
25. Siso S, Ferrer I, Pumarola M: Juvenile neuroaxonal dystrophy in a Rottweiler: accumulation of synaptic proteins in dystrophic axons, *Acta Neuropathol* 102:501-504, 2001.
26. Craig AM, Blythe LL, Lassen ED, et al: Variations of serum vitamin E, cholesterol, and total serum lipid concentrations in horses during a 72-hour period, *Am J Vet Res* 50:1527-1531, 1989.

27. Blythe LL, Craig AM: Equine degenerative myeloencephalopathy. II. Diagnosis and treatment, *Compend Contin Educ Pract Vet* 14:1633-1636, 1992.
28. Roneus BO, Hakkarainen RV, Lindholm CA, et al: Vitamin E requirements of adult Standardbred horses evaluated by tissue depletion and repletion, *Equine Vet J* 18:50-58, 1986.
29. Beech J: Equine degenerative myeloencephalopathy, *Vet Clin North Am Equine Pract* 3:379-383, 1987.

Equine Protozoal Myeloencephalitis

1. Rooney JR, Prickett ME, Delaney FM, et al: Focal myelitis-encephalitis in horses, *Cornell Vet* 60:494-501, 1969.
2. Beech J, Dodd DC: Toxoplasma-like encephalomyelitis in the horse, *Vet Pathol* 11:87-96, 1974.
3. Cusick PK, Sells DM, Hamilton DP, et al: Toxoplasmosis in two horses, *J Am Vet Med Assoc* 164:77-80, 1974.
4. Dubey JP, Davis GW, Koestner A, et al: Equine encephalomyelitis due to a protozoan parasite resembling, *Toxoplasma gondii, J Am Vet Med Assoc* 165:249-255, 1974.
5. Dubey JP: A review of *Sarcocystis* of domestic animals and other coccidia of cats and dogs, *J Am Vet Med Assoc* 169:1061-1078, 1976.
6. Dubey JP, Davis SW, Speer CA, et al: *Sarcocystis neurona* n. sp. (Protozoa: *Apicomplexa*), the etiologic agent of equine protozoal myeloencephalitis, *J Parasitol* 77:212-218, 1991.
7. Marsh AE, Denver M, Hill FI, et al: Detection of *Sarcocystis neurona* in the brain of a Grant's zebra *(Equus burchelli bohmi), J Zoo Wildl Med* 31:82-86, 2000.
8. Dubey JP, Benson J, Larson MA: Clinical *Sarcocystis neurona* encephalomyelitis in a domestic cat following routine surgery, *Vet Parasitol* 112:261-267, 2003.
9. Forest TW, Abou-Madi N, Summers BA, et al: *Sarcocystis neurona*-like encephalitis in a Canada lynx *(Felis lynx canadensis), J Zoo Wildl Med* 31:383-387, 2000.
10. Lindsay DS, Thomas NJ, Dubey JP: Biological characterization of *Sarcocystis neurona* isolated from a Southern sea otter *(Enhydra lutris nereis), Int J Parasitol* 30:617-624, 2000.
11. Dubey JR, Rosypal AC, Rosenthal BM, et al: *Sarcocystis neurona* infections in sea otter *(Enhydra lutris)*: evidence for natural infections with sarcocysts and transmission of infection to opossums *(Didelphis virginiana), J Parasitol* 87:1387-1393, 2001.
12. Dubey JR, Johnson GC, Bermudez A, et al: Neural sarcocystosis in a straw-necked ibis *(Carphibis spinicollis)* associated with a *Sarcocystis neurona*-like organism and description of muscular sarcocysts of an unidentified *Sarcocystis* species, *J Parasitol* 87:1317-1322, 2001.
13. Dubey JP, Hamir AN, Niezgoda M, et al: A *Sarcocystis neurona*-like organism associated with encephalitis in a striped skunk *(Mephitis mephitis), J Parasitol* 82:172-174, 1996.
14. Dubey JP, Hedstrom OR: Meningoencephalitis in mink associated with a *Sarcocystis neurona*-like organism, *J Vet Diagn Invest* 5:467-471, 1993.
15. Dubey JP, Hamir AN: Immunohistochemical confirmation of *Sarcocystis neurona* infections in raccoons, mink, cat, skunk, and pony, *J Parasitol* 86:1150-1152, 2000.
16. Daft B, Barr B, Collins N, et al: *Neospora* encephalomyelitis and polyradiculoneuritis in an aged mare with Cushing's disease, *Equine Vet J* 28:240-243, 1996.
17. Dubey J, Porterfield M: *Neosporum caninum (Apicomplexa)* in an aborted equine fetus, *J Parasitol* 76:732-734, 1990.
18. Hamir A, Tornquist S, Gerros T, et al: *Neospora caninum*-associated equine protozoal myeloencephalitis, *Vet Parasitol* 79:269-274, 1998.
19. Lindsay D, Steinberg H, Dubielzig R, et al: Central nervous system neosporosis in a foal, *J Vet Diagn Invest* 8:507-510, 1996.
20. Marsh AE, Barr BC, Madigan JE, et al: Neosporosis as a cause of equine protozoal myeloencephalitis, *J Am Vet Med Assoc* 209:1907-1913, 1996.
21. Gray M, Harmon B, Sales L, et al: Visceral neosporosis in a 10-year old horse, *J Vet Diagn Invest* 8:130-133, 1996.
22. Mayhew IG, de Lahunta A, Whitlock RH, et al: Spinal cord disease in the horse, *Cornell Vet* 6(Suppl):1-207, 1978.
23. Reed SM, Granstrom D, Rivas LJ et al: Results of cerebrospinal fluid analysis in 119 horses testing positive to the Western blot test on both serum and CSF to equine protozoal encephalomyelitis. In *Proceedings of the American Association of Equine Practitioners,* Vancouver BC, AEEP, Lexington, KY, 1994, p 199.
24. NAHMS: *Equine protozoal myeloencephalitis in the US,* Ft Collins, CO, 2000, USDA:APHIS:VS, CEAH, National Animal Health Monitoring System.
25. Saville W, Reed S, Morley P, et al: Analysis of risk factors for the development of equine protozoal myeloencephalitis in horses, *J Am Vet Med Assoc* 217:1174-1180, 2000.
26. Ronen N: Putative equine protozoal myeloencephalitis in an imported Arabian filly, *J S Afr Vet Assoc* 63:78-79, 1992.
27. Lam K, Watkins K, Chan C: First report of equine protozoal myeloencephalitis in Hong Kong, *Equine Vet Educ* 11:54-56, 1999.
28. Pitel PH, Pronost S, Gargala G, et al: Detection of *Sarcocystis neurona* antibodies in French horses with neurological signs, *Int J Parasitol* 32:481-485, 2002.
29. Goehring LS: Sloet van Oldruitenborgh-Oosterbaan MM: Equine protozoal myeloencephalitis in the Netherlands? An overview, *Tijdschr Diergeneeskd* 126:346-351, 2001.
30. Fayer R, Mayhew IG, Baird JD, et al: Epidemiology of equine protozoal myeloencephalitis in North America based on histologically confirmed cases, *J Vet Intern Med* 4:54-57, 1990.
31. Mayhew IG, deLahunta A, Whitlock RH, et al: Equine protozoal myeloencephalitis, *Proc Am Assoc Equine Pract* 22:107-114, AEEP, Lexington, KY 1976.
32. Boy MG, Galligan DT, Divers TJ: Protozoal encephalomyelitis in horses: 82 cases (1972-1986), *J Am Vet Med Assoc* 196:632-634, 1990.
33. Saville W: The epidemiology of equine protozoal myeloencephalitis (EPM), *Veterinary preventive medicine,* Columbus, 1998, Ohio State University.
34. Gray LC, Magdesian KG, Sturges BK, et al: Suspected protozoal myeloencephalitis in a two-month-old colt, *Vet Rec* 149:269-273, 2001.
35. MacKay RJ, Davis SW, Dubey JP: Equine protozoal myeloencephalitis, *Compend Contin Educ Pract Vet* 14:1359-1367, 1992.
36. Mullaney T, Murphy AJ, Kiupel M, et al: Evidence to support horses as natural intermediate hosts for *Sarcocystis neurona, Vet Parasitol* 133:27-36, 2005.
37. Fenger CK, Granstrom DE, Langemeier JL, et al: Epizootic of equine protozoal myeloencephalitis on a farm, *J Am Vet Med Assoc* 210:923-927, 1997.
38. Fenger CK: Equine protozoal myeloencephalitis, *Compend Contin Educ Pract Vet* 19:513-523, 1997.
39. Bentz BG, Granstrom D, Stamper S: Seroprevalence of antibodies to *Sarcocystis neurona* in horses residing in a county of southeastern Pennsylvania, *J Am Vet Med Assoc* 210:517-518, 1997.
40. Blythe LL, Granstrom DE, Hansen DE, et al: Seroprevalence of antibodies to *Sarcocystis neurona* in horses residing in Oregon, *J Am Vet Med Assoc* 210:525-527, 1997.
41. Saville WJ, Reed SM, Granstrom DE, et al: Prevalence of serum antibodies to *Sarcocystis neurona* in horses residing in Ohio, *J Am Vet Med Assoc* 210:519-524, 1997.
42. Rossano MG, Kaneene JB, Marteniuk JV, et al: The seroprevalence of antibodies to *Sarcocystis neurona* in Michigan equids, *Prev Vet Med* 48:113-128, 2001.

43. Tillotson K, McCue P, Granstron D, et al: Seroprevalence of antibodies to *Sarcocystis neurona* in horse residing in northern Colorado, *J Equine Vet Sci* 19:122-126, 1999.
44. Vardeleon D, Marsh AE, Thorne JG, et al: Prevalence of *Neospora hughesi* and *Sarcocystis neurona* antibodies in horses from various geographical locations, *Vet Parasitol* 95:273-282, 2001.
45. Duarte PC, Conrad PA, Wilson WD, et al: Risk of postnatal exposure to *Sarcocystis neurona* and *Neospora hughesi* in horses, *Am J Vet Res* 65:1047-1052, 2004.
46. Dubey J, Venturini M, Venturini L, et al: Prevalence of antibodies to *Sarcocystis neurona, Toxoplasma gondii*, and *Neospora caninum* in horses from Argentina, *Vet Parasitol* 86:59-62, 1999.
47. Dubey J, Kerber C, Granstrom D: Serologic prevalence of *Sarcocystis neurona, Toxoplasma gondii*, and *Neospora caninum* in horses in Brazil, *J Am Vet Med Assoc* 215:970-972, 1999.
48. Dubey J, Romand S, Thulliez P, et al: Prevalence of antibodies to *Neospora caninum* in horses in North America, *J Parasitol* 85:968-969, 1999.
49. Dubey JP, Speer CA, Fayer R: *Sarcocystosis of animals and man*, Boca Raton, FL, 1989, CRC Press.
50. Fayer R, Dubey JP: Comparative epidemiology of coccidia: clues to the etiology of equine protozoal myeloencephalitis, *Int J Parasitol* 17:615-620, 1987.
51. Davis SW, Daft BN, Dubey JP: *Sarcocystis neurona* cultured in vitro from a horse with equine protozoal myelitis, *Equine Vet J* 23:315-317, 1991.
52. Davis SW, Speer CA, Dubey JP: In vitro cultivation of *Sarcocystis neurona* from the spinal cord of a horse with equine protozoal myelitis, *J Parasitol* 77:789-792, 1991.
53. Granstrom DE, Alvarez JO, Dubey JP, et al: Equine protozoal myelitis in Panamanian horses and isolation of *Sarcocystis neurona*, *J Parasitol* 78:909-912, 1992.
54. Granstrom DE, MacPherson JM, Gajadhar AA, et al: Differentiation of *Sarcocystis neurona* from eight related coccidia by random amplified polymorphic DNA assay, *Mol Cell Probes* 8:353-356, 1994.
55. Marsh A, Johnson P, Ramos-Vara J, et al: Characterization of a *Sarcocystis neurona* isolate from a Missouri horse with equine protozoal myeloencephalitis, *Vet Parasitol* 95:143-154, 2001.
56. Hyun C, Gupta GD, Marsh AE: Sequence comparison of *Sarcocystis neurona* surface antigen from multiple isolates, *Vet Parasitol* 112:11-20, 2003.
57. Hoane JS, Morrow J, Saville WJ, et al: Enzyme-linked immunosorbent assays for detection of equine antibodies specific to *Sarcocystis neurona* surface antigens, *Clin Diagn Lab Immunol* 12:1050-1056, 2005.
58. Howe D, Gaji R, Marsh A, et al: Strains of *S. neurona* exhibit differences in their surface antigens, including the absence of the major surface antigen SnSAG1, *Int J Parasitol* 38:623-631, 2008.
59. Dubey J, Saville W, Lindsay D, et al: Completion of the life cycle of *Sarcocystis neurona*, *J Parasitol* 86:1276-1280, 2000.
60. Cheadle M, Tanhauser S, Dame J, et al: The nine-banded armadillo *(Dasypus novemcinctus)* is an intermediate host for *Sarcocystis neurona*, *Int J Parasitol* 31:330-335, 2001.
61. Cheadle M, Yowell C, Sellon D, et al: The striped skunk *(Mephitis mephitis)* is an intermediate host for *Sarcocystis neurona*, *Int J Parasitol* 31:843-849, 2001.
62. Dubey J, Saville W, Stanek J, et al: *Sarcocystis neurona* infections in raccoons *(Procyon lotori)*: evidence for natural infection with sarcocysts, transmission of infection to opossums *(Didelphis virginiana)*, and experimental induction of neurological disease in raccoons, *Vet Parasitol* 100:117-129, 2001.
63. Turay H, Barr B, Caldwell A, et al: *Sarcocystis neurona* reacting antibodies in Missouri feral domestic cats *(Felis domesticus)* and their role as an intermediate host, *Parasitol Res* 88:38-43, 2002.
64. Stanek J, Stich R, Dubey J, et al: Epidemiology of *Sarcocystis neurona* infections in domestic cats *(Felis domesticus)* and its association with equine protozoal myeloencephalitis (EPM), case farms and feral cats, from a mobile spay and neuter clinic, *Vet Parasitol* 117:239-249, 2003.
65. Cohen N, MacKay RJ, Toby E, et al: A multicenter case-control study of risk factors for equine protozoal myeloencephalitis, *J Am Vet Med Assoc* 231:1857-1863, 2007.
66. Mullany T, Murphy A, Kiupel M, et al: Evidence to support horses as natural intermediate hosts for *Sarcocystis neurona*, *Vet Parasitol* 133:27-36, 2005.
67. Box ED, Smith JH: The intermediate host spectrum in a *Sarcocystis* species of birds, *J Parasitol* 68:668-673, 1982.
68. Box E: Recovery of *Sarcocystis* sporocysts from feces after oral administration, *Proc Helminthol Soc Wash* 50:348-350, 1983.
69. McAllister M, Dubey J, Lindsay D, et al: Dogs are definitive hosts of *Neospora caninum*, *Int J Parasitol* 28:1473-1478, 1998.
70. Dubey J: Recent advances in *Neospora* and neosporosis, *Vet Parasitol* 84:349-367, 1999.
71. Sofaly CD, Reed SM, Gordon JC, et al: Experimental induction of equine protozoan myeloencephalitis (EPM) in the horse: effect of *Sarcocystis neurona* sporocyst inoculation dose on the development of clinical neurologic disease, *J Parasitol* 88: 1164-1170, 2002.
72. Saville W, Stich R, Reed S, et al: Utilization of stress in the development of an equine model for equine protozoal myeloencephalitis, *Vet Parasitol* 95:211-222, 2001.
73. Cutler T, MacKay R, Ginn P, et al: Immunoconversion against *Sarcocystis neurona* in normal and dexamethasone-treated horses challenged with *S. neurona* sporocysts, *Vet Parasitol* 95:197-210, 2001.
74. Njoku CJ, Saville WJ, Reed SM, et al: Reduced levels of nitric oxide metabolites in cerebrospinal fluid are associated with equine protozoal myeloencephalitis, *Clin Diagn Lab Immunol* 9:605-610, 2002.
75. Ellison SB, Greiner E, Brown KK, et al: Experimental infection of horses with culture-derived *Sarcocystis neurona* merozoites as a model for equine protozoal myeloencephalitis, *Int J Appl Res Vet Med* 2:79-89, 2004.
76. Sellon DC, Knowles DP, Greiner EC, et al: Infection of immunodeficient horses with *Sarcocystis neurona* does not result in neurologic disease, *Clin Diagn Lab Immunol* 11:1134-1139, 2004.
77. Rossano MG, Schott HC, Murphy AJ: Parasitemia in immunocompetent horses experimentally challenged with *S. neurona* sporocysts, *Vet Parasitol* 127:3-8, Leesburg, VA 2005.
78. Goehring L: Master's thesis, Virginia Polytechnic Institute.
79. Liang FT, Granstrom DE, Zhao XM, et al: Evidence that surface proteins Sn14 and S. neurona 16 of *Sarcocystis neurona* merozoites are involved in infection and immunity, *Infect Immun* 66:1834-1838, 1998.
80. Witonsky SG, Gogal RM, Duncan RB Jr, et al: Prevention of meningoencephalomyelitis due to *S. neurona* in mice is mediated by CD8 cells, *Int J Parsitol* 35:13-23, 2005.
81. Dubey JP, Lindsay DS: Isolation in immunodeficient mice of *S. neurona* from opossum *(Didelphis virginiana)* faeces, and its differentiation from *Sarcocystis falcatula*, *Int J Parasitol* 28:1823-1828, 1998.
82. Dunigan CE, Oglesbee MJ, Podell M, et al: Seizure activity associated with equine protozoal myeloencephalitis, *Prog Vet Neurol* 6:50-54, 1995.
83. MacKay R, Granstrom D, Saville W, et al: Equine protozoal myeloencephalitis, *Vet Clin North Am Equine Pract* 16:405-426, 2000.
84. Moore L, Johnson P, Messer N, et al: Management of headshaking in three horses by treatment for protozoal myeloencephalitis, *Vet Rec* 141:264-267, 1997.

85. Granstrom D, Dubey JP, Davis SW, et al: Equine protozoal myeloencephalitis: antigen analysis of cultured *Sarcocystis neurona* merozoites, *J Vet Diagn Invest* 5:88-90, 1993.
86. Granstrom DE: Diagnosis of equine protozoal myeloencephalitis: Western blot analysis, In *Proceedings of the American College of Veterinary Internal Medicine Forum*, San Diego, ACVIM, Denver 1993, pp 587-590.
87. Furr M: Antigen-specific antibodies in cerebrospinal fluid after intramuscular injection of ovalbumin in horses, *J Vet Intern Med* 16:588-592, 2002.
88. Andrews FA, Maddux JM, Faulk D: Total protein, albumin quotient, IgG and IgG index determinations for horse cerebrospinal fluid, *Prog Vet Neurol* 1:197-204, 1993.
89. Andrews FA, Geiser DR, Sommerdahl CDS, et al: Albumin quotient, IgG concentrations, and IgG index determinations in cerebrospinal fluid of neonatal foals, *Am J Vet Res* 55:741-745, 1994.
90. Furr M, MacKay R, Andrews F, et al: Clinical diagnosis of equine protozoal myeloencephalitis (EPM): ACVIM consensus statement, *J Vet Intern Med* 16:618-621, 2002.
91a. Furr M, Kennedy T, MacKay R, et al: Efficacy of ponazuril 15% oral paste as a treatment for equine protozoal myeloencephalitis, *J Vet Ther* 2:215-222, 2001.
91b. Rossano MG, Mansfield LS, Kaneene JB, et al: Improvement of Western blot test specificity for detecting equine serum antibodies to *Sarcocystis neurona*, *J Vet Diagn Invest* 12:28-32, 2000.
92. Duarte PC, Daft BM, Conrad PA, et al: Comparison of a serum indirect fluorescent antibody test with two Western blot tests for the diagnosis of equine protozoal myeloencephalitis, *J Vet Diagn Invest* 15:8-13, 2003.
93. Duarte PC, Daft BM, Conrad PA, et al: Evaluation and comparison of an indirect fluorescent antibody test for detection of antibodies to *Sarcocystis neurona*, using serum and cerebrospinal fluid of naturally and experimentally infected, and vaccinated horses, *J Parasitol* 90:379-386, 2004.
94. Granstrom DE: Equine protozoal myeloencephalitis testing: review of 1993 and 1994, *Proc Annu Conv Am Assoc Equine Pract* 41:218-219, 1995.
95. Saville WJ, Dubey JP, Oglesbee MJ, et al: Experimental infection of ponies with *Sarcocystis fayeri* and differentiation from *Sarcocystis neurona* infections in horses, *J Parasitol* 90:1487-1491, 2004.
96. Ellison SP, Kennedy T, Brown KK: Development of an ELISA to detect antibodies to rSAG1 in the horse, *J Appl Res Vet Med* 1:318-327, 2003.
97. Packham AE, Conrad PA, Wilson D, et al: Qualitative evaluation of selective tests for detection of *Neospora hughesi* antibodies in serum and cerebrospinal fluid of experimentally infected horses, *J Parasitol* 88:1239-1246, 2002.
98. MacKay RJ: Equine protozoal myeloencephalitis: treatment, prognosis and prevention, *Clin Tech Equine Pract* 5:9-16, 2006.
99. Bedford S, McDonnell S: Measurements of reproductive function in stallions treated with trimethoprim-sulfamethoxazole and pyrimethamine, *J Am Vet Med Assoc* 215:1317-1319, 1999.
100. Furr M, Kennedy T: Cerebrospinal fluid and serum concentrations of ponazuril in horses, *Vet Ther* 2:232-237, 2001.
101. Kennedy T, Campbell J, Selzer V: Safety of ponazuril 15% oral paste in horses, *Vet Ther* 2:223-231, 2001.
102. Welsh TH, Bryan TM, Johnson L, et al: Characterization of sperm and androgen production by testes from control and ponazuril-treated stallions, *Therio* 58:389-392, 2002.
103. Furr M: Unpublished observation, 2002.
104. Fenger CK: Treatment of equine protozoal myeloencephalitis, *Compend Contin Educ Pract Vet* 20:1154-1157, 1998.
105. Muller J, Naguleswarean A, Muller N, et al: *Neospora caninum*: functional inhibition of protein disulfide isomerase by the broad-spectrum anti-parasitic drug nitazoxanide and other thiazolides, *Exp Parasitol* 118:80-88, 2008.
106. Cheadle MA, Lindsay DS, Rowe S, et al: Prevalence of antibodies to *Neospora* sp. in horses from Alabama and characterization of an isolate recovered from a naturally infected horse, *Int J Parasitol* 29:1537-1543, 1999.
107. Mitchell SM, Zajac AM, Davis WL, et al: The effects of ponazuril on development of apicomplexans in vitro, *J Euk Micro* 52:231-235, 2005.
108. Darius AK, Mehlhorn H, Heydorn AO: Effects of toltrazuril and ponazuril on *Hammondia heydorni* (syn *Neospora caninum*) infections in mice, *Parasitol Res* 92:520-522, 2004.
109. Finno CJ, Aleman M, Pusterla N: Equine protozoal myeloencephalitis associated with neosporosis in 3 horses, *J Vet Intern Med* 21:1405-1408, 2007.
110. Friebe A, Siegling A, Friederichs S, et al: Effects of inactivated parapoxvirus ovis (orf virus) on human peripheral immune cells: induction of cytokine secretion in monocytes and Th1-like cells, *J Virol* 78:9400-9411, 2004.
111. Furr M, MacKenzie H, Dubey J, et al: Pretreatment of horses with ponazuril limits infection and neurologic signs resulting from *S. neurona*, *J Parasitol* 92:637-643, 2006.

Equine Herpesvirus-1 Myeloencephalopathy

1. Ostlund EN, Powell D, Bryans JT: Equine herpesvirus 1: a review, *Proceedings of the thirty-sixth annual convention of the American Association of Equine Practitioners*, Lexington, KY, 1990, pp 387-395.
2. Ostlund EN: The equine herpesviruses, *Vet Clin North Am Equine Pract* 9:283-294, 1993.
3. Powell DG: *Viral respiratory disease*, Philadelphia, 1992, WB Saunders.
4. Jackson TA, Osburn BI, Cordy DR, et al: *Equine herpesvirus 1 infection of horses: studies on the experimentally induced neurologic disease* 38:709-719, 1977.
5. Peet RL, Coackley W, Smith VW, et al: Equine abortion associated with herpesvirus, *Aust Vet J* 54:151, 1978.
6. Van Maanen C: Equine herpesvirus 1 and 4 infections: an update, *Vet Q* 24:58-78, 2002.
7. Reed SM, Toribio RE: Equine herpesvirus 1 and 4, *Vet Clin North Am Equine Pract* 20:631-642, 2004.
8. Patel JR, Heldens J: Equine herpesviruses 1 (EHV-1) and 4 (EHV-4)—epidemiology, disease and immunoprophylaxis: a brief review, *Vet J* 170:6-7, 2005.
9. McCartan CG, Russell MM, Wood JL, et al: Clinical, serological and virological characteristics of an outbreak of paresis and neonatal foal disease due to equine herpesvirus-1 on a stud farm, *Vet Rec* 136:7-12, 1995.
10. van Maanen C, Sloet van Oldruitenborgh-Oosterbaan MM, Damen EA, et al: Neurological disease associated with EHV-1-infection in a riding school: clinical and virological characteristics, *Equine Vet J* 33:191-196, 2001.
11. Henninger RW, Reed SM, Saville WJ, et al: Outbreak of neurologic disease caused by equine herpesvirus-1 at a university equestrian center, *J Vet Intern Med* 21:157-165, 2007.
12. Meyer H, Thein P, Hubert P: Characterization of two equine herpesvirus (EHV) isolates associated with neurological disorders in horses, *Zentralbl Veterinarmed B* 34:545-548, 1987.
13. Thein P, Darai G, Janssen W, et al: Recent information about the etiopathogenesis of paretic-paralytic forms of herpesvirus infection in horses, *Tierarztl Praxis* 21:445-450, 1993.
14. Wilson JH: Neurological syndrome of rhinopneumonitis, In *Proceedings of the ninth annual Veterinary Medicine Forum of the American College of Veterinary Internal Medicine*, 1991, San Diego, pp 419-421.
15. Slater JD, Borcers K, Thackray AM, et al: The trigeminal ganglion is a location for equine herpesvirus 1 latency and reactivation in the horse, *J Gen Virol* 75:2007-2016, 1994.
16. Crabb BS, Studdert MJ: Equine herpesviruses 4 (equine rhino pneumonitis virus) and 1 (equine abortion virus), *Adv Virus Res* 45:153-190, 1995.

17. Agius CT, Nagesha HS, Studdert MJ: Equine herpesvirus 5: comparisons with EHV2 (equine cytomegalovirus), cloning, and mapping of a new equine herpesvirus with a novel genome structure, *Virology* 191:176-186, 1992.
18. Browning GF, Ficorilli N, Studdert MJ: Asinine herpesvirus genomes: comparison with those of the equine herpesviruses, *Arch Virol* 101:183-190, 1988.
19. Crabb BS, Studdert MJ: Comparative studies of the proteins of equine herpesviruses 4 and 1 and asinine herpesvirus 3: antibody response of the natural hosts, *J Gen Virol* 71:2033-2041, 1990.
20. Crabb BS, Allen GP, Studdert MJ: Characterization of the major glycoproteins of equine herpesviruses 4 and 1 and asinine herpesvirus 3 using monoclonal antibodies, *J Gen Virol* 72:2075-2082, 1991.
21. Allen GP, Bryans JT: Molecular epizootiology, pathogenesis, and prophylaxis of equine herpesvirus-1 infections, *Prog Vet Microbiol Immunol* 2:78-144, 1986.
22. Patel JR, Edington N: The pathogenicity in mice of respiratory, abortion and paresis isolates of equine herpesvirus-1, *Vet Microbiol* 8:301-305, 1983.
23. Palfi V, Christensen LS: Analyses of restriction fragment patterns (RFPs) and pathogenicity in baby mice of equine herpesvirus 1 and 4 (EHV-1 and EHV-4) strains circulating in Danish horses, *Vet Microbiol* 47:199-204, 1995.
24. van Woensel PA, Goovaerts D, Markx D, et al: A mouse model for testing the pathogenicity of equine herpes virus-1 strains, *J Virol Methods* 54:39-49, 1995.
25. Chowdhury SI, Kubin G, Ludwig H: Equine herpesvirus type 1 (EHV-1) induced abortions and paralysis in a Lipizzaner stud: a contribution to the classification of equine herpesviruses, *Arch Virol* 90:273-288, 1986.
26. Nowotny N, Burtscher H, Burki F: Neuropathogenicity for suckling mice of equine herpesvirus 1 from the Lipizzan outbreak 1983 and of selected other EHV 1 strains, *Zentralbl Veterinarmed B* 34:441-448, 1987.
27. Nugent J, Birch-Machin I, Smith KC, et al: Analysis of equid herpesvirus 1 strain variation reveals a point mutation of the DNA polymerase strongly associated with neuropathogenic versus nonneuropathogenic disease outbreaks, *J Virol* 80:4047-4060, 2006.
28. Goodman LB, Loregian A, Perkins GA, et al: A point mutation in a herpesvirus polymerase determines neuropathogenicity, *PLoS Pathog* 3:e160, 2007.
29. Wernery U, Wade JF, Mumford JA, et al: *Equine infectious diseases VIII*, Dubai, 1999, R & W Publications.
30. Kydd JH, Smith KC, Hannant D, et al: Distribution of equid herpesvirus-1 (EHV-1) in respiratory tract associated lyphoid tissue: implications for cellular immunity, *Equine Vet J* 26:470-473, 1994.
31. Edington N, Welch HM, Griffiths L: The prevalence of latent equid herpesviruses in the tissues of 40 Abattoir horses, *Equine Vet J* 26:140-142, 1994.
32. Welch HM, Bridges CG, Lyon AM, et al: Latent equid herpesviruses 1 and 4: detection and distinction using the polymerase chain reaction and co-cultivation from lymphoid tissues, *J Gen Virol* 73:261-268, 1992.
33. Rappocciolo G, Birch J, Ellis SA: Down-regulation of MHC class I expression by equine herpesvirus-1, *J Gen Virol* 84:293-300, 2003.
34. Edington N, Bridges CG, Huckle A: Experimental reactivation of equid herpesvirus 1 (EHV 1) following the administration of corticosteroids, *Equine Vet J* 17:369-372, 1985.
35. Patel JR, Edington N, Mumford JA: Variation in cellular tropism between isolates of equine herpesvirus-1 in foals, *Arch Virol* 74:41-51, 1982.
36. Anonymous: EHV-1: a recurrent problem, *Vet Rec* 124:443-444, 1989.
37. Campbell TM, Studdert MJ: Equine herpesvirus type 1 (EHV 1), *Vet Bull* 53:135-146, 1983.
38. Saxegaard F: Isolation and identification of equine rhinopneumonitis virus (equine abortion virus) from cases of abortion and paralysis, *Nord Vet Med* 18:504-516, 1966.
39. Bitsch V, Dam A: Nervous disturbances in horses in relation to infection with equine rhinopneumonitis virus, *Acta Vet Scand* 12:134-136, 1971.
40. Dalsgaard H: Enzootic paresis as a consequence of outbreaks of rhinopneumonitis (virus abortion), *Medlemsbl Danske Dyrlaegeforen* 53:71-76, 1970.
41. Thein P: Infection of the central nervous system of horses with equine herpesvirus serotype 1, *J S Afr Vet Assoc* 52:239-241, 1981.
42. Dinter Z, Klingeborn B: Serological study of an outbreak of paresis due to equid herpesvirus 1 (EHV-1), *Vet Rec* 99:10-12, 1976.
43. Crowhurst FA, Dickinson G, Burrows R: An outbreak of paresis in mares and geldings associated with equid herpesvirus 1, *Vet Rec* 109:527-528, 1981.
44. Greenwood RE, Simson AR: Clinical report of a paralytic syndrome affecting stallions, mares and foals on a thoroughbred stud farm, *Equine Vet J* 12:113-117, 1980.
45. Whitwell KE, Blunden AS: Pathological findings in horses dying during an outbreak of the paralytic form of equid herpesvirus type 1 (EHV-1) infection, *Equine Vet J* 24:13-19, 1992.
46. Collins JD: Virus abortion outbreak in Ireland, *Vet Rec* 91:129, 1972.
47. Studdert MJ, Crabb BS, Ficorilli N: The molecular epidemiology of equine herpesvirus 1 (equine abortion virus) in Australia 1975 to 1989, *J Vet Med Sci* 54:207-211, 1992.
48. Studdert MJ, Fitzpatrick DR, Horner GW, et al: Molecular epidemiology and pathogenesis of some equine herpesvirus type 1 (equine abortion virus) and type 4 (equine rhinopneumonitis virus) isolates, *Aust Vet J* 61:345-348, 1984.
49. Batra SK, Jain NC, Tiwari SC: Isolation and characterization of "EHV-1" herpesvirus associated with paralysis in equines, *Indian J Anim Sci* 52:671-677, 1982.
50. Jackson T, Kendrick JW: Paralysis of horses associated with equine herpesvirus 1 infection, *J Am Vet Med Assoc* 158:1351-1357, 1971.
51. Jackson TA, Osburn BI, Cordy DR, et al: Equine herpesvirus 1 infection of horses: studies on the experimentally induced neurologic disease, *Am J Vet Res* 38:709-719, 1977.
52. Kohn CW, Fenner WR: Equine herpes myeloencephalopathy, *Vet Clin North Am Equine Pract* 3:405-419, 1987.
53. Liu IKM, Castleman W: Equine posterior paresis associated with equine herpesvirus 1 vaccine in California: a preliminary report, *J Equine Med Surg* 1:397-401, 1977.
54. Little PB, Thorsen J: Disseminated necrotizing myeloencephalitis: a herpes-associated neurological disease of horses, *Vet Pathol* 13:161-171, 1976.
55. Little PB, Thorsen J, Moran K: Virus involvement in equine paresis, *Vet Rec* 95:575, 1974.
56. Pursell AR, Sangster LT, Byars TD, et al: Neurologic disease induced by equine herpesvirus 1, *J Am Vet Med Assoc* 175:473-474, 1979.
57. Franklin TE, Daft BM, Silverman VJ, et al: Serological titers and clinical observations in equines suspected of being infected with EHV-1, *Calif Vet J* 39:22-24, 1985.
58. Charlton KM, Mitchell D, Girard A, et al: Meningoencephalomyelitis in horses associated with equine herpesvirus 1 infection, *Vet Pathol* 13:59-68, 1976.
59. Thomson GW, McCready R, Sanford E, et al: Case report: an outbreak of herpesvirus myeloencephalitis in vaccinated horses, *Can Vet J* 20:22-25, 1979.
60. Friday PA, Scarratt WK, Elvinger F, et al: Ataxia and paresis with equine herpesvirus type 1 infection in a herd of riding school horses, *J Vet Intern Med* 14:197-201, 2000.
61. Thorsen J, Little PB: Isolation of equine herpesvirus type 1 from a horse with an acute paralytic disease, *Can J Comp Med* 39:358-359, 1975.

62. Platt H, Singh H, Whitwell KE: Pathological observations on an outbreak of paralysis in broodmares, *Equine Vet J* 12:118-126, 1980.
63. Bryans JT, Allen GP: Equine viral rhinopneumonitis, *Rev Sci Tech* 5:837, 1986.
64. Hughes PE, Ryan CP, Carlson GP, et al: An epizootic of equine herpes virus-1 myeloencephalitis, *Unpublished observations*, 1987.
65. USDA-APHIS: Equine herpes virus myeloencephalopathy: a potentially emerging disease (website). www.aphis.usda.gov/vs/ceah/cei/taf/emergingdiseasenotice_files/ehv.pdf. Accessed June 4, 2007.
66. Allen GP, Breathnach CC: Quantification by real-time PCR of the magnitude and duration of leucocyte-associated viraemia in horses infected with neuropathogenic vs. non-neuropathogenic strains of EHV-1, *Equine Vet J* 38:252-257, 2006.
67. Stierstorfer B, Eichhorn W, Schmahl W, et al: Equine herpesvirus type 1 (EHV-1) myeloencephalopathy: a case report, *J Vet Med B Infect Dis Vet Public Health* 49:37-41, 2002.
68. Montali RJ, Allen GP, Bryans JT, et al: Equine herpesvirus type 1 abortion in an onager and suspected herpesvirus myelitis in a zebra, *J Am Vet Med Assoc* 187:1248-1249, 1985.
69. Kydd JH, Smith KC, Hannant D, et al: Distribution of equid herpesvirus-1 (EHV-1) in the respiratory tract of ponies: implications for vaccination strategies, *Equine Vet J* 26:466-469, 1994.
70. Scott JC, Dutta SK, Myrup AC: In vivo harboring of equine herpesvirus-1 in leukocyte populations and subpopulations and their quantitation from experimentally infected ponies, *Am J Vet Res* 44:1344-1348, 1983.
71. Bryans JT: On immunity to disease caused by equine herpesvirus 1, *J Am Vet Med Assoc* 155:294-300, 1969.
72. Edington N, Bridges CG, Patel JR: Endothelial cell infection and thrombosis in paralysis caused by equid herpesvirus-1: equine stroke, *Arch Virol* 90:111-124, 1986.
73. Edington N, Smyth B, Griffiths L: The role of endothelial cell infection in the endometrium, placenta and foetus of equid herpesvirus 1 (EHV-1) abortions, *J Comp Pathol* 104:379-387, 1991.
74. Mayhew IG: *Equine herpesvirus 1 (rhinopneumonitis) myeloencephalitis*, Philadelphia, 1989, Lea & Febiger.
75. Slater JD, Gibson JS, Barnett KC, et al: Chorioretinopathy associated with neuropathology following infection with equine herpesvirus-1, *Vet Rec* 131:237-239, 1992.
76. Slater JD, Borchers K, Thackray AM, et al: The trigeminal ganglion is a location for equine herpesvirus 1 latency and reactivation in the horse, *J Gen Virol* 75:2007-2016, 1994.
77. Slater JD, Borchers K, Field HJ: Equine herpesvirus-1: a neurotropic alphaherpesvirus, *Vet Rec* 135:239-240, 1994 (letter).
78. Chesters PM, Allsop R, Purewal A, et al: Detection of latency-associated transcripts of equid herpesvirus 1 in equine leukocytes but not in trigeminal ganglia, *J Virol* 71:3437-3443, 1997.
79. Taouji S, Collobert C, Gicquel B, et al: Detection and isolation of equine herpesviruses 1 and 4 from horses in Normandy: an autopsy study of tissue distribution in relation to vaccination status, *J Vet Med B Infect Dis Vet Public Health* 49:394-399, 2002.
80. Klingeborn B, Dinter Z: Measurement of neutralizing antibody to equid herpesvirus 1 by single radial hemolysis, *J Clin Microbiol* 7:495-496, 1978.
81. Klingeborn B, Dinter Z, Hughes RA: Antibody to neuritogenic myelin protein P2 in equine paresis due to equine herpesvirus 1, *Zentralbl Veterinarmed B* 30:137-140, 1983.
82. Braund KG, Brewer BD, Mayhew IG: *Equine herpesvirus type 1 infection*, Philadelphia, 1987, WB Saunders.
83. MacKay RJ, Mayhew IG: *Equine herpesvirus myeloencephalitis*, ed 4, Goleta, CA, 1991, American Veterinary Publications.
84. deLahunta A: *Equine herpesvirus 1: myeloencephalopathy and vasculitis*, Philadelphia, 1983, WB Saunders.
85. George LW: *Equine herpesvirus 1 myeloencephalitis (rhinopneumonitis myelitis)*, St Louis, 1990, CV Mosby.
86. Roberts RS: A paralytic syndrome in horses, *Vet Rec* 77:404-405, 1965.
87. Andrews FM, Granstrom D, Provenza M: Differentiation of neurologic diseases in the horse by the use of albumin quotient and IgG index determinations. In *Proceedings of the forty-first annual conference of the American Association of Equine Practitioners*, AEEP, Lexington, KY, 1995, pp 215-217.
88. Donaldson MT, Sweeney CR: Herpesvirus myeloencephalopathy in horses: 11 cases (1982-1996), *J Am Vet Med Assoc* 213:671-675, 1998.
89. Keane DP, Little PB, Wilkie BN, et al: Agents of equine viral encephalomyelitis: correlation of serum and cerebrospinal fluid antibodies, *Can J Vet Res* 52:229-235, 1988.
90. Mumford JA: The development of diagnostic techniques for equine viral diseases, *Vet Ann* 24:182-189, 1984.
91. Whitwell KE, Gower SM, Smith KC: An immunoperoxidase method applied to the diagnosis of equine herpesvirus abortion, using conventional and rapid microwave techniques, *Equine Vet J* 24:10-12, 1992.
92. Schmidt P, Meyer H, Hubert P, et al: In-situ hybridization for demonstration of equine herpesvirus type 1 DNA in paraffin wax-embedded tissues and its use in horses with disseminated necrotizing myeloencephalitis, *J Comp Pathol* 110:215-225, 1994.
93. Sinclair R, Mumford JA: Rapid detection of equine herpesvirus type-1 antigens in nasal swab specimens using an antigen capture enzyme-linked immunosorbent assay, *J Virol Methods* 39:299-310, 1992.
94. Sharma PC, Cullinane AA, Onions DE, et al: Diagnosis of equid herpesviruses-1 and -4 by polymerase chain reaction, *Equine Vet J* 24:20-25, 1992.
95. Lawrence GL, Gilkerson J, Love DN, et al: Rapid, single-step differentiation of equid herpesviruses 1 and 4 from clinical material using the polymerase chain reaction and virus-specific primers, *J Virol Methods* 47:59-72, 1994.
96. Ballagi-Pordany A, Klingeborn B, Flensburg J, et al: Equine herpesvirus type 1: detection of viral DNA sequences in aborted fetuses with the polymerase chain reaction, *Vet Microbiol* 22:373-381, 1990.
97. Kirisawa R, Endo A, Iwai H, et al: Detection and identification of equine herpesvirus-1 and -4 by polymerase chain reaction, *Vet Microbiol* 36:57-67, 1993.
98. Wagner WN, Bogdan J, Haines D, et al: Detection of equine herpesvirus and differentiation of equine herpesvirus type 1 from type 4 by the polymerase chain reaction, *Can J Microbiol* 38:1193-1196, 1992.
99. Richa GYP, Charan S: A dot immunobinding assay in comparison with the gel diffusion test for the detection of equine herpesvirus-1 antigen from field samples, *Rev Sci Tech* 12:923-930, 1993.
100. Valentine-Thon E: Quality control in nucleic acid testing: where do we stand?, *J Clin Virol* 25(Suppl 3):S13-S21, 2002.
101. Mumford JA, Edington N: EHV1 and equine paresis, *Vet Rec* 106:277, 1980:(letter).
102. Drummer HE, Reynolds A, Studdert MJ, et al: Application of an equine herpesvirus 1 (EHV1) type-specific ELISA to the management of an outbreak of EHV1 abortion, *Vet Rec* 136:579-581, 1995.
103. Crabb BS, MacPherson CM, Reubel GH, et al: A type-specific serological test to distinguish antibodies to equine herpesviruses 4 and 1, *Arch Virol* 140:245-258, 1995.
104. Crabb BS, Studdert MJ: Epitopes of glycoprotein G of equine herpesviruses 4 and 1 located near the C termini elicit type-specific antibody responses in the natural host, *J Virol* 69:6332-6338, 1993.

105. Blythe LL, Mattson DE, Lassen ED, et al: Antibodies against equine herpesvirus 1 in the cerebrospinal fluid in the horse, *Can Vet J* 26:218-220, 1985.
106. Smith KO, Galloway KS, Hodges SL, et al: Sensitivity of equine herpesviruses 1 and 3 in vitro to a new nucleoside analogue, 9-[[2-hydroxy-1-(hydroxymethyl) ethoxy] methyl] guanine, *Am J Vet Res* 44:1032-1035, 1983.
107. Murray MJ, del Piero F, Jeffrey SC, et al: Neonatal equine herpesvirus type 1 infection on a thoroughbred breeding farm, *J Vet Intern Med* 12:36-41, 1998.
108. Garre B, Shebany K, Gryspeerdt A, et al: Pharmacokinetics of acyclovir after intravenous infusion of acyclovir and after oral administration of acyclovir and its prodrug valacyclovir in healthy adult horses, *Antimicrob Agents Chemother* 51:4308-4314, 2007.
109. Maxwell LK, Bentz BG, Bourne DW, et al: Pharmacokinetics of valacyclovir in the adult horse, *J Vet Pharmacol Ther* 31:312-320, 2008.
110. de la Fuente R, Awan AR, Field HJ: The acyclic nucleoside analogue penciclovir is a potent inhibitor of equine herpesvirus type 1 (EHV-1) in tissue culture and in a murine model, *Antiviral Res* 18:77-89, 1992.
111. Smith KC, Tearle JP, Boyle MS, et al: Replication of equid herpesvirus-1 in the vaginal tunics of colts following local inoculation, *Res Vet Sci* 54:249-251, 1993.
112. Allen GP, Yeargan MR, Turtinen LW, et al: Molecular epizootiologic studies of equine herpesvirus-1 infections by restriction endonuclease fingerprinting of viral DNA, *Am J Vet Res* 44:263-271, 1983.
113. Mumford JA: Equid herpesvirus 1 (EHV 1) latency: more questions than answers, *Equine Vet J* 17:340-342, 1985:(editorial).
114. Eaglesome MD, Henry JN, McKnight JD: Equine herpesvirus 1 infection in mares vaccinated with a live-virus rhinopneumonitis vaccine attenuated in cell culture, *Can Vet J* 20:145-147, 1979.
115. Burrows R, Goodridge D, Denyer MS: Trials of an inactivated equid herpesvirus 1 vaccine: challenge with a subtype 1 virus, *Vet Rec* 114:369-374, 1984.
116. Burki F, Rossmanith W, Nowotny N, et al: Viraemia and abortions are not prevented by two commercial equine herpesvirus-1 vaccines after experimental challenge of horses, *Vet Q* 12:80-86, 1990.
117. Burki F, Nowotny N, Oulehla J, et al: Attempts to immunoprotect adult horses, specifically pregnant mares, with commercial vaccines against clinical disease induced by equine herpesvirus-1, *Zentralbl Veterinarmed B* 38:432-440, 1991.
118. Heldens JG, Hannant D, Cullinane AA, et al: Clinical and virological evaluation of the efficacy of an inactivated EHV1 and EHV4 whole virus vaccine (Duvaxyn EHV1,4): vaccination/challenge experiments in foals and pregnant mares, *Vaccine* 19:4307-4317, 2001.
119. Patel JR, Bateman H, Williams J, et al: Derivation and characterization of a live equid herpes virus-1 (EHV-1) vaccine to protect against abortion and respiratory disease due to EHV-1, *Vet Microbiol* 91:23-39, 2003.
120. Patel JR, Foldi J, Bateman H, et al: Equid herpesvirus (EHV-1) live vaccine strain C147: efficacy against respiratory diseases following EHV types 1 and 4 challenges, *Vet Microbiol* 92:1-17, 2003.
121. Patel JR, Didlick S, Bateman H: Efficacy of a live equine herpesvirus-1 (EHV-1) strain C147 vaccine in foals with maternally-derived antibody: protection against EHV-1 infection, *Equine Vet J* 36:447-451, 2004.

Polyneuritis Equi

1. Reed SM: Neuritis of the cauda equina: polyneuritis equi in the horse. In Proc J D Stewart Memorial Refresher Course for Veterinarians, Stephen Roberts Memorial Lectures, Sydney, 183:385-386, 1992.
2. Vatistas NJ, Mayhew IG, Whitwell KE, et al: Polyneuritis equi: a clinical review incorporating a case report of a horse displaying unconventional signs, *Prog Vet Neurol* 2:67-72, 1991.
3. Rousseaux CG, Futcher KG, Clark EG, et al: Cauda equina neuritis: a chronic idiopathic polyneuritis in two horses, *Can Vet J* 25:214-218, 1984.
4. Wright JA, Fordyce P, Edington N: Neuritis of the cauda equina in the horse, *J Comp Pathol* 97:667-675, 1987.
5. White PL, Genetzsky RM, Pohlenz JFI, et al: Neuritis of the cauda equina in a horse, *Compend Contin Educ Pract Vet* 6:S217-S224, 1984.
6. Scarratt WK, Jortner BS: Neuritis of the cauda equina in a yearling filly, *Compend Contin Educ Pract Vet* 7:S197-S202, 1985.
7. Milne FJ, Carbonell PL: Neuritis of the cauda equina of horses: a case report, *Equine Vet J* 2:179-182, 1970.
8. Mayhew J: *Large animal neurology*, Philadelphia, 2009, Wiley-Blackwell.
9. Greenwood AG, Barker J: Neuritis of the cauda equina in a horse, *Equine Vet J* 5:111-115, 1973.
10. Fordyce PS, Edington N, Bridges GC, et al: Use of an ELISA in the differential diagnosis of cauda equina neuritis and other equine neuropathies, *Equine Vet J* 19:55-59, 1987.
11. Cummings JF, deLahunta A, Timoney JF: Neuritis of the cauda equina, a chronic polyradiculoneuritis in the horse, *Acta Neuropathol* 46:17-24, 1979.
12. Beech J: Neuritis of the cauda equina, *Proc Am Assoc Equine Pract* 21:75-76, 1976.
13. Robinson NE, editor: *Current therapy in equine medicine*, ed 6, St Louis, 2009, WB Saunders.
14. Yvorchuk-St Jean K: Neuritis of the cauda equina, *Vet Clin North Am Equine Pract* 3:421-427, 1987.
15. Kobluk CN, Ames TR, Geor RJ, editors: *The horse: diseases and clinical management*, Philadelphia, 1995, WB Saunders.
16. Edington N, Wright JA, Patel JR, et al: Equine adenovirus 1 isolated from cauda equina neuritis, *Res Vet Sci* 37:252-254, 1984.
17. Kadlubowski M, Ingram PL: Circulating antibodies to the neuritogenic protein, P2, in neuritis of the cauda equina of the horse, *Nature* 293:299-300, 1981.
18. van Galen G, Cassart D, Sandersen C, et al: The composition of the inflammatory infiltrate in three cases of polyneuritis equi, *Equine Vet J* 40:185-188, 2008.
19. Klingeborn B, Dinter Z, Hughes RAC: Antibody to neuritogenic myelin protein P2 in equine paresis due to equine herpesvirus 1, *Zentralbl Veterinarmed B* 30:137-140, 1983.
20. Granstrom DE, Dubey JP, Giles RC, et al: Equine protozoal myeloencephalitis: biology and epidemiology. In Nakajima H, Plowright W, editors: *Refereed proceedings*, Newmarket, England, 1994, R & W Publications.
21. Jackson T, Kendrick JW: Paralysis of horses associated with equine herpesvirus 1 infection, *J Am Vet Med Assoc* 158:1351-1357, 1971.
22. Ostlund EN, Powell D, Bryans JT: Equine herpesvirus 1: a review, *Proc Am Assoc Equine Pract* 36:387-395, 1990.
23. Ostlund EN: The equine herpesviruses, *Vet Clin North Am Equine Pract* 9:283-294, 1993.
24. Wilson JH, Erickson DM: Neurological syndrome of rhinopneumonitis, *Proc Am Coll Vet Intern Med* 9:419-421, 1991.
25. Blunden AS, Khalil LF, Webbon PM: *Halicephalobus deletrix* infection in a horse, *Equine Vet J* 19:255, 1987.
26. Lester G: Parasitic encephalomyelitis in horses, *Compend Contin Educ Pract Vet* 14:1624-1630, 1992.
27. Mayhew IG, Brewer BD, Reinhard MK, et al: Verminous *(Strongylus vulgaris)* myelitis in a donkey, *Cornell Vet* 74:30-37, 1984.
28. Divers TJ, Cummings JF, Mohammed HO, et al: Equine motor neuron disease, *Proc Am Coll Vet Intern Med* 13:918-921, 1995.

Viral Encephalitis

1. Grady GF, Maxfield HK, Hildreth SW, et al: Eastern equine encephalitis in Massachusetts, 1957-1976: a prospective study centered upon analysis of mosquitoes, *Am J Epidemiol* 107:170-178, 1978.
2. Casal J: Antigenic variants of equine encephalitis virus, *J Exp Med* 119:547-565, 1964.
3. Hahn CS, Lustig S, Strauss EG, et al: Western equine encephalitis virus is a recombinant virus, *Proc Natl Acad Sci U S A* 85(16):5997-6001, 1988.
4. Trent DW, Grant JA: A comparison of new world alphaviruses in the western equine encephalomyelitis complex by immunochemical and oligonucleotide fingerprint techniques, *J Gen Virol* 47:261-282, 1980.
5. Calisher CH, Kinney RM, de Souza Lopes O, et al: Identification of a new Venezuelan equine encephalitis virus from Brazil, *Am J Trop Med Hyg* 31:1260-1272, 1982.
6. Martin DH, Dietz WH, Alvarez OJ, et al: Epidemiological significance of Venezuelan equine encephalomyelitis virus in vitro markers, *Am J Trop Med Hyg* 31:561-568, 1982.
7. Walton TE, Alvarez O, Buckwalter RM, et al: Experimental infection of horses with enzootic and epizootic strains of Venezuelan equine encephalomyelitis virus, *J Infect Dis* 128:271-282, 1973.
8. Dietz WH, Alvarez O, Martin DH, et al: Enzootic and epizootic Venezuelan equine encephalomyelitis virus in horses infected by peripheral and intrathecal routes, *J Infect Dis* 137:227-237, 1978.
9. Udall DH: A report on the outbreak of "cerebro-spinal meningitis" (encephalitis) in horses in Kansas and Nebraska, *Cornell Vet* 3:17-43, 1913.
10. Meyer KF, Haring CM, Howitt B: Newer knowledge of neurotropic virus infections of horses, *JAMA* 79:376-389, 1931.
11. Reimann CA, Hayes EB, DiGuiseppi C, et al: Epidemiology of neuroinvasive arboviral disease in the United States, 1999-2007, *Am J Trop Med Hyg* 79(6):974-979, 2008.
12. TenBroeck C, Merrill MH: A serological difference between eastern and western equine encephalomyelitis virus, *Proc Soc Exp Biol Med* 31:217-220, 1933.
13. Records E, Vawter LR: Equine encephalomyelitis cross-immunity in horses between western and eastern strains of virus, *J Am Vet Med Assoc* 85:89-95, 1934.
14. Records E, Vawter LR: Equine encephalomyelitis cross-immunity in horses between western and eastern strains of virus: supplemental report, *J Am Vet Med Assoc* 86:764-772, 1935.
15. Hoff GL, Bigler WJ, Buff EE, et al: Occurrence and distribution of western equine encephalomyelitis in Florida, *J Am Vet Med Assoc* 172:351-352, 1978.
16. Goldfield M: Arbovirus infection of animals in New Jersey, *J Am Vet Med Assoc* 153:1780-1787, 1968.
17. Shahan MS, Giltner LT: A review of the epizootiology of equine encephalomyelitis in the United States, *J Am Vet Med Assoc* 197:279-287, 1945.
18. Kissling RE, Chamberlain RW: Venezuelan equine encephalitis, *Adv Vet Sci Comp Med* 11:65-84, 1967.
19. Kissling RE, Chamberlain RW, Nelson DB, et al: Venezuelan equine encephalomyelitis in horses, *Am J Hyg* 63:274-287, 1956.
20. Gilyard RT: A clinical study of Venezuelan virus equine encephalomyelitis in Trinidad, BWI, *J Am Vet Med Assoc* 106:267-277, 1945.
21. Young NA, Johnson KM: Antigenic variants of Venezuelan equine encephalitis virus: their geographic distribution and epidemiologic significance, *Am J Epidemiol* 89:286-307, 1969.
22. Scherer WF, Anderson K, Pancake BA, et al: Search for epizootic-like Venezuelan encephalitis virus at enzootic habitats in Guatemala during 1969-1971, *Am J Epidemiol* 103:576-588, 1976.
23. Scherer WF, Madalengoitia J, Flores W, et al: Ecologic studies of Venezuelan encephalitis virus in Peru during 1970-1971, *Am J Epidemiol* 101:347-355, 1975.
24. Sudia WD, Fernandez L, Newhouse VF, et al: Arbovirus vector ecology studies in Mexico during the 1972 Venezuelan equine encephalitis outbreak, *Am J Epidemiol* 101:51-58, 1975.
25. Sudia WD, Newhouse VF: Epidemic Venezuelan equine encephalitis in North America: a summary of virus-vector-host relationships, *Am J Epidemiol* 101:1-13, 1975.
26. Sudia WD, Newhouse VF, Beadle ID, et al: Epidemic Venezuelan equine encephalitis in North America in 1971: vector studies, *Am J Epidemiol* 101:17-35, 1975.
27. Sudia WD, McLean RG, Newhouse VF, et al: Epidemic Venezuelan equine encephalitis in North America in 1971: vertebrate field studies, *Am J Epidemiol* 101:36-50, 1975.
28. Monath TP, Sabattini MS, Pauli R, et al: Arbovirus investigations in Argentina, 1977-1980. IV. Serologic surveys and sentinel equine program, *Am J Trop Med Hyg* 34:966-975, 1985.
29. Dietz WHJ, Galindo P, Johnson KM: Eastern equine encephalomyelitis in Panama: the epidemiology of the 1973 epizootic, *Am J Trop Med Hyg* 29:133-140, 1980.
30. Srihongse S, Grayson MA, Morris CD, et al: Eastern equine encephalomyelitis in upstate New York: studies of a 1976 epizootic by modified serologic technique, hemagglutination reduction, for rapid detection of virus infections, *Am J Trop Med Hyg* 27:1240-1245, 1978.
31. Bigler WJ, Lassing EB, Buff EE, et al: Endemic eastern equine encephalomyelitis in Florida: a twenty-year analysis, 1955-1974, *Am J Trop Med Hyg* 25:884-890, 1976.
32. Bast TF, Whitney E, Benach JL: Considerations on the ecology of several arboviruses in eastern Long Island, *Am J Trop Med Hyg* 22:109-115, 1973.
33. Bryant ES, Anderson CR, Van der Heide L: An epizootic of eastern equine encephalomyelitis in Connecticut, *Avian Dis* 17:861-867, 1973.
34. Morgante O, Vance HN, Shemanchuk JA, et al: Epizootic of western encephalomyelitis virus infection in equines in Alberta in 1965, *Can J Comp Med* 32:403-408, 1968.
35. Ellis RA: Emergency measures and mosquito control during the 1975 western encephalomyelitis outbreak in Manitoba, *Can J Public Health* 67(Suppl 1):59-60, 1976.
36. Donogh NR: Public information on western encephalomyelitis and emergency mosquito control in Manitoba: 1975, *Can J Public Health* 67(Suppl 1):61-62, 1976.
37. Lillie LE, Wong FC, Drysdale RA: Equine epizootic of western encephalomyelitis in Manitoba: 1975, *Can J Public Health* 67(Suppl 1):21-27, 1976.
38. Potter ME, Currier RW, Pearson JE, et al: Western equine encephalomyelitis in horses in the northern Red River Valley, *J Am Vet Med Assoc* 170:1396-1399, 1977.
39. Morier L, Cantelar N, Soler M: Infection of a poikilothermic cell line (XL-2) with eastern equine encephalitis and western equine encephalitis viruses, *J Med Virol* 21:277-281, 1987.
40. Carneiro V, Cunha R: Equine encephalomyelitis in Brazil, *Arch Inst Biol Andina* 14:157-194, 1943.
41. Meyer KF, Wood F, Haring CM: Susceptibility of non-immune hyperimmunized horses and goats to eastern, western and Argentine virus of equine encephalomyelitis, *Proc Soc Exp Biol Med* 32:56-58, 1934.
42. Livesay HR: Isolation of eastern equine encephalitis virus from naturally infected monkey *(Macacus philippensis)*, *J Infect Dis* 84:306-309, 1949.
43. Gibbs EPJ: Equine viral encephalitis, *Equine Vet J* 8:66-71, 1976.
44. Holden P: Recovery of Western equine encephalomyelitis virus from naturally infected English sparrows of New Jersey, *Proc Soc Exp Biol Med* 88:490-492, 1955.

45. Keane DP, Little PB, Wilkie BN, et al: Agents of equine viral encephalomyelitis: correlation of serum and cerebrospinal fluid antibodies, *Can J Vet Res* 52:229-235, 1988.
46. Sellers RF: Weather, host and vector: their interplay in the spread of insect-borne animal virus diseases, *J Hyg (Lond)* 85:65-102, 1980.
47. Shahan MS, Giltner LT: Equine encephalomyelitis studies. I. Cross-immunity tests between eastern and Western types of virus, *J Am Vet Med Assoc* 86:7664-7672, 1935.
48. Smart DL, Trainer DO: Serologic evidence of Venezuelan equine encephalitis in some wild and domestic populations of Southern Texas, *J Wildl Dis* 11:195-200, 1975.
49. McLean RG, Frier G, Parham GL, et al: Investigations of the vertebrate hosts of eastern equine encephalitis during an epizootic in Michigan, 1980, *Am J Trop Med Hyg* 34:1190-1202, 1985.
50. Sudia WD, Stamm DD, Chamberlain RW, et al: Transmission of eastern equine encephalomyelitis to horses by *Aedes sollicitans* mosquitoes, *Am J Trop Med Hyg* 5:802-808, 1956.
51. Crans WJ, McNelly J, Schulze TL, et al: Isolation of eastern equine encephalitis virus from *Aedes sollicitans* during an epizootic in Southern New Jersey, *J Am Mosq Control Assoc* 2:68-72, 1986.
52. Hayes RO, Wallis RC: An ecology of Western equine encephalomyelitis in the Eastern United States, *Adv Virus Res* 21:37-83, 1977.
53. Syverton JT, Berry GP: The tick as a vector for the virus disease equine encephalomyelitis, *J Bacteriol* 33:60, 1937.
54. Kitselman CH, Grundman AW: Equine encephalomyelitis virus isolated from naturally infected *Triatoma sanguisuga*, *Kans Agric Exp Station Tech Bull* 50:15, 1940.
55. Hardy JL: The ecology of Western equine encephalomyelitis virus in the central valley of California, 1945-1985, *Am J Trop Med Hyg* 37(Suppl 3):18S-32S, 1987.
56. Hayes RO, Francy DB, Lazuick JS: Role of the cliff swallow bug *(Oeciacus vicarius)* in the natural cycle of a Western equine encephalitis-related alphavirus, *J Entomol* 14:257-262, 1977.
57. Vawter LR, Records E: Respiratory infection in equine encephalomyelitis, *Science* 78:41-42, 1933.
58. Chamberlain RW: Vector relationships of the arthropod-borne encephalitides in North America, *Ann N Y Acad Sci* 70:312-319, 1958.
59. Ross WA, Kaneene JB: Evaluation of outbreaks of disease attributable to eastern equine encephalitis virus in horses, *J Am Vet Med Assoc* 208(12):1988-1997, 1996.
60. Whitley RJ: Viral encephalitis, *N Engl J Med* 323:242-250, 1990.
61. Gahlinger PM, Reeves WC, Milby MM: Air conditioning and television as protective factors in arboviral encephalitis risk, *Am J Trop Med Hyg* 35:601-610, 1986.
62. McLintock J: The arbovirus problem in Canada, *Can J Public Health* 67(Suppl 1):8-12, 1980.
63. Parker RL, Dean PB, Zehmer RB: Public health aspects of Venezuelan equine encephalitis, *J Am Vet Med Assoc* 162:777-778, 1973.
64. Gardner CL, Burke CW, Tesfay MZ, et al: eastern and Venezuelan equine encephalitis viruses differ in their ability to infect dendritic cells and macrophages: impact of altered cell tropism on pathogenesis, *J Virol* 82(21):10634-10646, 2008.
65. Pursell AR, Mitchell FE, Seibold HR: Naturally occurring and experimentally induced eastern encephalomyelitis in calves, *J Am Vet Med Assoc* 169:1101-1103, 1976.
66. Giltner LT, Shahan MS: Transmission of infectious equine encephalomyelitis in mammals and birds, *Science* 78:63-64, 1933.
67. Karsted L, Hanson RP: Natural and experimental infections in swine with the virus of eastern equine encephalomyelitis, *J Infect Dis* 105:293-296, 1959.
68. Pursell AR, Peckham JC, Cole JR, et al: Naturally occurring and artificially induced eastern encephalomyelitis in pigs, *J Am Vet Med Assoc* 161:1143-1146, 1972.
69. Byrne RH, French GR, Yancy FS, et al: Clinical and immunologic interrelationship among Venezuelan, eastern, and Western equine encephalomyelitis viruses in burros, *Am J Vet Res* 25:24-31, 1964.
70. Binn LN, Sponseller ML, Wooding WL, et al: Efficacy of an attenuated Western encephalitis vaccine in equine animals, *Am J Vet Res* 27:1599-1604, 1966.
71. Henderson BE, Chappell WA, Johnston JG, et al: Experimental infection of horses with three strains of Venezuelan equine encephalomyelitis, *Am J Epidemiol* 93:194-205, 1971.
72. Wilson JH, Rubin HL, Lane TJ, et al: A survey of eastern equine encephalomyelitis in Florida horses: prevalence, economic impact, and management practices, 1982-1983, *Prev Vet Med* 4:261-271, 1986.
73. Doby PB, Schnurrenberger PR, Martin RJ, et al: Western encephalitis in Illinois horses and ponies, *J Am Vet Med Assoc* 148:422-427, 1966.
74. Sponseller ML, Binn LN, Wooding WL, et al: Field strains of Western encephalitis virus in ponies: virologic, clinical, and pathologic observations, *Am J Vet Res* 27:1591-1598, 1966.
75. Cox HR, Philip CB, Marsh H, et al: Observations incident to an outbreak of equine encephalomyelitis in the Bitterroot Valley of Western Montana, *J Am Vet Med Assoc* 94:225-232, 1938.
76. Calisher CH, Emerson JK, Muth DJ, et al: Serodiagnosis of Western equine encephalitis virus infections: relationships of antibody titer and test to observed onset of clinical illness, *J Am Vet Med Assoc* 183:438-440, 1983.
77. Calisher CH, Mahmud MI, el Kafrawi AO, et al: Rapid and specific serodiagnosis of Western equine encephalitis virus infection in horses, *Am J Vet Res* 47:1296-1299, 1986.
78. Scott TW, Olson JG, All BP, et al: Detection of eastern equine encephalomyelitis virus antigen in equine brain tissue by enzyme-linked immunosorbent assay, *Am J Vet Res* 49:1716-1718, 1988.
79. Monath TP, McLean RG, Cropp CB, et al: Diagnosis of eastern equine encephalomyelitis by immunofluorescent staining of brain tissue, *Am J Vet Res* 42:1418-1421, 1981.
80. Ferguson JA, Reeves WC, Hardy JL: Studies on immunity to alphaviruses in foals, *Am J Vet Res* 40:5-10, 1979.
81. Roberts ED, Sanmartin C, Payan J: Neuropathologic changes in 15 horses with naturally occurring Venezuelan equine encephalomyelitis, *Am J Vet Res* 31:1224-1229, 1970.
82. Monlux WS, Luedke AJ: Brain and spinal cord lesions in horses inoculated with Venezuelan equine encephalomyelitis virus (epidemic American and Trinidad strains), *Am J Vet Res* 34:465-473, 1973.
83. Hurst EW: The histology of equine encephalomyelitis, *J Exp Med* 59:529-542, 1934.
84. Patterson JS, Maes RK, Mullaney TP, et al: Immunohistochemical diagnosis of eastern equine encephalomyelitis, *J Vet Diagn Invest* 8(2):156-160, 1996.
85. Devine EH, Byrne RJ: A laboratory confirmed case of viral encephalitis (equine type) in a horse in which the animal completely recovered from the disease, *Cornell Vet* 50:494-497, 1960.
86. Eldridge BF: Strategies for surveillance, prevention, and control of arbovirus diseases in Western North America, *Am J Trop Med Hyg* 37(Suppl):77S-86S, 1987.
87. Spertzel RO, Kahn DE: Safety and efficacy of an attenuated Venezuelan equine encephalomyelitis vaccine for use in equidae, *J Am Vet Med Assoc* 20:128-130, 1971.
88. Byrne RJ: The control of eastern and Western arboviralence pH alomyelitis of horses, In *Proceedings of the third Conference on Equine Infectious Diseases*, Basel Switzerland, 1972, pp 115-123.

89. Gochenour WS, Berge TO, Gleiser CA, et al: Immunization of burros with living Venezuelan equine encephalomyelitis virus, *Am J Hyg* 75:351-362, 1962.
90. Berge T, Banks IS, Tigertt WD: Attenuation of Venezuelan equine encephalomyelitis virus by in vitro cultivation in guinea-pig heart cells, *Am J Hyg* 73:209-218, 1961.
91. Ferguson JA, Reeves WC, Milby MM, et al: Study of homologous and heterologous antibody responses in California horses vaccinated with attenuated Venezuelan equine encephalomyelitis vaccine (strain TC-83), *Am J Vet Res* 39:371-376, 1978.
92. Baker EF, Sasso DR, Maness K: Venezuelan equine encephalomyelitis vaccine (strain TC-83): a field study, *Am J Vet Res* 39:1627-1631, 1978.
93. Walton TE, Jochim MM, Barber TL, et al: Cross-protective immunity between equine encephalomyelitis viruses in equids, *Am J Vet Res* 50:1442-1446, 1989.
94. Jochim MM, Barber TL: Immune response of horses after simultaneous or sequential vaccination against eastern, Western, and Venezuelan equine encephalomyelitis, *J Am Vet Med Assoc* 165:621-625, 1974.
95. Barber TL, Walton TE, Lewis KJ: Efficacy of trivalent inactivated encephalomyelitis virus vaccine in horses, *Am J Vet Res* 39:621-625, 1978.
96. Vanderwangen LC, Pearson JL, Franti CE, et al: A field study of persistence of antibodies in California horses vaccinated against Western, eastern and Venezuelan equine encephalomyelitis,, *Am J Vet Res* 36:1567-1571, 1975.
97. Calisher CH, Sasso DR, Sather GE: Possible evidence for interference with Venezuelan equine encephalitis virus vaccination of equines by pre-existing antibody to eastern or Western equine encephalitis virus, or both, *Appl Microbiol* 26:485-488, 1973.
98. Ferguson JA, Reeves WC, Hardy JL: Antibody studies in ponies vaccinated with Venezuelan equine encephalomyelitis (strain TC-83) and other alphavirus vaccines, *Am J Vet Res* 38:425-430, 1977.
99. Morgan DO, Bryans JT, Mock RE: Immunoglobulins produced by the antigenized equine fetus, *J Reprod Fertil Suppl* 23:735-738, 1975.
100. Waldridge BM, Wenzel JG, Ellis AC et al: Serologic responses to eastern and Western equine encephalomyelitis vaccination in previously vaccinated horses, Vet Ther 4(3):242-248
101. Parkin WE: The occurrence and effects of the local strains of the California encephalitis group of viruses in domestic mammals of Florida, *Am J Trop Med Hyg* 22:788-795, 1973.
102. Artsob H, Wright R, Shipp L, et al: California encephalitis virus activity in mosquitoes and horses in Southern Ontario, 1975, *Can J Microbiol* 24:1544-1547, 1978.
103. Calisher CH, Monath TP, Sabattini MS, et al: A newly recognized vesiculovirus, Calchaqui virus, and subtypes of Melao and Maguari viruses from Argentina, with serologic evidence for infections of humans and horses, *Am J Trop Med Hyg* 36:114-119, 1987.
104. Campbell GL, Reeves WC, Hardy JL, et al: Distribution of neutralizing antibodies to California and Bunyamwera serogroup viruses in horses and rodents in California, *Am J Trop Med Hyg* 42:282-290, 1990.
105. Clark GG, Crabbs CL, Bailey CL, et al: Identification of *Aedes campestris* from New Mexico: with notes on the isolation of Western equine encephalitis and other arboviruses, *J Am Mosq Control Assoc* 2:529-534, 1986.
106a. Lynch JA, Binnington BD, Artsob H: California serogroup virus infection in a horse with encephalitis, *J Am Vet Med Assoc* 186:389, 1985.
106b. McFarlane BL, Embree JE, Embil JA, et al: Antibodies to snowshoe hare virus of the California group in the snowshoe hare *(Lepus americanus)* and domestic animal populations of Prince Edward Island, *Can J Microbiol* 27:1224-1227, 1981.
107. Emmons RW, Woodie JD, Laub RL, et al: Main Drain virus as a cause of equine encephalomyelitis, *J Am Vet Med Assoc* 183:555-558, 1983.
108. Kokernot RH, Hayes J, Will RL, et al: Arbovirus studies in the Ohio-Mississippi basin, 1964-1967. II. St Louis encephalitis virus, *Am J Trop Med Hyg* 18:750-761, 1969.
109. Bailey CL, Eldridge BF, Hayes DE, et al: Isolation of St Louis encephalitis virus from overwintering *Culex pipiens* mosquitoes, *Science* 199:1346-1349, 1978.
110. Little PB, Thorsen J, Moore W, et al: Powassan viral encephalitis: a review and experimental studies in the horse and rabbit, *Vet Pathol* 22:500-507, 1985.
111. Campbell J, Hore DE: Isolation of Murray Valley encephalitis virus from sentinel chickens, *Aust Vet J* 51:1-3, 1975.
112. Kay BH, Young PL, Hall RA, et al: Experimental infection with Murray Valley encephalitis: pigs, cattle, sheep, dogs, rabbits, chickens, and macropods, *Aust J Exp Biol Med Sci* 63:109-126, 1985.
113. Kay BH, Pollitt CC, Fanning ID, et al: The experimental infection of horses with Murray Valley encephalitis and Ross River viruses, *Aust Vet J* 64:52-55, 1987.
114. Gard GP: Association of Australian arboviruses with nervous disease in horses, *Aust Vet J* 53:61-66, 1977.
115. McLean RG, Calisher CH, Parham GL: Isolation of Cache Valley virus and detection of antibody for selected arboviruses in Michigan horses in 1980, *Am J Vet Res* 48(7):1039-1041, 1987.
116. Heath SE, Arsob H, Bell RJ, et al: Equine encephalitis caused by snowshoe hare (California serogroup) virus, *Can Vet J* 30:669-671, 1989.
117. Nelson DM, Gardner IA, Chiles RF, et al: Prevalence of antibodies against Saint Louis encephalitis and Jamestown Canyon viruses in California horses, *Comp Immunol Microbiol Infect Dis* 27:209-215, 2004.
118. Sahu SP, Landgraf J, Wineland N, et al: Isolation of Jamestown Canyon virus (California virus group) from vesicular lesions of a horse, *J Vet Diagn Invest* 12:80-83, 2000.
119. Hooper PT, Williamson MM: Hendra and Nipah virus infections, *Vet Clin North Am Equine Pract* 16:597-603, 2000.
120. Howell PG, Groenewald D, Visage CW, et al: The classification of seven serotypes of equine encephalosis virus and the prevalence of homologous antibody in horses in South Africa, *Onderstepoort J Vet Res* 69:79-93, 2002.
121. Paweska JT, Venter GJ: Vector competence of *Culicoides* species and the seroprevalence of homologous neutralizing antibody in horses for six serotypes of equine encephalosis virus (EEV) in South Africa, *Med Vet Entomol* 18:398-407, 2004.
122. Sellon DC, Long MT, editors: *Equine infectious diseases*, St Louis, 2007, WB Saunders.
123. Sauder C, Staeheli P: Rat model of Borna disease virus transmission: epidemiological implications, *J Virol* 77:12886, 2003.
124. Stitz L, Bilzer T, Planz O: The immunopathogenesis of Borna disease virus infection, *Front Biosci* 1:d541-555, 2002.
125. Timoney PJ, Donnelly WJC, Clements LO, et al: Encephalitis caused by louping ill virus in a group of horses in Ireland, *Equine Vet J* 8:113-117, 1976.
126. Timoney PJ: Susceptibility of the horse to experimental inoculation with louping ill virus, *J Comp Pathol* 90:73-86, 1980.
127. Sabattini MS, Monath TP, Mitchell CJ, et al: Arbovirus investigations in Argentina, 1977-1980. I. Historical aspects and description of study sites, *Am J Trop Med Hyg* 34:937-944, 1985.
128. Narayan O, Herzog S, Frese K, et al: Pathogenesis of Borna disease in rats: immune-mediated viral ophthalmoencephalopathy causing blindness and behavioral abnormalities, *J Infect Dis* 148:305-315, 1983.
129. Karabatsos N, Lewis AL, Calisher CH, et al: Identification of Highlands J virus from a Florida horse, *Am J Trop Med Hyg* 40:228-231, 1989.

130. Robin Y, Bourdin P, Le Gonidec E, et al: Semliki forest virus encephalomyelitis in Senegal, *Ann Inst Pasteur Microbiol* 125A:235-241, 1974.
131. Matsumura T, Goto H, Shimizu K, et al: Prevalence and distribution of antibodies to Getah and Japanese encephalitis viruses in horses raised in Hokkaido, *Nippon Juigaku Zasshi* 44:967-970, 1982.

Flavivirus Encephalitis

1. Overstreet M: Patient education series. West Nile virus, *Nursing* 35:64, 2005.
2. Kraftcheck DJ, et al: Ontario's 2003 West Nile virus public education campaign: was anybody listening?, *Can Commun Dis Rep* 29:189-194, 2003.
3. Center for Disease Control: Arboviral information sheet, 1999.
4. Monath TP, editor: *The arboviruses: epidemiology and ecology*, Boca Raton, FL, 1989, CRC Press, pp 59-88.
5. Hall RA, Scherret JH, MacKenzie JS: Kunjin virus: an Australian variant of West Nile?, *Ann N Y Acad Sci* 951:153-160, 2001.
6. MacKenzie JS: Emerging zoonotic encephalitis viruses: lessons from Southeast Asia and Oceania, *J Neurovirol* 11:434-440, 2005.
7. MacKenzie JS, Lindsay MD, Coelen RJ, et al: Arboviruses causing human disease in the Australasian zoogeographic region, *Arch Virol* 136:447-467, 1994.
8. MacKenzie JS, Smith DW, Broom AK, et al: Australian encephalitis in Western Australia, 1978-1991, *Med J Aust* 158:591-595, 1993.
9. Williamson F: Man against insect. III. Walter Reed v yellow fever, *Nurs Times* 70:1202-1203, 1974.
10. Rice CM, Lenches EM, Eddy SM, et al: Nucleotide sequence of yellow fever virus: implications for flavivirus gene expression and evolution, *Science* 229:726-735, 1985.
11. Lanciotti RS, et al: Origin of the West Nile virus responsible for an outbreak of encephalitis in the Northeastern United States, *Science* 286:2333-2337, 1999.
12. Wengler G, Wengler G: Cell-associated West Nile flavivirus is covered with E+pre-M protein heterodimers which are destroyed and reorganized by proteolytic cleavage during virus release, *J Virol* 63:2521-2526, 1989.
13. Grun JB, Brinton MA: Separation of functional West Nile virus replication complexes from intracellular membrane fragments, *J Gen Virol* 69(Pt 12):3121-3127, 1988.
14. Wengler G, Wengler G, Nowak T, et al: Analysis of the influence of proteolytic cleavage on the structural organization of the surface of the West Nile flavivirus leads to the isolation of a protease-resistant E protein oligomer from the viral surface, *Virology* 160:210-219, 1987.
15. Nowak T, Wengler G: Analysis of disulfides present in the membrane proteins of the West Nile flavivirus, *Virology* 156:127-137, 1987.
16. Castle E, Nowak T, Leidner U, et al: Sequence analysis of the viral core protein and the membrane-associated proteins V1 and NV2 of the flavivirus West Nile virus and of the genome sequence for these proteins, *Virology* 145:227-236, 1985.
17. Wengler G, Castle E, Leidner U, et al: Sequence analysis of the membrane protein V3 of the flavivirus West Nile virus and of its gene, *Virology* 147:264-274, 1985.
18. Hayes CG: West Nile virus: Uganda, 1937, to New York City, 1999, *Ann N Y Acad Sci* 951:25-37, 2001.
19. Turell MJ, O'Guinn M, Oliver J: Potential for New York mosquitoes to transmit West Nile virus, *Am J Trop Med Hyg* 62: 413-414, 2000.
20. McLean RG, Ubico SR, Bourne D, et al: West Nile virus in livestock and wildlife, *Curr Top Microbiol Immunol* 267:271-308, 2002.
21. Komar N, Panella NA, Boyce E: Exposure of domestic mammals to West Nile virus during an outbreak of human encephalitis, New York City, 1999, *Emerg Infect Dis* 7:736-738, 2001.
22. Komar N, Lanciotti R, Bowen R, et al: Detection of West Nile virus in oral and cloacal swabs collected from bird carcasses, *Emerg Infect Dis* 8:741-742, 2002.
23. Komar N, Langevin S, Hinten S, et al: Experimental infection of North American birds with the New York 1999 strain of West Nile virus, *Emerg Infect Dis* 9:311-322, 2003.
24. Hayes EB, Komar N, Nasci RS, et al: Epidemiology and transmission dynamics of West Nile virus disease, *Emerg Infect Dis* 11:1167-1173, 2005.
25. Hindiyeh M, Shulman LM, Mendelson E, et al: Isolation and characterization of West Nile virus from the blood of viremic patients during the 2000 outbreak in Israel, *Emerg Infect Dis* 7:748-750, 2001.
26. Investigations of West Nile virus infections in recipients of blood transfusions, *MMWR Morb Mortal Wkly Rep* 51:973-974, 2002.
27. Possible West Nile virus transmission to an infant through breast-feeding—Michigan, 2002, *MMWR Morb Mortal Wkly Rep* 51:877-878, 2002.
28. Update: investigations of West Nile virus infections in recipients of organ transplantation and blood transfusion, *MMWR Morb Mortal Wkly Rep* 51:833-836, 2002.
29. Investigation of blood transfusion recipients with West Nile virus infections, *MMWR Morb Mortal Wkly Rep* 51:823, 2002.
30. Mayer V, Rajcani J: Study of the virulence of tick-borne encephalitis virus. VI, *Intracerebral infection of monkeys with clones experimentally attenuated virus Acta Virol* 11:321-333, 1967.
31. Intrauterine West Nile virus infection—New York, 2002, *MMWR Morb Mortal Wkly Rep* 51:1135-1136, 2002.
32. Mayer V, Rajcani J: Study of the virulence of tick-borne encephalitis virus. VI. Intracerebral infection of monkeys with clones experimentally attenuated virus, *Acta Virol* 11:321-333, 1967.
33. Update: West Nile virus activity—United States, 2005, *MMWR Morb Mortal Wkly Rep* 54:964-965, 2005.
34. Drebot MA, Artsob H: West Nile virus. Update for family physicians, *Can Fam Physician* 51:1094-1099, 2005.
35. Cruz L, Cardenas VM, Abarca M, et al: Short report: serological evidence of West Nile virus activity in El Salvador, *Am J Trop Med Hyg* 72:612-615, 2005.
36. Dauphin G, Zientara S, Zeller H, et al: West Nile: worldwide current situation in animals and humans, *Comp Immunol Microbiol Infect Dis* 27:343-355, 2004.
37. Dupuis AP, Marra PP, Kramer LD: Serologic evidence of West Nile virus transmission, Jamaica, West Indies, *Emerg Infect Dis* 9:860-863, 2003.
38. Granwehr BP, et al: West Nile virus: where are we now?, *Lancet Infect Dis* 4:547-556, 2004.
39. Rappole JH, Derrickson SR, Hubalek Z: Migratory birds and spread of West Nile virus in the Western Hemisphere, *Emerg Infect Dis* 6:319-328, 2000.
40. Hayes EB, Gubler DJ: West Nile Virus: epidemiology and clinical features of an emerging epidemic in the United States, *Annu Rev Med*, 57:139-154, 2006.
41. Beasley DW, Davis CT, Estrada-Franco J, et al: Genome sequence and attenuating mutations in West Nile virus isolate from Mexico, *Emerg Infect Dis* 10:2221-2224, 2004.
42. Baqar S, Hayes CG, Murphy JR, et al: Vertical transmission of West Nile virus by *Culex* and *Aedes* species mosquitoes, *Am J Trop Med Hyg* 48:757-762, 1993.
43. Ahmed T, Hayes CG, Baqar S: Comparison of vector competence for West Nile virus of colonized populations of *Culex tritaeniorhynchus* from Southern Asia and the Far East, *Southeast Asian J Trop Med Public Health* 10:498-504, 1979.

44. Hindiyeh M, Shulman LM, Mendelson E, et al: Isolation and characterization of West Nile virus from the blood of viremic patients during the 2000 outbreak in Israel, *Emerg Infect Dis* 7:748-750, 2001.
45. Cornel AJ, Jupp PG: Comparison of three methods for determining transmission rates in vector competence studies with *Culex univittatus* and West Nile and Sindbis viruses, *J Am Mosq Control Assoc* 5:70-72, 1989.
46. Turell MJ, O'Guinn ML, Dohm DJ, et al: Vector competence of North American mosquitoes (Diptera: *Culicidae*) for West Nile virus, *J Med Entomol* 38:130-134, 2001.
47. Kulasekera VL, Kramer L, Nasci RS, et al: West Nile virus infection in mosquitoes, birds, horses, and humans, Staten Island, New York, 2000, *Emerg Infect Dis* 7:722-725, 2001.
48. Update: surveillance for West Nile virus in overwintering mosquitoes—New York, 2000, *MMWR Morb Mortal Wkly Rep* 49:178-179, 2000.
49. Komar N: West Nile virus: epidemiology and ecology in North America, *Adv Virus Res* 61:185-234, 2003.
50. Hayes CG, Basit A, Bagar S, et al: Vector competence of *Culex tritaeniorhynchus* (Diptera: *Culicidae*) for West Nile virus, *J Med Entomol* 17:172-177, 1980.
51. Sardelis MR, Turell MJ, Dohm DJ, et al: Vector competence of selected North American *Culex* and *Coquillettidia* mosquitoes for West Nile virus, *Emerg Infect Dis* 7:1018-1022, 2001.
52. Turell MJ, O'Guinn ML, Dohm DJ, et al: Vector competence of *Culex tarsalis* from Orange County, California, for West Nile virus, *Vector Borne Zoonotic Dis* 2:193-196, 2002.
53. Reisen WK, Fang Y, Martinez VM: Avian host and mosquito (Diptera: *Culicidae*) vector competence determine the efficiency of West Nile and St Louis encephalitis virus transmission, *J Med Entomol* 42:367-375, 2005.
54. Mans NZ, Yurgionas SE, Garvin MC, et al: West Nile virus in mosquitoes of Northern Ohio, 2001-2002, *Am J Trop Med Hyg* 70:562-565, 2004.
55. Blackmore CG, Stark LM, Jeter WC, et al: Surveillance results from the first West Nile virus transmission season in Florida, 2001, *Am J Trop Med Hyg* 69:141-150, 2003.
56. Godsey MS Jr, Blackmore MS, Panella NA, et al: West Nile virus epizootiology in the Southeastern United States, 2001, *Vector Borne Zoonotic Dis* 5:82-89, 2005.
57. Hribar LJ, Vlach JJ, Demay DJ, et al: Mosquitoes infected with West Nile virus in the Florida Keys, Monroe County, Florida, USA, *J Med Entomol* 40:361-363, 2003.
58. Rutledge CR, Day JF, Lord CC, et al: West Nile virus infection rates in *Culex nigripalpus* (Diptera: *Culicidae*) do not reflect transmission rates in Florida, *J Med Entomol* 40:253-258, 2003.
59. Zyzak M, Loyless T, Cope S, et al: Seasonal abundance of *Culex nigripalpus* Theobald and *Culex salinarius* Coquillett in north Florida, USA, *J Vector Ecol* 27:155-162, 2002.
60. Tesh RB, Parsons R, Siirin M, et al: Year-round West Nile virus activity, Gulf Coast region, Texas and Louisiana, *Emerg Infect Dis* 10:1649-1652, 2004.
61. Lillibridge KM, Parsons R, Randle Y, et al: The 2002 introduction of West Nile virus into Harris County, Texas, an area historically endemic for St Louis encephalitis, *Am J Trop Med Hyg* 70:676-681, 2004.
62. Sardelis MR, Turell MJ, Dohm DJ, et al: Vector competence of selected North American *Culex* and *Coquillettidia* mosquitoes for West Nile virus, *Emerg Infect Dis* 7:1018-1022, 2001.
63. Sardelis MR, Turell MJ, O'Guinn ML, et al: Vector competence of three North American strains of *Aedes albopictus* for West Nile virus, *J Am Mosq Control Assoc* 18:284-289, 2002.
64. Turell MJ, Dohm DJ, Sardelis MR, et al: An update on the potential of north American mosquitoes (Diptera: *Culicidae*) to transmit West Nile Virus, *J Med Entomol* 42:57-62, 2005.
65. Southam CH, Moore AE: Induced virus infections in man by the Egypt isolate of West Nile Virus, *Am J Trop Med Hyg* 3:19-50, 1954.
66. Smith TL, Hayes EB, O'Leary DR, et al: West Nile virus activity—United States, January 1-December 1, 2005, *MMWR Morb Mortal Wkly Rep* 54:1253-1256, 2005.
67. Blackmore CG, Stark LM, Jeter WC, et al: Surveillance results from the first West Nile virus transmission season in Florida, 2001, *Am J Trop Med Hyg* 69:141-150, 2003.
68. Romi R, Pontuale G, Clufolini MG, et al: Potential vectors of West Nile virus following an equine disease outbreak in Italy, *Med Vet Entomol* 18:14-19, 2004.
69. Gingrich JB, Casillas L: Selected mosquito vectors of West Nile virus: comparison of their ecological dynamics in four woodland and marsh habitats in Delaware, *J Am Mosq Control Assoc* 20:138-145, 2004.
70. Gingrich JB, Williams GM: Host-feeding patterns of suspected West Nile virus mosquito vectors in Delaware, 2001-2002, *J Am Mosq Control Assoc* 21:194-200, 2005.
71. Durand B, Chevalier V, Pouillot R, et al: West Nile virus outbreak in horses, southern France, 2000: results of a serosurvey, *Emerg Infect Dis* 8:777-782, 2002.
72. Kramer LD, Bernard KA: West Nile virus infection in birds and mammals, *Ann N Y Acad Sci* 951:84-93, 2001.
73. West Nile virus activity—United States, 2005, *MMWR Morb Mortal Wkly Rep* 54:769-770, 2005.
74. Petersen LR, Marfin AA: West Nile virus: a primer for the clinician, *Ann Intern Med* 137:173-179, 2002.
75. Weiss D, Kellachan J, Tan C, et al: Clinical findings of West Nile virus infection in hospitalized patients, New York and New Jersey, 2000, *Emerg Infect Dis* 7:654-658, 2001.
76. Update: West Nile Virus activity—Eastern United States, 2000, *MMWR Morb Mortal Wkly Rep* 49:1044-1047, 2000.
77. Outbreak of West Nile-like viral encephalitis—New York, 1999, *MMWR Morb Mortal Wkly Rep* 48:845-849, 1999.
78. Davidson AH, Traub-Dargatz JL, Rodeheaver RM, et al: Immunologic responses to West Nile virus in vaccinated and clinically affected horses, *J Am Vet Med Assoc* 226:240-245, 2005.
79. Schuler LA, Khaitsa ML, Dyer NW, et al: Evaluation of an outbreak of West Nile virus infection in horses: 569 cases (2002), *J Am Vet Med Assoc* 225:1084-1089, 2004.
80. Guarner J, Shieh WJ, Hunter S, et al: Clinicopathologic study and laboratory diagnosis of 23 cases with West Nile virus encephalomyelitis, *Hum Pathol* 35:983-990, 2004.
81. Jacobson ER, Ginn PE, Troutman JM, et al: West Nile virus infection in farmed American alligators *(Alligator mississippiensis)* in Florida, *J Wildl Dis* 41:96-106, 2005.
82. Heinz-Taheny KM, Andrews JJ, Kinsel MJ, et al: West Nile virus infection in free-ranging squirrels in Illinois, *J Vet Diagn Invest* 16:186-190, 2004.
83. Kiupel M, Simmons HA, Fitzgerald SD, et al: West Nile virus infection in eastern fox squirrels *(Sciurus niger)*, *Vet Pathol* 40:703-707, 2003.
84. Jacobson ER, Ginn PE, Troutman JM, et al: West Nile virus infection in farmed American alligato rs *(Alligator mississippiensis)* in Florida, *J Wildl Dis* 41:96-106, 2005.
85. Kutzler MA, Bildfell RJ, Gardner-Graff KK, et al: West Nile virus infection in two alpacas, *J Am Vet Med Assoc* 225:921-924, 2004:880.
86. Yaeger M, Yoon KJ, Schwartz K, et al: West Nile virus meningoencephalitis in a Suri alpaca and Suffolk ewe, *J Vet Diagn Invest* 16:64-66, 2004.
87. Porter MB, Long MT, Getman LM, et al: West Nile virus encephalomyelitis in horses: 46 cases (2001), *J Am Vet Med Assoc* 222:1241-1247, 2003.
88. Ostlund EN, Crom RL, Thomsen BV: West Nile virus: epidemiology, pathogenesis, immunologic response, 2002. In Proceedings American College of Veterinary Internal Medicine Forum, Denver, ACVIM.

89. Cantile C, Del Piero F, Di Guardo G, et al: Pathologic and immunohistochemical findings in naturally occurring West Nile virus infection in horses, *Vet Pathol* 38:414-421, 2001.
90. Snook CS, Hyman SS, Del Piero F, et al: West Nile virus encephalomyelitis in eight horses, *J Am Vet Med Assoc* 218:1576-1579, 2001.
91. Cantile C, Di Guardo G, Eleni C, et al: Clinical and neuropathological features of West Nile virus equine encephalomyelitis in Italy, *Equine Vet J* 32:31-35, 2000.
92. Desai A, Shankar SK, Ravi V, et al: Japanese encephalitis virus antigen in the human brain and its topographic distribution, *Acta Neuropathol* 89:368-373, 1995.
93. Rosemberg S: Neuropathology of S. Paulo south coast epidemic encephalitis *(Rocio flavivirus)*, *J Neurol Sci* 45:1-12, 1980.
94. Joubert L, Oudar J, Hannoun C, et al: Experimental reproduction of meningo-encephalomyelitis of horses with West Nile arbovirus. III. Relations between virology, serology, and anatomo-clinical evolution. Epidemiological and prophylactic consequences, *Bull Acad Vet Fr* 44:159-167, 1971.
95. Oudar J, Joubert L, Lapras M, et al: Experimental reproduction of meningo-encephalomyelitis of horses with West Nile arbovirus. II. Anatomo-clinical study, *Bull Acad Vet Fr* 44:147-158, 1971.
96. Tamalet J, Toga M, Chippaux-Hyppolite C, et al: Experimental encephalitis caused by West-Nile virus in mice: ultrastructural aspects of the central nervous system, *C R Acad Sci Hebd Seances Acad Sci D* 269:668-671, 1969.
97. Gilroy J: *Basic neurology*, ed 3, New York, 2000, McGraw Hill Professional.
98. Guillon JC, Oudar J, Joubert L, et al: Histological lesions of the nervous system in West Nile virus infection in horses, *Ann Inst Pasteur (Paris)* 114:539-550, 1968.
99. Tiroumourougane SV, Raghava P, Srinivasan S: Japanese viral encephalitis, *Postgrad Med J* 78:205-215, 2002.
100. Ostlund EN, Crom RL, Pedersen DD, et al: Equine West Nile encephalitis, *United States Emerg Infect Dis* 7:665-669, 2001.
101. Oudar J, Joubert L, Lapras M, et al: Experimental reproduction of meningo-encephalomyelitis of horses with West Nile arbovirus. II. Anatomo-clinical study, *Bull Acad Vet Fr* 44:147-158, 1971.
102. Joubert L, Oudar J, Hannoun C, et al: Epidemiology of the West Nile virus: study of a focus in Camargue. IV. Meningo-encephalomyelitis of the horse, *Ann Inst Pasteur (Paris)* 118:239-247, 1970.
103. Ogata A, Tashiro K, Nukuzuma S, et al: A rat model of Parkinson's disease induced by Japanese encephalitis virus, *J Neurovirol* 3:141-147, 1997.
104. Asher DM: Movement disorders in rhesus monkeys after infection with tick-borne encephalitis virus, *Adv Neurol* 10:277-289, 1975.
105. Mayhew J: *Large animal neurology*, Philadelphia, 2009, Wiley-Blackwell.
106. Shrestha B, Gottlieb D, Diamond MS: Infection and injury of neurons by West Nile encephalitis virus, *J Virol* 77:13203-13213, 2003.
107. Shrestha B, Diamond MS: Role of CD8+ T cells in control of West Nile virus infection, *J Virol* 78:8312-8321, 2004.
108. Wang Y, Lobigs M, Lee E, et al: CD8+ T cells mediate recovery and immunopathology in West Nile virus encephalitis, *J Virol* 77:13323-13334, 2003.
109. Takashima I: *Japanese encephalitis. Manual of standards for diagnostic tests and vaccines*, ed 4, Paris, 2001, Office International des Epizooties, 607-614.
110. Gould DJ, Byrne RJ, Hayes DE: Experimental infection of horses with Japanese encephalitis virus by mosquito bits, *Am J Trop Med Hyg* 13:742-746, 1964.
111. Grosenbaugh DA, Backus CS, Karaca K, et al: The anamnestic serologic response to vaccination with a canarypox virus-vectored recombinant West Nile virus (WNV) vaccine in horses previously vaccinated with an inactivated WNV vaccine, *Vet Ther* 5:251-257, 2004.
112. Guthrie AJ, Howell PG, Gardner IA, et al: West Nile virus infection of Thoroughbred horses in South Africa (2000-2001), *Equine Vet J* 35:601-605, 2003.
113. Pantheir R, Hannoun C, Oudar J, et al: Isolation of West Nile virus in a Camargue horse with encephalomyelitis, *C R Acad Sci Hebd Seances Acad Sci D* 262:1308-1310, 1966.
114. Schuler LA, Khaitsa ML, Dyer NW, et al: Evaluation of an outbreak of West Nile virus infection in horses: 569 cases (2002), *J Am Vet Med Assoc* 225:1084-1089, 2004.
115. Petersen LR, Marfin AA: West Nile virus: a primer for the clinician, *Ann Intern Med* 137:173-179, 2002.
116. Porter MB: Immunoglobulin M-capture enzyme-linked immunosorbent assay testing of cerebrospinal fluid and serum from horses exposed to West Nile virus by vaccination or natural infection, *J Vet Intern Med* 18:866-870, 2004.
117. Wamsley HL, Alleman AR, Porter MB: Findings in cerebrospinal fluids of horses infected with West Nile virus: 30 cases (2001), *J Am Vet Med Assoc* 221:1303-1305, 2002.
118. Cernescu C, Ruta SM, Tardei G, et al: A high number of severe neurologic clinical forms during an epidemic of West Nile virus infection, *Rom J Virol* 48:13-25, 1997.
119. Jeha LE, Sila CA, Lederman RJ, et al: West Nile virus infection: a new acute paralytic illness, *Neurology* 61:55-59, 2003.
120. Ostlund EN, Andresen JE, Andresen M: West Nile encephalitis, *Vet Clin North Am Equine Pract* 16:427-441, 2000.
121. Davidson AH, Traub-Dargatz JL, Rodeheaver RM, et al: Immunologic responses to West Nile virus in vaccinated and clinically affected horses, *J Am Vet Med Assoc* 226:240-245, 2005.
122. Johnson DJ, Ostlund EN, Pedersen DD, et al: Detection of North American West Nile virus in animal tissue by a reverse transcription-nested polymerase chain reaction assay, *Emerg Infect Dis* 7:739-741, 2001.
123. Tewari D, Kim H, Feria W, et al: Detection of West Nile virus using formalin fixed paraffin embedded tissues in crows and horses: quantification of viral transcripts by real-time RT-PCR, *J Clin Virol* 30:320-325, 2004.
124. Kolman JM: Serologic examination of some domestic animals from South Moravia on the presence of antibodies to selected arboviruses of the A, B, California and Bunyamwera groups, *Folia Parasitol (Praha)* 20:353-360, 1973.
125. Bonaduce A, Compagnucci M, Bonaduce D, et al: Studies on the occurrence and distribution of HI antibodies against some arboviruses in the serum of domestic mammals in Puglia, *Folia Vet Lat* 7:145-157, 1977.
126. Matsumura T, Goto H, Shimizu K, et al: Prevalence and distribution of antibodies to Getah and Japanese encephalitis viruses in horses raised in Hokkaido, *Nippon Juigaku Zasshi* 44:967-970, 1982.
127. Shrestha B, Gottlieb D, Diamond MS: Infection and injury of neurons by West Nile encephalitis virus, *J Virol* 77:13203-13213, 2003.
128. Kamalov NI, Novozhilova AP, Kreichman GS, et al: Morphological features of cell death in various types of acute tick-borne encephalitis, *Neurosci Behav Physiol* 29:449-453, 1999.
129. Ogata A, Tashiro K, Nukuzuma S, et al: A rat model of Parkinson's disease induced by Japanese encephalitis virus, *J Neurovirol* 3:141-147, 1997.
130. Schlesinger JJ, Chapman S, Nestorowicz A, et al: Replication of yellow fever virus in the mouse central nervous system: comparison of neuroadapted and non-neuroadapted virus and partial sequence analysis of the neuroadapted strain, *J Gen Virol* 77(Pt 6):1277-1285, 1996.

131. Shahar A, Lustig S, Akov Y, et al: Spinal cord slices with attached dorsal root ganglia: a culture model for the study of pathogenicity of encephalitic viruses, *Adv Exp Med Biol* 296:111-119, 1991.
132. Scholle F, Mason PW: West Nile virus replication interferes with both poly(I: C)-induced interferon gene transcription and response to interferon treatment, *Virology* 342(1):77-87, 2005.
133. Engle MJ, Diamond MS: Antibody prophylaxis and therapy against West Nile virus infection in wild-type and immunodeficient mice, *J Virol* 77:12941-12949, 2003.
134. Anderson JF, Rahal JJ: Efficacy of interferon alpha-2b and ribavirin against West Nile virus in vitro, *Emerg Infect Dis* 8:107-108, 2002.
135. Leis AA, Stokic DS: Neuromuscular manifestations of human West Nile Virus infection, *Curr Treat Options Neurol* 7:15-22, 2005.
136. Roos KL: West Nile encephalitis and myelitis, *Curr Opin Neurol* 17:343-346, 2004.
137. Jackson AC: Therapy of West Nile virus infection, *Can J Neurol Sci* 31:131-134, 2004.
138. Ben-Nathan D, Lachmi B, Lustig S, et al: Protection by dehydroepiandrosterone in mice infected with viral encephalitis, *Arch Virol* 120:263-271, 1991.
139. Drebot MA, Artsob H: West Nile virus. Update for family physicians, *Can Fam Physician* 51:1094-1099, 2005.
140. Romero JR, Newland JG: Viral meningitis and encephalitis: traditional and emerging viral agents, *Semin Pediatr Infect Dis* 14:72-82, 2003.
141. Engle MJ, Diamond MS: Antibody prophylaxis and therapy against West Nile virus infection in wild-type and immunodeficient mice, *J Virol* 77:12941-12949, 2003.
142. Petersen LR, Marfin AA: West Nile virus: a primer for the clinician, *Ann Intern Med* 137:173-179, 2002.
143. Anderson JF, Rahal JJ: Efficacy of interferon alpha-2b and ribavirin against West Nile virus in vitro, *Emerg Infect Dis* 8:107-108, 2002.
144. Unpublished data, Long, 2009.
145. Seino KK, Long MT, Gibbs EPJ, et al: Comparative efficacies of three commercially available vaccines against West Nile virus (WNV) in a short-duration challenge trial involving an equine WNV encephalitis model, *Clin Vaccine Immunol* 14:1465-1471, 2007.
146. Crom RL: Update on current status of West Nile virus: equine cases of West Nile virus infection in 2001: 1 January through 20 November, Washington, DC, 2001, United States Department of Agriculture Animal and Plant Health Inspection Service.
147. Crom RL: Update on current status, Washington, DC, 2002, United States Department of Agriculture Animal and Plant Health Inspection Service.
148 Ostlund EN, Andresen JE, Andresen M: West Nile encephalitis, *Vet Clin North Am Equine Pract* 16:427-441, 2000.
149. Goto H: Efficacy of Japanese encephalitis vaccine in horses, *Equine Vet J* 8:126-127, 1976.
150. Minke JM, Audonnet JC, Fischer L: Equine viral vaccines: the past, present and future, *Vet Res* 35:425-443, 2004.
151. Konishi E, Shoda M, Ajiro N, et al: Development and evaluation of an enzyme-linked immunosorbent assay for quantifying antibodies to Japanese encephalitis virus nonstructural 1 protein to detect subclinical infections in vaccinated horses, *J Clin Microbiol* 42:5087-5093, 2004.
152. Konishi E, Shoda M, Kondo T: Prevalence of antibody to Japanese encephalitis virus nonstructural 1 protein among racehorses in Japan: indication of natural infection and need for continuous vaccination, *Vaccine* 22:1097-1103, 2004.
153. Lam KH, Ellis TM, Williams DT, et al: Japanese encephalitis in a racing thoroughbred gelding in Hong Kong, *Vet Rec* 157:168-173, 2005.
154. Long MT, Gibbs EPJ, Mellencamp MW, et al: Efficacy, duration, and onset of immunogenicity of a West Nile virus vaccine, live *Flavivirus chimera*, in horses with a clinical disease challenge model, *Equine Vet J* 39:491-497, 2007.

Rabies

1. Krebs JW, Strine TW, Smith JS, et al: Rabies surveillance in the United States during 1993, *J Am Vet Med Assoc* 205:1695, 1994.
2. Martin ML, Sedmak PA: Rabies. I. Epidemiology, pathogenesis, and diagnosis, *Compend Contin Educ Pract Vet* 5:521, 1983.
3. Mansmann RA, McAllister ES, Pratt PW, editors: *Equine medicine and surgery*, ed 3, Santa Barbara, CA, 1982, American Veterinary Publications.
4. Robinson NE, editor: *Current therapy in equine medicine*, ed 6, St Louis, 2009, WB Saunders.
5. Baer GM, editor: *The natural history of rabies* vol. 1New York, 1975, Academic Press.
6. West GP: Equine rabies, *Equine Vet J* 17:280, 1985.
7. Striegel P, Genetzky RM: Signs of rabies in horses: a clinical review, *Mod Vet Pract* 64:983, 1983.
8. Joyce JR, Russell LH: Clinical signs of rabies in horses, *Compend Contin Educ Pract Vet* 3:S56, 1981.
9. Smith JM, Cox JH: Central nervous system disease in adult horses. III. Differential diagnosis and comparison of common disorders, *Compend Contin Educ Pract Vet* 9:1042, 1987.
10. Sommardahl CS, Henton JE, Peterson MG: Rabies in a horse, *Vet Clin North Am Equine Pract* 12:11, 1990.
11. Siger L, Green SL, Merritt AM: Equine rabies with a prolonged course, *Vet Clin North Am Equine Pract* 11:6, 1989.
12. Mayhew J: *Large animal neurology*, Philadelphia, 2010, Wiley-Blackwell.
13. Smith BP, editor: *Large animal internal medicine*, ed 4, St Louis, 2009, Mosby.
14. Meyer EE, Morris PG, Elcock LH, et al: Hindlimb hyperesthesia associated with rabies in two horses, *J Am Vet Med Assoc* 188:629, 1986.

Equine Motor Neuron Disease

1. Cummings JF, de Lahunta A, George C, et al: Equine motor neuron disease: a preliminary report, *Cornell Vet* 80:357, 1990.
2. Divers TJ, Mohammed HO, Cummings JF, et al: Equine motor neuron disease: findings in 28 horses and proposal of a pathophysiological mechanism for the disease, *Equine Vet J* 26:409, 1994.
3. de la Rúa-Domènech R, Mohammed HO, Cumming JF, et al: Epidemiologic evidence for clustering of equine motor neuron disease in the US, *Am J Vet Res* 56:1433, 1995.
4. Sustronck B, Deprez B, van Roy M, et al: Equine motor neuron disease: the first confirmed case in Europe, *Vlaams Diergeneedkd Tijdschr* 62:40, 1993.
5. Gruys E, Beynen AC, Binkhorst GJ, et al: Neurodegeneratieve aandoeningen van het centraal zenuwstelsel bij het paard, *Tijdschr Diergeneeskd* 119:561, 1994.
6. Benders NA, Wijnberg ID, van der Kolk JH: Equine motor neuron disease: een overzicht aan de hand van een casus, *Tijdschr Diergeneeskd* 126:376, 2001.
7. Kuwamura M, Iwaki M, Yamate T, et al: The first case of equine motor neuron disease in Japan, *J Vet Med Sci* 56:195, 1994.
8. Divers TJ, Mohammed HO, Cummings JF: Equine motor neuron disease, *Vet Clin North Am Equine Pract* 13:97, 1997.
9. Divers TJ, de Lahunta A, Hintz HF, et al: Equine motor neuron disease, *Equine Vet Educ* 13:63, 2001.
10. van der Hoven R, Meijer AEFH, Breukink HJ, et al: Enzyme histochemistry on muscle biopsies as an aid in the diagnosis of disease of the equine neuromuscular system: a study of six cases, *Equine Vet J* 20:46, 1988.

11. de la Rúa-Domènech R, Mohammed HO, Cummings JF, et al: Incidence and risk factors of equine motor neuron disease: an ambidirectional study, *Neuroepidemiology* 14:54, 1995.
12. Valentine BA, de Lahunta A, George C, et al: Acquired equine motor neuron disease, *Vet Pathol* 31:130, 1994.
13. Green SL, Tolwani RJ: Animal models for motor neuron disease, *Lab Anim Sci* 49:480, 1999.
14. Mohammed HO, Cummings JF, Divers TJ, et al: Risk factors associated with equine motor neuron disease, *Neurology* 43:966, 1993.
15. de la Rúa-Domènech R, Mohammed HO, Cummings JF, et al: Intrinsic, management, and nutritional factors associated with equine motor neuron disease, *J Am Vet Med Assoc* 211:1261, 1997.
16. Jackson CA, Riis RC, Rebhun WC, et al: Ocular manifestations of equine motor neuron disease, *Proc Am Assoc Equine Pract* 41:225, 1995.
17. Riis RC, Jackson C, Rebhun W, et al: Ocular manifestations of equine motor neuron disease, *Equine Vet J* 31:99, 1999.
18. Divers TJ, Valentine BA, Jackson CA, et al: Simple and practical muscle biopsy test for equine motor neuron disease, *Proc Am Assoc Equine Pract* 42:180, 1996.
19. Polack EW, King JM, Cummings JF, et al: Quantitative assessment of motor neuron loss in equine motor neuron disease (EMND), *Equine Vet J* 30:256, 1998.
20. de la Rúa-Domènech R, Mohammed HO, Cummings JF, et al: Association between plasma vitamin E concentration and the risk of equine motor neuron disease, *Br Vet J* 154:203, 1997.
21. Polack EW, King JM, Cummings JF, et al: Concentrations of trace minerals in the spinal cord of horses with equine motor neuron disease, *Am J Vet Res* 61:609, 2000.
22. Rosen DR, Siddique T, Patterson D, et al: Mutations in Cu/Zn superoxide dismutase gene are associated with familial amyotrophic lateral sclerosis, *Nature* 362:59, 1993.
23. Pate Skene JH, Cleveland DW: Hypoxia and Lou Gehrig, *Nat Genet* 28:107, 2001.
24. Mayhew IG: Odds and SODs of equine motor neuron disease, *Equine Vet J* 26:342, 1994.
25. Oosthuyse B, Moons L, Storkebaum E, et al: Deletion of the hypoxia-response element in the vascular endothelial growth factor promoter causes motor neuron degeneration, *Nat Genet* 28:131, 2001.
26. Hahn CN, Mayhew IG: Equine neurodegenerative diseases: stressed neurons and other radical ideas, *Vet J* 154:173, 1997.
27. de la Rúa-Domènech R, Wiedmann M, Mohammed HO, et al: Equine motor neuron disease is not linked to Cu/Zn superoxide dismutase mutations: sequence analysis of the equine Cu/Zn superoxide cDNA, *Gene* 178:83, 1996.
28. Kyles KW, McGorum BC, Fintl C, et al: Electromyography under caudal epidural anaesthesia as an aid to the diagnosis of equine motor neuron disease, *Vet Rec* 148:536, 2001.
29. Jackson CA, de Lahunta A, Cummings JF, et al: Spinal accessory nerve biopsy as an ante mortem diagnostic test for equine motor neuron disease, *Equine Vet J* 28:215, 1996.
30. Sojka JE, Hope W, Pearson D: Lead toxicosis in 2 horses: similarity to equine degenerative lower motor neuron disease, *J Vet Intern Med* 10:420, 1996.

Tetanus

1. Humeau Y, Doussau F, Grant NJ, et al: How botulinum and tetanus neurotoxins block neurotransmitter release, *Biochimie* 82:427-446, 2000.
2. Hatheway CL: Toxigenic clostridia, *Clin Microbiol Rev* 3:66-98, 1990.
3. Eisel U, Jarausch W, Goretzki K, et al: Tetanus toxin: primary structure, expression in *E. coli*, and homology with botulinum toxins, *EMBO J* 5:2495-2502, 1986.
4. Schiavo G, Benfenati F, Poulain B, et al: Tetanus and botulinum-B neurotoxins block neurotransmitter release by proteolytic cleavage of synaptobrevin, *Nature* 359:832-835, 1992.
5. Bizzini B: Tetanus toxin, *Microbiol Rev* 43:224-240, 1979.
6. Helting TB, Parschat S, Engelhardt H: Structure of tetanus toxin. Demonstration and separation of a specific enzyme converting intracellular tetanus toxin to the extracellular form, *J Biol Chem* 254:10728-10733, 1979.
7. Schwab ME, Thoenen H: Selective binding, uptake, and retrograde transport of tetanus toxin by nerve terminals in the rat iris. An electron microscope study using colloidal gold as a tracer, *J Cell Biol* 77:1-13, 1978.
8. Poulain B: Molecular mechanism of action of tetanus toxin and botulinum neurotoxins, *Pathol Biol (Paris)* 42:173-182, 1994.
9. Montecucco C, Schiavo G: Structure and function of tetanus and botulinum neurotoxins, *Q Rev Biophys* 28:423-472, 1995.
10. Montecucco C, Papini E, Schiavo G: Bacterial protein toxins penetrate cells via a four-step mechanism, *FEBS Letters* 346:92-98, 1994.
11. Pellizzari R, Rossetto O, Lozzi L, et al: Structural determinants of the specificity for synaptic vesicle-associated membrane protein/synaptobrevin of tetanus and botulinum type B and G neurotoxins, *J Biol Chem* 271:20353-20358, 1996.
12. Blumenthal R, Habig WH: Mechanism of tetanolysin-induced membrane damage: studies with black lipid membranes, *J Bacteriol* 157:321-323, 1984.
13. van Galen G, Delguste C, Sandersen C, et al: Tetanus in the equine species: a retrospective study of 31 cases, *Tijdschr Diergeneeskd* 133:512-517, 2008.
14, Burkitt JM, Sturges BK, Jandrey KE, et al: Risk factors associated with outcome in dogs with tetanus: 38 cases (1987-2005), *J Am Vet Med Assoc* 230:76-83, 2007.
15. Laird WJ, Aaronson W, Silver RP, et al: Plasmid-associated toxigenicity in *Clostridium tetani*, *J Infect Dis* 142:623, 1980.
16. Heinig A: Experimental research on, immunity against tetanus after single immunization, *Arch Exp Veterinarmed* 8:394-403, 1954.
17. Holmes MA, Townsend HG, Kohler AK, et al: Immune responses to commercial equine vaccines against equine herpesvirus-1, equine influenza virus, eastern equine encephalomyelitis, and tetanus, *Vet Immunol Immunopathol* 111:67-80, 2006.
18. Green SL, Little CB, Baird JD, et al: Tetanus in the horse: a review of 20 cases (1970 to 1990), *J Vet Intern Med* 8:128-132, 1994.
19. Jansen BC, Knoetze PC: The immune response of horses to tetanus toxoid,, *Onderstepoort J Vet Res* 46:211-216, 1979.
20. Liefman CE: Combined active-passive immunization of horses against tetanus, *Aust Vet J* 56:119-122, 1980.
21. Messer NT, Johnson PJ: Serum hepatitis in two brood mares, *J Am Vet Med Assoc* 204:1790-1792, 1994.
22. Messer NT, Johnson PJ: Idiopathic acute hepatic disease in horses: 12 cases (1982-1992), *J Am Vet Med Assoc* 204:1934-1937, 1994.
23. Guglick MA, MacAllister CG, Ely RW, et al: Hepatic disease associated with administration of tetanus antitoxin in eight horses, *J Am Vet Med Assoc* 206:1737-1740, 1995.
24. Wilson WD, Mihalyi JE, Hussey S, et al: Passive transfer of maternal immunoglobulin isotype antibodies against tetanus and influenza and their effect on the response of foals to vaccination, *Equine Vet J* 33:644-650, 2001.

Botulism

1. Goldmann L, Ausiello DA, Arend W, et al: *Cecil textbook of medicine*, ed 23, Philadelphia, 2008, WB Saunders.

2. Mitten LA, Hinchcliff KW, Holcombe SJ, et al: Mechanical ventilation and management of botulism secondary to an injection abscess in an adult horse, *Equine Vet J* 26(5):420-423, 1994.
3. Sakaguchi G: *Clostridium botulinum* toxins, *Pharmacol Ther* 9:164-194, 1983.
4. Wang Y, Sugiyama H: Botulism in metronidazole-treated conventional adult mice challenged orogastrically with spores of *Clostridium botulinum* type A or B, *Infect Immunol* 46:715-719, 1984.
5. Whitlock RH: Botulism, *Vet Clin North Am Equine Pract* 13(1):107-129, 1997.
6. Smith BP, editor: *Large animal internal medicine*, ed 4, St Louis, 2009, Mosby.
7. Turton K, Chaddock JA, Acharya KA: Botulinum and tetanus neurotoxins: structure, function and therapeutic utility, *Trends Biochem Sci* 27(11):552-558, 2002.
8. Kinde H, Betty RL, Ardans A, et al: *Clostridium botulinum* type C intoxication associated with consumption of processed hay cubes in horses, *J Am Vet Med Assoc* 199:742-746, 1991.
9. Whitlock RH: Botulism type C: experimental and field cases in horses, *Proc Am Coll Vet Intern Med* 13:720-723, 1995.
10. Divers TJ, Bartholomew RC, Messick JB, et al: *Clostridium botulinum* type B toxicosis in a herd of cattle and a group of mules, *J Am Vet Med Assoc* 188(4):382-386, 1986.
11. Vaala WE: Diagnosis and treatment of *Clostridium botulinum* infection in foals: a review of 53 cases, *Proc Am Coll Vet Intern Med* 9:379-381, 1991.
12. Szabo EA, Pemberton JM, Gibson AM, et al: Application of PCR to a clinical and environmental investigation of a case of equine botulism, *J Clin Microbiol* 32:1986-1991, 1994.
13. Singh BR, Silva MA: Detection of botulinum neurotoxins using optical fiber-based biosensor, In Singh BR, Tu A, editors: *Natural toxins II*, New York, 1996, Plenum Press.
14. Szabo EA, Pemberton JM, Desmarchelier PM: Detection of the genes encoding botulism neurotoxin types A to E by the PCR, *Appl Environ Microbiol* 59:3011-3020, 1993.

Equine Grass Sickness (Equine Dysautonomia)

1. Tocher JF, Tocher JW, Brown W, et al: Grass sickness investigation report, *Vet Rec* 3:37, 1923.
2. Gruys E, Beynen AC, Binkhorst GJ, et al: Neurodegeneratieve aandoeningen van het centraal zenuwstelsel bij het paard, *Tijdschr Diergeneeskd* 119:561, 1994.
3. McCarthy HE, Proudman CJ, French NP: Epidemiology of equine grass sickness: a literature review (1909-1999), *Vet Rec* 149:293, 2001.
4. Uzal FA, Robles CA, Olaechea FV: Histopathological changes in the coeliaco-mesenteric ganglia of horses with "mal seco," a grass sickness-like syndrome, in Argentina, *Vet Rec* 130:244, 1992.
5. Cottrell DF, McGorum BC, Pearson GT: The neurology and enterology of equine grass sickness: a review of basic mechanisms,, *Neurogastroenterol Motil* 11:79, 1999.
6. Milne EM, Mayhew IG: Equine grass sickness: clinical findings and pathology. In Proceedings of the International Equine Neurology Conference, Cornell Press Ithaca, NY, 1997.
7. Hahn CN, Mayhew IG, de Lahunta A: Central neuropathology of equine grass sickness, *Acta Neuropathol* 102:153, 2001.
8. Prince D, Corcoran BM, Mayhew IG: Changes in nasal mucosal innervation in horses with grass sickness, *Equine Vet J* 35:60, 2003.
9. Gilmour JS: Observations on neuronal changes in grass sickness in horses, *Res Vet Sci* 15:197, 1973.
10. Wood JL, Doxey DL, Milne EM: A case-control study of grass sickness (equine dysautonomia) in the United Kingdom, *Vet J* 156:7, 1998.
11. Hunter LC, Poxton IR: Systemic antibodies to *Clostridium botulinum* type C: do they protect horses from grass sickness (dysautonomia)?, *Equine Vet J* 33:547, 2001.
12. Böhnel H, Wernery U, Gessler E: Two cases of equine grass sickness with evidence for soil-borne origin involving botulinum neurotoxin, *J Vet Med* 50:178, 2003.
13. McGorum BC, Kyles KWJ, Prince D, et al: Clinicopathological features consistent with both botulism and grass sickness in a foal, *Vet Rec* 152:334, 2003.
14. Hunter LC, Miller JK, Poxton IR: The association between *Clostridium botulinum* type C with equine grass sickness: a toxicoinfection,, *Equine Vet J* 31:492, 1999.
15. McGorum BC, Kirk J: Equine dysautonomia (grass sickness) is associated with altered plasma amino acid levels and depletion of plasma sulphur amino acids, *Equine Vet J* 33:473, 2001.
16. McGorum BC, Wilson R, Pirie RS, et al: Systemic concentration of antioxidants and biomarkers of macromolecular oxidative damage in horses with grass sickness, *Equine Vet J* 35:121, 2000.
17. Robb J, Doxey DL, Milne EM, et al: The isolation of potentially toxinogenic fungi from the environment of horses with grass sickness and mal seco,, *Equine Vet J* 52:541, 1997.
18. Scholes SFE, Vaillant C, Peacock P, et al: Diagnosis of grass sickness by ileal biopsy, *Vet Rec* 133:7, 1993.
19. Divers TJ: Comparing equine motor neuron disease (EMND) with equine grass sickness (EGS), *Equine Vet J* 31:90, 1999.

Lyme Disease In Horses

1. Chang YF, Novosol V, McDonough SP, et al: Experimental infection of ponies with *Borrelia burgdorferi* by exposure to *Ixodid* ticks, *Vet Pathol* 37:68-76, 2000.
2. Cohen ND, Heck FC, Heim B, et al: Seroprevalence of antibodies to *Borrelia burgdorferi* in a population of horses in central Texas, *J Am Vet Med Assoc* 201:1030-1034, 1992.
3. Butler CM, Houwers DJ, Jongejan F, et al: *Borrelia burgdorferi* infections with special reference to horses. A review, *Vet Q* 27:146-156, 2005.
4. Parker JL, White KK: Lyme borreliosis in cattle and horses: a review of the literature, *Cornell Vet* 82:253-274, 1992.
5. Stefancikova A, Adaszek L, Pet'ko B, et al: Serological evidence of *Borrelia burgdorferi* sensu lato in horses and cattle from Poland and diagnostic problems of Lyme borreliosis, *Ann Agric Environ Med* 15:37-43, 2008.
6. Bernard WV, Cohen D, Bosler E, et al: Serologic survey for *Borrelia burgdorferi* antibody in horses referred to a mid-Atlantic veterinary teaching hospital, *J Am Vet Med Assoc* 196:1255-1258, 1990.
7. Cohen D, Bosler EM, Bernard W, et al: Epidemiologic studies of Lyme disease in horses and their public health significance, *Ann N Y Acad Sci* 539:244-257, 1988.
8. Piesman J: Strategies for reducing the risk of Lyme borreliosis in North America, *Int J Med Microbiol* 296(Suppl 40):17-22, 2006.
9. Lane RS, Piesman J, Burgdorfer W: Lyme borreliosis: relation of its causative agent to its vectors and hosts in North America and Europe, *Annu Rev Entomol* 36:587-609, 1991.
10. Shapiro ED, Gerber MA: Lyme disease, *Clin Infect Dis* 31:533-542, 2000.
11. Gall Y, Pfister K: Survey on the subject of equine Lyme borreliosis, *Int J Med Microbiol* 296(Suppl 40):274-279, 2006.
12. Carter SD, May C, Barnes A, et al: *Borrelia burgdorferi* infection in UK horses, *Equine Vet J* 26:187-190, 1994.
13. Burgess EC, Mattison M: Encephalitis associated with *Borrelia burgdorferi* infection in a horse, *J Am Vet Med Assoc* 191:1457-1458, 1987.
14. Magnarelli LA, Ijdo JW, Van Andel AE, et al: Serologic confirmation of *Ehrlichia equi* and *Borrelia burgdorferi* infections in horses from the Northeastern United States, *J Am Vet Med Assoc* 217:1045-1050, 2000.

15. Johnson AL, Divers TJ, Chang YF: Validation of an in-clinic enzyme-linked immunosorbent assay kit for diagnosis of *Borrelia burgdorferi* infection in horses, *J Vet Diagn Invest* 20:321-324, 2008.
16. Nardelli DT, Callister SM, Schell RF: Lyme arthritis: current concepts and a change in paradigm, *Clin Vaccine Immunol* 15:21-34, 2008.
17. Puius YA, Kalish RA: Lyme arthritis: pathogenesis, clinical presentation, and management, *Infect Dis Clin North Am* 22(vii):289, 2008.
18. Chang YF, Ku YW, Chang CF, et al: Antibiotic treatment of experimentally *Borrelia burgdorferi*-infected ponies, *Vet Microbiol* 107:285-294, 2005.
19. Chang Y, Novosol V, McDonough SP, et al: Vaccination against Lyme disease with recombinant *Borrelia burgdorferi* outer-surface protein A (rOspA) in horses, *Vaccine* 18:540-548, 1999.

Head Shaking

1. Newton SA, Knottenbelt DC, Eldridge PR: Headshaking in horses: possible aetiopathogenesis suggested by the results of diagnostic tests and several treatment regimes used in 20 cases, *Equine Vet J* 32:208-216, 2000.
2. Madigan JE, Bell SA: Owner survey of headshaking in horses, *J Am Vet Med Assoc* 219:334-337, 2001.
3. Lane JG, Mair TS: Observations on headshaking in the horse, *Equine Vet J* 19:331-336, 1987.
4. Cook WR: Headshaking in horses: an afterword, *Compend Contin Educ Pract Vet* 14:1369-1371, 1992.
5. Cook WR: Headshaking in horses. I, *Vet Clin North Am Equine Pract* 1:9, 1979.
6. Mills DS, Cook S, Taylor K, et al: Analysis of the variations in clinical signs shown by 254 cases of equine headshaking, *Vet Rec* 150:236-240, 2002.
7. Madigan JE, Bell SA: Characterization of headshaking syndrome: 31 cases, *Equine Vet J Suppl* 27:28-29, 1998.
8. Madigan JE, Kortz G, Murphy C, et al: Photic headshaking in the horse: 7 cases, *Equine Vet J* 27:306-311, 1995.
9. Cook WR: Headshaking in horses. IV. Special diagnostic procedures, *Vet Clin North Am Equine Pract* 2:7, 1980.
10. Moore LA, Johnson PJ, Messer NT, et al: Management of headshaking in three horses by treatment for protozoal myeloencephalitis, *Vet Rec* 141:264-267, 1997.
11. Mair TS: Headshaking associated with *Trombicula autumnalis* larval infestation in two horses, *Equine Vet J* 26:244-245, 1994.
12. McGorum BC, Dixon PM: Vasomotor rhinitis with headshaking in a pony, *Equine Vet J* 22:220-222, 1990.
13. Kold SE, Ostblom LC, Philipsen HP: Headshaking caused by a maxillary osteoma in a horse, *Equine Vet J* 14:167-169, 1982.
14. Blythe LL, Watrous BJ, Pearson EG, et al: Otitis media/interna in the horse: a cause of head shaking and skull fractures, *Proc Am Assoc Equine Pract* 36:517-528, 1991.
15. Mair TS: Assessment of bilateral infra-orbital nerve blockade and bilateral infra-orbital neurectomy in the investigation and treatment of idiopathic headshaking, *Equine Vet J* 31:262-264, 1999.
16. Wilkins PA: Cyproheptadine: medical treatment for photic headshakers, *Compend Contin Educ Pract Vet* 19:98-99, 1997.
17. Devor M, Amir R, Rappaport ZH: Pathophysiology of trigeminal neuralgia: the ignition hypothesis, *Clin J Pain* 18:4-13, 2002.
18. Sindrup SH, Jensen TS: Pharmacotherapy of trigeminal neuralgia, *Clin J Pain* 18:22-27, 2002.
19. Mills DS, Cook S, Jones B: Reported response to treatment among 245 cases of equine headshaking, *Vet Rec* 150:311-313, 2002.
20. Mills DS, Taylor K: Field study of the efficacy of three types of nose net for the treatment of headshaking in horses, *Vet Rec* 152:41-44, 2003.

Verminous Encephalomyelitis

1. Anderson RC, Linder KE, Peregrine AS: *Halicephalobus gingivalis* (Stefanski, 1954) from a fatal infection in a horse in Ontario, Canada with comments on the validity of *H. deletrix* and a review of the genus, *Parasitology* 5:255-261, 1998.
2. Wilkins PA, Wacholder S, Nolan TJ, et al: Evidence for transmission of *Halicephalobus deletrix (H. gingivalis)* from dam to foal, *J Vet Intern Med* 15:412-417, 2001.
3. Blunden AS, Khalil LF, Webbon PM: *Halicephalobus deletrix* infection in a horse, *Equine Vet J* 19(3):255-260, 1987.
4. Kinde H, Mathews M, Ash L, et al: *Halicephalobus gingivalis (H. deletrix)* infection in two horses in southern California, *J Vet Diagn Invest* 12(2):162-165, 2000.
5. Spalding MG, Greiner EC, Green SL: *Halicephalobus* (Micronema) *deletrix* infection in two half-sibling foals, *J Am Vet Med Assoc* 196:1127, 1990.
6. Ruggles AJ, Beech J, Gillette DM, et al: Disseminated *Halicephalobus deletrix* infection in a horse, *J Am Vet Med Assoc* 203(4):550-552, 1993.
7. Rames DS, Miller DK, Barthel R, et al: Ocular *Halicephalobus* (syn. *Micronema) deletrix* in a horse, *Vet Pathol* 32(5):540-542, 1995.
8. Alstad AD, Berg IE, Samuel C: Disseminated *Micronema deletrix* infection in the horse, *J Am Vet Med Assoc* 174(3):264-266, 1979.
9. Angus KW, Roberts L, Archibald DRN, et al: *Halicephalobus deletrix* infection in a horse in Scotland, *Vet Rec* 21:495, 1992.
10. Bröjer JT, Parsons DA, Linder KE, et al: *Halicephalobus gingivalis* encephalomyelitis in a horse, *Can Vet J* 41(7):559-561, 2000.
11. Buergelt CD: *Halicephalobus (Micronema) deletrix* infection in the horse, *Vet Clin North Am Equine Pract* 13(4):7-12, 1991.
12. Cho DY, Hubbard RM, McCoy DJ, et al: *Micronema* granuloma in the gingival of a horse, *J Am Vet Med Assoc* 187(5):505-507, 1985.
13. Darien BJ, Belknap J, Nietfeld J: Cerebrospinal fluid changes in two horses with central nervous system nematodiasis *(Micronema deletrix)*, *J Vet Intern Med* 2(4):201-205, 1988.
14. Ferris DH, Levine ND, Beamer PD: *Micronema deletrix* in equine brain, *Am J Vet Res* 33(1):33-38, 1972.
15. Johnson JS, Hibler CP, Tillotson KM, et al: Radiculomeningomyelitis due to *Halicephalobus gingivalis* in a horse, *Vet Pathol* 38:559-561, 2001.
16. Jose-Cunilleras E, Kohn CW: Unpublished observations, 1999.
17. Jordan WH, Gaafar SM, Carlton WW: *Micronema deletrix* in the brain of a horse, *Vet Med Small Anim Clin* 70:707-709, 1975.
18. Powers RD, Benz GW: *Micronema deletrix* in the central nervous system of a horse, *J Am Coll Vet Med* 170(2):175-177, 1977.
19. Rubin HL, Woodward JC: Equine infection with *Micronema deletrix*, *J Am Vet Med Assoc* 165(3):256-258, 1974.
20. Frauenfelder HC, Kazacos KR, Lichtenfels JR: Cerebrospinal nematodiasis caused by a filariid in a horse, *J Am Vet Med Assoc* 177(4):359-362, 1980.
21. Little PB, Lwin US, Fretz P: Verminous encephalitis of horses: experimental induction with *Strongylus vulgaris* larvae, *Am J Vet Res* 35(12):1501-1510, 1974.
22. Mayhew IG, Brewer BD, Reinhard M, et al: Verminous *(Strongylus vulgaris)* myelitis in a donkey, *Cornell Vet* 74(1):30-37, 1984.

23. Mayhew IG, Lichtenfels JR, Greiner EC, et al: Migration of a spiruroid nematode through the brain of a horse, *J Am Vet Med Assoc* 180(11):1306-1311, 1982.
24. Wright JD, Kelly WR, Waddell AH, et al: Equine neural angiostrongylosis, *Aust Vet J* 68(2):58-60, 1991.
25. Hadlow WJ, Ward JK, Krinsky WL: Intracranial myiasis by *Hypoderma bovis (Linnaeus)* in a horse, *Cornell Vet* 67(2):272-281, 1977.
26. Baker DW, Monlux WS: Hypoderma myiasis in the horse: summary of a series of cases studied during spring and summer, 1939, *J Parasitol* 25(Suppl):16, 1939.
27. Olander HJ: The migration of *Hypoderma lineatum* in the brain of a horse: a case report and review, *Pathol Vet* 4:477-483, 1967.
28. Van Biervliet J, de Lahunta A, Ennulat D, et al: Acquired cervical scoliosis in six horses associated with dorsal grey column chronic myelitis, *Equine Vet J* 35:86-92, 2003.
29. Tanabe M, Kelly R, de Lahunta A, et al: Verminous encephalitis in a horse produced by nematodes in the family Protostrongylidae, *Vet Pathol* 44:119-122, 2007.
30. Johnson AL, de Lahunta A, Divers TJ: Acquired scoliosis in equids: case series and proposed pathogenesis, *Proc Amer Assoc Equine Pract* 54:192-197, 2008.
31. Innes JRM, Pillai CP: Kumri—so-called lumbar paralysis—of horses in Ceylon (India and Burma) and its identification with cerebrospinal nematodiasis, *Br Vet J* 3:233-235, 1955.
32. Yoshihara T, Oikawa M, Wada R, et al: A survey of filarial parasites in the peritoneal cavity of horses in Japan, *Bull Equine Res Inst—Japan* 25:25-28, 1988.
33. Mason KV: Canine neural angiostrongylosis: the clinical and therapeutic features of 55 natural cases, *Aust Vet J* 64(7):201-203, 1987.
34. Wijesundera WS, Chandrasekharan NV, Karunanayake EH: A sensitive polymerase chain reaction based assay for the detection of *Setaria digitata*: the causative organism of cerebrospinal nematodiasis in goats, sheep and horses, *Vet Parasitol* 81(3):225-233, 1999.
35. Dunn DG, Gardiner CH, Dralle KR, et al: Nodular granulomatous posthitis caused by *Halicephalobus* (syn *Micronema*) spp in a horse, *Vet Pathol* 30:207-208, 1993.
36. Mayhew J: *Large animal neurology*, Philadelphia, 2009, Wiley-Blackwell.
37. Lester G: Parasitic encephalomyelitis in horses, *Compend Contin Educ Pract Vet* 14(12):1624-1631, 1992.

Miscellaneous Neurologic Disorders

1. Tyler CM, Davis RE, Begg AP, et al: A survey of neurological diseases in horses, *Aust Vet J* 70:445-449, 1993.
2. Allen D, Swayne D, Belknap JK: Ganglioneuroma as a cause of small intestinal obstruction in the horse: a case report, *Cornell Vet* 79:133-141, 1989.
3. Porter BF, Storts RW, Payne HR, et al: Colonic ganglioneuromatosis in a horse, *Vet Pathol* 44:207-210, 2007.
4. Carrigan MJ, Higgins RJ, Carlson GP, et al: Equine papillary ependymoma, *Vet Pathol* 33:77-80, 1996.
5. Hayes HM, Priester WA Jr, Pendergrass TW: Occurrence of nervous-tissue tumors in cattle, horses, cats and dogs, *Int J Cancer* 15:39-47, 1975.
6. Heath SE, Peter AT, Janovitz EB, et al: Ependymoma of the neurohypophysis and hypernatremia in a horse, *J Am Vet Med Assoc* 207:738-741, 1995.
7. Szazados I: [Ependymoma as the cause of severe brain symptoms in a horse], *Dtsch Tierarztl Wochenschr* 80:57, 1973.
8. Pirie RS, Mayhew IG, Clarke CJ, et al: Ultrasonographic confirmation of a space-occupying lesion in the brain of a horse: choroid plexus papilloma, *Equine Vet J* 30:445-448, 1998.
9. Bistner S, Campbell RJ, Shaw D, et al: Neuroepithelial tumor of the optic nerve in a horse, *Cornell Vet* 73:30-40, 1983.
10. Eagle RC Jr, Font RL, Swerczek TW: Malignant medulloepithelioma of the optic nerve in a horse, *Vet Pathol* 15:488-494, 1978.
11. Bistner SI: Medullo-epithelioma of the iris and ciliary body in a horse, *Cornell Vet* 64:588-595, 1974.
12. Dopke C, Grone A, von Borstel M, et al: Metastatic esthesioneuroblastoma in a horse, *J Comp Pathol* 132:218-222, 2005.
13. Knottenbelt DC, Hetzel U, Roberts V: Primary intraocular primitive neuroectodermal tumor (retinoblastoma) causing unilateral blindness in a gelding, *Vet Ophthalmol* 10:348-356, 2007.
14. Riis RC, Scherlie PH Jr, Rebhun WC: Intraocular medulloepithelioma in a horse, *Equine Vet J Suppl* :66-68, 1990.
15. Szymanski CM: Malignant teratoid medulloepithelioma in a horse, *J Am Vet Med Assoc* 190:301-302, 1987.
16. Ueda Y, Senba H, Nishimura T, et al: Ocular medulloepithelioma in a thoroughbred, *Equine Vet J* 25:558-561, 1993.
17. Yamate J, Izawa T, Ogata K, et al: Olfactory neuroblastoma in a horse, *J Vet Med Sci* 68:495-498, 2006.
18. Fankhauser R, Luginbuhl H, McGrath JT: Tumours of the nervous system, *Bull World Health Organ* 50:53-69, 1974.
19. Holshuh HJ, Howard EB: Pineoblastoma, a primitive neuroectodermal tumor in the brain of a horse, *Vet Pathol* 19:567-569, 1982.
20. Gelatt KN, Leipold HW, Finocchio EJ, et al: Optic disc astrocytoma in a horse, *Can Vet J* 12:53-55, 1971.
21. Pascoe PJ: Colic in a mare caused by a colonic neurofibroma, *Can Vet J* 23:24-27, 1982.
22. Pascoe RR, Summers PM: Clinical survey of tumours and tumour-like lesions in horses in south east Queensland, *Equine Vet J* 13:235-239, 1981.
23. Schoniger S, Summers B: Localized, plexiform, diffuse and other variants of neurofibroma in twelve dogs, two horses and a chicken, *Vet Pathol* , 2009.
24. Spritz RA, Itin PH, Gutmann DH: Piebaldism and neurofibromatosis type 1: horses of very different colors, *J Invest Dermatol* 122:xxxiv-xxxv, 2004.
25. Strubbe DT: Periocular neurofibrosarcoma in a horse, *Vet Ophthalmol* 4:237-241, 2001.
26. van den Top JG, de Heer N, Klein WR, et al: Penile and preputial tumours in the horse: a retrospective study of 114 affected horses, *Equine Vet J* 40:528-532, 2008.
27. Andreasen CB, Hedstrom OR, Allison P: Mediastinal Schwannoma in a horse-cytologic, histologic, and immunochemical evaluation, *Vet Clin Pathol* 22:54-59, 1993.
28. Williamson LH, Farrell RL: Intracranial schwannoma in a horse, *Cornell Vet* 80:135-141, 1990.
29. Kreeger JM, Templer A, Tumquist SE, et al: Paranasal meningioma in a horse, *J Vet Diagn Invest* 14:322-325, 2002.
30. McEntee M, Summers BA, de Lahunta A, et al: Meningocerebral hemangiomatosis resembling Sturge-Weber disease in a horse, *Acta Neuropathol* 74:405-410, 1987.
31. Lester GD, MacKay RJ, Smith-Meyer B: Primary meningeal lymphoma in a horse, *J Am Vet Med Assoc* 201:1219-1221, 1992.
32. Mayhew IG, MacKay RJ: The nervous system. In Mansmann RA, McAllister ES, editors: *Equine medicine and surgery*, 3 ed, Goleta, CA, 1982, American Veterinary Publictions, pp 1159-1252.
33. Duff S: Cholesterinic granulomas in horses, *Vet Rec* 135:288, 1994.
34. Jackson CA, deLahunta A, Dykes NL, et al: Neurological manifestation of cholesterinic granulomas in three horses, *Vet Rec* 135:228-230, 1994.
35. Johnson PJ, Lin TL, Jennings DP: Diffuse cerebral encephalopathy associated with hydrocephalus and cholesterinic granulomas in a horse, *J Am Vet Med Assoc* 203:694-697, 1993.

36. Vanschandevijl K, Gielen I, Nollet H, et al: Computed tomography-guided brain biopsy for in vivo diagnosis of a cholesterinic granuloma in a horse, *J Am Vet Med Assoc* 233:950-954, 2008.
37. Vink-Nooteboom M, Junker K, van den Ingh TS, et al: Computed tomography of cholesterinic granulomas in the choroid plexus of horses, *Vet Radiol Ultrasound* 39:512-516, 1998.
38. Ivoghli B, Emady M, Rezakhani A: Motor paralysis associated with cholesteatoma in a mare, *Vet Med Small Anim Clin* 72:602-604, 1977.
39. Maxwell HA: So-called cholesteatoma in a horse, *Cornell Vet* 38:102, 1948.
40. Rooney JR: Cerebral cholesteatoma, *Mod Vet Pract* 60:726, 1979.
41. Sundberg JP, Burnstein T, Page EH, et al: Neoplasms of Equidae, *J Am Vet Med Assoc* 170:150-152, 1977.
42. Sullivan ND: The nervous system. In: Jubb KVF, In Kennedy PC, Palmer N, editors: *Pathology of Domestic Animals*, 3 ed, Orlando, FL, 1985, Academic Press, pp 201-338.
43. Kannegieter NJ, Alley MR: Ataxia due to lymphosarcoma in a young horse, *Aust Vet J* 64:377-379, 1987.
44. Morrison LR, Freel K, Henderson I, et al: Lymphoproliferative disease with features of lymphoma in the central nervous system of a horse, *J Comp Pathol* 139:256-261, 2008.
45. Shamis LD, Everitt JI, Baker GJ: Lymphosarcoma as the cause of ataxia in a horse, *J Am Vet Med Assoc* 184:1517-1518, 1984.
46. Williams MA, Welles EG, Gailor RJ, et al: Lymphosarcoma associated with neurological signs and abnormal cerebrospinal fluid in two horses, *Prog Vet Neurol* 3:51-56, 1992.
47. Zeman DH, Snider TG 3rd, McClure JJ: Vertebral lymphosarcoma as the cause of hind limb paresis in a horse, *J Vet Diagn Invest* 1:187-188, 1989.
48. Hartmann E, Baumgartner W, Hungerland C: [Spinal lymphosarcoma in a foal], *Tierarztl Prax* 16:175-178, 1988.
49. Schott HC, Major MD, Grant BD, et al: Melanoma as a cause of spinal cord compression in two horses, *J Am Vet Med Assoc* 196:1820-1822, 1990.
50. Traver DS, Moore JN, Thornburg LP, et al: Epidural melanoma causing posterior paresis in a horse, *J Am Vet Med Assoc* 170:1400-1403, 1977.
51. Covington AL, Magdesian KG, Madigan JE, et al: Recurrent esophageal obstruction and dysphagia due to a brainstem melanoma in a horse, *J Vet Intern Med* 18:245-247, 2004.
52. Kirker-Head CA, Loeffler D, Held JP: Pelvic limb lameness due to malignant melanoma in a horse, *J Am Vet Med Assoc* 186:1215-1217, 1985.
53. Ladd SM, Crisman MV, Duncan R, et al: Central nervous system hemangiosarcoma in a horse, *J Vet Intern Med* 19:914-916, 2005.
54. Berry S: Spinal cord compression secondary to hemangiosarcoma in a saddlebred stallion, *Can Vet J* 40:886-887, 1999.
55. Van Biervliet J, Alcaraz A, Jackson CA, et al: Extradural undifferentiated sarcoma causing spinal cord compression in 2 horses, *J Vet Intern Med* 18:248-251, 2004.
56. D'Angelo A, Bertuglia A, Capucchio MT, et al: Central vestibular syndrome due to a squamous cell carcinoma in a horse, *Vet Rec* 161:314-316, 2007.
57. Patterson LJ, May SA, Baker JR: Skeletal metastasis of a penile squamous cell carcinoma, *Vet Rec* 126:579-580, 1990.
58. Spoormakers TJ, Ij J, Sloet van Oldruitenborgh-Oosterbaan MM: Neurological signs in a horse due to metastases of an intestinal adenocarcinoma, *Vet Q* 23:49-50, 2001.
59. Wright JA, Giles CJ: Diffuse carcinomatosis involving the meninges of a horse, *Equine Vet J* 18:147-150, 1986.
60. Davis JL, Gilger BC, Spaulding K, et al: Nasal adenocarcinoma with diffuse metastases involving the orbit, cerebrum, and multiple cranial nerves in a horse, *J Am Vet Med Assoc* 221:1460-1463, 2002:1420.
61. Martens J, Rosenbruch M: [Hypophyseal adenocarcinoma in a horse. A case study], *Tierarztl Prax* 12:354-358, 1984.
62. Reynolds BL, Stedham MA, Lawrence JM 3rd, et al: Adenocarcinoma of the frontal sinus with extension to the brain in a horse, *J Am Vet Med Assoc* 174:734-736, 1979.
63. Livesey MA, Wilkie IW: Focal and multifocal osteosarcoma in two foals, *Equine Vet J* 18:407-410, 1986.
64. Harada K, Uozumi T, Kuwabara S, et al: [Plasma cell tumor of the parieto-occipital bone; a case report], *No Shinkei Geka* 19:1067-1071, 1991.
65. Drew RA, Greatorex JC: Vertebral plasma cell myeloma causing posterior paralysis in a horse, *Equine Vet J* 6:131-134, 1974.
66. Brownie CF, Cullen J: Characterization of experimentally induced equine leukoencephalomalacia (ELEM) in ponies (Equus caballus): preliminary report, *Vet Hum Toxicol* 29:34-38, 1987.
67. Christley RM, Begg AP, Hutchins DR, et al: Leukoencephalomalacia in horses, *Aust Vet J* 70:225-226, 1993.
68. Kellerman TS, Marasas WF, Thiel PG, et al: Leukoencephalomalacia in two horses induced by oral dosing of fumonisin B1, *Onderstepoort J Vet Res* 57:269-275, 1990.
69. Lock TF: Leukoencephalomalacia in two quarter horses, *Mod Vet Pract* 55:464, 1974.
70. Marasas WF, Kellerman TS, Gelderblom WC, et al: Leukoencephalomalacia in a horse induced by fumonisin B1 isolated from Fusarium moniliforme, *Onderstepoort J Vet Res* 55:197-203, 1988.
71. Marasas WF, Kellerman TS, Pienaar JG, et al: Leukoencephalomalacia: a mycotoxicosis of Equidae caused by Fusarium moniliforme Sheldon, *Onderstepoort J Vet Res* 43:113-122, 1976.
72. Naranjo Cerrillo G, Soler Rodriguez F, Gomez Gordo L, et al: Clinical and pathological aspects of an outbreak of equine leukoencephalomalacia in Spain, *Zentralbl Veterinarmed A* 43:467-472, 1996.
73. Pienaar JG, Kellerman TS, Marasas WF: Field outbreaks of leukoencephalomalacia in horses consuming maize infected by *Fusarium verticillioides* (= *F. moniliforme*) in South Africa, *J S Afr Vet Assoc* 52:21-24, 1981.
74. Porter JK, Voss KA, Bacon CW, et al: Effects of Fusarium moniliforme and corn associated with equine leukoencephalomalacia on rat neurotransmitters and metabolites, *Proc Soc Exp Biol Med* 194:265-269, 1990.
75. Rosiles MR, Bautista J, Fuentes VO, et al: An outbreak of equine leukoencephalomalacia at Oaxaca, Mexico, associated with fumonisin B1, *Zentralbl Veterinarmed A* 45:299-302, 1998.
76. Ross PF, Ledet AE, Owens DL, et al: Experimental equine leukoencephalomalacia, toxic hepatosis, and encephalopathy caused by corn naturally contaminated with fumonisins, *J Vet Diagn Invest* 5:69-74, 1993.
77. Ross PF, Nelson PE, Owens DL, et al: Fumonisin B2 in cultured Fusarium proliferatum, M-6104, causes equine leukoencephalomalacia, *J Vet Diagn Invest* 6:263-265, 1994.
78. Ross PF, Rice LG, Reagor JC, et al: Fumonisin B1 concentrations in feeds from 45 confirmed equine leukoencephalomalacia cases, *J Vet Diagn Invest* 3:238-241, 1991.
79. Uhlinger C: Clinical and epidemiologic features of an epizootic of equine leukoencephalomalacia, *J Am Vet Med Assoc* 198:126-128, 1991.
80. Uhlinger C: Leukoencephalomalacia, *Vet Clin North Am Equine Pract* 13:13-20, 1997.
81. Voss KA, Norred WP, Plattner RD, et al: Hepatotoxicity and renal toxicity in rats of corn samples associated with field cases of equine leukoencephalomalacia, *Food Chem Toxicol* 27:89-96, 1989.
82. Wilkins PA, Vaala WE, Zivotofsky D, et al: A herd outbreak of equine leukoencephalomalacia, *Cornell Vet* 84:53-59, 1994.

83. Wilson BJ, Maronpot RR, Hildebrandt PK: Equine leukoencephalomalacia, *J Am Vet Med Assoc* 163:1293-1295, 1973.
84. Wilson TM, Nelson PE, Marasas WF, et al: A mycological evaluation and in vivo toxicity evaluation of feed from 41 farms with equine leukoencephalomalacia, *J Vet Diagn Invest* 2:352-354, 1990.
85. Wilson TM, Ross PF, Nelson PE: Fumonisin mycotoxins and equine leukoencephalomalacia, *J Am Vet Med Assoc* 198:1104-1105, 1991.
86. Wilson TM, Ross PF, Owens DL, et al: Experimental reproduction of ELEM. A study to determine the minimum toxic dose in ponies, *Mycopathologia* 117:115-120, 1992.
87. Wilson TM, Ross PF, Rice LG, et al: Fumonisin B1 levels associated with an epizootic of equine leukoencephalomalacia, *J Vet Diagn Invest* 2:213-216, 1990.
88. Wohlsein P, Hinrichs U, Brandt K, et al: [Leukoencephalomalacia in two horses-moldy corn poisoning in Germany?], *Tierarztl Prax* 23:582-587, 1995.
89. Cordy DR: Nigropallidal encephalomalacia in horses associated with ingestion of yellow star thistle, *J Neuropathol Exp Neurol* 13:330-342, 1954.
90. Farrell RK, Sande RD, Lincoln SD: Nigropallidal encephalomalacia in a horse, *J Am Vet Med Assoc* 158:1201-1204, 1971.
91. Fowler ME: Nigropallidal encephalomalacia in the horse, *J Am Vet Med Assoc* 147:607-616, 1965.
92. Gard GP, De Sarem WG, Ahrens PJ: Nigropallidal encephalomalacia in horses in New South Wales, *Aust Vet J* 49:107-108, 1973.
93. Larson KA, Young S: Nigropallidal encephalomalacia in horses in Colorado, *J Am Vet Med Assoc* 156:626-628, 1970.
94. Moret S, Populin T, Conte LS, et al: HPLC determination of free nitrogenous compounds of Centaurea solstitialis (Asteraceae), the cause of equine nigropallidal encephalomalacia, *Toxicon* 46:651-657, 2005.
95. Roy DN, Peyton DH, Spencer PS: Isolation and identification of two potent neurotoxins, aspartic acid and glutamic acid, from yellow star thistle (Centaurea solstitialis), *Nat Toxins* 3:174-180, 1995.
96. Sanders SG, Tucker RL, Bagley RS, et al: Magnetic resonance imaging features of equine nigropallidal encephalomalacia, *Vet Radiol Ultrasound* 42:291-296, 2001.
97. Young S, Brown WW, Klinger B: Nigropallidal encephalomalacia in horses caused by ingestion of weeds of the genus Centaurea, *J Am Vet Med Assoc* 157:1602-1605, 1970.
98. Young S, Brown WW, Klinger B: Nigropallidal encephalomalacia in horses fed Russian knapweed-Centaurea repens L, *Am J Vet Res* 31:1393-1404, 1970.
99. Baird JD, Arroyo LG, Vengust M, et al: Adverse extrapyramidal effects in four horse given fluphenazine decanoate, *J Am Vet Med Assoc* 229:104-110, 2006.
100. Brashier M: Fluphenazine-induced extrapyramidal side effects in a horse, *Vet Clin North Am Equine Pract* 22:e37-45, 2006.
101. Brewer BD, Hines MT, Stewart JT, et al: Fluphenazine induced Parkinson-like syndrome in a horse, *Equine Vet J* 22:136-137, 1990.
102. Kauffman VG, Soma L, Divers TJ, et al: Extrapyramidal side effects caused by fluphenazine decanoate in a horse, *J Am Vet Med Assoc* 195:1128-1130, 1989.
103. Rodriguez-Palacios A, Quesada R, Baird J, et al: Presumptive fluphenazine-induced hepatitis and urticaria in a horse, *J Vet Intern Med* 21:336-339, 2007.
104. Bertone JJ, Horspool LJI: Drugs and dosages for use in equines. In Bertone JJ, Horspool LJI, editors: *Equine Clinical Pharmacology*, Edinburgh, 2004, WB Saunders Co, pp 367-380.

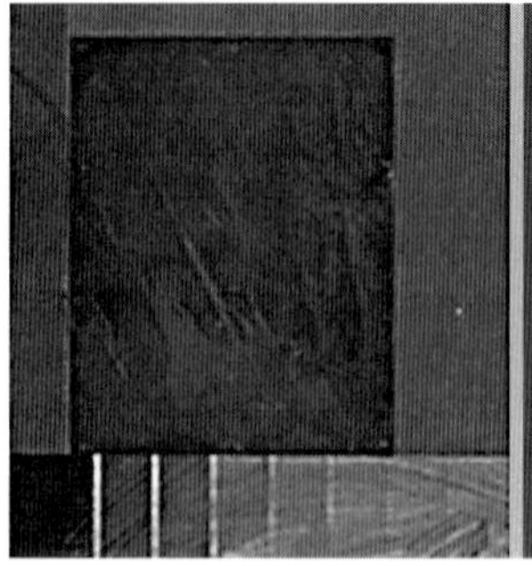

Disorders of the Skin

CHAPTER 13

*Christine A. Rees**

BASIC STRUCTURE AND FUNCTION OF THE SKIN

The skin is the largest and one of the most important organ systems within the body. Without skin a human being or animal would die. The functions of the skin are:

1. An enclosing barrier that prevents water, electrolytes, and macromolecules from being lost and provides internal support for various organs within the body
2. A storage reservoir for vitamins, fats, carbohydrates, electrolytes, water, proteins, and other materials
3. A protective barrier against chemicals and physical factors such as heat, cold, microbiologic organisms, and ultraviolet light (melanocytes)
4. A sensory organ for heat, cold, touch, pain, pressure, and itch
5. A regulator of body temperature through the hair coat
6. A regulator of blood pressure by changes in peripheral vasculature
7. A producer of keratinized structures such as hair, hooves, horn, and the uppermost layer of the epidermis
8. A secretory and excretory organ for apocrine and sebaceous glands that includes antimicrobial factors
9. A provider of flexibility, elasticity, or toughness to allow for shape and form
10. An immunosurveillance organ through keratinocytes, lymphocytes, and Langerhans cells
11. An indicator of general health (e.g., icteric skin can indicate hepatic dysfunction)[1]

GROSS ANATOMY

Skin

Skin thickness varies between 1 to 5 mm depending on the body location. The skin thickness is greatest at the dorsum and the proximal extremities and gets thinner ventrally and distally down the extremities. Skin is thickest on the forehead, dorsal neck, dorsal thorax, and base of the tail. The skin is thinnest on the ears and in the axillary, inguinal, and perianal areas.[2,3]

The skin consists of two main layers: the epidermis and dermis. The epidermis consists of the basal, spinous, granular, clear, and horny layers. Each layer has different types of cells and differs in function. The basal layer consists of a single column of cells that are attached to the basement membrane. Typical basal keratinocytes have an oval nucleus, prominent nucleolus or nucleoli, and little heterochromatin. The basal keratinocytes contain melanosomes; various metabolic and synthesizing organelles such as mitochondria, lysosomes, rough endoplasmic reticula, and Golgi complexes; and cytoskeletal structures such as keratin intermediate filaments, microfilaments, and microtubules. Structures such as desmosomes and hemidesmosomes that help form the attachment and help to shape the basal layer are also present.[4,5]

The spinous layer of the epidermis comprises two to four layers. The cells become progressively differentiated as they move outward toward the skin surface. The spinous layer cells first appear polyhedral and then become more flattened as they develop and move outward. The spinous cells contain cellular organelles and keratin filaments. The cells of the uppermost one to two layers of the granular layer contain small, oval, membrane-bound organelles (300 nm) with alternating lamellae called lamellar granules (membrane-coating granules, keratinosomes, Odland bodies) formed in the Golgi region. They contain polar lipids such as phospholipids, glycosphingolipids, free sterols, and so-called probarrier lipids and hydrolytic enzymes that convert the probarrier lipids into stacks of neutral lipid-rich lamellae that assemble in the intercellular space, coat the surfaces of the cornified cells, and provide a barrier to the permeation of the skin. The spinous cells have abundant desmosomes that consist of adhesion plaques and submembranous plaques involved in cell cohesion.[4,5]

The granular layer consists of highly differentiated cells that are flattened polyhedrons with keratohyalin granules. In this layer of the skin, dephosphorylation and proteinolysis activate filaggrin, which cross-links and bundles with keratin filaments into large macrofilaments. Filaggrin is broken down in the stratum corneum to free amino acids important for the proper hydration of the epidermis. Lamellar granules present in the granular layer aggregate beneath the plasma membrane and fuse with it, opening a channel for the release of granule

*The editors acknowledge and appreciate the contributions of Karen A. Moriello, Douglas J. DeBoer, and Susan D. Semrad, former authors of this chapter. Their work has been incorporated into this edition.

contents such as polysaccharides, glycoproteins, acid hydrolases, acid lipase, and probarrier lipids into the intercellular spaces. After release, polar lipids are remodeled into hydrophobic, neutral, lipid-rich lamellae that form an effective barrier. A dense layer of highly cross-linked proteins is deposited inside the inner leaflet of the membrane. Together with the membrane, this boundary is called the cornified cell envelope, a rigid structure that resists degradation and is rich is glutamyl-lysine isopeptide cross-links. At the uppermost aspect of this layer, substances such as keratins, filaggrin, and the cornified cell envelope are passed on to the cornified cell layer.[4,5]

The cornified layer contains the largest and most numerous cells of any zone in the epidermis. Cells are large, flattened, and polyhedral; overlap with the margins; and associate through interlocking ridges and modified desmosomes. The contents of the cell are limited primarily to disulfide-bonded keratin filaments, highly cross-linked bundles of macrofilaments, and filaggrin. The compact organization of the proteins becomes looser toward the outer epidermal surface. The breakdown of filaggrin to its constituent amino acids in the outer cell layers accounts for the greater water-holding capacity of the cells and the more diffuse organization of the filaments. Uricanic acid is degraded from filaggrin with histidase and absorbs ultraviolet light. Therefore uricanic acid is important in ultraviolet light protection. The pyrrolidone carboxylic acid derived from glutamine is hygroscopic and helps to keep the skin hydrated even in a dry environment. The preserved trilaminar plasma membrane outside the cornified cell envelope becomes discontinuous and desquamates toward the upper portion of the cornified layer so that the envelope serves as the real cell membrane.[4,5]

The dermis contains a variety of cells that are essential for the skin to function normally. The dermis contains cellular elements such as fibroblasts, macrophages, histiocytes, eosinophils, and mast cells in the fibrous matrix and nonfibrous matrix. The fibrous matrix consists of collagen and elastic fibers. The nonfibrous matrix consists of glycosaminoglycans and proteoglycans. The blood vessels, nerves, lymphatics, hair, and sebaceous and apocrine glands are found within the dermis. The sebaceous and apocrine glands in the horse are larger and more numerous compared with those in other large animal species.[4,5]

The area that separates the epidermis from the dermis is known as the basement membrane zone. This layer of the skin functions as a scaffold for organization (important for growth and differentiation of keratinocytes) and repair (speeds up reepithelization), acts to regulate selective permeability by only allowing passage of molecules of the correct charge and molecular size, provides a physical intercellular barrier (tumor containment), and links epithelia to their underlying matrices. The basement membrane consists of structures such as tonofilaments, hemidesmosomes, laminin, fibronectin, proteins such as collagen, laminin-like molecules such as entactin and nidogen, anionic glycosaminoglycans such as heparin sulfate, anchoring fibrils, oxytalan filaments, elaunin fibers, microthread-like filamentous threadwork, and large glycoproteins such as fibrillin.[5]

Hair

The hair tends to cycle in a specific manner. Initially, hairs are in the growing or anagen phase, progressing through an intermediate or catagen phase into a resting or telogen phase (Figure 13-1). The time period that hairs are in the catagen phase is short, and finding hairs in this stage of the cycle is difficult using a trichogram (plucking hairs and looking at them under the microscope). A variety of conditions including temperature, photoperiod, genetics, and hormones can affect the hair cycle.[1,6]

The hair follicles are located within the dermis and are associated with sebaceous and apocrine glands. Hairs are important in thermoregulation, protection of the skin from external factors, and as an ornament to attract other animals. The types of hairs found in equine skin are simple primary hairs. Horse hairs tend not to shed at once. Instead their hair sheds in patches or in a mosaic pattern.[1]

Ambient temperature affects the texture of the hairs. In warm temperatures the hair coat comprises thick, medullated hairs. Piloerection of hairs occurs to aid in cooling the body. In contrast, in cold temperatures the coat comprises longer, finer, and poorly medullated fibers. This type of hair coat provides more insulation from cold. The hairs of the fetlock, mane, and tail do not shed as do the other hairs on the horse.[1]

Additional Skin-Related Structures

The horse and other Equidae have skin structures unique to these species, including the ergot, chestnut, and hoof. The ergot is a small mass of cornified tissue located in a tuft of hair on the flexor surface of the fetlock. The ergot is a vestige of the second and fourth digits of extinct Equidae. The chestnut refers to a mass of horny tissue on the medial surface of the radius and is believed to be a vestige of the first digit. The hoof is the horny covering over the distal end of the third digit. The hoof includes the frog, important for shock absorption and stimulation of blood flow to the foot, and other components that provide a firm structure to facilitate motion.

HISTORY

A patient history of the horse can provide the clinician with useful clues to help determine the underlying cause of a dermatologic problem. Figure 13-2 is an example of a form with different types of dermatologic questions. For example, most allergies produce the clinical sign of pruritus. The owner may notice the horse rubbing, scratching, licking, or chewing, or physical examination may reveal evidence of pruritus (i.e., broken hairs and excoriations). Pruritus does not confirm a diagnosis of allergic disease. Other conditions such as parasitic infestation or secondary bacterial or fungal skin infection may be pruritic. These differential diagnoses may be ruled out by performing the diagnostic tests discussed later in this chapter.

Insect allergies and atopy frequently recur seasonally. However, in the warm climates of the United States, some horses may have year-round or nonseasonal pruritus with insect allergies or atopy. The practitioner should also include food allergy on the list of differential diagnoses for horses with nonseasonal pruritus.

Questions concerning whether other horses in the stabling or pasture facility have dermatologic lesions may be important. Similarly, knowing if grooming aids (brushes, combs, etc.) are used on more than one horse is important. Pruritus that affects multiple animals may indicate the possibility of a parasitic or infectious process.

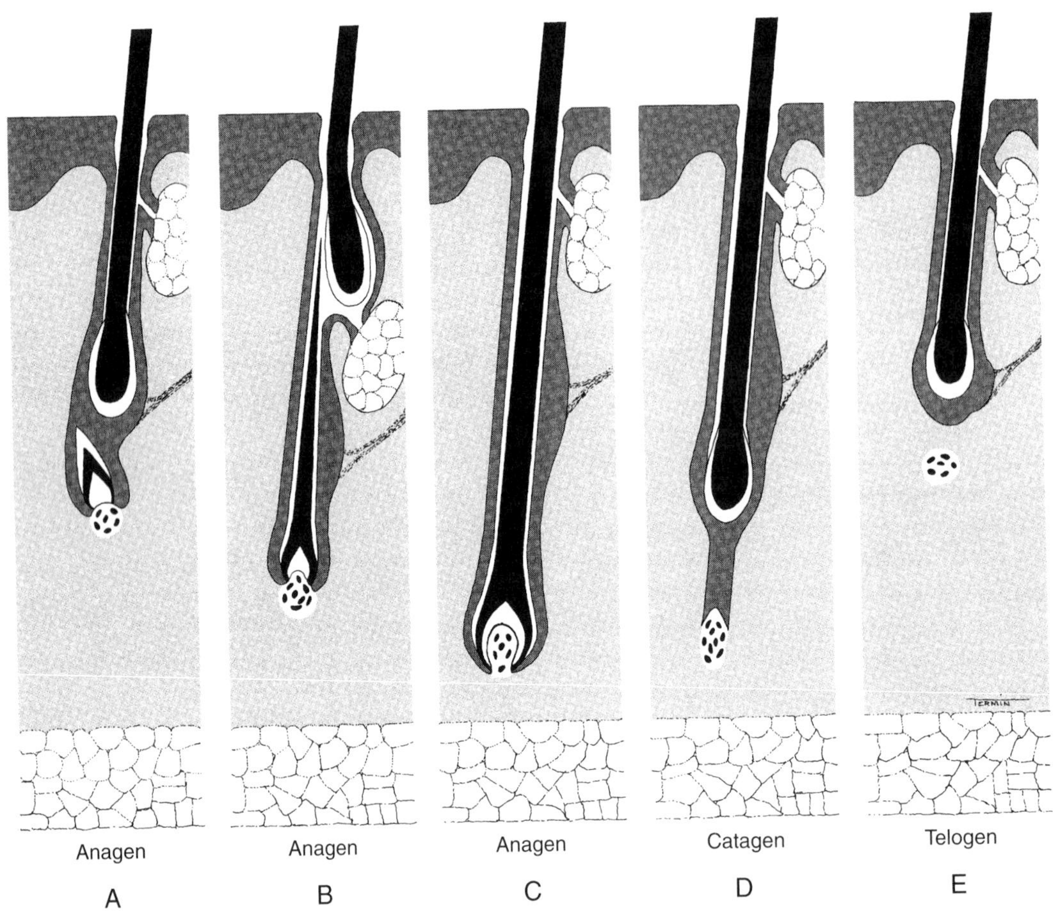

FIGURE 13-1 Phases in the life cycle of a hair. **A,** Anagen begins with the renewal of the intimate relationship between the papilla and the undifferentiated cells that partially enclose it. **B,** As anagen proceeds, matrix cells generate a new hair that pushes upward toward the surface and in the process dislodges the old club hair. **C,** Mature anagen hair follicle consists of infundibular, isthmus, and inferior segments. **D,** During catagen, the entire inferior segment of the follicle shrivels upward as a thin cord of epithelial cells and is followed upward by the papilla. **E,** During telogen, the club hair rests in its cornified sac at the level of the hair erector muscle. (From Moschella SL, Herley HJ: *Dermatology,* ed 3, Philadelphia, 1992, WB Saunders.)

Response to previous therapy is another useful historical clue. The practitioner should determine the dose and frequency of medication administration. If the appropriate drug or drug dose is not used, then the patient may not respond.

Other factors to consider include feed, stabling environment, and supplements or other medications (e.g., wormers, sprays, shampoos) used regularly. If any of these factors changed before the development of the dermatologic lesions, then the change may be related to the problem in the horse.

PHYSICAL EXAMINATION

The examiner should consider the type of skin lesions and lesion distribution when performing a physical examination on the equine patient with dermatologic disease. Pustules and vesicles are fragile skin lesions that are not found easily and are most common in bacterial or autoimmune skin diseases. Pustules and vesicles are considered primary lesions. Other examples of primary lesions include papules, wheals or hives, erythema, and nodules. Secondary lesions commonly observed in horses may include scale, crusts, excoriations, fistulae, ulcers, necrosis, hyperpigmentation, hypopigmentation, lichenification, hyperhidrosis, and scars.

The location of lesions is important because certain dermatologic conditions tend to occur on certain areas of the body. This tendency is especially true with parasitic hypersensitivity reactions because certain parasites have a predilection for certain areas of the body.[7] For example, pinworms tend to cause intense pruritus of the tailhead, and black flies tend to have a predilection for the head, ears, and ventral abdomen. More detailed information concerning insect feeding preferences is covered in the insect hypersensitivity section. The horse should be examined for evidence of external parasites such as ticks or flies.

The clinician should always perform a thorough physical examination, including determining the temperature, heart rate, and respiratory rate. If abnormalities in any of these parameters exist, then the horse may have a systemic disease or more than one medical problem. For the health of the animal, exploring and treating all possible medical problems is important.

EQUINE DERMATOLOGY HISTORY FORM

Date __________

Age when purchased __________

What is this horse's use? __________

What is your complaint about the horse's skin? __________

Age of horse? __________ Age when skin problem started? __________

Where on the body did the problem start? __________

What did the skin problem look like initially? __________

How has it spread or changed? __________

Is the problem continual or intermittent? __________

What season did the problem start? __________

Is the problem seasonal or year-round? __________

If seasonal, what seasons is the disease present? __________

Does the horse itch? __________ If so, where? __________

Do any horses in contact with the affected horse have skin problems? __________

If so, are they similar or different from this horse's problem? __________

Do any people in contact with the horse have skin problems? __________

Do you use insect control? __________ If so, describe. __________

Do any relatives of this horse have skin problems? __________ If yes, explain. __________

Please list any injectable, oral, or topical medications that have been used to treat the problem (veterinary or "home remedies"): __________

Did any help the condition? __________ If yes, which ones? __________

Did any aggravate the condition? __________ If yes, which ones? __________

Describe the environment where the horse is kept: Indoors __________

__________ Outdoors __________

What is the horse fed? __________

What feed additives do you use? __________

What is your deworming schedule? __________

Did the horse receive ivermectin? __________ If so, when? __________

List any other major medical problems or drugs that the horse received: __________

List any additional information you feel is relevant to the skin disease: __________

FIGURE 13-2 Sample equine history form.

COMMON CAUSES OF PRURITIC DERMATOSES

Pruritus is the sensation to rub, lick, scratch, or chew.[8] Horses most commonly rub the skin and hair coat when they are pruritic (Figure 13-3). Clinical evidence that a horse is pruritic may include the presence of broken hairs, excoriations, hemorrhagic crust, alopecia, lichenification (thickening of the skin), and hyperpigmentation. Lichenification and hyperpigmentation occur most commonly after chronic inflammation and pruritus.

Conditions that tend to be pruritic include parasite infestations such as lice, mites, ticks, *Onchocerca* spp., *Habronema* spp., and pinworms or allergic reactions such as insect hypersensitivity, food allergy, contact allergy, and atopy. Occasionally, pruritus occurs with bacterial or fungal infections.

Parasitic Skin Diseases

LICE (PEDICULOSIS)

Two types of lice may be found on horses. Biting lice feed on epidermal debris, whereas sucking lice feed on blood and lymph. *Haematopinus asini,* the sucking louse of horses, most commonly infests the mane and tail and the hairs behind the fetlock and pastern. The biting louse, *Damalinia equi,* tends to feed on the dorsolateral trunk.

Lice are host-specific and complete their entire life cycle on the host. Female lice attach their eggs to hairs. In cool, moist environments, lice can live for 2 to 3 weeks; they live only a few days off of the host. Lice infestations are transmitted by direct or indirect contact. Brushes, combs, and tack serve as fomites for transmission of lice. Adult horses may act as asymptomatic reservoirs for infection.

Lice infestations can occur year round, but they are more common in the winter in northern climates. Cooler skin and hair coat temperatures are more favorable for development of eggs within the female, oviposition, and egg development.[9] Skin temperatures on the legs of horses, with the possible exception of Draft-breed horses, are too cold for louse development.

Lice infestation has no age, breed, or sex predilection in horses. Affected horses tend to be restless and have a poor appetite. They have a dry, dull hair coat with patchy areas of hair loss and excoriation. The coat may appear moist and have a sour or mousy odor. Skin fasciculation may be the only evidence of early infestations in foals. Some horses may be asymptomatic carriers that are identified only when foals or other susceptible animals become infested. Heavy infestations of sucking lice may cause anemia or severe debilitation.

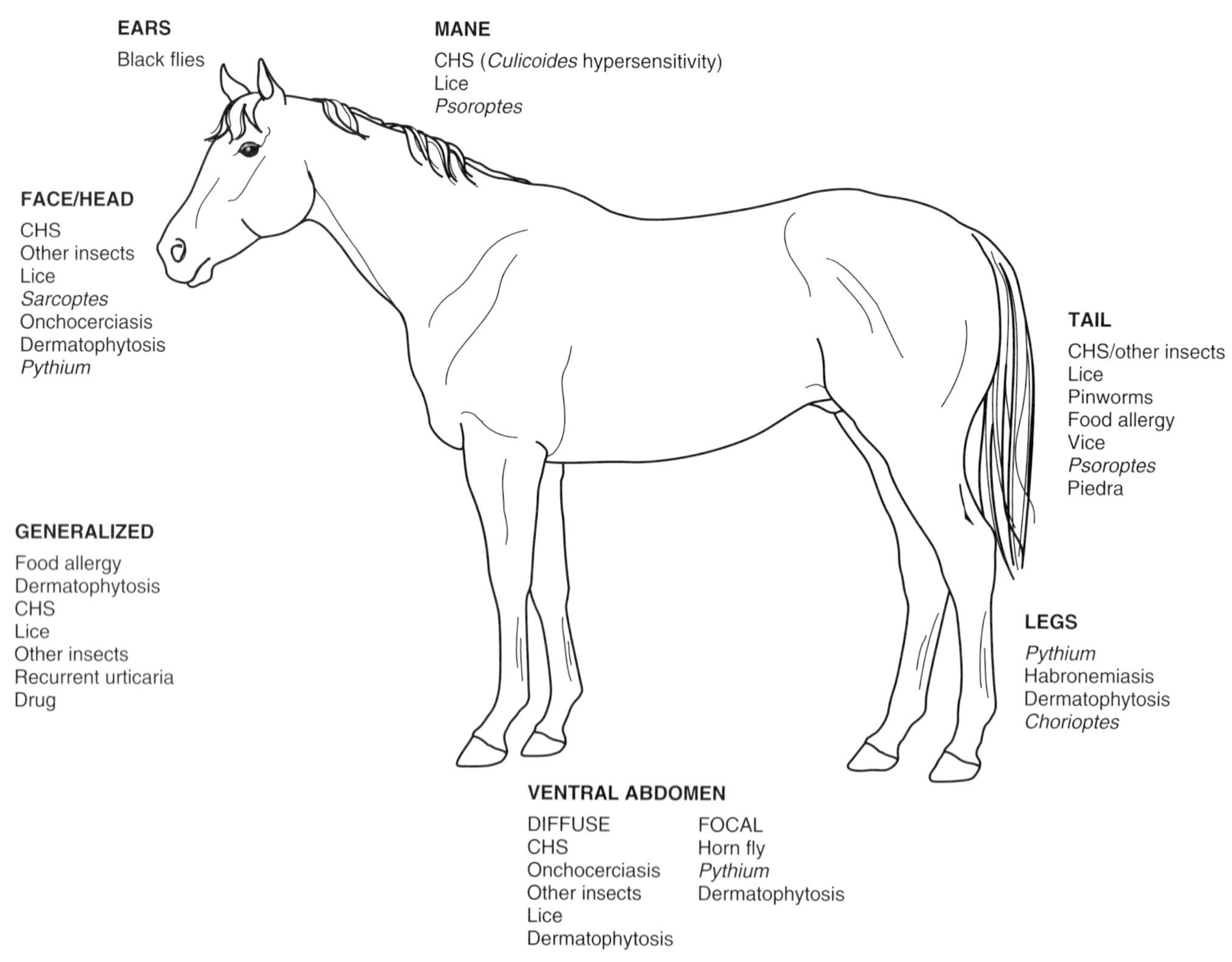

FIGURE 13-3 Regional pruritus: differential diagnosis of pruritic skin diseases.

The diagnosis of lice infestations is made by demonstration of adults or eggs or both on the hairs. Sometimes, lice cannot be visualized easily in direct light. In these circumstances the veterinarian may need to comb the hair coat with a fine-toothed comb to find the lice. Skin biopsies may reveal a nonspecific superficial perivascular eosinophilic dermatitis with or without intraepidermal microabscesses.[1]

When managing a lice infestation, the veterinarian should treat all animals on the premises. Ivermectin at 200 μg/kg orally every 2 weeks for three treatments is effective for treating sucking lice. Biting lice do not respond to ivermectin treatment, and thus one should treat affected horses with other medications, such as dips. Common types of dip may be used to treat sucking and biting lice infestations include lime sulfur, pyrethrins, methoxychlor, malathion, coumaphos, crotoxyphos, pyrethroids, lindane, permethrin, selenium sulfide, imidacloprid, phoxim, and fipronil.[10-12] Lime sulfur and pyrethrin dips have fewer associated adverse reactions in horses than do other dip treatments. All products should be used according to label directions. None of these treatments affect lice eggs, and two to three repeat applications of the dip are recommended at 2-week intervals. For optimal efficacy, one should treat the whole body of the horse when applying the dips. Other precautions include cleaning and disinfecting all tack and grooming supplies (brushes and combs), decontaminating the stabling area using a commercial premise spray used to kill fleas because lice may survive for days to weeks in the environment, and, although reinfestation is difficult to prevent, treating animals returning from shows, breeding farms, or training facilities prophylactically.

MITES (MANGE)

A variety of mites may infest horses. *Sarcoptes scabiei* var. *equi* (scabies, head mange), *Chorioptes equi* (leg mange), *Psoroptes equi* (body mange), *Pyemotes tritici* (straw itch mite), and *Trombicula* and *Eutrombicula* species (chiggers) are species associated with equine pruritic skin disease.[7] The pruritus accompanying a mite infestation results from a combination of mechanical irritation and hypersensitivity to the mite and by-products of the mite (i.e., feces).[13] The primary skin lesion from a mite infestation is a maculopapular eruption. These skin lesions are often difficult to find with chronic infestations.

Sarcoptes scabiei In the United States, *S. scabiei* infestations in horses are a reportable disease.[7] This mite is highly contagious and infests horses and transiently infests human beings (self-limiting disease) in contact with parasitized horses. This parasite is capable of surviving off the host for up to 3 weeks, and transmission of scabies by fomites or in the environment is possible. Scabies mites burrow in the superficial epidermis and lay their eggs. In early infestations, mites are found in highest concentration around the head and neck. These mites seem to prefer the ears on horses. As disease progresses, mites usually spread over the entire body. A scabies infestation in a horse results in intense pruritus and generalized scaling and crusting with excoriations and lichenification. A secondary skin infection may result from the pruritus. One may elicit the itch-scratch reflex by scratching the horse over the withers, causing the horse to tuck its nose close to its chest and make smacking noises and exaggerated lip movements. This reflex suggests scabies but is not diagnostic, and one may elicit the reflex in some normal horses.[14] The scabies mite is circular with short legs, a terminal anus, and long unjointed pedicles. Unfortunately, as in other species, the scabies mites are difficult to find on skin scrapings. Therefore a negative skin scraping does not ensure that the horse does not have scabies.

Ivermectin at a dose of 200 μg/kg orally is effective for treating horses with scabies. As in other species, the practitioner should repeat ivermectin treatment at 2-week intervals for a total of two to three treatments. Within 2 weeks the eggs hatch and new adult mites are present. Topical treatments such as lime sulfur dip, lindane, coumaphos, diazinon, malathion, or toxaphene also have been used. The practitioner should dip horses every 7 to 10 days for three to six treatments, treat all horses in contact with the infested horse, and decontaminate fomites (e.g., tack, brushes) and the environment.

Chorioptes equi *Chorioptes equi* mites are host-specific and do not parasitize human beings (Figure 13-4). Unlike the scabies mite, infestation with *C. equi* is not a reportable condition. *C. equi* mites spend their entire life cycle on the host feeding on epidermal debris. Preferred feeding sites include the distal limbs and perineum. Infested horses exhibit intense pruritus with stomping of feet and rubbing of the perineal area. Skin lesions include alopecia, erythema, and crusting of the pasterns, fetlocks, or perineum. Draft-breed horses or other horses with feathered fetlocks are predisposed to *C. equi*. The mite tends to be more common in the winter months. *C. equi* should be included in the list of differential diagnoses for horses with pastern dermatitis or greasy heel. Treatment of this mite is the same as for *S. scabiei*. However, ivermectin-resistant *C. equi* mites have been reported, and topical dip therapy may be indicated if the horse does not respond to oral therapy. If

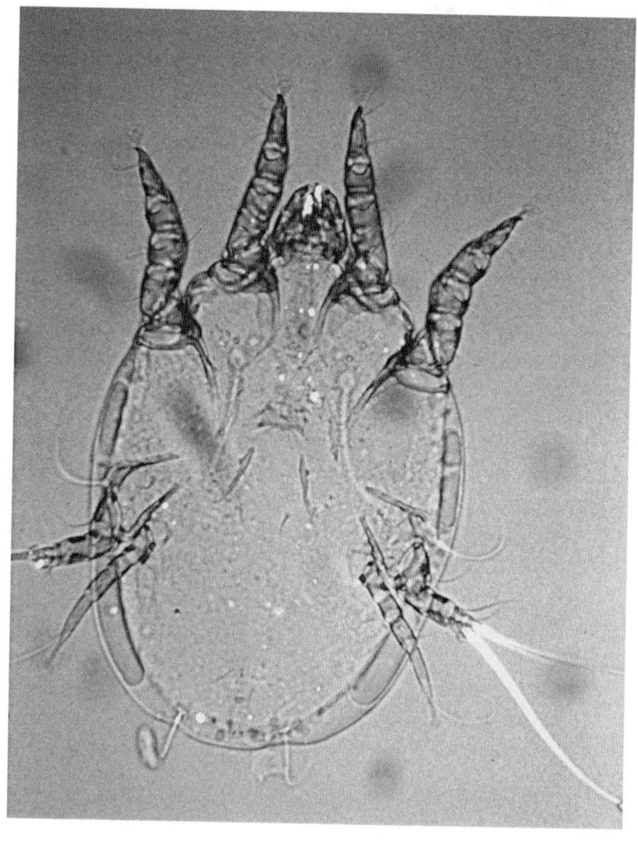

FIGURE 13-4 *Chorioptes* mite.

a topical medication is used, clipping the hair around the fetlocks and pasterns to ensure optimal contact of the dip with the skin and mites is advisable.

Psoroptee equi *Psoroptes equi* mite infestations are a reportable condition in horses in the United States. *P. equi* mites are highly contagious to other horses but do not infest human beings. These mites do not burrow but live on the skin surface. They are biting mites that feed on serum and cellular components. Transmission of *P. equi* mites is by direct contact and exposure to fomites. Mite infestations tend to begin on the forelock, mane, and tail and spread to the trunk. These mites have been known to infest the ear canal and cause otitis externa. Affected horses typically show head shaking or rubbing. As with many other mites, pruritus results in alopecia, papule, oozing crusts, excoriations, and ulcers on the skin. The intensity of pruritus varies. History and clinical signs suggest the diagnosis of *P. equi* mange. Skin scrapings are required to diagnose this condition definitively. *P. equi* has an oval body with segmented pedicles. Treatment for *P. equi* infection is similar to that described for sarcoptic mange.

Trombiculidiasis Trombiculidiasis (chiggers, red bugs, harvest mites) is caused by an infestation with larvae of free-living adult mites (genus *Eutrombicula* or *Neotrombicula*). Larvae are most prevalent in grasses, forests, or swamps in late summer and fall. Small rodents are the natural host. Pathognomonic skin lesions are papules or wheals with a small orange or red dot (trombiculid larvae) in the center. Trombiculidiasis is seasonal, but the seasonality varies with genus and species. *Eutrombicula alfreddugesi* is active in the late spring and peaks midsummer, whereas *Neotrombicula automnalis* is most active from the late summer to midautumn.[10] Larvae feed on the host in the late afternoon and early evening. Areas of the body most commonly infested are the face, muzzle, distal limbs, ventral thorax, and abdomen. The diagnosis is based on observation of the distinctive lesion with the larvae approximately 0.2 to 0.4 mm in size, oval in shape with six legs, in the center of the skin lesion. Trombiculidiasis is a self-limiting disease. Some horses are uncomfortable with this mite infestation and should be treated. Recommended treatments include lime sulfur dip, permethrin, pyrethrin, cypermethrin, and phoxim sprays or dips as a one-time treatment in association with prednisolone at a dose of 0.5 mg/kg orally for 3 to 5 days.

Pyemotes tritici *Pyemotes tritici* (straw itch mite) normally parasitizes the larvae of grain insects. Occasionally this mite parasitizes human beings and horses.[15] Infestation in horses occurs from contaminated hay fed in overhead racks. The mite produces a maculopapular crusted eruption on the head, neck, and trunk that is only occasionally pruritic. The diagnosis is based on history and clinical examination. This disease is self-limiting, and the owner should remove contaminated forage or feed the horse from the ground until all contaminated forage has been consumed. Infestations from fomites or hay fed on the ground have not been reported.

Dermanyssus gallinae The nymphs and adults of the poultry mite, *Dermanyssus gallinae,* will occasionally parasitize the horse. This mite feeds at night. The adults are oval, 0.6 to 1 mm long with eight long legs. The color of the mites is white, gray, or black. However, after the poultry mite consumes a blood meal the color turns to red.

This mite causes pruritic papules and crust of the head and legs of horses. Skin scrapings and tape preparations at night yield the best chance of obtaining the mite. Routine mite treatments that were discussed previously are also beneficial for treating this mite. However, with the poultry mite, one needs to treat the environment and remove the bird nests from the stable or eliminate the horse's contact with poultry.[10]

Demodicosis Demodicosis is a rare equine skin condition. Two species of *Demodex* can infest horses (i.e., *D. equi* and *D. caballi*), and each affects different areas of the body. *D. equi* affects the body, whereas *D. caballi* prefers the eyelids and muzzle. Clinically these horses have one or more alopecic or scaling areas of the body. The most common areas of the body affected in horses with demodex are the face, neck, and sometimes shoulders. The diagnosis is based on skin scrapings. Demodex mites are easily found on skin scrapings. Several different treatment options exist for treating equine demodex. Treatment with 2% trichlorfon topically every other day has been used with success. Daily ivermectin or dormectin has also been used with some success. Amitraz is contraindicated because this drug causes colic in horses. Regardless of the treatment used, one needs to identify and treat the underlying cause for the demodicosis. The most common underlying causes for equine demodicosis are chronic glucocorticoid use and equine Cushing's disease (pituitary pars intermedia dysfunction).[10,12]

General Comments Regardless of the type of mite present on the horse, skin scrapings should be part of the diagnostic workup. With the exception of lice and trombiculid larvae that can be seen with the naked eye, one can diagnose mite infestations best by microscopic examination of skin scraping samples.

Ticks

Ticks are an important ectoparasite in the horse because of their potential role in disease transmission, including a variety of viral, protozoal, rickettsial, and bacterial infections. Tick infestations are most common in the spring and summer.

Argasid ticks lay eggs in cracks and crevices in the environment, and immature ticks infect hosts after hatching. Larvae and nymphs suck blood and lymph and then drop off to develop into adults. These ticks infest barns, sheds, and other areas where animals are found. In horses, *Otobius megnini* (spinose ear tick) tends to infest the ears and ear canal. Clinical signs of infestation include otitis externa, head tilt, head shaking, ear rubbing, and occasionally aural hematomas.

Dermacentor, Ixodes, and *Amblyomma* species are the most common ixodid ticks of horses. These ticks are found outdoors and have complicated life cycles in which all stages of the life cycle are parasitic. The severity of clinical signs depends on the density of the infestation and whether the horse develops a hypersensitivity reaction to the bites. Infestations occur most commonly on the ears, face, neck, groin, distal limbs, and tail. Early lesions consist of papular to pustular eruptions that rapidly develop into crusts, erosions, ulcers, and hair loss. Hypersensitivity reactions may be local or general. Local responses appear as nodules that develop at the site of the tick bite. Although the pathogenesis is unknown, cutaneous basophil hypersensitivity is believed to be involved.[16] Systemic reactions are characterized by whole-body urticaria or multifocal urticarial plaques. In Australia, a hypersensitivity reaction to *Boophilus microplus* has been observed in sensitized horses.[17] Intense pruritus, papules, and wheals develop as soon as 30 minutes after ticks begin to feed.

A definitive diagnosis is made by observation of ticks attached to the horse or in the ear canal. Treatment aims at

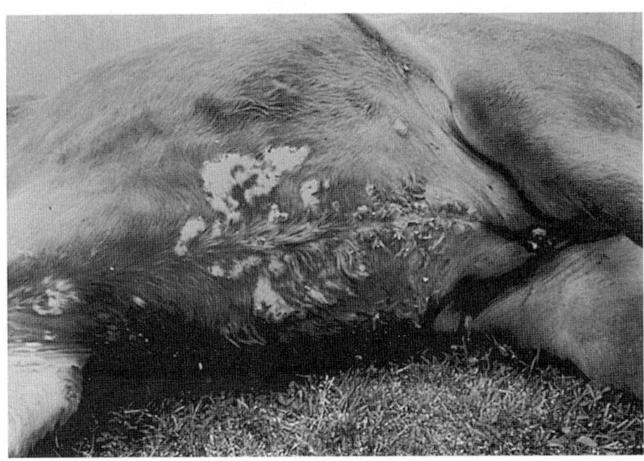

FIGURE 13-5 Ventral midline dermatitis caused by onchocerciasis.

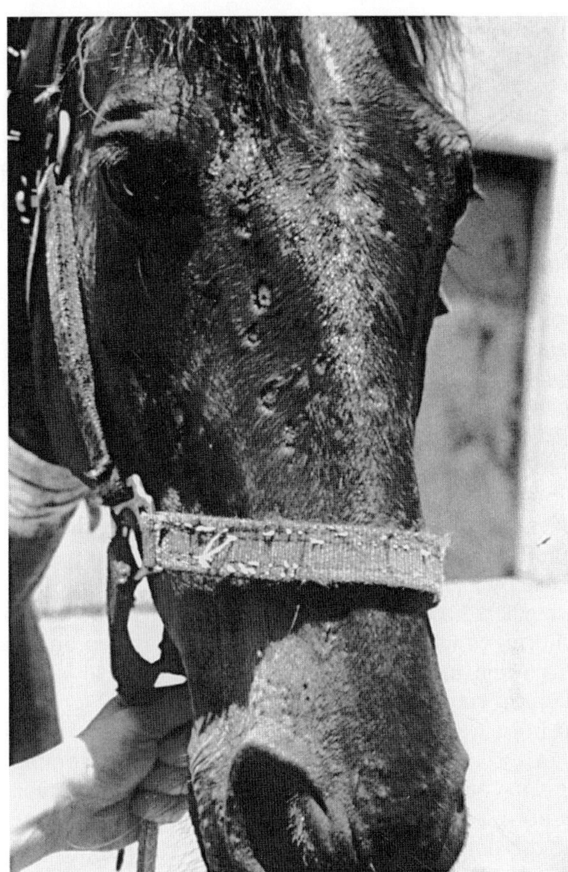

FIGURE 13-6 Equine onchocercosis.

killing ticks on the horse. The practitioner should apply pyrethrin or pyrethroid sponge-on dips to the body of the horse, taking extra care to soak skinfold areas. Usually, only one treatment is necessary unless reinfestation occurs. Resistance to insecticides can occur rapidly, and knowledge of local resistance patterns is important. Infestations of *O. megnini* require mechanical removal of as many ticks as possible. One part rotenone and three parts mineral oil applied twice weekly is an effective otic parasiticide for horses. The author has used a commercially available pyrethrin otic preparation (Otomite Plus, Vibac, Fort Worth, Tex.) for small animals in horse ears with success. Ivermectin also has been shown to be effective in treating ticks at a dose of 200 μg/kg orally.

Onchocerciasis Onchocerciasis is a nonseasonal skin disease of the horse caused by the parasite *Onchocerca cervicalis*. This nematode lives in the ligamentum nuchae and produces microfilariae that migrate to the skin and are ingested by the intermediate host, *Culicoides* species. Microfilarial populations in the skin vary, and the highest concentrations occur in the dermis of the face, neck, and ventral midline, especially the umbilicus (Figure 13-5).[18] Microfilarial populations vary seasonally and are highest in the spring, which interestingly is the peak season for the *Culicoides* vector.[19] Microfilariae are more superficial in the dermis during the spring and summer months. Clinical signs of onchocerciasis are believed to be caused by an idiosyncratic hypersensitivity reaction to one or more microfilarial antigens because many horses that have circulating microfilariae do not have any gross skin or ocular lesions.[20] Whether the reaction is directed only at dying or dead microfilariae is unknown.

Onchocerciasis has no breed or sex predilection and usually affects horses 4 years of age and older. Clinical signs are nonseasonal but may be worse in the spring and summer, most likely because of the added irritation from the vector. Lesions may occur on the face and neck, on the ventral chest and abdomen, or in all these areas.[21,22] Early lesions begin as a thinning hair coat. As the disease progresses, lesions may vary from focal to generalized areas of alopecia, scaling, crusting, and plaques. Affected areas may be severely excoriated, ulcerated, oozing, and lichenified. Annular lesions in the center of the forehead suggest the disease (Figure 13-6). Leukoderma usually develops at the site of lesions and is irreversible. Ocular lesions include sclerosing keratitis, vitiligo of the bulbar conjunctiva, white nodules in the pigmented conjunctiva, uveitis, and a crescent-shaped patch of depigmentation bordering the optic disk.[23]

The practitioner may make a presumptive diagnosis of onchocerciasis by demonstrating the microfilariae in the skin of animals with compatible historical and clinical findings. Skin scrapings and direct blood smears are often negative. One can demonstrate microfilariae most reliably with a mince preparation or via histologic examination of skin from a biopsy specimen.[22] Mince preparations require a 4- or 6-mm punch specimen of tissue obtained from the ventral abdomen. One places the tissue specimen in a Petri dish with a small amount of physiologic saline, minces it with a scalpel blade or razor, and incubates it at room temperature for 30 to 60 minutes. The specimen can then be examined microscopically for evidence of the rapid motion of the microfilariae. Skin biopsies reveal a superficial perivascular eosinophilic dermatitis. Often, microfilariae are visible in the superficial dermis.[7]

Ivermectin at a dose of 200 μg/kg orally is the treatment of choice.[7,21,24] A single dose often produces remission of clinical signs within 2 to 3 weeks. However, some horses require two to three monthly treatments before clinical signs resolve. Approximately 25% of horses have an adverse reaction, such as ventral midline edema or pruritus, which occurs 1 to 10 days after treatment. In rare cases, severe umbilical and eyelid edema and fever may occur. In confirmed cases of onchocerciasis, one should perform a thorough ocular examination to look for any signs of eye disease associated with onchocerciasis. Anecdotal reports suggest treatment may precipitate an episode of uveitis.

Prednisolone at a dose of 0.5 mg/kg orally may be necessary in the first week of treatment to prevent exacerbation of skin and ocular lesions as a result of massive destruction of microfilariae but is not routinely recommended. Indications include the development of ventral midline edema, pruritus, and fever. None of the currently available anthelmintics kill adult parasites in the ligamentaum nuchae, and affected individuals require periodic retreatment with ivermectin when clinical signs recur. The prevalence of cutaneous onchocerciasis has decreased significantly with the advent of routine dewormings with ivermectin.

Habronemiasis Cutaneous habronemiasis is a common nodular skin disease caused by three species of nematodes: *Habronema muscae, H. majus (H. microstoma),* and *Draschia megastoma (H. megastoma).* The housefly is an intermediate host for *H. muscae* and *D. megastoma,* whereas the stable fly is the intermediate host for *H. microstoma.* The normal life cycle for these parasites is similar. Adult nematodes live in the stomach and produce larvae. Larvae are passed in the feces and ingested by maggots of the foregoing intermediate hosts. The intermediate host deposits infective larvae near the mouth of the horse, which swallows them. Cutaneous habronemiasis occurs when intermediate hosts deposit infective larvae on skin, open wounds, or chronically wet areas.

A horse with cutaneous habronemiasis has ulcerative nodules in the spring and summer that partially or completely regress in the winter. A recent study suggests that Arabians, gray horses, and horses with diluted color (i.e., palomino, buckskin, dun) may be predisposed to developing cutaneous habronemiasis.[25] Interestingly, in this same study, Thoroughbred horses were the most underrespresented breed of horse for cutaneous habronemiais. No breed, sex, or age predilection exists. Some horses may be predisposed to cutaneous habronemiasis, exhibiting clinical signs each year, whereas other horses on the same premises never develop this condition.

Skin lesions of habronemiasis occur most commonly on the legs, urethral process of the penis, prepuce, medial canthus of the eye, or any area of trauma to the skin. Other areas that may be infected include the conjunctival sac, the lacrimal duct, and the third eyelid. Single or multiple nodules may be present. In most cases, pruritus is present, presumably due to a hypersensitivity reaction to the parasite. The intensity of pruritus may vary from mild to severe. In severe cases in which ocular lesions are present the horse can suffer from photophobia, epiphora, and chemosis. Dysuria can occur when lesions affect the urtheral process.

Lesions often are ulcerated and appear similar to exuberant granulation tissue. Yellow granules approximately 1 mm in diameter may be present.[26,27] Microscopic examination of these granules does not reveal branching hyphae such as one frequently observes with granules from pythiosis or zygomycosis lesions.

Differential diagnoses for cutaneous habronemiasis include bacterial granuloma, fungal granuloma, pythiosis, exuberant granulation tissue, squamous cell carcinoma, and equine sarcoid. *Habronema* spp. may be present concurrently with other dermatologic conditions, and biopsy is important for a complete and definitive diagnosis.

The diagnosis is based on history, physical examination, cytologic examination, and biopsy of lesions. Cytologic examination of exudate sometimes reveals the presence of nematode larvae. These larvae are large (3 mm by 60 μm), with a spiny tail, and are usually motile. Skin biopsies reveal a nodular to diffuse granulomatous dermatitis with large numbers of mast cells and eosinophils. Foci of coagulation necrosis are characteristic.[28,29] Sometimes this area of necrosis contains cross-sections of larvae.

Treatment of cutaneous habronemiasis should include control of the associated hypersensitivity reaction and elimination of the parasite. Treating horses with ivermectin alone is not always effective. The author and co-workers examined 14 horses between 1988 and 1998 that had been treated with ivermectin in the preceding month and had intralesional habronema larvae present on biopsy. Similarly, 5 of 31 horses treated with ivermectin for habronemiasis required an additional treatment 2 to 4 weeks later.[30] One may treat the hypersensitivity reaction with systemic corticosteroids such as prednisolone at a dosage of 1 mg/kg once daily for 10 to 14 days with a gradual decrease over an additional 2-week period. Corticosteroids and dimethyl sulfoxide (DMSO) are often combined with fenthion, thiabendazole, ronnel, or trichlorfon in a variety of topical preparations for treatment of habronemiasis.[29] Some more common topical lesional medications include (1) 1 oz dexamethasone (2 mg/ml) in 1 oz 90% DMSO and 1 oz 20% fenthion; (2) 3 oz 90% DMSO in 15 ml dexamethasone (2 mg/ml), 40 ml nitrofurazone solution, and 1 oz trichlorfon powder; and (3) 30 ml 20% fenthion, ¾ lb petrolatum (heated), 10 mg triamcinolone acetonide powder, and 90 ml 90% DMSO. Ivermectin is sometimes used concurrently with these topical medications. Unfortunately, fenthion is no longer commercially available in the United States. Another systemic medication besides ivermectin that has been used to treat habronemiasis is moxidectin at 400 μg/kg. This drug is active against *Habronema* spp. in the stomach. A more recent study suggested that topical triamcinolone ointment or a preparation containing 50 mg dexamethasone, 500 g nitrofuraxone, 60 g of 90% DMSO solution, and 1.4 g of ivermectin paste may be an effective alternative treatment for equine cutaneous habronemiasis. With these treatments the skin lesions healed within 7 to 42 days with a mean of 19.3 days in 25 out of 26 horses.[25]

The practitioner may treat conjunctival habronemiasis with topical echothiophate drops three times a day to kill larvae in combination with an ophthalmic ointment that contains dexamethasone and an antibiotic. Other ocular treatments include neomycin, polymyxin B, and dexamethasone applied three to four times daily to the ocular lesions until healed. If corneal ulcers are present, then this triple antibiotic preparation without the steroid is used until the ulcer is healed. After the corneal ulcer is healed, an opthalmic dexamethasone ointment is used. Most ocular lesions heal within 5 to 18 days, with a mean of 8.2 days.[25]

Fly control is an essential part of treatment. Oil-based fly sprays tend to last longer than water-based fly sprays. Products that contain permethrin are effective.

Prognosis for horses with habronemiasis is good with appropriate and timely treatment. The veterinarian should warn the owner that habronemiasis may recur in subsequent years. Fly control is essential to preventing recurrence. Regular collection and stacking of manure will also help with preventing recurrence.

Pinworms Equine pinworms, *Oxyuris equi,* cause intense anal pruritus. Adult pinworms are found in the colon. The female worm migrates down the gastrointestinal tract and deposits eggs around the anus. These eggs are cemented to the skin with a thick, sticky, yellow-gray substance. Horses develop perianal pruritus as a result of this sticky substance, which contains the eggs. In severe infestations, horses may develop vague abdominal discomfort. This abdominal discomfort results directly from inflammation of the cecal and colonic mucosa in response to third- and fourth-stage pinworm larvae.[31]

Eggs develop to the infective stage within a 4- to 5-day period. At this time the cement substance cracks and dries and then detaches from the skin as flakes. These flakes contain a large number of eggs that adhere to walls, buckets, and other objects in the environment.

Because ova of *O. equi* are not often observed on routine fecal flotation, a diagnosis of pinworms is based on clinical signs and identification of pinworm eggs on cellophane tape preparations. A piece of clear adhesive tape is pressed to the skin around the anus. One removes the tape and places it on a slide for microscopic examination for oval ova with an operculum or plug at one end.

O. equi infection is treated easily with a variety of anthelmintic agents. Anecdotal reports exist of occasional resistance to ivermectin and pyrantel; these horses respond to treatment with fenbendazole. One may treat the horse once with fenbendazole and remove it from the environment for 1 month. (Pinworms can survive in the environment under ideal conditions for up to 1 month.) Alternatively, one may treat horses with fenbendazole three times at 2- to 3-week intervals.

ALLERGIES

Insect Hypersensitivity

Insect hypersensitivity is a common cause of skin disease in the horse. Mosquitoes and species of *Culicoides* (biting midges, "sweet itch"), *Simulium* (black flies), *Tabanus* (horse flies), *Chrysops* (deer flies), *Stomoxys calcitrans* (stable flies), *Haematobia* (horn flies), *Musca* (houseflies), bees, and wasps cause skin lesions in horses.[7]

Insect hypersensitivity reactions are seasonal in colder climates, can be nonseasonal in warmer climates, and may affect any age, sex, or breed of horse. This dermatologic condition may have an inherited component, but specifics of these claims have not been verified. The distribution of skin lesions varies and may depend on the type of insect involved. Certain insects have preferred feeding sites.[7,32] The black fly tends to feed on the head, ears, and ventral abdomen. Black flies may produce a generalized pattern of ventral midline edema. Stable flies prefer feeding on the lower legs but also have been known to feed on the ventral abdomen, chest, and back. The location for *Culicoides* spp. feeding is species dependent. Classically, *Culicoides* spp. feed on the dorsal surface of the horse (especially the mane and tail areas), face, and ears (Figure 13-7). In Florida, some *Culicoides* spp. prefer feeding on the lower legs, ventral trunk, and neck. Horn flies feed on the ventrum around the umbilicus (Figure 13-8). Mosquitoes prefer feeding on the lateral aspects of the body.

A few insects bite anywhere on the body and do not prefer a specific location. Examples include deer flies, horse flies, houseflies, bees, and wasps.

Some insects require a specific environment to propagate. Knowledge of these requirements may be helpful in establishing insect control programs. *Culicoides* spp. and mosquitoes prefer freestanding stagnant water for propagation. In contrast, black flies prefer moving water such as a stream, brook, or river. Horn flies are obligate parasites of cattle that require fresh cattle feces for reproduction. Several species of insects, including stable flies and houseflies, prefer decaying vegetation or manure for reproduction. They tend to be a bigger problem when sanitation practices at the stabling facility are problematic.

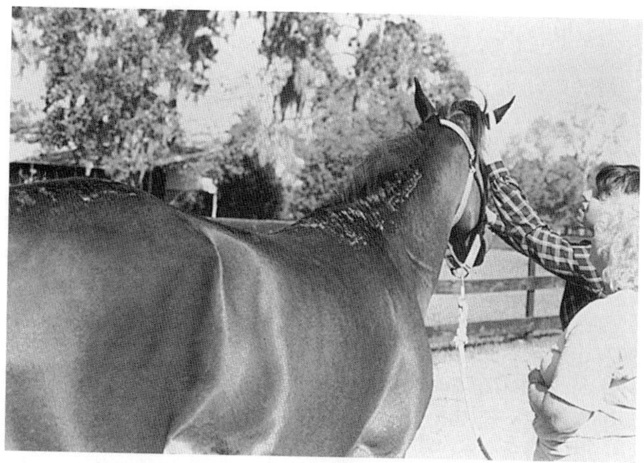

FIGURE 13-7 Two-year-old horse with *Culicoides* hypersensitivity.

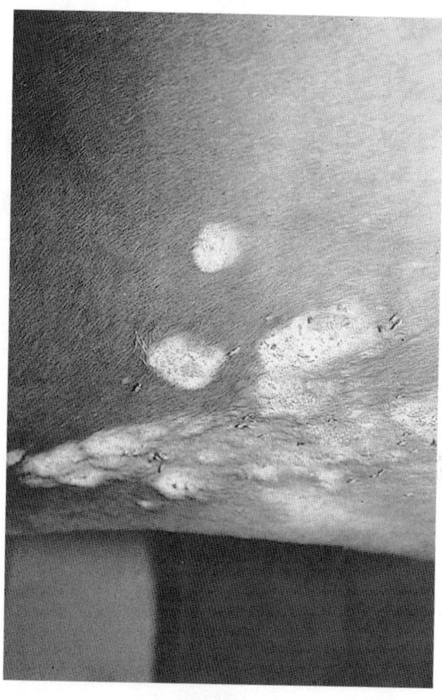

FIGURE 13-8 Alopecia with some crusting around the umbilicus on a horse with horn fly infestation.

The time of day that an insect prefers to feed also differs between species. Horseflies, stable flies, black flies, and horn flies are usually active during the daylight hours. More specifically, black flies feed in the morning and late afternoon. Mosquitoes and most *Culicoides* spp. are active at night. Mosquitoes are most active at dusk and the first 2 hours after sunset. If the time of feeding is known for the potential offending insect, then the horse may be stalled during peak feeding hours to limit exposure.

Types of dermatologic lesions seen with equine insect hypersensitivity include pruritus, alopecia, excoriations, and lichenification. A generalized papular-crusted eruption also may occur.

The diagnosis of insect hypersensitivity is based on a compatible history, physical findings, and elimination of other causes of pruritus in the horse. Skin scrapings show no abnormalities. Skin biopsies may reveal the presence of a superficial or deep perivascular eosinophilic dermatitis with epidermal spongiosis (intercellular edema of the epidermis), necrosis, and collagen degeneration. Intradermal skin testing is useful for diagnosing insect hypersensitivity.[21] Some insect allergens are inconsistently available (e.g., *Culicoides* spp.), and purchase of insect allergens for the nonspecialist veterinarian may be cost prohibitive. Fortunately, therapy and environmental control measures are similar for most biting and flying insects, and therefore confirming the diagnosis by intradermal skin testing may not be crucial.

Treatment of insect hypersensitivity involves insect control and judicious use of glucocorticoids.[21] Boxes 13-1 to 13-3 summarize recommendations. Ideally, owners should stable horses during the target peak feeding period for insects and should screen windows with a small-meshed screen and spray with a residual parasiticide. If possible, bedding areas for flies (e.g., standing water, manure) should be eliminated. Spraying horses with residual insecticides (e.g., pyrethrins or pyrethroids) is useful, and sprays containing permethrin and pyrproxifen (Knock-Out Spray, Vibrac, Fort Worth, Tex.) are effective for treating horses with *Culicoides* spp. hypersensitivity. Anecdotal reports suggest that weekly application of fipronil (Frontline, Merial, Iselin, N.J.) may be useful for treating horses with *Culicoides* spp. hypersensitivity. Avon Skin So Soft bath oil (Avon Products, Inc., New York, N.Y.) mixed in equal volumes with water has been used to repel insects in horses. However, this product with should be used with care because contact dermatitis has been reported. One should follow label recommendations with changes depending on the response of the individual horse. Cattle tags impregnated with insecticide may be helpful if attached to manes, tails, or halters.

Anecdotal reports suggest the importance of applying repellents and insecticide sprays to the horse when the skin is cool and dry, which may minimize development of sensitivity reactions to products by limiting percutaneous absorption. Many horses are sensitive to petroleum-based products and develop erythematous skin and hair loss in areas where the insecticide, fly wipe, or bath oil has been applied to the skin. If a horse has a history of this type of reaction, performing an open patch test with any new product before applying the spray over the entire body is advisable. The practitioner applies a small amount of the test substance to an area of skin and observes the site for 72 hours for signs of erythema, swelling,

BOX 13-1

PRIMARY MANAGEMENT STRATEGIES FOR COMMON EQUINE PESTS

1. Stabling
   - Tabanids: diurnal and crepuscular periods
   - Black flies: diurnal and crepuscular periods
   - Biting midges: under fans; nocturnal and crepuscular periods
2. Exclusion devices
   - Black flies: ear nets
   - Houseflies: facemasks
   - Face flies: facemasks
3. Hay and manure management
   - Stable flies: particularly hay in pastures
   - Houseflies: general sanitation
4. Cattle management
   - Horn flies: control pest on natural host
   - Face flies: undisturbed cattle manure requisite for larval development
5. Water management
   - Mosquitoes: only certain species
   - Biting midges: only certain species
6. Source identification and removal
   - Straw itch: normally infested hay
   - Blister beetle: normally products containing alfalfa
7. Restricted grazing or movement
   - Chiggers: erratic distribution in spring or fall
   - Ticks: mowing and understory control also helpful
   - Tabanids: allow horses to escape from wooded areas
   - Poultry pests (sticktight fleas and lice): separate horses from poultry

From Robinson NE, editor: *Current therapy in equine medicine*, ed 6, St. Louis, 2009, Saunders.

BOX 13-2

GENERAL INSECTICIDE TYPES USED FOR EQUINE PESTS*

Insecticides

Face flies
Facultative myiasis
Horn flies
Houseflies
Lice
Mosquitoes
Sticktight fleas
Poultry lice
Ticks

Repellents

Black flies
Biting midges
Chiggers
Horseflies

Insecticides and Repellents

Biting midges
Black flies
Chiggers
Facultative myiasis
Mosquitoes
Stable flies
Ticks

Premise Treatment

Houseflies
Mosquitoes
Stable flies

Modified from Robinson NE, editor: *Current therapy in equine medicine*, ed 6, St. Louis, 2009, Saunders.
*Categories may overlap because of differences in management systems or life cycles of different species.

BOX 13-3

PESTICIDES RECOMMENDED FOR EXTERNAL PARASITE CONTROL ON HORSES*

Residual Insecticides

Pyrethroids

Cypermethrin
Fenvalerate
Permethrin
Resmethrin
Tetramethrin
S-Bioallethrin
Sumethrin

Organophosphates

Coumaphos
Dichlorvos
Malathion
Tetrachlorvinphos

Organochlorines

Lindane
Methoxychlor

Other Compounds

Repellents

MGK 326 *di-N-propyl isocinchomeronate*
Stabilene: *butoxy polypropylene glycol*

Botanicals

Pyrethrins (also insecticidal)
Synergists
Piperonyl butoxide *5-((2-(2-butoxyethoxy) ethoxy)methyl)-6-propyl; 1,3- benzodioxole*
MGK 264 *N-octyl bicycloheptene dicarboximide*

From Robinson NE, editor: *Current therapy in equine medicine,* ed 6, Philadelphia, 2009, Saunders.
*Categories may overlap; for example, some pyrethrins are also insecticidal, and some pyrethroids are repellent. William B. Warner and Roger O. Drummond assisted in compiling this list.

and hair loss. Fly masks or fly sheets are useful adjunct therapy for control of insects.

In many cases, insect control alone is insufficient to alleviate discomfort and clinical signs. Hydroxyzine hydrochloride may be beneficial in some horses with insect hypersensitivity when administered orally at a dose of 200 to 500 mg every 8 to 12 hours.[33] This drug also has been useful in managing insect-induced urticaria. Side effects associated with hydroxyzine in horses include sedation or hyperactivity. If the horse does not respond after hydroxyzine administration, one may try systemic corticosteroids. The recommended dosage for prednisolone is 1 mg/kg orally administered daily until the pruritus is relieved (usually 1 to 2 weeks); the dose is then tapered to the lowest effective every-other-day dose.

Anecdotal reports suggest that a DMSO dervivative, methylsulfonyl methane, may be effective as an aid to relieve pruritus associated with equine insect hypersensitivity. This medication is available as a powder to be sprinkled on food and should be used according to label directions.

Fatty acids have been recommended for control of pruritus associated with insect hypersensitivity.[21,33] The effectiveness of this therapy may depend on dose and fatty acid source. One study in Florida used flaxseed oil in horses with *Culicoides* spp. hypersensitivity and found no benefit in decreasing pruritus.[34] A study in Canada demonstrated that flaxseed meal was beneficial in treating pruritus in horses with *Culicoides* spp. hypersensitivity.[35] These apparently disparate results may be explained by geographic factors or the source of flaxseed.

Food Allergy

Documented cases of feed-related hypersensitivity are rare in horses, and most information on this condition is based on anecdotal reports. Food hypersentitivity refers to an immune-mediated adverse reaction to a feedstuff unrelated to any physiologic effect of the feed. The pathogenesis of dietary hypersensitivity in horses is understood poorly but is believed to involve type I, type II, and type IV hypersensitivity reactions. The skin, respiratory tract, and gastrointestinal tract may be affected. The most commonly incriminated foods include potatoes, malt, beet pulp, buckwheat, fish meal, wheat, alfalfa, red and white clover, St. John's wort, chicory, glucose, barley, bran, oats, and tonics.[34]

Dermatologic manifestations of food allergy include generalized pruritus with or without papules, urticaria, and pruritus ani. Flatulence, loose stools, heaves, or asthma may accompany skin lesions.

The diagnosis is made by eliminating the more common causes of pruritus in horses and by positive response to a food elimination trial (Figure 13-9). Hypoallergenic diets are individualized for each patient, and obtaining a thorough dietary history from the owner is critical. One must identify any change in the diet (vitamin supplements, grains, hays). A practical approach is to start by eliminating any supplements and concentrates from the diet. The trial should not include dusty feedstuffs because some horses can develop inhalant allergy to feedstuffs. The horse should be fed oats and grass hay for 4 to 8 weeks and observed whether a decrease in pruritus occurs. In the South, coastal Bermuda grass hay tends to be less allergenic than other types of hay. If the horse is notably less pruritic, one should reinstitute the previous diet to confirm that the pruritus is caused by a food allergy and that improvement was not coincidental. If food allergy is present, pruritus will return, and one should reinstitute the hypoallergenic diet until clinical signs subside. The offending substance is identified by reintroducing one dietary item at a time each week and observing the horse for recurrence of clinical signs.

Contact Allergy

True contact allergies are rare in horses, perhaps in part because the hair coat acts as a protective barrier. Irritant contact reactions are more common (see the following discussion). Contact allergies, when they occur, are type IV hypersensitivity reactions. Potential allergens are usually small molecules that penetrate the skin, bind to dermal collagen or carrier proteins,

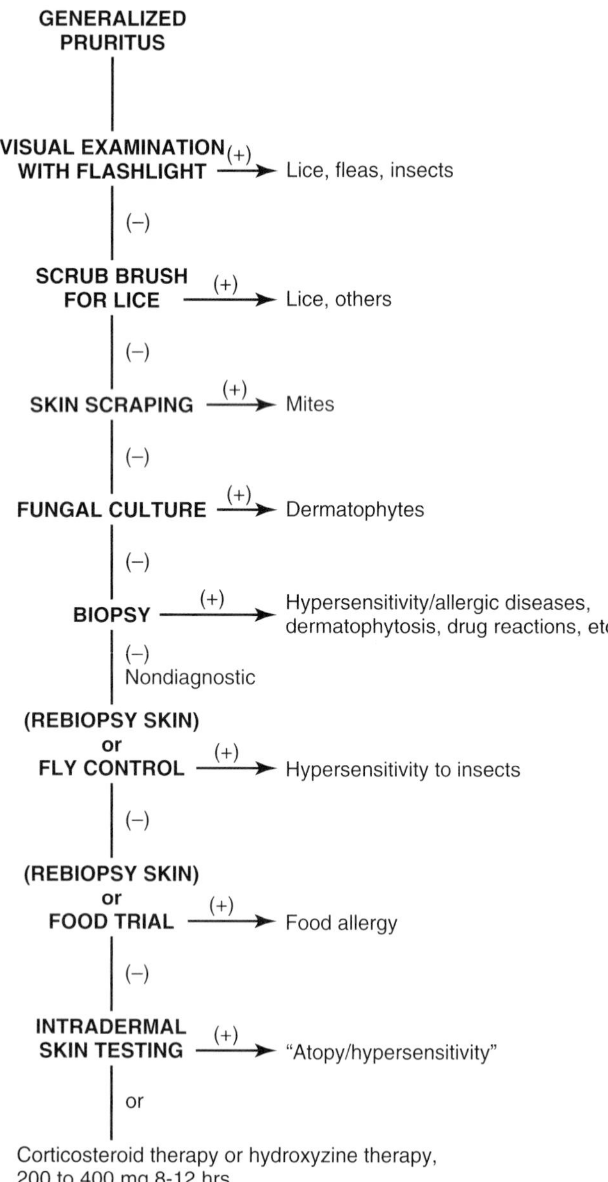

FIGURE 13-9 Flowchart for diagnosis of equine pruritic skin diseases.

and are taken up by antigen-presenting cells (Langerhans cells) in the dermis. On re-exposure, an inflammatory response occurs that results in skin disease. Development of allergic contact reactions usually takes months to years.

Contact reactions most likely are related to pasture plants, changes in bedding material, insect repellents, topical medication, and tack items.[1,36] Parasiticides and bath oils applied as insect repellents are the most commonly identified causes of contact allergy. Repeated application of chemicals to the coat of sweating horses may lead to development of a contact allergy by compromising the protective barrier of the skin.

Clinical signs of contact allergy vary and depend on the duration of the allergic reaction. Erythema, swelling, oozing, pain, or pruritus develops within 2 to 3 days of application of the offending substance. If untreated, lesions often progress over weeks or months to alopecia, lichenification, and crusting. The distribution of the lesions may suggest the cause: legs (plants, bedding), face and muzzle (plants, bedding), face and trunk (tack), and face, ear, neck, and trunk (insect repellents).[1]

A definitive diagnosis is based on provocative exposure or patch testing. Provocative exposure requires avoiding the suspect substance for 10 days or until lesions resolve, re-exposing the horse to the substance, and noting recurrence of lesions or clinical signs over the next 7 to 10 days.[1] Provocative testing does not distinguish between an irritant reaction and an allergic reaction but does identify the offending substance. Patch testing requires the application of the suspect substance to an area of the skin for 48 to 72 hours. Plant material, bedding, or other particulate matter does not adhere well to the skin and is tested best under an occlusive dressing (closed patch test). For each test substance, one clips a 3-cm^2 area of hair on the thorax or dorsum, applies a small amount of the suspect substance to the skin, and covers the site with a gauze sponge bandage for 48 to 72 hours. A control site should also be bandaged. On removing the bandages, the area is assessed for erythema, swelling, induration, pain, and exudation. Biopsies of the control should be obtained and the site or sites tested for histologic confirmation of the diagnosis. One may apply liquid substances to the skin daily and avoid using an occlusive bandage.

Successful treatment requires accurate identification of the offending substance and avoidance. If identification is not possible, one may prescribe short-term systemic corticosteroid therapy and mild cleansing shampoos.

ATOPY

Atopy is an inherited dermatologic or respiratory condition in horses. Horses with atopy develop senstitizing antibodies, immunoglobulin E, to offending allergens. Allergens that have been implicated in this problem include molds, grasses, trees, fabrics, and dust. One or more of these allergens may be involved in an individual horse.[37]

Sensitizing antibodies cross-link mast cells, triggering release of inflammatory mediators with resultant inflammation in the affected target organ (i.e., skin or respiratory tract). In skin, pruritus is the end result.[33,37]

Arabian and Thoroughbred horses appear to be predisposed to develop atopy.[33] This breed predisposition suggests equine atopy may be an inherited condition. In one report a stallion and five of his offspring had atopy-induced urticaria.[38] A more recent California study further substantiates the idea that equine atopy is inherited.[39] According to this report, Thoroughbreds accounted for 25% of the horses with atopy. Interestingly, male horses were twice as likely to develop atopy when compared with female horses. The exact mode of inheritance and importance of this more recent sex difference is not known.

Atopy in horses is characterized as a seasonal to nonseasonal pruritic skin disease. Several types of skin lesions are observable, including alopecia, excoriations, crusts, scales, erythema, and hives (urticaria).[40] Urticaria is not always pruritic in horses. A tentative diagnosis of atopy can be made after eliminating other causes of pruritus and on positive response to exogenous corticosteroids.

The most effective way to confirm a diagnosis of equine atopy is by intradermal skin testing. One sedates the horse with xylazine at 0.05 mg/kg intravenously and clips a rectangular area on the lateral aspect of the neck. One then injects allergens known to cause allergic problems in a particular geographic area intradermally and denotes each site of allergen injection on the skin by a dot made with permanent marker. The practitioner reads the test at specific time intervals after injection—15 minutes, 30 minutes, 4 to 6 hours, and 24 hours—then compares the negative (sterile saline) and positive (histamine 1:100,000 weight to volume) control reactions to reactions of the various allergens. The negative control is assigned an arbitrary grade of 0 and the positive control a grade of 4. One considers size of the wheal, firmness, redness, and shape when grading individual allergen reactions. Reactions greater than or equal to 2 are considered potentially significant. The history, clinical signs, and pollination times must be considered in the final determination of whether individual reactions are significant.

Certain allergens tend to cause many false-positive reactions, including alfalfa, corn, corn smut, grain dust, grain smut, black ants, mosquitoes, fire ants, *Rhizopus* spp., *Penicillium* spp., sheep wool epithelium, English plantain, red mulberry, black willow, mesquite, and dock sorrel. If a reaction occurs with one of these allergens and is inconsistent with the history and physical examination findings, it is probably an irritant reaction.

Horses with laminitis tend to have hyperresponsive immune systems and may be more likely to have false-positive skin test reactions than normal horses.[41] If the horse has had laminitis, skin test results should be interpreted with care.

Drugs such as corticosteroids, antihistamines, fatty acids, and those that affect vasodilation such as acepromazine may interfere with skin test results and cause false-negative reactions. To prevent this situation from occurring, one should observe drug withdrawal times. Exact withdrawal times are extrapolated from small animal medicine and applied to horses. Administering long-acting injectable corticosteroids should be avoided for 3 months before skin testing, oral or injectable dexamethasone for at least 1 month before skin testing, and antihistamines for 7 to 10 days before testing. A withdrawal time of 7 days is recommended for acepromazine.

Serum allergy testing has been recommended for diagnosis of atopy in horses. However, recent studies question the validity of this test. One study compared test results of three different serum allergy tests with intradermal skin test results in the same animal.[42] None of the three serum allergy tests reliably detected allergen hypersensitivity compared with results of the intradermal skin test. Serum allergy tests were not as sensitive as intradermal skin tests. At this time, in human and veterinary medicine, intradermal skin testing is considered the gold standard for confirming a diagnosis of atopy.[37]

Treatment of atopy should include hyposensitization whenever possible. The offending allergens are administered at a set amount and time to the horse. Many horses are treated with a maintenance schedule of 1 ml of a 20,000 protein nitrogen unit aqueous solution administered subcutaneously every 3 weeks. The exact mechanism of action for hyposensitization therapy is not known. Human beings with allergies tend to have a higher proportion of type 1 T helper cells compared with type 2 T helper cells.[43] After hyposensitization therapy the T helper cell populations shift toward normal. Other theories suggest that blocking antibodies are produced with hyposensitization. Regardless of the exact mechanism of action, hyposensitization therapy has been effective in human beings for more than 30 years.[44] The percentage of horses that respond to therapy varies and is thought to be similar to that in small animal medicine (59% to 86% effective).[44,45] Hyposensitization therapy may take 1 to 12 months (average 3 to 6 months) before it starts to work. One may use corticosteroids, antihistamines, and fatty acids in the period between initiation of hyposensitization therapy and expected response.

Corticosteroids are a mainstay of therapy for allergies but have been associated with a variety of adverse effects, including polyuria, polydipsia, increased suspectibility to infection, mood changes, elevations in liver enzymes, and laminitis.[46] The most commonly used corticosteroids in equine dermatology are prednisolone and dexamethasone. The dosage for prednisolone for treating atopy is 0.5 to 1.5 mg/kg daily as an induction dose (usually 4 to 14 days) tapered to 0.2 to 0.5 mg/kg every 48 hours for maintenance or 200 to 400 mg/500-kg horse every 24 hours. Prednisone is absorbed poorly from the intestine of many horses after oral administration and should not be used. The recommended dosage for dexamethasone is 0.04 to 0.2 mg/kg administered orally, intramuscularly, or intravenously every 24 to 48 hours for 4 to 7 days, decreasing to a maintance dose of 0.01 to 0.02 mg/kg every 48 hours. Another dosage for dexamethasone for treating atopy is 0.05 to 0.1 mg/kg every 24 hours either oral or injected intramuscularly or intravenously. Although the injectable dexamethasone has been used orally, the bioavailability of the injectable form of dexamethasone orally is only 60% to 70% of the injectable route. A tablet form for dexamethasone is available and appears to be effective.[39] Several antihistamines have been recommended for treating equine atopy.[39] Hydroxyzine is recommended at 200 to 400 mg orally, regardless of body mass, every 12 hours orally, 1.5 mg/kg orally every 8 to 12 hours, or 200 to 500 mg/500 kg orally every 8 to 12 hours. Other antihistamines that have been used include chlorpheniramine maleate (0.26 mg/kg every 12 hours orally), diphenhydramine (0.75 to 1 mg/kg every 12 hours orally), doxepin hydrochloride (300 to 400 mg every 12 hours or 0.5 to 0.75 mg/kg every 12 hours or 300 to 600 mg/500-kg horse orally every 12 hours), and pyrilamine maleate (0.8 to 1.32 mg/kg intravenously, intramuscularly, or subcutaneously; may be repeated in 6 to 12 hours if needed). The author has used all of these medications in horses and believes that hydroxyzine and chlorpheniramine maleate work most consistently in horses. Side effects associated with antihistamine use include sedation and behavior changes.

Fatty acids can act synergistically with steroids and antihistamines to decrease inflammation. Ω-3 and Ω-6 fatty acids seem to be most beneficial. They shift products of the arachidonic acid cascade from more inflammatory to less inflammatory mediators.[47]

Many fatty acid supplements are currently available, including Derm Caps ES (DVM Pharmaceuticals, Miami, Fla.), Derm Caps 100 (DVM Pharmaceuticals), Glänzen 3 (Horse Tech, Lawrence, Iowa), and Platinum Performance (Platinum Performance, Inc., Buellton, Calif.). The first two products are available as a capsule or liquid, whereas the last product is a powder to be sprinkled on food.

Dosage varies according to the fatty acid product used. The dosage for Derm Caps ES is five capsules every 12 hours; the dosage for Derm Caps 100 is two to three capsules every 12 hours. The dosage for the Glanzen 3 is 2- to 6-oz powder sprinkled on the food per day (not to exceed 6 oz per day). This product also contains biotin and other vitamins and minerals. The Platinum Performance is used according to label directions.

Topical treatments may be a useful adjunct therapy for horses with atopy. Various shampoos, lotions, and sprays marketed for use in small animals may be of benefit in horses. Antipruritic ingredients may include oatmeal, aloe, pramoxine, and hydrocortisone. Combination products may be most effective. The author prefers the Relief products marketed by DVM Pharmaceuticals of Miami, Florida, that contain oatmeal and pramoxine. These products may be used daily or weekly.

CUTANEOUS DRUG REACTIONS

Cutaneous drug reactions in horses are rare and can mimic any known skin disease. Drug reactions are believed to involve type I, II, III, or IV hypersensitivity reactions. Any therapeutic agent administered by any route may cause a drug reaction. The most commonly incriminated drugs are penicillin, streptomycin, oxytetracycline, neomycin, chloramphenicol, sulfonamides, phenothiazines, phenylbutazone, guaifenesin, aspirin, and glucocorticoids. Clinical signs vary, and pruritus may or may not be present. Urticaria is a commonly observed skin reaction. Less commonly, mucocutaneous ulceration or vesiculation may be present.

The diagnosis of a drug reaction depends on an accurate medication history. Skin biopsies may be helpful in supporting a clinical diagnosis. The most commonly reported patterns of inflammation are perivascular dermatitis and intraepidermal or subepidermal vesicular dermatitis.[1] One can confirm the diagnosis by provocative challenge, but this may lead to anaphylaxis or death and therefore is not recommended.

Treatment requires removal of the offending drug, symptomatic therapy, and avoiding related compounds. Drugs reactions, in general, do not respond well to glucocorticoids. A drug reaction usually subsides within 2 to 3 weeks but may last for months.

CAUSES OF PRURITUS: CRUSTING AND EXFOLIATIVE DERMATOSES

Dermatophytosis and bacterial skin infections may cause pruritus in horses. They are recognized more commonly in the field as crusting or exfoliative dermatoses.

Common Causes of Scaling and Crusting Dermatoses

Exfoliative dermatoses in horses have a wide range of causes. Historical and physical findings are important in differentiating these diseases. To make a diagnosis in difficult cases may require skin scrapings, fungal cultures, bacterial cultures, mince preparations of crusts for cytologic examination of dermatophilosis, and skin biopsies. If cost constraints are present the most useful diagnostic test is a carefully obtained skin biopsy. Not scrubbing or preparing the skin in any way before obtaining skin biopsy specimens is critical. In addition, one should take extreme care to collect the crust when obtaining a skin biopsy from a horse with exfoliative skin disease. In many instances, one obtains the causative agent or evidence of a definitive diagnosis from histopathologic examination of the crust. Figure 13-10 shows a simplified approach to the diagnosis of exfoliative dermatoses.

Infectious Causes of Exfoliation

DERMATOPHILOSIS (RAIN SCALD)

Dermatophilosis is a bacterial skin disease of horses and other large animals caused by the gram-positive, facultative anaerobic actinomycete *Dermatophilus congolensis*. The normal habitat of the organism is unknown, but the organism is thought to exist in a quiescent state on carrier animals until conditions are optimal for proliferation.[48] Whether carrier animals act as reservoirs of infection for other animals is unknown. However, one recent report suggests that dermatophilosis in horses can be zoonotic. In this report, a young girl riding a horse that had dermatophilosis contracted the bacteria and needed to be treated for this infection.[49]

The development of lesions depends on chronic moisture and skin damage.[1,48] The organism cannot penetrate intact healthy skin, and moisture is required for release of zoospores. The skin can be damaged from chronic maceration caused by moisture, biting flies, vegetation, or underlying pruritic skin diseases. Chronic moisture is more conducive to the growth of the organism than intermittent but heavy rainfall. When these two prerequisites (moisture and trauma) are met, the organism multiplies. Moisture induces release of infective, motile, flagellated zoospores. These organisms are attracted to low concentrations of carbon dioxide and repelled by high concentrations of carbon dioxide. As the organism multiplies and inflammatory cells migrate into the area the carbon dioxide concentration in the skin increases and zoospores migrate toward the surface of the skin in search of a more suitable environment. The organism again multiplies and numbers increase. This cycle repeats until layering, crusting, and matting of the hair coat results. Zoospores remain viable in crusts at ambient temperatures of 28° to 31° C for up to 42 months.[48]

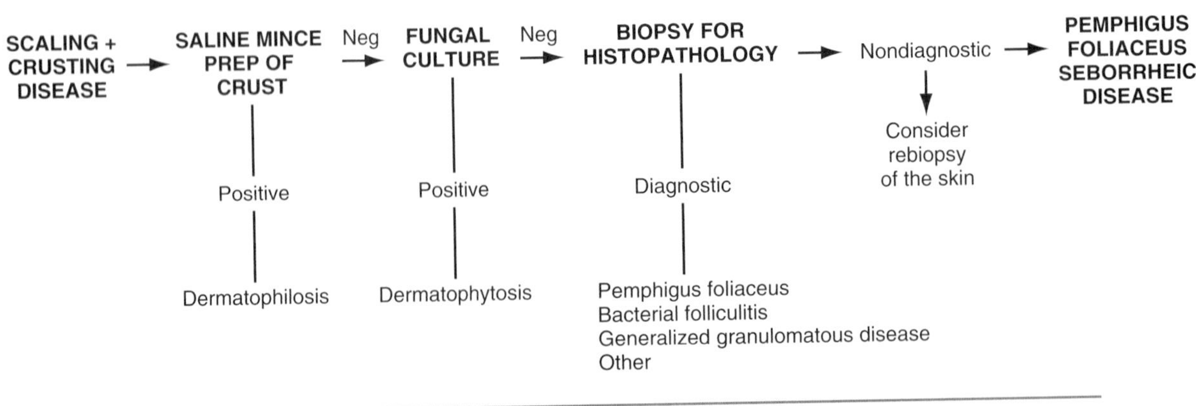

FIGURE 13-10 Flowchart for diagnosis of equine scaling and crusting diseases.

Clinical signs of dermatophilosis can develop within 24 hours. The disease has a follicular orientation, and lesions appear as crusted, moist mats of hair that can resemble small paintbrushes. Under fresh crusts, the skin is soft, exudative, and yellow-tinged. Exudative crusted lesions tend to occur on the back, gluteal area, face, neck, and distal extremities (Figure 13-11). Lesions on the limbs may cause pain, swelling, and erythema, especially in white or lightly pigmented areas. Racehorses or horses in training commonly develop abrasions on the cranial surface of the hindlegs. These lesions are prime sites for infection. Severely affected horses may be febrile, depressed, lethargic, and anorectic and have a regional lymphadenopathy.

Dermatophilosis is diagnosed by demonstration of the organism by cytologic examination of the crust or by histologic examination of a skin biopsy specimen. Dermatophilosis preparations can be made from dried or fresh crusts or from direct smears of exudate. Dried crusts are finely minced in a few drops of sterile saline, allowing the preparation to dry for 45 minutes and then staining it. A fast Giemsa, Diff Quik, or Gram stain can be used for direct smears or dried mince preparations. The organism is visualized best under 1000× oil immersion and appears as fine-branching multiseptate hyphae with transverse and longitudinally arranged cocci (railroad track appearance; Figure 13-12). When a skin biopsy is collected from a horse with suspected dermatophilosis, submitting a specimen with the crust attached to the skin or hairs is important. Key histologic findings include folliculitis, intraepidermal pustules, intradermal edema, and alternating layers of parakeratotic (epidermal cells with retained nuclei) and orthokeratotic (keratinized epidermal cells without nuclei) hyperkeratosis with leukocyte debris.[44] The organism is oftent found only in crusts.

The practitioner may treat horses with mild infections with topical therapy alone. One should gently soak and remove crusts using a mild antibacterial shampoo such as chlorhexidine or benzoyl peroxide. Some horses for which this treatment is difficult or painful may require sedation. One should dry the horse with towels and apply a topical antibacterial sponge-on dip (chlorhexidine 1:32 dilution of 2% stock solution or lime sulfur 1:32 dilution of stock solution). Another option is a commercially prepared chlorhexidene 2% lotion (Resi-Chlor, Vibrac, Fort Worth, Tex.). This formulation is a leave-on product with residual properties. Daily shampoo therapy should continue for 5 to 7 days until healing is evident then twice weekly until all lesions have resolved. Horses with lesions on the muzzle may benefit from a topical cream with or without corticosteroids. Severely affected animals may benefit greatly from systemic antibiotics, such as procaine penicillin at 22,000 IU/kg intramuscularly twice daily for 5 to 7 days. Trimethoprim sulfa (TMS) at 10 to 15 mg/kg orally twice daily for 5 to 7 days also may be effective. In either case, one should eliminate exposure to excessive moisture and skin trauma. However, some cases of dermatophilosis do not appear to be responsive to TMS. In these cases, doxycyline at a dose of 10 mg/kg every 12 hours with food has been used and appears to be effective. In vivo sensitivity results suggest that doxycyline is a reasonable option for refractory cases of dermatophilosis.[50]

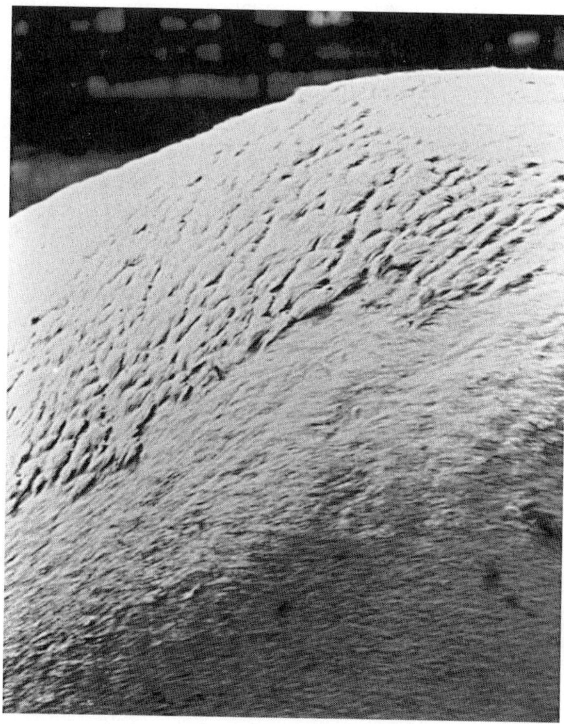

FIGURE 13-11 Horse with matting of coat caused by dermatophilosis.

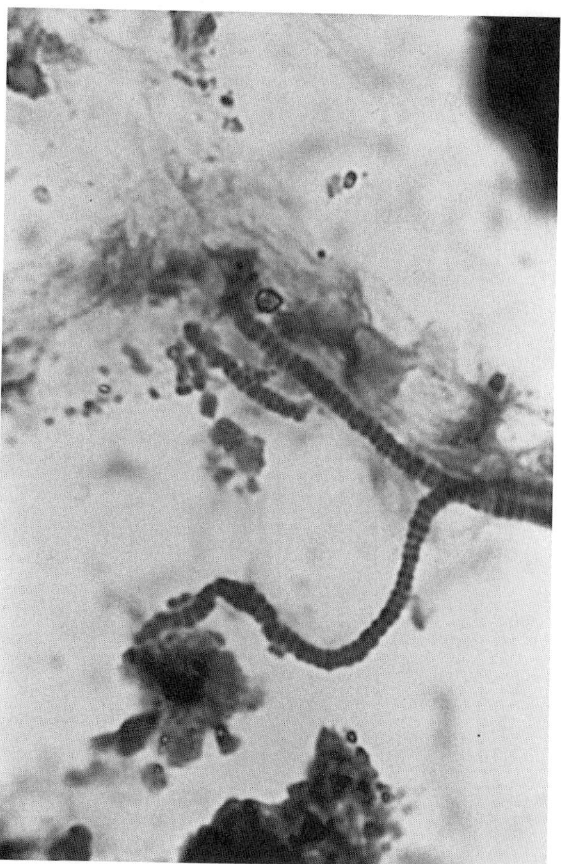

FIGURE 13-12 Microscopic appearance of *Dermatophilus congolensis*.

DERMATOPHYTOSIS (RINGWORM)

Dermatophytosis is the most common contagious skin disease in the horse. *Trichophyton equinum, T. mentagrophytes, Microsporum gypseum*, and *M. canis* are the most frequent isolates.[51] The infection is self-limiting but may affect the function of the horse seriously and is of zoonotic importance.

Dermatophytes are transmitted by direct contact with an infected host or by indirect contact with contaminated fomites or the environment. Illness, poor nutrition, overcrowding, age (young or old immunosuppressed individuals), and stress predispose horses to infection. Chronic moisture from sweating or the environment damages the protective barrier of the skin, enhancing the opportunity for infection. When fungal spores contact the hair coat, the spores may be removed mechanically, may be unable to compete with the normal flora of the skin, or may remain on the coat in a dormant state until conditions are optimal for infection. Dermatophytes invade keratin of the epidermis and hair with the aid of enzymes that are allergenic to the host. Dermatophytosis is considered a biologic contact dermatitis.[51] The incubation period is usually several weeks. During this time, fungi invade the epidermal keratin, hair follicles, and the hair shaft itself. The epidermis responds to the intruder by increasing epidermal cell turnover in an effort to remove the fungi mechanically. Clinically the response is scaling. Hair shaft integrity is compromised, and hairs fall out or are fractured easily, resulting in areas of alopecia characteristic of the disease. Infection is eliminated from a particular hair on shedding or as it enters the telogen stage, or the dermatophyte elicits an inflammatory response.

Clinical signs of dermatophytosis, including pain and pruritus, vary. The infection is follicular in distribution, and early lesions often begin as a papular eruption with erect hairs (Figure 13-13). Urticarial eruption may occur 24 to 72 hours before the owner notices the papules.[52] Lesions rapidly progress to crusted papules that spread circumferentially. The classic lesion is a circular patch of alopecia with stubbly hairs on the margin and variable amounts of scaling (Figure 13-14). Erythema and hyperpigmentation may be present. In rare instances, dermatophytosis may cause generalized scaling without significant hair loss. If the dermatophytosis causes follicular rupture, nodules, and ulcers, or a kerion reaction (inflammatory dermatophyte infection that may resemble an abscess) may develop. Lesions are most common in areas where tack contacts the skin but may be limited to the posterior pastern. Rarely, dermatophytes can cause coronary band disease.[53]

The diagnosis is made by demonstration and identification of the organism. Wood's lamp examinations are not useful for logistic reasons and, more importantly, because few cases of equine dermatophytosis are caused by *M. canis*. Direct examination of hair and scale is useful but requires special training. The most reliable tests are fungal culture and skin biopsy. The details of superficial fungal culture techniques have been reviewed elsewhere.[1,27] One should collect hairs for culture from the periphery of a newly developing lesion. Avoiding areas that may have been treated previously is critical. One should wipe the area gently with an alcohol swab before collecting hair samples to minimize growth of contaminants, should pluck hairs in the direction of growth, and transport them to the laboratory or clinic in a paper envelope for inoculation on dermatophyte test medium or Sab-Duets plates (Bacti-Labs, Mountain View, Calif.), the commercial fungal culture media preferred by most veterinary dermatologists. Each plate contains Sabouraud's glucose medium and dermatophyte test medium. Using both media plates greatly enhances the culturing of suspect organisms. *Trichophyton* spp. isolation improves if a few drops of B vitamin complex is added to the surface of the media and the plate is incubated at 37° C. Because *T. equinum* is supposed to be one of the more common equine dermatophytes, one should add the B vitamin complex to all equine fungal cultures. One should select skin biopsy sites with care and should not scrub or wipe the area before sampling. Early lesions with crusts are ideal. Histologic findings include folliculitis, perifolliculitis, and furunculosis; superficial perivascular dermatitis with ortho- or parakeratosis; and intraepidermal vesicular or pustular dermatitis. Septate fungal hyphae and oval spores may be present in the superficial keratin or hair follicle.[1]

Dermatophytosis is a self-limiting disease, and most cases heal spontaneously within 1 to 6 months. Treatment is strongly advised to minimize contagion to other animals and human beings. In horses, antifungal shampoos and sponge-on dips are the treatment of choice. The author has found the most effective topical treatment combination to be weekly

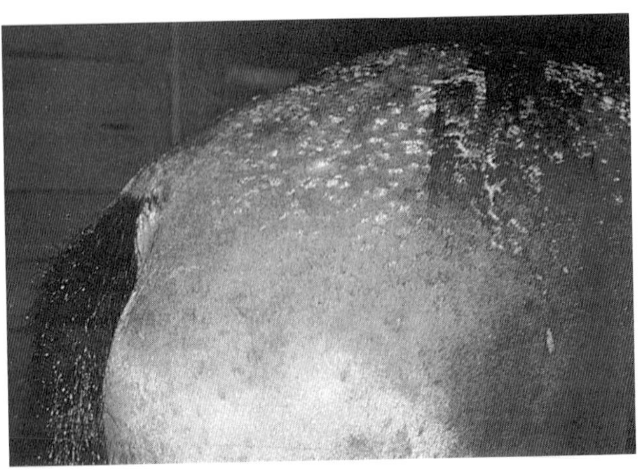

FIGURE 13-13 Dermatophytosis. The papular eruption on the advancing edge of lesions is notable.

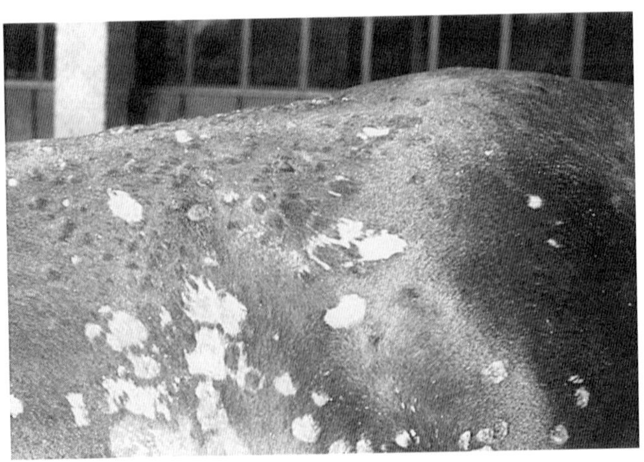

FIGURE 13-14 Classic signs of dermatophytosis (ringworm).

bathing with a shampoo that contains 2% miconazole followed by a lime sulfur dip (Lym-Dyp; DVM Pharmaceuticals, Miami, Fla.), or lime sulfur dip (DermPet, Potomac, Md.) for 4 to 8 weeks. Another alternative is a miconazole and chlorhexidene shampoo (Malaseb; DVM Pharmaceuticals) followed by a micronazole and chlorhexidene rinse (Malaseb rinse, DVM Pharmaceuticals, Miami, FL). A less-expensive topical alternative that has been used is a dilute bleach solution (1:10 in water). This bleach solution is messy, odiferous, and staining. Systemic antifungal drugs, such as griseofulvin (50 mg/kg orally once daily or 100 mg/kg once daily for 7 to 10 days) or itraconazole (5 to 10 mg/kg orally once daily) are effective but expensive. Alternatively, intravenous injections of 20% sodium iodine or 250 ml/500-kg horse every 7 days for one to two treatments has also been used. This treatment is contraindicated in pregnant mares given that sodium iodine systemically has been shown to induce abortion.[53] In instances in which treating an infected herd is necessary or desirable, itraconazole at 5 to 10 mg/kg orally once daily for 15 days aborts the infection. Concurrent topical therapy with lime sulfur is necessary.

Elimination of dermatophytosis from single or multiple horse barns requires elimination of the organism from infected hosts and decontamination of the environment. Box 13-4 summarizes one approach to treatment. Commercial antifungal vaccines for equine dermatophytosis are not available in the United States. Autogenous vaccines are not recommended at this time because of lack of information on their efficacy and potential for serious adverse effects, including sterile abscesses, hypersensitivity reactions, generalized anaphylaxis, and death.

BOX 13-4

TREATMENT OF EQUINE DERMATOPHYTOSIS (RINGWORM, FUNGUS) IN MULTIPLE HORSES

In the treatment of ringworm or superficial fungal infections of the skin, one must accomplish three things:

1. Kill the fungus on the animal to stop progression of the disease.
2. Kill the fungus on the animal to prevent spread to other animals, human beings, and the environment.
3. Decontaminate the environment.

The following suggestions have been helpful when treating outbreaks in the multiple-horse barn. Fungal infections may take 6 to 8 weeks to heal completely.

1. Isolate all affected horses from normal horses.
2. Treat the barn by cleaning out all bedding and spraying stalls and exposed surfaces with 1:10 dilution of household bleach.
3. Treat all affected horses daily with lime sulfur sponge-on preparations (4 oz/gal) for 7 days and then once weekly. Treating the entire body of each horse, not just the affected areas, is vital. One should allow sponge-on preparations to dry on the horse and should not bathe horses between treatments.
4. Use individual brushes and tack for each horse. Disinfect brushes and tack frequently. Do not transfer equipment between horses.
5. Blankets should be disinfected with household bleach twice weekly or more often. Not using blankets or sheets is best to prevent enhancing the spread of the lesions.
6. Ideally, the persons who handle affected horses should not handle normal horses. If this precaution is not possible, one should handle normal horses first and then affected horses. Washing thoroughly between animals with a chlorhexidine scrub is important.
7. Ringworm is contagious to other animals and human beings; handlers should be careful to wash thoroughly and report the development of any lesions. If possible, handlers should wear gloves when handling affected horses.
8. Ideally, horses affected with ringworm should be rested from training or riding until lesions are gone. Continued riding or training may contribute to skin microtrauma and spread of infection.

Modified from client education handouts used at the College of Veterinary Medicine, University of Florida, and the School of Veterinary Medicine, University of Wisconsin.

BACTERIAL INFECTIONS

Bacterial folliculitis in horses is caused most commonly by *Staphyloccoccus* spp. *Streptococcus* spp. infections also may occur. Infections most frequently occur in the summer when heat, moisture, increased insect populations, and increased use of the horse act in concert as predisposing factors.

The pathogenesis of bacterial folliculitis in the horse is similar to that in other animals. The causative agents are normally found on the host; when the natural protective barrier of the skin is compromised, bacteria invade and multiply within hair follicles. Infection results in inflammation, destruction of the hair follicle, and shedding of the hair. As the infection spreads, lesions enlarge. If hair follicles rupture, furunculosis and deep pyoderma may result.

Clinically, bacterial folliculitis may be indistinguishable from dermatophytosis. Bacterial lesions are much more likely to be painful and are only rarely pruritic. Infection is most common in the saddle and tack area but may be limited to the pastern area. Deep pyoderma of the tail base also occurs.

The definitive diagnosis is made best by cytologic examination, bacterial culture, and skin biopsy. Differentiating bacterial folliculitis from dermatophytosis is important. Skin biopsy reveals varying degrees of folliculitis, intraepidermal pustules, and perivascular inflammation. Neutrophils are the primary inflammatory cell. Keratinocytes often show intracellular edema; parakeratosis and orthokeratosis are common in the crust. Special stains often reveal bacteria within the crusts and hair follicles.

Treatment depends on severity of the clinical signs. Mild infections may be self-limiting but benefit from topical therapy. Severe cases require daily topical antibacterial shampoos with benzoyl peroxide or chlorhexidine and oral antibiotics. Ideally, systemic antibiotic therapy should be based on results of culture and sensitivity testing, but procaine penicillin at 22,000 IU/kg intramuscularly every 12 hours until resolution of clinical signs is usually effective.[1] A minimum of 10 to 14 days of therapy is recommended.

Nutritional Causes of Exfoliation

Nutritional deficiencies are rare in horses, and much of this information has been extrapolated from work in other species or experimentally induced deficiencies.

PROTEIN

Protein deficiency may occur in horses with fever, dysphagia, burns, proteinuria, liver disease, gastrointestinal diseases, or any disease in which metabolic demand increases and production of protein decreases. The skin uses 25% to 30% of the daily protein intake for hair production and maintenance of the epidermis,[54] a requirement that may increase fivefold in disease states. In experimental deficiencies created in ruminants and laboratory animals, protein-deficient animals develop dry, dull, brittle, thin hair. Prolonged shedding also occurs.[1] Presumably, horses with protein-deficient diets would exhibit similar clinical signs.

ZINC

Naturally occurring zinc deficiencies have not been reported in horses. Classically this deficiency appears as crusting skin disease. Experimentally induced zinc deficiencies in foals resulted in alopecia, dense scaling on the lower limb that progressed to the trunk, inappetence, decreased growth rate, and decreased tissue and serum zinc concentrations.[1] The definitive diagnosis is made by observing histologic lesions compatible with zinc deficiency (diffuse epidermal and follicular parakeratosis) and response to oral supplementation with zinc sulfate at 10 mg/kg once daily. A significant response usually occurs within 2 to 3 weeks, and therapy may or may not be lifelong.

IODINE

Suspected iodism caused by excessive supplementation therapeutically or in feeds has been reported in horses.[55] Noncutaneous signs include cough, lacrimation, nasal discharge, and joint pain. Severe dry seborrhea with or without dorsal alopecia is also present. No treatment is necessary, and horses recover spontaneously on removal of the source of excess iodine.

Parasitic Causes of Exfoliation

Insect hypersensitivities (discussed earlier) are the most common parasitic cause of exfoliation in horses. The major differentiating feature is the presence of pruritus, lack of a circumferentially spreading lesion, and the absence of pain. Skin biopsy findings of superficial or deep eosinophilic perivascular dermatitis with or without collagen degeneration suggest insect hypersensitivity.

Immunologic Causes of Exfoliation: Pemphigus Foliaceus

Pemphigus foliaceus (PF) is a rare autoimmune skin disease that results in severe crusting and matting of the hair coat. An autoantibody against the glycocalyx of keratinocytes results in the release and activation of keratinocyte proteolytic enzymes into the intercellular space. The glycocalyx is hydrolyzed and intercellular cohesion is lost, leading to acantholysis.[56]

Pemphigus foliaceus has no age or sex predilection. Previous reports suggest that Appaloosa horses appear to be predisposed to developing PF.[57] However, a recent California study suggests that no breed predispostion is involved for horses developing PF. Interestingly, this same study found a statistically significant number of horses developed PF between September and February.[58] The occurrence of seasonality being associated with the development of PF has suggested that an insect hypersensitivity (especially black flies or *Simuliidae* spp.) may play an important role. Another interesting finding was the development of a drug induced PF in one horse treated with trimethoprim sulfa. In humans, thiol group or sulfur molecule has been shown to trigger PF. The sulfa drugs and their metabolites bind to cell membranes as haptens to change conformation of cell-surface antigens. This change causes an inadequate cell adhesion and results in acantholysis.[59,60]

Lesions usually begin on the face and limbs and may take weeks or months before becoming generalized. In some horses the disease affects only the coronary band. One rarely observes the primary lesion, a subcorneal pustule, because of the hair coat of the horse. The most common clinical presentation is severe matting and crusting of the coat with oozing of serum from the skin (Figure 13-15). Most horses are depressed and show signs of systemic illness. Swelling and pain of the distal extremities, in addition to lameness, are common. Pruritus and pain on the trunk, ventral edema, and regional or generalized lymphadenopathy vary. The California PF study found that the most common early clinical sign was edema of the distal legs and ventral abdomen. In the past, the edema was thought to be caused by hypoproteinemia.[58] However, none of the horses with edema also had hypoproteinemia.

The definitive diagnosis is made by routine histologic examination of a skin biopsy specimen. Submitting a skin biopsy with intact crusts attached to the underlying skin or hairs is critical. Histologically, PF is characterized by intragranular to subcorneal acantholysis. One often observes layered rafts of acantholytic cells within crusts interspersed among neutophils.[52] According to one study, approximately one third of the horses with PF will have a predominance of eosinophils in the inflammatory infiltrate.[57] Direct immunofluorescence is unreliable but, if positive, reveals diffuse intercellular fluorescence. One may make a tentative diagnosis of PF based on impression smears of the content of intact pustules or the underside of exudative crusts (Figure 13-16). Rafts of deeply basophilic acantholytic cells and nondegenerate neutrophils are highly suggestive of this disease.

Treatment recommendations vary depending on the age of onset for the PF. PF in horses less than 1 year of age is usually self-limiting. Spontaneous remission is common in foals, and they often do not require long-term therapy. Because treatment is difficult and often unrewarding in adults, many owners elect euthanasia.

When the owner elects to treat the horse, remission and control of the disease is induced with prednisolone at 1 mg/kg orally every 12 hours until no new lesions develop, which usually occurs within 7 to 10 days, at which point alternate-day therapy continues at the same dose. A recommended immunosuppressive dose for dexamethasone is 0.05 to 0.1 mg/kg/day or 20 to 40 mg per horse per day. Chrysotherapy (gold salts) has been used in horses but is expensive.[21,62] One administers two doses of aurothioglucose (Solganal; Schering Corp., Kenilworth, N.J.) 1 week apart intramuscularly, 20 and 40 mg, respectively. If no adverse effects (stomatitis, urticaria, sloughing of skin, blood dyscrasia) are observed, then one begins weekly therapy at 1 mg/kg intramuscularly until observing a response (6 to 12 weeks). Maintenance therapy is tailored to the individual animal, which may involve biweekly or monthly

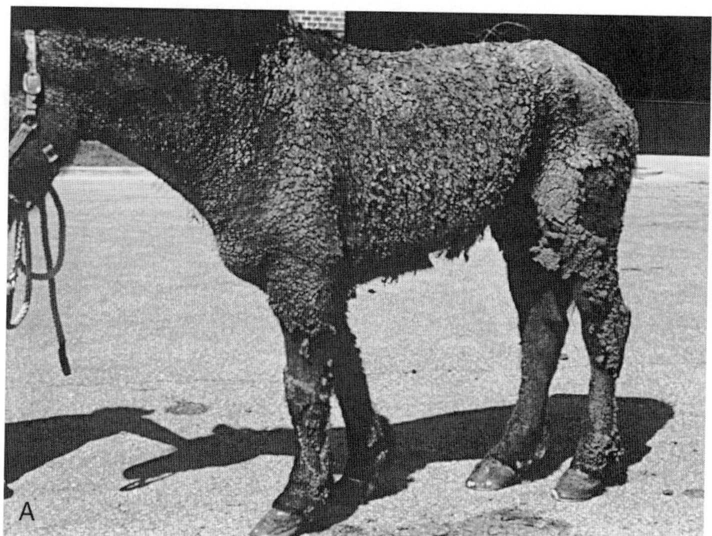

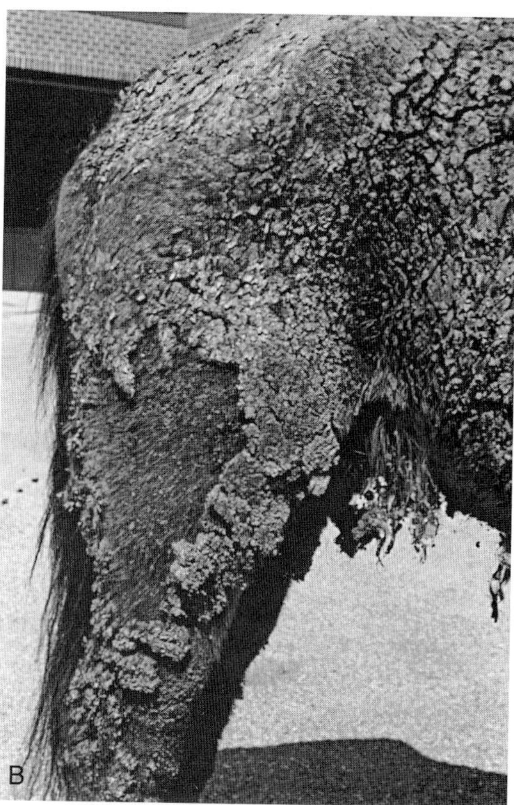

FIGURE 13-15 **A,** Pemphigus foliaceus in a horse. **B,** Skin with significant crusting.

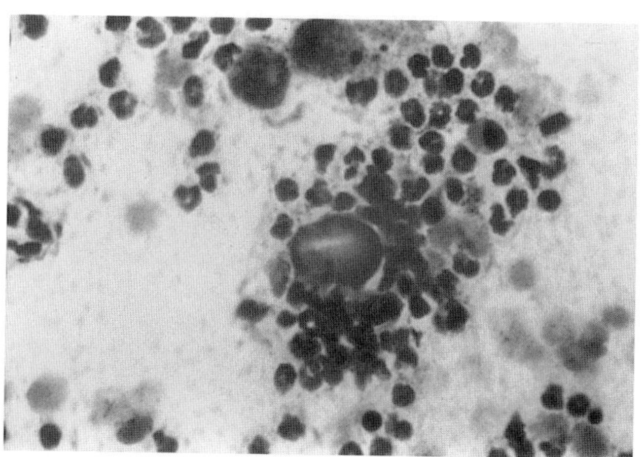

FIGURE 13-16 Cytologic appearance of a touch preparation from a lesion of pemphigus. Rounded cells (acanthocytes) are notable.

therapy. Complete remission of clinical signs may not be possible to achieve even with combination therapy. The most common adverse effects of aurothioglucose therapy in human beings, dogs, and cats are immune-mediated thrombocytopenia and proteinuria. Presumably, these effects could occur in the horse. Weekly monitoring of a complete blood count and urinalysis is recommended for the first month and then monthly if no abnormalities are observed. Aurothioglucose is no longer commercially available. Antedoctal reports suggest that a different gold salt, gold sodium thiomalate (Myochrysine: Merck and Co., White house Station, NJ) may be used in place of the aurothioglucose. The dose and contraindications appear to be the same for both drugs. Azathioprine has also been used as a steroid sparing drug to treat equine PF. The dose for azathioprine is 1 mg/kg/day orally for 14 days then every other day or 2.2 mg/kg every other day orally.

The survival rate for PF-treated horses is reported to be 46% (20 horses total in study). Therefore a guarded prognosis should be given to owners who have horses diagnosed with PF.[58]

Irritant Contact Dermatitis

Irritant contact dermatitis is fairly common in horses. This reaction differs from allergic contact dermatitis because the offending substance invariably causes a reaction if left in contact with the skin; prior sensitization is not needed.

The mechanism of irritant contact reaction depends on the causative chemical, but moisture and tissue maceration are important predisposing factors. Common irritating substances include feces, urine, wound secretions, caustic substances, crude oil, diesel oil, turpentine, blisters, leg sweats, improperly used insecticides, fly wipes, concentrated disinfectants, irritating plants, and soiled bedding.[1]

No age, sex, or breed predilection exists for irritant contact dermatitis.[1,21,63] Direct contact with the offending substance is required for irritant reactions to occur. Acute lesions are often erythematous, vesiculated, erosive or ulcerated, and painful. As the condition continues, necrosis, crusting, scaling, and hair loss occur. Leukoderma and leukotrichia are common and may be permanent. Prutitus and pain vary.

The diagnosis is determined from the history, clinical signs, and inspection of the environment of the horse. Provocative testing is useful in identifying and confirming the causative agent, as long as the risk is minimal to the horse.

Histologic examination of skin reveals necrosis, spongiotic vesicles, and ulceration.

Treatment requires identification and removal of the offending substance. One should wash affected areas daily with copious amounts of water and apply topical 0.5% chlorhexidine soaks. Astringent topical solutions, for example, aluminum acetate (Domeboro, available as an over-the-counter preparation), may be beneficial but often cause pain or delay wound healing. Topical antimicrobial creams free of corticosteroids may promote healing. Healing is usually rapid once the irritant is removed.

Allergic Contact Dermatitis

Allergic contact dermatitis has been discussed. An important note is that allergic contact dermatitis may cause scaling and crusting in addition to pruritus. Lesions are usually distributed in a pattern that reflects the offending substance.

Photodermatitis

Photodermatitis is caused directly by sunburn or indirectly by photoallergy or photosensitization.

SUNBURN

Sunburn is a phototoxic reaction caused by excessive exposure to ultraviolet B light. Horses with white or light skin or hair are at risk. Affected areas become erythematous and scaly. If sunburn is severe, necrosis and exudation may occur. The diagnosis is based on history and clinical signs. Topical glucocorticoid creams alleviate pain, but excessive use has the potential to cause minor adverse effects (depigmentation, failure, or slowing of hair regrowth) or possibly serious adverse effects (laminitis) because these drugs are absorbed systemically. Stabling horses during periods of intense sunlight and application of water-repellent sunscreens may be helpful.

PHOTOALLERGY

Photoallergy is believed to be caused by contact with a chemical or plant (species unknown) and ultraviolet light. The condition is observed most commonly on white muzzles and extremities of horses housed on pasture containing clover, particularly alsike clover. Erythema, vesicles, and crusts develop. The diagnosis is determined by clinical findings. If one cannot identify the offending substance and remove it from the environment, then horses should be stabled during daylight, if possible, to minimize exposure to the offending substance.

PHOTOSENSITIZATION

Photosensitization may develop as a result of hepatogenous photosensitization, aberrant pigmentation formation, or ingestion, injection, or topical application of a primary photodynamic agent.[1,4] Examples of plants known to cause primary photosensitization in horses include St. John's wort, buckwheat, perennial rye grass, and burr trefoil. Chemicals that may cause primary photosensitization include phenothiazine, thiazide, acriflavine, rose bengal, methylene blue, sulfonamides, and tetracyclines. Plants, fungi, infection, neoplasms, and certain chemicals have been associated with hepatogenous photosensitization in horses. Plants that may cause equine hepatogenous photosensitization are burning bush or fireweed, ngaio tree, rape or kale, heliotrope, ragworts, tarweed or fiddleneck, and *Crotalaria* (rattleweed). Fungi that can induce hepatogenous photosensitization in horses include blue-green algae and *Phomopsis leptostromiformis* (on lupins). A detailed discussion on the pathogenesis of liver disease and its association with cutaneous photosensitization is included elsewhere in this text.

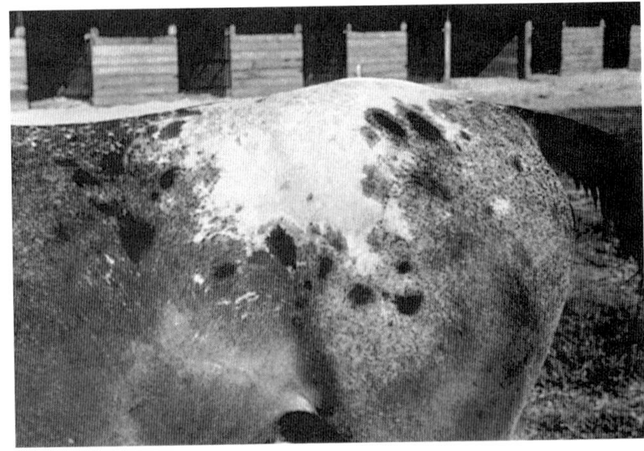

FIGURE 13-17 Horse with photosensitization.

Regardless of the source of the photodynamic agent, the pathophysiologic nature of skin disease is similar. Photodynamic agents are deposited in the skin and absorb energy when exposed to sunlight. These molecules are elevated to a high-energy state and, in the presence of oxygen, produce free radicals that damage cell membranes. Lysosomes and other organelles release hydrolytic enzymes and other mediators of inflammation.

Lesions are most common in white or lightly pigmented areas but have been observed to extend into dark-colored areas.[1] Eyelids, lips, face, perineum, and coronary bands are commonly affected. Usually an acute onset of erythema, edema, pruritus, and pain occurs. Vesicles and bullae may develop (Figure 13-17). Necrosis, ulceration, and crusting often occur.

The diagnosis is based on clinical signs, history, and laboratory tests. One should perform liver function tests regardless of whether the horse is showing clinical signs of hepatic disease.

Treatment requires identification of the underlying cause. Prognosis varies in horses with liver disease. Therapy requires removal of the offending substance, avoidance of sunlight, and topical or systemic glucocorticoids.[1]

Seborrhea and Localized Disorders of Keratinization as Causes of Scaling and Crusting

SEBORRHEA

Seborrhea is a descriptive term for excessive scaling and crusting. The condition may or may not result from excessive sebum production. Most seborrheic skin conditions are secondary, resulting from dermatophytosis, dermatophilosis, or parasitic or bacterial skin diseases. The natural response of the skin to insult is proliferation as a mechanism by which to remove an offending organism or as a result of inflammation. Primary seborrhea is a disorder of keratinization in which epidermal cell turnover time and basal cell proliferation increase. Genetic factors may control these mechanisms. Secondary seborrhea, the most common form of seborrhea, can occur in any inflammatory, infectious, or parasitic disease.

Idiopathic or primary seborrhea in horses may be generalized or localized to the tail and mane. No age, sex, or breed predilection exists. Generalized seborrhea appears clinically as diffuse matting of the coat. The texture of the coat may be oily and thick; adherent crusts may be removed easily. Oily or dry scales are present at the base of the hairs. Lesions are usually generalized and involve the face and legs (Figure 13-18). The animal is odoriferous and is not usually pruritic. Seborrhea of the mane and tail is common and characterized by crusts or scales attached to the bases of hairs. Pain and inflammation are generally absent.

Primary seborrhea is a diagnosis of exclusion. Severe generalized seborrhea must be differentiated from PF. One should perform skin scrapings, fungal cultures, dermatophilosis preparations, and skin biopsies on all suspected cases. Skin biopsies may help in determining whether primary or secondary seborrhea is present.[64] In early cases of generalized equine seborrhea involving little secondary inflammation, skin biopsy findings strongly suggest a primary keratinization disorder. The noncornified epidermis is not hyperplastic (thickened), but a significant orthokeratotic hyperkeratosis is attached to an epidermis of normal thickness. The superficial dermis shows only a noncornified epidermis, suggesting a keratinization defect. In horses with secondary inflammation or in which the seborrheic condition is more long standing, one may not interpret the biopsy findings as easily. The cornified epidermis is acanthotic (thickened) with significant orthokeratosis or parakeratotic hyperkeratosis. Superficial perivascular inflammation is often present in the superficial dermis.

Treatment of seborrhea involves eliminating the predisposing cause. Primary seborrhea is usually incurable, and management is symptomatic with topical therapy. The owner can usually manage a seborrheic condition satisfactorily with antiseborrheic shampoos. The owner should wash the horse with a cleansing shampoo before using a medicated shampoo. This treatment removes excess dirt and scale, improves efficacy of the medicated shampoo, and decreases the amount of medicated shampoo needed, minimizing potential for a contact reaction. The owner may use several brands of shampoo before finding a suitable shampoo for an individual patient. In general, dry seborrhea responds best to sulfur-based shampoos and oily seborrhea to tar-based shampoos. Benzoyl peroxide shampoos also work well in cases of oily seborrhea. Antiseborrheic shampoos formulated for small animals work well for horses but may be expensive. The owner should avoid human shampoos because these products are often more expensive than veterinary products and lather excessively, making rinsing difficult. Owners should allow the antiseborrheic shampoo to contact the coat for 10 to 15 minutes before rinsing. Thoroughly rinsing the horse is important, especially in the axillary and inguinal region, because shampoo residues irritate the skin. Initially, owners may need to shampoo the horse daily for 1 to 2 weeks. After the coat of the horse is normal, the owner may decrease shampooing to twice a week but must realize that therapy is lifelong. If shampoo therapy dries the coat and worsens dry seborrhea, then the owner may use a moisturizing spray or lotion.

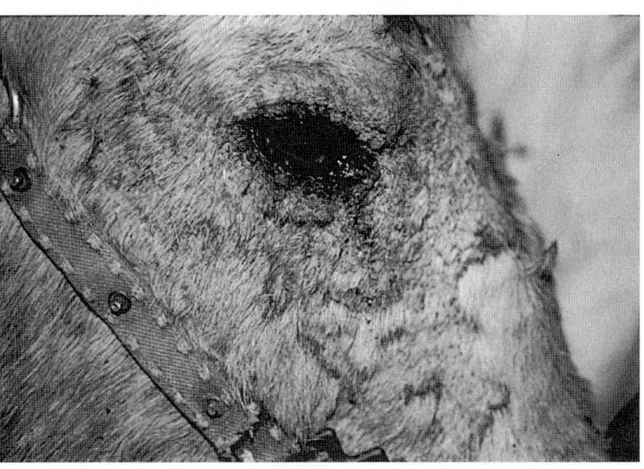

FIGURE 13-18 Horse with primary seborrhea.

CANNON KERATOSIS

Cannon keratosis is an idiopathic skin disease characterized by the presence of plaques and patches of hyperkeratosis on the cranial aspect of the rear cannon bones.[1,21] This disorder of keratinization is uncommon and does not appear to have any recognized age, breed, or sex predilection. Clinically, well-circumscribed plaques of tightly adherent crusts and scales with or without alopecia develop over the cranial surface of the rear cannon bones. The lesions are not pruritic.

The diagnosis is usually made by clinical examination and confirmed by skin biopsy. Differentiating cannon keratosis from dermatophilosis and dermatophytosis is important. Treatment consists of antiseborrheic shampoos. Topical glucocorticoids may be useful. Topical vitamin A cream (tretinoin [Rein-A cream 0.1%; Ortho Pharmaceutical Corp., Raritan, N.J.]) may be beneficial in removing crusts and plaques.

LINEAR KERATOSIS

Linear keratosis is an uncommon idiopathic disorder of keratinization.[1,21] The disease appears to be heritable, especially in Quarter Horses. Lesions develop between 1 and 5 years of age. One or more painless, nonpruritic unilateral, vertically oriented bands of alopecia and hyperkeratosis develop on the neck or lateral thorax. Lesions vary in size, ranging between 0.25 to 3.5 cm in width and 5 to 70 cm in length. Early lesions may begin as coalescing groups of papules. Lesions are not painful or pruritic.

The diagnosis usually is based on clinical signs alone. Skin biopsy reveals regular, irregular, or papillated epidermal hyperplasia with significant compact orthokeratotic hyperkeratosis.[64] Superficial perivascular dermatitis may or may not be present. If the linear keratosis does not interfere with the function of the horse, no treatment is necessary; surgical excision of small lesions may be curative. Topical vitamin A cream or salicylic cream may be useful in nonsurgical cases. These agents are keratolytic and may decrease the height, width, or thickness of the keratosis, allowing the horse to be used. Owners should not breed affected animals.

Idiopathic Causes of Scaling and Crusting

EQUINE EXFOLIATIVE EOSINOPHILIC DERMATITIS AND STOMATITIS

Equine exfoliative eosinophilic dermatitis and stomatitis is an idiopathic disease of horses characterized by ulcerative stomatitis, severe wasting, significant exfoliation, and eosinophil infiltration of the skin.[1,21,65] The disease is also called multisystemic eosinophilic epitheliotrophic disease. No age, sex, or breed predilection exists, but lesions tend to occur more commonly in the winter than other times of the year.

Early lesions begin as scaling, crusting, exudation, and fissuring at the coronary band. Oral ulcers are usually present at this stage. Over several weeks a generalized exfoliative dermatosis develops. Hairs are epilated easily, and alopecia with multifocal areas of ulceration and exudation develops. The horse may be pruritic. Affected horses without ulcerative stomatitis have a good appetite and may even be ravenous but exhibit rapid, severe weight loss. Some horses have concurrent protein-losing enteropathy or malabsorption syndrome.

The definitive diagnosis is based on the history, physical examination, and skin biopsy. Ruling out PF and bullous pemphigoid is important. The chronic wasting nature of the disease and multisystemic signs are key to making a diagnosis. Laboratory features include hypoalbuminemia, hypoproteinemia, impaired small intestinal carbohydrate absorption, and increased activities of gamma-glutamyltransferase, serum alkaline phosphatase, and bile duct isoenzymes. A superficial and deep eosinophilic and lymphoplasmacytic dermatitis with irregular epidermal hyperplasia is present.[65,66] Exocytosis of eosinophils and lymphocytes and necrosis of keratinocytes occurs.[1,65,66] Perivascular collagen degeneration, lymphoid nodules, and a lichenoid inflammatory infiltrate may be present. Eosinophilic infiltrates of the pancreas, salivary glands, oral cavity, and gastrointestinal tract are common. Peripheral eosinophilia is usually absent.

Two horses have responded to dexamethasone at 0.2 mg/kg intramuscularly for the first 5 days, followed by prednisolone at 0.5 mg/kg orally every 12 hours for 7 days, and then 1.0 mg/kg every 24 hours for a week, followed by alternate-day therapy.[1,65,66] However, most horses respond poorly to systemic glucocorticoids, and the prognosis is grave. A single horse with this disease showed a partial response to hydroxyurea and dexamethasone therapy.[67]

GENERALIZED GRANULOMATOUS DERMATITIS (EQUINE SARCOIDOSIS)

Generalized granulomatous disease is a rare idiopathic skin disease characterized by exfoliation, severe wasting, and granulomatous inflammation of multiple organ systems.[21,68] This disease has also been called equine sarcoidosis because it resembles sarcoidosis of human beings. One should avoid using this term because of possible confusion with sarcoid tumors. The cause of the disease is unknown. The disease may represent an abnormal host reaction to an infectious agent or allergen[21] or a nonmalignant neoplastic proliferation of cells.

No breed, age, or sex predilection exists for this condition. The skin disease begins as scaling, crusting, and alopecia on the face, limbs, and trunk (Figure 13-19). Clinical signs rapidly become generalized. Occasionally the disease is focal or multifocal in distribution.[21] Peripheral lymphadenopathy may develop concurrently with weight loss, muscle wasting, anorexia, exercise intolerance, and fever.

The definitive diagnosis is made by skin biopsy.[21] Perifollicular and middermal noncaseating granulomatous dermatitis occurs frequently with multinucleated giant cells. Neutrophils, lymphocytes, and plasma cells are present in small numbers. Granulomata are present in the superficial portion of the dermis. Granulomatous infiltrates also occur in other organs, including the lymph nodes, lung, gastrointestinal organs, liver, and spleen. A complete blood count reveals leukocytosis, increased fibrinogen, and hyperglobulinemia. Anemia caused by chronic infection may be present.

The prognosis is grave, and no treatment exists. Horses are usually euthanized within several months. Large doses of prednisolone (2 mg/kg orally every 24 hours) may be beneficial in the early stage of the disease. Occasionally, spontaneous remission may occur.

DISEASES CHARACTERIZED BY PAPULES AND NODULES

Many diseases are associated with single or multiple nodules in the skin of horses. Making a definitive diagnosis based on history and clinical signs alone is almost impossible. The most useful and cost-effective diagnostic test is a skin biopsy. Figure 13-20 illustrates a diagnostic algorithm for equine nodular skin disease.

INFECTIOUS CAUSES OF NODULES

BACTERIAL GRANULOMATA (BOTRYOMYCOSIS)

Botryo- is a prefix that means "grapelike." Horses affected with botryomycosis have clusters of nodular, grapelike lesions. Many species of bacteria have been associated with bacterial granulomata in horses; however, the most commonly isolated organism for equine bacterial granulomata is *Staphylococcus* spp.

Bacterial granulomata begin as traumatic injuries to the skin during which an infectious organism is inoculated into the dermis. A granulomatous reaction develops because the organism is capable of eliciting a response from the host, but the host is only able to contain the infection and not eradicate it. Bacterial granulomata develop in areas of previous trauma and are common on the limbs and scrotum. Poorly circumscribed, firm, draining lesions may or may not be painful. The center of the lesion may be ulcerated. In some cases, variable numbers of white to yellow pieces of particulate matter resembling grains of sand (tissue grains) may be present in the exudate.[68]

Confirmation of the diagnosis is made by skin biopsy, and identification of the causative organism is confirmed by bacterial or fungal culture. Histologic examination of a skin biopsy

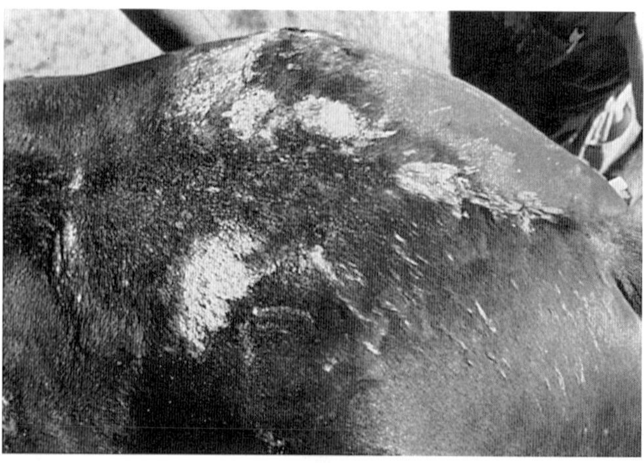

FIGURE 13-19 Horse with generalized granulomatous dermatitis. (Courtesy A. A. Stannard, University of California at Davis.)

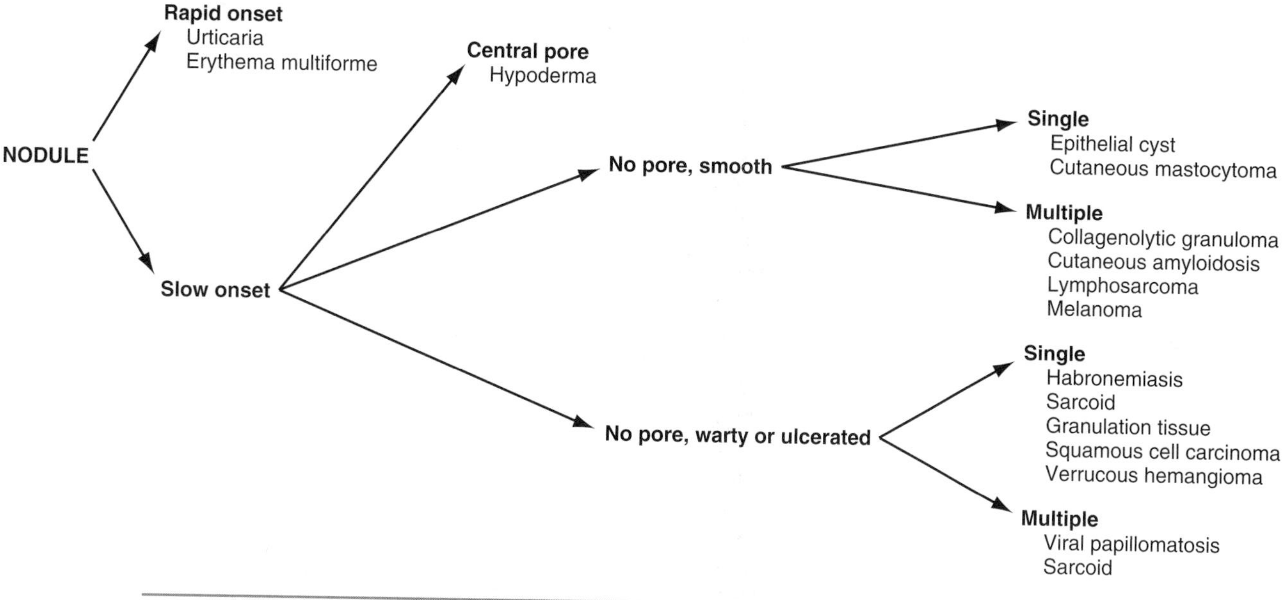

FIGURE 13-20 Flowchart for equine nodular dermatitis.

reveals nodular to diffuse pyogranulomatous inflammation with or without tissue grains. One may observe bacteria.

Surgical excision or radical debulking followed by long-term antibiotic therapy based on culture and sensitivity has been the most successful treatment for bacterial granulomata.[27,68] Organisms may be difficult to isolate from biopsy tissue samples, and submission of large wedges of tissue obtained at the time of surgery is recommended. If possible, tissue should be obtained to submit for aerobic, anaerobic, and deep fungal culture from the deepest portion of the lesion to increase the likelihood of isolating an infectious agent.

CORYNEBACTERIAL INFECTIONS

Corynebacterium spp. are gram-positive pleomorphic rods that are associated with two clinical syndromes in horses: abscesses and ulcerative lymphangititis.[27,48,69]

Abscesses Corynebacterial abscesses occur frequently in the horse in the western United States. Lesions tend to be seasonal, occurring most commonly during the summer and fall concurrent with peak fly season, especially in dry dusty conditions. The organism is believed to be transmitted by flies, particularly horn flies. For unknown reasons, fly bites are susceptible to infection.

Lesions develop slowly and may be single or multiple. The pectoral and ventral abdominal areas are affected most commonly. These abscesses drain a creamy to caseous material that may be whitish to greenish. Pitting edema, ventral midline dermatitis, depression, fever, and lameness may be present. The course of the disease may be chronic, and recurrent internal abscesses are frequent.

The diagnosis is based on the season and the appearance of the abscess and exudate. Because identifying the organism on cytologic examination of exudate may be difficult, a culture is always recommended.

Treatment is protracted and is complicated by the limited response of the organism to systemic antibiotics. The veterinarian should allow the abscess to mature and then surgically incise and drain it.[27] Systemic antibiotic use before abscess rupture may be followed by recurrence of the abscess on discontinuation of the drug. If drainage cannot be accomplished, large doses of procaine penicillin (50,000 IU/kg intramuscularly every 12 hours) for up to 6 months may be curative.[27,48,68,69] Toxoids and bacterins have not been useful.

Ulcerative Lymphangitis Ulcerative lymphangitis is an infection of the cutaneous lymphatics caused most commonly by *Corynebacterium pseudotuberculosis*. Infection is believed to begin by wound contamination. The disease occurs infrequently today.

No age, sex, or breed predilection exists. Lesions usually develop on the hindlimbs, especially at the fetlocks. Hard to fluctuant chains of nodules that abscess, ulcerate, and drain occur most commonly. Old lesions heal within 1 to 2 weeks, but new lesions develop.[1] The affected limb may be swollen and painful, and the horse may be depressed. Regional lymphatics appear corded. In chronic cases, permanent thickening of the tissue surrounding the regional lymphatics is common.

The diagnosis is based on the appearance of the lesion and identification of the organism. Direct smears of the exudate stained with a fast Giemsa or Gram stain and a culture and sensitivity usually confirm the diagnosis.

The practitioner must initiate treatment rapidly to prevent permanent debilitation and disfigurement. In early cases, hydrotherapy, exercise, surgical drainage, and large doses of procaine penicillin (20,000 to 80,000 IU/kg intramuscularly every 12 hours) for at least 30 days after clinical normalcy may be curative.[68] Nonsteroidal anti-inflammatory drugs may be beneficial. If the area becomes fibrotic and joint motion is restricted, then the prognosis is poor.

MYCETOMATA

Mycetomata (Table 13-1) are chronic subcutaneous infections characterized by swelling, draining tracts, and tissue granules. Filamentous bacteria or eumycetic fungi (fungi that inhabit

TABLE 13-1

Fungal Diseases of Horses

Disease	Common Causative Agents	Clinical Signs
SUPERFICIAL INFECTIONS		
Dermatophytosis	*Microsporum* and *Trichophyton* spp.	Circular patches or hair loss, crusting and scaling, urticaria, papules
Piedra	*Piedraia* spp. or *Trichosporon beigelii*	Black or white filamentous nodules on hair shaft
INTERMEDIATE INFECTIONS		
Sporotrichosis	*Sporothrix schenckii*	Papules and nodules occur along lymphatics; nodules may ulcerate, become thickened, and drain a thick brown-to red-colored exudate
Phaeohyphomycosis (chronic, subcutaneous fungal infection caused by pigmented opportunistic fungi)	*Hormodendrum, Drechslera, Phialophora, Curvularia, Cladosporium*	Single or multiple nodules; lesions may be grossly or microscopically pigmented, nonpruritic, nonpainful, and cool to the touch
Mycetoma (chronic subcutaneous infection)	Filamentous bacterial organisms and opportunistic fungi	Single or multiple nodular lesions are present; ulcerated, draining tracts are common; mycetomata discharge tissue grains in contrast to phaeohyphomycosis, which does not

the soil or vegetation) may cause mycetomata. The most common fungal organisms that cause mycetomata in horses are *Curvularia geniculata* and *Pseudallescheria boydii*. The most common bacteria isolated from equine mycetomata are *Actinobacillus* spp., *Nocardia* spp., and *Actinomyces* spp. Regardless of causative agent the organism usually gains entrance to the body through traumatic inoculation. As with other granulomatous reactions the body is able to recognize the intruder and isolate it but not to eliminate it.

Single or multiple nodules of varying sizes can occur almost anywhere on the body of the horse. The nodules often are pigmented and ulcerated and may discharge tissue grains (small sandlike particles). The tissue grains are believed to be masses of hyphae from the organism. Gross examination of the cut surface often reveals dark-brown pigment or granules scattered in yellow to pink tissue.

Distinguishing clinically among bacterial or fungal mycetomata or any number of other causes of lumps in the skin is impossible. A definitive diagnosis requires an excisional or wedge biopsy of a lesion. Histologic examination shows diffuse to nodular pyogranulomatous to granulomatous inflammation surrounding septate branching hyphae. Tissue grains are often visible microscopically. The hyphae contained in tissue grains or tissue may be pigmented or nonpigmented. Fungi are cultured best from tissue grains and, occasionally, exudate. If possible, surgical excision is curative.[27] Antibiotic therapy is usually ineffective, especially for fungal mycetomata.

Phaeohyphomycosis

Phaeohyphomycosis (see Table 13-1), sometimes known as chromomycosis, is a chronic subcutaneous and occasionally systemic infection caused by pigmented opportunistic fungi, such as *Hormodendrum, Drechslera, Phialophora, Curvularia*, and *Cladosporium* species. Many of the organisms that cause fungal mycetomata can cause phaeohyphomycosis. The distinguishing difference is the lack of tissue grains. Pigmented fungi (dematiaceous fungi) causing this disease are soil and vegetative saprophytes that gain entrance into the body via a wound or abrasion. The body is not able to eliminate the organism, which proliferates in tissues. Immunosuppression may be a predisposing factor.

Lesions appear anywhere on the body and may be single or multiple. Some lesions are pigmented deeply on gross examination, or pigmentation is only a microscopic feature. Nodules vary in size and are cool, nonpainful, and nonpruritic. Regional granulomatous dermatitis may be present.

The definitive diagnosis is made by histologic examination of an excised nodule. Skin biopsy reveals suppurative to granulomatous dermatitis with pigmented septate hyphae. Observation of pigmented septate hyphae in the skin indicates opportunistic invasion of the tissue. Fungal culture of tissue samples is necessary to identify the organism. An important note is that growth of these organisms is slow, often requiring weeks, and a reference laboratory is able to culture the organism best.

Excision is the only effective treatment but may be impractical when numerous lesions are present. These organisms are not susceptible to commonly used systemic or topical antifungal agents. However, the author has treated an affected dog successfully with itraconazole. The recommended dosage is 3 mg/kg orally every 12 hours for 1 month beyond when the skin appears normal (usually 4 to 12 months). Ketoconazole therapy is not recommended in the horse because of poor bioavailability after oral administration. Even when the solution is acidified with hydrochloric acid, bioavailability is approximately 23%.

Sporotrichosis

Sporotrichosis (see Table 13-1) is a fungal disease caused by *Sporothrix schenckii*, a dimorphic aerobic fungus. The organism is a soil and plant saprophyte that lives in decaying vegetation and gains entrance via traumatic inoculation, especially from puncture wounds.

In horses the cutaneous lymphatic form is most common.[70,71] Early lesions begin as papules that may exude a seropurulent material. Nodules are most common on the thigh or proximal foreleg and chest. If the immune system does not eliminate the organism, hard subcutaneous nodules develop along the lymphatics draining the area. The lymphatics become corded and drain thick, brown to red exudate. Regional lymph nodes are not involved. Occasionally, only a solitary nodule develops. The disease rarely becomes systemic.

The definitive diagnosis is determined by demonstration of the organism via cytologic examination of exudate, culture of tissue or exudate, or skin biopsy. The organism appears as a cigar-shaped yeast in macrophages and neutrophils on Giemsa-stained smears. Histologic examination of tissue reveals nodular to diffuse, suppurative to granulomatous dermatitis. Intraepidermal microabscesses may be visible. The yeast is rarely seen in tissue sections. The number of organisms present in the tissue may vary, and repeat cultures are often necessary.

Sodium iodide (20% solution) has been successful for treating sporotrichosis in horses.[21,71] A loading dose of 20 to 40 mg/kg is administered intravenously for 2 to 5 days, followed by once daily oral therapy (20 to 40 mg/kg) until all clinical lesions are gone. One should administer therapy for at least 3 weeks after lesions disappear. Sodium iodide may be given orally via syringe or mixed in sweet feed. Topical hot packs of 20% sodium iodide may be used on open wounds. Iodism (see the previous discussion) may develop and may require temporary discontinuation of therapy. Iodines cause abortion and should not be used in pregnant mares.[21]

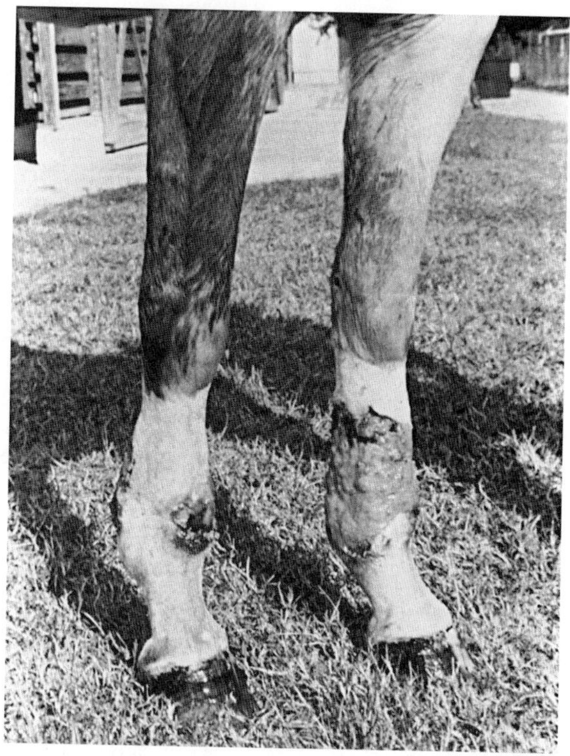

FIGURE 13-21 Horse with bilateral pythiosis on the legs.

Pythiosis (Phycomycosis, Florida Leeches, Gulf Coast Fungus, and Swamp Cancer)

Pythiosis is caused by an aquatic fungus, *Pythium insidiosum,* common in the Gulf Coast region of the United States, South America, and Australia. This organism is a plant parasite that normally lives on aquatic vegetation or organic debris. Damaged animal tissue is chemotactic for the organism, and the fungus probably gains entrance into animal tissue via wounds in prolonged contact with contaminated water.[72]

The disease commonly affects ventral body areas, including legs, abdomen, and chest (Figure 13-21), and also may involve nasal tissue. Wire cuts, puncture wounds, and ventral midline dermatitis caused by horn flies or *Culicoides* gnats are prime locations. Early signs of fungal invasion include single or multiple minute foci of necrosis that progress rapidly into circular, ulcerative, granulomatous masses with serosanguinous discharges. These masses are intensely pruritic and are often hemorrhagic from self-trauma. Thick, sticky material exudes from the wound. This discharge often contains "kunkers," hard, gritty, white to yellow masses that develop in tissue tracts and are considered a hallmark of this disease. These granules branch macroscopically, distinguishing them from granules observed in other skin diseases. Kunkers are composed of fungal hyphae, host exudate, and protein. Lameness, regional lymph node involvement, anemia, and hypoproteinemia are common noncutaneous findings. Anemia and hypoproteinemia develop after blood loss and serum exudation from the mass. Occasionally the disease may become systemic. The disease is not a known zoonosis, but protective latex gloves should be worn when examining patients.

Pythiosis is difficult to differentiate from habronemiasis, exuberant granulation tissue, bacterial granulomata, and invasive squamous cell carcinoma. A definitive diagnosis requires biopsy, culture, and cytologic examination of exudate and kunkers. One should submit tissue specimens and kunkers for histologic examination. Common findings include pyogranulomatous inflammation with large numbers of eosinophils. If hyphae are visible, they are 2.6 to 6.4 μm in diameter, thick-walled, and irregular.[1] Pythiosis can be grown on fungal culture medium and requires incubation in a vegetable extract agar. A laboratory familiar with appropriate isolation techniques is able best to culture it. One should collect kunkers, wash them in sterile saline, and embed them deeply in the media. Occasionally, the disease can be diagnosed by cytologic inspection of the kunkers. One macerates and minces small kunkers with a scalpel, places the material on hydroxide, and stains it with India ink. Hyphae appear as black, broad, thick-walled branching structures. Recent advances in enzyme-linked immunosorbent assays and molecular techniques offer a better potential for organism detection and identification.[73]

The prognosis is poor because treatment is difficult. With early diagnosis, surgical excision may be possible. However, relapses are common, and repeated excision may be required. One should monitor surgical sites closely for evidence of recurrence manifesting as focal areas of edema in the granulation tissue with dark hemorrhagic patches 1 to 5 mm in diameter and serosanguinous discharge.

Systemic antifungal drugs are not effective in treating this disease.[72,74] Systemic amphotericin B (Fungizone IV; Bristol-Myers Squibb, New Brunswick, N.J.) combined with topical amphotericin B may be curative in rare, isolated cases. Amphotericin B is administered at a dose of 0.3 mg/kg in 5% dextrose intravenously daily until reaching a total dose of 350 mg. One then administers this dose on alternate days until the horse is cured. In addition, one treats lesions topically with gauze dressing soaked in an amphotericin B and DMSO solution (50 mg amphotericin B, 10 ml sterile water, and 10 ml DMSO). One may also inject amphotericin B into the lesions. Amphotericin B is nephrotoxic, and serum creatinine and serum urea nitrogen concentrations and hydration should be monitored daily. Immunotherapy with phenolized, ultrasonicated proportion from fungal culture is reportedly curative if administered early in the course of the disease. In a small number of cases, vaccine administration resulted in a decrease in the size of the lesion. This therapy may be of benefit if used preoperatively to enhance complete removal of the infected tissue. Unfortunately the vaccine is not commercially available. Because of the cost of medical or surgical therapy the risks of treatment, and because of the high probability that excision is incomplete, owners often elect euthanasia.

Parasitic Causes of Nodules

A variety of parasites may infest equine skin and cause cutaneous nodules. Some of the more common causes of parasitic nodules in the horse are warbles, cutaneous habronemiasis, and ticks. The last two have been discussed previously and are not covered in this section.

Warbles occasionally occur in horses and are caused by a larval stage of *Hypoderma bovis* and *Hypoderma lineatum*. In horses, larvae do not usually complete their life cycle.[24] Horses that develop infestation are usually pastured or housed with cattle. Adult flies lay eggs on the hairs, and larvae migrate toward the skin surface and eventually penetrate the skin. Once in the body of the host, the larvae migrate to reach the subcutaneous tissues of the neck and trunk. A swelling develops at the site of the larvae, which eventually becomes perforated as a breathing pore is formed. Nodules are visible most commonly over the withers, and almost all develop a breathing pore. The nodules are often painful. Spontaneous rupture may cause anaphylaxis.[24] Occasionally, aberrant migration causes neurologic signs.

The presence of dorsal swelling or a nodule with a breathing pore is diagnostic. The major differential consideration is collagenolytic granuloma; however, these nodules lack a breathing pore. Hypodermiasis is treated by gently enlarging the breathing pore surgically and removing the grub, removing the entire nodule surgically, or allowing the grub to fall out spontaneously. In areas of high occurrence, one may use pour-on insecticides as a preventative. Horses should be treated at the same time of year as affected cattle are treated in the area.

Urticaria

Urticaria is a nodular skin disease of horses characterized by wheals, edema, and often pruritus (Figure 13-22) and most commonly is caused by a type I hypersensitivity reaction. However, urticaria may also result from nonimmunologic factors such as pressure, sunlight, heat, exercise, stress, and drugs. Prerace stress, insect or arthropod bites, bacterial infections, topical parasiticides, systemic drugs (penicillin, phenylbutazone, aspirin, guaifenesin, phenothiazine, quinidine, streptomycin, oxytetracyline), feedstuffs, soaps, leather conditioners, vaccines, snake bites, inhalants, and plants can cause urticaria in horses. In the author's experience, urticaria is a common manifestation of insect hypersensitivity and atopy. Mosquito swarmings commonly result in urticaria.

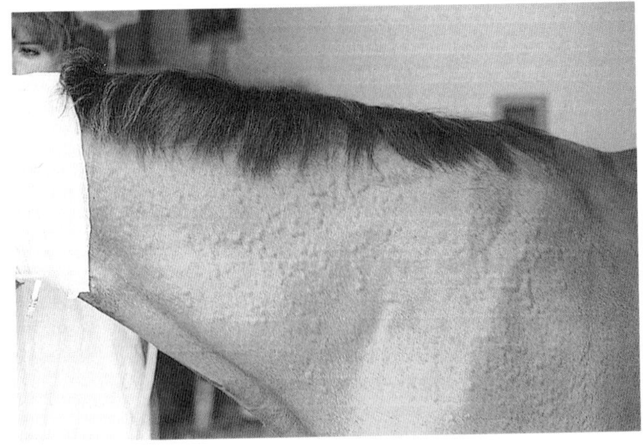

FIGURE 13-22 Urticaria in a horse following administration of penicillin.

No age, sex, or breed predilection exists for urticaria. Lesions may develop rapidly or slowly and may be localized or generalized. Lesions are raised, cool to the touch, pit when depressed, and may or may not exude serum or blood. Pruritus varies. In rare instances, lesions may coalesce to form bizarre patterns.

Although urticaria is usually recognizable, its cause can be difficult to identify. The cause of an acute urticaria episode (<6 weeks in duration) is much more likely to be identified than the cause of a chronic episode (>6 weeks in duration). A detailed history is critical. Important questions to answer are listed in Box 13-5.

In cases in which lesions are bizarre in appearance, chronic, or exudative, one should perform a skin biopsy to rule out other causes of nodular disease. Typical histologic findings for urticaria include vasodilation, edema in the dermis, and mild to moderate eosinophilic perivascular inflammation. Complete blood cell counts and serum chemistry profiles are rarely useful. Before beginning expensive or involved diagnostic testing, one should be sure to rule out the possibility of allergic reactions to shampoos, tack cleaners, soaps, and so forth. All horses with chronic urticaria should undergo a food trial, be moved to a new environment for 5 to 7 days, and undergo a program of insect control before being referred for intradermal skin testing. Intradermal skin testing is the best method for identifying the cause of allergic inhalant dermatitis. Horses should not receive antihistamines or tranquilizers for 1 week or corticosteroids for 4 weeks before intradermal skin testing.

Treatment is aimed at eliminating the underlying cause, if possible. Hydroxyzine at 200 to 400 mg orally every 12 hours is effective in eliminating urticarial swellings in most horses with acute or chronic urticaria.[35] Transient sedation of several days may occur with this drug. If the horse is nonresponsive to hydroxyzine, prednisolone at 1 mg/kg or dexamethasone at 0.02 to 0.1 mg/kg orally, intravenously, or intramuscularly may be beneficial on a short-term (<1 week) basis.

BOX 13-5

QUESTIONS USED TO DIAGNOSE URTICARIA

1. Is this a corticosteroid-responsive urticaria? A positive answer would indicate an allergic cause such as atopy, insect hypersensitivity, or food allergy.
2. Does the development of the lesion correlate with the administration of systemic drugs or the application of topical medications? A positive answer would suggest a drug reaction.
3. Does the application of fly repellent aggravate or alleviate the urticaria? Worsening of the urticaria suggests an allergic contact reaction, whereas alleviation suggests an insect hypersensitivity.
4. Do the lesions resolve with stabling the horse for 24 to 48 hours or moving to a new environment? A positive answer would suggest an environmental cause of the urticaria (molds, inhaled dust from bedding, hay, feedstuffs, feathers from roosting birds).
5. Do lesions improve if the horse is moved off pasture? A positive answer would suggest plant antigen as a cause of the urticaria.
6. Do the lesions improve if the feed is changed? Improvement in clinical signs suggests an ingested allergen or inhaled allergen from feedstuffs.

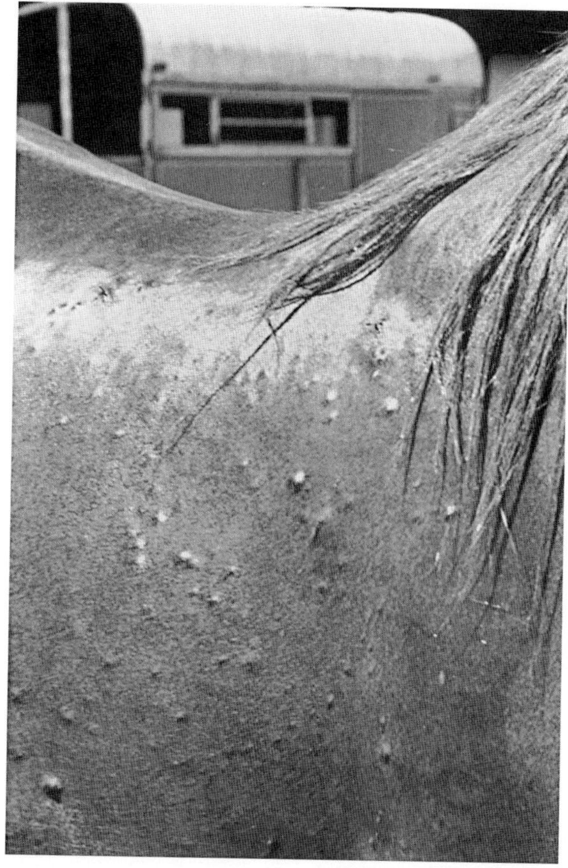

FIGURE 13-23 Horse with multiple eosinophilic granuloma.

Idiopathic Inflammatory Causes of Nodules

EOSINOPHILIC COLLAGENOLYTIC GRANULOMA (NODULAR COLLAGENOLYTIC GRANULOMA AND NODULAR NECROBIOSIS)

Eosinophilic collagenolytic granuloma are a frequent cause of nodules in the skin of horses. The exact cause of these lesions is unknown, but they may result from a hypersensitivity reaction to insect bites.[1] Lesions, however, have been reported to develop spontaneously or as a result of trauma, suggesting multiple causes.[75] Regional variability in the occurrence of lesions has been noted.

These lesions have no sex, breed, or age predilection but occur most commonly in warmer months. They may be single or multiple and vary greatly in size (0.5 to 10 cm in diameter). The nodules may occur anywhere on the body but are most common on the neck, withers, and dorsal trunk (Figure 13-23). Individual lesions are rounded, well circumscribed, firm, haired, nonpainful, and nonpruritic. Owners of horses with seasonal problems have reported that early lesions are often soft and fluctuant and develop into firm masses over weeks to months. If lesions are under the saddle, then the horse may exhibit pain.

The definitive diagnosis is made by skin biopsy. Histologic examination of tissue reveals multifocal areas of collagen degeneration surrounded by granulomatous eosinophilic inflammation. Chronic lesions may have significant dystrophic mineralization.[64]

Solitary lesions that do not cause the horse discomfort require no treatment. Problem lesions respond to excision or sublesional injections of triamcinolone acetonide (3 to 5 mg per lesion) or methylprednisolone acetate (5 to 10 mg per lesion).[1] One should inject no more than 20 mg per horse of triamcinolone acetonide because of the danger of laminitis. Horses with multiple lesions may be treated with prednisolone orally at 1 mg/kg once daily for 2 to 3 weeks. After lesions have resolved, the dose of prednisolone should be tapered and discontinued over a 5- to 10-day period. Horses with seasonal recurrences in which insect hypersensitivity is involved and documented via intradermal skin testing might benefit from hyposensitization to insects.

EQUINE AXILLARY NODULAR NECROSIS

Equine axillary nodular necrosis is a rare idiopathic skin disease of horses. The disease is similar to equine eosinophilic granuloma with collagen degeneration, except that the lesions are localized to the axillary region.[29]

The condition has no known age, sex, or breed predilection. Clinically, single or multiple nodules develop unilaterally in the axillae. The nodules are painless, nonpruritic, haired, well-circumscribed firm masses that vary in size from 0.5 to 4.0 cm or greater in diameter. Multiple lesions tend to be arranged in a row.

Skin biopsy is diagnostic. Biopsy findings include pyogranulomatous, eosinophilic dermatitis with foci of coagulation necrosis. Collagen degeneration is not a common finding.

Treatment is the same as that for equine eosinophilic granuloma. Corticosteroids often do not work well, and surgical excision may be necessary. Lesions tend to recur.

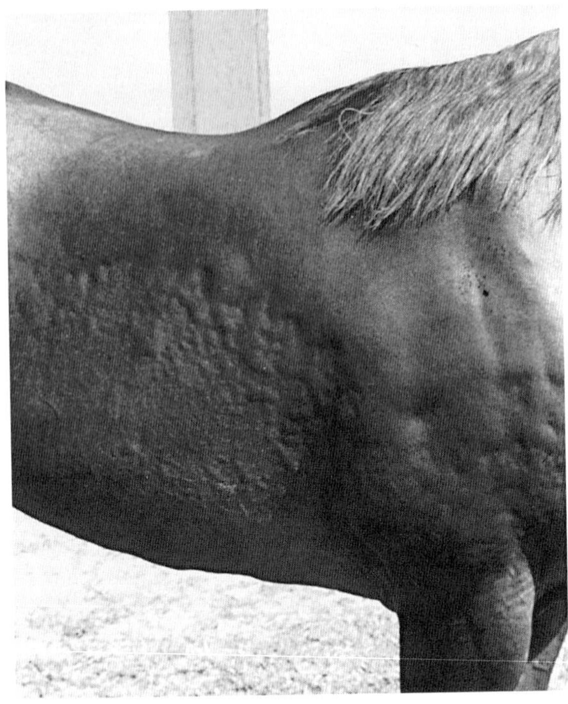

FIGURE 13-24 Horse with unilateral papular dermatitis. (Courtesy V. Fadock, University of Florida.)

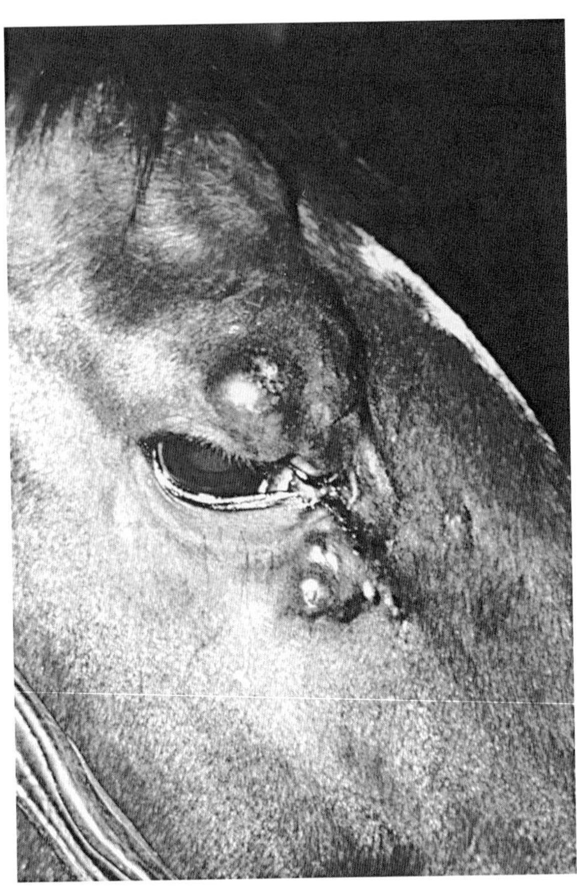

FIGURE 13-25 Fibroblastic (proliferative) sarcoid.

EQUINE UNILATERAL PAPULAR DERMATOSIS

Equine unilateral papular dermatosis is a rare idiopathic skin disorder of horses.[76] This disease has been seen in several breeds of horses but may be more common in Quarter Horses. Lesions develop in the warm months and are characterized by the unilateral development of multiple (30-300) papules and nodules on the trunk (Figure 13-24). Lesions are firm, well circumscribed, nonpainful, and nonpruritic.

The diagnosis is made by skin biopsy. Histologic examination of tissue reveals eosinophilic folliculitis and furunculosis. Spontaneous remission may occur; otherwise, prednisolone at 1 mg/kg orally once daily for 2 to 3 weeks is recommended until nodules resolve. Relapses may occur.

Neoplastic Causes of Nodules

Reviewing all of the neoplastic skin conditions of horses is beyond the scope of this chapter. Only the skin tumors of horses that commonly masquerade as nodules are discussed: sarcoids, melanomas, mast cell tumors, and cutaneous lymphoma. One can diagnose some cutaneous neoplasms via exfoliative cytologic examination, but biopsy is the diagnostic test of choice.

SARCOIDS

Sarcoids are the most common skin neoplasms in horses, accounting for up to one third of all reported tumors in horses. Sarcoids are locally invasive fibroblastic neoplasms.[21,27,77-79]

The cause of equine sarcoids is controversial; currently the papovavirus is believed to be involved in the development of lesions.[27,76,77] Polymerase chain reaction nucleotide sequences strongly suggest that equine sarcoids are caused by bovine papillomavirus types 1 and 2.[78] Evidence for this suggestion includes the clinical observations that lesions often develop in areas of previous trauma, lesions may spread to other areas on the same horse or to other horses, epizootics of equine sarcoid have been described, and autotransmission is possible under experimental conditions. Equine sarcoids were produced in donkeys inoculated experimentally with bovine papillomavirus. A predisposition or susceptibility also appears to play a part in the pathogenesis. Equine sarcoids occur with increased incidence in certain families, and a genetic link with specific major histocompatibility complex genes (W13 MHC class II antigen) has been demonstrated. Exposure to the virus and genetic susceptibility are probably required for a horse to develop sarcoids.

No sex or breed predilection exists, but greater than 70% of sarcoids develop in horses less than 4 years of age. They may arise spontaneously or at a site of previous trauma and may occur anywhere on the body. Sarcoids have a predilection for the head, ears, and limbs. One third of affected horses have multiple lesions.

Equine sarcoids may be classified as nodular sarcoids, fibroblastic sarcoids (Figure 13-25), verrucous sarcoids, occult or flat sarcoids (Figure 13-26), malevolent sarcoids, and mixed sarcoids. Each type of sarcoid differs clinically in its morphologic appearance and lesion location.[21] Nodular sarcoids are firm, raised, circular nodules that are 5 to 20 mm in diameter and tend to occur on the sheath or groin areas and the eyelids. Fibroblastic sarcoids resemble proud flesh (proliferative, fleshy, and ulcerated lesion) and are usually located around the groin, lower limbs, coronet, and eyelid. Verrucous sarcoids

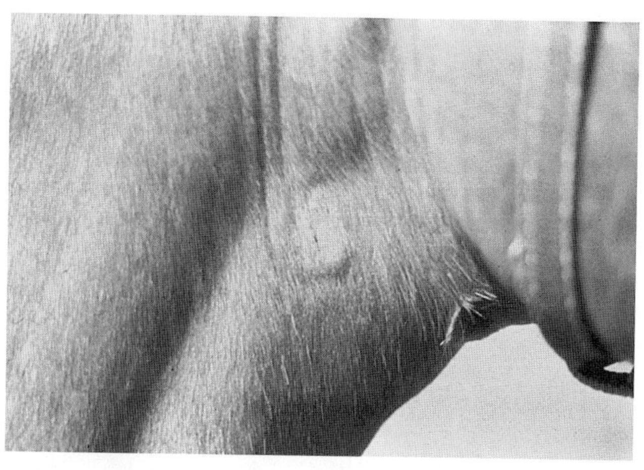

FIGURE 13-26 Flat sarcoid.

are warty and tend to occur on the face, body, and sheath or groin areas. Occult sarcoids normally appear as flat, circular, hyperkeratotic areas. Occult sarcoids may also appear as one or more small nodules 2 to 5 mm in diameter. The typical lesion location for occult sarcoids is the neck, mouth, eyes, and the medial aspects of the forearm and thigh. Malevolent sarcoids are locally invasive tumors with multiple nodules and a fibroblastic character. Some malevolent sarcoids infiltrate lymphatics and produce a cordlike appearance. Although local lymph nodes are enlarged, no evidence of sarcoid tumor has been detected within the lymph nodes themselves. Mixed sarcoids consist of sarcoid lesions that appear as a confluence of several different types of sarcoids. Mixed sarcoids contain verrucous- or occult-type tissue along with fibroblastic- or nodular-appearing tissue. This type of sarcoid is more common in long-standing sarcoid lesions or lesions that have experienced minor trauma.

A skin biopsy is the only way to diagnose an equine sarcoid definitively. Flat or small verrucous forms may become more aggressive after a biopsy. For this reason, some veterinarians are reluctant to take a biopsy sample of these lesions.

The histologic pattern observed with equine sarcoids is a fibroblastic proliferation of cells that form whorls or interlacing bundles.[64] The usual overall orientation of this proliferation is perpendicular to the basement membrane, but exceptions exist. The epidermis, when present, is hyperplastic with characteristic elongated rete ridges, but normal or even atrophic epidermis with significant hyperkeratosis can occur (flat sarcoids).

Several different treatments are described for managing equine sarcoids.[21,79] Previous experience suggests that the best treatment for occult and verrucous sarcoids is benign neglect. These types of sarcoids become more aggressive after biopsies have been performed. For fibroblastic sarcoids the treatment of choice is cryotherapy along with surgical debulking of the tumor. The inclusion of cryotherapy in the treatment regimen is associated with a lower rate of recurrence than with surgery alone (30% to 40% recurrence rate for cryosurgery versus 50% to 64% recurrence rate with traditional surgery). Adverse effects associated with cryosurgery include swelling, hyperemia, hemorrhage, necrosis, and local edema after treatment. Average healing time after cryosurgery is 2.4 months, with a range of 1 to 3.5 months. Cryotherapy usually destroys hair follicles in the treated area, and hair regrowth is white. If cortical bone accidentally freezes, then the strength of the bone may decrease by 70%. For lesions around the eyes, recommended treatment is surgical debulking of the tumor followed by injections with bacille Calmette-Guérin (BCG) vaccine or mycobacterial cell wall products. BCG vaccine is thought to work by stimulating the immune response of the host to sarcoid cells. Mycobacterial antigens are thought to stimulate host lymphocytes and also may stimulate an increase in natural killer cells. The tumor is injected with BCG vaccine every 2 to 3 weeks for four treatments. One should pretreat horses with flunixin meglumine and prednisolone 30 minutes before using BCG vaccine to help reduce the risk of anaphylaxis.

Local radiation therapy using a variety of implants also has been recommended for treating equine sarcoids. This form of treatment is limited to smaller lesions because radiation does not effectively penetrate deeper skin lesions. Relapse rates with this form of therapy vary from 0% to 50%. Some disadvantages of radiation therapy are that the horse must be kept in a radiation-approved area, and cost may be significant if the tumor is large.

Cisplatin (Platinol; Bristol-Myers Squibb, Princeton, N.J.) in oil has recently been described as a treatment for horses with sarcoids. This treatment may be up to 100% effective but requires multiple intralesional injections. Emulsions are made of equal volumes of an aqueous solution of 1 mg cisplatin per milliliter of sesame or almond oil. A dose of 1 mg cisplatin per cubic centimeter of tumor is suggested. With denser sarcoid tumors, injecting cisplatin solution into the tumor may be difficult. Precautions recommended when using cisplatin include wearing gloves and protective clothing. One should place all material in a biohazard container after use and should use a Luer-Lok syringe and extension set to help minimize potential human exposure. Local skin reactions may occur when citsplatin contacts the skin and mucous membranes and, if this occurs, the area should be thoroughly washed with soap and water. One should avoid using cisplatin in patients with renal impairment or in breeding animals. Cisplatin is associated with teratogenic and embryotoxic reactions in mice and azoospermia and impaired spermatogenesis in human beings.

Another recently described therapy for equine sarcoids is a topical treatment known as Xxterra (Larson Laboratories, Fort Collins, Colo.).[76] This product contains a caustic substance and an extract of the bloodroot plant. Native Americans have used the bloodroot plant to treat a variety of conditions including warts. This product is thought to work by changing the antigenicity of the sarcoids so that the body recognizes these cells as foreign and produces antibodies against them. One applies Xxterra (while wearing gloves) to the sarcoid lesion and places a bandage over it for 4 days. If the sarcoid has not sloughed by 4 days, the treatment should be repeated. If one cannot bandage the area with the sarcoid, then the product should be applied to the sarcoid daily for 4 days or until sloughing occurs. Interestingly, when this product was applied to normal skin nothing happened, but when the product was applied to a sarcoid, the skin became inflamed and the sarcoid sloughed. An exception to this rule is pigmented skin. If freckles are present on the skin, Xxterra may react with them. Horses with mixed coat colors or Paint Horses have not had problems with this tissue reaction. Application of Xxterra to the ears may result in crinkling of the ears. If this reaction would be an unsatisfactory side effect for the owner, then a different treatment should be used. In addition, the veterinarian should warn owners that the treated area may ooze a purulent material and become malodorous, which often occurs before the tissue sloughs.

Other therapies for equine sarcoids that have been used with success are limited in their use because of expense and availability. Examples of such treatments include radiofrequency-induced hyperthermia, carbon dioxide laser surgery, and immunotherapy using a tumor vaccine. With time, these therapeutic options may become more readily available and accepted.

Regardless of the form of therapy chosen the client needs to be aware that sarcoid tumors tend to recur. Verrucous or flat tumors are best left untreated.

MELANOMAS

Melanomas may arise from dermal melanocytes or melanoblasts and may be benign or malignant. These tumors occur most commonly in older horses of Arabian and Percheron breeding. The relationship between development of melanomas and gray coat color is recognized widely.[80] Melanomas appear to occur exclusively in horses that are gray or become dapple-gray with age. Up to 80% of gray horses more than 15 years of age are estimated to have melanomas.[81]

Lesions may be solitary or multiple and occur most commonly on the perineum or ventral surface of the tail. Tumors are usually firm and nodular and may be hairless and ulcerated. They are almost always black. Vitiligo may precede the development of the lesions.[80] Three growth patterns have been described: (1) slow growth without metastasis, (2) slow growth with sudden metastasis, and (3) rapid growth and malignancy from the onset.

The diagnosis is usually based on clinical signs. Biopsy is not usually needed to confirm the diagnosis unless the lesion is bizarre in appearance.

No treatment is needed unless the melanoma interferes with function. Cimetidine (Tagamet; GlaxoSmithKline, Middlesex, United Kingdom) at 2.5 mg/kg every 8 hours has been reported to cause partial to complete regression of some melanomas. The number and size of the melanomas decreased by 50% to 90% in horses treated for 3 months. After tumors have regressed, daily maintenance therapy at 1.6 mg/kg orally once daily is recommended.[82]

MASTOCYTOMA (MAST CELL TUMOR)

Mast cell tumors are uncommon in horses. Equine mast cell tumors are five times more common in males than females. Arabian Horses appear to be predisposed to developing mast cell tumors. The breed that is least predisposed to developing mast cell tumors is the Thoroughbred.[1,29] No age predilection exists for equine mast cell tumors.

Two distinct types of mast cell tumors in horses are a hyperplastic type and a neoplastic type. Most equine mast cell tumors are hyperplastic. Clinically, two forms of equine mast cell tumors exist.[1] The most common form is a single cutaneous nodule, often located on the head (Figure 13-27). Nodules range in size from 2 to 20 cm in diameter. The surface of the nodules may be normal, hairless, or ulcerated. Alternatively, mast cell tumors may cause diffuse swelling on a lower extremity, usually below the carpus or hock. The swelling is firm, and the overlying skin is normal in appearance. Radiographs of the limb commonly show multifocal areas of soft tissue mineralization.[64]

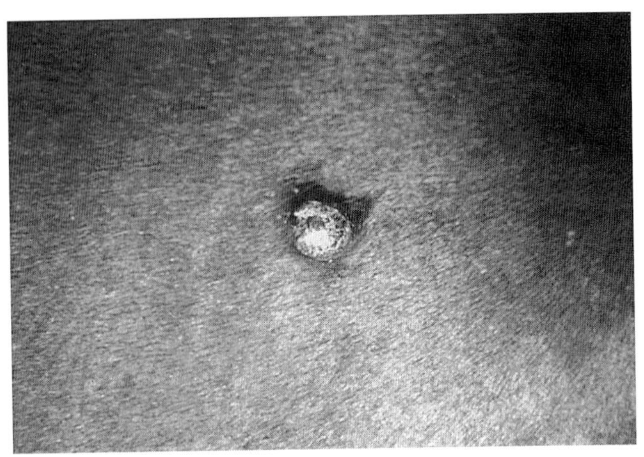

FIGURE 13-27 Hyperplastic mast cell tumor in a horse.

The diagnosis is determined by biopsy. Diffuse to nodular proliferations of mast cells occur in the dermis. Tumor cells may be well differentiated or more atypical. Tissue eosinophilia, collagen degeneration, and dystrophic mineralization occur commonly in horses.

One may treat solitary tumors by excision, with sublesional triamcinolone acetonide (5 to 10 mg per lesion), or with cryosurgery. Spontaneous remission may occur after incomplete excision or in young horses. Metastasis has not been reported.[29]

CUTANEOUS LYMPHOMA

Systemic cutaneous lymphoma is discussed in detail in Chapter 14. Cutaneous lymphoma is rare in horses.[75,83] No age, sex, or breed predilection exists for this tumor. Lesions develop slowly or rapidly. They may occur anywhere on the body, but the trunk and neck are affected most commonly. Individual lesions may be firm or fluctuant, resembling urticaria. The overlying skin is usually normal. Involvement of internal organs may occur.

A definitive diagnosis is made by histologic examination of a skin biopsy. One should submit several representative tissue samples for examination. Histologically, lymphosarcoma is characterized by diffuse dermal and subcutaneous infiltration of malignant lymphocytes.[1]

If the owners want to pursue treatment, several options are available. Prednisolone at 1 mg/kg orally once daily for 7 days and then every other day has been used successfully. In addition, PEG-l-asparaginase at 10,000 IU/m^2 once weekly may be beneficial, although expensive. Recently, low-dose cyclophosphamide and immunization with vaccinia virus–infected autologous tumor cells was successful in inducing a 19-month remission in a 13-year old horse; however, this therapy is experimental.[84]

PSEUDOLYMPHOMA

Pseudolymphomata are common in horses compared with lymphomata.[1] Differentiating the two diseases is important because the prognosis for pseudolymphoma is excellent.

Pseudolymphomata are nodular to papular lesions that develop in the skin as a result of chronic antigenic stimulation. The most common antigenic stimuli are believed to be insect bites and drug reactions. Lesions occur most commonly in late summer and fall and are usually solitary but may be multiple.[1,83] Pseudolymphomata usually occur on the head and trunk. Individual lesions are firm, raised, and haired.

A definitive diagnosis is made by a skin biopsy. Histologic examination of tissue shows dense dermal and subcutaneous infiltration of lymphocytes, histiocytes, plasma cells, and eosinophils. Lymphoid nodules and eosinophils are present and are an important aid in the differentiation of pseudolymphoma from lymphoma.[64,83]

Pseudolymphomata often spontaneously regress but may be excised surgically or injected sublesionally with triamcinolone acetonide at 3 to 5 mg per lesion, not to exceed a total dose of 15 to 20 mg.[83]

Congenital Causes of Nodules

DERMOID CYSTS

A dermoid cyst is a tumor of developmental origin consisting of a wall of fibrous tissue lined with stratified epithelium containing hair follicles, sweat glands, sebaceous glands, nerves, or any combination of these. Dermoid cysts may be congenital or hereditary, have been reported in horses 6 months to 9 years of age, and are common in Thoroughbreds.[85] They occur frequently on the dorsal midline between the rump and withers. The cysts appear as soft, fluctuant swellings with normal overlying skin. The diagnosis is made by histologic examination after excision.

ATHEROMA (FALSE NOSTRIL CYST)

An atheroma is a cyst in the false nostril. These lesions are believed to develop from hair follicle retention cysts or from displaced germ material.[82] Atheromata are present at birth, are usually unilateral, and enlarge with time. They are not usually noticeable until they enlarge to greater than 2 cm. The tumor is firm on palpation but is rarely painful.

The diagnosis is based on clinical signs. Treatment is not necessary unless the tumor compromises breathing or the owner is disturbed by the lesion. Surgical excision is the treatment of choice, but one must take care to remove the entire cyst, lest recurrence or chronic drainage occur.

DISORDERS OF PIGMENTATION

Skin and hair color depend on melanin production in the skin. Melanocytes produce pigment at the dermal-epidermal junction and in the outer root sheath of the hair follicle. The ratio is one melanocyte for every 10 to 20 keratinocytes. Melanin pigments have a wide range of colors, including black-brown eumelanins, yellow-red pheomelanins, and a range of intermediate pigments. Special tyrosinase-rich organelles called melanosomes, which are found in the cytoplasm of melanocytes, produce melanin pigment. Tyrosine is converted to dopa, which is oxidized to dopaquinone. The copper-containing enzyme tyrosinase catalyzes both reactions. Subsequent intermediate products polymerize, eventually forming melanin. Melanocytes secrete or inject melanosomes into adjacent keratinocytes. Production of melanin is controlled by genetics, hormones, local keratinocytes, and Langerhans cells. Ultraviolet light, inflammation, byproducts of the arachidonic acid cycle, androgens, estrogen, glucocorticoids, and thyroid hormone also may influence pigmentation.[83]

The number, size, type, and distribution of melanosomes determines skin and hair color. Melanosomes are responsible for coat color, photoprotection, free radical scavenging, and heat conservation.

Causes of Hyperpigmentation

Hyperpigmentation is almost always an acquired change. The skin and hair may become hyperpigmented. The usual cause of localized or patchy hyperpigmentation is chronic inflammation or irritation. Macular patches of noninflammatory hyperpigmentation, called lentigo, can occur in horses. Lentigo occurs most frequently at mucocutaneous junctions. The most important differential diagnosis for lentigo is cutaneous melanoma. A skin biopsy of the affected area is the most useful diagnostic test. Generalized hyperpigmentation of the coat or skin has not been reported; however, if observed, the condition may suggest an underlying hormonal disorder.

Causes of Hypopigmentation

Hypopigmentation is a decrease in normal melanin pigmentation. Depigmentation specifically refers to a loss of preexisting melanin. Leukoderma and leukotrichia are clinical terms used to describe the loss of color in skin and hair, respectively. Amelanosis is a total lack of melanin.

ALBINISM AND LETHAL WHITE FOAL DISEASE

Albinism is rare in horses and is transmitted by an autosomal dominant gene. Affected animals have white skin and hair, hypopigmented irides, and photophobia. Lethal white foal disease has two forms. One form is caused by an autosomal dominant gene characterized by early embryonic death in the homozygous state. The second form results from breeding of two overo Paint Horses and is an autosomal recessive disorder. Affected foals are characterized by a white hair coat and congenital ileocolonic aganglionosis.

LEUKODERMA

Leukoderma develops in areas of previous trauma or inflammation and may be temporary or permanent. Affected areas appear normal but depigmented. Leukoderma occurs commonly in horses with onchocerciasis, lupus erythematosus, pressure sores, ventral midline dermatitis, viral skin diseases, freezing, burns, or sun damage (Figure 13-28). Leukoderma can result from the contact of skin with chemicals that inhibit or interfere with melanogenesis, such as phenol and rubber products containing monobenzyl ether or hydroquinone.

The diagnosis is usually made by clinical signs, but elliptic biopsy of the junction of the pigmented and nonpigmented area confirms the diagnosis. Leukoderma causes no discomfort to the horse, but it may be a source of great agitation to the owner. No treatment is known.

VITILIGO OF ARABIAN HORSES (ARABIAN FADING SYNDROME AND PINKY SYNDROME)

The term vitiligo refers to an idiopathic acquired depigmentation. Leukoderma develops in areas with no known history of previous trauma. Vitiligo can occur in any age, sex, or breed of horse but is most common in the Arabian (Figure 13-29).[1] Vitiligo appears to be more common in pregnant or postpartum mares, suggesting a hormonal or stress influence. In addition, the condition may be hereditary.[85]

With vitiligo, annular areas of depigmentation develop symmetrically on the muzzle, face, lips, and periocular areas.

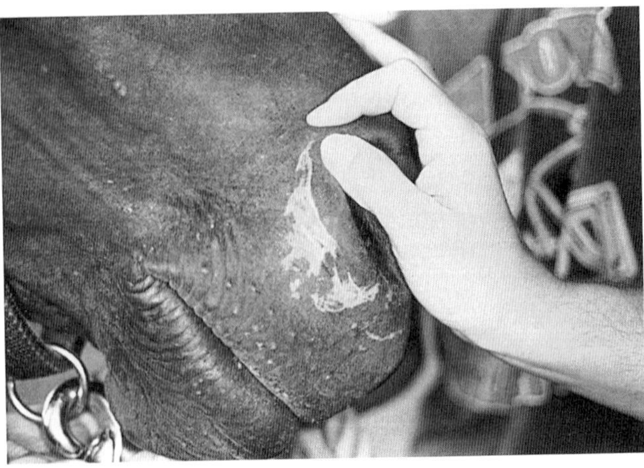

FIGURE 13-28 Idiopathic leukoderma in a horse.

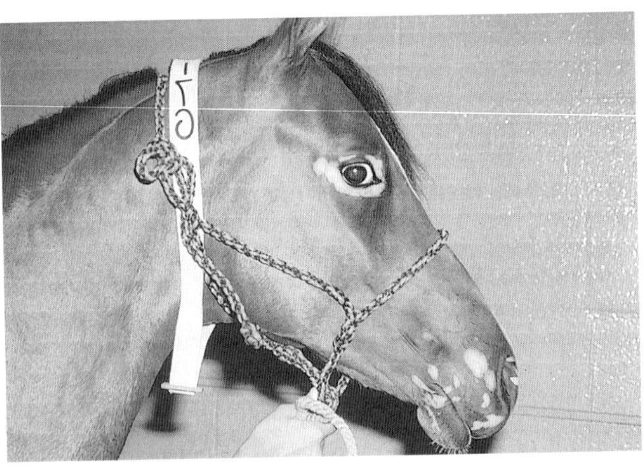

FIGURE 13-29 Horse with Arabian fading syndrome. Depigmented areas on the face are notable.

Depigmentation also can occur at the mucocutaneous junctions of the genital and anal area. Areas of depigmentation vary between 1 mm to 2 to 3 cm in size, and spots may become confluent at the mucocutaneous junctions. Depigmentation may wax and wane, and rarely the skin repigments completely within 1 to 2 years.

History, physical examination, and skin biopsy are diagnostic. Skin biopsy shows complete absence of epidermal melanin and lack of an inflammatory infiltrate. Success of treatment with topical glucocorticoids and vitamin-mineral supplementation (i.e., copper) is unpredictable. The practitioner should consider the condition untreatable, and owners should not breed affected animals because the condition is heritable and is considered a flaw. More practically, these areas are prone to sunburn and may predispose the horse to squamous cell carcinoma.

LEUKOTRICHIA

Leukotrichia is an acquired loss of pigment in hairs that occurs most commonly in areas of previous trauma or inflammation. Leukotrichia may also occur at the site of previous injections of epinephrine with or without lidocaine.

Reticulated leukotrichia is an inherited disorder of Quarter Horses, Thoroughbreds, and Standardbreds[1,85,86] (Figure 13-30).

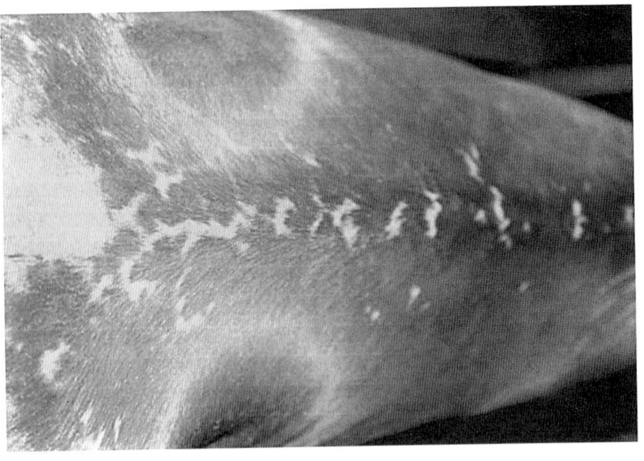

FIGURE 13-30 Reticulated leukotrichia in a Quarter Horse.

The condition has no sex predilection. Affected horses begin to show clinical signs as yearlings. Linear crusts in a netlike to crosshatched design develop over the dorsum from the withers to the tailhead region. Crusts are shed and after the temporary alopecia resolves, new hair growth is white. The underlying skin is normal, and leukotrichia is permanent. Leukotrichia causes no discomfort to the horse or interference with training or use of the animal. No therapy is available, and owners should not breed affected animals because leukotrichia is considered a breed flaw.

Spotted leukotrichia is a similar condition observed most commonly in Arabian Horses.[1,85,86] Permanent spots of leukotrichia develop over the hindquarters and trunk. Occasionally, lesions resolve spontaneously. No treatment is known, and owners should not breed affected animals because the condition is a breed flaw.

Hyperesthetic leukotrichia is a rare disease reported only in California.[87] Single or multiple crusts that are intensely painful characterize this disorder. Lesions develop on the dorsal midline from the withers to the tailhead. Within a few weeks, white hairs develop in the areas of crusting. The intense pain and crusting may last weeks to months. Eventually, lesions subside, but leukotrichia is permanent. Skin biopsy shows significant subepidermal and intraepidermal edema. No treatment is known, and large doses of glucocorticoids have not been of value.

DISCOID LUPUS ERYTHEMATOSUS

Discoid lupus erythematosus is a rare skin disease in horses that is believed to be a variant of systemic lupus erythematosus. Affected horses develop areas of patchy erythema, crusting alopecia, and scaling on the face, ears, and neck.[1] Leukoderma and leukotrichia may be present.

The diagnostic test of choice is a skin biopsy. The skin biopsy reveals an interface dermatitis (hydropic or lichenoid or both). Focal hydropic degeneration of basal epidermal cells, pigmentary incontinence (pigment granules in the dermis or in dermal macrophages), and focal thickening of the basement membrane are important histologic features. Direct immunofluorescence testing may show a linear deposition of immunoglobulins at the basement membrane zone. This test is not reliable and is not recommended as a substitute for a routine histopathologic study.

Discoid lupus erythematosus is treated on an individual basis. Ideally the owner should stable the horse during the hours of strong sunlight because sunlight aggravates the disease.[1] Topical sunscreens and topical glucocorticoids, for example, 0.1% betamethasone 17-valerate, may be beneficial. Severe or refractory cases of discoid lupus erythematosus may require immunosuppressive doses of oral prednisolone (see the section on pemphigus foliaceus).

DISORDERS OF COLLAGEN FORMATION

Hereditary equine dermal asthenia (HERDA) and hyperelastosis cutis are defects in collagen. HERDA is an autosomal recessive trait[91] that occurs primarily in cutting horse strains of Quarter Horses and horses of Quarter Horse lineage (Paints and Appaloosas).[4,88-90] A similar condition has been described in an Arabian cross-breed, a Thoroughbred gelding, a Hanoverian foal, and a Haflinger horse. Male and female horses are affected equally. Foals are born with abnormal collagen, but the condition may take months to years before becoming clinically apparent to the owner.

Clinical signs include loose skin that is hyperextensible, hyperfragile, and easily torn and that exhibits impaired healing (Figures 13-31 and 13-32). The most common lesions in affected horses are seromas or hematomas, open wounds, sloughing skin, and loose easily tented skin that does not return to its original position. Lesions may be solitary or multiple, and the most common lesion location is the dorsal body surface. Affected horses rarely, if ever, exhibit hypermobility of the joints. Occassionally, owners complain that the horse develops hematomas and subcutaneous abscesses.

The diagnosis is based on clinical signs, physical examination, and skin biopies. The most common histologic findings are an absent or greatly diminished deep dermal collagen layer. Other changes that may occur are thinning of the dermis and thinning, fragmented, and disordered collagen fibers. Zonal dermal seperation is a distinctive histopathologic lesion associated with hyperelastosis cutis in the Quarter Horse.[90] The presence of tightly grouped thin and shortened collagen fibers arranged in clusters in the deep dermis is typical of HERDA.[91] Trichrome, acid orcein-Giemsa and immunohistochemical stains for collagen I and II showed no consistent abnormalities compared with control horses. In addition, no abnormalities were noted on electron microscopy. Therefore the diagnosis of HERDA relies on clinical presentation and may be supported by suggstive histopathologic lesions.

No treatment for hyperelastosis cutis is available. Owners should attempt to minimize trauma to affected horses and promptly treat secondary infections. Most affected horses are euthanized because their fragile skin impairs their usefulness. Owners should remove sires and dams of affected horses from the breeding stock.

HAIR ABNORMALITIES

Horses have simple hair follicles, which are accompanied by a sebaceous and sweat gland and an arrector pili muscle. Photoperiods and ambient temperature predominantly govern the hair cycle. Nutrition, hormone, genetics, and general well-being also may influence hair growth. Hair replacement in the horse occurs in a random pattern (mosaic) with the exception of the coarse permanent hair of the mane, tail, and fetlock.

Chemical and Plant Causes of Coat Abnormalities

SELENIUM TOXICOSIS

Selenium is a trace mineral found in high concentrations in the Great Plains and Rocky Mountain areas of the United States. Toxicosis occurs when high levels of selenium in the soil are concentrated in selenium-concentrating plants. Interestingly, many of these plants grow selectively in selenium-rich soil and can contain up to several thousand parts per million of selenium. Selenium toxicosis may also occur when water contains 0.1 to 0.2 ppm selenium or feed contains greater than 5 ppm.[1] The exact mechanism of action is unknown, but selenium is believed to interfere with oxidative enzyme systems that possess sulfur-containing amino acids by displacing the sulfur groups. Selenium is substituted for sulfur in sulfur-containing amino acids. Keratinization of the hoof and hair are especially affected by the defective amino acids.

Selenium toxicosis occurs in any age, breed, or sex of animal but is most common in horses on pasture.[92] Early lesions begin as lameness and soreness of the coronary band and feet. The hindfeet usually are affected first. The coronary band and hoof develop cracks and separation and eventually the hoof may slough. The hair coat becomes rough, and generalized

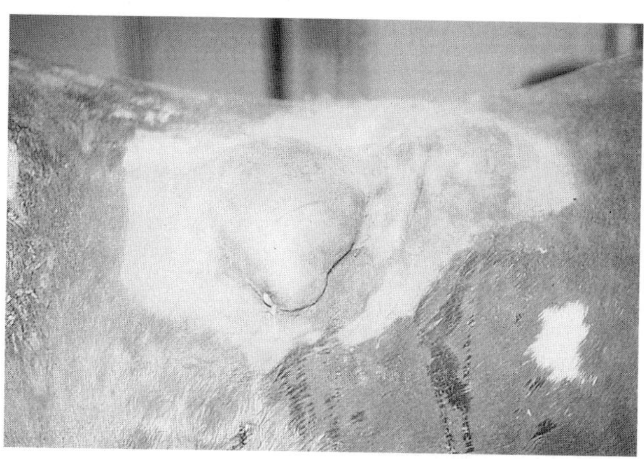

FIGURE 13-31 Horse with severe hyperelastosis cutis.

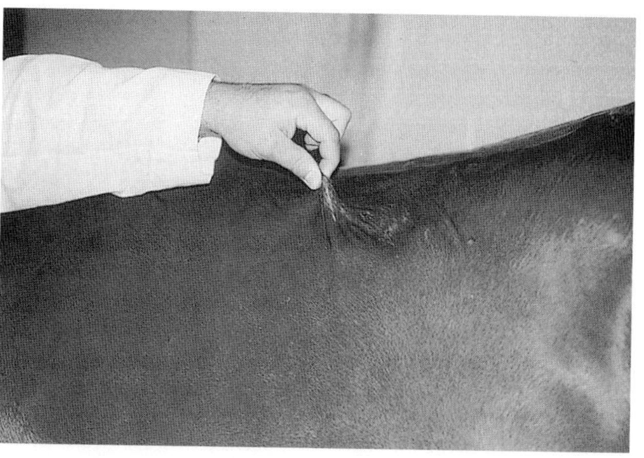

FIGURE 13-32 Horse with mild hyperelastosis cutis.

epilation of the long hairs of the mane and tail occurs. Generalized alopecia may be visible.

A definitive diagnosis is made by history, clinical signs, and tissue analysis for selenium levels. Selenium in excess of 1 to 4 ppm from blood, 11 to 45 ppm for hair, and 8 to 20 ppm for the hoof indicates chronic toxicity. Identifying and removing the exogenous source of selenium is critical. Treatment of individual animals is frustrating because of the prolonged recovery period. Chronically affected animals have a 50% chance of recovery. A high-protein diet rich in sulfa-containing amino acids and 2 to 3 mg orally per day of DL-methionine may be beneficial. Naphthalene orally at 4 to 5 g per adult horse also may be of benefit. The horse should receive one cycle of treatment: 5 days of naphthalene, stop for 5 days, and 5 days of naphthalene treatment. Inorganic arsenic at 5 ppm in drinking water or salt with 35 to 40 ppm arsenic may protect the sulfur-containing structures of the body.[92]

ARSENIC POISONING

Arsenic is commonly found in some parasiticidal dips, weed and orchard sprays, insect baits, and arsenic-containing medications. Arsenic is a general tissue poison, and 1 to 5 mg/kg may be toxic to horses.[21] Signs of arsenic toxicosis include gastrointestinal disturbances, weight loss, and a dry, dull, easily epilated hair coat. Some horse may develop a long shaggy coat with severe seborrhea.

The diagnosis is based on history of ingestion of arsenic or an arsenic-containing compound and clinical signs. A definitive diagnosis may be difficult because the test of choice is the measurement of arsenic levels in kidney or liver (>10 ppm).[1,21]

Treatment of arsenic toxicity is complicated by the peracute nature of the disease. One should wash off topically absorbable arsenic and should empty the digestive tract of the horse with the aid of laxatives. Orally administered sodium thiosulfate at 50 to 75 g every 6 to 8 hours binds unabsorbed arsenic. Intraveously administered sodium thiosulfate at 25 to 30 g of a 20% solution in distilled water may counterabsorb arsenic. Dimercaprol (British AntiLewisite [BAL] in oil) is the classic antidote for arsenic toxicity and is effective if administered within hours of ingestion. Initial treatment is 5 mg/kg intramuscularly and then 3 mg/kg every 6 hours for the first day, followed by a dosage of 1 mg/kg intramuscularly every 6 hours for the next 48 hours. Intramuscular injections are painful.[21] One must identify the source of arsenic and eliminate it.

MERCURY POISONING

Mercury poisoning occurs when the horse ingests feed contaminated with fungicide or absorbs or ingests mercury from counterirritants.[1] Affected horses may have gastrointestinal disorders, depression, anorexia, weight loss, and emaciation. Generalized alopecia with subsequent loss of mane and tail hairs is common. The diagnosis is complicated because the sample of choice is kidney tissue, where mercury is concentrated. Orally administered potassium iodide at 4 g per day for 14 days may be beneficial in treating affected horses.[82]

LEUCENOSIS POISONING

Leucenosis is a toxicosis resulting from the ingestion of plants of the genus *Leucaena*.[1,21] In the United States, these plants are found in Hawaii. This plant contains a toxic amino acid (mimosine) that is a potent depilatory agent.

Horses with this toxicosis show a gradual loss of the mane, tail, and fetlock hairs. Severely intoxicated animals may undergo complete hair loss 7 to 14 days after exposure. Laminitis and hoof dystrophies have been reported.[1,21]

The diagnosis is based on history and clinical signs. One treats affected horses symptomatically after preventing further exposure to the plants. Ferrous sulfate 1% added to the feed may benefit affected horses and limit further hoof damage.[1]

Hair Follicle Abnormalities

MANE AND TAIL DYSTROPHY

Mane and tail dystrophy may be congenital or acquired. Whether the condition is hereditary is unknown. Affected horses (juvenile or adult) have short, brittle, dull hairs on the mane and tail. No treatment is known, but the condition does not affect the health or function of the horse.

BLACK AND WHITE FOLLICLE DYSTROPHY

Affected horses (juvenile and adult) have abnormal hairs growing in patches of white- or black-haired areas. These hairs are short, brittle, and dull. Affected areas may be hypotrichotic. No treatment is available.

CURLY COAT

Curly coat is a hereditary condition of Percherons, Missouri Fox Trotters, and Bashkin Horse breeds that is inherited as an autosomal recessive trait. Clinically affected horses have unusually curly coats.

Endocrine Causes of Hair Abnormalities

HYPERADRENOCORTICISM

Equine hyperadrenocorticism secondary to pituitary pars intermedia dysfunction is discussed in detail in the chapter of this text on Disorders of the Endocrine System. Abnormal pituitary function results in abnormal secretion of numerous hormones.[21,93] Clinical signs are most common in older horses (12 to 15 years old or older), [21,93,94] but the condition is reported occasionally in horses 7 to 10 years of age. The first clinical sign noted by an owner is often a rapid regrowth of long hair after the shedding season or failure to shed the coat (Figure 13-33). The coat becomes shaggy, and body hairs can reach lengths of 10 to 12 cm. Interestingly, mane, tail, and fetlock hairs are unaffected. Secondary seborrhea may develop. Affected horses may be predisposed to dermatophytosis, dermatophilosis, or secondary bacterial pyoderma. Nondermatologic signs include polydipsia, polyuria, muscle wasting, lethargy, weight loss, pendulous abdomen, laminitis, and flaccid muscles. Neurologic disorders and blindness may develop.

The diagnosis is based on clinical signs and laboratory test results.[94-97] Complete blood counts often reveal neutrophilia, lymphopenia, and eosinopenia. Urinalysis may reveal a low specific gravity and occasionally glucosuria. A serum chemistry panel may reveal any combination of the following: hyperglycemia, hypercholesterolemia, and lipemia.[94] The definitive diagnosis and treatment of pituitary pars intermedia dysfunction in horses is discussed elsewhere in this text.

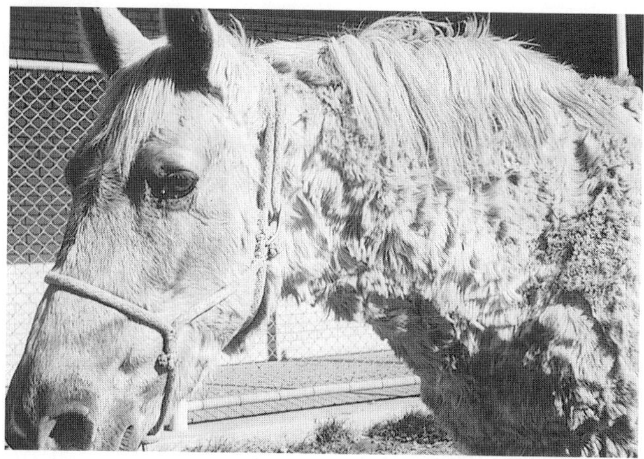

FIGURE 13-33 Horse with pituitary pars intermedia dysfunction. The long hair coat did not shed in the spring.

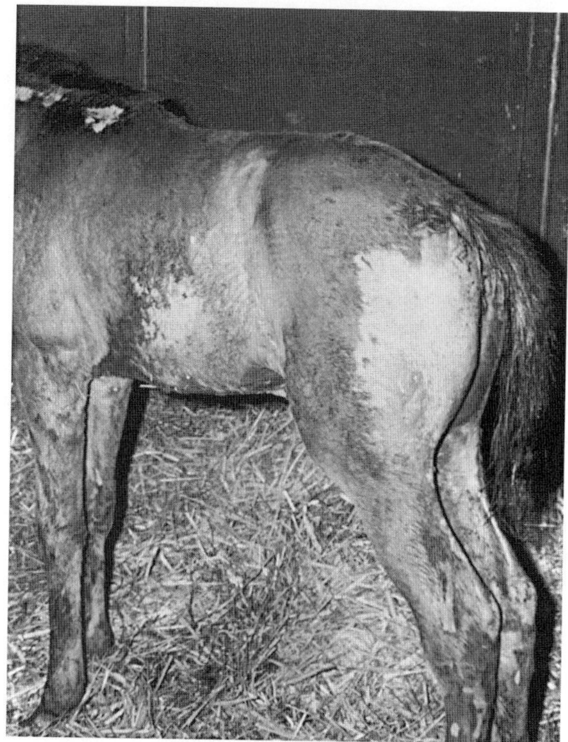

FIGURE 13-34 Foal with telogen effluvium after illness.

HYPOTHYROIDISM

Hypothyroidism in the horse is rare, and much of the information on this endocrinopathy is anecdotal.[98-100] Horses with naturally occurring hypothyroidism reportedly have a wide range of clinical signs, including loss of mane and tail hairs, muscle weakness, hyperpigmentaion, seborrhea, lethargy, poor performance, infertility, agalactia, myxedema, and dry, dull, brittle hair. The diagnosis and treatment of equine hypothyroidism is discussed in this text in the chapter on Disorders of the Endocrine System.

Miscellaneous Disorders Affecting the Hair Coat

ANAGEN DEFLUXION AND TELOGEN DEFLUXION

Anagen defluxion refers to a condition in which a disease or drug interferes with anagen hair growth resulting in abnormal hairs or hair shaft abnormalities or both. Hair loss occurs within days of the insult or drug. The condition occurs most commonly in horses with high fevers, systemic illnesses, or malnutrition[21] (Figure 13-34). Typically the mane and tail are not affected.

Telogen defluxion refers to a condition in which a stressful situation causes the sudden cessation of anagen hair growth and the sudden synchrony of many hair follicles in the telogen hair cycle stage.[21] Two to three months later a sudden shedding and a wave of new hair growth occur.

These conditions cannot be distinguished clinically. The diagnosis is based on examining the hair shaft of easily epilated hairs. Anagen defluxion is characterized by dysplastic hairs, the hair shaft may be weak or narrow, and the root end contains a root sheath. Telogen defluxion is characterized by uniform hairs with no shaft abnormalities and a nonpigmented root end lacking a root sheath. Both conditions resolve spontaneously when the animal recovers from the predisposing condition.

TRICHORRHEXIS NODOSA

Trichorrhexis nodosa is an acquired hair shaft disorder of horses caused by physical or chemical trauma.[86] Overzealous grooming, shampoos, pesticides, alcohol, or solvents are the most common causes. The lesions are visible without magnification and appear as small white to gray nodules on the hair shaft. The hair shaft fractures and breaks easily at these sites. Microscopically, affected hairs have the appearance of two brooms shoved together. Therapy consists of identifying and eliminating the trauma.

PIEDRA

Piedra is a rare superficial fungal disease of horses that causes nodules on the hair shaft. Black or white filamentous nodules consisting of tightly packed hyphae are most commonly visible on the mane and tail. Affected hairs break at the site of infection. A definitive diagnosis is made by fungal culture and microscopic identification of the agent *Piedraia* sp. or *Trichosporon beigelii*. Treatment of affected horses includes clipping the hair and applying topical fungicides.

ABNORMAL SHEDDING: PHOTOPERIOD AND TEMPERATURE RELATED SHEDDING

Most horses have a spring and fall shed. Abnormal shedding in horses may result in large areas of alopecia.[86] Large areas of hair loss may develop on the face, shoulders, or even over the entire body. The pathogenesis is unknown. Skin biopsy is recommended to eliminate infectious or parasitic causes of hair loss. Skin biopsy is normal and shows normal hair follicles in various stages of development. Horses spontaneously recover in up to 3 months.[87]

ALOPECIA AREATA

Alopecia areata is a rare idiopathic skin disease of horses characterized by focal areas of alopecia.[85] Lesions may be single or multiple, and the underlying skin is otherwise normal. If and when hair regrows, it may be a different color. The diagnosis is made by biopsy. Classically, in early lesions, skin biopsy shows an accumulation of lymphoid cells around the proximal end of the anagen hair follicles.[86] This change is diagnostic but may require numerous biopsies before being observed. Prognosis is uncertain. In human beings, alopecia areata may resolve spontaneously in 3 to 5 years. Whether spontaneous resolution occurs in horses is unknown.

MUCOCUTANEOUS VESICULAR DISEASES

A vesicle is an elevated, fluctuant, fluid-filled lesion of less than 1 cm in size. A vesicular eruption suggests a viral, autoimmune, or irritant cause. In horses, vesicles are transient because the epidermis is thin, and these lesions rupture easily. Erosions or ulcerations are often the first clue that a vesicle-producing disease is present. Additionally, vesicular diseases may masquerade as pustular eruptions. Vesicles in horses rapidly fill with inflammatory cells, making them indistinguishable from frank pustules. In rare instances, horses may develop bullae (>1 cm in diameter) or large vesicles. Occasionally, bullae fill with blood and are red-purple.

Viral Causes of Vesicular Eruptions

EQUINE HERPES COITAL EXANTHEMA

Coital exanthema is a rare contagious venereal disease of horses cause by equine herpesvirus type 3, which occurs worldwide. The disease is transmitted via coitus, insects, fomites, and inhalation. Early lesions begin as papules that rapidly progress to vesicles or bullae or pustules on the vulva or perineum of mares and the penis and prepuce of stallions.[4] Vesicles and bullae also may be present in the mouth or nostril or on the lips. Affected areas commonly become eroded and ulcerative. Lesions are more often pruritic rather than painful. Depigmentation often occurs in areas where lesions have developed and healed. Stress may precipitate recurrences.

The diagnosis is based on the appearance of lesions on the vulva, perineum, penis, or prepuce; skin biopsy; and virus isolation. Histologic findings include hyperplastic superficial and deep perivascular dermatitis with ballooning degeneration and eosinophilic intranuclear inclusion bodies.

Treatment is symptomatic, but corticosteroids are contraindicated. Owners should isolate affected horses and remove broodmares and stallions from the breeding program for a minimum of 4 weeks. The disease has no known effect on fertility.

VESICULAR STOMATITIS (SORE NOSE AND SORE MOUTH)

Vesicular stomatitis is caused by a rhabdovirus with two major serotypes: New Jersey and Indiana.[21] The disease affects horses, cattle, and swine and is enzootic in North, Central, and South America. In North America the disease is reportable.

The disease has a seasonal occurrence in summer and fall and is believed to be transmitted to horses by insect bites. Within a group of horses, however, the disease may be transmitted via direct contact. The incubation period is short (24 to 72 hours), and lesions may last for only 3 to 4 days. Infected horses rapidly develop vesicles up to 2 cm in diameter in the mouth and on the lips. These lesions rupture, leaving large painful erosions and ulcers. Affected animals salivate profusely, and fever and anorexia are common. Rarely, lesions develop on the hooves, prepuce, and teats.

Confirmation of the diagnosis is obtained by serologic examination. Histologic findings are nonspecific and include a hyperplastic epidermis, intercellular and intracellular edema of the epidermis, reticular degeneration, spongiotic microvesicles, and focal necrosis. Superficial and deep perivascular dermatitis is present.

Owners should feed affected horses a soft gruel until oral lesions heal, usually within a few days. Permanent depigmentation may occur in areas of former ulceration. Infection results in immunity for up to 6 months.

HORSEPOX

Horsepox is uncommon and has been reported only in Europe. Horsepox is a benign disease, caused by an unclassified poxvirus.

The virus gains access to the body by the respiratory tract or the skin.[101] Systemic spread occurs by the lymphatics. Poxvirus inoculated into the skin may multiply locally, directly enter the blood, and create a primary viremia. The virus causes degenerative changes in the epithelium as a result of virus replication and results in development of vesicular lesions. Poxviruses also cause epithelial hyperplasia by stimulating host-cell DNA synthesis before the onset of cytoplasmic virus-related DNA replication. Ischemia and necrosis occur in the dermis and subcutaneous areas as a result of vascular damage.

Clinical lesions of equine poxvirus infections develop as follows. An erythematous maculopapular eruption develops, followed by the development of vesicles. This stage is transient and may not be observed. Vesicles develop into umbilicated pustules with a depressed center and a raised erythematous border. When the pustule ruptures a crust develops and the lesion heals, often with scarring.

Horsepox may affect horses of any age. The disease is transmitted by direct contact with an infected host or with contaminated grooming tools or tack. Lesions of horsepox are typically vesicles and umbilicated pustules with crusts. Three clinical presentations (oral, leg, and vulvar) have been described.[64] Oral horsepox (buccal horsepox, contagious pustular stomatitis) is characterized by the development of lesions on the inner lips and buccal mucosa. In severe forms, pox lesions may develop in the pharynx, larynx, nostrils, or all of these sites. Leg pox usually develops on the pasterns and fetlocks and often is confused with "scratches" or "greasy heel." Pain and lameness are common. Vulvar pox (genital horsepox) is uncommon, occurring predominantly in severely affected animals. One may observe pyrexia and anorexia early in the course of the three forms of horsepox.

The diagnosis is based on history and clinical signs and confirmed by histologic examination. Intracytoplasmic inclusion bodies demonstrated by routine histopathologic examination of tissue or electron microscopy are diagnostic. Other findings include ballooning degeneration of the epidermis (stratum spinosum), reticular degeneration, acantholysis (loss of cohesion of cell in the granular area), intraepidermal microvesicles, a superficial and deep perivascular dermatitis, and intraepidermal microabscesses and pustules.

Treatment is symptomatic. Most horses recover in 2 to 4 weeks. Occasionally the disease is fatal in severely affected young horses. Recovery produces lifelong immunity. This disease affects human beings and cattle.

Autoimmune Diseases Causing Vesicular Lesions

Bullous pemphigoid is a rare autoimmune skin disease of horses characterized by the development of vesicles and ulceration of the oral mucosa and occasionally the skin. Bullous pemphigoid is caused by production of an autoantibody (pemphigoid antibody) against a component in the basement membrane of the skin and mucous membranes.[56] The pemphigoid antibody binds to the basement membrane zone and complement fixation occurs, resulting in production of inflammatory mediators chemotactic for neutrophils and eosinophils. These cells release proteolytic enzymes that disrupt the dermal-epidermal cohesion; separation occurs, and a vesicle forms.

In horses, vesicles and bullae develop at the mucocutaneous junction in the inguinal region or in the oral cavity.[85] Skin lesions occur in the axilla and groin. Vesicles and bullae rupture easily and are often crusted and secondarily infected with bacteria. Pain, pruritus, anorexia, fever, and salivation are common.

A definitive diagnosis is made by eliminating other causes of vesicular lesions from the differential list and by skin biopsy. Biopsy of a vesicle or intact bullae is essential; biopsy of crusted or ulcerative lesions will be nondiagnostic. Bullous pemphigoid is characterized by subepidermal vacuolar alterations and subepidermal clefts and vesicles.[1] Neutrophilic and eosinophilic infiltration of the superficial epidermis is common. If direct immunofluorescence testing is performed and the results are positive, one observes a linear deposition of immunoglobulin at the basement membrane zone. Direct immunofluorescence testing is not recommended.

There are few reports of the treatment of bullous pemphigoid in horses.[1,57,85] Treatments have included an initial large dose of prednisolone (1 mg/kg orally every 12 hours) or dexamethasone (0.2 mg/kg orally every 24 hours) to induce remission. After the arrest of new lesion development and healing, one institutes maintenance therapy with alternate-day administration of glucocorticoids at the smallest effective dose. Therapy must be individualized and will most likely be lifelong. The use of adjuvant therapy (e.g., gold salts or azathioprine) has not been reported in horses with bullous pemphigoid but may be useful.

Irritant and Toxic Causes of Mucocutaneous Vesicles

Irritant reactions, toxic chemicals, or allergic reaction to drugs may result in oral mucocutaneous vesicles. One should suspect these causes when lesions develop acutely in the absence of signs of systemic illness, in single animals within a herd, or in horses receiving medications or counterirritants. Mercurial compounds (commonly used in counterirritants) can also cause generalized hair loss, lameness, and emaciation in chronically intoxicated animals. Creosol and cantharidin beetles are common causes of oral ulcers. Foreign bodies such as grass awns may cause mucocutaneous ulceration and vesicles.

Vasculitis

Oral ulcers may develop in horses with vasculitis (see the section on Vasculitis and Purpura Hemorrhagica).

Necrotizing Skin Disorders

Necrotizing skin diseases develop from a wide range of causes. The unifying characteristic is that each of these diseases may cause local or widespread full-thickness death of the skin, sloughing of tissue, ulceration, and exudation. A definitive diagnosis of the underlying cause may be difficult in some cases.

Decubital Ulcers (Pressure Sores, Setfasts, Saddle Galls, and Saddle Sores)

Decubital ulcers or sores are caused by prolonged application of pressure to an area. Thin and emaciated animals are at greatest risk for development of decubital ulcers.

Pressure sores may develop from poorly fitting tack on the back, neck, or girth of the horse; from recumbency during surgery, even while on suitable bedding; and from casts, leg wraps, or elastic bandages that have become wet or are unevenly wrapped, too tight, or ill fitting. The amount of pressure required to create a decubital ulcer is not great. Tack and saddles may cause lesions over bony prominences or other areas subjected to extended pressure. Capillary circulation is stopped or severely limited, resulting in tissue anoxia and retention of metabolic wastes with tissue damage and death. Most lesions begin as small areas of tissue necrosis and progress to areas of ulceration. Secondary infections are common.[1]

Clinically, early lesions begin with hair loss, swelling, and erythema. A red-purple area of tissue discoloration may be visible. Within a few days, oozing, necrosis, and ulceration become visible. In severe cases the skin loses its elasticity, subcutaneous tissues slough, and the skin may harden. Strands of living tissue may be attached to necrotic tissue. Lesions are often malodorous. Healed lesions tend to scar, and leukotrichia or leukoderma are common sequela.[82]

The diagnosis is based on history and clinical examination. Areas of skin that have lost sensation or have a parchmentlike feel should be suspect.

Treatment of these lesions is difficult. Because of significant capillary and venous congestion, systemic antibiotics are often not effective.[1,82] Wounds are managed best topically. One should clean the wounds daily with copious amounts of water to remove tissue debris and stimulate circulation and should use topical antibiotic creams or ointments (i.e., iodine and chlorhexidine) to prevent secondary infection and to prevent the wound from becoming desiccated. Re-epithelialization and wound healing greatly improve with the use of surgical dressings, but bandaging some lesions may be difficult. Surgical débridement and skin grafting may be indicated in some cases.

Gangrene

Gangrene is a clinical term used to describe wet or dry tissue necrosis. Gangrene may result from external pressure, severe edema, burns, frostbite, snake bites, vasculitis, ergotism, fescue toxicosis, or bacterial or viral infections.[1] The characteristic lesion results from occlusion of the venous or arterial blood supply.

Dry gangrene occurs when the arterial blood supply to an area is occluded but the venous or lymphatic drainage is intact.

Wet or moist gangrene is caused by occlusion or impairment of lymphatic and venous drainage plus putrefaction caused by a bacterial infection. Lesions of dry gangrene are dry, leathery, discolored, sunken, and cold to the touch. The skin may take a long time to slough. Lesions of wet gangrene are swollen, discolored, and malodorous.

The diagnosis is most often made by clinical examination and confirmed by biopsy. One must identify and treat the primary cause of gangrene.

Thermal Injuries

BURNS

Excessive heat (burns) can occur from barn fires, brush fires, accidental spillage of hot solutions, lightning, electrocution, rope burns, counterirritants, or radiation. Barn fires cause most burns in horses.

Large thermal injuries in horses are difficult to manage.[21,102-104] The large surface area of the burn dramatically increases the potential for fluid, electrolyte, and caloric losses. Burns on 50% or more of the body are usually fatal, but this depends on the depth of the burn.[93,95] Massive wound contamination is almost impossible to prevent because of the impossibility of maintaining a sterile environment.[21,101] Horses require long-term restraint to prevent continued trauma; wounds are often pruritic, and self-mutilation is common.[103] Burned horses are frequently disfigured, preventing them from returning to full function.

Burns are classified by the depth of the injury.[21,102-104] First-degree burns involve only the most superficial layers of the epidermis. These burns are characterized by erythema, edema, desquamation of superficial layers of the skin, and pain. The germinal layer of the epidermis is spared, and these burns heal without complication.[21] Second-degree burns involve the entire epidermis and may be superficial or deep. Superficial second-degree burns involve the stratum corneum, stratum granulosum, and a few cells of the basal layer. Deep second-degree burns involve all layers of the epidermis. Clinically, these burns are characterized by erythema, edema at the epidermal-dermal junction, necrosis of the epidermis, accumulation of white blood cells at the basal layer of the burn, eschar (slough produced by a thermal burn) formation, and minimal pain. The only germinal cells spared are those within the ducts of sweat glands and hair follicles. Second-degree burns heal well with good wound care.[21] Third-degree burns are characterized by loss of epidermal and dermal components. Fluid loss occurs, along with significant cellular response at the margins and deeper tissue, eschar formation, lack of pain, shock, wound infection, and possible bacteremia and septicemia. Healing is by contraction and epithelization and occurs only from the wound margins. Infection and problems with wound healing frequently complicate these burns.[21] Fourth-degree burns involve all the skin and underlying muscle, bone, and ligaments.

Burns cause local and systemic effects.[21,27,103,104] Local tissue damage results from massive protein coagulation and cellular death. In the immediate area of the burn, arteries and venules constrict and capillary beds dilate. Capillary wall permeability increases in response to vasoactive amines released as a result of tissue damage and inflammation.[104] These vascular responses result in fluid, protein, and inflammatory cells accumulating in the wound. Vascular sludging, thrombosis, and dermal ischemia occur, resulting in further tissue damage. The tissue ischemia continues for 24 to 48 hours after the injury and is believed to be caused by the local release of thromboxane A_2.[21,104] Lipid layers in the skin are destroyed, and a fourfold increase in the loss of fluid occurs. Fluid losses result in increased heat loss from evaporation and an increased metabolic rate. The full extent and depth of the burn may not be evident for several days. Neutrophil function and chemotaxis greatly decrease, predisposing the wound to local infection, bacteremia, and septicemia. The following microorganisms frequently colonize burns: *Pseudomonas aeruginosa, Staphylococcus, Escherichia coli, Klebsiella* spp., nonhemolytic *Streptococcus* spp., *Proteus* spp., *Clostridium* spp., and *Candida* spp.[21,101-103] Systemic effects are life-threatening and include hypovolemia, fluid and electrolyte losses, protein loss, pulmonary edema, anemia, increased basal metabolic rate, increased caloric needs, and depressed cell-mediated and humoral immune responses. Hypovolemia exacerbates a decrease in cardiac output after a circulating myocardial-depressant factor.[27]

The practitioner should treat first-degree burns and superficial second-degree burns immediately with ice or cold water to prevent further tissue necrosis.[21,101] One should apply aloe vera cream or a water-soluble antibacterial cream to the wound to prevent infection. In addition, nonsteroidal analgesics should be administered to alleviate pain and to help reduce dermal ischemia. Aspirin at 10 to 20 mg/kg orally once or twice daily decreases thromboxane production, may halt further dermal ischemia, and may be the initial drug of choice.[21]

Deep second-degree burns are initially treated as described previously; however, these burns tend to form blisters that should be left intact as long as possible because the vesicular fluid is a good medium for reepithelialization.[21,102,103] One should trim ruptured blisters, clean the area with copious amounts of water, and cover the wound with an antibacterial dressing or xenograft or allow an eschar to form.[21,102-104] The bandage should allow drainage and should be changed at least daily.

Full-thickness burns (third and fourth degree) are treated by occlusive dressing (closed technique), eschar production (exposure technique), continuous wet dressings (semiopen technique), or excision and grafting technniques.[104] The most practical therapy for large burns in horses is the semiopen method, leaving the eschar intact with continuous application of moist bandages and antibacterial agents. The moist dressings help prevent heat and moisture loss from the eschar, provide protection of the eschar, and help prevent bacterial invasion in the wound.

Routine use of systemic antibiotics is not recommended in burn patients. Short-term systemic antibiotics may be useful in the initial 3 to 5 days after the burn to minimize bacterial colonization of burns and systemic sepsis.[104] In the absence of sepsis, systemic antibiotics are contraindicated. Extensive use of antibiotics may cause altered microbial flora in the gut and in mucous membranes, which may predispose the patient to infections from antibiotic-resistant gram-negative bacteria or from fungi.[105] Topical medications should be water-based, should be applied and removed easily, should not interfere with wound healing, and should be excreted or metabolized readily. Silver sulfadiazine and aloe vera are effective. Silver sulfadiazine is effective against gram-negative bacteria, causes no discomfort to the horse, penetrates eschar, and has a 24-hour duration of action. Aloe vera is reported to relieve pain, decrease inflammation, stimulate cell growth, and kill bacteria and fungi. Aloe vera is most useful in the early treatment of wounds. Several excellent references for further information on long-term medical and surgical management of horses with large thermal burns are available.[21,102-104]

FROSTBITE

Frostbite occurs when tissue is exposed to extreme cold. Sick, debilitated, and neonatal animals are at increased risk. Cold temperatures inhibit cell metabolism and cause tissue dehydration, cell disruption by ice crystals, ischemia, and vascular damage. The most commonly affected areas are the glans penis, ear tips, coronary bands, and heels.[1] The initial lesion of frostbite is paleness of the skin. Erythema, scaling, and hair loss follow. Pigment loss may occur. In severe cases, necrosis and dry gangrene occur.

Mild cases of frostbite do not require treatment. More severe cases require rapid thawing in warm water (41° to 44° C).[1] After rewarming, one should apply antibiotic ointments without steroids to the area. In severe cases with necrosis and sloughing, topical wet soaks and symptomatic therapy with antibiotics may be needed to prevent sepsis. One should not attempt surgical débridement until an obvious demarcation is present between viable and nonviable tissue. Previously frostbitten areas may be more susceptible to cold injury.

Chemical Toxicosis

In addition to causing disorders of the hair coat, selenosis may result in necrosis and sloughing of the hoof (see the section Chemical and Plant Causes of Coat Abnormalities).

Stachybotryotoxicosis

Stachybotryotoxicosis is a mycotoxicosis caused by the toxins of the fungus *Stachybotrys atra*.[1] This fungus grows on hay and straw and produces toxins referred to as macrocytic trichothecenes. These toxins cause bone marrow suppression, profound neutropenia, thrombocytopenia, and necrotic-ulcerative lesions of the skin and mucous membranes.

Commonly, lesions begin at the mucocutaneous junction as focal areas of necrosis and ulceration. Petechiae, ulcers, large areas of necrosis, catarrhal rhinitis, suppurative rhinopharyngitis, and laryngitis follow. Skin lesions occur as early as 24 hours after ingestion of the toxin. Systemic signs include lethargy, anorexia, weight loss, hyperactivity, proprioceptive deficits, colic, muscular stiffness, and second-degree atrioventricular block. Affected animal develops hemorrhagic diathesis, hemorrhagic enteritis, and septicemia and die.

The diagnosis is based on history, clinical signs, and finding the toxin in the feed. If one recognizes toxicosis early in the course of the disease, withdrawal of affected feed has resulted in resolution of signs. Animals with extensive lesions and chronic exposure have a poor prognosis.

Bites and Stings of Venomous Insects, Spiders, and Reptiles

Many species of snakes, spiders, and insects have venomous bites and stings. Except for snake bites, these animals lack sufficient quantity of venom to cause more than transient pain or local inflammation. Venoms contain a variety of substances, including enzymes, peptides, polypeptides, amines, and glycosides, which act locally by causing tissue necrosis and vascular thrombosis and hemorrhage or systemically by causing widespread hemolysis and neurotoxicity.

SNAKE BITE

Of the poisonous snakes in the United States, bites from rattlesnakes, water moccasins, and copperheads occur most commonly in horses.[106] The venom from snakes is hemotoxic and proteolytic and produces extreme local swelling with significant tissue and red blood cell destruction.

Most bites occur in the spring and summer. Horses are most commonly bitten on the nose, head, neck, and legs. Snake bites may or may not involve envenomation and may be dry or wet. Bites in which no venom is injected swell minimally and are only slightly painful (dry bite). When envenomation occurs (wet bite), rapid swelling, pain, and local hemorrhage develop, usually within 60 minutes of the bite. Fang marks are often difficult to find because of tissue swelling. Edema, erythema, and tissue necrosis develop over days, and the skin may slough (Figure 13-35). Bites occurring on the face or head are serious because of the risk of respiratory and nasal edema. If respiratory distress is severe, the horse may need a tracheotomy.

Snake bites should be treated symptomatically. One should clean the wound and provide hydrotherapy with cold water to minimize swelling. If swelling is already present, warm hydrotherapy may stimulate circulation and removal of tissue edema. Whether hydrotherapy increases the absorption of venom in the early stages of the bite is unknown, however. Broad-spectrum antibiotics are indicated to prevent secondary infection. The use of glucocorticoids is controversial but may be beneficial in decreasing inflammation and pain. Nonsteroidal anti-inflammatory agents also may be beneficial. Surgical débridement and wound closure may be necessary if severe necrosis and sloughing occur. Although specific antivenoms are available, they are of limited use. Maximal benefit is attained only when they are administered within hours of the bite. Additionally, the volume of antivenom necessary to treat snake bites in horses may be cost prohibitive.

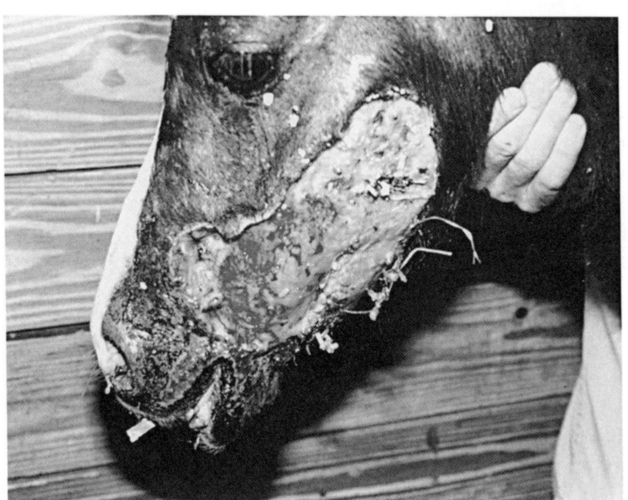

FIGURE 13-35 Face of a horse after being bitten by an Eastern diamondback rattlesnake.

FIRE ANT BITES

Fire ants, *Solenopsis* spp., are common in the southern United States. Single or small numbers of stings are acutely painful and rapidly develop into a pustule or crust. Horses are bitten most commonly on the legs, nose, and ventrum, but massive exposure can occur if the horse rolls on an anthill and is bitten by hundreds or thousands of ants. Complications of massive exposure include infection, anaphylactic shock, bronchospasms, and sloughing of the epidermis. Single or multiple small numbers of solitary stings usually require little or no treatment. Applying an antibiotic ointment to minimize the chance of myiasis is prudent; otherwise, wounds heal without complication. If massive exposure has occurred, one may need to use systemic antibiotics and nonsteroidal anti-inflammatory drugs to decrease pain and swelling.

SPIDER BITES

Black, brown, and red widow spiders (*Latrodectus* spp.) and the brown recluse *(Loxosceles reclusa)* spider are common in America. In Australia the black house spider *(Ixeuticus)* causes painful bites.[106] Spider bites are characterized by hot, edematous, painful swellings in the area of the bite. The brown recluse spider has a dermal necrotoxin that may cause severe dermal necrosis, but this has not been reported in horses.

Treatment is symptomatic. Cold ice packs applied to the area, and systemic glucocorticoids or antihistamines, or both, may be helpful. Spraying the environment of the horse with a parasiticide is important. Owners should remove discarded furniture, newspapers, old cloths, and trash from the premises because these are favorite living areas for venomous spiders.

VASCULITIS AND PURPURA HEMORRHAGICA

Vasculitis is an inflammatory reaction occurring in the wall of the blood vessel (Figure 13-36). Vasculitides are classified by inflammatory cell type. Neutrophilic vasculitides are subdivided further into leukocytoclastic (neutrophil nuclei undergo karyorrhexis) or nonleukocytoclastic.

The immunologic mechanisms involved are typically type I and type II hypersensitivity reactions.[21] Equine viral arteritis, equine influenza, *C. pseudotuberculosis,* and *Streptococcus* spp. (especially *S. zooepidemicus* subsp. *equi*) infections may result in vasculitis.[35] Vasculitis also may occur after *Rhodococcus equi* pneumonia, cholangiohepatitis, and some antibiotic treatments. The underlying cause is often not identified.

Idiopathic vasculitis has no known breed, sex, or age predilection. The most common locations for lesions are the distal limbs, ears, lips, and periocular areas.[1] Oral ulcers and bullae may be present. Skin lesions consist of purpura, edema, and erythema. Systemic signs may include pyrexia, depression, anorexia, weight loss, and lameness.

Purpura hemorrhagica is an acute noncontagious disease of horses characterized by extensive edema and hemorrhage of the subcutaneous tissue. Hemorrhage in the mucosae and viscera are common. Most cases occur after strangles or equine influenza.[1] Clinical signs usually develop within 2 to 4 weeks of the respiratory infection. Urticaria followed by pitting edema of the distal limbs, head, and ventral abdomen is common. Severe edema of the head may compromise breathing.[17] Tissue exudation and sloughing may occur. Pain and pruritus are rare. Affected horses usually are depressed, reluctant to move, and often anorectic.

The diagnosis of vasculitis is made by skin biopsy. Obtaining skin biopsy specimens from lesions 8 to 24 hours of age is important because these lesions tend to have the most diagnostic changes. Lesions more than 24 hours old may be nondiagnostic because of intense secondary cellular infiltrates or necrosis. Skin biospy reveals neutrophilic, eosinophilic, lymphocytic, or mixed cellular infiltrates in the vessel wall. Fibrinoid degeneration and hemorrhage are common.[64] Direct immunofluorescence testing is occasionally useful as an adjunctive diagnostic aid.

Prognosis for horses with vasculitis is unpredictable.[27] Therapy of vasculitis is discussed elsewhere in this text.

PANNICULITIS AND FAT NECROSIS

Panniculitis refers to inflammation of the subcutaneous fat. This condition is rare in horses and results from widespread death of lipocytes. Fat cells are vulnerable to trauma, ischemia, and neighboring inflammation. When lipocytes are damaged, lipid is released and undergoes hydrolysis into glycerol and fatty acids. Fatty acids are potent inflammatory agents that elicit further inflammatory reactions.[21]

Panniculitis may be precipitated by a wide range of causes, including trauma, infections, autoimmune disease, pancreatic disease, glucocorticoid therapy, vasculitis, vitamin E deficiency, and idiopathic causes. In the horse, few cases have been reported, and the causes of those were obscure. Vitamin E deficiency was suspected in a few horses.[76]

Clinically, horses with panniculitis show deep-seated nodules and plaques.[21] Lesions may be single or multiple and vary in size. Nodules may be hard and well-defined or soft and ill-defined. Initially, lesions are not fixed to the overlying

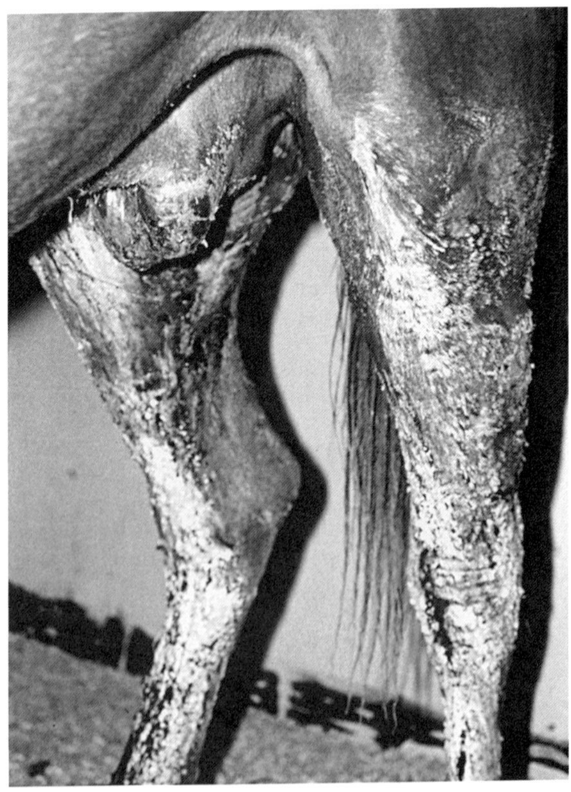

FIGURE 13-36 Horse with vasculitis resulting from strangles.

skin, but as the disease progresses, nodules become cystic and rupture onto the skin surface. The ulcerating nodules drain a yellow to brown to bloody oily material. Pain varies. Healed lesions may leave depressed scars. Affected animals may be febrile, depressed, lethargic, and anorectic.

A definitive diagnosis is made by skin biopsy. Samples should be obtained for histopathologic evaluation by deep excisional biopsy using a scalpel blade because skin biopsy punches do not obtain sufficiently deep samples to be diagnostic. One should request special stains (i.e., periodic acid–Schiff, Gomori's methenamine silver, Brown and Brenn) for causative agent. Skin biopsy reveals lobular to diffuse pyogranulomatous inflammation in the panniculitis.

The practitioner should identify and treat underlying causes appropriately. Idiopathic panniculitis may respond well to prednisolone at 1 to 2 mg/kg orally once daily for 7 to 14 days or to a single treatment of dexamethasone at 20 to 30 mg intramuscularly.[21,76] Clinical improvement usually occurs within 7 to 14 days. Relapses occur, and the horse may require lifelong therapy.

DERMATOSIS OF THE LOWER LIMB

Skin diseases of the lower limbs of horses are common dermatologic problems. These diseases may be extensions of generalized dermatoses or unique clinical syndromes.

Infectious Diseases of the Lower Limb

BACTERIAL PASTERN FOLLICULITIS

Bacterial folliculitis of the pastern is caused by *Staphylococcus aureus*, *Staphylococcus hyicus*, or β-hemolytic streptococci.[82,106] This disease is considered a primary pyoderma, but the mechanism by which organisms initiate the disease is unknown.

Lesions are limited to the posterior aspect of the pastern and fetlock region and may affect single or multiple limbs. The initial lesion consists of papules and pustules that eventually coalesce and produce large areas of ulceration and suppuration. The disease is not associated with systemic signs.

The diagnosis is based on clinical signs, skin scrapings, cytologic examination of the exudate, Gram stain, and bacterial culture and sensitivity. Cytologic examination of pustule contents usually reveals large numbers of neutrophils engulfing bacteria.

Sedation may be necessary for initial treatment because lesions are painful.[106] One should clip hair from affected areas and wash the area daily in an antimicrobial scrub or shampoo (e.g., chlorhexidine shampoo or scrub) and should apply an appropriate antibiotic ointment without corticosteroids twice daily. Systemic antibiotic therapy is not usually necessary.

ULCERATIVE LYMPHANGITIS

Ulcerative lymphangitis is a bacterial infection of the cutaneous lymphatics of horses. Lesions are most common on the hindlegs, especially distal to the hock, and consist of hard to fluctuant nodules that abscess, ulcerate, and drain pus. Individual nodules may heal, but new lesions develop. Cording of the regional lymphatics, edema, and fibrosis are common. Regional lymph nodes usually are not involved.

A definitive diagnosis is based on direct smear, Gram stain, and culture of a nodule. Skin biopsy reveals superficial and deep perivascular dermatitis that may be suppurative or pyogranulomatous. Special stains (Brown and Brenn, and Gram) may reveal the organism.

If one treats the disease early, therapy may be effective and may prevent permanent disfigurement and debilitation. The drug of choice pending culture and sensitivity is procaine penicillin 20,000 to 80,000 IU/kg intramuscularly every 12 hours for 30 days or longer. Adjunct hydrotherapy may be beneficial. After fibrosis develops, prognosis is poor.[106] One should clean the affected area daily with copious amounts of water and wash it with an antimicrobial scrub (e.g., chlorhexidine).

VIRAL PAPILLOMATOSIS

Equine viral papillomatosis (warts) is caused by a DNA papovavirus.[101] Viral papillomatosis is common in horses and occurs most frequently in horses less than 3 years of age. No sex or breed predilection exists. Transmission appears to be by direct contact. Groups of young horses are often affected more frequently than horses of the same age housed individually. Lesions are most common on the muzzle, genitalia, and distal legs and are usually multiple and resemble papillomatosis of other species.

A definitive diagnosis is made by skin biopsy. Epithelial proliferation without connective tissue proliferation is typical.

Benign neglect is the best treatment for these lesions; spontaneous remission almost always occurs. One should consider surgical removal only when the lesion interferes with function. Anecdotal reports that surgical removal or damage to part of the lesion induces remission of the lesion are unproven.[83] In fact, controlled studies suggest that such intervention might increase the duration of the lesions.[83,106] Efficacy of autogenous vaccines is unproven.

SPOROTRICHOSIS

The dimorphic fungus S. *schenckii* causes sporotrichosis, which was discussed in detail under Infectious Causes of Nodules.

A cutaneous lymphatic form of sporotrichosis may localize to the distal extremities of horses. The lymphatics become corded, and large nodules ulcerate and drain a thick brown-red discharge. Regional lymph nodes are not involved. Edema is rare. Diagnosis and treatment have been discussed previously.

Parasitic Diseases of the Lower Limb

The common parasitic diseases of horses have been discussed previously (see Parasitic Skin Diseases). Infestations of lice, *Chorioptes* spp., and chiggers are the most common parasitic dermatoses that cause lower limb pruritus.

Neoplastic and Nonneoplastic Proliferation Diseases of the Lower Limbs

KELOIDS

A keloid is a nonneoplastic fibroblastic response that occurs on the pastern of horses. Clinically the keloid resembles a cluster of grapes. A definitive diagnosis is determined by biopsy. These lesions do not respond to surgical excision, and in fact surgery may exacerbate them.[21,106] The best treatment for keloids is by intralesional injection of triamcinolone acetonide (not to exceed 20 mg per horse). Unfortunately, most lesions are so massive that response to therapy is poor.

HEMANGIOMATA

Hemangiomata are benign tumors of the endothelial cells of blood vessels. Lesions occur most commonly in horses less than 1 year of age, and some horses are born with them.[83] Hemangiomata tend to be solitary tumors occurring on the distal limbs. The clinical appearance varies and may be circumscribed, nodular, firm to fluctuant, blue to black in color, dermal or subcutaneous, hyperkeratotic, or verrucous. Ulceration and bleeding are common.

Confirmation of the diagnosis is made by skin biopsy, which reveals proliferation of blood-filled vascular spaces lined by single layers of well-differentiated endothelial cells.[37,83] Equine hemangiomata are characterized by a multinodular capillary hemangioma with hyperplasia and hyperkeratosis of the overlying epidermis.

Surgical excision is the treatment of choice. Equine verrucous hemangioma is difficult to excise, and cryosurgery may be beneficial. Recurrence is common.

Autoimmune Diseases of the Lower Limbs

PEMPHIGUS FOLIACEUS

Pemphigus foliaceus was discussed under Immunologic Causes of Exfoliation. In some horses the condition affects only the coronary band.[1] The coronary band of all four limbs is crumbly, degenerating, and exudative. Pain, lameness, and edema of the lower limb may occur.

SYSTEMIC LUPUS ERYTHEMATOSUS

Systemic lupus erythematosus is a multisystemic autoimmune disease that is rare in horses. Profound lymphedema of the lower limbs may be the only clinical sign. The disease is treated with immunosuppressive doses of prednisolone (2 mg/kg orally every 12 hours). The prognosis is grave.

VASCULITIS

Vasculitis was discussed earlier under Vasculitis and Purpura Hemorrhagica. In some horses, cutaneous vasculitis is restricted to the white skin of the pasterns and face of horses in the summer.[1] Characteric lesions are erythema, swelling, pain, and exudation, and lesions may resemble photodermatitis, which suggests a photoinduced cause. Edema of the pastern and face is significant.

LEUKOCYTOCLASTIC VASCULITIS

Leukocytoclastic vasculitis or photoaggravated vasculitis is a relatively common but poorly understood disease.[80] Immune deposits (immunoglobulin G or complement component 3 or both) around the vessel walls have been detected in early skin lesions using direct immunofluorescence. The fact that unpigmented skin appears to be affected suggests a role of ultraviolet light in the development of this dermatologic problem. Drug reactions may play a role and a recent report suggested that *Staphlycoccus* spp. bacterial infection as an underlying cause. This dermatologic condition generally affects mature horses. The skin lesions are confined to the lower limb (Figure 13-37). A lack of pigment in the affected area is the most common finding, but pigmented skin has also been reportedly diagnosed with this condition. Lesions are usually multiple and well marked. Initially, erythema and exudation occur, which progresses to crusting and open sores or ulcerated areas. The affected area may ooze, and swelling is present. Chronic cases may develop a rough or "warty" surface. This condition is more painful than pruritic. The diagnosis for this condition is made by skin biopsy. On histopathologic examination, leukocytoclastic skin lesions will have inflammation around the blood vessels with blood vessel degeneration and clost involving the small vessels in the superficial dermis. Treatment consists of systemic corticosteroids at relatively high doses for 1 week and reduced doses for another 4 to 6 weeks. A reduction in ultraviolet light exposure by bandaging the affected leg or stabling the horse indoors during daylight hours or both is thought to be beneficial. Application of sun block (minimal sun protection factor of 20) is thought to be beneficial.

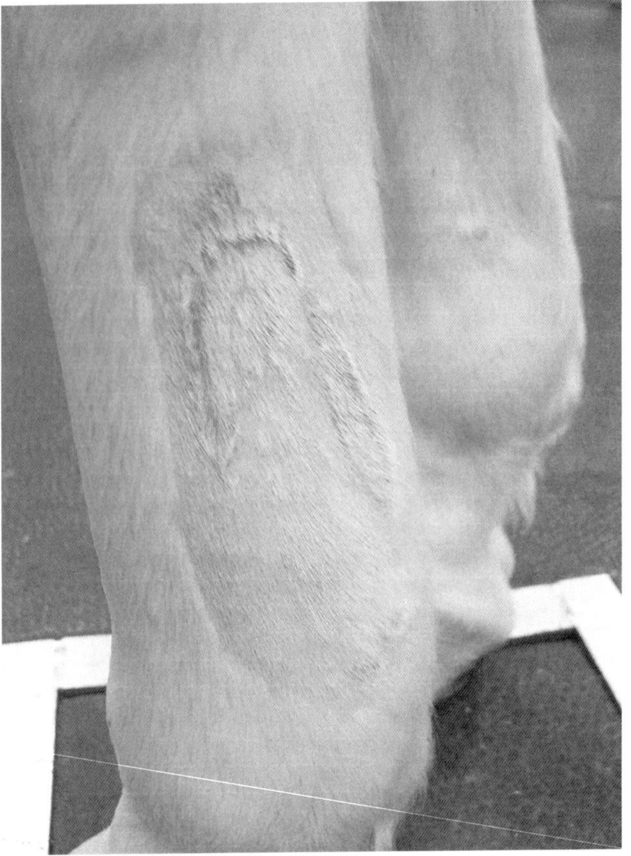

FIGURE 13-37 Horse with leukocytoclastic vasculitis.

PASTERN DERMATITIS (GREASY HEEL AND SCRATCHES)

Skin disease of the lower limbs is a common and frustrating problem in horses. Pastern dermatitis, scratches, greasy heel, and mud fever are colloquial terms for a moist exudative dermatitis of the caudal heel and pastern area. The reader should remember that these terms are nonspecific and describe a variety of inflammatory skin conditions of the lower limbs of horses.

The pathogenesis of this syndrome is not understood completely. The initial lesion may be a primary infection or may follow a predisposing factor such as PF or mites. Horses with long fetlock hair or horses housed in muddy paddocks, unsanitary conditions, or rough stubbly pasture are at risk for

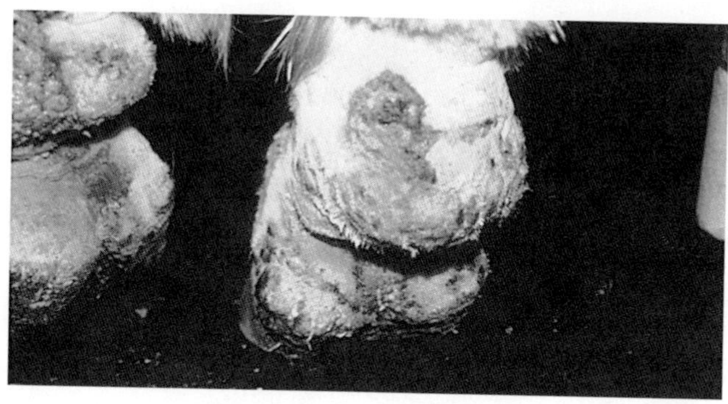

FIGURE 13-38 Pastern dermatitis.

pastern dermatitis. The problem is common in horses worked on tracks consisting of grit particles, which can cause microtrauma to the skin.

Clinical signs depend greatly on whether the condition is acute or chronic and whether the owner has treated the lesions. Many horse owners do not recognize the acute development of skin diseases, minimizing the opportunity to identify the underlying cause. To complicate matters further, many owners treat these lesions before seeking veterinary care. Many common over-the-counter medications can induce irritant or allergic reactions, making distinguishing between these reactions and the original skin disease almost impossible.

Regardless of the cause, clinical signs are similar (Figure 13-38).[106] Acute lesions usually begin at the heel. Pain, swelling, moist exudation, and hair loss are common. As the disease process continues, lesions spread proximally and anteriorly. Matting of the hair occurs, and the horse may be noticeably lame. Crusting is common. If the underlying disease process involves a vasculitis, ulceration may be present. If the disease is left untreated, a foul odor develops. Because of the constant flexion in the area, fissures often develop. In Draft horses, vegetative granulomatous growths commonly result. Lesions may occur on one or multiple limbs or just on extremities with white markings.

A definitive diagnosis requires a complete medical history. Liver function tests are essential in any horse in which the lesions are limited to the unpigmented areas of the skin. One should perform *Dermatophilus* preparations, fungal cultures, and skin scrapings in all cases. In horses with long hairs on the fetlocks, the hair should be combed thoroughly with a fine-toothed metal comb, which is often the only successful method for finding lice. In difficult cases, tissue samples should be submitted for bacterial or fungal culture.

Correct therapy requires identifying the underlying cause. The reader can find specific therapy for most of the diseases elsewhere in this chapter or in the references. In all cases, one should clip the long hairs of the fetlock area and thoroughly wash the affected area with an antimicrobial scrub (e.g., 2% chlorhexidine). Iodine preparations should be avoided because they can be irritating. One should remove all crusts and exudation, daily if necessary, and should avoid exposing the horse to moistures and irritants. Horses with idiopathic greasy heel often respond well to cleaning of the area, improved hygiene of the stall, and systemic corticosteroid therapy (assuming bacteria are not the cause). Large doses of prednisolone (e.g., 1 mg/kg orally once daily) may be necessary to induce remission of clinical signs. One should not decrease the dose of glucocorticoids too rapidly or relapse may occur. If oral prednisolone does not induce remission, dexamethasone at 0.02 to 0.04 mg/kg orally once daily for 3 to 5 days may be effective.

SYSTEMIC DISEASES WITH CUTANEOUS MANIFESTATIONS

Reviewing all the skin diseases that may have systemic clinical signs is beyond the scope of this chapter. The author has made an effort to include the most common systemic findings in this chapter. Table 13-2 provides a brief summary.

TABLE 13-2

Skin Diseases with Systemic Manifestations

Disease	Cutaneous Signs	Systemic Signs
ENVIRONMENTAL		
Gangrene	Wet: moist swelling, discoloration, malodorous, tissue decomposition Dry: dry, discolored, leathery skin	Depends on underlying cause; fever
Burns	Superficial: erythema, edema, pain, vesicles Deep: necrosis, ulceration, anesthesia, scarring	Shock, respiratory compromise
Selenosis	Painful coronary band, sloughing and necrosis of hoof, rough hair coat, progressive loss of long hairs of mane and tail	Lameness, weight loss
Arsenic poisoning	Severe seborrhea, ulcer, nonhealing wounds, hypertrichosis	Gastroenteritis, emaciation, variable appetite
Mercury poisoning	Progressive alopecia	Gastroenteritis, lameness, emaciation
Iodism	Severe dry seborrhea with or without hair loss	Cough, variable appetite, joint pain, seromucoid nasal discharge, lacrimation
Hepatogenous photosensitization	Erythema, edema, pruritus, pain, in white or light-skinned area; vesicles and bullae may progress to oozing, necrosis, and sloughing	Acute: hepatic encephalopathy, icterus, depression, decreased appetite Chronic: weight loss, depression neurologic signs
Ergotism	Swelling of coronary band, necrosis of feet, sloughing of ears, tail, feet	Lameness of hind legs, fever, weight loss, poor appetite
Leucenosis	Hoof dystrophies, shedding of hair	Laminitis, lameness
Hairy vetch toxicosis	Cutaneous plaques and papules that ooze yellow pus; pruritus; hair loss	Conjunctivitis, anorexia, pyrexia, weight loss
BACTERIAL DISEASES		
Strangles	Limb edema; edema of lips, eyelids; petechial hemorrhages of mucous membranes and sclera	History of acute contagious upper respiratory infection; pyrexia, mucopurulent nasal discharge; abscesses in the mandibular or retropharyngeal lymph nodes
Corynebacterium pseudotuberculosis abscesses	Single or multiple deep abscesses that develop slowly or rapidly; 50% occurring in the pectoral or ventral abdominal area; ventral midline edema	Pitting edema, depression, fever, lameness, internal abscess, prolonged fever, abortion
Dermatophilosis	Exudative crusted lesions on dorsal trunk, face, pastern, or coronets	Depression, fever, lethargy, poor appetite, weight loss, lymphadenopathy; lesions on legs may cause edema, pain, and lameness.
Actinobacillosis	Thick-walled abscess of soft tissue	In newborn foals, disease is a highly fatal septicemic disease, and skin lesions are rare.
Clostridial infections	Malignant edema: swelling at site of infection, pitting edema, local erythema; skin may become hot to touch, painful, or slough; crepitus Blackleg: hot, painful, swelling that progresses to a cold painful swelling with edema and subcutaneous emphysema	High fever, anorexia, muscle tremors, acute death possible within 24-48 hours
Glanders (farcy) *Burkholderia mallei* (not in United States)	Subcutaneous nodules begin most commonly on medial aspect of hock; lesions rapidly ulcerate and drain a honey-colored material; lymphadenopathy and cording of lymphatics is common	Respiratory infection that rapidly leads to death
FUNGAL DISEASE		
Histoplasma farciminosa (epizootic lymphangitis)	Unilateral nodules on face, head, neck and occasionally trunk; nodules initially are firm but rupture and exude light-green, blood-tinged exudate; large ulcer may form and lesions may spread bilaterally	Lacrimation, conjunctivitis, and respiratory signs may occur

TABLE 13-2

Skin Diseases with Systemic Manifestations—cont'd		
Disease	**Cutaneous Signs**	**Systemic Signs**
PARASITES		
Lice	Pruritus, scaling, alopecia	Anemia in severe infestations with sucking lice
Black flies	Painful papules, and wheals that may become vesicular, hemorrhagic, and necrotic; lesion may be localized to ears or intermandibular areas	Toxin in bite can cause increased capillary permeability; depression, weakness, staggers, tachypnea, tachycardia, weak pulse, shock, and possible death
IMMUNE-MEDIATED DISEASES		
Atopy	Chronic pruritic urticaria, excoriations, alopecia, lichenification	Respiratory difficulty, especially on expiration
Pemphigus foliaceus	Crusts, scales, oozing, annular eruption, matting of the coat; lesions may be limited to coronary band	Depression, weight loss, poor appetite, pyrexia
Bullous pemphigoid	Vesicles and bullae in mouth, groin, and axilla; crusts, ulcers	Anorexia, depression, fever
Systemic lupus erythematosus	Lymphedema, panniculitis, alopecia, leukoderma; scaling of face, neck, and trunk	Polyarthritis, thrombocytopenia, proteinuria, fever, depression, weight loss
Transfusion reactions and graft-versus-host disease (may occur in horse after unmatched blood transfusion)	Exfoliative to ulcerative dermatitis, ulcerative stomatitis	Diarrhea, increased heart and respiratory rates, lacrimation, muscle fasciculation
Erythema multiforme	Symmetric maculopapular lesions, urticaria that results in annular arciform or polycyclic shapes; wheals that do not disappear	Occurs after pregnancy, drugs, neoplasia, connective tissue disease, and infections or may be idiopathic
Vasculitis	Purpura, edema, erythema, necrosis, crusts; purpura hemorrhagica causes edema and hemorrhagic swelling in tissue, mucosa, and viscera	May occur after strangles or influenza; depression, fever, reluctance to move, colic, diarrhea
Equine exfoliative eosinophilic dermatitis and stomatitis	Scaling and crusting that progress to generalized exfoliation, alopecia, ulceration, and exudation; variable pruritus	Severe, progressive weight loss; no diarrhea, ravenous appetite
Equine cutaneous amyloidosis	Papules, nodules, and plaques over the head and neck that develop rapidly	Diffuse nodules in upper respiratory tract may cause severe dyspnea
ENDOCRINE DISEASES		
Hypothyroidism	Dull rough hair coat, delayed shedding of coat, edema of face and limb	Anecdotal reports of laminitis, infertility, anhidrosis, anemia, myopathy; weight gain and decreased food intake; skeletal limb disorders have been reported in foals
Pituitary paors intermedia dysfunction	Long shaggy hair that fails to shed; mane and tail are unaffected	Polydipsia, polyuria, muscle wasting, weight loss, lethargy, swayback appearance, pendulous abdomen, blindness, chronic infections, neurologic disorders or signs
SWEAT GLAND DISORDERS		
Anhidrosis	Acute episode: none Chronic: dry hair coat, excessive scaling, partial alopecia, pruritus	Acute: labored breathing, fever, flared nostrils, lack of sweating, collapse, death Chronic: polydipsia, polyuria, poor appetite, loss of body condition
MISCELLANEOUS DISEASES		
Panniculitis	Firm to fluctuant nodules most commonly found on trunk in subcutaneous tissue that ruptures and drains an oily yellow-brown to bloody discharge	Anorexia, depression, lethargy, pyrexia
NEOPLASTIC DISEASES		
Hemangioma and hemangiosarcoma	Two types: (1) well-circumscribed nodules that are blue-black in appearance; (2) dark hyperkeratotic and verrucous lesions that bleed easily	Anemia
Lymphosarcoma	Single or multiple dermal-to-subcutaneous nodules, especially on trunk	Internal organ involvement; usually fatal

REFERENCES

1. Scott DW: *Large animal dermatology*, Philadelphia, 1988, WB Saunders.
2. Talukdar AH, Calhoun ML, Stinson AW, et al: Microscopic anatomy of the skin of the horse, *Am J Vet Res* 33:2365, 1972.
3. Sisson S, Grossman JD: *Anatomy of domestic animals*, Philadelphia, 1975, WB Saunders.
4. Fitzpatrick TB, Eisen AZ, Wolff K, et al: *Dermatology in general medicine*, ed 3, New York, 1993, McGraw-Hill.
5. Suter MM, Crameri FM, Olivry T, et al: Keratinocyte biology and pathology, *Vet Dermatol* 8(2):67-100, 1997.
6. Rook AJ, Walton GS, editors: *Comparative physiology and pathology of the skin*, Blackwell, 1965, Oxford.
7. Perris EE: Parasitic dermatoses that cause pruritus in horses, *Vet Clin North Am Equine Pract* 11(April):11-28, 1995.
8. Ettinger SJ, Feldman: *EC, Textbook of veterinary internal medicine*, ed 6, St. Louis, 2005, Saunders.
9. Murray MD: Influence of skin temperature on populations of Linognathus pedialis, *Aust J Zool* 8:357, 1960.
10. Bergvall K: Advances in acquisition, identification and treatment of equine parasites, *Clinc Tech Equine Pract* 4:296-301, 2005.
11. Hugnet C, Cadore JL, Bourdoiseaq G: Intert du fiprinol a 0.25 pour cent anspray dans le traitement de la philtirose, *Vet Equine* 31: 65-68, 1999.
12. Littlewood JD: Control of ectoparasites in horses, *Pract* 21:418-424, 1999.
13. Martineau GP: Pathophysiology of sarcoptic mange in swine, part 2, *Compend Cont Educ Pract Vet* 9:F93, 1987.
14. ARCO, In Hayes MH, editor: New York, 1968, Veterinary notes for horse owners.
15. Kunkle GA, Greiner EC: Dermatitis in horses and man caused by straw itch mite, *Am J Vet Med Assoc* 181:467, 1982.
16. Dvorak HF: Cutaneous basophil hypersensitivity, *J Allergy Clin Immunol* 58:229, 1976.
17. Pascoe RR: The nature and treatment of skin conditions observed in horses in Queensland, *Aust Vet J* 49:35, 1979.
18. Rabalasis FC, Votava CL: Cutaneous distribution of Onchocerca cervicalis in horses, *Am J Vet Res* 35:1369, 1974.
19. Foil L, Foil C: Parasitic skin diseases, *Vet Clin North Am Equine Pract* 5:529, 1983.
20. Stannard AA, Cello RM: Onchocerca cervicalis infection in horses from the western United States, *Am J Vet Res* 36:1029, 1975.
21. Robinson NE, Sprayberry KA, editors: *Current therapy in equine medicine*, ed 6, St. Louis, 2009, Saunders.
22. Fadok VA, Mullowney PC: Dermatologic diseases of horses. 1. Parasitic dermatoses of the horse, *Compend Cont Educ Pract Vet* 5:S615, 1983.
23. Lavach JP: *Large animal opththalmology*, St Louis, 1989, Mosby-Year Book.
24. Anderson RR: The use of ivermectin in horses: research and clinical observations, *Compend Cont Educ Pract Vet* 6:S516, 1984.
25. Pusterla N, Watson JL, Wilson WD, et al: Cutaneous and ocular habronemiasis in horses: 63 cases, *Am Vet Med Assoc* 222:978-982, 1985-2002:2003.
26. Vasey JR, et al: Equine cutaneous habronemiasis, *Compend Contin Educ Pract Vet* 3:S290-S295, 1981.
27. PT Colahan, IG Mayhew, AM Merritt, editors: *Equine medicine and surgery*, SGoleta, Calif, 1991, American Veterinary Publications.
28. Stannard AA: Nodular diseases, *Vet Dermatol* 11:179-186, 2000.
29. Mathison PT: Eosinophilic nodular dermatoses, *Vet Clin North Am Equine Pract* 11 (April):83-86, 1995.
30. Herd RP, Donham JC: Efficacy of ivermectin against "summer sores" due to Draschia and Habronema infection in horses. Proceedings of the twenty-sixth annual meeting of the Association of Veterinary Parasitologists, July 19-20, 1981, St Louis. p 8.
31. Bowman DD: Helminths. In Bowman DD, editor: *Georgis' parasitology for veterinarians*, ed 7, Philadelphia, 1999, WB Saunders.
32. Greiner EC: Entomologic evaluation of insect hypersensitivity in horses, *Vet Clin North Am Equine Pract* 11 (April):29-46, 1995.
33. Rosenkrantz W, Griffin C: Treatment of equine urticaria and pruritus with hyposensitization and antihistamines. Proceedings of the annual meeting of the American Academy of Veterinary Dermatology and the American College of Veterinary Dermatology, New Orleans, 1986.
34. Friberg CA, Logas D: Treatment of Culicoides hypersensitive horses with high-dose n-3 fatty acids: a double-blinded crossover study, *Vet Dermatol* 10:117-122, 1999.
35. O'Neill W, McKee S, Clarke AF: Flaxseed as a Potential Treatment for Allergic Skin Disease in Horses, Nutraceutical Alliance Research Web site: http://www.nutraceuticalalliance.com/ research_flaxseed3.htm.
36. Ackermann LJ: *Practical equine dermatology*, Philadelphia, 1988, WB Saunders.
37. Fadok VA: Overview of equine pruritus, *Vet Clin North Am Equine Pract* 11:1-10, 1995.
38. Rees CA: Response to immunotherapy in six related horses with urticaria secondary to atopy, *J Am Vet Med Assoc* 218: 753-755, 2001.
39. White SD: Advances in equine atopic dermatitis:serologic and intradermal allergy testing. Clin Tech, *Equine Pract* 4:311-313, 2005.
40. Fadok VA: Overview of equine papular and nodular dermatoses, *Vet Clin North Am Equine Pract* 11:61-74, 1995.
41. Wagner IP, Rees CA, Dunstan RW, et al: Evaluation of systemic immunologic hypersensitivity after intradermal testing in horses with chronic laminitis, *Am J Vet Res* 3:279-283, 2003.
42. Lorch G, Hillier A, Kwochka KW, et al: Comparison of immediate intradermal test reactivity with serum IgE quantitation by use of radioallergosorbent test and two ELISA in horses with and without atopy, *J Am Vet Med Assoc* 218:1314-1322, 2001.
43. Magnan AO, Mely LG, Camilla CA, et al: Assessment of Th1/ Th2 paradigm in whole blood in atopy and asthma: increased IFN-gamma producing CD8 (+) T cells in asthma, *Am J Respir Crit Care Med* 161:1790-1796, 2000.
44. Karl S, Ring J: Pro and contra of specific hyposensitization, *Eur J Dermatol* 9:325-331, 1999.
45. Kwochka KW, Willemse T, Tscharner CV, et al: *Advances in veterinary dermatology*, ed 3, Boston, 1998, Butterworth Heinemann.
46. Plumb DC, editor: *Veterinary drug handbook*, ed 3, Ames, Iowa, 1999, Iowa State University Press.
47. White P: Essential fatty acids: use in management of canine atopy, *Compend Cont Educ Pract Vet* 15:451, 1993.
48. Lloyd DH, Sellers KC: *Dermatophilosis infection in domestic animals and man*, New York, 1976, Academic Press.
49. Burd EM, Juzych LA, Rudrik JT, et al: Pustular dermatitis cause by Dermatophilus congolensis, *J Clin Microbiol* 45:1650-1658, 2007.
50. Hermoso MJ, Arenas A, Rey J, et al: In vitro study of Dermatophilus congolensis antimicrobial inhibitory and bacteriocidal concentrations, *Br Vet J* 150:189-196, 1994.
51. Mackie RM, editor: *Current perspectives in immunodermatology*, Edinburgh, 1984, Churchill Livingstone.
52. Stannard AA: Alopecia in the horse: an overview, *Vet Dermatol* 11:191-203, 2000.
53. White SD: Equine bacterial and fungal diseases. A diagnostic and therapeutic update, *Clin Tech Equine Pract* 4:302-310, 2005.

54. Buffington CAT: Nutrition and the skin. In *Proceedings of the eleventh annual KalKan Symposium*, Columbus, Ohio, 1987, Ohio State University, p 11.
55. Fadok VA, Wild S: Suspect cutaneous iodism in a horse, *J Am Vet Med Assoc* 183:1104, 1983.
56. Halliwell REW, Gorman NTL: *Veterinary clinical immunology*, Philadelphia, 1989, WB Saunders.
57. Scott DW, Walton DK, Slater MR: Immune-mediated dermatoses in domestic animals: ten years after, part 2, *Compend Cont Educ Pract Vet* 9:S39, 1987.
58. Vandenabeele SIJ, White SD, Affolter VK, et al: Pemphigus foliaceous in the horses: a retrospective study of 20 cases, *Vet Dermatol* 15:381-388, 2004.
59. Brenner S, Wolf R, Ruocoo V: Drug-induced pemphigus, *Clin Dermatol* 11:501-505, 1993.
60. Brenner S, Bialy-Golan A: Ruoccov: Drug-induced pemphigus, *Clin Dermatol* 16:393-397, 1998.
61. Peroni DL, Stanely S, Kollias-Baker C, et al: Prednisone per os is likely to have limited efficacy in horses, *Equine Vet J* 34: 283-287, 2002.
62. Manning T, Sweeny C: Immune-mediated equine skin disease, *Compend Cont Educ Pract Vet* 12:979, 1986.
63. Mullowney PC: Dermatologic diseases of horses. 4. Environmental, congenital and neoplastic diseases, *Compend Cont Educ Pract Vet* 7:S22, 1985.
64. Jubb KV, Kennedy J, editors: ed 3, *Pathology of domestic animals* vol. 1, New York, 1985, Academic Press.
65. Wilkie JSN, Yager JA, Nation PN: Chronic eosinphilic dermatitis: a manifestation of a multisystemic, eosinophilic, epitheliotropic disease in five horses, *Vet Pathol* 22:297, 1985.
66. Lindberg R: Clinical and pathophysiological features of granulomatosis in the horse, *Zentralbl Vet Med Assoc* 32:536, 1985.
67. Hillyer MH, Mair TS: Multisystemic eosinophilic epitheliotrophic disease in a horse: attempted treatment with hydroxy urea and dexamethason, *Vet Rec* 130:392, 1992.
68. Kerdel FA, Moschella S: Sarcoidosis: an updated review, *J Am Acad Dermatol* 11:1, 1984.
69. Mullowney PC, Fadok VA: Dermatological diseases of horses. Part 2. Bacterial and viral diseases, *Compend Cont Educ Pract Vet* 6:S16, 1984.
70. Miers KC, Ley WB: Corynebacterium pseudotuberculosis infection in the horse: study of 117 clinical cases and consideration of etiopathogenesis, *J Am Vet Med Assoc* 117:250, 1980.
71. Blackford J: Superficial and deep mycoses in horses, *Vet Clin North Am Large Anim Pract* 6:47, 1984.
72. Mullowney PC, Fadok VA: Dermatologic diseases of horses. 3. Fungal skin diseases, *Compend Cont Educ Pract Vet* 6:S324, 1984.
73. Hubert JD, Grooters AM: Treatment of equine phytiosis, *Compen Contin Edu Pract Vet* 24:812-815, 2002.
74. Miller RI, Campbell RSF: The comparative pathology of equine cutaneous phycomycosis, *Vet Pathol* 21:325, 1984.
75. Chaffin MK, Schumacher J, McMullan WC: Cutaneous pythiosis in the horse, *Vet Clin North Am Equine Pract* 11: 91-103, 1995.
76. Thomsett LR: Noninfectious skin diseases of horses, *Vet Clin North Am Large Anim Pract* 6:57, 1984.
77. Sullins KE, Lavach JD, Roberts SM, et al: Equine sarcoid, *Equine Pract* 8:21-27, 1986.
78. Lazary S, Gerber H, Glatt PA: Equine leukocyte antigens in sarcoid affected horses, *Equine Vet J* 17:283, 1985.
79. Otten N, von Tscharner C, Lazary S, et al: DNA of bovine papillomavirsu type 1 and 2 in equine sarcoids: PCR detection and direct sequencing, *Arch Virol* 132:121, 1993.
80. Pascoe RRR, Knottenbelt DC: Neoplastic conditions. In Pascoe RR, Knottenbelt DC, editors: *Manual of equine dermatology*, London, 1999, WB Saunders.
81. Tuthill RE, Clark WH: Jr., Levene, A: Equine melanotic disease: a unique model for human dermal melanocytic disease (abstract), *Lab Invest* 46:85A, 1982.
82. Stannard AA, Pulley LT: Tumors of the skin and soft tissue. In Moulton JE, editor: *Tumors in domestic animals* vol. 2, Berkeley, 1978, University of California Press.
83. Goetz TE: Cimetidine for treatment of melanoma in three horses, *J Am Vet Med Assoc* 196:449, 1990.
84. Sheahan BJ, Atkins GJ, Russell RJ, O'Connor JP: Histiolymphocytic lymphosarcoma in the subcutis of two horses, *Vet Pathol* 17:123, 1980.
85. Gallagher RD, Ziola B, Chelack BJ: Immunotherapy of equine cutaneous lymphosarcoma using low dose cyclophosphamide and autologous tumor cells infected with vaccinia virus, *Can Vet J* 34:371, 1993.
86. Pascoe RR, Summers RM: Clinical survey of tumors and tumor-like lesions in horses in southeast Queensland, *Equine Vet J* 13:235, 1981.
87. Pascoe RR: *Equine dermatoses (no. 22), Post Graduate Foundation in Veterinary Science*. Sydney, Australia, 1981, University of Sydney.
88. Lerner DJ, McCracken MD: Hyperelastosis cutis in 2 horses, *J Equine Med Surg* 2:350-352, 1978.
89. Hardy MH, Fischer KRS, Vrablic OE, et al: An inherited connective tissue disease in the horse, *Lab Invest* 59:253-262, 1988.
90. Bridges CH, McMullan WC: Dermatosparaxis in Quarter horses. In *Proceedings of the thirty-fifth annual meeting of the American College of Veterinary Pathologists*, Toronto, November 12-16, 1984, Canada, p 22.
91. White SD, Affolter VK, Bannasch DL, et al: Hereditary equine regional dermal asthenia ('hyperelastosis cutis') in 50 horses: clinical, histological, immunohistological and ultrastructual findings, *Vet Dermatol* 15:207-217, 2004.
92. Brounts SH, Rashimir-Raven M, Black SS: Zonal dermal seperation: a distinctive histopathological lesion associated with hyperelastosis cutis in a Quarter horse, *Vet Dermatol* 12:219-223, 2001.
93. Jones RJ: Toxicity of Leucaena leucocephala, *Aust Vet J* 54:387, 1978.
94. Feld JR, Wolf C: Cushing's syndrome in a horse, *Equine Vet J* 20:301-304, 1988.
95. vander Kolk H: Diagnosis of equine hyperadrenocorticism, *Equine Pract* 17:24-27, 1995.
96. Kolk JH, Van der Kalsbeek HC, Wensing T, et al: Urinary concentration of corticoids in normal horses and horses with hyperadrenocorticism, *Res Vet Sci* 56:126-128, 1994.
97. Auer DE, Wilson RG, Groenendick S, et al: Glucose metabolism in a pony with a tumour of the pituitary gland pars intermedia, *Aust Vet J* 64:379-382, 1987.
98. Munoz MC, Doresle F, Ferrer O, et al: Pergolide treatment for Cushing's syndrome in a horse, *Vet Rec* 139:41-43, 1996.
99. Shaver JR, Fretz P, Doige CE, et al: Skeletal manifestations of suspected hypothyroidism in two foals, *J Equine Med Surg* 3:269, 1979.
100. Vivrette SL: Skeletal disease of a hypothyroid foal, *Cornell Vet* 74:373, 1984.
101. Howard JC, editor: *Current veterinary therapy*, Philadelphia, 1981, WB Saunders, food animal practice.
102. Gillespie JH, Timoney JF: *Hagen and Bruner's infectious diseases of domestic animals*, Ithaca, New York, 1981, Cornell University Press.
103. Geiser DR, Walker RD: Management of large animal thermal injuries, *Compend Cont Educ Pract Vet* 7:S69, 1985.
104. Fox SM: Management of a large thermal lesion in a horse, *Compend Cont Educ Pract Vet* 10:88, 1988.
105. Asch MJ, Meserol PM, Mason AD Jr, et al: Systemic and pulmonary hemodynamic changes accompanying thermal injuries, *Ann Surg* 178:218, 1973.
106. Swaim SF, Lee AH: Topical wound medications: a review, *J Am Vet Med Assoc* 190:588, 1988.

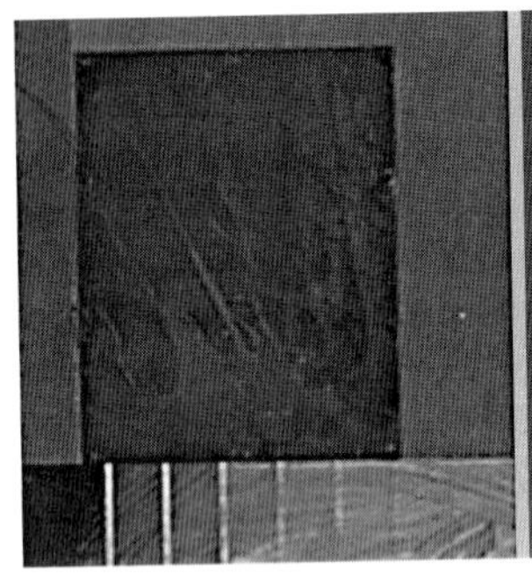

Disorders of the Hematopoietic System

CHAPTER 14

Debra C. Sellon, L. Nicki Wise

The hematopoietic system includes the blood and blood-forming tissues of the body. Peripheral blood cells are essential for tissue oxygenation, immune surveillance and clearance of foreign antigens, coagulation, and inflammatory reactions. Because of the interactions of blood with other body tissues and organs, alterations in blood parameters often reflect dysfunctions elsewhere in the body, and evaluation of the blood and its constituents has become an essential component of many diagnostic efforts.

This chapter discusses the basics of hematopoiesis and hematopoietic metabolism as they relate to specific disease conditions in the horse. Included is a discussion of the erythron, leukon, platelets, and hemostatic mechanisms of the horse.

ERYTHRON

Erythropoietic tissue of the bone marrow and the circulating erythrocytes may be referred to as the *erythron,* to emphasize their organlike function. Erythrocytes are essential for delivery of oxygen to all tissues of the body. The complex maturation and development of erythrocytes and their pivotal role in survival of all body tissues make them uniquely reflective of many pathologic conditions. An understanding of the erythron and its responses to perturbations in homeostatic mechanisms throughout the body can provide the astute clinician with invaluable clues in unraveling difficult diagnostic dilemmas.

Physiology

Erythropoiesis refers to the process of development and maturation of erythrocytes. Knowledge of the metabolic processes of these cells is critical to understanding pathologic processes that interfere with their primary function of tissue oxygenation.

In the fetus, the cellular elements of blood are produced almost exclusively in the liver and spleen. As the body matures and differentiates in utero, hematopoiesis gradually shifts to the marrow cavities so that at birth the bone marrow is the main organ of hematopoiesis. As an animal ages, bone marrow hematopoiesis decreases and fat infiltrates much of the previously active marrow. In the older adult animal, active hematopoiesis is limited to the marrow of the vertebrae, ribs, sternum, skull, and pelvis, as well as to the epiphyseal marrow of the humerus and femur.

Erythrocyte production begins from a pluripotent colony-forming unit stem cell capable of differentiating into erythroid-, myeloid-, megakaryocytoid-, or lymphoid-producing cell lines. The stem cell is capable of self-renewal to provide a continuing supply of pluripotent stem cells. The direction of differentiation is determined in part by the types and quantities of cytokine mediators to which the stem cell is exposed at the time it begins to divide. The exact combinations of mediators necessary to direct differentiation into each line are not understood entirely. In erythrocyte development the stem cell undergoes sequential mitotic divisions to produce the committed erythrocyte progenitor burst-forming unit, followed by erythroid colony-forming units. These two stages are capable of limited replicative self-renewal but are committed ultimately to differentiate into erythrocytes (Figure 14-1). Burst-promoting activity depends on the presence of various cytokines, including interleukin 3 (IL-3), IL-4, and granulocyte-macrophage colony-stimulating factor. The erythroid colony-forming unit cell is the immediate precursor stage of the first morphologically recognizable erythrocyte precursor, the proerythroblast.

Initial stages of erythrocyte development depend greatly on the presence of the glycoprotein hormone erythropoietin, which the kidney produces in response to renal hypoxia and is an absolute requirement for erythrocyte progenitor cell maturation and differentiation. The absence of erythropoietin, as in patients with chronic renal disease, is associated with potentially severe nonregenerative anemia. Erythrocytosis, an increase in the circulating red blood cell (RBC) mass, is associated with excess secretion of erythropoietin in certain disease conditions.

Bone marrow proerythrocytes undergo four successive divisions followed by a period of maturation to produce 16 erythrocytes. Sequential divisions produce basophilic erythroblasts, polychromatophilic erythroblasts I and II, and orthochromic erythroblasts. The orthochromic erythroblast becomes a reticulocyte by ejecting its nucleus. Reticulocyte production requires approximately 72 hours; 24 to 48 hours later the reticulocyte will have matured into an erythrocyte.

Iron is an essential component for hemoglobin synthesis and thus for erythropoiesis. The diet of the horse normally contains an abundance of readily available iron. Absorption is most efficient in the duodenum but may occur at almost any part of the gastrointestinal tract. The amount of iron

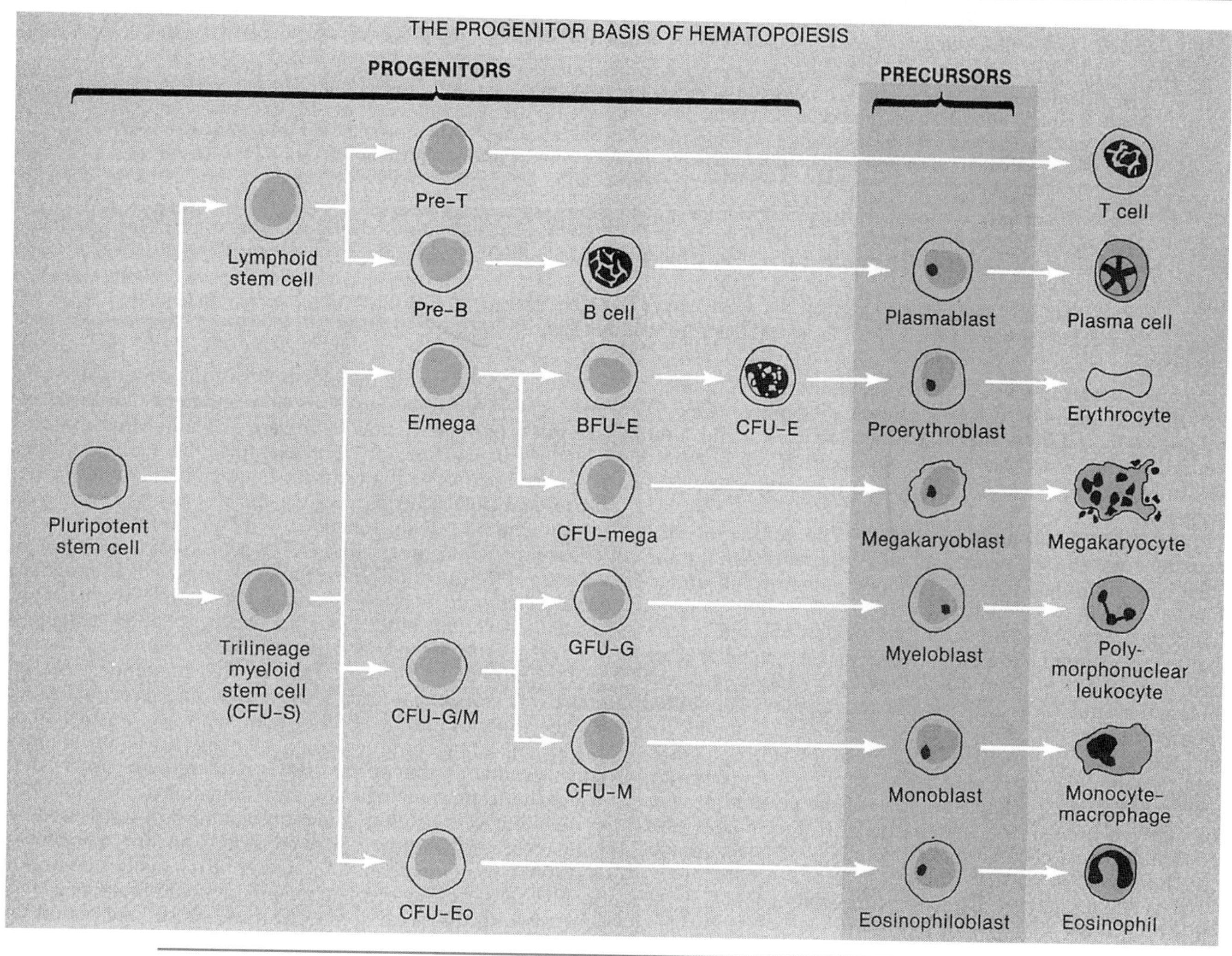

FIGURE 14-1 Schematic representation of the progenitor basis of hematopoiesis. Maturation is depicted from left to right with circulating blood cells as the final product on the far right of the drawing. Progressive amplification of progenitors and precursors as they mature and differentiate is not shown. *CFU-S,* Colony-forming unit, spleen; *CFU-G/M,* CFU-granulocyte/macrophage; *CFU-Eo,* CFU-eosinophil; *BFU-E,* burst-forming unit, erythroid; *CFU-mega,* CFU-megakaryocyte; *CFU-G,* CFU-granulocyte; *CFU-M,* CFU-monocyte; *CFU-E,* CFU-erythrocyte. (From Wyngaarden JB, Smith LH, editors: *Cecil textbook of medicine,* ed 18, Philadelphia, 1988, WB Saunders.)

absorbed from the gastrointestinal tract varies with the systemic iron status of the animal. Absorption increases in iron-depleted animals and decreases in animals with ample iron stores. Unabsorbed iron passes through the remainder of the tract and is lost in feces. Horses, especially young foals, supplemented with excessive dietary iron can develop hemochromatosis, hepatic cirrhosis, and liver failure.[1-4]

After absorption the blood transports iron complexed with the protein transferrin. In the liver, spleen, and bone marrow, iron is transferred to molecules of the storage protein ferritin. Approximately 30% of body iron is present in the storage proteins ferritin and hemosiderin (a complex aggregation of ferritin molecules). Only minute amounts of iron are complexed to the transport protein transferrin at any given time. Minor quantities of iron are also present in myoglobin and various electron transport molecules and enzymes. The hemoglobin of senescent erythrocytes removed from the peripheral circulation is degraded in cells of the mononuclear phagocyte system in the spleen, liver, and bone marrow. Iron ultimately is recycled to the bone marrow or liver to be used in synthesis of hemoglobin for new erythrocytes. Almost 70% of total body iron is present in hemoglobin.

Hemoglobin is synthesized in the mitochondria of the developing erythroblast and consists of four polypeptide chains (two α and two β in the adult) and a heme moiety. Heme is the functional portion of the hemoglobin molecule and contains an iron atom held in place by the four pyrrole rings of a porphyrin molecule. The iron in hemoglobin must be in the ferrous form (Fe^{2+}) to bind oxygen reversibly. Heme iron oxidized to the ferric form (Fe^{3+}) forms methemoglobin, and the molecule is no longer capable of transporting oxygen.

The normal life span of equine erythrocytes in circulation is approximately 150 days.[5,6] Mononuclear phagocytes of the spleen, liver, and bone marrow remove senescent RBCs from circulation. Transferrin transports released iron to RBC precursors in the marrow. Heme in phagocytic cells undergoes enzymatic degradation to biliverdin and then bilirubin. Phagocytic cells release unconjugated bilirubin into the circulation, where it binds to plasma albumin. Hepatocytes take up unconjugated bilirubin, which is conjugated and excreted via the bile into the gastrointestinal tract, where it is converted to urobilinogen and then stercobilin. Intravascular or extravascular hemolysis often results in increased serum unconjugated bilirubin concentrations.

During intravascular hemolysis, ruptured erythrocytes release hemoglobin, which combines with haptoglobin, an acute phase protein normally present in plasma, to be carried back to the liver, where hemoglobin is converted to bilirubin and excreted. If the level of hemoglobin exceeds the carrier capacity of hemoglobin, then the result is free hemoglobin in the plasma. Free plasma hemoglobin is filtered readily across the renal glomerulus and reabsorbed by renal tubular epithelial cells. Hemoglobin and other related pigment molecules, including myoglobin, are potentially nephrotoxic, and excessive intravascular hemolysis may result in acute renal failure.

The mature erythrocyte is an anucleate cell incapable of de novo protein synthesis to replace enzymes or other proteins that have been used during normal metabolism. Binding, transport, and delivery of oxygen to tissues does not require energy expenditure by the erythrocyte, but maintaining iron and various cellular proteins in a reduced state essential for proper function does require energy. Maintenance of appropriate electrolyte gradients across the RBC membrane also requires energy. Glucose is the main in vivo energy source for erythrocytes. RBCs differ from other cell types in the absence of the Krebs (tricarboxylic acid) cycle. Glucose must be metabolized via the anaerobic glycolytic (Embden-Meyerhof) pathway or via the hexose monophosphate shunt. The enzymes involved in these metabolic pathways are critical to RBC survival and rare hereditary deficiencies have been described in the horse. The deficiencies of either glucose-6-phospahte dehydrogenase (G6PD) or flavin adenine dinucleotide (FAD) resulted in hemolytic anemia and persistent methemoglobinemia, respectively.[7,8]

The body must maintain iron, hemoglobin, some critical RBC enzymes, and several membrane proteins in a reduced form for appropriate activity. High intracellular concentrations of glutathione (GSH), a sulfhydryl-containing tripeptide, are important for reduction of sulfhydryl groups of hemoglobin and other erythrocyte proteins. Reduction reactions involve the conversion of GSH to its oxidized form (GSSG), which then is returned to the reduced form (GSH) by the action of GSH reductase. When the functional ferrous form of iron (Fe^{2+}) in hemoglobin is oxidized to the ferric form (Fe^{3+}), the resulting methemoglobin is incapable of carrying oxygen. Small amounts of methemoglobin (1% to 2% of total hemoglobin) are produced normally in erythrocytes. This methemoglobin is reduced to functional hemoglobin primarily via the action of the enzyme methemoglobin reductase.

EVALUATION OF THE ERYTHRON

Laboratory evaluation of the blood and bone marrow provides diagnostic clues that may aid the practitioner in diagnosing and treating a variety of disorders. Knowing the tests that are available and developing an understanding of how and why they are performed aids one in interpreting the results.

PERIPHERAL BLOOD EVALUATION

Most clinical laboratories now use automated cell counters for evaluation of peripheral blood. These counters are capable of determining RBC counts, hemoglobin, packed cell volume (PCV), and various erythrocyte indices. Tables 14-1 and 14-2 list normal values for the horse.[9,10] These values are intended as guidelines only. Each laboratory should establish its own normal values for each species.

Red blood cell count, hemoglobin, and PCV are the most frequently used parameters for assessing the quantity of erythrocytes in circulation. In the normal horse, hemoglobin concentration is approximately one third of the PCV. This value increases in horses with intravascular hemolysis and hemoglobinemia. RBC count, hemoglobin concentration, and PCV decrease rapidly during the first weeks of life in the equine neonate. This decrease has been attributed to decreased erythrocyte production, a shorter RBC life span in the neonate, and hemodilution. During this period, mean RBC volume also decreases to the point that cells would be classified as *microcytic* if compared with normal adult values.[11]

Evaluation of RBC indices can be helpful in characterizing anemia. If these parameters are not included in automated

TABLE 14-1

Reference Ranges for Equine Hematologic Parameters*

Parameter	Units	Light Horse†	Draft Horse‡	Miniature Horse§	Donkey¶
RBC count	$10^6/\mu l$	6.0-10.0	5.5-9.5	4.3-10.3	4.7-9.0
Hemoglobin	g/dl	12.0-17.0	8.0-14.0	9.0-16.0	9.5-16.5
PCV	%	32-50	24-44	24-42	28-47
MCV	fl	42-58	—	38-61	46-67
MCH	µg	15-20	—	14-23	16-23
MCHC	g/dl	32-38	—	33-40	32-36

RBC, Red blood cell; *PCV,* packed cell volume; *MCV,* mean corpuscular volume; *MCH,* mean corpuscular hemoglobin; *MCHC,* mean corpuscular hemoglobin concentration.
*Numbers are for comparison only. Each laboratory should establish its own normal values.
†North Carolina State University Clinical Pathology Laboratory equine reference values.
‡Data from Jain N: *Schalm's veterinary hematology,* ed 4, Philadelphia, 1986, Lea & Febiger.
§Data from Harvey R, Hambright M, Rowe L: Clinical biochemical and hematologic values of the American Miniature Horse: reference values, *Am J Vet Res* 45:987, 1984.
¶Data from Zinkl J, Mae D, Merida P, et al: Reference ranges and the influence of age and sex on hematologic and serum biochemical values in donkeys *(Equus asinus), Am J Vet Res* 51:408, 1990.

TABLE 14-2

Influence of Breed on Normal Erythron Values (Mean ± Standard Deviation) in Adult Horses

Breed	RBC (× 10^6/μl)	HGB (g/dl)	PCV (%)	MCV (fl)	MCH (pg)	MCHC (%)
Thoroughbred	9.35 ± 1.05	14.8 ± 1.3	41.7 ± 3.8	44.7 ± 3.4	15.9 ± 1.4	35.8 ± 1.4
Standardbred	8.37 ± 1.02	13.6 ± 1.6	38.3 ± 3.5	46.1 ± 4.0	16.3 ± 1.4	35.5 ± 1.6
Quarter Horse	8.26 ± 1.02	13.3 ± 1.6	38.0 ± 4.0	46.2 ± 3.9	16.1 ± 1.7	34.9 ± 1.6
Appaloosa	8.60 ± 1.11	13.3 ± 1.6	38.4 ± 4.7	44.8 ± 4.4	15.5 ± 1.3	34.5 ± 0.8
Arabian	8.41 ±1.21	13.8 ± 2.1	39.3 ± 5.0	46.9 ± 1.9	16.4 ± 0.9	34.9 ± 1.0
Clydesdale	7.30 ± 0.87	12.4 ± 1.1	33.0 ± 3.0	44.6	—	38.1
Percheron	7.39 ± 1.08	11.7 ± 1.4	—	—	—	—
Mixed cold-blooded	7.76 ± 1.23	—	33.0 ± 7.0	42.3	—	—

From Moms DD: Review of anemia in horses. I. Clinical signs, laboratory findings and diagnosis, *Vet Clin North Am Equine Pract* 11:27-34, 1989; modified from Jain NC, editor: *Schalm's veterinary hematology,* ed 4, Philadelphia, 1986, Lea & Febiger.

RBC, Red blood cell; *Hgb,* hemoglobin; *PCV,* packed cell volume; *MCV,* mean corpuscular volume; *MCH,* mean corpuscular hemoglobin; *MCHC,* mean corpuscular hemoglobin concentration.

blood analyses, then they may be calculated from the PCV, RBC count (in millions), and hemoglobin (in g/dl) as presented in Box 14-1. Some automated cell counters also report RBC distribution width.

Peripheral blood evaluation is not complete without a thorough examination of a stained blood smear to assess erythrocyte morphology. The normal equine erythrocyte is a biconcave disc; however, in contrast to other species, most equine RBCs lack distinct central pallor. Equine RBCs normally exhibit a strong tendency toward rouleau formation, a coinlike stacking or grouping of erythrocytes. This tendency causes equine erythrocytes to sediment rapidly after collection, and one should mix all samples thoroughly, immediately before any evaluation. Excellent pictures of normal and abnormal equine erythrocyte morphologic condition are available in a variety of texts, and the reader is referred to those to aid in recognition of the following cell types[12,13]:

Poikilocyte: Any abnormally shaped erythrocyte. Poikilocytosis usually is reserved for description of RBCs that exhibit a variety of morphologies. If one particular shape predominates, then one should use a more specific description.

Anisocytosis: A variability in the size of erythrocytes, usually associated with an increased RBC distribution width.

Polychromasia: A variability in the color of erythrocytes usually caused by a variable hemoglobin and RNA content.

Spherocyte: Spherical erythrocyte observed in some horses with immune-mediated hemolysis.

Echinocyte: Burr cell with short, regularly spaced spicules projecting from the RBC surface. Echinocytes may be associated with uremia.

Acanthocyte: Spur cell with irregularly shaped spicules extending from the RBC surface. Acanthocytes may be associated with liver disease or gastrointestinal malabsorption.

Elliptocyte: Ellipsoid or oval erythrocyte found in animals with iron deficiency or myelophthisic anemia.

Leptocyte: Thin, flat RBC frequently associated with hepatic disease or iron deficiency.

Codocyte: Target cell with a dense central area of hemoglobin surrounded by a pale zone. Codocytes may be associated with hypochromic anemias or hepatic disease.

BOX 14-1

EVALUATION OF RED BLOOD CELL INDICES: CALCULATION FROM THE PACKED CELL VOLUME, RED BLOOD CELL COUNT (MILLIONS), AND HEMOGLOBIN (G/DL)

$$MCV = \frac{PCV \times 10}{RBC\ count}$$

Expressed as femtoliters (fl)

Increased in some horses with regenerative anemia

Decreased with iron deficiency anemia

Increased in older horses*

$$MCV = \frac{hemoglobin \times 10}{RBC\ count}$$

Expressed as picograms (pg)

Increased with intravascular hemolysis

Decreased with iron deficiency anemia

$$MCHC = \frac{hemoglobin \times 100}{PCV}$$

Expressed as grams per deciliter (g/dl)

Increased with intravascular hemolysis

Decreased with iron deficiency anemia

*Data From McFarlane D, Sellon DC, Gaffney D, et al: Hematologic and serum biochemical variables and plasma corticotropin concentration in healthy aged horses, *Am J Vet Res* 59:1247, 1998.

RBC, Red blood cell; *PCV,* packed cell volume; *MCV,* mean corpuscular volume; *MCHC,* mean corpuscular hemoglobin concentration.

Howell-Jolly bodies: Basophilic nuclear remnants seen in the cytoplasm of erythrocytes. Approximately 10 in 10,000 erythrocytes contain Howell-Jolly bodies in the normal horse.[13]

Heinz bodies: Oxidized precipitated hemoglobin indicating oxidative damage to the RBC, usually resulting in intravascular or extravascular hemolysis. One may see Heinz bodies best using new methylene blue stain but may observe them in smears using Wright's stain as round structures protruding from the edge of the RBC membrane.

Occasionally, specialized tests of erythrocyte function or stability are indicated. Osmotic fragility tests measure the resistance of erythrocytes to in vitro hemolysis when incubated in increasingly hypotonic sodium chloride (NaCl) solutions. Erythrocytes from horses with immune-mediated hemolytic anemia (IMHA) frequently are more fragile than RBCs from normal horses.[14,15] The direct antiglobulin or Coombs' test is also helpful for diagnosing IMHA. Coombs' test detects immunoglobulin (Ig) or complement on the surface of circulating erythrocytes. The Coombs' reagent should contain antisera to immunoglobulin G (IgG), immunoglobulin M (IgM), and the third component of complement (C3). One incubates washed erythrocytes from the patient with Coombs' reagent and observes for agglutination. The cells can be incubated at 10° C to detect cold reactive antibodies or at 30° C to detect warm reactive antibodies.[13] Because agglutination is the end point of the direct Coombs' test, autoagglutination of blood is considered diagnostic of immune mediated hemolysis. One must differentiate autoagglutination from rouleau formation by dilution of an RBC suspension with isotonic saline. Saline disperses rouleau formation but does not affect true autoagglutination. The indirect Coombs' test detects the presence of circulating anti-RBC antibody in the serum by incubating patient serum with normal equine erythrocytes and monitoring for agglutination.

BONE MARROW EVALUATION

Examination of the bone marrow of a horse is indicated if one identifies or suspects a disorder of the hematopoietic system but cannot diagnose it from information gathered by history, physical examination, and routine laboratory tests.[16] Bone marrow aspirates or core biopsies may be useful in characterizing anemias, evaluating iron stores, or explaining quantitative or qualitative abnormalities of blood cells.

One may collect equine bone marrow aspirates or biopsies from the sternum,[16-18] tuber coxae,[16,19] or proximal ribs.[16,20] The sternal aspirates are obtained from the ventral midline between the front legs. This site is preferable in most horses because hematopoietic activity persists throughout life, bones are not covered by a large muscle mass, and the marrow cavity is covered by only a thin layer of bone.[16] One may attempt an aspirate of the tuber coxae in young horses by directing the needle toward the opposite coxofemoral joint. The costal marrow is collected from the proximal portion of an easily palpable cranial rib, usually beneath the latissimus dorsi and serratus posticus muscles.[20] Any large-gauge (16 gauge or larger) bone marrow needle with stylet can be used to collect marrow aspirates. The needle should be at least 2 inches long. The veterinarian clips the appropriate area and surgically scrubs it, injects a small amount of local anesthetic into the subcutaneous and periosteal tissues, and makes a stab incision through the skin and subcutaneous fascia. Forcing the bone marrow needle through the bone and into the marrow cavity may require considerable pressure and rotational movement.

The veterinarian removes the stylet from the needle; uses a sterile syringe containing a small quantity of anticoagulant to aspirate red-colored marrow, discontinuing aspiration when blood is visible in the hub of the syringe; withdraws the needle; and smears marrow from the hub of the syringe and the needle on glass microscope slides as for blood smears. Alternatively, one injects the marrow sample into a Petri dish. On visualization, the clinician transfers spicules to a glass slide for staining. One may obtain core marrow biopsies using a 10-gauge Jamshidi needle and fixing the sample for routine histopathologic analysis.[16,21]

Marrow samples should first be examined at low magnification for evidence of cellularity, distribution of fat cells, and heterogeneity of progenitor cell populations. At higher magnification, one may evaluate individual progenitor series and estimate a bone marrow myeloid-to-erythroid ratio (M:E) by counting 500 to 800 cells.[12] Descriptions and pictures of bone marrow progenitor cells are reported elsewhere, and the reader is referred to these for identification of cell types present in bone marrow aspirates or biopsies.[12,13,19] Normal M:E in the horse has been reported to range between 0.5 and 3.76.[17,18,20] Ratios of less than 0.5 are considered indicative of erythrocyte regeneration or myeloid suppression.[22] Special histochemical stains for iron (Prussian blue stain) are available to evaluate peripheral iron stores in the horse.[23] In many horses with of hemolytic anemia, bone marrow macrophages may be visible with phagocytosed RBCs.

Myelophthisis is a reduction in the cellular elements in the bone marrow, frequently a result of myelofibrosis, proliferation of fibrous tissue in the marrow. Myelodysplasia implies accumulation of abnormal cells in the bone marrow. These cells are often not dysplastic in the truest sense of the word but rather result from myeloproliferative neoplasia.

IRON STATUS EVALUATION

Adult horses do not often develop abnormalities in iron status because iron is readily available in most forages and horses have a natural ability to store iron. However, evaluation of systemic iron status may aid in characterizing hematologic abnormalities, especially in the investigation of anemias. Several laboratory parameters can aid in the identification and classification of abnormalities of iron metabolism. The peripheral blood smear may provide initial clues. Microcytic, hypochromic erythrocytes often are seen in animals with disturbances of iron metabolism. One may confirm these observations by calculating the mean corpuscular volume (MCV) and mean corpuscular hemoglobin concentration (MCHC) of peripheral blood erythrocytes. Measurement of serum ferritin provides a reliable index of stored hepatic and splenic iron in the horse. Serum ferritin concentration in 28 normal horses was 152 ± 54.6 ng/ml. A bone marrow aspirate examined after special iron stains is also an excellent means of assessing the pool of storage iron. Serum iron concentration reflects the total quantity of transport iron in the plasma (i.e., the quantity of iron bound to transferrin). Normal equine values of 120 ± 5.0 μg/dl[24] and 108 μg/dl[25] have been reported. The total iron-binding capacity (TIBC) reflects the amount of iron that plasma transferrin could bind if fully saturated. Normal TIBC in the horse has been reported as 388 ± 8.1 μg/dl.[24] One calculates the percentage of transferrin saturation from the serum iron concentration and the TIBC. Percentage transferrin saturation is normally approximately 30%. Serum iron concentration increases dramatically for 48 to 72 hours after administration of corticosteroids, but TIBC and serum ferritin concentrations do not.[26]

In healthy foals at birth, serum iron and ferritin concentrations are lower than those of adult horses but very rapidly increase over the first 24 hours of life to levels greater than that of adults because of absorption of colostral iron. This is accompanied by a very high-percent saturation of transferrin with iron.[11,27] The high transferrin saturation makes foals quite susceptible to iron toxicity in the first 24 to 72 hours of life. A small amount of orally administered iron can be absorbed and exceed the iron-binding capacity of serum with free or unbound iron reaching tissues, especially the liver, resulting in acute hepatic failure.[28] Iron, ferritin, and transferrin saturation values gradually decrease to less than normal adult concentrations, reaching a minimum concentration at 3 weeks and returning to normal adult values by 6 months of age. The PCV of neonatal foals correlates closely with these changes: PCV is relatively high in the first few days of life followed by a decrease in PCV to less than adult values by 2 weeks of age. Iron supplementation does not change these hematologic parameters.

Disorders of the Erythron

ERYTHROCYTOSIS

Erythrocytosis or polycythemia is a real or apparent increase in the circulating RBC mass and may be classified as *relative,* caused by a decrease in plasma volume, or *absolute,* caused by a real increase in RBC numbers. Animals with persistent erythrocytosis have muddy red to blue mucous membranes, prolonged capillary refill time, weakness, lethargy, and exercise intolerance. Despite the large RBC mass in the circulation, oxygen delivery to the peripheral tissues often decreases because of increased blood viscosity and sludging in small vessels. Persistent erythrocytosis may lead to complications including hypertension, tissue hypoxia, thrombosis, and hemorrhage.[29]

Relative Erythrocytosis Relative erythrocytosis or polycythemia may occur because of hemoconcentration or splenic contraction. Hemoconcentration occurs when total plasma volume decreases without any change in total RBC numbers in circulation. Clinical dehydration is usually evident, with slow capillary refill time, dry mucous membranes, and prolonged skin tenting. Dehydration may occur with excessive water losses accompanying diuresis, diarrhea, or excessive sweating, as well as with decreased water intake. Endotoxic shock results in dehydration and hemoconcentration by causing a shift of water from plasma to the interstitial space. An increase in total plasma protein usually accompanies relative erythrocytosis caused by hemoconcentration. An exception to this occurs with concurrent loss of protein and body water (e.g., in horses with severe protein-losing diarrhea or glomerulonephritis). In these horses, total plasma protein may be normal or decreased in the presence of a high PCV. The PCV of hemoconcentrated horses usually returns to normal after intravenous fluid therapy, unless water losses continue.

The spleen of the resting horse may harbor up to one third of the total circulating erythrocyte volume. Exercise, endogenous epinephrine release caused by excitement or stress, and exogenous epinephrine administration results in splenic contraction that may increase the PCV by as much as 50%.[30-33] This relative erythrocytosis is not accompanied by a significant increase in total plasma protein. If the horse is allowed to relax in a nonstressful environment, then PCV usually returns to normal within a few hours.

Absolute Erythrocytosis Absolute erythrocytosis occurs when increased erythropoiesis causes an increase in PCV, RBC count, and hemoglobin concentration. Plasma volume and plasma protein concentration remain normal.

Primary absolute erythrocytosis (including polycythemia vera) is rare and considered a myeloproliferative disorder of the bone marrow.[29] Serum erythropoietin concentrations are decreased to normal and Pa_{O_2} is normal. This condition may be accompanied by thrombocytosis or leukocytosis. Severe erythrocytosis has been described in two horses with normal serum erythropoietin levels.[29,34]

Secondary absolute erythrocytosis may be appropriate or inappropriate, depending on the presence or absence, respectively, of tissue hypoxia. Appropriate secondary absolute erythrocytosis is associated with increased circulating erythropoietin levels caused by chronic hypoxia from right-to-left shunting of blood in the heart or great vessels, chronic pulmonary disease, or adaptation to high altitude. The most common cardiac anomalies associated with erythrocytosis are complex defects such as tetralogy or pentalogy of Fallot, although a number of other defects, including ventricular septal defect, eventually may result in right-to-left shunting and secondary erythrocytosis.[35] Horses with this condition frequently have cyanotic mucous membranes and an audible heart murmur. One can document chronic hypoxia by measuring the Pa_{O_2}. Oxygen saturation concentrations of less than 92% usually are required for stimulation of erythropoiesis.[29,36] One may confirm the diagnosis with cardiac radiography, ultrasonography, angiocardiography, or cardiac catheterization with blood gas and pressure analyses.

Erythrocytosis is rare in horses with chronic lung disease. Auscultation of animals with chronic lung disease severe enough to result in hypoxia likely would reveal abnormal lung sounds such as wheezes and crackles. Thoracic radiographs aid in assessing the extent and severity of the problem. One should direct treatment of these animals toward correction or alleviation of the primary problem. If this is not possible, then periodic phlebotomy and removal of several liters of blood helps decrease blood viscosity and may improve the quality of life of these horses.

Inappropriate secondary absolute erythrocytosis occurs after increased erythropoietin or other hormone release in the absence of tissue hypoxia. Although reported in horses with metastatic carcinoma and thoracic lymphoma,[37,38] this condition is most common in horses with hepatic neoplasms or renal abnormalities. These animals have a normal or nearly normal Pa_{O_2}. In human beings, hydronephrosis, renal cysts, and embryonal nephromata have been associated most frequently with this paraneoplastic syndrome. In the horse, secondary absolute erythrocytosis has been described in association with hepatocellular carcinoma and hepatoblastoma. All affected horses have been less than 3 years of age, and concurrent elevations in serum erythropoietin concentrations, α-fetoprotein concentrations, or both have been described.[39-41] These horses had a persistently elevated PCV that did not decrease with intravenous fluid therapy, normal plasma protein concentrations, and mild to moderate elevations in hepatic enzymes. A horse with erythrocytosis that occurred after metastatic carcinoma also has been described.

Most horses with primary or secondary erythrocytosis have a guarded to poor prognosis. If an underlying disease exists, then one should treat it appropriately. Intermittent phlebotomy may provide supportive therapy.[29]

ANEMIA

Anemia is a decrease in the circulating RBC mass caused by an imbalance in the rate of loss or destruction of erythrocytes and the rate of their production in the bone marrow. Anemia is not considered a primary diagnosis but rather a hematologic abnormality resulting from an underlying disease process. Anemia is defined most frequently as a decrease in PCV or RBC numbers. Hemoglobin also is decreased, except in cases of intravascular hemolysis. A systematic approach to characterization of the anemia can provide valuable clues in the diagnosis of an underlying disease process. All anemias may be classified as *regenerative* or *nonregenerative* based on bone marrow response to the decrease in circulating RBC mass. Regenerative anemia results from loss of intact erythrocytes from circulation (hemorrhage) or accelerated destruction of RBCs (hemolysis) and is characterized by an increase in effective erythropoiesis in the bone marrow. Nonregenerative anemia occurs after systemic abnormalities or because of intrinsic bone marrow disease and results from a lack of appropriate marrow erythropoiesis in response to normal or accelerated RBC senescence or destruction.

Anemia also may be characterized on the basis of erythrocyte size (MCV) and hemoglobin content (MCHC). Normocytic normochromic anemia accompanies many chronic systemic disease processes, including renal and hepatic failure, endocrine abnormalities, neoplastic conditions, and chronic infections. Microcytic hypochromic anemia (low MCV and MCHC) is associated classically with iron deficiency anemia. Small erythrocytes, characterized by a low MCV, are normal in foals. Macrocytic anemia (increased MCV) occasionally occurs in horses after a severe hemolytic or hemorrhagic crisis. Large erythrocytes, characterized by a high MCV, are normal in older horses, especially those over 20 years of age.

Clinical signs of severe anemia relate to decreased tissue oxygenation and the physiologic compensatory mechanisms intended to alleviate this hypoxia. Signs include pallor of the mucous membranes, tachycardia, polypnea, weakness, lethargy, and a systolic heart murmur caused by decreased viscosity and increased turbulence of the blood as it flows through the heart and great vessels. Horses with mild to moderate anemia may have no obvious clinical signs or may have only lethargy and slightly pale mucous membranes. Other clinical signs, including fever, icterus, and hemoglobinuria, may be present in anemic horses and reflect the primary pathophysiologic process involved.

Regenerative Anemia When erythrocytes are lost from the circulation at an accelerated rate by hemorrhage or hemolysis, the bone marrow responds by increasing its rate of erythrocyte production and release into the peripheral circulation. Documentation of an active regenerative response is important in diagnosis and prognosis of many cases of anemia. An increase in the number of reticulocytes in the peripheral circulation and an increase in the MCV are considered accurate indicators of a regenerative response in the bone marrow of most species. Unfortunately, in the horse, reticulocytes are not routinely released into the peripheral circulation, even during a strong regenerative bone marrow response. An equine-specific, automated hematology instrument that was used in a horse with severe hemolytic anemia revealed the presence of a low level of reticulocytes in the peripheral circulation. This analysis was based on detection of nucleic acids within the RBCs by flow cytometry.[42,43] Increases in MCV are inconsistent but tend to be slightly more common after hemolysis than after acute blood loss.[44-46] A slight anisocytosis that is quantitatively assessed through changes in RBC distribution width can be observed in equine peripheral blood after acute hemorrhage or hemolysis.[46-48]

Because of the difficulty in documenting a regenerative bone marrow response with conventional methods, several erythrocyte parameters have been investigated as markers of RBC regeneration in the equid.[49-51] G6PD, creatine,[49] and adenosine-5-triphosphate[52] increase in equine erythrocytes during a regenerative response, but tests for these are not available in most veterinary laboratories. The most practical, reliable method of assessing the erythrocyte regenerative response in an anemic horse, aside from serial PCV analysis, is bone marrow analysis. A bone marrow M:E of less than 0.5 is considered evidence of erythrocyte regeneration.[22] Reticulocyte counts in the bone marrow are also indicative of a regenerative response in the horse. Normal equine bone marrow contains approximately 3% reticulocytes, but this may increase to as high as 66% in response to severe blood loss.[21,22]

Hemorrhage Blood loss anemia may develop acutely or chronically. In many cases the source of the hemorrhage is obvious but in others is not. Internal hemorrhage (into body cavities) permits the body to reuse blood components. Approximately two thirds of the erythrocytes lost into the abdomen or thorax are autotransfused back into the circulation within 24 to 72 hours. The other one third are lysed or phagocytized, and the iron and protein are reused. External hemorrhage (including hemorrhage into the gastrointestinal tract) prevents reuse of these components. Accelerated bone marrow erythropoiesis is usually evident by 3 days after acute hemorrhage and is maximal by 7 days.[12] Box 14-2 lists differential diagnoses for blood loss in the horse.

Clinical signs of hemorrhage in the horse vary depending on the duration and severity of blood loss. Horses may lose up to one third (approximately 10 to 12 L) of their blood volume acutely without dying. Acute loss of large quantities of blood results in severe hypovolemic shock with tachycardia, polypnea, pale mucous membranes, poor venous distention, weakness, and oliguria. Initially, RBC parameters in the remaining circulating blood appear normal because all blood components have been lost in equal volumes. Physiologic compensatory mechanisms induce redistribution of interstitial fluid into the vasculature and eventually result in decreased RBC numbers and total protein in the peripheral blood. This redistribution may take up to 24 hours after acute hemorrhage. The difficulty in estimating the severity of blood loss during the first 24 hours after hemorrhage is compounded by the many erythrocytes that can be stored in the equine spleen and released into the circulation as a consequence of endogenous catecholamine release. After vascular equilibration, hematologic parameters should reveal a decrease in PCV, total RBC count, and hemoglobin with no change in associated RBC indices (MCV, MCHC, and MCH). Anemia caused by hemorrhage usually is accompanied by panhypoproteinemia because of significant loss of plasma proteins. A neutrophilic leukocytosis commonly is apparent by 3 hours after hemorrhage; platelets may increase as well if they have not been consumed by excessive coagulation.[12]

One may diagnose blood loss into the thoracic cavity by thoracic radiography, ultrasound, or thoracocentesis and may diagnose blood loss into the abdominal cavity by ultrasound or abdominocentesis. Horses with severe hemorrhage into the

BOX 14-2

DIFFERENTIAL DIAGNOSES FOR BLOOD LOSS IN THE HORSE

Epistaxis

- Guttural pouch mycosis
- Pulmonary abscess
- Exercise-induced pulmonary hemorrhage
- Ethmoid hematoma
- Paranasal sinus abscess or infection
- Traumatic nasogastric intubation
- Upper respiratory tract neoplasm
- Coagulopathy
- Trauma
- Pneumonia/pleuritis
- Hemothorax
- Thoracic trauma
    - Fractured rib
    - Lacerated heart or vessels
- Ruptured pulmonary abscess
- Ruptured great vessel
- Neoplasia
- Coagulopathy

Hematuria

- Pyelonephritis
- Cystitis/urolithiasis
- Neoplasia
- Trauma
- Urethral ulceration
- Coagulopathy

Hemoperitoneum

- Trauma
    - Splenic rupture
    - Hepatic rupture
- Mesenteric vessel rupture
- Verminous arteritis
- Uterine artery rupture
- Abdominal abscess
- Neoplasia
- Coagulopathy

Gastrointestinal Hemorrhage

- Ulcerations
- Nonsteroidal antiinflammatory drug (NSAID) toxicity
- Parasites
    - *Strongylus vulgaris*
    - Small strongyles
- Granulomatous intestinal disease
    - Histoplasmosis
    - Tuberculosis
    - Granulomatous enteritis
- Neoplasia
    - Squamous cell carcinoma
    - Lymphosarcoma
- Coagulopathy

External Hemorrhage

- Trauma
- Surgical complication
- Coagulopathy
- External parasites

abdominal cavity may exhibit signs of colic or abdominal discomfort. One may differentiate intra-abdominal hemorrhage from inadvertent splenic aspiration or laceration of a subcutaneous blood vessel by the presence of erythrophagocytosis and absence of platelets and may differentiate recent hemorrhage into the abdominal cavity from diapedesis across compromised bowel or old hemorrhage by the presence of platelets in fresh blood. One may observe gastrointestinal blood loss as melena or hematochezia. More commonly, gastrointestinal hemorrhage is not severe enough to result in these overt signs, and feces appear normal.

Brood mares in the periparturient period can suffer from rupture of the middle uterine, utero-ovarian, or external iliac arteries.[53,54] The ruptured vessel can lead to blood loss into the peritoneal cavity, into the broad ligament or serosa of the uterus, or into the lumen of the uterus iteslf.[55] This condition should be considered possible in any mare up to 48 hours after foaling exhibiting the aforementioned clinical signs of acute blood loss, as well as lethargy, colic, and sweating. Older mares[53,56,57] or multiparous mares[58] are at the greatest risk and a link between age and declining serum copper concentrations, vascular degeneration, and fatal hemorrhage has been proposed.[54] Therapy for hemorrhage discussed in the following sections pertains to this form of hemorrhage as well. Oxytocin can also be used to enhance uterine involution.

Effective treatment of acute blood loss anemia must begin with finding and eliminating the source of hemorrhage. In many animals, this source is readily apparent, and direct pressure or surgical ligation of ruptured vessels is indicated. Internal hemorrhage or postpartum hemorrhage is more difficult to control because immediate surgery to access the site of hemorrhage is usually not an option. In horses with acute severe hemorrhage the administration of isotonic crystalline intravenous fluids may aid tissue oxygenation by increasing peripheral blood volume and perfusion pressures. Administration of hypertonic saline solution (4 to 5 ml/kg of 7.5% NaCl) or hydroxyethyl starch (5 to 10 ml/kg) may be beneficial for rapid volume expansion after achieving adequate hemostasis.[59] However, volume expansion has the potential risk of exacerbating hemorrhage if one cannot achieve hemostasis. Use of hypertonic or colloidal solutions should be followed by administration of appropriate isotonic crystalline fluid therapy.

Polymerized ultrapurified bovine hemoglobin is an alternative oxygen-carrying fluid that has been administered to horses, including postpartum mares, in lieu of whole blood transfusion.[60,61] Although expensive and used with variable success, this product has the advantages of compatibility without crossmatching and long shelf life.

Naloxone, a μ-specific opioid antagonist, has been recommended for use in horses with acute hemorrhage. Evidence suggests that endogenous opioids are involved in the pathophysiology of shock and that administration of naloxone may decrease some of the associated cardiovascular derangements.[62]

Aminocaproic acid is an antifibrinolytic drug that has been used in human patients to reduce hemorrhage during various surgical procedures. In horses, it has been suggested that aminocaproic acid may be useful if a hyperfibrinolytic state exists.[63] This drug has been used to treat mares suffering from periparturient hemorrhage.[55] Pharmacokinetic studies in the horse suggest that a loading dose of 70 mg/kg intravenously (diluted in 1 L of saline and given over 20 minutes) followed by a constant-rate infusion at 15 mg/kg/hr is safe and achieves target blood concentrations. However, clinical efficacy research is lacking.[64]

The Chinese herb Yunnan Baiyao has been used with some evidence of efficacy in human patients with hemorrhage. The mechanism of action for this inexpensive herb is unclear but proposed effects include decreased bleeding and clotting times, platelet effect, and vasoconstriction. The drug decreased template bleeding times and activated clotting times in anesthetized ponies,[65] and it is advocated as an adjunctive treatment protocol for mares with periparturient hemorrhage.[55] A dose of 8 mg/kg orally every 6 hours has been suggested, but clinical trials are needed.

If 20% to 30% of the total blood volume is lost acutely, then blood transfusion from a compatible donor horse is indicated. More detailed discussion of the principles of blood and blood product therapy occur later in this chapter. Hemorrhage into a large body cavity frequently is followed by autotransfusion of erythrocytes back into the peripheral circulation. Therefore one should not remove blood from these spaces unless necessary to stop continued bleeding (because the blood is interfering with vital organ function) or to lavage potentially septic sites.

Horses with subacute hemorrhage (over a few days) usually begin to show clinical signs of severe anemia when the PCV declines to 15% to 20%. The same clinical signs may not be noticeable in horses with chronic blood loss (over weeks to months) until the PCV reaches 12% or less. Blood lactate concentration and central venous pressure may be used as indicators of the need for transfusion or to monitor cardiovascular responses to transfusion in horses with acute blood loss. Increased blood lactate concentrations and decreased central venous pressures are early indicators of blood loss. Post-transfusion, the pressures and blood lactate concentrations should rapidly return to near normal.[66] Because these laboratory parameters are so variable and potentially misleading, one should base treatment decisions on the clinical signs in the individual patient and not necessarily on defined target clinical laboratory parameters.

A horse with subacute to chronic blood loss anemia severe enough to result in peripheral tissue hypoxia as a result of inadequate RBC mass to supply needed oxygen exhibits tachycardia, polypnea, pale mucous membranes, weakness and lethargy, and possibly a mild to moderate systolic heart murmur caused by reduced viscosity and increased turbulence of the blood. If these signs are severe, then blood transfusion is indicated. As with acute hemorrhage, one must identify the source of the blood loss.

Other treatment is supportive and should be designed to eliminate the primary problem. If external blood loss has occurred over weeks to months, then body iron stores may be depleted, a particularly common problem with chronic gastrointestinal bleeding. Depletion of iron slows or stops effective bone marrow erythropoiesis so that these animals have laboratory parameters typical of iron deficiency anemia. One may identify low serum iron, low marrow iron stores, and increased TIBC, accompanying a hypochromic, microcytic anemia. Dietary iron may be supplemented orally with ferrous sulfate at a dose of 2 mg/kg body mass. One should not administer iron dextran parentally to horses because it has been associated with sudden death in this species. If iron must be administered intravenously, then iron cacodylate solutions are available.

Administration of human recombinant erythropoietin to horses results in increased RBC mass and tissue oxygenation.[67] After experimentally induced anemia, horses receiving concurrent recombinant erythropoietin and iron supplementation had RBC counts and reticulocyte parameters that indicated enhanced regeneration.[43] However, repeated administration of human recombinant erythropoietin may result in production of antibodies against the drug that cross-react with, and inhibit the activity of, naturally produced equine erythropoietin. The end result is a potentially fatal nonregenerative aplastic anemia that persists until antibody levels are depleted.

Because of the lack of peripheral signs of a bone marrow regenerative response in the horse, accurately assessing the regenerative efforts of bone marrow after hemorrhage may be difficult. One may evaluate serial bone marrow aspirates if this information is critical, but in most cases, monitoring increases in PCV over time is adequate. After experimental phlebotomy to mimic blood loss anemia in the horse, PCV increased approximately 0.672% per day, more slowly than in other species.[52] Experimentally, the bone marrow erythroid response peaked at 9 days after phlebotomy, coinciding with the lowest marrow M:E ratio. Regeneration of the erythroid compartment was incomplete 31 days after hemorrhage.[68]

Hemolysis Intravascular or extravascular destruction of erythrocytes can occur in a variety of disorders. During intravascular hemolysis, hemoglobin released from destroyed erythrocytes combines with plasma haptoglobin, and tissue mononuclear phagocytes remove the haptoglobin-hemoglobin complex. Plasma haptoglobin levels decrease as intravascular hemolysis increases.[69,70] When plasma haptoglobin binding is exceeded, free hemoglobin accumulates in the plasma and is eliminated via the kidneys. Thus the hallmarks of intravascular hemolysis are hemoglobinemia and hemoglobinuria. Horses recovering from a severe hemolytic episode are more likely to have a demonstrable increase in MCV than are horses recovering from acute blood loss.[44,45,71]

The most common causes of hemolysis in horses are immune-mediated disease, oxidant-induced damage to erythrocytes, and infectious diseases. However, acute hemolytic anemia of adult horses has been associated with a wide variety of pathologic conditions (Box 14-3). Dimethyl sulfoxide administered intravenously at concentrations of 50% or greater results in severe intravascular hemolysis.[72] Hemolytic-uremic syndrome is characterized by acute renal failure, microangiopathic hemolytic anemia, and intravascular coagulation. Erythrocytes become damaged as they pass between fibrin strands deposited in the lumen of small renal vessels. Thrombocytopenia may occur concurrently.[73,74] Hemolysis has been reported in horses ingesting leaves of the northern red oak *(Quercus rubra* L. var. *borealis)*. Other associated clinical signs included abdominal pain, constipation, and increased coagulation times.[75] Administration of significantly hypotonic or

BOX 14-3

DIFFERENTIAL DIAGNOSES FOR HEMOLYSIS IN THE HORSE

Infectious Diseases

Piroplasmosis
Equine infectious anemia (EIA)

Immune-Mediated Disease

Autoimmune disease
Bacterial infection
 Clostridium perfringens
 Streptococcal infections
Viral infection
 EIA
Neoplasia
 Lymphosarcoma
Drug reaction
 Penicillin
Neonatal isoerythrolysis

Oxidative Injury

Phenothiazine
Onion
Red maple leaf
Familial methemoglobinemia

Iatrogenic Conditions

Hypotonic solutions
Hypertonic saline

Miscellaneous Conditions

Hepatic disease
Hemolytic uremic syndrome
Disseminated intravascular coagulation (DIC)

Other Toxicities

Intravenous dimethyl sulfoxide
Bacterial toxins (Clostridium)
Oak
Burn injury

hypertonic solutions to horses also may result in intravascular hemolysis. All these conditions are uncommon in the horse.

Immune-Mediated Hemolytic Anemia Immune-mediated hemolytic anemia develops when an animal produces antibodies that attach to the surface of RBCs. Primary IMHA is an autoimmune process in which antibodies are directed against surface antigens and occurs when a normally suppressed B-lymphocyte clone proliferates and produces an antibody directed against normal RBCs.[76] Secondary IMHA is more common than true autoimmune disease. Antibodies attach to the surface of erythrocytes for several possible reasons: (1) alterations in the RBC membrane produced by a primary viral, bacterial, or neoplastic disease process; (2) antigen-antibody complex deposition on the surface of RBCs; or (3) drugs that cause immunoproteins to react indirectly with RBCs.

Drug-induced immune-mediated hemolysis may occur via three mechanisms[77]:

1. The drug may combine with RBC membranes and may be recognized as foreign by the body. An antibody to this new antigen develops and destroys the drug-coated erythrocytes. These animals have a positive direct Coombs' test.
2. The drug may complex with a carrier molecule in the blood and induce an immune response, and the drug-carrier-antibody complex attaches to RBC membranes in a complement-mediated process that leads to hemolysis.
3. Occasionally, a drug may induce true autoantibody production that leads to RBC destruction.

Antibody-coated RBCs are unable to pass through the microcirculation of the spleen, become sequestered there, and are destroyed or phagocytized. If RBC membrane is lost in excess of intracellular contents, then spherocytes with an increased osmotic fragility form. Most immune-mediated hemolysis is extravascular; however, if the antibody fixes and activates complement, then intravascular complement-mediated hemolysis may result.[13]

IMHA may be classified as *warm* or *cold hemagglutinin disease* based on the optimal temperature at which the autoantibody agglutinates the host RBCs. Many clinical pathologists believe that these designations can be arbitrary and reflect an in vitro phenomenon rather than in vivo pathogenesis. Classically, in cold hemagglutinin disease, the antibody involved is IgM, complement is activated, and the liver is the primary site of removal of injured RBCs from the circulation. In warm hemagglutinin disease, IgG more commonly is involved, and the spleen is the primary site of RBC sequestration.[13,78,79] Warm hemagglutinins are frequently incomplete (i.e., they do not cause autoagglutination).[78] Warm[80,81] and cold[78,82] hemagglutinin anemia have been described in the horse.

Primary and secondary IMHA are uncommon in the adult horse.[48] Onset of disease is usually insidious, and many horses have fever, lethargy, and weight loss or have signs referable to a primary disease process. Routine hematologic and biochemical analyses frequently reveal decreased RBC numbers, spherocytosis, increased MCV, anisocytosis, and an increased total and indirect bilirubin. Most cases of immune-mediated hemolysis involve extravascular RBC destruction; however, if intravascular hemolysis is occurring, then hemoglobinuria will occur. One confirms the diagnosis by documenting a regenerative erythropoietic response in the bone marrow, increased erythrocyte fragility in hypotonic saline, autoagglutination, and a positive direct antiglobulin or Coombs' test. The Coombs' reagent used should contain antisera to IgG, IgM, and C3. One must differentiate autoagglutination from rouleau formation by dilution of a cell suspension with isotonic saline. Saline disperses rouleau formation but does not affect true autoagglutination. Flow cytometry has been used to confirm a diagnosis of IMHA in an affected horse by identifying and quantifying the amount of erythrocyte surface-bound antibody.[83]

In human beings, IMHA has been associated with lymphoreticular neoplasms, a variety of viral and bacterial diseases, inflammatory or granulomatous diseases, and generalized autoimmune disorders such as systemic lupus erythematosus. One may have difficulty distinguishing between primary autoimmune hemolytic anemia (AIHA), in which autoantibodies are directed against an abnormal epitope on the erythrocyte membrane, and nonspecific immune complex deposition on the surface of erythrocytes, usually occurring via attachment to Fc or complement receptors. In the horse, immune-mediated hemolysis has been reported in association with *Clostridium perfringens* septicemia and myositis,[42,48,79] an unclassified respiratory infection,[48] purpura hemorrhagica,[82,84] a streptococcal abscess,[82] and lymphosarcoma.[14,82,84] Regardless of the exact sequence of events leading to antibody deposition on the surface of erythrocytes, affected horses show clinical signs similar to those described for primary AIHA, and clinical pathologic data and diagnosis are similar.

IMHA that occurs after treatment with penicillin has been documented in horses.[85-88] Most affected horses have not been hemoglobinuric, indicating predominantly extravascular hemolysis. IMHA in the horse also has been associated with administration of trimethoprim-sulfamethoxazole.[89] Although not documented as causing immune-mediated hemolysis in the horse, drugs that have caused this problem in other species include tetracycline, rifampin, cephalosporins, chlorpromazine, and various nonsteroidal anti-inflammatory drugs (NSAIDs). In all reported cases of drug-induced IMHA in horses, the problem has resolved with discontinuation of administration of the offending therapeutic agent and appropriate supportive care.

Neonatal isoerythrolysis is an important form of immune-mediated hemolysis in the foal[90] and is discussed in detail elsewhere in this text.

Immune-mediated anemia resulting in intravascular and extravascular hemolysis may be present in horses with equine infectious anemia (EIA) (see the following discussion). Infected horses may have a positive result on the Coombs' test or exhibit autoagglutination, especially during acute disease. Immune-mediated anemia also has been described in a horse with systemic lupus erythrematosus.[91]

Therapy of immune-mediated hemolysis is similar regardless of the initiating factor (or factors) involved. One should discontinue any previously administered drug and treat specific underlying primary disease processes. If hemolysis is severe and life threatening, then the veterinarian should administer blood transfusions from a compatible donor (see the discussion on blood transfusion). If the horse has severe intravascular hemolysis with hemoglobinuria, then one should initiate intravenous fluid therapy to protect against pigment-induced nephropathy.

Several cases of immune-mediated hemolysis in the horse have been at least transiently responsive to corticosteroid therapy.[14,48,80] One horse experienced complete disease remission after a 10-week regimen of glucocorticoids.[76] Parenterally administered corticosteroids are recommended initially, and dexamethasone is probably the drug of choice. One should titrate the amount and frequency of administration to the response of the individual animal, but an initial dose of 30 to 40 mg dexamethasone may be tried in an adult horse. Ideally, administration of corticosteroids in the morning minimizes interference with the circadian rhythm of endogenous corticosteroid release from the adrenal gland. However, in an acute hemolytic crisis, twice-daily administration of dexamethasone is recommended until RBC numbers cease to decline. After stabilization, one should decrease corticosteroid doses to once daily, then every other day, and gradually discontinue the therapy. If the horse requires long-term therapy, then one may administer prednisolone orally with a declining every-other-day dosage. Potential complications of corticosteroid therapy in the horse include laminitis and secondary infections. Exacerbation of primary infectious conditions also may occur in cases of secondary autoimmune hemolysis treated with corticosteroids. Caution is recommended, especially when using corticosteroids at a high dose or for a prolonged period. One horse with IMHA refractory to corticosteroid therapy was treated successfully with cyclophosphamide at 1.1 mg/kg intramuscularly once daily and azathioprine at 1.1 mg/kg intramuscularly once daily.[92]

Oxidative injury to RBCs is evident from Heinz body formation, hemolytic anemia, and methemoglobinemia. Heinz bodies are aggregations of oxidized precipitated hemoglobin. They are small, round, blue-black, refractile granules near the cellular margin of erythrocytes stained with new methylene blue.[93] Heinz bodies damage the erythrocyte membrane, disturbing intracellular tonicity and resulting in rupture of the cell (intravascular hemolysis). Cells of the mononuclear-phagocyte system of the spleen and liver may recognize damaged RBC membranes as abnormal and remove the RBCs from the peripheral circulation (extravascular hemolysis). One mechanism by which the RBCs protect themselves is through the production of reduced nicotinamide adenine dinucleotide phosphate (NADPH) via the pentose pathway. Several enzymes are essential to this pathway, including the rate-controlling enzyme G6PD.

Oxidation of iron in the hemoglobin molecule from the normal ferrous state (Fe^{2+}) to the ferric state (Fe^{3+}) forms methemoglobin. Erythrocytes normally produce methemoglobin, which cellular enzymes like FAD rapidly convert back to hemoglobin. In addition, cellular GSH acts to decrease the amount of methemoglobin formed by competing with hemoglobin for oxidizing agents.[94]

Methemoglobin is incapable of carrying oxygen, and excessive accumulation results in a brownish discoloration of blood. Methemoglobin formation alone does not result in hemolysis,[95] but toxins simultaneously may oxidize the sulfhydryl groups of the globin moiety of methemoglobin. This oxidation causes methemoglobin denaturation and precipitation, Heinz body formation, and intravascular hemolysis. Pathologic methemoglobin accumulation in the blood most frequently results from exposure to an oxidative toxin that overwhelms the protective mechanisms of the body but also may result from a decreased rate of reduction of physiologically produced methemoglobin.

The aforementioned enzymes involved in erythrocyte metabolism are essential, and a deficiency of any of these enzymes can cause a decrease in the erythrocyte life span and a form of anemia. Several genetic alterations that lead to these deficiencies have been identified in human beings and dogs; however, only three have been identified in the horse thus far, and all result in clinical signs typical of oxidative RBC injury.

A deficiency of G6PD in human beings is the result of a well-described X-linked genetic mutation that is relatively common. When subjected to oxidative insult, affected individuals develop hemolytic anemia and hyperbilirubinemia.[96] A 6-month-old American Saddlebred colt was diagnosed with this disorder via a series of tests including G6PD assays, electron microscopy, and numerous other erythrocyte assays. The colt had no history of exposure to exogenous oxidants but was suffering from a significant dermatitis. This was assumed to be the source of endogenous oxidants, and the hemolytic anemia improved as the dermatitis resolved. Management of these cases may simply include prevention of inflammation and other forms of oxidative stress. Although most clinicians believe that this disorder is inherited in horses as it is in human beings, this has not been confirmed.[7]

Two adult horses, a Spanish Mustang and a Kentucky Mountain Saddle Horse, were diagnosed with FAD deficiencies through a series of tests including flavin assays. Both horses had persistent methemoglobinemia, eccentrocytosis, and pyknocytosis on laboratory analysis. Hemoglobin crystals were identified in the Mustang. Neither horse was profoundly anemic nor were exogenous oxidants identified.[8]

Familial methemoglobinemia and hemolytic anemia caused by decreased erythrocyte GSH reductase and intracellular GSH have been described in two Trotter mares.[97] These mares displayed findings similar to those with FAD deficiency.

Acute hemolytic anemia and methemoglobinemia can develop in horses after ingestion of wilted red maple *(Acer rubrum)* leaves.[71,98-101] The toxic principle is uncertain, but gallic acid, a strong oxidant, has been implicated in conjunction with another unidentified agent.[102] Freshly harvested leaves are not dangerous but become toxic when dried and remain so for at least 30 days. Overnight freezing of the leaves does not affect toxicity. Affected horses present most commonly in late summer and fall, often with brownish discoloration of the blood (massive methemoglobinemia) and peracute death within 12 to 18 hours of exposure. A more prolonged hemolytic syndrome characterized by icterus, methemoglobinemia, hemoglobinuria, bilirubinemia, bilirubinuria, fever, and possibly death may occur 5 days or more after ingestion of wilted leaves. Horses may initially present for evaluation of colic.[101] Laboratory evaluation of horses with the hemolytic syndrome of red maple leaf toxicosis frequently reveals Heinz body anemia, depletion of RBC-reduced GSH, and increased RBC osmotic fragility.[99] Normal methemoglobin concentration in equine blood is 1.77% of total hemoglobin.[97] Horses with red maple leaf toxicosis may have methemoglobin concentrations of close to 50% of total hemoglobin.[100]

Treatment of horses with red maple leaf toxicity includes eliminating access to the toxic leaves, whole blood or packed cell transfusions as needed, and general nursing care. The veterinarian should treat all exposed animals with activated charcoal via nasogastric tube to decrease absorption of toxin, even if several days have elapsed since exposure. Massive intravascular hemolysis may result in pigment-induced nephropathy. Fluid diuresis is indicated to prevent or treat this complication. One should use potentially nephrotoxic drugs with caution. Some clinicians have suggested dexamethasone administration to stabilize cellular membranes, but administration of corticosteroids is associated with an increased mortality rate in affected horses.[98,101,103] Methylene blue therapy has been attempted in some horses without success.[71] Because methylene blue may potentiate hemolysis, its use is not advisable. Two horses with severe hemolysis and methemoglobinemia caused by ingestion of red maple leaves were treated with large doses of ascorbic acid (vitamin C), but administration of this drug is not significantly associated with survival.[101,103] Ascorbic acid is thought to convert methemoglobin to reduced hemoglobin and may supplement endogenous protective mechanisms.[104] One may give adult horses a dose of ascorbic acid at 30 mg/kg twice daily in intravenous fluids.[103]

Prognosis for horses with red maple leaf toxicosis is guarded to poor and is not associated with initial physical examination findings or laboratory abnormalities at the time of presentation.[101] Horses are at risk for pigment nephropathy and acute anuric renal failure, colic, diarrhea, and laminitis.[100] Mortality rates have been reported at approximately 60%.

Outbreaks of Heinz body anemia have been reported in horses with access to unharvested onions[105] or overgrazed pasture covered with wild onions *(Allium canadense)*.[93] The toxic principle in onions is *n*-propyl disulfide. Treatment should include removal from access to the plants, activated charcoal via nasogastric tube to reduce absorption of the toxin, and blood transfusions and supportive care as indicated.

Heinz body anemia in horses also has been reported after phenothiazine administration. Toxicity appears to depend on individual susceptibility and some as yet unidentified environmental factors. Groups of animals may be affected at a dose that is generally considered safe, and animals in poor condition may be more susceptible to toxicity.[106] Although a 30-g dose for a 1000-lb horse is considered safe, one report described poisoning in six of nine horses treated with 25 g of phenothiazine.[107] Because phenothiazine is no longer widely used as an equine anthelmintic, reports of its toxicity are becoming rare.

Nitrate poisoning is associated with methemoglobin formation in horses but only rarely with intravascular hemolysis. Although it has been speculated that the horse might be more susceptible to nitrate poisoning than other simple-stomach species because the cecum and colon provide an optimal environment for microbial reduction of nitrate to nitrite,[71,108,109] nitrate toxicity appears to be extremely rare in horses.

Heinz body anemia has been reported in one horse with lymphosarcoma.[110] The authors could not confirm access to known oxidative toxins and presumed the anemia to be caused by the neoplastic process by an unidentified mechanism. Several horses that endured severe subcutaneous burns developed intravascular hemolytic anemia because of oxidative damage to RBCs. The mechanism of the damage to the RBC is not fully understood but does seem to correlate with severity of burns.[111]

Equine infectious anemia virus (EIAV) is a viral disease of horses known colloquially in the United States as *swamp fever* because of its high prevalence in Gulf Coast states where climatic conditions are favorable for transmission. The causative agent is a member of the lentivirus genus of the family Retroviridae. Infected horses may have one of three clinical syndromes: (1) acute infection, (2) chronic infection, or (3) inapparent carrier.[112,113]

Acutely infected horses show fever, lethargy, and anorexia within 30 days of exposure. The most consistent hematologic abnormality in these horses is thrombocytopenia, although anemia also may be present. Many acutely infected animals show few if any recognizable clinical signs, and definitive diagnosis may be difficult because some of these horses are not yet seropositive. Most horses seroconvert by 40 days after infection.

The horse chronically infected with EIAV has classic signs of recurrent fever, weight loss, ventral edema, and anemia. These animals are seropositive by the agar gel immunodiffusion (AGID or Coggins) test or by competitive enzyme-linked immunosorbent assay (C-ELISA). Each cycle of disease is associated with the emergence of a new antigenic strain of the virus, temporary evasion of the host immune response, and replication of the virus to high titer.

The anemia from which the disease derives its name results from intravascular and extravascular hemolysis of complement-coated RBCs and an impaired bone marrow response.[114-117] Each febrile episode is associated with thrombocytopenia, but platelet counts rebound rapidly as temperature returns to normal. Thrombocytopenia may result from immune[118] or nonimmune[119] platelet destruction or decreased platelet production in the bone marrow.[120]

Most EIAV seropositive horses are clinically normal and never show any recognizable clinical signs. However, they have immune-related blood abnormalities (hyperglobulinemia, decreased percentage of $CD5^+$ and $CD4^+$ lymphocytes) consistent with ongoing viral activity.[121] These animals are inapparent carriers of the virus and remain infected for life. They have circulating infectious virus in their blood and remain a threat to other horses for the rest of their lives. Regardless of disease stage (acute, chronic, or inapparent carrier), virus is found in vivo primarily in tissue macrophages and endothelial cells.[122-124]

Transmission of EIAV occurs predominantly by the intermittent feeding of hematophagous insects such as horseflies and deerflies. Flies are strictly mechanical vectors, and virus does not appear to survive more than 30 to 120 minutes on their mouthparts. Chances of transmission are greatest when flies feed on horses undergoing a febrile, viremic episode. However, horseflies can transmit virus from inapparent carrier horses to uninfected animals under field conditions, so all seropositive horses must be considered infectious for life.

EIAV also can be transmitted iatrogenically with blood product transfusions and previously used or improperly sterilized needles, surgical instruments, tattooing instruments, dental equipment, or any other blood-contaminated materials. Virus occasionally is transmitted across the placental barrier from an infected mare to its foal. Mares experiencing a febrile episode during gestation are more likely to give birth to infected foals than are asymptomatic mares. Of foals born to chronic carrier mares, approximately 10% are virus and antibody positive.[125,126] Virus transmission to foals may occur by ingestion of colostrum and milk from infected mares.[126,127] Foals born to antibody-positive mares usually are seropositive for EIAV at 24 hours of age because of absorption of colostral immunoglobulins. This colostral immunity is usually undetectable by 6 months of age.[126,127]

The Coggins test and C-ELISA are recognized by the U.S. Department of Agriculture as valid and reliable for the diagnosis of EIAV. Good correlation has been reported between Coggins test results and C-ELISA results.[128] A few horses have been identified, however, with consistently negative or equivocal AGID results that were proved subsequently to be infected.[129,130]

No specific antiviral therapy for EIAV is available. Treatment of an animal requires supportive therapy as indicated during febrile episodes. Minimizing environmental stress may be helpful in decreasing the severity and recurrence of clinical signs. All EIA reactor horses (seropositive) must be permanently identified using the National Uniform Tag code number assigned by the United States Department of Agriculture (USDA) to the state in which the reactor was tested, followed by the letter "A". A hot brand, chemical brand, freeze-marking, or lip tattoo may be used and must be applied by a USDA representative. Brands must be at least 2 inches high and applied to the left shoulder or left side of the neck. Lip tattoos should not be less than 1 inch high and ¾ inches wide and should be applied to the inner surface of the upper lip of the reactor. Reactor horses must be separated from other horses by quarantine at the premises of origin, euthanasia, or movement to a federally approved diagnostic or research facility. The ramining horses on the premises must be serologically tested for EIA with repeat testing at 30 to 60 day intervals until no new cases are found. The premises are released from quarantine when all tests have been negative for a minimum of 60 days after the last reactor equid was removed.[131]

Federal law prohibits interstate travel of horses that have tested positive for EIAV. Interstate movement of infected horses is allowed under three conditions: (1) back to the farm of origin, (2) to slaughter, and (3) to a diagnostic laboratory or approved research facility. Before interstate movement, reactors must be identified officially using the national uniform tag code number assigned by the U.S. Department of Agriculture to the state in which the reactor was tested, followed by the letter *A*. A hot iron, chemical brand, or freeze-marking may be used. Markings must be at least 2 inches high and applied to the left shoulder or left side of the neck.

Despite the significant decline in the incidence of EIAV in the United States since these control measures were implemented in the mid-1970s, propagating epizootics still occur.[132] Veterinarians should advise horse owners to do the following:

1. Require a negative EIAV test as part of every prepurchase examination.
2. Require all new arrivals on a farm to have documentation of a recent negative EIAV test, and test all horses on the farm annually.
3. Practice excellent fly control.
4. Encourage all events involving the congregation of horses to require documentation of a recent negative EIAV test.
5. Thoroughly disinfect any surgical items contacting equine blood before use on another horse.
6. Do not share or reuse needles and syringes between horses.

Equine piroplasmosis results from infection with one or both of two species of hemoprotozoan parasite: *Babesia caballi* and *B. equi*. These intraerythrocytic parasites are found in subtropical locales and transmitted predominantly by tick vectors. Although classified in the genus *Babesia*, *B. equi* may be related more closely to the theilerial organisms.[133] *Babesia equi* undergoes some developmental stages in lymphocytes and apparently lacks transovarial tick transmission typical of most *Babesia* organisms. Iatrogenic transmission has occurred through administration of contaminated blood products and use of unsterilized or shared needles or surgical instruments.

Piroplasmosis is only enzootic in those areas where the tick vector can survive the winter such as South and Central America, the Caribbean, and areas within Africa, Europe, and the Middle East. *Babesia caballi* infection has previously been diagnosed in horses in Florida and is spread by the tropical horse tick *Dermacentor nitens*. In the United States, *D. nitens* has been found in southeastern Florida and occasionally in Texas. Only rarely has *B. equi* infection been confirmed in horses in the United States, and none of the ticks commonly found in this country are known to transmit this organism. The United States is currently considered *Babesia* free. Horses raised in *Babesia*-endemic areas frequently are infected with the organisms without ever showing recognizable clinical signs. Clinically recovered horses remain infected, asymptomatic carriers of the organism as well, and stress may precipitate clinical relapse. Horses with *B. caballi* infection may clear the organism spontaneously after 12 to 42 months, whereas horses infected by *B. equi* do not appear to clear the organism spontaneously.[134] Infected animals develop a strong active immunity that depends on the continuing presence of the organism (premunity). They may be reinfected readily, soon after the organism is eliminated from the body. An infected dam will passively transfer antibodies to offspring but antibody levels are undetectable by 63 to 77 days of age.[135] No evidence of cross-protection exists between the two species of *Babesia*.[136]

Previously unexposed adult horses develop clinical signs of disease within 1 to 4 weeks of exposure. The horse may have fever, depression, dyspnea, pale or icteric mucous membranes, ecchymoses of the nictitating membrane, constipation, colic, and dependent edema. As anemia worsens, affected horses may develop diarrhea. Massive intravascular destruction of parasitized erythrocytes occasionally occurs, resulting in hemoglobinuria. Cardiac arrhythmias may develop as a result of myocardial damage.[137] Clinical disease with *B. caballi* lasts a few days to a few weeks, and mortality is usually low. Horses infected with *B. equi* generally have a more severe clinical course and may die within 24 to 48 hours of initial signs.

Diagnosis can be made by identification of the *Babesia* organism in blood smears stained with a Giemsa-type stain. The absence of *Babesia* organisms in the peripheral blood does not exclude the diagnosis of piroplasmosis because parasitemia may be brief and occur before the onset of recognizable clinical signs. Several diagnostic tests are also available. A complement fixation (CF) test was previously recommended as a means of identifying both the actively infected and the carriers. The indirect fluorescent antibody (IFA) test is a more sensitive test than the CF test, especially for latent infections.[138] However, the most sensitive test, and therefore the most appropriate test for screening asymptomatic carriers, is the competitive inhibition enzyme-linked immunosorbent assay (CI-ELISA).[139] Because native horses in the United States are rarely infected with this organism, the United States has instituted strict regulations for import of horses from endemic areas. Before import, all horses must undergo mandatory testing by the Animal and Plant Health Inspection Servise using the CI-ELISA. This test is considered the standard for identification of inapparent carriers and is now commercially available to horse owners and veterinarians.[140] The World Organization for Animal Health lists the ELISA and IFA tests as prescribed tests for equine piroplasmosis with the CF test as an alternative test.

Treatment of piroplasmosis varies depending on the location of the horse and the desired goal of treatment. In animals that reside in *Babesia*-endemic areas, suppressing clinical signs without eliminating the organism from the body is desirable, because premunition depends on the continued presence of the parasite at low levels. Clinical signs exhibited by carriers usually subside after one intramuscular injection of imidocarb dipropionate (Burroughs Wellcome Co., Research Triangle Park, N.C.) at 2.2 mg/kg. Owners who wish to move their horses to or enter *Babesia*-free areas should isolate them from all tick vectors and should have them treated to eliminate the organism. Administration of imidocarb dipropionate organism for treatment of *B. caballi* has shown variable results. Elimination of the organism was achieved at 2 mg/kg intramuscularly once daily for 2 days.[141] However, recent research has shown that long-term elimination was not achieved with doses as high as 4.7 mg/kg every 72 hours for five doses.[142] *B. equi* is a more difficult organism to eliminate from the horse, and four doses of imidocarb at 4 mg/kg intramuscularly at 72-hour intervals had variable efficacy in eliminating the carrier state.[143-145] In one study by Frerichs, Allen, and Holbrook,[144] the foregoing treatment regimen successfully cleared 13 of 14 horses of the infection, whereas in a more recent study by Kuttler, Zaugg, and Gipson,[143] this treatment regimen cleared none of nine geldings of infection. This wide difference in efficacy may be because of strain differences in drug susceptibility. Potential adverse effects of imidocarb administration include salivation, restlessness, colic, and gastrointestinal tract hypermotility. Donkeys appear to be sensitive to the toxic effects of imidocarb, and eight donkeys treated with the drug died.[144] Although the antitheilerial drug buparvaquone at 4 to 6 mg/kg intravenously or intramuscularly is therapeutically effective in horses acutely infected with *B. equi,* it is not consistent in clearing infection in carrier horses.[146]

Severe Hepatic Disease Acute intravascular hemolysis and anemia may develop in the terminal stages of acute or chronic hepatic failure in horses and is characterized by hemoglobinemia, hemoglobinuria, and icterus.[147] Onset and progression are rapid, and the condition is usually fatal; however, signs of hemolysis may subside if the liver disease is treated sucessfully.[148] Affected erythrocytes have increased osmotic fragility. Hemolysis may result from decreased structural integrity of the erythrocyte membrane caused by alterations in exchangeable RBC membrane lipoproteins and the effect of bile acids on erythrocyte metabolism during liver failure.[13]

Microangiopathic Hemolysis This disorder occurs after thrombosis or fibrinoid change within the lumen of small blood vessels,[149] is typical of chronic disseminated intravascular coagulation (DIC), and has been reported in horses.[73] The resulting hemolysis is usually mild.

Nonregenerative Anemia A variety of intrinsic or extrinsic factors may suppress normal bone marrow erythropoiesis, resulting in anemia caused by a failure to replace senescent RBCs adequately as they are removed from circulation (Box 14-4). The most common disorders associated with nonregenerative anemia in the horse are iron deficiency; chronic inflammatory, endocrine, or neoplastic diseases; and generalized bone marrow failure. Dietary factors often are incriminated in these abnormalities but only rarely are involved. Severe protein deprivation may result in decreased erythropoiesis as the body becomes deficient in synthesizing hemoglobin and

BOX 14-4

DIFFERENTIAL DIAGNOSES FOR NONREGENERATIVE ANEMIA IN THE HORSE

Iron Deficiency

Chronic hemorrhage
Nutritional deficiency (rare)

Chronic Disease

Chronic infection/inflammation
- Pleuritis/pneumonia
- Peritonitis/enteritis
- Bacterial endocarditis
- Internal abscess
- Chronic viral disease (e.g., equine infectious anemia [EIA])

Neoplasia
Endocrine disorders

Bone Marrow Failure

Myelophthisis
Myeloproliferative disease
Bone marrow toxins
- Phenylbutazone
- Chloramphenicol

Radiation
Idiopathic pancytopenia

Miscellaneous Conditions

Administration of human recombinant erythropoietin
Chronic hepatic disease
Chronic renal disease
Recent hemorrhage or hemolysis

other cellular proteins. Folic acid and cobalamin (vitamin B_{12}) deficiencies cause macrocytic hypochromic anemia in human beings, but they are associated rarely with anemia in domestic animals, including the horse. Horses do not have an absolute dietary requirement for vitamin B_{12}, which is produced by bacterial action in the gut and absorbed from the lower gastrointestinal tract.[150] Anemia associated with hypothyroidism is thought to be functional, following a lowered metabolic rate. Normocytic normochromic anemia responsive only to thyroid replacement therapy has been reported in one horse.[151]

Iron Deficiency Iron deficiency in the horse is associated only rarely with low dietary iron intake or absorption. More commonly, iron deficiency results from chronic external blood loss. In initial stages of iron deficiency, the only detectable abnormalities reflect decreased iron storage pools: a low serum ferritin concentration and decreased stainable iron in the bone marrow. Progression of the condition affects erythropoiesis adversely. These animals have a decrease in the percentage saturation of plasma transferrin, an increased TIBC, and increased numbers of hypochromic erythrocytes (decreased MCHC). Fulminant iron deficiency anemia leads to abnormal development of erythrocytes in the bone marrow late in the maturation process. Cells continue to divide in the late rubricyte stage, without sufficient iron to continue heme synthesis. The result is the release of small cells with decreased hemoglobin concentration into the peripheral circulation (decreased MCHC and MCV).

Treatment of iron deficiency anemia should concentrate initially on the identification and elimination of the source of chronic iron loss. In the horse, occult blood loss occurs most frequently from the gastrointestinal tract and may be verified with a fecal occult blood test. Chronic gastrointestinal ulceration after phenylbutazone administration is a well-recognized phenomenon and is more frequent and severe in ponies than in horses. Gastrointestinal parasites, especially *Strongylus vulgaris* and small strongyles, occasionally may result in chronic blood loss and subsequent iron deficiency. Many iron-containing hematinics are available commercially, and oral supplementation with a product containing ferrous sulfate is probably best. Parenteral iron dextran solutions have been associated with fatal anaphylactoid reactions in horses. If parenteral administration is essential, then 1 g of iron cacodylate administered intravenously for an adult horse generally is considered safe.

Neonatal foals in the first few days of life have high serum iron concentrations and a high percentage saturation of transferrin.[11,27] As a result they are quite susceptible to iron toxicity if they receive oral or intravenous supplements. Administration of oral digestive inoculants containing ferrous fumarate to neonatal foals was associated with a fatal toxic hepatopathy characterized by icterus, hepatic atrophy, bile duct hyperplasia, lobular necrosis, and intrahepatic cholestasis.[2,28] Researchers have concluded that little beneficial effect occurs on hematologic variables when giving healthy foals oral iron supplementation.[152]

In contrast, older foals may be more susceptible than adults to the development of iron deficiency anemia because of their naturally lower levels of iron during growth (after the first week of life). In a survey of iron status in hospitalized horses, only six animals with iron deficiency were identified on the basis of low serum ferritin and serum iron concentrations. All six were foals younger than 5 weeks of age.[153] Foals, although technically iron deficient, rarely develop anemia as a result. A severe anemia attributed to a significant iron deficiency was identified in a foal that concurrently suffered from septicemia.[154] The source of the deficiency was not identified and considered mulitfactorial, including lack of access to dirt and pasture and low dietary iron intake.

Chronic Disease Chronic inflammatory conditions and neoplasms frequently are associated with a mild to moderate normocytic, normochromic, nonregenerative anemia. This anemia has been attributed to several abnormalities. A block of iron released from reticuloendothelial storage (ferritin and hemosiderin) results in an unavailability of iron for heme synthesis. Horses with anemia of chronic disease typically have a decreased serum iron concentration, normal to decreased TIBC, decreased transferrin saturation with iron, normal to increased serum ferritin concentration, and normal to increased bone marrow storage iron. In addition to altered iron mobilization, a defective response of the bone marrow to circulating erythropoietin and a decrease in RBC life span during many chronic diseases are apparent. The anemia of chronic disease rarely is associated with clinical signs of decreased tissue oxygenation. Therapy is directed at the primary disease process. Oral iron supplementation is not indicated because systemic iron stores are usually normal to increased.

Bone Marrow Suppression Anemia caused by selective bone marrow suppression of erythropoiesis is unusual in the horse. Selective erythroid hypoplasia has been reported as a sequela to administration of recombinant human erythropoietin to horses.[155,156] Anemia is thought to result from production of antibodies that cross-react with erythropoietin, inhibiting erythropoiesis. Treatment is with blood transfusions and corticosteroids. Prognosis for recovery is fair to guarded.

Pancytopenia (decreased circulating erythrocytes, leukocytes, and platelets) has been described in horses with aplastic bone marrow disorders [157-159] and with myelophthisic diseases. Myelophthisis is a reduction in the cellular elements of the bone marrow, frequently a result of metastatic neoplasia or myelofibrosis, a proliferation of fibrous tissue in the marrow. Myelodysplasia implies accumulation of abnormal cells in the bone marrow. These cells are not usually dysplastic in the truest sense of the word, but rather they result from myeloproliferative neoplasia. Hematopoietic neoplasia is rare in the horse and is discussed in more detail later in this chapter. These conditions usually result in concurrent anemia, leukopenia, and thrombocytopenia. Diagnosis is by identification of abnormal cells in bone marrow aspirates.

Bone marrow from horses with aplastic anemia is generally devoid of hematopoietic precursor cells because of a congenital or acquired failure of stem cell function. Acquired aplasia may be associated with bacterial and viral infections, chronic renal or hepatic disease, neoplasia, irradiation, or drug therapy. In most cases a predisposing factor is not identified.[157-162] Because of the shorter life spans of the cells, leukopenia and thrombocytopenia usually precede anemia.[12] Diagnosis depends on bone marrow biopsy. If one cannot obtain adequate marrow by serial aspirates, then one must obtain a core biopsy sample. Hypoplastic marrow is yellow because of fatty infiltration with a mixture of cell types, but the number of erythroid, myeloid, and megakaryocytoid cells is decreased.[12] Aplastic anemia is thought to be an autoimmune disorder in some cases, and some horses have apparently benefited from therapy with corticosteroids and anabolic steroids.[157] These drugs stimulate erythropoietin production and increase sensitivity of the stem cell receptors to erythropoietin.

Temporary or permanent bone marrow aplasia has been associated with the administration of a variety of drugs in other species. Transient hypoplastic anemia after phenylbutazone administration has been reported in one horse.[82] Aplastic anemia has been induced experimentally by feeding of trichloroethylene-extracted soybean oil meal to horses or by irradiation.[163] Chloramphenicol produces transient and irreversible forms of bone marrow dysfunction in human beings, and similar reactions are possible in other species. One always should handle chloramphenicol with caution because human toxic reactions appear to be idiosyncratic and may be associated with absorption of low amounts of the drug. Any ongoing drug therapy should be discontinued in horses with aplastic anemia, and supportive therapy should be administered. Some cases of drug-induced bone marrow failure are temporary, and hematopoietic function returns to normal with time if secondary complications are not severe. One may administer compatible whole blood transfusions to horses with severe anemia or thrombocytopenia, and systemic antibiotics and strict isolation from other animals may be considered for horses with severe leukopenia.

Bone marrow erythropoiesis frequently is suppressed in horses with chronic renal disease. Suppression generally is attributed to a decrease in erythropoietin production by the kidneys. Recombinant erythropoietin has been used successfully in cats and human beings with severe anemia associated with renal disease.

LEUKON

The leukon consists of circulating leukocytes, their precursor cells, and the tissues that produce them. This includes the granulocytes (neutrophils, eosinophils, and basophils), monocytes and macrophages, and lymphocytes. The leukon provides the primary effector cells for immune surveillance and clearance. This discussion provides a brief description of the production of these cells and their quantitative abnormalities in peripheral blood. Excellent pictures of the various developmental stages of equine leukocytes in the bone marrow and peripheral blood are available in other texts, and the reader is referred to these for identification of cell types.[12,13]

NEUTROPHILS

PHYSIOLOGY

Granulocytes and mononuclear phagocytes originate from a common committed progenitor cell in the bone marrow. Under the influence of cytokines—including granulocyte-macrophage colony-stimulating factor, monocyte colony-stimulating factor, granulocyte colony-stimulating factor (G-CSF), and various interleukins—this stem cell proceeds along a path to granulocyte or monocyte production. Cytokine signals for constitutive leukocyte production differ from those during periods of increased demand for specific cell types. The progenitor cell undergoes successive mitotic divisions from myeloblast (the first recognizable precursor of neutrophils) to promyelocyte and myelocyte. Mitosis does not occur as the cell matures from metamyelocyte to band cell to mature neutrophil. Mature neutrophils are stored in the bone marrow until needed. The peripheral neutrophil pool is equally divided between circulating cells and cells adhered to the endothelium of small vessels (the marginated pool).[164] Circulating neutrophils have a half-life of 10 $^1/_2$ hours in the horse[165] and eventually migrate into peripheral tissues, where they live several more days.

Neutrophils alter their distribution between storage, circulating, and marginating pools in response to various endogenous and exogenous stimuli. The marginating neutrophils are mobilized into the circulating pool in response to exercise, epinephrine, or stress. Glucocorticoids increase the rate of neutrophil egress from the bone marrow storage pool and decrease egress from the circulation.[166,167]

Neutrophils are attracted to sites of infection and inflammation by soluble chemotactic factors released during proinflammatory reactions. Neutrophils ingest and kill invading microorganisms and release additional factors that further propagate inflammation at the site of tissue injury.

The morphology of neutrophils on a stained smear of blood or body fluids (e.g., peritoneal or pleural fluid) aids in interpretation of the significance and severity of many disorders. Toxic changes in circulating neutrophils occur in response to inflammation and include cytoplasmic basophilia, cytoplasmic granulation and vacuolation, and appearance of Döhle's bodies (slate gray inclusions caused by retention and aggregation of rough endoplasmic reticulum).[13] Degenerative changes result from altered cell membrane permeability and include hydropic degeneration of the nucleus and a spreading out of the nuclear chromatin so that it more completely fills up the cytoplasm of the cell. Aged neutrophils may exhibit hypersegmented, pyknotic nuclei with round, tightly clumped chromatin. Aged neutrophils most commonly are visible in tissue fluids. Idiopathic hypersegmentation of blood neutrophils of one Quarter Horse, unrelated to any clinical disease, has been described.[168]

DISORDERS OF NEUTROPHILS

Neutropenia Neutropenia is a decrease in the number of circulating neutrophils and may be acute (occurring transiently over 24 to 48 hours) or chronic (lasting several days to months). Acute neutropenia most commonly results from a shift of neutrophils from circulating to marginating pools. Endotoxin is a potent stimulus for margination of circulating neutrophils with sequestration in pulmonary capillaries.[164] Experimentally, administration of endotoxin to horses results in neutropenia within 90 minutes and return to baseline numbers within 6 to 18 hours.[169] Endotoxemia is probably the common denominator in the neutropenia associated with various equine gastrointestinal disturbances including strangulating obstruction, peritonitis, enteritis, and salmonellosis. Neutropenia is a common finding in acute septicemia in the adult and is considered an aid for diagnosis of sepsis in the neonate.[170] A variety of bacterial, rickettsial, and viral disorders also may be associated with neutropenia in the horse.

Chronic neutropenia may result from increased peripheral use of neutrophils or decreased bone marrow production. Neutropenia may accompany severe infectious or inflammatory diseases such as pleuritis, pneumonia, peritonitis, internal abscessation, enteritis, burns, vasculitis, or immune-mediated diseases. Neutropenia caused by increased use often is accompanied by appearance of immature cells in circulation. As tissue demand increases, the bone marrow releases progressively more immature band cells into circulation.[12] This regenerative left shift is an appropriate response to high tissue demand for neutrophils. In animals with a degenerative left shift, the number of immature band cells or metamyelocytes in circulation exceeds the number of mature neutrophils because tissue use exceeds the capacity of the bone marrow to increase production.[13] A degenerative left shift is considered a poor prognostic indicator.

Neutropenia caused by bone marrow suppression may occur in horses with pancytopenia from a variety of causes (discussed previously). Myeloproliferative disorders including granulocytic leukemia also may result in chronic neutropenia.[171] Alloimmune neonatal neutropenia (ANN), an immune-mediated neutropenia in newborn foals, has been described in several breeds.[172-174] This disease is confirmed by flow cytometric identification of increased neutrophil surface-bound antibody. Affected foals require treatment with prophylactic antibiotics during the recovery period. They may also benefit from administration of G-CSF as described below. The neutrophil count generally returns to normal within 1 month. A syndrome of neutropenia and thrombocytopenia is described in related Standardbreds. A heritable cyclic neutropenia was suspected. Most affected horses died from complications of infectious diseases, thrombocytopenia, or both.[175]

Administration of canine or bovine recombinant G-CSF to normal newborn foals results in a profound increase in blood neutrophil count after a single subcutaneous injection of 6 μg/kg.[174,176,177] The factor may also benefit foals recovering from septicemia. Recombinant G-CSF is reported to improve recovery of adult horses when administered after experimental bowel resection.[178]

Neutrophilia Many of the same disorders associated with neutropenia may be associated alternatively with neutrophilia. Endogenous or exogenous glucocorticoids or epinephrine, excitement, exercise, or stress may result in neutrophilia.[13,179] Any infections or inflammatory process in any part of the body may result in neutrophilia. Many neoplastic conditions also are accompanied by peripheral neutrophilia. A rebound neutrophilia is common in later stages of endotoxemia.

The balance between bone marrow production and tissue use determines the magnitude of a neutrophilic response. A regenerative left shift is not uncommon in animals with neutrophilia because of excessive tissue demand. A severe neutrophilia with significant left shift including metamyelocytes and myelocytes indicates serious inflammatory disease and is termed a *leukemoid response* because of its similarity to granulocytic leukemia.[12]

Eosinophils

Eosinophils arise from the same bone marrow precursor as neutrophils and mononuclear phagocytes. They may be distinguished first from neutrophils at the early myelocyte stage and eventually develop characteristic bright red–staining cytoplasmic granules. IL-5 is critical in the differentiation and maturation of eosinophils. The prominent cytoplasmic granules of eosinophils contain a variety of substances, including major basic protein, peroxidase, and various hydrolytic enzymes. Eosinophils are important in parasite immunity and are involved in some hypersensitivity reactions. Eosinopenia may result from acute infections, corticosteroid or epinephrine administration or release, or stress. Peripheral eosinophilia most commonly results from parasitic infections, including habronemiasis, strongylosis, and pediculosis. Occasionally, allergic reactions also may result in peripheral eosinophilia. Eosinophilic myeloproliferative disease has been described in the horse.[180] A marked eosinophilia also has been seen in horses with lymphosarcoma and transitional cell carcinoma.[181]

Basophils

Basophils also originate from the common granulocyte-macrophage precursor cell and mature into cells with basophilic cytoplasmic granules. They are the least common of the circulating granulocytes, and basopenia is not clinically significant. Basophils live in the blood approximately 6 hours and then migrate into tissues, where they exist another 10 to 12 days.[13] Basophils are involved in mediating some hypersensitivity reactions. Increased numbers of circulating basophils may occur with allergic, inflammatory, or neoplastic diseases or in association with lipemia.

Mononuclear Phagocytes

Monoblasts are the first recognizable bone marrow precursors of peripheral blood monocytes, originating from a pluripotent marrow precursor. After progressing through the promonocyte stage, monocytes are released into the peripheral blood where they circulate for a few days before migrating into tissues to mature into tissue macrophages. The role of mononuclear phagocytes in orchestrating immune and inflammatory reactions has long been underplayed. These cells are critical in regulating inflammation through release of proinflammatory cytokines such as tumor necrosis factor (TNF), IL-1, and platelet-activating factor. Mononuclear phagocytes phagocytose microbial organisms, particulate debris, and possibly neoplastic cells. They process these foreign antigens and present them to T lymphocytes in a form that initiates specific immune responses. They produce cytokines, including granulocyte-macrophage colony-stimulating factor, that are critical for regulation of hematopoiesis. They are responsible for removal of senescent cells and activated coagulation factors from circulation. Quantitative abnormalities of monocytes rarely are encountered in equine medicine, but monocytosis may be observed in some cases of chronic inflammation.

Lymphocytes

Lymphocytes are the primary mediators of humoral and cell-mediated immune responses. They originate from an uncommitted bone marrow progenitor cell that is capable of differentiating into a committed lymphopoietic precursor or a granulocyte-macrophage precursor cell. Committed lymphopoietic progenitor cells differentiate into T lymphocytes that mature during migration through the thymus or B cells that appear to differentiate in the marrow and then migrate to lymph nodes. Circulating lymphocytes are predominantly T cells and represent only a small fraction of the total lymphocyte pool. Most lymphocytes reside in the spleen, lymph nodes, and other lymphoid tissue of the body.

The spleen contains the greatest number of lymphocytes in the adult horse. The spleen plays a major role in immune defense. The large number of phagocytic cells in the spleen facilitates filtering of senescent blood cells, particulate debris, and microorganisms from the blood. Hemoglobin is degraded, and iron is stored in splenic phagocytes pending reuse for erythropoiesis. The spleen is also important as a reservoir of RBCs and platelets, as discussed previously.

Lymphopenia is associated with glucocorticoid administration, stress, many viral infections, and combined immunodeficiency of Arabian foals. Lymphocytosis is associated with epinephrine administration, excitement, exercise, lymphocytic leukemia, and chronic immune stimulation. As horses age, the number of lymphocytes in their peripheral blood gradually decreases.[182,183]

Hematopoietic Neoplasia

MYELOID NEOPLASIA

Neoplasia that results in unregulated proliferation of leukocytes can be categorized as myeloid neoplasia and lymphoid neoplasia. Lymphoid forms, including lymphosarcoma, are more common. Myeloid neoplasia is characterized by uncontrolled proliferation of one or more marrow-derived blood cell lines. When neoplastic cells are observed in peripheral circulation, the disease process is termed *leukemia*. Forms of myeloid neoplasia that have been described in the horse include acute and chronic granulocytic leukemia,[171,184,185] myeloblastic leukemia,[186] myelomonocytic leukemia,[187-190] monocytic leukemia,[191] eosinophilic myeloproliferative disorder,[180] and malignant histiocytosis.[192] Regardless of the involved cell line, the eventual outcome is significant myelophthisis with loss of normal marrow elements.

No age predilection is apparent for equine myeloid neoplasia.[171,180] Common clinical signs include depression, weight loss, edema, anemia, and mucosal petechial hemorrhages. Fever,[180,187,189,190] peripheral lymphadenopathy,[187,190] nonhealing wounds,[185] hemorrhagic diathesis,[180] and oral ulcers [187,188] were identified in some of the horses.

Most affected horses are anemic and thrombocytopenic; total white blood cell counts may be decreased, normal, or increased. Common clinical signs and hematologic parameters can be explained by severe destruction of normal bone marrow resulting in inadequate production of erythrocytes, platelets, and normal leukocytes. This predisposes affected horses to hemorrhagic diathesis, infection, and inadequate oxygenation of tissues.

Definitive diagnosis can often be made by observation of abnormal cells on a peripheral blood smear. Abnormal leukocytes typically predominate in bone marrow aspirates and may be identified in peripheral lymph node aspirates. Acute leukemia is defined as more than 20% blast cells in the peripheral circulation, whereas chronic leukemias lack a significant number of blast forms in the blood.[185] Exact identification of cell type can be difficult because of abnormal cellular architecture in neoplastic cells. As a result, additional staining and cytochemical analysis is often needed for a specific diagnosis.

The cause of myeloid neoplasia remains uncertain. Treatment with cytotoxic[190] drugs and with steroids[186,184] has been attempted in affected horses with no success. Appropriate long-term combination chemotherapy protocols have not been attempted. Compared with lymphoid neoplasia, presentation of clinical signs as a result of myeloid neoplasia is often acute and patients rarely survive for more than a few weeks after diagnosis. Horses that suffer from forms that are better differentiated tend to have a longer duration of clinical signs before presentation, but unfortunately the prognosis remains the same.[193] Postmortem examinations have revealed the presence of abnormal leukocytes within various organs, most commonly the liver and spleen.

LYMPHOID NEOPLASIA

The most common type of neoplasia to involve the equine hemolymphatic system is lymphosarcoma.[194] Four anatomic forms have been described (generalized, intestinal, mediastinal, and cutaneous) based on the major site of tumor involvement[194,195]; however, the forms overlap substantially, both clinically and pathologically. Rarely, horses can develop lymphocytic leukemia either as a primary neoplastic condition or, much more commonly, as a sequela to lymphosarcoma that has metastasized to the marrow.[193]

The typical age of onset of lymphoid neoplasia in horses is between 5 and 10 years,[196] although lymphosarcoma has been documented in horses ranging in age from birth through 25 years.[197-199] No breed or gender predilection exists. The incidence of disease is unknown; however, reported prevalence of affected horses at autopsy is between 2% and 5%, and less than 3% of all tumors are classified as *lymphoma*.[200] Lymphocytic or lymphoblastic leukemia is quite rare in horses, so conclusions regarding age, breed, and gender predilections are difficult to interpret.[193,201-203]

Cause and Pathogenesis A viral cause of equine lymphosarcoma has not been documented[204,205]; however, one report describes viruslike particles in the lymph node of a foal with lymphosarcoma that died shortly after birth.[199] A congenital or genetic predisposition is possible, because tumors were observed in an aborted fetus and in two horses less than 1 year of age.[206] Clinical signs and laboratory changes of lymphosarcoma generally are caused by loss of normal organ and tissue function after infiltration by lymphocytes or physical obstruction by tumor masses or the excessive generation of tumor cell cytokines.[206] Data on immunophenotyping of equine lymphosarcoma are conflicting. Histologic examination of tumor cells typically reveals a heterogeneous cell population. Previous research indicates that the majority of equine lymphoma is B-cell lymphoma, with many of these described as T-cell rich B-cell lymphomas. A more recent report suggested the opposite: T-cell lymphoma is more prevalent that B-cell lymphoma.[206] Anatomically, T-cell lymphoma is commonly associated with mediastinal tumors and B-cell tumors tend to be more multicentric. Too few cases of lymphocytic leukemia have been described to draw accurate conclusions regarding cytologic classification, but T-cell lymphoma tends to predominate.

Decreased serum concentrations of IgM and other indications of immunosuppression have been observed in horses with lymphosarcoma.[207-210] A decreased serum IgM concentration is defined as ≤23 mg/dl. A recent study found that IgM concentrations should not be used as a screening test for equine lymphoma because of extremely poor sensitivity.[211] Other neoplastic lymphocytes may arise from autoreactive B-cell clones that produce antibodies responsible for gammopathies and immune-mediated cytopenias. Neoplastic proliferation of large granular lymphocytes with natural killer cell activity was described in one horse.[212]

Clinical Signs and Laboratory Findings Lymphosarcoma most commonly presents as a chronic, progressive disease with a sudden onset of more significant clinical signs. The most common clinical signs of lymphosarcoma are chronic weight loss, ventral subcutaneous edema, and regional lymphadenopathy.[213,214] Peripheral lymphadenopathy is not observed frequently. Other clinical manifestations are highly variable depending on the organs involved and the duration of the disease process. Sudden death was attributed to thoracic lymphoma in one racing Standardbred.[215]

Lymphosarcoma involving the thoracic cavity may cause tachypnea, dyspnea, cough, and pleural effusion.[197,216,217] Lymphoma should also be considered in horses with recurrent pleural effusion.[218] Ultrasound and thoracic radiography can be useful for the diagnosis if tumors are located in an area that is amenable to imaging with these modalities. If pleural effusion is present, then one frequently identifies neoplastic lymphocytes by routine cytologic evaluation of fluid obtained by thoracocentesis.[183]

If cytologic findings are nondiagnostic but indicative of thoracic lymphoma, then immunophenotyping of the fluid may be performed to identify markers of lymphosarcoma.[218]

Alimentary lymphoma, the most common intestinal neoplasia of horses,[195] causes clinical signs consistent with an infiltrative, inflammatory disorder of the gastrointestinal tract including weight loss, recurrent colic, and diarrhea.[219-221] Weight loss can often be attributed to malabsorptive disease, as well as to the negative energy balance caused by chronic, systemic inflammation.

The regional or generalized occurrence of multiple subcutaneous nodules with histopathologic characteristics of lymphosarcoma, unassociated with other lesions of lymphosarcoma, has been reported in horses.[194,222] Nodules may appear suddenly, grow slowly, remain static or regress, and recur at a later time. Hormonal factors including estrous cycle, pregnancy, lactation, and foaling may influence this cutaneous form of lymphosarcoma. In one horse, cutaneous lymphosarcoma cells were positive for progesterone receptors, and lesions regressed completely after surgical removal of an ovarian tumor.[223]

Tumor masses in localized areas may result in clinical signs referable to dysfunction of involved and adjacent tissues and organs.[204,213,216,224-229] Pharyngeal and laryngeal masses may result in dysphagia and unresponsive nasal discharge. Ocular lymphosarcoma may manifest as uveitis or as infiltrates in palpebral conjunctiva, eyelids, third eyelid, at the corneoscleral junction, or in the retrobulbar area.[230] Lymphosarcoma of the central nervous system may result in ataxia and cranial nerve deficits.[204,229,231] Other manifestations of lymphoma include parotid gland, uterine, bladder, epididymal, and periarticular tumors.[232-236] Angiotrophic T-cell lymphoma, which is characterized by proliferation of neoplastic lymphocytes within the lumen of small vessels, was identified in a Thoroughbred mare with a history of anemia but no abnormalities in the circulating leukocyte examination.[237]

The laboratory findings in horses with lymphosarcoma are highly variable. Hematologic indications of chronic inflammatory disease are common, including neutrophilic leukocytosis, nonresponsive anemia, hyperfibrinogenemia, thrombocytopenia, and hypergammaglobulinemia.[206,214,216] Anemia may result from immune-mediated destruction, decreased production because of some degree of myelophthisis, or a combination of both.[206] Horses with lymphocytic leukemia have lymphocytosis and circulating, neoplastic lymphocytes.[221,238-241]

The total plasma protein concentration may be low, normal, or elevated, but the albumin-to-globulin ratio often is reduced, particularly with gastrointestinal involvement.[221,242] The ventral edema observed does not always result from hypoalbuminemia and is more likely caused by lymphatic stasis or obstruction.[206] Protein electrophoresis produces variable results, with the possibility of either polyclonal or monoclonal gammopathy. Polyclonal gammopathies are nonspecific and may be due in part to the production of acute phase proteins, Ig, tumor cytokines, or secondary infection. A mild increase in liver-derived serum enzymes may occur with hepatic involvement. Hyperbilirubinemia usually is caused by anorexia or hemolysis.

A variety of paraneoplastic syndromes have been identified in association with equine lymphosarcoma. Hypercalcemia occasionally is reported.[226,243-245] Pseudohyperparathyroidism, resulting in hypercalcemic nephropathy and polyuria or polydipsia, has been reported in a horse with splenic lymphosarcoma.[246] In some patients, Coombs'-positive IMHA, immune-mediated thrombocytopenia (IMTP), or both may occur.[14,84,247] Hypereosinophilia has been reported in one pony with intestinal lymphosarcoma.[181] Concurrent intestinal lymphosarcoma and eosinophilic epitheliotrophic disease have been reported in a Paso Fino mare.[248] These two cases suggest the possibility that clonal proliferation of lymphocytes occasionally may result in hypersecretion of IL-5 with subsequent eosinophil activation. A case of thoracic lymphoma resulted in paraneoplastic polycythemia because of erythropoietin gene expression from the tumor cells.[38] Paraneoplastic pruritus and alopecia also has been described in a horse with lymphosarcoma.[243]

Diagnosis The diagnosis of lymphosarcoma is confirmed by demonstration of neoplastic lymphocytes in affected tissue. Histologic examination of a biopsy from a tumor mass or affected lymph node is the most reliable method, and excisional biopsies are much preferred over needle biopsies or aspirates. Without lymph nodes or other masses accessible for biopsy, antemortem diagnosis is often difficult.[14,197,228,249] Diagnosis is only rarely possible on a peripheral blood smear[238,240] and generally requires careful cytologic evaluation of bone marrow, pleural effusion, or peritoneal fluid.[216,250,251] Between 38% and 50% of horses with the alimentary form of lymphoma have evidence of neoplastic cells on abdominocentesis.[252,253] The clinician rarely is able to locate neoplastic lymphocytes by transcutaneous liver biopsy[254]; however, laparoscopy may be used to visualize a mass for biopsy more clearly.[197] Although the lymphocyte count more commonly is normal or reduced in horses with lymphoma, the presence of atypical or obviously neoplastic lymphocytes on a peripheral blood smear occurs in 30% to 50% of cases.*

One may palpate splenic enlargement, internal lymphadenopathy, or abdominal masses on rectal examination. The character of these masses can then be defined further through ultrasonography.[256] Abdominocentesis may reveal inflammatory changes in the fluid (increased nucleated cell count and protein concentration), but identifying neoplastic cells in abdominal fluid of horses with alimentary or abdominal lymphosarcoma is not common.

Radiography and ultrasonography may be useful in locating and perhaps enabling biopsies of masses in the thorax or abdomen. Often, diagnosis of lymphosarcoma is possible only by exploratory laparotomy or postmortem examination.[14,219,228,249]

The morphologic condition of neoplastic lymphocytes in horses is highly variable.[198] On cytologic preparations they often appear as large lymphoid cells with a variable nucleus-to-cytoplasm ratio, multiple nucleoli, nuclear chromatic clumping, cytoplasmic basophilia, and vacuolation. Mitotic figures and binucleate cells may be visible. The cytologic diagnosis of lymphosarcoma is best left to those experienced in evaluation of equine fluid specimens, because normal reactive lymphocytes and mesothelial cells may be difficult to distinguish from well-differentiated neoplastic cells. Histologically, the

*References: 14, 207, 214, 238, 254, and 255.

neoplastic cellular morphology also varies, but destruction of normal tissue architecture by a population of lymphoid cells aids the diagnosis. More advanced diagnostic techniques may be used to specifically analyze the neoplastic cell line and its immunologic characteristics. These tests include cytochemical staining, immunophenotyping using both flow cytometry and immunohistochemistry, and immunologic function testing.[193]

Treatment Clinical experience in treating horses with lymphosarcoma is limited, because horses tend to be greatly debilitated by the time of diagnosis. Resection of localized tumors may be curative or at least significantly prolong survival.[257] Several solitary tumors located in areas such as the perineum and the nasal cavity have been treated successfully with high-dose radiation.[258] Remission of generalized disease can be transiently achieved through the use of cytotoxic drugs, immunomodulators, and immunosuppressants.

Chemotherapeutic regimens and dosages have been adapted from human and small animal oncology and are now being used with some success in the equine lymphoma patient. Controlled clinical research supporting the use of these drugs is lacking, but case reports and anecdotal evidence support their use where appropriate. The drugs are dosed on a square meter calculation of body surface area, and the protocols generally use a combination of cytotoxic and immunosuppressive drugs administered over several weeks to months depending on the severity. Most commonly used protocols include cytosine arabinoside, cyclophosphamide, vincristine, chlorambucil, doxorubicin, L-asparaginase, and prednisolone.[218,259] One report suggests a remission rate of as high as 50% for several months to a year in horses diagnosed with multicentric lymphoma using a protocol of prednisolone, vincristine, and cytosine arabinoside.[259] Immunosuppressive doses of dexamethasone have also been effective in reducing the size of some tumors and severity of clinical signs for up to 18 months.[247] The cutaneous form of lymphosarcoma is often responsive to corticosteroid and progestin therapy or a combination of low-dose cyclophosphamide and immunotherapy with an autologous tumor cell vaccine.[260] However, abrupt discontinuation or insufficient duration of therapy may result in recurrence of cutaneous lesions in a more aggressive and rapidly progressive form.[261] Treatment of lymphocytic leukemia with the aforementioned therapies has been less rewarding. These drugs are typically very expensive, and remission has not been established in the horse with any of various reported protocols.

The prognosis for equine generalized lymphosarcoma is grave for long-term survival. Most horses die or are euthanized within 6 months of diagnosis; however, with increased use of chemotherapy in the horse, these survival times may begin to increase. Horses with lymphocytic leukemia typically do not survive for more than several weeks after a diagnosis regardless of treatment strategy.[193]

Plasma Cell Myeloma

Plasma cell myeloma (multiple myeloma), characterized by proliferation of neoplastic plasma cells in the bone marrow, spleen, liver, and lymph nodes, is rare in horses. Clinical signs include weight loss, weakness, recurrent fever, ventral edema, hemorrhage, lameness, and posterior paralysis.[262-266] Recurrent infections secondary to the lack of normal immunoglobulins are not uncommon. Renal failure has also been described in affected horses. In human beings and dogs, skeletal pain and pathologic fractures result from neoplastic invasion of bone that causes osteolytic "punched-out" lesions[267,268]; osteolysis, however, does not occur consistently in horses.

Laboratory findings include anemia, hypercalcemia, azotemia, and hyperproteinemia with monoclonal gammopathy. A diagnosis of plasma cell myeloma should be considered in horses that demonstrate hypercalcemia with normal parathyroid hormone (PTH), elevated parathyroid hormone–related protein (PTH-rP), and hyperglobulinemia.[269] Light-chain proteinuria is variable. If any degree of lameness is noted, then radiographs of the affected limb are warranted. Criteria for diagnosis of plasma cell myeloma include plasmacytosis in the bone marrow or a soft tissue lesion, evidence of invasiveness, and the presence of monoclonal gammopathy or light-chain proteinuria.[267] The degree of plasmacytosis observed in the bone marrow is variable, because marrow involvement may be focal rather than diffuse. Examination of multiple samples from different areas of marrow are recommended whenever possible. If protein electrophoresis yields nonspecific results, then it is recommended to perform radioimmunodiffusion to quantify specific Ig classes.[269] AL amyloidosis, which is commonly associated with multiple myeloma in human beings, was diagnosed in one horse with concurrent multiple myeloma.[270]

Histologic and clinicopathologic findings in some horses with multiple myeloma can be quite similar to those of lymphosarcoma; therefore achieving a definitive diagnosis may be difficult.[271,272] Of the 15 horses with plasma cell myeloma described to date in the literature, none have been successfully treated. Horses typically survive for no more than 2 years after initial diagnosis. Management of horses with multiple myeloma generally includes careful monitoring and treatment of recurrent infections as needed.[273]

PLATELETS

Platelets are circulating anucleate fragments of bone marrow megakaryocytes that are essential for the formation of primary hemostatic plugs. Platelets adhere to injured vascular endothelium, release substances that initiate and propagate hemostatic events, and provide a phospholipid surface for activation of several coagulation factors.[274] Platelets also are important proinflammatory elements that interact with endothelium, mononuclear phagocytes, neutrophils, and fibroblasts in initiation and propagation of inflammation.

Physiology

Platelets ultimately originate from the same pluripotent stem cell as erythrocytes and leukocytes. This stem cell undergoes successive divisions, becoming progressively more differentiated. The colony-forming unit megakaryocytoid cell is committed fully to platelet production. Polyploid megakaryoblasts double their DNA content by a process of endomitosis, becoming megakaryocytes, the largest of the hematopoietic cells of the bone marrow, within 5 days. The highly compartmentalized cytoplasm of the megakaryocyte ultimately disintegrates to release up to 8000 platelets into the peripheral circulation. Various cytokines, including IL-3, thrombopoietin, and IL-6, are essential for this process of differentiation, maturation, and release.

The mature platelet is a complex anucleate cell fragment that accumulates many substances in a variety of secretory granules. These include dense bodies containing adenosine diphosphate (ADP), adenosine triphosphate (ATP), calcium, and serotonin; α-granules that accumulate various procoagulant factors, albumin, platelet-derived growth factor, thrombospondin, and platelet factor 4; and lysosomal granules with acid hydrolases.[274] Glycoprotein receptor molecules are embedded in the external lipid bilayer membrane and interact with extracellular proteins that mediate platelet adhesion and aggregation. The external lipid membrane of the platelet invaginates into the interior to form a complex canalicular system important for secretory function. A second internal membrane system, the dense tubular system, supplies enzymes for arachidonic acid metabolism and is involved in sequestration and release of calcium.[275]

When a circulating platelet contacts exposed vascular subendothelial collagen, platelet surface receptors recognize and attach to the damaged endothelium in a process known as *adhesion*. Normal adhesion requires von Willebrand's factor (vWF), a glycoprotein found in vascular endothelium and platelets and present in plasma as a multimolecular complex with coagulation factor VIII. (The role of vWF in platelet adhesion is separate from the role of factor VIII in secondary hemostasis, which is discussed later. The two activities are referred to as *VIII:vWF* for the platelet adhesion mediated by vWF and as *VIII:C* for the coagulative protein.) The glycoprotein P-selectin is another essential platelet surface receptor that is involved in primary hemostasis by enhancing interactions between platelets, endothelial cells, and leukocytes. Expression of P-selectin offers a possible platelet surface marker for platelet activation.[276]

Adhesion of platelets attracts additional platelets in a process known as *aggregation*. Primary aggregation is reversible and not associated with platelet degranulation. Irreversible secondary aggregation begins with release of ADP from platelet granules and production of thromboxane A_2 (TXA_2) via metabolism of arachidonic acid in the platelet membrane. Substances that promote aggregation usually do so by decreasing the concentration of intracellular cyclic adenosine monophosphate by inhibiting adenylate cyclase or by stimulating phosphodiesterase.[274] Equine platelets exhibit reversible aggregation when exposed to serotonin and arachidonic acid and exhibit irreversible aggregation when exposed to ADP.[277] Platelet-platelet bridging requires fibrinogen attachment to a newly exposed binding site on activated platelets.[275] Thrombospondin, a glycoprotein released from platelet α-granules, is also integral in the platelet aggregation response. Platelet aggregation is responsible for formation of the initial hemostatic plug (primary hemostasis) at any site of vascular injury.

Arachidonic acid release from the membranes of the platelet-dense tubular network and its subsequent metabolism are critical to platelet aggregation. Arachidonic acid is a polyunsaturated fatty acid normally attached to the second glycerol carbon atom of many membrane glycerophospholipids. Arachidonic acid may be released by the direct action of phospholipase A_2 or by the sequential actions of phospholipase C and diglyceride lipase. Free arachidonic acid is metabolized via a cyclooxygenase pathway to form prostaglandins and TXA_2 or via a lipoxygenase pathway to form various eicosanoids. TXA_2 is a potent platelet activator, stimulating platelet aggregation and vasoconstriction. Although platelets preferentially produce TXA_2 via the cyclooxygenase pathway, vascular endothelial cells produce prostacyclin (prostaglandin I_2), a potent inhibitor of platelet aggregation and a strong vasodilator. The balance between TXA_2 production by platelets and prostacyclin production by vascular endothelium appears to regulate platelet aggregation in vivo.[274,275]

As with erythrocytes, platelets can be sequestered in the spleen and splenic contraction can increase the number of circulating platelets by 30% to 50%. In horses, splenectomy results in substantial and persistent increases in platelet counts.[13] Normal equine platelets have a life span of 4 to 5 days.[278] As platelets age, tissue macrophages of the spleen, liver, and bone marrow remove them from circulation.[279]

Disorders of Platelets

THROMBOCYTOPENIA

Thrombocytopenia is a decrease in the number of circulating platelets. Normal platelet counts in the horse are slightly less than in other species, with higher counts in horses younger than 3 years of age and in male horses.[280] Most laboratories define thrombocytopenia in the horse as a peripheral platelet count of less than 100,000 per microliter. Clinical signs of thrombocytopenia in the horse reflect abnormal primary hemostasis and include petechial and ecchymotic hemorrhages of mucosal membranes, epistaxis, increased bleeding after venipuncture, melena, or hyphema.[281-286] Clinical bleeding usually is associated with platelet counts of less than 30,000 per microliter. Decreased numbers of circulating platelets can result from decreased production of platelets in the bone marrow, increased destruction of platelets, sequestration of platelets, or increased use of platelets during processes of coagulation (Box 14-5).

Proper sample collection and platelet counting is essential before one can make a diagnosis of true thrombocytopenia in a horse.[279] One can obtain an accurate platelet count in most horses from a blood sample obtained with ethylenediamine tetraacetic acid (EDTA) as the anticoagulant. However, the platelets of some horses consistently clump in EDTA, resulting in an inaccurate count or pseudothrombocytopenia.[287] An experienced technician always should examine a stained blood smear visually to assess the presence of platelet clumps. Platelet clumping may occur as a result of in vivo or in vitro platelet activation.[279] When in doubt, reassessing the platelet count in a blood sample anticoagulated with sodium citrate instead of EDTA is advisable. Platelet clumping and pseudothrombocytopenia also have been described in equine blood samples collected using low–molecular-weight heparin as an anticoagulant.[288]

Decreased Platelet Production Thrombocytopenia only infrequently results from decreased platelet production.[289] Primary bone marrow disease is diagnosed by bone marrow analysis, and caution must be used when interpreting megakaryocyte numbers from equine bone marrow aspirates. Megakaryocytes may be absent or present in low numbers in aspirates, even though adequate numbers are present in the intact marrow, possibly because of trapping of these large cells within the subendothelial layer of marrow sinuses. Bone marrow core biopsies are preferred for adequate evaluation of megakaryocyte numbers in the horse. Flow cytometric enumeration of thiazole orange–positive platelets in peripheral blood may be useful as a noninvasive test to assess platelet production.[290]

Because of the short life span of platelets in the peripheral circulation, thrombocytopenia is a common abnormality in animals with generalized bone marrow suppression of any

BOX 14-5

DIFFERENTIAL DIAGNOSES FOR THROMBOCYTOPENIA IN THE HORSE

Decreased Platelet Production

- Hereditary defects
- Myelophthisis
- Myeloproliferative disease
- Idiopathic pancytopenia
- Myelosuppressive drugs
  - Phenylbutazone
  - Chloramphenicol
  - Estrogens
  - Trichlorethylene-extracted soybean meal
- Irradiation

Increased Platelet Use

- Intravascular coagulation
  - Disseminated intravascular coagulation (DIC)
  - Localized
    - Hemolytic uremic syndrome
    - Hemangioma
- Hemorrhage
- Thrombosis

Platelet Sequestration

- Splenomegaly

Increased Platelet Destruction

- Infectious diseases
  - Equine infectious anemia (EIA)
  - *Anaplasma phagocytophilum*
- Immune-mediated diseases
  - Autoimmune disease
  - Systemic lupus erythematosus
  - Idiopathic disease
  - Secondary disease
  - Neoplasia (lymphosarcoma)
  - Bacterial infection
  - Viral infection
  - Drugs
  - Neonatal alloimmune disease
- Drugs or toxins
- Snakebites

Laboratory Error

cause. Thrombocytopenia with dramatically decreased bone marrow megakaryocyte numbers has been reported in horses with a variety of myeloproliferative disorders.[171,180,187,264] Thrombocytopenia also is recognized in horses with idiopathic pancytopenia[156,160] and drug- or toxin-induced myelosuppression.

A syndrome of neutropenia and thrombocytopenia has been described in related Standardbreds. A heritable cyclic neutropenia was suspected. Most affected horses died from complications of infectious diseases, thrombocytopenia, or both.[175]

Increased Platelet Destruction A variety of pathophysiologic events may increase the rate at which platelets are removed from circulation. Most of these disorders are accompanied by a compensatory bone marrow megakaryocytosis best identified with core marrow biopsies. Immunoglobulin deposition on the surface of platelets is the most common cause of accelerated platelet destruction. Cells of the mononuclear phagocyte system, especially splenic macrophages and hepatic Kupffer's cells, remove antibody-coated platelets from circulation. Nonimmune mechanisms of accelerated platelet destruction include drug- or toxin-induced platelet damage and snake bites. Thrombocytopenia of controversial cause has been described in human beings and horses receiving heparin therapy.[291,292]

Immune-Mediated Thrombocytopenia. Most cases of idiopathic thrombocytopenia in the horse likely are the result of an immune-mediated increase in platelet destruction. The initiating factors of this condition often are not identified, but immune-mediated destruction of platelets may be associated with viral or bacterial infections, neoplastic conditions such as lymphosarcoma, and with other immunemediated disorders, including IMHA, glomerulonephritis, and systemic vasculitis.[281] Circulating platelets from human beings with IMTP have increased quantities of surface-bound IgG, IgM, or complement.[293-295] The mechanics of antibody attachment to platelets are similar to those described for IMHA. True autoantibodies may be produced against normal platelet surface antigens or against novel platelet antigens that have developed in response to a primary disease process. Circulating immune complexes may attach to platelets nonspecifically via Fc or complement receptors. Antibodies also may be directed against foreign molecules, such as drugs, that have attached themselves to platelet membranes. Regardless of the source of the antibody, mononuclear phagocytes remove Ig-coated platelets from the circulation, principally in the spleen and liver.[296]

Horses with IMTP may have petechial and ecchymotic hemorrhages of mucosal membranes, epistaxis, increased bleeding after venipuncture, melena, or hyphema.[281-286] Clinical bleeding usually is associated with platelet counts of less than 30,000 per microliter. Patient history and a careful physical examination are critical for identifying underlying disease. An AGID or Coggins test for EIA is indicated. One should evaluate other coagulation parameters, including prothrombin time (PT) and partial thromboplastin time (PTT), to identify complex coagulative defects such as those seen with DIC (discussed in a subsequent section). A bone marrow analysis usually reveals normal to increased numbers of megakaryocytes. However, if antibodies against platelet membranes cross-react with megakaryocyte membrane antigens, megakaryocytes may be decreased or absent in the bone marrow.[297]

Confirmation of IMTP in horses can be difficult, requiring demonstration of increased quantities of platelet-bound antibody. This can be accomplished by measuring platelet factor 3 or by performing flow cytometry. Platelet factor 3 is a platelet membrane phospholipid released when platelets are injured. Addition of patient plasma containing released platelet factor 3 to platelet-rich plasma from a normal horse results in accelerated clotting of the sample. Unfortunately, this test is difficult to perform consistently, results vary, and most veterinary laboratories do not offer the assay. Direct fluorescent antibody testing and flow cytometric assay for platelet surface IgG and IgM have been described in horses with IMTP.[117,298] Direct and indirect immunoradiometric assays and an indirect enzyme-linked immunosorbent assay (ELISA) for detection of platelet-bound antibody also have been described.[299,300] These tests are not widely available, however, and require careful control and interpretation. In the absence of an easy, accurate, and reliable method for definitive diagnosis of IMTP in the horse, one may make a presumptive diagnosis in horses with a low platelet count, normal coagulation parameters (PT and PTT), and no evidence of excessive consumption of platelets (i.e., DIC).

Any current medication being administered to horses suspected of having IMTP should be discontinued immediately. If life-threatening hemorrhage is occurring, then transfusions of fresh whole blood or platelet-rich plasma are indicated. Most horses respond to therapy with parenterally administered corticosteroids.[281,285] Corticosteroids appear to act by suppressing the phagocytic activity of mononuclear phagocytes, inhibiting antibody synthesis, increasing effective platelet production, and reducing capillary fragility. One should tailor the corticosteroid dose and route of administration to the individual patient to achieve the best results with the lowest possible dose. Horses with IMTP have been reported to respond to dexamethasone at 0.1 mg/kg intravenously or intramuscularly twice daily.[282,285] One always should taper corticosteroid administration gradually to once-daily morning administration to decrease interference with endogenous corticosteroid release. If long-term maintenance therapy is necessary, every-other-day or every-third-day administration of the lowest effective dose is indicated. Maintenance therapy may be oral or parenteral. Potential complications associated with corticosteroid administration in the horse include laminitis, secondary infections, and iatrogenic hyperadrenocorticism.

Occasionally, horses with IMTP fail to respond to parenteral corticosteroid therapy. Two such horses responded favorably to azathioprine at 3.0 mg/kg orally once daily.[286] However, a recent study on the pharmacokinetic properties of azathioprine indicates that the drug has poor bioavailability in the horse when administered orally at the previously recommended dose and that clinical trials for efficacy are needed.[301] Azathioprine has been used in human beings and dogs with IMTP and acts as an immunosuppressive agent interfering with humoral and cell-mediated immune function. Vincristine is a vinca alkaloid used to treat refractory IMTP in human beings. Vincristine therapy was successful in treating one horse with idiopathic IMTP[302] and unsuccessful in treating another.[286] Alternative treatments for IMTP that have been effective in other species include danazol (a synthetic analog of androgenic steroids and progesterone), gamma globulin infusions, and splenectomy.[303]

Neonatal alloimmune thrombocytopenia has been described in horse and mule foals.[299,300,304] A syndrome of presumptive neonatal alloimmune thrombocytopenia, mucosal erosions, and skin lesions has been described in foals of several breeds. These foals respond to supportive care with judicious administration of corticosteroids and transfusions of platelet-rich plasma. Long-term prognosis is good, but platelet counts can take 30 days or longer to stabilize at more than 10,000 per microliter.

Equine Infectious Anemia Virus. Acute febrile episodes of EIAV are accompanied by a sharp decline in platelet count followed by a rapid rebound as fever and viremia resolve. This thrombocytopenia is probably multifactorial in origin. Circulating platelets have increased quantities of IgG and IgM on the surface[117] and show evidence of in vivo activation, possibly indicating enhanced nonimmune-mediated destruction of platelets.[118] Bone marrow megakaryocytes are not infected during acute disease[117]; however, evidence exists of decreased bone marrow production of platelets in horses with EIA, possibly because of altered cytokine production in the bone marrow.[119,305,306] The thrombocytopenia of EIAV may contribute to petechia and ecchymoses but rarely is associated with a severe bleeding diathesis. EIAV is discussed in detail in previous sections.

Equine Granulocytic Ehrlichiosis. Infection with the obligate, intracellular, rickettsia *Anaplasma phagocytophilum* (formerly *Ehrlichia equi*) can result in a syndrome of fever, anorexia, depression, petechia and ecchymoses, icterus, ventral edema, and ataxia lasting 3 to 16 days. Involuntary recumbency with seizurelike activity was observed in a horse diagnosed with anaplasmosis.[307] Consistent hematologic abnormalities regardless of clinical presentation include thrombocytopenia, leukopenia, and mild anemia.[308,309] Clinical signs are more severe in adult horses than in those younger than 4 years of age. Foals younger than 1 year of age often experience only fever.[309,310] Most infected horses originate from the foothills of northern California, but infections also have been diagnosed in horses from other parts of the country.[310,311] Most cases of ehrlichiosis occur in late fall, winter, and spring, and the disease is known to be transmitted by several species of the *Ixodes* spp. tick. Tick control is recommended for prevention of disease in endemic areas.

Granular inclusion bodies may be visible in the cytoplasm of neutrophils and eosinophils during routine cytologic examination using any Wright's or Giemsa type of stain. One may see inclusion bodies best under oil immersion, and they appear as pleomorphic, blue-gray to dark-blue spoke-wheel shapes.[309] Inclusion bodies represent a cluster of coccobacillary organisms, varying in size between 0.2 to 5 μm in diameter, within cytoplasmic membrane-bound vacuoles. The appearance of cytoplasmic inclusion bodies correlates closely with the onset of fever, and they remain visible for approximately 10 days.[308]

Serologic diagnosis using the IFA test has historically been the standard method for diagnosis of equine anaplasmosis.[312] However, as many as 50% of normal horses in endemic areas of California have antibodies against the organism.[313] A polymerase chain reaction (PCR) test to detect the organism's DNA offers a means to confirm a diagnosis early in the course of the disease with comparatively high sensitivity and specificity. Animals that are experimentally infected become PCR positive on approximately the fifth day after infection but do not show clinical signs until day 7. Seroconversion occurs quickly after clinical signs become apparent at approximately days 12 to 16. Extrapolating the results of this study to clinical situations suggests that PCR is likely to be positive before onset of clinical signs and that IFA should be performed early with suspicion of disease so that seroconversion can be accurately assessed.[312]

Mortality is rare in horses with ehrlichiosis; most untreated animals recover over 2 weeks and acquire a sound immunity against reinfection for at least 2 years.[308,309] Death, when it occurs, is usually associated with secondary infections that are the result of immunosuppression or trauma because of ataxia.[314] One experimentally infected horse died with signs consistent with systemic inflammatory response syndrome, shock, and DIC.[315] Treatment with oxytetracycline at 7 mg/kg intravenously once or twice daily for up to 7 days may hasten recovery. One should provide supportive therapy, including intravenous fluids, leg wraps, and stall confinement for the severely ataxic horse, as indicated.[308,309,311] In animals that die or are killed, necropsy lesions include petechial and ecchymotic hemorrhages, edema, and icterus. Histologically, small arteries and veins are inflamed, and mild inflammatory vascular or interstitial lesions may be present in kidneys, heart, brain, and lungs.[308]

Increased Platelet Use Rapid use of circulating platelets occasionally occurs and may be appropriate, as in the case of massive trauma or external hemorrhage, or inappropriate, as in some cases of systemic or localized activation of hemostatic mechanisms. Thrombocytopenia accompanying hemorrhage or trauma is usually mild to moderate and rapidly reversible. DIC is a complex disorder of hemostasis resulting from widespread systemic activation of coagulation mechanisms. This microvascular coagulation rapidly uses circulating platelets, and thrombocytopenia is a common result. Affected animals have a variety of other abnormalities detectable by routine coagulation testing. Horses with DIC and normal platelet counts may have abnormal platelet function, inhibiting the use of those platelets. In one study of horses presented to a veterinary referral hospital, DIC after gastrointestinal or inflammatory diseases was the most common cause of thrombocytopenia.[289] In horses evaluated for colitis, approximately half of the horses had platelet counts less than 100,000,[316] and in horses that underwent surgery for correction of a large colon torsion, a decreased platelet count was significantly associated with increased mortality.[317,318] The section on DIC provides more information on the pathophysiology, diagnosis, and treatment of this disorder.

Localized activation of coagulation may occur in some disease conditions, including neoplasia and renal disease. Thrombocytopenia has been reported accompanying hemangiosarcoma in the horse[319-321] and is associated with vascular tumors in human beings and dogs.[322,323] Hemolytic uremic syndrome is an unusual condition in the horse characterized by acute renal failure with microangiopathic intravascular hemolysis and disseminated or renal intravascular coagulation. Thrombocytopenia is a common finding in affected horses.[73,74]

Thrombocytosis

Thrombocytosis is an increase in the number of circulating platelets. Increased bone marrow production of megakaryocytes may occur as a primary myeloproliferative disorder or in association with other neoplastic conditions, including polycythemia vera. Thrombocytosis more commonly is associated with acute or chronic inflammatory disorders or follows acute hemorrhage.[324] Mild thrombocytosis also may occur during and immediately after exercise or excitement caused by splenic contraction and release of sequestered platelets into the peripheral circulation. Thrombocytosis is usually asymptomatic, and specific therapy is not indicated. Thrombocytosis rarely may be associated with venous thrombotic tendencies, and one may consider anticoagulation therapy in these cases.

Functional Defects of Platelets

Functional defects of platelets can result in clinical signs similar to those of thrombocytopenic patients, despite a normal to increased platelet count. The most widely used laboratory tests to assess platelet function are bleeding time and platelet aggregation studies. Bleeding time depends on the number and function of platelets, the level of vWF, and vascular integrity. One performs the test by inverting the lower lip and making a vertical incision 1 mm deep by 5 mm long, with a template bleeding time device (Surgicutt, International Technidyne Corp., Edison, N.J.). After 30 seconds the blood is removed with Whatman filter paper. Then the previous step is repeated every 15 seconds until one no longer detects blood on the filter paper, and the total time is recorded.[325] Alternatively, one may make an incision on the caudolateral aspect of the foreleg with proximal venostasis using a sphygmomanometer cuff above the carpus.[326,327] The site should be shaved before testing. Normal bleeding time varies, depending on the technique and site of incision, and one must establish the time for each technique. The veterinarian should evaluate a normal control horse concurrently with the patient. A platelet aggregometer can be used to measure the aggregation of platelets in response to ADP, serotonin, epinephrine, arachidonic acid, thrombin, ristocetin, collagen, and collagen-related peptide.[328-330] One should collect whole blood samples with sodium citrate as an anticoagulant and prepare platelet-rich plasma by centrifugation.

Congenital defects in platelet function are rare but have been identified in horses. Glanzmann thrombasthenia is a rare, heritable platelet disorder that has been thoroughly described in human beings and dogs. Four horses including a Standardbred,[331] an Oldenburg,[332] a Quarter Horse, and a Thoroughbred cross[333] have been diagnosed with the condition. The platelet dysfunction was due to an amino acid change in the gene for the platelet fibrinogen receptor, integrin αIIb β_3.[334] Horses present for clinical bleeding, most commonly in the form of epistaxis. Platelet count and coagulation times are normal, whereas mucosal bleeding time is significantly prolonged and clot retraction is markedly reduced. Results of aggregometry testing are consistent with an inability of the platelets to bind to fibrinogen; flow cytometry reveals decreased surface integrin αIIb β_3.[332,333] Treatment was attempted in these horses with tapering doses of dexamethasone with no apparent change in the occasional bleeding and laboratory abnormalities.

Another heritable thrombasthenia caused by a platelet fibrinogen-binding defect has been identified in a population of Thoroughbreds.[330,335,336] The clinical condition was identified in a mare and its offspring, prompting a survey of a population of Thoroughbreds in that area. The syndrome observed in the Thoroughbred mare and its filly resembled Glanzmann thrombasthenia in clinical presentation and basic laboratory analysis. However, aggregometry and flow cytometry results differ in that platelets of the affected horses bind in reduced amounts to fibrinogen in the presence of thrombin.[336] Aggregometry often demonstrates the inability of the platelets to bind in the presence of collagen.[330] Although the genetic basis of this disorder remains unclear, a secretion defect is believed to be related to either abnormal platelet granule contents or intracellular signaling. The population study reported an incidence of 0.7% (3/444 horses) of this disorder, yet none of the horses in the screening program exhibited clinical signs. When appropriate, flow cytometry should be used to screen for this heritable disease.[335]

Researchers have described von Willebrand's disease in the horse.[337] Because the disease is not an inherent platelet defect, it is discussed later in this chapter (with hereditary defects of coagulation).

Acquired platelet functional defects may be associated with uremia, acute myelodysplastic diseases, and dysproteinemias, as well as after the administration of various drugs. Abnormal responses to platelet aggregating agents and increased bleeding time have been described in normal human and equine neonates,[325,329] and neonatal foals may have an increased susceptibility to platelet-associated hemorrhagic diathesis.

Many human beings and animals with uremia exhibit abnormal hemostasis, most of which is attributable to abnormal platelet function and likely is caused by abnormalities in the biochemical processes necessary for platelet aggregation and granule release. Human beings with myeloproliferative and lymphoproliferative disorders may have abnormal platelet shapes and decreased aggregation and secretion.[338] Dysproteinemia in these patients may result in platelet dysfunction when abnormal proteins coat platelets or endothelium and interfere with normal adhesion and aggregation. A hemorrhagic diathesis caused by platelet dysfunction has been described in one horse with monoclonal gammopathy and lymphoproliferative disease.[271]

Drugs used in equine medicine and associated with abnormalities of platelet function in human beings include penicillins, cephalosporins, quinidine, chlorpromazine, halothane, and NSAIDs.[338] NSAIDs act by inhibiting cyclooxygenase, an enzyme critical for the formation of prostaglandins, prostacyclins, and thromboxane from arachidonic acid. As previously discussed, TXA_2 is a strong stimulus for platelet aggregation and release reactions and is a potent vasoconstrictor. Aspirin covalently acetylates cyclooxygenase, and because platelets are anucleate cells, they are incapable of producing new enzyme. The result is an irreversible inhibition of platelet cyclooxygenase that can be corrected only when the body clears aspirin from the circulation and the bone marrow releases new platelets. In contrast, other NSAIDs produce only a temporary inhibition of cyclooxygenase by reversibly binding to the enzyme. Template bleeding time is prolonged in horses that have received aspirin, phenylbutazone, or flunixin meglumine.[327,328,339,340] The effect is most pronounced after aspirin therapy, and a dosage of 17 mg/kg once daily for 3 days increases bleeding time for at least 3 days after discontinuation of therapy.[327] The minimal effective dose of aspirin to decrease thromboxane generation is 5 mg/kg; the duration of decrease is dose dependent.[341]

HEMOSTASIS

The vascular system provides a closed conduit for the circulation of fluid and cellular components of blood. Exchange of substances across the vessel surfaces is controlled carefully. The body must repair any disruption in the closed network of blood vessels rapidly and efficiently to prevent excessive loss of critical blood elements into the extravascular environment. This repair process requires interaction between the injured vessel wall, platelets, and soluble proteins and accessory molecules in the blood. The end result is a stable fibrin mesh that prevents loss of blood while the vascular endothelium regenerates. When endothelium has been repaired, fibrinolytic reactions occur to remove fibrin and re-establish vessel patency. A careful balance of coagulative and fibrinolytic processes must occur to maintain optimal circulatory capacity without loss of blood. The body also must control procoagulative forces carefully to prevent inappropriate activation that might result in thrombosis of normal vessels with subsequent tissue and organ ischemia.

PHYSIOLOGY

Primary hemostasis is the process of platelet interaction with the vessel wall to achieve a temporary plug of the vascular defect. Secondary hemostasis involves the interaction of soluble coagulation factors to produce a stable fibrin mesh that reinforces the platelet plug. The body carefully regulates hemostatic mechanisms via an intricate network of positive and negative feedback with inhibitors and potentiators of coagulation and fibrinolysis.

The initial vascular response to injury is intense vasoconstriction to divert blood from the site. Anticoagulative processes associated with vascular endothelium, including synthesis of prostacyclin and plasminogen activators and uptake and degradation of proaggregating molecules,[13] prevent the interaction of normal intact vascular endothelium with circulating platelets. Exposure of subendothelial collagen at the site of vascular injury triggers platelet adherence with interaction between endothelial vWF and platelet receptors. The function of platelets in primary hemostasis has been discussed in detail already. Platelet adhesion stimulates a release reaction involving platelet secretory granules. Contents of these granules (including ADP, ATP, serotonin, platelet factors 3 and 4, TXA_2, and acid hydrolases) attract other platelets in a process of irreversible platelet aggregation at the site of vascular injury. Platelet aggregation provides a favorable environment for accumulation and activation of the intrinsic and extrinsic coagulation systems.

The classic coagulation pathway has traditionally offered a concept of hemostasis based on and under the control of protein coagulation factors. The system involves sequential activation of inactive precursor factors (Table 14-3) by limited proteolysis (Figure 14-2). Activated factors are indicated by the letter *a* after their numeric designation. Most coagulation factors are classified as *serine proteases* because of a critical serine residue at the active site of the enzyme. This serine is exposed after cleavage of a short peptide during activation of factor precursors.

Although commonly discussed as separate pathways, intrinsic and extrinsic coagulation cascades interact at many levels and are considered more accurately as part of one highly complex system. For the sake of simplicity, however, they are

TABLE 14-3

Coagulation Factors

Factor	Synonym
I	Fibrinogen
II	Prothrombin
III	Tissue factor, tissue thromboplastin
IV	Calcium
V	Proaccelerin, labile factor
VI	Not assigned
VII	Proconvertin, stable factor
VIII	Antihemophilic factor
IX	Christmas factor
X	Stuart-Prower factor
XI	Plasma thromboplastin antecedent
XII	Hageman factor
XIII	Fibrin-stabilizing factor
Prekallikrein	Fletcher factor
High-molecular-weight kininogen	Fitzgerald factor

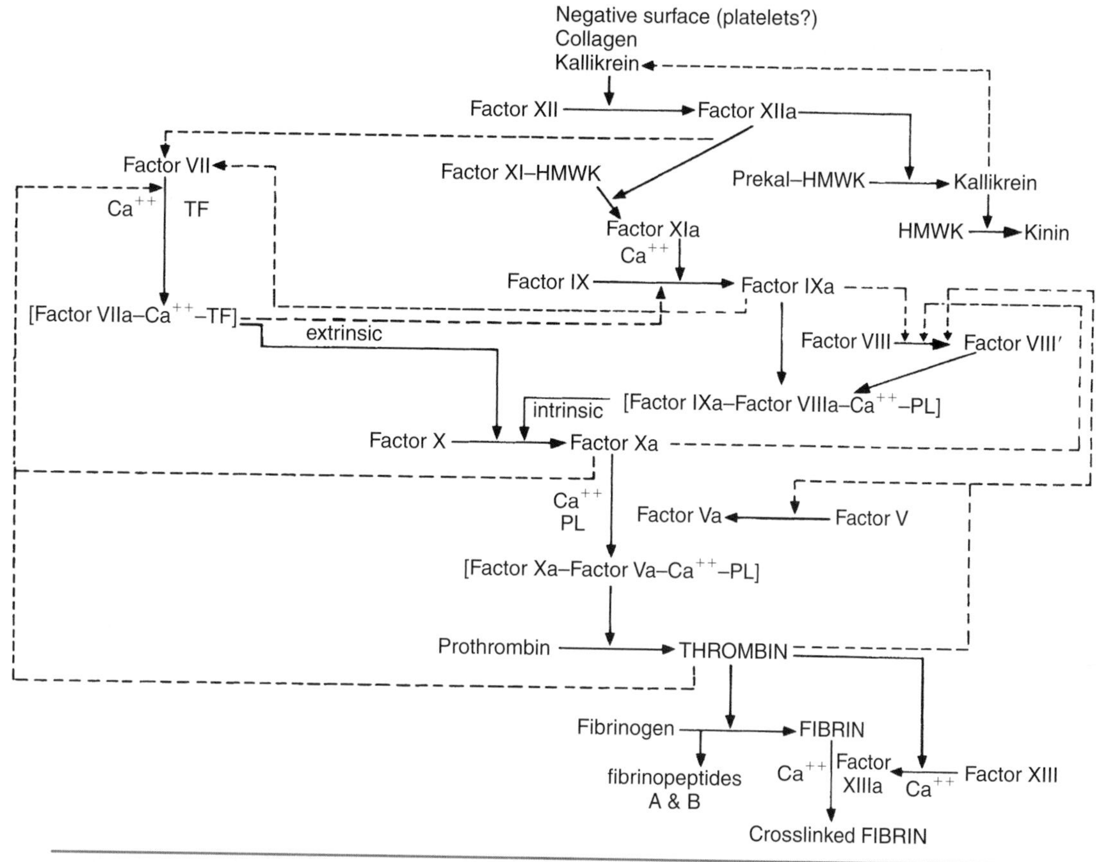

FIGURE 14-2 Schematic representation of blood coagulation showing the numerous interactions between coagulation factors in the classic extrinsic and intrinsic pathways. *Arrow,* Primary action; *dashed arrow,* actions of secondary importance; *a,* activated form; *HMWK,* high-molecular-weight kininogen; *TF,* tissue factor; *PL,* phospholipids; *Prekal,* prekallikrein. (From Morris DD: Recognition and management of disseminated intravascular coagulation in horses, *Vet Clin North Am Equine Pract* 4:115-143, 1988.)

discussed separately. The liver produces most soluble coagulation factors. Mononuclear phagocytes are responsible for clearing activated clotting factors from the circulation.

Contact of soluble coagulation factors with negatively charged subendothelial collagen and with the various products of the platelet release reaction initiates the intrinsic coagulation system. This initial contact phase (see Table 14-3) requires interaction of coagulation factor XII, high-molecular-weight kininogen (HMWK), and prekallikrein to accelerate production of the activated form of factor XII (designated *XIIa*). Factor XIIa in turn catalyzes the limited proteolysis of factor XI to XIa. Elements of the contact phase reaction are also capable of inducing parallel pro-inflammatory reactions by initiating kinin and complement cascades. The importance of this contact phase reaction to in vivo coagulation is questionable. Human beings and animals with hereditary deficiencies of the proteins involved in this reaction (factor XII, HMWK, or prekallikrein) rarely show any clinical bleeding tendencies. In contrast, deficiency of almost any other coagulation factor, including factor XI, results in profound hemorrhagic tendencies.

Factor XIa, in the presence of calcium, activates factor IX. Factor IXa forms a molecular complex with factor VIIIa and calcium on a phospholipid membrane surface to catalyze the conversion of factor X to Xa. Platelet membranes are thought to provide the phospholipid surface for this reaction. Activation of factor X is the point of interaction between the extrinsic and intrinsic systems.

The extrinsic coagulation system begins with formation of a molecular complex between tissue factor (TF; thromboplastin), factor VIIa, and calcium ions on a platelet phospholipid surface to catalyze the conversion of factor X to Xa. Factor Xa is capable of activating factor VII to VIIa in a feedback loop that increases the production of both. In a slower reaction that appears to be important in vivo, the TF VIIa-calcium complex is also capable of activating factor IX.[342] TF is present in virtually every tissue of the body, and a variety of insults can initiate the extrinsic coagulation system, including vascular endothelial damage, endotoxin, antigen-antibody complexes, RBC hemolysis, and local areas of tissue necrosis.

Formation of factor Xa marks the beginning of what classically is termed the *common pathway of coagulation.* Factor Xa complexes with factor Va and calcium on a phospholipid membrane to convert prothrombin to thrombin enzymatically. Thrombin in turn is the catalyst for formation of fibrin from fibrinogen. Thrombin is also important in the activation of factors V, VIII:C, and XIII, forming positive feedback loops that potentiate the coagulative process and promote platelet aggregation. Fibrin monomers aggregate, and factor XIIIa catalyzes, the formation of covalent cross-linkages between the monomers to stabilize the clot.

The cascade concept of the physiology of hemostasis has recently been revisited because several disease processes cannot be adequately explained. Many experts now believe that coagulation should be viewed as three overlapping steps termed *initiation, amplification,* and *propagation.*[343] This series of events is dependent on two cells: the TF-bearing cell located extravascularly and the platelet. In a normal physiologic state, coagulation is prevented until necessary by limiting contact of these two cell types. Once an injury to a vessel has occurred, the two come into contact and the process of coagulation begins.

Initiation begins as a vessel is damaged, plasma is exuded, and it comes in contact with the TF-bearing extravascular cells. Factor VIIa binds to TF and after activation by several proteases forms a factor VIIa-TF complex. This complex in turn activates factors X and IX. Factor Xa goes on to activate factor Va, and together this prothrombinase complex, located on the surface of TF-bearing cells, forms small amounts of thrombin. If factor Xa leaves the cell surface, then it is quickly inhibited. In contrast, factor IXa can move from cell to cell without rapid inhibition.

The amplification phase also involves the aforementioned damage to the vessel that is significant enough to allow exudation of platelets and factorVIII-vWF into the extravascular space. Platelets adhere to the extravascular matrix and interact with the small amount of thrombin that was produced on the surface of the TF-bearing cells. This thrombin enhances platelet adhesion, activates other platelets, and activates factors Va and VIIIa on the platelet surface. This activation allows vWF to be released, further enhancing platelet adhesion and aggregation. These activated platelets with factors Va and VIIIa bound to their surfaces are the basis for the propagation phase.

Propagation involves the formation of two additional complexes. Factor IXa that was activated by the factor VII-TF complex during the initiation phase, binds to activated platelets. Factor IXa then forms a complex (tenase complex) with factor VIIIa already on the platelet cell surface. This complex activates factor Xa that is present on the platelet surface. Factor Xa then forms a complex with already platelet bound factor Va (prothrombinase complex) that causes a marked increase in thrombin formation (enough to bind fibrinogen and form a clot).[343]

Inhibitors of procoagulative elements in part maintain a balance between clot formation at sites of vascular injury and pathologic thrombosis. Several physiologically important systems for in vivo procoagulant inhibition have been described. The most important of these is plasma antithrombin III (AT III), responsible for 50% to 75% of plasma antithrombin activity. AT III inhibits all serine proteases generated during the coagulation process, including thrombin; factors Xa, IXa, XIa, and XIIa; plasmin; kallikrein; and the anticoagulants protein C and protein S. Heparin interacts with AT III, causing a conformational change that increases the activity of AT III 1000-fold.[344]

Tissue factor pathway inhibitor (TFPI) is a protein that reversibly inhibits factor Xa and then as a complex with Xa, can inhibit the factor VII-TF complex at the level of the endothelial cell. Another of the main anticoagulative systems involves protein C, protein S, and thrombomodulin. As the primary clot is formed, small pieces of thrombin are lost within the vasculature. When this thrombin comes in contact with an intact endothelial cell, it binds to thrombomodulin, which in turn activates proteins C and S. These vitamin K–dependent serine proteases act to inactivate factors Va and VIIIa and prevent inappropriate clotting. This system acts mainly on endothelial cells rather than platelets.[345]

The fibrinolytic system is responsible for eventual remodeling and removal of a stable fibrin clot to restore blood flow (Figure 14-3). Because small amounts of fibrin production

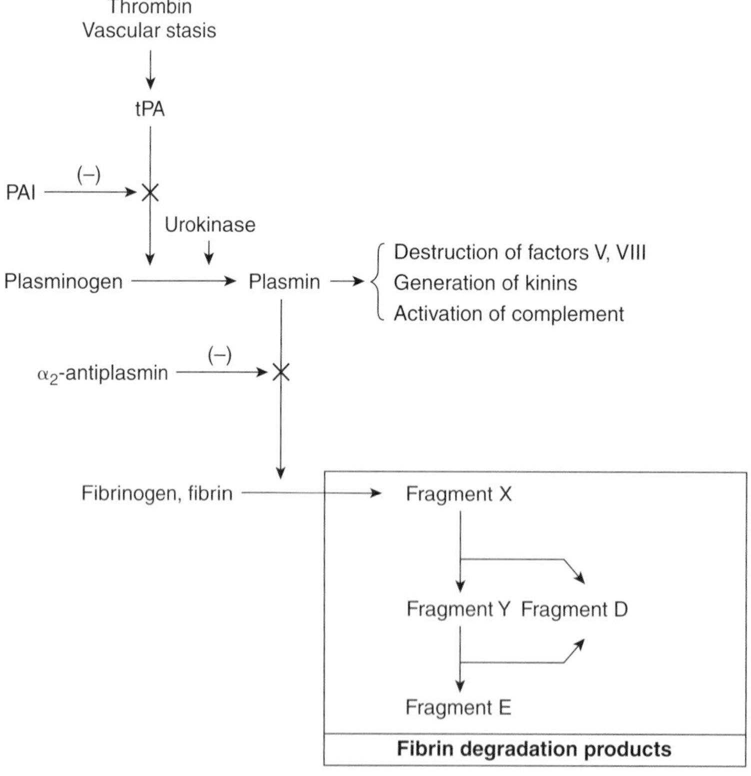

FIGURE 14-3 Major fibrinolytic reactions (see text for details). A negative sign (–) indicates inhibition of a specific reaction. *TPA,* Tissue plasminogen activator; *PAI,* plasminogen activator inhibitor. (From Kobluk CN, Ames TR, Geor RJ: *The horse: diseases and clinical management,* Philadelphia, 1995, WB Saunders.)

and subsequent fibrinolysis occur continuously in vivo, the body must maintain a delicate balance between procoagulant and fibrinolytic processes to prevent widespread thrombosis or hemorrhage. The principal enzyme of the fibrinolytic system is plasmin, normally present in plasma as an inactive precursor, plasminogen. Plasminogen is converted to plasmin proteolytically by endothelial tissue plasminogen activator, an enzyme present in most normal and neoplastic tissue. Endothelial cells adjacent to clot formations release tissue plasminogen activator in response to vascular stasis and a high local concentration of thrombin. Released tissue plasminogen activator has a high affinity for fibrin, localizing it to the adjacent clot for plasminogen activation. Circulating antiplasmins, the most important of which is α_2-antiplasmin, rapidly inactivate circulating plasmin. Plasmin bound to fibrin is much less accessible for inactivation because plasmin interactions with fibrin obscure binding sites for inhibitors.[346]

Plasminogen also may be activated during the contact phase of the intrinsic coagulation system. Factor XIIa and HMWK interact with prekallikrein to produce kallikrein. Kallikrein activates urokinase, which in turn converts plasminogen to plasmin.[347] Because plasmin can activate factor XII, a potential feedback loop amplification exists. The importance of contact phase activation in vivo is questionable, however.

Plasmin is a serine protease with a high affinity for fibrinogen and fibrin, degrading them into fibrin degradation products (FDPs). Plasmin also may aid in degradation of factors V, VIII, IX, and XI. Fibrin and fibrinogen are split into the clinically significant FDPs including D-dimers, as well as fragments X,Y,O, and E. Increases in the circulating concentrations of these fragments can be attributed to ongoing fibrinolysis. The mononuclear phagocytes of the liver clear FDPs from the circulation.

Evaluation of Hemostasis

Disorders of hemostasis usually may be classified based on clinical signs as abnormalities of primary or secondary hemostasis. Abnormalities of primary hemostasis include vascular diseases and changes in the number or function of platelets. Affected horses usually have signs of mucosal bleeding, petechia and ecchymoses, epistaxis, hyphema, or melena. Platelet function tests were discussed previously. Diagnosis of the vasculitides is discussed in another section.

Disorders of secondary hemostasis usually involve abnormalities in quantity or function of the soluble coagulation factors and present as spontaneous or excessive hemorrhage in response to surgery or trauma. These horses may have hemorrhage into body cavities, hematoma formation, hemarthroses, prolonged bleeding after venipuncture, or external hemorrhage. Most coagulation tests measure the time necessary for clot formation under various circumstances. Coagulation times tend to be longer in horses than in human beings or other domestic animals.[348] Table 14-4 lists some laboratory tests used to assess equine hemostatic function with normal reference values.

Activated clotting time measures the time to clot formation on activation of whole blood by contact with diatomaceous earth. This process bypasses the contact phase of coagulation and is useful in evaluating deficiencies of factors VIII and IX, prothrombin, and fibrinogen. Abnormalities of factor VII and platelets do not appear to alter the activated clotting time.[348] One collects blood directly into a tube containing diatomaceous earth, mixes, incubates the contents at 37° or 38° C, and measures the time until clot formation.

PTT and activated partial thromboplastin time (APTT) measure the activity of factors XII, XI, X, IX, VIII, and V, prothrombin, and fibrinogen. The PTT test is performed by adding platelet-poor plasma to a glass tube containing phospholipid emulsion and calcium and determining the time to

TABLE 14-4

Reference Ranges for Equine Hemostatic Values*

Parameter	Units	Value	Reference
Platelet count	per μl	75,000-300,000	NCSU†
Fibrinogen	g/dl	<400	NCSU
PT	seconds	8.5-9.9	NCSU
APTT	seconds	30-44	NCSU
FDPs	mg/dl	<20	NCSU
AT III	% PNEP	63-131	Johnstone et al.‡
AT III	% PNHP	218 ± 18	Bernard et al.§
Plasminogen	% PNEP	64.6-155.9	Welles et al.‖
Protein C	% PNEP	104.5 ±13.8	Welles et al.¶

PT, Prothrombin time; *APTT,* activated partial thromboplastin time; *FDPs,* fibrin degradation products; *AT III,* antithrombin III; *PNEP,* pooled normal equine plasma; *PNHP,* pooled normal human plasma.

*These numbers are for reference only. Each laboratory should establish its own normal equine values.

†Data from *NCSU,* North Carolina State University College of Veterinary Medicine Clinical Pathology Laboratory normal equine reference values;

‡Johnstone IB, Physick-Sheard P, Crane S: Breed, age, and gender differences in plasma antithrombin-III activity in clinically normal young horses, *Am J Vet Res* 50:1751, 1989;

§Bernard W, Morris DD, Divers TJ, et al: Plasma antithrombin-III values in healthy horses: effect of sex and/or breed, *Am J Vet Res* 48:866, 1987;

‖Welles EG, Prasse KW, Duncan A: Chromogenic assay for equine plasminogen, *Am J Vet Res* 51:1080, 1990;

¶Welles EG, Prasse KW, Duncan A, et al: Antigenic assay for protein C determination in horses, *Am J Vet Res* 51:1075, 1990.

clot formation. One performs the APTT test similarly, except an activating agent is added. PT, also known as *one-stage PT*, measures the function of the extrinsic and common coagulation pathways, including factors V, VII, and X, prothrombin, and fibrinogen. In this test, platelet-poor plasma is mixed with thromboplastin and calcium and the time to clot formation is determined. One may use citrated whole blood or plasma for accurate measurement of PT up to 3 days after collection. A control sample from a clinically normal horse should accompany the patient's sample.[349] Commercially available tests for measurement of PT have been evaluated in horses and found to be accurate when the manufacturer's guidelines were followed and the appropriate reagent was used.[350] In horses with colic, APTT is more reliably elevated and more markedly changed than any of the other routine coagulation tests.[351,352] A prolonged APTT at admission is associated with a negative prognosis.[353] Thrombin time (TT) measures the time to clot formation after addition of thrombin to citrated plasma. TT is only prolonged with abnormalities in fibrinogen quantity or function or in the presence of thrombin inhibitors.

Most commonly, FDPs are measured in the serum using antibody-coated latex beads and monitoring macroscopic agglutination. This test reflects only the presence of D and E fragments. One must collect blood into a special tube containing thrombin and a protease inhibitor (ThromboWellcotest; Burroughs Wellcome Co., Research Triangle Park, N.C.). Commercially available latex agglutination kits for FDPs are not suitable for use in the horse.[353] However, D-dimers, a fibrinogen degradation product, can be measured reliably in horses using latex agglutination kits. An increase in D-dimers occurs in horses with colic,[317,352] laminitis,[354] jugular vein thrombosis, and DIC[355] and may indicate a risk factor for development of a coagulopathy.

Fibrinogen concentration may be easily estimated by refractometer as the difference between plasma protein concentration at room temperature and the concentration after heating plasma to 56° to 58° C for 3 minutes and centrifugation to remove precipitated fibrinogen. Alternatively, fibrinogen may be estimated from the thrombin clot time, which is inversely proportional to the fibrinogen concentration, or by immunologic assays.

Tests for plasma AT III measure the presence or the activity of the protein. Because inactive AT III antigen may be present, functional tests are preferable. Assays of AT III activity are clotting or chromogenic tests that measure residual thrombin activity after one adds the patient sample to a known quantity of thrombin. Normal AT III activity in the horse has been reported as 218% of normal human pooled plasma[356] and 63% to 131% of normal equine pooled plasma.[357,358] Widespread in vivo activation of coagulation is the most common cause of decreased plasma AT III activity. This is reliably observed in horses with gastrointestinal disease[317] and is a negative prognostic indicator for some populations of horses.[359,360] Decreased activity has been associated with protein-losing enteropathies or nephropathies and liver disease. Decreased AT III activity has been attributed to consumption of AT III, but the decrease may actually be the result of the loss of albumin or decreased production as seen with liver disease.[361] AT III's role as an acute phase protein in the horse is controversial.[351,352] Increased AT III activity has rarely been reported in horses with hepatic disease.[358]

Specialized assays for various components of the equine procoagulative and fibrinolytic systems have been described and are available only at specialized laboratories. These include assays for thrombin-antithrombin complexes (TAT),[317] protein C,[362] plasminogen,[363]α_2-antitrypsin,[364] vWF,[337] and factor VIII:C.[365] Mean platelet component (MPC) is a measure of platelet density that reliably decreases when platelets become activated and degranulate. This test was found to be an indicator of platelet activation in both adult horses and ill neonates.[366]

Hereditary Disorders of Hemostasis

Inherited disorders of hemostasis are most common in purebred animals that have been highly inbred. Many of these disorders are inherited in an autosomal recessive fashion; both parents must be carriers of the disorder to produce clinically affected offspring. For practitioners to be able to differentiate between inherited and acquired disorders of hemostasis is essential to advise owners appropriately. Inherited disorders are potentially treatable, but they are incurable. Owners should not use affected animals and their carrier parents as breeding stock. Practitioners see most animals with inherited bleeding problems when they are still young. Owners frequently complain of inappropriate bleeding in response to trauma or surgery or apparently spontaneous external hemorrhage or hematoma formation. As with any inherited defect, one should obtain a careful history and examine the patient and any close relatives, including siblings and parents, if possible. Most inherited defects result from a single-factor abnormality. Routine coagulation studies may narrow the differential diagnoses for these bleeding disorders, but confirmation of diagnosis usually requires specialized tests. In contrast, most acquired defects of hemostasis are characterized by multiple-factor abnormalities, frequently with a severe underlying systemic disorder.

VON WILLEBRAND'S DISEASE

von Willebrand's factor is a glycoprotein of plasma, platelets, and endothelium required for platelet adhesion to exposed subendothelium and subsequent normal platelet plug formation. In plasma, vWF is bound in a multimolecular complex to coagulation factor VIII. Quantitative or qualitative abnormalities of vWF result in spontaneous bleeding from mucosal surfaces and excessive bleeding after surgery or trauma. Researchers have reported von Willebrand's disease in a Quarter Horse filly[337] that presented for episodes of oral bleeding, conjunctival hemorrhage, and prolonged bleeding at injection sites, as well as in a Thoroughbred mare and foal that presented for episodes of epistaxis. Routine complete blood count (CBC), including platelet count and coagulation times were within normal limits. Another 8-day-old Quarter Horse foal had a fever and numerous focal swellings at various sites around its body. This foal was persistently anemic and hypoproteinemic despite repeated transfusions and at necropsy was found to have significant hemarthrosis and secondary infection.[367] The ELISA for vWF is a sensitive and rapid means for diagnosis of this deficiency. Ristocetin, a co-factor involved in platelet aggregation, is deficient in human beings suffering from type II vWD. This specific deficiency was also identified in the aforementioned related Thoroughbreds.[368] This condition is heritable in human beings and dogs, and reports indicate the same is true in horses. Owners should not use affected animals for breeding.

FACTOR VIII DEFICIENCY

Classic hemophilia (factor VIII deficiency, hemophilia A) is the most commonly reported inherited defect of hemostasis in the horse. Hemophilia has been diagnosed in Thoroughbred, Standardbred, Quarter Horse, and Arabian colts[365,369-376] with severe spontaneous hemorrhage or excessive hemorrhage related to surgery or mild trauma. Coagulation testing reveals abnormal function of the intrinsic coagulation system, with a prolonged APTT and a normal PT. Diagnosis is confirmed by measuring factor VIII:C activity in plasma. In human beings the severity of clinical signs varies inversely with this value, and the same appears to be true for affected horses. In severely affected horses, factor VIII activity is less than 10% of normal equine plasma.[365,371,373] A less severely affected colt that survived castration and was undiagnosed until 3 years of age had a factor VIII activity of 20% to 30%.[375] As in human, canine, and feline hemophilia, equine factor VIII deficiency is transmitted as an X-linked recessive trait.[370] Carrier mares transmit the defect to 50% of male offspring on average. Carrier female horses usually have a factor VIII:C activity of approximately 50% of normal, although this value may vary widely and even overlap normal values. No cure exists for hemophilia, and the disease is progressively debilitating and potentially lethal. Affected human beings are treated with repeated transfusions of fresh plasma and factor concentrates. Factor IX and XI deficiencies have been reported in one Arabian foal with concurrent factor VIII deficiency.[372]

COAGULATION FACTOR ABNORMALITIES

In the classic pathway, initiation of the intrinsic coagulation system involves interaction of factor XII, prekallikrein, and HMWK ultimately to activate factor XI. This process usually begins with contact between factor XII and negatively charged molecules such as subendothelium or collagen. Prekallikrein deficiency has been diagnosed in families of Belgian horses[377] and American Miniature Horses.[378] Plasma prekallikrein deficiency is characterized by prolonged APTT with a normal PT. Affected horses may or may not show clinical signs of a bleeding tendency.[377,378] Confirmation of diagnosis is by demonstrating low prekallikrein activity with normal activity of other intrinsic coagulation factors. One also can correct the prolonged APTT by extended incubation with a contact activator.[377,378] In human beings, prekallikrein deficiency is inherited as an autosomal recessive or autosomal dominant trait.[379] The mode of inheritance in horses has not been confirmed, but appearance of the defect in multiple members of some equine families strongly suggests that it is an inherited disorder in this species as well. A similar defect in the contact phase of coagulation, not thought to result from prekallikrein deficiency, was diagnosed in one Quarter Horse gelding with prolonged APTT and normal PT.[380] Researchers did not observe a clinical bleeding problem in association with this defect.

Acquired Disorders of Hemostasis

VASCULITIS

Vasculitis, inflammation of blood vessels, may occur as a primary disease process but more commonly is encountered as a secondary complication of infectious, immunologic, toxic, or neoplastic disorders.[381] Hypersensitivity vasculitides are characterized by predominant involvement of small blood vessels in the skin. In most cases the postcapillary venules are involved. The most common inflammatory pattern is leukocytoclasis, defined by the presence of neutrophilic nuclear debris in and around the involved vessels. Vessel wall necrosis and fibrinoid changes occur.

Clinical signs depend on the type of vessel affected and the severity of the inflammatory response. Vascular occlusion may result in tissue ischemia and necrosis. Increased vascular permeability results in hemorrhage and edema as fluid and cellular constituents of the blood escape into the extravascular space. In horses, vasculitis is characterized by well-demarcated areas of cutaneous edema that may involve any portion of the body.[382] The distal extremities and ventral body wall are affected most commonly, and the edematous area is often hot and painful. Affected horses generally are depressed and reluctant to move. Hyperemia, petechial and ecchymotic hemorrhages, and ulcerations are commonly present on mucous membranes of the mouth, nose, and vulva. Other clinical signs may reflect edema, hemorrhage, and infarction in other body systems. Lameness, colic, diarrhea, dyspnea, or ataxia can result from involvement of vessels in joints, muscles, gastrointestinal tract, respiratory tract, and central nervous system. Subclinical renal disease may occur. Secondary complications such as laminitis, thrombophlebitis, and localized infections are common. Affected skin often weeps serum and eventually sloughs.

The underlying disease, length of illness, other organ involvement, and secondary complications usually determine hematologic and serum biochemical findings in vasculitis; none are characteristic. Neutrophilia, mild anemia, hyperglobulinemia, and hyperfibrinogenemia usually accompany chronic inflammation. The platelet count is often normal to increased but can be low because of a concomitant consumptive coagulopathy or IMTP. With renal involvement, serum creatinine may be elevated or urinalysis may reveal hematuria or proteinuria or both.

INFECTIOUS DISEASES

Infectious diseases associated with vasculitis and subsequent petechiation, ecchymoses, and dependent edema include EIAV, equine granulocytic ehrlichiosis, and equine viral arteritis (EVA). All three diseases may result in thrombocytopenia, although this is somewhat less common with EVA. The first two are discussed in detail elsewhere in this chapter; a discussion of EVA follows.

An arterivirus of the family Arteriviridae causes EVA. The disease can be characterized by fever, chemosis, lacrimation, rhinitis, focal dermatitis, ventral edema, and occasionally abortion.[383,384] However, many infected horses do not show recognizable clinical signs.

Horses become infected by aerosol or venereal contact with an infected animal. The virus replicates in the intima and media of most arteries, resulting in an inflammatory reaction and cellular influx.[385] Although mares and geldings generally clear the disease, stallions may become asymptomatic carriers of the disease, harboring virus in the accessory sex glands[383,386] and transmitting infection to previously unexposed mares. Infected mares usually make an uneventful recovery from EVA and eliminate the virus from the body. Abortion may occur during or shortly after acute illness or asymptomatic infection as a result of myometrial necrosis and edema leading to placental separation and fetal death.[387] Not all infected mares abort, however, and the incidence of abortion may be strain dependent.[388]

One confirms diagnosis of EVA in mares by serum neutralization assay, demonstrating a fourfold or greater rise in titer between acute and convalescent serum samples. EVA titer may remain elevated for a long time after natural infection, and recovered mares are considered immune to further infection.

Diagnosis of persistently infected, asymptomatic, nonvaccinated stallions depends on a positive serum neutralization test of greater than 1:4, with either isolation of the virus from semen samples or demonstration of seroconversion of an otherwise unexposed mare within 2 weeks of breeding to the suspect stallion.[389] Diagnosis of abortion caused by EVA requires virus isolation from the fetus or the placenta. Recent seroconversion in the mare is highly supportive of a diagnosis of EVA abortion.

A modified live virus vaccine is available but should be reserved for use only in breeding animals.[388] It should be administered annually to mares while open and to stallions or teasers 3 to 4 weeks before the breeding season.[390] Vaccinates should be isolated for 21 days after vaccination because of virus shedding during this time frame. Infections caused by the vaccinate strain cannot be distinguished from natural infection. Most breeding facilities require a negative serologic result before acceptance of semen, stallions, or broodmares. Any breeding animal that may be potentially exported must have a negative serologic test followed by an appropriate vaccination record before export.[391] Vaccine records should be carefully managed as to provide protection and allow accurate diagnostic testing.[392,393] One may offer supportive care to acutely infected animals and should isolate them from uninfected animals, especially pregnant mares.

IMMUNOLOGIC DISEASES

Most noninfectious cases of vasculitis in the horse are thought to be immune mediated. Small cutaneous vessels most commonly are affected, resulting in edema that may progress to skin infarctions, necrosis, and exudation.[381] The best characterized of these disorders is purpura hemorrhagica after *Streptococcus equi* subsp. *equi* infection. However, vasculitides of undetermined cause also have been described in the horse.[284,394] Most of these cases appear to have an immune-mediated cause. The antigenic stimulus of hypersensitivity vasculitis is usually a microbe, drug, toxin, or foreign or endogenous protein. The deposition of circulating immune complexes with subsequent vessel wall damage is probably the major event in the pathogenesis of these vasculitic syndromes. Soluble immune complexes, formed in moderate antigen excess, become deposited in blood vessel walls in areas of increased permeability. Deposited immune complexes activate complement with resulting formation of C5a, a potent chemotactic factor for neutrophils. Infiltrating neutrophils release lysosomal and other cytoplasmic enzymes such as elastase and collagenase that directly damage vessel walls. The net effect is vessel wall leakage and luminal compromise, resulting in edema, hemorrhage, thrombosis, and ischemic changes in supplied tissues.

Aside from vessel wall necrosis, vasculitis results in vascular dysfunction characterized by a net increase in vasoconstriction and platelet aggregation, which contribute to tissue ischemia.[395] The diseased endothelium releases endothelin, a polypeptide that causes contraction of underlying smooth muscle[396] and produces fewer dilator substances such as endothelial-derived relaxing factor.[397] Injury to the vessel wall also results in diminished prostacyclin production, which usually serves to maintain vasodilation and platelet nonreactivity.[267] Thus endothelial dysfunction contributes ultimately to vessel failure after vasculitis.

The factors that determine which individuals develop hypersensitivity vasculitis remain undefined. Genetic predisposition, altered immunoregulatory mechanisms, and the amount, relative size, and type of complement components in circulating immune complexes are important in determining the potential risk of developing vasculitis (because these factors determine how quickly the mononuclear phagocyte system clears immune complexes).[398] Perhaps even more significant in this potential risk are genetic and acquired differences in the number and activity of receptors for complement and IgG on erythrocytes and macrophages. The difference can affect immune complex handling and distribution greatly.[399,400] Receptors for complement and the Fc of IgG mediate immune complex transport to and removal by the macrophages of the mononuclear phagocyte system. Physical factors such as turbulence of blood flow, hydrostatic pressure within vessels, and previous endothelial damage likely determine the size, type, and location of blood vessels involved in vasculitis. Researchers believe that the propensity for lesion formation in the skin of dependent body portions likely is caused by the hydrostatic pressure in affected postcapillary venules in these areas.[267]

DIAGNOSIS

The diagnosis of vasculitis depends on demonstration of typical histologic changes (e.g., leukocytoclasis, fibrinoid necrosis) in involved vessels. One should obtain full-thickness punch biopsies (6 mm in diameter) of skin in an affected area and preserve it in 10% formalin for histopathologic study. The skin in the designated area may be clipped but not scrubbed before sampling. One can process the samples saved in Michel's transport medium subsequently for immunofluorescence analysis to detect immune complexes.[401] Multiple biopsies from various sites are optimal in reaching a diagnosis, because distribution of histologic lesions and immune complexes is patchy. However, affected skin is often on the distal limbs where risk increases for cellulitis or exuberant granulation tissue. The irregular distribution of histologic lesions, coupled with difficulty in obtaining biopsies, makes the definitive diagnosis of vasculitis difficult. Often a diagnosis of vasculitis is based on history, clinical signs, and response to therapy.

Purpura hemorrhagica is a syndrome of cutaneous vasculitis that can develop several weeks after infection with *Streptococcus equi* subsp. *equi, S. equi* subsp. *zooepidemicus,* influenza virus, *Corynebacterium pseudotuberculosis,* or equine herpesvirus. Purpura hemorrhagica also has been described as an adverse side effect of antistreptococcal vaccination in the horse. Purpura hemorrhagica after infection with *S. equi* subsp. *equi* has been attributed to deposition of circulating immune complexes consisting of IgA and *S. equi* subsp. *equi* M protein in small subcutaneous vessels.[402] In approximately 30% of affected horses, no viral, bacterial, or vaccine cause is identified.[381,403] Horses are often febrile with ventral edema, especially of the distal limbs. Affected animals frequently have great pain and are reluctant to move. Petechia and ecchymoses may be present on oral, nasal, and conjunctival mucous membranes. Extensive skin necrosis and sloughing often follow severe swelling. A more severe infarctive form of purpura has also been described.[404] Affected horses develop areas of infarcted skin, as well as areas of ischemic damage in the intestines, kidneys, and skeletal muscles. Reports show increased mortality with this form and indicate that older horses repeatedly vaccinated or exposed to *S. equi* subsp. *equi* may be at an increased risk of developing the syndrome.

Horses with purpura hemorrhagica are not usually thrombocytopenic but frequently have laboratory evidence of chronic inflammatory disease, including increased fibrinogen and total plasma protein, as well as neutrophilia.[381] Careful monitoring of physical examination parameters and lab values is important to rapidly identify changes in the disease including kidney and skeletal muscle involvement.[404] If *S. equi* subsp. *equi* is the possible inciting cause, then M protein titers can be measured. Titers in horses suffering from *S. equi* subsp. *equi*–induced purpura are often very high, but lower titers can be hard to interpret in horses that have been exposed to or vaccinated against the organism.[405] Cutaneous biopsy of affected areas may confirm the diagnosis. Histopathologically, a leukocytoclastic vasculitis characterized by neutrophilic accumulation in and around small dermal and subcutaneous vessels occurs.

TREATMENT

The aims in the therapy of equine vasculitic syndromes are (1) to remove the antigenic stimulus if possible, (2) to reduce vessel wall inflammation, (3) to normalize the immune response, and (4) to provide supportive care. Regardless of the cause, vasculitis in horses generally warrants aggressive nursing care, which one should institute immediately. Hydrotherapy can minimize edema, and pressure wraps are useful on the limbs. Animals that become severely depressed and fail to drink or those with dysphagia caused by pharyngeal edema require fluids, intravenously or via nasogastric tube. A tracheostomy may be necessary in horses with stridor and dyspnea that occurs after edema of the upper respiratory tract. Phenylbutazone, flunixin meglumine, or other NSAIDs are indicated to reduce vascular inflammation and provide analgesia. The disease also may warrant corticosteroid administration. Long-term antimicrobial therapy is indicated to reduce the incidence or severity of cellulitis or other septic sequelae.[403]

Because no treatment effectively eliminates EIA or EVA from the body, neither disease warrants specific therapy. Although equine anaplasmosis spontaneously resolves, elimination of the organism by oxytetracycline therapy considerably shortens the clinical course of disease.

When the cause is unknown, vasculitis can be difficult to treat because the antigenic stimulus remains undefined and may not be eliminated easily. One should discontinue administration of any drug being used at the time that signs occur. A thorough search for an underlying infection or neoplasia is warranted. Horses with a recent history of strangles or that have been exposed to the disease should receive procaine penicillin G at 22,000 U/kg intramuscularly twice daily or potassium penicillin G intravenously four times daily for at least 2 weeks. One should drain accessible abscesses and examine and culture the guttural pouches via endoscopy. Even though the sensitizing infection usually has resolved by the time signs of purpura hemorrhagica occur, ongoing sepsis and antigen production prolong the allergic vasculitis. Although the use of corticosteroids for treating hypersensitivity vasculitis was once controversial,[267] research and clinical experience suggest that horses with purpura hemorrhagica or idiopathic vasculitic syndromes respond favorably to corticosteroid therapy. Of the 53 cases documented, all were treated with corticosteroids, resulting in a 93% recovery rate.[381,403]

Mild cases of vasculitis may resolve without immunosuppressive therapy, but life-threatening edema involving the upper respiratory tract or causing organ system dysfunction necessitates early aggressive corticosteroid treatment. One should administer dexamethasone (0.05 to 0.2 mg/kg intravenously, intramuscularly, or orally once or twice daily) at the dose and rate necessary to reduce edema. Prednisolone may be substituted at 0.5 to 1.0 mg/kg orally twice daily for dexamethasone, but prednisone should not be used because it has poor oral absorption in the horse. After edema and hemorrhages start to resolve, one may reduce the corticosteroid dose gradually (by 10% to 15% every 1 to 2 days) while carefully monitoring the horse for relapse. It is not uncommon for horses with purpura hemorrhagica to require corticosteroid and antibiotic therapy for a period of 4 to 6 weeks before edema permanently resolves.

Occasionally, horses suffer disease flare-ups that require the corticosteroid dose to be increased over the previously efficacious level. In these instances, flunixin meglumine may enhance steroid efficacy. Antimicrobials are indicated throughout the period of systemic corticosteroid administration to reduce the incidence and severity of secondary sepsis.

PROGNOSIS

The prognosis for vasculitis depends on the initiating disease process. With early aggressive therapy and supportive care, most horses recover from purpura hemorrhagica within 4 weeks, although numerous sequelae may prolong the convalescence. A 93% recovery rate was reported in one study[403]; however, horses that suffer from the severe infarctive form carry a much poorer prognosis for recovery.[404] Dermal infarction in the distal limbs often leads to skin sloughing followed by exuberant granulation tissue and may require excision followed by skin grafting. Laminitis and various infections such as cellulitis, pneumonia, colitis, and thrombophlebitis are common and may be related to long-term corticosteroid therapy.

EVA and equine anaplasmosis carry a good prognosis, and disease confers some immunity to reinfection. Horses with EIA are infected persistently and may suffer recurrent clinical relapses. Horses with idiopathic vasculitic syndromes have an unpredictable response to therapy, and some have a poor prognosis. Inadequate resolution of hypersensitivity vasculitis in human beings usually is caused by failure to identify the antigenic stimulus or completely eliminate it from the body.[267]Although in most horses remission is spontaneous, some have debilitating cutaneous disease or develop systemic necrotizing vasculitis with a poor prognosis.

THROMBOCYTOPENIA

When circulating platelet counts decrease to less than 30,000 per microliter, a bleeding diathesis frequently occurs. Affected horses have petechial and ecchymotic hemorrhages of mucosal membranes, epistaxis, increased bleeding after venipuncture, melena, or hyphema.[281-286] Similar signs may occur in horses with platelet function defects. Disorders involving alterations in platelet number or function are described in previous sections.

VITAMIN K DEFICIENCY

Vitamin K is a fat-soluble vitamin essential for a final step, γ-carboxylation, in the hepatic synthesis of many coagulation factors. The serine proteases, including factors II, VII, IX, and

X, require γ-carboxylation of glutamate before they are biologically functional. Vitamin K deficiency results in a gradual decrease in functional coagulation factors in circulation that ultimately can end in a clinical syndrome of inappropriate bleeding. The rapidity with which coagulation factor concentrations in circulation decline depends largely on the half-life of those factors in circulation. Factor VII has a plasma half-life in the dog of 4 to 6 hours (compared with 41, 14, and 16 hours for factors II, IX, and X, respectively) and reaches a critical concentration in the circulation more rapidly than other vitamin K–dependent factors.[406] As a result, coagulation studies early in the course of vitamin K deficiency may reveal abnormalities in the extrinsic coagulation system (prolonged PT) with a normal intrinsic system (normal APTT). As the condition progresses, however, extrinsic and intrinsic coagulation parameters are abnormal.

All green leafy feeds, including hay and fresh pasture, contain high concentrations of vitamin K. For this reason, foals before weaning have decreased vitamin K levels as compared with adult horses.[407] Researchers also believe that vitamin K is synthesized by the intestinal microflora of many species. As a result, vitamin K deficiency only rarely results from an absolute deficiency of the nutrient in the diet. More commonly, deficiency results from an inability of the horse to absorb or use dietary vitamin K. Chronic intestinal malabsorption of lipids can result in clinical bleeding problems. One may assess dietary fat absorption by feeding 150,000 IU of vitamin A (another fat-soluble vitamin) in corn oil with grain and measuring increases in serum vitamin A concentration.[408] Concentrations should double over 12 to 24 hours. Fat absorption depends on bile acid secretion from the liver, and chronic cholestatic disorders also can result in decreased vitamin K absorption.

Antagonism of vitamin K by warfarin or other dicumarol derivatives is a more common clinical problem than is absolute vitamin-K deficiency. The dicumarol derivative warfarin has been advocated as an oral anticoagulant for use in horses with navicular disease[409] or jugular thrombophlebitis.[410] Warfarin also is the active ingredient in many rodenticides, and accidental exposure to toxic doses of the compound is possible. Warfarin is an effective antagonist of vitamin K and inhibits the production of functional coagulation factors II, VII, IX, and X. Warfarin therapy may begin with a daily dose of 0.018 mg/kg orally and increase in increments of 20% to achieve the desired therapeutic effect,[409] which usually results in a final dose of 0.012 to 0.75 mg/kg daily.

Concurrent administration of other drugs, especially phenylbutazone, may increase the risk of warfarin-induced hemorrhage. Phenylbutazone acts by competing with warfarin for binding sites on plasma albumin, increasing the concentration of free warfarin in circulation. Similarly, hypoalbuminemia can increase the risk of warfarin toxicosis. Thyroxin and corticosteroids lower the necessary therapeutic dose of warfarin by enhancing receptor affinity and increasing clotting factor catabolism. Rapid withdrawal of drugs that induce hepatic microsomal enzyme metabolism, such as rifampin, chloramphenicol, and barbiturates, also can potentiate toxicosis because these drugs enhance warfarin metabolism.

Because factor VII has the shortest half-life of the vitamin K–dependent factors, warfarin affects the extrinsic coagulation system more rapidly than the intrinsic system, and determination of PT is the most commonly used method for monitoring the effectiveness of warfarin anticoagulative therapy. An increase in PT of 1.5 to 2.5 times baseline is recommended as a therapeutic goal of warfarin anticoagulation.[410,411]

Toxic doses of warfarin result in spontaneous hemorrhage that may be life threatening. One makes a diagnosis of warfarin toxicity based on a history of exposure, clinical evidence of hemorrhage (bleeding from body orifices or into body cavities, hematoma formation, or clinical pathologic indications of blood loss anemia), prolonged PT or PTT with normal platelet count and fibrinogen and FDP concentrations, and response to exogenous vitamin K administration.[412]

Because warfarin interferes with the final stages of clotting factor synthesis, administration of vitamin K_1 at up to 1.0 mg/kg subcutaneously rapidly reverses toxicity.[410] One may repeat this dose every 4 to 6 hours until PT returns to normal, followed by daily monitoring for 3 to 4 days.[413] PT returns to normal approximately 5 days after the last dose of warfarin without administration of supportive therapy; administration of vitamin K_1 results in a return of PT to baseline within 24 hours.[413,414] In horses with severe bleeding, one should administer whole blood transfusions concurrently to replace plasma clotting factors. The horse should improve within 1 to 2 hours. One may administer smaller doses of vitamin K_1 orally, concurrent with warfarin, to titrate the anticoagulant effects of the latter.[415]

Second-generation anticoagulant rodenticides such as brodifacoum have a prolonged half-life (1.2 days) and lower median lethal dose compared with warfarin.[415] As a result, their potential for adverse effects are greater. History of exposure is important because therapy requires prolonged antidotal therapy.[416] Aggressive symptomatic and supportive therapy is often unsuccessful.[417]

Toxicosis caused by ingestion of moldy sweet clover (*Melilotus* spp.) hay is reported in all herbivores.[418] White sweet clover (*Melilotus alba*) and yellow sweet clover (*M. officinalis*) contain coumarin. When sweet clover hay is cured improperly, numerous fungi (e.g., *Penicillium, Mucor*) propagate; these fungi convert coumarin to 4-hydroxycoumarin, which condenses to dicumarol.[419] Animals that ingest sufficient quantities of moldy hay develop severe coagulation dysfunction within 2 to 7 days with internal and external hemorrhaging.[42] Continued ingestion of moldy hay can result in a lethal hemorrhagic crisis. One should consider toxicity as a diagnosis in horses with history of access to moldy sweet clover hay and can confirm the diagnosis with coagulation tests described previously for warfarin toxicosis. Suspect hay should be destroyed because toxic concentrations of dicumarol may remain for up to 4 years.[419]

One may treat clinical bleeding episodes resulting from inadequate vitamin K and subsequent deficiency in the levels of vitamin K–dependent coagulation factors in circulation with parenteral vitamin K_1 (phylloquinone) injections at a dosage of 0.3 to 0.5 mg/kg. Subcutaneous injection is recommended because intravenous administration has resulted in a high incidence of adverse reactions in other species. One ultimately must address underlying gastrointestinal or hepatic disorders as well. Parenterally administered vitamin K_3 (menadione sodium bisulfite) is nephrotoxic in horses at the manufacturer's recommended dose and should not be administered.[421] Horses that receive vitamin K_3 may show signs of colic, hematuria, azotemia, and electrolyte abnormalities consistent with acute renal failure.

Hepatic Diseases

Severe hepatic disease often is associated with hemorrhagic tendencies caused by decreased production of coagulation factors II, V, VII, IX, and X and fibrinogen. Impairment of bile acid secretion may impair absorption of the fat-soluble vitamins, resulting in decreased production of the vitamin K–dependent clotting factors. Hepatic Kupffer's cells are responsible for removal of many activated coagulation factors and FDPs from the circulation. Increased circulating FDPs inhibit normal platelet function and generation of fibrin. These abnormalities may combine to initiate DIC. A severe bleeding diathesis is a poor prognostic indicator in horses with hepatic disease.

Drug-Induced Alterations in Hemostasis

A variety of pharmaceutic agents can alter hemostatic mechanisms. Incorrect or poorly monitored administration of these agents may result in hemorrhagic tendencies in the horse.

ASPIRIN

Aspirin causes an irreversible inhibition of platelet function. The mechanisms and implications of this effect are discussed in previous sections.

HEPARIN

Heparin is a mucopolysaccharide complex of variable molecular weight that potentiates the activity of AT III in neutralizing coagulation factor X and increasing the rate of inactivation of other serine proteases (factors II, IX, XI, and XII).[422,423] Potentiation of AT III activity is attributed primarily to lower-molecular-weight forms of the molecule that inhibit factors X and XII, with minimal inhibitory effects on thrombin and factors IX and XI.[423] Heparin has been advocated for maintenance of the patency of indwelling catheters, prophylaxis for venous thrombosis and laminitis, anticoagulation of whole blood transfusions, prevention of postoperative peritoneal adhesions, and treatment and prevention of DIC.[422,424-427] Efficacy remains controversial with reports supporting and denying the effects of heparin.[428,429]

Bleeding complications associated with unfractionated heparin therapy are uncommon, but administration of protamine sulfate at up to 1 mg for every 90 to 100 U of heparin has been recommended in horses with heparin-associated hemorrhage.[422] Protamine sulfate forms a stable salt with heparin and with soluble fibrinogen monomers. If the FDP concentration increases in a patient, then precipitation of these salts may result in intravascular infarction, and use of protamine sulfate is contraindicated.

The most pronounced adverse effect associated with unfractionated heparin administration in the horse is a significant reduction in the circulating RBC mass.[291,430] Doses of 160 to 320 U/kg subcutaneously twice daily for nine doses resulted in a significant decrease in RBC numbers, PCV, and total hemoglobin, and an increase in MCV, with a rapid return of values to baseline after discontinuation of therapy.[291] Because heparin is known to increase the activity of mononuclear phagocytes, decreased RBC numbers originally were hypothesized to result from an enhanced phagocytosis of erythrocytes.[430] However, decreased RBC numbers now are thought to result primarily from in vivo erythrocyte agglutination.[431,432] One can reverse this agglutination in vitro by adding a trypsin solution to the RBC suspension. Decreases in RBC numbers and increases in MCV associated with heparin administration are most likely artifactual, resulting from the measurement of multiple agglutinated cells as single units.[432] Unfractionated heparin administration in horses (160 U/kg subcutaneously twice daily) also has been associated with development of large plaques of painful edema.[433]

Low-molecular-weight heparin (LMWH) is derived from unfractionated heparin by solvent extraction or gel filtration. The resulting drug is made up of smaller molecules and has more reliable anticoagulant properties, better bioavailability, and a longer half-life in human beings.[434] The pharmacokinetic properties of LMWH have been studied in the horse, and appropriate dosages have been identified.[435] An injection of 50 IU/kg of LMWH once daily was compared with unfractionated heparin at tapering dosages between 150 to 100 IU/kg twice daily in horses with colic.[436] Significantly more jugular vein problems were observed in horses receiving unfractionated heparin and adverse effects, including decreased PCV and prolonged APTT and TT, were markedly increased in the unfractionated group as compared with the LMWH group. Efficacy trials for the use of LMWH in prevention and treatment of hypercoagulability are lacking, but LMWH may offer fewer adverse effects as compared with horses treated with the unfractionated form. The use of this drug is often confounded by its expense in the horse.

Disseminated Intravascular Coagulation

DIC is a condition of pathologic activation of coagulative and fibrinolytic systems, ultimately leading to microvascular ischemia and secondary organ dysfunction. Human research indicates that the inflammatory cytokine cascade that results from massive trauma or sepsis is intimately associated with the development of a hypercoagulable state that can ultimately lead to DIC.[437] DIC may be acute or chronic, systemic or localized, and frequently is characterized by severe hemorrhage caused by consumption of coagulation factors, but it also may manifest as a pronounced thrombotic tendency due to a hypercoagulable state. The type and severity of clinical signs depend on the initial stimulus for pathologic systemic coagulation activation, the duration and extent of activation, the availability of coagulation factors, and the relative strengths of activation of procoagulant and fibrinolytic forces. The final result in horses with severe DIC is often widespread ischemic organ failure, severe hemorrhage, and death.

DIC is not considered a primary diagnosis and occurs after a variety of disorders triggered by many different mechanisms. In the horse, DIC most commonly is associated with gastrointestinal disease or sepsis.[438-448] The common initiating factor in most cases is endotoxin, the external lipopolysaccharide cell wall of gram-negative bacteria. Endotoxin can activate factor XII directly to initiate the intrinsic coagulation pathway and may cause widespread damage to vascular endothelium, exposing subendothelial collagen and releasing tissue thromboplastin to trigger the coagulation pathways. Endotoxin damages platelets, inducing aggregation and activation, and exposing platelet factor 3. Other conditions associated with DIC include intravascular hemolysis, bacteremia (gram positive or gram negative), viremia, neoplasia, circulating immune complexes, immune thrombocytopenia, fetal death in utero, burns, hepatic disease, renal disease, and vasculitides. Virtually any primary disease process may initiate DIC by injury to blood cells, increasing the availability of phospholipid surfaces, injury to vascular endothelium, or tissue injury and subsequent release of thromboplastin.[449]

As widespread activation of proinflammatory pathways occurs, kinins are generated and the complement cascade is stimulated.[449] Cytokines involved in the activation of this cascade include TNF-α, IL-1, IL-6, and IL-8.[450] Factor XIIa is responsible for initiating kinin formation by activating kallikrein, which in turn proteolytically converts HMWK to kinins. Bradykinin, the most physiologically important of the kinins, enhances vascular permeability, dilates some blood vessels, and stimulates migration of leukocytes into the extravascular space.[451] Plasmin activates the complement cascade and induces neutrophil chemotaxis, increases vascular permeability, and destroys RBCs and platelets, releasing membrane phospholipoprotein and ADP to act as procoagulants. Complement products can activate factor XII.

In response to endotoxin, mononuclear phagocytes release procoagulant substances including TF, platelet activating factor, TNF, and IL-1.[452] These phagocytic cells are responsible for removal of activated clotting factors and FDPs from the circulation. Massive concentrations of activated clotting factors or FDPs, or impairment of phagocytic function, can lead to abnormally high levels of either element in the blood. Activated clotting factors then remain available for continued coagulative events. Elevated FDP levels in the peripheral circulation can inhibit fibrin monomer polymerization and thrombin formation and also coat platelet membranes, interfering with aggregation.

The clinical signs associated with DIC in the horse vary widely and reflect the primary disease process, the duration and severity of coagulation activation, and the balance between procoagulant and fibrinolytic forces. Horses seldom show severe bleeding diathesis after DIC, and less severe forms of DIC in which the horse may be in a subclinical hypercoagulable state may go unnoticed. Careful clinical examination may reveal petechia and ecchymoses of mucous membranes and prolonged bleeding from venipuncture sites. Many horses exhibit an increased tendency to venous thrombosis after venipuncture.[442] Other clinical signs may reflect organ dysfunction after microvascular thrombosis and tissue ischemia. In the kidney, organ dysfunction may occur as tubulointerstitial disease and acute renal failure. In the foot, DIC may contribute to digital ischemia and laminitis[424,425,438,442]; however, experimentally induced laminitis was not associated with significant changes in hemostatic parameters.[364] Many horses with DIC have clinical signs reflecting poor peripheral perfusion and shock, including prolonged capillary refill time, cool extremities, and tachycardia, which may result from the primary disease process or occur after DIC-induced microvascular occlusion and inflammation.

Diagnosis of DIC depends on the results of a variety of tests assessing the quantity and function of coagulative substances. The most commonly evaluated parameters in horses are platelet count and function, PT, PTT, activated clotting time, and FDPs. Platelet counts usually are decreased in horses with DIC.[439-442,444,447] In horses with normal platelet counts, platelet function frequently is impaired.[438] Although coagulation times may be shorter early in the disease, rarely does one examine horses at this time. Most horses have reached a stage of hemorrhagic tendency, largely because of consumption of coagulative elements, by the time DIC is recognizable. These patients have increased PT, PTT, and activated clotting time. Because DIC accelerates fibrinolytic processes, elevations in circulating FDPs and D-dimers occur commonly.[438,442,444,447] In contrast to other species, horses with DIC commonly have normal to increased fibrinogen concentrations.[352,438,442,447] Fibrinogen acts as an acute phase reactant protein in the horse, and inflammation, which accompanies most cases of DIC in the horse, stimulates accelerated hepatic production.

Several other laboratory tests may aid in diagnosis of DIC in the horse. Decreased plasma AT III concentrations are considered a sensitive indicator of DIC in human beings.[453] Because AT III is bound irreversibly to serine proteases in the plasma, AT III is consumed rapidly during pathologic intravascular coagulation. AT III activity has been shown to decline in horses with experimentally induced large colon torsion.[445] This decline was reversible in horses that survived and persisted in horses that died. In horses with naturally occurring colic or acute colitis, plasma AT III activity is decreased significantly.[357,439,440] One does not always find decreases in AT III activity, however, and normal activity has been reported in ponies with coagulopathy after equine ehrlichial colitis.[443] Because AT III is a small protein, it may be lost from circulation in most disease conditions associated with hypoalbuminemia, including protein-losing enteropathies and nephropathies.[454] Increased plasma AT III activity has been associated with hepatic disease in the horse.[357]

Assays for equine α_2-antiplasmin, plasminogen, and protein C have been described, and normal values have been reported.[362-364] Plasma α_2-antiplasmin concentrations were decreased in ponies with coagulopathy after equine ehrlichial colitis. Plasminogen concentrations were increased in these ponies, possibly indicating a role of plasminogen as an acute phase reactant.[443] Plasma protein C concentrations may be decreased in human beings with DIC.[455] One may determine individual coagulation factor levels, but such determination rarely provides more information than PT or PTT.

Diagnostic criteria for DIC in the horse have not been defined rigidly. One must assess each patient in the light of the severity and duration of underlying disease processes, clinical appearance, and laboratory hemostatic values. Subclinical DIC may be documented with laboratory evaluation of animals that have no overt clinical signs of pathologic coagulopathy. Multiple hemostatic abnormalities in an animal with thrombotic or hemorrhagic tendencies strongly suggest DIC. Regardless of the definition of DIC, if a high index of suspicion exists, attempted therapy is warranted.

The therapeutic plan for horses with DIC must focus on treatment of the primary underlying disease process. Only by removing the pathologic stimulus for coagulation can procoagulant and fibrinolytic mechanisms be rebalanced effectively. One should administer supportive therapy for shock, decreased tissue perfusion, and acid-base and electrolyte abnormalities. If endotoxemia contributes to the disease process, then one should administer NSAIDs. Low-dose flunixin meglumine therapy (0.25 mg/kg intravenously three times daily) is effective in inhibiting endotoxin-induced cyclooxygenase activity.[456] One should treat animals with sepsis with appropriate antimicrobial agents. Fresh platelet-rich plasma can be introduced intravenously to horses with life-threatening hemorrhage after DIC. Fresh plasma resupplies soluble coagulation factors, and normal platelets may restore primary hemostatic mechanisms. The recommended dose of plasma for use in DIC in other species is typically 10 to 20 ml/kg or 5 to 10 L in the average horse, which is expensive. Because knowledge regarding the efficacy of this treatment is limited, few patients undergo such aggressive therapy. Administration of whole blood or blood products remains controversial in the treatment of patients with DIC because of the potential for worsening the coagulopathy on administration of fresh coagulation factors. One must consider this possibility, but in the face of life-threatening hemorrhage, benefits may outweigh risks.

Heparin therapy has been advocated for treatment of DIC in other species. Because heparin acts as an anticoagulant by complexing with AT III to inhibit serine proteases, AT III levels must be normal to achieve any benefits from heparin therapy. Heparin administration is controversial in the horse.[422,424-429] As discussed previously in this chapter, the use of LMWH has been advocated over unfractionated heparin because of a tendency for unfractionated heparin to cause erythrocyte agglutination and anemia in vivo.[291,432] The recommended dosage of LMWH is 50 to 100 IU/kg for dalteparin and 40 to 80 IU/kg for enoxaparin subcutaneously once daily.[435]

Aspirin, as mentioned previously, acts as an irreversible inhibitor of platelet cyclooxygenase, which leads to a decreased platelet aggregation. It has been used in horses in a hypercoagulable state. Aspirin can be given at 20 mg/kg either orally once daily or every other day; it can be given rectally once daily when oral administration is contraindicated. Adverse effects can include bleeding because of platelet dysfunction or gastrointestinal ulceration.[457]

Pentoxifylline and other methylxanthine derivatives are effective in decreasing the production of inflammatory cytokines, including TNF-α, IL-1, and IL-6, as well as increasing RBC flexibility.[458] This drug acts as a nonspecific phosphodiesterase inhibitor and may be helpful in decreasing clinical platelet activation in the horse.[459] Administration at 10 mg/kg orally twice daily yields appropriate plasma levels; however, long-term administration might require increasing dosages as the clinical response decreases with ongoing treatment.[458]

Other drugs, including etamsylate and recombinant hirudin, have been used successfully in other species for their antithrombogenic effects.[460,461] Initial investigation of these drugs in horses have yielded promising results, but further research is required.

Early recognition of DIC and aggressive therapy of underlying disease conditions remain the most effective treatments for the horse with pathologic coagulopathy. Understanding the pathogenesis and diagnosis of DIC will aid the practitioner in this process.

Thrombosis and Thrombophlebitis

A thrombus is an intravascular accumulation of fibrin, platelets, and leukocytes that usually occurs at a site of endothelial damage. Three factors may predispose a horse to vascular thrombosis: (1) vascular endothelial injury, (2) vascular stasis or slowing of blood flow, and (3) abnormalities of coagulation processes. After vascular damage, thrombus formation is the normal end result of procoagulative forces. However, pathologic or abnormal thrombus formation may occur in patients with an imbalance of procoagulative and fibrinolytic forces, as in DIC.

The horse appears to be particularly prone to superficial vein thrombosis during periods of systemic activation of coagulation. Jugular vein thrombosis may occur in these animals after a single, apparently atraumatic, venipuncture. Jugular catheter associated thrombophlebitis has been linked to several risk factors including catheter material and experience of the person placing the catheter,[462,463] but most risk factors are related to the patient. Studies suggest that endotoxemic horses and septicemic horses have an increased susceptibility to thrombosis at the site of indwelling venous catheters.[464] Bilateral jugular vein thrombosis leads to increased intravascular pressures proximal to the thrombus formation and severe edema of the head. This edema may impair respiratory function, necessitating tracheostomy. If one suspects that sepsis is contributing to thrombus formation, then appropriate antibiotic therapy should be initiated. If hypercoagulation may be a predisposing factor for thrombosis, then aspirin administration at 20 mg/kg every other day may be beneficial to inhibit platelet aggregation and release reactions.[338,341] Hot compresses and hydrotherapy may improve collateral blood flow and decrease inflammation at the site of thrombosis. The thrombus eventually should recanalize, and venous flow should return. One may assess recanalization and the size of the thrombus with ultrasound examination of blood flow through the affected vessel.[465] If an underlying disease process is present, then primary care should be directed at correcting this disorder. In horses with unilateral jugular vein thrombosis, one should protect patency of the opposite jugular vein by minimizing prothrombotic trauma to that vessel, including venipuncture or catheter placement.

BLOOD AND BLOOD COMPONENT THERAPY

Treatment of a variety of equine disorders involves administration of whole blood, plasma, or other blood constituents. One must base therapeutic decisions on clinical signs, laboratory parameters, availability of suitable donor services, and economic considerations.

Whole Blood Transfusion

One most commonly administers blood transfusions to horses with anemia severe enough to impair tissue oxygenation. Tachycardia, tachypnea, lethargy, weakness, cool extremities, and pale mucous membranes indicate significant tissue hypoxia and may occur at a PCV as high as 18 or as low as 10, depending on the rapidity of erythrocyte loss. Chronic anemias allow for physiologic adaptation to the low circulating RBC numbers, and severe clinical signs may not be apparent until the PCV is extremely low. Fresh whole blood transfusions also may be indicated in horses with severe hemorrhage associated with DIC to renew supplies of soluble coagulation factors and platelets.

Donor animals should lack detectable circulating alloantibodies against erythrocyte antigens that might be present in the recipient.[466,467] One can use crossmatching to detect existing antibody before transfusion. EDTA-anticoagulated blood and serum should be collected from the recipient and from several potential donor horses. The major crossmatch checks for compatibility between donor RBCs and any alloantibody that might be present in patient serum. The minor crossmatch assesses compatibility between alloantibody that might be present in donor serum and patient RBCs.[13] Both tests are important before transfusion of whole blood; the minor crossmatch is most critical when one contemplates plasma transfusion.

Transfusion of RBCs may sensitize the recipient to produce alloantibody against any incompatible erythrocyte antigens present in donor blood. For this reason, one should consider routine use of donors that are negative for factors Aa and Qa to prevent the inadvertent sensitization of brood mares against the two most common alloantigens involved in neonatal isoerythrolysis, Aa and Qa.

If crossmatching is not possible, unmatched transfusion for critical patients can be considered. One must weigh the potential adverse effects of a transfusion reaction against the potential benefits to the patient. Most horses without previous transfusions may safely receive a single transfusion or multiple transfusions over 3 to 4 days from an unmatched donor. Chances of an adverse reaction increase when either donors or recipients are mares that have been bred previously. For this reason, male horses or female horses that have never been pregnant are preferred as donor animals for unmatched transfusions.

One safely may remove 5 to 10 L of blood from most adult donor horses. All equipment used for blood or blood product collection and administration should be sterile, and all procedures should be performed with strict attention to aseptic technique. Stock solutions of acid citrate dextrose anticoagulant are available commercially. Alternatively, one may use sodium citrate as an anticoagulant, mixing one part of a 3.2% sodium citrate solution to nine parts whole blood. Plastic blood collection bags with premeasured anticoagulant are convenient and effective for use with horses. Equine RBCs are stable for 35 days after collection when collected and stored in commercially available bags using citrate phosphate dextrose (CPD) as the anticoagulant.[468]

The volume of blood administered to a patient depends on the severity of RBC depletion and the total blood volume. A recommended formula for calculating this is as follows[329]:

$$\text{Body mass (kg)} \times \text{blood volume (ml/kg)} \\ \times [(\text{PCV desired} - \text{PCV observed})/\text{PCV of donor blood}]$$

Normal blood volume in adult horses is approximately 72 ml/kg.[469] In neonates, blood volume is 151 ml/kg, decreasing to 93 ml/kg at 4 weeks, 82 ml/kg at 12 weeks, and adult values by 4 to 6 months of age.[470] Transfused RBCs survive less than 1 week in the horse, sometimes less than 2 days, and multiple transfusions may be necessary to maintain a patient until bone marrow production can exceed the rate of peripheral RBC destruction or loss.[471]

Blood products should be administered through an intravenous system with an in-line filter. Even with crossmatching of donor and recipient, one should administer the initial 25 to 50 ml of transfused blood slowly over 15 to 30 minutes with close monitoring of patient heart rate, respiratory rate, and behavior. If these parameters remain stable, then the remainder of the transfusion can be administered at a rate of 15 to 25 ml/kg/hr. One should give transfusions to horses with suspected or confirmed endotoxemia or septicemia more cautiously.

Several adverse reactions, immediate or delayed, may be associated with administration of blood or blood components. Mild reactions such as development of urticaria and tachycardia often occur.[472] More severe reactions are characterized by increases in heart and respiratory rates, dyspnea, fever, trembling, weakness, hypotension, diarrhea, abdominal pain, anaphylaxis, shock, or pulmonary edema. Acute hemolytic reactions with hemoglobinemia and hemoglobinuria result from transfusions from a donor with an incompatible blood type. DIC may accompany severe acute hemolysis. One should discontinue the transfusion immediately and administer supportive therapy. Intravenous crystalline fluids improve peripheral circulation and maintain renal perfusion. NSAIDs may decrease inflammatory reactions.

Febrile reactions are not uncommon during or immediately after transfusions and may result from incompatible leukocyte or platelet antigens or presence of pyrogens in the transfused blood. One should discontinue transfusions if clinical signs are severe. NSAIDs may help in decreasing the febrile response.

Occasionally, blood products become contaminated with bacteria or bacterial products, and their administration can result in severe septicemia and endotoxemia. Affected animals develop uncontrollable shaking, hypotension, weakness, tachycardia, tachypnea, and collapse. If this occurs, the transfusion should be discontinued immediately, supportive care should be provided, and the blood being administered should be cultured. A Gram stain may reveal bacteria if contamination is severe. In this case, one should institute appropriate antibiotic therapy. NSAIDs may help in alleviating the adverse effects of endotoxin.

More delayed reactions to transfusion include transmission of infectious diseases and allosensitization of the recipient. One should test all donor horses regularly for EIAV. Other infectious agents potentially transmittable via blood transfusions include *Anaplasma phagocytophilum* and the equine herpesviruses (EHV). Mares that receive blood transfusions are at risk for producing foals that develop neonatal isoerythrolysis later in life.

Plasma Transfusion

Plasma transfusion is indicated in horses with hypoproteinemia sufficient to result in significant fluid loss from the blood to the extravascular space and also is indicated for foals with failure of passive transfer (discussed previously in the text), replacement of some coagulation factors (II, V, VII, X, XIII), reversal of warfarin toxicity, endotoxemia-septicemia, and in some cases of DIC. Selection of donor animals, administration of plasma, and potential adverse reactions are similar to those described for whole blood transfusions. One may estimate the volume (in milliliters) to be administered to a hypoproteinemic horse from the following:

$$\text{Body mass (kg)} \times \text{blood volume (ml/kg)} \\ \times \frac{(\text{albumin desired - albumin observed})}{\text{albumin concentration of donor}}$$

Plasma volume in adult horses is estimated as 48 ml/kg.[469] In neonates, plasma volume is approximately 95 ml/kg, decreasing to 62 ml/kg at 4 weeks, 53 ml/kg at 12 weeks, and adult values by 4 to 6 months of age.[470] The observed increase in plasma protein after plasma transfusions is often not as great as would be predicted from this formula and most likely is caused by equilibration of administered blood proteins between intravascular and extravascular spaces.

Plasma transfusions should be administered cautiously in the same manner as whole blood transfusions. Severe anaphylaxis is possible, but most reactions are mild and include only urticaria and edema of the face and limbs. Patients should be monitored for these signs, as well as for increased heart rate, increased respiratory rate, sweating, colic, and agitation. Another less common reaction to plasma that has been described is fatal serum hepatitis. The four horses described had received plasma transfusions at 41 to 60 days before demonstration of clinical signs consistent with severe liver disease. This study estimated the prevalence of this complication to be 0.4% of horses older than 1 year of age receiving plasma transfusions.[473]

Plasma from suitable donors is commercially available. Large equine practices may consider the purchase of plasmapheresis equipment, capable of economically preparing large quantities of pure plasma. One also may prepare plasma by allowing erythrocytes in whole blood to settle by gravity or, preferably, by centrifugation. The plasma is then removed in an aseptic manner and administered through an intravenous system with an in-line filter. Compared with gravity flow, automated plasmapheresis is the preferred method of plasma collection; the effect on hematologic and coagulation factors is mild and of no consequence to the recepient.[474,475]

Blood Component Therapy

Continuous-flow centrifugation hemapheresis has been used extensively in human medicine to produce relatively pure blood components for administration to patients needing replacement of one specific blood constituent. This technique is being used increasingly in veterinary medicine and is the preferred method for equine plasma collection. Blood removed from one jugular vein of a donor horse circulates in a closed loop through the blood separation device, with collection of desired blood components and return of unwanted components to the donor via the opposite jugular vein.[476,477] By altering the centrifugal force of the collection device, one may collect plasma, RBCs, leukocytes, or platelets preferentially.[478]

Collection of leukocyte and platelet-rich fractions from horses has been described.[476,478] Platelet transfusions may be indicated in selected horses with thrombocytopenia. Leukocyte transfusions have been beneficial in septic human neonates, and the feasibility and efficacy of granulocyte transfusions in the equine neonate have been investigated.[478,479]

REFERENCES

1. Arnbjerg J: Poisoning in animals due to oral application of iron with a description of a case in a horse, *Nord Vet Med* 33:71, 1981.
2. Divers TJ, Warner A, Vaala WE, et al: Toxic hepatic failure in newborn foals, *J Am Vet Med Assoc* 183:1407, 1983.
3. Edens LM, Robertson JL, Feldman BF: Cholestatic hepatopathy, thrombocytopenia and lymphopenia associated with iron toxicity in a Thoroughbred gelding, *Equine Vet J* 25:81, 1993.
4. Lavoie JP, Teuscher E: Massive iron overload and liver fibrosis resembling haemochromatosis in a racing pony, *Equine Vet J* 25:552, 1993.
5. Cornelius C, Kaneko J, Benson D, et al: Erythrocyte survival studies in the horse, using glycine-2-C14, *Am J Vet Res* 21:1123, 1960.
6. Marcilese N, Figueiras H, Kremenchuzky S: Red cell survival time in the horse, determined with di-isopropyl-phosphorodluoridate-P32, *Am J Physiol* 211:281, 1966.
7. Stockham SL, Harvey JW, Kinden DA: Equine glucose-6-phosphate dehydrogenase deficiency, *Vet Pathol* 31:518-527, 1994.
8. Harvey JW, Stockham SL, Scott MA, et al: Methemoglobinemia and eccentrocytosis in equine erythrocyte flavin adenine dinucleotide deficiency, *Vet Pathol* 40:632-642, 2003.
9. Harvey R, Hambright M, Rowe L: Clinical biochemical and hematologic values of the American Miniature Horse: reference values, *Am J Vet Res* 45:987, 1984.
10. Zinkl J, Mae D, Merida P, et al: Reference ranges and the influence of age and sex on hematologic and serum biochemical values in donkeys *(Equus asinus)*, *Am J Vet Res* 51:408, 1990.
11. Harvey J, Asquith R, McNulty P, et al: Haematology of foals up to one year old, *Equine Vet J* 16:347, 1984.
12. Latimer KS, Mahaffey EA, Prasse KW: *Duncan and Prasse's veterinary laboratory medicine*, ed 4, Ames, Iowa, 2003, Iowa State University Press.
13. Feldman BF, Zinkl JG, Jain NC: *Schalm's veterinary hematology*, ed 5, Philadelphia, 2000, Lippincott Williams & Wilkins.
14. Reef V, Dyson S, Beech J: Lymphosarcoma and associated immune-mediated hemolytic anemia and thrombocytopenia in horses, *J Am Vet Med Assoc* 184:313, 1984.
15. Perk K, Frei Y, Herz A: Osmotic fragility of red blood cells of young and mature domestic laboratory animals, *Am J Vet Res* 25:1241, 1964.
16. Russell KE, Sellon DC, Grindem CB: Bone marrow in horses: indications, sample handling, and complications, *Compend Contin Educ Pract Vet* 16:1359, 1994.
17. Franken P, Wensing T, Schotman A: The bone marrow of the horse. I. The techniques of sampling and examination and values of normal warm-blooded horses, *Zentralbl Veterinarmed A* 29:16, 1982.
18. Franken P, Wensing T, Schotman A: The bone marrow of the horse. I. Warm-blooded horses with anaemia, *Zentralbl Veterinarmed A* 29:23, 1982.
19. Tschudi P, Archer R, Gerber H: The cells of equine blood and their development, *Equine Vet J* 7:141, 1975.
20. Calhoun M: A cytological study of the costal marrow. III. Hemograms of the horse and cow, *Am J Vet Res* 16:297, 1955.
21. Tablin F, Weiss L: Equine bone marrow: a quantitative analysis of erythroid maturation, *Anat Rec* 213:202, 1985.
22. Schalm O: Equine hematology. IV. Erythroid marrow cytology in response to anemia, *Vet Clin North Am Equine Pract* 2:35, 1980.
23. Tschudi P, Archer R, Gerber H: Cytochemical staining of equine blood and bone marrow cells, *Equine Vet J* 9:205, 1977.
24. Smith J, Moore K, Cipriano J, et al: Serum ferritin as a measure of stored iron in horses, *J Nutr* 114:677, 1984.
25. Osbaldiston G, Griffith P: Serum iron levels in normal and anemic horses, *Can Vet J* 13:105, 1972.
26. Smith J, DeBowes R, Cipriano J: Exogenous corticosteroids increase serum iron concentrations in mature horses and ponies, *J Am Vet Med Assoc* 133:1296, 1986.
27. Harvey JW, Asquith RL, Sussman WA, et al: Serum ferritin, serum iron, and erythrocyte values in foals, *Am J Vet Res* 48:1348, 1987.
28. Mullaney TP, Brown CM: Iron toxicity in neonatal foals, *Equine Vet J* 20:119, 1988.
29. McFarlane D, Sellon DC, Parker B: Primary erythrocytosis in a 2-year-old Arabian gelding, *J Vet Intern Med* 12:384, 1998.
30. Torton M, Schalm O: Influence of the equine spleen on rapid changes in the concentration of erythrocytes in peripheral blood, *Am J Vet Res* 25:500, 1964.
31. Archer R, Clabby J: The effect of excitation and exertion on the circulation blood of horses, *Vet Rec* 77:689, 1965.
32. Keenan D: Changes in packed cell volume of horses during races, *Aust Vet Pract* 10:125, 1980.
33. Dalton R: The significance of variations with activity and sedation in the haematocrit, plasma protein concentration and erythrocyte sedimentation rate of horses, *Br Vet J* 128:439, 1972.
34. Beech J, Bloom JC, Hodge TG: Erythrocytosis in a horse, *J Am Vet Med Assoc* 184:986, 1984.
35. Bayly WM, Reed SM, Leathers CW, et al: Multiple congenital heart anomalies in five Arabian foals, *J Am Vet Med Assoc* 181:684, 1982.

36. Berlin NI: Diagnosis and classification of the polycythemias, *Semin Hematol* 12:339, 1975.
37. Cook T, Divers TJ, Rowland PH: Hypercalcaemia and erythrocytosis in a mare associated with a metastatic carcinoma, *Equine Vet J* 27:316, 1995.
38. Koch TG, Wen X, Bienzle D: Lymphoma, erythrocytosis, and tumor erythropoietin gene expression in a horse, *J Vet Intern Med* 20(5):1251-1255, 2006.
39. Lennox TJ, Wilson JH, Hayden DW, et al: Hepatoblastoma with erythrocytosis in a young female horse, *J Am Vet Med Assoc* 216:718, 2000.
40. Roby KA, Beech J, Bloom JC, et al: Hepatocellular carcinoma associated with erythrocytosis and hypoglycemia in a yearling filly, *J Am Vet Med Assoc* 196:465, 1990.
41. Jeffcott LB: Primary liver-cell carcinoma in a young Thoroughbred horse, *J Pathol* 97:394, 1969.
42. Weiss DJ, Moritz A: Equine immune-mediated hemolytic anemia associated with *Clostridium perfringens* infection, *Vet Clin Pathol* 32(1):22-26, 2003.
43. Cooper C, Sears W, Bienzle D: Reticulocyte changes after experimental anemia and erythropoietin treatment of horses, *J Appl Physiol* 99:915-921, 2005.
44. Lumsden HJ, Valli VE, McSherry BJ, et al: The kinetics of hematopoiesis in the light horse. III. The hematological response to hemolytic anemia, *Can J Comp Med* 39:332, 1975.
45. Lumsden JH, Valli VE, McSherry BJ, et al: The kinetics of hematopoiesis in the light horse. II. The hematological response to hemorrhagic anemia, *Can J Comp Med* 39:324, 1975.
46. Radin M, Eubank M, Weiser M: Electronic measurement of erythrocyte volume and volume heterogeneity in horses during erythrocyte regeneration associated with experimental anemias, *Vet Pathol* 23:656, 1986.
47. Easley JR: Erythrogram and red cell distribution width of Equidae with experimentally induced anemia, *Am J Vet Res* 46:2378, 1985.
48. Weiser G, Kohn C, Vachon A: Erythrocyte volume distribution analysis and hematologic changes in two horses with immune-mediated hemolytic anemia, *Vet Pathol* 20:424, 1983.
49. Shull R: Biochemical changes in equine erythrocytes during experimental regenerative anemia, *Cornell Vet* 71:280, 1981.
50. Wu MJ, Feldman BF, Zinkl JG, et al: Using red blood cell creatine concentration to evaluate the equine erythropoietic response, *Am J Vet Res* 44:1427, 1983.
51. Kaneko JJ, Tanaka S, Nakajima H, et al: Enzymes of equine erythrocytes: changes during equine infectious anemia, *Am J Vet Res* 30:543, 1969.
52. Smith JE, Agar NS: Studies on erythrocyte metabolism following acute blood loss in the horse, *Equine Vet J* 8:34, 1976.
53. Rooney JR: Internal haemorrhage related to gestation in the mare, *Cornell Vet* 54:11, 1964.
54. Lofstedt R: Haemorrhage associated with pregnancy and parturition, *Equine Vet Educ* 6:138, 1994.
55. Scoggin CF, McCue PM: How to assess and stabilize a mare suspected of periparturient hemorrhage in the field, *Proceedings Am Assn Eq Pract* 53:342-348, 2007.
56. Pascoe RR: Rupture of the utero-ovarian or middle uterine artery in the mare at or near parturition, *Vet Rec* 104:77, 1979.
57. Stowe HD: Effects of age and impending parturition upon serum copper of Thoroughbred mares, *J Nutr* 95:179, 1968.
58. Arnold CE, Payne M, Thompson JA, et al: Periparturient hemorrhage in mares: 73 cases (1998-2005), *J Am Vet Med Assoc* 232:1345-1351, 2008.
59. Moon PF, Snyder JR, Haskins SC, et al: Effects of a highly concentrated hypertonic saline-dextran volume expander on cardiopulmonary function in anesthetized normovolemic horses, *Am J Vet Res* 52:1611, 1991.
60. Belgrave RL, Hines MT, Keegan RD, et al: Effects of a polymerized ultrapurified bovine hemoglobin blood substitute administered to ponies with normovolemic anemia, *J Vet Intern Med* 16:396, 2002.
61. Maxson AD, Giger U, Sweeney CR, et al: Use of a bovine hemoglobin preparation in the treatment of cyclic ovarian hemorrhage in a miniature horse, *J Am Vet Med Assoc* 203:1308, 1993.
62. Weld JM, Kamerling SG, Combie JD, et al: The effects of naloxone on endotoxic and hemorrhagic shock in horses, *Res Commun Chem Pathol Pharmacol* 44:227-238, 1984.
63. Heidmann P, Tornquist SJ, Qu A, et al: Laboratory measures of hemostasis and fibrinolysis after intravenous administration of epsilon-aminocaproic acid in clinically normal horses and ponies, *Am J Vet Res* 66:313-318, 2005.
64. Ross J, Dallap BL, Dolente BA, et al: Pharmacokinetics and pharmacodynamics of epsilon-aminocaproic acid in horses, *Am J Vet Res* 68:1016-1021, 2007.
65. Graham L, Farnsworth K, Cary J: The effect of Yunnan baiyao on the template bleeding time and activated clotting time in healthy halothane anesthetized ponies. In Proceedings of the Eighth International Veterinary Emergency Critical Care Society Symposium, San Antonio, Tex, 2002.
66. Magdesian KG, Fielding CL, Rhodes DM, et al: Changes in central venous pressure and blood lactate concentration in response to acute blood loss in horses, *J Am Vet Med Assoc* 229:1458-1462, 2006.
67. McKeever K, Kirby K, Hinchcliff KW: Effects of erythropoietin on plasma and red cell volume Vo_2 max and hemodynamics in exercising horses [abstract], *Med Sci Sports Exerc* 25:S23, 1993.
68. Malikides N, Kessell A, Hodgson JL, et al: Bone marrow response to large volume blood collection in the horse, *Res Vet Sci* 67:285, 1999.
69. Allen B, Archer RK: Haptoglobins in the horse, *Vet Rec* 89:106, 1971.
70. McGuire T, Henson J: The detection of intravascular haemolysis in the horse, *Br Vet J* 125:v-vi, 1969.
71. Tennant B, Dill SG, Glickman LT, et al: Acute hemolytic anemia, methemoglobinemia, and Heinz body formation associated with ingestion of red maple leaves by horses, *J Am Vet Med Assoc* 179:143, 1981.
72. Alsup EM, DeBowes RM: Dimethyl sulfoxide, *J Am Vet Med Assoc* 185:1011, 1984.
73. MacLachlan N, Divers T: Hemolytic anemia and fibrinoid change of renal vessels in a horse, *J Am Vet Med Assoc* 181:716, 1982.
74. Morris CF, Robertson JL, Mann PC, et al: Hemolytic uremic-like syndrome in two horses, *J Am Vet Med Assoc* 191:1453, 1987.
75. Duncan S: Oak leaf poisoning in two horses, *Cornell Vet* 51:159, 1961.
76. Beck DJ: A case of primary autoimmune haemolytic anaemia in a pony, *Equine Vet J* 22:292, 1990.
77. Dodds W: Autoimmune hemolytic disease and other causes of immune-mediated anemia: an overview, *J Am Anim Hosp Assoc* 13:437, 1977.
78. Moriarty K, Brown M, Sutton R: An anaemic state in a horse associated with a cold-acting antibody, *N Z Vet J* 24:85, 1976.
79. Reef VB: *Clostridium perfringens* cellulitis and immune-mediated hemolytic anemia in a horse, *J Am Vet Med Assoc* 182:251, 1983.
80. Anderson L: Idiopathic auto-immune haemolytic anaemia in a horse, *N Z Vet J* 22:102, 1974.
81. Sutton R, Pearce H, Kelley C, et al: Auto-immune haemolytic anaemia in a horse, *N Z Vet J* 26:311, 1978.
82. Kitchen H, Krehbiel JD: Proceedings of the First International Symposium on Equine Hematology, East Lansing, MI, 1975, American Assoc Equine Practitioners.
83. Davis EG, Wilkerson MJ, Rush BR: Flow cytometry: clinical applications in equine medicine, *J Vet Intern Med* 16:404-410, 2002.

84. Farrelly B, Collins J, Collins S: Autoimmune haemolytic anaemia (AHA) in the horse, *Ir Vet J* 20:42, 1977.
85. Blue J, Dinsmore R, Anderson K: Immune-mediated hemolytic anemia induced by penicillin in horses, *Cornell Vet* 77:263, 1987.
86. McConnico RS, Roberts MC, Tompkins M: Penicillin-induced immune-mediated hemolytic anemia in a horse, *J Am Vet Med Assoc* 201:1402, 1992.
87. Step DL, Blue JT, Dill SG: Penicillin-induced hemolytic anemia and acute hepatic failure following treatment of tetanus in a horse, *Cornell Vet* 81:13, 1991.
88. Robbins RL, Wallace SS, Brunner CJ, et al: Immune-mediated haemolytic disease after penicillin therapy in a horse, *Equine Vet J* 25:462, 1993.
89. Thomas HL, Livesey MA: Immune-mediated hemolytic anemia associated with trimethoprim-sulphamethoxazole administration in a horse, *Can Vet J* 39:171, 1998.
90. Bailey E: Prevalence of anti-red blood cell antibodies in the serum and colostrum of mares and its relationship to neonatal isoerythrolysis, *Am J Vet Res* 43:1982, 1917.
91. Geor RJ, Clark EG, Haines DM, et al: Systemic lupus erythematosus in a filly, *J Am Vet Med Assoc* 197:1489, 1990.
92. Messer NT, Arnold K: Immune-mediated hemolytic anemia in a horse, *J Am Vet Med Assoc* 198:1415, 1991.
93. Pierce KR, Joyce JR, England RB, et al: Acute hemolytic anemia caused by wild onion poisoning in horses, *J Am Vet Med Assoc* 160:323, 1972.
94. Fettman M: Comparative aspects of glutathione metabolism affecting individual susceptibility to oxidant injury, *Compend Contin Educ Pract Vet* 13:1079, 1991.
95. Clark B, Morrissey R: Relation of methemoglobin to hemolysis, *Blood* 6:532, 1951.
96. Harvey JW: Pathogenesis, laboratory diagnosis, and clinical implications of erythrocyte enzyme deficiencies in dogs, cats and horses, *Vet Clin Pathol* 35:144-156, 2006.
97. Dixon PM, McPherson EA, Muir A: Familial methaemoglobinaemia and haemolytic anaemia in the horse associated with decreased erythrocytic glutathione reductase and glutathione, *Equine Vet J* 9:198, 1977.
98. Divers TJ, George LW, George JW: Hemolytic anemia in horses after the ingestion of red maple leaves, *J Am Vet Med Assoc* 180:300, 1982.
99. George LW, Divers TJ, Mahaffey EA, et al: Heinz body anemia and methemoglobinemia in ponies given red maple (*Acer rubrum* L.) leaves, *Vet Pathol* 19:521, 1982.
100. Corriher CA, Parviainen AKJ, Gibbons DS, et al: Equine red maple leaf toxicosis, *Compend Contin Educ Pract Vet* 21:74, 1999.
101. Alward A, Corriher CA, Barton MH, et al: Red maple *(Acer rubrum)* leaf toxicosis in horses: a retrospective study of 32 cases, *J Vet Intern Med* 20:1197-1201, 2006.
102. Boyer JD, Breeden DC, Brown DL: Isolation, identification, and characterization of compounds from *Acer rubrum* capable of oxidizing equine erythrocytes, *Am J Vet Res* 63:604-610, 2002.
103. McConnico R, Brownie C: The use of ascorbic acid in the treatment of 2 cases of red maple *(Acer rubrum)*—poisoned horses, *Cornell Vet* 82:293, 1992.
104. Cullison R: Acetaminophen toxicosis in small animals: clinical signs, mode of action, and treatment, *Compend Contin Educ Pract Vet* 6:315, 1984.
105. Thorp F, Harsefield G: Onion poisoning in horses, *J Am Vet Med Assoc* 94:52, 1939.
106. McSherry B, Roe C, Milne F: The hematology of phenothiazine poisoning in horses, *Can Vet J* 7:3, 1966.
107. Purchase H: Phenothiazine poisoning in a Thoroughbred racing stable, *J S Afr Vet Med Assoc* 32:403, 1961.
108. Wright M, Davison K: Nitrate accumulation in crops and nitrate poisoning in animals, *Adv in Agronomy* 16:197, 1964.
109. Davidson W, Doughty J, Bolton J: Nitrate poisoning of livestock, *Can J Comp Med* 5:303, 1941.
110. Rollins JB, Wigton DH, Clement TH: Heinz body anemia associated with lymphosarcoma in a horse, *Vet Clin North Am Equine Pract* 13:20, 1991.
111. Norman TE, Chaffin MK, Johnson MC, et al: Intravascular hemolysis associated with severe cutaneous burn injuries in five horses, *J Am Vet Med Assoc* 226:2039-2043, 2005.
112. Clabough D: Equine infectious anemia: the clinical signs, transmission, and diagnostic procedures, *Vet Med* 85:1007, 1990.
113. Clabough D: The immunopathogenesis and control of equine infectious anemia, *Vet Med* 85:1020, 1990.
114. McGuire TC, Henson JB, Quist SE: Viral-induced hemolysis in equine infectious anemia, *Am J Vet Res* 30:2091, 1969.
115. McGuire TC, Henson JB, Quist SE: Impaired bone marrow response in equine infectious anemia, *Am J Vet Res* 30:2099, 1969.
116. Sentsui H, Kono Y: Complement-mediated hemolysis of horse erythrocytes treated with equine infectious anemia virus, *Arch Virol* 95:53, 1987.
117. Perryman LE, O'Rourke KI, McGuire TC: Immune responses are required to terminate viremia in equine infectious anemia lentivirus infection, *J Virol* 62:3073, 1988.
118. Clabough DL, Gebhard D, Flaherty MT, et al: Immune-mediated thrombocytopenia in horses infected with equine infectious anemia virus, *J Virol* 65:6242, 1991.
119. Russell KE, Perkins PC, Hoffman MR, et al: Platelets from thrombocytopenic ponies acutely infected with equine infectious anemia virus are activated in vivo and hypofunctional, *Virology* 259:7, 1999.
120. Crawford TB, Wardrop KJ, Tornquist SJ, et al: A primary production deficit in the thrombocytopenia of equine infectious anemia, *J Virol* 70:7842, 1996.
121. Russell KE, Walker KM, Miller RT, et al: Hyperglobulinemia and lymphocyte subset changes in naturally infected, inapparent carriers of equine infectious anemia virus, *Am J Vet Res* 59:1009, 1998.
122. Oaks JL, McGuire TC, Ulibarri C, et al: Equine infectious anemia virus is found in tissue macrophages during subclinical infection, *J Virol* 72:7263, 1998.
123. Oaks JL, Ulibarri C, Crawford TB: Endothelial cell infection in vivo by equine infectious anaemia virus, *J Gen Virol* 80:2393, 1999.
124. Clabough D, Perry S, Coggins L, et al: Wild-type equine infectious anemia virus replicates in vivo predominantly in tissue macrophages, not in peripheral blood monocytes, *J Virol* 66:5906, 1992.
125. Kemen MJ Jr, Coggins L: Equine infectious anemia: transmission from infected mares to foals, *J Am Vet Med Assoc* 161:496, 1972.
126. Burns SJ: Equine infectious anemia: plasma clearance times of passively transferred antibody in foals, *J Am Vet Med Assoc* 164:64, 1974.
127. Tashjian R: Transmission and clinical evaluation of an equine infectious anemia herd and their offspring over a 13-year period, *J Am Vet Med Assoc* 184:282, 1984.
128. Burki F, Rossmanith E: Comparative evaluation of the agar gel immunodiffusion test and two commercial ELISA kits for the serodiagnosis of equine infectious anemia, *Zentralbl Veterinarmed A* 37:448, 1990.
129. Issel CJ, Adams WV Jr: Detection of equine infectious anemia virus in a horse with an equivocal agar gel immunodiffusion test reaction, *J Am Vet Med Assoc* 180:276, 1982.
130. McConnell S, Katada M, Darnton S: Occult equine infectious anemia in an immunosuppressed serologically negative mare, *Vet Clin North Am Equine Pract* 5:32, 1983.
131. Tashjian RJ, editor: *Equine infectious anemia: a review of policies, programs, and future objectives*, Amarillo, Tex, 1985, American Quarter Horse Association.

132. Hall RF, Pursell AR, Cole JR Jr, et al: A propagating epizootic of equine infectious anemia on a horse farm, *J Am Vet Med Assoc* 193:1082, 1988.
133. Moltinann H, Melhourn H, Schein G: Ultrastructural study of the development of *Babesia equi* (Coccidia: Piroplasmia) in the salivary glands of its vector ticks, *J Protozool* 30:218, 1983.
134. Holbrook AA: Biology of equine piroplasmosis, *J Am Vet Med Assoc* 155:453, 1969.
135. Kumar S, Kumar R, Gupta AK, et al: Passive transfer of *Theileria equi* antibodies to neonate foals of immune tolerant mares, *Vet Parasitol* 151:80-85, 2008.
136. Taylor WM, Bryant JE, Anderson JB, et al: Equine piroplasmosis in the United States—a review, *J Am Vet Med Assoc* 155:915, 1969.
137. Diana A, Guglielmini C, Candini D, et al: Cardiac arrhythmias associated with piroplasmosis in the horse: a case report, *Vet J* 174:193-195, 2007.
138. Ogunremi O, Halbert G, Mainar-Jaime R, et al: Accuracy of an indirect fluorescent-antibody test and of a complement-fixation test for the diagnosis of *Babesia caballi* in field samples from horses, *Prev Vet Med* 83:41-51, 2008.
139. Knowles DP, Perryman LE, McElwain TF, et al: Conserved recombinant antigens of *Anaplasma marginale* and *Babesia equi* for serologic diagnosis, *Vet Parasitol* 57:93-96, 1995.
140. Brüning A: Equine piroplasmosis an update on diagnosis, treatment and prevention, *Br Vet J* 152:139-151, 1996.
141. Kirkham WW: The treatment of equine babesiosis, *J Am Vet Med Assoc* 155:457, 1969.
142. Butler CM, Nijhof AM, van der Kolk JH, et al: Repeated high dose imidocarb dipropionate treatment did not eliminate *Babesia caballi* from naturally infected horses as determined by PCR-reverse line blot hybridization, *Vet Parasitol* 151:320-322, 2008.
143. Kuttler KL, Zaugg JL, Gipson CA: Imidocarb and parvaquone in the treatment of piroplasmosis *(Babesia equi)* in equids, *Am J Vet Res* 48:1613, 1987.
144. Frerichs WM, Allen PC, Holbrook AA: Equine piroplasmosis *(Babesia equi)*: therapeutic trials of imidocarb dihydrochloride in horses and donkeys, *Vet Rec* 93:73, 1973.
145. Singh B, Banerjee D, Guatam O: Comparative efficacy of diminazene diaceturate and imidocarb dipropionate against *B. equi* infection in donkeys, *Vet Parasitol* 7:173, 1980.
146. Zaugg JL, Lane VM: Evaluations of buparvaquone as a treatment for equine babesiosis *(Babesia equi)*, *Am J Vet Res* 50:782, 1989.
147. Tennant B, Evans C, Kaneko J, et al: Intravascular hemolysis associated with hepatic failure in the horse, *Calif Vet J* 26:15, 1972.
148. Ramaiah SK, Harvey JW, Giguère S, et al: Intravascular hemolysis associated with liver disease in a horse with marked neutrophil hypersegmentation, *J Vet Intern Med* 17:360-363, 2003.
149. Colman RW, Hirsch J, Marder VJ, et al: *Hemostasis and thrombosis: basic principles and clinical practice*, ed 2, Philadelphia, 1987, JB Lippincott.
150. Stillions M, Teeter S, Nelson W: Utilization of dietary B_{12} and cobalt by mature horses, *J Anim Sci* 32:252, 1971.
151. Waldron-Mease E: Hypothyroidism and myopathy in racing Thoroughbreds and Standardbreds, *J Equine Med Surg* 3:124, 1979.
152. Kohn CW, Jacobs RM, Knight D, et al: Microcytosis, hypoferremia, hypoferritemia, and hypertransferrinemia in Standardbred foals from birth to 4 months of age, *Am J Vet Res* 51:1198, 1990.
153. Smith JE, Cipriano JE, DeBowes R, et al: Iron deficiency and pseudo-iron deficiency in hospitalized horses, *J Am Vet Med Assoc* 188:285, 1986.
154. Fleming KA, Barton MH, Latimer KS: Iron deficiency anemia in a neonatal foal, *J Vet Intern Med* 20:1495-1498, 2006.
155. Woods PR, Campbell G, Cowell RL: Nonregenerative anemia associated with administration of recombinant human erythropoietin in a Thoroughbred racehorse, *Equine Vet J* 29:326, 1997.
156. Piercy RJ, Swardson CJ, Hinchcliff KW: Erythroid hypoplasia and anemia following administration of recombinant human erythropoietin to two horses, *J Am Vet Med Assoc* 212:244, 1998.
157. Lavoie JP, Morris DD, Zinkl JG, et al: Pancytopenia caused by bone marrow aplasia in a horse, *J Am Vet Med Assoc* 191:1462, 1987.
158. Archer R, Miller W: A case of idiopathic hypoplastic anaemia in a two-year-old Thoroughbred filly, *Vet Rec* 77:538, 1965.
159. Ward M, Mountan P, Dodds W: Severe idiopathic refractory anemia and leukopenia in a horse, *Calif Vet J* 4:19, 1982.
160. Angel KL, Spano JS, Schumacher J, et al: Myelophthisic pancytopenia in a pony mare, *J Am Vet Med Assoc* 198:1039, 1991.
161. Berggren PC: Aplastic anemia in a horse, *J Am Vet Med Assoc* 179:1400, 1981.
162. Milne EM, Pyrah ITG, Smith KC, et al: Aplastic anemia in a Clydesdale foal: a case report, *J Equine Vet Sci* 15:129, 1995.
163. Archer R, Jeffcott L: *Comparative clinical hematology*, Oxford, 1977, Blackwell Scientific.
164. Athens J, Haab O, Raab S, et al: Leukokinetic studies. IV. The total blood, circulating, and marginal granulocyte pools and the granulocyte turnover rate in normal subjects, *J Clin Invest* 40:989, 1961.
165. Carakostas MC, Moore WE, Smith JE: Intravascular neutrophilic granulocyte kinetics in horses, *Am J Vet Res* 42:623, 1981.
166. Carakostas MC, Moore WE, Smith JE, et al: Effects of etiocholanolone and prednisolone on intravascular granulocyte kinetics in horses, *Am J Vet Res* 42:626, 1981.
167. Dale D, Fauci A, Wolff S: Alternate day prednisone: leukocyte kinetics and susceptibility to infections, *N Engl J Med* 291:1154, 1974.
168. Prasse KW, George LW, Whitlock RH: Idiopathic hypersegmentation of neutrophils in a horse, *J Am Vet Med Assoc* 178:303, 1981.
169. Ward DS, Fessler JF, Bottoms GD, et al: Equine endotoxemia: cardiovascular, eicosanoid, hematologic, blood chemical, and plasma enzyme alterations, *Am J Vet Res* 48:1150, 1987.
170. Brewer BD, Koterba AM: Development of a scoring system for the early diagnosis of equine neonatal sepsis, *Equine Vet J* 20:18, 1988.
171. Searcy G, Orr J: Chronic granlulocytic leukemia in a horse, *Can Vet J* 22:148, 1981.
172. Jain NC, Vegad JL, Kono CS: Methods for detection of immune-mediated neutropenia in horses, using antineutrophil serum of rabbit origin, *Am J Vet Res* 51:1026, 1990.
173. Leidl W, Cwik S, Schmid D: Neonatal isoimmune leukopenia in foals, *Berl Munch Tierarztl Wochenschr* 93:141, 1980.
174. Davis EG, Rush B, Bain F, Clark-Price S, et al: Neonatal neutropenia in an Arabian foal, *Equine Vet J* 35:517-520, 2003.
175. Kohn C, Couto G, Swardson S, et al: Myeloid hypoplasia in related Standardbreds, *J Vet Intern Med* 6:133, 1992.
176. Madigan JE, Zinkl JG, Fridmann DM, et al: Preliminary studies of recombinant bovine granulocyte colony stimulating factor on haematological values in normal neonatal foals, *Equine Vet J* 26:159, 1994.
177. Zinkl JG, Madigan JE, Fridmann DM, et al: Haematological, bone marrow and clinical chemical changes in neonatal foals given canine recombinant granulocyte-colony stimulating factor, *Equine Vet J* 26:313, 1994.
178. Sullivan KE, Snyder JR, Madigan JE, et al: Effects of perioperative granulocyte colony stimulating factor in horses with large colon ischemia, *Vet Surg* 22:343, 1994.

179. Burguez PN, Ousey J, Cash RS, et al: Changes in blood neutrophil and lymphocyte counts following administration of cortisol to horses and foals, *Equine Vet J* 15:58, 1983.
180. Morris DD, Bloom JC, Roby KA, et al: Eosinophilic myeloproliferative disorder in a horse, *J Am Vet Med Assoc* 185:993, 1984.
181. Duckett WM, Matthews HK: Hypereosinophilia in a horse with intestinal lymphosarcoma, *Can Vet J* 38:719, 1997.
182. McFarlane D, Sellon DC, Gaffney D, et al: Hematologic and serum biochemical variables and plasma corticotropin concentration in healthy aged horses, *Am J Vet Res* 59:1247, 1998.
183. McFarlane D, Sellon DC, Gibbs SA: Age-related quantitative alterations in lymphocyte subsets and immunoglobulin isotypes in healthy horses, *Am J Vet Res* 62:1413, 2001.
184. Ringger NC, Edens L, Bain P, et al: Acute myelogenous leukaemia in a mare, *Aust Vet J* 75:329-331, 1997.
185. Johansson AM, Skidell J, Lilliehöök I, et al: Chronic granulocytic leukemia in a horse, *J Vet Intern Med* 21:1126-1129, 2007.
186. Clark P, Cornelisse CJ, Schott HC, et al: Myeloblastic leukaemia in a Morgan horse mare, *Equine Vet J* 31:446-448, 1999.
187. Brumbaugh GW, Stitzel KA, Zinkl JG, et al: Myelomonocytic myeloproliferative diseases in a horse, *J Am Vet Med Assoc* 180:313, 1982.
188. Boudreaux MK, Blue JT, Durham SK, et al: Intravascular leukostasis in a horse with myelomonocytic leukemia, *Vet Pathol* 21:544, 1984.
189. Blue J, Perdrizet J, Brown E: Pulmonary aspergillosis in a horse with myelomonocytic leukemia, *J Am Vet Med Assoc* 190:1562, 1987.
190. Spier SJ, Madewell BR, Zinkl JG, et al: Acute myelomonocytic leukemia in a horse, *J Am Vet Med Assoc* 188:861, 1986.
191. Burkhardt E, Saldern FV, Huskamp B: Monocytic leukemia in a horse, *Vet Pathol* 21:394, 1984.
192. Lester GD, Alleman AR, Raskin RE, et al: Pancytopenia secondary to lymphoid leukemia in three horses, *J Vet Intern Med* 7:360-363, 1993.
193. McClure JT: Leukoproliferative disorders in horses, *Vet Clin North Am Equine Pract* 16:165-182, 2000.
194. Theilen GH, Madewell BR: *Veterinary cancer medicine*, Philadelphia, 1979, Lea & Febiger.
195. van den Hoven R, Franken P: Clinical aspects of lymphosarcoma in the horse, *Equine Vet J* 15:49, 1983.
196. Neufeld JL: Lymphosarcoma in the horse: a review, *Can Vet J* 14:129, 1973.
197. Mackey VS, Wheat JD: Reflections on the diagnostic approach to multicentric lymphosarcoma in an aged Arabian mare, *Equine Vet J* 17:467, 1985.
198. Haley PJ, Spraker T: Lymphosarcoma in an aborted equine fetus, *Vet Pathol* 20:647, 1983.
199. Tomlinson MJ, Doster AR, Wright ER: Lymphosarcoma with virus-like particles in a neonatal foal, *Vet Pathol* 16:629, 1983.
200. Savage CJ: Lymphoproliferative and myeloproliferative disorders, *Vet Clin North Am Equine Pract* 14:563-578, 1998.
201. Dascanio JJ, Zhang CH, Antczak DF, et al: Differentiation of chronic lymphocytic leukemia in the horse. A report of two cases, *J Vet Intern Med* 6:225-229, 1992.
202. McClure JT, Young KM, Fiste M, et al: Immunophenotypic classification of leukemia in 3 horses, *J Vet Intern Med* 15:144-152, 2001.
203. Rendle DI, Durham AE, Thompson JC, et al: Clinical, immunophenotypic and functional characterization of T-cell leukaemia in six horses, *Equine Vet J* 39:522-528, 2007.
204. Kannegieter NJ, Alley MR: Ataxia due to lymphosarcoma in a young horse, *Aust Vet J* 64:377, 1987.
205. Marayama K, Swearingen GR, Dmochowsku L, et al: Herpes type virus and type C particles in spontaneous equine lymphoma. In Proceedings of the Twenty-Eighth Annual Meeting of the Electron Microscope Society Of America, 1970, p 162.
206. Meyer J, DeLay J, Bienzle D: Clinical, laboratory, and histopathologic features of equine lymphoma, *Vet Pathol* 43:914-924, 2006.
207. Perryman LE, Wyatt CR, Magnuson NS: Biochemical and functional characterization of lymphocytes from a horse with lymphosarcoma and IgM deficiency, *Comp Immunol Microbiol Infect Dis* 7:53, 1984.
208. Dopson LC, Reed SM, Roth JA, et al: Immunosuppression associated with lymphosarcoma in 2 horses, *J Am Vet Med Assoc* 182:1239, 1983.
209. Furr MO, Crisman MV, Robertson J, et al: Immunodeficiency associated with lymphosarcoma in a horse, *J Am Vet Med Assoc* 201:307, 1992.
210. Ansar Ahmed S, Furr M, Chickering WR, et al: Immunologic studies of a horse with lymphosarcoma, *Vet Immunol Immunopathol* 38:229, 1993.
211. Perkins GA, Nydam DV, Flaminio MJ, et al: Serum IgM concentrations in normal, fit horses and horses with lymphoma or other medical conditions, *J Vet Intern Med* 17:337-342, 2003.
212. Grindem CB, Roberts MC, McEntee MF: Large granular lymphocyte tumour in a horse, *Vet Pathol* 26:86, 1989.
213. Rebhun WC, Bertone AL: Equine lymphosarcoma, *J Am Vet Med Assoc* 184:720, 1984.
214. Schalm OW: Lymphosarcoma in the horse, *Vet Clin North Am Equine Pract* 3:23, 1981.
215. Lawn K: Sudden death due to thoracic lymphoma in a Standardbred racing horse, *Can Vet J* 46:528-529, 2005.
216. Mair TS, Lane JG, Laucke VM: Clinicopathological features of lymphosarcoma involving the thoracic cavity in the horse, *Equine Vet J* 17:428, 1985.
217. Garber JL, Reef VB, Reimer JM: Sonographic findings in horses with mediastinal lymphosarcoma: 13 cases (1985-1992), *J Am Vet Med Assoc* 205:1432, 1994.
218. Saulez MN, Schlipf JW, Cebra CK, et al: Use of chemotherapy for treatment of a mixed cell thoracic lymphoma in a horse, *J Am Vet Med Assoc* 224:733-738, 2004.
219. Bertone AL, Yovich JV, McIlwraith CW: Surgical resection of intestinal lymphosarcoma in a mare, *Compend Contin Educ Pract Vet* 7:S506, 1985.
220. Traub-Dargatz JL, Bayly WM, Reed SM, et al: Intraabdominal neoplasia as a cause of chronic weight loss in the horse, *Compend Contin Educ Pract Vet* 5:S526, 1983.
221. Wiseman A, Petrie L, Murray M: Diarrhea in the horse as a result of alimentary lymphosarcoma, *Vet Rec* 95:454, 1974.
222. Sheahan BJ, Atkins GJ, Russell RJ, et al: Histiolymphocytic lymphosarcoma in the subcutis of two horses, *Vet Pathol* 17:123, 1980.
223. Henson KL, Alleman AR, Cutler TJ, et al: Regression of subcutaneous lymphoma following removal of an ovarian granulosa theca cell tumor in a horse, *J Am Vet Med Assoc* 212:1419, 1998.
224. Lane PC: Palatine lymphosarcoma in two horses, *Equine Vet J* 17:465, 1985.
225. Adams R, Calderwood-Mays MB, Peyton LC: Malignant lymphoma in three horses with ulcerative pharyngitis, *J Am Vet Med Assoc* 193:674, 1988.
226. Esplin DJ, Taylor JL: Hypercalcemia in a horse with lymphosarcoma, *J Am Vet Med Assoc* 170:180, 1977.
227. Murphy CJ, Lavoie JP, Groff J, et al: Bilateral eyelid swelling attributable to lymphosarcoma in the horse, *J Am Vet Med Assoc* 194:939, 1989.
228. Rousseaux CG, Doige CE, Tuddenham TJ: Epidural lymphosarcoma with myelomalacia in a seven-year-old Arabian gelding, *Can Vet J* 30:751, 1989.
229. Shamis LB, Everitt JI, Baker GJ: Lymphosarcoma as the cause of ataxia in a horse, *J Am Vet Med Assoc* 184:1517, 1984.
230. Rebhun WC, Del Piero F: Ocular lesions in horses with lymphosarcoma: 21 cases (1977-1997), *J Am Vet Med Assoc* 212:852, 1998.

231. Lester GD, MacKay RJ, Smith-Meyer B: Primary meningeal lymphoma in a horse, *J Am Vet Med Assoc* 201:1219, 1992.
232. Freeman SL, England GC, Bjornson S, et al: Uterine T cell lymphoma in a mare, with multicentric involvement, *Vet Rec* 141:391-393, 1997.
233. Held JP, McCracken MD, Toal R, et al: Epididymal swelling attributable to generalized lymphosarcoma in a stallion, *J Am Vet Med Assoc* 201:1913-1915, 1992.
234. Coumbe KM: Primary parotid lymphoma in a 10 year old Hanoverian gelding, *Eq Vet Educ* 6:91-94, 1994.
235. Sweeney RW, Hamir AN, Fisher RR: Lymphosarcoma with urinary bladder infiltration in a horse, *J Am Vet Med Assoc* 199:1177-1178, 1991.
236. Gerard MP, Healy LN, Bowman KF, et al: Cutaneous lymphoma with extensive periarticular involvement in a horse, *J Am Vet Med Assoc* 213:391-393, 1998.
237. Raidal SL, Clark P, Raidal SR: Angiotrophic T-cell lymphoma as a cause of regenerative anemia in a horse, *J Vet Intern Med* 20:1009-1013, 2006.
238. Madewell BR, Carlson GP, MacLachlan NJ, et al: Lymphosarcoma with leukemia in a horse, *Am J Vet Res* 43:807, 1982.
239. Roberts MC: A case of primary lymphoid leukaemia in a horse, *Equine Vet J* 9:216, 1977.
240. Bernard WV, Sweeney CR, Morris CR, et al: Primary lymphocytic leukemia in a horse, *Vet Clin North Am Equine Pract* 10:24, 1988.
241. Green PD, Donovan LA: Lymphosarcoma in a horse, *Can Vet J* 18:257, 1977.
242. Roberts MC, Pinsent PJN: Malabsorption in the horse associated with alimentary lymphosarcoma, *Equine Vet J* 7:166, 1975.
243. Finley MR, Rebhun WC, Dee A, et al: Paraneoplastic pruritus and alopecia in a horse with diffuse lymphoma, *J Am Vet Med Assoc* 213:102, 1998.
244. Mair TS, Yeo SP, Lucke VM: Hypercalcaemia and soft tissue mineralization associated with lymphosarcoma in two horses, *Vet Rec* 126:99, 1990.
245. Moore BR, Weisbrode SE, Biller DS, et al: Metacarpal fracture associated with lymphosarcoma-induced osteolysis in a horse, *J Am Vet Med Assoc* 207:208, 1995.
246. Marr CM, Love S, Pirie HM: Clinical, ultrasonographic and pathological findings in a horse with splenic lymphosarcoma and pseudohyperparathyroidism, *Equine Vet J* 21:221, 1989.
247. Robinson NE, editor: *Current therapy in equine medicine*, ed 6, St Louis, 2009, WB Saunders.
248. La Perle KM, Piercy RJ, Long JF, et al: Multisystemic, eosinophilic, epitheliotropic disease with intestinal lymphosarcoma in a horse, *Vet Pathol* 35:144, 1998.
249. McConnel S, Katada M, Fiske RA, et al: Equine lymphosarcoma diagnosed as equine infectious anemia in a young horse, *Equine Vet J* 14:160, 1982.
250. Lock PF, Macy DW: Equine ovarian lymphosarcoma, *J Am Vet Med Assoc* 175:72, 1979.
251. Thatcher CD, Roussel AJ, Chickering WR, et al: Pleural effusion with thoracic lymphosarcoma in a mare, *Compend Contin Educ Pract Vet* 7:S726, 1985.
252. Taylor SD, Pusterla N, Vaughan B, et al: Intestinal neoplasia in horses, *J Vet Intern Med* 20:1429-1436, 2006.
253. Zicker SC, Wilson WD, Medearis I: Differentiation between intra-abdominal neoplasms and abscesses in horses, using clinical and laboratory data: 40 cases (1973-1988), *J Am Vet Med Assoc* 196:1130-1134, 1990.
254. Hambright MB, Meuten DJ, Scrutchfield WL: Equine lymphosarcoma, *Compend Contin Educ Pract Vet* 5:S53, 1983.
255. Allen BV, Wannop CC, Wright IM: Multicentric lymphosarcoma with lymphoblastic leukemia in a young horse, *Vet Rec* 115:130, 1984.
256. Chaffin MK, Schmitz DG, Brumbaugh GW, et al: Ultrasonographic characteristics of splenic and hepatic lymphosarcoma in three horses, *J Am Vet Med Assoc* 201:743, 1992.
257. Dabareiner RM, Sullins KE, Goodrich LR: Large colon resection for treatment of lymphosarcoma in two horses, *J Am Vet Med Assoc* 208:895, 1996.
258. Henson FMD, Dixon PM, Dobson JM: Treatment of 4 cases of equine lymphoma with megavoltage radiation, *Equine Vet Educ* 16:312-314, 2004.
259. Mair TS, Couto CG: The use of cytotoxic drugs in equine practice, *Equine Vet Educ* 18:149-156, 2006.
260. Gollagher RD, Zoila B, Chelack BJ, et al: Immunotherapy of equine cutaneous lymphosarcoma using low dose cyclophosphamide and autologous tumor cells infected with vaccinia virus, *Can Vet J* 34:371-373, 1993.
261. Littlewood JD, Whitwell KE, Day MJ: Equine cutaneous lymphoma: a case report, *Vet Dermatol* 6:105, 1995.
262. Cornelius CE, Goodbary RF, Kennedy PC: Plasma cell myelomatosis in a horse, *Cornell Vet* 49:478, 1959.
263. Drew RA, Greatorex JC: Vertebral plasma cell myeloma causing posterior paralysis in a horse, *Equine Vet J* 6:131, 1974.
264. Henry M, Prasse K, White S: Hemorrhagic diathesis caused by multiple myeloma in a three-month-old foal, *J Am Vet Med Assoc* 194:392, 1989.
265. MacAllister C, Qualls C, Ryler L, et al: Multiple myeloma in a horse, *J Am Vet Med Assoc* 191:337, 1987.
266. Markel MD, Dorr TE: Multiple myeloma in a horse, *J Am Vet Med Assoc* 188:621, 1986.
267. Goldman L, Ausiello DA, editors: *Cecil textbook of medicine*, ed 23, Philadelphia, 2008, WB Saunders.
268. Seide RK, Jacobs RM, Dobblestein TN, et al: Characterization of a homogenous paraprotein from a horse with spontaneous multiple myeloma syndrome, *Vet Immunol Immunopathol* 17:69, 1987.
269. Barton MH, Sharma P, LeRoy BE, et al: Hypercalcemia and high serum parathyroid hormone-related protein concentration in a horse with multiple myeloma, *J Am Vet Med Assoc* 225:409-413, 2004.
270. Kim DY, Taylor HW, Eades SC, et al: Systemic AL amyloidosis associated with multiple myeloma in a horse, *Vet Pathol* 42:81-84, 2005.
271. Jacobs RM, Kociba GJ, Ruoff WW: Monoclonal gammopathy in a horse with defective hemostasis, *Vet Pathol* 20:643, 1983.
272. Thrall MA: Lymphoproliferative disorders: lymphocytic leukemia and plasma cell myeloma, *Vet Clin North Am Small Anim Pract* 11:321, 1981.
273. Pusterla N, Stacy BA, Vernau W, et al: Immunoglobulin A monoclonal gammopathy in two horses with multiple myeloma, *Vet Rec* 155:19-23, 2004.
274. Jackson M: Platelet physiology and platelet function: inhibition by aspirin, *Compend Contin Educ Pract Vet* 9:627, 1987.
275. Gerrard J: Platelet aggregation: cellular regulation and physiologic role, *Hosp Pract* 23:89, 1988.
276. Segura D, Monreal L, Perez-Pujol S, et al: Assessment of platelet function in horses: ultrastructure, flow cytometry, and perfusion techniques, *J Vet Intern Med* 20(3):581-588, 2006.
277. Meyers KM, Lindner C, Grant B: Characterization of the equine platelet aggregation response, *Am J Vet Res* 40:260, 1979.
278. Coyne CP, Kelly AB, Hornof WJ, et al: Radiolabeling of equine platelets in plasma with 111-In-(2-mercaptopyridine-N-oxide) and their in vivo survival, *Am J Vet Res* 48:385, 1987.
279. Sellon DC, Grindem CB: Quantitative platelet abnormalities in horses, *Compend Contin Educ Pract Vet* 16:1335, 1994.
280. Finocchio E, Coffman J, Osbaldiston G: Platelet counts in horses, *Cornell Vet* 60:518, 1960.
281. Byars TD, Greene CE: Idiopathic thrombocytopenic purpura in the horse, *J Am Vet Med Assoc* 180:1422, 1982.
282. Larson VL, Perman V, Stevens JB: Idiopathic thrombocytopenic purpura in two horses, *J Am Vet Med Assoc* 183:328, 1983.

283. Sockett DC, Traub-Dargatz J, Weiser MG: Immune-mediated hemolytic anemia and thrombocytopenia in a foal, *J Am Vet Med Assoc* 190:308, 1987.
284. Werner LL, Gross TL, Hillidge CJ: Acute necrotizing vasculitis and thrombocytopenia in a horse, *J Am Vet Med Assoc* 185:87, 1984.
285. Morris DD, Whitlock RH: Relapsing idiopathic thrombocytopenia in a horse, *Equine Vet J* 15:73, 1983.
286. Humber KA, Beech J, Cudd TA, et al: Azathioprine for treatment of immune-mediated thrombocytopenia in two horses, *J Am Vet Med Assoc* 199:591, 1991.
287. Hinchcliff KW, Kociba GJ, Mitten L: EDTA-dependent pseudothrombocytopenia in a horse, *J Am Vet Med Assoc* 203:1715, 1993.
288. Kingston JK, Bayly WM, Sellon DC, et al: Effects of sodium citrate, low molecular weight heparin, and prostaglandin E1 on aggregation, fibrinogen binding, and enumeration of equine platelets, *Am J Vet Res* 62:547, 2001.
289. Sellon DC, Levine J, Millikin E, et al: Thrombocytopenia in horses: 35 cases (1989-1994), *J Vet Intern Med* 10:127, 1996.
290. Russell KE, Perkins PC, Grindem CB, et al: Flow cytometric method for detecting thiazole orange-positive (reticulated) platelets in thrombocytopenic horses, *Am J Vet Res* 58:1092, 1997.
291. Duncan SG, Meyers KM, Reed SM: Reduction of the red blood cell mass of horses: toxic effect of heparin anticoagulant therapy, *Am J Vet Res* 44:2271, 1983.
292. Bell W: Thrombocytopenia occurring during heparin therapy, *N Engl J Med* 295:276, 1976.
293. Myers T, Kim B, Steiner M, et al: Platelet-associated complement C3 in immune thrombocytopenic purpura, *Blood* 59:1023, 1982.
294. Nel JD, Stevens K, Mouton A, et al: Platelet-bound IgM in autoimmune thrombocytopenia, *Blood* 61:119, 1983.
295. Court WS, Bozeman JM, Soong SJ, et al: Platelet surface-bound IgG in patients with immune and nonimmune thrombocytopenia, *Blood* 69:278, 1987.
296. Neiman J, Mant M, Shnitka T: Phagocytosis of platelets by Kupffer cells in immune thrombocytopenia, *Arch Pathol Lab Med* 111:563, 1987.
297. Hoffman R, Zaknoen S, Yang H, et al: An antibody cytotoxic to megakaryocyte progenitor cells in a patient with immune throbocytopenic purpura, *N Engl J Med* 312:1170, 1985.
298. McGurrin MK, Arroyo LG, Bienzle D: Flow cytometric detection of platelet-bound antibody in three horses with immune-mediated thrombocytopenia, *J Am Vet Med Assoc* 224:83-87, 2004.
299. Buechner-Maxwell V, Scott MA, Godber L, et al: Neonatal alloimmune thrombocytopenia in a Quarter Horse foal, *J Vet Intern Med* 11:304, 1997.
300. Ramirez S, Gaunt SD, McClure JJ, et al: Detection and effects on platelet function of antiplatelet antibody in mule foals with experimentally induced neonatal alloimmune thrombocytopenia, *J Vet Intern Med* 13:534, 1999.
301. White SD, Maxwell LK, Szabo NJ, et al: Pharmacokinetics of azathioprine following single-dose intravenous and oral administration and effects of azathioprine following chronic oral administration in horses, *Am J Vet Res* 66:1578-1583, 2005.
302. Fey K, Sasse HL: Relapsing immune-mediated thrombocytopenia of unknown origin in a stallion, *Equine Vet Educ* 10:127, 1998.
303. Sellon DC: Thrombocytopenia in horses, *J Vet Intern Med* 10:133, 1998.
304. Traub-Dargatz JL, McClure JJ, Koch C, et al: Neonatal isoerythrolysis in mule foals, *J Am Vet Med Assoc* 206:67, 1995.
305. Tornquist SJ, Crawford TB: Suppression of megakaryocyte colony growth by plasma from foals infected with equine infectious anemia virus, *Blood* 90:2357, 1997.
306. Wardrop KJ, Baszler TV, Reilich E, et al: A morphometric study of bone marrow megakaryocytes in foals infected with equine infectious anemia virus, *Vet Pathol* 33:222, 1996.
307. Nolen-Walston RD, D'Oench SM, Hanelt LM, Sharkey LC, et al: Acute recumbency associated with *Anaplasma phagocytophilum* infection in a horse, *J Am Vet Med Assoc* 224(12):1964-1966, 2004.
308. Gribble DH: Equine ehrlichiosis, *J Am Vet Med Assoc* 155:462, 1969.
309. Madigan JE, Gribble D: Equine ehrlichiosis in northern California: 49 cases (1968-1981), *J Am Vet Med Assoc* 190:445, 1987.
310. Ziemer EL, Keenan DP, Madigan JE: *Ehrlichia equi* infection in a foal, *J Am Vet Med Assoc* 190:199, 1987.
311. Brewer BD, Harvey JW, Mayhew IG, et al: Ehrlichiosis in a Florida horse, *J Am Vet Med Assoc* 185:446, 1984.
312. Franzén P, Aspan A, Egenvall A, et al: Acute clinical, hematologic, serologic, and polymerase chain reaction findings in horses experimentally infected with a European strain of *Anaplasma phagocytophilum*, *J Vet Intern Med* 19:232-239, 2005.
313. Madigan JE, Gribble D: Equine ehrlichiosis in northern California: 49 cases (1968-1981), *J Am Vet Med Assoc* 190:445-448, 1987.
314. Madigan JE, Pusterla N: Ehrlichial diseases, *Vet Clin North Am Equine Pract* 16:487-499, 2000.
315. Franzén P, Berg AL, Aspan A, et al: Death of a horse infected experimentally with *Anaplasma phagocytophilum*, *Vet Rec* 160:122-125, 2007.
316. Dolente BA, Wilkins PA, Boston RC: Clinicopathologic evidence of disseminated intravascular coagulation in horses with acute colitis, *J Am Vet Med Assoc* 220:1034-1038, 2002.
317. Dallap BL: Coagulopathy in the equine critical care patient, *Vet Clin North Am Equine Pract* 20:231-251, 2004.
318. Dallap B, Dolente B, Boston R: Coagulation profiles in 27 horses with large colon volvulus. In Proceedings of the Eleventh Annual Veterinary Meeting of the American College of Veterinary Surgeons, Chicago, 2001, p 4.
319. Valentine BA, Ross CE, Bump JL, et al: Intramuscular hemangiosarcoma with pulmonary metastasis in a horse, *J Am Vet Med Assoc* 188:628, 1986.
320. Waugh S, Long G, Uriah L: Metastatic hemangiosarcoma in the equine: report of 2 cases, *J Equine Med Surg* 1:311, 1977.
321. Johns I, Stephen JO, Del Piero F, et al: Hemangiosarcoma in 11 young horses, *J Vet Intern Med* 19:564-570, 2005.
322. Hargis AM, Feldman BF: Evaluation of hemostatic defects secondary to vascular tumors in dogs: 11 cases (1983-1988), *J Am Vet Med Assoc* 198:891, 1991.
323. Shim WK: Hemangiomas of infancy complicated by thrombocytopenia, *Am J Surg* 116:896, 1968.
324. Sellon DC, Levine JF, Palmer K, et al: Thrombocytosis in 24 horses (1989-1994), *J Vet Intern Med* 11:24, 1997.
325. Clemmons RM, Dorsey-Lee MR, Gorman NT, et al: Haemostatic mechanisms of the newborn foal: reduced platelet responsiveness, *Equine Vet J* 16:353, 1984.
326. Cambridge H, Lees P, Hooke RE, et al: Antithrombotic actions of aspirin in the horse, *Equine Vet J* 23:123, 1991.
327. Kopp KJ, Moore JN, Byars TD, et al: Template bleeding time and thromboxane generation in the horse: effects of three non-steroidal anti-inflammatory drugs, *Equine Vet J* 17:322, 1985.
328. Meyers KM, Lindner C, Katz J, et al: Phenylbutazone inhibition of equine platelet function, *Am J Vet Res* 40:265, 1979.
329. Koterba A, Drummond W, Kosch P, editors: *Equine clinical neonatology*, Philadelphia, 1990, Lea & Febiger.
330. Fry MM, Walker NJ, Blevins GM, et al: Platelet function defect in a Thoroughbred filly, *J Vet Intern Med* 19:359-362, 2005.
331. Sutherland RJ, Cambridge H, Bolton JR: Functional and morphological studies on blood platelets in a thrombasthenic horse, *Aust Vet J* 66:366-370, 1989.
332. Macieira S, Rivard GE, Champagne J, et al: Glanzmann thrombasthenia in an Oldenbourg filly, *Vet Clin Pathol* 36:204-208, 2007.

333. Livesey L, Christopherson P, Hammond A, et al: Platelet dysfunction (Glanzmann's thrombasthenia) in horses, *J Vet Intern Med* 19:917-919, 2005.
334. Christopherson PW, Insalaco TA, van Santen VL, et al: Characterization of the cDNA encoding alphaIIb and beta3 in normal horses and two horses with Glanzmann thrombasthenia, *Vet Pathol* 43:78-82, 2006.
335. Norris J, Pratt S, Auh J-H, et al: Investigation of a novel, heritable bleeding diathesis of Thoroughbred horses and development of a screening assay, *J Vet Intern Med* 20:1450-1456, 2006.
336. Norris JW, Pratt SM, Hunter JF, et al: Prevalence of reduced fibrinogen binding to platelets in a population of Thoroughbreds, *Am J Vet Res* 68:716-721, 2007.
337. Brooks M, Leith GS, Allen AK, et al: Bleeding disorder (von Willebrand disease) in a Quarter Horse, *J Am Vet Med Assoc* 198:114, 1991.
338. George J, Shattil S: The clinical importance of acquired abnormalities of platelet function, *N Engl J Med* 324:27, 1991.
339. Judson D, Barton M: Effect of aspirin on haemostasis in the horse, *Res Vet Sci* 30:241, 1981.
340. Trujillo O, Rios A, Maldonado R, et al: Effect of oral administration of acetylsalicylic acid on haemostasis in the horse, *Equine Vet J* 13:205, 1981.
341. Baxter GM, Moore JN: Effect of aspirin on ex vivo generation of thromboxane in healthy horses, *Am J Vet Res* 48:13, 1987.
342. Osterud B, Rapaport S: Activation of factor IX by the reaction product of tissue factor and factor VII: additional pathway for initiating blood coagulation, *Proc Natl Acad Sci U S A* 74:5, 1977.
343. Hoffman M, Monroe DM 3rd: A cell-based model of hemostasis, *Thromb Haemost* 85:958-965, 2001.
344. Rosenberg R, Lam L: Correlation between structure and function of heparin, *Proc Natl Acad Sci U S A* 76:1218, 1979.
345. Hoffman M: Remodeling the blood coagulation cascade, *J Thromb Thrombolysis* 16:17-20, 2003.
346. Christensen U, Clemmensen I: Kinetic properties of the primary inhibitor of plasmin from human plasma, *Biochem J* 163:389, 1977.
347. Morris DD: Recognition and management of disseminated intravascular coagulation in horses, *Vet Clin North Am Large Anim Pract* 4:115, 1988.
348. Rawlings CA, Byars TD, Van Noy MK, et al: Activated coagulation test in normal and heparinized ponies and horses, *Am J Vet Res* 36:711, 1975.
349. Wagner AE: Transport of plasma for prothrombin time testing in monitoring warfarin therapy in the horse, *J Am Vet Med Assoc* 178:306, 1981.
350. Mischke R, Junker J, Deegen E: Sensitivity of commercial prothrombin time reagents to detect coagulation factor deficiencies in equine plasma, *Vet J* 171:114-119, 2006.
351. Topper MJ, Prasse KW: Analysis of coagulation proteins as acute-phase reactants in horses with colic, *Am J Vet Res* 59:542-545, 1998.
352. Feige K, Kästner SB, Dempfle CE, et al: Changes in coagulation and markers of fibrinolysis in horses undergoing colic surgery, *J Vet Med A Physiol Pathol Clin Med* 50:30-36, 2003.
353. Stokol T, Erb HN, De Wilde L, et al: Evaluation of latex agglutination kits for detection of fibrin(ogen) degradation products and D-dimer in healthy horses and horses with severe colic, *Vet Clin Pathol* 34:375-382, 2005.
354. Weiss DJ, Geor RJ, Burger K: Effects of pentoxifylline on hemorheologic alterations induced by incremental treadmill exercise in Thoroughbreds, *Am J Vet Res* 57(9):1364-1368, 1996.
355. Stern-Balestra E: *Bestimmung von löslichen Fibrinkomplexen beim Pferd als Möglichkeit der Diagnostik einer aktivierten Blutgerinnung, doctoral thesis*, Zurich, Switzerland, 2000, University of Zurich.
356. Bernard W, Morris DD, Divers TJ, et al: Plasma antithrombin-III values in healthy horses: effect of sex and/or breed, *Am J Vet Res* 48:866, 1987.
357. Johnstone IB, Physick-Sheard P, Crane S: Breed, age, and gender differences in plasma antithrombin-III activity in clinically normal young horses, *Am J Vet Res* 50:1751, 1989.
358. Johnstone I, Petersen D, Crane S: Antithrombin III: (AT III) activity in plasmas from normal and diseased horses, and in normal canine, bovine and human plasmas: *Vet Clin Pathol* 16:14, 1987.
359. Johnstone I, Crane S: Haemostatic abnormalities in horses with colic—their prognostic value, *Equine Vet J* 18:271-274, 1986.
360. Holland M, Kelly A, Snyder J, et al: Antithrombin III activity in horses with large colon torsion, *Am J Vet Res* 47:897-900, 1986.
361. Asakura H, Ontachi Y, Mizutni T, et al: Decreased plasma activity of antithrombin or protein C is not due to consumption coagulopathy in septic patients with disseminated intravascular coagulation, *Eur J Haematol* 67:170-175, 2001.
362. Welles EG, Prasse KW, Duncan A, et al: Antigenic assay for protein C determination in horses, *Am J Vet Res* 51:1075, 1990.
363. Welles EG, Prasse KW, Duncan A: Chromogenic assay for equine plasminogen, *Am J Vet Res* 51:1080, 1990.
364. Prasse KW, Allen D Jr, Moore JN, et al: Evaluation of coagulation and fibrinolysis during the prodromal stages of carbohydrate-induced acute laminitis in horses, *Am J Vet Res* 51:1990, 1950.
365. Littlewood JD, Bevan SA, Corke MJ, Haemophilia A: (classic haemophilia, factor VIII deficiency) in a Thoroughbred colt foal, *Equine Vet J* 23:70, 1991.
366. Segura D, Monreal L, Armengou L, et al: Mean platelet component as an indicator of platelet activation in foals and adult horses, *J Vet Intern Med* 21:1076-1082, 2007.
367. Laan TTJM, Goehring LS: Sloet van Oldruitenborgh-Oosterbaan MM: Von Willebrand's disease in an eight-day-old quarter horse foal, *Vet Rec* 157:322-324, 2005.
368. Rathgeber RA, Brooks MB, Bain FT, et al: von Willebrand disease in a Thoroughbred mare and foal, *J Vet Intern Med* 15:63, 2001.
369. Archer R: True haemophilia (haemophilia A) in a Thoroughbred foal, *Vet Rec* 73:338, 1961.
370. Archer RK, Allen BV: True haemophilia in horses, *Vet Rec* 91:655, 1972.
371. Feldman B, Giacopuzzi R: Hemophilia A: (factor VIII deficiency) in a colt, *Vet Clin North Am Equine Pract* 4:24, 1982.
372. Hinton M, Jones DR, Lewis IM, et al: A clotting defect in an Arab colt foal, *Equine Vet J* 9:1, 1977.
373. Henninger RW: Hemophilia A in two related quarter horse colts, *J Am Vet Med Assoc* 193:91, 1988.
374. Sanger V, Mairs R, Trapp A: Hemophilia in a foal, *J Am Vet Med Assoc* 144:259, 1964.
375. Mills J, Bolton J: Haemophilia A in a 3-year-old Thoroughbred horse, *Aust Vet J* 60:63, 1983.
376. Hutchins D, Lepherd E, Crook I: A case of equine haemophilia, *Aust Vet J* 43:83, 1967.
377. Geor RJ, Jackson ML, Lewis KD, et al: Prekallikrein deficiency in a family of Belgian horses, *J Am Vet Med Assoc* 197:741, 1990.
378. Turrentine MA, Sculley PW, Green EM, et al: Prekallikrein deficiency in a family of miniature horses, *Am J Vet Res* 47:2464, 1986.
379. Williams W, Beutler E, Erslev A, et al: *Hematology*, ed 4, New York, 1990, McGraw Hill.
380. Ainsworth DM, Dodds WJ, Brown CM: Deficiency of the contact phase of intrinsic coagulation in a horse, *J Am Vet Med Assoc* 187:71, 1985.

381. Morris DD: Cutaneous vasculitis in horses: 19 cases (1978-1985), *J Am Vet Med Assoc* 191:460, 1987.
382. Morris DD: Vasculitis in horses. In *Proceedings of the Fourth Scientific Forum of the American College of Veterinary Internal Medicine,* Washington, DC, 1990, p 3.
383. Huntington P, Ellis P, Forman A, et al: Equine viral arteritis, *Aust Vet J* 67:429, 1990.
384. Traub-Dargatz J, Ralston S, Collins J, et al: Equine viral arteritis, *Compend Contin Educ Pract Vet* 7:S490, 1985.
385. Crawford T, Henson J: Immunofluorescent, light microscopic and immunologic studies of equine viral arteritis. In *Proceedings of the Third International Conference on Equine Infectious Diseases,* Basel, Switzerland, 1972, S. Karger Press, Basel, Switzerland, p 282.
386. Neu S, Timoney P, McCollum W: Persistent infection of the reproductive tract in stallions experimentally infected with equine arteritis virus. In *Proceedings of the International Conference on Equine Infectious Diseases,* Lexington, Ky, 1988, University Press of Kentucky, Lexington, KY, p 149.
387. Coignoul FL, Cheville NF: Pathology of maternal genital tract, placenta, and fetus in equine viral arteritis, *Vet Pathol* 21:333, 1984.
388. Timoney PJ, McCollum WH, Roberts AW, et al: Status of equine viral arteritis in Kentucky, *J Am Vet Med Assoc* 191(36):1987, 1985.
389. Timoney P, McCollum W, Roberts A, et al: Demonstration of the carrier state in naturally acquired equine arteritis virus infection in the stallion, *Res Vet Sci* 41:279, 1986.
390. Timoney P J: Equine viral arteritis in perspective: fact vs. fiction. In *Proceedings of the Sixth World Equine Veterinary Congress,* September 30-October 3, 1999, pp 167-170.
391. Timoney PJ: The increasing significance of international trade in equids and its influence on the spread of infectious diseases, *Ann N Y Acad Sci* 916:55-60, 2000.
392. Timoney PJ, McCollum WH, Vickers ML: The rationale for greater national control of EVA, *Equine Dis Q* 7:2-3, 1998.
393. Glaser AL, Rottier PJM, Horzinek MC, et al: Equine arteritis virus: a review of clinical features and management aspects, *Vet Q* 18:95-99, 1996.
394. Morris DD, Miller WH Jr, Goldschmidt MH, et al: Chronic necrotizing vasculitis in a horse, *J Am Vet Med Assoc* 183:579, 1983.
395. Conn DT: Update on systemic necrotizing vasculitis, *Mayo Clin Proc* 4:535, 1989.
396. Yanagisawa M, Kurihara H, Kimura S, et al: A novel potent vasoconstrictor peptide produced by vascular endothelial cells, *Nature* 332:411, 1988.
397. Vanhoutte PM: The endothelium-modulator of vascular smooth-muscle tone, *N Engl J Med* 319:512, 1988.
398. Schifferli JA, Ng YC, Peters DK: The role of complement and its receptor in the elimination of immune complexes, *N Engl J Med* 315:488, 1986.
399. Smiley JD, Moore SE: Southwestern Internal Medicine Conference: role of complement and IgG-Fc receptor functions, *Am J Med Sci* 298:257, 1989.
400. Fearon DT: Complement, C receptors, and immune complex disease, *Hosp Pract* 23:63, 1988.
401. Caciolo PL, Hurvitz AI, Nesbitt GH: Michel's medium as a preservative for immunofluorescent staining of cutaneous biopsy specimen in dogs and cats, *Am J Vet Res* 45:128, 1984.
402. Galan JE, Timoney JF: Immune complexes in purpura hemorrhagica of the horse contain IgA and M antigen of *Streptococcus equi, J Immunol* 135:3134, 1985.
403. Pusterla N, Watson JL, Affolter VK, et al: Purpura haemorrhagica in 53 horses, *Vet Rec* 153(4):118-121, 2003.
404. Kaese HJ, Valberg SJ, Hayden DW, et al: Infarctive purpura hemorrhagica in five horses, *J Am Vet Med Assoc* 226: 1893-1898, 2005.
405. Waller AS, Jolley KA: Getting a grip on strangles: recent progress towards improved diagnostics and vaccines, *Vet J* 173:492-501, 2007.
406. Ettinger SJ, Feldman EC, editors: *Textbook of veterinary internal medicine,* ed 6, St Louis, 2005, WB Saunders.
407. Siciliano PD, Warren LK, Lawrence LM: Changes in vitamin K status of growing horses, *J Equine Vet Sci* 20:726-729, 2000.
408. Ralston S: Equine clinical nutrition: specific problems and solutions, *Compend Contin Educ Pract Vet* 10:357, 1988.
409. Colles CM: A preliminary report on the use of warfarin in the treatment of navicular disease, *Equine Vet J* 11:187, 1979.
410. Scott EA, Byars TD, Lamar AM: Warfarin anticoagulation in the horse, *J Am Vet Med Assoc* 177:1146, 1980.
411. Scott EA, Sandler GA, Byars TD: Warfarin: effects on anticoagulant, hematologic, and blood enzyme values in normal ponies, *Am J Vet Res* 40:142, 1979.
412. Vrins A, Carlson G, Feldman B: Warfarin: a review with emphasis on its use in the horse, *Can Vet J* 24:211, 1983.
413. Byars TD, Greene CE, Kemp DT: Antidotal effect of vitamin K1 against warfarin-induced anticoagulation in horses, *Am J Vet Res* 47:2309, 1986.
414. Scott EA, Sandler GA, Byars TD: Warfarin: effects of intravenous loading doses and vitamin K on warfarin anticoagulation in the pony, *Am J Vet Res* 39:1978, 1888.
415. Boermans HJ, Johnstone I, Black WD, et al: Clinical signs, laboratory changes and toxicokinetics of brodifacoum in the horse, *Can J Vet Res* 55:21, 1991.
416. McConnico RS, Copedge K, Bischoff KL: Brodifacoum toxicosis in two horses, *J Am Vet Med Assoc* 211:882, 1997.
417. Ayala I, Rodriguez J, Martos N, et al: Fatal brodifaccum poisoning in a pony. *Can Vet J,* 48:627-629, 2007.
418. Blood DC, Radostits OM, Arundel JH, et al: *Veterinary medicine,* ed 7, Philadelphia, 1989, Balliere Tindall.
419. Burrows GE, Tyrl RJ: Plants causing sudden death in livestock, *Vet Clin North Am Food Anim Pract* 5:263, 1989.
420. Osweiler GD, Rurh LP: Plants affecting blood coagulation: In Howard JS, editor: *Current veterinary therapy food animal practice,* ed 2, Philadelphia, 1986, WB Saunders.
421. Rebhun WC, Tennant BC, Dill SG, et al: Vitamin K_3-induced renal toxicosis in the horse, *J Am Vet Med Assoc* 184:1237, 1984.
422. Byars TD, Wilson RC: Clinical pharmacology of heparin, *J Am Vet Med Assoc* 178:739, 1981.
423. MacHarg MA, Becht JL: The pharmacology of heparin prophylaxis, *J Am Vet Med Assoc* 183:129, 1983.
424. Hood D: Current concepts of the physiopathology of laminitis. *Proc Am Assoc Eq Pract* 25: 13-20, 1979.
425. Hood D, Gremmel S, Amoss M: Equine laminitis. III. Coagulation dysfunction in the developmental and acute disease, *J Equine Med Surg* 3:355, 1979.
426. Parker J, Fubini S, Car B, et al: Prevention of intrabdominal adhesions in ponies by low dose heparin therapy, *Vet Surg* 16:459, 1987.
427. Moore BR, Hinchcliff KW: Heparin: a review of its pharmacology and therapeutic use in horses, *J Vet Intern Med* 8:26-35, 1994.
428. Belknap JK, Moore JN: Evaluation of heparin for prophylaxis of equine laminitis: 71 cases (1980-1986), *J Am Vet Med Assoc* 195:505, 1989.
429. Young D, Richardson D, Markel D: The effect of low dose heparin therapy on complication and survival rates in horses following exploratory celiotomy, *Equine Vet J Suppl* 7:91, 1989.
430. Engelking LR, Mariner JC: Enhanced biliary bilirubin excretion after heparin-induced erythrocyte mass depletion, *Am J Vet Res* 46:2175, 1985.
431. Mahaffey EA, Moore JN: Erythrocyte agglutination associated with heparin treatment in three horses, *J Am Vet Med Assoc* 189:1478, 1986.
432. Moore JN, Mahaffey EA, Zboran M: Heparin-induced agglutination of erythrocytes in horses, *Am J Vet Res* 48:68, 1987.

433. Moore J, Colicchio M, Darien B: Effects of heparin on coagulation times and plasma antithrombin III in normal horses, *Symp Equine Colic Res* 2:347, 1986.
434. Weitz JI: Low-molecular-weight heparins, *N Engl J Med* 337(10):688-698, 1997.
435. Schwarzwald C, Fiege K, Wunderli-Allenspach H, et al: Comparison of pharmacokinetic variables for two low molecular weight heparins after subcutaneous administration of a single dose to horses, *Am J Vet Res* 63:868-873, 2002.
436. Feige K, Schwarzwald CC, Bombeli T: Comparison of unfractioned and low molecular weight heparin for prophylaxis of coagulopathies in 52 horses with colic: a randomized double-blind clinical trial, *Equine Vet J* 35:506-513, 2003.
437. Marshall J: Inflammation, coagulopathy, and the pathogenesis of multiple organ dysfunction syndrome, *Crit Care Med* 29(Suppl 7):S99-S104, 2001.
438. Johnstone I, Blackwell T: Disseminated intravascular coagulation in a horse with postpartum ulcerative colitis and laminitis, *Can Vet J* 25:195, 1984.
439. Johnstone IB, Crane S: Hemostatic abnormalities in equine colic, *Am J Vet Res* 47:356, 1986.
440. Johnstone IB, Crane S: Haemostatic abnormalities in horses with colic—their prognostic value, *Equine Vet J* 18:271, 1986.
441. Johnstone IB, McAndrew KH, Baird JD: Early detection and successful reversal of disseminated intravascular coagulation in a Thoroughbred mare presented with a history of diarrhea and colic, *Equine Vet J* 18:337, 1986.
442. Morris DD, Beech J: Disseminated intravascular coagulation in six horses, *J Am Vet Med Assoc* 183:1067, 1983.
443. Morris DD, Messick J, Whitlock RH, et al: Effect of equine ehrlichial colitis on the hemostatic system in ponies, *Am J Vet Res* 49:1030, 1988.
444. Morris D, Vaala W, Sartin E: Protein-losing enteropathy in a yearling filly with subclinical disseminated intravascular coagulation and autoimmune hemolytic disease, *Compend Contin Educ Pract Vet* 4:S542, 1982.
445. Holland M, Kelly AB, Snyder JR, et al: Antithrombin III activity in horses with large colon torsion, *Am J Vet Res* 47:897, 1986.
446. Lavoie JP, Madigan JE, Cullor JS, et al: Haemodynamic, pathological, haematological and behavioural changes during endotoxin infusion in equine neonates, *Equine Vet J* 22:23, 1990.
447. Pablo LS, Purohit RC, Teer PA, et al: Disseminated intravascular coagulation in experimental intestinal strangulation obstruction in ponies, *Am J Vet Res* 44:2115, 1983.
448. Meyers K, Reed S, Keck M, et al: Circulating endotoxin-like substance(s) and altered hemostasis in horses with gastrointestinal disorders: an interim report, *Am J Vet Res* 43:2233, 1982.
449. Feldman B: Disseminated intravascular coagulation, *Compend Contin Educ Pract Vet* 3:46, 1981.
450. van der Poll T, de Jonge E, Levi M: Regulatory role of cytokines in disseminated intravascular coagulation, *Semin Thromb Hemost* 27:639-651, 2001.
451. Habal F, Movat H: Kininogens of human plasma, *Semin Thromb Hemost* 3:27, 1976.
452. Henry MM, Moore JN: Clinical relevance of monocyte procoagulant activity in horses with colic, *J Am Vet Med Assoc* 198:843, 1991.
453. Bick R, Bick M, Fekete L: Antithrombin III patterns in disseminated intravascular coagulation, *Am J Clin Pathol* 73:577, 1980.
454. Green RA, Kabel AL: Hypercoagulable state in three dogs with nephrotic syndrome: role of acquired antithrombin III deficiency, *J Am Vet Med Assoc* 181:914, 1982.
455. Clouse L, Camp P: The regulation of hemostasis: the protein C system, *N Engl J Med* 314:1298, 1986.
456. Semrad SD, Hardee GE, Hardee MM, et al: Low dose flunixin meglumine: effects on eicosanoid production and clinical signs induced by experimental endotoxaemia in horses, *Equine Vet J* 19:201, 1987.
457. Broome TA, Brown MP, Gronwall RR, et al: Pharmacokinetics and plasma concentrations of acetylsalicylic acid after intravenous, rectal, and intragastric administration to horses, *Can J Vet Res* 67:297-230.
458. Liska DA, Akucewich LH, Marsella R, et al: Pharmacokinetics of pentoxifylline and its 5-hydroxyhexyl metabolite after oral and intravenous administration of pentoxifylline to healthy adult horses, *Am J Vet Res* 67:1621-1627, 2006.
459. Dunkel B, Rickards KJ, Page CP, et al: Phosphodiesterase isoenzymes in equine platelets and their influence on platelet adhesion, *Am J Vet Res* 68:1354-1360, 2007.
460. Segura D, Monreal L, Pérez-Pujol S, et al: Effects of etamsylate on equine platelets: in vitro and in vivo studies, *Vet J* 174:325-329, 2007.
461. Feige K, Dennler M, Kästner SB, et al: Pharmacokinetics of recombinant hirudin in healthy horses, *Equine Vet J* 36:135-141, 2004.
462. Spurlock SL, Spurlock GH: Risk factors of catheter-related complications, *Compend Contin Educ Pract Vet* 12:214-245, 1990.
463. Armstrong CW, Mayhall CG, Miller KB, et al: Prospective study of catheter placement and other factors for infection of hyperalimentation catheters, *J Infect Dis* 154:808-814, 1986.
464. Dolente BA, Beech J, Lindborg S, et al: Evaluation of risk factors for development of catheter-associated jugular thrombophlebitis in horses: 50 cases (1993-1998), *J Am Vet Med Assoc* 227:1134-1141, 2005.
465. Gardner SY, Reef VB, Spencer PA: Ultrasonographic evaluation of horses with thrombophlebitis of the jugular vein: 46 cases (1985-1988), *J Am Vet Med Assoc* 199:370, 1991.
466. Stormont C, Suzuki Y, Rhode E: Serology of horse blood groups, *Cornell Vet* 54:439, 1964.
467. Stormont CJ: Blood groups in animals, *J Am Vet Med Assoc* 181:1120, 1982.
468. Niinistö K, Raekallio M, Sankari S: Storage of equine red blood cells as a concentrate, *Vet J* 176:227-231, 2008.
469. Carlson GP, Rumbaugh GE, Harrold D: Physiologic alterations in the horse produced by food and water deprivation during periods of high environmental temperatures, *Am J Vet Res* 40:982, 1979.
470. Spensley MS, Carlson GP, Harrold D: Plasma, red blood cell, total blood, and extracellular fluid volumes in healthy horse foals during growth, *Am J Vet Res* 48:1703, 1987.
471. Kallfelz FA, Whitlock RH, Schultz RD: Survival of 59Fe-labeled erythrocytes in crosstransfused equine blood, *Am J Vet Res* 39:617, 1978.
472. Hurcombe SD, Mudge MC, Hinchcliff KW: Clinical and clinicopathologic variables in adult horses receiving blood transfusions: 31 cases (1999-2005), *J Am Vet Med Assoc* 231:267-274, 2007.
473. Aleman M, Nieto JE, Carr EA, et al: Serum hepatitis associated with commercial plasma transfusion in horses, *J Vet Intern Med* 19:120-122, 2005.
474. Feige K, Ehrat FB, Kästner SB, et al: The effects of automated plasmapheresis on clinical, haematological, biochemical and coagulation variables in horses, *Vet J* 169:102-107, 2005.
475. Feige K, Ehrat FB, Kästner SB, et al: Automated plasmapheresis compared with other plasma collection methods in the horse, *J Vet Med A Physiol Pathol Clin Med* 50:185-189, 2003.
476. Gordon BJ, Latimer KS, Murray CM, et al: Evaluation of leukapheresis and thrombocytapheresis in the horse, *Am J Vet Res* 47:997, 1986.
477. Gordon BJ, Latimer KS, Murray CM, et al: Continuous-flow centrifugation hemapheresis in the horse, *Am J Vet Res* 47:342, 1986.
478. Morris DD, Bruce J, Gaulin G, et al: Evaluation of granulocyte transfusion in healthy neonatal pony foals, *Am J Vet Res* 48:1187, 1987.
479. Morris DD: Blood products in large animal medicine: a comparative account of current and future technology, *Equine Vet J* 19:272, 1987.

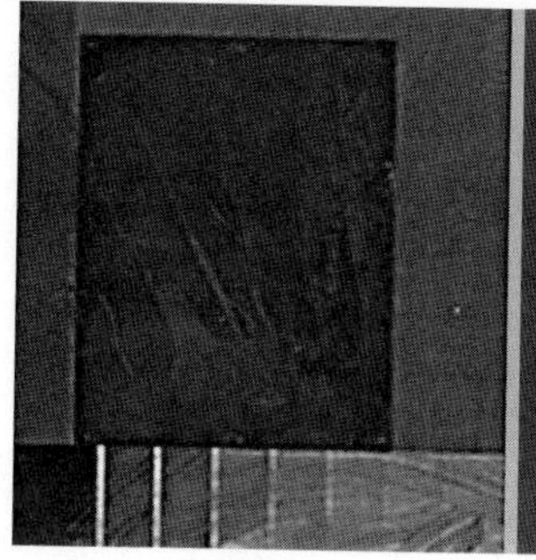

Disorders of the Gastrointestinal System*

CHAPTER

15

EXAMINATION FOR DISORDERS OF THE GASTROINTESTINAL TRACT

L. Chris Sanchez

PHYSICAL EXAMINATION

Examination of patients with disease of the gastrointestinal tract must include evaluation of the metabolic and cardiovascular status of the patient, because acute conditions of the proximal or distal intestinal tract can lead to endotoxemia and sepsis. Examination of the cardiovascular system (heart, peripheral pulse, and mucous membranes), lungs, and abdomen is essential to detect clinical signs of systemic inflammation from endotoxemia, coagulation disorders, dehydration, ileus, shock, and other abnormalities resulting from injury to the small or large intestine. Clinical signs of systemic inflammation from endotoxemia and sepsis are described elsewhere in this chapter.

One performs the physical examination of the abdomen primarily by auscultation, transabdominal ballottement, and transrectal palpation. Abdominal distention often indicates distention of the large intestine; however, small intestinal distention also can cause visible abdominal distention if a large proportion of the small intestine is involved. Abdominal palpation can be performed in neonatal foals; after several weeks of age, however, the abdominal wall is too rigid to allow effective palpation of intra-abdominal structures.

Abdominal auscultation is particularly useful for assessing the motility of the large intestine. Progressive motility of the small intestine, conversely, is difficult to distinguish by auscultation from nonprogressive motility. The distinct character of the borborygmi produced during propulsive contractions of the cecum and ascending colon allows evaluation of the frequency and strength of retropulsion and propulsion. Propulsive contractions of the cecum and ventral colon occur every 3 to 4 minutes and give rise to prolonged rushing sounds heard over long segments of intestine. Retropulsive sounds presumably are similar to propulsive sounds, but they occur less frequently. Distinguishing between propulsion and retropulsion is not important clinically because both types of contractions signify normal motility. Interhaustral and intrahaustral mixing contractions produce nonspecific sounds of fluid and ingesta movement that are difficult to distinguish from other borborygmi, such as small intestinal contractions or spasmodic contractions.[1]

Auscultation over the right flank and proceeding along the caudal edge of the costal margin toward the xiphoid allows evaluation of the cecal borborygmi. Auscultation over a similar area on the left side allows evaluation of the pelvic flexure and ascending colon. Typical progressive borborygmi heard every 3 to 4 minutes on both sides of the abdomen indicate normal motility of the cecum and ascending colon. Less frequent progressive sounds may indicate a pathologic condition of the large intestine or may result from anorexia, nervousness (sympathetic tone), or pharmacologic inhibition of motility (i.e., α_2-adrenergic agonists such as xylazine).[2-5] Absolute absence of any auscultable borborygmi suggests abnormal motility and indicates ileus resulting from a serious pathologic condition but is not specific to any segment of the intestine.[3,6] If borborygmi are audible but progressive sounds are not detectable, determining whether a significant abnormality exists is difficult.[6] Borborygmi heard more frequently than normal may result from increased motility following feeding; from excessive stimulation from irritation, distention, or inflammation; or after administration of parasympathomimetic drugs such as neostigmine. Large intestinal motility increases in the early stages of intestinal distention regardless of the site.[7] Mild inflammation or irritation of the large intestinal mucosa also can stimulate motility.[3] Parasympathomimetic drugs stimulate contractions and auscultable borborygmi in the large intestine; however, an increase in parasympathetic tone may result in segmental contractions, which actually inhibit progressive motility.[2]

One can detect sand or gravel in the large intestinal ingesta by auscultation behind the xiphoid process. It is possible to hear sand or gravel particles grinding together during

*The authors wish to acknowledge the work of former contributors to the following sections: Examination for Disorders of the Gastrointestinal Tract, Jennifer L. Davis and Samuel L. Jones; Pathophysiology of Diarrhea, Rebecca S. McConnico; Gastrointestinal Ileus, Guy D. Lester; Esophageal Diseases, Samuel L. Jones, Anthony T. Blikslager; Duodentitis, Rebecca S. McConnico; Diseases Associated with Malabsorption and Maldigestion, Malcolm C. Roberts; Ischemic Disorders of the Intestinal Tract, Samuel L. Jones; Obstructive Disorders of the Gastrointestinal Tract, Samuel L. Jones; Peritonitis, Charles Dickinson.

progressive contractions of the ascending colon. In one study characteristic sounds were heard on auscultation (5 minutes' duration) after daily administration of sand to healthy horses, none of which developed clinical signs of colic or diarrhea.[8] If the frequency of progressive contractions is low or absent, detecting sand by auscultation is difficult.

Percussion of the abdomen during auscultation can reveal gas in the large intestine. The characteristic *ping* produced by simultaneous digital percussion and auscultation over a gas-filled viscus often is associated with abnormal accumulation of gas under pressure. This technique is particularly useful in foals, ponies, and miniature horses because of the limitations of rectal palpation.

Transabdominal ballottement can be used to detect large, firm masses or an abnormal volume of peritoneal fluid (PF). The usefulness of this technique is usually limited to animals too small to palpate rectally. One can detect soft tissue masses or fetuses by bumping the structures with a hand or fist. If excessive PF is present, a fluid wave can be generated by ballottement; however, this technique is not as useful in horses older than 4 weeks because the abdominal wall is rigid.

Transrectal palpation is the most specific physical examination technique for investigation of intestinal disease and is particularly valuable when evaluating obstructive diseases.[9,10] The primary objectives of transrectal palpation are to assess the size, consistency, and position of the segments of the large intestine; to determine the presence of any distention of the small intestine; and to detect intra-abdominal masses. Evaluation of the wall thickness and texture and the mesenteric structures (blood and lymphatic vessels and lymph nodes) also may aid in diagnosis of large intestinal disease. The interpretation of transrectal palpation findings in light of clinical signs and laboratory results is an important diagnostic aid for developing appropriate treatment strategies for intestinal diseases manifested by abdominal pain. Enlargement of one or more segments of large intestine detected by transrectal palpation provides evidence of obstruction at or distal to the enlarged segment. By systematically evaluating each segment, one can determine the site of obstruction. Obstruction of the pelvic flexure, for instance, results in enlargement of the pelvic flexure and ventral colon, but the dorsal and descending colons are of normal size. Enlargement of a segment of the large intestine usually is accompanied by abnormal consistency of the contents. It is possible to distinguish among gas, fluid, and ingesta and to detect foreign bodies in palpable segments. Accumulation of gas and fluid suggests complete and acute obstruction, whereas accumulation of ingesta suggests chronic and incomplete obstruction. Accumulation of fluid usually indicates ileus. The practitioner must evaluate the consistency of the contents in light of the size of the segment; ingesta in the ventral colon of a dehydrated patient may be firm, but the size of the ventral colon will be normal. Conversely, if the ingesta is firm because of a distal obstruction, the ventral colon will be enlarged.

Displacement of a segment of the large intestine may create an obstruction detectable by enlargement of the segment and accumulation of gas and fluid, even if the site of obstruction is not palpable. Torsion of the ascending colon at the sternal and diaphragmatic flexures results in acute accumulation of gas and fluid proximal to the torsion, causing distention of the left dorsal and ventral colons. Depending on the degree of torsion, the position of the ventral and dorsal colons may not be significantly abnormal. Displacement of a segment of large intestine often results in incomplete obstruction, and the diagnosis relies solely on detection of the displaced segment in an abnormal position. The position of the displaced segment may not be palpable, and the diagnosis then relies on the inability to find the segment in a normal position. One must take care to ensure that the segment that appears to be displaced is not in a normal position but has become too small to palpate because of a decrease in the volume of ingesta. The cecum, right dorsal and ventral colons, pelvic flexure, and descending colon are palpable in most horses. One should palpate the nephrosplenic space to detect the presence of intestine, usually pelvic flexure, entrapped within the ligament.

Small intestine is not normally palpable in the horse. Distention indicates ileus with gas or fluid retention, usually following a strangulating or nonstrangulating obstruction. Strangulating obstructions result from conditions such as volvulus or torsion, lipoma, and entrapments. Such conditions often are accompanied by severe pain, dehydration, PF changes, and a varying degree of gastric fluid accumulation. The small intestine in these cases is turgid and firm on palpation. One should assess the mesentery and wall thickness in the same manner as for large intestinal disorders. Careful palpation of the inguinal rings in stallions with small intestinal distention is crucial for determining inguinal herniation.

Evaluation of the wall thickness and mesenteric vessels can reveal venous congestion (mural edema and enlarged blood and lymphatic vessels) or inflammation (mural edema with normal vessels). Disruption of arterial blood flow does not cause venous congestion, but the arterial pulse is not detectable. Mesenteric tears may not be palpable, but the entrapped ischemic intestinal segment may be thickened with edema. It is possible to detect acute or chronic inflammation with cellular infiltration of the intestinal wall as thickening of the wall without edema; enlargement of mesenteric lymph nodes also may be noted. One should interpret abnormalities in the wall or vessels in light of the size, consistency, and position of the segment of intestine and the clinical signs. Several conditions involving small intestinal strangulating lesions do not necessarily cause abnormal rectal examination findings until the disease has been present for an extended time. These conditions include diaphragmatic herniae and epiploic foramen entrapments. PF analysis can be normal in these cases as well because the fluid is trapped in the thorax or cranial abdomen.

Nonstrangulating causes of small intestinal distention can be divided further into intraluminal and extraluminal obstructions. Ileal impactions are probably the most common cause of intraluminal obstruction, and on rare occasions the impaction can be palpated in the upper right quadrant, near the ileocecal opening. Intraluminal masses caused by lymphoma, eosinophilic enteritis, foreign bodies, or ascarid impactions often lead to small intestinal distention and are usually indistinguishable from one another on the basis of palpation alone. Small intestine in these cases can be moderately to severely distended, depending on the degree of obstruction. Extraluminal obstructions include abdominal masses, abscesses or tumors, and large colon displacement. One should always palpate the rest of the abdomen carefully to help rule out these causes. Some cases of small intestinal distention result from a physiologic rather than a mechanical obstruction. Ileus may result postoperatively or after inflammatory diseases of the bowel (proximal enteritis) or peritoneal cavity (peritonitis).

The bowel is usually mildly to moderately distended and almost always is accompanied by significant amounts of accumulated gastric fluid.

The small colon is easily distinguishable by the presence of normal fecal balls and an antimesenteric band. In cases of impaction of the small colon, a long, hard, tubelike structure is present in the caudal abdomen, and the band is palpable along the length. Fluid stool is often present in the rectum in these cases, as is tenesmus, and the rectal mucosa is often edematous and occasionally roughened. One can detect and carefully evaluate rectal tears by palpation. Also detectable are mural masses in palpable segments of intestine or mesentery; however, if a mass causes obstruction, it is possible to detect the result of the obstruction in proximal segments of intestine even if the mass is unreachable. Palpation of the mesenteric vessels may reveal thickening and thrombosis, which can lead to ischemia or infarction.

One can perform visual inspection of the mucosa of the rectum and descending colon with a speculum or flexible endoscope and also can evaluate rectal tears or perforations, mural masses, strictures, or mucosal inflammation. One can also perform guided biopsy of the mucosa or masses. The obvious limitations are the amount of fecal material, which can interfere with the examination, and the distance of the lesion of interest from the anus. These techniques offer little advantage over palpation in many cases, unless the patient is too small to palpate.

Examination of the oral cavity in cases of dysphagia or weight loss is a necessary part of the physical examination. One should adequately sedate the horse and use a full-mouth speculum to allow palpation and visualization of all parts of the oral cavity. One should examine the area for abnormal dentition, foreign bodies, fractures, abscesses, and ulceration.

The presence of fluid accumulation in the stomach indicates a decrease or absence in propulsive motions of the small intestine or obstruction of gastric outflow. Decreased small intestinal motility may result from a functional or mechanical blockage. Masses, feed impactions, or strictures in the pylorus or in the proximal duodenum may obstruct gastric outflow. One routinely assesses fluid accumulation in the stomach by siphoning off the gastric contents with a nasogastric tube and examining the fluid for amount, color, and any particular odor. Normal fluid is green and may contain foamy saliva. The volume obtained by gastric lavage is usually less than 4 L. Large volumes of fluid (≥8 to 10 L) accumulate in the stomach of horses with proximal enteritis, and the fluid is foul smelling and often has an orange to yellow discoloration. If proximal enteritis is suspected, the fluid can be submitted for culture and Gram staining. *Salmonella* sp. and *Clostridium* sp. have been cultured in some cases. Patients with postoperative ileus also frequently accumulate large amounts of gastric fluid. Horses with strangulating obstructions or luminal obstructions often accumulate moderate amounts of gastric fluid, but the amount is generally less than in horses with proximal enteritis or postoperative ileus. Hemorrhage in the gastric fluid usually indicates devitalized small intestine, stomach wall, or severe gastric ulceration. Fluid with large amounts of food material can indicate a gastric impaction, and one should lavage the stomach until no more ingesta can be obtained. Horses and foals with chronic gastric ulceration in the glandular mucosa of the stomach or in the duodenum may develop strictures and have accumulated fluid in the stomach. Endoscopy or contrast radiography aids in diagnosing gastric outflow obstruction.

DIAGNOSTIC EVALUATION

Clinical Pathology

Evaluation of the hemogram is essential when assessing conditions of the gastrointestinal tract. However, hematologic alterations associated with diseases of the gastrointestinal tract are often nonspecific, reflecting systemic response to inflammation, endotoxemia, or sepsis. Neutrophilic leukocytosis and normochromic, normocytic anemia with or without hyperfibrinogenemia commonly are associated with chronic inflammatory conditions of the intestine. Anemia from chronic blood loss occurs infrequently in adult horses because of the large iron stores and high concentrations of iron in their diet; anemia usually follows chronic inflammation, as do alterations in the leukon and plasma fibrinogen concentrations. Plasma protein concentrations vary depending on gastrointestinal losses of albumin and globulin and elevation of globulin concentration from antigenic stimulation. Protein-losing enteropathies may manifest predominantly as a hypoalbuminemia or as a panhypoproteinemia. Immunoglobulin quantification can be useful in selected cases; immunosuppression with low immunoglobulin M concentration has been shown to occur in some cases of lymphosarcoma.[11] Parasitic infections, especially strongylosis, may be characterized by elevated serum immunoglobulin G(T) concentration.[12]

Significant alterations of the hemogram do not accompany acute disease of the intestine unless severe inflammation, dehydration, endotoxemia, or sepsis is present. During the early stages of endotoxemia, elevations in circulating concentrations of inflammatory mediators, epinephrine, and cortisol produce characteristic changes in the hemogram. Leukopenia, with neutropenia and a left shift, toxic changes in the neutrophil cytoplasm, and lymphopenia commonly occur.[13] Hemoconcentration and hyperfibrinogenemia are also common. Thrombocytopenia and other coagulopathies are also features of endotoxemia. Indeed, thrombocytopenia may be the earliest indicator of sepsis.[14] Endotoxemia and circulating mediators of inflammation activate the coagulation cascade, causing a hypercoagulable state that can lead to consumption of coagulation factors and coagulation defects manifested as elevated prothrombin time, partial thromboplastin time, fibrin degradation products, and bleeding time and reduced activity of antithrombin III.[15-17] Neutrophilic leukocytosis occurs during the later stages of endotoxemia.[15]

The most common serum biochemical abnormalities with diseases of the large or small intestine are electrolyte imbalances. Serum calcium concentrations are often low with strangulating obstructions and acute inflammatory diseases.[18] Inflammation of the mucosa can severely disrupt electrolyte fluxes. Diarrhea or gastric reflux greatly exacerbates the loss of sodium, potassium, calcium, magnesium, and bicarbonate. Hypoxia and cellular damage caused by ischemia of the intestine may be reflected by an elevated serum phosphate concentration resulting from phosphate leakage from damaged cells.[19] Ischemia and cellular hypoxia in any segment of the intestine also causes a shift in energy metabolism to anaerobic glycolysis, resulting in increased production of lactate and elevated serum lactate concentration. Reduced perfusion of peripheral tissues from hypotensive shock and intestinal ischemia can cause elevations in serum lactate. However, obstruction of the intestine during ischemia may result in absorption of lactate from the lumen.[20,21] Anion gap is an indirect measurement of organic acid production during states of tissue hypoxia and is a reasonable estimate of serum lactate concentration.[21] Metabolic acidosis may accompany lactic acidemia, but an inconsistent association exists between the two, especially when mixed acid-base imbalances are present.[21,22] Elevations of hepatic enzymes, specifically γ-glutamyltransferase, may occur with large colon displacements, duodenal strictures, or anterior enteritis. An elevated γ-glutamyltransferase is more suggestive of a right dorsal displacement than a left dorsal displacement.[23]

Relative polycythemia from hemoconcentration or splenic contraction and changes in red blood cell deformability from hypoxia or hypocalcemia may increase blood viscosity. Blood viscosity increases in patients with acute obstructive disease. Hyperviscosity reduces perfusion of capillary beds, thereby exacerbating ischemia and tissue hypoxia.[24] Hyperviscosity is one manifestation (along with lactic acidemia, coagulopathies, and clinical signs of shock) of the pathophysiologic events that take place during acute inflammatory or vascular injury to the large intestine. Laboratory tests designed to reflect the systemic effects of endotoxemia, ischemia, sepsis, and shock are important to design therapeutic strategies and monitor response to therapy.

PERITONEAL FLUID

Abdominocentesis and analysis of PF are diagnostic techniques performed on many patients with disease of the gastrointestinal tract. The veterinarian can quantitate cytologic examination of PF; white blood cell and red blood cell counts; protein, fibrinogen, lactate, phosphate, and glucose concentrations; lactate dehydrogenase, creatine kinase, and alkaline phosphatase activity; and pH. The results of PF analysis may help establish a specific diagnosis and, more important, may reflect inflammatory, vascular, or ischemic injury to the intestine requiring surgical intervention.

PF reflects a sequence of events that takes place during acute vascular injury to the intestine. The PF protein concentration first increases, followed by an increase in the red blood cell count and fibrinogen concentration. A transudative process resulting from vascular congestion and increased endothelial permeability allows small macromolecules (albumin) to escape into the PF, followed by larger macromolecules (globulin and fibrinogen), and finally diapedesis of cells (red blood cells, and then white blood cells).[25,26] If ischemic inflammation of the intestine and visceral peritonitis occurs, an exudative process ensues. Severe inflammation of the intestine and visceral peritoneum causes large quantities of protein and white blood cells, primarily neutrophils, to escape into the PF.[24,26] As damage to the bowel progresses, the protein concentration and red blood cell and white blood cell counts continue to rise. As the degree of irreversible damage to the intestine increases, the PF characteristics become more exudative.[25,26] Eventually, bacteria begin to translocate across the intestinal wall and appear in the PF as the mucosal barrier breaks down. Neutrophils predominate, their cytoplasm becomes granulated, and Döhle's bodies often are visible. If perforation occurs, bacteria and particles of ingesta appear in the PF, and the neutrophils become degenerate (i.e., pyknotic), with karyorrhexis, karyolysis, and smudge cells.

Elevated PF protein concentration is a sensitive indicator of early inflammation, whereas elevated red blood cell counts in the presence of normal white blood cell counts suggest vascular damage without significant tissue ischemia.[26] Of note, the anticoagulant potassium EDTA, but not lithium heparin, can cause an increase in total protein as measured by refractometer, relative to the value obtained from the same sample without anticoagulant.[27] Elevation of the white blood cell count usually indicates severe tissue inflammation or intestinal injury.[20] The gross color of the PF can be helpful in detecting injury and necrosis of the intestine. A serosanguinous appearance indicates vascular injury, whereas orange or brown-red indicates necrosis with the release of pigments such as hemosiderin. Serial samples of PF are most useful in determining the nature and extent of damage to the intestine, but in many cases of ischemia, irreversible tissue damage has occurred by the time PF abnormalities appear.

Tissue hypoxia and ischemia cause a rapid elevation of PF lactate dehydrogenase, creatine kinase, and alkaline phosphatase activity and lactate concentration.[20,21,28,29] Phosphate concentration increases when cellular disruption occurs.[19] PF enzyme activities, phosphate, and lactate concentration increase faster and higher than serum activities.[19-21,28,29] PF pH and glucose concentration tend to decrease during intestinal ischemia but are not as low as in septic peritonitis.[30] Although biochemical alterations may be early indicators of intestinal ischemia and necrosis, they are nonspecific and offer no advantage over conventional methods of PF analysis in many cases. PF alkaline phosphatase has been shown to arise predominantly from degenerating white blood cells, and elevations of other enzyme activities may occur with many inflammatory diseases.[28] Thus the specificity of many tests performed on PF is questionable. However, in selected cases in which conventional PF analysis and physical examination do not provide sufficient information to develop a treatment plan, biochemical analysis of the PF may be useful.

Cytologically examined cells of the PF may reflect chronic inflammatory conditions of the large intestine, especially eosinophilic or lymphocytic processes.[31] Infectious and inflammatory conditions often cause increases in the neutrophil count and may be indistinguishable unless bacteria are visible. One also may detect neoplastic diseases by PF examination. Chronic infection and inflammation may be associated with elevated PF protein and fibrinogen concentrations. Culture of PF usually is required to distinguish bacterial infections from noninfectious inflammation unless bacteria are visible on cytologic examination. However, culture of PF is often unrewarding because factors that are found in inflammatory PF inhibit bacterial growth, and leukocytes phagocytose many bacteria in the PF.[32] Decreases in PF glucose concentrations (<30 mg/dl), and pH (<7.3) are early indicators of a septic process. The glucose concentration and pH in the PF should approximately equal the blood glucose concentration and pH. A PF fibrinogen concentration greater than 200 mg/dl also indicates bacterial infection.[33]

FECAL EXAMINATION

Gross examination of the feces can provide information about digestion and transit time in the large intestine. Large fiber particles in the feces represent poor mastication or poor digestion in the large intestine. Small, mucus-covered, hard fecal balls indicate prolonged transit through the descending colon, whereas increased fluidity implies decreased transit time. Feces containing sand or gravel are not necessarily abnormal. However, a significant amount of sand implies that large quantities are present in the colon. Frank blood indicates substantial bleeding into the distal colon (right dorsal colon, small colon, or both) resulting from mucosal damage.

Laboratory analysis of the feces is performed frequently in cases of diarrhea. Fecal cytologic examination and tests for occult blood detect mucosal inflammation, erosion, or ulceration. Severe inflammatory diseases in human beings, invasive bacterial infections in particular, have been shown to increase the shedding of leukocytes in the feces. A higher percentage of horses with salmonellosis and diarrhea have fecal leukocyte counts greater than 10 cells per high power field than horses with negative fecal cultures for *Salmonella.* These results suggest that high fecal leukocyte counts indicate salmonellosis in horses with diarrhea. However, the specificity of this test is probably low. Low fecal leukocyte counts do not rule out salmonellosis.[34]

Fecal occult blood tests detect blood in the feces, presumably from erosion or ulceration of the mucosa, but do not distinguish the source of the blood. Large volumes of blood (1 to 2 L) given by nasogastric tube were required to produce a positive test for occult blood in the feces, but the amount of blood originating from the large intestine required to produce a positive test is unknown. A positive test implies significant hemorrhage into the gastrointestinal tract. Newer, more sensitive tests detect not only occult blood but also degraded blood and may be useful to determine the site and quantity of blood loss.[35] However, large-scale evaluation of these tests is as yet unavailable.

Bacteriologic examination of the fecal flora has been used to quantitate specific bacterial species in the feces of horses with diarrhea. Quantitation of clostridial species may be beneficial in diagnosing clostridial infection of the large intestine.[36] Tests to detect clostridial toxins in intestinal contents or feces are important to determine whether clostridia cultured from the feces are causing disease. The most common bacterial pathogens isolated from the feces of horses are *Salmonella* sp. and *Clostridium* sp. The number of *Salmonella* organisms isolated from the feces of horses with clinical salmonellosis is usually higher than from horses with asymptomatic infections. However, the volume of feces in many cases of acute diarrhea is high, and the concentration of *Salmonella* organisms may be lower than would be expected, accounting for many false-negative fecal cultures. The sensitivity of fecal cultures for detecting *Salmonella* infection may be as low as 20%. Culture of five consecutive daily fecal samples is recommended to increase the sensitivity of the test. Because salmonellae are intracellular organisms, culture of rectal scrapings or a rectal biopsy sample, along with fecal material, may increase the sensitivity of culture for detecting *Salmonella* infection to 50%.[37] One can perform a polymerase chain reaction assay on fecal samples to detect DNA from *Salmonella* sp. The polymerase chain reaction test is more sensitive than culture and is frequently positive in clinically normal horses that continuously shed small amounts of bacteria. Polymerase chain reaction or immunologic tests also may detect *Clostridium perfringens* and *Clostridium difficile* exotoxins in the feces.

Qualitative fecal examination is a technique to detect nematode and cestode ova, protozoan oocysts, parasitic larvae, and protozoan trophozoites. A direct smear of fecal material is a rapid method to screen feces for ova and oocysts, to detect parasite larvae and trophozoites, and to observe motility of ciliates and parasite larvae. Fecal flotation is a more sensitive technique for isolating and detecting ova and oocysts because the eggs are concentrated from the sample. Zinc sulfate and sucrose solutions often are used to concentrate less dense ova and oocysts. Zinc sulfate produces less distortion of trophozoites and larvae than sucrose solutions. Fecal sedimentation is particularly appropriate for ciliates, *Giardia* organisms, and trichomonads. Quantitative techniques such as the Cornell-McMaster method allow estimation of the number of eggs per gram of feces and are most appropriate in monitoring parasite control programs.[38]

Radiography

Survey radiography of the normal esophagus is usually unrewarding but may be useful in horses with esophageal obstructions to determine the extent and location of the obstruction. It is possible to detect foreign bodies or soft tissue masses and, in cases of esophageal rupture, free air and ingesta in the tissues surrounding the esophagus. Pneumomediastinum also may be observed.[39] Thoracic radiographs may be necessary to detect intrathoracic esophageal obstructions, megaesophagus, or cranial mediastinal masses causing extraluminal obstruction. One may use barium swallows or double-contrast esophagrams after resolution of the obstruction to determine whether a stricture, diverticulum, or other underlying disorder is present.[40] Barium sulfate is the usual contrast medium and can be administered orally by way of a dose syringe or nasogastric tube (50 to 100 ml of a 40% barium sulfate suspension or barium paste). Oral administration is preferred for evaluation of swallowing and lesions in the proximal esophagus. Administration of contrast using a nasogastric tube (preferably cuffed) allows for delivery of larger volumes of barium (up to 500 ml) but should be performed without sedation if possible. Administration of contrast material can be followed with air insufflation to create a double-contrast effect. If rupture of the esophagus is suspected or if the contrast material is likely to be aspirated, iodinated organic compounds in an aqueous solution should be used as contrast material.[39] Contrast radiography may be the most definitive method for the diagnosis of primary megaesophagus or other functional disorders such as autonomic dysautonomia (grass sickness) affecting the esophagus.[40] When interpreting esophageal radiographs, the veterinarian should take particular care if the horse is sedated. Acepromazine or detomidine administration causes esophageal dilation in normal horses, especially after passage of a nasogastric tube.[41]

Radiography of the adult equine abdomen is an effective technique in detecting radiodense material in the large intestine, such as enteroliths, sand, and metallic objects.[42,43] One survey demonstrated that radiography has 76.9% sensitivity and 94.4% specificity for diagnosing enterolithiasis.[42] Radiography also can be a useful tool for detecting sand accumulation in the colon that causes diarrhea or impactions (Figure 15-1) and for monitoring resolution in medically treated horses.[44] Recently, an objective scoring system demonstrated greater efficacy and less interobserver variability than a subjective assessment of radiographic sand accumulation in horses with or without a clinical diagnosis of sand colic.[45] The large size and density of the adult abdomen precludes evaluation of soft tissue structures because the detail and contrast of the radiographs are usually poor. One is more likely to obtain diagnostically useful abdominal radiographs from small ponies

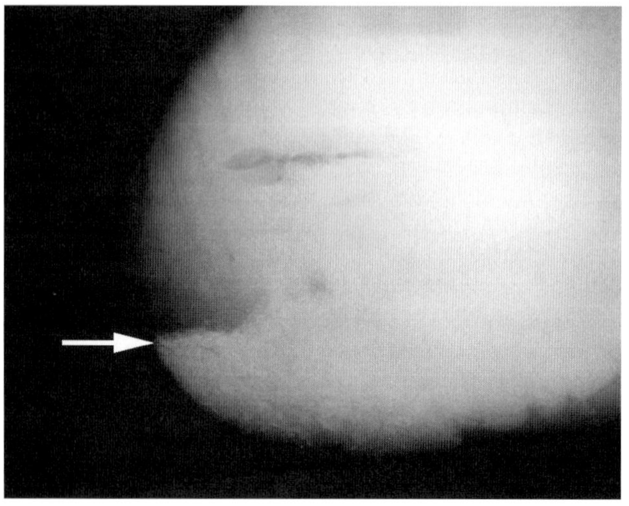

FIGURE 15-1 Radiograph of the cranioventral abdominal region of a weanling colt with diarrhea. The radiopaque accumulation of sand *(arrow)* in the sternal flexure of the ventral colon is notable.

and miniature horses than from full-size adult horses. Accumulation of gas is visible on radiographs of adult horses, but distinguishing normal intestinal gas from obstruction is often difficult. Horses should be fasted for 24 to 48 hours to reduce the amount of ingesta in the large intestine before radiography, if clinically warranted.

Abdominal radiography is more useful in foals than in adult horses. Radiographs are more detailed, and contrast can be good. Radiographic evidence of gas distention in the large intestine may indicate large intestinal obstruction, and radiographic signs of displacement are often diagnostic. Radiography allows the diagnosis of impactions, intussusceptions, foreign bodies, and other disorders. Functional ileus may be difficult to distinguish from mechanical obstruction.[46,47] Administration of contrast (barium sulfate 30% at 5 ml/kg) through a nasogastric tube increases the diagnostic capabilities of radiography and is especially useful for diagnosis of gastric outflow obstruction in the older foal.[48] Gastric ulceration also is recognizable with contrast radiography in the foal, although this is not as accurate a method as endoscopy.[49] Contrast administered retrograde through a 24-F Foley catheter inserted into the rectum at a dose of up to 20 ml/kg has excellent potential for diagnosing disorders of the small colon, transverse colon, and large colon in foals.[50]

Ultrasonography

Ultrasonographic evaluation of the abdomen can add valuable information in cases of acute or chronic gastrointestinal disease. Examination of the adult horse requires a 2.5- to 5.0-MHz transducer at minimum. Sector, linear, or curved linear transducers may be used. Clipping of the hair over the area to be examined, along with the application of isopropyl alcohol and ultrasound coupling gel, enhances evaluation. However, a functional exam is often performed with alcohol alone and no clipping of the hair.

To evaluate the abdomen adequately, one must know the anatomic location and normal appearance of the individual organs. In the left cranial abdomen, it is possible to assess the greater curvature of the stomach between the eleventh and thirteenth intercostal space, and the spleen and the large splenic vein can be used as landmarks. Cases of gastric dilation from gas or impaction appear as an enlargement of the viewing area to cover more than five rib spaces.[51] The veterinarian also can evaluate the stomach for intramural or extramural masses such as abscesses or for squamous cell carcinoma.[52] The lesser curvature is not routinely visible. Assessment of the small intestine should include evaluation for changes in thickness, motility, location, and visibility. Small intestinal loops are easily found in the left lower quadrant of the abdomen, but these normally are visible in other locations. One can visualize the duodenum consistently on the right side of the abdomen deep to the liver in the tenth to twelfth intercostal space or deep to the right kidney at the fifteenth to sixteenth intercostal space. Mural thickening (>4 mm) may occur with edema, infiltrative or proliferative diseases, enteritis, and paralytic or mechanical ileus. Thickening of the small intestinal wall in neonatal foals, with or without the presence of intramural gas shadows, should raise suspicions of clostridial enteritis. One can assess motility by monitoring a specific area for contractions over time.

Ultrasonography can be an accurate method of distinguishing strangulating disorders of the small intestine from nonstrangulating disorders. Strangulated small intestine has thicker walls and a larger diameter than typically observed in nonstrangulating disorders. Strangulating lesions have decreased motility in the incarcerated segments, with normal motility elsewhere.[53] Cases of paralytic ileus or nonstrangulating obstruction have a diffusely decreased peristalsis but not to the degree observed with strangulating lesions.[51,53]

Ultrasonography may be used to diagnose some specific lesions of the small intestinal tract. Ascarids may be visible in foals in cases of ascarid impaction,[51] and epiploic foramen entrapments are identified as edematous loops of small intestine found in the right cranial abdomen.[54] The veterinarian may note small intestinal intussusceptions as targetlike lesions when viewed in cross sections.[55] The presence of bowel loops, stomach, or liver in the thoracic cavity indicates the presence of herniation through the diaphragm and should be confirmed using radiography or surgical exploration.

Evaluation of the large intestine may be difficult because of the large amounts of gas within the lumen. It is also extremely difficult to reliably differentiate between specific segments of the colon ultrasonographically.[56] However, certain disorders are readily identifiable through ultrasonography. The nephrosplenic ligament area can be assessed for bowel entrapment in the left paralumbar fossa. In cases of entrapment the spleen will be pulled away from the body wall, and fluid or gas shadows will be observable dorsal to the spleen, obscuring the kidney, which is normally adjacent and abaxial to the spleen.[57] Small colon, small intestine, or pneumoperitoneum also may produce a gas shadow and obscure the kidney from view.[51]

Sand impactions may appear as hyperechoic bands on the ventral abdominal wall,[51] but ultrasound does not describe the extent of sand accumulation as well as radiographic assessment.[58] Ileocecal and cecocolic intussusceptions may be visible in the upper right paralumbar fossa.[59] In cases of colitis large, fluid-filled colons may be visible with or without intramural edema. The right dorsal colon is consistently located abaxial to the liver, within the right thirteenth to fifteenth intercostal space, and may be thickened (>5 mm) in cases of right dorsal colitis. Ultrasound also can be a useful tool for evaluating changes in motility over time in a given location.[60]

Evaluation of the abdomen always should include assessment of the peritoneal space for any evidence of an increased amount of PF or increased cellularity of the fluid, as indicated by an increase in echogenicity. Ultrasonography also can be useful in determining the ideal location for abdominocentesis. One also should evaluate the liver, kidneys, and spleen to detect any choleliths, nephroliths, masses, abscesses, or enlargement. Identifying abscesses or tumors not associated with visceral organs may be difficult and depends on their location and surrounding structures.

Nuclear Scintigraphy

Although more commonly used to diagnose lameness and musculoskeletal problems, nuclear scintigraphy has several uses in the evaluation of the gastrointestinal tract. Proper isolation protocols and waste disposal techniques must be strictly observed.

The procedure requires special gamma cameras and the injection of radioactive materials into the bloodstream. One of two methods may be used: injection of technetium-99m methylene diphosphonate (99mTc-MDP) directly into the blood or injection of 99mTc-labeled leukocytes.[61] The principle of nuclear scintigraphy then lies in increased uptake of the dye or the white blood cells into areas of inflammation. One of the most common uses of nuclear scintigraphy in evaluating the gastrointestinal tract is diagnosis of dental disease. Scintigraphy using 99mTc-MDP proved to be more sensitive in cases of dental disease than was radiography. Scintigraphy was slightly less specific, however, and therefore should be used with radiography or computed tomography for ultimate accuracy.[62] Scintigraphy using radiolabeled white blood cells can support a diagnosis of right dorsal colitis in the horse.[63] Images taken of the abdomen 20 hours after injection showed an increased linear uptake of leukocytes in the region of the right dorsal colon in horses with right dorsal colitis compared with normal horses. Other uses of nuclear scintigraphy include evaluation of metastasis of abdominal tumors to bony areas, assessment of biliary kinetics, and determination of liquid- and solid-phase gastric emptying.[62-64]

Advanced Imaging

Computed tomography (CT) is becoming increasingly available, and as such, various references are currently available describing the normal anatomy of the equine head as imaged with this modality.[65,66] CT is extremely useful to evaluate dental disease as well as tumors and masses of the head, larynx, pharynx, and proximal esophagus.[67,68] CT also has promise for evaluating abdominal disorders in foals. Most equipment can accommodate animals up to 400 lb. Restrictions of CT as a diagnostic aid include expense, availability, and weight and size limitation.

Endoscopy

Endoscopic examination of the gastrointestinal tract begins with evaluation of the pharyngeal area for any signs of collapse or dysfunction. One should evaluate the ability of the horse to swallow. The floor of the pharynx should be clean and free of feed material and foreign bodies. The oral cavity should be examined with the horse under heavy sedation or anesthesia and with the help of a full-mouth speculum. One can examine the teeth for any irregularities, obvious cavities, sharp points, or hooks and the hard and soft palates for completeness and any evidence of ulceration, masses, or foreign bodies.

A 3-m flexible endoscope should be used to examine the esophagus, which is accomplished best by passing the endoscope into the stomach and viewing the esophagus as one withdraws the endoscope while dilating the lumen with air. The esophageal mucosa normally should be a glistening, light pink color. Ulceration can occur with cases of choke or reflux esophagitis or in horses that have had an indwelling nasogastric tube. Erosions may be punctate, linear, or circumferential. One should evaluate carefully for any ulcers to ensure that no areas of perforation through the entire thickness of the esophageal wall exist. Distinguishing normal peristaltic contractions from areas of stricture requires observation of the area and its motility over time. Diverticula also may be noted as outpouchings of the mucosa, sometimes associated with a stricture distally. Megaesophagus, although rare, appears as a generalized dilation of the esophagus. Endoscopy may reveal food or foreign body impactions. The veterinarian always should re-evaluate the esophagus after removing any obstruction to detect the presence of complications (ulceration, rupture) or initiating causes (strictures, diverticula, and masses).

A 3-m flexible endoscope also allows examination of the stomach. The horse should be fasted for at least 12 hours before endoscopy. One can examine the cardia and fundus easily, as well as the margo plicatus. With complete emptying of the stomach (aided with gastric lavage, if necessary), one can also can evaluate the pylorus and proximal duodenum. The squamous mucosa should resemble the esophageal mucosa. The glandular mucosa should be glistening red and may have a reticulated pattern. The veterinarian should carefully examine it for evidence of ulceration or masses. Transendoscopic biopsy material can be easily obtained from esophageal, pharyngeal, or gastric masses, and because the biopsy size will be small, several samples should be taken for histopathologic examination. A complete description of gastroscopy and evaluation of gastric and gastroduodenal ulceration is available later in this chapter.

Tests of Absorption and Digestion

D-Glucose or D-xylose absorption tests are useful in determining malabsorption of carbohydrates from the small intestine in horses. The protocol for absorption tests using either carbohydrate is similar. The horse should be fasted for 18 to 24 hours before testing. Increased periods of fasting actually have been shown to decrease absorption of D-xylose and interfere with results.[69] A dosage of 0.5 to 1 g/kg of D-glucose or D-xylose is administered through a nasogastric tube. Administration of sedatives may falsely increase the blood glucose levels and interfere with gastrointestinal transit times. Blood samples are collected to measure glucose or xylose concentrations at 0, 30, 60, 90, 120, 150, 180, 210, and 240 minutes after administration. Additional samples can be taken up to 6 hours after dosing if the results are questionable. One should measure glucose in blood samples collected with sodium fluoride as an anticoagulant and measure xylose in samples collected in heparinized plasma.

A normal D-glucose absorption test, also known as an *oral glucose tolerance test,* should have a peak between 90 and 120 minutes, and this peak should be greater than 85% above the resting glucose value.[70] *Complete malabsorption* is defined as a peak less than 15% above the resting levels, and *partial malabsorption* is defined as a peak between 15% and 85% above the resting level. It is important to remember that gastric emptying, gastrointestinal transit time, length of fasting, cellular uptake and metabolism, age, diet, and endocrine function influence glucose absorption curves.[70,71] Malabsorption demonstrated by the oral glucose tolerance test is sensitive but not specific. Diseases that may cause a lowered or delayed peak include infiltrative lymphosarcoma, inflammatory bowel disease (lymphocytic-plasmacytic or eosinophilic), cyathostomiasis, chronic colitis (*Salmonella* sp.), multisystemic eosinophilic epitheliotropic disease, food allergies, and small intestinal bacterial overgrowth.[72] D-Xylose absorption tests have some advantages over the oral glucose tolerance test because xylose is not metabolized in the small intestinal mucosa and insulin does not influence its absorption. Gastric and intestinal motility, intraluminal bacterial overgrowth, and renal function still influence xylose absorption because the kidneys clear xylose.[72] The other main drawback to D-xylose is that it is generally available only in research settings. However, xylose measurements are available at many major universities. A normal D-xylose absorption curve should peak between 20 and 25 mg/dl at 60 to 120 minutes after dosing.[73] Decreased xylose absorption can occur in horses with inflammatory bowel disease, lymphosarcoma, multisystemic eosinophilic epitheliotropic disease, cyathostomiasis, extensive small intestinal resections, and any cause of villous atrophy.[72]

Maldigestion is a common occurrence in foals with diarrhea. Bacteria (especially *Clostridium* sp.) and viruses (especially rotavirus or coronavirus) may invade and destroy the villous epithelial cells that manufacture lactase and other disaccharidases, resulting in an inability to digest lactose. In this case continued ingestion of the mare's milk may cause an osmotic diarrhea, which may exacerbate the underlying enterocolitis. The veterinarian can perform lactose tolerance testing to assess the degree of maldigestion by administering D-lactose at 1 g/kg as a 20% solution via nasogastric tube and measure glucose concentrations in the blood at 0, 30, 60, 90, 120, 150, 180, 210, and 240 minutes. A normal curve shows doubling of glucose levels compared with baseline by 60 minutes after administration.[74]

Evaluation of Gastric Emptying

Assessment of gastric emptying may be useful in cases of gastric and esophageal ulceration, pyloric stenosis, proximal enteritis, and potentially postoperative ileus. However, accurate measurement of gastric emptying can be difficult to assess.

Multiple diagnostic imaging techniques have been used to study gastric emptying times. Contrast radiography can be used to assess gastric emptying in foals. In the normal foal barium remains in the stomach for varying amounts of time, but a significant amount should be gone within 2 hours.[48] Gastric emptying of solid, nondigestible, radiopaque markers also has been used in adult horses and ponies, but the results were variable and unpredictable even in the normal horse.[75] Nuclear scintigraphy is used commonly in human beings to measure gastric emptying and can be used in horses when available. The technique for measurement of liquid gastric emptying requires oral administration of 99mTc pentenate (10 mCi) and serial images taken of the cranial abdomen. The tracer is usually not visible 1 hour after administration in normal horses.[64] An adaptation of this methodology can be used for measurement of solid phase emptying of a 99m Tc–labeled pelleted ration.[76]

Alternatively, if nuclear scintigraphy is not available, acetaminophen absorption testing can be used as an indirect determination of liquid gastric emptying.[77,78] This test is performed by administering 20 mg/kg of acetaminophen orally and measuring subsequent blood values, then calculating the time to reach maximum serum concentrations and the absorption constant. In human beings the proximal small intestine absorbs almost all of the acetaminophen.[79] The median time to reach peak plasma levels using acetaminophen absorption in horses was 47.7 minutes.[77]

The 13C-octane acid breath test offers an easy, noninvasive method of determining gastric emptying of solids.[76,80] This test is performed by feeding a standard 13C-labeled test meal, and then collecting breath samples using a modified mask. The breath is then analyzed for the ratio of the novel isotope, 13:CO_2, to the normally produced 12:CO_2.

HISTOPATHOLOGIC EXAMINATION

It is often necessary to perform a histopathologic examination of tissues from the intestine to diagnose chronic inflammatory, infiltrative, or neoplastic conditions, and such examination can be useful in evaluating the extent of injury after obstruction or ischemia. Rectal mucosal biopsies are easy to collect, with few complications. However, to collect a full-thickness biopsy of the intestine requires a surgical approach (flank or ventral midline approach). Laparoscopy offers a safer technique to observe the large intestine and other abdominal structures.[81] The practitioner can obtain biopsies of masses, lymph nodes, and mesentery or intestinal serosa using laparoscopy and mucosal biopsies of the upper gastrointestinal tract using endoscopy.

LAPAROSCOPY

Other diagnostic tools, specifically laparoscopy and CT, are available but require specialized equipment and personnel with specific training. Flexible or rigid endoscopes used for laparoscopic evaluation of the abdomen allow for visualization of visceral organs and potentially for collection of biopsy material from masses or organs. Full-thickness biopsies of the intestines are not routinely possible through the laparoscope and usually require flank or ventral midline laparotomy. The laparoscopic procedure can be done with the horse standing or recumbent. Advantages of this technique over a flank or ventral midline celiotomy include smaller incisions, shorter healing time, and shorter procedure time. Disadvantages include the large amount of equipment needed, the high degree of skill involved, and the limitation as a diagnostic modality, rather than a treatment.[82] Clinical applications of diagnostic laparoscopy include the correction of rectal tears; percutaneous abscess drainage, assessment of adhesions, displacements, and integrity of the serosa of various bowel segments; and biopsy of abdominal masses.[81]

PATHOPHYSIOLOGY OF GASTROINTESTINAL INFLAMMATION

Samuel L. Jones

The inflammatory response of the gastrointestinal tract is a mechanism ultimately aimed at eliminating pathogens, initiating tissue repair, and restoring the gastrointestinal barrier. Blood flow is altered, endothelial permeability increases, cells are rapidly recruited into the tissue, plasma protein cascades are activated, and myriad soluble products are released that coordinate the response, trigger innate and adaptive immunity, and mobilize reparative elements. Although the cellular and vascular response and the secreted mediators of inflammation are important for killing pathogens and limiting invasion of injured tissues by commensal organisms, they can be quite damaging to host cells and proteins if not tightly regulated. Thus if the inciting stimulus is not eliminated quickly, then the inflammatory response itself will cause significant tissue injury. The mechanism regulating inflammation has been the focus of much research to identify therapeutic targets to modulate the damage to host tissues that occurs in many gastrointestinal diseases. Recent work has provided some of the molecular and cellular details of this complex physiology and has led to novel therapeutic strategies for treating inflammation.

INITIATION OF THE INFLAMMATORY RESPONSE

EPITHELIUM

The gastrointestinal epithelium interfaces with a luminal environment that is inhabited by potentially hostile microbial organisms. The epithelium presents a physical barrier to invasion by the flora of the gastrointestinal tract, consisting of the apical cellular membrane, intercellular tight junctions (the permeability of which is highly regulated), and a secreted layer of mucus. When invading pathogens breach the mucosal barrier, potent soluble and neural signals are generated that initiate an inflammatory response.[1] The epithelium can be conceptualized as a sensory organ that detects pathogen invasion to trigger an appropriate host defense and reparative response.

Noninfectious mucosal injury or invasion of epithelial cells by pathogenic organisms such as *Salmonella* activates the synthesis of pro-inflammatory chemokines (chemoattractants) by epithelial cells that triggers a robust influx of neutrophils into the tissue within hours of the damage.[1] Of the chemoattractants produced by epithelium, interleukin-8 (IL-8) has a particularly important role in initiating inflammation by recruiting neutrophils from blood[2-4] and regulating neutrophil migration through tissue matrix adjacent to epithelium.[5,6] Complement fragments such as C5a and bacteria-derived formylated chemotactic peptides also act as potent "end target" chemoattractants that are fully capable of stimulating a robust inflammatory response in the intestine if the epithelial barrier permits invasion of bacteria or the diffusion of bacterial peptides across the mucosa.

Epithelial cells activated during infection produce cytokines such as tumor necrosis factor α (TNF-α), arachidonic acid metabolites, and other pro-inflammatory mediators that activate recruited leukocytes.[7] Microbial products, particularly lipopolysaccharide and other bacterial cell wall components and microbial nucleic acids, are potent activators of leukocytes recruited into the tissue.[8] Mast cells are key sentinel leukocytes that sense microbial invasion, releasing TNF-α that appears to be a critical initiator and regulator of the cellular phase of inflammation.[9] Once the inflammatory response has been initiated, TNF-α; IL-1β; and other pro-inflammatory products of neutrophils, monocytes, mast cells, and epithelial cells amplify the inflammatory response.

The enteric nervous system has a key role in sensing and regulating inflammatory responses in the intestine. For example, *Clostridium difficile* toxin A activates a neural pathway that triggers mast cell degranulation and neutrophil influx into the tissue.[10,11] Blockade of this neural pathway is sufficient to abolish the profound inflammatory response induced by toxin A as well as many of the effects of toxin A on enterocyte secretion. Other pathogens and immune-mediated hypersensitivity reactions similarly stimulate inflammation by mechanisms that involve the enteric nervous system. Thus the epithelium interacts in a highly complex manner with the intestinal milieu, the enteric nervous system, and inflammatory cells to regulate the tissue response to injury and infection.

MACROPHAGES

Resident macrophages located in the lamina propria, submucosa, and intestinal lymphoid organs are among the first cells beyond the epithelium to respond to infection or injury. Macrophages are activated by microbial products by way of pattern recognition receptors and begin to produce pro-inflammatory molecules important for recruiting and activating neutrophils and monocytes. Pattern recognition receptors recognize microbial molecules such as lipopolysaccharide, lipoproteins, flagellin, peptidoglycan, and nucleic acids to signal the invasion by pathogens.[8] Of the pattern recognition receptors, the lipopolysaccharide (LPS) receptor complex is perhaps the best defined. LPS activates macrophages by way of the CD14-Toll-like receptor 4 complex to initiate transcription of the inflammatory cytokines TNF-α and IL-1β, which synergize with LPS to amplify the macrophage response.[8] LPS, particularly in concert with inflammatory cytokines, stimulates macrophages to produce copious amounts of nitric oxide, which is both microbicidal and vasoactive.[12] Nitric oxide and other nitrogen radicals react with reactive oxygen intermediates (ROIs) generated by the activated oxidase complex to produce some of the most toxic molecules of the host defense system: the peroxynitrites.[12] IL-8 is produced as well to recruit neutrophils. As the response progresses, other inflammatory mediators, particularly the arachidonic acid–derived lipids dependent on inflammation-induced cyclooxygenase-2 and 5-lipoxygenase activity, are produced that have potent vasoactive and pro-inflammatory effects through the activation of endothelial cells, neutrophils, and platelets.[13]

VASCULAR RESPONSE DURING INFLAMMATION

Four important changes occur in the intestinal vasculature during inflammation: (1) alteration of blood flow; (2) increased vascular permeability; (3) increased adhesiveness of endothelial cells, leukocytes, and platelets; and (4) exposure of the basement membrane and activation of the complement, contact, and coagulation cascades.

A wide range of mediators alter blood flow during inflammation in the intestinal tract, ranging from gases such as nitric oxide (a major vasodilator of the intestinal vasculature) to lipids (prostaglandins, leukotrienes, thromboxanes, and platelet-activating factor [PAF]), cytokines, bradykinin, histamine, and others. The major sources for these mediators include activated leukocytes, endothelial cells, epithelial cells, and fibroblasts. The primary determinant of blood flow early in inflammation is vascular caliber, which initially decreases in arterioles but then quickly changes to vasodilation coincident with opening of new capillary beds, increasing net blood flow. The increase in blood flow is relatively short lived, as the viscosity of the blood increases because of fluid loss and tissue edema resulting from leaky capillaries. Leukocyte margination, platelet adhesion to endothelial cells and exposed matrix, and areas of coagulation protein accumulation further decrease local circulation.

Increased vascular permeability is initially caused by inflammatory mediator actions on the endothelial cells. Histamine, leukotrienes, PAF, prostaglandins, bradykinin, and other mediators stimulate endothelial cell contraction, and interendothelial gaps form.[14,15] This stage of increased vascular permeability is readily reversible. Concurrently, mediators such as the cytokines TNF-α and IL-1β induce a structural reorganization of the interendothelial junctions, resulting in frank discontinuities in the endothelial monolayer.[16] Cytokines also stimulate endothelial cells to express adhesion molecules that support adhesion of leukocytes and platelets,[17] leading to the next and perhaps most devastating event. Leukocytes (primarily neutrophils) and platelets adhere to exposed basement membranes and activated endothelial cells. Adherent neutrophils and platelets are then exposed to the mediators of inflammation present in the surrounding milieu, which activates the cells to release oxidants and proteases (particularly elastase) that injure the endothelium and have the potential to cause irreparable harm to the microvasculature.[18-20] Marginated neutrophils begin to transmigrate between endothelial cells (as described in later sections), which, if in sufficiently large numbers, disrupt the integrity of the interendothelial junctions, worsening the vascular leakage.[19]

These stages of enhanced vascular permeability can be conceptualized as a mechanism to allow plasma proteins to enter the tissues and to potentiate the critical influx of leukocytes into tissues. However, if they are not regulated precisely, alterations in both hydrostatic and oncotic forces and irreversible damage to the vascular bed may have devastating consequences. Moreover, inappropriate activation of plasma protein cascades and leukocytes by activated endothelium and exposed matrix proteins can contribute to systemic inflammation (systemic inflammatory response syndrome, or SIRS; see the section on gastrointestinal ileus for more information) characterized by hypotension, generalized vascular leak syndrome, and multiorgan dysfunction, which may be fatal. Phosphodiesterase inhibitors reduce endothelial permeability in ischemia-reperfusion injury and other models of inflammation-induced vascular leakage[21,22] by increasing endothelial tight junction integrity and thus may be a viable therapeutic strategy to prevent or reduce the permeability alterations associated with inflammation.

CELLULAR EFFECTORS OF INFLAMMATION

Endothelial Cells

Endothelial cells respond to products of activated epithelial cells and macrophages in the intestinal tissue to recruit cells and humoral mediators of inflammation into the tissue. Activated endothelial cells display a range of molecules critical for neutrophil and platelet adhesion. The role of endothelial cells in mediating neutrophil recruitment is discussed in more detail later in this chapter. Intercellular permeability is increased to expose basement membrane proteins that trigger humoral defense systems (complement, coagulation, and contact system cascades) and to provide access for these macromolecules to the tissue. Endothelial cells are an important source of inflammatory mediators that amplify the response and vasoactive substances (particularly nitric oxide) altering blood flow.

Neutrophils

RECRUITMENT

Infection or injury to the gastrointestinal mucosa causes an influx of leukocytes from the blood that lay the foundation of the inflammatory response. Neutrophils, the first to arrive during inflammation, have a dominant role in the acute response. Within minutes neutrophils are recruited into the tissue, where they are activated to release products that not only are lethal to pathogens and pro-inflammatory but also may damage host cells and tissues.[23] Not surprisingly, much attention has been paid to the role of neutrophils in the pathophysiology of many inflammatory conditions.[24] Neutrophil depletion is protective in many models of gastrointestinal inflammatory disease. Of interest to clinicians, blockade of neutrophil migration into inflamed tissues prevents many of the pathophysiologic events associated with infectious enteritis, ischemia-reperfusion injury, and other gastrointestinal diseases.[18,25-29]

Neutrophil transendothelial migration is a multistep process that is temporally and spatially regulated and has a degree of cell type specificity (Figure 15-2). The predominant sites of neutrophil transendothelial migration are in the postcapillary venules and, in some tissues, capillaries. Endothelial cells in these vessels respond to cytokines and other soluble signals by expressing molecules that promote neutrophil adhesion and transmigration, including selectins and counter receptors for integrins. As neutrophils flow through these vessels, they are first tethered to activated endothelium. Tethering is mediated by selectin molecules expressed on neutrophils (L-selectin) and on activated endothelial cells (P- and E-selectins), which bind to PSGL-1, ESL-1, and other mucin counter-receptors.[30,31] The function of tethering is to increase the exposure of the neutrophil to activating chemokines presented on the surface of the endothelial cells.

Stimulation of neutrophils by IL-8 and other chemokines activate the second step of transendothelial migration. Chemokine binding to their receptors on the neutrophil generates signals that activate the binding of integrin adhesion receptors to their ligands, called *intracellular adhesion molecules* (ICAMs)

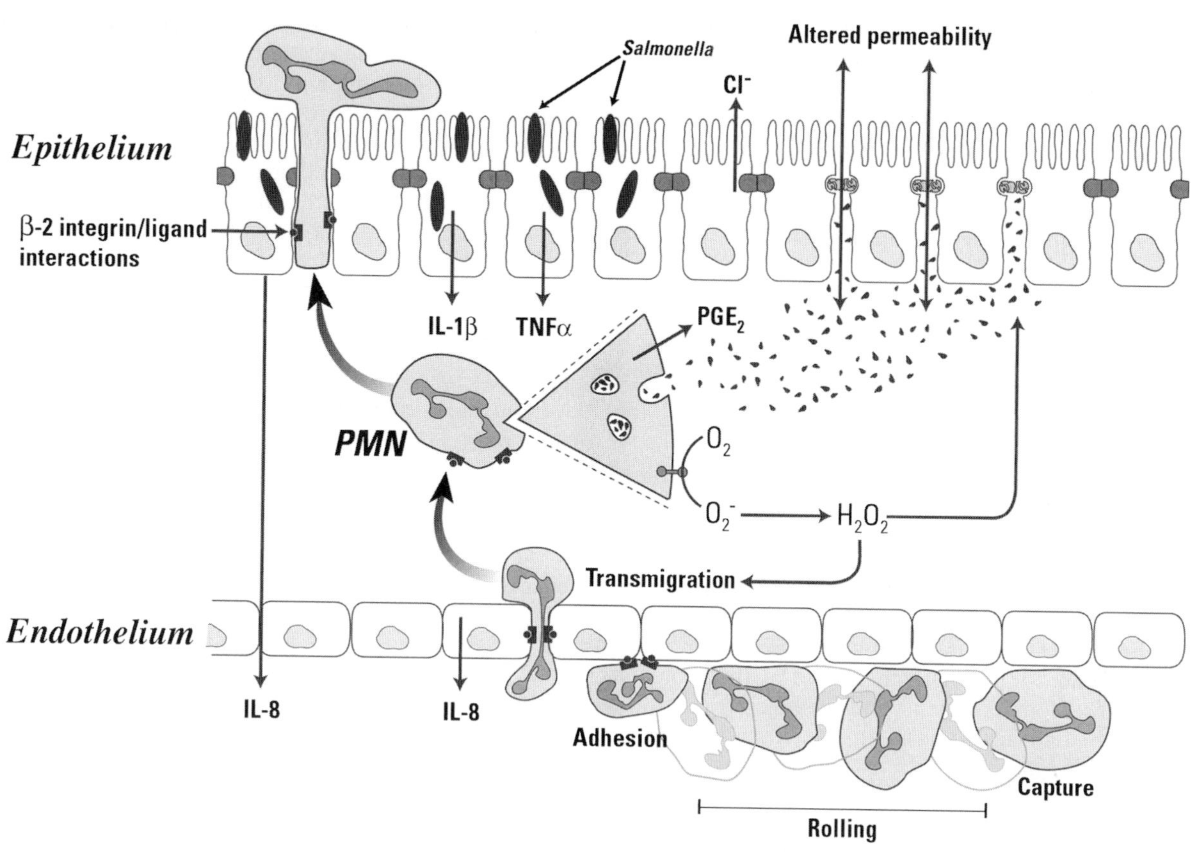

FIGURE 15-2 Depiction of neutrophil responses during intestinal inflammation in response to salmonella infection. Salmonellae infect epithelial cells, stimulating the production of chemokines (interleukin-8 [IL-8]), cytokines (IL-1β and tumor necrosis factor-α [TNF-α]), and other proinflammatory mediators. Endothelial cells stimulated by inflammatory mediators produce chemoattactants (such as IL-8) and display adhesion molecules that promote neutophil emigration. The three steps of neutophil (polymorphonuclear [PMN]) emigration—capture/rolling (mediated by selectins), adhesion (mediated by β_2 integrins), and transendothelial migration (mediated by integrins and platelet/endothelial cellular adhesion molecule [PECAM])—occur on activated endothelium. Chemoattractant molecules such as IL-8 trigger neutrophil emigration. In inflamed tissues cytokines (IL-1β and TNF-α) and a variety of other pro-inflammatory mediators stimulate the neutrophil oxidase complex to produce reactive oxygen intermediates (ROIs; O_2- and H_2O_2 and their derivatives). Activated neutrophils degranulate to release proteases and other hydrolases, cationic peptides (defensins), myeloperoxidase, and other products into the tissue. Activated neutophils synthesize a variety of inflammatory mediators, including prostaglandins (PGE_2) that modulate the inflammatory response. The products of activated neutrophils (ROIs, proteases, and mediators) stimulate epithelial secretion and alter tight junction permeability, promoting diarrhea. Neutrophils eventually migrate across the infected epithelium by a mechanism that involves integrins, disrupting tight junction integrity and increasing permeability to bacterial products, thus exacerbating the inflammatory response.

or *vascular cell adhesion molecules* (VCAMs), expressed on endothelial cells in inflamed mucosa. Integrin ligation to ICAMs arrests the tethered neutrophils, resulting in firm adhesion to the endothelium. Of the integrins expressed on neutrophils, the β2 integrins have a particularly important role in transendothelial migration. Calves and people with the disorder leukocyte adhesion deficiency (LAD) illustrate the requirement for β2 integrin-mediated adhesion in neutrophil function. LAD is a result of an autosomal recessive trait resulting in the lack of the β2 integrin expression. The neutrophils from affected individuals cannot migrate into most tissues and do not function normally, resulting in poor tissue healing and profound susceptibility to infection, especially at epithelial barriers.[32,33] Other integrins also have a role in transendothelial migration. β1 Integrins mediate transendothelial migration in some cells and seem to be particularly important for mediating emigration of monocytes into many tissues.[34]

Following this firm adhesion step, neutrophils migrate through the endothelium along a chemotactic gradient of IL-8 and other chemoattractants, such as C5a and LTB4.[3,19,35] Neutrophils migrate across the endothelial monolayer at intercellular junctions by way of a mechanism involving a series of integrin-ligand interactions mediated by both β2 and β1 integrins and other adhesion molecules[31] that is generally capable of maintaining the integrity of the endothelial barrier.[36] However, massive flux of neutrophils through the endothelium alter endothelial tight junctions and injure the basement membrane, resulting in increased endothelial permeability to molecules as large as plasma proteins and even endothelial cell detachment from the basement membrane.[19,20] Nonintegrin molecules such as platelet-endothelial cell adhesion molecules (PECAMa) also are involved in transendothelial migration of neutrophils.[31] Homotypic binding of PECAMs on adjacent endothelial cells form part of the intercellular junction. Neutrophils express an integrin of the β3 family that can bind PECAM, and through sequential binding of β3 integrins to PECAM, the neutrophil can "unzip" the intercellular junction and migrate through, closing it behind itself.

ACTIVATION

A key feature of neutrophils and other leukocytes is the requirement for integrin-mediated adhesion to extracellular matrix (ECM) proteins or other cells to achieve an optimal effector phenotype.[37] Critical components of the ECM in inflamed tissues include fibronectin, fibrinogen, and vitronectin, deposited in tissues as a result of plasma leakage and by synthesis of new proteins by stromal cells and resident macrophages in response to inflammatory mediator activation. The changing composition of the matrix proteins deposited in tissues during inflammation serves as a cue as to the nature of the tissue environment for recruited inflammatory cells as they become activated. Individual gene expression studies have demonstrated that adhesion to matrix proteins induces the expression of cytokines and chemokines and their receptors, arachidonic acid–derived lipid mediator synthases, metalloproteinases, growth factors, transcription factors, and other genes that influence the differentiation and activation of inflammatory cells.[38] Reactive oxygen intermediate production, phagocytosis, degranulation, and other effector functions stimulated by inflammatory mediators and bacterial products are optimal only when neutrophils are adherent to the ECM.[37] Adhesion to distinct ECM proteins selectively activates signaling pathways and gene expression of neutrophils, monocytes, and other leukocytes with differing abilities to promote certain functions such that the composition of ECM in many ways controls the development of the ultimate effector phenotype. Thus integrin-mediated adhesion provides a mechanism whereby neutrophils and other leukocytes can sense the complex tissue environment and respond appropriately.

Of the activators of neutrophils at sites of inflammation, complement (C3-opsonized particles), cytokines (TNF-α and IL-1β), PAF, immune complexes, and bacterial products are among the most potent stimuli. Other mediators produced during inflammation may modify neutrophil activity, particularly formylated bacterial peptides, chemokines, complement fragments (C5a), leukotriene B_4 (LTB_4), and prostaglandins. Activated neutrophils are highly phagocytic; produce large amounts of ROI; degranulate to release myeloperoxidase, cationic antimicrobial peptides (defensins), serine proteases (mainly elastase), and metalloproteinases; and secrete inflammatory mediators (TNF-α, IL-1β, prostaglandins, leukotrienes, and others) (see Figure 15-2).

Mast Cells

Mast cells strategically reside in mucosal tissues, including the submucosa and lamina propria of the gastrointestinal tract, and constitute a crucial first line of defense at epithelial barriers. However, they are also important effector cells of the pathophysiology of inflammatory gastrointestinal diseases.[39] Experimental depletion of mast cells, genetic deficiency in the development of mast cells, or pharmacologic stabilization of mast cells to prevent degranulation all have a protective effect in a variety of models of gastrointestinal inflammatory disease, including dextran- or trinitrobenzenesulfonic acid–induced colitis[40,41], ischemia-reperfusion injury,[42,43] and immediate hypersensitivity responses.[44]

Mast cells are activated by a wide variety of microbial products and host-derived mediators.[45] Among the activators of mast cells, the so-called anaphylatoxins (complement fragments C3a, C5a, and C4a) are extremely potent stimuli causing release of mediators of inflammation. In addition, mast cells are the primary effector cells of IgE-mediated anaphylaxis (Type I hypersensitivity reactions) by virtue of their high affinity receptors for IgE. Cross-linking of receptor-bound IgE on mast cell surface by antigens (i.e., food antigens) causes rapid degranulation, resulting in the explosive release of granule contents.[46] Neural pathways in the intestine also regulate mast cells. Mast cells respond to enteric pathogen invasion via neural reflexes that stimulate the release of inflammatory mediators.

Activated mast cells release preformed histamine, 5-HT, proteases, heparin, and cytokines from granules. Activation also stimulates de novo synthesis of a range of inflammatory mediators, including prostaglandins, PAF, and leukotrienes. Transcription of a number of peptide mediators, such as the cytokines TNF-α and IL-1β among many others, also increases upon stimulation of mast cells. Mast cell products have profound effects on the vasculature, increasing endothelial permeability and causing vasodilation.[47] Moreover, mast cell–derived mediators markedly enhance epithelial secretion by a mechanism that involves the activation of neural pathways and direct stimulation of epithelial cells.[46] In particular, the mast cell granule protease tryptase operating via the protease-activated receptor-2 is a key regulator of gastrointestinal physiologic responses during inflammation, including epithelial secretion and intercellular junction integrity, motility, and pain responses.[48,49] Mast cell products significantly alter intestinal motility, generally increasing transit and expulsion of intestinal contents. Mast cell–derived leukotrienes and TNF-α also have a crucial role in host defense against bacterial pathogens, acting to recruit and activate neutrophils,[50,51] and are crucial players in the mechanism regulating dendritic cell function and adaptive immune responses.[52]

Mast cells have a newly identified role in host defense and inflammatory responses to bacterial pathogens.[9] Their role is in part due to the release of pro-inflammatory mediators during bacterial infection, which is critical for recruiting and activating other innate host defense cells such as neutrophils. However, mast cells are also phagocytic, have microbicidal properties, and can act as antigen presenting cells to the adaptive immune system.[9] The role for mast cells in host protective responses appears to be as a sensor of bacterial invasion. Unlike IgE-mediated responses, bacterial products seem to elicit a highly regulated and selective response from mast cells.

HUMORAL MEDIATORS OF INFLAMMATION

Complement

The complement cascade is a fundamental part of the inflammatory response. Activation of the complement cascade, either by immune complexes (classical pathway) or by bacteria or bacterial products, polysaccharides, viruses, fungi, or host cells (alternative pathway), results in the deposition of complement proteins on the activating surface and the release of soluble proteolytic fragments of several complement components.[53] In particular, activation of either pathway results in the deposition of various fragments of the complement protein C3, which are potent activators of neutrophils and monocytes.[53] Opsonization of particles with C3 fragments constitutes a major mechanism of target recognition and phagocyte activation.[54] During the activation of the complement cascade culminating in deposition of C3, soluble fragments of C3 (C3a), C5 (C5a), and C4 (C4a) are liberated. These fragments, termed *anaphylatoxins,* have potent effects on tissues and cells during inflammation. Perhaps most notably, they are chemotactic for neutrophils (particularly C5a), activate neutrophil and mast cell degranulation, and stimulate reactive oxygen metabolite release from neutrophils.[53] The termination of the complement cascade results in the formation of a membrane attack complex in membranes at the site of complement activation. If this occurs on host cells such as endothelium, the cell may be irreversibly injured. Although the primary source of complement is plasma, epithelial cells of the gastrointestinal tract also produce C3, suggesting that local production and activation of the complement cascade during inflammation occurs in intestinal tissues.

It is clear that if the regulatory mechanisms of the complement cascade fail, then the inflammatory response may be inappropriate and tissue injury can occur. The role of complement in gastrointestinal inflammation has been most extensively studied in models of ischemia-reperfusion injury. Activation of the complement cascades has a major role in altered endothelial and epithelial permeability in these models. Several lines of evidence support the importance of complement in intestinal injury. Mice deficient in C3 or C4 are protected against ischemia-reperfusion injury.[55] Moreover, administration of monoclonal antibodies against C5 reduced local and remote injury and inflammation during intestinal reperfusion injury in a rat model.[56] Administration of a soluble form of complement receptor 1, a regulatory protein that halts the complement cascade by dissociating C3 and C5 on host cell membranes, reduced mucosal permeability, neutrophil influx, and leukotriene B4 production during ischemia-reperfusion injury in rats and mice.[55,57] Although neutrophils and mast cells mediate many of the pathophysiologic effects of the complement cascade, the membrane attack complex may have a primary role in altered vascular permeability during ischemia-reperfusion injury.[58]

Contact System

The contact system of plasma is initiated by four components: Hageman factor (HF), prekallikrein, Factor XI, and high-molecular-weight kininogen. HF is a large plasma glycoprotein that binds avidly to negatively charged surfaces.[59] Bacterial cell walls, vascular basement membranes, heparin, glucosaminoglycans, and other negatively charged surfaces in the intestine capture HF and the other three important initiators of the contact system in a large multimolecular complex. Of the surfaces that bind HF, the ECM is an extremely potent activator of the contact system. Once bound, HF is converted to HF-α, which cleaves prekallikrein to kallikrein and Factor XI to Factor XIa. The ultimate result is further cleavage of HF by kallikrein and triggering of the contact system cascade, activation of intrinsic coagulation by Factor XIa, activation of the alternative pathway by HF, and proteolytic cleavage of high-molecular-weight kininogen by kallikrein, releasing biologically active kinins.

The products of the contact system, particularly bradykinin, have several important biologic properties that drive many of the vascular and leukocyte responses during inflammation.[59] Bradykinin induces endothelial cell contracture and intracellular tight junction alterations that increase vascular permeability to fluid and macromolecules. Bradykinin also affects vascular smooth muscle contracture, resulting in either vasoconstriction or vasodilation, depending on the location. Bradykinin also increases intestinal motility, enhances chloride secretion by the intestinal mucosa, and intensifies gastrointestinal pain. In neutrophils kinins stimulate the release of many inflammatory mediators, including cytokines, prostaglandins, leukotrienes, and reactive oxygen intermediates.[60] Kallikrein cleaves C5 to release C5a, a potent chemotactic factor for neutrophils, and thus has a role in recruiting and activating inflammatory leukocytes.

The plasma kallikrein-bradykinin system is activated in a variety of acute and chronic inflammatory diseases of the gastrointestinal tract.[61,62] Recent evidence has demonstrated that blockade of the pathophysiologic effects of bradykinin has clinical applications. Oral or intravenous administration of the bradykinin receptor antagonist icatibant reduces the clinical signs, onset of diarrhea, and many of the histopathologic changes in experimental models of colitis in mice.[63] Inhibition of kallikrein by oral administration of P8720 attenuated the intestinal inflammation, clinical score, and systemic manifestations in a model of chronic granulomatous enterocolitis.[62] Thus the contact system is a viable therapeutic target for inflammatory diseases of the intestine.

Tissue Injury During Inflammation

Changes in blood flow to the mucosa and other regions of the intestine that reduce perfusion of the tissues can potentiate the initial damage caused by infection or injury. For example, reperfusion of ischemic tissues is associated with platelet and neutrophil clumping in the small vessels of the mucosa, which can impede blood flow.[64] Platelets are activated and adhere to exposed basement membrane and activated endothelial cells and provide a surface for leukocyte adhesion. The accumulation of platelets and leukocytes can significantly reduce vessel diameter and blood flow while potentiating local coagulation and thrombus formation.

Soluble mediators released by activated leukocytes and endothelial cells also affect blood flow. Histamine and the vasoactive lipids derived from arachidonic acid (leukotrienes, prostaglandins, thromboxane, prostacycline, and PAF) have a prominent role in regulating local perfusion during inflammation and may have systemic effects on blood flow as well. Procoagulant mediators released by inflammatory cells in response to the inflammatory process (i.e., tissue factor produced by macrophages or endothelial cells), exposed basement membrane proteins, and bacterial components can trigger the contact system and the coagulation and complement cascades, the products of which affect blood flow. Nitric oxide, whether produced by endothelial cells or leukocytes (macrophages), is a potent regulator of blood flow and has a significant role in the control of perfusion during inflammation.[65] Many of the mediators that affect perfusion also affect endothelial permeability, altering osmotic and hydrostatic balance and tissue edema. In extreme cases local and systemic coagulopathies initiated by vascular injury and absorption of microbial products and inflammatory mediators induce a hypercoagulable state, leading to microthrombus formation, which can reduce blood flow or macrothrombus formation, causing tissue infarction.

The cellular mediators of inflammation have the potential to inflict severe injury to intestinal tissues. Neutrophils have an important role in the pathophysiology of many intestinal diseases, including ischemia-reperfusion injury,[18,25] infectious enterocolitis,[26,28,66] nonsteroidal anti-inflammatory drug–induced mucosal ulceration,[29] and others. Depletion of neutrophils, blockade of their emigration into tissues, or inhibition of neutrophil activation reduces the severity of these and other inflammatory diseases.[67] Thus many anti-inflammatory therapies are emerging that specifically target neutrophil adhesion, migration, and activation.

Migration of neutrophils through endothelium during emigration into inflamed tissues is remarkable in that the permeability of the endothelial monolayer is preserved under most circumstances. However, there is a limit above which neutrophil migration alters the permeability characteristics of the endothelium. The effect is in part physical in that the mere movement of large numbers of neutrophils through the endothelium is sufficient to mechanically disrupt the tight junctions and in part due to toxic products of neutrophils that damage endothelial cells and basement membranes.[64,68] Serine proteases (particularly elastase) and metalloproteinases released by degranulating neutrophils liquefy tissue matrix proteins and cleave cell surface proteins that make up endothelial intercellular junctions to ease neutrophil migration to the site of infection.[23] These degradative enzymes are particularly damaging to basement membranes and the cellular barriers of the endothelium, thus contributing to vascular permeability (and local tissue edema) and thrombosis. The permeability may be affected to the extent that not only water but also macromolecules (e.g., albumin, matrix proteins, complement) leak into the interstitium. Blockade of neutrophil adhesion to endothelium with anti-β2 integrin antibodies has a sparing effect on the microvasculature in experimental intestinal ischemia-reperfusion injury, reducing the alterations in vascular permeability and histopathologic evidence of microvascular damage.[64]

Similar to the endothelium of inflamed tissues, massive neutrophil transmigration occurs across the epithelium in response to infection or injury. Neutrophil transepithelial migration increases epithelial permeability by disrupting tight junctions.[68] Like the endothelium, neutrophils disrupt the epithelial barrier mechanically as they migrate through (see Figure 15-2). Proteases, particularly elastase, degrade basement membrane components and tight junction proteins. Protease activated receptor-2 activated by neutrophil granule serine proteases alter epithelial and endothelial tight junction integrity. Pro-inflammatory products of activated neutrophils (TNF-α and IFN-γ) increase tight junction permeability by direct effects on enterocytes. Prostaglandins released by activated neutrophils stimulate epithelial secretion, thus contributing to diarrhea. Subepithelial accumulation of neutrophils can lead to de-adhesion of the epithelial cells from the basement membrane and mild to severe ulceration. The physiologic result of the effects of neutrophils and their products on the epithelial barrier includes protein-losing enteropathy and absorption of bacterial cell wall constituents, which potentiates the local and systemic inflammatory responses.

Neutrophils in inflamed tissues stimulated by potent host-derived activators (such as IL-1β and TNF-α) and bacterial products (LPS) release copious amounts of reactive oxygen intermediates (see Figure 15-2). Although these oxygen and oxyhalide radicals are important for killing pathogens, they are also potentially toxic to epithelial and endothelial cells and matrix proteins. Reactive nitrogen intermediates (RNIs), produced primarily by macrophages during inflammation, combine with ROI to form peroxynitrites, which are particularly toxic.[12] In addition to injury to mucosal tissues, ROI also have an as yet ill-defined role in recruiting and activating neutrophils, thereby potentiating the inflammatory response.[69] In support of the role of ROI in inflammatory diseases of the gastrointestinal tract, administration of inhibitors of ROI production or pharmacologic ROI scavengers can be protective in many models of reperfusion injury or enterocolitis. Many therapies are aimed at inhibiting neutrophil activation, and effector functions in tissues have been evaluated for use in intestinal diseases. Phosphodiesterase inhibitors, by causing cyclic adenosine monophosphate (cAMP) accumulation in neutrophils, are anti-inflammatory by virtue of their ability to suppress neutrophil activation and ROI production. New phosphodiesterase inhibitors selective for the predominant neutrophil isoform of phosphodiesterase hold promise for use in many inflammatory diseases.

Subepithelial mast cells also have an important role in altering epithelial permeability in inflamed intestine. During the intestinal hypersensitivity response subepithelial mast cell release of mast cell protease tryptase by degranulation increases epithelial permeability via an effect on tight junctions.[44,70,71] This alteration in tight junction permeability results in enhanced transepithelial flux of macromolecules, including proteins and bacterial products. Cytokines released by mast cells and phagocytes also regulate tight junction permeability. IL-4, a product of mast cells and macrophages, has been demonstrated to increase epithelial permeability.[72] Moreover, TNF-α and IFNγ, products of many inflammatory cells, synergistically increase tight junction permeability.[73]

PATHOPHYSIOLOGY OF DIARRHEA

L. Chris Sanchez

Acute equine colitis causes rapid, severe debilitation and death in horses (more than 90% of untreated horses die or require euthanasia).[1] Since 1919 several reports have described a number of acute diarrheal conditions in the horse that appear to share a common characteristic clinical presentation.[2] Diarrhea associated with acute equine colitis occurs sporadically and is characterized by intraluminal sequestration of fluid; moderate to severe colic (abdominal pain); and profuse watery diarrhea with resultant endotoxemia, leukopenia, and hypovolemia.[3,4] Causes of acute colitis and therapeutic options are discussed elsewhere in this chapter.

Although the mechanisms responsible for the fluid losses are not known, inflammatory cells may play an integral role because this condition is characterized by large numbers of granulocytes infiltrating the large intestinal mucosa.[5-9] Equine cecal and colonic tissues collected during the acute stages of experimentally induced acute equine colitis

(Potomac horse fever, lincomycin with and without *Clostridium* spp. inoculation, nonsteroidal anti-inflammatory drug administration) reveal the presence of numerous neutrophils and eosinophils in the lamina propria and submucosa.[5,8,10,11] Granulocyte-derived reactive oxygen intermediates are crucial to antimicrobial defenses in the gut and stimulate chloride and water secretion by interactions with enterocytes.[12,13] Normal equine intestinal tissue is unique compared with that in most other mammalian species for a preponderance of eosinophils located in the intestinal mucosa and submucosa.[14,15] Production of ROIs by stimulated phagocytic granulocytes following mucosal barrier disruption may be responsible for the massive fluid secretory response that occurs during the early stages of acute equine colitis.

Colitis refers to inflammation and mucosal injury of the colon and cecum (typhlocolitis) that may occur in response to a number of causes.[16] The cause of the colonic injury may be well-defined such as in naturally occurring infectious or experimentally induced colitis. However, many cases of human and animal diarrhea have a speculative or unknown diagnosis or no diagnosis. Irrespective of the underlying or initiating cause of colonic injury, the colon apparently has a limited repertoire of responses to damage because most forms of colitis demonstrate similarities in histopathologic appearance and clinical presentation. Various degrees of mucosal erosion and ulceration, submucosal and mucosal edema, goblet cell depletion, and presence of an inflammatory cellular infiltrate within the mucosa and submucosa are common to many types of human and animal colitis.[15,16] Characteristic clinical manifestations include intraluminal fluid sequestration; abdominal discomfort; hypovolemia; and most often profuse, watery diarrhea.

PATHOPHYSIOLOGY OF COLITIS

Large bowel diarrhea results from abnormal fluid and ion transport by cecal and colonic mucosa. Loss of fluid by the large intestine can result from malabsorptive or hypersecretory processes and is often a combination of the two.[17] Colonic secretory processes are a function of the crypt epithelium, whereas absorptive processes are limited to surface epithelial cells.[18,19] Under normal baseline conditions an underlying secretion by crypt epithelium is masked by a greater rate of surface epithelial cell absorption. Abnormal forces influencing the rates of secretion and absorption can result in massive, uncontrolled secretion and malabsorption by large intestinal mucosal epithelial cells, leading to rapid dehydration and death.[17-19]

Two intracellular processes control colonic secretion: the cyclic nucleotide cAMP and cyclic guanosine monophosphate (cGMP) and the calcium system.[20,21] Agents may activate adenyl cyclase (vasoactive intestinal peptide, prostaglandin E2 [PGE_2]) or guanyl cyclase (bacterial enterotoxins) and induce increases in cAMP or cGMP, respectively. This reaction causes phosphorylation of specific protein kinases that induce the actual apical and basolateral membrane transport events. Increases in intracellular free calcium may arise from cyclic nucleotide–dependent release of stored calcium within the cell or from increased calcium entry across the cell membrane.[17-19] Calcium may act through calmodulin, which then can activate membrane-phosphorylating protein kinases.

At least four central systems control intestinal secretion: (1) the hormonal system, (2) the enteric nervous system, (3) bacterial enterotoxins, and (4) the immune system.[21,22] Hormonal control of colonic electrolyte transport is exerted primarily through the renin-angiotensin-aldosterone axis.[23] The enteric nervous system controls transport through three separate components: (1) extrinsic nerves of the parasympathetic and sympathetic pathways; (2) intrinsic ganglia and nerves, which secrete a variety of neurotransmitters, including peptides; and (3) neuroendocrine cells (intraepithelial lymphocytes) that reside in the epithelium and release messengers onto the epithelial cells in a paracrine manner.[17,21-23] Many bacterial enterotoxins can induce intestinal secretion by cAMP or cGMP signal transduction.[24] Bacterial enterotoxins can stimulate release of mediators (such as substance P) from primary afferent neurons, which then affect enteric neurons, often propagating neurogenic inflammation.[25]

Preformed inflammatory mediators such as histamine, serotonin, or adenosine and newly synthesized mediators such as prostaglandins, leukotrienes, PAF, various cytokines, the inducible form of nitric oxide, and reactive oxygen metabolites can initiate intestinal secretion by directly stimulating the enterocyte and by acting on enteric nerves indirectly to induce neurotransmitter-mediator intestinal secretion.[22] For instance, when added to the T84 colonic cell line, the known mast cell mediators histamine, adenosine, and PGD_2 induce chloride secretion.[26,27] Prostaglandins of the E and F series can cause an increase in chloride secretion in intact tissue and isolated colonic cells.[28,29] Leukotrienes, PAF, and a number of cytokines have been shown to have no effect on T84 cell secretion but have a significant effect on electrolyte transport in intact tissue, suggesting that intermediate cell types may be involved in these secretory responses.[30-32]

The epithelial cell chloride secretory response occurs via prostaglandin- and adenosine-mediated increases in cellular cAMP, whereas histamine acts by H_1 receptor induction of phosphatidylinositol turnover, production of inositol triphosphate, and mobilization of intracellular calcium stores.[22] Lipoxygenase products (leukotrienes) are capable of activating a colonic secretory response and do not appear to involve the cyclic nucleotides or calcium ions.[30] Phagocyte-derived reactive oxygen mediators (ROMs) can induce colonic electrolyte secretion in vitro, suggesting that oxidants may contribute directly to the diarrhea associated with colitis.[33] Reactive oxygen species initiate the secretory response by increasing cellular cAMP or stimulating mesenchymal release of PGE_2 or prostacyclin, which in turn stimulates the epithelial cell or enteric neuron, respectively.[33-36] Sodium nitroprusside, an exogenous source of nitric oxide, stimulated an increase in chloride secretion in rat colon that was mediated by cyclooxygenase products and enteric neurons.[37] Table 15-1 summarizes inflammatory mediator–induced epithelial cell chloride secretion.

ROLE OF INFLAMMATORY CELLS

Acute colitis rarely develops as a result of a simple cause or effect phenomenon but instead is influenced by many extrinsic and intrinsic host and microorganism factors. Inflammatory mediators released from mast cells and monocytic or granulocytic phagocytes cause intestinal chloride and water secretion and inhibit neutral sodium and chloride absorption.[21,22,52] Inflammatory cells, particularly the phagocytic granulocytes, play an important role in mucosal pathophysiology in cases of colitis.[13,53] Large numbers of these cells are observed on histopathologic examination of tissues from human and animal cases of colitis. Products of cell activation stimulate direct and

TABLE 15-1

Inflammatory Mediators that Stimulate Epithelial Cell Chloride Secretion

Mediator	Action	Reference
Prostaglandin E_2	Increases Cl secretion	38
	Decreases neutral NaCl absorption	
Vasoactive intestinal peptide	Increases cAMP-mediated NaCl secretion	39
	Activates cholinergic nerves	40
Endotoxin	Increases Na absorption	41
	Increases cell membrane permeability	
Serotonin	Increases fluid and electrolyte secretion	42
Interferon-γ	Decreases tight junctions and causes increase in cell membrane permeability	43
Interleukin-1 and interleukin-1β	Increase prostaglandins E_2 and $F_1\alpha$ and thromboxane B_2.	44
Histamine (H_1)	Increases Cl secretion via Ca-mediated pathways	26,45
Bradykinin	Increases Cl secretion through prostaglandin-mediated pathways	46,47
Reactive oxygen mediators	Increase Cl secretion	33, 48
Thromboxanes	Increase Cl secretion	49
	Decrease neutral NaCl absorption	
Lipoxygenase products	Increase Cl secretion via prostaglandin-mediated pathways	50
Platelet-activating factor	Increases Isc (Cl secretion)	51
Adenosine	Increases Cl secretion	27

cAMP, Cyclic adenosine monophosphate.

indirect secretory responses in intestinal cells and tissues.[21,22] Products of phagocyte secretion may amplify the inflammatory signal or have effects on other target cells in intestine such as enterocytes and smooth muscle cells.

ROLE OF PHAGOCYTE-DERIVED REACTIVE OXYGEN METABOLITES

The nicotinamide adenine dinucleotide phosphate (NADPH)-oxidase system of phagocytes (neutrophils, eosinophils, monocytes/macrophages) is a potent inducer of superoxide radicals used as a host defense mechanism to kill invading microorganisms.[13] During inappropriate stimulation such as inflammation, trauma, or ischemia followed by reperfusion, increased levels of toxic oxygen species are produced, causing damage to host tissues. Engagement of any of several receptor and nonreceptor types including phagocytosis mediators, chemotactic agents, various cytokines, and microbial products can stimulate phagocytes.[13] Resident phagocytes or those recruited to colonic mucosa early in the disease process are considered to augment mechanisms causing fluid and electrolyte secretory processes, a so-called amplification process.[54,55]

Activation of the respiratory burst results in the production and release of large amounts of superoxide anion (O_2^-) and H_2O_2.[56] In addition to these ROMs, activated phagocytes secrete peroxidase enzyme (myeloperoxidase from neutrophils and eosinophil peroxidase from eosinophils) into the extracellular space. The peroxidases catalyze the oxidation of Cl– by H_2O_2 to yield HOCl, the active ingredient in household bleach products. The peroxidase-H_2O_2-halide system is the most cytotoxic system of the phagocytes; HOCl is 100 to 1000 times more toxic than O_2^- or H_2O_2. HOCl is a nonspecific oxidizing and chlorinating agent that reacts rapidly with a variety of biologic compounds, including deoxyribonucleic acid (DNA), sulfhydryls, nucleotides, amino acids, and other nitrogen-containing compounds. HOCl reacts rapidly with primary amines to produce the cytotoxic N-chloramines. The mechanisms by which these substances damage cells and tissue remain speculative, but possibilities include direct sulfhydryl oxidation, hemoprotein inactivation, protein and amino acid degradation, and inactivation of metabolic co-factors of DNA.[57] Luminal perfusion of specific ROMs increased mucosal permeability, and serosal application caused increases in Cl– secretion in vitro.[58] Tissue myeloperoxidase activity, an index of tissue granulocyte infiltration, is used clinically and experimentally to assess degree of intestinal inflammation.[59] Myeloperoxidase activity is elevated in acute flare-ups of human inflammatory bowel disease and various animal models of acute colitis.[59-61] The acute inflammatory response in these conditions is characterized predominantly by neutrophils, the predominant source of myeloperoxidase activity. However, this assay measures total hemoprotein peroxidase, which includes monocyte and eosinophil peroxidase in addition to neutrophils.[62] Moreover, levels of peroxidase activity in equine circulating eosinophils are greater than in circulating neutrophils,[63] and this may apply to resident tissue eosinophils as well.

Arachidonic acid metabolites are thought to play a role in intestinal inflammation in diarrheal disease.[22] Elevated levels of these intermediate metabolites have been demonstrated in natural disease and experimental models of colitis and appear to parallel increases in ROMs in inflamed intestine.[64] Addition of H_2O_2 or HOCl to rat colonic tissue in Ussing chambers induces PGE_2 release and active Cl– secretion.[36,65] Prostaglandins can stimulate increases in Cl– secretion in intact intestinal tissue[35,65,66] and in isolated colonic T84 cells.[34,36] Interactions between ROMs and mesenchymal release of PGE_2/PGI_2 may be relevant to the mechanisms producing the diarrheic condition. Fibroblasts co-cultured or juxtaposed to colonic T84 cells greatly increased the Cl– secretory response to H_2O_2 in vitro through the release of PGE_2.[34] In addition, equine colonic mucosa has an increased sensitivity to endogenously released prostaglandin by exhibiting a significant secretory response under in vitro conditions.[67]

ROLE OF ENDOTOXIN, MALNUTRITION, IMMUNODEFICIENCY, AND INTESTINAL MICROFLORA

ENDOTOXIN

Endotoxin, the LPS component of the outer cell wall of gram negative bacteria, is present in large quantities in the large intestine of healthy horses.[63,67] The intact bowel forms an effective barrier to the transport of significant amounts of these highly antigenic toxins, but the diseased gut absorbs these macromolecules in large amounts, causing the subsequent adverse systemic effects that are often life threatening.[68] A complete review of endotoxemia and systemic inflammatory response syndrome (SIRS) is presented later in this chapter.

Endotoxins trigger mucosal immune cells and subsequent release of inflammatory mediators in cases of colitis. The first report of experimentally induced endotoxemia described clinical signs and hematologic findings that closely paralleled those reported for severe colitis in horses.[69] Studies in which endotoxin was administered intravenously in human beings and laboratory animals caused significant dose-related gastrointestinal changes, ranging from mild diarrhea to bloody, watery diarrhea.[70,71] In vitro studies on the effects of endotoxin on intestinal water and electrolyte transport in adult male rats showed a significant decrease in net colonic sodium absorption and increased colonic permeability.[41] In animal models of protein energy deficiency, endotoxin-induced mortality increased compared with that of well-nourished control animals. Endotoxin depresses lymphocyte responses to specific mitogens.[72] Thus the adverse effects of malnutrition and endotoxin are mutually aggravating. In horses endotoxin negatively affects gastrointestinal motility, including in the cecum and right ventral colon, and perfusion.[73]

IMMUNODEFICIENCY

The importance of a normal immune system to the defense of the mucosal surface of the gastrointestinal tract is evident in the immunosuppressed state. Primary immunodeficiencies affecting the gastrointestinal tract are well documented. Common agammaglobulinemia is the most frequently reported gastrointestinal disease and causes B cell deficiency–associated giardiasis in other species.[74] In horses severe combined immunodeficiency can result in diarrhea secondary to adenovirus, coronavirus, and *Cryptosporidium* infection.[75,76] Interestingly, selective immunoglobulin A (IgA) deficiency rarely results in intestinal disease because of a speculated increase in mucosal IgM response. However, combined IgA and IgM deficiencies with a higher incidence of intestinal disease occur. A selective deficiency of secretory IgA has been associated with intestinal candidiasis in other species. Certain mucosal pathogens may enhance their pathogenicity by producing IgA proteases.[74] Acquired immunodeficiency or immunosuppression in adults can result from infectious diseases (particularly viral), nutritional deficiencies, aging phenomenon, and drugs (corticosteroids, azathioprine, cyclophosphamide). Chronic salmonellosis was documented secondary to adult-onset B cell deficiency in a Quarter Horse.[77]

NUTRITIONAL DEFICIENCIES

Nutrition is a critical determinant of immunocompetence and risk of illness.[78] Impaired systemic and mucosal immunity contributes to an increased frequency and severity of intestinal infections observed in cases of undernourishment. Abnormalities occur in cell-mediated immunity, complement system, phagocytic function, mucosal secretory antibody response, and antibody affinity. Morbidity caused by diarrheal disease is increased particularly among individuals with stunted growth rate because of malnourishment.[79] The critical role of several vitamins and minerals in immunocompetence has been substantiated in animals deprived of one dietary element and findings in human patients with single-nutrient deficiency. Nutritional deficiency can cause increased colonization of the intestine with microorganisms, alter the symbiotic characteristics of resident intestinal bacterial populations, and impair defenses of the gastrointestinal tract, allowing increased risk of systemic spread of infection and absorption of macromolecules (in particular, endotoxin).

INTESTINAL MICROFLORAE

Indigenous microflorae greatly impede colonization of the gastrointestinal mucosa by pathogenic organisms. The ability of a potential pathogen to initiate an infection depends on its ability to breach the mucosal epithelial barrier. Resident microbes protect against pathogens by producing bacteriocidal substances and competing for available mucosal sites and nutrients.[80] In addition, microflorae are important for development of the adaptive immune system.[81] Alterations in the gastrointestinal microflorae, or their interaction with the innate immune response, can lead to disorders such as inflammatory bowel disease and the irritable bowel syndrome in humans.[82] In fact, hyper-responsiveness to commensal bacteria appears vital to the development of inflammatory bowel disease in humans.[83] Whether a similar association is present in horses is currently unknown.

FACTORS AFFECTING MOTILITY

Disturbances in motility patterns occur during inflammatory diseases of the colon, but the role of motility alterations in the pathogenesis of diarrhea remains unclear. Invasive bacteria cause characteristic motor patterns in the colon consisting of rapid bursts of motor activity that appear to decrease transit time through the large intestine. The result is reduced clearance of bacteria from the large intestine, which may contribute to the virulence of the organism.[84] Absorption of endotoxin and the release of inflammatory mediators such as prostaglandins disrupt the motility patterns of the large intestine, resulting in less-coordinated contractions, and may contribute to the alterations in motility seen with invasive bacteria. Although the effect of endotoxin and prostaglandins on transit time is not profound, the disruption of coordinated activity may play a role in causing diarrhea.[85] Thorough mixing and prolonged retention time of ingesta are important not only in microbial digestion of nutrients but also in absorption of microbial byproducts and fluid.[23] The ingesta is viscous and therefore must be mixed to bring luminal ingesta in contact with the mucosa for absorption.[86] In addition, poor mixing increases the thickness of the unstirred layer, decreasing contact of ingesta with the mucosa and decreasing absorption.[23]

Progressive motility must be present, however, if a diarrheal state is to occur.[23] Ileus may be accompanied by increased fluid in the lumen of the large intestine, but without progressive motility the fluid is not passed. Frequently, acute colitis causes a period of ileus characterized by scant stool. Diarrhea is apparent only when motility returns and the ingesta is passed. Increased progressive motility has been suggested to cause diarrhea by decreasing transit time and is thought to play a role in irritant catharsis and in the mechanism of action of some laxatives.[87] Irritation and distention increase motility and may well decrease transit time, but increased secretion also is thought to contribute to diarrhea caused by these substances.[88]

PATHOPHYSIOLOGY OF MUCOSAL INJURY AND REPAIR

Anthony T. Blikslager

MUCOSAL BARRIER FUNCTION

To gain an appreciation of the mechanisms whereby the mucosa is injured and subsequently repaired, it is important to understand how the integrity of the mucosa is physiologically regulated. Regulation of mucosal integrity is referred to as *mucosal barrier function,* which is vital because it prevents bacteria and associated toxins from gaining access to subepithelial tissues and the circulation. However, the mucosa has two conflicting functions: It must serve as a protective barrier while continuing to absorb solutes necessary to maintain well-being of the host. This conflict is most notable at the intercellular (paracellular) space, which allows passage of select solutes and water[1-4] but which does not admit large molecules, including bacterial toxins.[5] The paracellular space is almost exclusively regulated by the tight junction,[6] which is the interepithelial junction at the apical-most aspect of paracellular space. Although these tight junctions were originally viewed as inert cellular adhesion sites, it has become clear in recent years that tight junction permeability is dependent on tissue-specific molecular structure and regulated by a complex array of intracellular proteins and the cytoskeleton. Tight junctions consist of a group of transmembrane proteins that interdigitate from adjacent cells. Although occludin was originally thought to be the predominant tight junction transmembrane protein, a group of proteins termed *claudins* appear to "fine tune" the function of the tight junction. For example, select claudins are responsible for the relative porosity of the barrier to select electrolytes based on their charge within the paracellular space.[7] These transmembrane proteins interact with the cytoskeleton via a series of intracellular proteins, including zonula occludens (ZO)-1, ZO-2, ZO-3, cingulin, and others.[8] In addition, local regulatory proteins such as the small GTPase Rho are critical to tight junction function. In general, the relative contractile state of the actin cytoskeleton determines the degree to which tight junctions are open or closed, but the complexities of regulation of this process are poorly understood.[9,10]

The most sensitive measure of mucosal barrier function is transepithelial electrical resistance, which is measured by mounting mucosa in an in vitro system called an Ussing chamber. This measurement is largely a reflection of the permeability of mucosa to ions.[11,12] There are two routes ions may follow when traversing epithelium: transcellular and paracellular.[5] Since cell membranes have a resistance to passive flow of ions 1.5 to 3 log units greater than that of the epithelium as a whole, measurements of transepithelial resistance largely reflect the resistance of the paracellular space and in particular the tight junctions that regulate paracellular flow of ions.[12] Because tight junctions differ in structure from different portions of the mucosa,[13] measurements of transepithelial resistance reflect the net resistance of epithelium of variable permeability within a given tissue. For example, tight junctions in the intestinal glandular structures called *crypts* are leakier than those in the surface epithelium because of fewer and less-organized tight junction strands.[11,14] Conversely, surface epithelium has a greater number of well-organized tight junction strands that result in epithelium with a relatively high resistance.[11] This correlates well with the absorptive function of epithelium located on the mucosal surface and the secretory function of crypt epithelium. Structure of tight junctions also varies with the segment of intestine. For example, tight junctions have more strands in the ileum than the jejunum, which is reflected by a higher transepithelial resistance in the ileum.[15] In addition, cells are more closely apposed at the level of the tight junction within the colon. This is in keeping with the largely absorptive role of the colon and is advantageous given the hostile microbial environment of the colon.

Gastric Mucosal Barrier Function

There are four regions of the stomach, based on the type of mucosal lining (in an orad to aborad order): nonglandular stratified squamous epithelium, cardiac epithelium, proper gastric mucosa, and pyloric mucosa.[16] Stratified squamous epithelium has distinct differences in terms of barrier function compared with the remainder of the gastrointestinal tract. This epithelium has baseline transepithelial resistance measurements of approximately 2000 to 3000 $\Omega \cdot cm^2$, which is an order of magnitude higher than the adjacent cardiac mucosa.[17,18] Thus the stratified squamous mucosa is exceptionally impermeable. This is the only mechanism this mucosa has to defend itself against injury. The stratified squamous epithelium consists of four layers: the outer *stratum corneum, stratum transitionale, stratum spinosum,* and the basal *stratum germinativum.* However, not all layers contribute equally to barrier function, which is largely composed of interepithelial tight junctions in the *stratum corneum,* and mucosubstances secreted by the *stratum spinosum.*[17,19] The relative impermeability of stratified squamous mucosa can be demonstrated by the effects of HCl on this type of epithelium in vitro, which has very little effect until it reaches a pH of 2.5 or below.[18] Thus, although the majority of the literature on equine ulceration pertains to the effects of HCl and inhibitors of HCl secretion,[20-23] other factors may be critical to the development of gastric ulcer disease.

The site of HCl secretion (proper gastric mucosa) is also protected from so-called back-diffusion of H^+ ions by a relatively high transepithelial electrical resistance (compared with cardiac mucosa), but there are also a number of other critical mechanisms to prevent acid injury. The gastric mucosa secretes both mucus and bicarbonate, which together form a HCO_3^--containing gel that titrates acid before it reaches the lumen.[11,24] The mucus layer is principally formed by glycoproteins (mucins) secreted by goblet cells but also includes other gastric secretions and sloughed epithelial cells. Mucins consist of core peptides with a series of densely packed O-linked polysaccharide side-chains that, once secreted, become hydrated and form a viscoelastic gel. However, the mucus layer does not form an absolute barrier to back-diffusion of acid. Thus, for acid that does back diffuse into the gastric mucosa, epithelial Na^+/H^+ exchangers are capable of expelling H^+ once the cell reaches a critical pH.[11]

Recent studies have renewed interest in the protective mechanisms of mucus because of the discovery of a group of compounds secreted by goblet cells called the *trefoil peptides*. The name of these peptides is derived from a highly conserved cloverleaf structural motif, which confers substantial resistance to degradation by proteases, including pepsin. There are three known members of this group, pS2, spasmolytic polypeptide (SP), and intestinal trefoil factor (ITF), the latter of which is solely secreted by goblet cells in the small and large intestine. Both pS2 and SP are secreted by goblet cells within the stomach and are believed to intercalate with mucus glycoproteins, possibly contributing to the barrier properties of mucus.[25] These peptides also play a critical role in repair of injured mucosa.

ADAPTIVE CYTOPROTECTION

An additional mucosal function that serves to reduce the level of injury is adaptive cytoprotection, wherein application of topical irritants to gastric mucosa results in subsequent protection of mucosa in response to repeated exposure to damaging agents. For example, pretreatment with 10% ethanol protected against mucosal damage in response to subsequent application of absolute ethanol, and this effect was abolished by treatment with the cyclooxygenase (COX) inhibitor indomethacin.[26] The cytoprotective effects of prostaglandins have been demonstrated directly in studies wherein pre-administration of prostaglandins protected gastric mucosa from damage by agents such as concentrated hydrochloric acid and hypertonic saline.[27] Prostaglandins appear to be cytoprotective in the stomach at doses lower than those used to inhibit gastric acid secretion, ruling out a simple antacid mechanism.[28] Although not fully characterized, cytoprotection has been attributed in part to prostaglandin-stimulated mucus production.[29] An associated beneficial effect of prostaglandins is the increased production of bicarbonate, which is trapped within mucus on the surface of the mucosa.[30,31] Interestingly, PGE_2 appears to lose its cytoprotective activity in the presence of the mucolytic agent *N*-acetylcysteine. Attention has also been directed at enhanced mucosal blood flow as a potential mechanism for prostaglandin-mediated cytoprotection. For example, pretreatment with prostaglandin I_2 (PGI_2) protected against ethanol-induced mucosal damage as a result of increased mucosal blood flow.[32] In addition, PGE_2, which is also cytoprotective despite the fact that it does not increase blood flow, prevents vascular stasis associated with irritant-induced vascular damage by inhibiting neutrophil adherence to damaged endothelium.[33,34]

Sensory nerves distributed throughout gastrointestinal mucosa have also been implicated in cytoprotective mechanisms. As an example of their importance in mucosal cytoprotection, pretreatment of newborn rats with capsaicin (which dose-dependently destroys sensory nerves) renders the mature rats more susceptible to gastric injury.[35] Alternatively, use of a low dose of capsaicin, which stimulates rather than destroys sensory nerves, protects gastric mucosa against injurious agents.[36,37] Sensory nerves contain neuropeptides such as calcitonin-gene related peptide (CGRP) and substance P, which may play a protective role via vascular mechanisms. For instance, CGRP stimulates increased gastric blood flow, which is theorized to reduce injury in much the same way as prostaglandins. In fact, recent studies suggest that the roles of prostaglandins and CGRP in gastric cytoprotection are intimately intertwined. In particular, PGI_2 is believed to sensitize sensory nerves following treatment with a mild irritant, with resultant increases in CGRP release and mucosal flow. Similar studies have shown that antagonists of CGRP inhibit the cytoprotective action of PGE_2.[38] Another neural mediator, nitric oxide, has also been implicated in adaptive cytoprotection. Interestingly, nitric oxide has a number of actions that are similar to those of prostaglandins, including maintenance of mucosal blood flow.[39]

INTESTINAL BARRIER FUNCTION

Regulation of barrier function in the intestine is not as well characterized as that of the stomach, although mechanisms of barrier function, including secretion of mucus and regulation of mucosal blood flow, are presumed to be similar. The proximal duodenum also has to protect itself from acid damage as it receives gastric contents, and this involves secretion of mucus and bicarbonate in much the same way as the stomach. One other mechanism that helps both the stomach and the intestine to maintain mucosal barrier function is the speed with which the mucosa repairs. Thus, for a defect to develop in the mucosal barrier, injurious factors have to outpace mucosal recovery. Such recovery initially involves epithelial migration across denuded regions of basement membrane (restitution).[25] This process is so rapid that epithelial defects may be resurfaced within minutes. For example, in bile salt–injured equine colon, denuded surface mucosa was completely covered by restituting epithelium within 180 minutes.[40] In the small intestine intestinal villi greatly amplify the surface area of the mucosal luminal surface, which in turn takes far longer to resurface with restituting epithelium once it has become denuded.[41] However, intestinal villi are able to dramatically reduce the denuded surface area by contracting.[42]

MECHANISMS OF GASTRIC INJURY

Stratified Squamous Mucosal Ulceration

Although the stratified squamous epithelium is relatively impermeable to HCl, there are a number of factors that can dramatically enhance the damaging effects of HCl in this epithelium. In particular, bile salts and short chain fatty acids (SCFAs) are capable of breaking down the squamous epithelial barrier at an acid pH, thereby exposing deep layers to HCl, with subsequent development of ulceration.[18,43] Relatively high concentrations of SCFA normally exist within the equine stomach as a result of microbial fermentation.[17] These weak acids penetrate squamous mucosa and appear to damage Na^+ transport activity principally located in the stratum germinativum. Bile salts also may be present in the proximal stomach as a result of reflux from the duodenum. Although such reflux has a relatively high pH, it appears that bile salts adhere to stratified squamous epithelium, becoming lipid soluble and triggering damage once the pH falls below 4.[44] Diet and management (e.g., periods of fasting) also play crucial roles in the development of conditions conducive to gastric ulceration. Typically, there is a pH gradation in horses from proximal to distal compartments of the stomach, with the lowest pH values in the distal stomach.[45] However, during periods of fasting, this stratification is disrupted such that low pH values may be recorded in the proximal stomach.[46] Fasting conditions also increase the concentration of duodenal contents within the proximal stomach, particularly bile.[44]

Ulceration of Proper Gastric Mucosa

Proper gastric mucosa is exposed to injurious agents, including pepsin, bile, and acid. The latter is constantly secreted by parietal cells in the horse as an adaptation to near-continuous intake of roughage,[16] but it is tightly regulated by enterochromaffin-like (ECL) cells within the proper gastric mucosa and G- and D-cells, which are present within the pyloric mucosa. Acid secretion is amplified by ECL-released histamine, which interacts with H_2 receptors on parietal cells, and G-cells, which release the prosecretory hormone gastrin. A combination of histamine and gastrin can have a synergistic effect on parietal cell gastric secretion, because these mediators have distinct receptors and second messengers. On the other hand, D-cells are sensitive to an acidic environment and release somatostatin, which inhibits acid secretion.[47] Nonetheless, gastric mucosa may be exposed to acid for prolonged periods of time, particularly in horses that are extensively meal fed and which do not have the benefit of roughage, which tends to buffer stomach contents.[44,47]

Aside from peptic ulceration, induced by combinations of acid and pepsin, research in the human field has revealed the tremendous importance of *Helicobacter pylori* in inducing ulceration. Infection with this organism has the effect of raising gastric pH because of disruption of gastric glands, but it also induces an inflammatory reaction that causes damage.[48] However, to date there is very little evidence that this organism is involved in gastric ulcers in horses. In the absence of a known role for infectious agents in gastric ulceration in animals, ulceration likely develops from injurious factors similar to those found in the proximal stomach, including gastric acid and bile. However, some factors that are important to induction of squamous epithelial ulceration may not be important in development of proper gastric mucosal ulceration. For example, feed deprivation and intensive training reproducibly induce squamous epithelial ulceration in horses but have little effect on proper gastric mucosa in horses.[49] Gastric acid likely plays a key role, whereas other factors, such as nonsteroidal anti-inflammatory drugs (NSAIDs), serve to reduce gastric defense mechanisms. In particular, inhibition of prostaglandin production would reduce mucus and bicarbonate secretion while also reducing gastric mucosal blood flow.[50] Some of the NSAIDs also have a topical irritant effect, although this appears to be of minor significance, because the route of administration (oral or parenteral) seems to have little influence on development of ulceration.[51]

The source of prostaglandins responsible for gastric protection was originally assumed to be COX-1, because this COX isoform is constitutively expressed in gastric mucosa, whereas COX-2 is not expressed in the stomach unless it is induced by inflammatory mediators. However, mice in which the COX-1 gene has been knocked out fail to develop spontaneous gastric lesions,[52] possibly because of compensatory increases in prostaglandin production by COX-2.[53] This concept supports recent data indicating that inhibition of both COX isoforms is required to induce gastric ulceration.[54] From a clinical perspective this data indicates that drugs selective for either COX-1 or COX-2 may be less ulcerogenic in the horse because they allow the uninhibited COX isoforms to continue to produce protective prostanoids. Because COX-2 elaborates prostaglandins induced by inflammatory stimuli, preferential or selective inhibitors of COX-2 may be particularly useful because of their ability to serve as anti-inflammatory agents that are less ulcerogenic.[55]

INTESTINAL ISCHEMIA AND REPERFUSION INJURY

The most notable cause of intestinal mucosal injury in horses, particularly those suffering from colic, is ischemia. Initially, it seems intuitive that reducing gastrointestinal blood supply would injure the mucosa. However, the anatomy of the gastrointestinal tract and the differing structure of the intestinal mucosa at various anatomic locations have a significant influence on the extent of mucosal injury. Furthermore, ischemic injury may be induced by several mechanisms, including occlusion of arterial supply by a thrombus, strangulation of intestinal vasculature, and generalized reduction in blood flow associated with various shock states. In addition, a number of seemingly distinct mechanisms of intestinal injury, such as intestinal distention, also trigger mucosal injury via an ischemic mechanism. Finally, reperfusion injury may also influence the extent of mucosal injury following an ischemic episode, and it has been proposed as a potential site of therapeutic intervention.[56,57] Thus it is critical that the mechanisms of ischemia-reperfusion injury be understood in order to develop an understanding of the severity of various clinical conditions and begin to formulate a therapeutic approach to diseases characterized by this devastating form of injury.

Regulation of Intestinal Blood Flow

The intestinal circulation is capable of closely regulating blood flow during periods of low systemic perfusion pressure.[58,59] Local regulation of resistance vessels within the microvasculature is particularly prominent; metabolic end products of ATP cause continued dilation of resistance vessels despite reductions in systemic arterial pressure. This results in continued perfusion of gastrointestinal tissues during the early stages of shock; other organs, such as skeletal muscle, undergo massive shunting of blood as a result of marked increases in the resistance of resistance vessels. The reasons for these differences in regulation are not entirely clear but may be related to the relatively high level of energy required to fuel the intestinal mucosa and the serious systemic effects of breaches in the mucosal barrier. However, as blood flow falls below a critical level, regulatory systems are no longer effective and oxygen uptake by the gastrointestinal tissue decreases, culminating in tissue damage.[58]

The villus tip is the most susceptible region affected by hypoxia in the equine small intestine, largely because of the countercurrent exchange mechanism of blood flow in the small intestinal villus.[58] This countercurrent exchange mechanism is attributable to the vascular architecture, which consists of a central arteriole that courses up the core villus, arborizes at the tip, and is drained by venules coursing down the periphery of the villus.[60] As oxygenated blood flows into the central arteriole, oxygen tends to diffuse across to the adjacent venules, which are flowing in the opposite direction. This series of events takes place along the length of the villus, resulting in a villus tip that is relatively hypoxic even under normal conditions. Furthermore, when blood flow is reduced, as occurs in hypovolemic or septic shock, the countercurrent exchange of oxygen is enhanced, and the tip becomes absolutely hypoxic.[58] This mechanism might explain why the small intestinal mucosa is more susceptible to ischemic injury, compared with the colon, which has no villi. For example, the duration required to produce severe morphologic damage to the equine colon is approximately 25% longer than that required to produce similar damage to the small intestine.[61]

Ischemic Epithelial Injury

Intestinal mucosal epithelium is very susceptible to hypoxia because of the relatively high level of energy required to fuel the Na^+/K^+-ATPase that directly or indirectly regulates ion and nutrient flux. The first biochemical event to occur during hypoxia is a loss of oxidative phosphorylation. The resulting diminished ATP concentration causes failure of the energy-dependent Na^+/K^+-ATPase, resulting in accumulation of sodium and subsequently intracellular water. The pH of the cytosol drops as lactic acid and inorganic phosphates accumulate from anaerobic glycolysis. The falling pH damages cell membranes, including lysosomal membranes, resulting in the release and activation of lysosomal enzymes into the cytosol, further damaging cellular membranes. Damage to the cell membrane allows the accumulation of high concentrations of calcium in the cytosol, which activates calcium-dependent degradative enzymes.[62] These events result in cytoplasmic blebbing of the basal membrane, with subsequent detachment of cells from the underlying basement membrane.

Recent studies on epithelial injury during ischemia suggest that the majority of epithelial cells undergo programmed cell death (apoptosis) during ischemia and reperfusion rather than necrosis, allowing retention of reusable components of irreversibly injured cells.[63] In one study 80% of detached epithelium during small intestinal ischemia-reperfusion underwent apoptosis.[64] Although the most obvious result of apoptosis is loss of surface epithelium, a number of cells on the lower portion of the villus (in the small intestine) and cells within the crypts may also undergo apoptosis that only becomes evident up to 24 hours following reperfusion of ischemic tissue.[65]

TABLE 15-2

Grading System for Ischemia-Reperfusion Injury in Small Intestinal Mucosa

Grade	Description
1	Separation of epithelium at the tip of the villus, creating a small space between epithelium and basement membrane called Grüenhagen's space
2	Loss of epithelium from the tip of the villus
3	Loss of epithelium from the upper third of the villus
4	Complete loss of villus epithelium
5	Injury or loss of epithelium within the crypt in addition to complete loss of villus epithelium

Adapted from Chiu CJ, McArdle AH, Brown R, et al: Intestinal mucosal lesion in low-flow states. 1. A morphological, hemodynamic, and metabolic reappraisal, *Arch Surg* 101:478–483, 1970.

Morphologic changes observed in ischemic-injured small intestinal mucosa follow a similar sequence regardless of whether injury is induced by ischemia alone or ischemia-reperfusion (Table 15-2).[66] Initially, epithelium separates from the underlying basement membrane, forming a fluid-filled space termed *Grüenhagen's space* (Figure 15-3). The mechanism of fluid accumulation in this space is not entirely understood but may result from continued epithelial absorption of NaCl and water, before it has fully detached from neighboring epithelial cells. This fluid accumulation likely exacerbates epithelial separation from the basement membrane. Subsequently, epithelium progressively sloughs from the tip of the villus toward the crypts, which are the last component of the intestinal mucosa to become injured.[67-69] This likely relates to the vascular architecture, because crypts receive a blood supply that is separate from the vasculature involved in the villous countercurrent exchange mechanism. The early morphologic changes observed in the equine large colon during ischemia are somewhat different from those described in the equine small intestine because of the lack of intestinal villi. However, as might be expected, the more superficially located surface cells are sloughed before those in crypts.[61,70] The orderly progression of tissue injury has been used by one group of investigators to accurately predict survival in horses with large colon volvulus. Biopsies were taken from the pelvic flexure, which accurately reflects mucosal changes along the length of the colon,[71] and histologically examined for the width of the crypts and intercrypt interstitial space. The latter measurements were expressed as an interstitium:crypt width (I:C) ratio. Nonviable colon was defined as that which had greater than 60% loss of crypt and an I:C ratio greater than 3. Using this methodology, survival was correctly predicted in 94% of horses.[72]

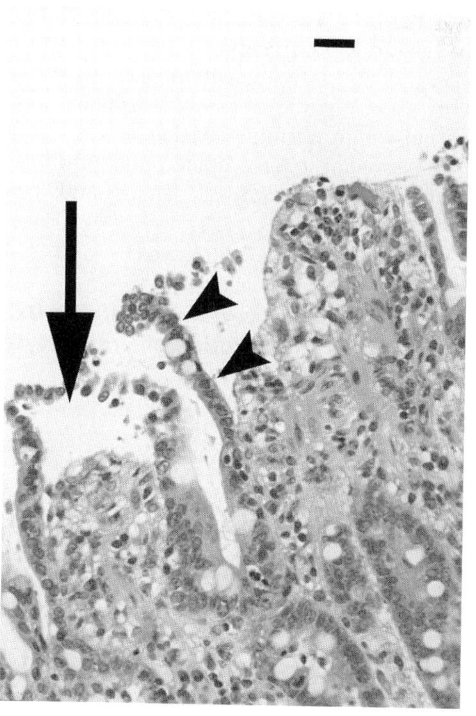

FIGURE 15-3 Histologic appearance of Grüenhagen's space in ischemic injured ileal mucosa. Note separation of epithelium at the tip of the villus from its basement membrane, creating a space *(arrows)*. Epithelium subsequently sloughs into the lumen *(arrowheads)*. 1 cm bar = 100 μm

Strangulating Obstruction

Since the dramatic decline in *Strongylus vulgaris*–induced colic, which was frequently associated with infarction of intestinal arterial blood supply,[73] the vast majority of ischemic lesions are associated with strangulating obstruction. Therefore it is important to consider mechanisms of ischemic injury in horses with naturally occurring strangulating lesions. The majority of experimental work has assessed either complete ischemia (complete occlusion of the arterial blood supply)[61] or low-flow ischemia (reduction of arterial blood flow).[74,75] However, during intestinal strangulation a disparity between the degree of occlusion of the veins and arteries occurs whereby veins are occluded before arteries because of differences in compliance of vascular walls. Thus strangulating lesions are typically hemorrhagic (hemorrhagic strangulating obstruction) because the arteries continue to supply blood to tissues that have little or no venous drainage. This results in ischemic injury, as previously outlined, but also in tremendous congestion of the tissues. Such hemorrhagic congestion has two opposing effects: It disrupts tissue architecture, including the mucosa and its epithelium, but it continues to provide oxygenated blood to the tissues during much of the ischemic episode. In contrast, when strangulation results in sudden cessation of arterial blood flow (ischemic strangulating obstruction), tissues appear pale, and the mucosa rapidly degenerates because of a complete lack of oxygenated blood.[69] From a clinical standpoint, this makes it difficult to assess the degree of mucosal injury in horses with strangulating injuries, because intestine that may look nonviable (dark red) may in fact have less mucosal injury than that of ischemic strangulated intestine.[76]

An additional consideration in clinical strangulating obstruction is the degree of ischemia that may be induced by intestinal distention. For example, experimental distention (18 cm of H_2O for 2 hours) and decompression (2 hours) of jejunum resulted in a significant increase in microvascular permeability and a significant decrease in tissue oxygenation similar to that which would be expected with low-flow ischemia.[77,78] In particular, microscopic evaluation of vasculature revealed capillary endothelial cell damage and local edema formation.[79] These data suggest that distended intestine proximal to an obstruction may undergo mucosal injury despite its relatively normal appearance. Indeed, in one study intraluminal pressures greater than 15 cm H_2O in naturally occurring cases of colic correlated with a poor prognosis for survival.[80]

Reperfusion Injury

Although it has recently been taken for granted that reperfusion of ischemic tissues results in exacerbation of mucosal injury, it should be remembered that mechanisms underlying intestinal reperfusion injury have been largely defined in laboratory animals under specific conditions.[81-85] On the other hand, studies on reperfusion injury in horses have had some conflicting results.[67,75,86] This may be attributable to the way in which the studies have been performed. In particular, the type of ischemia used in most laboratory animal studies has been low-flow ischemia (in which the blood flow is typically reduced to 20% of baseline flow), whereas studies in horses have used a number of different ischemic models, including various types of strangulating obstruction. Although strangulating obstruction is of great clinical relevance, this type of ischemic insult is less likely to develop into reperfusion injury.[67,87,88] Conversely, low-flow ischemia appears to prime tissues for subsequent injury once the tissue is reperfused, and there is considerable evidence to support the presence of reperfusion injury in horses following low-flow ischemia.[74,75,79,89] Nonetheless, low-flow ischemia may not be a common clinical entity.

In addition to the type of ischemia, there are other factors involved in priming tissues for reperfusion injury, including species and anatomic-specific variation in oxidant enzyme and neutrophil levels (Table 15-3). For example, the foal appears to have very low levels of small intestinal xanthine oxidase, an enzyme that has been shown to play a critical role in triggering reperfusion injury in laboratory animals,[83,84,95] whereas adult levels are much greater, particularly in the proximal small intestine.[94] In addition, horses appear to have low numbers of resident neutrophils in the intestinal mucosa,[96] and it is this population of neutrophils (rather than those recruited from the circulation) that appear to be most critical for induction

TABLE 15-3

Comparison of Mean Levels of Xanthine Oxidase/Xanthine Dehydrogenase (XO/XDH) and Myeloperoxidase (as an Indication of Granulocyte Numbers) in the Small Intestine of Various Species

Species	Intestinal Segment	Total XO/ XDH (mU/g Tissue)	Myeloperoxidase (U/g Tissue)	Reference
Cat (adult)	Jejunum	80	12	86, 90
	Ileum	NR	NR	
Rat (adult)	Jejunum	405-523	1.9	91, 92
	Ileum	150	NR	91, 93
Pig (6-8 weeks)	Jejunum	3.4 (0)*	NR	91
	Ileum	0.4 (0.9)*	2.2	91
Horse (adult)	Jejunum	100-131 (60)†	0.02	94, 91
	Ileum	30-48 (0)†	0.1	91

*XO/ XDH in the neonatal piglet.
†XO/ XDH in the foal.
NR, Not reported.

of reperfusion injury.[85] However, studies demonstrating reperfusion injury in the equine colon following low-flow ischemia have shown significant accumulation of neutrophils within the mucosa.[74] Therefore a complete understanding of mechanisms of neutrophilic infiltration and the mechanisms whereby they damage tissue will require further study.

Reperfusion injury is initiated during ischemia when the enzyme xanthine dehydrogenase is converted to xanthine oxidase, and its substrate, hypoxanthine, accumulates simultaneously as a result of adenosine triphosphate (ATP) utilization (Figure 15-4).[56,97] However, there is little xanthine oxidase activity during ischemia, because oxygen is required as an electron acceptor. During reperfusion xanthine oxidase rapidly degrades hypoxanthine in the presence of oxygen, producing the superoxide radical as a by-product.[56] The superoxide radical contributes to oxidative tissue damage and, most important, activates neutrophil chemoattractants.[83,84] Thus inhibition of xanthine oxidase in feline studies of intestinal ischemia/-reperfusion injury prevents infiltration of neutrophils and subsequent mucosal injury.[82,83] However, inhibition of xanthine oxidase has had no effect on ischemia/-reperfusion injury in equine small intestine[86] and colon,[98] suggesting that either reperfusion injury is simply a continuation of injury initiated during ischemia, as suggested in some equine studies,[62] or that the classic reperfusion injury pathway is activated by alternate sources of ROMs. The latter has been suggested by studies in feline models of ischemia/-reperfusion injury, in which the source of a significant proportion of ROMs is unknown, and independent of xanthine oxidase and neutrophils.[82]

In a veterinary review of the pathogenesis of intestinal reperfusion injury in the horse, the concept of a therapeutic window wherein treatment of reperfusion injury would be beneficial was suggested.[56] The basis of this concept is that there are certain conditions under which ischemic injury is minimal and that tissues are severely damaged during reperfusion.[87] Thus, under conditions of low-flow ischemia, very little injury is demonstrated during 3 hours of ischemia, but remarkable injury occurs during 1 hour of reperfusion.[82-84]

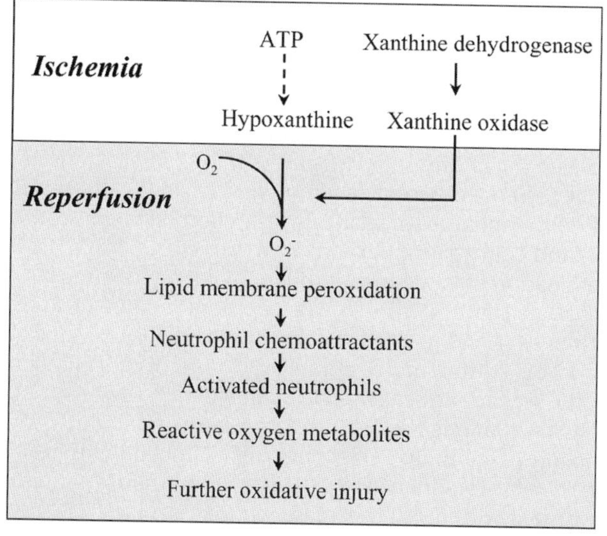

FIGURE 15-4 Intestinal reperfusion injury cascade. Reperfusion injury is initiated by elaboration of superoxide by metabolism of hypoxanthine by xanthine oxidase and subsequent infiltration of neutrophils.

However, a therapeutic window may not exist under conditions of strangulating obstruction wherein severe injury occurs during ischemia and minimal injury occurs during reperfusion.[91] This in turn greatly reduces the clinician's ability to ameliorate ischemia- reperfusion injury with treatments such as anti-oxidants at the time of reperfusion.

MECHANISMS OF GASTROINTESTINAL MUCOSAL REPAIR

Gastric Reparative Mechanisms

Mechanisms of gastric repair are highly dependent on the extent of injury. For instance, superficial erosions can be rapidly covered by migration of epithelium adjacent to the wound, a process termed *epithelial restitution.* However, ulceration (full thickness disruption of mucosa and penetration of the muscularis mucosa) requires repair of submucosal vasculature and ECM. This is initiated by formation of granulation tissue, which supplies connective tissue elements and microvasculature necessary for mucosal reconstruction. Connective tissue elements include proliferating fibroblasts that accompany newly produced capillaries that form from proliferating endothelium. Recent studies indicate that nitric oxide is critical to both of these processes,[39,99] which likely explains the reparative properties of nitric oxide in the stomach.[100]

Once an adequate granulation bed has been formed, newly proliferated epithelium at the edge of the wound begins to migrate across the wound. In addition, gastric glands at the base of the ulcer begin to bud and migrate across the granulation bed in a tubular fashion.[101] Epidermal growth factor is expressed by repairing epithelium and appears to facilitate these processes.[102] In addition, these events are facilitated by a mucoid cap, which retains reparative factors and serum adjacent to the wound bed.[50] Once the ulcer crater has been filled with granulation tissue and the wound has been re-epithelialized, the subepithelial tissue remodels by altering the type and amount of collagen. Despite the remodeling process, ulcers tend to recur at sites of previous ulceration, and there is the concern that this remodeling can result in excessive deposition of collagen and fibrosis.[25]

Intestinal Reparative Mechanisms

Reparative mechanisms are similar in the intestine, except that in the small intestine mucosal villi contribute to mucosal repair. Once intestinal epithelium is disrupted, there are two events that occur almost immediately to reduce the size of the denuded portion of the villus: contraction of the villus and epithelial restitution (Figure 15-5). For example, in porcine ileum subjected to 2 hours of ischemia, villi were 60% of their former height and 50% of the denuded villous surface area was covered in flattened epithelium within 6 hours.[41] Villous contraction appears to be regulated by enteric nerves, because inhibition of enteric nerve conduction prevents villous shortening after injury. The contractile component of the villus is a network of myofibroblasts distributed throughout the lamina propria of the villus and along the central lacteal. Inhibition of villus contraction results in retarded epithelial repair because of the larger denuded surface that remains to be covered by migrating epithelium compared with similarly injured villi that have contracted.[42] Prostaglandin E_2 has also been implicated

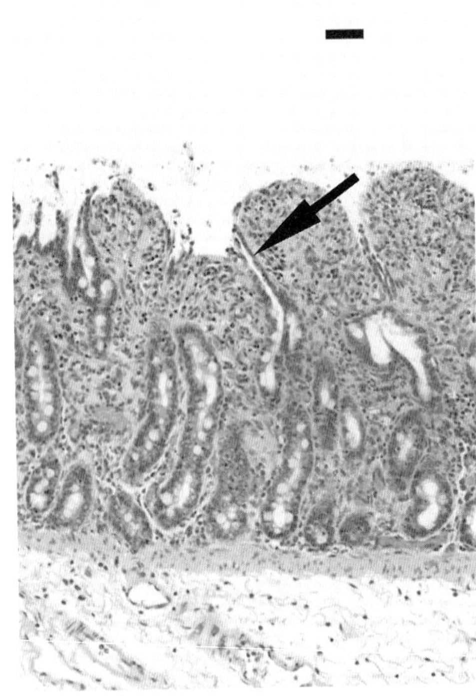

FIGURE 15-5 Histologic appearance of repairing intestinal mucosa 6 hours after a 2-hour ischemic episode. Note blunting of the villus, attributable to villous contraction, and evidence of epithelial restitution *(arrows)*. 1 cm bar = 100 μm

in regulating villous contraction, because application of PGE_2 resulted in villus contraction when perfused through normal rat ileum.[103] As villi contract, assuming there is an intact basement membrane, epithelium from the margins of the wound migrates in a centripetal direction to resurface toward the tip of the villus.[42] The process of restitution is similar in denuded colonic mucosa, except that it may proceed more rapidly because of the lack of villi.[41] Epithelial restitution is solely a migratory event that does not depend on provision of new enterocytes by proliferation. Cellular migration is initiated by extension of cellular lamellipodia that receive signals from the basement membrane via integrins. Intracellular signaling converges on the actin cytoskeleton, which is responsible for movement of lamellipodia. Specific components of the basement membrane appear to be critical to the migratory process. For example, application of antibodies to collagen types III and IV, which are important components of intestinal mucosal basement membrane, impeded epithelial restitution.[104,105] Other elements of the basement membrane, including proteoglycans, hyaluronic acid, and noncollagenous proteins such as fibronectin and laminin, may also provide important signals.[106] These subepithelial matrix components that facilitate restitution may form the basis for clinical treatments designed to speed up the repair process, analogous to administration of matrix components to horses with articular cartilage damage.

Although epithelial restitution results in gross closure of previously denuded regions of gastrointestinal mucosa, closure of interepithelial spaces is ultimately required to restore normal epithelial barrier resistance.[107] Because the tight junction is principally responsible for regulating the permeability of the interepithelial space, it is likely that repair and closure of this structure is critical to restore intestinal barrier function. Recent research indicates that prostaglandins play a vital role in recovery of tight junction resistance,[108] indicating that administration of nonselective COX inhibitors to horses with colic, particularly those recovering from strangulating obstruction, may be deleterious. Therefore judicious use of NSAIDs is appropriate until more selective drugs that allow continued production of reparative prostaglandins are available for use in horses in this country. Recent studies have shown that NSAIDs preferential for COX-2 allow for optimal repair of injured intestine as compared to traditional nonselective NSAIDs.[55]

Once the epithelial barrier has been restored, normal mucosal architecture must be re-established to allow normal gut absorptive and digestive function. In porcine ileum subjected to 2 hours of ischemia, the epithelial barrier was restored within 18 hours, but villi were contracted and covered in epithelium with a squamous appearance. Restoration of normal villus architecture required an additional 4 days.[41] The flattened villus epithelium that characterizes restitution is replaced by newly proliferated crypt epithelium. Under normal circumstances, new enterocytes are formed by division of stem cells, of which there are approximately four at the base of each mucosal crypt. Newly divided enterocytes migrate from the crypt onto the villus.[108] During migration enterocytes differentiate and acquire specific absorptive and digestive functions. Fully differentiated enterocytes reside on the upper third of the villus for 2 to 3 days and are then sloughed into the intestinal lumen.[109] This process is accelerated during mucosal repair, which requires increased proliferative rates. Increased proliferation may be stimulated within 12 to 18 hours by a variety of locally available gut-derived factors, including luminal nutrients, polyamines, and growth factors.[41] The return of the normal leaflike shape of the villus occurs subsequent to the appearance of normal columnar epithelium.

MEDIATORS OF REPAIR

PROSTAGLANDINS

Although prostaglandins have been strongly implicated in mucosal cytoprotective function, relatively few studies have assessed their importance in mucosal repair. One study implicated prostaglandins in growth factor–stimulated restitution,[110] but a more prominent role of prostaglandins in mucosal repair is their ability to close interepithelial tight junctions.[107,111,112] For instance, ischemic-injured small intestine rapidly recovers barrier function (as measured in vitro as transepithelial resistance) in the presence of prostaglandins I_2 and E_2, despite the fact that these prostanoids have relatively little effect on villous contraction and epithelial restitution. However, electron-microscopic examination of tissues reveals dilation of tight junctions in tissues treated with NSAIDs,[112] whereas those additionally treated with prostaglandins have closely apposed tight junctions (Figure 15-6). Prostaglandins stimulate closure of tight junctions via the second messengers cAMP and Ca^{2+},[105] which, interestingly, were among the first mediators found to modulate tight junction permeability.[113,114] Such tight junction closure is of considerable importance to patients with intestinal injury that are treated with NSAIDs because reduced prostaglandin levels may result in increased intestinal permeability. For example, in a study on ischemic-injured porcine ileum, treatment with the NSAID indomethacin resulted in a significant increase in intestinal permeability to inulin and LPS compared with tissues that were additionally treated with PGI_2 and PGE_2.[107]

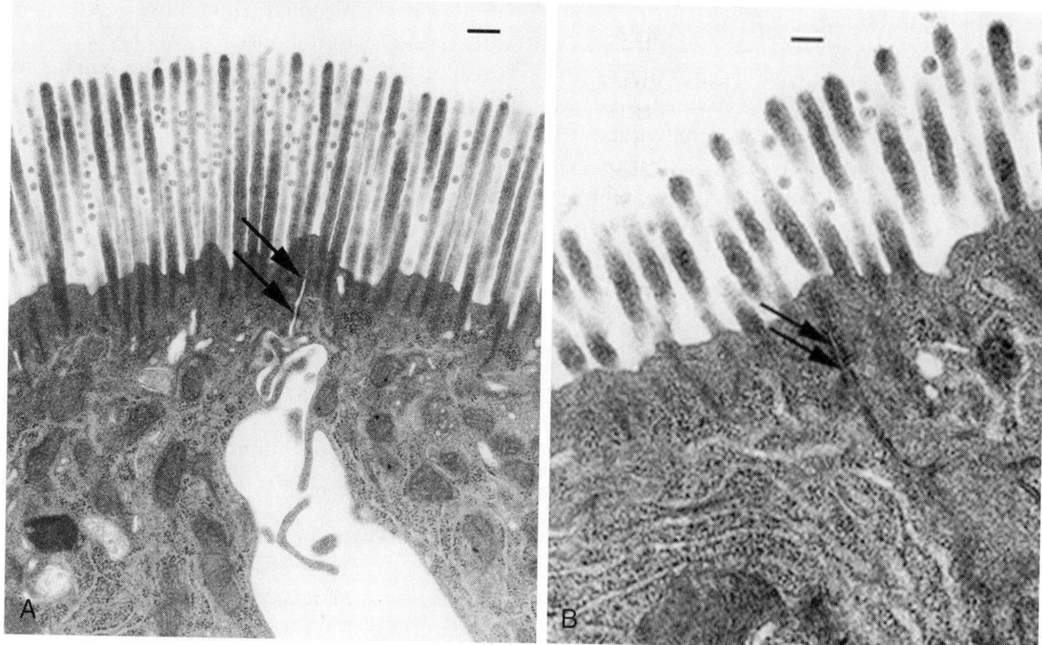

FIGURE 15-6 Ultrastructural appearance of repairing ischemic-injured mucosa. **A,** Restituting epithelium 2 hours after a 1-hour ischemic episode in the presence of the nonselective COX inhibitor indomethacin. Note dilation of the interepithelial space and the apical tight junction *(arrows),* which correlates with a "leaky" intestinal barrier. **B,** Similar restituting epithelium that has been additionally treated with PGE_2 and PGI_2. Note the close apposition of the tight junction *(arrows)* and the interepithelial space correlated with normalization of intestinal barrier function. 1 cm bar = 6 μm.

Polyamines

The process of restitution is absolutely dependent on a group of compounds called *polyamines.*[115,116] The rate-limiting enzyme in the formation of the polyamines spermine, spermidine, and putrescine is ornithine decarboxylase (ODC). In rats with stress-induced duodenal ulcers, systemic administration of the ODC inhibitor α-difluoromethyl ornithine significantly reduced polyamine levels and markedly reduced epithelial restitution. Furthermore, intragastric treatment of these same rats with putrescine, spermidine, and spermine prevented the delayed mucosal repair induced by α-difluoromethyl ornithine.[115] Interestingly, gastric tissue levels of ODC were increased in rats with stress-induced gastric ulcers, suggesting that polyamine production is enhanced during tissue injury and may contribute to the normal rapid rate of epithelial restitution.[117]

The mechanisms whereby polyamines stimulate epithelial restitution are not clear. McCormack et al. hypothesized that polyamines increased transglutaminase activity, an enzyme that catalyzes the cross-linking of cytoskeletal and basement membrane proteins.[118] Further investigation of the role of polyamines in IEC-6 cell migration showed that depletion of polyamines resulted in disruption of the cytoskeleton and reduced the physical extension of lamellipodia.[119] More recent studies have clarified this pathway. In particular, it has been shown that polyamines regulate cytoskeletal cellular migration via activation of the small GTPase Rho-A by elevating intracellular Ca^{2+} levels. These elevations in Ca^{2+} result from polyamine regulation of expression of voltage-gated K^+ channels and altered membrane electrical potential.[120]

Polyamines also play a role in the normal physiologic regulation of crypt cell proliferation and differentiation.[121,122] Polyamines are produced by fully differentiated enterocytes at the villous tip and may reach the crypt either within sloughed luminal epithelium or via local villous circulation.[123] After intestinal injury polyamines appear to stimulate enhanced proliferation by increasing the expression of proto-oncogenes, which control the cell cycle.[124] The mechanism whereby polyamines influence gene expression likely relates to the cationic nature of these compounds, which may influence the tertiary structure of negatively charged DNA and ribonucleic acid (RNA).[115]

GROWTH FACTORS

Locally produced growth factors, including epidermal growth factor (EGF), transforming growth factor (TGF)-α, TGF-β, and hepatocyte growth factor (HGF), have the ability to modulate mucosal recovery. The most important of these growth factors in early mucosal repair events is TGF-β, which is a potent stimulus of epithelial restitution and modulator of the ECM.[25] Neutralization of TGF-β retards epithelial migration in vitro, and it appears that TGF-β may serve as a point of convergence for mediators of restitution, because neutralizing TGF-β also inhibits the effects of other peptides. However, TGF-β paradoxically inhibits epithelial proliferation, thereby reducing the supply of new enterocytes for mucosal repair. Conversely, EGF, produced by the salivary glands and duodenal Brunner's glands, and the related TGF-α, produced by small intestinal enterocytes, are potent stimulants of enterocyte proliferation. These growth factors share approximately 30% of their amino acid structure, bind to the same receptor on the basolateral surface of enterocytes, and are not related to TGF-β.[125] The physiologic role of EGF is somewhat difficult to discern because it is present in the intestinal lumen, with no apparent access to its basally located receptor.[126] However, it has been proposed that EGF acts as a "surveillance agent" that gains access to its receptor during epithelial injury (when the EGF receptor would likely be exposed) to stimulate proliferation.[126] TGF-α presumably has a similar role, but it is present in greater concentrations in the small intestine because it is produced by differentiated villous enterocytes. The mature peptide is cleaved from the extracellular component of the transmembrane TGF-α precursor and released into the lumen.[125]

Trefoil Peptides

Another group of proreparative peptides that are locally produced within the gastrointestinal tract are the trefoil peptides. Under physiologic conditions trefoil peptides are secreted by mucus-producing cells at distinct anatomic sites. For example, the trefoil peptide pS2 is produced by gastric epithelium, whereas ITF is produced by small and large intestinal mucosa.[127] However, any of the trefoil peptides may be upregulated within repairing epithelium regardless of anatomic site.[25,128] In addition, trefoil peptides have the ability to induce their own expression, amplifying the level of these reparative factors at sites of mucosal repair.[129] Trefoil peptides are the most potent stimulants of epithelial migration in vitro, and their effects are independent of growth factors, including TGF-β.[130] However, recent evidence suggests that EGF receptor activation is required for induction of pS2 and another of the trefoil peptides termed *spasmolytic peptide* in gastric epithelium in vitro. The importance of trefoil peptides to the mucosal repair response in vivo is illustrated by gene knockout studies, in which mice deficient in ITF have dramatically reduced ability to repair intestinal injury.[131] In fact, detergent-induced mucosal injury was lethal because of a lack of restitution as compared with wildtype mice that fully recovered from similar mucosal injury. The fact that restitution was restored by administration of ITF has important therapeutic implications. The mechanism whereby trefoil peptides stimulate epithelial migration is yet to be fully characterized, but it appears to involve translocation of the adherens junction protein E-cadherin, thereby allowing cells to become untethered from neighboring cells.[25]

Intestinal Nutrients

The principal metabolic fuel of enterocytes is glutamine, and for colonocytes it is butyrate. However, recent studies suggest that glutamine and butyrate have more specific proliferative actions aside from their role as nutrients. For example, in the piglet IPEC-J2 enterocyte cell line, glutamine enhanced gene transcription by increasing mitogen-activated protein kinase activity.[132,133] Similarly, butyrate stimulated mucosal growth following colonic infusion in the rat.[134] Because of such growth-promoting actions, glutamine was shown to prevent intestinal mucosal atrophy and dysfunction that accompanies starvation[135,136] and long-term total parental nutrition.[137,138] Additionally, glutamine improves function of transplanted small intestine[139,140] and protects intestinal mucosa from injury if administered before chemotherapy[141] and radiation.[142,143] Intestinal nutrients may also synergize with other proliferative agents. For example, administration of glutamine and TGF-α to porcine ileum that had been subjected to 2 hours of ischemia resulted in a synergistic increase in mitogen-activated protein kinase activity, enterocyte proliferation, and villous surface area.[41] Although there has been a concern that such early return to normal surface area may result in dysfunctional mucosal digestive and absorptive function because of resurfacing denuded mucosa with immature epithelium, nutrients and growth factors also appear to promote early differentiation. In the case of glutamine and TGF-α restoration of postischemic small intestine, rapid recovery of digestive enzymes was also documented.[144]

GASTROINTESTINAL ILEUS

L. Chris Sanchez

Effective gastrointestinal motility involves a complex interaction among the enteric nervous system, muscular wall, and luminal contents. Additional factors that influence the net transit of digesta include gravity, the volume and viscosity of the contents, and pressure gradients created by simultaneous contraction and relaxation of adjacent segments of bowel. Casual use of the term *intestinal motility* in veterinary medicine often underestimates the complexity of the processes involved in the transit of intestinal contents. This is particularly true when the term is used to describe the frequency and or intensity of intestinal sounds, or borborygmi. The existence of borborygmi does not always equate with progressive movement of intestinal contents.

Disruption to normal motility occurs commonly in horses for a variety of reasons. Examples of diseases in which altered motility may be present include grass sickness, gastroduodenal ulceration, intraluminal obstruction or impaction, excessive wall distention, strangulating obstruction, peritonitis, and inflammatory disorders such as duodenitis proximal jejunits and colitis. Ineffective intestinal motility is also a feature of several neonatal diseases, including prematurity, systemic sepsis, and perinatal asphyxia. Certain parasitic infections, electrolyte derangements, and endotoxemia can modify digesta transit in horses of all ages. General anesthesia and specific sedatives, such as xylazine, romifidine, and detomidine, also disturb motility.

MANIFESTATIONS OF ILEUS

The inhibition of propulsive bowel activity usually is referred to as *ileus*. Ileus is ascribed most frequently to the condition that occurs after laparotomy and is termed *simple* or *uncomplicated postoperative ileus (POI)*. The term *complicated* or *paralytic ileus* describes intestinal motility disturbed for longer periods after surgery. POI in horses is associated most commonly with surgery of the small intestine, particularly after resection and anastomosis,[1,2] and can have a negative effect on short-term postoperative survival.[3-6] Motility dysfunction likely is present in all horses after laparotomy, but many are affected subclinically and require minimal or no specific intervention. In symptomatic animals clinical signs are apparent shortly after recovery and include colic, tachycardia, dehydration, decreased borborygmi and fecal output, and sequestration of fluid within the stomach. Rectal examination and ultrasound reveal small intestinal distention with rare or absent wall movement. The severity and duration of intestinal stasis varies, lasting from minutes to days.

A specific motility disorder involving the cecum or ileocecocolic region occurs sporadically in horses.[7-9] The condition most commonly occurs after general anesthesia and extra-abdominal surgery, particularly orthopedic and upper airway procedures, and therefore often is categorized as a form of POI. Other cases occur spontaneously, often in animals with painful primary conditions such as uveitis or septic tenosynovitis. In a study of 114 horses diagnosed with cecal impaction, 12 were hospitalized for a condition other than colic at the time of diagnosis and 9 others were being treated with phenylbutazone, most for a musculoskeletal injury.[10] Eight of the 114 horses had undergone general anesthesia in the 8 days preceding diagnosis. The syndrome is frustrating in that clinical signs are often subtle unless cecal perforation has occurred. In horses with a cecal emptying defect after anesthesia, overt signs are usually apparent 3 to 5 days after the procedure. The earliest detectable signs include depression and a reduction in feed intake and fecal output. Ineffective emptying results in overfilling of the cecum with moist contents, which is manifested by signs of mild to moderate colic. If the condition is recognized late or untreated, the cecum may rupture and result in fatal peritonitis.

PHYSIOLOGY

Current understanding of motility throughout the equine gastrointestinal tract is remarkably limited, and much of our presumptive knowledge comes from work in other species. The enteric nervous system is involved in all aspects of motility, either directly via neurotransmitters or indirectly via interstitial cells of Cajal (ICC), immune, or endocrine regulation. The inherent rhythmicity of electric activity in the intestine is controlled by the ICC, specialized cells that are electrically coupled to myocytes via gap junctions.[11] These cells are responsible for generating and propagating slow wave activity and hence are deemed the pacemaker cells of the intestine. A decrease in ICC density has been observed in horses with obstructive disorders of the large intestine[12] and in the ileum and pelvic flexure of horses diagnosed with equine grass sickness (dysautonomia),[13] although such a decrease was not evident in a horse with dysautonomia that recovered.[14] This alteration in ICC infrastructure appears to result in reduced slow wave activity in vitro.[15]

The enteric nervous system primarily controls and coordinates intestinal contraction. A combination of central and autonomic innervation influences events, but contraction does not require external neural input. The parasympathetic supply to the gastrointestinal tract is via the vagus and pelvic nerves, and the sympathetic supply is through postganglionic fibers of the cranial and caudal mesenteric plexuses. A complex network of interneurons within each plexus integrates and amplifies neural input; the intensity and frequency of resultant smooth muscle contractions are proportional to the amount of sympathetic and parasympathetic input. Additional binding sites for a number of other endogenous chemicals, including dopamine, motilin, and serotonin, exist within the enteric nervous system and on smooth muscle cells.[16] Acetylcholine is the dominant excitatory neurotransmitter in the gastrointestinal tract and exerts its action through muscarinic type 2 receptors on smooth muscle cells. Sympathetic fibers innervating the gastrointestinal tract are adrenergic, postganglionic fibers with cell bodies located in the prevertebral ganglia. Activation of α_2-adrenergic receptors on cholinergic neurons within enteric ganglia inhibits the release of acetylcholine and therefore reduces intestinal contraction. β_1-, β_2-, and β-atypical receptors are directly inhibitory to the intestinal smooth muscle.[17] Inhibitory nonadrenergic, noncholinergic neurotransmitters include ATP, vasoactive intestinal peptide, and nitric oxide.[18,19] These neurotransmitters are critical for mediating descending inhibition during peristalsis and receptive relaxation. Substance P is a nonadrenergic, noncholinergic neurotransmitter that may be involved in contraction of the large colon.[20,21]

The rate and force of intestinal contractions along the small intestine and large colon of the horse are important determinants of intestinal motility; of even greater importance to the net propulsion of digesta are the cyclical patterns of contractile activity. These patterns are known as the small intestinal and colonic migrating motility (or myoelectric) complexes (MMCs).[22,23] The colonic complex usually originates in the right ventral colon and variably traverses the ascending and descending colons. Many of these complexes are related temporally to a specialized motility event of the ileum, the migrating action potential complex.[24]

PATHOPHYSIOLOGY

Inflammation

Local inflammation within the intestinal muscularis and inhibitory neural events are important initiators of intestinal ileus.[25,26] Intestinal inflammation not only is important in primary intestinal diseases in horses, such as duodenitis-proximal jejunitis and colitis, but also is induced after simple intestinal handling during laparotomy. In rodents simple intestinal manipulation causes a cascade of inflammation within the muscularis that results in leukocyte infiltration and subsequent suppression of muscle contractility. The inflammatory response to bowel manipulation is not limited to the affected tissue but can also result in global inflammation and ileus throughout the gastrointestinal tract.[27]

The associated inflammatory events are extremely complex, involving a milieu of pro-inflammatory cytokines, prostaglandins, and leukocytes. Depletion or inactivation of muscularis macrophage function can prevent inflammation associated with intestinal manipulation and associated decreased contractility.[28] Mast cell activation is involved in intestinal manipulation-associated POI in humans.[29] Inflammation associated with colonic manipulation may involve gut-derived bacterial products.[30] Another factor in the development of intestinal stasis after inflammation is the local overproduction of nitric oxide caused by the upregulation of inducible nitric oxide synthase (iNOS) by resident macrophages.[31] iNOS upregulation was important for initiation of the inflammatory response and inhibition of motility. Nitric oxide is a key inhibitory neurotransmitter of the nonadrenergic, noncholinergic system.[19]

In the horse significant neutrophilic inflammation is apparent in jejunum from clinical cases necessitating resection and following a period of recovery in jejunum subjected to 1 or 2 hours of ischemia.[32] The ischemic tissue also had evidence of leukocyte activation, as demonstrated by calprotectin-positive cells in associated tissue histologically.

Drugs

The inhibitory effects of α_2-adrenergic agonists such as xylazine and detomidine on duodenal, cecal, and large colon motility are well described, because these drugs activate presynaptic receptors within the enteric nervous system.[33-39] Intravenously administered xylazine inhibits cecal and large colon motility for 20 to 30 minutes without seriously disrupting small intestinal myoelectric activity, and detomidine can reduce large intestinal myoelectric activity for up to 3 hours. Detomidine decreases duodenal motility in a dose-dependent fashion.[40] The α_2-antagonist yohimbine has a weak but positive effect on cecal emptying in normal ponies, suggesting that normal motility is under constant α_2-adrenergic tone.[34]

Several opioid agonists also have documented inhibitory effects on equine gastrointestinal motility at both a central and peripheral level. Morphine decreased frequency of defecation and fecal moisture content and increased gastrointestinal transit time in normal horses at a dose of 0.5 mg/kg twice daily for 6 days.[41] Single doses of fentanyl or morphine decreased jejunal and colonic MMC activity in ponies, whereas the antagonist naloxone elicited increased propulsive activity in the colon.[42] Fentanyl administered as an intravenous constant-rate infusion did not have an apparent deleterious effect on duodenal motility.[43] Butorphanol, an opioid agonist-antagonist, decreases myoelectrical activity in the jejunum but not pelvic flexure.[44] In another series of experiments, butorphanol alone did not decrease gastric or duodenal motility,[45] but administration in combination with xylazine resulted in a synergistic inhibitory effect that was more pronounced than that obtained by administration of xylazine alone.[39] Administration of butorphanol as a constant-rate infusion appears to have minimal to no effect on global gastrointestinal[46,47] or duodenal motility.[48]

N-butylscopolammonium bromide appears to cause a profound but very short-lived negative effect on duodenal motility, but this effect was not significant between groups.[48] Atropine is a postganglionic blocking agent that binds to muscarinic receptors. When administered at 0.04 mg/kg, atropine inhibits individual small intestinal, cecal, and colonic contractions for about 120 minutes but supresses small intestinal and colonic migrating complexes for up to 8 hours.[49]

Neural Reflexes

Neural reflexes also may mediate inhibition of motility associated with peritoneal inflammation and abdominal pain.[50,51] The afferent segment is composed partly of capsaicin-sensitive visceral afferent C fibers that terminate in the dorsal horn of the spinal cord, where they can activate inhibitory sympathetic fibers or synapse directly on the sympathetic ganglia. Consequently, the efferent limb of the reflex expresses increased sympathetic outflow, primarily mediated through stimulation of α_2-adrenoreceptors, and inhibition of acetylcholine release, which provides the rationale for α_2-blockade in treating ileus. Intraluminal infusion of capsaicin before abdominal surgery ameliorated the severity of POI in experimental rats. This finding highlights the importance of visceral afferent fibers in the development of POI.[52] Decreasing postoperative inflammation and pain decreases the risk of gastrointestinal ileus in many species in both experimental and clinical studies.

Distention

Ileus also can occur in association with intestinal obstruction or displacement. Mild to moderate distention of the bowel, such as that occurring in the early stages of an intraluminal obstruction, evokes an increase in local contractile activity.[53,54] Excessive distention results in inhibition of motility within the distended segment of bowel. Intestinal stasis is not always detrimental and under certain conditions may be protective. Repeated distention for determination of nociceptive threshold has also resulted in an overall decrease in duodenal motility over time, irrespective of other interventions.[43,48]

Endotoxin

Endotoxemia is a clinical feature of many diseases of the equine gastrointestinal tract, and endotoxins independently can exert a negative effect on intestinal motility and transit.[55] A variety of mediators likely are involved, but activation of α_2-adrenoreceptors and production of prostanoids appear to be important because pretreatment with yohimbine or NSAIDs (phenylbutazone or flunixin), respectively, ameliorates the inhibitory effects of experimental endotoxin infusion.[56-59] Pretreatment with metocolopromide or cisapride had a similar effect.[60,61] Endotoxin infusion induced an inflammatory response in the intestine of rats that mimicked the response induced by handling during laparotomy.[62] The similarity of the responses was highlighted in a recent study demonstrating that prior exposure of the muscularis to endotoxin protected the intestine from the effects of manipulation.[63] In rats colonic manipulation alone causes transference of intraluminal LPS to the muscularis, which likely contributes to the global gastrointestinal inflammatory response and decrease in contractility associated with tissue manipulation.[30] In response to endotoxin alone, the inflammatory response within the jejunal muscularis is predominantly monocytic, whereas the response to polymicrobial sepsis is predominantly neutrophilic.[64]

Other Effects

The pathophysiology of cecal emptying defect is not known. This syndrome may best mimic POI in human beings, which is generally considered a large intestinal disorder. An important difference in horses is that laparotomy is a rare predisposing factor, and most cases occur in horses undergoing routine extra-abdominal surgical procedures. Thus whether it should truly be classified as a form of POI is subject to debate. General anesthesia itself is a potent inhibitor of gastrointestinal motility in horses, but these effects are short-lived and reversible within hours of anesthetic withdrawal.[23] The return of normal motility in horses after experimental ileus was most delayed in the cecum, suggesting that this may be a common site of ileus in horses.[65] A link between routine postoperative medications, such as phenylbutazone and aminoglycoside antibiotics, has been suspected but not established. An inhibitory effect of NSAIDs on large colon contractility has been demonstrated using in vitro techniques.[66] Primary sympathetic overstimulation could be involved because many of the affected animals are young male horses or animals with painful diseases.

The duration of surgery influences the development of small intestinal POI but not cecal emptying dysfunction.[9,67] Technique may have a weak influence on small intestinal POI after jejunojejunostomy. The duration of intestinal ileus was shorter in animals that received a side-to-side stapled anastomosis than those that had a hand sewn end-to-end procedure.[3] The duration of ileus after stapled end-to-end anastomosis was not different from that after either procedure. Jejunocecostomy more commonly results in POI than other types of small intestinal resection and anastomosis, whether related to diseases necessitating this procedure or the procedure itself.[68]

Other reported risk factors for the development of POI include age (>10 years), small intestinal resection and anastomosis, breed (Arabians had a greater risk than other breeds), and duration of surgery.[67] A prospective study found small intestinal lesion, high packed cell volume and duration of anesthesia to increase the risk of POI, whereas performance of a pelvic flexure enterotomy and intraoperative administration of lidocaine may have a modest protective effect against POI.[69]

DIAGNOSIS

The diagnosis of ileus is based on history and physical examination findings. Case inclusion criteria for clinical studies of POI have varied.[67-70] Important tests include determination of heart rate and rhythm, auscultation and percussion of the abdomen, rectal palpation, and passage of a nasogastric tube. A complete blood count with fibrinogen estimation and cytologic analysis of PF may improve the accuracy of diagnosis. Affected animals have varying signs of abdominal discomfort from mild to severe because of accumulation of fluid in the small or large intestine. Decompression of the stomach is important diagnostically and therapeutically in horses with POI after intestinal surgery. Failure to relieve pain with gastric decompression could point toward mechanical obstruction, severe inflammation of the intestine, or peritonitis. Most animals with ileus are depressed and have reduced fecal output and intestinal borborygmi. Intestinal sounds must be interpreted with caution, however, because the presence of borborygmi does not always equate to progressive intestinal motility and may merely reflect local, nonpropagated contractions. Food intake, or the lack thereof, can also significantly alter gastrointestinal sounds.[71]

Rectal palpation findings in cases of persistent POI or duodenitis-proximal jejunitis are usually nonspecific but may include dilated, fluid-filled loops of small intestine. The clinician occasionally can palpate roughened peritoneal surfaces if peritonitis is present. Cecal distention with digesta can be palpated in horses with advanced cecal dysfunction. Distinguishing functional ileus from mechanical obstruction is important and can be difficult, but horses with mechanical obstruction typically have sustained high volumes of gastric reflux that vary little over time and abdominal pain that is typically not relieved by gastric decompression. Abdominal ultrasound in horses with ileus typically reveals mild to moderately fluid-filled hypomotile to amotile small intestine, without alteration in the amount or character of PF or small intestinal wall thickness. Horses with reflux from other causes (peritonitis, mechanical obstruction) will have changes reflective of their disease process. This differentiation is important for appropriate case management because horses with a mechanical obstruction often need either primary or repeat laparotomy, which should not be delayed.

TREATMENT

The management of intestinal ileus depends on the segment of gastrointestinal tract involved. Therapy for ileus of the proximal gastrointestinal tract involves a combination of gastric decompression, fluid and electrolyte therapy, analgesic therapy, and anti-inflammatory drug therapy. Electrolyte therapy is critical, particularly for maintaining adequate extracellular concentrations of potassium, calcium, and magnesium. Calculation of the volume of fluid to be administered should include maintenance requirements plus an estimate of losses, especially those lost through gastric decompression. The clinician should consider parenteral provision of calories when feed has been withheld for more than 96 hours, particularly after surgery. Hand walking also may provide some benefit to these animals but is not likely to have a direct effect on intestinal motility.

One should either avoid the previously mentioned drugs, which can have an inhibitory effect on motility, or use them sparingly. Fluid therapy is the key component in managing cecal emptying defect, usually in combination with lubricants or laxatives, such as mineral oil or magnesium sulfate, and with careful use of anti-inflammatory drugs. Horses with primary cecal impaction or impaction caused by an emptying defect may require surgery to prevent fatal rupture. The surgical management of these cases is controversial and may include typhlotomy alone, typhlotomy with a bypass procedure such as ileocolic or jejunocolic anastomosis, or a bypass without typhlotomy.[72] Most horses that undergo simple typhlotomy have an uneventful recovery.[73] In a large retrospective study 44 of 54 horses treated medically survived to discharge, and 37 of 49 horses treated surgically were allowed to recover, 35 of which survived to discharge.[10] Ileocolostomy was performed in only two of the 37 horses treated surgically (one of which survived to discharge), with the remainder receiving typhlotomy without bypass. Survival to 1 year was not statistically different between horses treated medically (18 of 19) and those treated surgically (25 of 28), although six horses had a recurrence of cecal impaction.[10]

Experimental and anecdotal evidence provides a strong rationale for using anti-inflammatory drugs to prevent and treat gastrointestinal ileus, particularly in animals that may have endotoxemia.[74] Flunixin meglumine is used widely in equine practice as an analgesic and anti-inflammatory agent, and it ameliorates many of the adverse systemic effects of endotoxin, particularly those on the cardiovascular system. A potential negative effect of NSAIDs on large intestinal contractility has been suggested. A differential effect on contractility between selective and nonselective COX inhibitors is currently unknown. Broad-spectrum antimicrobials are indicated when sepsis is suspected or for the compromised immune system, as in cases of moderate to severe endotoxemia. Theoretical concerns have been raised regarding the use of aminoglycoside antibiotics in animals with ileus. High concentrations of aminoglycoside antimicrobials inhibited intestinal contractions in exposed sections of intestine in vitro, but this inhibitory effect is unlikely to occur at clinically relevant doses.[75]

Motility-enhancing drugs have been advocated to treat gastrointestinal ileus. Unfortunately, information directly pertinent to horses is limited and must be extrapolated cautiously from that of other species because of the differences in intestinal anatomy and physiology. Prokinetic drugs potentially can shorten the length of hospitalization, thereby reducing the cost of treatment and the number of potential complications, such as weight loss, thrombophlebitis, and laminitis. Experimental evidence indicates that prokinetic drugs can minimize the development of postoperative abdominal adhesions.[76] Most prokinetic drugs require a healthy gut wall to enhance intestinal contraction, and downregulation of motilin receptors has been demonstrated in the inflamed equine jejunum.[77] Therefore one should not assume that many of these drugs would be effective in the presence of an inflammatory injury such as that which can occur after intestinal manipulation at surgery or that associated with duodenitis-proximal jejunitis.

Cholinomimetics

Bethanechol is a parasympathomimetic agent that acts at the level of the myenteric plexus and directly on intestinal smooth cells through muscarinic receptors. In the horse this effect is mediated predominantly by the M_3 receptor, but the M_2 receptor may also play a role.[78] Bethanechol is a synthetic ester of acetylcholine and is not degraded by anticholinesterase. Bethanechol has cholinergic side effects, including abdominal discomfort, sweating, and salivation, although these are minimal when the drug is administered subcutaneously or orally at 0.025 mg/kg body mass. Bethanechol has efficacy in diseases that involve abnormal gastric emptying and delayed small intestinal transit and has been shown to increase gastric contractility and hasten the emptying of liquid and solid phase markers from the stomach of normal horses.[79] Bethanechol also increases the strength and duration of wall contractions in the cecum and right ventral colon and consequently speeds up cecal emptying.[34]

Neostigmine increases receptor concentration of acetylcholine by inhibiting cholinesterase. The drug (0.022 to 0.025 mg/kg intravenously) promotes cecal and colonic contractile activity and hastens the emptying of radiolabeled markers from the cecum.[34] Neostigmine has been used to manage small intestinal ileus, but it significantly delayed the emptying of 6-mm beads from the stomach of normal adult horses.[80]

Benzamides and Dopamine Antagonists

Metoclopramide acts principally as a 5-hydroxytryptamine 4-receptor (5HT-4) agonist and 5HT-3 receptor antagonist. In contrast to newer generation benzamides, metoclopramide is also an antagonist at dopamine 1 (DA_1) and 2 (DA_2) receptors. Antagonism of prejunctional DA_2 receptors facilitates acetylcholine release and smooth muscle contraction. Metoclopramide crosses the blood-brain barrier, where its antagonist properties on central DA_2 receptors can result in extrapyramidal signs, including seizure. Metoclopramide increased contractility of muscle strips in vitro in the pyloric antrum, proximal duodenum, and midjejunum.[81] Those in vitro data support previous work in which metoclopramide administration restored gastroduodenal coordination of motility in a model of POI.[82] In another study metoclopramide had no effect on jejunal or pelvic flexure myoelectrical activity.[44] Constant intravenous infusion (0.04 mg/kg/hr) of metoclopramide was well tolerated in a population of postoperative horses and significantly decreased the volume and duration of gastric reflux over control and intermittent drug infusion groups.[83]

Cisapride is a second-generation benzamide that acts as a 5HT-4 agonist and 5HT-3 receptor antagonist but is without antidopaminergic action. Stimulation of 5HT-4 receptors within the enteric nervous system enhances release of acetylcholine from the myenteric plexus. Several reports suggest the efficacy of cisapride in managing intestinal disease in horses, including the resolution of persistent large colon impaction, treatment of equine grass sickness, and as a preventative for POI in horses after small intestinal surgery (0.1 mg/kg body mass intramuscularly during the postoperative period).[84-87] The horse erratically absorbs tablets administered rectally, but a method for preparing a parenteral form of the drug from tablets has been described.[88] Cisapride has the potential to cause adverse cardiac side effects mediated through blockage of the rapid component of the delayed rectifier potassium current that include lengthening of the QT interval and development of torsades de pointes, a potentially fatal arrhythmia.[89] These adverse effects have resulted in withdrawal of the drug in the United States but have not been reported in the horse.

Tegaserod, a 5HT-4 agonist, has been shown to increase pelvic flexure smooth muscle contractility (0.27 mg/kg PO)[90] and hasten gastrointestinal transit time (0.02 mg/kg intravenously) in healthy horses.[91] It has not, to the author's knowledge, yet been objectively evaluated in abnormal horses but may prove useful. In humans this drug was marketed for women with constipation-predominant or mixed symptom irritable bowel syndrome and demonstrated clear benefits in quality of life and gastrointestinal syptoms, but it is currently available only in a restricted fashion because of its association with ischemic colitis and cardiovascular disease.[92]

Domperidone acts as a competitive antagonist at peripheral DA_2 receptors. The drug is a therapeutic agent (1.1 mg/kg/day) for mares grazing endophyte-infected tall fescue, principally because of drug-enhanced prolactin release. The potential prokinetic effects of domperidone have not been studied extensively in horses, but a modest efficacy of domperidone (0.2 mg/kg intravenously) has been demonstrated in experimental ileus in ponies.[84]

Antimicrobials

Erythromycin, a macrolide antibiotic, is a direct motilin receptor agonist on smooth muscle cells and also may act within the enteric nervous system to facilitate the release of acetylcholine and motilin. Erythromycin displaces motilin from its receptor in the equine duodenum, jejunum, cecum, and pelvic flexure.[93] Erythromycin enhances gastric emptying in normal horses but has a more pronounced effect on the hindgut.[79,94] Erythromycin lactobionate (1.0 mg/kg IV) hastens cecal emptying in normal animals and induces colonic MMC-like activity across the colon. Administration often is associated with defecation and abdominal discomfort. The prokinetic effect of erythromycin apparent in the ileum, cecum, and pelvic flexure documented in normal horses was reduced in the immediate postoperative period.[95] Similarly, luminal distention and decompression resulted in inflammation and a decreased response to erythromycin.[96] A decrease in motilin receptors in response to luminal distention has been documented in the equine jejunum,[77] and this may explain the difference in response between normal and clinically affected horses. Repeated dosing can cause downregulation of motilin receptors in other species.[97] Because erythromycin can induce diarrhea in adults, it should not be administered over many days.

Potassium penicillin (20 million IU intravenously to adult horses) can stimulate defecation and increase myoelectrical activity in the cecum and pelvic flexure, and these effects are not produced by an equimolar amount of potassium ion given intravenously as potassium chloride.[98]

Opioid and α2-Adrenoreceptor Antagonists

Naloxone (0.05 mg/kg intravenously) induces contractile activity in the cecum and left colon.[42] Defecation commonly follows administration of naloxone within 15 to 20 minutes.

N-methylnaltrexone increases jejunal and pelvic flexure contractility in vitro[99] and has been shown to prevent the negative effects of morphine on fecal output and intestinal transit time when administered concurrently.[100]

α_2-Adrenoreceptor antagonists such as yohimbine or tolazoline counteract increased sympathetic outflow in response to nociceptive stimulation. Yohimbine infusion (75 μg/kg) also may attenuate the negative effects of endotoxin on motility.[56,58]

Local Anesthetics

The use of intravenous lidocaine as a prokinetic has gained tremendous popularity and was reported to be the agent most commonly used by equine surgeons for POI following most gastrointestinal lesions.[101] Lidocaine may exert prokinetic effects by suppressing primary afferent neurons, thereby limiting reflex efferent inhibition of motility.[102] Other proposed mechanisms of action include anti-inflammatory properties, potentially through NF-κβ signaling[103] or improving mucosal repair.[104] Intravenous lidocaine can also exert analgesic effects, although it was shown to alter somatic but not visceral antinociception in clinically normal horses in one study.[105] Lidocaine increased contractile activity in isolated strips of proximal duodenum in vitro.[81] The most commonly cited dosage is a 1.3 mg/kg bolus, typically over 15 minutes, followed by 0.05 mg/kg/min constant-rate infusion. This dosage did not alter MMC duration or spiking activity, nor did it reset the MMC in the jejunum in clinically normal horses[106] or significantly alter a variety of indicators of POI after colic surgery.[107] In another study significantly more horses with POI stopped refluxing within 30 hours following the institution of lidocaine infusion, relative to saline infusion.[108] Lidocaine infusion can be associated with reversible side effects that include muscle fasciculations, ataxia, and seizure. Consequently, the rate of infusion requires close monitoring. Prolonged infusion of lidocaine in the horse appears safe, although accumulation of the GX metabolite has been documented.[109]

ENDOTOXEMIA

Katharina L. Lohmann, Michelle Henry Barton

Endotoxemia is literally defined as the presence of endotoxin in the bloodstream. Most often, however, the term is used to refer to the associated clinical manifestations caused by an excessive and unbalanced inflammatory reaction. Endotoxemia is not a disease in its own right but rather a complication of many septic and nonseptic disease processes affecting horses and other animals. Its diagnosis and management must therefore be discussed in the context of underlying primary pathologic conditions.

In its pathophysiologic consequences the innate immune response to endotoxin (LPS) is similar to the response to other stimuli (e.g., bacterial infection, viral infection, severe trauma). Moreover, the clinical presentation and clinical pathologic abnormalities of patients suffering from severe systemic inflammation are consistent regardless of the etiologic cause, and outcome may be predicted more accurately by the severity of the inflammatory response than the nature of the inciting insult.[1] In 1992, therefore, the term *systemic inflammatory response syndrome* (SIRS) was introduced in a consensus statement of chest physicians and critical care physicians to account for these similarities and provide a case definition for clinical and research purposes. Fairly soon thereafter, however, the 1992 SIRS definition was criticized as being too sensitive while providing little specificity,[2] and its usefulness for clinical practice was challenged because it failed to predict outcome and to discriminate patients at a high risk of morbidity and mortality.[3] The definition of *SIRS* may therefore be valuable from a conceptual standpoint, but it has little value in daily clinical practice.

Sepsis was defined as the systemic inflammatory response to infection, and *septic shock* as "sepsis-induced hypotension, persisting despite adequate fluid resuscitation, along with the presence of hypoperfusion abnormalities or organ dysfunction."[1] According to these definitions the diagnosis of *sepsis* requires documentation of infection by culture in addition to two or more of the following findings: hypothermia or hyperthermia; tachycardia; tachypnea or hypocapnia; and leukocytosis, leukopenia, or an increased proportion of immature leukocyte forms.

Organ failure is a common sequela of endotoxic or septic shock, and the term *multiple organ dysfunction syndrome* describes insufficiency of two or more organ systems, as evident by clinical or clinicopathologic changes. In horses the laminae of the feet should be included in the list of organs susceptible to failure.

ENDOTOXIN

German scientist Richard Pfeiffer (1858–1945), in working with *Vibrio cholerae*, first described endotoxin as a toxin "closely attached to, and probably integral of, the bacterial body."[4] He observed this toxin to be distinct from the actively secreted, heat-labile, and proteinaceous bacterial exotoxins. Endotoxin later was found to be a heat-stable LPS structure, and the terms *endotoxin* and *LPS* now are often used interchangeably.

LPS is a major structural cell wall component of all gram negative bacteria, including noninfectious species (Figure 15-7). With 3 to 4 × 10^6 molecules per cell, LPS makes up about 75% of the outer layer of the outer cell membrane and is a key functional molecule for the bacterial outer membrane, serving as a permeability barrier against external noxious agents. The LPS molecule consists of four domains, which are essential for

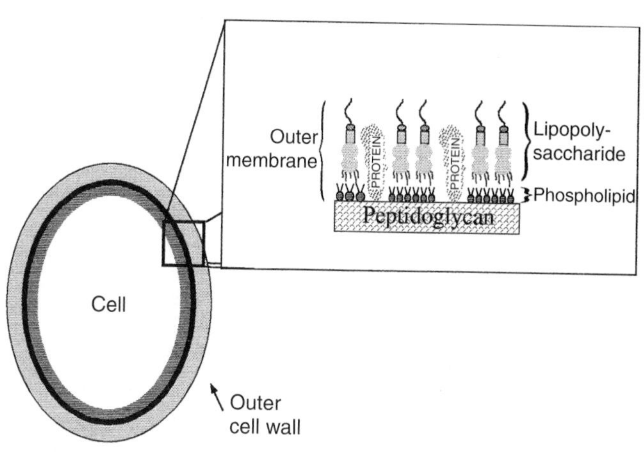

FIGURE 15-7 Lipopolysaccharide.

the virulence of gram negative bacteria.[5] Three of the domains (inner core, outer core, and O-specific chain) represent the hydrophilic polysaccharide portion of the molecule, whereas the lipid A portion represents the hydrophobic lipid portion (Figure 15-8). Combined, these domains confer the overall amphiphilic properties of the molecule that lead to the formation of micellar aggregates in aqueous solutions.

O-specific chains (also called O-antigen polysaccharides or O-chains) are characteristic of any given type of LPS and show enormous structural variability among bacterial serotypes.[6] O-chains are synthesized by addition of preformed oligosaccharide blocks to a growing polymer chain and therefore have a repetitive structure. O-specific chains determine part of the immunospecificity of bacterial cells[5] and, on interaction with the host immune system, serve as antigens for the production of species-specific antibodies.[7] O-specific chains are further responsible for the smooth appearance of gram negative bacterial colonies on culture plates,[5] and LPS molecules containing an O-chain are termed *smooth lipopolysaccharide*.

The inner (lipid A-proximal) and outer (O-chain-proximal) core oligosaccharide portion is more conserved among different strains of gram negative bacteria than the O-specific chain.[6] The core of all LPS molecules contains the unusual sugar KDO (3-deoxy-D-manno-oct-2-ulopyranosonic acid), which links the core region to the lipid A molecule. Synthesis of a minimal core is essential for the survival of bacteria,[5] and the smallest naturally occurring LPS structure consists of lipid A and KDO.[8] In contrast to the S-form colonies, colonies of gram negative bacteria with LPS molecules that lack the O-specific chain but contain a core region show a rough appearance on culture plates. Rough LPS molecules are denoted further as Ra, Rb, and so on to indicate the length of the core region. In Re-LPS (also called *deep rough LPS*), the core region is reduced to a KDO residue. Remutants often are used to raise antibodies against the core region in an attempt to provide cross-protection against a variety of bacterial species. The lipid A portion, which serves to anchor the LPS molecule in the bacterial outer membrane, has been identified as the toxic principle of LPS,[9] and its structure is highly conserved among gram negative bacteria. The common structure shared by lipid A molecules is a 1,4′-bisphosphorylated β1,6-linked D-glucosamine disaccharide backbone (lipid A backbone), which is acylated by up to six fatty acids.[6] Figure 15-9 shows the acylation pattern for *Escherichia coli* LPS. Variation in the lipid A structure between gram negative bacteria affects the number, length, and position of fatty acids and the backbone structure and the substitution of phosphate by other polar groups.[7]

CAUSES OF ENDOTOXEMIA IN HORSES

According to its nature as a structural cell wall component, the presence of endotoxin implies the presence of gram negative bacteria as a source. Depending on the nature of the underlying disease, these bacteria may circulate in the bloodstream in their intact form (i.e., bacteremia), may be confined to a localized infectious process, or may be part of the endogenous bacterial florae colonizing the gastrointestinal tract. In any of these scenarios endotoxin molecules are released as a byproduct of bacterial growth and in large numbers on bacterial cell death.[10] Common infectious conditions associated with endotoxemia in horses include neonatal gram negative sepsis, bacterial pneumonia and pleuropneumonia, endometritis, peritonitis, and infectious colitis with bacteria such as *Salmonella* spp. that are not part of the normal intestinal florae. In one study, for example, endotoxin was detectable in plasma of 50% of foals evaluated for presumed sepsis.[11]

The term *translocation* describes entry of endogenous bacteria and bacterial products from the gastrointestinal tract into tissues and the systemic circulation.[12] The natural intestinal flora of horses consists mainly of gram negative, anaerobic bacteria, and thus large amounts of endotoxin normally exist in the lumen of the equine intestinal tract.[13] Even in healthy horses small amounts of endotoxin probably cross the intact mucosal barrier and reach the portal circulation and the liver.[14] These molecules are cleared, however, by the mononuclear phagocytic system in the liver and lead only to a localized and restricted activation of the host immune system.

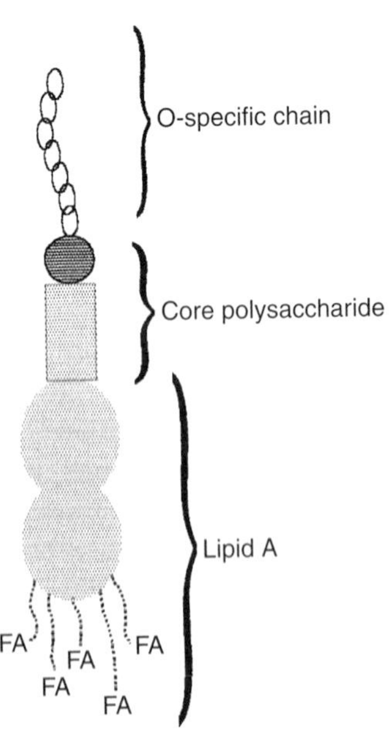

FIGURE 15-8 Three domains of the lipopolysaccharide molecule.

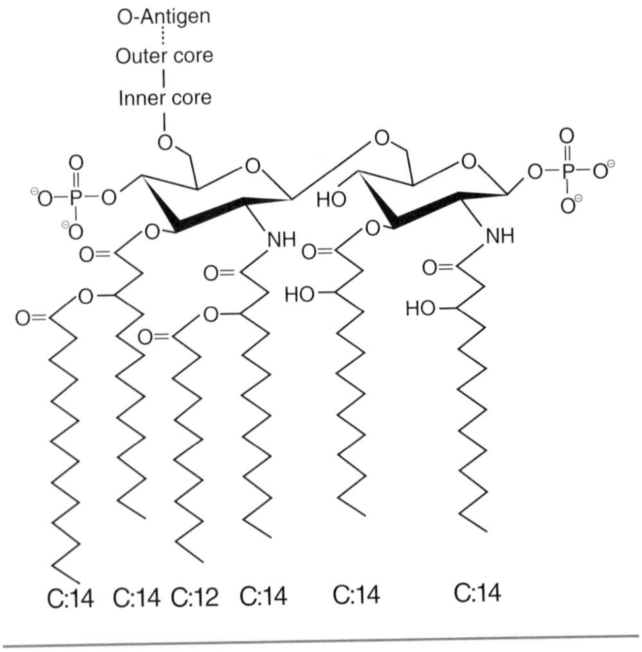

FIGURE 15-9 Acylation pattern for *Escherichia coli* LPS.

For endotoxin translocation to become detrimental, excessive amounts have to cross the intestinal barrier and overwhelm the mononuclear phagocytic system, or the capacity of the liver to detoxify lipopolysaccharide must be compromised. The latter may be a concern in conditions such as hepatitis, cholangiohepatitis, or portosystemic shunting of blood.

Permeability of the intestinal mucosal barrier frequently increases in cases of acute gastrointestinal disease. Colic patients are prime candidates to develop endotoxemia, and plasma endotoxin was detectable in 10% to 40% of colic patients on admission.[15,16] The studies differed in their inclusion criteria, and the higher percentage of horses testing positive for plasma endotoxin was observed when only patients presenting for surgical intervention were evaluated.[16] Aside from gastrointestinal rupture, increased permeability to intact bacteria or free endotoxin molecules is thought to be associated most commonly with ischemic insults such as strangulating obstruction and bowel infarction; severe inflammation, as in proximal enteritis and colitis; bacterial overgrowth; and intraluminal acidosis, which occurs with grain overload.[17,18] One study, however, found no difference in plasma endotoxin detection among disease groups, therefore emphasizing the fact that any disease of the abdominal cavity can induce endotoxemia in horses. In the same study endotoxin was approximately three times more likely to be detected in PF as opposed to plasma samples. Similarly, higher cytokine concentrations have been measured in PF than in plasma. The likely explanation for these findings is a local inflammatory response in the peritoneal cavity elicited by translocated bacteria or LPS molecules before their absorption into the systemic circulation.[15]

Although gastrointestinal disease is likely the most important cause of endotoxin translocation in horses, other conditions may also result in translocation of endotoxin and bacteria. In experimental studies using laboratory animals, entry of gut-associated bacteria into the lymphatic system was demonstrated after hypovolemic shock, burn injuries, trauma, malnutrition, and starvation.[19-21] Furthermore, endotoxin itself caused bacterial translocation into mesenteric lymph nodes after intraperitoneal administration to mice.[22] These findings have received much attention in the literature concerning human patients because they serve to explain cases of endotoxic shock in the absence of demonstrable bacterial infection. The veterinarian should keep in mind the possibility of translocation when evaluating cases of presumed SIRS in horses, in which bacterial infection or gastrointestinal disease cannot be demonstrated. Endotoxin translocation also may be associated with strenuous exercise, which results in reduced splanchnic blood flow, hypoxemia, and a higher body temperature. In fit racehorses a significantly increased mean plasma LPS concentration was found after racing, whereas antilipopolysaccharide immunoglobulin G levels were decreased. Fit horses showed significantly higher antilipopolysaccharide immunoglobulin G concentrations at rest than sedentary controls, suggesting leakage of small amounts of endotoxin from the intestinal lumen during training and racing.[23] A study in endurance horses demonstrated detectable LPS concentration in approximately 50% of horses, and correlation between plasma endotoxin and lactate concentration suggested that plasma endotoxin concentration may be reflective of the vigor of exercise.[24] Surprisingly, the latter study failed to show a correlation between plasma endotoxin concentration and levels of inflammatory mediators such as TNF-α and IL-6,[24] such that the clinical significance of endotoxin translocation during exercise requires further investigation. At least experimentally, however, alterations in innate immune function during and after strenuous exercise in horses have been demonstrated.[25]

MECHANISMS OF CELLULAR ACTIVATION BY LIPOPOLYSACCHARIDE

The initiating event in the pathophysiology of endotoxemia is the activation of LPS-responsive cells by endotoxin, resulting in altered cellular functions and increased expression of inflammatory mediators. Immune cells such as macrophages respond to minute amounts of LPS, which usually allows them to eliminate gram negative bacteria and free LPS molecules efficiently. An important factor in the exquisite sensitivity to LPS is the presence of LPS-binding protein (LBP).[6] LBP is an approximately 60-kd plasma glycoprotein[26] that is synthesized primarily by hepatocytes[27] and belongs to the family of lipid transfer/LBPs. LBP is an acute phase protein, and inflammatory agents and cytokines such as IL-1 increase LBP plasma concentration tenfold to 100-fold within 24 to 48 hours of an inflammatory stimulus.[28,29] The main function of LBP is to transfer LPS to endotoxin-responsive cells, which include mononuclear phagocytes, neutrophils, lymphocytes, and endothelial cells. The importance of a highly sensitive response to LPS for protection against gram negative bacterial infection is demonstrated in experiments using LBP knockout mice—that is, mice that lack the LBP gene and are therefore unable to synthesize LBP. Although these animals are resistant to the effects of purified LPS, they are unable to control infection with viable bacteria and rapidly succumb.[30] Despite its crucial importance for an effective host defense, LBP is not essential for LPS-receptor interaction per se, because high concentrations of LPS can activate cells in the absence of LBP.[31]

Aside from its role as a catalyst of cellular activation by LPS, LBP has opsonizing activity[32] and participates in the phagocytosis of LPS by macrophages and neutrophils.[33,34] Although phagocytosis of LPS is receptor dependent, it appears to be uncoupled from intracellular signaling events and occurs in the absence of cell activation.[5] LBP further catalyzes transfer of LPS to lipoproteins such as high-density lipoprotein, which neutralizes LPS activity.[35] This detoxifying effect may become important when large amounts of LPS are present. A protective effect of LBP against LPS challenge and infection has been demonstrated in a murine model of septic shock,[36] and further studies investigating potential therapeutic use of LBP are under way. More recently, LBP has also been investigated as a diagnostic and prognostic indicator in human patients, where it may differentiate between SIRS and sepsis and predict outcome of septic patients.[29] One study investigating serum amyloid A and LBP in horses with colic[37] found no correlation between serum concentration of LBP with outcome, type of disease process, or affected portion of the gastrointestinal tract.

The most important LPS receptors known to date are cluster differentiation antigen 14 (CD14) [31] and Toll-like receptor 4 (TLR-4).[38] Both are classified as pattern recognition receptors,[39] which means that they recognize LPS as a structural motif common to all gram negative bacteria. CD14 is a 53-kd protein that in its membrane-bound form (mCD14) is inserted into the cell membrane via a glycosyl-phosphatidyl-inositol anchor.[40] CD14 is expressed primarily on monocytes and tissue macrophages and to a lesser extent on neutrophils.[41] CD14 also is found in a soluble form (sCD14)[42] that can bind to cell types lacking CD14, such as endothelial cells, and make them LPS-responsive. In addition to this pro-inflammatory effect, high concentrations of sCD14 can sequester and neutralize LPS.[43] The amount of circulating sCD14 greatly increases during inflammation, which makes it a useful marker of acute and chronic inflammation.[41]

Although CD14 is known to be crucial for cellular activation, it cannot transmit signals to the inside of the cell because it lacks a transmembrane domain. The missing link between CD14 and the cytosolic environment is a Toll-like receptor in association with the molecule MD-2.[44] The name *Toll-like receptor* stems from the homology of the mammalian receptor with a receptor type in *Drosophila* (Toll) that is important for dorsoventral orientation and immune responses in the fly. A number of Toll-like receptors have been identified in mammalian species so far, but TLR4 appears to be the receptor subtype most important for LPS signaling.[38] The importance of CD14 and TLR4 in the cellular response to LPS has been demonstrated in a number of experiments. Mice deficient in CD14 are incapable of mounting a normal inflammatory response to LPS,[43] whereas mutation or deletion of the gene encoding for TLR4 causes LPS hyporesponsiveness.[45-47]

After binding of LPS to cellular receptors, TLR4 undergoes oligomerization and recruits downstream adaptor proteins in order to activate intracellular signaling pathways.[48] Signaling pathways are characterized by sequential phosphorylation and thereby activation of enzymatic activities, and ultimately result in the alterations of cellular metabolism known as *cell activation*. A typical result of intracellular signaling is the activation of transcription factors—that is, proteins that bind to DNA and promote gene transcription. Translational mechanisms are activated in a similar manner.

TLR4-dependent cell signaling pathways can be differentiated according to the use of adaptor proteins that bind to the intracellular domain of TLR4.[48] The MyD88 (myeloid differentiation primary response gene 88)-dependent pathway results in activation of IKK (Iκβ kinase) and MAPK (mitogen-activated protein kinase) pathways and ultimately in expression of pro-inflammatory cytokine genes. IKK activates the well-described transcription factor NF-κβ by phosphorylating an inhibitor protein complex (IκB) that sequesters and inactivates NF-κβ in the cytoplasm. On phosphorylation IκB is ubiquitinated and degraded, and NF-κβ is translocated to the nucleus, where it unfolds its activity.[49] The MyD88-independent pathway, on the other hand, is activated by interaction of TLR4 with the adaptor protein TRIF (Toll-interleukin-1 receptor domain-containing adaptor inducing interferon-β). While the MyD88-independent pathway also activates MAPK and NF-κβ (in addition to a transcription factor called *IRF3),* this pathway primarily results in activation of type I interferons, which are important for antiviral and antibacterial responses.[48] Despite the characterization of seemingly separate and "ordered" pathways, one should recognize that interaction and synergy between pathways is likely to occur. Similarly, inhibitory pathways are required for regulation of the cell response and can target multiple levels of TLR4 signaling.[48] The potential manipulation of signaling pathways for therapeutic use in septic patients is under investigation.

INFLAMMATORY MEDIATORS

Although endotoxin can exert some direct effects, cytokines are a primary mediator of LPS effects. Cytokines are glycoprotein molecules that regulate inflammatory and immune responses by acting as a signal between cells.[50] Cytokines of major interest in the pathogenesis of endotoxemia include TNF-α, the interleukins, chemokines, and growth factors such as granulocyte-monocyte colony-stimulating factor. TNF-α is thought of as the most "proximal" cytokine released in response to LPS. Studies corroborate this by showing that administration of recombinant TNF-α mimics the effects of LPS[51] and that antibodies directed against TNF-α protect against the lethal effects of endotoxin.[52] Increased plasma activity of TNF is associated with increased mortality in equine patients with acute gastrointestinal disease and in septic neonates.[15] Despite being a structurally diverse group of proteins, cytokines share several characteristics that allow them to execute their complex functions in the inflammatory response.[50] Any individual cytokine generally is produced by several different cell types, can act on different cell types, and has multiple effects on any given cell. Furthermore, cytokine effects are redundant, meaning that different cytokines can share the same effect. In endotoxemia this is particularly true for the effects of IL-1 and TNF-α.[53] Many of the biologic activities of cytokines in vivo result from synergistic or antagonistic actions involving two or more cytokines.[54] Within itself the cytokine response is highly regulated: Cytokines induce or suppress synthesis of other cytokines, including their own (feedback regulation); regulate expression of cytokine receptors; and regulate cytokine activities. Additional regulatory mechanisms include the release of specific cytokine inhibitors such as soluble IL-1 and TNF-α receptors; cytokine receptor antagonists such as IL-1 receptor antagonist; and anti-inflammatory cytokines, including IL-10, IL-4, IL-13, and TGF-β. Glucocorticoids, which are produced increasingly in response to endotoxin, also inhibit the production of cytokines.[55] During a "controlled" inflammatory response, therefore, cytokine secretion is a self-limited event, whereas excessive stimulation of cytokine production can lead to the perpetuation of the inflammatory response even after the initial stimulus has been removed. Aberrations from the controlled, self-regulated inflammatory response have been described as predominantly pro-inflammatory (SIRS), anti-inflammatory or hypoinflammatory (compensatory anti-inflammatory response syndrome or CARS), or combined (mixed antagonist response syndrome) responses.[56] That these responses may not represent a continuum in response to infection was demonstrated in a recent study investigating cytokine profiles in an experimental model of sepsis.[57] Here, increased plasma concentration of anti-inflammatory mediators such as IL-1 receptor antagonist and IL-10 in the early phase of sepsis predicted early mortality almost as accurately as the typical pro-inflammatory cytokines such as IL-6. Cytokine profiles failed to predict mortality in the later stages of sepsis, thereby suggesting that late outcome is not "preprogrammed" early on in the disease. A progression from pro-inflammatory (SIRS) to anti-inflammatory (CARS), as previously proposed, could not be demonstrated.[57] The authors concluded that use of biomarkers may be helpful in determining the inflammatory status of clinical patients suffering from sepsis and that the success of treatments aimed at suppressing or stimulating immune responses may depend on the individual patient's inflammatory profile.

Interestingly, tolerance to endotoxin develops after repeated exposure to LPS.[19] Tolerance can be demonstrated in vitro and in vivo and encompasses decreased production of cytokines and a diminished clinical response.[19,58] Tolerance may be a protective mechanism and was shown to reduce mortality in some experimental models; however, impaired resistance to infectious processes was demonstrated by other investigators.[59] Mechanisms that likely are responsible for the development of endotoxin tolerance include receptor downregulation,[60] downregulation of intracellular signaling pathways,[59,61] and mediators such as glucocorticoids and IL-10.[59] The development of endotoxin tolerance in horses has been reported.[62,63] More recently, the term "cellular reprogramming" has been introduced to describe altered inflammatory cell functions in septic and SIRS patients. This term better accounts for the observation that cellular LPS-sensing ability appears to be maintained while intracellular signaling and thereby cytokine production is modified toward an anti- rather than pro-inflammatory response.[59]

Aside from cytokines, a number of other molecules function as inflammatory mediators in the pathogenesis of endotoxemia, the synthesis and release of which are stimulated by endotoxin and by cytokines. These mediators include the arachidonic acid metabolites or prostanoids, PAF, oxygen-derived free radicals, nitric oxide, histamine, kinins, and complement components. Table 15-4 summarizes the origins, targets, and effects of the most important inflammatory mediators involved in the pathogenesis of endotoxemia. Figure 15-10 shows the pathways of arachidonic acid metabolism by COX and lipoxygenase. COX products are the prostaglandins (PGs), prostacyclin (PGI_2) and thromboxanes, and the lipoxygenase produces the leukotrienes.

PATHOGENESIS

The innate immune response to LPS is an efficient defense mechanism that provides maintenance of homeostasis and therefore health in the face of an almost continuous exposure to microorganisms and their products.[5] Detrimental

TABLE 15-4

Important Mediators of the Systemic Inflammatory Response to Endotoxin

Mediator	Origin	Effects
Tumor necrosis factor	Macrophages	Induces synthesis of TNF, IL-1, IL-6, and GM-CSF
	Monocytes	Activates neutrophils
	Neutrophils	Activates fibrinolysis and coagulation
	CD4+ T cells	Activates contact and complement system
	Natural killer cells	Induces a catabolic state
		Induces insulin resistance
		Is a pyrogen (direct action and via IL-1 induction)
Interleukin-1	Activated macrophages	Induces synthesis of TNF, IL-1, IL-6, PGI_2, PAF, and GM-CSF
	Endothelial cells	Activates pyrogen
	Fibroblasts	Induces malaise
	Dendritic cells	Activates neutrophils and chemotaxis
	Lymphocytes	Activates fibrinolysis and coagulation
	Keratinocytes	Activates contact and complement system
		Induces acute phase response
		Increases activity of lipoprotein lipase
		Mobilizes amino acids
		Induces muscle proteolysis
Interleukin-6	Activated macrophages	Induces acute phase response
	Fibroblasts	Induces stress response
	Keratinocytes	Is a weak pyrogen
	T lymphocytes	
Interleukin-8	Macrophages	Activates neutrophils and chemotaxis
	Endothelial cells	
Thromboxane A2	Platelets	Induces vasoconstriction
		Activates platelet aggregation
Prostaglandin E2	Most nucleated cells	Induces vasodilation
		Activates platelet aggregation
		Induces fever
Prostaglandin I2	Vascular endothelial cells	Induces vasodilation
		Inhibits platelet aggregation

Continued

TABLE 15-4

Important Mediators of the Systemic Inflammatory Response to Endotoxin—cont'd

Mediator	Origin	Effects
Platelet-activating factor	Macrophages	Activates platelet aggregation
	Platelets	Activates macrophages and neutrophils
	Neutrophils	Induces hypotension
	Mast cells	Increases vascular permeability
	Eosinophils	Aids recruitment of leukocytes
		Induces visceral smooth muscle contraction
		Is a negative inotrope and arrhythmogenic
		Induces ileus
Prostaglandin $F_2\alpha$	Most nucleated cells	Induces vascoconstriction
		Activates luteolysis
Leukotriene B_4	Most nucleated cells	Is a chemoattractant
		Promotes neutrophil interaction with endothelial cells
Leukotrienes C_4, D_4, E_4	Most nucleated cells	Increase vascular permeability
		Induce bronchoconstriction
		Induce vasoconstriction
Kinins	Produced from serum precursors	Increase vascular permeability
		Induce smooth muscle contraction cause pain
Complement components (C3a, C5a)	—	Activate neutrophils and chemotaxis
		Induce smooth muscle constriction
		Induce mast cell degranulation
		Induce release of histamine and serotonin
		Increase vascular permeability
Oxygen-derived free radicals	Macrophages	Damage cell membranes
	Neutrophils	Inactive enzymes
		Damage tissues
Granulocyte- monocyte colony- stimulating factor	—	Induces rebound neutrophilia

TNF, Tumor necrosis factor; IL, interleukin; GM-CSF, granulocyte-monocyte colony-stimulating factor; PG, prostaglandin; PAF, platelet-activating factor.

consequences of this immune response occur only if excessive and uncontrolled mediator output results in endothelial damage, neutrophil-mediated tissue damage, and uncontrolled activation of the coagulation and fibrinolytic cascades and the complement system. Ultimately, the combination of these events culminates in cardiovascular instability, impaired hemostasis, organ failure, shock, and death. The following discussion addresses the various pathophysiologic events in the development of endotoxemia and shock and the role of inflammatory mediators.

Endothelial Dysfunction and Damage

Normal endothelium plays an important role in regulating blood pressure and regional tissue perfusion and provides an anticoagulant surface. Endothelial dysfunction and damage result in a decreased responsiveness to vasoactive agents (vasoplegia), increased vascular permeability, and a tendency for clot formation in the microvasculature. If the basement membrane and underlying matrix are compromised, microvascular hemorrhage can occur. Endothelial cell damage is primarily neutrophil-mediated. More specifically, damage is caused by oxygen-derived free radicals, which are produced within endothelial cells through reactions involving neutrophil-derived elastase and hydrogen peroxide molecules, endothelial cell enzymes such as xanthine oxidase, and endothelial cytosolic iron. The hypochloric anion radical ($HO^{\cdot}$) is thought to be responsible most directly for endothelial cell cytotoxicity. Nitric oxide, which is produced by constitutively expressed nitric oxide synthase in endothelial cells and scavenges superoxide radicals in a reaction to form peroxynitrite, may afford protection from oxygen radical–induced endothelial cell damage. Variations in the ability to produce nitric oxide may explain

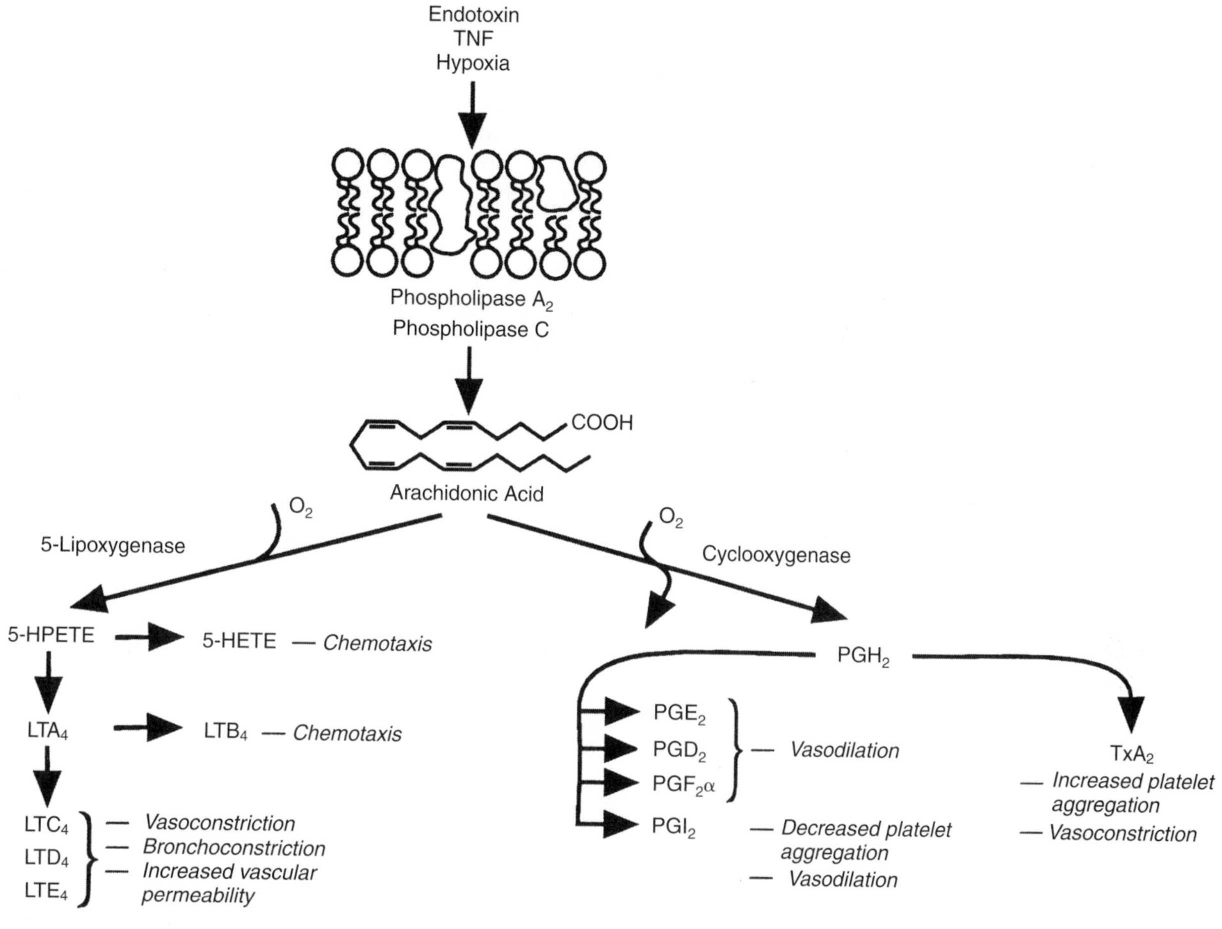

FIGURE 15-10 Pathways of arachidonic acid metabolism by cyclooxygenase and lipoxygenase.

why vascular beds in different organs vary in their susceptibility to neutrophil-mediated damage.[64] Excessive production of nitric oxide by an inducible form of nitric oxide synthase (iNOS), however, contributes to tissue damage, and increased peroxynitrite concentrations may be responsible in part for PAF-induced increases in vascular permeability.[65] In addition to oxygen-derived free radicals, activated neutrophils release matrix metalloproteinases, which contribute to tissue damage.[55] Vascular endothelial cells are further susceptible to direct effects of various cytokines, most prominently TNF-α and IL-1. These cytokines are thought to cause damage via the induction of COX activity and production of prostanoids and through generation of free radicals. Endothelial cell damage in response to endotoxin infusion and the association with leukocyte attachment have been demonstrated in horses.[66]

Neutrophil Activation, Margination, and Transmigration

Neutrophil activation by LPS and cytokines results in stimulation of phagocytosis and the respiratory burst, release of lysosomal enzymes and inflammatory mediators, and expression of adhesion molecules. Perhaps the single most specific clinicopathologic indicator of endotoxemia is pronounced neutropenia,[67] which temporally correlates with peak plasma concentrations of TNF.[68] Neutropenia is caused primarily by margination of neutrophils in the vasculature, especially of the lungs,[69] whereas significant loss through active migration into peripheral tissues likely is limited to the presence of a localized source of infection. In fact, neutrophils exposed to endotoxin or inflammatory mediators exhibit reduced capacity to respond to chemotactic stimuli and extravasate.[69] Margination is made possible by adhesion molecules on endothelial cells and leukocytes that interact and allow sticking of leukocytes to the endothelial lining of blood vessels. The details of neutrophil margination and transmigration are reviewed in several excellent texts.[50,70] Recent evidence demonstrates a role for TLR-4 in neutrophil margination in the lung microvasculature during endotoxemia, and suggests that activation and TLR-4 expression of endothelial cells may be more important than that of circulating neutrophils.[69] While neutrophil activation during infections provides the body with an effective defense system against microbial invaders, margination and reduced migratory ability of neutrophils during endotoxemia results in the accumulation of activated cells at the endothelial surface. These cells are then positioned to effect endothelial injury, increase vascular permeability, and in some cases cause parenchymal cell death and organ dysfunction.[71] In addition, inhibition of transmigration deprives the body of phagocytic cells at sites of infection, resulting in reduced ability to fight bacterial infection.

This latter complication of endotoxemia may have significant clinical impact, because defective neutrophil recruitment has been demonstrated at low endotoxin doses that do not yet result in tissue damage.[71,72] In human patients endotoxemia and impaired neutrophil migration have been associated with infectious complications of surgical procedures.[71] Decreased phagocytic function and oxidative burst activity have also been suggested in sick and septic hospitalized foals,[73,74] where a beneficial effect of plasma transfusion on neutrophil function could be demonstrated. The mechanisms of migration inhibition during endotoxemia are incompletely understood but may include occupation of neutrophil chemotactic receptors by cytokines and complement components, resulting in an inability of activated cells to respond to a chemotactic gradient.[71] Rebound neutrophilia, which is observed frequently following episodes of endotoxemia, is caused by neutrophil release from the bone marrow reserve pool and by stimulation of myeloid cell proliferation via granulocyte-macrophage colony-stimulating factor and is mediated primarily by TNF and IL-1.[53]

Coagulopathy and Disseminated Intravascular Coagulation

In health coagulation and fibrinolysis underlie stringent control mechanisms that allow appropriate clot formation and their resolution. Coagulopathies frequently are observed in horses with colic[17,75,76] and foals with sepsis[11] and are likely attributable to endotoxemia. In human medicine virtually all septic patients are considered to have some degree of coagulopathy, which may range from subclinical abnormalities of the clotting profile to fulminant disseminated intravascular coagulation (DIC).[77,78] DIC results from a widespread activation of the coagulation and fibrinolytic systems and failure of their control mechanisms. Ultimately, this leads to disseminated fibrin deposition in the microvasculature, consumption of platelets and clotting factors, and accumulation of fibrin degradation products (FDPs). Depending on the underlying disease process and the relative impairment of the coagulation and fibrinolytic systems, DIC can manifest as a diffuse thrombotic syndrome leading to ischemic organ failure, a fibrinolytic syndrome with uncontrolled hemorrhage, or a combination of both.[79] A procoagulant state characterized by clinicopathologic abnormalities of the clotting profile precedes DIC.

The intrinsic and extrinsic arms of the coagulation cascade are activated in endotoxemia. The intrinsic pathway is initiated by activation of coagulation factor XII (HF), prekallikrein, and high-molecular-weight kininogen, which compose the contact system.[19] Although direct activation of coagulation factor XII by endotoxin has been demonstrated,[80] the extrinsic pathway likely is more important for the development of coagulopathy in endotoxemia and sepsis.[19] Activation of the extrinsic pathway depends on the interaction of coagulation factor VII with tissue factor, which is the only coagulation factor not constitutively present in blood. Tissue factor is present in subendothelial tissues and is exposed on vascular injury but also is expressed on endothelial cells and mononuclear phagocytes in response to LPS.[81,82] Increased expression of monocyte tissue factor (also described as increased procoagulant activity) was found to be associated significantly with coagulopathy and poor prognosis in horses with colic.[83] Furthermore, LPS-induced tissue factor expression by equine peritoneal macrophages may be associated with the development of intra-abdominal adhesions.[62]

Regulatory mechanisms of the coagulation cascade include tissue factor pathway inhibitor, antithrombin III (AT III), and the protein C system.[19] Protein C acts as an anticoagulant by inactivating clotting factors V and VIII and promotes fibrinolysis by inactivating plasminogen activator inhibitor (PAI).[84] Protein C activation by thrombin-thrombomodulin complexes is important for the anticoagulative properties of normal endothelium,[19] and downregulation of endothelial thrombomodulin expression by TNF and IL-1 along with decreased expression of AT III and tissue factor pathway inhibitor by damaged endothelial cells contribute to the procoagulant state in endotoxemia and sepsis.[85-87] In addition, activation of vascular endothelial cells leads to a loss of prostacyclin and nitric oxide production and an increased release of thromboxane A_2 (TXA_2). As a result, platelets are stimulated to aggregate and release TXA_2 and PAF, thereby further promoting clot formation.[18]

The crucial step in the fibrinolytic cascade is the conversion of plasminogen to plasmin, a fibrin-degrading enzyme.[19] Tissue-type (tPA) and urokinase-type (uPA) plasminogen activator are the major initiators of fibrinolysis, whereas PAI and α2-antiplasmin are the main regulatory components.[88,89] TNF and IL-1 have been shown to induce the release of uPA and tPA and the synthesis of PAI.[19] Activation of fibrinolysis leads to consumption of α2-antiplasmin and accumulation of FDPs, which if present in high concentrations can interfere with platelet aggregation, fibrin polymerization, and thrombin formation and can promote bleeding. Additionally, FDPs mediate an increase in vascular permeability. LPS infusion in rabbits[90] and human beings[91] resulted in an early increase in plasma tPA activity, followed by a later profound rise in PAI activity and fall in tPA activity. Increased plasma PAI concentrations also were found in horses with colic compared with controls.[92,93] Thus although fibrinolysis may compensate initially for accelerated coagulation, its subsequent inhibition contributes to clot formation.

Cross-activation between the inflammatory and coagulation cascades plays an important role in endotoxemia and sepsis, and presence of coagulopathies has been associated with an increased risk of organ failure and poor outcome in septic human patients.[77,78] Interestingly, activated protein C, an anticoagulant, is the only new treatment shown to reduce mortality in septic human patients.[94] Activated protein C reduces inflammation by inhibiting leukocyte activation and cytokine production and was shown to lower plasma concentration of IL-6.[94] Although bleeding complications were increased in treated patients, incidence of severe bleeding was not increased significantly.

Complement Activation

Activation of the complement system in endotoxemia occurs via the alternative pathway through interaction with LPS. Increased concentrations of plasmin and kallikrein (caused by activation of the fibrinolytic and contact system) further promote this pathway by directly activating complement factors C3a and C5a. Aside from being key molecules in the complement cascade, C3a and C5a are anaphylatoxins and cause an increase in vascular permeability via mast cell degranulation. C5a further activates the lipoxygenase pathway in neutrophils and monocytes, acts as a chemotaxin for leukocytes and monocytes, and promotes neutrophil adhesion to endothelial cells.

Acute Phase Response

In response to acute inflammation, synthesis and secretion of a number of proteins called the *acute phase proteins* increases in hepatocytes, whereas synthesis of albumin decreases. The primary function of this acute phase response may be to suppress and contain inflammatory processes.[55] IL-6 and IL-1 are the most important cytokines that induce the acute phase response,[95] which typically begins within a few hours of the insult and subsides within 24 to 48 hours,[50] unless the initiating cause persists. In horses fibrinogen (the most commonly evaluated acute phase protein), haptoglobin, transferrin, ferritin, ceruloplasmin, coagulation factor VIII:C, serum amyloid A, C-reactive protein, α1-acid glycoprotein, and phospholipase A2 are considered part of the acute phase response.[96] Serum amyloid A has been evaluated in several studies and was found to be a sensitive indicator of experimentally induced inflammation.[97] Although serum amyloid A is a nonspecific indicator of inflammation, its measurement may be helpful in the diagnosis of inflammatory gastrointestinal disease,[37] neonatal weakness and diarrhea,[98] and various infectious diseases. A commercially available turbidometric immunoassay for human serum amyloid A was reliable in measuring equine serum amyloid A in one study.[99]

The effect of acute inflammation on the serum concentration of several coagulation factors must be considered when evaluating coagulation profiles. Serum fibrinogen concentration is determined primarily by the acute phase response, although fibrinogen is consumed increasingly on activation of the clotting cascade.

Hemodynamic Changes, Development of Shock, and Organ Failure

Shock is characterized by a loss of homeostasis attributable to breakdown of hemodynamic control mechanisms, decreases in cardiac output and the effective circulating volume, and inadequate perfusion of vital organs. Shock caused by endotoxemia is classified as distributive shock[100] and is largely initiated by vascular dysfunction in the periphery. Peripheral vascular beds are of major importance for the regulation of local tissue perfusion and affect systemic blood pressure by regulating total peripheral resistance. Normally, vascular smooth muscle tone is regulated by endothelin-1 (vasoconstriction), nitric oxide, and prostacyclin (vasodilation) released from vascular endothelial cells.[19] As mentioned before, detrimental effects of nitric oxide are attributable to overproduction of nitric oxide by iNOS in macrophages and other cell types, rather than endothelial-derived nitric oxide. Peripheral vasomotor effects of endotoxin manifest as vasodilation and vasoplegia and are mediated by PGI_2, nitric oxide, and mediators such as bradykinin. Widespread vasodilation leads to vascular blood pooling, decentralization of blood flow, decreased venous return, and in effect decreased effective circulating volume and cardiac output.[100] Compensatory responses in the form of an initial hyperdynamic phase include tachycardia, increased cardiac output and central venous pressure, pulmonary hypertension, peripheral vasoconstriction, and increased peripheral vascular resistance.[100-102]

The early vasoconstrictive phase corresponds to an increased serum concentration of TXA_2,[18] but additional vasoconstrictors such as arginine vasopressin, angiotensin II, serotonin, endothelin, and norepinephrine likely are implicated in the pathogenesis of shock and organ failure.[55] With progression of disease the animal enters a stage of decompensated shock and progressive systemic hypotension, which corresponds to increased plasma concentrations of prostacyclin, PGE2, and bradykinin.[18,55] Inadequate blood flow and oxygen delivery to tissues caused by hypotension are confounded by direct myocardial suppression via nitric oxide,[100] increased vascular permeability,[18] intravascular microthrombosis, and impaired tissue oxygen extraction[100] and results in progressive metabolic acidosis and inhibition of normal cellular metabolism.

CLINICAL SIGNS AND DIAGNOSIS

Quantification of endotoxin in plasma samples is possible. The Limulus amebocyte lysate assay is an activity assay based on the endotoxin-sensitive hemolymph coagulation cascade in the horseshoe crab *Limulus polyphemus*. In Limulus this reaction is thought to be a defense mechanism against gram negative infection.[103] Although frequently used as a research tool, the assay is not convenient enough to become a routine clinical test. The clinician therefore must appreciate the primary disease processes associated with a high risk of endotoxemia and rely on clinical signs and clinicopathologic data to achieve a diagnosis. In a survey of board-certified internists and surgeons concerning endotoxemia in horses, colitis and enteritis, small intestinal strangulation and obstruction, retained placenta and metritis in mares, grain overload, and pleuropneumonia were among the most frequently cited conditions associated with endotoxemia.[104] In some cases, endotoxemia may be the first indication of disease or may be the most overt of otherwise subtle clinical manifestations. With colitis or proximal enteritis, for example, one may detect signs of endotoxemia before the development of colic, diarrhea, or gastric reflux, which more specifically indicate the nature of the primary illness. Presence of neutropenia should always prompt the clinician to investigate causes of endotoxemia, including septic processes.

In vivo LPS challenge experiments in horses clearly show that many of the clinical signs associated with acute gastrointestinal disease and sepsis are attributable to endotoxemia. On administration of sublethal doses of LPS, the clinical response can be divided into the early hyperdynamic and the later hypodynamic or shock phases. Clinical signs during the first phase, which begins within 15 to 45 minutes after LPS administration, include anorexia, yawning, sweating, depression, evidence of abdominal discomfort, muscle fasciculations, and recumbency. Heart and respiratory rates increase, and decreased borborygmi suggest ileus. Hyperemia of the mucous membranes and an accelerated capillary refill time indicate the hyperdynamic state.[67] If large amounts of LPS are administered or if exposure is ongoing, depression worsens progressively, anorexia persists, and feces develop diarrheic character. Signs of colic typically abate after the initial stage. Fever develops as a result of direct action of TNF on the thermoregulatory center and IL-1–induced local production of PGE2 in or near the hypothalamus.[105,106] Because of compromised peripheral perfusion, mucous membrane color changes to brick red or purple, a dark "toxic" line appears, and capillary refill time is prolonged.[67] Inadequate peripheral perfusion and compromised organ function finally characterize the hypodynamic shock phase. Body temperature may become subnormal, and the skin, especially on extremities, is cool to the touch. The arterial pulse weakens and venous fill is decreased. Vascular endothelial damage and increased capillary permeability result in a muddy mucous membrane color and diffuse scleral reddening. Similar changes are evident in horses suffering from endotoxemia associated with natural disease. In the previously mentioned survey,[104] tachycardia, fever, abnormal mucous membrane color, and increased capillary refill time were named by most specialists as indicating endotoxemia.

Hemostatic abnormalities can manifest in the form of thrombosis, such as of the jugular vein, or increased bleeding tendency with mucosal petechiation or ecchymoses and prolonged bleeding from venipuncture sites.[79] Bleeding also may occur in the form of spontaneous epistaxis or prolonged hemorrhage after nasogastric intubation.[18] Additional clinical signs typically reflect the development of organ failure. Renal failure and laminitis[104] appear to be common complications of endotoxemia in horses, and endotoxemia was identified as the only clinical condition significantly associated with the development of acute laminitis in one retrospective case-control study of horses admitted to a referral center.[107] Other potential complications include liver failure,[79] respiratory failure, colic and ischemia-induced gastrointestinal ulceration,[18] cardiac failure, and abortion in pregnant mares.[108,109] Renal failure results from ischemic cortical necrosis and acute tubular necrosis caused by coagulopathy-induced afferent arteriolar obstruction. Clinical signs may include oliguria, anuria, or hematuria caused by renal infarction. Laminitis may lead to lameness, increased digital arterial pulsation, increased warmth of the hoof wall, and sensitivity to hoof tester pressure. The exact nature of the association between endotoxemia and laminitis is not understood, and, interestingly, experimental endotoxin infusion does not reliably induce laminitis. Studies have shown, however, that endotoxin administration decreases digital blood flow and laminar perfusion[110] coincident with increased plasma concentrations of 5-hydroxytryptamine and thromboxane B_2.[111] In addition, in vitro vascular reactivity of digital vessels is altered following sublethal endotoxin administration to horses.[112] In addition to the response to circulating mediators, LPS exposure also alters the production of vasoactive mediators by digital vascular endothelial cells.[113] Alterations in vascular reactivity are therefore likely responsible for development of laminitis in endotoxemia; however, other mechanisms may apply depending on the underlying clinical disease.

CLINICAL PATHOLOGIC TESTING

Alterations in the hemogram and serum biochemical profile mainly reflect the underlying disease process and the occurrence of organ failure. Leukopenia caused by neutropenia may be the most specific indicator of acute bacterial sepsis or endotoxemia.[67] In prolonged cases an increased proportion of immature neutrophil forms (bands), and toxic changes are observed. Toxic changes resulting from neutrophil activation include vacuolation, cytoplasmic granulation, basophilic cytoplasm, and Döhle's bodies. Because neutropenia occurs early in the development of endotoxemia, it also may be a useful parameter for monitoring horses at risk.[67] On recovery neutropenia typically is followed by a pronounced rebound neutrophilia.

An elevated hematocrit and total serum protein concentration are frequently interpreted as evidence of dehydration; however, splenic contraction caused by increased sympathetic stimulation, increased production of acute phase proteins, or protein losses also influence these parameters. Hyperproteinemia may be observed as a result of increases in the fibrinogen or globulin concentration, and determination of protein fractions, including protein electrophoresis, is indicated in hyperproteinemic patients. Hypoproteinemia and hypoalbuminemia can occur because of loss via the gastrointestinal or urinary tract or with pleural or peritoneal cavity effusion. Increased vascular permeability and edema formation contribute to hypoproteinemia.

Serum electrolyte abnormalities primarily depend on the nature and duration of underlying disease processes and need to be evaluated individually. Common sources of electrolyte loss are gastrointestinal secretions, urine, and sweat; however, severe effusion into body cavities may contribute. In anorexic patients lack of dietary intake is a confounding factor that warrants consideration. In human patients gram negative sepsis frequently is associated with hypocalcemia, more specifically a decrease in serum ionized calcium concentration. Endotoxin is thought to be a causative factor, and proposed mechanisms include acquired parathyroid gland insufficiency, dietary vitamin D deficiency, impaired calcium mobilization, and renal 1-hydroxylase insufficiency leading to decreased 1,25-hydroxylation of vitamin D. Hypocalcemia in septic human patients was associated with hypotension and poor outcome.[114] In horses with surgically managed gastrointestinal disease, decreased serum ionized calcium concentration was a common finding and was most severe in patients with strangulating or nonstrangulating infarctions. In some horses ionized calcium concentration decreased further throughout surgery. Treatment with calcium gluconate resulted in normalization of serum ionized calcium concentrations in all cases.[115]

Septic neonatal patients are frequently hypoglycemic, which may be attributable to decreased oral intake, generally increased metabolism, glucose use by the infecting bacteria, inhibition of gluconeogenesis by endotoxin, and insulin-like activity produced by macrophages.[18] Interestingly, experimental endotoxin administration results in transient hyperglycemia in adult horses,[101] whereas profound hypoglycemia occurs in foals.[116] Because of the high incidence of coagulopathies in endotoxemic and septic patients, clinicians should consider monitoring coagulation parameters. The most significant changes can be expected with severe inflammatory disease such as colitis,[75,76] devitalized intestine as with strangulating obstruction,[76,117] and with increased duration of disease. In 30 horses with acute gastrointestinal disease, coagulation profiles were considered normal in only two horses.[75] Although coagulation times may be shortened during the procoagulant state, commonly observed abnormalities with developing DIC include an increased concentration of FDPs and soluble fibrin monomer, prolonged prothrombin time indicative of factor VII consumption, prolonged activated partial thromboplastin time indicative of factor VIII:C and IX consumption, prolonged thrombin time, decreased AT III activity, thrombocytopenia, and decreased protein C and plasminogen activities. Fibrinogen concentration appears to reflect the acute phase response rather than coagulation abnormalities in horses and is frequently increased.[83] Some clinicians make a diagnosis of DIC if three or more coagulation parameters (specifically AT III, FDPs, platelet count, prothrombin time, and activated partial thromboplastin time) are abnormal,[117] whereas others require overt clinical signs of hemorrhage and concomitant thrombosis in addition to classic laboratory findings.[76] The prognostic value of coagulation parameters has been evaluated.[17,76,93] Overall, persistence or worsening of abnormalities in the face of treatment appears to be more indicative of poor outcome than alterations in any specific parameter. In one study decreased serum AT III concentration was the parameter most commonly associated with fatal outcome in mature horses with colic.[75]

Clinical pathologic parameters are also helpful in identifying potential underlying diseases and monitoring organ function. Serum creatinine and urea nitrogen concentration in combination with urinalysis parameters are usually monitored as indicators of renal function, whereas serum activity of liver enzymes, serum indirect and direct bilirubin concentration, serum bile acids, and blood ammonia are useful indicators of liver function. One should evaluate arterial blood gases in patients with primary respiratory disease or with clinical evidence of respiratory failure and in profoundly depressed, recumbent patients, especially neonates. Hypoxemia observed in response to endotoxin infusion is thought to be caused by an increase in ventilation-perfusion mismatch rather than pulmonary edema, as occurs in human patients with acute respiratory distress syndrome. Pulmonary edema may occur in patients with associated sepsis or complications such as DIC.[118]

MANAGEMENT

The ideal treatment for endotoxemia is prevention. Recognition and close monitoring of patients at risk are crucial because doing so allows institution of timely, possibly proactive treatment, which may reverse the effects of endotoxin before the inflammatory response has developed a dynamic of its own. Unfortunately, endotoxemia can develop rapidly, and horses are exquisitely sensitive to the effects of endotoxin; therefore many equine patients are not presented for evaluation until they have reached more severe stages of endotoxemia or shock. Prognosis and patient outcome then frequently depend on the severity of complications associated with endotoxemia.[18]

Treatment of endotoxemia involves multiple aspects, and the following strategies have been proposed:[119]

- Inhibition of endotoxin release into the circulation
- Scavenging of LPS molecules to prevent direct effects and interaction with inflammatory cells
- Inhibition of cellular activation by LPS
- Inhibition of mediator synthesis
- Interference with the effects of inflammatory mediators
- General supportive care

In addition, treatment must also address the primary disease process as well as any complications.

When evaluating reports concerning the efficacy of any one treatment, the clinician should keep in mind differences in underlying disease processes and the complexity of the inflammatory cascade. A "one for all" treatment most likely will not be found; similarly, any one treatment can address only a few pathophysiologic aspects of endotoxemia at most. In human septic patients many treatments that showed initial promise for improving patient outcome failed to show benefit in larger populations, although benefit for certain subgroups of patients was sometimes demonstrated. Understanding the rationale for different treatment strategies is therefore important to be able to tailor treatment to the needs of the patient. In the following sections discussion will focus on treatments that have been evaluated for use in horses, while mention is also made of studies in other species, where applicable.

Inhibition of Endotoxin Release into the Circulation

Inhibition of endotoxin release requires identification and removal of its source. Therefore whenever endotoxemia is evident, the clinician should strive to reach a diagnosis of the underlying disease and ascertain whether ischemic or inflamed bowel or a gram negative septic process is present. Aside from history, physical examination, and routine laboratory testing, evaluation may include exploratory laparotomy in colic patients, radiographic and ultrasonographic evaluation of the pleural and peritoneal cavity, ultrasonographic evaluation of umbilical remnants in neonatal foals, evaluation of passive transfer and calculation of a sepsis score in foals, and repeated culturing of blood or other specimens. Identification of responsible microorganisms and their antimicrobial sensitivity spectrum is a crucial step toward effective therapy; however, one should not necessarily delay treatment to obtain culture results. Specimen containers with antimicrobial removal devices may be useful in cases for which initiation of treatment precedes specimen collection. Once a diagnosis is reached, appropriate measures to correct the primary disease process must be taken. Examples are removal of devitalized sections of bowel or infected umbilical remnants, drainage of infected pleural or PF, and gastric lavage followed by administration of mineral oil or intestinal adsorbants in cases of grain overload. Di-tri-octahedral smectite (Biosponge™, Platinum Performance Inc., Buellton, California) was shown to remove endotoxin in an in vitro assay[120] and may be useful in preventing endotoxemia of intestinal origin. Septic processes must be addressed with appropriate antimicrobial therapy, and principles of antimicrobial therapy should be followed. Regarding endotoxemia specifically, antimicrobial therapy has been suggested to increase the amount of circulating endotoxin by inducing endotoxin release on cell death of gram negative bacteria. An in vitro study comparing endotoxin release and inflammatory mediator activity among antimicrobials commonly used to treat *E. coli* septicemia in foals evaluated amikacin, ampicillin, amikacin plus ampicillin, ceftiofur, and imipenem. Although these antimicrobials showed no difference in the ability to kill bacteria, amikacin and the amikacin-ampicillin combination resulted in the lowest, and ceftiofur in the greatest, release of endotoxin. Endotoxin release appeared to be dose dependent in that lesser amounts were released at higher antimicrobial concentrations.[121] On the basis of these results and clinical experience, combining antimicrobial therapy with endotoxin-binding agents such as polymyxin B may be beneficial, especially when using β-lactam antimicrobials.

Scavenging of Lipopolysaccharide Molecules

Endotoxin typically has a short plasma half-life and is removed rapidly by mononuclear phagocytes or neutralized by binding to serum proteins and lipoproteins. Many conditions responsible for the development of endotoxemia in horses, however, may be associated with an ongoing release of endotoxin. Examples include severe gastrointestinal inflammation as in proximal enteritis or colitis, grain overload, or uncontrolled sepsis. Therapy directed against endotoxin itself may be able to interrupt the continuous activation of the inflammatory cascade in these cases. Further benefits of anti-endotoxin treatment may be derived if large amounts of endotoxin have been released before the inciting cause can be addressed.

IMMUNOTHERAPY

An important consideration regarding the efficacy of immunotherapy is the region of the LPS molecule against which antibodies are raised. The O-chain of LPS acts as a potent antigen on infection with gram negative bacteria;[7] however, antibodies directed against the O-chain are serotype specific and cannot afford significant cross-protection against heterologous bacterial strains. The core and lipid A region, both of which show a much higher degree of homology between LPS derived from different bacterial strains, offer a more promising target for immunotherapy. Active immunization against endotoxin has been reported for horses. Vaccination with a bacterin-toxoid vaccine prepared from rough mutants of *Salmonella typhimurium* or *S. enteritidis* protected horses against homologous and heterologous endotoxin challenge[122,123] and carbohydrate overload.[132] Despite these encouraging results and the current availability of a vaccine for use in horses (Endovac-Equi, Immvac Inc., Columbus, Missouri), active immunization against endotoxin does not appear to be a common practice. In comparison, passive immunization with antilipopolysaccharide antibodies is used widely. Rough bacterial mutants, most commonly J5 of *E. coli* O111:B4 and *S. minnesota* Re595, are used to immunize donor horses and subsequently prepare serum or plasma products. Proposed mechanisms of action after binding of the antibodies to LPS include steric blockade of lipid A interaction with cellular receptors and enhanced bacterial clearance by opsonization.[124-126] Studies concerning the efficacy of antibody administration in equine patients vary in their results. Beneficial effects have been described in experimental models of endotoxemia, acute gastrointestinal disease, and neonates with sepsis,[123,127-130] whereas in other studies antibodies failed to protect foals and horses against endotoxin effects.[131-133] Furthermore, administration of a *S. typhimurium* antiserum to foals was associated with an increased respiratory rate and higher serum activities of IL-6 and TNF.[131]

Various equine serum and plasma products are commercially available. An antiserum raised against the LPS-core of *S. typhimurium* (Endoserum®, Immvac Inc., Columbus, Missouri) is available for administration to endotoxemic horses at a recommended dose of 1.5 ml/kg body mass. Diluting the serum tenfold to 20-fold in crystalloid intravenous solutions, administering it slowly over 1 to 2 hours, and monitoring the patient for adverse reactions is advisable. Although the product is marketed for use in foals with failure of passive transfer, adverse effects have been reported,[131] and one should use caution when administering it to neonates. Plasma from donors inoculated with J5 (*E. coli*) and *S. typhimurium* (Re mutant) is available under a California license (Equiplas J®, Plasvacc USA Inc, Templeton, California). The manufacturer recommends administration of at least 1 to 2 L in cases of endotoxemia. In addition, hyperimmune plasma, which has a guaranteed minimum immunoglobulin G content but does not contain specific antiendotoxin antibodies (Hi-Gamm Equi, Lake Immunogenics, Inc., Ontario, New York; Equiplas and Equiplas Plus, Plasvacc USA Inc,), is marketed for treatment of failure of passive transfer, and many clinicians use it to treat endotoxemia and sepsis. In addition to antibodies and protein, plasma contains active constituents such as complement components, fibronectin, clotting factors, and AT III[128] and therefore may be particularly useful in patients with endotoxemia-induced coagulopathy. Volumes of 2 to 10 ml/kg body mass of hyperimmune plasma have been recommended for use in endotoxemic patients.[55,134]

POLYMYXIN B

Polymyxin B is a cationic polypeptide antibiotic that binds to the anionic lipid A portion of LPS and neutralizes its endotoxin capacity.[135] At dosages required for antimicrobial activity, polymyxin B carries the risk of respiratory paralysis and ototoxic, nephrotoxic, and neurotoxic side effects; however, a much lower dose is required for endotoxin-binding activity. The effects of polymyxin B in horses have been evaluated in different experimental models.[131,135,136] In an in vivo study in foals, treatment with polymyxin B at a dosage of 6000 U/kg body mass before infusion with *S. typhimurium* LPS resulted in significantly less severe elevations of body temperature, respiratory rate, and serum activities of TNF and IL-6 compared with untreated controls.[131] Similarly, polymyxin B treatment of adult horses given endotoxin significantly ameliorated clinical signs and decreased plasma TNF activity.[137] In the latter study benefits of treatment were also evident at lower dosages of polymyxin B (1000 and 5000 U/kg body mass) and administration of polymyxin B 1 hour after the start of endotoxin infusion. Conversely, polymyxin B failed to ameliorate clinical signs of endotoxemia or prevent the development of coagulopathy, acidosis, lameness, and shock in experimental carbohydrate overload.[138] Side effects suggestive of neurotoxicity appeared after repeated administration of 5 mg/kg body mass (36,000 U/kg) and in milder form 2.5 mg/kg body mass (18,000 U/kg) polymyxin B. Nephrotoxicity was not observed. Currently, use of polymyxin B in equine patients is recommended at dosages of 1000 to 6000 U/kg body mass every 8 to 12 hours.[139,140] Treatment should be initiated as early in the disease process as possible because the beneficial effects of LPS scavenging may be limited to the first 24 to 48 hours after the onset of endotoxemia, before endotoxin tolerance develops. Side effects in the form of neuromuscular blockade and apnea, which necessitate slow infusion of the drug in human patients, have not been observed in horses. Therefore the entire dose can be administered as a slow bolus. If treating horses with hypovolemia, dehydration, or azotemia, the clinician should attempt to improve peripheral tissue perfusion, minimize the polymyxin B dose, and closely monitor patients for nephrotoxicity. Close monitoring is also important if medications such as aminoglycoside antibiotics, which share a similar spectrum of potential side effects, are administered concurrently. Azotemic neonates have been reported to be more susceptible to the nephrotoxic effects of polymyxin B than adult horses.[137]

In an attempt to decrease the risk for adverse effects while preserving LPS-neutralizing ability, a conjugate of polymyxin B with dextran has been developed.[141] In conjugated form, polymyxin B is prevented from extravasation into tissues, where it exerts toxic effects by interaction with cell membranes. In addition, conjugation increases the residence time of polymyxin B in the circulation and therefore should prolong the antiendotoxic effect. The polymyxin B–dextran combination was evaluated at a total dose of 5 mg/kg body mass of polymyxin B in 6.6 g/kg body mass dextran given 15 minutes before administration of endotoxin in horses.[142] Treatment was found to block the development of tachycardia, tachypnea, fever, and neutropenia completely and to prevent increases in serum concentrations of TNF, IL-6, TXB_2 (a TXA_2 metabolite), and the prostacyclin metabolite 6-keto-$PGF_1\alpha$. Although mild adverse effects in the form of tachypnea, sweating, and increased systolic blood pressure were observed, these were transient and could be prevented by pretreatment with ketoprofen. To the author's knowledge, the polymyxin B–dextran combination is not commercially available at this time.

NATURAL ENDOTOXIN-BINDING SUBSTANCES

Natural endotoxin-binding proteins such as LBP, lipoproteins, and sCD14 have been evaluated experimentally. Results of these studies are somewhat contradictory, and detrimental effects occurred in some cases.[143] A protein receiving much attention regarding potential therapeutic efficacy is the bactericidal permeability-increasing protein (BPI). This protein is structurally similar to LBP but is expressed exclusively in myeloid precursors of polymorphonuclear leukocytes.[144] BPI is stored in primary granules of mature neutrophils and during inflammation is expressed on their cell membranes and secreted into the extracellular environment.[145] BPI has an even higher affinity for LPS than LBP[146] and shows antibacterial activity specific for gram negative bacteria.[5] Binding of BPI to the gram negative bacterial membrane results in growth arrest and is an important factor in the antibacterial activity of intact neutrophils. Furthermore, BPI binding disrupts normal membrane organization and makes bacteria more susceptible to hydrophobic substances, including antimicrobials.[147] Experimentally, recombinant BPI protects against the toxic and lethal effects of isolated LPS and intact gram negative bacteria, and clinical trials in human patients show promising results regarding its therapeutic use.[148] The biology and potential use of BPI in horses has not been evaluated.

Phospholipid emulsions have recently been evaluated for treatment of experimentally induced endotoxemia in horses. Phospholipid infusion improved clinical parameters, ameliorated neutropenia, and reduced inflammatory mediator production in response to an endotoxin challenge.[149,150] Because hemolysis was a complication of phospholipid infusion in some horses in these studies, optimization of dose and time of administration will be necessary before evaluating this treatment for potential clinical use.

Inhibition of Cellular Activation by Lipopolysaccharide

Treatments aimed at inhibiting LPS interaction with cells or turning off intracellular signaling pathways are under investigation. Nontoxic LPS or lipid A structures can act as endotoxin antagonists, if they competitively inhibit binding to LBP or cellular receptors or inhibit cellular activation by other mechanisms. Of the potential antagonists that have been evaluated experimentally, LPS and lipid A of the phototrophic bacterium *Rhodobacter sphaeroides* and the synthetic compounds E5531 and E5564 have been most promising.[150-156] Unfortunately, species differences exist regarding cellular response to these structures, and *R. sphaeroides* LPS as well as E5531 have been found to have agonist activity in equine cells.[157,158] In cell transfection experiments, TLR4 was shown to be responsible for this phenotypic variation with regard to *R. sphaeroides* LPS.[159] Given these results, any future potential LPS antagonists must be evaluated in equine systems.

Inhibition of Mediator Synthesis

NONSTEROIDAL ANTI-INFLAMMATORY DRUGS

NSAIDs are probably the most commonly used drugs to treat endotoxemia in horses. The rationale for their use is inhibition of COX and thereby inhibition of prostanoid production (see Figure 15-10). Additional beneficial effects may include scavenging of oxygen-derived free radicals and iron chelation; however, side effects may occur at dosages required to achieve these effects.[160] Prostanoids have been identified as important mediators in the inflammatory response in a number of studies, and inhibition of their synthesis is associated with beneficial effects. Generally speaking, two COX isoforms are recognized: constitutively expressed COX-1 and inducible COX-2. Upregulation of COX-2 expression results from various pro-inflammatory stimuli, including LPS, TNF α, and IL-1.[161] Constitutively expressed COX products are likely important for maintenance of homeostasis, whereas increased production of prostanoids by COX-2 is thought to be responsible for detrimental effects during inflammation and shock. Research has focused on the development of selective COX-2 inhibitors, and firocoxib (Equioxx®, Merial Ltd., Duluth, Georgia) has been approved for treatment of osteoarthritis in horses. This drug has not been evaluated critically for treatment of endotoxemia.

In horses the most commonly used NSAID to treat endotoxemia is flunixin meglumine. Beneficial effects of flunixin meglumine have been described in experimental models of endotoxemia[162-164] and in clinical cases. In equine colic patients treatment with flunixin meglumine before exploratory surgery resulted in reduced plasma concentrations of TXB_2 and PGE_2 and had a favorable effect on cardiovascular parameters.[165] Flunixin meglumine was shown further to maintain cardiac output and systemic arterial blood pressure, improve blood flow to vital organs, reduce pulmonary endothelial damage, and improve survival on endotoxin challenge.[66,166-168] Conversely, in vitro studies have suggested that flunixin meglumine impairs recovery of intestinal barrier function in intestinal segments subjected to ischemia-reperfusion injury and may increase mucosal permeability to LPS.[169,170] This effect may be reduced or eliminated by concurrent administration of continuous-rate infusion of lidocaine.

NSAID use in horses carries the risk of side effects, the most significant of which is the development of gastrointestinal ulceration and renal papillary necrosis (renal crest necrosis). Differences may exist among NSAIDs in their propensity to induce adverse effects,[171] but all NSAIDs must be used cautiously. A concern about NSAID use specifically in colic patients is the masking of cardiovascular effects of endotoxin, which are used to determine the necessity of surgical exploration.[172] For these reasons a reduced dose of flunixin meglumine (0.25 mg/kg body mass thrice daily) has been suggested and is used widely in horses.[104] At this dosage flunixin meglumine inhibits eicosanoid synthesis efficiently in an in vivo model of endotoxemia.[173] Reduction of clinical signs, however, was dose dependent, and lower doses provide minimal, if any, analgesia (see Chapter 4 for further discussion of NSAID therapy in horses). Therefore the veterinarian should choose the appropriate dose of any NSAID after carefully considering the circumstances of each case.

Some researchers have suggested that ketoprofen offers superior effects because of a proposed dual inhibitory effect on COX and lipoxygenase and may carry a decreased risk of adverse effects compared with flunixin meglumine and phenylbutazone. A comparison of cytokine and eicosanoid production by LPS-stimulated isolated monocytes in vitro, however, showed no significant difference between horses pretreated with flunixin meglumine (1.1 mg/kg body mass) or ketoprofen (2.2 mg/kg body mass), respectively.[174]

Eltenac has been evaluated in an experimental endotoxemia model in horses.[175] Given 15 minutes before LPS infusion, eltenac at a dose of 0.5 mg/kg protected against changes in clinical, hemodynamic, and hematologic parameters and blunted the LPS-induced rise in plasma cytokine concentrations in comparison with controls. Some parameters, however, including heart rate, leukocyte count, lactate concentration, and plasma TNF activity, were not improved. Ibuprofen may have beneficial effects superior to those of the other NSAIDs because it may be possible to achieve tissue concentrations safely that allow iron chelation to occur. According to a study in healthy foals, dosages of ibuprofen up to 25 mg/kg every 8 hours can be given safely for up to 6 days.[160]

CORTICOSTEROIDS

The use of corticosteroids for anti-inflammatory therapy in sepsis and endotoxemia has been controversial in human and equine patients, and beneficial effects superior to the ones achieved by NSAIDs have not been demonstrated consistently. Corticosteroids inhibit the activity of phospholipase A_2 and the release of arachidonic acid from cell membrane phospholipids, as well as the production of TNF, IL-1, and IL-6 in response to a LPS stimulus. Experimentally, beneficial effects of dexamethasone in equine endotoxemia have been demonstrated.[176,177] To inhibit TNF production by equine peritoneal macrophages, however, the required concentration of dexamethasone was high and corresponded to an in vivo dosage (approximately 3 mg/kg body mass) greatly exceeding current recommendations.[176] Although single doses of corticosteroids are unlikely to carry a disproportionate risk of adverse effects, the clinician should consider the suggested association of laminitis with corticosteroid use in horses. In cases of sepsis immunosuppressive effects could also be detrimental.

In human patients with certain types of septic shock, dysfunction of the hypothalamic-pituitary-adrenal axis has been recognized and successfully treated with hydrocortisone replacement therapy.[178] Hypothalamic-pituitary-adrenal axis dysfunction has been suggested to occur in septic foals;[179] however, the use of low-dose corticosteroids for this indication remains to be investigated in horses.

PENTOXIFYLLINE

Pentoxifylline, a methylxanthine derivative and phosphodiesterase inhibitor, has been suggested for use in endotoxemia because of its effects on neutrophil function and its ability to inhibit the production of various cytokines, interferons, and thromboplastin. Decreased production of TNF, IL-6, TXB_2, and thromboplastin in response to endotoxin was shown in an equine ex vivo model.[180] In horses given endotoxin followed by treatment with pentoxifylline (7.5 mg/kg body mass followed by continuous infusion of 3 mg/kg/hr for 3 hours), however, only minimal beneficial effects were observed.[181] Treatment significantly improved body temperature, respiratory rate, and whole blood recalcification time, but no effect was observed regarding heart rate, blood pressure, leukocyte count, plasma fibrinogen concentration, and serum cytokine concentrations. The conclusion was that benefits of treatment with pentoxifylline might be restricted to administration of high bolus doses or continuous infusion early in the pathophysiologic process. In an in vivo endotoxemia model in horses, the combination of pentoxifylline (8 mg/kg body mass) and flunixin meglumine (1.1 mg/kg body mass) was found to have greater benefit than each treatment on its own.[182] Because of its rheologic properties (i.e., the ability to increase erythrocyte deformability and microvascular blood flow), pentoxifylline has been suggested for use in endotoxemic patients showing evidence of laminitis; however, no effect on blood flow to the hoof was demonstrated after administration to healthy horses.[183] An intravenous preparation of pentoxifylline is not commercially available.

ANTIOXIDANTS

Dimethyl sulfoxide (DMSO) is used by some clinicians in an attempt to scavenge oxygen-derived radicals. The treatment may be most appropriate in cases of ischemia-induced intestinal damage and associated reperfusion injury. However, DMSO failed to show beneficial effects in an experimental model of intestinal ischemia when administered on reperfusion of the ischemic intestine.[184] DMSO at a dose of 1 g/kg body mass was shown to increase mucosal loss after ischemia and reperfusion of the large colon,[185] and hence a reduced dose of 0.1 g/kg body mass has been proposed for cases of intestinal ischemia. DMSO failed to show significant benefit in an experimental model of endotoxemia in horses, although it ameliorated the effect on fever.[186] For intravenous administration, DMSO should be diluted in polyionic solutions to a concentration not exceeding 10%. Oral administration of a 10% to 20% solution via nasogastric intubation is also possible. Aside from DMSO the xanthine oxidase inhibitor allopurinol has been suggested as a treatment to prevent oxygen radical–induced tissue damage. During periods of ischemia tissue xanthine dehydrogenase is converted to xanthine oxidase, which on reperfusion catalyzes the generation of superoxide radicals.[187,188] Evaluation in horses showed beneficial effects of 5 mg allopurinol per kilogram body mass administered 12 hours before endotoxin challenge.[189] In another study mucosal damage attributable to oxygen-derived free radicals was not attenuated by allopurinol in an experimental ischemia-reperfusion model.[185]

LIDOCAINE

Lidocaine given intravenously has been suggested as an anti-inflammatory, analgesic, and prokinetic agent, and some clinicians use it to treat colic and laminitis in horses. In an experimental endotoxemia model in rabbits, lidocaine inhibited hemodynamic and cytokine responses to endotoxin profoundly if given immediately after LPS infusion.[190] Lidocaine further ameliorated the inhibitory effects of flunixin on recovery of mucosal barrier function following ischemic injury in equine small intestine.[191] Use of lidocaine therefore may have merit in endotoxemic patients. A common regimen for lidocaine use in horses is administration of an initial bolus (1.3 mg/kg body mass) followed by continuous infusion at a rate of 0.05 mg/kg/min. The veterinarian should monitor patients for toxic neurologic effects associated with a lidocaine overdose.

ω-3 FATTY ACIDS

High concentrations of ω-3 fatty acids can alter the phospholipid composition of cellular membranes toward a decreased ratio of ω-6 to ω-3 and thereby can affect membrane functions such as phagocytosis, receptor binding, and activities of membrane-bound enzymes.[67] Most important for the treatment of endotoxemia, ω-3 fatty acid incorporation into cell membranes decreases the availability of arachidonic acid (an ω-6 fatty acid) for eicosanoid synthesis[192] and provides alternative substrates. Metabolism of ω-3 fatty acids via the COX and lipoxygenase pathway leads to the production of 3-series prostaglandins and 5-series leukotrienes, which have less biologic activity than their 2-series and 4-series counterparts derived from arachidonic acid. Aside from these mechanisms, ω-3 fatty acids prevent LPS-induced upregulation of CD14 in monocytic cells and therefore may be able to block transmembrane signaling of LPS.[193] Cells from horses given linseed oil (high in ω-3 fatty acids) for 8 weeks before blood collection showed significantly decreased expression of procoagulant activity, TXB_2, and TNF in response to LPS stimulation.[194,195] In an in vivo experimental model of endotoxemia in horses, treatment resulted in prolonged activated partial thromboplastin time and whole blood recalcification time, suggesting an anticoagulant effect; however, a significant beneficial effect on clinical response and serum eicosanoid concentrations was not observed.[196] Because dietary addition of ω-3 fatty acids requires several weeks of treatment, intravenous infusion was evaluated and shown to alter the composition of cell membrane phospholipids rapidly.[197] Further evaluation of this treatment for use in horses is necessary before specific dosage recommendations can be made.

Interference with the Effects of Specific Inflammatory Mediators

ANTIBODIES DIRECTED AGAINST TUMOR NECROSIS FACTOR

Monoclonal and polyclonal antibodies against equine TNF have been evaluated in horses.[198-200] Administration of a monoclonal antibody preparation before LPS infusion resulted in significantly reduced plasma TNF activity, improved clinical abnormality scores, lower heart rate, and higher leukocyte count compared with controls.[199] Furthermore, plasma concentrations of lactate and 6-keto-PGF1α were reduced significantly, whereas TXA_2 production was not affected.[198] In another study[200] administration of a rabbit polyclonal antibody against recombinant human TNF did not improve clinical and hematologic parameters when given shortly (15 minutes) after LPS infusion, although inhibition of TNF activity was present in vitro.[200,201] Findings in horses are in agreement with studies in other species and suggest that beneficial effects of TNF inhibition may be limited to administration before LPS exposure. Widespread clinical use therefore is unlikely to become feasible. Clinical trials in septic human patients have not shown significant benefits of TNF antibody treatment.[202,203]

PLATELET-ACTIVATING FACTOR RECEPTOR ANTAGONISTS

The effects of selective PAF receptor antagonists have been evaluated. PAF is implicated in the development of systemic hypotension,[204] LPS-induced platelet aggregation,[205] ileus,[206] and increased vascular permeability[207] and may mediate recruitment of leukocytes to inflamed tissues.[208,209] A study in horses using the PAF receptor antagonist SRI 63-441 before LPS infusion showed significant decreases in heart rate and shorter elevation of lactate concentrations in response to the treatment. Although not statistically significant, additional beneficial effects included delayed onset of fever, a shortened period of neutropenia, and reduced maximal platelet aggregation.[210]

Supportive Care

FLUID THERAPY AND CARDIOVASCULAR SUPPORT

Fluid therapy is a mainstay of therapy of most endotoxemic patients suffering from the cardiovascular effects of systemic inflammation. Many endotoxemic equine patients will further require fluid therapy for treatment of the underlying disease process and correction of dehydration and electrolyte and acid-base abnormalities. Principles of fluid therapy are discussed elsewhere in this text.

Patients with severe hypovolemia and shock present management challenges, especially because increased vascular permeability in endotoxemic patients requires careful consideration of fluid therapy plans. A rapid increase in total body fluid volume may be detrimental in patients with compromised cardiac and peripheral vasomotor function and may increase the severity of vascular pooling in peripheral organs. In these patients hypertonic solutions or colloids may be more appropriate means of stabilization than large volumes of crystalloid solutions. Hypertonic saline solution (7.5% sodium chloride) is the most commonly used hypertonic solution in horses and has beneficial effects in endotoxemic patients.[211] A dose of 4 ml/kg is recommended, which should be given as a bolus infusion over 10 to 15 minutes, followed by administration of an isotonic solution to restore total body fluid volume. The clinician should use hypertonic saline with caution in patients with sodium or chloride derangements and should monitor serum electrolyte concentrations in the case of repeated administration. Improvement of the cardiovascular status in response to fluid therapy is indicated by normalization of heart rate, mucous membrane color, and capillary refill time. Failure of urination to occur despite appropriate fluid resuscitation should result in critical evaluation of renal function. In one recent study small volume resuscitation with hypertonic saline plus hetastarch failed to alleviate hemodynamic responses in experimental endotoxin infusion in horses.[212]

Plasma is an ideal colloid and should be administered to maintain a serum total protein concentration above 4.2 g/dl.[134] To raise plasma protein concentration and colloid osmotic pressure significantly, however, horses often require large volumes of plasma (7 to 10 L or more in a 450-kg horse), and alternative colloids should be considered. High-molecular-weight polymers are thought to provide superior oncotic effects in cases of sepsis and endotoxemia, when vascular permeability is increased. Hetastarch, or hydroxyethyl starch (Hespan), is commercially available as a 6% solution in 0.9% sodium chloride. Hetastarch molecules have very high molecular weight, and degradation must occur before renal excretion.[213] These properties result in a longer plasma half-life and prolonged oncotic effects compared with other colloids; persistence of the oncotic effect for 24 hours was observed in hypoproteinemic horses.[214] A dosage of 5 to 15 ml/kg given by slow intravenous infusion along with an equal or greater volume of crystalloid fluids has been recommended.[213,215] In human patients prolonged activated partial thromboplastin time, decreased factor VIII activity, and decreased serum fibrinogen concentration have been described in association with hetastarch use.[216] In the limited number of equine studies, bleeding times were not affected;[217,218] however, patients treated with hetastarch should be monitored for coagulopathy.

Metabolic acidosis in endotoxic shock is attributable to lactic acidemia and inadequate tissue perfusion.[219] Acid-base balance often improves considerably after fluid resuscitation (preferably with alkalinizing solutions such as lactated Ringer's solution) alone; however, additional sodium bicarbonate may be required in cases in which serum bicarbonate concentration remains below 15 mEq/L.

Foals with sepsis are frequently hypoglycemic, and 5% dextrose solutions are useful as initial resuscitation fluids. The clinician should reduce the glucose concentration of intravenous solutions according to the blood glucose concentration to avoid prolonged hyperglycemia. Administration of hyperimmune plasma (20 to 40 ml/kg body mass) is highly recommended in foals with evidence of partial or complete failure of passive transfer.

One should consider positive inotropic and vasomotor agents in patients with persistently inadequate tissue perfusion. Lower dosages of dopamine (0.5 to 2 μg/kg/min) result in vasodilation of the renal, mesenteric, coronary, and intracerebral vasculature via dopaminergic effects, whereas higher dosages (up to 10 μg/kg/min) also exert stimulation of α_1-adrenergic receptors, resulting in increased myocardial contractility and heart rate.[220] Dobutamine is a direct α_1-adrenergic agonist and does not appear to have significant vasodilator properties. Dosages for dobutamine of 1 to 5 μg/kg/min as a continuous intravenous infusion have been recommended for use in horses. In addition, norepinephrine was evaluated in hypotensive critically ill foals that were refractory to the effects of dopamine and dobutamine.[221] At dosages up to 1.5 μg/kg/min administered concurrently with dobutamine, six out of seven foals showed an increase in mean arterial pressure, and all foals had increased urine output. Because of the risk of cardiac side effects, close monitoring of heart rate and rhythm should accompany infusion of inotropes. Indirect blood pressure measurements using a tail cuff may be used to monitor the effects of treatment.

MANAGEMENT OF COAGULOPATHY

More frequently than overt thrombosis or bleeding attributable to DIC, hemostatic abnormalities occur in the form of alterations in the coagulation profile. A procoagulant state with shortened bleeding times or prolonged bleeding times caused by consumption of clotting factors may be evident. One should address abnormalities in the coagulation profile as early as possible but especially if they persist more than 24 hours after initiation of therapy. Because of the complex interactions of coagulation and fibrinolysis during endotoxemia, it might be necessary to combine anticoagulant therapy with the administration of fresh frozen plasma to replace clotting and fibrinolytic factors. Heparin acts as an anticoagulant by activation of AT III and subsequent inhibition of thrombin, release of tissue factor pathway inhibitor from endothelial cells, and inhibition of platelet aggregation.[222] Because endogenous AT III levels frequently are decreased in patients with coagulopathy, addition of heparin to fresh frozen plasma may be the most effective route of administration. An initial dose of 100 IU/kg body mass followed by 40 to 80 IU/kg body mass thrice daily has been recommended.[134] Anemia caused by erythrocyte agglutination occurs in some patients during therapy with unfractionated heparin[223,224] but typically resolves within 96 hours if therapy is discontinued.[134] Because of the risk of microthrombosis associated with erythrocyte agglutination, use of low-molecular-weight heparin (50 IU/kg body mass subcutaneously every 24 hours) has been recommended[225] but may be cost prohibitive. Aspirin can be given orally (10 to 20 mg/kg body mass, every 48 hours), which irreversibly inhibits platelet COX activity, to inhibit platelet aggregation and microthrombosis. Platelet hyperaggregability has been implicated in the pathogenesis of carbohydrate-induced laminitis,[226] and heparin and aspirin have been recommended to prevent development of laminitis. In an in vitro study, however, aspirin did not inhibit endotoxin-induced platelet aggregation.[227]

OTHER CONSIDERATIONS

Luteolysis caused by increased concentrations of $PGF_2\alpha$ may lead to pregnancy loss in endotoxemic mares before day 55 of pregnancy (see Chapter 18).[228] Daily administration of altrenogest (Regu-Mate, Hoechst-Roussel Agri-Vet, Somerville, New Jersey) at a dose of 44 mg orally consistently prevented fetal loss in mares if administered until day 70 of pregnancy.[108] Treatment with flunixin meglumine, by blockade of $PGF_2\alpha$ release,[109] also may contribute to the maintenance of pregnancy in endotoxemic mares. The pathogenesis of fetal loss and abortion caused by endotoxemia, surgery, or systemic disease later in gestation is not understood completely. Proposed mechanisms include direct effects on the fetus, placental function, or placental progesterone production.[229]

Decreased nitric oxide production by vascular endothelial cells in response to endotoxin has been suggested as a mechanism for vasoconstriction and decreased blood flow leading to laminitis (see Chapter 11);[230] however, use of nitric oxide donors remains controversial. Maintenance of adequate peripheral perfusion and anticoagulant and anti-inflammatory therapy may be helpful in preventing and treating laminitis caused by endotoxemia.

SUMMARY

Although the innate immune response to endotoxin (LPS) is crucially important for the preservation of homeostasis and health, large amounts of endotoxin can evoke an excessive and uncontrolled inflammatory response and result in a dysfunction of hemostatic and circulatory control mechanisms, loss of vascular integrity, and finally tissue damage and organ failure. Conditions commonly associated with the development of endotoxemia in horses are acute gastrointestinal diseases, especially of ischemic and severe inflammatory nature, and localized or generalized infections. Although measuring endotoxin concentrations in equine plasma is possible, a diagnosis of endotoxemia is typically based on clinical signs and clinicopathologic data. Successful treatment of endotoxemia requires resolution of the primary disease process in addition to neutralization of circulating endotoxin, interference with the activities of inflammatory mediators, and general supportive care. Newer treatments, such as blockade of endotoxin interaction with cells or interruption of cell signaling pathways, are under investigation. Possible sequelae of endotoxemia include DIC, multiple organ failure, circulatory failure, and death. Frequently, the outcome of conditions associated with endotoxemia in horses depends on the severity of associated complications (e.g., renal compromise and laminitis).

ORAL DISEASES*

L. Chris Sanchez

The word *mouth* is used commonly to signify the first part of the alimentary canal or the entrance to it.[1] The mouth is bounded laterally by the cheeks, dorsally by the palate, and ventrally by the body of the mandible and by the mylohyoideus muscles. The caudal margin is the soft palate. The mouth of the horse is long and cylindric, and when the lips are closed, the contained structures almost fill the cavity. A small space remains between the root of the tongue and the epiglottis and is termed the *oropharynx.* The cavity of the mouth is subdivided into sections by the teeth. The space external to the teeth and enclosed by the lips is termed the *vesicle of the mouth,* and in the resting state the lateral margins of the vesicle (i.e., the buccal mucosa) are in close contact with the cheek teeth. Caudally, the external space communicates with the pharynx through the aditus pharyngis. The mucous membrane of the mouth is continuous at the margin of the lips with the skin and during life is chiefly pink but can be more or less pigmented, depending on the skin color and the breed type.

MORPHOLOGY AND FUNCTION

The lips are two muscular membranous folds that unite at angles close to the first cheek teeth. Each lip presents an outer and an inner surface. The upper lip has a shallow median furrow (philtrum); the lower lip has a rounded prominence or chin (mentum). The internal surface is covered with a thick mucous membrane that contains small, pitted surfaces that are the openings of the ducts of the labial glands. Small folds of the mucous membrane called the *frenula labii* pass from the lips to the gum.

The free border of the lip is dense and bears short, stiff hairs. The arteries of the mouth are derived from the maxillary, mandibular, labial, and sphenopalatine arteries of the major palatine artery. The veins drain chiefly to the lingual facial vein. Sensory nerves originate from the trigeminal nerve (cranial nerve V) and the motor nerves from the facial nerve (VII). The cheeks spread back from the lips and from both sides of the mouth and are attached to the alveolar borders of the bones of the jaws. The cheeks are composed of skin and muscular and glandular layers and then the internal mucous membrane. The skin is thin and pliable. In contrast, the oral mucous membrane is dense and in many areas of the oral cavity is attached firmly to the periosteum so that construction of oral mucosal flaps can be achieved only by horizontal division of the periosteal attachment. Such a feature is important in reconstructive techniques applied to the oral cavity. The blood supply to the cheeks comes from the facial and buccal arteries and the sensory nerves from the trigeminal and motor nerves from the facial nerve.

The hard palate (palatum durum) is bounded rostrally and laterally by the alveolar arches and is continuous with the soft palate caudally. The hard palate has a central raphe that divides the surface into two equal portions. From the line of the rostral cheek tooth, the hard palate is concave to the line of the caudal cheek tooth. Paired transverse ridges (approximately 18) traverse the concavity and have their free edges directed caudally. The incisive duct is a small tube of mucous membrane that extends obliquely through the palatine fissure. The dorsal component communicates by a slitlike opening in the rostral portion of the ventral nasal meatus, and its palatine end is blind and lies in the submucosa of the palate. When stallions display their flehmen response, watery secretions enter the nose from the glands of the vomeronasal duct. To what extent these secretions aid in pheromone reception is not known.[2]

That portion of the palatine mucosa immediately behind the incisor teeth frequently is swollen (lampas) during eruption of the permanent teeth. This swelling is physiologic and not pathologic.

The tongue is situated on the floor of the mouth between the bodies of the mandible and is supported by the sling formed by the mylohyoideus muscles. The root of the tongue is attached to the hyoid bone, soft palate, and pharynx. The upper surface and the rostral portion of the tongue are free; the body of the tongue has three surfaces. The apex of the tongue is spatulate and has a rounded border. The mucous membrane adheres intimately to the adjacent structure and on the dorsum is dense and thick. From the lower surface of the free part of the tongue, a fold of mucous membrane passes to the floor of the mouth, forming the lingual frenulum. Caudally, a fold passes on each side of the dorsum to join the soft palate, forming the palatoglossal arch. Dorsally from the soft palate, the palatopharyngeal arch attaches and circumvents the aditus laryngis and attaches to the roof of the nasopharynx. The mucous membrane of the tongue presents four kinds of papillae:

1. Filiform papillae are fine threadlike projections across the dorsum of the tongue. They are absent on the root of the tongue and are small on the rostral portion of the tongue.
2. The fungiform papillae are larger and easily seen at the rounded free end. They occur principally on the lateral portion of the tongue.
3. Vallate papillae are usually two or three in number and are found on the caudal portion of the dorsum of the tongue. The free surface bears numerous small, round secondary papillae.
4. Foliate papillae are situated rostral to the palatoglossal arches of the soft palate, where they form a rounded eminence about 2 or 3 cm in length marked by transverse fissures.

Foliate, vallate, and fungiform papillae are covered with taste buds and secondary papillae.

*Previous version by Samuel L. Jones.

The lingual and sublingual arteries supply the tongue from the linguofacial trunk and matching veins. The linguofacial trunk drains into the linguofacial vein. The lingual muscles are innervated by the hypoglossal nerve (XII), and the sensory supply is from the lingual and glossopharyngeal (IX) nerves.

EQUINE DENTITION

The formula for the deciduous teeth of the horse is 2 times I3-3 C0-0 P3-3 for a total of 24. The permanent dental formula is 2 times I3-3 C1-1 P3-3 or P4-3 M3-3 for a total of 40 or 42. In the mare the canine teeth are usually small or do not erupt, hence reducing the number to 36 or 38. The first premolar tooth (wolf tooth) is often absent and has been reported as occurring in only 20% of the upper dentition of Thoroughbreds.[3] The teeth of the horse are complex in shape and are compounded of different materials (dentin, cementum, and enamel). They function as grinding blades to masticate and macerate cellulose food in the important first stage of the digestive process. The cheek teeth in the horse are a well-documented feature of the evolution of *Equus caballus*.

Deciduous Teeth

The first incisor is present at birth or the first week of life. The second incisor erupts at 4 to 6 weeks of age; the third incisor, at 6 to 9 months of age; the first and second premolars, at birth to 2 weeks of age; and the third premolar, 3 months of age.

Permanent Teeth

The eruption times for the permanent teeth are as follows: first incisor, 2 ½ years of age; second incisor, 3 ½ years of age; third incisor, 4 ½ years of age; the canine tooth, 4 to 5 years of age; the first premolar (wolf tooth), 5 to 6 months of age; the second premolar, 2½ years of age; the third premolar, 3 years of age; the fourth premolar, 4 years of age; the first molar, 10 to 12 months of age; the second molar, 2 years of age; and the third molar, 3½ to 4 years of age. This eruption sequence clearly indicates that the eruption of the second and third permanent premolar teeth gives the potential for dental impaction.

The modern horse has six incisor teeth in each jaw that are placed close together so that the labile edges form a semicircle. The occlusal surface has a deep enamel invagination (infundibulum) that is filled only partially with cementum. As the incisor teeth wear, a characteristic pattern forms in which the infundibulum is surrounded by rings of enamel, dentin, enamel, and crown cementum in a concentric pattern. Each incisor tooth tapers from a broad crown to a narrow root so that as the midportion of the incisor is exposed to wear, the cross-sectional diameters are about equal; that is, at 14 years of age, the central incisor tooth of the horse has an occlusal surface that is an equilateral triangle. Observations on the state of eruption, the angles of incidence of the incisor teeth, and the pattern of the occlusal surfaces are used as guides for aging of horses. The canine teeth are simple teeth without complex crowns and are curved. The crown is compressed and is smooth on its labial aspect but carries two ridges on its lingual aspect. No occlusal contact occurs between the upper and lower canine teeth.

When erupted, the six cheek teeth of the horse function as a single unit in the mastication of food. Each arcade consists of three premolar and three molar teeth. The maxillary arcade is slightly curved, and the teeth have a square occlusal surface. The occlusal surfaces of the mandibular teeth are more oblong, and each arcade is straighter. The horse is anisognathic; that is, the distance between the mandibular teeth is narrower (one third) than the distance between the upper cheek teeth. This anatomic arrangement affects the inclination of the dental arcade as the jaws slide across each other in the food preparation process. The unworn upper cheek tooth presents a surface with two undulating and narrow ridges, one of which is lateral and the other medial. On the rostral and lingual side of the medial style is an extra hillock. The central portion of these surfaces is indented by two depressions that are comparable with, but much deeper than, the infundibula of the incisor teeth. When the teeth have been subjected to wear, the enamel that closed the ridges is worn through and the underlying dentin appears on the surface. Thus after a time the chewing surface displays a complicated pattern that may be likened to the outline of an ornate letter *B*, the upright stroke of the *B* being on the lingual aspect. Dentin supports the enamel internally, cementum supports the enamel lakes, and the peripheral cementum fills in the spaces between the teeth so that all six teeth may function as a single unit (i.e., the dental arcade). Transverse ridges cross each tooth so that the whole maxillary arcade consists of a serrated edge. The serrations are formed so that a valley is present at the area of contact with adjacent teeth. These serrations match fitting serrations on the mandibular arcade. One should note that the mediolateral mandibular motion that occurs while the horse is chewing pellets does not provide full occlusal contact as it does when the horse is chewing hay.[4]

The true roots of the cheek teeth are short compared with the total length of the tooth. Cheek teeth have three roots: two small lateral roots and one large medial root. By custom, that portion of the crown embedded within the dental alveolus is referred to as the *reserve crown*, and the term *root* is confined to the area of the tooth that is comparatively short and enamel free. Wear on the tooth gradually exposes the reserve crown, and the roots lengthen. In an adult 1000-lb horse, the maxillary cheek teeth are between 8 and 8.5 cm in length. Dental wear accounts for erosion and loss of tooth substance at a rate of 2 mm annually. The pulp chambers of the teeth are also complex. The incisors and canines have a single pulp chamber. The mandibular cheek teeth have two roots and two separate pulp chambers. The maxillary cheek teeth, although they have three roots, have in fact five pulp chambers.

As occlusal wear proceeds, deposition of secondary dentin within the pulp chambers protects the chambers (e.g., the dental star, medial to the infundibulum on the incisor teeth). In the mandibular cheek teeth, the transverse folding of the enamel anlage (during morphogenesis of the tooth) does not take place, and the occlusal surface is a simple surface of central dentin surrounded by enamel. Each tooth then is conformed to a single arcade by the presence of peripheral crown cementum.

MOUTH DISEASES

The oral cavity and oropharynx are subject to a variety of diseases. However, many conditions affecting the first portion of the alimentary system produce the same clinical signs, regardless of their cause. The clinical signs may include inappetence or reluctance to eat, pain on eating or swallowing,

TABLE 15-5

Correlation Between Dental Disease and Dental Therapy

Age	Examine for	Necessary Dentistry
2-3 years	1. First premolar vestige (wolf teeth)	1. Remove wolf teeth if present.
	2. First deciduous premolar (upper and lower)	2. Remove deciduous teeth if ready; if not, file off corners and points of premolars
	3. Hard swelling on ventral surface of mandible beneath first premolar	3. Obtain X-ray film; extract retained temporary premolar if present
	4. Cuts or abrasions on inside of cheek in region of the second premolars and molars	4. Lightly float or dress all molars and premolars if necessary
	5. Sharp protuberances on all premolars and molars	5. Rasp protuberances down to level of other teeth in arcade
3-4 years	1. (1), (2), (4), and (5) above	1. (1), (2), (4), and (5) above
	2. Second deciduous premolar (upper and lower)	2. Remove if present and ready
4-5 years	1. (1), (4), and (5) above	1. (1), (4), and (5) above
	2. Third deciduous premolar	2. Remove if present and ready
5 years and older	1. (1), (4), and (5) above	1. (1), (4), and (5) above
	2. Uneven growth and "wavy" arcade	2. Straighten if interfering with mastication
	3. Unusually long molars and premolars	3. Unusually long molars and premolars may have to be cut if they cannot be filed down

From Baker GJ: Diseases of the teeth. In Colohan PT, Mayhew IG, Merritt AM, et al, editors: *Equine medicine and surgery*, ed 4, vol 1, Goleta, Calif, 1991, American Veterinary Publications.

oral swelling, oral discharge, and fetid breath. Affected animals may show some interest in food but hesitate to eat it. Salivation may be excessive and contaminated with purulent exudate or blood. The occurrence of bruxism (i.e., grinding of teeth) can indicate discomfort in other areas of the alimentary tract; for example, bruxism and frothing oral saliva are characteristic features of gastric ulceration in the foal. The clinician should be aware that considerable weight loss can occur rapidly with the inability to feed and swallow. Diseases that result in denervation of the pharynx and inappropriate swallowing can have the complication of aspiration pneumonia.

Examination and Clinical Signs

After performing a complete physical examination and ascertaining the history, the clinician should approach examination of the mouth systematically in all cases. One can examine a considerable portion of the mouth and teeth from the outside by palpation of the structures through the folds of the cheek. Most horses allow a cursory oral examination without sedation or the use of an oral speculum. In many cases, however, a detailed oral examination is best achieved by sedation and the use of an oral speculum and a light source. The clinician should irrigate the mouth to wash out retained food material before inspecting and palpating the lips, cheeks, teeth, and gums.

The classic signs of dental disease in the horse include difficulty and slowness in feeding, with a progressive unthriftiness and loss of body condition. In some instances the horse may quid (i.e., drop poorly masticated food boluses from the mouth), and halitosis may be obvious. Additional problems reported by owners include bitting and riding problems and headshaking or head shyness. Facial or mandibular swelling may occur. Nasal discharge can result from dental disease associated with maxillary sinus empyema. Mandibular fistulae frequently are caused by lower cheek tooth apical infections. Some correlation exists between the age of the animal and clinical signs (Table 15-5).

Ancillary Diagnostic Techniques

Ancillary aids for a complete examination of the oral cavity of the horse include radiology, endoscopic examination, fluoroscopy, biopsy, and culture. The clinician always should take care during endoscopic evaluation of the oral cavity using a flexible endoscope. The author recommends sedation and the use of an oral speculum to prevent inadvertent mastication of the endoscope. If general anesthesia is used as part of the diagnostic workup, then endoscopic evaluation of the oral cavity is much easier. In selected cases advanced imaging technologies such as computed tomography, magnetic resonance imaging, or nuclear scintigraphy may be beneficial.

DYSPHAGIA

Clinical Signs and Diagnosis

The lips of the horse are mobile and prehensile. In many ways they function like the tip of the elephant's trunk in that they test, manipulate, and sample the environment for potential nutritive value. Consequently, loss of motor function (e.g., facial palsy) affects the efficiency of the prehensile system. The lips grasp food in grazing or browsing, and the incisor teeth section the food. With mastication and lubrication with saliva, the bolus of food forms and is manipulated from side to side across the mouth, assisted by the tight cheeks of the horse and the palatine ridges. Swallowing begins as the food bolus contacts the base of the tongue and the pharyngeal walls. During swallowing the soft palate elevates to close the nasopharynx, the base of the tongue elevates, and the hyoid bone and the larynx move rostrally following contraction of the hyoid muscles. During this process the rima glottidis closes, and the epiglottis tilts dorsally and caudally to protect the airway so that food is swept through lateral food channels around the sides of the larynx into the laryngoesophagus. Fluoroscopic studies in nursing foals in the dorsoventral view showed that contact occurs between the lateral food channels in the midline so that in outline the food bolus achieves a bow-tie shape.[5]

Dysphagia is defined as the difficulty or inability to swallow. Anatomic classifications for dysphagia include prepharyngeal, pharyngeal, and esophageal (postpharyngeal) dysphagias. The site of the cause for dysphagia influences the clinical signs. Prepharyngeal dysphagia is characterized by dropping food (quidding) or water from the mouth, reluctance to chew, hypersalivation, or abnormalities in prehension. Pharyngeal and esophageal dysphagias are characterized by coughing; nasal discharge containing saliva, water, or food material; gagging; anxiousness; and neck extension during attempts to swallow. The following section describes esophageal dysphagia in more detail. Causes of dysphagia can be divided into four types: painful, muscular, neurologic, or obstructive (Table 15-6). Pain and obstruction cause dysphagia by interfering with the mechanics of prehension, bolus formation and transfer to the pharynx, and deglutition. Muscular and neurologic causes of dysphagia impede prehension and swallowing by affecting the motor function of the lingual or buccal musculature, muscles of mastication (temporal and masseters), and pharyngeal and cranial esophageal muscles. Sensory loss to the lips, buccal mucous membranes, pharynx, or tongue also may cause dysphagia. Neurologic causes of dysphagia may affect the forebrain, brainstem, or peripheral nerves that control prehension (cranial nerves Vm, Vs, VII, and XII), transfer of the food bolus to the pharynx (cranial nerves Vs and XII), and swallowing (cranial nerves IX and X). The latter point was classical thinking, but recent evidence suggests that although stimulation of cranial nerve IX stimulates swallowing, bilateral blockade of that nerve is not necessary for normal swallowing of either liquid or solid material.[6]

Diagnosis of the cause of dysphagia is based on physical examination, including a careful oral examination; neurologic examination; clinical signs; and endoscopy of the pharynx, esophagus, and guttural pouches. Radiology may be useful to assess the bony structures of the head and throat. Ultrasonography is valuable for examining the retropharyngeal space and esophagus to detect and evaluate masses. One may detect pharyngeal or esophageal causes of dysphagia with routine endoscopic examination or with contrast radiography. Although endoscopy can also be used to assess deglutition, it is important to remember that sedation adversely affects the deglutition mechanism. One may assess deglutition using fluoroscopy[7] or manometry,[8] but these techniques require specialized equipment. Specific diagnostic procedures for nonalimentary causes of dysphagia are covered elsewhere in this text (see Chapter 3).

Management

Specific treatments aimed at resolving the underlying disorder causing dysphagia are discussed in detail elsewhere. Most horses with dysphagia should not eat roughage with long fiber length (hay or grass). Dietary modifications that promote swallowing, such as feeding slurries made from complete pelleted feeds, may be sufficient to manage some cases of partial dysphagia. Care must be taken to prevent or avoid aspiration pneumonia in horses with pharyngeal or esophageal dysphagia. Affected foals can be managed by feeding mare's milk or a suitable substitute through a nasogastric tube. The clinician also may administer pellet slurries or formulated liquid diets through a nasogastric tube to older horses. Prolonged nutritional management of dysphagic horses may require extraoral feeding using a tube placed through an esophagostomy.[9]

Formulated pelleted diets are often easy to administer through a tube as slurry and are balanced to meet the nutritional requirements for healthy horses. Sufficient quantities must be fed to deliver adequate calories (16 to 17 Mcal/day for a 500-kg horse). Adjustments may be necessary for horses that are cachectic or have extra metabolic demand (e.g., pregnancy). Adding corn oil to the ration (1 cup every 12 or 24 hours) is a common method of increasing fed calories. Liquid diets also have been used for enteral feeding[10] but may not be tolerated as well as pelleted diets. Regardless of the method of nutritional management, the clinician must monitor and replace salivary losses of electrolytes. Saliva contains high concentrations of Na, K, and Cl. A group of ponies with experimental esophagostomies[11] and a horse with esophageal squamous cell carcinoma[12] were fed a complete pelleted diet through esophagostomy tubes but developed metabolic acidosis, hyponatremia, and hypochloremia, apparently because of salivary losses. Surprisingly, salivary losses of potassium did not result in hypokalemia in these cases, presumably because of replacement in the diet. However, if the diet is deficient in potassium, hypokalemia may result. Electrolyte replacement often can be accomplished by adding NaCl and KCl to the diet. Horses can be maintained for months with frequent feedings through an esophagostomy tube.[12] Parenteral nutrition (total or partial) may be useful in the short term but is not often feasible for long-term management.

DENTAL DISEASES

Eruption Disorders

Tooth eruption is a complex phenomenon involving the interplay of dental morphogenesis and those vascular forces responsible for creating the eruption pathway. These changes are responsible for osteitis and bone remodeling within the maxilla and mandible. Young horses frequently show symmetric bony swelling resulting from these eruption cysts. In some cases additional clinical signs of nasal obstruction with respiratory stridor or nasal discharges may be apparent.

Pathologic problems associated with maleruption include a variety of dental diseases.[13] Oral trauma can displace or damage erupting teeth or the permanent tooth buds. As a result, teeth may be displaced and erupt in abnormal positions or may have abnormal shapes. Supernumerary teeth, incisors and molars, can develop as well as palatal displacement of impacted teeth (maxillary P3-3, or third cheek tooth). In almost all of these conditions, some form of surgical treatment is necessary, but depending on the number and location, conservative theapy can be successful.[14]

Significant evidence from the location of apical osteitis in diseased teeth confirms that dental impaction is a major cause of dental disease in the horse. In a series of 142 extracted teeth,

TABLE 15-6

Differential Diagnoses for Dysphagia

Class of Dysphagia	Differential Diagnoses
Painful	Tooth root abscess or periodontal disease
	Broken teeth
	Abnormal dentition or wear
	Stomatitis, glossitis, or pharyngitis
	Nonsteroidal anti-inflammatory drug toxicity
	Chemical irritation
	Thrush (candidiasis)
	Influenza
	Streptococcus equi subsp. *equi*
	Vesicular stomatitis virus
	Actinobacillus lignieresii
	Buccal, gingival, or glossal trauma (bits or chains)
	Foreign bodies
	Retropharyngeal lymphadenopathy or abscess
	Mandibular trauma
	Temposohyoid osteoarthropathy
	Temporomandibular osteopathy
Muscular	Hyperkalemic periodic paralysis
	Nutritional myopathy (white muscle disease)
	Polysaccharide storage disease
	Glycogen branching enzyme deficiency
	Masseter myositis
	Hypocalcemia tetany or eclampsia
	Myotonia
	Rectus capitis ventralis rupture
	White snakeroot toxicity
	Megaesophagus
Obstructive	Retropharyngeal abscess and lymphadenopathy
	Oral, pharyngeal, retropharyngeal, laryngeal, or esophageal malformations, injury, edema, or neoplasia
	Pharyngeal or epiglottic cysts
	Pharyngeal abscess or foreign body
	Dorsal displacement of the soft palate
	Rostral displacement of the palatopharyngeal arch
	Cleft palate
	Guttural pouch tympany or empyema
	Follicular pharyngitis
	Esophageal obstruction
	Pharyngeal cicatrix

Continued

TABLE 15-6

Differential Diagnoses for Dysphagia—cont'd

Class of Dysphagia	Differential Diagnoses
Neurologic forebrain disease; generalized neuropathy; disorders of cranial nerves V, VII, IX, X, or XII	Retropharyngeal abscess or neoplasia
	Guttural pouch empyema, mycosis, or neoplasia
	Temporohyoid osteoarthropathy
	Lead poisoning
	Petrous temporal bone osteomyelitis or fracture
	Botulism
	Yellow star thistle toxicity
	Viral encephalitis
	Cerebral edema
	Cerebral or brainstem hemorrhage
	Intracranial masses (hematoma, neoplasia, abscess)
	Meningitis
	Verminous encephalitis
	Equine protozoal myeloencephalitis
	Equine herpesvirus 1
	Equine dysautonomia
	Hepatoencephalopathy
	Tetanus
	Polyneuritis equi

63 were P3-3 or P4-4 (cheek tooth 2 or 3, respectively).[15] Early observations had indicated that the first molar (M1, or cheek tooth 4) was the most commonly diseased tooth, and an "open infundibulum" in this tooth has been suggested as the cause.[16] In a later study the mandibular cheek teeth 2 and 3 were the most commonly affected, whereas cheek teeth 2 and 4 were most commonly affected in the maxillary arcade, which was the more commonly affected arcade.[17] Studies on cementogenesis of the maxillary cheek teeth have shown, however, that in fact most maxillary cheek teeth have a greater or lesser degree of hypoplasia of cementum within the enamel lakes and that this "lesion" rarely expands into the pulp. The central infundibular hole is the site of its vascular supply to the unerupted cement lake. On those occasions in which caries of cementum occurs (i.e., secondary inflammatory disease and acid necrosis of the cementum), apical osteitis may develop.

Dental Decay

Pulpitis is key to the pathogenesis of dental decay in the horse. The initiation of inflammatory pulp changes may be a sequela to dental impaction or dental caries or may result from fracture of a tooth. If the onset of the inflammatory process is slow, then formation of secondary dentin within the pulp chambers may protect the pulp and the tooth. Secondary dentin formation occurs from stimulation of odontoblasts within the pulp chamber. Such changes are the normal process of protection during dental wear and attrition as crown substances wear away and the reserve crown comes into wear. In acute disease, however, this defense mechanism is ineffective, and the changes that occur and that are sequelae to pulpitis reflect the location of each affected tooth. For example, pulpitis and apical osteitis of the third mandibular cheek tooth most commonly results in the development of a mandibular dental fistula. Pulpitis of the third maxillary cheek tooth, however, results in an inflammatory disease within the rostral maxillary sinus and in development of chronic maxillary sinus empyema.

Oblique radiographs greatly assist the diagnosis of dental decay by demonstrating sinus tract formation, sequestration of bone, mandibular osteitis, hyperplasia of cementum, and new bone formation (so-called alveolar periosteitis).[18] Nuclear scintigraphy and computed tomography can aid in an accurate diangosis.[19,20] The management of dental decay in the horse usually involves surgical extraction of the diseased tooth. In some cases one can use apicoectomy and retrograde endodontic techniques to save the diseased tooth. The clinician must take care, however, in selection of patients. In most cases of apical osteitis in the horse that result from dental impaction, immature root structures make achieving an apical seal of the exposed pulp difficult.

PERIODONTAL DISEASE

Gingival hyperemia and inflammation occur during the eruption of the permanent teeth and are common causes of a sore mouth in young horses (particularly 3-year-olds as the first dental caps loosen). Such periodontal changes usually resolve as the permanent dental arcade is established. During normal mastication the shearing forces generated by the occlusal contact of the cheek teeth essentially clean the teeth of plaque and effectively inhibit deposition of dental calculus. Wherever occlusal contact is ineffective, periodontal changes and calculus buildup occur; for example, the deposition of calculus on the canine teeth of mature geldings and stallions is common. Routine dental prophylaxis forms an important component of maintaining normal occlusal contact, and for this reason arcade irregularities that result in enamel point formation on the buccal edges of the maxillary cheek teeth and the lingual edges of the mandibular cheek teeth should be removed. The clinician should remove these edges annually in horses that are at grass and twice yearly in young horses, aged horses, and stabled horses. Horses at grass have been shown to have a greater range of occlusal contact and therefore better periodontal hygiene than stabled horses. In stabled horses the range of occlusal contact is narrower, and the formation of enamel points occurs more frequently with subsequent buccal ulceration and the initiation of a cycle of altered occlusal contact and hence irregular arcade formation. This process leads to severe forms of periodontal disease and wave mouth formation.

Periodontal disease occurs with abnormal occlusal contact and initiation of the cycle of irregular wear and abnormal contact. Such changes progress to loss of alveolar bone, gross periodontal sepsis, and loss of tooth support. In this sense periodontal disease truly is the scourge of the equine mouth and results in tooth loss.[21]

CONGENITAL AND DEVELOPMENTAL ABNORMALITIES

Cleft Palate

Palatine clefts may result from an inherited defect and are caused by failure of the transverse palatal folds to fuse in the oral cavity. Harelip accompanies few palatine clefts in the horse. The degree of palatine clefting depends on the stage at which interruption in the fusion of the palatopalatal folds occurs. Toxic or teratogenic effects are documented in other species, but little data are available in the horse.

In recent years treatment for repair of uncomplicated palatine defects has been recommended, but the prognosis is generally poor because of the considerable nursing care required and the high incidence of surgical failures. One should emphasize early surgery and the use of mandibular symphysiotomy in affording surgical exposure. The combination of mandibular symphysiotomy and transhyoid pharyngotomy to approach the caudal margins of the soft palate affords surgical access, and mucosal flaps can be constructed to repair the defects. However, the incidence of surgical breakdown is high, and healing by first intention is the exception rather than the rule. A recent surgical report documented the successful closure of a median cleft of the lower lip and mandible in a donkey.[22]

Campylorhinus Lateralis

Foals born with a severely deviated premaxilla and palate have a wry nose. Good functional and cosmetic outcome can be achieved with surgical correction.[23] Circumstantial evidence indicates that such a defect has a genetic cause, and the defect occurs most frequently in the Arabian breed.

Cysts

Other developmental abnormalities are subepiglottic cysts resulting from cystic distortion of remnants of the thyroglossal duct, which may cause dyspnea and choking in foals. Surgical removal of these cysts results in normal function.

Parrot Mouth

The most significant developmental defect of dental origin is a maxilla that is longer than the mandible (i.e., parrot mouth). An overbite of 2 cm in the incisor arcade may be present in a horse with a mismatch of less than 1 cm between the first upper and lower cheek teeth. Parrot mouth and monkey or sow mouth are thought to be inherited conditions. Some correction of minor incisor malocclusion occurs up to 5 years of age. Recognition and detection of parrot mouth are important in the examination of potential breeding stock. Surgical attempts to inhibit overgrowth of the premaxilla by wiring or by the application of dental bite plate procedures have been documented.[24]

Oral Wounds

As has been indicated, the horse is by nature a curious animal that uses its lips as a means of exploring a variety of objects. Wounds of the lips, incisive bone, and the mandibular incisor area occur commonly in the horse and usually result from the horse getting the lips, jaw, or teeth caught in feeding buckets, in fence posts, or in halters or having a segment of tongue encircled with hair in tail chewing. As the horse panics and pulls away from its oral entrapment, considerable trauma can occur to the lips, teeth, and gums.

Most wounds heal satisfactorily, provided one finds them early and observes the basic principles of wound hygiene, excision of necrotic tissue, and wound closure. One must ensure that oral mucosal defects are closed and that effective oral seals are made before external wounds are closed. In some cases offering specially constructed diets or even feeding the horse by nasogastric tube or esophagostomy during the healing processes may be necessary.

STOMATITIS AND GLOSSITIS

Foreign body penetration of the tongue, cheek, or palate has been reported in grazing and browsing horses, particularly horses that have certain hay sources containing desiccated barley awns or yellow bristle grass.[25] Other plant material and grass awns also occasionally may penetrate the tongue, gingiva, or cheek, causing inflammation or abscesses. Metallic foreign bodies have been reported in the tongue, and a history of feeding hay or the use of cable-framed tractor tires was often reported as part of the history.[26] Ulcerative stomatitis also results from the toxicity of phenylbutazone therapy.[27] Vesicular stomatitis is a highly contagious viral blistering disease described in more detail elsewhere. Treatment of glossitis and stomatitis primarily aims at removing the inciting cause. *Actinobacillus lignieresii,* the causative agent of actinobacillosis, has been isolated and identified from ulcers on the free border of the soft palate and oral and laryngeal granulomata. The bacterium also was reported in a sublingual caruncle in a horse with a greatly swollen tongue.[28] Therapy with 150 ml of 20% sodium iodide and 5 g of ampicillin every 8 to 12 hours effected a clinical cure.

SALIVARY GLANDS

Function

Saliva is important for lubricating and softening food material. The horse has paired parotid, mandibular, and polystomatic sublingual salivary glands. The parotid gland is the largest of the salivary glands in the horse and is situated in the space between the ramus of the mandible and the wing of the atlas. The parotid duct is formed at the ventral part of the gland near the facial crest by the union of three or four smaller ducts. The duct leaves the gland above the linguofacial vein, crosses the tendon of the sternocephalicus muscle, and enters the mouth obliquely in the cheek opposite the third upper cheek tooth. The parotic duct orifice is small, but some dilation of the duct and a circular mucous fold (the parotid papillae) exist at this point. The mandibular gland is smaller than the parotid gland and extends from the atlantal fossa to the basihyoid bone. For the most part the mandibular gland is covered by the parotid gland and the lower jaw. The mandibular duct is formed by the union of a number of small duct radicles that emerge along the concave edge of the gland and run rostral to the border of the mouth opposite the canine tooth.

The orifice is at the end of a sublingual caruncle. The mandibular gland possesses serous, mucous, and mixed alveolar glandular components. The parotid gland is a compound alveolar serous gland. The parotid salivary gland can secrete saliva to yield rates of 50 ml/min, and a total daily parotid secretion can be as much as 12 L in a 500-kg horse. Parotid secretion occurs only during mastication, and administration of atropine or anesthesia of the oral mucosa can block secretion. Parotid saliva is hypotonic compared with plasma, but at high rates of flow, concentrations of sodium, chloride, and bicarbonate ions increase.

Salivary Gland Disorders

Parotid saliva of the horse has a high concentration of calcium, and occasionally calculi (sialoliths) form within the duct radicles of the parotid salivary gland.[29] Congenital parotid duct atresia, acquired stricture from trauma to the duct, or obstruction by plant material (e.g., sticks or foxtails and other seeds) also may occur. The clinical signs of sialolithiasis or other forms of ductule obstruction include a fluid swelling in the form of a mucocele proximal to the stone and occasionally inflammation of the parotid gland. Ultrasonography is useful to diagnose salivary mucoceles and to detect foreign bodies or sialoliths. Measurement of electrolyte concentrations in aspirates from suspected mucoceles might be helpful to distinguish them from hematomas. Salivary potassium and calcium concentrations are higher than those in plasma. Treatment may require surgical removal of the stone or plant material in the case of sialolithiasis or foreign body obstructions. Other causes of obstruction may require resection of the affected portion of the duct or chemical ablation of the gland.[30]

Primary sialoadenitis is unusual but can occur in one or both glands. The condition is painful and may be associated with a fever and anorexia. Secondary sialoadenitis is more common and usually is associated with trauma. Infectious sialoadenitis resulting from *Corynebacterium pseudotuberculosis*[31] or other bacterial pathogens also may occur. Diagnosis is by physical examination and identification of an enlarged edematous parotid gland tissue on ultrasonographic examination. Culture and cytologic examination of aspirates may be useful for diagnostic purposes. Treatment is usually palliative, consisting of NSAIDs. Appropriate antibiotic therapy is indicated as directed by culture and sensitivity results.

Chemical irritation, glossitis, stomatitis, or other causes of prepharyngeal dysphagia cause ptyalism, or excessive salivation, in horses. Specific therapy for the ptyalism usually is not required as long as salivary losses are not excessive, resulting in dehydration and electrolyte imbalances. Ingestion of the fungal toxin slaframine also causes hypersalivation in horses.[32] The fungus *Rhizoctonia leguminicola,* which produces slaframine, causes black patch disease in red clover. Slaframine is a parasympathomimetic compound that stimulates exocrine secretion in the parotid gland. Slaframine toxicosis most commonly occurs in the spring or early summer and rarely requires treatment other than removal from the pasture. Mowing removes the source in most cases because regrowth in pastures often has less fungal contamination.[33]

ESOPHAGEAL DISEASES

L. Chris Sanchez

ANATOMY AND FUNCTION

The esophagus is a musculomembranous tube that originates from the pharynx dorsal to the larynx and terminates at the cardia of the stomach.[1] In adult Thoroughbreds the esophagus is approximately 120 cm long. The cervical portion is approximately 70 cm long; the thoracic portion, approximately 50 cm long; and the short abdominal portion, only approximately 2 cm long. The cervical esophagus generally lies dorsal and to the left of the trachea in the cervical region. In the thorax the esophagus courses through the mediastinum lying dorsal to the trachea and crosses to the right of the aortic arch dorsal to the heart base.

The esophagus has no digestive or absorptive functions and serves as a conduit to the stomach for food, water, and salivary secretions. The esophageal mucosa is a keratinized stratified squamous epithelium.[1] The submucosa contains elastic fibers that contribute to the longitudinal folds of the esophagus and confer elasticity to the esophageal wall. A transition occurs in the muscle type composing the tunica muscularis from striated skeletal muscle in the proximal two thirds of the esophagus to smooth muscle in the distal third. In the proximal esophagus the skeletal muscle layers spiral across one another at angles. Within the smooth muscle layers of the distal esophagus the outer layer becomes more longitudinal, whereas the inner layer thickens and becomes circular. The wall of the terminal esophagus can be 1 to 2 cm thick. Deep cervical fascia, pleura, and peritoneum contribute to the thin fibrous tunica adventitia of the esophagus. Motor innervation to the striated skeletal muscle of the esophagus includes the pharyngeal and esophageal branches of the vagus nerve, which originate in the nucleus ambiguus of the medulla oblongata. Parasympathetic fibers of the vagus nerve supply the smooth muscle of the distal esophagus. Sympathetic innervation of the esophagus is minimal.

Passage of ingesta through the esophagus can be considered part of the swallowing process, which consists of oral, pharyngeal, and esophageal stages. The oral stage is voluntary and involves transport of the food bolus from the mouth into the oropharynx. During the involuntary pharyngeal stage, the food bolus is forced through the momentarily relaxed upper esophageal sphincter by simultaneous contractions of the pharyngeal muscles. In the esophageal phase of swallowing, the upper esophageal sphincter closes immediately, the lower esophageal sphincter opens, and esophageal peristalsis propels the bolus into the stomach.[2] Unlike a food bolus, liquids do not require peristalsis to reach the lower esophageal sphincter and may precede the food bolus during swallowing.

The upper esophageal sphincter prevents esophagopharyngeal reflux during swallowing and air distention of the esophagus during inspiration. Upper esophageal pressure increases in response to pressure from a food bolus and to increased intraluminal acidity, as would occur with gastroesophageal reflux. The lower esophageal sphincter is a smooth muscle located at the gastroesophageal junction that is morphologically ill defined but forms an effective functional barrier.[2] The lower esophageal sphincter is normally closed in response to gastric distention to restrict gastroesophageal reflux. Relaxation of the lower esophageal sphincter permits passage of ingested material from the esophagus to the stomach. Distention of the stomach with ingesta mechanically constricts the lower esophageal sphincter. Gastric distention also triggers a vagal reflex that increases lower esophageal sphincter tone, a safety mechanism against gastroesophageal reflux. The mechanical and vagal mechanisms that promote lower esophageal sphincter tone prevent spontaneous decompression of the stomach, which, along with a lack of a vomiting reflex in the horse, increases the risk of gastric rupture during episodes of severe distention.

A wide variety of congenital and acquired disorders of the esophagus have been described in horses. These are summarized in Table 15-7 and discussed in detail in the next sections.

ESOPHAGEAL OBSTRUCTION

Esophageal obstruction has many causes (Table 15-8) and most often is manifested clinically by impaction of food material and resulting esophageal dysphagia. Esophageal obstruction may be caused by primary impactions (simple choke) of roughage, particularly leafy alfalfa hay, coarse grass hay, bedding, and even grass.[3] Prior esophageal trauma or poor mastication caused by dental abnormalities may predispose horses to primary esophageal impaction.[16] Wolfing or gulping food may precipitate primary impactions, particularly if the horse is exhausted or mildly dehydrated after a long ride or is weakened from chronic debilitation. Impactions also may result from disorders that physically impede the passage of food material and fluid by narrowing the luminal diameter, reduce the compliance of the esophageal wall, or alter the conformation of the esophageal wall such that food material accumulates in a pocket or diverticulum. Foreign bodies, intramural or extramural masses, or acquired or congenital anomalies cause these so-called secondary impactions. Intramural causes of esophageal obstruction include tumors (squamous cell carcinoma), strictures, diverticula, and cysts.[6,16,26,34,42,53-56] Mediastinal or cervical masses (tumors or abscesses) may cause extramural obstructions. Congenital anomalies are covered in detail later.

Clinical Signs and Diagnosis

The clinician must perform a thorough physical examination, including a complete oral and neurologic examination, to help rule out causes of dysphagia and nasal discharge other than esophageal obstruction. The clinical signs associated with esophageal obstructions are related to dysphagia.[57] Horses with esophageal obstruction are often anxious and stand with their neck extended. They may gag or retch, particularly with acute proximal obstructions. Bilateral frothy nasal discharge containing saliva, water, and food material; coughing; odynophagia; and ptyalism are characteristic clinical signs, the severity of which varies with the degree and location of the obstruction. Distention in the jugular furrow may be evident at the site of obstruction. Other clinical signs related to regurgitation of saliva, water, and food material may be observed, such as dehydration, electrolyte or acid-base imbalances, weight loss, and aspiration pneumonia. In extreme cases pressure necrosis from the impaction or trauma to the esophagus may cause esophageal rupture. If the rupture is in the cervical esophagus, crepitus or cellulitis may be evident along with signs of systemic inflammation. Thoracic auscultation is important to determine whether aspiration pneumonia is present. Intrathoracic esophageal rupture may result in pleuritis and its associated clinical signs.

Passage of a nasogastric tube is an effective way to detect and localize an obstruction but provides little information about the nature of the obstruction or the condition of the esophagus. The most direct method for diagnosis of esophageal obstructions is endoscopic examination. Most cases of esophageal obstruction occur at sites of natural narrowing of the esophageal lumen, such as the cervical esophagus, the thoracic inlet, base of the heart, or the terminal esophagus; thus an endoscope longer than 1 m may be necessary for complete evaluation. Endoscopic evaluation is useful before relief of an impaction to localize the obstruction and to investigate the nature of the impaction if a foreign body is suspected. Foreign bodies may be retrievable through transendoscopic tethering.[58] The veterinarian can obtain critical diagnostic and prognostic information after resolution of the impaction. Assessing the affected esophagus for mucosal ulceration, rupture, masses, strictures, diverticula, and signs of functional abnormalities is important (Figures 15-11 and 15-12).

Ultrasonography of the cervical region is useful not only to confirm a cervical esophageal impaction but also to provide critical information about the location and extent of the impaction and esophageal wall thickness and integrity. Ultrasonography may provide information about the cause.[35] Radiographic assessment of the esophagus can confirm the presence of esophageal obstruction when the affected area cannot be adequately viewed using endoscopy. Impacted food material in the esophagus can be detected by its typical granular pattern, and gas accumulation is often visible proximal to the obstruction. Air or barium contrast radiographic studies are most useful for evaluating the esophagus after relief of the impaction if a stricture is suspected. It is often easier to detect esophageal dilation, diverticula, rupture, functional disorder (megaesophagus), or luminal narrowing caused by extraluminal compression by using contrast radiographic studies instead of endoscopy (Figure 15-13).[59-61] One should take care when interpreting radiographic studies in sedated horses, particularly after passage of a nasogastric tube or other esophageal manipulations that may contribute to esophageal dilation.[62]

TABLE 15-7

Esophageal Disorders of Horses

Disorder	Presenting Complaints	Diagnosis	Treatment	Selected References
ACQUIRED DISORDERS				
Choke	Nasal discharge of saliva and food; retching; excessive salivation; cough; sweating; extension of head and neck	Passage of a nasogastric tube; endoscopy	Medical and surgical treatment options as described in text	3-5
Foreign bodies	Acute or recurrent choke	Endoscopy; radiography	Manual retrieval or removal; endoscopic removal; surgery	6-10
External compression	Acute or recurrent choke.	Endoscopy; radiography; ultrasound	Removal of the obstructive mass	11
Muscular hypertrophy	No clinical signs observed in most affected horses; may predispose to esophageal diverticula	Incidental finding at necropsy	None	12
Gastroesophageal reflux disease	Inappetence; bruxism; ptyalism; colic; gastric reflux; weight loss; exercise intolerance	Esophageal and gastric endoscopy	Correct primary problem; decrease gastric acidity; gastric protectants; surgery	13-15
Stricture	Recurrent choke; weight loss	Endoscopy; contrast radiography	Bougienage; surgery	16-25
Diverticula*	Recurrent choke; weight loss	Endoscopy; contrast radiography	Surgery	24,26-29
Perforation, trauma	Salivation; bruxism; cough; nasal discharge; sepsis	Endoscopy	Enteral feeding; supportive care	30,31
Megaesophagus*	Recurrent choke; intermittent food and saliva from nares; pneumonia; weight loss; colic	Endoscopy; contrast radiography	Nutritional modification as described in text	32, 33
Neoplasia	Recurrent choke; weight loss	Endoscopy; biopsy	Surgical resection	34,35
Granulation tissue	Recurrent choke; swelling in the region of the cervical esophagus	Endoscopy; biopsy	Laser surgical resection	36
CONGENITAL DISORDERS				
Tubular duplication of the esophagus	Young horse; mass caudal to mandible; dyspnea; dysphagia; nasal regurgitation of food and saliva	Radiography and ultrasonography of mass; endoscopy; contrast radiography	Surgical excision	37,38
Cystic duplication of the esophagus	Young horse; mass in cervical or throatlatch area; recurrent choke; bruxism; excessive salivation; nasal regurgitation of saliva and feed; weight loss	Endoscopy; ultrasonography; aspiration of cyst; contrast radiography	Surgical excision; marsupialization of cyst	39-41
Vascular ring anomaly	Cervical swelling after introduction to solid feed; chronic respiratory disease	Endoscopy; contrast radiography; computed tomography; magnetic resonance imaging	Surgical correction	42-49
Congenital stenosis	Nasal regurgitation of milk; cough	Endoscopy; contrast radiography	Dietary management as described in text	50
Ectasia	Nasal regurgitation of milk	Histologic evaluation	None described	51,52

*May occur as congenital or acquired lesions.

TABLE 15-8

Causes of Complete or Partial Esophageal Obstruction in the Horse

Category	Differential	Examples
Intraluminal	Foreign body	Apples, potatoes
	Feed material	
Extramural	Neoplasia	Squamous cell carcinoma, lymphoma
	Vascular ring anomaly	Persistent right aortic arch
	Granuloma	
Intramural	Esophageal abscess	
	Granuloma	
	Neoplasia	Squamous cell carcinoma, leiomyosarcoma
	Cysts	Intramural cysts, duplication cysts
	Diverticula	
	Stenosis	
Functional disorders	Dehydration	
	Exhaustion	
	Pharmacologic	Acepromazine, detomidine
	Primary megaesophagus	Congenital ectasia
	Esophagitis	
	Autonomic dysautonomia	
	Vagal neuropathies	

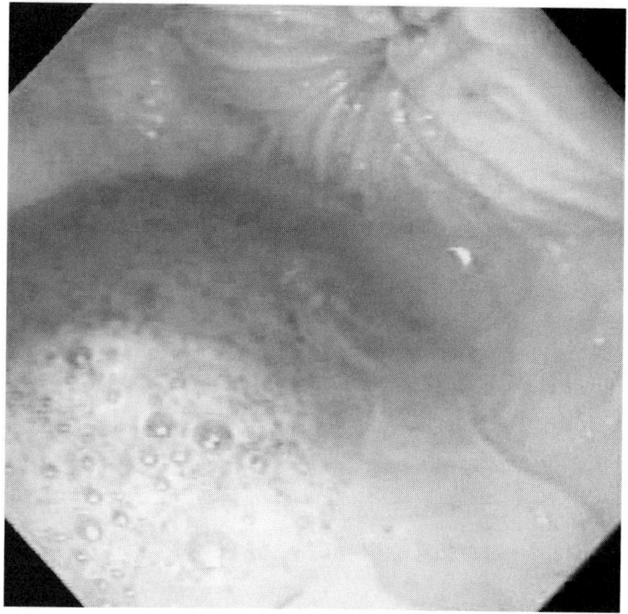

FIGURE 15-11 Endoscopic view of the cervical esophagus in an adult horse 6 months after an episode of choke that caused circumferential ulceration of the esophageal mucosa. The area of luminal narrowing (stricture) is at the upper right of the image, and the proximal dilation forms an outpouching of the esophageal wall. A contrast esophagram revealed that the outpouching was a pulsion diverticulum.

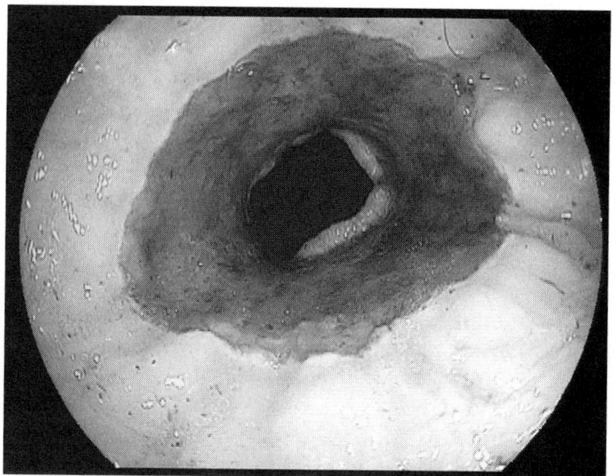

FIGURE 15-12 Endoscopic view of the proximal esophagus in a yearling filly with recurrent esophageal obstruction. Circumferential mucosal ulceration is evident proximal to incomplete stricture formation.

Treatment

The primary goal of treatment for esophageal impaction is to relieve the obstruction. A variety of approaches have been described, ranging from minimal conservative therapy to aggressive intervention. Parenteral administration of acepromazine (0.05 mg/kg intravenously), xylazine (0.25 to 0.5 mg/kg intravenously) or detomidine (0.01 to 0.02 mg/kg intravenously), oxytocin (0.11 to 0.22 IU/kg intramuscularly), and esophageal instillation of lidocaine (30 to 60 ml of 1% lidocaine) may reduce esophageal spasms caused by pain or may decrease esophageal tone.[4,62,63] Some clinicians advocate parasympatholytic drugs such as atropine (0.02 mg/kg intravenously) to reduce salivary secretions and lessen the risk of aspiration. However, undesirable effects of atropine, including excessive drying of the impaction and inhibition of distal gastrointestinal motility, may preclude its use.

In many horses with esophageal obstruction secondary to a feed impaction, the problem may be resolved with conservative management. To facilitate examination, relieve anxiety, and relax the esophagus, the clinician should begin by sedating the horse. Then, the clinician passes a stomach tube to confirm the diagnosis. When an obstruction is encountered, gentle pressure is applied in an attempt to dislodge and move distally the offending feed material. If the choke is not easily dislodged with gentle pressure, the tube is removed. Appropriate sedatives (e.g., xylazine, detomidine, acepromazine), anti-inflammatory-analgesic (e.g. flunixin, butorphanol), and smooth muscle-relaxing drugs (e.g., oxytocin) are administered. The horse is moved to an unbedded stall with absolutely no food or water within reach and is muzzled if

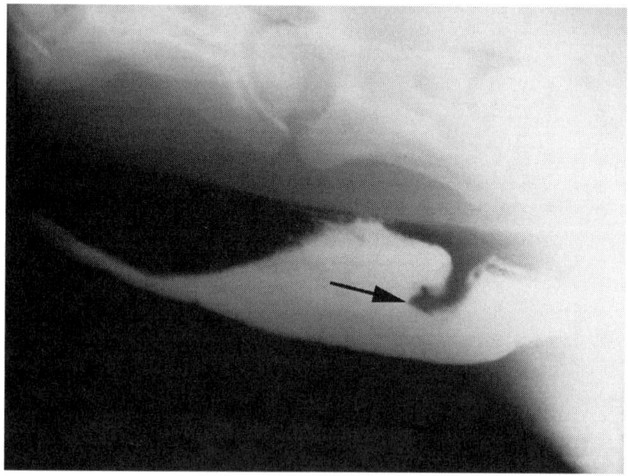

FIGURE 15-13 Contrast esophagram in a horse with circumferential esophageal stricture *(arrow)* and a pulsion diverticulum proximal to the stricture.

necessary. The horse is left alone in the stall for several hours. If there is evidence of dehydration, appropriate intravenous fluid therapy is provided. If there is evidence of aspiration pneumonia, appropriate intravenous antimicrobial therapy is provided. Upon re-examination, a stomach tube is passed and gentle pressure is again applied to the area of obstruction. In most horses the impaction will have softened and can be easily dislodged, if it has not resolved already, with minimal pressure from the stomach tube.

Some clinicians prefer a more interventional approach to resolution of an impaction, and some impactions are severe enough to require physical dispersal of the material.[4] A nasogastric tube can be used to displace the impacted material along with external massage if the obstruction is in the cervical region. Often, carefully lavaging the esophagus with water using an uncuffed or a cuffed nasogastric tube while the head is lowered is necessary to aid in breaking up the impaction. Some clinicians advocate a dual tube method, whereby a tube is placed through each nasal passage into the esophagus for ingress and egress of the lavage fluid. Because of the risk of aspiration of water and food material, esophageal lavage sometimes is done under general anesthesia with a cuffed nasotracheal tube.

In refractory cases intravenous administration of isotonic fluid containing 0.9% NaCl and KCl (10 to 20 mEq/L) for 24 hours at a rate of 50 to 100 ml/kg/day along with esophageal relaxants such as oxytocin may promote hydration and softening of the impaction and help prevent or alleviate any electrolyte or acid-base imbalances resulting from salivary losses of chloride, sodium, and potassium.[64] Oxytocin may or may not provide a direct effect for the resolution of an esophageal obstruction. Oxytocin reduced area under the curve for esophageal smooth muscle strip contractions but had no effect on skeletal muscle strips in vitro.[65] In one in vivo report, oxytocin administration resulted in decreased esophageal tone in the proximal esophagus (aborad to larynx and thoracic inlet).[63] However, in another study oxytocin administration did not affect esophageal manometric recordings.[66] Rarely, esophageal obstruction ultimately may require esophagotomy to relieve the impaction. Strict restriction of food and water, including access to bedding material, must be enforced until the obstruction is resolved and the esophagus has regained function. Surgical removal of esophageal foreign bodies can be considered if the size or orientation of the object is such that transendoscopic retrieval is considered unlikely to be successful.[6,7] In one report an intraluminal mass composed of exuberant granulation tissue was removed through serial transendoscopic ND:Yag laser ablation.[36]

Systemic effects of dysphagia associated with esophageal impaction include dehydration, hyponatremia, hypochloremia, and metabolic alkalosis from prolonged loss of salivary free water and electrolytes.[64] If the duration of a complete esophageal obstruction is 48 hours or longer, the clinician should correct dehydration and electrolyte and acid-base imbalances. One can restore fluid and electrolyte balance with oral electrolyte solutions if the patient is less than 6% to 7% dehydrated and the esophageal obstruction is resolved. In horses that are greater than 6% to 7% dehydrated or those that have a refractory obstruction or moderate to severe electrolyte imbalances, intravenous fluid therapy with solutions containing 0.9% NaCl and KCl (10 to 20 mEq/L) may be required.

The clinician should perform esophageal endoscopy after relief of the impaction to determine whether any complications of the impaction have developed or if a primary cause of the obstruction is present. Endoscopic examination is critical to determine the postobstruction treatment plan and for follow-up evaluation of esophageal healing. One should reevaluate the horse every 2 to 4 weeks after resolution of the impaction if esophageal dilation or mucosal injury is evident. Additional evaluation using radiography may be warranted to assess motility and transit times.

Dilation proximal to the site of obstruction, mucosal injury from trauma, stricture formation, formation of a diverticulum, megaesophagus, and esophagitis are sequelae to esophageal obstruction that predispose patients to re-obstruction. Underlying functional or morphologic abnormalities were much more likely in cases of recurrent, relative to first time, obstruction in a retrospective study.[3]

The rate of re-obstruction may be as high as 37%. Depending on the duration of the obstruction and the degree of trauma or dilation, the risk of re-obstruction is high for 24 to 48 hours or longer; thus food should be withheld for at least 24 to 48 hours after resolution of the obstruction. Sucralfate (20 mg/kg orally every 6 hours) may hasten healing if esophageal ulceration is evident, but the efficacy of sucralfate for this purpose is not established. Some clinicians suggest that administration of an NSAID such as flunixin meglumine (1 mg/kg orally or intravenously every 12 hours) or phenylbutazone (1 to 2 mg/kg orally or intravenously every 12 to 24 hours) for 2 to 4 weeks after resolution of the impaction may reduce the development of strictures. Judicious use of NSAIDs is recommended to prevent NSAID-induced worsening of esophageal mucosal injury. Orally administered NSAIDs are not recommended if esophagitis is present. After 48 to 72 hours or when the esophageal mucosa has recovered as assessed by endoscopy, the horse can be fed soft food (e.g., moistened pellets and bran mashes). One can return the patient gradually to a high-quality roughage diet over 7 to 21 days, depending on the degree of esophageal damage induced by the impaction and the nature of any underlying disease. The prognosis for survival is good (78% to 88%), but some horses may require permanent dietary modification if chronic obstruction persists.[3,16]

Aspiration pneumonia is a potential complication in every case of esophageal obstruction, and perforation is possible with severe or prolonged obstruction. In one report duration of obstruction before presentation was a good predictor of pneumonia, whereas endoscopic evidence of tracheal food contamination was not.[3] Thus administration of broad-spectrum antibiotics that are effective against gram positive and gram negative organisms, including metronidazole for anaerobes, is highly recommended if the duration of obstruction is either unknown or prolonged or if aspiration is at all suspected. A subsequent section describes treatment of esophageal perforation or rupture.

ESOPHAGITIS

Esophagitis refers to a clinical syndrome of esophageal inflammation that may or may not be ulcerative. The major protective mechanisms of the esophageal mucosa include salivary and food material buffers, normal peristaltic motility, and the barrier formed by the gastroesophageal sphincter. Reflux esophagitis is caused by repeated episodes of gastric fluid regurgitation into the distal esophagus and subsequent chemical injury to the mucosa.[67] Esophageal mucosal ulceration also can occur if the clearance of gastric fluid from the esophagus is delayed, such as in functional disorders of the esophagus. Like ulceration of the squamous portion of the stomach in horses, gastric acid and bile salt chemical injury is a major mechanism of esophageal squamous epithelial ulceration.[67,68] Reflux esophagitis may occur along with gastric ulcer disease, motility disorders, increased gastric volume from gastric outflow obstructions, gastric paresis, intestinal ileus, or impaired lower esophageal sphincter function.[55,67] Other causes of esophagitis in horses include trauma (e.g., foreign bodies, food impactions, nasogastric tubes), infection (e.g., mural abscesses), or chemical injury (e.g., pharmaceuticals, cantharidin) (Figure 15-14).[7,8,30,69]

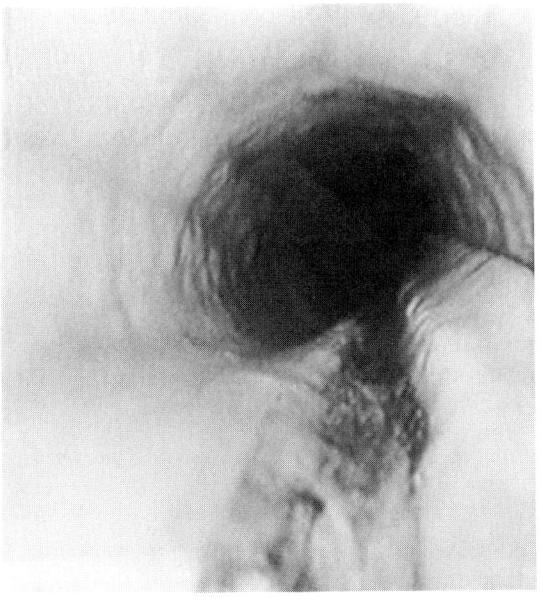

FIGURE 15-14 Endoscopic view of the cervical esophagus of a horse that had repeated passages of a stiff nasogastric tube. The deep, linear ulceration of the esophageal mucosa is notable.

Clinical Signs and Diagnosis

The clinical signs of esophagitis are nonspecific and similar to those of esophageal obstruction and gastric ulceration. Gagging or discomfort when swallowing may be evident, along with hypersalivation and bruxism. Esophageal (postpharyngeal) dysphagia may be evident. Partial or complete anorexia may occur, such that horses with chronic esophagitis may have significant weight loss. Esophageal hypomotility dysfunction caused by the inflammatory process may result in esophageal impaction. Clinical signs of underlying diseases that predispose to esophagitis may predominate or mask the signs of esophagitis. Horses with gastrointestinal motility disorders such as proximal enteritis or gastric outflow obstruction are at a high risk of developing reflux esophagitis because of the presence of gastric acid and bile salts in the fluid reflux. Foals with obstructive gastroduodenal ulcer disease commonly have reflux esophagitis.

Diagnosis requires endoscopic examination of the esophagus. Diffuse, patchy, linear, or coalescing erosion or ulcerations may be evident (see Figure 15-14), as well as significant edema or hyperemia. It is important to determine whether an underlying disease, such as infection, neoplasia, esophageal strictures, or diverticula, is present. In addition, the clinician must examine the stomach to determine whether the esophagitis is associated with gastritis, gastric outflow obstruction, or gastric ulcer disease. Contrast radiography may be helpful to detect esophageal ulceration and is useful to assess esophageal motility and transit time.[60]

Treatment

The principles of therapy for reflux esophagitis include control of gastric acidity, mucosal protection, and correction of any underlying disorder contributing to gastroesophageal reflux. Reduction of gastric acid production with proton pump antagonists such as omeprazole or H_2 histamine receptor blockers such as ranitidine is critical for resolution of esophagitis. Some clinicians advocate using sucralfate to promote healing of ulcerated esophageal mucosa. However, the ability of sucralfate to bind ulcerated esophageal mucosa and hasten esophageal ulcer healing has not been established.

Horses with reflux esophagitis following delayed gastric outflow caused by gastroduodenal ulcer disease, gastric paresis, or proximal enteritis may benefit from prokinetic drugs that act on the proximal gastrointestinal tract. Metoclopramide (0.02 to 0.1 mg/kg subcutaneously every 4 to 12 hours) reduces gastroesophageal reflux by increasing lower esophageal sphincter tone, gastric emptying, and gastroduodenal coordination. The clinician should exercise caution when giving metoclopramide to horses because they are prone to extrapyramidal neurologic side effects of the drug. Cholinergic drugs such as bethanechol (0.025 to 0.035 mg/kg subcutaneously every 4 to 24 hours or 0.035 to 0.045 mg/kg orally every 6 to 8 hours) may improve gastric emptying and are effective for treating reflux esophagitis. The clinician should take care to rule out a physical obstruction before using prokinetic drugs. For esophagitis from trauma or pressure injury after esophageal impaction, judicious use of NSAIDs may be warranted to reduce esophageal inflammation and pain.

Dietary modification may be necessary for patients with esophagitis, depending on the degree of ulceration or if motility is impaired. Horses with mild esophagitis should be fed frequent small meals of moistened pellets and fresh grass. Severe esophagitis may necessitate withholding food and imposing complete esophageal rest for several days. Although the prognosis for esophagitis is good in the absence of underlying disease, the risk of stricture formation is high if severe circumferential or coalescing ulcerations are present. Esophagitis from severe trauma or infection may lead to stricture formation.

MOTILITY DISORDERS

Motility dysfunction of the equine esophagus most commonly is caused by hypomotility resulting in esophageal dilation (ectasia) or megaesophagus. Although megaesophagus in horses usually is acquired, reports indicate that idiopathic megaesophagus in young horses may be congenital.[32,33,51,52,70] Acquired megaesophagus in horses may be a consequence of chronic or recurrent esophageal obstruction.[16,55] Esophageal impactions of a short duration cause a proximal dilation of the esophagus that is generally reversible.[60] However, if the duration of the obstruction is long enough, the motility of the esophagus proximal to the site of obstruction may be impaired permanently. Other causes of acquired megaesophagus include extra-esophageal obstruction by tumors or abscesses, pleuropneumonia, and vascular ring anomalies.[16,42] A retrospective report of horses with megaesophagus reveals an overrepresentation of Friesian horses (14 of 18 cases), suggesting the possibility of a predisposition for esophageal disorders in this breed.[32] The authors state that preliminary pedigree analyses suggest the possibility of a recessive pattern of inheritance.[32]

Megaesophagus also may result from neurologic, neuromuscular, and muscular disorders. Neurologic diseases that cause vagal neuropathy (e.g., equine protozoal myeloencephalitis, equine herpesvirus myeloencephalitis, idiopathic vagal neuropathy) have been associated with megaesophagus in horses. Pleuropneumonia may be associated with a vagal neuropathy resulting in megaesophagus. Megaesophagus is an early sign of equine dysautonomia[71] and may be observable in patients with botulism. Myasthenia gravis is a well-known cause of megaesophagus in nonequine species but has not been reported in horses. Also in other species electrolyte disorders, cachexia, primary myopathies, myositis, and Addison's disease may affect esophageal motility but have not been associated with megaesophagus in horses. One can induce iatrogenic megaesophagus by the α_2-adrenergic agonist detomidine, but this is transient and reversible.[62,72] Acepromazine, detomidine, and a combination of xylazine and butorphanol can alter proximal esophageal motility by disrupting coordinated peristalsis and decreasing spontaneous swallowing, but only acepromazine affected the manometric profile of the distal esophagus.[66] None of these drugs altered contractility of isolated esophageal smooth or striated muscle strips in vitro.[65] Nonetheless, the use of these drugs may complicate clinical evaluation of esophageal motility. Esophageal disorders, including megaesophagus, esophageal diverticulum, and esophageal rupture, appear to be more common in young Friesian horses, suggesting the possibility of a genetic predisposition in this breed.

Esophageal inflammation, particularly reflux esophagitis, may affect motility and cause megaesophagus. However, because esophageal hypomotility affects the tone and function of the lower esophageal sphincter, reflux esophagitis also may be a complication of a primary functional disorder. Thus assessing esophageal motility in horses with esophagitis that is not responding appropriately to treatment is important.

Clinical Signs and Diagnosis

Along with a complete physical examination, the clinician should perform a careful neurologic examination to help rule out primary neurologic causes of megaesophagus. Because esophageal hypomotility is a functional obstruction, the clinical signs of esophageal hypomotility or megaesophagus are similar to those of esophageal obstruction. Unlike mechanical obstruction the onset of clinical signs is insidious rather than acute. The clinical signs include those associated with esophageal dysphagia.[33,42,51,52,55,70] The cervical esophagus may be dilated enough to be evident externally. Weight loss is a common sign. Signs attributable to an underlying disease may be evident.

Diagnosis of esophageal hypomotility requires transit studies. One can measure the transit time of a bolus from the cervical esophagus to the stomach by fluoroscopy or contrast radiography.[60,71] Other signs of esophageal hypomotility and megaesophagus include pooling of contrast material and an absence of peristaltic constrictions.[55,60,70,71] Endoscopy may reveal a dilated esophagus and an absence of peristaltic waves.[55,70] Evidence of underlying disease causing obstruction or esophageal dilation may be apparent.[16,55] One should evaluate the esophagus for evidence of esophagitis that is causing esophageal motility dysfunction or is a result of impaired esophageal clearance of gastric fluid. Esophageal manometry may be useful to document abnormal postdeglutition contraction pressures, contraction time, and propagation times but is not often available for routine clinical application.[70,73] One should perform other diagnostic tests, such as a complete blood count and chemistry, to help determine a possible underlying cause. Cerebral spinal fluid analysis may be indicated to rule out neurologic disorders. Specialized testing such as electromyography may also be indicated to detect neuromuscular disorders.

Treatment

Treatment of esophageal hypomotility or megaesophagus should aim at treating the underlying cause. Dietary modification should aim at improving esophageal transit of food. The horse should be fed slurries of pellets from an elevated position to promote transit by gravity flow. Metoclopramide or bethanechol may benefit patients with reflux esophagitis associated with megaesophagus by increasing lower esophageal tone, gastric emptying, and reducing gastroesophageal reflux. The prognosis depends on the underlying cause and the degree of dilation. Although many cases of megaesophagus associated with reflux esophagitis respond well to treatment, many other forms of megaesophagus, including congenital megaesophagus, have a poor prognosis.

ESOPHAGEAL STRICTURE

Strictures most commonly are caused by pressure necrosis from esophageal impactions that induce circumferential erosion or ulceration of the esophageal mucosa, although esophageal injury caused by oral administration of corrosive medicinal agents and trauma to the neck may also result in stricture formation.[17] Congenital strictures also have been reported.[74]

Strictures caused by mucosal and submucosal trauma are termed *esophageal webs* or *rings*. Strictures may also originate in the muscular layers and adventitia of the esophagus (mural strictures) or in all of the layers of the esophagus (annular stenosis).[18,74] Horses with these lesions have a presentation similar to those with simple obstructions, because strictures result in partial obstruction and impaction of food material in the lumen. Endoscopy can be used to detect esophageal webs or rings (see Figures 15-11 and 15-12), whereas identification of mural strictures or annular stenosis may require a double-contrast esophogram (see Figure 15-13). In a retrospective study of horses with esophageal stricture following simple obstruction, maximal reduction in esophageal lumen diameter occurred within 30 days of the esophageal obstruction. Although surgery has been used to relieve such strictures, initial medical management is warranted because strictures may resolve with conservative therapy, and the esophagus continues to remodel for up to 60 days following ulceration. In one report seven horses with esophageal obstruction-induced stricture were treated conservatively by feeding a slurry diet and administering anti-inflammatory and antimicrobial medications, and five of seven were clinically normal within 60 days.[17] One of the five successfully treated horses had a 10-cm area of circumferential ulceration, suggesting that the potential exists for extensive mucosal injury to resolve without permanent stricture formation.

If resolution of strictures within 60 days is insufficient, the veterinarian should investigate other methods to increase esophageal diameter. Bougienage and balloon dilation have been used successfully in small animal patients and human beings and with variable results in horses.[19-21]The technique involves passage of a tubular dilatable instrument down the esophagus and stretching of the stricture. One may perform the technique by passing a nasogastric tube with an inflatable cuff. However, the procedure must be performed frequently to have any success, and horses may not tolerate it well.[74] Alternatively, a number of surgical techniques have been used to resolve strictures, including resection and anastomosis,[75,76] temporary esophagostomy with fenestration of the stricture,[18] esophagomyotomy for strictures of the muscularis and adventitia,[22,77] and patch grafting with local musculature.[23] However, such surgeries are fraught with complications, largely because of the propensity of the traumatized esophagus to restricture.[16,17] The esophagus lacks a serosal layer and does not rapidly form a fibrin seal as does the remainder of the intestinal tract, so anastomoses tend to leak.[76] In addition, tension on the esophagus during swallowing and movement of the neck impairs healing of anastomoses.[18,75] In spite of these difficulties, the long-term prognosis for horses with chronic esophageal strictures treated surgically is better than for those treated nonsurgically.[16] Two recent reviews describe surgical approaches to the esophagus in detail.[24,78]

ESOPHAGEAL DIVERTICULA

Two types of diverticula are traction (true) diverticula and pulsion (false) diverticula. Traction diverticula result from wounding and subsequent contraction of periesophageal tissues, with resultant tenting of the wall of the esophagus. Pulsion diverticula arise from protrusion of esophageal mucosa through defects in the muscular wall of the esophagus and usually result from trauma or acute changes in intraluminal pressure.[74] Traction diverticula appear as a dilation with a broad neck on contrast esophagography, whereas pulsion diverticula typically have a flask shape with a small neck on an esophagram (see Figure 15-13).[26,27] Although traction diverticula are usually asymptomatic and of little clinical significance, pulsion diverticula may fill with feed material, ultimately leading to esophageal obstruction and rupture.[9,27,28]

A movable mass in the midcervical region may be noticeable before onset of complete obstruction.[74] Pulsion diverticula may be corrected surgically by inverting or resecting prolapsed mucosa and closing the defect in the wall of the esophagus.[26-28] Inversion of excessive mucosa may reduce the diameter of the esophageal lumen and predispose horses to esophageal obstruction and therefore should be reserved for small diverticula.[26]

CONGENITAL DISORDERS

Congenital disorders of the esophagus are rare. Reported congenital abnormalities include congenital stenosis,[50] persistent right aortic arch,[42-47] other vascular anomalies,[48] esophageal duplication cysts,[37,39,40] intramural inclusion cysts,[41,56] and idiopathic megaesophagus.[33,51,52] In the one report of congenital stenosis, double-contrast radiography revealed concentric narrowing of the thoracic esophagus in the absence of any vascular abnormalities at the base of the heart. Successful treatment included having the foal stand with the forelimbs elevated off the ground following each feeding.[50]

Persistent right aortic arch is a congenital anomaly in which the right fourth aortic arch becomes the definitive aorta instead of the left aortic arch, which results in constriction of the esophagus by the ligamentum arteriosum as it extends between the anomalous right aorta and the left pulmonary artery.[49] Clinical signs may include those associated with esophageal (postpharyngeal) dysphagia, drooling, and distention of the cervical esophagus resulting from partial obstruction of the thoracic esophagus.[42,43] Endoscopic examination typically reveals dilation of the esophagus cranial to the obstruction, with evidence of diffuse esophagitis. Surgical treatment of persistent right aortic arch has been reported in foals, with varying degrees of success.[43,45,47] In one report, preoperative computed tomography was used to identify the exact anatomic location of the offending lesion and guide the surgical approach.[47]

Esophageal duplication cysts and intramural inclusion cysts cause typical signs of esophageal obstruction, including salivation, esophageal dysphagia, and swelling of the cervical esophagus as the cysts enlarge.[37,39,41] Such signs can make them difficult to differentiate from other forms of esophageal obstruction (choke). Endoscopic examination may reveal compression of the esophageal lumen and communication with the esophageal lumen if it exists.

Ultrasonographic examination may be the most useful method of antemortem diagnosis if the cyst is in the cervical esophagus. Examination of an aspirate of the mass may aid in the diagnosis by revealing the presence of keratinized squamous cells.[39,41] Surgical treatments have included complete surgical resection and surgical marsupialization.[37,39,41] The latter appears to be more successful and results in fewer complications.[37,41] Complications of surgical resection include laryngeal hemiplegia following surgical trauma to the recurrent laryngeal nerve in the region of the esophagus and esophageal fistula formation.[41]

Esophageal Perforation

Perforation typically occurs in the cervical region in response to external trauma, necrosis of the esophageal wall caused by a food impaction, or rupture of an esophageal lesion such as an impacted diverticulum. The esophagus is particularly vulnerable to external trauma in the distal third of the neck because only a thin layer of muscle covers it at this point.[79] Iatrogenic perforation may occur in response to excessive force with a stomach tube against an obstruction or a compromised region of the esophagus.[30] Esophageal perforations may be open or closed and tend to cause extensive cellulitis and necrosis of tissues surrounding the wound because of drainage of saliva and feed material within fascial planes. Systemic inflammation resulting from septic cellulitis may occur. Closed perforations of the esophagus are particularly troublesome because food material, water, saliva, and air may migrate to the mediastinum and pleural space via fascial planes.[30,79] Because of the leakage of air into the tissues surrounding the rupture, extensive subcutaneous and fascial emphysema frequently develops and is usually evident clinically and on cervical radiographs. Pneumomediastinum and pneumothorax are potentially fatal complications of esophageal ruptures. If the esophagus ruptures into the mediastinum, horses usually exhibit signs of acute systemic inflammatory response syndrome that may be mistaken for colic.

Treatment should include converting closed perforations to open perforations if possible,[80] extensive débridement and lavage of affected tissues, broad spectrum antibiotics, tetanus prophylaxis, and esophageal rest. The clinician may achieve the latter by placing a feeding tube into the esophagus via the wound. Alternatively, one may place a nasogastric tube using a small tube (12-F diameter).[30] For open perforations, once the wound has granulated and contracted to a small size, peroral feeding may be attempted.[79] Extensive loss of saliva via esophageal wounds may lead to hyponatremia and hypochloremia. In addition, transient metabolic acidosis occurs because of salivary bicarbonate loss, followed by progressive metabolic alkalosis.[64] Although reports of esophageal wounds healing well by second intention exist, healing time is prolonged.[81] In addition, some perforations never completely heal and form permanent esophagocutaneous fistulae that may require surgical correction. The development of esophageal strictures is not common because wounds are usually linear and not circumferential. However, traction diverticula may develop. Other complications of esophageal wounds include Horner's syndrome and left laryngeal hemiplegia.[79]

In a retrospective study on esophageal disorders, only 2 of 11 horses with esophageal perforations survived over the long term;[16] in a report of esophageal trauma following nasogastric intubation, four of five horses were euthanized.[30] The prognosis is therefore poor in horses with esophageal perforations, largely because of the extent of cellulitis, tissue necrosis, shock, and local wound complications.

DISEASES OF THE STOMACH

L. Chris Sanchez

The availability of specialized endoscopic equipment allowing visual inspection of the entire adult equine stomach and proximal duodenum is now commonplace for veterinarians in referral and select ambulatory settings. Thus veterinarians, owners, and trainers are increasingly aware of gastric disease in horses.

GASTRODUODENAL ULCERATION

Peptic ulcer disease is defined as erosions or ulcers of any portion of the gastrointestinal tract normally exposed to acid.[1] Mucosal damage can include inflammation, erosion (disruption of the superficial mucosa), and ulceration (penetration of the submucosa). In severe cases full-thickness ulceration can occur, resulting in perforation. The proximal (orad) portion of the equine stomach is lined by stratified squamous mucosa similar to that lining the esophagus. This proximal portion is also commonly termed the *nonglandular region* of the stomach. The distal (aborad) portion of the stomach is lined with glandular mucosa, and the distinct junction between the two regions is deemed the *margo plicatus*. Ulceration can occur in either or both gastric regions, although different clinical syndromes and pathophysiologic mechanisms apply. As a result, the broad term *equine gastric ulcer syndrome* (EGUS) has been used to encompass the wide array of associated clinical syndromes.[2] EGUS develops in horses of all ages and is arguably the most clinically and economically important disorder of the equine stomach.

Prevalence

The prevalence of gastric ulceration has been reported for a variety of breeds and usages; however, most current data involve Thoroughbreds or Standardbreds in race training. The prevalence of squamous ulceration in horses in race training varies between 70% to 95%[3-11] and can be as high as 100% when limited to animals actively racing.[7] In recent years horses performing in other disciplines have also been evaluated, including active show horses (58% prevalence),[12] endurance horses (67%),[13] western performance horses (40%),[14] Thoroughbred broodmares (67% pregnant; 77% nonpregnant),[15] and nonracing performance horses (17% precompetition; 56% postcompetition).[16] In one large retrospective study (3715 adult horses from 1924-1996) evaluating incidence of gastric ulceration identified at necropsy, an overall prevalence of 10.3% was found, with the highest prevalence in Thoroughbreds (including Arabians) and Standardbred trotters (19%).[17] Horses in a university riding program also demonstrated a low squamous ulceration prevalence (11%).[18] Approximately 49% of horses seen in a referral hospital for colic had evidence of gastric ulceration.[19] The reported prevalence of gastric ulceration in foals varies between 25% to 57%.[20-22]

Many earlier studies investigating the prevalence of gastric ulceration do not differentiate between nonglandular and glandular lesions, and many evaluate only the nonglandular region of the stomach, but this trend is changing. In a recent study of 162 horses in a hospital setting, 58% had antral or pyloric erosions or ulcerations, 58% had squamous mucosal lesions, and 8% had lesions involving the glandular body.[23] In other studies 56% of Thoroughbreds in which the pylorus was examined had glandular ulceration,[9] and 47% of racehorses (Thoroughbred and Standardbred) in which the pylorus was evaluated had ulceration in that location.[11] In the former study[9] all horses with glandular lesions also had squamous disease, whereas such an association was not seen in the latter study.[11] In endurance horses with a 67% overall lesion prevalence, 57% had squamous ulceration, whereas 27% had glandular disease.[13] In a postmortem evaluation, lesions were most commonly located in the squamous mucosa along the margo plicatus, followed by the glandular body, proximal squamous mucosa, and antrum.[17]

Pathophysiology

An imbalance between inciting and protective factors in the mucosal environment can result in ulcer formation.[24,25] The major intrinsic factors promoting ulcer formation include hydrochloric acid (HCl), bile acids, and pepsin, with HCl the predominant factor. Various intrinsic factors protect against ulcer formation, such as the mucus-bicarbonate layer, maintenance of adequate mucosal blood flow, mucosal prostaglandin E_2 and epidermal growth factor production, and gastroduodenal motility. In humans extrinsic ulcerogenic factors include NSAIDs; *Helicobacter pylori;* stress; changes in diet; and gastrointestinal disorders, especially those resulting in delayed gastric emptying.[1] In human neonates physiologic stress associated with a major primary illness seems to be strongly associated with gastric ulcers.[26] Many of the other factors mentioned previously are believed to be important in horses, but clear evidence of an infectious agent has not yet been identified in horses or foals with EGUS.[27,28] Recently, the possibility of *Helicobacter* infection in horses has re-emerged with the identification of polymerase chain reaction (PCR) products consistent with *Helicobacter*-like bacteria in horses with and without gastric lesions[29,30] and a new species, *Helicobacter equorum*, identified in horse feces.[31] Serum antibodies against *H. pylori* appear common in postsuckling foals and their dams.[32] However, *H. equorum* did not colonize the equine stomach in an experimental model,[33] and a true link between *Helicobacter* infection and any form of EGUS remains elusive.

The specific factors involved in injury as well as protective mechanisms vary among regions of the proximal gastrointestinal tract, and a thorough review of mucosal injury and repair is presented elsewhere in this chapter. The pathophysiology of squamous mucosal ulceration in the horse appears similar to that seen in gastroesophageal reflux disease (GERD) in human beings and ulceration of the nonglandular mucosa in pigs. Excessive acid exposure is the predominant mechanism responsible for squamous mucosal ulceration, although many details remain unclear.[34] Hydrochloric acid is secreted by parietal cells in the gastric glands via a hydrogen-potassium adenosine triphosphatase (H^+, K^+-ATPase) pump on the luminal side. Horses secrete acid continuously, and measured pH of equine gastric contents is variable from less than 2 to greater than 6, depending on the horse's dietary state (fed versus fasted).[35,36] A protocol of repeated 24-hour periods of fasting and feeding induces squamous erosion and ulceration.[37] Because this protocol results in periods of prolonged gastric acidity (pH < 2.0) and concurrent administration of the histamine$_2$ (H_2) receptor antagonist ranitidine reduces lesion severity, it supports the role of acid exposure in the pathogenesis of squamous ulcer disease.

Several peptides can stimulate or inhibit the secretion of acid by the parietal cell. The predominant stimuli to hydrochloric acid secretion are gastrin, histamine, and acetylcholine via the vagus nerve.[1] Gastrin is released by G cells within the antral mucosa, and histamine is released by mast cells and ECL cells in the gastric gland. Histamine binds to type 2 receptors on the parietal cell membrane, causing an increase in cyclic adenosine monophosphate (cAMP), resulting in phosphorylation of enzymes that activate the proton pump. Gastrin and acetylcholine can act via calcium-mediated intracellular pathways and also stimulate histamine release directly.[38] Isolated equine parietal cells respond maximally to histamine stimulation and only minimally to carbachol and pentagastrin.[39] In vivo, histamine or pentagastrin infusion can stimulate similar maximal acid output.[40] Interestingly, pentagastrin stimulation also induces a marked duodenal secretion of a sodium chloride-rich fluid, which can reflux back into the stomach under fasting conditions.[40] Gastrin release is primarily controlled by gastrin-releasing peptide (GRP), which is stimulated by gastric distention and increased luminal pH, but the interaction between gastrin and histamine has not been fully elucidated in the horse.

Gastric acid secretion by parietal cells is primarily inhibited by somatostatin, released by fundic and antral D cells. The inhibitory effect of somatostatin is primarily paracrine, but plasma levels of somatostatin negatively correlate with gastric luminal acidity.[41] Gastric acid secretion also is inhibited by epidermal growth factor (EGF), a peptide produced in saliva.[42]

Foals can produce significant amounts of gastric acid by the second day of life, with consistent periods of acidity (pH $<$ 2.0) in clinically normal animals.[43,44] In one study foals tended to have a high gastric pH at day 1 of age,[43] but in a study of critically ill foals, some foals demonstrated periods of gastric acidity on the first day of life.[45] Suckling was associated with an immediate rise in gastric pH, whereas periods of rest during which foals did not suck for more than 20 minutes were associated with prolonged periods of acidity.[44] Premature human infants are capable of gastric acid production at 28 weeks of gestation.[46] In sheep abomasal pH begins to drop at approximately 125 days of gestation but does not reach values normal for adult sheep (2.5) until after birth, which corresponds to the presence of H+/K+/ATPase mRNA, present in the fetal fundus by 125 days of gestation and rising to adult levels until after birth.[47] This observed increase in acid secretion corresponds to an increase in bioactive serum gastrin. Only one of seven premature foals demonstrated an acidic pH recording in a study of gastric pH profiles in critically ill foals.[45] Although multiple factors were likely involved in those foals, the true ontogeny of gastric acid production in foals is currently unknown.

Equine squamous mucosa is very thin at birth but becomes hyperplastic and parakeratotic within days (Figure 15-15).[48]

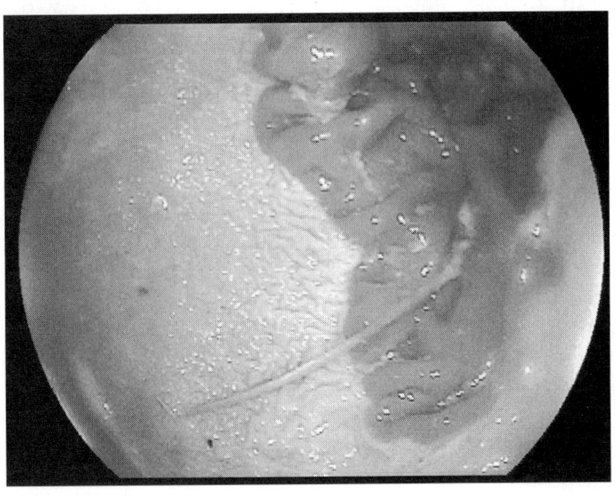

FIGURE 15-15 Endoscopic image of the greater curvature of the stomach in a 3-day-old Thoroughbred colt.

The parallel between decreasing pH and proliferation of squamous epithelium correlates with that seen in other species.[49] The combination of a relatively thin gastric epithelium with a high acid output may leave neonatal foals susceptible to ulcer formation at a very young age. In addition, one must remember the difference in normal appearance of the squamous mucosa when interpreting gastric endoscopy in a neonatal population.

In esophageal squamous mucosa, intercellular tight junctions and bicarbonate secretion are the major factors involved in protection against acid injury in other species, although squamous bicarbonate secretion has not been documented in the horse.[50-52] The principal barrier is a glycoconjugate substance secreted by cells in the *stratum spinosum,* with a contribution from the tight junctions in the *stratum corneum*.[52] This barrier function is considered weak at best, and thus a functioning lower esophageal sphincter, normal salivary flow, and salivary mucins contribute to the prevention of acid injury in human GERD. In horses a mechanical barrier like the lower esophageal sphincter is not available to protect the gastric squamous mucosa from acid exposure. The squamous mucosa adjacent to the margo plicatus, especially along the lesser curvature, likely receives regular exposure to acidic gastric contents. Recently, surface mucus demonstrating cross-reactivity to a mixture of anti-human MUC5AC (a mucin gene) antibodies has been identified in both the glandular and nonglandular regions of healthy equine gastric mucosa.[53]

Bile salts and pepsin have been implicated as contributing factors to ulcer disease in many species. In rabbit esophageal mucosa, bile salt absorption occurs and is directly correlated with mucosal barrier disruption.[54] The unconjugated bile salts cholate and deoxycholate have a pK_a of 5 and 5.3, respectively, and therefore cannot remain in solution and cause mucosal damage in the presence of acid. Alternatively, the conjugated bile salt taurocholate (pK_a 1.9) can cause mucosal injury in either the ionized salt form at pH 7 or the nonionized acid form at pH 1-2.[54] In the pig bile salts or acid alone causes squamous mucosal damage, whereas a combination of the two result in extensive damage in vitro.[55] In the horse a similar synergistically damaging effect was found with the addition of bile salts and acid (pH 2.5) to stratified squamous mucosa in vitro in one study.[56] In addition, the investigators were able to document levels of both bile salts and acid sufficient to cause mucosal damage in gastric contents within 14 hours of feed deprivation. This is not surprising, given that duodenogastric reflux occurs normally in the horse.[40] In a separate in vitro study of equine squamous mucosa, prolonged exposure to acid alone (pH 1.5) had a damaging effect, and synergism with exposure to a combination of acid and pepsin or taurocholate was not found.[57] The lack of synergism is likely due to the lower pH used in this study and stresses the importance of acid exposure in squamous ulcer disease. The effect of acid has been consistent among studies. In addition, several volatile fatty acids (acetic, butyric, and proprionic), which had previously been documented in gastric contents of horses fed hay or hay and grain diets, decreased nonglandular mucosal barrier function.[58,59] Lactic acid exposure alone does not appear to alter nonglandular mucosal bioelectric properties.[60]

Pepsinogens are secreted primarily by chief cells, although secretion by neck cells, cardiac glands, and antral pyloric glands also occurs.[61] In an acidic environment (pH <3.0), pepsinogen is converted to the active pepsin. Although the proteolytic activity of pepsin is normally directed toward dietary protein, it can also act on the gastric mucosa.[62]

Several mechanisms help protect the glandular mucosa from acid injury. The mucus-bicarbonate layer serves to titrate H^+ ion from the gastric lumen to CO_2 and H_2O. Cellular restitution and prostaglandins of the E series, which enhance mucosal blood flow and mucus-bicarbonate secretion in the glandular mucosa, have not been documented in squamous epithelium.[34,51] Of these mechanisms mucosal blood flow is likely the most important contributor to overall gastric mucosal health. Nitric oxide is a key regulator of mucosal blood flow and prostaglandin synthesis and thus may play a role in mucosal protection.[63]

Overall, acid remains the major contributing factor to nonglandular mucosal damage, although other factors, such as pepsin and bile salts, may play an important role as well, either in the initiation or perpetuation of disease.

Risk Factors

Many aspects of diet and management have been associated with the development of nonglandular ulceration in adult horses, several of which have already been discussed with reference to pathophysiology. These include diet, feeding patterns, exercise, stall confinement, transportation, and administration of NSAIDs.

Horses in race training have a high incidence of gastric ulceration and are frequently fed high-concentrate, low-roughage diets. A diet high in concentrate and either high or low in forage, in conjunction with stall confinement but no exercise, was shown to induce nonglandular ulceration within 2 weeks.[64] In one study higher volatile fatty acid concentrations, higher gastric juice pH, and lower number and severity of nonglandular ulceration were documented after feeding an alfalfa hay-grain diet when compared to a bromegrass hay diet.[58] However, many factors differed between the diets, such as digestible energy, bulk, crude protein, and mineral content (especially calcium). These findings were recently supported by a study in which an alfalfa hay/pelleted concentrate diet significantly reduced ulcer severity scores and prevented ulcer development relative to a coastal hay-concentrate diet in horses managed with dry lot housing and regular exercise.[65] Intermittent feeding has clearly been shown to induce nonglandular ulceration and is a consistent model of ulcer induction.[36,37,66]

The pathophysiologic correlation between exercise and squamous ulcer disease has not yet been defined, despite the high prevalence of ulceration in performance horses. Nonglandular ulceration can develop within 8 days of exercise varying from light halter to active race training[67], and time in work was found to be a risk factor for squamous ulceration in racing Thoroughbreds.[68] Elevations in postfeeding serum gastrin concentration have been demonstrated after treadmill exercise.[69] During treadmill exercise at gaits faster than a walk, proximal gastric size decreases in conjunction with an increase in intra-abdominal pressure, resulting in a simultaneous decrease in proximal gastric pH.[70] Both proximal gastric size and pH return to baseline levels as soon as the horse returned to a walk, and the resultant theory was that gastric contracture could result in increased acid exposure to the squamous mucosa by raising the level of liquid gastric contents.

Stall confinement[66] and transport[71] have been shown to induce nonglandular ulceration. However, a distinct mechanism for either of these factors has not been definitively determined. A recent study did not detect a difference in pH in the proximal or ventral stomach in response to three different environmental situations (stall confinement alone in a barn, stall confinement with a horse in an adjacent stall, and paddock turnout with a companion horse), each for 24 hours.[72] This work suggests that increased acid exposure to the proximal stomach alone is not causative.

Several studies have failed to document a correlation between NSAID administration and naturally occurring ulcer disease.[3,4,6,7,17] However, NSAID administration is a well-known cause of gastric ulceration under experimental conditions.[73-77] NSAID-related ulceration is typically described as predominantly glandular in nature, although nonglandular ulceration can also occur by a mechanism that has not yet been fully characterized. NSAIDs cause a decrease in prostaglandin E_2 synthesis caused by inhibition of the COX pathway. Therefore a resultant decrease in glandular mucosal protection, most notably by way of decreased mucosal blood flow and mucus production, is the most likely mechanism of action. In one study, however, phenylbutazone administration resulted in ulceration of the glandular mucosa at the pyloric antrum but did not significantly alter mucosal prostaglandin E_2 concentration.[75]

Other risk factors associated with gastric ulceration include gender and age, and the reported prevalence of gastric ulcers has increased over time. In one study the frequency of gastric ulceration increased from less than 6% before 1945 to approximately 18% after 1975.[17] The association between sex or age and ulceration has not been consistent among studies.[7,9,10,17,78] Crib biting has also been discussed as a risk factor.[68,79] In one study difficulty maintaining weight and playing of a radio were also associated with risk of ulceration.[68] Although the former is easily explained, the latter certainly requires further investigation. In foals risk factors are less clearly defined and will be discussed along with the clinical syndrome in each age group.

Clinical Syndrome: Neonatal foals

Clinical signs typically associated with gastric ulceration in foals include poor appetite, diarrhea, and colic. Many foals probably never exhibit clinical signs, and some do not exhibit clinical signs until ulceration is severe or fatal perforation has occurred. Glandular ulceration is typically considered the most clinically significant type of disease in this population.

The physiologic stress of a concurrent illness has been associated with gastric ulceration in foals. Retrospectively, 14 (23%) of 61 foals up to 85 days of age with a clinical disorder were found to have lesions in the gastric glandular mucosa,[22] and prospectively 8 (40%) of 20 foals up to 30 days of age with a clinical disorder had glandular ulceration.[80] By contrast, only 4% to 9% of clinically normal foals examined in endoscopic surveys had lesions observed in the gastric glandular mucosa.[21,81]

Critically ill neonatal foals can have a markedly different pH profile compared with that seen in clinically normal foals, possibly because of alterations in gastric motility and acid secretion.[45] Gastric ulceration was not identified in any animals at necropsy in that study; however, ulceration has been documented in a similar population.[20] Thus factors other than acid exposure, most notably mucosal perfusion, may play an important role in the so-called stress-related ulceration seen in neonates. Gastric ulceration and rupture in the hospitalized neonatal population appears to occur less often now than in previous reports, despite a decline in the use of ulcer prophylaxis in one hospital.[82] Advances in overall neonatal care, especially supportive care, have likely contributed to this decline.

One recent report evaluated the use of gastric tonometry as a measurement of mucosal perfusion in neonatal foals.[83] However, despite investigations into the effect of age, feeding, and omeprazole administration, the reference interval in foals appears too wide to warrant clinical application of this tool to evaluate the relationship between ulceration and mucosal perfusion in foals.

Clinical Syndrome: Sucklings and Weanlings

In suckling foals younger than 50 days old, lesions typically originate in the squamous mucosa adjacent to the margo plicatus along the greater curvature. Such lesions can be seen in foals as young as 2 days of age and have been observed in 50% of foals younger than 50 days old. Histologic examination of these lesions has revealed disruption of the epithelial layers of the mucosa and a neutrophilic infiltration. Another phenomenon that occurs in young foals is the shedding, or desquamation, of squamous epithelium, which appears as flakes or sheets of epithelium. Desquamation occurs without ulceration in up to 80% of foals less than 35 days of age, and this process is not typically associated with clinical signs.[21,22,81]

In older foals lesions become more prevalent in the squamous mucosa, particularly along the lesser curvature.[80] Lesions also are found in the squamous mucosa of the fundus and adjacent to the margo plicatus. These lesions can be very severe and are often associated with clinical signs such as diarrhea, poor appetite, and poor growth and body condition. Diarrhea is the most frequent sign in symptomatic foals with squamous mucosal lesions and is associated with more diffuse erosion or ulceration of the squamous mucosa than occurs in asymptomatic foals. In some foals poor growth, rough hair coat, a potbelly appearance, or all of these occur in conjunction with moderate to severe squamous mucosal ulceration. In cases with severe or diffuse squamous ulceration, bruxism or colic may occur.

Gastroduodenal ulcer disease (GDUD) occurs almost exclusively in suckling and early weanling foals. Clinical signs of duodenal ulceration are similar to that described for gastric ulceration (bruxism, colic, ptyalism, diarrhea), but the consequences are often more severe. Lesions occur primarily in the proximal duodenum, ranging from diffuse inflammation to severe ulceration, but affected foals typically have severe squamous or glandular ulceration as well (Figure 15-16). Foals with duodenal ulceration often have delayed gastric emptying and may have gastroesophageal reflux. Potential complications include gastric or duodenal rupture, pyloric or duodenal stricture (Figure 15-17), and ascending cholangitis. Severe squamous and esophageal ulceration and aspiration pneumonia can occur secondary to gastroesophageal reflux.[24,84-87]

The GDUD syndrome can occur in outbreaks and is most commonly identified in intensive breeding operations. The cause of duodenal lesions in foals is not known. One theory is that the problem begins with diffuse duodenal inflammation that can coalesce down to a focal area of ulceration.[88] A temporal relationship between GDUD and rotaviral diarrhea has been suggested, but an infectious etiology remains unproven. Although lesion location and severity associated with rotaviral

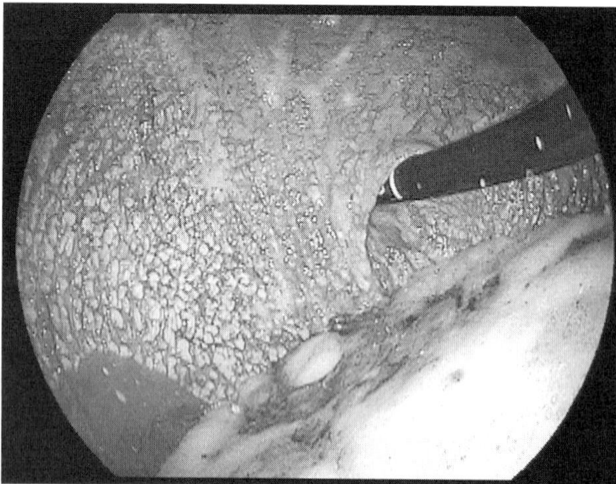

FIGURE 15-16 Endoscopic image of the lesser curvature in a 3-month-old foal diagnosed with gastroduodenal ulcer disease and a gastric outflow obstruction.

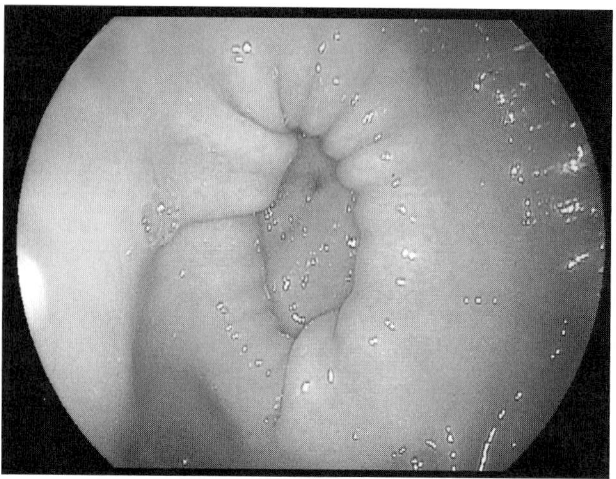

FIGURE 15-17 Endoscopic image of the pylorus in the foal depicted in Figure 2, 2 months after surgery. Note the extremely small pyloric opening, which had formed a mechanical obstruction to gastric outflow.

infection varies among species, duodenal ulceration has not been reported.[89]

Clinical Syndrome: Yearlings and Adult Horses

Clinical signs attributable to EGUS in older horses are variable and classically include anorexia and chronic or intermittent colic of varying severity.[90] Many horses with endoscopic evidence of disease may appear to be clinically normal or have vague signs that include decreased consumption of concentrates, postprandial episodes of colic, poor performance or failure to train up to expectations, poor hair coat, and decreased condition or failure to thrive. Diarrhea is not typically associated with gastric ulceration in adult horses, although ulceration can occur concurrently with other causes of diarrhea. Neither presence nor type of clinical signs was correlated with prevalence or severity of ulceration.[9] Horses actively racing appear more likely to have squamous ulceration than those solely in training.[7,10] In some studies of horses in race training, neither prevalence nor severity of ulceration was associated with age or sex,[9,10,78] whereas in others ulcer severity increased with age.[7,91]

Lesions occur predominantly in the squamous mucosa, particularly adjacent to the margo plicatus, but glandular and antral involvement has become increasingly apparent.[9,23] In severe cases lesions can extend dorsally into the squamous fundus. Clinically relevant lesions typically affect a greater portion of the squamous mucosa and can be deep enough to cause bleeding, but a correlation between lesion severity and clinical signs is often not apparent. Bleeding from ulcers in the gastric squamous mucosa is typically not associated with anemia or hypoproteinemia.

Diagnosis

Although a diagnosis of EGUS can be suspected on the basis of clinical signs and response to treatment, the only current method of confirmation is gastroendoscopy, which can easily be performed in the standing horse or foal with mild sedation. In adult horses a 3-meter endoscope allows for visual inspection of the entire stomach, pylorus, and proximal duodenum. Shorter scopes will permit examination of the gastric body and fundus but not the pyloric antrum in most cases. Recent work detailing the prevalence of glandular and antral disease, often in the absence of squamous disease, underscores the importance of performing a thorough examination. A maximum external diameter of 9 mm should be used for neonatal foals. Numerous scoring systems for lesion severity have been described, but a recent consensus has been published by the Equine Gastric Ulcer Council[2] (Table 15-9). This system appears to be accurate and more user-friendly than previous systems.[92] Urine[93] and blood[94] sucrose absorption testing have recently been evaluated as a measure of gastric mucosal permeability in horses with EGUS. Also, serum α_1-antitrypsin was detectable more frequently in foals with gastric ulceration than normal foals.[95] These blood tests may provide economical, less invasive screening tools, but further evaluation of sensitivity and specificity is necessary before widespread use.

TABLE 15-9

Equine Gastric Ulcer Syndrome Lesion Scoring System[2]

Lesion Grade	Description
Grade 0	Intact epithelium with no appearance of hyperemia or hyperkeratosis
Grade 1	Intact mucosa with areas of reddening or hyperkeratosis (squamous)
Grade 2	Small single or multifocal lesions
Grade 3	Large single or multifocal lesions or extensive superficial lesions
Grade 4	Extensive lesions with areas of deep ulceration

Duodenal ulceration can be difficult to confirm. Duodenoscopy is the most specific means of diagnosis, although the procedure is more difficult than gastroscopy. Additionally, an endoscope at least 200 cm in length is needed for foals up to 5 to 7 months old, and a longer endoscope usually is required for older animals. Diffuse reddening or inflammation may be the only recognizable lesion in cases of early duodenal disease. In older foals with GDUD, detection of gastric outflow obstruction is critical to the therapeutic plan and appropriate prognosis. Abdominal radiography without contrast in foals with outflow obstruction typically reveals a distinctly enlarged, gas-filled stomach. Liquid barium contrast will either have markedly delayed (with incomplete obstruction) or no (complete obstruction) outflow. Clinically, foals with outflow obstruction will develop reflux after suckling or marked reflux even with limited to no suckling if the duodenal obstruction is distal to the common bile duct.

Treatment

Multiple pharmacologic treatments have been suggested for the treatment of EGUS. Because acid has been implicated as the most important pathophysiologic component of squamous ulcer disease, most anti-ulcer therapy centers on suppression or neutralization of gastric acid. Severity and location of gastric lesions and severity and duration of clinical signs as well as medication cost can play a role in the therapeutic management of EGUS (Table 15-10).

If gastroendoscopy is unavailable, some guidelines to therapy can be employed, but the efficacy of the treatment will be based on clinical signs, which are often vague or nonspecific. Signs of colic or diarrhea that result from gastric ulcers often resolve within 48 hours. Improvements in appetite, bodily condition, and attitude can be noted within 1 to 3 weeks. If improvement in clinical signs is not observed, either treatment has not been effective or gastric ulceration was not the primary problem. Typically, a treatment period of at least 2 to 4 weeks, followed by prophylaxis depending on the animal's exercise and environmental status, is recommended.

The principal therapeutic options for ulcer treatment include H_2 antagonists (cimetidine, ranitidine, famotidine, nizatidine), proton pump inhibitors (PPIs; omeprazole, pantoprazole, rabeprazole, esomeprazole), the mucosal adherent sucralfate, and antacids.

The H_2 antagonists suppress hydrochloric acid secretion through competitive inhibition of the parietal cell histamine receptor that can be partially overcome with exogenous pentagastrin.[96] Use of H_2 antagonists has been successful in raising gastric pH and resolving gastric lesions in both foals and adult horses.[44,85,97] Clinical and experimental evidence has demonstrated greater individual variability with lower dosages of H_2 antagonists.[98] Thus dosage recommendations are based on levels necessary to increase gastric pH and promote ulcer healing in a majority of horses. Commonly recommended dosages are 20 to 30 mg/kg orally every 8 hours or 6.6 mg/kg intravenously every 6 hours for cimetidine and 6.6 mg/kg orally every 8 hours or 1.5 to 2 mg/kg intravenously every 6 hours for ranitidine. Famotidine has been used less extensively in the horse, but a dose of 10 to 15 mg/kg/day has been recommended. Although clinically normal foals respond predictably to ranitidine,[44] sick neonates have shown variability in pH response to intravenous ranitidine, with a much shorter duration of action and, in some cases, no noticeable response.[45] Currently, cimetidine and ranitidine are available in injectable, tablet, and liquid forms. Famotidine and nizatidine are available in tablets. Omeprazole appears more effective for ulcer healing than either ranitidine or cimetidine.[99,100]

PPIs block secretion of H^+ at the parietal cell membrane by irreversibly binding to the H^+, K^+-ATPase proton pump of the cell. These agents have a prolonged antisecretory effect, which allows for once-daily dosing. Omeprazole, the first PPI to be developed, is the only currently approved agent for the treatment of EGUS. Several studies have documented the safety of oral omeprazole in foals and adult horses.[101,102] Omeprazole has demonstrated efficacy in the healing of NSAID-induced ulcers in horses as well naturally occurring cases of EGUS.[103,104] Omeprazole has been shown to eliminate or reduce the severity of gastric ulcers in Thoroughbreds maintained in race training.[105] The available equine preparation of omeprazole (GastroGard™, Merial, Ltd., Duluth, GA) is recommended at a dose of 4 mg/kg orally every 24 hours for ulcer healing (Figures 15-18 to 15-20). An increase in gastric pH and a decrease in acid output are evident 5 to 8 hours after omeprazole paste

TABLE 15-10

Therapeutic Options for the Treatment of Equine Gastric Ulcer System

Drug	Dose (mg/kg)	Dosing Interval (hours)	Route of Administration
Ranitidine	6.6	8	PO
Ranitidine	1.5-2	6	IV, IM
Cimetidine	20-25	8	PO
Cimetidine	6.6	6	IV, IM
Omeprazole	0.5	24	IV
Omeprazole	1-2 (prevention)	24	PO
Omeprazole	4 (treatment)	24	PO
Pantoprazole	1.5	24	IV, PO
Sucralfate	20-40	8	PO

PO, Per os (by mouth); *IV,* intravenous; *IM,* intramuscular.

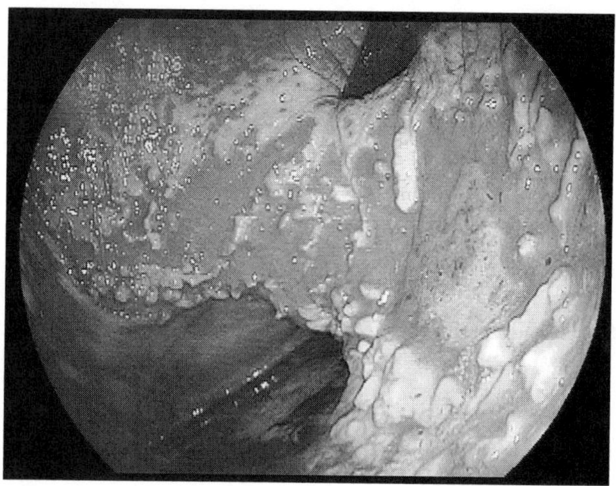

FIGURE 15-18 Endoscopic image of the lesser curvature of the stomach in a 17-year-old Quarter Horse diagnosed with severe gastric ulceration.

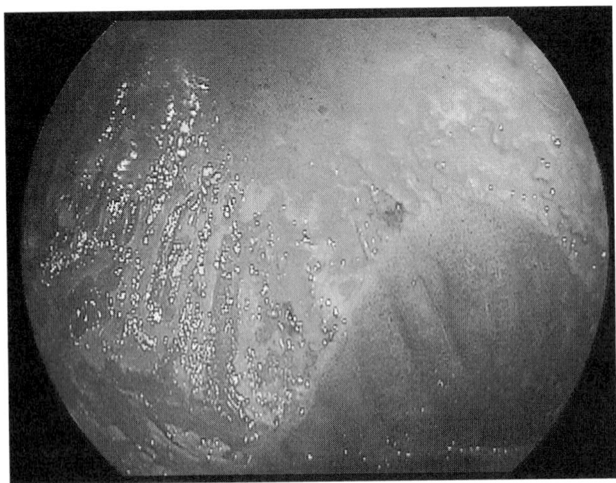

FIGURE 15-19 Greater curvature viewed endoscopically in the horse depicted in Figure 15-18.

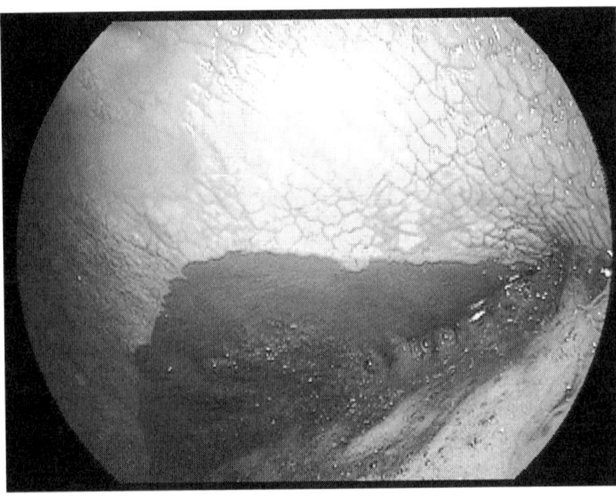

FIGURE 15-20 Endoscopic image of the greater curvature in the horse depicted in Figures 15-18 and 15-19 after 1 week of omeprazole (4 mg/kg PO every 24 hours) therapy.

administration.[106] Treatment with 1, 2, or 4 mg/kg orally every 24 hours has been shown to decrease or prevent disease or the recurrence of disease in animals maintained in training.[67,107-109] Omeprazole (4 mg/kg) also has demonstrated efficacy in raising intragastric pH in clinically normal[110] or critically ill[111] foals and in ulcer healing in foals.[103]

Because the powder form of omeprazole is rapidly degraded in an acidic environment, an enteric-coated capsule (as used in the human preparation) or a specially formulated paste must be used to allow delivery of the active drug to the small intestine for absorption. Compounded preparations have shown limited to no efficacy in pharmacodynamic and clinical trials,[112,113] and the proprietary formulation of omeprazole was the only product (including buffers, H_2-receptor antagonists, sucralfate, and compounded preparations) that decreased the odds of gastric ulceration in a population of racehorses.[114] Omeprazole appears to be more effective in ulcer healing than either ranitidine or cimetidine.[99,100] A compounded intravenous preparation of omeprazole (0.5 mg/kg) increases gastric juice pH and decreases the number of nonglandular lesions in horses.[115] From a regulatory standpoint, omeprazole (4 mg/kg/day orally) does not appear to affect quantitative measurements of performance in Standardbreds.[116]

Other PPIs have been recently developed for use in humans, including rabeprazole, lansoprazole, esomeprazole, and pantoprazole. In the treatment of GERD in humans, esomeprazole has demonstrated a higher rate of healing at 4 and 8 weeks when compared with omeprazole, but rabeprazole, lansoprazole, and pantoprazole have similar efficacy.[117] Pantoprazole given by either intravenous or intragastric routes (1.5 mg/kg) raised intragastric pH in clinically normal neonatal foals.[118]

Sucralfate is effective in the treatment of peptic ulcers and prevention of so-called stress-induced ulcers in humans. The mechanism of action likely involves adherence to ulcerated mucosa, stimulation of mucus secretion, enhanced prostaglandin E synthesis, and increased concentration of growth factor at the site of ulceration, although the prostaglandin effects may not play an important role in ulcer healing.[119] These are all factors relevant to glandular mucosa, and the efficacy of sucralfate in treating ulcers in the equine gastric squamous mucosa remains undetermined. In one study sucralfate did not promote subclinical ulcer healing in foals, relative to corn syrup.[120] In another, simultaneous sucralfate administration significantly reduced the total area of oral ulceration and gastric epithelial necrosis experimentally induced by phenylbutazone but did not significantly reduce the number of squamous or glandular ulcers in foals.[121] In humans sucralfate provides protection against stress-induced ulcers with a decreased risk of pathogenic gastric colonization.[122] Sucralfate should be given at a dosage of 10 to 20 mg/kg every 6 to 8 hours. The efficacy of sucralfate in an alkaline pH is controversial but appears likely.[123-125]

The use of antacids in the treatment of gastric ulcers has not been critically examined in the horse. Research in horses has shown that 30g aluminum hydroxide/15 g magnesium hydroxide will result in an increase in gastric pH above 4 for approximately 2 hours.[126] Thus, although antacids may be useful for the treatment of ulcers in horses, a dose of approximately 180 to 200 ml at least every 4 hours is necessary for a standard adult horse.

The use of synthetic prostaglandin E_1 analogs, such as misoprostol, has been effective in the treatment of gastric and duodenal ulcers in humans, and the proposed mechanism of action involves both inhibition of gastric acid secretion and mucosal cytoprotection.[127] In horses misoprostol (5 μg/kg) increases gastric pH[128] and ameliorates deleterious effects of flunixin on mucosal recovery after ischemic injury in vitro.[129] Misoprostol is contraindicated in pregnant mares.

Prokinetic drugs should be considered in foals with duodenal disease, gastroesophageal reflux, and when delayed gastric emptying without a physical obstruction is suspected. Bethanechol and erythromycin increase the rate of gastric emptying in horses.[130] In cases of acute gastric atony, bethanechol 0.025 to 0.030 mg/kg, administered subcutaneously every 3 to 4 hours, has been effective in promoting gastric motility and emptying, followed by oral maintenance dosages of 0.35 to 0.45 mg/kg three to four times daily. Adverse effects can include diarrhea, inappetence, salivation, and colic, but at the dosages stated, adverse effects have been infrequent and mild. A complete review of ileus and prokinetic therapy is available elsewhere in this chapter.

For foals with severe GDUD that have developed duodenal stricture, surgical therapy is necessary.[84,131] These animals require a serious financial commitment because intensive perioperative medical therapy is critical for a successful outcome. Prognosis in two recent abstracts has improved over that previously reported. In one, 98% of surgically treated foals survived to discharge from the hospital, with 68% survival 8 months following discharge from the hospital.[132] In that study, of the surviving Thoroughbreds of racing age, 71% had started a race. In another, short-term survival was reported as 80% for those foals treated surgically and 50% for those treated medically.[133] A variety of nutraceuticals are currently marketed for the treatment and prevention of EGUS, but as of this writing no objective data are available regarding their efficacy.

Prevention

Because gastric perforation resulting from glandular ulcer disease has been reported in hospitalized neonates, many clinicians routinely use prophylactic anti-ulcer therapy in this population. Because some critically ill foals have a predominantly alkaline gastric pH profile, and because gastric acidity may be protective against bacterial translocation in neonates, the need for prophylactic ulcer therapy is controversial. In critically ill human neonates, although intravenous ranitidine therapy raises gastric pH and gastric bacterial colonization, it does not increase the risk of sepsis.[134] In a retrospective study of 85 hospitalized foals younger than 30 days of age, no difference in the frequency of gastric ulceration at necropsy was found between those foals that received prophylactic treatment for gastric ulcers and those that did not.[82] Because of the retrospective nature of that study, specific details regarding lesion location and severity were not available; however, none of the foals in the study died as a result of gastric ulcer disease. Thus many clinicians no longer recommend routine ulcer prophylaxis in all ill neonates. Possible exceptions include foals requiring significant doses of NSAIDs for painful orthopedic disorders.

In adults dietary and environmental management can help prevent gastric ulceration. Pasture turnout and continuous access to high-quality forage, especially alfalfa, are currently recommended. For horses at high risk, the best proven pharmacologic approach to prevention involves administration of omeprazole (1 to 2 mg/kg orally every 24 hours).[100,107-109]

OTHER DISORDERS OF THE STOMACH

Pyloric Obstruction and Delayed Gastric Emptying

Pyloric stenosis is a structural resistance to gastric outflow. Congenital pyloric stenosis has been reported in foals and one yearling and results from hypertrophy of the pyloric musculature.[135-137] Acquired pyloric stenosis can result from neoplasia or duodenal ulceration.[138-141] Clinical signs depend on the degree of obstruction but include abdominal pain, salivation, and teeth grinding. Complete or near-complete obstruction can result in gastric reflux and reflux esophagitis. In foals with congenital pyloric hypertrophy, clinical signs may begin with the consumption of solid feed. In foals a presumptive diagnosis can be made using gastric endoscopy and radiography (plain and contrast studies). Depending on the cause and severity of disease, gastric endoscopy may provide a presumptive diagnosis in the adult horse. Measurement of gastric emptying can aid the diagnosis. Several methods of measurement are currently available, including nuclear scintigraphy, acetaminophen absorption, and postconsumption [^{13}C]-octanoic acid blood or breath testing.[130,142,143] During an exploratory laparotomy, a distended stomach and thickened pylorus are accompanied by a relatively empty intestinal tract.

If complete obstruction is not present, medical therapy with a prokinetic such as bethanecol can increase the rate of gastric emptying.[130] Phenylbutazone and cisapride have also been shown to attenuate the delay in gastric emptying caused by endotoxin administration.[142,144] Surgical repair is necessary for definitive treatment of complete or near-complete obstruction and consists of either gastroenterostomy or pyloroplasty.[84,131] Pyloric-duodenal intussusception has been reported in an adult horse with colic.[145]

Gastric Dilation and Rupture

Gastric dilation can be classified as primary, secondary, or idiopathic. Causes of primary gastric dilation include gastric impaction, grain engorgement, excessive water intake after exercise, aerophagia, and parasitism.[141,146] Secondary gastric dilation is more common and can result from primary intestinal ileus or small or large intestinal obstruction. Time to development of gastric reflux is proportional to the distance to the intestinal segment involved, with duodenal obstruction resulting in reflux within 4 hours.[147] Clinical signs of gastric dilation include those associated with acute colic and, in severe cases, ingesta appearing at the nares. Associated laboratory abnormalities include hemoconcentration, hypokalemia, and hypochloremia.[141]

The most common cause of gastric rupture in horses varies between reports. In a retrospective study of 54 horses, gastric rupture occurred most commonly as a secondary phenomenon (65%), usually caused by small intestinal obstruction, with primary gastric dilation and idiopathic rupture occurring almost equally (15% and 17%, respectively).[146] In another retrospective study of 50 horses in combination with a search of the Veterinary Medical Database, 60% of the gastric rupture cases were classified as idiopathic.[148] Risk factors for gastric rupture include feeding grass hay, not feeding grain, gelding, and a nonautomatic water source.[146,148] Nasogastric intubation does not preclude the possibility of gastric rupture, and the amount of reflux obtained before rupture is highly variable.[146] Because of the retrospective nature of these reports, one cannot rule out confounding factors with certainty.

Regardless of the initiating cause, gastric rupture usually occurs along the greater curvature. In horses with rupture resulting from gastric dilation, tears in the seromuscular layer are frequently larger than the corresponding tears in the mucosal layer, indicating that the seromuscularis likely weakens and tears before the mucosa.[146,148] In contrast, horses with gastric rupture secondary to gastric ulceration usually demonstrate full-thickness tears of equal size in all layers. Gastric rupture is usually fatal because of the widespread contamination of the peritoneal cavity, septic peritonitis, and septic shock. Initial clinical signs vary with the primary disease; however, when rupture occurs, horses that had been in pain may exhibit signs of relief. Subsequent signs, including tachypnea, tachycardia, sweating, and muscle fasciculations are consistent with peritonitis and shock. Surgical repair is thus limited but has been reported for partial-thickness tears[149] and, in one case of a combined tear of the mucosa and muscularis with only a focal serosal tear, a full-thickness repair was performed with a favorable outcome.[150]

Gastric Impaction

Gastric impaction can result in either acute or chronic signs of colic in the horse. Although a specific cause is not always evident, ingestion of coarse roughage (e.g., straw bedding, poor-quality forage), foreign objects (e.g., rubber fencing material), and feed that may swell after ingestion or improper mastication (e.g., persimmon seeds, mesquite beans, wheat, barley, sugar beet pulp) have been implicated.[151-154] Possible predisposing factors include poor dentition, poor mastication and rapid consumption of feedstuffs, and inadequate water consumption. Clinical signs vary, from anorexia and weight loss to those consistent with severe abdominal pain. In severe cases spontaneous reflux may occur, with gastric contents visible at the nares. If the horse suffers from acute severe abdominal pain, a diagnosis is often made during exploratory celiotomy. In horses that do not exhibit signs of colic warranting surgical intervention, an endoscopic finding of a full stomach after a normally adequate fast (18 to 24 hours) can often confirm the diagnosis. Abdominal radiographs are reserved for smaller horses and ponies. In addition to pain management, specific treatment consists of gastric lavage via nasogastric intubation or massage and injection of fluid to soften the impaction during laparotomy.[151-153]

Miscellaneous Causes of Gastritis

Nonulcerative gastritis rarely appears to be a clinical problem in the horse, but it has been reported at necropsy in a large retrospective study.[17] Emphysematous gastritis caused by *Clostridium perfringens*[155] and *Clostridium septicum*[156] has been reported.

DUODENTITIS-PROXIMAL JEJUNITIS

Laura H. Javsicas

Duodenitis-proximal jejunitis (DPJ) is an inflammatory condition affecting the upper small intestine and resulting in distention, abdominal pain, gastric reflux caused by excessive fluid and electrolyte secretion, and increased PF protein concentration without a significant elevated nucleated cell count. Other terms for this condition are *anterior enteritis* and *proximal enteritis*. Clinical signs of DPJ mimic those of a small intestinal obstruction; thus distinguishing between the two syndromes is important. The clinical syndrome of DPJ was well described in the 1980s,[1-4] but the severity of clinical signs, especially duration of disease, is variable. Although not typical, DPJ can occur in conjunction with gastritis, ileitis, typhlitis, and colitis.

PATHOPHYSIOLOGY

Typical pathologic findings in horses with DPJ include involvement of the duodenum and usually the proximal jejunum.[4] The ileum and large colon usually are determined to be grossly normal. Gastric distention is a common finding and is thought to be caused by hypersecretory mechanisms in the proximal small intestine and a functional ileus of affected enteric segments. The small intestine may be 5 to 7 cm in diameter because of fluid distention with malodorous, red to brown-red intraluminal fluid accumulation. Duodenal (and jejunal) serosal surfaces may have varying degrees and distribution of bright red to dark red petechial and ecchymotic hemorrhages and yellow to white streaks. The enteric mucosal surfaces are usually hyperemic and have varying degrees of petechiation and ulceration.

Microscopically, the most severe lesions have been located in the duodenum and proximal jejunum but may extend proximally to the gastric mucosa and aborally to the large intestinal mucosa and submucosa.[4] Microscopic lesions consist of varying degrees of mucosal and submucosal hyperemia and edema. More severe lesions include villous degeneration with necrosis and, more severely, sloughing of villous epithelium. The lamina propria, mucosa, and submucosa may have varying degrees of granulocyte infiltration (predominantly neutrophils), and the muscular layers and serosal surfaces contain small hemorrhages. Proximal small intestinal serosal fibrinopurulent exudate is a common finding in the more severe cases; therefore the term *hemorrhagic fibrinonecrotic duodenitis-proximal jejunitis* has been suggested as a more descriptive name for this syndrome.

Horses with DPJ often have evidence of multiple organ involvement and can have hepatic changes including hepatocellular vacuolization, cholestasis, inflammatory infiltrate (either in association with centrilobular necrosis or periportal), and biliary hyperplasia.[5] Hepatic disease is thought to result from ascending infection by way of the common bile duct, local absorption of endotoxin via the portal circulation, systemic consequences of endotoxin absorption, metabolic imbalances such as acidemia, and hypoperfusion or hypovolemia.

In most cases an underlying etiology cannot be determined. In some cases *Salmonella* spp. or *Clostridium* spp. can be isolated from culture of gastric reflux. Salmonellosis has never been consistently identified in a majority of cases, and many horses with documented infections by these organisms do not develop DPJ. Recently, toxigenic strains of *Clostridium difficile* were isolated from the reflux of five out of five horses with DPJ and none of six control horses with other causes of nasogastric reflux.[6] Further investigation of this organism is clearly warranted. Another suspected infectious agent is *Fusarium* spp.[7] A recent dietary change with an abrupt increase in dietary concentrate level has been suggested to predispose a horse to developing DPJ because of intraluminal microbial imbalances. Feeding and grazing practices have been shown to be different between horses with DPJ and those with other forms of colic or lameness. In one report horses with DPJ were fed significantly more grain and were more likely to have grazed pasture, but these associations were not deemed strong enough to allow clinical application to differentiate DPJ from other causes of colic.[8]

Two intracellular processes control intestinal secretion: the cyclic nucleotide (cyclic adenosine monophosphate and cyclic guanosine monophosphate) and calcium systems.[9] Inflammatory mediators, microorganisms, and toxins can activate adenyl cyclase (vasoactive intestinal peptide, prostaglandin E_2) or guanyl cyclase (bacterial enterotoxins) and induce increases in cyclic adenosine monophosphate and cyclic guanosine monophosphate, respectively. This reaction causes phosphorylation of specific protein kinases, which induce the actual mucosal membrane transport events. Increases in intracellular free calcium may arise from cyclic nucleotide-dependent release of stored calcium within the cell or from increased calcium entry across the cell membrane. Calcium may act through calmodulin, which then can activate membrane-phosphorylating protein kinases. The net effect is increased movement of sodium and chloride into the mucosal cell from the interstitium, with secretion of sodium and chloride into the intestinal lumen. Water follows the directional flux of sodium and chloride through highly permeable intercellular spaces. Several bacterial toxins and endogenous mediators can cause active secretion and contribute to a synergistic mucosal secretory response. Passive secretion of protein-rich fluid into the lumen occurs after damage to the mucosal epithelium, capillary endothelium, and submucosal inflammation in the proximal small intestine. The clinically relevant events that result from active and passive fluid secretion are proximal small intestinal distention and nasogastric reflux, dehydration, and circulatory shock.[10]

The concentration of protein in the PF from horses with DPJ is usually higher than in horses with small intestinal obstruction. A disproportionate increase in total protein concentration relative to nucleated cell count occurs, probably by leakage of blood or plasma into the peritoneal cavity without a significant stimulus for leukocyte chemotaxis. Suggested mechanisms for increased abdominal fluid protein concentration include serositis associated with inflamed intestine and small intestinal distention causing passive congestion and increased capillary hydrostatic pressure of visceral peritoneal vessels.[11] Small intestinal ileus is another hallmark sign of DPJ, and the pathophysiology is complicated, involving primary and secondary dysfunction of the central, autonomic, and enteric nervous systems and their purported roles in governing intestinal motility. Primary role players in DPJ-associated ileus include peritoneal inflammation, inflammatory cell migration/activation within the muscularis, small intestinal mechanical distention, and endotoxin absorption. Further detail regarding the effect of inflammation on small intestinal motility is provided elsewhere in this chapter.

CLINICAL AND CLINICOPATHOLOGIC SIGNS

The veterinarian has the challenge of differentiating horses with DPJ from horses with small intestinal obstructive lesions so as to avoid surgical intervention. Although there are differences between DPJ and small intestinal obstructive lesions, there is no single distinguishing feature and all information must be considered collectively. Horses with obstructive lesions of the small intestine usually show consistent signs of abdominal pain until the affected viscus is repaired surgically or ruptures. In contrast, signs of acute abdominal pain typically subside after gastric decompression and volume replacement in horses with DPJ. They are replaced by signs of lethargy and general malaise. On rectal examination the degree of small intestinal distention may be subjectively less with DPJ than with obstructive lesions, particularly following gastric decompression. Although the color and odor of gastric reflux can be similar, horses with DPJ tend to have a larger volume (≥4 to 20 L with each decompressive effort) of reflux than horses with obstructive lesions. Horses with DPJ often have a temperature of 38.6° to 39.1° C (101.5° to 102.5° F), whereas horses with obstructive lesions are typically normothermic or hypothermic. DPJ-affected horses typically are dehydrated and have brick-red mucous membranes, lethargy, decreased to absent borborygmi, prolonged capillary refill time, tachycardia (≥60 beats/min), and tachypnea.

Typical clinical laboratory findings include an increased packed cell volume and total plasma protein reflective of volume depletion and a normal, decreased, or increased peripheral white blood cell count.[1,4] Abnormalities in the leukogram are more common in horses with DPJ than with an acute obstructive lesion. In addition, hyponatremia, hypochloremia, hypokalemia, prerenal azotemia, and elevated hepatic enzymes (γ-glutamyl transferase [GGT], alanine transaminase [AST], and alkaline phosphatase [AP]) are often evident.[5] The loss of enteric bicarbonate through evacuation of enterogastric reflux and hyperlactemia from poor tissue perfusion and hypovolemia can lead to metabolic acidosis with a high anion gap.

PF analysis may be helpful in distinguishing DPJ from an obstructive lesion. The typical findings with DPJ include an increased PF protein concentration (often ≥3.5 g/dl) and a mild to moderate elevation of the peritoneal white blood cell count, although the count usually is less than 10,000 cells per microliter. The disproportionate increase in PF total protein compared with peritoneal nucleated cell count may be due to leakage of blood or plasma without a marked leucotactic response.[4] The PF is usually yellow and turbid, but in severe cases diapedesis can occur, resulting in a serosanguinous color. Strangulating lesions typically result in more severe changes in the PF. Serosanguinous PF with increased protein, white blood cells, and red blood cells is typical. Horses with intraluminal obstructions such as ileal impactions typically have grossly normal PF with a mildly elevated protein resulting from intestinal distention.[1,4,10]

Abdominal ultrasound findings can help support a diagnosis of DPJ and allow evaluation of the small intestinal diameter and wall thickness as well as the PF volume and character. Ultrasonographic findings in horses with DPJ typically include gastric distention, duodenal distention, and segments of small intestine containing hypoechoic to anechoic fluid. The wall of the small intestine can be normal or thickened with time. Peristalis can be decreased, normal, or increased. Differentiation from a small intestinal obstructive lesion remains difficult. More long-standing obstructions typically result in increased wall thickness, sedimentation of ingesta within the small intestinal lumen, and distended small intestine proximal to the lesion with collapsed intestine distally.[12,13]

A definitive diagnosis of DPJ is made in most cases by gross examination of the duodenum and proximal jejunum at surgery or at necropsy, but the diagnosis is typically suspected on the basis of clinical and clinicopathologic signs and response to therapy.

TREATMENT

Horses with DPJ appear to share a common characteristic clinical presentation, and the mechanisms leading to electrolyte imbalances, fluid loss, ileus, and endotoxemia and septicemia are similar. Treatment regimens are supportive and provide plasma volume replacement, analgesic and anti-inflammatory therapy, gastric decompression, anti-endotoxin therapy, antimicrobial therapy if indicated, nutritional support, and nursing care.

Gastric Decompression

Although the signs of abdominal pain usually resolve after gastric decompression, most horses remain severely lethargic. Without periodic removal of fluid that accumulates in the proximal intestinal tract, signs of abdominal pain usually recur. Horses with DPJ often require gastric decompression at 2-hour intervals, with 2 to 10 L of fluid recovered each time. Nasogastric tubes left in place for long periods cause varying degrees of pharyngitis (Figure 15-21), laryngitis, and esophagitis, and maintenance of an indwelling nasogastric tube may further delay gastric emptying.[10,14,15]

Fluid Support

Aggressive intravenous polyionic fluid therapy should be instituted immediately in a horse with suspected DPJ. The veterinarian should calculate the total fluid deficit on the basis of clinical assessment of dehydration (e.g., for 8% or moderate dehydration, 0.08 × 450 kg body mass = 36 L) and should administer replacement fluids rapidly (up to 6 to 10 L per hour for a 450-kg adult horse). Placement of a second, large-bore (10- or 12- gauge) intravenous catheter can aid in rapid administration of large volumes of fluid during the initial resuscitation. Administering intravenous hypertonic saline (7%) may be useful to treat hypovolemic shock in horses with severe circulatory shock. The use of 1 to 2 L of hypertonic saline (7% NaCl) improved cardiac output in horses with hemorrhagic shock and in a model of equine endotoxemia.[16,17] If this treatment option is chosen, intravenous administration of replacement isotonic fluids must follow immediately to maintain tissue integrity. Horses with significant volumes of gastric reflux should not be allowed to ingest foodstuffs or liquids orally.

Once replacement fluids have been administered and the horse is well hydrated, one should administer maintenance fluid amounts, which may be as high as 120 ml/kg/day. Unfortunately, the intravenous fluid therapy itself may accelerate the flux of fluid from the vasculature into the intestinal lumen because of a reduction in intravascular oncotic pressure and an increased capillary perfusion pressure, which can result in an increased volume of gastrointestinal reflux. However, the veterinarian should not consider reducing the volume of intravenous fluid therapy because excessive fluid losses continue to occur. One should monitor plasma protein concentration, overall hydration, and the volume of reflux and then determine the rate of intravenous fluid administration. Ongoing fluid losses should be calculated by measuring the volume of net reflux in a graduated bucket. Close monitoring of "ins and outs" allows adjustment of the rate of fluid administration to ensure that adequate volumes are given to account for correction of the initial fluid deficit, maintenance requirements, and ongoing losses from reflux. The clinical response, as measured by improved hydration status, decreased nasogastric reflux, improved attitude, and improvement in values reflecting kidney function (decreased blood urea nitrogen and creatinine), correlates with improvement of intestinal damage.

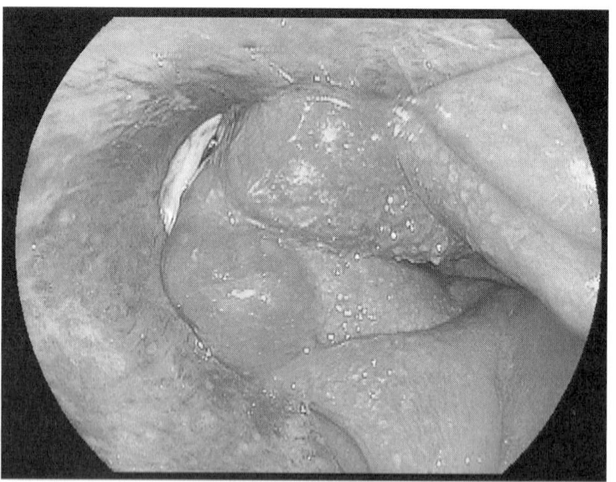

FIGURE 15-21 Endoscopic image from a 15-year-old Quarter Horse gelding. The horse was diagnosed with duodenitis-proximal jejunitis (DPJ) and developed mild respiratory stridor and gagging and wretching behavior after an indwelling nasogastric tube had been in place for 48 hours to allow for intermittent drainage of gastric reflux. The horse responded well to medical therapy for DPJ and pharyngitis-esophagitis.

Oncotic Support

Horses with DPJ that continue to reflux large volumes of enterogastric fluid frequently for more than 36 to 48 hours may experience protein loss from the inflamed and disrupted intestinal mucosal barrier and from systemic protein catabolism. Decreased colloid oncotic pressure leads to decreased effective circulating fluid volume and edema. Total plasma protein may decline to below 4 g/dl, and the albumin may decrease to below 2.0 g/dl. Fresh or thawed frozen plasma is ideal for replacement of functional proteins. One should consider treatment with intravenous plasma therapy or a combination of plasma and synthetic colloid (e.g., hydroxyethyl starch (Hetastarch [6%], Abbott Laboratories, North Chicago, Illinois) as soon as a consistent decline in total plasma protein or albumin is evident or if the horse is developing dependent edema. Fresh plasma (preferred) or fresh frozen plasma is the treatment of choice if coagulation disorders accompany protein loss. An average-size horse (450 kg) requires 6 to 10 L of plasma (albumin 3.0 g/dl) or synthetic colloid to improve plasma oncotic pressure. Administration of additional aliquots of 2 to 10 L of a balanced colloidal solution may be necessary if the DPJ crisis continues. In addition to albumin (the major colloid component), plasma contains other components that provide overall systemic support (e.g., fibronectins, complement inhibitors, elastase and proteinase inhibitors, antithrombin III). One may administer a 6% solution of hydroxyethyl starch at 5 to 10 ml/kg/day. Because of the large size of the starch molecules, this solution is an effective plasma volume expander, resulting in sustained dose-dependent decreases in packed cell volume and plasma protein concentration with increased oncotic pressure. The cost of an appropriate amount of commercial plasma or synthetic colloid solution for treatment of adult horses with DPJ may be prohibitive but can be life saving.

Anti-endotoxin

Horses with enteritis frequently absorb large amounts of endotoxin from the disrupted intestinal mucosal barrier, thereby putting these horses at a high risk for laminitis. One should monitor digital pulses frequently until systemic signs of enteritis have abated (e.g., fever, leukopenia) and even for several days beyond this point. Treatment to combat endotoxemia is critical, and several therapeutic approaches are available. Choice of treatment options is based on severity of disease, renal function, hydration status, and economics. Endotoxemia and systemic inflammatory response syndrome are discussed elsewhere in this chapter.

Anti-inflammatory and Analgesic

NSAIDs are the most frequently used group of drugs for treatment of abdominal pain in horses (flunixin meglumine 0.25-1.1 mg/kg intravenously every 8-12 hours, with the higher dose given only at the least frequent interval). These agents also have beneficial anti-inflammatory and anti-endotoxic effects. The clinician must weigh the benefit of these drugs against their negative effects on gastrointestinal mucosa and renal function. Another popular analgesic option is butorphanol, an opioid agonist-antagonist, given at 0.02 to 0.1 mg/kg intramuscularly every 6 to 8 hours or as a constant-rate infusion at 13 μg/kg/h.[18] This route appears to have minimal effects on gastrointestinal motility.

Antimicrobial

Because *Clostridium* spp. are suspected as a causative agent of DPJ, penicillin, metronidazole, or both are often administered to affected horses. However, the veterinarian should consider broad spectrum antimicrobial coverage for horses with DPJ and significant leukopenia. An aminoglycoside or enrofloxacin can be added to the penicillin therapy, although the potential adverse effects of aminoglycosides on renal function should be noted.

Nutritional Support

The veterinarian should consider the nutritional needs of horses with DPJ. Most horses have a total body protein loss on account of cachexia and a protein-losing enteropathy. Total parenteral nutrition may be indicated in horses that remain anorectic for more than 3 to 4 days. Parenterally administered solutions containing glucose, balanced amino acid solutions, lipid emulsions, balanced electrolyte and trace minerals, and vitamins have been administered to adult horses with small intestinal ileus or enterocolitis. Based on a small number of horses, this therapy has proved promising in terms of minimizing protein losses and decreasing the duration of illness. Postoperative parenteral nutrition ameliorates clinicopathologic evidence of starvation following small intestinal resection and anastamosis in adult horses.[19] Providing for part of the nutritional requirements of the horse (8000 to 12,000 kcal/day) is possible with glucose–amino acid solutions, which are of moderate cost. It is reasonable to suppose that providing nutritional support to an anorectic, severely ill horse will facilitate healing and even shorten the duration of illness. Thus the overall cost of providing parenteral nutritional supplementation to horses with DPJ may be offset by quicker recovery and diminished requirements for other, expensive treatments, but further data are necessary to accurately assess this point.

Prokinetics

Normal (healthy) intestine is necessary for optimal performance of most prokinetic agents in horses. Many motility-modifying agents likely are ineffective in cases of DPJ. Inflamed jejunal tissue has been shown to have downregulation and decreased production of motilin receptors, which may alter the prokinetic response to erythromycin.[20] However, some benefit may come of the judicious use of prokinetic agents in inflammatory conditions of the equine intestine, particularly if the agent provides additional effects such as analgesia. Lidocaine has shown particular promise for this use. Although the exact mechanism of action is unknown, the beneficial effects in horses with ileus are likely due to anti-inflammatory effects because a direct prokinetic effect has not been demonstrated.[21] In horses with nasogastric reflux attributable to postoperative ileus or enteritis, a constant-rate infusion of lidocaine was shown to reduce the hourly volume of reflux and shorten the time to cessation of reflux compared with saline.[22] A 2 mg/kg loading dose over 15 minutes followed by 50 μg/kg/min has been recommended.[23] Prokinetic therapy with erythromycin lactobionate, metaclopromide, or bethanechol can also be considered.[24,25] Motility-modifying agents and the influence of inflammation on their effects are discussed elsewhere in this chapter.

Surgical Therapy

Medical therapy is sufficient in most cases of DPJ, but in those cases in which the horse continues to produce copious enterogastric reflux despite aggressive medical treatment, or when a mechanical obstruction cannot be satisfactorily ruled out, surgery may be considered as an option. Refractory cases have improved with surgical intervention; however, some horses with refractory DPJ have been observed to recover after prolonged (up to 20 days) supportive care and gastric decompression. The decision as to when to intervene surgically often is difficult. Surgery may be necessary to determine the extent of gross pathologic condition and intestinal distention and to perform intestinal bypass so as to direct enterogastric reflux toward the cecum and colon. For a horse exhibiting abdominal discomfort with small intestinal distention palpable per rectum that produces more than 2 L of gastric reflux, the veterinarian should recommend referral to an appropriate surgical facility. Typically, the main determinants for surgical intervention are degree and duration of abdominal pain, PF analysis, and results of (often repeated) rectal palpation and ultrasonography.

Short-term mortality rates have been reported to be 37% for horses in which manual evacuation of the small intestine into the cecum was performed surgically, compared with 40% for horses that received medical treatment.[26] A 95% recovery rate was reported in horses with DPJ that underwent laparotomy and manual evacuation of the small intestine into the cecum, combined with treatment for *Clostridium perfringens* consisting of intravenous metrondiazole and intramuscular procaine penicillin.[27] Drawbacks of surgery include the expense, risks of anesthesia, prolonged return to training, and risk of incisional complications. However, when an obstruction cannot be ruled out, these concerns are of minor consequence.[10]

PROGNOSIS

Survival rates for DPJ range between 25%[2] to 94%.[1,4] At present the survival of horses with DPJ that undergo surgery is much greater than previously described, and certainly greater than that of horses with small intestinal obstruction that do not have surgery.[26,27] Horses with DPJ that receive appropriate therapy have a reasonably good chance of making a full recovery, and recurrence is rare. Horses that continue to have frequent episodes of voluminous nasogastric reflux and systemic signs of endotoxemia and septicemia have a poorer prognosis for recovery. Frequent complications of DPJ include laminitis, thrombophlebitis, and weight loss. In one study, survival was significantly less (45.5%) in horses that developed laminitis than in horses without laminitis (68.7%).[24] There appears to be geographic variation in the severity and prognosis for DPJ, with horses in the southeastern United States most severely affected.

DISEASES ASSOCIATED WITH MALABSORPTION AND MALDIGESTION

L. Chris Sanchez

Malabsorption and maldigestion are commonly recognized clinical problems in humans and small animals and documented clinical entities in horses. The term *malabsorption* implies impairment of digestive and absorptive processes arising from functional or structural disorders of the small intestine and related organs, including the pancreas, liver, and biliary tract. The condition can affect absorption of carbohydrates; proteins; fats; vitamins; minerals; and, to a lesser extent, water and electrolytes. In horses the resulting pathophysiologic changes may influence large intestinal function adversely through alterations in the substrate presented for fermentation or through direct infiltration of the large colon.

Differentiation among carbohydrate, protein, or fat malabsorption is not possible in the horse because of its herbivorous diet and the contribution of large intestinal functions. The rarity of pancreatic problems, such as exocrine pancreatic insufficiency, in horses along with their herbivorous diet makes maldigestion less problematic. However, maldigestion can certainly contribute to chronic weight loss in horses with severe infiltrative small intestinal disease and exacerbate diarrhea in the suckling foal through reduced intestinal bile salt concentrations from hepatic or ileal dysfunction.

Malabsorption is not synonymous with diarrhea, although diarrhea may be a feature. Adult horses rarely exhibit diarrhea with small intestinal problems unless large intestinal involvement is concomitant. Chronic diarrhea is predominantly a large intestinal disorder that reflects an overload of water and electrolytes and thus may be considered a state of impaired absorption. Primary small intestinal disease is more likely in neonates and young foals. For example, acquired small intestinal brush border lactase deficiency may result in increased lactose fermentation in the large intestine and induction of osmotic diarrhea.[1]

CLINICAL ASSESSMENT

Physical Examination

The principal concern of the owner is weight loss and poor condition of the horse. Many clinical examination findings, except for body condition, may appear within normal limits. Investigation of weight loss, with clinical pathologic findings, helps eliminate other, more commonly encountered causes of wasting.

Malabsorption is associated with pathologic conditions of the small intestine characterized by substantial reduction of the available absorptive surface area. By virtue of the extent of the morphologic changes, interference with digestive processes occurs, although maldigestion may be difficult to confirm in the absence of assessment measures. The small bowel problem may alter the composition and availability of substrate presented for fermentation in the large intestine. Clinical signs may be modified or accentuated if involvement of the large intestine is concomitant. Diarrhea indicates significant alterations in bidirectional fluid and electrolyte fluxes and in large intestinal transit.

Clinical Pathology

No characteristic clinical pathologic profile of malabsorption exists. The syndrome tends to cause anemia (normocytic, normochromic) and neutrophilia. Hemolytic or macrocytic anemia and thrombocytopenia have been observed in alimentary lymphosarcoma. Lymphocytosis (leukemia) rarely is encountered. Peripheral eosinophilia is uncommon even with widespread tissue eosinophilia. Many animals are hypoalbuminemic and hypoproteinemic; horses with alimentary lymphosarcoma may exhibit hyperproteinemia and hypergammaglobulinemia. Serum or plasma may be lipemic. The clinician may find elevated hepatic and biliary tract enzymes (γ-glutamyltransferase and alkaline phosphatase) in multisystemic conditions such as multisystemic eosinophilic epitheliotropic disease (MEED). Abdominocentesis can aid in the diagnosis of alimentary lymphosarcoma but rarely in the granulomatous conditions.

Table 15-11 lists the clinical and clinicopathologic features of the diseases most commonly associated with malabsorption.

Ultrasonography

Ultrasonographic examination of the abdomen can yield information on intestinal distention, wall thickness, and unexplained masses detected on rectal palpation. This can be helpful in the determination of small and large intestinal involvement. One should also note the amount and character of free PF and examine all abdominal organs in an effort to detect evidence of multisystemic involvement.

Gross and Microscopic Pathology

Rectal biopsy is easy to perform and may reveal cellular infiltration that could be present at more proximal locations. However, interpretation is frequently equivocal. In one retrospective study inflammatory bowel disease was diagnosed on the basis of rectal biopsy specimens in approximately 50% of cases.[2] In that report simple proctitis (neutrophils in the crypt or surface epithelium) was associated with inflammatory disorders, whereas only mild scattered neutrophil infiltration was seen in controls. Rectal biopsy aided in the diagnosis of three of seven horses with lymphocytic-plasmacytic enterocolitis[3] and one of two horses with eosinophilic enterocolitis.[4]

Table 15-12 presents the pathologic features of the diseases most commonly associated with malabsorption. In the same animal the extent and severity of pathologic changes vary in

TABLE 15-11

Predominant Clinical and Clinicopathologic Features of Horses with Proliferative and Inflammatory Bowel Diseases

Condition	Breed	Age Range	Clinical Signs	Dermatitis/ Coronitis	Hematology	Chemistry	Absorption Tests
Alimentary lymphosarcoma	None	2 yr to aged; Majority ≤4 yr	Weight loss, poor appetite, edema, depression, occadional fever, occasional diarrhea or colic	+ /– Scurfy skin	Anemia, neutrophilia; lymphocytosis rare	Decreased albumin; TP normal to increased; increased globulin	Reduced absorption; partial to complete mal-absorption
Granulomatous enteritis	Standardbred	1-6 yr; Majority ≤3 yr	Severe wasting, edema, variable appetite, depression, infrequent diarrhea, occasional slight fever	+ /– Scurfy skin; severe lesions rare	Anemia; Leukocytes normal to slightly increased or decreased	Decreased albumin; TP normal to decreased; GGT normal, ALP normal to increased	Reduced absorption; partial to complete mal-absorption
Multisystemic eosinophilic epitheliotropic disease	Standardbred, Thoroughbred	1 yr to aged; Majority ≤4 yr	Severe wasting, edema, appetite poor to ravenous, slight fever, diarrhea or soft feces common, rare colic, depression, oral ulcers	+ +++ Severe skin lesions and ulcerative coronitis prominent	Anemia rare to slight; neutrophilia and eosinophilia rare	Decreased albumin; TP normal to decreased; GGT and ALP normal to increased	Delayed absorption (peak shifted to right); reduced or normal peak concen-tration
Lymphocytic-plasmacytic enterocolitis	None	3 yr to aged	Inappetence, depression, colic, edema		Normal	Decreased albumin and TP; increased fibrinogen	Inadequate absorption or delayed peak
Proliferative enteropathy	None	3-8 months; sporadic reports older	Depression, colic, diarrhea, edema, appetite often normal, concurrent infection	+ /- Scurfy skin	Anemia, leukocytosis	Decreased albumin and TP; Increased CPK	Often normal

**GGT*, γ-Glutamyltransferase; *ALP*, alkaline phosphatase; *CPK*, creatine phosphokinase; *none, no* predominant breed.

TABLE 15-12

Pathologic Features of Proliferative and Inflammatory Bowel Diseases of Horses

Condition		Small Intestine	Large Intestine	Other Organs/Systems
Alimentary lymphosarcoma	G	**Constant**; extensive thickening, thickened mucosa, fissures, serosal plaques, nodules, congestion	**Infrequent**; unremarkable to thickened segments	MLNs massively enlarged; occasional enlargement of other LN
	H	Villous atrophy (partial to total); crypts disappear with hyperplasia; infiltrate of pleomorphic lymphoid cells, plasma cells; transmural	Nothing evident to diffuse mucosal infiltration	Extensive infiltration of MLNs; moderate in other LNs (liver, spleen, stomach rare)
Granulomatous enteritis	G	**Constant**; thickened wall and mucosa, fissures, widespread ulceration (tiny ulcers)	**Common**, generally discrete	MLNs enlarged, edematous; stomach commonly affected (generally discrete); liver/pancreas rare
	H	Villous atrophy (partial to total), crypt hyperplasia and abscesses, diffuse granulomatous inflammation; mononuclear cells (lymphoid), giant cells, epithelioid foci; lymphangiectasia	Similar infiltrate usually discrete; mucosa, submucoa	Similar infiltrate; stomach discrete; MLNs discrete to florid macrophage infiltration; diffuse cortical hyperplasia
Multisystemic eosinophilic epitheliotropic disease	G	**Common**; diffusely thickened, especially proximal duodenum and distal ileum; serosal nodules or granularity; ulceration	**Constant**; severe; segmental or multifocal granuloma; mucosal (predominantly) and transmural thickening; extensive ulcers	MLNs and other LNs enlarged; stomach and esophagus commonly affected; liver/pancreas commonly affected; may be hyperkeratotic; Skin: exudative dermatitis, ulcerative coronitis
	H	Villous atrophy rare; lymphocytic and eosinophilic infiltration most severe in cranial duodenum, ileum, ileocecal junction; infiltrate more widespread than gross lesions	Segmental/multifocal lesions, severe infiltration, reactive fibrosis, tissue eosinophilia, walled-off granulomata, central necrotic core of eosinophilic material	Similar infiltration with fibrosis of MLNs, liver, pancreas; skin: acanthosis, hyperkeratosis, diffuse infiltrate of eosinophils, lymphoctytes in dermis; focal eosinophilic accumulations
Lymphocytic-plasmacytic enterocolitis	G	**Constant**; mucosal/ submucosal edema; prominent folds	**Common**; edema, congestion, areas of mucosal ulceration	MLNs enlarged
	H	Villous blunting to atrophy; moderate to severe infiltration of lymphocytes, plasma cells; edema, dilated lymphatics	Similar infiltrate, less remarkable	Minimal evidence
Proliferative enteropathy	G	**Constant**; significant mucosal thickening, corrugated appearance from proximal jejunum to distal ileum	**Uncommon**; submucosal edema	MLNs unremarkable
	H	Villous shortening, severe hyperplasia of crypt epithelium, small curved bacteria in apical cytoplasm, mononuclear infiltrate	No evidence	No evidence

G, Gross pathologic findings; *H*, histopathologic findings; *MLNs*, mesenteric lymph nodes; *LNs*, lymph nodes

different regions of the small and large intestines, thus influencing the severity of clinical signs and abnormalities present, if any, in tests of intestinal function. Early diagnosis remains a challenge, and even multiple intestinal biopsies taken at exploratory laparotomy may prove unhelpful.

Biopsies of skin, liver, lymph node, or lung may reveal evidence of multisystemic disease and can easily be obtained in the standing horse, with organ biopsies typically obtained with ultrasonographic guidance. One can obtain intestinal and lymph node biopsies during a standing laparotomy. Exploratory laparotomy facilitates rigorous inspection of the gastrointestinal tract and associated organs to obtain multiple biopsies from intestinal sites and lymph nodes. Cost and potential postoperative complications may limit surgical procedures for diagnosis. Laparoscopy may provide an alternative means to facilitate biopsy of certain tissues but is typically more helpful from a diagnostic rather than a therapeutic standpoint. From this perspective, the veterinarian should consider surgical exploration as an option early in the process rather than as a last resort.

TESTS OF INTESTINAL FUNCTION

Intestinal function tests are a practical and inexpensive means to assess the absorptive capability of the small intestine. For clinical practice purposes this is limited to carbohydrate absorption tests, which are easy to perform. The noninvasive breath hydrogen test used to assess carbohydrate malabsorption in human beings has not proved reliable in equine studies.[5] Abnormality of carbohydrate absorption has become an important precept on which to base a diagnosis of malabsorption in the horse. However, results of the oral glucose tolerance test (OGTT) or D-xylose absorption test require cautious interpretation. Pathologic changes in the mucosa and submucosa must be extensive and widely distributed to greatly affect the peak plasma concentration and shape of the curve. Many commercial laboratories conduct xylose assays, and glucose concentrations are routinely monitored in most referral and many primary care facilities.

Oral Glucose Tolerance Test

The OGTT is typically performed by administering 1 g of glucose per kg of body weight as a 20% solution through a nasogastric tube following an overnight fast (14-16 hours).[6] Blood is collected into heparinized tubes before glucose administration and at 30-minute intervals for 180 minutes; if possible, the test is continued at 60-minute intervals until 360 minutes have elapsed. An alternative protocol is to continue sampling at 30-minute intervals for 240 minutes. Food is withheld during the sampling period, but water is allowed at all times. Maximum plasma glucose level (>85% baseline) is reached by 120 minutes in healthy horses.[6,7]

The immediate dietary history, gastric emptying rate, intestinal transit, age, and hormonal effects of the horse influence glucose peak and curve shape. Prolonged fasting (≥24 hours) results in a delayed and slightly lower peak plasma glucose concentration.[8] Higher glucose peaks are recorded from healthy animals eating grass or hay than from those eating concentrates[9] and from horses fed a pasture (clover and kikuyu) versus stable (oat hay, complete feed, and alfalfa/oat chaff) diet.[10] Results from the OGTT can also be affected by the content of nonstructural carbohydrate and fat in the diet[11] and other disorders, such as polysaccharide storage myopathy.[12]

In one report of 42 mature horses with chronic weight loss, a normal OGTT (peak glucose concentration at 120 minutes >85% baseline) was not associated with abnormal small intestinal morphology in any of the five horses in which it was documented. When peak glucose concentration was between 15% and 85% of baseline at 120 minutes (considered partial malabsorption), approximately 72% had small intestinal infiltrative disease, and when peak concentration at 120 minutes was less than 15% above baseline (total malabsorption), all had severe small intestinal infiltrative disease.[7] However, other reports have documented horses with flat OGTT curves that subsequently showed more normal OGTT responses and resolved clinical condition[13] and poor diagnostic sensitivity of carbohydrate absorption tests to detect small intestinal involvement in horses with chronic diarrhea and predominantly large intestinal problems.[14] Thus an abnormal absorption test and weight loss can occur in the horse as a transient event and without significant morphologic changes in the small intestine.

D-Xylose Absorption Test

The D-xylose absorption test is performed in the same manner as the OGTT, except 0.5 g D-xylose per kilogram of body weight is administered as a 10% solution through a nasogastric tube. The pretest period of fasting and timing of sample collection is identical. Before collecting the samples, the veterinarian should contact the laboratory to ensure that heparinzed plasma is acceptable. Plasma D-xylose should peak between 20 and 25 mg/dl between 60 and 90 minutes after administration, with occasional peaks as late as 120 minutes.[15,16]

D-xylose absorption testing is not confounded by hormonal effects or mucosal metabolism, as is glucose, but is altered by diet, length of fasting (which could also be influenced by recent appetite or degree of cachexia), and age. Horses fed a high-energy (e.g., oat chaff, oats, and corn) diet had a lower mean peak plasma D-xylose concentration (14.1 versus 24.9 mg/dl) than those consuming a low-energy (alfalfa chaff) diet.[10] Healthy mares fasted for up to 96 hours had flatter curves and a slower decrease in plasma xylose than when fasted for 12 to 36 hours.[15] Kinetic analysis indicates that prolonged food deprivation does not alter renal or nonrenal excretion of D-xylose; thus the effect of fasting on the curve is likely related to intestinal transit, small intestinal absorption, or both.[17,18] Ponies may have lower peak D-xylose concentrations than horses, although the range is wide and diagnostic discriminatory cutoff points for peak plasma xylose concentrations have not been determined. Foals normally have a higher mean peak xylose concentration at 1 and 2 months of age, but mean peak falls to a level similar to that seen in adults by 3 months of age.[19] Gastric emptying rate, intestinal motility, intraluminal bacterial overgrowth, and renal clearance can affect curve shape.

D-Xylose, a pentose sugar, is absorbed unchanged by the duodenum and jejunum in other species. The intestinal sugar active transport system has a low affinity for D-xylose in the equine jejunum in vitro; hence D-xylose absorption likely occurs primarily by convection or diffusion.[20] Thus an abnormal D-xylose absorption test likely indicates abnormal mucosal surface area or permeability. Such an abnormality, represented by a flat curve or delayed absorption, has been observed with most examples of chronic inflammatory bowel disease, parasitism, and idiopathic villous atrophy.[21,22] Abnormal absorption curves have been detected in the absence of small intestinal histologic changes,[23] and interpretation is clouded further by findings from small intestinal resection studies in healthy ponies. One study demonstrated a progressive decline in mean peak xylose concentration after 70% distal small intestinal resection in ponies, despite their normal clinical appearance and absence of diarrhea.[24] In another study a similar decline in peak xylose concentration following extensive (≥60%) small intestinal resection was accompanied by weight loss, diarrhea, and ill thrift.[25]

Peak xylose concentrations were much lower in horses with granulomatous enteritis than those with eosinophilic granulomatosis (EG), whereas in EG the absorption curve shifted to the right, with the peak occurring at 240 minutes.[26] This is not surprising given the typical lesion distribution with these disorders. As with the OGTT, results of the xylose absorption test can improve after therapy.[27]

Lactose Absorption

Milk intolerance is well documented in children and can result from primary or secondary lactase (neutral β-galactosidase) deficiency. Secondary lactase deficiency can occur when a small intestinal disorder, typically rotavirus, damages the epithelial cells, resulting in decreased brush border disaccharidase activity. Such an association has been reported secondary to clostridial enteritis in the foal.[28] In horses lactase activity peaks at birth and declines slowly, such that activity is approximately 50% at 2 years of age and rapidly decelerates after 3 years of age; it is barely detectable by 4 years of age.[29] The oral lactose tolerance test is performed in foals after a 4-hour fast, with a standard dose of 1 g/kg lactose monohydrate given through a nasogastric tube as a 20% solution. Blood sampling is performed in the same manner as for the OGTT. Plasma glucose typically peaks 1 hour after lactose administration, with a range from 30 to 90 minutes, with a mean increase of 77 mg/dl and a 35 mg/dl increase covering two standard deviations.[30] It should be noted that older foals (12 weeks) had a more significant increase in plasma glucose relative to 1-week-old foals.

Nuclear Medicine

Scintigraphy with radiolabeled leukocytes (technetium-99m-labeled hexamethyl-propyleneamine oxime (^{99m}Tc-HMPAO) was recently used to evaluate 17 horses with suspected intestinal malabsorption.[31] In that report the investigators were able to detect intestinal inflammation in 12 of 17 horses, and increased intestinal uptake was not evident in any of the control horses. Corroborating histopathologic results were not available for all cases; this technique was not able to differentiate between type or location of disease, nor did it indicate prognosis.

DISEASES ASSOCIATED WITH MALABSORPTION AND MALDIGESTION

The clinical signs of chronic wasting and poor body condition, although nonspecific for a diagnosis of malabsorption ante mortem, can be attributed to proliferative or inflammatory intestinal disorders, often collectively referred to as *chronic inflammatory bowel diseases* (CIBD).[22] Summaries of the characteristic clinicopathologic and pathologic findings for each disease are presented in Tables 15-11 and 15-12, respectively.

Alimentary Lymphosarcoma

Alimentary lymphosarcoma of the horse may represent a primary neoplasia of the gut-associated lymphoid tissue with significant cellular infiltration of the small intestine and associated lymph nodes with minimal large intestinal or systemic involvement. Case series and pathology reports indicate that young horses 2 to 4 years of age primarily are affected, although the age range can be broad.[32-34] No breed or sex predilection has been documented, and disease prevalence is unknown. Despite the progressive nature of lymphomata, onset of clinical signs can be rapid, and the animal may become acutely ill. As with all adult cases of CIBD, antemortem diagnosis is by a process of exclusion and usually is confirmed post mortem. Frequent abnormalities include anemia, thrombocytopenia, neutrophilia or neutropenia, and hypoalbuminemia with hyperglobulinemia, resulting in either a normal or elevated serum protein. Lymphocytosis is rare. Intra-abdominal masses, mainly enlarged mesenteric lymph nodes, may be rectally palpated. Abdominocentesis and rectal biopsy can provide a diagnosis but are not sensitive indicators of disease. Carbohydrate absorption tests usually reveal partial to total malabsorption indicative of the severely reduced surface area resulting from significant villous atrophy and the extensive mucosal or transmural infiltration. Early confirmation of a suspected diagnosis necessitates exploratory laparotomy to obtain multiple intestinal and lymph node biopsies if the results of rectal biopsy or abdominocentesis are normal. Prognosis is poor, especially insofar as most horses are presented in an advanced state of disease. Immunosuppressive drugs or chemotherapy may afford temporary improvement, but long-term outcome is unaffected. A detailed discussion of lymphosarcoma is included in Chapter 14.

Granulomatous Enteritis

Granulomatous enteritis was first described as a chronic wasting condition in 1974[35]; 9 of 10 horses were young Standardbreds. Most affected horses are 2 to 3 years of age. Case reports from many countries revealed a predominance of Standardbred over Thoroughbreds by three to one.[26,36] Some of the Standardbreds were related, implicating a genetic predisposition, but this has not been proved. Prevalence is low. The condition is sporadic and has an insidious onset, and the course can be protracted. Significant diagnostic features include anemia, slight increases or decreases in white blood cell counts, hypoalbuminemia, normal serum protein or hypoproteinemia, occasional increases in serum alkaline phosphatase activity, normal serum γ-glutamyltransferase activity, and enlarged mesenteric lymph nodes on rectal palpation. Partial or complete malabsorption is typically documented by carbohydrate absorption testing. The low proportion of horses exhibiting diarrhea can be attributed to the preferential distribution of inflammatory infiltration in the small intestine.[37] Rectal biopsy can be a useful aid to diagnosis.[2]

The cause of granulomatous enteritis is unknown. Several infectious agents have been implicated, including *Mycobacterium avium*.[38] The condition may represent a granulomatous hypersensitivity reaction. Immune-mediated responses to dietary, parasitic, or bacterial antigens may be important initiating factors.[22] Six cases purported to represent granulomatous enteritis were linked to environmental contamination with aluminum,[39] although problems existed regarding the case definition, data, and interpretation.[40]

Treatment of horses with granulomatous enteritis with a variety of drugs, particularly corticosteroids, has not affected the long-term outcome in the majority of cases.[41] Prolonged (i.e., 5 months) corticosteroid administration produced clinical remission and a favorable athletic outcome in a 6-year-old Standardbred gelding based on improvement in clinical signs and in D-xylose absorption.[27] Surgery may be indicated with localized disease. Two young horses underwent resection of the thickened terminal small intestine; one horse died 4 months after surgery, and the other remained clinically normal for at least 10 years.[36]

Multisystemic Eosinophilic Epitheliotropic Disease

MEED encompasses disorders characterized by a predominant eosinophilic infiltrate in the gastrointestinal tract, associated lymph nodes, liver, pancreas, skin, and other structures and accompanied by some degree of malabsorption and enteric protein loss. The disorders include chronic eosinophilic gastroenteritis,[42] eosinophilic granulomatosis,[26] chronic eosinophilic dermatitis,[43] and probably basophilic enterocolitis.[44]

Although prevalence is low, MEED appears to be more common than granulomatous enteritis. Most affected horses are 2 to 4 years of age, and Standardbreds and Thoroughbreds are reported to predominate. The condition is sporadic and has an insidious onset and often a protracted course (i.e., 1 to 10 months). Diarrhea is common. Severe skin lesions with exudative dermatitis and ulcerative coronitis are prominent and frequently are the principal presenting complaint. Despite extensive tissue eosinophilia, systemic eosinophilia is rare and hematologic values are usually unremarkable. Notable features include hypoalbuminemia and elevations in serum γ-glutamyltransferase and alkaline phosphatase activities. Most reports of carbohydrate absorption test findings indicate a reduced or normal peak concentration delayed to at least 180 minutes. Morphologic changes are less pronounced in the small intestine than in the large intestine,[26] and small intestinal lesions predominate segmentally in the proximal duodenum and distal ileum. Furthermore, significant hyperkeratosis of the fundic region may contribute to gastric muscle contractile disruption. Diarrhea can be a consequence of the severe segmental or multifocal granulomatous lesions in the large intestine, with mucosal and transmural thickening and extensive ulceration. Abundant fibrosis is a feature of all affected tissues.

The cause of MEED is unknown and could represent a chronic, ongoing, immediate hypersensitivity reaction against undefined antigens ingested or excreted into the lumen from parasitic, bacterial, or dietary sources. Infectious agents have not been identified.[42,43] Eosinophilia is a feature of parasitism in the equine intestinal tract, although nematodes rarely have been identified in any lesions of MEED.[42,45] However, failure to detect larval structures in these lesions may be attributable to the chronicity of the disease and destruction of the parasites in tissue.[36] Biopsies of the rectal mucosa[2] or of the skin, liver, intestinal tract, and lymph nodes may assist in diagnosis. Unlike the other conditions, MEED has definitive liver and pancreatic involvement; thus maldigestion may contribute to the wasting disease.

Treatment has been attempted with a variety of drugs, including antibiotics, corticosteroids, and anthelmintics with larvicidal activity. Although some horses improve briefly, the long-term prognosis is poor.

Eosinophilic Enterocolitis

Idiopathic eosinophilic enterocolitis affects segmental lesions in the small or large intestine, inducing signs of colic, and often requires surgical intervention.[36,46,47] This problem may not involve evidence of malabsorption and does not have multisystem involvement. Because the problem is often associated with signs of colic and not signs of malabsorption, eosinophilic enterocolitis differs from the other conditions discussed in this section and is often diagnosed at the time of surgery. It carries a much better prognosis than the other inflammatory bowel diseases.

Lymphocytic-Plasmacytic Enterocolitis

The morphologic findings in lymphocytic-plasmacytic enterocolitis reflect the predominant infiltrative cellular elements of this rarely encountered condition. No specific clinical or clinicopathologic features differentiate this condition ante mortem from other inflammatory diseases of adult horses. In a retrospective study of 14 horses, carbohydrate absorption was abnormal or delayed in 9 of 12 horses, consistent with the predominance of small intestinal pathologic changes.[3] Rectal biopsies were abnormal in three of seven horses, two of which were reported as having lymphocytic-plasmacytic proctitis. Prognosis is poor. Treatment has been unsuccessful, probably because of the advanced nature of the condition at the beginning of treatment.

Proliferative Enteropathy

Proliferative enteropathy (PE) typically affects weanling foals between 3 to 8 months of age and has been reported in North America, Europe, and Australia, causing disease in individuals or outbreaks of multiple affected animals on the same premise.[48-59] PE has been reported uncommonly in yearlings and adult horses.[57,60] The disease affects many other species, especially swine, and is caused by *Lawsonia intracellularis*, an obligate intracellular bacterium found in the cytoplasm of proliferative crypt epithelial cells of the jejunum and ileum.[51,57,59] The condition in a foal was described first as intestinal adenomatosis,[61] but later work confirmed that intestines from an affected foal contained *L. intracellularis*.[51]

Clinical signs include depression, rapid and significant weight loss, edema, diarrhea, and colic.[57] Poor body condition, a rough hair coat, and potbelly appearance are also reported. It is important to remember that not all clinical signs are present in all cases, and diarrhea has been noted in only approximately half of reported cases. Other problems often were concurrent, including respiratory tract infection, dermatitis, intestinal parasitism, and gastric ulceration. The most significant laboratory finding is profound hypoproteinemia, predominantly characterized by hypoalbuminemia, but panhypoproteinemia can also occur.[48,52,57] Leukocytosis and hyperfibrinogenemia are also common, with occasional alterations in electrolytes (hyponatremia, hypokalemia, hypochloremia) and elevated serum creatine kinase concentrations. Abdominal ultrasound commonly reveals increased small intestinal mural thickness.[48,52] Colloid oncotic pressure is typically low, if measured.[48]

One can suspect PE based on clinical signs and severe hypoalbuminemia in a weanling foal with exclusion of common enteric infections. Fecal PCR for bacterial DNA or serum immunofluorescence assay or immunoperoxidase monolayer assay (IMPA) for antibodies against the organism can provide additional support for the diagnosis. The IMPA may be more sensitive, and typically titers greater than or equal to 1:60 are considered positive.[60] Submission of both tests is recommended; although both tests are quite specific, both also lack sensitivity, especially early in the course of disease (serology) or with prior antimicrobial therapy (fecal PCR).[48,57] Notably, fecal PCR can become negative in affected foals within 4 days of antimicrobial therapy.[58] PE is not typically associated with abnormal carbohydrate absorption test results.[57,58] In cases with diarrhea, infectious causes should be ruled out. A definitive postmortem diagnosis can be confirmed by identifying characteristic mural thickening and intracellular bacteria within the apical cytoplasm of proliferating crypt epithelial cells using silver stains, PCR, or immunohistochemical testing.[57]

Reported antimicrobial therapy includes eythromycin, alone or with rifampin, azithromycin, clarithromyxin, oxytetracycline, doxycycline, metronidazole, or chloramphenicol.[48,57,62] Recent reports appear to favor the use of intravenous oxytetracycline, followed by oral doxycycline, with apparent success.[48,62] Duration of therapy is typically 2 to 4 weeks. Affected foals often need supportive therapy, including crystalloid fluid and electrolyte replacement and often colloid support with either hydroxyethyl starch or plasma. NSAID therapy can be used as needed for significant pyrexia. Corticosteroid therapy is not indicated because inflammation is not a significant pathologic finding. Response to therapy has been good, with reported survival rates between 82% and 93%.[48,57,62] Rapid improvement in clinical signs, even within 24 hours, preceded the rise in plasma protein concentration.

The source of infection is typically not determined. In some epidemiological investigations, close proximity to swine operations was apparent, but in most such an association was not evident.[52,57] Comparisons of epidemiologic findings from the swine disease indicated that overcrowding, feed changes, antibiotic usage, and mixing and transportation were potential risk factors at two of the farms in one study, and recent weaning appears to be a common risk factor.[57]

Other Conditions

Abnormal D-xylose absorption has also been noted in association with AA amyloid-associated gastroenteropathy in an 18-year-old Morgan stallion[63] and a horse with a gastric mass and secondary small intestinal villous atrophy.[64]

MANAGEMENT, THERAPY, AND OUTCOME

The chronic wasting horse with suspected malabsorption and probable enteric protein loss has at best a guarded to poor prognosis, with the exception of those suffering from PE. Prognosis may be improved through early and aggressive investigation to achieve a diagnosis. In the short term intravenous infusion of plasma or colloids, with or without fluids and electrolytes, may be necessary to stabilize the profoundly hypoalbuminemic patient. Prognosis is much worse for the horse that is inappetent. Prolonged intensive total parenteral nutrition, oral alimentation, or both may not be a realistic course of action. The owner must be cognizant from the start that the outcome may not be altered, even after protracted therapy; only a few case reports of successful responses with long-term follow-up have been documented.

Nutrition

Some level of digestive and absorptive capability remains in the diseased small intestine. Interval feeding of small quantities of easily digestible food may be beneficial. Diet should include feeds with a high fiber content to favor large intestinal fermentation, including grass hay and access to pasture complemented by high-fiber rations based on beet pulp and soybean hulls, which are commercially available in many complete pelleted feeds. Energy intake can be increased through feeding high-energy dense fats that provide 2.25 times more calories than carbohydrates. Most affected horses should tolerate high fat (5% to 10%) processed feeds containing vegetable oils or rice bran (up to 20% of the concentrate mix, equivalent to 8% vegetable oil) to achieve the higher-fat composition. The transition to a higher-fat concentrate should be gradual. Even in healthy animals that can eat up to 20% added fat, appetite may decrease as the percentage increases, and fecal consistency may change. Clearly, the objective for the horse with suspected malabsorption is to sustain, and preferably increase, dietary intake, value, and efficiency.

The owner of an affected horse must be prepared to experiment with feeds, be patient, and keep records. Exposure to a feed component may contribute to the problem as an allergen eliciting a hypersensitivity reaction. Identifying the potential allergen through immunologic testing or by stepwise removal and outcome assessment over a longer period may be difficult. The clinician should give immunosuppressive drugs early in the process.

Drug Therapy

Immunosuppressive agents have produced the most promising responses to ameliorate the effects of conditions associated with malabsorption, particularly CIBD. Short-duration, and in some cases more prolonged and sustained, improvements in body condition, weight gain, demeanor, energy, and activity levels have occurred following corticosteroid administration. Treatment should begin as early as possible. The clinician should follow initial parenteral (intramuscular or intravenous) loading doses of dexamethasone (sodium phosphate) with a series of depot injections or orally administered prednisolone on a tapered-dose protocol over a period of months. Interval low-dose therapy may be necessary if clinical signs return after treatment ends. The clinician should use the lowest dose that effectively controls the clinical signs for alternate-day therapy. Clinical benefits far outweigh concerns over potential adverse effects. Chemotherapeutic agents such as vincristine, cytosine, cyclophosphamide, and hydroxyurea have been tried in a few cases of CIBD or lymphosarcoma with no apparent success, probably because of the advanced stage of the disease when treatment was initiated and the dose selected.

Surgery

Resection of a segment of intestine that is edematous, hemorrhagic, or constricted is an option in localized forms of CIBD,[46,47] particularly if gross changes are not discernible in adjacent or distant parts of the intestinal tract—that is, malabsorption is not a feature. Long-term outcome has been favorable. Removal of a substantial proportion of the diseased small intestine may be indicated in a horse with malabsorption, considering that resection of 70% distal small intestine was performed in healthy animals without inducing adverse effects.[24] However, because pathologic changes may exist in normal-appearing small or large intestine that is not resected or biopsied, the prognosis remains guarded. Two young horses with granulomatous enteritis had the thickened terminal small intestine resected with positive outcomes; one survived 4 months, the other has a follow-up extending more than 10 years.[36]

INFLAMMATORY DISEASES OF THE GASTROINTESTINAL TRACT CAUSING DIARRHEA

Samuel L. Jones

Acute diarrhea caused by colitis in adult or young horses is a potentially life-threatening disorder with a variety of possible etiologies (Table 15-13) characterized by hypersecretion of fluid, motility disturbances, and an impaired mucosal barrier resulting from direct injury or inflammation. Many of the clinical and clinicopathological features are similar regardless of the underlying cause. Severe dehydration with profound electrolyte abnormalities is common, as is systemic inflammation secondary to absorption of endotoxin or other bacterial products through compromised gastrointestinal mucosa. Severe cases may be complicated by serosal inflammation and mural ischemia and infarction as a direct extension of mucosal inflammation or secondary to coaglopathies. The diagnostic approach for horses with acute diarrhea is aimed at determining the underlying etiology but must be accompanied by clinical and laboratory assessment of hydration, electrolyte and acid base balance, organ function, and evaluation of the degree of systemic inflammation and the integrity of the intestinal wall. The therapeutic approach for horses with colitis, regardless of cause, consists primarily of controlling local and systemic inflammation, maintaining fluid and electrolyte balance, and promoting mucosal repair. In addition, some horses with acute colitis require specific therapy aimed at the underlying etiology.

INFECTIOUS DISEASES

SALMONELLOSIS

PATHOGENESIS

Salmonella enterica is a species of gram negative facultatively anaerobic bacteria that is a common gastrointestinal pathogen in horses. Many serovars of *S. enterica* have been reported to infect horses, but those classified in group B appear to be more commonly associated with disease than those in other groups. Group B includes *S. enterica var. typhimurium* and *S. enterica var. agona,* two of the species most frequently isolated from horses.[1-3] *S. enterica var. typhimurium* is the most pathogenic serotype in horses and is associated with a higher case fatality rate than other serovars of *S. enterica.*[1] The number of horses that are inapparently infected with and actively shed *S. enterica* in their feces has been reported to be as high as 10% to 20%, but actual prevalence of *S. enterica* shedding in the general horse population is likely to be much lower, less than 2%.[4] Horses shedding *S. enterica* are a potential source of infection to susceptible horses,[1,5] as are environmental reservoirs.[6-8] For these reasons salmonellosis is one of the most common nosocomial diseases in horses. Nosocomial salmonellosis significantly affects morbidity and mortality in hospitalized horses.[9] The emergence of multidrug resistance in equine *S. enterica* isolates has been a cause of concern because of the importance of salmonellosis as a nosocomial disease and because a number of serovars of *S. enterica* are significant zoonotic pathogens.[7,10,13]

TABLE 15-13

Differentials and Diagnosis of Some Causes of Acute Diarrhea in Adult Horses

Category	Differentials	Diagnosis
Infectious	Salmonellosis	Fecal culture (5 consecutive) Fecal PCR
	Clostridium perfringens	Quantitative fecal culture Fecal toxin immunoassay or PCR
	Clostridium difficile	Fecal culture Fecal toxin immunoassay or PCR
	Lawsonia intracellularis	Serology Fecal PCR Small intestinal ultrasound Histopathology
	Neoristicii risticii	Fecal or blood PCR Serology
Parasitic	Strongylosis	Fecal egg counts Cranial mesenteric artery palpation Serum IgG(T)
	Cyathostomiasis	Fecal egg count Rectal biopsy Cecal or colonic biopsy
Toxic	NSAID	History and clinical signs Right dorsal colon ultrasonography Laparoscopy or laparotomy
	Cantharidin	History of exposure Fecal or urine cantharidin concentrations
	Arsenic	History of exposure Fecal, blood, urine, or tissue arsenic concentrations
Miscellaneous	Carbohydrate overload	History of inappropriate ingestion of carbohydrate Blood lactate concentration
	Sand enteropathy	Auscultation of ventral colon Fecal sand content Abdominal radiography

PCR, Polymerase chain reaction; *NSAID,* nonsteroidal anti-inflammatory drug.

The virulence of the bacteria varies tremendously with serotype and even among strains of the same serotype. In part, this is due to the important role of host susceptibility in the pathogenicity of particular organisms. The infective dose is generally on the order of millions of organisms inoculated orally, but various environmental and host factors can reduce the infective dose to a few thousand or even hundreds of organisms.[14-16] Environmental factors or stresses that increase susceptibility to *S. enterica* infection are not well defined, but it is known that high ambient temperature, for example, can greatly increase the prevalence of salmonellosis in horses.[6,15,16] Indeed, the peak incidence of salmonellosis in horses occurs in late summer and fall.[6,15,16] Other environmental and host factors that increase the risk of or are associated with salmonellosis or shedding of *S. enterica* organisms in feces include transportation, antibiotic administration before or during hospitalization, gastrointestinal or abdominal surgery, general anesthesia, preexisting gastrointestinal disease (e.g., colic, diarrhea), presence of leukopenia or laminitis during hospitalization, prolonged hospital stay, change in diet, and immunosuppression.[1,8,16-18] Interestingly, foals with gastrointestinal disease are more likely to shed *S. enterica* organisms than are adult horses with gastrointestinal disease.[17]

Host factors that restrict gastrointestinal colonization and invasion by pathogens include gastric pH, commensal gastrointestinal flora, gastrointestinal motility, the mucosal barrier, and mucosal immunity.[1,19] Gastric acidity is an important defense mechanism for preventing live organisms from reaching the intestine.[19] Altering the gastric pH, with histamine H_2 receptor antagonists, for example, may increase susceptibility to infection. Gastrointestinal flora inhibit the proliferation and colonization of *S. enterica* by secreting bacteriocins, short-chain fatty acids (SCFAs), and other substances that are toxic to *S. enterica*.[19] In addition, elements of the normal flora compete for nutrients and space, especially on the mucosa.[19] Being predominantly anaerobic, the normal flora maintain a low oxidation-reduction potential in the environment of the large intestine, which inhibits the growth of many bacterial pathogens.[20] The importance of normal host gastrointestinal ecology is illustrated by the fact that disturbances of the colonic flora with antibiotics, changes in feed, ileus, or other underlying gastrointestinal disease markedly increases the susceptibility of the host to infection by *S. enterica,* often resulting in serious disease.

The immune status of the host may be one of the most important factors determining not only the susceptibility to *S. enterica* infections but also the degree of invasion and subsequent outcome of the infection. Local immunity, such as mucosal antibody secretion and enterocyte-derived cationic peptides, prevents colonization of the mucosa.[19,21,22] Opsonizing antibodies and activation of the complement cascade are important in fighting systemic invasion by *S. enterica* by increasing the efficiency of phagocytosis and by direct bactericidal activity. Humoral immunity, however, is often ineffective in preventing disease and dissemination once invasion occurs and *S. enterica* has established in its intracellular niche. Following invasion, *S. enterica* is capable of surviving and multiplying within macrophages, rendering humoral (noncellular) immune systems ineffective.[23,24] Specific cellular immunity may be the most effective defense mechanism in the host arsenal against dissemination and systemic infection by *S. enterica*.[20,24] Protective immunity in horses and calves may be induced by oral inoculation with small numbers of virulent organisms, but the duration of the immunity is not known.[25,26] Oral and parenteral vaccines using killed or attenuated organisms and bacterial products have been promising but are effective only against homologous organisms and are usually not cross-protective among different serogroups.[25-27]

In adult horses *S. enterica* primarily infects the cecum and proximal colon, causing enterocolitis, with limited likelihood of dissemination beyond the intestine. In foals, however, salmonellosis is often associated with septicemia. The ability of *S. enterica* to cause enterocolitis depends on the ability of the bacteria to invade the gastrointestinal mucosa.[19,23] Invasion of the gastrointestinal mucosa occurs preferentially through specialized enterocytes called *M cells* that overlay intestinal lymphoid tissues such as Peyer's patches in nonequine species. M cells are exploited by a variety of enteric pathogens during infection of intestinal tissue.[28] Invasion of the epithelium occurs by self-induced uptake via the apical membrane of the M cell, often killing the cell in the process.[23] *S. enterica* then invades neighboring cells via the basolateral membrane, eventually spreading the destruction of the epithelium beyond the principal area of attack. Virulent *S. enterica* have a well-developed invasion mechanism that involves the generation of an apparatus called a Type III secretory system that enables virulence gene products to be injected directly into enterocytes.[29] Virulence proteins injected by *S. enterica* into enterocytes engage the cellular machinery and induce the cell to engulf the bacteria by macropinocytosis. *S. enterica* virulence gene products also induce enterocyte chloride and fluid secretion and upregulate enterocyte transcription of inflammatory cytokines (TNF-α and IL-1β) and chemokines that trigger a mucosal inflammatory response.[23,29,30]

Once *S. enterica* has invaded the mucosa, the organisms are quickly phagocytosed by macrophages and dendritic cells in the lamina propria and in lymphoid tissues. The ability of *S. enterica* to disseminate systemically and cause enteric fever is associated with the ability to survive and proliferate in macrophages. Indeed, phagocytes have an important role in dissemination to blood, lymph nodes, liver, and spleen.[31] The majority of *S. enterica* in the blood and tissues of animals infected with a strain of *S. enterica* that is competent to cause enteric fever are within phagocytic cells.[31] In adult horses with salmonellosis, dissemination appears to be limited to the intestine and mesenteric lymph nodes, and *S. enterica* is rarely cultured from blood. However, in foals and in some adults, *S. enterica* causes an enteric fever–like disease with dissemination to mesenteric lymph nodes, liver, spleen, and blood.

Specific virulence gene clusters called *pathogenicity islands* encoded on the chromosome or on plasmids confer the main virulence traits of *S. enterica*: invasion, enteropathogenesis, intracellular survival, and proliferation.[23] Some of the genes encoded within these islands or virulence factors are sensors that signal to the bacteria that it has entered an intracellular environment and turn on other genes required for intracellular survival. Others, such as invasion genes, are transported from the bacteria and injected into macrophage cytosol by a Type III secretory system apparatus to prevent phagosome-lysosome fusion and subvert other essential macrophage-killing mechanisms. Virulent *S. enterica* may also possess multiple genes that enable adhesion to target cells or confer resistance to reactive oxygen and nitrogen metabolites, perhaps the most lethal antimicrobial mechanisms of macrophages.[32]

Diarrhea associated with salmonellosis has multiple causes. A *S. enterica* cytotoxin inhibits protein synthesis in mucosal cells, causing morphologic damage and altered permeability.[34] Virulent *S. enterica* also produce an enterotoxin that is similar to the heat-labile (LT) toxin produced by *E. coli*.[34,35] This enterotoxin contributes to, but is not required, in the pathogenesis of diarrhea.[36,37] *S. enterica* enterotoxin increases secretion of chloride and water by colonic mucosal cells in many species, including horses, by increasing intracellular cAMP concentrations.[34,35,38]

The ability of virulent *S. enterica* to cause diarrhea appears to be most closely associated with the ability to invade enterocytes and to trigger an inflammatory reaction in the intestinal tissue.[23,39] Gene products injected into enterocyte cytosol by the Type III secretory system of invading *S. enterica* stimulate chloride and fluid secretion.[29] *S. enterica* invasion of enterocytes is also a potent activator of inflammatory chemokine and cytokine production, resulting in the recruitment of leukocytes, particularly neutrophils, and activation of resident macrophages and mast cells. Products of these activated leukocytes, including prostaglandins, leukotrienes, reactive oxygen metabolites, and histamine, are potent stimulators of chloride secretion in the colon of many species.[19,40-42] The enteric nervous system integrates the diverse processes of pathogen recognition, triggering of the inflammatory response, and induction of enterocyte fluid secretion.[42]

Many of the inflammatory mediators studied stimulate colonic secretion by prostaglandin-dependent mechanisms, resulting in either increased intracellular cAMP or calcium concentrations, or both, in mucosal cells.[40] In addition, these mediators and the enteric nervous system may stimulate secretion by prostaglandin-independent mechanisms, inhibit sodium and water absorption, cause motility disturbances, and potentiate tissue injury, all of which enhance the pathogenicity and dissemination of *S. enterica* and contribute to the pathogenesis of diarrhea.[40,42] Neutrophils recruited to the mucosa by signals generated by the infected enterocytes physically contribute to mucosal injury by producing a variety of products that are lethal to pathogens but are also toxic to host cells.[43,44] Moreover, neutrophils attracted to infected epithelial cells accumulate beneath the monolayer, lifting it off the basement membrane in sheets. Neutrophils also migrate across the epithelial monolayer in potentially massive numbers—enough to be detectable in feces as a marker of inflammatory diarrhea. Although the transepithelial migration of neutrophils has a benefit, positioning the host defense cell at the apical membrane to ward off attacks by invading bacteria, the mechanical disruption to the epithelial barrier may be significant enough to increase the permeability to macromolecules, bacterial products, and even bacteria.[44] Potentially massive losses of electrolytes, water, and protein can occur, depending on bacterial and host factors. Perhaps most devastatingly, mucosal injury and altered permeability allow systemic absorption of bacterial products and dissemination of bacteria, resulting in life-threatening sepsis.

CLINICAL SIGNS AND DIAGNOSIS

Four clinical syndromes of *S. enterica* infection have been documented clinically and reproduced experimentally in horses: (1) inapparent infections with latent or active carrier states; (2) depression, fever, anorexia, and neutropenia without diarrhea or colic; (3) fulminant or peracute enterocolitis with diarrhea; and (4) septicemia (enteric fever) with or without diarrhea.[45] Inapparent infections can be activated to clinical disease in compromised horses, such as horses with colic or horses being treated with antibiotics, causing mild to severe enterocolitis. In addition, latent infections (nonshedding) can become active infections (shedding) under certain conditions, such as transportation stress and antibiotic treatment. Horses with depression, anorexia, fever, and neutropenia without diarrhea generally have a good prognosis and recover in several days without specific treatment.[45] The septicemic form is mostly restricted to neonatal foals and is uncommon in adult horses. The focus of this discussion is acute enterocolitis.

Acute enterocolitis is characterized by severe fibrinonecrotic typhlocolitis, with interstitial edema and variable degrees of intramural vascular thrombosis that may progress to infarction.[1] Severe ulceration of the large intestinal mucosa may occur, with serosal ecchymoses and congestion. The earliest signs of enterocolitis are usually fever and anorexia.[1,16] Signs of colic may be seen early in the course of the disease, especially if ileus is present. Clinical signs of endotoxemia are common, and range from fever, elevated heart and respiratory rates, poor peripheral perfusion, and ileus to fulminant and rapidly progressive signs of endotoxemic shock. Oral mucous membranes are often pale with perigingival hyperemia (a toxic rim) but may be brick red or cyanotic, with prolonged capillary refill time. Weakness, muscle fasciculations, cold extremities, and other signs suggestive of hypotensive shock; synchronous diaphragmatic flutter; abdominal pain; and marked metabolic and electrolyte abnormalities may be noted in severe cases of enterocolitis. Signs of mild dehydration may be observed before diarrhea is seen. Once diarrhea is evident, dehydration may rapidly become severe. Occasionally, horses die peracutely, without developing diarrhea.

Diarrhea may not occur for several days, but usually is evident by 24 to 48 hours after the onset of fever.[1,16] The duration of diarrhea may be days to weeks. The character of the first diarrheal feces is usually watery, with particles of roughage, but may rapidly become fluid without solid material. Finding frank blood and fibrin in the feces is unusual. The volume of feces is often large, with frequent defecation. Straining or signs of colic may be observed when the patient is defecating, and rectal prolapse may occasionally occur. Persistent straining and rectal prolapse may be a sign of colonic infarction. Abdominal borborygmi are often absent early in the course of the disease because of ileus but become evident later, usually when diarrhea begins. Fluid and gas sounds are commonly ausculted, but normal progressive motility is less frequently heard than normally. Transrectal palpation may reveal edematous rectal and colonic mucosa and fluid-filled colon and cecum. Gastric reflux may be obtained, especially early in the course, when ileus is evident.

Hematologic abnormalities early in the course of the disease include moderate to severe neutropenia, lymphopenia, and leukopenia, a mild to moderate left shift, and toxic changes in the neutrophils.[1,16] Thrombocytopenia, moderate to severe hemoconcentration, and hyperfibrinogenemia are also common. Neutropenia is an early but nonspecific indicator of salmonellosis, often occurring concurrently with the onset of fever.[1] Later in the course of disease, neutrophilic leukocytosis may be seen, indicating recovery. A degenerating left shift, with metamyelocytes and myelocytes seen in the peripheral blood, is a poor prognostic sign.

Serum biochemical analysis may reveal azotemia, increases in serum sorbitol dehydrogenase and γ-glutamine aminotransferase activity, and increased blood lactic acid concentration. Azotemia is often prerenal, but acute hemodynamic renal failure may be seen in severely dehydrated, endotoxemic, or septic patients. Indeed, elevation of creatinine concentration is a poor prognostic indicator in horses with acute colitis.[46] Hemodynamic renal disease may be complicated by toxic injury caused by administration of nephrotoxic drugs. Hyponatremia may also contribute to prerenal azotemia. Elevations in hepatocellular enzymes are usually mild and reflect damage to the hepatocytes from absorbed toxins such as endotoxin and from poor perfusion resulting from hypotensive shock, dehydration, or both. Lactic acidemia may be present, reflecting poor tissue perfusion. Plasma protein rapidly drops, as protein is lost in the gastrointestinal tract, causing moderate to severe hypoalbuminemia and hypoglobulinemia. Peripheral or organ edema (vascular leak syndrome) may occur if hypoproteinemia is severe, coupled with systemic inflammation-induced increases in endothelial permeability.

Hypokalemia, hyponatremia, hypochloridemia, and hypocalcemia are common electrolyte abnormalities in patients with enterocolitis. Metabolic acidosis may also be present and DIC is common. Urinalysis may reveal isosthenuria, proteinuria, hematuria, cylindruria, or glucosuria if hemodynamic or toxic renal injury is present. The number of leukocytes in the feces is usually elevated, and occult blood may be detected. PF is usually normal except when severe mural inflammation or colonic infarction occurs.

S. enterica in feces is routinely detected by analyzing five daily cultures of large samples (10-30 g) of feces using enrichment techniques.[1,47,48] However, the sensitivity of fecal culture can be as low as 30% to 50%, even if several fecal samples collected daily are cultured.[48] Concurrent culture of rectal biopsy specimens and feces increases the sensitivity of culture techniques to 60% to 75%.[48] Currently, the PCR test is the most sensitive and rapid way to detect *S. enterica* in feces. A single PCR test applied early in the course of disease is a more sensitive test for the presence of *S. enterica* than repeated fecal cultures,[49,50] with as high as 100% sensitivity and 98% specificity for detection of organisms in some reports.[51] Although detection of *S. enterica* organisms in feces does not prove a diagnosis of salmonellosis, the positive predictive value of either a positive PCR or culture result is high in horses with compatible clinical signs. Culture of peripheral blood may allow isolation of the organism if bacteremia or septicemia is present, but blood cultures are not a sensitive test for salmonellosis in adult horses. However foals are more likely than adults to become septicemic and culture of blood is recommended in all foals with signs of sepsis. Increased numbers of fecal leukocytes suggest an invasive process in the colon but are not specific for salmonellosis.

Early in the course of the disease, dehydration, electrolyte and acid-base imbalances, endotoxemia, and sepsis may be life threatening. Aggressive treatment during the acute stages to replace fluids lost in the diarrhea and to control sepsis and endotoxemia is often effective in controlling the primary disease. Weight loss and hypoproteinemia are often severe. Possible complications include multiorgan dysfunction, vascular leak syndrome with peripheral and organ edema, laminitis, acute renal failure, venous thrombosis and septic phlebitis, irreversible protein-losing enteropathy or chronic malabsorption, pulmonary aspergillosis, and gastrointestinal infarction. The reader is referred to Chapter 7 and the section on endotoxemia in this chapter for additional information regarding treatment of horses with severe endotoxemia and SIRS.

In many instances horses recover from acute salmonellosis with aggressive treatment, only to succumb to complications of the disease, which partially explains the high fatality rate of equine salmonellosis compared with that of human salmonellosis. Chronic, mild to moderate diarrhea is occasionally seen in horses after a bout of severe salmonellosis, usually with protein-losing enteropathy. If the chronic diarrhea persists beyond 4 to 5 weeks after the onset of signs, the prognosis for recovery is poor.[16]

Potomac Horse Fever

PATHOGENESIS

Potomac horse fever is caused by the obligate intracellular rickettsial organism *Neorickettsia risticii* (formerly called *Ehrlichia risticii*).[52,53-56] The disease is most common from late summer to early fall, with a peak incidence in July and August.[53,54] Potomac horse fever was first described in the Northeastern United States but has since been described now in most areas of the continental United States, with a particularly high prevalence in the Northeast and Midwest. The geographical distribution is characterized by a significantly higher percentage of cases found along waterways and rivers.[53,54] The disease occurs sporadically, both temporally and geographically, and can affect any age group of horses. The case fatality rate ranges between 5% to 30%.[53]

Transmission of *N. risticii* has been reproduced experimentally by oral, intramuscular, intradermal, subcutaneous, and intravenous routes.[53,57] Attempts to transmit the disease experimentally with ticks *(Dermacentor variablis)* or biting flies (*Stomoxys calcitrans*) were unsuccessful.[58,59] Recently, *N. risticii* was found to infect virgulate cercariae, larval stages of trematodes that use operculate freshwater snails of the family *Pleuroceridae* (*Juga* spp. in California and *Elimia* spp. in Ohio and Pennsylvania), as intermediate hosts in their life cycle.[60-63] Infected virgulate cercariae have been identified in aquatic snails collected in other parts of the world as well.[64] Although the trematode species infected with *N. risticii* remain to be definitively identified, at least two species have been identified as potential vectors,[65] and at least two potential definitive hosts were identified when *N. risticii* DNA was detected in the blood, liver, or spleen of 23 of 53 little and big brown bats harboring gravid trematodes in their intestinal tracts.[66]

Aquatic snails release large numbers of infected cercariae into water, where they seek their next intermediate host—any of a variety of aquatic insects.[63,67] Successful transmission of *N. risticii* to horses was accomplished experimentally using trematode stages collected from *Juga yrekaensis* snails.[68] The number of PCR-positive snails in endemic regions corresponds to the seasonal incidence of Potomac horse fever and may be as high as 26%.[69] However, preliminary studies suggest that *N. risticii* may in fact be naturally transmitted to horses through the ingestion of caddisflies and mayflies.[63,70]

The pathogenesis of *N. risticii* is not completely understood. The organism infects and survives in monocytes and monocyte-derived leukocytes and can be found in blood monocytes during natural infections, but the sequence of events resulting in enterocolitis remains open to speculation. The organism appears first to infect blood monocytes in experimentally infected horses, which may be the vehicle of organ infection.[55,71] However, it is unclear whether leukocytes of the monocytic lineage or epithelial cells are infected first in naturally infected horses. The target organ is the gastrointestinal mucosa, with the most severe lesions found in the large intestine.[71,72] Infection of human colonic cells in vitro does not cause major cytopathologic effects for several days.[73] Disruption of the microvilli in the region of the plasma membrane where sodium chloride channels are located has been observed in human colonic cell cultures.[73] Infection in horses is associated with variable degrees of morphologic damage.[71,72] Mild morphologic damage and mononuclear cell infiltration of the lamina propria occur early during the infection, but fibrinous, necrotizing typhlocolitis with severe mucosal ulceration and inflammation of the lamina propria may occur later in the disease. Vasculitis and intravascular coagulation are consistent features in the large intestine, with perivascular edema.[72] *N. risticii* can be observed in mucosal cells and macrophages and mast cells of the lamina propria.[71,72] *N. risticii* can survive and multiply in macrophages by inhibiting the production of reactive oxygen intermediates and avoiding lysosomal digestion by blocking phagosome-lysosome fusion.[74-76]

Some researchers have suggested that impaired sodium chloride absorption in the colon contributes to diarrhea in infected horses and may be related to destruction of the enterocyte membrane structure in the region of sodium chloride channels.[73,77] Direct injury to the mucosa by *N. risticii* and colonic inflammation are likely to be prominent features leading to diarrhea, especially later in the disease.[72] Loss of fluid, protein, and electrolyte is likely due to mucosal injury and effects on enterocyte fluid secretion caused by the inflammatory response. Like other inflammatory conditions of the colon, systemic inflammation caused by absorption of bacteria and bacterial products is a potential complication of *N. risticii* infections if mucosal injury is severe, which contributes to the clinical signs seen during the disease.

CLINICAL SIGNS AND DIAGNOSIS

N. risticii infection is clinically similar to other forms of enterocolitis and is characterized by anorexia, depression, and fever.[53,72,78] Experimental infections produce a biphasic fever wherein the second febrile phase occurs 6 to 7 days after the first.[78,79] Decreased gastrointestinal motility, manifested as reduced borborygmi, occurs during the early stages, before the onset of diarrhea. Diarrhea is seen in 75% of cases, and occurs 2 days after the second fever episode during experimental infections.[78,79] The diarrhea can be moderate to severe and dehydrating. Ileus can develop at any stage of the disease and can cause signs of moderate to severe colic. Systemic signs of endotoxemia, shock, and peripheral edema may occur and are similar to those described for salmonellosis. Experimental and natural infection with *N. risticii* can cause abortion of infected fetuses in pregnant mares.[80,81] Laminitis is a complication in 20% to 30% of naturally occurring cases and is often severe.[54] Other complications include protein-losing enteropathy, thrombosis, and renal failure, as described for salmonellosis.

Hematologic abnormalities reflect endotoxemia, dehydration, and sepsis and are essentially identical to those described for salmonellosis. Neutropenia with a left shift is a consistent feature and occurs concurrently with or soon after the onset of diarrhea.[79] Thrombocytopenia is common and often severe.[79] Neutrophilic leukocytosis occurs later in the course of the disease. Hyperfibrinogenemia is usually more pronounced than that seen with salmonellosis. Serum electrolyte, acid-base, and biochemical abnormalities are also similar to those described for salmonellosis. Coagulopathies are commonly seen during *N. risticii* infection and reflect activation of coagulation pathways. DIC is not uncommon and may be the cause of the high frequency of laminitis associated with *N. risticii* infection.[82]

Diagnosis of *N. risticii* infection cannot be based solely on clinical signs because the disease is clinically similar to other forms of enterocolitis. However, in endemic areas, acute colitis is likely to be caused by *N. risticii*, and thus the clinical signs of acute inflammatory colitis may in fact have a high predictive value in these areas. Serologic evidence of infection, such as rising antibody titers to *N. risticii* detected by indirect immunofluorescence (IFA) or enzyme-linked immunosorbent assay (ELISA) in paired serum samples, may be helpful in establishing a diagnosis.[54,83] Care should be taken when interpreting the IFA serologic test for *N. risticii* because the test appears to have a high false-positive rate.[84] Culture of the organism from blood is possible but difficult and is generally useful only in the research laboratory. Recently developed PCR tests for *N. risticii* DNA are rapid, highly sensitive (as sensitive as culture), and specific tests for *N. risticii* infection that can be applied to blood or feces.[85-87]

PREVENTION

Prevention of the disease by reducing exposure to the etiologic organism is difficult because the mode of transmission is not known. A killed vaccine has been developed that is relatively effective in preventing clinical illness other than fever in 80% of experimentally challenged horses using the vaccine strain. However, field studies suggest the vaccine has limited benefit for preventing natural infection or decreasing its severity.[88,89] Vaccine failures have been attributed to strain differences in antigenicity or to poor antibody responses to the vaccine.[88,89]

EQUINE INTESTINAL CLOSTRIDIOSIS

PATHOGENESIS

Clostridiosis is an important cause of acute enterocolitis in foals and adult horses. *Clostridium perfringens* and *Clostridium difficile* are most commonly associated with intestinal clostridiosis in horses, but other clostridial species, including *Clostridium septicum, Clostridicum cadaveris,* and *Clostridium sordelli* have also been isolated from horses with enterocolitis.[90-95] In horses of all ages, clostridial enterocolitis appears to be a common antibiotic-associated and nosocomial cause of enterocolitis.[94,96,97] Hemorrhagic enterocolitis caused by *C. perfringens* in neonatal foals is a distinct clinical entity and will be discussed in more detail elsewhere. This discussion focuses on adult intestinal clostridiosis. The reader is referred to Chapter 21 for information regarding the disease in foals.

Clostridium organisms are obligate anaerobic to aerotolerant spore-forming gram positive rods that are ubiquitous in the environment in the spore form.[95] They are elements of the normal flora of horses of all ages and are among the first bacteria acquired after birth. However, *Clostridium* organisms inhabiting the gastrointestinal tract are normally found in very low numbers and do not produce enterotoxins. Clostridiosis is associated with an increase in the number of a particular species of *Clostridia* in the gastrointestinal tract and, perhaps most important, exotoxin production. Although the conditions resulting in exotoxin production are not fully understood, several factors increase clostridial numbers in the gastrointestinal tract. Dietary factors affect the numbers of *Clostridium* species shed in horse feces.[90] Experimental induction of colic has been shown to increase fecal shedding of *Clostridium* species in the absence of diarrhea.[98] Antibiotics, particularly those administered orally or recycled via the enterohepatic system, have been shown to increase the recovery of *Clostridia* colony-forming units in equine feces and clinical clostridiosis.[91,93,99-101] Indeed, clostridiosis associated with *C. difficile* is likely to be the most important cause of antibiotic-induced enterocolitis in the horse.

Clostridium perfringens *C. perfringens* includes many genetically distinct strains of variable virulence that produce one or more of a large group of exotoxins. The pattern of exotoxin production is used to classify *C. perfringens* into five types: A, B, C, D, and E. *C. perfringens* type A is the most common clostridial isolate from healthy and diarrheic horses of all ages. *Clostridium perfringens* types A, B, C, and D have all been associated with hemorrhagic enteritis in foals younger than 10 days of age, with type C being the most common cause in North America.

The primary toxin produced by *C. perfringens* type A is α-toxin (phospholipase C), which interferes with glucose uptake and energy production and activates arachidonic acid metabolism and signaling pathways in enterocytes.[95] Oral administration of α-toxin does not cause tissue necrosis but causes increased secretion by small intestinal mucosal cells.[24,102] The β toxin of types B and C is a cytotoxin that causes enterocyte necrosis, ulceration, and ultimately severe intestinal inflammation and hemorrhage.[24,95] A novel toxin designated β_2 may also have a role in *C. perfringens* enterocolitis.[103] The biologic activity of the β_2 toxin is similar to that of β toxin, but β_2 toxin is not related to β toxin in its genetic sequence. The β_2 toxin was prevalent in two groups of horses with acute enterocolitis but not in healthy horses.[104] The β_2 toxin is predominantly associated with *C. perfringens* that would have otherwise been classified as type A but that may in fact represent a previously undescribed type.

Virulent strains of *C. perfringens* type A and, to a lesser extent, type C may produce enterotoxin. Enterotoxin is a cytotoxin that inserts into cell membranes to form pores, which alter permeability to water and macromolecules and ultimately lead to cellular necrosis.[105] Massive desquamation of the intestinal mucosa that is a result of enterotoxin cytotoxicity triggers an inflammatory response, intestinal edema, mural hemorrhage, and systemic inflammation.[106] Enterotoxin also alters tight junction integrity, resulting in increased paracellular permeability by a noncytotoxic mechanism.[107]

Clostridium difficile *C. difficile* produces several toxins, only two of which, toxin A and toxin B, have been studied in detail. Toxin B is a potent cytotoxin in vitro, but its role in enterocolitis is less clear than that of toxin A. Toxin B does not induce fluid secretion, inflammation, or characteristic alterations in intestinal morphology. *C. difficile* toxin A is an enterotoxin that induces an inflammatory response with hypersecretory diarrhea.[108] Toxin A induces neutrophil influx into intestinal tissue, mast cell degranulation, and secretion of prostaglandins, histamine, cytokines, and 5-HT by these activated leukocytes.[108-110] The products of neutrophils and mast cells have a significant role in the vasodilatory and secretory responses in the intestine during *C. difficile* infection.

The enteric nervous system (ENS) is central to the induction of intestinal inflammation and mucosal secretion by toxin A. A model for toxin A–induced secretory diarrhea has emerged in which toxin A stimulates substance P–containing afferent sensory nerve fibers, which in turn stimulate mast cell degranulation, recruitment and activation of polymorphonuclear leukocyte (PMN), and vasodilation.[111-113] Toxin A–induced stimulation of enterocyte secretion can occur via secretomotor neuronal stimulation by substance P–containing sensory neurons or products of mast cells and PMN. Mast cell degranulation, PMN influx, and enterocyte secretion are all abolished by neural blockade or depletion of substance P. How toxin A triggers the sensory component of the ENS remains unknown, but it is likely that toxin A–induced necrosis of enterocytes exposes afferent neurons to the noxious milieu of the intestinal contents.

CLINICAL SIGNS AND DIAGNOSIS

Equine intestinal clostridiosis is clinically similar to other forms of acute enterocolitis in horses.[90,95] Although the clinical course is usually acute, peracute colitis with rapid death may occur. Occasionally, a milder, more prolonged clinical course is seen. Fever, anorexia, and depression may be observed before the onset of gastrointestinal signs, but the absence of prodromal signs is more common. Signs of endotoxemia and shock may accompany acute signs of colic and severe, dehydrating diarrhea. Diarrhea may not be profuse but is usually dark and foul. Like the clinical signs, hematologic and serum biochemical abnormalities are similar to those associated with other forms of enterocolitis and reflect fluid, protein, and electrolyte loss and systemic inflammation resulting from endotoxemia. Neutropenia, leukopenia, and hemoconcentration are common. Hypoproteinemia may be profound. Hyponatremia, hypokalemia, hypochloremia, hypocalcemia, and a mixed prerenal-renal azotemia are often noted, as well as metabolic acidosis and coagulopathies. Serum concentrations of hepatocellular enzymes, such as sorbitol dehydrogenase, may be elevated, and liver function may be reduced.

Preliminary diagnosis of equine intestinal clostridiosis caused by *C. perfringens* is based on the isolation of greater than 100 colony-forming units (CFU) of *C. perfringens* type A per gram of feces from patients with diarrhea and signs suggestive of toxemia.[90,114] Similar criteria are used to screen human patients for *C. perfringens* type A infection. Normal horses shed less than 100 CFU/g of feces, and usually horses with intestinal clostridiosis shed greater than 10^6 CFU/g.[90,114] However, identification of high numbers of *Clostridium* organisms in the feces does not prove infection. Detection of *C. perfringens* toxins in feces or intestinal contents in horses with high numbers of fecal CFU and clinical signs of enterocolitis is more conclusive evidence of an enterotoxigenic infection than that based on culture alone.[95] Immunoassays are available that are primarily designed to detect *C. perfringens* enterotoxin.[95] However, the reliability (specificity) of some immunoassays for diagnosis of *C. perfringens* infection has come into question. Recently, PCR multiplex and gene probe assays have been developed for detection of the major lethal toxins in bacterial isolates or fecal samples to determine the pattern of toxin production and are currently the preferred methods of detection.[115-117]

Like *C. perfringens*, diagnosis of *C. difficile* infection depends on culture of the organism from feces and identification of toxins in the feces. Bacterial culture of *C. difficile* may be difficult, and therefore it is an insensitive diagnostic test in horses.[118,119] Enrichment techniques and culture of multiple fecal samples may be required.[119,120] Detection of toxin A or B (or both) in feces by cell cytotoxicity assay or immunoassay is the preferred test for diagnosis of *C. difficile* infection in humans.[95] These tests are more sensitive than bacterial culture for identifying *C. difficile* infection in adult horses.[118,119] Sensitive PCR methods may also be used to identify genes for toxins A and B in fecal samples from diarrheic horses.[95]

PROLIFERATIVE ENTEROPATHY

PATHOGENESIS

Proliferative enteropathy is a chronic hyperplastic disorder of the small intestine that has been described in a wide variety of mammalian and avian species.[121,122] The only etiologic agent identified to date that induces PE is the obligate intracellular pathogen *Lawsonia intracellularis*.[122,123] The pig is the most frequently naturally affected species. However, reports of equine PE associated with *L. intracellularis* have increased in recent years.[124-127] The relatedness of the strains of *L. intracellularis* causing PE in pigs and horses or even among other affected species is not known. There appears to be no host restriction because hamsters and other rodents can be infected with porcine strains of *L. intracellularis*. Before 2000 there were sporadic reports of PE in the literature describing isolated cases in horses.[125-127] Since 2000 outbreaks on breeding farms have been described in Canada and anecdotally reported in the U.S.[128]

Although the epidemiology of PE is not known specifically for horses, in other species the mode of transmission is fecal-oral, and large numbers of organisms can be shed in feces of infected animals.[122] Affected animals shedding the organism in the feces serve as a source of infection for herd mates. It is possible that nonequine species serve as reservoirs contributing to outbreaks on horse farms. Factors that increase the risk of PE in pigs include overcrowding, ration changes, transport, and weaning.[122,123] Like pigs, horses are affected as weanlings. Factors associated with weaning and other stresses may affect immunity and increase susceptibility to infection. The incubation period is 2 to 3 weeks in nonequine species and is presumed to be similar in horses.

Experimental *L. intracellularis* infection produces characteristic pathologic lesions in pigs and hamsters that are identical to lesions in horses with PE.[122,123] A profound hyperplasia of the mucosa associated with proliferation of crypt epithelium and crypt hyperplasia is induced locally in infected islands of tissue that eventually extend to the entire distal jejunum and ileum. *L. intracellularis* preferentially infects proliferating cells, thus the tropism for the crypt epithelium. Infected cells proliferate far more rapidly than uninfected cells, suggesting that *L. intracellularis* directly induces the proliferative response. However, the molecular basis for enhanced proliferation is not known. *L. intracellularis* penetrates epithelial cells in a membrane-bound vesicle but eventually escapes the vacuole and is found free in the cytoplasm, concentrated at the apical pole of the cell.

The gross pathologic lesions of equine PE are quite characteristic.[124-127] Lesions may be segmental and are most commonly found in the ileum and terminal jejunum in horses. However, the duodenum may also be affected. Severe mucosal hypertrophy is often observed but may wane during the chronic stages of the disease. The mucosa may become corrugated with focal erosions or ulcers. Submucosal edema is often easily identified on cut sections of affected segments. Moderate to severe crypt hyperplasia with atrophy of intestinal villi is a consistent feature. Hyperplastic crypts are branched and may herniate into the submucosa. Necrosis, edema of the submucosal and lamina propria, hemorrhage, mononuclear inflammation, and muscular hypertrophy have been reported in affected intestinal segments but are not consistent. Special stains such as silver stain are required to detect intracellular organisms. The organisms are curved or comma-shaped rods found clustered in the apical cytoplasm of hyperplastic crypt epithelium.

The proliferative response of the intestinal mucosa alters absorption of nutrients and fluid secretion by disrupting the architecture of the villi and by altering the maturation of epithelial cells into absorptive cells, accounting for the secretory diarrhea and often severe weight loss.[121,123] The combined effects of the inflammatory response and malabsorption may account for the clinically observed protein-losing enteropathy.

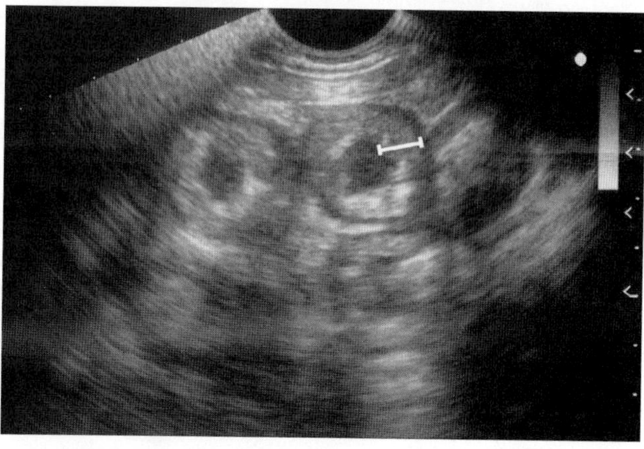

FIGURE 15-22 Ultrasonogram of the small intestine in a weanling foal with weight loss, diarrhea, and hypoproteinemia. Note the extreme mural thickening of the small intestine *(bar)* typical of proliferative enteropathy.

CLINICAL SIGNS AND DIAGNOSIS

Weanling foals 4 to 6 months of age are most commonly affected.[124-127] The clinical signs of PE include ill thrift, weight loss, peripheral edema, diarrhea, and colic.[124-127] The diarrhea is usually in the form of soft feces but may be profuse and watery. Some foals with mild diarrhea have black, tarry feces. Secondary complications such as gastric ulceration, bronchopneumonia, and parasitism may occur concurrently with the PE. Clinicopathologic features include mild to moderate anemia, moderate to severe hypoalbuminemia (often <2 g/dl), hypoglobulinemia, neutrophilic leukocytosis, and hyperfibrinogenemia. Creatine kinase activities may be elevated in affected foals. Prerenal azotemia and electrolyte imbalances such as hyponatremia may be associated with diarrhea. PF analysis is usually unremarkable. Ultrasonographic examination of the small intestine often reveals marked thickening of the intestinal wall (Figure 15-22). Intestinal edema may be evident as a hypoechoic appearance to one or more layers of the intestinal wall.

Methods for antemortem diagnosis include serologic analysis of *L. intracellularis* antibodies and PCR analysis of feces.[124] Serologic analysis using an indirect immunofluorescent antibody test may be the most useful single test available. The PCR test is very specific, but the sensitivity may be low as a result of sporadic shedding of organisms at the time clinical signs are evident. By the time clinical signs appear, 90% of pigs are serologically positive for anti–*L. intracellularis* IgG.[129] In contrast, only 37% of pigs had positive fecal PCR tests.[129] Of the seven foals tested in an outbreak of equine PE,[124] four foals with confirmed disease and three with suspected PE had serologic titers against *L. intracellularis* of 1:30 or greater. In contrast, serum samples collected from 72 foals before the outbreak were negative for *L. intracellularis* antibodies. Fecal PCR for *L. intracellularis* was positive in 6 of 18 foals tested, and half of the serologically positive foals had negative fecal PCR tests. Many clinicians combine serologic analysis with fecal PCR testing to increase the sensitivity and specificity of these diagnostic methods. Isolation and culture of the organism require cell culture techniques that are not widely available. Thus no practical method for culturing the organism from feces or tissues is available for clinical use.

Definitive diagnosis requires histopathologic examination of affected tissues.[121] Diagnosis is based on typical histopathologic findings of mucosal hypertrophy and submucosal edema and identification of small, curved, rod-shaped intracellular bacteria at the apical pole of epithelial cells in affected segments of intestine. Special stains such as Warthin-Starry silver stain are required to detect the bacteria in histopathologic specimens. PCR analysis of affected intestinal tissue is a very specific test for the presence of *L. intracellularis* and, unlike fecal PCR analysis, appears to be quite sensitive.[130]

Strongylosis

PATHOGENESIS

Strongyle infections in horses are caused by two groups of nematodes: large and small strongyles (see the section on cyathostomiasis). Large strongyles that are pathogenic in horses include *Strongylus vulgaris, Strongylus edentatus,* and *Strongylus equinus.* Of these species *S. vulgaris* is by far the most important cause of disease in the large intestine and in fact is the most pathogenic parasitic infection in horses.[131] *S. vulgaris* infection in horses is manifested clinically by two forms, causing acute and chronic disease.[131] The age and resistance of the host, the infective dose, and the size and function of the affected arteries influence the type and degree of disease that occurs. Sudden ingestion of large numbers of infective larvae by a naive host causes acute strongylosis, whereas ingestion of fewer infective larvae over a long period of time by an older, more resistant host causes chronic strongylosis. Acute strongylosis is more likely to cause colic than diarrhea and may be rapidly fatal. Chronic strongylosis tends to cause debilitation and signs of colic but may also cause diarrhea.

Diarrhea associated with acute strongylosis occurs within several days of infection and is likely to be caused by migration of the larvae through the intestinal wall. Fourth-stage larvae migrate through the mucosa and submucosa into the arterioles of the intestine, causing mural edema, hemorrhage, and infiltration of inflammatory cells.[131,132] Increased secretion and decreased absorption of fluid and electrolytes, stimulated by inflammatory mediators such as prostaglandins and histamine, may play a role in the diarrhea induced by *S. vulgaris.* Interstitial edema and damage to the interstitial matrix and mucosa may occur as a result of inflammation and migration of the parasites, causing increased secretion of fluid and albumin loss. Abnormal gastrointestinal motility may also play a role in the development of diarrhea. Migration of larvae through the intestinal wall early in the course of infection affects myoelectrical activity and motility in the large intestine and may affect retention of ingesta and absorption of fluid.[133,134] The cause of death in acute strongylosis has not been addressed, but it may be related to massive migration through the vasculature, causing thrombosis with ischemia and infarction of the intestine.

Chronic strongylosis causes typical verminous arteritis and is more commonly associated with natural infections in horses than acute strongylosis.[131] Lesions of the large intestinal vasculature caused by migration of larvae through the intima are characterized by thrombus formation, narrowing of the arterial lumen, fibrosis, and thickening of the arterial wall.[131,132] Embolization may occur, causing acute segmental infarction of the large intestine, but more commonly, reduced blood flow without embolization causes ischemia and occasionally infarction.[132,135] Postmortem examination of horses with colonic infarction failed to reveal embolization as the cause in the majority of cases.[135] Reduced blood flow in the tissues of the intestine usually results from narrowing of the arterial lumen by the thrombus and formation of microthrombi at sites independent of the parasites. Release of vasoconstrictive inflammatory mediators, such as leukotrienes, from platelets, neutrophils, and eosinophils, as well as elaboration of parasitic antigens or toxins, may cause vasoconstriction and ischemia.[136] Horses with experimental strongylosis had a 50% reduction of blood flow in the colonic vasculature.[137]

Clearly, reduced blood flow is an important effect of chronic strongylosis, but the relationship between blood flow and diarrhea is unclear. Disrupted motility resulting from ischemia may lead to diarrhea by reducing the retention of ingesta and absorption of fluid. Acute infarction and mucosal ulceration cause severe, chronic diarrhea in naturally infected horses.[138] Release of inflammatory mediators, such as prostaglandins, histamine, and kinins, from inflammatory cells associated with thrombi and inflamed intestine may also affect secretion, absorption, and motility, leading to diarrhea.

CLINICAL SIGNS AND DIAGNOSIS

The clinical signs of acute strongylosis caused by *S. vulgaris* infection include depression, moderate to severe colic, and fever.[139] Diarrhea is less often a feature of acute strongylosis than colic.[131] Most cases of acute strongylosis occur in young naïve horses that are introduced to an infested environment or are inoculated experimentally with infective larvae. This form of strongylosis is not often recognized naturally. Chronic strongylosis, however, is most commonly observed as a natural syndrome. Weight loss or poor weight gain; chronic, intermittent colic; fever; poor appetite; and diarrhea are frequently observed.[131,132] Diarrhea may be profuse and watery, or the feces may be soft but of normal volume. Transrectal palpation may reveal thickening and fremitus in the cranial mesenteric artery. Young horses are most commonly affected, but older horses may also be affected. Horses with acute infarction or large intestinal ulceration secondary to chronic strongylosis may have signs of severe abdominal pain, sepsis, and endotoxemia, and profuse, watery diarrhea is common.

Hematologic abnormalities associated with strongylosis include neutrophilic leukocytosis and eosinophilia.[139-141] Neutrophilia appears to be an early event during the course of the disease, and eosinophilia tends to appear later.[139,141] Hyperfibrinogenemia may also occur, especially later in the course of the disease. Serum α- and β-globulin and IgG(T) concentrations are characteristically elevated.[140-142] Horses with chronic ulcerative colitis secondary to strongylosis may develop severe hypoalbuminemia.[138] PF analysis may reveal an elevated protein concentration and eosinophilia.[140,141] Tentative diagnosis is based on clinical signs, hematologic abnormalities, and PF analysis. Elevated serum α- and β-globulin concentrations and IgG(T) concentration support the diagnosis.[142] Fecal analysis may reveal strongyle eggs, but fecal egg counts are often unreliable because nonpatent larvae cause the disease.

PREVENTION

Appropriate preventive measures are important in controlling this disease, including such management procedures as preventing overcrowding, reducing exposure of susceptible individuals, and instituting proper deworming schedules. Ivermectin is the preferred anthelmintic used to control strongylosis in horses. Monitoring fecal egg counts as a means of evaluating the efficacy of parasite control measures is recommended.

Cyathostomiasis

PATHOGENESIS

Infection with small strongyles (cyathostomiasis) is well recognized as a cause of diarrhea and large intestinal disease in horses of all ages.[143-148] Clinical disease is caused by intramural larval stages of more than 50 species of small strongyles (cyathastomes). The cyathostome life cycle requires migration by fourth-stage larvae through the mucosa of the large intestine and may include a period of hypobiosis, during which the larvae remain encysted within the mucosal layer of the large intestine.[143] After a period of hypobiosis, the larvae emerge in response to a largely unknown stimulus. Most cases occur when larval emergence takes place, classically in the late winter and spring in the northern temperate zones and in the late fall or winter months in the southeastern U.S. and subtropical regions.[143] Sudden emergence of encysted larvae causes mucosal injury, ulceration, and an inflammatory reaction that are largely responsible for the clinical disease.[143,149] However, migration of the larvae as they penetrate the mucosa affects motility patterns and can cause inflammation that may contribute to diarrhea.[149] Chronic, eosinophilic, granulomatous colitis and diarrhea with histopathologic evidence of hypobiotic cyathostome larvae in the large intestine has been reported in two horses during a period in which emergence of larvae would not be expected to occur (early winter).[143]

Natural emergence of cyathostome larvae causes fibrinous inflammation of the large intestine, focal necrosis, mural hemorrhage, and ulceration of the large intestinal mucosa, which may even result in bleeding into the lumen.[132,149] Mild to moderate eosinophilic and mononuclear inflammation of the lamina propria is seen.[132,149] Moderate to severe interstitial edema is frequently observed.[132,149] Colonic inflammation and interstitial edema may contribute to diarrhea, in conjunction with the loss of the mucosal barrier, by causing increased active and passive secretion of fluid, electrolytes, and protein. Protein loss is often significant, resulting in profound hypoalbuminemia and interstitial edema of skin and other organs. Chronic granulomatous colitis has been reported to occur in response to encysted larvae and may cause diarrhea by increased secretion secondary to granulomatous inflammation or disruption of the interstitium by granulomatous infiltration. Administration of an anthelmintic to horses with a heavy load of encysted larvae may also cause rapid larval death and acute and often severe inflammation similar to natural emergence.

CLINICAL SIGNS AND DIAGNOSIS

Cyathostomiasis may be the most commonly identified cause of chronic diarrhea in the horse.[150-152] However, an acute syndrome has also been associated with cyathostomiasis.[148] Clinical signs of cyathostomiasis characterized by moderate to severe weight loss or poor weight gain, ill thrift, ventral edema, intermittent fever, and intermittent mild colic.[143-148,152] Acute onset of diarrhea is typically profuse and progresses to chronic diarrhea that is often mild and the consistency of bovine feces and may be intermittent.[143-148,152] Appetite is usually normal, but some affected horses have a ravenous appetite. Transrectal palpation usually does not reveal any abnormalities. Horses of any age may be affected, and clinical signs are more common during periods of emergence of larvae, corresponding to late winter and spring in northern temperate zones. The deworming history may appear to be adequate.

Neutrophilic leukocytosis is typically evident, but the white blood cell count may be normal.[143-148] Profound hypoalbuminemia is a characteristic feature of cyathostomiasis, manifested clinically by ventral edema. Plasma α- and β-globulin concentrations may be elevated, which can result in a normal total plasma protein concentration in spite of hypoalbuminemia.[144-146] The serum IgG(T) concentration, however, has been reported to be normal, which may help distinguish cyathostomiasis from *S. vulgaris* infection.[143,145,146] PF analysis does not usually reveal any abnormalities, in contrast to horses with *S. vulgaris* infection. Fecal analysis may be unrewarding because the infection is often not patent when clinical signs are apparent. Measurement of plasma fructosamine may provide a measure of protein catabolism or protein loss in the absence of hypoalbuminemia.[152,153] Plasma fructosamine concentrations are significantly lower in horses with experimental cyathostomiasis than in normal controls,[152,153] suggesting that this test may be a useful diagnostic tool. However, the test has not yet been validated in naturally occurring cases, and neither the specificity nor the sensitivity is known. Rectal scrapings or rectal mucosal biopsies may reveal evidence of cyathostome larvae.[143,146] Definitive diagnosis usually requires microscopic examination of biopsy specimens of the cecum and ascending colon, collected by laparotomy. Examination of biopsy specimens collected from the small intestine is recommended to rule out other causes of weight loss and diarrhea. Appropriate diagnostic tests, such as culture of feces for pathogenic bacteria, should be included in the workup to further rule out other causes.

PREVENTION

Preventive measures are appropriate for other horses on the premises known to have a problem with cyathostomiasis. These include frequent deworming (every 6 weeks) during times of high infectivity (spring and summer in the north and fall, winter, and early spring in the south) to eliminate parasites before they become patent.[143] Because of high levels of resistance to benzimidazoles, avermectins (ivermectin or moxidectin) are often the drugs of choice for cyathostome control.[154-156] Resistance to ivermectin has been demonstrated, but the prevalence of ivermectin resistance appears to remain low.[154] Although daily pyrantel pamoate administration has also been reported to effectively reduce worm burdens and pasture infectivity in young and mature horses,[157] cyathostome resistance has been reported and is a concern for the use of this drug as a routine preventive anthelmintic.[155,158,159] Because of the rapid emergence of resistant strains to even ivermectin, targeted treatment, based on fecal egg counts and careful monitoring for the development of resistance to any anthelmintics used for cyathostome control, is warranted.[159]

TOXICOLOGIC DISEASES

Antibiotic-Associated Diarrhea

PATHOGENESIS

Antibiotic-associated diarrhea has been reported in many species, including horses.[160] Certain antibiotics, such as trimethoprim-sulfonamide combinations, erythromycin, penicillins, tetracyclines, clindamycin, and lincomycin, are associated with naturally occurring and experimental enterocolitis syndromes in horses.[91,160-163] In some cases, such as those seen with trimethoprim-sulfonamide combinations, the geographical incidence of antibiotic-associated diarrhea appears to differ markedly.

C. perfringens, C. difficile, and serovars of *S. enterica* are apparently the most common causes of antibiotic-associated diarrhea in horses. Outbreaks of *C. difficile* have been reported in hospitalized horses being treated with antibiotics.[93,97] In Sweden accidental erythromycin ingestion has been associated with *C. difficile* enterocolitis in mares in which their foals were being treated for *R. equi.*[100,162,164] Tetracycline administration has been associated with an increase in the numbers of gram negative enteric bacteria and *C. perfringens* in the feces of horses as well as reactivation of salmonellosis and prolongation of fecal shedding of serovars of *S. enterica.*[90,165]

The most common mechanism by which antibiotics cause diarrhea is disruption of the gastrointestinal flora. The normal large intestinal flora, composed of mainly obligate anaerobes and streptococci, protects the host from pathogenic bacteria by colonization resistance.[20] Ecologic factors play an important role in colonization resistance. For example, surface bacteria in the large intestine interact with receptors on the mucosal cells, facilitating adherence to the mucosa.[20,166] In doing so, the normal organisms compete more successfully for this important niche. Competition for space and nutrients is an important means of preventing colonization and proliferation of pathogenic bacteria.[19,20,166] In addition, anaerobic bacteria produce short-chain fatty acids and other metabolites that are toxic to facultative anaerobic bacteria, especially in the conditions of the large intestine.[19,20,166] Organisms of the normal flora produce bacteriocins that inhibit growth of potential pathogens.[19]

Antibiotics that deplete the population of obligate anaerobes and streptococci efficiently decrease colonization resistance.[19] Production of fatty acids is diminished, and competition for space and nutrients is reduced. As a result, gram negative enteric bacteria, such as *S. enterica var typhimurim,* are able to proliferate. In addition, pathogenic anaerobes normally found in low numbers can proliferate. Antibiotic-resistant strains of bacteria, especially gram negative enteric bacteria and possibly clostridia, may be selected by antibiotic administration, allowing proliferation of pathogenic bacteria resistant to many antibiotics.[167] Obligate anaerobic commensal organisms, perhaps the most critical group of microbes for maintaining colonization resistance, are usually susceptible to macrolides, tetracyclines, β-lactams, and lincomamides, which may explain the high incidence of diarrhea associated with the administration of these antibiotics.[95]

In addition to reduction of colonization resistance, depletion of the normal anaerobic microbial population in the intestine decreases carbohydrate fermentation and production of SCFAs, which contributes to the pathogenesis of antibiotic-associated diarrhea by decreasing absorption of sodium and water by the colonic mucosa.[168] Ampicillin decreases colonic fermentation of carbohydrates in humans.[169] Human patients with antibiotic-associated diarrhea have markedly impaired colonic fermentation and very low production of SCFAs.[170] Erythromycin, ampicillin, or metronidazole treatment is associated with decreased production of SCFA in patients with and without diarrhea.[170] Absorption of sodium and water is stimulated by absorption of SCFA in the equine colon, suggesting that reduction of colonic SCFA content by antibiotic-induced depletion of anaerobic flora has similar effects in horses as in humans.[168]

Broad spectrum antibiotics exert a more profound effect on the gastrointestinal flora than narrow-spectrum antibiotics.[171] Antibiotics administered orally, especially those that are poorly absorbed, are more likely to cause diarrhea than parenterally administered antibiotics.[171] For instance, clindamycin is less likely to cause diarrhea in humans when administered intravenously than when administered orally.[171] Antibiotics with extensive enterohepatic circulation, such as tetracyclines and erythromycin, are excreted in high concentrations in the bile and are more commonly associated with diarrhea than antibiotics that do not undergo enterohepatic circulation.[171]

Antibiotics may cause diarrhea by other means than by disrupting the normal flora. Direct toxic effects may play a role in producing irritation, increasing secretion, and disrupting motility patterns. Tetracyclines are irritating to the gastrointestinal mucosa and may cause inflammation and increase secretion.[171] Erythromycin has been shown to interact with smooth muscle cells, stimulating gastrointestinal motility.[171,172] Normal peristalsis plays an important role in suppressing the population size of potentially pathogenic bacteria. Normally, bacteria that are prevented from adhering to the mucosa by colonization resistance are swept aborally by peristalsis and excreted in the feces. Disruption of normal motility patterns may prevent clearance of pathogenic bacteria, contributing to the colonization of mucosal surfaces.

CLINICAL SIGNS AND DIAGNOSIS

Diarrhea induced by antibiotics usually occurs within 7 days of initiation of antibiotic administration but may occur several days after cessation of antibiotic treatment. The clinical syndrome of antibiotic-associated diarrhea varies from mild diarrhea to fulminant enterocolitis with severe diarrhea. Mild diarrhea is common, especially in foals receiving erythromycin, trimethoprim-sulfa combinations, or rifampin[162,173] and are usually not clinically significant. However, acute, severe enterocolitis can occur in horses of all ages receiving antibiotics and can be life threatening. Clinical signs are identical to those resulting from other causes of acute enterocolitis. Severe, dehydrating diarrhea; endotoxemia; sepsis; and shock may occur. Hemoconcentration, neutropenia, hypoproteinemia, and electrolyte and acid-base imbalances are common. Severe hyponatremia may occur in foals with antibiotic-associated diarrhea, especially if trimethoprim-sulfa and rifampin combinations are the cause.[173] More detailed descriptions of the clinical and laboratory findings were given earlier. Diagnosis is presumptive because definitive diagnosis of antibiotic-associated diarrhea is impossible. Fecal culture or PCR testing may reveal *S. enterica* or *Clostridium* spp. infection.

Nonsteroidal Anti-inflammatory Drugs

PATHOGENESIS

Toxicity resulting from NSAID administration has been well documented in several species, including horses, and is discussed in Chapter 4.[174-180] In horses and humans NSAID toxicity is manifested by renal and gastrointestinal disease. Foals are considered to be more susceptible than adult horses to gastrointestinal disease secondary to NSAID administration, and ponies may be more susceptible than horses. NSAID toxicity varies primarily as a result of properties that influence distribution to sensitive tissues and relative selectivity for COX-1 or COX-2. All nonselective NSAIDs are capable of inducing gastrointestinal and renal damage at toxic concentrations. Aspirin has been suggested to be more toxic than other NSAIDs because it irreversibly inactivates COX by acetylation, whereas other NSAIDs reversibly inhibit COX.[174] Phenylbutazone is the drug most commonly reported to cause gastrointestinal toxicity in horses, perhaps because of its widespread usage by veterinarians and horse owners or perhaps because of bona fide differences in toxicity in horses compared with other nonselective NSAIDs. Acute phenylbutazone toxicity in horses resulting from overdose is characterized by mucosal ulceration throughout the gastrointestinal tract, oral ulceration, renal papillary necrosis, vasculopathy, thrombosis, and protein-losing enteropathy with hypoalbuminemia.[176-178] COX-2–selective NSAIDs appear to be much less toxic in the equine gastrointestinal tract.[181,182] The focus of this discussion is on the toxic effects of NSAIDs on the large intestine, but this necessarily includes elements of upper gastrointestinal and renal disease.

Horses with large intestinal disease resulting from NSAID toxicity generally are receiving inappropriately large doses or have underlying disorders that predispose the large intestine to the toxic effects of NSAIDs even at appropriate dosages. The dosage regimen recommended for phenylbutazone (4.4 mg/kg every 12 hours for 1 day, and then 2.2 mg/kg every 12 hours) is considered safe. Experimental studies in horses, however, have shown toxicity to occur when amounts exceeding the recommended dosage (6.6 mg/kg/day) is administered for several days.[176,177] Most reported cases of phenylbutazone toxicosis occurred in horses receiving higher-than-recommended dosages.[178,180,183] Regardless, administration of phenylbutazone at the recommended dosage has been reported to cause a significant decrease in plasma protein concentration and gastrointestinal disease.[177,184] Moreover, signs of NSAID toxicity have been reported in normovolemic horses treated with appropriate doses of phenylbutazone.[184,185] Dehydration, sepsis, endotoxemia, and other conditions that alter hemodynamic homeostasis exacerbate renal and gastrointestinal toxicity of NSAIDs.[174] Underlying inflammation of the intestinal tissues may increase the likelihood of gastrointestinal ulceration resulting from NSAIDs.

Gastrointestinal disease induced by NSAIDs is manifested by mucosal ulceration, inflammation, bleeding, and protein-losing enteropathy.[176,177,180,184] In addition to direct effects on the mucosal barrier, NSAID administration causes an acute relapse of preexisting colonic inflammatory disease and worsens colonic inflammation in humans with inflammatory bowel disease.[174,186,187]

It is not clear whether the aforementioned NSAID effects occur in horses. The mechanism by which NSAIDs induce mucosal damage is probably multifactorial. Direct irritation may play a role in oral and gastric irritation and ulceration; however, parenteral administration of NSAIDs produces oral and gastric ulceration as well. Inhibition of prostaglandin synthesis by inhibition of both COX-1 and COX-2 appears to be the most important mechanism of mucosal injury. Prostaglandins, particularly PGE_2 and PGI_2, are critical for mucosal health and repair after injury.[188,189] PGE_2 increases mucosal blood flow; increases secretion of mucus, water, and bicarbonate; increases mucosal cell turnover rate and migration; stimulates adenyl cyclase activity; and exerts other protective effects in the gastric mucosa of several species.[174,188,189] Perhaps most important, PGE_2 and PGI_2 have roles in maintaining epithelial tight junction integrity, which is indispensable for mucosal barrier function and repair after mucosal injury.[188]

In spite of the overwhelming amount of information about the role of prostaglandins in maintaining the mucosal barrier in other species and clear clinical and experimental evidence that NSAIDs injure the equine colonic mucosa, the role of prostaglandins in mucosal protection in the equine colon is not yet well defined. Inhibition of COX-1 and COX-2 in equine colonic mucosa with flunixin meglumine results in reduced electrical resistance of the mucosa and increased permeability to macromolecules in vitro,[190] suggesting that flunixin treatment disrupts the epithelial tight junctions in the equine colon. This was correlated with a profound inhibition of PGE_2 and PGI_2 concentrations in the treated tissues. Administration of a PGE_2 analog prevents the gastrointestinal manifestations of phenylbutazone-toxicosis in ponies.[177]

Recent development of NSAIDs that specifically inhibit COX-2 have markedly reduced the frequency and severity of gastrointestinal side effects in humans taking NSAIDs for chronic musculoskeletal conditions.[191] COX-2–specific NSAIDs such as firocoxib hold promise for use in horses to treat arthritis[192] and other conditions, with reduced incidence of toxicity. For example, the relatively COX-2–specific inhibitors meloxicam and firocoxib are less harmful to equine intestinal mucosa than flunixin meglumine in vitro.[181,182] Moreover, COX-2–selective inhibitors are significantly more permissive than flunixin for recovery of the mucosa in equine ischemic-injured intestinal tissues; in fact, recovery is no different than that for control tissues.[181,182]

NSAID-induced mucosal injury is associated with a marked inflammatory response to microbial products exposed to the lamina propria.[193] This inflammation exacerbates mucosal dysfunction and injury associated with NSAID toxicity. For example, depletion of neutrophils or blockade of neutrophil influx into gastrointestinal tissues or inhibition of neutrophil activation and release of toxic products prevents many of the pathophysiologic effects of NSAID toxicity in the gastrointestinal tract.[194-197] The inflammatory response alone may result in moderate to severe gastrointestinal ulceration, mural vascular thrombosis and edema, fluid secretion, protein-losing enteropathy, and mucosal hemorrhage.

CLINICAL SIGNS AND DIAGNOSIS

NSAID colitis manifests as two clinical syndromes: right dorsal ulcerative colitis (RDUC) and generalized NSAID toxicity. As its name implies, RDUC is a disorder isolated to the right dorsal segment of the large intestine.[179,180,185] The most prominent clinical signs of RDUC are anorexia, lethargy, and colic. Anorexia, depression, diarrhea, fever, and signs of endotoxemia may also be features. If RDUC is chronic, weight loss, intermittent colic, lethargy, anorexia, and ventral edema are common clinical signs with soft and unformed feces. Ulceration of the right dorsal colonic mucosa results in protein-losing enteropathy and significant hypoproteinemia attributable mainly to hypoalbuminemia. Hypoproteinemia may be one of the earliest clinical manifestations of RDUC and can be sufficiently severe to cause peripheral (usually ventral) edema. In some cases, dehydration, electrolyte abnormalities, neutropenia or anemia, azotemia, and biochemical abnormalities may be noted if the ulceration and diarrhea are severe or if systemic inflammation is present.

Clinical signs of generalized NSAID toxicity vary from mild diarrhea with no systemic signs to severe dehydrating diarrhea with anorexia, fever, depression, peripheral edema, oral ulceration, and colic.[177,178,183]

Clinical signs of systemic inflammation caused by endotoxemia may occur, manifested as poor peripheral perfusion, tachycardia and tachypnea, weakness, trembling, and cyanotic or hyperemic oral mucous membranes. Hematuria or oliguria may be present with renal involvement. Complications associated with other forms of severe enterocolitis, such as laminitis, thrombophlebitis, and severe weight loss, may occur.

Although phenylbutazone has been associated specifically with bone marrow depression resulting in abnormalities in one or more blood cell lines,[198] hematologic abnormalities of generalized NSAID toxicity are usually nonspecific and include neutropenia with a left shift or leukocytosis and hemoconcentration. Serum biochemical analysis is characterized by profound hypoproteinemia, hyponatremia, and metabolic acidosis.[183,184] Hypocalcemia, hypokalemia, hypochloremia, and elevated hepatocellular enzyme activities may also be seen. Hypoproteinemia may occur without signs of diarrhea. Azotemia may be prerenal as a result of dehydration, but it is frequently caused by renal failure that results from a combination of hemodynamic effects of NSAIDs and direct toxic renal injury. Urinalysis frequently reveals hematuria, proteinuria, cylindruria, and isosthenuria. Fecal occult blood is frequently detected.

Diagnosis of either form of NSAID colitis is often presumptive, with a history of overdose of NSAIDs being strong evidence of NSAID toxicity. But as discussed earlier, toxicity may occur with dosage regimens that are not considered inappropriate, particularly if the horse experiences a concurrent period of dehydration. Ultrasonographic examination of the right dorsal colon can be used to confirm a diagnosis of RDUC, but the sensitivity of this method appears to be low.[199] Ultrasonography (3.5-5 MHz transducer at the right twelth through fifteenth intercostal spaces below the margin of the lung axial to the liver) may reveal a thickened right dorsal colon (>0.5 cm) and evidence of colonic edema in horses with RDUC.[199,200] Nuclear scintigraphy of horses after infusion with technetium-99–labeled white blood cells can be used to document inflammation of the right dorsal colon.[201] Laparotomy or laparoscopic examination of the right dorsal colon may be required for definitive diagnosis of RDUC. Other causes of enterocolitis, such as salmonellosis, Potomac horse fever, clostridiosis, and antibiotic-associated diarrhea, must be ruled out.

Cantharidin Toxicity

PATHOGENESIS

Cantharidin is the toxic substance found in beetles of the genus *Epicauta,* commonly known as *blister beetles.*[202-204] Ingestion of the beetles causes release of the toxin and absorption through the gastrointestinal tract. Transcutaneous absorption may occur but appears to be rare in horses.[203] Blister beetles feed on the flowers of alfalfa and may be incorporated into processed alfalfa hay if the hay is cut and processed simultaneously, as by crimping.[202-204] The beetles often swarm, and large numbers of beetles may be found in relatively small portions of hay. The lethal dose of cantharidin is less than 1 mg/kg, but the concentration of cantharidin varies among species of blister beetles and between sexes.[202,203] As many as 100 to as few as six beetles may be lethal. Usually, only one or a few horses fed contaminated hay will ingest beetles because the beetles are concentrated in a small portion of the hay. However, outbreaks involving many horses on a farm have occurred. Most cases have occurred in Texas and Oklahoma, but horses in other states may be affected as well, especially if hay is imported from states where blister beetles are common. Peak incidence is in late summer and fall.[205] The fatality rate may be 50% or greater,[202,206] but if the patient survives several days, recovery is probable.

Cantharidin is absorbed from the gastrointestinal tract and excreted by the kidneys. Cantharidin is a potent irritant, causing acantholysis and vesicle formation when applied topically.[202,204,206] The chemical is thought to disrupt oxidative metabolism in the mitochondria, causing mitochondrial swelling, plasma membrane damage, and changes in membrane permeability.[202] The mucosa of the gastrointestinal tract is most commonly affected in horses because they ingest the toxin. Cell swelling and necrosis occur, resulting in mucosal ulceration. Oral, esophageal, gastric, and small and large intestinal ulceration have been observed in natural and experimental canthariasis.[202,204,206] Severe fibrinous to pseudomembranous inflammation and submucosal edema of the intestine have also been reported. Diarrhea probably results from the severe ulceration and inflammation of the large intestine, causing increased secretion of water, electrolytes, and protein and decreased absorption of fluid. Large volumes of fluid and protein are lost in the gastrointestinal tract, causing hemoconcentration and profound hypoalbuminemia in some affected horses.[202,203,206]

Cystitis and myocarditis occur in natural and experimentally induced cases of cantharidin toxicity.[202,204,206] The toxin is excreted by the kidneys, and high concentrations of cantharidin in the urine induce cystitis. Occasionally, hemorrhagic cystitis may occur, resulting in hematuria or frank hemorrhage into the bladder.[202] The cause of myocarditis and myocardial necrosis is unknown but may be a direct effect of toxin on the myocardium. Increased plasma creatine kinase activity is often observed and has been postulated to arise from the damaged myocardium.[202,203] Affected horses have a characteristically stiff gait, but histopathologic evidence of skeletal muscle injury that explains the elevated plasma creatine kinase activity has not been observed.[203] The kidneys are often pale, swollen, and moist, with occasional infarcts.[204]

Hypocalcemia and hypomagnesemia are biochemical features of cantharidin toxicity in horses that have not been explained.[202,203,206] Hypocalcemia may result from hypoalbuminemia, but the ionized calcium concentration is often decreased, indicating that hypoalbuminemia is not responsible for the hypocalcemia.[203]

CLINICAL SIGNS AND DIAGNOSIS

Cantharidin toxicity can cause a range of clinical signs, from mild depression and abdominal discomfort to fulminant signs of toxemia and rapid death, depending on the ingested dose of toxin.[202,203,206] Most commonly, clinical signs include depression, sweating, irritability, abdominal pain, elevated heart and respiratory rates, fever, polyuria, polydipsia, and profuse diarrhea.[202,203,206] Blood is rarely seen in the feces. Stranguria and pollakiuria are common.[202] Signs of hypocalcemia include synchronous diaphragmatic flutter and tremors. A stiff and stilted gait may be evident. Neurologic signs such as head pressing, swaying, and disorientation may be noted.[206] Signs of systemic inflammation resulting from endotoxemia may be seen in severe cases. Some horses develop severe depression and toxemia and may die within hours of ingesting cantharidin without developing diarrhea.[202,206]

Hematologic abnormalities include hemoconcentration and neutrophilic leukocytosis.[202,203] Occasionally, neutropenia and leukopenia may accompany endotoxemia. Serum biochemical analysis usually reveals increased creatine kinase activity, hypocalcemia, and hypoalbuminemia.[202,203] Biochemical abnormalities include hypocalcemia (both ionized and total calcium concentrations), hypomagnesemia, and azotemia.[202,203,206] Urine specific gravity is characteristically in the hyposthenuric range.[202,203] Microscopic hematuria and mild proteinuria may be evident. Fecal occult blood is often present, but hematochezia is unusual.

A tentative diagnosis can be made on the basis of clinical signs and identification of blister beetles in the hay. Determining the species of the insects may be necessary to estimate the amount of cantharidin ingested. All species of *Epicauta* contain cantharidin, but some have small amounts. Definitive diagnosis requires the measurement of the cantharidin concentration in gastric or intestinal contents and urine.[202,205]

Arsenic Toxicosis

PATHOGENESIS

Arsenic toxicosis is an unusual cause of diarrhea in horses, resulting from ingestion of arsenic-containing herbicides, insecticides, and other pest-control products contaminating water or roughage used as a food source.[207] The toxicity of arsenic depends on the valence of the element.[207,208] Arsenate may be reduced to arsenite in mammalian systems.[208] Arsenite is thought to be more toxic than arsenate and less rapidly excreted in urine.[208] Arsenate and arsenite uncouple oxidative phosphorylation, leading to breakdown of energy metabolism in the cells of many tissues.[208] Widespread cellular injury and death occur rapidly during acute arsenic toxicosis. Multiorgan failure is usually the result. In fact, cardiomyopathy and pulmonary disease are common causes of death in humans.[209] Damage to the large intestine is probably due in part to direct cellular toxicity and corrosion by the compound. However, vasculitis is a hallmark of the disease in humans and horses and is thought to be the most important mechanism of large intestinal disease in humans.[207,210] Acute hemorrhagic colitis is a feature of arsenic toxicosis, with severe mural edema and mucosal ulceration.[207] Profuse hemorrhagic diarrhea and abdominal pain result. Chronic arsenic toxicity can occur but appears to be rare in horses.

CLINICAL SIGNS AND DIAGNOSIS

Depression, weakness, abdominal pain, hemorrhagic diarrhea, and shock are characteristic of acute arsenic toxicosis in horses.[207] Death may occur before diarrhea is evident. Initial clinical signs may be difficult to distinguish from other peracute forms of colitis and are related to endotoxic shock, metabolic disturbances, and dehydration. Later, cardiac arrhythmias, pulmonary edema, acute renal failure, and neurologic deficits (ataxia and stupor) may develop.[207] Anuria or polyuria may be observed. Hemolytic anemia caused by preferential binding of arsenic compounds to red blood cells is a feature of arsenic poisoning in humans.[209] Hematologic abnormalities resulting from injury to bone marrow cells and ongoing hemolysis may be seen after the peracute stage. Leukopenia and thrombocytopenia have been described in human patients.[209] Serum biochemical analysis may reveal azotemia, hepatocellular enzyme activities higher than generally attributed to endotoxemia, and increased creatine kinase activity.[207] Urine specific gravity may be in the isosthenuric range, with hematuria, cylindruria, and proteinuria evident by urinalysis.

Diagnosis may be possible by measuring blood and urine arsenic concentration, but these tests may not be diagnostic. Postmortem diagnosis is confirmed by measuring arsenic concentrations in liver and kidney samples.[207] History of exposure and clinical signs remain the primary means of diagnosis.

MISCELLANEOUS DISORDERS OF THE LARGE INTESTINE

Intestinal Anaphylaxis

PATHOGENESIS

Severe intestinal anaphylaxis is a syndrome in horses characterized by peracute, rapidly fatal colitis.[211] The severe syndrome is clinically and pathologically similar to other known causes of peracute colitis, such as salmonellosis, clostridiosis, and antibiotic-associated diarrhea. Some cases are less severe and manifest as mild to moderate diarrhea or colic (or both). The syndrome of intestinal anaphylaxis can be produced by either an IgE-mediated Type I hypersensitivity or an IgE-independent anaphylactoid reaction.[212,213] Intestinal anaphylaxis is usually induced by local gastrointestinal exposure to a food, environmental, drug, or other allergen [212,214] but may also occur with systemic exposure to an allergen.[215-217] Massive mast cell degranulation, secretion of inflammatory mediators, and activation of enteric neural reflexes in the intestine causes profound alterations in blood flow, increased vascular permeability and interstitial edema, recruitment of neutrophils, altered motility, mucosal injury, absorption of microbial products, and mucosal hypersecretion.[218-222] Systemic signs may be caused by the anaphylactic reaction or may be associated with systemic inflammation triggered by microbial products (endotoxin) absorbed through the injured and hyperpermeable mucosa.

Intestinal anaphylaxis in horses may be a peracute, fulminant enterocolitis with endotoxemia that may be fatal.[211,223] This form is characterized by severe intramural edema and hemorrhagic inflammation of the large intestine, often producing submucosal thickening on the order of many centimeters. Vascular thrombosis may be widespread, with mucosal and serosal petechia and ecchymoses. Less severe forms of intestinal anaphylaxis may manifest as patchy areas of intestinal edema and congestion.[215] Diarrhea results from intestinal inflammation initiated by the type I hypersensitivity response. Many of the mediators of type I hypersensitivity, such as histamine and 5-HT, have well-documented stimulatory effects on mucosal secretory activity, vascular and epithelial permeability, and motility[218-220] in the intestine. Systemic inflammation resulting from endotoxemia may be overwhelming once the mucosal barrier breaks down. Infarction of intestinal segments and other organs may result from intravascular coagulation. Ileus, abdominal distention, and moderate to severe abdominal pain may result from motility disturbances and infarction of the large intestine.

CLINICAL SIGNS AND DIAGNOSIS

The clinical signs are similar to those described for other forms of peracute colitis. However, the severity may be variable, manifesting as colic or moderate diarrhea. Characteristically, severe shock, signs of systemic inflammation resulting from endotoxemia, and severe metabolic disturbances are observed.[211,223] Heart and respiratory rates may be markedly elevated, with other signs of cardiovascular collapse, such as weak and thready peripheral pulses and peripheral vasoconstriction. However, peripheral vasodilation may be seen later in the course of disease. Dark red, muddy, or cyanotic mucous membranes with a prolonged capillary refill time are consistent with sepsis. Borborygmi are usually absent, and abdominal tympany may be heard on percussion, secondary to ileus. Moderate to severe colic may accompany ileus. Severe diarrhea is possible, but death may occur before diarrhea is evident. Multiorgan failure resulting from DIC is not unusual. The rapid onset of weakness, staggering, and trembling commonly precedes death. The syndrome may cause death in 4 to 24 hours.

Hematologic abnormalities include severe neutropenia and leukopenia, thrombocytopenia, and hemoconcentration.[211] Serum biochemical alterations include hyponatremia, hypokalemia, hypocalcemia, and severe metabolic acidosis. Blood urea nitrogen and creatinine may be elevated from prerenal or renal azotemia. If acute renal failure occurs, hyperkalemia may result. Hepatocellular enzyme activity may be increased on account of endotoxemia. Severe coagulopathies are common, resulting in prolonged coagulation times, decreased antithrombin III activity, and increased plasma concentration of fibrin degradation products. Analysis of PF may be valuable because infarction of the large intestine is not unusual. Protein concentration and the white blood cell count may be elevated. Red blood cell counts are less likely to be elevated because infarction, rather than strangulation, of the intestine occurs.

Diagnosis is based on clinical signs, postmortem findings, and exclusion of other causes. Cultures and toxicologic analysis of fecal samples and gastrointestinal tissues fail to demonstrate a clear cause. Other diagnostic tests are also inconclusive. If an antigen is suspected as the trigger of the anaphylaxis, a Prausnitz-Kustner passive cutaneous anaphylaxis sensitization test can confirm the presence of antigen-specific IgE in the patient serum.[215]

Carbohydrate Overload

PATHOGENESIS

Overeating of soluble carbohydrates, especially so-called hot grains such as corn, overwhelms the digestive capability of the small intestine, resulting in a high percentage of soluble carbohydrates entering the large intestine. The amount of soluble carbohydrates that will produce diarrhea varies according to the previous dietary history of the individual. Horses fed diets higher in soluble carbohydrates are more resistant to the deleterious effects of carbohydrate overload. Gradual accommodation to a diet high in carbohydrates can be accomplished over several weeks. However, horses fed an unusually large amount of grains or other form of soluble carbohydrates often develop diarrhea and may, depending on the amount ingested, develop severe colitis, systemic inflammation resulting from endotoxemia, metabolic acidosis, and laminitis.[224-227]

The pathogenesis of colitis from carbohydrate overload is primarily due to the toxic effects on the microbial flora in the large intestine.[225] A sudden delivery of soluble carbohydrates to the large intestine causes rapid fermentation by gram positive lactic acid–producing bacteria and a sudden increase in organic acid production.[226] The cecal pH level rapidly decreases, and the lactic acid concentration rapidly increases.[226] Rapid organic acid production overwhelms the buffering capacity of the large intestine, not only by directly depleting the buffers found in the contents but also by reducing the efficiency of buffer secretion. Bicarbonate secretion is linked to absorption of volatile fatty acids, which are produced in low amounts by fermentation of soluble carbohydrates. The contents of the large intestine become profoundly acidic, resulting in unfavorable conditions for the microbial flora. Lactic acid–producing bacteria flourish, whereas the gram negative bacteria, especially the *Enterobacteriaceae*, are killed in large numbers by the acids. Large quantities of endotoxin are released from the dying bacteria.[226]

The osmotic load from lactic acid produced in the large intestine is an important factor in the development of diarrhea because organic acids such as lactic acid are poorly absorbed. Mild cases of carbohydrate overload may result purely from osmotic diarrhea. In more severe cases the acidic contents of the large intestine are toxic to the mucosa, causing necrosis of the mucosal tissues similar to that seen in ruminal acidosis. Mucosal ulceration allows absorption of large quantities of endotoxin and lactic acid produced by the massive die-off of acid-intolerant microbes and fermentation of soluble carbohydrates, normally poorly absorbed by intact mucosa.[227] Systemic inflammation resulting from endotoxemia may be overwhelming, and profound metabolic acidosis may occur. Secretory diarrhea caused by the direct effects of acid luminal contents on the mucosa, as well as the effects of inflammatory mediators on enterocyte secretion, worsens the acidosis and dehydration. Systemic inflammation resulting from endotoxemia, along with intestinal inflammation, adversely affects intestinal motility, and ileus develops. Ileus and gas production from fermentation of carbohydrates may cause severe distention of the large intestine and signs of abdominal pain. Laminitis is a frequent complication of endotoxemia and lactic acidosis. In fact, carbohydrate overload is used to induce laminitis as an experimental model because of the consistency of the laminitis produced.[225-227]

CLINICAL SIGNS AND DIAGNOSIS

Clinical signs of colitis from carbohydrate overload can vary according to the amount of carbohydrate ingested and accommodation of the flora to a high carbohydrate diet. Mild cases may result in a transient osmotic diarrhea, with no systemic effects. Severe cases are characterized by signs similar to those described for other forms of colitis, including abdominal pain, moderate to severe diarrhea, and dehydration. Signs of endotoxemia and sepsis are frequently present in severe cases. Elevated heart and respiratory rates are common, with peripheral vasoconstriction early in the disease, followed by peripheral vasodilation as the disease progresses. Depression may be profound as a result of metabolic acidosis and endotoxemia. Abdominal auscultation and percussion may reveal ileus and intestinal tympany. Nasogastric intubation may yield significant gastric acidic reflux. Particles of grain may be noted in the gastric reflux and the feces if grain overload is the source of the carbohydrate overload. Laminitis may complicate both mild and severe cases of carbohydrate overload, especially if the animal has had previous bouts of laminitis.

Hematologic abnormalities include neutropenia and leukopenia. Severe dehydration may result in profound hemoconcentration. Protein loss later in the course of disease may result in hypoproteinemia. Serum biochemical abnormalities include azotemia, elevated hepatocellular enzyme activity, hyponatremia, and hypokalemia. Severe hypocalcemia and metabolic acidosis are characteristic of the disease. Serum lactate concentrations are elevated in the absence of evidence of intestinal strangulation or infarction. PF analysis often reveals no abnormalities.

Sand Enteropathy

Sand enteropathy is described in more detail under the heading of Obstructive Diseases, because acute obstruction is often associated with abnormally large amounts of sand in the large intestine.[228] However, chronic sand-induced diarrhea is a distinct syndrome that can occur at any age as a result of the abnormal accumulation of sand in the large intestine.[229,230] Chronic diarrhea and signs of colic may be seen without obstruction. The pathogenesis of sand accumulation in individual horses, other than simple ingestion of large quantities, is unclear, as described elsewhere in this chapter. Presumably, the sand causes irritation and may disrupt motility, leading to diarrhea. The diarrhea is usually not severe and dehydrating and may be intermittent. Weight loss is characteristic and can be severe in some cases.[229] Complications may occur, such as peritonitis and acute obstruction.[229]

Diagnosis is usually based on the presence of abnormal amounts of sand in the feces. Because sand-induced chronic diarrhea is primarily associated with sand accumulation in the ventral colon, auscultation of the ventral abdomen immediately behind the xiphoid process may reveal characteristic sand sounds.[231] This technique is sensitive only if peristalsis is present. Ultrasonography may also be useful to identify sand in the ventral colon, but it is not useful to quantitate the amount of sand. Occasionally, radiography may be required to detect sand in the colon.[229]

PRINCIPLES OF THERAPY FOR ACUTE DIARRHEA

The principles of therapy for acute diarrhea resulting from colitis are similar regardless of the cause and include replacement of fluid and electrolyte losses, control of colonic inflammation, reduction of fluid secretion, promotion of mucosal repair, control of endotoxemia and sepsis, and re-establishment of normal flora. The purpose of this section is to review the principles of therapy, with references to specific therapies for particular etiologies as they arise.

Fluid Replacement and Circulatory Support

Replacement of fluid and electrolyte losses is of primary concern in treating horses with salmonellosis. Depending on the severity of the disease, fluid losses may be minimal or massive. Fluid and electrolytes can be administered orally or intravenously. Some horses with mild to moderate diarrhea may maintain hydration and electrolyte balance by consuming water and electrolytes voluntarily. Fresh water and water containing electrolytes should be available in all cases. In many instances, periodic nasogastric intubation and administration of water and electrolytes through the tube may be sufficient to maintain hydration.[232] In severe cases indwelling nasogastric tubes can be maintained, and up to 8 L of fluid can be administered by the tube every 20 to 30 minutes, if ileus is not evident. However, intravenous administration of fluids is preferred in most cases, requiring significant quantities of fluid to replace and maintain hydration and electrolyte balance.[233] It is not unusual for patients with severe diarrhea to require large volumes (50-100 L/day) of intravenous fluids to maintain hydration. Frequent monitoring of packed cell volume, serum electrolyte concentration, venous blood gases or total serum carbon dioxide, blood urea nitrogen and creatinine, urine protein and cytology, and body weight is important to monitor hydration, electrolyte and acid-base balance, and renal function.

Isotonic sodium chloride or lactated Ringer's solution is frequently used to restore and maintain fluid and electrolyte balance. Potassium chloride can be added to the fluids and administered at a rate up to 0.5 to 1.0 mEq/kg/hr. Generally, a rate of less than 0.5 mEq/kg/hr is used. Hypertonic NaCl solutions (1-2 L of 5% or 7.5% NaCl) have been used in horses that are severely hyponatremic (<120 mEq/dL). Hypertonic solutions should not be administered to severely dehydrated horses, but they have been used clinically without complication and with considerable beneficial effect in patients with hemodynamic shock resulting from sepsis. The beneficial effects of hypertonic NaCl are short-lived (30 to 60 minutes). Isotonic solutions should be administered concurrently or immediately after administration of hypertonic NaCl solutions. Isotonic (1.3%) or hypertonic (5.0%) sodium bicarbonate solutions are used to correct metabolic acidosis. Prolonged administration of sodium-containing fluids may promote diuresis and renal water loss or accumulation of peripheral edema and should be used conservatively when a relative free water loss is noted. Administration of isotonic dextrose (5%) or 2.5% dextrose/0.45% NaCl solutions may be beneficial when free water loss (relative sodium excess) is evident.

Many horses with acute colitis are concurrently hypoproteinemic because of gastrointestinal losses and are absorbing bacterial products that induce a systemic inflammatory response. Thus plasma oncotic pressures are abnormally low in the face of increased vascular permeability. Interstitial edema formation is a clinical problem in these patients, which contributes to organ dysfunction. Crystalloid fluids, although critical for replacing water and electrolyte losses resulting from diarrhea, may actually contribute to a decline in plasma oncotic pressure as a result of hemodilution.[234,235] Administration of colloid solutions is helpful for volume expansion and maintenance of plasma oncotic pressures, which improve tissue perfusion and oxygenation and organ function in hypovolemic, hypotensive, and hypoproteinemic patients with or without SIRS.[236] Colloids are more effective than crystalloid fluids at expanding plasma volume, thus requiring smaller volumes. Moreover, the effect of colloid volume expansion is longer lasting than crystalloid fluid volume expansion, because colloids are better retained in the vasculature.[235,236] Natural colloids, such as plasma and purified albumin, are commonly used. In addition to its beneficial colloidal properties, plasma harvested from donor horses immunized with rough mutants of *E. coli* (J5) or *S. enterica var typhimurium* may have other benefits for treatment of endotoxemia resulting from gastrointestinal disease.[237,238] Large volumes (6-8 L/day) may be required to significantly increase and maintain plasma protein concentration. Synthetic colloids such as dextrans, starches, or polymerized hemoglobin are also available for use in the horse. Hydroxyethyl starch (Hetastarch; 5 to 10 ml/kg of a 6% solution) increases colloidal oncotic pressures for up to 24 hours in hypoproteinemic horses[234] and has beneficial effects on cardiac output and other cardiorespiratory parameters, vascular permeability, interstitial fluid content, and tissue perfusion in models of hypoproteinemia and SIRS.[236] However, infusion of such solutions may be associated with renal failure in human patients with sepsis,[239] so this fluid should be used with caution in horses with sepsis. When synthetic colloids or even natural colloids are being administered, it may be more practical to monitor plasma oncotic pressure rather than plasma protein concentrations as a means of assessing the need for plasma or other colloid administration.[234] Hetastarch may prolong bleeding times by altering von Willebrand's factor (vWF) function; thus this synthetic colloid should be used cautiously in horses with suspected coagulopathies, active hemorrhage, or other bleeding problems.[235]

Inflammation

Control of colonic inflammation and secretion is a difficult and poorly studied aspect of equine acute colitis. The role of inflammation and mediators such as prostaglandins as a cause of fluid loss is well known during *S. enterica* and clostridial infection of the intestinal tract.[19,39,39,108-110,240,241] COX inhibitors (NSAIDs) have antisecretory effects on the inflamed intestinal tract,[242,243] including in the equine colon.[244,245] NSAIDs are commonly administered to horses with salmonellosis and other forms of colitis to reduce inflammation-associated fluid secretion. However, prostaglandins such as PGE_2 and PGI_2 are also have cytoprotective effects on gastrointestinal mucosa and are critical for mucosal repair.[188,242] NSAIDs used pharmacologically to inhibit colonic inflammation and secretion may in fact be detrimental to mucosal integrity and healing if not used judiciously in inflammatory diarrheal diseases. NSAIDs exacerbate colonic inflammation in humans with inflammatory colitis, impede mucosal healing in several models of mucosal injury, and have well-documented detrimental effects on colonic mucosa in horses.[176,186,188,242] In addition to toxicity to the colonic mucosa, gastric ulceration is not unusual in horses with enterocolitis and may be related to treatment with NSAIDs. Although the use of COX-2–selective NSAIDs should, in theory, be less likely to harm or impede repair of the colonic mucosal in patients with colonic inflammation causing diarrhea, the safety and efficacy of these medications has not been evaluated in this application. In addition, the prothrombotic adverse effects of COX-2 selective drugs[246] suggest that very cautious use of highly COX-2–selective medications is warranted in patients with systemic inflammation at risk for thrombosis (e.g., endotoxemia and sepsis).

In addition to NSAIDs, other drugs are occasionally used as anti-inflammatory and antisecretory therapy. Bismuth subsalicylate is commonly used in adults and foals with diarrhea. The volume required for any effect in adults with colitis is quite high (1-4 L by nasogastric tube every 4-8 hours), which often precludes its use. Metronidazole has beneficial effects in experimental models of gastrointestinal inflammation, including NSAID toxicity,[193] and may be useful for treating horses with colitis; however, evidence supporting its use is lacking. Orally administered bismuth subsalicylate solutions are often used to decrease inflammation and secretion in the colon. In adult horses the volume of solution necessary to be beneficial is large (3 to 4 L, every 4 to 6 hours). Often the solution is administered twice daily instead of four to six times daily. If a beneficial effect is not achieved within 3 to 4 days of treatment, administration of bismuth subsalicylate solution should be discontinued. More frequent administration can be accomplished in foals, and clinical improvement is more often seen in foals than in adult horses.

In light of the role of reactive oxygen metabolites in colonic inflammation, free radical scavengers have been advocated to reduce the effects of these molecules. Sulfasalazine metabolites have been shown to reduce reactive oxygen metabolite–induced colonic inflammation in other species,[193] and sulfasalazine has been used to treat chronic inflammatory disease in horses but has not been used to treat acute colitis. The only free radical scavenger commonly used in horses with colitis is dimethyl sulfoxide (DMSO, 0.1 to 1.0 g/kg intravenously every 12 to 24 hours in a 10% solution), but evidence of efficacy is lacking.

SIRS associated with endotoxemia and sepsis frequently occurs in patients with salmonellosis. The principles of therapy for endotoxemia and sepsis are covered in detail elsewhere in this chapter. Oral administration of activated charcoal and mineral oil is commonly used to reduce absorption of endotoxin in horses with colitis. Low doses of NSAIDs (such as flunixin meglumine, 0.1 to 0.25 mg/kg intravenously every 6 to 8 hours) inhibit eicosanoid synthesis induced by endotoxin. In addition, NSAIDs are administered to prevent laminitis resulting from endotoxemia, a devastating complication of salmonellosis. It is important to remember that prostaglandins are important for mucosal healing and may worsen mucosal injury in colitis. It is generally believed that the benefits of low doses of NSAIDs administered to horses with SIRS outweigh the risks of worsening gastrointestinal damage, but judicious use is recommended.

Mucosal Repair and Protection

Sucralfate (20 mg/kg by mouth every 6 hours) has been advocated to aid in healing of the colonic mucosa in patients with NSAID toxicity. There is evidence in experimental phenylbutazone toxicosis in foals suggesting that sucralfate administration lessens ulceration and other histopathologic lesions throughout the alimentary tract and lessens protein loss.[247] However, there is no evidence supporting the use of sucralfate to treat colonic ulceration in adult horses.

Misoprostol (5 μg/kg by mouth every 12 hours or 2 μg/kg by mouth every 6 to 8 hours) and other synthetic PGE analogs enhance mucosal healing in the intestine and promote recovery in experimental models of colitis.[248] Misoprostol may be particularly useful for treating NSAID toxicity, either the generalized form or RDUC. However, the efficacy of misoprostol in hastening mucosal healing is clinically unproven in equine colitis. The primary drawbacks of prostaglandin analogs such as misoprostol are the adverse effects of the drug, including abdominal cramping, diarrhea, sweating, and abortion in pregnant mares.

Psyllium mucilloid can be added to the diet (5 tablespoons every 12 to 24 hours) to increase the production of SCFAs in the colon. Amylase-resistant fermentable fiber such as psyllium is hydrolyzed by colonic bacteria to SCFAs such as butyrate, which represent a major energy source for colonocytes. Butyrate and other SCFAs hasten epithelial maturation and stimulate salt (and thus fluid) absorption in the colon, improve the clinical course of ulcerative colitis, and hasten colon healing.[249] Psyllium is itself a source of butyrate in the colon and also promotes the movement of amylase-sensitive carbohydrates into the distal colon, which are then fermented to SCFAs. Thus psyllium is thought to be clinically useful for promoting mucosal healing in colitis.

Pain Control

Many horses with salmonellosis or other forms of colitis have mild to severe signs of abdominal pain caused by gas and fluid distention of the colon, colonic ischemia, or infarction. Analgesia can be accomplished with NSAIDs such as flunixin, but the potential for worsening mucosal injury or nephrotoxicity may prevent the use of analgesic doses, especially in horses with suspected NSAID toxicity. Newer NSAIDs that specifically target COX-2 with minimal inhibition of COX-1 may be useful analgesics that spare the gastrointestinal mucosa. For example, meloxicam and firocoxib have analgesic properties in horses in experimental models of ischemic colic and spare the intestinal mucosa from the detrimental effects associated with nonselective COX inhibitor treatment.[182,250]

Xylazine or detomidine may provide temporary relief of pain. Butorphanol is a useful analgesic that can be administered either intramuscularly (0.05 to 0.1 mg/kg IM every 6 to 8 hours) or as a continuous infusion. An infusion rate of 13.2 μg/kg/hr in isotonic crystalloid fluid such as lactated Ringers' solution is often effective.[251] Continuous-rate infusion of lidocaine (1.3 mg/kg, IV loading dose administered slowly over 5 minutes followed by 3 mg/kg/hr infusion in isotonic crystalloid fluids) can provide analgesia, anti-inflammatory activity, and prokinetic benefits.[252,253]

Antibiotics

NEUTROPENIA

Broad spectrum antibiotic treatment is often recommended in neutropenic horses or horses with signs of septicemia. Neutropenia is associated with an increased risk of sepsis, septicemia, and septic complications, such as septic phlebitis and infection of surgical sites.[254-262] Sepsis, bacteremia, and septicemia are complications of enterocolitis that may be caused by *S. enterica*, *Clostridium* organisms, or other pathogenic enteric bacteria or by toxic or inflammatory injury to the colonic mucosa that breaks down the barrier, allowing absorption of microbial molecules that trigger inflammation or invasion of microbes into tissues and blood. Neutropenia weakens host defenses to render horses susceptible to infection and dissemination of organisms that breach the mucosal barrier. Although most attempts to culture bacteria from the blood of adult horses with colitis fail to insolate organisms, no detailed studies have been undertaken to determine the prevalence of bacteremia or septicemia in these patients. Disseminated aspergillosis has been reported in horses as a complication of acute colitis, demonstrating the potential for systemic infections with rarely pathogenic organisms stemming from colonic mucosal injury in the face of potential immunosuppression resulting from neutropenia.[263,264] Broad spectrum antibiotics lessen septic complications in human patients. However, evidence supporting this principle in horses with colitis is lacking.

SALMONELLOSIS

Treatment with antibiotics is controversial in horses with salmonellosis. Treatment with antibiotics is not thought to alter the course of the enterocolitis, but it may lessen dissemination and severity of disease. Treatment with antibiotics directly targeted at *S. enterica* is often reserved for patients with the enteric fever (septicemia) form of salmonellosis, documented with positive blood cultures. However, some clinicians treat all cases of salmonellosis with targeted antibiotic therapy. Lipid-soluble antibiotics are ideally suited for *S. enterica* infections because the bacteria persist intracellularly. Enrofloxacin (5 mg/kg/day IV), chloramphenicol (50 mg/kg , PO every 6 hours), and cephalosporins (ceftiofur 10 to 20 mg/kg, IVevery 12 hours) are preferred antibiotics for treatment of salmonellosis depending on the antimicrobial sensitivity of the isolate.

POTOMAC HORSE FEVER

As with other causes of enterocolitis, the use of antibiotics is controversial. The risk of inducing salmonellosis or other forms of antibiotic-induced diarrhea and the difficulty of diagnosing the etiology of diarrheal diseases demand judicious use of antibiotics.[54] However, in patients in which the likelihood of *N. risticii* infection is high, treatment with antibiotics is often indicated before definitive diagnosis. Lipid-soluble drugs are preferred because the organism can live within cells. Oxytetracycline (6.6 mg/kg/day, IV), doxycycline (10 mg/kg, PO every 12 hours), trimethoprim-sulfadiazine (5 mg/kg trimethoprim, PO or IV every 8 to 2 hours, and 25 mg/kg sulfadiazine every 8 to 12 hours), or erythromycin-rifampin (30 mg/kg, PO every 12 hours, and 5 mg/kg, PO every 12 hours, respectively) have been used effectively to treat clinical cases.[54,265-267] The tetracyclines appear to be the most effective antibiotics for treatment of Potomac horse fever and are considered the treatment of choice. Treatment is most successful if initiated before the onset of diarrhea.[54,266]

CLOSTRIDIOSIS

If antibiotics are being administered at the onset of enterocolitis, they should be discontinued if possible. Specific treatment with metronidazole (15 mg/kg, PO every 8 hours) is effective for treating clostridiosis in humans and appears to be effective in horses.[95,268] Metronidazole resistance in clinical isolates of *C. difficile* has been reported in one outbreak but appears to be rare in most human and equine cases.[269] Metronidazole-resistant isolates were sensitive to vancomycin, which may be effective for treating clinical cases if metronidazole resistance is suspected. However, metronidazole remains the treatment of choice. *C. perfringens* type C antitoxin has been recommended for treatment of neonatal clostridiosis, but there is no evidence of its efficacy.[270] Antitoxin preparations are not generally advocated for use in adult horses with clostridiosis.

PROLIFERATIVE ENTEROPATHY

L. intracellularis is susceptible to a variety of antibiotics in vitro, including chlortetracycline, erythromycin, penicillin, difloxacin, and ampicillin.[271] Lipid-soluble antibiotics with a large volume of distribution are usually chosen to treat PE because *L. intracellularis* is an intracellular organism. Erythromycin estolate (15 to 25 mg/kg, PO every 6 to 8 hours) alone or in combination with rifampin (5 mg/kg, PO every 12 hours) is the most commonly reported efficacious treatment for PE.[124] Chloramphenicol (50 mg/kg PO every 6 hours) has also been reported to be effective if erythromycin worsens the diarrhea.[124] Anecdotal reports suggest that administration of oxytetracycline, doxycycline, or both is also quite effective. Supportive care, including maintenance of hydration and electrolyte balance and plasma or colloid administration to increase colloid oncotic pressure in hypoalbuminemic patients, is also indicated. Affected foals are treated until clinical signs, hypoproteinemia, and ultrasonographic evidence of intestinal thickening resolve. The prognosis depends on the duration of the disease and the degree of fibrosis and destruction of the intestinal architecture.

Anticoagulation

Hypercoagulability is a common complication of enterocolitis, associated with systemic inflammation resulting from endotoxemia. Administration of heparin (20 to 80 IU/kg, SC or IV every 6 to 12 hours) may prevent thrombosis in these patients, provided antithrombin III concentrations are adequate in the plasma. Concentrated sources of antithrombin III are not available for use in horses, but whole plasma may provide an important source. Treatment with heparin is thought to decrease thrombosis, especially of the jugular vein, a serious complication of salmonellosis. Low-dose aspirin treatment (10 mg/kg, PO every 24 to 48 hours) in conjunction with heparin treatment may provide added benefit by irreversibly inhibiting platelet function.[272] Heparin and aspirin may have protective effects on the digital lamina.[272,273] Heparin may enhance the phagocytic activity of the reticuloendothelial system by enhancing the efficiency of opsonins such as fibronectin and immunoglobulin, thereby stimulating phagocytosis of products of coagulation and possibly other particles, including bacteria.[274,275]

Probiotics

SALMONELLOSIS

Maintenance of the bacterial flora and antagonism of pathogenic bacteria such as *S. enterica* in the gastrointestinal tract are important defense mechanisms preventing colonization by pathogenic bacteria. The use of probiotic preparations containing beneficial bacteria prevents colonization of pathogenic bacteria, including *S. enterica var. gallisepticum,* in poultry.[276] Little work has been done to investigate the efficacy of these products in preventing salmonellosis in horses, but ongoing studies may provide important information in this regard. Probiotic and other preparations designed to restore normal flora to the gastrointestinal tract, such as fecal suspensions, sour milk, and yogurt, have been used clinically to shorten the course of salmonellosis, with variable results. Therefore prevention of infection by using probiotic agents and other means is important. Exposure of susceptible horses to *S. enterica* should be avoided, but this is a difficult task, especially because inapparent infections are common and the bacteria are ubiquitous in the environment. Prophylactic use of probiotic preparations, judicious use of antibiotics in susceptible horses, control of environmental conditions such as temperature, and restricted exposure to pathogenic bacteria are important factors to control clinical salmonellosis.

CLOSTRIDIOSIS

Because altered large intestinal flora appears to play an important role in the pathogenesis of equine intestinal clostridiosis or any antibiotic-associated diarrhea, probiotic preparations have been advocated to treat affected horses.[277] Sour milk, a product containing lactose-producing *Streptococcus* species, appears to markedly improve the clinical course in horses suspected of having *C. perfringens* type A infection.[90] Sour milk may benefit the patient by altering the flora and antagonizing enterotoxigenic *C. perfringens* type A, but it is also reported to be bactericidal against *C. perfringens* type A.[90] Preparations of *Saccharomyces boulardi* are effective for reducing diarrhea and the frequency of *C. difficile* recurrence in humans[95] and decreasing the duration and severity of disease in horses with colitis.[278] *Lactobacillus* preparations have a protective effect in humans and decrease the severity and duration of antibiotic-associated diarrhea.[279,280] However, evidence of their clinical usefulness in horses is lacking.

Absorbent Powders and Mineral Oil

Absorbent powders are often used to reduce the bioactivity and absorption of bacterial toxins produced by bacterial or toxic metabolites produced by bacteria and other microorganisms (e.g., lactic acid in grain overload). Activated charcoal is indicated in cases of intoxication by arsenic and grain overload. Activated charcoal may also be administered in an attempt to reduce absorption of endotoxin and other pro-inflammatory microbial molecules in inflammatory colitis. Mineral oil may be useful to reduce absorption of cantharidin in patients with blister beetle poisoning. DTO smectite powder (Bio-Sponge™, Platinum Performance, Buellton, Calif) binds *C. difficile* and *C. perfringens* exotoxins in vitro[281,282] and may be useful for treating intestinal clostridiosis in horses. DTO smectite is available as a powder or paste and should be administered according to the manufacturer's instructions for 3 to 5 days.

Nutrition

Good nursing care and adequate nutrition are vital to the treatment of horses with salmonellosis. Salmonellosis and other severe forms of inflammatory colitis are catabolic diseases that increase caloric requirements. Normal intake of roughage to provide energy may be inadequate; however, feeding of grains should be avoided to prevent delivery of highly fermentable carbohydrate to the colon. Dietary management usually consists of restricting or eliminating long-stem roughage (hay) from the diet and feeding exclusively a complete pelleted diet (at least 30% dietary fiber). The rationale behind this recommendation is to reduce the mechanical and physiologic load on the colon. Frequent meals (4 to 6 times a day) are recommended. Corn oil (1 cup every 12 to 24 hours) can be added to the pellets to increase the caloric intake without adding roughage or grain. It is important to note that if a horse with colitis refuses to eat pelleted feed, then high-quality grass hay should be fed. In anorectic or severely catabolic patients, enteral and parenteral nutrition (total and partial) has been used successfully to provide calories and nutritional support.

Specific Therapies

STRONGYLOSIS

Treatment of *S. vulgaris* infection requires treatment of the migrating parasite larvae and the lesions produced by the parasite. Fenbendazole (10 mg/kg, PO every 24 hours for 3 days, or 10 mg/kg, PO every 24 hours for 5 days) and ivermectin (200 mg/kg PO) are effective in killing fourth-stage larvae.[131] Other anthelmintics may also be effective when given at higher doses than those required to kill adult worms. The efficacy of these anthelmintics against larvae within thrombi is not known.

Thrombolytic and antithrombotic therapy has been advocated in horses with suspected strongylosis.[131,138] Heparin (20 to 80 IU, IV or SC every 6 to 12 hours) may be administered as an anticoagulant. High-molecular-weight heparin causes anemia by inducing aggregation of red blood cells, which is an undesirable effect in sepsis. Low-molecular-weight heparins appear to be less likely to have this effect in horses. Aspirin (10 to 30 mg/kg, PO every 12 to 48 hours) is usually combined with heparin to inhibit platelet adhesion. Aspirin may also inhibit release of platelet products, such as thromboxane, that affect the motility of the large intestine. Low-molecular-weight dextrans have been advocated as antithrombotics that act by inhibiting platelet function and coagulation.[138,236] The clinical efficacy of dextran administration appears to be good, but no controlled studies have been performed.

CYATHOSTOMIASIS

Anthelmintic administration is usually the only treatment necessary for mild to moderate cases of cyathostomiasis treated early in the course of the disease (within 1 to 3 weeks of onset). Fenbendazole is effective against many larval stages, but resistance is high in some populations. Although the reported efficacy of ivermectin is variable against certain stages,[283] one study reported an overall efficacy of 75%.[286] Currently, fenbendazole (7.5 to 10 mg/kg, PO every 24 hours for 5 days) followed on day 6 by ivermectin (200 mg/kg PO) is the most commonly advocated treatment regimen.[143,285] Moxidectin (400 μg/kg PO every 24 hours) may also be effective against adult organisms and L_3 and L_4 larval stages[286] and may be useful for treating cyathostomiasis. Anti-inflammatory therapy may also be beneficial, especially in severe or refractory cases or before treatment with larvicidal medications. Pretreatment with dexamethasone or prednisolone is indicated before anthelmintic administration if heavy larval loads are suspected to prevent an acute exacerbation of the disease by rapid death of encysted larvae. Larvacidal treatment with moxidectin appears to be less likely than fenbendazole to result in tissue inflammation resulting from larval death.[287] NSAID administration may have limited value, but dexamethasone appears to be efficacious in refractory cases when used in conjunction with larvicidal anthelmintics.[143,146] Bismuth subsalicylate is often administered orally as an antisecretory agent in young animals. Supportive care may be necessary in severe cases, particularly if hypoproteinemia is severe. Administration of intravenous crystalloid fluids and plasma or other colloids is occasionally required. Proper nutritional support is also important.

CANTHARIDIN

Supportive care is the most important principle of therapy for cantharidin toxicity. Intravenous fluid administration, maintenance of electrolyte balance (especially calcium), and prevention of further renal and urinary tract damage is important.[202,206] Diuresis by intravenous fluid administration is often sufficient to prevent renal failure. Furosemide is often administered after rehydration of the patient to further promote diuresis and to decrease the concentration of the toxin in the urine, which may ameliorate some of the effects on the urinary tract mucosa.[202] Diuresis has also been suggested to increase clearance of the toxin, but no evidence for this has been found. Judicious use of NSAIDs may be necessary to control abdominal pain but should be reserved until the patient is rehydrated and renal failure has been ruled out. Cantharidin is lipid-soluble; therefore oral administration of mineral oil may prevent further absorption of the toxin.[202] Activated charcoal is often administered with the mineral oil.

ARSENIC TOXICITY

Reduction of arsenic absorption by administration of cathartics such as mineral oil, magnesium sulfate slurries, and activated charcoal by nasogastric tube should be initiated immediately.[207] Chelation therapy with sodium thiosulfate 920 to 30 g in 300 mL of water (administered orally) and dimercaprol (BAL; 3 mg/kg, PO every 4 hours) is indicated.[207] Dimercaprol is a specific antidote for trivalent arsenicals, but its efficacy in horses is questionable. Intravenous fluid administration may help treat shock, replace fluid lost in feces, and promote diuresis but should be monitored carefully because pulmonary edema is a frequent complication. More specific treatment of renal, cardiac, pulmonary, or neurologic disease may be required.

INTESTINAL ANAPHYLAXIS

Treatment of intestinal anaphylaxis is in principle similar to treatment of other forms of colitis, but it is often unsuccessful, owing to the rapidly progressive nature of the syndrome.[211,216,223] Inclusion of heparin in the intravenous fluids (20 to 80 IU/kg, IV every 8 to 12 hours) may help prevent vascular thrombosis. Administration of hypertonic saline solutions or colloids may prove useful during initial periods of shock. Early treatment with prednisolone sodium succinate (10 to 20 mg/kg IV) or dexamethasone (0.1 to 0.2 mg/kg, IV) may be essential for successful treatment.[211]

CARBOHYDRATE OVERLOAD

Mild cases of carbohydrate overload may not require treatment other than exclusion of grains from the diet for several days to weeks and gradual reintroduction of grain into the diet later if extra energy is needed. Patients showing signs of colic or diarrhea without other systemic signs may benefit from administration of mineral oil, charcoal, and fluids through a nasogastric tube. Lavage of residual carbohydrate from the stomach may also be accomplished with the nasogastric tube. Often, NSAIDs such as phenylbutazone (2.2 to 4.4 mg/kg/day, IV) or flunixin meglumine (1 mg/kg, IV) are administered to prevent laminitis. Phenoxybenzamine and heparin given before the onset of laminitis may prevent or decrease the severity of laminitis.[273,288]

More severe cases with dehydrating diarrhea, systemic signs of endotoxemia, or metabolic acidosis require intravenous fluid support to maintain water, electrolyte, and acid-base balance in addition to the previously mentioned treatments. Large amounts of bicarbonate-containing solutions may be required. Care should be taken when administering hypertonic bicarbonate solutions because many patients may already be hyperosmotic as a result of lactic acidemia. Isotonic sodium bicarbonate 1.3% may be useful in the hyperosmotic patient. Careful attention to calcium balance is also important because severe hypocalcemia may occur. Aggressive therapy for systemic inflammation resulting from endotoxemia should be instituted. Intravenous broad spectrum antibiotics are administered to combat bacteremia and septicemia, which frequently complicate carbohydrate overload–induced colitis.

In extreme cases, especially if the patient has ingested a very large quantity of grain, surgical removal of the grain from the large intestine may be indicated, especially if surgery can be accomplished before the onset of severe clinical signs. However, administration of oral cathartics, such as magnesium sulfate slurries or mineral oil, or a combination of these is often sufficient to clear the carbohydrate from the large intestine before fermentation, mucosal damage, and absorption of endotoxin and lactic acid occur. Oral administration of activated charcoal may prevent absorption of endotoxin by binding the molecules in the lumen of the bowel. In any case, feeding of the source of the soluble carbohydrate, such as grains, should be discontinued. Low carbohydrate and protein roughage such as grass or oat hays should be fed until the microbial flora recovers. Oral administration of probiotic preparations containing lactobacillus is contraindicated; however, other sources of normal equine large intestinal microbial flora, such as fecal extracts from normal feces or *S. boulardi,* may be useful to reintroduce appropriate microorganisms. Complications from laminitis and sepsis are common and often cause death.

SAND ENTEROPATHY

Treatment requires removal of the sand from the gastrointestinal tract, as described elsewhere in this chapter, using psyllium products and magnesium sulfate slurries administered orally. Analgesics may be required initially to relieve pain and stimulate appetite. A diet high in roughage often stimulates further passage of sand. Treatment may require several weeks to remove as much sand as possible. Prevention of the disease is important, and recurrence is not unusual.

ISCHEMIC DISORDERS OF THE INTESTINAL TRACT

Anthony T. Blikslager

STRANGULATING OBSTRUCTION

Pathophysiology

Strangulation obstruction of the intestine is characterized by simultaneous occlusion of the intestinal lumen and its blood supply. Although strangulation of the intestinal lumen results in clinical signs similar to those of simple obstruction, occlusion of the blood supply results in a more rapid deterioration of the intestinal mucosa and subsequent onset of sepsis. Although there has been a great deal of recent interest in the relevance and treatment of intestinal reperfusion injury,[1-3] the lesion that develops during strangulation is often severe, leaving little viable bowel for further injury during reperfusion.[2] Although extensive lengths of strangulated small intestine may be resected, strangulation of the large colon presents a much greater treatment dilemma because strangulated intestine usually extends beyond the limits of surgical resection.[4] Therefore horses with large intestinal strangulation are often recovered with extensive intestinal injury left in place. Thus subtle degrees of reperfusion injury may be very important in horses with large colon disease, warranting further work in this area in an attempt to reduce mortality.[3]

Strangulating obstruction may be divided into hemorrhagic and ischemic forms.[5,6] In hemorrhagic strangulating obstruction, which is most common, the veins become occluded before the arteries because of the greater stiffness of arterial walls. This lesion is noted by a darkened appearance in affected bowel and increased thickness as blood is pumped into the lesion. Ischemic strangulating obstruction occurs if the intestine is twisted tightly enough to simultaneously occlude both arteries and veins. In the case of the colon, some researchers suggest that this may be determined by how much ingesta is in the colon, because intestinal contents may prevent the intestine from twisting tightly.[7] Tissue involved in ischemic strangulating obstruction appears pale and of normal or reduced thickness because of a complete lack of blood flow (Figure 15-23). Bowel peripheral to strangulating lesions may also become injured as a result of distention, which reduces mural blood flow once it reaches critical levels. Furthermore, as this intestine is decompressed, it may also undergo reperfusion injury.[8-10]

SMALL INTESTINAL STRANGULATION

Clinical Signs

Horses with small intestinal strangulating obstruction typically have moderate to severe signs of abdominal pain that is only intermittently responsive to analgesic medications. During the latter stages of the disease process, horses may not experience much pain but rather become profoundly depressed as affected intestine necroses. Affected horses have progressive signs of sepsis, including congested mucous membranes, delayed capillary refill time, and an elevated heart rate (>60 beats/min in most cases). In addition, reflux is typically obtained after passage of a stomach tube, and loops of distended small intestine are usually detected on rectal palpation of the abdomen.[11] However, these latter findings are variable, depending on the duration and location of the obstruction. For example, horses with ileal obstructions tend to reflux later in the course of the disease process than horses with jejunal obstructions. Furthermore, a horse that has an entrapment of small intestine in the epiploic foramen or a rent in the proximal small intestinal mesentery may not have palpable loops of small intestine because of the cranial location of these structures.[12] Abdominocentesis can provide critical information on the integrity of the intestine and is indicated in horses with suspected strangulation of the small intestine.[11] A horse that has signs compatible with a small intestinal obstruction and also has serosanguinous abdominal fluid with an elevated protein level (>2.5mg/dl) is likely to require surgery, although these cases must be differentiated from proximal enteritis. In general, horses with small intestinal strangulation show continued signs of abdominal pain, whereas horses with proximal enteritis (discussed earlier in this chapter) tend to be depressed after initial episodes of mild abdominal pain.[13] In addition, horses with small intestinal strangulation continue to clinically deteriorate despite appropriate medical therapy and begin to show elevated white blood cell counts (>10,000 cells/μl) in the abdominal fluid, likely as the duration of strangulation increases. However, there are cases in which small intestinal strangulation and proximal enteritis cannot be not readily distinguished, at which point surgery may be elected rather than prolonging the decision to perform abdominal exploration on a horse with a potential strangulating lesion.[13]

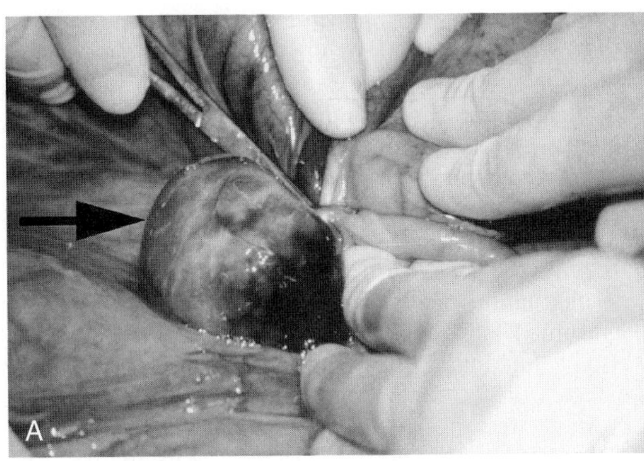

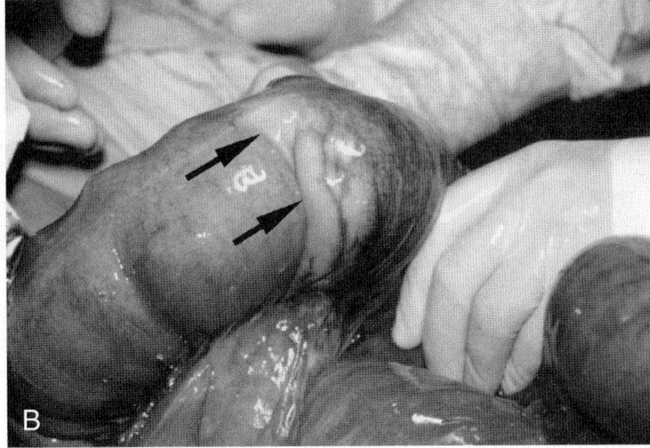

FIGURE 15-23 Ischemic strangulating obstruction of the small colon by a mesenteric lipoma. **A,** Note the lipoma *(arrow),* which has tightly encircled a segment of small colon. **B,** After resection of the lipoma, a pale area of strangulated small colon is clearly demarcated *(arrows),* the appearance of which is consistent with ischemic strangulating obstruction.

PROGNOSIS

The prognosis for survival in horses with small intestinal strangulating lesions is generally lower than for most forms of colic.[14] However, recent studies indicate that more than 80% of horses with small intestinal strangulating lesions will be discharged from the hospital.[15] Nonetheless, owners should be warned that the long-term survival rates are substantially reduced to below 70%,[16] in part because of long-term complications such as adhesions.[18,19] In addition, the prognosis is particularly low for some forms of strangulation, including entrapment of small intestine within a mesenteric rent.[19]

EPIPLOIC FORAMEN ENTRAPMENT

The epiploic foramen is a potential opening (because the walls of the foramen are usually in contact) to the omental bursa located within the right cranial quadrant of the abdomen. It is bounded dorsally by the caudate process of the liver and caudal vena cava and ventrally by the pancreas, the hepatoduodenal ligament, and the portal vein.[12] Intestine may enter the foramen from the visceral surface of the liver toward the right body wall or the opposite direction. Studies differ as to which is the most common form. In the case of entrapments that enter the foramen in a left-to-right direction, the omental bursa is ruptured as the intestine migrates through the epiploic foramen, which may contribute to the intra-abdominal hemorrhage often seen with this condition. Clinical signs include acute onset of severe colic with examination findings compatible with small intestinal obstruction. A recent study has shown that the stereotypic behavior of crib biting is a significant risk factor for epiploic foramen entrapment.[20] The reason for this is unclear but may be attributable to changes in abdominal pressure as the horse prepares the esophagus to ingest air. Other risk factors include increased height of the horse and previous colic surgery.[20] The condition was once believed to be more prevalent in older horses,[12] but this has since been refuted by more recent studies.[21] However, the disease has also been recognized in foals as young as 4 months of age.[22] The diagnosis is definitively made at surgery, although ultrasonographic findings of distended loops of edematous small intestine adjacent to the right middle body wall are suggestive of epiploic foramen entrapment.[12] In general, thickened, amotile intestine on ultrasonographic examination is highly predictive for small intestinal strangulating obstruction.[23] Small intestine entrapped in the epiploic foramen may be limited to a portion of the intestinal wall (parietal hernia),[24] and the large colon may become entrapped within the epiploic foramen.[25] In treating epiploic foramen entrapment, the epiploic foramen must not be enlarged either by blunt force or with a sharp instrument, because rupture of the vena cava or portal vein and fatal hemorrhage may occur. Prognosis has substantially improved over the last decade, with current short-term survival rates (discharge from the hospital) ranging because 74%[26] to 79%.[12] Preoperative abdominocentesis has been consistently found to be the most predictive test of postoperative survival.[12,26]

STRANGULATION BY PEDUNCULATED MESENTERIC LIPOMA

As horses age, lipomas form between the leaves of the mesentery and develop mesenteric stalks as the weight of the lipoma tugs on the mesentery. The stalk of the lipoma may subsequently wrap around a loop of small intestine or small colon, causing strangulation. Strangulating lipomas should be suspected in aged (>15 years) geldings with acute colic referable to the small intestinal tract.[27,28] Ponies also appear to be at risk for developing disease,[28] suggesting alterations in fat metabolism may predispose certain horses to development of mesenteric lipomas. The diagnosis is usually made at surgery, although on rare occasions a lipoma can be palpated rectally.[29] Treatment involves surgical resection of the lipoma and strangulated bowel, although strangulated intestine is not always nonviable.[27] Studies indicate that approximately 50%[28] to 78%[27] of horses are discharged from the hospital after surgical treatment.

SMALL INTESTINAL VOLVULUS

A volvulus is a twist along the axis of the mesentery, whereas torsion is a twist along the longitudinal axis of the intestine. Small intestinal volvulus is theoretically initiated by a change in local peristalsis, or the occurrence of a lesion around which the intestine and its mesentery may twist (e.g., an ascarid impaction).[11] It is reportedly one of the most commonly diagnosed causes of small intestinal obstruction in foals.[30,31] It has been theorized that young foals may be at risk for small intestinal volvulus because of changing feed habits and adaptation to a bulkier adult diet. Onset of acute, severe colic; a distended abdomen; and radiographic evidence of multiple loops of distended small intestine in a young foal would be suggestive of small intestinal volvulus. However, it is not possible to differentiate volvulus from other causes of small intestinal obstruction preoperatively. In adult horses volvulus frequently occurs in association with another disease process, during which small intestinal obstruction results in distention and subsequent rotation of the small intestina around the root of the mesentery. Although any segment of the small intestine may be involved, the distal jejunum and ileum are most frequently affected because of their relatively longer mesenteries.[11] The diagnosis is made at surgery by palpating a twist at the origin of the cranial mesenteric artery. Treatment includes resection of devitalized bowel, which may not be an option because of the extent of small intestinal involvement (similar to large colon volvulus). Prognosis is based on the extent of small intestine involved and its appearance after surgical correction of the lesion. In general, horses in which more than 50% of the small intestine is devitalized are considered to have a grave prognosis.[32]

Strangulation by Way of Mesenteric or Ligamentous Rents

There a number of structures that, when torn, may incarcerate a segment of intestine (typically the small intestine), including intestinal mesentery,[19] the gastrosplenic ligament,[33] the broad ligament,[34] and the cecocolic ligament.[35] Horses with such incarcerations exhibit presenting signs typical of a horse with strangulating small intestine, including moderate to severe signs of abdominal pain, endotoxemia, absent gastrointestinal sounds, distended small intestine on rectal palpation, nasogastric reflux, and serosanguinous abdominal fluid. However, the prognosis for many of these cases appears to be lower than for horses with other types of small intestinal strangulations. For example, in horses with small intestine entrapped in a mesenteric rent, only 7 of 15 horses were discharged from the hospital, and only 2 of 5 horses for which follow-up information was available survived long term (>5 months).[19] Poor outcome may result from the difficulty in unentrapping incarcerated intestine, the degree of hemorrhage, and the length of intestine affected.

Inguinal Hernia

Inguinal hernias are more common in Standardbred and Tennessee Walking horses that tend to have congenitally large inguinal canals.[11] Inguinal hernias may also occur in neonatal foals but differ from hernias in mature horses in that they are typically nonstrangulating. The nature of the hernia (direct versus indirect) is determined on the basis of the integrity of the parietal vaginal tunic. In horses in which the bowel remains within the parietal vaginal tunic, the hernia is referred to as *indirect* because, strictly speaking, the bowel remains within the peritoneal cavity. Direct hernias are those in which strangulated bowel ruptures through the parietal vaginal tunic and occupies a subcutaneous location. These direct hernias most commonly occur in foals and should be suspected when a congenital inguinal hernia is associated with colic, swelling that extends from the inguinal region of the prepuce, and intestine that may be palpated subcutaneously.[36,37] Although most congenital indirect inguinal hernias resolve with repeated manual reduction or application of a diaper, surgical intervention is recommended for congenial direct hernias.[36]

Historical findings in horses with strangulating inguinal hernias include acute onset of colic in a stallion that had recently been used for breeding. A cardinal sign of inguinal herniation is a cool, enlarged testicle on one side of the scrotum (Figure 15-24).[38,39] However, inguinal hernias have also been reported in geldings.[40] Inguinal hernias can also be detected on rectal palpation, and manipulation of herniated bowel per rectum can be used to reduce a hernia but is not recommended because of the risk of rectal tears. In many cases the short segment of herniated intestine will markedly improve in appearance once it has been reduced and can sometimes be left unresected.[41] The affected testicle will be congested because of vascular compromise within the spermatic cord, and although it may remain viable, it is generally recommended that it be resected.[41] The prognosis in adult horses is good, with up to 75% of horses surviving to 6 months of age.[39] Horses that have been treated for inguinal hernias may be used for breeding. In these horses the remaining testicle will have increased sperm production, although an increased number of sperm abnormalities will be noticed after surgery because of edema and increased temperature of the scrotum.

Strangulating Umbilical Hernias

Although umbilical hernias are common in foals, strangulation of herniated bowel is rare. In one study 6 of 147 (4%) horses with umbilical hernias had incarcerated intestine.[42] Clinical signs include a warm, swollen, firm, and painful hernia sac associated with signs of colic. The affected segment of bowel is usually small intestine, but herniation of cecum or large colon has also been reported.[43] In rare cases a hernia that involves only part of the intestinal wall may be found; this is termed a *Richter's hernia*. In foals that have a Richter's hernia, an enterocutaneous fistula may develop.[43] In one study 13 of 13 foals with strangulating umbilical hernias survived to discharge, although at least three were lost to long-term complications.[43]

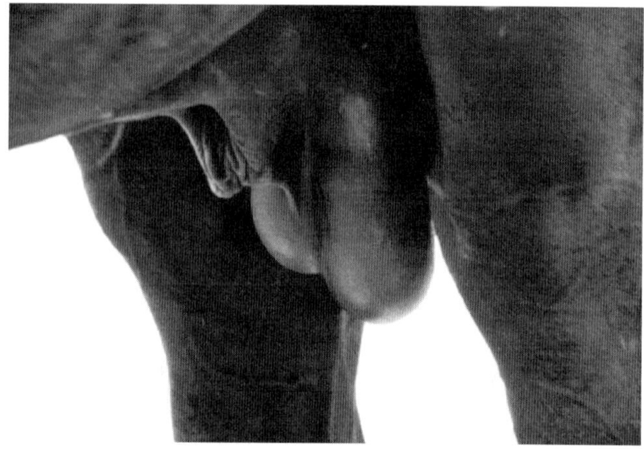

FIGURE 15-24 Inguinal hernia in a horse with colic. Note the enlarged testicle, which has compromised venous drainage because of herniated small intestine within the inguinal canal.

Intussusceptions

An intussusception involves a segment of bowel (intussusceptum) that invaginates into an adjacent aboral segment of bowel (intussuscipiens). The reason for such invagination is not always clear, but it may involve a lesion at the leading edge of the intussusception, including small masses, foreign bodies, or parasites. In particular, tapeworms *(Anoplocephala perfoliata)* have been implicated.[44] Ileocecal intussusceptions are the most common intestinal intussusceptions in the horse and typically affect young animals. In one study evaluating 26 cases of ileocecal intussusception, the median age of the horses was 1 year old.[45] Acute ileocecal intussusceptions are those in which the horses has a duration of colic of less than 24 hours and involve variable lengths of intestine, which ranged in one study from 6 cm to 457 cm in length. In acute cases the involved segment of ileum typically has a compromised blood supply. Chronic ileocecal intussusceptions typically involve short segments of ileum (up to 10 cm in length), and the ileal blood supply is frequently intact.[45] Abdominocentesis results are variable because strangulated bowel is contained within the adjacent bowel. There is often evidence of obstruction of the small intestine, including nasogastric reflux and multiple distended loops of small intestine on rectal palpation. Horses with chronic ileocecal intussusceptions have mild, intermittent colic, often without evidence of small intestinal obstruction. In one study a mass was palpated in the region of the cecal base in approximately 50% of cases.[44] Transabdominal ultrasound may be helpful in discerning the nature of the mass. The intussusception has a characteristic target appearance on cross section.[46] Other segments of the small intestine may also be intussuscepted, including the jejunum (Figure 15-25). In one study of 11 jejunojejunal intussusceptions, the length of bowel involved ranged between 0.4 to 9.1 m.[47] Attempts at reducing intussusceptions at surgery are usually futile because of intramural swelling of affected bowel. Jejunojejunal intussusceptions should be resected.

For acute ileocecal intussusceptions the small intestine should be transected as far distally as possible, and a jejunocecal anastomosis should be performed. In cases with particularly long intussusceptions (up to 10 m has been reported), an intracecal resection may be attempted.[48] For horses with chronic ileocecal intussusceptions, a jejunocecal bypass without small intestinal transection should be performed. The prognosis is good for horses with chronic ileocecal intussusceptions and guarded to poor for horses with acute ileocecal intussusceptions, depending on the length of bowel involved.[45]

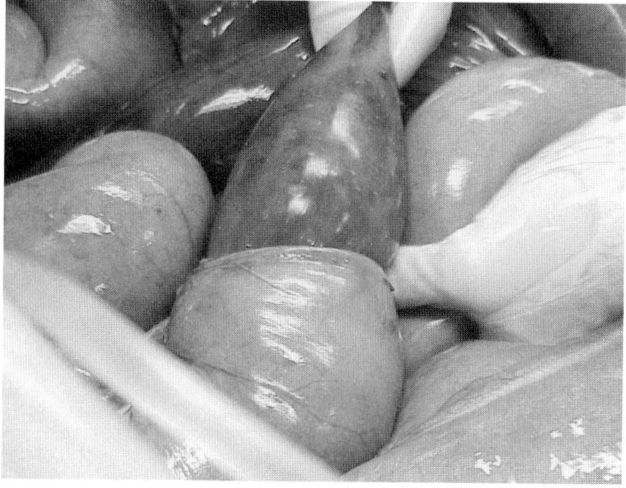

FIGURE 15-25 Jejunojejunal intussusception in a horse with colic. Note the intussusceptum, which has become ischemic as a result of invagination of intestine and its mesenteric blood supply into the intussuscipiens.

Diaphragmatic Hernias

Herniation of intestine through a rent in the diaphragm is rare in the horse. Any segment of bowel may be involved, although small intestine is most frequently herniated.[49] Diaphragmatic rents may be congenital or acquired, but acquired hernias are more common.[49] Congenital rents may result from incomplete fusion of any of the four embryonic components of the diaphragm: pleuroperitoneal membranes, transverse septum, body wall, and esophageal mesentery.[49] In addition, abdominal compression of the foal at parturition may result in a congenital hernia.[49] Acquired hernias are presumed to result from trauma to the chest or a sudden increase in intra-abdominal pressure, such as might occur during parturition, distention of the abdomen, a sudden fall, and strenuous exercise.[50] Hernias have been located in a number of different locations, although large congenital hernias are typically present at the ventral-most aspect of the diaphragm and most acquired hernias are located at the junction of the muscular and tendinous portions of the diaphragm.[49] A peritoneopericardial hernia has been documented in at least one horse.[51]

The clinical signs are usually associated with intestinal obstruction rather than respiratory distress.[50] However, careful auscultation may reveal an area of decreased lung sounds associated with obstructed intestine and increased fluid within the chest cavity.[52] Such signs may prompt thoracic radiography or ultrasound, both of which can be used to make a diagnosis. Auscultation may also reveal thoracic intestinal sounds, but it is typically not possible to differentiate these from sounds referred from the abdomen. In one report, two of three horses diagnosed with small intestinal strangulation by diaphragmatic hernia had respiratory acidemia, attributable to decreased ventilation.[53] Treatment of horses with diaphragmatic hernia is fraught with complications because of the need to reduce and resect strangulated bowel and the need to repair the defect in the diaphragm.[54,55] Because dorsal defects in the diaphragm are among the most common forms of diaphragmatic defect, it may not be possible to close the diaphragmatic hernia by way of the approach used for abdominal exploratory. However, because herniation is likely to recur,[54] it is appropriate to schedule a second surgery using an appropriate approach to resolve the diaphragmatic defect.

LARGE COLON VOLVULUS

Clinical Signs

Horses with large colon volvulus have rapid onset of severe, unrelenting abdominal pain. Postpartum broodmares appear to be at risk for this form of colic.[4] Once the large colon is strangulated (>270-degree volvulus), gas distention is marked, leading to gross distention of the abdomen, compromised respiration as the distended bowel presses up against the diaphragm, and visceral pooling of blood as the caudal vena cava is compressed. Horses with this condition are frequently refractory to even the most potent of analgesics. These horses may prefer to lie in dorsal recumbency, presumably to take weight off the strangulated colon. An abbreviated physical examination is warranted in these cases because the time from the onset of strangulation to surgical correction is critical. Under experimental conditions the colon is irreversibly damaged within 3 to 4 hours of a 360-degree volvulus of the entire colon.[56] Despite severe pain and hypovolemia, horses may have a paradoxically low heart rate, possibly related to increased vagal tone. In addition, results of abdominocentesis often do not indicate the degree of colonic compromise,[4,57] and in many cases it is not worth attempting to obtain abdominal fluid because of extreme colonic distention.[58] Rectal palpation reveals severe gas distention of the large colon, frequently associated with colonic bands traversing the abdomen. In many cases colonic distention restricts access to the abdomen beyond the pelvic brim. A recent study has shown that plasma lactate levels below 6.0 mmol/L had a sensitivity of 84% and a specificity of 83% in predicting survival in horses with large colon volvulus.[59]

Surgical Findings

At surgery the volvulus is typically located at the mesenteric attachment of the colon to the dorsal body wall, and the most common direction of the twist is dorsomedial when the right ventral colon is used as a reference point.[4] However, the colon may twist in the opposite direction, twist greater than 360 degrees (up to 720 degrees has been reported), or twist at the level of the diaphragmatic and sternal flexures.[4] In all cases the colon should be decompressed as much as possible, and in many cases a colonic evacuation by way of a pelvic flexure enterotomy will greatly aid correction of the volvulus. After correction of the volvulus, a determination must be made as to whether the colon has been irreversibly injured. This should be based on mucosal color and bleeding (if an enterotomy has been performed), palpation of a pulse in the colonic arteries, serosal color, and appearance of colonic motility.[7] If the colon is judged to be irreversibly damaged, the feasibility of a large colon resection can be considered. Although 95% of the colon can be resected (that part of the colon distal to the level of the cecocolic fold), damage from the volvulus usually exceeds that which can be resected. In these cases surgeons may elect to resect as much damaged bowel as possible or advise euthanasia.[7]

Prognosis

The prognosis is guarded to poor because of the rapid onset of this disease. In one study the survival rate was 35%.[57] In a more recent report, the survival rate was 36% for horses with 360-degree volvulus of the large colon compared with 71% for horses with 270-degree volvulus.[4] Postoperative complications include hypovolemic and endotoxemic shock, extensive loss of circulating protein, DIC, and laminitis. In addition, large colon volvulus has a propensity to recur. Although one study documented a recurrence rate of less than 5%,[57] some authors believe recurrence may be as high as 50%.[7] Therefore methods to prevent recurrence should be considered in patients at risk for recurrence, particularly broodmares that tend to suffer from the disease recurrently during the foaling season.[60,61]

Other Causes of Large Intestinal Ischemia

Intussusceptions

The most common intussusceptions of the large intestine are cecocecal and cecocolic intussusceptions (Figure 15-26).[62,63] Both are likely attributable to the same disease process, with variable inversion of the cecum. These conditions tend to occur in young horses (63% were younger than 3 years old in one study) and may be associated with intestinal tapeworms.[63] Horses are seen with highly variable clinical signs, including acute, severe colic; intermittent pain over a number of days; and chronic weight loss.[63] These variable presentations likely relate to the degree to which the cecum has intussuscepted. Initially, the cecal tip inverts, creating a cecocecal intussusception, which does not obstruct the flow of ingesta. As the intussusception progresses, the cecum inverts into the right ventral colon (cecocolic intussusception), which obstructs the flow of ingesta and often causes severe colic. The cause of abdominal pain is often difficult to differentiate in these cases, although it is sometimes possible to detect a mass on the right side of the abdomen by either rectal palpation or ultrasound examination.[62,63] Treatment involves manual surgical reduction by retracting the intussusceptum directly[62] or by way of an enterotomy in the right ventral colon.[64] However, sometimes the cecum cannot be readily reduced because of severe thickening, and in other cases surgical procedures result in fatal contamination. For example, in one report 8 of 11 horses were euthanized in the perioperative period because of complications,[62] and in another report 12 of 30 horses were euthanized either before or during surgery. The latter included all of the horses with chronic disease because of irreversible changes to the cecum.[63] However, one recent report on cecocolic intussusceptions indicated that 7 of 8 horses that underwent right ventral colon enterotomy and cecal resection survived long

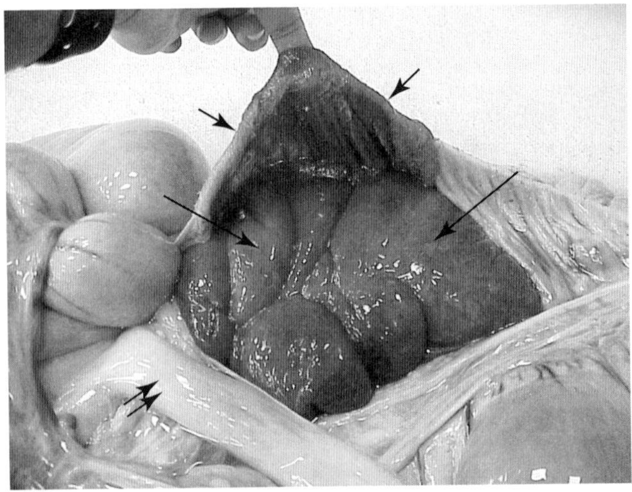

FIGURE 15-26 Cecocolic intussusception in a horse with colic. An enterotomy has been made in the right ventral colon *(short arrows)* to reveal an intussuscepted cecum *(arrows)*. Although this picture was taken at necropsy, an enterotomy such as the one shown in this figure can be used to exteriorize and resect the majority of the compromised cecum. Note the ileum adjacent to the colon *(double arrow)*.

term,[64] suggesting that continued improvements in surgical techniques may improve the prognosis.

Colocolic intussusceptions are exceptionally rare but have reportedly affected the pelvic flexure and the left colons.[65-68] Although the condition is reportedly more common in young horses,[66-68] older horses may be affected.[65] Clinical findings may include a palpable mass on the left side of the abdomen.[66] Ultrasonography may also be useful. Treatment requires manual reduction of the intussusception at surgery[66,68] or resection of affected bowel.[65] Because the left colons can be extensively exteriorized and manipulated at surgery,[65-68] the prognosis is fair.

RECTAL PROLAPSE

Rectal prolapse may occur secondary to any disease that causes tenesmus, including diarrhea, rectal neoplasia, and parasitism,[69] or prolapse can occur secondary to elevations in intra-abdominal pressure during parturition or episodes of coughing.[70,71] Rectal prolapses are classified into four categories (Table 15-14) depending on the extent of prolapsed tissue and the level of severity.[72] Type I rectal prolapse is most common and characterized by a doughnut-shaped prolapse of rectal mucosa and submucosa (Figure 15-27). Type II prolapses involve full-thickness rectal tissue, whereas type III prolapses additionally have invagination of small colon into the rectum.

TABLE 15-14

Classification of Rectal prolapse

Grade	Description	Prognosis
I	Prolapse of rectal mucosa	Good
II	Prolapse of full-thickness rectum	Fair
III	Grade 2 prolapse with additional protrusion of small colon	Guarded
IV	Intussusception of rectum and small colon through the anus	Poor

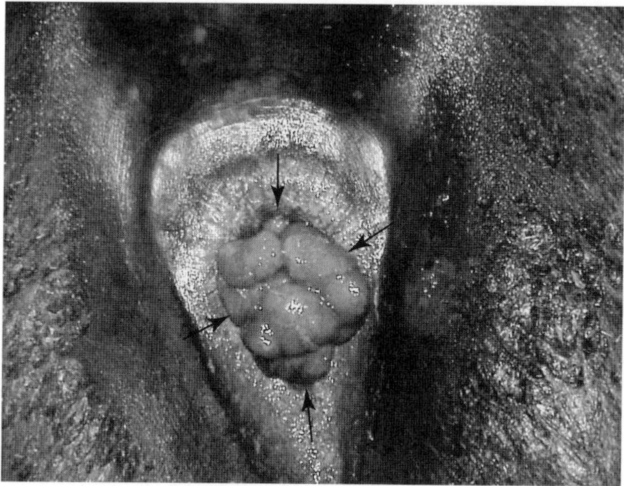

FIGURE 15-27 Type I rectal prolapse in a horse. Note circumferential protrusion of partial thickness rectal tissue *(arrows)* that is becoming congested as a result of pressure from the surrounding anus.

Type IV prolapses involve intussusception of proximal rectum or small colon through the anus in the absence of prolapse of tissue at the mucocutaneous junction at the anus.[72] These can be differentiated from other forms of prolapse by their appearance and a palpable trench between prolapsed tissue and the anus.

In type I prolapses most frequently seen in horses with diarrhea, the rectal mucosa becomes irritated and protrudes intermittently during episodes of tenesmus. If tenesmus persists, rectal mucosa can remain prolapsed. Rectal mucosa rapidly becomes congested and edematous under these conditions, which should be treated with osmotic agents such as glycerin or magnesium sulfate and by massaging and reducing the prolapse.[73] A purse-string suture may be necessary to keep the mucosa inside the rectum. Topical application of lidocaine solution or jelly, epidural anesthesia, and sedation may help reduce tenesmus that incites and exacerbates rectal prolapse. Similar treatments can be applied with type II rectal prolapses. However, these more severe prolapses may not be reducible without surgical resection of mucosa and submucosa from the prolapsed bowel.[69,73]

Type III and type IV rectal prolapses are more serious injuries because the small colon is involved.[74] In horses with type III prolapses, an abdominocentesis should be performed to determine if the injury to the small colon has resulted in peritonitis. The small colon component should be reduced manually if possible, whereas prolapsed rectal tissue typically requires mucosal or submucosal resection. Surgical exploration of the abdomen should be performed to determine the status of the small colon, although serial abdominocenteses can be used in lieu of surgery to detect progressive necrosis of bowel. Type IV prolapses are seen most commonly in horses with dystocia.[72] These prolapses are almost always fatal because of stretching and tearing of mesenteric vasculature, with subsequent infarction of affected bowel. Therefore euthanasia is usually warranted on the basis of physical examination findings. However, confirmation of severe small colonic injury requires abdominal exploration using either a midline approach or laparoscopy.[75] It is conceivable that a horse with compromised small colon could undergo a colostomy of the proximal small colon, but the compromised small colon will typically necrose beyond that which can be resected using a midline abdominal approach.[73]

NONSTRANGULATING INFARCTION

Nonstrangulating infarction occurs secondary to cranial mesenteric arteritis caused by migration of *Strongylus vulgaris*[76] and has become a relatively rare disorder since the advent of broad spectrum anthelmintics. Although thromboemboli have been implicated in the pathogenesis of this disease, careful dissection of naturally occurring lesions has not revealed the presence of thrombi at the site of intestinal infarctions in most cases.[76] These findings suggest that vasospasm plays an important role in this disease.[11] Clinical signs are highly variable, depending on the extent to which arterial flow is reduced and the segment of intestine affected. Any segment of intestine supplied by the cranial mesenteric artery or one of its major branches may be affected, but the distal small intestine and large colon are more commonly involved.[76] There are no clinical variables that can be used to reliably differentiate this disease from strangulating obstruction.[76] In some cases massive infarction results in acute, severe colic.[76]

Occasionally, an abnormal mass and fremitus may be detected on rectal palpation of the root of the cranial mesenteric artery. This disease should be considered a differential diagnosis in horses with a history of inadequate anthelmintic treatment and the presence of intermittent colic that is difficult to localize. Although fecal parasite egg counts should be performed, they are not indicative of the degree of parasitic infestation.

In addition to routine treatment of colic, dehydration, and endotoxemia, medical treatment may include aspirin (20 mg/kg/day) to decrease thrombosis.[11] Definitive diagnosis requires surgical exploration. However, these cases are difficult to treat because of the patchy distribution of the lesions and the possibility of lesions extending beyond the limits of surgical resection. In addition, further infarction may occur after surgery. The prognosis is fair for horses with intermittent mild episodes of colic that may be amenable to medical therapy but poor in horses that require surgical intervention.[11,76]

OBSTRUCTIVE DISORDERS OF THE GASTROINTESTINAL TRACT

Anthony T. Blikslager

APPROACH TO THE HORSE WITH COLIC

Clinical management of colic is distinctly different from management of many other clinical syndromes because the initial focus is not on defining the definitive diagnosis but rather on determining whether the horse requires surgical exploration. Therefore the clinician must collect a series of historical and physical examination findings and decide whether these findings warrant medical management or whether referral and potential surgical exploration of the abdomen are necessary because of a suspected obstructive or ischemic lesion. For example, a horse may exhibit presenting signs of severe abdominal pain, poor cardiovascular status, and abdominal distention that may be compatible with an extensive list of differential diagnoses and, more important, may indicate the need for abdominal exploration to minimize the extent of intestinal injury. The speed with which this clinical decision can be made has a tremendous impact on the well-being of the patient,[1,2] because delaying surgical exploration of a horse with ongoing intestinal injury exacerbates shock induced largely by microbial toxins such as LPS traversing damaged mucosa, and this in turn correlates with mortality.[3]

History

The initial clinical step in treating horses with colic is taking a thorough history. However, it may be necessary to delay this until after the physical examination and initial treatment because management of abdominal pain takes precedence. The vital components of the history that should be obtained before examination and treatment, if possible, are the duration and severity of colic symptoms, analgesics already administered, and a history of any adverse drug reactions. The two most critical factors from a history that would support a decision to refer and potentially surgically explore a horse with colic are the duration of signs[2] and the extent of pain.[4] The latter is deduced by asking the owner about the presence and frequency of pawing, looking at the flanks, rolling, repeatedly going down and getting back up, and posturing as if to lie down or urinate, in addition to other clinical evidence of pain. Other important components of the history that should be obtained to ascertain the reason for the colic are listed in Table 15-15.

Physical Examination Findings

Just as the clinician may need to postpone the complete history to allow rapid treatment of the colic, so must the clinician be able to alter the extent of the physical examination in order to treat the horse in a timely fashion. The most critical examination finding is the horse's heart rate, because this has repeatedly been shown to reflect the level of pain and provide an excellent assessment of the cardiovascular status of the horse. The heart rate is likely the single most reliable predictor of the need for surgery and survival.[5] Because analgesic treatments can dramatically alter the heart rate, it should be obtained, if at all possible, before administration of analgesics. Other components of the examination are specifically designed to provide additional information on the cardiopulmonary status of the horse (quality of the pulse, mucous membrane color, capillary refill time, respiratory rate, and full auscultation of the chest) and the nature of any intestinal obstruction that the horse might have (auscultation of gastrointestinal sounds, per rectal palpation of the abdomen, and presence of nasogastric reflux). Although there are classic presentations for horses with obstructions of either the small or large intestine (Table 15-16), clinical presentations of the various types of intestinal obstructions vary. For example, a horse that has a small intestinal obstruction may have several loops of distended small intestine without any evidence of nasogastric reflux, depending on the site of the obstruction (distal versus proximal), the extent of obstruction, and the duration of obstruction. Other examples include horses with large colon obstruction, which may have reflux because of direct compression of the small intestine by distended colon or because of tension on the duodenocolic ligament. The most useful diagnostic means to determine the type of intestinal obstruction is rectal palpation of the abdomen.[4] However, only approximately one third of the abdomen can be reached by way of the rectum, and this may be substantially less in very large or heavily pregnant horses. Nonetheless, it is worthwhile to try to determine the type of obstruction the horse has (i.e., small intestine versus large intestine and simple obstruction versus strangulating obstruction) because this information can be very helpful in determining the prognosis. In one study interns and residents at a veterinary teaching hospital were able to predict the type of lesion with a specificity exceeding 90%.[6] This in turn can be very helpful in educating the client about the potential findings in surgery and the likelihood that the horse will survive.

Management of Abdominal Pain

Before considering ways to manage signs of colic, the clinician should remember that such signs are very poorly localized. Therefore, although colic is most frequently associated with intestinal disease, dysfunction of other organ systems, including urinary obstruction,[7,8] biliary obstruction,[9] uterine torsion or tears,[10,11] ovarian artery hemorrhage,[10] and neurologic disease should be considered as differential diagnoses.[12] However, the duration and severity of colic signs are excellent

TABLE 15-15

History Findings and Their Relevance to Colic and Its Prevention

	Risk for Colic	Potential Mechanisms
Feeding	Recent change in feed	Alteration in fluid flux or fermentation in the large colon
	Coastal Bermuda hay with a high fiber content	Obstruction of ileum by fine, fibrous hay
	Feeding round bales	Poor-quality hay
	Feeding off the ground	Horses may ingest sand in some regions of the country
	Excessive concentrate	Alteration in fluid flux or fermentation in the large colon
	Large infrequent meals	Alteration in fluid flux or fermentation in the large colon
	Bolting feed	Large boluses of feed entering the esophagus and stomach
Environment	Excessive time in stall	Insufficient intake of roughage Insufficient exercise
	Insufficient access to water	Dehydration
Exercise	Exercise-induced exhaustion	Dehydration Reduced gastrointestinal motility
Preventive care	Insufficient dental care	Poor mastication of feed
	Insufficient anthelmintic treatment	Large parasite burden
Medication	Excessive administration of NSAIDs	Mucosal damage, particularly in the stomach and colon
Previous medical history	Colic surgery	Adhesions Anastomotic obstruction

TABLE 15-16

Indications for Surgery in Patients with Colic According to Their Clinical Signs

Indication	Clinical Signs
Refractory pain	Repeated episodes of pain despite treatment with analgesics Violent episodes of pain Persistently elevated heart rate (>48 beats/min)
Sepsis in the face of colic	Persistently elevated heart rate Weak peripheral pulse Abnormal mucous membrane color (pale, hyperemic, purple) Delayed capillary refill time (>2 seconds)
Evidence of a refractory small intestinal obstruction	Refractory pain Nasogastric reflux Distended loops of small intestine on rectal palpation
Evidence of a refractory large intestinal obstruction	Refractory pain Abdominal distention Distended large colon on rectal palpation Tight band(s) on rectal palpation
Evidence of devitalized bowel	Sepsis Abnormal abdominocentesis (TP >2.5 g/dl, TNCC >10,000/μl)

TNCC, Total nucleated cell count;
TN, total protein

TABLE 15-17

Analgesics Commonly Used to Treat Colic in Horses

Drug	Dosage	Amount for an Adult Horse
Butylscopolamin	0.3 mg/kg	150-170 mg
Xylazine	0.3 – 0.5 mg/kg prn	150-250 mg
Detomidine	0.01-0.02 mg/kg prn	5-10 mg
Butorphanol	0.01-0.02 mg/kg prn	5-10 mg
Flunixin	0.25-1.1 mg/kg every 8-12 hr*	125-500 mg

PRN, As needed.
*The longer treatment interval corresponds to the higher dose, whereas lower doses may be given more frequently

predictors of whether a horse requires surgical exploration of the abdomen. In fact, refractory pain supersedes all other predictors of the need for surgery in the colic patient. Once signs of colic have been recognized and categorized as to their severity, it is critical to rapidly and effectively nullify signs of pain, for the well-being of the horse and to reduce the owner's anxiety. In addition, it is becoming increasingly clear that pain is best managed before it becomes severe.[13] There are several classes of analgesics readily available for treatment of horses with colic (Table 15-17), including spasmolytics (N-butylscopolamine), α_2-agonists (xylazine, detomidine), opiates (butorphanol), and NSAIDs (e.g., flunixin meglumine). Although much of this information is very familiar to most practitioners, a couple of points should be emphasized. The short-duration drugs N-butylscopolamine, xylazine, and butorphanol, which provide analgesia either directly (xylazine and butorphanol) or indirectly (through cessation of intestinal spasm; N-butylscopolamine) for approximately 30 to 45 minutes, allow the veterinarian to determine if pain is recurrent within the time period of the typical examination. Alternatively, flunixin meglumine is not as potent as an analgesic, but its duration is much longer. In fact, the clinician should closely adhere to its treatment interval to prevent deleterious effects on gastrointestinal mucosa and the kidneys.[14,15] The recent discovery of two isoforms of COX, the enzyme inhibited by NSAIDs, has provided drugs that can more selectively inhibit pro-inflammatory COX-2, while permitting continued constitutive production of prostanoids. This may be advantageous in horses with colic, particularly in light of recent evidence of reduced intestinal recovery from an ischemic event when subjects were treated with flunixin compared with a drug that is more selective for COX-2.[16] The α_2-agonist detomidine should be reserved for horses with severe, unrelenting pain because of its tremendous potency in horses.[17] In addition, it should be remembered that α_2-agonists reduce the heart rate associated with a transient increase in blood pressure,[18,19] thereby reducing the predictive value of the heart rate and pulse pressure.

Clinical Pathology

The most useful clinical pathologic tests are the packed cell volume and total protein because they can be used to substantiate clinical estimates of dehydration and correlate strongly with prognosis.[2,20,21] A biochemical profile is useful for assessing electrolyte imbalances and kidney and liver function, whereas blood gas analysis can be used to assess acid-base status. Horses with colic most frequently show evidence of metabolic acidosis, associated with hypovolemia or endotoxemia, but other abnormalities, such as metabolic alkalosis in association with extensive loss or sequestration of stomach Cl^-, may be noted. Metabolic acidosis has been further investigated in horses with colic by measuring blood lactate, which is now an option in many laboratories.[22] Lactate levels have also been inferred from measurement of the anion gap, although one study noted that lactate in horses with colic did not account for the entire anion gap.[22] Lactate levels and anion gap closely correlate with the level of intestinal injury and the prognosis for survival.[20,23,24]

Other key components of the clinical pathologic evaluation of horses with colic are the abdominocentesis and complete blood count. Regarding the latter, the total white blood cell and differential counts can provide crucial evidence of colic attributable to colitis (leukopenia, neutropenia, and a left shift) rather than an obstruction (highly variable complete blood count findings). PF can be very helpful in determining the integrity of the intestine. Specifically, as the intestine becomes progressively devitalized, the PF will become serosanguinous as red blood cells are leaked into the abdomen, followed by an elevation in the total protein (>2.5g/dl) and progressive increases in total nucleated cell count (>10,000 cells/ µl). However, these findings do not always correlate well with the condition of the intestine, particularly in horses with large colon volvulus. For example, in a study of 57 horses with large colon volvulus, the average total protein (2.5 g/dl) and total nucleated cell count (1000 cells/µl) were normal despite the fact that only 36% with a 360-degree volvulus survived.[25] This may occur because the development of severe mucosal injury following large colon volvulus is rapid and may not allow sufficient time for protein and leukocytes to equilibrate with the abdominal fluid before the horse dies.[26]

Investigators have attempted to take all the variables routinely assessed during evaluation of horses for colic and develop models that can be used to accurately predict the need for surgery and the prognosis for life.[2,27-30] However, none of these models has taken the place of clinical decision making, although these predictive studies have added tremendously to our understanding of the importance of some prognostic factors, particularly those reflecting cardiovascular function.

SMALL INTESTINAL SIMPLE OBSTRUCTION

Simple obstruction involves intestinal obstruction of the lumen without obstruction of vascular flow. However, because there is a tremendous volume of fluid that enters the small intestinal lumen on a daily basis,[31,32] the obstructed intestine tends to become distended, which in turn may cause reduced mural blood flow.[33] Ultimately, such distention can result in necrosis of tissues, particularly in the immediate vicinity of the obstruction.[34] There are relatively few causes of simple obstruction in the small intestine, and the incidence of these types of obstruction is low (approximately 3% of all referred horses in one large hospital-based study).[5] However, in some geographic regions this type of obstruction is prevalent. For example, in the southeastern United States, ileal impactions are relatively common.[35,36]

Ascarid Impactions

Impactions caused by *Parascaris equorum* typically occur in foals younger than 6 months of age that have been on a poor deworming program and have a heavy parasite burden. Products that cause sudden ascarid death, including organophosphates, ivermectin, and pyrantel pamoate, have been incriminated in triggering acute intestinal obstruction by dead parasites.[37] This is a particular problem with ascarids because of the relatively large size of the adult parasite. Clinical signs include acute onset of colic after administration of an anthelmintic and signs compatible with small intestinal obstruction, including nasogastric reflux. Occasionally, dead parasites are present in the reflux. The onset of the disease varies according to the degree of obstruction.[37] A tentative diagnosis may be made on the basis of the history and signs referable to small intestinal obstruction. Abdominal radiographs and ultrasound may indicate the presence of multiple loops of distended small intestine but are not required if clinical signs indicate the immediate need for surgery. Initial medical treatment should include treatment of hypovolemic shock resulting from sequestration of fluid in the small intestine. Surgical treatment typically involves an enterotomy made over the intraluminal impaction and removal of ascarids. The prognosis is fair in cases that are rapidly addressed but poor in foals with evidence of hypovolemia and septic shock. In a recent study long-term survival of 25 affected horses was 33%.[37]

Ileal Impaction

Ileal impactions occur most commonly in adult horses in the southeastern United States. Although feeding of coastal Bermuda hay has been implicated in this regional distribution, it has been difficult to separate geographical location from regional hay sources as risk factors.[38] Nonetheless, it is likely that feeding suboptimal-quality coastal Bermuda hay puts horses at risk for ileal impaction, most likely because when the fiber content of this particular type of hay is high, the fibers are thin and most likely prematurely swallowed. The relationship between fiber content and eating patterns is theoretical and remains to be proved. In addition, sudden changes in feed from an alternative type of hay to coastal Bermuda hay likely put a horse at risk for ileal impaction.[38] Studies in the U.K. have revealed tapeworm infection as an important risk factor for ileal impaction. Based on risk analysis, the data suggested that more than 80% of the ileal impaction cases studied were associated with serologic or fecal evidence of tapeworm infection.[39] Because of the poor sensitivity of fecal analysis for tapeworms, a serologic test (ELISA) has been developed by Proudman et al. with a sensitivity of approximately 70% and a specificity of 95%.[40]

Clinical signs of horses with ileal impaction are typical for a horse with small intestinal obstruction, including onset of moderate to severe colic and rectally palpable loops of distended small intestine as the condition progresses. Because the ileum is the distal-most aspect of the small intestinal tract, nasogastric reflux may take a considerable time to develop and is found in approximately 50% of horses requiring surgical correction of impacted ileum.[35,41] The diagnosis is usually made at surgery, although an impacted ileum may on occasion be palpated rectally.[36] Multiple loops of distended small intestine frequently make the impaction difficult to palpate. Ileal impactions may resolve with medical treatment[36] but frequently require surgical intervention (Figure 15-28). At surgery fluids can be directly infused into the mass, allowing the surgeon to break down the impaction. Dioctyl sodium sulfosuccinate (DSS) may be included in the infused fluid to aid in disruption of the mass. Extensive small intestinal distention and intraoperative manipulation of the ileum may lead to postoperative ileus,[42] but recent studies indicate that this complication is less frequent as the duration of disease before admission has decreased.[35] However, an enterotomy should be considered to evacuate impacted intestinal contents and reduce manipulation. Recent studies indicate that the prognosis for survival is good.[35,36]

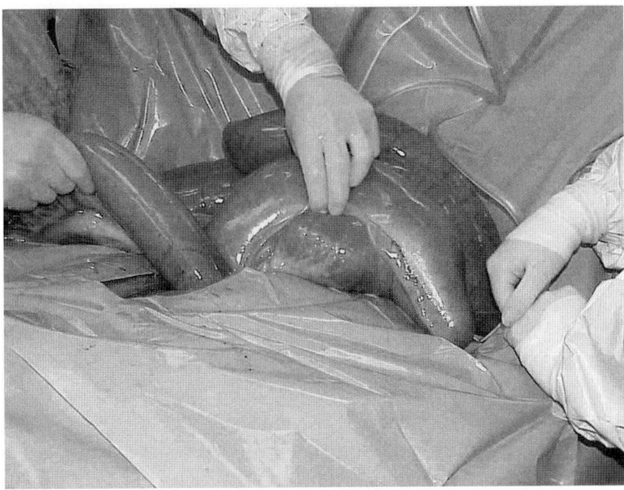

FIGURE 15-28 Intraoperative view of an ileal impaction. Note the distended appearance of the ileum as it courses toward the cecal base.

Ileal Hypertrophy

Ileal hypertrophy is a disorder in which the muscular layers (both circular and longitudinal) of the ileum thicken for unknown reasons (idiopathic) or secondary to an incomplete or functional obstruction. For idiopathic cases proposed mechanisms include parasympathetic neural dysfunction resulting in chronically increased muscle tone and subsequent hypertrophy of the muscular layers of the ileal wall. Such neural dysfunction possibly results from parasite migration.[43] Alternative hypotheses include chronic increases in the muscular tone of the ileocecal valve, leading to muscular hypertrophy of the ileum as it contracts against a partially occluded ileocecal valve. The jejunum may also be hypertrophied, either alone or in combination with the ileum.[43] Clinical signs include chronic intermittent colic as the ileum hypertrophies and gradually occludes the lumen. In one study partial anorexia and chronic weight loss (1 to 6 months) were documented in 45% of the horses, most likely because of intermittent colic and reduced appetite.[43] Because the ileal mucosa is not affected by this condition, there is no reason to believe that these horses experience malabsorption of nutrients. The diagnosis is usually made at surgery, although the hypertophied ileum may be palpated rectally in some cases.[43] For treatment an ileocecal or jejunocecal anastomosis to bypass the hypertrophied ileum is performed. Without surgical bypass intermittent colic persists, and the thickened ileum may ultimately rupture.[43] The prognosis is fair with surgical treatment.[44]

Secondary ileal hypertrophy is most commonly noted in horses that have previously had colic surgery and that may have a partial or functional obstruction at an anastomotic site. For example, in one case report a horse developed ileal hypertrophy after surgical correction of an ileocecal intussusception.[45] Ileal hypertrophy was also noted in a horse in which an ileocolic anastomosis was incorrectly orientated during surgical treatment of a cecal impaction.[46] Horses are typically re-examined for recurrence of colic in these cases. Surgical therapy is directed at addressing the cause of small intestinal obstruction and resecting hypertrophied intestine.

Meckel's Diverticulum

Meckel's diverticulum is an embryonic remnant of the vitelloumbilical duct, which fails to completely atrophy and becomes a blind pouch projecting from the antimesenteric border of the ileum.[47,48] However, similar diverticulae have also been noted in the jejunum.[49] These diverticulae may become impacted, resulting in partial luminal obstruction, or may wrap around an adjacent segment of intestine, causing strangulation.[47] Occasionally, an associated mesodiverticular band may course from the diverticulum to the umbilical remnant and serve as a point around which small intestine may become strangulated. Mesodiverticular bands may also originate from the embryonic ventral mesentery and attach to the antimesenteric surface of the bowel, thereby forming a potential space within which intestine may become entrapped.[50] Clinical signs range from chronic colic, for an impacted Meckel's diverticulum, to acute, severe colic if a mesodiverticular band strangulates intestine. The diagnosis is made at surgery, and treatment requires resection of the diverticulum and any associated bands.[50] The prognosis is good for horses with simple impaction of a Meckel's diverticulum and guarded for horses with an associated small intestinal strangulation.[50]

Adhesions

Adhesions of one segment of bowel to another or of a segment of intestine to other organs and the body wall typically occur after abdominal surgery and may be clinically silent, cause chronic colic attributable to partial obstruction, or result in acute obstruction. These differing clinical syndromes are attributable to the type of adhesions that develop. For example, a fibrous adhesion that does not by itself obstruct the intestinal lumen might serve as the pivot point for a volvulus, whereas an adhesion between adjacent segments of the intestinal tract may create a hairpin turn that causes chronic partial obstruction.[51] The number of adhesions that develop may also vary dramatically from horse to horse. Some horses may develop a single adhesion adjacent an anastomotic site or a discrete segment of injured intestine, whereas other horses may develop diffuse adhesions involving multiple segments of intestine, likely because of widespread inflammatory disease at the time of the original surgery.

The mechanisms whereby adhesions develop are complex, but they likely involve initial injury to the serosa initiated by intestinal ischemia, reperfusion injury, and luminal distention.[52] Such injury involves infiltration of neutrophils into the serosa, accompanied by loss of mesothelial cells (Figure 15-29). In one study assessing the margins of resected small intestine, extensive neutrophil infiltration was documented in the serosa, particularly in the proximal resection margin that had been distended before correction of a variety of strangulating lesions.[53] Regions of serosal injury and inflammation subsequently undergo reparative events similar to those of any wound, including local production of fibrin, de novo synthesis of collagen by infiltrating fibroblasts, and ultimately maturation and remodeling of fibrous tissue. Unfortunately, during this process fibrin may result in injured intestinal surfaces adhering to adjacent injured bowel or an adjacent organ. Once a fibrinous adhesion has developed, new collagen synthesis may result in a permanent fibrous adhesion. Alternatively, fibrinous exudate may be lysed by proteases released by local phagocytes, thereby reversing the adhesive process. Thus formation of adhesions may be viewed as an imbalance of fibrin deposition and fibrinolysis.[54]

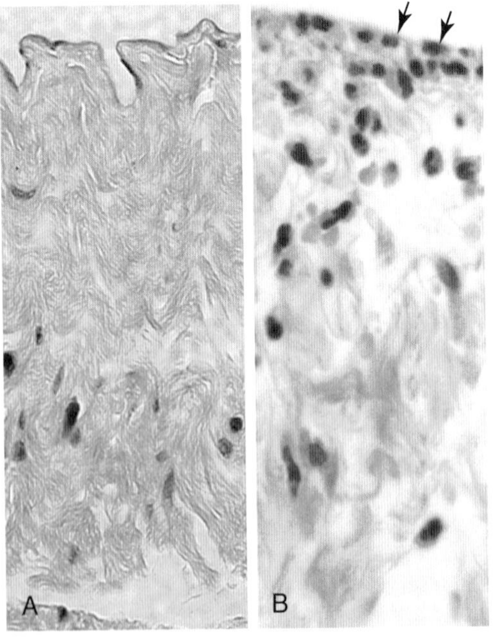

FIGURE 15-29 Histologic appearance of the serosa of equine jejunum. **A,** Normal intestine, with a clearly distinguishable layer of mesothelial cells. **B,** Jejunum after 2 hours of ischemia and 18 hours of reperfusion, showing complete loss of mesothelial cells and dense infiltration of neutrophils *(arrows).*

Prevention of adhesions relies on inhibition of the mechanisms involved in adhesion formation, including reduction of serosal injury with early intervention and good surgical technique, reduction of inflammation by administration of anti-inflammatory medications, physical separation of inflamed serosal surfaces (e.g., carboxymethylcellulose, hyaluronan),[55-57] and pharmacologic modulation of fibrinous adhesion formation (e.g., heparin[58]). In addition, early return of motility in the small intestine after surgery may reduce contact time between inflamed surfaces of intestine, thereby reducing the chances of adhesion formation.[54]

Horses at greatest risk of developing adhesions after colic surgery appear to be those that have small intestinal disease.[51,59] For example, in one study of horses undergoing surgical correction of small intestinal obstruction, 22% developed a surgical lesion associated with adhesions. However, foals appear to have an increased incidence of adhesions compared with mature horses, regardless of the nature of the abdominal surgery.[51] For example, one study indicated that 17% of foals developed lesions attributable to adhesions regardless of the type of the initial surgery.[60] Studies conflict as to whether the degree of surgical intervention influences adhesion formation,[51] but horses that require enterotomy or resection and anastomosis were found to be at greatest risk of developing adhesions in one study.[59] As an indication of the importance of postoperative adhesion formation, adhesions were among the most important reasons for repeat laparotomy in postoperative colic patients.[59,61]

Clinical signs in horses with adhesions are highly variable, depending on whether the adhesion is causing partial obstruction, complete luminal obstruction, or involvement of intestinal vasculature. However, adhesions would be an important differential for intermittent colic in the postoperative period, particularly if such colic was not relieved by nasogastric decompression of the stomach. Continued intermittent colic should prompt abdominocentesis to determine if there is evidence of septic peritonitis, which may contribute to adhesion formation. Placement of a large-bore drain and peritoneal lavage (Figure 15-30) will help resolve peritonitis and may reduce adhesion formation by reducing intra-abdominal inflammation. If postoperative colic persists, repeat laparotomy or laparoscopy may be elected. In one study on adhesions, 70% of repeat laparotomies were performed within 60 days, suggesting that surgical colic attributable to adhesions typically occurs within two months of an initial surgical procedure. Unfortunately, the prognosis for horses with colic attributable to adhesions is low, with only 16% of horses surviving adhesion-induced colic in one study.[51]

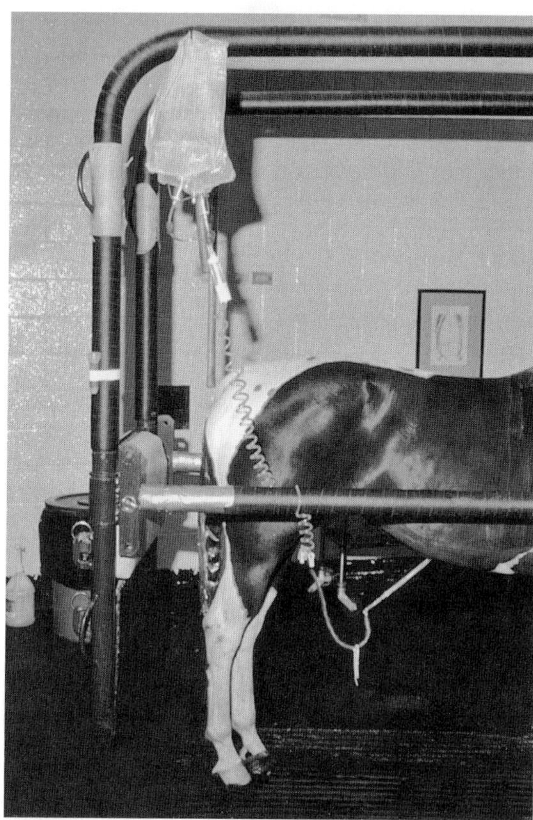

FIGURE 15-30 Peritoneal lavage in a horse. Note the use of an intravenous administration set and a large-bore catheter placed in the dependent portion of the abdomen adjacent to the ventral midline incision.

Postoperative Ileus

The definition of *ileus* is intestinal obstruction, which includes both physical and functional obstructions. However, in veterinary medicine the term is typically used to designate a lack of progressive aboral propulsion of ingesta resulting in functional obstruction.[62] The diagnosis of postoperative ileus is typically based on the presence of excessive nasogastric reflux and may occur after any abdominal exploratory procedure. However, horses undergoing surgery for strangulating small intestinal lesions or small intestinal obstructive lesions such as an ileal impaction are at greatest risk.[42] Recently, the syndrome of postoperative ileus in horses has been broadened to include those horses that may have delayed transit of ingesta through the large intestine after surgery. This large intestinal ileus may follow any type of surgery, particularly horses that have had orthopedic surgery, and is characterized by reduced fecal output (<three piles of manure/day) rather than excessive nasogastric reflux.[62] However, horses with excessive nasogastric reflux are unlikely to have normal fecal output, so the distinction between these two manifestations of ileus is not absolute.

Mechanisms involved in precipitating postoperative ileus characterized by small intestinal dysfunction likely involve local inflammation, reduced coordination of progressive motility, and increased sympathetic tone. A recent series of studies in the rat has shown that surgical manipulation of intestine results in delayed transit time associated with infiltration of neutrophils into intestinal longitudinal muscle and upregulation of inducible nitric oxide synthase and COX-2.[63-65] The mechanisms in the horse may be similar in that extensive manipulation of the intestine resulted in abnormal intestinal motility in ponies,[66] and prostanoids and nitric oxide have been shown to alter or reduce intestinal motility in horses.[67-69]

Clinical signs of postoperative ileus subsequent to colic surgery include evidence of abdominal pain, increased heart rate, reduced gastrointestinal sounds, and reflux of fluid through a nasogastric tube. A sudden increase in the heart rate of a postoperative patient following colic surgery should prompt immediate nasogastric intubation to decompress the stomach. Treatment should include attempts at refluxing the horse at frequent intervals, rather than relying on passive flow of reflux. In addition, administration of intravenous should account for the horse's maintenance requirement (50 ml/kg/day, approximately 1L/hr in the average horse) and fluid losses resulting from reflux. In practice, this requires frequent monitoring of packed cell volume and total protein to ensure that the horse remains well hydrated. Although there have been concerns that overhydrating horses may contribute to increased nasogastric reflux,[42] it is critical to keep horses well hydrated to prevent hypovolemic shock. Additionally, electrolytes should be frequently monitored, particularly in light of their potential role in smooth muscle contraction and nerve excitability. Because of the important role of inflammation in postoperative ileus, including elaboration of COX-2–produced prostanoids,[70] administration of NSAIDs is indicated. This is particularly true if postoperative ileus is associated with endotoxemia because LPS-induced prostanoid production disrupts propulsive motility in horses.[71,72] Interestingly, phenylbutazone was more effective than flunixin meglumine at reducing the deleterious actions of LPS on intestinal motility.[73] However, caution should be exercised when administering NSAIDs in patients with postoperative ileus in light of research suggesting that complete inhibition of prostanoid production can alter motility patterns in normal equine intestine.[68] The advent of selective COX-2 inhibitors may provide optimal anti-inflammatory treatment in the future.[74]

Other treatments aimed at specifically modulating intestinal motility include lidocaine (bolus of 1.3 mg/kg followed by 0.05 mg/kg/min for 24 hours), erythromycin (0.5-1.0 mg/kg slow intravenous infusion in 1 L saline every 6 hours), and metoclopramide (0.04 mg/kg/hr).[66,75,76] The mechanisms of lidocaine action may include inhibition of sensory nerve activity within the wall of the intestine, reduction of postoperative pain, and novel anti-inflammatory activity. However, the presence and clinical relevance of these mechanisms in the horse remain to be determined. Nonetheless, there is good evidence to show the action of lidocaine on sensory nerves in models of diarrheal disease, suggesting distinct mechanism of action for systemic administration of local anesthetics.[77] Metoclopramide may stimulate intestinal motility by several mechanisms, including dopamine receptor blockade, cholinergic stimulation, and adrenergic blockade.[66] Although this drug has been shown to be beneficial for reversing postoperative ileus in both clinical patients and research animals, it has central nervous system excitatory side effects in the horse that make its use difficult. Nonetheless, administration of metoclopramide to horses with postoperative ileus resulted in a significantly reduced duration of reflux and shorter postoperative hospital stays compared with horses not receiving this drug.[76] In addition, constant infusion of metoclopramide was shown to be superior to intermittent infusion in the same study.

Recent in vitro studies indicate that metoclopramide effectively increases smooth muscle contractile activity throughout the small intestine tract.[75] Similarly, the motilin agonist erythromycin had stimulatory effects on equine small intestine, although the results were not uniform throughout the small intestine. In particular, erythromycin stimulated contractile activity in the longitudinal muscle of the pyloric antrum but inhibited contractile activity in this segment of the gastrointestinal tract.[75] The latter may be attributable to activation of motilin receptors on inhibitory nerves and may result in enhanced gastric emptying. In vivo studies on erythromycin confirmed the stimulatory action of this drug on the distal small intestine and indicated that this drug also stimulates contractile activity in the cecum and pelvic flexure. However, this was dependent on the temporal association with surgery. In particular, erythromycin stimulated contractile activity in the postoperative period in the ileum and pelvic flexure but not the cecum,[78] which suggests that this drug may be useful for treatment of select cases of postoperative ileus.

For horses with presumed ileus of the large colon, signs included reduced fecal output (<three piles of manure/day), reduced gastrointestinal sounds, variable presence of colic, and occasionally a palpable impaction of the cecum or large colon. Risk factors for this syndrome include orthopedic surgery; length of the operative period; and, most important, inadequate treatment with phenylbutazone, presumably as a result of insufficient control of postoperative pain.[62] Although treatment of large colon impaction in the postoperative period is typically uncomplicated, cecal impaction is rapidly fatal in many horses because of the difficulty in recognizing horses that have cecal dysfunction. Therefore close attention should be paid to fecal production and optimal analgesic treatment in any horse after an orthopedic procedure.[62] It is likely that other painful procedures, including ophthalmologic procedures, also place horses at risk of developing ileus of the large intestine.

LARGE INTESTINAL SIMPLE OBSTRUCTION

Simple obstructions of the large intestine, such as impaction, tend to have a more gradual onset than those of the small intestine, although horses may experience acute and severe pain with some forms of colon displacement. In fact, some of these cases mimic and may progress toward large colon volvulus. Medical therapy is frequently successful in correcting large colon impactions. However, cecal impactions present much more of a dilemma because of the greater propensity of this organ to rupture, the relative difficulty of surgically manipulating the cecum, and the onset of cecal dysfunction that may prevent the cecum from emptying after surgical resolution of impaction.

Cecal Impaction

Cecal impaction may be divided into two syndromes: primary cecal impactions that result from excessive accumulation of ingesta in the cecum and secondary cecal impactions that develop while a horse is being treated for a separate problem.[79,80] Although primary impactions typically consist of impacted, relatively dry fecal material and secondary cecal impactions tend to have very fluid contents, there is considerable overlap between the two syndromes, and each case must be approached carefully. In horses with primary cecal impactions, there is a gradual onset of abdominal pain over a number of days reminiscent of the development of a large colon impaction. Cecal impactions should be differentiated from large colon impactions on the basis of rectal palpation findings. Cecal impactions have a propensity to rupture before the development of severe abdominal pain or systemic deterioration and therefore must be closely monitored.[79] Secondary cecal impactions typically develop after unrelated surgical procedures that result in postoperative pain (particularly orthopedic surgeries).[80] Secondary cecal impactions may be even more difficult to detect because postoperative depression and decreased fecal output may be attributed to the operative procedure rather than colic. By the time horses with secondary cecal impactions show noticeable signs of colic, the cecum may be close to rupture. In many cases there will be no signs of impending rupture.[80] Therefore the feed intake and manure production of all horses that undergo surgery in which considerable postoperative pain may develop should be closely monitored. A recent study indicated that horses producing less than three piles of manure daily in the postoperative period are at risk of developing a large intestinal impaction. Furthermore, horses that underwent prolonged (>1 hour) orthopedic surgery that received inadequate treatment with phenylbutazone were at considerable risk of reduced postoperative fecal output.[62] This is in contrast to statements indicating that NSAIDs may place horses at risk of impaction, which appear to be based largely on clinical impressions rather than risk analysis.[80]

The diagnosis of primary cecal impaction is based on rectal palpation of a firm, impacted cecum. In some cases cecal impactions may be difficult to differentiate from large colon impactions. However, careful palpation will reveal the inability to move the hand completely dorsal to the impacted viscus because of the cecum's attachment to the dorsal body wall. Treatment for horses with primary cecal impactions may include initial medical therapy, including aggressive administration of intravenous fluids and judicious use of analgesics.[80] However, if the cecum is grossly distended or if medical therapy has no effect within a reasonable period of time, surgical evacuation of the cecum by way of a typhlotomy is indicated.[79] The question of whether to bypass the cecum, because of postoperative cecal dysfunction and recurrence of impaction, led to techniques such as ileocolostomy to prevent ingesta from reaching the cecum. However, a recent study including a large number of cases suggests this is not necessary, possibly because of improvements in recognition and medical treatment of horses with colic.[81]

In horses that develop secondary cecal impactions, diagnosis is based on palpation of a markedly distended cecum filled with semifluid intestinal contents. The nature of the contents is likely related to the more rapid progression of this disease compared with that of primary cecal impaction. Surgery should not be delayed because of the risk of cecal rupture.[82] Following typhlotomy, aggressive medical management of the inciting cause of the impaction (such as orthopedic pain) should be addressed.

The prognosis is good for surgical treatment of all cecal impactions. However, fatalities may result from cecal rupture during prolonged medical treatment or during surgical manipulation. This complication can be avoided by early intervention. In a recent report assessing 114 horses, approximately 90% of those with long-term follow-up information available 1 year later survived regardless of whether they were treated medically or surgically.[81] However, a separate report indicated that all horses with cecal impaction secondary to another disease process had cecal rupture without any signs of impending rupture.[80]

Large Colon Impaction

Ingesta impactions of the large colon occur at sites of anatomic reductions in luminal diameter, particularly the pelvic flexure and the right dorsal colon.[83] Although there are a number of reported risk factors, most have not been proved. However, a sudden restriction in exercise associated with musculoskeletal injury appears to be frequently associated with onset of impaction.[84] A further consideration is equine feeding regimes, which usually entail twice-daily feeding of concentrate. Such regimens result in large fluxes of fluid into and out of the colon, associated with readily fermentable carbohydrate in the colon and subsequent increases in serum aldosterone, respectively. These fluid fluxes, which may cause dehydration of ingesta during aldosterone-stimulated net fluid flux out of the colon, may be prevented with frequent small feedings.[32]

Impaction of the ascending colon can be induced by the drug amitraz, an acaricide associated with clinical cases of colon impaction.[85,86] The importance of this is that it provides some clues as to the pathogenesis of large colon impaction. In particular, amitraz appears to alter pelvic flexure pacemaker activity, resulting in uncoordinated motility patterns between the left ventral and left dorsal colon and excessive retention of ingesta. Absorption of water from the ingesta increases with retention time, dehydrating the contents of the colon and resulting in impaction. It is conceivable that parasite migration in the region of a pacemaker may have a similar action.[87] Other factors implicated in large colon impaction include limited exercise, poor dentition, coarse roughage, and dehydration.

Clinical signs of large colon impaction include slow onset of mild colic. Fecal production is reduced, and the feces are often hard, dry, and mucus-covered because of delayed transit time. The heart rate may be mildly elevated during episodes of pain but is often normal. Signs of abdominal pain are typically well controlled with administration of analgesics but become increasingly more severe and refractory if the impaction does not resolve. The diagnosis is based on rectal palpation of a firm mass in the large colon. However, the extent of the impaction may be underestimated by rectal palpation alone because much of the colon remains out of reach.[83] Adjacent colon may be distended if the impaction has resulted in complete obstruction. Initial medical treatment should be attempted. Intermittent abdominal pain is controlled with administration of analgesics (flunixin meglumine, 0.25 to 1.1 mg/kg IV every 6 to 12 hours; butorphanol, 0.05 to 0.1 mg/kg IV every 6 to 8 hours; xylazine, 0.3 to 0.5 mg/kg IV as needed). Administration of oral laxatives such as mineral oil (2 to 4 L by nasogastric tube every 12 to 24 hours) and the anionic surfactant dioctyl sodium sulfosuccinate (DSS, 6 to 12 g/500 kg diluted in 2 to 4 L of water by nasogastric tube every 12 to 24 hours) are commonly used to soften the impaction. Saline cathartics such as magnesium sulfate (0.1 mg/kg in 2 to 4 L by nasogastric tube) may also be useful. Access to feed should not be permitted. For impactions that persist aggressive oral and intravenous fluid therapy (twofold to fourfold the maintenance fluid requirement) should be instituted.[83] If the impaction remains unresolved, the horse's pain becomes uncontrollable, or extensive gas distention of the colon occurs, surgery is indicated. In addition, abdominal fluid can be serially monitored to determine the onset of intestinal compromise.[83] At surgery the contents of the colon are evacuated by way of a pelvic flexure enterotomy. The prognosis is good for horses in which impactions resolve medically (95% long-term survival in one study) and fair in horses that require surgical intervention (58% long-term survival in the same study).[84]

Enteroliths

Enteroliths are mineralized masses typically composed of ammonium magnesium phosphate (struvite).[88] However, magnesium vivianite has also been identified in enteroliths, along with variable quantities of Na, S, K, and Ca. The formation of Mg-based minerals is puzzling because of the relative abundance of Ca in colonic fluids, which would favor the formation of Ca-phosphates (apatite) rather than struvite.[89] However, elevated dietary intake of magnesium and protein may play a role. Many horses that develop enteroliths live in California and are fed a diet consisting mainly of alfalfa hay. Analysis of this hay has revealed a concentration of magnesium approximately six times the daily requirements of the horse.[90] Furthermore, the high protein concentration in alfalfa hay may contribute to calculi formation by increasing the ammonia nitrogen load in the large intestine. Enteroliths most commonly form around a nucleus of silicon dioxide (a flintlike stone), but nidi have included nails, rope, and hair that have been ingested.[88] Enteroliths are usually found in the right dorsal and transverse colons.[90] Although enterolithiasis has a wide geographic distribution, horses in California have the highest incidence. In one California study, horses with enterolithiasis represented 28% of the surgical colic population, and Arabians, Morgans, American Saddlebreds, and donkeys were at greatest risk of this disease.[91] In a study of enterolithiasis in Texas, risk factors also included feeding of alfalfa hay and Arabian breed. However, in that study miniature horses were also found to be at risk.[92] Horses with enteroliths are rarely younger than 4 years old,[90] although an enterolith in an 11-month-old miniature horse was recently reported.[93]

Enterolithiasis is characterized by episodic, mild to moderate, intermittent abdominal pain.[90] Progressive anorexia and depression may develop. The amount of pain depends on the degree of obstruction and amount of distention. Partial luminal obstruction allows the passage of scant, pasty feces. Heart rate is variable and dependent on the degree of pain. In some cases an enterolith is forced into the small colon, where it causes acute small colon obstruction. Enteroliths may be diagnosed by abdominal radiography or at surgery. On rare occasions an enterolith may be palpated rectally, particularly if it is present in the distal small colon.

In general, surgery is required for these cases, although there are reports of enteroliths being retrieved rectally. In fact, in one study 14% of horses that required treatment of enterolithiasis had a history of passing an enterolith in the feces.[91] However, enteroliths are typically located in the right dorsal colon, transverse colon, or small colon. At surgery the enterolith is gently pushed toward a pelvic flexure enterotomy, but removal frequently requires a separate right dorsal colon enterotomy to prevent rupture of the colon. After removal of an enterolith, further exploration must be conducted to determine if other enteroliths are present. Solitary enteroliths are usually round, whereas multiple enteroliths have flat sides. The prognosis is good (92% 1-year survival in one study on 900 cases),[91] unless the colon is ruptured during removal of an enterolith. In one recent study rupture occurred in 15% of cases.[91]

Sand Impactions of the Large Colon

Sand impactions are common in horses with access to sandy soils, particularly horses whose feed is placed on the ground. Some horses, especially foals, deliberately eat sand. Fine sand tends to accumulate in the ventral colon, whereas coarse sand may accumulate in the dorsal colon.[94,95] However, individual differences in colonic function may contribute to accumulation of sand because some horses can clear consumed sand, whereas others cannot. Distention resulting from the impaction itself, or gas proximal to the impaction, causes abdominal pain. In addition, sand may trigger diarrhea, presumably as a result of irritation of the colonic mucosa.[96] In horses with sand impactions, clinical signs are similar to those of horses with large colon impactions.[94] Sand may be found in the feces, and auscultation of the ventral abdomen may reveal sounds of sand moving within the large colon.[97] The diagnosis is definitively made at surgery but may be tentatively based on clinical signs compatible with a large colon impaction and evidence of sand in the feces. To determine the presence of sand, several fecal balls are placed in a rectal palpation sleeve or other container, which is subsequently filled with water. If sand is present, it will accumulate at the bottom of the container. In addition, mineral opacity may be detected within the colon on abdominal radiographs, particularly in foals, ponies, and small horses.[95] Abdominal paracentesis typically yields normal fluid and poses some risk because large quantities of sand in the ventral colon make inadvertent perforation of the colon more likely.[95] PF is often normal but may have an elevated protein concentration.

Initially, medical therapy is warranted. Administration of *Psyllium hydrophilia* mucilloid (0.25 to 0.5 kg/500 kg in 4 to 8 L of water by stomach tube) may facilitate passage of sand. This should be administered rapidly because it will form a viscous gel. Therefore an alternative method of administration is to mix psyllium with 2 L of mineral oil, which will not form a gel and can be pumped easily through a nasogastric tube. Between 2 and 4 L of water is then pumped through the tube. The psyllium leaves the oil phase and mixes with the water, forming a gel within the stomach. Psyllium is thought to act by stimulating motility or agglutinating the sand. However, a recent experimental study failed to show a benefit of this treatment.[98] If a severe impaction is present, the psyllium should not be given until the impaction is softened by administrating intravenous or oral fluids and other laxatives. Perforation is a potential complication in horses with sand impactions because the sand stretches and irritates the intestinal wall and causes inflammation. Therefore if colic becomes intractable, surgical evacuation of the large colon should be performed. The prognosis is generally regarded as good.[94,95]

Large Colon Displacement

Displacement of the ascending colon is a common cause of large intestinal obstruction. The ascending colon is freely movable except for the right dorsal and ventral colons. Contact with adjacent viscera and the abdominal wall tends to inhibit movement of the ascending colon from a normal position; however, accumulation of gas and fluid or ingesta may cause the colon to migrate.[99] Feeding behavior, including feeding of large concentrate meals, likely plays a role in initiating displacement of the large colon. In particular, large concentrate meals increase the rate of passage of ingesta, allowing a greater percentage of soluble carbohydrates to reach the large intestine.[31] This in turn increases the rate of fermentation and the amount of gas and volatile fatty acids that are produced. The production of large amounts of volatile fatty acids stimulates the secretion of large volumes of fluid into the colon.[100] The association between feeding concentrate and development of displacements of the large colon is illustrated by studies indicating that ascending colon displacement is more prevalent in horses fed a high-concentrate, low-roughage diet.[101] Abnormal motility patterns of the ascending colon have also been suggested to contribute to the development of colonic displacement. Feeding stimulates colonic motility by way of the gastrocolic reflex, but large meals may alter normal motility patterns and concurrently allow rapid accumulation of gas and fluid resulting from fermentation.[31,102] Migration of parasite larvae (strongyles) through the intestinal wall have also been shown to alter colonic motility patterns.[103] Other experimental studies have shown that *Strongylus vulgaris* infection results in reduced blood flow to segments of the large intestine without necessarily causing infarction. Electrical activity of the colon and cecocolic junction increases after infection with *S. vulgaris* and cyathostome larvae, probably reflecting a direct effect of migration through the intestine and an early response to reduced blood flow.[103]

Displacements of the ascending colon are generally divided into three types: left dorsal displacement, right dorsal displacement, and retroflexion.[104] Left dorsal displacement is characterized by entrapment of the ascending colon in the renosplenic space. The colon is often twisted 180 degrees, such that the left ventral colon is situated in a dorsal position relative to the left dorsal colon. The entrapped portion may be only the pelvic flexure or may involve a large portion of the ascending colon, with the pelvic flexure situated near the diaphragm. The colon may become entrapped by migrating dorsally between the left abdominal wall and the spleen or may migrate in a caudodorsal direction over the nephrosplenic ligament.[104] Occasionally, the ascending colon can be palpated between the spleen and abdominal wall, lending support to the first mechanism of displacement. Gastric distention is thought to predispose horses to left dorsal displacement of the ascending colon by displacing the spleen medially, allowing the colon room to migrate along the abdominal wall.[104] Right dorsal displacement begins by movement of the colon cranially, either medial (medial flexion) or lateral (lateral flexion) to the cecum. According to one author, the proportion of right dorsal displacements with medial versus lateral flexion is approximately 1:15.[104] In either case the pelvic flexure ends up adjacent to the diaphragm. Retroflexion of the ascending colon occurs by movement of the pelvic flexure cranially without movement of the sternal or diaphragmatic flexures.

Displacement of the ascending colon partially obstructs the lumen, resulting in accumulation of gas or ingesta and causing distention. The distention may be exacerbated by the secretion of fluid in response to the distention.[105] Tension and stretch of the visceral wall are important sources of the pain associated with colonic displacement. Tension on mesenteric attachments and the root of the mesentery by the enlarged colon may also cause pain.[99] Ischemia is rarely associated with nonstrangulating displacement of the colon. However, vascular congestion and edema are often seen in the displaced segments of colon, resulting from increased hydrostatic pressure from reduced venous outflow. Morphologic damage to the tissues is usually minor.

Clinically, displacement of the ascending colon is characterized by intermittent signs of mild to moderate abdominal pain of acute onset. However, an insidious onset of colic may also be noted.[104] Dehydration may be noted if the duration of the displacement is prolonged. The heart rate may be elevated during periods of abdominal pain but is often normal. Abdominal distention may be present if the colon is enlarged by gas, fluid, or ingesta. Fecal production is reduced as progressive motility of the large intestine is absent. Left dorsal displacements are often diagnosed by rectal palpation. The left ventral colon can be felt in a dorsal position and is often filled with gas. The ascending colon can be traced to the nephrosplenic space, and the spleen may be displaced medially. Alternatively, a tentative diagnosis can be reached using abdominal ultrasonography.[106] The spleen can be visualized on the left side of the abdomen, but the left kidney will be obscured by gas-distended bowel. Evaluation of this technique indicates that there are very few instances of false-positive results, although false-negative results may occasionally occur.[106] A definitive diagnosis therefore may require surgery. Right dorsal displacements are characterized by the presence of the distended ventral colon running across the pelvic inlet and may be felt between the cecum and the body wall if a lateral flexion is present. The pelvic flexure is usually not palpable. Retroflexion of the ascending colon may produce a palpable kink in the colon. If the displaced colons are not distended by gas in the instance of right dorsal displacement and retroflexion, the ascending colon may not be palpable and is conspicuous by its absence from a normal position. PF may be increased in amount, but the color, protein concentration, and white blood cell count are usually normal. However, as the displaced segment becomes edematous, fluid leaking through the serosa into the PF increases the protein concentration.

Surgical correction of colon displacement is the most effective means of resolving this disorder. However, nonsurgical intervention has been successful in select cases of nephrosplenic entrapment of the large colon.[106-108] If such manipulations are to be attempted, the clinician must be certain of a diagnosis. The horse is anesthetized and placed in right lateral recumbency. The horse is rotated up to dorsal recumbency, rocked back and forth for 5 to 10 minutes, and then rolled down into left lateral recumbancy.[109] The nephrosplenic space should be rectally palpated to determine whether the entrapment has been relieved before recovering the horse from anesthesia. Phenylephrine (3 to 6 μg/kg/min over 15 minutes) may be administered to decrease the size of the spleen.[110] More recently, phenylephrine has been used in conjunction with 30 to 45 minutes of exercise to successfully reduce nephrosplenic entrapments in 4 of 6 horses.[26] The authors suggested that the technique be used on horses with mild to moderate colonic distention, particularly when there are severe financial constraints. There are anecdotal reports of fatal internal hemorrhage caused by rupture of large blood vessels after treatment of older horses with phenylephrine, and the drug should probably be used with caution in horses older than 15 years.

There are a number of cases in which nonsurgical interventions do not correct the problem and others in which nonsurgical manipulations correct the entrapment but result in large colon volvulus or displacement. These horses should undergo surgery promptly. The prognosis for horses with large colon displacement is good. In one study of horses with nephrosplenic entrapment of the large colon, survival was in excess of 90%.[108] A number of horses will suffer recurrence of nephrosplenic entrapment of the colon. Currently, the least invasive method of preventing this complication is laparoscopic closure of the nephrosplenic space.[111]

Foreign Body and Fecalith Obstruction

Foreign material such as bedding, rope, plastic, fence material, and feedbags can cause obstruction and may be ingested, particularly by young horses. These foreign bodies may result in impaction with ingesta and distention of the intestine, typically in the transverse or descending colon. Young horses are usually affected. In one study the obstructing mass could be rectally palpated in three of six horses.[112] Fecaliths are common in ponies, miniature horses, and foals (Figure 15-31).[113] Older horses with poor dentition may also be predisposed to fecaliths because of the inability to fully masticate fibrous feed material. Fecaliths commonly cause obstruction in the descending colon and may cause tenesmus.[112] Other clinical signs are similar to those of enterolithiasis. Abdominal radiography may be useful in smaller patients to identify the obstruction, especially if gas distention around the foreign body or fecalith provides contrast. Surgical treatment is usually required.

Mural Masses and Strictures

Mural masses such as abscesses, tumors (adenocarcinoma, lymphosarcoma), granulomas, and hematomas (Figure 15-32) can cause luminal obstruction and impaction, typically in older horses. Impaction may result from obstruction of the lumen or impaired motility in the segment of intestine with the mass. Abscesses may originate from the lumen of the intestine, or may extend from the mesentery or mesenteric lymph nodes. Intramural hematomas form most commonly in the descending colon and cause acute abdominal pain.[114] Once the acute pain caused by the hematoma subsides, impaction proximal to the hematoma develops as a result of impaired motility through the affected portion of the colon. Trauma, ulceration of the mucosa, and parasitic damage are speculated causes of intramural hematomas.[114,115] Stricture of the large intestine occurs when fibrous tissue forms in a circular pattern around or within the intestine, reducing the luminal diameter and the ability of the wall to stretch. Strictures may be congenital or secondary to peritonitis, previous abdominal surgery, or inflammatory bowel disease.[116] In a report of 11 horses with inflammatory

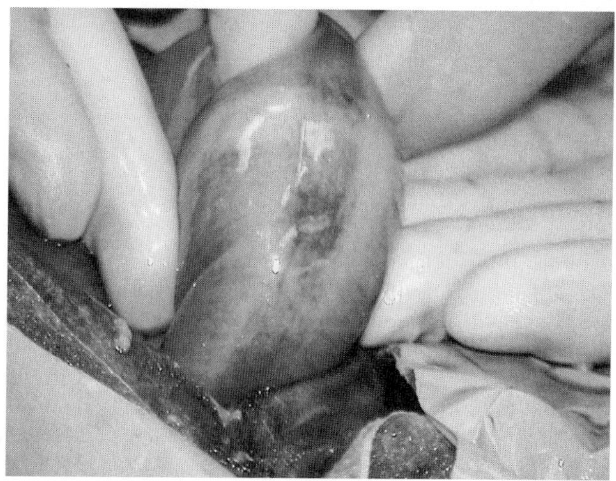

FIGURE 15-31 Fecalith in the small colon of a miniature horse. Note the mass being grasped by the surgeon. The small colon is distended, so that haustra cannot be identified. However, the antimesenteric tenia of the small colon is clearly visible.

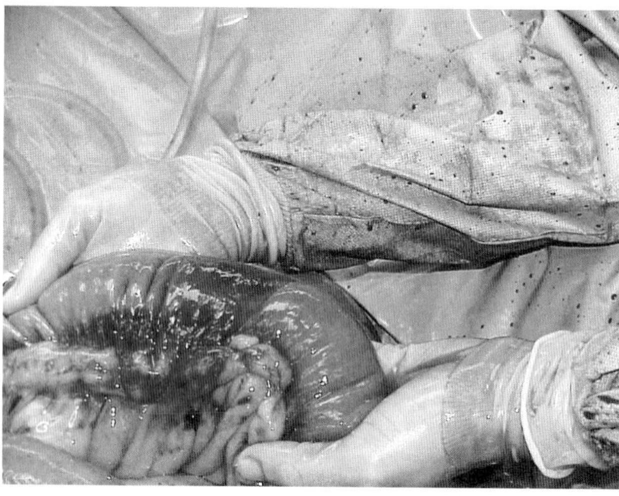

FIGURE 15-32 Intramural hematoma of unknown origin in the small colon of a horse taken to surgery for persistent signs of colic. The lack of a complete physical obstruction at this site was suggestive of a functional obstruction at the site of the hematoma.

bowel disease, 6 horses had strictures, 4 of which were in the small intestine and 2 of which were in the large colon.[116]

Clinical signs vary according to the degree of luminal obstruction. Partial obstruction and impaction tend to produce mild to moderate abdominal pain of insidious onset. Mural hematomas tend to produce signs of acute abdominal pain.[114,115] Rectal palpation of the abdomen may reveal the presence of a mass or simply the impacted segment, without the mass itself being felt. Fever, weight loss, and anorexia may be noted if an abscess or tumor is the cause. An elevated white blood cell count; hyperfibrinogenemia; hyperglobulinemia; or normocytic, normochromic anemia may be seen with abscesses or tumors. PF may reflect the cause of the mass. Tumor cells may infrequently be seen. Evidence of inflammation with bacteria may be noted if the cause of colic is an abscess or granuloma, in which case the fluid should be cultured. Hematomas may cause hemorrhage into the PF. Treatment usually requires surgical resection of the mass. Abscesses may be treated with appropriate antibiotics if the impaction can be resolved medically with oral or intravenous analgesics and laxatives. *Streptococcus* spp., *Actinomyces pyogenes, Corynebacterium pseudotuberculosis, R. equi*, anaerobic bacteria, and gram negative enteric organisms are commonly involved in abscesses.

Small Colon Impaction

Small colon impaction is distinct from other forms of impaction in its predispositions and clinical appearance. In one study the key risk factor for impaction of this segment of the intestine was diarrhea.[117] This paradoxical finding may be explained by edema of the colonic mucosa associated with proinflammatory causes of diarrheal disease that is usually noted in the ascending colon but may extend into the transverse and small colons. Once diarrheal disease is initiated, large volumes of ingesta are rapidly expelled from the ascending colon into the small colon, which has a far smaller diameter, especially if it is edmematous. This may result in the initial appearance of diarrhea, followed by intermittent episodes of colic that may be explained by impaction. The most important point to remember is that horses should be closely assessed for impaction even if diarrheal disease is present. Other parameters that are typically helpful for assessing the severity of colic, such as heart rate, were not predictive of obstruction in horses with small colon impaction.[117] Horses may be treated medically during the early stages with fluids, laxatives, and analgesics. The key clinical sign that indicates the need for surgery appears to be abdominal distention, associated with distention of the large colon. Other clinical signs, such as elevations in heart rate and refractory colic, are less pronounced in this disease. Postdiarrheal disease is not the only form of small colon impaction. These impactions can be formed as simple collections of ingesta or in response to luminal narrowing.

Atresia Coli

Atresia of a segment of the colon is a rare congenital abnormality in horses.[118] The heritability and causes of the condition are unknown. One potential mechanism for development of the lesion is intestinal ischemia during fetal life, which secondarily results in necrosis of a segment of intestine.[118] Clinical signs include a failure to pass meconium and colic within the first 12 to 24 hours of life. Secondary abdominal distention results from complete intestinal obstruction, and abdominal radiographs may reveal gas-distended colon. The diagnosis is made at surgery. Any portion of the colon may be absent, but the distal segment of the large colon or the proximal small colon (or both) is usually most severely affected. If sufficient tissue is present, anastomosis to the proximal blind end of the colon may be attempted.[118] The prognosis depends on the segment of the colon that is absent but is usually poor because of an absence of distal colon.

Ileocolonic Aganglionosis

Ileocolonic aganglionosis, commonly known as *overo lethal white syndrome* (OLWS), occurs in white foals with overo-spotted parents. Affected foals are either completely white or have very little pigmented hair around the muzzle, base of the tail, or hooves. They are homozygous for an abnormal endothelin receptor B (EDNRB) gene that results in altered neural crest cell migration or survival, which affects progenitor cells for melanocytes and intestinal ganglia.[119,120] Most, but not all, heterozygotes have a frame overo phenotype.[121] Rarely, an OLWS-affected foal may be born to a solid-colored mare. Homozygous foals have aganglionosis of the submucosal and myenteric ganglia of the distal portion of the ileum and large intestine.[122] This results in a foal that appears normal at birth but develops signs of intestinal ileus and colic within 12 to 24 hours. The eyes are blue, and the skin is pink. A genetic test is available to identify horses that are heterozygous for the defective EDNRB gene.

NEOPLASIA OF THE ALIMENTARY TRACT

Dana N. Zimmel

Neoplasia in the alimentary tract of the horse is uncommon.[1] Primary and metastatic neoplasia can affect multiple locations within the oral cavity and gastrointestinal tract (Boxes 15-1 and 15-2). Neoplasia is not limited to geriatric horses. The

BOX 15-1

NEOPLASIA OF THE ORAL CAVITY

Odontogenic Tumors (Originates from Dental Tissue)[2]

Ameloblastoma
Ameloblastic odontoma
Cementoma[3]
Complex odontoma
Compound odontoma
Fibro-myxoma
Odontoblasoma

Osteogenic Tumors (Originates from Bone)[2]

Leiomyosarcoma[4]
Myxoma
Osteoma
Osteosarcoma

Soft Tissue Tumors[2]

Epulis
Fibrous dysplasia
Hemangiosarcoma[5]
Juvenile ossifying fibroma
Melanoma
Papilloma
Sarcoid
Salivary adenocarcinoma
Squamous cell carcinoma

Tongue

Chondrosarcoma[6]
Lymphosarcoma[7]
Multiple myleoma[8]
Rhabdomyosarcoma[9]
Paraneoplastic bullous stomatitis[10]

BOX 15-2

NEOPLASIA OF THE GASTROINTESTINAL TRACT

Esophagus

Squamous cell carcinoma[11,12]

Stomach

Adenocarcinoma[13]
Gastric polyp[14]
Leiomyosarcoma[15]
Lymphoma (lymphosarcoma)[16,17]
Squamous cell carcinoma[11,18,19]

Small Intestine

Adenocarcinoma[20-22]
Adenomatous polyposis[23]
Ganglioneuroma[24]
Intestinal carcinoid[25]
Leiomyoma[26-28]
Leiomyosarcoma[29]
Lipoma[30]
Lymphoma (lymphosarcoma)[31]
Neurofibroma[32]

Cecum

Adenocarcinoma[33]
Intestinal myxosarcoma[34]
Stromal tumor[35]

Large Colon

Adenocarcinoma[36-38]
Lipomatosis[39]
Lymphoma (lymphosarcoma)[40]
Neurofibroma[41]

Small Colon

Lipoma[30,42]
Lipomatosis[39]
Leiomyoma[43,44]

Rectum

Leiomyosarcoma[45]
Lipoma[46]
Lymphoma (lymphosarcoma)[47]
Polyps[48]

Peritoneum

Disseminated leiomyomatosis[49]
Mesothelioma[50-52]
Omental fibrosarcoma[53]

average age of horses with squamous cell carcinoma is 8.6 to 14.6 years.[54,55] The alimentary form of lymphoma occurs most commonly in horses younger than 5 years of age.[56] One recent study found that the Arabian breed is 4.5-fold more likely to have intestinal neoplasia than other breeds.[20] Identification of benign versus malignant tumors is imperative to justify treatment and predict survival.

CLINICAL SIGNS

The clinical signs associated with alimentary neoplasia are related to the tumor location. Clinical signs of oral neoplasia include enlargement or ulceration of the mandible or maxilla.[57] Neoplasia of the tongue results in weight loss, quidding, dysphagia, halitosis, and nasal discharge containing feed material.[7, 8, 9] Tumors of the esophagus cause dysphagia, ptyalism, choke, intermittent colic, fever, weight loss, and halitosis.[11,58,59] Gastric neoplasia may be associated with abnormal chewing and swallowing behavior, anorexia, weight loss, abdominal distention, and intermittent fever.[18] Abdominal neoplasia has been implicated in 4% of horses with intermittent or chronic colic.[60,61] Altered stool character, ventral edema, and recurrent fever have been associated with intestinal neoplasia.[56] Weight loss is the most common clinical sign of horses with intestinal neoplasia.[20] Acute signs of abdominal discomfort may occur with intestinal obstructions resulting from malignant and benign neoplastic disease.

Paraneoplastic syndromes do occur in the horse. The most common syndromes described are cancer cachexia, ectopic hormone production, anemia, leukocytosis, thrombocytopenia, hypergammaglobulinemia, fever, and neurologic abnormalities.[62] Horses with cancer cachexia have profound weight loss despite adequate consumption of calories.

DIAGNOSTIC EVALUATION

Diagnosis of alimentary neoplasia can be challenging. Data collected from a complete blood count, biochemistry panel, and urinalysis may support the diagnosis of neoplasia but rarely confirms it. Normocytic normochromic anemia is indicative of chronic disease and is the most likely cause of anemia associated with neoplasia. Blood loss anemia (through the gastrointestinal tract) and immune-mediated hemolytic anemia (lymphoma)[63] are less frequent causes of anemia associated with abdominal neoplasia. Peripheral eosinophilia has been reported in association with multisystemic eosinophilic, epitheliotropic disease with lymphoma.[16] Leukocytosis and hyperfibrinogenemia are common findings.

Serum chemistry can confirm hypoalbuminemia caused by inflammation of the bowel wall. Hyperglobulinemia can be characterized with serum electrophoresis. This test is nonspecific for chronic inflammation. A few cases of lymphoma have been identified with monoclonal spikes in globulins.[64] Ectopic hormone production may result in hypercalcemina (calcium >14 mg/dl). Hypercalcemia has been associated with alimentary neoplasms such as lymphoma, multiple myleoma, carcinomas, and ameloblastoma.[54,65] Hypoglycemia (blood glucose <70 mg/dl) can occur with neoplasia of the pancreas or liver.[54]

Rectal examination may reveal an abdominal mass, thickening of the intestinal wall, lymph node enlargement, or a gritty texture in horses with carcinomatosis.[54] Lymphoma can be detected using rectal biopsy in some cases.[47] A fecal occult blood test is nonspecific for neoplastic disease, but it can detect blood loss through the gastrointestinal tract. Occasionally, abdominocentesis may be used to identify neoplasia if the tumor exfoliates cells into the abdomen. Squamous cell carcinoma, adenocarcinoma, and mesothelioma have been detected in PF.[11,50,51,66] It is common for the PF to be characterized as an inflammatory exudate or modified transudate without any neoplastic cells present. Hemoperitoneum is attributed to neoplasia in 18% of cases in a retrospective study of 67 horses. The neoplastic conditions identified included granulosa cell ovarian tumors (three); metastatic melanoma (two); multicentric hemangiosarcoma (two); and one case each of metastatic squamous cell carcinoma, splenic lymphoma, ovarian lymphosarcoma, pheochromocytoma, and a neuroendocrine tumor.[67,68] Abdominocentesis accurately predicted neoplasia in 11 of 25 cases in another study.[69] D-xylose absorption tests can be used to identify malabsorptive diseases that can include lymphoma.[47,70]

Specific immunoglobulin testing for IgM deficiency may aid in the diagnosis of lymphoma.[71] DNA cell cycle analysis of suspect neoplastic cells has been used to detect lymphoma in equine patients confirmed to have the disease. This method of evaluating fluid or tissues aspirates may increase the accuracy with which neoplasia is diagnosed in the future.[72]

A complete evaluation of the oral cavity may include using a full-mouth speculum, radiographs, endoscopy of the pharynx, and biopsy. Evaluation of the esophagus and stomach with a 3-meter endoscope may aid in the identification of intraluminal masses. Pleuroscopy has been used to biopsy extraluminal masses surrounding the esophagus. Contrast radiography can assist in the diagnosis of neoplasia within the wall or outside of the esophagus.[58,73] Ultrasonography of the stomach, small intestine, cecum, and large colon is useful in detecting intestinal wall thickness, abdominal masses, and excessive PF.[74] Irregular cauliflower-like masses can be visualized on the body wall and are consistent with peritoneal mesothelioma.[33] Identification of neoplasia in the liver, kidney, or spleen may support the finding of metastasis to other parts of the gastrointestinal tract or lymph nodes. Laparoscopy and exploratory laparotomy are often required to obtain a final diagnosis.[75]

SPECIFIC NEOPLASIA

Lymphoma (Lymphosarcoma)

Lymphoma, the most common neoplasia in the horse, has been divided into four categories.[20] Only the intestinal-alimentary form is discussed in this section. Lymphosarcoma is discussed in detail in Chapter 14. The condition was once called *lymphosarcoma,* but oncologists today prefer *lymphoma* because there is no benign form of this disease.[54] Lymphoma originates from lymphoid tissue and predominantly affects the small intestinal and intestinal lymph nodes. Chronic weight loss resulting from malabsorption, intermittent colic, and fever is the most common clinical finding.[76,31] Chronic diarrhea has been reported in some cases.[77] Paraneoplastic pruritus and alopecia have been identified in one case of diffuse lymphoma.[78] Peripheral lymphadenopathy is not generally noted, but enlargement of the intestinal lymph nodes may be evident on rectal examination.[56] Immunohistochemical staining can classify most tumors as of T-cell or B-cell origin, which may be helpful in determining prognosis.[79] Large colon resection for treatment of lymphoma has increased short-term survival in two horses.[40] The use of chemotherapy in two pregnant mares extended their lives long enough for normal parturition.[80,81]

Squamous Cell Carcinoma

Squamous cell carcinoma is a malignant tumor of the gastrointestinal epithelium. It is the second most common neoplasia in the horse and the most common oral neoplasia; however, the incidence of occurrence is rare.[11,18,59] In the oral cavity squamous cell carcinoma may affect the lips, tongue, hard palate, pharynx, and oral mucosa.[82,83] Treatment for squamous cell carcinoma in the oral cavity may involve surgical resection, iridium-192 brachytherapy, 5-fluorouracil, or intralesional cisplatin or carboplatin.[2,84-86] The prognosis for survival is good if complete removal of the tumor is possible. One report of reoccurring squamous cell carcinoma on the lip with metastasis to the lymph nodes was successfully treated with piroxicam over 58 months.[87] Metastasis beyond the regional lymph nodes is rare for oral squamous cell carcinoma.

Squamous cell carcinoma is the most common tumor of the stomach and esophagus.[12,18] It can invade these areas and metastasize to the lymph nodes and lungs. Abnormal masses were palpated on rectal examination in four of five horses with gastric squamous cell carcinoma.[18] Hypertrophic osteopathy secondary to gastric squamous cell carcinoma has been documented in one horse.[88] Treatment by surgical resection is not possible in most cases.[54]

Adenocarcinoma

Adenocarcinoma is a malignant tumor that can occur in the small intestine, cecum, and large colon.[13,21] The tumor arises from the glandular crypts of the gastrointestinal tract. It has been reported in middle-aged and older horses. Metastasis to the lymph nodes, liver, and lungs can occur. Intestinal adenocarcinoma has been reported to metastasize to the bone and was diagnosed with Tc-99m hydroxymethylene diphosphate.[33,36] In a study of 34 cases of intestinal neoplasia, 11 (32%) were adenocarcinomas with 9 (82%) involving the small intestine. After surgical removal only three horses survived to discharge. Only one horse survived longer than 5 years.[20] The short-term prognosis for resectable adenocarcinoma is fair, and the long-term prognosis is poor.[37]

Leiomyosarcoma

Leiomyosarcoma is a malignant tumor of the smooth muscle lining the gastrointestinal tract. It has been reported in the stomach, small intestine, and rectum.[15,26,27,45,69] In one case report gastroscopy could not identify a gastric mural mass found during exploratory surgery. Another report describes a favorable outcome for surgical resection of a leiomyosarcoma that was protruding from the anal sphincter in a 4-year-old Quarter Horse.[45] Prognosis for survival is favorable if surgical resection is possible. There is a single case review of a leiomyosarcoma invading the mandible and maxilla.[4]

Leiomyoma

Leiomyoma is a benign tumor of the smooth muscle of the gastrointestinal tract. It can occur in the stomach, small intestine, omentum, and small colon.[42,44,89] Clinical signs are consistent with intestinal obstruction. Surgical resection and anastomosis of the affected portion of the intestine has been performed without complications.

Lipoma

Lipoma is a benign tumor that occurs in older horses (10 to 26 years) and arises from mesenteric adipocytes. The tumor grows on a stalk that wraps around the intestine, causing a strangulating lesion of the intestine or an intestinal obstruction. Intestinal injury has resulted from lipomas strangulating the small intestine, small colon, and rectum. Long-term survival with surgical resection and anastomosis is reported to be 50%.[30,90,91]

Oral Neoplasia

Oral cavity neoplasia may involve the dental tissue (odontogenic tumors), bone (osteogenic tumors), or soft tissues (see Box 15-1). Ameloblastoma occurs in horses older than 10 years of age, and it mainly affects the mandible. Ameloblastic odontoma affects younger horses and usually involves the maxilla. Both are benign but locally invasive. Radiographs may aid in differentiation between an ameloblastoma (radiolucent lesion) and ameloblastic odontoma (radiolucent lesion with partially mineralized density). Regardless of the type, the best treatment option is surgical resection, radiation therapy, or both.[57] Teletherapy could be used to treat oral neoplasia.[92,93] Teletherapy is the practice of radiation used at a distance of 80 to 100 cm from the target tissue using a linear accelerator or cobalt-60 source.

Juvenile mandibular ossifying fibroma occurs in the rostral mandible of young horses between the age of 2 months and 2 years. It may cause significant distortion of the bone. Surgical excision of the mass has a good prognosis if diagnosed early.[94,95]

Melanomas, sarcoids, squamous cell carcinoma, and oral papilloma occur on the mouth and lips. Melanomas rarely metastasize, but they are commonly found in the parotid salivary glands and lymph nodes. Sarcoids are the most common skin tumor that can involve the mouth. Ulcerations of the buccal mucosa are difficult to treat. Intralesional cisplatin, cryosurgery, radiation, and laser excision have been tried with limited success.[2] Equine papilloma virus is responsible for the common skin wart that is found on the lips and muzzle of young horses. These lesions are self-limiting, but they can be removed with cryosurgery or excision.

PERITONITIS

Laura H. Javsicas

STRUCTURE AND FUNCTION

A number of detailed and informative reviews describe the anatomy, physiology, and pathophysiology of the equine peritoneum.[1-4] The peritoneum consists of a single layer of mesothelial cells. The mesothelial lining of the diaphragm, abdominal walls, and pelvic cavity is termed *parietal peritoneum*. The visceral peritoneum forms the serosal surfaces of the intra-abdominal organs. Caudally, the peritoneum reflects over the surfaces of the pelvic organs (portions of the urogenital tract and rectum), excluding them from the peritoneal space and defining the retroperitoneal space. The peritoneal space communicates with the lumen of the uterus (and thus the external environment) by way of the fallopian tubes in females. In males the peritoneum forms a true blind sac. The vascular supply and nervous innervation of the visceral peritoneum are supplied by the splanchnic vessels and visceral autonomic nerves, respectively. Branches of the intercostal, lumbar, and iliac arteries supply the parietal peritoneum, and the phrenic and intercostal nerves provide nervous innervation. The clinical relevance is that inflammation of the parietal peritoneum is perceived as somatic pain, resulting in a splinted abdominal wall, pain on external palpation, and reluctance to move.

The peritoneal lining functions as a semipermeable barrier to the diffusion of water and low-molecular-weight solutes between the blood and the abdominal cavity.[2] The peritoneum secretes a serous fluid that lubricates the abdominal cavity, inhibits adhesion formation, and has minor antibacterial properties.[2,3] Macrophages, mast cells, mesothelial cells, and lymphocytes provide immune function within the peritoneum.[1,3] The peritoneal surface maintains a high level of fibrinolytic activity through the production of plasminogen activators by mesothelial cells. This function, with the lubricant properties of the PF, helps maintain gliding surfaces within the peritoneum and prevent adhesion formation. PF produced by the mesothelium tends to move ventrally and cranially, aided largely by diaphragmatic movement. PF, waste products, and foreign material exit the peritoneal cavity to enter the lymphatic system through diffusely distributed subendothelial pores or by way of the large diaphragmatic stomata, depending on particle size. Large molecules and particles greater than approximately 40,000 MW (such as bacteria) exit through the diaphragmatic stomata and ultimately enter the thoracic duct.

The term *peritonitis* refers to inflammation of the mesothelial lining of the peritoneal cavity.

ETIOPATHOGENESIS

Peritonitis can occur in association with any insult—mechanical, chemical, or infectious—that results in disruption or irritation of the peritoneal lining, inflammation or infection of abdominal organs, or compromise of the intestinal wall.[1-4] Common mechanical injuries include blunt or perforating trauma to the abdominal wall, breeding and foaling accidents, and abdominal surgery. A variety of iatrogenic insults can cause peritonitis, such as abdominocentesis, enterocentesis, splenic puncture, bowel trocharization, liver biopsy, uterine biopsy, castration, and rectal tear. Chemical insults of endogenous origin include blood, urine, pancreatic enzymes, bile, gastric juice, chyme, and chyle. Talc, contrast agents, antibiotics, and lavage solutions are additional examples of chemical insults. Traumatic events often involve bacterial contamination at the time of injury, and mechanical and chemical injuries can become infected secondarily.

The most common manifestation of peritonitis is acute, diffuse, septic peritonitis following inflammation, vascular insult, perforation, or surgical manipulation (e.g., enterotomy, resection, anastomosis) of the gastrointestinal tract. The septic process in such cases involves mixed bacteria of gastrointestinal origin. Penetrating abdominal wounds also result in mixed infections. Less commonly, singular bacterial forms gain access to the peritoneum through hematogenous spread or extension from a contiguous organ or through the female genital tract. Primary monomicrobial infections have been reported involving *Streptococcus equi* subsp. *equi*,[5,6] *S. equi* subsp. *zooepidemicus*,[7] *R. equi*,[6] and *Corynebacterium pseudotuberculosis*.[7,8] Several case series involving peritonitis associated with *Actinobacillus equuli* have been reported.[9-11] Initial reports of *A. equuli* peritonitis originated solely in Australia, but recent cases have been reported from the United States[12,13] and New Zealand.[14] Septicemia, septic omphalophlebitis, ascending urinary tract infections, and uterine infections are additional causes of monomicrobial infection.

Most cases of trauma or intestinal perforation result in contamination of the peritoneum with large numbers of many types of bacteria. The intestinal tract contains a mixed population of bacteria, and the quantity of bacteria and prevalence of anaerobic species increase in the distal segments. Not surprisingly, mortality associated with contamination from the lower bowel is high. Hirsch and Jang[15] reported isolation of an infective agent from exudative equine PF in approximately 25% of attempts. Obligate anaerobic bacteria were cultured most frequently, followed by members of the Enterobacteriaceae family (predominantly *Escherichia coli*). Penicillin-resistant *Bacteroides fragilis* was isolated between 10% to 20% of cases. In another study in which bacteria were identified in equine abdominal fluid by cytologic examination or culture, *E. coli* was the organism most commonly isolated.[16] In human beings and laboratory animals, despite the variety of organisms initially introduced by polymicrobial contamination, established infections are characterized by only a few types of bacteria, which are often gram negative aerobes and anaerobic bacteria.[3] This selectivity occurs through the processes of selective reduction of bacterial populations and bacterial synergism. An example of synergism in human beings and laboratory animals is peritonitis involving *E. coli* and *B. fragilus*. The presence of each organism is beneficial to the survival of the other, and each is important in the overall pathogenesis of the disease. *E. coli* is associated with septicemia and early mortality, whereas *B. fragilis* infection tends to result in chronic abscessation with delayed morbidity and mortality.[3]

Other causes of equine peritonitis include parasites, viral disorders (influenza, EVA, EIA, African horse sickness),[6] and neoplasia.[3,17] Verminous arteritis caused by strongylosis can lead to vascular damage (thromboembolism, infarction) to the intestine.[3] The activities of strongyles, ascarids, and tapeworms can result in perforation of the bowel and damage to other abdominal organs. There has been one report of septic peritonitis resulting from colonic perforation associated with aberrant migration of *Gastrophilus intestinalis* larvae.[18]

Biologic events resulting from contamination of the abdomen or injury to the mesothelial cells include release of catecholamines, histamine, and serotonin from peritoneal mast cells; vasodilation and hyperemia; increase in peritoneal vascular permeability; secretion of protein-rich fluid into the peritoneum; transformation of mesothelial cells into macrophages; and influx of polymorphonuclear cells, humoral opsonins, natural antibodies, and serum complement into the peritoneal cavity.[1-4] Other possible events include depression of the peritoneal fibrinolytic activity, fibrin deposits on the peritoneal surface, and inflammatory- and sympathetic-mediated ileus. These processes serve to confine contamination and infection and, with clean, minimally invasive procedures such as enterocentesis or trocharization, are effective. However, with greater severity of peritoneal contamination or irritation, these processes are magnified and become deleterious. Consequences include hypovolemia, hypoproteinemia, gastrointestinal ileus, ischemia of the bowel wall with subsequent absorption of bacteria and toxins, and ultimately adhesion and abscess formation. Equine peritoneal macrophages release a multitude of inflammatory mediators when exposed to bacterial LPS,[19] and endotoxemia contributes to the clinical picture. A complete review of endotoxemia is presented earlier in this chapter.

A complete pathologic description of peritonitis includes origin (primary or secondary), onset (peracute, acute, chronic), distribution (localized versus diffuse), and presence of bacteria (septic versus nonseptic).[1] Clinically, viewing the pathogenesis of peritonitis as a series of stages is useful.[3] The contamination stage, lasting 3 to 6 hours, involves introduction of bacteria into the peritoneum and initiation of the acute inflammatory response previously described. If the organisms are not eliminated, the process evolves to the stage of acute diffuse peritonitis as, regardless of the location of the initial contamination, bacteria spread throughout the peritoneum within several hours. The stage of acute diffuse peritonitis lasts up to 5 days. The inflammatory response persists and escalates with continued exudation of proteinaceous fluid and influx of inflammatory cells. Offending organisms are delivered to the lymphatic system and may be eliminated by the immune system. Alternatively, organisms can gain access to the systemic circulation in sufficient numbers to result in clinically relevant bacteremia. Following polymicrobial contamination of the peritoneum in human beings and laboratory animals, *E. coli* bacteremia commonly occurs.[20] This stage of the disease process is associated with the highest mortality rate because of the effects of severe peritoneal inflammation, endotoxemia, and sepsis. If the animal survives this stage but fails to eliminate infection from the peritoneal cavity, the disease enters a transitional phase referred to as the *acute adhesive* (or *localizing*) *stage,* which typically occurs 4 to 10 days after the initial insult. Neutrophils are still active, macrophages are increasing in numbers, and fibrin aggregates are being organized or lysed. If infection persists beyond this point, organization of fibrin proceeds and organisms become isolated from host defenses. At this point the disease process enters the stage of chronic abscessation. This stage can begin as early as 8 days after inoculation and persist indefinitely.

CLINICAL SIGNS

Clinical signs of peritonitis depend on the primary disease process, the duration of the problem, and the extent of peritoneal inflammation. Localized peritonitis may have few or no systemic manifestations, whereas severe localized or generalized peritonitis often is accompanied by severe toxemia, septicemia, or both. Septic peritonitis usually causes more severe clinical signs because of the systemic inflammatory response and endotoxemia. Most clinical signs are nonspecific and include fever, depression, inappetence, decreased borborygmi, and dehydration. Additional signs, reported in 30 horses (2 months to 16 years of age) with peritonitis, were colic, ileus, weight loss, and diarrhea.[5]

Horses with peracute peritonitis, as occurs with rupture of the bowel or rectal tear, have severe toxemia, weakness, depression or severe colic, tachycardia, tachypnea, and circulatory failure. Fever may not be present, depending on the degree of shock. Typical clinical findings include sweating, pawing, muscle fasciculations, weak peripheral pulses, red to purple mucous membranes, prolonged capillary refill time, and decreased skin elasticity. Parietal pain, characterized by reluctance to move, splinting of the abdominal wall, and sensitivity to external abdominal pressure, occurs in some acute cases. Urination or defecation may be painful for the horse; therefore urine and fecal retention may be evident on rectal examination. Palpation of the abdomen externally may elicit flinching, aversion movements, or groaning. With extensive abdominal fecal contamination, rectal examination may reveal grittiness of the serosal and parietal surface of the peritoneum because of fibrin deposition.

In horses with more chronic peritonitis, clinical signs include chronic or intermittent colic, depression, anorexia, weight loss, intermittent fever, ventral edema, exercise intolerance, decreased or absent intestinal sounds, and mild dehydration. Heart rate and respiratory rate may be normal. Fecal output may be normal; however, horses with chronic diarrhea and weight loss have been reported. Rectal examination findings may include pain on palpation of fibrinous or fibrous adhesions, intestinal impaction or distention following ileus and dehydration, an abdominal mass (abscess or neoplasia), or an impression of bowel floating in fluid. In many cases no abnormalities are evident on rectal examination.[5]

In cases of *A. equuli* peritonitis, clinical signs in most horses included depression, inappetence, lethargy, and mild to moderate abdominal pain acutely or weight loss in a chronic form.[9,10] Postpartum mares with peritonitis secondary to a uterine perforation typically exhibit fever and depression, with or without abdominal pain. Septic tenosynovitis of the tarsal sheath secondary to bacterial peritonitis resulting from gastrointestinal perforation was recently reported.[21] Foals with peritonitis usually exhibit signs of colic (acute or chronic) and are febrile, depressed, and inappetent. In young foals peritonitis can cause rapid metabolic deterioration, and determination and correction of the primary problem require immediate attention. In older foals peritonitis may occur insidiously in association with *S. equi* subsp. *equi* or *R. equi* infections.

CLINICOPATHOLOGIC FINDINGS

Hematology and Serum Chemistry

Clinicopathologic abnormalities vary depending on the time of onset and severity of peritonitis. In the acute stage of septic peritonitis, leukopenia, hemoconcentration, metabolic acidemia, and azotemia predominate. After several days leukocytosis and hyperfibrinogenemia are more typical. Plasma protein concentration varies depending on the hydration status, degree of exudation into the peritoneum, and type of underlying problem. In chronic peritonitis hyperproteinemia with hyperglobulinemia may be present. Though not widely available for clinical use, serum concentrations of amyloid A, an acute-phase protein, were significantly higher in horses with colic caused by inflammatory conditions, including peritonitis, compared with those that had colic caused by other conditions.[22] Neonates with uroperitoneum tend to develop azotemia, hyponatremia, hypochloremia, hyperkalemia, and acidemia. Foals with septic peritonitis in either the acute or chronic stage have clinicopathologic profiles similar to those of their adult cohorts.

Peritoneal Fluid

Abnormalities in the composition of PF occur with peritoneal inflammation, and PF analysis is principal to the diagnosis of peritonitis. Fluid should be collected in a tube containing EDTA for cytologic analysis, a sterile tube for culture, and a tube containing lithium heparin (or the anticoagulant preferred by the specific laboratory) for biochemical analysis. The clinician should evaluate PF routinely as to color, turbidity, total protein, white blood cell count and differential, and the presence of bacteria as determined by Gram stain. Normal PF is clear and straw-colored and does not coagulate spontaneously. PF becomes turbid when increased numbers of white blood cells and concentration of protein are present. Pink or red fluid indicates free hemoglobin or hemorrhage. Blood introduced into the PF iatrogenically in some cases may be differentiated from blood resulting from internal hemorrhage on the basis of the presence of platelets and hematocrit. Fluid with iatrogenic blood contamination contains platelets, whereas fluid with blood following internal hemorrhage or diapedesis often does not have platelets. Blood contamination resulting from splenic puncture often results in the packed cell volume of the sample being greater than that of the peripheral blood. Large volumes of dark brown or green fluid with a fetid odor, especially if obtained from several sites, strongly suggest bowel rupture. However, the clinician should perform cytologic examination to confirm rupture versus enterocentesis.

Because the concentration of polymorphonuclear and mononuclear cells in PF varies widely, results typically support a number of disorders rather than a specific diagnosis. Normal equine PF contains fewer than 5000 nucleated cells per microliter.[23] White blood cell counts in acute peritonitis (100,000/μL) are reported to be higher than those in chronic peritonitis (20,000 to 60,000/μL).[5,23,24] However, this is not always the case, and the white blood cell count depends most on the cause of the peritonitis and does not always correlate with disease severity or prognosis. The PF white blood cell count can be greater than 100,000/μL following enterocentesis, with no clinical signs or problem.[25] Conversely, peritoneal white blood cell counts of fewer than 100,000/μL may be found in foals or horses with intra-abdominal abscesses.[26] The peritoneal white blood cell count can increase to greater than 150,000/μL after celiotomy[27] and can be higher if an enterotomy is done. Postoperatively, the white blood cell count normally continues to decline and returns to near normal by 5 to 7 days. Failure of the white blood cell count to decrease suggests peritonitis resulting from a postoperative complication. Finally, PF white blood cell counts greater than 500,000/μL indicate severe focal or generalized peritoneal sepsis. The distribution of polymorphonuclear and mononuclear cells varies in normal PF, but polymorphonuclear cells usually predominate.[23] With acute peritonitis polymorphonuclear cells typically increase to a greater degree than mononuclear cells, but this depends on the cause. In horses with gastrointestinal disease and endotoxemia, the number of peritoneal mononuclear cells increases, as does transformation of mesothelial cells to macrophages. In chronic cases transforming mesothelial cells may be easily mistaken for neoplastic cells, which can make diagnosis difficult.

Normal PF protein concentration is less than 1.5 g/dl.[23] Protein concentrations between 1.5 g/dl and 2.5 g/dl can be difficult to interpret, but levels greater than 2.5 g/dl should be considered abnormally elevated. Fibrinogen concentration increases with inflammation, and levels greater than 10 mg/dl in the PF suggest an acute inflammatory process.[28] Fibrinogen content will also increase as a result of blood contamination.

The presence of free and phagocytosed bacteria in PF indicates generalized suppuration, abscessation, or compromised bowel. If numerous microorganisms of mixed types are observed free in the PF, especially in conjunction with plant material, bowel rupture likely has occurred. The presence of toxic or degenerate neutrophils and bacteria within polymorphonuclear cells helps distinguish PF from intestinal contents in such cases. Fluid obtained from enterocentesis is largely devoid of white blood cells but is discolored and contains mixed microorganisms and plant material. Bacterial contamination of a sample can occur during collection of the sample, and iatrogenic contamination of a sample can result in free and intracellular bacteria, particularly if processing is delayed. In such cases the bacterial numbers are few, and the neutrophils appear healthy. In some cases of gastrointestinal perforation, the luminal material, inflammatory cells, and protein may be sequestered by the omentum and further contained by fibrinous adhesions. Abdominal fluid obtained from standard ventral paracentesis may have low cellularity and protein content but large numbers of mixed bacteria, which indicates bowel rupture. Examples include gastric rupture along the greater curvature of the stomach between the omental layers (omental bursa) and perforated gastric or duodenal ulcers in foals. Correlating all cytologic findings with clinical and clinicopathologic findings is important for interpreting the results of PF cytologic examination.

Biochemical analysis of PF may be useful in detecting sepsis when cytologic examination and culture are negative or otherwise unavailable. In a prospective study PF pH and glucose concentrations from horses with septic peritonitis were significantly lower than those from horses with nonseptic peritonitis and healthy horses.[29] PF pH values below 7.3, glucose counts below 30 mg/dl, and fibrinogen concentration greater than 200 mg/dl were considered highly predictive of septic peritonitis. Serum to peritoneal glucose concentration differences of greater than 50 mg/dl were considered the most diagnostically useful test for septic peritonitis in the study. Although not validated in horses with peritonitis, PF lactate levels can be expected to increase as a result of septic peritonitis, and the blood to peritoneal lactate concentration difference may prove to have diagnostic significance. In a small study in dogs, a blood-to-fluid lactate difference equal to or less than 2.0 mmol/L was shown to be 100% sensitive and specific for a diagnosis of septic peritonitis.[30] Increased activities of alkaline phosphatase, lactic dehydrogenase, creatine kinase, aspartate aminotransferase, tumor necrosis factor, and interleukin-6 have been measured in the PF of horses with abdominal disorders, but the diagnostic and prognostic implications of the presence or absence of these enzymes and analytes is limited.[28,29,31]

One should submit PF samples in appropriate media (i.e., Port-A-Cul Vial, BBL Microbiology System) for aerobic and anaerobic cultures in an attempt to identify the pathogenic organism or organisms. Obligate anaerobic bacteria such as *Bacteroides* spp. are difficult to culture because the sample must be collected, transported, and cultured under strict anaerobic conditions. Frequently, bacterial cultures are negative when bacteria are present in PF. To enhance recovery of bacteria, one can inoculate PF into blood culture medium (i.e., Septi-Chek Columbia, Hoffmann-LaRoche Inc., Nutley, New Jersey), and if the horse has received antimicrobial treatment, one first should pass fluid through an antimicrobial removal device (i.e., A.R.D., Becton Dickinson & Co., Cockeysville, Md).

TREATMENT

Early and aggressive therapy is required if treatment of peritonitis is to be successful. The goals of treatment are to resolve the primary problem, minimize the inflammatory response, and prevent long-term complications. In the acute phase the clinician gives primary consideration to the arrest of endotoxic, septic, or hypovolemic shock; correction of metabolic and electrolyte abnormalities and dehydration; and management of pain. In the absence of blood gas and electrolyte determinations, adequate volumes of a balanced electrolyte solution are required to correct dehydration and support the cardiovascular system. If the plasma protein concentration of the horse is less than 4.0 g/dl, the clinician should consider administration of plasma or synthetic colloids.

Flunixin meglumine should be administered for its local and systemic anti-inflammatory effects. Dosages vary depending on the severity of peritonitis, degree of toxemia, severity of pain, and hydration status of the horse and range between 0.25 mg/kg intramuscularly or intravenously every 6 to 10 hours to 1.0 mg/kg intramuscularly or intravenously every 12 hours. The higher dosage provides greater visceral analgesia, whereas the lower dosage is effective in modifying the effects of experimental endotoxemia.[6,32] In addition to analgesic and general anti-inflammatory effect, flunixin meglumine may be effective in retarding adhesion formation.[33] Heparin therapy has been recommended to prevent adhesion formation and to render bacteria more susceptible to cellular and noncellular clearing mechanisms. In experimental models using laboratory animals, heparin therapy was associated with decreased adhesions in septic peritonitis.[34] In the horse information specifically related to peritonitis is lacking, but results following ischemia-reperfusion injury are mixed. One study demonstrated a decrease in adhesion formation with heparin therapy,[35] whereas another study showed no benefit in foals.[33] Low-molecular-weight heparin has been evaluated in horses and was shown to decrease the adverse effects associated with unfractionated heparin, including decreased packed cell volume and prolongation of activated partial thromboplastin time (aPTT) and thrombin time (TT).[36] Suggested dosages for unfractionated[35] and low-molecular-weight heparin have been described.[37]

The clinician should initiate antimicrobial therapy after making a diagnosis of peritonitis and before the results of peritoneal culture are available, because of the delay in obtaining results and the likelihood of a negative culture even in the face of peritoneal sepsis. Thus one should assume mixed infection with gram negative and gram positive aerobic and anaerobic bacteria. Intravenous administration of antimicrobials is preferred over oral or intramuscular routes in acute, diffuse, septic peritonitis because more reliable concentrations of drug are achieved in the tissues and PF than otherwise would be obtained in horses with hypovolemia or decreased intestinal motility.[38] The combination of a β-lactam antibiotic with an aminoglycoside, such as potassium penicillin (22,000 to 44,000 IU/kg intravenously every 6 hours) combined with gentamicin (6.6 mg/kg every 24 hours), is appropriate in most circumstances. Metronidazole (15-25 mg/kg orally every 12 hours) can be added to the regimen given the strong possibility of infection involving penicillin-resistant *B. fragilis*. One can modify this antimicrobial regimen when culture and antimicrobial sensitivity results become available. Peritonitis caused by *A. equuli* usually is manifested as a diffuse, suppurative peritoneal exudate.[10] These infections generally respond well to combination therapy with penicillin, either alone or in combination with gentamicin. Aminoglycosides and NSAIDs have the potential to induce acute renal tubular damage, particularly with concurrent dehydration and decreased renal perfusion. Therefore adequate restoration and maintenance of hydration and monitoring of renal function are important. Monitoring of white blood cell count, plasma fibrinogen, and abdominal fluid analysis often guide duration of therapy. Horses with abdominal abscessation resulting from monomicrobial infections typically require weeks to months of therapy, whereas polymicrobial infection may require many months of antibiotic treatment. Further details regarding principles of antimicrobial therapy are provided elsewhere in this text.

Abdominal drainage and lavage can help remove excess fluid, foreign materials, fibrin, and bacterial products from horses with peritonitis, and postoperative lavage decreases the incidence of experimentally induced abdominal adhesions.[39] Open surgical exploration provides the most effective and thorough examination of all peritoneal surfaces and is recommended if gastrointestinal perforation or ischemia is suspected or in any other case in which correction of a primary lesion is indicated. A ventral abdominal drain can be placed either at the time of surgery or in the standing horse with sedation and local anesthesia. Techniques have been described in detail elsewhere.[40,41]

Peritoneal lavage is typically performed with 10 to 20 L of a balanced isotonic electrolyte solution (such as lactated Ringer's solution or Normosol-R) twice a day for 3 to 5 days, until the lavage solution becomes clear, or until the catheter becomes clogged with fibrin or omentum. Hypertonic solutions are not recommended because they can result in fluid shifts into the peritoneum. The addition of povidone iodine to a balanced solution should also be avoided because concentrations as low as 3% can induce peritoneal inflammation.[42] Other agents, such as antibiotics or heparin, have been suggested as components of the lavage solution, but data demonstrating their benefit are not currently available. Active (or closed suction) abdominal drains have also been advocated, with benefits and potential complications similar to those of other methods.[41] Lavage with a plain isotonic solution did not alter the pharmacokinetics of gentamicin administered systemically.[43] Thus alteration of antimicrobial dosing does not appear necessary if lavage with plain solutions is part of the therapeutic regimen. Complications associated with the use of abdominal drains or repeated peritoneal drainage include retrograde infection, local irritation, pneumoperitoneum, and subcutaneous seepage around the drain with resultant cellulitis. If the patient is hypovolemic or hypoproteinemic, the clinician should consider volume replacement and administration of plasma or synthetic colloids before removing large quantities of fluid from the abdomen.

For horses with suspected parasitic involvement, the clinician should give larvicidal doses of an anthelmintic once the condition of the horse is stabilized. Ivermectin, moxidectin, fenbendazole, and thiabendazole have been recommended as larvacidal therapies.

The decision to perform surgery rather than treat medically is controversial in horses with peritonitis and should be made on a case-by-case basis. Although surgical exploration may allow diagnosis and resolution of the inciting cause and more thorough lavage of the abdomen, the risks of anesthesia, possible additional cost of surgery, and potential for a delayed return to performance may be significant. In a recent study of horses and foals with peritonitis, survival to discharge without surgery was associated with lack of signs of abdominal pain, normal or improved rectal temperature, normal or improved borborygmi, normal fecal production, no abnormal findings on rectal palpation, no nasogastric reflux, and yellow-orange PF.[44] A retrospective comparison of medical and surgical treatment of postpartum mares with peritonitis secondary to a uterine tear found no significant differences among admission variables, survival rate, hospital bill, duration of hospital stay, and likelihood to foal after discharge. A limitation of this study is the ability to definitively diganose a uterine tear in those mares treated medically; if a tear was not palpable, the diagnosis was based on exclusion of other causes.[45]

PROGNOSIS

The prognosis is grave for peritonitis associated with gastrointestinal rupture. Reported survival rates for horses with peritonitis vary but can be as high as 59.7%[16] to 78%.[44] In the study with a 78% overall survival rate, 68% of horses treated medically survived. Some of the variability in reported survival percentages can be related to inclusion criteria, mainly whether or not horses with gastrointestinal rupture were included. Septic peritonitis following abdominal surgery has been associated with high mortality (56%) in some studies,[16] whereas no difference in short-term survival was seen in another study.[46] Peritonitis associated with *A. equuli* carries a very favorable prognosis, and all horses in these reports responded to medical therapy if it was attempted.[9-11]

REFERENCES

Examination for Disorders of the Gastrointestinal Tract

1. Sellers A, Lowe J: Visualization of auscultation sounds of the large intestine, *Proceedings of the Annual Convention of the American Association of Equine Practitioners* 29:359-364, 1983.
2. Argenzio RA: Functions of the equine large intestine and their interrelationship in disease, *Cornell Vet* 65:303-330, 1975.
3. Adams SB: Equine intestinal motility: an overview of normal activity, changes in disease, and effects of drug administration, *Proc Am Assoc Equine Pract* 33:539-553, 1987.
4. Lester GD, Merritt AM, Neuwirth L, Vetro-Widenhouse T, Steible C, Rice B: Effect of alpha 2-adrenergic, cholinergic, and nonsteroidal anti-inflammatory drugs on myoelectric activity of ileum, cecum, and right ventral colon and on cecal emptying of radiolabeled markers in clinically normal ponies, *Am J Vet Res* 59:320-327, 1998.
5. Naylor JM, Poirier KL, Hamilton DL, Dowling PM: The effects of feeding and fasting on gastrointestinal sounds in adult horses, *J Vet Intern Med* 20:1408-1413, 2006.
6. Parry BW, Anderson GA, Gay CC: Prognosis in equine colic: a study of individual variables used in case assessment, *Equine Vet J* 15:337-344, 1983.
7. King JN, Gerring EL: Observations on the colic motor complex in a pony with a small intestinal obstruction, *Equine Vet J Suppl* :43-45, 1989.
8. Ragle CA, Meagher DM, Schrader JL, Honnas CM: Abdominal auscultation in the detection of experimentally induced gastrointestinal sand accumulation, *J Vet Intern Med* 3:12-14, 1989.
9. Adams SB, McIlwraith CW: Abdominal crisis in the horse: a comparison of presurgical evaluation with surgical findings and results, *Vet Surg* 7:63-69, 1978.
10. Blikslager AT, Roberts MC: Accuracy of clinicians in predicting site and type of lesion as well as outcome in horses with colic, *J Am Vet Med Assoc* 207:1444-1447, 1995.
11. Dopson LC, Reed SM, Roth JA, Perryman LE, Hitchcock P: Immunosuppression associated with lymphosarcoma in two horses, *J Am Vet Med Assoc* 182:1239-1241, 1983.
12. Patton S, Mock RE, Drudge JH, Morgan D: Increase of immunoglobulin T concentration in ponies as a response to experimental infection with the nematode Strongylus vulgaris, *Am J Vet Res* 39:19-23, 1978.
13. Feldman RG: The hemogram: a key to seeing beyond the signs of colic, *Vet Med* 83:935-938, 1988.
14. Poskitt TR, Poskitt PK: Thrombocytopenia of sepsis. The role of circulating IgG-containing immune complexes, *Arch Intern Med* 145:891-894, 1985.
15. Duncan SG, Meyers KM, Reed SM, Grant B: Alterations in coagulation and hemograms of horses given endotoxins for 24 hours via hepatic portal infusions, *Am J Vet Res* 46: 1287-1293, 1985.
16. Johnstone IB, Crane S: Hemostatic abnormalities in equine colic, *Am J Vet Res* 47:356-358, 1986.
17. Holland M, Kelly AB, Snyder JR, et al: Antithrombin III activity in horses with large colon torsion, *Am J Vet Res* 47:897-900, 1986.
18. Dart AJ, Snyder JR, Spier SJ, Sullivan KE: Ionized calcium concentration in horses with surgically managed gastrointestinal disease: 147 cases (1988-1990), *J Am Vet Med Assoc* 201:1244-1248, 1992.
19. Arden WA, Stick JA: Serum and peritoneal fluid phosphate concentrations as predictors of major intestinal injury associated with equine colic, *J Am Vet Med Assoc* 193:927-931, 1988.
20. Moore JN, Owen RR, Lumsden JH: Clinical evaluation of blood lactate levels in equine colic, *Equine Vet J* 8:49-54, 1976.
21. Gossett KA, Cleghorn B, Martin GS, Church GE: Correlation between anion gap, blood L lactate concentration and survival in horses, *Equine Vet J* 19:29-30, 1987.
22. Gossett KA, Cleghorn B, Adams R, et al: Contribution of whole blood L-lactate, pyruvate, D-lactate, acetoacetate, and 3-hydroxybutyrate concentrations to the plasma anion gap in horses with intestinal disorders, *Am J Vet Res* 48:72-75, 1987.
23. Gardner RB, Nydam DV, Mohammed HO, et al: Serum gamma glutamyl transferase activity in horses with right or left dorsal displacements of the large colon, *J Vet Intern Med* 19:761-764, 2005.
24. Andrews FM, Hamlin RL, Stalnaker PS: Blood viscosity in horses with colic, *J Vet Intern Med* 4:183-186, 1990.
25. Johnston JK, Morris DD: Comparison of duodenitis proximal jejunitis and small intestinal-obstruction in horses: 68 cases (1977-1985), *J Am Vet Med Assoc* 191:849-854, 1987.
26. Hunt E, Tennant B, Whitlock RH: Interpretation of peritoneal fluid erythrocyte counts in horses with abdominal disease, *Proc Equine Colic Res Symp* 2, 168-174, 1986.
27. Estepa JC, Lopez I, Mayer-Valor R, et al: The influence of anticoagulants on the measurement of total protein concentration in equine PF, *Res Vet Sci* 80:5-10, 2006.
28. Turner A, McIlwraith C, Trotter G, Wagner A: Biochemical analysis of serum and peritoneal fluid in experimental colonic infarction in horses, *Proceedings of the equine colic research symposium* 1984:79-87, September 28-30, 1982.
29. Latson KM, Nieto JE, Beldomenico PM, Snyder JR: Evaluation of peritoneal fluid lactate as a marker of intestinal ischaemia in equine colic, *Equine Vet J* 37:342-346, 2005.
30. Parry BW: Use of clinical pathology in evaluation of horses with colic, *Vet Clin N Am Equine Pract* 3:529-542, 1987.
31. Bach LG, Ricketts SW: Paracentesis as an aid to the diagnosis of abdominal disease in the horse, *Equine Vet J* 6:116-121, 1974.
32. Rumbaugh GE, Smith BP, Carlson GP: Internal abdominal abscesses in the horse: a study of 25 cases, *J Am Vet Med Assoc* 172:304-309, 1978.
33. Van Hoogmoed L, Rodger LD, Spier SJ, et al: Evaluation of peritoneal fluid pH, glucose concentration, and lactate dehydrogenase activity for detection of septic peritonitis in horses, *J Am Vet Med Assoc* 214:1032-1036, 1999.
34. Morris DD, Whitlock RH, Palmer JE: Fecal leukocytes and epithelial cells in horses with diarrhea, *Cornell Vet* 73:265-274, 1983.
35. Pearson EG, Smith BB, McKim JM: Fecal blood determinations and interpretations, *Proc Am Assoc Equine Pract* 33:77-81, 1987.
36. Wierup M, DiPietro JA: Bacteriologic examination of equine fecal flora as a diagnostic tool for equine intestinal clostridiosis, *Am J Vet Res* 42:2167-2169, 1981.
37. Palmer JE, Whitlock RH, Benson CE, et al: Comparison of rectal mucosal cultures and fecal cultures in detecting Salmonella infection in horses and cattle, *Am J Vet Res* 46:697-698, 1985.
38. Georgi JR: Antemortem diagnosis, In Georgi JR, Theodorides VJ, Georgi ME, editors: *Parasitology for veterinarians*, Philadelphia, 1985, pp 1-344, Saunders.
39. Alexander JE: Radiologic findings in equine choke, *J Am Vet Med Assoc* 151:47-53, 1967.
40. Greet TR: Observations on the potential role of oesophageal radiography in the horse, *Equine Vet J* 14:73-79, 1982.
41. King JN, Davies JV, Gerring EL: Contrast radiography of the equine oesophagus: effect of spasmolytic agents and passage of a nasogastric tube, *Equine Vet J* 22:133-135, 1990.
42. Yarbrough TB, Langer DL, Snyder JR, et al: Abdominal radiography for diagnosis of enterolithiasis in horses: 141 cases (1990-1992), *J Am Vet Med Assoc* 205:592-595, 1994.
43. Fischer AT: Advances in diagnostic techniques for horses with colic, *Vet Clin N Am-Equine Pract* 13:203-219, 1997.
44. Ruohoniemi M, Kaikkonen R, Raekallio M, Luukkanen L: Abdominal radiography in monitoring the resolution of sand accumulations from the large colon of horses treated medically, *Equine Vet J* 33:59-64, 2001.

45. Keppie NJ, Rosenstein DS, Holcombe SJ, Schott HC: Objective radiographic assessment of abdominal sand accumulation in horses, *Vet Radiol & Ultrasound* 49:122-128, 2008.
46. Cudd TA, Toal RL, Embertson RM: The use of clinical findings, abdominocentiesis, and abdominal radiographs in assessing surgical versus nonsurgical abdominal disease in the foal, *Proc Am Assoc Equine Pract* 33:41-53, 1987.
47. Lester GD, Lester NV: Abdominal and thoracic radiography in the neonate, *Vet Clin N Am Equine Pract* 17:19-46, 2001.
48. Campbell ML, Ackerman N, Peyton LC: Radiographic gastrointestinal anatomy of the foal, *Vet Radiol* 25:194-204, 1984.
49. Traub JL, Gallina AM, Grant BD, et al: Phenylbutazone toxicosis in the foal, *Am J Vet Res* 44:1410-1418, 1983.
50. Fischer AT, Yarbrough TY: Retrograde contrast radiography of the distal portions of the intestinal tract in foals, *J Am Vet Med Assoc* 207:734-737, 1995.
51. Fontaine GL, Hanson RR, Rodgerson DH, Steiger R: Ultrasound evaluation of equine gastrointestinal disorders, *Compendium on Continuing Education for the Practicing Veterinarian* 21:253-262, 1999.
52. Hillyer M: The use of ultrasonography in the diagnosis of abdominal tumours in the horse, *Equine Vet Educ* 6:273-278, 1994.
53. Klohnen A, Vachon AM, Fischer AT: Use of diagnostic ultrasonography in horses with signs of acute abdominal pain, *J Am Vet Med Assoc* 209:1597-1601, 1996.
54. Vachon AM, Fischer AT: Small intestinal herniation through the epiploic foramen: 53 cases (1987-1993), *Equine Vet J* 27:373-380, 1995.
55. Bernard WV, Reef VB, Reimer JM, et al: Ultrasonographic diagnosis of small-intestinal intussusception in three foals, *J Am Vet Med Assoc* 194:395-397, 1989.
56. Hendrickson EH, Malone ED, Sage AM: Identification of normal parameters for ultrasonographic examination of the equine large colon and cecum, *Can Vet J* 48:289-291, 2007.
57. Santschi EM, Slone DE Jr, Frank WM: Use of ultrasound in horses for diagnosis of left dorsal displacement of the large colon and monitoring its nonsurgical correction, *Vet Surg* 22:281-284, 1993.
58. Korolainen R, Ruohoniemi M: Reliability of ultrasonography compared to radiography in revealing intestinal sand accumulations in horses, *Equine Vet J* 34:499-504, 2002.
59. Mcgladdery AJ: Ultrasonographic diagnosis of intussusceptions in foals and yearlings, *Proc Am Assoc Equine Pract* 36:239-240, 1990.
60. Sasaki N, Murata A, Lee I, Yamada H: Evaluation of equine cecal motility by ausculation, ultrasonography and electrointestinography after jejunocecostomy, *Res Vet Sci* 84:305-310, 2008.
61. Butson RJ, Webbon PM, Fairbairn SM: 99Tcm-HMPAO labelled leucocytes and their biodistribution in the horse: a preliminary investigation, *Equine Vet J* 27:313-315, 1995.
62. Weller R, Cauvin ER, Bowen IM, May SA: Comparison of radiography, scintigraphy and ultrasonography in the diagnosis of a case of temporomandibular joint arthropathy in a horse, *Vet Rec* 144:377-379, 1999.
63. East LM, Trumble TN, Steyn PF, et al: The application of technetium-99m hexamethylpropyleneamine oxime (99mTc-HMPAO) labeled white blood cells for the diagnosis of right dorsal ulcerative colitis in two horses, *Vet Radiol Ultrasound* 41:360-364, 2000.
64. Lohmann KL, Roussel AJ, Cohen ND, et al: Comparison of nuclear scintigraphy and acetaminophen absorption as a means of studying gastric emptying in horses, *Am J Vet Res* 61:310-315, 2000.
65. Smallwood JE, Wood BC, Taylor WE, Tate LP Jr: Anatomic reference for computed tomography of the head of the foal, *Vet Radiol Ultrasound* 43:99-117, 2002.
66. Morrow KL, Park RD, Spurgeon TL, et al: Computed tomographic imaging of the equine head, *Vet Radiol Ultrasound* 41:491-497, 2000.
67. Tietje S, Becker M, Bockenhoff G: Computed tomographic evaluation of head diseases in the horse: 15 cases, *Equine Vet J* 28:98-105, 1996.
68. Tucker RL, Farrell E: Computed tomography and magnetic resonance imaging of the equine head, *Vet Clin N Am Equine Pract* 17:131-144, 2001.
69. Freeman DE, Ferrante PL, Kronfeld DS, Chalupa W: Effect of food deprivation on D-xylose absorption test results in mares, *Am J Vet Res* 50:1609-1612, 1989.
70. Mair TS, Hillyer MH, Taylor FG, Pearson GR: Small intestinal malabsorption in the horse: an assessment of the specificity of the oral glucose tolerance test, *Equine Vet J* 23:344-346, 1991.
71. Murphy D, Reid SW, Love S: The effect of age and diet on the oral glucose tolerance test in ponies, *Equine Vet J* 29:467-470, 1997.
72. Roberts MC: Small intestinal malabsorption in horses, *Equine Veterinary Education* 12:214-219, 2000.
73. Roberts MC, Norman P: A re-evaluation of the D (+) xylose absorption test in the horse, *Equine Vet J* 11:239-243, 1979.
74. Roberts MC: Carbohydrate digestion and absorption studies in the horse, *Res Vet Sci* 18:64-69, 1975.
75. Baker SJ, Gerring EL: Gastric emptying of solid, nondigestible, radiopaque markers in ponies, *Res Vet Sci* 56:386-388, 1994.
76. Sutton DG, Bahr A, Preston T, et al: Validation of the 13C-octanoic acid breath test for measurement of equine gastric emptying rate of solids using radioscintigraphy, *Equine Vet J* 35:27-33, 2003.
77. Lohmann KL, Bahr A, Cohen ND, et al: Evaluation of acetaminophen absorption in horses with experimentally induced delayed gastric emptying, *Am J Vet Res* 63:170-174, 2002.
78. Doherty TJ, Andrews FM, Provenza MK, Frazier DL: Acetaminophen as a marker of gastric emptying in ponies, *Equine Vet J* 30:349-351, 1998.
79. Clements JA, Heading RC, Nimmo WS, Prescott LF: Kinetics of acetaminophen absorption and gastric emptying in man, *Clin PharmacolTher* 24:420-431, 1978.
80. Wyse CA, Murphy DM, Preston T, et al: The(13)C-octanoic acid breath test for detection of effects of meal composition on the rate of solid-phase gastric emptying in ponies, *Res Vet Sci* 71:81-83, 2001.
81. Trostle S: Gastrointestinal endoscopic surgery, *Vet Clin N Am Equine Pract* 16:329-341, 2000.
82. Hendrickson DA, Wilson DG: Instrumentation and techniques for laparoscopic and thoracoscopic surgery in the horse, *Vet Clin North Am Equine Pract* 12:235-259, 1996.

Pathophysiology of Gastrointestinal Inflammation

1. Kagnoff MF, Eckmann L: Epithelial cells as sensors for microbial infection, *J Clin Invest* 100:6-XXX, 1997.
2. Harada A, Sekido N, Akahoshi T, et al: Essential involvement of interleukin-8 (IL-8) in acute inflammation, *J Leukoc Biol* 56:559-XXX, 1994.
3. Huber AR, Kunkel SL, Todd RF III, et al: Regulation of transendothelial neutrophil migration by endogenous interleukin-8, *Science* 254, 1991:99-XXX, 1991.
4. Ina K, Kusugami K, Yamaguchi T, et al: Mucosal interleukin-8 is involved in neutrophil migration and binding to extracellular matrix in inflammatory bowel disease, *Am J Gastroenterol* 92:1342-XXX, 1997.
5. McCormick BA, Colgan SP, lp-Archer CP, et al: Salmonella typhimurium attachment to human intestinal epithelial monolayers: transcellular signalling to subepithelial neutrophils, *J Cell Biol* 123:895-XXX, 1993.
6. McCormick BA, Miller SI, Carnes D, et al: Transepithelial signaling to neutrophils by salmonellae: a novel virulence mechanism for gastroenteritis, *Infection & Immunity* 63:2302-XXX, 1995.

7. Jung HC, Eckmann L, Yang SK, et al: A distinct array of proinflammatory cytokines is expressed in human colon epithelial cells in response to bacterial invasion, *J Clin Invest* 95:55-XXX, 1995.
8. Akira S: Toll-like receptors and innate immunity, *Adv Immunol* 78:1-XXX, 2001.
9. Malaviya R, Abraham SN: Mast cell modulation of immune responses to bacteria, *Immunol Rev* 179:16-24, 2001:16-XXX, 2001.
10. Pothoulakis CI, Castagliuolo JT, LaMont A, et al: CP-96,345, a substance P antagonist, inhibits rat intestinal responses to Clostridium difficile toxin A but not cholera toxin, 1994, *Proceedings of the National Academy of Sciences of the United States of America*, 91:947-XXX.
11. Castagliuolo I, LaMont JT, Letourneau R, et al: Neuronal involvement in the intestinal effects of Clostridium difficile toxin A and Vibrio cholerae enterotoxin in rat ileum. [see comments], *Gastroenterology* 107:657-XXX, 1994.
12. Bogdan C, Rollinghoff M, Diefenbach A: Reactive oxygen and reactive nitrogen intermediates in innate and specific immunity, *Curr Opin Immunol* 12:64-XXX, 2000.
13. Blikslager AT, Moeser AJ, Gookin JL, et al: Restoration of barrier function in injured intestinal mucosa, *Physiol Rev* 87:545-XXX, 2007.
14. Joris I, Cuenoud HF, Doern GV, et al: Capillary leakage in inflammation. A study by vascular labeling, *Am J Pathol* 137:1353-XXX, 1990.
15. Joris I, Majno G, Corey EJ, et al: The mechanism of vascular leakage induced by leukotriene E4. Endothelial contraction, *Am J Pathol* 126:19-XXX, 1987.
16. Brett J, Gerlach H, NawrothP, et al: Tumor necrosis factor/cachectin increases permeability of endothelial cell monolayers by a mechanism involving regulatory G proteins, *J Exp Med* 169:1977-XXX, 1989.
17. Springer TA: Traffic signals for lymphocyte recirculation and leukocyte emigration: the multistep paradigm, *Cell* 76:301-XXX, 1994.
18. Hernandez LA, Grisham MB, Twohig B, et al: Role of neutrophils in ischemia-reperfusion-induced microvascular injury, *Am J Physiol* 253:H699-H703, 1987.
19. Rosengren S, Olofsson AM, von Andrian UH, et al: Leukotriene B4-induced neutrophil-mediated endothelial leakage in vitro and in vivo, *J Appl Physiol* 71:1322-XXX, 1991.
20. Harlan JM, Killen PD, Harker LA, et al: Neutrophil-mediated endothelial injury in vitro mechanisms of cell detachment, *J Clin Invest* 68:1394-XXX, 1981.
21. Coe DA, Freischlag JA, Johnson D, et al: Pentoxifylline prevents endothelial damage due to ischemia and reperfusion injury, *J Surg Res* 67:21-XXX, 1997.
22. Nakagawa K, Miller FN, Knott AW, et al: Pentoxifylline inhibits FMLP-induced macromolecular leakage, *Am J Physiol* 269:H239-H245, 1995.
23. Nathan C: Neutrophils and immunity: challenges and opportunities, *Nat Rev Immunol* 6:173–XXX, 2006.
24. Dallegri F, Ottonello L: Tissue injury in neutrophilic inflammation, *Inflamm Res* 46:382–XXX, 1997.
25. Kubes P, Hunter J, Granger DN: Ischemia/reperfusion-induced feline intestinal dysfunction: importance of granulocyte recruitment, *Gastroenterology* 103:807–XXX, 1992.
26. Kelly CP, Becker S, Linevsky JK, et al: Neutrophil recruitment in Clostridium difficile toxin A enteritis in the rabbit, *J Clin Invest* 93:1257, 1994.
27. Giannella RA: Importance of the intestinal inflammatory reaction in salmonella- mediated intestinal secretion, *Infect Immun* 23:140-XXX, 1979.
28. Elliott E, Li Z, Bell C, et al: Modulation of host response to Escherichia coli o157:H7 infection by anti-CD18 antibody in rabbits, *Gastroenterology* 106:1554-XXX, 1994.
29. Wallace JL, Keenan CM, Granger DN: Gastric ulceration induced by nonsteroidal anti-inflammatory drugs is a neutrophil-dependent process, *Am J Physiol* 259:G462-G467, 1990.
30. Ley K, Tedder TF: Leukocyte interactions with vascular endothelium. New insights into selectin-mediated attachment and rolling, *J Immunol* 155:525-XXX, 1995.
31. Brown EJ, Lindberg FP: Leucocyte adhesion molecules in host defence against infection, *Ann Med* 28:201-XXX, 1996.
32. Nagahata H, Kehrli ME Jr, Murata H, et al: Neurtrophil function and pathologic findings in Holstein calves with leukocyte adhesion deficiency, *Am J Vet Res* 55:40-XXX, 1994.
33. Anderson DC, Springer TA: Leukocyte adhesion deficiency: an inherited defect in the Mac-1, LFA-1, and p150,95 glycoproteins, *Ann Rev Med* 38:175-194, 1987.
34. Issekutz AC, Issekutz TB: Monocyte migration to arthritis in the rat utilizes both CD11/CD18 and very late activation antigen 4 integrin mechanisms, *J Exp Med* 181:1197-XXX, 1995.
35. Shuster DE, Kehrli ME Jr, Ackermann MR: Neutrophilia in mice that lack the murine IL-8 receptor homolog, *Science* 269:1590-XXX, 1995.
36. Huang AJ, Furie MB, Nicholson SC, et al: Effects of human neutrophil chemotaxis across human endothelial cell monolayers on the permeability of these monolayers to ions and macromolecules, *J Cell Physiol* 135:355-XXX, 1988.
37. Berton G, Yan SR, Fumagalli L, et al: Neutrophil activation by adhesion: mechanisms and pathophysiological implications, *Int J Clin Lab Res* 26:160-XXX, 1996.
38. Rosales C, Juliano RL: Signal transduction by cell adhesion receptors in leukocytes, *J Leukoc Biol* 57:189-XXX, 1995.
39. Wershil BK: IX. Mast cell-deficient mice and intestinal biology, *Am J Physiol Gastrointest Liver Physiol* 278:G343-G348, 2000.
40. Araki Y, Andoh A, Fujiyama Y, et al: Development of dextran sulphate sodium-induced experimental colitis is suppressed in genetically mast cell-deficient Ws/Ws rats, *Clin Exp Immunol* 119:264-XXX, 2000.
41. Stein J, Ries J, Barrett KE: Disruption of intestinal barrier function associated with experimental colitis: possible role of mast cells, *Am J Physiol* 274:G203-G209, 1998.
42. Andoh A, Kimura T, Fukuda M, et al: Rapid intestinal ischaemia-reperfusion injury is suppressed in genetically mast cell-deficient Ws/Ws rats, *Clin Exp Immunol* 116:90-XXX, 1999.
43. Kimura T, Fujiyama Y, Sasaki M, et al: The role of mucosal mast cell degranulation and free-radical generation in intestinal ischaemia-reperfusion injury in rats, *Eur J Gastroenterol Hepatol* 10:659-XXX, 1998.
44. Yang PC, Berin MC, Yu L, et al: Mucosal pathophysiology and inflammatory changes in the late phase of the intestinal allergic reaction in the rat, *Am J Pathol* 158:681–XXX, 2001.
45. Galli SJ, Maurer M, Lantz CS: Mast cells as sentinels of innate immunity, *Curr Opin Immunol* 11:53-XXX, 1999.
46. Castro GA, Harari Y, Russell D: Mediators of anaphylaxis-induced ion transport changes in small intestine, *Am J Physiol* 253:G540-G548, 1987.
47. Metcalfe DD, Baram D, Mekori YA: Mast cells, *Physiol Rev* 77:1033-XXX, 1997.
48. Kawabata A, Matsunami M, Sekiguchi F: Gastrointestinal roles for proteinase-activated receptors in health and disease, *Br J Pharmacol* 153(Suppl 1):S230-S240, 2008:Epub; 2007 Nov 12: S230-S240.
49. Bueno L, Fioramonti J: Protease-activated receptor 2 and gut permeability: a review, *Neurogastroenterol Motil* 20:580-XXX, 2008.
50. Malaviya R, Ikeda T, Ross E, et al: Mast cell modulation of neutrophil influx and bacterial clearance at sites of infection through TNF-alpha, *Nature* 381, 1996:77-XXX, 1996.
51. Malaviya R, Abraham SN: Role of mast cell leukotrienes in neutrophil recruitment and bacterial clearance in infectious peritonitis, *J Leukoc Biol* 67:841-XXX, 2000.

52. McLachlan JB, Shelburne CP, Hart JP, et al: Mast cell activators: a new class of highly effective vaccine adjuvants, *Nat Med* 14:536-XXX, 2008.
53. Gallin JI, Goldstein IM, Snyderman R, editors: *Inflammation: basic principles and clinical correlates*, New York, 2008, Raven Press.
54. Brown EJ: Complement receptors and phagocytosis, *Curr Opin Immunol* 3:76-XXX, 1991.
55. Williams JP, Pechet TT, Weiser MR, et al: Intestinal reperfusion injury is mediated by IgM and complement, *J Appl Physiol* 86:938-XXX, 1999.
56. Wada K, Montalto MC, Stahl GL: Inhibition of complement C5 reduces local and remote organ injury after intestinal ischemia/reperfusion in the rat, *Gastroenterology* 120:126-XXX, 2001.
57. Eror AT, Stojadinovic A, Starnes BW, et al: Antiinflammatory effects of soluble complement receptor type 1 promote rapid recovery of ischemia/reperfusion injury in rat small intestine, *Clin Immunol* 90:266-XXX, 1999.
58. Austen WG Jr, Kyriakides C, Favuzza J, et al: Intestinal ischemia-reperfusion injury is mediated by the membrane attack complex, *Surgery* 126:343-XXX, 1999.
59. Cochrane CG, Griffin JH: The biochemistry and pathophysiology of the contact system of plasma, *Adv Immunol* 33:241-306, 1982.
60. Bockmann S, Paegelow I: Kinins and kinin receptors: importance for the activation of leukocytes, *J Leukoc Biol* 68:587-XXX, 2000.
61. Stadnicki A, Sartor RB, Janardham R, et al: Kallikrein-kininogen system activation and bradykinin (B2) receptors in indomethacin induced enterocolitis in genetically susceptible Lewis rats, *Gut* 43:365-XXX, 1998.
62. Stadnicki A, Sartor RB, Janardham R, et al: Specific inhibition of plasma kallikrein modulates chronic granulomatous intestinal and systemic inflammation in genetically susceptible rats, *FASEB J* 12:325-XXX, 1998.
63. Arai Y, Takanashi H, Kitagawa H, et al: Effect of icatibant, a bradykinin B2 receptor antagonist, on the development of experimental ulcerative colitis in mice, *Dig Dis Sci* 44:845-XXX, 1999.
64. Thiagarajan RR, Winn RK, Harlan JM: The role of leukocyte and endothelial adhesion molecules in ischemia-reperfusion injury, *Thromb Haemost* 78:310-XXX, 1997.
65. Mashimo H, Goyal RK: Lessons from genetically engineered animal models. IV. Nitric oxide synthase gene knockout mice, *Am J Physiol* 277:G745-G750, 1999.
66. Giannella RA, Drake KW: Effect of purified Escherichia coli heat-stable enterotoxin on intestinal cyclic nucleotide metabolism and fluid secretion, *Infect Immun* 24:19-XXX, 1979.
67. Brown E: Neutrophil adhesion and the therapy of inflammation, *Semin Hematol* 34:319-XXX, 1997.
68. Edens HA, Parkos CA: Modulation of epithelial and endothelial paracellular permeability by leukocytes, *Adv Drug Deliv Rev* 41:315-XXX, 2000.
69. Suzuki M, Asako H, Kubes P, et al: Neutrophil-derived oxidants promote leukocyte adherence in postcapillary venules, *Microvasc Res* 42:125-XXX, 1991.
70. Scudamore CL, Thornton EM, McMillan L, et al: Release of the mucosal mast cell granule chymase, rat mast cell protease-II, during anaphylaxis is associated with the rapid development of paracellular permeability to macromolecules in rat jejunum, *J Exp Med* 182:1871-XXX, 1995.
71. Scudamore CL, Jepson MA, Hirst BH, et al: The rat mucosal mast cell chymase, RMCP-II, alters epithelial cell monolayer permeability in association with altered distribution of the tight junction proteins ZO-1 and occludin, *Eur J Cell Biol* 75:321-XXX, 1998.
72. Colgan SP, Resnick MB, Parkos CA, et al: IL-4 directly modulates function of a model human intestinal epithelium, *J Immunol* 153:2122-XXX, 1994.
73. Mullin JM, Snock KV: Effect of tumor necrosis factor on epithelial tight junctions and transepithelial permeability, *Cancer Res* 50:2172-XXX, 1990.

Pathophysiology of Diarrhea

1. White NA: *The equine acute abdomen*, Philadelphia, 1990, Lea & Febiger.
2. Graham R, Hill FHD, Hill JF: Bacteriologic studies of a peracute disorder of horses and mules, *J Am Vet Med Assoc* 56:378-597, 1919.
3. Whitlock RH: Colitis: differential diagnosis and treatment, *Equine Vet J* 18:278-283, 1986.
4. Merritt AM, Bolton JR, Cimprich R: Differential diagnosis of diarrhoea in horses over six months of age, *J S Afr Vet Assoc* 46:73-76, 1975.
5. Johnson CM, Cullen JM, Roberts MC: Morphologic characterization of castor oil-induced colitis in ponies, *Vet Pathol* 30:248-255, 1993.
6. Roberts MC, Clarke LL, Johnson CM: Castor-oil induced diarrhoea in ponies: a model for acute colitis, *Equine Vet J Suppl* : 60-67, 1989.
7. Rikihisa Y, Johnson GC, Wang YZ, et al: Loss of absorptive-capacity for sodium and chloride in the colon causes diarrhea in Potomac horse fever, *Res Vet Sci* 52:353-362, 1992.
8. Cordes DO, Perry BD, Rikihisa Y, Chickering WR: Enterocolitis caused by Ehrlichia Sp. in the horse (Potomac horse fever), *Vet Patho* 23:471-477, 1986.
9. Umemura T, Ohishi H, Ikemoto Y, et al: Histopathology of colitis X in the horse, *Nippon Juigaku Zasshi* 44:717-724, 1982.
10. Ochoa R, Kern SR: The effects of Clostridium perfringens type A enterotoxin in Shetland ponies: clinical, morphologic and clinicopathologic changes, *Vet Pathol* 17:738-747, 1980.
11. Lees P, Higgins AJ: Effects of a phenylbutazone paste in ponies: model of acute nonimmune inflammation, *Am J Vet Res* 47:2359-2363, 1986.
12. Keshavarzian A, Morgan G, Sedghi S, Gordon JH, Doria M: Role of reactive oxygen metabolites in experimental colitis, *Gut* 31:786-790, 1990.
13. Weiss SJ: Tissue destruction by neutrophils, *N Engl J Med* 320:365-376, 1989.
14. Rooney JR, Bryans JT, Prickett ME, Zent WW: Exhaustion shock in the horse, *Cornell Vet* 56:220-235, 1966.
15. Meschter CL, Tyler DE, White NA, Moore J: Histologic findings in the gastrointestinal tract of horses with colic, *Am J Vet Res* 47:598-606, 1986.
16. Guerrant RL, Bobak DA: Bacterial and protozoal gastroenteritis, *N Engl J Med* 325:327-340, 1991.
17. Argenzio RA: Pathophysiology of diarrhea. In Anderson NV, editor: *Veterinary gatroenterology*, Philadelphia, 1992, Lea & Febiger.
18. Field M, Rao MC, Chang EB: Intestinal electrolyte transport and diarrheal disease (2), *N Engl J Med* 321:879-883, 1989.
19. Field M, Rao MC, Chang EB: Intestinal electrolyte transport and diarrheal disease (1), *N Engl J Med* 321:800-806, 1989.
20. Musch MW, Kachur JF, Miller RJ, Field M, Stoff JS: Bradykinin-stimulated electrolyte secretion in rabbit and guinea pig intestine. Involvement of arachidonic acid metabolites, *J Clin Invest* 71:1073-1083, 1983.
21. Perdue MH, McKay DM: Integrative immunophysiology in the intestinal mucosa, *Am J Physiol* 267:G151-G165, 1994.
22. Field M, Frizzell RA, Powell DW: *Handbook of physiology: the gastrointestinal system*, Rockville, Md, 1991, American Physiology Society.
23. Argenzio RA: Physiology of diarrhea—large intestine, *J Am Vet Med Assoc* 173:667-672, 1978.

24. Field M, Graf LH Jr, Laird WJ, Smith PL: Heat-stable enterotoxin of Escherichia coli: in vitro effects on guanylate cyclase activity, cyclic GMP concentration, and ion transport in small intestine, *Proc Natl Acad Sci USA* 75:2800-2804, 1978.
25. Mantyh CR, Pappas TN, Lapp JA, et al: Substance P activation of enteric neurons in response to intraluminal Clostridium difficile toxin A in the rat ileum, *Gastroenterology* 111: 1272-1280, 1996.
26. Wasserman SI, Barrett KE, Huott PA, et al: Immune-related intestinal Cl- secretion. I. Effect of histamine on the T84 cell line, *Am J Physiol* 254:C53-C62, 1988.
27. Barrett KE, Cohn JA, Huott PA, et al: Immune-related intestinal chloride secretion. II. Effect of adenosine on T84 cell line, *Am J Physiol* 258:C902–C912, 1990.
28. Racusen LC, Binder HJ: Effect of prostaglandin on ion transport across isolated colonic mucosa, *Dig Dis Sci* 25:900-904, 1980.
29. Weymer A, Huott P, Liu W, McRoberts JA, Dharmsathaphorn K: Chloride secretory mechanism induced by prostaglandin E_1 in a colonic epithelial cell line, *J Clin Invest* 76:1828-1836, 1985.
30. Jett MF, Marshall P, Fondacaro JD, Smith PL: Action of peptidoleukotrienes on ion transport in rabbit distal colon in vitro, *J Pharmacol Exp Ther* 257:698-705, 1991.
31. Hanglow AC, Bienenstock J, Perdue MH: Effects of platelet-activating factor on ion transport in isolated rat jejunum, *Am J Physiol* 257:G845-G850, 1989.
32. Chang EB, Musch MW, Mayer L: Interleukins 1 and 3 stimulate anion secretion in chicken intestine, *Gastroenterology* 98: 1518-1524, 1990.
33. Grisham MB, Gaginella TS, von Ritter C, Tamai H, Be RM, Granger DN: Effects of neutrophil-derived oxidants on intestinal permeability, electrolyte transport, and epithelial cell viability, *Inflammation* 14:531-542, 1990.
34. Berschneider HM, Powell DW: Fibroblasts modulate intestinal secretory responses to inflammatory mediators, *J Clin Invest* 89:484-489, 1992.
35. Tamai H, Kachur JF, Baron DA, Grisham MB, Gaginella TS: Monochloramine, a neutrophil-derived oxidant, stimulates rat colonic secretion, *J Pharmacol Exp Ther* 257:887-894, 1991.
36. Tamai H, Gaginella TS, Kachur JF, Musch MW, Chang EB: Ca-mediated stimulation of Cl secretion by reactive oxygen metabolites in human colonic T84 cells, *J Clin Invest* 89:301-307, 1992.
37. Wilson KT, Xie Y, Musch MW, Chang EB: Sodium nitroprusside stimulates anion secretion and inhibits sodium chloride absorption in rat colon, *J Pharmacol Exp Ther* 266:224-230, 1993.
38. Crowe SE, Sestini P, Perdue MH: Allergic reactions of rat jejunal mucosa. Ion transport responses to luminal antigen and inflammatory mediators, *Gastroenterology* 99:74-82, 1990.
39. Frizzell RA, Koch MJ, Schultz SG: Ion transport by rabbit colon. I. Active and passive components, *J Membr Biol* 27:297-316, 1976.
40. Donowitz M, Welsh MJ: Regulation of mammalian small intestinal electrolyte secretion. In Johnson LR, editor: *Physiology of the gastrointestinal tract*, New York, 1987, Raven Press.
41. Ciancio MJ, Vitiritti L, Dhar A, Chang EB: Endotoxin-induced alterations in rat colonic water and electrolyte transport, *Gastroenterology* 103:1437-1443, 1992.
42. Donowitz M, Asarkof N, Pike G: Calcium dependence of serotonin-induced changes in rabbit ileal electrolyte transport, *J Clin Invest* 66:341-352, 1980.
43. Madara JL, Stafford J: Interferon-gamma directly affects barrier function of cultured intestinal epithelial monolayers, *J Clin Invest* 83:724-727, 1989.
44. Hinterleitner TA, Berschneider HM, Powell DS: Fibroblast-mediated Cl secretion by T84 cells is amplified by interleukin-1beta, *Gastroenterology* 100:A90, 1991.
45. Hardcastle J, Hardcastle PT: The secretory actions of histamine in rat small intestine, *J Physiol* 388:521-532, 1987.
46. Tien XY, Wallace LJ, Kachur JF, et al: Characterization of Ile, Ser-bradykinin-induced changes in short-circuit current across rat colon, *J Pharmacol Exp Ther* 254:1063-1067, 1990.
47. Warhurst G, Lees M, Higgs NB, Turnberg LA: Site and mechanisms of action of kinins in rat ileal mucosa, *Am J Physiol* 252:G293-G300, 1987.
48. Klebanoff SJ: Phagocytic cells: products of oxygen metabolism. In Gallin JI, Goldstein IM, editors: *Inflammation: basic principles and clinical correlates*, New York, 1988, Raven Press.
49. Powell DW: Epithelial secretory responses to inflammation. Platelet activating factor and reactive oxygen metabolites, *Ann N Y Acad Sci* 664:232-247, 1992, Perth, Western Australia.
50. Field M, Musch MW, Miller RL, Goetzl EJ: Regulation of epithelial electrolyte transport by metabolites of arachidonic acid, *J Allergy Clin Immunol* 74:382-385, 1984.
51. Kubes P, Suzuki M, Granger DN: Modulation of PAF-induced leukocyte adherence and increased microvascular permeability, *Am J Physiol* 259:G859-G864, 1990.
52. Perdue MH, Masson S, Wershil BK, Galli SJ: Role of mast cells in ion transport abnormalities associated with intestinal anaphylaxis. Correction of the diminished secretory response in genetically mast cell-deficient W/Wv mice by bone marrow transplantation, *J Clin Invest* 87:687-693, 1991.
53. Verspaget HW, Mulder TP, van dS V, Pena AS, Lamers CB: Reactive oxygen metabolites and colitis: a disturbed balance between damage and protection. A selective review, *Scand J Gastroenterol Suppl* 188:44-51, 1991.
54. Buell MG, Berin MC: Neutrophil-independence of the initiation of colonic injury. Comparison of results from three models of experimental colitis in the rat, *Dig Dis Sci* 39:2575-2588, 1994.
55. Kubes P, Hunter J, Granger DN: Ischemia/reperfusion-induced feline intestinal dysfunction: importance of granulocyte recruitment, *Gastroenterology* 103:807-812, 1992.
56. Petrone WF, English DK, Wong K, McCord JM: Free radicals and inflammation: superoxide-dependent activation of a neutrophil chemotactic factor in plasma, *Proc Natl Acad Sci U S A* 77:1159-1163, 1980.
57. Granger RN, Rutili G: Neutrophil-mediated mucosal injury: role of reactive oxygen metabolites, *Dig Dis Sci* 33:6S-15S, 1988.
58. Miller MJ, Zhang XJ, Barkemeyer B, et al: Rabbit gut permeability in response to histamine chloramines and chemotactic peptide, *Gastroenterology* 103:1537-1546, 1992.
59. Krawisz JE, Sharon P, Stenson WF: Quantitative assay for acute intestinal inflammation based on myeloperoxidase activity. Assessment of inflammation in rat and hamster models, *Gastroenterology* 87:1344-1350, 1984.
60. Wardle TD, Hall L, Turnberg LA: Inter-relationships between inflammatory mediators released from colonic mucosa in ulcerative colitis and their effects on colonic secretion, *Gut* 34:503-508, 1993.
61. McConnico RS, Roberts MC, Poston MB: The interrelationship between arachidonic acid and reactive oxygen metabolites with neutrophilic infiltration in the large intestine in a pony model of acute colitis, *Proc ACVIM Forum* 12:A1016, 1994.
62. Grisham MB, Benoit JN, Granger DN: Assessment of leukocyte involvement during ischemia and reperfusion of intestine, *Methods Enzymol* 186:729-742, 1990.
63. Moore JN, Morris DD: Endotoxemia and septicemia in horses: experimental and clinical correlates, *J Am Vet Med Assoc* 200:1903-1914, 1992.
64. Hinterleitner TA, Powell DW: Immune system control of intestinal ion transport, *Proc Soc Exp Biol Med* 197:249-260, 1991.
65. Karayalcin SS, Sturbaum CW, Wachsman JT, et al: Hydrogen peroxide stimulates rat colonic prostaglandin production and alters electrolyte transport, *J Clin Invest* 86:60-68, 1990.

66. Bern MJ, Sturbaum CW, Karayalcin SS, Berschneider HM, Wachsman JT, Powell DW: Immune system control of rat and rabbit colonic electrolyte transport. Role of prostaglandins and enteric nervous system, *J Clin Invest* 83:1810-1820, 1989.
67. Clarke LL, Argenzio RA: NaCl transport across equine proximal colon and the effect of endogenous prostanoids, *Am J Physiol* 259:G62-G69, 1990.
68. van Deventer SJ, ten Cate JW, Tytgat GN: Intestinal endotoxemia. Clinical significance, *Gastroenterology* 94:825-831, 1988.
69. Carroll EJ, Schalm OW, Wheat JD: Endotomemia in a horse, *J Am Vet Med Assoc* 146:1300-1303, 1965.
70. Schmall LM, Argenzio RA, Whipp SC: Effects of intravenous Escherichia coli endotoxin on gastrointestinal function in the pony, *Proc Equine Colic Res Symp* 1:157-164, 1982.
71. Hinshaw LB: Application of animal shock models to the human, *Circ Shock* 17:205-212, 1985.
72. Deitch EA, Xu DZ, Qi L, et al: Protein malnutrition alone and in combination with endotoxin impairs systemic and gut-associated immunity, *JPEN J Parenter Enteral Nutr* 16:25-31, 1992.
73. Eades SC, Moore JN: Blockade of endotoxin-induced cecal hypoperfusion and ileus with an alpha 2 antagonist in horses, *Am J Vet Res* 54:586-590, 1993.
74. Katz AJ, Rosen FS. Gastro intestinal complications of immuno deficiency syndromes. Porter, Ruth and Julie Knight (Ed.).Ciba Foundation Symposium, Vol 46 Immunology of the Gut. London, England, April 26-28, 1976. Viii+376P.Illus.Elsevier/Excerpta Medica/North-Holland: Amsterdam, Netherlands; Elsevier-North-Holland, Inc: New York, 1977; 243-261
75. Mair TS, Taylor FG, Harbour DA, Pearson GR: Concurrent cryptosporidium and coronavirus infections in an Arabian foal with combined immunodeficiency syndrome, *Vet Rec* 126:127-130, 1990.
76. Bjorneby JM, Leach DR, Perryman LE: Persistent cryptosporidiosis in horses with severe combined immunodeficiency, *Infect Immun* 59:3823-3826, 1991.
77. MacLeay JM, Ames TR, Hayden DW, Tumas DB: Acquired B lymphocyte deficiency and chronic enterocolitis in a 3-year-old quarter horse, *Vet Immunol Immunopathol* 57:49-57, 1997.
78. Chandra RK, Kumari S: Nutrition and immunity: an overview, *J Nutr* 124:S1433-S1435, 1994.
79. Chandra RK: Nutrition and the immune system from birth to old age, *Eur J Clin Nutr* 56:S73-S76, 2002.
80. Lotz M, Menard S, Hornef M: Innate immune recognition on the intestinal mucosa, *Int J Med Microbiol* 297:379-392, 2007.
81. Tlaskalovb-Hogenovb H, Stepbnkovb R, Hudcovic T, et al: Commensal bacteria (normal microflora), mucosal immunity and chronic inflammatory and autoimmune diseases, *Immunol Letters* 93:97-108, 2004.
82. Othman M, Aguero R, Lin HC: Alterations in intestinal microbial flora and human disease, *Curr Opin Gastroenterol* 24:11-16, 2008.
83. Duchmann R, Schmitt E, Knolle P, et al: Tolerance towards resident intestinal flora in mice is abrogated in experimental colitis and restored by treatment with interleukin-10 or antibodies to interleukin-12, *Eur J Immunol* 26:934-938, 1996.
84. O'Loughlin EV, Scott RB, Gall DG: Pathophysiology of infectious diarrhea: changes in intestinal structure and function, *J Pediatr Gastroenterol Nutr* 12:5-20, 1991.
85. King JN, Gerring EL: The action of low dose endotoxin on equine bowel motility, *Equine Vet J* 23:11-17, 1991.
86. Read NW: Colon: relationship between epithelial transport and motility, *Pharmacology* 36(suppl 1):120-125, 1988.
87. Adams SB: Equine intestinal motility: an overview of normal activity, changes in disease, and effects of drug administration, *Proc Am Assoc Equine Pract* 33:539-553, 1987.
88. Ewe K: Intestinal transport in constipation and diarrhoea, *Pharmacology* 36(Suppl 1):73-84, 1988.

Pathophysiology of Mucosal Injury and Repair

1. Pappenheimer JR: Paracellular intestinal absorption of glucose, creatinine, and mannitol in normal animals: relation to body size, *Am J Physiol* 259:G290-G299, 1990.
2. Pappenheimer JR: Physiological regulation of epithelial junctions in intestinal epithelia, *Acta Physiol Scand Suppl* 571:43-51, 1988.
3. Pappenheimer JR: Physiological regulation of transepithelial impedance in the intestinal mucosa of rats and hamsters, *J Membr Biol* 100:137-148, 1987.
4. Pappenheimer JR, Reiss KZ: Contribution of solvent drag through intercellular junctions to absorption of nutrients by the small intestine of the rat, *J Membr Biol* 100:123-136, 1987.
5. Madara JL: Warner-Lambert/Parke-Davis Award lecture. Pathobiology of the intestinal epithelial barrier, *Am J Pathol* 137:1273-1281, 1990.
6. Madara JL: Review article: Pathobiology of neutrophil interactions with intestinal epithelia, *Aliment Pharmacol Ther* 11(Suppl 3):57-62, 1997.
7. Van Itallie CM, Anderson JM: Claudins and epithelial paracellular transport, *Annu Rev Physiol* 68:403-429, 2006.
8. Itoh M, Furuse M, Morita K, et al: Direct binding of three tight junction-associated MAGUKs, ZO-1, ZO-2, and ZO-3, with the COOH termini of claudins, *J Cell Biol* 147:1351-1363, 1999.
9. Karczewski J, Groot J: Molecular physiology and pathophysiology of tight junctions III. Tight junction regulation by intracellular messengers: differences in response within and between epithelia, *Am J Physiol Gastrointest Liver Physiol* 279:G660-G665, 2000.
10. Mitic LL, Van Itallie CM, Anderson JM: Molecular physiology and pathophysiology of tight junctions I. Tight junction structure and function: lessons from mutant animals and proteins, *Am J Physiol Gastrointest Liver Physiol* 279:G250-G254, 2000.
11. Johnson LR, editor: *Physiology of the gastrointestinal tract*, New York, 1994, Raven Press.
12. Madara JL: Loosening tight junctions. Lessons from the intestine, *J Clin Invest* 83:1089-1094, 1989.
13. Madara JL, Marcial MA: Structural correlates of intestinal tight-junction permeability, *Kroc Found Ser* 17:77-100, 1984.
14. Tice LW, Carter RL, Cahill MB: Changes in tight junctions of rat intestinal crypt cells associated with changes in their mitotic activity, *Tissue Cell* 11:293-316, 1979.
15. Marcial MA, Carlson SL, Madara JL: Partitioning of paracellular conductance along the ileal crypt-villus axis: a hypothesis based on structural analysis with detailed consideration of tight junction structure-function relationships, *J Membr Biol* 80:59-70, 1984.
16. Stevens CE, Hume ID: *Comparative physiology of the vertebrate digestive system*, New York, 1995, Cambridge University Press.
17. Argenzio RA: Comparative pathophysiology of nonglandular ulcer disease: a review of experimental studies, *Equine Vet J Suppl* 29:19-23, 1999.
18. Argenzio RA: Mechanisms of acid injury in porcine gastroesophageal mucosa, *Am J Vet Res* 57:564-573, 1996.
19. Murray MJ, Mahaffey EA: Age-related characteristics of gastric squamous epithelial mucosa in foals, *Equine Vet J* 25:514-517, 1993.
20. Andrews FM, Sifferman RL, Bernard W, et al: Efficacy of omeprazole paste in the treatment and prevention of gastric ulcers in horses, *Equine Vet J* (Suppl 29):81-86, 1999.
21. Vatistas NJ, Snyder JR, Nieto J, et al: Acceptability of a paste formulation and efficacy of high dose omeprazole in healing gastric ulcers in horses maintained in race training, *Equine Vet J Suppl* 29:71-76, 1999.
22. Murray MJ: Suppression of gastric acidity in horses, *J Am Vet Med Assoc* 211:37-40, 1997.

23. Campbell-Thompson ML, Merritt AM: Basal and pentagastrin-stimulated gastric secretion in young horses, *Am J Physiol* 259:R1259-R1266, 1990.
24. Schreiber S, Nguyen TH, Stuben M, Scheid P: Demonstration of a pH gradient in the gastric gland of the acid-secreting guinea pig mucosa, *Am J Physiol Gastrointest Liver Physiol* 279:G597-G604, 2000.
25. Podolsky DK: Mucosal immunity and inflammation. V. Innate mechanisms of mucosal defense and repair: the best offense is a good defense, *Am J Physiol* 277:G495-G499, 1999.
26. Robert A, Nezamis JE, Lancaster C, et al: Mild irritants prevent gastric necrosis through "adaptive cytoprotection" mediated by prostaglandins, *Am J Physiol* 245:G113-G121, 1983.
27. Robert A: Cytoprotection by prostaglandins in rats. Prevention of gastric necrosis produced by alcohol, HCl, NaOH, hypertonic NaCl, and thermal injury, *Gastroenterology* 77:433-443, 1979.
28. Robert A: Prostaglandins: effects on the gastrointestinal tract, *Clin Physiol Biochem* 2:61-69, 1984.
29. Ruppin H, Person B, Robert A, Domschke W: Gastric cytoprotection in man by prostaglandin E_2, *Scand J Gastroenterol* 16:647-652, 1981.
30. Mutoh H, Ota S, Hiraishi H, et al: Adaptive cytoprotection in cultured rat gastric mucus-producing cells. Role of mucus and prostaglandin synthesis, *Dig Dis Sci* 40:872-878, 1995.
31. Wallace JL: Increased resistance of the rat gastric mucosa to hemorrhagic damage after exposure to an irritant. Role of the "mucoid cap" and prostaglandin synthesis, *Gastroenterology* 94:22–32, 1988.
32. Konturek SJ, Robert A: Cytoprotection of canine gastric mucosa by prostacyclin: possible mediation by increased mucosal blood flow, *Digestion* 25:155-163, 1982.
33. Leung FW, Robert A, Guth PH: Gastric mucosal blood flow in rats after administration of 16,16-dimethyl prostaglandin E2 at a cytoprotective dose, *Gastroenterology* 88:1948-1953, 1985.
34. Asako H, Kubes P, Wallace J, et al: Modulation of leukocyte adhesion in rat mesenteric venules by aspirin and salicylate, *Gastroenterology* 103:146-152, 1992.
35. Holzer P, Sametz W: Gastric mucosal protection against ulcerogenic factors in the rat mediated by capsaicin-sensitive afferent neurons, *Gastroenterology* 91:975-981, 1986.
36. Holzer P, Pabst MA, Lippe IT, et al: Afferent nerve-mediated protection against deep mucosal damage in the rat stomach, *Gastroenterology* 98:838-848, 1990.
37. Holzer P, Pabst MA, Lippe IT: Intragastric capsaicin protects against aspirin-induced lesion formation and bleeding in the rat gastric mucosa, *Gastroenterology* 96:1425-1433, 1989.
38. Merchant NB, Dempsey DT, Grabowski MW, et al: Capsaicin-induced gastric mucosal hyperemia and protection: the role of calcitonin gene-related peptide, *Surgery* 116:419-425, 1994.
39. Wallace JL, Miller MJ: Nitric oxide in mucosal defense: a little goes a long way, *Gastroenterology* 119:512-520, 2000.
40. Campbell NB, Jones SL, Blikslager AT: The effects of cyclo-oxygenase inhibitors on bile-injured and normal equine colon, *Equine Vet J* 34:493-498, 2002.
41. Blikslager AT, Rhoads JM, Bristol DG, et al: Glutamine and transforming growth factor-alpha stimulate extracellular regulated kinases and enhance recovery of villous surface area in porcine ischemic-injured intestine, *Surgery* 125:186-194, 1999.
42. Moore R, Carlson S, Madara JL: Villus contraction aids repair of intestinal epithelium after injury, *Am J Physiol* 257:G274-G283, 1989.
43. Lang J, Blikslager A, Regina D, et al: Synergistic effect of hydrochloric acid and bile acids on the pars esophageal mucosa of the porcine stomach, *Am J Vet Res* 59:1170-1176, 1998.
44. Berschneider HM, Blikslager AT, Roberts MC: Role of duodenal reflux in nonglandular gastric ulcer disease of the mature horse, *Equine Vet J Suppl* 29:24-29, 1999.
45. Baker SJ, Gerring EL: Technique for prolonged, minimally invasive monitoring of intragastric pH in ponies, *Am J Vet Res* 54:1725-1734, 1993.
46. Murray MJ: Equine model of inducing ulceration in alimentary squamous epithelial mucosa, *Dig Dis Sci* 39:2530-2535, 1994.
47. Merritt AM: Normal equine gastroduodenal secretion and motility, *Equine Vet J Suppl* 29:7-13, 1999.
48. Peek RMJ IV: Helicobacter pylori strain-specific activation of signal transduction cascades related to gastric inflammation, *Am J Physiol Gastrointest Liver Physiol* 280:G525-G530, 2001.
49. Murray MJ: Pathophysiology of peptic disorders in foals and horses: a review, *Equine Vet J Suppl* 29:14-18, 1999.
50. Wallace JL: Nonsteroidal anti-inflammatory drugs and gastroenteropathy: the second hundred years, *Gastroenterology* 112:1000-1016, 1997.
51. Henry D, Dobson A, Turner C: Variability in the risk of major gastrointestinal complications from nonaspirin nonsteroidal anti-inflammatory drugs, *Gastroenterology* 105:1078-1088, 1993.
52. Langenbach R, Morham SG, Tiano HF, et al: Prostaglandin synthase 1 gene disruption in mice reduces arachidonic acid-induced inflammation and indomethacin-induced gastric ulceration, *Cell* 83:483-492, 1995.
53. Smith WL, Langenbach R: Why there are two cyclooxygenase isozymes, *J Clin Invest* 107:1491-1495, 2001.
54. Wallace JL, McKnight W, Reuter BK, Vergnolle N: NSAID-Induced gastric damage in rats: requirement for inhibition of both cyclooxygenase 1 and 2, *Gastroenterology* 119:706-714, 2000.
55. Little D, Brown SA, Campbell NB, et al: Effects of the cycooxygenase inhibitor meloxicam on recovery of ischemia-injured jejunum, *Am J Vet Res* 68:614-624, 2007.
56. Moore RM, Muir WW, Granger DN: Mechanisms of gastrointestinal ischemia-reperfusion injury and potential therapeutic interventions: a review and its implications in the horse, *J Vet Intern Med* 9:115-132, 1995.
57. Moore RM: Clinical relevance of intestinal reperfusion injury in horses, *J Am Vet Med Assoc* 211:1362-1366, 1997.
58. Shepherd AP, Granger DN, editors: *Physiology of intestinal circulation*, New York, 2001, Raven Press.
59. Bulkley GB, Kvietys PR, Parks DA, et al: Relationship of blood flow and oxygen consumption to ischemic injury in the canine small intestine, *Gastroenterology* 89:852-857, 1985.
60. Dart AJ, Snyder JR, Julian D, Hinds DM: Microvascular circulation of the small intestine in horses, *Am J Vet Res* 53:995-1000, 1992.
61. Snyder JR, Olander HJ, Pascoe JR, et al: Morphologic alterations observed during experimental ischemia of the equine large colon, *Am J Vet Res* 49:801-809, 1988.
62. McAnulty JF, Stone WC, Darien BJ: The effects of ischemia and reperfusion on mucosal respiratory function, adenosine triphosphate, electrolyte, and water content in the ascending colon of ponies, *Vet Surg* 26:172-181, 1997.
63. Noda T, Iwakiri R, Fujimoto K, et al: Programmed cell death induced by ischemia-reperfusion in rat intestinal mucosa, *Am J Physiol* 274:G270-G276, 1998.
64. Ikeda H, Suzuki Y, Suzuki M, et al: Apoptosis is a major mode of cell death caused by ischaemia and ischaemia/reperfusion injury to the rat intestinal epithelium, *Gut* 42:530-537, 1998.
65. Coopersmith CM, O'Donnell D, Gordon JI: Bcl-2 inhibits ischemia-reperfusion-induced apoptosis in the intestinal epithelium of transgenic mice, *Am J Physiol* 276:G677-G686, 1999.

66. Chiu CJ, McArdle AH, Brown R, et al: Intestinal mucosal lesion in low-flow states. I. A morphological, hemodynamic, and metabolic reappraisal, *Arch Surg* 101:478-483, 1970.
67. Laws EG, Freeman DE: Significance of reperfusion injury after venous strangulation obstruction of equine jejunum, *J Invest Surg* 8:263-270, 1995.
68. Arden WA, Slocombe RF, Stick JA, Parks AH: Morphologic and ultrastructural evaluation of effect of ischemia and dimethyl sulfoxide on equine jejunum, *Am J Vet Res* 51:1784-1791, 1990.
69. Meschter CL, Tyler DE, White NA, Moore J: Histologic findings in the gastrointestinal tract of horses with colic, *Am J Vet Res* 47:598-606, 1986.
70. Meschter CL, Craig D, Hackett R: Histopathological and ultrastructural changes in simulated large colonic torsion and reperfusion in ponies, *Equine Vet J* 23:426-433, 1991.
71. van Hoogmoed L, Snyder JR, Pascoe JR, Olander HJ: Evaluation of uniformity of morphological injury of the large colon following severe colonic torsion, *Equine Vet J Suppl* 32:98-100, 2000.
72. van Hoogmoed L, Snyder JR, Pascoe JR, Olander H: Use of pelvic flexure biopsies to predict survival after large colon torsion in horses, *Vet Surg* 29:572-577, 2000.
73. White NA, Moore JN, Douglas M: SEM study of Strongylus vulgaris larva-induced arteritis in the pony, *Equine Vet J* 15:349-353, 1983.
74. Moore RM, Bertone AL, Bailey MQ, et al: Neutrophil accumulation in the large colon of horses during low-flow ischemia and reperfusion, *Am J Vet Res* 55:1454-1463, 1994.
75. Moore RM, Bertone AL, Muir WW, et al: Histopathologic evidence of reperfusion injury in the large colon of horses after low-flow ischemia, *Am J Vet Res* 55:1434-1443, 1994.
76. Gerard MP, Blikslager AT, Roberts MC, et al: The characteristics of intestinal injury peripheral to strangulating obstruction lesions in the equine small intestine, *Equine Vet J* 31:331–335, 1999.
77. Dabareiner RM, White NA, Donaldson LL: Effects of intraluminal distention and decompression on microvascular permeability and hemodynamics of the equine jejunum, *Am J Vet Res* 62:225-236, 2001.
78. Dabareiner RM, Sullins KE, Snyder JR, et al: Evaluation of the microcirculation of the equine small intestine after intraluminal distention and subsequent decompression, *Am J Vet Res* 54:1673-1682, 1993.
79. Dabareiner RM, Snyder JR, White NA, et al: Microvascular permeability and endothelial cell morphology associated with low-flow ischemia/reperfusion injury in the equine jejunum, *Am J Vet Res* 56:639-648, 1995.
80. Allen DJ, White NA, Tyler DE: Factors for prognostic use in equine obstructive small intestinal disease, *J Am Vet Med Assoc* 189:777-780, 1986.
81. Schoenberg MH, Poch B, Younes M, et al: Involvement of neutrophils in postischaemic damage to the small intestine, *Gut* 32:905-912, 1991.
82. Nilsson UA, Schoenberg MH, Aneman A, et al: Free radicals and pathogenesis during ischemia and reperfusion of the cat small intestine, *Gastroenterology* 106:629-636, 1994.
83. Grisham MB, Hernandez LA, Granger DN: Xanthine oxidase and neutrophil infiltration in intestinal ischemia, *Am J Physiol* 251:G567-G574, 1986.
84. Granger DN: Role of xanthine oxidase and granulocytes in ischemia-reperfusion injury, *Am J Physiol* 255:H1269-H1275, 1988.
85. Kubes P, Hunter J, Granger DN: Ischemia/reperfusion-induced feline intestinal dysfunction: importance of granulocyte recruitment, *Gastroenterology* 103:807-812, 1992.
86. Horne MM, Pascoe PJ, Ducharme NG, et al: Attempts to modify reperfusion injury of equine jejunal mucosa using dimethylsulfoxide, allopurinol, and intraluminal oxygen, *Vet Surg* 23:241-249, 1994.
87. Park PO, Haglund U, Bulkley GB, Falt K: The sequence of development of intestinal tissue injury after strangulation ischemia and reperfusion, *Surgery* 107:574-580, 1990.
88. Haglund U: Gut ischaemia, *Gut* 35:S73-S76, 1994.
89. Dabareiner RM, Snyder JR, Sullins KE, et al: Evaluation of the microcirculation of the equine jejunum and ascending colon after ischemia and reperfusion, *Am J Vet Res* 54:1683-1692, 1993.
90. Granger DN: Role of xanthine oxidase and granulocytes in ischemia-reperfusion injury, *Am J Physiol* 255:H1269-H1275, 1988.
91. Blikslager AT, Roberts MC, Rhoads JM, et al: Is reperfusion injury an important cause of mucosal damage after porcine intestinal ischemia? *Surgery* 121:526-534, 1997.
92. Musemeche CA, Pizzini RP, Andrassy RJ: Intestinal ischemia in the newborn: the role of intestinal maturation, *J Surg Res* 55:595-598, 1993.
93. Kanwar S, Kubes P: Mast cells contribute to ischemia-reperfusion-induced granulocyte infiltration and intestinal dysfunction, *Am J Physiol* 267:G316-G321, 1994.
94. Prichard M, Ducharme NG, Wilkins PA, et al: Xanthine oxidase formation during experimental ischemia of the equine small intestine, *Can J Vet Res* 55:310-314, 1991.
95. Grisham MB, Granger DN: Neutrophil-mediated mucosal injury. Role of reactive oxygen metabolites, *Dig Dis Sci* 33: 6S-15S, 1988.
96. Blikslager AT, Roberts MC, Gerard MP, Argenzio RA: How important is intestinal reperfusion injury in horses?, *J Am Vet Med Assoc* 211:1387-1389, 1997.
97. Parks DA, Williams TK, Beckman JS: Conversion of xanthine dehydrogenase to oxidase in ischemic rat intestine: a reevaluation, *Am J Physiol* 254:G768-G774, 1988.
98. Moore RM, Muir WW, Bertone AL, et al: Effects of dimethyl sulfoxide, allopurinol, 21-aminosteroid U-74389G, and manganese chloride on low-flow ischemia and reperfusion of the large colon in horses, *Am J Vet Res* 56:671-687, 1995.
99. Schaffer MR, Efron PA, Thornton FJ, et al: Nitric oxide, an autocrine regulator of wound fibroblast synthetic function, *J Immunol* 158:2375-2381, 1997.
100. Konturek SJ, Brzozowski T, Majka J, et al: Inhibition of nitric oxide synthase delays healing of chronic gastric ulcers, *Eur J Pharmacol* 239:215-217, 1993.
101. Tarnawski A, Tanoue K, Santos AM, Sarfeh IJ: Cellular and molecular mechanisms of gastric ulcer healing. Is the quality of mucosal scar affected by treatment?, *Scand J Gastroenterol Suppl* 210:9-14, 1995.
102. Tarnawski A, Stachura J, Durbin T, et al: Increased expression of epidermal growth factor receptor during gastric ulcer healing in rats, *Gastroenterology* 102:695-698, 1992.
103. Erickson RA: 16,16-Dimethyl prostaglandin E_2 induces villus contraction in rats without affecting intestinal restitution, *Gastroenterology* 99:708-716, 1990.
104. Moore R, Madara JL, MacLeod RJ: Enterocytes adhere preferentially to collagen IV in a differentially regulated divalent cation-dependent manner, *Am J Physiol* 266:G1099-G1107, 1994.
105. Moore R, Madri J, Carlson S, Madara JL: Collagens facilitate epithelial migration in restitution of native guinea pig intestinal epithelium, *Gastroenterology* 102:119-130, 1992.
106. McCormack SA, Viar MJ, Johnson LR: Migration of IEC-6 cells: a model for mucosal healing, *Am J Physiol* 263:G426-G435, 1992.
107. Blikslager AT, Roberts MC, Rhoads JM, Argenzio RA: Prostaglandins I_2 and E_2 have a synergistic role in rescuing epithelial barrier function in porcine ileum, *J Clin Invest* 100:1928-1933, 1997.
108. Bjerknes M, Cheng H: Clonal analysis of mouse intestinal epithelial progenitors, *Gastroenterology* 116:7-14, 1999.

109. Jankowski JA, Goodlad RA, Wright NA: Maintenance of normal intestinal mucosa: function, structure, and adaptation, *Gut* 35:S1-S4, 1994.
110. Zushi S: Role of prostaglandins in intestinal epithelial restitution stimulated by growth factors, *Am J Physiol* 270: G757-G762, 1996.
111. Blikslager AT, Roberts MC, Young KM, et al: Genistein augments prostaglandin-induced recovery of barrier function in ischemia-injured porcine ileum, *Am J Physiol Gastrointest Liver Physiol* 278:G207-G216, 2000.
112. Moeser AJ, Haskell MM, Shifflett DE, et al: ClC-2 chloride secretion mediates prostaglandin-induced revoerry of barrier function in ischemia-injured porcine ileum, *Gastroenterology* 127:802-815, 2004.
113. Duffey ME, Hainau B, Ho S, Bentzel CJ: Regulation of epithelial tight junction permeability by cyclic AMP, *Nature* 294:451-453, 1981.
114. Palant CE, Duffey ME, Mookerjee BK, et al: Ca^{2+} regulation of tight-junction permeability and structure in Necturus gallbladder, *Am J Physiol* 245:C203-C212, 1983.
115. Wang JY, Johnson LR: Luminal polyamines substitute for tissue polyamines in duodenal mucosal repair after stress in rats, *Gastroenterology* 102:1109-1117, 1992.
116. Wang JY, Johnson LR: Polyamines and ornithine decarboxylase during repair of duodenal mucosa after stress in rats, *Gastroenterology* 100:333-343, 1991.
117. Wang JY, Johnson LR: Role of ornithine decarboxylase in repair of gastric mucosal stress ulcers, *Am J Physiol* 258:G78-G85, 1990.
118. McCormack SA, Wang JY, Viar MJ, et al: Polyamines influence transglutaminase activity and cell migration in two cell lines, *Am J Physiol* 267:C706-C714, 1994.
119. McCormack SA, Wang JY, Johnson LR: Polyamine deficiency causes reorganization of F-actin and tropomyosin in IEC-6 cells, *Am J Physiol* 267:C715-C722, 1994.
120. Rao JN, Li L, Golovina VA, Platoshyn O, et al: Ca^{2+}-RhoA signaling pathway required for polyamine-dependent intestinal epithelial cell migration, *Am J Physiol Cell Physiol* 280:C993-1007, 2001.
121. Ray RM, McCormack SA, Johnson LR: Polyamine depletion arrests growth of IEC-6 and $Caco_2$ cells by different mechanisms, *Am J Physiol Gastrointest Liver Physiol* 281:G37-G43, 2001.
122. Ray RM, Zimmerman BJ, McCormack SA, et al: Polyamine depletion arrests cell cycle and induces inhibitors p21(Waf1/Cip1), p27(Kip1), and p53 in IEC-6 cells, *Am J Physiol* 276:C684-C691, 1999.
123. Johnson LR, Tseng CC, Wang P, et al: Mucosal ornithine decarboxylase in the small intestine: localization and stimulation, *Am J Physiol* 256:G624-G630, 1989.
124. Wang JY, Johnson LR: Expression of protooncogenes c-fos and c-myc in healing of gastric mucosal stress ulcers, *Am J Physiol* 266:G878-G886, 1994.
125. Barnard JA, Beauchamp RD, Russell WE, et al: Epidermal growth factor-related peptides and their relevance to gastrointestinal pathophysiology, *Gastroenterology* 108:564-580, 1995.
126. Playford RJ, Wright NA: Why is epidermal growth factor present in the gut lumen?, *Gut* 38:303-305, 1996.
127. Blikslager AT, Roberts MC: Mechanisms of intestinal mucosal repair, *J Am Vet Med Assoc* 211:1437-1441, 1997.
128. Khulusi S, Hanby AM, Marrero JM, et al: Expression of trefoil peptides pS2 and human spasmolytic polypeptide in gastric metaplasia at the margin of duodenal ulcers, *Gut* 37:205-209, 1995.
129. Taupin D, Wu DC, Jeon WK, et al: The trefoil gene family are coordinately expressed immediate-early genes: EGF receptor- and MAP kinase-dependent interregulation, *J Clin Invest* 103:R31-R38, 1999.
130. Goke M, Zuk A, Podolsky DK: Regulation and function of extracellular matrix intestinal epithelial restitution in vitro, *Am J Physiol* 271:G729-G740, 1996.
131. Mashimo H, Wu DC, Podolsky DK, Fishman MC: Impaired defense of intestinal mucosa in mice lacking intestinal trefoil factor, *Science* 274:262-265, 1996.
132. Rhoads JM, Argenzio RA, Chen W, et al: Glutamine metabolism stimulates intestinal cell MAPKs by a cAMP- inhibitable, Raf-independent mechanism, *Gastroenterology* 118:90-100, 2000.
133. Rhoads JM, Argenzio RA, Chen W, et al: L-glutamine stimulates intestinal cell proliferation and activates mitogen-activated protein kinases, *Am J Physiol* 272:G943-G953, 1997.
134. Kripke SA, Fox AD, Berman JM, et al: Stimulation of intestinal mucosal growth with intracolonic infusion of short-chain fatty acids, *J Parenter Enteral Nutr* 13:109-116, 1989.
135. Inoue Y, Grant JP, Snyder PJ: Effect of glutamine-supplemented total parenteral nutrition on recovery of the small intestine after starvation atrophy, *J Parenter Enteral Nutr* 17:165-170, 1993.
136. Souba WW, Herskowitz K, Salloum RM, et al: Gut glutamine metabolism, *J Parenter Enteral Nutr* 14:45S-50S, 1990.
137. Platell C, McCauley R, McCulloch R, Hall J: The influence of parenteral glutamine and branched-chain amino acids on total parenteral nutrition-induced atrophy of the gut, *J Parenter Enteral Nutr* 17:348-354, 1993.
138. Tremel H, Kienle B, Weilemann LS, et al: Glutamine dipeptide-supplemented parenteral nutrition maintains intestinal function in the critically ill, *Gastroenterology* 107:1595-1601, 1994.
139. Frankel WL, Zhang W, Afonso J, et al: Glutamine enhancement of structure and function in transplanted small intestine in the rat, *J Parenter Enteral Nutr* 17:47-55, 1993.
140. Zhang W, Frankel WL, Singh A, et al: Improvement of structure and function in orthotopic small bowel transplantation in the rat by glutamine, *Transplantation* 56:512-517, 1993.
141. Fox AD, Kripke SA, De Paula J, et al: Effect of a glutamine-supplemented enteral diet on methotrexate-induced enterocolitis, *J Parenter Enteral Nutr* 12:325-331, 1988.
142. Klimberg VS, Salloum RM, Kasper M, et al: Oral glutamine accelerates healing of the small intestine and improves outcome after whole abdominal radiation, *Arch Surg* 125: 1040-1045, 1990.
143. Klimberg VS, Souba WW, Dolson DJ, et al: Prophylactic glutamine protects the intestinal mucosa from radiation injury, *Cancer* 66:62-68, 1990.
144. Ahdieh N, Blikslager AT, Bhat BG, et al: L-glutamine and transforming growth factor-alpha enhance recovery of monoacylglycerol acyltransferase and diacylglycerol acyltransferase activity in porcine postischemic ileum, *Pediatr Res* 43:227-233, 1998.

Gastrointestinal Ileus

1. Adams SB: Recognition and management of ileus, *Vet Clin N Am Equine Pract* 4:91-104, 1988.
2. Becht JL, Richardson DW: Ileus in the horse: clinical significance and management, *Proc Am Assoc Equine Pract* 27:291–297, 1981.
3. Semevolos SA, Ducharme NG, Hackett RP: Clinical assessment and outcome of three techniques for jejunal resection and anastomosis in horses: 59 cases (1989-2000), *J Am Vet Med Assoc* 220:215-218, 2002.
4. van den BR, van der Velden MA: Short-and long-term evaluation of surgical treatment of strangulating obstructions of the small intestine in horses: a review of 224 cases, *Vet Q* 23: 109-115, 2001.
5. Morton AJ, Blikslager AT: Surgical and postoperative factors influencing short-term survival of horses following small intestinal resection: 92 cases (1994-2001), *Equine Vet J* 34: 450-454, 2002.

6. Mair TS, Smith LJ: Survival and complication rates in 300 horses undergoing surgical treatment of colic. Part 2: Short-term complications, *Equine Vet J* 37:303-309, 2005.
7. Campbell ML, Colahan PC, Brown MP, et al: Cecal impaction in the horse, *J Am Vet Med Assoc* 184:950-952, 1984.
8. Ross MW, Martin BB, Donawick WJ: Cecal perforation in the horse, *J Am Vet Med Assoc* 187:249-253, 1985.
9. Hilbert BJ, Little CB, Bolton JR, McGill CA: Caecal overload and rupture in the horse, *Aust Vet J* 64:85-86, 1987.
10. Plummer AE, Rakestraw PC, Hardy J, Lee RM: Outcome of medical and surgical treatment of cecal impaction in horses: 114 cases (1994-2004), *J Am Vet Med Assoc* 231:1378-1385, 2007.
11. Horowitz B, Ward SM, Sanders KM: Cellular and molecular basis for electrical rhythmicity in gastrointestinal muscles, *Annu Rev Physiol* 61:19-43, 1999.
12. Fintl C, Hudson NP, Mayhew IG, et al: Interstitial cells of Cajal (ICC) in equine colic: an immunohistochemical study of horses with obstructive disorders of the small and large intestines, *Equine Vet J* 36:474-479, 2004.
13. Hudson N, Mayhew I, Pearson G: A reduction in interstitial cells of Cajal in horses with equine dysautonomia (grass sickness), *Auton Neurosci* 92:37-44, 2001.
14. Milne EM, Fintl C, Hudson NP, et al: Observations on the interstitial cells of Cajal and neurons in a recovered case of equine dysautonomia (grass sickness), *J Comp Pathol* 133: 33-40, 2005.
15. Hudson N, Mayhew I, Pearson G: Presence of in vitro electrical activity in the ileum of horses with enteric nervous system pathology: equine dysautonomia (grass sickness), *Auton Neurosci* 99:119-126, 2002.
16. Bertaccini G, Coruzzi G: Receptors in the gastrointestinal tract, *Pharmacol Res Commun* 19:87-118, 1987.
17. Re G, Belloli C, Badino P, et al: Identification of beta-adrenergic receptor subtypes mediating relaxation in isolated equine ileum, *Am J Vet Res* 58:621-625, 1997.
18. Malone ED, Kannan MS, Brown DR, et al: Adrenergic, cholinergic, and nonadrenergic-noncholinergic intrinsic innervation of the jejunum in horses, *Am J Vet Res* 60:898-904, 1999.
19. Rakestraw PC, Snyder JR, Woliner MJ, et al: Involvement of nitric oxide in inhibitory neuromuscular transmission in equine jejunum, *Am J Vet Res* 57:1206-1213, 1996.
20. Sellers AF, Lowe JE, Cummings JF: Trials of serotonin, substance P and alpha 2-adrenergic receptor effects on the equine large colon, *Cornell Vet* 75:319-323, 1985.
21. Sonea IM, Wilson DV, Bowker RM, Robinson NE: Tachykinin receptors in the equine pelvic flexure, *Equine Vet J* 29:306-312, 1997.
22. Merritt AM, Panzer RB, Lester GD, Burrow JA: Equine pelvic flexure myoelectric activity during fed and fasted states, *Am J Physiol* 269:G262-G268, 1995.
23. Lester GD, Bolton JR, Cullen LK, Thurgate SM: Effects of general anesthesia on myoelectric activity of the intestine in horses, *Am J Vet Res* 53:1553-1557, 1992.
24. Ross MW, Cullen KK, Rutkowski JA: Myoelectric activity of the ileum, cecum, and right ventral colon in ponies during interdigestive, nonfeeding, and digestive periods, *Am J Vet Res* 51:561-566, 1990.
25. Kalff JC, Carlos TM, Schraut WH, et al: Surgically induced leukocytic infiltrates within the rat intestinal muscularis mediate postoperative ileus, *Gastroenterology* 117:378-387, 1999.
26. Turler A, Moore BA, Pezzone MA, et al: Colonic postoperative inflammatory ileus in the rat, *Ann Surg* 236:56-66, 2002.
27. Schwarz NT, Kalff JC, Turler A, et al: Selective jejunal manipulation causes postoperative pan-enteric inflammation and dysmotility, *Gastroenterology* 126:159-169, 2004.
28. Wehner S, Behrendt FF, Lyutenski BN, et al: Inhibition of macrophage function prevents intestinal inflammation and postoperative ileus in rodents, *Gut* 56:176-185, 2007.
29. The FO, Bennink RJ, Ankum WM, et al: Intestinal handling-induced mast cell activation and inflammation in human postoperative ileus, *Gut* 57:33-40, 2008.
30. Turler A, Schnurr C, Nakao A, et al: Endogenous endotoxin participates in causing a panenteric inflammatory ileus after colonic surgery, *Ann Surg* 245:734-744, 2007.
31. Kalff JC, Schraut WH, Billiar TR, Simmons RL, Bauer AJ: Role of inducible nitric oxide synthase in postoperative intestinal smooth muscle dysfunction in rodents, *Gastroenterology* 118:316-327, 2000.
32. Little D, Tomlinson JE, Blikslager AT: Post operative neutrophilic inflammation in equine small intestine after manipulation and ischaemia, *Equine Vet J* 37:329-335, 2005.
33. Roger T, Ruckebusch Y: Colonic alpha 2-adrenoceptor-mediated responses in the pony, *J Vet Pharmacol Ther* 10:310-318, 1987.
34. Lester GD, Merritt AM, Neuwirth L, et al: Effect of alpha 2-adrenergic, cholinergic, and nonsteroidal anti-inflammatory drugs on myoelectric activity of ileum, cecum, and right ventral colon and on cecal emptying of radiolabeled markers in clinically normal ponies, *Am J Vet Res* 59:320-327, 1998.
35. Merritt AM, Campbell-Thompson ML, Lowrey S: Effect of xylazine treatment on equine proximal gastrointestinal tract myoelectrical activity, *Am J Vet Res* 50:945-949, 1989.
36. Clark ES, Thompson SA, Becht JL, et al: Effects of xylazine on cecal mechanical activity and cecal blood flow in healthy horses, *Am J Vet Res* 49:720-723, 1988.
37. Adams SB, Lamar CH, Masty J: Motility of the distal portion of the jejunum and pelvic flexure in ponies: effects of six drugs, *Am J Vet Res* 45:795-799, 1984.
38. Rutkowski JA, Ross MW, Cullen K: Effects of xylazine and/or butorphanol or neostigmine on myoelectric activity of the cecum and right ventral colon in female ponies, *Am J Vet Res* 50:1096-1101, 1989.
39. Merritt AM, Burrow JA, Hartless CS: Effect of xylazine, detomidine, and a combination of xylazine and butorphanol on equine duodenal motility, *Am J Vet Res* 59:619-623, 1998.
40. Elfenbein JR, Sanchez LC, Robertson SA, et al: Effect of detomidine on visceral and somatic nociception and duodenal motility in conscious adult horses, *Vet Anaesth Analg*, 36:162-172: 2009.
41. Boscan P, Van Hoogmoed LM, Farver TB, Snyder JR: Evaluation of the effects of the opioid agonist morphine on gastrointestinal tract function in horses, *Am J Vet Res* 67:992-997, 2006.
42. Roger T, Bardon T, Ruckebusch Y: Colonic motor responses in the pony: relevance of colonic stimulation by opiate antagonists, *Am J Vet Res* 46:31-35, 1985.
43. Sanchez LC, Robertson SA, Maxwell LK, et al: Effect of fentanyl on visceral and somatic nociception in conscious horses, *J Vet Intern.Med* 21:1067-1075, 2007.
44. Sojka JE, Adams SB, Lamar CH, Eller LL: Effect of butorphanol, pentazocine, meperidine, or metoclopramide on intestinal motility in female ponies, *Am J Vet Res* 49:527-529, 1988.
45. Merritt AM, Campbell-Thompson ML, Lowrey S: Effect of butorphanol on equine antroduodenal motility, *Equine Vet J Suppl* :21-23, 1989.
46. Sellon DC, Roberts MC, Blikslager AT, et al: Effects of continuous rate intravenous infusion of butorphanol on physiologic and outcome variables in horses after celiotomy, *J Vet Intern Med* 18:555-563, 2004.
47. Sellon DC, Monroe VL, Roberts MC, Papich MG: Pharmacokinetics and adverse effects of butorphanol administered by single intravenous injection or continuous intravenous infusion in horses, *Am J Vet Res* 62:183-189, 2001.

48. Sanchez LC, Elfenbein JR, Robertson SA: Effect of acepromazine, butorphanol, or N-butylscopolammonium bromide on visceral and somatic nociception and duodenal motility in conscious horses, *Am J Vet Res* 69:579–585, 2008.
49. Lester GD: *The development and application of a computer system for the recording and analysis of intestinal myoelectrical activity in the horse*, 1990, Murdoch University.
50. Sjoqvist A, Hallerback B, Glise H: Reflex adrenergic inhibition of colonic motility in anesthetized rat caused by nociceptive stimuli of peritoneum. An alpha 2-adrenoceptor-mediated response, *Dig Dis Sci* 30:749-754, 1985.
51. Pairet M, Ruckebusch Y: On the relevance of non-steroidal anti-inflammatory drugs in the prevention of paralytic ileus in rodents, *J Pharm Pharmacol* 41:757-761, 1989.
52. Zittel TT, Meile T, Huge A, et al: Preoperative intraluminal application of capsaicin increases postoperative gastric and colonic motility in rats, *J Gastrointest Surg* 5:503-513, 2001.
53. Lowe JE, Sellers AF, Brondum J: Equine pelvic flexure impaction. A model used to evaluate motor events and compare drug response, *Cornell Vet* 70:401-412, 1980.
54. MacHarg MA, Adams SB, Lamar CH, Becht JL: Electromyographic, myomechanical, and intraluminal pressure changes associated with acute extraluminal obstruction of the jejunum in conscious ponies, *Am J Vet Res* 47:7-11, 1986.
55. King JN, Gerring EL: The action of low dose endotoxin on equine bowel motility, *Equine Vet J* 23:11-17, 1991.
56. Eades SC, Moore JN: Blockade of endotoxin-induced cecal hypoperfusion and ileus with an alpha 2 antagonist in horses, *Am J Vet Res* 54:586-590, 1993.
57. King JN, Gerring EL: Antagonism of endotoxin-induced disruption of equine bowel motility by flunixin and phenylbutazone, *Equine Vet J Suppl* :38-42, 1989.
58. Meisler SD, Doherty TJ, Andrews FM, et al: Yohimbine ameliorates the effects of endotoxin on gastric emptying of the liquid marker acetaminophen in horses, *Can J Vet Res* 64:208-211, 2000.
59. Valk N, Doherty TJ, Blackford JT, et al: Phenylbutazone prevents the endotoxin-induced delay in gastric emptying in horses, *Can J Vet Res* 62:214-217, 1998.
60. Valk N, Doherty TJ, Blackford JT, et al: Effect of cisapride on gastric emptying in horses following endotoxin treatment, *Equine Vet J* 30:344-348, 1998.
61. Doherty TJ, Andrews FM, Abraha TW, et al: Metoclopramide ameliorates the effects of endotoxin on gastric emptying of acetaminophen in horses, *Can J Vet Res* 63:37-40, 1999.
62. Eskandari MK, Kalff JC, Billiar TR, et al: Lipopolysaccharide activates the muscularis macrophage network and suppresses circular smooth muscle activity, *Am J Physiol* 273:G727-G734, 1997.
63. Schwarz NT, Engel B, Eskandari MK, et al: Lipopolysaccharide preconditioning and cross-tolerance: the induction of protective mechanisms for rat intestinal ileus, *Gastroenterology* 123:586-598, 2002.
64. Overhaus M, Togel S, Pezzone MA, Bauer AJ: Mechanisms of polymicrobial sepsis-induced ileus, *Am J Physiol Gastrointest Liver Physiol* 287:G685-G694, 2004.
65. Hooper RN, Roussel AJ, Cohen ND: Erythromycin stimulates myoelectric activity in the ileum and pelvic flexure of horses in the post-operative period, *Proc Equine Colic Res Symp* 6:42, 1998.
66. Van Hoogmoed L, Rakestraw PC, Snyder JR, Harmon FA: In vitro effects of nonsteroidal anti-inflammatory agents and prostaglandins I2, E2, and F2alpha on contractility of taenia of the large colon of horses, *Am J Vet Res* 60:1004-1009, 1999.
67. Roussel AJ Jr, Cohen ND, Hooper RN, Rakestraw PC: Risk factors associated with development of postoperative ileus in horses, *J Am Vet Med Assoc* 219:72-78, 2001.
68. Freeman DE, Hammock P, Baker GJ, et al: Short- and long-term survival and prevalence of postoperative ileus after small intestinal surgery in the horse, *Equine Vet J Suppl* :42-51, 2000.
69. Cohen ND, Lester GD, Sanchez LC, et al: Evaluation of risk factors associated with development of postoperative ileus in horses, *J Am Vet Med Assoc* 225:1070-1078, 2004.
70. Blikslager AT, Bowman KF, Levine JF, et al: Evaluation of factors associated with postoperative ileus in horses: 31 cases (1990-1992), *J Am Vet Med Assoc* 205:1748-1752, 1994.
71. Naylor JM, Poirier KL, Hamilton DL, Dowling PM: The effects of feeding and fasting on gastrointestinal sounds in adult horses, *J Vet Intern Med* 20:1408-1413, 2006.
72. Gerard MP, Bowman KF, Blikslager AT, et al: Jejunocolostomy or ileocolostomy for treatment of cecal impaction in horses: nine cases, *J Am Vet Med Assoc* 1996(209):1287-1290, 1985-1995.
73. Roberts CT, Slone DE: Caecal impactions managed surgically by typhlotomy in 10 cases (1988-1998), *Equine Vet J Suppl* :74-76, 2000.
74. Collins SM: The immunomodulation of enteric neuromuscular function: implications for motility and inflammatory disorders, *Gastroenterology* 111:1683-1699, 1996.
75. Paradelis AG: Inhibition of the pendular movements of the intestine by aminoglycoside antibiotics, *Methods Find Exp Clin Pharmacol* 3:173-177, 1981.
76. Sparnon AL, Spitz L: Pharmacological manipulation of postoperative intestinal adhesions, *Aust N Z J Surg* 59:725-729, 1989.
77. Koenig JB, Sawhney S, Cote N, LaMarre J: Effect of intraluminal distension or ischemic strangulation obstruction of the equine jejunum on jejunal motilin receptors and binding of erythromycin lactobionate, *Am J Vet Res* 67:815-820, 2006.
78. Marti M, Mevissen M, Althaus H, Steiner A: In vitro effects of bethanechol on equine gastrointestinal contractility and functional characterization of involved muscarinic receptor subtypes, *J Vet Pharmacol Ther* 28:565-574, 2005.
79. Ringger NC, Lester GD, Neuwirth L, et al: Effect of bethanechol or erythromycin on gastric emptying in horses, *Am J Vet Res* 57:1771-1775, 1996.
80. Adams SB, MacHarg MA: Neostigmine methylsulfate delays gastric emptying of particulate markers in horses, *Am J Vet Res* 46:2498-2499, 1985.
81. Nieto JE, Rakestraw PC, Snyder JR, Vatistas NJ: In vitro effects of erythromycin, lidocaine, and metoclopramide on smooth muscle from the pyloric antrum, proximal portion of the duodenum, and middle portion of the jejunum of horses, *Am J Vet Res* 61:413-419, 2000.
82. Gerring EE, Hunt JM: Pathophysiology of equine postoperative ileus: effect of adrenergic blockade, parasympathetic stimulation and metoclopramide in an experimental model, *Equine Vet J* 18:249-255, 1986.
83. Dart AJ, Peauroi JR, Hodgson DR, Pascoe JR: Efficacy of metoclopramide for treatment of ileus in horses following small intestinal surgery: 70 cases (1989-1992), *Aust Vet J* 74:280-284, 1996.
84. Gerring EL, King JN: Cisapride in the prophylaxis of equine post operative ileus, *Equine Vet J* (Suppl):52-55, 1989.
85. Milne EM, Doxey DL, Woodman MP, et al: An evaluation of the use of cisapride in horses with chronic grass sickness (equine dysautonomia), *Br Vet J* 152:537-549, 1996.
86. Steinebach MA, Cole D: Use of cisapride in the resolution of pelvic flexure impaction in a horse, *Can Vet J* 36:624-625, 1995.
87. Valden MA, Klein WR: The effects of cisapride on the restoration of gut motility after surgery of the small intestine in horses: a clinical trial, *Vet Q* 15:175-179, 1993.
88. Cable CS, Ball MA, Schwark WS, et al: Preparation of a parenteral formulation of cisapride from propulsid tablets and pharmacokinetic analysis after its intravenous administration, *J Equine Vet Sci* 18:616-621, 1999.

89. Cubeddu LX: QT prolongation and fatal arrhythmias: a review of clinical implications and effects of drugs, *Am J Ther* 10:452-457, 2003.
90. Delco ML, Nieto JE, Craigmill AL, et al: Pharmacokinetics and in vitro effects of tegaserod, a serotonin 5-hydroxytryptamine 4 (5-HT4) receptor agonist with prokinetic activity in horses, *Vet Ther* 8:77-87, 2007.
91. Lippold BS, Hildebrand J, Straub R: Tegaserod (HTF 919) stimulates gut motility in normal horses, *Equine Vet J* 36:622-627, 2004.
92. Hammerle CW, Surawicz CM: Updates on treatment of irritable bowel syndrome, *World J Gastroenterol* 14:2639-2649, 2008.
93. Koenig JB, Cote N, LaMarre J, et al: Binding of radiolabeled porcine motilin and erythromycin lactobionate to smooth muscle membranes in various segments of the equine gastrointestinal tract, *Am J Vet Res* 63:1545-1550, 2002.
94. Lester GD, Merritt AM, Neuwirth L, Vetro-Widenhouse T, Steible C, Rice B: Effect of erythromycin lactobionate on myoelectric activity of ileum, cecum, and right ventral colon, and cecal emptying of radiolabeled markers in clinically normal ponies, *Am J Vet Res* 59:328-334, 1998.
95. Roussel AJ, Hooper RN, Cohen ND, et al: Prokinetic effects of erythromycin on the ileum, cecum, and pelvic flexure of horses during the postoperative period, *Am J Vet Res* 61:420-424, 2000.
96. Nieto JE, Van Hoogmoed LM, Spier SJ, et al: Use of an extracorporeal circuit to evaluate effects of intraluminal distention and decompression on the equine jejunum, *Am J Vet Res* 63:267-275, 2002.
97. Bologna SD, Hasler WL, Owyang C: Down-regulation of motilin receptors on rabbit colon myocytes by chronic oral erythromycin, *J Pharmacol Exp Ther* 266:852-856, 1993.
98. Roussel AJ, Hooper RN, Cohen ND, et al: Evaluation of the effects of penicillin G potassium and potassium chloride on the motility of the large intestine in horses, *Am J Vet Res* 64:1360-1363, 2003.
99. Van Hoogmoed LM, Boscan PL: In vitro evaluation of the effect of the opioid antagonist N-methylnaltrexone on motility of the equine jejunum and pelvic flexure, *Equine Vet J* 37:325-328, 2005.
100. Boscan P, Van Hoogmoed LM, Pypendop BH, et al: Pharmacokinetics of the opioid antagonist N-methylnaltrexone and evaluation of its effects on gastrointestinal tract function in horses treated or not treated with morphine, *Am J Vet Res* 67:998-1004, 2006.
101. Van Hoogmoed LM, Nieto JE, Snyder JR, Harmon FA: Survey of prokinetic use in horses with gastrointestinal injury, *Vet Surg* 33:279-285, 2004.
102. Rimback G, Cassuto J, Tollesson PO: Treatment of postoperative paralytic ileus by intravenous lidocaine infusion, *Anesthesia Analgesia* 70:414-419, 1990.
103. Lahat A, Horin SB, Lang A, Fudim E, Picard O, Chowers Y: Lidocaine down-regulates nuclear factor-kappaB signalling and inhibits cytokine production and T cell proliferation, *Clin Exp Immunol* 152:320-327, 2008.
104. Cook VL, Jones SJ, McDowell M, Campbell NB, Davis JL, Blikslager AT: Attenuation of ischaemic injury in the equine jejunum by administration of systemic lidocaine, *Equine Vet J*, Jun; 40(4):353-357, 2008.
105. Robertson SA, Sanchez LC, Merritt AM, Doherty TJ: Effect of systemic lidocaine on visceral and somatic nociception in conscious horses, *Equine Vet J* 37:122-127, 2005.
106. Milligan M, Beard W, Kukanich B, et al: The effect of lidocaine on postoperative jejunal motility in normal horses, *Vet Surg* 36:214-220, 2007.
107. Brianceau P, Chevalier H, Karas A, et al: Intravenous lidocaine and small-intestinal size, abdominal fluid, and outcome after colic surgery in horses, *J Vet Intern Med* 16:736-741, 2002.
108. Malone E, Ensink J, Turner T, et al: Intravenous continuous infusion of lidocaine for treatment of equine ileus, *Vet Surg* 35:60-66, 2006.
109. Dickey EJ, McKenzie Iii HC, Brown JA, de Solis CN: Serum concentrations of lidocaine and its metabolites after prolonged infusion in healthy horses, *Equine Vet J*, Jun; 40(4):353-357, 2008.

Endotoxemia

1. American College of Chest Physicians/Society of Critical Care Medicine Consensus Conference: Definitions for sepsis and organ failure and guidelines for the use of innovative therapies in sepsis, *Crit Care Med* 20(6):864-874, 1992.
2. Vincent J-L, Dear SIRS: I'm sorry to say that I don't like you, *Crit Care Med* 25:372-374, 1997.
3. Opal SM: The uncertain value of the definition for SIRS. Systemic inflammatory response syndrome, *Chest* 113:1442-1443, 1998.
4. Pfeiffer R: Untersuchungen ueber das Choleragift, *Z Hyg* 11:393-412, 1892.
5. Brade H, Opal SM, Vogel SN, et al: *Endotoxin in health and disease*, New York, 1999, Marcel Dekker.
6. Rietschel ET, Wagner H, editors: *Pathology of septic shock*, Berlin, 1996, Springer.
7. Zahringer U, Lindner B, Rietschel ET: Molecular structure of lipid A, the endotoxic center of bacterial lipopolysaccharides, *Adv Carbohydr Chem Biochem* 50:211-276, 1994.
8. Poxton IR: Antibodies to lipopolysaccharide, *J Immunol Methods* 186(1):1-15, 1995.
9. Galanos C, Luderitz O, Rietschel ET, et al: Synthetic and natural Escherichia coli free lipid A express identical endotoxic activities, *Eur J Biochem* 148(1):1-5, 1985.
10. Bradley SG: Cellular and molecular mechanisms of action of bacterial endotoxins, *Annu Rev Microbiol* 33:67-94, 1979.
11. Barton MH, Morris DD, Norton N, et al: Hemostatic and fibrinolytic indices in neonatal foals with presumed septicemia, *J Vet Intern Med* 12(1):26-35, 1998.
12. Alexander JW, Boyce ST, Babcock GF, et al: The process of microbial translocation, *Ann Surg* 212(4):496-510, 1990.
13. Moore JN, Garner HE, Berg JN, et al: Intracecal endotoxin and lactate during the onset of equine laminitis: a preliminary report, *Am J Vet Res* 40(5):722-723, 1979.
14. Triger DR, Boyer TD, Levin J: Portal and systemic bacteraemia and endotoxaemia in liver disease, *Gut* 19:935-939, 1978.
15. Barton MH, Collatos C: Tumor necrosis factor and interleukin-6 activity and endotoxin concentration in PF and blood of horses with acute abdominal disease, *J Vet Intern Med* 13(5):457-464, 1999.
16. Steverink PJGM, Sturk A, Rutten VPMG, et al: Endotoxin, interleukin-6 and tumor necrosis factor concentrations in equine acute abdominal disease: relation to clinical outcome, *J Endotoxin Res* 2:289-299, 1995.
17. Henry MM, Moore JN: Whole blood re-calcification time in equine colic, *Equine Vet J* 23(4):303-308, 1991.
18. Morris DD: Endotoxemia in horses: a review of cellular and humoral mediators involved in its pathogenesis, *J Vet Intern Med* 5(3):167-181, 1991.
19. Schlag G, Redl H, editors: *Shock, sepsis, and organ failure: scavenging of nitric oxide and inhibition of its production*, Berlin, 1999, Springer.
20. Deitch EA, Maejima K, Berg R: Effect of oral antibiotics and bacterial overgrowth on the translocation of the GI tract microflora in burned rats, *J Trauma* 25(5):385-392, 1985.
21. Deitch EA, Winterton J, Berg R: Effect of starvation, malnutrition, and trauma on the gastrointestinal tract flora and bacterial translocation, *Arch Surg* 122(9):1019-1024, 1987.
22. Deitch EA, Berg R, Specian R: Endotoxin promotes the translocation of bacteria from the gut, *Arch Surg* 122(2):185-190, 1987.

23. Baker B, Gaffin SL, Wells M, et al: Endotoxaemia in racehorses following exertion, *J S Afr Vet Assoc* 59(2):63-66, 1988.
24. Barton MH, Williamson L, Jacks S, Norton N: Effects on plasma endotoxin and eicosanoid concentrations and serum cytokine activities in horses competing in a 48-, 83-, or 159-km endurance ride under similar terrain and weather conditions, *Am J Vet Res* 64(6):754-761, 2003.
25. Donovan DC, Jackson CA, Colahan PT, et al: Assessment of exercise-induced alterations in neutrophil function in horses, *Am J Vet Res* 68(11):1198-1204, 2007.
26. Tobias PS, Soldau K, Ulevitch RJ: Isolation of a lipopolysaccharide-binding acute phase reactant from rabbit serum, *J Exp Med* 164(3):777-793, 1986.
27. Ramadori G, Meyer zum Buschenfelde KH, Tobias PS, et al: Biosynthesis of lipopolysaccharide-binding protein in rabbit hepatocytes, *Pathobiology* 58(2):89-94, 1990.
28. Schumann RR, Leong SR, Flaggs GW, et al: Structure and function of lipopolysaccharide binding protein, *Science* 249(4975):1429-1431, 1990.
29. Zweigner J, Schumann RR, Weber JR: The role of lipopolysaccharide-binding protein in modulating the innate immune response, *Microbes and Infection* 8:946-952, 2006.
30. Jack RS, Fan X, Bernheiden M, et al: Lipopolysaccharide-binding protein is required to combat a murine gram-negative bacterial infection, *Nature* 389(6652):742-745, 1997.
31. Wright SD, Ramos RA, Tobias PS, et al: CD14, a receptor for complexes of lipopolysaccharide (LPS) and LPS binding protein, *Science* 249(4975):1431-1433, 1990.
32. Wright SD, Tobias PS, Ulevitch RJ, et al: Lipopolysaccharide (LPS) binding protein opsonizes LPS-bearing particles for recognition by a novel receptor on macrophages, *J Exp Med* 170(4):1231-1241, 1989.
33. Schiff DE, Kline L, Soldau K, et al: Phagocytosis of gram-negative bacteria by a unique CD14-dependent mechanism, *J Leukoc Biol* 62(6):786-794, 1997.
34. Grunwald U, Fan X, Jack RS, et al: Monocytes can phagocytose gram-negative bacteria by a CD14-dependent mechanism, *J Immunol* 157(9):4119-4125, 1996.
35. Wurfel MM, Hailman E, Wright SD: Soluble CD14 acts as a shuttle in the neutralization of lipopolysaccharide (LPS) by LPS-binding protein and reconstituted high density lipoprotein, *J Exp Med* 181(5):1743-1754, 1995.
36. Lamping N, Dettmer R, Schroder NW, et al: LPS-binding protein protects mice from septic shock caused by LPS or gram-negative bacteria, *J Clin Invest* 101(10):2065-2071, 1998.
37. Vandenplas ML, Moore JN, Barton MH, et al: Concentrations of serum amyloid A and lipopolysaccharide-binding protein in horses with colic, *Am J Vet Res* 66(9):1509-1516, 2005.
38. Chow JC, Young DW, Golenbock DT, et al: Toll-like receptor-4 mediates lipopolysaccharide-induced signal transduction, *J Biol Chem* 274(16):10689-10692, 1999.
39. Janeway CA: Jr: The immune system evolved to discriminate infectious nonself from noninfectious self, *Immunol Today* 13(1):11-16, 1992.
40. Haziot A, Chen S, Ferrero E, et al: The monocyte differentiation antigen, CD14, is anchored to the cell membrane by a phosphatidylinositol linkage, *J Immunol* 141(2):547-552, 1988.
41. Stelter F: Structure/function relationships of CD14, *Chem Immunol* 74:25-41, 2000.
42. Durieux JJ, Vita N, Popescu O, et al: The two soluble forms of the lipopolysaccharide receptor, CD14: characterization and release by normal human monocytes, *Eur J Immunol* 24(9):2006-2012, 1994.
43. Jack RS: Introduction: hunting devils, *Chem Immunol* 74:1-4, 2000.
44. Shimazu R, Akashi S, Ogata H, et al: MD-2, a molecule that confers lipopolysaccharide responsiveness on Toll-like receptor 4, *J Exp Med* 189(11):1777-1782, 1999.
45. Poltorak A, He X, Smirnova I, et al: Defective LPS signaling in C3H/HeJ and C57BL/10ScCr mice: mutations in Tlr4 gene, *Science* 282(5396):2085-2088, 1998.
46. Qureshi ST, Lariviere L, Leveque G, et al: Endotoxin-tolerant mice have mutations in Toll-like receptor 4 (Tlr4), *J Exp Med* 189(4):615-625, 1999.
47. Arbour NC, Lorenz E, Schutte BC, et al: TLR4 mutations are associated with endotoxin hyporesponsiveness in humans, *Nat Genet* 25(2):187-191, 2000.
48. Lu Y-C, Yeh W-C, Ohashi PS: LPS/TLR4 signal transduction pathway, *Cytokine* 42:145-151, 2008.
49. Maniatis T: Catalysis by a multiprotein IkappaB kinase complex, *Science* 278(5339):818-819, 1997.
50. Tizard IR: *Veterinary immunology: an introduction*, ed 8, St Louis, 2008, Saunders.
51. Beutler B, Cerami A: Cachectin and tumour necrosis factor as two sides of the same biological coin, *Nature* 320(6063):584-588, 1986.
52. Beutler B, Milsark IW, Cerami AC: Passive immunization against cachectin/tumor necrosis factor protects mice from lethal effect of endotoxin, *Science* 229(4716):869-871, 1985.
53. Le J, Vilcek J: Biology of disease; tumor necrosis factor and interleukin 1: cytokines with multiple overlapping biological activities, *Lab Invest* 56:234-248, 1987.
54. Le JM, Vilcek J: Interleukin 6: a multifunctional cytokine regulating immune reactions and the acute phase protein response, *Lab Invest* 61(6):588-602, 1989.
55. MacKay RJ: Treatment of endotoxemia and SIRS, *Proceedings of the nineteenth American College of Veterinary Internal Medicine Forum*, Denver, May 23-26, 2001, Colo.
56. Bone RC: Sir Isaac Newton, sepsis, SIRS, and CARS, *Crit Care Med* 24(7):1125-1128, 1996.
57. Osuchowski MF, Welch K, Siddiqui J, Remick DG: Circulating cytokine/inhibitor profiles reshape the understanding of the SIRS/CARS continnuum in sepsis and predict mortality, *J Immunol* 177:1967-1974, 2006.
58. Mengozzi M, Ghezzi P: Cytokine down-regulation in endotoxin tolerance, *Eur Cytokine Netw* 4(2):89-98, 1993.
59. Cavaillon J-M, Adib-Conquy M: Bench-to-bedside review: Endotoxin tolerance as a model of leukocyte reprogramming in sepsis, *Crit Care* 10(5):233, 2006.
60. Nomura F, Akashi S, Sakao Y, et al: Cutting edge: endotoxin tolerance in mouse peritoneal macrophages correlates with down-regulation of surface Toll-like receptor 4 expression, *J Immunol* 164(7):3476-3479, 2000.
61. Heagy W, Hansen C, Nieman K, et al: Impaired mitogen-activated protein kinase activation and altered cytokine secretion in endotoxin-tolerant human monocytes, *J Trauma* 49(5):806-814, 2000.
62. Barton MH, Collatos C, Moore JN: Endotoxin induced expression of tumour necrosis factor, tissue factor and plasminogen activator inhibitor activity by peritoneal macrophages, *Equine Vet J* 28(5):382-389, 1996.
63. Allen GK, Campbell-Beggs C, Robinson JA, et al: Induction of early-phase endotoxin tolerance in horses, *Equine Vet J* 28(4):269-274, 1996.
64. Lentsch AB, Ward PA: Regulation of inflammatory vascular damage, *J Pathol* 190(3):343-348, 2000.
65. Klabunde RE, Anderson DE: Role of NO and ROS in platelet activating factor-induced microvascular leakage, *FASEB J* 15:A47, 2001.
66. Turek JJ, Templeton CB, Bottoms GD, et al: Flunixin meglumine attenuation of endotoxin-induced damage to the cardiopulmonary vascular endothelium of the pony, *Am J Vet Res* 46(3):591-596, 1985.
67. Barton MH: Endotoxemia. In White NA, Moore JN, editors: *Current techniques in equine surgery and lameness*, ed 2, Philadelphia, 1998, Saunders.

68. Morris DD, Crowe N, Moore JN: Correlation of clinical and laboratory data with serum tumor necrosis factor activity in horses with experimentally induced endotoxemia, *Am J Vet Res* 51(12):1935-1940, 1990.
69. Andonegui G, Goyert SM, Kubes P: Lipopolysaccharide-induced leukocyte-endothelial cell interactions: a role for CD14 versus toll-like receptor 4 within microvessels, *J Immunol* 169:2111-2119, 2002.
70. Meager A: Cytokine regulation of cellular adhesion molecule expression in inflammation, *Cytokine Growth Factor Rev* 10(1):27-39, 1999.
71. Wagner JG, Roth RA: Neutrophil migration during endotoxemia, *J Leukocyte Biol* 66:10-24, 1999.
72. Wagner JG, Harkema JR, Roth RA: Temporal relationship between intravenous and intratracheal administrations of lipopolysaccharide (LPS) on pulmonary neutrophil (PMN) recruitment, *Am J Respir Crit Care Med* 153:A837, 1996:(abstract).
73. Gardner AB, Nydam DV, Luna JA, et al: Serum opsonization capacity, phagocytosis, and oxidative burst activity in neonatal foals in the intensive care unit, *J Vet Intern Med* 21(4):797-805, 2007.
74. McTaggart C, Penhale J, Raidala SL: Effect of plasma transfusion on neutrophil function in healthy and septic foals, *Aust Vet H* 83(8):499-505, 2005.
75. Johnstone IB, Crane S: Hemostatic abnormalities in equine colic, *Am J Vet Res* 47(2):356-358, 1986.
76. Prasse KW, Topper MJ, Moore JN, et al: Analysis of hemostasis in horses with colic, *J Am Vet Med Assoc* 203(5):685-693, 1993.
77. Levi M, de Jonge E, van der PollSepsis T: Disseminated Intravascular Coagulation, *J Throm Thrombolysis* 16:43-47, 2003.
78. Amaral A, Opal SM, Vincent JL: Coagulation in sepsis, *Intensive Care Med* 30:1032-1040, 2004.
79. Morris DD: Recognition and management of disseminated intravascular coagulation in horses, *Vet Clin North Am Equine Pract* 4(1):115-143, 1988.
80. Kalter ES, Daha MR, ten Cate JW, et al: Activation and inhibition of Hageman factor-dependent pathways and the complement system in uncomplicated bacteremia or bacterial shock, *J Infect Dis* 151(6):1019-1027, 1985.
81. Lyberg T: Clinical significance of increased thromboplastin activity on the monocyte surface: a brief review, *Haemostasis* 14(5):430-439, 1984.
82. Drake TA, Cheng J, Chang A, et al: Expression of tissue factor, thrombomodulin, and E-selectin in baboons with lethal Escherichia coli sepsis, *Am J Pathol* 142(5):1458-1470, 1993.
83. Henry MM, Moore JN: Clinical relevance of monocyte procoagulant activity in horses with colic, *J Am Vet Med Assoc* 198(5):843-848, 1991.
84. Welles EG, Prasse KW, Moore JN: Use of newly developed assays for protein C and plasminogen in horses with signs of colic, *Am J Vet Res* 52(2):345-351, 1991.
85. Nawroth PP, Stern DM: Modulation of endothelial cell hemostatic properties by tumor necrosis factor, *J Exp Med* 163(3):740-745, 1986.
86. Pober JS, Gimbrone MA Jr, Lapierre LA, et al: Overlapping patterns of activation of human endothelial cells by interleukin 1, tumor necrosis factor, and immune interferon, *J Immunol* 137(6):1893-1896, 1986.
87. Hack CE, Zeerleder S: The endothelium in sepsis: source of and a target for inflammation, *Crit Care Med* 29(suppl 7):S21-S27, 2001.
88. Kruithof EK: Plasminogen activator inhibitors: a review, *Enzyme* 40(2-3):113-121, 1988.
89. Travis J, Salvesen GS: Human plasma proteinase inhibitors, *Annu Rev Biochem* 52:655-709, 1983.
90. Krishnamurti C, Barr CF, Hassett MA, et al: Plasminogen activator inhibitor: a regulator of ancrod-induced fibrin deposition in rabbits, *Blood* 69(3):798-803, 1987.
91. Suffredini AF, Harpel PC, Parrillo JE: Promotion and subsequent inhibition of plasminogen activation after administration of intravenous endotoxin to normal subjects, *N Engl J Med* 320(18):1165-1172, 1989.
92. Collatos C, Barton MH, Schleef R, et al: Regulation of equine fibrinolysis in blood and peritoneal fluid based on a study of colic cases and induced endotoxaemia, *Equine Vet J* 26(6):474-481, 1994.
93. Collatos C, Barton MH, Prasse KW, et al: Intravascular and peritoneal coagulation and fibrinolysis in horses with acute gastrointestinal tract diseases, *J Am Vet Med Assoc* 207(4):465-470, 1995.
94. Bernard GR, Vincent JL, Laterre PF, et al: Efficacy and safety of recombinant human activated protein C for severe sepsis, *N Engl J Med* 344:699-709, 2001.
95. Ramadori G, Christ B: Cytokines and the hepatic acute-phase response, *Semin Liver Dis* 19(2):141-155, 1999.
96. Topper MJ, Prasse KW: Analysis of coagulation proteins as acute-phase reactants in horses with colic, *Am J Vet Res* 59(5):542-545, 1998.
97. Nunokawa Y, Fujunaga T, Taira T, et al: Evaluation of serum amyloid A protein as an acute-phase reactive protein in horses, *J Vet Med Sci* 55(6):1011-1016, 1993.
98. Hultén C, Demmers S: Serum amyloid A (SAA) as an aid in the management of infectious disease in the foal: comparison with total leucocyte count, neutrophil count and fibrinogen, *Equine Vet J* 34(7):693-698, 2002.
99. Jacobsen S, Kjelgaard-Hansen M: Hagbard Petersen H, Jensen AL: Evaluation of a commercially available human serum amyloid A (SAA) turbidometric immunoassay for determination of equine SAA concentrations, *Vet J* 172(2):315-319, 2006.
100. Muir WW: Shock, *Compend Cont Educ Pract Vet* 20(5):549-566, 1998.
101. Burrows GE: Escherichia coli endotoxemia in the conscious pony, *Am J Vet Res* 32(2):243-248, 1971.
102. Clark ES, Collatos C: Hypoperfusion of the small intestine during slow infusion of a low dosage of endotoxin in anesthetized horses, *Cornell Vet* 80(2):163-172, 1990.
103. Armstrong GP: Cellular and humoral immunity in the horseshoe crab. In Gupta AP, editor: *Limulus polyphemus: immunology of insects and other arthropods*, Boca Raton, Fla, 1991, CRC Press.
104. Shuster R, Traub-Dargatz J, Baxter G: Survey of diplomates of the American College of Veterinary Internal Medicine and the American College of Veterinary Surgeons regarding clinical aspects and treatment of endotoxemia in horses, *J Am Vet Med Assoc* 210(1):87-92, 1997.
105. Dinarello CA, Cannon JG, Wolff SM, et al: Tumor necrosis factor (cachectin) is an endogenous pyrogen and induces production of interleukin 1, *J Exp Med* 163(6):1433-1450, 1986.
106. Coceani F, Bishai I, Dinarello CA, et al: Prostaglandin E2 and thromboxane B2 in cerebrospinal fluid of afebrile and febrile cat, *Am J Physiol* 244(6):R785-R793, 1983.
107. Parsons CS, Orsini JA, Krafty R, et al: Risk factors for development of acute laminitis in horses during hospitalization: 73 cases (1997-2004), *J Am Vet Med Assoc* 230(6):885-889, 2007.
108. Daels PF, Stabenfeldt GH, Hughes JP, et al: Evaluation of progesterone deficiency as a cause of fetal death in mares with experimentally induced endotoxemia, *Am J Vet Res* 52(2):282-288, 1991.
109. Daels PF, Stabenfeldt GH, Hughes JP, et al: Effects of flunixin meglumine on endotoxin-induced prostaglandin F2 alpha secretion during early pregnancy in mares, *Am J Vet Res* 52(2):276-281, 1991.

110. Ingle-Fehr JE, Baxter GM: Evaluation of digital and laminar blood flow in horses given a low dose of endotoxin, *Am J Vet Res* 59(2):192-196, 1998.
111. Menzies-Gow NJ, Bailey SR, Katz LM, et al: Endotoxin-induced digital vasoconstriction in horses: associated changes in plasma concentrations of vasoconstrictor mediators, *Equine Vet J* 36(3):273-278, 2004.
112. Zerpa H, Verga Fm Vasquez J, et al: Effect of sublethal endotoxemia on in vitro digital vascular reactivity in horses, *J Am Vet Med Assoc* 52:67-73, 2005.
113. Menzies-Gow NJ, Bailey SR, Berhane Y, et al: Evaluation of the induction of vasoactive mediators from equine digital vein endothelial cells by endotoxin, *Am J Vet Res* 69(3):349-355, 2008.
114. Zaloga GP, Chernow B: The multifactorial basis for hypocalcemia during sepsis: studies of the parathyroid hormone-vitamin D axis, *Ann Intern Med* 107(1):36-41, 1987.
115. Dart AJ, Snyder JR, Spier SJ, et al: Ionized calcium concentration in horses with surgically managed gastrointestinal disease: 147 cases (1988-1990), *J Am Vet Med Assoc* 201(8):1244-1248, 1992.
116. Lavoie JP, Madigan JE, Cullor JS, et al: Haemodynamic, pathological, haematological and behavioural changes during endotoxin infusion in equine neonates, *Equine Vet J* 22(1): 23-29, 1990.
117. Welch RD, Watkins JP, Taylor TS, et al: Disseminated intravascular coagulation associated with colic in 23 horses (1984-1989), *J Vet Intern Med* 6(1):29-35, 1992.
118. Olson NC: Effects of endotoxin on lung water, hemodynamics, and gas exchange in anesthetized ponies, *Am J Vet Res* 46(11):2288-2293, 1985.
119. Moore JN, Barton MH: An update on endotoxemia part 2: treatment and the way ahead, *Equine Vet Educ* 11(1):30-34, 1999.
120. Weese JS, Cote NM, DeGannes RVG: Evaluation of in vitro properties of di-tri-octahedral smectite on clostridial toxins and growth, *Equine Vet J* 35(7):638-641, 2003.
121. Bentley AP, Barton MH, Norton N, et al: Antimicrobial-induced endotoxin and cytokine activity in an in vitro model of septicemia in foals, *Am J Vet Res* 63(5):660-668, 2002.
122. Sprouse RF, Garner HE, Lager K: Protection of ponies from heterologous and homologous endotoxin challenges via Salmonella typhimurium bacterin-toxoid, *Equine Pract* 11(2):34-40, 1989.
123. Garner HE, Sprouse RF, Green EM: Active and passive immunization for blockade of endotoxemia. *Proceedings of the thirty-first annual convention of the American Association of Equine Practitioners*, Toronto, 1985, Canada.
124. Ziegler EJ, Fisher CJ Jr, Sprung CL, et al: Treatment of gram-negative bacteremia and septic shock with HA-1A human monoclonal antibody against endotoxin: a randomized, doubleblind, placebo-controlled trial, The HA-1A Sepsis Study Group, *N Engl J Med* 324(7):429-436, 1991.
125. Ziegler EJ, McCutchan JA, Fierer J, et al: Treatment of gram-negative bacteremia and shock with human antiserum to a mutant Escherichia coli, *N Engl J Med* 307(20):1225-1230, 1982.
126. Sakulramrung R, Domingue GJ: Cross-reactive immunoprotective antibodies to Escherichia coli O111 rough mutant J5, *J Infect Dis* 151(6):995-1004, 1985.
127. Garner HE, Sprouse RF, Lager K: Cross-protection of ponies from sublethal Escherichia coli endotoxemia by Salmonella typhimurium antiserum, *Equine Pract* 10(4):10-17, 1988.
128. Spier SJ, Lavoie JP, Cullor JS, et al: Protection against clinical endotoxemia in horses by using plasma containing antibody to an Rc mutant E. coli (J5), *Circ Shock* 28(3):235-248, 1989.
129. Gaffin SL, Baker B, DuPreez J, et al: Prophylaxis and therapy with anti-endotoxin hyperimmune serum against gastroenteritis and endotoxemia in horses. *Proceedings of the twenty-eighth annual convention of the American Association of Equine Practitioners*, Atlanta, 1982, Ga.
130. Peek SF, Semrad S, McGuirk SM, et al: Prognostic value of clinicopathologic variables obtained at admission and effect of antiendotoxin plasma on survival in septic and critically ill foals, *J Vet Int Med* 20:569-574, 2006.
131. Durando MM, MacKay RJ, Linda S, et al: Effects of polymyxin B and Salmonella typhimurium antiserum on horses given endotoxin intravenously, *Am J Vet Res* 55(7):921-927, 1994.
132. Morris DD, Whitlock RH, Corbeil LB: Endotoxemia in horses: protection provided by antiserum to core lipopolysaccharide, *Am J Vet Res* 47(3):544-550, 1986.
133. Morris DD, Whitlock RH: Therapy of suspected septicemia in neonatal foals using plasma-containing antibodies to core lipopolysaccharide (LPS), *J Vet Intern Med* 1(4):175-182, 1987.
134. Cohen ND, Divers T: Acute colitis in horses. 2. Initial management, *Compend Cont Educ Pract Vet* 20:228-234, 1998.
135. Coyne CP, Fenwick BW: Inhibition of lipopolysaccharide-induced macrophage tumor necrosis factor-alpha synthesis by polymyxin B sulfate, *Am J Vet Res* 54(2):305-314, 1993.
136. Parviainen AK, Barton MH, Norton NN: Evaluation of polymyxin B in an ex vivo model of endotoxemia in horses, *Am J Vet Res* 62(1):72-76, 2001.
137. Barton MH: Use of polymyxin B for treatment of endotoxemia in horses, *Compend Cont Educ Pract Vet* 11:1056-1059, 2000.
138. Raisbeck MF, Garner HE, Osweiler GD: Effects of polymyxin B on selected features of equine carbohydrate overload, *Vet Hum Toxicol* 31(5):422-426, 1989.
139. Barton MH, Parviainen AK: *Use of polymyxin B for equine endotoxemia. Proceedings of the American College of Veterinary Internal Medicine Forum*, Seattle, May 25-28, 2000, Wash.
140. Morresey PR, MacKay RJ: Endotoxin-neutralizing activity of polymyxin B in blood after IV administration in horses, *Am J Vet Res* 67:642-647, 2006.
141. Coyne CP, Moritz JT, Fenwick BW: Inhibition of lipopolysaccharide-induced TNF-alpha production by semisynthetic polymyxin-B conjugated dextran, *Biotechnol Ther* 5(3-4):137-162, 1994.
142. MacKay RJ, Clark CK, Logdberg L, et al: Effect of a conjugate of polymyxin B-dextran 70 in horses with experimentally induced endotoxemia, *Am J Vet Res* 60(1):68-75, 1999.
143. Hellman J, Warren HS: Antiendotoxin strategies, *Infect Dis Clin N Am* 13(2):371-386, 1999.
144. Weiss J, Olsson I: Cellular and subcellular localization of the bactericidal/permeability-increasing protein of neutrophils, *Blood* 69(2):652-659, 1987.
145. Weersink AJ, van Kessel KP, van den Tol ME, et al: Human granulocytes express a 55-kDa lipopolysaccharide-binding protein on the cell surface that is identical to the bactericidal/permeability-increasing protein, *J Immunol* 150(1):253-263, 1993.
146. Abrahamson SL, Wu HM, Williams RE, et al: Biochemical characterization of recombinant fusions of lipopolysaccharide binding protein and bactericidal/permeability-increasing protein: implications in biological activity, *J Biol Chem* 272(4):2149-2155, 1997.
147. Vaara M: Lipid A: target for antibacterial drugs, *Science* 274(5289):939-940, 1996.
148. Levin M, Quint PA, Goldstein B, et al: Recombinant bactericidal/permeability-increasing protein (rBPI21) as adjunctive treatment for children with severe meningococcal sepsis: a randomised trial, rBPI21 Meningococcal Sepsis Study Group, *Lancet* 356(9234):961-967, 2000.
149. Winchell WW, Hardy J, Levine DM, et al: Effect of administration of a phospholipid emulsion on the initial response of horses administered endotoxin, *Am J Vet Res* 63(10):1370-1378, 2002.
150. Moore JN, Norton N, Barton MH, et al: Rapid infusion of a phospholipid emulsion attentuates the effects of endotoxaemia in horses, *Equine Vet J* 39(3):243-248, 2007.

151. Lei MG, Qureshi N, Morrison DC: Lipopolysaccharide (LPS) binding to 73-kDa and 38-kDa surface proteins on lymphoreticular cells: preferential inhibition of LPS binding to the former by Rhodopseudomonas sphaeroides lipid A, *Immunol Lett* 36(3):245-250, 1993.
152. Golenbock DT, Hampton RY, Qureshi N, et al: Lipid A-like molecules that antagonize the effects of endotoxins on human monocytes, *J Biol Chem* 266(29):19490-19498, 1991.
153. Zuckerman SH, Qureshi N: In vivo inhibition of lipopolysaccharide-induced lethality and tumor necrosis factor synthesis by Rhodobacter sphaeroides diphosphoryl lipid A is dependent on corticosterone induction, *Infect Immun* 60(7):2581-2587, 1992.
154. Christ WJ, Asano O, Robidoux AL, et al: E5531, a pure endotoxin antagonist of high potency, *Science* 268(5207):80-83, 1995.
155. Bunnell E, Lynn M, Habet K, et al: A lipid A analog, E5531, blocks the endotoxin response in human volunteers with experimental endotoxemia, *Crit Care Med* 28(8):2713-2720, 2000.
156. Rossignol DP, Lynn M: Antagonism of in vivo and ex vivo response to endotoxin by E5564, a synthetic lipid A analogue, *J Endotoxin Res* 8(6):483-488, 2002.
157. Lohmann KL, Vandenplas M, Barton MH, Moore JN: Lipopolysaccharide from Rhodobacter sphaeroides is an agonist in equine cells, *J Endotoxin Res* 9(1):33-37, 2003.
158. Bryant CE, Oullette A, Lohmann K, et al: The cellular Toll-like receptor 4 antagonist E5531 can act as an agonist in horse whole blood, *Vet Immunol Immunopathol* 116(3-4):182-189, 2007.
159. Lohmann KL, Vandenplas ML, Barton MH, et al: The equine TLR4/MD-2 complex mediates recognition of lipopolysaccharide from Rhodobacter sphaeroides as an agonist *J Endotoxin Res* 13(4):235-242, 2007.
160. Breuhaus BA, DeGraves FJ, Honore EK, et al: Pharmacokinetics of ibuprofen after intravenous and oral administration and assessment of safety of administration to healthy foals, *Am J Vet Res* 60(9):1066-1073, 1999.
161. Fink MP: Eicosanoids and platelet activating factor in the pathogenesis of sepsis and organ dysfunction. In Williams JG, editor: *Multiple organ dysfunction syndrome: examining the role of eicosanoids and procoagulants*, Austin, Tex, 1996, RG Landes.
162. Ewert KM, Fessler JF, Templeton CB, et al: Endotoxin-induced hematologic and blood chemical changes in ponies: effects of flunixin meglumine, dexamethasone, and prednisolone, *Am J Vet Res* 46(1):24-30, 1985.
163. Moore JN, Garner HE, Shapland JE, et al: Prevention of endotoxin-induced arterial hypoxaemia and lactic acidosis with flunixin meglumine in the conscious pony, *Equine Vet J* 13(2):95-98, 1981.
164. Moore JN, Hardee MM, Hardee GE: Modulation of arachidonic acid metabolism in endotoxic horses: comparison of flunixin meglumine, phenylbutazone, and a selective thromboxane synthetase inhibitor, *Am J Vet Res* 47(1):110-113, 1986.
165. Gerdemann R, Deegen E, Kietzmann M, et al: [Effect of flunixin meglumine on plasma prostanoid concentrations in horses with colic in the perioperative period], *Dtsch Tierarztl Wochenschr* 104(9):365-368, 1997.
166. Templeton CB, Bottoms GD, Fessler JF, et al: Effects of repeated endotoxin injections on prostanoids, hemodynamics, endothelial cells, and survival in ponies, *Circ Shock* 16(3):253-264, 1985.
167. Bottoms GD, Fessler JF, Roesel OF, et al: Endotoxin-induced hemodynamic changes in ponies: effects of flunixin meglumine, *Am J Vet Res* 42(9):1514-1518, 1981.
168. Fessler JF, Bottoms GD, Roesel OF, et al: Endotoxin-induced change in hemograms, plasma enzymes, and blood chemical values in anesthetized ponies: effects of flunixin meglumine, *Am J Vet Res* 43(1):140-144, 1982.
169. Tomlinson JE, Blikslager AT: Effects of cyclooxygenase inhibitors flunixin and deracoxib on permeability of ischaemic-injured equine jejunum, *Equine Vet J* 37(1):75-80, 2005.
170. Little D, Brown SA, Campbell NB, et al: Effects of cyclooxygenase inhibitor meloxicam on recovery of ischemia-injured equine jejunum, *Am J Vet Res* 68(6):614-624, 2007.
171. MacAllister CG, Morgan SJ, Borne AT, et al: Comparison of adverse effects of phenylbutazone, flunixin meglumine, and ketoprofen in horses, *J Am Vet Med Assoc* 202(1):71-77, 1993.
172. King JN, Gerring EL: Antagonism of endotoxin-induced disruption of equine bowel motility by flunixin and phenylbutazone, *Equine Vet J* (Suppl 7):38-42, 1989.
173. Semrad SD, Hardee GE, Hardee MM, et al: Low dose flunixin meglumine: effects on eicosanoid production and clinical signs induced by experimental endotoxaemia in horses, *Equine Vet J* 19(3):201-206, 1987.
174. Jackman BR, Moore JN, Barton MH, et al: Comparison of the effects of ketoprofen and flunixin meglumine on the in vitro response of equine peripheral blood monocytes to bacterial endotoxin, *Can J Vet Res* 58(2):138-143, 1994.
175. MacKay RJ, Daniels CA, Bleyaert HF, et al: Effect of eltenac in horses with induced endotoxaemia, *Equine Vet J* Suppl 32:26-31, 2000.
176. Morris DD, Moore JN, Crowe N, et al: Dexamethasone reduces endotoxin-induced tumor necrosis factor activity production in vitro by equine peritoneal macrophages, *Cornell Vet* 81(3):267-276, 1991.
177. Frauenfelder HC, Fessler JF, Moore AB, et al: Effects of dexamethasone on endotoxin shock in the anesthetized pony: hematologic, blood gas, and coagulation changes, *Am J Vet Res* 43(3):405-411, 1982.
178. Annane D: Corticosteroids for septic shock, *Crit Care Med* 29(Suppl 7):S117-S120, 2001.
179. Gold JR, Divers TJ, Barton MH, et al: Plasma adrenocorticotropin, cortisol, and adrenocorticotropin/cortisol ratios in septic and normal-term foals, *J Vet Intern Med* 21(4):791-796, 2007.
180. Barton MH, Moore JN: Pentoxifylline inhibits mediator synthesis in an equine in vitro whole blood model of endotoxemia, *Circ Shock* 44(4):216-220, 1994.
181. Barton MH, Moore JN, Norton N: Effects of pentoxifylline infusion on response of horses to in vivo challenge exposure with endotoxin, *Am J Vet Res* 58(11):1300-1307, 1997.
182. Baskett A, Barton MH, Norton N, et al: Effect of pentoxifylline, flunixin meglumine, and their combination on a model of endotoxemia in horses, *Am J Vet Res* 58(11):1291-1299, 1997.
183. Ingle-Fehr JE, Baxter GM: The effect of oral isoxsuprine and pentoxifylline on digital and laminar blood flow in healthy horses, *Vet Surg* 28(3):154-160, 1999.
184. Arden WA, Slocombe RF, Stick JA, et al: Morphologic and ultrastructural evaluation of effect of ischemia and dimethyl sulfoxide on equine jejunum, *Am J Vet Res* 51(11):1784-1791, 1990.
185. Moore RM, Muir WW, Bertone AL, et al: Effects of dimethyl sulfoxide, allopurinol, 21-aminosteroid U-74389G, and manganese chloride on low-flow ischemia and reperfusion of the large colon in horses, *Am J Vet Res* 56(5):671-687, 1995.
186. Kelmer G, Doherty TJ, Elliott S, et al: Evaluation of dimethyl sulphoxide effects on initial response to endotoxin in the horse, *Equine Vet J*, Jun; 40(4): 358-363, 2008.
187. Weisiger RA: Oxygen radicals and ischemic tissue injury, *Gastroenterology* 90(2):494-496, 1986.
188. Grisham MB, Hernandez LA, Granger DN: Xanthine oxidase and neutrophil infiltration in intestinal ischemia, *Am J Physiol* 251(4 Pt 1):G567-G574, 1986.

189. Lochner F, Sangiah S, Burrows G, et al: Effects of allopurinol in experimental endotoxin shock in horses, *Res Vet Sci* 47(2):178-184, 1989.
190. Taniguchi T, Shibata K, Yamamoto K, et al: Effects of lidocaine administration on hemodynamics and cytokine responses to endotoxemia in rabbits, *Crit Care Med* 28(3):755-759, 2000.
191. Cook VL, Jones Shults J, McDowell M, et al: Attenuation of ischaemic injury in the equine jejunum by administration of systemic lidocaine, *Equine Vet J*, Jun; 40(4):358-363, 2008.
192. Carrick JB, McCann ME: The effect of short-term administration of omega 3 fatty acids on endotoxemia, *Proceedings of the American College of Veterinary Internal Medicine Forum*, 1997:Lake Buena Vista, Fla.
193. Chu AJ, Walton MA, Prasad JK, et al: Blockade by polyunsaturated n-3 fatty acids of endotoxin-induced monocytic tissue factor activation is mediated by the depressed receptor expression in THP-1 cells, *J Surg Res* 87(2):217-224, 1999.
194. Morris DD, Henry MM, Moore JN, et al: Effect of dietary alpha-linolenic acid on endotoxin-induced production of tumor necrosis factor by peritoneal macrophages in horses, *Am J Vet Res* 52(4):528-532, 1991.
195. Henry MM, Moore JN, Feldman EB, et al: Effect of dietary alpha-linolenic acid on equine monocyte procoagulant activity and eicosanoid synthesis, *Circ Shock* 32(3):173-188, 1990.
196. Henry MM, Moore JN, Fischer JK: Influence of an omega-3 fatty acid-enriched ration on in vivo responses of horses to endotoxin, *Am J Vet Res* 52(4):523-527, 1991.
197. McCann ME, Moore JN, Carrick JB, et al: Effect of intravenous infusion of omega-3 and omega-6 lipid emulsions on equine monocyte fatty acid composition and inflammatory mediator production in vitro, *Shock* 14(2):222-228, 2000.
198. Cargile JL, MacKay RJ, Dankert JR, et al: Effects of tumor necrosis factor blockade on interleukin 6, lactate, thromboxane, and prostacyclin responses in miniature horses given endotoxin, *Am J Vet Res* 56(11):1445-1450, 1995.
199. Cargile JL, MacKay RJ, Dankert JR, et al: Effect of treatment with a monoclonal antibody against equine tumor necrosis factor (TNF) on clinical, hematologic, and circulating TNF responses of miniature horses given endotoxin, *Am J Vet Res* 56(11):1451-1459, 1995.
200. Barton MH, Bruce EH, Moore JN, et al: Effect of tumor necrosis factor antibody given to horses during early experimentally induced endotoxemia, *Am J Vet Res* 59(6):792-797, 1998.
201. MacKay RJ, Socher SH: Anti-equine tumor necrosis factor (TNF) activity of antisera raised against human TNF-alpha and peptide segments of human TNF-alpha, *Am J Vet Res* 53(6):921-924, 1992.
202. Abraham E, Wunderink R, Silverman H, et al: Efficacy and safety of monoclonal antibody to human tumor necrosis factor alpha in patients with sepsis syndrome: a randomized, controlled, double-blind, multicenter clinical trial, TNF-alpha MAb Sepsis Study Group, *JAMA* 273(12):934-941, 1995.
203. Fisher CJ Jr, Opal SM, Dhainaut JF, et al: Influence of an anti-tumor necrosis factor monoclonal antibody on cytokine levels in patients with sepsis, The CB0006 Sepsis Syndrome Study Group, *Crit Care Med* 21(3):318-327, 1993.
204. Wilson DV, Eberhart SW, Robinson NE, et al: Cardiovascular responses to exogenous platelet-activating factor (PAF) in anesthetized ponies, and the effects of a PAF antagonist, WEB 2086, *Am J Vet Res* 54(2):274-279, 1993.
205. Jarvis GE, Evans RJ: Platelet-activating factor and not thromboxane A_2 is an important mediator of endotoxin-induced platelet aggregation in equine heparinised whole blood in vitro, *Blood Coagul Fibrinolysis* 7(2):194-198, 1996.
206. King JN, Gerring EL: Antagonism of endotoxin-induced disruption of equine gastrointestinal motility with the platelet-activating factor antagonist WEB 2086, *J Vet Pharmacol Ther* 13(4):333-339, 1990.
207. Mills PC, Ng JC, Seawright AA, et al: Kinetics, dose response, tachyphylaxis and cross-tachyphylaxis of vascular leakage induced by endotoxin, zymosan-activated plasma and platelet-activating factor in the horse, *J Vet Pharmacol Ther* 18(3):204-209, 1995.
208. Dawson J, Lees P, Sedgwick AD: Platelet activating factor as a mediator of equine cell locomotion, *Vet Res Commun* 12(2-3):101-107, 1988.
209. Foster AP, Lees P, Cunningham FM: Platelet activating factor is a mediator of equine neutrophil and eosinophil migration in vitro, *Res Vet Sci* 53(2):223-229, 1992.
210. Carrick JB, Morris DD, Moore JN: Administration of a receptor antagonist for platelet-activating factor during equine endotoxaemia, *Equine Vet J* 25(2):152-157, 1993.
211. Bertone JJ, Gossett KA, Shoemaker KE, et al: Effect of hypertonic vs isotonic saline solution on responses to sublethal Escherichia coli endotoxemia in horses, *Am J Vet Res* 51(7):999-1007, 1990.
212. Pantaleon LG, Furr MO, McKenzie HC II, Donaldson L: Cardiovascular and pulmonary effects of hetastarch plus hypertonic saline solutions during experimental endotoxemia in anesthetized horses, *J Vet Int Med* 20(6):1422-1428, 2006.
213. McFarlane D: Hetastarch: a synthetic colloid with potential in equine patients, *Compend Cont Educ Pract Vet* 21(9): 867-877, 1999.
214. Jones PA, Bain FT, Byars TD, et al: Effect of hydroxyethyl starch infusion on colloid oncotic pressure in hypoproteinemic horses, *J Am Vet Med Assoc* 218(7):1130-1135, 2001.
215. Cohen ND, Divers T: Equine colitis, *Proceedings of the fifteenth American College of Veterinary Internal Medicine Forum*, 1997:Lake Buena Vista, Fla.
216. Turkan H, Ural A, Beyan C, et al: Effects of hydroxyethyl starch on blood coagulation profile, *Eur J Anaesthesiol* 16(3):156-159, 1999.
217. Jones PA, Tomasic M, Gentry PA: Oncotic, hemodilutional, and hemostatic effects of isotonic saline and hydroxyethyl starch solutions in clinically normal ponies, *Am J Vet Res* 58(5):541-548, 1997.
218. Meister D, Hermann M, Mathis GA: Kinetics of hydroxyethyl starch in horses, *Schweiz Arch Tierheilkd* 134(7):329-339, 1992.
219. Moore JN, Garner HE, Shapland JE, et al: Lactic acidosis and arterial hypoxemia during sublethal endotoxemia in conscious ponies, *Am J Vet Res* 41(10):1696-1698, 1980.
220. Hosgood G: Pharmacologic features and physiologic effects of dopamine, *J Am Vet Med Assoc* 197(9):1209-1211, 1990.
221. Corley KT, McKenzie HC, Amoroso LM, et al: Initial experience with norepinephrine infusion in hypotensive critically ill foals, *J Vet Emerg Crit Care* 10(4):267-276, 2000.
222. Moore BR, Hinchcliff KW: Heparin: a review of its pharmacology and therapeutic use in horses, *J Vet Intern Med* 8(1):26-35, 1994.
223. Mahaffey EA, Moore JN: Erythrocyte agglutination associated with heparin treatment in three horses, *J Am Vet Med Assoc* 189(11):1478-1480, 1986.
224. Moore JN, Mahaffey EA, Zboran M: Heparin-induced agglutination of erythrocytes in horses, *Am J Vet Res* 48(1):68-71, 1987.
225. Monreal L, Villatoro AJ, Monreal M, et al: Comparison of the effects of low-molecular-weight and unfractioned heparin in horses, *Am J Vet Res* 56(10):1281-1285, 1995.
226. Weiss DJ, Evanson OA, McClenahan D, et al: Evaluation of platelet activation and platelet-neutrophil aggregates in ponies with alimentary laminitis, *Am J Vet Res* 58(12): 1376-1380, 1997.
227. Jarvis GE, Evans RJ: Endotoxin-induced platelet aggregation in heparinised equine whole blood in vitro, *Res Vet Sci* 57(3):317-324, 1994.

228. Daels PF, Starr M, Kindahl H, et al: Effect of Salmonella typhimurium endotoxin on PGF-2 alpha release and fetal death in the mare, *J Reprod Fertil Suppl* 35:485-492, 1987.
229. Youngquist RS, Threlfall W, editors: *Current therapy in large animal theriogenology*, ed 2, St Louis, 2007, Saunders.
230. Baxter GM: Alterations of endothelium-dependent digital vascular responses in horses given low-dose endotoxin, *Vet Surg* 24(2):87-96, 1995.

Oral Diseases

1. Getty R, editor: *Sisson and Grossman's the anatomy of domestic animals*, Philadelphia, 1975, Saunders.
2. Lindsay FE, Burton FL: Observational study of "urine testing" in the horse and donkey stallion, *Equine Vet J* 15:330-336, 1983.
3. Harvey CE: *Veterinary dentistry*, Philadelphia, 1985, Saunders.
4. Bonin SJ, Clayton HM, Lanovaz JL, Johnston T: Comparison of mandibular motion in horses chewing hay and pellets, *Equine Vet J* 39:258-262, 2007.
5. Baker GJ: Fluroscopic investigations of swallowing in the horse, *Vet Radiol* 23:84-88, 1982.
6. Klebe EA, Holcombe SJ, Rosenstein D, et al: The effect of bilateral glossopharyngeal nerve anaesthesia on swallowing in horses, *Equine Vet J* 37:65-69, 2005.
7. Heffron CJ, Baker GJ, Lee R: Fluoroscopic Investigation of Pharyngeal Function in the Horse, *Equine Veterinary Journal* 11:148-152, 1979.
8. Clark ES, Morris DD, Whitlock RH: Esophageal dysfunction in a weanling thoroughbred, *Cornell Vet* 77:151-160, 1987.
9. Freeman DE, Naylor JM: Cervical esophagostomy to permit extraoral feeding of the horse, *J Am Vet Med Assoc* 172:314-320, 1978.
10. Sweeney RW, Hansen TO: Use of a liquid diet as the sole source of nutrition in six dysphagic horses and as a dietary supplement in seven hypophagic horses, *J Am Vet Med Assoc* 197:1030-1032, 1990.
11. Stick JA, Robinson NE, Krehbiel JD: Acid-base and electrolyte alterations associated with salivary loss in the pony, *Am J Vet Res* 42:733-737, 1981.
12. Jones SL, Zimmel D, Tate LP, Campbell N, et al: Case presentation: dysphagia caused by squamous cell carcinoma in two horses, *Compend Cont Educ Pract Vet* 23:1020-1024, 2001.
13. Dixon PM, Tremaine WH, Pickles K, et al: Equine dental disease part 2: a long-term study of 400 cases: disorders of development and eruption and variations in position of the cheek teeth, *Equine Vet J* 31:519-528, 1999.
14. Quinn GC, Tremaine WH, Lane JG: Supernumerary cheek teeth (n = 24): clinical features, diagnosis, treatment and outcome in 15 horses, *Equine Vet J* 37:505-509, 2005.
15. Colahan PC, Mayhew IG, Merrit AM, et al: Equine medicine and surgery, American Veterinary Publications, *Goleta, Calif,* 1991.
16. Hormeyr CB: Comparative dental pathology (with particular reference to caries and paradental disease in the horse and the dog), *J S Afr Vet Med Assoc* 29:471-475, 1960.
17. Dixon PM, Tremaine WH, Pickles K, et al: Equine dental disease part 4: a long-term study of 400 cases: apical infections of cheek teeth, *Equine Vet J* 32:182-194, 2000.
18. Baker GJ: Some aspects of equine dental radiology, *Equine Vet J* 3:46-51, 1971.
19. Weller R, Livesey L, Maierl J, et al: Comparison of radiography and scintigraphy in the diagnosis of dental disorders in the horse, *Equine Vet J* 33:49-58, 2001.
20. Tietje S, Becker M, Bockenhoff G: Computed tomographic evaluation of head diseases in the horse: 15 cases, *Equine Vet J* 28:98-105, 1996.
21. Baker GJ: Some aspects of equine dental decay, *Equine Vet J* 6:127-130, 1974.
22. Farmand M, Stohler T: The median cleft of the lower lip and mandible and its surgical correction in a donkey, *Equine Vet J* 22:298-301, 1990.
23. Schumacher J, Brink P, Easley J, Pollock P: Surgical correction of wry nose in four horses, *Vet Surg* 37:142-148, 2008.
24. Gift LJ, DeBowes RM, Clem MF, et al: Brachygnathia in horses: 20 cases (1979-1989), *J Am Vet Med Assoc* (200):715-719, 1992.
25. Bankowski RA, Wichmann RW, Stuart EE: Stomatitis of cattle and horses due to yellow bristle grass (Setaria lutescens), *J Am Vet Med Assoc* 129:149-152, 1956.
26. Pusterla N, Latson KM, Wilson WD, Whitcomb MB: Metallic foreign bodies in the tongues of 16 horses, *Vet Rec* 159:485-488, 2006.
27. Snow DH, Bogan JA, Douglas TA, Thompson H: Phenylbutazone toxicity in ponies, *Vet Rec* 105:26-30, 1979.
28. Baum KH, Shin SJ, Rebhun WC, Patten VH: Isolation of Actinobacillus-Lignieresii from Enlarged Tongue of A Horse, *J Am Vet Med Assoc* 185:792-793, 1984.
29. Freestone JF, Seahorn TL: Miscellaneous conditions of the equine head, *Vet Clin North Am Equine Pract* 9:235-242, 1993.
30. Schmotzer WB, Hultgren BD, Huber MJ, et al: Chemical involution of the equine parotid salivary gland, *Vet Surg* 20:128-132, 1991.
31. Aleman M, Spier SJ, Wilson WD, Doherr M: Corynebacterium pseudotuberculosis infection in horses: 538 cases (1982-1993), *J Am Vet Med Assoc* 209:804-809, 1996.
32. Sockett DC, Baker JC, Stowe CM: Slaframine (Rhizoctonia leguminicola) intoxication in horses, *J Am Vet Med Assoc* 181:606, 1982.
33. Plumlee KH, Galey FD: Neurotoxic mycotoxins: a review of fungal toxins that cause neurological disease in large animals, *J Vet Intern Med* 8:49-54, 1994.

Esophageal Diseases

1. Getty R, editor: *Sisson and Grossman's the anatomy of domestic animals*, Philadelphia, 1975, Saunders.
2. Smith BP: *Large animal internal medicine*, ed 4, St Louis, 2008, Mosby.
3. Feige K, Schwarzwald C, Furst A, Kaser-Hotz B: Esophageal obstruction in horses: a retrospective study of 34 cases, *Can Vet J* 41:207-210, 2000.
4. Hillyer M: Management of oesophageal obstruction ('choke') in horses, In *Practice* 17:450-Jun; 40(4):353-357, 2008.
5. Duncanson GR: Equine oesophageal obstruction: a long term study of 60 cases, *Equine Vet Educ* 8, 2006:336-240.
6. Jansson N: Foreign body obstruction of the esophagus in a foal, *Compendium Equine* 1:147-150, 2006.
7. Meagher DM, Spier S: Foreign-body obstruction in the cervical esophagus of the horse - A case-report, *J Equine Vet Sci* 9:137-140, 1989.
8. Appt SA, Moll HD, Scarratt WK, Sysel AM: Esophageal foreign body obstruction in a Mustang, *Equine Practice* 18:8-11, 1996.
9. MacDonald MH, Richardson DW, Morse CC: Esophageal phytobezoar in a horse, *J Am Vet Med Assoc* 191:1455-1456, 1987.
10. Baird AN, True CK: Fragments of nasogastric tubes as esophageal foreign bodies in two horses, *J Am Vet Med Assoc* 194:1068-1070, 1989.
11. Adams R, Nicon A, Hager D: Use of intraoperative ultrasonography to identify a cervical foreign body: A case report, *Vet Surg* 16:384-388, 1987.
12. Benders NA, Veldhuis Kroeze EJ, van der Kolk JH: Idiopathic muscular hypertrophy of the oesophagus in the horse: a retrospective study of 31 cases, *Equine Vet J* 36:46-50, 2004.
13. Becht JL, Byars TD: Gastroduodenal ulceration in foals, *Equine Vet J* 18:307-312, 1986.
14. Baker SJ, Johnson PJ, David A, et al: Idiopathic gastroesophageal reflux disease in an adult horse, *J Am Vet Med Assoc* 224:1967-1970, 2004:1931.

15. Sandin A, Skidell J, Haggstrom J, et al: Postmortem findings of gastric ulcers in Swedish horses older than age one year: a retrospective study of 3715 horses, *Equine Vet J* 2000(32):36-42, 1924-1996.
16. Craig DR, Shivy DR, Pankowski RL, Erb HN: Esophageal disorders in 61 horses. Results of nonsurgical and surgical management, *Vet Surg* 18:432-438, 1989.
17. Todhunter RJ, Stick JA, Trotter GW, Boles C: Medical management of esophageal stricture in seven horses, *J Am Vet Med Assoc* 185:784-787, 1984.
18. Craig D, Todhunter R: Surgical repair of an esophageal stricture in a horse, *Vet Surg* 16:251-254, 1987.
19. Tillotson K, Traub-Dargatz JL, Twedt D: Balloon dilation of an oesophageal stricture in a one-month-old Appaloosa colt, *Equine Veterinary Education* 15:67-71, 2003.
20. Borchers-Collyer P, Wong D, Sponseller B, Sponseller B: Esophageal strictures, *Compendium Equine* 2:144-156, 2007.
21. Knottenbelt DC, Harrison LJ, Peacock PJ: Conservative treatment of oesophageal stricture in five foals, *Vet Rec* 131:27-30, 1992.
22. Wagner PC, Rantanen NW: Myotomy as a treatment for esophageal stricture in a horse, *Equine Practice* 2:40-45, 1980.
23. Hoffer RE, Barber SM, Kallfelz FA, Petro SP: Esophageal patch grafting as a treatment for esophageal stricture in a horse, *J Am Vet Med Assoc* 171:350-354, 1977.
24. Waguespack RW, Bolt DM, Hubert JD: Esophageal strictures and diverticula, *Compendium Equine* 2:194-206, 2007.
25. Lillich JD, Frees KE, Warrington K, et al: Esophagomyotomy and esophagopexy to create a diverticulum for treatment of chronic esophageal stricture in 2 horses, *Vet Surg* 30:449-453, 2001.
26. Hackett RP, Dyer RM, Hoffer RE: Surgical correction of esophageal diverticulum in a horse, *J Am Vet Med Assoc* 173:998-1000, 1978.
27. Ford TS, Schumacher J, Chaffin MK, et al: Surgical repair of an intrathoracic esophageal pulsion diverticulum in a horse, *Vet Surg* 20:316-319, 1991.
28. Frauenfelder HC, Adams SB: Esophageal diverticulectomy in a horse, *J Am Vet Med Assoc* 180:771-772, 1982.
29. Gonzalez M, Swor TM, Hines MT: Perforated epiphrenic diverticulum with secondary septic pleuritis in two horses, *Equine Vet Educ* 20:194-200, 2008.
30. Hardy J, Stewart RH, Beard WL, Yvorchuk-St-Jean K: Complications of nasogastric intubation in horses: nine cases, *J Am Vet Med Assoc* 1992(201):483-486, 1987-1989.
31. Golenz MR, Knight DA, Yvorchuk-St Jean KE: Use of a human enteral feeding preparation for treatment of hyperlipemia and nutritional support during healing of an esophageal laceration in a miniature horse, *J Am Vet Med Assoc* 200:951-953, 1992.
32. Broekman LE, Kuiper D: Megaesophagus in the horse. A short review of the literature and 18 own cases, *Vet Q* 24:199-202, 2002.
33. Bowman KF, Vaughan JT, Quick CB, Hankes GH, Redding RW, Purohit RC, Rumph PF, Powers RD, Harper NK: Megaesophagus in a colt, *J Am Vet Med Assoc* 172:334-337, 1978.
34. Green S, Green EM, Aronson E: Squamous-cell carcinoma - an unusual cause of choke in a horse, *Modern Veterinary Practice* 67:870-875, 1986.
35. Jones SL, Zimmel D, Tate LP, et al: Case presentation: dysphagia caused by squamous cell carcinoma in two horses, *Compend Cont Educ Pract Vet* 23:1020-1024, 2001.
36. Erkert RS, MacAllister CG, Higbee R, et al: Use of a neodymium: yttrium-aluminum-garnet laser to remove exuberant granulation tissue from the esophagus of a horse, *J Am Vet Med Assoc* 221:403-407, 2002:368.
37. Gaughan EM, Gift LJ, Frank RK: Tubular duplication of the cervical portion of the esophagus in a foal, *J Am Vet Med.Assoc* 201:748-750, 1992.
38. Swanstrom OG, Dade AA: Reduplication of the esophageal lumen in a quarter horse filly, *Vet Med Small Anim Clin* 74: 75-76, 1979.
39. Orsini JA, Sepesy L, Donawick WJ, McDevitt D: Esophageal duplication cyst as a cause of choke in the horse, *J Am Vet Med Assoc* 193:474-476, 1988.
40. Peek SF, De Lahunta A, Hackett RP: Combined oesophageal and tracheal duplication cyst in an Arabian filly, *Equine Vet J* 27:475-478, 1995.
41. Sams AE, Weldon AD, Rakestraw P: Surgical treatment of intramural esophageal inclusion cysts in three horses, *Vet Surg* 22:135-139, 1993.
42. Butt TD, MacDonald DG, Crawford WH, Dechant JE: Persistent right aortic arch in a yearling horse, *Can Vet J* 39:714-715, 1998.
43. Mackey VS, Large SM, Breznock EM, Arnold JS: Surgical correction of a persistent right aortic arch in a foal, *Veterinary Surgery* 15:325-328, 1986.
44. Bartels JE, Vaughan JT: Persistent right aortic arch in the horse, *J Am Vet Med Assoc* 154:406-409, 1969.
45. Petrick SW, Roos CJ, van Niekerk J: Persistent right aortic arch in a horse, *J S Afr Vet Assoc* 49:355-358, 1978.
46. van der Linde-Sipman JS, Goedegebuure SA, Kroneman J: Persistent right aortic arch associated with a persistent left ductus arteriosus and an interventricular septal defect in a horse, *Tijdschr Diergeneeskd* (Suppl 94):104, 1979.
47. Bauer S, Livesey MA, Bjorling DE, Darien BJ: Computed tomography assisted surgical correction of persistent right aortic arch in a neonatal foal, *Equine Vet Educ* 8:40-46, 2006.
48. Smith TR: Unusual vascular ring anomaly in a foal, *Can Vet J* 45:1016-1018, 2004.
49. Grevemeyer B, Kainer RA, Morgan JP: Persistent right aortic arch in foals, *Compend Equine* 3:95-102, 2008.
50. Clabough DL, Roberts MC, Robertson I: Probable congenital esophageal stenosis in a thoroughbred foal, *J Am Vet Med.Assoc* 199:483-485, 1991.
51. Barber SM, Mclaughlin BG, Fretz PB: Esophageal ectasia in a quarterhorse colt, *Can Vet J Rev Vet Can* 24:46-49, 1983.
52. Rohrbach BW: Congenital esophageal ectasia in a thoroughbred foal, *J Am Vet Med Assoc* 177:65-67, 1980.
53. Roberts MC, Kelly WR: Squamous cell carcinoma of the lower cervical oesophagus in a pony, *Equine Vet J* 11:199-201, 1979.
54. Moore JN, Kintner LD: Recurrent esophageal obstruction due to squamous cell carcinoma in a horse, *Cornell Vet* 66:590-597, 1976.
55. Murray MJ, Ball MM, Parker GA: Megaesophagus and aspiration pneumonia secondary to gastric ulceration in a foal, *J Am Vet Med Assoc* 192:381-383, 1988.
56. Scott EA, Snoy P, Prasse KW, Hoffman PE, Thrall DE: Intramural esophageal cyst in a horse, *J Am Vet Med Assoc* 171:652-654, 1977.
57. MacKay RJ: On the true definition of dysphagia, *Compend Cont Educ Pract Vet* 23:1024-1028, 2001.
58. Traver DS, Egger E, Moore JN: Retrieval of an esophageal foreign body in a horse, *Vet Med Small Anim Clin* 73:783-785, 1978.
59. Alexander JE: Radiologic findings in equine choke, *J Am Vet Med Assoc* 151:47-53, 1967.
60. Greet TR: Observations on the potential role of oesophageal radiography in the horse, *Equine Vet J* 14:73-79, 1982.
61. Quick CB, Rendano VT: Equine radiology: the esophagus, *Mod Vet Pract* 59:625-631, 1978.
62. King JN, Davies JV, Gerring EL: Contrast radiography of the equine oesophagus: effect of spasmolytic agents and passage of a nasogastric tube, *Equine Vet J* 22:133-135, 1990.
63. Meyer GA, Rashmir-Raven A, Helms RJ, Brashier M: The effect of oxytocin on contractility of the equine oesophagus: a potential treatment for oesophageal obstruction, *Equine Vet J* 32:151-155, 2000.

64. Stick JA, Robinson NE, Krehbiel JD: Acid-base and electrolyte alterations associated with salivary loss in the pony, *Am J Vet Res* 42:733-737, 1981.
65. Wooldridge AA, Eades SC, Hosgood GL, Moore RM: In vitro effects of oxytocin, acepromazine, detomidine, xylazine, butorphanol, terbutaline, isoproterenol, and dantrolene on smooth and skeletal muscles of the equine esophagus, *Am J Vet Res* 63:1732-1737, 2002.
66. Wooldridge AA, Eades SC, Hosgood GL, Moore RM: Effects of treatment with oxytocin, xylazine butorphanol, guaifenesin, acepromazine, and detomidine on esophageal manometric pressure in conscious horses, *Am J Vet Res* 63:1738-1744, 2002.
67. Kumar V, Fausto N, Abbas A: *Robbins and Cotran pathologic basis of disease*, ed 7, Philadelphia, 2005, Saunders.
68. Lang J, Blikslager A, Regina D, et al: Synergistic effect of hydrochloric acid and bile acids on the pars esophageal mucosa of the porcine stomach, *Am J Vet Res* 59:1170-1176, 1998.
69. Schoeb TR, Panciera RJ: Pathology of blister beetle (Epicauta) poisoning in horses, *Vet Pathol* 16:18-31, 1979.
70. Clark ES, Morris DD, Whitlock RH: Esophageal dysfunction in a weanling thoroughbred, *Cornell Vet* 77:151-160, 1987.
71. Greet TR, Whitwell KE: Barium swallow as an aid to the diagnosis of grass sickness, *Equine Vet J* 18:294-297, 1986.
72. Watson TD, Sullivan M: Effects of detomidine on equine oesophageal function as studied by contrast radiography, *Vet Rec* 129:67-69, 1991.
73. Clark ES, Morris DD, Whitlock RH: Esophageal manometry in horses, cows, and sheep during deglutition, *Am J Vet Res* 48:547-551, 1987.
74. Auer JA, Stick JA: *Equine surgery*, ed 3, St Louis, 2005, Saunders.
75. Suann CJ: Oesophageal resection and anastomosis as a treatment for oesophageal stricture in the horse, *Equine Vet J* 14:163-164, 1982.
76. Gideon L: Esophageal anastomosis in two foals, *J Am Vet Med Assoc* 184:1146-1148, 1984.
77. Nixon AJ, Aanes WA, Nelson AW, Messer NT: Esophagomyotomy for relief of an intrathoracic esophageal stricture in a horse, *J Am Vet Med Assoc* 183:794-796, 1983.
78. Freeman DE: Surgery for obstruction of the equine oesophagus and trachea, *Equine Veterinary Education* 17:135-141, 2005.
79. Freeman DE: Wounds of the esophagus and trachea, *Vet Clin North Am Equine Pract* 5:683-693, 1989.
80. Digby NJ, Burguez PN: Traumatic oesophageal rupture in the horse, *Equine Vet J* 14:169-170, 1982.
81. Lunn DP, Peel JE: Successful treatment of traumatic oesophageal rupture with severe cellulitis in a mare, *Vet Rec* 116:544-545, 1985.

Diseases of the Stomach

1. Mertz HR, Walsh JH: Peptic ulcer pathophysiology, *Med Clin North Am* 75:799-814, 1991.
2. Andrews FM, Bernard WV, Byars TD, et al: Recommendations for the diagnosis and treatment of equine gastric ulcer syndrome (EGUS), *Equine Vet Educ* 1:122-134, 1999.
3. Hammond CJ, Mason DK, Watkins KL: Gastric ulceration in mature thoroughbred horses, *Equine Vet J* 18:284-287, 1986.
4. Vatistas NJ, Snyder JR, Carlson G, et al: Epidemiological study of gastric ulceration in the thoroughbred racehorse: 202 horses 1992-1993, *Proc Am Assoc Equine Pract* 40:125-126, 1994.
5. Vatistas NJ, Snyder JR, Carlson G, et al: Cross-sectional study of gastric ulcers of the squamous mucosa in thoroughbred racehorses, *Equine Vet J Suppl* :34-39, 1999.
6. Murray MJ, Grodinsky C, Anderson CW, et al: Gastric ulcers in horses: a comparison of endoscopic findings in horses with and without clinical signs, *Equine Vet J Suppl* :68-72, 1989.
7. Murray MJ, Schusser GF, Pipers FS, Gross SJ: Factors associated with gastric lesions in thoroughbred racehorses, *Equine Vet J* 28:368-374, 1996.
8. Orsini JA, Pipers FS: Endoscopic evaluation of the relationship between training, racing, and gastric ulcers, *Vet Surg* 26:424, 1997.
9. Bell RJW, Kingston JK, Mogg TD, Perkins NR: The prevalence of gastric ulceration in racehorses in New Zealand, *N Z Vet J* 55:13-18, 2007.
10. Jonsson H, Egenvall A: Prevalence of gastric ulceration in Swedish Standardbreds in race training, *Equine Vet J* 38:209-213, 2006.
11. Begg LM, O'Sullivan CB: The prevalence and distribution of gastric ulceration in 345 racehorses, *Austr Vet J* 81:199-201, 2003.
12. McClure SR, Glickman LT, Glickman NW: Prevalence of gastric ulcers in show horses, *J Am Vet Med Assoc* 215:1130-1133, 1999.
13. Nieto JE, Snyder JR, Beldomenico P, et al: Prevalence of gastric ulcers in endurance horses: a preliminary report, *Vet J* 167:33-37, 2004.
14. Bertone J: Prevalence of gastric ulcers in elite, heavy use western performance horses, *J Vet Intern Med*, 2000:14.
15. Jeune S, Nieto J, Dechant J, Snyder J: Prevalence of gastric ulcers in Thoroughbred broodmares in pasture, *Proceedings of the 52nd Annual Convention of the American Association of Equine Practitioners*, Texas, USA, 2-6 December, 2006, San Antonio, 264.
16. Hartmann AM, Frankeny RL: A preliminary investigation into the association between competition and gastric ulcer formation in non-racing performance horses, *J Equine Vet Sci* 23:560-561, 2003.
17. Sandin A, Skidell J, Haggstrom J, Nilsson G: Postmortem findings of gastric ulcers in Swedish horses older than age one year: a retrospective study of 3715 horses, *Equine Vet J* 2000(32): 36-42, 1924-1996.
18. Chameroy KA, Nadeau JA, Bushmich SL, et al: Prevalence of non-glandular gastric ulcers in horses involved in a university riding program, *Prevalence of non-glandular gastric ulcers in horses involved in a university riding program* 26:207-211, 2006.
19. Dukti SA, Perkins S, Murphy J, et al: Prevalence of gastric squamous ulceration in horses with abdominal pain, *Equine Vet J* 38:347-349, 2006.
20. Wilson JH: Gastric and duodenal ulcers in foals: A retrospective study, *Proc Equine Colic Res Symp 2nd* :126-128, 1986.
21. Murray MJ, Grodinsky C, Cowles RR, et al: Endoscopic evaluation of changes in gastric lesions of Thoroughbred foals, *J Am Vet Med Assoc* 196:1623-1627, 1990.
22. Murray MJ: Endoscopic appearance of gastric lesions in foals: 94 cases (1987-1988), *J Am Vet Med Assoc* 195:1135-1141, 1989.
23. Murray MJ, Nout YS, Ward DL: Endoscopic findings of the gastric antrum and pylorus in horses: 162 cases (1996-2000), *J Vet Intern Med* 15:401-406, 2001.
24. Nappert G, Vrins A, Larybyere M: Gastroduodenal ulceration in foals, *Comp Contin Ed* 11:338-345, 1989.
25. Murray MJ, Grodinsky C: Regional gastric pH measurement in horses and foals, *Equine Vet J* (Suppl):73-76, 1989.
26. Nord KS: Peptic ulcer disease in the pediatric population, *Pediatr Clin North Am* 35:117-140, 1988.
27. Green EM, Sprouse RF, Jones BD: Is *Helicobacter (Campylobacter) pylori* associated with gastritis/ulcer disease in asymptomatic foals? *Proc Equine Colic Res Symp* 4:27, 1991.
28. Murray MJ: Aetiopathogenesis and treatment of peptic ulcer in the horse: a comparative review, *Equine Vet J Suppl* 13:63-74, 1992.

29. Scott DR, Marcus EA, Shirazi-Beechey SSP, et al: Evidence of Helicobacter infection in the horse, *Proc Am Soc Micro*:56, 2001.
30. Contreras M, Morales A, Garcia-Amado MA, De Vera M, Bermudez V, Gueneau P: Detection of Helicobacter-like DNA in the gastric mucosa of Thoroughbred horses, *Lett Appl Microbiol* 45:553-557, 2007.
31. Moyaert H, Decostere A, Vandamme P, et al: Helicobacter equorum sp nov., a urease-negative Helicobacter species isolated from horse faeces, *Internat Jl Sys Evol Microbiol* 57:213-218, 2007.
32. Scott D, Marcus E, Smith S, et al: A longitudinal sero-epidemiological study of Helicobacter infection in the horse, *Abstr Gen Meeting Am Soc Microbio* 103:26, 2003.
33. Moyaert A, Decostere A, Pasmans F, et al: Acute in vivo interactions of Helicobacter equorum with its equine host, *Equine Vet J* 39:370-372, 2007.
34. Argenzio RA: Comparative pathophysiology of nonglandular ulcer disease: a review of experimental studies, *Equine Vet J Suppl* :19-23, 1999.
35. Campbell-Thompson ML, Merritt AM: Basal and pentagastrin-stimulated gastric secretion in young horses, *Am J Physiol* 259:R1259-R1266, 1990.
36. Murray MJ, Schusser GF: Measurement of 24-h gastric pH using an indwelling pH electrode in horses unfed, fed and treated with ranitidine, *Equine Vet J* 25:417-421, 1993.
37. Murray MJ: Equine model of inducing ulceration in alimentary squamous epithelial mucosa, *Dig Dis Sci* 39:2530-2535, 1994.
38. Wolfe MM, Soll AH: The physiology of gastric acid secretion, *N Engl J Med* 319:1707-1715, 1988.
39. Campbell-Thompson M: Secretagogue-induced [14C] aminopyrine uptake in isolated equine parietal cells, *Am J Vet Res* 55:132-137, 1994.
40. Kitchen DL, Burrow JA, Heartless CS, Merritt AM: Effect of pyloric blockade and infusion of histamine or pentagastrin on gastric secretion in horses, *Am J Vet Res* 61:1133-1139, 2000.
41. Schubert ML, Edwards NF, Makhlouf GM: Regulation of gastric somatostatin secretion in the mouse by luminal acidity: a local feedback mechanism, *Gastroenterology* 94:317-322, 1988.
42. Lewis JJ, Goldenring JR, Asher VA, Modlin IM: Effects of epidermal growth factor on signal transduction in rabbit parietal cells, *Am J Physiol* 258:G476-G483, 1990.
43. Baker SJ, Gerring EL: Gastric pH monitoring in healthy, suckling pony foals, *Am J Vet Res* 54:959-964, 1993.
44. Sanchez LC, Lester GD, Merritt AM: Effect of ranitidine on intragastric pH in clinically normal neonatal foals, *J Am Vet Med Assoc* 212:1407-1412, 1998.
45. Sanchez LC, Lester GD, Merritt AM: Intragastric pH in critically ill neonatal foals and the effect of ranitidine, *J Am Vet Med Assoc* 218:907-911, 2001.
46. Kuusela AL: Long-term gastric pH monitoring for determining optimal dose of ranitidine for critically ill preterm and term neonates, *Arch Dis Child Fetal Neonatal Ed* 78:F151-F153, 1998.
47. Read MA, Chick P, Hardy KJ, Shulkes A: Ontogeny of gastrin, somatostatin, and the H+/K(+)-ATPase in the ovine fetus, *Endocrinology* 130:1688-1697, 1992.
48. Murray MJ, Mahaffey EA: Age-related characteristics of gastric squamous epithelial mucosa in foals, *Equine Vet J* 25:514-517, 1993.
49. De Backer A, Haentjens P, Willems G: Hydrochloric acid. A trigger of cell proliferation in the esophagus of dogs, *Dig Dis Sci* 30:884-890, 1985.
50. Tobey NA, Orlando RC: Mechanisms of acid injury to rabbit esophageal epithelium. Role of basolateral cell membrane acidification, *Gastroenterology* 101:1220-1228, 1991.
51. Orlando RC: Esophageal epithelial defense against acid injury, *J Clin Gastroenterol* 13(Suppl 2):S1-S5, 1991.
52. Orlando RC, Lacy ER, Tobey NA, Cowart K: Barriers to paracellular permeability in rabbit esophageal epithelium, *Gastroenterology* 102:910-923, 1992.
53. Bullimore SR, Corfield AP, Hicks SJ, et al: Surface mucus in the non-glandular region of the equine stomach, *Research in Veterinary Science* 70:149-155, 2001.
54. Lillemoe KD, Gadacz TR, Harmon JW: Bile absorption occurs during disruption of the esophageal mucosal barrier, *J Surg Res* 35:57-62, 1983.
55. Lang J, Blikslager A, Regina D, Eisemann J, Argenzio R: Synergistic effect of hydrochloric acid and bile acids on the pars esophageal mucosa of the porcine stomach, *Am J Vet Res* 59:1170-1176, 1998.
56. Berschneider HM, Blikslager AT, Roberts MC: Role of duodenal reflux in nonglandular gastric ulcer disease of the mature horse, *Equine Vet J Suppl* :24-29, 1999.
57. Widenhouse TV, Lester GD, Merritt AM: The effect of hydrochloric acid, pepsin, or taurocholate on the bioelectric properties of gastric squamous mucosa in horses, *Am J Vet Res*, May; 63(5):744-749, 2002.
58. Nadeau JA, Andrews FM, Mathew AG, et al: Evaluation of diet as a cause of gastric ulcers in horses, *Am J Vet Res* 61:784-790, 2000.
59. Nadeau JA, Andrews FM, Patton CS, et al: Effects of hydrochloric, acetic, butyric, and propionic acids on pathogenesis of ulcers in the nonglandular portion of the stomach of horses, *Am Jl Vet Res* 64:404-412, 2003.
60. Andrews FM, Buchanan BR, Elliott SB, et al: In vitro effects of hydrochloric and lactic acids on bioelectric properties of equine gastric squamous mucosa, *Equine Vet J*, Jun; 40(4): 301-305, 2008.
61. Muller MJ, Defize J, Hunt RH: Control of pepsinogen synthesis and secretion, *Gastroenterol Clin North Am* 19:27-40, 1990.
62. Hirschowitz BI: Pepsinogen, *Postgrad Med J* 60:743-750, 1984.
63. Konturek PC, Brzozowski T, Sliwowski Z, et al: Involvement of nitric oxide and prostaglandins in gastroprotection induced by bacterial lipopolysaccharide, *Scand J Gastroenterol* 33:691-700, 1998.
64. McGowan CM, McGowan TW, Andrews FM, Al Jassim RAM: Induction and recovery of dietary induced gastric ulcers in horses, Induction and recovery of dietary induced gastric ulcers in horses *J vet med* 21:603, 2007.
65. Lybbert T, Gibbs P, Cohen N, et al: Feeding alfalfa hay to exercising horses reduces the severity of gastric squamous mucosal ulceration, *Proc Am Assoc Equine Pract* 53:525-526, 2007.
66. Murray MJ, Eichorn ES: Effects of intermittent feed deprivation, intermittent feed deprivation with ranitidine administration, and stall confinement with ad libitum access to hay on gastric ulceration in horses, *Am J Vet Res* 57:1599-1603, 1996.
67. White G, McClure SR, Sifferman R, et al: Effects of short-term light to heavy exercise on gastric ulcer development in horses and efficacy of omeprazole paste in preventing gastric ulceration, *J Am Vet Med Assoc* 230:1680-1682, 2007.
68. Lester GD, Robertson ID, Secombe C: Risk factors for gastric ulceration in thoroughbred racehorses, *Proc Am Assoc Equine Pract* 53:529, 2007.
69. Furr M, Taylor L, Kronfeld D: The effects of exercise training on serum gastrin responses in the horse, *Cornell Vet* 84:41-45, 1994.
70. Lorenzo-Figueras M, Merritt AM: Effects of exercise on gastric volume and pH in the proximal portion of the stomach of horses, *Am J Vet Res* 63:1481-1487, 2002.
71. McClure SR, Carithers DS, Gross SJ, Murray MJ: Gastric ulcer development in horses in a simulated show or training environment, *J Am Vet Med Assoc* 227:775-777, 2005.

72. Husted L, Sanchez LC, Olsen SN, et al: Effect of paddock vs. stall housing on 24 hour gastric pH within the proximal and ventral equine stomach, *Equine Vet J*, 2008.
73. Collins LG, Tyler DE: Phenylbutazone toxicosis in the horse: a clinical study, *J Am Vet Med Assoc* 184:699-703, 1984.
74. Collins LG, Tyler DE: Experimentally induced phenylbutazone toxicosis in ponies: description of the syndrome and its prevention with synthetic prostaglandin E_2, *Am J Vet Res* 46:1605-1615, 1985.
75. Meschter CL, Gilbert M, Krook L, et al: The effects of phenylbutazone on the morphology and prostaglandin concentrations of the pyloric mucosa of the equine stomach, *Vet Pathol* 27:244-253, 1990.
76. MacKay RJ, French TW, Nguyen HT, Mayhew IG: Effects of large doses of phenylbutazone administration to horses, *Am J Vet Res* 44:774-780, 1983.
77. MacAllister CG, Morgan SJ, Borne AT, Pollet RA: Comparison of adverse effects of phenylbutazone, flunixin meglumine, and ketoprofen in horses, *J Am Vet Med Assoc* 202:71-77, 1993.
78. Roy MA, Vrins A, Beauchamp G, Doucet MY: Prevalence of ulcers of the squamous gastric mucosa in Standardbred horses, *J Vet Intern Med* 19:744-750, 2005.
79. Nicol CJ, Davidson HPD, Harris PA, et al: Study of crib-biting and gastric inflammation and ulceration in young horses, *Vet Rec* 151:658-662, 2002.
80. Furr MO, Murray MJ, Ferguson DC: The effects of stress on gastric ulceration, T3, T4, reverse T3 and cortisol in neonatal foals, *Equine Vet J* 24:37-40, 1992.
81. Murray MJ, Murray CM, Sweeney HJ, et al: Prevalence of gastric lesions in foals without signs of gastric disease: an endoscopic survey, *Equine Vet J* 22:6-8, 1990.
82. Barr BS, Wilkins PA, Del Piero F, Palmer JE: Is prophylaxis for gastric ulcers necessary in critically ill equine neonates?: A retrospective study of necropsy cases 1989-1999, *J Vet Intern Med* 14(3):328, 2000.
83. Sanchez LC, Giguere S, Javsicas LH, et al: Effect of age, feeding, and omeprazole administration on gastric tonometry in healthy neonatal foals, *J Vet Intern Med* 22:406-410, 2008.
84. Orsini JA, Donawick WJ: Surgical treatment of gastroduodenal obstructions in foals, *Vet Surg* 15:205-213, 1986.
85. Becht JL, Byars TD: Gastroduodenal ulceration in foals, *Equine Vet J* 18:307-312, 1986.
86. Campbell-Thompson ML, Merritt AM: Gastroduodenal ulceration in foals, *Proc Am Assoc Equine Pract* 33:29-40, 1987.
87. Murray MJ, Ball MM, Parker GA: Megaesophagus and aspiration pneumonia secondary to gastric ulceration in a foal, *J Am Vet Med Assoc* 192:381-383, 1988.
88. GD Lester/AM Merritt, personal communication, 2002.
89. Morris AP, Estes MK: Microbes and microbial toxins: paradigms for microbial-mucosal interactions. VIII. Pathological consequences of rotavirus infection and its enterotoxin, *Am J Physiol Gastrointest Liver Physiol* 281:G303-G310, 2001.
90. Murray MJ: Gastric ulceration in horses: 91 cases (1987-1990), *J Am Vet Med Assoc* 201:117-120, 1992.
91. Rabuffo TS, Orsini JA, Sullivan E, et al: Associations between age or sex and prevalence of gastric ulceration in Standardbred racehorses in training, *J Am Vet Assoc* 221:1156-1159, 2002.
92. Bell RJW, Kingston JK, Mogg TD: A comparison of two scoring systems for endoscopic grading of gastric ulceration in horses, *N Z Vety J* 55:19-22, 2007.
93. O'Conner MS, Steiner JM, Roussel AJ, et al: Evaluation of urine sucrose concentration for detection of gastric ulcers in horses, *Am J Vet Res* 65:31-39, 2004.
94. Hewetson M, Cohen ND, Love S, et al: Sucrose concentration in blood: a new method for assessment of gastric permeability in horses with gastric ulceration, *J Vet Intern Med* 20:388-394, 2006.
95. Taharaguchi S, Nagano A, Okai K, et al: Detection of an isoform of alpha(1)-antitrypsin in serum samples from foals with gastric ulcers, *Vet Rec* 161:338-342, 2007.
96. Campbell-Thompson ML, Merritt AM: Effect of ranitidine on gastric acid secretion in young male horses, *Am J Vet Res* 48:1511-1515, 1987.
97. Furr MO, Murray MJ: Treatment of gastric ulcers in horses with histamine type 2 receptor antagonists, *Equine Vet J Suppl* :77-79, 1989.
98. Murray MJ, Grodinsky C: The effects of famotidine, ranitidine and magnesium hydroxide/aluminium hydroxide on gastric fluid pH in adult horses, *Equine Vet J* (Suppl):52-55, 1992.
99. Lester GD, Smith RL, Robertson ID: Effects of treatment with omeprazole or ranitidine on gastric squamous ulceration in racing Thoroughbreds, *J Am Vet Med Assoc* 227:1636-1639, 2005.
100. Nieto JE, Spier SJ, Van Hoogmoed L, et al: Comparison of omeprazole and cimetidine in healing of gastric ulcers and prevention of recurrence in horses, *Equine Vet Educ* 13:260-264, 2001.
101. Plue RE, Wall HG, Daurio C, et al: Safety of omeprazole paste in foals and mature horses, *Equine Vet J* Suppl:63-66, 1999.
102. Murray MJ, Eichorn ES, Holste JE, et al: Safety, acceptability and endoscopic findings in foals and yearling horses treated with a paste formulation of omeprazole for twenty-eight days, *Equine Vet J* Suppl:67-70, 1999.
103. MacAllister CG, Sifferman RL, McClure SR, et al: Effects of omeprazole paste on healing of spontaneous gastric ulcers in horses and foals: a field trial, *Equine Vet J* Suppl:77-80, 1999.
104. Murray MJ, Haven ML, Eichorn ES, et al: Effects of omeprazole on healing of naturally-occurring gastric ulcers in thoroughbred racehorses, *Equine Vet J* 29:425-429, 1997.
105. Vatistas NJ, Snyder JR, Nieto J, et al: Acceptability of a paste formulation and efficacy of high dose omeprazole in healing gastric ulcers in horses maintained in race training, *Equine Vet J* Suppl:71-76, 1999.
106. Daurio CP, Holste JE, Andrews FM, Merritt AM, Blackford JT, Dolz F, Thompson DR: Effect of omeprazole paste on gastric acid secretion in horses, *Equine Vet J* (Suppl):59-62, 1999.
107. Andrews FM, Sifferman RL, Bernard W, et al: Efficacy of omeprazole paste in the treatment and prevention of gastric ulcers in horses, *Equine Vet J* (Suppl):81-86, 1999.
108. McClure SR, White GW, Sifferman RL, et al: Efficacy of omeprazole paste for prevention of gastric ulcers in horses in race training, *J Am Vet Med Assoc* 226:1681-1684, 2005.
109. McClure SR, White GW, Sifferman RL, et al: Efficacy of omeprazole paste for prevention of recurrence of gastric ulcers in horses in race training, *J Am Vet Med Assoc* 226:1685-1688, 2005.
110. Sanchez LC, Murray MJ, Merritt AM: Effect of omeprazole paste on intragastric pH in clinically normal neonatal foals, *Am J Vet Res* 65:1039-1041, 2004.
111. Javsicas LH, Sanchez LC: The effect of omeprazole paste on intragastric pH in clinically ill neonatal foals, *Equine Vet J* 40:41-44, 2008.
112. Merritt AM, Sanchez LC, Burrow JA, et al: Effect of GastroGard and three compounded oral omeprazole preparations on 24 h intragastric pH in gastrically cannulated mature horses, *Equine Vet J* 35:691-695, 2003.
113. Nieto JE, Spier S, Pipers FS, et al: Comparison of paste and suspension formulations of omeprazole in the healing of gastric ulcers in racehorses in active training, *J Am Vet Med Assoc* 221:1139-1143, 2002.
114. Orsini JA, Haddock M, Stine L, et al: Odds of moderate or severe gastric ulceration in racehorses receiving antiulcer medications, *J Am Vet Med Assoc* 223:336-339, 2003.
115. Andrews FM, Frank N, Sommardahl CS, et al: Effects of intravenously administrated omeprazole on gastric juice pH and gastric ulcer scores in adult horses, *J Vet Intern Med* 20:1202-1206, 2006.

116. McKeever JM, McKeever KH, Albeirci JM, et al: Effect of omeprazole on markers of performance in gastric ulcer-free standardbred horses, *Equine Vet J* (Suppl):668-671, 2006.
117. Edwards SJ, Lind T, Lundell L: Systematic review of proton pump inhibitors for the acute treatment of reflux oesophagitis, *Aliment Pharmacol Ther* 15:1729-1736, 2001.
118. Ryan CA, Sanchez LC, Giguere S, Vickroy T: Pharmacokinetics and pharmacodynamics of pantoprazole in clinically normal neonatal foals, *Equine Vet J* 37:336-341, 2005.
119. Ogihara Y, Okabe S: Effect and mechanism of sucralfate on healing of acetic acid-induced gastric ulcers in rats, *J Physiol Pharmacol* 44:109-118, 1993.
120. Borne AT, MacAllister CG: Effect of sucralfate on healing of subclinical gastric ulcers in foals, *J Am Vet Med Assoc* 202:1465-1468, 1993.
121. Geor RJ, Petrie L, Papich MG, Rousseaux C: The protective effects of sucralfate and ranitidine in foals experimentally intoxicated with phenylbutazone, *Can J Vet Res* 53:231-238, 1989.
122. Ephgrave KS, Kleiman-Wexler R, Pfaller M, et al: Effects of sucralfate vs antacids on gastric pathogens: results of a double-blind clinical trial, *Arch Surg* 133:251-257, 1998.
123. Danesh BJ, Duncan A, Russell RI: Is an acid pH medium required for the protective effect of sucralfate against mucosal injury? *Am J Med* 83:11-13, 1987.
124. Konturek SJ, Brzozowski T, Mach T, et al: Importance of an acid milieu in the sucralfate-induced gastroprotection against ethanol damage, *Scand J Gastroenterol* 24:807-812, 1989.
125. Danesh JZ, Duncan A, Russell RI, Mitchell G: Effect of intragastric pH on mucosal protective action of sucralfate, *Gut* 29:1379-1385, 1988.
126. Clark CK, Merritt AM, Burrow JA, Steible CK: Effect of aluminum hydroxide/magnesium hydroxide antacid and bismuth subsalicylate on gastric pH in horses, *J Am Vet Med Assoc* 208:1687-1691, 1996.
127. Leandro G, Pilotto A, Franceschi M, et al: Prevention of acute NSAID-related gastroduodenal damage: a meta-analysis of controlled clinical trials, *Dig Dis Sci* 46:1924-1936, 2001.
128. Sangiah S, MacAllister CC, Amouzadeh HR: Effects of misoprostol and omeprazole on basal gastric pH and free acid content in horses, *Res Vet Sci* 47:350-354, 1989.
129. Tomlinson JE, Blikslager AT: Effects of cyclooxygenase inhibitors flunixin and deracoxib on permeability of ischaemic-injured equine jejunum, *Equine Vet J* 37:75-80, 2005.
130. Ringger NC, Lester GD, Neuwirth L, et al: Effect of bethanechol or erythromycin on gastric emptying in horses, *Am J Vet Res* 57:1771-1775, 1996.
131. Campbell-Thompson ML, Brown MP, Slone DE, et al: Gastroenterostomy for treatment of gastroduodenal ulcer disease in 14 foals, *J Am Vet Med Assoc* 188:840-844, 1986.
132. Zedler ST, Embertson RM: Surgical resolution of gastric outflow obstruction in the horse, *Proc Equine Colic Res Symp* 8:196-198, 2005.
133. Elfenbein JR, Sanchez LC: Gastroduodenal ulcer disease in foals: 30 cases (1986-2006), *Proc Equine Colic Res Symp* 9, 158-159, 2008.
134. Cothran DS, Borowitz SM, Sutphen JL, et al: Alteration of normal gastric flora in neonates receiving ranitidine, *J Perinatol* 17:383-388, 1997.
135. Munroe GA: Pyloric stenosis in a yearling with an incidental finding of Capillaria hepatica in the liver, *Equine Vet J* 16:221-222, 1984.
136. Barth AD, Barber SM, McKenzie NT: Pyloric stenosis in a foal, *Can Vet J* 21:234-236, 1980.
137. Crowhurst RC, Simpson DJ, McEnery RJ, Greenwood RE: Intestinal surgery in the foal, *J S Afr Vet Assoc* 46:59-67, 1975.
138. Church S, Baker JR, May SA: Gastric retention associated with acquired pyloric stenosis in a gelding, *Equine Vet J* 18: 332-334, 1986.
139. McGill CA, Bolton JR: Gastric retention associated with a pyloric mass in two horses, *Aust Vet J* 61:190-191, 1984.
140. Laing JA, Hutchins DR: Acquired pyloric stenosis and gastric retention in a mare, *Aust Vet J* 69:68-69, 1992.
141. Campbell-Thompson ML, Merritt AM: Alimentary system: diseases of the stomach. In Colahan PT, Mayhew IG, Merritt AM, Moore JN, editors: *Equine medicine and surgery*, St Louis, 1999, Mosby, pp 699-715.
142. Valk N, Doherty TJ, Blackford JT, et al: Effect of cisapride on gastric emptying in horses following endotoxin treatment, *Equine Vet J* 30:344-348, 1998.
143. Wyse C, Murphey D, Preston T, et al: Use of the [^{13}C]octanoic acid breath test for assessment of gastric emptying in ponies: A preliminary study, *Proc Equine Colic Res Symp* (6th), 1998:40.
144. Valk N, Doherty TJ, Blackford JT, et al: Phenylbutazone prevents the endotoxin-induced delay in gastric emptying in horses, *Can J Vet Res* 62:214-217, 1998.
145. Buchanan BR, Sommardahl CS, Moore RR, Donnell RL: What is your diagnosis? Pyloric-duodenal intussusception, *J Am Vet Med Assoc* 228:1339-1340, 2006.
146. Todhunter RJ, Erb HN, Roth L: Gastric rupture in horses: a review of 54 cases, *Equine Vet J* 18:288-293, 1986.
147. Puotunen-Reinert A, Huskamp B: Experimantal duodenal obstruction in the horse, *Vet Surg* 15:420-428, 1986.
148. Kiper ML, Traub-Dargatz J, Curtis CR: Gastric rupture in horses: 50 cases (1979-1987), *J Am Vet Med Assoc* 196:333-336, 1990.
149. Steenhaut M, Vlaminck K, Gasthuys F: Surgical repair of a partial gastric rupture in a horse, *Equine Vet.J* 18:331-332, 1986.
150. Hogan PM, Bramlage LR, Pierce SW: Repair of a full-thickness gastric rupture in a horse, *J Am Vet Med Assoc* 207:338-340, 1995.
151. Owen RA, Jagger DW, Jagger F: Two cases of equine primary gastric impaction, *Vet Rec* 121:102-105, 1987.
152. Barclay WP, Foerner JJ, Phillips TN, MacHarg MA: Primary gastric impaction in the horse, *J Am Vet Med Assoc* 181:682-683, 1982.
153. Honnas CM, Schumacher J: Primary gastric impaction in a pony, *J Am Vet Med Assoc* 187:501-502, 1985.
154. Kellam LL, Johnson PJ, Kramer J, Keegan KG: Gastric impaction and obstruction of the small intestine associated with persimmon phytobezoar in a horse, *J Am Vet Med Assoc* 216:1279-1281, 2000.
155. Weldon AD, Rowland PH, Rebhun WC: Emphysematous gastritis in a horse, *Cornell Vet* 81:51-58, 1991.
156. Delesalle C, Deprez P, Vanbrantegem L, et al: Emphysematous gastritis associated with Clostridium septicum in a horse, *J Vet Intern Med* 17:115-118, 2003.

Duodentitis-Proximal Jejunitis

1. Seahorn TL, Cornick JL, Cohen ND: Prognostic indicators for horses with duodenitis-proximal jejunitis: 75 Horses (1985-1989), *J Vet Intern Med* 6:307-311, 1992.
2. White NA, Tyler DE, Blackwell RB, Allen D: Hemorrhagic fibrinonecrotic duodenitis-proximal jejunitis in horses: 20 cases (1977-1984), *J Am Vet Med Assoc* 190:311-315, 1987.
3. Blackwell RB, White NA: Duodenitis-proximal jejunitis in the horse, *Proc Equine Colic Res Symp* 1:106, 1982.
4. Johnston JK, Morris DD: Comparison of duodenitis proximal jejunitis and small intestinal-obstruction in horses: 68 cases (1977-1985), *J Am Vet Med Assoc* 191:849-854, 1987.
5. Davis JL, Blikslager AT, Catto K, Jones SL: A retrospective analysis of hepatic injury in horses with proximal enteritis (1984-2002), *J Vet Intern Med* 17:896-901, 2003.

6. Arroyo LG, Staempfli H, Rousseau JD, Weese JS: Culture evaluation of Clostridium spp. in the nasogastric reflux of horses with duodenitis proximal jejunitis, *Proc Equine Colic Res Symp* 8:51-52, 2005.
7. Schumacher J, Mullen J, Shelby R, et al: An investigation of the role of fusarium-moniliforme in duodenitis proximal jejunitis of horses, *Vet Human Toxicol* 37:39-45, 1995.
8. Cohen ND, Toby E, Roussel AJ, et al: Are feeding practices associated with duodenitis-proximal jejunitis?, *Equine Vet J* 38:526-531, 2006.
9. Perdue MH, McKay DM: Integrative immunophysiology in the intestinal mucosa, *Am J Physiol* 267:G151-G165, 1994.
10. Freeman DE: Duodenitis-proximal jejunitis, *Equine Vet Educ* 12:322-332, 2000.
11. Morris DD, Johnston JK: Peritoneal fluid constituents in horses with colic due to small intestinal disease, *Proc Equine Colic Res Symp* 2, 1986.
12. Reef VB, editor: *Equine diagnostic ultrasound*, Philadelphia, 1998, Saunders.
13. Desrochers AM: Abdominal ultrasonography of normal and colicky adult horses, *Proc AAEP Focus on Colic* :20-26, 2005.
14. Lammers TW, Roussel AJ, Boothe DM, Cohen ND: Effect of an indwelling nasogastric tube on gastric emptying rates of liquids in horses, *Am J Vet Res* 66:642-645, 2005.
15. Cruz AM, Li R, Kenney DG, Monteith G: Effects of indwelling nasogastric intubation on gastric emptying of a liquid marker in horses, *Am J Vet Res* 67:1100-1104, 2006.
16. Schmall LM, Muir WW, Robertson JT: Haemodynamic effects of small volume hypertonic saline in experimentally induced haemorrhagic shock, *Equine Vet J* 22:273-277, 1990.
17. Bertone JJ, Gossett KA, Shoemaker KE, et al: Effect of hypertonic vs isotonic saline solution on responses to sublethal Escherichia coli endotoxemia in horses, *Am J Vet Res* 51:999-1007, 1990.
18. Sellon DC, Roberts MC, Blikslager AT, et al: Effects of continuous rate intravenous infusion of butorphanol on physiologic and outcome variables in horses after celiotomy, *J Vet Intern Med* 18:555-563, 2004.
19. Durham AE, Phillips TJ, Walmsley JP, Newton JR: Nutritional and clinicopathological effects of post operative parenteral nutrition following small intestinal resection and anastomosis in the mature horse, *Equine Vet J* 36:390-396, 2004.
20. Koenig JB, Sawhney S, Cote N, LaMarre J: Effect of intraluminal distension or ischemic strangulation obstruction of the equine jejunum on jejunal motilin receptors and binding of erythromycin lactobionate, *Am J Vet Res* 67:815-820, 2006.
21. Cook VL, Blikslager AT: Use of systemically administered lidocaine in horses with gastrointestinal tract disease, *J Am Vet Med Assoc* 232:1144-1148, 2008.
22. Malone E, Ensink J, Turner T, et al: Intravenous continuous infusion of lidocaine for treatment of equine ileus, *Vet Surg* 35:60-66, 2006.
23. Cohen ND, Lester GD, Sanchez LC, et al: Evaluation of risk factors associated with development of postoperative ileus in horses, *J Am Vet Med.Assoc* 225:1070-1078, 2004.
24. Cohen ND, Faber NA, Brumbaugh GW: Use of bethanechol and metoclopramide in horses with duodenitis proximal jejunitis: 13 cases (1987-1993), *J Equine Vet Sci* 15:492-494, 1995.
25. Paradis MR: Prokinetic drugs in the treatment of proximal enteritis, *Compend Cont Educ Pract Vet* 21:1147-1149, 1999.
26. Leeth B, Robertson JT: A retrospective comparison of surgical to medical management of proximal enteritis in the horse, *Proc Am Assoc Equine Pract* 34:69-79, 1989.
27. Edwards GB: Duodenitis-proximal jejunitis (anterior enteritis) as a surgical problem, *Equine Vet Educ* 12:318-321, 2000.

Diseases Associated with Malabsorption and Maldigestion

1. Roberts MC, Kidder DE, Hill FW: Small intestinal beta-galactosidase activity in the horse, *Gut* 14:535-540, 1973.
2. Lindberg R, Nygren A, Persson SG: Rectal biopsy diagnosis in horses with clinical signs of intestinal disorders: a retrospective study of 116 cases, *Equine Vet J* 28:275-284, 1996.
3. Kemper DL, Perkins GA, Schumacher J, et al: Equine lymphocytic-plasmacytic enterocolitis: a retrospective study of 14 cases, *Equine Vet J* Suppl :108-112, 2000.
4. Gibson KT, Alders RG: Eosinophilic enterocolitis and dermatitis in two horses, *Equine Vet J* 19:247-252, 1987.
5. Murphy D, Reid SWJ, Love S: Breath hydrogen measurement in ponies: a preliminary study, *Res Vet Sci* 65:47-51, 1998.
6. Roberts MC, Hill FW: The oral glucose tolerance test in the horse, *Equine Vet J* 5:171-173, 1973.
7. Mair TS, Hillyer MH, Taylor FG, Pearson GR: Small intestinal malabsorption in the horse: an assessment of the specificity of the oral glucose tolerance test, *Equine Vet J* 23:344-346, 1991.
8. Breukink HJ: Oral mono- and disaccharide tolerance tests in ponies, *Am J Vet Res* 35:1523-1527, 1974.
9. Murphy D, Reid SW, Love S: The effect of age and diet on the oral glucose tolerance test in ponies, *Equine Vet J* 29:467-470, 1997.
10. Jacobs KA, Norman P, Hodgson DRG, Cymbaluk N: Effect of diet on the oral D-xylose absorption test in the horse, *Am J Vet Res* 43:1856-1858, 1982.
11. Pratt SE, Geor RJ, McCutcheon LJ: Effects of dietary energy source and physical conditioning on insulin sensitivity and glucose tolerance in standardbred horses, *Equine Vet J* Suppl :579-584, 2006.
12. De La Corte FD, Valberg SJ, MacLeay JM, Williamson SE, Mickelson JR: Glucose uptake in horses with polysaccharide storage myopathy, *Am J Vet Res* 60:458-462, 1999.
13. Church S, Middleton DJ: Transient glucose malabsorption in two horses: fact or artefact? *Austr Vet J* 75:716-718, 1997.
14. Love S, Mair TS, Hillyer MH: Chronic diarrhea in adult horses: a review of 51 referred cases, *Vet Rec* 130:217-219, 1992.
15. Freeman DE, Ferrante PL, Kronfeld DS, Chalupa W: Effect of food deprivation on D-xylose absorption test results in mares, *Am J Vet Res* 50:1609-1612, 1989.
16. Bolton JR, Merritt AM, Cimprich RE, et al: Normal and abnormal xylose absorption in the horse, *Cornell Vet* 66:183-197, 1976.
17. Ferrante PL, Freeman DE, Ramberg CF, Kronfeld DS: Kinetic-analysis of D-xylose distribution after intravenous administration to mares, *Am J Vet Res* 54:147-151, 1993.
18. Ferrante PL, Freeman DE, Ramberg CF, Kronfeld DS: Kinetic analysis of D-xylose absorption after its intragastric administration to mares deprived of food, *Am J Vet Res* 54:2110-2114, 1993.
19. Merritt T, Mallonee PG, Merritt AM: D-Xylose absorption in the growing foal, *Equine Vet J* 18:298-300, 1986.
20. Freeman DE: In vitro concentrative accumulation of D-xylose by jejunum from horses and rabbits, *Am J Vet Res* 54:965-969, 1993.
21. Brown CM: The diagnostic value of the D-xylose absorption test in horses with unexplained chronic weight loss, *Br Vet J* 148:41-44, 1992.
22. Roberts MC: Malabsorption syndromes in the horse, *Compend ContEduc Pract Vetn* 7:S637-S646, 1985.
23. Roberts MC: Small intestinal malabsorption in horses, *Equine Vet Educ* 12:214-219, 2000.
24. Haven M, Roberts M, Argenzio R, et al: Intestinal adaptation following 70% small bowel resection in the horse, *Pferdeheilkunde* :86-87, 1992.
25. Tate LP Jr, Ralston SL, Koch CM, Everitt JI: Effects of extensive resection of the small intestine in the pony, *Am J Vet Res* 44:1187-1191, 1983.
26. Lindberg R, Persson SG, Jones B, et al: Clinical and pathophysiological features of granulomatous enteritis and eosinophilic granulomatosis in the horse, *Zentralbl Veterinarmed A* 32:526-539, 1985.

27. Duryea JH, Ainsworth DM, Mauldin EA, et al: Clinical remission of granulomatous enteritis in a standardbred gelding following long-term dexamethasone administration, *Equine Vet J* 29:164-167, 1997.
28. Weese JS, Parsons DA, Staempfli HR: Association of Clostridium difficile with enterocolitis and lactose intolerance in a foal, *J Am Vet Med Assoc* 214(205):229-232, 1999.
29. Roberts MC: The development and distribution of mucosal enzymes in the small intestine of the fetus and young foal, *J Reprod Fertil* Suppl :717-723, 1975.
30. Martens RJ, Malone PS, Brust DM: Oral lactose tolerance test in foals: technique and normal values, *Am J Vet Res* 46:2163-2165, 1985.
31. Menzies-Gow NJ, Weller R, Bowen IM, et al: Use of nuclear scintigraphy with 99mTc-HMPAO-labelled leucocytes to assess small intestinal malabsorption in 17 horses, *Vet Rec* 153:457-462, 2003.
32. Roberts MC, Pinsent PJ: Malabsorption in the horse associated with alimentary lymphosarcoma, *Equine Vet J* 7:166-172, 1975.
33. van den HR, Franken P: Clinical aspects of lymphosarcoma in the horse: a clinical report of 16 cases, *Equine Vet J* 15:49-53, 1983.
34. Platt H: Alimentary lymphomas in the horse, *J Comp Pathol* 97:1-10, 1987.
35. Cimprich RE: Equine granulomatous enteritis, *Vet Pathol* 11:535-547, 1974.
36. Schumacher J, Edwards JF, Cohen ND: Chronic idiopathic inflammatory bowel diseases of the horse, *J Vet Intern Med* 14:258-265, 2000.
37. Lindberg R: Pathology of equine granulomatous enteritis, *J Comp Pathol* 94:233-247, 1984.
38. Merritt AM, Cimprich RE, Beech J: Granulomatous enteritis in nine horses, *J Am Vet Med Assoc* 169:603-609, 1976.
39. Fogarty U, Perl D, Good P, et al: A cluster of equine granulomatous enteritis cases: the link with aluminium, *Vet Hum Toxicol* 40:297-305, 1998.
40. Collery P, McElroy M, Sammin D, White P: Equine granulomatous enteritis linked with aluminum?, *Vet Hum Toxicol* 41:49-50, 1999.
41. Meuten DJ, Butler DG, Thomson GW, Lumsden JH: Chronic enteritis associated with malabsorption and protein-losing enteropathy in horse, *J Am Vet Med Assoc* 172:326-333, 1978.
42. Pass DA, Bolton JR: Chronic eosinophilic gastroenteritis in the horse, *Vet Pathol* 19:486-496, 1982.
43. Nimmo Wilkie JS, Yager JA, Nation PN, et al: Chronic eosinophilic dermatitis: a manifestation of a multisystemic, eosinophilic, epitheliotropic disease in five horses, *Vet Pathol* 22:297-305, 1985.
44. Pass DA, Bolton JR, Mills JN: Basophilic enterocolitis in a horse, *Vet Pathol* 21:362-364, 1984.
45. Platt H: Chronic inflammatory and lymphoproliferative lesions of the equine small intestine, *J Comp Pathol* 96: 671-684, 1986.
46. Edwards GB, Kelly DF, Proudman CJ: Segmental eosinophilic colitis: a review of 22 cases, *Equine Vet J* Suppl :86-93, 2000.
47. Scott EA, Heidel JR, Snyder SP, et al: Inflammatory bowel disease in horses: 11 cases (1988-1998), *J Am Vet Med Assoc* 214:1527-1530, 1999.
48. Sampieri F, Hinchcliff KW, Toribio RE: Tetracycline therapy of Lawsonia intracellularis enteropathy in foals, *Equine Vet J* 38:89-92, 2006.
49. Schumacher J, Schumacher J, Rolsma M, Brock KV, Gebhart CJ: Surgical and medical treatment of an Arabian filly with proliferative enteropathy caused by Lawsonia intracellularis, *J Vet Intern Med* 14:630-632, 2000.
50. Bihr TP: Protein-losing enteropathy caused by Lawsonia intracellularis in a weanling foal, *Can Vet J-Rev VetCan* 44:65-66, 2003.
51. Williams NM, Harrison LR, Gebhart CJ: Proliferative enteropathy in a foal caused by Lawsonia intracellularis-like bacterium, *J Vet Diagn Invest* 8:254-256, 1996.
52. McGurrin MK, Vengust M, Arroyo LG, Baird JD: An outbreak of Lawsonia intracellularis infection in a standardbred herd in Ontario, *Can Vet J* 48:927-930, 2007.
53. McClintock SA, Collins AM: Lawsonia intracellularis proliferative enteropathy in a weanling foal in Australia, *Austr Vet J* 82:750-752, 2004.
54. Frank N, Fishman CE, Gebhart CJ, Levy M: Lawsonia intracellularis proliferative enteropathy in a weanling foal, *Equine Vet J* 30:549-552, 1998.
55. Brees DJ, Sondhoff AH, Kluge JP, et al: Lawsonia intracellularis-like organism infection in a miniature foal, *J Am Vet Med Assoc* 215:511-514, 1999.
56. Smith DGE: Identification of equine proliferative enteropathy, *Equine Vet J* 30:452-453, 1998.
57. Lavoie JP, Drolet R, Parsons D, et al: Equine proliferative enteropathy: a cause of weight loss, colic, diarrhoea and hypoproteinaemia in foals on three breeding farms in Canada, *Equine Vet J* 32:418-425, 2000.
58. Dauvillier J, Picandet V, Harel J, et al: Diagnostic and epidemiological features of Lawsonia intracellularis enteropathy in 2 foals, *Can Vet J* 47:689-691, 2006.
59. Cooper DM, Swanson DL, Gebhart CJ: Diagnosis of proliferative enteritis in frozen and formalin-fixed, paraffin-embedded tissues from a hamster, horse, deer and ostrich using a Lawsonia intracellularis-specific multiplex PCR assay, *Vet Microbiol* 54:47-62, 1997.
60. Wilson JH, Gebhart CJ: Lawsonia proliferative enteropathy in foals: clinical features and piglet parallels, *Proc AAEP Focus on the first year of life* , 2008.
61. Duhamel GE, Wheeldon EB: Intestinal adenomatosis in a foal, *Vet Pathol* 19:447-450, 1982.
62. Frazer ML: How to diagnose and treat Lawsonia intracellularis, *Proc Am Assoc Equine Pract* 53:236-239, 2007.
63. Hayden DW, Johnson KH, Wolf CB, Westermark P: AA amyloid-associated gastroenteropathy in a horse, *J Comp Pathol* 98:195-204, 1988.
64. MacKay RJ, Iverson WO, Merritt AM: Exuberant granulation tissue in the stomach of a horse, *Equine Vet J* 13:119-122, 1981.

Inflammatory Diseases of the Gastrointestinal Tract Causing Diarrhea

1. Smith BP: Salmonella infection in horses, *Comp Cont Ed Pract Vet* 3:S4-S17, 1981.
2. Smith BP, Reina-Guerra M, Hardy AJ: Prevalence and epizootiology of equine salmonellosis, *J Am Vet Med Assoc* 172: 353-356, 1978.
3. Donahue JM: Emergence of antibiotic-resistant Salmonella agona in horses in Kentucky, *J Am Vet Med Assoc* 188:592, 1986.
4. Traub-Dargatz JL, Garber LP, Fedorka-Cray PJ, Ladely S, Ferris KE: Fecal shedding of Salmonella spp by horses in the United States during 1998 and 1999 and detection of Salmonella spp in grain and concentrate sources on equine operations, *J Am Vet Med Assoc* 217:226, 2000.
5. Traub-Dargatz JL, Salman MD, Jones RL: Epidemiologic study of salmonellae shedding in the feces of horses and potential risk factors for development of the infection in hospitalized horses, *J Am Vet Med Assoc* 196:1617, 1990.
6. House JK, Mainar-Jaime RC, Smith BP, House AM, Kamiya DY: Risk factors for nosocomial Salmonella infection among hospitalized horses, *J Am Vet Med Assoc* 214:1511, 1999.
7. Schott HC, Ewart SL, Walker RD, et al: An outbreak of salmonellosis among horses at a veterinary teaching hospital, *J Am Vet Med Assoc* 218:1152, 2001.

8. Tillotson K, Savage CJ, Salman MD, et al: Outbreak of Salmonella infantis infection in a large animal veterinary teaching hospital, *J Am Vet Med Assoc* 211:1554, 1997.
9. Mainar-Jaime RC, House JK, Smith BP, et al: Influence of fecal shedding of Salmonella organisms on mortality in hospitalized horses, *J Am Vet Med Assoc* 213:1162, 1998.
10. Hartmann FA, Callan RJ, McGuirk SM, West SE: Control of an outbreak of salmonellosis caused by drug-resistant Salmonella anatum in horses at a veterinary hospital and measures to prevent future infections, *J Am Vet Med Assoc* 209: 629, 1996.
11. Bucknell DG, Gasser RB, Irving A, Whithear K: Antimicrobial resistance in Salmonella and Escherichia coli isolated from horses, *Austr Vet J* 75:355, 1997.
12. Hartmann FA, West SE: Utilization of both phenotypic and molecular analyses to investigate an outbreak of multidrug-resistant Salmonella anatum in horses, *Can J Vet Res* 61:173, 1997.
13. Dargatz DA, Traub-Dargatz JL: Multidrug-resistant Salmonella and nosocomial infections, *Vet Clin North Am Equine Pract* 20:587, 2004.
14. Smith BP: Understanding the role of endotoxins in gram-negative sepsis, *Vet Med* 12:1148, 1986.
15. Carter JD, Hird DW, Farver TB, Hjerpe CA: Salmonellosis in hospitalized horses: seasonality and case fatality rates, *J Am Vet Med Assoc* 188:163, 1986.
16. Morse EV, Duncan MA, Page EA, Fessler JF: Salmonellosis in Equidae: a study of 23 cases, *Cornell Vet* 66:198, 1976.
17. Ernst NS, Hernandez JA, MacKay RJ, et al: Risk factors associated with fecal Salmonella shedding among hospitalized horses with signs of gastrointestinal tract disease, *J Am Vet Med Assoc* 225:275, 2004.
18. Kim LM, Morley PS, Traub-Dargatz JL, et al: Factors associated with Salmonella shedding among equine colic patients at a veterinary teaching hospital, *J Am Vet Med Assoc* 218:740, 2001.
19. Giannella RA: Pathogenesis of acute bacterial diarrheal disorders, *Annu Rev Med* 32:341, 1981.
20. Biberstein EL, Zee YC, editors: *Review of veterinary microbiology*, Boston, 1991, Blackwell Scientific.
21. Selsted ME, Miller SI, Henschen AH, Ouellette AJ: Enteric defensins: antibiotic peptide components of intestinal host defense, *J Cell Biol* 118:929, 1992.
22. Brandtzaeg P, Baekkevold ES, Farstad IN, et al: Regional specialization in the mucosal immune system: what happens in the microcompartments?, *Immunol Today* 20:141, 1999.
23. Ohl ME, Miller SI: Salmonella: a model for bacterial pathogenesis, *Annu Rev Med* 52:259, 2001.
24. Gyles CL, Thoen: *CO, Pathogenesis of bacterial infections in animals.* Ames, Iowa, 2001, Iowa University Press.
25. Moore JN, White NA, Becht JL, editors: *Proceedings of the first Equine Colic Symposium*, Lawrenceville, NJ, 1982, Veterinary Learning Systems.
26. Smith BP, Reina-Guerra M, Hoiseth SK, et al: Aromatic-dependent Salmonella typhimurium as modified live vaccines for calves, *Am J Vet Res* 45:59, 1984.
27. Sheoran AS, Timoney JF, Tinge SA, et al: Intranasal immunogenicity of a Delta cya Delta crp-pabA mutant of Salmonella enterica serotype Typhimurium for the horse, *Vaccine* 19:3787, 2001.
28. Sansonetti PJ, Phalipon A: M cells as ports of entry for enteroinvasive pathogens: mechanisms of interaction, consequences for the disease process, *Semin Immunol* 11:193, 1999.
29. Galan JE, Collmer A: Type III secretion machines: Bacterial devices for protein delivery into host cells, *Science* 284:1322, 1999.
30. Kagnoff MF, Eckmann L: Epithelial cells as sensors for microbial infection, *J Clin Invest* 100:6, 1997.
31. Vazquez-Torres A, Jones-Carson J, Baumler AJ, et al: Extraintestinal dissemination of Salmonella by CD18-expressing phagocytes, *Nature* 401:804, 1999.
32. Vazquez-Torres A, Fang FC: Oxygen-dependent anti-Salmonella activity of macrophages, *Trends Microbiol* 9:29, 2001.
33. Koo FC, Peterson JW, Houston CW, Molina NC: Pathogenesis of experimental salmonellosis: inhibition of protein synthesis by cytotoxin, *Infect Immun* 43:93, 1984.
34. Giannella RA, Gots RE, Charney AN, et al: Pathogenesis of Salmonella-mediated intestinal fluid secretion. Activation of adenylate cyclase and inhibition by indomethacin, *Gastroenterology* 69:1238, 1975.
35. Peterson JW, Molina NC, Houston CW, Fader RC: Elevated cAMP in intestinal epithelial cells during experimental cholera and salmonellosis, *Toxicon* 21:761, 1983.
36. Chopra AK, Huang JH, Xu X, et al: Role of Salmonella enterotoxin in overall virulence of the organism, *Microb Pathog* 27:155, 1999.
37. Watson PR, Galyov EE, Paulin SM, et al: Mutation of invH, but not stn, reduces Salmonella-induced enteritis in cattle, *Infect Immun* 66:1432, 1998.
38. Murray MJ: Enterotoxin activity of a Salmonella typhimurium of equine origin in vivo in rabbits and the effect of Salmonella culture lysates and cholera toxin on equine colonic mucosa in vitro, *Am J Vet Res* 47:769, 1986.
39. Giannella RA: Importance of the intestinal inflammatory reaction in salmonella-mediated intestinal secretion, *Infect Immun* 23:140, 1979.
40. O'Loughlin EV, Scott RB, Gall DG: Pathophysiology of infectious diarrhea: changes in intestinal structure and function, *J Pediatr Gastroenterol Nutr* 12:5, 1991.
41. Murray MJ: Digestive physiology of the large intestine in adult horses. Part II: Pathophysiology of colitis, *Comp Cont Educ Pract Vet* 10:1309, 1988.
42. Powell DW: Neuroimmunophysiology of the gastrointestinal mucosa: implications for inflammatory diseases, *Trans Am Clin Climatol Assoc* 106:124, 1994.
43. McCormick BA, Miller SI, Carnes D, Madara JL: Transepithelial signaling to neutrophils by salmonellae: a novel virulence mechanism for gastroenteritis, *Infection & Immunity* 63:2302, 1995.
44. Madara JL: Review article: Pathobiology of neutrophil interactions with intestinal epithelia, *Alimentary Pharmacology & Therapeutics* 11(Suppl 3):57, 2000.
45. Smith BP, Reina-Guerra M, Hardy AJ, Habasha F: Equine salmonellosis: experimental production of four syndromes, *Am J Vet Res* 40:1072, 1979.
46. Cohen ND, Woods AM: Characteristics and risk factors for failure to survive of horses with acute diarrhea: 122 cases (1990-1996), *J Am Vet Med Assoc* 214:382, 1999.
47. van Duijkeren E, Flemming C, van Oldruitenborgh-Oosterbaan MS, et al: Diagnosing salmonellosis in horses. Culturing of multiple versus single faecal samples, *Vet Q* 17:63, 1995.
48. Palmer JE, Whitlock RH, Benson CE, et al: Comparison of rectal mucosal cultures and fecal cultures in detecting Salmonella infection in horses and cattle, *Am J Vet Res* 46:697, 1985.
49. Cohen ND, Martin LJ, Simpson RB, Wallis DE, Neibergs HL: Comparison of polymerase chain reaction and microbiological culture for detection of salmonellae in equine feces and environmental samples, *Am J Vet Res* 57:780, 1996.
50. Amavisit P, Browning GF, Lightfoot D, et al: Rapid PCR detection of Salmonella in horse faecal samples, *Vet Microbiol* 79:63, 2001.
51. Kurowski PB, Traub-Dargatz JL, Morley PS, Gentry-Weeks CR: Detection of Salmonella spp in fecal specimens by use of real-time polymerase chain reaction assay, *Am J Vet Res* 63:1265, 2002.

52. Dumler JS, Barbet AF, Bekker CP, et al: Reorganization of genera in the families Rickettsiaceae and Anaplasmataceae in the order Rickettsiales: unification of some species of Ehrlichia with Anaplasma, Cowdria with Ehrlichia and Ehrlichia with Neorickettsia, descriptions of six new species combinations and designation of Ehrlichia equi and 'HGE agent' as subjective synonyms of Ehrlichia phagocytophila, *Int J Syst Evol Microbiol* 51:2145, 2001.
53. Palmer JE: Potomac horse fever, *Vet Clin North Am Equine Pract* 9:399, 1993.
54. Mulville P: Equine monocytic ehrlichiosis (Potomac horse fever): a review, *Equine Vet J* 23:400, 1991.
55. Dutta SK, Myrup AC, Rice RM, et al: Experimental reproduction of Potomac horse fever in horses with a newly isolated Ehrlichia organism, *J Clin Microbiol* 22:265, 1985.
56. Rikihisa Y, Perry BD: Causative ehrlichial organisms in Potomac horse fever, *Infect Immun* 49:513, 1985.
57. Madigan JE, Pusterla N: Ehrlichial diseases, *Vet Clin North Am Equine Pract* 16(ix):487, 2000.
58. Levine JF, Levy MG, Nicholson WL, Gager RB: Attempted Ehrlichia risticii transmission with Dermacentor variabilis (Acari: Ixodidae), *J Med Entomol* 27:931, 1990.
59. Burg JG, Roberts AW, Williams NM, et al: Attempted transmission of Ehrlichia risticii (Rickettsiaceae) with Stomoxys calcitrans (Diptera: Muscidae), *J Med Entomol* 27:874, 1990.
60. Reubel GH, Barlough JE, Madigan JE: Production and characterization of Ehrlichia risticii, the agent of Potomac horse fever, from snails (Pleuroceridae: Juga spp.) in aquarium culture and genetic comparison to equine strains, *J Clin Microbiol* 36:1501, 1998.
61. Barlough JE, Reubel GH, Madigan JE, et al: Detection of Ehrlichia risticii, the agent of Potomac horse fever, in freshwater stream snails (Pleuroceridae: Juga spp.) from northern California, *Appl Environ Microbiol* 64:2888, 1998.
62. Kanter M, Mott J, Ohashi N, et al: Analysis of 16S rRNA and 51-kilodalton antigen gene and transmission in mice of Ehrlichia risticii in virgulate trematodes from Elimia livescens snails in Ohio, *J Clin Microbiol* 38:3349, 2000.
63. Mott J, Muramatsu Y, Seaton E, et al: Molecular analysis of Neorickettsia risticii in adult aquatic insects in Pennsylvania, in horses infected by ingestion of insects, and isolated in cell culture, *J Clin Microbiol* 40:690, 2002.
64. Park BK, Kim MJ, Kim EH, et al: Identification of trematode cercariae carrying Neorickettsia risticii in freshwater stream snails, *Ann N Y Acad Sci* 990:239-247, 2003.
65. Pusterla N, Johnson EM, Chae JS, Madigan JE: Digenetic trematodes, Acanthatrium sp. and Lecithodendrium sp, as vectors of Neorickettsia risticii, the agent of Potomac horse fever, *J Helminthol* 77:335, 2003.
66. Gibson KE, Rikihisa Y, Zhang C, Martin C: Neorickettsia risticii is vertically transmitted in the trematode Acanthatrium oregonense and horizontally transmitted to bats, *Environ. Microbiol* 7:203, 2005.
67. Chae JS, Pusterla N, Johnson E, et al: Infection of aquatic insects with trematode metacercariae carrying Ehrlichia risticii, the cause of Potomac horse fever, *J Med Entomol* 37:619, 2000.
68. Pusterla N, Madigan JE, Chae JS, et al: Helminthic transmission and isolation of Ehrlichia risticii, the causative agent of Potomac horse fever, by using trematode stages from freshwater stream snails, *J Clin Microbiol* 38:1293, 2000.
69. Pusterla N, Johnson E, Chae J, et al: Infection rate of Ehrlichia risticii, the agent of Potomac horse fever, in freshwater stream snails (Juga yrekaensis) from northern California, *Vet Parasitol* 92:151, 2000.
70. Madigan JE, Pusterla N, Johnson E, et al: Transmission of Ehrlichia risticii, the agent of Potomac horse fever, using naturally infected aquatic insects and helminth vectors: preliminary report, *Equine Vet J* 32:275, 2000.
71. Rikihisa Y, Perry BD, Cordes DO: Ultrastructural study of ehrlichial organisms in the large colons of ponies infected with Potomac horse fever, *Infect Immun* 49:505, 1985.
72. Cordes DO, Perry BD, Rikihisa Y, Chickering WR: Enterocolitis caused by Ehrlichia sp. in the horse (Potomac horse fever), *Vet Pathol* 23:471, 1986.
73. Rikihisa Y: Growth of Ehrlichia risticii in human colonic epithelial cells, *Ann N Y Acad Sci* 590:104, 1990.
74. Williams NM, Cross RJ, Timoney PJ: Respiratory burst activity associated with phagocytosis of Ehrlichia risticii by mouse peritoneal macrophages, *Res Vet Sci* 57:194, 1994.
75. Williams NM, Timoney PJ: In vitro killing of Ehrlichia risticii by activated and immune mouse peritoneal macrophages, *Infect Immun* 61:861, 1993.
76. Wells MY, Rikihisa Y: Lack of lysosomal fusion with phagosomes containing Ehrlichia risticii in P388D1 cells: abrogation of inhibition with oxytetracycline, *Infect Immun* 56:3209, 1988.
77. Moore JN, White S, Morris DD, editors: *Proceedings of the third equine colic symposium*, Lawrenceville, NJ, 1988, Veterinary Learning Systems.
78. Dutta SK, Penney BE, Myrup AC, et al: Disease features in horses with induced equine monocytic ehrlichiosis (Potomac horse fever), *Am J Vet Res* 49:1747, 1988.
79. Ziemer EL, Whitlock RH, Palmer JE, Spencer PA: Clinical and hematologic variables in ponies with experimentally induced equine ehrlichial colitis (Potomac horse fever), *Am J Vet Res* 48:63, 1987.
80. Long MT, Goetz TE, Kakoma I, et al: Evaluation of fetal infection and abortion in pregnant ponies experimentally infected with Ehrlichia risticii, *Am J Vet Res* 56:1307, 1995.
81. Long MT, Goetz TE, Whiteley HE, et al: Identification of Ehrlichia risticii as the causative agent of two equine abortions following natural maternal infection, *J Vet Diagn Invest* 7:201, 1995.
82. Morris DD, Messick J, Whitlock RH, et al: Effect of equine ehrlichial colitis on the hemostatic system in ponies, *Am J Vet Res* 49:1030, 1988.
83. Dutta SK, Rice RM, Hughes TD, et al: Detection of serum antibodies against Ehrlichia risticii in Potomac horse fever by enzyme-linked immunosorbent assay, *Vet Immunol Immunopathol* 14:85, 1987.
84. Madigan JE, Rikihisa Y, Palmer JE, et al: Evidence for a high rate of false-positive results with the indirect fluorescent antibody test for Ehrlichia risticii antibody in horses, *J Am Vet Med Assoc* 207:1448, 1995.
85. Pusterla N, Leutenegger CM, Sigrist B, et al: Detection and quantitation of Ehrlichia risticii genomic DNA in infected horses and snails by real-time PCR, *Vet Parasitol* 90:129, 2000.
86. Mott J, Rikihisa Y, Zhang Y, et al: Comparison of PCR and culture to the indirect fluorescent-antibody test for diagnosis of Potomac horse fever, *J Clin Microbiol* 35:2215, 1997.
87. Biswas B, Mukherjee D, Mattingly-Napier BL, Dutta SK: Diagnostic application of polymerase chain reaction for detection of Ehrlichia risticii in equine monocytic ehrlichiosis (Potomac horse fever), *J Clin Microbiol* 29:2228, 1991.
88. Atwill ER, Mohammed HO: Evaluation of vaccination of horses as a strategy to control equine monocytic ehrlichiosis, *J Am Vet Med Assoc* 208:1290, 1996.
89. Dutta SK, Vemulapalli R, Biswas B: Association of deficiency in antibody response to vaccine and heterogeneity of Ehrlichia risticii strains with Potomac horse fever vaccine failure in horses, *J Clin Microbiol* 36:506, 1998.
90. Wierup M: Equine intestinal clostridiosis. An acute disease in horses associated with high intestinal counts of Clostridium perfringens type A, *Acta Vet Scand* Suppl 1 , 1977.
91. Prescott JF, Staempfli HR, Barker IK, et al: A method for reproducing fatal idiopathic colitis (colitis X) in ponies and isolation of a clostridium as a possible agent, *Equine Vet J* 20:417, 1988.

92. Jones RL, Adney WS, Alexander AF, et al: Hemorrhagic necrotizing enterocolitis associated with Clostridium difficile infection in four foals, *J Am Vet Med Assoc* 193:76, 1988.
93. Madewell BR, Tang YJ, Jang S, et al: Apparent outbreaks of Clostridium difficile-associated diarrhea in horses in a veterinary medical teaching hospital, *J Vet Diagn Invest* 7:343, 1995.
94. Weese JS, Staempfli HR, Prescott JF: A prospective study of the roles of clostridium difficile and enterotoxigenic Clostridium perfringens in equine diarrhoea, *Equine Vet J* 33:403, 2001.
95. Jones RL: Clostridial enterocolitis, *Vet Clin North Am Equine Pract* 16:471, 2000.
96. Donaldson MT, Palmer JE: Prevalence of Clostridium perfringens enterotoxin and Clostridium difficile toxin A in feces of horses with diarrhea and colic, *J Am Vet Med Assoc* 215:358, 1999.
97. Baverud V, Gustaffsson A, Franklin A, et al: Clostridium difficile associated with acute colitis in mature horses treated with antibiotics, *Equine Vet J* 29:279, 1997.
98. Linerode PA, Goode RL: The effect of colic on the microbial activity of the equine intestine, *Proc Am Assoc Equine Pract* 16:219, 1970.
99. White G, Prior SD: Comparative effects of oral administration of trimethoprim/sulphadiazine or oxytetracycline on the faecal flora of horses, *Vet Rec* 111:316, 1982.
100. Baverud V, Franklin A, Gunnarsson A, et al: Clostridium difficile associated with acute colitis in mares when their foals are treated with erythromycin and rifampicin for Rhodococcus equi pneumonia, *Equine Vet J* 30:482, 1998.
101. Staempfli HR, Prescott JF, Brash ML: Lincomycin-induced severe colitis in ponies: association with Clostridium cadaveris, *Can J Vet Res* 56:168, 1992.
102. Samuel SC, Hancock P, Leigh DA: An investigation into Clostridium perfringens enterotoxin-associated diarrhoea, *J Hosp Infect* 18:219, 1991.
103. Gibert M, Jolivet-Reynaud C, Popoff MR, Jolivet-Renaud C: Beta$_2$ toxin, a novel toxin produced by Clostridium perfringens, *Gene* 203:65, 1997.
104. Herholz C, Miserez R, Nicolet J, et al: Prevalence of beta$_2$-toxigenic Clostridium perfringens in horses with intestinal disorders, *J Clin Microbiol* 37:358, 1999.
105. McClane BA: An overview of Clostridium perfringens enterotoxin, *Toxicon* 34:1335, 1996.
106. Ochoa R, Kern SR: The effects of Clostridium perfringens type A enterotoxin in Shetland ponies-clinical, morphologic and clinicopathologic changes, *Vet Pathol* 17:738, 1980.
107. Sarker MR, Singh U, McClane BA: An update on Clostridium perfringens enterotoxin, *J Nat Toxins* 9:251, 2000.
108. Kelly CP, LaMont JT: Clostridium difficile infection, *Ann Rev Med* 49:375, 1998.
109. Wershil BK, Castagliuolo I, Pothoulakis C: Direct evidence of mast cell involvement in Clostridium difficile toxin A-induced enteritis in mice, *Gastroenterology* 114:956, 1998.
110. Kelly CP, Becker S, Linevsky JK, et al: Neutrophil recruitment in Clostridium difficile toxin A enteritis in the rabbit, *J Clin Invest* 93:1257, 1994.
111. Castagliuolo I, LaMont JT, Letourneau R, Kelly C, O'Keane JC, Jaffer A, Theoharides TC, Pothoulakis C: Neuronal involvement in the intestinal effects of Clostridium difficile toxin A and Vibrio cholerae enterotoxin in rat ileum, *Gastroenterology* 107:657, 1994.
112. Castagliuolo I, Keates AC, Qiu B, et al: Increased substance P responses in dorsal root ganglia and intestinal macrophages during Clostridium difficile toxin A enteritis in rats, *Proc Nat Acad Sci U S A* 94:4788, 1997.
113. Pothoulakis C, Castagliuolo I, LaMont JT, et al: CP-96,345, a substance P antagonist, inhibits rat intestinal responses to Clostridium difficile toxin A but not cholera toxin, *Proc Nat Acad Sci U S A* 91:947, 1994.
114. Wierup M, DiPietro JA: Bacteriologic examination of equine fecal flora as a diagnostic tool for equine intestinal clostridiosis, *Am J Vet Res* 42:2167, 1981.
115. Daube G, Simon P, Limbourg B, et al: Hybridization of 2,659 Clostridium perfringens isolates with gene probes for seven toxins (alpha, beta, epsilon, iota, theta, mu, and enterotoxin) and for sialidase, *Am J Vet Res* 57:496, 1996.
116. Netherwood T, Wood JL, Mumford JA, Chanter N: Molecular analysis of the virulence determinants of Clostridium perfringens associated with foal diarrhoea, *Vet J* 155:289, 1998.
117. Meer RR, Songer JG: Multiplex polymerase chain reaction assay for genotyping Clostridium perfringens, *Am J Vet Res* 58:702, 1997.
118. Weese JS, Staempfli HR, Prescott JF: Survival of Clostridium difficile and its toxins in equine feces: implications for diagnostic test selection and interpretation, *J Vet Diagn Invest* 12:332, 2000.
119. Jones RL: Diagnostic procedures for isolation and characterization of Clostridium difficile associated with enterocolitis in foals, *J Vet Diagn Invest* 1:84, 1989.
120. Marler LM, Siders JA, Wolters LC, et al: Comparison of five cultural procedures for isolation of Clostridium difficile from stools, *J Clin Microbiol* 30:514, 1992.
121. Cooper DM, Gebhart CJ: Comparative aspects of proliferative enteritis, *J Am Vet Med Assoc* 212:1446, 1998.
122. Lawson GH, Gebhart CJ: Proliferative enteropathy, *J Comp Pathol* 122:77, 2000.
123. Smith DG, Lawson GH: Lawsonia intracellularis: getting inside the pathogenesis of proliferative enteropathy, *Vet Microbiol* 82:331, 2001.
124. Lavoie JP, Drolet R, Parsons D, et al: Equine proliferative enteropathy: a cause of weight loss, colic, diarrhoea and hypoproteinaemia in foals on three breeding farms in Canada, *Equine Vet J* 32:418, 2000.
125. Williams NM, Harrison LR, Gebhart CJ: Proliferative enteropathy in a foal caused by Lawsonia intracellularis-like bacterium, *J Vet Diagn Invest* 8:254, 1996.
126. Brees DJ, Sondhoff AH, Kluge JP, et al: Lawsonia intracellularis-like organism infection in a miniature foal, *J Am Vet Med Assoc* 215(511):483, 1999.
127. Frank N, Fishman CE, Gebhart CJ, Levy M: Lawsonia intracellularis proliferative enteropathy in a weanling foal, *Equine Vet J* 30:549, 1998.
128. McGurrin MK, Vengust M, Arroyo LG, Baird JD: An outbreak of Lawsonia intracellularis infection in a standardbred herd in Ontario, *Can Vet J* 48:927, 2007.
129. Knittel JP, Jordan DM, Schwartz KJ, et al: Evaluation of antemortem polymerase chain reaction and serologic methods for detection of Lawsonia intracellularis-exposed pigs, *Am J Vet Res* 59:722, 1998.
130. Cooper DM, Swanson DL, Gebhart CJ: Diagnosis of proliferative enteritis in frozen and formalin-fixed, paraffin-embedded tissues from a hamster, horse, deer and ostrich using a Lawsonia intracellularis-specific multiplex PCR assay, *Vet Microbiol* 54:47, 1997.
131. Drudge JH: Clinical aspects of Strongylus vulgaris infection in the horse. Emphasis on diagnosis, chemotherapy, and prophylaxis, *Vet Clin North Am Large Anim Pract* 1:251, 1979.
132. Owen J, Slocombe D: Pathogenesis of helminths in equines, *Vet Parasitol* 18:139, 1985.
133. Bueno L, Ruckebusch Y, Dorchies P: Disturbances of digestive motility in horses associated with strongyle infection, *Vet Parasitol* 5:253, 1979.
134. Lester GD, Bolton JR, Cambridge H, Thurgate S: The effect of Strongylus vulgaris larvae on equine intestinal myoelectrical activity, *Equine Vet J* (Suppl 8), 1989.
135. White NA: Intestinal infarction associated with mesenteric vascular thrombotic disease in the horse, *J Am Vet Med Assoc* 178:259, 1981.

136. Becht JL: The role of parasites in colic, *Proc Am Assoc Equine Pract* 33:301, 1987.
137. Sellers AF, Lowe JE, Drost CJ, et al: Retropulsion-propulsion in equine large colon, *Am J Vet Res* 43:390, 1982.
138. Greatorex JC: Diarrhoea in horses associated with ulceration of the colon and caecum resulting from S vulgaris larval migration, *Vet Rec* 97:221, 1975.
139. Patton S, Drudge JH: Clinical response of pony foals experimentally infected with Strongylus vulgaris, *Am J Vet Res* 38:2059, 1977.
140. Amborski GF, Bello TR, Torbert BJ: Host response to experimentally induced infections of strongylus vulgaris in parasite-free and naturally infected ponies, *Am J Vet Res* 35:1181, 1974.
141. Klei TR, Torbert BJ, Ochoa R, Bello TR: Morphologic and clinicopathologic changes following Strongylus vulgaris infections of immune and nonimmune ponies, *Am J Vet Res* 43:1300, 1982.
142. Patton S, Mock RE, Drudge JH, Morgan D: Increase of immunoglobulin T concentration in ponies as a response to experimental infection with the nematode Strongylus vulgaris, *Am J Vet Res* 39:19, 1978.
143. Lyons ET, Drudge JH, Tolliver SC: Larval cyathostomiasis, *Vet Clin North Am Equine Pract* 16:501, 2000.
144. Chiejina SN, Mason JA: Immature stages of Trichonema spp as a cause of diarrhoea in adult horses in spring, *Vet Rec* 100:360, 1977.
145. Giles CJ, Urquhart KA, Longstaffe JA: Larval cyathostomiasis (immature trichonema-induced enteropathy): a report of 15 clinical cases, *Equine Vet J* 17:196, 1985.
146. Church S, Kelly DF, Obwolo MJ: Diagnosis and successful treatment of diarrhoea in horses caused by immature small strongyles apparently insusceptible to anthelmintics, *Equine Vet J* 18:401, 1986.
147. Mair TS: Recurrent diarrhoea in aged ponies associated with larval cyathostomiasis, *Equine Vet J* 25:161, 1993.
148. Mair TS: Outbreak of larval cyathostomiasis among a group of yearling and two-year-old horses, *Vet Rec* 135:598, 1994.
149. Love S, Murphy D, Mellor D: Pathogenicity of cyathostome infection, *Vet Parasitol* 85:113, 1999.
150. Love S, Mair TS, Hillyer MH: Chronic diarrhoea in adult horses: a review of 51 referred cases, *Vet Rec* 130:217, 1992.
151. Mair TS, de Westerlaken LV, Cripps PJ, Love S: Diarrhoea in adult horses: a survey of clinical cases and an assessment of some prognostic indices, *Vet Rec* 126:479, 1990.
152. Murphy D, Love S: The pathogenic effects of experimental cyathostome infections in ponies, *Vet Parasitol* 70:99, 1997.
153. Murphy D, Reid SW, Graham PA, Love S: Fructosamine measurement in ponies: validation and response following experimental cyathostome infection, *Res Vet Sci* 63:113, 1997.
154. Klei TR, Rehbein S, Visser M, et al: Re-evaluation of ivermectin efficacy against equine gastrointestinal parasites, *Vet Parasitol* 98:315, 2001.
155. Tarigo-Martinie JL, Wyatt AR, Kaplan RM: Prevalence and clinical implications of anthelmintic resistance in cyathostomes of horses, *J Am Vet Med Assoc* 218:1957, 2001.
156. Jacobs DE, Hutchinson MJ, Parker L, Gibbons LM: Equine cyathostome infection: suppression of faecal egg output with moxidectin, *Vet Rec* 137:545, 1995.
157. Monahan CM, Chapman MR, Taylor HW, et al: Experimental cyathostome challenge of ponies maintained with or without benefit of daily pyrantel tartrate feed additive: comparison of parasite burdens, immunity and colonic pathology, *Vet Parasitol* 74:229, 1998.
158. Chapman MR, French DD, Monahan CM, Klei TR: Identification and characterization of a pyrantel pamoate resistant cyathostome population, *Vet Parasitol* 66:205, 1996.
159. Little D, Flowers JR, Hammerberg BH, Gardner SY: Management of drug-resistant cyathostominosis on a breeding farm in central North Carolina, *Equine Vet J* 35:246, 2003.
160. Andersson G, Ekman L, Mansson I, et al: Lethal compications following administration of oxytetracycline in the horse, *Nord Vet Med* 23:2, 1971.
161. Raisbeck MF, Holt GR, Osweiler GD: Lincomycin-associated colitis in horses, *J Am Vet Med Assoc* 179:362, 1981.
162. Stratton-Phelps M, Wilson WD, Gardner IA: Risk of adverse effects in pneumonic foals treated with erythromycin versus other antibiotics: 143 cases (1986-1996), *J Am Vet Med Assoc* 217:68, 2000.
163. Wilson DA, MacFadden KE, Green EM, et al: Case control and historical cohort study of diarrhea associated with administration of trimethoprim-potentiated sulphonamides to horses and ponies, *J Vet Intern Med* 10:258, 1996.
164. Gustafsson A, Baverud V, Gunnarsson A, et al: The association of erythromycin ethylsuccinate with acute colitis in horses in Sweden, *Equine Ve J* 29:314, 1997.
165. Owen RA, Fullerton J, Barnum DA: Effects of transportation, surgery, and antibiotic therapy in ponies infected with Salmonella, *Am J Vet Res* 44:46, 1983.
166. Borriello SP: The influence of the normal flora on Clostridium difficile colonisation of the gut, *Ann Med* 22:61, 1990.
167. Owen R, Fullerton JN, Tizard IR, et al: Studies on experimental enteric salmonellosis in ponies, *Can J Comp Med* 43:247, 1979.
168. Argenzio RA: Physiology of diarrhea—large intestine, *J Am Vet Med Assoc* 173:667, 1978.
169. Rao SS, Edwards CA, Austen CJ, et al: Impaired colonic fermentation of carbohydrate after ampicillin, *Gastroenterology* 94:928, 1988.
170. Clausen MR, Bonnen H, Tvede M, Mortensen PB: Colonic fermentation to short-chain fatty acids is decreased in antibiotic-associated diarrhea, *Gastroenterology* 101:1497, 1991.
171. Grossman RF: The relationship of absorption characteristics and gastrointestinal side effects of oral antimicrobial agents, *Clin Ther* 13:189, 1991.
172. Roussel AJ, Hooper RN, Cohen ND, et al: Prokinetic effects of erythromycin on the ileum, cecum, and pelvic flexure of horses during the postoperative period, *Am J Vet Res* 61:420, 2000.
173. Lakritz J, Madigan J, Carlson GP: Hypovolemic hyponatremia and signs of neurologic disease associated with diarrhea in a foal, *J Am Vet Med Assoc* 200:1114, 1992.
174. Kore AM: Toxicology of nonsteroidal antiinflammatory drugs, *Vet Clin North Am Small Anim Pract* 20:419, 1990.
175. Gibson GR, Whitacre EB, Ricotti CA: Colitis induced by nonsteroidal anti-inflammatory drugs. Report of four cases and review of the literature, *Arch Intern Med* 152:625, 1992.
176. Meschter CL, Gilbert M, Krook L, Maylin G, Corradino R: The effects of phenylbutazone on the intestinal mucosa of the horse: a morphological, ultrastructural and biochemical study, *Equine Vet J* 22:255, 1990.
177. Collins LG, Tyler DE: Experimentally induced phenylbutazone toxicosis in ponies: description of the syndrome and its prevention with synthetic prostaglandin E_2, *Am J Vet Res* 46:1605, 1985.
178. Collins LG, Tyler DE: Phenylbutazone toxicosis in the horse: a clinical study, *J Am Vet Med Assoc* 184:699, 1984.
179. Karcher LF, Dill SG, Anderson WI, King JM: Right dorsal colitis, *J Vet Intern Med* 4:247, 1990.
180. Hough ME, Steel CM, Bolton JR, Yovich JV: Ulceration and stricture of the right dorsal colon after phenylbutazone administration in four horses, *Austr Vet J* 77:785, 1999.
181. Little D, Brown SA, Campbell NB, et al: Effects of the cyclooxygenase inhibitor meloxicam on recovery of ischemia-injured equine jejunum, *Am J Vet Res* 68:614, 2007.

182. Cook, V.L., C.T. Meyers, N.B. Campbell, and A.T. Blikslager. 2008. Effect of firocoxib or flunixin meglumine on recovery of ischemic-injured equine jejunum, *Am J Vet Res Aug:*70(8): 992-1000, 2009.
183. Murray MJ: Phenylbutazone toxicity in a horse, *Comp Cont Ed Pract Vet* 7:S389-S394, 1985.
184. Lees P, Creed RF, Gerring EE, et al: Biochemical and haematological effects of phenylbutazone in horses, *Equine Vet J* 15:158, 1983.
185. Cohen ND, Carter GK, Mealey RH, Taylor TS: Medical management of right dorsal colitis in 5 horses: a retrospective study (1987-1993), *J Vet Intern Med* 9:272, 1995.
186. Kaufmann HJ, Taubin HL: Nonsteroidal anti-inflammatory drugs activate quiescent inflammatory bowel disease, *Ann Intern Med* 107:513, 1987.
187. Hovde O, Farup PG: NSAID-induced irreversible exacerbation of ulcerative colitis, *J Clin Gastroenterol* 15:160, 1992.
188. Blikslager AT, Roberts MC: Mechanisms of intestinal mucosal repair, *J Am Vet. Med Assoc* 211:1437, 1998.
189. Semble EL, Wu WC: Prostaglandins in the gut and their relationship to non-steroidal anti-inflammatory drugs, *Baillieres Clin Rheumatol* 3:247, 1989.
190. Campbell NB, Jones SL, Blikslager AT: The effects of cyclo-oxygenase inhibitors on bile-injured and normal equine colon, *Equine Vet J* 34:493, 2002.
191. Jones SL, Blikslager AT: The future of antiinflammatory therapy, *Vet Clin North Am Equine Pract* 17:245, 2001.
192. Doucet MY, Bertone AL, Hendrickson D, et al: Comparison of efficacy and safety of paste formulations of firocoxib and phenylbutazone in horses with naturally occurring osteoarthritis, *J Am Vet Med Assoc* 232:91, 2008.
193. Yamada T, Deitch E, Specian RD, et al: Mechanisms of acute and chronic intestinal inflammation induced by indomethacin, *Inflammation* 17:641, 1993.
194. Beck PL, Xavier R, Lu N, et al: Mechanisms of NSAID-induced gastrointestinal injury defined using mutant mice, *Gastroenterology* 119:699, 2000.
195. Wallace JL, Granger DN: Pathogenesis of NSAID gastropathy: are neutrophils the culprits?, *Trends Pharm Sci* 13:129, 1992.
196. Morise Z, Komatsu S, Fuseler JW, et al: ICAM-1 and P-selectin expression in a model of NSAID-induced gastropathy, *Am J Physiol* 274:G246-G252, 1998.
197. Wallace JL, Keenan CM, Granger DN: Gastric ulceration induced by nonsteroidal anti-inflammatory drugs is a neutrophil-dependent process, *Am J Physiol* 259:G462-G467, 1990.
198. Brune K, Beck WS: Towards safer nonsteroidal anti-inflammatory drugs, *Agents Actions Suppl* 32(13):13-25, 1991.
199. Davis JL, Gardner SY, Jones SL, et al: Pharmacokinetics of azithromycin in foals after i.v. and oral dose and disposition into phagocytes, *J Vet Pharmacol Ther* 25:99, 2002.
200. Cohen ND, Mealey RH, Chaffin MK, Carter GK: The recognition and medical management of right dorsal colitis in horses, *Vet Med* 9:687, 1995.
201. East LM, Trumble TN, Steyn PF, et al: The application of technetium-99m hexamethylpropyleneamine oxime (99mTc-HMPAO) labeled white blood cells for the diagnosis of right dorsal ulcerative colitis in two horses, *Vet Radiol Ultrasound* 41:360, 2000.
202. Schmitz DG: Cantharidin toxicosis in horses, *J Vet Intern Med* 3:208, 1989.
203. Shawley RV, Rolf LLJ: Experimental cantharidiasis in the horse, *Am J Vet Res* 45:2261, 1984.
204. Schoeb TR, Panciera RJ: Pathology of blister beetle (Epicauta) poisoning in horses, *Vet Pathol* 16:18, 1979.
205. Ray AC, Kyle AL, Murphy MJ, Reagor JC: Etiologic agents, incidence, and improved diagnostic methods of cantharidin toxicosis in horses, *Am J Vet Res* 50:187, 1989.
206. Helman RG, Edwards WC: Clinical features of blister beetle poisoning in equids: 70 cases (1983-1996), *J Am Vet Med Assoc* 211:1018, 1997.
207. Osweiler GD, Carron JL, Buck WB: *Clinical and diagnostic veterinary toxicology*, Dubuque, Iowa, 1985, Kendal Hunt, p. 253.
208. Tamaki S, Frankenberger WTJ: Environmental biochemistry of arsenic, *Rev Environ Contam Toxicol* 124:79, 1992.
209. Goldman L, Ausiello DA, Arend W, et al: *Cecil Textbook of medicine*, ed 23, Philadelphia, 2008, Saunders.
210. Mack RB: Gee, honey, why does the iced tea have a garlic taste? Arsenic intoxication, *N C Med J* 44:753, 1983.
211. Olson NE: Acute diarrheal disease in the horse, *J Am Vet Med Assoc* 148:418, 1966.
212. Wershil BK, Walker WA: The mucosal barrier, IgE-mediated gastrointestinal events, and eosinophilic gastroenteritis, *Gastroenterol Clin North Am* 21:387, 1992.
213. Strobel S: IgE-mediated (and food-induced) intestinal disease, *Clin Exp Allergy* 25(Suppl 1):3, 1995.
214. Ohtsuka Y, Naito K, Yamashiro Y, et al: Induction of anaphylaxis in mouse intestine by orally administered antigen and its prevention with soluble high affinity receptor for IgE, *Pediatr Res* 45:300, 1999.
215. Zimmel DN, Blikslager AT, Jones SL, et al: Vaccine-associated anaphylactic-like reaction in a horse, *Comp Cont Ed Pract Vet* 1:81, 2000.
216. Mansmann RA: Equine anaphylaxis, *J Am Vet Med Assoc* 161:438, 1972.
217. McGavin MD, Gronwall RR, Mia AS: Pathologic changes in experimental equine anaphylaxis, *J Am Vet Med Assoc* 160:1632, 1972.
218. Stenton GR, Vliagoftis H, Befus AD: Role of intestinal mast cells in modulating gastrointestinal pathophysiology, *Ann Allergy Asthma Immunol* 81:1, 1998.
219. Mourad FH, O'Donnell LJ, Ogutu E, et al: Role of 5-hydroxytryptamine in intestinal water and electrolyte movement during gut anaphylaxis, *Gut* 36:553, 1995.
220. Catto-Smith AG, Patrick MK, Hardin JA, Gall DG: Intestinal anaphylaxis in the rat: mediators responsible for the ion transport abnormalities, *Agents Actions* 28:185, 1989.
221. Scott RB, Diamant SC, Gall DG: Motility effects of intestinal anaphylaxis in the rat, *Am J Physiol* 255:G505-G511, 1988.
222. Baron DA, Baird AW, Cuthbert AW, Margolius HS: Intestinal anaphylaxis: rapid changes in mucosal ion transport and morphology, *Am J Physiol* 254:G307-G314, 1988.
223. Rooney JR, Bryans JT, Prickett ME, Zent WW: Exhaustion shock in the horse, *Cornell Vet* 56:220, 1966.
224. Garner HE, Hutcheson DP, Coffman JR, Hahn AW, Salem C: Lactic acidosis: a factor associated with equine laminitis, *J Anim Sci* 45:1037, 1977.
225. Garner HE, Moore JN, Johnson JH, et al: Changes in the caecal flora associated with the onset of laminitis, *Equine Vet J* 10:249, 1978.
226. Moore JN, Garner HE, Berg JN, Sprouse RF: Intracecal endotoxin and lactate during the onset of equine laminitis: a preliminary report, *Am J Vet Res* 40:722, 1979.
227. Sprouse RF, Garner HE, Green EM: Plasma endotoxin levels in horses subjected to carbohydrate induced laminitis, *Equine Vet J* 19:25, 1987.
228. Ragle CA, Meagher DM, Lacroix CA, Honnas CM: Surgical treatment of sand colic. Results in 40 horses, *Vet Surg* 18:48, 1989.
229. Bertone JJ, Traub-Dargatz JL, Wrigley RW, et al: Diarrhea associated with sand in the gastrointestinal tract of horses, *J Am Vet Med Assoc* 193:1409, 1988.
230. Ramey DW, Reinertson EL: Sand-induced diarrhea in a foal, *J Am Vet Med Assoc* 185:537, 1984.
231. Ragle CA, Meagher DM, Schrader JL, Honnas CM: Abdominal auscultation in the detection of experimentally induced gastrointestinal sand accumulation, *J Vet Intern Med* 3:12, 1989.

232. McGuinness SG, Mansmann RA, Breuhaus BA: Nasogastric electrolyte replacement in horses, *Comp Cont Educ Pract Vet* 18:942, 1996.
233. Cohen ND, Divers TJ: Acute colitis in horses. II. Initial management, *Comp Cont Educ Pract Vet* 20:228, 1998.
234. Jones PA, Bain FT, Byars TD, et al: Effect of hydroxyethyl starch infusion on colloid oncotic pressure in hypoproteinemic horses, *J Am Vet Med Assoc* 218:1130, 2001.
235. Jones PA, Tomasic M, Gentry PA: Oncotic, hemodilutional, and hemostatic effects of isotonic saline and hydroxyethyl starch solutions in clinically normal ponies, *Am J Vet Res* 58:541, 1997.
236. Roberts JS, Bratton SL: Colloid volume expanders. Problems, pitfalls and possibilities, *Drugs* 55:621, 1998.
237. Tyler JW, Cullor JS, Spier SJ, Smith BP: Immunity targeting common core antigens of gram-negative bacteria, *J Vet Intern Med* 4:17, 1990.
238. Spier SJ, Lavoie JP, Cullor JS, et al: Protection against clinical endotoxemia in horses by using plasma containing antibody to an Rc mutant E. coli (J5), *Circ Shock* 28:235, 1989.
239. Wiedermann CJ: Systematic review of randomized clinical trials on the use of hydroxyethyl starch for fluid management in sepsis, *BMC Emerg Med* 8(1):1, 2008.
240. Duebbert IE, Peterson JW: Enterotoxin-induced fluid accumulation during experimental salmonellosis and cholera: involvement of prostaglandin synthesis by intestinal cells, *Toxicon* 23:157, 1985.
241. Clarke LL, Argenzio RA: NaCl transport across equine proximal colon and the effect of endogenous prostanoids, *Am J Physiol* 259:G62-G69, 1990.
242. Blikslager AT, Moeser AJ, Gookin JL, et al: Restoration of barrier function in injured intestinal mucosa, *Physiol Rev* 87:545, 2007.
243. Perdue MH, McKay DM: Integrative immunophysiology in the intestinal mucosa, *Am J Physiol* 267:G151-G165, 1994.
244. Freeman DE, Inoue OJ, Eurell TE: Effects of flunixin meglumine on short circuit current in equine colonic mucosa in vitro, *Am J Vet Res* 58:915, 1997.
245. Richter RA, Freeman DE, Wallig M, Whittem T, Baker GJ: In vitro anion transport alterations and apoptosis induced by phenylbutazone in the right dorsal colon of ponies, *Am J Vet Res* 63:934, 2002.
246. Joshi GP, Gertler R, Fricker R: Cardiovascular thromboembolic adverse effects associated with cyclooxygenase-2 selective inhibitors and nonselective antiinflammatory drugs, *Anesth Analg* 105:1793, 2007.
247. Geor RJ, Petrie L, Papich MG, Rousseaux C: The protective effects of sucralfate and ranitidine in foals experimentally intoxicated with phenylbutazone, *Can J Vet Res* 53:231, 1989.
248. Fedorak RN, Empey LR, MacArthur C, Jewell LD: Misoprostol provides a colonic mucosal protective effect during acetic acid-induced colitis in rats, *Gastroenterology* 98:615, 1990.
249. Wachtershauser A, Stein J: Rationale for the luminal provision of butyrate in intestinal diseases, *Eur J Nutr* 39:164, 2000.
250. Rhoads JM, Chen W, Gookin J, et al: Arginine stimulates intestinal cell migration through a focal adhesion kinase dependent mechanism, *Gut* 53:514, 2004.
251. Sellon DC, Monroe VL, Roberts MC, Papich MG: Pharmacokinetics and adverse effects of butorphanol administered by single intravenous injection or continuous intravenous infusion in horses, *Am J Vet Res* 62:183, 2001.
252. Cook VL, Blikslager AT: Use of systemically administered lidocaine in horses with gastrointestinal tract disease, *J Am Vet Med Assoc* 232:1144, 2008.
253. Cook VL, Jones SJ, McDowell M, et al: Attenuation of ischaemic injury in the equine jejunum by administration of systemic lidocaine, *Equine Vet J* 40:353, 2008.
254. Crosby WH: How many "polys" are enough?, *Arch Intern Med* 123:722, 1969.
255. Verdrengh M, Tarkowski A: Role of neutrophils in experimental septicemia and septic arthritis induced by Staphylococcus aureus, *Infect Immun* 65:2517, 1997.
256. Conlan JW: Critical roles of neutrophils in host defense against experimental systemic infections of mice by Listeria monocytogenes, Salmonella typhimurium, and Yersinia enterocolitica, *Infect Immun* 65:630, 1997.
257. Bodey GP, Rodriguez V, Chang HY: Fever and infection in leukemic patients: a study of 494 consecutive patients, *Cancer* 41:1610, 1978.
258. Bodey GP, Buckley M, Sathe YS, Freireich EJ: Quantitative relationships between circulating leukocytes and infection in patients with acute leukemia, *Ann Intern Med* 64:328, 1966.
259. Pizzo PA: Management of fever in patients with cancer and treatment-induced neutropenia, *N Engl J Med* 328:1323, 1993.
260. Engels EA, Ellis CA, Supran SE, et al: Early infection in bone marrow transplantation: quantitative study of clinical factors that affect risk, *Clin Infect Dis* 28:256, 1999.
261. Li Y, Karlin A, Loike JD, Silverstein SC: Determination of the critical concentration of neutrophils required to block bacterial growth in tissues, *J Exp Med* 200:613, 2004.
262. Li Y, Karlin A, Loike JD, Silverstein SC: A critical concentration of neutrophils is required for effective bacterial killing in suspension, *Proc Nat Acad Sci U S A* 99:8289, 2002.
263. Tunev SS, Ehrhart EJ, Jensen HE, et al: Necrotizing mycotic vasculitis with cerebral infarction caused by Aspergillus niger in a horse with acute typholocolitis, *Vet Pathol* 36:347, 1999.
264. Sweeney CR, Habecker PL: Pulmonary aspergillosis in horses: 29 cases (1974-1997), *J Am Vet Med Assoc* 214:808, 1999.
265. Rikihisa Y, Jiang BM: Effect of antibiotics on clinical, pathologic and immunologic responses in murine Potomac horse fever: protective effects of doxycycline, *Vet Microbiol* 19:253, 1989.
266. Palmer JE, Benson CE, Whitlock RH: Effect of treatment with oxytetracycline during the acute stages of experimentally induced equine ehrlichial colitis in ponies, *Am J Vet Res* 53:2300, 1992.
267. Palmer JE, Benson CE: Effect of treatment with erythromycin and rifampin during the acute stages of experimentally induced equine ehrlichial colitis in ponies, *Am J Vet Res* 53:2071, 1992.
268. McGorum BC, Dixon PM, Smith DG: Use of metronidazole in equine acute idiopathic toxaemic colitis, *Vet Rec* 142:635, 1998.
269. Jang SS, Hansen LM, Breher JE, et al: Antimicrobial susceptibilities of equine isolates of Clostridium difficile and molecular characterization of metronidazole-resistant strains, *Clin Infect Dis* 25(Suppl 2):S266-S267, 1997.
270. MacKay RJ: Equine neonatal clostridiosis: Treatment and prevention, *Comp Cont Ed Pract Vet* 23:280, 2001.
271. McOrist S, Mackie RA, Lawson GH: Antimicrobial susceptibility of ileal symbiont intracellularis isolated from pigs with proliferative enteropathy, *J Clin Microbiol* 33:1314, 1995.
272. Cambridge H, Lees P, Hooke RE, Russell CS: Antithrombotic actions of aspirin in the horse, *Equine Vet J* 23:123, 1991.
273. Belknap JK, Moore JN: Evaluation of heparin for prophylaxis of equine laminitis: 71 cases (1980-1986), *J Am Vet Med Assoc* 195:505, 1989.
274. van de Water L, Schroeder S, Crenshaw EB, Hynes RO: Phagocytosis of gelatin-latex particles by a murine macrophage line is dependent on fibronectin and heparin, *J Cell Biol* 90:32, 1981.
275. Doran JE, Mansberger AR, Edmondson HT, Reese AC: Cold insoluble globulin and heparin interactions in phagocytosis by macrophage monolayers: mechanism of heparin enhancement, *J Reticuloendothel Soc* 29:285, 1981.

276. Fuller R: Probiotics in man and animals, *J Appl Bacteriol* 66:365, 1989.
277. Traub-Dargatz JL, Jones RL: Clostridia-associated enterocolitis in adult horses and foals, *Vet Clin North Am Equine Pract* 9:411, 1993.
278. Desrochers AM, Dolente BA, Roy MF, et al: Efficacy of Saccharomyces boulardii for treatment of horses with acute enterocolitis, *J Am Vet Med Assoc* 227:954, 2005.
279. Wunderlich PF, Braun L, Fumagalli I, et al: Double-blind report on the efficacy of lactic acid-producing Enterococcus SF68 in the prevention of antibiotic-associated diarrhoea and in the treatment of acute diarrhoea, *J Int Med Res* 17:333, 1989.
280. Siitonen S, Vapaatalo H, Salminen S, et al: Effect of Lactobacillus GG yoghurt in prevention of antibiotic associated diarrhoea, *Ann Med* 22:57, 1990.
281. Lawler JB, Hassel DM, Magnuson RJ, et al: Adsorptive effects of di-tri-octahedral smectite on Clostridium perfringens alpha, beta, and beta-2 exotoxins and equine colostral antibodies, *Am J Vet Res* 69:233, 2008.
282. Weese JS, Cote NM, deGannes RV: Evaluation of in vitro properties of di-tri-octahedral smectite on clostridial toxins and growth, *Equine Vet J* 35:638, 2003.
283. Xiao L, Herd RP, Majewski GA: Comparative efficacy of moxidectin and ivermectin against hypobiotic and encysted cyathostomes and other equine parasites, *Vet Parasitol* 53:83, 1994.
284. Love S, Duncan JL, Parry JM, Grimshaw WT: Efficacy of oral ivermectin paste against mucosal stages of cyathostomes, *Vet Rec* 136:18, 1995.
285. Duncan JL, Bairden K, Abbott EM: Elimination of mucosal cyathostome larvae by five daily treatments with fenbendazole, *Vet Rec* 142:268, 1998.
286. Hutchens DE, Paul AJ: Moxidectin: Spectrum of activity and uses in an equine anthelmintic program, *Comp Cont Ed Pract Vet* 22:373, 2000.
287. Steinbach T, Bauer C, Sasse H, et al: Small strongyle infection: consequences of larvicidal treatment of horses with fenbendazole and moxidectin, *Vet Parasitol* 139:115, 2006.
288. Hood DM, Stephen KA, Amoss MS: The use of alpha and beta adrenergic blockade as a preventive in the carbohdrate model of laminitis, *Proceedings First Equine Endotoxin Laminitis Symposium* 1:141, 1982.

Ischemic Disorders of the Intestinal Tract

1. Laws EG, Freeman DE: Significance of reperfusion injury after venous strangulation obstruction of equine jejunum, *J Invest Surg* 8:263-270, 1995.
2. Blikslager AT, Roberts MC, Gerard MP, Argenzio RA: How important is intestinal reperfusion injury in horses? *J Am Vet Med Assoc* 211:1387-1389, 1997.
3. Moore RM: Clinical relevance of intestinal reperfusion injury in horses, *J Am Vet Med Assoc* 211:1362-1366, 1997.
4. Snyder JR, Pascoe JR, Olander HJ, et al: Strangulating volvulus of the ascending colon in horses, *J Am Vet Med Assoc* 195:757-764, 1989.
5. White NA, Moore JN, Trim CM: Mucosal alterations in experimentally induced small intestinal strangulation obstruction in ponies, *Am J Vet Res* 41:193-198, 1980.
6. Meschter CL, Tyler DE, White NA, Moore J: Histologic findings in the gastrointestinal tract of horses with colic, *Am J Vet Res* 47:598-606, 1986.
7. Hughes FE, Slone DEJ: Large colon resection, *Vet Clin North Am Equine Pract* 13:341-350, 1997.
8. Dabareiner RM, Sullins KE, Snyder JR, et al: Evaluation of the microcirculation of the equine small intestine after intraluminal distention and subsequent decompression, *Am J Vet Res* 54:1673-1682, 1993.
9. Freeman DE, Koch DB, Boles CL: Mesodiverticular bands as a cause of small intestinal strangulation and volvulus in the horse, *J Am Vet Med Assoc* 175:1089-1094, 1979.
10. Lundin C, Sullins KE, White NA, et al: Induction of peritoneal adhesions with small intestinal ischaemia and distention in the foal, *Equine Vet J* 21:451-458, 1989.
11. White NA, editor: *The equine acute abdomen*, Philadelphia, 1990, Lea & Febiger.
12. Vachon AM, Fischer AT: Small intestinal herniation through the epiploic foramen: 53 cases (1987-1993), *Equine Vet J* 27:373-380, 1995.
13. Freeman DE: Duodenitis-proximal jejunitis, *Equine Vet Educ* 12:322-332, 2000.
14. White NA, Lessard P: Risk factors and clinical signs associated with cases of equine colic, *Proc Am Assoc Equine Pract* 32: 637-644, 1986.
15. Mair TS, Smith LJ: Survival and complication rates in 300 horses undergoing surgical treatment of colic. Part 1: Short-term survival following a single laparotomy, *Equine Vet J* 37:296-302, 2005.
16. Freeman DE, Hammock P, Baker GJ, et al: Short- and long-term survival and prevalence of postoperative ileus after small intestinal surgery in the horse, *Equine Vet J Suppl* 32:42-51, 2000.
17. MacDonald MH, Pascoe JR, Stover SM, Meagher DM: Survival after small intestine resection and anastomosis in horses, *Vet Surg* 18:415-423, 1989.
18. Proudman CJ, Edwards GB, Barnes J, French NR: Factors affecting long-term survival of horses recovering from surgery of the small intestine, *Equine Vet J* 37:360-365, 2005.
19. Gayle JM, Blikslager AT, Bowman KF: Mesenteric rents as a source of small intestinal strangulation in horses: 15 cases (1990-1997), *J Am Vet Med Assoc* 216:1446-1449, 2000.
20. Archer DC, Pinchbeck GK, French NP, Proudman CJ: Risk factors for epiploic foramen entrapment colic: an international study, *Equine Vet J*, (Jan 11) [Epub ahead of print], 2008.
21. Age distributions of horses with strangulation of the small intestine by a lipoma or in the epiploic foramen: 46 cases (1994-2000), *J Am Vet Med Assoc* 219:87-89, 2001.
22. Murray RC, Gaughan EM, Debowes RM, et al: Incarceration of the jejunum in the epiploic foramen of a four month old foal, *Cornell Vet* 84:47-51, 1994.
23. Klohnen A, Vachon AM, Fischer AT Jr: Use of diagnostic ultrasonography in horses with signs of acute abdominal pain, *J Am Vet Med Assoc* 209:1597-1601, 1996.
24. Hammock PD, Freeman DE, Magid JH, Foreman JH: Parietal hernia of the small intestine into the epiploic foramen of a horse, *J Am Vet Med Assoc* 214:1354-1355, 1999.
25. Foerner JJ, Ringle MJ, Junkins DS, et al: Transection of the pelvic flexure to reduce incarceration of the large colon through the epiploic foramen in a horse, *J Am Vet Med Assoc* 203:1312-1313, 1993.
26. Engelbert TA, Tate LPJ, Bowman KF, Bristol DG: Incarceration of the small intestine in the epiploic foramen. Report of 19 cases (1983-1992), *Vet Surg* 22:57-61, 1993.
27. Blikslager AT, Bowman KF, Haven ML, et al: Pedunculated lipomas as a cause of intestinal obstruction in horses: 17 cases (1983-1990), *J Am Vet Med Assoc* 201:1249-1252, 1992.
28. Edwards GB, Proudman CJ: An analysis of 75 cases of intestinal obstruction caused by pedunculated lipomas, *Equine Vet J* 26:18-21, 1994.
29. Mason TA: Strangulation of the rectum of a horse by the pedicle of a mesenteric lipoma, *Equine Vet J* 10:269, 1978.
30. Orsini JA: Abdominal surgery in foals, *Vet Clin North Am Equine Pract* 13:393-413, 1997.
31. Crowhurst RC, Simpson DJ, McEnery RJ, Greenwood RE: Intestinal surgery in the foal, *J S Afr Vet Assoc* 46:59-67, 1975.

32. Tate LPJ, Ralston SL, Koch CM, Everitt JI: Effects of extensive resection of the small intestine in the pony, *Am J Vet Res* 44:1187-1191, 1983.
33. Yovich JV, Stashak TS, Bertone AL: Incarceration of small intestine through rents in the gastrosplenic ligament in the horse, *Vet Surg* 14:303-306, 1985.
34. Becht JL, McIlwraith CW: Jejunal displacement through the mesometrium in a pregnant mare, *J Am Vet Med Assoc* 177:436, 1980.
35. Gayle JM, MacHarg MA, Smallwood JE: Strangulating obstruction caused by intestinal herniation through the proximal aspect of the cecocolic fold in 9 horses, *Vet Surg* 30:40-43, 2001.
36. Spurlock GH, Robertson JT: Congenital inguinal hernias associated with a rent in the common vaginal tunic in five foals, *J Am Vet Med Assoc* 193:1087-1088, 1988.
37. van der Velden MA: Ruptured inguinal hernia in new-born colt foals: a review of 14 cases, *Equine Vet J* 20:178-181, 1988.
38. Schneider RK, Milne DW, Kohn CW: Acquired inguinal hernia in the horse: a review of 27 cases, *J Am Vet Med Assoc* 180:317-320, 1982.
39. van der Velden MA: Surgical treatment of acquired inguinal hernia in the horse: a review of 51 cases, *Equine Vet J* 20:173-177, 1988.
40. van der Velden MA, Stolk PW: Different types of inguinal herniation in two stallions and a gelding, *Vet Q* 12:46-50, 1990.
41. Freeman DE: Surgery of the small intestine, *Vet Clin North Am Equine Pract* 13:261-301, 1997.
42. Freeman DE, Orsini JA, Harrison IW, et al: Complications of umbilical hernias in horses: 13 cases (1972-1986), *J Am Vet Med Assoc* 192:804-807, 1988.
43. Markel MD, Pascoe JR, Sams AE: Strangulated umbilical hernias in horses: 13 cases (1974-1985), *J Am Vet Med Assoc* 190:692-694, 1987.
44. Edwards GB: Surgical management of intussusception in the horse, *Equine Vet J* 18:313-321, 1986.
45. Ford TS, Freeman DE, Ross MW, et al: Ileocecal intussusception in horses: 26 cases (1981-1988), *J Am Vet Med Assoc* 196:121-126, 1990.
46. Bernard WV, Reef VB, Reimer JM, et al: Ultrasonographic diagnosis of small-intestinal intussusception in three foals, *J Am Vet Med Assoc* 194:395-397, 1989.
47. Gift LJ, Gaughan EM, Debowes RM, et al: Jejunal intussusception in adult horses: 11 cases (1981-1991), *J Am Vet Med Assoc* 202:110-112, 1993.
48. Beard WL, Byrne BA, Henninger RW: Ileocecal intussusception corrected by resection within the cecum in two horses, *J Am Vet Med Assoc* 200:1978-1980, 1992.
49. Bristol DG: Diaphragmatic hernias in horses and cattle, *Comp Contin Educ Pract Vet* 8:S407-S411, 1986.
50. Wimberly HC, Andrews EJ, Haschek WM: Diaphragmatic hernias in the horse: a review of the literature and an analysis of six additional cases, *J Am Vet Med Assoc* 170:1404-1407, 1977.
51. Orsini JA, Koch C, Stewart B: Peritoneopericardial hernia in a horse, *J Am Vet Med Assoc* 179:907-910, 1981.
52. Everett KA, Chaffin MK, Brinsko SP: Diaphragmatic herniation as a cause of lethargy and exercise intolerance in a mare, *Cornell Vet* 82:217-223, 1992.
53. Santschi EM, Juzwiak JS, Moll HD, Slone DE: Diaphragmatic hernia repair in three young horses, *Vet Surg* 26:242-245, 1997.
54. Dabareiner RM, White NA: Surgical repair of a diaphragmatic hernia in a racehorse, *J Am Vet Med Assoc* 214(1496):1517-1518, 1999.
55. Wimberly HC, Andrews EJ, Haschek WM: Diaphragmatic hernias in the horse: a review of the literature and an analysis of six additional cases, *J Am Vet Med Assoc* 170:1404-1407, 1977.
56. Snyder JR, Olander HJ, Pascoe JR, et al: Morphologic alterations observed during experimental ischemia of the equine large colon, *Am J Vet Res* 49:801-809, 1988.
57. Harrison IW: Equine large intestinal volvulus. A review of 124 cases, *Vet Surg* 17:77-81, 1988.
58. Johnston JK, Freeman DE: Diseases and surgery of the large colon, *Vet Clin North Am Equine Pract* 13:317-340, 1997.
59. Johnston K, Holcombe SJ, Hauptman JG: Plasma lactate as a predictor of colonic viability and survival after 360 degrees volvulus of the ascending colon in horses, *Vet Surg* 36:563-567, 2007.
60. Hance SR: Colopexy, *Vet Clin North Am Equine Pract* 13:351-358, 1997.
61. Hance SR, Embertson RM: Colopexy in broodmares: 44 cases (1986-1990), *J Am Vet Med Assoc* 201:782-787, 1992.
62. Gaughan EM, Hackett RP: Cecocolic intussusception in horses: 11 cases (1979-1989), *J Am Vet Med Assoc* 197:1373-1375, 1990.
63. Martin BBJ, Freeman DE, Ross MW, et al: Cecocolic and cecocecal intussusception in horses: 30 cases (1976-1996), *J Am Vet Med Assoc* 214:80-84, 1999.
64. Hubert JD, Hardy J, Holcombe SJ: Moore RM: Cecal amputation via a right ventral colon enterotomy for correction of nonreducible cecocolic intussusception in 8 horses, *Vet Surg* 29:317-325, 2000.
65. Robertson JT, Tate LPJ: Resection of intussuscepted large colon in a horse, *J Am Vet Med Assoc* 181:927-928, 1982.
66. Dyson S, Orsini J: Intussusception of the large colon in a horse, *J Am Vet Med Assoc* 182:720, 1983.
67. Wilson DG, Wilson WD, Reinertson EL: Intussusception of the left dorsal colon in a horse, *J Am Vet Med Assoc* 183:464-465, 1983.
68. Meagher DM, Stirk AJ: Intussusception of the colon in a filly, *Mod Vet Pract* 55:951-952, 1974.
69. Turner TA, Fessler JF: Rectal prolapse in the horse, *J Am Vet Med Assoc* 177:1028-1032, 1980.
70. Snyder JR, Pascoe JR, Williams JW: Rectal prolapse and cystic calculus in a burro, *J Am Vet Med Assoc* 187:421-422, 1985.
71. Blythman WG: Rectal prolapse in a foaling mare, *Vet Rec* 122:471-472, 1988.
72. Rick MC: Management of rectal injuries, *Vet Clin North Am Equine Pract* 5:407-428, 1989.
73. Auer JA, Stick JA, editors: *Equine surgery*, ed 3, St Louis, 2005, Saunders.
74. Jacobs KA, Barber SM, Leach DH: Disruption to the blood supply to the small colon following rectal prolapse and small colon intussusception in a mare, *Can Vet J* 23:132, 1982.
75. Ragle CA, Southwood LL, Galuppo LD, Howlett MR: Laparoscopic diagnosis of ischemic necrosis of the descending colon after rectal prolapse and rupture of the mesocolon in two postpartum mares, *J Am Vet Med Assoc* 210:1646-1648, 1997.
76. White NA: Intestinal infarction associated with mesenteric vascular thrombotic disease in the horse, *J Am Vet Med Assoc* 178:259-262, 1981.

Obstructive Disorders of the Gastrointestinal Tract

1. Fischer AT: Jr: Diagnostic and prognostic procedures for equine colic surgery, *Vet Clin North Am Equine Pract* 5:335-350, 1989.
2. Proudman CJ, Edwards GB, Barnes J, French NR: Factors affecting long-term survival of horses recovering from surgery of the small intestine, *Equine Vet J* 37:360-365, 2005.
3. King JN, Gerring EL: Detection of endotoxin in cases of equine colic, *Vet Rec* 123:269-271, 1988.
4. White NA, Elward A, Moga KS, et al: Use of web-based data collection to evaluate analgesic administration and the decision for surgery in horses with colic, *Equine Vet J* 37:347-350, 2005.

5. White NA, Lessard P: Risk factors and clinical signs associated with cases of equine colic, *32nd American Association of Equine Practitioners Annual Convention* 32:637-644, 1986.
6. Blikslager AT, Roberts MC: Accuracy of clinicians in predicting site and type of lesion as well as outcome in horses with colic, *J Am Vet Med Assoc* 207:1444-1447, 1995.
7. Vacek JR, MacHarg MA, Phillips TN, et al: Struvite urethral calculus in a three-month-old thoroughbred colt, *Cornell Vet* 82:275-279, 1992.
8. Laverty S, Pascoe JR, Ling GV, et al: Urolithiasis in 68 horses, *Vet Surg* 21:56-62, 1992.
9. Johnston JK, Divers TJ, Reef VB, Acland H: Cholelithiasis in horses: ten cases (1982-1986), *J Am Vet Med Assoc* 194:405-409, 1989.
10. Boening KJ, Leendertse IP: Review of 115 cases of colic in the pregnant mare, *Equine Vet J* 25:518-521, 1993.
11. Pascoe JR, Meagher DM, Wheat JD: Surgical management of uterine torsion in the mare: a review of 26 cases, *J Am Vet Med Assoc* 179:351-354, 1981.
12. Green SL, Smith LL, Vernau W, Beacock SM: Rabies in horses: 21 cases (1970-1990), *J Am Vet Med Assoc* 200:1133-1137, 1992.
13. Muir WW III, Woolf CJ: Mechanisms of pain and their therapeutic implications, *J Am Vet Med Assoc* 219:1346-1356, 2001.
14. Freeman DE: Gastrointestinal pharmacology, *Vet Clin North Am Equine Pract* 15(vii):535-559, 1999.
15. Kallings P: Nonsteroidal anti-inflammatory drugs, *Vet Clin North Am Equine Pract* 9:523-541, 1993.
16. Little D, Brown SA, Campbell NB, et al: Effects of the cyclooxygenase inhibitor meloxicam on recovery of ischemia-injured equine jejunum, *Am J Vet Res* 68:614-624, 2007.
17. England GC, Clarke KW: Alpha $_2$ adrenoceptor agonists in the horse: a review, *Br Vet J* 152:641-657, 1996.
18. Yamashita K, Tsubakishita S, Futaok S, et al: Cardiovascular effects of medetomidine, detomidine and xylazine in horses, *J Vet Med Sci* 62:1025-1032, 2000.
19. Wagner AE, Muir WW III, Hinchcliff KW: Cardiovascular effects of xylazine and detomidine in horses, *Am J Vet Res* 52:651-657, 1991.
20. Parry BW, Anderson GA, Gay CC: Prognosis in equine colic: a study of individual variables used in case assessment, *Equine Vet J* 15:337-344, 1983.
21. Puotunen-Reinert A: Study of variables commonly used in examination of equine colic cases to assess prognostic value, *Equine Vet J* 18:275-277, 1986.
22. Moore JN, Owen RR, Lumsden JH: Clinical evaluation of blood lactate levels in equine colic, *Equine Vet J* 8:49-54, 1976.
23. Johnston K, Holcombe SJ, Hauptman JG: Plasma lactate as a predictor of colonic viability and survival after 360 degrees volvulus of the ascending colon in horses, *Vet Surg* 36:563-567, 2007.
24. Bristol DG: The anion gap as a prognostic indicator in horses with abdominal pain, *J Am Vet Med Assoc* 181:63-65, 1982.
25. Snyder JR, Pascoe JR, Olander HJ, et al: Strangulating volvulus of the ascending colon in horses, *J Am Vet Med Assoc* 195:757-764, 1989.
26. Johnston JK, Freeman DE: Diseases and surgery of the large colon, *Vet Clin North Am Equine Pract* 13:317-340, 1997.
27. Proudman CJ, Edwards GB, Barnes J, French NP: Modelling long-term survival of horses following surgery for large intestinal disease, *Equine Vet J* 37:366-370, 2005.
28. Reeves MJ, Curtis CR, Salman MD, et al: Multivariable prediction model for the need for surgery in horses with colic, *Am J Vet Res* 52:1903-1907, 1991.
29. Reeves MJ, Curtis CR, Salman MD, Hilbert BJ: Prognosis in equine colic patients using multivariable analysis, *Can J Vet Res* 53:87-94, 1989.
30. Orsini JA, Elser AH, Galligan DT, et al: Prognostic index for acute abdominal crisis (colic) in horses, *Am J Vet Res* 49:1969-1971, 1988.
31. Clarke LL, Roberts MC, Argenzio RA: Feeding and digestive problems in horses. Physiologic responses to a concentrated meal, *Vet Clin North Am Equine Pract* 6:433-450, 1990.
32. Clarke LL, Argenzio RA, Roberts MC: Effect of meal feeding on plasma volume and urinary electrolyte clearance in ponies, *Am J Vet Res* 51:571-576, 1990.
33. Dabareiner RM, Sullins KE, Snyder JR, et al: Evaluation of the microcirculation of the equine small intestine after intraluminal distention and subsequent decompression, *Am J Vet Res* 54:1673-1682, 1993.
34. Allen DJ, White NA, Tyler DE: Morphologic effects of experimental distention of equine small intestine, *Vet Surg* 17: 10-14, 1988.
35. Hanson RR, Wright JC, Schumacher J, et al: Surgical reduction of ileal impactions in the horse: 28 cases, *Vet Surg* 27:555-560, 1998.
36. Hanson RR, Schumacher J, Humburg J, Dunkerley SC: Medical treatment of horses with ileal impactions: 10 cases (1990-1994), *J Am Vet Med Assoc* 208:898-900, 1996.
37. Cribb NC, Cote NM, Bouré LP, Peregrine AS: Acute small intestinal obstruction associated with Parascaris equorum infection in young horses: 25 cases (1985-2004), *N Z Vet J* 54:338-343, 2006.
38. Parks AHA, Allen D: *The purported role of coastal Bermuda hay in the etiology of ileal impactions: results of a questionnaire (abstract). 6th Equine Colic Research Symposium*, 1998, University of Georgia, p. 37.
39. Proudman CJ, French NP, Trees AJ: Tapeworm infection is a significant risk factor for spasmodic colic and ileal impaction colic in the horse, *Equine Vet J* 30:194-199, 1998.
40. Proudman CJ, Trees AJ: Use of excretory/secretory antigens for the serodiagnosis of Anoplocephala perfoliata cestodosis, *Vet Parasitol* 61:239-247, 1996.
41. Parks AH, Doran RE, White NA, et al: Ileal impaction in the horse: 75 cases, *Cornell Vet* 79:83-91, 1989.
42. Blikslager AT, Bowman KF, Levine JF, et al: Evaluation of factors associated with postoperative ileus in horses: 31 cases (1990-1992), *J Am Vet Med Assoc* 205:1748-1752, 1994.
43. Chaffin MK, Fuenteabla IC, Schumacher J, et al: Idiopathic muscular hypertrophy of the equine small intestine: 11 cases (1980-1991), *Equine Vet J* 24:372-378, 1992.
44. Edwards GB: Obstruction of the ileum in the horse: a report of 27 clinical cases, *Equine Vet J* 13:158-166, 1981.
45. Mair TS, Lucke VM: Ileal muscular hypertrophy and rupture in a pony three years after surgery for ileocaecal intussusception, *Vet Rec* 146:472-473, 2000.
46. Gerard MP, Bowman KF, Blikslager AT, et al: Jejunocolostomy or ileocolostomy for treatment of cecal impaction in horses: nine cases (1985-1995), *J Am Vet Med Assoc* 209:1287-1290, 1996.
47. Hooper RN: Small intestinal strangulation caused by Meckel's diverticulum in a horse, *J Am Vet Med Assoc* 194:943-944, 1989.
48. Grant BD, Tennant B: Volvulus associated with Meckel's diverticulum in the horse, *J Am Vet Med Assoc* 162:550-551, 1973.
49. Yovich JV, Horney FD: Congenital jejunal diverticulum in a foal, *J Am Vet Med Assoc* 183:1092, 1983.
50. Freeman DE, Koch DB, Boles CL: Mesodiverticular bands as a cause of small intestinal strangulation and volvulus in the horse, *J Am Vet Med Assoc* 175:1089-1094, 1979.
51. Baxter GM, Broome TE, Moore JN: Abdominal adhesions after small intestinal surgery in the horse, *Vet Surg* 18:409-414, 1989.

52. Lundin C, Sullins KE, White NA, et al: Induction of peritoneal adhesions with small intestinal ischaemia and distention in the foal, *Equine Vet J* 21:451-458, 1989.
53. Gerard MP, Blikslager AT, Roberts MC, et al: The characteristics of intestinal injury peripheral to strangulating obstruction lesions in the equine small intestine, *Equine Vet J* 31:331-335, 1999.
54. Southwood LL, Baxter GM: Current concepts in management of abdominal adhesions, *Vet Clin North Am Equine Pract* 13:415-435, 1997.
55. Hay WP, Mueller PO, Harmon B, Amoroso L: One percent sodium carboxymethylcellulose prevents experimentally induced abdominal adhesions in horses, *Vet Surg* 30:223-227, 2001.
56. Mueller PO, Harmon BG, Hay WP, Amoroso LM: Effect of carboxymethylcellulose and a hyaluronate-carboxymethylcellulose membrane on healing of intestinal anastomoses in horses, *Am J Vet Res* 61:369-374, 2000.
57. Mueller PO, Hunt RJ, Allen D, et al: Intraperitoneal use of sodium carboxymethylcellulose in horses undergoing exploratory celiotomy, *Vet Surg* 24:112-117, 1995.
58. Parker JE, Fubini SL, Car BD, Erb HN: Prevention of intraabdominal adhesions in ponies by low-dose heparin therapy, *Vet Surg* 16:459-462, 1987.
59. Phillips TJ, Walmsley JP: Retrospective analysis of the results of 151 exploratory laparotomies in horses with gastrointestinal disease, *Equine Vet J* 25:427-431, 1993.
60. Vatistas NJ, Snyder JR, Wilson WD, et al: Surgical treatment for colic in the foal (67 cases): 1980-1992, *Equine Vet J* 28:139-145, 1996.
61. Parker JE, Fubini SL, Todhunter RJ: Retrospective evaluation of repeat celiotomy in 53 horses with acute gastrointestinal disease, *Vet Surg* 18:424-431, 1989.
62. Little D, Redding WR, Blikslager AT: Risk factors for reduced postoperative fecal output in horses: 37 cases (1997-1998), *J Am Vet Med Assoc* 218:414-420, 2001.
63. Türler A, Kalff JC, Moore BA, et al: Leukocyte-derived inducible nitric oxide synthase mediates murine postoperative ileus, *Ann Surg* 244:220-229, 2006.
64. Kalff JC, Schraut WH, Billiar TR, et al: Role of inducible nitric oxide synthase in postoperative intestinal smooth muscle dysfunction in rodents, *Gastroenterology* 118:316-327, 2000.
65. Kalff JC, Carlos TM, Schraut WH, et al: Surgically induced leukocytic infiltrates within the rat intestinal muscularis mediate postoperative ileus, *Gastroenterology* 117:378-387, 1999.
66. Gerring EE, Hunt JM: Pathophysiology of equine postoperative ileus: effect of adrenergic blockade, parasympathetic stimulation and metoclopramide in an experimental model, *Equine Vet J* 18:249-255, 1986.
67. Hunt JM, Gerring EL: The effect of prostaglandin E_1 on motility of the equine gut, *J Vet Pharmacol Ther* 8:165-173, 1985.
68. Van Hoogmoed LM, Snyder JR, Harmon F: In vitro investigation of the effect of prostaglandins and nonsteroidal anti-inflammatory drugs on contractile activity of the equine smooth muscle of the dorsal colon, ventral colon, and pelvic flexure, *Am J Vet Res* 61:1259-1266, 2000.
69. Van Hoogmoed LM, Rakestraw PC, Snyder JR, Harmon FA: Evaluation of nitric oxide as an inhibitory neurotransmitter in the equine ventral colon, *Am J Vet Res* 61:64-68, 2000.
70. Schwarz NT, Kalff JC, Turler A, et al: Prostanoid production via COX-2 as a causative mechanism of rodent postoperative ileus, *Gastroenterology* 121:1354-1371, 2001.
71. King JN, Gerring EL: The action of low dose endotoxin on equine bowel motility, *Equine Vet J* 23:11-17, 1991.
72. Gerring EL: Sir Frederick Hobday Memorial Lecture. All wind and water: some progress in the study of equine gut motility, *Equine Vet J* 23:81-85, 1991.
73. King JN, Gerring EL: Antagonism of endotoxin-induced disruption of equine bowel motility by flunixin and phenylbutazone, *Equine Vet J* (Suppl):38-42, 1989.
74. Blikslager AT: Cyclooxygenase inhibitors in equine practice, *Comp Contin Educ Pract Vet* 21:548-550, 1999.
75. Nieto JE, Rakestraw PC, Snyder JR, Vatistas NJ: In vitro effects of erythromycin, lidocaine, and metoclopramide on smooth muscle from the pyloric antrum, proximal portion of the duodenum, and middle portion of the jejunum of horses, *Am J Vet Res* 61:413-419, 2000.
76. Dart AJ, Peauroi JR, Hodgson DR, Pascoe JR: Efficacy of metoclopramide for treatment of ileus in horses following small intestinal surgery: 70 cases (1989-1992), *Austr Vet J* 74:280-284, 1996.
77. Lundgren O, Peregrin AT, Persson K, et al: Role of the enteric nervous system in the fluid and electrolyte secretion of rotavirus diarrhea, *Science* 287:491-495, 2000.
78. Roussel AJ, Hooper RN, Cohen ND, et al: Prokinetic effects of erythromycin on the ileum, cecum, and pelvic flexure of horses during the postoperative period, *Am J Vet Res* 61:420-424, 2000.
79. Campbell ML, Colahan PC, Brown MP, et al: Cecal impaction in the horse, *J Am Vet Med Assoc* 184:950-952, 1984.
80. Dart AJ, Hodgson DR, Snyder JR: Caecal disease in equids, *Austr Vet J* 75:552-557, 1997.
81. Plummer AE, Rakestraw PC, Hardy J, Lee RM: Outcome of medical and surgical treatment of cecal impaction in horses: 114 cases (1994-2004), *J Am Vet Med Assoc* 231:1378-1385, 2007.
82. Dabareiner RM, White NA: Diseases and surgery of the cecum, *Vet Clin North Am Equine Pract* 13:303-315, 1997.
83. White NA, Dabareiner RM: Treatment of impaction colics, *Vet Clin North Am Equine Pract* 13:243-259, 1997.
84. Dabareiner RM, White NA: Large colon impaction in horses: 147 cases (1985-1991), *J Am Vet Med Assoc* 206:679-685, 1995.
85. Roberts MC, Argenzio A: Effects of amitraz, several opiate derivatives and anticholinergic agents on intestinal transit in ponies, *Equine Vet J* 18:256-260, 1986.
86. Roberts MC, Seawright AA: Experimental studies of drug-induced impaction colic in the horse, *Equine Vet J* 15:222-228, 1983.
87. Sellers AF, Lowe JE, Drost CJ, et al: Retropulsion-propulsion in equine large colon, *Am J Vet Res* 43:390-396, 1982.
88. Blue MG, Wittkopp RW: Clinical and structural features of equine enteroliths, *J Am Vet Med Assoc* 179:79-82, 1981.
89. Hassel DM, Schiffman PS, Snyder JR: Petrographic and geochemic evaluation of equine enteroliths, *Am J Vet Res* 62:350-358, 2001.
90. Lloyd K, Hintz HF, Wheat JD, Schryver HF: Enteroliths in horses, *Cornell Vet* 77:172-186, 1987.
91. Hassel DM, Langer DL, Snyder JR, et al: Evaluation of enterolithiasis in equids: 900 cases (1973-1996), *J Am Vet Med Assoc* 214:233-237, 1999.
92. Cohen ND, Vontur CA, Rakestraw PC: Risk factors for enterolithiasis among horses in Texas, *J Am Vet Med Assoc* 216:1787-1794, 2000.
93. Peloso JG, Coatney RW, Caron JP, Steficek BA: Obstructive enterolith in an 11-month-old miniature horse, *J Am Vet Med Assoc* 201:1745-1746, 1992.
94. Specht TE, Colahan PT: Surgical treatment of sand colic in equids: 48 cases (1978-1985), *J Am Vet Med Assoc* 193:1560-1564, 1988.
95. Ragle CA, Meagher DM, Lacroix CA, Honnas CM: Surgical treatment of sand colic. Results in 40 horses, *Vet Surg* 18:48-51, 1989.
96. Bertone JJ, Traub-Dargatz JL, Wrigley RW, et al: Diarrhea associated with sand in the gastrointestinal tract of horses, *J Am Vet Med Assoc* 193:1409-1412, 1988.
97. Ragle CA, Meagher DM, Schrader JL, Honnas CM: Abdominal auscultation in the detection of experimentally induced gastrointestinal sand accumulation, *J Vet Intern Med* 3:12-14, 1989.

98. Hammock PD, Freeman DE, Baker GJ: Failure of psyllium mucilloid to hasten evaluation of sand from the equine large intestine, *Vet Surg* 27:547-554, 1998.
99. Hackett RP: Nonstrangulated colonic displacement in horses, *J Am Vet Med Assoc* 182:235-240, 1983.
100. Argenzio RA: Functions of the equine large intestine and their interrelationship in disease, *Cornell Vet* 65:303-330, 1975.
101. Morris D, Moore J, Ward S: Comparisons of age, breed, history and management in 229 horses with colic, *Equine Vet J* (Suppl 7):129-133, 1986.
102. Ruckebusch Y: Motor functions of the intestine, *Adv Vet Sci Comp Med* 25:345-369, 1981.
103. Lester GD, Bolton JR, Cambridge H, Thurgate S: The effect of Strongylus vulgaris larvae on equine intestinal myoelectrical activity, *Equine Vet J* Suppl 7:8-13, 1989.
104. Huskamp B: Displacement of the large colon. In Robinson NE, editor: *Current therapy in equine medicine*, Philadelphia, 1987, Saunders, pp 60-65.
105. Bury KD, McClure RL, Wright HK: Reversal of colonic net absorption to net secretion with increased intraluminal pressure, *Arch Surg* 108:854-857, 1974.
106. Santschi EM, Slone DEJ, Frank WM: Use of ultrasound in horses for diagnosis of left dorsal displacement of the large colon and monitoring its nonsurgical correction, *Vet Surg* 22:281-284, 1993.
107. Sivula NJ: Renosplenic entrapment of the large colon in horses: 33 cases (1984-1989), *J Am Vet Med Assoc* 199:244-246, 1991.
108. Baird AN, Cohen ND, Taylor TS, et al: Renosplenic entrapment of the large colon in horses: 57 cases (1983-1988), *J Am Vet Med Assoc* 198:1423-1426, 1991.
109. Kalsbeek HC: Further experiences with non-surgical correction of nephrosplenic entrapment of the left colon in the horse, *Equine Vet J* 21:442-443, 1989.
110. Hardy J, Bednarski RM, Biller DS: Effect of phenylephrine on hemodynamics and splenic dimensions in horses, *Am J Vet Res* 55:1570-1578, 1994.
111. Röcken M, Schubert C, Mosel G, Litzke LF: Indications, surgical technique, and long-term experience with laparoscopic closure of the nephrosplenic space in standing horses, *Vet Surg* 34:637-641, 2005.
112. Gay CC, Speirs VC, Christie BA, et al: Foreign body obstruction of the small colon in six horses, *Equine Vet J* 11:60-63, 1979.
113. McClure JT, Kobluk C, Voller K, et al: Fecalith impaction in four miniature foals, *J Am Vet Med Assoc* 200:205-207, 1992.
114. Speirs VC, van Veenendaal JC, Christie BA, et al: Obstruction of the small colon by intramural haematoma in three horses, *Austr Vet J* 57:88-90, 1981.
115. Pearson H, Waterman AE: Submucosal haematoma as a cause of obstruction of the small colon in the horse: a review of four cases, *Equine Vet J* 18:340-341, 1986.
116. Scott EA, Heidel JR, Snyder SP, et al: Inflammatory bowel disease in horses: 11 cases (1988-1998), *J Am Vet Med Assoc* 214:1527-1530, 1999.
117. Frederico LM, Jones SL, Blikslager AT: Predisposing factors for small colon impaction in horses and outcome of medical and surgical treatment: 44 cases (1999-2004), *J Am Vet Med Assoc15* 229:1612-1616, 2006.
118. Benamou A, Blikslager AT, Sellon D: Intestinal atresia in horses, *Comp Contin Educ Pract Vet* 17:1510-1517, 1995.
119. Santschi EM, Purdy AK, Valberg SJ, et al: Endothelin receptor B polymorphism associated with lethal whit efoal syndrome in horses, *Mamm Genome* 9:306-309, 1998.
120. Metallinos DL, Bowling AT, Rine J: A missense mutation in the Endothelin-B receptor gene is associated with lethal white foal syndrome: an equine version of Hirschprung disease, *Mamm Genome* 9:426-431, 1998.
121. Santschi EM, Vrotsos PD, Purdy AK, et al: Incidence of the endothelin receptor B mutation that causes lethal white foal syndrome in white-patterned horses, *Am J Vet Res* 62:97-103, 2001.
122. Hultgren BD: Ileocolonic aganglionosis in white progeny of overo spotted horses, *J Am Vet Med Assoc* 180:289-292, 1982.

Neoplasia of the Alimentary Tract

1. Pascoe RR, Summers PM: Clinical survey of tumors and tumor-like lesions in horses in South East Queensland, *Equine Vet Jl* 13:235-239, 1981.
2. Baker GJ, Easley J, editors: *Equine dentistry*, ed 2, London, 2004, Saunders.
3. Kreutzer R, Wohlsein P, Staszyk C, et al: Dental benign cementomas in three horses, *Vet Pathol* 44:533-536, 2007.
4. MacGillivray KC, Graham TD, Parente EJ: Multicentric leiomyosarcoma in a young male horse, *J Am Vet Med Assoc* 223(986):1017-1986, 2003:1021.
5. Dunkel BM, Del Piero E, Kraus BM, et al: Congenital cutaneous, oral, and periarticular hemangiosarcoma in a 9-day-old rocky mountain horse, *J Vet Intern Med* 18:252-255, 2004.
6. Wilson GJ, Anthony ND: Chondrosarcoma of the tongue of a horse, *Austr Vet J* 85:163-165, 2007.
7. Rhind SM, Dixon PM: T cell-rich B cell lymphosarcoma in the tongue of a horse, *Vet Rec* 145:554-555, 1999.
8. Markel MD, Dorr TE: Multiple myeloma in a horse, *J Am Vet Med Assoc* 188:621-622, 1986.
9. Hanson PD, Frisbie DD, Dubielzig RR, Markel MD: Rhabdomyosarcoma of the Tongue in A Horse, *J Am Vet Med Assoc* 202:1281-1284, 1993.
10. Williams MA, Dowling PM, Angarano DW, et al: Paraneoplastic bullous stomatitis in a horse, *J Am Vet Med Assoc* 207:331-334, 1995.
11. McKenzie EC, Mills JN, Bolton JR: Gastric squamous cell carcinoma in three horses, *Austr Vet J* 75:480-483, 1997.
12. Campbellbeggs CL, Kiper ML, Macallister C, et al: Use of esophagoscopy in the diagnosis of esophageal squamous-cell carcinoma in a horse, *J Am Vet Med Assoc* 202:617-618, 1993.
13. Patton KM, Peek SF, Valentine BA: Gastric adenocarcinoma in a horse with portal vein metastasis and thrombosis: a novel cause of hepatic encephalopathy, *Vet Pathol* 43:565-569, 2006.
14. Morse CC, Richardson DW: Gastric hyperplastic polyp in a horse, *J Comp Pathol* 99:337-342, 1988.
15. Boy MG, Palmer JE, Heyer G, Hamir AN: Gastric leiomyosarcoma in a horse, *J Am Vet Med Assoc* 200:1363-1364, 1992.
16. La Perle KM, Piercy RJ, Long JF, et al: Multisystemic, eosinophilic, epitheliotropic disease with intestinal lymphosarcoma in a horse, *Vet Pathol* 35:144-146, 1998.
17. Asahina M, Murakami K, Ajito T, et al: An immunohistochemical study of an equine B-cell lymphoma, *J Comp Pathol* 111:445-451, 1994.
18. Olsen SN: Squamous-cell carcinoma of the equinestomach: a report of 5 cases, *Vety Rec* 131:170-173, 1992.
19. Tennant B, Keirn DR, White KK, et al: 6 Cases of squamous-cell carcinoma of the stomach of the horse, *Equine Vet Jl* 14:238-243, 1982.
20. Taylor SD, Pusterla N, Vaughan B, et al: Intestinal neoplasia in horses, *J Vet Intern Med* 20:1429-1436, 2006.
21. Honnas CM, Snyder JR, Olander HJ, Wheat JD: Small intestinal adenocarcinoma in a horse, *J Am Vet Med Assoc* 191:845-846, 1987.
22. Moran JAM, Lemberger K, Cadore JL, Lepage OM: Small intestine adenocarcinoma in conjunction with multiple adenomas causing acute colic in a horse, *J Vet Diagn Invest* 20:121-124, 2008.

23. Patterson-Kane JC, Sanchez LC, Mackay RJ, et al: Small intestinal adenomatous polyposis resulting in protein-losing enteropathy in a horse, *Vet Pathol* 37:82-85, 2000.
24. Allen D, Swayne D, Belknap JK: Ganglioneuroma as a cause of small intestinal obstruction in the horse: a case report, *Cornell Vet* 79:133-141, 1989.
25. Orsini JA, Orsini PG, Sepesy L, et al: Intestinal carcinoid in a mare: an etiologic consideration for chronic colic in horses, *J Am Vet Med Assoc* 193:87-88, 1988.
26. Hanes GE, Robertson JT: Leiomyoma of the small intestine in a horse, *J Am Vet Med Assoc* 182:1398, 1983.
27. Collier MA, Trent AM: Jejunal intussusception associated with leiomyoma in an aged horse, *J Am Vet Med Assoc* 182:819-821, 1983.
28. Kasper C, Doran R: Duodenal leiomyoma associated with colic in a 2-year-old horse, *J Am Vet Med Assoc* 202:769-770, 1993.
29. Mair TS, Taylor FGR, Brown PJ: Leiomyosarcoma of the duodenum in 2 horses, *J Comp Pathol* 102:119-123, 1990.
30. Blikslager AT, Bowman KF, Haven ML, et al: Pedunculated lipomas as a cause of intestinal obstruction in horses: 17 cases (1983-1990), *J Am Vet Med Assoc* 201:1249-1252, 1992.
31. Hoven R, Franken P: Clinical aspects of lymphosarcoma in the horse: a clinical report of 16 cases, *Equine Vet J* 15:49-53, 1983.
32. Kirchhof N, Scheidemann W, Baumgartner W: Multiple peripheral nerve sheath tumors in the small intestine of a horse, *Vet Pathol* 33:727-730, 1996.
33. Kirchhof N, Steinhauer D, Fey K: Equine adenocarcinomas of the large intestine with osseous metaplasia, *J Comp Pathol* 114:451-456, 1996.
34. Edens LM, Taylor DD, Murray MJ, et al: Intestinal myxosarcoma in a thoroughbred mare, *Cornell Vet* 82:163-167, 1992.
35. Hafner S, Harmon BG, King T: Gastrointestinal stromal tumors of the equine cecum, *Vet Pathol* 38:242-246, 2001.
36. Rottman JB, Roberts MC, Cullen JM: Colonic adenocarcinoma with osseous metaplasia in a horse, *J Am Vet Med Assoc* 198:657-659, 1991.
37. Roy MF, Parente EJ, Donaldson MT, et al: Successful treatment of a colonic adenocarcinoma in a horse, *Equine Vet J* 34:102-104, 2002.
38. Harvey-Micay J: Intestinal adenocarcinoma causing recurrent colic in the horse, *Can Vet Jl-Rev Vet Can* 40:729-730, 1999.
39. Henry GA, Yamini B: Equine colonic lipomatosis, *J Vet Diagn Invest* 7:578-580, 1995.
40. Dabareiner RM, Sullins KE, Goodrich LR: Large colon resection for treatment of lymphosarcoma in two horses, *J Am Vet Med Assoc* 208:895-897, 1996.
41. Pascoe PJ: Colic in a mare caused by a colonic neurofibroma, *Can Vet J-Rev Vet Can* 23:24-247, 1982.
42. Edwards GB, Proudman CJ: An analysis of 75 cases of intestinal obstruction caused by pedunculated lipomas, *Equine Vet J* 26:18-21, 1994.
43. Mair TS, Davies EV, Lucke VM: Small colon intussusception associated with an intralumenal leiomyoma in a pony, *Vet Rec* 130:403-404, 1992.
44. Haven ML, Rottman JB, Bowman KF: Leiomyoma of the small colon in a horse, *Vet Surg* 20:320-322, 1991.
45. Clem MF, Debowes RM, Leipold HW: Rectal leiomyosarcoma in a horse, *J Am Vet Med Assoc* 191:229-230, 1987.
46. Mason TA: Strangulation of rectum of a horse by pedicle of a mesenteric lipoma, *Equine Vet J* 10:269, 1978.
47. Lindberg R, Nygren A, Persson SGB: Rectal biopsy diagnosis in horses with clinical signs of intestinal disorders: a retrospective study of 116 cases, *Equine Vet J* 28:275-284, 1996.
48. DeBowes RM: Standing rectal and tail surgery, *Vet Clin North Am Equine Pract* :649-667, 1991;December.
49. Johnson PJ, Wilson DA, Turk JR, et al: Disseminated peritoneal leiomyomatosis in a horse, *J Am Vet Med Assoc* 205:725-728, 1994.
50. Ricketts SW, Peace CK: A case of peritoneal mesothelioma in a thoroughbred mare, *Equine Vet J* 8:78-80, 1976.
51. Harps O, Brumhard J, Bartmann CP, Hinrichs U: [Ascites as a result of peritoneal mesotheliomas in a horse], *Tierarztl Prax* 24:270-274, 1996.
52. LaCarrubba AM, Johnson PJ, Whitney MS, Miller MA, Lattimer JC: Hypoglycemia and tumor lysis syndrome associated with peritoneal mesothelioma in a horse, *J Vet Intern Med* 20:1018-1022, 2006.
53. Harvey KA, Morris DD, Saik JE, Donawick WJ: Omental fibrosarcoma in a horse, *J Am Vet Med Assoc* 191:335-336, 1987.
54. East LM, Savage CJ: Abdominal neoplasia (excluding urogenital tract), *Vet Clin North Am Equine Pract* 14:475-493, 1998.
55. McFadden KEPL: Clinical manifestation of squamous cell carcinoma in horses, *Compend Contin Educ Prac Vet* 13:669-677, 1991.
56. Smith BP, editor: *Large animal internal medicine*, ed 4, St Louis, 2008, Mosby.
57. Robinson NE, editor: *Current therapy in equine medicine*, ed 6, St Louis, 2009, Saunders.
58. Ford TS, Vaala WE, Sweeney CR, et al: Pleuroscopic diagnosis of gastroesophageal squamous-cell carcinoma in a horse, *J Am Vet Med Assoc* 190, 1987:1556-1158.
59. Moore JN, Kintner LD: Recurrent esophageal obstruction due to squamous-cell carcinoma in a horse, *Cornell Vet* 66:590-597, 1976.
60. Mair TS, Hillyer MH: Chronic colic in the mature horse: a retrospective review of 106 cases, *Equine Vet J* 29:415-420, 1997.
61. Hillyer MH, Mair TS: Recurrent colic in the mature horse: a retrospective review of 58 cases, *Equine Vet J* 29:421-424, 1997.
62. Ogilvie GK: Paraneoplastic syndromes, *Vet Clin North Am Equine Pract* 14:439-449, 1998.
63. Reef VB, Dyson SS, Beech J: Lymphosarcoma and associated immune-mediated hemolytic-anemia and thrombocytopenia in horses, *J Am Vet Med Assoc* 184:313-317, 1984.
64. Dascanio JJ, Zhang CH, Antczak DF, et al: Differentiation of chronic lymphocytic-leukemia in the horse: a report of 2 cases, *J Vet Intern Med* 6:225-229, 1992.
65. Mccoy DJ, Beasley R: Hypercalcemia Associated with Malignancy in A Horse, *J Am Vet Med Assoc* 189:87-89, 1986.
66. Fulton IC, Brown CM, Yamini B: Adenocarcinoma of intestinal origin in a horse: diagnosis by abdominocentesis and laparoscopy, *Equine Vet J* 22:447-448, 1990.
67. Dechant JE, Nieto JE, Le Jeune SS: Hemoperitoneum in horses: 67 cases (1989-2004), *J Am Vet Med Assoc* 229:253-258, 2006.
68. Southwood LL, Schott HC, Henry CJ, et al: Disseminated hemangiosarcoma in the horse: 35 cases, *J Vet Intern Med* 14:105-109, 2000.
69. Zicker SC, Wilson WD, Medearis I: Differentiation between intraabdominal neoplasms and abscesses in horses, using clinical and laboratory data: 40 cases (1973-1988), *J Am Vet Med Assoc* 196:1130-1134, 1990.
70. Roberts MC, Pinsent PJ: Malabsorption in the horse associated with alimentary lymphosarcoma, *Equine Vet J* 7:166-172, 1975.
71. Perkins GA, Nydam DV, Flaminio MJBE, Ainsworth DM: Serum IgM concentrations in normal, fit horses and horses with lymphoma or other medical conditions, *J Vet Intern Med* 17:337-342, 2003.
72. Davis EG, Wilkerson MJ, Rush BR: Flow cytometry: Clinical applications in equine medicine, *J Vet Intern Med* 16:404-410, 2002.
73. Wrigley RH, Gay CC, Lording P, Haywood RN: Pleural effusion associated with squamous-cell carcinoma of the stomach of a horse, *Equine Vet J* 13:99-102, 1981.
74. Klohnen A, Vachon AM, Fischer AT: Use of diagnostic ultrasonography in horses with signs of acute abdominal pain, *J Am Vet Med Assoc* 209:1597-1601, 1996.

75. Pearson H, Pinsent PJ, Denny HR, Waterman A: The indications for equine laparotomy: an analysis of 140 cases, *Equine Vet J* 7:131-136, 1975.
76. Rebhun WC, Bertone A: Equine lymphosarcoma, *J Am Vet Med Assoc* 184:720-721, 1984.
77. Wiseman A, Petrie L, Murray M: Diarrhea in horse as a result of alimentary lymphosarcoma, *Vet Rec* 95:454-457, 1974.
78. Finley MR, Rebhun WC, Dee A, Langsetmo I: Paraneoplastic pruritus and alopecia in a horse with diffuse lymphoma, *J Am Vet Med Assoc* 213:102-104, 1998.
79. Meyer J, Delay J, Bienzle D: Clinical, laboratory, and histopathologic features of equine lymphoma, *Vet Pathol* 43:914-924, 2006.
80. Mair TS, Couto CG: The use of cytotoxic drugs in equine practice, *Equine Vet Educ* 18:149-156, 2006.
81. Saulez MN, Schlipf JW, Cebra CK, et al: Use of chemotherapy for treatment of a mixed-cell thoracic lymphoma in a horse, *J Am Vet Med Assoc* 224:733-738, 2004.
82. Tuckey JC, Hilbert BJ, Beetson S, Adkins A: Squamous-cell carcinoma of the pharyngeal wall in a horse, *Austr Vet J* 72:227, 1995.
83. Schuh JCL: Squamous-cell carcinoma of the oral, pharyngeal and nasal-mucosa in the horse, *Vet Pathol* 23:205-207, 1986.
84. Paterson S: Treatment of superficial ulcerative squamous cell carcinoma in three horses with topical 5-fluorouracil, *Vet Rec* 141:626-628, 1997.
85. Theon AP, Pascoe JR, Carlson GP, Krag DN: Intratumoral chemotherapy with cisplatin in oily emulsion in horses, *J Am Vet Med Assoc* 202:261-267, 1993.
86. Orsini JA, Nunamaker DM, Jones CJ, Acland HM: Excision of oral squamous-cell carcinoma in a horse, *Vet Surg* 20:264-266, 1991.
87. Moore AS, Beam SL, Rassnick KM, Provost R: Long-term control of mucocutaneous squamous cell carcinoma and metastases in a horse using piroxicam, *Equine Vet J* 35:715-718, 2003.
88. Schleining JA, Voss ED: Hypertrophy osteopathy secondary to gastric squamous cell carcinoma in a horse, *Equine Vet Educ* 16:304-307, 2004.
89. Schaudien D, Muller JMV, Baumgartner W: Omental leiomyoma in a male adult horse, *Vet Pathol* 44:722-726, 2007.
90. Dart AJ, Snyder JR, Pascoe JR: Extensive resection and anastomosis of the descending (small) colon in a mare following strangulation by a mesenteric lipoma, *Austr Vet J* 68:61-64, 1991.
91. Riley E, Martindale A, Maran B, et al: Small colon lipomatosis resulting in refractory small colon impaction in a Tennessee Walking Horse, *Equine Vet Educ* 19:484-487, 2007.
92. Henson FMD, Dixon K, Dobson JM: Treatment of 4 cases of equine lymphoma with megavoltage radiation, *Equine Veterinary Educ* 16:312-314, 2004.
93. Henson FMD, Dobson JM: Use of radiation therapy in the treatment of equine neoplasia, *Equine Vet Educ* 16:315-318, 2004.
94. Morse CC, Saik JE, Richardson DW, et al: Equine juvenile mandibular ossifying fibroma, *Vet Pathol* 25:415-421, 1988.
95. Brounts SH, Hawkins JE, Lescun TB, et al: Surgical management of compound odontoma in two horses, *J Am Vet Med Assoc* 225:1423-1427, 2004.

Periotonitis

1. Smith BP: *Large animal internal medicine*, ed 4, St Louis, 2008, Mosby.
2. Hosgood G: Peritonitis .1. A review of the pathophysiology and diagnosis, *Aust Vet Pract* 16:184-190, 1986.
3. Kobluk CN, Ames TR, Geor RJ: *The horse: diseases and clinical management*, Philadelphia, 1995, Saunders.
4. Colahan PT, Mayhew IG, Merritt AM, et al: *Equine medicine and surgery*, St Louis, 1999, Mosby.
5. Dyson S: Review of 30 cases of peritonitis in the horse, *Equine Vet J* 15:25-30, 1983.
6. Semrad SD, Hardee GE, Hardee MM, Moore JN: Flunixin meglumine given in small doses: pharmacokinetics and prostaglandin inhibition in healthy horses, *Am J Vet Res* 46:2474-2479, 1985.
7. Zicker SC, Wilson WD, Medearis I: Differentiation between intra-abdominal neoplasms and abscesses in horses, using clinical and laboratory data: 40 cases (1973-1988), *J Am Vet Med Assoc* 196:1130-1134, 1990.
8. Pratt SM, Spier SJ, Carroll SP, et al: Evaluation of clinical characteristics, diagnostic test results, and outcome in horses with internal infection caused by Corynebacterium pseudotuberculosis: 30 cases (1995-2003), *J Am Vet Med Assoc* 227:441-448, 2005.
9. Golland LC, Hodgson DR, Hodgson JL, et al: Peritonitis associated with Actinobacillus equuli in horses: 15 cases (1982-1992), *J Am Vet Med Assoc* 205:340-343, 1994.
10. Matthews S, Dart AJ, Dowling BA, et al: Peritonitis associated with Actinobacillus equuli in horses: 51 cases, *Austr Vet J* 79:536-539, 2001.
11. Gay CC, Lording PM: Peritonitis in horses associated with Actinobacillus equuli, *Austr Vet J* 56:296-300, 1980.
12. Stewart AJ: Actinobacillus pleuritis and peritonitis in a quarter horse mare, *Vet Clin North Am Equine Pract* 22:e77-e93, 2006.
13. Patterson-Kane JC, Donahue JM, Harrison LR: Septicemia and peritonitis due to Actinobacillus equuli infection in an adult horse, *Vet Pathol* 38:230-232, 2001.
14. Mogg TD, Dykgraaf S: Actinobacillus peritonitis in a Warmblood gelding, *Vet Clin North Am Equine Pract* 22:e9-16, 2006.
15. Hirsh DC, Jang SS: Antimicrobic susceptibility of bacterial pathogens from horses, *Vet Clin North Am Equine Pract* 3:181-190, 1987.
16. Hawkins JF, Bowman KF, Roberts MC, Cowen P: Peritonitis in horses: 67 cases (1985-1990), *J Am Vet Med Assoc* 203:284-288, 1993.
17. Wallace SS, Jayo MJ, Maddux JM, et al: Mesothelioma in a horse, *Compend Cont Educ Pract Vet* 9:210-216, 1987.
18. Lapointe JM, Celeste C, Villeneuve A: Septic peritonitis due to colonic perforation associated with aberrant migration of a Gasterophilus intestinalis larva in a horse, *Vet Pathol* 40:338-339, 2003.
19. Morris DD, Henry MM, Moore JN, Fischer K: Effect of dietary linolenic acid on endotoxin-induced thromboxane and prostacyclin production by equine peritoneal macrophages, *Circ Shock* 29:311-318, 1989.
20. Polk HC: *Clinical surgery international: infection and the surgical patient*, ed 4, New York, 1982, Churchill Livingstone.
21. Archer DC, Clegg PD, Edwards GB: Septic tenosynovitis of the tarsal sheath of an Arab gelding and suspected sepsis of the lateral digital flexor tendon subsequent to bacterial peritonitis, *Vet Rec* 155:485-489, 2004.
22. Vandenplas ML, Moore JN, Barton MH, et al: Concentrations of serum amyloid A and lipopolysaccharide-binding protein in horses with colic, *Am J Vet Res* 66:1509-1516, 2005.
23. Brownlow MA, Hutchins DR, Johnston KG: Reference values for equine peritoneal fluid, *Equine Vet J* 13:127-130, 1981.
24. West J: Diagnostic cytology in the equine species: overview, effusions (peritoneal, pleural and synovial joint) and transtracheal wash, *Proc Am Assoc Equine Pract* 30:169-201, 1984.
25. Schumacher J, Spano JS, Moll HD: Effects of enterocentesis on PF constituents in the horse, *J Am Vet Med Assoc* 186:1301-1303, 1985.
26. Rumbaugh GE, Smith BP, Carlson GP: Internal abdominal abscesses in the horse: a study of 25 cases, *J Am Vet Med Assoc* 172:304-309, 1978.
27. Blackford JT, Schneiter HL, VanSteenehouse JL: Equine peritoneal fluid analysis following celiotomy, *Proc Equine Colic Res Symp* 3:130, 1986.

28. Nelson AW: Analysis of equine peritoneal fluid, *Vet Clin North Am Large Anim Pract* 1:267-274, 1979.
29. Van Hoogmoed L, Rodger LD, Spier SJ, et al: Evaluation of peritoneal fluid pH, glucose concentration, and lactate dehydrogenase activity for detection of septic peritonitis in horses, *J Am Vet Med Assoc* 214:1032-1036, 1999.
30. Bonczynski JJ, Ludwig LL, Barton LJ, et al: Comparison of peritoneal fluid and peripheral blood pH, bicarbonate, glucose, and lactate concentration as a diagnostic tool for septic peritonitis in dogs and cats, *Vet Surg* 32:161-166, 2003.
31. Barton MH, Collatos C: Tumor necrosis factor and interleukin-6 activity and endotoxin concentration in peritoneal fluid and blood of horses with acute abdominal disease, *J Vet Intern Med* 13:457-464, 1999.
32. Semrad SD, Hardee GE, Hardee MM, Moore JN: Low dose flunixin meglumine: effects on eicosanoid production and clinical signs induced by experimental endotoxaemia in horses, *Equine Vet J* 19:201-206, 1987.
33. Sullins KE, White NA, Lundin CS, et al: Prevention of ischaemia-induced small intestinal adhesions in foals, *Equine Vet J* 36:370-375, 2004.
34. Hau T, Simmons RL: Heparin in the treatment of experimental peritonitis, *Ann Surg* 187:294-298, 1978.
35. Parker JE, Fubini SL, Car BD, Erb HN: Prevention of intraabdominal adhesions in ponies by low-dose heparin therapy, *Vet Surg* 16:459-462, 1987.
36. Feige K, Schwarzwald CC, Bombeli T: Comparison of unfractioned and low molecular weight heparin for prophylaxis of coagulopathies in 52 horses with colic: a randomised double-blind clinical trial, *Equine Vet J* 35:506-513, 2003.
37. Schwarzwald CC, Feige K, Wunderli-Allenspach H, Braun U: Comparison of pharmacokinetic variables for two low-molecular-weight heparins after subcutaneous administration of a single dose to horses, *Am J Vet Res* 63:868-873, 2002.
38. Kunesh JP: Therapeutic strategies involving antimicrobial treatment of large animals with peritonitis, *J Am Vet Med Assoc* 185:1222-1225, 1984.
39. Hague BA, Honnas CM, Berridge BR, Easter JL: Evaluation of postoperative peritoneal lavage in standing horses for prevention of experimentally induced abdominal adhesions, *Vet Surg* 27:122-126, 1998.
40. Davis JL: Treatment of peritonitis, *Vet Clin North Am Equine Pract* 19:765-778, 2003.
41. Nieto JE, Snyder JR, Vatistas NJ, et al: Use of an active intra-abdominal drain in 67 horses, *Vet Surg* 32:1-7, 2003.
42. Schneider RK, Meyer DJ, Embertson RM, et al: Response of pony peritoneum to four peritoneal lavage solutions, *Am J Vet Res* 49:889-894, 1988.
43. Easter JL, Hague BA, Brumbaugh GW, et al: Effects of postoperative peritoneal lavage on pharmacokinetics of gentamicin in horses after celiotomy, *Am J Vet Res* 58:1166-1170, 1997.
44. Southwood LL, Russell G: The use of clinical findings in the identification of equine peritonitis cases that respond favorably to medical therapy, *J Vet Emerg Crit Care* 17:382-390, 2007.
45. Javsicas LH, Slovis NM, Freeman DE, Giguere S: Peritonitis secondary to uterine tears in postpartum mares: retrospective comparison of surgical versus medical treatment, *Proc Equine Colic Res Symp* 9, 2008.
46. Mair TS, Smith LJ: Survival and complication rates in 300 horses undergoing surgical treatment of colic. Part 4: Early (acute) relaparotomy, *Equine Vet J* 37:315-318, 2005.

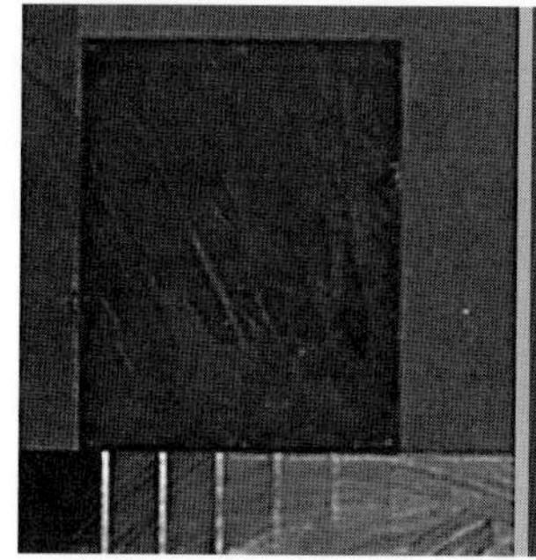

DISORDERS OF THE LIVER

CHAPTER 16

Michelle Henry Barton

NORMAL LIVER

ANATOMY

The liver is the largest organ in the body, constituting approximately 1% of the body weight in the adult horse.[1] The location of the liver between the gastrointestinal tract and the heart is functionally suited for its metabolic, secretory, excretory, and storage properties. In the normal horse, the liver lies mostly to the right of the median, is completely contained within the rib cage, and does not contact the ventral abdominal floor. The most cranial portion of the liver is located in the ventral third of the sixth to seventh intercostal spaces and extends caudad to the right kidney (fifteenth rib). In disease processes resulting in hepatomegaly, and in the normal equine neonate, the liver may extend beyond the caudal border of the last rib. Right liver lobe atrophy has been described as an uncommon normal anatomic variation in adult horses. However, in 1994 it was hypothesized that right hepatic lobe atrophy in horses is a pathologic condition resulting from long-term compression of the right lobe of the liver by abnormal distension of the right dorsal colon and base of the cecum.[2]

The equine liver consists of two surfaces, diaphragmatic and visceral, and is divided by fissures into four lobes: right, left, quadrate, and caudate. The visceral surface of the liver in situ is malleable and contains impressions of the organs with which it is in contact. The visceral surface also contains the hilum, or *porta* (door), of the liver, through which blood vessels, lymphatics, and nerves enter, and the hepatic duct exits. In the horse, six ligaments secure the liver in the abdominal cavity.[1] The *coronary ligament* has two laminae, right and left, which attach the diaphragmatic surface of the liver to the caudal vena cava and the abdominal esophagus. The two laminae of the coronary ligament unite ventrally to form the *falciform ligament.* The falciform ligament, a remnant of the fetal ventral mesentery that extends from the diaphragm to the umbilicus, attaches the quadrate and left lobes to the sternal diaphragm and ventral abdominal floor. The *round ligament,* the remnant of the fetal umbilical vein, is contained within the free border of the falciform ligament. The right and left *triangular ligaments* attach the dorsal right lobe to the right costal diaphragm and the dorsal left lobe to the tendinous center of the diaphragm. The *hepatorenal ligament* connects the caudate process of the quadrate lobe to the right kidney and the base of the cecum.

HISTOLOGY

At the hilum of the liver, a tree of connective tissue consisting of collagen and fibroblasts enters the hepatic parenchyma. The parenchymal cells, or hepatocytes, compose approximately 50% to 60% of the mass of the liver and are epithelial cells.[3,4] The hepatocytes are arranged in rows, or cords, at least two cells thick that anastomose to form blood passageways called *sinusoids* (Figure 16-1). Hepatic sinusoids are larger than capillaries and are lined with endothelial cells and Kupffer's cells. Kupffer's cells are tissue-fixed macrophages and are estimated to make up 20% of the mass of the liver.[4] The endothelial cells make up approximately 20% of the mass of the liver.[4] A cleft, called the *space of Disse,* lies between the hepatocytes and the cells lining the sinusoids. The space of Disse contains fluid similar to the composition of blood but does not contain erythrocytes.

The afferent hepatic blood vessels, bile ducts, lymphatics, and nerves follow the branching connective tissue tree into the hepatic parenchyma. The liver receives approximately one third of the cardiac output. Two entirely separate sources of blood supply the liver and empty into the hepatic sinusoids: the portal vein and the hepatic artery. The portal vein contains poorly oxygenated blood that carries nutrients absorbed from the gastrointestinal tract to the liver for storage, metabolism, transformation, or packaging for export to other tissues. The hepatic artery contains oxygen-rich blood to support the metabolic and energy-generating activities of the liver. The sinusoids drain into terminal hepatic venules or central veins, which connect with the hepatic vein and caudal vena cava.

The space between contiguous hepatocytes in a cord forms a bile canaliculus through which bile excreted by the hepatocytes drains into bile ductules and ducts. The bile canaliculi thus are formed solely by the cell membranes of the hepatocytes. The bile ductules and ducts are lined with cuboidal and columnar epithelial cells, respectively, that make up approximately 7% of the mass of the liver.[4] The bile ducts run in the connective tissue tree, adjacent to branches of the portal vein and hepatic artery, to form a distinct portal tract, radicle, canal, or triad (see Figure 16-1). The bile ducts converge at the hilum to form the *hepatic duct,* which drains into the duodenum just distal to the pylorus. Because the horse does not have a gallbladder or a sphincter at the entry site of the hepatic duct into the intestine, the bile is unconcentrated and

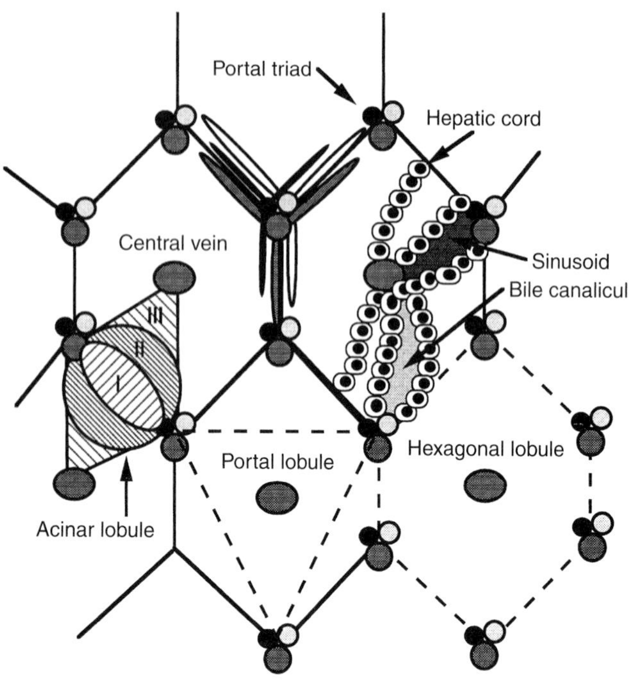

FIGURE 16-1 Histology of the liver. Roman numerals *I, II,* and *III* represent zones 1, 2, and 3, respectively, of the acinar lobule.

flows continuously in a direction opposite that of the blood flow in the portal vein and hepatic artery.[1]

The liver can be divided anatomically or functionally into lobules to facilitate histopathologic description of lesions[3] (see Figure 16-1). The classic hepatic lobule is delineated by abundant interlobular connective tissue that in cross-section roughly appears hexagonal. Three to eight portal tracts define the corners of the hexagon with a central vein in the center of the lobule. In contrast, the portal lobule is a functional unit describing the exocrine duties of the liver. Central veins define the three corners of the portal lobule, with a portal tract situated in the center. The acinus lobules describe the vascular supply to the hepatic parenchyma, divided according to the tissue oxygen content. Zone I of the acinus lobule is located immediately adjacent to branching hepatic arteries and portal veins, is the most metabolically active zone, and receives the best oxygen supply. Zone III is located adjacent to central veins, has high mixed-function oxidase activity, is least favorably situated with respect to oxygen content, and thus is most susceptible to toxic and hypoxic damage. Zone II is situated between zones I and III.

Physiology

The liver is the main organ involved in the regulation of nutrient distribution.[5] The majority of nutrients absorbed from the gastrointestinal tract pass directly to the liver via the portal circulation. The incoming nutrients are metabolized for energy, transformed to other nutrient classes, packaged and exported to peripheral tissues, or stored by the liver. The liver is capable of adjusting to the carbohydrate, protein, and lipid load from the gastrointestinal tract, as well as maintaining consistent blood levels of nutrients between feedings and in response to special needs. In addition to its role in nutrient metabolism and homeostasis, the liver is involved in excretion (bile), detoxification and metabolism of endogenous and exogenous substances, and hematopoiesis.[4]

Protein Metabolism

Amino acids, which are transported to the liver via the portal or hepatic blood, may be used in the biosynthesis of intrinsic hepatocellular proteins, plasma proteins, porphyrins, polyamines, purines, and pyrimidines.[5] The liver synthesizes 90% of the plasma proteins, including albumin, factors involved in coagulation and fibrinolysis (fibrinogen and factors II, V, VII-XIII; antithrombin III; protein C; plasminogen; plasminogen activator inhibitor; α_2-antiplasmin; α_2-macroglobulin; and α_1-antitrypsin), transport proteins (haptoglobin, transferrin, ceruloplasmin, hormone transport proteins), and acute phase reactant proteins (α- and β-globulins).[4] The liver is the only site of synthesis of albumin and fibrinogen.

The liver is also capable of transamination, or the reversible transfer of an amino group on one amino acid to an α-keto acid, thus forming a new amino acid and a new keto acid. If the liver receives an excess of amino acids or if carbohydrates are unavailable as an energy source, then the liver deaminates the amino acids and converts them to pyruvate, acetoacetate, and intermediates of the tricarboxylic acid cycle[5] (Figure 16-2). These intermediates may be oxidized for energy or used as precursors in *gluconeogenesis,* the synthesis of glucose from noncarbohydrate precursors. Endogenous and exogenous glucocorticoids, glucagon, and thyroid hormone act directly on the liver to increase gluconeogenesis[6] (Figure 16-3). Simultaneously, glucocorticoids indirectly influence liver gluconeogenesis by promoting peripheral protein catabolism, thus increasing the availability of amino acids. Insulin inhibits gluconeogenesis in the liver.[6]

In addition to protein synthesis and gluconeogenesis, the liver plays an important role in eliminating the major toxic by-product of amino acid catabolism, *ammonia.*[5,7] Tissues and intestinal microflora generate ammonia, which is subsequently released into the circulation. One method by which the liver, as well as certain peripheral tissues, eliminates ammonia is by synthesizing nonessential amino acids from α-keto acids and ammonia in a reversal of deamination. A fundamental reaction in the synthesis of nonessential amino acids is the formation of *glutamate* from α-ketoglutarate and ammonia (Figure 16-4). Subsequently, glutamate is used in transamination reactions to form other amino acids. Glutamate also participates in the conversion of cytotoxic free ammonia into a nontoxic transport form, *glutamine.* Glutamine may be delivered to the kidney, converted back to free ammonia and excreted, or delivered to the liver for urea synthesis.

The liver has sole responsibility for converting free ammonia or glutamine into *urea,* the principal form of amino group nitrogen excretion by mammals.[4] Urea is formed by the irreversible condensation of two ammonia molecules with carbon dioxide (see Figure 16-4). The reaction takes place in the hepatocyte mitochondria via the Krebs-Henseleit cycle.[5] The newly formed urea is released from the hepatocyte, secreted into the sinusoidal blood, and transported to the kidney as *blood urea nitrogen* (BUN) for excretion.

CARBOHYDRATE METABOLISM

The liver is responsible for the synthesis, storage, and release of glucose.[5] Monosaccharides absorbed from the gastrointestinal tract are delivered via portal blood to the liver. In the

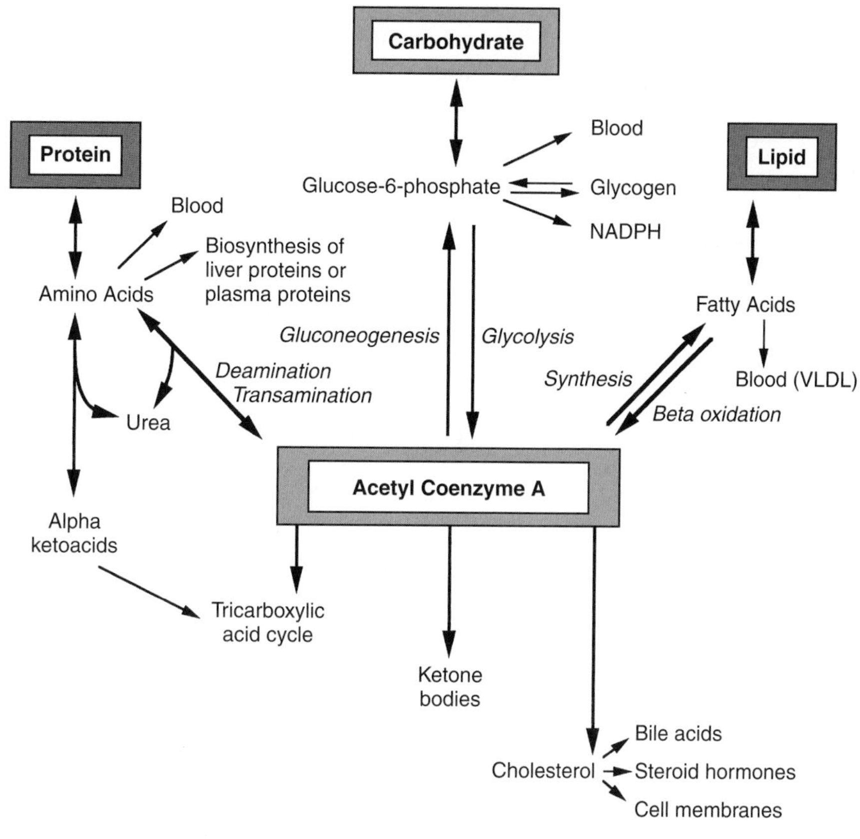

FIGURE 16-2 Role of the liver in the metabolism of nutrients. *VLDL,* very-low-density lipoprotein; *NADPH,* nicotinamide adenine dinucleotide phosphate.

hepatocyte the majority of glucose is phosphorylated to *glucose-6-phosphate* by the enzyme hexokinase (see Figure 16-2). The remaining glucose is released into the systemic circulation. Other monosaccharides (fructose, galactose) are phosphorylated and converted in the liver to glucose-6-phosphate. The majority of glucose-6-phosphate is converted to glycogen for storage. A small amount of glucose-6-phosphate is oxidized to form adenosine triphosphate, although the major source of adenosine triphosphate in the liver is amino acid and fatty acid oxidation. Approximately half of the liver glucose enters the phosphogluconate pathway for generation of nicotinamide adenine dinucleotide phosphate, which is required as a reducing agent in the biosynthesis of fatty acids and cholesterol. Glucocorticoids, catecholamines, glucagon, and thyroid hormone increase gluconeogenesis and glycogenolysis in the liver, while insulin inhibits gluconeogenesis[6] (see Figure 16-3).

LIPID METABOLISM

Short-chain fatty acids (fewer than 10 carbon atoms) can be absorbed directly from the gastrointestinal tract, bound to albumin, and delivered to the liver via the portal circulation.[5] However, the majority of short-chain fatty acids are incorporated into phospholipid or triglyceride by the intestinal epithelium and transported to the liver via the portal blood. The remaining fatty acids absorbed from the gastrointestinal tract are transported as triglyceride in *chylomicrons*. After formation in the intestinal epithelial cells and absorption into lymphatics, chylomicrons enter the systemic circulation via the thoracic duct and subsequently are delivered to the liver. The liver also may take up albumin-bound fatty acids released from adipose tissue.

The fate of fatty acids in the liver depends on the state of energy demand, the rate of fatty acid delivery, and hormonal influences. The primary role of the liver in lipid metabolism is to esterify free fatty acids into triglycerides for export to other tissues[5] (see Figure 16-3). The triglycerides are packaged with protein, carbohydrate, and cholesterol in the endoplasmic reticulum of the hepatocyte into *very-low-density lipoproteins* (VLDLs), which primarily contain triglyceride, and *high-density lipoproteins* (HDLs), which primarily contain protein and phospholipid.[8] The VLDLs and HDLs are released into the hepatic sinusoids. Once the VLDLs are in the systemic circulation, the adipose tissue takes them up or endothelial cell lipases alter their composition by removing triglyceride, forming *intermediate-* and *low-density lipoproteins*.

In addition to exporting plasma lipoprotein, the liver can oxidize free fatty acids for energy to acetyl coenzyme A (acetyl CoA), a fundamental compound in the tricarboxylic acid cycle (see Figure 16-2). The acetyl CoA thus formed also may be used in the synthesis of other fatty acids, cholesterol, steroids, and ketone bodies, acetoacetate, and β-hydroxybutyrate.[5] Furthermore, through the synthesis of acetyl CoA from glucose and most amino acids, the liver is capable of converting carbohydrates and proteins into lipids. Ketone bodies can be exported from the liver and used for energy by peripheral tissues, especially the brain, when glucose is deficient. However, overproduction of ketone bodies can be detrimental, resulting in ketoacidosis.[8]

Insulin and glucocorticoids closely regulate lipid metabolism[6] (see Figure 16-3). Glucocorticoids function primarily to

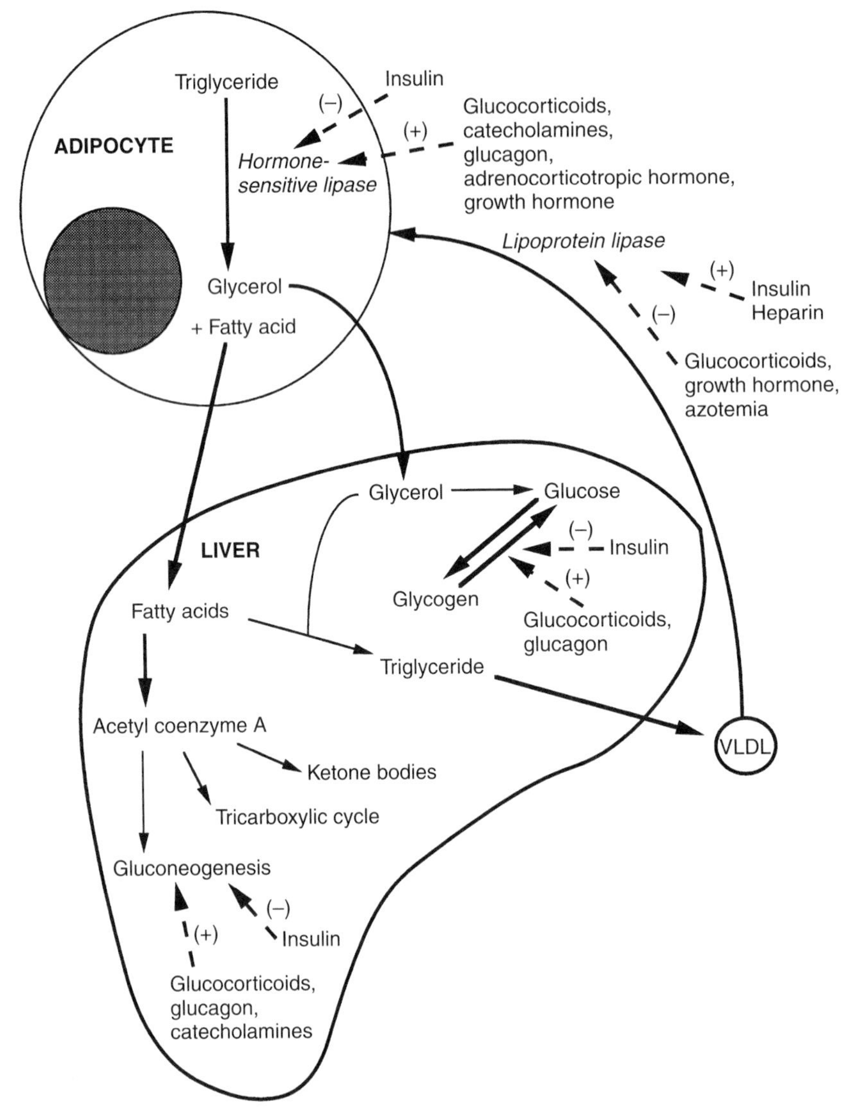

FIGURE 16-3 Hormonal control of metabolism. –, inhibitory effect; +, stimulatory effect.

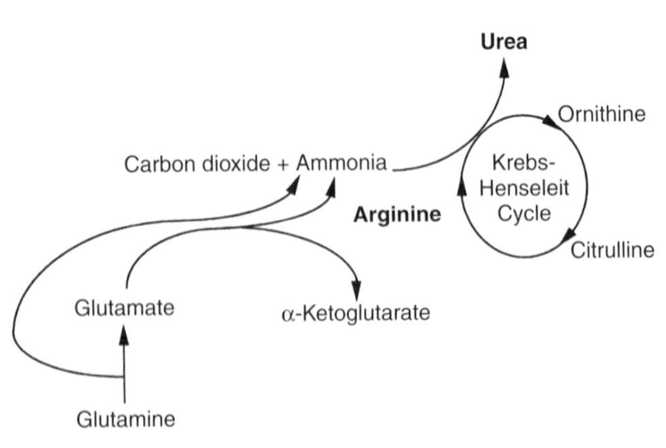

FIGURE 16-4 The urea cycle.

increase fatty acid mobilization from the periphery, whereas insulin decreases adipose tissue release of fatty acids by activating lipoprotein lipase and inhibiting hormone-sensitive lipase. Insulin acts on the liver to increase fatty acid synthesis from glucose.

EXCRETION OF BILE

Bile consists of several components, including conjugated bilirubin, bile acids, cholesterol, lecithin, water, and electrolytes.[4] Bile is released by hepatocytes into the bile canaliculi where water diffuses passively. Bile then is transported by large bile ducts and the hepatic duct to the intestine. Water and electrolyte exchange takes place between the bile and the bile duct epithelium; however, isotonicity is maintained. Because the horse does not have a gallbladder or a sphincter at the site of entry of the hepatic duct into the duodenum, the bile is unconcentrated and flow is continuous.[1]

Bile acids compose 90% of the organic portion of bile.[9] Bile acids are amphoteric molecules that act as detergents. These detergents facilitate the excretion of cholesterol and phospholipid from the liver into bile and facilitate the absorption of lipids

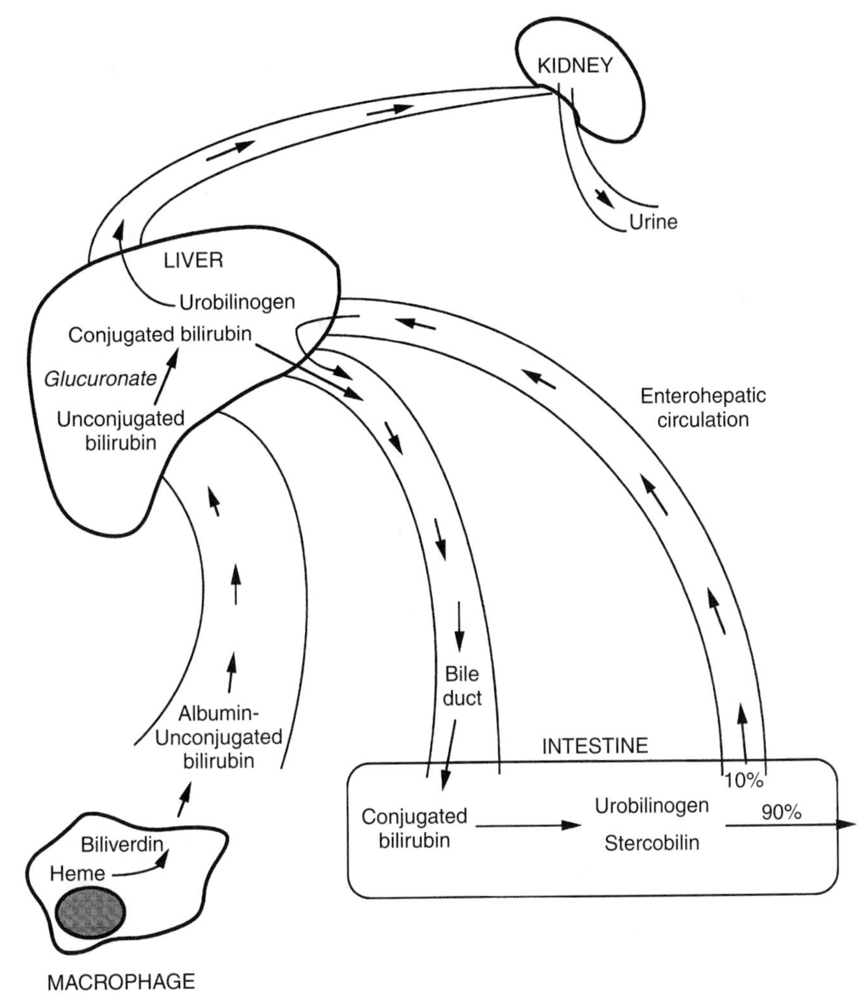

FIGURE 16-5 Metabolism and excretion of bile.

and lipid-soluble compounds (vitamins A, D, E, and K) from the intestinal tract. The principal *primary bile acids* (i.e., nondegraded) in the horse are *cholate* and *chenodeoxycholate,* both of which are conjugated with taurine.[9] Once secreted into the lumen of the intestinal tract, cholate and chenodeoxycholate may be reabsorbed or degraded by bacteria, forming the *secondary bile acids, deoxycholate* or *lithocholate,* respectively. More than 95% of the conjugated bile acids excreted in bile and released into the intestinal lumen are reabsorbed by the ileum and returned to the liver via the *enterohepatic circulation.* Deoxycholate acts as a normal bile acid and can undergo enterohepatic circulation, whereas lithocholate is only reabsorbed once. Bile acids are estimated to be recycled at least 38 times a day in healthy ponies.[9]

Bilirubin is the breakdown product of tetrapyrroles that function as electron transport pigments.[4] The majority of bilirubin is formed from hemoglobin and myoglobin, but nonheme pigments such as the cytochromes also serve as a source of bilirubin. Macrophages in the spleen, bone marrow, and liver (Kupffer's cells) engulf the pigments first, convert it to biliverdin (Figure 16-5), and then convert biliverdin to bilirubin and release it from the cell as free, insoluble bilirubin. This form of bilirubin also is referred to as *indirect-reacting* or *unconjugated bilirubin.* Unconjugated bilirubin is bound with albumin in the plasma to decrease its hydrophobicity and is delivered to the liver. At the surface of the hepatocyte, the bilirubin is transferred from albumin to *ligandin,* an intrahepatic transport and storage protein.[4,9] Within the hepatocyte, the bilirubin is conjugated with glucuronide in the endoplasmic reticulum. *Conjugated bilirubin,* also called *direct-reacting bilirubin,* is water soluble and is excreted into the bile canaliculi. Under normal circumstances, little conjugated bilirubin escapes into the general circulation.

Microflora in the intestinal tract reduce conjugated bilirubin to *urobilinogen* and *stercobilin* (see Figure 16-5), which impart a yellow-brown color to feces. In herbivores, the presence of chlorophyll pigments in the feces masks the color of urobilinogen.[10] Only in the neonatal herbivore receiving a milk diet are the feces yellow. Urobilinogen is absorbed by the intestinal mucosa and transported back to the liver via the enterohepatic circulation. A small amount of conjugated bilirubin in the intestinal lumen is hydrolyzed to unconjugated bilirubin and subsequently is reabsorbed. The liver extracts most of the urobilinogen; however, a small amount spills over into the urine. Urobilinogen is concentrated in the normally alkaline urine of horses and thus is detectable.[10]

DETOXIFICATION

The liver is responsible for the *biotransformation* of numerous endogenous and exogenous compounds. Biotransformation involves a series of enzymatic reactions that alter the physical properties or activity of compounds. Biotransformation occurs in two phases.[11] In phase 1, polar groups are added to the compound or existing polar groups are exposed by oxidation, hydroxylation, deamination, or reduction. In phase 2, the product of phase 1 is conjugated, usually with glucuronate or sulfate. Substrates for detoxification usually are water insoluble and biotransformation renders them more susceptible to renal or biliary excretion.[4,12] Examples of endogenous substances biotransformed by the liver include ammonia, bilirubin, and steroid hormones (estrogen, cortisol, aldosterone). The liver biotransforms countless exogenous substances, including many drugs, plant toxins, insecticides, and mercaptans.

Phase 1 of biotransformation occurs primarily on the enzyme-bound systems of the endoplasmic reticulum, called *microsomes*.[4,12] Most of these enzymes are iron-containing enzymes of the P-450 system, thus named because they absorb light at 450 nm. The P-450 enzymes are also called *mixed function oxidases*. Some substrates, referred to as *inducers*, are capable of saturating the enzymes involved in biotransformation. Enzyme saturation and induction causes hypertrophy of the endoplasmic reticulum and all contained enzymes, thus accelerating substance removal rates. Inducers not only accelerate their own removal rate but also may accelerate the biotransformation of other endogenous and exogenous substances. Examples of enzyme inducers are the barbiturates, phenylbutazone, and chlorinated hydrocarbons. Other agents presented for biotransformation, including chloramphenicol, cimetidine, organophosphates, morphine, and quinidine, may inhibit microsomal enzymes thus prolonging the effect of other substrates. Hepatic biotransformation sometimes results in the formation of a toxic metabolite from a nontoxic parent compound examples being aspirin and halothane.[12]

MONONUCLEAR PHAGOCYTE SYSTEM

Hepatic macrophages, or Kupffer's cells, make up a major portion of the mononuclear phagocyte system. Cells of the mononuclear phagocyte system are derived from bone marrow myeloid progenitors and serve two main functions: (1) phagocytosis and (2) to act as antigen-processing cells for lymphocytes. Kupffer's cells respond to opsonins and synthesize a vast array of inflammatory mediators, including interleukins, tumor necrosis factor (TNF), and eicosanoids. Unlike other macrophages in the mononuclear phagocyte system, Kupffer's cells function mainly in phagocytosis and are located strategically along the hepatic sinusoids, where portal blood can be cleansed, for example, of bacterial endotoxin, before exposure to the hepatocytes and subsequently the systemic circulation.[13] Kupffer's cells also help cleanse systemic blood entering via the hepatic artery by removing *fibrin degradation products (FDPs)*, tissue plasminogen activators, hemoglobin, microbes, foreign antigens, and other particulate debris.

MISCELLANEOUS FUNCTIONS

The liver serves as a storage site for several vitamins and trace minerals, including vitamins A, D, and B_{12}; copper; and iron. Vitamin D is first converted in the liver to 25-hydroxycholecalciferol and exported to the kidney, where it is transformed into 1,25-dihydroxycholecalciferol, the active form of the vitamin.[6] In the fetus the liver is involved in *hematopoiesis*.[4] In the adult the bone marrow serves as the primary site for hematopoiesis; however, the liver may serve as an extramedullary site of hematopoiesis under intense conditions of erythrocyte regeneration or if a large portion of the bone marrow is destroyed.

HEPATIC INSUFFICIENCY

DEFINITION

Hepatic insufficiency or failure refers to the inability of the liver to perform its normal functions properly. Because the liver is involved in such a diverse array of physiologic activities, any pathologic process may hinder one or several functions without impeding others. Furthermore, most hepatic functions are not impaired until greater than 80% of the hepatic mass is lost.[4,8,10] The liver also has the capability to regenerate under certain conditions. If hepatocyte loss is gradual and regeneration parallels destruction, then hepatic failure does not necessarily ensue. Thus hepatic disease may be present without accompanying hepatic failure. Consequently, hepatic disease does not always manifest clinically.

PATTERNS AND PATHOLOGY OF HEPATIC INJURY

The severity of the accompanying clinical signs and the course of hepatic disease vary depending on the pattern, location, rate, and extent of hepatic damage. Hepatic injury may be reversible (fatty degeneration, cloudy swelling), irreversible (necrosis), focal or zonal, generalized, acute, chronic, inflammatory, anatomic, or functional.

ACUTE FOCAL OR MULTIFOCAL HEPATIC INJURY

Focal hepatic injury occurs with uniform damage to one small area of the liver. Examples of focal hepatic injury include hepatic abscesses, solitary infarctions, and neoplastic growths. Because adequate hepatic reserve exists in the unaffected regions, clinical signs of hepatic failure rarely accompany focal hepatic injury, although evidence of hepatic disease may be demonstrable.[11] Acute multifocal hepatic injury is more likely to result in clinically significant hepatic disease. Acute hepatic injury may be degenerative, necrotizing, or inflammatory. Hepatic *degeneration* refers to a toxic or immunologic insult that causes hepatocytes to swell and take on an edematous appearance.[14] *Ballooning degeneration* is used to describe irregularly clumped cytoplasm with large clear areas.[14] If biliary material has been retained, then the hepatocytes appear foamy and swollen *(foamy degeneration)*. *Ischemic coagulative necrosis* refers to poorly stained and mummified hepatocytes with lysed nuclei, whereas *lytic necrosis* describes osmotically swollen and ruptured cells.[14] Necrosis of contiguous hepatocytes that spans adjacent lobules in a portal to portal, portal to central, or central to central fashion is called *bridging necrosis*.[14]

Hepatic injury may be zonal, that is, affecting certain zones of the liver uniformly throughout the entire organ.[11] The liver often appears pale with an enhanced lobular pattern on the cut surface. The two most common types of zonal hepatic injury are centrilobular and periacinar. In *centrilobular zonal injury*, the area adjacent to the central veins (zone III) is uniformly affected, whereas in *periacinar* or *(paracentral) zonal injury*, cellular degeneration involves only a wedge around the central vein (see Figure 16-1). Hepatocytes in these locations are most susceptible to anoxic damage, because the normal oxygen tension is lowest and mixed function oxidase activity is the greatest in these areas. Examples of disease states resulting in centrilobular injury are severe acute anemia, passive congestion caused by congestive heart failure *(nutmeg liver)*, and toxic hepatopathies.

Periportal (zone I acinar lobular) injury is rare but may occur with infarction of hepatic vessels, as may occur during verminous arteritis, or exposure to toxins that do not require metabolism by mixed function oxidases (e.g., phosphorus).

ACUTE GENERALIZED HEPATIC INJURY

Acute generalized hepatic injury is often accompanied by clinical signs of hepatic failure, with the extent of damage dictating the severity of the clinical signs.[11] Typically, the liver appears pale and enlarged and is often friable. Acute generalized hepatic injury may be the result of infection, necrosis, inflammation, or hepatotoxic agents.[4] Bacterial or viral infections, parasitic infestations, or immune disorders may cause acute generalized necrosis or inflammation. Despite its cause, any process that results in an inflammatory response in the hepatic parenchyma is referred to as *hepatitis*. Acute inflammation most commonly accompanies necrosis and is characterized by the presence of neutrophils and lymphocytes in the areas of cell death or surrounding portal triads. An inflammatory process primarily involving the biliary system is called *cholangitis,* usually the result of ascending infection from the intestinal tract or after cholestasis.

CHRONIC GENERALIZED HEPATIC INJURY

Chronic hepatic injury is accompanied by clinical signs of hepatic failure when greater than 80% of the hepatic mass is destroyed or replaced by fibrosis.[4,8] Fibrosis, the presence of collagen and fibroblasts, occurs when the rate of ongoing necrosis exceeds the rate of regeneration. Typically, the liver appears smaller than normal. Fibrosis commonly follows conditions resulting in chronic hypoxia, chronic inflammation, chronic cholangitis or cholestasis, metastatic neoplasia, trauma, or ingestion of antimitotic agents such as plants containing pyrrolizidine alkaloids. *Cirrhosis,* or an *end-stage liver disease,* refers to chronic hepatic disease characterized by the presence of widespread fibrosis, nodular regeneration, and biliary hyperplasia.[11] *Nodular regeneration,* or islands of hepatocytes, occurs when the normal architecture and blood supply of the liver are disrupted or destroyed by the presence of fibrosis. *Bridging fibrosis* implies fibrosis that extends from one portal area to another or from portal areas to central areas.[14] The cause of biliary hyperplasia during chronic liver disease is unknown. One form of chronic hepatic disease, called *chronic active hepatitis* (CAH), is characterized by the presence of cirrhosis plus an acute inflammatory response.[11]

ANATOMIC OR FUNCTIONAL INJURY

Anatomic or functional shunts cause liver injury by anoxic damage. Additionally, if blood habitually bypasses the liver, then the liver cannot perform its normal metabolic regulatory or detoxifying functions; thus clinical signs of hepatic failure become imminent. Anatomic shunts can be either congenital or acquired, intrahepatic or extrahepatic.

Clinical Signs of Hepatic Insufficiency

The clinical signs of hepatic insufficiency are highly variable, nonspecific, and depend on the extent and duration of hepatic disease (Box 16-1). Usually, greater than 80% of the liver mass must be lost before clinical signs become apparent, regardless of the cause of hepatic disease. Thus despite the duration of hepatic disease, the onset of clinical signs is often abrupt. The most common clinical signs of hepatic insufficiency in horses are depression, anorexia, colic, hepatic encephalopathy (HE), weight loss, and icterus.[15-17] Less commonly reported clinical signs include hepatogenic photosensitization, diarrhea, abdominal pain, bilateral laryngeal paralysis, and hemorrhagic diathesis. Rarely reported clinical signs of hepatic insufficiency in horses are ascites, dependent abdominal edema, steatorrhea, tenesmus, generalized seborrhea, pruritus, endotoxic shock, polydipsia, and hemolysis. The appearance of specific clinical signs of hepatic disease often reflects the type of hepatic function (or functions) that is altered.

BOX 16-1

CLINICAL SIGNS OF LIVER DISEASE

Common Signs

Depression
Anorexia
Colic
Hepatic encephalopathy (HE)
Weight loss
Icterus

Less Common Signs

Photosensitization
Diarrhea
Bilateral laryngeal paralysis
Bleeding
Ascites
Dependent edema

Rare Signs

Steatorrhea
Tenesmus
Generalized seborrhea
Pruritus
Endotoxic shock
Polydipsia
Pigmenturia (yellow-brown with bilirubinuria; red-brown with hemoglobinuria)

HEPATIC ENCEPHALOPATHY

Hepatic encephalopathy (HE) is a complex clinical syndrome characterized by abnormal mental status that accompanies severe hepatic insufficiency.[18-20] Clinical signs are widely variable but represent manifestations of augmented neuronal inhibition. This syndrome occurs in patients with advanced decompensated liver disease of all types and may be a feature of acute, subacute, or chronic hepatocellular disease. HE generally is considered to be a potentially reversible metabolic encephalopathy.[19] Whether multiple episodes of HE could lead to irreversible neuronal damage is uncertain.

Clinical Signs No specific features of HE allow this syndrome to be distinguished from other causes of cerebral dysfunction. The earliest phase of HE is probably missed in most equine patients because it represents minimal behavioral changes with subtle impairment of intellect because of bilateral forebrain dysfunction[21] (stage I; Table 16-1). In humans, these early signs are more apparent to close friends and family members than to a physician. As encephalopathy progresses, motor function, intellectual abilities, and consciousness become impaired; generally at this stage (corresponding to

TABLE 16-1

Clinical Stages of Hepatic Encephalopathy

Stage	Mental Status
I	Mild confusion, decreased attention, slowed ability to perform mental tasks, irritability
II	Drowsiness, lethargy, obvious personality changes, inappropriate behavior, disorientation
III	Somnolent but rousable, marked confusion, amnesia, occasional aggressive uncontrolled behavior
IV	Coma

Adapted from Gammel SH, Jones EA: Hepatic encephalopathy, Med Clin North Am 73:793–813, 1989.

stage II) horses become obviously affected. Clinical signs include depression, head pressing, circling, mild ataxia, aimless walking, persistent yawning, and other manifestations of inappropriate behavior. Somnolence develops. Next the horse is rousable but responds minimally or excessively to the usual stimuli. At this stage (III) the horse often manifests aggressive or violent behavior interspersed with periods of stupor. Finally, consciousness fades, the horse becomes recumbent, and coma ensues. Occasionally seizures occur during the later stages of HE, but in general they are atypical. The severity of encephalopathy corresponds to the degree of hepatic dysfunction; however, neither of these parameters correlates with type or reversibility of the underlying hepatic disease.

Cause and Pathophysiology By definition, the cause of HE is insufficient hepatocellular function, irrespective of the cause of the liver disease. That is, a normally functioning liver is necessary to maintain normal brain neuron and astrocyte function. With acute liver disease, HE is primarily caused by astrocyte swelling, acute cytotoxic cerebral edema, and intracranial hypertension. In chronic hepatic disease, HE develops more insidiously. Astrocytes are swollen but also show evidence of Alzheimer type II changes.[22] Whether acute or chronic in nature, the precise pathogenesis of HE remains unclear, and considering the numerous proposed hypotheses, the cause is almost certainly multifactorial. The following mechanisms have been suggested for the development of HE and any or all may be involved to greater or lesser degree:

1. Gastrointestinal-derived neurotoxins
2. Augmented activity of gamma-aminobutyric acid (GABA) in the brain
3. Altered expression of benzodiazepine receptors
4. Increased neurosteroid synthesis
5. False neurotransmitter accumulation after plasma amino acid imbalance
6. Increased blood manganese concentrations
7. Increased inflammatory mediator expression, principally cytokines
8. Increased permeability of the blood-brain barrier and cerebral hypertension
9. Impaired central nervous system (CNS) energy metabolism

Perhaps the oldest and most "predominant" hypothesis for HE involves the accumulation of toxic materials in the blood (derived from the metabolism of nitrogenous substrates in the gastrointestinal tract) that bypass the liver through functional or anatomic shunts.[18,21,23] Accordingly, HE may be caused primarily by failure of the liver to adequately remove certain substances from the blood that have the direct or indirect ability to modulate function of the CNS. Ammonia, after the degradation of amino acids, amines, and purines by enteric bacteria, has been supported widely as a major neurotoxin of hepatic disease.[22,23-25] In patients with liver failure, ammonia is insufficiently metabolized through the urea cycle; thus plasma concentrations increase, and ammonia enters the CNS, where it may cause encephalopathy.[23,26] Evidence also points to zinc deficiency, which is important for the urea cycle, in the pathogenesis of HE.[27]

Ammonia has a toxic effect on cell membrane neurons by inhibition of the Na,K-dependent adenosine triphosphatase activity in nerve cell membranes, causing depletion of adenosine triphosphate.[25,27] Hyperammonemia also is associated with a disturbance in CNS energy production caused by alterations in the tricarboxylic acid cycle that result in a decrease in α-ketoglutarate formation and increased synthesis of glutamine.[28] Astrocytes in the brain also detoxify ammonia by synthesizing glutamine through amidation of glutamate. Glutamine accumulation in astrocytes is a major cause of cell swelling and generation of cerebral edema in acute fulminate hepatic failure.[22,27] Another effect of prolonged exposure to ammonia to neuron tissue is depletion of glutamate and downregulation of glutamate receptors. Because glutamate is the major excitatory neurotransmitter on the mammalian brain, in acute liver failure, increased synaptic release of glutamate results in overactivation of glutamate receptors with resultant hyperexcitatory clinical signs. In chronic hepatic failure, downregulation of glutamate receptor activity likely contributes to the decreased excitatory transmission in HE. Hyperammonemia also induces nitric oxide and reactive oxygen species generation, which leads to accumulation of peroxides, oxidative stress, and nerve cell damage. These cumulative effects of ammonia on neural tissue certainly play an important role in the pathogenesis of HE. Experimentally, ammonia can induce encephalopathy[29]; because of congenital enzyme deficiencies, children with hyperammonemia have encephalopathy.[24] Furthermore, therapy aimed at reducing the absorption of ammonia from the intestine tends to ameliorate HE.[21] Although older clinical studies argued against the role of ammonia in the pathogenesis of HE because plasma ammonia concentrations correlated poorly with the severity of HE,[19,30] more recent reviews demonstrate that blood ammonia levels correlate strongly with the severity of HE.[31] Thus the actions of ammonia on the CNS are complex, and ammonia likely is involved in, but is not solely responsible for, HE.

The synergistic neurotoxins hypothesis for the pathogenesis of HE implicates not only ammonia but also other gut-derived neurotoxins, specifically mercaptans, short-chain fatty acids, and phenols.[21] Members of each of these classes of substances are increased in the blood of patients with hepatic failure in concentrations that alone are insufficient to induce encephalopathy. However, the combination of some or all of them may induce encephalopathy by their synergistic actions and by augmenting endogenous metabolic abnormalities,[21] mostly centering around inhibition of brain Na^+,K^+-ATPase with subsequent impaired neurotransmission.[19]As with ammonia, blood and brain concentrations of mercaptans correlate poorly with the stage of HE.[32]

Another popular theory regarding the pathogenesis of HE involves augmented activity of inhibitory neurotransmitter systems, GABA-benzodiazepine and serotonin, and depression of the function of the excitatory glutamatergic system.[27] Hyperammonemia has been shown to increase GABAergic tone in patients with liver disease.[22] When released from presynaptic neurons, GABA binds to specific receptors on postsynaptic neurons, resulting in increased chloride ion conductance across the postsynaptic neural membrane, membrane hyperpolarization, and generation of an inhibitory postsynaptic potential.[33] The GABA receptor is a chloride ionophore supramolecular complex that has interactive binding sites for three classes of synergistic ligands: (1) GABA and agonists, (2) benzodiazepines, and (3) barbiturates.[19,34] The binding of benzodiazepine or a barbiturate on its binding site of the GABA receptor potentiates GABA-induced sedation. The GABA hypothesis of HE originally was based on a series of observations using a model of HE in rabbits in which increased GABA-like activity was identified in the serum and cerebral spinal fluid (CSF) along with an increased density of GABA receptors.[33]

Increased brain levels of natural benzodiazepines probably constitute one mechanism for the increased GABAergic tone in HE.[27] Ammonia, which acts synergistically with natural benzodiazepines, also may enhance GABAergic neurotransmission. Agonists of benzodiazepine increase the frequency of GABA-induced chloride channel openings, and barbiturates lengthen the average time that channels are open.[35] Results of studies using electrophysiologic and in vitro techniques to study an animal model of HE provide strong evidence for a functional increase in GABAergic tone that is mediated allosterically through the benzodiazepine receptor by an endogenous diazepam-like substance.[36,37] Clinical studies that showed improved consciousness and reduced electroencephalogram changes of HE in patients treated with the benzodiazepine receptor antagonist flumazenil support this suggestion.[38,39] Neurosteroids also may affect GABAergic tone through benzodiazepine receptors. Activation of benzodiazepam receptors in liver failure facilitates the entry of cholesterol into astrocyte mitochondria, where synthesis of neurosteroids such as tetrahydroprogesterone and tetrahydrodeoxycorticosterone occurs. These substances are potent positive allosteric modulators of GABA receptors that can induce profound sedation and behavioral changes.[40]

A separate hypothesis holds that during liver failure, true neurotransmitters in the CNS such as norepinephrine and dopamine become depleted and that false neurotransmitters, especially octopamine and phenylethanolamine, increase.[20,41] The net neurophysiologic effect of such changes is reduced neuronal excitation and increased neural inhibition. The mechanism of this effect is related to the increased serum concentrations of aromatic amino acids (AAA; phenylalanine, tyrosine, tryptophan) and decreased concentrations of branched-chain amino acids (BCAAs; valine, leucine, isoleucine) that occur in liver failure.[42,43] Serum glucagon increases in hepatic failure, leading to muscle catabolism and release of amino acids. However, hepatic metabolism of AAAs is reduced, and because BCAAs are metabolized by muscle and adipose tissue, a relative increase in AAAs and a decrease in BCAAs occurs. The decreased plasma BCAA-to-AAA ratio during liver failure and increased brain glutamine concentration (presumably a consequence of ammonia retention) are considered to promote an influx of AAA into the brain and an efflux of glutamine from the brain by exchange transport processes at the blood-brain barrier.[19] Phenylalanine can compete with tyrosine for tyrosine hydroxylase, resulting in decreased production of dopamine[43] (Figure 16-6). The displaced tyrosine may be decarboxylated to tyramine, then converted to the false neurotransmitter, octopamine. Accumulated tyrosine also competes for dopamine β-oxidase and reduces the formation of norepinephrine. Phenylalanine and tryptophan in the CNS are ultimately converted to phenylethanolamine and serotonin, a false neurotransmitter and a neuroinhibitor, respectively. Tryptophan is also metabolized to serotonin and oxindole, which has a strong sedative effect.[27]

Consistent with this theory are the observations of increased serum concentrations of AAAs accompanied by increased CSF concentrations of octopamine, serotonin, and phenylethanolamine in patients with HE.[41] However, octopamine alone cannot induce encephalopathy and the plasma BCAA-to-AAA ratio correlates poorly with HE in human beings.[44] Controlled clinical trials of oral or intravenous BCAA therapy demonstrate inconsistent amelioration of signs of HE.[43,45]

Manganese is a trace element that is excreted by the liver. Patients with chronic liver disease have increased blood and brain concentrations of manganese. Chronic exposure to manganese causes neuronal and glial loss and Alzheimer type II changes in astrocytes.[31]

A recent hypothesis on the pathophysiology of HE centers on the role of inflammatory mediators in brain injury. Central to this hypothesis is the fact that human patients with acute liver failure are more likely to progress to severe HE if they concurrently have evidence of a systemic inflammatory response.[22] A variety of stimuli are capable of inducing astrocytes and microglial cells in the brain, as well as peripherally located mononuclear cells, to release inflammatory mediators. Several studies have demonstrated significantly increased levels of the cytokine, tumor necrosis factor α (TNF-α), in patients with both acute and chronic liver disease. Furthermore, TNF concentrations correlate with the severity of HE and prognosis, and therapeutic strategies aimed at reducing TNF levels ameliorate HE.[31] Several key mechanisms whereby increased TNF concentrations have been shown to be involved in the pathogenesis of HE include increasing ammonia diffusion into the brain, inhibition of astrocyte uptake of glutamate and inhibition of glutamate synthetase, increased expression of benzodiazepine receptors in the brain, and increasing brain capillary fluid leakage and cerebral edema formation. It has also been demonstrated that excess manganese potentiates the production of TNF in microglia.[31]

Finally, alterations in cerebral blood flow and blood-brain barrier permeability leading to cerebral hypertension and edema and changes in cerebral metabolism are present in patients with HE. Although the mechanisms responsible for these changes are not fully known, changes in astrocyte function, either directly or indirectly by increased blood ammonia concentrations, are likely to be involved.[22]

Diagnosis The diagnosis of HE is based on the presence of neurologic signs of cerebral dysfunction in a horse, with physical examination and laboratory findings compatible with liver disease (see Diagnosis and Laboratory Findings of Hepatic Insufficiency). Other possible causes for the neurologic signs should be excluded because no specific features of HE allow one to distinguish this syndrome definitively from other encephalopathies. A partial list of conditions to be ruled out includes trauma, viral encephalomyelitis, rabies, moldy corn toxicity (leukoencephalomalacia), brain abscess, equine protozoal myeloencephalitis, parasite larval migrans, blister beetle toxicosis, organophosphate toxicity, nigropallidal

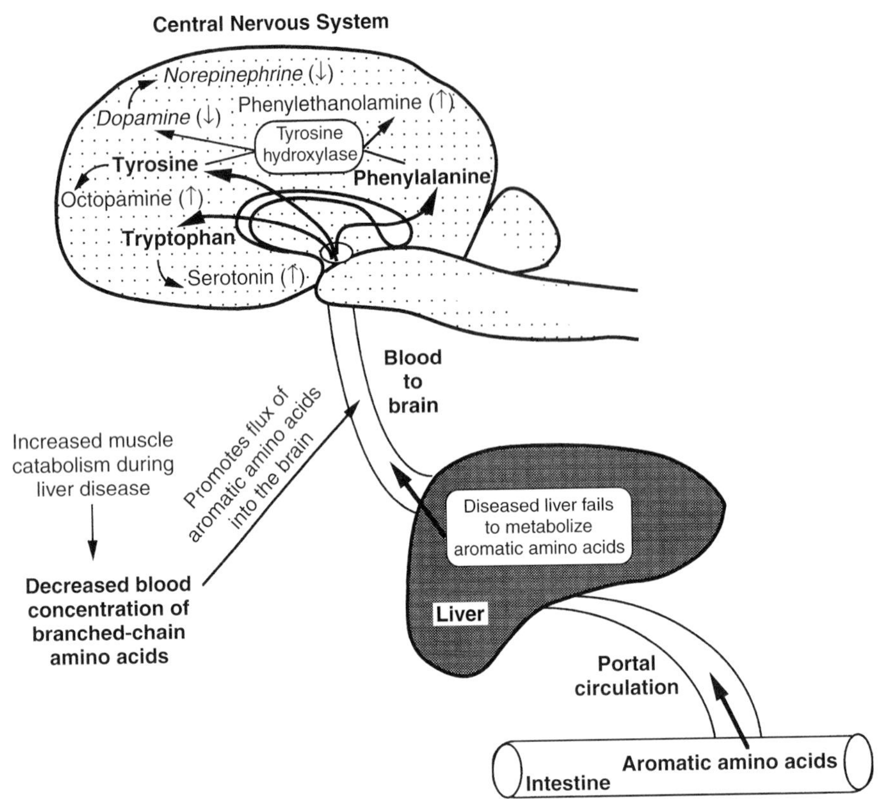

FIGURE 16-6 Role of aromatic amino acids in the brain in hepatic encephalopathy. Aromatic amino acids (tryptophan, tyrosine, phenylalanine) enter the central nervous system (CNS), where they are metabolized, altering the balance of neurotransmitters. True neurotransmitters (dopamine, norepinephrine) decrease *(arrow down),* while "false" neurotransmitters (octopamine, phenylethanolamine) increase *(arrow up).* The net effect is increased neuronal inhibition and reduced neuronal excitation.

encephalomalacia, botulism, fluphenazine or other sedative overdose, and heavy metal toxicosis. Many of these conditions have other characteristic clinical signs, the absence of which would exclude them from the differential diagnosis. Access to potential toxins or drugs should be carefully gleaned from the history.

Serum electrolyte analysis, calcium and creatinine values, and a complete blood count (CBC) may aid in ruling out other encephalopathies. Serology for the viral encephalitides and toxicologic screening for organophosphates and heavy metals may be appropriate. CSF analysis may be indicated if other causes of encephalopathy are highly suspect. The CSF is normal in horses with HE. In human beings, electroencephalogram changes of symmetrical generalized slowing of cerebral electrical activity are sensitive indicators of HE; however, they are not specific for this disorder because other metabolic encephalopathies can cause similar abnormalities.[18] Visual evoked potentials are superior to conventional electroencephalogram in terms of specificity and ease of quantitation.[46] An average visual evoked potential reflects the pattern and magnitude of postsynaptic neuronal activity evoked by a visual afferent stimulus. Hepatoencephalopathy in humans is attended by a distinctively abnormal visual evoked potential trace; however, this testing would be technically difficult in horses and has not been explored. As a general rule, the brain shows no definite light or electron microscopic structural changes; however, some patients with hepatic cirrhosis and portosystemic shunts have an increase in the number and size of astrocytes (Alzheimer type II) in the gray matter of the cerebrum and cerebellum.[19] These changes appear to be reversible and specific for portosystemic shunting of blood. The relevance of these changes, if any, to behavioral dysfunction of HE is unknown.

ICTERUS

Icterus, or *jaundice,* is caused by *hyperbilirubinemia* with subsequent deposition of the pigment in tissues causing yellow discoloration. Icterus is most apparent in nonpigmented skin; mucous membranes, especially the vulvar mucosa; and the sclerae. Approximately 10% to 15% of horses normally have slightly yellow sclerae. Disease states that result in hyperbilirubinemia can be categorized as follows: increased production of bilirubin, impaired hepatic uptake or conjugation of bilirubin, and impaired excretion of bilirubin.[8] Increased production of bilirubin occurs with hemolysis, both intravascular and extravascular, and after reabsorption of erythrocytes after massive intracorporeal hemorrhage. This form of hyperbilirubinemia, often called *hemolytic* or *prehepatic icterus,* occurs despite a normally functioning liver, because the rate of bilirubin production by the reticuloendothelial system temporarily exceeds the ability of the liver to conjugate and excrete. Classically, this form of icterus is caused by the increased concentration of unconjugated bilirubin in the blood. However, on occasion the concentration of conjugated bilirubin also mildly increases in the blood because of hepatic spillover when the liver processes the excessive bilirubin or the enterohepatic circulation reabsorbs it. The rate and extent of erythrocyte destruction and the rate of uptake of bilirubin determine the presence and intensity of hemolytic icterus by the liver.

Impaired uptake and conjugation of bilirubin also result in increased blood levels of unconjugated bilirubin with subsequent icterus. This form of icterus is referred to as *retention* or *hepatic icterus* and is the most common form in horses with liver disease, usually the result of acute hepatocellular disease.[8,10] In horses the presence of icterus is highly inconsistent with chronic hepatocellular disease.[9,17] In addition to hepatocellular disease, certain drugs, anorexia, or prematurity can impede bilirubin uptake and conjugation by hepatocytes, despite an otherwise normally functioning liver.[4,8-10] Steroids can inhibit bilirubin uptake in all species. Heparin administration to horses sometimes results in icterus and is believed to be caused in part by impaired uptake of bilirubin by hepatocytes.[9] Anorexia in horses causes variable degrees of hyperbilirubinemia and may be related to the half-life of ligandin.[9,10] Ligandin is the intrahepatic protein responsible for extracting unconjugated bilirubin from albumin in the sinusoidal blood. The half-life of ligandin is relatively short (days) and starvation in other species reduces the store of ligandin in the hepatocytes, thus impeding bilirubin uptake.[4] Premature and neonatal foals are also more susceptible to retention icterus, in the absence of hepatic disease. The cause of icterus in equine neonates is presumably a result of lower hepatocellular ligandin concentrations, compared with the adult.[47] In human beings, inherited or congenital deficiencies in enzymes responsible for conjugation (bilirubin-uridine diphosphate glucuronyl transferase) may result in intermittent or persistent icterus (Gilbert's syndrome or Crigler-Najjar syndrome type II) that often is not recognized until the patient is several years of age. The icterus occurs without other clinical or laboratory evidence of liver diease.[48] Persistent hyperbilirubinemia without anorexia, hemolysis, or evidence of acquired liver disease was reported in an otherwise healthy 4-year-old Thoroughbred gelding.[48] Conjugated bilirubin concentrations were normal, but total serum bilirubin concentrations ranged from 9.0 to 12.3 mg/dl during a 2.5-year monitoring period. The case most closely resembled Gilbert's syndrome.

If the excretion of conjugated bilirubin into the biliary tract is impeded, *regurgitation icterus* occurs.[8] Blockage of bile flow with resultant regurgitation icterus can accompany cholangitis, hepatitis, obstructive cholelithiasis, neoplastic infiltration, fibrosis, or hyperplasia of the biliary tract. Because conjugated bilirubin is water soluble, this form of icterus may be accompanied by bilirubinuria.

In hepatocellular disease, icterus most often is the result of a combined increase in both unconjugated and conjugated bilirubin.[8] Of the two fractions, the majority of the increase in the total bilirubin is from unconjugated bilirubin. Increases in the conjugated fraction greater than 25% of the total are usually indicative of hepatocellular disease, and increases greater than 30% are usually indicative of cholestasis.[10]

WEIGHT LOSS

Significant weight loss and failure to thrive are most consistently present during chronic hepatic insufficiency. However, chronic liver disease may be present without apparent weight loss. Weight loss is due to anorexia and the loss of normal hepatocellular metabolic activities.

HEPATOGENIC PHOTOSENSITIZATION

Photosensitization refers to abnormally heightened reactivity of the skin to ultraviolet sunlight because of the increased blood concentration of a photodynamic agent. In the case of hepatogenic photosensitization, the photodynamic agent is *phylloerythrin*. Phylloerythrin is normally formed in the gastrointestinal tract as a result of bacterial degradation of chlorophyll and is absorbed into the general circulation, conjugated, and excreted by the liver.[49] During hepatic insufficiency, the blood concentrations of this photodynamic agent are increased. Subsequent exposure of phylloerythrin to ultraviolet light causes activation of electrons within the molecule to an excited state, with resultant free radical formation. The local production of free radicals causes cell membrane damage and necrosis. Unpigmented areas most efficiently absorb ultraviolet light; thus the lesions of photosensitization are restricted to white skin. The skin first appears erythematous and edematous. Pruritus, pain, vesiculation, ulceration, necrosis, and sloughing may ensue.

COLIC, DIARRHEA, TENESMUS, ASCITES, STEATORRHEA

Abdominal pain associated with acute hepatocellular disease may be a result of acute hepatic swelling, or biliary obstruction (cholelithiasis).[4,50] Signs of anterior abdominal pain include anorexia, bruxism, sitting like a dog, recumbency, and rolling up onto the dorsum. Palpation over the last few ribs (especially on the right) or immediately caudal to the last rib may elicit a pain response. Alternations in intestinal motility also may cause concurrent signs of colic with liver disease. McGorum et al.[17] reported that 10 of 25 horses with liver disease and signs of colic had clinically significant gastric impactions. Of the horses with gastric impactions, seven also had signs of HE; none of these horses survived.

Diarrhea infrequently may accompany chronic hepatic insufficiency in horses.[51]Alterations in the intestinal microflora, portal hypertension, and deficiency of bile acids may be involved in the pathogenesis.[4] Though uncommon in horses, portal hypertension can lead to increased hydrostatic and oncotic pressure in the intestinal mucosa, with resultant water and protein loss into the lumen of the bowel and the peritoneal cavity (ascites). Tenesmus may be the result of constipation but has also been reported to be a sign of hepatoencephalopathy.[17]

Decreased excretion of bile may result in lipid malabsorption and excessive amounts of fat in the feces, or *steatorrhea*,[4] which subsequently may cause osmotic diarrhea. Because the normal equine diet is low in fat, steatorrhea is rare in horses. Chronic cholestasis may cause clay-colored feces because of lack of fecal urobilinogen and stercobilin. This coloration rarely is observed in adult herbivores, because the normal fecal color is generated primarily by plant chlorophylls and not by bilirubin metabolites.[10]

HEMORRHAGIC DIATHESIS

Because the liver is responsible for the synthesis of numerous factors involved in coagulation and fibrinolysis, abnormal hemostasis may be a sequela to hepatic insufficiency. Clinical signs may vary from petechial or ecchymotic hemorrhages to hemorrhage after trauma or venipuncture to spontaneous hemorrhage (epistaxis, melena, hemoptysis, hematuria, or hematomas).[4,8,10,21,52] Especially sensitive to hepatic disease is the synthesis of fibrinogen and the vitamin K–dependent factors (II, VII, IX, X, and protein C), which have short half-lives. Factor VII has a half-life of only 4 to 5 hours. Other vitamin K–dependent factors and fibrinogen have half-lives in the range of 4 to 5 days. Because vitamin K is fat soluble and requires bile acids for proper absorption from the intestinal tract, vitamin K–dependent factors are affected particularly during hepatic insufficiency when bile excretion is decreased.

During hepatic insufficiency, the synthesis of protein C and antithrombin III may be altered. Decreased plasma concentrations of these two anticoagulants would result in uncontrolled clot formation and consumption of other coagulation factors. In chronic hepatic disease the plasma concentration of protein C is normal or decreased; however, antithrombin III may be normal, increased, or decreased.[21] Pregnant women with fatty livers have decreased antithrombin III activity, but patients with biliary cirrhosis or biliary obstruction have increased antithrombin III activity.[21] Horses with liver disease have increased antithrombin III activity and theoretically should tend to bleed.[53] Alterations in the factors controlling fibrinolysis vary in chronic liver disease.[21] Conditions that promote fibrinolysis—such as increased plasminogen and plasminogen activator, or decreased plasminogen activator inhibitor, α_2-antiplasmin, and α_2-macroglobulin—result in bleeding tendencies. Conditions that aid thrombus formation, such as decreased plasminogen, further promote consumptive coagulopathy. The fibrinolytic factors have not been evaluated in horses with liver disease.

Finally, the liver plays an important role in balancing normal hemostasis by Kupffer's cell removal of activated coagulation factors and FDPs from the general circulation.[21] Failure to remove activated coagulation factors further promotes coagulation, and FDPs interfere with platelet function and fibrin clot formation.

FEVER

Horses with hepatic abscesses, acute hepatitis, CAH, obstructive cholelithiasis, fatty liver failure, or neoplasia may have constant or intermittent fevers.[50,54-59]

HEMOLYSIS

Hemolysis is a rarely seen but grave prognostic indicator of fulminant hepatic failure in horses.[15] The exact cause of hemolysis is not known but is believed to be the result of increased erythrocyte fragility.

PRURITUS AND SEBORRHEA

Retention of bile acids and accumulation in the skin may cause pruritus and seborrhea. This finding is rarely reported in horses.[15,60]

EDEMA

Hypoalbuminemia and water retention can occur with chronic liver failure and may result in dependent edema. Because the half-life of albumin is long (19 to 20 days) in the horse, edema is a rare clinical sign.[61] Ponies with hyperlipemia may develop dependent abdominal edema after vascular thrombosis.[58] Dependent abdominal edema also may form if significant portal hypertension and ascites exist.

ENDOTOXEMIA

The Kupffer's cell plays an important role in removing bacterial endotoxin that is normally absorbed from the lumen of the intestinal tract and carried to the liver via the portal circulation.[13] Failure of Kupffer's cell phagocytosis of endotoxin may result in clinical and laboratory evidence of endotoxemia.

POLYDIPSIA, POLYURIA, AND THE HEPATORENAL SYNDROME

Alterations in renal function, including deranged sodium concentrations, impaired water excretion, and urine-concentrating ability, may accompany severe liver disease.[4,21] Sodium retention results from increased blood aldosterone concentrations because of failure of hepatic biotransformation and a decrease in the effective circulating blood volume as a result of portal hypertension and hypoalbuminemia. Sodium retention raises the osmolality of the extracellular fluid, thereby stimulating the thirst center. Polydipsia has been reported in horses with chronic liver disease.[62,63] Despite the potential increase in exchangeable sodium, the serum sodium concentration is usually normal or decreased, as a result of superimposed water retention. The mechanism for water retention is multifactorial, but increased antidiuretic hormone, reduced effective circulating volume, and altered renal prostaglandin synthesis are most likely involved.[21] Sometimes the urine-concentrating ability is impaired because of reduced medullary interstitial urea, the net effect being polyuria, isosthenuria, or both.

Hepatorenal syndrome is characterized by acute azotemia and anuria and may occur in ponies with hyperlipemia and hepatic lipidosis (see Hyperlipemia and Hepatic Lipidosis). The pathogenesis is obscure, but speculative causes include reduced effective circulating volume, decreased hepatic inactivation of renin, and endotoxemia.[21]

Diagnosis and Laboratory Findings of Hepatic Insufficiency

Historical information (as discussed in the section on Specific Hepatic Diseases) may be useful in the diagnosis of certain types of hepatic insufficiency. Nonspecific clinical signs and variable laboratory findings confound the definitive diagnosis of hepatic disease in horses. Paramount to the laboratory diagnosis of hepatic insufficiency in horses is knowledge of the sensitivity and specificity of the tests (Table 16-2). Because massive hepatic disease must be present before alterations are seen with some laboratory tests, and because different liver functions are variably altered by disease, the specificity of the laboratory diagnosis of hepatic disease increases with the magnitude of abnormal findings. Laboratory findings also may be useful for therapeutic and prognostic considerations.

EVALUATION OF BILIRUBIN

Serum bilirubin concentration is not a sensitive indicator of liver disease in horses. In one report on serum biochemical changes in horses with liver disease, only one fourth of the cases had increased serum bilirubin concentrations.[17] The *total bilirubin* concentration in the blood, as determined by the van den Bergh test, is a combination of both unconjugated and conjugated bilirubin. Because the diagnostic value of the bilirubin concentration, when used for evaluation of hepatic disease, depends on which subfraction is increased, the concentrations of both unconjugated and conjugated bilirubin must be determined.

The serum bilirubin concentration is stable for several days, if the sample is protected against sunlight.[10] The total bilirubin concentration is determined first in a chromogenic

TABLE 16-2

Clinical Pathology of Liver Disease in Horses

Test	Aberration	Normal Value
SPECIFIC INDICATORS OF LIVER DISEASE		
Serum sorbitol dehydrogenase (SDH)	Increases	<8 U/L
Serum γ-glutamyltransferase (GGT)	Increases	<25 U/L
Serum bile acids concentration	Increases	<15 μmol/L
Arginase (ARG)	Increases	
Glutamate dehydrogenase (GLDH)	Increases	
Direct bilirubin	>25% of total	0-0.4 mg/dl (0-6.8 μmol/L)
Ammonia	Increases	(laboratory dependent)
BSP half-life	Prolonged	2.8 ± 0.5 min
Branched chain: aromatic amino acid ratio	Decreases	3.5-4.5
Urine bilirubin	Increases	
NONSPECIFIC INDICATORS OF LIVER DISEASE		
Total bilirubin	Increases	
Indirect bilirubin	Increases	
Lactate dehydrogenase-5 (LDH-5)	Increases	
Aspartate aminotransferase (AST)	Increases	
Alanine aminotransferase (ALT)	Increases	
Alkaline phosphatase (ALP)	Increases	
Blood urea nitrogen (BUN)	Decreases	
Globulins	Increases	
Albumin	Decreases	
Glucose	Decreases	
Prothrombin time (PT)	Prolonged	
Activated partial thromboplastin time (APTT)	Prolonged	
Triglyceride	Increases	
White blood cell count	Increases with infection or inflammation; decreases with endotoxemia	

assay by reaction for 30 minutes with a diazo reagent (sulfanilic acid and sodium nitrite) and methyl alcohol.[10] *Conjugated* or *direct-reacting bilirubin* is similarly determined over 5 minutes, without the addition of methyl alcohol. The amount of *unconjugated bilirubin* can then be determined by the difference between the total bilirubin concentration and the direct-reacting bilirubin. Because the unconjugated fraction is determined arithmetically, it is appropriately called *indirect-reacting bilirubin*. In normal horses, the total bilirubin concentration is in the range of 0.2 to 5.0 mg/dl (3.4 to 85.5 μmol/L) with conjugated bilirubin in the range between 0.0 to 0.4 mg/dl (0 to 6.8 μmol/L).[8] As discussed previously, increases in the unconjugated bilirubin fraction may occur without hepatic disease. Hemolysis, anorexia, intestinal obstruction, cardiac insufficiency, Gilbert's syndrome, and the administration of certain drugs (steroids, heparin, halothane) may cause an increase in the unconjugated bilirubin concentration.[9] If the unconjugated bilirubin concentration is increased, then the erythron should be concurrently evaluated to rule out hemolysis as the causative factor. Hemolysis may cause the unconjugated bilirubin concentration to rise as high as 80 mg/dl (1368 μmol/L).[10] Complete anorexia can cause an increase in the unconjugated bilirubin concentration within 12 hours; however, it is unlikely to rise greater than 6 to 8 mg/dl (102.6 to 136.8 μmol/L) in horses suffering purely from anorexia,[10] although values as high as 10.5 mg/dl have been reported in anorexic horses.[60] Finally, the age of the horse and concurrent drug therapy must be considered. Neonates normally have more unconjugated bilirubin than adults. The higher bilirubin concentration in foals most likely is caused by the turnover of fetal hemoglobin to adult hemoglobin and the deficiency of liver-binding and conjugating enzymes compared with the adult.[47] In the absence of liver disease, prematurity or illness in foals can further increase the unconjugated bilirubin fraction.

Keeping the foregoing limitations of interpretation in mind, increases in the unconjugated bilirubin fraction in horses with hepatic disease are most likely to occur with acute hepatocellular disease.[8-10] Rarely does the unconjugated bilirubin fraction in acute hepatic disease exceed 25 mg/dl (427.5 μmol/L).[10] An increase in the bilirubin concentration may be indicative of hepatic disease but not necessarily hepatic failure. Furthermore, a normal bilirubin value, as commonly occurs in chronic hepatic disease, does not necessarily preclude the diagnosis of hepatic insufficiency.

An increase in the conjugated bilirubin fraction in horses more reliably is indicative of hepatic disease.[8-10] If the conjugated bilirubin concentration is greater than 25% of the total bilirubin value, then hepatocellular disease should be suspected. If the conjugated bilirubin concentration is greater than 30% of the total value, then cholestasis should be suspected.[10] Conjugated bilirubin is water soluble and detectable in the urine of horses only if blood concentrations become sufficiently increased to surpass the renal threshold.[10] Therefore when urine tests positive for the presence of bilirubin, cholestatic disease should be suspected. Urine dipstick analysis is less sensitive than analysis with a diazo tablet.[10] Urobilinogen may be detected by dipstick analysis of normal horse urine, and its presence indicates a patent bile duct.[10] Because urobilinogen is highly unstable, it must be determined on a fresh urine sample. Dilute or acidic urine may interfere with accurate determination of urobilinogen. Reagent strips are not sensitive enough to detect the absence of urobilinogen; therefore Ehrlich's reagent must be used. The absence of urobilinogen does not necessarily indicate liver disease, but it may be compatible with failure of excretion of bilirubin into the intestine, biliary obstruction, failure of intestinal bacterial reduction (diarrhea, overuse of oral antimicrobials), or failure to reabsorb it from the ileum.[4] Increased concentrations of urobilinogen in the urine may be caused by the increased production of urobilinogen by intestinal bacteria, failure of the liver to remove it from the enterohepatic circulation, portosystemic shunting, or spillover after severe hemolysis.[4]

SERUM BILE ACID CONCENTRATION

The enterohepatic circulation normally removes greater than 90% of bile acids. Thus the blood concentration of bile acids may be increased with liver disease, and quantitation provides an excellent screen of liver failure and has essentially replaced foreign dye clearance (e.g., bromosulphthalein) as a functional test of the liver.[9,63,64] Serum bile acids are stable for at least 1 month if stored at -20° C and are measured by radioimmunoassay or by an enzymatic colorimetric method. The concentration of total serum bile acids is not affected by short-term fasting (<14 hours) but may be increased by more prolonged fasting.[65] The major serum bile acids in horses include ursodeoxycholic acid, chenodeoxycholic acid, and deoxycholic acid, but the exact composition of serum bile acids varies markedly among normal horses.[66] Reported normal mean values for horses and ponies as determined by radioimmunoassay are 8.2+/-1.6 μmol/L (n = 9)[63] and 5.3+/-6.5 μmol/L (n = 51)[64] and 5.0+/-28.0 μmol/L[66] for the colorimetric method. Increased serum bile acid concentrations are highly specific for the presence of liver disease (may increase within 24 to 48 hours after onset of hepatic disease) but are not specific for the type of liver disease.[9,67] Because bile acids are 90% restricted to the enterohepatic circulation, increases in the blood may occur as a result of shunting or decreased blood flow to the liver (first-pass effect), failure of the liver to remove bile acids from the enterohepatic circulation, failure of the hepatocytes to conjugate the bile acids for excretion, or failure of excretion with subsequent regurgitation of the bile acids into the blood (biliary obstruction). Increases in the primary (nondegraded) bile acids cholate and chenodeoxycholate account for most of the increase in total serum bile acids concentration in horses with liver disease.[66] In relation to the severity of liver disease, a significant shift in composition of serum bile acid profile from taurocholate to free unconjugated cholate also occurs. This finding suggests that hepatocellular excretion, and not resorption, is the most sensitive step in the enterohepatic circulation of bile acids in horses.[66]

Fasting for longer than 3 days in mature horses caused an increase in the serum bile acid concentration of three times over baseline values.[65] Ligation of the bile duct caused a sixfold increase in serum bile acid concentration compared with fasted horses.[65] Carbon tetrachloride toxicity resulted in a threefold increase compared with fasted horses.[65] Concentrations of serum bile acids greater than 50 μmol/L in horses with pyrrolizidine toxicosis were associated with a grave prognosis.[63] A value less than 20 μmol/L appears to be a good predictor in ruling out significant functional liver disease and should be included in the evaluation of horses suspected to have hepatic disease.[64] Serum bile acid concentrations greater than 20 μmol/L appear to be indicative of chronic liver disease but are less effective in detecting acute hepatic disease.[64] It is important to note that, compared with mature horses, serum bile acids concentrations are higher in healthy neonatal foals during the first month of life and frequently exceed 20 μmol/L.[68] Bile acid concentrations are highest in biliary obstructive diseases and portosystemic shunts.

TESTS OF PROTEIN SYNTHESIS

The blood concentrations of protein or amino acids relate not only to the rate of synthesis by the liver but also to their half-life in the circulation. The half-life of albumin in horses is long (19 to 20 days); thus a decrease in the albumin concentration is rarely detectable until greater than 80% of the liver mass is lost for more than 3 weeks.[8,10,17,61] It is unusual for the total serum protein concentration to decrease to less than 5 g/dl (50 g/L) in chronic liver disease.[13] Hypoalbuminemia is a nonspecific finding in chronic liver disease, because it may occur secondary to endoparasitism, nephrosis, malnutrition, malabsorption, circulatory failure, and many other chronic diseases.[10,61]

The globulin fraction often is increased in chronic hepatic disease as a result of decreased Kupffer's cell mass. Loss of Kupffer's cell function may result in wider dissemination of enteric-derived foreign antigens. Plasma cells respond to the general increased antigen load, resulting in polyclonal gammopathy.[4,8,10] Although the globulin fraction may be increased, it is a nonspecific finding with chronic hepatic disease, because polyclonal gammopathy can occur after numerous chronic diseases. The α-and β-globulins may also increase with chronic liver disease. A decreased serum albumin concentration concurrent with an increased globulin concentration in chronic hepatic disease causes the total plasma protein or serum protein to appear normal. Thus serum protein fractionation is paramount. Protein electrophoresis most accurately determines fractionation of the components making up the total serum protein concentration.[8]

The blood concentration of amino acids may be increased after acute hepatocellular necrosis or during protein catabolic states such as illness or starvation, in response to insulin or glucagon.[4] Fractionation of the blood amino acids and determination of the BCAA-to-AAA ratio is rarely done in clinical practice but is more useful than evaluating either fraction separately (see Hepatic Encephalopathy). Decreases in this ratio indicate hepatic insufficiency.[42] The risk of clinical signs of HE may be projected from the BCAA-to-AAA (phenylalanine, tyrosine) ratio. A normal ratio falls between 3.5 and 4.5. The risk of HE is low, medium, or high if the ratio is 3.0 to 3.5, 2.5 to 3.0, and less than 2.5, respectively.[42]

Because the liver is primarily responsible for removing *ammonia* from the circulation and converting it to urea for renal excretion, increases in the blood ammonia concentration or a decrease in the BUN concentration (<9 mg/dl; 6.43 mmol/L) may be indicative of chronic hepatocellular disease.[8,13,17] Daily blood ammonia levels vary widely in normal horses.[16] The compounding effects of ammonia-generating and urea-using bacteria in the gastrointestinal tract, ammonia generation with blood storage, as well as the effects of the ration may partly account for these fluctuations. In ethylenediaminetetraacetic acid (EDTA), whole blood can be refrigerated for up to 6 hours without a significant increase in ammonia content.[69] The effect of the ration and handling can be evaluated by concurrently determining the blood ammonia concentration of a stable mate receiving a similar ration. Oral ammonia challenge tests have not been fully evaluated in horses; however, the sensitivity of the oral challenge test may be decreased because of the effect of enteric bacteria. Normal values for ammonia for horses vary among laboratories but have been reported in the range of 13 to 108 μg/dl (7.63-63.42 μmol/L).[15]

No correlation exists between the blood ammonia concentration and the severity of liver disease in horses, but increased blood ammonia concentration is significantly correlated with the presence of liver disease, hepatoencephalopathy, or both.[16,17] Although hyperammonemia appears to be a sensitive indicator of liver disease in the horse, it is not specific for liver disease. Encephalopathy associated with hyperammonemia without concurrent evidence of liver disease has been reported in horses with acute gastrointestinal disease.[70,71] Hyperammonemia has also been reported as a fatal heritable disorder in Morgan foals and is believed to be caused by a defective mitochondrial transporter protein involved in urea synthesis.[72] The syndrome may be accompanied by mild to moderate increases in serum liver enzyme activities.

Because the liver is also responsible for the synthesis of certain coagulation factors, evaluation of hemostatic function may be useful. Changes in hemostatic function values are not specific for liver disease and must be evaluated in light of the other laboratory findings. The vitamin K–dependent factor with the shortest half-life is factor VII; thus abnormalities are frequently first observed in the *prothrombin time (PT)*.[16] However, adequate evaluation of hemostatic function necessitates determination of the *activated partial thromboplastin time* (APTT), the *fibrinogen* and FDP concentrations, and a platelet count. In one retrospective clinical review, almost half of the horses with liver disease had either an abnormally prolonged PT or APTT.[17] Typically, a 50% to 70% decrease in the blood concentration of the coagulation factors is necessary before a change in these clotting time–based assays is detectable.[8] Daily variation in the normal values for clotting times also hinders accurate detection of the abnormal. The clotting times may be standardized more appropriately if one concurrently determines a clotting assay on a normal horse. If the ratio of clotting time (PT or APTT) of the patient with possible hepatic disease to the normal horse's value is greater than 1.3, then the test may be interpreted as abnormal.[73] The sensitivity of coagulation factor deficiency during hepatic insufficiency may be increased by diluting the plasma[74] or by determining the concentration of specific factors, by either clot-based, chromogenic, or radioimmunologic assays. These later assays are not widely available.

Hypofibrinogenemia cannot be accurately detected by the heat block precipitation method, the most common method for determination of the plasma fibrinogen concentration.[8] Clotting assays using thrombin more accurately determine the fibrinogen concentration. Fibrinogen concentrations less than 100 mg/dl (1 g/L) indicate either decreased production or increased consumption of fibrinogen. The FDP concentration, as determined by latex agglutination, may be increased during hepatic insufficiency owing to decreased removal by Kupffer's cells. Concentrations of FDPs greater than 16 μg/dl are indicative of increased production or reduced removal. The plasma concentration of several factors acting as anticoagulants or involved in fibrinolysis also may be altered in chronic liver failure (see Hemorrhagic Diathesis). Tests for these factors are primarily limited to academic and research institutions.

Thrombocytopenia with associated petechiae or nasal mucosal bleeding has been reported in horses with liver disease; therefore in possible cases of liver disease, platelet counts should also be evaluated before invasive diagnostic or therapeutic techniques.[16]

TESTS OF CARBOHYDRATE METABOLISM

Changes in the blood glucose concentration rarely occur in horses with liver insufficiency.[13,17] Hyperglycemia may occur with stress-associated catecholamine and glucocorticoid release. Hypoglycemia (glucose <60 mg/dl; 3.33 mmol/L) may occur in acute massive hepatic failure but is more likely in chronic liver disease as anorexia progresses, glycogen stores are depleted, and gluconeogenesis and glycolysis are impaired by increased glucagon concentrations. If glucose is administered, then blood glucose levels often remain abnormally increased, indicating tissue insulin resistance.[20] Insulin receptor number and binding affinity for insulin are diminished in human beings with chronic liver disease. Changes in the blood glucose concentration are not specific for liver disease and must be evaluated in the light of other laboratory findings.

TESTS OF LIPID METABOLISM

The concentration of blood triglycerides may become increased during hepatic insufficiency because of increased mobilization from adipose tissue to support energy-requiring processes and a decreased clearance by the liver.[4,10] In contrast, the VLDL and esterified cholesterol blood concentrations may be decreased because of failure of liver synthesis. Compared with other species, equids are thought to possess a greater clearance capacity for triglycerides and a greater hepatic exporting capacity for VLDL. Thus changes in the blood VLDL, esterified cholesterol, or triglyceride concentrations rarely occur in horses.[10] An exception to this is the marked increase in blood triglyceride levels that occurs with hyperlipidemia syndrome in ponies and Miniature horses (see Hyperlipidemia and Hepatic Lipidosis). Because nonhepatic diseases may alter blood lipid concentrations, these tests are neither sensitive nor specific for liver disease in horses.[10] The blood cholesterol and triglyceride concentrations are normally higher in neonates, compared with adults.[47]

Increased mobilization of triglycerides and fatty acid oxidation by the liver may result in increased production of *ketone bodies,* acetoacetate, and β-hydroxybutyric acid.[5] Although peripheral tissues may use ketone bodies for energy, these compounds are weak acids and increased levels in the blood may result in ketoacidosis. The pathway for ketone formation is poorly developed in horses. Ketoacidosis is less common in horses than in other species.[10] Ketoacidosis should be suspected in horses that are acidemic and have an abnormally high anion gap. Ketones may be quantitated in the blood or urine. Because the renal threshold of ketone bodies is low, ketonuria usually precedes ketonemia. Routine urine dipsticks only detect acetoacetate.[10]

LIVER ENZYMES

Acute hepatocellular necrosis or changes in hepatocyte membrane permeability result in the release of soluble cytosolic enzymes into the sinusoidal blood. Thus increased blood activity of these cytosolic enzymes may be indicative of active hepatic disease. Caution must be exercised when evaluating increases in these enzymes because not all are liver specific. Furthermore, some of these hepatocellular enzymes may be increased because of induction by drugs. Most of these enzymes are quantitated colorimetrically; thus hemolysis or lipemia may interfere with accurate evaluation. Furthermore, wide variation in values can exist because of age differences, stage of hepatic disease, and laboratory methodology. In horses the following cytosolic enzymes are liver specific and are not inducible: *sorbitol dehydrogenase (SDH; iditol dehydrogenase), arginase (ARG),* ornithine carbamoyltransferase, and *glutamate dehydrogenase (GLDH)*.[8,10] Although increases in these enzymes in the blood are highly specific for hepatocellular disease, they are not specific for the type of disease. Significant increases occur after acute hepatic necrosis. Mild increases in these enzymes may occur after hepatic hypoxemia or toxemia resulting from endotoxemia, septicemia, transient intestinal disease, hyperthermia, or administration of certain drugs (benzimidazole anthelmintics).[8,10,13]

SDH has been widely used in the evaluation of acute liver disease in horses.[13,47,75] The short half-life of this liver cytosolic enzyme makes it ideal for the evaluation of acute ongoing disease, because values usually return to baseline within 3 to 5 days after a transient hepatic insult.[60] Its short half-life necessitates analysis within hours of collection. Storage of serum in the freezer (−15° C) or refrigerator results in losses of approximately 1.0% and 3.5%, respectively, of SDH activity per day.[76] Although mild variations exist between laboratories, the normal blood activity of SDH in horses is usually less than 8 U/L.[15] Foals 2 to 4 weeks of age may have SDH activity slightly greater than those of adult horses.[47,75] Increases in SDH have been reported after prolonged halothane anesthesia in horses.[77] ARG is used in the Krebs-Henseleit cycle for urea synthesis. It is found in highest activity in hepatocytes, although minute amounts also exist in renal tissue, brain, skin, testicles, and erythrocytes. Increases in ARG are most indicative of acute hepatic necrosis. Like SDH, ARG has a very short half-life. GLDH is found in hepatocytes, renal tissue, brain, muscle, and intestinal cells. Like SDH and ARG, GLDH has the highest tissue activity in the liver, and increases of this enzyme in the blood can be considered specific for acute liver disease. The half-life of GLDH is 14 hours.

Other cytosolic enzymes include *aspartate aminotransferase (AST), alkaline phosphatase (ALP), lactate dehydrogenase (LDH), alanine aminotransferase (ALT),* and *isocitrate dehydrogenase (ICD).* These enzymes are also found with high activity in other tissues, or are inducible. Thus increases in these enzymes are *not specific* for liver disease in horses. Because some of these enzymes are frequently reported in equine biochemical profiles, they may serve as a crude indicator of liver disease; however, the limitations of their usefulness must be recognized.

AST, formerly glutamic oxaloacetic transaminase (GOT), is a cytosolic- and mitochondrial-bound enzyme that catalyzes the reaction responsible for aspartate biosynthesis from carbohydrate.[8] Basically, all cells contain AST, but liver and skeletal muscle cells contain the highest activity. Cardiac muscle, erythrocytes, intestinal cells, and the kidney also are sources of AST. Hemolysis and lipemia will falsely increase the value of AST.[8] Increases are most frequently associated with muscle damage but may be seen after acute hepatic necrosis. Often the AST activity is normal in chronic hepatic disease.[13] The half-life of AST is long, and thus it may take longer than 2 weeks for the blood activity to decrease after acute hepatic disease. The AST value is most useful when analyzed with other tissue-specific enzymes. For instance, if a muscle-specific enzyme, such as creatine kinase, also is increased, then an increase in AST most likely has its origin in muscle. Serial AST and SDH values can be useful for the determination of ongoing hepatic disease. If the SDH and AST values were initially increased, but subsequent evaluation reveals a normal or decreasing SDH and elevated AST, then a favorable prognosis is indicated, because hepatic necrosis is most likely subsiding. The normal serum activity of AST is 98 to 278 U/L.[15] ICD has a distribution similar to AST.

ALT, formerly glutamic pyruvic transaminase (GPT), is responsible for alanine synthesis from carbohydrate.[8] Increases may be evident with acute hepatic disease, but myositis will also increase blood levels. Hemolysis will falsely increase the value of this enzyme, and microsomal enzyme inducers (i.e., glucocorticoids) will increase its production and release in the absence of liver disease. This enzyme is not useful for predicting liver disease in horses.[8]

ALP catalyzes the hydrolysis of monophosphate esters. This enzyme is bound to the mitochondrial membrane and thus does not leak into the blood with changes in cell membrane permeability or necrosis. Cholestasis and certain drugs, including glucocorticoids, primidone, and phenobarbital, will induce production and release of ALP. The ALP value most likely is to be increased in chronic or cholestatic liver diseases rather than acute or hepatocellular disease. Other tissues in addition to the liver contain ALP, including bone, intestine, kidney, placenta, and leukocytes, thus increases are not necessarily indicative of cholestasis. Because of increased osteoblastic activity, foals have ALP values two to three times those of adults.[10] Pregnancy, hemolysis, and gastrointestinal disease will also cause increases in ALP.

LDH is the name for five major isoenzymes located in liver, muscle, erythrocytes, intestinal cells, and renal tissue. Increases in LDH are not liver specific unless the isoenzyme activity is determined. Isoenzyme 5 (LDH-5) is a useful indicator of acute hepatocellular disease in horses because values typically return to baseline within 4 days after a transient hepatic insult.[60,78] LDH-5 is also present in muscle, so increased serum LDH-5 activity is specific for hepatic disease if other indicators of muscle damage (i.e., creatine kinase) are normal.[79] LDH-5 is stable at room temperature for 36 hours.

γ-Glutamyltransferase (GGT) is involved in glutathione metabolism and transfer of glutamyl groups.[8] GGT primarily is associated with microsomal membranes in the biliary epithelium. Cholestasis induces production and release of GGT. Renal tubule cells contain GGT, but this source is released into urine. The only other potentially significant source of GGT in the blood is pancreatic in origin. Because pancreatic disease is rare in horses, the blood activity of GGT is considered specific for hepatic disease in horses. Some clinicians consider GGT to be the single test of highest sensitivity when evaluating horses for evidence of liver disease.[60] The half-life of GGT is approximately 3 days; GGT is stable in serum for 2 days at room temperature or for 30 days if frozen. Mild increases may be evident after acute hepatocellular necrosis and may continue to rise for 1 to 2 weeks despite improvement in clinical signs.[60] Increases are more persistent in chronic disease, especially with cholestasis.[13] Foals 2 weeks to 1 month old may have greater GGT values than adults.[47,75] The wider variation in younger horses reflects the degree and extent of hepatic maturation. Normal values for GGT in adult horses typically are less than 30 U/L[15] but may be greater in racing Thoroughbreds, healthy donkeys, burros, and asses.[80] In chronic, nonactive hepatic fibrosis and focal hepatic disease, GGT may not be significantly increased. Increased serum GGT activity has been reported in horses with cholestasis secondary to colonic displacement.[79]

In summary, evaluation for liver disease in horses should include quantitation of at least SDH or ARG, and GGT. However, one should not interpret normal values for these liver enzymes as absence of liver disease.

CLEARANCE OF PHARMACEUTICALS

In addition to clearance of endogenous substances from the blood, liver function can be evaluated after injection of an exogenous substance. One such exogenous substance that is removed by the liver, conjugated, and excreted into bile is *bromsulphalein* (BSP).[10] After intravenous injection of 2.2 mg

BSP per kilogram body weight, a clearance half-life is determined by periodically obtaining heparinized blood samples over 12 to 15 minutes. One should exercise caution when injecting BSP, because it can be thrombogenic and irritating if administered perivascularly. Blood samples for BSP quantitation should be collected from a site other than the injection site. Suggested collection times are 3, 6, 9, 12, and 15 minutes after injection. Collection of plasma at the suggested times is not crucial; however, recording the exact times at which the samples were obtained is important to ensure accurate determination of the half-life. The half-life of BSP, thus the rate of extraction by the liver, is determined by plotting the plasma concentrations against the collection times on semi-log paper. The normal half-life of BSP in horses is 2.8 to 0.5 minutes.[10]

The BSP half-life is prolonged when greater than 50% of the hepatic function is lost.[8,10] This function test is useful in horses, especially to distinguish hepatoencephalopathy from other causes of abnormal behavior or cerebral signs, and to test liver function in chronic liver disease when bilirubin, SDH, and GGT blood levels may be normal. Proper interpretation of the BSP half-life must take into account the state of hepatic blood and bile flow and the bilirubin and albumin concentrations.[8] If the hepatic blood flow is decreased significantly, as may occur with hepatic congestion or portosystemic shunts, then the rate of delivery of BSP to the liver will be decreased; thus the half-life of BSP in the plasma will be prolonged. Because BSP is bound to albumin for delivery to the liver, if the blood concentration of albumin is markedly decreased, then a higher proportion of unbound BSP will be delivered to the hepatocytes; thus the half-life of BSP will be shortened.[8] If the blood concentration of bilirubin is increased greatly, then the bilirubin will compete with the BSP for binding sites and conjugating enzymes in the liver; thus the apparent half-life of BSP is prolonged. If significant cholestasis is present, then the BSP excreted into the biliary tract will be reabsorbed into the circulation, causing an apparent prolongation of its clearance. Therefore although a BSP clearance test is very useful as a test of hepatic function, one must interpret the results in light of these limitations. Furthermore, because pharmaceutical-grade BSP is no longer commercially available, this test is basically limited to academic and research institutions. Quantitation of serum bile acids concentration has essentially replaced BSP clearance as an indicator of hepatic function.

The determination of the BSP clearance time has been suggested to be more useful for detecting liver disease than the BSP half-life.[81] It has also been suggested that the proportionality transfer constants of clearance may be more useful in predicting hepatic disease than the BSP half-life alone.[82] The clearance time is the amount of dye irreversibly removed from the plasma per unit time. A dose of 5 mg BSP per kilogram of body weight is given intravenously, and heparinized blood samples are obtained 2, 5, 10, 15, 25, and 30 minutes after injection. The BSP clearance time in fed normal horses is 10 ml/min/kg and 6 ml/min/kg for horses fasted 3 days.[81]

The *indocyanine green* (ICG; Beckmann & Dickinson, Baltimore, Md.) clearance test has replaced the BSP clearance test in human beings.[4] Basically, the procedure and the limitations are the same as the BSP clearance test. The ICD clearance time in fed horses is 3.5 to 0.67 ml/min/kg, and 1.6 to 0.57 ml/min/kg for fasted horses.[81] Although the clearance of ICG is an excellent predictor of hepatic blood flow and extraction rates, its current expense precludes its routine use in horses. Another disadvantage is that quantitation requires a spectrophotometer that reads infrared wavelengths. These limitations have hindered evaluation of ICG clearance times as a diagnostic test of liver insufficiency in horses.

The hepatic clearance of the radiopharmaceutical technetium 99m-mebrofenin is used in human beings and small animals to assess hepatic function. In horses, the plasma clearance of technetium 99m-mebrofenin is not affected by withholding feed.[83]

OTHER NONSPECIFIC LABORATORY FINDINGS

Increased formation and release of acidic metabolic products, including ketone bodies, lactate, pyruvate, and amino acids, contribute to acidemia. Other factors that may contribute to acidemia include diarrhea and loss of renal acidification because of impaired urea synthesis. Anorexia may predispose to hypokalemia.

Although infrequently reported in horses, aldosterone and water retention may cause deranged concentrations of sodium and isosthenuria (see polydipsia, polyuria, and the hepatorenal syndrome). Azotemia may occur with hyperlipemia.[62]

Cholangiohepatitis, CAH, or a focal hepatic abscess may cause an inflammatory leukogram, anemia of chronic disease, and hyperfibrinogenemia.[59] Primary polycythemia has been reported in horses with hepatocellular carcinoma and hepatoblastoma.[84-86] Because fibrinogen is synthesized by the liver, widespread chronic hepatitis may mask an increase in this acute phase reactant protein.

DIAGNOSTIC IMAGING OF THE LIVER

Ultrasonography is a safe, noninvasive imaging technique that uses the reflection of high-frequency sound waves from tissue interfaces to produce a visual image. Liver ultrasonography in horses is limited by the ribs, the depth and size of the liver, and its anatomic location deep to the diaphragm and lungs.[74] Mechanical sector or linear array scanners with 3.0-MHz crystals are most effective.[74] Ultrasonography can be used to assess the right and left sides of the liver, and the liver shape, size, position, and texture. Hepatic vein walls are less echogenic than portal vein walls, and the biliary system is not normally visible. Ultrasonography is most useful for determining the general size of the liver; changes in the hepatic parenchyma, including abscesses, cysts, and neoplastic masses; and detecting dilated bile ducts or obstructions with choleliths. The common bile duct cannot be seen in a horse. Abnormal intra- or extrahepatic blood flow or vasculature may be detectable. Ultrasonography is also useful for guiding biopsy instruments into the liver (see Liver Biopsy).

Radionucleotide imaging also may be used to detect alterations in the hepatic parenchyma or blood flow.[87] Radionucleotide scanning noninvasively evaluates function and yields structural information. Two radionucleotide scanning techniques are available to evaluate the liver: liver scan and biliary scan. In the liver scan, a technetium 99m–labeled sulfur colloid is injected intravenously. Technetium-99m is a gamma-emitting radioactive compound that is detected in the body by a gamma camera. After injection, Kupffer's cells phagocytose the technetium 99m sulfur colloid. Subsequent scanning with the gamma camera detects the radioactive emissions from the technetium 99m and resolves them into a two-dimensional image. Thus alterations in blood flow (portosystemic shunt) or hepatic masses such as abscesses, cysts, and neoplasia may be detectable. In the biliary scan, technetium 99m–labeled iminodiacetic acid is injected intravenously. The iminodiacetic acid is extracted by the hepatocytes, conjugated, and excreted in the bile.[88] Subsequent scanning images the biliary system and may be useful for the detection of biliary obstruction, including atresia, cholangitis, and cholelithiasis. Because radionucleotide imaging is somewhat expensive and requires a large gamma camera, this procedure is limited to research and academic institutions.

Operative mesenteric portography can be performed when a portosystemic shunt is suspected. In this procedure, a celiotomy is performed, radiopaque material is injected into a mesenteric vein, and rapid, sequential survey radiographs are obtained. Simultaneous opacification of the portal vein, azygous vein, and caudal vena cava or lack of filling of the intrahepatic portal system is indicative of portosystemic shunting.[87]

LIVER BIOPSY

A liver biopsy can yield important diagnostic and prognostic information. In a retrospective study of 73 horses with liver disease, a scoring system that graded the degree of fibrosis, reversible and irreversible cytopathology, inflammation, haemosiderosis, and bile duct proliferation was useful in predicting long-term survival.[89] A liver biopsy is performed at the right twelfth to fourteenth intercostal spaces at the intersection of a line drawn from the tuber coxae to a point midway between the elbow and the point of the shoulder. The procedure must be performed in a sterile manner. The area is clipped, aseptically prepared, injected with local-acting anesthetic subcutaneously, and a stab incision is made with a no. 15 scalpel blade. A Tru-Cut (Baxter-Travenol, St Louis) or Franklin-modified Vim-Silverman (Mueller & Co, Chicago, IL) biopsy instrument is inserted and directed craniad and ventrad through the diaphragm into the liver. Semiautomatic biospy instruments (EZ Core, Products Group International, Lyons, CO) and automatic biopsy guns (ProMag 2.2 Biopsy System, Manan Medical Products, Northbrook, IL) equipped with 14-gauge, 16-cm needles are very helpful for a quick and accurate liver biopsy. Samples should immediately be placed in formalin for histopathologic evaluation and, if necessary, in transport media for culture of micro-organisms. Precautions to consider before performing the procedure include the risk of hemorrhage, pneumothorax, and peritonitis from bile leakage and colon or abscess puncture, as well as spread from infectious hepatitis. These complications may be reduced by performing a hemostasis profile to assess the risk of hemorrhage and by using ultrasonography to guide needle placement. Although subclinical coagulopathy has been frequently reported in horses with liver disease, clinically significant or fatal hemorrhage after performing a liver biopsy is rarely reported.[16,17]

SUMMARY OF DIAGNOSTIC PROCEDURES

The most useful diagnostic tests for evaluation of hepatic disease in horses are quantitation of SDH, GGT, and serum bile acids. In the face of clinically significant liver disease, at least one of the three former serum tests typically is abnormal. Although less useful in horses, additional tests of liver disease may include quantitation of bilirubin, ALP, AST, albumin, fibrinogen, globulins, glucose, esterified triglycerides, ammonia, BUN, BSP clearance, and amino acids. Serial testing of these indices may increase their diagnostic and prognostic value. Abnormal laboratory findings should be further investigated with ultrasonography and biopsy, after evaluation of a hemostasis profile.

TREATMENT OF HEPATIC INSUFFICIENCY

Management techniques for hepatic insufficiency are largely supportive. (Therapies for specific liver diseases are discussed in more detail under Specific Hepatic Diseases.) The basic goal of treatment is to maintain the animal until enough liver regenerates to provide adequate function. Patients with severe hepatic fibrosis respond poorly because adequate regeneration often is not possible. Horses with signs of HE that are agitated, restless, or uncontrollable must be sedated to enable therapy; however, any medication should be used judiciously because most tranquilizers are metabolized by the liver or potentiate the abnormal neural function of HE. *Xylazine* or *detomidine* in small doses are safest and most effective in these instances. Use of diazepam is contraindicated because it enhances the effect of GABA on central inhibitory neurons and may exacerbate signs of HE.[27] Intravenous fluids should correct fluid deficit and acid-base or electrolyte imbalances. Because most horses with HE are anorectic and blood glucose may be decreased, continuous intravenous infusion of 5% dextrose at a rate of 2 ml/kg/hr can be beneficial.[90] If continued more than 24 to 48 hours, then 2.5% to 5.0% dextrose in half-strength saline or lactated Ringer's solution should be substituted. In human beings, volume expansion with 0.9% saline solution enhances urinary ammonia excretion.[91] If bicarbonate therapy is necessary to treat acidotic patients with hyperammonemia, then the rate of administration should be monitored carefully, because too rapid of a rate may increase blood levels of ammonia.[27] Hypokalemia or alkalosis result in increased renal production of ammonia and increased diffusion of ammonia into the CNS; thus treatment with potassium or acidifying fluids may be beneficial.[92]

Therapy should also be directed at reducing the production of toxic protein metabolites by enteric bacteria or by interfering with their absorption. The administration of *mineral oil* or magnesium sulfate per nasogastric tube is safe and aids in reducing toxin absorption. HE in human beings with acute fulminant hepatic failure is almost always associated with cerebral edema. Thus recommendations for treatment of severe acute HE in human beings include elective hyperventilation; elective moderate hypothermia; use of mannitol (0.5 to 1 g/kg body weight); hypertonic saline infusion; antioxidants such as acetylcystiene, selenium, and vitamin E (25 IU/kg/day PO); and extracorporeal liver support devices.[93,94]

Methods to reduce the production of ammonia and other enteric toxins include the oral administration of antibiotics (neomycin, metronidazole, rifaximin, vancomycin)[91] or lactulose or lactitol (not available in the United States).[92] In horses, *neomycin* has been recommended at a dosage of 10 to 100 mg/kg PO every 6 hours.[55,80] This treatment significantly alters the gastrointestinal flora, may cause diarrhea in some horses, and may predispose horses to salmonellosis because most *Salmonella* spp. are not sensitive to neomycin. However, in one retrospective study in horses with liver disease, oral neomycin therapy subjectively was more helpful that lactulose in alleviating signs of HE.[17] *Lactulose*, a syrup containing lactose and other disaccharides, passes through the upper small intestine and is metabolized by ileal and colonic bacteria to organic acids, thereby reducing luminal pH. Proposed beneficial mechanisms of action of lactulose include increased bacterial assimilation of ammonia, decreased ammonia production, ammonia trapping in the bowel lumen, enteric microflora changes, and osmotic catharsis.[19,95] A dose of 0.3

ml/kg of lactulose syrup every 6 hours per nasogastric tube has been recommended for horses[80]; however, this therapy is expensive and may cause diarrhea. In human beings, lactulose also may be given as an enema when the oral route is unavailable.[93] When given orally three times a day at 333 mg/kg of body weight, lactulose (Duphalac, Solvay Pharmaceuticals, Marietta, GA) significantly decreased blood ammonia values in healthy adult horses.[95] None of the horses developed diarrhea, although one horse foundered on the sixth day of treatment. Fecal pH did not decrease. As an alternative or adjunct to antimicrobials or lactulose, one may attempt modification of intestinal flora with probiotics, such as *Lactobacillus acidophilus* or *Enterococcus faecium*.[92] Many clinicians prefer not to use oral antimicrobials or lactulose but to rely on institution of a low-protein diet. Oral and intravenous formulations of *BCAAs* are commercially available for use in horses (BCAA Equine Sports Inc, Lake Forest, IL; Baxter Healthcare Corp, Deerfield, IL), but controlled clinical trials in human beings have not shown this form of therapy to consistently ameliorate the signs of HE.[43]

A number of experimental drugs have been studied in human beings and may have a future role in management of HE in horses. Regimens to stimulate hepatic regeneration include insulin and glucagon[96] and cytosolic extracts from regenerating liver.[97] None have been shown to be definitively effective in human beings. As discussed previously, benzodiazepine receptor antagonists have been suggested to induce clinical and electrophysiologic remissions of HE in human beings with both acute and chronic liver failure.[19,98] This neuropharmacologic approach to treatment of HE holds great promise, although it may not be economically feasible in horses. In human beings with HE, treatment with *flumazenil*, a benzodiazepine antagonist and *bromocriptine*, a dopamine agonist, have provided either short-term or inconsistent results.[93,99] Zinc, levocarnitine, and ornithine aspartate enhance ureagenesis and also may reduce blood ammonia concentrations.[91-93] These treatments have not been evaluated in the horse.

Anti-inflammatory drugs may be beneficial and include *flunixin meglumine, dimethyl sulfoxide* (DMSO), and pentoxifylline. DMSO (0.5 to 1 gm/kg body weight, given intravenously diluted to 10% for 3 to 5 days) may help dissolve intrabiliary sludge or small calcium bilirubinate stones. *Pentoxifylline* has been shown to reduce hepatic fibrosis in human beings[100] and may be given to horses at 8 mg/kg every 8 to 12 hours. *Colchicine*, an antigout drug, and *cyclosporine*, a potent T helper cell immunosuppressant have been used to slow hepatic fibrosis in dogs and people.[101] These drugs have not been fully evaluated in horses; however, colchicine has been ineffective in cases of pyrrolizidine alkaloid toxicity.[101]

If any drugs are to be administered to a horse with hepatic insufficiency, it may be necessary to alter dosage. Alterations in hepatic blood flow, albumin, and biotransformation during hepatic insufficiency may prolong the half-life, as well as the dosage interval. Drugs that rely heavily on the liver for metabolism and excretion, such as chloramphenicol, erythromycin, and corticosteroids, should be avoided.[12]

Once the appetite returns, a horse with HE or chronic liver disease is best managed by dietary manipulation. The ration should be high in carbohydrates and low in protein, with the protein source optimally rich in BCAAs. A mixture of two parts beet pulp and one part cracked corn in molasses can be fed at a rate of 2.5 kg/100 kg body weight per day divided into six or more feedings.[80] Sorghum, bran, or milo can be substituted for the beet pulp. Multiple small feedings are optimal in horses with liver disease because of impaired gluconeogenesis. Oat hay is the best roughage, followed by other types of grass hay.[90] Horses should be encouraged to graze grass pastures provided they are protected from the sun. Alfalfa and legumes should be avoided because of their high protein content; however, any caloric intake is important in liver failure and should be allowed even if it includes legumes. Oats, soybean meal, and fat should be avoided.[102] Vitamins B_1, K_1, and folic acid should be administered parenterally on a weekly basis. Vitamin-K therapy is most useful when cholestasis is present.[4]

Prognosis

The prognosis for hepatic insufficiency in horses depends on the severity and type of the underlying disease. Horses with focal or mild to moderate acute hepatic disease have the best chance for hepatic regeneration; thus they have a guarded to fair prognosis if adequate and appropriate supportive care is given. Patients with severe hepatic fibrosis and chronic liver disease have a poorer prognosis because of their inability to compensate for lost hepatic function. Regardless of the cause of liver disease, the presence of severe encephalopathy, intravascular hemolysis, profound acidosis, clinical signs of coagulopathy, diarrhea, bilateral laryngeal paralysis, markedly increased serum bile acid concentration, BSP half-life greater than 10 minutes, decreased serum albumin, and histologic evidence of bridging fibrosis have all been associated independently with a poor to grave prognosis. If a horse survives more than 5 days after an acute transient hepatic insult, then the prognosis is fair. Decreasing blood levels of SBA, GLDL, and GGT are more likely to occur in horses that survive.[16] Therapy is generally unrewarding in horses with severe hepatic fibrosis.

SPECIFIC HEPATIC DISEASES

The wide variety of clinical signs with hepatic disease, coupled with the fact that the majority of the hepatic parenchyma must be affected before function is lost, makes the clinical distinction between acute and chronic liver disease a challenge. The onset of signs may be sudden, even with chronic disease. A history of progressive weight loss or "failure to thrive" may indicate chronicity. Although no single blood test is specific for distinguishing acute from chronic hepatic disease, the presence of hyperglobulinemia or hypoalbuminemia may suggest chronicity. Histopathologically, the hallmark evidence of chronicity is the presence of fibrosis. For the purpose of discussion of specific hepatic disorders in the following sections, diseases have been classified as either *acute* or *chronic* based on the known cause of the disease (Box 16-2).

Acute Hepatic Diseases

THEILER'S DISEASE

Sir Arnold Theiler's first described this disease in South Africa in 1918 after vaccination of horses against African horse sickness with both live virus and equine-origin antiserum.[103] In 1934 and 1937, a similar disease was described in the United States after vaccination of horses against western equine encephalomyelitis using live virus and equine-origin antiserum.[56,104,105] Despite numerous accounts of this syndrome, the exact cause of Theiler's disease remains unclear. Today this disease is one of the most commonly described causes of acute hepatic failure

BOX 16-2

LIVER DISEASES OF HORSES

Acute Disease

- Theiler's disease (Serum-associated hepatitis)
- Hyperlipemia
- Tyzzer's disease
- Infectious necrotic hepatitis (Black disease)
- Cholangiohepatitis
- Acute biliary obstruction
  - Cholelithiasis
  - Colon displacement
  - Hepatic torsion
- Parasitic hepatitis
  - *Parascaris equorum*
  - Large strongyles
  - *Echinococcus granulosa*
  - Schistosoma
- Toxic hepatopathy
  - Plants
  - Mycotoxins
  - Chemicals
  - Drugs
  - Iron
- Viral hepatitis
  - Equine infectious anemia (EIA)
  - Equine herpesvirus-1 (EHV-1)
  - Equine viral arteritis (EVA)
  - Giant cell hepatopathy

Chronic Disease

- Pyrrolizidine alkaloid toxicity
- Clover poisoning
- Chronic active hepatitis (CAH)
- Cholelithiasis
- Gastroduodenal obstruction
- Abscess
- Neoplasia
  - Metastatic infiltration of the liver
  - Cholangiocarcinoma
  - Hepatocellular carcinoma
  - Hepatoblastoma
  - Mixed hamartoma
- Amyloidosis
- Chronic hypoxia

Congenital or Heritable Disease

- Portosystemic shunt
- Biliary atresia
- Hyperammonemia of Morgans
- Glycogen branching enzyme deficiency

in horses.[15,56,106-108] Theiler's disease is also referred to as *acute hepatic necrosis, serum-associated hepatitis,* and *serum sickness.*

Clinical Signs Theiler's disease is limited to adult horses, although one report describes subclinical disease in a 2-month-old foal.[107] The onset of clinical signs of hepatic failure in Theiler's disease is acute to subacute and often rapidly progresses over 2 to 7 days. Most horses are anorectic and icteric; HE is reported in the majority of the cases.[56,106,107] Sudden death, photodermatitis, hemorrhagic diathesis, fever, dependent edema, colic, and bilirubinuria may be present.[56,106,107] Although uncommon, some horses with Theiler's disease have an insidious history of chronic weight loss.

Epidemiology and Pathogenesis The disease typically occurs sporadically, but outbreaks involving multiple horses on a single farm over several months have been reported.[56,106,107] A pattern of seasonality may occur, with a larger percentage of cases presenting in summer and fall.[56,106,107] Frequently, horses with Theiler's disease have received an equine-origin biologic antiserum 4 to 10 weeks before the onset of hepatic failure, hence the name *serum-associated hepatitis.* Equine-origin biologic antiserums that have been associated with Theiler's disease include vaccines or antisera for African horse sickness, eastern and western encephalomyelitis, *Bacillus anthracis,* tetanus antitoxin, *Clostridium perfringens, C. botulinum, Streptococcus equi,* subsp. *equi,* influenza, equine herpesvirus type 1 (EHV-1), pregnant mare's serum, and plasma.[13,56,106,107,109] Some reports suggest lactating broodmares given tetanus antitoxin after parturition are particularly prone to Theiler's disease.[106-108]

Reports of outbreaks in association with parenteral injection of homologous live virus vaccine or antiserum suggest an infectious blood-borne viral cause.[56] The history, onset, clinical signs, and histopathologic findings of Theiler's disease appear most similar to hepatitis B virus in human beings. Hepatitis B virus is present in all body fluids and excreta and is transmitted primarily by parenteral injection.[20] Viral surface antigen or antibody to viral core protein is detectable in 75% to 90% of human patients with hepatitis B.[20] Newer techniques that detect viral deoxyribonucleic acid (*DNA*) are even more sensitive and specific tests of infection. To date these assays have been negative in horses with Theiler's disease. Furthermore, viral isolation on horses with Theiler's disease has been unsuccessful, the disease has not been transmitted experimentally by blood or tissue inoculation, and a large percentage of horses with Theiler's disease do not have a recent history of receiving an equine-origin biologic antiserum.[110,111] The sum of these negative findings does not exclude the possibility of a viral cause; however, if such a cause exists, then other modes of transmission, infection, and establishment of disease must also exist.

Other suggested causes of Theiler's disease include exposure to hepatotoxic substances, such as mycotoxins (aflatoxin and rubratoxin), plant toxins (pyrrolizidine alkaloids, alsike clover), drugs, or chemicals.[13,108] However, these causes have not been uniformly demonstrable and usually are considered separate disease entities.

Aside from widespread tissue icterus, pathologic findings are limited to the liver. The liver appears smaller than normal, but it may be large in peracute cases. Although not pathognomonic, the histopathologic findings in Theiler's disease consistently include widespread centrilobular to midzonal hepatocellular necrosis with hemorrhage (Figure 16-7),[110] which helps distinguish it from acute pyrrolizidine alkaloid toxicity, which has predominantly periportal changes. Moderate to severe centrilobular hepatocyte vacuolar (fatty) change and granular swelling, hemosiderosis, and bile casts may be seen.[106] A mild inflammatory infiltrate, primarily monocytes and lymphocytes, is present in portal triads. The occasional finding of mild to moderate biliary hyperplasia and fibroblastic infiltration is evidence of a more chronic disease course than the clinical signs alone would suggest.[110]

Diagnosis Recent inoculation with an equine-origin biologic antiserum, coupled with an abrupt onset of clinical signs

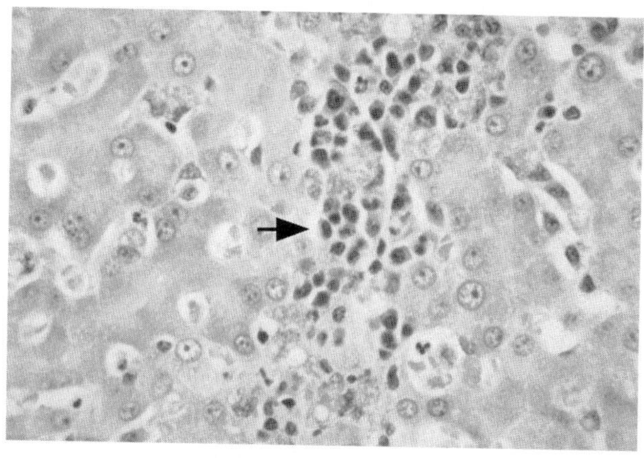

FIGURE 16-7 Histopathology of the liver: Theiler's disease. Note the central area of hepatic necrosis *(arrow)*.

and laboratory evidence of hepatic insufficiency, strongly suggests Theiler's disease. No single laboratory test is diagnostic. Bilirubinemia and bilirubinuria are usually present. Liver enzymes, including SDH, ARG, and AST, are increased. The BSP half-life, PT, and APTT are often prolonged, and blood ammonia concentrations are increased. Acidosis, leukocytosis, polycythemia, and increases in serum creatine kinase activity have also been reported.[106-108] Hemolysis may occur terminally. The histopathologic findings on a liver biopsy (see previous pathogenesis section) offer the strongest diagnostic evidence of Theiler's disease.

Treatment No specific treatment for Theiler's disease exists aside from general supportive care for hepatic insufficiency (see Treatment of Hepatic Insufficiency).

Prognosis and Client Education The prognosis is poor to grave in horses with severe HE, hemorrhage, or hemolysis. Horses that survive longer than 1 week usually recover completely, although death or progressive weight loss have been reported during the ensuing months.[107] A favorable prognosis is warranted if serial SDH activities are decreasing or clinical signs are waning. Increased serum activity of GGT may be sustained for several weeks, despite clinical improvement and long-term survival.[106] No preventative exists, aside from the judicious use of equine-origin antiserum.

BACTERIAL HEPATITIS

Tyzzer's Disease *Clostridium piliforme* (formerly, *Bacillus piliforme*) is a motile, spore-forming, obligate intracytoplasmic bacterium that causes acute necrotizing hepatitis. The disease was first described by E. E. Tyzzer's in 1917 in a colony of waltzing mice.[112] The first documented outbreak in foals occurred in Kentucky on a single farm between 1964 and 1973, fatally infecting 23 foals.[113]

Clinical Signs In horses, Tyzzer's disease is limited to foals between 7 and 42 days of age.[114-116] The clinical signs are usually nonspecific and include loss of a suckle reflex, depression progressing to recumbency, fever, tachypnea, tachycardia, icterus, petechiation, diarrhea, dehydration, shock, seizures, and coma.[113-118] Often the foals are found dead without premonitory signs.

Epidemiology and Pathogenesis Outbreaks of Tyzzer's disease are sporadic; thus the disease is not believed to be contagious.[116] Seasonality has not been demonstrated. The disease has been reported in the United States, Canada, South Africa, England, New England, and Australia.[116,117] Mice with Tyzzer's disease are infected by an oral route perinatally, with clinical signs and death occurring between 6 and 44 days of age.[117] *C. piliforme* is excreted in the feces of clinically healthy horses and can survive in the soil for at least 1 year.[115,117] Foals are infected by eating contaminated feces of their dams or by ingesting contaminated soil.[115] The bacteria replicate in the intestinal epithelium and reach the liver and heart by way of the lymphatics and blood supply.[115] In rodents and rabbits, administration of corticosteroids or sulfonamides may induce active disease.[117] The presence of antibody to the flagella of *C. piliforme* in the serum of healthy horses suggests that *exposure* to *C. piliforme* is not uncommon.[119]

C. piliforme causes acute multifocal hepatitis and enteritis. Grossly, the liver is swollen with 1- to 5-mm white foci scattered throughout the parenchyma. Tissues are icteric and petechial hemorrhages are present in many tissues. Microscopically, the foci are areas of coagulative necrosis with an associated inflammatory infiltrate consisting of neutrophils, macrophages, and lymphocytes. The organisms, best demonstrated at the periphery of the lesions by Warthin-Starry or Dietrerle's silver stains, appear as long bacilli organized in bundles. In addition to hepatitis, enterocolitis, myositis, pleural effusion, pulmonary congestion and edema, and lymphoid necrosis or depletion may be present.[116,117]

Diagnosis The peracute onset and nonspecific signs confound antemortem diagnosis of Tyzzer's disease. Hematologic study may reveal hemoconcentration, leukopenia or leukocytosis, a left shift, and toxic neutrophils.[114-117] Other nonspecific laboratory findings include hyperfibrinogenemia, acidosis, hyperkalemia or hypokalemia, and profound hypoglycemia.[114-118,120] Liver enzymes are increased, including SDH, GGT, AST, ALP, and LDH-5.[114-118]

The definitive diagnosis is determined at necropsy by demonstration of the organism intracytoplasmically using silver stains or by polymerase chain reaction (PCR) analysis.[120] *C. piliforme* is fastidious and can only be grown in living tissue, such as embryonated chick eggs.[120] Positive serology may be supportive evidence for exposure.[119] Differential diagnosis for hepatic disease in foals includes iron hepatotoxicity, perinatal EHV-1, bacteremia, atresia of the bile duct, and portosystemic shunt.

Treatment Tyzzer's disease is highly fatal in foals. In rodents and rabbits, *C. piliforme* is sensitive to penicillin, tetracycline, erythromycin, and streptomycin. Rare reports exist of successful treatment of foals with Tyzzer's disease using penicillin, TMS, and partial parential nutrition.[114,120]

Prognosis and Client Education Tyzzer's disease in foals is considered highly fatal. No preventative exists.

INFECTIOUS NECROTIC HEPATITIS

Clostridium novyi type B is the cause of *infectious necrotic hepatitis* or *black disease*. The disease is most common in sheep and cattle, but several cases have been documented in horses.[54,121-124]

Clinical Signs The onset of disease may be peracute with sudden death. Acute signs are progressive over 24 to 72 hours and include depression, reluctance to move, fever, icterus, ataxia, colic, petechiae, periods of recumbency, tachycardia, and tachypnea.[54,121-124] Some affected horses remain standing until a short time before death.

Epidemiology and Pathogenesis Reported cases of infectious necrotic hepatitis in horses have occurred in or adjacent to areas with a large population of sheep.[54,121-124] In sheep and cattle, infectious necrotic hepatitis is the result of multiplication of *C. novyi* in areas of liver compromised by the migration of *Fasciola hepatica*. This fluke normally does not infest horses, but migration of any parasite through the liver may predispose the animal to infectious necrotic hepatitis. Some horses with infectious necrotic hepatitis had parasitic infestations, although migrating parasites in the liver at the time of necropsy was not evident. The onset of disease in one case occurred 48 hours after administration of mebendazole.[54]

The carcass blackens rapidly after death from engorgement of subcutaneous blood vessels; hence the name *black disease*. Often, necropsy findings include serosanguineous effusion in the pericardial sac and the thoracic and abdominal cavities, widespread hemorrhages and icterus, and multifocal areas (1 to 2 mm) of coagulative hepatic necrosis. Smears or histologic sections of the hepatic lesions reveal large numbers of gram-positive rods.

Diagnosis The acute and nonspecific nature of this disease makes antemortem diagnosis improbable. Liver-specific enzymes and bilirubin are mildly to moderately increased.[54,121,124] An abdominocentesis was performed on one horse and revealed serosanguineous peritonitis.[54] Definitive diagnosis is based on positive staining with fluorescein conjugated antiserum specific for *C. novyi* or isolation of the organism at necropsy.[121,124] The organism is difficult to isolate and requires rapid tissue sampling and anaerobic conditions.

Treatment Treatment with high doses of penicillin or ampicillin is indicated, in addition to general supportive care for hepatic insufficiency.

Prognosis and Client Education Most reported cases of infectious necrotic hepatitis in horses were fatal.

MISCELLANEOUS CAUSES OF BACTERIAL HEPATITIS

Primary bacterial hepatitis is rare in adult horses. Bacterial septicemia in neonates may result in multifocal hepatitis, although clinical signs of hepatic failure rarely accompany the disease. Bacterial endotoxin, released during acute fulminant gram-negative infection or absorbed from the gastrointestinal tract after mural damage, may cause hepatic ischemia indirectly through hemodynamic alternations. Because Kupffer's cells normally phagocytose endotoxin, bombardment of the liver with endotoxin may temporarily impede the function of Kupffer's cells.

Primary bacterial cholangiohepatitis has been reported in horses, although more commonly it is secondary.[50,125-128] *Secondary cholangiohepatitis* in horses is a sequela to biliary stasis, cholelithiasis, CAH, hepatic neoplasia, pancreatitis, intestinal parasitism, intestinal obstruction, and proximal enteritis.[129] Clinical signs include anorexia, colic, fever, and icterus; HE may be present. Laboratory abnormalities may include leukocytosis; toxemia; hyperfibrinogenemia; and increased activity of SDH, ARG, GGT; increased direct-reacting bilirubin; and evidence of septic or nonseptic peritonitis.[126,128] Definitive diagnosis is based on histopathologic findings on liver biopsy and bacterial isolation. Isolates are most commonly enteric organisms such as *Salmonella* spp., *Escherichia coli, Citrobacter, Klebsiella, Aeromonas,* and *Acinetobacter* spp.[126-128] Treatment includes general supportive care for hepatic failure (see Treatment of Hepatic Insufficiency) and 4 to 6 weeks of antimicrobial therapy. The antimicrobial therapy should be based on culture and sensitivity results. Recommended antimicrobials for bacterial cholangiohepatitis in horses include trimethoprim-sulfonamide, ceftiofur, enrofloxacin, penicillin and gentamicin, ampicillin, and chloramphenicol.[50,125-128]

VIRAL HEPATITIS

Equine Herpesvirus Infection in Foals Pregnant mares infected with EHV-1 may abort in the third trimester or deliver stillborn or weak foals. Some foals may appear normal at birth but develop clinical signs of respiratory distress, icterus, fever, and severe depression.[130,131] Secondary bacterial septicemia is common. Despite profound hepatic necrosis in herpesvirus-positive foals, serum enzyme activities were not significantly different from premature foals or foals with septicemia.[131] Pathologic lesions of aborted fetuses or neonatal foals are similar and include severe pulmonary congestion, pneumonitis, bronchiolitis, hyaline membrane disease, and intralobular coagulative hepatocellular necrosis.[130,131] Intranuclear, acidophilic inclusions are present in hepatocytes and biliary epithelium. General supportive care and prophylactic administration of broad-spectrum antimicrobials are indicated. The prognosis is poor to grave. Most affected foals die within a few days of birth. Vaccination of pregnant mares is only partially efficacious for prevention.

Equine Infectious Anemia The causative organism of equine infectious anemia is a retrovirus that has a tropism for mononuclear phagocytes.[132] Although cyclic fever, anemia, icterus, edema, and weight loss are the systemic manifestations of the disease, the Kupffer's cells in the liver are a major site of infection. Icterus is due to increased erythrocyte destruction, as well as acute hepatic necrosis.

Equine Viral Arteritis This disease is caused by a member of the Arteriviridae family and typically is manifest clinically by depression, fever, acute upper respiratory tract infection, abortion, petechiation, and edema. After ingestion or inhalation, viral septicemia leads to vascular damage. Overt clinical signs of hepatic disease are rare, but vascular damage in the liver may cause icterus.[133]

Giant Cell Hepatopathy A disease similar to human neonatal hepatitis has been reported in aborted midterm fetuses.[134] Histologically, disorganization of hepatic cords, multifocal necrosis, a mild mononuclear cell infiltrate, and a large hepatocyte syncytium with 8 to 10 nuclei exist. The cause in horses and human beings is unknown but is presumably viral. Viral and bacterial isolation, viral immunofluorescence, and serologic testing have been unsuccessful in horses. Giant cell hepatopathy was reported in one foal with prolonged neonatal isoerythrolysis.[134]

PARASITIC HEPATITIS

Parasitic infestation may cause focal hepatic disease but rarely overt hepatic insufficiency. After their ingestion, as embryonated eggs, larvae of *Parascaris equorum,* hatch in the small intestine, and then migrate through the liver and lungs. Focal or diffuse hepatic fibrosis may result.[80] Migration of *Strongylus edentatus* or *S. equinus* through the hepatic portal veins may cause focal hepatitis, subcapsular hemorrhage, and edema, followed by focal parenchymal fibrosis and capsular fibrin deposits.[80] Focal hepatic infarcts may occur secondary to thrombotic emboli because of migrating *S. vulgaris* in mesenteric arteries. Protozoal schizonts consistent with a *Sarcocystis* spp. other than *S. neurona* were reported at necropsy in the liver of a horse with concurrent bacterial osteomyelitis, a plasma cell tumor of the maxilla, and hepatic salmonellosis.[135] The canine cestode, *Echinococcus granulosa,* may form hydatid (larval) cysts in the liver, which are usually an incidental finding.[136,137]

Fibrosing granulomas were found in the liver, intestinal and diaphragmatic serosae, and lung of several horses submitted for necropsy.[138] The granulomas consisted of dense fibrous tissue surrounding a necrotic, laminated, mineralized center. The periphery of the granuloma contained a small rim of inflammatory cells. The typical architecture of the granulomas, combined with the finding of a residual eggshell typical of *Schistosoma* (a trematode) in one horse, lead to the conclusion that the granulomas were caused by chronic schistosomiasis. Although the granulomas were considered to be incidental findings of undetermined origin in most of the horses, they caused liver failure in one horse.

TOXIC HEPATOPATHY

Numerous chemicals, drugs, mycotoxins, and plant toxins are hepatotoxic, but these rarely cause acute hepatic failure in horses. Clinical signs and routine laboratory diagnostic tests will not distinguish between these toxins; thus diagnosis largely relies on exclusion of other causes, history of exposure, and in some cases, documentation of the toxin in the blood or liver. Some substances cause fatty change, cloudy swelling, necrosis, mild inflammatory infiltration, and fibrosis, primarily in the centrilobular location where the oxygen tension is lowest. Other substances cause the same lesions periportally, in the area of initial exposure. Some substances are directly hepatotoxic, whereas others require biotransformation by the liver to toxic metabolites.

Hepatotoxic Plants Plants best known for causing hepatic disease in horses are those containing pyrrolizidine alkaloids. Although pyrrolizidine alkaloid toxicity can cause acute hepatic necrosis, it more often results in hepatic fibrosis (and is discussed as a separate entity under Chronic Hepatic Diseases). Other plants that have been reported to cause hepatic necrosis in horses in North America include kleingrass *(Panicum coloratum, P. dichotomiflorum),* lantana, lechuguilla *(Agave lechuguilla),* alsike clover *(Trifolium hybridum),* whitebrush (*Lippia* spp.), sneezeweed (*Helenium* spp.), blue green algae (*Microcystis* and *Nodularia* spp.), lupine (*Lupine* spp.), ryegrass, and some poisonous mushrooms (*Amanita* and *Galerina* spp.).[101]

Chemical Hepatotoxins Horses are rarely exposed to hepatotoxic chemicals in sufficient amounts to induce hepatic failure. Potential hepatotoxic chemicals include arsenic (pesticide), carbon tetrachloride (fumigant), chlorinated hydrocarbons (insecticide), carbon disulphide (botacide), pentachlorophenols (wood preservative, herbicide, fungicide), phenol (disinfectant, wood preservative), phosphorus (fertilizer), polybrominated biphenyl (fire retardant), and paraquat (herbicide).[80] All of these cause centrilobular necrosis, except phosphorus, which causes primarily periportal changes.

Drugs Pharmaceutical agents can have a wide range of effects on the liver depending on the drug type, dose, frequency, duration, and route of administration; age of the animal; diet; and concurrent treatment.[139] The hepatic damage may be acute or chronic, cholestatic, zonal, vascular, or hypersensitivity mediated. Certain drugs alter hepatocellular permeability without visible injury or loss of function.

Drugs that are intrinsically hepatotoxic reproducibly cause hepatocellular necrosis.[20,80] Examples of intrinsic hepatotoxic drugs that cause zonal centrilobular necrosis include carbon disulfide and carbon tetrachloride.[80] These drugs cause hepatocellular damage in a dose-related manner, and toxicity often results in hepatic failure. Anabolic steroids cause cholestasis with little or no evidence of hepatic damage or inflammation, resulting in mild icterus, which is completely and rapidly reversible once the drug is discontinued.[20,139] Phenothiazines and macrolide antibiotics (erythromycin) cause cholestatic injury, which is accompanied by significant hepatocellular necrosis and periportal inflammation.[20] Recovery is usually expected after discontinuation of the drug. Some drugs, such as tetracycline, cause fatty infiltration of the liver but rarely cause liver dysfunction.

Idiosyncratic hepatotoxicity has been reported after administration of erythromycin, rifampin, tetracycline, isoniazid, halothane, fluothane, phenothiazines, dantrolene, diazepam, sulfonamides, phenobarbital, phenytoin, and aspirin.[20,80,101] Injury varies from mild focal hepatitis to massive necrosis. Idiosyncratic hepatopathy has a low incidence, is not dose related, and often resolves on discontinuation of the drug. Rarely, progressive liver failure ensues. Some idiosyncratic drug hepatopathies may have a pathogenesis similar to drug allergy; others may be related to biotransformation properties of the liver. For example, if an individual has enhanced biotransformation of a certain drug and the metabolite of the drug is more cytotoxic than the original unaltered drug, then hepatic damage may ensue.

Finally, some drugs induce increased hepatic enzyme activities or alter hepatocellular permeability but do not cause significant hepatic damage or clinical signs. Examples include benzimidazole anthelmintics, phenobarbital, phenylbutazone, and corticosteroids. Compared with humans and dogs, corticosteroids are apparently less likely to cause hepatopathy in horses; however, one report describes steroid hepatopathy in a horse that received an overdose of triamcinolone for treatment of pruritus.[140] Three weeks after the overdose, the horse developed muscle wasting, depression, polydipsia, and laminitis. Mature neutrophilia, lymphopenia, hyperglycemia, increased serum activities of AST and GGT, and multizonal hepatocellular vacuolation were reported.

Iron Toxicity Acute, fatal toxic hepatopathy was reported in numerous newborn foals given an oral microbial inoculum.[51] The syndrome is reproducible if *ferrous fumarate* is given orally.[141] The incidence of hepatic failure was highest when the foals were given the inoculum before nursing. Colostrum contains abundant vitamin E, an essential cofactor for glutathione. Glutathione protects against free radical damage, a proposed mechanism for iron toxicity. Thus presumably, foals that are given iron supplements before ingesting colostrum are most susceptible to iron toxicity.[141] This is exacerbated by high serum iron concentrations and high percent saturation of transferrin in foals during the first few 24 hours of life. Supplementation of iron during this time period results in excessive free iron and increased risk of fatal hepatotoxicity.

Clinical signs include HE, icterus, and peracute death. Laboratory abnormalities include increased blood levels of bilirubin, SDH, GGT, and ammonia, and reduced BCAA-to-AAA ratio, decreased glucose, and prolonged PT. At necropsy the liver was abnormally small; histologic study revealed massive hepatic necrosis with blood-filled reticula. Some livers had mild biliary hyperplasia and periportal fibrosis. Supportive therapy may prolong life, but most foals with iron hepatotoxicosis die. Those foals that survived recovered fully.

Adult horses are less susceptible to iron toxicitiy; however, rare cases of haemochromatosis have been reported.[142,143] Haemochromatosis is characterized by tissue damage and dysfunction caused by deposition of hemosiderin in parenchymal cells.[142] Haemochromatosis was diagnosed in three adult horses by histopathology and use of Prussian blue stain, which detects iron deposition (hemosiderin pigment).[142] Excessive dietary iron was not apparent. All three of the horses had signs and laboratory evidence of liver disease. Serum iron concentration was normal, and there was no evidence of saturation of the iron transport system in the serum. Haemochromatosis was accompanied by bile duct hyperplasia and hepatic fibrosis. All three horses died or were euthanized because of deterioration. Haemochromatosis was diagnosed in a pony receiving approximately four times the daily recommended amount of iron.[143] The diagnosis was confirmed by histopathology (severe periportal fibrosis, hemosiderosis, biliary hyperplasia) and increased serum and liver concentrations of iron.

Mycotoxins Mycotoxicosis is more common in ruminants than in horses. The two most common mycotoxins affecting horses are *aflatoxin,* produced by the molds *Aspergillus flavus* and *Aspergillus parasiticus,* and *rubratoxin,* produced by the mold *Penicillium rubrum. Aspergillus* spp. grow on a wide variety of feedstuffs if the temperature, moisture, and carbohydrate content are sufficient.[80] Aflatoxins impair protein synthesis and carbohydrate metabolism.

The degree of hepatic damage and extent of clinical signs depend on the duration and extent of exposure to the mycotoxin. Most horses refuse to eat moldy feed; thus hepatic failure is uncommon. Pathologic findings include hepatocellular necrosis, fatty change, biliary hyperplasia, periportal fibrosis, and megalocytosis. No specific treatment for aflatoxicosis exists. Administration of activated charcoal or a cathartic shortly after ingestion may impede absorption. Avoiding moldy feed best prevents mycotoxicosis.

Fumonisin B1, the mycotoxin of *Fusarium moniliforme,* is most frequently associated with contaminated corn and causes leukoencephalomalacia in horses. The mycotoxin also causes hepatocellular necrosis and periportal fibrosis. Although most horses with leukoencephalomalacia have hepatic disease, signs of leukoencephalopathy predominate and hepatic failure is rare. Recovery from hepatic disease is more likely than from the neurologic disease.

ACUTE BILIARY OBSTRUCTION

Acute obstruction of the common bile duct causes icterus and signs of abdominal pain. Acute biliary occlusion may occur secondary to cholelithiasis (see Cholelithiasis) or colon displacement. Intense icterus, colic, and increased levels of direct bilirubin (>85.5 μmol/L), GGT (>400 U/L), and bile acids (>150 U/L) were reported in two horses with acute colon displacements.[79] These abnormalities quickly abated after surgical correction of the displaced colon. In a comparative study of cases of colon displacement, 49% of horses with a right dorsal colon displacement had increased GGT, compared with 2% of horses with a left dorsal displacement.[144] Torsion of the left lobe of the liver was the cause of acute colic, hepatic congestion, necrosis, and focal hepatitis in a 14-year-old Arabian gelding.[145] Resection of the affected lobe resulted in complete recovery.

HYPERLIPEMIA AND HEPATIC LIPIDOSIS

Hyperlipemia, defined as a serum triglyceride concentration in excess of 500 mg/dl, occurs primarily in ponies and Miniature Horses and donkeys and may lead to fatty infiltration of the liver, often accompanied by clinical signs of liver disease and a poor prognosis. *Hyperlipidemia* refers to an increase in serum triglyceride concentration (generally less than 500 mg/dl) without grossly lactescent blood or fatty infiltration of the liver. Obesity, stress, inability to satisfy metabolic energy demands, and hormonal imbalance are the major precipitating factors for hyperlipemia.[146-151]

Epidemiology and Clinical Signs Ponies (especially Shetland ponies and mare ponies), Miniature Horses, and donkeys are most susceptible to hyperlipemia. Rarely, other breeds, such as the Quarter Horse, Paso Fino, and Tennessee Walking Horse may be affected. Affected ponies are usually obese, have a recent history of stress or weight loss, and are in late gestation or early lactation during the winter months.[58] In Miniature Horses and donkeys, hyperlipemia can occur at any age and frequently develops as a sequela to an underlying primary illness lasting several days. The most commonly reported primary diseases predisposing Miniature Horses to hyperlipemia are enterocolitis, endotoxemia, parasitism, pituitary dysfunction, azotemia, and neonatal septicemia.[150,151] The onset of clinical signs of hyperlipemia is often acute and includes icterus, anorexia, weakness, severe depression, ataxia, muscular weakness, recumbency, diarrhea, mild colic, fever, and dependent edema.[58,146,148] In severe cases, clinical signs of hepatic failure may prevail (see Clinical Signs of Hepatic Insufficiency). Sudden death because of hepatic rupture may occur.[147] Signs of predisposing primary disease in Miniature Horses may overshadow signs of hyperlipemia.

Pathogenesis The liver serves a unique role in energy homeostasis (see Physiology), especially in large animals in which volatile fatty acids, and not glucose, are a major energy source. Glucose is primarily manufactured in the liver from fatty acids and amino acids and is stored as glycogen for future use. If intake is decreased or energy demands are increased, then glycogen stores become depleted and the major source of energy is provided by fatty acid oxidation. Obesity sets the stage for hyperlipemia by providing excessive adipose tissue stores of fatty acids, available for immediate and rapid mobilization. Fatty acid mobilization is usually first triggered by a stress or inability to maintain energy homeostasis. Concurrent or underlying primary diseases such as enterocolitis, azotemia, infection, parasitism, or neoplasia, as well as any stressful event, such as transport or weaning, may precipitate fatty acid mobilization. Stress increases the release of catecholamines and glucocorticoids, which stimulate fatty acid release from the adipose tissue. A negative energy balance, as may occur during late gestation, early lactation, starvation, or secondary to anorexia induced by some other primary disease, exacerbates hyperlipemia by further promoting fatty acid mobilization.

After lipolysis of adipose tissue triglyceride occurs, free fatty acids, nonesterified fatty acids, and glycerol are released into the blood. Glyceride, fatty acids bound to albumin, and nonesterified fatty acids are carried to the liver, where the glyceride is converted to glucose. In the liver, free fatty acids may be oxidized to acetyl CoA and used in the tricarboxylic acid cycle, used in gluconeogenesis, resynthesized to triglycerides and stored in the liver, or used to make triglycerides that are released into the sinusoidal blood as VLDLs (see Figure 16-3). Ponies with hyperlipemia have larger-diameter VLDLs containing greater concentrations of triglycerides than normal ponies.[152,153] Thus hyperlipemia in ponies and Miniature Horses is from efficient hepatic synthesis of triglycerides from mobilized free fatty acids, with subsequent secretion of triglyceride-laden VLDL into the blood. Endothelial lipoprotein lipase is the rate-limiting enzyme responsible for the removal of VLDL from the blood back into adipose tissue. In hyperlipemic ponies, the activity of lipoprotein lipase is not impaired and in fact is increased several fold.[167,168] Thus it is the overproduction of VLDL by the liver, not impairment of their removal, which is primarily responsible for hyperlipidemia in ponies. [152,153]

If the oxaloacetate supply is limited when free fatty acids are mobilized to the liver, acetyl CoA is shuttled away from the tricarboxylic acid cycle and used to make ketone bodies. Because the equine liver is quite efficient in synthesizing triglycerides and exporting VLDL, hepatic lipidosis and ketosis are less common than in other species.[149] However, if fatty acid mobilization and synthesis of triglycerides exceed oxidation and VLDL secretion, then hepatic lipidosis ensues. Fat infiltration disrupts hepatic function, and excessive amounts of fat in the liver can result in hepatic failure and even hepatic rupture.[147]

Hormonal factors may contribute to the development of hyperlipemia and hepatic lipidosis. Insulin normally impedes the development of hyperlipemia by inhibiting tissue hormone-sensitive lipase, the enzyme responsible for lipolysis of adipose tissue. Insulin also curtails the development of hyperlipemia by stimulating gluconeogenesis in the liver and by activating lipoprotein lipase, the enzyme responsible for uptake of VLDL by adipose tissue. Despite often-normal insulin levels, ponies appear to have tissue insulin insensitivity compared with horses.[147] Fasting in donkeys has been shown to cause a reduction in tissue sensitivity to insulin.[154] Glucocorticoids, catecholamines, adrenocorticotropic hormone, thyroid stimulating hormone, growth hormone, antidiuretic hormone, and progesterone may contribute to the development of hyperlipemia by opposing the biologic actions of insulin (see Figure 16-3). This may account for the high incidence of hyperlipemia during periods of increased cortisol levels (stress, pituitary adenoma, late pregnancy) and increased progesterone (pregnancy). In ponies, norepinephrine linearly stimulates the release of free fatty acids from adipose tissue, an effect that does not occur in horses.[155] Considering the unique effects of insulin and catecholamines on fat metabolism in ponies, it is not surprising that ponies are more susceptible than horses to the development of hyperlipemia.

Vascular thrombosis can occur secondary to hyperlipemia and fat embolism and may be seen in the lung, kidney, brain, and subcutaneous vessels. Subcutaneous thrombosis causes dependent edema. Renal nephrosis and necrotizing pancreatitis are sometimes present.[58,147] Renal disease most likely is a sequela of occlusive thrombosis. The exact cause of pancreatitis is not known; however, hyperlipemia precedes pancreatitis. Researchers speculate that excessive lipid is deposited in and around the pancreas, which is subsequently hydrolyzed by pancreatic lipase and released as free fatty acids. Free (unbound to albumin) fatty acids are cytotoxic; when the albumin-binding capacity is exceeded, pancreatic vascular injury occurs.[156]

Azotemia prevents lipid removal from the blood by inhibiting lipoprotein lipase. The degree of hyperlipidemia is directly correlated with the degree of azotemia.[157] Almost half of hyperlipemic Miniature Horses are azotemic.[150,151] Compared with ponies and Miniature Horses, hyperlipemia rarely develops in horses, though *hyperlipidemia* (triglyceride <500 mg/dl) may develop during azotemia.[148,157] Mild hepatic lipidosis may ensue, but hyperlipidemia rarely results in clinically recognizable disease.

Diagnosis Hyperlipemia should be considered in the differential diagnosis for any obese pony or Miniature Horse with clinical signs of severe depression, anorexia, ataxia, and icterus. The normal triglyceride level in horses and ponies should be less than 85 mg/dl but may be up to 290 mg/dl in healthy donkeys and up to 250 mg/dl in healthy pregnant pony mares.[153] In hyperlipemia, the blood grossly appears opalescent (Figure 16-8) and the concentrations of all lipids are increased, especially triglycerides (>500 mg/dl), nonesterified fatty acids, and VLDLs. Laboratory evidence of hepatic disease may include increased serum activity of SDH, GGT, increased concentrations of serum bile acids, bilirubin, and ammonia, as well as decreased glucose, BUN, and albumin.[146] In hyperlipemic Miniature Horses, only about half of affected patients have significant hepatic impairment.[150] The BSP half-life is prolonged. Oral and intravenous glucose challenge tests may reveal glucose intolerance because of insulin insensitivity. Metabolic acidosis is frequent, and ketoacidosis should be suspected if the anion gap is increased. Lipemia may increase serum creatinine values falsely and interfere with accurate determination of other serum chemistries. A definitive diagnosis of hepatic lipidosis is confirmed by the concurrent demonstration of increased blood concentrations of lipid, laboratory evidence of hepatic dysfunction, and ultrasonographic or histopathologic findings of fatty infiltration in the liver (Figure 16-9). The serum concentrations of creatinine and electrolytes should be determined as an adjunct to therapy. Because of the incidence of hyperlipemia in ill Miniature Horses and donkeys, monitoring blood triglyceride levels would facilitate early recognition of hyperlipidemia in these patients.

Necropsy findings in affected ponies include widespread fatty change in the liver, skeletal muscle, kidney, adrenal cortex, and myocardium.[58,147] The liver and kidney are enlarged, yellow, friable, and greasy. One of every five ponies with hepatic lipidosis has a ruptured liver.[147] Microscopically, hepatocytes are engorged with lipid. The nucleus is often displaced, and hepatocellular necrosis may ensue.

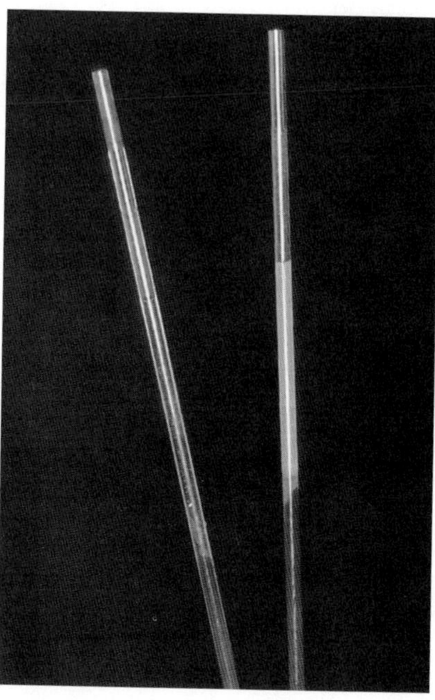

FIGURE 16-8 Hyperlipemia. The spin hematocrit tube on the right is from a miniature horse with hyperlipemia. The hematocrit tube on the left is from an unaffected horse.

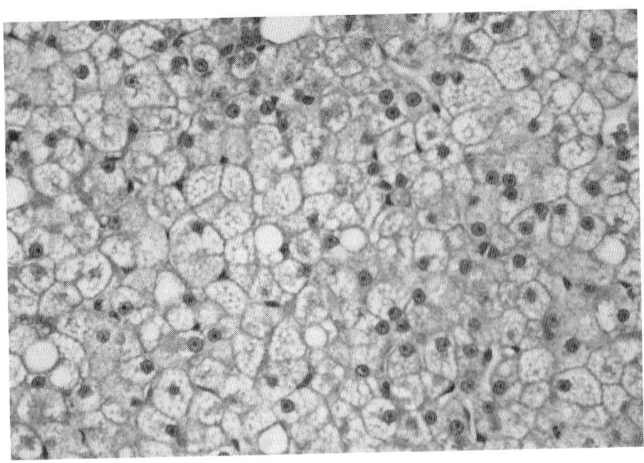

FIGURE 16-9 Histopathology of the liver: fatty liver.

Treatment The major therapeutic objectives for hyperlipemia and hepatic lipidosis include the following:

1. Treatment of hepatic disease
2. Improvement of energy intake and balance
3. Elimination of stress or treatment of concurrent disease
4. Inhibition of fat mobilization from adipose tissue
5. Increased triglyceride uptake by peripheral tissues

Treatment of hepatic failure is addressed elsewhere (see Treatment of Hepatic Insufficiency). Concentrated carbohydrate feed, such as molasses-coated grain and high-quality pasture or hay, should be encouraged. Anorectic ponies should receive 5% dextrose as a continuous infusion at a rate of 2 ml/kg/hour, and enteral nutrition should be attempted. NutriFoal, NutriPrime (KenVet, Ashland, OH), and Osmolyte HN (Ross Laboratory, Columbus, OH) have successfully been used as sources of enteral nutrition in hyperlipemic Miniature Horses.[150] If enteral nutrition is not possible, then partial parenteral nutrition should be provided with equal volumes of 50% dextrose and 8.5% amino acids.[150] Monitoring blood glucose concentrations closely is mandatory, because some ponies have glucose intolerance (and excessive glucose will worsen acidosis and induce hypokalemia). Weaning suckling foals may help reduce stress and the energy demand imposed on lactating mares. Concurrent diseases amenable to therapy, such as parasitism, chronic infection, and musculoskeletal disease, should be appropriately treated with anthelmintics, antimicrobials and anti-inflammatory agents, or analgesics, respectively.

In addition to supplying immediate energy, glucose therapy stimulates the release of insulin. Concurrent carbohydrate and insulin administration have been used successfully to manage hyperlipemia in ponies.[146,158] The following regimen has been suggested for a 200-kg pony[158]: On day 1 the patient is administered 30 IU of protamine zinc insulin IM and 100 g of glucose orally (both twice daily). On day 2 the patient is administered 15 IU of insulin intramuscularly, twice daily, and 100 g of galactose once. Galactose is slowly converted to glucose; thus lactic acid production is minimized. This regimen may be continued for 3 days. Blood glucose and insulin concentrations should be closely monitored. Insulin treatment may not lower triglyceride levels, but it may help control hyperglycemia if partial parenteral nutrition is provided.[150] Nicotinic acid, thought to act by inhibiting hormone-sensitive lipase, has been used in cattle with fatty liver; however, nicotinic acid has not been evaluated in ponies with hepatic lipidosis.

Heparin potentiates the activity of lipoprotein lipase and may increase triglyceride removal from the blood. However, because lipoprotein lipase activity is already at maximum rate in affected ponies, whether or not heparin provides additional benefit is questionable.[153] Recommended dosages range between 40 to 250 IU/kg twice daily.[146,158] Because of the potential for hemorrhage, heparin therapy should be used with discretion and monitored by daily hemostatic testing. If azotemia, acidosis, and electrolyte abnormalities are present, then appropriate fluid therapy is suggested.

Lipotropic agents such as choline and methionine are unlikely to be useful in horses with hyperlipemia, because triglyceride synthesis in the liver is usually sufficient.

Prognosis and Client Education The prognosis for hyperlipemia in equids is poor. Mortality has been estimated to occur in 60% to 100% of affected ponies.[146,147] Survival rate is reportedly better in Miniature Horses, and death often results from the underlying disease and not fatty liver failure.[150,151] Most Miniature Horses with blood triglyceride levels less than 1200 mg/dl survive.[151] Prevention is achieved best by providing appropriate nutrition without inducing obesity while avoiding stress and practicing good routine health care.

Chronic Hepatic Diseases

The distinction between acute and chronic hepatic disease is difficult. Often horses with chronic liver disease display abrupt onset of signs. With the possible exception of hyperglobulinemia, no serum biochemical parameters reliably distinguish acute from chronic hepatocellular disease. Regardless of the cause or site of injury, histopathologic evidence of fibrosis develops only after chronic injury.[159] The following diseases are classified as chronic based on the presence of fibrosis in the liver or because the cause is known to result in gradual hepatic dysfunction.

CHRONIC MEGALOCYTIC HEPATOPATHY

Megalocytic hepatopathy occurs worldwide and is the most common cause of chronic liver failure in horses in certain parts of the United States.[15] It is caused by the ingestion of *pyrrolizidine alkaloid*–containing plants. The intoxication typically results in the delayed onset of chronic, progressive liver failure.

Clinical Signs The development of clinical signs of liver disease is usually delayed 4 weeks to 12 months after the consumption of pyrrolizidine alkaloid–containing plants. However, individual differences in susceptibility occur (not all horses consuming the plants develop clinical signs).[160] The onset of obvious hepatic failure, characterized by HE and photosensitization, usually is abrupt and occurs late in the disease despite the time interval since ingestion. Premonitory signs of insidious onset may include anorexia, weight loss, exercise intolerance, and mild to moderate icterus. Diarrhea, edema, polydipsia, pruritus, laryngeal hemiparalysis, and hemolysis also have been reported to occur late in the disease.[63,80,160] Sometimes oral ulcers and halitosis develop.[161] Although uncommon, if sufficient consumption occurs during a single exposure, then abortion or clinical signs of liver disease may develop acutely.

Epidemiology and Pathogenesis Numerous species of pyrrolizidine alkaloid–containing plants exist (Table 16-3).

TABLE 16-3

Pyrrolizidine Alkaloid–Containing Plants		
Species Name	**Common Name**	**Alkaloids**
Senecio jacobea	Tansy or common ragwort, stinking Willie	Jacobine, jacodine, senecionine
Senecio riddellii	Reddell's groundsel	Ridelline
Senecio longilobus	Threadleaf groundsel	Longilobine
Senecio vulgaris	Common groundsel	Senecionine, seneciphylline, retrorsine
Senecio spartioides	Broom groundsel	Seneciphylline
Senecio integerrimus	Lamb's tongue groundsel	Intergerrimine
Amsinckia intermedia	Fiddleneck, fireweed, tarweed	
Crotalaria species	Rattlebox	Monocrotaline, fulvine, crispatine
Echium plantagineum	Viper's bugloss	
Heliotropium europaeum	Common heliotrope or potato weed	Heliotrine, lasiocarpine

In the United States, *Senecio jacobea,* and *S. vulgaris* are found primarily along the Pacific Coast and in the western states, *Amsinckia intermedia* in the West, and *Crotalaria sagittalis* (Figure 16-10), *Crotalaria spectabilis,* and *Heliotropium europaeum* primarily in the Southeast.

Pyrrolizidine alkaloid–containing plants are not palatable, and horses will not typically consume them unless pastures are heavily contaminated or no alternative feed source exits. Some herbicides may increase palatability.[80] Pyrrolizidine alkaloids are stable, and much intoxication occurs after ingestion of contaminated hay, pellets, or grain. *S. vulgaris* is a common contaminant in alfalfa hay, especially at the first cutting. Not all parts of the plant contain pyrrolizidine alkaloids, and the concentration may vary with the season.[133] *Amsinckia* and *Crotalaria* spp. concentrate pyrrolizidine alkaloids in their seeds; thus intoxication may occur after ingestion of contaminated oat hay or grain screenings.[80]

Horses and cattle are relatively sensitive to pyrrolizidine alkaloid intoxication compared with goats and sheep. Consumption of the plants at a dose of 2% to 5% of the body weight, fed at one time or over a few days, can result in acute toxicity.[80] The effects of pyrrolizidine alkaloids are cumulative; thus it is more common for toxicity to occur after chronic low-level exposure. Hundreds of different pyrrolizidine alkaloids exist, but only a few have proved to be toxic (see Table 16-3). The toxic pyrrolizidine alkaloids vary among plants, but they all cause the same basic lesion. Ingested pyrrolizidine alkaloids are carried to the liver via the portal circulation and are metabolized by the microsomal enzymes to toxic pyrrole derivatives.[161] Drugs that induce microsomal enzymes, such as mixed function oxidases, will increase the toxicity of pyrrolizidine alkaloids. The pyrroles are chemically highly reactive and capable of alkylating nucleic acids and protein; consequently the pyrroles inhibit cellular replication and protein synthesis. Because the cells cannot divide, hepatocytes enlarge, forming *megalocytes*. When the megalocytes die, fibrosis ensues. When fibrosis becomes extensive, the liver shrinks, develops a firm texture, and failure is inevitable.

Hepatocytes surrounding the portal triads are usually affected first. When acute massive consumption exists, extensive centrilobular hepatocellular necrosis occurs. Fibrosis around the portal vessels can cause portal hypertension, ascites, and diarrhea. Endothelial cell swelling in the portal vein

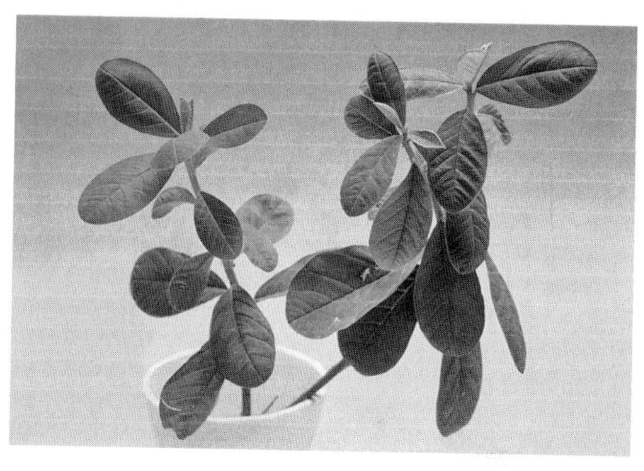

FIGURE 16-10 Picture of *Crotalaria* spp. plant containing toxic pyrrolizidine alkaloids. (Courtesy Susan White.)

is especially common with *Crotalaria* spp., further promoting veno-occlusion. Despite periportal fibrosis and veno-occlusion, portal hypertension rarely develops in horses, although it is a common manifestation of pyrrolizidine alkaloid toxicity in cattle.[80] Additional pathologic findings include myocardial necrosis, colitis, widespread hemorrhages, and adrenal cortical hypertrophy.[63] The toxic pyrrolizidine alkaloid in *Crotalaria* spp., monocrotaline, also is pneumonotoxic and may cause hydrothorax, pulmonary edema, epithelialization, and pulmonary arteritis.[161]

Pyrrolizidine alkaloids are rapidly excreted in body fluids such as milk and urine, and they can pass the placenta.[161] A report describes pyrrolizidine alkaloid toxicosis in a 2-month-old foal with a dam that consumed pyrrolizidine alkaloid–containing plants during pregnancy.[162]

Diagnosis A presumptive diagnosis of megalocytic hepatopathy can be made from history of exposure to pyrrolizidine alkaloids, clinical signs, and laboratory evidence of hepatic disease. Early in the disease, SDH and AST may be increased, but by the time clinical signs develop, these enzymes are often normal or only mildly increased. Because fibrosis occurs periportally, GGT, ALP, and serum bile acids concentration are persistently increased. Bilirubin may be increased and the BCAA-to-AAA ratio may be decreased.[163] The BSP half-life is prolonged and serum bile acids are usually increased late in the disease.[63]

A definitive diagnosis of pyrrolizidine alkaloid intoxication requires a liver biopsy. The histopathologic findings of megalocytosis, biliary hyperplasia, and fibrosis are essentially pathognomonic. Pyrrolizidine alkalosis must be distinguished from aflatoxicosis and alsike clover toxicity. The latter two toxicities are rare compared with pyrrolizidine alkaloids and cause periportal fibrosis and biliary epithelial hyperplasia without megalocytosis. Pyrrolizidine alkaloids can be detected in feed by high-performance liquid chromatography.[63] Some pyrrolizidine alkaloids can be identified in liver tissue. Unfortunately, because of the prolonged delay in development of clinical signs, often the original source of contamination remains unidentified.

Treatment and Prognosis No specific antidote for pyrrolizidine alkaloid intoxication exists. Despite general supportive care, death usually occurs within 10 days of the onset of obvious clinical signs of hepatic failure. A serum bile acid concentration greater than 50 μmol/L is suggestive of a grave prognosis.[63] Because regeneration is not possible, if extensive megalocytosis and fibrosis are present, then treatment is not warranted. Treatment with BCAA may decrease the severity of neurologic signs but does not prevent death.[63] If clinical signs or histologic changes are mild, then a low-protein (grass or oat hay), high-energy (molasses concentrate grain) ration may be beneficial.

Attention should be directed toward asymptomatic horses that also may have consumed the plants. The source of contamination should be identified by locating the plant in hayfields or pasture or by analysis of feed. Progress can be monitored by serial liver enzyme quantitation and biopsies. Serum GGT activity may be helpful in detecting subclinical cases of pyrrolizidine alkaloid toxicity.[164]

CLOVER POISONING

Alsike clover *(Trifolium hybridum)* and red clover *(Trifolium pratense)* poisoning rarely occurs in horses pastured or fed hay containing these types of clover.[165-167] Both photodermatitis and liver disease have been reported. Signs of liver disease may become apparent after 2 weeks of consumption and when the diet consists of at least 20% of clover.[165] The likelihood of poisoning reportedly is greater when the pasture is heavily covered with the clover in full bloom during wet seasons. Although the toxic principle is not known, the disease is characterized histopathologically by the presence of biliary hyperplasia and periportal fibrosis. Minimal parenchymal lesions distinguish alsike clover poisoning from pyrrolizidine alkaloid toxicity.

CHRONIC ACTIVE HEPATITIS

Chronic active hepatitis in horses is an idiopathic, chronic, progressive hepatopathy characterized histopathologically by biliary hyperplasia, with concomitant periportal or biliary inflammation (or both) and associated hepatocellular damage.

Clinical Signs The onset of clinical signs of CAH is insidious. Signs are compatible with progressive liver failure and include depression, exercise intolerance, weight loss, anorexia, colic, icterus, and fever. The signs may be intermittent. Although uncommon, some horses with CAH have moist exfoliative coronary dermatitis.[59]

Cause and Pathogenesis The exact cause of CAH in horses is not known. A similar syndrome occurs in human beings and has been linked to autoimmune disease, chronic hepatitis B virus infection, non-A and non-B (viral) hepatitis, Wilson's disease, α_1-antitrypsin deficiency, and drug allergy.[168] Human beings with autoimmune-associated CAH often have marked polyclonal gammopathy and hepatic actin, smooth muscle, and antinuclear antibodies.[168] Histologic study of the liver reveals mononuclear and plasma cell infiltrates, large areas of necrosis, and fibrosis. Extrahepatic signs of autoimmune disease, including dermatitis, arthritis, and glomerulonephritis, may be present. Some horses with CAH have polyclonal gammopathy, but this is a nonspecific finding in many types of chronic hepatic disease and is not necessarily indicative of autoimmunity. Occasionally, horses with CAH have predominantly plasma and mononuclear cell infiltrates in the liver, suggesting heightened humoral activity. The presence of coronary dermatitis in horses with CAH may be a manifestation of autoimmune disease, although this has not been confirmed by immunohistologic staining. No reports have surfaced of antinuclear antibodies in horses with CAH. In addition, viral hepatitis, Wilson's disease, and α_1-antitrypsin deficiency have not been documented in these animals. Idiosyncratic drug hypersensitivity has been reported in horses, although not as a consistent feature of CAH.

In addition to the possibility of an autoimmune or hypersensitivity reaction, CAH in horses may be a manifestation of chronic cholangitis. Many horses with CAH have a suppurative inflammatory response involving the biliary system, in addition to periportal inflammation and hepatocellular necrosis.[59] Often the cholangiohepatitis is accompanied by biliary hyperplasia, fibrosis, and cholestasis. In some cases, coliform organisms have been isolated from the liver, suggestive of ascending infection from the gastrointestinal tract. In a large number of horses, histopathologic evidence of fibrosis, acute inflammation, and hepatocellular necrosis is seen, but no specific cause can be determined.

Diagnosis The diagnostic criteria for CAH in human beings include abnormally increased serum transaminase activity for longer than 6 months, abnormal immunologic findings, and characteristic histopathologic findings.[168] In horses, serum SDH and AST activity may be mildly increased, but GGT and ALP are often markedly increased in CAH. The serum bile acid, total protein, and bilirubin (especially the direct-reacting fraction) concentrations may be increased. Bilirubinuria may be present, and the BSP half-life is usually prolonged. Hematology may reveal an inflammatory leukogram, with or without a left shift.[59] Immunodiagnostics, including antinuclear antibody titer and anti-immunoglobulin immunofluorescent staining of skin lesions, may help confirm an autoimmune phenomenon.

In the face of clinical signs and the demonstration of significant laboratory findings indicative of liver disease, a liver biopsy should be obtained (see Liver Biopsy). A sample should be submitted for histopathologic examination and for bacterial isolation and antimicrobial sensitivity testing. The definitive diagnosis of CAH depends on the presence of characteristic histopathologic findings. Progressive periportal hepatocellular necrosis obscures and distorts the limiting plate, the cord of hepatocytes that surrounds the portal triad. As this destructive process continues, bands of necrotic hepatocytes and inflammatory cells connect one liver lobule to another or extend from the portal tract to the central vein. This feature is called *bridging necrosis*. As bridging necrosis progresses, fibrosis and cirrhosis prevail. Mononuclear cells may be the predominant inflammatory infiltrate; however, neutrophils predominate if cholangiohepatitis is a feature. Biliary hyperplasia may be evidence of concurrent cholangiohepatitis.

Treatment General supportive care for hepatic failure (see Treatment of Hepatic Insufficiency) is indicated whenever clinical signs are apparent. Specific therapy for CAH depends on the histopathologic findings. If the liver biopsy reveals abundant plasma cells, or other diagnostic tests suggest autoimmune or hypersensitivity disease, then corticosteroid therapy may be beneficial. In human beings with autoimmune-associated CAH, corticosteroids improve appetite and attitude, reduce inflammation and serum transaminase activity, and hinder fibrosis. Despite short-term improvement, corticosteroids do not alter survival time and the long-term prognosis remains poor. In horses, initial treatment with dexamethasone at 0.05 to 0.1 mg/kg/day for 4 to 7 days, followed by a gradual reduction in dose over 2 to 3 weeks, has been suggested.[80] Additional treatment with prednisolone (1 mg/kg/day) may be necessary for several weeks. In human beings, azathioprine (2 mg/kg every 24 hours) has also been used to control cases refractory to steroids,[168] although recent studies suggest that oral bioavailability of this drug in the horse is quite low, ranging between 1% to 7%.[169] If the liver biopsy reveals cholangitis, then long-term (4 to 6 weeks) antimicrobial therapy is indicated. The choice of antimicrobial is best determined by culture and sensitivity results. Antimicrobials that are excreted in bile, such as chloramphenicol, ceftiofur, ampicillin, or broad-spectrum antimicrobials such as penicillin and gentamicin, are recommended. The decision for corticosteroid therapy should be carefully scrutinized in these cases of CAH.

Prognosis The prognosis for CAH is variable, depending on the cause and duration of disease. The presence of cirrhosis warrants a grave prognosis.

CHOLELITHIASIS

Cholelithiasis, or the formation of biliary calculi, occasionally results in hepatocellular disease in horses. A *cholelith* is a calculi that develops anywhere along the biliary pathway. A *hepatolith* and *choledocholith* refer to calculi within intrahepatic ducts and the common bile duct, respectively. Hepatic failure and clinical signs occur when multiple stones are present or when they occlude the common bile duct.

Clinical Signs Cholelithiasis occurs most commonly in adult, middle-aged horses (6 to 15 years old), although horses as young as 3 years old have been affected.[50,125,170] Broodmares may be predisposed.[125] The most frequently reported clinical signs include icterus, abdominal pain, fever, depression, and weight loss.[50,125,170-172] Signs of hepatic failure, such as photosensitization, petechial hemorrhages, diarrhea, and HE, have been reported less frequently.[50,125,170-172] Clinical signs are often intermittent unless the common bile duct is occluded, whereupon persistent abdominal pain prevails.

Pathogenesis The initial step in the formation of a cholelith is precipitation or aggregation of normally soluble constituents of bile: bilirubin, cholesterol, or bile acids. In human beings, 75% of bile stones are composed principally of cholesterol and 25% are composed principally of calcium bilirubinate. The majority of calcium bilirubinate choleliths in human beings are associated with bacterial cholangitis.[4,173] Most choleliths in horses consist principally of calcium bilirubinate and are associated with cholangitis.[50,125,170]

The exact sequence of events leading to precipitation of bilirubin in bile is not entirely known; however, soluble, conjugated bilirubin becomes unconjugated by the enzyme α-glucuronidase and combines with calcium, a normal constituent of bile, to form calcium bilirubinate. Excessive formation of unconjugated bilirubin causes the formation of columnar complexes of calcium bilirubinate that subsequently precipitate. The bile duct epithelium, hepatocytes, and certain bacteria synthesize β-glucuronidase. The concentration of β-glucuronidase is normally very low in bile, and an inhibitor, glucaro-1,4-lactone, is usually present.

Whether bacterial, biliary, or hepatic in origin, increased bile concentration of β-glucuronidase has been demonstrated in human beings with obstructive cholangitis.[4] Because most choleliths in horses are composed of calcium bilirubinate and many affected horses with cholelithiasis have documented bacterial cholangitis, it seems logical that cholelith formation in horses most likely occurs subsequent to bacterial infection. Furthermore, because enteric organisms are isolated most commonly from horses with cholelithiasis, infection presumably ascends from the intestinal tract. Horses may be more prone to ascending infection because they lack an exit port sphincter to prevent backflow of intestinal contents into the biliary tree. If bile flow is decreased for any reason, then retrograde flow and infection are likely. However, the correlation of infection with cholelithiasis in horses does not necessarily prove causation. Another plausible explanation is the initial presence of a stone, precipitating cholestasis and subsequent infection. Despite its origin, cholangitis is the likely cause of fever. Chronic cholestasis because of the presence of choleliths results in increased biliary pressure, a likely cause of abdominal discomfort. If biliary pressure is not resolved, then pressure-induced periportal hepatocellular necrosis with subsequent fibrosis ensues.

At necropsy, tissues are icteric and the liver is mottled in appearance. The liver appears enlarged after acute biliary obstruction, and it appears shrunken and firm with chronic cholestasis. Choleliths range in size, are single or multiple in number, usually green-brown in color (bilirubinate), and smooth textured. Histopathologic study reveals periportal hepatocellular necrosis, fibrosis, biliary stasis, and biliary hyperplasia. Suppurative cholangitis is often present. Organisms isolated from the liver or bile consist predominately of gram-negative coliforms, though *Enterococcus* spp. has also been reported.[50,125,170] Nonobstructive choleliths are subclinical and only recognized at necropsy.

Diagnosis Cholelithiasis should be considered in the differential diagnosis in any horse with a history of fever, icterus, and abdominal pain, especially if accompanied by signs of hepatic failure. Hematology often reveals leukocytosis because of mature neutrophilia, especially if cholangitis is present.[50,125,170] Other nonspecific but frequent findings include hyperproteinemia and hyperfibrinogenemia.[50,125,170] The most common abnormal laboratory findings that suggest cholestatic liver disease include markedly increased GGT (>15 times normal); increased serum bile acids concentration; hyperbilirubinemia, with the direct-reacting fraction greater than 25% of the total value; and bilirubinuria.* Although not liver specific, ALP often is increased greatly. Less commonly, SDH, ARG, AST, and LDH-5 are mildly to moderately increased and clotting times and the BSP half-life are prolonged.[50,125,170-172,174] Affected horses frequently have nonseptic peritonitis or peritoneal transudate.[170]

*References: 50, 125, 170, 171, 173, and 174.

Although no single blood test was specific for cholelithiasis, hepatic ultrasonography or biopsy accurately predicted a diagnosis of cholelithiasis in all cases reviewed.[170] In retrospective studies of cholelithiasis, 75% of the cases had visibly dilated bile ducts, which appear as thin-walled, anechoic structures.[50,125,170,175] This finding contrasts with normal horses, in which the bile ducts are not detectable. Dilatation of intrahepatic biliary radicals lying adjacent to portal venous structures may be evident.[175] The liver may appear enlarged with increased echogenicity. Hepatoliths, which are observed in 60% of cases, are found most frequently at the level of the right sixth to seventh intercostal space,[50,125,170,175] appear as hyperechoic foci within the bile ducts, and may cast acoustic shades (Figure 16-11). Determination of obstruction of the common bile duct in horses is difficult, because the common bile duct cannot be seen by transabdominal ultrasonography. Hepatobiliary scintigraphy may be useful to document obstruction of biliary excretion.[176] Otherwise, choledocholiths can only be detected via palpation during exploratory celiotomy.

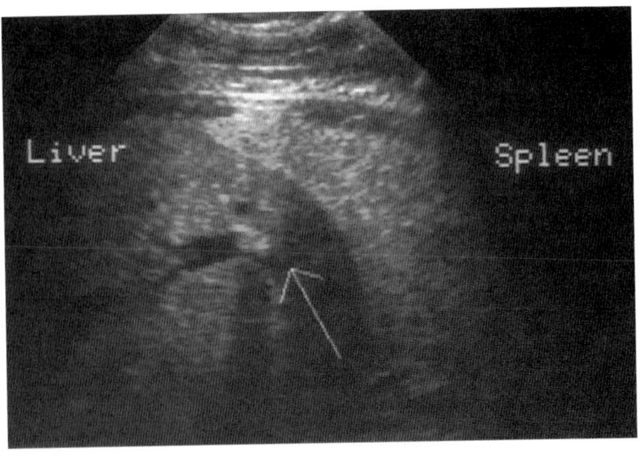

FIGURE 16-11 Ultrasound image of the liver showing a hepatolith *(arrow)* casting an acoustic shadow in a dilated bile duct in a horse with obstructive cholelithiasis.

Obtaining a liver biopsy is useful for diagnostic, therapeutic, and prognostic purposes. The histopathologic findings of periportal fibrosis, biliary stasis and hyperplasia, and cholangitis are not pathognomonic for cholelithiasis; however, a liver biopsy may help rule out other causes of biliary stasis such as CAH or megalocytic hepatopathy. Concentric fibrosis around intrahepatic bile ducts is strong evidence of occlusion of the common bile duct (Figure 16-12).

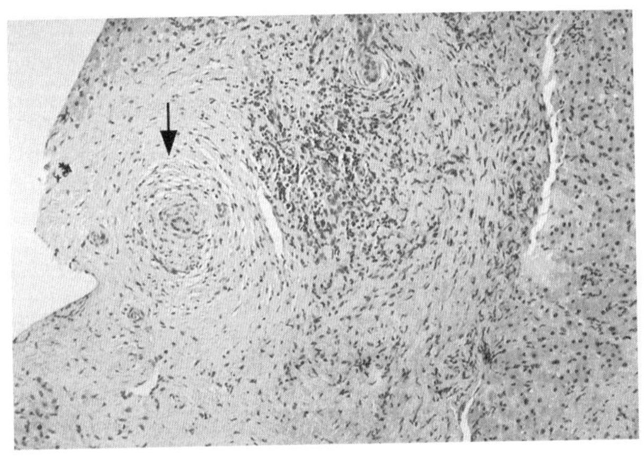

FIGURE 16-12 Histopathology of the liver: concentric fibrosis *(arrow)* around a bile duct characteristic of obstruction of the common bile duct.

Treatment If clinical signs of liver failure are present, general supportive care should be provided (see Treatment of Hepatic Insufficiency). Long-term (4-6 weeks) treatment with antimicrobials is indicated. Antimicrobial selection should be guided by clinical response and by bacterial isolation and sensitivity results obtained either via a liver biopsy or culture of the bile or cholelith obtained at surgery. Penicillin-gentamicin, ceftiofur, chloramphenicol, ampicillin, enrofloxacin, metronidazole, and trimethoprim-sulfonamide have been used successfully[50,125,170]; however, recent reports indicate resistance of isolates from affected horses to trimethoprim-sulfonamide.[170] Antimicrobial therapy should be continued until complete resolution of clinical signs and laboratory evidence of inflammation. It has been suggested that antimicrobial therapy should be continued until the serum GGT activity is normal.[125]

Dissolution of cholesterol choleliths in human beings has been successful with long-term administration of bile acids.[20] Because choleliths in horses are composed primarily of biliary pigments, treatment with bile acids would most likely be unavailing and potentially harmful. Evidence indicates that DMSO dissolves calcium bilirubinate stones in human beings; thus its use may be beneficial to horses with cholelithiasis.[125] Use of other anti-inflammatory drugs, such as flunixin meglumine, may help speed resolution of hepatic and biliary inflammation and thus restore biliary excretion.

Surgical intervention may be necessary if the common bile duct is occluded. The decision for surgery is difficult because no direct way exists to determine the extent of occlusion of the common bile duct in horses. In one report, horses with discrete occlusive choledocholiths had persistent fever; more persistent, though mild and intermittent, abdominal pain; and significantly greater serum bile acid concentrations than did horses that were managed successfully with medical therapy.[170] Although cholelithotripsy may be accomplished in human beings percutaneously, via endoscopy or laparotomy, exploratory laparotomy currently is the only available means for reducing a common bile duct obstruction in horses. Choledocholithotripsy (the crushing of choleliths in the bile ducts) and choledochotomy (surgical formation of an opening into the bile duct) have been performed successfully in the horse.[173,177,178] In one recent report on horses, external massage of the common bile duct, without choledochotomy, successfully dislodged choledocholiths into the duodenum in all of the cases in which it was attempted.[170] If multiple hepatoliths are distributed throughout the biliary tree, then these cannot be readily removed by surgery.

Prognosis The prognosis of cholelithiasis depends on the extent of hepatic fibrosis, severity of clinical signs, and number and location of choleliths. Extensive or bridging fibrosis, multiple choleliths accompanied by clinical signs of hepatic failure, hepatic atrophy, and severe HE warrant a poor to grave prognosis.[50,125,170] Reports of resolution of extensive fibrosis exist after re-establishment of bile flow; thus one should not consider the presence of extensive fibrosis alone to be lethal.[170,179] In contrast to reports of 30% survival for equine cholelithiasis,[50] recent reviews indicate 77% to 85% survival with medical or medical and surgical treatment.[125,170] If obstruction of the bile duct requires a choledochotomy, then the prognosis is guarded because of limited access to the bile duct in a horse and the risk of choleperitoneum.

CHRONIC CHOLANGIOHEPATITIS AND BILIARY FIBROSIS

Chronic cholangiohepatitis and biliary fibrosis most commonly are associated with CAH, cholelithiasis, and pancreatitis. Liver failure rarely results from primary idiopathic cholangitis or biliary fibrosis.[56] Therapy is supportive. Treatment of bacterial cholangiohepatitis is discussed elsewhere (see Bacterial Hepatitis, Chronic Active Hepatitis, and Cholelithiasis). The prognosis depends on the degree of fibrosis. Extensive fibrosis warrants a poor prognosis, although reports of reversal of hepatic fibrosis exist, especially on relief of the obstruction in cholestatic diseases.[179]

NEONATAL ACQUIRED BILIARY OBSTRUCTION

Healing duodenal ulcers located adjacent to the hepatopancreatic ampulla in neonatal foals may result in extrahepatic biliary stenosis.[15,180] Clinical signs are compatible with gastroduodenal obstruction and include reduced suckling reflex, depression, prolonged recumbency, colic, bruxism, and firm feces. Nasogastric intubation often produces voluminous reflux. Duodenal stenosis may be confirmed radiographically by delayed gastric emptying of barium sulfate. One should consider a diagnosis of biliary stenosis if the serum levels of conjugated bilirubin and GGT are increased or if nuclear scintigraphy indicates delayed biliary excretion. Cholangiohepatitis may develop because of chronic cholestasis and may be confirmed by histopathologic examination of a liver biopsy. One must differentiate acquired biliary stenosis from congenital biliary atresia (discussed later in this chapter). Successful surgical correction of acquired biliary stenosis secondary to duodenal stricture has been described.[180]

Chronic cholangiohepatitis without biliary stenosis, another potential sequela to duodenitis or duodenal ulceration, should be considered in icteric foals with increased serum conjugated bilirubin and GGT.[15] The diagnosis is confirmed by histopathologic examination. Treatment should consist of long-term antimicrobial therapy directed by bacterial isolation and sensitivity results (see Bacterial Hepatitis).

HEPATIC ABSCESSATION

Liver abscessation is uncommon in horses. Clinical signs of hepatic abscessation depend on the extent and location of the abscess or abscesses; however, abscesses are unlikely to result in hepatic failure. Small solitary abscesses or multifocal microabscesses usually remain subclinical. Larger abscesses may be accompanied by weight loss, intermittent fever, and anorexia.

Hepatic abscessation in foals may be hematogenous in origin as a sequela to bacteremia or ascending through the umbilical vein as a sequela to omphalophlebitis.[181] In the adult, bacteremia is uncommon, and hepatic infection or abscessation more likely originates in the intestinal lumen and ascends the bile duct or originates in the intestinal wall or mesenteric lymph nodes and is carried to the liver via the portal blood. The latter is a likely sequela to primary abdominal or mesenteric abscessation because of *Streptococcus equi* subsp. *equi*. In one retrospective study of abdominal abscesses in horses, only two of 25 horses had solely hepatic abscesses, although some horses had abscesses involving several abdominal structures.[182] In a description of three adult horses with hepatic abscesses, disease was postulated to result from primary inflammatory bowel disease, as a sequelae to abdominal surgery, and secondary to penetration of a foreign body from the colon.[183] Laboratory diagnosis of hepatic abscessation is difficult. Smaller abscesses may not result in sufficient hepatocellular damage to impede liver function. Laboratory abnormalities characteristic of chronic inflammation and infection, including anemia of chronic disease, hyperfibrinogenemia, hypergammaglobulinemia, and mature neutrophilia, may occur with larger abscesses. Increased serum activity of liver-specific cytosolic enzymes or serum bile acids concentration rarely occurs unless liver abscessation is extensive. Ultrasonography of the liver may reveal focal changes in echogenicity. A liver biopsy should be guided by ultrasound to avoid penetration of the abscess. One should direct long-term antimicrobial therapy by culture and sensitivity results. Common isolates from abdominal abscesses in horses include *S. equi*, sups. *equi, S. equi* subsp. *zooepidemicus,* and *Corynebacterium pseudotuberculosis*.[182]

HEPATIC NEOPLASIA

Primary hepatic neoplasia is rare in horses. A retrospective survey in 1952 indicated that hepatic tumors accounted for only 1% of all equine neoplasms.[184] Of the documented primary hepatic neoplasms in horses (cholangiocarcinoma, hepatocellular carcinoma, hepatoblastoma, and mixed hamartoma), cholangiocarcinoma is the most common.[57,85,86,184-188] Hepatic neoplasia in horses is more likely to occur after metastasis of some other primary tumor, especially lymphosarcoma.[74] Because clinical signs of hepatic failure usually are not apparent and laboratory findings are nonspecifically indicative of chronic inflammatory disease, antemortem diagnosis of hepatic neoplasia is difficult.

In one report, *cholangiocarcinoma* accounted for 9 of 10 primary liver neoplasms in horses.[184] Cholangiocarcinoma originates from the bile duct epithelium and is distinguished from hepatocellular carcinoma by its tendency to form multiple foci, its firm texture, and a whitish color produced by abundant fibrous stroma. The primary mass is typically solitary, with multiple intrahepatic secondaries. Extrahepatic metastasis is common, with transperitoneal lymphatic spread to the peritoneum and diaphragm and hematogenous spread to the lungs.[186] In human beings, dogs, and cats, a causative relationship appears to exist between cholangiocarcinoma and liver fluke infestation or a history of biliary tract disease.[186] A report describes cholangiocarcinoma in a horse after treatment for prolonged septic cholangiohepatitis.[176] Aberrant expression of the protein products of the tumor suppressor gene, p53, was reported at necropsy in one horse with cholangiocarcinoma.[189] Loss of function of p53 has been described in other types of carcinomas and may have contributed to malignancy. Microscopically, cholangiocarcinoma is adenocarcinomatous, producing cuboidal or columnar-lined ductules and acini. The neoplastic bile ducts do not contain bile but may contain mucus.

The clinical presentation and progression of cholangiocarcinoma in horses is not well documented, but this disorder appears to be more common in older horses.[184] One case report describes a 10-year-old mixed-breed horse in which the presenting signs included anorexia, weight loss, pyrexia, mild icterus, tachypnea, severe dependent edema, and abdominal distention.[188] Abnormal clinicopathologic findings included mature neutrophilia; hyperfibrinogenemia; anemia; moderately increased serum bilirubin, GGT, and SDH; and nonseptic peritonitis and pleuritis. Neoplastic cells were not detected in the body cavity effusions. Definitive antemortem diagnosis of cholangiocarcinoma was made by histopathologic examination of a liver biopsy. Necropsy revealed multiple extrahepatic metastases on the serosal surfaces of the intestine and spleen, diaphragm, omentum, pleural surfaces, and lung.

Hepatocellular carcinoma, or hepatoma, has been reported in several horses, the majority of which were less than 3 years of age.[84-86,187] Hepatocellular carcinomas are usually solitary and multilobulated. Extrahepatic metastasis occurs transperitoneally and hematogenously to lungs. Microscopically, the neoplastic cells resemble hepatocytes and retain cord arrangement. However, the normal liver architecture is lost, and sometimes the cells are difficult to differentiate. Mitotic figures are uncommon. Possible causative factors in other species include heredity, parasitism, chemical and plant carcinogens, and viral hepatitis.[186]

Reported clinical signs of hepatocellular carcinoma in horses include depression, anorexia, weight loss, intermittent diarrhea, and abdominal distention.[84-86,187] Abnormal laboratory findings included absolute erythrocytosis; persistent hypoglycemia; sanguineous peritoneal effusion; and increased serum SDH, GGT, LAP, and indirect-reacting bilirubin. In one case, absolute erythrocytosis was attributed to erythropoietin secretion by the carcinoma (inappropriate secondary erythrocytosis).[86] The same horse had a high serum concentration of α-fetoprotein, a globulin normally synthesized only by embryonic fetal liver cells that is commonly detectable in human patients with hepatocellular carcinoma.

Two case reports describe malignant *hepatoblastoma* in young horses.[57,190] Hepatoblastoma is an embryonic tumor of the liver with a wide range of histologic patterns that include both epithelial and mesenchymal elements. Clinical signs included emaciation, pyrexia, and pleural effusion. Laboratory abnormalities included mature neutrophilia, erythrocytosis with normal erythropoietin levels, hypergammaglobulinemia, hyperfibrinogenemia, and increased serum activity of GGT and ASP. In one of the cases, transabdominal ultrasonography identified abnormal hepatic architecture. Increased serum α-fetoprotein may serve as a tumor marker but cannot be used alone to confirm a diagnosis.[190]

A *mixed hamartoma* was described in the liver of a late-term aborted equine fetus.[203] Histologically, the lesion appeared to be a proliferation of large hepatocyte-like cells with eccentric nuclei and voluminous cytoplasm, abnormal bile ducts, and fibroblastic fibrocystic interstitial tissue, with complete lack of structural organization.

HEPATIC AMYLOIDOSIS

Amyloidosis refers to a group of diseases that are characterized by the extracellular deposition of a proteinaceous fibril substance, *amyloid,* in the tissues. Amyloid deposits are composed of nonbranching fibrils in β-pleated sheet conformation formed by the proteolytic cleavage of precursor proteins by the mononuclear phagocyte system. Depending on the organ of deposition, amyloid distorts normal tissue architecture and may lead to functional impairment. In horses, the liver and spleen are the most common organs involved in systemic amyloidosis.[191] Two forms of systemic amyloidosis exist and are distinguished by the type of precursor protein and subsequent protein fibril. The precursor in *reactive* or *secondary* systemic amyloidosis is serum amyloid protein AA, an acute phase protein produced by hepatocytes in response to chronic infection or inflammation. The AA fibrils are identified in tissues by green birefringence in polarized light, after staining with Congo red, which is lost after treatment with potassium permanganate. Most often in horses, hepatic amyloid deposits are AA fibrils and have been associated with severe parasitism or chronic infection and inflammation.[191,192] One horse in which the liver was the principal organ of amyloid deposition presented for evaluation of chronic weight loss.[192] An antemortem diagnosis of hepatic amyloidosis was not made; however, laboratory abnormalities included severe hypoalbuminemia, polyclonal gammopathy, and large numbers of ascarid and strongylid eggs in the feces. Histopathologically, the liver revealed extracellular deposits of AA amyloid periportally and adjacent to the sinusoids in the space of Disse. The amyloid deposits were accompanied by hepatocytic atrophy and a mild mononuclear cell infiltrate.

Systemic primary, immunocytic, or *idiopathic amyloidosis* is caused by the deposition of amyloid light chain fibrils. The precursor proteins in primary amyloidosis are the variable region of immunoglobulin light chains. The amyloid fibrils also stain with Congo red, but staining is retained after potassium permanganate treatment. *Local immunocytic amyloidosis,* with deposition in the upper respiratory mucosa or skin, is more common in horses than systemic primary amyloidosis. However, at least one reported case of systemic primary amyloidosis in a 14-year-old Thoroughbred mare with chronic weight loss and cutaneous nodules exists.[193] Amyloid deposits were identified in the liver, myocardium, spleen, gastrointestinal mucosa, pulmonary interstitium, pancreas, and arterial walls.

CHRONIC HYPOXEMIA

Right-sided heart failure causes the pressure in the caudal vena cava to rise. Retrograde pressure increases in the hepatic central veins, causing hypoxemia and pressure necrosis of the adjacent hepatocytes. Chronic passive congestion may cause fatty change, atrophy, and fibrosis.

Congenital or Heritable Abnormalities

PORTOSYSTEMIC SHUNT

Portosystemic shunts may be intrahepatic or extrahepatic, congenital or acquired. Few reports have documented congenital extrahepatic portosystemic shunts in foals.[87,194] The vascular shunts allow blood within the portal system to bypass the liver and drain into the systemic circulation, directly or indirectly, via the caudal vena cava or the azygous vein. In the reported cases, age at presentation varied between 2 and 6 months. Vague intermittent neurologic signs of blindness, ataxia, and severe depression were consistent with HE. Growth appeared to be stunted. These clinical signs are caused by the altered hepatic blood flow and hepatic insufficiency secondary to hepatocellular atrophy.

Laboratory abnormalities in the reported cases varied, but the most consistent findings included a decreased BUN, prolonged BSP half-life, and increased blood ammonia concentration. Liver biopsies revealed hepatocellular atrophy and necrosis, fibrosis, and biliary hyperplasia.[87] Antemortem diagnosis was confirmed by operative mesenteric portography or nuclear scintigraphy (see Diagnostic Imaging of the Liver). Surgical correction was attempted unsuccessfully in one case.[195] Necropsy examination revealed small, firm livers. The location of the shunt (or shunts) in reported cases varied, but all were extrahepatic, involving a direct connection between the mesenteric veins and the caudal vena cava. Alzheimer type II astrocytes were visible in the brain in one case and were consistent with HE.[194]

Acquired portosystemic shunts are rare in horses. One report describes an 11-year-old Thoroughbred with HE that subsequently was determined to have a functional portosystemic shunt secondary to vascular thrombosis of the portal vein.[195]

BILIARY ATRESIA

At least two cases of extrahepatic biliary atresia in foals have been documented.[196,197] An antemortem diagnosis was not possible in either case; however, veterinary attention was sought at 4 weeks of age in both foals for anorexia, depression, lethargy, poor weight gain, colic, polydipsia, polyuria, pyrexia, and icterus. Laboratory evaluation of one of the foals was consistent with biliary obstruction, as indicated by a mildly increased serum activity of SDH and markedly increased activity of GGT and conjugated bilirubin.[196] Necropsy of both foals revealed a large, firm liver. Although not specifically documented in one case, both the entrance to the bile duct and the main bile duct were absent in the other foal.[196] Histologically, both livers appeared similar and consistent with extrahepatic biliary atresia. Bile canaliculi were present and distended, with associated degenerative hepatocytes. Biliary proliferation was extensive and surrounded by fibrous tissue with interdispersed islands of hepatocytes. No bile was found in the proliferative bile ducts, and the portal triad ducts were absent.

In horses, extrahepatic biliary atresia is believed to be congenital. In human beings, other possible causes include neonatal sclerosing cholangiohepatitis, excretion of a biliary toxin, deficit of bile flow in utero, or lumen destruction because of ductal vascular insufficiency.[197] Despite the cause, extrahepatic biliary atresia induces intrahepatic biliary hypertrophy, an abortive attempt to establish continuity. The biliary hypertrophy displaces hepatocytes, causing periportal and perilobular hepatocellular degeneration, fibrous replacement, and ultimately, loss of normal hepatic architecture. Although an antemortem diagnosis was not possible in either equine case, hepatobiliary scintigraphy (see Diagnostic Imaging of the Liver) successfully detected total biliary obstruction in a neonatal lamb with biliary atresia.[88]

SEROUS CYSTS

Serous hepatic cysts have been reported and usually are an incidental finding at necropsy.[11]

GLYCOGEN BRANCHING ENZYME DEFICIENCY

Autosomal recessive inheritance of glycogen branching enzyme deficiency has been reported in Quarter Horse foals (see the chapter on Musculoskeletal Diseases for a detailed discussion). The nonsense mutation of the affected gene, glycogen branching enzyme 1, prevents synthesis of functional enzyme. Affected foals died before 2 months of age. Clinical signs vary from stillbirth, seizures, and persistent recumbency to cardiac or respiratory failure. Leukopenia, intermittent hypoglycemia, increased creatine kinase, GGT, and AST are common laboratory findings. Histopathology of the liver demonstrates abnormal periodic acid–Schiff (PAS) positive globular or crystalline intracellular inclusions and reduced glycogen branching enzyme activity.[198]

REFERENCES

1. Getty R, editor: *Sisson's and Grossman's the anatomy of domestic animals*, Philadelphia, 1975, WB Saunders.
2. Jakowski R: Right hepatic lobe atrophy in horses: 17 cases (1983-1993), *J Am Vet Med Assoc* 204:1057, 1994.
3. Ham AW: Pancreas, liver and galbladder. In *Histology*, ed 7, Philadelphia, 1974, W.B. Saunders.
4. Sodeman WA, Sodeman TM, editors: *Sodeman's pathologic physiology: mechanisms of disease*, Philadelphia, 1985, WB Saunders.
5. Lehninger AL: *Biochemistry*, New York, 1975, Worth Publishers Inc.
6. Guyton AC, Hall JE: *Textbook of medical physiology*, ed 10, Philadelphia, 2006, WB Saunders.
7. McDermott WV: Metabolism and toxicity of ammonia, *N Engl J Med* 257:1076, 1957.
8. Duncan JR, Prasse KW: *Veterinary laboratory medicine*, Ames, IA, 1986, Iowa University Press.
9. Engelking LR: Evaluation of equine bilirubin and bile acid metabolism, *Compend Contin Educ Pract Vet* 11:328, 1989.
10. Coles EG: *Veterinary clinical pathology*, Philadelphia, 1988, WB Saunders.
11. Thompson RG, editor: *Special veterinary pathology*, Philadelphia, 1988, BC Decker Inc.
12. Papich MG, Davis LE: Drugs and the liver, *Veterinary clinics of North American, small animal practice*, vol. 15, Philadelphia, 1985, WB Saunders.
13. Reed S, Andrews FM: The biochemical evaluation of liver function in the horse. In *Proceedings of the thirty-second annual convention of the American Association of Equine Practitioners*, 1986, Nashville, TN, p 81, AAEP, Lexington, KY.
14. Kumar V, Fausto N, Abbas A, editors: *Robbins pathologic basis of disease*, ed 7, Philadelphia, 2005, WB Saunders.
15. Divers TJ: Liver disease and liver failure in horses. In *Proceedings of the twenty-ninth American Association of Equine Practitioners*, Las Vegas:213, 1983, AAEP, Lexington, KY.
16. West H: Clinical and pathological studies in horses with hepatic disease, *Equine Vet J* 28:146, 1996.
17. McGorum B, Murphy D, Love S, et al: Clinicopathological features of equine primary hepatic disease: a review of 50 cases, *Vet Rec* 145:134, 1999.
18. Fraser CL, Arieff AI: Hepatic encephalopathy, *N Engl J Med* 313:865, 1985.
19. Gammal SH, Jones EA: Hepatic encephalopathy, *Med Clin North Am* 73:793, 1989.
20. Goldman L, Ausiello DA, Arend W, et al: *Cecil textbook of medicine*, ed 23, Philadelphia, 2008, WB Saunders.
21. Schiff L, Schiff ER, editors: *Disease of the liver*, Philadelphia, 1987, JB Lippincott.
22. Shawcross D, Jalan R: The pathophysiologic basis of hepatic encephalopathy: central role for ammonia and inflammation, *Cell Mol Life Sci* 62:2295, 2005.
23. Lockwood AH, MacDonald JM, Reiman RE, et al: The dynamics of ammonia metabolism in man. Effects of liver disease and hyperammonemia, *J Clin Invest* 63:449, 1979.
24. Flannery DB, Hsia YE, Wolf B: Current status of hyperammonemia syndromes, *Hepatology* 2:495, 1982.
25. Bode J, Schafer K: Pathophysiology of chronic hepatic encephalopathy, *Hepatogasteroentology* 32:259, 1985.
26. McCandless DW, editor: *Cerebral energy metabolism and metabolic energy*, New York, 1985, Plenum.
27. Albrecht J, Jones E: Hepatic encephalopathy: molecular mechanisms underlying the clinical syndrome, *J Neurol Sci* 170:138, 1999.

28. Bessman SP, Bessman AN: The cerebral and peripheral uptake of ammonia in liver disease with a hypothesis for the mechanism of hepatic coma, *J Clin Invest* 34:622, 1975.
29. Pappas SC, Ferenci P, Scafer DF, et al: Visual evoked potentials in rabbit model of hepatic encephalopathy. II. Comparison of hyperammonemic encephalopathy, postictal coma and coma induced by synergic neurotoxins, *Gastroenterology* 86:546, 1984.
30. Cohn R, Castell DO: The effect of acute hyperammonemia on the encephalogram, *J Lab Clin Med* 68:195, 1966.
31. Odeh M: Pathogenesis of hepatic encephalopathy: the tumour necrosis factor alpha theory, *Eur J Clin Invest* 37:291, 2007.
32. Record CO, Mardini H, Bartlett K: Blood and brain mercaptan concentrations in hepatic encephalopathy, *Hepatology* 2:144, 1982.
33. Jones EA, Schafer DF, Ferenci P, et al: The neurobiology of hepatic encephalopathy, *Hepatology* 4:1235, 1984.
34. Tallman JF, Gallager DW: The GABA-ergic system: a locus of benzodiazepine action, *Annu Rev Neurosci* 8:21, 1985.
35. Study R, Barker J: Diazepam and (–) pentobarbitol: fluctuation analysis reveals different mechanisms for potentiation of gamma-aminobutyric acid responses in cultured central neurons, *Proc Natl Acad Sci U S* A77:7486, 1981.
36. Basile AS, Gammal SH, Mullen KD: Differential responsiveness of cerebellar Purkinje neurons to GABA and benzodiazepine ligands in an animal model of hepatic encephalopathy in man, *J Neurosci* 8:2414, 1988.
37. Bassett ML, Mullen K, Skolnick P, et al: Amelioration of hepatic encephalopathy by pharmacologic antagonism of the GABA-benzodiazepine receptor complex in a rabbit model of fulminant heptic failure, *Gastroenterology* 93:1069, 1987.
38. Ferenci P, Jones EA, Hanbauer I: Lack of evidence for impaired dopamine receptor function in experimental hepatic coma in the rabbit, *J Neurosci* 65:60, 1986.
39. Lock B, Pandit K: Is flumanzenil an effective treatment for hepatic encephalopathy, *Ann Emerg Med* 47:286, 2006.
40. Ahboucha S, Butterworth R: The neurosteroid system: an emerging therapeutic target for hepatic encephalopathy, *Metab Brain Dis* 22:291, 2007.
41. Fischer JE, Baldessarine RJ: False neurotransmitters in hepatic failure, *Lancet* 2:75, 1971.
42. Gulick BA, Rogers QR, Knight HD: Plasma amino acid patterns in horses with hepatic disease. In *Proceedings of the twenty-fourth annual convention of the American Association of Equine Practitioners*, 1978, St Louis, p 517, AAEP, Lexington, Ky.
43. Alexander WF, Spinder E, Harty RF, et al: The usefulness of branched chain fatty acids with acute or chronic hepatic encephalopathy, *Am J Gastroenterol* 84:91, 1989.
44. Morgan MY, Milson PJ, Sherlock S: Plasma ratio of valine, leucine, and isoleucine to phenylalanine, tyrosine in liver disease, *Gut* 19:1068, 1978.
45. Bianchi G, Marocchi R, Agostini F, et al: Update on nutritional supplementation with branched chained amino acids, *Curr Opin Clin Nutr Metab Care* 8:83, 2005.
46. Schafer DF, Fowler JM, Jone EA: Colonic bacteria: a source of gamma-aminobutyric acid in blood, *Proc Soc Exp Biol Med* 167:301, 1981.
47. Bauer JE, Asquith RL, Kivipelto J: Serum biochemical indicators of liver function in neonatal foals, *Am J Vet Res* 50:2037, 1989.
48. Divers T, Schappel K, Sweeney R, et al: Persistent hyperbilirubinemia in a healthy thoroughbred horse, *Cornell Vet* 83:237, 1993.
49. Scott DW: *Large animal dermatology*, Philadelphia, 1988, WB Saunders.
50. Johnston JK, Divers TJ, Reef VB, et al: Cholelithiasis in horses: ten cases (1982-1986), *J Am Vet Med Assoc* 194:405, 1989.
51. Divers TJ, Warner A, Vaala WE, et al: Toxic hepatic failure in newborn foals, *J Am Vet Med Assoc* 183:1407, 1983.
52. Jubb KVF, Kennedy PJ, Palmer N, editors: *Pathology of domestic animals*, Orlando, FL, 1985, Academic Press.
53. Johnstone IB: Antithrombin III activity in normal and diseased horses, *Vet Clin Pathol* 17:20, 1988.
54. Gay CC, Lording PM, McNeil P, et al: Infectious necrotic hepatitis (Black disease) in a horse, *Equine Vet J* 12:27, 1980.
55. Tennant BC, Hornbuckle WE: Diseases of the liver. In Anderson NV, editor: *Veterinary gastroenterology*, Philadelphia, 1980, Lea & Febiger.
56. Tennant B: Acute hepatitis in horses: problems of differentiating toxic and infectious causes in the adult. In *Proceedings of the twenty-fourth annual convention of the American Association of Equine Practitioners*, 1978, St Louis, p 465, AAEP, Lexington, Ky.
57. Prater PE, Patton CS, Held JP: Pleural effusion resulting from malignant hepatoblastoma in a horse, *J Am Vet Med Assoc* 194:383, 1989.
58. Gay CC, Sullivan ND, Wilkinson JS, et al: Hyperlipaemia in ponies, *Aust Vet J* 54:459, 1978.
59. Carlson GP: Chronic active hepatitis in horses. In Proceedings from the seventh annual veterinary forum of the American College of Veterinary Internal Medicine, printed by Omnipress, Madison, Wisc 1989, p 595, ACVIM.
60. Divers T: Biochemical diagnosis of hepatic disease and dysfunction in the horse, *Vet Clin North Am Equine Pract* 15:15, 1993.
61. Pearson EG: Hypoalbuminemia in horses, *Compend Contin Educ Pract Vet* 12:555, 1990.
62. Robinson NE, editor: *Current therapy in equine medicine*, ed 9, St Louis, 2009, WB Saunders.
63. Mendle VE: Pyrrolizidine alkaloid-induced liver disease in horses: an early diagnosis, *Am J Vet Res* 49:572, 1988.
64. Pearson EW, Craig AM: Serum bile acids for diagnosis of chronic liver disease in horses. Proceeding from the fourth annual veterinary medical forum of the American College Veterinary Internal Medicine, printed by Ominpress, Madison, Wisc 1986, pp 10-71, ACVIM.
65. Hoffman WE, Baker G, Rieser S, et al: Alterations in selected serum biochemical constituents in equids after induced hepatic disease, *Am J Vet Res* 48:1343, 1987.
66. Kaneko J, Rudolph W, Wilson D, et al: Bile acid fractionations by high performance liquid chromatography in equine liver disease, *Vet Res Commun* 16:161, 1992.
67. West HJ: Evaluation of total plasma bile acid concentration for the diagnosis of hepatobiliary disease in horses, *Res Vet Sci* 46:264, 1989.
68. Barton M, LeRoy B: Serum bile acids concentrations in healthy and clinical ill neonatal foals, *J Vet Intern Med* 21:508, 2007.
69. Lindner A, Bauer S: Effect of temperature, duration of storage and sampling procedure on ammonia concentration in equine blood plasma, *Eur J Clin Chem Clin Biochem* 31:473, 1993.
70. Hasel K, Summers B, deLahunta A: Encephalopathy with idiopathic hyperammonaemia and Alzheimer type II astrocytes in Equidae, *Equine Vet J* 31:478, 1999.
71. Peek S, Divers T, Jackson C: Hyperammonaemia associated with encephalopathy and abdominal pain without evidence of liver disease in four mature horses, *Equine Vet J* 29:70, 1997.
72. McConnico R, Duckett W, Wood P: Persistent hyperammonemia in two related Morgan Weanlings, *J Vet Intern Med* 11:264, 1997.
73. Feldman BF: Acquired disorders of hemostasis. In *Proceedings of the Seventh Annual Veterinary Medical Forum of the American College of Veterinary Internal Medicine,* printed by Ominpress, Madison, Wisc 1989, p 33, ACVIM.
74. Rantanen NW: Diseases of the liver, *Diagnostic ultrasound*, Philadelphia, 1986, WB Saunders.
75. Gossett KA, French DD: Effect of age on liver enzyme activities in serum of healthy quarter horses, *Am J Vet Res* 45:354, 1984.

76. Sherman K, Wells R, Mattiacci M: Lability of sorbitol dehydrogenase in refrigerated and frozen horse serum, *J Equine Vet Sci* 11:176, 1991.
77. Steffey E, Giri S, Dunlop C, et al: Biochemical and haematological changes following prolonged halothane anaesthesia in horses, *Equine Vet J* 25:338, 1993.
78. Bernard W, Divers TJ, Ziemer E: Isoenzyme 5 of lactate dehydrogenase as an indicator of equine hepatocellular disease, *Vet Clin Pathol* 17:19, 1988.
79. Divers T: Diagnosis of hepatic disease and dysfunction in the horse. In *Proceedings of the tenth annual veterinary medical forum of the American College of Veterinary Internal Medicine,* 1992, San Diego, CA, p 430, printed by Ominpress, Madison, Wisc; published by ACVIM.
80. Smith B, editor: *Large animal internal medicine*, ed 3, St Louis, 2003, Mosby.
81. Engelking LR, Answer MS, Lofstedt J: Hepatobiliary transport of indocyanine green and bromosulphthalein in fed and fasted horses, *Am J Vet Res* 46:2278, 1985.
82. West HJ: Clearance of bromosulphthalein from plasma as a measure of hepatic function in normal horses and in horses with liver disease, *Res Vet Sci* 44:343, 1988.
83. Morandi F, Frank N, Avenell J, et al: Quantitative assessment of hepatic function by means of ^{99m}Tc mebrofenin in healthy horses, *J Vet Intern Med* 19:751, 2005.
84. Lennox T, Wilson J, Hayden DW, et al: Hepatoblastoma with erythrocytosis in a young female horse, *J Am Vet Med Assoc* 216:718, 2000.
85. Jeffcott LB: Primary liver-cell carcinoma in a young thoroughbred horse, *J Pathol* 97:394, 1968.
86. Roby AA, Beech J, Bloom JC, et al: Hepatocellular carcinoma associated with erythrocytosis and hypoglycemia in a yearling, *J Am Vet Med Assoc* 196:465, 1990.
87. Buonanno AM, Carlson GP, Kantrowitz B: Clinical and diagnostic features of portosytemic shunt in a foal, *J Am Vet Med Assoc* 192:387, 1988.
88. Lofstedt J, Koblik PD, Jakowski RM, et al: Use of hepatobiliary scintigraphy to diagnose bile duct atresia in a lamb, *J Am Vet Med Assoc* 193:95, 1988.
89. Durhman A, Smith K, Newton J, et al: Development and application of a scoring system for prognostic evaluation of equine liver biopsies, *Equine Vet J* 35:534, 2003.
90. Mansmann RA, McAllister ES, Pratt PW, editors: *Equine medicine and surgery*, Santa Barbara, CA, 1982, American Veterinary Publication.
91. Rothenberg M, Keeffe E: Antibiotics in the management of hepatic encephalopathy: an evidence based review, *Rev Gastroerntrol Disord* 5:26, 2005.
92. Gerber T, Schomerus H: Hepatic encephalopathy in liver cirrhosis, *Drugs* 60:1353, 2000.
93. Riordan S, Williams R: Treatment of hepatic encephalopathy, *N Engl J Med* 337:473, 1997.
94. Tofteng F, Larsen F: Management of patients with fulminant hepatic failure and brain edema, *Metab Brain Dis* 19:207, 2004.
95. Scarratt W, Warnick L: Effects of oral administration of lactulose in healthy horses, *J Equine Vet Sci* 18:405, 1998.
96. Farivar M, Wands JR, Isselbacher KJ, et al: Beneficial effects of insulin and glucagon in fulminant murine viral hepatitis, *Lancet* 1:696, 1979.
97. Ohkawa M, Hayashi H, Chaudry IH, et al: Effects of regenerating liver cytosol on drug-induced hepatic failure, *Surgery* 97:455, 1985.
98. Ferenci P, Grimm G, Meryn S, et al: Successful long-term treatment of portal-systemic encephalopathy by the benzodiazepam antagonist flumazenil, *Gastroenterology* 96:240, 1989.
99. King Han M, Hyzy R: Advances in critical care management of hepatic failure and insufficiency, *Crit Care Med* 34:S225, 2006.
100. Windmeier C, Gressner A: Pharmacological aspects of pentoxifylline with emphasis on its inhibitory actions on hepatic fibrogenesis, *Gen Pharmacol* 29:181, 1997.
101. Pearson E: Liver disease in the mature horse, *Equine Vet J* 11:87, 1999.
102. Ralston S: Nutrition for clinically ill horses, *J Equine Vet Sci* 17:632, 1997.
103. Theiler A: Acute liver atrophy and parenchymatous hepatitis in horses. In *Proceeding from the fifth and sixth Res Dir Vet Res Dept Agr Union, S Africa* :9, 1917.
104. Madsen DE: Equine encephalomyelitis, *Utah Acad Sci Arts Letter* 11:95, 1934.
105. Marsh H: Supplementary note to article on equine encephalomyelitis, *J Am Vet Med Assoc* 91:330, 1937.
106. Guglick M, MacAllister C, Ely R, et al: Hepatic disease associated with administration of tetanus antitoxin in eight horses, *J Am Vet Med Assoc* 206:1737, 1995.
107. Messer N, Johnson P: Idiopathic acute hepatic disease in horses: 12 cases (1982-1992), *J Am Vet Med Assoc* 204:1934, 1994.
108. Messer N, Johnson P: Serum hepatitis in two brood mares, *J Am Vet Med Assoc* 204:1790, 1994.
109. Aleman M, Nieto J, Carr E, et al: Serum hepatitis associated with commercial plasma transfusion in horses, *J Vet Intern Med* 1:2005, 2005.
110. Robinson M, Gopinth C, Hughes DL: Histopathology of acute hepatitis in the horse, *J Comp Pathol* 85:111, 1975.
111. Thomsett LR: Acute hepatic failure in a horse, *Equine Vet J* 3:15, 1971.
112. Tyzzer EE: A fatal disease of Japanese Waltzing Mice caused by a spore-bearing bacillus, *J Med Res* 37:307, 1917.
113. Swerczek TW, Crowe MW, Prickett ME, et al: Focal bacterial hepatitis in foals, *Mod Vet Pract* 54:66, 1973.
114. Peek S, Byars T, Rueve E: Neonatal hepatic failure in a Thoroughbred foal: successful treatment of a case of presumptive Tyzzer's disease, *Equine Vet J* 6:307, 1994.
115. Sigurdardottir O: *Clostridium piliforme* infection (Tyzzer's disease) in a foal: a case report and literature survey, *Nord Vet Med* 110:79, 1998.
116. Humber KA, Sweeney RW, Saik JE, et al: Clinical and clinicopathologic findings in two foals infected with Bacillus piliformis, *J Am Vet Med Assoc* 193:1425, 1988.
117. Turk MA, Gallina AM, Perryman LE: *Bacillus piliformis* infection (Tyzzer's disease) in foals in northwest United States: a retrospective study of 21 cases, *J Am Vet Med Assoc* 178:279, 1981.
118. Carrigan MJ, Pedrana RG, McKibbin AW: Tyzzer's disease in foals, *Aust Vet J* 61:199, 1984.
119. Hook R, Riley L, Franklin C, et al: Seroanalysis of Tyzzer's disease in horses: implications that multiple strains can infect Equidae, *Equine Vet J* 27:8, 1995.
120. Borchers A, Madgesian K, Halland S, et al: Successful treatment and polymerase chain reaction (PCR) confirmation of Tyzzer's disease in a foal and clinical and pathologic characteristics in 6 additional foals (1986-2005), *J Vet Intern Med* 20:1212, 2006.
121. Sweeney HJ, Greg A: Infectious necrotic hepatitis in a horse, *Equine Vet J* 18:150, 1986.
122. Hollingsworth TC, Green VJ: Focal necrotizing hepatitis caused by *Clostridium novyi* in a horse, *Aust Vet J* 54:48, 1978.
123. Dumaresq JA: A case of black disease in the horse, *Aust Vet J* 15:53, 1939.
124. Oaks J, Kanaly T, Fiser T, et al: Apparent *Clostridium haemolyticum/ Clostridum novyi* infection and exotoxemia in two horses, *J Vet Diagn Invest* 9:324, 1997.
125. Peek S, Divers T: Medical treatment of cholangiohepatitis and cholelithiasis in mature horses: 9 cases (1991-1998), *Equine Vet J* 32:301, 2000.

126. Schulz KS, Simmons TR, Johnson R: Primary cholangiohepatitis in a horse, *Cornell Vet* 80:35, 1990.
127. Thornberg LP, Kintner LD: Cholangiohepatitis in a horse, *Vet Med Small Anim Clin* 75:1895, 1980.
128. Clabough D, Duckett W: Septic cholangitis and peritonitis in a gelding, *J AmVet Med Assoc* 200:1521, 1992.
129. Davis J, Blikslager A, Catto K, et al: A retrospective analysis of hepatic injury in horses with proximal enteritis (1984-2002), *J Vet Intern Med* 17:896, 2003.
130. Hartley WJ, Dixon RJ: An outbreak of foal perinatal mortality due to equid herpesvirus type 1: pathologic observations, *Equine Vet J* 11:214, 1979.
131. Perkins G, Ainsworthy D, Erb H, et al: Clinical, haematological and biochemical findings in foals with neonatal Equine herpesvirus-I infection compared with septic and premature foals, *Equine Vet J* 31:422, 1999.
132. Clabough D: Equine infectious anemia: the clinical signs, transmission, and diagnostic procedures, *Vet Med* 85:1007, 1990.
133. Blood DC, Radostits OM: *Veterinary medicine a textbook of the diseases of cattle, sheep, pigs, goats, and horses*, ed 7, Philadelphia, 1989, Bailler Tindall.
134. Car BD, Anderson WI: Giant cell hepatopathy in 3 aborted midterm equine fetuses, *Vet Pathol* 25:389, 1988.
135. Davis C, Barr B, Pascoe J, et al: Hepatic sarcocystosis in a horse, *J Parasitol* 85:965, 1999.
136. Hoberg E, Miller S, Brown M: *Echinococcus granulosus* (*Taeniidae*) and autochothonous echinococcosis in a North American horse, *J Parasitol* 80:141, 1994.
137. Benhazim A, Harmon B, Roberson E, et al: Hydatid disease in a horse, *J Am Vet Med Assoc* 200:958, 1992.
138. Buergelt C, Greiner E: Fibrosing granulomas in the equine liver and peritoneum: a retrospective morphologic study, *J Vet Diagn Invest* 7:102, 1995.
139. Adam SE: A review of drug hepatopathy in animals, *Vet Bull* 42:683, 1972.
140. Cohen N, Carter G: Steroid hepatopathy in a horse with glucocorticoid-induced hyperadrenocorticism, *J Am Vet Med Assoc* 200:1682, 1992.
141. Mullaney TP: Iron toxicity in neonatal foals, *Equine Vet J* 20:119, 1988.
142. Pearson E, Hedstrom O, Poppenga R: Hepatic cirrhosis and hemochromatosis in three horses, *J Am Vet Med Assoc* 204:1053, 1994.
143. Lavoie J, Teuscher E: Massive iron overload and liver fibrosis resembling haemochromatosis in a racing pony, *Equine Vet J* 25:552, 1993.
144. Gardner R, Nydam D, Mohammed H, et al: Serum gamma glutamyl transferase activity in horses with right or left dorsal displacements of the large colon, *J Vet Intern Med* 19:761, 2005.
145. Turner T, Brown C, Wilson J, et al: Hepatic lobe torsion as a cause of colic in a horse, *Vet Surg* 22:301, 1993.
146. Naylor NJ: Treatment and diagnosis of hyperlipemia and hyperlipidemia. In *Proceedings from the American College of Veterinary Internal Medicine Medical Forum*, Salt Lake City, 1982, p 47.
147. Jeffcott LB, Field JR: Current concepts of hyperlipemia in horses and ponies, *Vet Rec* 116:461, 1985.
148. Field JR: Hyperlipemia in a Quarter horse, *Compend Contin Educ Pract Vet* 10:218, 1988.
149. Bauer JE: Plasma lipids and lipoproteins of fasted ponies, *Am J Vet Res* 44:379, 1983.
150. Moore B, Abood S, Hinchcliff K: Hyperlipemia in 9 Miniature Horses and Miniature Donkeys, *J Vet Intern Med* 8:376, 1994.
151. Mogg T, Palmer J: Hyperlipidemia, hyperlipemia, and hepatic lipidosis in American Miniature Horses: 23 cases (1990-1994), *J Am Vet Med Assoc* 207:604, 1995.
152. Watson T, Burns L, Love S, et al: Plasma lipids, lipoproteins, and post heparin lipases in ponies with hyperlipidemia, *Equine Vet J* 24:341, 1992.
153. Watson T, Love S: Equine hyperlipidemia, *Compend Contin Educ Pract Vet* 16:89, 1994.
154. Forhead A, Dobson H: Plasma glucose and cortisol responses to exogenous insulin in fasted donkeys, *Res Vet Sci* 62:265, 1997.
155. Breidenbach A, Fuhrmann H, Deegen E, et al: Studies on equine lipid metabolism 2, lipolytic activities of plasma and tissue lipases in large horses and ponies, *Zentralbl Veterinarmed A* 46:39, 1999.
156. Kirk RW, editor: *Current therapy ix small animal practice*, Philadelphia, 1986, WB Saunders.
157. Naylor JM, Kronfeld DS, Acland H: Hyperlipemia in horses: effects of undernutrition and disease, *Am J Vet Res* 41:899, 1980.
158. Wensing TH, Schotman AJ, Kroneman J: Effect of treatment with glucose, galactose, and insulin in hyperlipemia in ponies, *Tijdschr Diergeneeskd* 99:919, 1974.
159. Friedman S: The cellular basis of hepatic fibrosis, *N Engl J Med* 328:1993, 1828.
160. Giles CJ: Outbreak of ragwort *(S. jacobaea)* poisoning in horses, *Equine Vet J* 3, 1983.
161. McLean EK: The toxic actions of pyrrolizidine (Senecio) alkaloids, *Pharm Res* 22:429, 1970.
162. Small A, Kelly W, Seawright A, et al: Pyrrolizidine alkaloidosis in a 2 month old foal, *J Vet Med* 40:213, 1993.
163. Lessard P, Wilson WD, Alander HJ, et al: Clinicopathologic study of horses surviving pyrrolizidine alkaloid toxicosis, *Am J Vet Res* 47:1776, 1986.
164. Curran J, Sutherland R, Peet R: A screening test for subclinical liver diseases in horses affected by pyrrolizidine alkaloid toxicosis, *Aust Vet J* 74:236, 1996.
165. Talcott P: Alsike clover and red clover poisonings in horses. In *Proceedings from the eighteenth annual veterinary medical forum of the American College of Veterinary Internal Medicine*, 2000, Seattle, WA, p 161.
166. Nation P: Hepatic disease in Alberta horses: a retrospective study of "alsike clover poisoning," *Can Vet J* 32:602, 1991.
167. Colon J, Jackson C: Hepatic dysfunction and photodermatitis secondary to alsike clover poisoning, *Compend Contin Educ Pract Vet* 189:1022, 1996.
168. Krawitt E: Autoimmune hepatitis, *N Engl J Med* 334:897, 1996.
169. White SD, Maxwell LK, Hawkins JL, et al: Pharmacokinetics of azathioprine following single-dose intravenous and oral administration and effects of azathioprine following chronic oral administration in horses, *Am J Vet Res* 66:1578-1583, 2005.
170. Barton M: Cholelithiasis in horses. In *Proceedings from the seventeenth annual veterinary medical forum of the American College of Veterinary Internal Medicine*, Chicago, 1999.
171. Scarratt WK, Fessler RL: Cholelithiasis and biliary obstruction in a horse, *Compend Contin Educ Pract Vet* 7:s428, 1985.
172. McDole MC: Cholelithiasis in a horse, *Vet Clin North Am Equine Pract* 2:37, 1980.
173. Roussel AJ, Becht JL, Adams SB: Choledocholithiasis in a horse, *Cornell Vet* 74:166, 1984.
174. Leur RJvd, Kroneman J: Three cases of cholelithiasis and biliary fibrosis in the horse, *Equine Vet J* 14:251, 1982.
175. Reef V, Johnston J, Divers T, et al: Ultrasonographic findings in horses with cholestasis: eight cases (1985-1987), *J Am Vet Med Assoc* 196:1836, 1990.
176. Durando M, McKay RJ, Staller G, et al: Septic cholangiohepatitis and cholangiocarcinoma in a horse, *J Am Vet Med Assoc* 206:1018, 1995.
177. Green DS, Davies JV: Successful choledocholithotomy in a horse, *Equine Vet J* 21:464, 1989.

178. Tulleners ER, Becht JL, Richardson DW, et al: Choledocholithotripsy in a mare, *J Am Vet Med Assoc* 186:1317, 1985.
179. Bonis P, Friedman S, Kaplan M: Is liver fibrosis reversible? *N Engl J Med* 344:452, 2001.
180. Orsini JA, Donawick WJ: Hepaticojejunostomy for treatment of common hepatic duct obstructions associated with duodenal stenosis in two foals, *Vet Surg* 18:34, 1989.
181. Reef VB, Collatos C, Spencer PA, et al: Clinical, ultrasonographic, and surgical findings in foals with umbilical remnant infections, *J Am Vet Med Assoc* 69, 1989.
182. Rumbaugh GE, Smith BP, Carlson GP: Internal abdominal abscesses in horses: a study of 25 cases, *J Am Vet Med Assoc* 172:304, 1978.
183. Sellon DC, Spaulding K, Breuhaus BA, et al: Hepatic abscesses in three horses, *J Am Vet Med Assoc* 216:882-887, 2000.
184. Tamaschke C: Beitrage zur vergleichenden onlologie der haussaugtiere, *Wiss Z Humboldt Univ [Math Naturwiss]* 1:37, 1952.
185. Roperto F, Galati P: Mixed hamartoma of the liver in an equine fetus, *Equine Vet J* 16:218, 1984.
186. Moulton JE: *Tumors in domestic animals*, ed 2, Los Angeles, 1978, University of California Press.
187. Kanemaru T, Oikaura MI, Yoshihara T: Post-mortem findings of hepatocellular carcinoma in a racehorse, *Exp Reports on Equine Health Lab* 15:8, Tokyo: Equine Health Laboratory, Japan Racing Assoc, 1964-1979.
188. Mueller PO, Morris DD, Carmichael KP, et al: Cholangiocarcinoma in a horse, *J Am Vet Med Assoc* 201:899, 1992.
189. Sironi G, Riccaboni P: A case of equine cholangiocarcinoma displaying aberrant expression of p53 protein, *Vet Rec* 141:77, 1997.
190. Lennox T, Wilson J, Hayden D, et al: Hepatoblastoma with erythrocytosis in a young female horse, *J Am Vet Med Assoc* 216:718, 2000.
191. Andel AC, Gruys E, Kroneman J: Amyloid in the horse: a report of nine cases, *Equine Vet J* 20:277, 1988.
192. Vanhooser SL, Reinemeyer CR, Held JP: Hepatic AA amyloidosis associated with severe strongylosis in a horse, *Equine Vet J* 20:274, 1988.
193. Hawthorne TB, Bolon B, Meyer DJ: Systemic amyloidosis in a mare, *J Am Vet Med Assoc* 196:323, 1990.
194. Lindsay WA, Ryder JK, Beck KA, et al: Hepatic encephalopathy caused by a portacaval shunt in a foal, *Vet Med* 83:798, 1988.
195. Beech J: Portal vein anomaly and hepatic encephalopathy in a horse, *J Am Vet Med Assoc* 170:164, 1977.
196. Leur RJvd: Biliary atresia in a foal, *Equine Vet J* 14:91, 1982.
197. Witzleben CL, Buck BE, Schnaufer BE, et al: Studies on the pathogenesis of biliary atresia, *Lab Invest* 38:525, 1978.
198. Valberg S, Ward T, Rush B, et al: Glycogen branching enzyme deficiency in quarter horse foals, *J Vet Intern Med* 15:572, 2001.

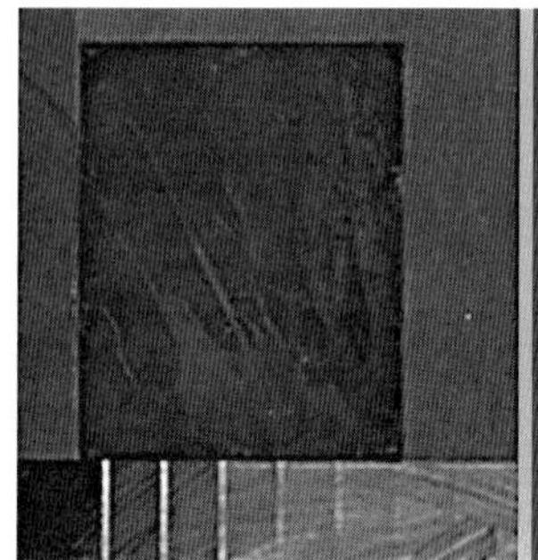

EQUINE OPHTHALMOLOGY

CHAPTER 17

David A. Wilkie

EXAMINATION

The equine eye presents particular challenges for diagnostic and therapeutic approaches. However, the basic principles of a complete ophthalmic examination hold true. Box 17-1 lists the equipment required for a routine ophthalmic examination. One should perform the initial ophthalmic examination in a well-lighted environment and before tranquilization. The examiner assesses facial, orbital, and eyelid symmetry; looks for ocular discharge (serous, mucoid, mucopurulent) or blepharospasm; and evaluates the cranial nerves, specifically cranial nerves II through VII. A complete ophthalmic examination includes assessment of pupillary light and menace response, maze testing, globe position and mobility, sensation of ocular and adnexal structures, and eyelid position and function. To evaluate direct and consensual pupillary light responses accurately often requires a bright focal light source (3.5-V halogen) and a darkened examination area.

Further examination or therapy may require some form of tranquilization, regional nerve blocks, and topical anesthesia. Detomidine (Dormosedan, Pfizer Animal Health, Exton, Pa.) administered intravenously at 0.01 to 0.02 mg/kg or xylazine (Rompun, Haver-Lockhart, Shawnee, KS) at 0.5 to 1.0 mg/kg combined with butorphanol tartrate (Torbugesic, Bristol Laboratories, Inc., Evansville, Ind.) at 0.01 mg/kg administered intravenously provide a synergistic analgesic effect and facilitate examination, sample collection, intraocular pressure determination, nasolacrimal irrigation, lavage tube placement, and minor surgical procedures. If one intends to determine intraocular pressure (IOP), it is important to note that intravenous administration of xylazine significantly lowers the IOP.[1]

Sensory innervation of the globe and adnexa is from the trigeminal nerve (cranial nerve V), and motor innervation is from the facial nerve (cranial nerve VII). The ophthalmic nerves blocked most frequently are the auriculopalpebral branch of cranial nerve VII and the supraorbital (frontal) branch of cranial nerve V. Blocking of these nerves provides akinesia and anesthesia of the superior eyelid, respectively. One can palpate the auriculopalpebral nerve as it courses over the zygomatic arch in the area of the temporofrontal suture. Using a 25-gauge, $^5/_8$-inch needle, one blocks the nerve by injecting 3 to 5 ml of mepivacaine (Carbocaine, Winthrop Laboratories, New York, N.Y.) over the zygomatic arch in this area. One blocks the supraorbital nerve as it emerges from the supraorbital foramen of the frontal bone by palpating the foramen, inserting a 25-gauge, $^5/_8$-inch needle into the foramen, and injecting 2.0 ml of mepivacaine; one infuses another 1 to 2 ml subcutaneously while removing the needle. Additional sensory nerves that are occasionally blocked include the infratrochlear, lacrimal, and zygomatic branches of cranial nerve V.[2] Alternatively, local infiltration of anesthetic can be used to provide anesthesia of a specific area. Finally, a retrobulbar nerve block may be performed for standing surgical procedures or to assist with general anesthesia. A retrobulbar block is performed using an 8-mm spinal needle. The needle is placed posterior to the dorsal bony orbital arch and directed ventrally and posterior to the globe. When the needle comes into contact with the dorsal rectus muscle of the eye, the globe will be seen to deviate dorsally. The needle is advanced just past the dorsal rectus muscle into the orbital muscle cone, and 5 to 8 ml of carbocaine is injected.

A complete ophthalmic examination can now be performed (see Box 17-1). The practitioner should obtain samples for bacterial or fungal culture or evaluation of tear production before instilling any topical solution or ointment on the eye. Aqueous production of tears is measured by using commercially available Schirmer tear test strips, with normal wetting being 20 mm or greater in 30 seconds. For a complete ophthalmic examination, the pupil should be dilated. This is performed using 1% tropicamide (Mydriacyl® Alcon Laboratories, Fort Worth, Texas) and will take 15 to 20 minutes for adequate dilation. Failure to dilate the pupil will result in abnormalities of the lens and posterior segment being overlooked. Using a bright focal light source, the practitioner now examines the conjunctiva, nictitans, cornea, anterior chamber, iris, pupil, and lens. The practitioner evaluates the ocular media (cornea, aqueous humor, lens, and vitreous) for clarity and transparency; assesses the position and size of the lens, shape and mobility of the pupil, and appearance of the corpora nigra; and examines the eye for irregularities, vascularization, and pigmentation. Although it is possible to examine the whole anterior segment using a Finoff transilluminator with or without magnification, a new handheld monocular slit lamp that attaches to an otoscope or ophthalmoscope handle is available (HSL-10, Heine, United States). The handheld slit lamp provides magnification and an appreciation for depth

BOX 17-1

EQUIPMENT FOR BASIC EQUINE OPHTHALMIC EXAMINATION

Bright, focal light source: 3.5-V halogen light with Finoff illuminator

Direct ophthalmoscope

Indirect 20-D 5× lens

Handheld slit lamp: HSL-10 attaches to direct ophthalmoscope handle (Heine, United States)

Magnifying loupe, 2×-4×

Dressing forceps

Open-ended urinary catheter (3.5 French) for nasolacrimal catheterization

No. 5 French catheter for cannulation of nasolacrimal duct at nares

Sterile fluorescein strips

Sterile rose bengal strips

Schirmer tear test strips

Sterile culture swabs

Kimura spatula for obtaining cytologic sample

Glass slides

Sterile eyewash

Proparacaine 0.5% (Alcaine): topical anesthetic

Tropicamide 1% (Mydriacyl): short-acting dilating agent

Sedation: Xylazine (Rompun)

Butorphanol tartrate (Torbugesic)

Detomidine (Dormosedan)

Mepivacaine (Carbocaine): local nerve blocks

Modified from Wilkie DA: Ophthalmic procedures and surgery in the standing horse, Vet Clin North Am Equine Pract 7:535–547, 1991.

and three-dimensional anatomy from the anterior vitreous forward. Fluorescein staining of the cornea detects the presence of corneal ulceration, and the appearance of fluorescein at the nares indicates a patent nasolacrimal system. Some ophthalmologists also use rose bengal to stain the cornea. Rose bengal will stain damaged or devitalized corneal epithelial cells and may be more sensitive than flourescein for early fungal or herpetic disease. After instillation of topical anesthesia (proparacaine 0.5%, Alcaine, Alcon Laboratories, Fort Worth, Texas), the clinician can cannulate the nasolacrimal puncta using a 3.5F urinary catheter and irrigate the nasolacrimal system. Alternatively, one can irrigate the nasolacrimal system in retrograde fashion, cannulating the duct using a 5F catheter at the nasal opening. Using thumb forceps, one can grasp the nictitans and examine the palpebral and bulbar surfaces for foreign bodies, mass lesions, or other abnormalities. Conjunctival and corneal cells are collected for cytologic study using a Kimura spatula after administration of topical anesthesia. If available, Tonopen Vet (Reichert Ophthalmic Depew, N.Y.) can be used to determine ocular pressure.

To examine the posterior segments of the eye (vitreous, optic nerve, retinal blood vessels, and tapetal and nontapetal fundus), the clinician should perform both direct and indirect ophthalmoscopy. A new monocular indirect ophthalmoscope, the PanOptic ophthalmoscope (Welch Allyn Inc., Skaneateles Falls, N.Y.) allows those more familiar with the technique of direct examination to perform indirect ophthalmoscopy. The clinician evaluates the size and color of the optic nerve, number and size of retinal blood vessels, pigmentation of the nontapetal fundus, the presence or absence of hyporeflective or hyper-reflective changes of the tapetal fundus and the vitreous for opacities or degeneration.

OCULAR ULTRASONOGRAPHY

Technique

Ocular ultrasonography is performed directly through the cornea or the eyelids or by using an offset device. The optimal transducer for ocular ultrasonography is a 10- to 20-MHz probe, but one can use a 5- to 7.5-MHz probe. Ultrasound biomicroscopy (UBM) can be performed using 25- to-100 MHz probes, allowing detailed imaging of the cornea, limbus, iridocorneal angle, and anterior uvea. Sedation, auriculopalpebral nerve block, and topical anesthesia generally are required. Sterile, water-soluble lubricating jelly works well as a contact material, provided one irrigates the cornea afterward.

Normal Anatomy

With use of a 5- to 7.5-MHz probe, the cornea and a portion of the anterior chamber are lost in the near artifact unless an offset device is used. With a probe of 10 MHz or higher, the anterior chamber and cornea can be visualized. The anterior and posterior lens capsules are visible as an echodense line at the 12 and 6 o'clock positions, whereas the remainder of the normal lens is anechoic. The iris, corpora nigra, and ciliary body are often visible. The vitreous body is normally anechoic. The posterior eye wall is visible as a concave echodensity, with the optic nerve head visible as an echodense area at the posterior pole with an anechoic optic nerve posteriorly. The orbital contents are best visualized using a 7.5-MHz transducer to evaluate the extraocular muscle cone, optic nerve, and associated structures.

Indications

Ocular ultrasound is indicated for evaluation of intraocular contents when one or more of the ocular transmitting media are opaque, including opacification of the cornea, aqueous and vitreous humors, and the lens. The most common indications for ocular ultrasound are in eyes with a cataract to evaluate for a retinal detachment, after traumatic hyphema to assess posterior segment damage, or in eyes with severe corneal opacification. In addition, ocular ultrasound can be used to evaluate the orbit in instances of exophthalmos or orbital trauma. UBM can be used to determine depth of a corneal lesion such as a squamous cell carcinoma or to examine an anterior uveal mass for extent of involvement.

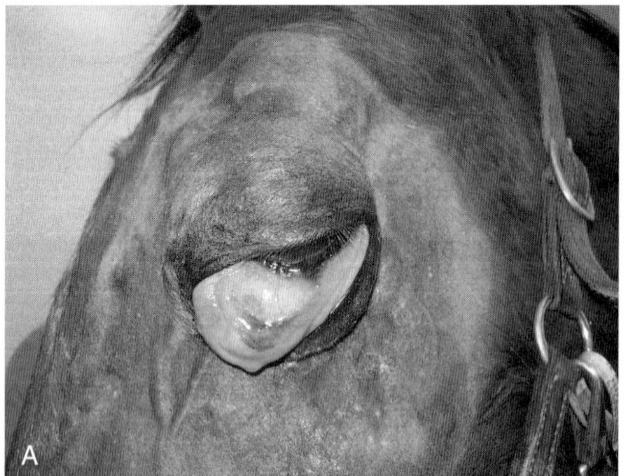

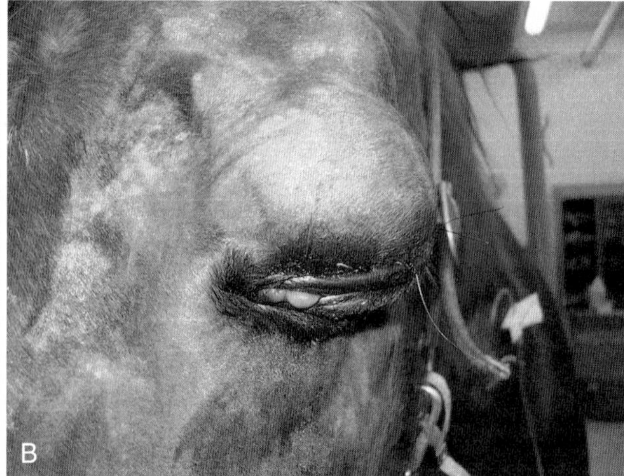

FIGURE 17-1 A, Severe blepharoedema associated with facial trauma. **B,** A temporary tarsorraphy was performed standing to prevent exposure and dessication of the cornea and conjunctiva.

EYELIDS

Congenital

Diseases of the equine eyelid are common. Congenital lesions include coloboma, agenesis, dermoid, and entropion.[3,4] Of these, entropion is the only frequently occurring disease. Entropion is inward rolling of the eyelid margin that results in facial hairs coming into contact with the cornea, leading to irritation, conjunctivitis, and possibly secondary corneal ulceration. Causes include prematurity or dehydration in foals with enophthalmos, ocular pain resulting in spastic entropion, and primary conformational problems. Manual reduction and frequent topical ocular lubrication with artificial tear ointment is the initial treatment of choice and may be the only treatment required in some foals, especially if the entropion follows dehydration. If the entropion is severe or does not respond to manipulation, the clinician may place two or three temporary vertical everting mattress sutures to position the eyelid correctly.[3] It is important to avoid overcorrection, which could lead to the inability to close the eyelids during blinking. Suture placement is at and perpendicular to the eyelid margin, tacking this to the periocular skin over the orbital rim. Monofilament, 3–0 to 5–0 nylon suture is preferrable; the sutures are removed after 10 to 14 days. The clinician must treat associated corneal disease to prevent secondary infection and subsequent scar formation. Entropion requiring more aggressive surgical intervention in the form of skin excision is rare. Severe or recurrent entropion is correctable by excising an elliptic portion of eyelid skin in the affected area and reapposing the skin edges (Hotz-Celsus procedure).

Acquired

Common acquired conditions involving the equine eyelid include trauma and neoplasia.

TRAUMA

Eyelid trauma includes contusions and lacerations.[5] Commonly associated with eyelid trauma are corneal abrasions or lacerations; anterior uveitis; and, if the trauma involves the medial canthus, nasolacrimal system damage. Eyelid contusions often result in blepharoedema and hemorrhage. Although mild blepharoedema does not require therapy, recovery can be hastened by using systemic flunixin meglumine (Banamine, Schering Corp., Kenilworth, New Jersey), cold compresses in the acute phase, and warm compresses beginning the day after the injury. In additon to the aformentioned therapy, severe blepharoedema may also require a temporary tarsorraphy and elevation of the head to protect the tissues and resolve the swelling (Figure 17-1).

Eyelid lacerations are more serious and usually require immediate therapy (Figure 17-2). The vascular supply to the eyelid is extensive, and many apparent avascular segments of eyelid recover after repair. If possible, primary wound closure is preferable. It is important to remove all debris from the wound before closure, disinfect the eyelid surface and adjacent tissues with a 1:25 to 1:50 dilution of povidone-iodine solution, avoid excessive tissue débridement, and under no circumstances amputate a pedicle of eyelid. Loss of eyelid margin, whether iatrogenic or the result of trauma, leads to severe, chronic corneal irritation; vascularization; ulceration; and fibrosis (Figure 17-3). In addition, reconstructing an eyelid margin from the adjacent skin after amputation of the normal eyelid margin is difficult.

One should suture lacerated eyelids using a two-layer closure, ensuring accurate anatomic apposition of the wound edges and eyelid margin. Minor surgical repairs can be performed using sedation and local nerve blocks, but the horse may require general anesthesia if the injury is severe. First, suture the deeper, conjunctival layer using 5-0 to 6-0 absorbable suture in a horizontal mattress pattern beginning away from and working toward the eyelid margin, taking care to avoid penetrating the conjunctiva so that the suture does not come into contact with the cornea. The practitioner then closes the skin with 5–0 to 6–0 nonabsorbable monofilament suture. The eyelid margin is the most important part of wound closure and is closed first to ensure accurate apposition. The author prefers to use a cruciate suture pattern at the eyelid margin and a simple interrupted pattern for the remainder of the skin closure. Failure to perform a two-layer closure or achieve precise apposition of the eyelid margin may result

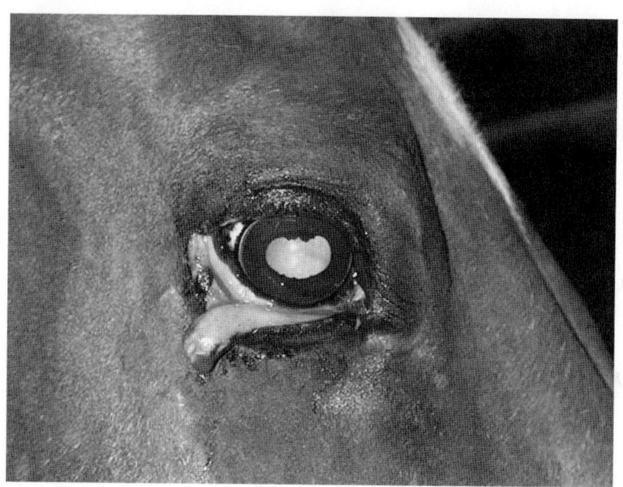

FIGURE 17-2 Tramatic laceration of the inferior lateral eyelid margin.

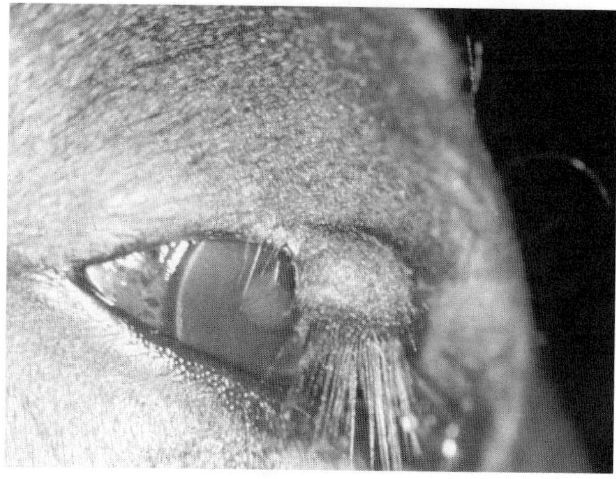

FIGURE 17-3 Failure to repair a superior eyelid lacretaion has resulted in contracture of the pedicle and exposure of the cornea.

in ulcerative keratitis or other secondary complications.[6] Postoperative therapy includes administration of antibiotics for 5 to 7 days for systemic effect; tetanus toxoid; warm, moist compresses; and flunixin meglumine if inflammation and swelling are a problem. Topical medication is not required for eyelid injuries unless corneal or anterior segment damage accompanies the injury. The practitioner must evaluate eyelid function, and the eyelid must provide adequate protection to the cornea. If the blink response is impaired, the cornea should be protected with topical lubricants as often as possible. Advanced blepharoplastic techniques for repair of severe eyelid trauma with resulting loss of tissue are beyond the scope of this chapter but are discussed in detail elsewhere.[3]

NEOPLASIA

The most common neoplasms of the equine eyelid are sarcoid and squamous cell carcinoma. In addition, melanoma, mast cell tumor, lymphosarcoma, basal cell carcinoma, and papilloma can affect the eyelid (Figure 17-4). The differential diagnosis for eyelid neoplasms includes parasitic diseases such as ocular habronemiasis and other causes of granulomatous skin disease. Treatment of eyelid neoplasia depends on the location, size, tumor type, age and purpose of the horse, cost, surgical skill, and equipment available. Treatment modalities include surgical excision, radiation therapy, intralesional chemotherapy, hyperthermia, immunotherapy, cryosurgery, or a combination of these. The aim of therapy is to eliminate or halt progression of the tumor while maintaining eyelid function and preserving the eye and vision. Complete excision with primary closure is the optimal treatment but often cannot be achieved because of limitations on availability of tissue for reconstruction and the extensive and aggressive nature of many eyelid neoplasms. If the veterinarian cannot appose eyelid margins after tumor excision, more involved blepharoplastic techniques, such as advancement skin flaps, may be indicated (Figure 17-5).

Squamous Cell Carcinoma Squamous cell carcinoma (SCC) involving the eyelid is usually erosive and ulcerative.[5] The medial canthus is the most common site of origin (see Figure 17-6). Invasion of adjacent soft and bony orbital tissue is possible if the disease is untreated. Treatment of ocular SCC is discussed in detail in the sections on conjunctiva and third eyelid.

Sarcoid Periocular sarcoid is the second most common eyelid neoplasm of the horse. The average age of an affected horse is 4 years, and smooth and warty sarcoids occur. Orbital invasion and bony involvement are possible. Surgical excision is associated with frequent recurrence and often is combined with cryosurgery, hyperthermia, chemotherapy, or irradiation to ensure complete tumor destruction. Of all treatment modalities, radiation is the most expensive and yields the best overall success.[7]

Intralesional immunotherapy with cell wall extracts of bacillus Calmette-Guérin (BCG) in oil has been used effectively in repeated injections 3 weeks apart. A total of four doses usually is required for complete tumor regression, with the overall response reported to be 69%, provided the injection was intralesional.[7] Injection of cell wall extracts of BCG is associated with local inflammation and tumor necrosis. During this period of inflammation, the clinician must protect the globe to prevent corneal desiccation or ulceration. The use of live BCG organisms or whole killed organisms has been associated with anaphylactic reaction and death and is discouraged. Adverse systemic reactions to cell wall extracts of BCG are rare, but premedication with systemic corticosteroids is advised.

Intralesional chemotherapy with cisplatin in an oil-water emulsion has been reported to result in regression of equine sarcoid.[8] A series of four injections, spaced 2 weeks apart, with a mean dose of cisplatin of 0.97 mg/cm^3 of tumor mass resulted in tumor regression in all treated horses. In addition, 87% of horses treated for sarcoids were relapse free at a 1-year follow-up. A larger study of intralesional cisplatin reported a cure rate of 96.3% for sarcoids and 88% for SCC at 4 years after treatment. [9]

CONJUNCTIVA AND THIRD EYELID

The conjunctiva is divided into bulbar and palpebral surfaces. The conjunctiva merges with the cornea at the limbus, with the eyelid at the eyelid margin, and the bulbar and palpebral conjunctiva join to form the fornix. The conjunctiva has normal resident bacterial and fungal populations. The most common isolates from the equine conjunctiva vary according to

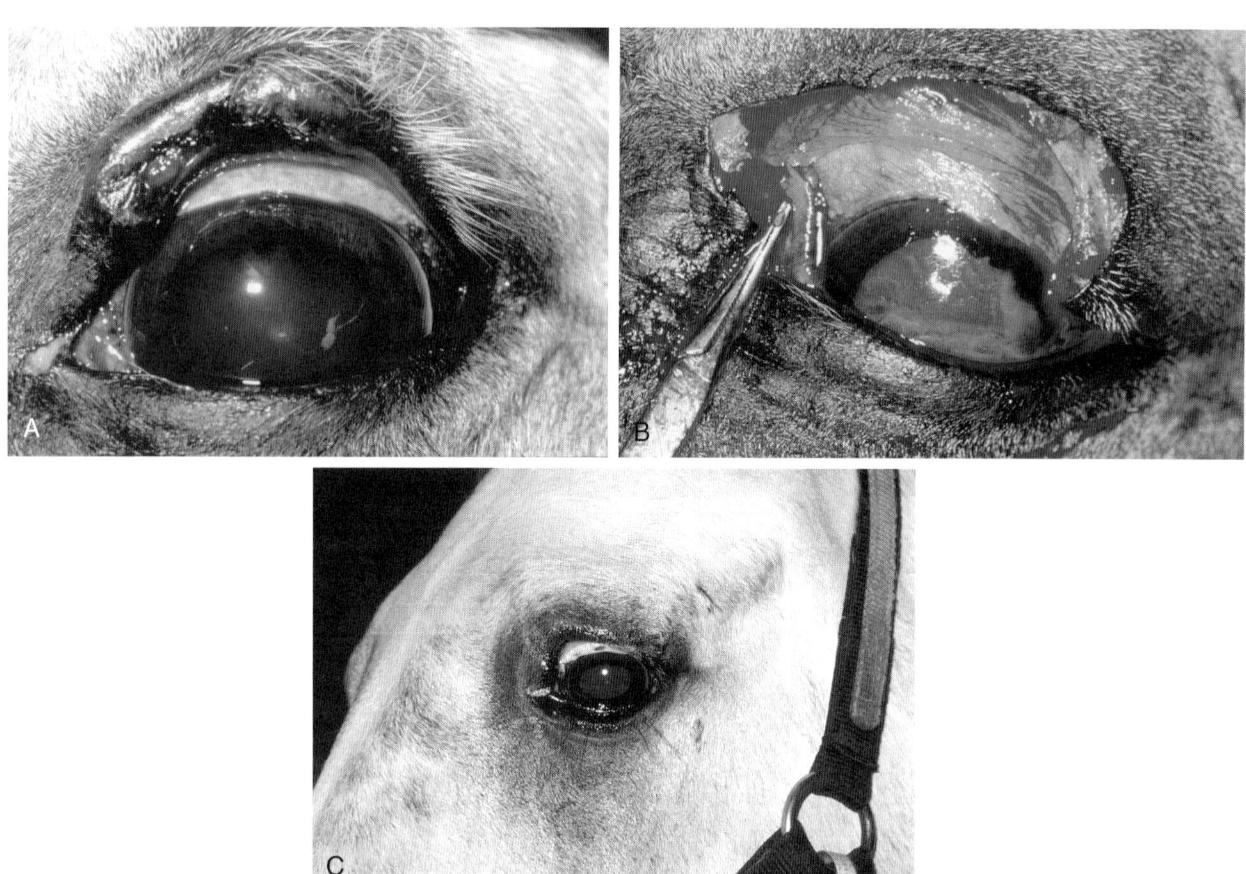

FIGURE 17-4 **A,** Melanoma of the superior eyelid. **B,** An excisional biopsy is performed, and the resulting defect cannot be closed by primary closure of the eyelid margins. **C,** An advancement graft is performed to reconstruct the superior eyelid.

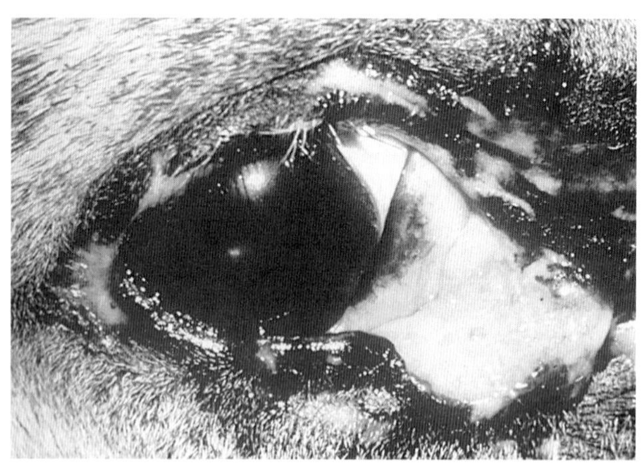

FIGURE 17-5 Squamous cell carcinoma involving the medial canthus and inferior eyelid of a 19-year-old Appaloosa.

geography, season of the year, and investigator.[10-12] In general, isolates of gram positive organisms—*Corynebacterium, Bacillus, Staphylococcus,* and *Streptomyces*—are more common than gram negative organisms from normal equine conjunctiva.[11] Fungi are isolated more commonly in the summer and autumn and have been reported to be present in 95% of normal horse conjunctiva samples.[12] In addition, fungi are isolated more frequently from stabled horses, which likely relates to the immediate environmental and husbandry conditions.[11]

Congenital diseases of the equine conjunctiva are uncommon, conjunctival dermoid being the most common congenital abnormality. A dermoid is a congenital tumor of skin and associated glands, hair, and hair follicles that can affect the cornea and adjacent conjunctiva. A dermoid that is irritating the globe or adnexa should be surgically removed by superficial keratectomy or conjunctivectomy.

Unlike the small animal patient, horses rarely acquire infectious conjunctivitis. Organisms reported to result in infectious conjunctivitis in the horse include equine herpesvirus type 2,[13] *Mycoplasma* spp., *Chlamydia, Moraxella equi,* and mycotic and viral agents.[3]

Foreign bodies and trauma are common causes of conjunctival irritation and damage and often are associated with concurrent eyelid and corneal injuries. The clinician directs treatment to eliminate the cause, treat any conjunctival or associated eyelid or corneal damage, and prevent secondary infection. A complete ophthalmic examination is necessary in all animals with evidence of ocular trauma. Conjunctival foreign bodies should be considered in any horse with a recurrent corneal erosion, ocular pain, or conjunctivitis. The clinician should examine the superior and inferior fornices and the bulbar and palpebral surface of the nictitans after topical administration of 0.5% proparacaine. Magnification is essential to detect foreign bodies. In addition, irrigation of the nasolacrimal system may yield foreign material associated with chronic conjunctivitis or dacryocystitis.

Severe chemosis with conjunctival prolapse and exposure may result from self-trauma, especially associated with being recumbent for a prolonged time. Treatment includes systemic anti-inflammatory drugs; artificial tear ointment to protect exposed conjunctiva; elevation of the head; and, in severe cases, repositioning of the conjunctiva and a temporary tarsorraphy until the swelling resolves (see Figure 17-1).

Parasites

Common parasites of the equine conjunctiva include *Thelazia lacrymalis*, *Habronema* spp., and *Onchocerca cervicalis*.[14] In a necropsy sample the prevalence of *Thelazia* organisms in the conjunctival sac of horses is highest in young animals, with 43% of 1- to 4-year-old horses being affected.[15] In most instances infection is not associated with clinical signs, but chronic conjunctivitis, seromucoid discharge, and conjunctival nodules can occur.[3] The adult parasite may be visible on ophthalmic examination of the cornea and conjunctival fornix, and larvae may be visible on examination of centrifuged samples of nasolacrimal washes. Treatment includes removal of the adult worms, irrigation of the nasolacrimal system, topical corticosteroids to reduce inflammation, and fly control. The topical organophosphates echothiophate, 0.03% to 0.06% every 12 hours, or isoflurophate, 0.025% every 24 hours for 7 days, have been reported to kill the parasite.[16] Systemic treatment with fenbendazole at 10 mg/kg orally every 24 hours for 5 days also is reported to be effective against *Thelazia* organisms.[17]

Ocular manifestations of equine cutaneous habronemiasis result when the house or stable fly deposits the larvae of the *Habronema* spp. on or around the eye.[3,18,19] The resulting granuloma is associated with inflammation, intense pruritus, and epiphora. Yellow, caseous granules are notable throughout the granulation tissue. Histologically, eosinophils and mast cells predominate. Diagnosis is based on clinical signs, location, season of the year, and histologic findings. Clinical appearance can simulate squamous cell carcinoma. Histologically, the differential diagnosis is equine cutaneous mastocytosis.[3,19] Ocular lesions are most common at the medial canthus and may involve the skin, nasolacrimal duct, third eyelid, or conjunctiva. Treatment of equine cutaneous habronemiasis varies, and no single treatment is routinely successful.[18] Surgical excision, cryosurgery, local and systemic corticosteroid therapy, systemic ivermectin (single dose, 0.2 mg/kg intramuscularly), various larvicidal treatments in the form of topical and systemic organophosphates, and various topical formulations containing ronnel or metrifonate with a dimethyl sulfoxide vehicle are used[3,18,19] (Table 17-1). Dimethyl sulfoxide serves as a vehicle and has anti-inflammatory effects, possibly related to its ability to detoxify hydroxyl radicals generated by neutrophils. The aim of therapy is to kill the larvae while controlling the resulting inflammation. In addition, fly control is an essential part of an overall management program.

The blood-sucking midge *Culicoides nubeculosus* transmits *O. cervicalis* microfilariae. After transmission the immature microfilariae migrate through lymphatics and can travel to ocular and adnexal tissues. The prevalence of equine onchocerciasis increases with age, with an overall prevalence of 50% to 60%.[14,20-22] The prevalence of onchocerciasis on histologic examination of the lateral bulbar conjunctiva is 10.8%. The presence of conjunctival microfilaria does not correlate with clinical abnormalities. Ocular onchocerciasis has been proposed as a cause of keratitis, conjunctivitis, equine recurrent uveitis, and depigmentation of the temporal bulbar conjunctiva.[22] The pathogenesis is thought to involve the death of the microfilariae, release of antigens, and development of hypersensitivity in susceptible horses. Treatment is indicated in those horses with active conjunctivitis, keratitis, or uveitis attributable to onchocerciasis and includes anti-inflammatory agents such as topical corticosteroids and systemic flunixin meglumine; topical echothiophate iodide 0.025%; and systemic diethylcarbamazine, levamisole, or ivermectin[3] (Table 17-2).

TABLE 17-1

Topical Preparations Used to Treat Equine Cutaneous Habronemiasis

Ingredients	Amount
Ronnel solution (33%)[13]	60 ml
Thiabendazole (33%)[13]	120 g
9-Fluoroprednisolone acetate[13]	60 mg
Dimethyl phthalate (24%)[13]	30 ml
Dimethyl sulfoxide[13]	500 ml
Nitrofurantoin ointment[14]	225 g
Ronnel solution[14]	20 ml
Dimethyl sulfoxide[14]	20 ml
Dexamethasone solution[14]	20 ml
Nitrofurazone ointment (0.2%)[15]	135 g
Trichlorfon (12.3%)[15]	30 ml
Dexamethasone (2 mg/ml)[15]	30 ml
Dimethyl sulfoxide[15]	30 ml

TABLE 17-2

Systemic Treatment of Ocular Onchocerciasis

Drug	Dose
Diethylcarbamazine	4.4-6.6 mg/kg/day orally for 21 days
Levamisole	1.1 mg/kg/day orally for 7 days
Ivermectin	0.2-0.5 mg/kg intramuscularly

Neoplasia

Neoplasms affecting the conjunctiva and third eyelid include SCC, lymphosarcoma, melanocytoma, mastocytoma, hemangioma, and angiosarcoma.[3,16] Diagnosis and characterization of adnexal neoplasms are based on history, signalment, location, appearance, and histopathologic examination. Routine surgical biopsy is performed with sedation, local nerve blocks, and topical anesthesia. Most adnexal neoplasms are benign or locally invasive, the exception being ocular angiosarcoma, which is reported to have a high incidence of metastasis.[23] Treatment of adnexal neoplasms varies according to tumor type, location, and size; use of the animal; treatment modalities

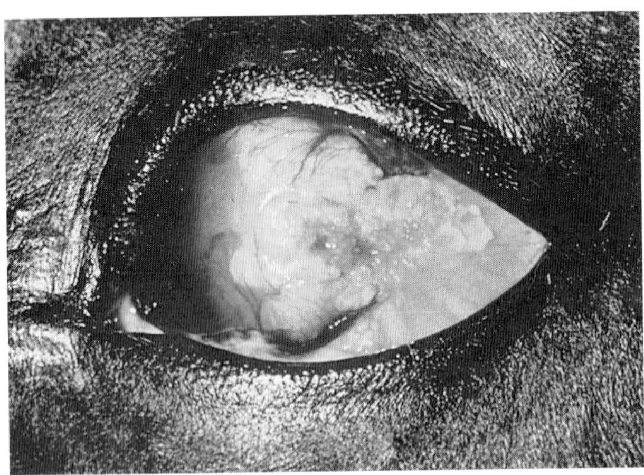

FIGURE 17-6 Squamous cell carcinoma affecting the temporal conjunctiva, limbus, and cornea.

available; and cost. The aim of treatment is to eliminate the tumor, restore normal anatomy, and maintain function of the eye and associated structures.

SCC is the most common tumor of the equine eye and adnexa (Figure 17-6). Involvement can be unilateral or bilateral, with the third eyelid and medial canthus affected most frequently.[16,24] Involvement of the corneal limbus, sclera, conjunctiva, and other adnexal structures also has been reported.[16,24,25]

The mean age of onset for SCC is 9.8 years for all horses compared with 3.8 years for ocular sarcoidosis.[25] The incidence of ocular SCC is higher in draft-breed horses and Appaloosas than in light horses,[26,27] and sexually intact males and females have a decreased incidence.[26] Adnexal hypopigmentation and increased exposure to actinic radiation[25,26] are hypothesized to predispose horses to develop ocular SCC.

Ocular SCC is malignant and locally invasive with the potential to metastasize.[22,28] Metastases to local and cranial mediastinal lymph nodes, parotid salivary glands, and the thoracic cavity occur in 10% to 15% of patients.[27]

Treatment of ocular SCC varies and must be designed for the individual patient. Surgical excision,[25] radiofrequency hyperthermia,[29] cryotherapy,[30] immunotherapy,[30] radiation therapy,[25,28-30] intralesional chemotherapy,[8,31] laser surgery,[5] or a combination of these[29,30] have been used with success. Location, size, and depth of the tumor; visual status; financial commitment; purpose of the animal; and the presence or absence of metastatic disease influence the choice of therapy.

If possible, complete surgical excision is curative and is the preferred therapy. Difficulty arises with surgical excision when preservation of the globe and ocular and adnexal anatomy and function are required. Complete excision of the third eyelid is possible and often can be performed using sedation and local nerve blocks. To prevent possible herniation of the orbital fat, the clinician should appose the bulbar and palpebral margins of the third eyelid conjunctiva after excision using 5–0 to 6–0 absorbable suture in a simple continuous pattern.

Most SCCs are radiosensitive and can be treated successfully with sources of β- or γ-radiation. The major disadvantage of less expensive modes of radiation therapy, such as strontium 90 (^{90}Sr), a source of β-radiation, is the size limit of tumor amenable to treatment. With ^{90}Sr, for example, half the β-radiation produced is lost after passage through 1 mm of soft tissue. Thus the practitioner should limit treatment to lesions less than 2 mm deep, such as corneal, scleral, or superficial conjunctival SCCs. Radiation is most appropriate as an adjunct therapy after surgical removal of a corneal or conjunctival SCC. When used appropriately, ^{90}Sr can achieve a nonrecurrence rate for SCC of 87.5% after 2 years.[32]

The use of interstitial radiotherapy for periocular SCC has been reported.[29,32] Radioactive gold seeds (^{198}Au) were used to impart a medium-energy γ-ray (0.41 MeV) with a half-life of 93.3 hours for a total recommended dose of 5000 rad.[29] Success rates of 80% at 1 year and 70% at 2 years are reported.[32] Disadvantages of radioactive implants are their substantial cost, their limited availability, the risks associated with human exposure, and the licensing restrictions on their handling.[29] Secondary complications of interstitial radiation therapy include temporary corneal opacity, local necrosis, hair loss, damage to normal structures, and local depigmentation.[29,32] Although no retinal or lens changes have been reported after interstitial radiation treatment, the practitioner should consider the possibility of photoreceptor damage and cataractogenesis following radiation therapy.

Radiofrequency hyperthermia involves the passage of a radiofrequency (2 MHz) electric current between two electrodes. Tissue between these probes offers resistance, resulting in thermal energy being transferred to the tissue. Tissue temperature increases to 50° C in a 1-cm^2 area,[29] with malignant cells exhibiting a greater sensitivity to thermal energy than normal cells. The practitioner should not use topical radiofrequency hyperthermia as the only mode of treatment for tumors extending deeper than 3 mm or those greater than 4 to 5 cm in diameter. Superficial eyelid SCCs or corneal and conjunctival SCCs are most appropriate for treatment using radiofrequency hyperthermia. The practitioner should be careful not to overlap the fields of exposure, especially in corneal tumors, because this creates a risk of excessive necrosis of normal tissue.[33]

Cryosurgery using nitrous oxide (–80° C) or liquid nitrogen (–185° C) in a single freeze- or double freeze-thaw cycle results in tissue destruction. Cryodestruction is most often indicated for treatment of eyelid SCCs. Associated local depigmentation of skin and hair may occur in the treated area. The practitioner should use thermocouples, and tissue temperatures of –25° C are optimal.

Intralesional chemotherapy with cisplatin or bleomycin in an oil-water emulsion has been reported to result in regression of equine SCC. Treatment is the same as previously described for eyelid sarcoidosis. Of those horses with adnexal SCC treated with intralesional cisplatin, 65% to 93% were relapse free at 1 year.[8,31] A second study reported a success of 88% at 4 years.[9]

Regardless of the treatment used, frequent and continued follow-up examinations result in the greatest long-term success in managing ocular and periocular SCC. Recurrence may happen at the initial site of involvement and must be distinguished from granulation tissue associated with the previous treatment. In addition, the practitioner must monitor other sites and the opposite eye for the development of new SCC lesions.

NASOLACRIMAL SYSTEM

The nasolacrimal system consists of the superior and inferior puncta and canaliculi, nasolacrimal sac, nasolacrimal duct, and nasal punctum located on the floor of the nasal vestibule.[34] The nasolacrimal system serves to carry tears from the medial canthus of the eye to the nasal vestibule. Abnormalities of the nasolacrimal system result in epiphora, an overflow of tears, following an impairment in drainage of tears. Epiphora can be serous, mucoid, or mucopurulent and must be differentiated from reflex lacrimation resulting from ocular irritation or inflammation. Examination of the nasolacrimal system includes placement of fluorescein stain in the conjunctival cul-de-sac and observing its appearance at the nasal opening. The nasolacrimal system can be irrigated antegrade from the eyelid punctum or retrograde from the nasal punctum. The practitioner applies topical anesthetic (0.5% proparacaine) to the eye and places a 3.5F open-ended feline urinary catheter in the superior punctum. Sterile eyewash or saline (10 to 20 ml) is used to irrigate the system, and fluid is observed passing out of first the inferior punctum and subsequently the nasal punctum. If performing retrograde irrigation from the nasal punctum, the practitioner uses a 5F or 6F urinary catheter and increases the volume of irrigating solution. Radiographic imaging of the nasolacrimal duct, dacryocystorhinography, can be performed using contrast material injected into the duct from the superior eyelid punctum.[3,34]Lateral and oblique radiographic views are best, and useful contrast materials include 60% barium sulfate (Novapaque, Picker Corp., Cleveland, Ohio) and 31% diatrizoate meglumine and diatrizoate sodium (Renovist II, Bristol-Myers Squibb, Princeton, N.J.). Indications for dacryocystorhinography include chronic epiphora, inability to irrigate the nasolacrimal duct, suspicion of a nasolacrimal foreign body, and evaluation of the nasolacrimal duct for congenital or acquired abnormalities. The nasolacrimal duct can also be imaged using a computed tomography (CT) scanner.

Abnormalities of the nasolacrimal system can be congenital or acquired. In the horse the most common congenital abnormality is atresia of the distal portion of the nasolacrimal duct and the nasal punctum, which results in mucoid epiphora at 3 to 4 months of age.[3,35]Additional congenital abnormalities include atresia of an eyelid punctum, abnormal placement of an eyelid punctum, and multiple nasal openings.[3,16] Whether these conditions are inherited is unknown. To correct an atretic nasal opening, the clinician passes a catheter from the inferior eyelid punctum to the level of the atresia. The clinician then palpates the end of the catheter in the nasal vestibule and makes an incision through the nasal mucosa overlying the catheter, exposing the catheter. The clinician then brings the tubing out the nasal opening and, along with the portion of tubing from the inferior punctum, sutures it to the skin of the face. The tubing is left in place for 3 to 4 weeks, and topical broad spectrum ophthalmic antibiotic solution is administered during this time.

Acquired conditions of the nasolacrimal system include dacryocystitis, foreign body obstruction, trauma, and involvement secondarily in neoplastic or inflammatory conditions of the medial canthus. Dacryocystitis appears as a mucopurulent ocular discharge without associated ocular inflammation. Dacryocystitis and foreign body obstructions are treated by nasolacrimal irrigation, as previously described, and bacterial and fungal culture with or without the aid of radiographic or CT evaluation. Topical broad spectrum ophthalmic antibiotic solution is administered after irrigation. Topical corticosteroids or systemic nonsteroidal anti-inflammatory drugs (NSAIDs) can also be used to help control swelling and inflammation. Traumatic or other damage to the nasolacrimal duct is best repaired at the time of injury, and placement of a tube in the nasolacrimal duct for 3 to 4 weeks to maintain patency while healing occurs is recommended. Surgical repair of the nasolacrimal duct is a referral procedure and requires general anesthesia. If the nasolacrimal duct cannot be made patent, treatment is symptomatic therapy for the epiphora or surgical trephination (conjunctivorhinotomy) to create a new outflow pathway for the tears.

CORNEA

Anatomy and Physiology

The cornea consists of the epithelium, stroma, Descemet's membrane, and endothelium. The epithelium is 7 to 15 cells thick and is replaced every 7 to 10 days. The corneal endothelium is a monolayer of cells with little to no regenerative capacity. Damage to the endothelium is therefore of great significance, because complete repair is often not possible and results in permanent corneal edema. The cornea is transparent and avascular and is supplied with sensory nerves from the ophthalmic branch of the trigeminal nerve. The epithelium and anterior stroma are innervated richly with sensory nerves, whereas the middle and inner cornea is less well supplied. Nutrition and waste removal are carried out by the tear film, aqueous humor, and diffusion to and from the scleral and conjunctival blood vessels. The cornea is maintained in a state of deturgescence by the mechanical barrier and pump mechanisms of the epithelium and endothelium. Interference with these barriers results in corneal edema, with endothelial damage being the more significant. Chronic irritation of the cornea results in superficial vascularization, whereas inflammation of the anterior uvea results in deep corneal vascularization. Corneal pigmentation often follows vascularization. Cellular infiltration of the cornea occurs in neoplastic, infectious, and inflammatory disease. All of these processes can occur alone or in combination, resulting in an alteration of corneal transparency. In addition, scar formation and noncellular infiltrates such as mineral and phospholipid deposits (corneal degeneration) alter corneal transparency. Establishing the cause of these changes and, if possible, eliminating the cause are essential.

Ulcerative Diseases

Corneal ulceration is perhaps the most frustrating and potentially devastating disease of the equine eye. Of all species commonly treated in veterinary ophthalmology, the cornea of the horse is the slowest to heal, is the most likely to become infected, and has the poorest prognosis for outcome. In addition, the size and temperament of the animal make frequent treatment difficult for owner and veterinarian. In most instances corneal ulceration results from an initial trauma, but secondary infection is common, especially in eyes treated with topical corticosteroids after ulceration.

CLINICAL SIGNS AND DIAGNOSIS

A corneal ulcer is a break in the corneal epithelium. Clinically, ulceration results in lacrimation, blepharospasm, photophobia, conjunctival hyperemia, corneal edema, and possibly miosis and aqueous flare. The diagnosis of a corneal ulcer is based on these clinical signs and fluorescein staining of the cornea. The underlying stroma retains the fluorescein stain and appears green. Before instilling any therapeutic or diagnostic agents in the eye, the veterinarian should submit bacterial and fungal culture samples from all corneal ulcers in the horse and should obtain culture samples from the margin of the ulcer. After obtaining culture samples and staining the cornea with fluorescein, the veterinarian applies topical anesthetic and obtains a scraping from the ulcer for cytologic examination. The cells are placed on a glass slide and stained to allow examination for bacteria, fungal hyphae, and cell type. Gram and Giemsa stains work well for examination. The presence of gram negative rods indicates the possibility of an infection with *Pseudomonas* spp., whereas cocci are suggestive of *Streptococcus* spp., a frequent and severe corneal pathogen. The presence of fungal hyphae is pathognomonic for mycotic keratitis, with *Aspergillus* spp. and *Fusarium* spp. being the most frequent corneal pathogens. Mixed bacterial and fungal infections are common.

A corneal ulcer is characterized according to size, depth, and the presence or absence of cellular infiltration. In addition, the veterinarian examines the anterior chamber for anterior uveitis. With all corneal ulcers, attempting to establish the cause of the ulceration and eliminate it is esssential (Figure 17-7). The veterinarian examines the palpebral conjunctiva and bulbar surface of the nictitans for the presence of a foreign body, evaluates the blink response and tear film, and obtains a complete history regarding trauma and previous medication. Topical corticosteroids should not be administered in the presence of a corneal ulcer, and a history of previous topical corticosteroid therapy increases the likelihood of infectious, especially fungal, keratitis.

Some specific types of corneal ulcers in the horse include indolent ulcers,[36] ulcers with eosinophilic cellular infiltrate,[37] collagenase and mycotic ulcers, and possibly viral ulcerative keratitis.[3,16]

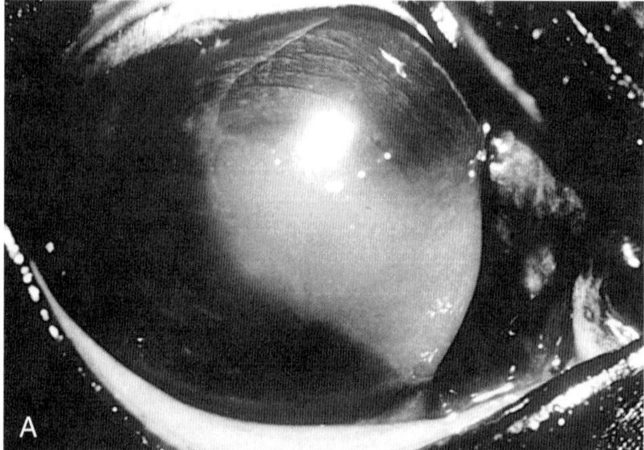

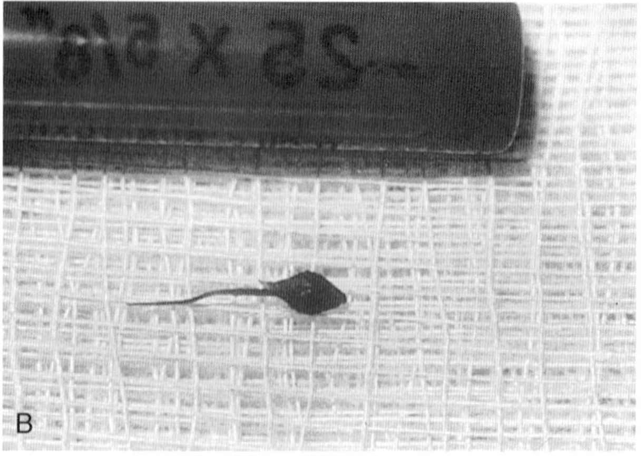

FIGURE 17-7 A, Chronic, superficial corneal ulcer. The shape and orientation of the corneal ulcer suggest a foreign body on the bulbar surface of the nictitans. **B,** Foreign body removed after examination of the bulbar surface of the nictitans.

ROUTINE TREATMENT

Treatment of an uncomplicated corneal ulcer involves controlling pain and inflammation, eliminating or preventing infection, and preventing secondary complications (Table 17-3). Healing occurs by migration and mitosis of the adjacent epithelial cells and, depending on the size of the ulcer, should be complete in 2 to 6 days for an uncomplicated corneal ulcer. Complicated corneal ulcers are those that fail to heal in an appropriate time, are secondarily infected, have an ongoing source of irritation or reulceration, have a collagenase component, are associated with corneal vascularization, or are worsening despite appropriate treatment.

If miosis is evident, the clinician can admininster topical atropine 1% to dilate the pupil, decrease the pain of anterior uveitis, and prevent posterior synechiae formation. Topical atropine is used as needed to dilate the pupil, but treatment frequency should not exceed 4 times daily. All topical ophthalmic medications are absorbed and have systemic effects, and topical atropine can result in colic following ileus. While administering topical atropine, the clinician should evaluate intestinal motility by auscultation, and the owner should observe for fresh fecal material in the stall every day. Systemic flunixin meglumine is indicated to suppress inflammation and control pain associated with a corneal ulcer, which in combination with topical atropine helps dilate the pupil.

Topical broad spectrum antibiotics such as neomycin-bacitracin-polymyxin B ophthalmic are the initial antibiotics of choice. Ointments are preferred for their ease of administration and prolonged corneal contact time. Frequency of administration varies according to severity of the disease. When topical antibiotics are used prophylactically for an uncomplicated corneal ulcer treatment, administration three or four times daily is sufficient, but in severe infectious keratitis, therapy might be hourly. If infection with *Pseudomonas* spp. is suspected, topical gentamicin, polymyxin B, tobramycin, or preferably ciprofloxacin or ofloxacin is indicated every 2 to 4 hours. Although gram positive organisms predominate initially in equine infectious keratitis, intensive topical antimicrobial therapy results in a significant shift to gram negative organisms and a change in susceptibility patterns.[38,39] Additional treatment varies according to the type and severity of the ulcer (see the section on complicated ulcerative diseases). Topical corticosteroids should not be administered to a horse with a corneal ulcer.

COMPLICATED ULCERATIVE DISEASES

Complicated corneal ulcers are those that require treatment over and above routine ulcer management, are infected, exhibit chronicity or recurrence, are in imminent danger of perforation, or have a collagenase component (Figure 17-8). Secondary infection of a corneal ulcer is suggested by increasing pain, corneal edema, interstitial keratitis associated with an

TABLE 17-3

Commonly Used Ophthalmic Medications

Route	Category	Drug	Indication	Dose*
TOPICAL				
	Antibiotics	Gentamicin	Corneal ulceration	q2-6h
		Neomycin-bacitracin-polymyxin B	Corneal ulceration	q2-6h
		Ciprofloxacin	Corneal ulceration	q2-6h
		Ocufloxacin	Corneal ulceration	q2-6h
		Tobramycin 0.3% (Tobrex)	Corneal ulceration	q2-6h
	Antifungals	Natamycin (Natacyn)	Corneal ulceration with suspected fungal keratitis	q2-4h
		1% Miconazole IV, topical	Corneal ulceration with suspected fungal keratitis	q2-4h
		1% Voriconazole		
		Intraconazole/DMSO		q2-4h
	Anti-inflammatories			
	Corticosteroids	1.0% Prednisolone acetate (Econopred Plus)		1-6/day
		0.1% Dexamethasone solution (Decadron)		1-6/day
		0.05% Dexamethasone ointment (Decadron)		1-6/day
	Nonsteroidal	0.03% Flurbiprofen (Ocufen)		4/day
		0.1% Diclofenac		q1-4/day
		1.0% Suprofen (Profenal)		4/day
	Parsympatholytics	Tropicamide 1%	Diagnostic agent to dilate the pupil	single dose
		Atropine 1%	Therapeutic agent to dilate the pupil long term	1-4 day
SUBCONJUNCTIVAL (Do not exceed a volume of 1.0 ml)	Anti-inflammatories	Dexamethasone acetate		10-15 mg
		Betamethasone		5-15 mg
SYSTEMIC				
	Anti-inflammatories	Flunixin meglumine	Extra- or intraocular inflammation	1.1mg/kg PO,IM,IV q12-24h
		Phenylbutazone	Extra- or intraocular inflammation	2-4mg/kg PO q12-24h
		Aspirin	Extra- or intraocular inflammation	25 mg/kg PO q12-24h
	Antifungal	Fluconazole	Fungal keratitis	1 mg/kg PO q12h x 12d Then q24h x 7d

*PO, Orally; IM, intramuscularly; IV, intravenously

increase in stromal inflammatory cells, corneal vascularization, purulent discharge, severe anterior uveitis, and stromal necrosis and liquefaction.

In many instances, complicated corneal ulcers require frequent and prolonged therapy, and some form of medication delivery system is indicated to ensure adequate treatment. Use of subpalpebral and nasolacrimal medication delivery systems has been described previously.[40] The author prefers to use the commercially available Mila lavage catheter (Mila International, Inc., Erlanger, KY.). When a lavage catheter is used, it should be kept clean and medication should be delivered to the eye slowly using air to push the medication through the tubing. Medication used with a subpalpebral lavage system must be in solution, not ointment. The volume of medication used at each treatment time should be 0.1 to 0.2 ml, and air must be used to deliver this medication to the eye. The use of irrigating solution to deliver the medication dilutes the medication. Once daily the system should be irrigated with sterile eyewash to ensure its patency and to rinse away mucus buildup.

Complications from a subpalpebral lavage system include trauma during tube placement, improper placement of the catheter or foot plate, irritation to the cornea from the tubing, and migration of the tubing. Observation of the medication reaching the cornea always is essential. Improper placement or migration of the tube may result in delivery of medication to the subcutaneous tissues and severe irritation. If corneal trauma occurs, the clinician must remove the tube and replace it or find an alternative means of medication. Many complicated corneal ulcers require a combination of surgical and medical therapy to improve the likelihood of a successful outcome.

INDOLENT CORNEAL ULCERATION

Indolent corneal ulcers are by definition chronic and superficial.[36,41] Indolent ulcers often have a rim of loose or detached epithelium at the margin, are associated with focal corneal edema and moderate discomfort, and elicit minimal corneal vascularization. As with all chronic corneal ulceration, the veterinarian must examine the eyelids, conjunctiva, and third eyelid thoroughly for the presence of foreign bodies, ectopic cilia, or other abnormality that might result in persistent ulceration.

The cause of indolent ulcers is suspected to be a failure in the attachment of the corneal epithelium to the underlying basement membrane. This attachment normally develops after epithelial migration and mitosis in the repair of a corneal ulcer. A basement membrane abnormality is suspected to be the underlying problem.

Treatment of indolent corneal ulcers includes removal of abnormal, loose epithelium and facilitation of epithelial attachment. After sedation, auriculopalpebral nerve block, and topical anesthesia, the veterinarian débrides the loose epithelial margins of the indolent ulcer to the point of normal attachment using a cotton swab or cilia forceps. A superficial linear keratotomy using a 25-gauge needle may facilitate healing in some instances but will also expose the corneal stroma and increase the potential for infectious keratitis. A linear keratotomy is performed using the beveled edge of the needle to create a series of superficial, parallel horizontal and vertical grooves in the cornea 0.5 to 1.0 mm apart that extend through the basement membrane and need be only deep enough to be visualized.

These areas serve as attachment sites for the migrating epithelium, shortening the healing time. Topical tetracycline has been shown to shorten time to healing for indolent ulcers in other species and is indicated every 6 to 8 hours. Tetracycline works not as an antimicrobial but as a matrix metalloproteinase inhibitor and anti-inflammatory. Topical, broad spectrum antibiotics are administered every 6 hours for prophylaxis, and if miosis is present, atropine 1% is used as needed to dilate the pupil. Systemic NSAIDs improve patient comfort. Topical soft contact lenses or hyperosmotics have been advocated for indolent corneal ulceration but are of no benefit in the author's opinion, and topical corticosteroids are contraindicated. A superficial keratectomy or a conjunctival pedicle graft or both can be used for indolent ulcers that fail to respond to débridement and superficial linear keratotomy. Corneal sequestration is also possible in the horse and will appear as an indolent-like ulcer that fails to respond to therapy. A superficial keratectomy is indicated in the case of corneal sequestration.

SUPERFICIAL PUNCTATE KERATITIS

Superficial punctate keratitis is characterized by multifocal, lacelike epithelial to subepithelial corneal opacities, some of which may be flourescein positive, with mild corneal edema. Blepharospasm may be evident, but many horses are asymptomatic. The cause is unknown, but viral agents, specifically equine herpesvirus type 1, onchocerciasis, and immune-mediated causes, have been proposed.[5,13,16]

Treatment recommendations vary and include topical antibiotic and corticosteroid application three to four times daily, topical cyclosporin A,[46] topical antiviral therapy, or a combination of these. Although the condition may respond to topical corticosteroids, recurrence is common, and extreme caution is essential when using topical corticosteroids. Topical ophthalmic antiviral agents (idoxuridine and trifluridine) or cyclosporin are administered every 6 to 8 hours and are the treatment of choice for most ophthalmologists.

EOSINOPHILIC KERATOCONJUNCTIVITIS

Presenting symptoms of eosinophilic keratitis include blepharospasm, chemosis, and conjunctivitis, but the hallmark feature is a yellow-white caseous plaque adhering to the limbal cornea with perilesional edema and corneal ulceration[37,43] (Figure 17-9). Similar caseous material may also be found adhering to areas of ulcerated conjunctiva. Cytologically, the caseous material is predominantly eosinophils with a few mast cells.[37] The lesion may be unilateral or bilateral, and more than one lesion may be present within an eye. The condition appears seasonally, presenting in the spring and summer. The diagnosis is based on clinical signs, season of the year, and cytologic examination.

Untreated, eosinophilic keratoconjunctivitis is a chronic disease with healing by vascularization and scarring over several months. During this time secondary infection and acute exacerbation are possible. Treatment with topical corticosteroids has been described as reducing clinical signs, but mean time to resolution was 64 days, which is not significantly greater than without treatment.[37] In addition, secondary bacterial or

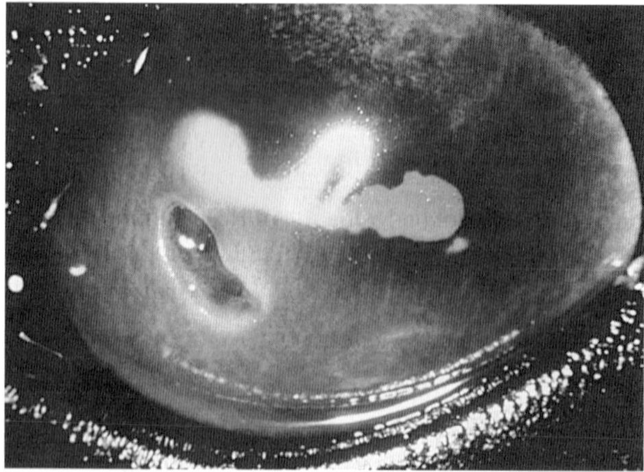

FIGURE 17-8 Deep corneal ulcer and descemetocele with associated focal corneal edema and miosis.

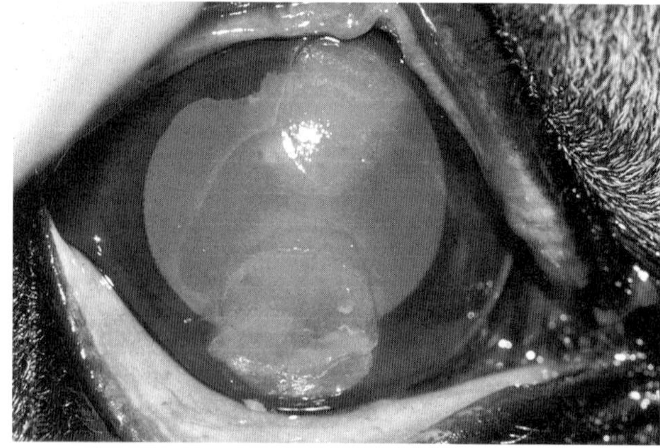

FIGURE 17-9 Two areas of ulcerative keratitis are present, each adjacent to the corneoscleral junction. Cytology revealed large numbers of eosinophils.

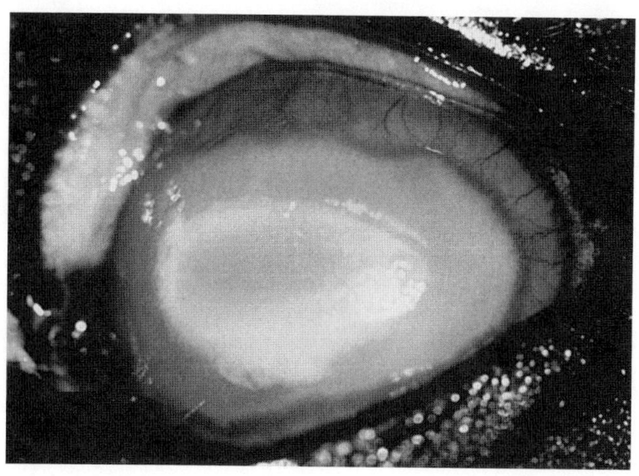

FIGURE 17-10 Mycotic keratitis. Deep corneal vascularization, stromal edema, and cellular infiltration resulted from infection with *Aspergillus* spp.

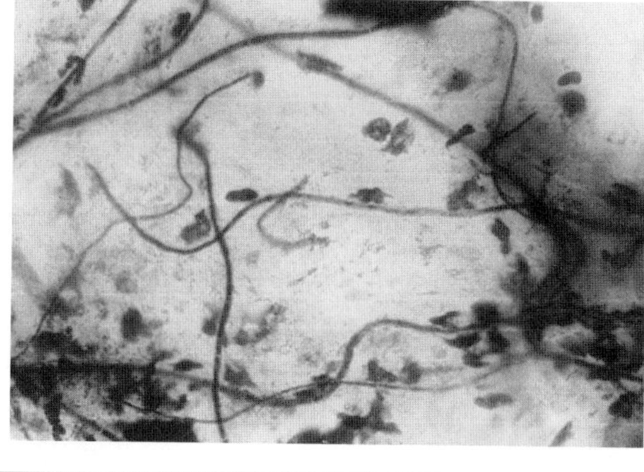

FIGURE 17-11 Corneal cytologic sample from horse with a combined infection of *Aspergillus* spp. and *Streptococcus* spp. Filamentous hyphae and bacteria are present in the sample.

fungal infectious keratitis is a risk with the use of topical corticosteroids. Topical lodoxamide 0.1% (Alomide, Alcon Laboratories) every 6 to 8 hours is the treatment of choice, along with fly control using fly masks. Superficial keratectomy also may be of benefit in resolving eosinophilic keratoconjunctivitis.

MYCOTIC KERATITIS

The clinician must consider all chronic corneal ulcers and ulcers that have been treated with topical corticosteroids as mycotic ulcers until proved otherwise. Keratomycosis is more common in the summer months and in warm climates.[44] Mycotic ulcers often have multifocal areas of cellular infiltrate and colonies of fungal organisms (Figure 17-10) that appear as white lesions deep in the corneal stroma adjacent to the ulcer and often appear 7 to 10 days after initial ulceration. These infiltrates are often fluorescein negative as the overlying epithelium heals, resulting in a corneal stromal abscess. Diagnosis of mycotic keratitis is based on history; clinical signs; cytologic examination; culture; and, if possible, histopathologic examination of a biopsy sample (Figure 17-11). Failure to see fungal elements on cytologic examination or culture does not rule out mycotic keratitis. The most common isolate for eyes with keratomycosis is *Aspergillus* spp.[44] *Fusarium* spp., *Penicillium* spp., and *Candida albicans* also are associated with keratomycosis. If the cause is in doubt, treating the horse for fungal infection is appropriate.

In eyes in which mycotic keratitis is suspected or documented, topical antifungals are indicated in addition to routine ulcer management. The only approved ophthalmic antifungal is natamycin 5% suspension (Natacyn, Alcon Laboratories), but it is costly and has limited efficacy. Although not approved for ophthalmic use, the imidazole antibiotics (miconazole, ketoconazole, fluconazole, voriconazole) may have the best efficacy for the treatment of keratomycosis.[44] Miconazole 1% can be compounded as a solution or ointment and administered every 2 to 4 hours topically for mycotic keratitis. An itraconazole–dimethyl sulfoxide ointment also has been used topically to treat keratomycosis.[45] In addition, dilute povidone-iodine solution is fungicidal and can be applied to the cornea with a cotton swab once every 1 to 2 days. Iodine is irritating to corneal and conjunctival tissues and should be irrigated from the conjunctival cul-de-sac after application. All topical antifungal medications have limited ability to penetrate intact corneal epithelium, although miconazole is better than most. If the lesion is fluorescein negative, débriding the epithelium before medicating may be necessary (see the section on corneal stromal abscess). Topical antifungal medication must be administered for a minimum of 3 to 4 weeks along with concurrent routine topical and systemic corneal ulcer management. Dermal antifungal preparations are not appropriate for topical use in the eye, but human vaginal antifungal preparations may be administered as a last resort.

Recently, use of the systemic antimycotic agent fluconazole has been evaluated.[46] In the author's opinion, oral administration of fluconazole (Diflucan, Pfizer Roerig, New York, N.Y.) at 1 mg/kg every 12 hours for 14 days and then every 24 hours for 7 days is associated with significant improvement and resolution of early keratomycosis and corneal stromal abscessation after fungal infection. In addition, topical 1% voriconazole has been evaulated for use in horses, and the author's clinical experience suggests that this is the current topical antifungal of choice.[47]

Many mycotic corneal ulcers are managed best using a combination of surgical and medical management.[16] Surgical débridement in the form of a partial- or full-thickness keratectomy may help remove much or all of the infected corneal stroma, respectively; is performed under general anesthesia; and requires microsurgical instrumentation and magnification. For a partial-thickness keratectomy, the clinician may manage the resulting ulcer medically or, more appropriately, may suture a conjunctival pedicle graft[3,48,49] to the ulcer to aid in healing. The corneal vascularization provided by a conjunctival graft facilitates healing. One can perform a penetrating keratoplasty with a corneal transplant for deeper lesions[50] (see the section on corneal surgery). Most mycotic corneal ulcers and abscesses ultimately vascularize and scar to some degree, regardless of the treatment method. Topical corticosteroids have little if any effect on corneal scar formation and are not indicated, even after resolution of keratomycosis, because the possibility of sequestered organisms exists with subsequent exacerbation.

COLLAGENASE ULCERS

Keratomalacia, or corneal melting, results from host-derived collagenase (from neutrophils and keratocytes) and bacterial enzymes such as those produced by *Pseudomonas aeruginosa*

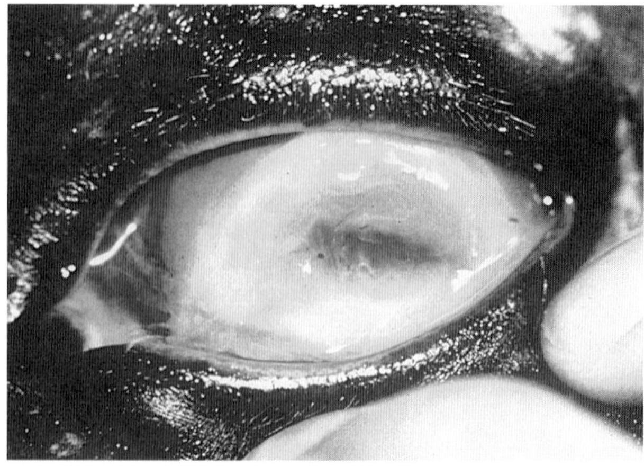

FIGURE 17-12 Severe melting caused by collagenase ulcer following infection with *Pseudomonas aeruginosa.* Corneal malacia surrounds a large descemetocele.

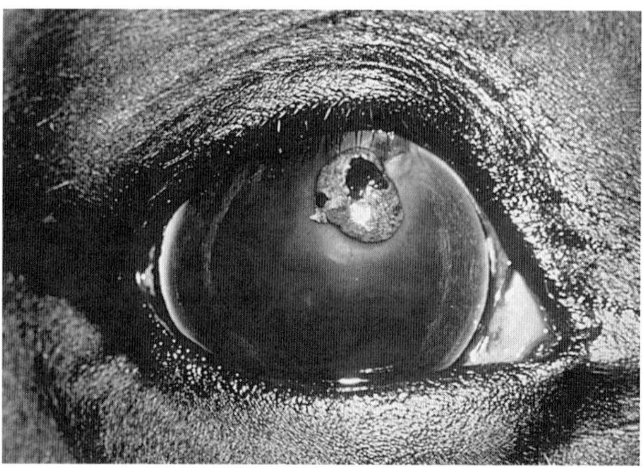

FIGURE 17-13 Corneal perforation with associated hyphema and iris prolapse.

or β-hemolytic *Streptococcus* spp.[51] Collagenase ulcers progress rapidly and can result in corneal perforation within 24 hours (Figure 17-12). Samples should be obtained for bacterial and fungal culture and cytologic examination. Cytologic examination must include Gram staining to examine for the presence of gram negative rods suggesting *Pseudomonas* spp. or gram positive cocci suggesting β-hemolytic *Streptococcus* spp. The topical antibiotics of choice for collagenase ulcers are ciprofloxacin (Ciloxan, Alcon Laboratories, Fort Worth, Tex.)[38,51] or ofloxacin (Ocuflox, Allergan Inc.) every 2 hours. Topical tetracycline every 4 to 6 hours or oral doxycycline may be of benefit because they inhibit matrix metalloproteinases that are activated in keratomalacia. Topical autologous serum may also inhibit corneal malacia and can be administered every 2 to 4 hours. Serum must be collected and handled in a sterile manner and replaced every 24 to 48 hours to prevent contamination. In addition, débridement of the malacic cornea and a conjunctival pedicle graft or penetrating keratoplasty often are indicated to repair the defect, aid in healing, and prevent corneal perforation.

DESCEMETOCELE

Descemet's membrane is the basement membrane of the endothelium and the last barrier to corneal perforation. Descemet's membrane does not stain with fluorescein and appears as a clearing in the center of an otherwise edematous corneal ulcer (see Figure 17-8). As with all corneal ulcers in the horse, routine diagnostic procedures for a descemetocele include culture and cytologic examination. A descemetocele is a surgical emergency and likely requires referral to a veterinary ophthalmologist. Surgical management is designed to provide support to the weakened cornea, allowing blood vessels and fibroblasts to repair the damage. Support is achieved with a conjunctival graft or a lamellar or penetrating keratoplasty (see the section on corneal surgery). Routine treatment for a corneal ulcer follows surgery and is best delivered through a subpalpebral lavage system to avoid manipulation of the eyelids and corneal graft. The conjunctival graft may be débrided 6 to 8 weeks after surgery in an attempt to minimize scar formation by severing the blood supply to the graft tissue.

CORNEAL PERFORATION AND LACERATION

Causes of corneal perforation include rupture of a deep corneal ulcer or descemetocele and sharp and blunt trauma. Depending on the cause of the perforation and severity of the damage, treatment involves primary repair, an intraocular prosthesis, or enucleation. If the horse is to be referred for consultation and treatment, self-trauma can be prevented during transportation by using cradles or other protective devices and sedation as required. The prognosis after a penetrating injury varies depending on the cause, size of the wound, location, depth of penetration, intraocular damage, and the presence or absence of infection or retained foreign objects. In general, perforating corneal wounds in the horse have a grave prognosis for vision and a guarded prognosis for cosmesis. Such wounds always are associated with secondary anterior uveitis, iris prolapse, and possible lens perforation and rupture (Figure 17-13). Sequelae to a corneal perforation include corneal scar, anterior and posterior synechiae, cataract, glaucoma, retinal detachment, phthisis bulbi, blindness, and loss of the eye.

Primary repair of a corneal perforation is a referral procedure. Treatment includes repairing the rent, re-establishing the anterior chamber, preventing infection, and decreasing inflammation and pain. Removal of a penetrating object is best done at the time of repair. Tetanus toxoid is administered before repair. The aqueous humor, along with any retained foreign objects, should be cultured for aerobic bacteria and fungi. If iris tissue protrudes but appears viable and minimally contaminated, it can be replaced; however, contaminated, nonviable iris is amputated using electrocautery to minimize hemorrhage. If electrocautery is not available, one can perform sharp excision and control the bleeding. Intracamerally administered epinephrine, 1:10,000, can help control intraoperative bleeding and also facilitates pupil dilation. One can use a viscoelastic agent such as sodium hyaluronate to tamponade vessels in addition to maintaining the anterior chamber and manipulating tissues. If the lens capsule has ruptured secondary to trauma, the lens should be removed; lens protein is antigenic and may stimulate severe anterior uveitis. If it is possible to appose wound margins, the cornea is repaired with partial-thickness, simple interrupted or continuous 7–0 to 8–0 absorbable sutures. The anterior chamber is reformed with a balanced salt solution or, if this is unavailable, lactated Ringer's solution. Conjunctival grafts can be used to promote rapid corneal healing and vascularization and to provide support. If a portion of cornea is missing or the wound edges cannot be apposed, a corneal-scleral transposition or other type of graft procedure is required. After surgery, one administers topical broad spectrum antibiotics every 2 to 4 hours, uses topical atropine as needed, and administers systemic antibiotics and flunixin meglumine. Use of a subpalpebral lavage delivery system is indicated.

Blunt trauma, whether contusive, penetrating, or perforating, generally results in more severe ocular damage than injury from a sharp object[5] (Figure 17-14). In contrast to sharp perforating injuries, blunt trauma results in a rapid increase in IOP, an explosive rupture from the inside outward, and the expulsion of the intraocular contents. The resulting rent in the fibrous tunic is often large and irregular, and portions of the cornea or sclera may be lost. The typical wound is one that originates at the limbus, extending forward into the cornea and posterior into the sclera. If the posterior portion of the eye ruptures, the horse may show hyphema and decreased IOP and may require ocular ultrasound for accurate diagnosis.

Repair of these explosive ruptures is difficult, and the treatment of choice may be enucleation. If cosmetic repair is important, an intraocular silicone prosthesis may be used in some patients, provided enough tissue is left to close the fibrous tunic.[3] This procedure should be performed as soon as possible after injury. If the injury is chronic and atrophy of the globe has occurred, placement of an intraocular prosthesis is not possible. The only cosmetic alternative in these horses is an orbital prosthesis, which is expensive and time consuming and requires frequent maintenance on the part of the owner.[3]

CORNEAL SURGERY

Surgery in the form of a superficial keratectomy, conjunctival graft, or corneal graft may be indicated in addition to aggressive medical therapy for many complicated corneal ulcers.[53] Corneal surgery requires general anesthesia to optimize the outcome.

A superficial keratectomy provides a biopsy for histopathologic examination, débrides and debulks damaged and infected corneal stroma, and provides a bed for transplanting and suturing a conjunctival or corneal graft. A No. 64 Beaver blade or Martinez corneal dissector is used first to outline the area to be excised and then to undermine and remove the affected area of cornea. In general, 50% to 70% of the corneal thickness can be removed, but excision of 50% or more is an indication to reinforce the remaining cornea with a conjunctival or corneal lamellar graft. The normal equine cornea is 1.0 to 1.5 mm thick and is thinnest centrally. The cornea increases in thickness with disease because of edema, cellular infiltration, vascularization, and scar formation.

Conjunctival grafts include advancement, hood, bridge, pedicle, and complete conjunctival grafts.[48,49,52]The author prefers to perform a conjunctival pedicle graft for most focal corneal ulcers and uses the other types for more extensive lesions.[49] Before placement of a conjunctival graft, débridement of the affected cornea by superficial keratectomy is indicated. The bulbar conjunctiva is mobilized, leaving an intact blood supply. One should attempt to appose conjunctival and corneal epithelium at the edge of the graft and to place 7–0 to 8–0 Vicryl (polyglactin 910) sutures two thirds deep into healthy cornea. A continuous suture pattern, simple or double, works best and is associated with less graft retraction and dehiscence than a simple interrupted suture pattern for equine conjunctival grafts. Conjunctival grafts adhere to the underlying exposed corneal stroma, providing the blood supply and cells required to repair and rebuild the damaged cornea. Opacification of the graft site occurs but is generally less than what would have occurred without surgery. Opacification can be minimized by trimming the graft and severing its blood supply 6 to 8 weeks after the initial surgery.

Autologous and homologous lamellar corneal grafts, corneal-scleral transposition, deep lamellar keratectomy, and penetrating keratoplasty are more involved techniques reserved for the most severe corneal ulcers or for perforating corneal lesions. These are described elsewhere and are referral procedures.[53-55]

In addition to cornea and conjunctiva, other grafting materials, such as equine amnion and porcine collagen, have been used with success for management of equine corneal disease.[56] Nictitating membrane or third eyelid flaps are of little or no benefit for managing complicated and infected equine corneal disease and are contraindicated in many instances.

NONULCERATIVE DISEASES

Nonulcerative corneal diseases include corneal scar, corneal edema, stromal abscessation, cellular and noncellular infiltrates, immune keratitis, and nonulcerative keratouveitis.[57] Corneal scars are not painful, follow a history of corneal disease, and are associated with corneal vascularization. Topical corticosteroid therapy does not decrease corneal scarring significantly but does predispose the eye to infection and decreases healing in the event of a corneal ulcer. Tattooing of a corneal scar for ocular cosmesis is described[3,16] but not advised.

Cellular infiltration in the corneal stroma includes neoplastic and inflammatory cells. The most common corneal neoplasia is SCC (see the section on conjunctiva and third eyelid; see Figure 17-6). Corneal lymphosarcoma also occurs. Inflammatory cellular infiltration (neutrophils, lymphocytes, plasma cells, eosinophils) usually occurs in infectious keratitis (bacterial, mycotic) and is associated with corneal ulceration. However, a small, focal corneal ulcer can become infected and re-epithelialize, resulting in a corneal stromal abscess. In addition, inflammatory corneal infiltration occurs with equine

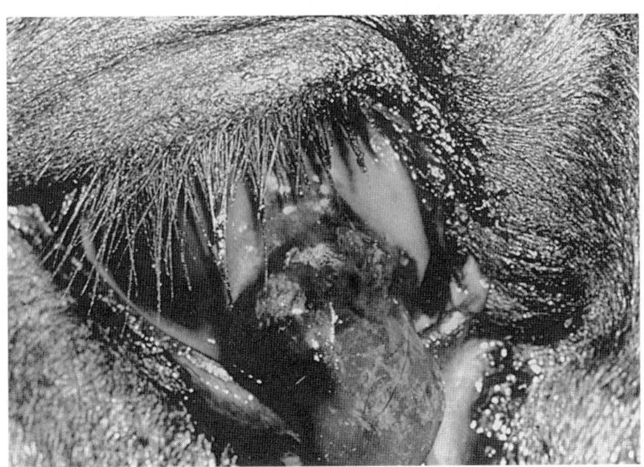

FIGURE 17-14 Corneal perforation following blunt trauma. The lesion is explosive and expulsive with loss of intraocular contents. Enucleation is the treatment of choice.

ocular onchocerciasis, immune keratitis, and nonulcerative keratouveitis.

Noncellular corneal infiltration or corneal degeneration is a sequela of previous corneal or limbal inflammation. Accumulations of mineral and phospholipids may remain within the corneal stroma after inflammation and appear as crystalline infiltration. Such accumulations are rare, generally are not painful, and do not require treatment. In some instances they predispose the eye to corneal ulceration and can be removed with a superficial keratectomy.[3]

CORNEAL EDEMA

Corneal edema, if not associated with a corneal ulcer (fluorescein negative), results from corneal endothelial damage. Blunt trauma to the globe can result in displacement of the corneal endothelium from the posterior surface of the cornea, which results in full-thickness, diffuse corneal edema and which may gravitate to the ventral cornea with time. In addition, diseases of the anterior uvea and aqueous humor, anterior uveitis and glaucoma, and anterior lens luxation can interfere with endothelial cell function, resulting in diffuse corneal edema. Although no specific treatment exists for corneal edema of endothelial origin, hyperosmotic agents such as sodium chloride 5% (Muro-128; Bausch and Lomb, Rochester, N.Y.) applied topically every 4 to 6 hours may decrease the severity of the edema and help prevent rupture of corneal bullae. In the author's opinion, this has only minimal efficacy. With time the corneal endothelium may reattach, or adjacent endothelial cells may hypertrophy, resulting in a decrease in corneal edema. While the edema is present, the cornea is compromised and at risk of ulceration. Topical corticosteroids are therefore contraindicated.

NONULCERATIVE KERATOUVEITIS

A condition consisting of interstitial keratitis with peripheral corneal vascularization, edema, and cellular infiltrate and anterior uveitis (miosis, aqueous flare, iritis) has been described in five horses.[57] The pathogenesis of nonulcerative keratouveitis is unknown, but anterior uveitis has been suggested to follow interstitial keratitis, and an immune-mediated mechanism is believed to be involved. No infectious or neoplastic process is apparent. Histologically, nonulcerative keratouveitis is characterized by vascularization, fibroblasts, and inflammatory cells, predominantly lymphocytes. No infectious agents are visible on light or transmission electron microscopy.

Treatment is similar to that for equine recurrent uveitis and involves suppression of inflammation and control of ocular pain. Topical and subconjunctival corticosteroids, topical NSAIDs, topical cyclosporin A,[42] topical mydriatic cycloplegics, and systemic NSAIDs effectively control the signs, but some level of long-term maintenance therapy usually is required.

The differential diagnoses for nonulcerative keratouveitis include corneal stromal abscess, equine ocular onchocerciasis, and neoplasia.

CORNEAL STROMAL ABSCESS

The usual cause of corneal stromal abscess formation is a focal, superficial corneal ulcer that allows opportunistic infection of the corneal stroma and then heals, trapping the microorganism. Topical antibiotic-corticosteroid therapy in eyes with corneal epithelial cell loss may predispose to stromal abscess formation.[3,58,59] The lesion results in discomfort apparent as photophobia, blepharospasm, and excessive lacrimation. A chronic, yellow-white, corneal stromal infiltrate with associated corneal edema and deep corneal vascularization is present.[58,59] Anterior uveitis may be present. Fluorescein staining of the cornea is often negative. Diagnosis is based on clinical signs. A corneal scraping should be obtained from the lesion, after removal of the overlying corneal epithelium, and submitted for cytologic examination, bacterial culture and sensitivity, and fungal culture. Gram positive cocci (*Streptococcus* and *Staphylococcus* spp.) are the predominant organisms recovered,[58] but fungal stromal abscesses also occur. Differential diagnosis includes nonulcerative keratouveitis.

If the overlying epithelium is intact, one can remove it before initiating treatment to facilitate penetration of antibiotics. The flouroquinolones, ciprofloxacin or ofloxacin, are the topical antibiotics of choice because they penetrate intact corneal epithelium; treatment every 4 hours is recommended pending culture and sensitivity results. In addition, some authors recommend subconjunctival injections of antibiotics.[3,58] If a mycotic stromal abscess is suspected, oral administration of fluconazole (Diflucan, Pfizer Roerig, New York, N.Y.) at 1 mg/kg every 12 hours for 14 days and then every 24 hours for 7 days is indicated.[46] Alternately, 1% voriconazole or an itraconazole-dimethyl sulfoxide ointment can be used topically.[45]

If anterior uveitis is present, topical atropine 1% is administered as needed to dilate the pupil, up to a maximum of 4 times a day. Systemic flunixin meglumine helps reduce ocular pain and secondary complications associated with inflammation. Topical corticosteroids are contraindicated. Resolution of the abscess requires 2 to 8 weeks, is associated with corneal vascularization, and results in corneal scar formation. In addition, the associated anterior uveitis may result in secondary intraocular complications.

A superficial keratectomy and conjunctival pedicle graft,[59] posterior lamellar keratoplasty,[60] or penetrating keratoplasty[50,55,61] is also appropriate and may result in a more rapid resolution and reduced corneal opacification than medical management alone. After performing a keratectomy, one should submit the excised corneal stroma for culture and cytologic or histopathologic examination, because the corneal stroma yields more diagnostic information than preoperative samples.[59]

EQUINE OCULAR ONCHOCERCIASIS

Onchcocerca cervicalis is a common equine parasite that has been implicated in conjunctivitis, peripheral keratitis, anterior uveitis, and peripapillary chorioretinitis. Corneal lesions result from *Onchocerca* microfilariae that migrate to and die in the corneal stroma and may incite an inflammatory response. The lesion begins peripherally at the temporal limbus but can extend axially. Interstitial keratitis, manifested as corneal edema, vascularization, and subepithelial focal corneal opacities, occurs and may be associated with temporal bulbar conjunctival vitiligo, conjunctivitis, and anterior uveitis. Diagnosis is based on history, clinical signs, and the presence of eosinophils on cytologic examination and microfilariae on conjunctival biopsy.[62] One can demonstrate microfilariae cytologically through a biopsy of temporal bulbar conjunctiva, placing the sample on a slide with warm saline and examining for the presence of motile microfilariae. The presence of microfilariae must be interpreted in conjunction with the clinical signs because microfilariae can be found in many horses without associated ocular disease.

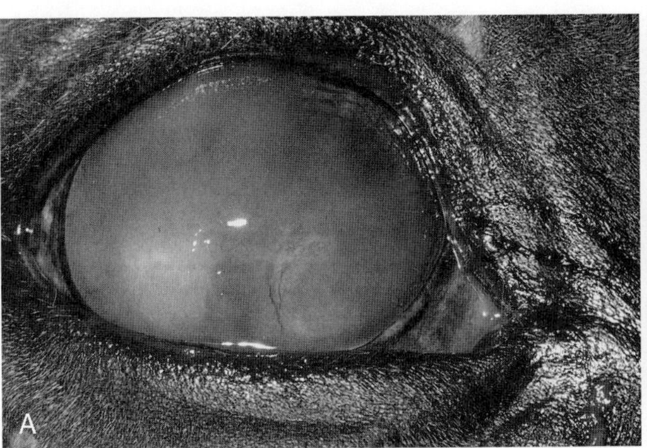

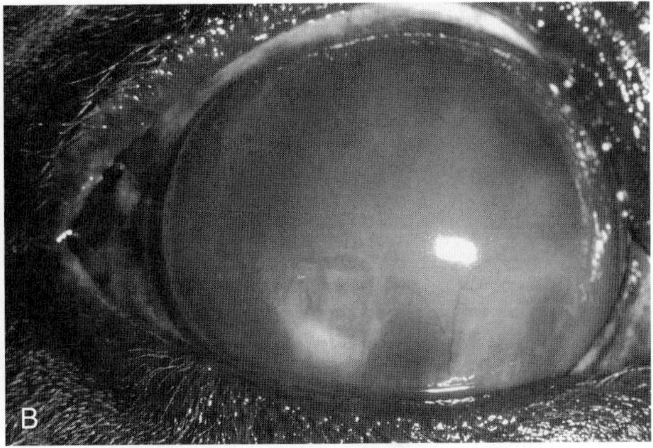

FIGURE 17-15 **A,** Presumed immune keratitis before treatment. **B,** The same eye 5 days after therapy with oral doxycycline.

Treatment includes suppression of ocular inflammation and microfilaricidal therapy (see Table 17-2). Topical corticosteroids and systemic phenylbutazone or flunixin meglumine control inflammation (see Table 17-3). If anterior uveitis is present, topical atropine 1% can be used as needed to dilate the pupil. Pretreatment with anti-inflammatory medications for 2 to 3 days before administration of microfilaricides is indicated to minimize the ocular response to the dying microfilariae.

BAND KERATOPATHY

Single or multiple linear streaks affecting one or both eyes in the horse have been described.[63] Histologically, these are areas of thinning of Descemet's membrane and may be congenital. The principle differential is a corneal stria following chronic glaucoma and enlargement of the globe with stretching of Descemet's membrane. Ophthalmic examination should reveal evidence of prior inflammation or glaucoma, and the clinician should assess vision and determine IOP.

OTHER KERATOPATHIES

In addition to the corneal diseases noted, there exists a keratitis that is presumed to be immune mediated. The keratitis presents with punctate to diffuse corneal involvement with mild to no discomfort. The cornea is flourescein negative, and no concurrent uveitis is observed. There is often a yellow-green color to the corneal stroma (Figure 17-15). Biopsy to date has revealed lymphocytic-plasmacytic keratitis, with no organisms identified. The keratitis has responded to topical corticosteroids, cyclosporin A, and systemic doxycycline, with each horse varied in its response to the form of therapy selected. In addition, the keratitis often recurs when therapy is stopped.

UVEA

Anatomy

The uvea is the middle, vascular tunic of the eye and comprises the anterior portion, the iris and ciliary body, and the posterior choroid. Histologically, the uvea contains blood vessels; pigment cells; smooth muscle; and in the horse, a noncellular, fibrous tapetum in the choroid. The uvea is the primary site of the blood-ocular barrier, which has importance in the formation of the aqueous humor, serves as a barrier to bloodborne materials, and is an immunologic barrier to the internal components of the eye. Inflammation disrupts this barrier (uveitis). Smooth muscles in the iris and ciliary body, under autonomic control, regulate pupil size and accommodate for near and far vision, respectively. In uveitis spasm of these muscles results in constriction of the pupil and pain, seen clinically as miosis and photophobia. The ciliary body is the source of aqueous humor, which supplies nutrition to the cornea and lens. Aqueous humor is produced by active and passive processes; its production is decreased by inflammation and by pharmacologic agents used in glaucoma therapy. The choroid supplies nutrition to the retina and also serves as a heat sink to protect the photoreceptors from the heat generated by light striking the retina. The tapetum, contained within the superior choroid, reflects light back across the retina, thereby maximizing the use of available light.

Abnormalities of the Pupil

The pupil of the horse is horizontally elliptic, with the dorsal and ventral margins having pigmented prominences termed *corpora nigra.* The pupillary light reflex in the horse is similar to that of other species with a direct and a consensual response. The afferent fibers of the pupillary light reflex are carried in cranial nerve II, and the efferent parasympathetic fibers are carried in cranial nerve III. Abnormalities in pupil response to a light stimulus result from afferent lesions involving the retina or optic nerve. Afferent abnormalities are associated with loss of vision in the affected eye. Efferent lesions are rare but include damage to cranial nerve III with an associated ventrolateral strabismus, abnormalities of the iris itself (as with synechiae), and glaucoma. It is important to differentiate excited horses with sympathetic override, weak light source, and improper examination technique from an abnormal pupillary light response.

Sympathetic nerve fibers supply the dilator muscles of the iris. These fibers travel in the spinal cord, emerge in the ventral nerve roots at first and second thoracic nerves, course through the thorax, run in association with the internal carotid artery, synapse at the cranial cervical sympathetic ganglion, and travel to the eye with the ocular arteries. Damage to the sympathetic fibers results in Horner's syndrome. Clinical signs include ptosis, miosis, enophthalmos, protrusion of the third eyelid, and sweating on the affected side of the face and neck.

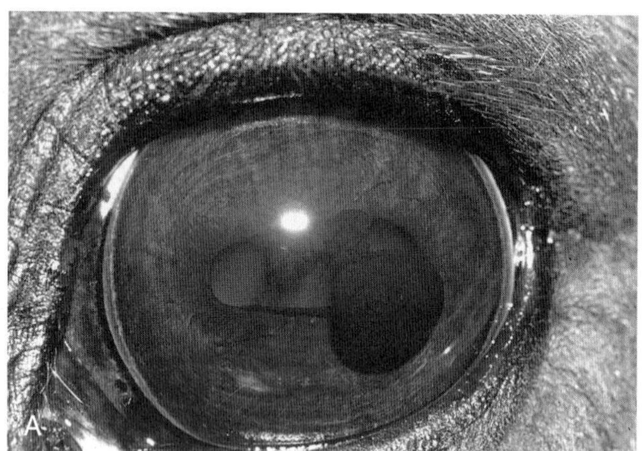
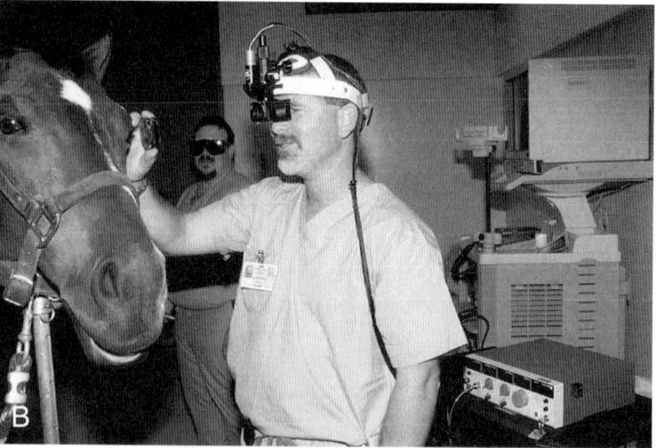
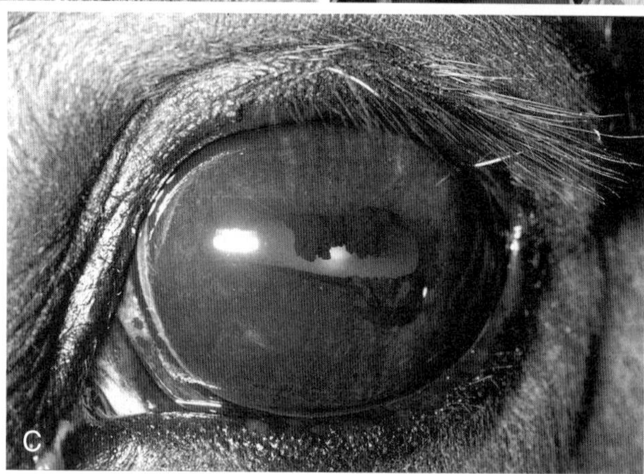

FIGURE 17-16 **A,** A heavily pigmented uveal cyst that is resulting in headshaking and shying behavior. **B,** Transcorneal laser ablation of the cyst is performed in the standing horse. **C,** The cyst immediately after laser ablation.

Treatment is directed toward the primary disease, if possible. In some horses the clinical signs of Horner's syndrome resolve without treatment.

Uveal Cysts

Cysts of the anterior uvea (iris, corpora nigra, and ciliary body) have been reported in the horse.[64,65] The cysts are usually heavily pigmented and may not transilluminate, making a uveal melanoma the most likely differential diagnosis. Ocular ultrasonography reveals these as cystic structures and confirms the diagnosis.

Treatment is not required unless the cysts are numerous or impair sight. One can collapse the cyst; aspirate it by paracentesis; or disrupt it using laser energy delivered transcorneally if this technology is available.[65] Diode laser energy (810 nm) can be delivered to the cyst through the cornea using an indirect ophthalmoscope and a 20-D condensing lens. One performs the procedure on the standing horse and photocoagulates the cyst wall, shrinking the cyst and preventing recurrence (Figure 17-16).

Anterior Segment Dysgenesis

Anterior segment dysgenesis has been described in the Rocky Mountain Horse, Kentucky Mountain Saddle Horse, and Mountain Pleasure Horse breeds. The abnormalities associated with this syndrome include macropalpebral fissure, megalocornea, ciliary body and peripheral retinal cysts, congenital miosis, iris stromal hypoplasia, iridocorneal angle abnormalities, cataract, retinal dysplasia, and retinal detachment.[66] The abnormalities appear linked to coat color, with the highest prevalence of abnormalities associated with chocolate coat and white mane and tail.

Uveitis

Uveitis is an inflammation of the iris and ciliary body (anterior) and choroid (posterior). Uveitis is a common manifestation of many ocular and systemic infectious and noninfectious diseases, and as such, an attempt to ascertain the cause is essential. Differentiating uveitis from other ophthalmic diseases resulting in a red and painful eye, such as glaucoma, corneal ulceration, and conjunctivitis, is also essential. Uveitis is reported as the leading cause of blindness in horses throughout the world.[4,5,16]

CLINICAL SIGNS

Acute inflammation of the anterior uvea results in spasm of the iris and ciliary muscles, which is apparent clinically as miosis and photophobia, and a breakdown in the blood-ocular barrier (Box 17-2). The primary mediators of intraocular inflammation are prostaglandins. Eyelids and conjunctiva may be swollen and hyperemic in the acute phase of anterior uveitis.

BOX 17-2

SIGNS OF ACUTE AND CHRONIC UVEITIS

Acute

Miosis
Photophobia
Blepharospasm
Eyelid swelling
Aqueous flare
Corneal edema
Chorioretinitis
Keratitic precipitates
Hypopyon
Hypotony

Chronic

Posterior synechiae
Cataract
Pigmentation of anterior lens capsule
Atrophy of corpora nigra
Glaucoma
Peripapillary depigmentation
Phthisis bulbi
Blindness
Lens luxation

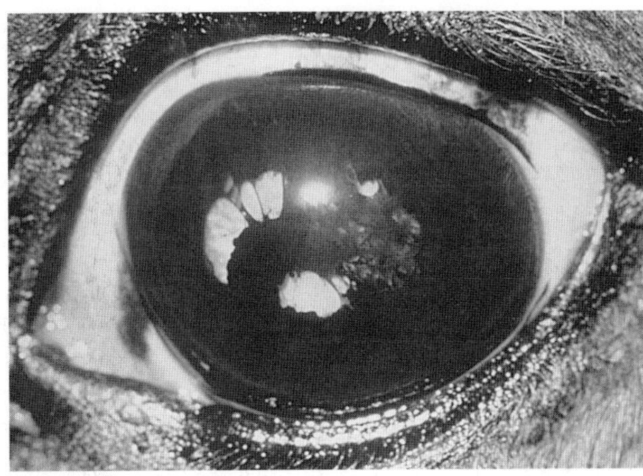

FIGURE 17-17 Numerous posterior synechiae and a cataract occur following chronic anterior uveitis. The corpora nigra are adhered to the anterior lens and result in distortion of the pupil margin.

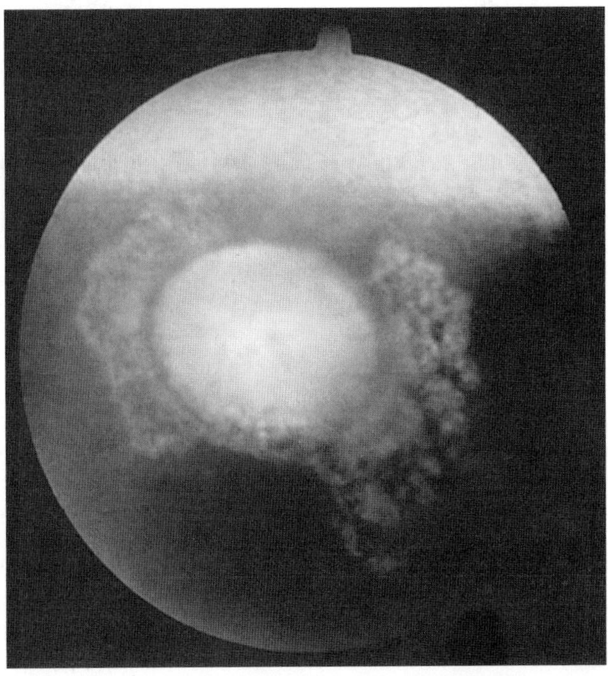

FIGURE 17-18 Peripapillary depigmentation, a so-called butterfly lesion, associated with the chorioretinitis of equine recurrent uveitis.

Protein and cells leak into the anterior chamber, resulting in aqueous flare, hypopyon, and keratitic precipitates. The cornea may show diffuse edema, and the IOP will be low in acute uveitis. Chronic inflammatory changes in the aqueous humor can result in secondary corneal endothelial and lens changes (e.g., corneal edema and cataract) and adhesions between the iris and adjacent lens or cornea, termed *synechiae* (Figure 17-17). The lens may stain a yellow color as a result of chronic serum leakage. The corpora nigra will atrophy with chronic uveitis, appearing abnormally small and smooth. Inflammation of the choroid, because of its close association with the retina, usually also involves the retina and is termed *chorioretinitis*. Chorioretinitis is diagnosed by direct or indirect ophthalmoscopy and results in retinal and subretinal transudate and exudate, retinal vascular changes, hemorrhage, retinal detachment, and retinal degeneration. The optic nerve may show hyperemia and later atrophy. Vitreal changes may be observed in association with posterior uveitis. This may include vitreous debris, cells, liquefaction, and yellow discoloration of the vitreous. Choroidal depigmentation and areas of repigmentation or pigment clumping may be present (Figure 17-18). Other chronic changes resulting from intraocular inflammation include secondary glaucoma, retinal detachment, blindness, and phthisis bulbi. The development of intraocular changes following uveitis is related directly to the duration and severity of the acute episode and is exacerbated by recurrent episodes of inflammation.

CAUSES

The causes of anterior and posterior uveitis include primary ophthalmic and systemic diseases.[1] Blunt or penetrating ocular trauma, intraocular neoplasia (primary or secondary), corneal ulceration, parasitic infiltration, and numerous systemic infectious diseases with associated septicemia, toxemia, immune-complex disease, and viremia are associated with uveitis. Of the systemic infectious diseases implicated in equine uveitis, infections of *Streptococcus equi* subsp. *equi* (strangles) and *Leptospira interrogans* serogroup *pomona*[68,69] and gram negative sepsis occur most commonly. In addition to a complete ophthalmic examination, evaluating the entire animal through a complete physical examination and appropriate laboratory testing is essential. A complete ophthalmic evaluation must include fluorescein staining of the cornea; penlight examination to evaluate pupil size, aqueous humor content, lens position, and transparency; and direct and consensual pupillary light responses. Direct (with or without indirect) ophthalmoscopic examination of the fundus is also essential. Failure to perform these routine diagnostic tests results in misdiagnosis and incorrect therapy and may result in a failure to consider and examine for systemic disease, thereby placing the health of the animal in jeopardy.

Primary ophthalmic diseases that result in anterior uveitis include corneal ulceration, lens-induced uveitis, intraocular neoplasia, and direct ocular trauma. Corneal ulceration results in secondary anterior uveitis through a reflex pathway involving the ophthalmic branch of cranial nerve V. Fluorescein staining of the cornea therefore is indicated in eyes with anterior uveitis. The lens is considered to be an immune-privileged site and as such is capable of stimulating an inflammatory reaction. Lens protein is exposed by traumatic rupture of the lens capsule or during the degenerative process of a hypermature cataract undergoing liquefaction and leakage. Either of these processes can lead to anterior uveitis, with rupture of the lens resulting in the more severe inflammation and frequently secondary glaucoma. Uveitis resulting from direct ocular trauma may be associated with rupture of the fibrous tunic of the eye, hyphema, lens luxation, corneal endothelial damage, retinal detachment, or proptosis. A complete ophthalmic examination is essential. If the anterior and posterior segments of the eye are not completely visible, then an ocular ultrasound examination is indicated, specifically to evaluate the position of the lens and retina and to look for changes in the echogenicity of the vitreous humor. In addition to a complete ophthalmic evaluation, the entire animal should be examined for signs of trauma to other body systems. Fractures and soft tissue damage of the head and neck, thoracic and abdominal trauma, fractures of the limbs, and neurologic changes involving the central nervous system are potential complications associated with ocular trauma.

Systemic diseases resulting in anterior and posterior uveitis are numerous and include bacteremia, septicemia, disseminated mycoses, and the syndrome of equine recurrent uveitis. Infection with *Borrelia burgdorferi* has been reported to result in arthritis and panuveitis in a pony.[69] Foals with neonatal septicemia are especially prone to anterior and posterior uveitis. The uveitis in these foals is usually sterile. Systemic antimicrobial, topical and systemic anti-inflammatory, and topical atropine 1% therapy are the treatments of choice. Copious fibrin production may result from anterior uveitis, especially in young foals, and can result in posterior synechia and opacification of the lens capsule. Intracameral tissue plasminogen activator, 25 to 75 μg administered in the first few days after fibrin formation, can result in complete lysis and resolution.

EQUINE RECURRENT UVEITIS

Equine recurrent uveitis (ERU; also known as *moon blindness* or *periodic ophthalmia*) is the most common cause of blindness in horses, with Appaloosas at increased risk.[68] ERU is an immune-mediated disease with numerous initiating or exacerbating factors[3,67,70] (Box 17-3). The clinical signs of ERU are similar to those of other causes of uveitis, the distinguishing feature being its recurrent nature. The frequency and severity of each recurrence vary greatly. Even in times of clinical quiescence, inflammation is believed to continue at a subclinical level, resulting in further intraocular damage. Diagnosis is based on history and clinical examination. Although serologic evaluation for *Leptospira* spp., *Brucella* spp., or *Toxoplasma* and conjunctival biopsies to evaluate for the presence of *O. cervicalis* have been advocated,[3] the results of these tests rarely alter individual therapy, in part because of the chronicity of the disease and because the inciting cause may have begun years before development of uveitis.

BOX 17-3

CAUSES IMPLICATED IN EQUINE RECURRENT UVEITIS

Leptospira interrogans serovar *pomona*

Onchocerca cervicalis

Toxoplasma sp.

Virus infection: adenovirus, influenza

Brucella spp.

Streptococcus spp.

Borrelia burgdorferi

Trauma

Other

Treatment of the individual horse is directed toward suppressing inflammation, controlling pain, and preventing sequelae. When the prevalence of ERU in a barn exceeds that which is normally expected, serologic testing and examination to attempt to determine the cause are indicated. Routine vaccination for *Leptospira* spp. is controversial and may be contraindicated in horses with active inflammation.

The prognosis for ERU varies according to the severity of uveitis, duration of episodes, response to treatment, and frequency of recurrence. Each episode results in some degree of intraocular damage, and damage to the corneal endothelium, lens, and retina is cumulative because repair of these tissues is difficult. In addition, damage often occurs at a subclinical level during the so-called inactive periods. Horses with evidence of previous uveitis, corneal edema, cataract, synechiae, pigment on the anterior lens capsule, atrophy of the corpora nigra, and degeneration of retina and optic nerve should be considered ophthalmologically unsound. All animals that have had an episode of acute uveitis should be considered at risk to develop chronic recurrent uveitis. All animals with chronic recurrent uveitis have a guarded prognosis for long-term maintenance of normal vision, with blindness often the result.

TREATMENT

The treatment of any uveitis, acute or chronic, involves specific therapy determined by the cause of the uveitis and nonspecific therapy designed to decrease inflammation, alleviate pain, and prevent further intraocular damage. The initiation of specific therapy depends on correctly identifying the cause, whether a primary ophthalmic disease or a systemic problem. Failure to control intraocular inflammation may lead to severe secondary ophthalmic complications such as glaucoma, synechiae, cataract, retinal detachment, phthisis bulbi, and blindness.

Nonspecific therapy includes topical and systemic corticosteroids and NSAIDs to decrease inflammation and atropine to dilate the pupil and decrease the pain of ciliary muscle spasm. Selection of medication, frequency of treatment, and route of administration depend on the cause and severity of the uveitis and whether the uveitis is anterior, posterior, or both.

Topical medications for treating anterior uveitis include atropine, corticosteroids, cyclosporin A, and NSAIDs. Topical atropine 1% is administered as needed to dilate the pupil, but generally not more than four times a day. The clinician should monitor intestinal motility because topical atropine can result in ileus and colic. Topical corticosteroids are useful, provided corneal ulceration is not present, as determined by fluorescein stain. Prednisolone acetate 1% ophthalmic is the corticosteroid of choice because it achieves the highest intraocular levels. Alternatively, dexamethasone 0.1% ophthalmic solution or 0.05% ointment may be used. Frequency of administration varies according to severity, with initial frequency being every 4 to 6 hours and subsequently decreased as the eye responds to therapy. Topical corticosteroid therapy should be continued for several weeks after resolution of clinical signs. In addition, subconjunctival corticosteroids have been advocated in severe cases of anterior uveitis[3,16] (see Table 17-3). Topical NSAIDs are available, but little information exists regarding their efficacy for treating ERU. The author's experience suggests some efficacy but significantly less clinical response than with topical corticosteroids. Topical NSAIDs can be used in horses with anterior uveitis and associated corneal ulceration with less risk than corticosteroids. Topical corticosteroids and NSAIDs have a synergistic effect and can be used in combination. Topical antibiotics are not required unless a corneal ulcer is present; corticosteroids then are contraindicated. Topical cyclosporin A 0.2% ointment (Optimmune, Schering-Plough, Kenilworth, New Jersey) may be efficacious for treating active uveitis and as a long-term treatment to decrease the frequency and severity of subsequent recurrences.[42] Unfortunately, although cyclosporine is the drug of choice, it has limited ability to penetrate the intact cornea and reach target tissues.

Systemic NSAIDs are used with topical therapy. Flunixin meglumine is the systemic NSAID of choice for acute ocular inflammation and can be used safely in the presence of corneal ulcer. Alternatively, phenylbutazone or aspirin can be used. Chronic oral administration of aspirin at 25 mg/kg every 24 to 48 hours has been advocated to decrease the frequency and severity of recurrent episodes of uveitis.[3] Horses with active uveitis should be confined in a darkened stall to decrease discomfort and limit exercise.

Recently, surgical management of ERU has been advocated. Surgeries include intravitreal or suprachoroidal placement of a sustained-release cylosporine-impregnated device[71-74] or vitrectomy.[75] Implantation of a 4-μg/day intravitreal cyclosporin A implant decreased the frequency and severity of recurrent uveitis episodes in 23 horses with a mean follow-up of 1 to 29 months (mean 10.5 ± SD 7.6 months).[71,74] Of the treated horses 18 of 23 (78.2%) had sight at the time of follow-up. Complications of the intravitreal cyclosporin A implant include glaucoma and retinal detachment, both of which may relate to ERU. Placement of a suprachoroidal implant is associated with less postsurgical complications than with the intravitreal device and is the current treatment of choice for many horses with ERU. Compared with suprachoroidal cyclosporin A implantation, pars plana vitrectomy is a more invasive surgery, requiring more instrumentation and expertise, and is often associated with significant postoperative vision-threatening complications. Pars plana vitrectomy does appear, however, to decrease the severity and frequency of ERU episodes.

Glaucoma

Glaucoma is an elevation of IOP to a level incompatible with the health of the eye. Equine glaucoma is secondary in virtually all cases, typically resulting from ERU.[76] The reported normal IOP in the horse varies according to the technique used and whether sedation is used, with sedation resulting in a decrease in IOP. One should perform an auriculopalpebral nerve block before determining IOP in the horse. Normal values are reported to range between 15 to 25 mm Hg. Measurement of IOP in the horse presents a challenge in that indentation tonometers, such as the Schiøtz, are not well suited for use in the horse. Applanation tonometers, especially portable devices such as the Tonopen Vet, are best suited for determining equine IOP. In the author's practice determination of IOP is a routine part of a complete equine ophthalmic examination. Before determining IOP in the horse, one should remember that intravenous administration of xylazine significantly lowers the IOP.[3]

Although congenital glaucoma (megaloglobus) has been reported in the horse, secondary glaucoma resulting from anterior uveitis, especially ERU, is the most common cause of equine glaucoma.[76] The clinical signs of glaucoma in the horse are often more subtle than those in other species. Acute glaucoma may result in pain (photophobia, blepharospasm, lacrimation), corneal edema, linear corneal opacities (striae), mydriasis (provided uveitis or posterior synechiae are not present), and decreased menace response. The linear opacities in equine glaucoma often extend from limbus to limbus and are areas of thinning of Descemet's membrane.[5] Similar linear opacities also occur in normal horses, have been termed *band* or *linear keratopathy*, and are not significant. In chronic glaucoma corneal edema and corneal striae may be visible. Enlargement of the globe (buphthalmos), retinal degeneration, and blindness also occur.

Unfortunately, most horses with glaucomatous eyes do not receive treatment until late in the disease, resulting in a poor response to therapy. Medical treatment of acute glaucoma involves topical agents such as timolol maleate 0.5% (Timoptic; Merck and Co., West Point, Pa.), dorzolamide 2% (Trusopt, Merck), and the combination of these two drugs (Cosopt; Merck).[77,78] These drugs are administered alone or in combination two to three times daily in an effort to reduce IOP by increasing the outflow and decreasing production of aqueous humor. Of all the topical glaucoma agents, timolol maleate and dorzolamide are most effective in the horse, and the combination is more effective than administration of the two drugs concomitantly.[77] Because of the large percentage of uveoscleral outflow in the horse, careful use of topical atropine may actually reduce IOP in some eyes.[79] Use of atropine is controversial, however. Topical corticosteroids, systemic flunixin meglumine, or combined therapy is indicated to control any concomitant inflammation or pain. Failure of topical therapy to control acute glaucoma indicates the need for surgical intervention.

Surgery for the acute glaucoma patient includes transscleral cyclocryosurgery or cyclophotocoagulation using a Nd:YAG or diode laser.[76,80-83] Both procedures are designed to reduce the production of aqueous humor and decrease IOP. Cyclophotocoagulation has fewer intraocular side effects than cyclocryosurgery and is the surgical treatment of choice. In a retrospective evaluation of 27 horses treated by transscleral diode laser cyclophotocoagulation, adjunct medical therapy was required for 90% of horses and vision was maintained in 64% with a mean follow-up of 33 months (7 to 69 months).[76] Surgical filtering procedures, designed to provide an alternative outflow pathway for aqueous humor, are generally unsuccessful in the horse.[5]

Treatment of chronic glaucoma is surgical and is designed to reduce discomfort. Enucleation or evisceration with insertion of an intraocular silicone prosthesis is the procedure of choice.[84]

HYPHEMA

Hyphema is blood in the anterior chamber of the eye (see Figure 17-13). As is true of bleeding into other body cavities, blood in the anterior chamber of the eye does not usually clot. It is important to remember that not all hyphema results from ocular trauma. One must consider systemic diseases that result in clotting disorders or intraocular inflammation.

If the hyphema is complete and precludes the evaluation of intraocular structures, ocular ultrasound is indicated to assess the lens position, retina, and posterior eye wall. The greatest resolution in ocular ultrasound is achieved with a 10- to 20-MHz or, if unavailable, a 7.5-MHz probe. One places the probe directly on the cornea or images through the eyelid or an offset device. Provided no other intraocular damage is evident, hyphema will resolve, often without significant sequelae. If associated intraocular damage has occurred, potential sequelae include cataract, posterior synechiae, glaucoma, retinal detachment, and blindness (Figure 17-19).

When hyphema results from a traumatic event, concurrent anterior uveitis is usually present. Although hyphema usually does not require therapy, the associated anterior uveitis does. As previously discussed, anterior uveitis is treated with topical atropine and systemic flunixin meglumine. If no corneal ulcer is associated with the hyphema, topical corticosteroids also may be administered. Resolution of hyphema may require 7 to 21 days; to decrease the incidence of rebleeding, the horse should not be exercised during this time. Surgical intervention to remove the hyphema rarely, if ever, is indicated. When lysis of a clot is beneficial, intracameral injection of tissue plasminogen activator (TPA; 25-75 μg; Activase, Genentech, Inc., South San Francisco, California) may be indicated.[85] Injection of TPA should not be performed until the cause of the hemorrhage is resolved and the vessel wall repair is complete, or rebleeding may occur. This generally happens 7 to 14 days after the initial bleeding episode.

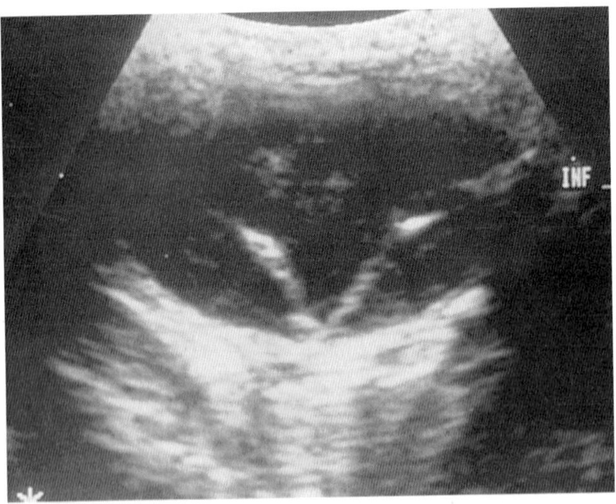

FIGURE 17-19 Ocular ultrasonography using a 7.5-MHz probe. A retinal detachment is visible with the retina remaining attached at the optic nerve and ciliary body.

LENS

The lens originates from surface ectoderm and is a clear, avascular, biconvex structure suspended posterior to the iris by lenticular zonules arising from the ciliary body. The lens depends on the aqueous and vitreous humors to supply nutrition and remove waste products. The lens should be examined in a darkened environment after dilation of the pupil with tropicamide 1.0% (Mydriacyl, Alcon Laboratories). Using a bright focal light source, one evaluates the lens for size, shape, location, and transparency. In addition, a new handheld, monocular slit lamp that attaches to an otoscope or ophthalmoscope handle is available (HSL-10) and provides magnification and an appreciation for depth and three-dimensional anatomy of the lens and anterior segment. Abnormalities of the lens include congenital malformations, cataract, and luxation.

CONGENITAL

Congenital disorders of the lens, other than cataract, are rare. Abnormalities of size (aphakia, microphakia), shape (coloboma, spherophakia), and location (luxation) generally are associated with other ocular abnormalities, such as microphthalmos, retinal dysplasia, and retinal detachment. These abnormalities can be unilateral or bilateral and may or may not be inherited. Treatment usually is not required except for cataract and luxation. Breeding of affected animals is discouraged.

CATARACTS

A cataract is any opacity, of any size, involving the lens or its capsule (Figures 17-20 and 17-21). Cataracts can be unilateral or bilateral and are classified according to location and degree of lens affected (Box 17-4). Classification helps determine the cause and likelihood of progression and helps the clinician follow progression. These terms are only descriptive and are

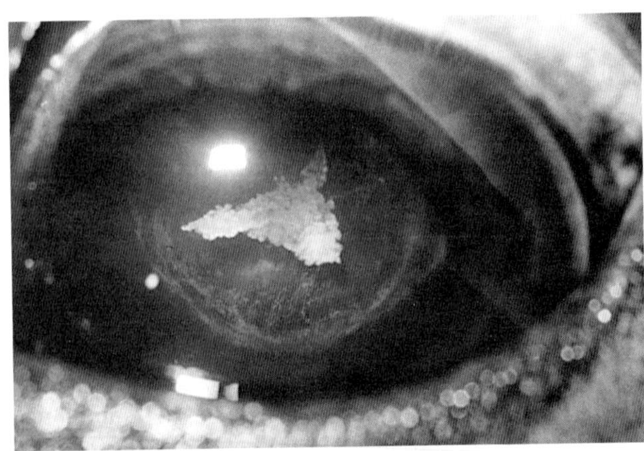

FIGURE 17-20 An incipient posterior cortical cataract.

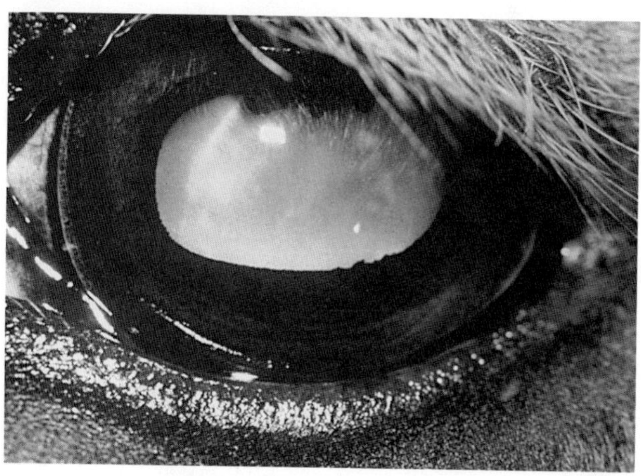

FIGURE 17-21 A mature cataract.

BOX 17-4

CHARACTERIZATION OF CATARACTS

Location
- Capsular
- Subcapsular
- Cortical
- Equatorial
- Axial
- Nuclear
- Anterior/posterior

Severity
- Incipient: earliest form; small vacuoles
- Immature: most of lens affected; fundus visible
- Mature: entire lens affected; fundus not visible
- Hypermature: liquefying lens fibers; leaking through lens capsule
- Morgagnian: entire cortex liquefied; nucleus settles ventrally

not mutually exclusive. For example, one such description might be an "anterior, cortical, axial, incipient cataract." In general, anterior, cortical, and equatorial cataracts are more likely to progress than are nuclear and posterior cataracts. In addition, cataracts are classified on the basis of age of onset and, if possible, cause. Classification by age of onset includes congenital, juvenile, adult, and senile cataracts. Congenital cataracts are the most common congenital ocular anomaly in the horse, can be unilateral or bilateral, and may affect only the nuclear portion of the lens.[86] Juvenile and adult cataracts, although acquired, are still heritable.

Although many causes of cataracts exist in other species, most causes have not been documented in the horse. Potential causes of cataract formation include inherited, inflammatory, traumatic, metabolic, toxic, and nutritional abnormalities. Suspected inherited cataracts have been reported in several breeds of horses (Belgian, Morgan) and are thought to occur in other breeds but are difficult to prove because of the small number of offspring produced. It is important to remember that inherited cataracts are not necessarily congenital and that not all congenital cataracts are inherited. In general, if the cause of a cataract cannot be determined and intraocular inflammation is not evident, breeding of the animal should be discouraged. The most common cause of cataract formation in the horse is ERU.

Treatment of cataracts, if required, is surgical. The decision to treat depends on the severity and cause of the cataract and the presence or absence of concomitant ocular disease. Cataracts that are unilateral or not sufficiently severe to interfere significantly with vision generally do not require treatment. Cataracts resulting from intraocular inflammation, such as those associated with ERU, may not be amenable to surgery. However, with the availabilty of a sustained-release cylosporine-impregnated device,[71-73] cataract surgery can be performed with or without a partial vitrectomy and implantation of a cyclosporin A device. Treatment of cataracts associated with abnormalities of the retina, such as retinal detachment or degeneration, is not indicated. If the cataracts are bilateral, interfere with vision, and do not result from ERU or other intraocular inflammation, then the lens and its anterior capsule can be surgically removed. Before cataract surgery, retinal anatomy and function should be evaluated using ocular ultrasound and electroretinography. One should operate on foals with congenital cataracts early (<6 months) to prevent possible deprivation amblyopia. Surgery is best performed using phacoemulsification.[5,87,88] An artificial intraocular lens implant (IOL) is now available for horses. Cataract extraction without implantation of an IOL results in a significant degree of postoperative hyperopia (farsightedness).[16] Implantation of an IOL is designed to correct this postoperative refractive error and restore the horse to emmetropia. Although use of an IOL is common in other species, it is only recent in the horse, and there is not sufficient information to discuss intraoperative and postoperative complications. Cataract surgery is a referral procedure.

Luxation

Lens luxation and subluxation can be congenital or acquired. Acquired lens luxation results from glaucoma and buphthalmos; trauma; or, most frequently, uveitis, especially ERU. Once luxated, the lens can be displaced anteriorly or posteriorly. A posteriorly luxated lens results in liquefaction of the vitreous from lens movement. The lens settles inferiorly, may or may not attach to the retina, and generally does not result in significant problems or require therapy. Anterior lens luxation results in anterior uveitis; trauma to the corneal endothelium, resulting in diffuse corneal edema; and obstruction of aqueous humor circulation, resulting in secondary glaucoma. Treatment of anterior lens luxation is surgical removal using an intracapsular extraction technique, provided the eye is visual. This is a referral procedure. In a blind, painful eye, enucleation or intrascleral prosthesis is the treatment of choice.

FUNDUS

The equine fundus is best examined in a darkened environment after mydriasis. Direct and indirect ophthalmoscopy are useful for examining the equine fundus, although direct ophthalmoscopy is preferable for examining the optic nerve and retinal blood vessels. Examination should include evaluation of the tapetal and nontapetal fundus, retina, retinal blood vessels, and optic nerve. Variations in the normal equine fundus are common, and familiarity with these variations is essential.[16,86,89,54] The horse has a periangiitic retina (partially vascularized) with 30 to 60 small retinal vessels radiating from the margin of the optic disc. These vessels are visible for a distance of one to two disc diameters. The remainder of the equine retina is avascular, being supplied from the underlying choroidal blood vessels. The optic disc is situated in the nontapetal fundus, is oval, and is salmon-pink. The fundus is divided into tapetal and nontapetal regions. The tapetum is situated in the dorsal fundus and is responsible for the characteristic yellow-green of this portion of the fundus. Variations in tapetal color are related to coat color and include yellow, orange, and blue-green.[16,86] The tapetum of the horse is fibrous and penetrated by small choroidal vessels that appear as dark dots in the tapetum, termed the *stars of Winslow*. The ventral, nontapetal fundus is generally dark brown or black but can appear lighter or nonpigmented depending on coat color.[16,86]

Abnormalities of the posterior segment can be congenital or acquired. Abnormalities on fundic examination include changes in size, shape, and color of the optic nerve and retinal vessels; elevation or depression of the optic nerve; hemorrhage; changes in tapetal reflectivity (hyper-reflective and hyporeflective), and changes in pigmentation. Hyperreflection abnormalities often indicate thinning or loss of retinal tissue. Hyporeflective changes can indicate an increase in tissue thickness resulting from cellular infiltrates, edema, or folding of the retina, as in retinal dysplasia. Inflammation can result in depigmentation and pigment clumping in the nontapetal fundus and hyperpigmentation in the tapetal fundus. Equine motor neuron disease has been described to result in a mosaic pattern of yellow-brown pigmentation in the tapetal fundus accompanied by a horizontal band of pigment at the tapetal-nontapetal junction.[90]

RETINA

Congenital Stationary Night Blindness

Equine night blindness is a bilateral, congenital, nonprogressive retinal disease of Appaloosas. The degree of visual disturbance varies among horses, with mildly affected horses exhibiting signs only in dark conditions, whereas severely affected horses are totally blind in the dark, exhibit apprehension in daylight, and may have a bilateral dorsomedial strabismus and nystagmus.[91] The diagnosis is based on history, breed of horse, clinical signs, and maze testing in illuminated and darkened environments, but it must be confirmed by electroretinogram because the fundic examination in affected horses is normal. Electroretinography demonstrates an almost purely negative waveform in the scotopic (dark-adapted) response, characteristic of equine night blindness.[91,92] The results of the electroretinogram indicate an abnormality in signal transmission from the photoreceptor cells to the inner retina.[91] Although the inheritance of equine night blindness in the Appaloosa is not defined completely, the disease is suspected to be an autosomal recessive disease. No treatment is available.

Chorioretinitis

Inflammation of the retina and choroid in the horse most often results from ERU and may be associated with concomitant optic neuritis. In addition, the vascular nature of the choroid results in susceptibility to bloodborne disease, as with bacteremia, septicemia, and viremia, and most often occurs in foals with pneumonia, strangles *(Streptococcus equi* subsp. *equi)*, and other severe infectious diseases. Inflammation of the anterior portions of the eye, anterior uveitis, often is associated with chorioretinitis. Treatment of chorioretinitis includes systemic therapy for the primary infectious disease, if present, and flunixin meglumine to decrease inflammation. Topical treatment is indicated only with anterior uveal involvement. The sequelae of chorioretinitis include retinal degeneration, retinal detachment, and optic nerve atrophy.

Retinal Detachment

Retinal detachment can be congenital or acquired, partial or complete (Figure 17-22). Because the equine retina depends almost totally on the underlying choroid for its blood supply, detachment results in rapid and severe retinal degeneration. Common causes of retinal detachment in the horse include an inherited abnormality (associated with retinal dysplasia), ERU, and trauma. Congenital retinal detachment often is associated with other ocular abnormalities. Hyphema may be associated with traumatic detachment, requiring ocular ultrasonography for definitive diagnosis. Treatment is limited to controlling the inciting disease and use of systemic anti-inflammatory drugs.

Photic Headshaking

A condition of headshaking induced by exposure to light and eliminated by blindfolding, darkened environment, and contact lenses has been reported in horses.[93,94] The problem usually occurs in the spring and summer; is exacerbated by exercise; and may be accompanied by sneezing, snorting, and nasal rubbing. Differential diagnoses for photic head shaking include middle ear disorders, ear mites, guttural pouch

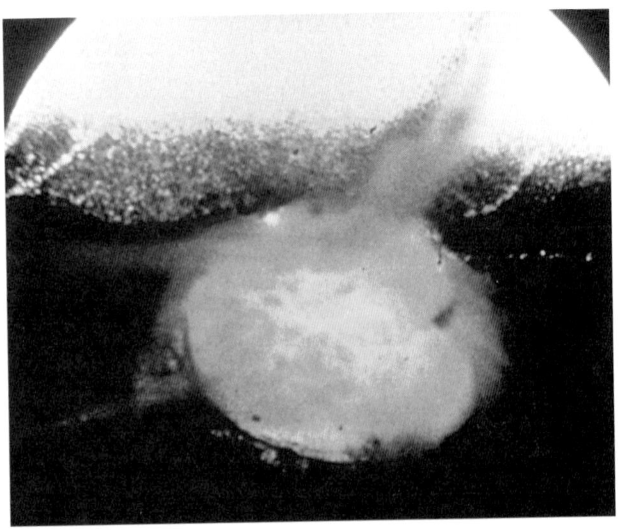

FIGURE 17-22 Gray folds of retina are visible overlying and adjacent to the optic nerve, indicating retinal detachment.

mycosis, other ocular disorders, and nasal and dental disease. Ophthalmic examination in these animals is normal. An optic-trigeminal response is hypothesized to occur with optic stimulation, resulting in referred stimulation in areas innervated by the trigeminal nerve.[93]

Treatment using cyproheptadine at 0.3 mg/kg (Sidmark Laboratories Inc., East Hanover, N.J.) orally every 12 hours has been effective in several horses.[93,94] Cyproheptadine is an antihistamine (histamine$_1$ blocker) and a serotonin antagonist and is hypothesized to work in photic headshaking by moderating the trigeminal nerve sensation, having a central effect on melatonin, or through anticholinergic activity.[93]

Equine Motor Neuron Disease

Equine motor neuron disease results from a dietary deficiency in the antioxidant vitamin E (See Chapter 12).[95,96] Ceroid-lipofuscin subsequently accumulates in the retinal pigment epithelium.[95] With ophthalmoscopy, this appears as irregular, sometimes linear accumulations of pigment in the tapetal and nontapetal retina (Figure 17-23). The ophthalmoscopic findings, along with appropriate musculoskeletal signs, highly suggest a diagnosis of equine motor neuron disease.

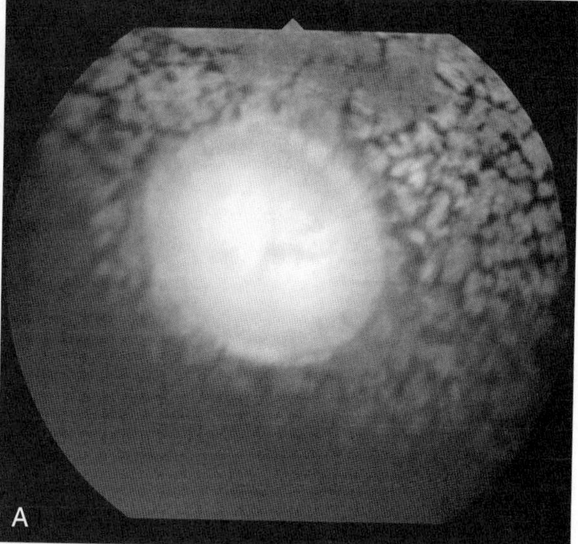

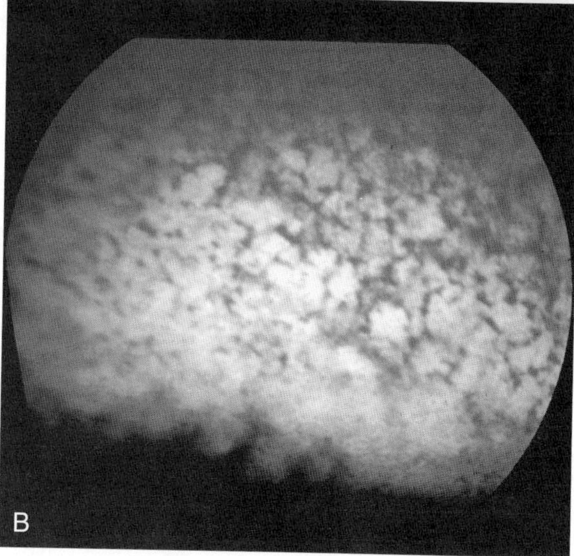

FIGURE 17-23 A, The optic nerve and peripapillary region of horse affected with equine motor neuron disease. The linear accumulations of pigment are ceroid-lipofuscin in the retinal pigment epithelium. **B,** Similar lesions are visible in the dorsal tapetal retina.

OPTIC NERVE

The equine optic nerve is oval, salmon-pink, and located in the nontapetal region of the fundus. Arterioles and venules (30 to 60) extend a short distance from the optic nerve into the surrounding peripapillary retina. On direct ophthalmoscopic examination the margin of the optic nerve is sharp and well defined, as are the retinal blood vessels. Often the nerve fiber layer of the retina is visible as linear white streaks radiating outward from the optic nerve. Congenital abnormalities of the optic nerve are rare and include coloboma and hypoplasia, which may occur alone or in association with other ocular congenital anomalies. Acquired abnormalities of the optic nerve may appear as indistinct margins, pallor, vascular attenuation, peripapillary depigmentation, edema, hemorrhage, or proliferative changes.

Optic Atrophy

Trauma to the head of the horse has been associated with acute unilateral or bilateral blindness resulting from optic nerve damage. The pupil in the affected eye is dilated, but the remainder of the ophthalmic examination may be normal initially. Occasionally, retinal hemorrhage and papilledema are present. Fundic examination 3 to 4 weeks after the traumatic episode reveals optic nerve pallor and absence of retinal blood vessels, indicating atrophy (Figure 17-24). The cause of this lesion is hypothesized to be stretching of the optic nerve with subsequent rupture of the optic nerve axons[97] or trauma from bony fractures adjacent to the optic nerve. A small number of these horses may benefit from systemic anti-inflammatory therapy in the acute phase. The prognosis, however, is guarded, and treatment usually is unrewarding. Optic nerve atrophy also is associated with ERU and results from chronic glaucoma.

Ischemic Optic Neuropathy

Ischemic optic neuropathy and resulting blindness are described as following treatment of guttural pouch mycosis by arterial occlusion (see Chapter 9). The horses are acutely blind, with a fixed and dilated pupil on the affected side immediately after surgery. Blindness is thought to result from ischemia and infarction of the optic nerve and its associated fibers. The initial fundic examination is normal, with abnormalities first seen 3 days after surgery. Indistinct optic disc margins suggesting papilledema or papillitis and raised, white lesions involving the optic nerve are the initial changes.

Optic Nerve Hypoplasia

Horses affected with optic nerve hypoplasia have visual impairment or blindness and slow to absent pupillary light reflexes.[16,86] The abnormality is congenital and can be unilateral or bilateral. Optic nerve hypoplasia may be associated with other ocular abnormalities, including cataracts, retinal detachment, and microphthalmos.[86] The optic disc appears

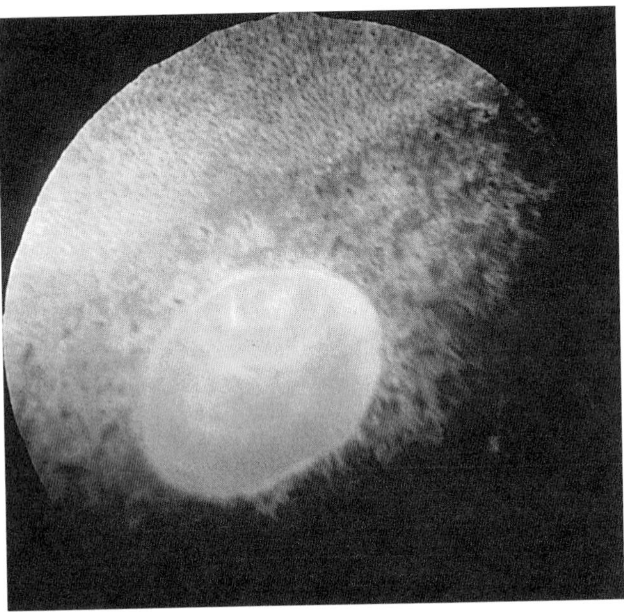

FIGURE 17-24 Severe optic nerve atrophy associated with head trauma. The optic nerve is pale, with loss of peripapillary retinal blood vessels. The horse is blind in the affected eye.

small and pale, with fewer retinal vessels than normal. Clinically, optic nerve hypoplasia can resemble acquired optic nerve atrophy. A definitive diagnosis can be made on histologic examination. No treatment is indicated, and although the definitive cause is not known, owners should not use the affected horse and possibly the sire and dam for breeding.

Other abnormalities of the optic nerve include bilateral optic neuropathy and blindness following severe hemorrhage[99]; proliferative optic neuropathy, as in aged horses[100]; neoplasia of the optic nerve[101]; and optic neuritis, which may be associated with ERU.

ORBIT

The horse has a complete bony orbital rim composed of the frontal, lacrimal, zygomatic, and temporal bones. The caudolateral and ventral walls of the equine orbit are fasciae. Abnormalities of the equine orbit usually result from trauma. The zygomatic arch and supraorbital process of the frontal bone and the medial orbital wall are most susceptible to injury. Damage to these areas can involve the supraorbital foramen and its associated nerve or the osseous portion of the nasolacrimal system, respectively.

The diagnosis of an orbital fracture is based on history, clinical signs, and radiographs. Radiographic evaluation of the equine orbit is technically difficult and often unrewarding. Oblique views, highlighting the area of greatest concern, usually are required. One must take care to evaluate the paranasal sinuses—the frontal, maxillary, and sphenopalatine—especially when subcutaneous emphysema is present.

Traumatic fractures of the orbit often are associated with concomitant injury of the globe and adnexa. Complete ophthalmic examination is essential and must include assessment of facial symmetry, vision (menace response, maze testing), pupillary light reflex, fluorescein staining for the presence of a corneal ulcer, examination of the anterior chamber for hyphema and anterior uveitis, fundic examination evaluating the retina and optic nerve, assessment of globe and eyelid mobility, and nasolacrimal irrigation. Head trauma in the horse has been reported to result in acute blindness with fixed, dilated pupils resulting from optic nerve compression, stretching, or avulsion. In those eyes in which ocular damage precludes examination of the posterior segment, ocular ultrasound examination is advised.

Blunt trauma to the orbit can result in a breakdown of the fibrous orbital septum and subsequent herniation of orbital fat. Clinically, the condition is a nonpainful swelling that appears at the time of, or following, orbital trauma and is best treated surgically, removing or replacing the herniated portion of the orbital fat pad and attempting to repair the rent in the septum.

Traumatic proptosis is rare in the horse because of the complete bony orbital rim. If the globe protrudes, it indicates severe head trauma, and thorough physical and neurologic examinations are required. Provided the optic nerve and extraocular muscles are intact, an exophthalmic globe should be replaced, a procedure that requires general anesthesia. After replacing the globe, one performs a temporary tarsorrhaphy to protect the eye until the swelling subsides. Systemic antibiotics and anti-inflammatory drugs are indicated to control postoperative complications.

Treatment of orbital trauma in the acute phase includes systemic anti-inflammatory therapy; systemic antibiotics, especially if a paranasal sinus is involved; and cold compresses. The anti-inflammatory drug of choice is systemic flunixin meglumine. Local therapy is required to manage corneal exposure, ulceration, and anterior uveitis. If eyelid movement is impaired because of neurologic dysfunction or swelling of the eyelids, the cornea must be protected from exposure and desiccation by using a topical, sterile ophthalmic lubricant applied as frequently as possible or, in the more severe cases, by using a temporary tarsorrhaphy. Topical broad spectrum antibiotics are indicated in horses with corneal ulceration, and atropine relieves the discomfort associated with anterior uveitis.

Although facial and orbital fractures in horses often heal without surgery, they may do so in a manner that results in deformity and interferes with the normal function of the eye and adnexa. Therefore surgical correction may be indicated, especially in those fractures that are displaced. Fractures that extend into a paranasal sinus must be considered as open fractures because these sinuses contain resident bacterial and fungal flora. Early repair is associated with a more favorable cosmetic result because skull fractures consolidate rapidly, and the resulting fibrous callus may interfere with surgical reduction. Generous skin flaps in the surgical approach are advised because fractures are often more extensive than initially thought. Excessive periosteal dissection is not recommended because periosteum provides stability and blood supply to the damaged area.

Orbital neoplasia is rare and may result in exophthalmos, strabismus, and vision and pupil abnormalities. Skull radiographs, orbital ultrasound, cytologic examination of a fine-needle aspirate, and histopathologic examination are useful in confirming the diagnosis. SCC, lymphosarcoma, adenocarcinoma, medulloepithelioma, melanoma, and tumors of neuroendocrine origin have been described.[102] Differential diagnoses include trauma and orbital abscess and cellulitis. Because most horses do not receive treatment until late in the course of disease, orbital exenteration is often the treatment of choice. If an orbital neurendocrine tumor is suspected, caution should be exercised during enucleation and exenteration because extensive intraoperative hemorrhage is frequent.

A technique for radical enucleation and exenteration with partial orbital rim resection, mesh skin expansion, and second intention healing has been described recently for extensive periocular tumors in horses.[103] This technique is indicated when skin is insufficient to complete a standard primary closure after surgical resection.

REFERENCES

1. van der Woerdt A, Gilger BC, Wilkie DA, et al: Effect of auriculopalpebral nerve block and intravenous administration of xylazine on intraocular pressure and corneal thickness in horses, *Am J Vet Res* 56:155-158, 1995.
2. Manning JP, St Clair LE: Palpebral, frontal, and zygomatic nerve blocks for examination of the equine eye, *Vet Med* 71:187-189, 1976.
3. Lavach JD: *Large animal ophthalmology*, St Louis, 1989, Mosby-Year Book.
4. Barnett KC, Crispin SM, Lavach JD, et al: *Color atlas and text of equine ophthalmology*, St Louis, 1995, Mosby-Wolfe.
5. Robinson NE, editor: *Current therapy in equine medicine*, ed 6, St Louis, 2009, Saunders.
6. van der Woerdt A, Wilkie DA, Gilger BC: Ulcerative keratitis secondary to single layer repair of a traumatic eyelid laceration in a horse, *Equine Pract* 18:33-39, 1996.
7. Knottenbelt DC, Kelly DF: The diagnosis and treatment of periorbital sarcoid in the horse: 445 cases from 1974 to 1999, *Vet Ophthalmol* 3:169-192, 2000.
8. Theon AP, Pascoe JR, Carlson GP, et al: Intratumoral chemotherapy with cisplatin in oily emulsion in horses, *J Am Vet Med Assoc* 202:261-267, 1993.
9. Theon AP, Wilson DW, Magdesian KG, et al: Long term outcome associated with intratumoral chemotherapy with cisplatin for cutaneous tumors in equidae: 573 cases (1995-2004), *J Am Vet Med Assoc* 230:1506-1513, 2007.
10. Whitley RD, Moore CP: Microbiology of the equine eye in health and disease, *Vet Clin North Am Large Anim Pract* 6: 451-466, 1984.
11. Moore CP, Heller N, Majors LJ, et al: Prevalence of ocular microorganisms in hospitalized and stabled horses, *Am J Vet Res* 49:773-777, 1988.
12. Samuelson DA, Andresen TL, Gwin RM: Conjunctival flora in horses, cattle, dogs, and cats, *J Am Vet Med Assoc* 184:1240-1242, 1984.
13. Collinson PN, O'Reilly JL, Ficorilli N, et al: Isolation of equine herpesvirus type 2 (equine gammaherpesvirus 2) from foals with keratoconjunctivitis, *J Am Vet Med Assoc* 205:329-331, 1994.
14. Moore CP, Sarazan RD, Whitley RD, et al: Equine ocular parasites: a review, *Equine Vet J* 2(suppl):76-79, 1983.
15. Lyons ET, Tolliver BS, Drudge JH, et al: Eyeworms (Thelazia lacrymalis) in one- to four-year-old thoroughbreds at necropsy in Kentucky (1984-1985), *Am J Vet Res* 47:315-316, 1986.
16. Gelatt KN, editor: *Veterinary ophthalmology*, ed 4, Philadelphia, 2007, Wiley-Blackwell.
17. Lyons ET, Drudge JH, Tolliver SC: Controlled tests with fenbendazole in equids: special interest on activity of multiple doses against natural infections of migratory stages of strongyles, *Am J Vet Res* 44:1058-1063, 1983.
18. Vasey JR: Equine cutaneous habronemiasis, *Compend Cont Educ Pract Vet* 3:290-294, 1981.
19. Rebhun WC, Mirro EJ, Georgi ME, et al: Habronemic blepharoconjunctivitis in horses, *J Am Vet Med Assoc* 179:469-472, 1981.
20. Cummings E, James ER: Prevalence of equine onchocerciasis in southeastern and midwestern United States, *J Am Vet Med Assoc* 186:1202-1203, 1985.
21. Lyons ET, Tolliver SC, Drudge JH, et al: Onchocerca spp: frequency in thoroughbreds at necropsy in Kentucky, *Am J Vet Res* 47:880-882, 1986.
22. Schmidt GM, Krehbiel JD, Coley SC, et al: Equine ocular onchocerciasis: histopathologic study, *Am J Vet Res* 43: 1371-1375, 1982.
23. Hacker DV, Moore PF, Buyukmichi NC: Ocular angiosarcoma in four horses, *J Am Vet Med Assoc* 189:200-203, 1986.
24. Dugan SJ, Roberts SM, Curtis CR, et al: Prognostic factors and survival of horses with ocular/adnexal squamous cell carcinoma: 147 cases (1978-1988), *J Am Vet Med Assoc* 198: 298-303, 1991.
25. Gelatt KN, Myers VS, Perman V, et al: Conjunctival squamous cell carcinoma in the horse, *J Am Vet Med Assoc* 168:617-620, 1974.
26. Dugan SJ, Curtis CR, Roberts SM, et al: Epidemiologic study of ocular/adnexal squamous cell carcinoma in horses, *J Am Vet Med Assoc* 198:251-256, 1991.
27. Schwink K: Factors influencing morbidity and outcome of equine ocular squamous cell carcinoma, San Francisco, 1985. In *Proceedings of the American College of Veterinary Ophthalmology*, pp 180.
28. Owen LN, Barnett KC: Treatment of equine squamous cell carcinoma of the conjunctiva using a strontium^{90} applicator, *Equine Vet J* 2(suppl):105-108, 1983.
29. Wilkie DA, Burt JK: Combined treatment of ocular squamous cell carcinoma in a horse, using radiofrequency hyperthermia and interstitial ^{198}Au implants, *J Am Vet Med Assoc* 196: 1831-1833, 1990.
30. Rebhun WC: Treatment of advanced squamous cell carcinomas involving the equine cornea, *Vet Surg* 19:297-302, 1990.
31. Theon AP, Pascoe JR, Madigan JE, et al: Comparison of intratumoral administration of cisplatin versus bleomycin for treatment of periocular squamous cell carcinomas in horses, *Am J Vet Res* 58:431-436, 1997.
32. Walker MA, Goble D, Geiser D: Two-year non-recurrence rates for equine ocular and periorbital squamous cell carcinoma following radiotherapy, *Vet Radiol* 27:146-149, 1986.
33. Grier RL, Brewer WG, Paul SR, et al: Treatment of bovine and equine ocular squamous cell carcinoma by radiofrequency hyperthermia, *J Am Vet Med Assoc* 177:55-61, 1980.
34. Latimer CA, Wyman M, Diesem CD, et al: Radiographic and gross anatomy of the nasolacrimal duct of the horse, *Am J Vet Res* 45:451-458, 1984.
35. Latimer CA, Wyman M: Atresia of the nasolacrimal duct in three horses, *J Am Vet Med Assoc* 184:989-992, 1984.
36. Cooley PL, Wyman M: Indolent-like corneal ulcers in 3 horses, *J Am Vet Med Assoc* 188:295-297, 1986.
37. Yamagata M, Wilkie DA: Gilger BC: Eosinophilic keratoconjunctivitis in seven horses, *J Am Vet Med Assoc* 209:1283-1286, 1996.
38. Moore CP, Collins BK, Fales WH: Antibacterial susceptibility patterns for microbial isolates associated with infectious keratitis in horses: 63 cases (1986-1994), *J Am Vet Med Assoc* 207:928-933, 1995.
39. Gemensky AJ, Wilkie DA, Kowalski J, et al: Changes in equine ocular bacterial and fungal flora following experimental application of topical antibiotic and antibiotic-corticosteroid ophthalmic preparations, *Am J Vet Res* 66:800-811, 2005.
40. Schoster JV: The assembly and placement of ocular lavage systems in horses, *Vet Med* 87:460-471, 1992.
41. Rebhun WC: Chronic corneal epithelial erosions in horses, *Vet Med Small Anim Clin* 78:1635-1639, 1983.
42. Gratzek AT, Kaswan RL, Martin CL, et al: Ophthalmic cyclosporine in equine keratitis and keratouveitis: 11 cases, *Equine Vet J* 27:327-333, 1995.

43. Ramsey DT, Whitley HE, Gerding PA, et al: Eosinophilic keratoconjunctivitis in a horse, *J Am Vet Med Assoc* 205: 1308-1311, 1994.
44. Coad CT, Robinson NM, Wilhelmus KR: Antifungal sensitivity testing for equine keratomycosis, *Am J Vet Res* 46:676-678, 1985.
45. Ball MA, Rebhun WC, Gaarder JE, et al: Evaluation of itraconazole-dimethyl sulfoxide ointment for treatment of keratomycosis in nine horses, *J Am Vet Med Assoc* 221:199-203, 1997.
46. Latimer FG, Colitz CMH, Campbell NB, et al: Pharmacokinetics of fluconazole following intravenous and oral administration and body fluid concentrations of fluconazole following repeated oral dosing in horses, *Am J Vet Res* 62:1606-1611, 2001.
47. Clode AB, Davis JL, Salmon J, et al: Evaluation of concentration of voriconazole in aqueous humor after topical and oral administration in horses, *Am J Vet Res* 67:296-301, 2006.
48. Holmberg DL: Conjunctival pedicle grafts used to repair corneal perforations in the horse, *Can Vet J* 22:86-89, 1981.
49. Hakanson N, Lorimer D, Merideth RE: Further comments on conjunctival pedicle grafting in the treatment of corneal ulcers in the dog and cat, *J Am Anim Hosp Assoc* 24-30:602, 1988.
50. Whittaker CJG, Smith PJ, Brooks DE, et al: Therapeutic penetrating keratoplasty for deep corneal stromal abscesses in eight horses, *Vet Comp Ophthalmol* 7:19-28, 1997.
51. Sweeney CR, Irby NL: Topical treatment of Pseudomonas sp. infected corneal ulcers in horses: 70 cases (1977-1994), *J Am Vet Med Assoc* 209:954-957, 1996.
52. Giuliano EA, Maggs DJ, Moore CP, et al: Inferomedial placement of a single-entry subpalpebral lavage tube for treatment of equine eye disease, *Vet Ophthalmol* 3:153-156, 2000.
53. Wilkie DA, Whittaker C: Surgery of the cornea, *Vet Clin North Am Small Anim Pract* 27:1067-1107, 1997.
54. Gilger BC, editor: *Equine ophthalmology*, St Louis, 2005, Saunders.
55. Brooks DE, Plummer CE, Kallberg ME, et al: Corneal transplantation for inflammatory keratopathies in the horse: Visual outcome in 206 cases, *Vet Ophthalmol* 11(208): 123-133, 1993-2007.
56. Lassaline ME, Brooks DE, Ollivier FJ, et al: Equine amniotic membrane transplantation for corneal ulceration and keratomalacia in three horses, *Vet Ophthalmol* 8:311-317, 2005.
57. Brooks DE, Millichamp NJ, Peterson MG, et al: Nonulcerative keratouveitis in five horses, *J Am Vet Med Assoc* 196: 1985-1991, 1990.
58. Rebhun WC: Corneal stromal abscesses in the horse, *J Am Vet Med Assoc* 181:677-679, 1982.
59. Hendrix DVH, Brooks DE, Smith PJ, et al: Corneal stromal abscesses in the horse: a review of 24 cases, *Equine Vet J* 27:440-447, 1995.
60. Andrew SE, Brooks DE, Biros DJ, et al: Posterior lamellar keratoplasty for treatment of deep stromal abscesses in nine horses, *Vet Ophthalmol* 3:99-104, 2000.
61. Andrew SE: *Corneal stromal abscess in a horse* 2:207-212, 1999.
62. Munger RJ: Equine onchocercal keratoconjunctivitis, *Equine Vet J* 2(suppl):65-69, 1983.
63. Walde I: Band opacities, *Equine Vet J Suppl* 2:32-41, 1983.
64. Dziezyc J, Samuelson DA, Merideth R: Ciliary cysts in three ponies, *Equine Vet J* 22:22-25, 1990.
65. Gilger BC, Davidson MG, Nadelstein B, et al: Neodymium: yttrium-aluminum-garnet laser treatment of cystic granula iridica in horses: 8 cases (1988-1996), *J Am Vet Med Assoc* 211:341-343, 1997.
66. Ramsey DT, Ewart SL, Render JA, et al: Congenital abnormalities of Rocky Mountain horses, *Vet Ophthalmol* 2:47-59, 1999.
67. Sillerud CL, Bey RF, Ball M, et al: Serologic correlation of suspected Leptospira interrogans serovar pomona–induced uveitis in a group of horses, *J Am Vet Med Assoc* 191:1576-1578, 1987.
68. Dwyer AE, Crockett RS, Kaslow CM: Association of leptospiral seroreactivity and breed with uveitis and blindness in horses: 372 cases (1986-1993), *J Am Vet Med Assoc* 207:1327-1331, 1995.
69. Burgess EC, Gillette D, Pickett JP: Arthritis and panuveitis as manifestations of Borrelia burgdorferi infection in a Wisconsin pony, *J Am Vet Med Assoc* 189:1340-1342, 1986.
70. Hines MT: Immunologically mediated ocular disease in the horse, *Vet Clin North Am Large Anim Pract* 6:501-512, 1984.
71. Gilger BC, Wilkie DA, Davidson MG, et al: Use of an intravitreal sustained-release cyclosporine delivery device for treatment of equine recurrent uveitis, *Am J Vet Res* 62:1892-1896, 2001.
72. Gilger BC, Malok E, Stewart T, et al: Long-term effect on the equine eye of an intravitreal device used for sustained release of cyclosporine A, *Vet Ophthalmol* 3:105-110, 2000.
73. Wilkie DA, Gemensky AJ, Norris KN, et al: Intravitreal cyclosporin A implantation for equine recurrent uveitis, *Vet Ophthalmol* 4:292, 2001.
74. Gilger BC, Salmon JH, Wilkie DA, et al: A novel bioerodible suprachoroidal cyclosporine implant for uveitis, *Invest Ophthalmol Vis Sci* 47:2596-2605, 2006.
75. Fruhauf B, Ohnesorge B, Deegen E, et al: Surgical management of equine recurrent uveitis with single port pars plana vitrectomy, *Vet Ophthalmol* 1:137-151, 1998.
76. Wilkie DA, Peckham ES, Paulic S, et al: Equine glaucoma and diode laser transscleral cyclophotocoagulation: 27 cases, *Vet Ophthalmol* 4:294, 2001.
77. Willis AM, Robbin TE, Hoshaw-Woodard S, et al: Effect of topical 2% dorzolamide HCL and 2% dorzolamide HCL-0.5% timolol maleate on intraocular pressure in normal horse eyes, *Am J Vet Res* 62:709-713, 2001.
78. van der Woerdt A, Wilkie DA, Gilger BC, et al: Effect of single and multiple dose timolol maleate 0.5% on intraocular pressure and pupil size in female horses, *Vet Ophthalmol* 3: 165-168, 2000.
79. Herring IP, Pickett P, Chanpagne ES, et al: Effect of topical 1% atropine on intraocular pressure in normal horses, *Vet Ophthalmol* 3:139-143, 2000.
80. Nasisse MP, Davidson MG, MacLachlan NJ, et al: Neodymium: yttrium, aluminum, and garnet laser energy delivered transsclerally to the ciliary body of dogs, *Am J Vet Res* 49: 1972-1978, 1972.
81. Miller TL, Willis AM, Wilkie DA, et al: Description of ciliary body anatomy and identification of sites for transscleral cyclophotocoagulation in the equine eye, *Vet Ophthalmol* 4:183-190, 2001.
82. Morreale RJ, Wilkie DA, Gemensky AJ, et al: Acute histologic effects of transcleral cyclophotocoagulation on the normal horse eye, *Vet Ophthalmol* 4:289, 2001.
83. Whigham HM, Brooks DE, Andrew SE, et al: Treatment of equine glaucoma by transscleral neodymium:yttrium aluminium garnet laser cyclophotocoagulation: a retrospective study of 23 eyes of 16 horses, *Vet Ophthalmol* 2:243-250, 1999.
84. Provost PJ, Ortenburger AI, Caron JP: Silicone ocular prosthesis in horses: 11 cases (1983-1987), *J Am Vet Med Assoc* 194(1764-1766):1989.
85. Martin C, Kaswan R, Gratzek A, et al: Ocular use of tissue plasminogen activator in companion animals, *Prog Vet Comp Ophthalmol* 3:29-36, 1993.

86. Munroe GA, Barnett KC: Congenital ocular disease in the foal, *Vet Clin North Am Large Anim Pract* 6:519-537, 1984.
87. Dziezyc J, Millichamp NJ, Keller C: Use of phacofragmentation for cataract removal in horses: 12 cases (1985-1989), *J Am Vet Med Assoc* 198(1774-1778), 1991.
88. Millichamp NJ, Dziezyc J: Cataract phacofragmentation in horses, *Vet Ophthalmol* 3:157-164, 2000.
89. Gelatt KN: Ophthalmoscopic studies in the normal and diseased ocular fundi of horses, *J Am Anim Hosp Assoc* 7:158-167, 1971.
90. Jackson CA, Riis RC, Rebhun WC, et al: Ocular manifestations of equine motor neuron disease, *Proc Am Assoc Equine Pract* 41:225, 1995.
91. Rebhun WC, Loew ER, Riis RC, et al: Clinical manifestations of night blindness in the Appaloosa horse, *Compend Cont Educ Pract Vet* 6:S103, 1984.
92. Witzel DA, Joyce JR, Smith EL: Electroretinography of congenital night blindness in an Appaloosa filly, *J Equine Med Surg* 1:226-230, 1977.
93. Madigan JE, Kortz G, Murphy C, et al: Photic headshaking in the horse: 7 cases, *Equine Vet J* 27:306-311, 1995.
94. Wilkins PA: Cyproheptadine: medical treatment for photic headshakers, *Compend Cont Educ* 19:98-102, 1997.
95. Riis RC, Jackson C, Rebhun W, et al: Ocular manifestations of equine motor neuron disease, *Equine Vet J* 31:99-110, 1999.
96. Riis RC, Divers TJ: Effect of vitamin E deficiency on horse retinas, *Vet Ophthalmol* 3:254, 2000.
97. Martin L, Kaswan R, Chapman W: Four cases of traumatic optic nerve blindness in the horse, *Equine Vet J* 18:133-137, 1986.
98. Hardy J, Robertson JT, Wilkie DA: Ischemic optic neuropathy and blindness after arterial occlusion for treatment of guttural pouch mycosis in two horses, *J Am Vet Med Assoc* 196:1631-1634, 1990.
99. Gelatt KN: Neuroretinopathy in horses, *J Equine Med Surg* 3:91-95, 1979.
100. Vestre WA, Turner TA, Carlton WW: Proliferative optic neuropathy in a horse, *J Am Vet Med Assoc* 181:490-491, 1982.
101. Bistner SI, Cambell RJ, Shaw D, et al: Neuroepithelial tumor of the optic nerve in a horse, *Cornell Vet* 73:30-34, 1983.
102. Basher AWP, Severin GA, Chavkin MJ, et al: Orbital neuroendocrine tumors in three horses, *J Am Vet Med Assoc* 210:668-671, 1997.
103. Beard WL, Wilkie DA: Partial orbital rim resection, mesh skin expansion, and second intention healing combined with enucleation or exenteration for extensive periocular tumors in horses, *Vet Ophthalmol* 5:23-28, 2002.

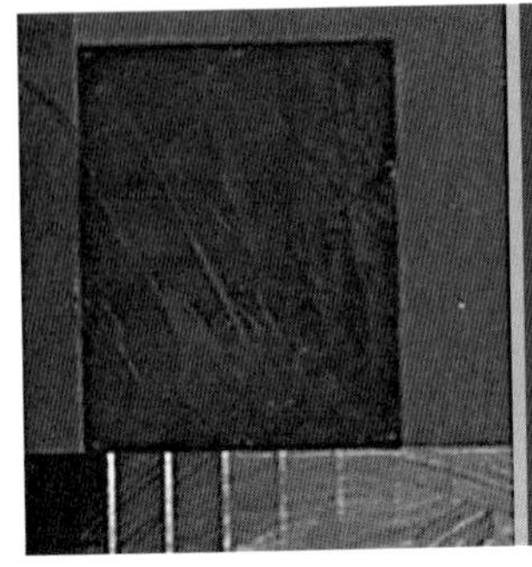

Disorders of the Reproductive Tract

CHAPTER 18

Grant Frazer

REPRODUCTIVE ANATOMY AND PHYSIOLOGY OF THE NONPREGNANT MARE

Daniel C. Sharp, Michael B. Porter

Equine reproductive physiology deviates from other domestic and companion animal models, often providing open-minded practitioners and researchers with a lifetime of challenges or frustrations, depending on their approach. This chapter presents the authors' current understanding of equine reproductive physiology set against a backdrop of accepted dogma for other species as often as appropriate.

SEASONAL REPRODUCTIVE CYCLE

A dominant and often troublesome feature of equine reproduction is the adherence to an annual rhythm of reproductive competence and incompetence. The annual reproductive cycle of mares reflects an evolutionary strategy to maximize survival of foals by programming the breeding season so that it is attuned to gestation length. Thus mares, with approximately 11 months' gestation, begin to breed in the midspring so as to time parturition in midspring. Therefore the mechanisms best able to regulate timing of the annual reproductive cycle are long-term and highly reliable. Nutritional and environmental temperature changes do not fit that requirement well. The four main phases of the annual reproductive rhythm are discussed in the subsequent sections.

Anestrus

Anestrus usually occurs during the shortest days of winter and is characterized by reproductive incompetence in most mares. Measurements of hypothalamic gonadotropin-releasing hormone (Gn-RH)[1-4] indicate a low hypothalamic Gn-RH content and secretion rate during anestrus. Pituitary gonadotropin secretion consequently is reduced, with low or undetectable circulating concentrations of luteinizing hormone (LH) and follicle-stimulating hormone (FSH).[5-7] Although pituitary stores of FSH appear to be adequate throughout anestrus,[8] this is not the case with LH. The messenger ribonucleic acid (mRNA) encoding LH subunit production becomes undetectable in pituitary tissue during anestrus.[9,10] Thus pituitary gonadotropins (FSH and LH) are low during anestrus because of suppression of the releasing signal from the hypothalamus (Gn-RH), plus inactivation of the gene encoding LH synthesis in the pituitary. The result is, not surprisingly, loss of function of the ovaries. Ovarian activity, including follicular development and hormone production, is minimal, with few follicles greater than 5 mm in diameter and undetectable circulating concentrations of estradiol and progesterone.

As might be expected from this reduction in circulating hormones, sexual receptivity in mares during anestrus tends to be reduced or lacking altogether. Given the lack of circulating hormones, the passivity of mares in response to teasing not surprisingly is highest in winter.[6]

Vernal (Springtime) Transition

The vernal transition of the annual reproductive cycle, which begins sometime around the first of the calendar year, is the most troublesome commercially. The first event in transition—likely the initiating one—is an increase in hypothalamic Gn-RH observable within 1 week after the winter solstice[2] or 2 weeks after exposure to an artificially increased photoperiod several weeks before the solstice (Figure 18-1).[11] Whether the increase in hypothalamic Gn-RH represents a response to increasing day length, refractoriness to short day length, or some other factor remains unresolved.

Hart, Squires, Imel, et al.[8] reported that the increased Gn-RH secretion shortly after the winter solstice leads to increased FSH secretion from available pituitary stores but that LH levels remain low. Sherman, Wolfe, Farmerie et al.[9] explained this phenomenon, stating that the mRNA encoding LH subunit synthesis was undetectable in the winter and early spring. The third major event during the vernal transition, after hypothalamic Gn-RH secretion and subsequent release of pituitary FSH stores, is follicular development. During vernal transition the size and number of manually detectable follicles increases.[12,13] The follicular population changes from only two or three small follicles (5 to 10 mm in diameter) to six or more midsize follicles (15 to 25 mm), with the diameter of the largest follicle exceeding 35 to 40 mm.[12] A major problem early in the breeding season is that many of these large vernal transition follicles do not ovulate. In ponies an average 3.5 ± 0.7 large (≥30 mm) anovulatory follicles develop in sequence before the first ovulation of the year.[6] These anovulatory vernal transition

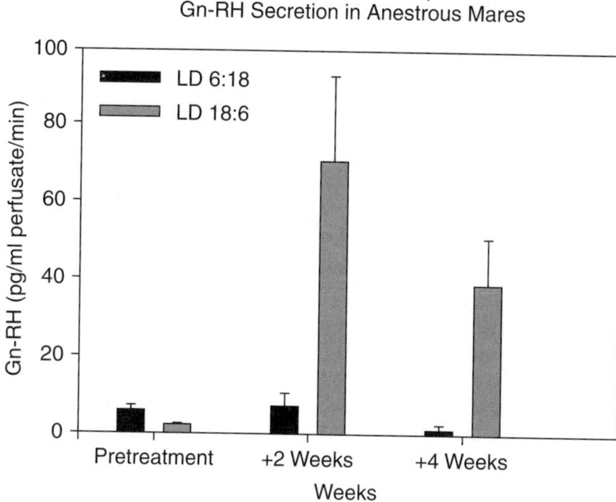

FIGURE 18-1 Gonadotropin-releasing hormone (Gn-RH) secretion (picograms per milliliter per minute, LS means ± SEM) as measured with push-pull perfusion of the pituitary in mares exposed to short photoperiod (LD 6:18, n = 4) and in mares exposed to long photoperiod (LD 18:6, n = 4) for 4 weeks. In the bars marked pretreatment, all mares had been exposed to LD 6:18. Subsequently, four mares were exposed to LD 18:6, and Gn-RH secretion was measured at 2-week intervals. Time of year the experiment was begun was December 1. Gn-RH was highly significantly elevated in mares after only 2 weeks of photostimulation.

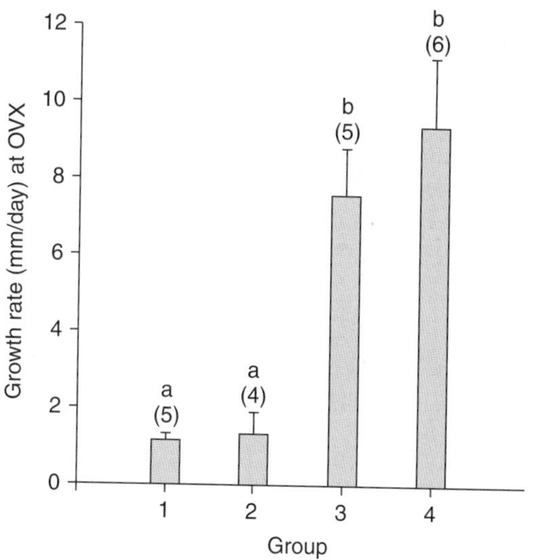

FIGURE 18-2 Growth rate (millimeters per day) of follicles during vernal transition. Groups represent mares at first, second, third, and fourth follicle of the year. (From Tucker KE, Cleaver BD, Sharp DC: Does resumption of follicular estradiol synthesis during vernal transition in mares involve a shift in steroidogenic pathways? *Biol Reprod* (suppl 1) 48:188, 1993.)

follicles are the cause of high reproductive inefficiency during the springtime, and it is impossible to discern, by palpation or ultrasound, whether they will be ovulatory. Consequently, many mares are sent to the stallion inappropriately, which adds to to the frustration and expense of breeding. Furthermore, mares with chronic failure of uterine clearance likely suffer most from such an inappropriate breeding, and the penalty to the breeder is often greater expense aimed at resolving uterine contamination.

The first several vernal transition follicles are different from fully functional follicles during the breeding season. Although they attain a diameter comparable with that of preovulatory follicles of the breeding season (>30 mm), they do so much more slowly. Careful tracking of follicles reveals that the first and second large follicle of the year grow at a rate of only 1 to 2 mm per day (Figure 18-2), compared with growth rates of about 10 mm per day for follicles that go on to ovulate.[14] Therefore one may assess the potential functional status of springtime follicles by frequently monitoring their growth.

The slower growth rate of vernal transition follicles reflects other metabolic deficiencies, including poor vascularity compared with that of ovulatory follicles and significantly smaller granulosa cell content.[15] The poor granulosa cell investment of early vernal transition follicles is significant in that the granulosa cell layer contributes substantially to the steroidogenic capabilities of the follicle. Thus steroid production by the early vernal transition follicles is limited. The follicles do not produce estradiol, as monitored by peripheral blood, follicular fluid, or in vitro production rate. Estradiol concentration is low or undetectable in peripheral plasma until 5 or 6 days before the first ovulation of the year.[7,14,16] One can measure circulating estradiol to discriminate between nonfunctional and functional (ovulatory) follicles.

When one of the sequential vernal transitional follicles acquires steroidogenic capability, the circulating estradiol increases significantly 5 to 6 days before the first ovulation of the year. The average date for the first ovulation of the year is consistent from year to year, and variance among mares in a population is low. Data collected from as far north as 43 degrees north latitude to as far south as 18 degrees north latitude have indicated an onset of the breeding season (date of first ovulation of the year) to be around the first week of April in mares and the second week of May for pony mares that have not been exposed to artificial lighting. Once the first ovulation of the year has occurred, vernal transition is completed and regular polyestrous cycles occur throughout the late spring and summer in unbred mares.

Renewed LH synthesis and secretion, also manifested by a large surge 5 to 6 days before the first ovulation of the year, is associated with the rise in estradiol. Sharp, Grubaugh, Davis et al.,[17] and Cleaver and Sharp[18] have demonstrated that administration of estrogen advances this secretion of LH in mares during early vernal transition, and Sharp, Wolfe, Cleaver et al.[10] further demonstrated that estrogen administration to ovariectomized mares at the same time of year stimulated the mRNA encoding for the LH α and β subunits. In other words, estrogen administration was associated with activation of the LH gene. However, as Freedman, Garcia, and Ginther[5] and Peltier, Robinson, and Sharp[7] have demonstrated, the increase in peripheral LH occurs at approximately the same time in mares with and without ovaries. Thus the role of estrogen in bringing about the resurgence of LH synthesis and secretion remains unclear. Furthermore, one must resist the temptation to use estrogen to hasten LH synthesis in mares during the early vernal transition because of the negative effects of estrogen on FSH secretion. The clinician may initiate LH synthesis only to find that it inhibits follicular development.

Breeding Season

The next section discusses the breeding season in detail. The breeding season is characterized by regularly recurring cycles of estrus and diestrus throughout the summer, unless pregnancy occurs.

Autumnal Transition

The transition from reproductive competence in the breeding season to reproductive quiescence characteristic of anestrus is perhaps the least understood part of the annual seasonal reproductive cycle in mares. The period of reproductive decline has a much greater variance during the fall than does the period of reproductive renewal in the spring. The variance is understandable from the evolutionary aspect, because mares likely faced little pressure to reproduce in the fall because their offspring would face more difficult survival at foaling the next year. Although this is an oversimplification, the autumnal transition may be characterized simply as the gradual loss of gonadotropic support for ovarian function, resulting in reduced follicular development. The final act of the autumnal transition may be development of a large preovulatory follicle that fails to ovulate.[19]

MORPHOLOGIC BEHAVIORAL AND HORMONAL CHANGES OF THE ESTROUS CYCLE

Estrus

Estrus, defined by receptivity of the mare to a stallion, is characterized by profound changes in the ovaries as follicles develop and in the uterus, cervix, and vagina as the developing follicles begin producing estrogen and by the occurrence of a prolonged surge or increase in LH.

BEHAVIOR

Understanding estrous behavior, as monitored by teasing with a stallion, is an important foundation to any breeding program. The word *estrus,* coined by Walter Heape,[20] is thought to come from the Greek word *Oestridae,* a genus of the gadfly, because locomotor activity of many female ungulates increases during estrus. Estrous behavior is associated temporally with increasing estrogen concentrations peripherally but also may be associated with the concomitant decline in progesterone levels. Support for the idea that estrogen may not be essential for estrous behavior comes from observations of estrous display in mares with inactive ovaries and from ovariectomized mares during anestrus.[21] The displays of estrous mares reflect a wide range of behaviors and extents, however, and successful breeding farms often owe their success in part to careful monitoring and record keeping for each mare. Among the signs observed during estrus are elevation of the tail in the presence of the stallion, eversion of the vulvar lips to expose the clitoris ("winking"), squatting with rotation of the pelvis, urination, and remaining calm (i.e., not moving away) in the immediate presence of a stallion. Recording behavioral signs tends to take the decision making out of the watching process and potentially provides a more precise record of progress through the estrous cycle.

OVARIAN MORPHOLOGY

Morphologic changes during estrus can be used to monitor the progress toward ovulation. The equine ovary is structurally different from that of other species in that the cortical elements containing the primordial follicles are located centrally in the ovary instead of peripherally, as in all other species that have been studied so far. This central position of potential ovulatory follicles presents a dilemma in that ovulation cannot occur at the site of follicle development. Most of the surface of the equine ovary is covered with mesothelium, which apparently does not allow the tissue remodeling required for rupture of the follicle. Instead, ovulation in the mare always occurs at a specific site, called the "ovulation fossa," which is located ventrally on the ovary. The bean shape of the equine ovary creates a recessed fossa area in which germinal epithelium is located. This inside-out structure of the mare's ovary likely contributes to some of the unusual aspects of the equine estrous cycle, including the period of prolonged estrus, the large preovulatory follicle size, and the prolonged increase in LH that precedes ovulation. A logical assumption is that the structure of the ovary led to co-evolution of a hypothalamic-pituitary axis that was able to present gonadotropins over a prolonged duration. The ovarian structure requires extensive tissue remodeling for a developing follicle to reach the restricted area of the fossa where it can ovulate. The extended gonadotropin secretion seems likely to be an important part of the tissue remodeling process that precedes rupture of the follicle. Administration of Gn-RH analog to stimulate endogenous LH release, or human chorionic gonadotropin (hCG; LH activity), results in increased levels of tissue remodeling enzymes in the follicle within 24 hours.[22] This prolonged process presents challenges to the breeder or veterinary practitioner who is attempting to schedule breeding at a time appropriate to the expected ovulation.

TUBULAR REPRODUCTIVE TRACT

Perhaps the two most prominent changes in the equine tubular reproductive tract are the appearance of the external portion of the cervix and the pattern of intrauterine edema as monitored with ultrasound. The vaginal portion of the cervix exhibits cyclic changes that reflect the rise and fall of estrogens and progesterone. During estrus the cervix becomes relaxed and droops toward the ventral floor of the anterior fornix, whereas in diestrus, under the influence of progesterone, the external cervical folds become more rigid and buttonlike, or "tight and white" in the vernacular. One can appreciate these changes by visual examination with a vaginal speculum.

Changes in intrauterine edema are evident, as monitored by ultrasound imaging, in the pattern of fluid (edema) present in the endometrial folds during estrus (Figure 18-3). The appearance of edema often is used to indicate estrus, but an important note is that the relationship between edema and ovulation is inverse. Edema is maximal several days before ovulation and then begins to dissipate. Ovulation occurs 3 to 4 days after peak edema scores are exhibited and the edema pattern is in the process of dissipation.[23] Because estrogen stimulates edema rapidly (within 6 hours), the presence of edema appears to be a useful indicator of estrogen secretion. However, dissipation of the edema is an active process, requiring the presence of ovaries, and likely involves progesterone as well. Far more intriguing, then, is the question of the mechanism of dissipation of edema. What is the purpose of edema

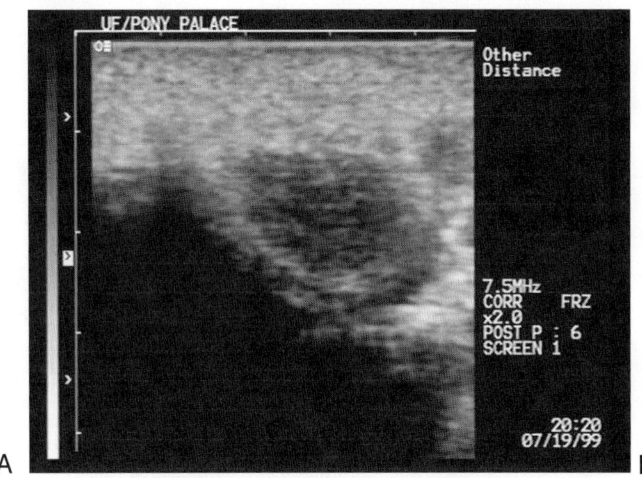

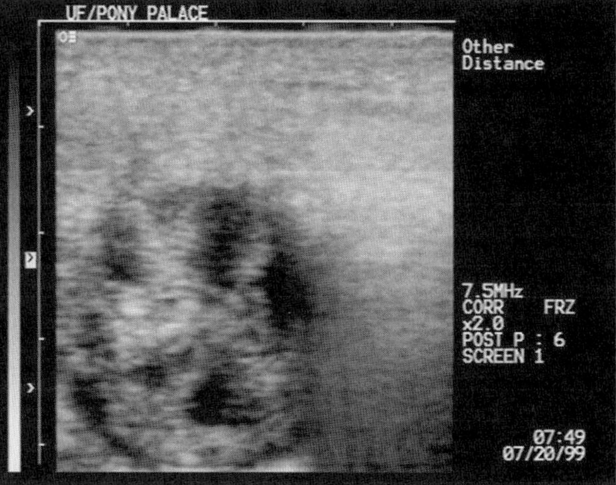

FIGURE 18-3 A, Portion of uterine horn showing edema score of 1 (relatively homogeneous pattern with little evidence of fluid). **B,** Portion of uterine horn showing edema score of 4 (marked heterogeneity with clear evidence of fluid-filled lacunae).

in the first place if an active process exists for its dissolution before ovulation?

HORMONES

Estrus in mares is characterized by increasing estrogen and a prolonged elevation in LH. The prolonged elevation of LH,[24] often reaching peak concentrations after ovulation, may reflect the need for extensive tissue remodeling of the ovaries for ovulation to occur. Estradiol reaches peak concentrations of greater than 30 to 40 pg/ml 2 to 3 days before ovulation. Evidence exists for a positive feedback effect of estradiol on LH,[25] but evidence also suggests that LH rises spontaneously after corpus luteum (CL) regression and the loss of progesterone negative feedback. This raises the question of whether estrogen positive feedback is necessary for the ovulatory increase in LH or whether it merely serves to enhance the default situation of elevated LH in the absence of progesterone.

DIESTRUS

Diestrus is essentially the polar opposite of estrus from the behavioral standpoint.

BEHAVIOR

Mares generally exhibit little or no interest in the approach of a stallion, and this often is manifested by violent demonstrations (e.g., kicking, switching of the tail, flattening of the ears, vocalizing) in a teasing situation. Rising progesterone concentrations are thought to play a role in the sexual nonreceptivity of mares. Although not critically determined, the sexually negative behavior of mares is widely assumed to be associated with progesterone concentrations greater than 1 ng/ml. Progesterone concentrations increase quickly after ovulation, reaching 1 ng/ml by 24 to 48 hours after ovulation, which coincides with the expected onset of diestrus.

OVARIAN MORPHOLOGY

The primary feature of ovarian morphology in diestrus is the presence of a CL within the ovary. Because of the inside-out structure of the ovary and the restriction of ovulation to the ovulation fossa, the CL remains almost entirely within the ovary and provides little evidence of its presence by transrectal palpation, which is not the case with ruminants. The advent of ultrasound imaging has improved diagnostic capabilities by enabling practitioners to visualize the CL.

HORMONES

Diestrus is dominated by elevated progesterone, with its negative feedback effect on LH secretion.

POSTPARTUM PERIOD

Immediately after expulsion of the fetus, the equine uterus begins the process of involution, and this continues for several days after passage of the placenta. During this time detection of fluid within the uterine lumen by ultrasound is not abnormal. However, the uterine fluid (lochia) and debris should dissipate 7 to 10 days after parturition in preparation for "foal heat" in the mare.[26] One should not detect fluid by ultrasound 10 to 14 days postpartum, and the uterus should be restored to nearly prepregnancy condition within 3 to 4 weeks.

Foal heat is defined as the first period of sexual receptivity after parturition and usually begins 7 to 9 days after foaling.[27] The first ovulation after foaling occurs on average at 9 days after foaling. Depending on the efficiency of uterine involution, the fertility of this foal heat varies. If significant fluid is present within the uterus at foal heat, breeding the mare is not recommended. In addition, studies regarding the effect of season on first postpartum ovulation suggest that mares that foal in January and February tend to have longer intervals from foaling to the first fertile ovulation than mares that foal in late spring.[28] After the foal heat most mares have a 30-day heat that occurs approximately 21 days after the foal heat and may represent a more fertile estrous cycle.

In addition to the effects of season, a condition known as *lactational anestrous* may develop immediately after foaling. In some cases the condition may persist until weaning (4 to 6 months). Determining whether the lactational anestrous results from the foal nursing or the time of year (seasonal) is important. Limited studies have been performed in which foals were removed from mares at varying time points after parturition. Research indicates that removal of the foal hastens the onset of estrus. Foal removal has been associated with elevated LH concentrations and increased ovarian follicle diameter.[29]

MARE BREEDING SOUNDNESS EXAMINATION

Nigel R. Perkins, John B. Chopin

Breeding soundness examination (BSE) of the mare may be performed for a variety of reasons, including prepurchase or prebreeding examinations to confirm the absence of detectable abnormalities involving the genital tract and examination of subfertile mares after unsuccessful breeding or tentative identification of a potential problem associated with the genital tract. Procedures that should be performed in all BSEs include perineal examination, rectal palpation, ultrasonography, vaginoscopy, and digital vaginal examination. Additional procedures may be considered depending on patient signalment, history, and initial findings of each individual.

IDENTIFICATION

Detailed identification of the mare is very important. The recording of acquired brands, tattoos, and detection of a microchip should all be considered to supplement the physical description or photographs.

SIGNALMENT AND HISTORY

History and signalment may suggest possible problems and guide the diagnostic approach (Table 18-1). The use of drugs during an athletic career can affect the horse's breeding future. The use of anabolic steroids can change behavior and external genitalia. There might also be a downregulating effect on the hypothalamic-pituitary-gonadal axis that has to reverse over time. The use of an anti-GnRH vaccine (Equity; Pfizer Animal Health, West Ryde, Australia) is an effective way to inhibit estrus behavior in fillies. Unfortunately a number of fillies have had prolonged ovarian inactivity into their breeding career.[1] The author had one cytogenetically normal mare that was retired from breeding with four seasons of ovarian inactivity after the use of the vaccine.

Breeding history should include detailed information from the immediate past, including information on the standard of breeding management and facilities. It is also valuable, though more difficult, to obtain historical information on the mare's entire breeding career.

BEHAVIOR

The season of the year should be considered when assessing behavior in the mare.[2] Assessing the mare's response to the teaser while in estrus is important for future breeding use. Shy or aggressive behavior toward the teaser by the mare while in physiological estrus might limit natural breeding options.

TABLE 18-1

Details of Information to be Gathered During History Taking

History	Comments
General health	Vaccination, deworming, foot care, dental care, nutritional history, systemic diseases, and management
Athletic	Level of activity, age at which athletic career ended, any known drug usage
Cycling	Length of estrus, expression of estrus, interovulatory interval
Breeding	Number of cycles bred, breeds per cycle, natural or artificial insemination, fertility of stallion, age at which the mare was last bred
Pregnancies	Number of diagnosed pregnancies and outcomes
Foaling	Any history of dystocia, type of management
Prior reproductive examinations	Diagnoses, treatment, management
Prior reproductive surgeries	Nature of surgery, date performed and outcome
Drug use during breeding season	Ovulation induction, estrous cycle manipulation

GENERAL PHYSICAL EXAMINATION

General observation of the mare while loose and being led to the stocks will allow assessment of behavior and preliminary assessment of condition and conformation. A brief general physical examination should be performed to ensure that the mare has no detectable condition that could interfere with an ability to conceive or carry a foal to term. The practitioner should inspect the mammary glands visually and with digital palpation for evidence of abnormalities such as mastitis, fibrosis, and neoplasia. In general, excessive body condition will not interfere with reproductive potential, whereas poor body condition may.

RESTRAINT

The mare must be adequately restrained before examination. What constitutes adequate restraint will depend on the nature of the mare, the skill and experience of the handler and veterinarian, procedures being performed, and the physical facilities available. Particular care must be exercised when performing a BSE on mares with little prior exposure to procedures such as transrectal palpation. Stocks should be used for restraint during a BSE. The primary function of stocks is to prevent the mare moving forward or to the side during the examination.

Chemical restraint is an effective and safe method in most cases for BSE procedures, particularly in those that are either less well tolerated or more prolonged. Chemical restraint may cause some degree of relaxation of the perineal region and alter assessment of vulval conformation in some cases. If possible, examination of vulval conformation should be made before sedation.

EXAMINATION OF EXTERNAL GENITALIA

The perineal region is inspected for indications of vulval discharge and gross abnormalities of the anogenital region. Vulval discharge or urine scalding of the inner thighs may suggest genital infection, urine pooling, or urinary incontinence. Clitoral enlargement may indicate prior exposure to androgens or progestagens or an intersex condition. Normal vulval lips are vertical, have good tone, and are in close apposition. The practitioner should gently part the vulval lips to determine if air is readily aspirated into the vagina. If there is poor vulval apposition or ready aspiration of air, then the mare may be prone to pneumovagina and at increased risk of ascending vaginitis.

Vulval integrity is important in the formation of an effective seal against contamination of the genital tract with air, urine, feces, and potential pathogens.[3] Vulval conformation is assessed by digital palpation adjacent to the vulval lips to locate the caudal bony pelvic brim. Pascoe's description of a Caslick index has been modified to produce a simple assessment technique for vulval conformation:[4]

- VC (vulval conformation) good: No Caslick is required. Dorsal commissure of the vulva is less than 4 cm above the bony pelvic brim, and vulval lips are within 10 degrees of vertical and form an effective seal.
- VC marginal: Caslick may be required. Dorsal commissure of the vulva is 4 to 7 cm above the bony pelvic brim, vulval lips are within 10 to 20 degrees of vertical, vulval lips are still forming an effective seal.
- VC poor: Caslick or some other corrective procedure is definitely required. Dorsal commissure of vulva is 5 to 9 cm or more above the bony pelvic brim, vulval lips are 30 degrees or more in front of vertical, and the vulval seal is less than effective.

TRANSRECTAL PALPATION AND ULTRASOUND EXAMINATION OF THE GENITAL TRACT

It is absolutely imperative that the nonpregnant status of the mare be confirmed before any procedure is performed that could threaten a pregnancy, even if the history suggests that she is not pregnant. Transrectal palpation of the genital tract is associated with some risk of rectal mucosal trauma and potentially laceration. The risk increases if excessive force is used, if palpation continues in the presence of pneumorectum, and if the mare strains excessively. Mild sedation to relieve the anxiety of the animal, especially with mares that are not accustomed to the experience, may be accomplished with an α-2 agonist (e.g., xylazine) with or without an opioid (e.g., butorphanol). Administration of N-butylscopolamine by intravenous injection several minutes before the examination may also help prevent straining, but it may interfere with assessment of uterine tone.

Palpation of the genital tract requires a methodical approach. The author usually locates the uterus and palpates structures in the following sequence: right uterine horn, right ovary, right uterine horn, left uterine horn, left ovary, left uterine horn, uterine body, cervix. Cervical size and consistency are assessed by pressing the cervix down against the pelvic floor. Cervical relaxation can most effectively be measured on a sliding scale, from 0% relaxed (i.e., tightly closed, tubular cervix) to 100% relaxed (i.e., indistinguishable from adjacent uterus).[5]

It is important to purposefully assess anatomic structures other than the genital tract as part of the palpation examination, including pelvis, intestines, lymph nodes, and bladder. Note the presence of soft tissue or bony changes that may narrow the luminal diameter of the pelvis. Possible causes include vaginal lacerations, hematoma, abscessation, neoplasia, and pelvic fracture.

Ultrasound examination should be considered a routine part of a reproductive tract examination. Ultrasound examination allows the use of electronic calipers for measuring structures and allows assessment of tissue and fluid characteristics. Table 18-2 presents comparative information on the application of palpation and ultrasound for assessing various genital tract structures.

TABLE 18-2

Application of Transrectal Palpation and Ultrasound of the Genital Tract for Assessing Various Parameters

Organ	Structure	Detail of assessment	Technique
Ovary	Ovary	Size, shape, presence of ovulation fossa	P, US
		Echotexture of contents	US
		Consistency of tissue	P
	Corpus haemorrhagicum	Presence	P, US
	Corpus luteum	Presence or absence, size, shape, echotexture	US
	Follicles	Size	P, US
		Shape, wall thickness and echotexture, echotexture of contents	US
		Turgidity	P
Uterus		Diameter, shape, tone, wall thickness, endometrial folds, luminal fluid (larger amounts)	P, US
		Wall echotexture, endometrial folds, luminal fluid volume and echotexture	US
Cervix		Length, width, depth	P, US
		Echotexture	US
		Relaxation	P
Vagina and vestibule		Fluid accumulation, gas (air) accumulation	P, US

P, Transrectal palpation; *US*, ultrasound.

The same basic approach is used for ultrasound examination as described previously for rectal examination. While holding a linear transrectal ultrasound probe, the practitioner extends the fingers beyond the ventral surface of the probe to assist in locating genital tract structures and to palpate uterine horns for assessing uterine tone. The uterine body is initially identified as a landmark by sweeping the probe from side to side in the anterior pelvis. The uterine body is then followed cranially to the bifurcation and the probe then swept out toward the right uterine horn and right ovary. Structures are examined in the same order as for palpation alone: right horn, right ovary, right horn, left horn, left ovary, left horn, uterine body, and cervix. As the probe is withdrawn into the pelvic cavity, the uterine body is examined by moving the probe from side to side.

A simple recording system should be used with defined abbreviations. This ensures that records can be understood at a later date and facilitates a common approach for use by multiple attending veterinarians. Uterine horn diameter should be measured about one third of the distance from the bifurcation, and uterine tone is recorded with presence of dilation and fluid. Endometrial folds can be assessed by gently palpating the uterus between fingers and thumb. The practitioner should assess the dimensions and shape of each ovary and ensure that the ovulation fossa is detectable (loss of ovulation fossa can be an early indicator of distortion of the normal ovarian shape caused by neoplasia). All follicles larger than about 15 mm in diameter are recorded individually, and smaller follicles are recorded as multiple small follicles. Loss of turgidity is recorded for preovulatory follicles (softness being a possible indicator of impending ovulation).

DIAGNOSIS OF OVARIAN PATHOLOGY

Abnormal ovarian enlargement should be suspected if an ovary is greater than 10 cm in diameter and the increased size cannot be attributed to recent ovulation or a follicle and persists for more than a month.[5,6] Large ovaries may be associated with physiologic causes (e.g., persistent follicles, hematoma, multiple CLs) or pathologic processes (e.g., neoplasia, abscess).

Neoplasia more commonly affects one ovary, although it can affect both, and typically results in a variable degree of alteration in ovarian size, shape, and consistency. There appears to be no consistent pattern in the change affecting a neoplastic ovary, with the exception of teratomas in which the diagnosis may be based on detection of germ tissues, including cartilage, hair, and bone. Other neoplasias may present as single large cystic or multicystic structures or even solid tissue. In many cases the diagnosis of ovarian neoplasia is based on persistent unilateral ovarian enlargement with obliteration of the ovulation fossa and an inactive or normally functioning contralateral ovary.[7,8] There might be a history of aberrant ovarian activity before the development of the tumor.[9] A granulosa cell tumor may produce varying levels of testosterone, estrogen, and inhibin[9,10] but rarely produce progesterone. The measurement of α-inhibin might be more accurate for diagnosis than measuring $\alpha\beta_A$-inhibin.[11]

Functional ovarian tumors such as granulosa-theca cell tumor (GTCT) may manifest as masculinization of appearance and behavior and increased plasma inhibin and testosterone concentrations.[12] The ultrasonographic appearance of the GTCT is characteristic, varying from uniformly dense to cystic.[13,14]

Anovulatory follicles often grow to an unusually large size and fill with blood, organizing into a structure with the ultrasonographic appearance of a hematoma that gradually recedes over time. Some of these structures appear to develop a thick rim of tissue resembling luteal tissue, with the mare entering a diestrus-like state. Others do not develop a thick rim of tissue, and the structure may appear to be inert. There is a lack of consensus regarding terminology, with some authors distinguishing anovulatory hemorrhagic follicles (no luteinization) from luteinized unruptured follicles (development of luteal rim). Others suggest that the two structures are variations of the same condition.[15] The condition appears to be more common in mares approaching winter anestrous and in pregnant mares under the influence of equine chorionic gonadotropin. Anovulatory follicles occur in 8% of all estrous cycles[16] but in 5% of estrous cycles in the early ovulatory season and 20% of estrous cycles in the late ovulatory season.[17] The ultrasonographic appearances of ovulatory and anovulatory follicles are largely the same.

Failure of the normal process of luteolysis may result in prolonged luteal maintenance. Diagnosis depends on confirmation of nonpregnant status and the presence of a CL for a period longer than the normal diestrus length. This condition, termed *pseudopregnancy,* must be differentiated from cases in which a mare is ovulating between examinations and exhibiting an apparently persistent CL. Luteolysis depends on prostaglandin (PG) release from the uterus,[18-20] which in turn might depend on a uterine clock being set for PG release. An ovulation during diestrus does not always set this clock, and the resultant CL can last for more than 2 months.[19,20] Other reasons for failure of luteolysis include release of PG when the CL is still immature and unable to respond to PG (before 6 days of age), failure of PG to be released at the proper time, and insignificant release of PG from the endometrium in mares with degenerative endometritis.[21]

Small cystic structures may be palpated or visualized ultrasonographically, adjacent to the ovary. These are typically incidental findings assumed to be cystic remnants of the mesonephric tubules and ducts. It is possible that these structures could interfere with gamete transport if they obstruct normal function of the ovarian bursa and infundibulum.

Very small and inactive ovaries may be secondary to seasonal anestrus, reproductive senescence in old mares, pituitary gland dysfunction, severe malnutrition, administration of anabolic steroids, administration of anti-GnRH vaccine, or congenital infertility resulting from sex chromosome abnormalities.[1,22] Sex chromosome abnormalities are often associated with hypoplasia or segmental aplasia of the tubular tract. Karyotyping may be used to further investigate such mares. Chromosomal abnormalities have also been reported from subfertile mares that have foaled previously and have no detectable abnormalities of the genital tract. In light of this fact, karyotyping may be considered in mares in which routine diagnostic procedures fail to explain subfertility.

Individuals with 63,X karotype tend to be small in stature, phenotypically female, with small uterus and ovaries, and no sexual behavior.[23-26] However, some might show irregular estrus behavior, and the uterus palpably and histologically can be within normal limits.[24,27] Plasma estrogen levels are low and plasma LH levels are normal to high.[24] Sex reversal is a disorder that occurs in horses and can have a variety of abnormalities.[28] The two most common forms of sex reversal are mare phenotype with male karyotype 64,XY and male phenotype with female karyotype 64,XX. There can be a wide phenotype variation with both conditions.[29,30]

X trisomy is relatively rare in the horse. The mare is infertile; shows estrus behavior and normal external genitalia; and is phenotypically female, with small, thin walled uterus and small hypoplastic ovaries.[23,25,31,32]

Mosaics and chimeras occur when the individual has more than one cell line with different chromosomal makeups. 63,X/64,XX mosaics are phenotypically female; the uterus varies in development, but ovaries may be small and nonfunctional. These horses may show estrus behaviour, an endometrial biopsy reveals glandular hypoplasia, and the clitoris may be enlarged.[23-25,26,33]

DIAGNOSIS OF UTERINE PATHOLOGY

ENDOMETRITIS

Ultrasonography is very useful for evaluating presence, quantity, and echotexture of uterine luminal fluid. Fluid echotexture is correlated with the amount of debris or white blood cell infiltration into the fluid and is more common in older mares.[34] Table 18-3 presents a grading system for recording uterine fluid echotexture.[35] The presence of grade I, II, or III fluid during any stage of the cycle indicates endometritis. The presence of fluid in diestrus results in a lower pregnancy rate and a higher embryo loss rate,[36] presumably caused by high levels of PGF_{2a} in the fluid from the neutrophils.[37] The presence of more than 2 cm of fluid in the lumen during estrus, the presence of fluid during diestrus, and fluid 72 hours after insemination are strong indicators of mare susceptibility to endometritis.[38] Table 18-4 presents a grading system for recording the volume of intrauterine fluid.

TABLE 18-3

Classification System for Recording Uterine Fluid Echotexture

Grade	Ultrasound Appearance	Gross Appearance
I	White (hyperechoic)	Thick and creamy
II	Light gray	Milky
III	Black with white specks	Obvious sediment in fluid
IV	Black (anechoic)	Clear fluid

TABLE 18-4

Grading System for Recording Volume of Intrauterine Fluid

Classification	Maximum Fluid Depth (mm)	Gross Description
VS (very small)	1 to 2	Barely detectable
S (small)	1 to 5	Often focal
M (moderate)	5 to 20	Obvious fluid
L (large)	>20	Immediately apparent

Complete absence of detectable uterine luminal fluid during estrus is associated with absence of cytologic inflammation in 99% of cases.[39] The significance of clear (grade IV) luminal fluid is less clear. Small or very small volumes of clear fluid during estrus are likely to be normal, particularly if present during early estrus before complete cervical relaxation and maximal uterine drainage. Large volumes of clear fluid during estrus, fluid that persists into late estrus, or smaller volumes during early diestrus suggest an increased predisposition to endometritis and reduced pregnancy rates compared with mares without fluid.[39-41] Luminal fluid visible more than 12 to 20 hours after breeding indicates mating-induced endometritis.[22,42] This condition has recently been reported in 10% to 15% of mares being bred on a commercial Thoroughbred stud farm.[43]

Discrete hyperechogenic reflections seen in the uterine lumen on ultrasonographic examination indicate air. Pneumouterus may be seen in normal mares soon after uterine treatment, insemination, or breeding but should not be seen more than hours after breeding or treatment. The presence of pneumouterus at times other than soon after breeding or uterine therapy indicates loss of integrity of physical barriers to contamination (vulva, vestibulovaginal sphincter, and cervix).

ENDOMETRIAL CYSTS

Circumscribed, discrete collections of clear fluid within the uterine lumen indicate endometrial cysts or a conceptus. Cysts may occur on the endometrial surface or within the endometrium. Cysts may be single, discrete structures closely resembling a conceptus or complex, compartmentalized structures with irregular borders. Cysts that protrude into or occlude the uterine lumen may reduce fertility by interfering with embryo mobility and maternal recognition of pregnancy.[36,44,45] Cysts within the endometrium may interfere with gland function.

Properties of an early conceptus that can be used to distinguish it from a cyst include the following: movement between days 10 through 16 post ovulation; spherical, symmetric appearance; rate of growth (cysts are assumed to grow little if at all); and appearance of the embryo proper after about day 20. In addition, there are palpable changes in the tract that are consistent with early pregnancy (e.g., increased uterine tone and closed, elongated cervix) that would not be expected to occur in a nonpregnant mare with endometrial or lymphatic cysts. Any association between cysts and reduced fertility remains unclear.[46] Large cysts or large numbers of cysts may interfere with embryonic movement, maternal recognition of pregnancy, and early placentation. Extensive glandular cystic change may also adversely affect uterine gland function and compromise establishment or normal development of pregnancy.

PYOMETRA

Pyometra is a chronic condition with mucoid or mucopurulent material within the uterine lumen, with or without cervical occlusion. The condition is not dependent on the presence of a CL, as it usually is in other species, and does not typically result in any systemic signs of illness. Pyometra may be mistaken for pregnancy on palpation as a result of fluid distention of the uterus but can be diagnosed effectively with ultrasound.[47]

Adhesions

Adhesions and scarring involving the endometrium may result from infusion of irritating solutions into the uterus and perhaps as a result of trauma associated with dystocia and its correction. Luminal adhesions involving the cervix have similar initiating causes. The role of chronic endometritis or iatrogenic causes such as mechanical curettage in uterine or cervical adhesions is less clear. Adhesions may reduce fertility by interfering with function of the uterotubal junction or with embryo movement and maternal recognition of pregnancy.[45]

Occlusive adhesions may result in accumulation of fluid in the proximal portions of the tubular tract, and this may be detected on palpation or ultrasound examination of the tract. More commonly, adhesions are detected during hysteroscopy.

Focal uterine lesions may respond well to surgical removal using a biopsy instrument or laser surgical equipment guided by hysteroscopy.[48] If the lesions are extensive or affecting the deeper layers of the endometrium, then the prognosis may be poor and treatment not warranted. Cervical adhesions are commonly managed by manual disruption and then repeated application of topical ointment containing antibiotic and steroid in an attempt to prevent recurrence. In many horses, cervical adhesions tend to recur once treatment stops.

Ventral Uterine Sacculation

Ventral sacculation is associated with a loss of normal muscular contractile activity in the uterine wall, with the uterine wall forming sacculations ventrally at the base of one or both uterine horns. The condition is more common in older, multiparous mares and may indicate increased risk of endometritis caused by loss of the normal contractile mechanisms responsible for expelling uterine luminal fluid. This may also be linked to mares that have a more ventral oriented uterus. When the uterocervical angle is more ventral than horizontal, the mare is more prone to fluid accumulation because of a reduced ability to clear fluid.[49]

Hygiene for Vaginal Procedures

Good hygienic practice is essential in performing any vaginal procedure and particularly those procedures that involve penetration of the cervix. This is perhaps the simplest and most fundamental principle of good reproductive practice. The practitioner should bandage the proximal portion of the tail or enclose it in a plastic sleeve and tie it to the mare's neck with a quick release knot; alternatively, an assistant may hold it out of the way. The perineal region should then be washed with water and detergent and rinsed thoroughly, preferably with a spray nozzle attached to a hose to deliver a constant supply of fresh clean water. The practitioner should then wipe just inside the vulval lips with damp cotton to remove any contaminating material; this is particularly important for mares with sloping vulval lips or if a rectal examination has just been performed. The presence of fecal matter in the dorsal vestibular area without a history of any invasive procedures indicates a failure of the vulvovestibular seal.

Use of sterile, plastic sleeves for vaginal procedures is ideal. A practical alternative used by the author is to keep, in a dust-free area, a zipper storage bag (e.g., Ziploc) containing clean plastic sleeves to be used for vaginal procedures only. A new sleeve is taken out carefully by grasping it only at the open end, or each sleeve is turned inside out immediately before putting it on to minimize the risk of contamination. Tearing off the fingers from a plastic sleeve and putting on a sterile, surgical glove can increase sensitivity and also facilitate cleanliness. Sterile lubricant and equipment should be used. The practitioner should be meticulous to prevent contamination of either equipment or sleeves and gloves during any procedure.

Vaginal Speculum Examination

A sterile, lubricated speculum is inserted into the vestibule in a slightly dorsal direction to avoid the urethral opening and pushed through the vulvovestibular sphincter, with sphincter integrity assessed as the speculum is inserted. Because they reduce the risk of iatrogenic infection, single-use, sterile, disposable specula are preferred over metal caslick specula for routine examinations. In some cases, a self-retaining metal caslick speculum may provide better visualization of the caudal vagina and vestibule.

Vaginoscopy is useful for detection of vaginal hyperemia, suppurative exudates, persistent hymen, urine pooling, varicose veins, vaginal trauma, rectovaginal defects, and cervical defects. Although examination with a vaginal speculum may be performed at any stage of the cycle, inspection of mares suspected of pooling urine is best performed during estrus because estrogenic relaxation of the genital tract and perineal region is maximal at this time.[50] Vaginal speculum examination is an important component of the BSE but should not be considered a routine procedure to be performed repeatedly in normal mares.

The timing of the vaginal examination in relation to the rectal examination is also important. Careful cleaning of the perineum is required if the vaginal examination follows the rectal examination. However, this slight disadvantage is offset by the advantage of doing the rectal ultrasound examination first to assess pneumovagina and pneumouterus. The presence of air in the vagina and uterus is difficult to interpret after a vaginal examination. However, if air is present before a vaginal examination, it may indicate vulvovestibular seal dysfunction. Repeated vaginoscopy may be associated with an increased risk of iatrogenic vaginitis and persistent infection. As a result, the author prefers to perform routine assessment of cervical relaxation by transrectal palpation.

Manual Examination of the Vagina and Cervix

Examination of the genital tract is incomplete without manual exploration of the vagina and cervix. The major benefit in this procedure is detection of cervical defects. Once the hand is inserted into the anterior vagina, the forefinger is placed into the cervical lumen and the thumb in the vaginal fornix. The hand is then rotated and the entire circumference of the cervix palpated between finger and thumb to feel for disruption in the cervix resulting from lacerations or damage to submucosal layers that might interfere with the ability of the cervix to close effectively. Cervical disruption is significant only if it prevents the cervix from forming an effective seal during diestrus and pregnancy. A partial tear involving the external os of the cervix may not require treatment if the cervix can still maintain an effective seal. For this reason, assessment of the severity of cervical disruption should be performed when the mare is in diestrus.[51] Alternatively, the diestrus tone can be duplicated by the administration of progesterone or progestagen for a few days to close the cervix.

Care should be taken while performing a manual examination of the vagina and cervix to take time to palpate the vaginal surface for problems such as rectovaginal fistulas, vaginal lacerations, and perivaginal hematoma or abscess formation. The examiner should also consider the length and diameter of the cervical canal in relation to the estrous stage of the mare. A tortuous canal might impair drainage. The older maiden mare, typically older than 10 years of age, can have a long, narrow cervix that is difficult to open and has poor drainage of uterine fluid.

Endometrial Culture and Cytology

The practitioner must not perform any procedure that involves penetrating the cervix of a mare unless the nonpregnant status of the mare has been confirmed by transrectal palpation, either alone or in combination with ultrasonography.

A variety of instruments and techniques have been described for culturing the genital tract. The lack of consistency in methodology has almost certainly contributed to the lack of consensus regarding the role and interpretation of genital tract cultures. Interestingly, in a group of mares infected with *Klebsiella,* the normal uterine swab was less sensitive at detecting infection (27/60) than use of a tampon (55/60).[52] A gynecologic brush was superior to a cotton swab or aspiration in the detection of endometritis. The cotton swab often produced a false-negative result.[53] In the author's experience, aspiration or analysis of a small volume saline lavage can sometimes yield more information than a cotton swab. Sterile digital sampling of the endometrium has been described as a quick stallside test for cytology.[54] Care should be taken not to collect neutrophils from caudal areas of the reproductive tract and interpret that as endometritis.

Cultures may be taken from multiple sites in the genital tract, including endometrium, cervix, vagina, clitoral fossa, and clitoral sinuses. The isolation of bacteria from the anterior vagina is associated with reduced fertility.[55] Genital tract culture performed to investigate possible endometritis or as part of a BSE should be taken from the endometrial lumen and not from the vagina or cervix. Endometrial culture should be performed before any other invasive procedure in a BSE to reduce the risk of inadvertent contamination of the uterine lumen before taking the culture sample.

A guarded culture rod should be used to minimize the risk of contamination with material from sites other than the uterine lumen.[56] Single- or double-guarded culture rods may be used. It is also possible to take an endometrial culture from a uterine biopsy sample as long as the culture sample is taken in a sterile manner and before placing the tissue into fixative. There is a lack of consensus on the optimal time of the cycle for obtaining endometrial culture and cytology samples. Some experts recommend performing endometrial cultures on the first or second day of estrus, when uterine secretions are increasing and the flushing action of the uterus is just beginning.[57,58]

Mares with endometritis have been reported to accumulate free luminal fluid in late diestrus, and this represents an alternative time for endometrial culture.[36] The practitioner should carry the guarded culture rod into the vagina and through the cervix beside one finger. The rod is then passed cranial to the finger, into the endometrial lumen, and the culture tip pushed through the guard and rolled against the endometrial surface for 30 to 60 seconds. The culture tip is withdrawn into the rod before withdrawing the culture rod to prevent contamination during removal from the genital tract.

The sample should be transferred onto the final growing medium immediately after the sample is obtained to allow quantification of colony numbers as an indication of severity of infection. When possible, quantification of colony growth should be performed because heavy growth after 24 to 48 hours' incubation is more meaningful than a few scattered colonies. If immediate plating is not possible, transfer the culture tip in a sterile manner into appropriate transport medium. Use of transport medium allows proliferation of some species and possibly reduced growth of others, so colony counts are not interpretable.

Interpretation of endometrial culture results is difficult. False-positive and false-negative results are common. Several recommendations can be made to minimize the likelihood of an erroneous interpretation. Culture results should be interpreted in conjunction with results of concurrent endometrial cytologic examination. In addition, the practitioner should consider whether the organisms recovered represent pure or mixed growth and whether growth can be considered heavy or light. Acute endometritis is more commonly associated with mixed bacterial growth on culture than pure growth.[59]

A wide range of organisms have been isolated from horses with acute endometritis. A combination of positive culture and evidence of inflammation on endometrial cytology is sufficient to diagnose endometritis and identify the organisms recovered as the causative agents. A positive bacterial culture in the absence of any cytologic evidence of inflammation is considered likely to be due to contamination during the culture procedure and does not indicate endometritis.

In the absence of cytologic evidence, it is particularly difficult to interpret culture results. Recovery of relatively pure or heavy cultures of the following organisms may be considered indicative of endometritis: β-hemolytic streptococci, hemolytic *Esherichia coli, Pseudomonas* spp., *Klebsiella* spp., and *Candida* spp.[60,61] Recovery of other organisms without concurrent cytologic information should be viewed with more suspicion.

Endometrial cytology is used by some practitioners as a rapid screening test for detection of endometrial inflammation in mares at the beginning of the breeding season or before breeding. When it was first described in the mare,[62] the detection of neutrophils was correlated with positive bacteriologic findings. When no or low numbers of neutrophils were detected, bacteriologic findings were more often negative.[62] Mares with cytologic evidence of inflammation had lower 28-day pregnancy rates than mares with normal cytologic results, irrespective of culture results. Day 28 pregnancy rates were also lower in mares that had bacteria isolated from their uterus even if cytologic results were normal.[63]

Numerous techniques have been described for collecting cytologic samples. The approach used by the author is simple, rapid, and feasible in busy clinical practice. A guarded culture rod with a snap-on cap (Kalayjian: Kalayjian Industries Inc., Long Beach, California) is used to collect a culture sample. The swab tip is withdrawn back into the sheath and the rod rolled against the endometrium to collect fluid and cells in the cap. After the rod is withdrawn from the mare, the cap can be cut off and tapped against a slide to make the smear from the small drop of fluid.[64] The smear is dried and stained using any commercial staining kit (e.g., Diff-Quik; (American Scientific Products, McGaw Park, Ill.). If no endometrial cells are seen on an initial inspection of the slide, the sample may not have been collected from the uterus and another sample should be taken. The presence of polymorphonucleocytes (PMNs) is generally believed to indicate bacterial endometritis, but the most appropriate methodology for quantifying PMNs remains subject to debate. Suggestions for criteria to diagnose endometrial inflammation include observation of more than 1 or 2 PMNs in five high-power microscope fields (400×) or more than 1 PMN per 10 endometrial cells in more than one area of the slide.[65,66] In most mares with endometritis, there are large numbers of PMNs evident on cytologic evaluation.

Endometrial Biopsy

Preparation for endometrial biopsy is the same as for culture or cytology. Diestral samples are generally preferred over estral samples because physiologic changes in the endometrium during estrus make the slides more difficult to interpret.[67,68] However, samples may be taken at any stage of the cycle as long as the information on the stage of cycle is provided and the person reading the slide has experience in assessing equine biopsy slides. In the absence of clinically detectable pathology involving the uterus, a single endometrial biopsy sample is representative of the entire endometrium.[69] However, another study found that even in clinically normal mares endometrial biopsy scores varied with the site selected.[70]

The sterile mare biopsy instrument is introduced into the uterine lumen guided by one hand placed in the vagina. The tip of the biopsy forceps might necessitate assistance through the cervix, especially with a biopsy procedure performed during diestrus. The traditional technique involves withdrawing the hand from the vagina and inserting it into the rectum. The instrument is directed to a specific site within the uterus, generally the base of one horn. The instrument is then turned on its side and the jaws gently opened. A portion of endometrium is pressed between the jaws using the index finger within the rectum and the jaws closed to remove the tissue sample.

A simpler vaginal technique is useful for collecting biopsy samples when there is no need to sample from a specific site.[67,68,71] The instrument is introduced into the uterine lumen, and the hand is left in the vagina with the index finger in the cervical lumen. The tip of the instrument is advanced about 2 to 3 cm into the uterine lumen with the jaws closed. The jaws are opened and the instrument advanced an additional 1 to 2 cm. The instrument can then be deviated slightly to one side and the jaws closed to collect a sample. The sample is taken from the cranial uterine body close to the bifurcation. This approach has the advantage of being quick and simple. It allows the operator to return for a second sample immediately if the first sample is too small, whereas the rectovaginal technique often results in gross contamination of the instrument and vulva during the procedure, making a second sample impossible unless the mare is cleaned again and a second sterile instrument is available.

The specimen is removed from the biopsy basket using a small-gauge needle and transferred to fixative solution, preferably Bouin's fixative or 10% buffered formalin. Samples placed into Bouin's fixative should be transferred to 10% formalin or 80% ethanol after 12 to 24 hours for optimal retention of cell detail and tissue integrity.[64]

There is a strong case to be made for clinicians to read slides from their own cases. Although expert assessment by a trained pathologist may better reflect histologic tissue changes, the clinician is in the best position to interpret histologic change in light of clinical and historical information about the mare. Training and practice will allow the clinician to detect most of the common pathologic changes seen in biopsy samples, although expert help should be sought if needed. The examination process should be methodical. The clinician must ensure that cellular characteristics are consistent with the stage of estrous cycle. Pathologic changes include inflammation, fibrosis, cystic glandular distention, and lymphatic stasis. Increasing numbers of inflammatory cells in the lamina propria indicate inflammation. Acute inflammation is associated with PMNs and an increased likelihood of positive endometrial culture. Increasing numbers of PMNs and their presence in deeper layers of the lamina propria indicate more severe inflammation. Chronic inflammatory change includes lymphocytes, plasma cells, eosinophils, and mast cells.

Endometrial fibrosis is a permanent degenerative change occurring around glands (fibrotic nests) or gland branches and also adjacent to the basement membrane of the luminal epithelium. Fibrosis often forms in concentric layers around gland branches or glands, and the number of layers of fibrosis is related to the severity of the degenerative change.[72] Fibrosis may be localized or diffuse, and the more widespread or severe the change, the more adverse the effect on gland function and fertility. These degenerative changes appear to be closely associated with age rather than parity.[34,73-75] Severe degenerative endometrial fibrosis can occur in the older maiden mare that has not had the challenges of pregnancy and exposure to semen.[74,75]

Cystic gland distention may be seen in normal mares during anestrus. When diagnosed in mares during the breeding season, it is considered a pathologic change and is associated with reduced fertility. Glandular fibrosis may also be associated with cystic distention of the affected glands. Extensive fibrosis interferes with uterine gland function and may result in early embryonic death.[76]

Endometrial atrophy is associated with an extremely poor breeding prognosis.[67,68] Large empty spaces on the biopsy slide must be interpreted with caution, because they may be artifacts associated with sample processing. If the spaces appear to be lined with an endothelial cell layer, this indicates lymphatic stasis. Widespread lymphatic stasis may be associated with reduced contractile capability within the uterus, a doughy feel to the uterus on transrectal palpation, and reduced fertility.[64]

Assessment of severity and distribution of pathologic changes allow the sample to be classified into one of four diagnostic and prognostic levels based on a modified version of the original three-level system proposed by Kenney.[72,77]

Category I: No significant changes in the endometrium and no treatment required; expected foaling rate of 80% to 90%.

Category IIA: Slight to moderate inflammatory change. Scattered fibrotic change may consist of either fibrosis around individual gland branches or fewer than two fibrotic nests per high-power field. There is moderate cystic glandular distention or extensive lymphatic stasis. If two or more of these changes are present in the same sample, the sample is classified as IIB. Expected foaling rates are 50% to 80%.

Category IIB: Inflammatory change is widespread and moderately severe. There is widespread fibrotic change or up to four fibrotic nests per high-power microscope field. Widespread, severe cystic glandular distention or lymphatic stasis is evident. If two or more of these changes are present, the sample is classified as III. Expected foaling rates are 10% to 50%.

Category III: The mare exhibits widespread, severe changes that are likely to be permanent and has an expected foaling rate of less than 10%.

Use of paired biopsy samples taken at the initial diagnostic workup and again 4 weeks after completion of treatment appears to improve the usefulness of the biopsy as a prognostic indicator of a mare's fertility.[74,75] Mares that were classified as grade III pretreatment and that improved to grade II after treatment achieved a foaling rate of 40%, whereas mares that were still grade III after treatment had a 0% foaling rate. This is likely to be a result of improvement in reversible pathologic changes.[74,75] This approach allows effective use of the grade III categorization on the follow-up biopsy to justify recommending that such mares be culled from the breeding program.

Uterine Endoscopic Examination: Hysteroscopy

Hysteroscopy allows direct visual inspection of the uterine lumen through a flexible fiberoptic endoscope. Hysteroscopy is indicated when other diagnostic procedures do not detect a cause for subfertility or to further examine a mare with a suspected uterine luminal lesion.[78,79]

Sedation is a useful restraint aid because the procedure is associated with mild discomfort. The perineum is prepared as for other vaginal or uterine procedures, and a sterilized endoscope is inserted in the vagina and manipulated through the cervix and into the uterus. The cervical lumen is then occluded, either by inserting 1 or 2 fingers into the cervix alongside the endoscope or by gently holding the external os of the cervix around the endoscope. The uterine lumen is distended with saline or water infused through a flexible catheter held adjacent to the endoscope or with air delivered through the endoscope. Endometrial folds should be assessed while the uterus is being distended because they flatten out and become difficult to distinguish in the fully distended uterus. The endoscope is then manipulated through the uterine lumen, allowing visualization of the entire endometrial surface, including the tips of the uterine horns and the two oviductal ostia. Hysteroscopy allows direct visualization of a variety of abnormal changes, including inflammation, polyps or neoplasia, cysts, adhesions, and severe scarring or fibrotic change. It can also aid in various procedures, including guided retrieval of foreign bodies and laser surgical management of conditions such as endometrial cysts or adhesions.

Excessive distention of the uterus may cause discomfort and an elevated heart rate and should be avoided.[80] Mares subjected to hysteroscopy appear to be at risk of developing subsequent endometritis.[80] Care should be taken to sterilize the equipment before use; the author suggests that mares be examined during the subsequent estrus period to check for evidence of endometritis.

HORMONAL ASSAYS

In the nonpregnant mare serum or plasma samples may be collected for measurement of a variety of reproductive hormone concentrations, including progesterone, estrogens, testosterone, inhibin, and gonadotropins. Other conditions that may have effects on cyclicity and fertility include abnormalities involving the thyroid and adrenal glands and pituitary pars intermedia dysfunction.

Progesterone is produced by ovarian luteal tissue. Serum progesterone concentrations are low during estrus and begin to rise 12 to 24 hours after ovulation, peaking between days 5 to 10 after ovulation.[81,82] Progesterone assays in nonpregnant mares can be used to assist in determining the stage of the cycle and to confirm that ovulation has occurred. They are also used as an indirect method of pregnancy diagnosis, but false-positive results are common.

Progesterone is necessary for pregnancy maintenance, and primary luteal insufficiency has been linked to pregnancy loss.[40,83,84] Low levels of progesterone are associated with increased pregnancy loss, and higher levels of progesterone are associated with successful pregnancies in mares that habitually aborted twins.[85] Older mares appear to require a higher level of progesterone to maintain pregnancy.[59] Progesterone levels on day 7 were significantly lower in mares with periovulatory intrauterine fluid accumulation and significantly lower in mares that underwent embryonic loss.[40] The presence of luminal fluid in diestrus was associated with a lower progesterone level and increased embryonic loss, indicating endometritis as a cause for lower progesterone levels[36]

Some researchers recommend that progesterone concentration in peripheral blood of pregnant mares be above 2.5 to 4 ng/ml for normal pregnancy maintenance.[86] Single samples of peripheral blood concentrations are difficult to interpret because repeated sampling of normal pregnant mares has shown that blood levels vary widely over short periods of time.[81,82]

Thyroid gland dysfunction has been linked to subfertility in mares with recommendations to measure total serum thyroxine (T4) or thyroxine response to administration of thyroid-stimulating hormone (TSH). Thyroxine is significantly affected by season and reproductive status.[87,88] Thyroxine is seasonally regulated when mares are kept on a constant energy balance out of season.[89] Although thyroidectomy of pony mares did not have any adverse effect on reproductive performance,[90] mares that continued to cycle out of season had higher levels of thyroxine than anestrous mares.[88,91] Mares with low thyroxine levels were more likely to enter anestrus after parturition.[88] There was no association between thyroxine level and pregnancy rate 15 to 16 days after ovulation.[92,93]

Ovarian neoplasia, particularly GTCTs, may be associated with increased production of testosterone and inhibin by the affected ovary. Serum inhibin concentration is elevated in approximately 90% of mares with a GTCT, and testosterone in about 50% to 60% of cases.[94] Functional GTCT cases almost invariably have a nonfunctional contralateral ovary and are anovulatory. Therefore a serum sample demonstrating high inhibin or testosterone and low progesterone concentrations is consistent with ovarian neoplasia. Normal ranges in nonpregnant mares for inhibin and testosterone are 0.1 to 0.7 ng/ml and less than 45 pg/ml, respectively.[12,94]

Horses with pituitary pars intermedia dysfunction often exhibit variable degrees of hirsutism with a range of other systemic signs. Diagnosis and treatment of this disorder are discussed in Chapter 20.

Measurement of estrogen concentration in blood, urine, feces, milk, and saliva has been used for monitoring the estrous cycle,[95] determining pregnancy status,[96-98] and monitoring fetal viability.[99] Peripheral blood estrogens may be either unconjugated or conjugated (bound to sulfates), and different forms of estrogens are found in the mare, particularly during pregnancy. Conjugated estrogens generally exist in the circulation at much higher concentrations than unconjugated forms, and measuring either estrone sulfate or total conjugated estrogens appears to offer the most use for the aforementioned indications mentioned. A dramatic increase in peripheral blood estrone sulfate concentrations occurs in pregnant mares after day 60 of pregnancy, whereas in fecal assays this increase may take up to 150 days to occur.[100,101] A rapid decline of estrone sulfate concentration in a pregnant mare may indicate loss of fetal viability.[99]

Equine chorionic gonadotropin (eCG) is a hormone produced from the formation of endometrial cups at around day 36 of gestation. It has a luteinizing effect on follicles to create accessory CLs to help maintain pregnancy until the placenta is fully formed. These follicles often luteinize without ovulating.[102] Pregnancy loss after day 35 can sometimes be associated with negative blood eCG, and the failure of endometrial cup formation is presumed to play an essential role in pregnancy maintenance. Pregnancy loss after day 35 may be associated with a positive eCG measurement, and affected mares often do not cycle properly because follicles fail to ovulate and luteinize. When ovulation does occur, the pregnancy rate is low, presumably because of a low-grade endometritis resulting from the presence of endometrial cups. The endometrial cups have a life span of about 100 days and are therefore nonfunctional after about 150 days gestation.[102] However, there have been reports of the prolonged survival of endometrial cups after abortion.[103,104] The endometrial cups lasted an average of 18 months but could last up to 30 months. This has implications into the next breeding season, and mares showing aberrant ovarian activity should be investigated for the possibility of persistent endometrial cups.

Measurement of serum or plasma concentrations of GnRH, gonadotropins (FSH and LH), and steroids appears to offer promise in the diagnostic assessment of the hypothalamic-pituitary-ovarian axis. The anterior pituitary gland produces FSH in response to GnRH release.[105,106] FSH is released in a bimodal pattern with peaks (35 ng/ml) in early and late diestrus. There are two major waves of follicular growth coincident with the two surges of FSH.[107] FSH starts to rise 4 to 5 days before an ovarian follicular wave. The peak of FSH is 3 days before the emergence of the wave, which then plateaus for 5 days.

GnRH release from the hypothalamus stimulates LH release from the pituitary gland,[108] although there is an association between releases of oxytocin in estrous mares and LH release, which suggests that repeated sexual stimulation might also increase LH and advance ovulation.[109] LH concentrations are low during the midluteal phase (5 ng/ml) but rise a few days before estrus after progesterone decreases (<1 ng/ml) because of luteolysis. LH peaks (45 ng/ml) during estrus at ovulation and returns to midluteal levels over a few days.[107]

Several issues must be addressed before such methodologies become either available or useful. Little information is available regarding the existence of abnormalities in the hypothalamic-pituitary-ovarian axis and either their relationship with subfertility or their detection by measurement of hormone concentrations. Assessment of the production and release of either GnRH or FSH and LH presents practical difficulties because this may require cannulation of the pituitary venous sinuses.[110] In addition, these hormones are released in a pulsatile manner, with pulse frequency and amplitude influencing function.[111,112] Finally, there are varying isoforms with differing bioactivity that may be difficult to distinguish on enzyme-linked immunosorbent assay (ELISA) or radioimmunoassay (RIA).[111,112]

Leptin is a protein synthesized by adipose (fat) tissue.[113-115] Leptin acts as negative feedback to brain centers to control obesity (satiety centers) in times of nutritional abundance.[113,114,116] During starvation reduced leptin levels cause changes in reproductive endocrinology that limit reproductive activity.[117] Short-term feed restriction (for 24 hours) significantly decreases leptin levels in mares but does not affect reproductive hormones.[118] There might be a seasonal influence on leptin levels because mares in good body condition experience a general decline in leptin concentrations during winter. The decline is not as great as that observed in mares in poor body condition, and the mares in good body condition continue to have estrous cycles through winter.[119]

Currently, measurement of these and other hormones of the central nervous system appears to be restricted to research applications. Measuring these products may offer considerable benefits in the future, but additional research and development are required before it can be of use to field practitioners.

MARE REPRODUCTIVE PATHOLOGY

Carlos R.F. Pinto, Dale L. Paccamonti

VULVA

The integrity of the vulvar lips and their anatomic relation to the perineal area and anus are essential components of a mare's fertility because they provide the first barrier to contamination between the external environment and the uterus. The endocrine patterns associated with each stage of the estrous cycle and pregnancy can influence the disposition of the vulva, affecting vulvar length and tone. In general, the vulva should have at least two thirds of its length below the pelvic brim, the slope of the vulva in relation to the vertical axis should not be greater than 10 degrees, and the vulvar lips should have an even and firm apposition. Absence (natural or acquired) of a normal perineal conformation can facilitate the entry of air (pneumovagina), feces, and potential pathogens into the reproductive tract, which jeopardizes the fertility of the mare.

Body Weight

Severe loss of body condition, as experienced by some pregnant mares not adequately supplemented during the winter, results in a sunken anus and an increased slope of the vulva. An apparently normal perineal conformation noted in mares in good body condition may become less than adequate if loss of body weight is extreme. Contamination of the vagina with feces during mid to late gestation may lead to ascending bacterial placentitis, one of the leading causes of abortion and neonatal septicemia in the United States.[1]

Parity and Age

Aging of the mare associated with repeated foaling can cause stretching and loss of tone of the perineal muscles that allow the vulva to form a barrier to external contamination and entry of air into the vagina. Injury to the mare during foaling aggravates this condition, resulting in loss of vulvar tone and apposition of the labia. Mares undergoing episiotomy also may have permanent damage to vulvar structures.

Caslick Vulvoplasty

Surgical closure of the dorsal part of the vulvar labia is intended to correct poor perineal conformation. By decreasing the length of the vulvar cleft, one decreases entry of air and potential pathogens into the vagina in a mare otherwise susceptible to pneumovagina, fecal contamination, and associated complications. It has been reported that Caslick-operated mares with poor perineal conformation that successfully foal should be resutured immediately after parturition to minimize the chances of uterine contamination and consequent endometritis. This preventive measure is believed to contribute to adequate pregnancy rates and maintenance of pregnancy until term.[2]

This procedure, however, is overused in mares in which such intervention is not warranted. Paradoxically, a mare with successive Caslick surgeries may experience considerable loss of vulvar tissue, thus generating an abnormal perineal conformation.

Another indirect complication associated with the Caslick vulvoplasty is the increased incidence of vulvar lacerations and dystocias in mares in which the vulva was not opened before foaling. Regardless of the originating cause, the Caslick operation is used to correct first-degree perineal laceration affecting only the perineal skin and vulvar mucosa. Second-degree (laceration of deeper tissues of the perineal body) and third-degree (a defect resulting in communication of the ventral rectum with the dorsal vagina) lacerations require more elaborate reconstructive surgery to correct.[3] As a rule, any corrective surgery of the perineal body and vulva should be delayed until inflammation and edema of the involved tissues have resolved. Mares with third-degree rectovestibular laceration invariably develop endometritis, but endometrial biopsy of mares affected with third-degree laceration have shown a rapid endometrial response to surgical repair of the laceration; mares can be artificially inseminated by 2 weeks after surgery.[4]

Equine Coital Exanthema

Equine coital exanthema is a venereal disease caused by equine herpesvirus type 3. Mares infected with equine coital exanthema develop pustules and ulcers in the vulvar mucosa and perineal area. Once the lesions start to heal (usually by 14 days after the onset of clinical signs), characteristic depigmented areas in the vulvar labia and perineal skin are visible.[5] Similarly to other herpesvirus-induced diseases, lifelong infection is the rule. Recrudescence may occur after stimuli such as stress, systemic disease, or trauma to the genital area. No specific treatment is recommended, other than disinfection of pustules and ulcers to prevent secondary bacterial infections during the acute phase. Natural service should be avoided while active lesions are present to prevent transmission of the disease. One can artificially inseminate affected mares during the symptomatic stage of the disease or wait until 6 weeks after complete healing of equine coital exanthema–associated lesions before natural service.

Neoplasia

Melanoma is the most common disease affecting the vulva, affecting 80% to 100% of adult gray horses and, less frequently, aging horses of other colors. Common sites for melanoma include the anus, perineum, and vulva. No effective treatment is available for melanomas; however, oral treatment with cimetidine (a histamine$_2$ antagonist) has been reported with variable success to result in partial or complete regression of melanocytic nodules.[6] Squamous cell carcinomas are less common than melanomas.

CLITORIS

The clitoris is enclosed in the clitoral fossa in the ventral part of the vulva but is rhythmically exposed after urination or teasing (winking) as a result of contractions of the vulvar constrictor muscle. The clitoris has several sinuses that contain a natural smegma. Whereas the lateral sinuses are shallow, the median sinuses are sufficiently deep to allow the growth of bacteria. The anatomy of the clitoris in the mare is particularly important because the clitoris is an important reservoir for the bacterium *Taylorella equigenitalis* in mares affected with contagious equine metritis. The disease is highly contagious, and the organism can be harbored in the clitoral fossa and sinuses (especially the median sinuses) for prolonged periods. To test a mare for contagious equine metritis, the practitioner should swab the median clitoral sinuses and then seed an Amies charcoal medium to be transported (preferably kept at 4° C) to a diagnostic laboratory.

Even in contagious equine metritis–free areas, it is important to remember that the clitoral sinuses may function as nidi for uterine infection, especially infection that was iatrogenically induced during diagnostic procedures of the reproductive tract or artificial insemination. Careful asepsis of the perineal and vulvar area, including the clitoral fossa, with a mild disinfectant before any invasive procedures are performed minimizes the risk of introducing potential pathogens into the uterus.

Congenital anomalies of the external genitalia occur in intersex animals that may have underdeveloped vulvar labia associated with an abnormally enlarged clitoris. Treating prepubertal mares with anabolic steroids may lead to enlargement of the clitoris, resulting in a partially and permanently exteriorized clitoris.

VAGINA

The vestibule is the area that separates the vulva and clitoris from the vagina proper. At the cranial border of the vestibule, where it meets the vagina, lies the vaginovestibular fold. This folded mucous membrane acts as the second and most important[7] physical barrier between the uterus and the external environment. In young horses the hymen is usually a weak membranous extension of the vaginovestibular fold. Occasionally, a persistent hymen may be present in a maiden mare. A manual examination of the vagina is usually sufficient to rupture the persistent hymen. Some mares with a persistent hymen may accumulate fluid in the vagina proper and uterus (mucometra). Once the persistent hymen is disrupted, evacuation of the fluid is uneventful.

Pneumovagina

Listening for an inrush of air into the vagina when one gently parts the vulvar labia can test the adequacy of the vaginovestibular fold as a physical barrier to external contaminants. A positive test (noticeable sound of air rushing in to the vagina) indicates that the vestibular fold is not properly restricting the vagina proper from the outside environment.

Improper functioning of the first barrier (vulva) and second barrier (vaginovestibular fold) may lead to the constant or frequent entry of air into the vagina. The condition may be exacerbated during estrus, when the perineal body is more relaxed than in other stages of the estrous cycle. Accumulation of small amounts of a frothy fluid in the cranial vagina may indicate pneumovagina, as may the presence of air in the uterus (pneumouterus) that is visible as hyperechoic particles between the endometrial folds during ultrasonographic examination.

In mares with severe alteration of the perineal conformation, vulvar closure using Caslick vulvoplasty may not correct the problem, and surgical reconstruction of the perineal body (perineoplasty) is recommended.

Urovagina

Urovagina, also known as *vesicovaginal reflux* or *urine pooling,* refers to the presence of urine in the cranial vagina and possibly in the uterus. As with pneumovagina, mares with marginal perineal conformation may be predisposed to accumulate urine in the vagina during estrus, when reproductive organs and the perineal body are relaxed. In older mares with splanchnoptosis, the reflux of urine into the genital tract may be permanent. Urovagina can cause vaginitis, cervicitis, and endometritis, which ultimately result in infertility. Perineoplasty and urethral extension are common surgical procedures to correct this condition.

Varicose Veins

During estrus and especially during pregnancy, varicose veins may develop in older mares. Varicose veins can be present in any part of the vagina; however, they often are found in the vaginovestibular area. Bleeding may occur after natural service or spontaneously during mid to late gestation. Occasionally, a persistent hemorrhage results in considerable blood loss; however, the condition usually subsides with the end of pregnancy. Cautery or ligation of varicose veins is warranted if hemorrhage is persistent or frequent.

Neoplasia

Vaginal neoplasms are not common in mares. Leiomyomas and squamous cell carcinoma have been reported.

Vaginitis

Minor tears, lacerations, and hematomas are common findings in the vaginas of mares after foaling. Medical treatment generally is not needed, and most mares do not show complications in the postpartum period. If more serious trauma occurs, the mare may develop vaginitis. Mares with extensive vaginitis or a large hematoma may show signs of pain and refuse to stand quietly to nurse the foal. Vaginal abscesses can develop when a vaginal laceration becomes infected. Clinical signs caused by swelling from a hematoma or abscess include stranguria and straining to defecate. Treatment with antibiotics and anti-inflammatory drugs is warranted when extensive vaginitis or abscesses are found in the vagina. An abscess impinging on the urethra or interfering with defecation may require drainage. Occasionally, vaginal trauma may result in adhesions that can interfere with uterine drainage.

Rectovaginal Fistulas

During parturition the foot of the foal may be directed toward the dorsal vagina or ventral rectum and if unattended may cause a third-degree perineal laceration. However, if the dystocia is corrected in time, the damage may be limited to a first- or second-degree rectovaginal tear or rectovaginal fistula. Surgical correction of the anatomic defect is necessary to restore fertility.

Breeding Trauma

Vaginal lacerations may occur during natural service when the stallion is disproportionately large compared with the mare. Depending on the location of the tear in relation to the peritoneal reflection, a vaginal tear may communicate with the peritoneal cavity, likely resulting in peritonitis, or may be retroperitoneal. Treatment includes broad spectrum antibiotics, anti-inflammatory drugs, and tetanus prophylaxis. Peritoneal lavage may be beneficial if the tear communicates with the peritoneal cavity. A breeding roll positioned under the tail of the mare and dorsal to the penis of the stallion prevents the stallion from inserting the full length of its penis into the vagina and consequently helps prevent mating-induced trauma.

CERVIX

The cervix is the last of the three physical barriers protecting the uterus from the external environment. Cyclic hormonal changes dictate the tonicity of the cervix. During estrus the cervix is relaxed and open. High concentrations of progesterone during diestrus or pregnancy cause the cervix to be tubular, firm, and tightly closed. These changes are readily palpable rectally. Moreover, a vaginal examination during estrus reveals the cervix positioned low in the cranial vagina and relaxed and easily dilated, allowing access to the uterus. During diestrus or pregnancy, a vaginal examination reveals a tightly closed cervical os, which is pale and positioned high off the floor of the vagina.

Cervicitis

Inflammation of the cervix often accompanies vaginitis or endometritis. Cervicitis usually occurs in the postpartum period, especially after a dystocia. Severe cervicitis associated with metritis also may occur in mares infected with organisms such as *T. equigenitalis* that cause copious purulent discharge.[8] Infusion of certain chemicals (e.g., chlorhexidine, strong iodine solutions) into the uterus to treat endometritis may irritate not only the endometrium but also the cervix and vaginal mucosa. If the practitioner intends to use such solutions, vaginal speculum examinations to assess the condition of the cervix are warranted between treatments.

Trauma

Although cervical lacerations can occur during natural service, these lesions are usually small and resolve without major consequences. Occasionally, maiden mares are found in estrus with a tightly closed cervix, which might suffer laceration during natural service, especially if the stallion is disproportionately larger than the mare. However, these tears are usually small and heal without further treatment. Most serious lacerations occur during parturition. They may result from normal parturition, or they may be iatrogenic, occurring during intervention to correct a dystocia by mutation or fetotomy. Although one should examine the cervix digitally after a difficult foaling or dystocia, especially if a fetotomy procedure is involved, the extent and severity of a cervical laceration are best evaluated once the cervical lesion is healed. The competency of the cervix should be evaluated during diestrus or when the mare is under the influence of exogenous progestagens so that its ability to close tightly can be verified. One can more easily diagnose transluminal adhesions and anatomic defects by digital examination of the cervix rather than by vaginoscopy. Because surgical correction is difficult and not always rewarding, the practitioner should take a biopsy sample of the uterus to assess the mare's ability to maintain a pregnancy before attempting surgical correction of a cervical laceration.

Polyps or Cysts

Occasionally, pedunculated cystlike structures are apparent on visual or manual examination of the cervix. These structures are attached to the cervical os or emanate from the cervical lumen and protrude into the vagina or uterine body. Although their cause is unknown, they do appear to be associated with infertility, and removal by laser or ligation is recommended.

UTERUS

Ventral Sacculations

Aside from changes associated with pregnancy, other pathologic conditions cause focal enlargements in the ventral portion of the uterus. These uterine changes usually are associated with increased age and parity and invariably are found at the base of one or both of the uterine horns, where pregnancies usually are established. Inexperienced palpators may mistake these enlargements for a pregnancy, especially if they do not use ultrasonography to confirm their palpation findings. Mechanisms contributing to formation of ventral uterine enlargements have been identified, including but not limited to endometrial atrophy, focal myometrial atonia, and lymphatic lacunae.[9] Furthermore, in older and multiparous mares the uterus may tilt ventrally in relation to the pelvic brim (uterine splanchnoptosis). Mares with ventral sacculations and uterine splanchnoptosis have a higher incidence of delayed uterine clearance than normal mares.[10]

Endometrosis

Endometrosis was once known as *chronic infiltrative endometritis* and currently refers to the presence of fibrosis in the stromal and periglandular compartments. The degree of endometrosis is associated closely with the ability of a mare to establish and maintain a healthful pregnancy until term. Parity and age contribute to degenerative changes occurring in the endometria of mares.[11]

Fibrotic changes may occur around the endometrial glands and in association with the basement membrane in the stratum compactum. The amount and pattern of distribution of the fibrotic tissue has been classified descriptively as slight, one to three layers of periglandular fibrosis; moderate, 4 to 10 layers; and severe, more than 10 layers of periglandular fibrosis.[12] Cystic glandular dilation is another manifestation of endometrosis. Periglandular fibrosis, glandular epithelial hypertrophy, or inadequate lymphatic drainage may lead to dilation of the endometrial glands.

Other degenerative alterations in the endometrium that lead to endometrosis include lymphatic lacunae and angiosis.[11,13] Lymphatic lacunae are histopathologic indications of lymphangiectasia. Angiosis (a vascular pathologic condition) is associated with aging and parity, especially in uteri with ventral sacculations and associated venous congestion, which are pathogenic factors for angiosis.[13] No treatments exist for these anatomic and vascular degenerative changes in the uterus. Mares with lymphatic lacunae and disseminated uterine angiosis are at risk for infertility caused by delayed uterine clearance and persistent mating-induced endometritis.[11,13]

Pregnancy loss attributed to endometrial fibrosis more commonly manifests during the embryonic period. The secretion of histotroph by the endometrium is critical for proper embryonic development. The area of the endometrium in immediate contact with the conceptus has been shown to undergo specific changes in glandular density on days 16 through 30 of gestation, a period during which embryonic loss is commonly diagnosed in mares with endometrosis.[14] If pregnancy continues to progress beyond the initial 30 days of gestation, abortion during the early fetal period may still occur if uterine fibrosis interferes with implantation of the placenta. Microcotyledonary attachments begin to develop by 80 to 120 days of gestation.[15] Ultrastructural evaluation of the placenta in mares with chronic degenerative endometritis (endometrosis) has shown a delay in microcotyledon development and a reduction in the number of microcotyledons and villi per surface area. Endometrial atrophy may not result in abortion but can influence fetal growth. Fetal weights in mares with degenerative endometritis were lower than in normal mares.[16] Evidence of endometrial atrophy may be evident on inspection of the placenta after delivery.[17]

Endometritis

Whereas endometriosis reflects chronic structural changes associated with age and parity, endometritis encompasses endometrial changes associated with acute or chronic inflammation. These changes are modulated by the action of a local immune system and influenced by the hormonal milieu. A transient endometritis normally occurs in all mares that were mated naturally or artificially inseminated. Mares mount an inflammatory reaction in response to the presence of semen in the uterus, but this apparently normal inflammatory response subsides (histologically) within 2 to 3 days. Detection of intrauterine fluid by ultrasonography per rectum 24 hours after mating suggests delayed clearance. Persistent mating-induced endometritis is a clinical entity that has been recognized as a major cause of infertility in mares.

Endometrial Biopsy

An endometrial biopsy often is considered a routine part of a complete BSE. Because an endometrial biopsy can aid in predicting the chances of a mare carrying a foal to term, one should consider the information provided by a biopsy before purchasing the horse or undertaking reproductive surgery such as repair of a cervical tear. Biopsies sometimes provide information that is useful in the diagnosis of infertility and may provide a basis for treatment. One must realize, however, that an endometrial biopsy alone is not the only, nor usually the most important, piece of information and must be considered in light of other information obtained from the history and reproductive examination.

Generally, a biopsy specimen is taken from a site at the base of one of the uterine horns. When procuring a biopsy, the practitioner should take care not to obtain tissue from a site near the internal cervical os. Glands are less dense near the cervix, making a biopsy obtained from that area less representative of the uterus and more difficult to interpret. Moreover, accidentally taking a biopsy sample from the cervix can result in adhesions.

A single biopsy long has been considered to be representative of the entire uterus; however, studies have shown that variation by as much as an entire category may exist among sites.[18] Therefore one first should perform a thorough examination by palpation and ultrasonography to determine whether any areas of the uterus appear to be abnormal. If one detects an abnormal area, one should obtain biopsy samples from the abnormal and the normal areas. Repeated or multiple biopsies do not significantly affect fertility. A mare may become pregnant when bred just a few days after taking of a biopsy specimen.[19]

Because the cervix is dilated easily, biopsy samples may be taken at any time during the year or during any stage of the estrous cycle. Some clinicians prefer to obtain a biopsy sample during diestrus, when the endometrial glands are under the influence of progesterone, whereas others recommend taking the sample during estrus because of the ease in passing the instrument through the cervix. One must relay all pertinent history, including the estrous stage during which the biopsy sample was obtained, to the pathologist reading the sample. Periglandular fibrosis may appear worse in biopsy samples taken during anestrus because of the sparseness of glands. In addition, biopsy samples taken during anestrus or transition may have evidence of increased inflammation because the cervix has been in a relaxed state for a prolonged period as a result of the absence of progesterone.

Endometrial biopsies are classified into four categories (I, IIA, IIB, III).[20] A mare with a category I biopsy has an essentially normal endometrium. The likelihood of the mare becoming pregnant and carrying a foal to term, estimated at 80% to 90%, depends more on broodmare management than on the inherent fertility of the mare. Mares with a category III biopsy have severe pathologic changes in the endometrium and an estimated 10% chance of carrying a foal to term even with good breeding management. Most mares are classified as a category IIA or IIB with an estimated 50% to 80% and 10% to 50% chance, respectively, of carrying a foal to term, reflecting a combination of management practices and the inherent fertility of the mare.

The pathologist usually provides a complete histopathologic description, but it is beneficial if the practitioner reviews the biopsy slide because this can be helpful in developing a therapeutic plan for the mare. The clinician's primary concern is the severity and distribution of inflammation and the presence of degenerative changes such as periglandular fibrosis, angiosis, and lymphatic lacunae (enlarged and dilated lymphatics). Degenerative changes carry a worse prognosis than inflammatory changes because they are considered to be permanent and progressive. No effective treatment for these conditions has been identified. The cause of such degenerative conditions is not known but widely presumed to be caused by repeated insults to the uterus. These conditions are more common in older mares.[11] Dilated lymphatics often indicate a uterine clearance problem. However, the practitioner can diagnose delayed clearance more reliably by ultrasonographic examination in the postmating period.

Although biopsy can reveal the presence of an inflammatory condition, other methods (e.g., examination of perineal conformation) are necessary to reveal the reason that the condition is present, and a culture is needed to identify the particular pathogen. A repeat biopsy after appropriate therapy may provide insight regarding the extent to which treatment was successful and aid in determining a prognosis for future fertility.[21]

ENDOMETRIAL CYSTS

Endometrial cysts often are cited as a cause of infertility; however, a clear cause-and-effect relationship has not been established. The proportion of mares with endometrial cysts increases with age. Mares older than 11 years of age are more than 4 times as likely to have endometrial cysts as are younger mares, and most mares older than 17 years of age have endometrial cysts. Reports that associate endometrial cysts with a lower pregnancy rate or increased embryonic loss fail to account for the effect of advancing age. When one controls for confounding effects such as parity and age, the assumption that cysts are causing infertility is not supportable. When confounding factors were accounted for in the analysis of nearly 300 mares, endometrial cysts did not have a statistically significant effect on establishing or maintaining pregnancy, although the time of initial pregnancy diagnosis was not controlled strictly.[22] Another report by a different group of researchers who did control the time of pregnancy diagnosis similarly found no difference in pregnancy loss between mares with cysts and those without, although mares with endometrial cysts tended to have a lower day-40 pregnancy rate. The effect of cysts on fertility appeared to be quantitative because an effect was not evident until a mare had numerous cysts or the cysts were large. However, even then the effect of endometrial cysts on fertility was much less than that with delayed uterine clearance or intrauterine fluid accumulation. A quantitative effect of endometrial cysts could be caused by interference with embryonic mobility. A well-known fact is that the equine embryo undergoes a period of mobility after entering the uterus, finally becoming fixed in place at approximately 16 or 17 days of gestation. If mobility is restricted during this period and the embryo is not permitted to come into contact with a sufficient portion of the endometrium, maternal recognition of pregnancy may not occur, resulting in luteolysis and embryonic loss.

Rather than viewing endometrial cysts as a cause of infertility, one should consider them as an indication of underlying pathologic changes in the uterus. Endometrial cysts are of lymphatic origin, and their occurrence may be associated with a disruption of lymphatic function.

Endometrial cysts are best diagnosed with ultrasonography. Cysts are identified as hypoechoic, immovable structures with a clear border, as opposed to intraluminal fluid, which is movable and has a less distinct shape or border. Endometrial cysts are usually multiple and most commonly found at the base of the uterine horns. Cysts may change in size and number between estrus and pregnancy.

Endometrial cysts can complicate a diagnosis of early pregnancy. An endometrial cyst is often similar in size and appearance to an early conceptus. Cysts that appear spherical often are shown to have a more irregular shape if the ultrasound probe can be reoriented in relation to the cyst. To make the diagnosis of early pregnancy easier and more reliable, the practitioner should record the size and location of endometrial cysts using a diagram or by storing ultrasonographic images during a prebreeding examination. Even so, it may be necessary to repeat the pregnancy examination or delay confirmation in some mares with endometrial cysts. In most cases of endometrial cysts, no treatment is necessary other than recording their size and location for future reference during pregnancy examination. However, if the cysts are sufficient in size or number such that they pose a potential threat to embryonic migration, treatment can be aimed at facilitating establishment of pregnancy by providing exogenous progestagen.

Progestagens, usually in the form of altrenogest (0.044 mg/kg/day, administered orally), can maintain pregnancy even when the signal for maternal recognition of pregnancy is lacking. Numerous studies have shown the ability of altrenogest to maintain pregnancy after luteolysis or in ovariectomized mares. It is important to note that if progestagen therapy is deemed necessary, the correct dose and frequency of administration are required, or the effort is wasted. For example, once-weekly injections of progesterone in oil or once-a-month administration of medroxyprogesterone are insufficient to maintain pregnancy and therefore would not be beneficial in mares with large or numerous endometrial cysts.

Alternatively, endometrial cysts may be removed surgically. Laser surgery is an ideal method if the equipment is available. Ligation and transection of the stalk of pedunculated cysts is an alternative. Merely puncturing and draining the cyst or incising its wall does not provide long-term remission.

Transluminal Adhesions

Severe infectious or chemically induced (e.g., after intrauterine infusion of irritating chemicals) endometritis may induce the formation of transluminal adhesions in the uterus. These lesions are asymptomatic and found during hysteroscopy. Uterine adhesions may cause the retention of endometrial secretions, resulting in mucometra or pyometra. Early embryonic motility, a phenomenon paramount for maternal recognition in horses, may be impaired by intraluminal adhesions. Treatment modalities include manual disruption of intraluminal adhesions or ablation by way of laser surgery.

Pyometra

Pyometra is an accumulation of purulent exudate in the uterus. Unlike cows, mares with pyometra do not necessarily have a persistent CL, and many may cycle normally. A cervical anatomic defect that prevents the clearance of fluid from the uterus may predispose mares to pyometra. However, this condition also can affect mares without an apparent anatomic defect in the reproductive tract. One can diagnose pyometra readily by transrectal ultrasonography when intraluminal fluid with moderate echogenicity is visible in the uterus. Because most mares with pyometra are brought to the veterinarian's attention at an advanced stage, degenerative changes such as endometrial atrophy may preclude mares from returning to normal fertility after treatment. A biopsy sample of the uterus should be examined before treatment to determine the prognosis for potential fertility. Although medical evacuation of the uterus may be attempted, hysterectomy is an option for mares refractory to treatment or with advanced degeneration of the endometrium (severe endometrosis).

Neoplasia

Uterine neoplasms are uncommon in mares. Leiomyomas, often referred to as *fibroids,* are benign mesenchymal neoplasms derived from smooth muscle and often are associated with the presence of fibrous tissue. Leiomyoma is the most common neoplasm affecting the uteri of mares; if the neoplasm is small, reproductive failure does not necessarily result. Leiomyosarcoma, lymphosarcoma, and adenocarcinoma are rare malignant neoplasms affecting mares.

Neoplasms affecting the equine uterus are usually discovered during rectal palpation and transrectal ultrasonography in broodmares during the breeding season. If a uterine neoplasm is suspected, the clinician should perform uterine endoscopy and take a biopsy sample of the tissue for final diagnosis. Surgical excision of neoplasms is indicated when extensive hemorrhage and endometritis are present or when the presence of the neoplasia would be incompatible with establishing a pregnancy. Prognosis for future fertility is reduced, but pregnancy has been reported in mares with partial hysterectomy.[23]

Uterine Lacerations

Uterine lacerations can occur during unattended or assisted parturition. Rectal and vaginal palpation and abdominocentesis aid in diagnosis.[24] Adhesions involving the serosal surface of the uterus may occur after cesarean section or uterine tears. No effective treatment, other than attempted surgical excision, exists once the adhesions form. Therefore the veterinarian should take steps to minimize the likelihood of adhesion formation, including daily palpation of the uterus after cesarean section.

Uterine Artery Rupture

Age and parity are contributing factors for mares at risk for uterine artery rupture.[25] Uterine vessels undergo extensive dynamic remodeling during pregnancy and the postpartum period, and this is thought to contribute to progressive degenerative vascular changes. If a mare survives an acute episode of rupture of the uterine artery, antimicrobial therapy is indicated to prevent the hematoma from becoming an abscess. Monitoring the mucous membranes and pulse for 30 minutes after foaling is indicated if the parturition was induced or assisted by a veterinarian and especially when an intervention to correct a dystocia is performed.[27] In mares that survive a ruptured uterine artery, fertility is not altered, but mares may suffer fatal hemorrhage during the subsequent parturition.

UTERINE TUBES

The function of uterine tubes is essential for normal fertility. The passage of equine embryos throughout the uterine tube is longer than for other domestic species, which underlines the importance of the tubal environment for normal fertility.

Mares are also unique in that unfertilized oocytes are retained in the uterine tubes and are not transported to the uterus. The mechanism accounting for this phenomenon (selective transport of fertilized versus unfertilized oocytes) has not yet been elucidated fully, but it appears to involve secretion of PGE_2. A healthy uterine tube responds to embryonic signals, resulting in proper timing of tubal transport. Diagnosis of pathologic conditions in the uterine tubes is difficult and often occurs only in postmortem examinations.

Postmortem examination of reproductive tracts revealed that salpingitis was common in mares; 37% had infundibulitis, 21% had ampullitis, and 9% had isthmitis. In that study 50% of mares were more than 15 years old, and 85% were older than 11 years of age. The infundibulum generally was found adhered to the uterus, mesovarium, or ovary. The incidence of adhesions on the right side was significantly higher than on the left side.[28]

Postmortem analysis of uterine tubes has suggested that tubal patency is not a major problem in mares. Oviductal obstructions are less common in the mare than in the cow, although masses of collagen have been found in the oviducts of young maiden mares and pregnant mares and were observed more often in mares more than 7 years old.[29] An examination of 700 postmortem specimens, primarily from mares older than 11 years of age, found that almost all oviducts were patent, although more than 40% had adhesions involving the infundibula.[28] Only one uterine tube was found to be occluded among 1248 pairs of uterine tubes that were flushed post mortem.[28,30] Based on these findings, diagnostic procedures to determine the patency of uterine tube in mares with unexplained infertility are not warranted.

OVARY

The presence of an enlarged ovary in a mare may be normal or an indication of a pathologic ovarian condition. Consideration of the various possibilities and careful diagnostic procedures are necessary so that normal ovaries are not surgically removed. A thorough history, including changes in behavior, estrous cycle characteristics, sexual behavior, and the last observed estrus, is important to consider. Ultrasonography, palpation, and hormonal assays are helpful in reaching an accurate diagnosis. In some mares sequential examinations are beneficial in determining changes in the size of ovaries or various structures on an ovary.

Discovery of an enlarged ovary may be an incidental finding during a normal reproductive examination or may be stimulated by specific clinical signs. Behavioral changes or signs of colic in a mare warrant examination of the reproductive tract, with special attention to the ovaries. Mares with a history of infertility often are suspected of having abnormalities of the ovaries and deserve a thorough examination before surgical removal of an enlarged ovary. The clinician must consider various factors, such as season and pregnancy status, when interpreting a finding of ovarian enlargement. Large ovaries may be normal during the transitional periods in the spring and fall and are expected during certain stages of gestation.

NEOPLASIA

Granulosa-theca cell tumors are the most common tumors of the reproductive tract in mares. They are benign sex-cord tumors that can occur in mares of any age and also have been reported in foals and pregnant mares. Although the granulosa and the theca interna cell layers may be involved, the granulosa cell layer most commonly is affected.

Behavioral changes are common in mares with granulosa cell tumors. Behavior may be stallionlike, or persistent estrus or anestrus may occur, depending on the steroid production of the tumor. In other cases of granulosa cell tumors, behavior may be unchanged yet the mare may be showing signs of abdominal discomfort, lameness, or anemia or other signs seemingly unrelated to the reproductive system. Stallionlike behavior is the most commonly reported behavioral change observed, possibly because the change from previous behavior is obvious to the owner and causes an increased challenge in handling the mare. In one report of 63 mares diagnosed with granulosa cell tumors, 20 exhibited anestrus, 14 were in persistent estrus, and 29 showed stallionlike behavior. Stallionlike behavior usually is associated with elevated serum testosterone. However, persistent estrus has not been correlated with elevated estrogen.

On rectal palpation the affected ovary is enlarged, whereas the contralateral ovary is typically small and inactive. Atrophy of the contralateral ovary can be misleading during winter anestrus, when ovaries are typically small and inactive. Atrophy of the contralateral ovary is not absolute. Although unusual, granulosa cell tumors have been reported in pregnant mares and in cyclic mares with a functional contralateral ovary and even in both ovaries.[31] The enlarged ovary may be smooth or knobby, hard or soft, and may feel as if multiple follicles are present. Typically, one cannot palpate the ovulation fossa on the enlarged ovary, although with any greatly enlarged ovary, the fossa may be difficult or impossible to palpate. Although uncommon, the occurrence of bilateral granulosa cell tumors have been reported.[31,32] In one report a mare developed a granulosa cell tumor in the contralateral ovary 4.5 years after the initially affected ovary was surgically removed.[32] Ultrasonographic evaluation often shows the classic multiloculated appearance. However, sometimes the tumor may appear solid or with larger cystlike hypoechoic areas.[33] Although ultrasonography is a useful adjunct, it may not yield a definitive diagnosis in many cases. The ultrasonographic image of granulosa cell tumors can be similar to that of other ovarian abnormalities, especially ovarian hematomas. A variety of reported appearances make diagnosis based solely on ultrasonography impossible in many instances.

Mares with granulosa cell tumors may have elevated concentrations of estrogen or testosterone, but progesterone is almost always less than 1 ng/ml. Measurement of estradiol is of limited value. Although testosterone often is elevated in mares with granulosa cell tumors exhibiting stallionlike behavior, testosterone is within normal limits in 10% to 50% of cases. Testosterone in normal cycling mares is approximately 45 pg/ml and often is greater than 100 pg/ml in mares with stallionlike behavior. McCue reported that only 54% of mares with granulosa cell tumors had elevated testosterone, yet 87% had elevated inhibin, leading to the conclusion that inhibin is a better indicator of the disease.[34] Inhibin suppresses FSH, which leads to a decline in follicular growth, thus explaining the profound negative feedback effect on the contralateral ovary.

Overall, the prognosis for life and reproductive function in a mare with a granulosa cell tumor is good. Depending on the time of year when the ovary is removed, the individual mare, and the length of time the tumor has been present, resumption of ovarian activity usually occurs 83 to 392 days after surgery, with a mean of 209 days. If the intended use of the mare is solely as a broodmare, a reproductive examination, including a uterine biopsy, is recommended before surgery.

Teratomas, although uncommon, are the second most common ovarian tumors. They contain at least two, if not all three, germinal layers. Most teratomas found in mares are benign. They usually contain hair and also may contain bone, teeth, and neural tissue. Teratomas are usually an incidental finding because most are small and do not often cause significant ovarian enlargement. However, on occasion, large teratomas develop that result in ovarian enlargement. Teratomas do not affect the estrous cycle and therefore lack obvious outward clinical signs.

Serous cystadenomas are neoplasms of epithelial origin usually found in older mares. These tumors do not metastasize. Although they have been found in mares with high plasma testosterone,[35] behavioral changes are not characteristic. The contralateral ovary is not affected, continues to have normal activity, and does not atrophy; and affected mares continue to cycle. On the affected ovary the ovulation fossa is not obliterated and is palpable.

Dysgerminomas are highly malignant tumors also of germ cell origin. They metastasize rapidly to the abdominal and thoracic cavities and are considered the counterpart of the testicular seminoma. Because of their nature, dysgerminomas can affect other organ systems, and cases have been reported of associated hypertrophic pulmonary osteoarthropathy.[36] Clinical signs on presentation therefore often are unrelated to the reproductive system. These tumors carry a poor prognosis.

Ovarian Abscess

Ovarian abscesses often are attributed to procedures involving puncture of the ovary, such as biopsy or follicle aspiration. As assisted reproductive techniques became more successful and therefore more popular, the incidence of ovarian abscesses was thought likely to increase. However, this has not proved to be the case. Moreover, not all ovarian abscesses can be attributed to iatrogenic causes. Ovarian abscesses have been reported in mares that have had no such procedures performed on them. In these cases they are likely caused by the hematogenous spread of bacteria or may be associated with strongyle migration.

Affected mares may be febrile and anorectic with an elevated white blood cell count. On ultrasonographic examination the enlarged ovary typically has a thick-walled, fluid-filled structure. The fluid is usually hyperechoic. Medical management with long-term antibiotic therapy has been successful in treating these cases. Surgical removal of the affected ovary is an alternative treatment, but one must take care that the abscess does not rupture in the abdominal cavity.

Ovarian Torsion

Ovarian torsion, a condition not uncommon in women, has been reported in a mare with a large GTCT that was showing signs of abdominal discomfort.[37] Ovarian torsion might be suspected in mares with known ovarian enlargement if sudden signs of abdominal pain develop.

Non-neoplastic Ovarian Enlargement

An ovarian hematoma forms as hemorrhage occurs into the previous follicular lumen after ovulation. On occasion this hemorrhage can be excessive, possibly because of an anticoagulant in follicular fluid. Hematomas can be large, up to 20 cm in diameter or more. They are able to produce progesterone and do not affect the estrous cycle. Although the ovulation fossa is still present, palpating it can be difficult if the hematoma is large. The ultrasonographic appearance varies, causing confusion with a granulosa cell tumor. Large, fluid-filled cavities may be observed, or the hematoma may have a more solid appearance, sometimes with fibrin strands. A trait that is sometimes useful in differentiating a hematoma from a granulosa cell tumor is the responsiveness to PG. Hematomas that are at least 5 or 6 days old often respond to PG by decreasing in size because of the luteolytic effect. Granulosa cell tumors do not respond to PG treatment with any change in size, shape, or ultrasonographic appearance. Because the follicle wall still undergoes luteinization despite the presence of the hematoma, cyclicity remains unaltered; thus normal fertility is not compromised. However, because of the presence of a hematoma, the enlargement of the ovary may persist for several estrous cycles even though the life span of the luteal tissue is normal. Because this structure is a postovulatory phenomenon, the oocyte has been released and the mare may become pregnant if she is mated.

Anovulatory follicles most commonly occur in mares near the end of the breeding season as they go through the autumn transition. These follicles grow to an unusually large size (70 to 100 mm) yet fail to ovulate. Instead, they fill with blood and develop a gelatinous consistency. A thick (compared with a normal follicle) wall commonly forms. The follicles become firmer and then regress over time, usually disappearing within a month. With ultrasonography free-floating echogenic spots are evident in the antrum of the follicle; these increase in number as the follicle grows. When the follicle stops growing, the contents become organized, with an echogenic appearance and fibrin strands. Formation of luteal tissue around the periphery of the anovulatory follicle is usually minimal in a true autumnal follicle that occurs at the end of the season. The cause of anovulatory follicles is unknown, although they are hypothesized to be caused by changes in the hormonal status of the mare that occur with autumn transition. This hypothesis does not explain the occasional occurrence of anovulatory follicles during the breeding season, however. Luteinized anovulatory follicles, although unusual during the ovulatory season, most often occur in older mares and may be associated with senility. Their response to PG varies.

During certain periods of gestation, ovarian enlargement is normal and should be expected. Ovarian enlargement is associated with increased follicular activity and subsequent ovulation (secondary CLs) or anovulatory luteinization (accessory CLs). An increase in follicular growth begins before day 20 of gestation. New CLs form at approximately day 40 of gestation. Corpora hemorrhagica and hemorrhagic follicles commonly occur from day 40 to day 60. Mares bred early in the season have greater follicular activity during the first 4 months of gestation than mares bred after July.

During the spring, as mares undergo transition from winter anestrus to the normal ovulatory season, they undergo periods of prolonged anovulatory follicular development. These periods are characterized by the development of numerous follicles, at times large, on either ovary or usually both ovaries. The follicles may persist for varying lengths of time and then regress, and new follicles develop. This period lasts for a variable time depending on the mare, photoperiod, and other undetermined factors. The ovaries can be large during this time and may be mistakenly called *cystic*. No treatment is necessary, although a combination of progesterone and estrogen often is used to suppress follicular activity in an attempt to hasten the onset of ovulation and normal cyclicity. The transition period ends with the first ovulation of the season, after which follicular activity and ovarian size return to normal.

Small and inactive ovaries normally are found in mares in deep anestrus, prepubertal mares, and pregnant mares in the last third of gestation when, curiously, the fetal gonads are larger than the ovaries of the dam. Mares subject to severe malnutrition, mares of advanced age, mares treated with anabolic steroids, and mares with chromosomal alterations leading to gonadal dysgenesis may have abnormally small and inactive ovaries.

ENDOMETRITIS AND UTERINE THERAPY

Nigel R. Perkins, John B. Chopin

Endometritis is a major problem facing stud veterinarians attempting to maximize per-cycle conception and foaling rates. An improved understanding of the pathogenesis of endometritis has resulted in more effective methods to minimize the impact on fertility. Endometritis has been categorized into persistent mating-induced endometritis, chronic infectious endometritis, chronic degenerative endometritis, and sexually transmitted diseases.[1-3]

Failure of mechanical clearance of fluid, debris, and inflammatory by-products from the uterine lumen is recognized as the major predisposing factor associated with development of infectious endometritis.[4-6] Spermatozoa incite a leucocytic response leading to endometritis[7] 4 to 24 hours after insemination.[8] Significant endometritis is still present 48 hours after either artificial insemination or natural mating, even in mares of normal fertility.[9] Seminal plasma plays an important role in downregulating of endometrial inflammatory reaction to spermatozoa after mating,[10,11] and its removal from the inseminate might cause the reaction to worsen. Seminal plasma does not prevent neutrophil chemotaxis[12] but appears to prevent neutrophils from binding to spermatozoa.[13,14]

Diagnosis of infectious endometritis is based on one or more of the following: ultrasound detection of echogenic uterine luminal fluid and acute inflammatory change on endometrial cytology or biopsy in conjunction with a positive endometrial culture. The condition may be suspected in mares with cervical, vaginal, or vulval discharge during estrus. Diagnosis of chronic degenerative endometritis is mainly based on observation of fibrotic changes in endometrial biopsy samples and is most commonly a condition of older mares. Mares may have a history of failing to conceive over successive cycles or seasons, recurrent or chronic endometritis, and pregnancy loss before 60 days.

Sexually transmitted diseases include contagious equine metritis (CEM; *T. equigenitalis*), *Pseudomonas aeruginosa*, and *Klebsiella pneumoniae*. Susceptible mares bred to a CEM-shedding stallion will usually show shortened interovulatory intervals with a copious mucopurulent genital tract discharge associated with vaginitis, cervicitis, and endometritis.[15-17] Diagnosis depends on recovery of the causative organism from culture samples obtained from the uterus, cervix, clitoral fossa, and clitoral sinuses.[18] The organism is difficult to culture and requires careful sampling, specific transport media, chilling during shipment, and appropriate incubation environment in a laboratory skilled at microbiologic procedures.[19] *P. aeruginosa* and *K. pneumoniae* are present in most equine breeding populations as occasional genital tract pathogens with the capability to be sexually transmitted. Diagnosis and treatment in the mare are as for other causes of infectious endometritis. Mares should be withheld from natural breeding until the infection is eliminated. The choice of uterine therapies for endometritis should be based on the same fundamental principles as for pharmacotherapy in other body systems. The anticipated therapeutic benefit should outweigh the potential risks associated with both the disease and the treatment being applied. Historical use of a particular treatment does not justify continued use unless it is accompanied by clear evidence documenting efficacy and safety. Many of the therapies described in this section are based on empirical evidence alone.

Drug preparations must be relatively nonirritating if they are to be used in the genital tract of the mare. Almost any substance, including physiologic saline, will induce an inflammatory response when introduced into the uterus of the mare.[20] This is particularly important when treatment is performed around the time of breeding because an inflammatory response that is severe and persists for longer than 5 days after ovulation is likely to interfere with embryo survival once the embryo enters the uterine lumen at about day 6 after ovulation.

ANTIBIOTICS

The use of antibiotics in the treatment and prevention of endometritis is largely based on empirical evidence. One early review showed no effect on the foaling rate with the use of intrauterine antibiotics.[21] A more recent study of a large number of mares showed a significant increase in fertility when antibiotics were used.[22] There appear to be relatively few pharmacokinetic studies on which to base recommendations regarding choice of drug, route, dose rate, and frequency of administration. Table 18-5 provides recommended doses for various preparations commonly infused into the uterus of the mare.

INTRAUTERINE VERSUS SYSTEMIC ANTIBIOTIC THERAPY

Antibiotics that have been recommended as possible systemic treatments for equine endometritis include amikacin sulfate, ampicillin trihydrate, gentamicin sulfate, procaine penicillin, and trimethoprim in combination with sulfadiazine. The use of a single dose of intrauterine antibiotics leads to levels in the reproductive tract that were higher at 12 and 24 hours than a single dose administered intravenously or intramuscularly.[23] After intrauterine administration, antibiotic levels peak in the tissue 1 hour after infusion and then decline steadily over 24 hours.[24] Systemic dosages, routes, and frequency of administration usually follow published guidelines for administration of these drugs for other conditions.[25]

Several advantages have been hypothesized to be associated with systemic antibiotic therapy as opposed to intrauterine infusion. Parenteral administration eliminates the risk of

TABLE 18-5

Recommended Doses of Intrauterine Drugs

Drug	Dose	Comment
Amikacin sulfate	1 to 2 g	Gram negative
Ampicillin	1 to 3 g	
Carbenicillin	2 to 6 g	*Pseudomonas*
Ceftiofur	1 g	Broad spectrum
Gentamicin sulfate	0.5 to 2 g	Excellent, gram negative
Kanamycin sulfate	1 to 2 g	*E. coli,* toxic to sperm
Neomycin	3 to 4 g	
Nitrofurazones	50 to 60 ml	Questionable efficacy
Oxytetracycline	1 to 5 g	Use povidone-based products only
Penicillin (Na or K salt)	5,000,000 IU	Streptococci
Penicillin G procaine	3 to 6,000,000 IU	Streptococci
Polymixin B	40,000 to 1,000,000 IU	
Ticarcillin	1 to 6 g	Streptococci, *E. coli, Pseudomonas,* poor against *Klebsiella*
Trimethoprim/sulfadiazine	120 mg	
COMBINATIONS		
Neomycin Polymixin B Furaltadone Penicillin (Na or K salt)	1 g 40,000 IU 600 mg 3 to 5,000,000 IU	
Neomycin Penicillin G procaine	2 g 3,000,000 IU	
Gentamicin sulfate Penicillin G procaine	0.5 to 2 g 3 to 6,000,000 IU	
ANTIFUNGAL THERAPIES		
Nystatin	250,000 to 1,000,000 IU	Mix with sterile water; precipitates in saline
Amphotericin B	200 to 250 mg	
Clotrimazole	300 to 600 mg	Every 2 to 3 days for 12 days
Clotrimazole	500 mg cream	Daily infusion for 1 week
Vinegar	2% solution	20 ml wine vinegar in 1l saline
Povidone-iodine	1 to 2 % solution	
IRRITANTS		
Chlorhexidine	1 to 2 % of stock solution	
DMSO	5% solution	Infuse 50 to 100 ml
EDTA-Tris	1.2 g EDTA plus 6.05 g Tris per 1 water	Titrate to pH 8.0 with glacial acetic acid; infuse, then wait 3 hr, then infuse antibiotic
Hydrogen peroxide	1:4 dilution with saline	
Kerosene	50 ml	Avoid reflux through cervix
Povidone-iodine	0.05% solution	
Saline	Variable volume	Consider warming to 45° to 50° C
Streptococcal cell free filtrate		

Adapted from Perkins N: Equine reproductive pharmacology, *Vet Clin North Am: Equine Pract* 15: 687–704, 1999.
DMSO, dimethyl sulfoxide; *EDTA,* ethylenediamine tetraacetic acid.

bacterial contamination of the reproductive tract, which is associated with repeated intrauterine infusions. Uterine tissue concentrations of ampicillin and enrofloxacin are reported to be higher than serum concentrations after systemic administration of the drugs by intravenous and oral routes.[26,27] Some drugs may be associated with an adverse local tissue reaction when administered into the uterine lumen and yet not have any adverse effect on uterine tissue when administered systemically. For example, intrauterine infusion of enrofloxacin has been linked to uterine pathology, including adhesion formation. Enrofloxacin has been associated with cartilage and skeletal damage in young, growing horses as well as joint effusion and mild cartilage lesions in adult horses after systemic use.[27] Nonetheless, mares receiving oral enrofloxacin (5 mg/kg b.i.d, for 21 days) had endometrial tissue concentrations higher than those observed in serum and all tissue levels of drug exceeded minimum inhibitory concentration (MIC) levels for common equine pathogens. Further work is required before this product can be recommended as a treatment for endometritis. Little documentation exists regarding the efficacy of systemic therapy in the treatment of endometritis. Some researchers have suggested that systemic therapy be considered when deeper layers of the uterus are infected or inflamed, as in the case of postpartum metritis.[1,20] The author routinely uses systemic antibiotic therapy only in mares that show systemic signs of illness associated with the reproductive tract. Most uterine infections in the mare are limited to the lumen and the superficial endometrium. Local uterine therapy by way of uterine infusion is favored in the treatment of such conditions because it is considered likely to result in high antibiotic levels within the lumen and superficial layers of the endometrium. In addition, uterine infusion of antibiotic is considered likely to be more economical than systemic therapy because doses and administration frequency are often lower than those used systemically.

Choice of Antibiotic

Factors to consider in the choice of antibiotic to use in the uterus include types of organisms isolated, antibiotic-sensitivity patterns of isolated organisms, and potential efficacy of the drug in the uterus. Antibiotic selection should be as specific as possible and based on microbiologic isolation of the etiologic organisms by uterine culture, followed by sensitivity testing.[28] The use of broad spectrum antibiotics in the absence of culture and sensitivity results is discouraged insofar as such indiscriminant use of antibiotics is likely to increase the risk of bacterial resistance and superinfection with different bacterial strains, fungi, or yeast.[20,29] Methicillin-resistant *Staphylococcus aureus* was isolated from several mares from one farm in Japan. The source of the infection was a cutaneous lesion on a stallion.[30] Fungi and yeast did not become more prevalent as causes of endometritis until the widespread use of intrauterine antibiotics in the mid-1950s.[29]

The use of antibiotic combinations is also discouraged because of the risk of incompatibilities resulting in reduced efficacy. An example is the suggested inactivation that is thought to occur when β-lactam antibiotics such as penicillin are combined with aminoglycosides such as gentamicin.[31] However, some experts argue that the first choice of antibiotic for intrauterine use should be a broad spectrum combination of drugs aimed at successfully treating all components of the mixed aerobic and anaerobic infections that commonly occur.[32] When culture and sensitivity results are not available, the choice of drug should be based on the expected bacterial organisms and their predicted antibiotic susceptibility patterns.[31]

Virtually any bacterial species could be isolated from acute endometritis, although certain bacterial isolates are considered to be more likely than others. Several studies have reported that between 70% and 80% of acute aerobic endometritis cases were associated with *Streptococcus zooepidemicus, E. coli, P. aeruginosa,* and *K. pneumoniae*.[31,33-35] Large-scale data from routine endometrial cultures in the U.K. appear to show a slightly different pattern of bacterial involvement.[25] Of 3414 isolates associated with cytologic evidence of endometritis, 38% were recovered in pure culture and 62% in mixed culture.[25] Streptococci were more likely to be isolated when there was clinical signs of endometritis, whereas *E. coli* was more likely when mares were presented for repeat breeding.[37] The role of anaerobic bacteria in endometritis remains unclear. One study has reported that 18 of 71 (25%) cases in which endometrial cytology and culture were positive grew an anaerobe only on culture. The most common anaerobe recovered was *Bacteroides fragilis*.[38] Others have suggested that anaerobes are unlikely to play a significant role in endometritis.[39] No single antimicrobial therapy is effective against all of the commonly isolated uterine pathogens. β-Lactam antibiotics (penicillins and cephalosporins) are very effective against streptococci. Synthetic penicillins such as ampicillin and ticarcillin are also effective against many strains of *E. coli* and *P. aeruginosa*. Aminoglycosides are used primarily in the treatment of gram negative organisms. Bacterial sensitivity patterns are often variable, particularly for gram negative organisms, and accurate prediction of sensitivity patterns is impossible in many cases.[31]

The difficulties described in identification of the etiologic agent in cases of endometritis, prediction of antibiotic sensitivities, and the time constraints of a short breeding season mean that in most cases broad spectrum antibiotics are used as a first-choice treatment. In many cases a broad spectrum of activity is achieved by using combinations of drugs. Commonly used broad spectrum antibiotics include ticarcillin-clavulanic acid, ampicillin, and drug combinations such as penicillin-aminoglycoside and penicillin-furaltadone-neomycin-polymixin B (Utrin Wash, Univet Ltd., Wedgewood Road, Bicester, U.K.). Recently, ceftiofur sodium (1 g by intrauterine administration daily for 3 successive days) was used in clinical trials as a broad spectrum intrauterine treatment for equine endometritis and was considered to be an effective and safe alternative to the combination of penicillin, neomycin, polymixin B, and furaltadone.[32]

Antibiotic Formulation, Treatment Frequency, and Volume

There is little evidence on which to base recommendations regarding dosage, formulation, volume of drug infused, diluent, and frequency of treatment. Dose regimens should be based on MIC data in conjunction with pharmacokinetic studies of drug disposition after intrauterine administration. In the absence of any data, it appears that dosages are based on the recommended parenteral dosage for the drug in question. In many cases the dose rate recommended for intrauterine use is lower than the systemic dose. Sometimes this is based on clinical evidence, and in others it appears to be more a response to convenience or cost. Use of a 2-g dose of amikacin sulfate administered by intrauterine infusion was reported to be associated with a higher cure rate than 0.5- or 1-g doses in mares experimentally inoculated with *K. pneumoniae*.[40] There was little difference in endometrial or uterine luminal amikacin concentrations in mares after infusion of 2 g versus 3 g, and both infusion doses resulted in endometrial levels within assumed therapeutic ranges for a 24-hour period.[24] This information suggests that the infusion dose of amikacin should be 2 g.

Intrauterine treatments are commonly performed every day or every second day for 3 to 7 days. Treatment is usually performed during estrus, largely because uterine defense mechanisms are more effective during estrus than diestrus. Treatments may proceed for 2 to 4 days after ovulation, provided the infused preparation results in little endometrial irritation. Once-daily treatment with 3 g ampicillin maintains uterine levels above MIC for common equine uterine pathogens for the entire 24-hour period between treatments.[41] Although frequency of treatment should be based on the length of time that the antibiotic remains active and above estimated MIC within the uterus, the fact remains that the standard daily or every-other-day treatments are likely to be based on convenience and practicality rather than science. It may not be necessary to maintain antibiotic levels above MIC for the entire time interval between successive treatments. Exposure of bacteria to large doses of antibiotic for brief periods of time reportedly increases the susceptibility of bacteria to leucocyte killing.[42] This may explain the success of a convenience-based treatment protocol that might not maintain antibiotic levels above MIC for the entire intertreatment interval. The volume of fluid infused into a mare's uterus with each treatment ranges between 30 and 250 ml. In most cases a sufficient volume of fluid should be used to obtain complete uterine coverage when infused.[28,34,43] The capacity of a typical nonpregnant mare's uterus is about 35 ml, whereas an older mare's uterus may hold 60 to 150 ml.[28,34]

Infusion of fluid volumes ranging between 30 to 250 ml may not result in uniform distribution of fluid within the uterine lumen. The majority of infused fluid pools in the uterine body and at the body-horn junctions.[44] Most cervical reflux was observed 10 to 15 minutes after infusion, which is consistent with endogenous oxytocin or PGF_2-α–stimulated uterine contractions. Larger volumes were more likely to result in reflux through the cervix. It appears likely that some of the benefit from infusing antibiotic into the uterus in volumes large enough to encourage cervical reflux is actually due to a lavage effect rather than a direct antibacterial effect.

Insoluble or irritant preparations are not recommended because they can cause chronic endometritis.[45] Drugs for uterine infusion are commonly diluted in either saline, balanced electrolyte solutions, or water for injection. Acidic drugs such as gentamicin and amikacin may be buffered by mixing equal volumes of antibiotic and 7.5% sodium bicarbonate before infusion into the uterus.[25] The choice of diluent may influence the pharmacokinetics of some drugs. Infusion of gentamicin into the uterus of cattle was followed by systemic absorption of more than 60% of the dose when the gentamicin was diluted in water, versus less than 20% of the dose when diluted with saline.[46] Procaine penicillin is discouraged for intrauterine administration owing to an early study based on hysteroscopy in which the endometrium was reported to be visibly covered with a white, chalky material, thought to be antibiotic, after infusion of ampicillin. The material was visible 3, 7, and 14 days after infusion.[47] Nonetheless, procaine penicillin is widely used as an intrauterine infusion and is commonly mixed with aminoglycosides, particularly gentamicin and neomycin. The use of procaine penicillin in the equine uterus requires additional investigation.

ANTIFUNGAL PREPARATIONS

Dilute povidone iodine or 2% vinegar (20 ml white vinegar in 1000 ml saline) has been proposed as an intrauterine therapy for fungal endometritis. A variety of antifungal medications have also been used as intrauterine treatments,[48] some of which are presented in Table 18-5. There appears to be little or no data on which to base recommendations regarding sensitivity patterns, dose rates, or frequency of treatment. Fungal endometritis has been reported as being difficult to treat, although this perception may be due in part to the use of ineffective or inappropriate treatments.[48,49]

A report using an instillation of 540 mg of lufenuron in 60 ml of saline after uterine lavage reported success of removal of fungal infection in 4 mares.[50]

ANTISEPTICS AND IRRITANTS

Antiseptic or irritant therapy has commonly been recommended for mares in which a diagnosis of endometritis has been made but no specific etiologic agent isolated or for aged, subfertile mares with distinct degenerative changes on endometrial biopsy. Irritants have been used to reduce the size of the uterus and increase uterine tone. Antibiotics are not useful in this manner unless they are irritating. In addition, irritants may decrease fluid viscosity within the uterus to aid in its expulsion. Irritant therapy has also been credited with stimulating a severe, acute inflammatory response within the endometrium, which may help resolve the chronic monocytic inflammation commonly associated with degenerative endometritis or endometrosis. Mechanical curettage has similar effects, although the technique is difficult because of the bicornuate nature of the equine uterus. The typical endometrial response to infusion of an irritant is a nonspecific inflammatory reaction with hyperemia and neutrophil influx. This is followed by a slower infiltration of mononuclear cells that peaks between 4 and 7 days after treatment. The duration of inflammation and the extent of tissue damage varies considerably among individual animals receiving the same treatment. Irritant therapy nonspecifically activates endometrial glands.[51] Excessive irritation of the endometrium, associated with too harsh or concentrated a solution, may result in worsening of the degenerative condition and even in adhesion formation. Threlfall has stated that chlorhexidine solution has a propensity to cause endometrial adhesions and severe reactions and should not be used within the uterus.[43] Recently, anecdotal evidence suggests that enrofloxacin administered as a uterine infusion in mares may be highly irritating, resulting in a severe inflammatory reaction with serosanguineous uterine fluid containing fibrin tags.

Povidone Iodine

Dilute povidone iodine solution is a commonly recommended intrauterine treatment because of its irritant, bactericidal, and fungicidal properties. Bactericidal activity of povidone-iodine is maintained in vitro down to concentrations of 0.01 to 0.005%, whereas more than 0.2% povidone iodine has been claimed to inhibit neutrophil migration.[52] Stock povidone-iodine solution, used in practices to disinfect surgical sites, is described as a solution containing 10% povidone iodine, equivalent to 1% available iodine.

Discussions regarding the safety of dilute povidone-iodine solutions in the mare exemplify the need for critical information on the uterine effects of all potential irritant therapies. Earlier studies found severe inflammatory responses in the endometrium after infusions of 2% or more povidone-iodine.[53,54] A similar study reported severe prolonged irritation of the endometrium after infusion of 1% povidone-iodine solution, with mares still showing evidence of inflammation at the conclusion of the study, 30 days after infusion.[55] Other researchers have reported resolution of inflammation on uterine biopsy within 6 days of uterine infusion of 0.05% povidone-iodine solution.[20] In addition, infusion of 1 L of 0.05% povidone-iodine into the uterus 4 hours after breeding had no adverse effect on pregnancy rates.[56] Recently, Bracher reported that infusion of 0.05% povidone-iodine solution into the uterus (alone or in combination with either dimethyl sulfoxide [DMSO] or collagenase) induced adhesions, ulceration of the endometrium, and severe stromal fibrosis and gland degeneration in three of five treated mares.[51] Individual mares may be hypersensitive to povidone-iodine solution. Asbury and Lyle[25] have suggested that if any signs of discomfort or irritation, either on clinical observation or examination with a vaginal speculum, are observed after povidone-iodine infusion genital tract should be flushed with saline and povidone-iodine therapy should be discontinued. The author suggests that povidone iodine solutions be avoided or used with caution until further information is available regarding its safety as a uterine therapy.

Hydrogen Peroxide

Hydrogen peroxide acts as an irritant and has been recommended as an alternative approach for treating intrauterine infections caused by *P. aeruginosa*. Hydrogen peroxide is an oxidizing agent that readily breaks down to release oxygen and water, accompanied by effervescence. It should be used only in mares during estrus.[57]

Tris-EDTA

Intrauterine infusion of Tris–ethylenediamine tetraacetic acid (EDTA) results in a degree of inflammation similar to that observed after saline infusion.[58] Tris-EDTA may have a potentiating effect on the antimicrobial activity of a variety of antibiotic and antibacterial solutions.[59] It may have direct antibacterial effects in some cases; in others it may cause a reduction in the MIC for some organisms in association with particular antibiotics, including penicillin, oxytetracycline, and gentamicin.

Chlorhexidine Gluconate

Chlorhexidine is a strong irritant with the potential to cause intrauterine adhesions and therefore has been disregarded for potential uterine therapy.[43] Pony mares tolerate uterine infusions of 0.25% chlorhexidine gluconate (Hibitane: Schering-Plough Animal Health, Upper Hutt, New Zealand; dilution of stock solution of 20% v:v BP in water) with little evidence of irritation on vaginal inspection, whereas dilutions of 0.5%, 1%, and 2% caused severe irritation in a number of mares treated.[60] A solution containing 100 μg/ml chlorhexidine gluconate exceeds the MIC for *Streptococcus equi* subsp. *zooepidemicus*, *P. aeruginosa*, *K. pnemoniae*, *Actinobacillus equlli*, and *Candida albicans*.[61] Infusion of this solution in a 200-ml volume on 3 successive days during estrus had no adverse effect on pregnancy rate when mares were given PGF_2-α 8 to 9 days after ovulation and bred at the successive estrus.[62] More research is needed regarding the safety and efficacy of chlorhexidine as a uterine therapy.

Dimethyl Sulfoxide

Dimethyl sulfxide causes an inflammatory response after intrauterine infusion.[51] Intrauterine DMSO may decrease endometrial biopsy classification scores by 1 or more points largely because of the reduction of periglandular fibrosis,[57] although others have reported that DMSO did not have any fibrolytic effect.[51,63] One mare in a treatment group receiving concentrated DMSO subsequently was found to have developed transluminal adhesions.[51] A clinical trial involving uterine infusion of DMSO into subfertile mares failed to detect any improvement in fertility after DMSO infusion.[57]

Kerosene

Kerosene has been used as an irritant therapy in the equine uterus for many years.[64] Recently, an experimental comparison evaluated the uterine response in subfertile mares to infusions of kerosene, dilute povidone-iodine, DMSO, and collagenase. The uterine response to kerosene, collagenase, and DMSO was similar, resembling that seen after mechanical curettage. Gross and histologic evidence of inflammation resolved within 14 to 21 days of infusion. Kerosene-treated mares differed from other treatment groups in having improved gland activity on uterine biopsy and higher pregnancy rates after breeding. Nine of 11 (82%) mares conceived, and 5 of 11 (45%) subsequently foaled. Bracher concluded that the increase in secretory activity of the glands observed after intrauterine infusion of kerosene was a major factor in achieving the higher conception and foaling rates.

The standard approach for infusing kerosene involves infusing 50 ml of commercial-grade kerosene into the uterine lumen during diestrus. Diestrus is preferred because the closed cervix is more likely to prevent reflux of kerosene into the vagina with resulting inflammation.[57] Alternatively, infusions during estrus should be followed by digital occlusion of the cervix for a short time to prevent vaginal reflux.

Saline

Saline is very useful as a means of flushing or mechanically removing fluid and debris from the uterus as well as stimulating the uterus to contract and expel contents. It irritates the endometrium and causes migration of PMN into the uterine lumen. Warmed saline results in rapid and transient enhancement of uterine tone in mares with atonic or atrophic uteri. Saline flushes on day 6 after ovulation result in luteolysis through endometrial PGF release.[25,43]

The use of saline to flush the uterus 4 to 6 hours after insemination might result in increased fertility compared with lavage at 18 to 20 hours after insemination. Unfortunately, low treatment numbers did not allow a significant result.[65] Lavage with lactated Ringer's solution can be performed immediately before insemination without affecting fertility provided that most of the fluid is removed first.[66]

PLASMA

Plasma may be beneficial in mares with chronic and chronic-active endometritis by providing immunoglobulins and complement, both important components in opsonization of bacteria within the uterus.[67-69] Suppression of uterine neutrophil function in susceptible mares is likely to be a result of the accumulation of fluid, debris, and bacteria that occurs secondary to an underlying failure of uterine mechanical clearance.[70] Treatment and prevention are therefore better aimed at aiding clearance than infusing plasma. This hypothesis is supported by studies failing to demonstrate any beneficial effect of plasma in susceptible mares.[71]

The use of plasma alone reduced inflammation but did not inhibit bacterial growth.[2] Pascoe recently described a large field study involving the routine postbreeding use of plasma in conjunction with antibiotics. A significant improvement in pregnancy rate was seen when plasma was infused into barren and lactating mares but not in maiden mares.[72] It is possible that plasma may be beneficial in foaling mares or in mares that do not have a mechanical clearance problem. Further work is needed to determine factors that may influence the effect of plasma in the uterus of the mare.

Autologous plasma is believed to be preferable to heterologous plasma because of the risk of hypersensitivity, anaphylaxis, or transfusion illness after heterologous plasma infusion. However, many mares have received heterologous plasma without experiencing any problems. Preparation of plasma requires aseptic withdrawal of venous blood into a heparin-based anticoagulant (typically 5-10 units heparin per ml of blood).[1] Because complement rapidly degrades at room temperature, separation of plasma should be rapid. Gravity sedimentation is acceptable but should be performed under refrigeration. Once separated, plasma should be infused immediately or stored frozen in 100-ml aliquots ready for thawing and infusion. Thawing must be performed in warm water or in a microwave on a low setting. Thawing at too high a temperature will result in denaturation of protein and loss of immunoglobulin activity. In field conditions preparation of plasma is invariably performed under conditions that are less than ideal. The author always combines field-derived plasma with broad spectrum antibiotic as a uterine infusion to minimize the risk of inadvertently introducing infectious organisms when infusing plasma.

UTEROTONICS

The importance of mechanical clearance of the uterus in resistance to bacterial infections has been clearly documented.[2,6,70,73,74] The inability to physically clear contaminating material from the uterus within a short period is believed to be the major factor resulting in mares being susceptible to chronic and recurrent uterine bacterial infection.[1] Some affected mares show decreased contractility of longitudinal muscles and decreased available intracellular calcium,[75] possibly as a result of a contractile defect in the myometrium of susceptible mares.[76] In addition, in the uterine fluid and endometrium of susceptible mares, there is a higher concentration of nitric oxide, which relaxes smooth muscle and will inhibit mechanical clearance.[77,78]

Treatments that help the uterus to physically clear bacteria, fluid, and associated inflammatory by-products and debris from the uterine lumen are critical to the effective treatment and prevention of infectious endometritis. Uterine lavage is very effective at removing material from the uterine lumen.

Pharmacologic therapies that induce uterine contractions include oxytocin and PGF_2-αand analogs.[79] The use of oxytocin improved fertility,[22,80] especially when combined with antibiotics.[22]

PGF_2-α or cloprostenol administered by intramuscular injection causes an increase in intrauterine pressure within 10 minutes, with contractions lasting for about 5 hours. Oxytocin produces a response within 60 seconds of intravenous administration, but contractions last only 40 to 60 minutes. Recently, investigators concluded that oxytocin was more effective than PG in clearing the uterus of colloid.[73] The same study also concluded that cloprostenol was more effective than PGF or fenprostalene, although all mares treated with PG analogs had an increased clearance of radiocolloids.[73]

Cloprostenol has also been recommended in favor of dinoprost in mares that have lymphatic stasis. Lymphatics drain particulate matter from the uterine lumen and reabsorb the intramural fluid that accumulates within the uterine wall during estrus.[74,81] Lymphatics drain dorsally into the vessels in the broad ligament and then into the iliac and aortic lymph nodes. Lymphatic vessels do not contain smooth muscle and therefore must rely on uterine contractions to push fluid dorsally within lymph vessels.[74]

PGs should not be administered more than 48 hours after ovulation to minimize the risk of inducing luteal regression. There was a reduction in progesterone production and pregnancy rate after the use of cloprostenol, but not oxytocin,[82] 24 hours after ovulation.

Concurrent medications may interfere with uterine clearance in susceptible mares. Phenylbutazone and acepromazine administration interfere with the clearance of uterine radiocolloid in susceptible mares. The effect is reversed with the administration of oxytocin.[74] Xylazine may be a preferable to acepromazine as a sedative for susceptible mares in the breeding shed because xylazine causes an increase in uterine pressure. In the event that mares receive either acepromazine or phenylbutazone around the time of breeding, consideration should be given to concurrent administration of oxytocin to assist in uterine clearance.

Intrauterine oxytocin administration increases intrauterine pressure but not as much as intramuscular or intravenous administration.[83] Preliminary studies involving the intrauterine administration of 10-mg doses of dinoprost suggest that it is effective at inducing uterine contractility.[2,84] The use of oxytocin and PG (or analogs) as aids for uterine clearance remains empirical. Doses of 10 to 25 IU oxytocin have been used to aid mechanical evacuation of the uterus. Little information exists regarding the most effective dose, route of administration, and frequency of administration. There is also a lack of information on the safety of these products when used around the time of breeding, although both products are commonly used during estrus, both before and after breeding. In addition, there is relatively little information on practical methods of identifying mares with delayed uterine clearance that is suitable for application in the field. The presence of ultrasonographically detectable uterine fluid appears to be an indicator of reduced clearance, particularly if it persists for more than 6 to 12 hours after mating.[3]

UTERINE LAVAGE

Uterine lavage is a traditional and highly effective method of removing fluid and associated debris from the lumen of the uterus. Uterine lavage is commonly performed both before and after breeding and is often combined with infusion of antibiotic, antiseptic, or other materials (e.g., plasma).[43] In addition, lavage is commonly applied in the early postpartum mare for the treatment of retained placenta, metritis, or both. Emptying the uterus of fluid before antibiotic infusion is likely to improve the efficacy of uterine antibiotic therapy by removing foreign material and inflammatory products from the lumen. This is likely to be more important for aminoglycoside and polymixin antibiotics, which bind to purulent material.[20]

Saline induces an inflammatory response within the uterus. Infusion of acidic saline resulted in an immediate release of endogenous PGF, whereas infusion of pH-neutral saline does not.[85] Heating lavage fluid to 45° to 50° C results in a rapid and transient increase in uterine contractility.[43]

Uterine lavage is normally performed with a Foley catheter or embryo transfer catheter with a large balloon cuff (75 ml). Fluid is infused until the uterus is distended (500 to 1000 ml), removed under gravity flow, and collected into a vessel to allow measurement of lavage and recovered volumes; the appearance of the recovered fluid is then assessed. The opacity of the recovered fluid is an indicator of the degree of inflammation present within the uterus and helps the clinician decide whether additional flushing is necessary. Lavage should be repeated until the recovered fluid is clear. There are no controlled studies documenting the efficacy of lavage as a treatment modality for endometritis.

ALTERNATIVE TREATMENTS

The use of lectins to bind to *Streptococcus* and prevent it from binding to the endometrium was somewhat successful with D-galNAc and D-(+)-mannose. However, it required exposure of the lectin to the bacteria before its introduction to the uterine environment.[86,87]

Corticosteroid treatment of endometritis in mares has yielded contradictory results. Administration of dexamethasone (40 μg/kg) for 3 days while mares received concurrent progesterone therapy resulted in worse disease symptoms than those observed in control mares or mares receiving dexamethasone and antibiotics.[88] However, in a separate study mares receiving prednisolone had no difference in response to therapy than normal mares. Mares with a history of endometritis had decreased uterine fluid that was clearer and had a lower cell count after insemination with frozen semen compared with untreated mares. The pregnancy rate in the treated barren mares was greater then in untreated barren mares.[89]

Immunizing mares against *S. equi* subsp. *zooepidemicus* reduced infection and inflammation when the uterus was experimentally infected with the same bacteria.[90] The use of an immunostimulant made from *Propionibacterium acnes* reduced the cytologic diagnosis of endometritis on subsequent estruses.[91,92] The conception rate was good, but unfortunately the control mares that still had a high level of endometritis were not bred as controls.[92] Another study found a reduction in the diagnosis of endometritis with the use of *P. acnes* injection, and mares were more likely to get pregnant after treatment.[93]

When susceptible mares with experimental endometritis were treated with fresh, frozen, or lysed leucocytes, they were able to clear bacteria significantly more quickly than the control mares.[94]

There is anecdotal evidence that magnesium sulfate may benefit some mares with endometritis. No fertility data have been published, but the few mares that were examined after being infused with 1 L of saline with 128 g of magnesium sulfate showed no evidence of permanent damage.[95,96]

When the mare is exposed to auditory and visual stimulus from the stallion or teaser male, there is a release of oxytocin and an increase in myometrial contractions.[97] The authors have used this with mares that show an adverse reaction to, or are dangerous with, repeated oxytocin injections. The mare can be run alongside the teaser male for the period of time that oxytocin release is needed, provided that the fences are sound and safe. In the authors' opinion, the stance that the mare adopts when she is teasing, wherein the caudal aspect of the pelvis tilts ventrally, might help in posturally draining the reproductive tract.

CONCLUSION

Successful treatment of acute or chronic infectious endometritis is based on elimination of the etiologic organism, reduction of any accompanying inflammation, correction of anatomic defects, and prevention of recurrence. Predisposing anatomic causes of endometritis such as poor vulval conformation, cervical or rectovestibular lacerations, and urine pooling must be corrected surgically before the application of therapies aimed at resolving endometritis. The most common routine procedure performed on broodmares is Caslick surgery. More extensive surgical procedures should be performed during the nonbreeding season to allow the mare time to recover before breeding.

The approach to uterine therapy depends on the diagnosis and presenting clinical signs. Infectious endometritis is managed by elimination of fluid and debris from the uterine lumen by lavage and administration of uterotonic agents followed by uterine infusion of a topical treatment (e.g., antibiotic, antifungal, antiseptic). Choice of uterine therapy, formulation, dose, volume infused, diluent, and treatment frequency must be determined after consideration of individual patient information. It is necessary to lavage the uterus on subsequent treatment visits only if the uterine lumen continues to accumulate fluid or if the lavage is being performed to stimulate uterine contractility.

Many treatments have been suggested for chronic degenerative endometritis (endometrosis), but consistently favorable results have not been reported. Mechanical and chemical curettage or irritant therapy are commonly employed in mares with this condition.

Topical treatment of the uterus must be accompanied by strict attention to hygiene. Attention must be paid to management principles if successful resolution of endometritis is to be accompanied by a reduction in the risk of recurrence and an optimal opportunity for pregnancy to be achieved.[20]

An area in which important advances have been made in the past several years is in our understanding and management of postmating endometritis. A transient and physiologic endometritis occurs after breeding because of the intrauterine deposition of semen.[1] In normal, fertile (resistant) mares, this transient inflammation resolves within 36 hours after mating. Contamination and inflammation of the uterus after breeding must be resolved before the embryo enters the uterine lumen at approximately 6 days after ovulation in the pregnant mare. Impaired physical clearance of bacteria, fluid, and inflammatory products is considered the primary factor responsible for susceptibility to persistent infectious endometritis.[1] Mares should be examined in early estrus using ultrasonography to evaluate the presence and echotexture of uterine luminal fluid. The presence of large volumes of echogenic fluid indicates acute endometritis, and it may be preferable to treat such mares aggressively through the estrus period and short cycle them to aim for breeding on the successive estrus. Large volumes of anechoic fluid in early estrus can be removed using uterine lavage with saline, followed by injection of oxytocin to prevent fluid accumulation recurring. Small to moderate volumes of fluid may be managed by oxytocin alone. It is useful to examine mares 20 minutes after administration of oxytocin to ensure that uterine fluid has been expelled. In some cases manual dilation of the cervix is needed to facilitate effective expulsion of fluid. Intrauterine infusion of antibiotic may be used in early estrus in an attempt to eliminate endometritis or reduce the risk of endometritis before breeding. Any product used for uterine lavage or instillation in the prebreeding or postbreeding estrous period should have minimal irritating effect on the endometrium. Physiologic saline, Dulbecco's phosphate buffered saline, or lactated Ringers' solution are believed to be associated with a reduced inflammatory response compared with water. Antibiotics should be chosen with care and antiseptics or irritants not used at all in this period. Ultrasound examinations may be continued through estrus right up to immediately before breeding, with the goal being to eliminate fluid from the lumen of the uterus before breeding.

There is general agreement that mares should be bred only once to minimize contamination of the uterus and genital tract. The use of ovulation induction agents such as hCG or synthetic GnRH should be considered routine for susceptible mares because they greatly improve the likelihood of a single breeding per ovulatory cycle. It is normal practice to aim for a single breeding in the period from 24 hours before ovulation to 12 hours after ovulation. Depending on stallion fertility, mares may be bred as early as 48 to 72 hours before ovulation without reduction in fertility. Recently, Pycock proposed that susceptible mares be bred only once, at least 24 hours before ovulation and perhaps earlier, assuming suitable stallion fertility.[98] This ensures that any contamination associated with breeding occurs at a time when circulating estrogen concentrations are maximal, progesterone concentrations are minimal, uterine defense mechanisms and physical drainage should be optimal, and there is more time available after breeding to implement uterine therapy before progesterone rises and the cervix begins to close after ovulation.

If breeding by artificial insemination, semen extender containing antibiotic should be added to the ejaculate and the extended semen allowed to stand undisturbed for a minimum of 15 minutes to allow elimination of possible pathogens from the ejaculate. Antibiotic-containing semen extender may be infused into the uterus of the mare immediately before natural breeding in an attempt to obtain a similar effect. Susceptible mares should be examined by ultrasound as early as 4 hours after breeding and preferably before 12 hours, again to check for accumulation of fluid.[56] This ensures that uterine fluid can be eliminated using lavage, uterotonics, or a combination of these treatments before the development of an inflammatory response or proliferation of potentially pathogenic organisms. Uterine infusion with broad spectrum antibiotics is performed about 20 minutes after administration of uterotonic. Pycock suggests using a small volume infusion (30 ml) for the postbreeding treatment because susceptible mares are expected to have clearance problems.[98]

Administration of oxytocin can be continued and the mare examined the following day to ensure that uterine fluid is not accumulating. If fluid is still present, the treatment approach (lavage, uterotonic, and infusion) can be repeated. Intrauterine treatment should not be continued past day 3 after ovulation in order to minimize the risk of endometrial inflammation persisting past day 5 or 6, when an embryo may be expected to be entering the uterus. Uterotonics should not be administered past day 2 after ovulation because the cervix is generally starting to close and uterine drainage is then inhibited. PGs should be used with care after ovulation because of the added risk of possible induction of luteal regression. The use of a single postbreeding uterine infusion of broad spectrum antibiotic in combination with uterotonic administration results in higher pregnancy rates in field trials than either antibiotic or uterotonic alone.[99]

The combination of prebreeding and very early postbreeding estral management, with the use of oxytocin, has greatly improved our ability to prepare an optimal uterine environment, both for breeding and for establishment of early pregnancy. Anecdotal reports support the use of systemic antibiotics and nonsteroidal anti-inflammatory drugs in susceptible mares after breeding as a possible way to reduce the risk of establishment of endometritis and endometrial PG release.[100,101] Such therapies remain unproven.

HORMONAL MANIPULATION OF THE MARE

Elizabeth Metcalf

Veterinarians attempt to alter the physiology or behavior of the mare through the administration of exogenous hormones. This chapter examines the effects of hormonal preparations administered to mares in an attempt to enhance their reproductive efficiency.

VERNAL TRANSITION

As day length increases, nonpregnant mares gradually emerge from a state of ovarian quiescence to regular cyclicity. Through activation of the hypothalamic-pineal-pituitary-ovarian axis, mares begin to show clinical signs of a prolonged estrous period followed at last by the first ovulation of the season. The first section of this chapter, Reproductive Anatomy and Physiology of the Nonpregnant Mare, presents more precise physiologic events of this period.

Many hormonal regimens aimed at shortening the interval to first ovulation have been examined. Increasing the exposure of a mare to light from 6 A.M. to 10 P.M. has proved a potent and effective means of shortening the time to first ovulation of the season. In an attempt to more effectively hasten the interval using exogenous hormonal manipulation, researchers have examined other preparations, including melatonin,[1] progestins[2] (plus estrogens),[3] and dopamine antagonists such as domperidone,[4-6] sulpiride,[6] and perphenazine.[7]

Although all regimens are effective at shortening the interval to first ovulation, none were more effective than progesterone alone.[6] Intravaginal pessaries impregnated with progesterone also have been successful in induction of cyclicity in anestrous mares.[8] The provision of good nutrition, especially in aged mares, may hasten the onset of the first ovulation,[9] possibly by involving hormones that are associated with digestive metabolism. Once a mare has entered the period of transitional estrus in the spring and has developed a 25-mm follicle, intramuscular administration of 12.5 mg eFSH (Bioniche) twice daily significantly hastens the time to first ovulation compared with untreated control mares (22.4 versus 10.9 days, $P < 0.05$) and increases the number of embryos recovered in treated mares.[10]

SYNCHRONIZING THE ESTROUS CYCLE

In the attempt to optimize breeding efficiency, the ability to predict estrus and ovulation becomes an important management tool. Although mares show variability in their response to hormonal treatment, the concept of fixed-timed insemination, or "appointment breeding" has proved successful in equine reproduction. The objective of most attempts to manipulate the timing of the estrous cycle of the mare is synchronization of a group of mares (e.g., in an embryo transfer program) or, more commonly, strategic management of insemination with shipped or frozen semen.

To manipulate the estrous cycle of the mare with some precision, one must understand the basic endocrine events of the normal 21- to 22-day cycle of the mare.[11] The day of ovulation is considered to be day 0 and is preceded by a period of estrogen domination (5 to 7 days). The high estrogen levels are responsible for the signs of behavioral estrus and the palpably decreased tone of the uterus and cervix. Under the influence of estrogen priming, a cascade of preovulatory events occurs in the hypothalamic-pituitary axis, culminating in a sharp increase in (LH) blood levels that ultimately results in ovulation. The diestrous phase is dominated by progesterone secretion from the resultant CL. This diestrous phase lasts 14 to 16 days. In the absence of maternal recognition of a pregnancy, endometrial prostaglandin F_2-α_α (PGF_2-$\alpha\alpha$) surges—possibly stimulated by, or at least coordinated with, oxytocin—cause luteolysis and regression of the CL. Concomitant with the decline in progesterone, estrogen levels begin to rise as a new cohort of follicles develops.

Most hormone regimens used to synchronize estrus are aimed at manipulating the luteal phase of the cycle. Perhaps the simplest method of synchronizing the cycle of a mare is through the use of synthetic preparations of PGF_2-α, which effectively and reliably shortens the cycle of the mare if used after the CL is well formed—after day 5 or 6 of the cycle. The mare returns to estrus within 3 to 5 days after administration of PGF_2-α and subsequent regression of the CL. Depending on the structures present on the ovary at the time of administration, the mare ovulates approximately 7 days later.[12] Although administration of PGF_2-α before day 5 is usually ineffective in returning a mare to estrus, treatment of mares with a PGF_2-α analog on day 0 (ovulation) or day 1 has an negative effect on the developing CL. Not only is the size and echogenicity of the CL reduced, but a transient yet also significant suppression in progesterone levels occurs. Most important, pregnancy rates may be lower in treated mares.[1,13,14]

A number of PGF_2-α preparations have been used successfully for luteolysis in the mare; some are associated with undesirable side effects, including profuse sweating, anxiety, diarrhea, and signs of colic. The severity of the side effects depends on the dose and preparation of PGF_2-α. A two-dose regimen at a much lower dose (0.5 mg PGF_2-α) is equally effective in inducing luteolysis as a higher single dose (50 mg PGF_2-α) but devoid of adverse effects.[15] Similarly, a single dose of 25 μg cloprostenol (Estrumate; Bayer Corp., Shawnee, Kan.), ⅒ of the previously recommended dose, is effective in inducing luteolysis and does not cause the adverse side effects.[16]

Treatment with progestins represents one of the oldest and most reliable means of synchronizing estrus in the mare, especially when coupled with appropriate light exposure and PGF_2-α administration. Progestins simulate the diestrous period of the estrous cycle. Repositol progesterone, progesterone in oil (Sigma Chemical Co., St. Louis, Mo.), or oral progestin compounds (altrenogest [Regumate, Intervet Inc. Millsboro, Del.]) are effective in suppressing estrous behavior but not necessarily follicular development or ovulation. Combining progesterone with estradiol 17B (called *P+ or P+E*) may be administered daily or as a 10-day repositol injection that will effectively suppress both estrus behavior and the formation of follicles. Treatment with these preparations is only effective, however, in synchronizing mares that are transitioning into regular cyclicity or cycling regularly; treatment is not effective in mares that remain in seasonal anestrus. Therefore examining the reproductive tract of the mare by transrectal palpation and ultrasound before initiating treatment is prudent. Ovaries in anestrous mares feel smooth, firm, and small on palpation. Their follicles are small, usually less than 10 mm in size on the ultrasound examination. Conversely, mares that are ready to begin regular cycles or are cycling regularly have larger, irregular-shaped ovaries of variable firmness, with multiple follicles greater than 10 mm in diameter, the presence of a CL, or both.

The oral progestin preparation altrenogest is perhaps still the most popular progestin compound for use in mares. Altrenogest is easy to administer, is not painful, and has few adverse effects. Fillies born to mares treated with altrenogest may reach puberty earlier than fillies from untreated mares and rarely are born with transiently enlarged clitorides. Injectable preparations of repositol altrenogest may be effective in suppressing estrus behavior but have not been thoroughly investigated for their ability to effectively synchronize estrus.

All progestin preparations should be used with caution in mares that are susceptible to delayed uterine clearance or uterine infections, for several reasons. Progestins increase the tone of the cervix, and their use may inhibit the physical clearance of fluid. Progestins also have been associated with lower immunoglobulin levels (especially IgG) in the uterus.[17] The combination of these adverse effects ultimately can lead to delayed uterine clearance, endometritis, pyometra, and other conditions.

When synchronizing mares, one should administer progestins for a minimum of 10 days in cycling mares and 14 days in transitional mares. On the last day of progestin treatment, a PGF_2-α injection may be administered to lyse any remaining CLs. As in treatment with PGs alone, the mare should come into heat 3 to 5 days after the last treatment and ovulate an average of 7 days after treatment, depending on the structures present on the ovary at the end of treatment.

INDUCING OVULATION

A number of agents that shorten the interval to ovulation in the mare have been used to induce ovulation. The most effective agents possess LH activity with varying degrees of FSH activity. Human chorionic gonadotrophin (Chroulon, Intervet), with its potent LH-like activity, is currently the least expensive and perhaps the most popular agent used for the induction of ovulation. Given intramuscularly, intravenously, or subcutaneously, hCG has been reported to be effective at doses ranging between 1000 to 5000 IU.[18]

Use of hCG in the mare has some limitations. First, with its repeated use, antibody development may occur.[19,20] Secondly, mare owners often complain about the apparent pain associated with administration of some hCG products. Finally, the reliability of hCG in its ability to hasten the interval to ovulation, especially in the older or compromised mare, has been questioned. Regardless of its potential disadvantages, hCG remains a popular, inexpensive, and effective means of inducing ovulation in most mares.

Synthetic GnRH analogs also have proved to be effective in inducing ovulation (deslorelin acetate [Ovuplant, Fort Dodge, Canada]; and buserelin [Buserelin, Intervet; neither is commercially available in the United States]).[21,22,23] The use of these agents may delay return to estrus by 1 or 2 days if the mare fails to conceive, but removal of the implant a few days after insertion can ameliorate this delay.[23] Injectable deslorelin is available through compounding companies in the U.S. The general impression of practitioners is that because these GnRH analogs are more reliable in inducing ovulation, especially in mares that are more prone to ovulation failure (e.g., older mares, mares in vernal transition, mares concomitantly treated with PG-inhibiting agents such as many anti-inflammatory drugs). Lastly, recombinant LH (rLH), administered at a dose of 750 μg, is an effective ovulation induction agent in the mare[24] and should be commercially available soon. Although the window of ovulation may not be as precisely synchronized as it is with deslorelin, rLH does not induce antibody production with repeated use.[24]

Ovulation induction agents are reliable and effective only if given at the appropriate time during estrus. If endometrial folds are apparent on the ultrasound examination and a dominant softening follicle is present, usually greater than 30 mm in diameter, then hCG, deslorelin acetate, and buserelin are expected to induce ovulation in an average of 36, 41 to 48,[18] and 24 to 48[22] hours, respectively, after administration. Samper reported that 98% of mares with maximal endometrial edema given hCG or deslorelin consistently ovulated within 48 hours of administration.[25] Most remarkably, most mares to which Ovuplant has been administered at the proper time, ovulate 38 plus or minus 2 hours later,[26] truly allowing appointment breeding.

SYNCHRONIZING ESTRUS AND OVULATION

Progestins can be used with estradiol-17-β to obtain greater synchrony in mares. Although not commercially available, biodegradable microspheres impregnated with progesterone (1.25 g) and estradiol (100 mg) also have been used to synchronize the estrous cycle of the mare[27-29]; they appear to suppress follicular development and ovulation. However, these drugs have been replaced to some extent by intravaginal devices (CIDR-B, InterAg, Hamilton, New Zealand) that contain progesterone; estradiol (10 mg) is administered at the time of insertion. Administration of a PGF_2-α analog is advised at the time of insert removal (12 to 14 days). Finally, an ovulation induction agent is administered when the dominant follicle reaches a size of 35 mm. This regimen nicely synchronizes ovulation and estrus[30]; however, neither these intravaginal devices nor the encapsulated microspheres currently are licensed for use in horses.

DELAYING ESTRUS AND OVULATION

Although most hormonal regimens act to hasten the interval to estrus and ovulation, there are occasional managerial reasons to delay estrus. Altrenogest was designed to prevent show mares from exhibiting estrous behavior, and it has proved to be effective in this regard, suppressing signs of estrus in 95% of mares that were given a daily dose of 0.044 mg/kg for 3 days.[31] In an attempt to find a more economic and less time-consuming means of suppressing estrous behavior in mares, progestin-estradiol implants (Synovex, Syntex Animal Health, Des Moines, Iowa) licensed for food animals have been investigated in mares. Although some mare owners report an improvement in the behavior of the mare, scientific reports have been less supportive of their use. McCue et al.[32] found that mares treated with these implants, even at 20 times the usual dose, did not show suppression of estrous behavior and cyclicity. Vanderwall et al[33] have examined the effect of oxytocin on luteolysis. Mares that received oxytocin (60 IU twice daily intramuscularly) on days 7 through 14 after ovulation demonstrated prolonged luteal function up to 30 days after ovulation, suggesting that oxytocin administration may offer a means of long-term suppression of estrus.

Immunization against gonadotrophin releasing factor (GnRF) is another effective means of estrus suppression in the mare. Mares vaccinated twice, 4 weeks apart, with a GnRF vaccine (Equity; Pfizer Animal Health, Sydney) did not return to estrus during that breeding season but returned to cyclicity the next year. Foaling rates were not significantly different than for control mares.[34] The vaccine is not yet commercially available worldwide.

Theoretically, if the LH surge has not occurred yet, oral progestin treatment should inhibit LH and delay ovulation. Altrenogest at label dose or double the label dose is effective in delaying ovulation compared with control mares as long as an ovulation induction agent has not been administered.[35] Intraluminal fluid retention, possibly caused by increased cervical tone, has been observed in some mares. Although this application is promising, results should be interpreted with caution because treated mares had lower pregnancy rates (although the difference was not statistically significant).

Delaying the interval to first ovulation of recently foaled mares results in higher pregnancy rates for the first heat cycle. Although the natural foal heat of a mare may be highly fertile, many early pregnancies are lost, likely because of an adverse uterine environment. To optimize the maintenance of those early pregnancies and yet still increase the reproductive efficiency of the mare by breeding her back as soon as possible, delay of the first postpartum interval to ovulation using a combination of progesterone and estradiol-17β (E2-17B; Sigma) in oil is beneficial. In an attempt to increase the fertility of foal heat breeding, Sexton and Bristol[36] reported that this protocol successfully delays the postpartum interval to first ovulation, thereby increasing the period of time for uterine involution and pregnancy rate.

SUPEROVULATION

In an effort to increase the number of offspring produced in the lifetime of a mare or in any given season, researchers have investigated numerous means of superovulating mares. Overall, attempts at reliable superovulation in mares have not been as successful as those in the food animal industry. An increased number of ovulations and embryos have been minimal. The administration of porcine FSH preparations is ineffective in mares, except at cost-prohibitive doses.[37] Stimulation of endogenous FSH secretion by indirect and direct immunization against inhibin has not resulted in a superovulatory response in mares.[38] The administration of equine pituitary extract preparations in research trials only increases the number of embryos recovered from 0.5 per cycle to 2.2 per cycle.[39,40] Promising results have been achieved with the use of equine FSH (eFSH) (Box 18-1). Treatment of cycling mares with eFSH in early diestrus (12.5 mg, administered twice daily) increased the pregnancy rate compared with untreated control mares (1.8 versus 0.6, respectively).[41] In another study, wherein Welsh et al. incorporated a "coast" period into the above experimental design, the ovulation and embryo recovery rate were 3.8 ± 1.2 ovulations and 1.7 ±1.4 embryos, respectively.[42]

Follicular stimulation through the use of eFSH has also been effective in the management of postpartum anestrus mares. In one study,[43] eFSH was administered to five mares with a history of lactational anestrus. After 5 to 10 days of twice-daily injections of 6.25 mg eFSH, all mares developed a preovulatory follicle, ovulated in response to hCG, and conceived.[43]

The efficacy of eFSH in stimulating early follicular development as well as shortening the interval to first ovulation during the spring transition has been evaluated. Administration of twice-daily injections of 12.5 mg eFSH resulted in ovulation in 80% of transitional mares. Multiple ovulations were induced in 40% of treated mares. The interval to first ovulation was 7.6 ± 2.4 days in treated mares versus 39.5 ± 17.2 days in control mares.[44]

Unfortunately, the continued commercial availability of purified eFSH is limited. Recombinant FSH (reFSH) stimulates follicular activity in the mare and may replace purified eFSH as it becomes commercially available.[45]

BOX 18-1

RECOMMENDED PROTOCOL FOR SUPEROVULATION IN MARES USING EFSH

1. Determine the day of ovulation.
2. Moniter follicular development in early diestrus.
3. Begin eFSH therapy (12.5 mg IM twice daily) when the largest follicle is 22 to 25 mm in diameter.
4. Administer cloprostenol (259 µg IM) on the second day of eFSH therapy
5. Discontinue eFSH treatment when follicle(s) are greater than 32 to 35 mm in diameter.
6. Administer hCG (2500 IU) to induce ovulation.
7. Breed or inseminate according to standard procedure.

eFSH, Equine follicle stimulating hormone; IM, intramuscular. Adapted from McCue PM, LeBlanc MM, Squires EL: eFSH in clinical equine practice. *Theriogenology* 68: 429-433, 2007.

TEASER MARES

For semen to be collected from most stallions, breeding facilities require at least one mare exhibiting behavioral estrus. Some stallions appear to prefer a particular mare or a certain color of mare, and therefore a variety of mares in heat is sometimes desirable for good libido. Thus the use of exogenous hormone regulation to encourage a mare to display signs of estrous behavior often becomes necessary.

One strategy for ensuring the availability of a teaser mare is to have a rotating supply of mares that are constantly short-cycled with PGF_2-α analogs. If the mare is injected with PGF_2-α 5 days after the cessation of behavioral estrus, in theory she will return to heat in a few days because the mature CL on her ovary will be lysed by the injection. Ideally, a minimum of two teaser mares suffices for this program. An additional benefit is that the fertility of the mare is unaffected by the PGs.

Administration of estrogen compounds causes some mares to exhibit estrous behavior. Estradiol cypionate (ECP, Upjohn), a long-acting estrogen, and estradiol-17β, a shorter-acting estrogen, have been investigated; the results of administration of either compound vary, especially over time and in particular with estradiol cypionate. The estrogen compounds are far more effective in ovariectomized mares than in intact mares because even the smallest amount of progestin secretion from the ovary inhibits signs of behavioral estrus. Interestingly, ovariectomized mares often demonstrate low-grade signs of heat even in the absence of exogenous hormonal administration. Theoretically, these signs are caused by the absence of ovarian progesterone and the continued secretion of estrogens from other sources, particularly the adrenal glands. Moreover, even the smallest amounts of circulating estrogens are postulated to cause some mares to show constant signs of estrus in the presence of a stallion. The long-term response of ovariectomized mares to exogenous estradiol-17β or estradiol cypionate has not been reliable, especially with administration of these hormones in increasing amounts and frequency. The hormones appear to reach a threshold at which the clinical response is contrary to the signs expected, and treated mares actually may show increased aggressiveness to stallions. Low doses (1 mg intramuscularly) of estradiol cypionate, administered every 2 to 3 weeks, appear to be most effective in preserving the ovariectimized teaser mares for many years of service. Old, anestrous mares often function as ideal teaser mares for some stallions. In the absence of functional ovarian secretion, the low levels of circulating estrogens may cause a mare to exhibit signs of estrous behavior continually. Unfortunately, a number of stallions appear uninterested in these old mares despite their overt display of heat.

MAINTENANCE OF PREGNANCY

Although the precise mechanism is unclear, progesterone supplementation in the form of injectable or oral preparations often is used to maintain pregnancy at all stages of gestation. Early pregnancy maintenance in the mare requires the function first of the primary CL (approximately 45 days) and then of the accessory CL (45 to 90 days or more). Regardless, some mares appear to require progesterone supplementation during this period; otherwise, they lose the pregnancy. Hormonal assays can sometimes be misleading because progestin levels in these mares may appear well within the normal range for mares that do not appear to require supplementation.

Some mares appear to require progesterone supplementation for maintenance of pregnancy in the later stages of gestation as well. Altrenogest may be effective in preserving the pregnancy in a compromised mare. In an experiment that examined the maintenance of pregnancy in mares suffering from experimentally induced endotoxemia, mares treated with oral altrenogest administered at twice the recommended dosage (0.088 mg/kg/day) suffered significantly fewer pregnancy losses than untreated mares.[46] Interestingly, in mares suffering from experimentally induced placentitis, a significant change in progesterone profiles was associated with fetal-placental compromise and pregnancy loss.[47] Separate studies demonstrate that the addition of oral altrenogest (0.088 mg/kg/day) to antibiotic treatment in mares with placentitis significantly reduces pregnancy loss.[48,49]

Rates of pregnancy loss appear higher in the Miniature Horse mare (25%)[50] than reported in larger breeds (<10%).[51] Moreover, unlike reports of studies on larger breeds, most pregnancy loss in the Miniature Horse mare occurs during late term.[50] Thus many Miniature Horse mares receive supplemental progesterone for the duration of their pregnancy. Some researchers speculate that placental insufficiency may contribute to the increased loss of pregnancy in this breed because the size of the foal often is larger with respect to its dam than in the larger breeds of horses.

DELAYED UTERINE CLEARANCE

Mating-induced endometritis is regarded as a normal transient physiologic event in the mare in response to sperm deposited in the uterus.[52] However, some mares are susceptible to delayed uterine clearance (DUC), especially older, multiparous mares in which the uterus lies well beneath the pelvic brim.[53] Small intramuscular or intravenous doses of oxytocin after warm saline lavage of the uterus have been especially beneficial in these susceptible mares.[54,55] The response to oxytocin appears to be greatest with administration just before ovulation.[56,57] Routine administration of exogenous oxytocin to mares immediately after insemination does not improve pregnancy rates.[58] Those mares with DUC in which intraluminal fluid remains or recurs despite multiple small doses of oxytocin may respond to carbetocin, a long-acting oxytocin analog. The duration of action of carbetocin is more than threefold longer than oxytocin.[59] In mares that appear to be unresponsive to tocolytic therapy, PGF_2-α analogs that exert a more sustained effect on uterine myometrial activity than oxytocin may promote uterine evacuation and enhanced lymphatic drainage.[60] The effect of periovulatory adminstration of PGF_2-α analogs on pregnancy rates has been controversial in the mare. The results from one study found that 250 μg closprostenol administered by intramuscular injection to mares on the day of ovulation resulted in lower pregnancy rates.[13] In contrast, Nie et al. reported that pregnancy rates are not affected by the administration of 20 IU oxytocin or 250 μg cloprostenol every 6 hours after ovulation if treated before the second day after ovulation.[61]

CERVICAL DILATION

One of the most frustrating conditions encountered when breeding mares is failure of cervical dilation during estrus. On transrectal palpation the cervix may feel toned instead of soft, as it should during estrus just before ovulation. Because previous damage to the cervix and the subsequent formation of adhesions can present a similar and confusing picture of failure of cervical relaxation, a thorough visual and manual cervical examination is prudent. In maiden mares inserting a finger through the cervix to act as a guide for the insemination pipette is often difficult. Although this condition does not prevent artificial insemination, it can prevent not only penetration of the cervix by the penis of the stallion but also the normal evacuation of fluid in the hours after breeding, thereby setting the stage for DUC and persistent endometritis. Although not objectively studied, this condition appears to affect older maiden mares more commonly. However, even normal maiden mares may not have the same degree of cervical relaxation during estrus that is typical of pluriparous mares. A synthetic PGE_1 analog, misoprostol (Cytotek; Searle Corp., Chicago, Ill.), has been used successfully in women for cervical dilation. This compound has not yet been evaluated objectively in horses and currently is not approved for veterinary use. However, many clinicians have seen some encouraging results, simply by covering the external cervix with PGE_1 cream several hours before cervical dilation is desired. If only PGE_1 tablets are available, practitioners have crushed 1 to 2 tablets (200 μg) and mixed them with a small amount of sterile lubricant before application. Digital insertion of a tablet into the external cervical os may be effective as well. Occasionally, veterinarians have used this preparation combined with other parturition induction agents when attempting to terminate a pregnancy prematurely. Again, only anecdotal reports of efficacy currently exist.

OVIDUCTAL AND UTERINE CONTRACTION

The early embryo secretes PGE_2, which is believed to play a role in the contractility of smooth muscle of the oviduct and to promote propulsion of the embryo through the oviduct.[62] PGE_2 is also secreted during the high mobility phase of the embryo and is suspected to stimulate uterine contraction and enhance uterine tone.[63] Laparoscopic application of PGE_2 along the serosal surface of the oviduct can modify embryo transport. Interestingly, not only is embryo transport hastened, but also unfertilized oocytes that are rarely recovered in the mare are transported to the uterus.[64]

The addition of PGE_2 to semen just before artificial insemination has increased pregnancy rates in mares bred with fertile semen but not with subfertile semen.[65] These results are disappointing because the addition of PGE_2 to semen is associated with higher fertility rates in other species.[66,67] The role of PGE_2 at the uterotubal junction (UTJ) of the mare has been speculated to affect spermatozoal selection. It was once believed that this selection at the UTJ was based on sperm morphology; however, motility of the spermatozoa may play a larger role in this selection process than initially suspected. Selection is an area of research that deserves continuing attention.

BREEDING MANAGEMENT TO OPTIMIZE PREGNANCY RATES

Elizabeth Metcalf

In the past foals were born only as a result of natural field breeding, but innovations in modern horse breeding, both an art and a science, have kept pace with advances in reproduction. Foals are now born as a result of more advanced procedures that include artificial insemination, oocyte transfer, embryo transfer, embryo splitting, intracytoplasmic sperm injection, gender selection, and cloning from a single cell. Furthermore, through improvements in cryogenic techniques, gametes and embryos may be preserved indefinitely. Veterinarians and scientists function primarily as facilitators of these processes that serve to preserve and perpetuate valuable genetic lines. The following sections examine the procedures currently used in equine private practice to facilitate the insemination of horses.

Although increasing the number of pregnancies produced per mare in a given year is possible through the techniques of embryo and oocyte transfer, pregnancy rates per cycle have not improved significantly from field breeding to artificial insemination. In the past decade many changes have been implemented in breeding facilities and include (but are not limited to) the housing of mares and stallions, the methods used for teasing mares and stallions, the design of the breeding shed, stallion and mare handling techniques, promoting appropriate behavior in the breeding shed, the processing of stallion semen, and the management of the mare population.

In an attempt to mimic the physical and physiologic events that occur in nature, breeders must understand not only equine behavior but also the processes of intromission, ejaculation, and eventually fertilization of the oocyte.

Although natural and artificial insemination of the mare entail deposition of semen within the uterus of the mare, natural service invokes several physiologic processes that are absent in artificial insemination.[1] When the penis of the stallion enters the vagina of the mare, several rhythmic pelvis thrusts occur before ejaculation directly into the uterine body. Not only does this action cause rapid vasodilation of blood vessels that supply the corpus spongiosum penis, resulting in the characteristic "belling" of the glans penis, but also it stimulates strong uterine contractions that in turn propel the deposited sperm toward the oviductal papillae of the mare. The engorged glans penis also may function as a physical barrier to prevent the immediate backflow of semen during ejaculation. Detumescence of the penis follows ejaculation, and the mare moves forward, out from under the stallion. This sequence of events may occur many times on a given day under natural conditions.

Fertilization of the oocyte in the mare takes place in the ampulla of the oviduct. Before this, the spermatozoa must undergo capacitation and the acrosome reaction, a complex series of events that results in remodeling of the sperm plasma membrane and release of specific enzymes that enable the sperm to penetrate the oocyte. Although capacitated sperm can be recovered from the uterus of the mare, uncapacitated sperm[2,3] are selected[4] to reside in the isthmus of the oviduct until the oocyte is present. Spermatozoa actually bind to oviductal epithelial cells, a process that appears to be enhanced in estrous mares but not in diestrous mares.[5] Abnormalities of this process may contribute to the subfertility of the mare or the stallion.

Mares with poor fertility have fewer sperm residing in the storage sites of the oviduct.[6] Stallions with poor fertility may have spermatozoa with inherent damage that prevents them from being selected to reside in the oviduct. The effect of this damage is more likely to be caused by poor binding capacity than poor motility or reduced sperm transport.[3] Spermatozoa survive in oviductal cell culture for at least 6 days,[7] which supports the report of a mare that became pregnant after a single mating 7 days before ovulation[8] and the study by Woods, Bergfelt, and Ginther[9] in which mares were bred successfully more than 6 days before ovulation. Conversely, an oocyte is viable in the oviduct for only a short time, perhaps as little as 12 hours,[10] as indicated by the low pregnancy rates of mares bred more than 12 hours after ovulation.[9,11,12] Capacitated spermatozoa therefore must be available for successful fertilization.

Before any type of insemination, the assessment of fertility of the mare and stallion is advisable. Many tests are available that evaluate the fertility of stallion semen, but the most informative measure is the per cycle conception or foaling rate. Although no single in vitro laboratory test correlates precisely with stallion fertility, stallions with semen that demonstrates a high percentage of morphologically normal, progressively motile spermatozoa with little reduction in motility over the first 24 hours of storage often prove to have better fertility than those with semen that lacks these attributes. The stability of chromatin structure is also correlated with stallion fertility, and therefore sperm chromatin structure assays may help in predicting fertility or diagnosing infertility. Other in vitro means of predicting stallion fertility include flow cytometric analysis of sperm membranes, cellular organelles, and viability; computer-assisted motility analysis; membrane "stress" tests; glass wool–Sephadex bead filtration; binding and penetration assays; and antisperm antibody assays (see discussion elsewhere in this chapter). These advanced tests are commercially available at several university teaching hospitals.

The fertility of the mare should also be evaluated. Too often the mare is selected as a broodmare candidate simply because of her availability. A BSE based on the age, history, and parity of the mare should be performed. The BSE may range from a rectal and ultrasonographic examination of the reproductive tract to a cytologic testing, culture, and biopsy of the endometrium to a videoendoscopic examination of the endometrium. Inclusion of an ultrasound examination at every rectal examination not only enhances the continual education of the veterinarian but also aids in the detection of many unpalpable changes. Most important, ultrasound examination ultimately enhances breeding efficiency and pregnancy rates by taking advanage of the most sophisticated tools available.

PREPARATION OF THE MARE FOR BREEDING

The ultimate goal of insemination is to provide semen in a time frame that coordinates the availability of capacitated spermatozoa with the arrival of the transported oocyte within the oviduct of the mare. Therefore the timing of insemination with ovulation is critical.

Mares in heat require daily examination. During the estrous phase of the heat cycle, the practitioner performs an ultrasound examination of the reproductive tract, which

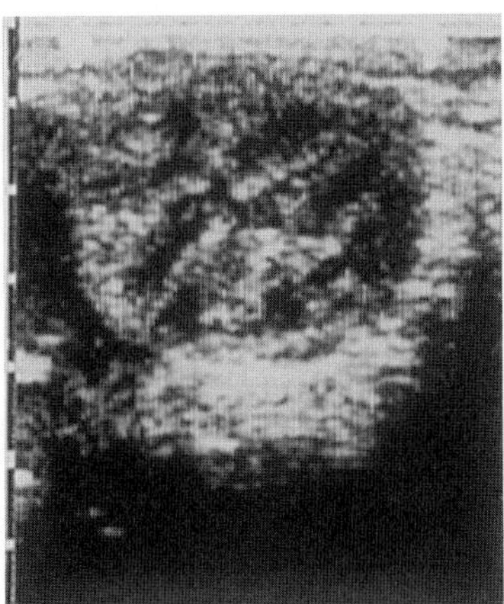

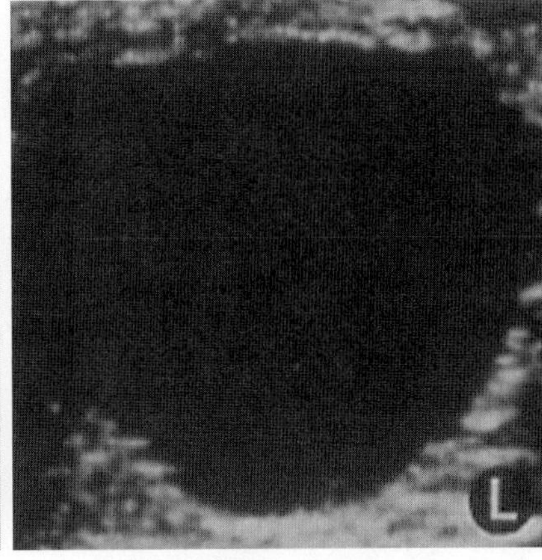

FIGURE 18-4 The appearance of a dominant, growing, softening follicle *(right)* and the classic spoke-wheel pattern of endometrial edema *(left)* indicate pending ovulation. (From Ginther OJ: *Reproductive biology of the mare,* ed 2, Cross Plains, Wisconsin, 1992, Equiservices.)

complements the results of the rectal examination. The appearance of a dominant, growing follicle and the classic spoke-wheel pattern of endometrial edema, which may be evaluated and quantified subjectively[13,14] and objectively,[15] indicates pending ovulation (Figure 18-4). The ultrasound examination also may demonstrate the presence of echogenic particles within the follicle and increasing echogenicity of its wall, both of which indicate impending ovulation within the next 24 hours.[16] Detection of a decrease in follicular pressure by measuring transrectal tonometry indicates pending ovulation.[17] Although the duration of heat in the mare may vary, most mares ovulate near the end of this estrous phase.[18] Follicular edema is less apparent on ultrasound examination just before ovulation. Because the timing of insemination with ovulation is so critical, the presence or absence of this edema can be a powerful tool to optimize pregnancy rates through the control of ovulation timing.

A number of agents are available that effectively shorten the interval to ovulation.[19-23] These agents include hCG, GnRH analogs (see the previous discussion of hormonal manipulation in this chapter), and rLH. These induction agents are reliable and effective if administered at the appropriate time during estrus. If endometrial folds are observed on the ultrasound examination and a dominant softening follicle is present, usually greater than 30 mm in diameter, one can expect hCG, deslorelin acetate (Ovuplant, 2.2 mg; Fort Dodge, Canada), and buserelin (Buserelin; Intervet, Millsboro, Del. [not commercially available in the United States]) to hasten ovulation on an average of 36,[19] 41 to 48,[19] and 24 to 48[13,20,24] hours, respectively, after administration. However, some disadvantages are associated with the use of an implanted pellet of deslorelin acetate. In mares implanted with deslorelin acetate, the interestrus interval may be prolonged on an average of 2 days because of a diestrous inhibition of pituitary FSH secretion.[25] Removal of the implant 2 days after administration appears to prevent the delay in return to estrus.

PASTURE BREEDING

Successful pasture breeding requires an understanding of equine social structure. Every time a new member is introduced to the herd, disruption of the social strata and a reorganization of the ranking occur. Theoretically, optimal field breeding management aims for a closed herd to minimize stress and enhance breeding efficiency.

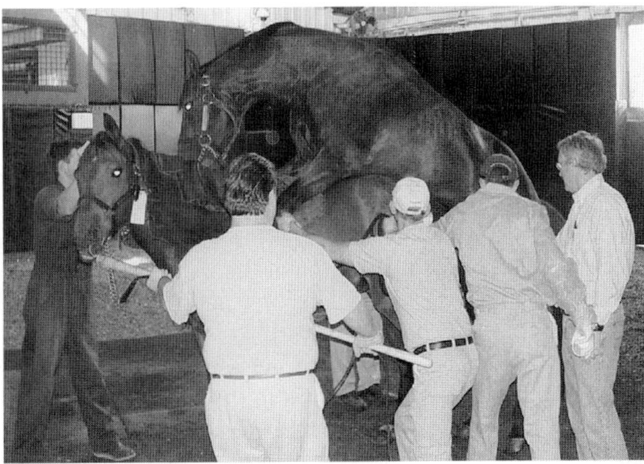

FIGURE 18-5 Breeding in-hand often requires more personnel to ensure safety of the horses and handlers.

Under field conditions mares in heat approach the stallion for teasing. If interested, a stallion may mount a mare numerous times with or without an erection; with or without copulation; and, most interesting, with or without ejaculation. This behavior rarely is sanctioned in breeding facilities because it often leads to undesirable behavior in breeding stock.

BREEDING IN HAND

Many breeding facilities continue to breed their stallions in hand, especially if the stallions belong to registries that do not allow registration of foals produced by artificial insemination. One perceived advantage to this management practice is that it may require fewer personnel or less time to breed the mare and therefore is less costly. However, this is not usually the case, for in-hand breeding poses far more risk to the mare, stallion, and handlers and therefore requires more personnel to ensure the safety of all involved (Figure 18-5). In-hand breeding also may require far more preparation of the mare

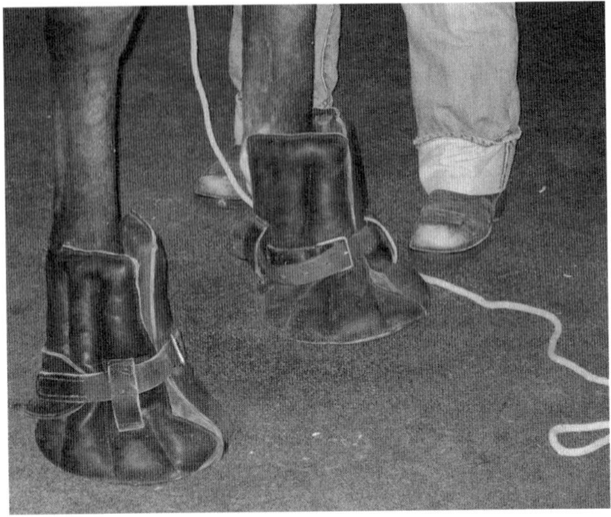

FIGURE 18-6 Padded boots cover the rear hooves of a mare to prevent injury to the stallion during breeding or semen collection.

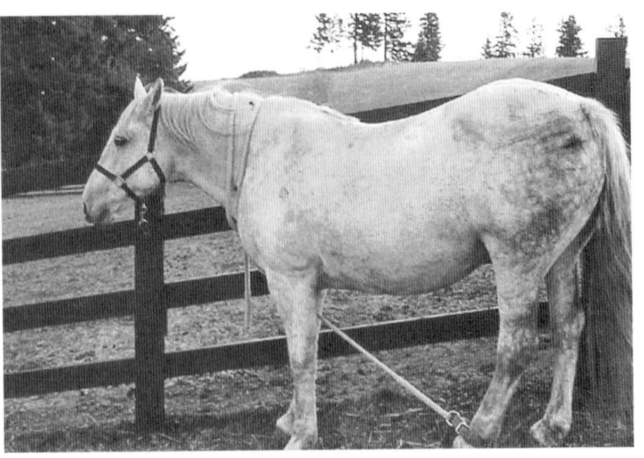

FIGURE 18-7 A simple yet effective hobble.

than artificial insemination, especially in the application of restraining devices or removal of the foal for breeding.

If breeding in hand, good communication among involved personnel is paramount to ensuring the safety of the horses. First, one prepares the mare in heat for natural cover by wrapping her tail to prevent laceration of the stallion's penis by the hair during breeding and washes her perineum with a mild soap, rinses it well, and dries it with a clean paper towel. One may apply a leather harness to her crest to allow the stallion to hold on to the mare securely without biting her during breeding. To protect the stallion from being kicked by the mare, padded hoof boots may be applied to the rear hooves (Figure 18-6) or hobbles may be fastened to the rear legs of the mare.

Desirable hobble attributes include comfort, ease of application, ease of removal (ensuring a quick release if needed), and simplicity so that the stallion cannot become entangled in the ropes or straps. Perhaps the simplest, safest, and most effective hobble design consists of two pieces of soft cotton rope that fit many different mares (Figure 18-7). The first cotton loop slips loosely around the neck of the mare to rest against the point of both shoulders. The second portion is a longer cotton rope attached to a padded leather anklet designed to fit snugly around the rear pastern of the mare. One straps the anklet around the left rear pastern, brings the left rear leg well under the body of the mare, pulls the rope gently between the front legs of the mare, and ties a quick-release knot just below the point of the shoulder on the left side. Additional restraint devices may be employed. A twitch may be applied just minutes before the stallion arrives, or the mare may be sedated. These additional restraints may inhibit the desired response, however, and the mare may fail to show signs of heat in response to the stallion.

All personnel stand on the left side of the horses, thereby allowing the horses to move unencumbered to the right if necessary. The mare handler steadies the mare as the stallion mounts and breeds her. The stallion handler is perhaps at the most risk during in-hand breeding (or semen collection) and therefore may direct the cover. Neither size nor strength is necessary in a stallion handler; rather a calm, firm, knowledgeable person fares the best in the breeding shed. The quality of the ejaculate often reflects the expertise of the stallion handler.

After ejaculation a variable latency period occurs until the stallion begins to dismount. In field breeding the mare initiates the dismount by moving away from the stallion. Patience and ingenuity are needed during in-hand breeding because theoretically the restrained mare cannot move. Because of the possibility that a mare may kick during the dismount, the heads of both horses are turned to the left simultaneously, causing their hind ends to move to the right and thereby creating an adequate space between them. If a dismount semen sample is required, expediency and experience are necessary to obtain it between the end of ejaculation and the dismount.

ARTIFICIAL INSEMINATION

Most equine breed registries, with the notable exception of the Jockey Club, not only sanction but also encourage the use of artificial insemination. The advantages to breeding horses by artificial insemination are numerous and range from increasing the safety of horses and their handlers to enhancing the value of the stallion by increasing the number of offspring produced yearly (Box 18-2). Use of frozen semen for insemination has additional advantages (Box 18-3). Although cryopreserved semen is an attractive alternative for many reasons, it also can require more intensive mare management and sometimes results in lower pregnancy rates.

In an attempt to mimic the events of natural mating and yet ensure minimal contamination of the reproductive tract of the mare during artificial insemination, the following techniques have been described.[27] The mare should be restrained properly, preferably in stocks to protect the inseminator. Other devices, such as a twitch, have been used effectively for restraint but are usually unnecessary. If chemical restraint is warranted, the use of α-agonists such as xylazine may be preferable to other agents because of their effect on contractility of the uterus while it is under the influence of estrogen, particularly in mares exhibiting DUC after insemination.[28] One bandages the tail of the mare, ties the tail so that it is not in contact with the vulva and perineum, washes the vulva well with liquid soap, and rinses the vulva thoroughly with water. The washing is repeated at least three times until the area appears to be free of any debris. The vulva and perineal area are then dried with a clean paper towel.

If cooled semen is being used, it is not necessary to warm it after removal from the storage container. If frozen semen is being used, it should be thawed in a water bath before insemination. Frozen semen is stored in liquid nitrogen at −196° C until ready for use, at which time the inseminator must follow the thawing and insemination instructions that accompany the frozen semen. Thawing protocols at high temperatures (50° to 75° C) require closer adherence to exact immersion times than do low temperatures (37° C). Depending on the cryopreservation techniques and sperm concentration per straw, a breeding dose may consist of a single straw (0.5 to 5.0 ml) or multiple straws.

The inseminator dons a sterile sleeve and grasps a sterile insemination pipette between thumb and palm to protect the tip in a sterile environment. If using 0.5-ml straws of frozen-thawed semen, the inseminator may use a sterile insemination gun instead of the pipette. Nonspermicidal sterile lubricant is applied sparingly to the sleeve covering the forefinger. Although labeled as nonspermicidal, some sterile lubricants have still been found to be detrimental to sperm motility and velocity.[26] The product Pre-Seed Equine™ (INGFertility Valleyford, Wash.) has been found to be less detrimental to stallion spermatozoa than Priority Care (First Priority, Elgin, Ill.), MiniLube™ (Minitube, Verona, Wis.), or EquiLube (Boehringer Ingelheim, St. Joseph, Mo.). Prepared semen should be contained in a nonspermicidal syringe and protected in the nonsterile hand from adverse environmental conditions such as ultraviolet light, cold, heat, and air.

The inseminator inserts the sleeved hand, continuing to protect the tip of the insemination pipette, through the lips of the vulva and into the vaginal vault and inserts one or two fingers through the cervical os. The finger (or fingers) then acts as a guide for advancement of the insemination pipette through the cervix approximately 1 cm into the uterus of the mare. If the advancement of the pipette has not encountered resistance once in the uterus, the inseminator can advance it carefully and gently into the desired uterine horn (usually ipsilateral to the developing follicle). This advancement is not always possible because of the amount of endometrial edema and folding, and the inseminator must take extreme care not to damage the endometrium. Once the pipette is satisfactorily in place, the inseminator depresses the plunger of the syringe and deposits the semen in the uterus. If resistance is encountered when depressing the plunger, the tip of the pipette may be obstructed by the endometrium and may require repositioning. A small amount of air may be introduced to clear the pipette. Massage of the vaginal vault during withdrawal of the inseminator's hand may stimulate uterine contraction and aid in propulsion of spermatozoa to the uterotubal junction.

BOX 18-2

ADVANTAGES OF ARTIFICIAL INSEMINATION USING COOLED SEMEN

- Allows many mares to be bred with a single ejaculate
- Prevents overuse of the stallion
- Enables mare owners to breed to any stallion regardless of distance, especially with cryopreserved semen
- Enhances and encourages genetic variability and hybrid vigor
- Controls management of the difficult breeder
- Reduces the chances of spread of infectious disease, venereal and systemic
- Reduces possibility of injury to mare and stallion
- Eliminates transportation and boarding expenses of the mare
- Allows evaluation of semen quality at each insemination
- Allows advance shipment of cryopreserved semen and increased availability
- May result in less variability in semen quality because of central processing station

BOX 18-3

ADDITIONAL ADVANTAGES TO USING CRYOPRESERVED SEMEN FOR INSEMINATION

- Ability to breed any stallion in the world, regardless of distance
- Ability to ship the semen well in advance of breeding so that it is available when needed
- Preservation of stallion genetics for many years
- Insurance against unavailability, injury, or death of the stallion
- Less variability of semen quality

SEMEN DEPOSITION

Although pregnancy rates appear to be independent of semen volume,[29] minute volumes and numbers of motile spermatozoa (as low as 1×10^6 motile sperm) deposited at the uterotubal junction (Figure 18-8) or within the oviduct have shown promising pregnancy results.[30-32] Furthermore, deep uterine insemination may enhance pregnancy rates under conditions of low sperm availability.[26] With the procedure described by

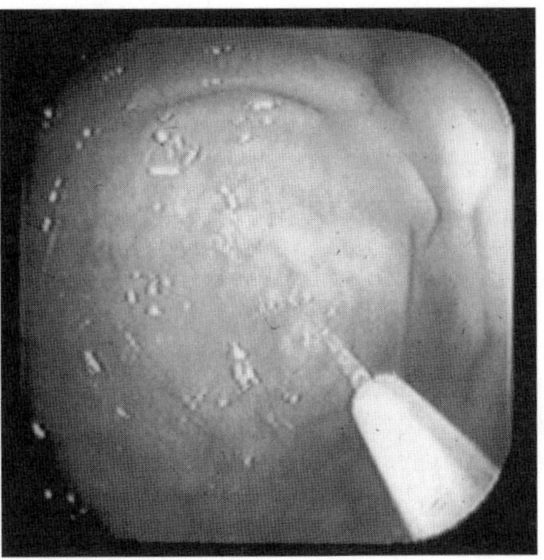

FIGURE 18-8 Through hysteroscopic insemination less than 0.25 ml of semen is deposited on the oviductal papilla. (Courtesy EL Squires, Colorado State University, Fort Collins, Col.)

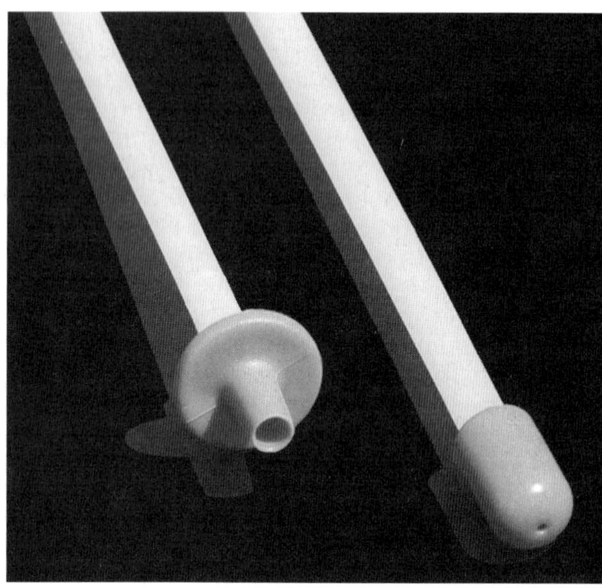

FIGURE 18-9 Specialized pipette for deep horn insemination. (Courtesy Minitube of America, Verona, Wis.).

Rigby,[33] the inseminator first passes the insemination pipette transcervically into the uterine body and then directs it into the uterine horn ipsilateral to the dominant follicle. Through transrectal manipulation the pipette is guided into the uterine horn by gently threading the uterus around the pipette. Specialized pipettes with palpable bulbs at the distal end have been designed for deep horn insemination in the mare (Figure 18-9). Because of the degree of edema of the mare endometrium during estrus, the inseminator must be careful not to damage the endometrium when using this technique.

OPTIMIZING PREGNANCY RATES

Insemination of mares with a minimum insemination dose of 500×10^6 progressively motile spermatozoa every other day has long been accepted as a means to maximize pregnancy rates.[34] Some stallions with apparently superior fertility may provide maximum pregnancy rates at much lower dosages. As with bulls, the minimal insemination dose for optimizing pregnancy rate appears highly male dependent.[35] However, as is not the case with bulls, no evidence currently suggests that increasing the insemination dose can compensate for morphologic defects in stallion sperm. Fortunately, the number of spermatazoa in a single ejaculate from a normal stallion far exceeds this dose, provided that the stallion is not suffering from overuse. Therefore, depending on the intensity of management, most breeding operations using in-hand breeding aim to cover mares shortly before ovulation or, if the stallion is not breeding other mares, every 48 hours while the mare is in standing heat. To prevent overuse of the stallion and to enhance pregnancy rates, mares should be examined with transrectal palpations and ultrasound at least every other day and should be bred when ovulation is expected within 24 to 48 hours. Postovulation breeding, although sometimes successful, more often is associated with embryos of inferior quality.[10,36-38]

In a breeding program that uses artificial insemination, the fertility of most stallion semen is greatest on the farm, followed by that of shipped cooled semen, with frozen semen being least fertile.[34] Exceptions to this rule invariably occur. Because the fertility of semen appears to be stallion dependent, good breeding management requires an awareness of the minimal insemination dose necessary to maximize pregnancy rates for each stallion. The aim in a cooled-semen insemination protocol is to provide a minimum insemination dose (500×10^6 progressively motile sperm) to be inseminated every other day before ovulation. The semen must be extended to 25 to 50×10^6 motile sperm per milliliter to achieve maximal pregnancy rates.[39] With highly fertile stallions, the minimum insemination dose necessary for optimal pregnancy rates may be much lower.

In an artificial insemination program that uses cooled shipped semen, often more than a single dose of semen is sent. Controversy exists regarding the fate of the unused doses: Should they remain in storage at 4° C, or should they be inseminated immediately into the mare? Supporters of the Equitainer (Hamilton-Thorne Research Inc., Danvers, Mass.) hypothesis argue that the sperm storage sites in the oviduct of the mare are filled with the first insemination and do not need to be replenished for at least 24 hours[40]; therefore using the mare as the incubator for the second dose is wasteful because the excess spermatozoa will be expelled. Those in favor of the mare as the optimal reservoir believe that although the motility of the second dose of semen fares well in the Equitainer, it does not necessarily reflect the fertility of this dose and therefore the sperm fare better in the mare.[41] The studies that have addressed this argument have used few stallions in the experimental design or have failed to take into account the interval from insemination to ovulation. In the study presented by Love et al.,[42] maintaining the fertility of the sperm when cooled at 5° C may yet again be stallion dependent; stallions with poor fertility appear to have more chromatin damage with cooling than stallions with good fertility. The most convincing evidence for sequential breedings arises in a studies by Heiskanen et al.[43,44] These researchers found that mares bred with semen stored at 5° C for up to 40 and 80 hours have pregnancy rates of 87% and 65%, respectively, thus demonstrating acceptable pregnancy rates with stored semen. Still, the optimal means for preserving the fertility of extra doses of semen remains a controversial subject, and the answer is not entirely clear, perhaps because the fertility varies among individual stallions and mares.

Occasionally, a suboptimal dose of semen arrives: the semen may be extended improperly, the sperm numbers may be low, or the motility or morphology may be poor. If the total volume of semen is not so great that it is expelled through the cervix on insemination, one should make every attempt to inseminate an optimal dose of semen for pregnancy. If the volume is too great, the semen may be centrifuged, but this may jeopardize the motility of the spermatazoa. Therefore reinseminating the mare 6 to 12 hours after the first insemination with a second dose is perhaps best in an attempt to cover her with an optimal dose over 24 hours.

Pregnancy rates with transported cooled semen are reported to range from less than 20% to greater than 80%.[45,46] Although dependent on the fertility of the mare and stallion, the extreme variability of the fertility rate often is due to other management factors, such as handling and management of the stallion, handling and management of the semen, extension of the semen, shipment of the semen, number of motile spermatazoa inseminated, management of the mare, preparation of the mare for breeding, insemination technique, handling of the semen during insemination, and postinsemination management of the mare. Therefore pregnancy rates reflect not only the fertility of the horses but also the expertise and conscientiousness of the personnel involved in this endeavor.

With cooled semen, insemination of mares within 24 hours before ovulation is recommended to allow ample time for capacitation of the spermatozoa and transport to the oviduct. If ovulation fails to occur in the expected time frame, reinsemination every 24 to 48 hours with at least 500×10^6 progressively motile spermatozoa should optimize pregnancy rates. However, repeated inoculation of the uterus with rebreeding can cause problems in mares that are susceptible to endometritis or DUC.

Pregnancy rates with frozen-thawed semen also demonstrate a wide range of success.[45] Cryopreserved semen from most stallions generally is believed to result in lower fertility rates than cooled semen, but this is not always the case. Frozen-thawed semen probably does not maintain viability within the mare as long as fresh or fresh-cooled semen.[47] This short viability may be due to the capacitation-like changes associated with frozen-thawed sperm.[7] Fewer spermatozoa are found bound to the oviduct of the mare after insemination with frozen-thawed semen. If indeed a selective mechanism exists for sperm-binding capacity within the oviduct and that sperm must be noncapacitated, irreversible damage during the process of freezing and thawing may cause spermatozoa to lose this binding ability.[47]

Per cycle pregnancy rates of 25% to 45% are typical[48-50] when breeding every 24 hours or after ovulation; high pregnancy rates (>70% per cycle) have been achieved with appointment breeding that includes preovulation and postovulation timed inseminations.[48-52] Predicting ovulation can be challenging, and management of mares to be inseminated with frozen semen is time consuming; however, timely treatment with an ovulation induction agent can ease management greatly. Not only do these agents reliably shorten the interval to ovulation, but also the window of ovulation is so small that far fewer examinations of the mare are necessary for success. Their use can curtail, if not eliminate, late-night breeding. Inseminations can be performed either at 24 and 40 hours or 36 and 44 hours after ovulation induction, with ovulation occurring between inseminations. This protocol allows insemination at specific times and eliminates more frequent examinations of the mare to determine if the mare has ovulated, and the single dose is then inseminated. The results of a recent retrospective study in which 876 mares were bred with frozen-thawed semen from 106 stallions revealed no significant difference in first-cycle pregnancy rates, seasonal pregnancy rates, or number of cycles per pregnancy between cooled and frozen semen shipped from one facility to a large number of mare owners (Table 18-6).[53] In this study inseminators were instructed to breed the mares with the frozen-thawed semen before and after ovulation and close to ovulation. In this instance management and selection of the stallions were optimal, and the stud farm was involved closely (through instruction and communication) with selection and insemination of the mares. Therefore management and selection of breeding stock may assume even greater importance when breeding with frozen semen.

The number of morphologically normal, progressively motile sperm (PMS) that yields optimal pregnancy rates with frozen-thawed semen is likely to be stallion and management dependent (Table 18-7). Vidament[54] examined more than 30,000 mare inseminations in the French National Stud and concluded that mares should be inseminated with a minimum of 750×10^6 total frozen-thawed sperm per cycle; doses consisting of a lower total number of total sperm were associated with lower per cycle pregnancy rates. Based on these results, this figure has been adopted and is currently recommended by the World Breeding Federation of Sporthorses. The number of motile frozen-thawed spermatozoa also affects pregnancy rates.[55] Per cycle pregnancy rates were significantly higher when the insemination dose of frozen-thawed semen was increased from $137\text{-}210 \times 10^6$ to $222\text{-}333 \times 10^6$ PMS (44% versus 73% respectively).[56] Significant differences in per cycle pregnancy rates were observed based on the insemination dose of frozen-thawed PMS; mares bred with $600\text{-}800 \times 10^6$ PMS had significantly higher per cycle pregnancy rates than mares bred with other doses.[52]

FUTURE TECHNIQUES

Procedures that were once considered to be advanced reproductive technology have become a routine part of many equine reproduction practices. These procedures include embryo transfer, gamete intrafallopian transfer, and cryopreservation

TABLE 18-6

Comparison of Field Fertility of Fresh and Frozen-Thawed Semen

	Cooled	Frozen
Number of stallions	16	100
Number of mares	850	641
First cycle conception rate (%)	59.4	51.3
Seasonal pregnancy rate	74.7	71.9

Data from Loomis PR: The equine frozen semen industry, *Anim Reprod Sci* 68:191–200, 2001.

TABLE 18-7

The Relationship Between Number of Progressively Motile Sperm (Frozen-Thawed) and per Cycle Pregnancy Rate

Total number PMS	Pregnant	Open	% Pregnant
<200	12	10	54.5[a]
200-400	66	28	70.2[a]
400-600	30	20	60[a]
600-800	60	8	88.2[b]
>800	44	34	56.4[a]

b is significantly different from *a* ($p < 0.02$)
PM, Progressively motile sperm.
Data from. Metcalf ES: Optimizing pregnancy rates using frozen-thawed equine semen. *Anim Reprod Sci* 89:297–299, 2005.

of spermatozoa and oocytes, to name a few. These techniques offer the possibility of preserving valuable lines that otherwise might be lost in breeding stock.

EQUINE EMBRYO TRANSFER

Elizabeth Metcalf

Unlike the stallion, the mare is limited in the number of offspring that she can produce in her lifetime. Embryo transfer offers a means for enhancing production of offspring from mares of superior genetic lines or that are incapable of carrying a foal to term. More specifically, this procedure offers the following advantages:

1. Embryo transfer allows a mare to remain in competition while still producing valuable offspring.
2. Embryo transfer allows production of offspring from mares suffering from pathologic conditions of the uterus severe enough to prevent carrying a foal to term.
3. Embryo transfer allows production of offspring from mares suffering from systemic illness that prevents them from carrying a foal to term.
4. Embryo transfer allows for production of offspring from mares with musculoskeletal disease in which their health may be jeopardized by carrying a pregnancy to term or delivering a foal (e.g., fractured pelvis or hip, severe arthritis).
5. Embryo transfer prevents risk of postfoaling complications in the valuable mare or older mare at risk.
6. Embryo transfer allows more than a single offspring to be born within a given year.
7. Immature (2-year-old) mares unable to carry a foal to term are capable of producing embryos that have a good survival rate in mature recipient mares.
8. In breed registries in which the value of the offspring often depends on a determined date of birth, embryo transfer allows mares that foal late in the season to produce an embryo for that year and yet also be prepared to be bred early on the subsequent season because they have been left open.
9. The procedure has proved invaluable in many research projects comparing effects on twins that arise from embryo splitting or double ovulation.

As breed registries have permitted registration of the foals produced by embryo transfer, the technique rapidly has become a routine procedure offered in many equine private practices. Although most practices do not maintain a herd of recipient mares and most small-scale mare owners do not provide enough recipients, the procedure of flushing embryos from donor mares and shipping the embryos to recipient mares at a distant location has grown in popularity. Still, despite the numerous advantages to transferring embryos, the procedure is an expensive endeavor that may cost in veterinary and mare care alone more than $10,000.[1] Coupled with the stud fee, these offspring, assuming the procedure is successful, are indeed valuable.

FACTORS AFFECTING SUCCESS RATES

Three major factors affect success rates in an embryo transfer program: the fertility of the mares (donor and recipient), the fertility of the semen, and the expertise of all technical and veterinary personnel. Best management practices optimize all three factors for success. All horses involved should receive a BSE, the extent of which depends on the age, history, and parity of the mares and the reproductive history of the stallion.

Fertility of the Donor Mare

The ideal candidate for a donor mare in an embryo transfer program is a 3- to 10-year-old, healthy, reproductively sound mare. Foss, Wirth, Schlitz et al.[2] reported high embryo recovery rates in show mares (84.2%) followed by an acceptable rate in multiparous, nonbarren mares (59.7%). However, mares with a history of infertility showed a significantly lower embryo recovery rate (30%). Unfortunately, the value of many mares is not realized until they are older, when superior performance of their offspring has been exhibited. The age of the mare appears to play a major role in fertility[3]; early loss of pregnancy is a common and frustrating problem encountered in older mares. Investigation into the causes of this age-associated infertility has led researchers to examine changes that occur in the reproductive tracts of aging mares: the uterine environment, the uterine tube environment, and ovarian function.

The numbers and quality of oocytes differ greatly between young and aged mares.[4] Oocytes from older mares (i.e., >20 years) have significantly more morphologic anomalies.[5] The clinical impression of many practitioners is that delayed development occurs in embryos obtained from older mares.[4,6] In evaluations of equine embryo quality and viability, not only have young mares (<10 years old) been reported to produce more embryos, but also the embryos that are recovered from them are of significantly superior quality compared with embryos from older mares.[7-9] Embryos are graded on the basis of morphologic characteristics and size (grade 1, excellent; grade 4, poor).[10] Transfer of grade 1 embryos results in significantly higher 50-day pregnancy rates (70% to 80%) than transfer of grade 4 embryos (30% to 40%).[9] Transferred embryos classified as grades 1 and 2 demonstrate significantly higher pregnancy rates than grade 3 embryos.[10] Embryo loss between 12 and 50 days of gestation was significantly greater with grade 2 embryos than with grade 1 embryos.[11]

Because the number of blastocysts recovered from the oviductal lumen 2 days after ovulation does not vary according to the age of the mare,[6,11] fertilization and early cleavage steps may not be the limiting factors in production of embryos in older mares. However, pregnancy rates at 4 days demonstrate a significant difference depending on mare age.[6,12] Although age-associated degenerative and inflammatory changes to the endometrium and its associated blood vessels are well documented and in some cases may contribute to lower foaling rates in old mares, the defect that causes early embryonic losses appears to occur before the mature blastocyst can be found within the uterus.[13] Early (2-day) pregnancy rates are not different depending on the age of the mare,[12] but 3-day pregnancy rates are decreased significantly in aged mares.[14] Day 4 embryos collected from the uterine tubes of old mares and transferred to the uteruses of young normal mares show significantly lower survival rates.[15]

Apparently, older mares require superior nutritional support, particularly during the vernal transition period to hasten the interval to ovulation.[16-19] Follicular development is prolonged in older mares, especially as they approach ovarian senescence.[20,21] The most common cause of early pregnancy loss in older mares appears to be an intrinsic defect within the oocyte itself or in the physiologic events that occur before the formation of a day 3 embryo. Other factors, such as failure of maternal recognition of pregnancy, immune-mediated causes, chromosomal aberrations, reaction to stress, nutrition, hormonal insufficiencies, and postovulatory insemination may play a role in early pregnancy loss and delayed embryonic development.[22]

Fertility of the Recipient Mare

A young, healthy, reproductively sound mare is the ideal candidate to act as an embryo recipient. Factors that further enhance success rates in the recipients include good nutrition, good general health care, minimal stress, and hormonal synchrony with the donor mare. Ideally, the recipient mare should ovulate during a period from 1 day (+1) before to as many as 6 days after (–6) the donor mare to optimize pregnancy rates.[23,24] Carnevale, Ramirez, Squires et al.[11] have reported that embryo loss rates are significantly higher in recipient mares that ovulate 7 days or more (–7) after the donor mare. The administration of PGF_2-α alone or with progestin compounds promotes synchrony between the ovulations of the donor and recipient mares.[25] Ovulation induction agents such as hCG or deslorelin may further enhance desired synchrony.

To eliminate the need for synchrony, many researchers have used ovariectomized recipient mares that have been treated with progestins alone or a combination of progestins and estrogen.[26-28] Although McKinnon, Squires, Carnevale et al.[28] found that pregnancy rates were similar between ovariectomized, progesterone-supplemented mares and synchronized recipients, results in the field have been unreliable using ovariectomized recipients, perhaps because ovariectomized mares that remain open for a season appear to be less optimal candidates for subsequent recipient seasons. From an economic standpoint, ovariectomized mares also require upward of 120 days of progestin supplementation.[29] Researchers also have evaluated the suitability of hormone-treated mares in the beginning of the transitional period as embryo recipients, but pregnancy rates are often not as high as those in recipients that are cycling regularly.[11]

Uterine tone at day 5 after recipient ovulation represents a useful predictive indicator of success in transfer. Recipient mares with good uterine tone 5 days after ovulation had significantly higher pregnancy rates at day 50 than mares with poor to fair uterine tone.[11] McCue, Vanderwall, Keith et al.[30] have shown that mares that qualify as recipients on the basis of uterine tone have significantly higher progesterone concentrations at day 5 than mares who failed to qualify. This finding is consistent with another study reported by Sevinga, Schukken, Hesselink et al.[31] that found that the size of the CL and progesterone production are higher at day 8 or 9 after ovulation in pregnant mares compared with nonpregnant mares.

Although veterinarians generally agree that the parturient mare determines the size of the foal at birth, research has demonstrated that choosing a recipient pony mare to deliver the foal of a donor Warmblood mare is unwise.[32] Allen[33] has demonstrated that the size of the recipient mare does affect the adult size of the offspring. Wilsher and Allen[34] split equine embryos and transferred these identical twins into recipient mares of varying heights. Although the donor mare appeared to determine the size of the foal at birth, the height of the adult horse appeared to depend on the size of the recipient mare. Therefore choosing donor and recipient mares of similar size is recommended.

Fertility of the Semen

The quality of semen affects the success rate of embryo recovery.[35] In general, the best results are obtained when the mare is inseminated with semen collected on the farm (or is bred under natural cover), followed by semen that is cooled and shipped to arrive within 24 hours of collection, followed by frozen semen.[25] High pregnancy rates have been demonstrated when the mares are inseminated before and after ovulation during a 12-hour period.[36] Results from an embryo transfer program in a private practice over a 2-year period of evaluation support this discrepancy in fertility based on the type of semen, with fresh, chilled, and frozen semen resulting in embryo recovery rates of 55%, 44%, and 32%, respectively.[24]

Expertise of the Veterinarian

The veterinarian's role is not only to determine the optimal time for breeding but also to recognize abnormalities as they arise. Abnormalities such as DUC[37] or hemorrhagic follicles can be detrimental to successful embryo recovery. The veterinarian also should be experienced in embryo recovery and transfer techniques to achieve the most successful pregnancy rates. Owners must have realistic expectations before embarking on this expensive endeavor. They must realize that even with a young, fertile mare bred with fertile semen and under the care of an experienced veterinarian, the best embryo recovery rates are only 70% to 80%. If semen shipped cooled or frozen is used, then the success rates are often lower.[38]

PROCEDURE FOR EMBRYO RECOVERY

Most embryo flushes are attempted on days 7 or 8, with the day that the donor ovulated designated as day 0. Day 0 is the first day that a corpus hemorrhagicum is visible on transrectal ultrasound examination, assuming that the mare has been examined at least daily. If the mare is examined more frequently, as is often the case when breeding with frozen semen, day 0 is still determined by the first appearance of the corpus hemorrhagicum. Occasionally, another question of ovulation may arise because of the presence of a hemorrhagic follicle; these anomalies occur more often in transitional and older mares. In these cases ovulation generally is believed not to have occurred.[39]

The developing embryo enters the uterus after day 5 at the morula or early blastocyst stage.[40] Enormous growth of the blastocyst and rapid expansion of the inner cavity, the blastocoele, occur during the next few days. Most embryos destined for transfer are flushed as expanded blastocysts (day 7 or 8) because they appear to optimize transfer pregnancy rates.[24,41,42]

One lavages the uterus of the donor serially with liters of Dulbecco's phosphate buffered saline or synthetic oviductal fluid warmed to 37° C (Figure 18-10). Antimicrobial agents and 1% fetal calf serum (FCS; Hyclone Laboratories, Logan, Utah) may be added to the lavage medium. Although many Foley-type catheters have been used for the lavage, a large-bore (8.0 mm) sterile silicone catheter (80 cm; Bivona ET flushing catheter; Western Veterinary Supply, Grapevine, Tex.) with

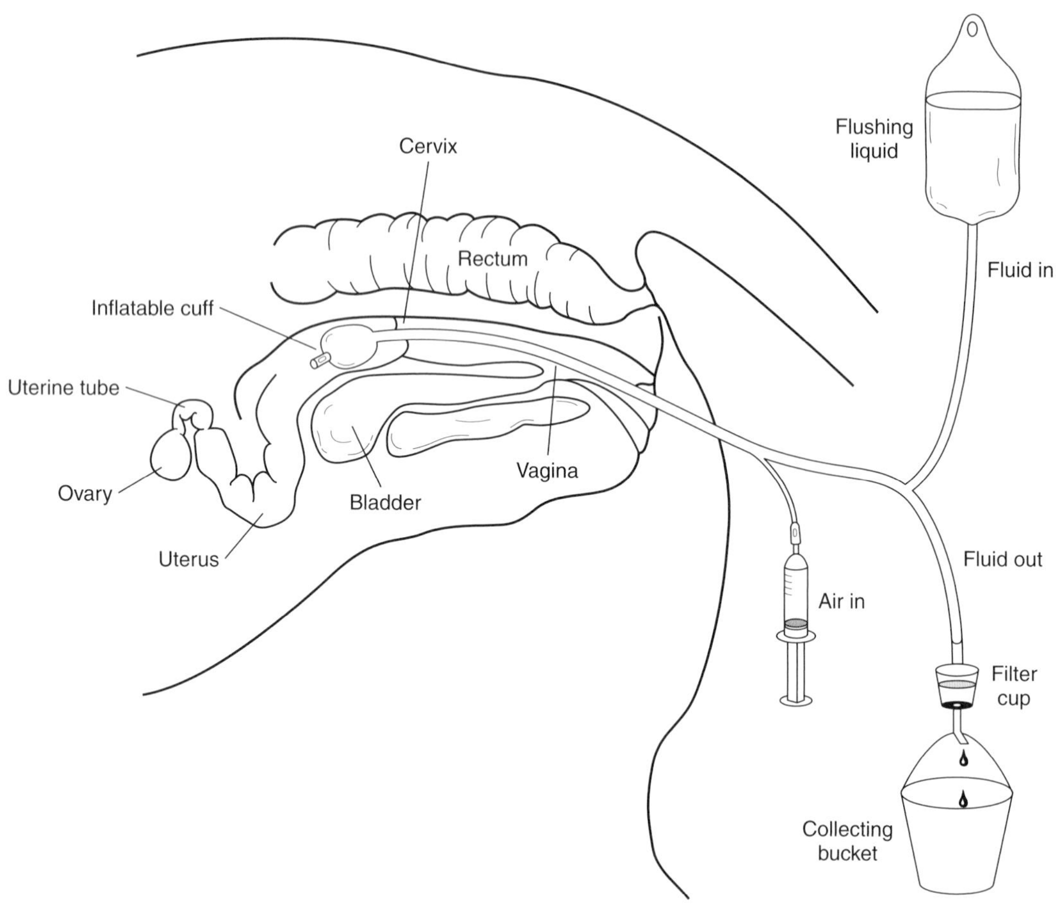

FIGURE 18-10 Embryo flushing: the inflated catheter seals the cervix. (Courtesy T. Ayres, Aurora, Ore.)

an inflatable cuff is often ideal for most donors presented in practice. The uteruses of some older or multiparous mares may require more than a single liter of fluid to distend the uterus. Likewise, the smaller uteruses of maiden mares may take less than 1 L for maximum distention. This often can be determined by the ease of fluid flow into the uterus. One evacuates the uterus by gravity flow and passes the recovered fluid through a sterile recovery cup lined with a 0.75-μm filter (Harvet, Spring Valley, Wisconsin). It is important to ensure that the cup does not run dry; a certain amount of fluid must remain in this cup at all times to bathe the embryo. Even though most embryos are recovered in the first flush, this procedure must be repeated two or three more times, with the recovered fluid measured on each flush so that most of the fluid has been recovered by the time that the procedure is complete. One performs transrectal massage of the uterus for the last two flushes, ensuring recovery of all fluid introduced into the uterus.

Once in the laboratory, the contents of the cup are swirled and then poured into search dishes that have been maintained at 37° C. The cup is rinsed with 20 ml of the remaining Dulbecco's phosphate buffered saline solution, which is then decanted into the search dishes. Using a stereoscopic microscope, usually at 15× magnification, one methodically seaches for the embryo. After finding it, one evaluates the embryo at higher magnification for age, size, and morphology and then washes it three times in lavage medium with 10% FCS in preparation for shipping or transfer. Antimicrobial agents often are added to this medium as well.

EMBRYO TRANSFER INTO THE RECIPIENT MARE

Surgical and nonsurgical techniques have been used successfully to transfer mare embryos. For many years surgical transfer by way of a standing flank laparotomy demonstrated the most favorable pregnancy rates. However, this procedure is more expensive, labor intensive, and time consuming for the veterinarian, and it poses a higher risk to the recipient mare. Over the past few years, nonsurgical transfer has been reported to achieve similar, if not superior, pregnancy rates for many clinicians.[2,38,43] This success rate appears to depend on the experience and expertise of the veterinarian performing the transfer.

One loads the embryo into a sterile 0.25-ml or 0.50-ml straw using a ureteral catheter adapter (Cook Urological, Spencer, Indiana) attached to a tuberculin syringe. The size of the straw depends on the size of the embryo. To ensure the midstraw location of the embryo at all times before transfer, one first loads the straw with lavage medium (10% FCS), then with an air pocket, then with medium (10% FCS) containing the embryo, then with another air pocket, and followed at last by medium (10% FCS). For nonsurgical transfer, the first fluid section must penetrate the wick of the straw to prevent loss of the contents of the straw by gravity. This sequence not only allows verification of the location of the embryo but also reduces the amount of fluid inoculated into the uterus of the mare on transfer.

The straw is loaded into a sterile insemination gun. Although several commercially available guns have been designed to fit the different sizes of straws, some veterinarians prefer to use a stainless steel reusable gun, and others prefer an intrauterine pipette for transfer of large embryos. Manipulation of the cervix or inoculation of the uterus during transfer long has been considered detrimental to a successful pregnancy. This invasion of the reproductive tract of a diestrus recipient mare also has been suspected potentially to lead to eventual regression of the CL through the release of PG, oxytocin, or both. Thus one must take many steps to preserve the CL and thus the transferred pregnancy.

Although studies have shown that no benefit accrues from treating the recipient mare with altrenogest (Regumate, Intervet Inc., Millsboro, Delaware) or flunixin meglumine (Banamine, Schering-Plough Animal Health, Union, N.J.), many practitioners continue to administer these drugs to mares before transfer of the embryo. Some also use a single intramuscular dose of procaine penicillin (Aquacillin, Vedco, St. Joseph, Missouri) for its antibiotic action, whereas others administer dexamethasone (Dexaject SP; Burns Veterinary Supply, Rockville Center, N.Y.) for its anti-inflammatory effects, terbutaline (Franck's Veterinary Pharmacy, Des Moines, Iowa) for its tocolytic action on the uterus, and propantheline bromide (Franck's) for transient relaxation of the rectum.[2]

Unfortunately, scientific data validating the merits of these therapies are lacking. Sedation of the recipient mare depends on her temperament and degree of discomfort during the procedure. Work by LeBlanc, DeLille, Cadario et al.[44] suggests that tranquilization using an α_2-agonist such as dormosedan may cause less stimulation of uterine contraction because the uterus of the recipient mare is under the influence of progesterone from the CL. When α_2-adrenoceptors predominate, they inhibit contractions.

One secures the loaded, sterile embryo transfer gun, perhaps shielded by a sterile outer guard sleeve, in the palm with the thumb; then applies a small amount of sterile lubricant; and inserts the hand and gun transvaginally. One digitally palpates the external cervical os and passes just the tip of the gun gently through the guard sleeve and then the remainder of the cervix. At this point, many prefer to deposit the embryo in the uterine body. If the veterinarian is planning to deposit the embryo in the uterine horn instead, he or she then inserts a well-lubricated arm into the rectum of the recipient, locates and grasps the uterine horn, and gently threads the tip of the gun into the uterine horn. Next, the veterinarian slowly depresses the plunger, releasing the embryo from the straw as the gun is withdrawn. Because of equine embryo mobility, into which horn the embryo is deposited does not matter.

Surgical transfer of an embryo is performed on a sedated recipient mare aseptically prepared for a routine flank incision. An inverted L or line block over the paralumbar fossa is generally used for local anesthesia. The surgeon exteriorizes the uterine horn of the mare and makes a small puncture with a cutting-edge suture needle. The surgeon then enlarges the hole slightly with iris forceps and inserts the sterile straw containing the embryo through the hole into the uterine lumen to deposit the embryo. The surgeon places the uterine horn back into the abdomen and then repairs the incision with a routine three-layer closure.

A developing embryonic vesicle can be detected by transrectal ultrasound examination as early as 5 days after transfer. If the embryonic vesicle is not visible at this time, the mare must be rechecked every 48 hours at least through day 16. Carnevale, Ramirez, Squires et al.[11] have shown that the presence or absence of an embryonic vesicle at 5 days is an important predictor of pregnancy loss by 50 days. Recipient mares in which the embryonic vesicle is large enough to be seen on the first pregnancy examination (usually 5 days) have fewer embryonic deaths than mares in which the vesicle is not seen until subsequent examinations. Ginther, Bergfelt, Leith et al.[45] support this theory; they also found that undersized embryonic vesicles are associated with a higher rate of pregnancy loss.

SHIPPING EMBRYOS

Carney, Squires, Cook et al.[46] have shown that no significant differences occur in pregnancy rates between mares that have embryos transferred immediately after collection and mares that receive cooled, transported embryos. The expense of maintaining open recipient mares is considerable, and a number of commercial recipient herds are now available to practitioners. Because most of these commercial herds have limited numbers of mares, having contracts signed and mares reserved early in the breeding season is important.

Preparing the embryo for shipping is uncomplicated. Most embryos in the United States are shipped in Ham's F-10 (Sigma Chemical Co., St. Louis, Mo.) medium buffered to an optimal pH with a mixture of 5% carbon dioxide, 5% oxygen, and 90% nitrogen gas.[47] The final preparation of the medium contains 10% FCS (filtered through a Millipore filter) and antimicrobial agents (usually a combination of penicillin and streptomycin). Although most larger commercial operations send the buffered medium on ice to the practitioner the day before the embryo flush, this transport medium is simple for the practitioner to make in the clinic, provided that a tank of the appropriate gas mixture is on hand.

Several other media are available for embryo transport that eliminate the need for the gas buffer of Ham's F-10, which is necessary to maintain the correct pH for embryo transport. Moussa, Duchamp, Bruyas et al.[48] reported that two commercially available embryo holding media (Emcare Holding Solution [ICP, Auckland, New Zealand] and ViGro [AB Technology, Pullman, Wash.]) appear to have an effect on embryo viability similar to the gas-buffered Ham's F-10 for 24-hour cooled storage of embryos. However, this study did not examine pregnancy rates after transfer. Fleury, Fleury, and Landim-Alvarenga[49] recently reported that using hydroxyethyl-piperazine ethane-sulfonate (HEPES)-buffered Ham's F-10 (with 0.4% bovine serum albumin [BSA]) for temporary storage of embryos gave 15-day pregnancy rates of greater than 75% in recipient mares. This medium also eliminates the need for incubation with the gases. In this experiment embryos were stored at ambient temperature, between 15° and 24° C, thereby eliminating the need for cooling as well.

The washed embryo is transferred using a sterile 0.25- or 0.5-ml straw to a 6-ml snap-top tube containing the transport medium. One tightly closes the top and places the tube in a larger tube (50-ml centrifuge tube) also filled with transport medium. One then places both tubes into an isothermalizer cup (37° C) and places that into an Equitainer (Hamilton-Thorne Research Inc., Danvers, Mass.) for shipment.

Some commercial operations with recipient herds prefer that the embryos be transported by commercial airlines in an attempt to minimize the time that the embryo spends outside of the uterus of the mare. Others believe that commercial transport companies that deliver the embryo within 24 hours are acceptable and that pregnancy rates do not differ between 12-hour and 24-hour shipment.[50] Foss[24] has shown that pregnancy rates do not differ between embryos transported by airlines and those transported by courier services. The largest factor in choosing the means of transportation is reliability of service. Whatever means of transporting the embryo that is ultimately chosen, the imperative is to ensure that the paperwork is filled out correctly and that the shipment is insured.

THE PREGNANT MARE

Grant S. Frazer

PHYSIOLOGY OF GESTATION

Maternal Recognition of Pregnancy

The zygote begins its journey down the oviduct once the oocyte has been fertilized, reaching the uterine horn by day 6.[1,2] Detailed descriptions of the early development of the equine embryo have been published and are beyond the scope of this text.[3,4] Early embryonic development in the horse is characterized by the formation of an unusual acellular glycoprotein "capsule" between the trophectoderm and the overlying zona pellucida. This structure is first detected between days 6 and 7 after ovulation and completely envelops the spherical conceptus until as late as day 23 of gestation.[5] Although the term *embryo* is used routinely to describe the early conceptus, it is important to understand that what is generally being discussed is the embryonic vesicle as well as the embryo itself. These two structures will ultimately develop into the fetal membranes and fetus, respectively. Embryonic development has progressed sufficiently by day 40 of gestation that the term *fetus* is used thereafter.[4]

The longitudinal arrangement of the endometrial folds may favor mobility of the spherical equine embryo.[4] After entering the tip of the uterine horn on day 6, the embryo moves down toward the body by day 8.[6,7] The intrauterine mobility phase continues until days 15 through 17, and during this period the embryo may move between horns 10 to 20 times each day.[2,4,7-9] If the pregnancy is to be maintained, the embryo must send a signal to the endometrium and prevent the cyclic release of the uterine luteolysin (PGF_2-α).[10] An embryo-derived factor is the most likely cause for the suppression of PGF_2-α release and interruption of the oxytocin– PGF_2-α interaction in mares during early pregnancy.[11,12] The mobility of the spherical equine conceptus is critical for blockage of luteolysis.[3] This is why large uterine cysts may cause pregnancy loss.[13-15] If the enlarging vesicle can not pass by a cyst, it may be unable to come into contact with all endometrial surfaces and thus inhibit PGF_2-α production.[16] Yet another unique feature of equine reproduction is the fact that the luteolysin is delivered to the ovary systemically.[17] Such delivery contrasts with the local countercurrent, utero-ovarian route in domestic ruminants in which intimate contact occurs between the ovarian artery and utero-ovarian vein.[18] The embryo typically becomes fixed at the base of one of the uterine horns, with the embryonic pole of the vesicle opposite the mesometrial attachment (antimesometrial).[19] An early vascular indicator of the future position of the embryo proper consists of a colored spot in the Doppler image of the endometrium, close to the wall of the embryonic pole. This finding may prove useful when differentiating between a cyst and a vesicle before the embryo proper becomes visible on the ultrasound image.[19,20] In postpartum mares the embryo usually becomes fixed in the more involuted horn.[21-23]

Placentation

The trophoblast cells of the early embryo are destined to form the absorptive placental contact with the endometrium.[4] The mare has a rather unique nondeciduate, epitheliochorial, diffuse, microcotyledonary placenta.[3,24-30] The entire maternal surface of the fetal membranes becomes covered with delicate microvilli (diffuse), which interdigitate with the proliferating luminal epithelial cells to form intricately branched microcotyledons.[25,26,28] The interdigitation tends to be deeper at the tip of the nongravid horn, and this may help explain the higher incidence of fetal membrane retention in that horn.[31] In a normal pregnancy the noninvasive allantochorion extends slowly to fill the uterus by days 80 through 85, and its microcotyledonary architecture, which provides both hemotrophic and histotrophic nutrition for the growing fetus, is not fully established until days 120 through 140.[2,28,32,33] During the second half of gestation, most of the mitotic activity is confined to the periphery of the microcotyledons, which are still growing.[33-36] Constant supplies of the principal vasculogenic and angiogenic factor (vascular endothelial growth factor) and its two main receptor molecules are available on both the maternal and fetal sides of the placental barrier throughout gestation in the mare. They are presumed to facilitate the continuing development of the extensive fetal and maternal capillary networks that are such prominent features within the microplacentomes of the diffuse, epitheliochorial equine placenta.[36,37]

Degenerative changes (endometrosis) in the maternal endometrium can adversely affect the ability of the microcotyledonary placenta to facilitate optimal hemotrophic nutrition and exchange of waste products.* If the pregnancy is maintained, dysfunctional placental attachment can lead to the birth of small, weak foals (intrauterine growth retardation) and may have detrimental consequences on the health and athletic performance of the mature horse.[28,36,45-48] Likewise, the presence of twin fetal sacs deprives variable areas of each allantochorion of the necessary endometrial contact to promote development of the diffuse microvilli. Failure of development of the microcotyledons results in the characteristic white, avillous portions on the maternal surface of aborted twin fetal membranes (see the section on early pregancy loss and abortion).[49,50] Although the histotrophic form of nutrition is likely to remain important throughout gestation, adequate hemotrophic nutrition is essential to support the rapid fetal growth that occurs during the latter part of gestation.† The morphology of endometrial blood vessels in uterine biopsy can vary considerably, depending on the age and reproductive status of the mare. In a recent study inflammatory vascular alterations were observed in 20.5%

*References 15, 28, 32, 33, 36, 38-45.

†References 2, 27, 28, 32, 35, 36, 38, 45

of the endometrial specimens examined.[36,44] Smaller and larger arterial and venous vessels demonstrated mild to severe degenerative lesions. Unaltered vessels were detected only in maiden mares.

The incidence and severity of angiosis increases with the number of previous pregnancies and with advancing age.[36,40,44] Changes in the endometrial vasculature of multiparous mares have been compared with the so-called pregnancy sclerosis of other species, with fraying and disruption of the membrana elastica interna, medial and adventitial elastosis and fibrosis, and calcification processes within the media.[40,44] Cycles of vascular growth during pregnancy and subsequent involution postpartum are thought to result in progressive degenerative vascular changes, as seen in multiparous mares. Aging processes, chronic inflammation, and short foaling intervals have been suggested as additional detrimental factors.[36,40,44] Severe angiosis is frequently combined with phlebectasia and lymphangiectasia, possibly indicating a reduced ability of the vessels to adapt to the varying demands of uterine circulation, with a decrease of uterine perfusion and lymph drainage. Angiosis in older, multiparous mares might therefore be intimately related to infertility, possibly because of detrimental effects on early embryo nourishment and subsequent placentation.[32,40,44,51]

Some interesting embryo transfer experiments have demonstrated the impact that uterine capacity—and placental area—can have on the size and birth weight of the foal.[52-56] In one study pony embryos were transferred into draft mare recipients, and then the genetic dams were permitted to carry a full sibling to term. The final experimental outcome was three pairs of sex-matched, full-sibling pony foals. The embryo transfer foals were all larger than their siblings at birth. Although the increased milk production of the draft mares may have explained the subsequent faster growth rates, it was noted that all three draft-gestated foals were still heavier at 4 years of age.[52] A similar embryo transfer experiment used a Thoroughbred-in-Pony (Tb-P) and Pony-in-Thoroughbred (P-Tb) comparison, with Thoroughbred-Thoroughbred and Pony-Pony transfers acting as controls.[54,56] The P-in-Tb foals were heavier than the Tb-in-P foals. Comparison of placental measurements (weight, volume, and surface area) confirmed the impact of nutrient supply on fetal growth and foal birth weight, and sudden mare weight loss in midgestation has also been shown to have detrimental effects on placental development.[33,35,53-56] These studies confirmed earlier work in which a Shetland pony mare was inseminated with Shire semen and a Shire mare was bred with Shetland pony semen. The foal out of the pony mare was 50% of the weight of the half sibling that was gestated in the Shire mare. The marked size discrepancy remained even after these half siblings reached maturity.[57]

Equids possess the unusual ability to interbreed freely among the phenotypically and karyotypically diverse member species of the genus to produce viable, but usually infertile, offspring.[58] The mule (female horse crossed with male donkey) is one example of this successful interbreeding. Even more amazing, mares and donkeys have been shown to be capable of carrying to term a range of true, xenogeneic extraspecies pregnancies created by embryo transfer. In these instances all of the allantochorion tissue is composed of foreign protein (see the following discussion of endometrial cups). Successful pregnancies include Przewalski's horse (*Equus prezwalskii;* 2n = 66) carried-in-horse and Grant's zebra (*E. burchelli;* 2n = 44) carried-in-horse (*E. caballus;* 2n = 64).[58]

Endocrinology

By day 35 a specialized, circumferential group of trophoblast cells (chorionic girdle) detach from the embryonic vesicle, and some successfully invade the endometrium.[2,3,59-63] Here they give rise to discrete aggregates of endocrinologically active tissue (endometrial cups).[2,59,60,64] These endometrial cups become visible by day 38 to 40 as a ring of small, pale plaques that surround the developing conceptus.[3,4,32] Because the maternal and fetal cells (sire contribution) have differing genotypes, the fetal antigens invoke a cell-mediated immune response.[4,65,66] The influx of lymphocytes creates a pronounced, localized immunologic reaction, and by day 120 of gestation the endometrial cups are sloughed.[32,65-68] The necrotic tissue and inspissated secretions form invaginations into the chorioallantois (allantoic pouches).[69] These structures can be seen on the allantoic surface of the fetal membranes after the mare has foaled.

The endometrial cups produce eCG—formerly known as *pregnant mare serum gonadotrophin* (PMSG). A large-molecular-weight glycoprotein, eCG has both FSH-like and LH-like activity.[70] Periodic surges (10 to 12 days apart) of pituitary FSH release drive a series of follicular waves on the equine ovary during early pregnancy.[2,32,71,72] The eCG promotes luteinization (and sometimes ovulation) of the dominant follicle in each wave.[3,32,73-75] These accessory (secondary) CLs augment the progesterone production from the original structure that developed at the time of conception. This process is critical to ensure pregnancy maintenance before the development of steroid production by the placenta.[2,3,32,76-79] The fully developed equine placenta produces significant quantities of progestins.[2,3,32] Pregnancy can be maintained in ovariectomized embryo transfer recipient mares provided that they receive an exogenous progestin supplement during the early period when CL progesterone is critical.[80] The need for progesterone therapy after day 100 of gestation is controversial and will be discussed later in this section.[2,81-83] High levels of eCG may be detected in the blood of pregnant mares from 40 to 120 days of gestation.[2] This forms the basis of the mare immunologic pregnancy (MIP) test. A positive MIP test can occur when a mare is no longer pregnant because pregnancy loss after days 35 to 40 will not eliminate the endometrial cups.[3] The endometrial cups can produce high levels of eCG in a mare that has suffered fetal loss during the second or third months of gestation.[84] This results in erratic estrous behavior, unreliable follicular development, luteinization of immature follicles, and unpredictable ovulation.[32,85]

Another unique feature of early gestation in the mare is an elevation in plasma conjugated estrogen levels associated with gonadotrophin stimulation of the luteal tissue.[3,74,86,87] A second, prolonged rise in estrogen levels begins by day 70, peaking around day 240, then gradually declining toward basal levels at term.[79,88,89] Peak estrogen levels range between 300 to 400 ng/ml.[79] These large quantities of estrogens are secreted by the fetoplacental unit after synthesis from precursors produced by the enlarged fetal gonads.[2,78,89-94] Bilateral fetal gonadectomy between days 197 and 253 of gestation causes a precipitous drop in plasma estrogen levels that then remains basal until small foals are spontaneously delivered in 70 to 97 days.[79] After day 220 the enlarged gonads gradually shrink into an insignificant size by birth.[95] Serum estrogens in the pregnant mare include estradiol, estrone, and the equine-specific steroid ring-B unsaturated estrogens—equilin and equilenin.[94,96-98]

Estrogen assays have been used by researchers to confirm pregnancy and fetal viability.[99-101]

Four separate components combine to produce the progesterone and biologically active 5α-reduced pregnanes needed to maintain pregnancy in the mare.[83,89,102] The primary CL is prolonged beyond its cyclical life span by the downregulation of endometrial oxytocin receptors to prevent activation of the luteolytic pathway. Its waning progesterone production is supplemented from day 40 of gestation by the formation of a series of accessory CLs that develop in the maternal ovaries as a result of the gonadotrophic actions of pituitary FSH and eCG.[102] The equine fetoplacental unit produces significant quantities of progesterone and C-21 progestagens.[2,76-79,89,103-105] The placenta (chorioallantois and endometrium) initially uses maternally derived cholesterol to metabolize into pregnenelone and then progesterone. A significant amount of progesterone originates from this source—starting from approximately day 70 of gestation.[76-79,89,105] In normal pregnant mares the circulating progesterone concentration starts to decline by 4 months of gestation, reaching baseline levels by day 180.[106] Progesterone may be undetectable at levels of less than 1 ng/ml.[83,89] Thus plasma progesterone-specific assays are of limited clinical value after midgestation.[83,89,107-109] The circulating progesterone concentration is no longer indicative of what is happening at the uterine level, where the placenta secretes progesterone and progestagens directly to the endometrium and underlying myometrium.[89,103-105,109] In the second half of gestation, most of the placental-derived progesterone is further metabolized into 5α-reduced pregnanes (5α-dihydroprogesterone or 5α-pregnane-3,20-dione; and 20α-5P or 20α-hydroxy-5α-pregnane-3-one; together with other 5α-reduced metabolites of progesterone and pregnenelone).[83,89,105,109-113] In the later part of gestation, it has been suggested that another steroid, perhaps 5α-pregnane-3,20-dione (5 αDHP) and not progesterone, is the important steroid precursor for the other progestin metabolites found in circulating plasma.[89,109,114] A precise biologic explanation for this mechanism has not been elucidated to date.

In the last months of gestation, the enlarging fetal adrenal gland secretes appreciable quantities of pregnenelone, which is then utilized by the placenta to synthesize progestagens.* Even at this late stage in equine gestation, there is insufficient adrenal 17α-hydroxylase activity to convert the pregnenelone into fetal cortisol, and thus it passes out in the umbilical vessels and is converted to 5α-reduced pregnanes in the placenta.† Thus, unlike the trend in ruminants, there is a significant increase in the mare's plasma progestagen concentrations during the last 4 to 6 weeks of gestation, followed by a precipitous drop in levels at the time of parturition.‡ A premature rise in progestins has been observed in mares with placentitis, and this phenomenon is thought to be associated with fetal stress and premature maturation of the pituitary adrenocortical axis.[54,116,121] When pony mares were subjected to intrafetal injections of adrenocorticotropic hormone (ACTH) at day 300 of gestation, maternal plasma progestagen concentrations increased significantly.[122]

Physiology of parturition in the mare does not follow the well-documented ruminant model.[123-125] The precise mechanism that couples the fetal hypothalamic-pituitary-adrenal axis in the foal that is carried to term is not known at this time, but it is invariably triggered when the fetus becomes fully mature.[83,89,126,127] In the mare the fetal cortisol level remains basal until the last 2 days of gestation, when a marked rise culminates in parturition.[47,127,128] Enhanced adrenocortical activity in the fetus is related to the onset of parturition in many species.[122,127] Final maturation of the fetus results in increased ACTH release from the pituitary and subsequent stimulation of the fetal adrenal cortex.[110,115,116,129,130] It is not until the maturing adrenal gland attains 17α-hydroxylase capacity that the high levels of pregnenelone are metabolized into fetal cortisol.[89,113,129] Disruption of these fetal maturational processes, with suppression of fetal adrenocortical activity, appears to play an integral part in the pathophysiology of fescue toxicosis.[118] The normal fetal maturational change (pregnenelone conversion into fetal cortisol) causes the maternal progestagen levels to plummet, with the result that there is a rising estrogen-to-progestagen ratio, and in the final hours estrogen ultimately becomes dominant in the preparturient mare.[79,120,131] Estrogens promote the synthesis of PGs and increase the number of both oxytocin receptors and myometrial gap junctions.[120,127] Studies with intrafetal injections of ACTH have indicated that both precocious maturation of the equine fetus and a significant reduction in gestational length is likely to be mediated through adrenal regulation of fetal maturation and production of maternal progestagens.[122] Follow-up work by Ousey, Rossdale et al. demonstrated that administration of high doses of maternal ACTH appears to accelerate fetal maturation and delivery in pony mares. Further work is required to establish the optimal gestational age and dosage for maternal ACTH administration before clinical recommendations can be given for this therapy.[132] These same workers are currently investigating early (day 315) use of dexamethasone to promote precocious fetal maturation and early delivery.[133] It was thought that there is little transplacental transfer of cortisol from the mare to the fetus because of the presence of a placental enzyme (11α-hydroxysteroid dehydrogenase), which converts cortisol to inactive cortisone.[83,134] However, the enzyme may not be 100% efficient, and some synthetic glucocorticoids may pass more readily.[83] This area warrants futher study, and the timing of the glucocorticoid treatment with respect to gestational age may be important.[83] A rise in fetal cortisol is definitely essential for final maturation, and foals that are delivered without adequate cortisol stimulation will usually fail to thrive and eventually die as a result of multiorgan failure.[83,126]

Relaxin is produced by the placental trophoblast cells, but current knowledge about relaxin activity in the pregnant mare is limited.[135,136] Relaxin levels may serve to keep the uterus quiescent until parturition is imminent.[135,137-139] Relaxin is thought to be involved in softening the pelvic ligaments to facilitate fetal passage. Mares may be seen to develop a relaxed croup just before foaling. The myometrium becomes more responsive to oxytocin and PG, and eventually the high concentrations of oxytocin and PGs may overcome the inhibitory effects of relaxin.* The sudden dominance of estrogen is thought to promote cervical production of PGE_2. PGF_2-α promotes myometrial contractility by acting on intracellular calcium, but PGE_2 promotes cervical relaxation.[83,146] The

*References 2, 89, 102, 109, 110, 113, 115-117.
†References 2, 47, 89, 109, 110, 112, 113, 117, 118.
‡References 79, 89, 103, 109, 110, 119, 120.

*References 115,120,124,137,138,140-145.

contracting myometrium forces the chorioallantoic sac against the softening cervix, and stage I of parturition ensues. The expulsive efforts during vaginal passage of the foal are driven by rising oxytocin and PG levels.[94,147-149] Oxytocin and PG levels reach peak concentrations during the expulsive (stage II) phase of parturition.[137,149,150] Maternal straining (contraction of the abdominal muscles) is almost always associated with large sustained uterine contractions.

In the last week before foaling, the prolactin concentration increases, and it is this hormone that drives mammary development and the initiation of lactation.[151,152] Prolactin (PRL) release from lactotrophs in the anterior pituitary is regulated by hypothalamic secretion of PRL-releasing factor. The PRL-inhibiting factor is thought to be dopamine.[153-156] Oxytocin is synthesized in the supraoptic and paraventricular nuclei of the hypothalamus. Milk is produced in the alveoli and expelled into the lactiferous ducts and teat cisterns when oxytocin causes contraction of the myoepithelial cells. Although it is assumed that nursing by the foal stimulates the release of oxytocin from the neurohypophysis, recent research has revealed that the process is more complicated in the mare.[149] A significant effect of suckling on oxytocin release by the mare was detected in only two of nine mares, when oxytocin concentrations were evaluated 0 to 3 minutes after suckling. When foals were prevented from sucking for 1 hour, by being either muzzled (n = 2) or separated from the mare (n = 2), there was no significant association between resumption of suckling and oxytocin release by the mare.[149]

Myometrial Activity

The myometrium of the uterus is composed of an inner circular and an outer longitudinal smooth muscle layer. This arrangement of muscle fibers permits regulation of luminal size (circular) and uterine length (longitudinal).[3] The uterus is palpably flaccid during and immediately after estrus and then increases in tone and becomes turgid if the mare is pregnant.[157,158] Myometrial activity is vitally important in the uterine clearance mechanism after breeding.[159,160] Uterine contractions also play an integral role during the embryo mobility phase.[157,161-164] Between at least day 9 and day 16 after ovulation, the spherical equine conceptus migrates continuously throughout the uterine lumen, propelled by peristaltic myometrial contractions.[3,9] This unusually long period of intrauterine movement ensures that the conceptus delivers its antiluteolytic signal to the entire endometrium. Conceptus mobility is high between day 10 and day 14 after ovulation but can be reduced immediately, and markedly, by an intravenous injection of flunixin meglumine. This suggests that PGs are the primary stimulus for the myometrial contractions that drive migration of the conceptus.[9] The embryo itself produces a myometrial stimulant, and the subsequent uterine contractions result in embryo mobility.[6,161] The conceptus produces estrogens by day 12, and these, along with embryonic production of PGE_2, are thought to play a role in stimulating uterine contractions and increasing uterine tone during the mobility phase.[165-170] Progesterone is vital for embryonic development, and it plays a role in the mobility, fixation, orientation, and maintenance of the equine conceptus.[171]

Because there is little, if any, progesterone in the maternal circulation during late gestation, the quiescence of the uterus is thought to be maintained by progestagens—uteroplacental metabolites of pregnenolone and progesterone.[83,109] These hormones are thought to play a significant role through a paracrine action within the fetus and uteroplacental tissues.[83] Administration of a progestagen (altrenogest) will prevent PG-induced abortion in the first trimester of pregnancy.[172] There is considerable controversy and confusion surrounding the use of progestagen supplementation in the later trimesters.[83] The cellular mechanisms involved in myometrial contractility have not been well characterized in the pregnant mare, and it may not be appropriate to extrapolate from studies in nonpregnant mares.[11,12,173-176] The classic theory in many species is that myometrial excitation and uterine contractility are suppressed by the so-called progesterone block.[177] Progesterone and progestagens were once assumed to be necessary for myometrial quiescence in the pregnant mare, and it was also thought that binding of 5α-dihydroprogesterone to endometrial progesterone receptors controlled uterine PG production and inhibited myometrial activity.[47,83,105,113,115,178] It is now known that 5α-dihydroprogesterone binds to uterine progesterone receptors more strongly than progesterone itself.[179] The oxytocin-neurophysin I gene is transcribed into mRNA in the endometrium of mares, and mRNA levels are negatively correlated with serum progesterone concentrations.[180] However, progestagens were ineffective at controlling myometrial contractility in vitro and did not inhibit the effects of oxytocin.[181,182] A pregnancy-induced inhibition of PGF_2-αrelease is not associated with suppression of oxytocin release or oxytocin receptor density, and an embryo-derived factor is thought to be the most likely cause for the suppression of PGF_2-α release and interruption of the oxytocin-PGF_2-α interaction in mares during early pregnancy.[11,12] An oncofetal protein that is found in the placenta has been shown to reduce oxytocin-induced myometrial contractions in vitro, and this protein may play a role in controlling myometrial quiescence in mares as well.[83,181] A reduction in circulating progestagen levels by experimental blockade with the 3β-hydroxysteroid dehydrogenase inhibitor (epostane) did not increase myometrial activity (labor) in late-gestation pony mares.[104,112] However, despite a paucity of evidence that a deficiency of fetoplacental progestagen production is a cause of pregnancy loss in the mare, exogenous progestagen therapy is widely used as a form of preventive insurance in the belief that it will promote uterine quiescence and guard against the possibility of pregnancy failure.[83,102,109] The progestagens may enhance the activity of the endometrial enzyme 15-hydroxyprostaglandin dehydrogenase and thus promote rapid metabolism of PGs into inactive metabolites.[83,105]

Electromyographic activity in the uterus of pregnant mares increases during the last week before foaling—even though the circulating progestagen levels are still quite high.[120,121,137,183] There is a progressive, reversible rise in myoelectrical activity at night in the last 6 days preceding parturition.[184] The endocrine profile of the periparturient mare is characterized by increasing concentrations of progestagens and decreasing estrogens.[89,131] Despite this decline, estrogens are essential for normal parturition in the mare. Recent work suggests that nightly elevations in estradiol-17β levels may bring about changes in the uteroplacental tissues that facilitate the PG and oxytocin release that is necessary to promote the onset of myometrial contractions.[83,131] Pashen and Allen showed that if the fetal gonads were removed, the pregnancy would continue, but there were weak ineffective myometrial contractions and significantly reduced PG production during labor.[79] The high levels of relaxin in the prepartúrient mare may act by inhibiting myometrial contractions until rising oxytocin and PG concentrations become overwhelming.[120,137] The number of oxytocin receptors and myometrial gap junctions may not increase until just before parturition in the mare.[120,137,181] At that time the myometrium becomes remarkably sensitive to even low doses of oxytocin.[185] A rapid membrane depolarization will result in the onset of strong, coordinated uterine contractions that characterize the first stage of labor. In the last 6 hours before rupture of the chorioallantois, a significant increase in PGF_2-α concentrations occurs before there is a significant increase in oxytocin concentration.[149] Even if the PGF_2-α concentrations are reduced by the cyclooxygenase inhibitor flunixin meglumine (1.1 mg/kg), oxytocin administration can still facilitate an expedient delivery.[150] Oxytocin levels in naturally foaling mares reach peak concentrations during the expulsive (stage II) phase of parturition.[137,149,150]

Teratogenesis

Little is known about the embryotoxic, and possible teratogenic, effects of chemicals, drugs, and other agents that may be administered to pregnant mares. Goiter has been reported in two newborn Arabian foals after the mares had been supplemented with excess iodine during the final 24 weeks of pregnancy.[186] Phenothiazines, thiabendazole, and organophosphate anthelmintics have been reported to cause pregnancy loss.[187] Likewise, Sudan grass or sorghum pastures have been reported to be toxic to the fetus.[187,188] In recent years more definitive documentation has become available with respect to the toxic effects of some medications. When griseofulvin was used to treat dermatomycosis in a mare during the second month of pregnancy, the mare carried a male foal to 331 days' gestation.[189] The foal showed bilateral microphthalmia, severe brachygnathia superior, and palatocheiloschisis. The lesions were incompatible with life, and the animal was euthanized.[189] Griseofulvin administration during pregnancy has been associated with similar lesions in other species. Given that the development of the eyes and facial bones in the horse occurs in the second month of pregnancy, the lesions described in this case most likely can be attributed to griseofulvin administration.[189] Three weak, recumbent neonatal foals with skin lesions, including a thin, wooly coat, were born to mares being treated for equine protozoal myeloencephalitis. The foals were anemic, leukopenic, azotemic, hyponatremic, and hyperkalemic.[190] The pregnant mares had received sulfadiazine or sulfamethoxazole-trimethoprim, pyrimethamine, folic acid, and vitamin E orally. Serum folate concentrations in the three foals and two mares were lower than those reported in the literature for clinically normal brood mares.[190] At necropsy each foal had lobulated kidneys with thin cortices and a pale medulla. The spleen and thymus were small. Histologic examination revealed marked epidermal necrosis without inflammatory cells, thin renal cortices, renal tubular nephrosis, lymphoid aplasia, and bone marrow aplasia and hypoplasia.[190] These observations indicated that oral administration of 2,4-diaminopyrimidines (pyrimethamine with or without trimethoprim), sulfonamides, and folic acid to mares during pregnancy is related to congenital defects in newborn foals.[190] Further investigations are warranted to ascertain the toxic agent and to determine at what stage of gestation the fetus is most vulnerable.

PREGNANCY DIAGNOSIS

Standard transrectal imaging technique will permit an experienced practitioner (using a 5-MHz ultrasound transducer under optimal lighting conditions) to detect up to 98% of embryos as early as day 11 after confirmation of ovulation.[191] The black (anechoic) spherical vesicle is characteristic of early equine pregnancy. Novices should realize that bright white (echoic) spots on the upper and lower surfaces of the black sphere are specular reflections generated by the ultrasound waves.[192] They also must appreciate that the equine embryo can be anywhere in the uterine lumen before fixation on day 16. Diagnostic errors can easily be made unless the entire length of both horns, and the uterine body down to the cervix, are meticulously searched during an ultrasonographic examination. Confirmation of mobility is useful in differentiating a vesicle from a cyst. At the time of fixation at the base of a uterine horn, the yolk sac has three germ layers (ectoderm, mesoderm, endoderm) near the embryonic pole, and only two layers (ectoderm and endoderm) at the opposite pole.[3,4] The difference in rigidity between the three-layered ventral wall, and the two-layered dorsal wall explains the characteristic guitar pick–shaped image on ultrasound by day 18.[3,4] The thickest portion of the yolk sac wall (embryonic pole) rotates to a ventral position. The change from the previous spherical shape is due to uterine turgidity and thickening of the dorsal uterine wall.[174] The increased uterine tone is responsible for the failure of the embryonic vesicle's diameter to enlarge between day 18 and 26, thus creating the classic growth profile that plateaus during this period.[4,191]

By day 21 the amniotic cavity has completely formed and the embryo itself can often be detected by ultrasound. The allantoic sac can be seen to be raising the embryo off the ventral floor by day 24. The embryo itself can be seen suspended on a thin echoic line that delineates the apposition of allantois and yolk sac.[4,191,193] This separating membrane tends to be horizontal and thus is a useful means for differentiating a singleton from twin embryonic vesicles. In the latter case the adjacent walls of the two vesicles tend to form a vertical separation. The primitive heartbeat can be detected between 22 and 25 days and is a useful indicator of embryonic viability. By day 40 the embryo (now fetus) has been elevated to the dorsal pole because the allantois has almost completely displaced the vestigial yolk sac. The membranes and blood vessels that separate the allantois and yolk sac give rise to the umbilical cord. The increasing size of the fetus causes the fetus and amniotic sac to gradually descend back to the floor of the chorioallantoic vesicle by day 48. The remnant of the yolk sac is incorporated into the umbilical cord. The site where the umbilical cord attaches to the chorioallantois identifies the horn and site where embryo fixation originally occurred. The dorsal attachment ensures that the developing fetus will not compress this vital area.[4]

Although ultrasonographic examinations have become standard practice for confirmation of pregnancy in mares, it is still essential that the veterinarian be competent at manual diagnosis. By 18 days after breeding, an experienced clinician may be able to perceive changes in uterine tone and consistency that, coupled with palpation of a narrow elongated cervix, are consistent with early pregnancy. However, it should be remembered that it is not uncommon for a persistent CL to provide a prolonged progesterone environment in a nonpregnant mare. It is important not to mistake the curvature at the base of the uterine horn for an embryonic vesicle.[3,158,194] An ultrasound image of the embryonic vesicle is required to definitively confirm pregnancy at this early stage. However, the gradually enlarging embryonic vesicle will eventually create a discernible ventral bulge that has been described as being the size of a hen's egg (day 30), goose's egg (day 35), and orange (days 40 to 45).[194,195] Because there is minimal dorsal distention at this stage of pregnancy, it is essential that the ventral aspect of each uterine horn be examined. Errors can be made if the fingers are not passed far enough around the cranial aspect of the uterine horn so as to reach well under the uterine body and horns.[194] A ventral bulge that is consistent with a 35- to 45-day pregnancy can be identified by the distinct margins that are palpable when the fingers are moved along the ventral aspect of the uterus. The conceptus becomes more oval as it expands during the third month of pregnancy. At 90 days the chorionic vesicle is comparable in size and shape to a football.[194,195] The mare's age and the number of previous foals will affect the rate of descent of the gravid uterus over the pelvic brim.[195,196] Positive pregnancy diagnosis becomes progressively more difficult as the large, heavy uterus descends into the abdominal cavity. Normal pregnant mares should have a thin, pliable uterine wall, whereas pyometra cases have a thickened uterine wall and viscous purulent fluid in the uterus. The fetus itself is not always palpable before 120 days of gestation, but after that time gentle ballottement will usually reveal the fetus.[194,195] Palpation of some part of the fetus should be able to confirm pregnancy status between 5 months and term.

Blood tests for pregnancy are sometimes indicated, especially in miniature breeds.[100] Measurement of eCG levels verifies that the mare has endometrial cups but does not guarantee that a viable fetus is still present.[3] With this caveat in mind, eCG is suitable for determining pregnancy status in miniature mares between 40 and 100 days after mating.[197] However, mares that have been diagnosed as pregnant should undergo a blood estrone sulfate test 100 or more days after mating to eliminate the possibility of a false-positive diagnosis. Large quantities of estrogen are secreted by the fetoplacental unit.[88,100] Measuring blood estrone sulfate levels is recommended as the method of choice for determining pregnancy status in miniature mares 100 or more days after mating.[198] Fecal estrone sulfate measurements provide a noninvasive alternative to blood testing from 150 days after mating. However, the discrimination between pregnant and nonpregnant levels of estrone sulfate is not as great in feces as it is in blood.[197] An early pregnancy factor (EPF) test has recently been reported to be useful to confirm pregnancy in the mare.[199] EPF is an immunosuppressive protein detected by a rosette inhibition test in the early pregnancy serum. EPF appears in the maternal blood circulation 24 to 72 hours after mating. It can be detected until the second trimester, and after that it disappears from the maternal serum.[199] Unfortunately, the early conception factor (ECF) assay test that has been marketed for horses has not proved to be a reliable method for detecting the presence of an embryo.[200,201]

MANAGEMENT OF TWINS

Monitoring Follicular Development and Ovulation

Most twin pregnancies arise from double ovulations.[202-205] There is a higher incidence of twin ovulations in some breeds (e.g., Thoroughbreds, Warmbloods), and mares that tend to double ovulate can be expected to do this frequently.[3,203,205-209] In one study of 1581 Thoroughbred mares, multiple ovulation occurred in 29.3% of cycles. Multiple ovulation incidence significantly ($p < 0.05$) increased with age (20.7% in 2- to 4-year-olds; 35.6% in 17- to 19-year-olds).[210] Double ovulations may occur on the same day or 2 days apart.[3,211] If a fertile stallion was used to breed the mare on the first ovulation, it is possible that viable sperm will still be present in the reproductive tract when the second oocyte arrives. This possibility must be remembered when scanning mares for pregnancy at 13 to 16 days. At that time it is good practice to scan the ovaries for evidence of luteal tissue from a second ovulation. In a large Thoroughbred study, 25.2% of multiple ovulations were apparent as multiple pregnancies and 37.8% as single pregnancies at 13 to 14 days after ovulation.[210] In another study of English Thoroughbreds, the rate of twin vesicles being present at days 13 through 16 after ovulation was reported as between 10.3% and 13.1%.[212] This was similar to a Swedish study (n = 430) wherein the frequency of twin vesicles at days 14 through 15 was 10.5%.[213]

In the past veterinarians often elected to discourage breeding of a mare when two large (>30-mm) follicles were palpated or to recheck the second follicle 10 to 12 hours after the first detected ovulation.[214] Because an ovulated oocyte is less likely to result in a viable embryo after this time, a delayed breeding could be performed in anticipation of the second ovulation. Today the preferred strategy is to breed all eligible mares—irrespective of the number of preovulatory follicles. The widespread adoption of early ultrasonographic pregnancy examinations has permitted the focus to be placed on embryonic vesicle reduction after the presence of a twin pregnancy is confirmed.[84,215]

Manual Reduction

The increasing size of the embryonic vesicle, coupled with the increasing tone of the early pregnant uterus, tends to fix the conceptus at the base of one uterine horn by day 16.[3] It is essential that the ultrasound scan of the uterus be thorough, with a complete examination of the length of both horns plus the uterine body as far back as the cervix. This is especially important before day 16 because the vesicle moves freely within the lumen of both horns and the uterine body.[211] If twin vesicles are detected, manually separating them before day 16 will be easier. Successful elimination of one vesicle is more likely at that time because the uterine walls are thin and minimal pressure is required to crush a vesicle.[215] A definite *pop* can often be felt when the vesicle ruptures, but success always should be confirmed by ultrasound. This sensation is attributable to the rupture of the embryonic capsule.[5,216]

The downside to this approach is that an early embryonic vesicle can easily be confused with an endometrial cyst. The embryo itself does not become readily identifiable until the fourth week of pregnancy. Thus it is good practice to note the size and location of any cysts at the time the mare is being examined for breeding. If there is no record of cyst size and location, then it is virtually impossible to tell early twin vesicles from a singleton and a cyst with a single examination. This is especially true insofar as asynchronous ovulations are likely to result in considerable size discrepancy between the two vesicles.[3] Under these circumstances it may be best to measure each suspect vesicle and note its location. A second scan in 1 or 2 days should note a size increase in any normally growing vesicle (approximately 4 mm per day).[191] Unfortunately, this delay may make separation of unilaterally fixed vesicles more difficult because of their ongoing growth and the increased uterine tone.

Manual reduction of bilaterally fixed vesicles requires less manipulation than with unilateral twins. It is a relatively easy procedure, and success rates exceeding 90% are not uncommon if the vesicle is crushed before day 16.[213,215,217,218] After fixation a success rate of 75% is still possible if the bilateral twin is crushed before day 30.[215] If the vesicles are unilaterally fixed, then the clinician should attempt to move the more proximal vesicle toward the tip of the uterine horn. At this location the manual reduction procedure is less likely to disrupt the remaining vesicle. The vesicle can be crushed by pinching it between the thumb and fingers. Alternatively, the vesicle is squeezed against the mare's pelvis until it ruptures. If the twins can be separated before crushing, then the success rate may be similar to that for reduction of bilateral twins.[219] If the unilateral twins cannot be separated or are greater than 20 days' gestation, then the success rate is lower.[84] Because of the extra pressure used to eliminate a twin vesicle after fixation, many clinicians administer anti-inflammatory medications and progestin therapy. When crushing is performed within 19 days of conception, significant changes in 15-ketodihydro-PGF ($_2$-α), cortisol, or progesterone plasma concentrations do not seem to occur.[220] The likelihood of success improves with experience.[215,218] If the unilateral vesicles are not detected until after day 20, manipulations can easily result in the disruption of both vesicles. The best option in these cases may be to wait and see whether natural reduction occurs.

Natural Reduction

There is negligible natural reduction of twins before day 15, when the vesicles are close to the end of their mobility phase.[215] Thus manual reduction is the treatment of choice if twins are diagnosed before fixation. Almost three quarters (70%) of twin embryonic vesicles become fixed unilaterally, with only 30% of twin vesicles becoming fixed bilaterally.[221,222] When twin vesicles are dissimilar in size, there appears to be a much higher incidence of unilateral fixation. The larger vesicle is thought to serve as an impediment to the continued mobility of the smaller vesicle.[4] Fortunately, natural reduction to a singleton is far more likely with unilaterally fixed vesicles. More than 80% of unilaterally fixed twins are likely to naturally reduce to a singleton, with over half of these occurring between days 16 and 20.[3,221,222] On the other hand, the majority of bilaterally fixed vesicles will continue to develop. The proposed mechanism for reduction has to do with loss of apposition between the embryo's trophoblastic surface and the endometrium, especially if the embryo proper is adjacent to another vesicle.[4,221,223]

Pregnancy Termination with Prostaglandin

The probability of natural reduction occurring decreases significantly by day 40.[215,224] If natural reduction does not occur, termination of the early pregnancy with a PG injection may be considered. This should lyse the CLs that resulted from the double ovulation, and the precipitous decline in progesterone will bring the mare back into estrus. However, treatment failures have been reported, and successful termination of the pregnancy should be confirmed by ultrasound.[225] Certainly, this treatment must be given before day 35 because once the endometrial cups begin to form, repeated PG injections may be necessary to terminate the pregnancy.[32,226] Owners should be aware that the mare is unlikely to return to normal ovulatory cycles until the cups are sloughed. In the interim they secrete eCG, a hormone that causes the development of accessory CLs.[3] The result is erratic estrous behavior, unreliable follicular development, and unpredictable ovulation.[32]

If a mare carries twins into the latter half of gestation, it is quite likely that abortion will occur between 7 and 9 months. Induced abortion is not without risk, and owners should be aware of the potential for dystocia, cervical lacerations, and fetal membrane retention.[215] Although several researchers have investigated induction of parturition at term, few protocols for early termination of an advanced pregnancy have been published.[215] The natural PG analog cloprostenol has been used at various doses and frequencies, but results are inconsistent with respect to efficiacy and duration to fetal expulsion.[172,215] Daels administered cloprostenol (250 μg) daily until fetal expulsion, or for up to 5 days in mares that were 98 to 153 days pregnant. Fetal expulsion occurred after 2 to 3 cloprostenol administrations.[172] Wolfsdorf used a higher dose of cloprostenol (375 μg IM) at 20-minute intervals for two doses, with repeated daily injections as necessary.[215,227] The addition of intracervical PGE on the second day may help dilate the cervix and hasten delivery.[215,228]

Transvaginal Ultrasound-Guided Twin Reduction

Even though the advent of transrectal ultrasonography has dramatically improved the ability of veterinarians to make an early diagnosis of twin pregnancies, diagnostic errors still occur.[229,230] This could be due to an early pregnancy diagnosis when the second vesicle was too small to detect; incomplete examination of the entire uterus; poor image quality; or an inability of the clinician to differentiate two embryonic vesicles that are closely apposed to each other.[230] If natural reduction does not occur or the diagnosis of twins is not confirmed until after 30 days, transvaginal aspiration of one vesicle is an option.[84,215,231] The results are best if the procedure is performed before day 35, preferably before day 25.[84,215,231] Although spontaneous reduction of twin pregnancies can occur even after day 40, the probability of this occurring is low.[50,224,232] Natural twin reduction is more likely to occur if an obvious size discrepancy between the two vesicles is present at this time.[215,221,223]

If a transvaginal reduction is to be attempted, the mare should be treated with flunixin meglumine. Many clinicians will also administer oral altrenogest. Because sedation causes significant uterine relaxation, most clinicians use a lidocaine enema to reduce straining.[233] The transvaginal aspiration technique employs a 5.0- or 7.5-MHz endovaginal curvilinear transducer. The transducer and casing should be cold-disinfected or sterilized before use. The assembled unit is then placed in a sterile transducer cover that has been filled with sterile lubricating gel. The transducer is advanced aseptically until it is seated lateral to the cervix. The clinician grasps the pregnancy rectally and advances a sterile, 60-cm, 18-gauge spinal needle with an echogenic tip along the needle guide in the transducer casing. A dotted line on the ultrasound screen can be used to select a path for the needle entry into the embryonic vesicle. A sharp jab of the needle penetrates the vaginal wall, peritoneal lining, uterus, and ultimately the allantoic or yolk sac. A 60-ml syringe is attached to the needle, and the embryonic fluid is aspirated. Aspiration should be stopped when there is a danger of damaging the adjacent vesicle of unicornuate twins. If a bilateral twin is being eliminated, the needle can be moved within the vesicle until all detectable fluid has been aspirated.[84,215] The success rate is better for bicornuate twin reductions.[233] Death of the remaining twin is most likely to occur within 2 weeks of the procedure. Although reports are scarce, preliminary data suggest that experienced operators may achieve a live singleton birth in about one third of cases.[215]

Craniocervical Dislocation

Results of postfixation twin reduction techniques have been inconsistent with regard to producing a single healthy foal. A craniocervical dislocation method recently was proposed. The procedure entails dislocating the first cervical vertebra from the cranium, disrupting the ligamentous attachments, and severing the spinal cord.[215] A transrectal approach may be performed on a sedated mare between 60 and 90 days. Propantheline bromide (30 mg IV) is recommended to relax the smooth muscles of the uterus and rectum, and flunixin meglumine (1 mg/kg) is administered to inhibit PG release. Daily altrenogest (0.088 mg/kg) is suggested for 3 to 4 weeks. A surgical procedure has been used on twin pregnancies of between 2 to 4 months' duration, when attempts at the technically difficult transrectal reduction have been unsuccessful.[215] This new technique enables the twin to be reduced before complete placenta formation has occurred, allowing the remaining fetus to use the entire endometrial surface and to grow to its full potential.[215]

Transcutaneous (Abdominal) Ultrasound-Guided Fetal Puncture

In advanced twin pregnancies (up to approximately 5.5 months), it is possible to attempt reduction by a transabdominal approach.* Fetal intracardiac injection of potassium chloride (KCl) is effective but requires accurate placement of the KCl into the fetal heart. Best results are obtained when the pregnancy is between 115 and 130 days.[236] At this stage experienced operators can achieve a 50% success rate.[219] Procaine penicillin G (PPG) can cause fetal death when injected into either the fetal thorax or abdomen, but the effect is not instantaneous. The advantage of the latter treatment is that it does not require precise placement of the injection into the fetal heart.[219,226] PPG also reduces the likelihood of bacterial infection, and the injection can be visualized on the ultrasound screen.[226] The author has managed a case that aborted the twins along with mucopurulent exudate, and it is likely that infection resulted from bacterial contamination at the time of the fetal injection. Mares should be started on oral altrenogest, systemic antibiotics, and flunixin meglumine on the day of the procedure. The antibiotic coverage and anti-inflammatory medication should be continued for 3 days.[84,226]

A 3.0-mHz transducer can be used to image the 90- to 130-day fetus in the caudal abdomen, just cranial to the udder, and best results may be obtained after day 115.[226,230] Once the mare has been sedated, the uterus will relax and the location of the fetuses will shift cranially. A sedative-analgesic combination that works well for this procedure is acepromazine (10 mg), xylazine (100 mg), and butorphanol (10 mg).[215,230] The smallest or most easily accessible fetus is selected for reduction. The ventral abdomen should be surgically prepared, and local anesthetic infiltrated at the puncture site. An 18-gauge, 8-inch spinal needle with stylet can be used for most fetal injections, but the length of the needle is detemined by the depth of the fetus from the abdominal wall.[215,226,230] Specialized needles with echogenic tips are available to provide better visualization via ultrasound.[219] Once the location of the selected twin's thorax is confirmed, the needle is introduced through the prepared skin, abdominal wall, and uterus. If PPG is to be injected, the needle may puncture either the fetal thorax or abdomen. Up to 20 ml is typically injected into the fetus.[219,230] Fetal death should be confirmed the next day.[226]

Although the benefits of supplemental progestin therapy are debatable, many clinicians suggest that the mare be medicated for at least 2 weeks if the initial twin reduction has been successful.[226,230] It is essential that fetal viability be checked regularly because supplemental progestin therapy may prevent elimination of the dead fetuses if both die.[237] Most abortions occur within 1 to 2 months after the reduction procedure.[84] If the operator is experienced in the technique, between 40% and 60% of cases can be expected to deliver a viable singleton foal.[215,219,230] The eliminated twin in these cases can be seen as a mummified remnant contained within an invaginated pouch that protrudes into the allantoic space of the viable foal's fetal membranes.[215,226,235] One theory for the loss of both twins after an intrafetal injection has to do with the presence of vascular anastomoses between the two fetoplacental units.[238] It has been suggested that circulation of either the injected solution or other tissue degradation products could result in the death of the adjoining twin fetus.[230] Small anastomosing vessels are present between twin vesicles as early as 40 to 60 days' gestation.[239]

Early Pregnancy Loss and Abortion

Embryonic Loss

Once conception has occurred, any pregnancy failure up to day 40 of gestation is defined as being early embryonic loss.[3] Between 10% and 15% of mares undergo embryonic loss or abortion at some time in gestation, and most of these losses occur during the first 40 days of gestation, when the primary CL is the sole source of progesterone.[102,212] However, all the available evidence suggests that untoward luteolysis is not common in this period, and the losses that do occur have other underlying causes.[102] In a study of 376 Thoroughbred pregnancies, 12.2% experienced embryonic loss within 45 days after ovulation,[240] whereas a much larger study (n = 3,373 mares) reported a loss of 7.2 to 8.0% by day 42.[212] Three quarters of the losses in the smaller study occurred between 16 and 25 days, and the loss was highest in previously barren mares, followed by aged mares (>15 years) and mares of more than 10 parities.[241] These results were similar to those reported in a Swedish study.[213] Increasing mare age was the single biggest limiting factor to an otherwise high rate of fertility in the larger study of

*References 84, 215, 219, 226, 234, 235.

well-managed English Thoroughbreds.[212] A higher embryonic loss may be expected in mares that are bred during the first postpartum estrus and in those with cysts in the uterus.[240]

Fertilization failure rates and embryonic losses are higher in aged mares.[242-246] It is not easy to differentiate between fertilization failure and embryonic loss before day 10 because this is the earliest stage of development wherein ultrasonographic detection is possible under ideal research conditions. Fertilization rates in young, well-managed mares may exceed 90% and appear to be over 80% in aged mares.[245,247] Oocytes from aged mares may be more likely to result in nonviable embryos because of inherent morphologic defects.[245,248] Carnevale transferred oocytes from young and aged mares into young recipients so that fertilization and early embryonic development occurred in an optimal oviductal environment. The day 12 pregnancy rate in the recipients that received the oocytes from aged mares was significantly less than that achieved with the younger mares' oocytes.[249] Research has shown that embryo recovery rates are considerably lower in aged mares and that there are significant losses occurring before day 14 of pregnancy.[243,250-252] The uterine environment may not be the only reason for subfertility in some mares. Embryos collected from normal mares resulted in similar pregnancy rates in both fertile and subfertile recipients (significant uterine pathology) at day 28.[253] In a reversal of study design, embryos were collected from the oviducts of normal and subfertile mares 4 days after ovulation, then transferred into normal recipients. Pregnancy rates were lower in those normal mares that received embryos from the subfertile donors.[250] Thus, although the uterine environment may have a delayed effect on embryonic and fetal loss, it appears that oocyte quality and oviductal influences play a significant role in the problem of subfertility and early embryonic loss in mares.[254] In practice, embryonic losses that may be detected between days 14 and 40 can range between 8% to 15% in young, well-managed mares to 25% or 30% in aged mares.[212,247,255] The presence of endometrial inflammation and uterine fluid accumulation will have a detrimental effect on early embryo survival and can markedly increase the likelihood of early pregnancy loss.[240,256,257]

Early Fetal Loss

Formation of the endometrial cups is a defining moment with regard to early pregnancy loss in mares. If the embryo dies before day 35, the chorionic girdle cells do not invade the endometrium and the endometrial cups do not form. These mares should return to normal estrous cycle activity and may be successfully bred again during the same breeding season. However, if the fetus is lost after day 40, the endometrial cups are irreversibly established.[3] Thus, if an assay for eCG (a MIP test) is performed after the endometrial cups form, a false-positive test for pregnancy will be obtained until the endometrial cups are sloughed between days 120 and 140 after the original conception occurred.[3] Retention of the endometrial cups after fetal loss results in erratic estrous behavior, unreliable follicular development, and unpredictable ovulation.[32] Thus this unique physiologic mechanism typically prevents mares suffering fetal loss after endometrial cup formation from being bred back during the current breeding season.[85]

A large study of Throughbred mares revealed an overall pregnancy loss of only 4% to 6% between day 40 and day 150 of gestation and then only a further 2% to 3% until term.[212] The exact mechanism that causes most pregnancy losses in the mare remains to be elucidated but may include chromosomal errors and endometrosis.[44,51,212,258] Beyond day 40 the secondary CLs receive powerful luteotrophic support from eCG, and from day 80 to day 100 until term the supply organ (placenta) and target tissues (endometrium and myometrium) are in direct contact with one another over their entire surfaces.[32,102] Little evidence suggests that a deficiency of progesterone production is a cause of pregnancy loss in the mare.[102] Certainly, fetal death may follow uteroplacental insufficiency, or an overwhelming sepsis.[212,258] In recent years there has been a broad consensus that the inflammatory mediator PGF_2-α may play an integral role in many cases.[107] It is well known that PGs are luteolytic.[3] Thus, in the first 70 to 80 days, when the pregnancy depends on progesterone production by the CLs (primary and accessory), it is especially susceptible to the luteolytic effects of PGs. However, it is important to remember that repeated exogenous PG injections may be required to electively terminate a pregnancy once the endometrial cups have formed. This is because some of the immature accessory CLs may not be sufficiently developed to respond to the first PG injection.[32] Another probable abortogenic feature of PGs may be myometrial hypermotility. This may be associated with placental inflammation or high systemic levels of PG.[259]

An early pregnancy may be lost subsequent to PG-induced luteal deficiency associated with endotoxemia.[260-262] The detrimental effect of the endotoxin could be prevented only if a cyclooxygenase inhibitor (flunixin meglumine) was administered before clinical signs of endotoxemia were evident.[82,261,263,264] Thus, although gram negative septicemia and endotoxemia associated with many gastrointestinal crises are known to result in elevated levels of inflammatory mediators, any pregnancy-sparing effect of PG inhibitors is likely to be effective only if anti-inflammatory agents such as flunixin meglumine are administered in the acute phase of the disease.[258] Because a healthy fetoplacental unit can produce enough progesterone to sustain the pregnancy after 80 days of gestation, the concept of prophylactic altrenogest past 3 months of gestation is controversial.[82,102,107,172,265]

Although recent in vitro studies suggest that progesterone may not be the primary regulator of myometrial quiescence, in situations where elevated PG levels are likely there appears to be adequate clinical justification at present to provide exogenous progestagen support for high-risk pregnant mares.[89,181] Based on our current knowledge, the administration of a double-dose (0.088 mg/kg/day) of altrenogest is suggested during the acute phase of a medical or surgical condition when PG levels are likely to be elevated.[182] If oral medication is not possible, short-term use of progesterone in oil (300 mg/day IV) is warranted. An intramuscular injection of a compounded long-acting progesterone formulation (BioRelease P4 LA 150) every 7 days may also be an efficacious and suitable alternative to currently available progesterone formulations that require daily administration.[266] Administration of supplemental progesterone is based on further work by Daels et al. demonstrating that progestin treatment could prevent PG-induced abortion at 3 to 5 months of gestation if a higher dose (0.088 mg altrenogest per kg) of progestin was administered.[82,172] Abortion did not occur in five of eight progesterone-treated mares and eight of eight altrenogest-treated mares, and endogenous PGF_2-α secretion was inhibited, compared with values in aborting mares.[172] It was concluded that circulating progestagen concentrations may play a role in the outcome of pregnancy during PG-induced abortion, as may occur after exposure to endotoxin.

It seems logical that separation of the chorioallantois from the endometrium will disrupt local endocrine function.[267] The fetoplacental unit does attempt to compensate for this placental dysfunction by increasing progesterone production.[89,268] However, endotoxemia may harm placental circulation and disrupt vital steroid metabolism within the fetoplacental unit.[269] Thus administration of flunixin meglumine to pregnant mares is indicated early in the course of any condition in which endotoxemia is possible.[263,270,272] If a mare develops a surgical colic condition during late pregnancy, the fetus is at risk not only from the maternal endotoxemia that can be associated with gastrointestinal crises but also from any maternal hypoxic episodes that may occur during anesthesia.[269,270,272,273] Acute enteritis or colitis in a pregnant mare can also result in abortion caused by the effects of endotoxemia.[272,273] Because maternal hypoxia is a risk factor for abortion, intraoperative hypoxia must be avoided if a pregnant mare requires surgery.[272] Approximately 16% to 20% of mares can be expected to abort after colic surgery, but superior intraoperative ventilatory techniques may reduce this risk.[272,273] Stage of gestation and duration of anesthesia are less critical factors if maternal oxygenation is adequate.[274] Apparently, aberrations in the cardiovascular and metabolic status of the mare and fetus are more detrimental to pregnancy maintenance than the actual medical or surgical condition.[271]

PLACENTITIS

Placentitis is a major cause of abortion in mares during the latter part of pregnancy.[229,275,276] Inflammation of the placenta can affect the interchange of gases, nutrients, and waste products along with disruption of both fetal metabolic and endocrinologic pathways.[277] The disease tends to be a sporadic, individual mare problem that seldom has any lasting effect on mare fertility.[278] Both bacterial (*S. zooepidemicus, Streptococcus equisimilis, E. coli, Enterobacter agglomerans, P. aeruginosa, K. pneumoniae)* and fungal (*Aspergillus* spp.) organisms may be incriminated.[49,196,267,279-283] Ascending infections are especially common, and these tend to result in a necrotizing, suppurative inflammation with detachment of the placenta in the area surrounding the cervical star.[283,284] The cervix is almost invariably softened, with purulent exudates draining into the vagina.[267,279,280] Thus this part of the fetal membranes should be closely examined whenever a mare aborts. The vestibular sphincter and vulvar lips are important barriers to ascending infections, and many aged mares require a Caslick procedure to reduce the likelihood of ascending infections. Hematogenous infection of the placenta is also possible.[279,280] *Leptospira* spp. induce a diffuse placentitis with large numbers of spirochetes in the placental tissues (see separate discussion).[285,286] A recent report incriminated *Rhodococcus equi* as the cause of placentitis that resulted in abortion.[287] *Mycoplasma* spp. have been associated with infertility, endometritis, vulvitis, and abortion in mares.[288]

A unique form of placentitis was reported as being a sporadic cause of abortion and weak foals in central Kentucky during the 1990s.[229,275,282,287,289-291] A review of nocardioform actinomycetes–related placentitis cases over a 9-year period (1990 to 1999) revealed that of the farms that had cases, 83% had two or fewer over the 9 years and 66% of the farms had only a single case during that time.[291] The number of nocardioform placentitis cases in central Kentucky has since decreased significantly, with only 93 cases being reported over six foaling seasons (2001-2007).[282] The causative organisms have recently been identified as *Crossiella equi* and *Amycolatopsis* spp.[289,292-294] These bacteria are responsible for nocardioform placentitis and are among the few actinomycetes known to cause disease in animals. Although numerous gram positive branching bacilli can be seen on histologic sections, the bacteria are seldom present in fetal tissue.[286,291,295] In vitro testing has demonstrated that the nocardioform bacteria are susceptible to sulfonamides and trimethoprim.[286] This combination is an ideal choice for systemic medication of a pregnant mare when placentitis is suspected because these antimicrobial agents are known to gain acceptable levels in the fetal fluids.[296-298]

Nocardioform placentitis was first diagnosed at the University of Kentucky in 1986 and has since been confirmed elsewhere in the United States and in other countries.[286,294,295,299,300] Although it has been suggested that the organism may gain access to the uterus at breeding, this unusual form of equine placentitis does not become apparent until the latter part of gestation.[278] The initial lesion is localized on the most dependent aspect of the chorion, in the cranioventral aspect of the uterine body, and then extends cranially onto the base of the horns and circumferentially around the placenta.[282,301] Outcomes vary from abortion to birth of a normal foal. Some foals are premature, whereas others are delivered at term but are either stillborn or weak and compromised, with an emaciated appearance.[282,286,301] Most affected mares appear normal, although many display signs of placentitis (premature mammary development and lactation).[278,286,291,301] Vaginal discharge is not a feature of this condition because the area around the cervical star is not involved. Once the fetus has been expelled, these mares rapidly clear the infection and experience no adverse effects on subsequent fertility.[286,291] When the fetal membranes are examined, there is an obvious line of demarcation between diseased and normal tissue, with the affected area being covered by a characteristic thick, brownish mucoid, viscous material.[286] The underlying chorionic villi are reduced in size and, in the central portion of the lesion, the chorionic surface may be completely denuded.[301]

A recent report from the University of Kentucky Livestock Disease Diagnostic Center suggests that two newly emerging abortigenic pathogens should be considered when placentitis is suspected.[282] Six cases of mycobacterial abortion and placentitis were confirmed by microbiologic, polymerase chain reaction (PCR), and histochemical staining procedures. The atypical mycobacteria were within the nontuberculous group and are classified as saprophytic and opportunistic microorganisms acquired from the environment (soil, water, decaying vegetation).[282] Gross lesions observed within the submitted cases varied from none to those of a "nocardioform-like" placentitis. Affected fetuses exhibited varying degrees of malnourishment and chronic placentitis. Several fetuses had granulomatous to pyogranulomatous pneumonia, and one fetus without pneumonia contained disseminated granulomas in various organs.[282] The other emerging organism is *Cellulosimicrobium cellulans,* a gram positive branching bacillus that is an opportunistic microorganism found in the soil.[282] The nine equine cases of abortion and placentitis resulting from *C. cellulans* described had nocardioform-like placentitis lesions as well as granulomatous pneumonia. Because atypical *Mycobacteria* and *C. cellulans* organisms can cause similar gross and histologic lesions within the fetus and placenta, they should be considered as differential diagnoses when encountering gross placental lesions suggestive of nocardioform placentitis.[282]

Placentitis continues to represent a significant problem and is a common cause of equine abortions.[282,283] Placental thickening and separation from the endometrium are consistent features in many abortions.[229] Placentitis is detrimental to the pregnancy not only because it disrupts nutrient exchange but also because of the inflammatory mediators (proinflammatory cytokines) that are released. The exact cause of fetal expulsion is not known, but ensuring myometrial quiescence is central to most therapeutic regimens.[184,302] Placentitis cases have substantially increased concentrations of PGF_2-α and PGE_2 in the allantoic fluid.[303,304] Thus anti-inflammatory medication (flunixin meglumine at 1.1 mg/kg; phenylbutazone at 4 mg/kg, every 12 hours) is indicated.[259,305] Placentitis associated with early abortions tends to be acute, with the fetus succumbing to bacteremia.[284] Broad spectrum antibiotics that have been recommended include trimethoprim-sulfadiazine (15-30 mg/kg PO every 12 hours), procaine penicillin (30,000 IU/kg/day) and gentamicin (6 mg/kg/day), and ceftiofur (1 to 5 mg/kg, every 12 hours).[259,297,298,305,306] Gentamicin was undetectable in the plasma of newborn foals after mares were treated with the antibiotic (6.6 mg/kg) an hour before parturition, and it was initially believed that gentamicin does not cross the placenta of mares at term.[307] More recently, Murchie et al. monitored drug concentrations in the allantoic fluid of pregnant pony mares using in vivo microdialysis to determine whether this method could detect allantoic concentrations of drugs in normal mares and those with placentitis.[308,309] Pharmacokinetic comparisons indicated that potassium penicillin G (22,000 IU/kg, administered 4 times daily) persists much longer in allantoic fluid than blood, whereas gentamicin (6.6 mg/kg/day) exhibited similar profiles in the two compartments. Flunixin meglumine (1 mg/kg b.i.d.) was not detected in allantoic fluid.[309] In infected mares penicillin G achieved a similar peak concentration in allantoic fluid, whereas peak gentamicin concentration appeared to be reduced relative to drug concentrations in noninfected mares. Thus penicillin G and gentamicin appear to undergo effective placental transfer in pregnant mares, but transplacental drug transfer may be altered selectively if active placental infection is present.[308,309]

If the localized production of high concentrations of PGs stimulates the formation of gap junctions, then the subsequent myometrial hypermotility may impede placental blood flow as the uterus contracts.[107,184,302,310] This will reduce fetal oxygenation and increase fetal stress. Because it is known that progesterone inhibits gap junction formation, it is clinically valid to conclude that progestin supplementation may be beneficial when uteroplacental inflammation is suspected. This is the rationale behind the current recommendation to treat suspected placentitis cases with a double dose of altrenogest (0.088 mg/kg/day).[107,259,268,305] Delaying premature labor long enough to allow accelerated fetal maturation to occur may improve foal survival rates.[283] The progestagens may also enhance the activity of the endometrial enzyme 15-hydroxyprostaglandin dehydrogenase and thus promote rapid metabolism of PGs into inactive metabolites.[83,89,105] Although altrenogest is not metabolized to 5α-pregnanes, both 5α-DHP and 3β-5P levels may be increased as a result of supplementation.[311] However, Ousey has suggested that progesterone supplementation may be contraindicated because high levels could inhibit the placental enzyme 3β-hydroxysteroid dehydrogenase.[83,89,114,312] This enzyme produces progesterone from pregnenolone, and thus inhibition could interfere with the normal fetoplacental steroidogenic pathway.[83,89] Thus at present this widely used therapy remains controversial, and even if it does no harm, the expense of long-term progestin supplementation may not be warranted in many cases.[83,102] Essentially, the use of hormone therapies is subjective and reflects, to a large extent, our lack of understanding about the endocrine relations among the mare, placenta, and fetus.[83,89,303] Recent studies suggest that measurement of relaxin levels may serve as a useful means of monitoring placental function and treatment efficacy in the mare.[313-315]

The rationale for other treatment regimens is based on extrapolations from the human-medicine literature and application of sound reasoning for the potential efficacy of a particular drug. Scientific investigation in this area is crucial. Many equine clinicians have been advocating the use of an oral β_2-sympathomimetic drug (clenbuterol) to suppress uterine motility.[259,305,316] In the United States the product is marketed as an oral formulation to treat chronic reactive airway obstruction. Research is needed to determine what oral dose of this bronchodilatory compound—if any—is actually effective on the gravid uterus. In countries where an intravenous formulation is available, a 300-μg intravenous dose of clenbuterol will reduce uterine tone for approximately 2 hours.[317-319] However, daily intravenous administration of clenbuterol to mares showing maximal milk calcium levels was not effective in preventing the onset of myometrial contractions and delivery in normal foaling mares at term.[320] The administration of pentoxyfylline (8.5 mg/kg PO b.i.d.) is recommended, on the basis of its use in treating tissue ischemia in humans and its ability to modulate the inflammatory process by downregulating proinflammatory cytokines.[259,283,297,305,321] Pentoxifylline increases erythrocyte flexibility. Inflammation-driven uterine hypermotility may impede circulation in the placental capillary bed, and it is thought that this drug may increase fetal oxygenation by facilitating blood flow.[322,323] Pentoxyfylline appears to have good uterine penetration and has been detected in the allantoic fluid of mares.[283,297,298,306] Despite these conflicting studies, data from a large field trial suggest that a multipronged approach (i.e., antibiotics, anti-inflammatory agents, altrenogest) to long-term therapy for placentitis may improve fetal survival and foal viability.[324]

Leptospirosis

Leptospirosis has been incriminated as a sporadic cause of placentitis, abortion, and premature births in horses.[229,275,290,325-337] Leptospiral infections may cause abortions in the latter part of gestation, generally with no premonitory clinical signs, and occasionally an infected premature or full-term weak, icteric foal.[325,327,330,331,333] The placenta is edematous, with a necrotic chorion covered with a mucoid exudate.[286] The gross placental lesions are associated with thrombosis, vasculitis, and inflammatory cell infiltrates. The spirochetes tend to be numerous and are readily demonstrated in the stroma and villi of the placenta.[333,338] A microscopic agglutination test (MAT) on fetal fluids (heart and body cavities) or maternal serum is likely to reveal a high titer (1:6400-1:819,200 or greater).[286,327] Leptospires may be detected in the fetus by the fluorescent antibody test (FAT), silver staining, or darkfield microscopy.[286,337] Immunohistochemistry is more sensitive than silver staining and more specific than serology (MAT).[337,339] The fetal kidney should be submitted for a FAT because this tissue yields the highest percentage of positive results and is also the best tissue for culture.[286,327] If urine is to be submitted from an infected mare (FAT or darkfield analysis), it is important to obtain collection instructions and an appropriate transport medium from the diagnostic laboratory.[286] The specimen must be obtained before any antimicrobial therapy has been administered.

In the genus *Leptospira,* the species *L. interrogans* contains several pathogenic serogroups (common antigens) and serovars (specific strain). Serogroups consist of closely related serovars. The predominant serovar affecting horses varies with country and region.[337] The *bratislava* serovar is most commonly isolated from aborted fetuses in Northern Ireland, but in central Kentucky most leptospiral abortions have been associated with the *pomona* serogroup, occasionally the *grippotyphosa* serogroup, and rarely the *hardjo* serogroup.[325,327,329] Equine leptospiral infections previously reported as being *L. pomona* are now thought to be more correctly identified as *L. interrogans* serogroup *pomona* serovar *kennewicki* and *L. kirschneri* serogroup *grippotyphosa* serovar *grippotyphosa.*[286,336,337,340] On the basis of recent serologic testing, those two serovars are thought to be responsible for 83% and 10% of leptospiral abortions, respectively.[337] In North America pregnant mares are considered to be incidental hosts that become infected after exposure from maintenance hosts (i.e., wildlife such as skunks and raccoons for *kennewicki* and *grippotyphosa* and cattle for *hardjo*).[286,325,327] Infected mares may shed leptospires in the urine for up to 14 weeks.[286,337] Thus therapy is aimed at prevention of urinary shedding and possibly prophylactic treatment of pregnant in-contact mares that have high titers.[286,337] A combination of penicillin (10,000 to 15,000 IU/kg, administered intramuscularly) and streptomycin (10 mg/kg administered intramuscularly) every 12 hours for a period of 1 week has been recommended, but streptomycin is no longer widely used in equine practice.[286,332,341] High doses of potassium penicillin G (20 million units, IV every 12 hours) may be effective in preventing infection of a fetus if the mare has a high titer, but this recommendation has not been validated in controlled studies.[337,341] The dosage and duration of treatment appear to be important. Oxytetracycline (5 to 10 mg/kg) has also been suggested, but it was less effective at preventing urinary shedding of leptospires in all cases tested (5 of 7 infected mares).[286,332,341] There is no approved vaccine available for the prevention of leptospirosis in horses in North America.[337] Attempts should be made to prevent direct contact between maintenance hosts and pregnant mares and also to prevent exposure to urine infected by these species (e.g., contaminated water and feed).[337] It may be prudent to vaccinate cattle with a multivalent vaccine if they are present on the same property as pregnant mares.[286]

Protozoal Abortion

There is limited information available on the association between equine *Neospora* infections and abortions.[342-345] However, the apicomplexan protozoan parasite *Neospora caninum* has been recognized as a major cause of abortion in cattle.[346] A recent European study documented the prevalence of antibodies against *Neospora* spp. in mares that recently aborted.[347] Using an agglutination test, researchers found that the number of animals with elevated (>80) anti–Neospora sp. antibody titer was higher in a group of 54 aborted mares than in a randomly chosen group of 121 mares ($p < 0.001$). *N. caninum* deoxyribonucleic acid (DNA) was found in 3 of 91 fetal brains, 2 of 77 fetal hearts, and 1 of 1 placenta and present in both brains and hearts of two fetuses.[347] The mere presence of the organism in an aborted fetus does not necessarily implicate it as being the cause of the abortion.[346] Antibodies to *Neospora* spp. were detected in the sera from 11.9% of 800 asymptomatic horses in Israel and from 37.5% of mares that aborted.[348] Antibodies to *Neospora* spp. have also been detected in mares in Brazil.[343] Further investigations will be needed to determine whether there is an association between equine reproductive failure and *Neospora* spp. infection.[342,343]

Mare Reproductive Loss Syndrome

In the spring of 2001, the equine breeding industry in central Kentucky was faced with a reproductive crisis that ultimately cost hundreds of millions of dollars, and the impact on the Thoroughbred industry is still being felt. Mares were foaling prematurely with premature separation of the chorioallantois (late-term "red bag" abortions). Many mares that were approximately 45 to 80 days pregnant suffered acute fetal loss, and most affected mares failed to resume normal cyclic activity until after the official breeding season had closed because endometrial cups had been formed before the occurrence of mare reproductive loss syndrome (MRLS). In addition, an unusual number of weak foals were born.[349,350] The Appalachian region to the north also reported a high number of similar cases. The author investigated more than 150 late-term abortions in southeast Ohio during the spring of 2001.[351] Reports of weather patterns and an unusually high emergence of Eastern tent caterpillars (ETCs; *Malacosoma americanum)* were identical in both the central Kentucky and southeast Ohio regions.[351,352] The epidemic that affected the horse industry in the Ohio Valley in late April and early May of 2001 and 2002 became known as MRLS.[349]

During the initial outbreak the state diagnostic laboratory was inundated with late-term aborted fetuses, and practitioners identified approximately 2000 early fetal losses.[353] Many of these were detected during what should have been a routine fetal gender determination. Fortunately, no contagious infectious cause was identified, and this newly recognized disease became self-limiting as the breeding season progressed. Veterinarians and scientists involved in the epidemic considered the possibility of mycotoxins, ergot alkaloids, phytoestrogens, and even cyanide from wild cherry tree foliage.[354-356] A temporal correlation was established between MRLS and the presence of ETCs was identified.[349,350,354,357-369] Mares inadvertently ingest ETCs when large numbers are present on pasture, hay, or in the water supply.[368] Abortions consistent with MRLS can be induced by oral administration of whole ETCs or their exoskeletons, which contain hairs (setae).[354,366,367] Setae embed into the submucosa of the gastrointestinal tract. Fetal loss occurs when bacteria from the alimentary tract (streptococci, actinobacilli) establish infection where the local immune system is compromised—the fetoplacental unit.[367-369] Management strategies for controlling ETC have been proposed to reduce the risk of MRLS.[353,362] A similar abortion syndrome in Australia is associated with ingestion of hairy processionary caterpillars *(Ochragaster lunifer).*[370]

Viral Abortions

Equine arteritis virus (EAV) and equine herpesvirus 1 (EHV1) are the most important causes of viral abortion in horses in the United States. Both viruses are associated with acute respiratory tract infection and are discussed in detail in Chapter 9.

EAV is transmitted through inhalation or venereally in the semen of asymptomatic ("shedder") stallions.[371-375] Abortion may occur if pregnant mares become infected in the later stage of gestation (5-10 months).[373,375-377] Clinical signs are variable but may include fever, conjunctivitis, nasal discharge, and dependent edema that is associated with the vasculitis.[374,377-379] Clinical signs are mild or subclinical in many horses and may be clinically indistinguishable from other respiratory infections.[380] Viral myometritis with degeneration of myocytes and infiltration of mononuclear cells leads to transplacental infection of the fetus.[381] Affected placentae are edematous, and degenerated fibroblasts may be observed in the subvillous layers.[381] Lesions in the fetal tissue include an atrophy of the lymphoid follicles in the spleen and lymph nodes with degenerated lymphocytes.[381] Immunofluorescence can detect EAV antigen in the myometrium and the endometrial glands in the dams, in the subvillous layer of the placentae, and in the aborted fetuses.[381] The virus may be recovered from the uterus and fetus, but the placenta is likely to yield the greatest amounts of the virus.[381] The disease may be controlled by an effective vaccination program and screening tests.[371]

Most abortions associated with herpesvirus are caused by EHV1, but occasional abortions are associated with EHV2, EHV4, and EHV5.[276,382] The number of abortions resulting from EHV1 infection has declined over the past 20 years, and isolated abortions, rather than abortion storms, are now a more common feature of this disease.[383] This is due to the widespread adoption of stringent vaccination programs in combination with improved management practices on broodmare farms.[384,385] Pregnant mares should be vaccinated with an approved vaccine at 5, 7, and 9 months of gestation. Many farms also vaccinate at 3 months. New arrivals should be isolated for 3 weeks, and groups of pregnant mares should be isolated by stage of gestation. It is especially important to segregate pregnant mares from weanlings and other horses.[386]

EHV1 can infect the fetus if a mare is viremic during pregnancy. The virus causes abortion as a result of the rapid detachment of the placenta.[387,388] Endothelial cells in the endometrium and allantochorion are often infected by the virus, with accompanying vascular lesions. The fetus can be infected by way of the chorionic vasculature or by inhalation of infected amniotic fluid.[389-391] Abortion may occur soon after the mare is infected or several weeks have elapsed. Therefore maternal serology is of little diagnostic value.[392] The aborted fetus will be fresh, with copious amounts of pleural and peritoneal fluid. The trachea may contain a fibrin clot. Small necrotic foci may be discernible on the swollen liver. A hyperplastic, necrotizing bronchiolitis may be seen in lung sections, and large intranuclear eosinophilic inclusion bodies are a characteristic histologic lesion. Although vaccination is widely practiced, owners should be aware that the protection is not absolute. If a pregnant mare is exposed to infected animals that have recently been to a show or that are returning from a training facility, it is possible that any protective immunity possibly conferred by the vaccine will be overwhelmed. Abortions have been associated with reactivation of latent virus that was induced by transport stress.[393] Therefore a history of regular vaccination of an aborting mare does not eliminate the possibility of a herpesvirus-related abortion. Neutralization and indirect immunofluorescence tests, as well as PCR and virus isolation, are used for EHV1 diagnostics. Antigen detection, in combination with virus isolation and PCR from fetal lungs, gives reliable results.[394] More detailed reviews have been published.[196,395]

A number of other acute viral infections have been associated with abortion in horses, especially if the horse suffers severe systemic illness at the time of initial infection. For example, mares may abort as a result of the systemic effects of acute infection with equine infectious anemia virus (EIAV), although it is not generally considered an abortigenic virus.[396] When widespread vaccination against West Nile virus was adopted in the United States, some suggested that the killed virus vaccine that was used might result in abortions, stillbirths, and deformities in foals. However, subsequent critical review clearly demonstrates that vaccination of pregnant mares during any period of gestation is not associated with an increased incidence of pregnancy loss.[397]

Noninfectious Causes of Abortion

TWINS

In North America the incidence of twin abortions has decreased significantly because of early intervention after ultrasonographic diagnosis of a multiple pregnancy.[84,215,229] Before the widespread adoption of this technology, twin abortions were a major cause of fetal loss.[49,50] A large European study (n = 12,648 pregnancies) of Thoroughbred mares revealed a twinning rate of 3.5%, with 443 twins and only two triplets.[398] The type of placentation in the mare (diffuse, microcotyledonary) makes it highly unlikely that a twin pregnancy will be carried to term. Obviously, there is a finite endometrial surface area available for allantochorion attachment. The more common unicornuate twin vesicles are a problem, because one conceptus is inevitably restricted to the proximal aspect of the gravid horn.[21,255] Thus the two conceptuses are literally in a deadly competition for adequate nourishment and subsequent placentation. If the twin pregnancy is maintained until the latter part of gestation, the nutrient demands of the rapidly growing fetuses outstrip the placental attachments. Fetal growth is such that nutrient demands may be met until the latter half of gestation, when the marked fetal development in the last trimester usually requires more exchange capability than the smaller placenta provides. The fetus becomes stressed as it becomes progressively emaciated and ultimately dies.[215,232] Death of one fetus or both fetuses is followed by abortion, with the characteristic avillous areas on the fetal membranes confirming the amount of placental disruption.[50,208,226,229] Affected mares develop premature mammary enlargement and may "run" milk before aborting.[50,399] Transabdominal ultrasonographic evaluation may be useful to confirm the diagnosis at this late stage.[226] Although the area of apposition of the two chorioallantoic membranes (twin membrane) may be seen, measurement of fetal thoracic diameters and heart rates can confirm the twin diagnosis.[226,232] Twin abortions in the last few months of gestation are likely to cause a dystocia. Bicornuate twins are more likely to survive because each membrane can attach to an entire horn and one side of the uterine body, but the resulting foals are likely to be stunted as a result of intrauterine growth retardation (IUGR).[4,50,215] The live birth of twin foals is extremely uncommon, and many of these neonates do not survive, with as few as 14% of surviving foals reaching the second week of neonatal life.[50,217] The mares are prone to fetal membrane retention and may be difficult to rebreed.

Thus it is not surprising that the equine breeding industry has always tried to prevent twin pregnancies. After such a diagnosis the owner is faced with three choices: attempt elimination of one fetus in utero, manage the pregnancy to term in the remote hope of two viable foals, or induce abortion.[226] Management of a twin pregnancy is discussed in more detail in a previous section.

UMBILICAL CORD COMPROMISE

On rare occasions, a large ossified remnant of the yolk sac may compromise blood flow through the umbilical cord and result in abortion.[400] The pathologic condition referred to as *umbilical cord torsion* may be defined as excessive twisting of the cord such that there is complete or partial occlusion of the umbilical vessels or urachus.[401] The two umbilical veins that return oxygenated blood from the placenta fuse within the distal aspect of the amniotic portion of the cord, and a single vein enters the fetal abdomen.[402] Strangulation may occur if the cord becomes tightly wrapped around a portion of the fetus. Pressure sites on or around fetal parts may be due to the effects of constriction by prolonged tension on a strangulated umbilical cord.[403] Affected fetuses are not usually expelled immediately after death, and thus some degree of tissue autolysis should be expected.[404]

The length of the equine umbilical cord in normal gestation can be quite variable, and factors that affect cord length and the number of twists present are unknown. Lethal umbilical torsion appears to be a sporadic condition with no apparent increased risk for future problems in mares that abort as a result of fetal complications.[405] Whitwell has shown that some mares have have three or more foals with abnormally long cords.[49] A Canadian study involving 93 Standardbreds did not demonstrate an effect of sire on cord length, and much larger studies will be required to ascertain whether genetics are involved.[29,406] Although the possibility of a heritable component for cord length cannot be discounted, a more plausible explanation may be that abnormally long cords are associated with the amount of fetal movement.[402]

Ultrasonographic studies of fetal mobility have helped explain the characteristic twisting that is a feature of the normal equine umbilical cord.[4,407-410] As is not the case with ruminants, the equine amnion floats freely within the allantoic fluid. Fetal rotation within the amniotic cavity and amniotic sac rotation within the allantoic cavity result in the characteristic twisting of the equine umbilical cord.[411,412] The lumen of both uterine horns becomes constricted (presumably by localized circular muscle contractions) between 5 and 7 months, and the allantoic fluid along with the fetus is contained within the confines of the uterine body.[4,407-409,412] What Ginther has described as the noncord horn remains closed, whereas the cord horn gradually permits the entry of the hindlimbs between 7 and 9 months. The limbs can enter the horn only when the fetus is in dorsal recumbency because the angle between the horn and body is so acute by this stage of gestation. Thereafter, the hindlimbs remain enclosed within the cord horn and the hooves extend to the horn tip by the tenth month.[4,407-409,412] It is interesting that the peak incidence of abortions due to umbilical torsions occurs when the hindlimbs can become permanently enclosed in the uterine horn. It may be that in some instances this prevents the unraveling of those critical few rotations that can lead to circulatory compromise. There is no doubt that a longer umbilical cord predisposes the fetus to this condition.

Reports from the United Kingdom suggest that with the decline in twin abortions, excessive twisting of the umbilical cord has become the most frequently made diagnosis in some laboratories. These abortions were associated with excessively long cords, with many over 80 cm in length.[276,413] Because spiraling of the equine cord (4 to 5 times over its length) is a normal feature, it is important to ensure that the cause of fetal demise was in fact due to vascular compromise.[402,411] Evidence of pathologic twisting with tension and compressive forces on the affected portion of the cord may include aneurysms, tearing of the intima of vessels, hemorrhage, thrombosis of vessels, blanched constricted areas, local edema, and urachal dilations of varying sizes. Inadequate perfusion can cause intravascular thrombosis in the peripheral tissues of the chorioallantois and possible necrosis of the aspect of the placenta that is most distant from the attachment of the cord (the cervical pole of the body segment).[402,404] These findings are by no means definitive, and there may be variability in interpretation among laboratories. Other considerations should include general agonal changes and the potential effects of cord tension when a live fetus is expelled. Whitwell's morphologic studies have established normal metrics for equine fetal membranes. The average length of the umbilical cord in a Thoroughbred is 55 cm (95% confidence interval; 36 to 83 cm; n = 143).[414]

Williams reviewed 168 cases of umbilical cord torsion from the University of Kentucky Livestock Disease Diagnostic Center, representing 6% of equine fetus submissions over a 5-year period.[415] The gestational age ranged between 5 to 10 months, with a mean of 7.5 months.[416] Umbilical cord length varied between 62 to 125 cm, with an average length of 96 cm. The cords tended to be highly twisted, with areas of constriction, edema, hemorrhage, and fluid-filled sacculations. The fetuses were slightly to moderately autolyzed, in a manner consistent with fetal death before abortion. Urinary bladder dilation was observed in some cases. The most consistent histopathologic finding was evidence of necrotic changes with secondary deposition of calcified material in the blood vessels of the chorioallantois.[405,417] A less common cause of abortion resulting from cord obstruction is when an excessively long amniotic portion of the cord becomes tightly wrapped around a portion of the fetus.[403,414,418] Although it may be more common for a fetal extremity to be involved, the author managed a case in a pony mare in which the tightly wrapped cord left a deep groove around the lumbar region, with evidence of local edema.[403]

GENDER DETERMINATION (FETAL SEXING)

The advent of fetal sexing has permitted early gender determination to influence the value of the pregnant mare. Factors that may vary depending on the predicted sex of the foal include choice of state for foaling, appraisals and insurance coverage, sales reserves, bookings for stallion service the next season, and retention or sale of the mare.[419] Accurate determination of the sex of the equine fetus can be made using either transrectal or transabdominal ultrasonography.[410,419-421] Fetal gender should be certified only when the identifying structures have been clearly delineated and the accuracy of the determination is guaranteed. Accurate determination of fetal sex may be difficult or impossible in some cases because of excessive mare or fetal movement or because the fetus is located too deeply to permit adequate imaging. Although tranquilization (e.g., xylazine and butorphanol tartrate) is sometimes used, it may cause the uterus to relax and drop away from the examiner.[419] A 5.0-MHz linear array transducer is adequate for transrectal gender determination, but a 3.5-MHz transducer will ensure the depth of penetration that is required to obtain transabdominal images.[191]

Gender determination is based on ultrasonographic assessment of the relative location of the genital tubercle, an embryologic structure that is initially located between the rear limbs in both sexes. The genital tubercle differentiates into either a clitoris or a penis and has an ultrasonographically distinctive, hyperechoic, bilobulated appearance in both sexes. Curren reported that the optimal time for gender determination is between days 59 and 68, and Holder concurs that a window between days 60 and 70 is ideal.[419,421] A second ideal period for gender determination may be between days 110 and 120, because the genitalia are now well developed and the fetus tends to be more accessible again. After this time the increasing depth of the uterus means that a diagnosis may not be possible if the fetus is in a anterior (cranial) presentation at the time of the examination.[419] If the transabdominal approach is used, the optimal window of time in both sexes is between days 100 and 220 of gestation.[410,420,421] Thereafter, it may become increasingly difficult to identify the anatomic structures required to make an accurate gender determination. Detailed instructions for fetal sexing by ultrasonography have been described.[410,419,420] Transabdominal gender identifications based on the presence of the penis or prepuce (or both) in males and mammary glands and teats or fetal gonads in females can be quite accurate.[421]

MONITORING FETAL WELL-BEING

Placentitis should be suspected in mares that develop premature mammary enlargement (with or without vulvar discharge). A reduction in plasma relaxin levels may indicate placental compromise because relaxin is produced by the equine placenta.[135,140-142,145,313,422-424] Low relaxin levels in late pregnancy have been associated with various causes of placental dysfunction, including fescue toxicosis, oliogohydramnios, and placentitis.[315] Measurement of an equine fetal protein and estrone sulfate levels in maternal plasma has not proved useful for early detection of fetal stress associated with medical and surgical colics.[99,100,425-428] Estrogens are produced from C19 precursors that are secreted by the gonads of a viable fetus and thus are unlikely to reflect fetal stress per se.[83] However, Riddle has reported that measurement of total estrogens can be useful for differentiating between a normal and a compromised fetus.[429] Before day 310 of gestation, total estrogen levels of less than 1000 ng/ml may be indicative of fetal stress, and mares with levels of less than 500 ng/ml are likely to have a severely compromised or dead fetus.[429]

It is important to remember that the circulating concentrations of hormones in maternal plasma generally represent a small percentage of the levels that are being metabolized by the fetus and uteroplacental tissues.[83,89,430] The definitive studies on mare progestagens (progestins) were performed using gas chromatography–mass spectrometry (GC-MS).[83,110,430] It is imperative that clincians appreciate that assays (e.g., RIA, ELISA) using an antibody raised against progesterone will usually cross-react with several of the progestagens but to a variable extent. Thus the value that is typically reported by the laboratory as being progesterone should actually be termed *total progestagens*. The level of cross-reactivity in a particular assay can cause substantial variation in the reported value.[83,430] Although placental pathology has been correlated with increased plasma progestin concentrations in some studies, others have not detected differences in plasma progestin concentrations in mares with impending abortion and mares with normal pregnancies when monthly blood sampling was performed.[46,83,110,121,430-433] Therefore it is recommended that serial samples (daily for 3 days, then weekly) be obtained from a mare in which the condition is suspected because doing so may help the clinician identify a clinically useful trend in progestagen concentrations.[83,99,259,277,430-434] Progestagen levels increase significantly in normal mares as gestation progresses, and concentrations in the maternal plasma may range between 5 to 50 ng/ml or even higher as mares approach term.[83,430] It is thought that chronic fetal stress may cause the elevated progesterone and pregnenolone levels (as well as those of several metabolites) that have been observed in mares with placentitis.[430,435]

Ousey has described three abnormal progestagen patterns that may be clinically useful: a rapid decline, precocious elevation, and failure to increase at term.[83,430] A rapid decline is consistent with fetal death or imminent fetal expulsion and may be seen after a uterine torsion or colic.[430,436] Pregnant mares that have experienced colic or uterine torsion and have progestagen levels below 2 ng/ml are at high risk for fetal loss.[99] Prolonged elevation of progestagens for several weeks before delivery (especially if earlier than 305 days' gestation) is consistent with metabolic activity in the fetus and uteroplacental tissues despite the presence of placental pathology.* Although typically small with poor skeletal development, foals born after being exposed to chronic fetal stress (placentitis) tend to exhibit precocious maturation—even when delivered several weeks early.[83,303,430,439] Analysis of specific progestagen profiles by GC-MS may differentiate mares with placentitis from those with villous poverty or placental edema.[83,430] If the total progestagen levels in maternal plasma fail to rise at term, fescue toxicosis (ergopeptine alkaloid-producing endophyte) is the most likely cause (see separate discussion).[83,118]

Transrectal ultrasonography provides an excellent assessment of the current status of the caudal allantochorion, and as such it is an invaluable aid when examining a mare in late pregnancy that exhibits signs of placentitis.[434,440,441] An image of the ventral placental tissues in the area adjacent to the cervical star provides the ability to accurately diagnose the early stages of ascending placentitis.[259,440,441] Experienced clinicians are able to observe abnormal tissue thickness and even evidence of placental separation with an associated pocket of inflammatory exudate. Early therapeutic intervention may provide the best chance for a successful outcome. In a normal placenta the chorioallantoic membrane and endometrium are intimately connected, making them ultrasonographically indistinguishable from each other. Thus a combined tissue measurement is used, and normal values for the combined thickness of the uterus and placenta (CTUP) have been established.[442] The amniotic membrane should not be included, and this should be remembered if the fetal limbs are active at the time of the examination. The area 1 to 2 inches cranial and ventral to the cervix provides the most consistent CTUP measurement in normal mares, and this is the recommended

*References 117,121,303,430,434,435,437,438.

site for any measurements. The ultrasound image should be frozen once the landmark vessel (a branch of the uterine artery) in the ventral uterine wall is located, and caliper measurements are taken from the inner surface of the ventral uterine vessel to the edge of the allantoic fluid.[259,440] Diagnostic accuracy can be improved by recording the average of at least three measurements. An increased CTUP at any point from midgestation until term indicates placental disruption and pending abortion.[431] Transrectal CTUP values indicative of placental pathology and impending abortion are greater than 8 mm (between days 271 and 300), greater than 10 mm (between days 301 and 330), and greater than 12 mm after day 330.[259,434,440,443,444]

It is important to employ strict hygienic procedures when performing a vaginal speculum examination on a mare with a high-risk pregnancy because the first two barriers to the pregnant uterus will be breached (i.e., vulvar lips, vestibular sphincter). Mares at risk for abortion often have a moist, hyperemic, relaxed cervix. Even if vaginal discharge has not been reported, many of these cases have a purulent cervical discharge if placentitis is present. However, whereas cervical softening and vaginal discharge may be present if the infection is localized around the cervical star, in the case of nocardioform placentitis the lesion does not involve the cervical star and vaginal discharge is conspicuously absent.[286,291,301] Thus, although transrectal ultrasound is an extremely useful aid in diagnosing ascending placentitis, the site of the nocardioform lesion makes it of limited diagnostic value in these cases.[316] Transabdominal examination of the ventral uterus may reveal separation of the chorioallantoic membrane from the uterine wall, often with evidence of inflammatory exudate accumulation between the two surfaces. Placentitis and associated placental edema will result in a thickened uteroplacental image. The uteroplacental thickness (CTUP) on a transabdominal ultrasound image should be between 7.1 ± 1.6 mm and 11.5 ± 2.4 mm.[440,445,446] If the uteroplacental thickness exceeds 2.0 cm in late gestation, placental pathology is likely to be present.[446,447]

Transabdominal ultrasonography of mares in late pregnancy has become a routine diagnostic aid for evaluating fetal well-being.[399,433,440,446,447] Although the 5.0-MHz linear array transducer is ideal for transrectal reproductive ultrasonography, its shallow depth of penetration (approximately 10 cm) limits its usefulness for transabdominal examinations in mares in late pregnancy. If the mare does not have a pronounced plaque of ventral edema, the 5.0-MHz transducer will often be sufficient to image the uteroplacental unit and some of the fetal fluids. Either a 3.5- or 2.5-MHz curved linear array or sector scanner transducer is best for transabdominal examinations because these can penetrate to a depth of 20 or 30 cm, respectively.[192,440,448] While the 70- to 90-day fetus may be imaged from the ventral abdomen, just cranial to the mammary gland, the late gestation gravid uterus extends along the ventral abdomen to the xiphoid.[399,440,445-449] By the ninth month of gestation, the fetus should be in anterior (cranial) presentation and dorsopubic or dorsolateral position.[4,408,449] Thus in late gestation the fetal head should be positioned near the mare's pelvis. An abnormal presentation or the presence of twins is possible if a fetal head is detected along the ventral abdomen during late gestation.[448] A more detailed examination is indicated in such cases. The posture of the extremities varies with fetal movement.[449]

A standardized methodology must be followed when scanning the uterus from the ventral abdomen, starting just cranial to the mare's mammary gland and moving cranially to locate the fetal thorax. The ribs cause multiple acoustic shadows that delineate the thoracic cavity. A complete examination of the fetus and uterus involves scanning cranially to the xiphoid in multiple parasagittal planes and then scanning from left to right sides of the abdomen in multiple transverse planes.[448] Transabdominal ultrasound examination is an important diagnostic tool when attempting to identify the presence of twin fetuses during late gestation. Identification of the nongravid horn can be useful to help rule out the possibility of twins. Obvious size discrepancy often serves as confirmation that twins are in fact present. In other cases one thoracic cavity does not contain a beating heart, confirming that one of the twins has already died.

In a normal pregnancy the majority of the fetal fluids are within the allantoic cavity. The amnion is imaged as a thin membrane that surrounds the fetus and lies in close contact with the fetus over much of its body. The amniotic membrane divides the imaged fetal fluid into two distinct cavities. It is most easily seen around the fetal neck, shoulder, thorax, and foreleg. The largest pocket of amniotic fluid is usually imaged at the point where the forelimb and neck meet the thorax.[448] The maximum vertical depth of amniotic and allantoic fluid and the quality of amniotic and allantoic fluid are useful guides to fetal well-being.[448] Any measurements of fluid depth should be made as perpendicular to the uteroplacental surface as possible.[447,448] In the normal equine pregnancy the maximum ventral fetal fluid pocket depth for amniotic fluid is 8 cm; it is 13 cm for allantoic fluid.[440,445,448] Extremes in either direction are not normal. Obviously deficient amounts of fetal fluid indicate placental dysfunction, and excessive amounts suggest a hydrops condition.[445,450] Fetal fluid quantities should be considered excessive if the maximal vertical amniotic fluid depth exceeds 14.9 cm or the maximum vertical allantoic fluid depth exceeds 22.1 cm.[448] The quality of the fetal fluid is scored from 0 (clear) to 3 (echogenic fluid with numerous particles).[447,448] It is not unusual for echogenic particles to be noted in the fetal fluids, especially during periods of fetal activity. These represent sloughed cells and proteinaceous debris. The fetal skin releases vernix as the pregnancy advances, and these free-floating particles can increase the cloudiness of the amniotic fluid.[440,446] Thus an increase in the number of echogenic particles in late gestation may not be abnormal.[447] However, if a high-risk pregnancy is being regularly monitored and a sudden increase in fluid turbidity (grade 3) is observed, the prognosis is not good.[446,447] The clinician should consider the possibility of inflammatory exudates, meconium passage by a compromised fetus, or even hemorrhage. It should be remembered that hippomanes (allantoic calculi) are a normal feature of the equine pregnancy. These structures may be observed on the ventral aspect of the allantoic cavity.[448]

An equine biophysical profile has been proposed as a guide to assessing fetal well-being and predicting perinatal morbidity and mortality.[440,446,447,451] Although a low score is definitely indicative of a negative outcome, higher scores do not guarantee the birth of a viable neonate.[448] Fetal breathing, heart rate and rhythm, fetal tone, and general activity are useful guides when evaluating fetal health and well-being. Therefore chemical sedation of the mare is not recommended because commonly used drugs are likely to induce fetal bradycardia and suppress normal fetal activity.[452,453] Fetal breathing is characterized by movement of the diaphragm between the thorax and abdomen, in conjunction with rib cage expansion—without any other movement by the fetus. Fetal breathing patterns should be monitored for at least 30 seconds.[440,448,454]

When fetal heart rate and rhythm is monitored, it is not appropriate to scan for only 10 or 15 seconds and then multiply by a correction factor to obtain the number of beats per minute. Beat-to-beat variations and observation of periodic accelerations are important. It is normal for the heart rate accelerations to occur in association with fetal activity. Multiple measurements of fetal heart rate and assessments of fetal heart rhythm should be made over a 30-minute period while evaluating the fetus, fetal fluids, and placenta.[440,448] Ideally, three measurements should be obtained with the fetus at rest and another three after periods of activity. It is difficult to accurately monitor the heart rate during periods of fetal activity, unless M-mode echocardiography equipment is available.[440,448,449] Fetal heart rates vary with the stage of gestation and the amount of fetal activity at the time of the examination.[440,455-457] The fetal heart beat is normally regular and will decrease from greater than 120 beats/min in midgestation to between 60 and 90 beats/min in late gestation.[440,445-447,449,455-459] Cardiac accelerations (20-40 beats/min above baseline) are normal if they are associated with fetal movement.[440,445,446,448] However, persistent tachycardia in the absence of fetal activity indicates fetal stress. A resting heart rate in excess of 104 beats/min indicates fetal stress in a late gestation fetus.[447,448] A heart rate of less than 57 beats/min in a fetus that is less than 330 days' gestation and a rate of less than 50 beats/min in a fetus older than 329 days' gestation should be considered abnormal.[447,448] A fetus suffering from hypoxia will have a slow heart rate, with minimal limb activity or fetal breathing, indicative of central nervous system depression.[446-449] However, if the condition is chronic and ischemic conditions are developing, the fetus will become tachycardic despite a lack of fetal activity. This is a prelude to fetal demise. In terminal cases extreme bradycardia ensues just before fetal death.[447,454] Whereas failure to observe fetal activity may be due to the stage of the normal rest-activity cycle, confirmation of a regularly beating heart at least confirms that the fetus is alive. This is a major advantage over transrectal fetal ballottement, wherein failure to detect movement can raise unnecessary concerns about fetal health.

If Doppler ultrasound equipment is available, the Doppler transducer is placed directly over the site where the best image was detected by the ultrasound scan. Tracings of fetal heart rate and rhythm can be recorded over time—usually intervals of 5 to 10 minutes.[460] This makes analysis easier and serves as a permanent record of the fetal status at the time of the recording. If there is some question about the presence of twins after a transabdominal ultrasound examination, fetal electrocardiogram (ECG) tracings may show two distinct fetal patterns.[458,459] Features of the ECG tracing that should be noted include fetal heart rate and rhythm, accelerations and decelerations, complex polarity changes, and beat-to-beat variation.[440,454] In the last weeks of pregnancy fetal foals usually have a baseline heart rate in the range of 60 to 75 beats per minute. Transient low heart rates of less than 60 beats/min are not uncommon. These troughs warrant concern only if they are not interspersed with accelerations. Likewise, transiently elevated rates in the order of 120 beats/min (occasionally >200 beats/min) are not abnormal provided that they return to baseline.[440,454] If the fetal heart rate is found to be less than 60 beats/min or greater than 120 beats/min during an observation period, then more frequent monitoring is justified to determine if the fetal is distressed. Beat-to-beat variations are normal, and a finding of no variability is an ominous sign. Maternal medications such as detomidine or butorphanol will reduce fetal heart rate variability transiently.[440,454]

The fetus is noted to have tone if it is observed to flex and extend the limbs, torso, or neck. Tone is poor or absent if the fetus appears flaccid.[440,447,448] Fetal movements include partial to full rotation around the long axis of the fetus as well as less marked activity such as extension and flexion of the extremities.[440,447,448] Fetal activity is rated on a scale from 0 to 3, with 3 being a very active fetus. A score of 0 indicates that no fetal movement was noted during the examination period.[447,448] Long periods without noticeable fetal activity are cause for concern and should be evaluated in conjunction with information about the fetal heart rate and rhythm. The fetus may be distressed, suffering from advanced hypoxia and central nervous system depression.[446,447]

Fetal aortic diameter is correlated with the weight of the pregnant mare, as well as the final neonatal foal weight.[440,445-447] Thus the pregnant mare's weight can be used to estimate what the fetal aortic diameter should be, using the regression equation ($Y = 0.00912 \times$ pregnant mare's weight in pounds + 12.46) where Y is the predicted fetal aortic diameter (mm).[447,448] The actual diameter of the fetal aorta should then be measured in the thoracic cavity, as close to the fetal heart as possible.[440,445,447] A smaller than predicted aortic diameter may indicate a dysmature or growth-retarded fetus (IUGR; intrauterine growth retardation) or twins. The maximal thoracic diameter is measured from the spine to the sternum over the caudal part of the thorax, and in a late gestation fetus it should be 18.4 ± 1.2 cm.[447,448] It has been correlated with fetal aortic diameter and neonatal foal weight in high-risk pregnancies.[447,448] Foal girth measurements and hip height are also correlated with fetal aortic diameter measurements.[446,448,461] Fetal biparietal measurements and orbital diameters have also been used to estimate fetal size.[440,448,461] Eye length (sclera to sclera) is a useful predictor of days before parturition in small ponies.[462] Decreased blood flow to the placental unit inhibits fetal growth, and some form of chronic placental insufficiency should be suspected when small fetal size is detected.

It is important to monitor fetal viability if a high-risk pregnancy is being maintained on altrenogest supplementation. Although most nonviable fetuses will be aborted, there are reports of a mummified fetus being retained when the mare was receiving long-term progestagen supplementation.[237]

COMPLICATIONS IN LATE GESTATION

Once confirmed to be at least 45 to 60 days pregnant, most mares can be expected to carry the fetus to term. The incidence of fetal loss after 100 to 120 days of gestation is low and accounts for only a small percentage of total pregnancy wastage. Fetal death and maceration is uncommon in the mare. However, the author has managed a case of macerated twins in a draft breed mare that suffered no ill effects systemically. The mare was evaluated only after the owner noticed a foul-smelling vaginal discharge.[463] Ventral body wall ruptures and uterine torsions are uncommon, and hydrops of the fetal membranes is an especially rare condition. Accurate diagnosis and appropriate management of these clinical cases can prevent the development of a life-threatening condition. If a ventral body wall rupture or uterine torsion is present, the birth of a viable foal may still be possible provided that the case is managed correctly.[464]

Hydrops of the Fetal Membranes

Hydrops is a condition of the last trimester, with the pregnancy developing normally until somewhere between 7.5 months and term. Hydrallantois and hydramnios are rare conditions that involve a pathologic accumulation of fluid within the allantoic and amniotic compartments, respectively. Normal volumes of allantoic fluid in mares vary from 8 to 18 L at term. In documented cases of hydrops, the allantoic fluid volume ranged from 110 to 230 L.[419] Just as with cows, hydrallantois accounts for most dropsical conditions in the mare.[465-468] The pathophysiology of hydrallantois in the cow has been related to an abnormality of placentation, whereas hydrops amnion has been associated with a fetal head anomaly that precludes swallowing.[195] Dysfunctional placentation may cause an increased production of transudate or disruption of transplacental fluid absorption. There does not appear to be any consistent abnormality of the fetus or fetal membranes that is characteristic of the condition in the mare.[469] In fact, a case at the University of Florida was confirmed to be hydrops amnion on the basis of analysis of fluid obtained through amniocentesis and allantocentesis, yet a viable foal was eventually delivered.[470] A mild diffuse placentitis or endometrial vasculitis has been incriminated in some cases.[419] In a report on 15 cases, all of the mares were pluriparous and ranged in age between 6 to 20 years.[419]

Generally, there is a sudden onset of abdominal distention, and walking becomes difficult.[470] The mare will exhibit variable degrees of colic. There is a progressive loss of appetite, and the mare may experience some difficulty in defecation. The increasing pressure on the diaphragm causes dyspnea, and the mucous membranes may appear cyanotic, especially when the mare is recumbent.[419] On physical examination the rectal temperature is normal, but the heart rate will be elevated. Rectal palpation reveals characteristic findings. Copious lubrication and extreme caution should be used because passage of the forearm will be impeded by pressure from the large fluid-filled uterus. The feces tend to be covered with mucus as a result of the prolonged passage through the lower gastrointestinal tract. The gross distention of the uterus means that the fetus is usually not palpable.[470] Failure to detect the fetus by external ballottement further supports the diagnosis. Transabdominal ultrasound may confirm the presence of excessive amounts of hyperechoic fluid.[470] A thorough examination from both sides of the abdomen should be performed to rule out the possibility of twins.[464]

Owners should be advised that this is a progressive condition and it is extremely unlikely that the mare will be able to sustain the pregnancy and deliver a live foal—although a recent report documented a case that was successfully managed until a viable foal was delivered at 321 days' gestation.[464,470] In that case the mare was provided with close monitoring of maternal and fetal health, in combination with supportive care that included a supportive belly-wrap, anti-inflammatory medication, and altrenogest. A partial drainage technique is sometimes used in an attempt to manage cases that were diagnosed within 2 to 4 weeks of term.[419] Affected mares receive abdominal support (belly band), intravenous fluids, broad spectrum antibiotics, and anti-inflammatory medication. The technique of slow, repeated drainage requires a major time commitment and would not be cost effective in many cases. Fetal death may occur as a result of placental separation. There also appears to be a considerable risk for iatrogenic fetal infection after contamination of the fetal fluids, despite attempts to perform the drainage technique in an aseptic manner. Thus, despite heroic attempts in valuable mares, the fetus is likely to be lost in cases of hydrallantois.[419]

In most cases induction of parturition may be advisable before the mare's condition deteriorates further. Continued abdominal enlargement will predispose the mare to prepubic tendon rupture,[470,471] and uterine rupture has also been reported.[472] Induction is not without risk (shock, dystocia), but the prognosis for survival of the mare is good provided that appropriate supportive therapy is instituted.[470] The prognosis for the mare's reproductive future may also be favorable provided that there are no untoward sequelae (cervical lacerations, retained fetal membranes, metritis). Application of PGE to the cervix before induction may facilitate atraumatic fetal extraction.[228,473] In one report six of eight mares that had previously developed a hydrops pregnancy subsequently became pregnant and delivered normal healthy foals at term.[419]

Before a therapeutic induction of parturition, the tail should be wrapped, the perineal area cleansed, and an indwelling intravenous catheter inserted. Large-volume intravenous fluid therapy may become necessary if hypovolemic shock develops as the allantoic fluid is discharged.[464] In some cases controlled drainage may be beneficial before inducing delivery. An added complication in hydrops cases is that the thickened, edematous chorioallantoic membrane may be difficult to rupture.[465] If digital pressure alone is unsuccessful, an endometrial biopsy forceps can be used to bite a piece out of the chorioallantois. Some authors report that the lack of pressure from the atonic uterine wall will result in minimal release of fetal fluid from the punctured chorioallantoic sac, but in the few cases that the author has been involved with there was a massive release of fluid once the chorioallantoic membrane was ruptured.[465,467] If insufficient fluid release occurs, a sterile nasogastric tube can be introduced into the uterus to begin controlled siphoning of fluid. An alternative technique is to introduce a thoracic trocar catheter through the cervix and employ a sharp puncture of the chorioallantois.[419] This approach permits the excess fluid to be removed by controlled drainage. Administration of intravenous fluids with gradual removal of the excess allantoic fluid will permit the mare's cardiovascular system to adapt. Both oxytocin and PG injections have been employed in an attempt to abort these cases.[465-467] Although oxytocin is widely considered to be the most efficacious method for routine induction of parturition, in hydrops cases the distended uterine musculature may not be able to contract effectively.[465,474] This uterine inertia is common, and gentle manual dilation of the cervix, or perhaps prior application of PGE, may be warranted.[473] Bain and Wolfsdorf have reported a smooth induction after two doses of cloprostenol administered 30 minutes apart.[419]

The abdominal musculature may be weakened by stretching, and thus the typical stage 2 abdominal press may be compromised. Malpositioning and malpostures are not uncommon. The fetus may need to be extracted by assisted vaginal delivery, but care should be taken so as not to traumatize the cervix by overzealous traction.[464] The expelled fetus will generally be alive, and humane euthanasia is warranted.

In one report at least 50% of foals had some malformation.[419] Additional oxytocin (1.0 IU per minute) should be added to the intravenous fluids to promote uterine involution. Retention of the fetal membranes should be expected, and appropriate treatment for removal of these membranes and prevention of the metritis-laminitis complex is indicated. Uterine involution should be monitored by transrectal palpation and ultrasonography.

Ventral Body Wall Hernias and Prepubic Tendon Rupture

Apart from those with pathologic pregnancies, mares with ventral body wall defects are generally close to term.[474,475] Damage to the abdominal sling of the pregnant mare may involve rupture of the transverse abdominis and oblique muscles, the rectus abdominus muscles, and the prepubic tendon.[476] In extreme cases the rupture may lead to hemorrhage, shock, and death.[477] The prepubic tendon attaches to the cranial border of the pubis, and lordosis occurs if the tendon is ruptured.[464,474,475] Although breed (draft-breed mares) and age (older mares) may predispose a mare to development of the condition, in most cases there is no apparent predisposing cause.[471,475,476] The extreme abdominal distention associated with the hydrops condition may cause rupture of the ventral musculotendinous support. Defects in the ventrolateral abdominal wall are more common than complete prepubic tendon rupture, and bilateral involvement of the abdominal wall seems to be most common.[471,475,476,478,479] In a retrospective study of 13 cases, only three were categorized as being caudal midline (prepubic tendon lesions), and all three had additional involvement of the body wall musculature.[475]

The most obvious clinical sign of an impending ventral body wall rupture is a thick plaque of ventral edema extending a variable distance cranial to the udder.[464,476] However, ventral edema may be a normal consequence of late pregnancy, and it can indicate external trauma. The author managed one case in which a large ventral swelling was associated with a massive hematoma that appeared to have originated from a kick. Mares in late pregnancy often develop a thick plaque of ventral edema that can extend from the udder to between the forelimbs. This is associated with the compressive weight of the gravid uterus on the venous and lymphatic drainage of the ventral abdomen. The presence of a hemorrhagic secretion in the mammary gland supports a diagnosis of tissue trauma rather than pregnancy edema.[475] Unilateral edema is more indicative of damage to the ventrolateral body wall, but it may be associated with partial rupture of the prepubic tendon.[464,476] The extreme pain that is associated with progressive enlargement of a ventral body wall rupture causes a marked tachycardia that may not be responsive to analgesics. Pregnant mares with a ruptured prepubic tendon or ventral abdominal wall show signs of colic and generally are reluctant to move. If the prepubic tendon is completely ruptured, the pelvis will be tilted such that the tailhead and tuber ischii are elevated, and a lordosis will be present.[464,471,475,476] The mammary gland is often displaced craniad and ventrad because of the loss of the caudal attachment to the pelvis. A rent in the abdominal musculature may be complicated by bowel incarceration.[464,471,475,476]

Confirmation of the tentative diagnosis is sometimes difficult. Because it is not always possible to be certain that a rupture has already occurred, mares with severe ventral edema should be confined to a stall, with exercise restricted to hand walking. Rectal palpation of the defect is usually not possible owing to the advanced stage of the pregnancy. External palpation is generally unrewarding because of the thickness of the edema, although some crepitation of the ventral abdominal wall may be noted. The mare is generally extremely sensitive and resists palpation of the area.[464,475,476] Ultrasonographic examination of the posterior aspect of the ventral abdomen may be useful in some cases and can detect the presence of a bowel segment.[448,464,475,477] Repture of the prepubic tendon can be identified as disruption of the tendon fibers immediately cranial to the pubis, whereas abdominal wall muscle tears are seen to be discrete tears within muscle fibers, often associated with hematomas.[475] An accurate assessment of the dimensions of the defect often cannot be made until the fetus and fetal fluids are expelled and the ventral edema has subsided.[464,476]

Depending on the degree of discomfort and stage of pregnancy, termination of the pregnancy may be the most humane treatment for the mare, given that further tissue damage is likely to occur to some degree until parturition. The possibility of a segment of intestine becoming incarcerated in the defect also should be considered.[476] In extreme cases the mare may eventually become recumbent, especially if there is a rapidly expanding body wall defect.[464,475] Owners should be aware that unless parturition is imminent, the prognosis for the foal is not good because fetal readiness for birth is difficult to predict.[475] Because the present fetus may well be the mare's last, owners often request that an attempt be made to maintain the pregnancy to term. In these cases the treatment is essentially supportive, and the prognosis for the foal is good.[475,476] Anti-inflammatory drugs will help alleviate the mare's discomfort. An abdominal sling (belly band) made of canvas or padded leather or a snug abdominal bandage help provide support for the ventral abdominal wall.[475,476] In the author's experience, abdominal bandages tend to be purely cosmetic because they soon stretch and thus provide minimal long-term support. If a sling is used, the area over the back must be well padded to prevent pressure necrosis because the purpose of this support is to transfer the weight of the gravid uterus to the vertebral column.[464,476] Reducing the bulk of the ration and feeding a mild laxative may help reduce the degree of abdominal exertion associated with defecation.[477]

Assistance with parturition should be available because the mare may experience difficulty in mounting sufficient abdominal pressure to expel the fetus.[471,475] However, one report suggests that some mares can position the foal and complete delivery unassisted.[475,476] Arrangements for an alternate source of colostrum should be made because ventral edema may prevent the foal from suckling. The owner should be informed that although in some cases surgical repair of the defect may be possible by mesh herniorrhaphy, rebreeding the mare may not always be advisable.[471,475,476] Some mares with small, unrepaired defects may subsequently foal without assistance, but the possibility that future pregnancies may exacerbate the condition should be considered.[477] Embryo transfer offers a viable alternative if this procedure is condoned by the relevant breed society.[475]

Uterine Torsion

Uterine torsion accounts for 5% to 10% of all complicated obstetric conditions in the mare.[480,481] Neither mare age nor parity appear to be significant risk factors.[482] The causes of uterine torsion in the mare are not well defined. The condition is much more common in cattle, and in that species a large term fetus has been implicated as a major risk factor. Most uterine torsions in cows occur at term and are thought to be a direct result of fetal positional changes during late first-stage and early second-stage labor.[483] A striking difference between the mare and the cow is that more than 50% of uterine torsions in mares occur before the end of gestation.[480] In the author's clinical experience, the vast majority occur before term, and cases may be seen as early as 8 months of gestation.[464] In fact, one recent report documented a case as early as 126 days of gestation.[484] A multicenter retrospective study of 63 cases reported that 59% of the mares were at less than 320 days of gestation.[482] Although Ginther et al. have shown that the fetus is locked into a dorsopubic position during the final months of gestation, it is still possible for the entire pregnancy (uterus and fetus) to rotate approximately 90 degrees on the lower maternal abdominal wall.[4] This occurs because any rotational movement of the caudal half of the fetus (pelvis and hindlimbs) by necessity will involve the close-fitting uterus. It seems likely that in extreme cases this rotating action can lead to a clinical uterine torsion.[230,419] Owners who work closely with their mares may observe excessive fetal movements in the flank area 1 or 2 days before. In a recent study 80% of term fetuses were in dorsosacral position when the uterine torsion was corrected. This suggests that fetal righting reflexes may have played a role in creating the torsion.[481] The author believes that vigorous fetal movements during the latter stages of gestation are likely to be a significant factor in the etiology of this condition in the mare.[419]

The clinical signs that attract the owner's attention are the result of abdominal pain.[464,485-488] These include restlessness, sweating, anorexia, frequent urination, sawhorse stance, looking at flanks, and kicking at the abdomen. When the veterinarian is first summoned, the signs may have been present for a period ranging between 2 hours to 3 days or more, especially if signs are intermittent and moderate.[464,486] In mares that are close to term, the owner may assume that the signs indicate impending parturition. In more extreme cases the signs are more severe and may be associated with concurrent involvement of the small or large colon.[482,484,487] Veterinarians should always consider the possibility of uterine torsion when a mare that is in the last trimester of gestation exhibits a mild, persistent colic. Delay in making a definitive diagnosis increases the likelihood of fetal compromise.[464] In one study of 63 cases, the mean time to admission was more than 20 hours.[482] Occasionally, the condition may remain undiagnosed for several weeks.[489] In these instances an owner may have attempted treatment with analgesics that were precribed for previous mild colic episodes.[464,485]

Rectal palpation is essential to determine whether a uterine torsion is present.[464,485] The author is of the opinion that all late pregnant mares that display signs of mild to moderate colic warrant a thorough rectal examination to rule out the possibility of uterine torsion. Although vaginal involvement in the torsion is very common in the cow, uterine torsions in the mare seldom cause detectable changes in the vagina.[464,483,486,489,490] Thus vaginal examination is generally not diagnostically useful. On rectal palpation the clinician should aim to carefully advance the forearm while palpating for a taut band on either side of the rectum. The ligament on the side of the torsion tends to be more caudal and is palpable as a tight vertical band. As the arm is advanced further, the opposite ligament will be palpable as it is pulled horizontally across the top of the uterus before being displaced ventrally.[464] An accurate examination of the broad ligaments will confirm the diagnosis, determine the direction of the torsion, and give some idea of the severity of the torsion.[419] One study (n = 54 mares) reported that 79% of referred cases were rotated no more than than 180 degrees, and 59% of cases involved clockwise torsion.[482] A transrectal ultrasound examination is useful to evaluate the condition of the fetal fluids and to note whether any placental detachment has occurred. The degree of uterine compromise can be gauged by noting the thickened uterine wall and distended vasculature. Compression of the veins and lymphatics occurs before occlusion of the arterial blood supply. Thus the initial changes will be associated with pooling of fluid within the uterine wall.[464] The compressive forces of the displaced broad ligaments may cause variable amounts of constriction of the small colon.[486,491]

Transabdominal ultrasonographic imaging may be used to assess fetal viability (heart rate and rhythm) and to evaluate the condition of the fetal fluid. Compression of the uterine blood supply can cause fetal hypoxia and a fetal stress response, especially in more advanced pregnancies. Abdominocentesis may provide prognostic information and guide the clinician in choosing a mode of correction.[492] Because it may be difficult to obtain peritoneal fluid from a mare in late gestation, transabdominal ultrasonography is sometimes useful in locating a pocket of fluid. Uterine rupture can be a complication of uterine torsion in the mare.[486,493] In the author's experience mild uterine torsions, or those of short duration, do not alter the color, cellularity, or total protein content of the peritoneal fluid.[492] Mares with severe or chronic uterine torsion may develop significant uterine compromise that results in changes in the composition of the peritoneal fluid. Any alterations in the composition of the peritoneal fluid may indicate the presence of a compromised or ruptured uterine wall or concurrent gastrointestinal involvement.[493] A flank laparoscopic examination can confirm the condition of the uterine wall.[494] This information will facilitate an informed choice of surgical approach or perhaps support a decision for euthanasia if economic considerations preclude surgical intervention.

The stage of gestation and the mare's heart rate are significant prognostic indicators for mare survival. A recent study reported that mares that died had significantly higher heart rates (mean 74 beats/min) at admission than survivors (mean 59 beats/min).[482] Increased fetal size and the weight of the gravid uterus make correction closer to term (>320 days) more difficult, and this may explain the poor mare survival rate (65%) when compared with cases in less advanced pregnancies (<320 days), wherein survival rates are excellent (97%).[482] Owners should be advised that fetal survival rates are not as good, but a similar effect of stage of gestation applies. The chances of the foal surviving exceed 70% if the mare is at less than 320 days' gestation, but only about 30% survive when mares are closer to term.[482]

If the mare is presented in stage I of labor and the cervix is sufficiently dilated to permit passage of a well-lubricated arm into the uterine body, then it may be possible to reach the fetus. It should be grasped ventrolaterally and then rocked back and forth until sufficient momentum is achieved to continue up in an arc. This manipulation should roll both fetus and uterus back into a normal position. Vandeplassche has reported that more than 80% of term torsions can be corrected in this manner.[196] Options for management of a preterm uterine torsion are rolling the mare, flank laparotomy, or a ventral midline celiotomy. In the controlled referral hospital environment, the method of correction is not associated with mare survival, but both rolling and midline celiotomy require general anesthesia and thus entail those additional risks.[482] There is a significant effect on foal survival if the mare is at less than 320 days' gestation, and employing the standing laparotomy approach should provide a significantly better prognosis compared with the ventral midline approach.[482] However, the final decision must be based on several factors, including the severity of pain being exhibited by the mare, client financial constraints, and surgeon preference. Ventral midline celiotomy does permit assessment of uterine viability and evaluation of the gastrointestinal tract.[464,482]

The anesthetized mare may be rolled in an attempt to rotate the mare's body around the stationary gravid uterus.[495] It is essential that the mare be placed in lateral recumbency on the side of the torsion.[419] The aim of the procedure is to roll the mare such that the pelvis "catches up" with the displaced uterus. Correction by rolling the mare is controversial.[464,477,486,496] Citations in the literature report on a limited number of cases.[480,487,496] Concerns with this approach include the following: unsuccessful attempts to correct the torsion will prolong its adverse effects; misdiagnosis of the direction of the torsion means that rolling the mare may make the condition worse; the condition of the uterus cannot be evaluated; and displacement of the colon may result.[464] In addition, a higher risk of placental detachment and uterine rupture has been reported.[477,479,487] Another concern is that if general anesthesia is induced under less than ideal conditions, maternal hypoxia may cause fatal complications in the already compromised fetus.[482,496]

In the standing flank approach, a grid incision is made on the same side as the direction of the torsion.[486] The torsion is corrected by placing the forearm under the uterus. The uterus and contents are rocked back and forth to gain momentum. A combination of lifting and rotating movements generally results in easy correction of the torsion.[419] The presence of a live fetus greatly facilitates the detorsion manipulations. More difficulty may be experienced in mares that are close to term, and this may justify the more expensive ventral midline celiotomy approach.[482] If the standing procedure is attempted, an incision in the opposite flank will permit a second surgeon to assist by gently pulling across the top of the uterus as it is elevated from below.[490] If the fetus is dead, the mare should abort naturally once the uterine torsion has been corrected, thereby removing the need for hysterotomy and any associated complications.[269,464,419] However, the mare should be closely monitored, and obstetric assistance must be available to correct any malposition or malposture. Mares experiencing intractable pain should receive general anesthesia during the operation.[480,486] A ventral midline celiotomy is also indicated when significant uterine compromise is a concern or another problem co-existing in the abdomen is suspected.[464,482]

The prognosis for mares with uterine torsion depends on the degree of vascular compromise. The severity and duration of the condition affect placental circulation and subsequent fetal viability.[464] In chronic cases in which there is significant uterine compromise, it is feasible to perform an ovariohysterectomy to salvage the mare for nonbreeding purposes.[485,489] It has been this author's experience that if the fetus is alive and the uterine wall is not severely congested and edematous, then the prognosis for both the mare's survival and for the birth of a live foal at term is good.[464,484] Progestin supplementation for 3 to 5 days after the manipulations involved in correcting a uterine torsion may be indicated to promote myometrial quiescence and thus maintenance of the placental attachment.[107] Although supplementation after a uterine torsion would be in the last 2 to 3 months of gestation, there are reports of mares retaining a nonviable fetus (one that died at 3 to 5 months' gestation) while receiving progestins.[237] Thus if progestin supplementation is administered to a mare after correction of a uterine torsion, it is prudent to monitor fetal viability at regular intervals.[464] There is probably little merit in continuing the supplementation once the mare has been discharged from the hospital. In one study 28 of 30 mares that were pregnant at the time of discharge subsequently delivered a live foal, and future fertility was good (24 of 29 were successfully rebred).[482]

Vaginal Hemorrhage

Visible blood on the tail hairs or hindlimbs of a pregnant mare warrants a careful examination. The integrity of placental attachment immediately cranial to the cervix should be evaluated using transrectal ultrasonography. A pocket of fluid may be evident if placental separation has occurred, and measurements of the CTUP should be made.[431,442] An increased CTUP measurement is a characteristic finding in cases of placentitis.[419] Because two of the three barriers protecting the fetus—vulvar lips, vestibular sphincter, and cervix—will be entered when performing a vaginal speculum examination, it is essential to ensure stringent hygiene.[497] Often, blood clots can be seen in the vestibule when the vulvar lips are parted. A sterile speculum should be covered with sterile lubricant and then gently inserted into the vagina. In some cases there may be evidence of a serosanguinous discharge from the cervical os. Mares that are aborting a twin pregnancy may also develop a bloody vaginal discharge. However, the practitioner should be aware that the most common source of vaginal hemorrhage in pregnant mares is from varicose veins in the hymenal remnants, not from an impending abortion. In many cases no blood is visible in the cranial vagina. If the cervix is closed, pale, and covered with tenacious mucus, it is unlikely that the blood is associated with fetoplacental unit. Although the blood could be associated with cystitis or urolithiasis, the source of the hemorrhage usually is varicose vessels in the remnants of the hymen at the level of the vestibular sphincter. It is not unusual to miss these as the speculum is inserted. Thus particular attention should be paid to this area as the speculum is withdrawn.[497]

Vaginal varicosities are most likely to occur in older, pluriparous mares during the latter months of gestation.[497,498] A large plexus of dilated veins can develop in the pedunculated mucosa at the level of the vestibulovaginal junction. The veins can become engorged from 1 to 2 cm during late gestation. If the vessels are ulcerated, there may be intermittent, mild episodes of bleeding from the ventral commissure of the vulva. An owner may report seeing large blood clots in the bedding when the mare is fed in the morning. Although this quantity may be alarming to an owner, it can be explained as merely representing the discharge of pooled blood while the mare was recumbent during the night.[497] Another explanation is that the pull of the rectal attachments when standing creates sufficient tension in the vaginal wall to control hemorrhage, whereas blood loss can occur when the mare is recumbent.[498] In more severe cases there may be dried blood on the perineum, tail hairs, and hindlimbs.[497] The author managed one case in which the red cell count and packed cell volume were subnormal, and there are reports in which the overt vaginal hemorrhage was sufficient to cause anemia.[498]

The etiology of vaginal varicosities in mares is unknown. The condition is not an uncommon complication of pregnancy in pluriparous women, and it has been proposed that a similar obstruction of venous return is responsible for the development of vaginal varicosities in the mare. Poor vulvar conformation, with cranial displacement of the perineum, may be involved in some cases.[497-499] It is possible that repeated stretching of the vestibulovaginal tissues and changes in the vulvar conformation of pluriparous mares create a physical impairment of venous return from the vestibular and vaginal components of the internal pudendal vein.[497-499] The dilated veins are generally located on the cranial aspect of the vestibular fold and on the dorsal aspect of the caudal vaginal wall. Thus vaginal varicosities can be easily missed when a tubular speculum is introduced, and they may not be evident during withdrawal. In some cases a trivalve metal Caslick speculum may provide better exposure so that the tissues of the vestibular-vaginal fold can be everted and fully explored.[497] If the diagnosis is still inconclusive, the next logical step in the physical examination is endoscopic visualization of the bladder. The clinician should first advance the flexible scope toward the cervix and then angle the lens back to better evaluate the cranial aspect of the vestibular-vaginal fold. If vaginal varicosities are present, usually no treatment is necessary, because the vessels will regress spontaneously after foaling (benign neglect).[497] However, if there is persistent or excessive hemorrhage or the owner is distressed, the offending vessels can be cauterized (diathermy) or ligated.[195,497,500] Locating the source of the bleeding can be difficult. Traction on the adjacent vaginal mucosa may arrest the bleeding and help identify the site in such cases. Submucosal resection of a pedunculated plexus of varicose veins has been reported to be successful.[497,498] Treatment is generally successful, and no recurrence has been reported.

It is important to consider bleeding from the urinary tract when vaginal hemorrhage is the presenting complaint. If an owner reports having seen bloody urine on the stall floor, it should be remembered that normal equine urine contains pyrocatechine. This oxidizing agent can cause urine to turn red-brown after exposure to air.[497] Hematuria can result from several disorders of the urinary tract.[501] If it is present throughout urination, the lesion is likely to be in the kidneys, ureters, or bladder. If the endoscopic examination has not identified vaginal varicosities as the source of the hemorrhage, the endoscope should be advanced down the urethra to visualize the bladder lumen (cystoscopy).[497] Although cystic uroliths are more common in male horses than in mares, a urolith may cause mucosal irritation and hemorrhage, resulting in hematuria.[502,503] Rectal palpation may reveal a firm mass in the bladder that can be imaged by ultrasonography. The pelvic portion of the urethra should also be palpated.[497] Although neoplasia of the urinary bladder is rare, mares are reported to be twice as likely as male horses to develop primary bladder tumors.[419,501,504] Squamous cell carcinoma is the most commonly reported bladder tumor, but transitional cell carcinomas can also occur. The condition has been reported as a cause of hematuria—often with blood clots.[505] A more detailed discussion of hematuria may be found elsewhere in this text.

FESCUE TOXICITY AND AGALACTIA

A wide range of reproductive problems (e.g., thickened placenta, abortion, prolonged gestation, dystocia, dead or weak foals, agalactia) have been attributed to the effects of the fungal endophyte (*Acremonium coenophialum*—now known as *Neothyphodium coenophialum*).[506-508] The endophyte produces a dopaminergic, vasoactive ergopeptine alkaloid (ergovaline).[506] This alkaloid disrupts the fetoplacental production of progestagens, but the precise mechanism has not been established.[116,118,509,510] Umbilical vein progestagen levels suggest that the disruption is not at the level of placental steroidogenesis—a remarkable observation when the fetal membranes are so edematous. Premature chorioallantoic separation and the failure of the membrane to rupture ("red bag") are attributable to the edematous splanchnic mesoderm.[506] ACTH, T4, triiodothyronine (T3), progestagen, and cortisol concentrations are lower in foals born to endophyte-exposed mares, suggesting that the effects are actually at the level of the fetal hypothalamo-pituitary axis, thyroid, and adrenal cortex.[118,511] This is likely to be the basis for the prolonged gestation and fetal dysmaturity that are associated with fescue toxicosis.[118,509] The ergovaline also inhibits prolactin secretion in affected mares by acting as a dopamine agonist at the maternal pituitary level.[154,155,510] Prolactin secretion can be inhibited experimentally by administering dopamine agonists such as bromocryptine.[156] Not only does such prolactin-inhibiting treatment of pregnant mares result in agalactia, but it also mimics the other symptoms of fescue toxicosis (thickened placenta, prolonged gestation, and dystocia).[156] An effect of fescue toxicosis in pregnant mares is a lowering of the circulating relaxin levels.[313] Clinical observations suggest that a one-time injection with fluphenazine improved pregnancy outcome by reducing the adverse effects of fescue toxicosis concomitant with a stabilization of plasma relaxin concentrations. (Caution should be exercised with administration of fluphenazine to horses because this drug may cause severe extrapyramidal neurologic signs). These data support the hypothesis that systemic relaxin may be a useful biochemical means of monitoring placental function and treatment efficacy in the mare.[313]

Because mares in late pregnancy are so susceptible to the toxic effects of ergopeptine alkaloids, they should not be permitted to graze in endophyte-infected tall fescue pasture or ingest hay derived from such pasture. Short-term exposure by mares at 300 days of gestation results in a significant decline in both prolactin and total progestagen concentrations within 48 hours. Fortunately, removal of pregnant mares (300 days' gestation) from infected pasture results in a significant increase in prolactin and progestagen levels within 3 days. This will prevent the development of the typical symptoms associated with fescue toxicosis.[118,509] Even when alternate feed sources are limited, every attempt should be made to remove pregnant mares from endophyte-infected fescue by 30 to 60 days before the expected foaling date. When this is not possible, prophylactic administration of the dopamine receptor antagonist domperidone (Equidone) at 1.1 mg/kg, administered orally, can prevent the negative effects of fescue toxicosis.[154-156,507,512-515]

INDUCTION OF PARTURITION

Induction of parturition may be indicated as a clinical management procedure for some high-risk pregnancies, including mares with hydrops, ruptured prepubic tendon, and ventral herniation. These mares often require assistance with delivery because the stage II abdominal press may be compromised.[464] The author does not believe that induction should be practiced for convenience alone.[516,517] Owners should be advised that complications such as dystocia, premature placental separation, fetal hypoxia, and dysmaturity are not uncommon sequelae of the induction procedure.[518-521] The aim of a controlled foaling is not only to deliver a viable fetus but also to prevent any injury to the mare that may compromise future fertility.[464]

Induced foalings are sometimes indicated to ensure that optimal veterinary assistance is available when complications are expected and to optimize resuscitation attempts when a compromised fetus has been monitored in utero. When fetal stress is detected in a high-risk pregnancy, the clinician is faced with the dilemma of inducing delivery and attempting supportive care in a neonatal intensive unit or leaving the compromised fetus in utero. Owners should be informed that delivery is indicated only if the probability of extrauterine survival exceeds that for continued maternal support. Experience suggests that an abnormal uterine environment is often more conducive to maintaining a fetal foal's life than a neonatal intensive care unit.[454] A fetus that has been exposed to an adverse uterine environment for some time may be more tolerant of premature delivery.[182] Many clinicians administer a dose of corticosteroids to the mare if premature delivery appears inevitable. This may stimulate surfactant production and promote accelerated maturation of the fetal lung.

The normal physiologic processes in the prepartum mare and fetus were discussed in a previous section. There is clear evidence that the fetal hypothalamic-pituitary-adrenal axis initiates the final stages of fetal maturation that initiates the hormonal cascade culminating in parturition.[89] Final maturation of the fetus results in increased ACTH release from the pituitary and subsequent stimulation of the fetal adrenal cortex.[89,110,115,116] It is not until the maturing adrenal gland attains 17α-hydroxylase capacity that the high levels of pregnenelone are metabolized into fetal cortisol.[89,113] These vital changes lead to a fetal cortisol rise in the last 2 or 3 days before birth, and thus the equine fetus is at a substantially increased risk of dysmaturity or prematurity if the induction is not carefully planned.[127,522] This planning has traditionally involved confirmation of gestation length, monitoring mammary development and milk or colostrum production, and ultimately evaluating the amount of cervical softening.[523] The fetus will usually be in the dorsopubic position, with neck and limbs flexed before induction. The incidence of posterior and transverse presentations is rare, but detection of these abnormalities by rectal palpation before induction would be reason to re-evaluate the induction plans. Delivery by cesarean section may be a more prudent course of action, especially with transverse presentations.

Gestation length is notoriously unpredictable in mares, and the greatest predictor of gestation length may be the mare herself.[524-526] Although the frequently recommended minimum gestation length for successful induction is 330 days, it must be remembered that many mares will carry a foal past 340 days and occasionally to 360 days and beyond.[3,523,525,527] There also appears to be some breed variability in gestation length, with the mean for Friesians reported as 332 days, Lipizzaners reported at 334 days, Andalusians reported at 337 days, and Arabians reported at 340 days.[526,528,529] In a retrospective study of Standardbred mares, the mean duration of gestation was 343.3 days, and it was significantly greater for colt fetuses (344.4 days) than for filly fetuses (342.2 days).[530] An average gestation length of 344.1 plus or minus 0.49 days was reported in a recent Thoroughbred study (n = 344 mares). Colt foal pregnancies were significantly longer (346.2 ± 0.72) than fillies (342.4 ± 0.65).[531] Colts were carried 1.5 days longer in a study of 495 Friesian mares.[528] The sire has been associated with duration of gestation; gestation after mating with certain sires was consistently less than 340 days in duration, whereas duration after mating with other sires was consistently more than 350 days.[528,530] Mares tend to carry foals longer if they are due to foal early in the season (shorter day length), whereas gestation length may be shorter if the foal is not due until longer days have arrived.[525,526,528-530,532,533] In Andalusians and Arabians, a delay of 1 month in breeding corresponded to a decrease of 3 days in the gestation length.[526] Placentitis and other placental pathology are often associated with precocious mammary gland development and premature changes in mammary secretion electrolyte concentrations. Milk electrolyte changes are unreliable for assessing fetal readiness for birth in abnormal pregnancies (e.g., placentitis, impending twin abortion). In these cases there may be elevated mammary secretion calcium concentrations (>10 mmol/L; >400 ppm; >40 mg/dl) before day 310 of gestation.[121]

Although mammary development is a useful sign of approaching parturition in normal mares, monitoring changes in mammary secretion electrolyte concentrations is the most reliable guide to imminent parturition.[534-538] An inversion in the sodium-to-potassium ratio, followed by a rapid rise in calcium (Ca) concentrations in the last 24 to 48 hours, has been correlated with fetal maturity in both mares and jennies.[536,539] Exact values may vary with the type of chemistry analyzer used by the diagnostic laboratory. In a normal term pregnancy, the combined mammary secretion levels of Ca (>40 mg/dl), potassium (>30 mEq/ml), and sodium (<30 mEq/ml) are indicative of fetal maturity.[536] Ca concentration of 10 mmol/L (40 mg/dl; 400 ppm) in mammary secretions is a reliable indicator of fetal "readiness for birth."[524,534,536,538,540] Several stallside tests are available that can measure the Ca ion (Ca^{++}) concentration in mammary secretions based on a colorimetric change of pads on a test strip. Water hardness kits are also useful for determining the concentration of Ca in mammary secretions.[522,540-544] These involve titration of a diluted sample until an indicator dye changes color, and although they are more labor intensive than the test strips, they are reported to provide a more reliable guide for predicting the onset of parturition within the next 24 hours.[544] However, it is important to ensure that the water hardness kit is measuring only Ca levels if it is being used to determine the safest time to induce parturition.[524] Many kits merely test for divalent cations, which include magnesium as well as Ca.[524] Because magnesium levels peak earlier than Ca levels, misleading information about fetal maturity may be obtained.[538,540] If the intent is merely to predict the onset of spontaneous parturition, the type of test is not as critical.[524]

A recent publication has questioned the interpretation of calcium carbonate ($CaCO_3$) test kit data that has formed the basis of recommendations that 200 or 250 ppm $CaCO_3$ be used as the benchmark for readiness for birth.[524,544,545] Paccamonti contends that because Ca in milk is not in the form of $CaCO_3$, any test that measures $CaCO_3$ levels in solution must be adjusted to account for this fact.[524] Because the molecular weight of $CaCO_3$ is 100 and that of Ca is only 40, the conversion factor is 2.5 (i.e., divide the $CaCO_3$ ppm by 2.5 to obtain

Ca ppm). Furthermore, because mammary secretions usually must be diluted before a water hardness test can be used to measure Ca, Paccamonti recommends that 1 ml of secretion be diluted in 4 ml of distilled water. Thus the final reading should be corrected by a factor of 5.[524] The division by 2.5 to convert $CaCO_3$ to Ca and the multiplication by 5 to correct for the dilution mean that the test result need only be doubled to provide an accurate level of Ca ppm. Using this logic, Paccamonti contends that the reports using 200 to 250 ppm $CaCO_3$ as an indication of readiness for birth are actually using Ca values of only 80 to 100 ppm.[524,544,545] However, if these values are corrected for the reported test dilution (1:6) factor, the $CaCO_3$ level being reported would have been 1400 to 1750 ppm (560 to 700 ppm Ca; 14 to 17.5 mmol/L). These corrected values are thus in excess of the 400 ppm (10 mmol/L) Ca concentrations reported by other researchers.[524,534-536,538,540] It is obviously important to keep these calculations in mind because water hardness kits may vary and technicians may use different dilutions. Inappropriate application of the math could lead to an erroneous conclusion about fetal maturity and subsequent induction of a premature foal.[524]

In general, mammary secretion Ca concentrations are more reliable for predicting when a mare is unlikely to spontaneously foal rather than for determining when she is likely to foal.[524,540] Ley used a water hardness kit and reported that $CaCO_3$ levels greater than 200 ppm (see preceding discussion) indicated a 54% probability of spontaneous foaling within 24 hours, 84% probability of spontaneous foaling within 2 days, and 97% probability of spontaneous foaling within 3 days. A small percentage of mares foaled within 24 hours despite a $CaCO_3$ level below 200 ppm.[544,545] However, using Paccamonti's logic, this equates to a corrected value of less than 560 ppm Ca^{2+}.[524] Because a value of 400 ppm Ca^{2+} indicates readiness for birth, it is not surprising that some of these mares foaled. Although the fetus initiates parturition, the mare appears to be able to regulate the actual timing of delivery.[517] Thus any untoward changes in the mare's environment may cause her to postpone the delivery and thus create discrepancies with predictions based on mammary secretion electrolyte concentrations. Ca levels can change rapidly during a single day. Thus testing secretions in the morning and evening may be useful. If a single test is to be performed, it is preferable to check the Ca levels late in the day.[524] Generally, the more rapid the rise in milk Ca levels, the more imminent is parturition. Primiparous mares can be especially difficult to monitor because no change in mammary secretion electrolyte composition may be detected until immediately before foaling.[522]

The presence of cervical softening has traditionally been suggested as a prerequisite for optimal induction of parturition in the mare, and in a recent study mares with a relaxed cervix before induction had a more rapid delivery.[474,523] The same study found that foals delivered from mares with a preinduction, relaxed cervix stood and nursed sooner and had fewer signs of intrapartum asphyxia (hypercapnia, maladjustment) than foals delivered from mares with a nondilated cervix. Mares that developed parturient complications (premature placental separation, dystocia) all had a closed cervix before induction.[474] The status of the cervix is controversial because earlier reports suggest that inductions may proceed successfully even though the cervix is tightly closed and covered with mucus.[518] A recent innovation has been the administration of intracervical PGE_2 (2.5 mg) before induction, but no difference was apparent in the mean interval from initial oxytocin treatment to rupture of the chorioallantois or to the delivery of the foal.[473] However, the impact on foal viability was positive in that foals delivered from PGE_2-treated mares suckled sooner. The application of intracervical PGE_2 may have some merit when terminating a pathologic pregnancy (e.g., hydrops) wherein the induction is known to be premature and is aimed at salvaging the breeding prospects of the mare.[228] Although there is no correlation between myometrial strip (in vitro) response to oxytocin treatment and gestational age, in the author's experience premature induction with oxytocin can take much longer (1-2 hours) than an induction in mares at term.[181,546] This is consistent with the belief that a critical sequence of hormonal changes are required before fetal expulsion can occur.[181] Because the aborted fetus will generally be alive and gasping for air, it is advisable to have ready some euthanasia solution with which to humanely destroy the nonviable neonate.

Several experimental protocols have been reported for induction of parturition in the term mare, including glucocorticoids,[133,518,520,547,548] PGs[518,520,536,549-554], and oxytocin.* High (100 mg/day) and repeated doses (administered intramuscularly daily for 4 days) are required for glucocorticoid induction because, as is not the case with ruminants, this regimen has limited efficacy in the mare.[518] However, a more recent study suggests that multiple injections of dexamethasone given to healthy mares at days 315 through 317 of gestation can induce precocious fetal maturation and delivery of viable foals within 5 to 7 days. The mares remained healthy, with no evidence of laminitis.[133] Further studies are needed to determine whether dexamethasone treatment can be used safely in mares with compromised pregnancies.[133] PG induction is not very efficient in the mare. The synthetic products (fenprostalene, fluprostenol, and prostalene) are more effective than natural PG, but results can be quite variable.[518,520,536,549-554] Oxytocin is the preferred drug for induction of parturition in the mare. A wide range of protocols have been suggested over the years, including a bolus dose (20-75 units), low doses (2.5-20 units) repeated every 15 minutes to effect, and as a slow intravenous drip of 60 to 120 units total (1.0 unit/min).[79,518,519,523,555-559] Recent work suggests that the choice of oxytocin regimen is less important for foal viability than appropriate case selection and adherence to criteria for induction.[474,522] A low-dose protocol has been recommended because it appears to work only in those mares that have a mature fetus.[185] Mares were diagnosed as being ready for birth by mammary secretion Ca strip test measurements. A single injection of 2.5 IU oxytocin (administered intravenously) was given between 1700 and 1900 hr and resulted in the delivery of a normal foal within 120 minutes in 95% of mares. In response to the first oxytocin injection, 24 of 38 (63%) treated mares foaled. Another 9 of 38 (24%) foaled the next evening in response to the second injection, and 3 of 38 (8%) in response to the third treatment. It was concluded that the major advantage of injecting a daily low dose of oxytocin appears to be that such a low dose induces delivery in only those mares that are carrying a mature fetus and are ready to foal. It has been proposed that this low-dose, early-evening oxytocin protocol could be used as a reliable method to induce parturition or to predict that the mare would not foal that night, if parturition did not occur within 2 hours of treatment.[185] However, even this promising

*References 185, 425, 473, 474, 518, 523, 555-558.

protocol has limitations because it is still possible to occasionally induce a mare to deliver a premature foal. Villani and Romano studied the effects of a daily oxytocin treatment (3.5 IU) on 174 full-term Standardbred mares that had mammary secretion Ca levels of greater than or equal to 200 ppm.[559] In this study 69% of the mares foaled within 2 hours of treatment (51.3% responded to the first oxytocin administration, 14.2% to the second, and 3.4% to the third). No significant difference between treated and control mares was observed in the gestational length (340 ± 8 days versus 337 ± 7 days), duration of foaling (10 ± 5.6 minutes versus 11 ± 4.9 minutes), incidence of dystocia (1.4% versus 1.7%), and failure of rupture of the allantochorion (0% versus 0.6%). No significant difference was observed in the incidence of placental retention between treated and control groups (8.1% versus 6.3%). Physical and behavioral characteristics were normal in foals of both groups. The authors concluded that daily injections of low doses of oxytocin in at-term mares showed only moderate efficacy for inducing parturition. However, the easy applicability and safety, for both mare and foal, of this method of foaling induction make it a useful tool to simplify the management of mares in commercial stud farms.[559]

Because most inductions will be performed because complications are expected, the clinician should be well prepared before administration of the induction agent (low-dose oxytocin).[524] Even if the induction is not being performed by an intravenous drip, it is recommended that an intravenous catheter be inserted. This will facilitate rapid induction of general anesthesia if obstetric difficulties ensue. A fully stocked obstetric kit and ample volumes of lubricant should be placed outside the stall. Neonatal resuscitation efforts should be anticipated, and appropriate supplies (e.g., oxygen delivery system) should be readily available. Premature separation of the placenta is not an uncommon complication of induced births. The clinician should immediately rupture the exposed chorioallantois and then assist with fetal delivery in conjunction with the mare's expulsive efforts. Overzealous traction at this time may cause a laceration of the cervix if it is not yet fully dilated. If necessary, an oxygen tube can be placed in the foal's nostril during the minute or two that may be required to complete the assisted delivery. Additional discussion of neonatal resuscitation and critical care is included in this text in Chapter 21.

OBSTETRICS

Management of the Pregnant Mare

A series of publications that discuss the effects of nutrition on various aspects of equine reproduction have recently been published.[560-563] Copper is an overemphasized factor in the etiopathogenesis of osteochondrosis lesions. Supplementation of pregnant mares with copper had no significant effect on the concentration of copper in the liver of foals at birth or on the frequency or severity of lesions in articular cartilage at 160 days of age.[564] Regular exercise and routine hoof maintenance are important for broodmares. A regular anthelmintic program is essential to ensure the mare's well-being. It will also reduce the exposure of the foal to parasite eggs in the mare's feces and the transmammary transfer of *Strongyloides westeri* larvae. Pregnant mares should be current for all vaccinations that are recommended for their particular geographical locations.[565,566] In North America it is especially important to advise owners about the importance of a regular vaccination program for equine herpesvirus. Owners and farm managers should be aware of the need to isolate pregnant mares from transient horses to reduce the risk of infectious disease, especially respiratory viral infections. A tetanus booster may be indicated 1 month before foaling. It is also recommended that the mare be transferred to the final foaling environment at least 1 month before the due date. Foals are born essentially agammaglobulinemic, and the neonate depends on passive transfer of colostral immunoglobulins to provide initial protection from environmental pathogens. If a vulvoplasty (Caslicks) has been performed, plans should be made to open this approximately 1 week earlier than the expected foaling date. If the mare has a history of a previous hemolytic foal (neonatal isoerythrolysis), plans should be made to prevent the neonate from suckling the mare until all the colostrum has been removed.

Those responsible for monitoring the foaling process should understand that mammary development, followed by distention and waxing of the teats and then relaxation of the perineal area, indicates approaching parturition in the mare. The use of mammary secretion electrolyte concentrations to predict foaling was discussed in a previous section. Although it is accepted that the fetus signals its readiness for birth, the mare can regulate the final timing of delivery.[83] Electronic monitoring systems that can be used to signal the start of parturition are also available. Inexperienced personnel should be counseled about normal foaling events and how to recognize when professional assistance is required. Inappropriate intervention by ill-informed individuals can jeopardize the foal's life and potentially cause life-threatening complications in the mare. Separation of the fetal membranes will deprive the fetus of oxygen, and this is the critical factor that must be considered when assessing an obstetric case that involves a live foal. Although most references suggest that fetal survival rates are very low if the foal is not delivered within 30 to 40 minutes of chorioallantoic rupture, one author reports having delivered live foals by cesarean section up to 90 minutes later.[567] These are cases that were promptly presented to the veterinary hospital and that had minimal—if any—vaginal intervention at the farm. It is likely that limited vaginal intervention is less disruptive to the placental attachment, and thus these foals are not deprived of their oxygen supply. Keeping the mare on her feet, and walking if necessary, may help to reduce straining while professional assistance is sought.

Normal Parturition

TERMINOLOGY

The terms *presentation, position,* and *posture* are used to describe the disposition of the fetus as it enters the vaginal canal. Often a fetus is described as having been malpresented or malpositioned when the only anomaly present is postural—the most common cause of dystocia in the mare.[568] To prevent confusion, Vandeplassche introduced the all-encompassing term *fetal maldisposition* to describe the combination of presentational, positional, and postural abnormalities that can contribute to a dystocia.[196] *Presentation* describes the aspect of the fetus that enters the vaginal canal first and also the orientation of the fetal spinal axis to that of the mare (anterior or posterior longitudinal; ventrotransverse or dorsotransverse). More recently, use of the terms *cranial* and *caudal presentation* has become more common. *Position* describes the relationship of the fetal dorsum (longitudinal) or head (transverse) to the quadrants of the mare's pelvis. The normal position for delivery is dorsosacral. A fetus that is still on its side would be right or left dorsoilial, and a fetus that is upside-down would be dorsopubic. The terms *right* and *left cephaloilial* refer to the position of the fetal head relative to the mare's pelvic walls, and they imply that a transverse presentation was present. Posture is purely fetal and describes the relationship of the extremities (head, neck, limbs) to the foal's body.[195,568]

FETAL KINETICS

Fetal mobility has been discussed with respect to umbilical cord torsion and abortion. Fetal rotation within the amniotic cavity and amniotic sac rotation within the allantoic cavity result in the characteristic twisting of the umbilical cord.[411,412] A highly efficient mechanism ultimately guides most equine fetuses into a cranial presentation.[4] Ultrasonographic studies have noted the percentage of anterior, posterior, and transverse presentations at 5 to 6 months to be 52%, 29%, and 19%, respectively, but the fetal presentation becomes predominantly anterior between 7 and 11 months.[408-412] Vandeplassche reported the incidence of anterior, posterior, and transverse presentations in the normal parturient mare population to be 98.9%, 1.0%, and 0.1%, respectively.[196,569] Ginther observed that muscular contractions close the lumen of both uterine horns between 5 and 7 months, and thus the allantoic fluid (with the fetus) is confined to the uterine body.[407,409,412] During this time the fetus positions itself so that its head end points toward the mare's cervix (cranial presentation).[407,408,410] It has been proposed that neurologic signals within the fetal inner ear may respond to the slope of the ventral uterine wall and guide the fetus to lie with its head elevated toward the cervix.[409] In most cases the noncord horn remains closed, whereas the cord horn gradually permits the entry of the hindlimbs between 7 and 9 months. The limbs can enter the horn only when the fetus is in dorsal recumbency because the angle between the horn and body is so acute by this stage of gestation. Thereafter, the hindlimbs remain enclosed within the cord horn and the hooves extend to the horn tip by the tenth month.[407-409,412] Thus the selective closing and opening of the uterine horns, with subsequent trapping of the hindlimbs, is believed to be a key feature of the mechanism that ultimately directs fetal orientation into cranial presentation.[408,409] Entrapment of the hindlimbs within the uterine horn generally means that the caudal portion of the anteriorly presented fetus will be lying in a dorsopubic, and occasionally dorsoilial, position.[409] Ginther's ultrasonographic investigations substantiate the classic radiographic study demonstrating that the full-term equine fetus is initially lying in a dorsopubic position with the head, neck, and forelimbs flexed.[570]

In early pregnancy the mesometrial attachments suspend the uterine horns so that they point cranially and dorsally, but by late gestation the horn containing the hindlimbs comes to rest on the dorsal surface of the uterine body, with the tip of the horn directed back toward the cervix.[4,408] The hooves and horn tip may be pushed so far caudally that they actually come to lie over the fetal head, meaning that when a rectal evaluation of a mare that is in late gestation is performed, the fetal hooves that are palpable may be attached to the hindlimbs. In some mares the vigorous, pistonlike thrusts of the hindlimbs in association with elevation of the fetal rump may push the hooves past the cervix into the rectogenital pouch.[4,408,409] This observation may explain the acute colic episodes that have been previously attributed to uterine dorsoretroflexion.[419] Although the caudal aspect of the fetus is intimately associated with the uterine wall, the cranial portion has room to rotate within the uterine body itself. Ultrasonographic studies on mares close to term (>330 days' gestation) have shown that the cranial half of the fetus was in dorsopubic position approximately 60% of the time and in dorsoilial position in about 40% of the time. The forelimbs and head were usually flexed (about 80%), but in the remainder the head or limbs were extended.[409] Postural changes are common, and thus rectal palpation before the onset of first-stage labor is not a good predictor of impending dystocia.[409,568] However, detection of a posterior or transverse presentation at this late stage is cause for concern, and appropriate plans should be made to manage the impending delivery.

STAGES OF PARTURITION

Behavioral changes that characterize the first stage of parturition include the mare looking at her flank, frequently lying down and getting up, stretching as if to urinate, and passing small amounts of feces. Patchy sweating may develop, and some mares will leak colostrum.[195,568] The restless behavior is similar to that of mild colic and is associated with the development of coordinated uterine contractions that increase uterine pressure and push the chorioallantoic sac (in the region of the cervical star) into the gradually dilating cervix. The increasing uterine tone during stage I of parturition may stimulate the fetus to extend its head and forelimbs up into the dilating pelvic canal.[4] Once the head and forelimbs are fully extended, they are unlikely to return to a flexed posture unless the foal reacts to manual intervention on the part of a foaling attendant. However, it is possible for the neck or a forelimb to develop a malposture if it is not correctly aligned when the mare begins an expulsive effort. Passage of the urinelike allantoic fluid ("water breaking") concludes the first stage of labor. Rupture of the chorioallantois and passage of the allantoic fluid does not occur until the fetlocks, or sometimes the knees, are at the level of the external cervical opening. If the chorioallantois doesn't rupture, further separation from the endometrium can result in a "red bag" delivery, with the velvety red membrane appearing at the vulvar lips. In a normal delivery the chorioallantois is thought to remain attached to the endometrium until after the foal is delivered.[568]

Failure of the chorioallantois to rupture is a common complication of induced parturition.[474] If this happens, continued separation from the endometrium will compromise transplacental oxygen exchange, and fetal hypoxia is likely.[568] Thus premature separation of the placenta is an emergency situation, and foaling attendants should be instructed to break the membrane and provide gentle traction in unison with the mare's expulsive efforts. Although the foal should be delivered as quickly as possible, injudicious traction at this time may cause a laceration in an incompletely dilated cervix.[568] Applying traction only in conjunction with the mare's expulsive efforts will reduce the likelihood of creating cervical trauma.

As parturition progresses, passage of the fetus into the pelvic inlet initiates a reflex release of oxytocin from the posterior pituitary (Ferguson reflex), thereby enhancing uterine contractility.[195] Stage II is characterized by strong abdominal contractions that provide the expulsive force necessary to expel the fetus. Most mares will assume lateral recumbency once active straining commences. Many get up once or twice during stage II labor in what is believed to be a further attempt to correctly position the fetus.[568] Appearance of the translucent fluid-filled amnion at the vulvar lips can be expected to occur within 5 minutes of rupture of the chorioallantois.[571] Any delay in the stage II expulsion process increases the likelihood of fetal asphyxia or neonatal problems associated with hypoxia caused by placental separation. At least one hoof should be visible within the amniotic sac, and the other should be located approximately 2 inches behind it. If everything is progressing normally, the soles of the hooves should face down toward the mare's hocks, and the foal's head should be resting between the carpi.[568]

By the time the nose has reached the vulva, the cranial half of the torso should have rotated from a dorsopubic to a dorsoilial position.[4] The mare probably assists the fetus to reposition itself by the characteristic side-to-side rolling each time she becomes recumbent.[568] It is likely that some dystocias involving fetal malposition and malposture are due to the failure of a compromised fetus to actively participate in the foaling process. Less vigorous or absent fetal righting reflexes early in the parturient process have been suggested by many authors as a cause of fetal maldisposition.[195,481,570] The observation that ventral deviation of the head and neck is more likely to be present if the fetus is in dorsoilial position than in dorsosacral position further substantiates the hypothesis that the fetal righting reflexes are compromised early in these cases.[481]

The second stage of labor in the mare is rapid, with the most forceful contractions occurring as the chest passes through the pelvic cavity. Most foals are delivered within 20 to 30 minutes after the chorioallantoic membrane ruptures. Primiparous dams generally require more time to expel the fetus than do multiparous dams.[195,571] The amniotic sac usually ruptures during these expulsive efforts.[568] However, the equine amniotic sac is not attached to the chorioallantois, as is the case with a ruminant placenta, and the foal sometimes may be delivered with a portion of the sac wrapped around its head.[571] Foaling attendants should be instructed to promptly free the foal's head from the amniotic sac to prevent suffocation. Active straining ceases once the foal's hips are delivered, and the mare will rest in lateral recumbency.[568] An active foal will extract the hindlimbs from the vagina as it struggles to stand. Stage III of parturition involves expulsion of the fetal membranes, which typically takes between 30 minutes and 3 hours.[195] Owners should be advised to seek veterinary assistance if passage of the membranes is delayed because life-threatening toxic metritis and laminitis are common sequelae of membrane retention.[568]

Etiology of Dystocia

The incidence of dystocia in the general horse population varies among breeds (Thoroughbreds: 4%, Shetland Ponies: 8%, draft breeds: 10%).[196] Dystocia is one of the few true emergencies in equine practice; literally, a matter of minutes can determine a successful outcome (i.e., the birth of a live foal).[568] Perinatal asphyxia associated with dystocia is a major cause of equine reproductive loss.[275,276] The long fetal extremities (limbs, neck) predispose the mare to foaling problems.[195,196,568] Alert, informed foaling attendants are essential to ensure that abnormalities are recognized early. Attendants should suspect that the mare is experiencing obstetric problems if either the first or the second stage of parturition is prolonged, or not progressive.[568] Signs that a mare may be in dystocia include the failure of any fetal parts, or of the amniotic membrane, to appear at the vulvar lips for a prolonged period after rupture of the chorioallantois; appearance of only one hoof at the vulva; hooves upside down at the vulva; hooves and nose in abnormal relationship; nose but not hooves at vulva.[571] The most common impediments to delivery are malpostures of the fetal extremities (head and neck, limbs).[481] An experienced foaling attendant may be able to correct minor problems and facilitate a successful delivery. However, inappropriate intervention can have potentially fatal consequences for the mare. Furthermore, obstetric manipulations can easily damage the uterus and cervix to the extent that the mare's reproductive future is jeopardized.[568]

Management of Dystocia

When attending to a mare in dystocia, the veterinarian should make a rapid assessment of the mare's general physical condition, noting, in particular, mucous membrane color and refill time (hemorrhage, dehydration, shock).[568] A mare that is aborting in late gestation may experience a dystocia because the dead fetus cannot participate in the delivery process. A malodorous discharge strongly suggests the presence of an emphysematous fetus. The perineal area should be inspected to determine the presence and nature of any vulvar discharge and the presence of fetal membranes and to identify any fetal extremities. Excessive hemorrhage or vulvar swelling may indicate that nonprofessional intervention has caused trauma to the reproductive tract. Occasionally, a mare will exhibit a rectal prolapse, an everted bladder, or intestinal loops protruding from the vulvar lips.[568] The intestines may be of fetal origin if there is incomplete closure of the ventral abdomen, but a ruptured vagina is more likely. In the later scenario the foal's foot may have ruptured the floor of the cranial vagina, but injudicious manipulations by an inexperienced attendant should not be discounted. If a rectal prolapse or the urinary bladder is evident, then an epidural anesthetic should be administered to prevent further straining. Alternately, the mare may be anesthetized to facilitate hoisting the hindquarters.[568] The advantage of this approach is that the straining can be stopped immediately. This is especially important if the prolapse involves an intussuscepted colon (type IV).[572,573] In these cases a palpable trench may extend several feet into the rectum, and avulsion of the mesentery can be a fatal complication that is not readily amenable to surgical correction.

The author considers stocks to be contraindicated when examining a foaling mare and prefers to perform the initial examination on a standing mare with no more restraint than a twitch or lip chain if her demeanor will permit this to be performed safely. The behavior of a mare in stage II labor is unpredictable and may be violent. It is important to ensure that the examination area is clean, with good footing. There should be ample space for the mare handler, obstetrician, and assistants to move to safety if necessary. Although most veterinary tranquilizers readily cross the placenta and can compromise the fetus, adequate restraint is essential for the safety of all concerned.[574] Sedation with tranquilizers may be necessary for some uncooperative mares, and in extremely intractable cases it may be preferable to anesthetize the mare with a short-acting combination. In these cases a hoist should be available because manipulating the foal is sometimes difficult when the mare is in lateral recumbency. Although not essential, an initial rectal examination may help the practitioner rule out the presence of a term uterine torsion and determine the condition of the uterine wall (tears, spasm). It also may-provide useful information regarding the disposition of the fetus. Before any vaginal examination the mare's tail should be wrapped and the perineal area thoroughly cleansed. The clinician's arms and hands should be scrubbed with disinfectant soap.[568] In a hospital environment the author also wears sterile rubber obstetric sleeves. Cleanliness and lubrication are the cornerstones of obstetrics.

The mare's vagina and cervix are easily traumatized by the friction associated with vaginal manipulations. Once the mucous membrane has been abraded, it is likely that adhesions and fibrosis will follow. Thus copious amounts of lubricant are vital to ensure that the soft tissues of the genital tract are not traumatized and thus preserve the mare's future fertility.[575] Lubricants include methyl cellulose, polyethylene polymer, white petrolatum combined with 10% boric acid, and mineral oil. Water-soluble lubricants are generally not as desirable, because they rapidly lose their lubricating abilities in the presence of fluids.[195] If a large volume of lubricant is to be pumped around the fetus, investigating the possibility of a uterine laceration is essential. In a referral situation the author routinely performs an abdominocentesis. Serosanguinous to sanguinous fluid that contains elevated total protein levels and an increased white blood cell count is highly suggestive of a uterine rupture.[492] If a uterine tear is unlikely, the author prefers to mix a polyethylene polymer powder with warm water and then use a clean stomach tube and pump to gently instill large volumes of lubricant into the uterine lumen.[575] This is repeated as often as necessary during the procedure to keep the fetus and reproductive tract coated with lubricant.

The vagina, cervix, and accessible parts of the uterus should be carefully explored to ascertain the source of any hemorrhage. Lacerations should be noted and their presence discussed with owners or the attending personnel before any veterinary manipulations are attempted. Occasionally, the cause of the dystocia is a pelvic deformity (e.g., callus). It is important to determine the degree of cervical dilation.[568] If the mare has been in labor for some time, it is possible that the uterus is relatively dry and tightly contracted around the fetus. This will make intrauterine manipulations much more difficult, especially because it becomes difficult to repel the fetus back into the uterus safely. If the uterus is contracted, warm lubricant tends to induce some uterine relaxation, and the volume expansion creates additional space in which to perform manipulations.[477,575] Myometrial contractions (uterine spasm) can be controlled by tocolytic drugs (isoxsuprine, clenbuterol) if they are available for veterinary use.[196] Although fetopelvic disproportion is uncommon in the mare, it can be a factor in some equine dystocias.[52,53,57,568] The disposition of the fetus should be noted and fetal viability determined. Care should be exercised because active fetal response to manipulations can easily complicate an initially simple dystocia.[568] Placement of a rope snare behind the ears and into the foal's mouth ensures that the clinician always has control of the head. This will facilitate correction of a potentially life-threatening development such as lateral deviation of the head and neck if the fetus pulls away from the clinician's manipulations.[568] If the snare is placed around the mandible, it is essential that only gentle traction be applied to guide the fetal head through the vaginal canal. Excessive force may cause a fracture of the mandible. When obvious fetal movement is absent, digital withdrawal may be initiated in response to pinching of the coronary band. Slight digital pressure over the eyelid onto the eyeball may arouse a response, as may stimulation of the tongue (swallowing). If the thorax can be reached, fetal heartbeat is definitive. In posteriorly presented cases the digital and anal reflexes are useful as indicators of fetal viability. Occasionally, it may be possible to reach the umbilical cord.[195]

The clinician should inform the owner of the various options, costs, and prognosis once the current status of the foal is known and the cause of the dystocia has been determined. Ensuring that the owner is aware of the potential complications that may arise is especially important because postpartum medical care can become quite expensive. If delivery of a live foal is anticipated, the clinician should consider the potential for fetal cardiovascular compromise before administering any tranquilizers to the mare.[568] Light sedation of the mare with acetylpromazine (2 to 3 mg/100 kg IV) has minimal effect on the foal and may be useful in some cases.[576] Xylazine is preferable to detomidine if the fetus is viable because its depressant effects are of much shorter duration.[576] However, neither xylazine nor detomidine should be used alone to sedate a dystocia case because some apparently sedated mares can become hypersensitive over the hindquarters.[453,576] The combination of xylazine and acepromazine provides good sedation in a quiet mare.[585] The author routinely uses a combination of xylazine (0.3 to 0.5 mg/kg IV) and butorphanol (0.01 to 0.02 mg/kg IV) for standing obstetric procedures if more sedation is required (e.g., fetotomy procedure). This provides good sedation and analgesia, and additional doses may be administered as necessary. Attendants are instructed to keep the lip chain loose and to tighten it only when instructed to do so. This will ensure that it retains its effectiveness when required to divert the mare's attention.[568] LeBlanc suggests a xylazine (1.1 mg/kg) and morphine (0.1 to 0.2 mg/kg) combination for sedation of fetotomy cases but cautions that gastrointestinal stasis is a frequent complication.[574] Although most dystocias can be resolved at the farm fairly quickly by brief manipulation and assisted vaginal delivery, the practitioner should consider the alternatives if resolution is likely to take more than 10 to 15 minutes. Prolonged, unproductive vaginal manipulations are contraindicated in equine obstetrics. Decisions on the next course of action should be based on the viability of the foal, the clinician's obstetric skills, the availability of equipment and facilities, and the financial constraints imposed by the owner.

An epidural does not prevent the mare's myometrial contractions or the abdominal press, and the time involved in administering an effective epidural anesthetic may make this form of restraint impractical when a live foal is present.[568,576] However, if the foal is dead, epidural anesthesia does reduce vaginal sensitivity and thus the mare's perception of vaginal manipulations (Ferguson reflex). Caudal epidural anesthesia should be used at the clinician's discretion, especially if general anesthesia or referral may become necessary. When an epidural is indicated, the author uses a combination of xylazine (0.17 mg/kg) and lidocaine (2 to 3 ml) diluted in saline, such that the final volume does not exceed 8 to 10 ml in order to reduce the likelihood of hindlimb weakness.[576,577] Excess volume can cause the mare to become ataxic. Short-term general anesthesia may be indicated when minor postural abnormalities are present and maternal expulsive efforts make correction difficult.[505] A xylazine (1.1 mg/kg IV) followed by ketamine (2.2 mg/kg IV) provides a general anesthetic with a smooth, short (10 to 15 minutes) duration. Addition of the central-acting muscle relaxant guaifenesin (1 L of a solution of 5% guaifenesin in 5% dextrose) can provide an additional 10 to 20 minutes for fetal manipulation.[576] In specialist equine hospitals that are located close to well-managed broodmare farms, the fetus is often still alive when the mare arrives.[567,578] A well-coordinated dystocia team that uses a defined protocol can minimize time spent nonproductively. Intrapartum intratracheal intubation and positive pressure ventilation of the fetus (ex utero intrapartum treatment [EXIT]) during resolution of the dystocia has been shown to improve survival rates. It should be remembered that positive pressure ventilation must be continued once begun because it promotes the conversion from fetal circulatory patterns to neonatal patterns, essentially eliminating the role of the umbilicus.[578] In referral hospitals it is common practice to anesthetize the mare after a brief vaginal intervention and then maintain the mare on halothane-oxygen with controlled ventilation. Because halothane anesthesia has been shown to compromise umbilical circulation, the concentration should be kept to a minimum if the foal is still alive.[496] Total intravenous anesthesia (the so-called triple drip of ketamine, xylazine, and guaifenesin) may be preferable until the foal has been delivered .[574] The mare should be ventilated with oxygen, and intravenous fluids should be administered as required. If the hind-end elevation technique is used, almost three quarters of such cases can be resolved by controlled vaginal delivery. However, if the fetus is still alive and has not been delivered within 15 minutes, an immediate cesarean section is performed—with a 30% foal survival rate possible, provided that the time from rupture of the chorioallantois to presentation at the veterinary hospital is minimal.[567,579] Fertility after cesarean section is quite good, and adverse reports probably pertain more to the extent of vaginal manipulation after surgery.[580,581] If a hoist is available in the field, hobbles can be placed on the hind pasterns and the hindquarters briefly elevated 1 to 2 feet. The combination of a relaxed uterus and the effects of gravity can facilitate fetal repulsion and manipulation. If attempts at mutation are successful, the mare should be lowered into lateral recumbency to permit extraction of the foal.[568] Prolonged dorsal recumbency results in compression of the aorta and vena cava and reduction in venous return, cardiac output, and blood pressure.[574] Hindlimb paresis may develop after prolonged hindquarter suspension and can complicate the recovery process. The use of pads to support the hindquarters will help take some weight off the limbs while the mare is suspended.

Mutation is an obstetric term that is used to describe manipulation of the fetal extremities, with correction of any positional abnormalities, such that assisted vaginal delivery can proceed.[195] Although extra space is available for manipulations when the fetus has been repelled into the uterus, the clinician should remain cognizant at all times that overzealous obstetric manipulations are a major cause of uterine rupture.* Repulsion of the fetus from the maternal pelvis is contraindicated if the uterus is contracted down around the fetus. In some cases pumping warm obstetric lubricant around the fetus induces some degree of uterine relaxation. In countries where they are legal, tocolytic agents are effective in relaxing a contracted uterus. If the fetus is dead, many cases may be amenable to correction by fetotomy provided that the clinician has the appropriate skills and equipment.[586-589] Although poor technique and inappropriate fetotomy cuts often lead to infertility, experienced clincians can rapidly resolve a dystocia while preserving the mare's future breeding potential.[586,589,590] The alternative is cesarean section.[578,579,591]

Traction must be applied with careful regard for both maternal and fetal well-being.[575,592] Traction applied entirely by hand often is all that is necessary. Obstetric straps or chains may provide a better grip. The author prefers to apply one loop above the fetlock, with a second loop encircling the pastern.[575] In assisted vaginal deliveries traction should be applied as an adjunct when the mare is exerting expulsive force and should be released when the dam stops straining, thereby permitting rest and recovery. This approach is critical to permit adequate dilation of the caudal reproductive tract.[575] Copious lubrication and slow traction with continuous monitoring of cervical dilation are especially important when a controlled vaginal delivery is performed on an anesthetized mare.[579] Excessive use of force may be associated with fetal fractures (ribs, vertebrae, and limbs) and maternal soft tissue trauma.[592] No more than two or three people (depending on size and strength) should apply traction to the fetus.[575]

CRANIAL (ANTERIOR) PRESENTATION

An anteriorly presented fetus that is in dorsosacral position with head and forelimbs extended should require minimal traction to complete the delivery, assuming that the vaginal canal is well lubricated. By ensuring that slightly more traction is applied to one limb than the other, the practitioner reduces the width of the fetus across the shoulders and can successfully deliver most cases. If progress is not being made, then all traction should stop and the vaginal canal must be fully explored.[575] There are three likely possibilities: elbow lock (incomplete extension of the forelimb); dog-sitting or hurdling posture; and, occasionally, a fetus that is too large. Absolute or relative fetopelvic disproportion is uncommon in the mare, even when the foal has been carried several weeks past the expected due date. In fact, some cases of prolonged gestation may involve a smaller than normal, dysmature fetus.[195,593] In a referral hospital study, fewer than 2% of dystocias were attributed to this condition.[481] It is significant, however, that approximately 30% of referral hospital dystocia cases are in primiparous mares.[481,569,571] Primiparous mares were disproportionately represented in a report on dystocia and neonatal asphyxia from the central Kentucky area.[229,594] Thus, although fetopelvic disproportion is not common in the mare, obstetric assistance (traction) is required much more often in primiparous mares.[196,594,595] Dystocia in these mares is further complicated by a tight vaginovestibular sphincter, which may predispose primiparous mares to lacerations and rectovaginal tears.[594] If copious lubrication and gentle traction do not help, cesarean section or partial fetotomy are the only alternatives.

Incomplete elbow extension may be unilateral or bilateral and should be suspected if the fetal muzzle lies at the same level as the hooves.[575] In this posture the fetal elbows will be tucked back under the shoulder joint, causing increased depth and width of the fetus within the maternal pelvic inlet. Correction involves repelling the fetal trunk so that the forelimbs can be extended and thus raise the elbows up over the floor of the pelvic inlet.[477]

In a dog-sitting or hurdling posture, there is either bilateral (dog-sitting posture) or unilateral (hurdling posture) hip flexion. This causes the fetal hooves (or hoof) to push against the pelvic brim during attempts at fetal extraction.[575] The

*References 195, 477, 491, 492, 419, 582-585.

unilateral posture is more common.[481] Severe trauma can be inflicted on the mare if this malposture is not recognized and inappropriate amounts of traction are applied. Thus it is important to stop all traction and repel the fetus enough to sweep the floor of the pelvic inlet. In extreme cases the hindlimb may actually extend under the fetus and up into the vagina.[481] Although the hindlimb may be successfully repelled if the fetus is alive, it is a difficult procedure and is associated with some risk of uterine laceration. Judicious use of a snare or fetatome may facilitate safe repulsion of the hindlimb by looping the pastern and using the instrument to repel the hoof away from the pelvic brim. Repulsion should not be attempted on a standing mare if the fetus is dead because the hindlimb may not return to its normal position.[586,588] In such cases the hoof of the flexed hindlimb can puncture the ventral uterine wall as the foal is being extracted. If a dog-sitting or hurdling foal is dead, it is recommended that general anesthesia and hoisting of the hindquarters be employed to reduce the risk of ventral uterine rupture.[596] In experienced hands partial fetotomy is a viable alternative to cesarean section.[586-588,590] A surgical alternative to a cesarean section involves manipulation of the hindlimb through a ventral midline celiotomy incision. An assistant may be able to extract the fetus through the vagina once the hindlimb has been grasped through the ventral incision. If successful, this technique will reduce the potential for contamination that may be associated with cesarean section. If a cesarean section is performed, some surgeons prefer to remove that portion of the foal that is protruding through the vulvar lips before withdrawing the hind end out through the surgical site.[419]

In a foot-nape posture one or both of the forelimbs is displaced over the foal's head and pushed against the roof of the vagina.[575] To correct this malposture the fetus must be repelled into the uterus by applying pressure to the head. Once the forelimbs have been replaced under the head, fetal extraction can proceed quite uneventfully.[575] If not corrected immediately, the mare's straining can cause the fetal hoof to lacerate the vaginal roof, and in extreme cases it can result in a rectovaginal fistula. A fistula is all that occurs if the foal withdraws its hoof from the rectum before delivery. A third-degree perineal laceration occurs if the strong expulsive efforts of the mare cause the limb that has penetrated the rectum to dissect through the caudal rectovaginal shelf and rupture through the anal sphincter, thereby creating a cloaca.[597-598]

Carpal flexion is a common cause of dystocia.[589,590] It may be unilateral or bilateral, and typically the affected carpus is located at the pelvic inlet.[575] To safely correct this malposture, the fetal body must first be repelled into the uterus. If the dystocia is prolonged, the amount of uterine contraction may preclude meaningful repulsion of the fetus back into the uterus. Because the fetus is likely to be dead in these cases, a relatively simple fetotomy cut can be made at the level of the distal row of carpal bones. This permits safe delivery of the foal without the need to traumatize the reproductive tract and generally facilitates extraction within minutes.[586,588,590] If the foal is alive, repulsion into the uterus will permit the flexed limb to be grasped at the level of the fetlock and pastern. By rotating the wrist, the obstetrician can rotate the carpus laterally while bringing the flexed fetlock medially and caudally into the birth canal. This maneuver allows maximal use of available space by obliquing the extremity through the pelvic inlet. The obstetrician should be aware that flexural deformities are considered to be the most common congenital anomaly of foals and that the rigid deformity often means that a cesarean section or fetotomy must be performed.[229,275,569,586-588] Limb contractures are generally bilateral. Contracture is more common in the forelimbs than the hindlimbs but can involve all four limbs.[569,575] Severely affected limbs cannot be straightened, and needless trauma can be inflicted on the genital tract by unrewarding attempts to manually correct the malposture. It is important that the clinician cup the hand over the bottom of the fetal hoof at all times while attempting to straighten the limb. Failure to do so may result in injury to the reproductive tract. Application of an obstetric chain or rope to the distal limb can be a useful aid. This permits traction to be applied to the distal limb while the hand covers and guides the hoof.[575]

The single most common abnormality in referral hospital dystocia populations is a reflected head and neck.[196,481,569,589] Unfortunately, these malpostures are often iatrogenic in that a viable fetus has pulled back from the initial vaginal intervention that aimed to correct a minor postural problem. If the mare strains while the foal's head is pulled back, it is possible for the muzzle to engage the wall or floor of the pelvic inlet. The mare's forceful expulsive efforts may then drive the head and neck ventrally, or laterally along the thorax, while the forelimbs are pushed further into the vaginal canal. Ventral or lateral displacements of the head and neck can be very difficult to correct. The length of the foal's neck often makes it impossible to reach the head. Inexperienced clinicians should consider referral as soon as the condition is diagnosed because prolonged unrewarding manipulations can easily jeopardize the mare's future fertility.[575,578] A relatively simple fetotomy cut can resolve these cases quite atraumatically if the fetus is dead when the veterinarian arrives. The author believes that this approach is preferable to prolonged—and often unsuccessful—attempts at manual correction of this extremely difficult malposture.[586,590] If the fetus is alive, an attempt can be made to place eye hooks or to loop a snare around the mandible. Some obstetricians even suggest applying a clamp on an ear to pull the head back enough to place a snare. The author prefers to use a snare whenever possible. If traction can be applied to the head, the foal's body must be carefully repelled while attempts are made to bring the head and neck around into a normal posture for delivery. Factors influencing the successful outcome include uterine tonicity, clinician arm length and skill, and the presence or absence of torticollis and facial scoliosis.[569,575] As with contracted tendons, it is essential that the practitioner consider the possibility of a wry neck. This condition is not amenable to correction by mutation, and needless trauma can be inflicted on the genital tract by unrewarding attempts at correction. Ventral deviation of the head is relatively easy to correct if the fetal nose is just below the brim of the pelvis (poll posture). It is generally easier to rotate the head laterally before attempting to bring the muzzle up over the pelvic brim. In more severe cases the neck is tucked down between the forelimbs and the head is often beyond reach (nape posture).[569,575] If attempts to reposition the head and neck are unsuccessful, then cesarean section or fetotomy are indicated.[579,586-588,590]

Shoulder flexion posture may be unilateral ("swimming" posture) or bilateral ("diving" posture).[569,575] To gain access to the retained limb, it is usually necessary to repel the head and neck into the uterus. An immediate cesarean section may be preferable if the foal is alive because correction of this malposture can be difficult and time-consuming. If this is not an option, it is recommended that a soft rope snare be placed on the fetal head (behind ears and into mouth) so that the head can be readily retrieved once the shoulder flexion has been corrected. If the limb can be reached, correction of this malposture is performed in two stages. Initially, the shoulder flexion is converted to a carpal flexion by grasping the limb in the area of the humerus and working down to the distal radius. The limb is then pulled caudally and medially as the fetal body is repelled. The carpus is then hooked over the brim of the pelvis to create a carpal flexion, which is then corrected as previously described. It must be remembered that it is not always possible to repel the head sufficiently to gain access to the retained forelimb. In these cases cesarean section is the only option for delivery of a live foal. If the fetus is dead, a fetotomy cut to remove the head and neck may provide sufficient room to correct the malposture.[586-588]

CAUDAL (POSTERIOR) PRESENTATION

A foal in posterior presentation will have the soles of the hooves facing up. Although the author has seen dystocias in which an anteriorly presented foal was in dorsopubic position with both forelimbs extended, this is a very unusual complication. Foaling attendants should be instructed to wash the mare's perineum and then to use a clean arm to check for the hocks somewhere in the vaginal canal. Gentle traction on the hindlimbs in conjunction with the mare's expulsive efforts may facilitate delivery of a live foal. However, approximately half of the fetuses may be malpositioned as well, and they often require veterinary assistance to permit an atraumatic delivery. Foals in caudal (posterior) presentation are more likely to be in dorsoilial position than foals in a cranial (anterior) presentation.[481] Although a normally positioned fetus in caudal presentation may not be particularly difficult to deliver, it is more likely to suffer hypoxia because of compression of the umbilical cord under the fetal thorax or because of premature rupture of the umbilical cord.[575] Although only about 1% of foals are presented posteriorly, this malpresentation accounts for between 14% and 16% of referral hospital dystocia cases because any postural abnormalities create a major complication.[196,481,569] Typically, both hindlimbs are involved, and these types of dystocia cases (hock flexion, hip flexion) are extremely difficult to correct under field conditions. Hock flexion malposture accounts for about one quarter of referred posterior cases.[196,481,569] Correction of a hock flexion is dangerous because of the risk of perforation of the dorsal aspect of the uterus. The fetus must be repelled into the uterus while one hock is pushed dorsolaterally and the distal limb is directed medially. The procedure for obliquing the extremity into the birth canal is similar to that previously described for correction of a carpal flexion. An obstetric chain or strap can be used to apply traction to the limb while the hoof is cupped in the hand. Straightening a flexed hock entails considerable risk because the hock is invariably forced against the dorsal uterine wall. When the uterus is contracted, there is a real possibility of causing a laceration or perforation. Cesarean section may be preferable for delivery of a live fetus. The author strongly believes that fetotomy is a safer procedure than attempts at mutation if the fetus is dead.[579,586-588] Approximately half of referred posterior presentation cases are breech (bilateral hip flexion posture).[196,481,569] A cesarean section is indicated if the fetus is alive because the manipulations involved in correcting this malposture are time consuming and extremely difficult. The comments for managing a hock flexion apply because if mutation is attempted, the hip flexion must first be converted into a flexed hock posture.[575] A key point is to remember to flex both hocks before attempting to straighten a limb. If one limb is extended into the vaginal canal while the other hip remains flexed, the fetal body will move back into the pelvic canal, and this will make it extremely difficult to access the retained limb.[593] If the fetus is dead, the author recommends attempting to convert the bilateral hip flexion into a hock flexion posture, followed by correction with two fetotomy cuts through the distal row of tarsal bones. This may be safer and less traumatic than attempting to straighten the limbs, provided that the clinician is experienced in the use of a fetatome.[587] Attempts to correct a bilateral hip flexion by fetotomy, without first creating a bilateral hock flexion, are often unrewarding because of the difficulty in correctly placing the fetotomy wire. Referral for cesarean section will often provide the best prognosis for future fertility in these cases.

TRANSVERSE PRESENTATION

Only about 1 in 1000 foals is presented transversely. Successful resolution of these dystocia cases requires a significant amount of obstetric experience, which explains why these rare presentations account for between 10% and 20% of referral hospital dystocia cases.[481,569,581] Most transverse presentations are ventral transverse, with the abdomen and limbs of the fetus presented toward the birth canal.[196,481,569] Although the widespread adoption of ultrasonography has markedly reduced the likelihood of a twin birth, this possibility must always be explored when more than two limbs are present in the birth canal.[229,275] In some instances it may be possible to repel the head and forequarters of the fetus while extending the two hindlimbs into the pelvic canal. If the manipulations are successful, the transverse presentation is thus converted into a posterior presentation for vaginal delivery. The likelihood of successfully resolving one of these cases is improved if the mare has been anesthetized and the hindquarters elevated.[575] Transverse presentations may be associated with flexural limb deformities, angular limb deformity, and spinal deformity. If the fetus is alive, the delivery method of choice is cesarean section.[579] Dorsal transverse presentations, with the spinal column of the fetus presented toward the birth canal, are very rare. These cases warrant an immediate referral for cesarean section, even if the foal is dead.[196,481,569] Although an experienced obstetrician may be able to deliver a transversely presented fetus by fetotomy, the owner should be advised that this will be a difficult and time-consuming procedure, with a high risk of trauma that will likely impede the mare's future fertility.[575,586-588]

FETAL ANOMALIES

Hydrocephalus is not uncommon in equine fetuses, especially in pony breeds.[196,481,569,599] The condition occurs when increased intracranial pressure causes the bones of the skull to enlarge, sometimes almost doubling the size of the head.[569] The skull is often very thin, and many affected foals can be delivered after incising the soft portion of the skull with a finger knife, allowing the skull to collapse.[586] The trunk of the hydrocephalic fetus is generally smaller than normal and seldom interferes with delivery.[575] If the enlarged cranium is bony, a fetotomy cut may be necessary to reduce the size of the head.[586-588]

CARE OF THE POSTPARTUM MARE

The fetal membranes should be examined as a matter of routine to ensure that they have been passed intact and to check for any placental anomalies that may indicate impending problems in the neonate. The chorioallantois often has tears that can be misleading, especially if the mare has trod on the membranes repeatedly. Examining the allantoic side of the membrane may be helpful in that the blood vessels can be pieced together and will give some idea as to whether a portion is actually missing.[30] Ideally, all foaling mares should receive a brief physical examination within 24 hours of parturition. If the mare's attitude is normal and she displays typical maternal behavior toward the foal, the udder should be checked and the perineal area inspected for evidence of trauma.[196] A detailed reproductive examination is usually unwarranted because it may unnecessarily disrupt the normal mare-foal bond that is developing at this time.[600] Routine postpartum use of oxytocin or PG (cloprostenol) therapy is not warranted because there is no apparent benefit for uterine involution in normally foaling mares.[601] All mares should receive a thorough reproductive examination at the foal heat.[477] Occasionally, an enlarged ovary is detected. This may be a GTCT that has enlarged during the course of the previous pregnancy. Prompt diagnosis and surgical intervention may permit the mare to resume normal cyclicity and conceive during the current breeding season.

Abdominal discomfort in the peripartum mare may be due to uterine contractions, especially if the mare has been treated with oxytocin to promote passage of the fetal membranes. However, other causes of abdominal pain should not be discounted.[493,602-604] When a postpartum mare displays abdominal discomfort, the author believes that abdominocentesis is indicated. The normal foaling process does not alter the composition of the peritoneal fluid from within the normal range. Even a dystocia does not necessarily cause significant changes in the peritoneal fluid. If an experienced obstetrician performs the vaginal manipulations or fetotomy, the fluid should remain normal.[493] If the peritoneal fluid is normal, the mare should be monitored closely for signs of clinical deterioration. Repeated abdominocentesis may be indicated when clinical signs suggest that a parturient-related abdominal lesion may be present because the peritoneal fluid constituents can change within hours.[493] A single elevated peritoneal fluid value (total protein, white cell count, or percent neutrophils) may be an incidental finding. Elevation of two or more values often signals the onset of clinical abnormalities. It has been the author's experience that if a postpartum peritoneal fluid sample has a total protein value above 3.0 g/dl, in conjunction with a white blood cell count greater than 15,000 cells/μl, and a white blood cell differential count greater than 80% neutrophils (especially if degenerative changes are present), then the presence of a potentially life-threatening lesion is likely.[493] The peritoneal fluid analysis should not be viewed in isolation and must be considered in conjunction with the history and clinical signs being exhibited by the mare. In the author's experience, detection of changes in the peritoneal fluid almost invariably indicates the presence of foaling-related trauma in either the reproductive or the gastrointestinal tract. An early diagnosis followed by appropriate medical or surgical intervention (or both) will often result in a favorable outcome. If treatment is not implemented until the affected mare has become depressed and febrile, with accompanying signs of shock and toxemia, the prognosis may be more guarded.

Periparturient Hemorrhage

The arterial supply to the uterus is supported by the mesometrium (broad ligament). The major blood supply to the uterus is from the uterine artery, a branch of the external iliac artery. It forms a cranial branch that supplies the proximal uterine horn and a caudal branch that supplies the distal uterine horn and uterine body. The smaller ovarian artery gives off a uterine branch that anastomoses in the proximal horn with the cranial vessels from the uterine artery. The urogenital artery is a branch off the internal pudendal artery, and it gives rise to the caudal uterine artery along with vessels to the rectum, ureter, bladder, urethra, and vagina. The caudal uterine artery supplies the lateral side of the cranial vagina and continues past the cervix to ramify on the uterine body, where it anastomoses with the caudal branch of the uterine artery.[3,605,606] Hemorrhage from these vessels, especially the large-diameter uterine artery, is a significant cause of periparturient colic signs and death in older multiparous mares.[195,419,583,604,605,607,608] However, a retrospective study of 73 cases suggests that periparturient hemorrhage can occur in mares of any age or parity, and the condition may occasionally occur before foaling.[609] In a study of 98 postpartum deaths, almost 40% were due to uterine artery rupture.[604] The rupture may be anywhere along the vessel and is typically 2 or 3 cm in length and oriented parallel to the long axis of the vessel. There generally is no evidence of a predisposing aneurysm.[604] An association with low serum copper levels has been proposed as a reason for vessel fragility in aged mares.[610]

There appears to be a predilection for right-side uterine vessel rupture. It has been suggested that the extent of cecal displacement of the gravid uterus to the left may be sufficient to place increased tension on the vessels in the right broad ligament.[604,608] Although the added stress of dystocia may increase the chances of arterial rupture, many cases occur in mares that appeared to have an uneventful delivery.[419,604] Hemorrhage from the hypertrophied vessels that supply the gravid uterus may be rapidly fatal, especially if the artery ruptures directly into the peritoneal cavity. The mare may be found dead or moribund with pale mucous membranes, tachycardia (up to 140 beats/min), and tachypnea. Heroic attempts to administer blood transfusions, plasma expanders, and associated fluid therapy may save the life of some valuable mares, but costs are often prohibitive.[321,419,477] If the bleeding is contained within the broad ligament, the mare may be trembling and will exhibit signs of extreme pain (anxiety, sweating, colic), presumably as a result of the stretching of the broad ligament as the hematoma develops.[477,583,604] The color of the mucous membranes may not change initially because of vascular compensation, and often these initial colic signs are mistaken for the typical discomfort experienced by postpartum mares as the uterus contracts. However, if significant hemorrhage is present, the color of the mucous membranes will eventually become pale and capillary refill will be delayed.[583] These mares must be monitored closely because the hematoma can subsequently rupture out of the mesometrium and lead to rapid exsanguinations.[608]

If a ruptured artery is suspected, the mare should not be disturbed any more than is necessary to perform an examination.[194] In many cases, postponing, or even forgoing, rectal palpation may be prudent. Although an internal examination will reveal valuable diagnostic information, transabdominal ultrasound, abdominocentesis, and a hemogram may be all that is necessary to confirm that an acute hemorrhagic episode has occurred.[196,477] Transabdominal ultrasonographic evaluation will reveal free blood in the abdominal cavity if the hematoma has torn the broad ligament.[321] If the broad ligament tears after a uterine artery rupture, a bloody tap invariably results, with an elevated red blood cell count in the peritoneal fluid.[492] The centrifuged sample will have a pink or hemolyzed appearance if hemoperitoneum is present. A smear that reveals phagocytosed erythrocytes indicates hemorrhage rather than contamination during sampling.[321] Even if a clot has contained most of the hemorrhage within the broad ligament, there is often considerable blood loss into the peritoneal cavity. The initial hemogram during an acute hemorrhagic episode can be confusing because the relative loss of erythrocytes and plasma may not alter the hematocrit immediately. Splenic contraction will also temporarily raise the hematocrit.[321] In the author's opinion, these mares should not be transported because movement could destabilize the clot and prove fatal. Any supportive therapy should be administered at the stall until the mare has stabilized. The foal should be kept safely nearby so that the mare does not become unduly distressed.

Most recommendations for the management of postpartum hemorrhage in mares are based on the collective wisdom of experienced clinicians and from methodologies that have been extrapolated from the human trauma literature. The approach taken will be governed by the facilities and expertise available and financial constraints. In some instances an extreme hypotensive state may actually offer the best chance for survival (conservative approach), whereas in other cases an attempt to restore intravascular pressures and circulatory volume could be indicated. The conservative approach is to confine the hypotensive mare to a dark, quiet stall with minimal disturbances. In some cases a platelet-fibrin plug allows the rent in the vessel to be sealed once the arterial pressure falls. Tranquilizers (especially acetylpromazine) should be used with caution because any induced drop in blood pressure may exacerbate the hypovolemic shock. Some clinicians employ hypotensive resuscitation by administering a vasodilating agent in conjunction with intravenous fluid therapy.[321] The idea in this instance is to provide lifesaving volume replacement while maintaining a low mean arterial pressure. In life-threatening situations anything that may stabilize the mare is worthwhile, but the clinician should consider the possibility of impeding resolution of the hematoma by rapid expansion of blood volume and elevation of blood pressure. The need to support cardiac output and ensure oxygen delivery must be balanced against the prospect of the increased arterial pressure promoting further hemorrhage.[321]

Although costly, an aggressive therapeutic approach can occasionally save the life of a valuable mare.[321,604,611] If a valuable mare presents in shock and appears to be deteriorating rapidly, a large intravenous catheter should be inserted and substantial fluid therapy begun. Whole blood transfusions must be given slowly and thus are of little benefit for resuscitative purposes when rapid volume expansion is required. One option is rapid administration of 2 to 3 L of hypertonic saline, followed with 10 to 20 L of lactated Ringer's solution over a period of 2 to 4 hours. An alternative to the hypertonic saline is the high oncotic pressure exerted by colloids (e.g., 3 L hydroxyethyl starch).[321] Synthetic oxygen-carrying fluids are commercially available but extremely expensive. Supplemental oxygen can be provided by nasal insufflation at a flow rate of 5 to 10 L/min. If the hematocrit continues to drop to under 15%, whole blood transfusions (6-8 L over several hours) may be warranted.[321] Benefits include provision of oxygen-carrying cells, clotting factors, and oncotic pressure (albumin).

A shock dose of corticosteroid is indicated. Because hemorrhagic shock can cause ischemic-reperfusion damage to the gut and lungs (multiple organ failure), broad spectrum antibiotics, antioxidant drugs, and anti-inflammatory medication may be warranted if the mare survives the initial hemorrhagic crisis.[321] Flunixin meglumine (1.1 mg/kg) is administered to reduce the inflammatory cascades activated by ischemia, and may help to alleviate the mare's discomfort. Low-dose (10 to 20 IU) oxytocin therapy may be useful to promote uterine involution and thereby reduce the weight supported by the ligaments. Higher doses should be avoided because an induced colic episode may precipitate a fatal hemorrhage. Antifibrinolytic drugs (aminocaproic acid, tranexamic acid) may assist with clot stabilization. Pentoxifylline increases erythrocyte flexibility and may increase oxygen delivery to ischemic tissues.[321] It should be remembered that there is little refereed veterinary literature to validate the use of some of these medications in the horse. For instance, a conjugated estrogen product has been proposed on the basis of its ability to shorten prolonged bleeding times in humans. However, the benefit, if any, would not be realized until several days after the crisis has passed. Likewise, anecdotal reports suggest that naloxone (8 mg) may be efficacious, but the concept has been extrapolated from small animals, and controlled equine studies are lacking.[321,419,477] A controversial historical therapy to promote hemostasis in the horse is the use of intravenous buffered 10% formalin. Advocates suggest that dilute formalin solutions could enhance the activation of the clotting cascade. However, recent controlled studies were not able to demonstrate an effect on coagulation parameters or template bleeding times in normal horses.[612] Broad spectrum antibiotics should be administered to prevent infection of the hematoma.[419]

If hemorrhage is contained within the wall of the uterus, the intramural hematoma may be an incidental finding at the foal heat examination. However, some mares may exhibit variable signs of abdominal discomfort, even to the extent of warranting an exploratory celiotomy.[419,597,613-615] If an endometrial laceration severs an artery in the uterine wall, substantial hemorrhage may ensue, often with blood escaping from the vagina. The mare should be confined to a stall and low-dose oxytocin therapy instituted. Uterine irrigation is contraindicated because it will disrupt clot formation and prolong the hemorrhagic episode. The internal pudendal artery, one of the terminal branches of the internal iliac artery, gives rise to the umbilical artery and the urogenital artery before terminating in branches to the perineal area and the vestibular bulb. The small cranial vesicular artery supplies the apex of the bladder before the remainder of the umbilical artery terminates into the cordlike round ligament of the bladder. The urogenital artery gives rise to a caudal uterine branch that runs cranially on the side of the vagina and ramifies with the caudal branch of the uterine artery on the body of the uterus. The urogenital artery also supplies branches to the rectum, ureter, caudal bladder, and urethra and continues as the vaginal artery to the caudal portion of the reproductive tract.[3,605,606] A hematoma arising from these vessels may dissect along the fascial plane within the pelvic cavity and present as a large unilateral vulvar swelling.[583] Affected mares typically will be experiencing violent colic. Abscessation of a retroperitoneal hematoma can become a life-threatening complication after a dystocia, and thus prophylactic broad spectrum antibiotic coverage is warranted.[604] Mares with an infected retroperitoneal hematoma develop signs of toxemia. In these cases the peritoneal fluid has an increased total protein content (3.0 to 5.0 g/dl) with a massive increase in the white blood cell count (often exceeding 100,000 cells/μl).[492]

Uterine Prolapse (Eversion)

Uterine prolapse, or eversion, is an uncommon complication of equine parturition that may occur up to several hours (and occasionally several days) after fetal delivery.[419,616] The condition may be complicated by bladder eversion (or prolapse), uterine rupture, or intestinal herniation and may be rapidly fatal if the uterine artery is ruptured.* If the mare is standing and personnel are available, instructions should be given to place the uterus in a large plastic bag and elevate it to the level of the vulva. This may prevent further damage to the endometrium and, more important, will relieve the tension on the uterine vessels.[616] Fluid therapy may be indicated, and any calcium deficit must be corrected. Epidural anesthesia may reduce the amount of reflex straining provoked by vaginal manipulations, but it will not eliminate the mare's strong abdominal press.[576] General anesthesia may be necessary if the mare exhibits violent discomfort or if straining is excessive. Any uterine lacerations should be closed with absorbable sutures. The well-lubricated uterus is then pushed back through the vagina with a kneading motion. The fingertips can easily damage the edematous tissue, and manipulating the uterus through a plastic bag will reduce the likelihood of a finger rupturing the wall.[477,617] Ultrasonography is useful to evaluate any suspicious contents. A trapped bladder may be aspirated through a large-diameter needle, but a loop of bowel may require a ventral midline celiotomy.[419]

The replaced uterus should be distended with sterile saline to ensure that the tips of both horns are fully extended. Repeated low doses (10 to 20 IU every 2 hours) of oxytocin should be administered to promote uterine involution. Failure to ensure complete extension of the uterine horns into a normal position within the abdomen may result in discomfort, straining, and recurrence of the prolapse.[477] Vulvar retention sutures should not be necessary provided that the uterus has been completely returned to its normal position, that the calcium deficit has been corrected, and that low-dose oxytocin therapy has been administered. Broad spectrum antibiotics, nonsteroidal anti-inflammatory drugs, and tetanus prophylaxis are indicated. The mare should be closely monitored for evidence of internal hemorrhage. Affected mares may exsanguinate after the uterus has been replaced. Ischemic damage to trapped bowel is a potential complication. The clinician should be cognizant of the potential risks of endometritis-metritis, septicemia, endotoxemia, and laminitis. Between 2 and 3 days of intrauterine therapy may be warranted, depending on the condition of the exposed endometrium.

Partial Inversion (Intussusception) of the Uterine Horn

Injudicious traction on a retained fetal membrane remnant may invert the tip of the uterine horn, and this may progress to complete uterine prolapse.[477] If only the horn is affected, compromised circulation and pressure on nerve endings may produce signs of abdominal discomfort. Thus the tips of both uterine horns should be rectally palpated when evaluating a postpartum colic case. The affected horn will be shorter than normal and extremely thickened.[196,419,618] Manual reduction by pressure from within the uterine lumen may be possible in some cases, and infusion of several liters of saline solution will usually ensure extension of the affected horn.[196] Oxytocin (10-20 IU) should then be administered and the fluid drained from the uterus as it contracts. Resolution of the problem should be confirmed by rectal palpation.

*References 195, 196, 419, 491, 584, 604.

Uterine Rupture

In any dystocia case there is a risk for iatrogenic tears, and the uterus should always be checked for any obvious lacerations immediately after extraction of the fetus. Early recognition is important because the prognosis is worse once peritonitis develops.[492,582,583,604,619] However, obstetric intervention is not always the cause of uterine tears. Occasionally, the foal's hoof may be forced through the dorsal uterine wall during the mare's expulsive efforts, and the mare may be found with a loop of bowel protruding through the vulvar lips.[419,491] The exposed bowel should be rinsed with sterile saline and replaced, but a ventral midline celiotomy may be warranted to fully evaluate intestinal damage and to repair the uterine laceration. A more common lesion in unassisted deliveries is a tear toward the tip of the gravid uterine horn.[619,620] Although the fetal hooves are covered with hard gel-like pads that presumably protect the placenta and uterine wall, the vigorous pistonlike thrusts of the hindlimbs may occasionally cause a rupture.[4,408,621] Affected mares generally experience bouts of colic and become depressed, febrile, and anorectic as peritonitis develops. The interval from occurrence of the tear to diagnosis and initiation of therapy has a marked impact on the prognosis for survival.* It may not be possible to ascertain uterine integrity by vaginal palpation alone.[583] The tips of the horns may be especially difficult to palpate from within the postpartum uterus. The changes in the peritoneal cavity depend on the duration of the condition, but generally one can expect to see serosanguinous to sanguinous fluid containing elevated total protein, increased white blood cell counts, and often extracellular and intracellular bacteria.[492,585,619,622] Laparoscopic evaluation of the uterus may confirm the diagnosis and provide useful information when determining the need for surgery.[623] Complete perforation of the uterine wall is not necessary for peritonitis to develop if traumatic obstetric manipulations have damaged the uterine wall.[624] However, recent research shows that even a fetotomy procedure does not alter the composition of the postpartum peritoneal fluid if it is performed correctly.[492]

If a uterine laceration is suspected (partial or full), the mare should receive systemic broad spectrum antibiotic coverage. Nonsteroidal anti-inflammatory medication may prevent the development of endotoxemia. Oxytocin therapy (10 to 20 IU every 2 hours) will promote uterine involution. The dose can be increased if the mare does not become uncomfortable. Fluid therapy should be administered as necessary, ensuring that calcium levels are within the normal range. Intensive medical management may suffice for small dorsal uterine tears, but most warrant suturing if costs are not a limitation.[619,620,622,623] Opinions vary on the need for, and usefulness of, peritoneal lavage.[619,623] Large full-thickness tears warrant surgical intervention. In some instances a laceration in the uterine body can be sutured blindly in situ, but often a ventral midline celiotomy is the preferred approach.[477,493,582,622]

*References 477, 492, 583, 604, 619, 620, 622.

Retained Fetal Membranes and Toxic Metritis

Once the umbilical cord ruptures, there is a sudden cessation in blood flow through the capillary network in the placenta.[195] This causes a reduction in the tissue volume of the microcotyledons, and the rhythmic tubocervical contraction waves cause the membrane tips to separate and invaginate into the horn. The ongoing tubocervical detachment process causes the membranes to be passed inside out, with the allantoic surface exposed. The membranes should be expelled within 3 hours after parturition, and the incidence of retention has been reported to range between 2% to 10% of foalings.[419,480,625,626] Membrane retention tends to be most commonly associated with the tip of the nongravid horn and appears to be associated with dysfunction of the initial separation process.[31] In circumstances wherein tissue inflammation is common (e.g., abortion, dystocia, cesarean section), it is more likely that membrane retention will occur. In these cases the endometrial edema may trap the microcotyledons within the endometrial crypts. Mares with membrane retention may have a significantly lower serum calcium level.[627] A recent study noted that the number of endometrial mast cells observed during the puerperal period is significantly lower in the endometrium of mares with retained fetal membranes.[628] It is likely that some dysfunction of the normal endocrine-related maturational processes within the microcotyledons is involved. One study suggests that there may be an association between inbreeding and the high incidence of fetal membrane retention in Friesian mares.[528,629]

Appropriate management of a mare with fetal membrane retention varies depending on the time since foaling.[630] Although some mares, especially those foaling in a natural environment, may not experience any complications, prophylactic medication is recommended under intensive husbandry conditions.[626,631] Bacterial contamination in this environment is highly likely. If a severe metritis develops, inflammation of the uterine wall permits bacteria and toxins to enter the systemic circulation, producing septicemia and endotoxemia.[624,632] Laminitis is a frequent sequela.[477] The approach to treating retained fetal membranes (RFMs) varies considerably, depending on the duration of membrane retention and the presence or absence of metritis with septicemia. In normal, unassisted foalings, one or two treatments with oxytocin may be all that is required to facilitate passage of the RFMs. The protruding placental remnants should be tied in a knot above the mare's hocks. An initial low dose (10 to 20 IU) of oxytocin is recommended because some postpartum mares are especially sensitive to this hormone and may experience a severe bout of colic within minutes of treatment. Higher doses are likely to be counterproductive because myometrial spasm will occur instead of the desired rhythmic tubocervical contractions. If colic does occur, the mare should be sedated so that she does not roll and possibly injure the neonate.[477] In these cases the next dosage of oxytocin should be reduced. Each mare's response to the initial treatment governs the subsequent dose recommendations of 10 to 20 IU incremental increases every 2 hours.

The author routinely distends the chorioallantoic sac with fluid after any obstetric procedure. This procedure, known as the *Burn's technique*, has promoted membrane expulsion (5 to 30 minutes) in most of the postdystocia mares that the author has managed. A major advantage is that expulsion of the intact fetal membranes will remove any contaminants that may have been introduced by the obstetric procedures.[633] The technique works only if a sterile nasogastric tube can be passed beyond the torn distal fragments and is best performed while the membranes are still fresh. In more protracted cases the rapidly autolyzing chorioallantois becomes friable and generally tears once the fluid pressure increases. To perform the procedure the exposed fetal membranes are held tightly around the tube while 12 to 15 L of solution are infused. The opening is then tied off with umbilical tape. The exact mechanism is unknown, but expansion of the uterine lumen may dilate the endometrial crypts such that the weight of the membranes can atraumatically pull the microcotyledons free. Endogenous oxytocin release can be supplemented to enhance uterine contractions.

Because the uterine response to oxytocin wanes during the postpartum period, the dose may be increased in small increments every 2 hours in mares that retain their fetal membranes despite the initial therapy. If a hospitalized mare is receiving intravenous fluids, each oxytocin treatment can be added to the fluid line. Another option is to add oxytocin to the fluid bag at a dose that is calculated on the basis of the flow rate (1 IU/min).[477] However, a disadvantage of this approach is that these fluids must be discarded if the mare becomes uncomfortable yet still requires rehydration. The calcium ion plays a vital role in myometrial contractility, and it is important to ensure that calcium levels are within the normal range.[538,634] Supplemental calcium can markedly expedite the rate of passage, which suggests that uterine hypomotility is a component in some of these cases.[626] Controlled exercise is often beneficial in promoting uterine involution but is not always feasible if the mare is hospitalized or is being kept in a stall while a compromised neonate is being medicated.

It is widely accepted that excessive traction on the fetal membranes is contraindicated, but a recent study suggests that cautious manual removal of the membranes may not be as deleterious as previously thought.[635] When the membranes are extracted by force there is inevitably disruption of the epithelial barrier, making the traumatized uterine lining more susceptible to bacterial invasion and the development of metritis.[632] Endometrial trauma is also likely to contribute to the development of periglandular fibrosis. It is not uncommon for the membrane tip to tear off and remain firmly attached within the nongravid horn.[31] Injudicious traction on the membranes can also cause an inversion of the tip of the uterine horn, and this can progress to a complete uterine prolapse.[477] If the fetal membranes have not been expelled after 2 days of supportive therapy, the autolytic tissue becomes less firmly embedded and a gentle twisting technique—with minimal traction—applied within the attached horn will often result in successful removal of the entire chorioallantois. In the author's experience, this procedure works best while the uterus is being distended during a uterine lavage. Recent studies suggest that a safe and potentially effective treatment for RFMs in mares may be intraplacental injections of collagenase.[636,637]

If the membranes have been retained for 6 to 8 hours when the mare is first examined, then systemic antibiotic therapy is indicated.[477] Drugs that have been recommended for systemic administration include ampicillin, gentamicin, kanamycin, penicillin, ticarcillin, and trimethoprim-sulfamethoxazole.[419] If a remnant is missing when the membranes are examined, then the approach to therapy should proceed as if the entire membrane were still present. Characteristic signs of toxic metritis are fever, depression, anorexia, tachycardia, and infected mucous membranes.[632] The foal will not be receiving adequate milk intake, and many of these mares will have bounding digital pulses and evidence of laminitis. Rectal palpation will reveal a large, thin-walled, atonic uterus that contains moderate to large amounts of fetid fluid.[477] A large volume of toxic, red-brown, watery fluid can accumulate within the pendulous postpartum uterus before any obvious vaginal discharge becomes evident. Often the history will reveal that the fetal membranes were discarded without being checked to ensure that they were passed intact.

Because the endometrium is likely to be necrotic, therapy should include broad spectrum antibiotics, anti-inflammatory drugs, and intravenous fluids if indicated. Tetanus prophylaxis is advisable. A combination of penicillin and gentamicin is widely used to provide broad spectrum systemic coverage, especially against the coliforms that frequently contribute to endotoxemia and laminitis.[638] Flunixin meglumine should be administered to ameliorate the effects of endotoxemia. It is commonly administered intravenously at a reduced dose (0.25 mg/kg) thrice daily.[477] Phenylbutazone (2 to 4 mg/kg) and provision of deep, soft bedding are useful to alleviate pain when laminitis appears to be imminent. Radiographs can be useful to monitor changes in the position of the pedal bone. Vasodilators such as acetylpromazine maleate may be administered by intramuscular injection (0.02-0.04 mg/kg every 4 to 6 hours).[638] Further discussion of the diagnosis and treatment of endotoxemia and laminitis are found in Chapter 15 and Chapter 11.

The uterus should be lavaged with sterile saline or very dilute ("weak tea") povidone-iodine solution. If povidone-iodine is used, the final concentration should not exceed 0.1%; this is equivalent to 10 ml of 10% povidone-iodine solution (e.g., Betadine) in 1 L of saline. If costs are a concern, 90 ml in a 9-L bucket of clean water may suffice. Extreme caution should be exercised to keep from puncturing the inflamed uterine wall with the tube. The lavage should be repeated until the returning fluid is relatively clear. The goal of therapy is to eliminate toxins and to prevent the rapid proliferation of bacteria—especially coliforms and possibly anaerobes. The administration of intrauterine antibiotics in the postpartum mare is controversial because little scientific validation has been performed. Intrauterine administration of antibiotics and antiseptics may depress the phagocytic activity of uterine neutrophils, and many chemicals are known to irritate the endometrium in mares being infused for endometritis.[419] The pharmacokinetic properties of each drug will influence its efficacy in the postpartum uterus. Most of the studies regarding intrauterine therapy in mares have addressed therapy for endometritis in nonparturient animals. The efficacy of antibiotic formulations in the presence of the mixed bacterial population and tissue debris associated with fetal membrane retention in the mare remains to be established. The antibiotic of choice should be added to a large infusion volume (2 to 3 L) to ensure uniform distribution across the inflamed endometrial surface once a lavage has removed the toxic fluid and necrotic debris. Unpublished microbiologic studies in the author's laboratory have demonstrated that many organisms cultured from metritis fluid are sensitive to amikacin.[639] Infusion of 2 g of this antibiotic after a uterine lavage is clinically effective. Polymixin B may have some merit because of its endotoxin-binding ability. Powdered and propylene glycol–based oxytetracycline formulations are known to be irritating when infused into the involuted uterus and therefore should be avoided.[187,640] Other antibiotics that have been suggested for postpartum intrauterine therapy include ampicillin (3 g), ticarcillin/clavulanic acid (1 to 3 g), and gentamicin (2 to 3 g).[419] In the author's unpublished studies, less than 60% of isolates from metritis fluid were sensitive to ampicillin.[639]

Gastrointestinal Complications

Prolonged straining during dystocia can lead to variable amounts of rectal mucosa being forced out through the anal sphincter (type I rectal prolapse). The tissue then becomes subject to trauma, contamination, and vascular compromise. If not promptly corrected, pressure from the anal sphincter will cause venous congestion and swelling. This promotes more straining, and the condition can deteriorate rapidly. A type II prolapse involves all or part of the ampulla recti.[419,598] An epidural anesthetic may help decrease straining. Topical glycerin or dextrose may be applied to the prolapsed tissue to reduce edema.[419,477] A purse-string suture can cause additional straining and will impede defecation.[419,641] Fecal softeners should be administered and the diet modified (e.g., pellets, pasture) to help produce soft feces.[419,642] Chronic prolapses may warrant surgical resection of the devitalized mucosal mass.[419,642] In a type III prolapse, there is a full-thickness rectal prolapse and an intussusception of the peritoneal rectum or small colon.[419] In a type IV prolapse the intussuscepted bowel protrudes through the anus such that there is a palpable trench that may extend several meters into the rectum, depending on the length of the intussusception.[419,572,573,641] Midventral celiotomy is usually necessary to reduce the intussusception, although some smaller prolapses will reduce after an attendant has extracted the foal.[419] The short mesentery that supports this section of bowel is often torn from the colon. Thus these cases have a guarded prognosis, dependent on the vascular integrity of the affected small colon. The author has seen this condition develop when as little as 6 to 10 inches of bowel appears to be prolapsed. The avulsion most likely occurs when the mare's intermittent straining forces an extra 4 to 6 inches of bowel in and out of the rectum. Thus it is imperative to prevent straining as soon as possible. If the foal has not yet been extracted, it may be best to immediately anesthetize the mare, then elevate the hindquarters before attempting to correct the cause of the dystocia.

In rectal prolapse cases that have been managed conservatively, one of the first postpartum clinical signs may be discomfort attributable to impaction colic. If avulsion of the mesocolon has occurred, ischemic necrosis of the affected bowel will cause a delayed peritonitis. Because early intervention is essential, sequential abdominocentesis is indicated when a type III or IV rectal prolapse is being conservatively managed. Initially, there may be negligible changes in the composition of the peritoneal fluid. However, if an avulsion has occurred, the compromised segment of bowel will soon lose its integrity and a massively increased white blood cell count can occur within 24 to 48 hours as peritonitis ensues.[492] Laparoscopic evaluation of the abdomen can provide an immediate assessment of bowel integrity and permit an accurate prognosis to be given to the owner.[494] The affected colon is not readily accessible for resection and anastomosis, so the prognosis in most cases is guarded.[642]

Variable degrees of uncomplicated impaction are not uncommon in the postparturient mare, possibly as a result of localized perineal pain causing reluctance to defecate.[477] Astute managers will note an absence of fecal matter in the stall. Treatment with fecal softeners (e.g., mineral oil) and analgesics generally corrects the problem. Laxative feeds (e.g., bran mash) are effective in reducing the incidence of constipation in foaling mares.[196] Postpartum mares appear to be at an increased risk for development of a large colon torsion.[273,604,643] This condition presents as an especially violent colic with readily discernible abdominal distention. Extensive ischemic damage affects the prognosis, but early surgical intervention can increase the survival rate.[583,644] Bruising of the abdominal viscera can occur during foaling, with subsequent development of moderate to severe signs of impaction colic and peritonitis.[419,583] Occasionally, the mesentery may be torn from a segment of intestine, leading to ischemic necrosis and peritonitis. An early diagnosis and prompt surgical intervention may save the mare's life.[492,494,602-604,645] A rent in the mesentery or broad ligament at the time of foaling may permit a segment of bowel to become incarcerated even weeks later.[270,597,603,604,646] Owners should be advised that surgical correction is feasible only if the segment of devitalized bowel is accessible.[270,603,645-647]

Although mares tend to reduce their feed intake in the days leading up to foaling, ensuring a reduction in the amount of available roughage may help reduce the incidence of bowel rupture.[196] The tip of the cecum is the most likely site of a foaling-related rupture in the alimentary tract. On rectal palpation the inflamed serosal surfaces will feel roughened, with a discernible crepitus. Abdominocentesis will reveal dark green-brown gastrointestinal fluid that contains plant material and massively increased neutrophil numbers. Humane euthanasia is indicated because the leaking ingesta incites a severe peritonitis with accompanying septic shock, and the condition is likely to be rapidly fatal.[419,604,648-652] Diaphragmatic herniation has been reported as a rare parturient complication in heavily pregnant mares.[491,653-655] Colic symptoms are attributable to strangulating obstruction or tension on the mesentery. Some mares may exhibit respiratory distress. Transthoracic ultrasonography can help confirm the presence of bowel within the thorax.[656] Surgical repair of the defect may not be possible, and assisted ventilation will be required.[654,655]

Vaginal Lacerations and Bladder Prolapse

Primiparous mares are especially susceptible to vaginal trauma. Vaginal lacerations are most likely to occur during injudicious attempts to relieve dystocia. Although most lacerations are retroperitoneal, they still may contribute to severe vaginitis, fibrosis, and possibly abscessation. If ventral trauma is present, a urinary catheter should be passed to check for urethral integrity. In some instances ligation of a severed artery will be necessary. Emollient creams, tetanus prophylaxis, broad spectrum antibiotics, and anti-inflammatory drugs are indicated. A major concern is the possibility of herniation of intestine into the vagina if the tear is located just caudal to the cervix in the vicinity of the urogenital pouch.[604,657] If eventration has occurred, the bowel should be cleansed and examined for evidence of vascular compromise. If the involved intestine appears to be grossly normal, it should be rinsed with sterile saline and returned to the abdominal cavity. If vascular compromise is detected at the time of the initial examination, then the prognosis is guarded and a ventral midline celiotomy to facilitate resection is warranted. A bladder prolapse occurs when the bladder is forced up through a vaginal laceration. The viscus rapidly becomes distended as a result of the continued accumulation of urine from the ureters and an inability to void urine because of kinking of the urethra. The edematous serosal surface of the bladder may protrude through the vulvar lips.[477] The exposed organ should be thoroughly cleansed, then gently returned the abdominal cavity. It may be necessary to administer an epidural and aspirate urine to facilitate replacement. If possible, the vaginal laceration should be sutured once any viscera have been returned to the abdominal cavity. In some cases the severity of the trauma precludes successful closure, and the wound must heal by second intention.[657] Placement of a Caslick suture reduces the possibility of bacterial aspiration. Mares may be cross-tied for several days to decrease the risk of eventration brought about by elevation of intraabdominal pressure as the mare lies down.[477] The mare should be treated for impending peritonitis (e.g., broad spectrum antibiotics, nonsteroidal anti-inflammatory drugs). Tetanus prophylaxis is indicated. If severe colic symptoms develop, bowel compromise should be suspected.[492]

Eversion of the Urinary Bladder

The mare's urethra has a large diameter, and occasionally the bladder may be everted up into the vagina after severe straining.[658] If the everted bladder protrudes through the vulvar lips, the exposed mucosal surface will rapidly become edematous, and urine may be seen to drip from the ventral surface. Closer inspection will reveal that the urine is dribbling from the exposed papilliform openings of the ureters on the dorsal surface of the neck of the bladder.[659] A lip chain and epidural may provide adequate restraint to facilitate replacement. The mucosal surface should be thoroughly cleansed and any defects repaired. Sterile lubricant should be applied and the friable organ gently massaged back through the urethra. In some instances it may be necessary to incise the urethral sphincter if the bladder mucosa is especially thickened.[659] This incision should be closed once the bladder has been replaced. A Foley catheter can be inserted to lavage the bladder lumen and ensure complete repositioning. Broad spectrum antibiotic coverage, nonsteroidal anti-inflammatory drugs, and tetanus prophylaxis are indicated.

Rupture of the Urinary Bladder

Occasionally, the bladder may rupture as a consequence of increased intra-abdominal pressure in the foaling mare or because of direct trauma during parturition.[660-662] Clinical signs are delayed and are associated with electrolyte imbalances. Affected mares may be depressed and inappetent, with failure to void urine. Clinical examination will reveal tachycardia, tachypnea, and decreased gastrointestinal activity. Blood chemistry will reveal elevated serum levels of creatinine, blood urea nitrogen, and potassium, in addition to decreased sodium and chloride levels. Evaluation of a peritoneal fluid sample helps confirm the diagnosis. The fluid will contain elevated urea and creatinine levels and calcium carbonate crystals.[660,661] Cystoscopy is useful to evaluate the size and extent of the bladder injury. Once the mare's medical condition has been stabilized, surgical repair is indicated.[597,660-662]

A standing vaginal approach eliminates the need for general anesthesia and allows excellent observation and repair of bladder tears in adult mares.[662]

Rectovaginal Fistulas and Perineal Lacerations

A first degree perineal laceration involves the mucous membrane of the vestibule and the skin of the vulvar lips. In second-degree perineal lacerations, the deeper tissues of the perineal body are involved. Both of these conditions may be associated with unassisted delivery of a large foal or may be a sequela of dystocia. The laceration may be amenable to immediate repair and placement of a Caslick suture, or the clinician may elect to wait until the wound has granulated. The mare should be treated with broad spectrum antibiotics, anti-inflammatory medication, and tetanus prophylaxis. Provision of a bran mash diet and administration of mineral oil may facilitate defecation during the initial inflammatory period.

Third-degree perineal lacerations generally occur during unassisted foalings when the fetal hoof catches on the vaginal roof at the vestibulovaginal junction. Forceful straining by the mare can drive the hoof through the rectovaginal shelf such that the fetal hoof comes to lie within the rectum. If the fetus is viable, it may remove the affected limb and delivery will proceed unimpeded; a rectovaginal fistula results. If the limb remains within the rectum, continued passage of the fetus causes the trapped limb to tear out the perineal body and anal sphincter. The resulting defect is called a *third-degree perineal laceration*. These injuries do not respond well to immediate surgical intervention, and the general recommendation is to wait 4 to 6 weeks before attempting reconstructive surgery.[597,658,663] In the interim the mare should be treated with broad spectrum antibiotics, anti-inflammatory medication, tetanus prophylaxis, and fecal softeners.

Grade IV (full-thickness) rectal tears that communicate directly with the peritoneal cavity have a poor prognosis and can occur as a result of parturition.[664,665] Tears tend to occur just cranial to the caudal peritoneal reflection. Such cases warrant immediate intervention, and the rectum should be packed to prevent abdominal contamination during transport to a referral hospital. A standing technique that permits an easy and effective stapled primary closure repair has been described.[664]

Perineal Bruising and Vulvar Hematomas

Much of the swelling after prolonged obstetric manipulations is edematous. Fecal softeners such as oral mineral oil and bran mash are recommended to ease the passage of feces through the swollen and bruised perineal area.[491,496] Hematomas in the vaginal wall and vulvar lips are not uncommon, especially in primiparous mares and mares that have delivered an extremely large foal. It is important to differentiate a bulging vestibular hematoma from an everted or prolapsed bladder.[196,605] Needle aspiration of vulvar hematomas is not recommended because of the risk of abscessation. Broad spectrum antibiotics and tetanus prophylaxis are indicated. Most hematomas will resolve uneventfully, but some vulvar, vaginal, or pelvic hematomas may warrant drainage in 7 to 10 days.[491]

Postpartum Eclampsia (Lactation Tetany)

Postpartum eclampsia, or lactation tetany, is extremely rare in mares but may occur in animals that are lactating heavily. The highest incidence is reported in draft breeds, but the author has encountered a case in a pony mare. Equine eclampsia is generally associated with some type of stress (e.g., change in surroundings). Early signs include restlessness, tachypnea, staring eyes, twitching, trembling, and clonic spasms (especially diaphragmatic). The clonic spasms gradually become more tonic, and eventually the mare may be unable to stand. The differential diagnosis is tetanus, but the nictitating membrane is not prolapsed. The condition responds well to intravenous calcium gluconate administration.[195]

ASSISTED REPRODUCTIVE TECHNIQUES

Elaine M. Carnevale, Marco A. Coutinho da Silva

ASSISTED REPRODUCTIVE TECHNIQUES FOR THE MARE

The development of new assisted reproductive techniques for the mare has allowed production of offspring from mares that are infertile using standard breeding techniques or embryo transfer.

Oocyte Transfer

Although the first successful oocyte transfer was performed in 1988, the technique was not used for commercial transfers until the late 1990s.[1-3] Oocyte transfer involves the transfer of an oocyte from a donor into the oviduct of a recipient; the recipient is inseminated within the uterus. Fertilization, embryo development, and fetal development occur within the recipient, thereby preventing problems associated with ovulation or the tubular genitalia of donors. The incidence of ovulatory failure increases with age and during the autumn months.[4,5] Prolonged exposure to an abnormal follicular environment results in aging and death of the oocyte. Some types of ovulatory failure can be detected with ultrasound as an atypical morphology of the follicle or ovulatory site. Mares that repeatedly fail to ovulate can provide oocytes for transfer successfully if oocytes are collected before deleterious changes occur within the follicle.[2]

Historically, the uterus has been considered the primary cause of reduced fertility in the mare. Mares with pyometra or persistent endometritis are expensive to treat and frequently do not provide embryos. Mares with cervical lacerations, cervical or uterine adhesions, or urine pooling often fail as embryo donors. Oviduct dysfunction is a major impediment to fertility, especially in aged mares. When the oviducts of old mares (>20 years) and young mares (2 to 9 years) were flushed between 1 and 4 days after ovulation, collection rates of recently ovulated oocytes or oviductal embryos were significantly higher in the young mares than in the old ones (26 of 27 [96%] versus 17 of 29 [59%], respectively).[6] In subfertile mares pathologic changes of the oviducts were imaged using scanning electron microscopy, and significantly fewer sperm were detected in the caudal isthmus in subfertile mares than in fertile mares. Few sperm found in the oviducts of subfertile mares were motile, whereas oviducts of the normal mares contained highly motile sperm.[7] Obstructions of the oviductal lumen are postulated to be the cause of subfertility in some mares. Globular masses composed of type I collagen were found more frequently in older than in younger mares.[8] Oviductal masses were found in the oviducts in 73% (16 of 22) of mares between 2 and 22 years of age; in a small number of mares (3 of 43), the masses occupied and distended the oviductal lumen and could have resulted in infertility. The equine embryo remains in the oviduct for 5 or 6 days before entering the uterus; therefore oviductal problems such as inflammation could affect embryo viability.[9]

Procedures for Oocyte Transfer

Requirements for oocyte donors are minimal. Uterine infections in donor mares should be treated to prevent introduction of a pathogen into the abdominal cavity during transvaginal oocyte collections. Donors should have regular estrous cycles with growth of a preovulatory follicle. The age of the donor affects success rates. When oocytes were collected from the follicles of young donors (6 to 10 years) and old donors (20 to 26 years) and transferred into the oviducts of young recipients (3 to 7 years), significantly more oocytes from young than old donors developed into embryonic vesicles (11 of 12 [92%] versus 8 of 26 [31%], respectively).[10] A higher incidence of morphologic anomalies was observed in oocytes from older than from younger mares.[11] Although younger mares are better candidates for oocyte donors, older (≥20 years) mares frequently are presented to commercial oocyte transfer programs, and pregnancies are obtainable through repeated transfers.[2]

Oocyte Collection

Currently, most oocytes are collected from preovulatory follicles between 24 and 36 hours after the administration of hCG (hCG; 1500 to 2500 IU, IV) or deslorelin (1.5 mg, IM) to the donor, with the oocytes collected between 18 and 20 hours before anticipated ovulation. Therefore oocytes are probably at metaphase I or II. Criteria for hCG administration are as follows: (1) a follicle greater than 35 mm in diameter, (2) relaxed cervical and uterine tone, and (3) uterine edema or estrous behavior for a minimum of 2 days. Some mares, especially old mares, do not consistently respond to hCG. In these cases the authors use a combination of deslorelin acetate, (1.5 mg intramuscularly) and hCG (2000 IU, IV), with hCG administered between 4 and 5 hours after deslorelin. Oocytes have been collected from the follicles of mares by laparotomy,[12] colpotomy,[13] flank puncture,[14,15] and ultrasound-guided follicular aspiration.[16,17] Currently, most laboratories collect oocytes through the flank or with ultrasound-guided punctures.

For the collection of oocytes using flank puncture, trocar is placed through the flank ipsilateral to the preovulatory follicle at approximately the position of the ovary. The ovary is manipulated by way of the rectum to position the preovulatory follicle against the end of the cannula. While stabilizing the ovary by way of the rectum, the clinician places a needle (12 to 17 gauge) through the cannula and into the follicular antrum and removes the follicular fluid and oocyte by gentle suction and lavage of the follicle. Transvaginal, ultrasound-guided follicular aspiration requires use of an ultrasound machine. Linear, curvilinear, and sector transducers have been used. The transducer is placed in a casing containing a needle guide. Rectal contractions may be minimized by administration of propanthelene bromide (0.04 mg/kg, IV)[2] or N-butylscopolamine or intrarectal use of lidocaine. The clinician applies a nontoxic lubricant to the transducer and positions it within the anterior vagina lateral to the posterior cervix and ipsilateral to the follicle to be aspirated. The follicle must be carefully positioned through transrectal manipulations with the follicular apex juxtaposed to the needle guide and advances the needle through the needle guide to puncture the vaginal and follicular walls. In the authors' laboratory, a 12-gauge double-lumen needle is used. The follicular fluid is aspirated from the follicle using a pump set at approximately 150 mm Hg or with suction from a large syringe. After removing the follicular fluid, the clinician lavages the lumen with between 50 and 100 ml of flushing liquid; typically modified Dulbecco's phosphate buffered solution or a sterile commercial embryo flush solution heparin (10 IU/ml) is added to the flush solution to prevent coagulation of blood in the aspirate. Oocytes were collected successfully from between 70% and 80% of the follicles in client donors.[2]

Oocyte Culture and Transfer

Oocytes are sensitive to temperature changes; therefore the clinician should warm media and equipment for handling the oocyte to 38.5° C. On collection the flushing solution is poured into large search dishes and examined under a dissecting microscope to locate the oocyte. One can transfer oocytes collected at least 30 hours after hCG administration to the donor immediately into a recipient's oviduct. Oocytes are usually collected 24 hours after administration to the donor and between 12 and 16 hours before transfer. Most oocytes are cultured in medium similar to that first described by Carnevale and Ginther.[10] The timing of oocyte collection (24 versus 36 hours after administration of hCG to donors) did not affect pregnancy rates.[18] A modification of these procedures was to collect oocytes 24 hours after hCG administration and immediately transfer them into the recipient's oviduct. Oocyte maturation was completed within the oviduct, and recipients were inseminated after oocyte maturation should have been completed, at 16 hours after transfer. Pregnancy rates were not statistically different for oocytes matured within the oviduct or within an incubator (43% versus 57%).[19]

Because the reproductive tract of the recipient provides the environment for sperm transport, fertilization, and embryo development, recipient mares should be young (optimally 4 to 10 years) and have normal reproductive tracts. Cyclic and noncyclic hormone-treated mares have been used as oocyte recipients. When cyclic mares are used, recipients are synchronized with the donor, and the recipient's own oocyte is removed by transvaginal or flank aspiration before transfer of the donor's oocytes.[20] Anestrus and early transitional mares are used as recipients during the nonovulatory season.[2,21] During the breeding season a high dose of a Gn-RH agonist (4.2 mg deslorelin acetate)[22] or injections of progesterone and estrogen (150 mg progesterone and 10 mg estradiol)[3] have been administered to reduce follicular development in potential recipients. The endocrine environment of the cyclic mare is imitated in the noncyclic recipient with administration of estradiol (1.5 to 5 mg daily for 3 to 7 days) before transfer.

Estradiol often is given to effect to obtain a recipient with a soft, open cervix and moderate endometrial edema. Progesterone (150 to 200 mg daily) or a progestin is administered after transfer. Pregnancies are maintained through the administration of exogenous progesterone or progestins.[2]

Because oocytes are transferred surgically, adequate exposure of the oviduct is essential, and mares with short, thick flanks or short, broad ligaments are not good candidates for recipients. Most oocyte transfers are performed through a standing flank laparotomy. Tranquilization, preparation, closure, and aftercare of recipients are similar to previously described methods for embryo transfer.[23] The authors generally use a fire-polished glass pipette to transfer oocytes. The oviductal os is located by following the outline of the oviduct along the external surface of the infundibulum. One identifies the end of the structure and inserts the pipette containing the oocyte into the os and carefully advances the pipette 2 to 3 cm. One deposits the oocyte and a minimal amount of medium (<0.1 ml) into the ampullar region of the oviduct, gently returns the ovary to the abdominal cavity, and closes the surgical site.

Insemination of Recipients

In a commercial oocyte transfer program, use of stallions with good fertility is essential for success; however, cooled, transported semen frequently is provided from stallions of variable fertility.[2,24] The equine oocyte remains viable for approximately 12 hours after a natural ovulation.[25] Because of this limited life span, recipients must be inseminated before or directly after oocyte transfer or both. Pregnancies have occurred when recipients were inseminated only before[26,27] or after[19] the transfer of oocytes. However, for most experimental transfers, recipients were inseminated before transfer (approximately 12 hours) and after transfer (approximately 2 hours) with a total of 2×10^9 motile sperm. In a commercial program using older donors and cooled semen from numerous stallions of variable fertility, pregnancy rates when recipients were inseminated before or before and after oocyte transfer were significantly higher than when recipients were inseminated only after transfer (18 of 45, 40%; 27 of 53, 51%; and 0 of 10, respectively).[24] The results suggest that insemination of a recipient only before transfer with at least 1×10^9 progressively motile sperm from a fertile stallion is sufficient. However, if fertility of the stallion is not optimal, insemination of the recipient before and after transfer could be beneficial.

After insemination and transfer, the uterus of the recipient should be examined with ultrasound to detect intrauterine fluid collections. One treats recipients with intrauterine fluid collections as one treats ovulating mares, with oxytocin or PGs to stimulate uterine contractions or with uterine lavage and infusion.

Success of Oocyte Transfer

Pregnancy rates for commercial transfers, using older donors and semen of variable quality, ranged between 27% to 40% per transfer.[2,24] In contrast, experimental transfers under similar conditions using oocytes from young mares and fertile stallions resulted in pregnancy rates between 54% and 83% per transfer.[24] However, one or more pregnancies were obtained for more than 80% of donors during the breeding season in a commercial oocyte transfer program.[2] All mares in the program had histories of reproductive failure in breeding and embryo transfer programs, with a mean of 7 years (range of 3 to 15 years) from the last successful pregnancy or embryo collection.[2]

In Vitro Maturation and Fertilization of Oocytes

In vitro fertilization is not repeatedly successful in the mare, with only two foals born after in vitro fertilization.[28,29] One problem in trying to study procedures such as in vitro fertilization in the horse is the paucity of equine oocytes. Oocytes often are collected from the preovulatory follicles of live mares. Collection of oocytes from small follicles during diestrus results in reduced collection rates compared with collection of oocytes from preovulatory follicles.[30] In one study,[26] oocytes were collected from small follicles and preovulatory follicles. Oocytes collected from small follicles were matured in vitro for 36 to 38 hours before transfer, whereas oocytes collected from preovulatory follicles were transferred immediately into a recipient's oviduct. Embryo development rates after transfers were 9% for in vitro maturation and 82% for in vivo. In contrast, some laboratories have been very successful in developing methods to collect and mature oocytes from small follicles. Colleoni and associates reported an oocyte recovery rate of 58%, or 11 oocytes per ovum pick-up session.[31]

Research involving oocytes from excised ovaries is aimed at developing a method to salvage gametes from the ovaries of valuable mares that have died or been euthanized. One can collect ovaries from mares immediately after death and ship them to a facility for oocyte recovery, maturation, and transfer. This technique was first attempted in 1999[2]; a pregnancy was established, which later underwent embryonic death. However, more recent attempts have resulted in pregnancies and healthy foals after shipment of ovaries from mares that were euthanized for various medical reasons.[32,33] In our laboratory we anticipate obtaining a late-term pregnancy or pregnancies from about one of four sets of ovaries that are shipped to the laboratory.

Cryopreservation of Oocytes and Embryos

Cryopreservation of the equine oocyte results in the preservation of female genetics, whereas cryopreservation of the embryo results in the preservation of the female and male genome. The first foal was produced from a cryopreserved embryo in 1982.[34] Procedures for embryo cryopreservation have been reviewed.[35] Cryopreservation of small embryos (morulae or early blastocysts) has consistently resulted in acceptable pregnancy rates close to 50%.[36,37] Cryopreservation of larger embryos (≥300 μm) is usually unsuccessful. Embryo collection is recommended on day 6 or 6½ after ovulation.[35] Embryo donors are examined twice daily for ovulation, or embryo collections are timed from administration of an ovulation-inducing agent.[38] In recent years vitrification procedures have been used to successfully cryopreserve small equine embryos.[38-40] Vitrification has the advantages over traditional slow-cooling methods of cryopreservation of being a rapid procedure (<15 min) that requires minimal equipment.

Although cryopreservation of the oocyte is difficult, successful fertilization of cryopreserved oocytes has been described.[41-43] In 2001 the first foals were born after cryopreservation of oocytes.[27] Clinical use of oocyte cryopreservation has not been reported.

ASSISTED REPRODUCTIVE TECHNIQUES FOR THE STALLION

Maximum fertility was obtained when fertile mares were inseminated every other day during estrus with 500×10^6 progressively motile sperm.[44] Insemination of low numbers of sperm would be beneficial for frozen semen that is of limited supply, semen from subfertile stallions with low sperm numbers, and insemination of sex-sorted sperm. The following discussion summarizes techniques for low-dose or assisted inseminations.

Deep Intrauterine Insemination

Uterine contractions move sperm into the tips of the uterine horns within 20 minutes of routine artifical insemination.[45] The aim of deep uterine insemination is to increase the number of sperm entering the oviduct ipsilateral to ovulation.[46-48] A flexible insemination pipette is passed through the cervix and into the uterine horn ipsilateral to the preovulatory follicle. One then uses rectal manipulation to position the catheter at the tip of the uterine horn where the sperm are deposited. Fresh, cooled, and sex-sorted sperm in volumes ranging from 0.2 to 1.0 ml of glucose milk extender have been used for deep intrauterine inseminations. Pregnancy rates after deep intrauterine inseminations with 5×10^6 progressively motile sperm were between 30% and 50%,[44,50] and inseminations with 25×10^6 progressively motile sperm ranged between 57% to 63%.[49,51] However, in the study by Woods, Rigby, Brinsko et al.,[51] control mares were inseminated with 25×10^6 progressively motile sperm in the uterine body, and pregnancy rates were not significantly different between standard and deep uterine inseminations. Because control inseminations were not done in many studies, the true benefit of deep uterine insemination has not been determined.

Hysteroscopic Insemination

Hysteroscopic insemination entails deposition of sperm directly onto the papilla of the uterotubal junction. A minute volume of extended sperm (approximately 0.05 to 0.25 ml) is desired for hysteroscopic insemination. Sperm are centrifuged through a density gradient to select a sperm population with a high percentage of motility. Numbers of fresh sperm inseminated ranged between 1 to 10×10^6 progressively motile sperm, with pregnancy rates between 40% to 75%.[50,52-54] Studies have been conducted using higher volumes[55] or lower sperm numbers[52]; however, fertility was reduced.

One aspirates semen into an equine gamete intrafallopian transfer (GIFT) catheter (Cook Veterinary Products) protected by an outer polypropylene cannula and loaded into the working channel of the videoendoscope. With a sterile gloved arm in the vagina of the mare, the operator guides the flexible endoscope (1.6 m in length) through the cervix and uterine lumen; directs the endoscope along the uterine horn ipsilateral to the preovulatory follicle; and on imaging the papilla of the uterotubal junction, extrudes the outer cannula and then the inner GIFT catheter containing the sperm suspension from the working channel of the endoscope. When the tip of the GIFT catheter touches the papilla, the operator bubbles the inseminate onto the surface of the papilla.[52]

Low-dose insemination with frozen-thawed sperm maximizes the use of a conventional dose of frozen sperm (800 to 1000×10^6 progressively motile sperm) by reducing the number of sperm needed for insemination. Using 5 or 10×10^6 frozen-thawed progressively motile sperm, different investigators obtained pregnancy rates between 33% and 47%.[53,56,57] Alvarenga, Trinque, Lima et al.[58] inseminated client mares with 100 to 150×10^6 frozen-thawed sperm from 15 Warmblood stallions and obtained an overall pregnancy rate of 57%, demonstrating that hysteroscopic insemination can be applied immediately in the horse industry. Current rates for sorting sperm into X or Y chromosome–bearing populations are approximately 10 million sperm per hour, meaning that low-dose inseminations are necessary for sex-sorted sperm. Several studies have been conducted using hysteroscopic insemination of sex-sorted sperm, resulting in pregnancy rates between 25% and 44%.[53,56]

Gamete Intrafallopian Transfer

GIFT involves transfer of oocytes and sperm into the recipient's oviduct. Compared with oocyte transfer, GIFT requires low numbers of sperm. The first successful GIFT in the horse was reported in 1998.[21] GIFT sperm are often selected through a density gradient to select a population with a high percentage of motile sperm, free of debris and seminal plasma, with 1 to 5×10^5 progressively motile sperm transferred with an oocyte into the recipient's oviduct. Optimal procedures for GIFT have probably not been established, although pregnancy rates between 27% to 82% have been reported.[19,59] GIFT is a potentially valuable technique to produce pregnancies from subfertile stallions, frozen semen, and sex-sorted sperm. However, the type of sperm and even extenders may have an effect on the success of GIFT. Pregnancy rates with GIFT were lower when cooled or frozen semen was used for GIFT (pregnancy rates of 25% and 8%, respectively) compared with pregnancy rates with fresh semen (82%).[60]

Intracytoplasmic Sperm Injection

Intracytoplasmic sperm injection (ICSI) has been successfully used for the assisted fertilization of equine oocytes. A single sperm is selected, aspirated into a fine-bore needle, and injected into a mature oocyte. The injected oocyte can be transferred into a receipient's oviduct or cultured to allow embryo development.[61] Cochrane et al reported the first successful ICSI of an equine oocyte that was matured in vitro. Foals have been produced by ICSI using oocytes matured in vivo or in vitro.[62,63] However, pregnancy rates per transferred oocyte were low (13% and 6%, respectively). Since that time, several investigators reported the in vitro production of blastocysts with higher efficiency,[64,65-67] and recently the clinical use of ICSI has been reported in the horse.[31,68]

The major clinical advantage of ISCI is that limited sperm numbers or poor-quality sperm can be used to produce offspring, and pregnancies have been obtained from epididymal or poor quality sperm.[31,68]

CONCLUSION

New assisted reproductive techniques have been developed that allow for the production of offspring from mares and stallions that would be considered subfertile or infertile using more standard breeding procedures. Although cost, expertise, and availability of these procedures may be limiting factors in their widespread use at this time, their clinical potential for the horse has been recognized.

THE STALLION

Juan C. Samper

ANATOMY AND PHYSIOLOGY OF THE STALLION

A breeding stallion is often the most significant financial asset of an equine breeding operation. A variety of factors may influence the future breeding potential of a colt as it is maturing. An understanding of the anatomy and physiology of the stallion assists the veterinarian in providing optimal monitoring, diagnostic, and therapeutic services to a farm.

REPRODUCTIVE PHYSIOLOGY

TESTICULAR DESCENT

Normal testicular descent into the scrotum occurs between the last 30 days of gestation and the first 10 days after birth. In some colts the testes may descend into the inguinal region and remain there for some time before fully descending. Androgen production by the developing fetal testis probably plays an important role,[1] as may müllerian inhibiting factor.[2] Traction of the gubernaculum, which attaches the caudal pole of the testis to the inguinal region, is believed to draw the developing testicle and epididymis into the inguinal ring.[3]

Failure of the testis to descend into a normal scrotal position is termed *cryptorchidism.* The left testis is retained more commonly in stallions. Cryptorchidism is diagnosed by manual palpation of scrotal contents. Rectal palpation and careful inguinal palpation may assist in identification of an abdominally or inguinally retained testis. In some instances heavy sedation of the stallion is necessary to permit careful examination of the area. Ultrasonography has been recommended as a useful diagnostic tool for such examinations as well.[4] In horses with bilaterally retained testicles or apparent geldings with stallionlike behavior, hormonal profiles may be useful in diagnosis of a retained testis. Measurement of testosterone levels has been suggested as a method to diagnose retained testicular tissue in an apparent gelding. A stimulation test using hCG increases the chances of detecting testosterone. To do this, one injects 5000 to 10,000 IU of hCG intravenously. Testosterone concentrations are determined before injection and 60 to 120 minutes later. A fivefold or greater increase in hormone indicates a retained testicle. However, false-negative results are possible. A single measurement of blood estrone sulfate concentration is a reliable indicator of the presence of testicular tissue, especially in colts older than 3 years of age.[5-7]

PUBERTY

Puberty is defined as the age at which a colt is able to mount, copulate, and successfully impregnate a mare and occurs during the second spring after the year of birth. Puberty should not be confused with sexual maturity, which occurs after the age of 5.

Puberty is probably regulated by the reactivation of the hypothalamic pulse generator, a group of cells located in the arcuate nucleus of the hypothalamus.[1] The pulsatile secretion of Gn-RH from the hypothalamus stimulates the secretion of LH and FSH from the anterior pituitary. Season, age, breed, nutritional status, and external hormones affect puberty, but in general puberty is complete by 18 to 24 months in the horse.[8]

ENDOCRINOLOGY

The pineal gland plays a significant role in the seasonality of the horse. The retina captures photoperiod information and transports it by way of nerve fibers to the pineal gland, which in turn inhibits the production of melatonin during long days. Low levels of circulating melatonin are consistent with higher levels of Gn-RH and gonadotropins. Stallions, in contrast to mares, do not undergo a complete reproductive quiescence and continue to produce sperm during the short photoperiodic days. The cause for this partial refractoriness of the stallion to changes in photoperiod is not well understood.

The hypothalamus, pituitary, and testes (hypothalamic-pituitary-gonadal axis) must work in synchrony for a stallion to be able to start and sustain sperm production. The primary role of the hypothalamus, located on the base of the brain, is the production of the 10-amino-acid peptide Gn-RH, which is secreted in multiple daily pulses and then transported via the hypothalamic-pituitary portal system to the anterior pituitary. In addition to melatonin-mediated stimulus, the hypothalamus responds to tactile, olfactory, and visual stimuli.[9]

The pituitary, which is connected to the hypothalamus by neural fibers, has two lobes. The anterior lobe possesses Gn-RH receptors. Gn-RH binds to these receptors and induces secretion of FSH or LH. The anterior pituitary gland also produces prolactin, the role of which is unclear in the stallion. FSH and LH act on the Sertoli's and Leydig's cells, respectively, stimulating production of steroids and other protein hormones. The peptide hormones inhibin and activin regulate FSH at the pituitary level. Testicular steroid hormones, mainly estradiol and testosterone, in turn have positive or negative feedback actions at the level of the pituitary on FSH and LH, respectively.

The complexity of the interaction among hormones has kept clinicians and researchers in the field of stallion andrology from being able to develop a test or a series of hormonal tests to predict or diagnose infertility or subfertility. Until such diagnostic methods become available, hormonal supplementation is strictly empirical and sometimes worsens or elicits a reproductive dysfunction in otherwise normal stallions.[9]

TESTICULAR CELLS

The endocrine role of the testes is to produce testosterone and estrone sulfate, whereas the exocrine role is to produce spermatozoa. The testicle is composed of 85% to 90% testicular parenchyma, of which seminiferous tubules comprise 70%. In turn, the seminiferous tubules are formed by Sertoli's and germinal cells. The interstitium, formed primarily by Leydig's cells and myoid cells, occupies close to 15% of the parenchyma.[10]

SERTOLI'S CELLS

Sertoli's cells, also known as *supportive cells,* contain the most testicular receptors for FSH. Some of the most important functions of the Sertoli's cell in the process of sperm maturation include the following:

1. Isolation of the advanced (haploid) stages of spermatogenesis by tight gap junctions forming the blood-testis barrier.
2. Production of androgen binding protein, activin, and inhibin. Androgen binding protein binds the bioactive form of testosterone, dihydrotestosterone, to maintain high levels of these products in the seminiferous tubules and epididymis. Activin and inhibin stimulate or suppress the release of FSH from the pituitary. The Sertoli's cells contribute to the regulation of Leydig's cell function and establish feedback mechanisms to the anterior pituitary primarily through the production of activin and inhibin. Sertoli's cells synthesize other proteins, such as SGP-2, ceruloplasmin, and transferrin, that are necessary to support spermatogenesis. Ceruloplasmin and transferrin act as carrier proteins for copper and iron, respectively, which are important regulators of spermatogenesis.
3. Germ cells begin the process of differentiation as large round cells on the basal compartment of the seminiferous tubule and approximately 55 days later finish as elongated cells in an adluminal position. This change in size, shape, and position occurs between two adjacent Sertoli's cells. The number of spermatogenic cells and ultimately the total sperm production of a given stallion are determined by the number of cells that can be accommodated between the tight gap junctions between two Sertoli's cells. Day length appears to be one of the most important factors in determining the number of Sertoli's cells per testis in adult stallions. Numbers of Sertoli's cells increase in young animals: 1 billion cells at 2 years of age, 2.8 billion at 3 years, and 3.6 billion after 4 to 5 years of age. The number of Sertoli's cells then decreases with advancing age.[11]

LEYDIG'S CELLS

The interstitial, or Leydig's, cells contain most of the testicular receptors for LH and are the main site of testosterone production. Testosterone concentration in the testicular microcirculation is at least 10 times higher than that in the general circulation. Through steroid production, Leydig's cells provide the feedback mechanisms on the pituitary necessary to maintain spermatogenesis, secondary sex characteristics, and libido. Season and not age appear to affect the testosterone production in adult stallions, which is mediated through a change in total number of Leydig's cells rather than total volume of cells per testis. Unlike Sertoli's cells, Leydig's cell numbers do not increase dramatically with age (1.4 billion at 2 years and 4.7 billion as a mature stallion). However, a significant increase in cell volume occurs that is regulated primarily by season.[12]

MYOID CELLS

The myoid cell has profound effects on germ cells and Leydig's cells primarily through the action of paracrine modulating factors. A paracrine modulating factor in the rat known as P-Mod-S is thought to stimulate or modulate some of the androgen binding protein functions. In addition, the myoid cells are responsible for the round architecture of the seminiferous tubule and probably for the intratesticular movement of sperm.

GERMINAL CELLS

Sperm is the final product of a 57-day process that starts at the base of the seminiferous tubule. Testicular volume has a direct correlation with the number of sperm that a normal stallion should be able to produce.[13]

SPERMATOGENESIS

Spermatogenesis is the series of chronologic changes that occur in the seminiferous tubule, transforming a large, round spermatogonium into a spermatozoon. This process in the stallion takes approximately 57 days and is not affected by frequency of ejaculation or season.[14]

The process starts when an A_1 stem cell spermatogonia undergoes mitosis, giving rise to (1) a second A_1 spermatogonia to maintain a constant population of stem cells and (2) an A_2 spermatogonia. In turn, the A_2 spermatogonia gives rise to A_3, A_3 to B_1, and B_1 to B_2. The entire process of spermatogenesis has been divided into three phases of similar length known as *spermatocytogenesis, meiotic divisions,* and *spermiogenesis.*

Spermatocytogenesis is characterized by the mitotic divisions of A and B spermatogonia. Meiotic divisions result in the formation of primary spermatocytes from B_2 spermatogonia and the subsequent formation of secondary spermatids. Leptotene spermatocytes that form immediately after the first meiotic division are hidden from the immune system by the hematotesticular barrier. Spermiogenesis is characterized by the transformation of round spermatogonia to elongated spermatids and ultimately to spermatozoa. During spermiogenesis the formation of the acrosome arises from the Golgi complex and the compaction of DNA, partly because of the expression of protamine genes at the spermatid stage. The end of spermatogenesis is characterized by spermiation, the release of the elongated spermatids or spermatozoa into the lumen of the seminiferous tubule.[15]

SEASONALITY

Although a reduction in testicular size, testicular volume, and daily sperm production during the nonbreeding season occur, the seasonal effect varies significantly between stallions and is not as significant as the effect on ovarian function in the mare. Stallions from which semen is collected throughout the year decrease their sperm output on the average by 1 to 2 billion during the nonbreeding season. In many of these stallions, libido is not affected adversely. Although the total number of sperm is affected, sperm morphology and motility remain unaltered, provided that stallions are maintained on a regular collection schedule. The effect of day length on sperm production can be explained by a decrease in serum LH during the nonbreeding season. This lack of stimulus to the Leydig's cell has a direct effect on intratesticular and extratesticular testosterone levels. Decreased testosterone concentration affects the number of Sertoli's cells and in turn the total number of germ cells that can be allocated between two Sertoli's cells.[16]

The effect of external lighting programs on spermatogenesis is uncertain. Burns and Douglas[17] reported increased sperm production and testicular size in stallions subjected to a lighting program but observed that this improvement was transitory, and in some cases detrimental, to stallion performance at the peak of the breeding season (April to May). Other investigators have found no detrimental effect on photostimulated stallions.[16,18] Several Thoroughbred breeding farms provide light to their stallions before the breeding season without significant reduction in conception rates.

Testicular Cell Interactions

Sertoli's, or nurse, cells have a direct interaction with germ cells, and Leydig's cells interact with Sertoli's and germinal cells through hormonal production. The myoid cell produces at least one paracrine factor that interacts directly with the Sertoli's cell. Paracrine and autocrine modulating factors, products of the peritubular cell, appear to have an effect on androgen binding protein function. In turn, the myoid cell is under regulatory influence of transforming growth factors α (stimulatory) and β (inhibitory). Other factors involved in cell-to-cell communication of the testicular cells include collagen, plasminogen activator, vitamin A, pyruvate, and carbohydrates.[19] Most of these products and mechanisms have not been investigated extensively in the stallion.

Epididymis

The specific absorptive and secretory functions of each segment of the stallion epididymis remain the subject of considerable debate and investigation. The histologic structure of the epididymis changes as it continues through its different regions, with epithelial height being greatest proximally and smooth muscle components greatest distally.[20] As spermatozoa are transported from the excurrent ducts into the head, along the body, and into the tail, they undergo a number of morphologic and physiologic changes that ultimately render them motile and fertile. Specific maturational changes include (1) the capacity for progressive motility, (2) shedding of the cytoplasmic droplet, (3) plasma and acrosomal membrane alterations, (4) DNA stabilization, and (5) metabolic changes.[21] The tail of the epididymis generally serves to store the matured spermatozoa. All these changes occur primarily at the level of the mid to distal corpus.[21,22]

Throughout the epididymis fluid resorption occurs at a steady rate and results in a significant increase in sperm concentration.[23] Whether stallions with high-volume ejaculates and poor sperm morphology have epidydimal dysfunction remains to be investigated.

External Genitalia

PENIS AND PREPUCE

The penis of the stallion is composed of a root, a body, and a glans penis and is musculocavernous. The penile base arises at the ischial arch in the form of two crura that fuse distally to form the single dorsal corpus cavernosum penis enclosed by a thick tunica albuginea. The corpus cavernosum, corpus spongiosum, and corpus spongiosum glandis are the three spaces that make up the erectile tissue of the penis. Engorgement of these spaces with blood from branches of the internal and external pudendal arteries and obturator arteries is responsible for erection. The cavernous spaces within the penis are continuous with the veins responsible for drainage. The corpus spongiosum originates in the pelvic area and surrounds the penile urethra within a groove on the ventral side of the penis and forms the corpus spongiosum glandis at the distal end of the penis.[24] The corpus spongiosum glandis is responsible for the distinct bell shape of the stallion penis after ejaculation.

The urethral process is distinctly visible at the center of the glans penis and is surrounded by an invagination known as the *fossa glandis*. Accumulations of smegma secretions, known as "beans" are predisposed in one or all of the diverticulae of the fossa glandis and urethral sinus. Careful examination and cleaning of this area are imperative during the reproductive evaluation of a stallion or before breeding.

The bulbospongiosus muscle located in the ventral aspect of the penis provides rhythmic contractions or pulsations to assist in moving the penile urethral contents (semen and urine) distally during ejaculation. Two retractor penis muscles also run ventrally along the length of the penis and are responsible for returning the penis to the sheath after detumescence.[25]

The prepuce is formed by a double fold of skin that is hairless and well supplied with sebaceous and sweat glands. The prepuce functions to contain and protect the nonerect penis. The external part of the prepuce, or sheath, begins at the scrotum and displays raphae that are continuous with the scrotal raphae. The internal layer of the prepuce extends caudally from the orifice to line the internal side of the sheath and then reflects cranially toward the orifice again before reflecting caudally to form the internal preputial fold and preputial ring. This additional internal fold allows the considerable lengthening (approximately 50%) of the penis during erection. During erection the preputial orifice is visible at the base of the penis just in front of the scrotum, and the preputial ring is visible at approximately the midshaft of the penis.[25]

One can best examine the penis and prepuce of a breeding stallion after teasing with an estrous mare, when one can observe the stallion drop the penis and attain a full erection.[26] The prepuce and penis should be free of vesicular, proliferative, or inflammatory lesions such as those found in horses with coital exanthema, squamous cell carcinoma, or cutaneous habronemiasis. Removal of smegma accumulations may be required for a complete examination of the skin surfaces.

SCROTUM

The scrotum is slightly pendulous and forms two distinct pouches that contain, protect, and thermoregulate the testes and epididymides. The testes are located in the scrotum to maintain testicular temperature at 3° to 5° C below the normal body temperature, which is a requirement for normal spermatogenesis.[19]

The scrotal wall consists of four layers: the skin, tunica dartos, scrotal fascia, and parietal vaginal tunic.[19,23] The scrotal skin is thin, generally hairless, and slightly oily, containing numerous sebaceous and sweat glands that assist in thermoregulation. The tunica dartos adheres to the scrotal skin and consists of muscular and fibroelastic tissue. The tunica dartos lines both scrotal pouches and extends into the median septum, which appears externally as the median rapha of the scrotum. The scrotal fascia is between the tunica dartos and parietal vaginal tunic and allows the testis and associated parietal tunic layer to move freely within the scrotum. The parietal vaginal tunic is the innermost layer and is an evagination of the parietal peritoneum through the inguinal rings that forms during testicular descent. This layer forms a sac that lines the scrotum and is apposed closely to the visceral vaginal tunic, the outer layer of the testis itself. The vaginal cavity is the space between the parietal and visceral layers of the vaginal tunic and normally contains a small amount of viscous fluid to allow some free movement of the testis within. The vaginal cavity is a potential space within which considerable fluid may accumulate.

The scrotum of the normal stallion should appear slightly pendulous, globular, and generally symmetric. One may observe normal variations in the positioning of the testes if one testis is anterior to or ventral to the other. The skin should have no evidence of trauma, scarring, or skin lesions. Palpation of the scrotum of a normal stallion reveals a thin and pliable covering that slides loosely and easily over the testicles and epididymides within.

TESTICLES

The testes of a normal stallion are palpable as two oval structures of nearly equal size lying horizontally within the scrotal pouches. Normal orientation of the testis is ascertained by palpation of the body of the epididymis, which is always dorsolateral to the testicle proper, and the tail of the epididymis and the ligament of the tail of the epididymis, which should be in a caudal position. The ligament is palpable as a fibrous nodule 5 to 19 mm in size that attaches the tail of the epididymis to the caudal pole of the testis. The ligament is particularly large in newborn colts and on palpation may be mistaken for a testis within the scrotum. Examination of a normal stallion may identify rotation of one or both testes, up to 180 degrees. Such rotations can be permanent, or the testis may rotate back and forth, usually with the stallion showing no outward signs of discomfort. A rotated testicle may have as much as a 40% reduction in blood flow.[19] Although this condition does not interfere with normal breeding by the stallion, it may be considered a criterion for failing a stallion during a BSE in some breed regulations. The presence of the condition must be clearly noted on the record, and the owner must be notified. Testis rotation should be differentiated from true testicular torsion in which stallions demonstrate signs of colic and for which palpation reveals a painful and swollen testicle.

Within the scrotum the testis is encapsulated by the tunica albuginea, a layer of tough collagenous tissue and smooth muscle that sends supportive trabeculae into the testicular parenchyma, dividing the testis into lobules. The muscular content of the tunica albuginea is thought to play a role in intratesticular sperm transport and determination of testicular tone.[23]

Testicular tone is described as the degree of turgidity of the testicle, which should be firm to turgid but resilient on palpation. Deviation from the normal toward a softer or firmer testis may be associated with degenerative, neoplastic, or traumatic conditions of the testis. Testicular degeneration is an acquired reversible or irreversible condition in which damage to the germinal epithelium results in eventual atrophy of the epithelium and an initial loss of testicular tone. As the disease progresses, the degenerating testicle becomes small and firm as fibrous tissue replaces testicular parenchyma.

Because testicular conditions may afflict only one testis, comparison of the size and consistency of the two testes of any individual stallion is imperative. Changes in testicular tone or consistency are best determined by sequential examinations of the stallion that allow the clinician to monitor the severity and rate of change as the disease progresses. Regular physical examinations of breeding stallions are an important part of routine stallion management and may allow early detection of problems that may affect fertility.

TESTICULAR SIZE AND VOLUME

Testicular size in stallions increases from the pubertal period to reach maximal size at the age of 5 to 6 years and is affected by breed, season, and age. Each testis of an adult stallion weighs between 150 and 300 g and measures 50 to 80 mm in width, 60 to 70 mm in height, and 80 to 140 mm in length, with breed being the biggest factor in determining size. Testicular volume correlates highly with daily sperm production and therefore is a useful predictor of the sperm-production potential of a stallion.[27]

To calculate the testicular volume, the clinician should obtain measurements of the length, width, and height of each testicle by calipers or ultrasound. Ultrasonographic measurements may be more accurate, although proper placement of the probe across the testis is critical to ensure that a cross-sectional image is obtained. Because a testis approximates the shape of an ellipsoid, the following formula converts length, width, and height measurements into testicular volume:

$$\text{Testis volume} = 0.5333 \times \text{H(cm)} \times \text{L(cm)} \times \text{W(cm)}$$

Love et al.[27] also recommend using this volume to predict the expected daily sperm output (DSO) of the stallion, using the following formula:

$$\text{Predicted DSO} = (0.024 \times \text{combined testicular volume}) - 0.76$$

Predicted DSO can be compared with actual DSO as estimated by semen collection during the routine BSE. A stallion in which actual DSO falls below that predicted for his testicular size requires further evaluation for disease conditions of the testes, epididymides, and accessory glands.

Testicular measurements are a useful and important part of the physical examination of any breeding stallion and can be used to predict sperm output and determine the size of the book for a given stallion. A stallion with small testicles will have lower sperm production and may need modification of the management strategies that result in optimization of the fertility of such a stallion.

EPIDIDYMIDES AND EXCURRENT DUCT SYSTEM

The epididymis is a single, highly convoluted duct approximately 70 m in length that has a grossly distinct head, body, and tail. The head of the epididymis is a flattened structure that lies dorsomedially along the cranial border of the testis and is attached closely to the testis. The body, or corpus, lies along the dorsolateral aspect of each testis and continues as the tail, or cauda, the large, prominent structure attached to the caudal pole of the testis. The deferent duct, the excretory duct for sperm, attaches to the tail of the corresponding epididymis, runs along the medial aspect of the testis, and ascends by way of the spermatic cord through the vaginal ring into the pelvis. Each deferent duct widens into its corresponding ampullary region and eventually terminates at the colliculus seminalis of the pelvic urethra. The colliculus seminalis is a rounded prominence situated on the dorsomedial wall of the urethra about 5 cm caudal to the urethral opening from the bladder. The colliculus is the common opening to the ampullae and the seminal vesicles. With care one can palpate all sections of the epididymis through the scrotal wall. However, the head of the epididymis may be difficult to ascertain because of its flattened nature and the close apposition of the cremaster muscle overlying it.[28]

SPERMATIC CORD

Each spermatic cord is enveloped in the parietal layer of the vaginal tunic, which extends distally from the internal inguinal ring. Within each cord are the corresponding deferent duct, testicular artery, testicular veins, lymphatic vessels, and nerves. The cremaster muscle is situated in the caudolateral borders of each spermatic cord. The testicular artery, a branch of the abdominal aorta, descends through the inguinal ring into the cranial border of the spermatic cord in a tortuous manner and divides near the testis into several branches to supply the testis and epididymis. These small branches, embedded in the tunica albuginea, enter the parenchyma by way of the trabeculae and septae of the testis. A corresponding network of veins leaves the testis and surrounds the testicular artery in a tortuous manner, forming the pampiniform plexus. This arrangement of artery and veins is responsible for much of the thermoregulation of the testis in the stallion when heat from the testicular arterial blood is transferred to the venous side, resulting in testicular arterial blood being several degrees cooler than systemic blood temperature. Abnormal distention of the veins of the pampiniform plexus is termed a *varicocele* and is an uncommon condition in stallions. Palpation of the spermatic cord of an affected stallion reveals the dilated and often tortuous vessels. Varicoceles are usually not painful but can result in fluid accumulation around the vaginal tunics, most often involve only one side of the spermatic cord, and usually are diagnosed by the observation of the dilation of the vessels from the pampiniform plexus with ultrasonography. The condition has been identified in stallions with normal semen parameters.[28]

ULTRASONOGRAPHIC EXAMINATION OF THE TESTICLES AND EPIDIDYMIS

Ultrasound examination of the testis and epididymis is a useful ancillary diagnostic tool that enables the clinician to assess palpable changes and to identify nonpalpable changes. Ultrasound is particularly useful in horses with generalized scrotal enlargement in which specific structures become difficult to palpate.

Examination is usually easier after semen collection, when the stallion is relaxed. A 5.0-, 7.5-, or 10.0-MHz linear array transducer is used.[9] The clinician usually begins the examination at the cranial end of the testis and slowly moves the probe caudally in a vertical position. Visualization of the scrotum reveals a thin, echogenic, uniform layer. Minimal, if any, fluid is visible between the scrotal skin and testicular parenchyma in the normal stallion. In the cranial third of the scrotum, the head of the epididymis, testicular parenchyma, blood vessels of the spermatic cord, and central vein are visible. As the probe is moved caudally, the central vein and spermatic cord vessels disappear and the head of the epididymis continues into the body of the epididymis. The head and body of the epididymis appear as heterogeneous areas just below the spermatic cord when the probe is positioned as described. As the probe continues further caudally, the body of the epididymis becomes indistinct.[29] With the exception of the central vein, the testicular parenchyma appears uniformly echogenic and homogenous. The central vein appears as a small anechoic area within the testicular parenchyma at the cranial third of the testis and should not be mistaken for a pathologic lesion. Dilation of the central vein may be visible in cases of varicocele or spermatic cord torsions and usually is accompanied by detectable dilations of the vessels of the spermatic cord. Well-defined and hypoechoic lesions within the parenchyma suggest testicular tumors.

After reaching the most caudal aspect of the testis, the clinician rotates the probe to face cranially in a vertical position and allow examination of the tail of the epididymis. This structure appears as a heterogeneous area, with a Swiss cheese–like appearance. Identification of the epididymal tail may assist in diagnosis of testicular rotations. In horses with 360-degree torsions, the tail of the epididymis, although in its caudal position, is more dorsal because of the tension on the ligament of the tail of the epididymis by the deferent duct.

The spermatic cord is most easily visualized by placing the probe horizontally across the cord, just proximal to the body of the testis. The arrangement of the pampiniform plexus results in the mottled, heterogeneous appearance of the spermatic cord, and the testicular artery and veins are identifiable in cross-sectional images.[29]

INTERNAL GENITALIA

ACCESSORY SEX GLANDS

The bulbourethral glands, prostate gland, and seminal vesicles collectively are referred to as the *accessory sex glands*. Their secretions produce the seminal plasma that makes up most of the ejaculate volume. The ampullae, which are dilations of the vas deferens before opening in the colliculus seminalis, are considered a storage place for sperm.

Although a short exposure to seminal plasma appears to be important for sperm function, long-term exposure to seminal plasma components may be detrimental to spermatozoa survival for some stallions. Artificial insemination programs deal with this potential detrimental effect by dilution of semen with extenders in fresh or fresh-chilled programs and by centrifugation to remove seminal plasma in frozen semen programs and some chilled-shipped programs. Seminal plasma appears to suppress the inflammatory response of the endometrium of the mare to sperm after insemination or natural mating. Although the functions of the specific components of the seminal plasma remain rather obscure, the fluid suspends the ejaculated sperm and also is thought to be a source of energy, protein, and other macromolecules required for sperm functions and metabolism.[30-32]

EXAMINATION AND ULTRASONOGRAPHY OF THE ACCESSORY SEX GLANDS

In some cases the reproductive examination of stallions should include rectal palpation and ultrasonography of the accessory sex glands.[33,34] Most stallions tolerate this procedure well with adequate restraint in stocks, and sedation is not usually necessary. Glands on sexually stimulated stallions are easier to palpate and visualize.

BULBOURETHRAL GLANDS

The bulbourethral glands, although not usually palpable rectally because of the urethralis and bulboglandularis muscles close to the ischiatic arch, are easy to evaluate by ultrasonography. Multiple ductules from the bulbourethral glands enter the medial aspect of the urethra distal to the prostatic ductules. Bulbourethral gland secretions compose most of the presperm or first fraction of the ejaculate and serve as a cleanser and pH stabilizer in the urethra before ejaculation. Using ultrasonography, one locates the bulbourethral glands 3 to 4 cm inside the anus off the midline, and in a stimulated stallion the glands appear as two distinct ovoid structures with multiple small hypoechoic spaces throughout the parenchyma.[33]

PROSTATE GLAND

In the stallion the prostate is formed by a central isthmus and two lateral lobes located on the caudolateral borders of each vesicular gland. Although not always palpable rectally, the prostate is lobulated or nodular and firm, distinguishing it from the smooth, thin-walled vesicular glands lying next to it. Each prostatic lobe measures 5 to 9 cm long, 2 to 6 cm wide, and 1 to 2 cm thick. Multiple ductules from the prostate enter the lumen of the urethra lateral to the colliculus seminalis. The secretions of the prostate contribute to the sperm-rich fraction of the ejaculate. The lobes of the prostate are easily identifiable with ultrasonography, with the two symmetric and homogeneously echogenic lobes distinctly visible lateral to the area in which the penile urethra merges with the neck of the bladder. Hypoechoic dilations within the gland parenchyma of each lobe are evident in a teased stallion.[33]

AMPULLAE

The ampullae are the enlarged distal portions of the deferent ducts measuring 1 to 2 cm in diameter and 10 to 25 cm in length. Palpable along the midline of the pelvic floor over the neck of the bladder, they converge caudally and pass beneath the prostate gland but lie dorsal to the pelvic urethra. At their distal ends they continue through the wall of the urethra, opening into the colliculus seminalis alongside the excretory ducts of the seminal vesicles. The ampullae, in addition to serving as a sperm storage area, have many branched tubular glands located within the thickened wall.[34]

Because of the longitudinal orientation of the ampullae, sometimes they are easier to find on rectal palpation. One can identify them by ultrasonography by their hypochoic central lumen surrounded by a uniformly echogenic wall and a hyperechogenic outer muscular layer. Orienting the transducer in a transverse position inside the rectum can provide a good cross-sectional image of the ampullae. The ampullae can be a common site for blockage because of sperm stasis. In these cases dilation of the lumen may or may not be visible. Stallions with such blockage usually have a history of infertility or subfertility and often display severe oligospermia or, in severe cases, complete azoospermia. When sperm are present, they have a variety of morphologic abnormalities, with predominantly tail-less heads; in some instances the ampullae are palpably enlarged. This condition may render a stallion virtually infertile if undiagnosed. Recommendations for treatment include ampullary massage by way of the rectum and repeated daily semen collection after injection of low doses of oxytocin or PG.[35]

SEMINAL VESICLES

The seminal vesicles or vesicular glands are paired, pyriform, and thin-walled structures lying lateral to the ampullae. On occasion they may extend far cranially to hang over the brim of the pelvis. Sexual stimulation results in dilation and elongation of the vesicular glands, up to 12 to 20 cm long and 5 cm in diameter. The distal ends of the glands converge, passing under the prostate as they lie parallel to the ampullae toward their termination at the urethra. The excurrent ducts of the vesicular glands open lateral to the excurrent ducts of the ampullae at the colliculus seminalis of the urethra. Secretions of the vesicular glands compose the gel fraction of the ejaculate. Higher gel volumes can be collected with pronounced sexual stimulation and season. The specific function of the gel fraction is unclear, and one should remove it when processing semen for evaluation or artificial insemination. Palpation of the vesicular glands may be easier after considerable teasing of the stallion with an estrous mare. The glands also are readily palpable in instances of pathologic enlargement.

With ultrasonography the vesicular glands appear in longitudinal section as flattened oval to triangular sacs, depending on the degree of sexual stimulation. A thin echogenic wall surrounds a generally uniformly anechoic lumen.[33] Increased echogenicity of vesicular gland fluid is associated with the highly viscous gel fraction produced by some stallions. The seminal vesicles are the glands that are most prone to bacterial infections. Diagnosis is based on the cytologic evaluation of the semen with presence of white blood cells.

EVALUATION OF THE PELVIC AND PENILE URETHRA

Although the pelvic urethra can be evaluated by transrectal ultrasonography, in most cases such evaluation is unrewarding. Endoscopic examination provides better information regarding the anatomic integrity of the urethra and its accessory structures. The procedure is performed by gently passing a 1-m endoscope with an outer diameter of 8 to 9 mm into the urethra of a sedated horse so that the penis is relaxed. The clinician applies gentle and constant pressure so as to pass 70 to 80 cm of the endoscope into the urethra.[36,37] Care must be taken not to inflate the bladder with too much air because of a slight risk of rupturing the bladder.

The bulbourethral gland ductules are grouped about 2.5 to 3 cm distal to the prostatic openings and are visible as two rows of 6 to 10 small openings dorsal and close to the midline. The prostatic ductules are arranged in a similar way to the bulbourethral and visible as two groups of small openings lateral to the ejaculatory orifices about 5 cm deeper. Just ventral and cranial to the colliculus, the openings of the urethral glands are visible laterally on the widened pelvic portion of the urethra, at the level of the prostatic gland openings.[36]

One can identify the colliculus seminalis as a rounded prominent structure found on the medial aspect of the dorsal wall of the urethra approximately 5 cm caudal to the internal opening of the urethra from the bladder. On either side of the colliculus is an ejaculatory duct orifice, a small slitlike diverticulum within which the ampullary ducts and ducts of the seminal vesicle open. By passing the endoscope into this orifice, one can visualize and evaluate the seminal vesicles.[36,37] Samples can be taken for culture with endoscopic culturettes if seminal vesiculitis is suspected.[38]

Endoscopic examination of the urethra is indicated in horses with hemospermia or in horses in which one suspects a pathologic condition of the accessory sex glands. In cases of hemospermia the bleeding area may be visualized with the endoscope. These lesions are most readily identified in the region of the ischiatic arch and distal urethra. One should take care to assess the urethral mucosa as the endoscope is passed forward because some irritation and erythema of the mucosal lining often results from the endoscopic examination.[38] A false diagnosis of urethritis may result if one assesses the mucosa while withdrawing the endoscope.

EVALUATION OF THE BREEDING STALLION

Equids in the wild are considered to be long-day seasonal breeders that live in a stable social group or harem. A free-running stallion interacts with a mare for hours or even days before copulation. In many management situations the domesticated stallion is restricted severely from its sociosexual activity. In general, breeding stallions are confined to a paddock or a box stall and do not have social interactions with other horses. In addition, mating and ejaculation often are permitted under only two conditions: hand mating at the convenience of the farm manager, allowing only a few minutes for stallion and mare interaction, or mounting of a mare or a phantom for artificial insemination purposes.

Perhaps the most remarkable difference in the breeding pattern, particularly with performance horses such as Thoroughbreds and Standardbreds, is the fact that most breedings are done during February to June, well in advance of the natural breeding season (May to September).

Behavior

NORMAL BEHAVIOR

Stallions display several behavioral responses during teasing and breeding. However, the intensity of the response, also known as *libido,* and the type of response depend greatly on breeding experience; management; and, in some cases, season. Olfactory, visual, and auditory stimuli also influence libido. Typically, a normal stallion that has never mated with a mare takes a longer time to mount but displays good libido. However, a stallion that has had a negative previous experience might show no interest in the mare or in mounting. Some of the typical normal responses by stallions when exposed to an estrous mare include vocalization, flehmen response, striking, nipping or biting, and sniffing or licking. A normal stallion should show interest in the mare and drop the penis within 1 to 2 minutes of exposure to a quiet mare in standing heat and should try to mount within the first 3 minutes. Once stallions are allowed to mount, they give several (five to eight) intravaginal thrusts, followed by three to five short thrusts immediately before ejaculation. Signs of ejaculation are rhythmic and frequent urethral pulsation, flagging of the tail, and a head relaxation. A single stallion tends to be consistent in its breeding behavior, provided that the conditions under which he usually mates are the same.[39]

ABNORMAL BEHAVIOR

Stallion behavioral dysfunction in many instances is difficult to define and is relative to the expectations of the breeding manager. A stallion that takes 30 minutes or more to mount and ejaculate or takes several mounts may be considered a problem in some intensive management situations. However, a stallion that takes several hours to achieve an erection, mount, and ejaculate may be considered normal if he breeds only two or three mares during the entire breeding season in pasture conditions.

A review of the incidence of problems in 250 stallions over a period of 5 years indicated that more than 50% of the cases had complaints related to poor libido or excessive aggressiveness. Of those, nearly half were described in stallions with no previous sexual experience. The rest were divided evenly between experienced stallions with low sexual interest and unruly and overly aggressive breeders. Mounting and erection dysfunction accounted for 11% of complaints, whereas ejaculatory problems accounted for 25% of the total cases. Other problems, such as self-mutilation and severe stereotypies that reportedly could be detrimental to fertility, accounted for 11% of the reported cases.[40]

DIAGNOSIS OF ABNORMAL BEHAVIOR

A normal stallion exposed to a mare in standing estrus should vocalize, sniff or nuzzle the mare, display the flehmen response by curling his upper lip, drop his penis, and achieve an erection within the first 3 minutes after initial exposure.[41] These precopulatory responses should be followed by mounting, intromission, and ejaculation. A normal, experienced stallion that is hand bred should require no more than 5 minutes from initial exposure to a mare until ejaculation. The frequency and intensity of the precopulatory responses are affected by management, breeding experience, and external stimuli. Stallions with no previous breeding experience are expected to be slower in mounting. However, interest in the mare and time to erection should be within normal limits. Once the novice stallion mounts, he soon gains confidence and ejaculation should occur following a normal thrusting pattern. After the first positive experience, time to mounting and to ejaculation should decrease. Novice stallions must be treated with patience, positive reinforcement, and perseverance. During this time unnecessary punishment and rough handling can aggravate a problem and may result in profound breeding disinterest. One should investigate any aberration in courtship or copulatory behavior carefully, always keeping in mind that sexual behavioral dysfunction is a problem with many possible causes involving management and the endocrine, cardiovascular, musculoskeletal, and nervous systems.[42]

LACK OF LIBIDO

Libido, defined as sexual drive or interest in breeding, is high in most stallions. Sexual stimuli and environmental factors profoundly affect libido in stallions. Low libido is apparent in improperly stimulated stallions. The best stimulus is a mare in standing heat. If this is not possible, an estrogenized ovariectomized mare may be used. Some stallions might have a preference for or an aversion to a particular color or type of mare.[42] Experienced stallions frequently are aroused by exposure to a breeding phantom. A novice stallion or one that has never mounted a breeding phantom cannot be expected to be stimulated positively by a dummy.

Lack of libido may be observed in experienced stallions toward the end of the breeding season, particularly in heavily used or overused animals. This problem is easily corrected by decreasing the frequency of service or collection.

Stallions that have been kicked by mares or negatively reinforced for displaying sexual behavior in shows or while performing at the track may have reduced sexual desire. Unfortunately, circulating levels of steroids or gonadotrophins are often poor predictors of libido.

Treatment of a stallion with low sexual drive is directed best at correction of the underlying problem. However, assessment of the nature of the problem is often difficult. One may try several alternatives, such as the following:

1. Change of stimulus mare or environment
2. Breeding or collecting another stallion in the presence of the low-libido animal
3. Intravenous administration of Gn-RH, 50 μg, 2 hours and 1 hour before breeding or of LH (hCG), 5000 to 10,000 IU, 1 hour before breeding
4. Single injection of a short-acting testosterone
5. Intravenous administration of diazepam at a dose of 0.05 mg/kg (maximum 20 mg) 10 to 15 minutes before breeding to reverse mild shyness in some stallions[9]

The efficacy of most of these treatments is empirical and requires further investigation; however, chronic administration of steroids, particularly androgens, is well documented to affect spermatogenesis negatively.[9] Therefore injection of stallions with exogenous steroids and particularly androgens to improve libido is not a recommended practice.

ERECTION FAILURE

The inability of a stallion to develop and maintain a normal erection despite normal libido suggests an anatomic rather than a psychogenic problem. The most common problems are vascular damage associated with traumatic injuries or neurologic problems associated with other penile or lumbosacral compromise.[43] Therapy of either problem, extrapolated from the human medicine literature, may be medical with injection of vasoactive drugs directly into the corpus cavernosum or surgical with penile implants. To date, no reports indicate that either procedure has been used in horses. No reports of dose or efficacy exist to support the use of sildenafil (Viagra) in these stallions; anecdotal reports of its use suggest that results are inconsistent.

EJACULATORY DYSFUNCTION

Some stallions show normal precopulatory behavior, mount, and copulate but fail to ejaculate. These stallions often attempt to ejaculate and may become exhausted or frustrated, becoming aggressive with the mare or handler. Before attempting to treat an ejaculatory dysfunction, the clinician must examine the horse for evidence of degenerative joint disease in the hocks, spine, vertebrae, and pelvis and for lesions or malformations in the hoof or foot abscesses. Recently, circulatory problems leading to iliac thrombosis have been reported to be associated with ejaculatory dysfunction.[26] Although difficult to diagnose, psychologic problems that can lead to ejaculatory dysfunction should always be considered when no organic causes account for the problem.[43] Often, typical behavior provides hints to the clinician about the psychogenic nature of the dysfunction. In most instances psychogenic ejaculatory dysfunction results from traumatic accidents associated with breeding. If the role of musculoskeletal pain in ejaculatory dysfunction is uncertain, the horse may be treated with 1 g of phenylbutazone every 12 hours for approximately 2 weeks. If the stallion refuses to ejaculate only under specific circumstances, such as into an artificial vagina (AV) or when breeding a mare, the systematic approach of a patient, knowledgeable, and creative person is important to determine the problem. A variety of behavioral and managerial aids have been used to help stallions ejaculate.[44] One should adapt these aids according to the physical condition of the stallion (i.e., stallions that cannot achieve a full erection; stallions that have difficulty mounting; stallions that refuse to ejaculate after normal erection, mounting, thrusting, and belling of the glans). Neither mounting nor full erection are necessary for ejaculation. Stallions that have difficulty mounting can be taught to ejaculate on the ground by stimulating the penis manually or with an AV. Stallions with erection problems can ejaculate, provided that proper stimulation is given to the penis. One can achieve proper stimulation to the penis by raising the temperature of the AV or by applying hot towels to the base of the penis during thrusting. It is also important to consider changes in footing and surroundings, stimulus mare, handler, and so forth before implementing pharmacologic therapy.[45]

Therapeutic regimens for ejaculatory dysfunction are empirical and include those already mentioned for the treatment of low-libido stallions. In addition, PGs, oxytocin, and xylazine have been used to aid stallions in the process of ejaculation. Oxytocin and PG also have been used to treat azoospermia caused by ampullary blockage.[46] The tricyclic antidepressant imipramine has been used orally to lower the threshold for ejaculation in stallions.[47] The doses for these products are discussed later in this chapter.

OTHER BEHAVIORAL PROBLEMS

In addition to the previously described problems, stallions may have other abnormal behavior and vices that could eventually limit their fertility. These problems include overaggressiveness and stereotypies such as weaving, cribbing, wall kicking, and stomping.

Overaggressiveness is managed best by a good stallion handler and patience; in most cases the problems can be corrected. Stable vices often can be solved or somewhat alleviated by putting a toy (rubber tire) or a companion animal (goat or sheep) in the stall with the stallion.

One of the most complex behavioral syndromes observed in stallions is self-mutilation. Self-mutilation in horses includes biting, stomping and kicking, rubbing, and lunging at objects. According to McDonnell, three distinct types of self-mutilation occur.[48] Type I represents a normal behavioral response to continuous or intermittent unrelieved physical discomfort. Type II, seen in stallions and geldings, can be recognized as self-directed intermale aggression. The behavior includes the elements and order of the natural interactive sequence typical of encounters between two stallions, except that the stallion himself is the target of his intermale behavior. Type III involves a more quiet, often rhythmically repetitive or methodical behavioral sequence of a stereotypy (e.g., nipping at various areas of the body in a relatively invarient pattern, stomping, kicking rhythmically against an object). Some researchers have speculated that self-mutilation has a genetic component. The prevalence of self-mutilation of one form or another has been observed in as many as 2% of domestic stallions.[49] Among and between stallions, self-mutilation varies in frequency and intensity and can reach levels that threaten the stallion's fertility and even his life.

Careful evaluation of the horse's behavior is often necessary to distinguish the specific type of self-mutilation that is occurring. Type I self-mutilation, in which physical discomfort is the root cause, can be eliminated by relieving the discomfort. For Type II and Type III, understanding of intermale interactive behavior of horses and the environmental factors that may trigger or exacerbate the self-mutilative form can be useful in guiding humane management or behavior modification. Pharmacologic interventions may be a useful adjunct to management and nutritional changes. The stallion compulsively nips or bites the chest, shoulder, or flank or aggressively kicks the walls. Although self-mutilation is limited to postpubertal horses, it is not limited to confined animals. In some animals the problem is exacerbated on presentation of a mare to a confined stallion or breeding in the presence of another stallion.[50] The compulsive behavior seems to be more dramatic during the breeding season.

Self-mutilation may be a problem exacerbated by olfactory stimuli. In most horses this behavior is triggered by smelling their own manure. The stallions often mistakenly recognize themselves as a threat, triggering the compulsive behavior. One must ensure that the horse does not develop the behavior out of frustration because of chronic pain, such as that caused by an inguinal testicle or chronic gastrointestinal ulcers.

Therapy of this complex syndrome depends on the type of self-mutilation and its underlying causes and may include pain management, surgery, regular exercise, stall toys, and companion animals. Products to reduce the olfactory sense can be used, and the level of energy in the diet can be reduced. Treatment with L-tryptophan in the grain may help some horses. Physical restraint such as head cradles or muzzles most likely will lead to development of another self-mutilating technique.[50] In extreme, inhumane, and refractory cases, castration of the stallion has eliminated the problem for type III self-mutilation but not for the other types. Therefore an accurate diagnosis is a critical component of the treatment protocol.

Semen Collection

In addition to appropriate libido and behavior, a stallion must have good mating ability and be able to deliver an ejaculate. Mating ability and semen quality may be influenced by hereditary or environmental factors or learned patterns that are influenced greatly by management. An integral part of the diagnostic workup on a stallion with known or suspected infertility is the collection of semen. The collection process is critical because improper technique may result in poor fertility or inferior semen quality.

SEMEN COLLECTION AREA

The area used for semen collection should be spacious; clean; and free of dust and distracting noises, animals, and persons. The size of the breeding shed should be designed with awareness for the space needed for animal and human safety in the event of an uncooperative mount mare or unruly stallion. Stallions with low libido or a reluctance to mount are frequently encouraged to mount a mare in estrus if the mare can be walked slowly forward or led in a large circle. There should be adequate space to permit safe handling of the stallion and mare. Additionally, the footing surface should afford the stallion good traction even when the flooring is wet.[9] Many stallions paw, strike, or kick out while teasing a mare or being washed or after dismounting. All loose dirt, stone dust, and shavings should be removed because some stallions paw debris and dust onto the washed, damp penis just before mounting. If the collection area is dusty, the area should be wetted regularly.

Collection of semen in an outside area is acceptable in most cases but sometimes compromises semen collection because of distractions by other animals, persons, and vehicles. Ambient temperature also may have a significant effect because it alters the rate at which the temperature of the AV declines during cold weather or adversely affects semen quality during hot weather. Semen collection in an outside, grassy area affords the stallion, mare, and handlers the best footing; is usually free of dust; and allows for plenty of space for safety. The distance from the semen collection area to the laboratory should be minimal.

SEMEN COLLECTION TECHNIQUES

One can collect semen from stallions by allowing natural breeding with the addition of a condom; using pharmacologic stimulation to promote ejaculation; manually manipulating the penis; or using an AV on the ground or on a mount. Under certain circumstances, it may be necessary to use any one of these methods. However, for routine collection of semen for commercial use, an AV or manual stimulation of the penis of the stallion are the methods of choice.[47,51]

Condom The stallion is fitted with a latex condom and allowed to breed the mare naturally. Immediately after ejaculation and when the stallion has withdrawn the penis from the vagina, the condom is retrieved. Semen collected using the condom method is contaminated heavily by bacteria and debris. This method also requires that a mount mare be in estrus and increases the risk of mare contamination of the penis by vaginal entry, urination, and defecation during natural breeding. Many stallions do not tolerate breeding while wearing a condom. Condom and semen loss are also common. However, a stallion accustomed to natural service occasionally may be intolerant of semen collection with an artificial vagina until adequately trained for this method of breeding.

Pharmacologically Induced Ejaculation Numerous schemes have been published for the ex copula ejaculation of stallions using xylazine, imipramine, xylazine and imipramine, and PG.[40,52-54] Semen collected in this fashion is of low volume and high concentration. One can use the resulting ejaculate for cryopreservation or artificial insemination of mares in a cooled-semen shipment program. Fertility with the fresh, cooled semen is normal. However, the inability to obtain ejaculates on a predictable schedule limits the commercial usefulness of these methods. In experimental ponies semen was collected in 10 of 24 attempts using imipramine and xylazine.[52] In selected cases in which the stallion is physically unable to mount and copulate, it is possible to obtain semen specimens with the aid of pharmacologic agents. Under farm conditions semen is obtained in 25% to 30% of attempts. Keeping the stallion quiet and undisturbed is important. Intravenous treatment should be given quietly. The intravenous administration of 2.0 mg/kg imipramine sometimes yields a successful result. The use of intravenous imipramine must be closely monitored because it has induced episodes of serious hallucination in stallions, with stallions hurting themselves trying to escape their confinement. If the drug does not induce erection and ejaculation in 10 to 15 minutes, xylazine is administered intravenously at the rate of 0.2 to 0.3 mg/kg. With imipramine and xylazine ejaculation occurs in association with erection and masturbation. If one uses xylazine alone to induce ejaculation, masturbation and erection do not occur in association with ejaculation.

Ejaculation usually occurs as the stallion enters a period of sedation or when he is recovering from the sedation. This method of semen collection was used in a cooled shipped-semen program for a stallion with severe tenosynovitis of a rear leg.[53] Although successful about 25% of the time, the procedure was time consuming and unpredictable for mare owners. Success rate may increase if the dosages are altered for individual stallions.

Manual Manipulation of the Penis Ejaculates collected by manual manipulation of the penis are similar to ejaculates collected in an AV. This method of collection has not received widespread acceptance because of the training and dexterity required by the person collecting semen from the horse. Many stallions fail to ejaculate unless trained for this method of collection.[44,51] A major advantage of this method of collection is that only one or two individuals are necessary for semen collection. The stallion is usually not in direct contact with a teaser mare. Specialized equipment or facilities are not necessary for semen collection by the manual stimulation method.

With manual stimulation of the glans penis for semen collection, the stallion remains standing on the ground or is trained to mount a phantom. The stallion may be trained for collection in his stall, an open barn aisle, or a corner of the breeding shed. An estrous mare is usually nearby, but mare stimulation for the stallion may need to be altered on the basis of stallion response. The horse is teased until erection occurs. The operator washes the penis of the stallion with warm water. Once full erection is achieved, the operator places a plastic sleeve or bag over the penis. The operator uses one hand to cup and stimulate the glans penis to achieve favorable thrusting and glans engorgement by the stallion. The operator uses the other to stimulate the base of the penis and urethra. The operator sometimes places a warm towel at the base of the penis to increase stimulation. Training a stallion for this method of collection may require considerable patience, although some stallions readily accept the procedure. Stallions trained for this method of semen collection become habituated to the routine of sights, sounds, and activities surrounding semen collection. These stallions may require little stimulation by a mare.

Ground Collection Ground collection may be particularly beneficial in stallions with tarsal arthritis, rear fetlock or tendon injury, laminitis, or hindlimb weakness associated with neurologic disease. The need for an estrous mare usually is eliminated, risk of injury to the horse by the mare is prevented, and one fewer handler is needed. This method of semen collection has been most useful on small farms that stand a stallion for artificial insemination and do not have adequate personnel and facilities for mare and stallion handling and collection.[9]

The semen can be collected in the breeding shed, barn aisle, or stall. The stallion is exposed to another horse that can stimulate the stallion to achieve an erection. The teaser animal may be free in a stall or 5 to 10 m away, being held on a lead shank. The penis of the stallion is washed with clear, warm water. With the stallion positioned against a smooth wall to prevent lateral movement or in front of a solid wall to prevent forward movement, the warm, lubricated AV is placed on the erect penis, and the stallion is encouraged to thrust into the AV. Once the stallion has engaged the AV, the collector uses the right hand to stimulate additional urethral pulsations while holding the AV against the abdomen of the stallion with the left hand. The stallion handler may help support the stallion by pushing against the shoulder of the stallion with the right hand. For safety reasons the person collecting the semen always should maintain shoulder contact with the stallion.

Stallions may stand on their rear legs or walk forward slowly while ejaculating or continue to stand with all four feet on the ground. The handler should not discourage the horse from walking forward or standing up. Once horses are trained in the procedure, they usually stand flat-footed with arched back and a head-down posture. At first application of the AV to the standing stallion, a few stallions may kick out or try to nip or bite at the handler. The veterinarian should inform the handler of the stallion and mare about likely responses before initiating this method of semen collection. After a successful collection, the procedure is repeated in 1 or 2 days, preferably in the same location with the same handler and collection person. A lightweight model of AV is recommended for this procedure.

The author has had good success by placing the chest of the stallion against a phantom when a stallion is not trained to mount. The thrusting into the AV usually causes the stallion to raise his front quarters, resulting in the collection on the mount.

Artificial Vagina Use of an AV is the most widely used method of semen collection. Many models of equine AVs are available. The device is fitted with a water jacket that allows for the passive control of the internal temperature of the liner, usually at 44° to 48° C. In most cases the internal diameter of the AV can be modified by the addition of water or air to the water jacket. The operator adds a lubricant manually to the innermost liner of the AV to alter the degree of friction during breeding. Lubricants containing bacteriostatic or spermicidal compounds are not recommended because they are detrimental to sperm motility and fertility.[55] In a recent study[56] Pre-Seed equine® was found to be the best type of lubricant, with the fewest effects on longevity of motility after 48 hours. The detrimental effects of other lubricants is most likely due to their high osmotic pressure or inadequate pH. Petroleum jelly may be used safely. Most commercially available AVs allow the incorporation of a filter into the semen collection system, if desired, so that one can remove dirt, debris, and gel from the semen sample. Otherwise, the entire ejaculate can be filtered after collection or the gel aspirated from the sample using a syringe. Most sperm losses during collection are accounted for by the filter and in the gel fraction of semen. Between 25% and 30% of the spermatozoa in an ejaculate can be lost in the gel and filter. Paper, polyester, or nylon filters can be used, with paper retaining the most sperm.[57]

Ideally, the AV should be constructed to maintain the desired temperature for a significant period of time, allow the direct ejaculation into the semen receptacle, and allow for ease of handling and manipulation by the operator. If the AV is large and heavy, the operator may have difficulty positioning it for tall stallions or holding it in place when the mount mare moves during collection. It is best for the collector to hold the AV in one hand at the appropriate position while using the other hand to deflect the base of the penis to the side of the phantom or mount mare. The arrangement is particularly helpful in stallions that thrust with significant force. Deflecting or stabilizing the base of the penis is stimulatory to most stallions and may help prevent penile accidents during collection.

Semen collection failures frequently are associated with inappropriate positioning of the AV for the particular stallion, an AV that has dropped in temperature below a critical point for the stallion, and the use of inadequate pressure in the AV (i.e., too loose or too tight). The operator should hold the device parallel to the ventral abdomen of the stallion and directly aligned with the base of the penis. By doing so, the operator prevents ventral or lateral bending of the penile shaft. In addition, the operator must ensure that the forceful thrusting of the stallion does not result in the forward movement of the AV because this will result in the stallion searching for the end of the AV and, in most cases, failing to ejaculate. In certain circumstances stallions having difficulty ejaculating into the AV necessitate elevating the internal temperature of the device to 50° C. However, the operator should make an effort to have the horse ejaculate directly into the semen receptacle or coned portion of the liner of the AV to prevent heat shock to the sperm. Sperm cells exposed to excess heat from the liner of the AV exhibit a circling type of motility, have reduced sperm longevity in raw and extended semen, and may be rendered infertile. Exposure of semen to elevated temperatures for as little as 10 to 20 seconds is sufficient to cause heat shock damage.

Selection of an Artificial Vagina All AVs used for semen collection from stallions are basically similar in that they have a water jacket that allows variation in the internal temperature and pressure of the AV liner. The specific characteristics of individual AV types vary in the overall length of the AV, its diameter, ease of filling the water jacket, ease of handling, weight of the AV, and location of ejaculation within the AV by the stallion. Commonly used AV models include the Missouri, Colorado, Hanover, Japanese HarVet, and Polish or-open ended models.[9,41]

Missouri Used commonly in the United States, the Missouri AV is inexpensive and easy to clean. It is not necessary to assemble this AV for each use because the water jacket is formed by two molded layers of latex rubber. A single rubber cone leads from the water jacket for attachment of a semen receptacle. The AV is held by a leather case with leather handle. Addition of water or air to the water jacket allows for adjustment in AV temperature and pressure. In most instances the glans penis of the stallion is beyond the warm water jacket at the time of ejaculation, which prevents heat shock damage to sperm. A clean plastic or glass bottle, a Whirl-Pak bag, or a disposable baby bottle liner can be attached to the AV for use as a semen receptacle. If desired, a filter can be incorporated into the semen receptacle.

Colorado The Colorado model of AV is substantially longer, larger in diameter, and heavier than other AVs when ready for use. The AV consists of a solid outer plastic casing and is assembled by adding two layers of rubber liners to the casing to form the water jacket. This AV maintains the working temperature for stallions for a significantly longer period. Because of the weight and size of this AV, some operators have difficulty holding it in the most appropriate position for some stallions and are unable to provide the necessary support for the stallion. A significant shortcoming of the Colorado model AV is that most stallions ejaculate midway along the length of the warm-water liner, exposing sperm cells to high temperatures. The operator must be extremely cautious when using this AV to prevent heat shock to sperm. Disposable filters and liners are available for the Colorado model AV to remove gel and reduce bacterial contamination from the rubber liners.

Hanover The Hanover model AV is used commonly in Europe, is shorter and smaller in diameter than the Colorado AV, and is made of a hard rubber casing and inner rubber liner. This AV should work well for most stallions. Ejaculation occurs at or near the end of the water jacket. Pressure of the Hanover model AV is critical. The AV has an eccentric opening. If the AV is too loose, the nonengorged glans can come through the ring and glans dilation occurs on the other side of the opening, which is very painful for the stallion.

Japanese Although the aluminium case Japanese AV is no longer commercially available in the United States, replacement latex liners are still available. The aluminum casing makes this a lightweight, easy-to-handle model, and most stallions ejaculate directly into the semen receptacle. The HarVet AV closely resembles the Japanese AV in its light weight and similar size with a plastic casing. This AV is designed to be used with disposable AV liners that form a semen receptacle at its distal end and therefore does not leak water, as the Japanese AV does.

Polish or Open-Ended Artificial Vagina The Polish model is substantially different from other models on the market. Using the open-ended AV, one can visualize the process of ejaculation and can collect individual jets of presperm, sperm-rich, or gel fraction of semen. This AV has been valuable in the diagnosis of hemospermia, urospermia, internal genital tract infections, and ejaculatory failure.[58] Additionally, this AV has been useful in obtaining semen for commercial use from stallions with hemospermia and urospermia, because most of these affected stallions ejaculate the blood or urine after the initial jets of sperm-rich semen. The open-ended AV also has been useful in cryopreservation programs to obtain sperm-rich and bacteria-free ejaculates from stallions. This method of collection is also used to obtain "clean" ejaculates from stallions that are untrained and intolerant of penile washing. The Polish AV also allows the use of high internal AV temperatures without the risk of sperm cell damage because the ejaculate usually is emitted directly into a funnel with an attached receptacle held by a second person.

Open-ended AVs are not currently available in the United States but can be made by hand from plastic or polyvinyl chloride tubing or by removing the coned portion of the Missouri model AV and using only the innermost rubber liner to form a water jacket.

To reduce the risk of chemical residue exposure of the semen from the AV liner cleaning process or to allow the use of the same AV by multiple stallions, sterile, plastic disposable liners have become commercially available for most types of AVs. However, many stallions object to these liners, and the number of mounts per ejaculation increases. Breakage of the plastic liner may occur during thrusting, and complete eversion of the liner may occur during dismount. If stallions ejaculate on first entry into an AV fitted with a disposable liner, the bacterial contamination of semen is reduced sharply. However, as the number of entries into the AV or the number of thrusts in the AV increases, the bacterial contamination of semen also increases.

The AV should be cleaned immediately after each use, rinsed thoroughly with hot water, and wiped clear of dirt, debris, and smegma. If disposable liners are not used, the rubber liners should be immersed in 70% alcohol for 1 hour or more, rinsed thoroughly with hot water, and hung in a dust-free, dry environment. Soaps and disinfectants should not be used on the rubber equipment to prevent the accumulation of chemical residue. If disposable AV liners are not used or the AV and its liners are not thoroughly cleaned, the AV may become contaminated by *Pseudomonas* spp., *Klebsiella* spp., *E. coli*, *T. equigenitalia*, or other harmful bacteria and therefore contaminate subsequent semen samples and inoculate the penile surface of the stallion. For these reasons many farms maintain an individual AV for each stallion at the breeding farm.

SELECTION OF A BREEDING MOUNT

Semen can be collected from the stallion while the stallion is mounted on a behaviorally estrous mare, phantom mare, or breeding mount or while the stallion is standing on the ground.

Live Mare Selection of a suitable mount mare frequently depends on the experience and breeding mannerisms of the stallion. For example, the inexperienced stallion may need to be taught to mount the mare from the rear quarters. This training requires a disciplined, cooperative mount that will tolerate being mounted from the side. Some stallions vocalize loudly in the breeding shed and may frighten maiden or timid mares. The mount mare needs to tolerate a certain amount of nipping and biting of the neck, shoulders, flank region, and hocks to be suitable for some stallions. Mares with foals at their sides are frequently protective of their foals and less cooperative than barren mares. The mount mare also should be an appropriate size match for the stallion. For routine breeding farm activities, the reliance on an estrous mare as a mount has significant shortcomings. Additionally, in a cooled, shipped semen program, the breeding farm may not have access to nonpregnant mares, particularly at the end of the breeding season. Therefore some breeding farms maintain one or more ovariectomized mares as mount mares. One should select from these ovariectomized mount mare candidates on the basis of their size, tolerant attitude toward handling, and their strong estrous behavioral signs as intact mares. A mare with gonadal dysgenesis (XO) may be a good mount mare candidate without requiring an ovariectomy. Most ovariectomized mares perform well as mount mares while being restrained with a twitch or lip chain placed on the upper gum. In some cases it may be necessary to administer a low dose of estradiol cypionate (0.5 to 2 mg) at intervals of 3 days to 3 weeks to maintain receptivity by the mare.

During the semen collection process, the mount mare usually is restrained using a twitch. Hobbles also may be applied to rear pasterns or hocks, but the novice stallion may become entangled in the hobbles if the collection procedure does not go as planned. The long tail hairs at the base of the mount mare should be wrapped to prevent the tail from interfering with deflection and entry of the penis into the AV.

Phantom Mare or Dummy Because of the lack of readily available mount animals, increased expertise required of an additional horse handler, and increased safety risks associated with use of a mount mare, many farms prefer to train the breeding stallions to mount a phantom or dummy mare for semen collection. Most stallions, including novice stallions, readily accept the phantom as a mount during semen collection. The working area around the phantom should be dust free and allow good footing by the stallion. Adequate space should surround the phantom for the safety of the handlers and to allow a teaser mare to be positioned alongside or in front of the phantom. Many stallions are trained to mount the phantom even when the teaser mare is not close to the phantom.

When the phantom is used to collect semen from a stallion, the stallion should approach the mount in a controlled fashion, mount the rear of the phantom, and use his forelimbs to stabilize himself by grasping the padded barrel of the mount. The operator should quickly deflect the penis to the side of the phantom. While on the left side of the stallion, the operator deflects and stabilizes the base of the penis with the right hand. This practice minimizes potential injury to the penis and prepuce during thrusting by the stallion. Some phantom mounts are fitted with a Colorado-type AV on the posterior end, which works well for some stallions and requires only one person for the collection procedure. However, some stallions need manual stimulation that is easier to provide when the operator has control of the AV. Stallions regularly used for live cover breedings can be difficult to train to accept the phantom as a suitable mount. For this reason, certain circumstances may require access to an estrous mare.

The breeding phantom usually is made of a hollow cylinder with closed ends. The barrel is covered with 1 to 2 inches of firm padding. The padded cylinder then is covered by a tough, nonabrasive cover that is free of wrinkles. Stallions that repeatedly mount and dismount a phantom abrade the medial aspects of the forearms and knees. The stallion should be taught to dismount the phantom in a controlled manner by backing off of the mount rather than making a side dismount. The diameter of the phantom's body should be 20 to 24 inches total. The legs of the phantom should be kept away from its mounting end to prevent injury to the hindlegs of the stallion during breeding and dismounting. The mount should be adjustable for height, and the angle of the phantom should be adjustable to accommodate older stallions, stallions with hock problems, and stallions of varying stature.[9,59]

Semen Collection Procedure Preparation and planning are the keys to the efficient collection of semen from stallions and to ensure proper handling of the semen immediately after collection. The laboratory should be prepared so that the equipment and any extenders used in semen handling after collection are clean and at the desired temperature (35° to 37° C). The AV should then be assembled and filled with warm water (usually at 48° to 52° C) because the AV equipment quickly drops in temperature during equilibration. The final temperature of the AV is adjusted, if necessary, to between 45° and 48° C for most stallions; the inner liner is lightly lubricated with a nonspermicidal lubricating gel; and the AV pressure is adjusted at this time.

A suitable area for semen collection should be selected. If an estrous mare is to be used as a mount mare, the tail should be wrapped and the perineal area washed to prevent undue contamination of the stallion's penis during mounting. With the mare adequately restrained, the stallion is brought into the collection area. Once the stallion has achieved full erection, the operator cleans the penis with clear, warm water; wipes the urethral diverticulae clean to reduce further bacterial contamination of the semen; and wipes the penis dry, if necessary, using a clean, soft towel.

The operator presents the stallion to the side of the mare and encourages him to mount after he has achieved a full erection and the mare has demonstrated her receptivity. For safety reasons the mare and stallion handlers should be on the same side of the mount mare as the individual collecting semen from the stallion. After the stallion has mounted, the operator directs the erect penis into the AV using the hand placed on the ventral surface of the penis. This hand continues to stabilize and deflect the base of the penis during thrusting and ejaculation. The operator should hold the AV to accommodate the stallion, which usually involves holding the AV parallel to the ventral abdominal wall of the stallion. Just before the stallion ejaculates, the operator can feel strong urethral pulsations with the right hand. Once ejaculation begins, the operator should tilt the AV downward to allow rapid entry of semen into the collection vessel to prevent heat shock to the sperm.

Semen collection from the stallion mounted on a phantom is done in the same manner. As soon as the stallion dismounts, the semen is taken to the laboratory for processing and evaluation. It is critical that the person who is collecting provide enough support to the stallion so that the operator is not pushed forward to the front end of the mare or phantom when the stallion is thrusting.

Semen Evaluation

Depending on the reason for semen collection and its ultimate purpose, the ejaculate must be handled, processed, and preserved in different ways. Evaluation of raw semen for a routine BSE or a prepurchase examination might require more detailed analysis than that done for semen collected regularly for an artificial insemination program at the farm. However, semen that will be processed for an artificial insemination program away from the site of collection requires different processing.

EVALUATION OF RAW SEMEN

The goal of most semen evaluations is to predict the fertilizing ability of a given ejaculate or the potential fertility of the animal undergoing the evaluation. However, the low predictive value and frequent lack of objectivity of traditional tests such as motility and morphology have led to the refinement of old techniques and the development of new methodologies for semen evaluation.[60] The standard evaluation of a given ejaculate involves the following:

1. Volume and color. One should record the color and volume (in ml) of the ejaculate. In general, the color of the ejaculate ranges from watery to creamy and depends on the sperm concentration per ml. Abnormal colors or volumes can indicate contamination of the ejaculate with blood, urine, or pus. Normal volumes of ejaculates range from 20 to 250 ml, with an average of 50 to 60 ml.[61] Factors that influence the volume are degree of sexual stimulation before collection, breeding conditions, and foreign material in the ejaculate. A large semen volume, however, in no way reflects the quality of the ejaculate. Low volumes of ejaculate with low sperm concentration in an otherwise normal stallion suggest an incomplete ejaculation, and another sample should be collected.
2. Sperm concentration. The number of sperm per ml must be accurately estimated in order to calculate total sperm numbers in the ejaculate as well as sperm available for insemination. Sperm concentration, or density, is reported in millions per ml. Average counts are between 100 and 300 million; however, it can range from less than 50 to over 500 million per ml, depending on the stallion and the frequency of collection. Although subject to as high as 10% variation, the Neubauer chamber or hemacytometer is regarded as the gold standard for evaluation of sperm concentration.[62] Even though the hemacytometer is regarded as the most accurate method to measure sperm concentration, it is time consuming and therefore not regularly used for routine counting of raw semen. Other systems, such as the SpermaCue, Equine Densimeter, or the Accucell, are used. With all these systems it is critical to have a very clean sample free of foreign particles, debris, or extender. All these systems are very accurate and repeatable at the 100 to 300 million sperm range; however, their accuracy diminishes out of this range.[62] Other methods for sperm counting are the computer-assisted sperm analysis (CASA) systems. In addition to providing sperm numbers, these systems report sperm motility and the number of fast-moving and progressively motile sperm. A fluorescence dye (propidium iodide) has been recently used to label and count sperm. The NucleoCounter SP-100 counts sperm cell nuclei stained with the DNA-specific fluorescent dye propidium iodide.[63]
3. Osmolarity and pH. Osmolarity of stallion semen ranges between 290 to 310 mOsm. Values greater than 350 mOsm may indicate urospermia, and one should measure the level of creatinine. Values less than 250 mOsm suggest water contamination, and values over 500 mOsm reflect possible lubricant contamination. Seminal pH ranges between 6.9 to 7.5, and values higher than those should warn the clinician that there may be extraneous material in the ejaculate or an infectious process in the reproductive tract of the stallion.
4. Spermatozoal motility. Sperm motility is a rough estimate of the percentage of viable sperm in the ejaculate. Several methods have been used to evaluate motility. First, visual motility is the most widely used assay for evaluating semen because of its simplicity and low cost. However, many factors greatly influence the evaluation: individual judgment, thickness of the sample, concentration of sperm in the ejaculate, degree of contamination, degree of agglutination, and temperature. For this reason, one should estimate motility by evaluating a number of fields in a 10-μl drop of well-mixed semen in a microscope with a heated stage.[41] Conversely, motility can be estimated by diluting a portion of the ejaculate with extender to a concentration of 25 to 50 × 10^6 sperm per milliliter.[64] Even under the most tightly controlled conditions, repeatability of visual motility is poor between technicians and laboratories. Visual motility estimates of freshly ejaculated stallion sperm have been reported to account for only 50% to 70% of the variation of fertility in that sample. The correlation is even worse ($r = 0.3$) when trying to predict fertility of a frozen-thawed sample of semen based on post-thaw motility.[65] CASA provides data on characteristics of sperm such as linear velocity, linearity, path velocity, and lateral head displacement that otherwise would be difficult to obtain. In addition, CASA provides information on sperm concentration and percentage of motile cells. Although analysis of sperm motion with a computer is more objective and provides a highly consistent way of evaluating spermatozoa, the fertility of stallion sperm is not well correlated with any of the sperm characteristics measured with these analyzers.[66]
5. Longevity of sperm motility. Duration of motility can be determined using raw, undiluted semen or extended semen. Dilution factor of semen to extender affects the longevity of sperm, so ratios of 1:3 to 1:4 are recommended. To evaluate longevity of motility, one should evaluate semen samples immediately after extension and at regular intervals thereafter for up to 96 hours.[64]
6. Sperm morphology. Several attempts have been made to try to correlate the percentage of morphologically normal sperm present in a given ejaculate with fertility.[67,68] However, because of the lack of consistency among clinicians in reporting sperm morphology, results have been inconclusive. Among the problems that clinicians encounter are the definition of normal and abnormal in light of the tremendous range of normality and the fact that little knowledge exists regarding specific sperm defects that interfere with fertility. This problem is even more vexing when a clinician is trying to interpret the results from a referring veterinarian or a veterinary technician. Some of these inconsistencies can be avoided by recording specific morphologic defects rather than grouping defects into primary and secondary because this last method erroneously assumes origin of sperm defects (i.e., testis and post-testicular, respectively). For any sperm morphology evaluation, a minimum of 200 cells should be counted. Normal sperm cells, as well as those with acrosomal, head, midpiece, droplets, and tail defects, should be recorded, with the specific type of defect noted for each part. Although only 200 cells are counted routinely, sperm cells with more than one defect should be

recorded as such to help the clinician evaluate the incidence of defects in a particular semen sample. One can evaluate cells as wet mounts under phase-contrast microscopy or differential interference contrast microscopy after fixation in buffered formal saline or 4% glutaraldehyde. If samples are to be preserved for longer periods of time, an antibiotic should be added to the fixative. Alternatively, cells can be evaluated after staining. One drop of semen is well mixed with the stain and then smeared on a glass slide. Common stains currently used include India ink, eosin-nigrosin, eosin–aniline blue, Giemsa, Wright's, and several others. The clinician should be aware that severe changes in the osmolarity of the stain as well as mechanical damage to the sperm could alter the normal morphology of the cells.

Additional morphologic information can be gained by performing scanning or transmission electron microscopy. Although these procedures are not recommended as a routine, they can prove valuable in cases of stallions with unexplained infertility.

ALTERNATIVE ASSAYS FOR SPERM EVALUATION

Other assays for evaluating sperm in stallion semen include the following:

1. Hypo-osmotic stress test. As with many other cells, when sperm with intact membranes are exposed to hypotonic solutions, the influx of water across the intact membrane causes swelling of the cell and is evident by a characteristic coiling of the tail.[69]
2. Flow cytometry. Flow cytometry now is used widely to evaluate stallion spermatozoa. This technique, based on labeling of sperm acrosomes or DNA with fluorescent dyes, has the advantage of analyzing a large population of cells, which in turn provides information on the distribution of acrosomal or chromatin integrity.[70-72]
3. Biochemical evaluation. Activity of enzymes such as aspartate aminotransferase, glutamine-oxaloacetic transaminase, lactate dehydrogenase, adenosine triphosphate, hyaluronidase, and acid and alkaline phosphatase are correlated positively with the number of sperm in the ejaculate. Because these enzymes are located mostly in the acrosome or midpiece, their activities—particularly those of glutamine-oxaloacetic transaminase, lactate dehydrogenase, and hyaluronidase—increase proportionally with the level of damage inflicted on the sperm. Therefore enzyme activities in the seminal plasma can be used as indicators of the degree of acrosomal or membrane damage.[73-75] Further research is needed in this area to establish normal enzyme activities in stallion seminal plasma. Levels of alkaline phosphatase can be used to determine excurrent duct blockage in azospermic stallions. Levels of over 10,000 Iu/L are indicative of epidydimal fluid contribution to the ejaculate.[76]

Preservation of Semen The specific processing of the ejaculate is determined by the length of time that the semen needs to be stored before insemination. Semen can be used fresh, cooled, or frozen.

Fresh Semen Semen that is collected and used immediately or up to 12 hours later need not be refrigerated and in most cases can be diluted with appropriate prewarmed extender at ratios of 1:1 to 1:4, depending on raw semen concentration and ejaculate volume. Immediately after extension, semen should be removed from the incubator and cooled to room temperature (15° to 20° C) without loss of its fertilizing potential. Raw semen may be used for artificial insemination within 30 minutes to 1 hour after collection, provided that it is kept at 37° C. Extension of all collected semen before insemination is highly recommended.[77]

Chilled Semen To retain its fertilization potential, semen that is going to be used 12 and up to 72 hours after collection should be cooled to 5° to 8° C. Besides storage temperature, the most important factors affecting the longevity of extended semen are semen quality, sperm concentration immediately after ejaculation, type of extender and antibiotic used, dilution rate, and cooling rate. Several systems of passive cooling for stallion semen are available; however, the Hamilton Thorne Equitainer system has proved to provide excellent cooling rates and is considered the most reliable method for shipping cooled semen. In addition to cooling the semen at an appropriate rate, the Equitainer maintains the semen at the desired temperature for up to 72 hours. Furthermore, the Equitainer II has been shown to be the most appropriate container to use if the container is likely to be subjected to freezing conditions for an extended time.[77]

Semen should be diluted at a ratio of 1:3 to 1:10, depending on the initial volume and concentration of the ejaculate. In general, the longevity of fresh cooled sperm is directly proportional to the dilution ratio, ensuring that the total dose has 1 billion sperm cells and concentrations between 25 million and 50 million sperm per ml.[77]

Idiosyncratic differences in individual stallion semen in tolerating the cooling process or to particular extenders or antibiotics are not uncommon. Although the factors that determine why the semen of some stallions does not preserve well are unknown, particular components in the seminal plasma, such as oxygen free radicals, are suspected of being involved. In fact, in some instances the longevity and fertility of some stallions can be significantly increased by removing the seminal plasma and resuspending the semen in the appropriate extender.[78]

When processing or evaluating shipped semen, one must remember the following:

1. Extenders should have an antibiotic. The combination of amikacin and potassium penicillin is popular and does not appear to interfere with fertility.
2. The modification of the traditional nonfat, dried milk solids–glucose extender may improve the semen quality of selected stallions, especially if all seminal plasma is removed.
3. The semen-to-extender dilution ratio may need to be altered for each individual ejaculate, with dilutions of 1:5 or greater not uncommon.
4. A commercial storage container should be selected in light of the transport time, method of shipment, and ambient temperatures to which the container will be exposed.
5. The use of nontraditional laboratory probes, such as the sperm chromatin structure assay, can provide meaningful information regarding the effects of semen storage on spermatozoal function.

A common practice for some breeding farms is to ship semen for two inseminations 12 hours apart. In recent years it has become evident that mammalian sperm, including stallion sperm, reaches the oviduct within a few hours after insemination and subsequently attaches to the oviductal epithelium and remains motile for at least 72 to 96 hours. This has led researchers to suggest that the oviduct of the mare is a better storage place than any of the transport systems available. Therefore using all available semen for insemination of the mare as soon as it arrives is highly recommended. However, one must take into account sperm quality and reproductive history of the mare to decide whether the mare's uterus can tolerate two inseminations.

Freezing Semen When the semen is intended to be inseminated more than 72 hours after collection, it must be frozen to retain some of its fertilizing potential. The only way to preserve sperm for long periods of time (i.e., for months or years) is cryopreservation or freezing. Different stallion semens tolerate the freezing and thawing process differently, and unfortunately, the number of motile sperm after thawing is a notoriously poor indicator of fertility of frozen-thawed semen.[78]

In general, the freezing process involves the collection of semen from the stallion, evaluation of the semen, dilution and centrifugation of the semen, and resuspension of the sperm in freezing extender. Unfortunately, frozen-thawed sperm appears to have a shorter life span in the reproductive tract of the mare than raw semen or fresh sperm. The reduced life span appears to be related partially to differences in calcium metabolism between fresh and frozen sperm.[79] Because of the apparent short life span of frozen semen, timing of insemination appears to be critical when using frozen semen.

Semen Processing for Freezing The equine frozen semen industry has made significant improvenents in the last decade. Although it is standard to freeze semen in 0.5-ml straws, the lack of a laboratory test that relates to fertility, and the inability of some stallions to tolerate the freezing and thawing process have been major obstacles in the refinement of freezing techniques.

Extenders for freezing stallion sperm must have energy and protein sources similar to those needed by fresh or cooled semen. However, in addition, freezing extenders must contain a cryoprotectant such as glycerol.[80,81]

Recently, a combination of a low level of glycerol (1%) combined with 4% dimethyl formamide has been used as a cryoprotectant for freezing stallion semen. Preliminary evidence indicates that stallions whose semen does not freeze well have better fertility and a reduced number of cycles per pregnancy when semen is frozen in this combination rather than on glycerol alone.[76] Semen that is intended for freezing should be processed as soon as possible. Although some semen holds up well after transportation, processing the semen more than 1 hour after collection is not advisable.

The raw semen from a stallion that is classified as a "good freezer" generally has a lower volume, higher motility, and higher number of total motile sperm than semen classified as a "poor freezers."[82] However, classification of stallion semen as a good or poor freezer based solely on the percentage of motile cells after thawing is risky. One should perform longevity of motility, detailed morphology, and in some cases acrosomal and flow cytometric evaluations to determine the quality of the semen before its commercial use.[83]

Processing an ejaculate for cryopreservation involves the following steps:

1. Collection and evaluation of the raw semen
2. Dilution of raw semen in a sugar- and protein-based extender
3. Centrifugation of extended semen and removal of the supernatant
4. Reconstitution of the pellet with freezing extender
5. Packaging of the sperm in an appropriate packaging system after adjusting suspension to the desired number of sperm per dose
6. Placement of straws in liquid nitrogen vapors or in a programmable freezer

Each frozen unit should be identified with at least the name and breed of the stallion, registration number for that breed, date of the freeze, and identification of the laboratory processing the semen.

Thawing and Evaluation The handling of frozen semen greatly depends on the recommendations given by the laboratory processing the semen and the type of package in which the semen is presented. In general, single 0.5-ml straws are thawed at 75° C for 7 seconds or at 38° C for at least 30 seconds. When an insemination dose consists of multiple 0.5-ml straws, the most common thawing protocol is 37° C for at least 30 seconds, making sure that the straws do not stick together during the thawing period. Frozen semen packed in 2.5-, 4-, or 5-ml straws should be thawed at 50° C for 40 to 45 seconds. Regardless of the thawing protocol or packaging system, the well-accepted fact is that once semen has been thawed, it should be inseminated almost immediately.[41]

Although the freezing procedure is simple, the evaluation after thawing and the prediction of the potential fertility of a given ejaculate after thawing are not so simple. Sperm quality has a profound effect on the pregnancy rates achieved with frozen-thawed semen. Motility after thawing, concentration per dose, morphology, and acrosome integrity are parameters one should evaluate to determine the quality of frozen semen. Unfortunately, a battery of tests, let alone a single test, cannot predict the fertility of frozen-thawed sperm so as to determine what is good and what is poor semen. In general, semen with higher motility is considered to be of better quality; unfortunately, this is not always the case. The motility of most stallion semen after thawing, regardless of the motility before freezing, is 30% to 45% less than for fresh sperm. But some stallion semen with motilities of less than 30% after thawing have acceptable pregnancy rates per cycle, whereas others with motilities greater than 40% have low pregnancy rates.[83,84]

MANAGEMENT OF THE BREEDING STALLION

One should consider many factors to optimize management of the breeding stallion, including feeding, exercise, and vaccination programs. Many management decisions are made on the basis of the number of mares that a stallion will breed in a season, breed, type of housing, and the method of breeding.

General Management

FEEDING PROGRAM

Successful breeding programs require a balanced feeding program. Overfeeding and oversupplementing of stallions are probably the most common forms of malnutrition in stallions. Obesity may adversely affect libido and mating ability. In general, the nutritional needs of a stallion during the breeding season do not appear to differ from those of maintenance. A maintenance ration consists of sufficient balanced nutrients to support normal, basic bodily functions. Adequate pasture or good-quality hay usually can meet these requirements. Free access to trace mineralized salt and fresh water ad libitum are also necessary. Grain as an energy supplement in cold weather or under certain stressful conditions also may be warranted. The size, condition, activity, and temperament of the stallion play a role in his nutritional needs.

The healthy stallion consumes 2% to 3% of his body weight daily. At least 50% of this should be in the form of roughage.[85] Stallions generally require 10% protein in their feed, with younger stallions requiring 12% to 14%.[86] Although micronutrients such as vitamins A and E, selenium, copper, and zinc play an important part in the successful completion of spermatogenesis, to date no evidence exists that any of these nutrients fed in excess increase sperm numbers or quality. However, recent evidence would suggest that feeding docosahexaenoic acid (DHA)–enriched nutriceuticals may have a significant effect on the quality of fresh, cooled, and frozen stallion semen.[87]

EXERCISE

Horses naturally are roaming and grazing animals. Exercise for stallions is an integral part of their management and affects their mental and reproductive well-being. The goal is to keep a stallion fit for the breeding shed, not the racetrack, so that he has a good attitude toward his daily duty (i.e., covering mares). The amount of exercise time must be tailored to the temperament and needs of the stallion. The owner should provide regular exercise to maximize the stallion's fertility and longevity, as well as physical and mental fitness. In addition, lack of exercise may lead to vices such as weaving, stall walking, or cribbing.[9]

Estimation of Stallion Book and Frequency of Service

A stallion usually is chosen as a breeding animal on the basis of pedigree, performance, and conformation. Little or no emphasis is placed on reproductive potential, and a significant number of stallions enter the breeding pool with poor or marginal fertility. A complete BSE on maiden stallions or a complete review of past reproductive performance for new stallions is an integral part of the management process. Information regarding the number of mares bred, number of covers made, pregnancy rate per cycle, and covers per pregnancy is helpful in evaluating reproductive efficiency. If a stallion has stood at stud in previous breeding seasons, collection of one or two ejaculates is sufficient to determine that his semen quality has not declined during his off time because of illness, trauma, or age.

Libido certainly can play a large role in determining the number of mares that a stallion can service during a breeding season. Libido, which is thought to be a genetically acquired trait, can be modified by handling and environmental conditions such as housing. Therefore testosterone levels and libido can be altered by exercise and interaction between stallions and mares. Many times, poor libido is a limiting factor in the number of mares that a stallion can cover. The number of covers that a stallion can make in a day varies with the individual stallion. Factors such as age, physical abnormalities, and testosterone levels play an important role. Some stallions can breed twice or thrice daily, 7 days a week, whereas some can cover only one mare a day.

The length of the breeding season also plays a role in the number of mares with which the stallion can mate. The Thoroughbred season is generally from February 15 to July 15. Therefore the number of mares that can be presented during this time is limited in a natural breeding program. In Warmblood stallions more than 500 mares can be bred with every-other-day collection of average-quality semen.

The age and physical condition of the stallion also must be considered. Stallions typically retire to stud at 3 to 5 years of age. Age influences reproductive capacity. Stallions reach puberty at 12 to 24 months of age but continue to mature and increase reproductive performance until at least 5 years of age or older. During the breeding season seasonal fluctuation of sperm production occurs.[88] In addition, physical problems, especially of the hind legs, may limit the number of mares that the stallion can mount and service. Furthermore, the quality of the book of mares that the stallion has for a particular year can have a significant effect on the number of mares that he can cover. For example, a stallion that has a book in which most of his mares are maiden or young foaling mares will be able to cover significantly more than one who is booked to a majority of old barren mares.

The effect that the reproductive potential of a stallion has on the overall breeding program is significantly more important than that of a single mare. However, for veterinarians and managers to understand the complex interactions among management, endocrinology, and the quality of the mares that a stallion breeds is imperative so that they can diagnose or treat infertility problems in the stallion.[9] One can estimate potential sperm production by using the combined testicular volume, as described in a previous section of this chapter.

Stallion as a Source of Disease Transmission

With increasing breeding management—that is, more mares bred to a stallion in a given year—the significance of venereally transmitted diseases in horses has gained importance. Thoroughbred stallions commonly may breed more than 100 mares by natural cover, and Standardbred or Warmblood stallions may breed twice that number or more in a single 5- to 6-month breeding season through artificial insemination. With the implementation of frozen semen technology, semen from virtually any country can spread disease in a country or continent far removed from the stallion's direct area of influence.

Veterinarians must be aware of the risk factors for disease transmission, diagnostic methods, and some management measures that can reduce the incidence of disease with its potentially devastating effects on fertility.[9]

RISK FACTORS

Several risk factors may increase the chances of disease transmission through semen:

1. Natural mating: Direct sexual contact may pose the greatest risk for venereally transmitted disease. All mares, particularly those with poor fertility histories, should be cultured before breeding. Stallions breeding by natural cover should be monitored regularly.
2. "Backyard stallions": Stallions that are not standing at a breeding farm tend to have lower numbers of mares per season and poorer reproductive management. Hygienic procedures in these cases often are neglected, and these stallions or mares can be carriers of infectious disease. These horses often are poorly housed, which can contribute to colonization of the penis by pathogenic bacteria.
3. Inconsistent breeding method: In breeds for which artificial insemination is allowed, a stallion commonly may

breed several mares by natural cover at the farm, under no veterinary supervision. The owner also may request that semen from the stallion be collected to be shipped to other mares. These inconsistent practices can increase the risk of a stallion becoming contaminated or of spreading microorganisms to several mares.

4. Artificial insemination: Artificial insemination has been advocated as a technique that greatly reduces the risk of disease transmission. Stallions breeding artificially could breed more than 200 mares during the year. These horses usually are scrutinized carefully for venereal diseases and are housed with other animals of similar health status. Other factors—such as the hygiene of the artificial vaginal, lubricants, collection bottles, dummy mount, teaser mare, and semen packing material—could serve as sources of contamination for venereal disease transmission. If cleanliness and hygiene factors are overlooked, the process of artificial insemination may serve as a multiplier of disease.[89]

TYPES OF DISEASE

The types of diseases that can be transmitted through semen include bacterial, viral, protozoal, and genetic.[9]

Bacterial Diseases The source of bacterial infections can be from the external or the internal genitalia.

External Bacterial Infections Virtually every stallion and all ejaculates have contaminants that could be potential pathogens in the mare because a variety of commensal bacteria inhabit the surface of the penis and prepuce. These bacteria constitute the normal flora of the penis and rarely produce genital infections in reproductively sound mares. One commonly can culture an unwashed stallion penis or fossa glandis and harvest myriad bacteria, including *E. coli*, *S. zooepidemicus*, *S. equisimilis*, *S. aureus*, *Bacillus* spp., *K. pneumoniae*, and *P. aeruginosa*.[90] However, when the normal bacterial flora is disrupted, potentially pathogenic bacteria, particularly *P. aeruginosa* and *K. pneumoniae*, can colonize the penis and prepuce. These organisms rarely produce clinical disease in stallions but can be transmitted to the genital tract of the mare at the time of breeding, resulting in infectious endometritis and associated subfertility. The factors that contribute to the colonization of the penis by these bacteria have not been determined clearly. Normal bacterial microflora of the external genitalia of the stallion may combat proliferation of pathogens, and frequent washing of the penis, especially with soaps, may remove these nonpathogenic resident bacteria, increasing the susceptibility of the penis and prepuce to colonization by pathogenic organisms.[91] Others dispute this concept, asserting that repeated washing of the external genitalia alone does not contribute to overgrowth of pathogenic microorganisms. The environment in which a stallion is housed may influence the type of organisms harbored on the external genitalia. The stallion also can acquire these organisms at the time of coitus with a mare that has a genital infection.[92]

One diagnoses pathogenic colonization of the stallion's penis first by careful evaluation of breeding records and early pregnancy diagnosis. A sudden and unexplained drop in pregnancy rates should warn the stallion manager about a possible problem. Definitive diagnosis is by isolation of the microorganism in culture. In addition, isolation of the same microorganism with a similar sensitivity pattern from the nonpregnant mares helps confirm the diagnosis.

Treatment of penile colonization depends on the type of bacteria and method of breeding. For stallions breeding by artificial insemination, a thorough penile wash before semen collection is recommended. One then dilutes the filtered semen with extender containing antibiotic to which the bacteria is sensitive. Incubation should be for at least 30 minutes before insemination. Operators thoroughly should wash and scrub each stallion breeding by natural cover and dry the penis after washing. After the stallion covers the mare, the operator lavages the uterus, infusing the mare with appropriate antibiotics between 4 and 6 hours after breeding.

Stallions with penile colonization by *Klebsiella* or *Pseudomonas* spp. can be washed with a weak solution of HCl or sodium hypochlorite. Systemic treatment is not recommended because it has proved unrewarding in most cases.[93]

Contagious Equine Metritis Contagious equine metritis, caused by the coccobacillus *T. equigenitalis*, is perhaps the only true venereal sexually transmissible disease in horses. CEM is an endemic disease in Europe and recently was diagnosed in the United States in several stallions with normal fertility and no clinical signs in them or in the mares that they have bred. The strain of the CEM, as well as its virulence, is still being investigated.[94] Stallions infected with CEM are asymptomatic carriers and harbor the organism in the urethral fossa, the urethra, or the sheath. Mares bred to infected stallions develop a severe purulent vaginitis, cervicitis, and endometritis. Infection in these mares appears to resolve, but they remain infected and the organism can be cultured from the clitoral fossa. Diagnosis of CEM is by culture of the organism. Amies medium supplemented with charcoal is recommended for transport of culture specimens. Swabs are plated on Columbia blood-chocolate agar at 37° C and 7% carbon dioxide. Because of the slow growth of *T. equigenitalis*, the possibility of false-negative results is high.[95]

Internal Bacterial Infections Although infections of the accessory sex glands are uncommon, unilateral or bilateral seminal vesiculitis can occur. Bacterial infection of the seminal vesicles is not accompanied by clinical signs except for white blood cells in the ejaculate.[7] In some stallions with seminal vesiculitis, the glands may be enlarged, firm, and painful on palpation if the condition is acute. One cannot consider gland size alone and the character of seminal vesicle fluid on ultrasound examination as accurate indicators of infection, because the glands vary in size and appearance within individual stallions and across breeds. Diagnosis of seminal vesiculitis is best made by rectal palpation, observation of large numbers of neutrophils in the semen, bacterial culture of semen, and endoscopy of the urethra and seminal vesicles. Direct culture of the seminal vesicles during endoscopy increases the clinician's confidence in the significance of organisms cultured. Treatment is difficult, and the prognosis is guarded. Reported treatments include systemic treatment with antibiotics or addition of extenders containing appropriate antibiotics to the semen of the affected stallion. Recently, endoscope-aided direct lavage followed by antibiotic instillation into the vesicular gland lumen has been advocated.

Bacterial infections of the accessory genital glands, epididymides, or testesare uncommon in stallions but are clinically important because of their persistent nature, tendency for venereal transmission, and detrimental effect on fertility of stallions. These infected stallions are usually identified by the presence of numerous neutrophils in their ejaculates, whereas other diagnostic procedures, such as ultrasound and endoscopy, are used to localize the site of infection. Treatment generally consists of combining local and systemic therapy.[41]

Viral Diseases Although many viruses can affect the reproductive performance of a stallion, only two are considered to be venereally transmissible. Equine herpesvirus 3, the causative agent for equine coital exanthema, and EAV, which is responsible for equine viral arteritis (EVA).

Equine Coital Exanthema Equine coital exanthema can be transmitted by the stallion to the mare or from the mare to the stallion. The disease is characterized by the formation of small (0.5- to 1-cm) blisterlike lesions on the penis and prepuce or on the perineal area of the mare. These lesions eventually break to form skin ulcers that usually resolve completely in 3 to 4 weeks, leaving some round white scars in the affected area. Sometimes mild fever and slight depression are apparent. The effect on fertility is not known, but stallions and mares during the acute phase of the disease should be rested sexually to prevent further spread of the disease.[89]

Equine Viral Arteritis EAV is a small RNA virus that can infect horses and donkeys and is thought to be present in most countries except Iceland and Japan. Presently, EAV is responsible for major restrictions in the international movement of horses and semen. Although most EAV infections are asymptomatic, acutely infected animals may develop a wide range of clinical signs, including fever, limb and ventral edema, depression, rhinitis, and conjunctivitis. The virus may cause abortion and has caused death in neonates. After natural EAV infection most horses develop a solid, long-term immunity to disease. Mares and geldings eliminate the virus within 60 days, but 30% to 60% of acutely infected stallions become persistently infected and maintain EAV within the reproductive tract, permanently shedding the virus in the semen and efficiently transmitting the virus through the semen.[96] Mares infected venereally may not have clinical signs, but they shed large amounts of virus in nasopharyngeal secretions and in urine, which may result in the lateral spread of infection by an aerosol route.

The consequences of venereally acquired infection are minimal, with no known effects on conception rate, but mares infected at later stages of gestation may abort. Identification of carrier stallions is crucial to control the dissemination of EAV. These animals are identified by serologic screening using a virus neutralization test. If the test is positive at a titer of 1:4 or higher, the stallion should be tested for persistent infection by virus isolation from the sperm-rich fraction of the ejaculate or by test mating. Shedding stallions should not be used for breeding or should be bred only to mares seropositive through natural infection or vaccination that are isolated subsequently from seronegative horses for 3 weeks after natural or artificial insemination.

One of the greatest risks of EAV infection is abortion, which may occur even if the mare had no clinical signs. In cases of natural exposure, the abortion rate has varied from less than 10% to more than 60% and can occur between 3 and 10 months of gestation. The abortions appear to result from the direct impairment of maternal fetal support and not from fetal infection.[96]

Although mares and geldings are able to eliminate virus from all body tissues by 60 days after infection, 30% to 60% of stallions become infected persistently. In these animals virus is maintained in the accessory organs of the reproductive tract, principally the ampullae of the vas deferens, and is shed constantly in the semen.[97] Three carrier states exist in the stallion: (1) a short-term state during convalescence (duration of several weeks), (2) a medium-term carrier state (lasting for 3 to 9 months), and (3) a long-term chronic condition that may persist for years after the initial infection. The development and maintenance of virus persistence depend in large part on the presence of testosterone. Persistently infected stallions that were castrated but given testosterone continued to shed virus, whereas those administered a placebo ceased virus shedding. In addition, virus could not be detected in geldings after 60 days after infection.[16] The ability of a large percentage of stallions to eliminate the virus effectively in time suggests that differences in the immune response of the host may be involved or that virus strains may have biologic differences influencing their ability to persist in the reproductive tract. Establishment of persistence may involve a multifactorial process, with dependence on host and viral factors.[96]

After clinical recovery from initial infection, no significant decrease in the fertility of shedding stallions occurs. Mares infected after service by a carrier stallion do not appear to have any related fertility problems during the same or subsequent years, and no reports indicate that mares becoming EAV carriers or chronic shedders or virus passage by the venereal route from a seropositive mare cause clinical disease or seroconversion in a stallion.[96]

The two major routes by which EAV is spread are aerosol transmission, generated by secretions (respiratory or urine) from acutely infected animals or by secretions from recent abortions, and venereal transmission, from the semen of a shedding stallion. Close contact between animals generally is required for efficient virus spread in aerosol transmission. Personnel and fomites may play a minor role in virus dissemination. Virus is viable in fresh, chilled, and frozen semen, and venereal transmission is efficient, with 85% to 100% of seronegative mares seroconverting after being bred to stallions shedding virus. In several cases outbreaks of clinical disease have been traced to a persistently infected stallion.[97]

Clinically, EVA resembles several other viral infections of horses, and a definitive diagnosis requires laboratory confirmation. Acute infections are diagnosed by virus isolation or by serologically identifying a fourfold or greater rise in neutralizing titer between acute and convalescent serum samples. In the case of abortion, one can attempt virus isolation from fetal and placental tissues or can demonstrate seroconversion in the mare. Persistent infection in stallions is diagnosed by first screening serum for antibody in a serum neutralization test. If the serum is seropositive at a titer of 1:4, one should perform virus isolation on the untreated, sperm-rich fraction of the ejaculate or should test-mate the stallion to seronegative mares and monitor them for seroconversion.

The method of choice for antibody detection is the serum neutralization test. Antibody titers develop 2 to 4 weeks after infection, are maximal at 2 to 4 months, and remain stable for several years. A titer of 1:4 or greater in duplicate sera is considered EAV seropositive. Semen from a seropositive stallion must be tested to determine the EVA status of the stallion as a carrier.[98] The current test for identifying virus in tissues and semen is virus isolation in cell culture. In EAV-related abortion the fetus and placenta contain large amounts of virus. Samples of placenta, spleen, lung, and kidney, along with fetal and placental fluids, must be collected in a sterile manner as soon as possible after the abortion occurred, chilled on ice, and submitted for virus isolation. One should obtain blood from the mare at the time of the abortion and 3 weeks later for testing by serum neutralization.[96]

After having determined that a stallion is seropositive at a titer of 1:4 in a serum neutralization test, one should collect a semen sample using an AV or a condom and a phantom or a teaser mare. If this is not possible, a dismount sample can be collected at the time of breeding; however, this is less satisfactory. The sample should be from the sperm-rich fraction of the full ejaculate and should be chilled immediately and shipped at 4° C to arrive at the diagnostic facility within 24 hours. If this is not possible, the sample should be frozen at below −20° C and shipped to the diagnostic facility under these conditions. Submission of two samples, collected the same day or on consecutive days, is recommended. The penis should not be washed with antiseptics or disinfectants before collection of the samples. Samples of commercial frozen semen also may be tested, but the sample must have at least 2 billion sperm cells to be representative. False-negative results have been reported because of the lack of seminal plasma in cryopreserved semen.[97]

Prevention and Control of Equine Viral Arteritis A modified live (ARVAC, Fort Dodge, Iowa) and a formalin-inactivated (ARTERVAC, Fort Dodge, Iowa) vaccine are available. Both vaccines induce virus-neutralizing antibodies, the presence of which correlates with protection from disease, abortion, and the development of persistent infection. EAV has a worldwide distribution, and its prevalence is increasing. As a consequence, an increasing number of EVA outbreaks are being reported. The trend is likely to continue unless action is taken to slow or halt the transmission of this agent through semen. The modified live virus vaccine (ARVAC) does not produce any adverse effects in stallions apart from a possible short-term abnormality of sperm morphology and a mild fever with no overt clinical signs. However, live virus can be isolated sporadically from the nasopharynx and blood after modified live virus vaccination. Serum neutralization antibody titers are induced within 5 to 8 days and persist for at least 2 years. The modified live virus protects against clinical disease and reduces the amount of virus shed from the respiratory tract in experimental infection. Horses in contact with and mares served by vaccinated stallions are not infected by EAV, and vaccinated mares experimentally challenged by artificial insemination are protected from clinical disease but not infection. In the field the modified live virus vaccine has been used to control EAV outbreaks in some states since 1984, but the vaccine is not licensed worldwide.[95]

EVA is entirely preventable if horse owners, breeders, and barn managers follow simple serosurveillance and hygiene procedures. Controlling the dissemination of EAV requires a concerted effort on the part of all those involved in the equine industry. The presence of neutralizing antibody that correlates well with protection from disease, abortion, and the development of persistent infection in stallions is evidence that a control program, once instituted, can be successful.

Protozoal Diseases *Trypanosoma equiperdum* is the causative agent for dourine, or mal du coit. The organism is not present in the United States or Europe but is still endemic in Africa and some areas in Asia and South America. *T. equiperdum* is perhaps the only protozoal organism that can be transmitted venereally. Tentative diagnosis is by the clinical manifestation of the disease, which includes intermittent fever, depression, progressive loss of body condition, and severe purulent discharge from the urethra. Definitive diagnosis is by complement fixation and culture.[95]

Other microorganisms with the potential to be transmitted venereally include *Chlamydia* spp. and *Mycoplasma* spp. Although both of these organisms have been isolated from the urethra of stallions, their effect on equine fertility is not well known. It is possible that these agents cause infertility in mares and stallions. *Candida* spp and *Aspergillus* spp., although not commonly present in semen or the genital tract of the stallion, can be potential pathogens, particularly in artificial insemination programs in which the hygiene of the collection and processing equipment is not well monitored.

Genetic Diseases One of the main reasons for stallions standing at stud is to produce offspring with their genetic attributes. However, sometimes stallions can be carriers of a hereditary condition that may be expressed in their foals when they are mated to certain mares. Perhaps the clearest example of the potential effect of the genetic effect is the Impressive syndrome of American Quarter Horses, in which thousands of mares were bred by one stallion, named Impressive, that transmitted the gene for hyperkalemic periodic paralysis (HYPP).

Conditions such as genetic mosaics (63 XO/64 XY or 65 XYY), certain sperm defects such as detached heads, and midpiece defects and testicular characteristics such as small testicular size or premature testicular degeneration are or could be transmitted genetically. Progress is being made in this area with the advances in the mapping of the Y chromosome.[99]

Other conditions that have been proved to have or are suspected of having a hereditary basis include combined immune deficiency in Arabians, umbilical and scrotal herniae, parrot mouth, cryptorchidism, and testicular rotation. The expression of any of these genetic traits can have profound and devastating effects on a breeding program. When such a condition is suspected, cytogenetic or molecular diagnostic procedures must be used to identify undesirable traits that will be expressed in the adult animal. In addition to HYPP, and with the availability of the equine genome, animals carrying the genes for other diseases, such as severe combined immunodeficiency disease (SCID) in Arabians, lethal white syndrome of frame overo Paint horses, and hereditary equine regional dermal asthenia (HERDA) in Quarter Horses, will be readily identified. [9]

The pivotal point in prevention and control of infectious disease is the identification of infected stallions and mares and the institution of management procedures to prevent the further spread of any disease to susceptible populations through the breeding of mares by natural service or artificial insemination. If a stallion proves to be a carrier, he should not be used for breeding through natural service or his semen should be treated with proper antibiotics in cases of bacterial disease. In the case of EVA a stallion might still be used, provided that the mare owners are informed that the stallion is a shedder so that they can take preventive measures, such as vaccinating the mares.

The option to use a particular stallion in a breeding facility may depend on the value of the stallion as a breeding animal and individual regional regulations. Whatever the case may be, all stallions should have a diagnosed status before each breeding season. Breeding managers and stallion owners must be aware that poor genital hygiene of a breeding stallion and the mares at the time of breeding greatly increases the chances of spreading disease from a stallion to a group of mares or from a mare to a stallion. Poor management, poor breeding records, and poor hygiene at the time of breeding are perhaps the most common reasons for venereal diseases, which can cause severe and irreversible problems in a breeding operation.

PATHOLOGIC CONDITIONS OF THE REPRODUCTIVE TRACT

Clinicians must be able to accurately identify pathologic conditions to make sound decisions regarding the therapy and management of stallions. Acquired conditions may be reversible by surgical or other therapeutic means, but diagnosis of irreversible or terminal conditions must be well substantiated because the conditions could have a significant effect on the budget of the breeding operation. Ethical considerations are also pertinent because some genetic diseases can have a significant effect on the breed as a whole.

Congenital Defects

For an individual to develop into a normal male the Y chromosome must be expressed. Horses with genetic abnormalities can vary in their genotype, anatomic features, and behavior.[100] The most common causes of congenital defects are hermaphroditism, XY sex reversal, and testicular feminization or androgen insensitivity.

Hermaphrodites are classified on the basis of the type of gonadal tissue present. True hermaphrodites have testicular and ovarian tissue,[100] whereas pseudohermaphrodites have testes (male pseudohermaphrodites) or ovaries (female pseudohermaphrodites), with various combinations of male and female internal reproductive organs.[101-104] Perhaps the most common of the intersexes is the male pseudohermaphrodite. For the veterinarian to examine a "mare" with a small vulva and an extremely large clitoris or what appears to be a glans penis is not uncommon. Behavior in these animals most likely depends on the gonadal tissue present.

Horses with XY sex reversal syndrome are characterized by female external genitalia but a normal 64XY karyotype.

Androgen insensitivity or testicular feminization syndrome is a well-characterized genetic disease in human beings and in some domestic species. Animals have a normal XY karyotype and male behavior but female genotype. The syndrome has two possible causes: a mutation at the level of the gene that codes for the androgen receptor or a deficiency in 5α-reductase, the enzyme responsible for conversion of testosterone to the active androgen dihydrotestosterone.[103] In either situation the reproductive tract is underdeveloped and only female genitalia are present.

Genetic defects can be tentatively diagnosed by visual inspection of the external genitalia, rectal palpation, and ultrasonography. However, a definitive diagnosis requires cytogenetic evaluation. Blood samples must be submitted in tubes with EDTA anticoagulant to the appropriate laboratory.

Segmental aplasia of the vas deferens or the epidydimal duct has also been reported recently.[105,106] Obviously, these conditions render the stallion sterile as a result of permanent azoospermia. A stallion recently was diagnosed with failure to mature sperm past the late spermatogonial stage because of a gene microdeletion in the Y chromosome.[107]

Diseases of the Scrotum

The scrotum in the horse is a pliable and thin-skinned pouch with a fine layer of short hair, numerous sweat glands, and the thick muscle layer (dartos). The scrotum is usually darkly pigmented. Functional integrity of the scrotum is vital because it is perhaps the most important structure regulating testicular temperature.[108] Abnormal conformation, absence, or increase in thickness can have a dramatic effect on spermatogenesis. The scrotum is easily accessible for examination by visual inspection and palpation. An absent or extremely small scrotum usually indicates a genetic abnormality such as bilateral cryptorchidism and intersex conditions. Any increases in the thickness of the scrotal wall, surface irregularities, or changes in skin should be recorded. Lesions of the scrotum can be physical or infectious in origin.

PHYSICAL PROBLEMS

Traumatic insults to the scrotum or the scrotal area and other inflammatory processes in the genital area often result in scrotal edema. The clinician must identify the cause or possible causes of the swelling to initiate adequate therapy. Chronic edema of the scrotum can result in abrasions or secondary lacerations and can be complicated further by cutaneous bacterial contamination. Differential diagnoses for scrotal swelling include systemic infectious processes, scrotal herniae, spermatic cord torsion, or hemorrhagic processes associated with the testicles or spermatic cords. One must be sure not to confuse primary edema of the scrotum with peritoneal fluid accumulation between the vaginal and parietal tunics of the testicle.[109] Ultrasonographic examination or fine-needle aspiration can be used for the differential diagnosis.

Therapy of scrotal edema should be directed toward removing the primary cause and controlling the inflammation with supportive therapy. Anti-inflammatory drugs, diuretics, and frequent cold-water therapy are measures aimed at re-establishing the circulation in the area. If the skin is broken, broad spectrum antibiotic therapy should be instituted. Gentle and continuous lubrication of the scrotum with emollients and a tetanus toxoid booster are recommended. Depending on the degree of involvement, unilateral or bilateral orchiectomy also may be indicated.[109]

INFECTIOUS CAUSES

Viral Causes Equine infectious anemia or diseases causing severe hypoproteinemia can cause scrotal edema. Hypoproteinemia is confirmed by analyzing levels of total protein in serum. The presence of the equine infectious anemia virus is demonstrated by agar gel immunodiffusion or Coggins test.

During the acute phase of EVA, male horses often display different degrees of lower abdominal edema that may involve the scrotum.

Neoplastic conditions of the scrotum that have been reported include melanomas and sarcoids. Melanomas have the characteristics of benign tumors of the dermis and epidermis but may become metastatic in some horses. Sarcoids are common nonmetastatic skin tumors. Both conditions are diagnosed by their general appearance; definitive diagnosis is made by histologic sections.[109]

Parasitic Causes Although *T. equiperdum*, the causative agent of dourine, is not present in North America, scrotal edema is a typical sign of the initial phases of this venereally transmitted disease.

Onchocerca cervicalis, a microfilaria, and summer sores caused by *Habronema* spp. are seldom a cause of scrotal dermatitis. These infections are transmitted by several species of flies and mosquitoes. Ivermectin therapy at regular intervals is recommended for treatment of these conditions.[110]

Bacterial Causes Scrotal infections most often result from secondary breaks in the skin caused by castrations, traumatic lacerations, or puncture wounds. Less often, infections of the scrotum can result from septic processes in the testis or peritoneum.[109] In addition to appropriate antibiotic therapy, continuous washing of the infected area, anti-inflammatory drugs, and supportive therapy should be implemented.

Diseases of the Testes

The four major cell types of the testis are Sertoli's, Leydig's, myoid, and germ cells. During the last month of gestation or first month of life in the normal horse, the gonads migrate through the inguinal canal into the scrotum. Because of this migration the testis is surrounded by the tunica vaginalis or peritoneum and the tunica albuginea or the capsule proper.

Abnormalities in sexual development often are expressed as testicular problems. Among the congenital testicular defects that have been reported in stallions are monorchidism, anorchidism, and polyorchidism, which are the absence of one or both testicles or the presence of more than two testes, respectively.[111]

ECTOPIC TESTIS

A gonad that fails to reach the scrotum and deviates from the normal path of descent is termed an *ectopic testis*. These testes may be subcutaneous in the inner thigh or abdominal or perineal region. Some authors report splenic-testicular fusion on the left side.

CRYPTORCHIDISM

In a cryptorchid animal one or both testicles are in an ectopic location for an adult animal, although the gonads remain in the normal path of testicular descent. Cryptorchid testes may be abdominal or inguinal. Because of the complexity of the process of testicular descent, the exact mechanism for the failure of normal gonadal migration is not well understood. Although cryptorchidism has been speculated to be a hereditary condition, none of 56 colts sired by a cryptorchid Quarter Horse had abnormalities in their testicular descent. If the condition is heritable, perhaps a gene with low penetrance controls the process or is associated with several autosomal genes, as has been shown in men. The incidence of the condition according to Stickle and Fessler[112] and Hayes[113] is believed to be between 15% and 20%. Prevalence is higher in Percherons, followed by Palominos and Quarter Horses. Prevalence in Thoroughbreds is lower than in other breeds.

The unilateral cryptorchid horse is easily diagnosed by palpation of the scrotal contents and the inguinal region. When the testis is closer to the internal inguinal ring, in an abdominal or ectopic location, diagnosis can be difficult. Although frequently unrewarding, rectal palpation and ultrasonography are used as diagnostic aids. The experienced clinician can locate the testis and epididymis in or around the internal inguinal ring just cranial to the pelvic brim slightly off the midline. When palpation and ultrasonography have failed to identify testicular tissue, hormonal assays should be performed. Circulating testosterone and estrone sulfate levels are of great diagnostic value. Because of the variation in baseline testosterone levels, the hormone should be measured after stimulation with 5000 to 10,000 IU of hCG.

Collection of serum samples immediately before stimulation and 30 and 60 minutes or 60 minutes and 4 hours after the injection is recommended. A twofold to threefold increase in the level of testosterone is diagnostic for testicular tissue. Although false-positive results are rare, false-negative results do occur in 5% to 10% of horses. A single measurement of estrone sulfate has been reported to be highly accurate for diagnosis of the condition in adult cryptorchids. In very young equids low hormonal levels should be interpreted carefully because false-negative results may be more common than in adult horses. The treatment for the condition is invariably castration.

GONADAL HYPOPLASIA

Small testes may result from a number of underlying complex processes such as spermatogenic arrest and germ cell deficiencies. Testicular hypoplasia is the failure of the gonads to reach their full adult size and must be differentiated from gonadal atrophy or testicular degeneration, which is the reduction in testicular size after the gonad has reached full adult size. The cause of the hypoplastic gonad is complex and is thought to be congenital or acquired. Although not clear for horses, a genetic component has been identified in other species.[114] In general, testicular hyperthermia, malnutrition, and endocrine imbalances, particularly in steroid-treated young stallions, can affect testicular size negatively. It is important to remember that the testicles do not start developing before 15 to 18 months and continue to increase in size until the age of 4 to 5 years. Testicular hypoplasia should not be confirmed before the stallion is 2 to 3 years old. The breeding of mares to stallions with hypoplastic gonads is discouraged; however, often because of the value or the performance record, animals with small testicular size are used at stud. In these cases implementation of managerial practices to maximize the reproductive performance of the animal is important and should include reducing the number of mares in the book and breeding mares only once when they are close to ovulation.

GONADAL ATROPHY

Also known as *testicular degeneration,* gonadal atrophy is found most commonly in the mature stallion and is a consequence of the disruption of the process of spermatogenesis. Atrophy and hypoplasia must be differentiated. A thorough reproductive examination and an accurate history are fundamental in differentiating the two conditions. One should note inconsistencies between sperm output and testicular size and patterns of agglutination of the sperm cells. Small testicular size in relation to the epididymis indicates atrophy. However, developmental abnormalities such as a small penis and enlarged inguinal rings associated with small testicular size often indicate hypoplasia. The veterinarian should know that atrophy or degeneration is an acquired condition that in some cases is reversible.

Testicular atrophy most commonly is caused by administration of anabolic steroids or other products, such as altrenogest, to colts or stallions during their racing or show careers. Although the negative effects of steroids on testicular function are considered to be reversible, a relationship is suspected between the length of exposure and the age at which the product is first administered. Therefore colts injected with anabolic steroids during their first year of life are at greater risk of having permanent damage of the testicular parenchyma. The detrimental effects on spermatogenesis are caused by an increase in the circulating levels of androgens, which in turn have a negative feedback on LH secretion by the pituitary with a consequent decline in endogenous testosterone. The reduction of endogenous testosterone reduces testicular function with a significant reduction in sperm production.

Hyperthermia or severe hypothermia caused by prolonged recumbency; trauma; torsions; infections with disruption of the blood-testis barrier and the consequent production of antisperm antibodies; inappropriate or prolonged steroid therapy, especially with testosterone or anabolic steroids; accumulations of fluids such as in hydroceles; and advanced age have been implicated as possible causes of testicular degeneration. Scrotal lesions that impair the normal testicular thermoregulation may be a significant factor causing gonadal atrophy. Other causes of testicular degeneration include radiation exposure; nutritional disorders, particularly those of vitamin A and zinc; and toxicity with heavy metals or nitrogen, phosphorus, and halogenated compounds.

In the initial phases of testicular degeneration, the testis feels softer. As the process becomes more chronic, the testicular tissue is replaced by connective tissue, making the testis feel firmer on palpation.

Leydig's and Sertoli's cells and spermatogonia and spermatozoa are more resistant to degeneration than cells of the intermediate stages of spermatogenesis; therefore semen analysis varies depending on the extent of damage.[115] In most cases gonadal atrophy does not affect libido.

Although not easy to do, the condition can be diagnosed by evaluating circulating levels of LH, FSH, testosterone, and total estrogens and inhibin. Elevated serum concentrations of FSH often indicate seminiferous epithelial damage,[9] whereas low levels of LH could indicate a pituitary problem. Evaluation of sperm production efficiency also can aid in the diagnosis of gonadal degeneration.

A degenerative process in the testicle often is reversible, provided that the causal factor is removed. The condition of hypogonadotropic hypogonadism in men is treated routinely with Gn-RH administered in a pulsatile manner. Anecdotal evidence suggests that similar conditions in stallions respond to Gn-RH therapy administered as subcutaneous osmotic minipumps. To date, no study indicates the benefit of Gn-RH therapy in stallions with poor-quality semen.[9]

TESTICULAR HYPERTROPHY AND HYPERPLASIA

Hypertrophy refers to a condition in which the individual cells of the testes increase in size. The most common cause of testicular hypertrophy is removal of one testis or the abdominal retention of one that triggers a compensatory growth of the contralateral gonad.

Hyperplasia refers to an increase in the number of cells and can be focal or generalized. Testicular hyperplasia is rare in stallions.

TESTICULAR NEOPLASIA

Among domestic species the stallion has a low incidence (4%) of testicular neoplasia.[116,117] Of 30 equine testicular neoplasias, McEntee reported that teratomas were the most common (37%), followed by interstitial cell tumors (30%), seminomas (23%), lipomata (7%), and mast cell tumors (3%).[116]

The cause of testicular tumors is not clear. Environmental and genetic factors may be important. Because of the alteration in temperature and hormone supply, cryptorchid stallions appear to have a higher incidence of germ cell tumors, particularly Leydig's cell tumors or seminomas, of the retained testis.[118] In general, equine testicular tumors have a low degree of metastatic activity; however, because of the potential of spreading to somatic organs, they are considered malignant. The incidence of regional lymph node involvement appears to be low compared with that of other domestic species.[119]

Diagnosis of testicular neoplasia if both testicles are in the scrotum is based on a careful examination of the suspect and the contralateral testis. One should palpate the scrotal contents and note soft spots, nodules, or asymmetry. Ultrasonographic examination is crucial for the identification of fluid-filled or solid nonpalpable lesions embedded deep in the testicular stroma. Spermiogram can be useful if the semen collected has a high incidence of abnormal spermatozoa combined with round spermatids and other testicular cells. Low sperm numbers but otherwise normal seminal parameters are common in horses with testicular neoplasia.[120]

A testicular tumor in an abdominal testicle is diagnosed by rectal palpation and ultrasonography, combined with endocrinologic tests. Depending on the size and location of the testicle, an inguinal, flank, or ventral midline incision is recommended. Abdominal tumors often are only an incidental finding during routine postmortem examinations.

The gross appearance of some tumors can help the clinician make a presumptive diagnosis. Leydig's (interstitial) cell tumors are usually soft, orange, and nodular, with no clear demarcation with the adjacent testicular tissue. Seminomas can vary in color from white to dark gray with a glistening appearance; the neoplastic area frequently bulges above the adjacent testicular tissue. Fluid-filled cysts often are present. Sertoli's cell tumors are usually firm and nodular and pale gray. Teratomas are easily identifiable by the presence of tissue of different origins (e.g., bone, hair). Ultimately, diagnosis is confirmed by histopathologic examination. Samples for histopathologic examination are obtained by fine-needle aspiration or testicular biopsy. Unilateral or bilateral orchiectomy is the treatment of choice regardless of the type of tumor. Ligation and removal of as much of the cord as possible is strongly recommended. If metastasis is suspected, excision of the adjacent lymph nodes is recommended.

ORCHITIS

An inflammatory process of the testicles is referred to as *orchitis*. The cause of orchitis in stallions may be bacterial, viral, parasitic, or aseptic after trauma. Orchitis can be primary or secondary as a postoperative complication of abdominal surgery. It is important to differentiate the condition from the more common periorchitis or scrotal edema, although the conditions may be present simultaneously. Bacterial orchitis in horses may be caused by *Brucella abortus*, *Actinobacillus equuli*, *Pseudomonas pseudomallei*, *S. zooepidemicus*, *S. equisimilis*, *Salmonella* spp., *E. coli*, and *Staphylococcus* spp.[116]

Parasitic orchitis is usually a sequela of migratory larvae of the parasite *Strongylus* spp.[121] The condition can affect descended or undescended testicles and the tunics and spermatic cords. A possible secondary lesion associated with the larvae is the condition known as focal lymphocytic orchitis, which occurs around the seminiferous tubules.[122] Focal lymphocytic orchitis is different from the condition of autoimmune orchitis reported for the mouse in which foci of lymphocytes are localized exclusively at the rete testis and efferent ductules. Initial diagnosis of the granulomatous-type lesions in the testicle caused by strongylosis sometimes can be done by ultrasonography; however, histopathologic identification is necessary for a definitive diagnosis. Regular deworming programs with ivermectin can help control this condition.

EVA and equine infectious anemia are the primary viral diseases that may affect the testis. The viral agents of equine infectious anemia and EVA are shed in the semen of affected stallions. Focal lymphocytic infiltrations may be observed in affected stallions.

As soon as spermatogonia enter the leptotene stage during the meiotic phase, they become isolated from the general immune system by tight junctions between adjacent Sertoli's cells. These gap junctions are known as the *blood-testis barrier*. A fine balance is maintained so that maturing spermatids can migrate toward the adluminal compartment without eliciting an immunologic response. In addition to the blood-testis barrier, local immunosuppresors are present in the testicular interstitium. Factors that disrupt the blood-testis barrier with the consequent formation of antisperm antibodies include tumors, trauma, biopsies, and testicular torsions of more than 360 degrees. The association between antisperm antibodies and infertility, although reported for the stallion, warrants further investigation.[123]

Diseases of the Epididymis

Problems that affect the epididymis can be grouped into congenital abnormalities and into infectious or physical causes. In the stallion a condition known as *blind-ending ductules* has been observed. If sufficient numbers of tubules are blocked, the condition may lead to spermiostasis with development of cystic dilations, formation of epidydimalsperm granulomas, and reduction of fertility. These cystic dilations may be diagnosed by palpation and ultrasonography.

Because the epididymis in the stallion is not fused completely with the testicle as in other species, a diagnosis of epididymal aplasia or agenesis is not uncommon. In some cases an abdominal testicle may have a caput attached with the corpus and cauda epididymis present in the scrotum. The inexperienced clinician sometimes mistakenly removes an epididymis and leaves the testicle in the inguinal canal or in the abdomen when performing a castration. Epididymal aplasia is rare in the stallion and if present is related to other anomalies of the wolffian duct system. One commonly detects spermatoceles and cystic dilations by palpation or ultrasonography. Other, less common conditions include adenomyosis and tumors.[124]

Bacteria or trauma to the scrotal area may cause inflammation of the epididymis, or epididymitis. Infectious epididymitis as a primary disease is rare in stallions and is considered a sequela to orchitis or to deep lacerations of the scrotal area. However, some authors report the presence of *S. zooepidemicus* in association with epididymal infection. Migration of *Strongylus edentatus* larvae also may cause epididymitis, with the consequent formation of granulomas.[125]

One confirms a diagnosis of epididymitis by palpation, ultrasonography, the presence of inflammatory cells in the ejaculate, or bacterial growth on culture.[126]

Other causes of epididymal dysfunction can be attributed to abnormal accumulation of sperm in the cauda epididymides or generalized dysfunction of the epididymal epithelium associated with deficiencies in electrolyte, protein, or steroid secretion or resorption. Such dysfunction would cause changes in pH and osmolarity that might adversely affect the ability of sperm cells to fertilize. This condition is diagnosed by frequent semen collections (twice daily for 7-10 days) and evaluation of sperm morphology and motility.

Diseases of the Spermatic Cord

Problems associated with the spermatic cord are limited to infections or vascular problems. Infectious processes of the cord result from larvae migration or secondary contamination with *Streptococcus* spp. after castration. Failure of the castration site to heal and continuous draining of purulent material with intermittent febrile periods often indicates an infection of the spermatic cord known also as *scirrhous cord* or *champignon*. Therapy includes opening the area and aggressive therapy with penicillin.

Vascular problems associated with the cord include torsion, varicoceles, and thrombosis.[127,128] Torsion of the cord is significant when the cord has rotated more than 180 degrees. Torsions of less than 180 degrees are an incidental finding and can be permanent or transient and are of little clinical significance. Torsions greater than 270 degrees are associated with scrotal swelling, severe pain, abnormal gaits, and colic symptoms and are considered an emergency. Diagnosis is by palpation and history, and torsion must be differentiated from scrotal herniae. If the tail of the epididymis is palpable, in torsions of 360 degrees the tail will be located in a dorsal position with respect to the normal stallion. The treatment of choice is hemiorchiectomy because the affected testicle will be nonfunctional. In addition, it is possible that immune-mediated infertility may result because of antisperm antibody production.[122]

Varicoceles and thrombosis of the spermatic cord are rare in stallions; however, they might interfere with testicular thermoregulation.[127] The presence of varicoceles is of questionable significance in the stallion and is diagnosed easily by ultrasonography. One must ensure that no adhesions of the spermatic cord occur because adhesions may result in fluid accumulation between the testicular tunics.[129] Thrombosis of the cord is a more serious condition. The clinical signs resemble those of higher-degree torsions, and unilateral castration is recommended.

Semen

Problems associated with semen may be divided into two distinct groups: (1) abnormalities of seminal fluids, such as volume, color, pH, and osmolarity, and (2) abnormalities of spermatozoa.

Abnormal volumes may be too small or too large. Extremely low volumes are associated with incomplete ejaculation or nonejaculation. Large volumes may be associated with extraneous fluids such as water, urine (urospermia), blood (hemospermia), or pus (pyospermia).[129]

Urospermia

Urine-contaminated semen is often readily detectable because of the typical change in color, odor, and increase in volume. However, when urine is not obvious but suspected to be a contaminant, the presence of urea nitrogen and creatinine in the semen are diagnostic of urospermia. The effect of urine on the sperm cells is not well documented. However, the reduction in motility and perhaps infertility is significant because of the effects of hyperosmotic medium and water removal from the sperm cells. Neurologic or behavioral dysfunctions have been associated with urospermia.[130] The author has observed several cases of urospermia associated with self-mutilating stallions. Pharmacologic therapy of the problem is purely empirical and limited to drugs that act to close the neck of the bladder such as β-blockers. A more common approach is to use managerial procedures such as collection of the semen directly into extender and immediate centrifugation. The ideal procedure is to fractionate the ejaculate during collection with an open-ended AV. In breeds for which artificial insemination is not allowed, extender may be infused into the uterus and flushed out 4 to 6 hours later.

HEMOSPERMIA

Lacerations of the penis and urethra can result in the presence of blood cells in the semen. Diagnosis is often obvious because of the pinkish or red color of the ejaculate. The presence of blood is believed to interfere with fertility, but there is no scientific evidence to confirm this clinical impression. However, stallions infected with *P. aeruginosa* may be at a higher risk for hemospermia.[131] Diagnosis is based on identification of the site of bleeding. If the bleeding site cannot be found externally, a common bleeding site is where the urethra folds over the ischium. Urethral bleeding can be diagnosed with a pediatric endoscope. The urethroscopy can be used to visualize the penile and pelvic urethra. If the source of bleeding can be identified in the urethra, a common approach to therapy is to rest the stallion so that cauterization takes place. Alternatively, a urethrostomy of the area is indicated sometimes until the urethra heals by second intention. Some of the management procedures described for urospermia also may be considered.

BACTERIOSPERMIA AND PYOSPERMIA

Every ejaculate contains a small amount of mixed bacteria, with no signs of inflammation. These bacteria are of little significance and should be interpreted in light of the fertility of the stallion. The presence of large numbers of white blood cells in the ejaculate usually indicates accessory sex gland infection. One should culture quantitative pre-ejaculatory and postejaculatory swabs and semen samples in an attempt to isolate the causative bacteria. If the clinician suspects that the stallion is the cause of bacteria-related fertility problems in a group of mares, it is important to culture the mares in an effort to identify the same bacteria in stallion and mares. Giemsa, Wright's, or Diff-Quik stains of the semen aid in identifying the type of white blood cell present.

SPERMATOZOAL PROBLEMS

Spermatozoal defects may be in number, motility, and morphology. Reduction in number, also known as *oligospermia,* can have several levels of severity, culminating in azoospermia, or the lack of sperm in the ejaculate. Poor motility is referred to as *asthenospermia,* whereas poor morphology is known as *teratospermia.* If the defects are in number, motility, and morphology simultaneously, the condition is described as *oligoteratoasthnospermia.* Testicular problems such as degeneration or hypoplasia; sperm stasis in the efferent ducts, epididymis, vas deferens, or ampullae; inadequate collection procedures or ejaculation failure; and increased frequency of ejaculation have a dramatic effect on the total number of sperm present in the ejaculate. Accurate assessment of the sperm production of the stallion and a good history are essential for diagnosis and prognosis of the condition.

Abnormal spermatozoal motility and morphology can result during the process of sperm formation and during post-testicular sperm transport, epididymal storage, and collection and handling. Improper handling procedures also may adversely affect the quality of a semen sample.

Stallion spermatozoa do not always display the same type of forward progressive motility as observed in human or ruminant sperm with a less linearity index. Sperm from some stallions may tend to swim in a wide circular pattern.[131] Backward motility, tight circular movement, or static motion (not bound to the glass slide) is considered abnormal. Midpiece and tail abnormalities—whether induced by cold shock or other mechanical means or as a direct result of spermatogenesis, spermiogenesis, and epididymal transport—are the most common causes of motility abnormalities.[129]

Every ejaculate contains some degree of sperm abnormalities, but in general normal stallions are expected to have at least 60% morphologically normal sperm. Spermatozoal morphology is evaluated by diluting raw semen in buffered formal saline under phase-contrast microscopy or under light microscopy using eosin-nigrosin or eosin–aniline blue stains (see the previous section).

DISEASES OF THE PREPUCE AND PENIS

PREPUCE

Preputial inflammation, or posthitis, may be traumatic or infectious. Regardless of the origin, inflammation of the prepuce invariably results in phimosis or paraphimosis, which is the ability to exteriorize or retract the penis, respectively. Inflammation caused by trauma, infection, or parasitic diseases should be differentiated from edema following priapism or penile paralysis. Traumatic injuries to the prepuce most commonly are associated with breeding accidents that can be prevented with proper breeding management practices.

Infectious, parasitic, and neoplastic preputial problems are similar to those affecting the scrotum and were described previously. Infections caused by equine herpesvirus 3 or coital exanthema are a common occurrence, as is colonization of the penis by gram negative bacteria. Congenital problems affecting the prepuce, penis, and scrotum often are linked to developmental abnormalities and are diagnosed easily.

PENIS

Penile Tumors The most common neoplasia affecting the penis is squamous cell carcinoma. Smegma accumulation on the penis may be a predisposing factor for this type of neoplasia.[132] The tumors start as small keratinized plaques that slowly progress into necrotic foci with foul-smelling material caused by secondary bacterial contamination. The papilloma virus was suggested recently as a predisposing factor, a hypothesis that warrants further investigation.[133] Conclusive diagnosis is based on histopathologic examination. The condition is treated with cryosurgery, reefing, or phallectomy.

Penile warts or squamous papillomas, sarcoids, melanomas, fibromas, and lipomas may occur on the penis. Cryotherapy or autogenous vaccines have been used with varying degrees of success to treat these conditions.

Penile Paralysis and Priapism Malnourished or exhausted horses, horses with neurologic disease, and those treated with phenothiazinic derivatives such as fluphenazine or acepromazine can sometimes lose tone of the retractor penis muscle that culminates in chronic relaxation of the penis, extensive penile edema, and secondary trauma.[134,135] Because venous return is impaired, the condition progresses to the development of ulcers, secondary bacterial contamination, and necrosis.

Treatment of the condition aims to restore the venous blood flow. Hydrotherapy; mechanical support of the penis; and application of topical emollients, anti-inflammatory drugs, and diuretics are recommended. In some instances flushing of the corpus cavernosum penis with heparinized saline or intracavernous injection of phenylephrine may aid in blood drainage and penile retraction. Traumatic accidents involving the penis are not uncommon. Cuts with mare tail hair, poorly constructed breeding phantoms with fixed AVs, and severe bending of the erect penis may result in laceration or abrasion varying from simple skin cuts to severe hematomas. These wounds are treated with supportive therapy or surgical intervention. Prevention of secondary contamination and adhesion formation is important.

Other mechanical problems observed in the penis and prepuce of stallions include fibrosis, strictures, or lacerations caused by the misuse of penile rings or brushes to dissuade the stallion from masturbation. The use of such instruments is inhumane and should be discouraged.

REFERENCES

Reproductive Anatomy and Physiology of the Nonpregnant Mare

1. Silvia PJ, Squires EL, Nett TM: Changes in the hypothalamic-hypophyseal axis of mares associated with seasonal reproductive recrudescence, *Biol Reprod* 35(4):897-905, 1986.
2. Silvia PJ, Johnson L, Fitzgerald BP: Changes in the hypothalamic-hypophyseal axis of mares in relation to the winter l, *J Reprod Fertil* 96(1):195-202, 1992.
3. Sharp DC, Grubaugh WR, Gum CG: Measurement of hypothalamic GnRH in mares using push-pull perfusion techniques. *Proceedings of the seventy-fifth annual meeting of the American Society of Animal Science*, Pullman, Wash, 1983.
4. Sharp DC, Grubaugh W: Seasonal patterns of GnRH secretion in the horses assessed by push-pull perfusion, *Biol Reprod* 34(suppl 1):143, 1986.
5. Freedman LJ, Garcia MC, Ginther OJ: Influence of photoperiod and ovaries on seasonal reproductive activity in mares, *Biol Reprod* 20:567-574, 1979.
6. Voss JL, McKinnen AO, editors: *Equine reproduction*, Philadelphia, 1993, Lea & Febiger.
7. Peltier MR, Robinson G, Sharp DC: Effects of melatonin implantation in pony mares. 1. Acute effects, *Theriogenology* 49:1115-1123, 1998.
8. Hart PJ, Squires EL, Imel KJ, et al: Seasonal variation in hypothalamic content of gonadotropin-releasing hormone (GnRH), pituitary receptors for GnRH, and pituitary content of luteinizing hormone and follicle stimulating hormone in the mare, *Biol Reprod* 30:1055-1062, 1984.
9. Sherman GB, Wolfe MW, Farmerie TA, et al: A single gene encodes the β subunits of equine luteinizing hormone and chorionic gonadotropin, *Mol Endocrinol* 6:951-959, 1992.
10. Sharp DC, Wolfe MW, Cleaver BD, et al: Effects of estradiol-17β administration on steady-state messenger ribonucleic acid (mRNA) encoding equine and LH/CGβ subunits in pituitaries of ovariectomized pony mares, *Theriogenology* 55:1083-1093, 2001.
11. Sharp DC, Grubaugh WR, Weithenauer J, et al: Exposure to long photoperiod results in increased GnRH secretion in anestrous pony mares, *Biol Reprod* 39(suppl 1):39, 1988.
12. Sharp DC, Ginther OJ: Induction of ovarian activity and estrous behavior in anestrous mares with light and temperature, *J Anim Sci* 41:1368-1372, 1975.
13. Davis SD, Sharp DC: Intra-follicular and peripheral steriod characteristics during vernal transition in the pony mare, *J Reprod Fertil* (suppl 44):333-340, 1991.
14. Tucker KE, Cleaver BD, Salute ME, et al: Relationship between IGF-1, 17αhydroxy progesterone and progesterone on estradiol 17β content in the equine follicle, *Biol Reprod* 46(suppl 1): 155, 1992.
15. Tucker KE, Cleaver BD, Sharp DC: Does resumption of follicular estradiol synthesis during vernal transition in mares involve a shift in steroidogenic pathways? *Biol Reprod* 48(suppl 1):188, 1993.
16. Davis SD, Sharp DC: Intrafollicular and peripheral steroid chara cteristics during vernal transition in the pony mare, *J Reprod Fertil* (suppl 44):333-340, 1992.
17. Sharp DC, Grubaugh WR, Davis SD, et al: Effects of steroid administration on luteinizing hormone and follicle stimulating hormone in ovariectomized pony mares in the springtime: pituitary responsiveness to gonadotropin releasing hormone (GnRH), circulating gonadotropin concentrations, and pituitary gonadotropin content, *Biol Reprod* 44:983-990, 1991.
18. Cleaver BD, Sharp DC: LH secretion in anestrous mares exposed to artificially lengthened photoperiod and treated with estradiol, *Biol Reprod Monog* (No. 1):449-457, 1995.
19. Ginther OJ: *Equiservices, Reproductive biology of the mare*, ed 2, Cross Plains, 1992, Wis.
20. Heape W: The "sexual season" of mammals and the relation of the "pro-oestrum" to menstruation, *Proc R Soc* 44:1-69, 1900.
21. Asa CS, Goldfoot DA, Garcia MC, et al: Sexual behavior in ovariectomized and seasonally anovulatory pony mares, *Horm Behav* 14:46-54, 1980.
22. Desvousges AL, Sharp DC, Smith MF, et al: The effect of hCG administration on matrix metalloproteinase II and steroidogenesis in transitional and preovulatory follicles of pony mares estradiol, *Biol Reprod* 64(suppl 1):164, 2001.
23. Pelehach L, Porter MB, Sharp DC: Relationship between uterine edema and estrogen in pony mares, *Biol Reprod* 60(suppl 1):206, 1999.
24. Porter MB, Cleaver BD, Peltier M, et al: Comparative study between pony mares and ewes evaluating gonadotrophic response to administration of gonadotrophin-releasing hormone, *J Reprod Fertil* 110:219-229, 1997.
25. Greaves HE, Kalariotes V, Cleaver BD, et al: Effects of ovarian input on GnRH and LH secretion immediately postovulation in pony mares, *Theriogenology* 55:1095-1106, 2001.
26. Vandeplassche M, Bouters R, Spincemaille J, et al: Observations on involution and puerperal endometritis in mares, *Irish Vet J* 37:126-162, 1983.
27. Ginther OJ: *Equiservices, Reproductive biology of the mare: basic and applied aspects*. Cross Plains, 1979, Wis.
28. Loy RG: Characteristics of postpartum reproduction in mares, *Vet Clin North Am Large Anim Pract* 2:345-359, 1980.
29. Turner DD, Garcia MC, Miller KF, et al: FSH and LH concentrations in periparturient mares, *J Reprod Fertil* (suppl 27):547-553, 1979.

Mare Breeding Soundness Examination

1. Robinson S, McKinnon A: Prolonged ovarian inactivity in broodmares temporally associated with administration of Equity, *Austr Equine Vet* 25(4):86-88, 2006.
2. Hughes J: Clinical examination of the brood mare, *J Repr Fertil* (suppl32):637, 1982.
3. Greenhoff G, Kenney R: Evaluation of reproductive status of nonpregnant mares, *Journal of American Veterinary Medical Association* 167(6):449-458, 1975.
4. Pascoe RR: Observations on the length and angle of declination of the vulva and its relation to fertility in the mare, *J Repr Fertil Supp* 27:299-305, 1979.

5. Hughes J, Stabenfeldt G, et al: The estrous cycle and selected functional and pathologic ovarian abnormalities in the mare, *Vet Clin North Am: Equine Pract* 2(2):225-239, 1980.
6. Carleton, C. (1996). Atypical, asymmetrical, but abnormal? Large ovary syndrome. *Proceedings of Mare Reproduction Symposium, Annual Conference for Theriogenology*, Society for Theriogenology.
7. Stabenfeldt G, Hughes J, et al: Clinical findings, pathological changes and endocrinological secretory patterns in mares with ovarian tumours, *J Reprod Fertil* (suppl 27):277-285, 1979.
8. Hinrichs K, Watson E, et al: Granulosa cell tumor in a mare with a functional contralateral ovary, *Journal of American Veterinary Medical Association* 197(8):1037-1038, 1990.
9. Chopin J, Chopin L, et al: Unusual ovarian activity in a mare preceding the development of an ovarian granulosa cell tumour, *Aust Vet J* 80(1&2):32-36, 2002.
10. Piquette G, Kenney R, et al: Equine granulosa-theca cell tumors express inhibin a- and b_A-subunit messenger ribonucleic acids and proteins, *Biol Reprod* 43:1050-1057, 1990.
11. Bailey M, Troedsson M, et al: Inhibin concentrations in mares with granulosa cell tumors, *Theriogenology* 57:1885-1895, 2002.
12. McCue P: *Diagnosis of ovarian abnormalities. Recent Advances in Equine Reproduction*, B. Ball. Ithaca, NY, 2000, International Veterinary Information Service, 1-7.
13. White R, Allen W: Use of ultrasound echography for the differential diagnosis of a granulosa cell tumour in a mare, *Equine Vet J* 17(5):401-402, 1985.
14. Hinrichs K, Hunt P: Ultrasound as an aid to diagnosis of granulosa cell tumour in the mare, *Equine Vet J* 22(2):99-103, 1990.
15. Samper J: *Equine breeding, management and artificial insemination*, ed 2, St Louis, 2009, Saunders.
16. McCue P, Squires E: Persistent anovulatory follicles in the mare, *Theriogenology* 58:541-543, 2002.
17. Ginther OJ, Gastal EL, et al: Incidence, Endocrinology, Vascularity, and Morphology of Hemorrhagic Anovulatory Follicles in Mares, *J Equine Vet J* 27(3):130-139, 2007.
18. Ginther O, First N: Maintenance of the corpus luteum in hysterectomized mares, *Am J Vet Res* 32(11):1687-1691, 1971.
19. Stabenfeldt G, Hughes J, et al: Spontaneous prolongation of luteal activity in the mare, *Equine Vet J* 6(4):158-163, 1974.
20. Stabenfeldt G, Hughes J, et al: The role of the uterus in ovarian control in the mare, *J Reprod Fertil* 3(7):343-351, 1974.
21. Neely D, Kindahl H, et al: Prostaglandin release patterns in the mare: physiological, pathophysiological, and therapeutic responses, *J Reprod Fertil* (suppl 27):181-189, 1979.
22. Robinson NE, editor: *Current therapy in equine medicine*, ed 6, St Louis, 2009, Saunders.
23. Chandley A, Fletcher J, et al: Chromosome abnormalities as a cause of infertility in mares, *J Reprod Fertil* (suppl 23): 377-383, 1975.
24. Hughes J, Benirschke K, et al: Gonadal dysgenesis in the mare, *J Reprod Fertil* (suppl 23):385-390, 1975.
25. Hughes J: Sex chromosome abnormalities, *J Reprod Fertil* (suppl32):642, 1982.
26. Long S: Chromosome anomalies and infertility in the mare, *Equine Vet J* 20(2):89-93, 1988.
27. Davies T: Turner's syndrome (Karyotype 63 XO) in a Thoroughbred mare, *Equine Vet Educ* 7(1):15-17, 1995.
28. McFeely R: A review of cytogenetics in equine reproduction, *J Vet Reprod Fertil* (suppl 23):371-374, 1975.
29. Buoen L, Zhang T, et al: SRY-negative, XX intersex horses: the need for pedigree studies to examine the mode of inheritance of the condition, *Equine Vet J* 32(1):78-81, 2000.
30. Bugno M, Klukowska J, et al: A sporadic case of the sex-reversed mare (64, XY; SRY-negative): molecular and cytogenetic studies of the Y chromosome, *Theriogenology* 59:1597-1603, 2003.
31. Makinen A, Hasegawa T, et al: Infertility in two mares with XY and XXX sex chromosomes, *Equine Vet J* 31(4):346-349, 1999.
32. Bugno M, Slota E, et al: Nonmosaic X trisomy, detected by chromosome painting, in an infertile mare, *Equine Vet J* 35(2):209-210, 2003.
33. Halnan C, Watson J: Detection by G- and C-band karyotyping of gonosome anomalies in horses of different breeds, *J Reprod Fertil* (suppl 32):626, 1982.
34. Carnevale E, Ginther O: Relationships of age to uterine function and reproductive efficiency in mares, *Theriogenology* 37:1101-1115, 1992.
35. McKinnon, A., E. Squires, et al (1987). Diagnostic ultrasonography of uterine pathology in the mare. *Proceedings of the Thirty-Third Annual Convention of the American Association of Equine Practitioners*.
36. Adams G, Kastelic J, et al: Effect of uterine inflammation and ultrasonically-detected uterine pathology on fertility in the mare, *J Reprod Fertil* (suppl 35):445-454, 1987.
37. Watson E, Stokes C, et al: Concentrations of uterine luminal prostaglandins in mares with acute and persistent endometritis, *Equine Vet J* 19(1):31-37, 1987.
38. Brinsko S, Rigby S, et al: A practical method for recognizing mares susceptible to post-breeding endometritis, *Am Assoc Equine Pract* 657-661, 2003.
39. Pycock J, Newcombe J: The relationship between intraluminal uterine fluid, endometritis, and pregnancy rate in the mare, *Equine Pract* 18(6):19-22, 1996.
40. Ginther O, Garcia M, et al: Embryonic loss in mares: pregnancy rate, length of interovulatory intervals, and progesterone concentrations associated with loss during days 11 to 15, *Theriogenology* 24(4):409-417, 1985.
41. Pycock, J. (1999). Management of the problem breeding mare. *Proceedings of the Annual Conference, Nashville, Tennessee, The Society for Theriogenology*.
42. Troedsson, M, Madill S (1999). Clinical examination of the reproductive tract of the mare. *Proceedings of the Annual Conference*, Nashville, Tennessee, The Society for Theriogenology.
43. Zent W, Troedsson H, et al: Postbreeding uterine fluid accumulation in a normal population of thoroughbred mares:a field study, *Am Assoc Equine Pract* 44:64-65, 1998.
44. Kenney R, Ganjam V: Selected pathological changes of the mare uterus and ovary, *J Reprod Fertil* (suppl23):335-339, 1975.
45. McDowell K, Sharp D, et al: Restricted conceptus mobility results in failure of pregnancy maintenance in mares, *Biol Reprod* 39:340-348, 1988.
46. Eilts B, Scholl D, et al: Prevalence of endometrial cysts and their effect on fertility, *Biol Reprod Monograph* 1:527-532, 1995.
47. Hughes J, Stabenfeldt G, et al: Pyometra in the mare, *J Reprod Fertil* (suppl 27):321-329, 1979.
48. Bracher V, Stone R, et al: Transendoscopic Nd:YAG laser surgery for treatment of intrauterine adhesions in 4 mares, *Equine Vet Educ* 6(1):22-26, 1994.
49. LeBlanc M, Neuwirth L, et al: Differences in uterine position of reproductively normal mares and those with delayed uterine clearance detected by scintigraphy, *Theriogenology* 50:49-54, 1998.
50. Easley K: Diagnosis and treatment of vesicovaginal reflux in the mare, *Vet Clin North Am: Equine Pract* 4:407-416, 1988.
51. Threlfall W: Broodmare uterine therapy, *Compend Cont Educ Pract Vet* 11:5246-5254, 1980.
52. Stratton L, Corstvet R, et al: Isolation of *Klebsiella pneumoniae* from the urogenital tract of experimentally infected mares, *J Reprod Fertil* (suppl27):317-320, 1979.

53. Alvarenga, M., M. Iawama de Mattos, et al. (1998). Comparison between the gynecological brush, cotton swab and aspiration technique for endometrial cytology in mares. *Proceedings for Annual Meeting*, Baltimore, Maryland, Society for Theriogenology.
54. Williams C: Crush-side cytology: an aid in evaluation of the uterine environment in the mare, *Aust Equine Vet* 23(3):149, 2004.
55. Millar R, Francis J: The relation of clinical and bacteriological findings to fertility in Thoroughbred mares, *Aust Vet J* 50:351-355, 1974.
56. Blanchard TL, Garcia MC, et al: Comparison of two techniques for obtaining endometrial bacteriologic cultures in the mare, *Theriogenology* 16(1):85-93, 1981.
57. Hughes, J. (1978). Reproductive panel discussion. *Proceedings for the Twenty-Fourth Annual Convention of the American Association of Equine Practitioners.*
58. Woolcock JB: Equine bacterial endometritis: diagnosis, interpretation, and treatment, *Vet Clin North Am: Equine Pract* 2(2):241-251, 1980.
59. Ricketts SW, Young A, et al: Uterine and clitoral cultures, In McKinnon AO, Voss JS, editors: *Equine Reproduction*, Philadelphia, 1993, Lea & Febiger, pp 234-245.
60. Conboy, H. (1978). Diagnosis and therapy of equine endometritis. *Proceedings of the Twenty-Fourth Annual Convention of the American Association of Equine Practitioners*, The American Association of Equine Practitioners.
61. McCue P, Hughes J, et al: Antimicrobial susceptibility patterns for equine endometrial isolates, *California Veterinarian* 45:23-26, 1991.
62. Knudsen O: Endometrial cytology as a diagnostic aid in mares, *Cornell Veterinarian* 54:415-422, 1964.
63. Riddle W, LeBlanc M, et al: Relationships between pregnancy rates, uterine cytology, and culture results in a Thoroughbred practice in central Kentucky, *Am Assoc Equine Pract* 51:2630, 2005.
64. LeBlanc M: Endometrial biopsy. In Colahan P, Mayhew I, Merritt A, Moore J, editors: *Equine Medicine and Surgery*, Goleta, Calif, 1991, American Veterinary Publications, Inc, pp 960-963.
65. Couto M, Hughes J: Technique and interpretation of cervical and endometrial cytology in the mare, *J Equine Vet Sci* 4:265-273, 1984.
66. Crickman J, Pugh D: Equine endometrial cytology: a review of techniques and interpretations, *Vet Med* 81:650, 1986.
67. Ricketts S: Endometrial biopsy as a guide to diagnosis of endometrial pathology in the mare, *J Reprod Fertil* (suppl 23):341-345, 1975.
68. Ricketts S: The technique and clinical application of endometrial biopsy in the mare, *Equine Vet J* 7(2):102-108, 1975.
69. Bergman, R. and R. Kenney: (1975). Representativeness of a uterine biopsy in the mare. *Proceedings of the Twenty-First Annual Convention of the American Association of Equine Practitioners*, American Association of Equine Practitioners.
70. Dybdal N, Daels P, et al: Investigation of the reliability of a single endometrial biopsy sample, with a note on the correlation between uterine cysts on biopsy grade, *J Reprod Fertil* (suppl 44):697, 1991.
71. Carleton C: Basic techniques for evaluating the subfertile mare, *Vet Med* 83:1253, 1988.
72. Kenney R: Prognostic value of endometrial biopsy of the mare, *J Reprod Fertil* (suppl 23):347-348, 1975.
73. Held J, Rohrbach B: Clinical significance of uterine biopsy results in the maiden and non-maiden mare, *J Reprod Fertil* (suppl 44):698-699, 1991.
74. Ricketts S, Alonso S: Assessment of the breeding prognosis of mares using paired endometrial biopsy techniques, *Equine Vet J* 23:185-188, 1991.
75. Ricketts S, Alonso S: The effect of age and parity on the development of equine chronic endometrial disease, *Equine Vet J* 23(3):189-192, 1991.
76. Kenney R: Cyclic and Pathologic Changes of the Mare Endometrium is Detected by Biopsy, with a Note on Early Embryonic Death, *J Am Vet Med Assoc* 172:241-262, 1978.
77. Youngquist RS, Threlfall W, editors: *Current therapy in large animal theriogenology*, ed 2, St Louis, 2007, Saunders.
78. Bracher V, Allen WR: Videoendoscopic evaluation of the mare's uterus: I. Findings in normal fertile mares, *Equine Vet J* 24:274-278, 1992.
79. Bracher V, Mathias S, et al: Videoendoscopic evaluation of the mare's uterus: II. Findings in subfertile mares, *Equine Vet J* 24(4):279-284, 1992.
80. Schiemann V: *Studies of uterine distension and development of intrauterine pressures during hysteroscopy in the horse*, Hannover, 2001, University of Hannover. Dr Met Vet.
81. Perkins N, Threlfall W, et al: Pulsatile secretion of luteinizing hormone and progesterone during the estrous cycle and early pregnancy, *Am J Vet Res* 54:1929-1934, 1993.
82. Perkins NR, Threlfall WR, et al: Absence of diurnal variation in serum progesterone concentrations in mares, *Theriogenology* 39(6):1353-1365, 1993.
83. Ginther O: Embryonic loss in mares: incidence, time of occurrence, and hormonal involvement, *Theriogenology* 23(1): 77-89, 1985.
84. Knowles J, Squires E, et al: Relationship of progesterone to early pregnancy loss in mares, *J Equine Vet Sci* 13(9):528-533, 1993.
85. Morgenthal J, van Niekerk C: Plasma progestagen levels in normal mares with luteal deficiency during early pregnancy, and in twinning habitual aborters, *J Reprod Fertil* (suppl 44): 728-729, 1991.
86. Shideler R, Squires E, et al: Progestagen therapy of ovariectomized pregnant mares, *J Reprod Fertil* (suppl 32):459-464, 1982.
87. Carleton, C.L., W.R. Threlfall, et al: (1998). Influence of season, age, and reproductive status on the levels of thyroxine (T4), triiodothyronine (T3), free T4 by dialysis (F4D), and free T3 (F3) in standard mares. *Proceedings for annual meeting. Baltimore*, Society for Theriogenology: 164.
88. Huszenicza G, Nagy P, et al: Relationship between thyroid function and seasonal reproductive activity in mares, *J Reprod Fertil* (suppl 56):163-172, 2000.
89. Buff PR, Messer Iv NT, et al: Seasonal and pulsatile dynamics of thyrotropin and leptin in mares maintained under a constant energy balance, *Dom Anim Endocrinol* 33(4):430-436, 2007.
90. Lowe J, Baldwin B, et al: Equine hypothyroidism: the long term effects of thyroidectomy on metabolism and growth in mares and stallions, *Cornell Vet* 64:276-295, 1974.
91. Fitzgerald B, Davison L: Thyroxine concentrations are elevated in mares which continue to exhibit estrous cycles during the nonbreeding season, *J Equine Vet Sci* 18(1):48-51, 1998.
92. Gutierrez C, Riddle T, et al: Equine thyroid hormone levels and pregnancy rates at 15 to 16 days post-ovulation, *Am Assoc Equine Pract* 46:319-320, 2000.
93. Gutierrez C, Riddle W, et al: Serum thyroxine concentrations and pregnancy rates 15 to 16 days after ovulation in broodmares, *J Am Vet Med Assoc* 220(1):64-66, 2002.
94. McCue P: Equine granulosa cell tumors, *Am Assoc Equine Pract*, 1992.
95. Allen W, Mathias S, et al: Serial measurement of peripheral oestrogen and progesterone concentrations in oestrous mares to determine optimum mating time and diagnose ovulation, *Equine Vet J* 27:460-464, 1995.
96. Daels PF, Ammon DC, et al: Urinary and plasma estrogen conjugates, estradiol and estrone concentrations in nonpregnant and early pregnant mares, *Theriogenology* 35(5):1001-1017, 1991.

97. Monfort SL, Arthur NP, et al: Monitoring ovarian function and pregnancy by evaluating excretion of urinary oestrogen conjugates in semi-free-ranging Przewalski's horses (Equus przewalskii), *J Reprod Fertil* 91(1):155-164, 1991.
98. Schwarzenberger F, Mostl E, et al: Faecal steroid analysis for non-invasive monitoring of reproductive status in farm, wild and zoo animals, *Anim Reprod Sci* 42(1-4):515-526, 1996.
99. Kasman L, Hughes J, et al: Estrone sulfate concentrations as an indicator of fetal demise in horses, *Am J Vet Res* 49:184-187, 1988.
100. Sist MD, Williams JF, et al: Pregnancy diagnosis in the mare by immunoassay of estrone sulfate in serum and milk, *J Equine Vet Sci* 7(1):20-23, 1987.
101. Henderson K, Perkins N, et al: Enzyme immunoassay of oestrone sulphate concentrations in faeces for non-invasive pregnancy determination in mares, *NZ Vet J* 47:61-66, 1999.
102. Allen WR: Hormonal control of early pregnancy in the mare, *Anim Reprod Sci* 7(1-3):283-304, 1984.
103. Steiner J, Antczak D, et al: Persistent endometrial cups, *Anim Reprod Sci* 94(1-4):274-275, 2006.
104. Allen W, Kolling M, et al: An interesting case of early pregnancy loss in a mare with persistent endometrial cups, *Equine Vet Educ* 19:539-544, 2007.
105. Evans M, Irvine C: Measurement of equine follicle stimulating hormone and luteinizing hormone: response of anestrous mares to gonadotropin releasing hormone, *Biol Reprod* 15:477-484, 1976.
106. Meinert C, Silva JFS, et al: Advancing the time of ovulation in the mare with a short-term implant releasing the GnRH analogue deslorelin, *Equine Vet J* 25(1):65-68, 1993.
107. Irvine C: Endocrinology of the estrous cycle of the mare: applications to embryo transfer, *Theriogenology* 15(1):85-104, 1981.
108. Ginther O, Wentworth B: Effect of a synthetic gonadotropin-releasing hormone on plasma concentrations of luteinizing hormone in ponies, *Am J Vet Res* 35(1):79-81, 1974.
109. Alexander S, Irvine C, et al: Is luteinizing hormone secretion modulated by endogenous oxytocin in the mare? Studies on the role of oxytocin and factors affecting its secretion in estrous mares, *Biol Reprod Monograph* 1:361-371, 1995.
110. Irvine CH, Alexander SL: A novel technique for measuring hypothalamic and pituitary hormone secretion rates from collection of pituitary venous effluent in the normal horse, *J Endocrinol* 113(2):183-192, 1987.
111. Alexander S, Irvine C, et al: Comparison by three different radioimmunoassay systems of the polymorphism of plasma FSH in mares in various reproductive states, *J Reprod Fertil* (suppl 35):9-18, 1987.
112. Alexander SL, Irvine CH: Secretion rates and short-term patterns of gonadotrophin-releasing hormone, FSH and LH throughout the periovulatory period in the mare, *J Endocrinol* 114(3):351-362, 1987.
113. Ahima R, Prabakaran D, et al: Role of leptin in the neuroendocrine response to fasting, *Nature* 382:250-252, 1996.
114. Cunningham M, Clifton D, et al: Leptin's action on the reproductive axis: perspectives and mechanisms, *Biol Reprod* 60:216-222, 1999.
115. Barb CR, Kraeling RR: Role of leptin in the regulation of gonadotropin secretion in farm animals, *Anim Reprod Sci* 82-83, 2004:155-167.
116. Smith G, Jackson L, et al: Leptin regulation of reproductive function and fertility, *Theriogenology* 57:73-86, 2002.
117. Barash I, Cheung C, et al: Leptin is a metabolic signal to the reproductive system, *Endocrinology* 137(7):3144-3147, 1996.
118. McManus C, Fitzgerald B: Effects of a single day of feed restriction on changes in serum leptin, gonadotropins, prolactin, and metabolites in aged and young mares, *Dom Anim Endocrinol* 19:1-13, 2000.
119. Gentry L, Thompson D Jr: The relationship between body condition, leptin, and reproductive and hormonal characteristics of mares during the seasonal anovulatory period, *Theriogenology* 58:563-566, 2002.

Mare Reproductive Pathology

1. Giles RC, Donahue JM, Hong CB, et al: Causes of abortion, stillbirth, and perinatal death in horses: 3,527 cases (1986-1991), *J Am Vet Med Assoc* 203:1170-1175, 1993.
2. Hemberg E, Lundeheim N, Einarsson S: Retrospective study on vulvar conformation in relation to endometrial cytology and fertility in thoroughbred mares, *J Vet Med Assoc Physiol Pathol Clin Med.* 52:474-477, 2005.
3. Trotter GW, McKinnon AO: Surgery for abnormal vulvar and perineal conformation in the mare, *Vet Clin North Am Equine Pract* 4:389-405, 1988.
4. Schumacher J, Schumacher J, Blanchard T: Comparison of endometrium before and after repair of third-degree rectovestibular lacerations in mares, *J Am Vet Med Assoc* 200:1336-1338, 1992.
5. Studdert MJ: Comparative aspects of equine herpes viruses, *Cornell Vet* 64:94-122, 1974.
6. Goetz TE, Ogilvie GK, Keegan KG, et al: Cimetidine for treatment of melanomas in three horses, *J Am Vet Med Assoc* 196:449-452, 1990.
7. Hinrichs K, Cummings MR, Sertich PL, et al: Clinical significance of aerobic bacterial flora of the uterus, vagina, vestibule, and clitoral fossa of clinically normal mares, *J Am Vet Med Assoc* 193:72-75, 1988.
8. Katz JB, Evans LE, Hutto DL, et al: Clinical, bacteriologic, serologic, and pathologic features of infections with atypical Taylorella equigenitalis in mares, *J Am Vet Med Assoc* 216:1945-1948, 2000.
9. Kenney RM, Ganjam VK: Selected pathological changes of the mare uterus and ovary, *J Reprod Fertil* (suppl 23):335-339, 1975.
10. Leblanc MM, Neuwirth L, Jones L, et al: Differences in uterine position of reproductively normal mares and those with delayed uterine clearance detected by scintigraphy, *Theriogenology* 50:49-54, 1998.
11. Ricketts SW, Alonso S: The effect of age and parity on the development of equine chronic endometrial disease, *Equine Vet J* 23:189-192, 1991.
12. Kenney RM: Cyclic and pathologic changes of the mare endometrium as detected by biopsy, with a note on early embryonic death, *J Am Vet Med Assoc* 172:241-262, 1978.
13. Gruninger B, Schoon HA, Schoon D, et al: Incidence and morphology of endometrial angiopathies in mares in relationship to age and parity, *J Comp Pathol* 119:293-309, 1998.
14. Lefranc AC, Allen WR: Endometrial gland surface density and hyperaemia of the endometrium during early pregnancy in the mare, *Equine Vet J* 39:511-515, 2007.
15. Bracher V, Mathias S, Stocker M, et al: Ultrastructural evaluation of placentation in mares with chronic degenerative endometritis. *Proceedings of second International Conference on Veterinary Perinatology*, Cambridge, England, July 13-15, 1990. pp 37.
16. Bracher V, Allen WR, McGladdery AJ, et al: Ultrastructural evaluation of naturally occurring and experimentally induced placental pathology in the mare. *Proceedings of the International Meeting on Disturbances in Equine Foetal Maturation: Comparative Aspects*, Naples, Fla, Jan 19-21, 1991. pp 34.
17. Asbury AC: Relationship of abnormality of the equine placenta to size, health and vigor of the foal. *Proceedings of the annual meeting of the Society of Theriogenology*, Orlando, Fla, 1988. pp 306-310.
18. Dybdal NO, Daels PF, Couto MA, et al: Investigation of the reliability of a single endometrial biopsy sample, with a note on the correlation between uterine cysts on biopsy grade, *J Reprod Fertil* (suppl 44):697, 1991.

19. Watson ED, Sertich PL: Effect of repeated collection of multiple endometrial biopsy specimens on subsequent pregnancy in mares, *J Am Vet Med Assoc* 201:438-440, 1992.
20. Youngquist RS, Threlfall W: *Current therapy in large animal theriogenology*, ed 2, St Louis, 2007, Saunders.
21. Ricketts SW, Alonso S: Assessment of the breeding prognosis of mares using paired endometrial biopsy techniques, *Equine Vet J* 23:185-188, 1991.
22. Eilts BE, Scholl DT, Paccamonti DL, et al: Prevalence of endometrial cysts and their effect on fertility, Biol Reprod Monogr 1, *Equine Reprod* 6:527-532, 1995.
23. Santschi EM, Slone DE: Successful pregnancy after partial hysterectomy in two mares, *J Am Vet Med Assoc* 205:1180-1182, 1994.
24. Frazer G, Burba D, Paccamonti D, et al: The effects of parturition and peripartum complications on the peritoneal-fluid composition of mares, *Theriogenology* 48:919-931, 1997.
25. Roberts SJ: *Veterinary obstetrics and genital diseases (theriogenology)*, ed 3, Woodstock, Vt, 1986, SJ Roberts.
26. Taylor EL, Sellon DC, Wardrop KJ, et al: Effects of intravenous administration of formaldehyde on platelet and coagulation variables in healthy horses, *Am J Vet Res* 61:1191-1196, 2000.
27. Perkins NR, Frazer GS: Reproductive emergencies in the mare, *Vet Clin North Am Equine Pract* 10:643-670, 1994.
28. Vandeplassche M, Henry M: Salpingitis in the mare, *Proc Am Assoc Equine Pract* 23:123-131, 1977.
29. Liu IKM, Lantz KC, Schlafke S, et al: Clinical observations of oviductal masses in the mare, *Proc Am Assoc Equine Pract* 37:41-45, 1990.
30. David JS: A survey of eggs in the oviducts of mares, *J Reprod Fertil* (suppl 23):513-517, 1975.
31. Turner TA, Manno B: Bilateral granulosa cell tumor in a mare, *J Am Vet Med Assoc* 182:713-714, 1983.
32. Frederico LM, Gerard MP, Pinto CR, Gradil CM: Bilateral occurrence of granulosa-theca cell tumors in an Arabian mare, *Can Vet J* 48:502-505, 2007.
33. McCue PM: Neoplasia of the female reproductive tract, *Vet Clin North Am Equine Pract* 14:505-515, 1998.
34. McCue PM: Equine granulosa cell tumors, *Proc Am Assoc Equine Pract* 38:587-593, 1992.
35. Hinrichs K, Frazer GS, deGannes RV, et al: Serous cystadenoma in a normally cyclic mare with high plasma testosterone values, *J Am Vet Med Assoc* 194:381-382, 1989.
36. Vanderkolk JH, Geelen SNJ, Jonker FH, et al: Hypertrophic osteopathy associated with ovarian-carcinoma in a mare, *Vet Rec* 143:172-173, 1998.
37. Sedrish SA, McClure JR, Pinto C, et al: Ovarian torsion associated with granulosa-theca cell tumor in a mare, *J Am Vet Med Assoc* 211:1152-1154, 1997.

ENDOMETRITIS AND UTERINE THERAPY

1. Robinson NE, editor: *Current therapy in equine medicine*, ed 6, St Louis, 2009, Saunders.
2. Troedsson M, Scott M, Liu I: Comparative treatment of mares susceptible to chronic uterine infection, *Am J Vet Res* 56: 468-472, 1995.
3. Troedsson M: Therapeutic considerations for mating induced endometritis, *Pferdeheilkunde* 13:516-520, 1997.
4. Troedsson M, Liu I: Uterine clearance of non-antigenic markers (51Cr) in response to a bacterial challenge in mares potentially susceptible and resistant to chronic uterine infections, *J Reprod Fertil* (suppl 44):283-288, 1991.
5. LeBlanc M, Neuwirth L, Asbury A, et al: Scintigraphic measurement of uterine clearance in normal mares and mares with recurrent endometritis, *Equine Vet J* 26:109-113, 1994.
6. LeBlanc M, Neuwirth L, Mauragis D: Oxytocin enhances clearance of radiocolloid from the uterine lumen of reproductively normal mares and mares susceptible to endometritis, *Equine Vet J* 26:279-282, 1994.
7. Kotilainen T, Huhtinen M, Katila T: Sperm-induced leukocytosis in the equine uterus, *Theriogenology* 41:629-636, 1994.
8. Katila T: Onset and duration of uterine inflammatory response of mares after insemination with fresh semen, *Biol Reprod Monograph* 1:515-517, 1995.
9. Nikolakopoulos E, Watson E: Does artificial insemination with chilled, extended semen reduce the antigenic challenge to the mare's uterus compared with natural service? *Theriogenology* 47:583-590, 1997.
10. Troedsson M, Lee C-S, Franklin R, et al: The role of seminal plasma in post-breeding uterine inflammation, *J Reprod Fertil* (suppl 56):341-349, 2000.
11. Troedsson M, Loset K, Alghamdi A, et al: Interaction between equine semen and the endometrium: the inflammatory response to semen, *Anim Reprod Sci* 68:273-278, 2001.
12. Fiala S, Pimentel C, Steiger K, et al: Effect of skim milk and seminal plasma uterine infusions in mares, *Theriogenology* 58:491-494, 2002.
13. Dahms B, Troedsson M: The effect of seminal plasma components on opsonisation and PMN-phagocytosis of equine spermatozoa, *Theriogenology* 58:457-460, 2002.
14. Troedsson M, Alghamdi A, Mattisen J: Equine seminal plasma protects the fertility of spermatozoa in an inflammed uterine environment, *Theriogenology* 58:453-456, 2002.
15. Day F, Crowhurst R, Simpson D, et al: An outbreak of contagious equine metritis in 1977 and its effect the following season, *J Reprod Fertil* (suppl 27):351-354, 1979.
16. Hazard G, Hughes K, Penson P: Contagious equine metritis in Australia, *J Reprod Fertil* (suppl 27):337-342, 1979.
17. Ricketts S, Rossdale P: Endometrial biopsy findings in mares with contagious equine metritis, *J Reprod Fertil* (suppl 27): 355-359, 1979.
18. Swerczek T: Contagious equine metritis-outbreak of the disease in Kentucky and laboratory methods for diagnosing the disease, *J Reprod Fertil Suppl* 27:361-365, 1979.
19. Powell D, Whitwell K: The epidemiology of contagious equine metritis (CEM) in England 1977-1978, *J Reprod Fertil Suppl* 27:331-335, 1979.
20. Brinsko S, Treatment of infectious infertility, *Proceedings of Mare Reproduction Symposium 1996*, Hastings, NE, pp. 150-155. (Society for Theriogenology)
21. Davis LE, Abbitt BA: Clinical pharmacology of antibacterial drugs in the uterus of the mare, *J Am Vet Med Assoc* 170: 204-207, 1970.
22. Pycock JF, Newcombe JR: Assessment of the effect of three treatments to remove intrauterine fluid on pregnancy rate in the mare, *Vet Rec* 138:320-323, 1996.
23. Locke TF: Distribution of antibiotics in the mare reproductive tract after various routes of administration, *J Reprod Fertil* (suppl 32):640, 1982.
24. Caudle A, Purswell B, Williams D, et al: Endometrial levels of amikacin in the mare after intrauterine infusion of amikacin sulphate, *Theriogenology* 19:433-439, 1983.
25. McKinnon A, Voss J, editors: *Equine reproduction*, Philadelphia, 1993, Wiley-Blackwell.
26. Arbeiter K, Awad-Maselmeh M, Kopschitz D, et al: Estimation of antibiotic levels in uterine tissue and blood plasma of the mare following parenteral administration of penicillin and ampicillin, *Wien Tierarztl Monaschr* 63:298-304, 1976.
27. Giguere S, Belanger M: Concentration of enrofloxacin in equine tissues after long term oral administration, *Vet Pharmacol Ther* 20:402-404, 1997.
28. Colahan PT, Merritt AM, Moore JN: *Equine medicine and surgery*, ed 5, St Louis, 1999, Mosby.
29. Farrelly B, Mullaney P: Cervical and uterine infection in Thoroughbred mares, *Irish Vet J* 18:201-212, 1964.
30. Anzai T, Kamada M, Kanemaru T: Isolation of methicillin-resistant *Staphylococcus aureus* (MRSA) from mares with metritis and its zooepidemiology, *J Equine Sci* 7:7-11, 1996.

31. McCue P, Hughes J, Jang S, Biberstein E: Antimicrobial susceptibility patterns for equine endometrial isolates, *Calif Vet* 45:23-26, 1991.
32. Ricketts S: Treatment of equine endometritis with intrauterine irrigations of ceftiofur sodium: a comparison with mares treated in a similar manner with a mixture of sodium benzylpenicillin, neomycin sulphate, polymixin B sulphate and furaltadone hydrochloride, *Pferdeheilkunde* 13:486-489, 1997.
33. Bain A: Estrus and infertility of the Thoroughbred mare in Australasia, *J Am Vet Med Assoc* :179-185, 1957.
34. Conboy H, Diagnosis and therapy of equine endometritis. In *Proceedings of the Twenty-Fourth Annual Convention of the American Association of Equine Practitioners*, pp. 165-171, 1978. The Association.
35. Dimock W, Bruner D: Barren broodmares, *Kentucky Agricultural Experimental Station Circular* 63:1-15, 1949.
36. Shin S, Lein D, Aronson A, Nusbaum S: The bacteriological culture of equine uterine contents, in-vitro sensitivity of organisms isolated and interpretation, *J Reprod Fertil Suppl* 27:307-315, 1979.
37. Albihn A, Baverud V, Magnusson U: Uterine microbiology and antimicrobial susceptibility in isolated bacteria from mares with fertility problems, *Acta Vet Scand* 44:121-129, 2003.
38. Ricketts SW, Mackintosh ME: Role of anaerobic bacteria in equine endometritis, *J Reprod Fertil Suppl* 35:343-351, 1987.
39. Purswell BJ, Ley WB, Sriranganathan N, Bowen JM: Aerobic and anaerobic bacterial flora in the postpartum mare, *J Equine Vet Sci* 9:141-144, 1989.
40. Gingerich D, Rourke J, Chatfield R, Strom P: Amikacin: a new aminoglycoside for treating equine metritis, *Vet Med Small Anim Clin* :787-793, 1983.
41. Love C, Strzemienski P, Kenney R: Endometrial concentrations of ampicillin in mares after intrauterine infusion of the drug, *Am J Vet Res* 51:197-199, 1990.
42. McDonald P, Wetherall B, Pruul H: Postantibiotic leukocyte enhancement-increased susceptibility of bacteria pretreated with antibioitcs to activity of leukocytes, *Rev Infect Dis* 3:38-44, 1981.
43. Threlfall W, Accurate diagnosis and appropriate therapy of uterine disease. In *Proceedings of Mare Reproduction Symposium*, Annual Conference for Theriogenology pp. 51-69. Society for Theriogenology, 1996.
44. Jones D: Fluid distribution and cervical loss following intrauterine infusion in the mare, *Equine Pract* 17:12-19, 1995.
45. Ricketts S: The barren mare: diagnosis, prognosis and treatment for genital abnormality, *Practice* 11:120-125, 1989.
46. Al-Guedawy SA, Vasquez L, Neff-Davis CA, et al: Effect of vehicle on intrauterine absorption of gentamicin in cattle, *Theriogenology* 19:771-778, 1983.
47. Mather E, Refsal K, Gustafsson B, et al: The use of fibre-optic techniques in clinical diagnosis and visual assessment of experimental intrauterine therapy in mares, *J Reprod Fertil* (suppl 27):293-297, 1979.
48. Dascanio J, Ley W, Schweizer C: How to diagnose and treat fungal endometritis, *Am Assoc Equine Pract* 46:316-318, 2000.
49. Dascanio J, Schweizer C, Ley W: Equine fungal endometritis, *Equine Vet Educ* 13:324-329, 2001.
50. Hess M, Parker N, Purswell B, Dascanio J: Use of lufenuron as a treatment for fungal endometritis in four mares, *J Am Vet Med Assoc* 221:266-267, 2002.
51. Bracher V: *Equine endometritis*, Cambridge, 1992, University of Cambridge.
52. Watson E: Effect of povidone-iodine on in vitro locomotion of equine neutrophils, *Equine Vet J* 19:226-228, 1987.
53. Bennett D, Poland H, Kaneps A, Snyder S: Histologic effect of infusion solutions on the equine endometrium, *Equine Pract* 3:37-44, 1981.
54. van Dyke E, Lange A: The detrimental affect of the use of iodine as an intrauterine instillation in mares, *J S Afr Vet Assoc* 57:205-210, 1986.
55. Olsen LM, Al-Bagdadi FK, Richardson GF, et al: A histological study of the effect of saline and povidone-iodine infusions on the equine endometrium, *Theriogenology* 37:1311-1325, 1992.
56. Brinsko SP, Varner DD, Blanchard TL: The effect of uterine lavage performed four hours post insemination on pregnancy rate in mares, *Theriogenology* 35:1111-1119, 1991.
57. Ley W: Treating endometrosis in mares, *Veterinary Medicine* 778-788, 1994.
58. Youngquist R, Blanchard T, Lapin D, et al: The effects of EDTA-Tris infusion on the equine endometrium, *Theriogenology* 22:593-599, 1984.
59. Ashworth C, Nelson D: Antimicrobial potentiation of irrigation solutions containing trisaminomethan-EDTA, *J Am Vet Med Assoc* 197:1513-1514, 1990.
60. Jackson P, Allen W, Ricketts S, Hall R: The irritancy of chlorhexidine gluconate in the genital tract of the mare, *Vet Rec* 105:122-124, 1979.
61. Freeman D, Momont H, Fahning M: Effectiveness and inflammatory response of antiseptics in the mare's uterus. In *Proceedings for the Annual Conference*, Society for Theriogenology. Hastings, NE pp. 365, 1987. The Society.
62. D Freeman, personal communication, 1998.
63. Frazer GS, Rossol TJ, Threlfall WR, Weisbrode SE: Histopathologic effects of dimethyl sulfoxide on equine endometrium, *Am J Vet Res* 49:1774-1781, 1988.
64. Bracher V, Neuschaefer A, Allen W: The effect of intra-uterine infusion of kerosene on the endometrium of mares, *J Reprod Fertil* (suppl 44):706-707, 1991.
65. Knutti B, Pycock J, van der Weijden G, Kupfer U: The influence of early postbreeding uterine lavage on pregnancy rate in mares with intrauterine fluid accumulation after breeding, *Equine V Educ*12:267-270, 2000.
66. Vanderwall D, Woods G: Effect on fertility of uterine lavage performed immediately prior to insemination in mares, *J Am Vet Med Assoc* 222:1108-1110, 2003.
67. Asbury A: Uterine defense mechanisms in the mare: the use of intrauterine plasma in the management of endometritis, *Theriogenology* 21:387-393, 1989.
68. Asbury A, Schultz K, Klesius P, et al: Factors affecting phagocytosis of bacteria by neutrophils in the mare's uterus, *J Reprod Fertil Suppl* 32:151-159, 1982.
69. Asbury AC: Uterine defense mechanisms in the mare: The use of intrauterine plasma in the management of endometritis, *Theriogenology* 21:387-393, 1984.
70. Troedsson MH, Liu IK, Ing M, et al: Multiple site electromyography recordings of uterine activity following an intrauterine bacterial challenge in mares susceptible and resistant to chronic uterine infection, *J Reprod Fertil* 99:307-313, 1993.
71. Adams G, Ginther O: Efficacy of intrauterine infusion of plasma for treament of infertility and endometritis in mares, *J Am Vet Med Assoc* 194:372-378, 1989.
72. Pascoe D: Effect of adding autologous plasma to an intrauterine antibiotic therapy after breeding on pregnancy rates in mares, *Biol Reprod Monogr* 1:539-543, 1995.
73. Combs GB, LeBlanc MM, Neuwirth L, Tran TQ: Effects of prostaglandin F2[alpha], cloprostenol and fenprostalene on uterine clearance of radiocolloid in the mare, *Theriogenology* 45:1449-1455, 1996.
74. LeBlanc M: Effects of oxytocin, prostaglandin and phenylbutazone on uterine clearance, *Pferdeheilkunde* 13:483, 1997.
75. Rigby S, Varner D, Blanchard T, et al, Intracellular Ca2+ and *in vitro* myometrial contractility of uterine muscle from mares susceptible to endometritis. In *Proceedings of the Annual Conference. Nashville*, Tennessee, pp. 34, 1999. The Society for Theriogenology.

76. Rigby S, Barhoumi R, et al: Mares with delayed uterine clearance have an intrinsic defect in myometrial function, *Bio Repro* 65:740-747, 2001.
77. Alghamdi A, Troedsson M: Concentration of nitric oxide in uterine secretion from mares susceptible and resistant to chronic post-breeding endometritis, *Theriogenology* 58: 445-448, 2002.
78. Alghamdi A, Foster D, Carlson C, Troedsson M: Nitric oxide levels and nitric oxide synthase expression in uterine samples from mares susceptible and resistant to persistent breeding-induced endometritis, *Am J Reprod Immunol* 53:230-237, 2005.
79. Cadario M, Thatcher M-J, LeBlanc M: Relationship between prostaglandin and uterine clearance of radiocolloid in the mare, *Biol Reprod Monograph* 1:495-500, 1995.
80. Rasch K, Schoon H, Sieme H, Klug E: Histomorphological endometrial status and influence of oxytocin on the uterine drainage and pregnancy rate in mares, *Equine Vet J* 28:455-460, 1996.
81. LeBlanc M, Johnson R, Calderwood Mays M, Valderrama C: Lymphatic clearance of india ink in reproductively normal mares and mares susceptible to endometritis, *Biol Reprod Monograph* 1:501-506, 1995.
82. Brendemuehl J: Effect of oxytocin and PGF2a on luteal formation, function, and pregnancy rates in mares, *Am Assoc Equine Pract* 47:239-241, 2001.
83. Sharpe KL, Eiler H, Hopkins FM: Absence of uterokinetic effects of prostaglandin F2[alpha] on oxytocin-reactive uterus in the mare, *Theriogenology* 30:887-892, 1988.
84. Sieme H, Schroter N, klug E, Schoon H: Influence of prostaglandin F2 alpha on conception rate of mares inseminated with chilled semen, *Pferdeheilkunde* 13:558, 1997.
85. Pascoe D: Single embryo reduction in the mare with twin conceptuses: studies of hormonal profiles and drug therapies using a physiological model, and manual and surgical reduction technique in vivo, 1985, University of California.
86. Ferreira-Dias G, Nequin L, King S: Displacement of *Streptococcus zooepidemicus* from equine uterine epithelium by N-acetyl-D-galactosamine in vitro, *J Equine Vet Sci* 13:489-492, 1993.
87. King S, Carnevale E, Nequin L, Crawford J: Inhibition of bacterial endometritis with mannose, *J Equine Vet Sci* 18:332-334, 1998.
88. McDonnell A, Watson E: The effects of dexamethasone sodium phosphate on mares with experimentally-induced endometritis, *J Equine Vet Sci* 13:202-206, 1993.
89. Dell'Aqua J Jr, Papa F, Lopes M, et al: Modulation of acute uterine inflammatory response after artificial insemination with equine frozen semen, *Animal Reproduction Science* 94:270-273, 2006.
90. Widders P, Warner S, Huntington P: Immunisation of mares to control endometritis caused by, *Streptococcus zooepidemicus. Res Vet Sci* 58:75-81, 1995.
91. Rogan D, Fumuso E, Rodriguez E, et al: Use of a mycobacterial cell wall extract (MCWE) in susceptible mares to clear experimentally induced endometritis with Streptococcus zooepidemicus, *J Equine Vet Sci* 27:112-117, 2007.
92. Zingher AC: Effects of immunostimulation with Propionibacterium acnes (EQSTIM-R) in mares cytologically positive for endometritis, *J Equine Vet Sci* 16:100-103, 1996.
93. Rohrbach B, Sheerin P, Steiner J, et al: Use of Propionibacterium acnes as adjunct therapy in treatment of persistent endometritis in the broodmare, *Anim Reprod Sci* 94:259-260, 2006.
94. Neves AP, Keller A, et al: Use of leukocytes as treatment for endometritis in mares experimentally infected with Streptococcus equi subsp. zooepidemicus, *Anim Reprod Sci* 97: 314-322, 2007.
95. Dascanio J, Parker N, Ley W, et al: Magnesium sulfate intrauterine therapy in the mare, *Equine Pract* 20:10-13, 1998.
96. Dascanio J, Parker N, Ley W, et al: Effect of magnesium sulfate on the equine endometrium. *Proceedings of the 42nd Annual Convention of the American Association of Equine Practitioners 42*, 148-149, 1996.
97. Madill S, Troedsson M, Alexander S, et al: Simultaneous recording of pituitary oxytocin secretion and myometrial activity in oestrous mares exposed to various breeding stimuli, *J Reprod Fertil Suppl* 56:351-361, 2000.
98. Pycock J, Management of the problem breeding mare. In *Proceedings for the Annual Conference, Society for Theriogenology*, 1999, Hastings, Neb, pp 79-89. Society for Theriogenology.
99. Pycock JF: A new approach to treatment of endometritis, *Equine Vet Educ* 6:36-38, 1994.
100. Douglas R, Luteal insufficiency, hypothyroidism and Cushings disease: what do we really know? In *Proceedings of 17th Equine Nutrition and Physiology Society*. University of Kentucky, 2001, pp 287-293. Equine Nutrition and Physiology Society.
101. Perkins N, The infertile mare: diagnosis, treatment and management. In *Proceedings for the Annual Conference of the New Zealand Veterinary Association*, 1995, pp. 47-64. (Massey University: Veterinary Continuing Education).

Hormonal Manipulation Of The Mare

1. Peltier MR, Robinson G, Sharp DC: Effects of melatonin implants in pony mares. 2. Long-term effects, *Theriogenology* 49:1125-1149, 1998.
2. Alexander SL, Irvine CHG: Control of the onset of the breeding season in the mare, its artificial regulation by progesterone treatment, *J Reprod Fertil* (suppl 44):307, 1991.
3. Wiepz GJ, Squires EL, Chapman PL: Effects of norgestomet, altrenogest and/or estradiol on follicular and hormonal characteristics of late transitional mares, *Theriogenology* 30:181-193, 1988.
4. McCue PM, Buchanan BR, Farquhar VJ, et al: Efficacy of domperidone on induction of ovulation in anestrous and transitional mares, *Proc Am Assoc Equine Pract* 45:217-218, 1999.
5. Brendemuehl JP, Cross DL: Effects of the dopamine antagonist domperidone on the vernal transition in seasonally anestrus mares. *Proceedings of the Seventh International Symposium on Equine Reproduction*, 1998, pp 47-48.
6. Daels PF: Management of spring transition. Proc Am Assoc Equine Pract (8th Annual Resort Symposium), 2006.
7. Bennett-Wimbush K, Loch WE, Plata-Madrid H, et al: The effects of perphenazine and bromocriptine on follicular dynamics and endocrine profiles in anestrous pony mares, *Theriogenology* 49:717-733, 1998.
8. Foglia RA, McCue PM, Squires EL et al: Stimulation of follicular development in transitional mares using a progesterone vaginal insert (CIDR-BO). *Proceedings of the annual conference of the Society for Theriogenology*, Nashville, Tenn, 1999. pp 33.
9. Carnevale EM, Thompson KN, King SS, et al: Effects of age and diet on the spring transition in mares, *Proc Am Assoc Equine Pract* 42:146-147, 1996.
10. Peres KR, Fernandes CB, Alvarenga MA, Landim-Alvarenga FC: Effect of eFSH on ovarian cyclicity and embryo preoduction of mares in spring transitional phase, *J Equine Vet Sci* 27(4): 176-180
11. Ginther OJ: *Reproductive biology of the mare: basic and applied aspects*, ed 2, Cross Plains, Wis, 1992, Equiservices.
12. Samper JC, Geertsema HP, Hearn P: Rate of luteolysis, folliculogenesis and interval to ovulation in mares treated with a prostaglandin analogue on day 6 or 10 of the estrous cycle, *Proc Am Assoc Equine Pract* 39:169-170, 1993.
13. Brendemuehl JP: Effect of oxytocin and PGF2a on luteal formation, function and pregnancy rates in mares, *Proc Am Assoc Equine Pract* 47:239-241, 2001.

14. Brendemuehl JP: Influence of oxytocin, PGF2a and cloprostenol administered in the immediate postovulatory period on luteal formation and function in the mare, Theriogenology (in press).
15. Irvine CH, McKeough VL, Turner JE, et al: Effectiveness of a two-dose regimen of prostaglandin administration in inducing luteolysis without adverse side effects in mares, *Equine Vet J* 34(2):191-194, 2002.
16. Nie GJ, Goodin AN, Braden TD, et al: How to reduce drug costs and side effects when using prostaglandins to short-cycle mares, *Proc Am Assoc Equine Pract* 50:396-398, 2004.
17. Asbury AC: Uterine defense mechanisms in the mare: the use of intrauterine plasma in the management of endometritis, *Theriogenology* 21:387-393, 1984.
18. McKinnon AO, Perriam WJ, Lescun TB, et al: Effect of a GnRH analogue (Ovuplant), hCG and dexamethasone on time to ovulation in cycling mare, *World Equine Vet Rev* 2(3):16-18, 1997.
19. Roser JF, Kiefer BL, Evans JW, et al: The development of antibodies to human chorionic gonadotrophin following its repeated injection in the cyclic mare, *J Reprod Fertil Suppl* 27:173-179, 1979.
20. Green JM, Raz T, Epp T, et al: Relationship between utero-ovarian parameters and the ovulatory response to human chorionic gonadotrophin (hCG) in mares, *Proc Am Assoc Equine Pract* 53:563-567, 2007.
21. Mumford EL, Squires EL, Jochle E, et al: Use of deslorelin short-term implants to induce ovulation in cycling mares during three consecutive estrous cycles, *Anim Reprod Sci* 39:129-140, 1995.
22. Barrier-Battut I, Le Poutre N, Trocherie E, et al: Use of buserelin to induce ovulation in the cyclic mare, *Theriogenology* 55:1679-1695, 2001.
23. McCue PM, Farquhar VJ, Squires EL: Effect of the GnRH agonist deslorelin acetate on pituitary function and follicular development in the mare, *Proc Am Assoc Equine Pract* 46: 355-356, 2000.
24. Niswender KD, Roser JF, Boime I, et al: Induction of ovulation in the mare with recombinant equine luteinizing hormone, *Proc Am Assoc Equine Pract* 52:189-191, 2006.
25. Samper JC: Ultrasonographic appearance and the pattern of uterine edema to time ovulation in mares, *Proc Am Assoc Equine Pract* 43:189-191, 1997.
26. Samper JC, Hankins K: Breeding mares with frozen semen in private practice, *Proc Am Assoc Equine Pract* 47:314-318, 2001.
27. Blanchard TJ, Varner DD, Burns PJ, et al: Regulation of estrus and ovulation in mares with progesterone or progesterone and estradiol biodegradable microspheres with or without PGF_2alpha, *Theriogenology* 38:1091-1106, 1992.
28. Fleury JJ, Costa-Neto JB, Burns PJ: Regulation of estrus and ovulation with progesterone and estradiol microspheres: effect of different doses of estradiol, *J Equine Vet Sci* 13: 525-528, 1993.
29. Jasko DF, Farlin ME, Hutchinson H, et al: Progesterone and estradiol in biodegradable microspheres for control of estrus and ovulation in mares, *Theriogenology* 40:465-478, 1993.
30. Klug E, Jochle W: Advances in synchronizing estrus and ovulations in the mare: a mini review, *J Equine Vet Sci* 21:474-479, 2001.
31. Paul JW, Rains JR, Lehman FD: Hoechst-Roussel Agri-Vet Company: the use and misuse of progestins in the mare, *Equine Pract* 17(3):21-22, 1995.
32. McCue PM, Lemons SS, Squires EL, et al: Efficacy of progesterone/ estradiol implants for suppression of estrus in the mare, *Proc Am Assoc Equine Pract* 42:195-196, 1996.
33. Vanderwall DK, Rasmussen DM, Woods GL: Effect of repeated administration of oxytocin during diestrus on duration of function of corpora lutea in mares, *J Am Vet Med Assoc* 231(12):1864-1867, 2007.
34. Card C, Raz T, Leheiget R, et al: GnRF immunization in mares: ovarian function, return to cyclicity, and fertility, *Proc Am Assoc Equine Pract* 53:576-577, 2007.
35. James AN, Vogelsang DW, Forrest GG, et al: Efficacy of short-term administration of altrenogest to postpone ovulation in mares, *J Equine Vet Sci* 18:329-331, 1998.
36. Sexton PE, Bristol FM: Uterine involution in mares treated with progesterone and estradiol-17B, *J Am Vet Med Assoc* 186(3):252-256, 1985.
37. Squires EL, Garcia RH, Ginther OJ, et al: Comparison of equine pituitary extract and follicle stimulating hormone for superovulating mares, *Theriogenology* 26:661-670, 1986.
38. McCue PM, Hughes JP, Lashley BL: Effect on ovulation rate of passive immunization of mares against inhibin, *Equine Vet J* 15(suppl):103-106, 1993.
39. Scoggin CF, Meira C, McCue PM, et al: Use of twice-daily step-down dosage of equine pituitary extract for induction of multiple ovulations in mares, *Theriogenology* 57:771, 2002:abstract.
40. Squires EL, McCue PM, Vanderwall D: The current status of equine embryo transfer, *Theriogenology* 51:91-104, 1999.
41. Squires EL, McCue PM, Niswender K, et al: A review on the use of eFSH to enhance reproductive performance, *Proc Am Assoc Equine Pract* 49:360-362, 2003.
42. Welsh SA, Denniston DJ, Hudson JJ, et al: Exogenous eFSH, follicle coasting, and hCG as a novel superovulation regimen in mares, *J Equine Vet Sci* 26:262-270, 2006.
43. McCue PM, LeBlanc MM, Squires EL: eFSH in clinical equine practice, *Theriogenology* 68(3):429-433, 2007.
44. Niswender KD, McCue PM, Squires EL: Effect of purified equine follicle-stimulating hormone on follicular development and ovulation in transitional mares, *J Equine Vet Sci* 24:37-39, 2004.
45. Niswender KD, Jennings M, Boime I, et al: In Vivo activity of recombinant equine follicle stimulating hormone in cycling mares, *Proc Am Assoc Equine Pract* 53:561-562, 2007.
46. Daels PF, Besognet B, Hansen B, et al: Effect of progesterone on prostaglandin F_2 alpha secretion and outcome of pregnancy during eleprostenol-induced abortion in mares, *Am J Vet Res* 57:1331-1337, 1996.
47. Morris S, Kelleman AA, Stawicki RJ, et al: Transrectal ultrasonography and plasma progestin profiles identifies feto-placental compromise in mares with experimentally induced placentitis, *Theriogenology* 67(4):681-691, 2007.
48. Baily CS, Macpherson ML, Graczyk J, et al: Treatment efficacy of trimethoprim sulfamethazole, pentoxyphylline and altrenogest in equine placentitis, *Theriogenoloy* 68:516-517, 2007.
49. MacPherson M: Identification and management of the high-risk pregnant mare, *Proc Am Assoc Equine Pract* 53:293-304, 2007.
50. Metcalf ES: Unpublished data, 2002.
51. Youngquist RS, Threlfall W, editors: *Current therapy in large animal theriogenology*, ed 2, St Louis, 2007, Saunders.
52. Troedsson MHT: Uterine response to semen deposition in the mare. *Proceedings of the Society for Theriogenology*, Nashville, Tenn, 1999. pp 130-135.
53. LeBlanc MM, Neuwirth L, Jones L, et al: Differences in uterine position of reproductively normal mares and those with delayed uterine clearance detected by scintigraphy, *Theriogenology* 50:49-54, 1998.
54. LeBlanc MM, Neuwirth L, Mauragis D, et al: Oxytocin enhances clearance of radiocolloid from the uterine lumen of reproductively normal mares and mares susceptible to endometritis, *Equine Vet J* 26:279-282, 1994.
55. Leblanc MM: Oxytocin: the new wonder drug for the treatment of endometritis? *Equine Vet Educ* 6:39-43, 1994.
56. Gutjahr S, Paccamonti DL, Pycock JF, et al: Effect of dose and day of treatment on uterine response to oxytocin in mares, *Theriogenology* 54:447-456, 2000.

57. Madill S, Troedsson MHT, Alexander SL, et al: Simultaneous recording of pituitary oxytocin and myometrial activity in estrous mares exposed to various breeding stimuli. *Proceedings of the International Symposium on Equine Reproduction*, Onderstepoort, South Africa, 1998. pp 93-94.
58. Rigby S, Hill J, Miller C, et al: Administration of oxytocin immediately following insemination does not improve pregnancy rates in mares bred by fertile or subfertile stallions, *Theriogenology* 51:1143-1150, 1999.
59. Handler J, Hoffman D, Weber F, et al: Oxytocin does not contribute to the effects of cervical dilation on progesyterone secretion and embryonic development in mares, *Theriogenology* 66(5):1397-1404, 2006.
60. Combs GB, LeBlanc MM, Neuwirth L, et al: Effects of prostaglandin F_2-α, cloprostenol and fenprostalene on uterine clearance of radio colloid in the mare, *Theriogenology* 45(4):1449-1455, 1996.
61. Nie GJ, Johnson KE, Wenzel J, et al: Effect of administering oxytocin or cloprostenol in the periovulatory period on pregnancy outcome and luteal function in mares, *Theriogenology* 60(6):1111-1118, 2003.
62. Weber JA, Freeman DA, Vanderwall DK, et al: Prostaglandin E_2 hastens oviductal transport of equine embryos, *Biol Reprod* 45:544-546, 1991.
63. Gastal MO, Gastal EL, Torres CAA, et al: Effect of PGE_2 on uterine contactility and tone in mares, *Theriogenology* 50:989-999, 1998.
64. Robinson SJ, Neal H, Allen WR: Modulation of oviductal transport in the mare by local application of prostaglandin E2. *Proceedings of the seventh International Symposium on Equine Reproduction*, Onderstepoort, South Africa, 1998. pp 153-154.
65. Woods J, Rigby S, Brinsko S, et al: Effect of intrauterine treatment with prostaglandin E2 prior to insemination of mares in the uterine horn or body, *Theriogenology* 53:1827-1836, 2000.
66. Dimov V, Georgiev F: Ram semen prostaglandin concentration and its effect on fertility, *J Anim Sci* 44:1050-1054, 1977.
67. Aitken RJ, Kelly RW: Analysis of the direct effects of prostaglandins on human sperm function, *J Reprod Fertil* 73:139-146, 1985.

Breeding Management to Optimize Pregnancy Rates

1. McDonnell SM: Bachelor and harem stallion behavior and endocrinology, Equine Reprod VI, *Biol Reprod Monogr* 1: 577-590, 1995.
2. Dobrinski I, Thomas P, B Ball: The oviductal sperm reservoir in the horse: functional aspects. *Proceedings of the Society for Theriogenology*, Kansas City, Mo, 1996. pp 265-270.
3. Dobrinski I, Thomas P, Smith T, et al: Sperm-oviduct interaction: role of sperm adhesion and effects of sperm cryopreservation. *Proceedings of the forty-second annual convention of the American Association of Equine Practitioners*, Denver, 1996. pp 144-145.
4. Thomas PGA, Ball BA, Miller PG, et al: A subpopulation of morphologically normal, motile spermatozoa attach to equine oviduct epithelial cells in vitro, *Biol Reprod* 51:303-309, 1994.
5. Thomas PGA, Ball BA, Brinsko SP: Interaction of equine spermatozoa with oviduct epithelial cell explants is affected by estrous cycle and anatomic origin of explant, *Biol Reprod* 51:222-228, 1994.
6. Scott MA, Overstreet JW: Sperm transport to the oviducts: abnormalities and their clinical implications. *Proceedings of the forty-first annual convention of the American Association of Equine Practitioners*, Lexington, Ky, 1995. pp 1-2.
7. Ellington JE, Ball BA, Blue BJ, et al: Capacitation-like membrane changes and prolonged viability in vitro of equine spermatozoa cultured with uterine tube epithelial cells, *Am J Vet Res* 54:1505-1510, 1993.
8. Newcombe JR: Conception in a mare to a single mating 7 days before ovulation, *Equine Vet Educ* 6(1):27-28, 1994.
9. Woods J, Bergfelt DR, Ginther OJ: Effects of time of insemination relative to ovulation on pregnancy rate and embryonic-loss rate in mares, *Equine Vet J* 22:410-415, 1990.
10. Ginther OJ: *Reproductive biology of the mare*, ed 2, Cross Plains, Wis, 1992, Equiservices.
11. Katila T, Koskinen E, Kuntsi H, et al: Fertility after post ovulatory insemination in mares. *Proceedings of the eleventh International Congress on Animal Reproduction and Artificial Insemination*, Dublin, Ireland, 1988. p 96.
12. Palmer E: Factors affecting stallion semen survival and fertility. *Proceedings of the tenth International Congress on Animal Reproduction and Artificial Insemination II*, 1984. pp 377-379.
13. Samper JC: Ultrasonographic appearance and the pattern of uterine edema to time ovulation in mares. *Proceedings of the forty-third annual convention of the American Association of Equine Practitioners*, Phoenix, Ariz, 1997. pp 189-191.
14. Samper JC: How to interpret endometrial edema in brood mares, *Proc Am Assoc Equine Pract* 53, 2007.
15. Bragg Wever ND, Pierson RA, Card CE: Relationship between estradiol 17-β abd endometrial echotexture during natural and hormonally manipulated estrus in mares, *Proc Am Assoc Equine Pract* 48:42-47, 2002.
16. Gastal EL, Gastal MO, Ginther OJ: Ultrasound follicular characteristics for predicting ovulation on the following day in mares, *Theriogenology* 49(1):257, 1998.
17. Bragg ND: Transrectal tonometric measurement of follicular softening and computer assisted ultrasound image analysis of follicular wall echotexture, *Proc Am Assoc Equine Pract* 47: 242-245, 2001.
18. Hughes JP, Stabenfeldt JH, Evans JW: Clinical and endocrine aspects of the estrous cycle of the mare. *Proceedings of the twenty-eighth annual convention of the American Association of Equine Practitioners*, 1972. pp 119-148.
19. McKinnon AO, Perriam WJ, Lescun TB, et al: Effect of a GnRH analogue (Ovuplant), hCG and dexamethasone on time to ovulation in cycling mare, *World Equine Vet Rev* 2(3):16-18, 1997.
20. Mumford EL, Squires EL, Jochle E, et al: Use of deslorelin short-term implants to induce ovulation in cycling mares during three consecutive estrous cycles, *Anim Reprod Sci* 39:129-140, 1995.
21. Farquhar VJ, McCue PM, Nett TM, et al: Effect of deslorelin acetate on gonadotrophin secretion and ovarian follicle development in cycling mares, *J Am Vet Med Assoc* 218: 749-752, 2001.
22. Barrier-Battut I, Le Poutre N, Trocherie E, et al: Use of buserelin to induce ovulation in the cyclic mare, *Theriogenology* 55:1679-1695, 2001.
23. Niswender
24. Samper JC, Hankins K: Breeding mares with frozen semen in private practice, *Proc Am Assoc Equine Pract* 47:314-318, 2001.
25. McCue PM, Farquhar VJ, Squires EL: Effect of the GnRH agonist deslorelin acetate on pituitary function and follicular development, *Proc Am Assoc Equine Pract* 46:355-356, 2000.
26. Samper JC: The effect of different lubricants on the longevity of motility and velocity of stallion spermatozoa, *Theriogenology* 68:496, 2007.
27. Samper JS, editor: *Equine breeding management and artificial insemination*, St Louis, 2000, Saunders.
28. LeBlanc MM, DeLille A, Cadario ME, et al: Tranquilization affects intrauterine pressure in mares administered oxytocin. *Proceedings of the forty-fourth annual convention of the American Association of Equine Practitioners*, Baltimore, 1998. pp 54-55.
29. Bedford SJ, Hinrichs K: The effect of insemination volume on pregnancy rates of pony mares, *Theriogenology* 42(4):571-578, 1994.

30. Manning ST, Bowman, PA, Fraser LM, et al: Development of hysteroscopic insemination of the uterine tube in the mare. *Proceedings of the forty-fourth annual convention of the American Association of Equine Practitioners*, Baltimore, 1998. pp 70-71.
31. Morris LH, Hunter ARHF, Allen WR: Hysteroscopic insemination of small numbers of spermatozoa at the uterotubal junction of preovulatory mares, *J Reprod Fertil* 118:95-100, 2000.
32. Squires EL, Lindsey AC, Buchanan BR: A method to obtain pregnancies in mares using minimal sperm numbers, *Proc Am Assoc Equine Pract* 46:335-337, 2000.
33. Rigby S: Oviductal sperm numbers following proximal uetrine horn or uterine body insemination. *Proceedings of the forty-sixth annual convention of the American Association of Equine Practitioners*, San Antonio, Tex, 2000. pp 332-334.
34. Youngquist RS, Threlfall W, editors: *Current therapy in large animal theriogenology*, ed 2, St Louis, 2007, Saunders.
35. denDaas N: Laboratory assessment of semen characteristics, *Anim Reprod Sci* 28:87-94, 1992.
36. Woods J, Bergfelt DR, Ginther OJ: Effects of time of insemination relative to ovulation on pregnancy rate and embryonic-loss rate in mares, *Equine Vet J* 22:410-415, 1990.
37. Huhtinen M, Koskinen E, Skidmore JA, et al: Recovery rate and quality of embryos from mares inseminated after ovulation, *Theriogenology* 45(4):719-726, 1996.
38. Katila T, Koskinen E, Kuntsi H, et al: Fertility after post ovulatory insemination in mares. *Proceedings of the eleventh International Congress on Animal Reproduction and Artificial Insemination*, 1998. pp 96.
39. Jasko DJ, Moran DM, Farlin ME, et al: Pregnancy rates utilizing fresh, cooled and frozen-thawed stallion semen. *Proceedings of the thirty-eighth annual convention of the American Association of Equine Practitioners*, Orlando, Fla, 1992. pp 649-660.
40. Squires EL, Brubake JK, McCue PM, et al: Effect of sperm number and frequency of insemination on fertility of mares inseminated with cooled semen, *Theriogenology* 49:743-749, 1998.
41. Shore MD, Macpherson ML, Combes GB, et al: Fertility comparison between breeding at 24 hours or at 24 and 48 hours after collection with cooled equine semen, *Theriogenology* 50:693-698, 1998.
42. Love CC, Thompson JA, Lowry VK, et al: The relationship between chromatin quality and fertility of chilled stallion sperm, *Proc Am Assoc Equine Pract* 47:229-231, 2001.
43. Heiskanen ML, Huhtinen M, Pirhonen A, et al: Insemination results with slow-cooled stallion semen stored for approximately 40 hours, *Acta Vet Scand* 35(3):257-262, 1994.
44. Heiskanen ML, Huhtinen M, Pirhonen A, et al: Insemination results with slow-cooled stallion semen stored for 70 or 80 hours, *Theriogenology* 42(6):1043-1051, 1994.
45. Metcalf L: Maximizing reproductive efficiency in private practice: the management of mares and the use of cryopreserved semen. *Proceedings of the Society for Theriogenology*, San Antonio, Tex, 1995. pp 155-159.
46. Metcalf ES: Pregnancy rates with cooled equine semen received in private practice, *Proc Am Assoc equine Pract* 44: 16-18, 1998.
47. Dobrinski I, Thomas PGA, Ball BA: Cryopreservation reduces the ability of equine spermatozoa to attach to oviductal epithelial cells and zonae pellucidae in vitro, *J Androl* 16: 536-542, 1995.
48. Vidament M, Dupere AM, Julienne P, et al: Equine frozen semen: freezability and fertility field results, *Theriogenology* 48(6):905-917, 1997.
49. Leipold SD, Graham JK, Squires EL, et al: Effect of spermatozoal concentration and number on fertility of frozen equine semen, *Theriogenology* 49:1537-1543, 1998.
50. Barbaracini S, Marchi V, Zavaglia G: Equine frozen semen results obtained in Italy during the 1994-1997 period, *Equine Vet Educ* 11(2):109-112, 1999.
51. Squires EL, Barabacini S, Necchi D, et al: Simplified strategy for insemination of mares with frozen semen, in *Proceedings Am Assoc Equine Pract* 49:353-356,2003.
52. Metcalf ES: Optimizing pregnancy rates using frozen-thawed equine semen, *Anim Reprod Sci* 89:297-2999, 2005.
53. Loomis PR: The equine frozen semen industry, *Anim Reprod Sci* 68:191-200, 2001.
54. Vidament M: French field results (1985-2005) on factors affecting fertility of frozen stallion semen, *Anim Reprod Sci* 89(1-4):115-136, 2005.
55. Samper JC, Hearn P, Ganheim A: Pregnancy rates and effect of extender on motility and acrosome status of frozen thawed stallion spermatozoa, *Proc Am Assoc Equine Pract* 40:41-42, 1994.
56. Volkmann DH, van Zyl D: Fertility of stallion semen frozen in 0.5-ml straws, *J Reprod Fertil* (suppl 35):143-148, 1987.

Equine Embryo Transfer

1. East LM: Equine embryo transfer: client and veterinary economics, *Equine Pract* 21(2):16-25, 1999.
2. Foss R, Wirth N, Schlitz P, et al: Nonsurgical embryo transfer in a private practice (1998), *Proc Am Assoc Equine Pract* 45: 210-212, 1999.
3. Woods GL, Baker CB, Baldwin JL, et al: Early pregnancy loss in broodmares, *J Reprod Fertil* (suppl 8):71-72, 1987.
4. Carnevale EM, Ginther OJ: Defective oocytes as a cause of subfertility in old mares, *Biol Reprod Monogr* 1:209-214, 1995.
5. Carnevale EM, Uson M, Bazzola JJ, et al: Comparison of oocytes from young and old mares with light and electron microscopy, *Theriogenology* 52:299, 1999:abstract.
6. Brinsko SP, Ball BA, Miller PG, et al: In vitro development of day 2 embryos obtained from young, fertile mares and aged, subfertile mares, *J Reprod Fertil* 102:371-378, 1994.
7. Carnevale EM, Ginther OJ: Reproductive function in old mares, *Proc Am Assoc Equine Pract* 40:15, 1994.
8. Vogelsang SG, Vogelsang MM: Influence of donor parity and age on the success of commercial equine embryo transfer, *Equine Vet J* (suppl 8):71-72, 1989.
9. Woods GL, Hillman RB, Schlafer DH: Recovery and evaluation of embryos from normal and infertile mares, *Cornell Vet* 76:386-394, 1986.
10. Squires EL: Embryo transfer, In McKinnon AO, Voss JL, editors: *Equine reproduction, Malvern, Penn*, , 1993, Lea & Febiger.
11. Carnevale EM, Ramirez RJ, Squires EL, et al: Factors affecting pregnancy rates and early embryonic death after equine embryo transfer, *Theriogenology* 54:965-979, 2000.
12. Ball BA, Little TV, Hillman RB, et al: Pregnancy rates at days 2 and 14 and estimated embryonic loss rates prior to day 14 in normal and subfertile mares, *Theriogenology* 26:611-619, 1986.
13. Ball BA, Hillman RB, Woods GL: Survival of equine embryos transferred to normal and subfertile mares, *Theriogenology* 28:167-174, 1987.
14. Carnevale EM, Griffin PG, Ginther OJ: Age-associated fertility before entry of embryos into the uterus of mares, *Equine Vet J* 15(suppl):31-35, 1993.
15. Ball BA, Little TV, Weber JA, et al: Survival of day-4 embryos from young, normal mares and aged, subfertile mares after transfer to normal recipient mares, *J Reprod Fertil* 85:187-194, 1989.
16. Carnevale EM, Thompson KN, King SS, et al: Effects of age and diet on the spring transition in mares, *Proc Am Assoc Equine Pract* 42:146-147, 1996.
17. Kubiak JR, Crawford BH, Squires EL, et al: The influence of energy intake and percentage of body fat on the reproductive performance of nonpregnant mares, *Theriogenology* 28:587-598, 1987.
18. Carnevale EM, Ginther OJ, Hermenet MJ: Age and pasture effects on vernal transition in mares, *Theriogenology* 47:1009-1018, 1996.
19. Spinelli V, Gastal MO, Gastal EL: Follicular activity in mares submitted to different nutritional diets, *Theriogenology* 57:627, 2002:abstract.

20. Carnevale EM, Bergfefelt DR, Ginther OJ: Aging effects on follicular activity and concentrations of FSH, LH and progesterone in mares, *Anim Repro Sci* 31:287-299, 1993.
21. Carnevale EM, Bergfefelt DR, Ginther OJ: Follicular activity and concentrations of FSH LH associated with senescence in mares, *Anim Repro Sci* 35:231-246, 1994.
22. Ginther OJ: *Reproductive biology of the mare: basic and applied aspects,* ed 2, Cross Plains, Wis, 1992, Equiservices.
23. Jacob JCF, Dominguew IB, Gastal EL, et al: The impact of degree of synchrony between donors and recipients in a commercial equine embryo transfer program, *Theriogenology* 57:545, 2002:abstract.
24. Foss R: Personal communication, 2002.
25. Youngquist RS, editor: *Current therapy in large animal theriogenology,* ed 2, St Louis, 2007, Saunders.
26. Hinriches K, Sertich PL, Palmer E, et al: Pregnancy in ovariectomised mares achieved by embryo transfer in ovariectomized mares treated with progesterone, *J Reprod Fertil* 80:395-401, 1987.
27. Hinrichs K, Sertich PL, Kenney RM: Use of altrenogest to prepare ovariectomized mares as embryo transfer recipients, *Theriogenology* 26:455-460, 1986.
28. McKinnon AO, Squires EL, Carnevale EM, et al: Ovariectomized steroid-treated mares as embryo transfer recipients and as a model to study the role of progestins in pregnancy maintenance, *Theriogenology* 29:1055-1063, 1988.
29. Lagneau D, Palmer E: Embryo transfer in anestrous recipient mares: attempts to reduce altrenogest administration period by treatment with pituitary extract, *Equine Vet J* 15(suppl): 107-111, 1993.
30. McCue PM, Vanderwall DK, Keith SL, et al: Equine embryo transfer: influence of endogenous progesterone concentration in recipients on pregnancy outcome, *Theriogenology* 51:267, 1999:abstract.
31. Sevinga M, Schukken YH, Hesselink JW, et al: Relationship between ultrasonic characteristics of the corpus luteum, plasma progesterone concentration and early pregnancy diagnosis in Fresian mares, *Theriogenology* 52:585-592, 1999.
32. Walton A, Hammond J: The maternal effects on growth and conformation in Shire horse-Shetland pony crosses, *Proc R Soc B* 125:311-335, 1938.
33. Allen WR: The physiology of later pregnancy in the mare. *Proceedings of the Equine Symposium and Society for Theriogenology*, Nov 28-Dec 2, 2000. pp 3-15.
34. Wilsher S, Allen WR: The influence of maternal size, age and parity on placental and fetal development in the horse, Proceedings of the 5th International Symp on Equine Embayo Transfer Editors: Katila T, Wade JF. R&W Publications, Newmarket, 2001, pp. 74-75.
35. Franc AT, Amann RP, Squires EL, et al: Motility and infertility of equine spermatozoa in milk extender over 24 hr at 20° C, *Theriogenology* 27:517-526, 1987.
36. Metcalf L: Maximizing reproductive efficiency in private practice: the management of mares and the use of cryopreserved semen. *Proceedings of the Society for Theriogenology*, San Antonio, Tex, 1995. pp 155-159.
37. Pycock JF, Newcombe JR: Endometritis, salpingitis and fertilisation rates after mating mares with a history of intrauterine intraluminal fluid accumulation, *Equine Vet J* 25(suppl): 109-112, 1997.
38. Squires EL, McCue PM, Vanderwall D: The current status of equine embryo transfer, *Theriogenology* 51:91-104, 1999.
39. McCue PM: Review of ovarian abnormalities in the mare, *Proc Am Assoc Equine Pract* 44:125-133, 1998.
40. Freeman DA, Weber JA, Geary RT, et al: Time of embryo transport through the mares's oviduct, *Theriogenology* 36: 823-830, 1991.
41. Squires EL, Seidel GE Jr: Collection and transfer of equine embryos, Animal Reproduction and Biotechnology Laboratory Bulletin No. 11, Fort Collins, 1995, Colorado State University.
42. Fleury JJ, Alvarenga MA: Effects of collection day on embryo recovery and pregnancy rates in a nonsurgical equine transfer program, *Theriogenology* 51:261, 1999:abstract.
43. Peres KR, Trinque CLN, Lima MM, et al: Non-surgical equine embryo transfer: a retrospective study, *Theriogenology* 57:558, 2002:abstract.
44. LeBlanc MM, DeLille A, Cadario ME, et al: Tranquilization affects intrauterine pressure in mares administered oxytocin, *Proc Am Assoc Equine Pract* 44:54-55, 1998.
45. Ginther OJ, Bergfelt DR, Leith GS, et al: Embryonic loss in mares: incidence and ultrasonic morphology, *Theriogenology* 24:73-86, 1985.
46. Carney NJ, Squires EL, Cook VM, et al: Comparison of pregnancy rates from transfer of fresh vs cooled transported equine embryos, *Theriogenology* 36:23-32, 1991.
47. Carnevale EM, Squires EL, McKinnon AO: Comparison of Ham's F10 with CO2 or Hepes buffer for storage of equine embryos at 5 C for 24 H, *J Anim Sci* 65:1775-1781, 1987.
48. Moussa M, Duchamp G, Bruyas JF, et al: Comparison of embryo quality of cooled stored equine embryos using 3 embryo holding solutions, *Theriogenology* 57:554, 2002:abstract.
49. Fleury JJ, Fleury PDC, Landim-Alvarenga FC: Storage of equine embryos in hepes-buffered Ham's F-10 at 15-18 degrees C for different periods of time: preliminary results, *Theriogenology* 51:261, 1999:abstract.
50. Squires EL, Cook VM, Jasko DJ, et al: Pregnancy rates after collection and shipment of equine embryos (1988-1991), *Proc Am Assoc Equine Pract* 38:609-618, 1992.

The Pregnant Mare

1. Betteridge KJ, et al: Development of horse embryos up to twenty-two days after ovulation: observations on fresh specimens, *J Anat* 135:191-209, 1982.
2. Allen WR: Fetomaternal interactions and influences during equine pregnancy, *Reproduction* 121(4):513-527, 2001.
3. Ginther OJ: *Reproductive biology of the mare: basic and applied aspects*, ed 2, Cross Plains, 1992, Wis, Equiservices.
4. Ginther OJ: Equine pregnancy: physical interactions between the uterus and conceptus, *Am Assoc Eq Pract* 44:73-104, 1998.
5. Stout TA, Meadows S, Allen WR: Stage-specific formation of the equine blastocyst capsule is instrumental to hatching and to embryonic survival in vivo, *Animal Reprod Sci* 87(3-4): 269-281, 2005.
6. Griffin PG, Ginther OJ: Effects of the embryo on uterine morphology and function in mares, *Anim Reprod Sci* 31:311-329, 1993.
7. Leith GS, Ginther OJ: Characterization of intrauterine mobility of the early conceptus, *Theriogenology* 22:401-408, 1984.
8. Ginther OJ: Mobility of the early equine conceptus, *Theriogenology* 19:603-611, 1983.
9. Stout TA, Allen WR: Role of prostaglandins in intrauterine migration of the equine conceptus, *Reproduction* 121(5):771-775, 2001.
10. Douglas RH, Ginther OJ: Concentration of prostaglandins F in uterine venous plasma of anaesthetized mares during the estrous cycle and early pregnancy, *Prostaglandins* 11:251-260, 1976.
11. Sharp DC, et al: Relationship between endometrial oxytocin receptors and oxytocin-induced prostaglandin F2 alpha release during the oestrous cycle and early pregnancy in pony mares, *J Repro Fertil* 109(1):137-144, 1997.
12. Starbuck GR, et al: Endometrial oxytocin receptor and uterine prostaglandin secretion in mares during the oestrous cycle and early pregnancy, *J Repro Fertil* 113(2):173-179, 1998.
13. Tannus RJ, Thun R: Influence of endometrial cysts on conception rate of mares, *Zentralblatt fur Veterinarmedizin -Reihe A* 42(4):275-283, 1995.

14. van Ittersum AR: [The electrosurgical treatment of endometrial cysts in the mare], *Tijdschr Diergeneeskd* 124(21):630-633, 1999.
15. Bracher V, Mathias S, Allen WR: Videoendoscopic examination of the mare's uterus. II. Findings in sub-fertile mares, *Equine Vet J* 24:279-284, 1992.
16. McDowell KJ, et al: Restricted conceptus mobility results in failure of pregnancy maintenance in mares, *Biol Reprod* 39:340-348, 1988.
17. Ginther OJ: Local versus systemic utero-ovarian relationships in farm animals, *Acta Vet Scand* (suppl 77):103-115, 1981.
18. Ginther OJ: Comparative anatomy of utero-ovarian vasculature, *Vet Scope* 20:3-17, 1976.
19. Silva LA, Ginther OJ: An early endometrial vascular indicator of completed orientation of the embryo and the role of dorsal endometrial encroachment in mares, *Biol Reprod* 74(2): 337-343, 2006.
20. Silva LA, et al: Changes in vascular perfusion of the endometrium in association with changes in location of the embryonic vesicle in mares 72:755-761, 2005.
21. Ginther OJ: Fixation and orientation of the early equine conceptus, *Theriogenology* 19:613-623, 1983.
22. Feo JC: Contralateral implantation in mares mated during post partum oestrus, *Vet Rec* 106:368, 1980.
23. Griffin PG, Ginther OJ: Uterine morphology and function in postpartum mares, *J Equine Vet Sci* 11:330-339, 1991.
24. Steven DH, Samuel CA: Anatomy of the placental barrier in the mare, *J Reprod Fertil* (suppl 23):579-582, 1975.
25. Samuel CA, Allen WR, Steven DH: Ultra-structural development of the equine placenta, *J Reprod Fert* (suppl 23):575-578, 1975.
26. Samuel CA, Allen WR, Steven DH: Studies on the equine placenta II. Ultrastructure of the placental barrier, *J Reprod Fertil* 48:257-264, 1976.
27. Samuel CA, Allen WR, Steven DH: Studies on the equine placenta III. Ultrastructure of the uterine glands and the overlying trophoblast, *J Reprod Fert* 51:433-437, 1977.
28. Wooding FBP, A.L. Fowden: Nutrient transfer across the equine placenta: correlation of structure and function, *Eq Vet J* 38(2):175-183, 2006.
29. Whitehead AE, Chenier TS, Foster RA: Placental characteristics of Standardbred mares. in American Association of Equine Practitioners, Seattle, 2005, Wash, The Association.
30. Whitwell KE, Jeffcott LB: Morphological studies on the fetal mambranes of the normal singleton foal at term, *ResVetSci* 14:44-55, 1975.
31. Vandeplassche M: Aetiology, pathogenesis and treatment of retained placenta in the mare, *Equine Vet Educ* 3:144, 1971.
32. Allen W, Kolling M, Wilsher S: An interesting case of early pregnancy loss in a mare with persistent endometrial cups, *Equine Vet Educ* 19:539-544, 2007.
33. Sibbons P: The role of stereology in the study of placental transfer between fetal foal and mare, *Equine Vet J* 38(2): 106-107, 2006.
34. Gerstenberg C, Allen WR, Stewart F: Cell proliferation patterns during development of the equine placenta, *J Repro Fertil* 117(1):143-152, 1999.
35. Wilsher S, Allen WR: Effects of a Streptococcus equi infection-mediated nutritional insult during mid-gestation in primiparous Thoroughbred fillies. Part 1: placental and fetal development, *Equine Vet J* 38(6):549-557, 2006.
36. Abd-Elnaeim MM, et al: Structural and haemovascular aspects of placental growth throughout gestation in young and aged mares, *Placenta* 27(11-12):1103-1113, 2006.
37. Allen WR, Gower S, Wilsher S: Immunohistochemical localization of vascular endothelial growth factor (VEGF) and its two receptors (Flt-I and KDR) in the endometrium and placenta of the mare during the oestrous cycle and pregnancy, *Reprod Domest Anim* 42(5):516-526, 2007.
38. Bracher V, Mathias S, Allen WR: Influence of chorionic degenerative endometritis (endometrosis) on placental development in the mare, *Equine Vet J* 28:180-188, 1996.
39. Kenny RM: In John P Hughes International Workshop on Equine Endometritis. 1993: *Equine Vet J*.
40. Schoon D, Schoon H-A, Klug E: Angiosis in the equine endometrium: pathogenesis and clinical correlations, *Pferdeheilkunde* 15:541-546, 1999.
41. Kenny RM: Cyclic and pathologic changes of the mare endometrium as detected by biopsy, with a note on early embryonic death, *J Am Vet Med Assoc* 172:241-262, 1978.
42. Doig PA, McKnight JD, Miller RB: The use of endometrial biopsy in the infertile mare, *Can Vet J* 22:72-76, 1981.
43. Gordon LR, Sartin EM: Endometrial biospsy as an aid to diagnosis and prognosis in equine infertility, *J Equine Med Surg* 2:328-336, 1978.
44. Gruninger B, et al: Incidence and morphology of endometrial angiopathies in mares in relationship to age and parity, *J Comp Pathol* 119(3):293-309, 1998.
45. Wilsher S, Allen WR: The effects of maternal age and parity on placental and fetal development in the mare, *Equine Vet J* 35(5):476-483, 2003.
46. Cotrill CM, et al: The placenta as a determinant of fetal wellbeing in normal and abnormal equine pregnancies, *J Reprod Fert* (suppl 44):591-601, 1991.
47. Allen WR: The physiology of later pregnancy in the mare, in The periparturient mare and neonate, San Antonio, Tex, 2000, Society for Theriogenology, pp 3-15.
48. Rossdale P, Ousey J: Fetal programming for athletic performance in the horse: potential effects of IUGR, *Equine Vet Educ* 14:98-112, 2002.
49. Whitwell KE: Investigations into fetal and neonatal losses in the horse, *Vet Clin North Am* 2:313-331, 1980.
50. Jeffcott LB, Whitwell KE: Twinning as a cause of fetal and neonatal loss in Thoroughbred mares, *J Comp Pathol* 83: 91-106, 1973.
51. Heilkenbrinker T, et al: [Examination of the appropriateness of anamnestic and clinical parameters for the prediction of the course of pregnancy under field conditions], *Dtsch Tierarztl Wochenschr* 104(8):313-316, 1997.
52. Tischner M, Klimczak M: The development of Polish ponies born after embryo transfer to large recipients, *Equine Vet J* (suppl 8):62-63, 1989.
53. Wilsher S, Allen WR: The influence of maternal size, age and parity on placental and fetal development in the horse, In Katila T, Wade J, editors: *Havemeyer Monograph* Vol. 3, New York, 2000, D R Havemeyer Foundation.
54. Allen WR, et al: The influence of maternal size on placental, fetal and postnatal growth in the horse. II. Endocrinology of pregnancy, *J Endocrinol* 172(2):237-246, 2002.
55. Allen WR, et al: The influence of maternal size on pre- and postnatal growth in the horse: III Postnatal growth, *Reproduction* 127(1):67-77, 2004.
56. Ousey JC, et al: Effects of manipulating intrauterine growth on post natal adrenocortical development and other parameters of maturity in neonatal foals, *Equine Vet J* 36(7):616-621, 2004.
57. Walton A, Hammond J: The maternal effects on growth and conformation in Shire horse-Shetland pony crosses, *Proc R Soc B* 125:311-335, 1938.
58. Allen WR, Short RV: Interspecific and extraspecific pregnancies in equids: anything goes, *J Heredity* 88(5):384-392, 1997.
59. Allen WR, Moor RM: The origin of the equine endometrial cups. I. Production of PMSG by fetal trophoblast cells, *J Reprod Fertil* 29:313-316, 1972.
60. Allen WR, Hamilton DW, Moor RM: The origin of equine endometrial cups. II. Invasion of the endometrium by trophoblast, *Anat Rec* 177:485-501, 1973.

61. Enders AC, Liu IKM: Lodgement of the equine blastocyst in the uterus from fixation through endometrial cup formation, *J Reprod Fert* (suppl 44):427-438, 1991.
62. Stewart F, Lennard SN, Allen WR: Mechanisms controlling formation of the quine chorionic girdle, *Biol Reprod* 1:151-159, 1995:Mono.
63. Enders AC, Liu IKM: Trophoblast-uterine interactions during equine chorionic girdle cell maturation, migration, and transformation, *Am J Anat* 192:366-381, 1991.
64. Hamilton DW, Allen WR, Moor RM: The origin of equine endometrial cups. III. Light and electron microscopic study of fully developed equine endometrial cups, *Anat Rec* 177:503-518, 1973.
65. Lunn P, Vagnoni KE, Ginther OJ: The equine immune response to endometrial cups, *J Reprod Immunol* 34:203-216, 1997.
66. Antczak DF, Allen WR: Maternal immunological recognition of pregnancy in equids, *J Reprod Fertil* (suppl 37):69-78, 1989.
67. Antczak DF, Allen WR: Invasive trophoblast in the genus *Equus*, *Ann Immunol* 135:301-351, 1984.
68. Allen WR: Immunological aspects of the endometrial cup reaction and the effect of xenogeneic pregnancy in horses and donkeys, *J Reprod Fertil* (suppl 31):57-94, 1982.
69. Clegg MT, Boda JM, Cole HH: The endometrial cups and allantochorionic pouches in the mare with emphasis on the source of equine gonadotrophin, *Endocrinology* 54:448-463, 1954.
70. Stewart F, Allen WR, Moor RM: Pregnant mare serum gonadotrophin: Ratio of follicle-stimulating hormone and luteinizing hormone activities measured by radioreceptor assay, *J Endocrinology* 71:371-382, 1976.
71. Evans MJ, Irvine CHG: Serum concentrations of FSH, LH and progesterone during the estrous cycle and early pregnancy in the mare, *J Reprod Fertil* (suppl 23):193-200, 1975.
72. Purcell SH, et al: Aspiration of oocytes from transitional, cycling, and pregnant mares, *Anim Reprod Sci* 100(3-4):291-300, 2007.
73. Urwin V, Allen WR: Pituitary and chorionic gonadotrophin control of ovarian function during early pregnancy in equids, *J Reprod Fertil* (suppl 32):371-382, 1982.
74. Bergfeldt DR, Pierson RA, Ginther OJ: Resurgence of the primary corpus luteum during pregnancy in the mare, *Anim Reprod Sci* 21:261-270, 1989.
75. Daels PF, Albrecht BA, Mohammed HO: Equine chorionic gonadotropin regulates luteal steroidogenesis in pregnant mares, *Biol Reprod* 59(5):1062-1068, 1998.
76. Holton DW, et al: Effect of ovariectomy on pregnancy in mares, *J Reprod Fertil* (suppl 27):457-463, 1979.
77. Bhavnani BR, Short RV, Solomon S: Formation of estrogens by the pregnant mare. II. Metabolism of 14C-acetate and 3H-cholesterol injected into the fetal circulation, *Endocrinology* 89:1152-1157, 1971.
78. Bhavnani BR, Short RV, Solomon S: Formation of estrogens by the pregnant mare. I. Metabolism of 7-3-H-dehydroisoandrosterone and 4-14 C-androstenedione injected into the umbilical vein, *Endocrinology* 85:1172-1179, 1969.
79. Pashen RL, Allen WR: The role of the fetal gonads and placenta in steroid production, maintenance of pregnancy and parturition in the mare, *J Reprod Fertil* (suppl 27):499-509, 1979.
80. Holtan DW, et al: Effect of ovariectomy on pregnancy in mares, *J Reprod Fertil* (suppl 27):457-463, 1975.
81. Holtan DW: Progestin therapy in mares with pregnancy complications: necessity and efficacy, *in Am Assoc Eq Pract* 1993.
82. Daels PF, et al: Efficacy of treatments to prevent abortion in pregnant mares at risk, *In Am Assoc Equine Pract* 40:31-32, 1994.
83. Ousey JC: Hormone profiles and treatments in the late pregnant mare, *Vet Clin North Am: Equine Pract* 22(3):727-747, 2006.
84. Macpherson ML, Reimer JM: Twin reduction in the mare: current options, *Animal Reprod Sci* :233-644, 2000:60-61.
85. Steiner J, et al: Persistent endometrial cups, *Ann Reprod Sci* 94:274-275, 2006.
86. Daels PF, et al: The corpus luteum: sources of estrogen during early pregnancy in the mare, *J Reprod Fertil* (suppl 44):501-508, 1991.
87. Squires EL, Garcia MC, Ginther OJ: Effects of pregnancy and hysterectomy on the ovaries of pony mares, *J Anim Sci* 38:823-830, 1974.
88. Cox JE: Estrone and equilin in the plasma of the pregnant mare, *J Reprod Fertil* (suppl 23):463-468, 1975.
89. Ousey JC: Peripartal endocrinology in the mare and foetus, *Reprod Domest Anim* 39(4):222-231, 2004.
90. Bhavnani BR, Short RV: Formation of steroids by the pregnant mare. IV. Metabolism of 14C-mevalonic acid and 3H-dehydroisoandrosterone injected into the fetal circulation, *Endocrinology* 92:1397-1404, 1973.
91. Tait AD, Santikarn LC, Allen WR: Identification of 3beta-hydroxy-5,7 androstadien-17-one as endogenous steroids in the fetal horse gonad, *J Endocrinology* 99:87-92, 1983.
92. Hay MF, Allen WR: An ultrastructural and histochemical study of the interstitial cells in the gonads of the fetal horse, *J Reprod Fertil* (suppl 23):557-561, 1975.
93. Merchant-Larios H: Ultrastructural events in horse gonadal morphogenesis, *J Reprod Fertil* (suppl 27):479-485, 1979.
94. Pashen RL: Maternal and fetal endocrinology during late pregnancy and parturition in the mare, *Equine Vet J* 16:233-238, 1984.
95. Walt ML, et al: Development of the equine ovary and ovulation fossa, *J Reprod Fert* (suppl 27):471-477, 1979.
96. Raeside JI, Liptrap RM: Patterns of urinary estrogen excretion in individual pregnant mares, *J Reprod Fertil* (suppl 23):469-475, 1975.
97. Lima SB, Verreschi IT, Ribeiro Neto LM: Reversed-phase liquid chromatographic method for estrogen determination in equine biological samples, *J Chrom Sci* 39(9):385-387, 2001.
98. Mostl E: The horse feto-placental unit, *Exp Clin Endocrinol* 102(3):166-168, 1994.
99. Santschi E, LeBlanc MM, Weston PG: Progestagen, oestrone sulphate and cortisol concentrations in pregnant mares during medical and surgical disease, *J Reprod Fertil* (suppl 44):627-634, 1991.
100. Stabenfeldt GH, et al: An oestrogen conjugate enzyme immunoassay for monitoring pregnancy in the mare: limitations of the assay between days 40 and 70 of gestation, *J Reprod Fertil* (suppl 44):37-44, 1991.
101. Terqui M, Palmer E: Oestrogen pattern during early pregnancy in the mare, *J Reprod Fert* 27:441-446, 1979.
102. Allen WR: Luteal deficiency and embryo mortality in the mare, *Reprod Domest Anim* 36(3-4):121-131, 2001.
103. Hamon M, et al: Production of 5-alpha-dihydroprogesterone during late pregnancy in the mare, *J Reprod Fertil* (suppl 44):529-535, 1991.
104. Fowden AL, Silver M: Effects of inhibiting 3beta-hydroxysteroid dehydrogenase on plasma progesterone and other steroids in the pregnant mare near term, *J Reprod Fertil* (suppl 35):539-545, 1987.
105. Han X, et al: Localisation of 15-hydroxy prostaglandin dehydrogenase (PGDH) and steroidogenic enzymes in the equine placenta, *Equine Vet J* 27(5):334-339, 1995.
106. Holtan DW, Nett TM, Estergreen VL: Plasma progestins in pregnant, postpartum and cycling mares, *J Anim Sci* 40:251-260, 1975.

107. Troedsson MHT: *Myometrial activity and progestin supplementation, in Periparturient mare and neonate*, San Antonio, Tex, 2000, Society for Theriogenology, p. 17-24.
108. Nagy P, et al: Progesterone determination in equine plasma using different immunoassays, *Acta Veterinaria Hungarica* 46(4):501-513, 1998.
109. Ousey J, et al: Ontogeny of uteroplacental progestagen production in pregnant mares during the second half of gestation, *Biol Reprod* 69:540-548, 2003.
110. Holton DW, et al: Plasma progestagens in the mare fetus and newborn foal, *J Reprod Fert* (suppl 44):517-528, 1991.
111. Schutzer WE, Holtan DW: Steroid transformations in pregnant mares: metabolism of exogenous progestins and unusual metabolic activity in vivo and in vitro, *Steroids* 61(2):94-949, 1996.
112. Arai KY, et al: Expression of inhibins, activins, insulin-like growth factor-I and steroidogenic enzymes in the equine placenta [electronic resource] 31:19-34, 2006.
113. Chavatte P, et al: Biosynthesis and possible biological roles of progestagens during equine pregnancy and in the newborn foal, *Equine Vet J* (suppl 24):89-95, 1997.
114. Schutzer WE, Kerby JL, Holtan DW: Differential effect of trilostane on the progestin milieu in the pregnant mare, *J Reprod Fertil* 107(2):241-248, 1996.
115. Thorburn GD: A speculative view of parturition in the mare, *Equine Vet J* (suppl 14):41-49, 1993.
116. Rossdale PD, et al: Increase in plasma progesterone concentrations in the mare after fetal injection with CRH, ACTH or betamethasone in late gestation, *Equine Vet J* 24:347-350, 1992.
117. Houghton E, et al: Plasma progestagen concentrations in the normal and dysmature newborn foal, *J Reprod Fertil* (suppl 44):609-617, 1991.
118. Brendemeuhl JP, et al: Plasma progestagen, tri-iodothyronine, and cortisol concentrations in postdate gestation foals exposed in utero to the tall fescue endophyte *Acremonium coenophialum*, *Biol Reprod* 1:53-59, 1995:Mono.
119. Holtan DW, Nett TM, Estergreen VL: Plasma progesterone in pregnant mares, *J Reprod Fertil* (suppl 23):419-424, 1975.
120. Haluska GJ, Currie WB: Variation in plasma concentrations of estradiol-17beta and their relationship to those of progesterone, 13,14-dihydro-15-keto-prostaglandin F-2alpha and oxytocin across pregnancy and at parturition in pony mares, *J Reprod Fertil* 84:635-646, 1988.
121. Rossdale PD, et al: Effects of placental pathology on maternal plasma progestagen and mammary secretion calcium concentrations and on neonatal adrenocortical function in the horse, *J Reprod Fertil* (suppl 44):579-590, 1991.
122. Ousey JC, et al: The effects of intrafetal ACTH administration on the outcome of pregnancy in the mare, *Reprod Fertil Dev* 10(4):359-367, 1998.
123. Liggins GC, et al: Parturition in the sheep, *Ciba Fdn Symp* 47:5-30, 1977.
124. Liggins GC, Thorburn GD: Role of the fetal pituitary-adrenal system and placenta in the initiation of parturition. In Lamming GE, editor: *Marshall's physiology of reproduction*, London, 1993, Chapman & Hall.
125. Liggins GC: Adrenocortical-related maturational events in the fetus, *Am J Obstet Gynecol* 126:931-939, 1976.
126. Rossdale PD, Ousey JC, Chavatte P: Readiness for birth: an endocrinological duet between fetal foal and mare, *Equine Vet J Suppl* (24):96-99, 1997.
127. Silver M: Prenatal maturation, the timing of birth and how it may be regulated in domestic animals, *Exp Physiol* 75:285-307, 1990.
128. Lovell JD, et al: Endocrine patterns of the mare at term, *J Reprod Fertil* (suppl 23):449-456, 1975.
129. Fowden A, Silver M: Comparative development of the pituitary-adrenal axis in the fetal foal and lamb, *Reprod Domest Anim* 30:170-177, 1995.
130. Cudd T, et al: Ontogeny and ultradian rhythms of adrenocorticotropin and cortisol in the late-gestation fetal horse, *J Endocrinol* 144:271-283, 1995.
131. O'Donnell LJ, et al: 24-hour secretion patterns of plasma oestradiol 17beta in pony mares in late gestation, *Reprod Domest Anim* 38:233-235, 2003.
132. Ousey JC, et al: Effects of maternally administered depot ACTH(1-24) on fetal maturation and the timing of parturition in the mare, *Equine Vet J* 32(6):489-496, 2000.
133. Ousey J, Koelling M, Allen W: The effects of maternal dexamethasone treatment on gestation length and foal maturation in Thoroughbred mares, *Anim Reprod Sci* 94:436-438, 2006.
134. Chavatte P, Rossdale P, Tait AD: 11beta-Hydroxysteroid dehydrogenase (11BHSD) in equine placenta, *In Am Assoc Equine Pract* 41:264-265, 1995.
135. Stewart DR, et al: Breed differences in circulating equine relaxin, *Biol Reprod* 46:648-652, 1992.
136. Klonish T, Hombach-Klonisch S: Review: relaxin expression at the feto-maternal interface, *Reprod Dom Anim* 35:149-152, 2000.
137. Haluska GJ, Lowe JE, Currie WB: Electromyographic properties of the myometrium correlated with the endocrinology of the pre-partum and post-partum periods and parturition in Pony mares, *J Reprod Fertil* (suppl 35):553-564, 1987.
138. Stewart DR, et al: Concentrations of 15-keto-13,14-dihydroprostaglandin F2alpha in the mare during spontaneous and oxytocin induced foaling, *Equine Vet J* 16:270-274, 1984.
139. Bryant-Greenwood GD: Relaxin as a new hormone, *Endocrine Rev* 3:62-90, 1982.
140. Stewart DR, et al: Determination of the source of equine relaxin, *Biol Reprod* 27:17-24, 1982.
141. Klonisch T, et al: Placental localization of relaxin in the pregnant mare, *Placenta* 18(2-3):121-128, 1997.
142. Stewart DR, Stabenfeldt GH: Relaxin activity in the pregnant mare, *Biol Reprod* 25:281-289, 1981.
143. Pashen RL, et al: Dehydroepiandrosterone synthesis by the fetal foal and its importance as an estrogen precursor, *J Reprod Fertil* (suppl 32):389-397, 1982.
144. Thorburn GD: The placenta, prostaglandins and parturition: a review, *Reprod Fertil Dev* 3:277-294, 1991.
145. Stewart DR, Stabenfeldt GH, Hughes JP: Relaxin activity in foaling mares, *J Reprod Fert* (suppl 32):603, 1982.
146. Silver M: Prostaglandins in maternal and fetal plasma, and in allantoic fluid during the second half of gestation in the mare, *J Reprod Fertil* 27:531-539, 1979.
147. Allen WE, Chard T, Forsling ML: Peripheral plasma levels of oxytocin and vasopressin in the mare during parturition, *J Endocrinol* 57:175-176, 1973.
148. Barnes RJ, et al: Fetal and maternal plasma concentrations of 13,14-dihydro-15-oxoprostaglandin F in mares during late pregnancy and at parturition, *J Endocrinol* 78:201-215, 1978.
149. Vivrette SL, et al: Oxytocin release and its relationship to dihydro-15-keto PGF2alpha and arginine vasopressin release during parturition and to suckling in postpartum mares, *J Reprod Fertil* 119(2):347-357, 2000.
150. Vivrette SL, et al: Effects of flunixin meglumine on pituitary effluent oxytocin, arginine vasopressin, and 15-ketodihydroprostaglandin F2a concentrations and clinical parturient events during oxytocin-induced parturition in mares, *Biol Reprod* 1:69-75, 1995:Mono.
151. Roser JF, et al: Plasma prolactin concentrations after oxytocin induction of parturition, *Dom Anim Endocrinol* 6:101-110, 1989.
152. Worthy K, et al: Plasma prolactin concentrations and cyclic activity in pony mares during parturition and early lactation, *J Reprod Fertil* 77:569-574, 1986.

153. Aurich C, Aurich JE, Parvizi N: Opioidergic inhibition of luteinising hormone and prolactin release changes during pregnancy in pony mares, *J Endocrinol* 169(3):511-518, 2001.
154. Strickland JR, et al: Effects of ergovaline, loline, and dopamine antagonists on rat pituitary cell prolactin release in vitro, *Am J Vet Res* 55(5):716-721, 1994.
155. Strickland JR, et al: The effect of alkaloids and seed extracts of endophyte-infected tall fescue on prolactin secretion in an in vitro rat pituitary perfusion system, *J Anim Sci* 70:2779-2786, 1992.
156. Ireland FW, et al: Effects of bromocryptine and perphenazine on prolactin and progesterone concentrations in pregnant pony mares during late gestation, *J Reprod Fertil* 92:179-186, 1991.
157. Bonafos LD, et al: Development of uterine tone in nonbred and pregnant mares, *Theriogenology* 42:1247-1255, 1994.
158. van Niekerk CH: Early clinical diagnosis of pregnancy in mares, *J So Afr Vet Med Assoc* 36:53-58, 1965.
159. Cadario ME, et al: Changes in intrauterine pressure after oxytocin administration in reproductively normal mares and in those with a delay in uterine clearance, *Theriogenology* 51(5):1017-1025, 1999.
160. Rasch K, et al: Histomorphological endometrial status and influence of oxytocin on the uterine drainage and pregnancy rate in mares, *Equine Vet J* 28(6):455-460, 1996.
161. Ginther OJ: Dynamic physical interactions between equine embryo and uterus, *Equine Vet J* (suppl 3):41-47, 1985.
162. Cross DT, Ginther OJ: Uterine contractions in nonpregnant and early pregnant mares and jennies as determined by ultrasonography, *J Anim Sci* 66:250-254, 1988.
163. Griffin PG, Ginther OJ: Uterine contractile activity in mares during the estrous cycle and early pregnancy, *Theriogenology* 34:47-56, 1990.
164. Leith GS, Ginther OJ: Mobility of the conceptus and uterine contractions in the mare, *Theriogenology* 22:401-408, 1985.
165. Hayes KEN, Ginther OJ: Role of progesterone and estrogen in development of uterine tone in mares, *Theriogenology* 25:581-590, 1986.
166. Gastal MO, et al: Transvaginal intrauterine injections in mares: Effect of prostaglandin E2, *Theriogenology* 49:258, 1998.
167. Watson ED, Sertich PL: Prostaglandin production by horse embryos and the effect of co-culture of embryos with endometrium from pregnant mares, *J Reprod Fertil* 8(7):331-336, 1989.
168. Zavy MT, et al: An investigation of the uterine luminal environment of non-pregnant and pregnant pony mares, *J Reprod Fertil* (suppl 27):403-411, 1979.
169. Bessent C, Cross DT, Ginther OJ: Effect of exogenous estradiol on the mobility and fixation of the early equine conceptus, *Anim Reprod Sci* 16:159-167, 1988.
170. Walters KW, Roser JF, Anderson GB: Maternal-conceptus signalling during early pregnancy in mares: oestrogen and insulin-like growth factor I, *Reproduction* 121(2):331-338, 2001.
171. Kastelic JP, Adams GP, Ginther OJ: Role of progesterone in the mobility, fixation, orientation and maintenance of the equine conceptus, *Theriogenology* 27:655-663, 1987.
172. Daels PF, et al: Effect of progesterone on prostaglandin F2 alpha secretion and outcome of pregnancy during cloprostenol-induced abortion in mares, *Am JVet Res* 57(9):1331-1337, 1996.
173. Vernon MW, et al: Prostaglandin in the equine endometrium: Steroid modulation and production capacities during the estrous cycle and early pregnancy, *Biol Reprod* 25:581-589, 1981.
174. Gastal MO, et al: Effect of oxytocin, prostaglandin F2 alpha, and clenbuterol on uterine dynamics in mares, *Theriogenology* 50(4):521-534, 1998.
175. Gutjahr S, et al: Effect of dose and day of treatment on uterine response to oxytocin in mares, *Theriogenology* 54(3):447-456, 2000.
176. Daels PF, et al: Endogenous prostaglandin secretion during cloprostenol-induced abortion in mares, *Ann Reprod Sci* 40:305-321, 1995.
177. Csapo AI: Progesterone "block"," *Am J Anat* 98:273-291, 1956.
178. Fowden AL, et al: Uteroplacental production of 5alpha-pregnane-3,20-dione (5alpha DHP) in pregnant mares, *Theriogenology* 58:821-824, 2002.
179. Chavatte-Palmer P, et al: Progesterone, oestrogen and glucocorticoid receptors in the uterus and mammary gland of mid-to late-gestation, *J Reprod Fertil* (suppl 56):661-672, 2000.
180. Behrendt-Adam CY, et al: Oxytocin-neurophysin I mRNA abundance in equine uterine endometrium, *Dom Anim Endocrinol* 16(3):183-192, 1999.
181. Ousey JC, et al: The effects of oxytocin and progestagens on myometrial contractility in vitro during equine pregnancy, *J Reprod Fertil* (suppl 56):681-691, 2000.
182. LeBlanc MM: Equine perinatology: what we know and what we need to know, *Anim Reprod Sci* 42:189-196, 1996.
183. Dudan FE, et al: Frequency distribution and daily rhythm of uterine electromyographic epochs of different duration in Pony mares in late gestation, *J Reprod Fert* (suppl 35):725-727, 1987.
184. McGlothlin JA, et al: Alteration in uterine contractility in mares with experimentally induced placentitis, *Reproduction* 127(1):57-66, 2004.
185. Camillo F, et al: Clinical studies on daily low dose oxytocin in mares at term, *Equine Vet J* 32(4):307-310, 2000.
186. Eroksuz H, et al: Equine goiter associated with excess dietary iodine, *Vet Hum Toxicol* 46(3):147-149, 2004.
187. Youngquist RS, Threlfall W, editors: *Current therapy in large animal theriogenology*, ed 2, St Louis, 2007, Saunders.
188. Pritchard JT, Voss JL: Fetal ankylosis in horses associated with hybrid Sudan pasture, *J Am Vet Med Assoc* 150:871-873, 1967.
189. Schutte JG, van den Ingh TS: Microphthalmia, brachygnathia superior, and palatocheiloschisis in a foal associated with griseofulvin administration to the mare during early pregnancy, *Vet Q* 19(2):58-60, 1997.
190. Toribio RE, et al: Congenital defects in newborn foals of mares treated for equine protozoal myeloencephalitis during pregnancy, *J Am Vet Med Assoc* 212(5):697-701, 1998.
191. Ginther OJ: *Ultrasonic imaging and animal reproduction: Book 2. Horses*, Cross Plains, Wis, 1995, Equiservices.
192. Ginther OJ: *Ultrasonic imaging and animal reproduction: Book 1. Fundamentals*, Cross Plains, Wis, 1995, Equiservices.
193. Enders AC, Liu IK: A unique exocelom-like space during early pregnancy in the horse, *Placenta* 21(5-6):575-583, 2000.
194. Colahan PT, Merritt AM, Moore JN, et al: *Equine medicine and surgery*, ed 5, St Louis, 1999, Mosby.
195. Roberts SJ: *Veterinary obstetrics and genital diseases (theriogenology)*, ed 3, 1986, Woodstock, Vt.
196. McKinnon AO, Voss JL, editors: *Equine reproduction*, Philadelphia, 1993, Lea & Febiger.
197. Henderson K, et al: Comparison of the merits of measuring equine chorionic gonadotrophin (eCG) and blood and faecal concentrations of oestrone sulphate for determining the pregnancy status of miniature horses, *Reprod Fertil Dev* 10(5):441-444, 1998.
198. Henderson K, Stewart J: A dipstick immunoassay to rapidly measure serum oestrone sulfate concentrations in horses, *Reprod Fertil Dev* 12(3-4):183-189, 2000.
199. Ohnuma K, et al: Study of early pregnancy factor (EPF) in equine (Equus caballus), *Am J Reprod Immunol (Copenhagen)* 43(3):174-179, 2000.

200. Parker E, Tibary A, Vanderwall DK: *Evaluation of a new early pregnancy test in mares.* 25:66-69, 2005.
201. Horteloup MP, Threlfall WR, Funk JA: The early conception factor (ECF) lateral flow assay for non-pregnancy determination in the mare, *Theriogenology* 64(5):1061-1071, 2005.
202. Meadows SJ, et al: Identical triplets in a thoroughbred mare, *Equine Vet J* 27(5):394-397, 1995.
203. Bruck I, Lehn-Jensen H, Yde G: Spontaneous multiple ovulation and development of multiple embryonic vesicles in a mare, *Equine Vet J* Suppl (25):63-68, 1997.
204. Short RV: Monozygotic triplets in the mare. [letter; comment], *Equine VetJ* 27(5):321, 1995.
205. Pascoe RR, Pascoe DR, Wilson MC: Influence of follicular status on twinning rate in mares, *J Reprod Fertil* (suppl 35):183-189, 1987.
206. Deskur S: Twinning in thoroughbred mares in Poland, *Theriogenology* 23:711, 1985.
207. Ginther OJ: Effect of reproductive status on twinning and on the side of ovulation and embryo attachment in mares, *Theriogenology* 20:383, 1983.
208. Merkt H, Jochle W: Abortions and twin pregnancies in Thoroughbreds: rate of occurence, treatments and prevention, *J Equine Vet Sci* 13:690-694, 1993.
209. Newcombe JR: Incidence of multiple ovulation and multiple pregnancy in mares, *Veterinary Record* 137(5):121-123, 1995.
210. Morel MC, Newcombe JR, Swindlehurst JC: The effect of age on multiple ovulation rates, multiple pregnancy rates and embryonic vesicle diameter in the mare, *Theriogenology* 63(9):2482-2493, 2005.
211. Ginther OJ: Twin embryos in the mare: I. From ovulation to fixation, *Equine Vet J* 21:166-170, 1989.
212. Allen WR, et al: Reproductive efficiency of Flatrace and National Hunt Thoroughbred mares and stallions in England, *Equine Vet J* 39(5):438-445, 2007.
213. Hemberg E, Lundeheim N, Einarsson S: Reproductive performance of Thoroughbred mares in Sweden, *Reprod Domest Anim* 39(2):81-85, 2004.
214. Ginther OJ, Douglas RH, Lawrence JR: Twinning in mares: A survey of veterinarians and analyses of theriogenology records, *Theriogenology* 18:333, 1982.
215. Wolfsdorf KE: Management of postfixation twins in mares, *Vet Clin North Am: Equine Pract* 22(3):713-725, 2006.
216. Ginther OJ: The twining problem: from breeding to day 16. In, *Am Assoc Equine Pract*, 29:11-26, 1983.
217. Pascoe RR: Methods for the treatment of twin pregnancy in the mare, *Equine Vet J* 15:40-42, 1983.
218. Pascoe DR, et al: Comparison of two techniques and three therapies for management of twin conceptuses by manual embryonic reduction, *J Reprod Fertil* (suppl 35):701-702, 1987.
219. McKinnon AO, Rantanen N, editors: *Equine diagnostic ultrasonography*, Baltimore, 1998, Williams & Wilkins.
220. Veronesi MC, et al: Plasma concentrations of 15-ketodihydro-PGF(2alpha), cortisol and progesterone during manual twin reduction in thoroughbred mares, *J Vet Med A Physiol Pathol Clin Med* 52(8):411-415, 2005.
221. Ginther OJ: Postfixation embryo reduction in unilateral and bilateral twins in mares, *Theriogenology* 22:11-26, 1984.
222. Ginther OJ: Twin embryos in mares II: post fixation embryo reduction, *Equine Vet J* 21:171-174, 1989.
223. Ginther OJ: The nature of embryo reduction in mares with twin conceptuses: Deprivation hypothesis, *Am J Vet Res* 50:45-53, 1989.
224. Ginther OJ: Twinning in mares: a review of recent studies, *J Equine Vet Sci* 2:127-135, 1982.
225. Watson ED, Nikolakopoulos E, Lawler DF: Case report: Survival and normal development of an embryo after prostaglandin treatment, *Equine Vet Educ* 9:283-285, 1997.
226. Gray GA, Dascanio JJ, Kolster KA: Theriogenology question of the month. What are the 3 management options for a mare with twin fetuses at this stage of gestation? *J Am Vet Med Assoc* 228(2):207-209, 2006.
227. Wolfsdorf K: Dose error in previous publication, *Personal communication* 2008.
228. Nie GJ, Barnes AJ: Use of prostaglandin E_1 to induce cervical relaxation in a maiden mare with post-breeding endometritis, *Equine Vet Educ* 15:221-224, 2003.
229. Giles RC, et al: Causes of abortion, stillbirth, and perinatal death in horses: 3,527 cases (1986-1991), *J Am Vet Med Assoc* 203(8):1170-1175, 1993.
230. Ball BA: Management of twin pregnancy in the mare: after endometrial cup formation. In Ball BA, editor: *Recent advances in equine theriogenology*, 2000, International Veterinary Information Service.
231. Mari G, et al: Reduction of twin pregnancy in the mare by transvaginal ultrasound-guided aspiration, *Reprod Domest Anim* 39(6):434-437, 2004.
232. Ginther OJ, Griffin PG: Natural outcome and ultrasonic identification of equine fetal twins, *Theriogenology* 41:1193-1199, 1994.
233. Bracher V, et al: Transvaginal ultrasound-guided twin reduction in the mare, *Vet Rec* 133:478-479, 1993.
234. Rantanen NW, Kincaid B: Ultrasound guided fetal cardiac puncture: a method of twin reduction in the mare, *Am Assoc Equine Pract* 34:173-179, 1988.
235. Ball BA, et al: Partial re-establishment of villous placentation after reduction of an equine co-twin by foetal cardiac puncture, *Equine Vet J* 25:336-338, 1993.
236. Rantanen NW: Ultrasound guided fetal cardiac puncture for twin reduction in mares, *Society for Theriogenology* 1990.
237. Barber JA, Troedsson MH: Mummified fetus in a mare, *J Am Vet Med Assoc* 208(9):1438-1440, 1996.
238. Jaszczak K, Parada R: Cytogenetic examination of horses from heterosexual twins, *Anim Sci Papers and reports* 17:115-121, 1999.
239. Pascoe DR, Stover SM: Surgical removal of one conceptus from 15 mares with twin conceptuses, *Vet Surg* 18:141-156, 1989.
240. Yang Y, Cho G: Factors concerning early embryonic death in Thoroughbred mares in South Korea, *J Vet Med Sci* 69(8):787-792, 2007.
241. Yang YJ, Cho GJ: Factors concerning early embryonic death in Thoroughbred mares in South Korea, *J Vet Med Sci* 69(8):787-792, 2007.
242. Woods GL, et al: Early pregnancy loss in brood mares, *J Reprod Fertil* (suppl 35):455-459, 1987.
243. Ball BA, et al: Pregnancy rates at Days 2 and 14 and estimated embryonic loss rates prior to day 14 in normal and subfertile mares, *Theriogenology* 26:611-619, 1986.
244. Brinsko SP, et al: In vitro development of Day 2 embryos obtained from young, fertile mares and aged, subfertile mares, *J Reprod Fertil* 102:371-378, 1994.
245. Carnevale EM, Griffin PG, Ginther OJ: Age-associated subfertility before entry of embryos into the uterus of mares, *Equine Vet J* (suppl 15):31-35, 1993.
246. Woods GL, et al: Selective oviductal transport and fertilization rate of equine embryos, *A Assoc Equine Pract* 37: 197-201,1991.
247. Vanderwall D: Early embryonic loss in the mare: Current perspectives, *Periparturient mare and neonate*, San Antonio, Tex, 2000, Society for Theriogenology.
248. Carnevale EM, et al: Comparison of oocytes from young and old mares with light and electron microscopy, *Theriogenology* 51:299, 1999.
249. Carnevale EM, Ginther OJ: Defective oocytes as a cause of subfertility in old mares, *Biol Reprod* 1:209-214, 1995:Mono.

250. Ball BA, et al: Survival of day-4 embryos from young, normal mares and aged, subfertile mares after transfer to normal recipient mares, *J Reprod Fertil* 85:187-194, 1989.
251. Vogelsang SG, Vogelsang MM: Influence of donor parity and age on the success of commercial equine embryo transfer, *Equine Vet J* (suppl 8):71-72, 1989.
252. Woods GL, Hillman RB, Schlafer DH: Recovery and evaluation of embryos from normal and infertile mares, *Cornell Vet* 76:386-394, 1986.
253. Ball BA, Hillman RB, Woods GL: Survival of equine embryos transferred to normal and subfertile mares, *Theriogenology* 28:167-174, 1987.
254. Squires EL, et al: Factors affecting reproductive efficiency in an equine embryo transfer programme, *J Reprod Fert* (suppl 32):409-414, 1982.
255. Morris LH, Allen WR: Reproductive efficiency of intensively managed Thoroughbred mares in Newmarket, *Equine Vet J* 34(1):51-60, 2002.
256. Adams AP, et al: Effect of uterine inflammation and ultrasonically-detected uterine pathology on fertility in the mare, *J Reprod Fert* (suppl 35):445-454, 1987.
257. Carnevale EM, Ginther OJ: Relationships of age to uterine function and reproductive efficiency in mares, *Theriogenology* 37:1101-1115, 1992.
258. Janosi S, et al: Endocrine and reproductive consequences of certain endotoxin-mediated diseases in farm mammals: a review, *Acta Veterinaria Hungarica* 46(1):71-84, 1998.
259. Troedsson MHT: Placental monitoring, *Periparturient mare and neonate*, San Antonio, Tex, 2000, Society for Theriogenology, pp 45-49.
260. Daels PF, et al: Effect of salmonella typhimurium endotoxin on PGF2alpha release and fetal death in the mare, *J Reprod Fertil* 35:485-492, 1987.
261. Daels PF, et al: The role of PGF_2-α in embryonic loss following systemic infusion of *Salmonella typhimurium* endotoxin in the mare and the protective action of altrenogest and flunixin meglumine. 11th International Congress on Animal Reproduction and Artificial Insemination. Dublin, 1988.
262. Daels PF, et al: Evaluation of progesterone deficiency as a cause of fetal death in mares with experimentally induced endotoxemia, *Am J Vet Res* 52:282-288, 1991.
263. Daels PF, et al: Effect of flunixin meglumine on endogenous prostaglandin F2 alpha secretion during cloprostenol-induced abortion in mares, *Am J Vet Res* 56(12):1603-1610, 1995.
264. Daels PF, et al: Effects of flunixin meglumine on endotoxin induced prostaglandin F2a secretion during early pregnancy in mares, *Am J Vet Res* 52:276-281, 1991.
265. McKinnon AO, et al: The inability of some synthetic progestagens to maintain pregnancy in the mare, *Equine Vet J* 32(1):83-85, 2000.
266. Vanderwall DK, Marquardt JL, Woods GL: Use of a compounded long-acting progesterone formulation for equine pregnancy maintenance, *J Equine Vet Sci* 27(2):62-66, 2007.
267. Whitwell KE: Infective placentitis in the mare, In, Powell DG (ed): Equine infectious diseases V: Proceedings of the 5th international conference. University Press of Kentucky, Lexington, Ky, 1988, pp. 172-180.
268. Santschi EM, LeBlanc MM: Fetal and placental conditions that cause high-risk pregnancy in mares, *Comp Cont Educ Pract Vet* 17:710-720, 1995.
269. Santschi EM, Slone D: Maternal conditions that cause high-risk pregnancy in mares, *Comp Cont Educ Pract Vet* 16:1481-1489, 1994.
270. Slone DE: Treatment of pregnant mares with colic: practical considerations and concerns, *Comp Cont Educ Pract Vet* 15:117-120, 1993.
271. White NA, Moore JN: *Current techniques in equine surgery and lameness*, Philadelphia, 1999, Saunders.
272. Santschi E, et al: Types of colic and frequency of postcolic abortion in pregnant mares: 105 cases (1984-1988), *J Am Vet Med Assoc* 199:374-377, 1991.
273. Boening KJ, Leendertse IP: Review of 115 cases of colic in the pregnant mare, *Equine Vet J* 25:518-521, 1993.
274. Fowden AL, et al: Equine uteroplacental metabolism at mid- and late gestation, *Exper Physiol* 85(5):539-545, 2000.
275. Hong CB, et al: Equine abortion and stillbirth in central Kentucky during 1988 and 1989 foaling seasons, *J Vet Diagn Invest* 5:560-566, 1993.
276. Smith KC, et al: A survey of equine abortion, stillbirth and neonatal death in the UK from 1988 to 1997, *Equine Vet J* 35(5):496-501, 2003.
277. Bucca S: Diagnosis of the compromised equine pregnancy, *Vet Clin North Am Equine Pract* 22(3):749-761, 2006.
278. Zent WW: Commentary, *Equine Dis Q* 7(3):1, 1999.
279. Platt H: Infection of the horse fetus, *J Reprod Fertil* (suppl 23):605-610, 1975.
280. Prickett ME: Abortion and placental lesions in the mare, *J Am Vet Med Assoc* 157:1465-1470, 1970.
281. Forster JL, et al: Absence of Chlamydia as an aetiological factor in aborting mares, *Vet Rec* 141(16):424, 1997.
282. Bryant UK: Equine placentitis: common causes and newly emerging pathogens, *Equine Dis Q* 17(2):4, 2008.
283. Macpherson M: Diagnosis and treatment of equine placentitis, *Vet Clin North Am Equine Pract* 22(3):763-776, 2006.
284. Mays M, LeBlanc MM, Paccamonti D: Route of fetal infection in a model of ascending placentitis, *Theriogenology* 58:791-792, 2002.
285. Hong CB: Equine placentitis, *Equine Dis Q* 1(3):4, 1993.
286. Donahue JM, N.M. Williams: Emergent causes of placentitis and abortion, *Vet Clin North Am* 16(3):443-456, 2000.
287. Patterson-Kane JC, Donahue JM, Harrison LR: Placentitis, fetal pneumonia, and abortion due to Rhodococcus equi infection in a Thoroughbred, *J Vet Diagn Invest* 14(2):157-159, 2002.
288. Tortschanoff M, et al: Phase and size variable surface-exposed proteins in equine genital mycoplasmas, *Vet Microbiol* 110 (3-4):301-306, 2005.
289. Labeda D, Donahue J, Williams N: *Amycolatopsis kentuckyensis* sp. nov., *Amycolatopsis lexingtonensis* sp. nov. and *Amycolatopsis pretoriensis* sp. nov., isolated from equine placentas, *Int J Syst Evol Microbiol* 53:1601-1605, 2003.
290. Hong CB, et al: Etiology and pathology of equine placentitis, *J Vet Diagn Invest* 5:56-63, 1993.
291. Williams NM, Donahue JM: Nocardioform placentitis, *Equine Dis Q* 9(1):5-6, 2000.
292. Javma: Scientists in pursuit of Kentucky racehorse disease, *J Am Vet Med Assoc* 220(4):438-441, 2002.
293. Donahue JM, et al: *Crossiella equi* sp. nov., isolated from equine placentas, *Int J Sys Evol Microbiol* 52:2169-2173, 2002.
294. Donahue JM, et al: *Crossiella equi* sp. nov., isolated from equine placentas, *Int J Systematic and Evolutionary Microbiol.* 52:2169-2173, 2002.
295. Christensen BW, et al: *Nocardioform placentitis* with isolation of *Amycolatopsis* spp in a Florida-bred mare, *J Am Vet Med Assoc* 228(8):1234-1239, 2006.
296. Sertich PL, Vaala WE: Concentrations of antibiotics in mares, foals and fetal fluids after antibiotic administration in late pregnancy, *American Association of Equine Practitioners* 38:727-733, 1992.
297. Graczyk J, et al: Treatment efficacy of trimethoprim sulfamethoxazole and pentoxifylline in equine placentitis, *Ann Reprod Sci* 94:434-435, 2006.
298. Rebello S, et al: Placental transfer of trimethoprim sulfamethoxazole and pentoxifylline in pony mares, *Ann Reprod Sci* 94:432-433, 2006.

299. Cattoli G, et al: First case of equine nocardioform placentitis caused by Crossiella equi in Europe 154:730-731, 2004.
300. Volkmann DH, et al: The first reported case of equine nocardioform placentitis in South Africa, *J S Afr Vet Assoc* 72(4):235-238, 2001.
301. Williams NM, Donahue JM: Placentitis in mares, *Equine Dis Q* 6(4):4, 1998.
302. Hendry JM, et al: Patterns of uterine myoelectrical activity in reproductively normal mares in late gestation and in mares with experimentally induced ascending placentitis, *Theriogenology* 58:853-855, 2002.
303. Stawicki RJ, Reubel H, Hansen PJ: Endocrinological findings in an experimental model of ascending placentitis in the mare, *Theriogenology* 58:849-852, 2002.
304. LeBlanc MM, et al: Premature delivery in ascending placentitis is associated with increased expression of placental cytokines and allantoic fluid prostaglandins E_2 and $F_{2}\alpha$, *Theriogenology* 58:841-844, 2002.
305. Macpherson ML: Treatment strategies for mares with placentitis, *Theriogenology* 64:528-534, 2005.
306. Rebello S, Macpherson M, Murchie T: The detection of placental drug transfer in equine allantoic fluid, *Theriogenology* 64(3):776-777, 2005.
307. Santschi EM, Papich MG: Pharmacokinetics of gentamicin in mares in late pregnancy and early lactation, *J Vet Pharmacol Ther* 23(6):359-363, 2000.
308. Murchie TA, et al: A microdialysis model to detect drugs in the allantoic fluid of pregnant pony mares. In Am Assoc Equine Pract, 49:118-119, 2003. New Orleans.
309. Murchie TA, et al: Continuous monitoring of penicillin G and gentamicin in allantoic fluid of pregnant pony mares by in vivo microdialysis, *Eq Vet J* 38(6):520-525, 2006.
310. Garfield RE, Kannan MS, Daniel EE: Gap junction formation in the myometrium: Control by estrogens, progesterone and prostaglandins, *Am J Physiol* 238:C81-C89, 1980.
311. Ousey JC, et al: Effects of progesterone administration to mares in late gestation, *Theriogenology* 58:793-795, 2002.
312. Chavatte P, Rossdale P, Tait A: Modulation of 3 beta-hydroxysteroid dehydrogenase (3 beta-HSD) activity in the equine placenta by pregnenolone and progesterone metabolites, *Equine Vet J* 27(5):342-347, 1995.
313. Ryan PL, et al: Systemic relaxin in pregnant pony mares grazed on endophyte-infected fescue: effects of fluphenazine treatment, *Theriogenology* 56(3):471-483, 2001.
314. Neumann JL, et al: Production and characterization of recombinant equine prorelaxin, *Domest Anim Endocrinol* 31(2):173-185, 2006.
315. Ryan PL, Vaala WE, Bagnell CA: Evidence that equine relaxin is a good indicator of placental insufficiency in the mare, *In Am Assoc Equine Pract* 44:62-63, 1998.
316. Zent WW, Williams NM, Donahue JM: Placentitis in central Kentucky broodmares, *Pferdeheilkunde* 15:630, 1991.
317. Card CE, Wood MR: Effects of acute administration of clenbuterol on uterine tone and equine fetal and maternal heart rates, *Biol Reprod* 1(1):7-11, 1995:Mono.
318. Bartmann CP, Klug E Deegen E. Periparturient colic in the mare. In Sixth Equine Colic Research Symposium. 1998. University of Georgia, 47.
319. Bostedt H: The use of beta2-mimetic agent (clenbuterol) in equine pregnancy disorders and obstetrics, *Tierarztl Prax* 16:57-59, 1988.
320. Palmer E, et al: Lack of effect of clenbuterol for delaying parturition in late pregnant mares, *Theriogenology* 58:797-799, 2002.
321. Sprayberry KA. Hemorrhage and hemorrhagic shock. In Bluegrass Equine Medicine and Critical Care Symposium. 1999. Lexington, KY.
322. Hoffman H, et al: Pentoxifylline decreases the incidence of multiple organ failure after major cardio-thoracic surgery, *Shock* 9(4):235-240, 1998.
323. Wattanasirichaigoon S, et al: Lisofylline ameliorates intestinal mucosal barrier dysfunction caused by ischemia and ischemia/reperfusion, *Shock* 11(4):269-275, 1999.
324. Troedsson MH, Zent WW: Clinical evaluation of the equine placenta as a method to successfully identify and treat mares with placentitis, *Workshop on the equine placenta*, Lexington, Ky, 2004, University of Kentucky Press.
325. Donahue JM, et al: Diagnosis and prevalence of leptospira infection in aborted and stillborn horses, *J Vet Diagn Invest* 3:148, 1991.
326. Donahoe JM, et al: Prevalence and serovars of leptospira involved in equine abortions in central Kentucky during the 1990 foaling season, *J Vet Diagn Invest* 4:279, 1992.
327. Donahue JM, et al: Prevalence and serovars of leptospira involved in equine abortions in central Kentucky during the 1991-1993 foaling seasons, *J Vet Diagn Invest* 7(1):87-91, 1995.
328. Ellis WA, O'Brien JJ: Leptospirosis in horses, In, Powell DG (ed): Equine infections diseases v: Proceedings of the 5th international conference. University Press of Kentucky, Lexington, Ky, 1988, pp. 168-171.
329. Ellis WA, Bryson DG, O'Brien JJ: Leptospiral infection in aborted equine foetuses, *Equine Vet J* 15:321, 1983.
330. Baird JD, Williams T, Claxton PD: A premature birth associated with Leptospira pomona infection in a mare, *Aust Vet J* 48:524, 1972.
331. Bernard WV, et al: Hematuria and leptospiruria in a foal, *J Am Vet Med Assoc* 203:276, 1993.
332. Bernard WV, et al: Leptospirosis on a central Kentucky horse farm: preventative measures following a case of abortion. In Am Assoc Equine Pract, 39:335-336, 1993. Lexington, Ky.
333. Hodgin EC, Miller DA, Lozano F: Leptospira abortion in horses, *J Vet Diagn Invest* 1:283, 1989.
334. Kitson-Piggot AW, Prescott JF: Leptospirosis in horses in Ontario, *Can J Vet Res* 51:448, 1987.
335. Tyndel PE: Probable leptospiral abortion in mares, *NZ Vet J* 25:401, 1977.
336. Sheoran AS, et al: Antibody isotypes in sera of equine fetuses aborted due to Leptospira interrogans serovar pomona-type kennewicki infection, *Vet Immunol Immunopathol* 77(3-4): 301-309, 2000.
337. Newman D, Donahue M: Equine leptospirosis, *Equine Dis Q* 16(3):4-5, 2007.
338. Poonacha KB, et al: Leptospirosis in equine fetuses, stillborn foals, and placentas, *Vet Pathol* 30:362, 1993.
339. Szeredi L, Haake DA: Immunohistochemical identification and pathologic findings in natural cases of equine abortion caused by leptospiral infection, *Vet Pathol* 43(5):755-761, 2006.
340. Lu KG, Morresey PR: Reproductive tract infections in horses, *Vet Clin North Am Equine Pract* 22(2):519-522, 2006.
341. Bernard WV: Leptospirosis, *Vet Clin North Am* 9:435-444, 1993.
342. Villalobos EMC, et al: Association between the presence of serum antibodies against Neospora spp. and fetal loss in equines, *Vet Parasitol* 142(3-4):372-375, 2006.
343. Locatelli-Dittrich R, et al: Investigation of Neospora sp. and Toxoplasma gondii antibodies in mares and in precolostral foals from Parana State, Southern Brazil, *Vet Parasitol* 135(3-4):215-221, 2006.
344. McDole MG, Gay JM: Seroprevalence of antibodies against Neospora caninum in diagnostic equine serum samples and their possible association with fetal loss 105:257-260, 2002.
345. Duarte PC, et al: Risk of transplacental transmission of Sarcocystis neurona and Neospora hughesi in California horses 90:1345-1351, 2004.
346. Doig P: Neosporosis in cattle, *Vet Clin North Am Food Anim Pract* 21(2):473-484, 2005.
347. Pitel PH, et al: Investigation of Neospora sp. antibodies in aborted mares from Normandy, France, *Vet Parasitol* 118 (1-2):1-6, 2003.

348. Kligler EB, et al: Seroprevalence of Neospora spp. among asymptomatic horses, aborted mares and horses demonstrating neurological signs in Israel, *Vet Parasitol* 148(2):109-113, 2007.
349. http://www.ca.uky.edu/gluck/MRLSindex.asp, Mare Reproductive Loss Syndrome (MRLS). 2008, Department of Veterinary Science, Gluck Center, University of Kentucky.
350. Dwyer RM, et al: Case-control study of factors associated with excessive proportions of early fetal losses associated with mare reproductive loss syndrome in central Kentucky during 2001, *J Am Vet Med Assoc* 222(5):613-619, 2003.
351. Frazer G: Mare reproductive loss syndrome in southeastern Ohio, Spring 2001. In *First Symposium on MRLS*, Lexington, Ky, 2003, Department of Veterinary Science, University of Kentucky Press.
352. Choate BA, Rieske LK: Life history and age-specific mortality of eastern tent caterpillar, *(Lepidoptera: Lasiocampidae). Ann Ent Soc Am* 98(4):496-502, 2005.
353. Moorehead JP, et al: Evaluation of early fetal losses on four equine farms in central Kentucky: 73 cases (2001), *J Am Vet Med Assoc* 220(12):1828-1830, 2002.
354. Sebastian M, et al: The mare reproductive loss syndrome and the eastern tent caterpillar: a toxicokinetic/statistical analysis with clinical, epidemiologic, and mechanistic implications, *Vet Ther* 4(4):324-339, 2003.
355. Taylor JR: Theory of ammonia toxicity as the mechanism of abortion in the mare reproductive loss syndrome, *J Eq Vet Sci* 22:237-239, 2002.
356. Swerczek TW: Saprotrophic fungi and bacteria and commensal bacteria that infect frost-damaged pastures may be contributing to gut microbial overgrowth and lesions associated with the mare reproductive loss syndrome, *J Equine Vet Sci* 22:234-237, 2002.
357. Dwyer RM, et al: An epidemiological investigation of mare reproductive loss syndrome: Breaking ground on a new disease. In Society for Veterinary Epidemiology and Preventive Medicine. 2002. Cambridge, England.
358. Cohen ND, et al: Descriptive epidemiology of late-term abortions associated with the mare reproductive loss syndrome in central Kentucky, *J Vet Diagn Invest* 15(3):295-297, 2003.
359. Cohen ND, et al: Case-control study of early-term abortions (early fetal losses) associated with mare reproductive loss syndrome in central Kentucky, *J Am Vet Med Assoc* 222(2):210-217, 2003.
360. Cohen ND, et al: Case-control study of late-term abortions associated with mare reproductive loss syndrome in central Kentucky, *J Am Vet Med Assoc* 222(2):199-209, 2003.
361. Cohen ND, et al: Temporality of early-term abortions associated with mare reproductive loss syndrome in horses, *Am J Vet Res* 66(10):1792-1797, 2005.
362. Potter DA, et al: Managing Eastern tent caterpillars *Malacosoma americanum* (F) on horse farms to reduce risk of mare reproductive loss syndrome, *Pest Manag Sci* 61(1):3-15, 2005.
363. Thompson JA, et al: Use of a Bayesian risk-mapping technique to estimate spatial risks for mare reproductive loss syndrome in Kentucky, *Am J Vet Res* 66(1):17-20, 2005.
364. http://www.ca.uky.edu/agc/pubs/sr/sr2003-1/sr2003-1.htm, *Proceedings of the first workshop on MRLS. 2003*, Department of Veterinary Science, University of Kentucky.
365. Seahorn JL, et al: Case-control study of factors associated with fibrinous pericarditis among horses in central Kentucky during spring 2001, *J Am Vet Med Assoc* 223(6):832-838, 2003.
366. Bernard WV, et al: Evaluation of early fetal loss induced by gavage with eastern tent caterpillars in pregnant mares, *J Am Vet Med Assoc* 225:717-721, 2004.
367. Webb BA, et al: Eastern tent caterpillars *(Malacosoma americanum)* cause mare reproductive loss syndrome, *J Insect Physiol* 50(2-3):185-193, 2004.
368. McDowell KJ: MRLS Update, *Equine Dis Q* 17(2):5, 2008.
369. Donahue JM, Sells SF, Bolin DC: Classification of *Actinobacillus* spp. isolates from horses involved in mare reproductive loss syndrome, *Am J Vet Res* 67(8):1426-1432, 2006.
370. Cawdell-Smith AJ, et al: Establishment of a link between processional caterpillars and pregnancy loss in Australian Mare. In *Proceedings of the Twentieth Symposium of the Equine Science Society*. 2007.
371. Metcalfe ES: The role of international transport of equine semen on disease transmission, *Ann Reprod Sci* 68:229-237, 2001.
372. Timoney PJ, McCollum WH: Equine viral arteritis: further characterization of the carrier state in stallions, *J Reprod Fertil* (suppl 56):3-11, 2000.
373. Balasuriya UB, et al: Serologic and molecular characterization of an abortigenic strain of equine arteritis virus isolated from infective frozen semen and an aborted equine fetus, *J Am Vet Med Assoc* 213(11):1586-1589, 1998.
374. Glaser AL, et al: Equine arteritis virus: a review of clinical features and management aspects, *Vet Q* 18(3):95-99, 1996.
375. Szeredi L, et al: Study on the epidemiology of equine arteritis virus infection with different diagnostic techniques by investigating 96 cases of equine abortion in Hungary 108:235-242, 2005.
376. MacLachlan NJ, et al: Fatal experimental equine arteritis virus infection of a pregnant mare: immunohistochemical staining of viral antigens, *J Vet Diagn Invest* 8(3):367-374, 1996.
377. Paweska JT: Effect of the South African asinine-94 strain of equine arteritis virus (EAV) in pregnant donkey mares and duration of maternal immunity in foals, *Onderstepoort J Vet Res* 64(2):147-152, 1997.
378. Timoney PJ, McCollum WH: Equine viral arteritis, *Can Vet J* 28:673-695, 1987.
379. Paweska JT, Henton MM, van der Lugt JJ: Experimental exposure of pregnant mares to the asinine-94 strain of equine arteritis virus, *J S Afr Assoc* 68(2):49-54, 1997.
380. Timoney PJ: Aspects of the occurrence, diagnosis and control of selected venereal diseases of the stallion. In Stallion Symposium. 1998. Baltimore: Society for Theriogenology.
381. Wada R, et al: Histopathological and immunofluorescent studies on transplacental infection in experimentally induced abortion by equine arteritis virus, *Zentralblatt Fuer Veterinaermedizin Reihe B* 43(2):65-74, 1996.
382. Leon A, Fortier G: Detection of equine herpesviruses in aborted fetuses by consensus PCR, *Vet Microbiol* 126(1-3):20-29, 2008.
383. Vickers ML: Equine herpes virus abortions, *Equine Dis Q* 10(1):3-4, 2001.
384. Kydd JH, Townsend HG, Hannant D: The equine immune response to equine herpesvirus-1: the virus and its vaccines, *Vet Immunol Immunopathol* 111(1-2):15-30, 2006.
385. Kydd J, Wattrang E, Hannant D: Pre-infection frequencies of equine herpesvirus-1 specific, cytotoxic T lymphocytes correlate with protection against abortion following experimental infection of pregnant mares, *Vet Immunol Immunopathol* 96:207-217, 2003.
386. Gilkerson JR, et al: Epidemiological studies of equine herpesvirus 1 (EHV-1) in Thoroughbred foals: a review of studies conducted in the Hunter Valley of New South Wales between 1995 and 1997, *Vet Microbiol* 68(1-2):15-25, 1999.
387. Smith KC, et al: Virulence of the V592 isolate of equid herpesvirus-1 in ponies, *J Comp Pathol* 122(4):288-297, 2000.
388. Smith KC, et al: Equine herpesvirus-1 abortion: atypical cases with lesions largely or wholly restricted to the placenta, *Equine Vet J* 36(1):79-82, 2004.
389. Smith KC, et al: Use of transabdominal ultrasound-guided amniocentesis for detection of equid herpesvirus 1-induced fetal infection in utero, *Am J Vet Res* 58(9):997-1002, 1997.
390. Smith KC, Mumford JA, Lakhani K: A comparison of equid herpesvirus-1 (EHV-1) vascular lesions in the early versus late pregnant equine uterus, *J Comp Pathol* 114(3):231-247, 1996.

391. Smith DJ, Hamblin AS, Edington N: Infection of endothelial cells with equine herpesvirus-1 (EHV-1) occurs where there is activation of putative adhesion molecules: a mechanism for transfer of virus, *Equine Vet J* 33(2):138-142, 2001.
392. Drummer HE, et al: Application of an equine herpesvirus 1 (EHV1) type-specific ELISA to the management of an outbreak of EHV1 abortion, *Vet Rec* 136(23):579-581, 1995.
393. van Maanen C, et al: An equine herpesvirus 1 (EHV1) abortion storm at a riding school, *Vet Q* 22(2):83-87, 2000.
394. Schroer U, et al: [Relevance of infection with equine herpesvirus 1 (EHV-1) in a German thoroughbred stud: vaccination, abortion and diagnosis], *Berl Munch Tierarztl Wochenschr* 113(2):53-539, 2000.
395. Ostlund EN: The equine herpesviruses, *Vet Clin North Am* 9:283-294, 1993.
396. Tashjian RJ: Transmission and clinical evaluation of an equine infectious anemia herd and their offspring over a 13-year period, *J Am Vet Med Assoc* 184:282-288, 1984.
397. Vest DJ, et al: Evaluation of administration of West Nile virus vaccine to pregnant broodmares, *J Am Vet Med Assoc* 225(12):1894-1897, 2004.
398. Wolc A, Bresinska A, Szwaczkowski T: Genetic and permanent environmental variability of twinning in Thoroughbred horses estimated via three threshold models, *J Anim Breed Genet* 123(3):186-190, 2006.
399. Pipers FS, Adams-Brendemeuhl CA: Techniques and applications of transabdominal ultrasonography in the pregnant mare, *J Am Vet Med Assoc* 185:766-771, 1994.
400. Cassar T, et al: Segmental ossification of involuted yolk sacs in equine umbilical cords, *Ann Reprod Sci* 94:439-442, 2006.
401. Williams N, et al: Equine placental pathology: Kentucky perspective. Powell DG, Furry D, Hale G (eds): Proceedings of a Workshop on the Equine Placenta. Lexington, KY. 2003.
402. Schlafer DH: The umbilical cord: lifeline to the outside world: structure, function, and pathology of the equine umbilical cord. Powell DG, Furry D, Hale G (eds): Proceedings of a Workshop on the Equine Placenta. Lexington, KY. 2003.
403. Frazer G: Umbilical cord compromise as a cause of abortion, *Equine Vet Educ* 19(11):535-537, 2007.
404. Whitwell KE: Equine placental pathology: the Newmarket perspective. Powell DG, Furry D, Hale G (eds): Proceedings of a Workshop on the Equine Placenta. Lexington, KY. 2003.
405. Williams NM: Umbilical cord torsion, *Equine Dis Q* 10(3):3-4, 2002.
406. Whitehe A, Foster R Chenier T. Placental characteristics of Standardbred mares. Powell DG, Furry D, Hale G (eds): Proceedings of a Workshop on the Equine Placenta. Lexington, KY. 2003.
407. Ginther OJ, Griffin PG, Equine fetal kinetics: presentation and location, *Theriogenology* 40:1-11, 1993.
408. Ginther OJ, Williams D, Curren S: Equine fetal kinetics: Entry and retention of fetal hind limbs in a uterine horn, *Theriogenology* 41:795-807, 1994.
409. Ginther OJ: Equine physical utero-fetal interactions: a challenge and wonder for the practitioner, *J Equine Vet Sci* 14:313-318, 1994.
410. Curren S, Ginther OJ: Ultrasonic fetal gender diagnosis during months 5 to 11 in mares, *Theriogenology* 40:1127-1135, 1993.
411. Vandeplassche M, Lauwers H: The twisted umbilical cord: an expression of kinesis of the equine fetus? *Anim Reprod Sci* 10:163-175, 1986.
412. Ginther OJ: Equine fetal kinetics: Allantoic-fluid shifts and uterine-horn closures, *Theriogenology* 40:241-256, 1993.
413. Ricketts SW, Barrelet A, Whitwell KE: A review of the causes of abortion in UK mares and means of diagnosis used in an equine studfarm practice in Newmarket, *Pferdeheikunde* 17:589-592, 2001.
414. Whitwell KE: Morphology and pathology of the equine umbilical cord, *J Reprod Fert* (suppl 23):599-603, 1975.
415. Williams, N. 2003.
416. Mizushima C: Late-term abortion associated with umbilical cord torsion in the mare: case report, *J Equine Vet Sci* 25:162-163, 2005.
417. Hong CB, et al: Equine abortion and stillbirth in central Kentucky during 1988 and 1989 foaling seasons, *J Vet Diagn Invest* 5(4):560-566, 1993.
418. Snider TA: Umbilical cord torsion and coiling as a cause of dystocia and intrauterine foal loss, *Equine Vet Educ* 19(11):532-534, 2007.
419. Holder RD: Equine fetal sexing. In Robinson NE, editor: *Current therapy in equine medicine Ed 5*, Philadelphia, 2002, Saunders.
420. Renaudin CD, Gillis CL, Tarantal AF: Transabdominal ultrasonographic determination of fetal gender in the horse during mid-gestation, *Equine Vet J* 31(6):483-487, 1999.
421. Bucca S: Equine fetal gender determination from mid- to advanced gestation by ultrasound, *Theriogenology* 64:568-571, 2005.
422. Ryan PL, et al: Relaxin as a biochemical marker of placental insufficiency in the horse: a review, *Pferdeheilkunde* 15:622-626, 1999.
423. Klonisch T, et al: Partial complementary deoxyribonucleic acid cloning of equine relaxin messenger ribonucleic acid, and its location within the equine placenta, *Biol Reprod* 52:1307-1315, 1995.
424. Stewart DR: Development of a homologous equine relaxin radioimmunoassay, *Endocrinology* 119:1100-1104, 1986.
425. Pashen RL, Allen WR, Endocrine changes after foetal gonadectomy and during normal and induced parturition in the mare, *Ann Reprod Sci* 2:271-288, 1979.
426. Raeside JI, Liptrap RM, Milne FJ: Relationship of fetal gonads to estrogen excretion by the pregnant mare, *Am J Vet Res* 34:843-845, 1973.
427. Barnes RJ, et al: Plasma progestagens and oestrogens in fetus and mother in late pregnancy, *J Reprod Fertil* (suppl 23):617-623, 1975.
428. Sorensen K, et al: Measurement and clinical significance of fetal protein in pregnant mare serum, *J Equine Vet Sci* 10:417-421, 1990.
429. Riddle T: Preparation of the mare for normal parturition. In Am Assoc Equine Pract, 49:1-5, 2003. New Orleans.
430. Ousey J, et al: Progestagen profiles during the last trimester of gestation in Thoroughbred mares with normal or compromised pregnancies, *Theriogenology* 63:1844-1856, 2005.
431. Troedsson MHT, et al: Transrectal ultrasonography of the placenta in normal mares and in mares with pending abortion: a field study, In *Am Assoc Equine Pract* 43:256-258, 1997.
432. Ousey J, et al: Plasma concentrations of progestagens, oestrone sulphate and prolactin in pregnant mares subjected to natural challenge with equid herpesvirus-1, *J Reprod Fertil* 35(suppl):519-528, 1987.
433. Vaala WE, Sertich PL: Management strategies for mares at risk for periparturient complications, *Vet Clin North Am* 10:237-265, 1994.
434. Morris S, et al: Transrectal ultrasonography and plasma progestin profiles identifies feto-placental compromise in mares with experimentally induced placentitis, *Theriogenology* 67(4):681-691, 2007.
435. van Niekerk C, Morgenthal J: Fetal loss and the effects of stress on plasma progestagen levels in pregnant Thoroughbred mares, *J Reprod Fertil* 32:453-457, 1982.
436. Ousey JC, et al: Ontogeny of uteroplacental progestagen production in pregnant mares during the second half of gestation, *Biol Reprod* 69(2):540-548, 2003.
437. Rossdale P, Ousey J, McGladdery A: A retrospective study of increased plasma progestagen concentrations in compromised neonatal foals, *Reprod Fertil Dev* 7(3):567-575, 1995.

438. Hoffman B, Gentz F, Failing K: Investigations into the course of progesterone, oestrogen and eCG concentrations during normal and impaired pregnancy in the mare, *Reprod Domest Anim* 31:717-723, 1996.
439. Ousey J, McGladdery A: Clinical diagnosis and treatment of problems in the late pregnant mare, *In Practice* 22:200-207, 2000.
440. Bucca S, et al: Assessment of feto-placental well-being in the mare from mid-gestation to term: transrectal and transabdominal ultrasonographic features, *Theriogenology* 64(3):542-557, 2005.
441. Kelleman A, et al: Evaluation of transrectal ultrasonographic combined thickness of the uterus and placenta (CTUP) in a model of induced ascending placentitis in late gestation in the pony mare, *Theriogenology* 58:845-848, 2002.
442. Renaudin CD, et al: Ultrasonographic evaluation of the equine placenta by transrectal and transabdominal approach in pregnant mares, *Theriogenology* 47:559-573, 1997.
443. Troedsson MH: Ultrasonographic evaluation of the equine placenta, *Pferdeheilkunde* 17:583-588, 2001.
444. Renaudin CD, et al: Transrectal ultrasonographic diagnosis of ascending placentitis in the mare: a report of two cases, *Equine Vet Educ* 11:69-74, 1999.
445. Reef VB, et al: Ultrasonographic evaluation of the fetus and intrauterine environment in healthy mares during late gestation, *Vet Radiol Ultrasound* 36:533-541, 1995.
446. Adams-Brendemeuhl CA, Pipers FS: Antepartum evaluation of the equine fetus, *J Reprod Fertil* (suppl 35):565-573, 1987.
447. Reef VB, et al: Ultrasonographic assessment of fetal well-being during late gestation: development of an equine biophysical profile, *Equine Vet J* 28:200-208, 1996.
448. Reef VB: *Equine diagnostic ultrasound*, Philadelphia, 1998, Saunders.
449. Reef VB, et al: Ultrasonographic assessment of fetal well-being during late gestation: A preliminary report on the development of an equine biophysical profile, *Equine Vet J* 28:200-208, 1995.
450. Sertich PL, et al: Hydrops amnii in a mare, *J Am Vet Med Assoc* 204:1-2, 1994.
451. Reef VB, et al: Transcutaneous ultrasonographic assessment of fetal well-being during late gestation: a preliminary report on the development of an equine biophysical profile, *In Am Assoc Equine Pract* 42:152-153 , 1996.
452. McGladdery AJ, Cottrill CM, Rossdale PD. Effects upon the fetus of sedative drugs administered to the mare. In Second International Conference on Veterinary Perinatology. 1990. Cambridge.
453. Luukkanen L, Katila T, Koskinen E: Some effects of multiple administration of detomidine during the last trimester of equine pregnancy, *Equine Vet J* 29(5):400-403, 1997.
454. Palmer J: Fetal monitoring, *Periparturient mare and neonate*, San Antonio, Tex, 2000, Society for Theriogenology, pp 39-43.
455. Hosaka F: Perinatal fetal heart rate changes and neonatal arrhythmias in the horse, *Jpn J Vet Res* 37:106, 1989.
456. Matsui K, et al: Alterations in the heart rate of Thoroughbred horse, pony, and Holstein cow through pre- and post-natal stages, *Jpn J Vet Sci* 46:505-509, 1984.
457. Pipers FS, et al: Ultrasonography as an adjunct to pregnancy assessments in the mare, *J Am Vet Med Assoc* 184:328-334, 1984.
458. Colles CM, Parks RD, May CJ: Fetal echocardiography in the mare, *Equine Vet J* 10:32-37, 1978.
459. Holmes JR, Darke PGG: Foetal electrocardiography in the mare, *Vet Rec* 82:651, 1968.
460. Yamamoto K, Yasuda J, Kimehiko T: Electrocardiography findings during parturition and blood gas tensions immediately after birth in thoroughbred foals, *Jpn J Vet Res* 39:143-157, 1991.
461. Renaudin CD, et al: Evaluation of equine fetal growth from day 100 of gestation to parturition by ultrasonography, *J Reprod Fertil* (suppl 56):651-660, 2000.
462. Turner RM, et al: Real-time ultrasound measure of the fetal eye (vitreous body) for prediction of parturition date in small ponies, *Theriogenology* 66(2):331-337, 2006.
463. Burns TE, Card CE: Fetal maceration and retention of fetal bones in a mare, *J Am Vet Med Assoc* 217(6):878-880, 2000.
464. Frazer GS, Emberstson R, Perkins NR: Complications of late gestation in the mare, *Equine Vet Educ* 9(6):306-311, 1997.
465. Vandeplassche M, et al: Dropsy of the fetal sacs in mares, *Vet Rec* 99:67-69, 1976.
466. Koterba A, Haibel G, Grimmet J: Respiratory distress in a premature foal secondary to hydrops allantois and placentitis, *Comp Cont Educ Pract Vet* 5:S121-S125, 1983.
467. Waelchli RO, Ehrensperger F: Two related cases of cerebellar abnormality in equine fetuses associated with hydrops of fetal membranes, *Vet Rec* 123:513-514, 1988.
468. Stich KL, Blanchard TL: *Hydrallantois in mares* 25:71-75, 2003.
469. Oppen T, Bartmann C: Two cases of hydroallantois in the mare, *Pferdeheilkunde* 17(6):593-596, 2001.
470. Christensen BW, et al: Management of hydrops amnion in a mare resulting in birth of a live foal, *J Am Vet Med Assoc* 228(8):1228-1233, 2006.
471. Hanson R, Todhunter R: Herniation of the abdominal wall in pregnant mares, *J Am Vet Med Assoc* 189:790-793, 1986.
472. Honnas C, et al: Hydramnios causing uterine rupture in a mare, *J Am Vet Med Assoc* 193:334-336, 1988.
473. Rigby S, et al: Use of prostaglandin E_2 to ripen the cervix of the mare prior to induction of parturition, *Theriogenology* 50(6):897-904, 1998.
474. Macpherson ML, et al: Three methods of oxytocin-induced parturition and their effects of foals, *J Am Vet Med Assoc* 210(6):799-803, 1997.
475. Ross J, Palmer JE, Wilkins PA: Body wall tears during late pregnancy in mares: 13 cases (1995-2006), *J Am Vet Med Assoc* 232(2):257-261, 2008.
476. Hendriks W, Stout T, van der Weijden G: Spinal trauma in a recently foaled Fresian mare as a complication of ventral abdominal rupture, *Equine Vet Educ* 19(5):247-250, 2007.
477. Perkins NR, Frazer GS: Reproductive emergencies in the mare, *Vet Clin N AmEq Pract* 10:643-670, 1994.
478. Meek DG, DeGrofft DL, Schneider EE: Surgical repair of similar parturition-induced midline ventral hernias in two mares: A comparison of results, *Vet Med Small Anim Clin* 72:1066-1074, 1977.
479. Adams SB: Rupture of the prepubic tendon in the mare, *Equine Pract* 1:17-19, 1979.
480. Vandeplassche M, et al: Some aspects of equine obstetrics, *Equine Vet J* 4:105-109, 1972.
481. Frazer GS, et al: Prevalence of fetal maldispositions in equine referral hospital dystocias, *Equine Vet J* 29(2):111-116, 1997.
482. Chaney KP, et al: The effect of uterine torsion on mare and foal survival: a retrospective study, 1985-2005, *Equine Vet J* 39(1):33-336, 2007.
483. Frazer GS, Perkins NR, Constable P: Bovine uterine torsions: 164 referral hospital cases, *Theriogenology* 46:739-793, 1996.
484. Ruffin DC, Schumacher J, Comer JS: Uterine torsion associated with small intestinal incarceration in a mare at 126 days of gestation, *J Am Vet Med Assoc* 207(3):329-330, 1995.
485. Doyle A, et al: Clinical signs and treatment of chronic uterine torsion in two mares, *J Am Vet Med Assoc* 220:349-353, 2002.
486. Pascoe J, Meagher D, Wheat J: Surgical management of uterine torsion in the mare: A review of 26 cases, *J Am Vet Med Assoc* 179:351-354, 1981.
487. Wichtel JJ, Reinertson E, Clark T: Nonsurgical correction of uterine torsion in seven mares, *J Am Vet Med Assoc* 193:337-338, 1988.

488. Barber SM: Torsion of the uterus: a cause of colic in the mare, *J Am Vet Med Assoc* 20:165-167, 1979.
489. Barber SM: Complications of chronic uterine torsion in a mare, *Can Vet J* 36(2):102-103, 1995.
490. Perkins NR, et al: Theriogenology question of the month: uterine torsion, *J Am Vet Med Assoc* 209:1395-1396, 1996.
491. Pascoe J, Pascoe R: Displacements, malpositions and miscellaneous injuries of the mare's urogenital tract, *Vet Clin North Am* 4:439, 1988.
492. Frazer GS, et al: The effects of parturition and peripartum complications on the peritoneal fluid composition of mares, *Theriogenology* 48:919-931, 1997.
493. Perkins NR, Robertson JT, Colon LA: Uterine torsion and uterine tear in a mare, *J Am Vet Med Assoc* 201:92-94, 1991.
494. Ragle CA, et al: Laparoscopic diagnosis of ischemic necrosis of the descending colon after rectal prolapse and rupture of the mesocolon in two postpartum mares, *J Am Vet Med Assoc* 210(11):1646-1648, 1997.
495. Bowen J, Gaboury C, Bousquet D: Non-surgical correction of a uterine torsion in the mare, *Vet Rec* 99:495-496, 1976.
496. Taylor PM: Anaesthesia for pregnant animals, *Equine Vet J* (suppl 24):1-6, 1997.
497. Frazer G: Differential diagnosis for vaginal hemorrhage in the mare, *Equine Vet Educ* 7(3):197-199, 2005.
498. White RAS, et al: Persistent vaginal haemorrhage in five mares caused by varicose veins of the vaginal wall, *Vet Rec* 115:263-264, 1984.
499. Pascoe RR: Observations on the length and angle of declination of the vulva and its relation to fertility in the mare, *J Reprod Fertil* (supp 27):299-305, 1979.
500. DeLuca C, Berry DB II, Dascanio JJ: Nd:YAG laser treatment of a vestibulovaginal varicosity in a 15-year-old pregnant mare, *J Equine Vet Sci* 27(5):217-220, 2007.
501. Schumacher J, Schumacher J, Schmitz D: Macroscopic haematuria of horses, *Equine Vet Educ* 14(4):201-210, 2002.
502. Laverty S, Pascoe JR, Ling GV: Urolithiasis in 68 horses, *Vet Surg* 21:56-62, 1992.
503. DeBowes RM, Nyrop KA, Boulton CH: Cystic calculi in the horse, *Comp Cont Educ Pract Vet* 6:S268-S273, 1984.
504. Gandini G, Pietra M, Cinotti S: Squamous cell carcinoma of the urinary bladder in a mare, *Equine Pract* 20:18-20, 1998.
505. Fischer AT, Spier S, Carlson GP: Neoplasia of the urinary bladder as a cause of hematuria, *J Am Vet Med Assoc* 186(12):1294-1296, 1985.
506. Brendemeuhl JP: Fescue and agalactia: pathophysiology, diagnosis and management, *Periparturient mare and neonate*, San Antonio, Tex, 2000, Society for Theriogenology, pp 25-32.
507. Cross DL, Redmond LM, Strickland JR: Equine fescue toxicosis: signs and solutions, *J Anim Sci* 73(3):899-908, 1995.
508. Putnam MR, et al: Effects of the fungal endophyte *Acremonium coenophialium* in fescue on pregnant mares and foal viability, *Am J Vet Res* 52:2071-2074, 1991.
509. Boosinger TR, et al: Effect of short-term exposure to, and removal from, the fescue endophyte *(Acremonium coenophialum)* on pregnant mares and foal viability, *Biol Reprod* (mono 1):61-67, 1995.
510. McCann SJ, et al: Influence of endophyte-infected tall fescue on serum prolactin and progesterone in gravid mares, *J Anim Sci* 70:217-223, 1992.
511. Boosinger TR, et al: Prolonged gestation, decreased triiodothyronine concentration, and thyroid gland histomorphologic features in newborn foals of mares grazing Acremonion coenophialum-infected fescue, *Am J Vet Res* 56(1):66-69, 1995.
512. Cross DL, et al: Clinical effects of domperidone on fescue toxicosis in pregnant mares, In *Am Assoc Equine Pract* 45:203-206, 1999.
513. Evans TJ, et al: A comparison of the relative efficacies of domperidone and reserpine in treating equine "Fescue Toxicosis." In *Am Assoc Equine Pract* 45:207-209, 1999.
514. Bennet-WimbushLoch KW: A preliminary study on the efficacy of fluphenazine as a treatment for fescue toxicosis in gravid pony mares, *J Eq Vet Sci* 18:169-173, 1998.
515. Redmond LM, et al: Efficacy of domperidone and sulpiride as treatments for fescue toxicosis in horses, *Am J Vet Res* 55:722-729, 1994.
516. Jochle W: Management and the hour of parturition in mares. (letter), *Vet Rec* 142(15):408, 1998.
517. Newcombe JR, Nout YS: Apparent effect of management on the hour of parturition in mares, *Vet Rec* 142(9):221-222, 1998.
518. Jeffcott LB, Rossdale PD: A critical review of current methods for induction of parturition in the mare, *Equine Vet J* 9:208-215, 1977.
519. Hillman RB: Induction of parturition in mares, *J Reprod Fertil* (suppl 23):641-644, 1975.
520. Alm CC, Sullivan JJ, First NL: The effect of corticosteroid (dexamethasone), progesterone, oestrogen and prostaglandin F2α on gestation length in normal and ovariectomized mares, *J Reprod Fertil* (suppl 23):637-640, 1975.
521. Duggan VE, et al: Influence of induction of parturition on the neonatal acute phase response in foals, *Theriogenology* 67(2):372-381, 2007.
522. Macpherson ML: Induction of parturition, *Periparturient mare and neonate symposium*, San Antonio, Tex, 2000, Society for Theriogenology, pp 51-58.
523. Purvis AD: The induction of labor in mares as a routine breeding farm procedure. In, *Ann Conv Am Assoc Equine Pract* 23:145, 1977.
524. Paccamonti DL: Milk electrolytes and induction of parturition, *Pferdeheilkunde* 17(6):616-618, 2001.
525. Giger R, Meier HP, Kupfer U: [Length of gestation of Freiberger mares with mule and horse foals], *Schweiz Arch Tierheilkd* 139(7):303-307, 1997.
526. Valera M, et al: Genetic study of gestation length in Andalusian and Arabian mares, *Anim Reprod Sci* 95(1-2):75-96, 2006.
527. Rossdale PD, Short RV: The time of foaling in Thoroughbred mares, *J Reprod Fertil* 13:341-343, 1967.
528. Sevinga M, et al: Retained placenta in Friesian mares: incidence, and potential risk factors with special emphasis on gestational length, *Theriogenology* 61(5):851-859, 2004.
529. Heidler B, et al: Body weight of mares and foals, estrous cycles and plasma glucose concentration in lactating and non-lactating Lipizzaner mares 61:883-893, 2004.
530. Marteniuk JV, et al: Association of sex of fetus, sire, month of conception, or year of foaling with duration of gestation in standardbred mares, *J Am Vet Med Assoc* 212(11):1743-1745, 1998.
531. Davies Morel MC, Newcombe JR, Holland SJ: Factors affecting gestation length in the Thoroughbred mare, *Anim Reprod Sci* 74(3-4):175-185, 2002.
532. Howell C, Rollins W: Environmental sources of gestation length in the mare, *J Anim Sci* 10:789-805, 1951.
533. Hodge SL, et al: Influence of photoperiod on the pregnant postpartum mare, *Am J Vet Res* 10:1752-1755, 1982.
534. Peaker M, et al: Changes in mammary development and the composition of secretion during late pregnancy in the mare, *J Reprod Fertil* (Suppl 27):555-561, 1979.
535. Leadon DP, Jeffcott LB, Rossdale PD: Mammary secretions in normal spontaneous and induced premature parturition in the mare, *Equine Vet J* 16:256, 1984.
536. Ousey J, Dudan F, Rossdale P: Preliminary studies of mammary secretions in the mare to access fetal readiness for birth, *Equine Vet J* 16:259-263, 1984.
537. Lloyd JW, et al: Use of a non-linear spline regression to model time-varying fluctuations in mammary-secretion element concentrations of periparturient mares in Michigan, USA, *Prev Vet Med* 43(3):211-222, 2000.

538. Rook JS, et al: Multi-element assay of mammary secretions and sera from periparturient mares by inductively coupled argon plasma emission spectroscopy, *Am J Vet Res* 58(4):376-378, 1997.
539. Carluccio A, et al: Electrolytes changes in mammary secretions before foaling in jennies, *Reprod Domest Anim* 43(2):162-165, 2008.
540. Ousey JC, Delclaux M, Rossdale PD: Evaluation of three strip tests for measuring electrolytes in mares' prepartum mammary secretions and for predicting parturition, *Equine Vet J* 21:196-200, 1989.
541. Camillo F, et al: Day-time management of the foaling mare: use of a rapid mammary Ca++ determination followed by a low dose of oxytocin, In *12th Int Cong Anim Reprod*, 1992.
542. Cash RSG, Ousey JC, Rossdale PD: Rapid strip test method to assist management of foaling mares, *Equine Vet J* 17:61, 1985.
543. Brook D: Evaluation of a new test kit for estimating the foaling time in the mare, *Equine Pract* 9:34, 1987.
544. Ley WB, et al: Daytime management of the mare. 1. Pre-foaling mammary secretions testing, *J Equine Vet Sci* :88-94, 1989.
545. Ley WB, et al: The sensitivity, specificity and predictive value of measuring calcium carbonate in mare's prepartum mammary secretion, *Theriogenology* 40:189-198, 1993.
546. Ousey JC, et al: The effects of oxytocin and progesterone on myometrial contractility in vitro during equine pregnancy. In *7th. International Symposium on Equine Reproduction* 1998.
547. Alm CC, Sullivan JJ: N.L. First: Induction of premature parturition by parenteral administration of dexamethasone in the mare, *J Am Vet Med Assoc* 165:721-722, 1974.
548. First NL, Alm CC: Dexamethasone-induced parturition in pony mares, *J Anim Sci* 44:1072, 1977.
549. Rossdale PD, Pashen RL, Jeffcott LB: The use of synthetic prostaglandin analogue (fluprostenol) to induce foaling, *J Reprod Fertil* (suppl. 27):521-529, 1979.
550. Pashen RL: Oxytocin: the induction agent of choice in the mare? *J Reprod Fertil* (suppl 32):645, 1982.
551. Ley WB, et al: Daytime foaling management of the mare 2: induction of parturition, *Equine Vet Sci* 9:95-99, 1989.
552. Ousey JC, et al: Effects of fluprostenol administration in mares during late pregnancy, *Equine Vet J* 16:264, 1984.
553. Bristol F: Induction of parturition in near-term mares by prostaglandin $F_2\alpha$. *J Reprod Fertil* (suppl 32):644, 1982.
554. Rossdale PD, Jeffcott LB, Allen WR: Foaling induced by a synthetic prostaglandin analogue (fluprostenol), *Vet Rec* 99:26, 1976.
555. Bennett DG: Artificially controlled versus spontaneous parturition in the mare, *Compend Cont Educ Pract Vet* 10:506-516, 1988.
556. Pashen RL: Low doses of oxytocin can induce foaling at term, *Equine Vet J* 12:85-87, 1980.
557. Hillman RB, Lesser MS: Induction of parturition. *Vet Clin North Am* 2:333-344, 1980.
558. Paccamonti DL: Elective termination of pregnancy in mares, *J Am Vet Med Assoc* 198:683-688, 1991.
559. Villani M, Romano G: Induction of parturition with daily low-dose oxytocin injections in pregnant mares at term: clinical applications and limitations, *Reprod Dom Anim* 43(4): 481-483, 2008.
560. van Niekerk FE, van Niekerk CH: The effect of dietary protein on reproduction in the mare. II. Growth of foals, body mass of mares and serum protein concentration of mares during the anovulatory, transitional and pregnant periods, *J S Afr Vet Assoc* 68(3):81-85, 1997.
561. van Niekerk FE, van Niekerk CH: The effect of dietary protein on reproduction in the mare. VII. Embryonic development, early embryonic death, foetal losses and their relationship with serum progestagen, *J S Afr Vet Assoc* 69(4):150-155, 1998.
562. van Niekerk FE, van Niekerk CH: The effect of dietary protein on reproduction in the mare. VI. Serum progestagen concentrations during pregnancy, *J SAfr Vet Assoc* 69(4):143-149, 1998.
563. van Niekerk FE, van Niekerk CH: The effect of dietary protein on reproduction in the mare. V. Endocrine changes and conception during the early post partum period, *J S Afr Vet Assoc* 69(3):81-88, 1998.
564. Gee EK, et al: Articular / epiphyseal osteochondrosis in Thoroughbred foals at 5 months of age: influences of growth of the foal and prenatal copper supplementation of the dam, *N Z Vet J* 53(6):448-456, 2005.
565. Barrandeguy M, et al: Prevention of rotavirus diarrhoea in foals by parenteral vaccination of the mares: field trial, *Dev Biol Stand* 92:253-257, 1998.
566. Becu T, Polledo G, Gaskin JM: Immunoprophylaxis of *Rhodococcus equi* pneumonia in foals, *Vet Microbiol* 56(3-4):193-204, 1997.
567. Embertson RM, et al: Hospital approach to dystocia in the mare, In *Am Assoc Equine Pract* 41:13-14 1995.
568. Frazer GS, Perkins NR, Embertson RM: Normal parturition and evaluation of the mare in dystocia, *Equine Vet Educ* 11(1):41-46, 1999.
569. Vandeplassche M: The pathogenesis of dystocia and fetal malformation in the horse, *J Reprod Fertil* (suppl 35):547-552, 1987.
570. Jeffcott LB, Rossdale P: A radiographic study of the fetus in late pregnancy and during foaling, *J Reprod Fertil* (suppl 27):563-569, 1979.
571. Ginther OJ, Williams D: On-the-farm incidence and nature of equine dystocias, *J Equine Vet Sci* 16:159-164, 1996.
572. Jacobs KA, Barber SM, Leach DH: Disruption of the blood supply to the small colon following rectal prolapse and small colon intussusception in a mare, *Can Vet J* 23:132-134, 1982.
573. Blythman WG: Rectal prolapse in a foaling mare, *Vet Rec* 5:471-472, 1988.
574. LeBlanc MM: Sedation and anesthesia of the parturient mare, *Periparturient mare and neonate*, San Antonio, Tex, 2000, Society for Theriogenology, pp 59-64.
575. Frazer GS, Perkins NR, Embertson RM: Correction of equine dystocia, *Equine Vet Educ* 11(1):48-53, 1999.
576. LeBlanc MM, Norman WM: Sedation and aneasthesia of the mare during obstetrical manipulations, In *Am Assoc Equine Pract* 38:619-622, 1992.
577. Grubb TL, Reibold TW, Huber MJ: Comparison of lidocaine, xylazine, and xylazine/lidocaine for caudal epidural analgesia in horses, *J Am Vet Med Assoc* 201:1187-1190, 1992.
578. Norton JL, et al: Retrospective study of dystocia in mares at a referral hospital, *Equine Vet J* 39(1):37-41, 2007.
579. Embertson RM: The indications and surgical techniques for cesarean section in the mare, *Equine Vet Educ* 4:31-36, 1992.
580. Byron CR, et al: Dystocia in a referral hospital setting: approach and results, *Equine Vet J* 35(1):82-85, 2003.
581. Maaskant A, et al: Prevalence, cause and outcome of dystocia in Friesian mares, in Br Equine Vet Assoc, Edinburgh, 2007, The Association.
582. Fisher AT, Phillips TN: Surgical repair of a ruptured uterus in five mares, *Equine Vet J* 18:153-155, 1986.
583. Rossdale PD: Differential diagnosis of postparturient hemorrhage in the mare, *Equine Vet Educ* 6:135-136, 1994.
584. Hooper RN, Blanchard TL, Taylor TS: Identifying and treating uterine prolapse and invagination of the uterine horn, *Vet Med* 88:60, 1991.
585. Brooks DE, McCoy DJ, Martin GS: Uterine rupture as a postpartum complication in two mares, *J Am Vet Med Assoc* 187:1377-1379, 1985.
586. Frazer GS: Fetotomy technique in the mare, *Equine Vet Educ* 13:195-203, 2001.

587. Frazer, G.S. Review of the use of fetotomy to resolve dystocia in the mare. In Am Assoc Equine Pract 43:262-268, 1997. Phoenix,.
588. Bierschwal CJ, deBois C: *The technique of fetotomy in large animals*, Bonner Springs, 1972, Kan, VM Publishing, pp 6-50.
589. Carluccio A, et al: Survival rate and short-term fertility rate associated with the use of fetotomy for resolution of dystocia in mares: 72 cases (1991-2005), *J Am Vet Med Assoc* 230(10):1502-1505, 2007.
590. Nimmo MR, et al: Fertility and complications after fetotomy in 20 brood mares (2001-2006), *Vet Surg* 36(8):771-774, 2007.
591. Byron C, et al: Dystocia in a referral hospital setting: approach and results, *Equine Vet J* 35(1):82-85, 2003.
592. Schambourg M, et al: Thoracic trauma in foals: post mortem findings, *Equine Vet J* 35(1):78-81, 2003.
593. Hillman RB: Dystocia management at the farm, *Periparturient mare and neonate symposium*, San Antonio, Tex, 2000, Society for Theriogenology, pp 65-71.
594. Jean D, et al: Thoracic trauma in newborn foals, *Equine Vet Journal* 31(2):149-152, 1999.
595. Vandeplassche M: Selected topics in equine obstetrics, *In Am Assoc Equine Pract* 38:623-628, 1992.
596. Baldwin JL, Cooper WL, Vanderwall DK: Dystocia due to anterior presentation with unilateral or bilateral hip flexion posture ("dog-sitting" presentation) in the mare: incidence, management, and outcomes, In *Am Assoc Equine Pract* 37:229-241, 1991.
597. Aanes WW: Surgical management of foaling injuries, *Vet Clin North Am* 4:417, 1988.
598. Auer JA, Stick JA, editors: *Equine Surgery*, ed 3, St Louis, 2006, Saunders.
599. Hodder AD, Ball BA: Theriogenology question of the month: hydrocephalus, *J Am Vet Med Assoc* 232(2):211-213, 2008.
600. Hausberger M, et al: First suckling: a crucial event for mother-young attachment? an experimental study in horses (Equus caballus), *J Comp Psychol* 121(1):109-112, 2007.
601. Gunduz MC, Kasikci G, Kaya HH: The effect of oxytocin and PGF(2alpha) on the uterine involution and pregnancy rates in postpartum Arabian mares, *Anim Reprod Sci* 104(2-4):257-263, 2008.
602. Dart AJ, Pascoe JR, Snyder JR: Mesenteric tears of the descending (small) colon as a postpartum complication in two mares, *J Am Vet Med Assoc* 199:1612-1615, 1991.
603. Livesey MA, Keller SD: Segmental ischemic necrosis following mesocolic rupture in postparturient mares, *Comp Cont Educ Pract Vet* 8:763-767, 1986.
604. Dwyer R: Postpartum deaths of mares, *Equine Dis Q* 2(1):5, 1993.
605. Lofstedt R: Haemorrhage associated with pregnancy and parturition, *Equine Vet Educ* 6:138-141, 1994.
606. Getty R: *Sisson and Grossman's the anatomy of the domestic animals*, ed 5, Philadelphia, 1975, Saunders.
607. Rooney JR: Internal hemorrhage related to gestation in the mare, *Cornell Vet* 54:11, 1964.
608. Pascoe R: Rupture of the utero-ovarian or middle uterine artery in the mare at or near parturition, *Vet Rec* 104:77, 1979.
609. Arnold C, et al: Periparturient hemorrhage in mares: 73 cases (1998-2005), *J Am Vet Med Assoc* 232(9):1345-1351, 2008.
610. Stowe HD: Effects of age and impending parturition upon serum copper of Thoroughbred mares, *J Nutr* 95:179-183, 1968.
611. Britt B: personal communication. 2002: Lexington, Ky.
612. Taylor EL, et al: Effects of intravenous administration of formaldehyde on platelet and coagulation variables in healthy horses, *Am J Vet Res* 61:1191-1196, 2000.
613. Shideler RK, et al: Uterine haematoma in a mare, *J Equine Vet Sci* 10:187-193, 1990.
614. Wenzel J, Caudle A, White N: Treating for uterine intramural haematoma in a horse, *Vet Med* 80:66-69, 1995.
615. Pycock JF: Uterine haematoma in 2 mares, *Equine Vet Educ* 6(3):132-134, 1994.
616. Causey R, Ruksznis D, Miles R: Field management of equine uterine prolapse in a Thoroughbred mare, *Equine Vet Educ* 19(5):254-259, 2007.
617. Kobluk CN, Ames TR, Geor RJ, editors: *The horse: disease and clinical management*, Philadelphia, 1996, Saunders.
618. Blanchard TL, et al: Identifying and treating uterine prolapse and invagination of the uterine horn, *Vet Med* 60, 1993.
619. Mogg TD, Hart J, Wearn J: Postpartum hemoperitoneum and septic peritonitis in a Thoroughbred mare, *Vet Clin North Am Equine Pract* 22(1):61-71, 2006.
620. Sutter WW, et al: Diagnosis and surgical treatment of uterine lacerations in mares (33 cases). In *Am Assoc Equine Practitioners*, New Orleans, 2003, AAEP.
621. Dascanio JJ, Ball BA, Hendrickson DA: Uterine tear without a corresponding placental lesion in a mare, *J Am Vet Med Assoc* 202:419-420, 1993.
622. Hooper RN, et al: Diagnosing and treating uterine ruptures in mares, *Vet Med* 88:263-270, 1993.
623. Hassel DM, Ragle CA: Laparoscopic diagnosis and conservative treatment of uterine tear in a mare, *J Am Vet Med Assoc* 205:1531-1536, 1994.
624. Blanchard TL, et al: Sequelae to percutaneous fetotomy in the mare, *J Am Vet Med Assoc* 182:1127, 1983.
625. Vandeplassche M, et al: Observations on involution and puerperal endometritis in mares, *Irish Vet J* 37:126, 1983.
626. Provencher R, et al: Retained fetal membranes in the mare: a retrospective study, *Can Vet J* 29:903-910, 1988.
627. Sevinga M, Barkema HW, Hesselink JW: Serum calcium and magnesium concentrations and the use of a calcium-magnesium-borogluconate solution in the treatment of Fresian mares with retained placenta, *Theriogenology* 57:941-947, 2002.
628. Welle MM, Audige L, Belz JP: The equine endometrial mast cell during the puerperal period: evaluation of mast cell numbers and types in comparison to other inflammatory changes, *Vet Pathol* 34(1):23-30, 1997.
629. Sevinga M, et al: Effect of inbreeding on the incidence of retained placenta in Friesian horses, *J Anim Sci* 82(4):982-986, 2004.
630. Blanchard TL, Varner DD: Therapy for retained placenta in the mare, *Equine Pract* 88:55-59, 1993.
631. Sertich PL: Periparturient emergencies, *Vet Clinics N Am* 10:19, 1994.
632. Blanchard TL, et al: Effect of intrauterine infusion of *Escherichia coli* endotoxin in postpartum pony mares, *Am J Vet Res* 46:2157-2162, 1985.
633. Burns SJ, et al: Management of retained placenta in mares, In *Am Assoc Equine Pract* 23:385, 1977.
634. Martin KL, et al: Calcium decreases and parathyroid hormone increases in serum of periparturient mares, *J Anim Sci* 74(4):834-839, 1996.
635. Sevinga M, Hesselink JW, Barkema HW: Reproductive performance of Fresian mares after retained placenta and manual removal of the placenta, *Theriogenology* 57(2):923-930, 2002.
636. Haffner JC, et al: Equine retained placenta: technique for and tolerance to umbilical artery injections of collagenase, *Theriogenology* 49(4):711-716, 1998.
637. Fecteau KA, Haffner JC, Eiler H: The potential of collagenase as a new therapy for separation of human retained placenta: hydrolytic potency on human, equine and bovine placentae, *Placenta* 19(5-6):379-383, 1998.
638. Blanchard T, et al: Management of dystocia in mares: retained placenta, metritis and laminitis, *Compend Cont Educ Pract Vet* 12:563, 1990.
639. Frazer, G.S., (unpublished observations). 2001.

640. Lock TF: Distribution of antibiotics in the mare reproductive tract after various routes of administration, *J Reprod Fertil* (suppl 32):640, 1982.
641. Turner TA, Fessler JF: Rectal prolapse in the horse, *J Am Vet Med Assoc* 177:1028-1032, 1980.
642. White N: *The equine acute abdomen*, Philadelphia, 1990, Lea & Febiger.
643. Hance SR, Emberstson RM: Colopexy in broodmares: 44 cases (1986-1990), *J Am Vet Med Assoc* 201:782-787, 1992.
644. Embertson R, et al: Large colon volvulus: surgical treatment of 204 horses (1986-1995). In *Am Assoc Equine Pract*, 1996.
645. Dart AJ, Pascoe J: Mesenteric tear of the distal jejunum as a periparturient complication in a mare, *Aust Vet J* 71:427-428, 1994.
646. Edwards GB: A review of 38 cases of small colon obstruction in the horse, *Equine Vet J* 13:S42-S50, 1992.
647. Zamos DT, et al: Segmental ischemic necrosis of the small intestine in two postparturient mares, *J Am Vet Med Assoc* 202:101-103, 1993.
648. Dart AJ, Hodgson DR, Snyder JR: Caecal disease in equids, *Aust Vet J* 75:552-557, 1997.
649. Donelan E, Sloss V: Two cases of rupture of the large intestine in the mare associated with unassisted parturition, *Aust Vet J* 48:413-414, 1972.
650. Voss JL: Rupture of the cecum and ventral colon of mares during parturition, *J Am Vet Med Assoc* 155:745-747, 1969.
651. Platt H: Caecal rupture in parturient mares, *J Comp Path* 93:343-346, 1983.
652. Littlejohn A, Ritchie J: Rupture of the caecum at parturition, *J S Afr Vet Assoc* 46:87, 1975.
653. Auer D, et al: Diaphragmatic rupture in a mare at parturition, *Equine Vet Educ* 17:331-333, 1985.
654. Bristol DG: Diaphragmatic hernias in horses and cattle, *Comp Cont Educ Pract Vet* 8:S407-S412, 1986.
655. Hance SR, Clem MF, DeBowes RM: Intra-abdominal hernias in horses, *Comp Cont Educ Pract Vet* 13:293-299, 1991.
656. Hartzband LE, Kerr DV, Morris EA: Ultrasonographic diagnosis of diaphragmatic rupture in a horse, *Vet Radiol* 31:42-44, 1990.
657. Tulleners E, Richardson D, Reid B: Vaginal evisceration of the small intestine in three mares, *J Am Vet Med Assoc* 186:385, 1985.
658. Singh PNS: Bugalia, Surgical management of a third degree perineal laceration and eversion of the bladder in a mare, *Vet Rec* 148(25):786-787, 2001.
659. Mansmann R, McAllister E, Pratt P, editors: *Equine medicine and surgery*, ed 3, Santa Barbara, 1981, American Veterinary Publications.
660. Nyrop KA, et al: Rupture of the urinary bladder in two postparturient mares, *Comp Contin Educ Pract Vet* 6:510-513, 1984.
661. Jones PA, Sertich PS, Johnston JK: Uroperitoneum associated with ruptured urinary bladder in a postpartum mare, *Aust Vet J* 74(5):354-358, 1996.
662. Rodgerson DH, et al: Standing surgical repair of cystorrhexis in two mares, *Vet Surg* 28(2):113-116, 1999.
663. Kasikci G, et al: A modified surgical technique for repairing third-degree perineal lacerations in mares, *Acta Vet Hung* 53(2):257-264, 2005.
664. Kay AT, et al: How to repair grade IV rectal tears in post-parturition mares, *American Association of Equine Practitioners*, Seattle, Wash 51:487-489, 2005, AAEP.
665. Welland LM: Transmural rectal intestinal evisceration associated with parturition in a primiparous mare, *Can Vet J* 44(9):740-742, 2003.

Assisted Reproductive Techniques

1. McKinnon AO, Carnevale EM, Squires EL, et al: Heterogenous and xenogenous fertilization of in vivo matured equine oocytes, *J Equine Vet Sci* 8:143-147, 1988.
2. Carnevale EM, Squires EL, Maclellan LJ, et al: Use of oocyte transfer in a commercial breeding program for mares with reproductive abnormalities, *J Am Vet Med Assoc* 218:87-91, 2001.
3. Hinrichs K, Provost PJ, Torello EM: Treatments resulting in pregnancy in nonovulating, hormone-treated oocyte recipient mares, *Theriogenology* 54:1285-1293, 2000.
4. Carnevale EM, Bergfelt DR, Ginther OJ: Follicular activity and concentrations of FSH and LH associated with senescence in mares, *Anim Reprod Sci* 35:231-246, 1994.
5. Rantanen NW, McKinnon AO, editors: *Equine diagnostic ultrasonography*, Baltimore, 1998, Williams & Wilkins.
6. Carnevale EM, Griffin PG, Ginther OJ: Age-associated subfertility before entry of embryos into the uterus in mares, *Equine Vet J Suppl* 5:31-35, 1993.
7. Scott MA, Liu IKM, Overstreet JW: Sperm transport to the oviducts: abnormalities and their clinical implications, *Proc Am Assoc Equine Pract* 41:1-2, 1995.
8. Liu IKM, Lantz KC, Schlafke S et al: Clinical observations of oviductal masses in the mare, *Proceedings of the thirtieth annual convention of the American Association of Equine Practitioners*, Lexington, Ky, 1990. pp 41-45.
9. Tsutsumi Y, Suzuki H, Takeda T, et al: Evidence of the origin of the gelatinous masses in the oviducts of mares, *J Reprod Fertil* 57:287-290, 1979.
10. Carnevale EM, Ginther OJ: Defective oocytes as a cause of subfertility in old mares, *Biol Reprod Monogr* 1:209-214, 1995.
11. Carnevale EM, Uson M, Bozzola JJ, et al: Comparison of ooyctes from young and old mares with light and electron microscopy, *Theriogenology* 51:299, 1999.
12. Vogelsang MM, Kraemer DC, Bowen MJ, et al: Recovery of equine follicular oocytes by surgical and non-surgical techniques, *Theriogenology* 25:208, 1986.
13. Hinrichs K, Kenney RM: A colpotomy procedure to increase oocyte recovery rates on aspiration of equine preovulatory follicles, *Teriogenology* 27:237, 1987:(abstract).
14. Hinrichs K, Kenney DF, Kenney RM: Aspiration of oocytes from mature and immature preovulatory follicles in the mare, *Theriogenology* 34:107-112, 1990.
15. Palmer E, Duchamp G, Bezard J, et al: Recovery of follicular fluid and oocytes of mares by non-surgical puncture of the preovulatory follicle, *Theriogenology* 25:178, 1986.
16. Cook NL, Squires EL, Ray BS, et al: Transvaginal ultrasound-guided follicular aspiration of equine oocytes, *J Equine Vet Sci* 15:71-74, 1993.
17. Carnevale EM, Ginther OJ: Use of a linear ultrasonic transducer for the transvaginal aspiration and transfer of oocytes in the mare, *J Equine Vet Sci* 13:331-333, 1993.
18. Hinrichs K, Betschart RW, McCue PM, et al: Effect of time of follicle aspiration on pregnancy rate after oocyte transfer in the mare, *J Reprod Fertil Suppl* 56:493-498, 2000.
19. Carnevale EM, Maclellan LM, Coutinho da Silva MA, et al: Comparison of culture and insemination techniques for equine oocyte transfer, *Theriogenology* 54:982-987, 2000.
20. Coutinho da Silva MA, Carnevale EM, Maclellan LJ, et al: Injection of blood into preovulatory follicles of equine oocyte transfer recipients does not prevent fertilization of the recipient's oocyte, *Theriogenology* 57:538, 2002.
21. Carnevale EM, Alvarenga MA, Squires EL et al: Use of noncycling mares as recipients for oocyte transfer and GIFT. *Proceedings of the annual conference of the Society for Theriogenology*, Nashville, Tenn, 1999. p 44.
22. Carnevale EM, Checura CH, Coutinho da Silva MA, et al: Use of deslorelin acetate to suppress follicular activity in mares used as recipients for oocyte transfer, *Theriogenology* 55:358, 2001.
23. Squires EL, Seidel GE: *Collection and transfer of equine embryos, Animal Reproduction and Biotechnology Laboratory Bulletin No. 08*, Fort Collins, 1995, Colorado State University.

24. Carnevale EM, Maclellan LJ, Coutinho da Silva MA, et al: Equine sperm-oocyte interaction: results after intraoviductal and intrauterine inseminations of recipients for oocyte transfer, *Anim Reprod Sci* 68:305-314, 2001.
25. Ginther OJ: *Reproductive biology of the mare*, ed 2, Cross Plains, Wis, 1992, Equiservices.
26. Scott TJ, Carnevale EM, Maclellan LJ, et al: Embryo development rates after transfer of oocytes matured in vivo, in vitro, or within oviducts of mares, *Theriogenology* 55:705-715, 2001.
27. Maclellan LJ, Carnevale EM, Coutinho da Silva MA, et al: Pregnancies from vitrified equine oocytes collected from superstimulated and non-stimulated mares, *Theriogenology* 58(5):911-919, 2002.
28. Palmer E, Bezard J, Magistrini M, et al: In vitro fertilization in the horse: a retrospective study, *J Reprod Fertil* 44:375-384, 1991.
29. Bezard J: In vitro fertilization in the mare. *Proceedings of the International Scientific Conference on Biotechnics in Horse Reproduction*, Crakow, Poland, 1992. p 12.
30. Franz LC, Squires EL, O'Donovan MK, et al: Collection and in vitro maturation of equine oocytes from estrus, diestrus and pregnant mares, *J Equine Vet Sci* 21:26-32, 2001.
31. Colleoni S, Barbacini S, Necchi D, et al: Application of ovum pick-up, intractyoplasmic sperm injection and embryo culture in equine practice, *Proc 53rd Annual Conf Am Assoc Equine Pract* :554, 2007.
32. Carnevale EM, Maclellan LJ, Coutinho da Silva MA, Squires EL: Pregnancies attained after collection and transfer of oocytes from ovaries of 5 euthanatized mares, *J Am Vet Med Assoc* 222:60-62, 2003.
33. Carnevale EM, Coutinho da Silva MA, Preis KA, et al: Establishment of pregnancies from oocytes collected from the ovaries of euthanatized mares, *Proc 50th Conv Am Assoc Equine Pract*:531-533, 2004.
34. Yamamoto Y, Oguri N, Tsutsumi Y, et al: Experiments in the freezing and storage of equine embryos, *J Reprod Fertil Suppl* 32:399-403, 1982.
35. Seidel GE Jr: Cryopreservation of equine embryos, *Vet Clin North Am Equine Pract* 12:85-99, 1996.
36. Slade NP, Takeda T, Squires EL, et al: A new procedure for the cryopreservation of equine embryos, *Theriogenology* 24:45-57, 1985.
37. Lascombes FA, Pashen RL: Results from embryo freezing and post ovulation breeding in a commercial embryo transfer programme, *Havemeyer Foundation Monograph Series No. 3: equine embryo transfer*, 2000.
38. Eldridge-Panuska WD, Caracciolo di Brienza V, Seidel GE Jr, et al: Establishment of pregnancies after serial dilution or vitrified equine embryos, *Theriogenology* 63:1308-1319, 2005.
39. Carnevale EM, Eldridge-Panuska WD, Caracciolo di Brienza V: How to collect and vitrify equine embryos for direct transfer, *Proc 50th Ann Conv Am Assoc Equine Pract* :402-405, 2004.
40. Hudson J, McCue PM, Carnevale EM, et al: The effects of cooling and vitrification of embryos from eFSH-treated mares on pregnancy rates after nonsurgical transfer, *J Equine Vet Sci* 26:51-54, 2006.
41. Maclellan LJ, Lane M, Sims MM, et al: Effect of sucrose or trehalose on vitrification of equine oocytes 12 h or 24 h after the onset of maturation, evaluated after ICSI, *Theriogenology* 55:310, 2001.
42. Vatja G: Vitrification of oocytes and embryos of domestic animals, *Anim Reprod Sci* :357-364, 2000:60/61.
43. Hochi S, Fujimoto T, Choi Y, et al: Cryopreservation of equine oocytes by 2-step freezing, *Theriogenology* 42:1085-1094, 1994.
44. Householder DD, Pickett BW, Voss JL, et al: Effect of extender, number of spermatozoa and hCG on equine fertility, *J Equine Vet Sci* 1:9-13, 1981.
45. Katila T, Sankari S, Makela O: Transport of spermatozoa in the reproductive tract of mares, *J Reprod Fertil Suppl* 56:571-578, 2000.
46. Rigby S, Derczo S, Brinsko S et al: Oviductal sperm numbers following proximal uterine horn or uterine body insemination, *Proc 46th Ann Conv Am Assoc Equine Pract,* San Antonio, Tex, Nov 26-29, 2000. pp 332-334.
47. Senger PL, Becker WC, Davidge ST, et al: Influence of cornual insemination on conception rates in dairy cattle, *J Anim Sci* 66:3010-3016, 1988.
48. Seidel GE Jr, Allen CH, Johnson LA, et al: Uterine inseminations of heifers with very low numbers of nonfrozen and sexed spermatozoa, *Theriogenology* 48:1255-1264, 1997.
49. Buchanan BR, Seidel GE Jr, McCue PM, et al: Insemination of mares with low numbers of either unsexed or sexed spermatozoa, *Theriogenology* 53:1333-1344, 2000.
50. Rigby SL, Lindsey AC, Brinsko SP, et al: Pregnancy rates in mares following hysteroscopic or rectally-guided utero-tubal insemination with low sperm numbers, *Anim Reprod Sci* 68:331-332, 2001.
51. Woods J, Rigby SL, Brinsko SP, et al: Effect of intrauterine treatment with prostaglandin E_2 before insemination of mares in the uterine horn or body, *Theriogenology* 53:1827-1836, 2000.
52. Morris LHA, Hunter RHF, Allen WR: Hysteroscopic insemination of small numbers of spermatozoa at the uterotubal junction of preovulatory mares, *J Reprod Fertil* 188:95-100, 2000.
53. Lindsey AC, Bruemmer JE, Squires EL: Low dose insemination of mares using non-sorted and sex-sorted sperm, *Anim Reprod Sci* 68:279-289, 2001.
54. Leao KM, Alvarenga MA, Puolli-Filho JN: Hysteroscopic insemination in mares with low sperm number, *Theriogenology* 57:381, 2002.
55. Manning ST, Bowman PA, Fraser LM et al: Development of hysteroscopic insemination of the uterine tube in the mare. *Proceedings of the annual meeting of Society for Theriogenology*, Baltimore, Md, 1998. pp 84-85.
56. Morris LHA, Allen WR: Hysteroscopic uterotubal insemination of mares with low numbers of spermatozoa, *Anim Reprod Sci* 68:330-331, 2001.
57. Alvarenga MA, Leao KM: Hysteroscopic insemination of mares with low number of frozen thawed spermatozoa selected by Percoll gradient. *Proceedings of the eighth International Symposium on Equine Reproduction*, Fort Collins, Colo, 2002.
58. Alvarenga MA, Trinque CC, Lima MM, et al: Utilization of hysteroscopy for the application of stallion frozen semen in commercial programs, *Rev Bras Reprod Anim* 25:361-362, 2001.
59. Coutinho da Silva MA, Carnevale EM, Maclellan LJ, et al: Embryo development rates after oocyte transfer comparing intrauterine or intraoviductal insemination and fresh or frozen semen in mares, *Theriogenology* 55:359, 2001.
60. Coutinho da Silva MA, Carnevale EM, Maclellan LJ, et al: Oocyte transfer in mares with intrauterine or intraoviductal insemination using fresh, cooled, and frozen stallion semen, *Theriogenology* 61:705-713, 2004.
61. Squires EL, Wilson JM, Kato H, et al: A pregnancy after intracytoplasmic sperm injection into equine oocyte matured in vitro, *Theriogenology* 45:306, 1996.
62. Cochran R, Meintjes M, Reggio B, et al: Live foals produced from sperm-injected oocytes derived from pregnant mares, *J Equine Vet Sci* 18:736-741, 1998.
63. McKinnon AO, Lacham-Kaplan O, Trounson AO: Pregnancies produced from fertile and infertile stallions by intracytoplasmic sperm injection (ICSI) of single frozen/thawed spermatozoa into in vivo matured mare oocytes, *J Reprod Fertil* (suppl 56):513-517, 2000.

64. Galli C, Crotti G, Duchi R, et al: Embryonic development of equine oocytes fertilized by ICSI, *Havemeyer Foundation Monograph Series No. 3: equine embryo transfer*, 2000.
65. Galli C, Maclellan LJ, Crotti G, et al: Development of equine oocytes matured in vitro in different media and fertilised by ICSI, *Theriogenology* 57:719, 2002.
66. Li X, Morris LHA, Allen WR: The development of blastocysts after intracytoplasmic sperm injection of equine oocytes, *Havemeyer Foundation Monograph Series No. 3: equine embryo transfer*, 2000.
67. Maclellan LJ, Sims MM, Squires EL: Effect of invasive adenylate cyclase during oocyte maturation on the development of equine embryos following ICSI, *Havemeyer Foundation Monograph Series No. 3: equine embryo transfer*, 2000.
68. Carnevale EM, Stokes JE, Squires EL, et al: Clinical use of intracytoplasmic sperm injection in horses, *Proc 53rd Conv Am Assoc Equine Pract* :560, 2007.

The Stallion

1. Levy JB, Husmann DA: The hormonal control of testicular descent, *J Androl* 16(6):459-463, 1995.
2. Johnson AD, Gomes WR, VanDenmark L, et al: *The testis*, New York, 1970, Academic Press.
3. Dyce KM, Sack WO, Wensing CJG: *Textbook of veterinary anatomy*, ed 3, St Louis, 2002, Saunders.
4. Jann HW, Rains JR: Diagnostic ultrasonography for evaluation of cryptorchidism in horses, *J Am Vet Med Assoc* 196:297, 1990.
5. Silberzahn P, Pouret E, Zwain I: Androgen and oestrogen response to a single injection of hCG in cryptorchid horses, *Equine Vet J* 21(2):126-129, 1989.
6. Cox JE: Experience with a diagnostic test for equine cryptorchidism, *Equine Vet J* 7:179-182, 1975.
7. Cox JE, Williams JH, Rowe PH, et al: Testosterone in normal, cryptorchid and castrated horses, *Equine Vet J* 5:85-90, 1973.
8. Johnson L, Varner DD, Thompson DL Jr: Effect of age and season on the establishment of spermatogenesis in the horse, *J Reprod Fertil* (suppl 44):87-97, 1991.
9. Samper J, editor: *Equine breeding management and artificial insemination*, ed 2, St Louis, 2009, Saunders.
10. Swierstra EE, Gebauer MR, Pickett BW: Reproductive physiology of the stallion. 1. Spermatogenesis and testis composition, *J Reprod Fertil* 40:113-123, 1974.
11. Hamilton DW, Greep RO, editors: *Handbook of physiology*, vol. 5, Washington, DC, 1975, American Physiological Society.
12. Johnson L, Thompson DL Jr: Seasonal variation in the total volume of Leydig cells in stallions is explained by variation in cell number rather than cell size, *Biol Reprod* 35:971-979, 1986.
13. Johnson L, Tatum ME: Temporal appeaiance of seasonal changes in numbers of Sertoli cells, Leydig cells, and germ cells in stallions, *Biol Reprod* 40:994-999, 1989.
14. Johnson L, Thompson DL Jr: Age-related and seasonal variation in the Sertoli cell population, daily sperm production and serum concentrations of follicle-stimulating hormone, luteinizing hormone and testosterone in stallions, *Biol Reprod* 29:777-789, 1983.
15. Cupps PT, editor: *Reproduction in domestic animals*, ed 4, New York, 1991, Academic Press.
16. Clay CM, Squires EL, Amann RP, et al: Influences of season and artificial photoperiod on stallions: luteinizing hormone, follicle-stimulating hormone and testosterone, *J Anim Sci* 66:1246-1255, 1988.
17. Burns PJ, Douglas RB: Effects of season, age and increased photoperiod on reproductive hormone concentrations and testicular diameters in thoroughbred stallions, *Equine Vet Sci* 4(5):202-208, 1987.
18. Clay CM, Squires EL, Amann RP, et al: Influences of season and artificial photoperiod on stallions: testicular size, seminal characteristics and sexual behavior, *J Anim Sci* 64:517-525, 1987.
19. Knobil E, Neill JD, editors: *The physiology of reproduction*, ed 2, New York, 1994, Raven Press.
20. Goyal HO: Morphology of the bovine epididymis, *Am J Anat* 172:155, 1985.
21. Amann RP: Function of the epididymis in bulls and rams, *J Reprod Fertil* 34:115, 1987.
22. Crabo B: Studies on the composition of epididymal content in bulls and boars, *Acta Vet Scand* 6:1-120, 1965.
23. Sack WO, editor: *Rooney's guide to the diseases of the horse*, ed 6, Ithaca, NY, 1991, Veterinary Textbooks.
24. Johnson L: Maturation of equine epididymal sperm, *Am J Vet Res* 41:1190-1196, 1980.
25. Getty R, editor: *Sisson and Grossman's the anatomy of the domestic animals*, ed 5, Philadelphia, 1975, Saunders.
26. Varner DD, Schumacher J, Blanchard T: *Diseases and management of breeding stallions*, American Veterinary Publications, Goleta, Calif, 1991.
27. Love CC, Garcia MC, Riera FR, et al: Use of testicular volume to predict daily sperm output in the stallion, *Proc Am Assoc Equine Pract* 36:15, 1990.
28. Little TV, Holyoak GR: Reproductive anatomy and physiology of the stallion. The veterinary clinics of North America, equine practice: stallion management, Saunders. Apr. 8(1): 1-29, 1992.
29. Love CC: Ultrasonographic evaluation of the testis, epididymis, and spermatic cord of the stallion, The veterinary clinics of North America, equine practice: stallion management, Saunders, Apr;8(1):167-182, 1992.
30. Gebauer MR, Pickett BW, Faulkner LC, et al: Reproductive physiology of the stallion. 7. Chemical characteristics of seminal plasma and spermatozoa, *J Anim Sci* 43:626-632, 1976.
31. Lindholmer CH: The importance of seminal plasma for human sperm motility, *Biol Reprod* 10:533-542, 1974.
32. Aurich JE: Seminal plasma affects membrane integrity and motility of equine spermatozoa after cryopreservation, *Theriogenology* 46(5):791-797, 1996.
33. Weber JA, Woods GL: Transrectal ultrasonography for the evaluation of stallion accesory sex glands. The veterinary clinics of North America, equine practice: stallion management, Saunders Apr 8(1):183-190, 1992.
34. Pozor AM, McDonnell SM: Ultrasound evaluation of stallion accessory sex glands, *Proceedings of the annual meeting for the Society for Theriogenology*, Kansas City, Mo, 1996. pp 294-297.
35. Love CC, Riera FL, Oristaglio RM et al: Sperm occluded (plugged) ampullae in the stallion, *Proceedings of the annual meeting of the Society for Theriogenology*, Kansas City, Mo, 1992. pp 117-123.
36. MacPherson ML: *Male genital endoscopy short course: advanced current topics in stallion veterinary practice*, Kennett Square, Penn, Oct 1997, New Bolton Center.
37. Sullins KE, Traub-Dargatz JL: Endoscopy of the equine urinary tract, *Compend Cont Educ Pract Vet* 6:663, 1984.
38. Traub-Dargatz JL, Brown CM, editors: *Equine endoscopy*, ed 2, St Louis, 1997, Mosby.
39. McDonnell SM: Normal and abnormal sexual behavior, *Vet Clin North Am Equine Pract* 8(1):71-89, 1992.
40. McDonnell SM: Ejaculation: physiology and dysfunction. The veterinary clinics of North America: equine practice, Saunders, Apr;8(1):57-70, 1992.
41. Kobluck CN, Ames TR, Geor RJ, editors: *The horse: diseases and clinical management*, Philadelphia, 1995, Saunders.
42. McDonnell SM: Stallion behavior and endocrinology. What do we really know? *Proceedings of the annual meeting of the American Association of Equine Practitioners*, Lexington, Ky, 1995.
43. McDonnell SM: Ejaculation: physiology and dysfunction, *Vet Clin North Am Equine Pract* 8(1):57-70, 1993.

44. McDonnell SM, Love CC: Manual stimulation collection of semen from stallions: training time, sexual behavior and semen, *Theriogenology* 33:1202, 1990.
45. Love CC: Semen collection techniques. The veterinary clinics of North America: equine practice, Saunders, Apr 8(1):111-128, 1992.
46. Love CC, Riera FL, Oristaglio RM et al: Sperm occluded (plugged) ampullae in the stallion, *Proceedings of the annual meeting of the Society for Theriogenology*, 1992. pp 117-123.
47. McDonnell SM, Garcia MC, Kenney RM, et al: Imipramine-induced erection, masturbation and ejaculation in male horses, *Pharmacol Biochem Behav* 27:187, 1987.
48. McDonnell Sm A: Practical review of self-mutilation in horses, *Anim Reprod Sci* 107:219-228, 2008.
49. Luescher UA, McKeown DB, Dean H: A cross-sectional study on compulsive behaviour (stable vices) in horses, *Eq Vet J* (suppl 27):14-18, 1998.
50. McDonnell SM, Diehl NK: Oristaglio Turner RM: Modification of unruly breeding behavior in stallions, *Compend Cont Educ Pract Vet* 17(3):411, 1994.
51. Crump J, Crump J: Stallion ejaculation by manual stimulation of the penis, *Theriogenology* 31:341, 1988.
52. McDonnell SM, Odion MJ: Imipramine and xylazine-induced ex copula ejaculation in stallions, *Theriogenology* 41:1005, 1994.
53. Turner RMO, McDonnell SM, Hawkins JF: Use of pharmacologically induced ejaculation to obtain semen from a stallion with a fractured radius, *J Am Vet Med Assoc* 206:1906, 1995.
54. McDonnell SM, Love CC: Xylazine-induced ex copula ejaculation in stallions, *Theriogenology* 36:73, 1991.
55. Froman DP, Amann RP: Inhibition of motility of bovine, canine and equine spermatozoa by artificial vagina lubricants, *Theriogenology* 20:357, 1983.
56. Samper JC, Garcia A: Post-thaw characteristics and fertility of stallion semen frozen in extenders with different cryoprotectants, *Ann Reprod Sci* 107:255, 2008.
57. Amann RP, Loomis PR, Pickett BW: Improved filter system for an equine artificial vagina, *Equine Vet Sci* 3:120, 1983.
58. Tischner M, Kosiniak K: Techniques for collection and storage of stallion semen with minimal secondary contamination, *Acta Vet Scand Suppl* 88:83, 1992.
59. Kenney RM, Cooper WL: Therapeutic use of a phantom for semen collection from a stallion, *J Am Vet Med Assoc* 165:706, 1994.
60. Jarrige R, Martin-Rosset W, editors: *Le Cheval. Reproduction, sélection, alimentation, exploitation*, Paris, 1984, INRA.
61. Pickett BW, Voss JL, Bowen RA et al: Seminal characteristics and total scrotal width (TSW) of normal and abnormal stallions, *Proceedings of the thirty-third annual convention of the American Association of Equine Practitioners*, San Diego, 1988. p 487.
62. Bailey E, Fenning N, Chamberlain S: Validation of sperm counting methods using limits of agreement, *J Andrology* 28:364, 2007.
63. Hansen C, Vermeiden T, Vermeiden JPW: Comparison of FACSCount AF system, improved Neubauer hemacytometer, Corning 254 photometer, SpermVision, UltiMate and NucleoCounter SP-100 for determination of sperm concentration of boar semen, *Theriogenology* 66:2188, 2006.
64. Varner DD, Blanchard TL, Love CL, et al: Effects of semen fractionation and dilution ratio on equine spermatozoal motility parameters, *Theriogenology* 28:709-723, 1987.
65. Samper JC, Hellander JC, Crabo BG: Relation between fertility of fresh and frozen stallion semen and its quality measured as sperm motility and with glass wool/Sephadex filters, *J Reprod Fertil Suppl* 44:107-114, 1991.
66. Amann RP: Computerized evaluation of stallion spermatozoa, *Proceedings of the thirty-third annual convention of the American Association of Equine Practitioners*, New Orleans, 1987. pp 453-473.
67. Jasko DJ, Lein DH, Foote RH: Determination of the relationship between sperm morphologic classifications and fertility in stallions: 66 cases (1987-1988), *J Am Vet Med Assoc* 197(3):389, 1990.
68. Voss JL, Pickett BW, Squires EL: Stallion spermatozoal morphology and motility and their relationship to fertility, *J Am Vet Med Assoc* 178(3):287, 1981.
69. Jeyendran RS, Vanderven HH, Zaneveld LJD: The hypoosmotic swelling test: an update, *Arch Androl* 29:105, 1992.
70. Magistrini M, Guitton E, Le Vern Y, et al: New staining methods for sperm evaluation estimated by microscopy and flow cytometry, *Theriogenology* 48:1129, 1997.
71. Evenson DP, Darzynkiewicz Z, Melamed MR: Relation of mammalian sperm chromatin heterogeneity to fertility, *Science* 210:1131, 1980.
72. Kenney RM, Evenson DP, Love CC, et al: Relationship between sperm chromatine structure, motility and morphology of ejaculated sperm and seasonal pregnancy rate, *Biol Reprod Monogr* 1:647, 1995.
73. Mann T: Studies on the metabolism of semen. 1. General aspects: occurrence and distribution of cytochrome, certain enzymes and co-enzymes, *J Biochem* 39:451, 1945.
74. Mann T: Studies on the metabolism of semen. 2. Glycolysis in spermatozoa, *J Biochem* 39:458, 1945.
75. Kosiniak K, Bittmar A: Prognosis of stallion semen freezability on the basis of biochemical tests, *J Reprod Fertil Suppl* 44:653, 1991.
76. Turner RM: Current techniques for evaluation of stallion fertility, *Clin Tech Eq Pract* 4:257, 2005.
77. Brinsko SP, Rowan KR, Varner DD, et al: Effects of transport container and ambient storage temperature on motion characteristics of equine spermatozoa, *Theriogenology* 53:1641-1655, 2000.
78. Padilla AW, Foote RH: Extender and centrifugation effects on the motility patterns of slow-cooled stallion spermatozoa, *J Anim Sci* 69:3308-3313, 1991.
79. Leopold S, Samper JC, Curtis E, et al: Effect of cryopreservation and oviductal cell-conditioned media on calcium flux in equine spermatozoa, *J Reprod Fertil Suppl* 56:431-445, 2000.
80. Wöckener A, Malmgrem L, Ob den Kamp B et al: Freezing of stallion semen: effects on sperm motility and morphology, *Proceedings of the twelfth International Congress on Animal Reproduction*, The Hague, The Netherlands, 1992.
81. Blach EL, Amann RP, Bowen RA, et al: Changes in quality of stallion spermatozoa during cryopreservation: plasma membrane integrity and motion characteristics, *Theriogenology* 31:283, 1989.
82. Samper JC, Hearn P, Ganheim A: Pregnancy rates and effect of extender and motility and acrosome status of frozen-thawed stallion spermatozoa, *Proceedings of the annual convention of the American Association of Equine Practitioners*, Vancouver, British Columbia, Canada, 1994. pp. 41-43.
83. Samper JC: Stallion semen cryopreservation: male factors affecting pregnancy rates, *Proceedings of the annual meeting of the Society for Theriogenology*, San Antonio, Texas, 1995. pp 160-165.
84. Graham JK, Kunze E, Hammerstedt RH: Analysis of sperm viability acrosomal integrity and mitochondrial function using flow cytometry, *Biol Reprod* 43:55, 1990.
85. National Research Council: *Nutrient requirements of horses*, Washington, DC, 1989, National Academy of Sciences, The Council.
86. Jackson SG: Feeding the stallion, *Proceedings of the Blue Grass Equine Reproduction Symposium*, Lexington, Ky, 2000.
87. Brinsko SP, Varner DD, Love CC, et al: Effect of feeding a DHA-enriched nutriceutical on the quality of fresh, cooled and frozen stallion semen, *Theriogenology* 63:1519-1527, 2005:15.

88. Burns PJ, Douglas RB: Effects of season, age and increased photoperiod on reproductive hormone concentrations and testicular diameters in thoroughbred stallions, *Equine Vet Sci* 4(5):202-208, 1987.
89. Blanchard Tl, Kenney RM, Timoney PJ: Venereal disease. Veterinary clinics of North America, equine practice, Saunders, Apr; 8(1):191-203, 1992.
90. Hoyumpa AH, McIntosh AL, Varner DD: Normal bacterial flora of equine semen: antibacterial effects of amikacin, penicillin, and an amikacin-penicillin combination in a seminal extenders, *Proceedings of the twelfth International Congress on Animal Reproduction*, The Hague, Netherlands, 1992. pp 1427-1429.
91. Bowen JM, Tobin N, Simpson RB: Effects of washing on the bacterial flora of the stallion's penis, *J Reprod Fertil Suppl* 32:41-46, 1982.
92. Varner DD: External and internal genital infections of stallions, *Proceedings of the Stallion Reproduction Symposium*, Society for Theriogenology, Baltimore, 1998. pp 84-94.
93. Kenney RM, Cummings MR: Potential control of stallion penile shedding of *Pseudomonas aureginosa* and Klebsiella pneumoniae, *Proceedings of the Symposium Voortplanting Pard*, Ghent, Belgium, 1990.
94. Deleted in pages.
95. Parlevliet JM, Bleumink-Plyum NMC, Houwers DJ: Epidemiological aspects of Tyllorela equigenitalis, *Theriogenology* 47:1169-1178, 1997.
96. Glazer AL, Chernside ED, Horzinek RE, et al: Equine arteritis virus, *Theriogenology* 47:1275-1295, 1997.
97. Timoney P, McCollum WH: Equine viral arteritis: essential facts about the disease, *Proc Am Assoc Equine Pract* 43:199, 1997.
98. Timoney PJ, McCollum WH, Murph TW, et al: The carrier state in equine arteritis virus infection in the stallion with specific emphasis on the venereal mode of virus transmission, *J Reprod Fertil Suppl* 35:95, 1987.
99. Chowdhary BP, Raudsepp T: The horse genome derby: racing from map to whole genome sequence, *Chromosome Res* 16:109, 2008.
100. Sommer MM, Meyers-WaUen VN: XX true hermaphroditism in a dog, *J Am Vet Med Assoc* 198(3):435-438, 1991.
101. Santen RJ, Swerdloff RS, editors: *Male reproductive dysfunction: diagnosis and management of hypogonadism, infertility and impotence*, New York, 1986, Marcel Dekker.
102. Card CE, Ball BA, Baxendell K, et al: Clinical features of persis tent mullerian duct syndrome (PMDS) in a horse, *J Androl* (Suppl 1), 1991.
103. Frandson RD, Epling GP, Davis RW: A case report: arrested testicular development in the horse, *J Am Vet Med Assoc* 137:255-257, 1960.
104. Sinclair AH, Berta P, Palmer MS, et al: A gene from the human sex-determining region encodes a protein with homology to a conserved DNA-binding motif, *Nature* 346:240, 1990.
105. Estrada A, Samper JC, Lillich JD, et al: EM.Azoospermia associated with bilateral segmental aplasia of the ductus deferens in a stallion, *J Am Vet Med Assoc* 222:1740-1742, 2003.
106. Blanchard TL, Woods JA, Brinsko SP: Theriogenology question of the month. Azoospermia attributable to bilateral epididymal hypoplasia, *J Am Vet Med Assoc* 217:825-826, 2000.
107. Samper JC, unpublished data
108. Robertson A, editor: Handbook on animal diseases in the tropics, Marcel Dekker (originally published in 1976), New York, 1986.
109. Blanchard TL, Bretzlaff KN: Identifying, treating, and preventing scrotal skin disorders of large animals, *Vet Med* 85:290-294, 1990.
110. DiPietro JA, Klie TR, French DD: Contemporary topics in equine parasitology, *Compend Cont Educ Pract Vet* 12:713, 1990.
111. Earnshaw RE: Polyorchidism, *Can J Comp Med* 23(2):66, 1959.
112. Stickle RL, Fessler JF: Retrospective study of 350 cases of equine cryptorchidism, *J Am Vet Med Assoc* 172:343-346, 1978.
113. Hayes HM: Epidemiological features of 5009 cases of equine cryptorchidism, *Equine Vet J* 18:467-471, 1986.
114. Arighi M, Bosu TK: Comparison of hormonal methods for diagnosis of cryptorchidism in horses, *J Equine Vet Sci* 9:20-26, 1989.
115. Johnson L, Thompson DL Jr: Age related and seasonal variation in the Sertoli cell population daily sperm production and serum concentrations of follicle-stimulated hormone luteinizing hormone and testosterone in stallions, *Biol Reprod* 29:777-789, 1983.
116. McEnteek: *Reproductive pathology of domestic animals*, Academic Press, San Diego, 1990, Mosby.
117. Caron JP, Barber SM, Bailey JV: Equine testicular neoplasia, *Compend Cont Educ Vet Pract* 7(1):S53-S59, 1985.
118. Smith BL, Morton LD, Watkins JP, et al: Malignant seminoma in a cryptorchid stallion, *J Am Vet Med Assoc* 195(6):775-776, 1989.
119. Pugh RCB: *Pathology of the testis*, Oxford, 1976, Blackwell.
120. Love CC, Garcia MC, Riera FR, et al: Use of testicular volume to predict daily sperm output in the stallion, *Proc Am Assoc Equine Pract* 36:15, 1991.
121. Smith JA: The occurrence of larvae of *Strongylus edentatus* in the testicles of stallions, *Vet Rec* 93:604-606, 1973.
122. Tung KSK: Pathogenesis of antoimmune orchitis, *Proceedings of the annual meeting of the Society for Theriogenology*, San Diego, Calif, 1991.
123. Boyle M: Immune related infertility in stallion? *Equine Vet J* 22:67-69, 1990.
124. Setchell BP: *The mammalian testis*, Ithaca, NY, 1978, Cornell University Press.
125. Kaufman DG, Nagler HM: Male infertility, *Urol Clin North Am* 16:489-498, 1987.
126. Held JP, Prater P, Toal RL, et al: Sperm granuloma in a stallion, *J Am Vet Med Assoc* 194:267-268, 1989.
127. Gerona GR, Sikes JO: Effects of elevated scrotum temperature onspermatogenesisandsemencharacteristics,*JDairySci*53:659, 1970.
128. Threlfall WR, Carleton CL, Robertson J, et al: Recurrent torsion of the spermatic cord and scrotal testis in a stallion, *J Am Vet Med Assoc* 196(10):1641-1643, 1990.
129. Amann RP: Function of the epididymis in bulls and rams, *J Reprod Fertil* 34:115, 1987.
130. Held JP, Vanhooser S, Prater P, et al: Impotence in a stallion with neuritis cauda equina: a case report, *J Equine Vet Sci* 9: 67-68, 1989.
131. McKinnon AO, Voss JL, Trotter GW, et al: Hemospermia of the stallion, *Equine Pract* 10(9):17-23, 1988.
132. Elce YA: The aetiopathogenesis of squamous cell carcinomas in horses. Where are we? *Equine Vet Educ* 21(1):17-18, 2009.
133. Smith MA, Levine DG, Getman LM, et al: Vulvar squamous cell carcinoma *in situ* within viral papillomas in an aged Quarter Horse mare, *Equine Vet Educ*. 21:11-16, 2009.
134. Pearson H, Weaver BMQ: Priapism after sedation, neurolept-analgesia and anaesthesia in the horse, *Equine Vet J* 10:85-90, 1978.
135. Klug E, Deegan E, Lazarz B, et al: Effect of adrenergic neurotransmitters upon the ejaculatory process in the stallion, *J Reprod Fertil Suppl* 32:31, 1982.

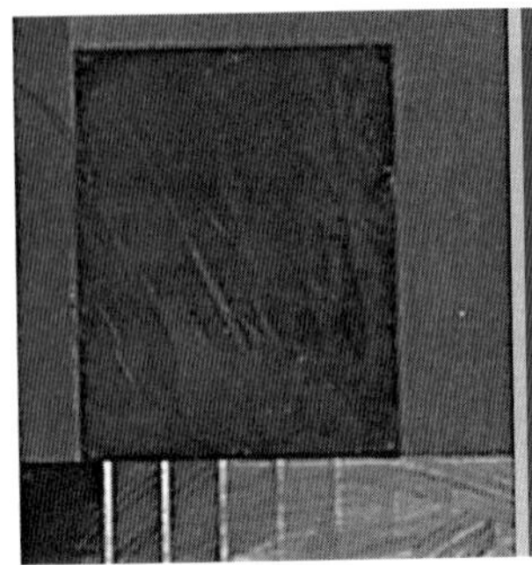

Disorders of the Urinary System

CHAPTER 19

Bryan Waldridge

ANATOMY AND DEVELOPMENT

Harold C. Schott II

ANATOMY

The urinary system of the horse, like that of most mammals, consists of paired kidneys and ureters, the bladder, and the urethra. With the exception of the abdominal portion of the urinary bladder, the entire urinary tract is located in the retroperitoneal space. In a newborn foal, each kidney weighs about 175 g. In an adult horse the left kidney weighs between 600 to 700 g, and the right kidney is usually 25 to 50 g heavier, although this is not a consistent finding, and one may observe the reverse relation.[1,2] Thus the kidneys account for approximately 0.65% to 0.75% and 0.27% to 0.37% of the total body mass of the foal and adult horse, respectively.[1,3] The right kidney is located immediately below the dorsal extent of the last two or three ribs and the first lumbar transverse process, is shaped like a horseshoe, and measures about 15 cm long, 15 cm wide, and 5 to 6 cm high (dorsal to ventral). Craniolaterally, the right kidney is embedded into the liver, and its more craniad position compared with the left kidney prevents it from being accessible on rectal palpation. Although not the classically bean-shaped organ found in human beings and small animals, the left kidney in the adult horse is more elongated than the right kidney, with the cranial pole at the level of the hilus of the right kidney; in equids, the left kidney is about 18 cm long, 10 to 12 cm wide, and 5 to 6 cm high. Because of its more caudal location, one routinely can palpate the caudoventral aspect of the left kidney during rectal examination. The blood supply to the kidneys comes from one or more renal arteries branching from the aorta. Accessory renal arteries (which generally enter caudally) may arise from the caudal mesenteric, testicular or ovarian, or deep circumflex iliac arteries.[1,2]

The ureters are 6 to 8 mm in diameter and travel about 70 cm to their insertions in the dorsal bladder neck or trigone, close to the urethra. The distal 5 to 7 cm of each ureter courses within the bladder wall. This intramural segment of the ureter functions as a one-way valve to prevent vesicoureteral reflux (VUR) with progressive bladder distention. The urinary bladder lies on the pelvic floor when empty but can increase in size and drop forward over the pelvic brim when filled with urine. The bladder can accommodate up to 3 to 4 L of urine before stimulation of micturition. In the foal the bladder is attached to the ventral abdominal wall by the urachus and remnants of the umbilical arteries. Consequently, when empty, the bladder is commonly a band-shaped structure in a neonatal foal. During the first few months of life, this ventral attachment loosens as the urachal remnant becomes the middle ligament and the umbilical arterial remnants become the round ligaments of the free border of the paired lateral ligaments of the bladder.[1]

The urethra is about 2 to 3 cm long in a mare and 75 to 90 cm long in a male. In the intact male the pelvic urethra, which is 10 to 12 cm long, widens in an elliptic pattern to a diameter of 5 cm across and 2 to 3 cm from dorsal to ventral. A rounded dorsal prominence, the colliculus seminalis, is located immediately caudal to the urethral orifice and is the site of the common openings of the ductus deferens and ducts of the seminal vesicles. The openings of the prostatic ducts are on two groups of small papillae lateral to the colliculus seminalis. Between 2 and 3 cm farther caudad, the ducts of the bulbourethral glands open in paired dorsal lines. The smaller openings of the ducts of the lateral urethral glands open at the same level on the lateral aspect of the urethra.[1]

A fibrous capsule that peels easily from the normal kidney covers the surface of each kidney. The equine kidney consists of an outer cortex slightly wider than the inner medulla. The cortex is dotted with dark spots—renal corpuscles or glomeruli within Bowman's capsules. In horses, the corticomedullary junction is less distinct than in other species and is typically a deep red that contrasts well against the paler medulla and red-brown cortex. This region undulates along renal pyramids (cortex) and renal columns (medulla). The pyramids are subdivisions of the renal parenchyma, which are separated by arcuate arteries at the level of the corticomedullary junction. The equine kidney contains a total of 40 to 60 pyramids arranged in four parallel rows. The renal pelvis is the dilated proximal portion of the ureter. Microscopic examination reveals numerous small openings of the collecting ducts (ducts of Bellini). Additionally, the renal pelvis and proximal ureter are lined with compound tubular mucous glands and goblet cells that secrete thick, viscid mucus usually found in the renal pelvis and urine of normal horses.[1,4]

The functional unit of the kidney is the nephron. Each nephron is composed of a renal corpuscle (glomerulus within

Bowman's capsule), a proximal tubule (convoluted and straight components), an intermediate tubule (loop of Henle), a distal convoluted tubule, a connecting tubule, and cortical, outer medullary, and inner medullary collecting ducts (Figure 19-1). The two populations of nephrons are (1) the superficial (or cortical) nephrons possessing short loops of Henle and (2) the juxtamedullary nephrons with long loops of Henle. Gradations exist between these two general categories of nephrons, as well as species variation in the ratio of short-looped nephrons to long ones. For example, human beings have seven times more short- than long-looped nephrons, whereas essentially 100% of nephrons in dogs and cats have long loops.[5] An early anatomic study found approximately 4 million glomeruli (nephrons) in the adult bovine kidney[6]; however, a recent study of kidney organogenesis using unbiased stereologic techniques to examine 45 equine left kidneys indicated that the left kidney of the horse may contain closer to 10 million glomeruli (for a total of 20 million in both kidneys).[7] The latter study also confirmed that the total number of glomeruli does not increase after birth despite continued growth of the kidney until about 1 year of age. At present, little information is available on the ratio of short- to long-looped nephrons in horses. Histologically, equine nephrons are similar to those of other mammalian species; however, the diameter and epithelial height of the tubule and collecting duct segments are comparatively larger. In addition, the equine macula densa (segment of the ascending loop of Henle that lies in close association with the juxtaglomerular apparatus of the afferent arteriole) appears more prominent than that of other mammals.[8] Whether or not these subtle histologic differences are accompanied by functional differences has not been investigated.

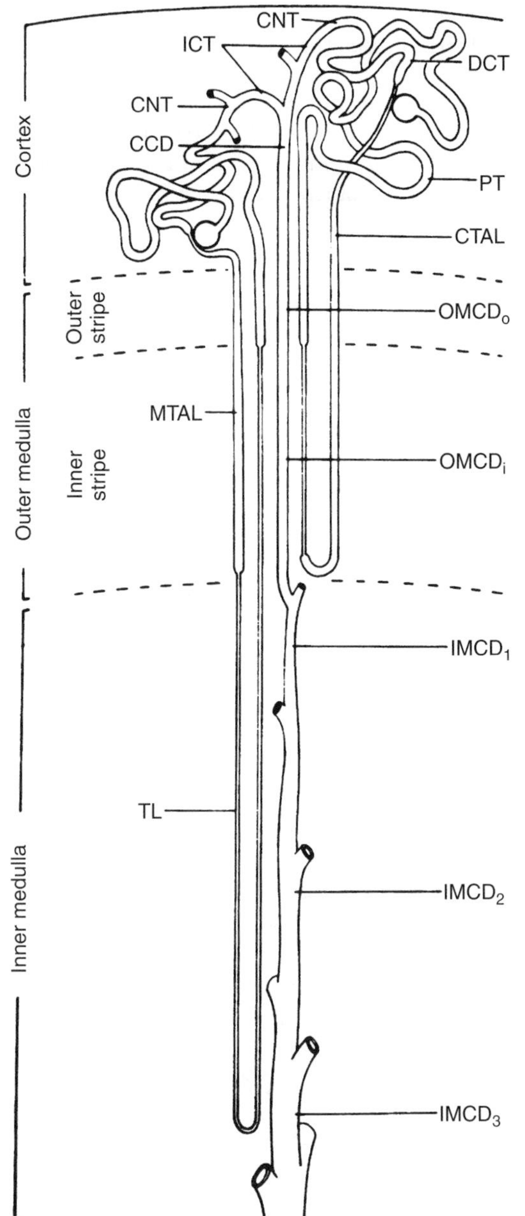

FIGURE 19-1 Diagram of a superficial and juxtamedullary nephron. *TL,* Thin limb of the loop of Henle; *MTAL,* medullary thick ascending limb (mTAL) of the loop of Henle; *CCD,* cortical collecting duct; *CNT,* connecting segment; *ICT,* initial collecting tubule; *DCT,* distal convoluted tubule; *PT,* proximal tubule; *CTAL,* cortical thick ascending limb of the loop of Henle; *OMCD$_0$,* collecting duct in outer stripe of outer medulla; *OMCD$_1$,* collecting duct in inner stripe of outer medulla; *IMCD$_1$,* outer third of inner medullary collecting duct; *IMCD$_2$,* middle third of inner medullary collecting duct; *IMCD$_3$,* inner third of inner medullary collecting duct. (From Brenner BM, Rector FC, editors: The kidney, ed 8, Philadelphia, 2008, WB Saunders.)

Relative to its size, the mammalian kidney has a richer innervation than almost any other organ.[9] Although the neuroanatomy of the equine kidney has not been well studied, autonomic nerves course from the aorticorenal and renal ganglia along the major renal vessels into the kidneys.[1] These nerves are predominantly sympathetic, because the kidneys appear to be poorly supplied by cholinergic nerves. Although the best-recognized effect of renal nerves is control of renal vascular resistance (for regulation of renal blood flow [RBF] over a wide range of perfusion pressures), the nerves also act directly on renal tubules and juxtaglomerular cells. For example, low-frequency stimulation of renal nerves (below the threshold for vasoconstriction) increases proximal tubular sodium reabsorption and renin release by activation of α_1-adrenoceptors.[10] In addition to α- and β-adrenoceptors, renal vasculature is rich in dopaminergic adrenoceptors, and activation of the latter, specifically dopamine type 1 receptors, leads to increased perfusion of the outer renal medulla. Presence of these receptors is the basis for use of dopamine, and more recently the DA-1 receptor agonist fenoldopam, in an attempt to improve RBF in acute renal failure (ARF) or to decrease the risk of radiocontrast nephropathy.[11-13] The administration of drugs also can activate renal adrenoceptors unintentionally. A common clinical example is the diuresis induced by administration of the α_2-agonists xylazine and detomidine. Although the diuresis has been attributed to a transient hyperglycemia and glucosuria, the latter is often absent.[14,15] An alternative explanation may be drug binding to α_2-adrenoceptors located on collecting duct epithelium. Activation of these receptors can lead to antagonism of the effects of antidiuretic hormone on cortical collecting ducts, which results in diuresis.[16] More recently, renal afferent nerves have been identified, and these nerves appear to play a role in the pathogenesis of hypertension in species affected by this disorder.[9]

Autonomic innervation of the ureters, bladder, and urethra is important to ureteral peristalsis and micturition. The equine ureteral smooth muscle contains α_1- and β_2-adrenoceptors, which induce contraction and relaxation, respectively, when activated by norepinephrine.[17] Recent studies of the innervation of the equine ureter demonstrated greater densities of adrenergic neurons in the proximal (renal pelvis) and intravesicular (bladder wall) portions of the ureter.[18] Increased densities in these regions are consistent with the suspected pacemaker activity of the renal pelvis, which initiates ureteral peristalsis and the sphincterlike function of the distal segment of the ureter. The sympathetic nerve supply to the urinary bladder is provided via the hypogastric nerve, with preganglionic fibers arriving from spinal segments L1 to L4 to synapse in the caudal mesenteric ganglion. Postganglionic fibers supply the bladder (β_2-adrenergic receptors) and proximal urethra (primarily α_1- and some α_2-adrenergic receptors).[19,20] In addition to adrenergic innervation, cholinergic and peptidergic nerve fibers also innervate the equine bladder.[21] Parasympathetic innervation originates in the sacral segments of the spinal cord, with neurons joining to form the pelvic nerve.[19,20] Many complex interneuronal connections exist between sympathetic and parasympathetic nerves in the wall of the bladder, along with small adrenergic cells that facilitate interaction between sympathetic and parasympathetic pathways.[22] As a result, complete denervation of the bladder is virtually impossible. Somatic innervation of the lower urinary tract is primarily to the striated muscle of the external urethral sphincter via a branch of the pudendal nerve, which originates from the sacral cord segments (S1 to S2).[1]

DEVELOPMENT

The embryonic upper urinary tract arises from bilateral primordial mesonephric ducts and intermediate mesoderm. The metanephric diverticulum originates from the caudal end of each mesonephric duct and develops craniad to become the ureter and renal pelvis. The advancing metanephric diverticuli collect about their ends intermediate mesoderm (metanephrogenic tissue), which becomes the collecting system and parenchyma of the mature kidney (Figure 19-2). The vascular supply is derived from a branch of the aorta (renal artery) that invades the metanephrogenic tissue. The urinary bladder develops as a dilated proximal portion of the allantois. The bladder is separated from the hindgut by the craniocaudad growth of the urorectal fold, which divides the rectum from the urogenital sinus. The latter structure gives rise to the urethra (Figure 19-3). The mesonephric and metanephric ducts initially open into the urogenital sinus, but as development continues, the distal segments of the mesonephric ducts are absorbed into the bladder wall and the openings of the

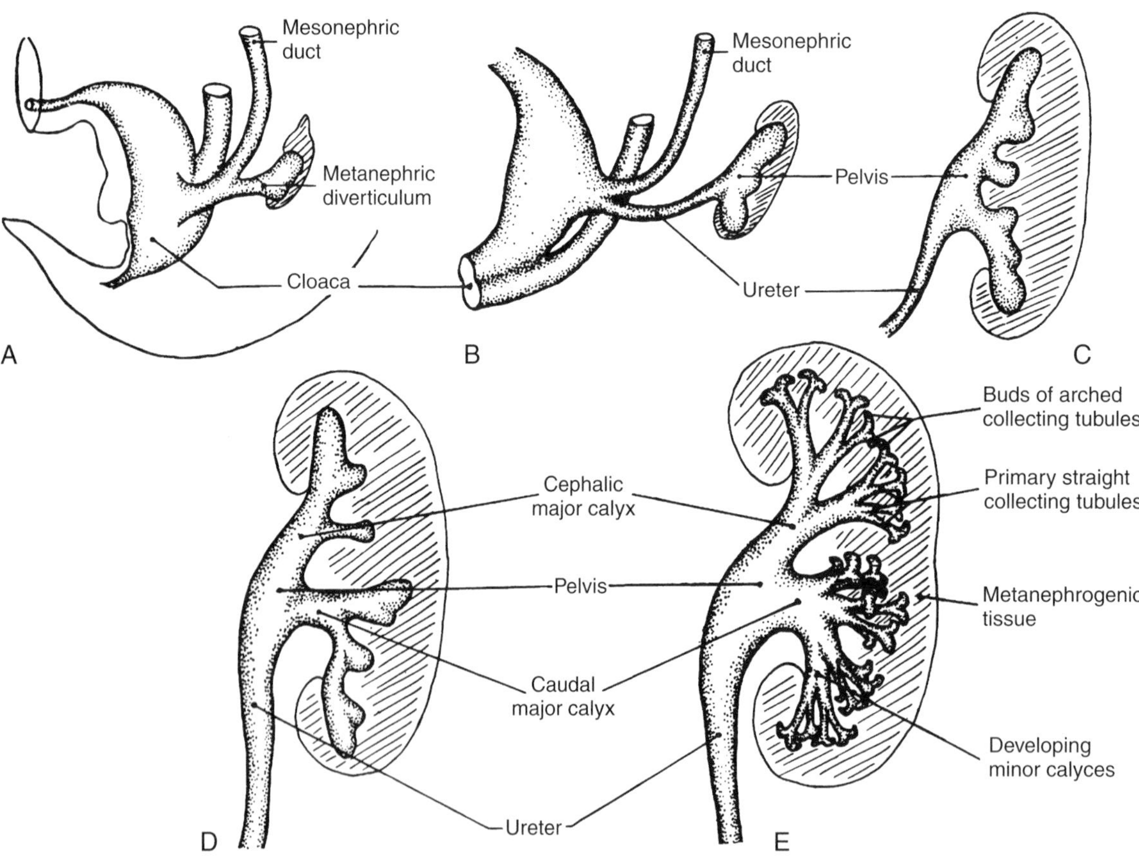

FIGURE 19-2 Progression of the differentiation and development of the metanephric diverticulum into the collecting system of the mature kidney. **A,** Metanephric diverticulum originates from the caudal end of the mesonephric duct. **B,** Metanephric diverticulum develops craniad, and intermediate mesoderm (metanephrogenic tissue, hatched lines) collects about its cranial end. **C** to **E,** The metanephric diverticulum becomes the ureter and renal pelvis, and the metanephrogenic tissue becomes the collecting system and parenchyma of the mature kidney. (From Carlson BM: Patten's foundations of embryology, ed 6, New York, 2003, McGraw-Hill.)

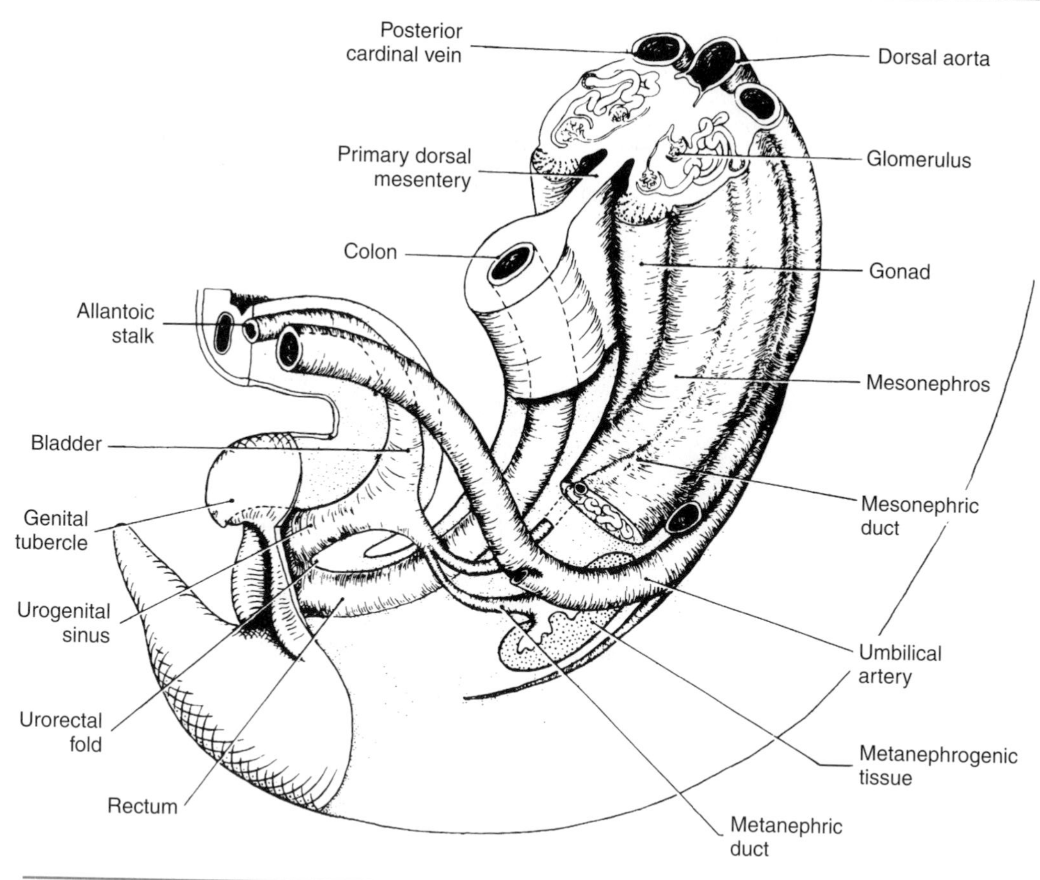

FIGURE 19-3 Developing urogenital tract of the young mammalian embryo. (From Carlson BM: Patten's foundations of embryology, ed 6, New York, 2003, McGraw-Hill.)

metanephric ducts are pulled craniad to their final site in the dorsal bladder neck.[23]

The fate of the mesonephric tubules (mesonephros) and mesonephric ducts varies with gender. Paired paramesonephric ducts (müllerian ducts) arise parallel to the mesonephric ducts in both sexes. In the female, the ducts fuse distally to become the vagina and uterine body, whereas proximally they remain separate to give rise to uterine horns and oviducts. The mesonephric ducts regress into vestigial remnants termed the *epoöphoron* proximally (near the ovaries) and *Gartner's canals* distally (near the vagina and uterus; Figure 19-4). In the male, sexual differentiation of the gonads and production of androgenic steroid hormones lead to regression of the müllerian ducts. The duct system of the male reproductive tract is appropriated from the mesonephros and mesonephric ducts (also termed *wolffian ducts*). Androgenic steroid hormones also stimulate these structures to develop into the seminiferous tubules, epididymis, and ductus deferens. The distal portion of the mesonephric duct becomes the ejaculatory duct, the terminal portion of the ductus deferens.[23]

DEVELOPMENTAL MALFORMATIONS OF THE URINARY TRACT

Anomalies of the urinary tract are uncommon in horses. A survey by Höflinger[24] revealed a similar frequency of unilateral renal agenesis (0.07%) in horses and human beings (0.10%).[5] In contrast, horseshoe kidneys (attached at the cranial or caudal poles) are the most common anomaly in human beings (0.25%) but rarely have been described in horses.[5,25]

Renal Agenesis, Hypoplasia, and Dysplasia

Renal agenesis, which may be unilateral or bilateral, results from failure of the metanephric duct to fuse with the metanephrogenic mesodermal tissue. Although unilateral anomalies have been described more frequently, this simply may reflect the incompatibility of bilateral agenesis with postnatal life.[24,26-28] Brown et al.[28] described a foal with bilateral renal agenesis in which severe azotemia was detected shortly after birth. Bilateral ureteral dysgenesis and cryptorchidism, agenesis of the right adrenal gland, and atresia ani accompanied the renal agenesis in this foal. Unilateral defects may be incidental findings in otherwise healthy horses[29] or may be detectable during examination of the reproductive tract, because many horses have associated anomalies of that system. Occasionally, unilateral agenesis may result in clinical renal disease if a problem arises in the contralateral kidney. Johnson et al.[27] described a 4-year-old Quarter Horse with unilateral renal agenesis and a ureterolith causing contralateral hydronephrosis. The gelding was presented for weight loss, pollakiuria, and stranguria. In addition to the renal anomaly, unilateral agenesis of the ipsilateral testicle also was found on necropsy. Renal agenesis may be a familial disorder in several species.[25,30] Although no information is

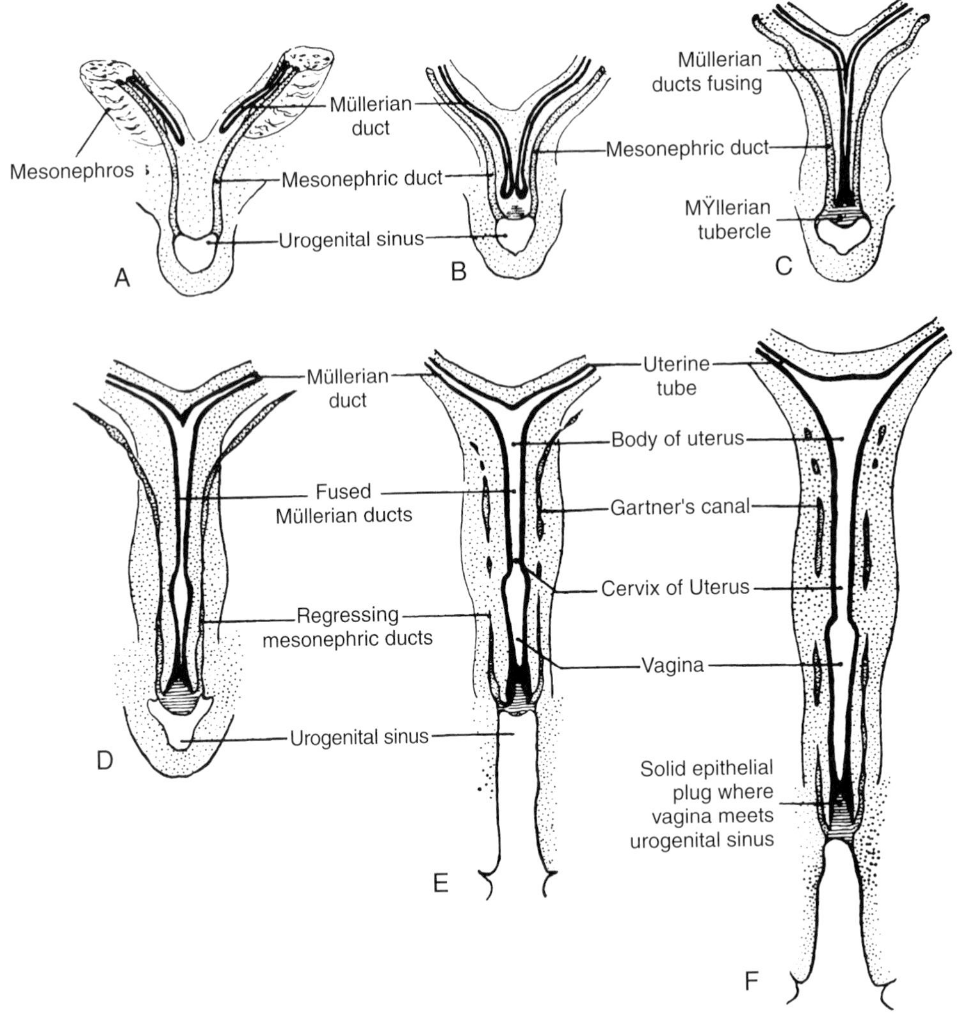

FIGURE 19-4 Development of the mesonephric tubules (mesonephros) and mesonephric ducts into the female reproductive tract. **A** and **B**, Paired paramesonephric ducts (müllerian ducts) arise parallel to the mesonephric ducts in both sexes. **C** to **E**, In females, the paramesonephric ducts fuse distally to become the vagina and uterine body but remain separate proximally to give rise to uterine horns. **D** and **E**, The mesonephric ducts regress into vestigial remnants termed *Gartner's canals.* (From Carlson BM: Patten's foundations of embryology, ed 6, New York, 2003, McGraw-Hill.)

available to suggest a hereditary basis in horses, one probably should discourage repeat matings after detecting such an anomaly.

One diagnoses renal hypoplasia when one kidney is at least 50% smaller than normal or when the total renal mass is decreased by more than one third.[25] Renal hypoplasia is a quantitative defect caused by a reduced mass of metanephrogenic tissue or by incomplete induction of nephron formation by the metanephric duct. The condition may be confused with renal dysplasia. Unilateral renal hypoplasia usually is associated with contralateral hypertrophy and normal renal function, whereas bilateral hypoplasia generally leads to chronic renal failure (CRF).[25,30] Andrews et al.[31] described bilateral renal hypoplasia in a foal presented after death and in three young horses with CRF that had poor growth from birth. Anomalies in these four horses were limited to the upper urinary tract.

Renal dysplasia is disorganized development of renal tissue caused by anomalous differentiation, intrauterine ureteral obstruction, fetal viral infection, or teratogens.[25,32] Bilateral dysplasia usually leads to renal failure. In general, dysplastic kidneys are normal in size unless concurrent hypoplasia exists or the animal lives for months to years before developing renal failure. Roberts and Kelly[33] reported a case of bilateral renal dysplasia in a 19-month-old pony gelding. The pony was presented for weight loss over a 3-month period, and clinicopathologic assessment revealed CRF. A small, firm, and nodular left kidney was palpable per rectum. At necropsy, the kidneys weighed 280 g each (33% smaller than normal for body weight) and were nodular. Renal dysplasia was suspected because glomeruli in the collapsed areas of the kidneys were small, tubules were immature, and inflammatory cells were scant. Six similar cases of bilateral renal dysplasia resulted in CRF in horses from 2 months to 7 years of age.[34-38] Small kidneys with increased echogenicity and an indistinct corticomedullary junction were typical ultrasonographic findings,[36-38] and these findings were corroborated by computed tomography in one Miniature Horse foal.[38] At necropsy, kidneys were typically small and

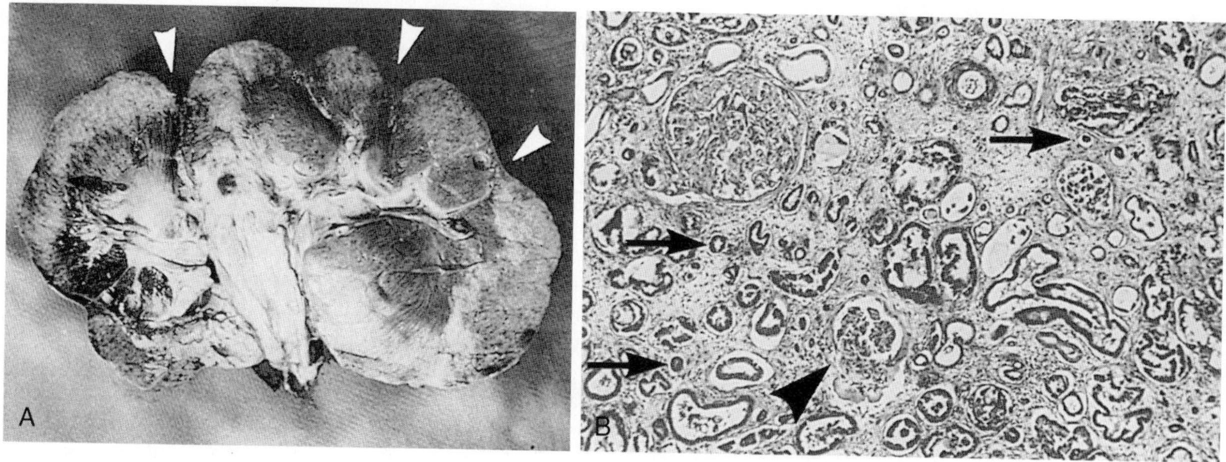

FIGURE 19-5 A, Longitudinal section of the right kidney from a 7-year-old Arabian gelding with renal dysplasia shows focal, irregular thinning of the cortex *(arrowheads)* resulting in a nodular surface and poor delineation of the corticomedullary junction. **B,** Histologic section of same kidney (Masson trichrome stain; original magnification ×35) reveals an immature glomerulus *(large arrowhead)* and primitive tubules *(arrows)* surrounded by persistent mesenchyme. (From Ronen N, van Amstel SR, Nesbit JW et al: Renal dysplasia in two adult horses: clinical and pathological aspects, Vet Rec 132:269, 1993.)

irregular, the cortex and medulla were not well-delineated, and immature glomeruli and primitive tubules were found on histologic examination (Figure 19-5). Renal dysplasia also may cause renal failure in neonates. For example, Zicker et al.[39] reported a case of renal dysplasia in a 2-day-old Quarter Horse foal presented for diarrhea and depression. Clinicopathologic assessment revealed azotemia, hyponatremia, hypochloremia, and urinary sodium wastage. At necropsy, the kidneys were normal in size (380 g), but histologic examination revealed immature glomeruli, hypoplastic tubules and vasa recta, and extensive myxomatous connective tissue occupying 90% of the total medullary volume. Finally, renal dysplasia also may be a unilateral problem that does not result in renal failure. Jones et al.[40] found ureteropelvic polyps to be the cause of unilateral hydronephrosis and renal dysplasia in a Trakehner colt. Poor growth and hematuria for several weeks were the presenting complaints. Renal function remained normal for 8 months after nephrectomy until the colt developed a severe bout of colic, prompting euthanasia. Ureteral obstruction by the polyps was the suggested cause of renal dysplasia, because urinary tract obstruction has been found in a large percentage of cases of human renal dysplasia.[32]

Renal Cysts

One or more renal cysts occasionally are discovered as incidental findings on necropsy examination. The cysts may arise from any portion of the nephron but more often occur in the cortex than in the medulla. The pathogenesis is not known, but a defect in the basement membrane that allows tubular dilation is suspected. Renal cysts vary in size from microscopic to as large as the organ itself and routinely have a clear to slightly opaque wall and contain a thin, clear fluid. Congenital cysts are differentiated easily from acquired cysts (after obstruction) by the extensive scarring that accompanies the latter. Renal cysts also may develop as a consequence of drug therapy (i.e., long-acting corticosteroids) or exposure to certain chemicals.[25,30]

Polycystic Kidney Disease, Glomerulocystic Disease, and Other Hereditary Nephropathies

Polycystic kidney disease (PKD) is a disorder in which numerous, variably sized cysts are found throughout the cortex and medulla. With glomerulocystic disease, cysts are microscopic and limited to Bowman's spaces. Cysts of the bile duct and pancreas also may occur with PKD, and both conditions have been described in stillbirths in many species, including foals.[25] The two major types of human PKD are (1) a rare congenital or infantile form inherited as an autosomal recessive trait (which may be found in stillbirths) and (2) a more common adult form inherited as an autosomal dominant trait that leads to renal insufficiency in later life in association with dramatically enlarged, cystic kidneys.[41,42] The latter form of PKD develops because of mutations in genes encoding for polycystins, integral membrane proteins responsible for cell-to-cell interaction.[43] Autosomal dominant PKD also has been documented in Persian cats and related breeds and in bull terriers.[44-46] The genetic defect in Persian cats is thought to be similar to the most common defect in human beings (PKD1 gene) and leads to end-stage renal disease by 3 to 10 years of age.[45] As in human beings, the disorder is detectable by renal ultrasonographic screening of juvenile cats and preventable by avoiding subsequent mating of affected animals. Nevertheless, because of heavy inbreeding the prevalence of PKD in Persian cats and related breeds is between 40% and 50%.[44,45]

Ramsey et al.[47] described polycystic kidneys in a 9-year-old Thoroughbred mare that exhibited anorexia and weight loss. Clinicopathologic assessment revealed CRF, and euthanasia was performed. At necropsy, the kidneys were grossly enlarged and each weighed 12 kg (Figure 19-6). A similar case of bilateral PKD was described in a 15-year-old pony with a 4-week history of hematuria and moderate weight loss. Evaluation revealed azotemia and presence of large masses in the

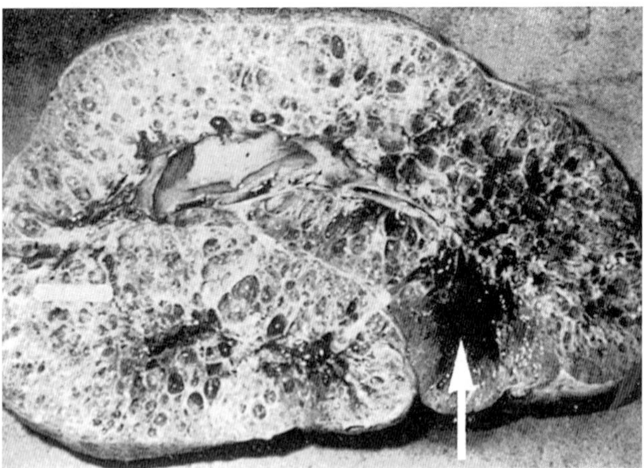

FIGURE 19-6 Longitudinal section of the left kidney (35 cm long, 25 cm wide, 20 cm deep, and weighing 12 kg) from a 9-year-old Thoroughbred mare with polycystic kidneys. A calculus is located in the renal pelvis, and the arrow demonstrates the only grossly normal-looking renal parenchyma. (From Ramsey G, Rothwell TLW, Gibson KT et al: Polycystic kidneys in an adult horse, Equine Vet J 19:243, 1987.)

area of both kidneys on rectal examination, and dramatically enlarged polycystic kidneys weighing 11.4 and 9.1 kg, respectively, were found at necropsy.[48] Bertone et al.[49] reported a third case of adult PKD in a 10-year-old Paint gelding with weight loss. The horse was mildly azotemic, and several 2- to 15-cm diameter cysts were imaged in both kidneys during ultrasonographic examination. In human beings, polycystic kidneys are believed to result in renal failure as cysts expand (sometimes under pressure) and compress adjacent normal renal tissue. Altered compliance of tubular basement membranes and proliferation of renal tubular epithelium result in outflow obstruction and proximal ballooning, leading to renal cyst formation.[42] In some human cases, pressure within cysts may be 5 to 10 times higher than surrounding interstitial tissue pressures. Bertone et al.[49] found no increase in pressure in several cysts catheterized percutaneously in a gelding with PKD, but differences in sodium concentrations suggested that the sampled cysts had arisen from different segments of the renal tubule. Euthanasia was performed after a prolonged hospital course (235 days), and the kidneys were not grossly enlarged except where distorted by large cysts. Although not well documented, PKD has been described anecdotally in two additional Paint horses, suggesting that an inherited form of PKD may occur in that breed. A recent report also documented PKD in an 11-year-old Andalusian gelding.[50]

In addition to PKD, a variety of other hereditary nephropathies have been described in human beings.[48] Similar disorders are starting to be recognized in domestic animals, including hereditary nephritis in bull terriers, Samoyeds, and English cocker spaniels. Analogous to Alport's syndrome in human beings, a defective molecular structure of type IV collagen, an important component of the glomerular basement membrane (GBM), appears to be the cause of hereditary nephritis in these dog breeds.[46] Similarly, a syndrome of renal tubular dysplasia with autosomal recessive pattern of inheritance recently has been described in a population of highly inbred Japanese black cattle,[51-53] as has a syndrome of suspected hereditary renal oxalosis in Beefmaster calves.[54] Similar hereditary nephropathies are likely to occur in horses; however, to date the only one documented is a syndrome of nephrogenic diabetes insipidus in Thoroughbreds.[55]

Vascular Anomalies

Anomalies of the vascular supply to the equine urinary tract are rare but may result in hematuria, hemoglobinuria, partial ureteral obstruction, or hydronephrosis.[30,56] Latimer, Magnus, and Duncan[57] described a distal aortic aneurysm and associated extrarenal arterioureteral fistula in a 5-month-old colt presented for intermittent hematuria, colic, and lameness. Partial ureteral obstruction and hydronephrosis were observed on the affected side. Intrarenal vascular anomalies, termed *renal arteriovenous malformations,* are similarly rare (reported frequency of 0.04% in human beings).[58] Interestingly, these vascular malformations may be silent until later in life, when varying degrees of hematuria and flank pain may ensue. The anomalous vessels are often tortuous and may be enlarged focally and devoid of elastic tissue. Hematuria and hemoglobinuria are thought to arise from areas where the anomalous vessels lie close to the collecting system.[58,59] With vascular anomalies, one should attempt to determine the extent of the defect (unilateral or bilateral) via ultrasonographic examination, contrast radiographic studies, or cystoscopy (visualization that hematuria is coming from only one ureteral orifice). When a unilateral defect is documented in the absence of azotemia, unilateral nephrectomy or selective renal embolization has been recommended to prevent possible fatal exsanguination through the urinary tract[56,57]; however, one may consider conservative treatment if the urinary tract bleeding is minor and has not resulted in anemia.

A large vascular anomaly resulting in transient hemoglobinuria has been reported in a Quarter Horse colt.[60] Over several weeks the large anomalous vascular structure (Figure 19-7) spontaneously filled with a thrombus so that specific treatment (a nephrectomy) was not pursued. Severe adult-onset, idiopathic renal hemorrhage also has been described in horses.[61] Whether this latter syndrome may have been a consequence of congenital renal vascular malformations has not been determined (see Hematuria section later in this chapter). Occasionally gross hematuria with passage of blood clots can accompany omphalitis or bladder rupture.[62] One usually can detect these problems during ultrasonographic examination of the umbilical structures and sometimes can image tissue echogenicity within the bladder that is attributable to a blood clot.

Pendulant Kidney

A pendulant kidney is a rare anomaly in the horse.[63] Rectal examination reveals an extremely mobile kidney attached to the dorsal body wall by a thin band of tissue. Although a pendulous kidney could result from extreme weight loss, hydronephrosis, or perirenal trauma, the condition usually is thought to be congenital. The abnormality is an incidental finding unless displacement or rotation leads to partial or complete ureteral obstruction. As an example, the author has palpated the entire right kidney of one mare immediately craniad of the pelvic canal, and ultrasonographic imaging revealed normal size and structure of the anomalously located kidney.

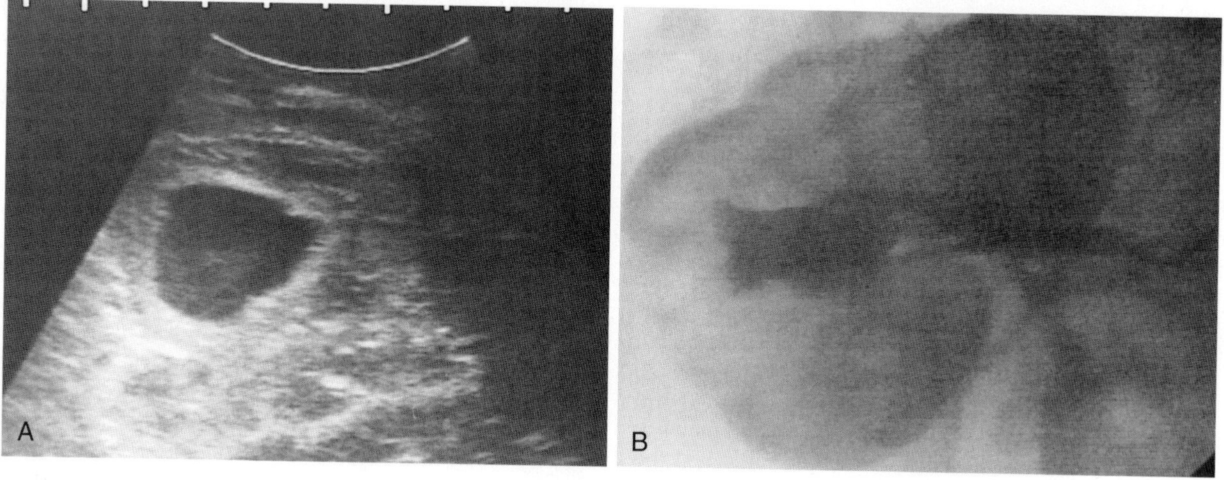

FIGURE 19-7 Ultrasonographic image of the right kidney of a 9-day-old Quarter Horse colt shows a 2×3-cm hypoechoic cavity on a dorsal oblique view. **A,** A swirling pattern, similar in appearance to blood in the ventricles of the heart, was consistent with an arteriovenous malformation. **B,** In a selective nephrogram of the right kidney of the same colt at 20 days of age, immediately after injection of contrast, a dilated vascular space was demonstrated (contrast appears dark because of reverse gray scale) and the renal cortical tissue abaxial to this structure appeared to have reduced capillary phase contrast. (From Schott HC, Barbee DD, Hines MT et al: Renal arteriovenous malformation in a Quarter horse foal, J Vet Intern Med 10:204, 1996.)

Ectopic Ureter

Although ureteral ectopia occurs rarely in the horse,[64] the condition is the most commonly reported developmental anomaly of the equine urinary tract.[64-82] Ectopic ureters may develop when (1) the ureteric bud (metanephric duct) fails to be incorporated into the urogenital sinus or fails to migrate craniad to the bladder neck or (2) the mesonephric duct fails to regress. In the former case, the ectopic ureter opens near the urethral papilla in females or into the pelvic urethra near the colliculus seminalis in males, whereas in the latter, the ureter may open anywhere along the vagina, cervix, or uterus (but only in females because this portion of the mesonephric duct becomes the wolffian duct system in males). In 118 reported cases of ectopic ureter in horses, 105 (89%) were females[65-68,72-77,79-82]; however, this sex distribution may reflect easier recognition in females of the presenting complaint of urinary incontinence rather than a true sex predilection. Incontinence is recognized more often in females because urine entering the pelvic urethra in males may pass retrograde into the bladder. Although a genetic predisposition for ectopic ureter exists for several dog breeds,[83] no breed predilection has been established in horses. However, Quarter Horses may be at greater risk because the condition has been reported in five Quarter Horses, three Standardbreds, two Thoroughbreds, two Appaloosas, an Arabian, a Clydesdale, a Shire, a Fresian, a Foxtrotter, and a Warmblood. The author also has seen the condition in two Quarter Horse fillies (one unilateral and one bilateral), yielding a total of 20 cases.

In horses with ureteral ectopia, urinary incontinence is generally apparent from birth, and affected animals are presented for extensive scalding of the hindlimbs. With unilateral ectopia, horses also void normally, because the other ureter enters the bladder in the appropriate location. Renal function is usually normal, but the affected ureter may be greatly dilated. Urine pooling in the vagina and uterus was a complicating factor in one case.[73] To determine the site of the ectopic ureteral orifice (or orifices), one initially visually examines the vestibule and vagina (using a blade speculum) to look for intermittent urine flow from the area of the urethral papilla. Ectopic ureteral openings usually are not apparent unless urine flow is visible. Endoscopy may be helpful in females (while inflating the vestibule and vagina with air and using a hand to form a seal at the vulva) and is required in males to visualize the ectopic ureteral opening. Intravesical placement of methylene blue dye was performed in one filly to provide evidence for ureteral ectopia. Continued dribbling of clear urine (from the ectopic ureter) followed by passage of blue, discolored urine indicated that only one ureter emptied into the bladder but provided no information on the location of the opening of the ectopic ureter.[66] Intravenous administration of dyes—including sodium fluorescein (10 mg/kg IV; yellow-green), indigotindisulfonate (indigo carmine, 0.25 mg/kg IV; blue-purple), azosulfamide (2.0 mg/kg IV; red), or phenolsulfonphthalein (1.0 mg/kg IV; red)—to discolor the urine may help locate ectopic ureteral openings.[84] Contrast radiography (excretory urography or retrograde contrast studies via catheterization of the bladder and ureters) has been used to detail renal architecture and the course of the ureters in some affected animals; however, results of intravenous urograms are frequently inconclusive in foals weighing more than 50 kg (contrast agent is poorly imaged). In a recent report, ultrasound-guided pyelography, in which contrast agent was injected directly into the renal pelvis using a spinal needle, proved to be a more effective technique than imaging after intravenous administration of contrast agent to detail the course of an ectopic ureter, and one should consider this technique in future cases.[82]

Treatment has included ureterocystostomy (surgical reimplantation of the ectopic ureter or ureters into the bladder) or unilateral nephrectomy. Before surgery, one must determine whether the condition is unilateral or bilateral, which side is affected if unilateral, and whether urinary tract infection

(UTI) is present. Further, one should attempt to rule out other anomalies, especially of the reproductive tract. If the problem is bilateral (8 of 20 cases), then one should establish the presence of a normal micturition response by measuring the intravesicular pressure response to progressive distention until the fluid infused is voided spontaneously. This procedure provides an estimate of bladder volume and ensures competency of the urethral sphincter before reimplantation. Among 14 cases in which surgical correction was pursued, ureterocystostomy was successful in establishing a functional urinary system in nine published cases* and one foal seen by the author, but four died of postoperative complications.[68,75,82] In contrast, all four cases treated by unilateral nephrectomy had a favorable outcome.[72,73,79] Because affected ureters often are dilated and tortuous, surgical reimplantation can be difficult and may not result in a functional ureteral orifice. Consequently, when the problem is unilateral, nephrectomy of the affected side may be the preferred treatment option.[85,86]

Ureteral Defects or Tears (Ureterorrhexis)

Retroperitoneal accumulation of urine and uroperitoneum has been described in seven foals with unilateral or bilateral ureteral defects[87-93] and has been observed in three additional foals by the author. These included seven male and three female foals of several breeds (five Standardbreds, two Thoroughbreds, one Belgian, one Oldenburg, and one Appaloosa). Clinical signs (decreased nursing, depression, abdominal distention, diarrhea, and muscle twitching or other signs of neuromuscular irritability) and clinicopathologic abnormalities (hyponatremia, hyperkalemia, hypochloremia, and azotemia) are similar to those in horses with bladder rupture but may have a slightly later onset (4 to 16 days of age). Mild protrusion of the vagina may occur in fillies in which the peritoneum has remained intact.[94] In affected foals, ultrasonographic examination may reveal dilation of the renal pelvis and affected ureter, as well as fluid accumulation around the kidneys or farther caudad within the retroperitoneal space. As with ectopic ureters, excretory urography generally has been an unrewarding diagnostic procedure, but contrast pyelography was used successfully to image leakage of contrast agent from a proximal ureteral defect in a recent report.[93] Contrast radiography has not been pursued routinely because exploratory celiotomy generally was performed shortly after a diagnosis of uroperitoneum. Catheterization of the ureters via a cystotomy and retrograde injection of methylene blue allowed localization of the defect (or defects), and surgical correction was performed successfully in four cases by suturing the defect around an indwelling catheter.[89,90,93] Although ascending UTI should be an expected complication with a stent, repair of a defect in one foal without use of an indwelling catheter resulted in further urine leakage from the ureter, prompting a nephrectomy 4 days after the initial surgery.[91] Of the remaining five foals, one died after three unsuccessful attempts at surgical repair,[88] and euthanasia was performed in four cases without attempting repair.[87,92]

At surgery or necropsy a single defect was found in six foals, whereas bilateral defects were found in four foals and multiple defects were apparent in one ureter. In most cases the defects have been located in the proximal third of the ureter near the kidney. Interestingly, distended, tortuous ureters, occasionally accompanied by hydronephrosis, also were described in three affected foals,[88,91,93] and distal obstruction of the ureters at the bladder was suspected in two of these cases, prompting ureteroneocystostomy. Although several reports suggest that these ureteral defects may be anomalies of development, the actual cause of these ureteral defects is not known. Traumatic disruption was suggested in the initial report in which histologic examination of the margins of the defect revealed hemorrhage and proliferation of immature connective tissue.[87] A traumatic cause was further supported by a subsequent report in which histologic examination of the defects revealed absence of transitional epithelium and inflammation in a foal that had been attacked by dogs.[92] Inflammation and granulation tissue also were visible in the apparently obstructed distal ureter in one of the foals with ureteral distention, again suggesting an acquired lesion. Blunt abdominal trauma, often sustained during automobile accidents, can cause retroperitoneal accumulation of urine and uroperitoneum in human beings.[95] Disruption of the ureter is usually near the kidney, and this complication of trauma may not be recognized for several days after injury. In one foal evaluated by the author, multiple rib fractures found at necropsy suggested that these ureteral tears actually could be a complication of foaling trauma.

*References 67, 68, 75, 76, 81, 82.

Rectourethral and Rectovaginal Fistulae

If the urorectal fold fails to separate completely the primitive hindgut from the urogenital sinus, then a rectourethral fistula may be found in a colt or a rectovaginal fistula or a persistent cloaca may be found in a filly.[96] These anomalies are rare in horses and when present usually are associated with atresia ani and other anomalies, including agenesis of the coccygeal vertebrae and tail, scoliosis, adherence of the tail to the anal sphincter area, angular limb deformities, and microphthalmia.[70,71,97-102] Affected foals usually are presented for atresia ani, although one also may observe signs of colic and straining. Evidence for a fistula is passage of fecal material from the vulva or urethra. In fillies one may detect rectovaginal fistulae by digital palpation of the dorsal vestibule and vagina, but in colts a definitive diagnosis usually requires contrast radiographic procedures such as a barium enema or a retrograde urethrogram (Figure 19-8). Surgical correction of atresia ani and fistulae has been performed successfully in several foals, but multiple surgical procedures may be required. Because ascending UTI may be a complication, one should submit a sample of urine collected via bladder catheterization (preferably during surgery) for bacterial culture.[96] In human beings the evidence suggests that these anomalies are hereditary, and in one report several foals born with atresia ani were sired by the same stallion.[97] Consequently, affected horses should not be used for breeding after surgical correction of the anomalies.

A urethrorectal fistula resulting in passage of urine from the anus also has been described in a 3-year-old Thoroughbred gelding.[103] The fistula in this gelding was thought to be acquired after trauma or straining because no other developmental problems were detected and the edges of the defect were irregular and inflamed when examined with a speculum inserted into the rectum.

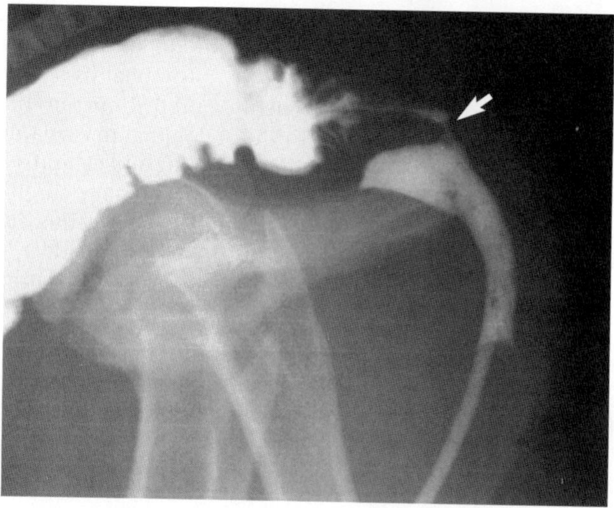

FIGURE 19-8 A positive contrast urethrogram in a 3-day-old burro that had atresia ani and intermittent passage of fecal material from the urethra. A catheter passed via the urethra and contrast agent injected into the catheter resulted in accumulation of a large amount of contrast agent in the rectum and a lesser amount in the intrapelvic portion of the urethra. A small amount of contrast agent is visible in the urethrorectal fistula *(arrow).*

Bladder Defects

Uroperitoneum may result from bladder rupture during parturition in foals (most commonly males)[104] or as a consequence of urachal leakage after infection of the umbilical structures.[105,106] In addition, Wellington described uroperitoneum in two foals that were full brothers.[107] Urine entered the abdomen from a dorsal defect in both colts, and smooth margins to the defects combined with a lack of appreciable inflammation provided evidence in favor of anomalous development rather than trauma. Other authors have suggested that some cases of uroperitoneum likely are associated with anomalous bladder defects because of the size, location, or lack of apparent inflammation of the margins of the defects.[70,108-111] For example, Bain[108] described uroperitoneum in a foal in which the ventral portion of the bladder was absent between the lateral ligaments (umbilical artery remnants) from the umbilicus to the urethra.

Anomalous fusion of the bladder to the inner umbilical ring (absence of the urachus) has been described in one foal.[112] The malformation precluded normal contraction and evacuation of the bladder, and a megavesica—a greatly enlarged bladder—developed. The clinical appearance was similar to that of uroperitoneum, and surgical separation of the bladder from the umbilical ring restored normal anatomic and functional integrity of the bladder. A similar case with a greatly distended bladder was reported in a foal evaluated for abdominal distention[70] that was attributed to an adhesion of the bladder to the urachus or umbilical remnant. An enlarged, flaccid bladder also was described in a foal undergoing exploratory celiotomy for suspected urinary tract disruption.[105] Adhesions to the abdominal wall were not reported, and the foal survived after the surgery during which 50% of the distended bladder was resected. In addition to bladder distention, persistent attachment of the bladder to the area of the umbilicus via a urachal remnant was reported to cause pollakiuria and dysuria in a 15-month-old Thoroughbred filly.[113] The author also has seen postpartum bladder rupture in a mare in which a persistent urachal attachment was suspected to be a contributing factor.

Excessive bladder distention or megavesica has been described further in four stillborn foals[114] and one neonatal foal.[115] In the latter foal and in another report,[116] chronic bladder distention appeared to lead to loss of smooth muscle in the dorsal bladder wall and replacement with collagen. The result was bladder rupture during parturition. Although these reports are similar to an early report by Rooney[104] describing the dorsal bladder wall as the anatomic weak link and likely area for rupture, they differ in that chronic distention of the bladder in utero with smooth muscle loss is not recognized in more typical bladder ruptures in neonatal foals. Why bladder distention should occur in utero without obstruction of the lower tract (not found in these cases) is not clear. Although an excessively long umbilical cord (longer than 85 cm) may lead to urachal obstruction,[114,117] urine produced in utero alternatively could drain into the amniotic cavity via the urethra. Thus this form of megavesica remains poorly characterized and poorly understood.

Bladder distention also is recognized in some foals with hypoxic-ischemic encephalopathy. Affected foals may posture to urinate frequently, and ultrasonographic examination may reveal an enlarged bladder or incomplete bladder emptying. In recumbent foals, one may note abdominal distention, and temporary use of an indwelling bladder catheter to keep the bladder empty is helpful; however, ascending UTI may be a complication. Cystometrography would be useful to assess detrusor function in affected foals, but no reports describe use of this diagnostic test in equine neonates. Although administration of cholinergic drugs (e.g., bethanechol) to improve detrusor function or α-adrenergic blockers (e.g., phenoxybenzamine, acepromazine) to decrease urethral sphincter tone has been described anecdotally to be of benefit, no reports describe the efficacy of these medications in foals with this problem.

Some neonatal foals examined for abdominal pain are apparently unable to urinate normally. Ultrasound examination will reveal a normal gastrointestinal tract and a greatly enlarged but intact urinary bladder. These foals can be treated with indwelling urinary catheters for 2 to 3 days along with phenazopyridine (4 mg/kg PO every 8 to 12 hours) for 5 to 7 days.[118] Phenazopyridine acts a local analgesic on the lower urinary tract and may relieve spasm or allow better relaxation of the bladder sphincters and promote normal micturition.

Patent Urachus

The urachus is the conduit through which fetal urine passes from the bladder into the allantoic cavity. Normally, the urachus closes at the time of parturition, but incomplete closure is the most common malformation of the equine urinary tract. Patent urachus occurs more commonly in foals than in other domestic species.[30] Greater than average length or partial torsion of the umbilical cord has been suggested to cause tension on the attachment of the umbilical cord to the body wall. The result is dilation of the urachus and subsequent failure to close at birth.[70,71,114,117,119] Patent urachus results in a persistently moist umbilicus after birth, from which urine may leak as drips or as a stream during micturition. One must distinguish this malformation from septic omphalitis, which also can result in urine leakage from the umbilicus within a few hours to days after birth. Ultrasound examination of the umbilical remnants is indicated to rule out or monitor for concurrent omphalophlebitis. Patent urachus has been referred to as a *congenital problem* and the latter as an *acquired problem*, but both may result in urine leakage from the urachus from birth. Neither is life threatening, but local sepsis often is accompanied by more severe illness, including septicemia or localized infection, particularly in joints.

The congenital patent urachus traditionally has been treated with frequent (two to four times daily) chemical cauterization of the urachus with swabs dipped in a concentrated phenol or 7% iodine solution or with silver nitrate applicators.[69] Because the urachus may close spontaneously in a number of cases, and because these agents desiccate and irritate tissue (and may predispose to infection), the rationale for this approach has been questioned.[119] In a study comparing the effects of disinfectant solutions on the bacterial flora of the umbilicus of normal foals, use of a 7% iodine solution was observed to cause rapid desiccation of the umbilical tissue and subsequent development of a patent urachus when the stump fell off a few days later.[120] Chlorhexidine diacetate (0.5%) appears to be more effective than 1% to 2% iodine solutions in reducing umbilical bacterial counts. Chlorhexidine is less irritating to tissue, binds to the stratum corneum, and has prolonged antiseptic effects.[120] The use of caustic or irritating solutions for routine umbilical dipping or treatment of patent urachus should probably be avoided because it may lead to localized necrosis and infection that may actually result in umbilical infections.

Consequently, in the absence of apparent infection, no local treatment may be indicated specifically, but affected foals frequently are given antibiotics prophylactically. For acquired patency (which may be associated with local infection, cachexia, or septicemia), broad spectrum antibiotic therapy is indicated, and resolution of the systemic disease may be accompanied by elimination of the umbilical infection and closure of the urachus. Most cases of patent urachus without septic omphalophlebitis will resolve with supportive care, routine umbilical disinfection, and antibiotic therapy. Empiric antibiotic therapy with antibiotics that are eliminated (and concentrated) in urine, such as potentiated sulfonamides, cephalosporins, aminoglycosides, or penicillins usually provides adequate antimicrobial protection with uncomplicated patent urachus in otherwise healthy foals. Chemical cauterization is contraindicated with local sepsis because it may increase the risk of urachal rupture and development of uroperitoneum.[121] If one observes no decrease in urine leakage after 5 to 7 days of medical therapy, or if ultrasonography reveals abnormalities of multiple structures in the umbilicus,[122,123] then surgical exploration and resection of the urachus and umbilical vessels may be indicated. In a retrospective study of 16 foals treated for sepsis of umbilical cord remnants, six of nine (67%) survived after surgical resection and antibiotic treatment, whereas only three of seven (43%) survived after antibiotic treatment alone.[124] Although this series of 16 foals often is cited in support of surgical intervention, one should note that the series studied a small number of foals and that the cases were evaluated over 10 years (1975-1985), during which time many aspects of neonatal care improved. In a more recent retrospective report of 33 foals with umbilical remnant infections, no difference in survival was observed between foals treated with antibiotics combined with surgical resection or with antibiotic therapy alone.[123] Further, emphasis was placed on the insensitivity of palpation of the umbilicus in detection of umbilical remnant infection (compared with ultrasonographic examination) and the poor outcome of cases in which the umbilical vein was involved. In addition to the possibility of omphalitis leading to urachal rupture and development of uroperitoneum, urachal leakage also may occur into the abdominal musculature and subcutaneous tissues and lead to swelling and cellulitis of the ventral abdominal wall.[125] Both instances require surgical intervention. Finally, trauma or tearing of the urachus also can lead to umbilical evagination of the urinary bladder,[126] which can result in partial or complete obstruction of urine flow, and surgical correction is indicated.

RENAL PHYSIOLOGY

Harold C. Schott II

The kidneys perform two essential functions in the maintenance of homeostasis: (1) elimination of nitrogenous and organic waste products and (2) control of body water content and ion composition. In addition, the kidneys are important endocrine organs that produce renin, erythropoietin, and the active form of vitamin D; they also play an important role in the degradation and excretion of a number of other hormones, including gastrin and parathormone. To gain an understanding of the pathophysiologic alterations associated with renal disorders in horses, one must first review some aspects of normal renal physiology in this species.

PRODUCTION AND ELIMINATION OF NITROGENOUS AND ORGANIC WASTES

The two most commonly recognized waste products excreted in urine are urea and creatinine (Cr), but many other nitrogenous or organic wastes are produced each day and subsequently are eliminated by the kidneys (Box 19-1).[1]

UREA METABOLISM

A molecule of urea is produced in the liver from two ammonium ions that are liberated during catabolism of amino acids. For each urea molecule the carbon atom is derived from bicarbonate. One ammonium ion is cleaved from an amino acid via an α-ketoglutarate–dependent transamination coupled to oxidative deamination of glutamate. The second ammonium ion is derived from aspartate in the urea cycle.[2] Urea synthesized in the liver is released into the blood, and clearance by the kidneys represents the major pathway (75% to 100%) of excretion. Extrarenal urea excretion includes losses in sweat and through the gastrointestinal tract. With normal intestinal function, enteric excretion is minimal because of enterohepatic recirculation (reabsorption of ammonia from the degradation of urea by bacterial ureases and subsequent reformation of urea in the liver).[3]

In human beings, inborn errors of metabolism leading to deficiency of a specific transaminase or of one of the five enzymes of the urea cycle can result in accumulation of ammonia and other intermediates of amino acid catabolism. These disorders typically are inherited as autosomal recessive traits, and the consequence is moderate to severe mental dysfunction because the accumulated intermediates can be toxic

BOX 19-1

COMPOUNDS EXCRETED BY THE KIDNEYS

Urea
Phenols
Indoles
Skatoles
Hormones
Polyamines
Trace elements
Serum proteases
Creatinine (Cr)
Pyridine derivatives
Guanidino compounds
β_2-Microglobulin
Hippurate esters
Aliphatic amines
Aromatic amines
Middle molecules

to the central nervous system (CNS; i.e., ammonia) or can act as false neurotransmitters (i.e., aromatic amines).[1] Because urea production is limited in these disorders, blood urea nitrogen (BUN) concentration is often low.[2] Although such defects in metabolism appear to be rare in domestic animals,[4] development of encephalopathy in association with hyperammonemia has been recognized in horses.[5,6] Furthermore, in one report of two related Morgan weanling fillies, persistent hyperammonemia was suspected to be caused by a defect in a mitochondrial ornithine transporter similar to an autosomal recessive syndrome of hyperornithinemia, hyperammonemia, and homocitrullinuria (HHH) in human beings.[7]

BUN concentration depends on age, diet, rate of urea production, and renal function. For example, a low BUN typically is found in neonatal foals after an anabolic demand for amino acids.[8] Investigations of nitrogen use in ponies have demonstrated that urea production is proportional to dietary protein content. Similarly, urinary urea excretion increases in proportion with urea production.[9,10] As a result, with increased levels of dietary protein or when urea is supplemented in the diet, BUN may increase twofold or greater.[11-13]

In human beings and small animals, BUN is routinely higher in samples collected postprandially because diets are typically high in protein.[3] Postprandial elevation of BUN has not been described in horses or other herbivores. However, fasting leads to enhanced protein catabolism to meet energy demands and increased BUN in horses.[14,15] In ponies, however, BUN decreases with fasting.[16] This opposite response suggests differences in the metabolic responses of horses and ponies to anorexia, consistent with a greater capacity of ponies to mobilize and use fat during starvation. Other causes of protein catabolism, including fever, infection, trauma, myositis, burns, and corticosteroid therapy, also can produce an increase in BUN.[3] Finally, a decrease in RBF or renal function produces an increase in BUN. The former may occur with dehydration or during periods of anesthesia or exercise; the latter is a reflection of renal disease.[3] With short bouts of moderate to intensive exercise, BUN often does not change[13,17]; however, during prolonged exercise BUN can increase by 50% or more because of the combined effects of decreased RBF and protein catabolism.[18,19]

Most renal nitrogen excretion occurs in the form of urea in urine. One must recognize that urea excretion is completely passive and that the high concentrations achieved in urine are merely a consequence of medullary tonicity produced by the countercurrent-multiplier function of the loop of Henle. Thus although variations in dietary protein intake lead to parallel changes in urea excretion, the idea that low-protein diets decrease the workload on the kidney is a fallacy.[3] Urinary urea nitrogen concentrations can vary from as low as 50 mg/dl in neonatal foals or horses with primary polydipsia to greater than 2500 mg/dl in normal horses on high-protein diets. Total daily urea excretion usually ranges between 100 and 300 g per day in horses with normal renal function.

Creatinine Metabolism

Cr is produced by the nonenzymatic, irreversible cyclization and dehydration of creatine. Three amino acids in the kidney, liver, and pancreas are indirectly responsible for its production; subsequently Cr is transported to other organs such as muscle and brain, where it is phosphorylated to store energy in the form of phosphocreatine.[3,20] In human beings, 1.5% to 2% of the creatine pool is converted to Cr daily and results in fairly constant excretion of Cr within a given individual.[3] With normal renal function, a direct relationship exists between daily Cr production, serum Cr concentration, and Cr excretion, all three being proportional to total muscle mass. The fact that Cr is 30% higher in male humans than in female humans and that urinary Cr excretion is correlated to body size across a wide range of animal species supports this relationship.[3,21] Cr is excreted principally in urine, but sweat and the gastrointestinal tract are secondary routes of excretion.[3] In contrast to urea, enterohepatic recycling of Cr does not occur, and the gastrointestinal tract may represent a major route of excretion when renal function is compromised. For example, in a group of azotemic human patients, between 15% and 65% of radiolabeled Cr was found to be excreted through the intestine.[22] Cr excreted by this route is degraded rapidly by bacteria so that little is found in feces.

Like BUN, Cr can vary with age, activity level, and renal function. In contrast, dietary protein intake has little influence on Cr in horses.[11] Newborn foals routinely have Cr values 30% to 50% higher than those measured in the mare, and values as high as 20 to 30 mg/dl have been measured in some premature or asphyxiated foals.[8] These high values may result from limited diffusion of Cr across the placenta. For example, the Cr in equine amniotic fluid collected at term is proportionately much greater than urea nitrogen concentration (Cr, 10.1 mg/dl; urea nitrogen, 38.8 mg/dl).[23] If the foal appears healthy and all other laboratory values are within reference ranges, then a Cr value in the range of 5 to 15 mg/dl should not cause alarm. In most healthy foals with normal renal function, Cr decreases to values below 3.0 mg/dl within the first 3 to 5 days of life.[22] After the first few days of life, Cr is usually lower in foals than in adults[12] because of the combined effect of rapid growth and the fact that skeletal muscle comprises a smaller percentage of body weight in foals than in adult horses. Other nonrenal factors that may influence Cr include fasting, rhabdomyolysis or muscle wasting caused by disease, and exercise. Although fasting can increase the measured value for Cr, a substantial portion of this increase actually is due to other compounds (possibly ketones) that increase during fasting and are measured as non-Cr chromagens in the commonly used Jaffe's colorimetric assay for Cr determination (see Examination of the Urinary System).[12,14,24] In contrast, the increase in Cr (up to 80% in some reports) associated with various types of exercise is likely the combined result of increased release of creatine from muscle and decreased urinary Cr excretion during the exercise bout.[12,14,17-19]

Cr is filtered freely at the glomerulus and is concentrated to values of 100 to 300 mg/dl in equine urine, which results in a total daily urine excretion of 15 to 25 g of Cr.[25,26] In comparison to urea, Cr excretion is responsible for only one tenth as much urinary nitrogen excretion. Minor species and sex differences have been reported for renal tubular handling of Cr, with a weak proximal tubular secretory mechanism in human beings and male dogs (accounting for 7% to 10% of total urinary Cr excretion).[3,20] To determine whether tubular secretion of Cr occurs in equine kidneys, Finco and Groves[27] fitted anesthetized ponies with ureteral catheters and performed simultaneous inulin and exogenous Cr clearance studies. Because inulin is filtered freely at the glomerulus and is neither secreted nor reabsorbed by renal tubules, inulin clearance (Cl_{In}) provides a standard of comparison for Cr clearance (Cl_{Cr}). Tubular secretion of Cr should result in a greater value for Cl_{Cr} than for Cl_{In}, whereas the opposite should occur with tubular reabsorption of Cr. To magnify any minor tubular secretion of Cr, stop-flow studies were performed by temporarily occluding the ureteral catheters. During obstruction, tubular lumen pressure increased and tubular flow decreased. As a consequence, fluid remained in contact with tubular epithelium for a prolonged period, enhancing local tubular secretory or resorptive processes. Analysis of a series of urine samples collected after release of ureteral occlusion revealed no differences in tubular handling of inulin or Cr, leading to the conclusion that Cr neither was reabsorbed nor secreted by equine kidneys. In contrast, simultaneous measurement of endogenous Cl_{Cr} and Cl_{In} in several horses with CRF (author's unpublished observations) has revealed higher values for Cl_{Cr}, indicating that tubular secretion of Cr may develop in horses as renal function declines (see the Chronic Renal Failure). Whether significant excretion of Cr occurs in sweat or through the gastrointestinal tract has not been investigated in horses.

Metabolism of Other Nitrogenous and Organic Compounds

Although the kidneys excrete a number of nitrogenous and organic wastes in addition to urea and Cr (see Box 19-1), these compounds are quantitatively unimportant in terms of nitrogen balance.[1] Two of the more commonly recognized molecules are ammonia and uric acid. In proximal tubular epithelial cells, ammonium ions and α-ketoglutarate are produced from glutamine. Subsequent metabolism of α-ketoglutarate results in generation of two bicarbonate molecules that are returned to the systemic circulation. Ammonium ions are secreted in exchange for sodium into the tubule lumen, where they remain trapped, because tubules are relatively impermeable to ammonium ions. Furthermore, because the pK_a for ammonia is greater than 9.0, most of the tubular ammonia remains in the form of ammonium ions, even in alkaline equine urine. Although ammonium ion excretion is of little significance in overall nitrogen excretion, it plays an important role in acid (hydrogen ion) excretion. In fact, glutamine metabolism and ammonium ion excretion can increase severalfold in response to metabolic acidosis.[28] Although urinary ammonium concentration is not measured routinely, one can estimate it because it is directly related to the urinary anion gap ($[Na^+ + K^+] - Cl^-$) in human patients with normal anion gap metabolic acidosis.[29] More important, impairment of this proximal tubular acid secretion pathway contributes to development of metabolic acidosis in patients with renal insufficiency.

Uric acid is a product of purine nucleotide degradation and is the major nitrogenous waste product formed in amphibians and reptiles. In mammals, however, uric acid excretion (mostly in the ionic form of urate) is unimportant in terms of overall nitrogen excretion.[1] Uric acid metabolism has received little attention in veterinary species with the exception of Dalmatian dogs. This breed exhibits high urate excretion rates and is predisposed to uric acid stone formation; however, this problem results from decreased hepatic uricase activity rather than any abnormality in renal urate handling.[30] Finally, hyperuricemia (leading to gout in human beings) also can be attributed to a lack of uricase activity in human tissues and greater renal reabsorption of urate compared with other mammalian species. Thus crystallization of urate in tissues appears to be limited to human beings.[1] Urate metabolism has been studied little in horses, although Keenan[17] observed that plasma concentrations increased dramatically in response to exercise (from <1 μmol/L at rest to 150 to 200 μmol/L 1 hour after racing) and that these increases were accompanied by a transient increase in urinary urate excretion (from <40 μmol/L at rest to 250 to 1270 μmol/L after racing).

The proximal tubule is also the major site of excretion (by tubular secretion) of a number of endogenous organic anions and cations.[1] The anions share the common pathway measured by p-aminohippurate clearance, the substance traditionally used to measure effective renal plasma flow (because more than 90% is excreted via this pathway). A number of exogenous compounds also are excreted via these pathways—acetazolamide, furosemide, probenecid, penicillin G, sulfadiazine, salicylate, atropine, cimetidine, and neostigmine. Thus administration of these compounds can interfere with tubular secretion of endogenous organic wastes or other exogenous products by healthy kidneys.[31] More importantly, the pharmacokinetic effects of these products vary widely in patients with renal insufficiency. Combined with the fact that anion binding to plasma proteins is decreased with azotemia, dosing protocols of many medications may need to be readjusted for patients with renal failure.

Body Water and Electrolyte Balance

Body Fluids: Volume and Composition

Water accounts for at least 60% of total body mass, equivalent to 300 L in a 500-kg horse.[1,29-34] About 200 L of total body water is intracellular fluid, and the remaining 100 L is extracellular fluid. Extracellular fluid is divided between plasma (4% to 6% of body mass, approximately 25 L), interstitial fluid and lymph (10% to 12% of body mass, approximately 45 L), and transcellular fluid (6% to 10% of body mass, approximately 30 L, most of which is in the lumen of the gastrointestinal tract). Despite significant differences in ion composition (Table 19-1), the extracellular fluid and intracellular fluid compartments exchange water freely to maintain osmotic equilibrium.[28]

From the values in Table 19-1 one can estimate the total amount of exchangeable sodium, potassium, and chloride in the body fluids of a 500-kg horse: approximately 16,000 mEq, approximately 28,800 mEq, and approximately 10,800 mEq, respectively (including gastrointestinal fluid ion contents). These values are accurate except for that of sodium, which may be twice as great; however, 40% to 50% is sequestered in bone and is not readily available to buffer sodium alterations in body fluids.[32-34] Thus the 16,000-mEq estimate is accurate for the exchangeable sodium content in body fluids. Similarly, one can estimate body fluid contents of calcium, magnesium, and phosphorus at approximately 1000 mEq (20 g), approximately 6875 mEq (84 g), and approximately 8150 mEq (140 g), respectively (excluding gastrointestinal fluid ion contents, because these vary with the amount and solubility of the dietary source). As for sodium, the values underestimate the total body content of calcium, magnesium, and phosphorus, because more than 99%, 70%, and 85% of these elements, respectively, are contained in the skeleton.[3]

Water Balance

Appropriate water balance maintains plasma osmolality in a narrow range (270 to 300 mOsm/kg) and is achieved by matching daily water intake with water loss.[35-37] Water is provided from three sources: (1) free water intake (drinking), (2) water in feed, and (3) metabolic water (Table 19-2). Horses consume most of the water by drinking (about 85%), but feed and metabolic water provide about 5% and 10% of daily water, respectively. Water can be lost by three routes: (1) in urine, (2) in feces, and (3) as insensible losses (evaporation) across the skin and respiratory tract (Table 19-3). Investigations of water balance have revealed a maintenance water requirement of 60 to 65 ml/kg/day or 27 to 30 L/day for a 500-kg horse.[35,38] These values are consistent with traditional recommendations that 5 to 10 gallons/day of fresh water be provided to a stabled horse under mild environmental conditions.[39] Urinary and

TABLE 19-1

Approximate Ionic Compositions (mEq/L) of Plasma, Interstitial Fluid, and Intracellular Fluid (Skeletal Muscle)

Electrolyte Cations	Plasma	Interstitial Fluid	Skeletal Muscle Cell
Na^+	140	143	10
K^+	4.0	4.1	142
Ca^{2+}	2.5	2.4	4.0
Mg^{2+}	1.1	1.1	34
Total	**147.6**	**150.6**	**190**
Anions			
Cl^-	100	113	4
HCO_3^-	25	28.2	12
$H_2PO_4^-$, HPO_4^{-2}	2.0	2.3	40
Protein	14	0.0	50
Other	6.6	7.1	84*
Total	**147.6**	**150.6**	**190**

Modified from Rose BD: *Clinical physiology of acid-base and electrolyte disorders,* ed 3, New York, 1989, McGraw-Hill.
*This largely represents organic phosphates such as adenosine triphosphate.

TABLE 19-2

Water Balance in Hay-Fed Horses in a Cool Climate

Water Intake (L)	Water Loss (L)
Consumption 23.6	Feces 14.0
Hay 1.1	Urine 4.9
Metabolic 2.7	Insensible 8.5
Total 27.4	Total 27.4

Data from Tasker JB: Fluid and electrolyte studies in the horse. 3. Intake and output of water, sodium, and potassium in normal horses, *Cornell Vet* 57:649, 1967.

TABLE 19-3

Water and Electrolyte Balance in Horses Receiving a Low-Sodium Diet (Alfalfa and Timothy Hay)

	Intake	Urinary Loss	Fecal Loss	Unmeasured*
Tasker†				
Water (L)	27.4	4.9	14	8.5 (31%)
Sodium (mEq)	329	7	116	206 (63%)
Potassium (mEq)	3930	2196	993	741 (19%)
Groenendyk, English, Abetz‡				
Water (L)	27.6§	9.9	7.2	10.5 (38%)
Sodium (mEq)	986	527	253	206 (21%)
Potassium (mEq)	3320	2661	504	155 (5%)
Chloride (mEq)	3008	2347	174	487 (16%)

*Unmeasured losses include insensible water losses and electrolyte losses thought to occur in sweat; value in parenthesis is the percentage represented by these unmeasured losses.
†Tasker JB: Fluid and electrolyte studies in the horse. 3. Intake and output of water, sodium, and potassium in normal horses, *Cornell Vet* 57:649, 1967.
‡Groenendyk S, English PB, Abetz I: External balance of water and electrolytes in the horse, *Equine Vet J* 20:189, 1988.
§Water intake includes imbibed water (23.6 L), water in feed (1.1 L), and metabolic water (2.9 L).

fecal water losses range between 20% to 55% and 30% to 55%, respectively, of the total daily water loss.[35,38,40,41] The remaining (insensible) loss accounted for up to 15% to 40% of daily water loss, despite mild ambient conditions and the lack of observed sweating in most studies of water balance.

Water drinking and urine production are the mechanisms by which water balance is finely tuned; however, they can vary widely between individual horses and also are affected by age, environmental conditions, level of exercise, and diet. Often, for example, neonatal foals consume milk in excess of 20% of their body mass daily,[42] which equates to fluid intake approaching 250 ml/kg/day. Water intake by horses increased 15% to 20% when ambient temperature increased from 13° to 25° C.[43] Under conditions of high ambient temperature and humidity, urine concentration also may increase to conserve water, whereas fecal water content tends to remain fairly stable, at about 75% of fecal weight. Exercising horses, especially endurance horses and racing horses treated with furosemide, can increase water consumption by 100% to 200% to replace body water lost in sweat (and urine). Horses and ponies on all-roughage diets also drink more and have greater daily fecal water loss (because of greater daily fecal volume) than animals fed a large amount of concentrate or complete pelleted diets.[40,41] Diets high in nitrogen (protein) and calcium, such as legume hays, typically increase urine volume by 50% or more and are associated with a similar increase in urinary nitrogen excretion. These diets are also more digestible so that fecal water excretion generally decreases because of a decrease in total fecal material.[9,14,40,41] Although high dietary levels of salt have been suggested to increase drinking and promote diuresis, no increase in water consumption or urine volume was observed in ponies fed 5 to 10 times the daily salt requirement (equivalent to about 350 g of sodium chloride [NaCl] for a 500-kg horse).[44] The effects of water access, continuous versus intermittent, have received less attention, although a recent study showed no difference in water balance in horses provided water three times daily compared with horses that had continuous access to water.[45] Furthermore, horses drink the most water within the hour after feeding,[46] and feral horses and ponies often drink only once or twice daily.[47] Thus horses are unlikely to require continuous access to water. An obvious exception is a patient with renal insufficiency that should have access to fresh water at all times.

Two main stimuli for thirst are (1) increased plasma osmolality and (2) hypovolemia or hypotension.[48] The former is mediated through osmoreceptors in the hypothalamus that have a high threshold for activation (about 295 mOsm/kg) in human beings. Hemodynamic stimuli are mediated by low- and high-pressure baroreceptors. Osmotic and hemodynamic stimuli can produce their dipsogenic effect in part by activating a local renin-angiotensin-aldosterone system in the CNS.[49,50]

Renal water reabsorption is controlled principally by the action of arginine vasopressin (antidiuretic hormone) on the collecting ducts.[51] Vasopressin is produced in the neurosecretory neurons of the supraoptic nuclei, packaged in granules, and transported down axons for storage in the neurohypophysis (pars nervosa or posterior pituitary). As for thirst, increases in plasma osmolality and hypovolemia or hypotension are the stimuli for vasopressin release. Osmoreceptors for vasopressin release also are located in the hypothalamus, adjacent to the osmoreceptors mediating thirst. Activation of these receptors is the signal for vasopressin release from the neurohypophysis. Furthermore, these osmoreceptors are not equally sensitive to all plasma solutes. For example, increases in plasma sodium concentration and infusion of mannitol are potent stimuli, whereas increases in plasma glucose and urea concentrations are weak stimuli. These differences have led to the suggestion that osmoreceptor activation is caused by an osmotic water shift that produces cell shrinkage (which would be greater for sodium and mannitol than for glucose or urea). Activation of osmoreceptors signaling vasopressin release also appears to have a threshold value; however, this threshold appears to vary highly between individuals. In addition, the threshold for vasopressin release in human beings is significantly lower (270 to 285 mOsm/kg) than that for thirst. Thus vasopressin release can be thought of as the initial line of defense against a mild increase in plasma osmolality, whereas thirst and drinking are secondary responses to even greater increases.

Studies in horses, ponies, and donkeys have demonstrated that increased plasma osmolality (induced by water deprivation or infusion of hypertonic saline) and hypovolemia (induced by furosemide administration) are stimuli for thirst.[45,51-55] Furthermore, after a period of water deprivation, dehydrated ponies, horses, and donkeys appear to be able to replace water deficits within 15 to 30 minutes of gaining access to water. The increases in plasma osmolality and vasopressin concentration associated with water deprivation also are corrected in this same period of time, indicating that imbibed water is absorbed rapidly from the gastrointestinal tract.[52] Although increases in plasma vasopressin concentration have been measured in horses and ponies during water deprivation,[52,56] vasopressin also appears to be a "stress hormone" in equids, because substantially greater concentrations (tenfold greater than those induced by water deprivation) have been measured after application of a nose twitch, nasogastric intubation, or exercise.[57,58] Thus increases in plasma vasopressin concentration after water deprivation would be expected to vary in horses, and separating osmotic effects from stress effects may be difficult sometimes.

Once released, vasopressin acts on V_2-receptors on the basolateral membrane of collecting duct epithelial cells, leading to insertion of water channels (transmembrane proteins) in the apical membrane.[48] These channels increase the water permeability of the apical membranes and lead to increased water reabsorption. Action of V_2-receptors is mediated by activation of adenylyl cyclase and a stimulatory transmembrane G protein. Interestingly, V_2-receptor activation can be antagonized by activation of adjacent α_2-adrenoceptors and by a prostaglandin E_2–mediated effect on an inhibitory G protein.[59,60] Although effects of these antagonists vary with species and have not yet been studied in horses, the diuresis associated with administration of α_2-agonists to horses [61,62] likely may be attributable to vasopressin antagonism at the collecting duct.

As mentioned previously, most water drinking in equids occurs periprandially; thus feeding practices affect timing of water intake.[46] If a horse eats a large meal once or twice daily, then both increased plasma sodium concentration and decreased plasma volume (because of a shift of fluid into the bowel) stimulate thirst and vasopressin release. The result is a simultaneous increase in water intake and a decrease in urine output.[63] In addition, hypovolemia further stimulates activation of the renin-angiotensin-aldosterone system, which leads to enhanced renal sodium conservation as an additional means of restoring plasma volume. Although the increase in plasma sodium concentration with meal feeding is rather small

(1% to 3%), the decrease in plasma volume is much greater (5% to 25%). The magnitude of this fluid shift (and the degree of activation of the renin-angiotensin-aldosterone system) can be attenuated largely by feeding small meals four to six times throughout the day.[64,65] Thus more frequent feeding causes less perturbation of body fluids and likely has a protective effect against development of some forms of colic.

Although balance of daily water intake and output is critical for maintenance of homeostasis, it warrants mention that equids tolerate water deprivation well.[66-72] For example, after horses were deprived of water for 72 hours (which resulted in body weight loss in excess of 10%), most of the weight lost (90% of which was assumed to be water) was recovered within the first hour of being provided access to water.[69] Similarly, even greater body weight losses (approaching 20%) induced by water deprivation and desert walking in donkeys and burros were replaced largely within the first few minutes after water was provided.[67,68] Thus in terms of water balance, equids (especially donkeys and burros) truly can be considered desert-adapted animals.[72,73] An important reason for their ability to tolerate water deprivation appears to be a substantial intestinal reserve of water and electrolytes that they call on during periods of dehydration for the maintenance of plasma volume.[74,75] Despite rapid fluid replacement by equids that have been dehydrated by water deprivation, horses that become dehydrated because of prolonged exercise or diarrheal disease (colitis) often do not drink. This behavior can be attributed to the fact that these conditions produce loss of body water and osmoles in the form of sweat or diarrhea. As a result, plasma osmolality does not increase and osmotic thirst stimulus is not produced. In human endurance athletes this state of mild to moderate dehydration that does not induce thirst has been called *voluntary* and *involuntary* dehydration,[76,77] and although less well-documented, a similar response appears to occur in endurance horses.[78] Another form of involuntary dehydration, which may be accompanied by increases in plasma osmolality and protein concentration, also has been described anecdotally in mares after foaling.

Electrolyte Balance

Intake and loss of electrolytes also must be matched appropriately to maintain body content of electrolytes within narrow ranges. This balance is most important for the exchangeable ions (Na^+, K^+, and Cl^-) because these have minimal tissue (skeletal) reserves that can be called on during times of need. An exception is the fluid and electrolyte reserve in the lumen of the gastrointestinal tract, which may be able to provide replacement of 10% or more of the body content of these electrolytes.[75] Three sources provide electrolytes: (1) feed, (2) water (usually minimal amounts), and (3) a number of dietary supplements. Electrolytes also can be lost by three routes: (1) in urine, (2) in feces, and (3) in sweat (insensible losses; see Table 19-3). Investigations of electrolyte balance have revealed that most horses that eat predominantly hay or pasture grass ingest excess potassium and chloride. In contrast, sodium intake varies and with some diets may be marginal.[35,37,38] A maintenance requirement for sodium of 0.4 to 0.8 mEq/kg/day or 200 to 400 mEq/day (6 to 12 g/day) for a 500-kg horse has been suggested[38,54]; however, exercising horses that may lose 500 to 1000 mEq of sodium per hour in sweat or are treated with furosemide have greater dietary requirements to replace such losses.[37] Thus addition of 50 to 75 g of common table salt (which provides 850 to 1275 mEq, because 1 g of NaCl provides approximately 17 mEq sodium) is a safe and economical method of providing daily supplemental sodium and chloride to athletic horses.

The data from the water and electrolyte balance studies performed by Tasker[35] and by Groenendyk, English, and Abetz[38] (see Table 19-3) provide a good illustration of the capacity of the equine kidneys to conserve sodium when dietary intake is low (see Tasker's data[35] at top) compared with when intake is unlimited (see Groenendyk, English, and Abetz's data[38] at bottom). Furthermore, these studies demonstrate that urinary excretion is the major route for loss of potassium and chloride. Although dietary intake of potassium is usually excessive, equine kidneys do not appear to have a great capacity to conserve potassium during periods of food and water deprivation or with anorexia associated with disease.[35,37,77] Thus urinary potassium concentration and total excretion can remain substantial in the face of decreased intake. Consequently, with decreased feed intake horses can develop significant total body potassium depletion and often benefit from supplemental dietary potassium (25 to 50 g per day of potassium chloride [KCl] provides 375 to 750 mEq, because 1 g KCl provides approximately 15 mEq of potassium).

In horses the stimuli for electrolyte intake (salt appetite) have received much less attention than stimuli for drinking. Houpt et al.[54] found that horses that had marginal sodium intake (250 mEq/day) and that were treated with furosemide ate more salt in the hours after treatment than did placebo-treated horses on the same diet; however, salt intake (which was comparable for eating salt from a block or drinking a 0.9% NaCl solution) was excessive in both treatment groups (in excess of 100 g). Thus salt appetite, unlike water intake, is less closely regulated to balance intake with losses. In fact, when salt is available ad libitum, horses appear to consume more than their maintenance needs. The excess is eliminated by increased urinary sodium excretion. Although this apparently excessive salt appetite may seem inappropriate, one could consider it advantageous for exercising horses, which have a much greater daily salt requirement.[79]

RENAL REGULATION OF BODY WATER CONTENT AND ION COMPOSITION

The kidneys are the organs responsible for fine-tuning body water content and ion composition within narrow ranges. The important components of renal regulation of water and ion content include RBF, glomerular filtration, and tubular modification of glomerular filtrate to produce the final urine.

Renal Blood Flow

At rest, the kidneys receive about 15% to 20% of the cardiac output, or about 7.5 to 10 L/min for an average-size horse.[80,81] This high tissue perfusion, 500 to 600 ml/min per 100 g of kidney compared with 50 to 100 ml/min per 100 g of brain tissue, is necessary for the kidney to function as an effective filter and as a regulator of extracellular fluid composition. Furthermore, tubular reabsorption of glomerular filtrate requires energy. Because more than 99% of the filtrate is reabsorbed, the metabolic rate of the kidney is high (second only to that of the heart), and despite the fact that the kidneys account for less than 1% of body weight, they are responsible for about 10% of whole body oxygen use.[1] Next, RBF is distributed preferentially to the renal cortex. In fact, renal medullary blood flow, which is derived largely via the vasa recta that arise from the efferent arterioles of juxtamedullary glomeruli, accounts for less than 20% of total RBF.[81] Consequently, the renal medullary tissue normally functions in a hypoxic environment. Medullary hypoxia has been described as "an inevitable accompaniment of efficient urinary concentration" as a consequence of countercurrent exchange.[82] Although the latter mechanism would suggest that oxygen tension should decrease progressively toward the inner medulla, the lowest values, often no greater than 10 mm Hg, are found in the inner portion of the outer medulla, termed the *inner stripe* (Figure 19-9).[83] This finding can be explained by the substantial metabolic activity of epithelial cells lining the medullary thick ascending limb (mTAL) of the loop of Henle in the inner stripe. The sodium-potassium-adenosine triphosphatase pumps (Na^+,K^+-ATPase) in the basal membrane of these cells are responsible for the greatest adenosine triphosphate (ATP) use (and thereby oxygen consumption) in the medulla.[84] The combined effects of low oxygen delivery and a high rate of use produce the lowest oxygen tension in the inner stripe. Fortunately, several "protective" mechanisms exist to preserve medullary blood flow and tissue oxygenation during periods of renal hypoperfusion and include a preferential reduction in cortical blood flow along with redistribution of RBF to the corticomedullary region, accumulation of adenosine with depletion of ATP, and production of prostaglandin E_2 (PGE_2) and prostaglandin I_2 (PGI_2) and nitric oxide.[82-84] Of clinical importance is that the use of nonsteroidal anti-inflammatory drugs (NSAIDs) in patients with poor renal perfusion can exacerbate tissue hypoxia because PGE_2 acts as a vasodilator and an inhibitor of Na^+,K^+-ATPase. In fact, the earliest lesions of analgesic nephropathy include degeneration and necrosis of mTAL cells before development of overt papillary necrosis.[84]

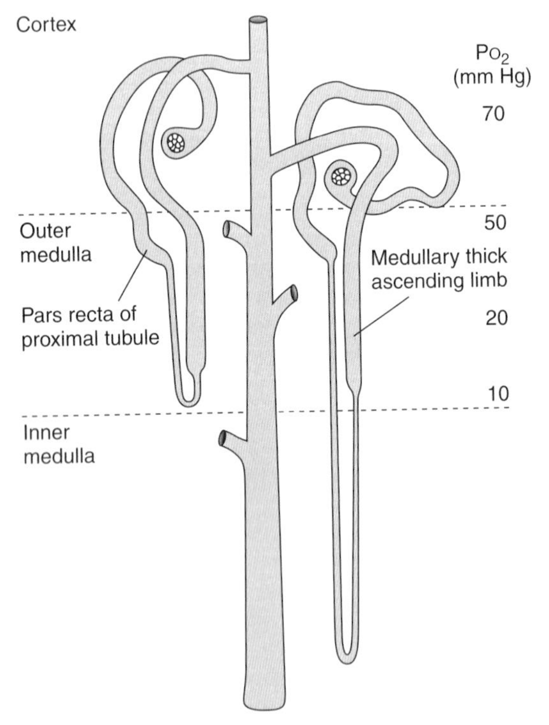

FIGURE 19-9 Schematic drawing of a nephron. In the outer medulla is the site of lowest intrarenal oxygen tension (Po_2), in the final (straight) portion of the proximal tubule and the medullary thick ascending limb (mTAL) of the loop of Henle. Limited medullary blood flow and high metabolic rates make these outer medullary nephron segments the most susceptible to damage during periods of renal hypoperfusion.

RBF of horses has been measured by a variety of techniques including p-aminohippurate clearance (Cl_{PAH}) by classic clearance techniques involving timed urine collections and by plasma disappearance curves, as well as clearance of radionuclides, microsphere injection, and use of ultrasonic Doppler flow probes placed around the renal artery (Table 19-4).[80,81,85-101] The latter technique does not provide absolute blood flow values but rather measures changes in RBF from a baseline value.[98] Recently, plasma disappearance curves for ^{131}I-orthoiodohippuric acid and 99mTc-mercaptoacetyltriglycine have been validated in normal horses in an attempt to establish radionuclide techniques for rapid and noninvasive measurement of RBF in hospitalized horses.[96,101] Although values for RBF determined by these radionuclide techniques compared well with previous data (Table 19-5), their future use in a clinical setting likely will remain limited because of moderate expense and the need to perform serial measurements to provide clinically relevant information in patients with reduced renal function.[113]

Intrinsic and extrinsic factors play a role in the control of RBF. The former include autoregulation and action of renal nerves; the latter include vasoconstrictors (catecholamines, renin-angiotensin system, arginine vasopressin) and vasodilators (prostaglandins, dopamine, atrial peptides, bradykinin, adenosine, and nitric oxide).[1] Although not unique to the kidney, autoregulation of blood flow is a physiologic response that maintains cortical RBF in the normal range through a rather wide range of perfusion pressures (75 to 180 mm Hg in human beings). This response is thought to be independent of neural or hormonal mechanisms and is attributed to a myogenic response to changes in arterial wall tension. The local action of renal nerves or release of vasoconstrictor substances leads to an increase in renal vascular resistance that may occur in response to disease states (hypovolemic or endotoxic shock), drugs (particularly anesthetic agents), or physical stress (exercise). RBF may or may not decrease, depending on the degree of vasoconstriction. For example, renal vascular resistance increases during low-intensity exercise to divert a greater portion of the cardiac output to the working muscles. Thus the fraction of cardiac output delivered to the kidneys decreases; however, because cardiac output also increases in response to exercise, total RBF remains unchanged.[93] In contrast, during halothane anesthesia in ponies, redistribution of cardiac output occurs without an increase in cardiac output. Under these circumstances, renal vasoconstriction is accompanied by a decrease in RBF to about 60% of the awake value at 1.0 to 1.5 minimal alveolar concentration of halothane. As the plane of anesthesia deepens (to 2.0 minimal alveolar concentration), a greater increase in renal vascular resistance (or degree of vasoconstriction) further decreases RBF to about 25% of the awake value, likely because of further vasodilatation of other vascular beds and a mild decrease in cardiac output.[89] Although RBF was not measured, results of a recent study of prolonged (18 hours) anesthesia with sevoflurane are of interest in terms of probable renal hypoperfusion and damage.[114] After 10 hours of anesthesia an increase in urine production

TABLE 19-4

Reported Values for Effective Renal Plasma Flow and Renal Blood Flow in Horses and Ponies

Number of Animals	Method[a]	Effective Renal Plasma Flow (Mean ± SD/SE ml/min/kg [Range])	Renal Blood Flow (RBF) (ml/min/kg)[b]	Reference
1 ♀ Horse	$Cl_{Diodrast}$	6.91 ± 0.81	13.2 ± 1.6	85
1 ♀ Pony	$Cl131_{I\text{-}o\text{-}HA}$	Bolus injection: 12.85 ± 1.81 Constant infusion: 11.45 ± 1.25	21.7 ± 3.1 19.4 ± 2.1	86[c]
3 ♀ Horses	$Cl131_{I\text{-}o\text{-}HA}$	Bolus injection: 11.97 ± 2.63 Constant infusion: 9.56 ± 1.84	20.2 ± 4.4 16.2 ± 3.1	
6 ♀ Ponies	Cl_{PAH}	12.09 ± 0.34 (7.86-21.62)	20.4 ± 0.6	87
2 ♀ Horses		9.59 ± 0.86 (4.75-19.78)	16.2 ± 1.4	
5 ♀/Gelding horses	$Cl131_{I\text{-}o\text{-}HA}$	8.24 ± 2.88 (5.66-12.89)	13.9 ± 4.9	88
8 ♀ Horses	Cl_{PAH}	Bolus injection: 12.0 ± 1.7	20.3 ± 2.9	91
4-Day-old foals		Bolus injection: 15.2 ± 1.5	25.7 ± 2.7	
5 Horses (3 ♂, 2 ♀)		Infusion (Cl-plasma): 18.2 ± 2.0	30.8 ± 3.4	
3 Ponies (1 ♂, 2 ♀)		Infusion (Cl-urine): 11.9 ± 1.9	20.1 ± 3.2	
6 ♀ Horses	Cl_{PAH}	8.5-10.8[d]	14.4-18.3	92
6 ♀ Horses	Cl_{PAH}	11.9 ± 1.0	20.0 ± 1.7	93
6 Horses[e]	$Cl131_{I\text{-}o\text{-}HA}$	6.26 (4.33-6.80)	10.58 (7.32-11.50)	94
8 ♀ Horses	Cl_{PAH} $Cl131_{I\text{-}o\text{-}HA}$	9.65 ± 0.84 (5.60-12.54) 11.32 ± 1.03 (7.82-15.71)	16.31 ± 1.42 19.14 ± 1.74	96
6 Pony foals (3 ♀, 3 ♂)	Cl_{PAH}	16.63 (15.61-17.26)	28.11	99
10 Horses (4 ♀, 6 gelding)	$Cl99_{mTc\text{-}MAG\text{-}3}$	7.92 ± 1.51 (5.58-10.62)	13.39 ± 2.55	100
4 Ponies[e]	Microspheres	—	208 ± 58[f,g]	81
11 Ponies[e]	Microspheres	—	548 ± 87[f]	80
8 Ponies[e]	Microspheres	—	483 ± 79[f]	89
11 Ponies[e]	Microspheres	—	670 ± 50[d,f]	90
3 Horses (♀, ♂, and gelding)	Microspheres	—	535 ± 93[f]	95
9 Horses[e]	Microspheres	—	589 ± 50[f]	97
4 Gelding ponies	Microspheres	–	428 ± 49[f]	101

[a]$Cl_{Diodrast}$, Clearance of 3,5-diiodo-4-pyridine-N-acetic acid; $Cl131_{I\text{-}o\text{-}HA}$, clearance of ^{131}I-*o*-iodohippurate; Cl_{PAH}, clearance of *p*-aminohippurate; $Cl99_{Tc\text{-}MAG3}$, clearance of 99mTc-mercaptoacetyltriglycine.
[b]RBF values presented have been calculated from effective renal plasma flow (ERPF) data using extraction ratios (ERs) of 0.80 for diodrast and 0.91 for ^{131}I-*o*-iodohippurate and *p*-aminohippurate: RBF = (ERPF/ER)/(1-hematocrit); hematocrit was assumed to be 0.35.
[c]Other horses and ponies also were studied after bolus injection of ^{131}I-*o*-iodohippurate and yielded ERPF values of 16.93 ± 6.05 and 10.65 ± 2.73 ml/min/kg for ponies and horses, respectively; these values corresponded to a RBF of 8.6 ± 10.2 ml/min/kg in ponies and 18.0 ± 4.6 ml/min/kg in horses.
[d]Values estimated from figure.
[e]Sex not reported.
[f]RBF values for microsphere studies are expressed in units of milliliters per minute per 100 g of kidney tissue; a value of 500 ml/min/100 g would correlate to an RBF value of 18 ml/min/kg (or 3.6 and 9 L/min for a 200-kg pony and a 500-kg horse, respectively).
[g]Values reported are for ponies under general anesthesia (halothane in oxygen); these authors also reported that renal medullary blood flow was 2.6% to 18.8% of total RBF in two ponies.

was accompanied by evidence of tubular dysfunction (e.g., glucosuria, enzymuria). Furthermore, microscopic lesions after anesthesia were limited to the more distal nephron (mTAL and distal tubule), providing support that these normally hypoxic nephron segments may be the first to succumb to prolonged hypoperfusion.

When RBF decreases, counteracting vasodilatory mediators usually are released in an attempt to ameliorate the decrease in RBF. The best studied of these vasodilatory mediators include renal prostaglandins (PGE_2 and PGI_2) and dopamine. Although the role of renal prostaglandins in the control of basal or resting RBF is thought to be insignificant, renal prostaglandins are important mediators of vasodilatation in response to a number of vasoconstrictive stimuli.[115] Furthermore, production of renal prostaglandins is several times greater in medullary tissue so that action of these mediators leads to a greater increase in inner cortical (region of juxtamedullary glomeruli) and medullary blood flow. As mentioned previously, one should not be surprised that the lesion associated with antagonism of prostanoid production by use of NSAIDs is medullary or

TABLE 19-5

Reported Values for Glomerular Filtration Rate in Horses and Ponies

Number of Animals	Method[a]	Glomerular Filtration Rate (GFR) (Mean ± SD/SE ml/min/kg [Range])	Cl_{crend}/Cl_{In} Ratio[a]	Reference
Not reported[b]	Cl_{In} Cl_{CRend}	0.83 ± 0.13[c,d] 0.85 ± 0.22[c,d]	1.02	85[b]
1 Horse[e]	Cl_{In}	1.4	—	85[b]
12 ♀ Horses	Cl_{In} Cl_{CRend}	1.66 ± 0.33[c] (1.17-2.28) 1.46 ± 0.24[c] (1.10-1.65)	0.88 ± 0.11	85
1 ♀ Pony	$Cl125_{I\text{-iothalamate}}$	Bolus injection: 5.43 (1 study) Constant infusion: 6.10 ± 1.27	— —	86[f]
3 ♀ Horses	$Cl125_{I\text{-iothalamate}}$	Bolus injection: 4.20 ± 1.13 Constant infusion: 3.14 ± 0.53		
13 Ponies[e] 9 (No NaCl supplement) 4 (NaCl supplement)	Cl_{CRend}	1.93 ± 0.37[c] (1.36-2.70) 2.06 ± 0.34[c] (1.64-2.70) 1.63 ± 0.27[c] (1.36-1.99)	—	102
7 ♀ Horses	Cl_{CRend}	3.68 ± 1.18[c] (2.07-4.99)	—	103
4 ♀ Horses	Cl_{In} Cl_{CRend}	1.65 ± 0.07[c] (1.34-2.04) 1.62 ± 0.03[c] (1.29-2.15)	0.96 ± 0.02	104
6 ♀ Ponies	Cl_{In} Cl_{CRend}	1.92 ± 0.06[c] (0.64-3.37) 2.24 ± 0.06[c] (1.04-4.15)	0.86[c]	87[g]
2 ♀ Horses	Cl_{In} Cl_{CRend}	1.86 ± 0.14[c] (0.71-3.68) 1.67 ± 0.13[c] (0.68-3.09)	1.11[c]	
12 ♀/Gelding horses	$Cl99m_{Tc\text{-}DTPA}$	1.93 ± 0.27 (1.39-2.53)	—	88
4 Gelding horses	Cl_{CRend}	1.34 ± 0.51[c] (1.01-2.10)	—	18
1 ♀ Pony	Cl_{CRend}	1.15 ± 0.08	—	105
4 Horses (1 gelding, 3 ♀)	Cl_{CRend}	1.45 ± 0.21[c]		
10 Gelding horses	Cl_{CRend}	1.88 ± 0.46	—	25
12 ♀ Horses	Cl_{CRend}	1.48 ± 0.04	—	106[h]
1 ♂ Pony	$Cl14_{C\text{-}In}$ Cl_{CRend}	1.74 ± 0.15 1.06 ± 0.10	0.61 ± 0.11	27[i]
4 Ponies (2 ♂, 2 ♀)	$Cl14_{C\text{-}In}$ Cl_{CRex}	1.66 ± 0.38[c] (1.34-2.22) 1.70 ± 0.39[c] (1.43-2.27)	1.02 ± 0.07[c]	
6 ♀ Horses	Cl_{CRend}	1.92 ± 0.51 (1.49-2.74)	—	26
2 ♀ Horses	Cl_{CRend}	Awake horses: 2.65[c] During anesthesia: 1.32[c] After anesthesia: 2.50[c]	—	107[j]
8 ♀ Horses	Cl_{In}	Bolus injection: 1.63 ± 0.33		91
4-Day-old foals	Cl_{CRend}	2.81 ± 0.55	1.00[c,k]	
5 Horse (3 ♂, 2 ♀) 3 Pony (1 ♂, 2 ♀)	Cl_{In}	Bolus injection: 2.30 ± 0.34 Infusion (Cl-plasma): 2.56 ± 0.30 Infusion (Cl-urine): 2.82 ± 0.32		
6 ♀ Horses	Cl_{CRex}	2.56 ± 0.60[c]	—	108
6 ♀ Horses	Cl_{In}	1.88 ± 0.67	—	93
8 ♀ Horses	Cl_{In} $Cl99m_{Tc\text{-}DTPA}$	1.83 ± 0.21 (0.89-2.95) 1.79 ± 0.18 (1.08-2.51)	—	96
12 ♀ Horses	Cl_{In} $Cl99m_{Tc\text{-}DTPA}$ $Cl99m_{Tc\text{-}DTPA(cam)}$	1.55 ± 0.04[c] (0.98-2.22) 1.47 ± 0.27[c] (0.91-1.82) 1.55 ± 0.22[c,l]	—	109

TABLE 19-5

Reported Values for Glomerular Filtration Rate in Horses and Ponies—cont'd

Number of Animals	Method[a]	Glomerular Filtration Rate (GFR) (Mean ± SD/SE ml/min/kg [Range])	Cl_{crend}/Cl_{In} Ratio[a]	Reference
30 Horses (7 ♂, 23 ♀)	Cl_{In}	1.73	1.03[c]	110
	Cl_{CRend}	1.79		
6 Pony foals (3 ♀, 3 ♂)	Cl_{In}	3.21 ± 0.36 (2.73-3.64)	0.60[c]	99
	Cl_{CRend}	1.92 ± 0.14 (1.60-2.14)		
5 Horses	$Cl99m_{Tc\text{-}DTPA}$	3.3 ± 0.4	—	111
6 ♀ Horses	Cl_{CRend}	1.20-1.87	—	112[a]

[a]Cl_{In}' Inulin clearance; Cl_{CRend}' endogenous creatinine clearance; $Cl125_{I\text{-}iothalamate}$' clearance of ^{125}I-iothalamate; $Cl99m_{Tc\text{-}DTPA}$' clearance of 99mTc-diethylenetriamine pentaacetic acid (99mTc-DTPA); $Cl14_{C\text{-}In}$' clearance of ^{14}C-inulin; Cl_{CRex}' exogenous creatinine clearance; $Cl99m_{Tc\text{-}DTPA(cam)}$' clearance of 99mTc-DTPA determined by serial imaging at the body surface with a gamma camera.
[b]Values taken from Knudsen.[85]
[c]Values presented have been calculated from original data.
[d]Low GFR values were attributed to rapidly declining plasma inulin concentrations (nonsteady state conditions) during the urine collection periods.
[e]Sex not reported.
[f]Other horses and ponies also were studied after bolus injection of ^{125}I-iothalamate and yielded GFR values of 5.39 ± 1.79 and 3.44 ± 1.11 ml/min/kg for ponies and horses, respectively.
[g]Attempts at measuring GFR by plasma disappearance after bolus injection of inulin were unsuccessful.
[h]Value presented is for control group; GFR was not different after phenylbutazone administration (1.36 ± 0.04 ml/min/kg) or phenylbutazone and furosemide administration (1.44 ± 0.12 ml/min/kg) but was reported to increase to 1.75 ± 0.16 ml/min/kg after water loading (25 L) and to 1.77 ± 0.18 ml/min/kg after water loading and phenylbutazone administration.
[i]Ponies were anesthetized during the studies.
[j]Mares studied before, during, and after 1.2 minimum alveolar concentration halothane anesthesia.
[k]Value calculated from urinary clearance values for inulin and creatinine (Cr).
[l]Despite correction for differences in depth (right kidney closer to lateral body surface than left kidney), the clearance of 99mTc-DTPA determined by serial imaging at the body surface with a gamma camera showed a greater (~60% total) GFR by the right kidney compared with the left kidney (~40% of total). Because similar differences have not been demonstrated in microsphere studies of renal blood flow (RBF) (in which both kidneys receive equal blood flow), this technique requires further refinement before it can be used to provide accurate measures of GFR in horses.

papillary necrosis.[116,117] With or without renal vasoconstriction, activation of dopamine receptors (DA_1 type) leads to renal vasodilatation. Because the receptors are located on most renal arterioles, blood flow increases in the renal cortex and the medulla. For this reason, dopamine infusions are touted to be of benefit in treating ARF because this catecholamine has been shown to increase RBF and urine output by 30% to 190% in normal horses.[98]

Glomerular Filtration

Approximately 20% of the blood entering the glomeruli passes through small pores in the filtration barrier into Bowman's capsule. The primary force driving filtration is glomerular capillary transmural hydraulic pressure. A relatively constant pressure across the glomerular capillary wall is maintained by greater resistance in the arteriole leaving the glomerulus (efferent arteriole) than in the arteriole entering the glomerulus (afferent arteriole). This difference in vascular resistance generates the hydraulic pressure that forces plasma water out of the glomerular capillaries.[1] The filtration barrier is made up of three layers: (1) endothelium of the glomerular capillaries, (2) basement membrane, and (3) foot processes of the epithelial cells (podocytes) lining Bowman's capsule. The pore size of the filtration barrier, about 8 to 10 nm in diameter, prevents filtration of cells and larger proteins. As a result, the fluid that enters Bowman's capsule is an ultrafiltrate that is essentially identical to plasma except that it has less than 0.05% of the protein content of plasma. Interestingly, the diameter of albumin is about 6 nm, so its size should not prevent filtration. Glycosaminoglycans containing heparin sulfate and sialic acid residues impart a significant negative charge to the filtration barrier. Thus charge repulsion of albumin (which is similarly negatively charged) may be more important than molecular size in preventing significant loss of albumin into the filtrate; however, metabolic disturbances (metabolic acidosis) can neutralize the glomerular charge barrier, and one can observe transient proteinuria in the absence of structural damage to the glomerular barrier.[118]

By definition, glomerular filtration rate (GFR) is the volume of plasma filtered per unit of time and commonly is described in milliliters per minute per kilogram of body mass. The GFR of horses and ponies ranges between 1.6 to 2.0 ml/kg/min, with some authors reporting slightly higher values for ponies. This range is similar to those of other animals and human beings. For a 500-kg horse this value equals 800 to 1000 ml per minute or about 1200 to 1400 L per day. This value represents filtration of the total plasma volume 60 to 70 times per day. Because urine production is about 10 L per day, more than 99% of the glomerular filtrate is reabsorbed.

Like RBF, GFR has been measured in horses by a variety of techniques, including Cl_{In} by classic clearance techniques, Cl_{Cr}, and clearance or plasma disappearance of radionuclides (see Table 19-5).* Plasma disappearance curves for 99mTc-diethylenetriamine pentaacetic acid (99mTc-DTPA) have been

*References 1, 25-27, 85-88, 91, 93, 96-110, 113-115, 119, 120.

documented to compare well in normal horses with Cl_{In} (the gold standard).[96] Although this technique is less expensive than ^{131}I-orthoiodohippuric acid clearance for estimating RBF,[113] clinical use is limited by availability of nuclear medicine capabilities and expense (because one must take multiple measurements to assess disease progression or response to treatment). Recently, Gleadhill et al.[120] described use of a three blood sample technique to estimate GFR by plasma disappearance of 99mTc-DTPA. Interestingly, rather than expressing GFR on the basis of per kilogram of body mass or a body surface area, they suggested that GFR should be compared with extracellular fluid volume. Because plasma activity of 99mTc-DTPA also can be used to estimate extracellular fluid volume, one can make this estimate of GFR using 99mTc-DTPA alone. Standardization of GFR based on extracellular fluid volume is attractive and warrants further consideration because it eliminates the effect of variable body composition (e.g., specifically differences in body fat) when expressing GFR based on body mass. The authors subsequently used this method to estimate the decrease in GFR accompanying exercise.[111]

The mechanisms responsible for control of RBF (autoregulation, neural input, hormonal factors) also play a role in control of GFR. In addition, GFR is affected further by factors such as plasma protein concentration (oncotic pressure) and alterations in the filtration barrier. As discussed previously, a balance exists between that action of vasoconstrictor and vasodilator substances during periods of decreased RBF. Interestingly, GFR decreases less than RBF with moderate to severe renal vasoconstriction. This sparing effect on GFR has long been attributed to greater vasoconstrictive effects of angiotensin II on efferent arterioles compared with afferent arterioles.[121] Such a response could increase the glomerular capillary transmural hydraulic pressure driving filtration and would be manifested by an increase in filtration fraction. In fact, the latter response has been documented in exercising horses.[93] More recently, however, other vasoconstrictors (endothelins) and vasodilators (endothelium-derived relaxing factors, nitric oxide) have been shown to play a role in the control of glomerular capillary hemodynamics and filtration so that a singular role for angiotensin II is likely an oversimplified explanation for the sparing effect on GFR.[122]

Renal Tubular Function

Once the glomerular filtrate enters the renal tubule, it is modified extensively in the process of becoming the final product excreted into the renal pelvis. A complete review of renal tubular function is beyond the scope of this text; however, a few general concepts warrant mention, and a number of specific aspects are addressed elsewhere in this chapter. First, most glucose, amino acid, electrolyte, and water reabsorption occurs across epithelial cells lining the proximal tubule; however, these substances are not all reabsorbed to the same extent. For example, this tubule segment is responsible for reabsorption of essentially all filtered glucose and amino acids, about 90% of filtered bicarbonate, about 70% of filtered sodium, and about 60% of filtered chloride.[28] Furthermore, at the end of the proximal tubule, fluid is no more concentrated than it was in Bowman's space. Tubular sodium concentration is unchanged, whereas tubular chloride concentration actually has increased (because of preferential bicarbonate reabsorption). Despite limited modification of these tubular fluid components, net reabsorption of between 60% and 80% of the total filtered load of sodium, chloride, and water occurs within the proximal tubule. Proximal tubular epithelial cells are also responsible for secretion of ammonium ions and a number of organic anions and cations, as described previously.

Tubular fluid passing into the loop of Henle becomes progressively more concentrated (hypertonic) as it travels to the inner medulla because the descending limb is permeable to water, urea, and electrolytes (the latter to a lesser degree).[28] In contrast, the ascending limb is relatively impermeable to water but actively reabsorbs sodium, chloride, and potassium via the apical $Na^+/K^+/2Cl^-$ co-transporter (blocked by furosemide), which is coupled to Na^+,K^+-ATPase on the basolateral membrane. As a result, fluid leaving this nephron segment is actually less concentrated (hypotonic) than the original filtrate. The loop of Henle is responsible for reabsorption of an additional 15% to 20% of filtered sodium and chloride, along with addition of urea to the tubular fluid. More important, the loop of Henle is responsible for generation of the medullary osmotic gradient via countercurrent multiplication. This function results from the combined effects of different permeability characteristics of the descending and ascending limbs of the loop of Henle and active removal of sodium and chloride in the ascending limb.

The distal tubule is quantitatively less important in reabsorption of electrolytes and water; however, the distal tubule is the nephron segment in which the final qualitative changes in urine occur.[28] For example, the distal tubule is an important site of calcium, potassium, and acid excretion. The latter two typically are exchanged for sodium under the influence of aldosterone. Tubule fluid passes from the distal tubule into the outer or cortical collecting ducts, which are impermeable to urea. In addition to further modification of fluid in the cortical collecting ducts, tubular urea concentration increases steadily as water is removed (under the influence of vasopressin) as fluid travels to the inner medulla. In contrast, in the absence of vasopressin (as with diabetes insipidus), the collecting ducts are impermeable to water and produce hypotonic urine. The collecting ducts remain impermeable to urea (which accounts for up to 50% of the osmoles in urine) except for the innermost medullary segments, which allow urea to be recycled into the interstitium for maintenance of the medullary osmotic gradient.

Reabsorption of glomerular filtrate by renal tubules requires a close association with the vascular system that carries reabsorbed solute and water to the circulation. Proximal tubules are adjacent to peritubular capillaries, which have a tremendous capacity to accommodate the massive flux of solute and water across proximal tubule epithelial cells. Equally important in maintenance of the medullary osmotic gradient are the vasa recta, hairpin capillaries that travel deep into the renal medulla in association with loops of Henle derived from the population of juxtamedullary nephrons. Blood flow through these capillaries is typically slow, allowing for countercurrent exchange of solute in the medullary interstitium, which is necessary for generation and maintenance of medullary hypertonicity. Urea leaving the descending limb of Henle and being recycled across the innermost portion of the medullary collecting duct is responsible for about half of this medullary hypertonicity.

These basic aspects of tubular function have a number of important clinical implications. First, proximal tubule epithelial cells have a high metabolic rate. Although most of the proximal tubule is in the more highly perfused renal cortex, renal hypoperfusion leads to a relative hypoxia surrounding these cells because of ongoing metabolic activity. Consequently, the proximal tubule is highly susceptible to injury when cortical blood flow is reduced (e.g., with hypovolemia or other states accompanied by a decrease in RBF). Second, as discussed previously, the renal medulla receives only a small fraction of the total RBF, leading to a normally hypoxic local environment. Thus any degree of renal hypoperfusion also is accompanied by exacerbation of medullary hypoxia, especially in the inner stripe because of the metabolic activity of epithelial cells lining the mTAL. In fact, in cases of ARF in human beings, histologic examination of renal tissue actually may show more severe lesions in the more distal nephron (mTAL) rather than in the proximal tubule.[123] Recognition of this more distal tubular damage has also led to consideration of therapeutic interventions to reduce damage to this nephron segment during periods of poor renal perfusion (e.g., continuous infusion of furosemide to decrease the metabolic activity of the mTAL). Third, despite the fact that the distal tubule and collecting ducts are responsible for reabsorption of less than 5% of the total glomerular filtrate, a decrease in reabsorption of only 1% to 2% can be quantitatively significant and can lead to dramatic polyuria (see Polyuria and Polydipsia, later in this chapter). Next, generation of a maximal medullary concentration gradient requires slow flow of tubular fluid for countercurrent multiplication and slow flow of blood through the vasa recta to maximize countercurrent exchange. Thus conditions that increase tubular flow rates (high-volume intravenous fluids) or increase vasa recta blood flow (endogenous PGE_2 and PGI_2 production consequent to renal hypoperfusion) compromise the medullary concentration gradient (partial medullary washout) and lead to production of more dilute urine with increased urinary sodium concentration (and excretion).

A final aspect of tubular function that appears to be unique to horses among the domestic species is excretion of calcium. Equine urine is well recognized as being cloudy and viscid. These qualities can be attributed to the large amount of calcium excreted in normal equine urine, largely in the form of calcium carbonate ($CaCO_3$) crystals, and mucus secreted by glands in the renal pelvis and proximal ureter that acts to "lubricate" the lower urinary tract to minimize adherence of crystal to the epithelium lining the ureters, bladder, and urethra. Although the nature of this unique tubular calcium excretion has been studied little in horses, one report of the role of vitamin D in calcium and phosphorous homeostasis in horses suggested that this vitamin-hormone was less important in horses than in other species.[124] This fascinating difference between horses and other species evaluated by large animal internists clearly warrants further investigation.

Excretion of Solute and Water

Renal function traditionally is thought of in terms of glomerular filtration, tubular modification of the filtered fluid, and excretion of the final urine. This concept accommodates excretion of nitrogenous and organic wastes and the major aspects of regulation of body water content and ionic balance. Urine concentration and volume also are affected by solute excretion, and another way to think about renal function is in terms of total solute and water excretion. For example, a horse could produce 6 L of urine daily with an osmolality of 900 mOsm/kg to excrete 5400 mOsm of solute or, if the solute load were doubled to 10,800 mOsm, then the horse could produce 12 L of urine with an osmolality of 900 mOsm/kg to eliminate the additional solute. Thus urine osmolality reflects the ability of the kidney to dilute or concentrate the final urine but does not necessarily provide an accurate estimate of the "quantitative ability" to excrete solute or retain water. One assesses these functions by calculating osmolal clearance (C_{osm}) and free water clearance (C_{H2O}).[28] Like other clearances, these calculations require measurement of urine flow (via timed urine collection) and measurement of plasma and urine osmolality.

These measures of renal solute and water handling are conceptualized by considering urine to have two components: (1) that which contains all the urinary solute in a solution that is isosmotic to plasma (C_{osm}, usually expressed in milliliters per minute or liters per day), and (2) that which contains free water without any solute (C_{H2O}, also expressed in milliliters per minute or liters per day). The sum of these two components is the actual urine flow rate in milliliters per minute or liters per day. Because urine is typically more concentrated than plasma, C_{H2O} typically has a negative value, indicating water conservation. In fact, the inverse of free water clearance is termed *renal water reabsorption.* Returning to the foregoing example, excretion of the 5400 mOsm would require production of 18 L of urine that is isosmotic with plasma (using a value of 300 mOsm/kg for plasma). However, because 6 L of concentrated urine actually was produced during the period measured, the kidneys quantitatively have reabsorbed 12 L of free water per day. In contrast, despite production of urine with an identical urine osmolality (900 mOsm/kg), excretion of 10,800 mOsm would require production of 36 L of urine isosmotic with plasma. Free water clearance would be 30 L per day (i.e., 30 L per day of free water would be reabsorbed by the kidneys). Thus although concentrated urine always will have a negative C_{H2O} value, indicating renal water reabsorption, and dilute urine always will have a positive value for C_{H2O}, indicating renal water excretion, quantitative assessment of renal solute and water handling requires measurement of osmolal and free water clearances.

Excretion of free water by the kidney occurs by generation of hypotonic tubule fluid in the ascending limb of the loop of Henle, and the amount or volume of free water produced depends on the amount of tubule fluid presented to that segment. Free water consequently is excreted by keeping the collecting ducts relatively impermeable to water (lack of vasopressin). Assessment of C_{H2O} is most helpful in patients with hyponatremia and hypo-osmolality that cannot be attributed to another primary disease process (diarrhea or bladder rupture). For hyponatremia to develop, water excretion must be defective. For example, hyponatremia can develop with prerenal failure (hypovolemia) or with oliguric renal failure after a reduction in GFR and the amount of filtrate presented to the loop of Henle. Hyponatremia and hypo-osmolality may also develop with use of loop diuretics, because less free water is generated in the ascending limb of the loop of Henle because of blockade of the apical $Na^+/K^+/2Cl^-$ co-transporter (smaller amounts of solute are removed). A final cause of true hyponatremia may be the syndrome of inappropriate vasopressin secretion or syndrome of inappropriate antidiuretic hormone secretion. Although the latter condition has not been documented in horses, occasionally it may play a role in the development of hyponatremia in a foal.[125]

EXAMINATION OF THE URINARY SYSTEM

Harold C. Schott II

HISTORY AND PHYSICAL EXAMINATION

To begin the evaluation of a horse with urinary tract disease, one should collect a complete history and perform a thorough physical examination. Important historical information includes duration and type of clinical signs, number of horses affected, diet, medications administered, and response to treatment. One also should assess water intake and urine output. For example, owners may mistake pollakiuria (frequent urination) for polyuria (increased urine production), and distinguishing between the two is helpful for forming a diagnostic plan. Pollakiuria frequently occurs in females during estrus or in either sex of horse with cystic calculi or cystitis. In contrast, polyuria more often accompanies renal disease, pituitary pars intermedia dysfunction (PPID), behavior problems (primary polydipsia), diabetes insipidus, or diabetes mellitus. Astute owners may note increased thirst after exercise or a change in urine character, such as a clearer stream, to support polydipsia and polyuria.

One can determine water intake over 24 hours by turning off any automatic-watering devices and providing a known volume of water to the horse.[1] Water intake can vary widely with environmental conditions, level of activity, and diet (see Renal Physiology) so that repeated measurements over several 24-hour periods may be more rewarding in documenting average daily water consumption. Urine output, which should range between 5 and 15 L in a horse with normal renal function, is more difficult to determine. One can apply a urine collection harness for 24-hour urine collections[2-5]; alternatively, one can use an indwelling Foley catheter attached to a collection apparatus to quantify urine output in mares. Although horses used for research tolerate these devices fairly well, the devices have limited application to clinical patients. One can construct a practical collection device for geldings and stallions by cutting off the bottom of a large plastic bottle, padding it, and fitting it over the prepuce. One covers the opening of the bottle with a rubber tube and clip; urine can be removed every few hours.[6] During the collection period, horses usually are tied or restrained in stocks to minimize interference with the collection device.

The most common presenting complaints for horses with urinary tract disease are weight loss and abnormal urination. Other clinical signs vary with the cause and site of the problem and may include fever, anorexia, depression, ventral edema, oral ulceration, excessive dental tartar, colic, or scalding or blood staining of the perineum or hindlimbs. Although lumbar pain and hindlimb lameness have been attributed to urinary tract disease, a musculoskeletal problem is the usual cause of these clinical signs. Decreased performance may be an early presenting complaint for renal disease, but poor performance likely results from changes associated with uremia (mild anemia and lethargy) rather than from renal pain. Occasionally a horse with urolithiasis or renal neoplasia may have a history of recurrent colic. Prolonged or repeated posturing to urinate and dysuria or hematuria would be important findings to implicate the urinary tract as the probable source of abdominal pain in such patients.

In addition to a thorough physical examination, one should include rectal palpation in the evaluation of all horses with suspected urinary tract disease. One should palpate the bladder to determine size, wall thickness, and presence of cystic calculi or mural masses. If the bladder is full, then one should palpate the bladder again after bladder catheterization or voiding. One can palpate the caudal pole of the left kidney for size and texture. The ureters generally are not palpable unless enlarged or obstructed by disease, but one should palpate the dorsal abdomen (retroperitoneal course of ureters) and trigone to determine if they are detectable. Dilation of a ureter may occur with pyelonephritis or ureterolithiasis; in mares, palpation of the distal ureters through the vaginal wall may be more rewarding. One also should palpate the reproductive tract to assess whether a reproductive problem could be causing the clinical signs.

HEMATOLOGY AND SERUM BIOCHEMISTRY

A complete blood count (CBC) that reveals an elevated white blood cell count and total protein or fibrinogen concentration would support an inflammatory or infectious disease process. One may observe mild anemia (packed cell volume [PCV], 20% to 30%) consequent to decreased erythropoietin production and a shortened red blood cell (RBC) life span in horses with CRF.

BUN and Cr concentrations are the most commonly used indices of renal function, specifically GFR.[7-9] One must remember that BUN and Cr do not increase until the majority of nephrons (generally considered about 75%) become nonfunctional.[10] Although this commonly used percentage is based on studies of partially nephrectomized laboratory animals, several clinical reports in which unilateral nephrectomy was used successfully to manage disorders of the upper urinary tract support a similar renal reserve capacity in horses.[11-15] In addition, renal function remained within normal ranges, and animals maintained body weight after experimental unilateral nephrectomy in ponies[16] and in horses.[17] Thus measurement of BUN and Cr is of little use in evaluating early or minor changes in GFR. Once elevated, however, small increases in BUN and Cr are more sensitive indicators of further deterioration in GFR, because one can interpret doubling of BUN or Cr as a 50% decline in remaining renal function (Figure 19-10).

Urea can be measured by a variety of methods, categorized broadly as direct or indirect analyses.[7,8] The direct method is the diacetyl monoxime reaction, in which urea reacts with diacetyl after hydrolysis of diacetyl monoxime to diacetyl and hydroxylamine. One determines urea concentration spectrophotometrically by measuring the yield of the yellow diazine reaction product. Indirect analysis is based on enzymatic conversion of urea to ammonia and carbonic acid by urease. Several methods exist for subsequently determining ammonia concentration, and the one used most often is the enzyme-coupled reaction with glutamate dehydrogenase. Although the term *BUN* is widely accepted, one must remember that the actual measurement reported is the urea concentration in serum or plasma.

Cr can also be assayed by several methods, but the one used most often is the Jaffe's reaction, which is a colorimetric assay based on the formation of a complex between Cr and alkaline

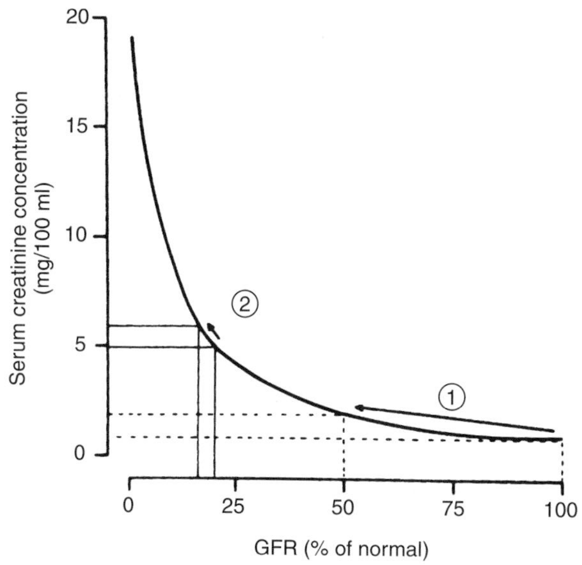

FIGURE 19-10 Relationship between glomerular filtration rate (GFR) and serum creatinine (Cr). When renal function is normal, a large decrease in GFR (as with acute renal failure) results in a minor increase in Cr *(arrow 1)*. In contrast, when renal function is decreased (as with chronic renal failure [CRF]), a much smaller decrease in GFR results in a similar increase in Cr *(arrow 2)*. (From Brenner BM, editor: Brenner and Rector's the kidney, ed 8, Philadelphia, 2008, WB Saunders.)

picrate.[7-9] Unfortunately, a number of other substances in plasma or serum contribute to the yellow color, which leads to a 20% overestimation of actual Cr in human beings and in horses.[18] These non-Cr chromagens include glucose, pyruvate, acetoacetate, fructose, uric acid, and ascorbic acid. Interference by non-Cr chromagens is greatest when Cr is in the normal range, which leads to a high coefficient of variation in repeated measurements of the same sample. With azotemia, Cr measurement by the Jaffe's reaction becomes more accurate because the contribution from non-Cr chromagens does not increase significantly (non-Cr chromagens are responsible for less than 5% of the color development when Cr is >5.0 mg/dl). Non-Cr chromagens do not interfere significantly with urine Cr measurement.

In addition to the factors discussed in the preceding section that influence urea and Cr metabolism (see Renal Physiology), spurious increases in Cr may be reported in various metabolic disorders or after administration of certain cephalosporin antibiotics.[8] When such increases in Cr are thought to be spurious, one can measure true Cr by several methods, which include use of an automated analyzer that distinguishes Cr and non-Cr chromagens by their different rates of color development or performance of the Cr imidohydrolase enzyme assay. The latter yields ammonia, which can be quantified by colorimetric methods. As an example, Cr measured by the Jaffe's reaction increased 16% after horses were fasted for 3 days; however, when serum was analyzed by the enzymatic method, no increase in Cr was detected.[18] In addition to spurious increases in Cr, other substances can cause spurious decreases in serum Cr. The most common one is bilirubin, which, when greater than 5.0 mg/dl, may decrease measured Cr by 0.1 to 0.5 mg/dl.[8]

The reporting of serum or plasma urea and Cr concentrations also varies between different countries. In the United States, BUN and Cr are reported in milligrams per deciliter, whereas in other parts of the world they are reported in standard international units of millimoles per liter and micromoles per liter, respectively. One can convert BUN from milligrams per deciliter to millimoles per liter and Cr from milligrams per deciliter to micromoles per liter by multiplying by 0.357 and 88, respectively.[8]

Azotemia is the term used to describe an elevation in BUN and Cr; thus it is strictly a laboratory abnormality. Azotemia can be prerenal in origin because of decreased renal perfusion, it may be attributable to primary renal disease, or may accompany obstructive diseases or disruption of the urinary tract (postrenal azotemia).[10,19] Thus one should interpret BUN and Cr in light of hydration status of the patient, presenting complaint, and physical findings. In general, animals with prerenal azotemia tend to have smaller increases in BUN and Cr than animals with intrinsic renal failure, whereas animals with postrenal failure may have the greatest degree of azotemia.[20] Unfortunately, BUN and Cr can cover a wide range of values for all three categories of azotemia; thus specific ranges do not identify the type of azotemia.[20-23] In an attempt to characterize azotemia better, use of the BUN-to-Cr ratio also has been examined. In theory the ratio should be higher for prerenal azotemia (because of increased reabsorption of urea with low tubule flow rates) and postrenal azotemia (because of preferential diffusion of urea across peritoneal membranes in cases of uroperitoneum) than for azotemia associated with intrinsic renal failure. As for categoric values for BUN and Cr, BUN-to-Cr ratios measured in azotemic dogs with naturally occurring diseases were distributed over wide, nondiscriminatory ranges for all three types of azotemia.[20,21] In horses the BUN-to-Cr ratio more often has been used to separate ARF from CRF. In the acute form of renal failure, Cr tends to increase proportionately more than BUN, leading to a BUN-to-Cr ratio of less than 10:1.[24] In contrast, with CRF, the BUN-to-Cr ratio often exceeds 10:1. Although a clear explanation for this difference has not been established, the difference may be related to different volumes of distribution for urea and Cr. Urea, a nonpolar molecule, diffuses freely into all body fluids, whereas Cr, a charged molecule, likely requires longer to diffuse out of the extracellular fluid space. Thus a sudden decrease in renal perfusion leads to a greater increase in Cr than in BUN. Muscle breakdown or damage, as with rhabdomyolysis, may be an additional factor contributing to the rapid increase in serum Cr. Furthermore, the BUN-to-Cr ratio value provides only a suggestion of the duration of azotemia in horses, because one can find exceptions for acute and CRF. Finally, the BUN-to-Cr ratio also may be useful in assessing adequacy of dietary protein intake in cases of CRF (see Chronic Renal Failure).[25]

The terms *prerenal azotemia* and *prerenal failure* describe the reversible increase in BUN and Cr associated with renal hypoperfusion.[10,19,23,26] Although these terms are entrenched firmly in human and veterinary medical literature, they likely contribute to the failure to recognize the renal damage that accompanies a number of medical and surgical conditions. Lack of recognition is attributable to the large renal functional reserve. In fact, in many cases of prerenal failure, one can demonstrate altered glomerular and tubule function by proteinuria and cast formation, impaired concentrating ability, and changes in electrolyte excretion.[27,28] Although such functional alterations are usually reversible, a degree of permanent nephron loss can occur and could explain the finding of microscopic evidence of renal disease in as many as one third of equine kidneys examined.[29] Thus considering prerenal failure as a transient and reversible period of compromised renal function that can lead to permanent but clinically silent decreased renal functional mass may be more appropriate. Furthermore, periods of decreased RBF or prerenal failure are accompanied by a number of compensatory renal responses that are mobilized to preserve RBF (autoregulatory response of the afferent arterioles) and GFR (increase in filtration fraction because of angiotensin II–mediated efferent arteriolar constriction). In addition, increased intrarenal production of vasodilatory prostaglandins (PGE_2 and PGI_2) is an important response to renal ischemia that maintains or even increases medullary blood flow (see Renal Physiology). Thus one also can consider prerenal failure as a period of decompensation from the numerous renal compensatory responses to hypoperfusion.[30]

Prerenal azotemia traditionally is differentiated from intrinsic renal failure by assessing urinary concentrating ability. With prerenal azotemia, maintenance of urinary concentrating ability is demonstrated by a urine specific gravity greater than 1.020 and urine osmolality exceeding 500 mOsm/kg. In contrast, urinary concentrating ability typically is lost with intrinsic renal failure, and urine specific gravity and osmolality are less than 1.020 and 500 mOsm/kg, respectively, in the face of dehydration.[31] Such assessment is challenging, however, because it is valid only when performed on urine collected before initiation of fluid therapy or administration of any of a number of medications (α_2-receptor agonists, furosemide) that can affect urine flow and concentration.[32-35] In addition to these measures of urinary concentrating ability, urine-to-serum ratios of osmolality, urea nitrogen and Cr concentrations, and fractional sodium clearance may provide useful information to differentiate prerenal azotemia from intrinsic renal failure (Table 19-6).[31,32] For example, urine-to-serum Cr ratios exceeding 50:1 (reflecting concentrated urine) and fractional sodium clearance values less than 1% (indicating adequate tubule function) would be expected in horses with prerenal azotemia, whereas ratios less than 37:1 and clearance values greater than 0.8% were reported in a group of horses determined to have primary renal disease.[31] Although these values can be helpful, the data in Table 19-6 illustrate that renal hypoperfusion is accompanied by a progressive loss of concentrating ability, because the ranges of these ratios tend to be lower for horses with prerenal azotemia than for clinically normal horses. Thus these data also support the concept that the progression from prerenal failure to intrinsic renal failure is associated with decompensation of the intrarenal responses to hypoperfusion.[30] Clinically, this decompensation is recognized as persistence of azotemia, whereas prerenal azotemia rapidly resolves (by 30% to 50% within 24 hours and completely by 72 hours) in response to fluid therapy and other supportive treatments.

In patients at risk for developing ARF, including horses with serious gastrointestinal disorders, or rhabdomyolysis and in those receiving nephrotoxic medications, serial assessment of urine specific gravity or osmolality, sodium concentration, and fractional sodium clearance may be useful in identifying significant changes in renal function before the onset of azotemia. Similarly, if one determines urine flow rate during a timed urine collection period, then assessment of renal water reabsorption (C_{H2O}; see Renal Physiology) can be a sensitive predictor of impending renal failure.[36-38] Unfortunately, monitoring of these parameters often is complicated by use of intravenous fluid support in such patients. Although intravenous fluids can complicate interpretation of many of these indexes of renal function, Roussel et al.[32] found that the urine-to-plasma osmolality ratio remained greater than 1.7:1 in healthy horses receiving 20 L of an intravenous polyionic solution over 4 hours. Thus serial measurement of urine specific gravity or osmolality may provide useful information for patients at high risk for ARF.

One usually considers a diagnosis of postrenal azotemia resulting from obstruction or disruption of the urinary tract based on clinical signs, including dysuria and renal colic. With bladder rupture, however, some affected foals and adult horses continue to void urine, although progressive abdominal distention usually accompanies development of uroperitoneum. One most often confirms urinary tract disruption by measuring a twofold or greater value for peritoneal fluid Cr concentration compared with Cr concentration. Occasionally in a foal with a urachal problem or a gelding with a disrupted urethra, postrenal azotemia may be accompanied by considerable swelling in the abdominal wall or in the prepuce, respectively.

In addition to screening for azotemia and concentrating ability, the laboratory database should include serum electrolyte, protein (albumin and globulin), and glucose concentrations, as well as muscle enzyme activity.[8,19,22-26] Hyponatremia and hypochloremia are common in horses with renal disease. Serum potassium concentration may be normal or may be elevated in cases of acute or CRF. Hyperkalemia is often most extreme and most serious with urinary tract disruption and uroperitoneum. Calcium and phosphorus concentrations vary in horses with renal disease. Hypercalcemia and hypophosphatemia often occur in horses with CRF, especially when they are fed alfalfa hay (see Chronic Renal Failure), whereas hypocalcemia and hyperphosphatemia are more common with ARF. With protein-losing glomerulopathies, albumin tends to be lost to a larger extent than the higher–molecular-weight globulin. One can find low total protein and albumin concentrations

TABLE 19-6

Diagnostic Indices that may be Useful for Separating Prerenal from Renal Azotemia in Horses

Diagnostic Index	Normal Horses	Prerenal Azotemia	Renal Azotemia
Urine osmolality (mOsm/kg)	727-145	458-961	226-495
Uosm/Posm	2.5-5.2	1.7-3.4	0.8-1.7
UUN/PUN	34.2-100.8	15.2-43.7	2.1-14.3
UCr/PCr	2.0-344.4	51.2-241.5	2.6-37.0
FCl_{Na}	0.01-0.70	0.02-0.50	0.80-10.10

Modified from Grossman BS, Brobst DF, Kramer JW et al: Urinary indices for differentiation of prerenal azotemia and renal azotemia in horses, *J Am Vet Med Assoc* 180:284, 1982.
Uosm, Urine osmolality; *Posm*, plasma osmolality; *UUN*, urine urea nitrogen; *PUN*, plasma urea nitrogen; *UCr*, urine creatinine; *PCr*, plasma creatinine; FCl_{Na}, fractional sodium clearance.

in severe cases of chronic renal disease, whereas other horses may have an increased globulin concentration consistent with a chronic inflammatory response. Hyperglycemia (values >150 to 175 mg/dl) after stress, exercise, sepsis, PPID, or diabetes mellitus can result in glucosuria.[39,40] Finally, when pigmenturia is a complaint, muscle enzyme activity measurements are helpful in differentiating myoglobinuria from hematuria or hemoglobinuria.

URINALYSIS

One should perform urinalysis whenever one suspects urinary tract disease. One can collect urine as a midstream catch during voiding, via urethral catheterization, or via cystocentesis in foals. Unlike cows, horses cannot be stimulated easily to urinate, but they often urinate within a few minutes after being placed in a freshly bedded stall. Manual compression of the bladder during rectal palpation may stimulate urination after the rectal examination is completed. One should evaluate color, clarity, odor, viscosity, and specific gravity at the time of collection.[41,42] Normal equine urine is pale yellow to deep tan and often is turbid because of the large amounts of $CaCO_3$ crystals and mucus. Urine appearance commonly changes during urination, especially toward the end of micturition, when more crystals tend to be voided. If pigmenturia or hematuria is present, then noting the timing and duration of passage of discolored urine may help localize the source. Pigmenturia throughout urination is most consistent with myonecrosis or a bladder or kidney lesion, whereas passage of discolored urine at the start or end of urination more often occurs with lesions of the urethra or accessory sex glands (see Hematuria).

Assessment of Urine Concentration

Urine specific gravity is a measure of the number of particles in urine and is a useful estimate of urine concentration. Although determination of specific gravity with a refractometer is quick and easy (reagent strips should not be used to measure specific gravity in horses),[41] one must recognize that urine concentration is determined most accurately by measurement of urine osmolality, because the presence of larger molecules in urine, such as glucose or proteins, leads to overestimation of urine concentration by assessment of specific gravity. Clinically, overestimation is a problem in patients with diabetes or heavy proteinuria.[43] Urine specific gravity is used to separate urine concentration into three categories: (1) urine that is more dilute than serum (hyposthenuria or specific gravity <1.008 and osmolality < 260 mOsm/kg); (2) urine and serum of similar osmolality (isosthenuria or specific gravity of 1.008 to 1.014 and osmolality of 260-300 mOsm/kg); and (3) urine that is more concentrated than serum (specific gravity >1.014 and osmolality >300 mOsm/kg). Although urine of most normal horses is concentrated (three to four times more concentrated than serum with specific gravity of 1.025 to 1.050 and an osmolality of 900-1200 mOsm/kg), occasionally a normal horse produces dilute or highly concentrated urine. For example, in response to water deprivation for 24 to 72 hours, horses with normal renal function often produce urine with a specific gravity greater than 1.045 and an osmolality greater than 1500 mOsm/kg.[44-46] In contrast, foals typically have hyposthenuric urine consequent to their mostly milk diet.[47] Although the constant polyuria decreases the ability of the neonate to generate a large osmotic gradient in the medullary interstitium, dehydrated foals still can produce urine with a specific gravity greater than 1.030. With chronic renal insufficiency the ability to produce concentrated (specific gravity >1.025) or dilute (specific gravity <1.008) urine is lost. Thus horses with CRF typically manifest isosthenuria. As discussed previously, urine specific gravity is helpful in differentiating prerenal from renal azotemia in horses that exhibit dehydration or shock after a number of disorders.

Reagent Strip Analysis

The pH of equine urine is usually alkaline (7.0 to 9.0 pH).[41,42,48] Vigorous exercise or bacteriuria can result in acidic pH. Bacteriuria can impart an ammonia odor to the urine secondary to breakdown of urea by bacteria with urease activity. Concentrate feeding generally decreases urine pH toward the neutral value.[48] Similarly, the more dilute the urine sample is, the closer the pH is to 7.0. The dilute urine produced by foals typically is neutral to mildly acidic and is relatively free of crystalline material. Interestingly, calcium oxalate crystals are more prevalent in urine of foals than in that of adults.[49] Occasionally, one detects aciduria in a dehydrated or anorectic horse. Although aciduria typically has been attributed to metabolic acidosis, many patients actually may have hypochloremic metabolic alkalosis accompanied by paradoxical aciduria. The mechanism for paradoxical aciduria is likely similar to that described in ruminants with abomasal outflow obstruction.[50] Briefly, after all chloride has been reabsorbed from the glomerular filtrate, further sodium reabsorption occurs by exchange with (excretion of) potassium or hydrogen ions. Thus paradoxical aciduria is most likely to occur with concomitant hypokalemia or whole-body potassium depletion.

Commercially available urine reagent strips can yield false-positive results for protein when one tests alkaline samples. Thus proteinuria can be assessed better by performing the semiquantitative sulfosalicylic acid precipitation test or by specific quantification with a colorimetric assay (e.g., the Coomassie brilliant blue dye method[51] or other assays that are used routinely on cerebrospinal fluid [CSF]). In normal mares a mean value of 3.2 mg/kg (1.6 g) per day and a range of 3.6 to 22.3 mg/kg (1.8 to 11.2 g) per day for urinary protein excretion have been reported by Schott, Hodgson, and Bayly[52] and by Kohn and Strasser,[53] respectively. These values translate into urinary protein concentrations of less than 100 mg/dl in most normal horses. Comparison of the quantitative protein result (milligrams per deciliter) to urine Cr concentration (milligrams per deciliter) in the form of a urine protein-to-Cr ratio also is recommended. This technique is more practical because it obviates timed urine collection. Although a normal range has not yet been reported for horses, values exceeding 1.0:1.0 and 3.5:1.0, respectively, are considered above normal for dogs[54] and indicate nephrotic range proteinuria in human beings.[8] Thus a urine protein-to-Cr ratio greater than 2:1 likely supports significant proteinuria in an equine patient. Proteinuria may occur with glomerular disease, bacteriuria, or pyuria or may transiently follow exercise.[52]

Normal equine urine should not contain glucose. Although the renal threshold for glucose has not been evaluated thoroughly in horses, an early study by Link[55] suggested that the threshold may be lower (about 150 mg/dl) than that of small animals and human beings. Thus glucosuria can accompany hyperglycemia associated with the causes described previously or with administration of dextrose-containing fluids or parenteral nutrition products.[39,40] In addition, glucosuria may accompany sedation with α_2-agonists or exogenous corticosteroid administration.[33,34] When one detects glucosuria in the absence of hyperglycemia, one should suspect primary tubule dysfunction. Glucosuria more often has been detected in horses with ARF (mostly in experimental models of nephrotoxicity) than in those with chronic renal disease. Unlike ruminants, ketones rarely are detected in equine urine, even in advanced catabolic states or with diabetes mellitus. A positive result for blood on a urine reagent strip can reflect the presence of hemoglobin, myoglobin, or intact RBCs in the urine sample. Evaluation of serum for hemolysis and of urine sediment for RBCs, combined with an ammonium sulfate precipitation test to detect myoglobin,[56] can be rewarding in differentiating between these pigments (see Hematuria). Finally, occasionally one detects bilirubinuria on reagent strip analysis of equine urine. Bilirubinuria is associated with intravascular hemolysis, hepatic necrosis, and obstructive hepatopathies. In most instances, one more commonly detects hemolysis and hepatic disease by abnormal biochemical data such as elevated serum bilirubin concentration and increased hepatic enzyme activity.

Sediment Examination

Sediment examination is probably the most underused diagnostic technique available for evaluation of urinary tract disorders in horses. In human beings, sediment examination has been demonstrated to be a useful predictor for occurrence and severity of ARF.[57] Unfortunately, a major limitation is that sediment should be examined within 30 to 60 minutes after collection. To perform sediment examination, 10 ml of fresh urine is centrifuged (usually in a conical plastic tube) at 1000 rpm for 3 to 5 minutes. The supernatant urine is discarded (or used for quantitative protein determination) and the pellet is resuspended in the few drops of urine remaining in the tube. A drop of sediment is transferred to a glass slide, and a coverslip is applied. One first examines the sediment at low power to evaluate for casts and subsequently at high power to quantify erythrocytes, leukocytes, and epithelial cells, as well as to determine whether bacteria are present. Casts are molds of Tamm-Horsfall glycoprotein and cells that form in tubules and subsequently pass into the bladder. They are rare in normal equine urine but may be associated with inflammatory or infectious processes. Casts are unstable in alkaline urine; thus one should evaluate sediment as soon as possible after collection to ensure accurate assessment. Fewer than five RBCs per high-power field should be seen in an atraumatically collected urine sample. Increased numbers of urinary RBCs can result from inflammation, infection, toxemia, neoplasia, or exercise (see Hematuria). Pyuria (more than 10 white blood cells per high-power field) most often is associated with infectious or inflammatory disorders; normal equine urine should have few bacteria, if any. The absence of bacteria on sediment examination does not rule out their presence, however, and bacterial culture of urine collected by catheterization or cystocentesis (foals) should be performed when one suspects cystitis or pyelonephritis. Finally, equine urine is rich in crystals. Most of these are $CaCO_3$ crystals of variable size, but calcium phosphate crystals and occasionally calcium oxalate crystals also are visible in normal equine urine (Figure 19-11).[41,42,58] Addition of a few drops of a 10% acetic acid solution may be necessary to dissolve crystals for accurate assessment of urine sediment.[41]

Enzymuria

Renal tubules are metabolically active, being responsible for absorption or excretion of a wide range of substances. Transport of these compounds is facilitated by a number of enzymes, which are found in large amounts in lysosomes within or in the brush borders of tubular epithelial cells. Regular turnover of these cells and release of endocytotic vesicles and lysosomes into the tubular lumen results in activity of enzymes in urine (enzymuria).[59] A number of substances that are filtered

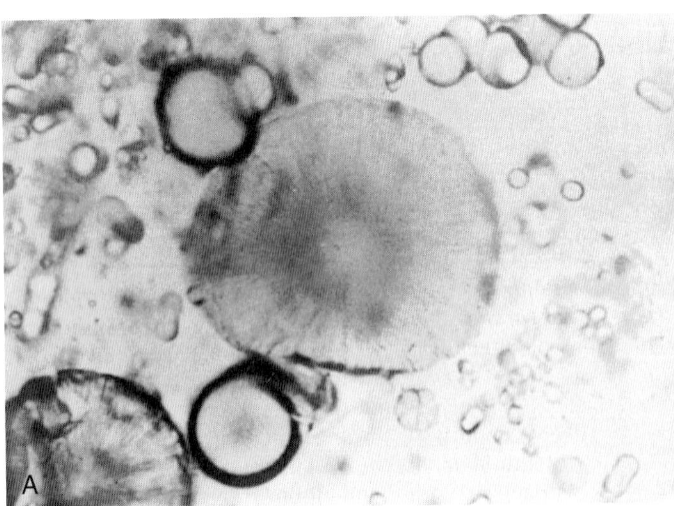

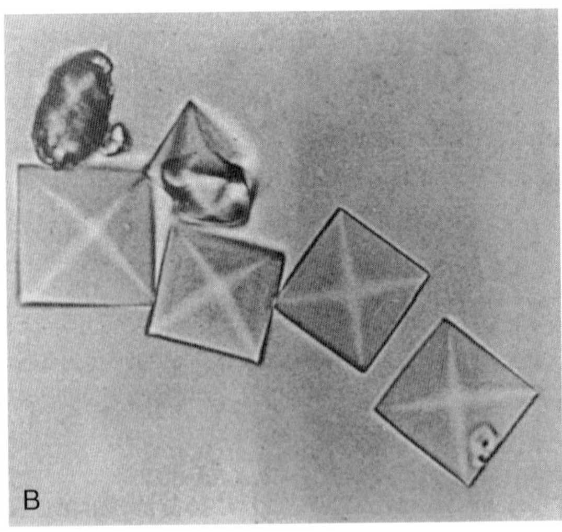

FIGURE 19-11 Crystals commonly observed in equine urine sediment (original magnification, ×160). **A,** Large, round calcium carbonate ($CaCO_3$) crystals (center and lower left) and smaller calcium phosphate crystals (oblong). **B,** Calcium oxalate dihydrate crystals. (Reproduced from Osborne CA, O'Brien TD, Ghobrial HK et al: Crystalluria: observations, interpretations, and misinterpretations, Vet Clin North Am Small Anim Pract 16:45, 1986.)

at the glomerulus (including bile acids, aminoglycoside and cephalosporin antibiotics, mannitol, dextrans, radiographic contrast media, and heavy metals) are taken up via endocytosis into proximal tubular epithelial cells. Endocytotic vesicles combine with lysosomes, and substances that are not broken down by lysosomal enzymes subsequently are extruded into the tubule lumen through evacuation of residual bodies.

Inflammation or necrosis of tubular epithelial cells results in elevated urinary activity of lysosomal and brush border enzymes. Because proximal tubular epithelial cells are the most metabolically active of all kidney cells, they are particularly susceptible to ischemic injury. Furthermore, they can be injured similarly by exposure to large quantities of nephrotoxins in glomerular filtrate. As a result, determination of the activities of certain urinary enzymes can provide evidence of tubular damage several days before azotemia may develop.[60-63] Additional contributors to increased urinary enzyme activity include (1) low–molecular-weight enzymes such as amylase that normally are filtered by glomeruli and reabsorbed in the proximal tubules, (2) postrenal genitourinary tract epithelia that usually contribute a negligible amount to the overall urinary enzyme activity (unless they become neoplastic), and (3) secretions from accessory sex glands. Contributions from the latter explain why intact males tend to have higher urinary activities of lactate dehydrogenase (LDH) and *N*-acetyl-β-D-glucosaminidase (NAG).

Although more than 40 enzymes have been detected in urine of different species, only a few appear to be of diagnostic relevance. To be of clinical use, a urinary enzyme must have measurable activity in the kidney; its activity must lie within a fairly narrow range in urine of healthy animals; it must be sufficiently large (molecular weight >60,000) so as not to be filtered freely across the glomerulus; and its activity must increase early enough during the course of renal injury to permit institution of corrective treatment. Finally, the activity of the urinary enzyme should remain fairly stable in urine for several days without the need for special processing. In human beings and dogs, a number of enzymes, including NAG, LDH, β-glucuronidase, alanine aminopeptidase, alkaline phosphatase (ALP), leucine aminopeptidase, γ-glutamyltransferase (GGT), and kallikrein have been demonstrated to be sensitive indicators of renal damage.[60-62,64,65] With respect to horses, normal values have been established for activities of GGT, ALP, NAG, LDH, and kallikrein.[66-70] Attempts to assay aspartate aminotransferase and alanine aminotransferase activities were unsuccessful in normal horse urine.[67]

ALP and GGT are membrane-associated enzymes found primarily in the brush border of the proximal tubular epithelium.[61-65,71] Their activity in distal tubular epithelium is negligible.[13] These enzymes have activity in other tissues, but because they are not filtered by the glomerulus, elevated activity in urine in the absence of significant proteinuria is presumed to originate from the kidneys. Measurable activity in normal urine is attributed to cell turnover.[61] LDH is a more ubiquitous tubular epithelial enzyme, being as active in the distal tubules and medullary papillae as in proximal tubular epithelium.[64-71] NAG is a proximal tubular lysosomal enzyme.[61-71] Only GGT, ALP, LDH, and NAG have been assayed in the urine of horses known to have, or thought to have, some form of renal dysfunction. Determination of NAG activity can be difficult in normal equine urine because of its alkalinity, and normal values may be less than detectable assay limits when one uses a spectrophotometric, rather than a fluorometric, method.[72-75] Published normal activities (expressed per gram of Cr) for these enzymes in equine urine are GGT: 0 to 25 IU/g Cr; ALP: 0 to 28 IU/g Cr; LDH: 0 to 12 IU/g Cr; and NAG: less than 1 IU/g Cr (<2 IU/L urine). Comparison with Cr concentration, which is relatively constant, results in less volume-related variation and allows interpretation of a randomly collected specimen (compared with a urine sample obtained during a timed collection period).[66,76,77]

Factors one must consider when measuring urinary enzyme activities include conditions under which the urine sample has been stored, urinary pH, diurnal variation, gender- and age-related variations, and other naturally occurring inhibitors or promoters of enzyme activity in urine (albumin, mucoproteins, proteolytic agents, amino acids, and ammonia). Although these factors have received limited study respecting equine urine, it has been documented that freezing can decrease activity of all enzymes, especially GGT. Furthermore, the colder the temperature, the more rapid the loss of enzyme activity.[66] To obtain the most accurate results, one should refrigerate samples (4° C) and assay them within 72 hours of collection. In species that have a slightly acidic or neutral urinary pH, assay of NAG is considered one of the most valuable diagnostic tests available. However, its activity appears to be susceptible to pH changes. In human beings receiving nephrotoxic medications, NAG activity in urine became undetectable at pH values greater than 8.[78] Similarly, NAG activities were undetectable (<2 IU/L) in urine of normal horses.[79] In a study of monensin toxicosis in horses, NAG activity increased as urinary pH decreased.[68] Certain amino acids and ammonia further act as inhibitors of lysosomal enzymes such as ALP and NAG in the urine of human beings, dogs, and rats,[80,81] and techniques have been developed to remove these agents from the urine by gel filtration before assay of their activity.[82]

Theoretically, assessment of changes in the urinary activity of selected enzymes may assist the clinician in identifying the segment of the nephron suffering the greatest dysfunction or damage. Although NAG, GGT, and ALP are associated primarily with proximal tubular epithelium, LDH usually is associated with distal tubular epithelial cells. Increases in urinary GGT and ALP activity have been induced experimentally in horses receiving gentamicin and neomycin for 5 to 10 days.[83,84] Increases also have been measured in horses with diarrhea, acute abdominal crises, and endotoxic shock. In the latter instances, enzymuria was assumed to indicate tubular damage after ischemia. Five consecutive days of furosemide administration also produced moderate increases in GGT and ALP activity, with ALP increasing more rapidly.[79] However, 48 hours of water deprivation failed to induce any changes in GGT, ALP, or LDH activity.[70] Similarly, no change in urinary LDH activity was observed in horses administered phenylbutazone (8.8 mg/kg PO) daily for 6 days.[70]

Although increases in urinary enzyme activities generally indicate acute tubular damage, one must interpret urine enzyme-to-Cr ratios carefully. Threshold values above which elevations are significant have not been well documented, although one study reported that a GGT/Cr value greater than 25 IU/g indicated tubular damage.[66] In contrast, in a study of gentamicin-induced nephrotoxicity in pony mares, Hinchcliff, McGuirk, and MacWilliams[83] measured GGT/Cr values exceeding 100 IU/g several days before measuring an increase in Cr concentration. Furthermore, one frequently may measure GGT/Cr values between 25 and 100 IU/g in horses receiving gentamicin at recommended doses. Similar to gentamicin pharmacokinetics, enzymuria in these horses has been highly variable; these horses have not been recognized to be at risk of developing ARF. Although enzymuria likely reflects a degree of tubular damage in these patients, one should interpret increases in GGT/Cr values between 25 and 100 IU/g with caution, whereas increases greater than 100 IU/g are more likely to be clinically significant.

Horses with chronic renal disease may have normal or reduced enzyme activities that reflect cellular changes that occur in the nephron in response to chronic inflammation. Just as BUN and Cr concentrations may be normal during the early stages of renal disease, urinary enzyme activities may not accurately reflect renal dysfunction later in the disease course when results of blood tests and urinalysis are more likely to be abnormal. A possible reason for this phenomenon is that substantial destruction of tubular epithelium occurring early in the disease leaves fewer epithelial cells to be an ongoing source of elevated enzyme activities. Alternatively, regenerating tubular epithelial cells may be more refractory to the effects of the toxin.

All in all, determination of urinary enzyme activities has failed to gain acceptance as a routine measure of renal tubular damage in most equine hospitals. This lack of acceptance can be attributed to the high sensitivity for detection of subclinical renal tubular damage. For example, although a urine GGT/Cr ratio elevated to a value of 75 supports tubular damage, it does not provide the clinician a quantifiable risk for development of ARF. Thus as a single measurement, the ratio is of limited use in deciding whether one should discontinue use of a nephrotoxic medication (e.g., gentamicin). In contrast, more dramatic elevations of the GGT/Cr ratio may precede development of azotemia and could be a useful warning that one may need to discontinue a medication or, at a minimum, prolong the dosing interval. Until values for urinary enzyme activities are reported for a larger number of equine patients with various diseases, the true value of assessing urinary enzyme activity will remain unclear.

Fractional Clearance of Electrolytes

Urinary electrolyte losses, which reflect tubular function, can be expressed as excretion rates (total amount of electrolyte excreted during a given time period, expressed as milliequivalents per minute) or as clearance rates. Determination of clearance rates uses the same clearance concept to measure GFR. In brief, a clearance rate (Cl_A) is a measure of the volume of plasma that is cleared completely of the substance in question (A) during a given time period. One calculates the Cl_A by performing a timed urine collection (to determine urine flow in milliliters per minute) and measuring the concentration of the desired substance in plasma and urine (Cr or inulin for determination of GFR)[8]:

$$ClA = (urine[A]/plasma[A]) \times urineflow$$

As with protein, urinary clearance of many substances, including electrolytes, often is compared with that of Cr.[8] Basically, a substance that is filtered mostly across the glomerulus but is neither reabsorbed nor secreted by renal tubules (inulin) will have a clearance rate similar to that of Cr. In contrast, a substance that is poorly filtered (larger molecule) or reabsorbed to a great extent by renal tubules (sodium or chloride) will have a lower clearance value than that of Cr. Similarly, clearance values for substances that are eliminated by filtration and tubular secretion (potassium) may exceed that measured for Cr. An advantage of comparing the clearance of a substance (A) to Cl_{Cr} (expressed as a fraction of Cl_{Cr}) is that it obviates the need to perform a timed urine collection, because the urine flow factor is cancelled out in the calculation:

$$\frac{Cl_A}{Cl_{Cr}} = \frac{\dfrac{urine[A]}{plasma[A]} \times \text{urine flow}}{\dfrac{urine[Cr]}{plasma[Cr]} \times \text{urine flow}}$$

that, by rearrangement and expression as a percentage becomes

$$\frac{Cl_A}{Cl_{Cr}} = \left[\frac{plasma[Cr]}{urine[Cr]} \times \frac{urine[A]}{plasma[A]}\right] \times 100$$

This calculation is called the *fractional Cr clearance value*.[8,85] More often, however, the term *fractional excretion* has been used to describe this value. Although most sources recommend that blood and urine samples be collected at the same time for determination of fractional clearance values, serum electrolyte and Cr concentrations are usually stable (except in patients with prerenal azotemia or ARF), so one can use blood values measured within a few days of the urine sample in the clearance calculations. Consequently, leaving a specimen cup for the client to use to collect a voided sample is acceptable and obviates bladder catheterization in many cases.

As previously discussed (see Renal Physiology), the equine kidneys function to conserve more than 99% of filtered sodium and chloride ions. In contrast, potassium ions are conserved poorly except during periods of whole-body potassium depletion (anorexia, prolonged exercise). Thus normal fractional clearance values are less than 1% for sodium but are considerably higher for potassium (Table 19-7).* Increases in fractional sodium and chloride clearance values may reflect an appropriate renal regulatory response to dietary excess, as with psychogenic salt consumption.[100] Alternatively, increases in fractional clearance values specifically for sodium and phosphorous also can be early indicators of renal tubule damage[31,83,97,101,102]; however, one must interpret results of these calculations in light of fluid therapy because fractional clearance values can be increased artifactually in horses receiving intravenous polyionic solutions.[31] Similarly, medication (furosemide) or light exercise also can result in increased urine flow and fractional sodium and chloride clearance values.[103]

The kidneys play an important role in equine calcium and phosphorus homeostasis, and renal loss of these ions varies with dietary intake. Thus fractional clearances of calcium and phosphorous also have been used to assess adequacy of dietary intake.† Although diet is evaluated more appropriately on a herd basis by analyses of hay and concentrates, fractional clearances may be useful in individual animals or when feed analysis is impractical (e.g., forage consists of pasture). Determination of fractional calcium and phosphorus clearances has received limited study with a focus on young racing horses.[92-94,104-106] For example, excessive dietary phosphorus intake (which can lead to nutritional secondary hyperparathyroidism) leads to increased fractional clearance of phosphorus. Evaluation of fractional calcium clearance is hampered by the fact that most of the calcium in equine urine is in the form of $CaCO_3$ crystals. To measure the urinary calcium concentration reliably, one must collect the entire contents of the bladder

*References 31, 42, 46, 53, 86-90, 95-99.

†References 87, 88, 90, 92-94, 96, 97, 104-106.

during voiding or via catheterization to ensure collection of the initial crystal-poor and final crystal-rich fractions. Subsequently, one treats a well-mixed aliquot of urine with acetic acid or nitric acid to solubilize the crystals.[97] In one report, fractional calcium and phosphorus clearance values greater than 2.5% and less than 4% were considered consistent with adequate dietary intake (adequate calcium intake with phosphorus intake that was not excessive).[93] Unfortunately, because the ranges for fractional calcium and phosphorus clearances can be wide in normal horses (see Table 19-7), measurement of these clearances may not be sensitive enough to detect minor dietary imbalances.

Determination of fractional electrolyte clearance values also has been advocated in the evaluation of horses with recurrent rhabdomyolysis.[91,107,108] Low sodium and potassium clearances have been reported in some affected horses. Whether these low fractional clearance values reflected total body electrolyte depletion (as a consequence of repeated bouts of exercise in hot weather or repeated furosemide administration) or a true physiologic predisposition to rhabdomyolysis was not determined. Nevertheless, low fractional clearance values document the need for electrolyte supplementation in equine athletes. Harris and Snow[107] also described another population of horses that exhibited recurrent rhabdomyolysis that had increased fractional phosphorus clearance and was reported to respond to dietary supplementation with ground limestone. Thus although determination of fractional electrolyte clearances may be helpful in the evaluation of horses with recurrent rhabdomyolysis, only a small portion of affected horses are likely to show significant clinical improvement in response to dietary electrolyte supplementation alone.

Finally, the methodology used to determine fractional electrolyte clearances should be standardized because several factors may lead to erroneous results. For example, a note of caution is warranted when ion-specific electrodes (instead of a flame photometer) are used to measure urinary potassium concentration, because components of animal urine can interfere with the ion-specific electrode and lead to spurious low values. One usually can avoid this problem by performing the analysis on urine diluted with water.[109] Next, as mentioned previously, light exercise may increase urine flow rate and sodium excretion.[103] Thus "spot" urine samples are best collected in the morning before feeding and exercise. Recently, McKenzie et al.[99] compared fractional electrolyte clearance values between single-sample spot urine collections to 24-hour volumetric urine collections over 3 days in horses receiving diets varying in cation-anion balance. They found substantial variation in fractional clearance values within individual horses over the 3-day study, despite feeding of a consistent diet. When they assessed the effect of the differing diets, fractional clearance

TABLE 19-7

Fractional Electrolyte Clearance Values for Horses and Ponies

Sodium	Potassium	Chloride	Phosphorus	Calcium	Reference
ADULTS					
0.16 ± 0.24	27.0 ± 14.6	0.17 ± 0.11	NR	NR	86*
0.02-1.00	15-65	0.04-1.60	0.00-0.50	NR	87
0.11-0.87	10.8-28.5	NR	0.07-0.74	NR	88
0.01-0.70	NR	NR	NR	NR	31
0.27 ± 0.02	38.52 ± 7.26	1.01 ± 0.24	NR	1.49 ± 1.58	89
0.0-0.46	23.9-75.1	0.48-1.64	0.04-0.16	NR	53
0.032-0.52	23.3-48.1†	0.59-1.86	0-20†	0.0-6.72†	90
0.034 ± 0.095	42.4 ± 9.8	0.352 ± 0.190	0.710 ± 0.250	NR	46
0.04-0.52	35-80	0.70-2.10	0.00-0.20	NR	91
0.0002-2.43	1.0-42.7‡	0.012-3.47	0.023-2.77	NR	42
NR	NR	NR	0.115-0.302	NR	92
NR	NR	NR	0.08-5.53†	2.10-4.60†	93
NR	NR	NR	0.61-0.75	11-33	94
FOALS					
0.31 ± 0.18	13.26 ± 4.49	0.42 ± 0.32	3.11 ± 3.81	2.85 ± 3.26	95
AFTER FUROSEMIDE ADMINISTRATION					
12.0	207	9.5			87

NR, Not reported.
*Values calculated from data provided.
†Fractional clearance of potassium may exceed upper limit on high potassium diets; a fractional clearance of phosphorus exceeding 4% suggests excessive dietary intake; a fractional clearance for calcium should exceed 2.5% with adequate intake.
‡Low range attributed to low urine potassium concentrations determined by ion-specific electrodes.
§Fractional clearance value for magnesium reported at 7 to 30.

values for sodium, potassium, and chloride were generally similar when calculated using urine electrolyte concentrations determined in spot urine samples or well-mixed 24-hour collection samples. However, they found greater variability with fractional clearance values for calcium and magnesium. The fact that they detected considerable variability should not be surprising when one remembers that fractional clearance values are a calculation using four measurements (Cr and electrolyte concentrations in plasma-serum and urine). Thus small variations in each measured value have the potential to magnify error in the final calculation. All in all, this study should serve as a reminder that determination of fractional electrolyte clearances is only one of the diagnostic tools one should use to evaluate patients with renal disease or recurrent rhabdomyolysis or to assess diet in a group of horses.

IMAGING TECHNIQUES

ULTRASONOGRAPHY

One can perform ultrasonographic examination of the urinary tract transrectally or transabdominally.[110-117] Bladder imaging is performed best transrectally using a 5-MHz probe. One must remember the character of equine urine while imaging the bladder; the urine will be an inhomogeneous, echogenic fluid because of the presence of mucus and crystals. The latter can appear as echogenic sediment in the ventral aspect of the bladder, and balloting the bladder may cause this echogenic material to swirl. One also can confirm the presence of a cystic calculus because calculi have a highly echogenic surface and produce an acoustic shadow (Figure 19-12). Similarly, one may image and palpate masses in the bladder wall during the examination.

The right kidney is triangular or horseshoe shaped and is imaged best transabdominally via the dorsolateral extent of the last two or three intercostal spaces (Figure 19-13, *A*). The left kidney is somewhat a more typical bean shape, lies deep to the spleen, and can be imaged via the last two intercostal spaces or via the paralumbar fossa. Because the left kidney is deeper than the right kidney, it can be difficult to image completely and is examined best with a 2.5- or 3-MHz probe (Figure 19-13, *B*). One should assess systematically the size and shape of both kidneys, architecture, and echogenicity of the parenchyma, including imaging the kidneys in dorsal, sagittal, transverse, and transverse oblique anatomic planes.[115] In a full-size horse the right kidney should not measure more than 15 cm in the longest axis, whereas the left kidney may measure up to 18 cm if imaged longitudinally.

In ARF the kidneys may be normal or enlarged, and abnormalities of parenchymal detail are not often detected. When present, abnormal findings may include perirenal edema, widening of the renal cortex, and loss of a distinct corticomedullary junction.[111,112,114,116-118] CRF can result in decreased kidney size, irregular surfaces, and increased echogenicity because of renal fibrosis. Cystic or mineralized areas in renal parenchyma can be associated with chronic renal disease or congenital anomalies. Although uncommonly recognized, distinct curvilinear hyperechoic bands in the outer renal medulla parallel to the corticomedullary junction have been imaged in foals and adults horses with renal disease attributable to acute or chronic phenylbutazone toxicity.[117,119,120] This finding, termed the *medullary rim sign,* is thought to result from

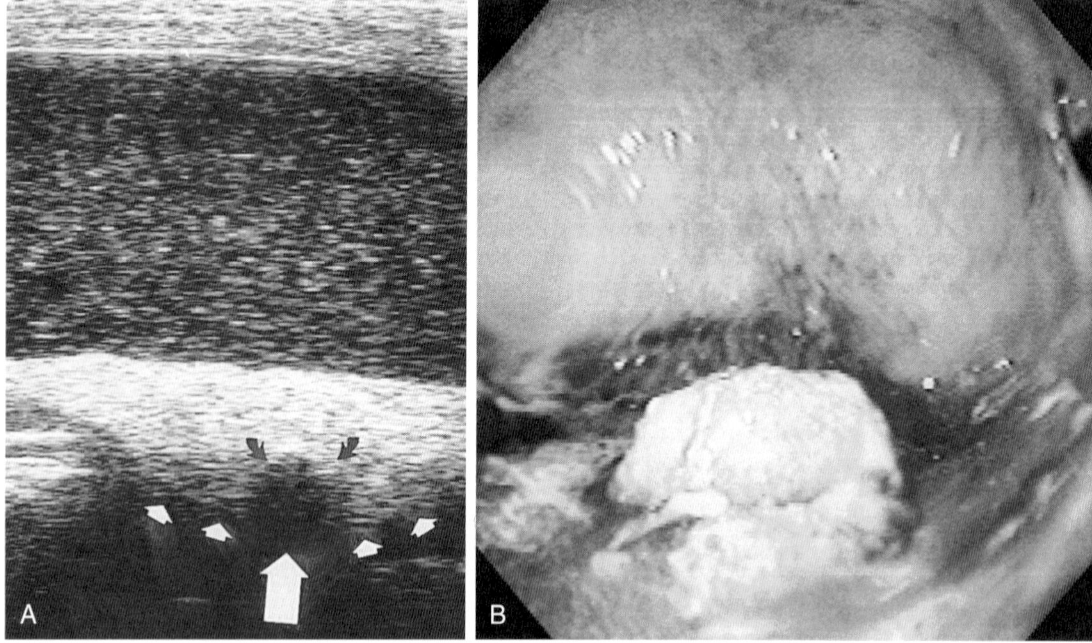

FIGURE 19-12 Transrectal ultrasonographic and cystoscopic images of the bladder of a Miniature Horse mare with recurrent cystitis and urolithiasis. **A,** The ultrasonographic image shows a layer of echogenic crystalline material in the ventral aspect of the bladder (small, white arrows outline ventral bladder wall) and presence of a small cystolith (outlined by small black arrows and large white arrow). **B,** After lavage of the urine sediment, cystoscopy confirmed presence of a small urolith, which was amenable to removal by digital manipulation.

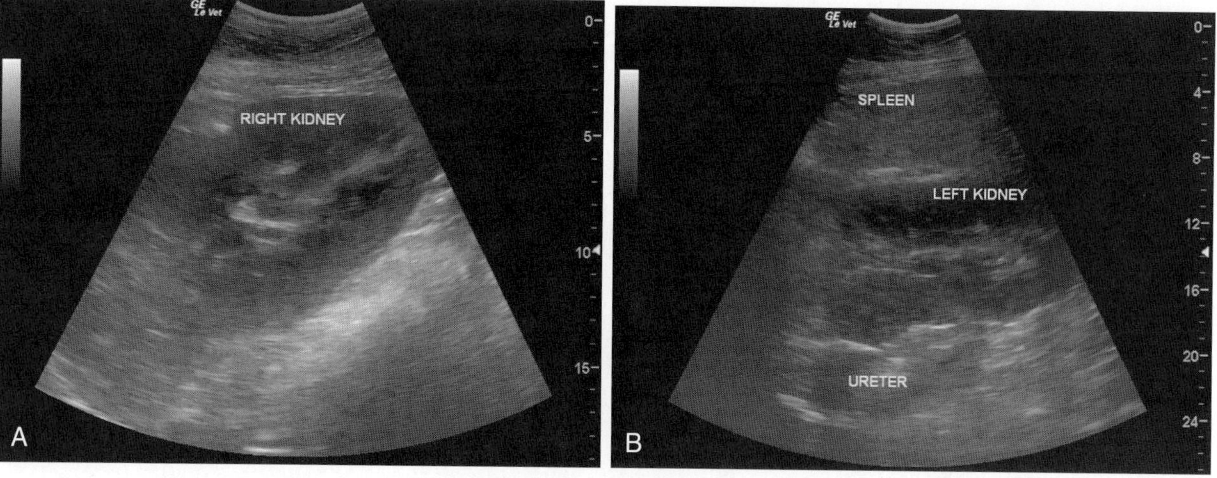

FIGURE 19-13 Transabdominal ultrasonographic image of a normal, **A,** right kidney and, **B,** left kidney. The renal medulla is more hypoechoic than the renal cortex, except for the renal pelvis, which varies in echogenicity. The left kidney is imaged deep to the spleen.

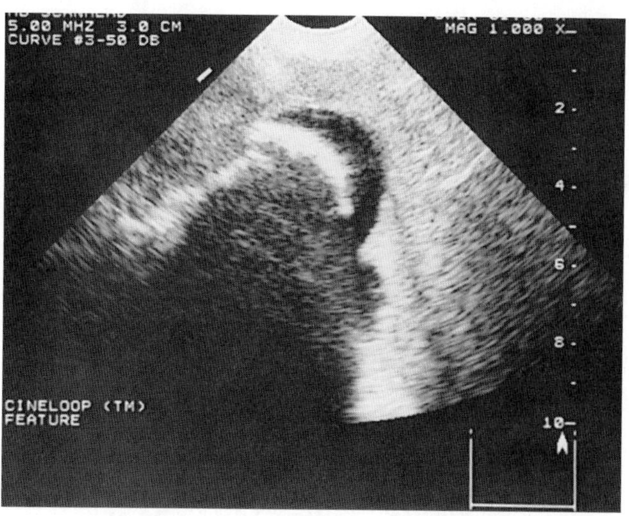

FIGURE 19-14 Transrectal ultrasonographic image of the left kidney of a mare with nephrolithiasis and hydronephrosis. The nephrolith has an echogenic surface and produces an acoustic shadow. The echolucent crescent moon-shaped structure is a fluid-filled remnant of the renal parenchyma, consistent with hydronephrosis.

damage (and possible secondary mineralization) to the inner stripe of the outer medulla, the location of highly metabolically active nephron segments including the distal extent of the proximal tubule and the thick ascending limb of the loop of Henle. Calculi in the renal pelvis generally cast an acoustic shadow and can result in hydronephrosis of the affected kidney (Figure 19-14).[111,112,114] Occasionally, one cannot image one or both kidneys because of a gas-filled bowel between the kidney and abdominal wall. Re-examination at a later time generally is required for successful imaging in such cases. In addition, administration of high rates of fluid therapy, especially in foals, can lead to iatrogenic pyelectasia (fluid distention of the renal pelvis).[117,121] One should use caution so as not to interpret this mild distention of the renal pelvis falsely as evidence of ureteral or lower urinary tract obstruction.

Radiography

Radiography rarely is used to evaluate urinary tract disease in adult horses. One usually can obtain diagnostic radiographs of the urinary tract only in foals or Miniature Horses. Excretory urography using intravenous contrast material or pyelography using contrast agent delivered into the renal pelvis under ultrasonographic guidance may be useful to identify a nonfunctional or hypoplastic kidney or an ectopic or torn ureter.[122,123] The latter procedure may be more rewarding, but both require general anesthesia to be performed safely. One also can use retrograde contrast studies to evaluate the ureters in mares[124]; however, they have been used most often in foals suspected of having an ectopic ureter or a ruptured bladder. Contrast radiographic studies also can help to identify strictures or masses in the urethra or bladder, but endoscopy is generally more useful for these problems. In small animals, abdominal survey radiographs are most useful for assessing kidney size and shape, whereas ultrasonography provides more information about parenchymal changes associated with renal disease.[125] Thus use of a standardized protocol for ultrasonographic evaluation of the equine kidneys should provide essentially the same amount of information as the combined use of survey radiography and ultrasonography in small animal patients.[115]

Nuclear Scintigraphy

Nuclear scintigraphy is an additional imaging modality often used to assess renal anatomy and function in human beings and small animals. One can use various radionuclides and pharmaceuticals, depending on the type of scintigraphic examination being pursued.[126-128] In fact, scintigraphy is used routinely for quantitative measurement of GFR in these species. Walsh and Royal[129] compared use of renal scintigraphy (using 99mTc-DTPA, which is similar to inulin in that it is neither secreted nor reabsorbed after filtration) for measurement of GFR in horses but found greater variability compared with GFR values measured by plasma disappearance of inulin or the same radionuclide (99mTc-DTPA).[129] Nevertheless, renal scintigraphy using 99mTc-DTPA can provide

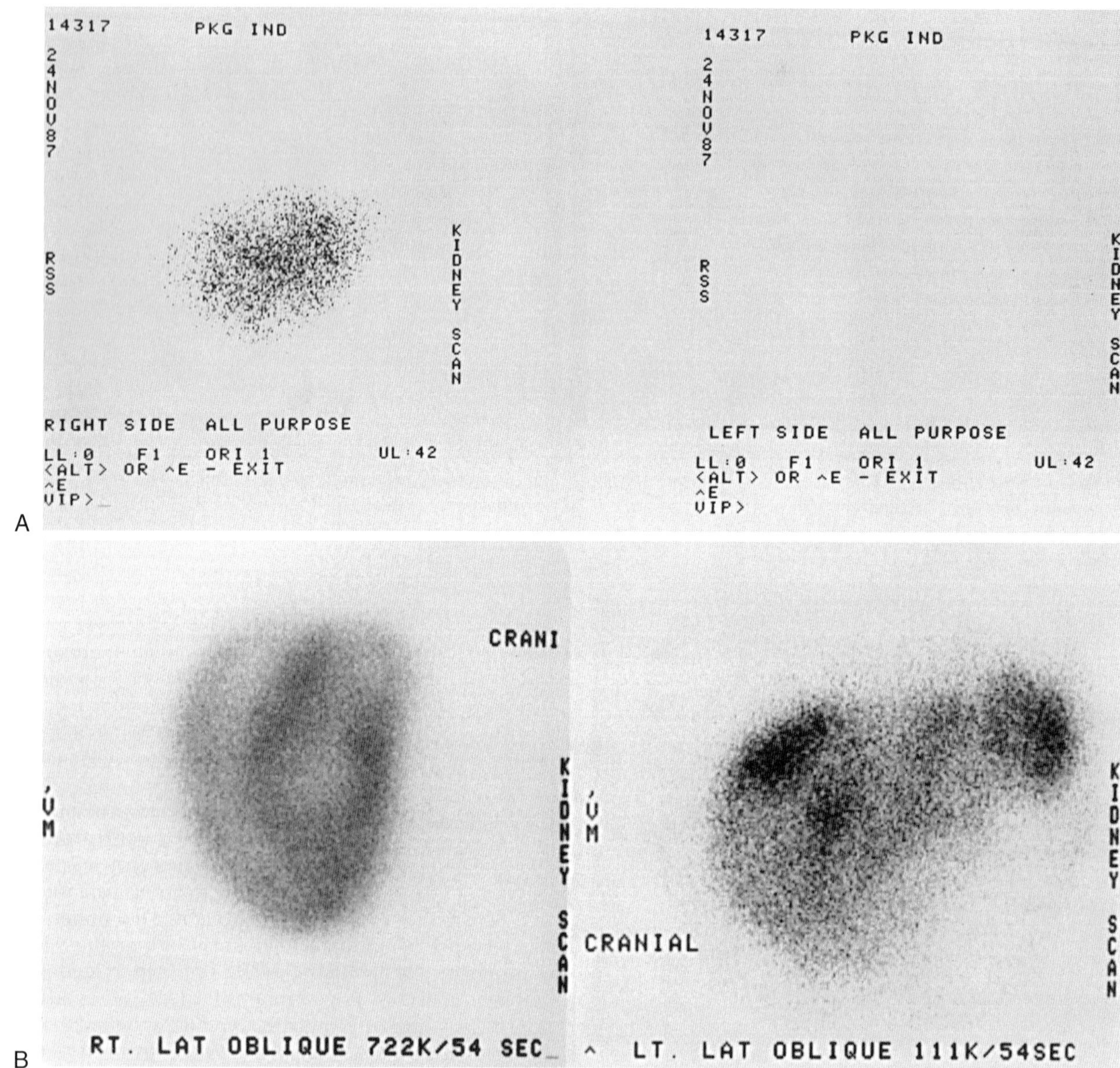

FIGURE 19-15 Renal scintigraphic images of horses with renal disease. **A,** Renal scintigraphic image using 99mTc-diethylenetriamine pentaacetic acid (99mTc-DTPA) revealed absence of functional left renal tissue, compared with an image of the right kidney, in a stallion with chronic renal failure (CRF). A nonfunctional hypoplastic left kidney was found on necropsy examination. **B,** Renal scintigraphic image using technetium-99m-glucoheptonate (99mTc-GH) in a gelding with unilateral left-sided pyelonephritis revealed inhomogeneous uptake of the radionuclide and lesser count emission over the same time compared with the normal right kidney. The scintigraphic study, which provided anatomic and functional information, supported pursuit of unilateral nephrectomy, rather than prolonged antibiotic administration, as the treatment of choice for this horse.

qualitative information about renal function and is the only method currently available for assessing split renal function (assessing individual kidney function) in horses. Renal scintigraphy also has been performed with 99mTc tagged to glucoheptonate (taken up by the proximal tubule epithelial cells to provide anatomic detail) or mercaptoacetyltriglycine (MAG_3, which is similar to p-aminohippurate because it is eliminated by proximal tubular secretion) to provide qualitative information about renal anatomy and function (Figure 19-15).[130,131] Thus one may use renal scintigraphy to document the presence of a functional kidney in horses when multiple ultrasonographic examinations have been complicated by interfering bowel or when one desires information about individual kidney function.

Endoscopy

Endoscopy of the urinary tract is a useful diagnostic aid when the complaint is abnormal urination.[41,132-134] A flexible endoscope with an outside diameter of 12 mm or less and a minimum length of 1 m is adequate for examination of the urethra and bladder of an adult horse of either sex.

One should sterilize the endoscope before endoscopy of the lower urinary tract. Tranquilization of the patient is recommended, and one should clean the distal end of the penis or the vulva thoroughly. The endoscope is passed as one passes a catheter, using the air control intermittently to inflate the urethra or bladder. Normal urethral mucosa is pale pink with longitudinal folds. When dilated with air the mucosa flattens and may appear redder than normal, and a prominent submucosal vascular pattern may be apparent. Passage of a catheter before endoscopy (for sample collection or to empty the bladder) can produce mild irritation and erythema of the urethral mucosa; therefore one should not mistake these findings for abnormal findings. The regions of the ischial arch (where the urethra begins to widen into the ampullar portion) and of the colliculus seminalis (in the roof of the pelvic urethra just distal to the urethral sphincter) should be examined closely, because these are common sites of posturination or postbreeding hemorrhage in geldings or stallions (see Hematuria). Subsequent passage of the endoscope through the urethral sphincter and air distention allows evaluation of the bladder for calculi, inflammation, and masses (see Figure 19-12). Viewing the ureteral openings in the dorsal aspect of the trigone can help determine the source of hematuria or pyuria (see Hematuria). A small volume of urine should pass from each ureteral opening approximately once each minute or more frequently if the horse is well hydrated or has been sedated with an α_2-agonist. One can perform ureteral catheterization to obtain urine samples from each kidney by passing sterile polyethylene tubing via the biopsy channel of the endoscope. Additionally, one can take biopsy samples of masses in the bladder or urethra.

SPECIALIZED DIAGNOSTIC TECHNIQUES

Ureteral Catheterization

With development of high-resolution videoendoscopic equipment, retrograde instrumentation of the bladder, ureter, and renal pelvis rapidly is replacing surgical exploration for diagnostic evaluation and therapeutic management of urinary tract disorders in human beings and dogs.[126,135-137] Similarly, retrograde ureteral catheterization and instrumentation can be a valuable technique for evaluation and treatment of horses with unilateral disorders of the upper urinary tract.[138-140] In addition to localization of unilateral renal hemorrhage, pyelonephritis, and neoplasia, ureteral catheterization further enables retrograde pyelography.[124] As mentioned previously, one may perform this technique successfully in male and female horses during cystoscopic examination.[41,132-134]

In mares, one also can catheterize the ureters manually without endoscopic guidance.[141] After preparation of the vulva, one catheterizes the bladder and drains the urine. One removes the bladder catheter and dilates the urethra manually until two fingers can be passed into the bladder. One can palpate the ureteral orifices dorsally as small, soft projections. When this is done, a catheter is placed between the fingertips, passed through the urethra, and directed into the ureter (Figure 19-16). A relatively rigid catheter with a rounded end (No. 8 to 10 French polypropylene catheter) facilitates passage into the ureter. After advancing the catheter 5 to 10 cm into the ureter, one attaches a syringe to the other end of the catheter and collects a urine sample. During sampling, the catheter is held in place and the ureteral opening is occluded with the fingertips to minimize loss of urine around the catheter.

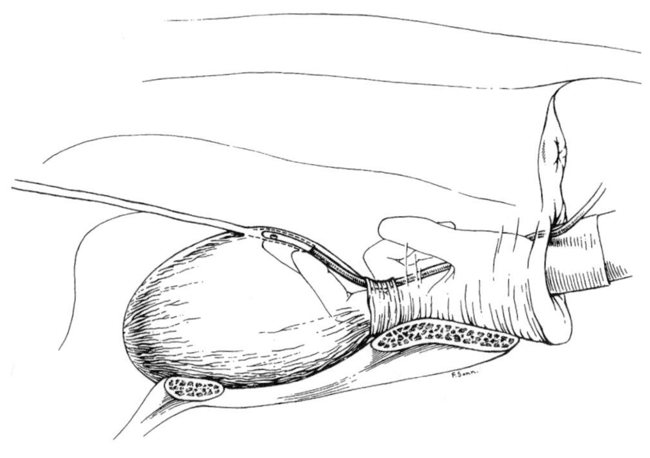

FIGURE 19-16 Manual placement of a polypropylene catheter into the ureter of a mare. (From Schott HC, Hodgson DR, Bayly WM: Ureteral catheterization in the horse, Equine Vet Educ 2:140, 1990.)

Water Deprivation and the Antidiuretic Hormone Challenge Test

Water deprivation is a simple test to determine whether hyposthenuric polyuria is caused by a behavior problem such as primary (psychogenic) polydipsia or results from central or nephrogenic diabetes insipidus.[6] One should not perform a water deprivation test in an animal that is clinically dehydrated or azotemic. A baseline urinalysis should be performed (sample collected by catheterization to empty the bladder at the start of the test), and BUN, Cr, and body weight should be measured before removal of water (food does not necessarily need to be removed, but this may help prevent gastrointestinal complications of water deprivation). One measures urine specific gravity and weight loss after 12 (usually overnight) and 24 hours. Horses with normal renal function typically produce urine with a specific gravity greater than 1.045 and an osmolality greater than 1500 mOsm/kg in response to water deprivation of 24 to 72 hours in duration.[44-46] Practically, one can stop the test when urine specific gravity reaches 1.025 or greater. Furthermore, the test should be stopped if more than 5% of body weight is lost or clinical evidence of dehydration becomes apparent. With long-standing primary polydipsia, affected horses may not be able to concentrate urine fully (to a specific gravity > 1.025) because of partial washout of the medullary interstitial osmotic gradient. Extending the test period beyond 24 hours for such patients offers little benefit; however, affected horses should respond more favorably to water deprivation (producing urine with a higher specific gravity) after a period of partial water deprivation (termed a *modified water deprivation test*) during which daily water intake is restricted to 40 ml/kg for several days, which should allow time for restoration of the medullary interstitial osmotic gradient.[6] Horses with central or nephrogenic diabetes insipidus cannot concentrate urine in response to a water deprivation test.[6,142-144] When one suspects these problems, patients should be monitored every few hours because significant dehydration may ensue within 6 hours of water deprivation.

In the absence of azotemia or clinical signs of early renal failure, inability to concentrate urine in response to water deprivation supports a diagnosis of diabetes insipidus; however, the test does not distinguish between the neurogenic and nephrogenic forms of the disorder. One can differentiate these by exogenous administration of vasopressin (antidiuretic hormone).[142-144] Currently, two approaches exist for performing an antidiuretic hormone challenge test. First, one can administer aqueous synthetic vasopressin (20 U/ml for intramuscular or subcutaneous injection) as an intravenous infusion (5 U [0.25 ml] added to 1 L of a 5% dextrose solution and administered IV at a rate of 2.5 mU/kg over 60 minutes [250 ml to a 500-kg horse]) or an intramuscular injection (0.5 U/kg). An increase in urine specific gravity to 1.020 or greater after 60 to 90 minutes would be the expected response, whereas failure to increase urine concentration would support nephrogenic diabetes insipidus. Second, one can use desmopressin acetate (DDAVP), a synthetic analog of arginine vasopressin. Administration of DDAVP is considered the safer diagnostic technique in small animals because the change in structure of this vasopressin analog has decreased pressor actions and less effect on visceral smooth muscle compared with an enhanced antidiuretic effect. One microgram of DDAVP has an antidiuretic activity of 4 U of arginine vasopressin. The author and co-workers recently validated the use of DDAVP as a replacement for the antidiuretic hormone challenge test in normal horses. In this study, the nasal spray form of DDAVP (0.1 mg/ml DDAVP) was diluted in sterile water and 0.05 μg/kg was administered intravenously (25 μg, equal to 100 U of antidiuretic activity, to a 500-kg horse) to horses that had polyuria induced by repeated nasogastric intubation with water for 3 days preceding DDAVP challenge. Urine was collected for 8 hours after DDAVP administration and an increase in urine specific gravity to values greater than 1.020 was observed from 2 to 7 hours after DDAVP administration (Figure 19-17).[145] Furthermore, DDAVP administration had no effect on heart rate or systemic blood pressures. These data demonstrate that intravenous administration of DDAVP is a safe and useful diagnostic tool for evaluation of horses with diabetes insipidus.

A final test for evaluating polyuria and polydipsia is an intravenous challenge with hypertonic saline (Hickey-Hare test).[146] The goal is to produce an increase in plasma osmolality, which should trigger release of endogenous vasopressin. One protocol for the test would be to measure plasma osmolality and endogenous vasopressin concentrations before and within 30 minutes after administration of 1 to 2 ml/kg of a 7.5% NaCl solution. A normal response, expected in horses with primary polydipsia, would be concurrent increases in plasma vasopressin concentration and urine specific gravity. Horses with nephrogenic diabetes insipidus also would respond with an increased plasma vasopressin concentration; those with neurogenic diabetes insipidus would not. Urine specific gravity would not be expected to increase in response to hypertonic saline administration with either form of diabetes insipidus. One could evaluate plasma vasopressin concentrations similarly before and at the end of a water deprivation test.[147,148] Unfortunately, however, assays for plasma vasopressin concentration are not currently available at commercial laboratories. Thus pursuit of this diagnostic test requires cooperation of a research laboratory.

Quantitative Measures of Renal Function

As mentioned previously, azotemia does not develop until more than 75% of nephrons cease to function; therefore measurement of BUN and Cr, although readily available, provides a poor reflection of smaller declines in renal function. A number of methods are available to quantitate renal function in horses.[41,149] Basically, these tests can be separated into plasma disappearance curves or clearance studies involving use of timed urine collections. Generation of plasma disappearance curves requires collection of an initial blood sample, intravenous administration of one of a number of compounds (inulin, Cr, sodium sulfanilate, phenolsulfonphthalein [phenol red], or radionuclides), and collection of another series of blood samples over the subsequent 60 to 90 minutes.[129,150-155] One can express results in terms of an elimination half-life in minutes or as clearance values in milliliters per kilogram per minute. Mean elimination half-lives of 39.5 ± 4.4, 32.8 ± 4.1, and 16.4 ± 2.3 minutes have been reported for sodium sulfanilate, 99mTc-MAG$_3$, and phenolsulfonphthalein, respectively, in healthy horses.[150,151,155] The difference in these values can be explained in part by the fact that 99mTc-MAG$_3$ and phenolsulfonphthalein are eliminated mostly by tubular secretion and consequently are cleared more rapidly from plasma than is sodium sulfanilate (eliminated mostly by glomerular filtration). Plasma elimination half-times are most useful when measured sequentially throughout the course of renal disease; for example, Bertone et al.[156] reported a progressive increase in the sodium sulfanilate elimination half-time from 90 to 150 minutes during a 240-day course of CRF in a horse with PKD.

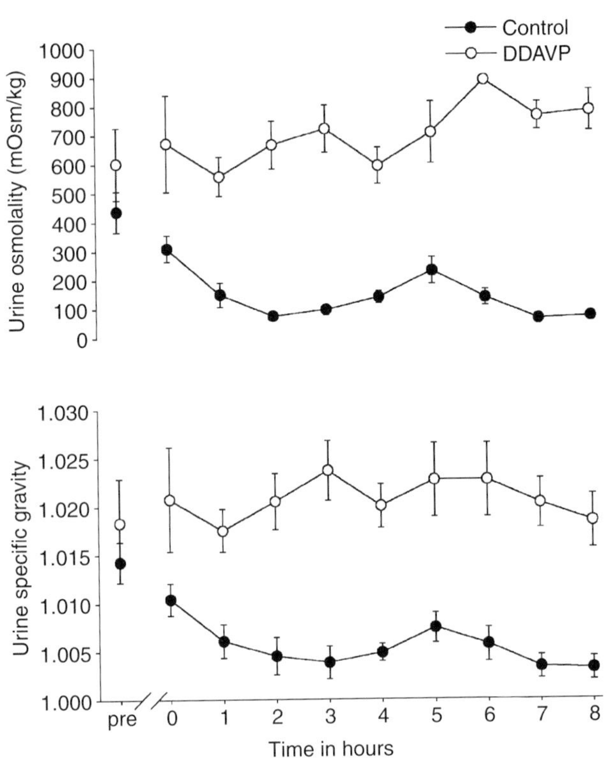

FIGURE 19-17 Urine osmolality and specific gravity in six horses administered 0.05 μg/kg desmopressin acetate (DDAVP) *(open circles)* or placebo *(filled circles)* intravenously at time 0. The horses had polyuria induced by repeated nasogastric intubation with water (40 ml/kg) twice daily for 3 days preceding DDAVP challenge and again 4 hours after administration of DDAVP. Urine was collected for 8 hours after treatment, and an increase in urine specific gravity to values greater than 1.020 was observed from 2 to 7 hours after DDAVP administration.[145]

When one uses plasma disappearance curves of a substance to estimate GFR, the compound being used must meet all the requirements of a filtration agent[152-154]: (1) no significant binding to plasma proteins, (2) ability to be filtered freely across the glomerulus, and (3) absence of tubular reabsorption or secretion. The gold standard compound is inulin. More traditionally, GFR has been measured by timed urine collection periods (to measure urine flow rate) and measurement of plasma and urine concentrations of a test compound that meets the listed requirements.[8,149] Several protocols exist for performing urine clearance studies. Ideally, the urine collection period should span 24 hours, although for practicality, one may use shorter collection periods.[6,149] For all protocols, one documents the bladder as being empty at the start of the collection period by catheterization or observation of voiding. All urine produced during the study period is collected and pooled into one sample. At the end of the collection period, the bladder should be emptied again via catheterization, the total volume of urine produced should be recorded, and an aliquot of the pooled urine sample should be assayed for the test substance. Similarly, one measures the concentration of the test substance in a blood sample collected near the midpoint of the urine collection period. For urine collections of 12 to 24 hours, endogenous Cr is the test substance used because it is the only one that does not have to be given by steady intravenous infusion during the collection period. GFR is calculated as the Cl_{Cr},

$$\mathrm{GFR} = \frac{\mathrm{urine[Cr]}}{\mathrm{plasma[Cr]}} \times \mathrm{urine\,flow}$$

with the modification that the result usually is divided by body mass (in kilograms) to express GFR in term of milliliters per minute per kilogram. Although endogenous Cr is a convenient test substance, its use typically underestimates GFR because non-Cr chromagens in serum artifactually increase the value in the denominator.[149] Similarly, significant tubular secretion of Cr can be one of the compensatory responses to renal failure. This can lead to overestimation of GFR calculated using endogenous Cl_{Cr}. Despite these limitations, the endogenous Cl_{Cr} technique for measurement of GFR can provide useful information, especially when it is performed on several occasions during the course of renal failure (see Chronic Renal Failure).

To avoid the limitations of endogenous Cl_{Cr} as a measure of GFR, one can administer a number of filtration markers (inulin, Cr, radionuclides) as an intravenous infusion throughout the urine collection period.[153,154,157-162] One starts the infusion as a bolus to increase the plasma concentration of the test substance to the desired level (e.g., the desired plasma concentration for exogenous Cr is 5 to 10 mg/dl, to minimize the influence of non-Cr chromagens) and subsequently continues a steady infusion throughout the remainder of the collection period. One usually performs this type of study for a shorter period with the horse restrained in stocks. One should empty the bladder of the horse at the start of the study and collect urine after two or three 30-minute intervals. One should pass a catheter and empty the bladder completely at the end of each 30-minute period. Alternatively, an indwelling bladder catheter can be used for the entire collection. After urine volumes are measured, an aliquot of each urine sample is assayed and a blood sample is collected at the midpoint of each urine collection period for the test substance; then the GFR is calculated as the mean value for the two or three collection periods. For all practical purposes, these types of GFR measurements (with the exception of exogenous Cl_{Cr}) usually are limited to research studies, because commercial laboratories do not offer inulin assays. One also can use this shorter protocol for GFR determination using endogenous Cr as the test substance, without the need for an intravenous infusion. (The results of a number of studies measuring GFR in normal horses are presented in the previous section of this chapter; see Renal Physiology.)

Renal Biopsy

Renal biopsy is a useful diagnostic technique for identifying the affected region of the nephron, the type of lesion, and the chronicity and severity of disease.[8,163-166] Although biopsy is a safe procedure when performed with ultrasonographic guidance, it has risks, including perirenal hemorrhage or hematuria and, less commonly, penetration of bowel. In human beings, perinephric hematomas are common and have been detected in 57% to 85% of patients the day after biopsy. Microscopic hematuria occurs in virtually all patients for the first couple of days after biopsy, and gross hematuria occurs in 5% to 10% of patients. Most of these complications are inconsequential, but in 1% to 3% of patients the complications have resulted in the need for postbiopsy transfusions.[8] Similarly, in a group of seven normal horses subjected to renal biopsy, postbiopsy macroscopic and microscopic hematuria occurred in five animals. Furthermore, perirenal hemorrhage was a prominent finding during necropsy examination of five of these animals (including one examined 27 days after biopsy tissue was collected).[166] Thus renal biopsies remain controversial in human and equine renal failure patients.[167-169] Renal biopsies should be approached with caution and are indicated only when the results would alter the therapeutic plan or prognosis. Information about the effect of renal biopsy results on therapy and outcome of renal disease in human beings is limited; however, in one prospective study, biopsy results were found to influence physicians' decisions on about half of cases when the technique was performed.[170] In general, renal biopsy is pursued more aggressively in human beings with acute renal insufficiency than in those with chronic renal insufficiency, especially when it is difficult to determine the type of renal disease based on results of urinalysis and sediment examination.[8] In the equine patient, one performs a renal biopsy with the horse sedated and restrained in a stocks. Penetration of the needle (a Tru-Cut biopsy needle or, preferably, a triggered biopsy device) into the renal parenchyma is imaged sonographically by triangulating the ultrasound beam with the biopsy instrument and the kidney or by determination of the site and depth of biopsy needle placement via ultrasonographic imaging immediately before biopsy. One should place the tissue collected in formalin for histopathologic and electron microscopic evaluation. Additional samples can be collected for bacterial culture and for immunofluorescence testing (placed in Michel's transport medium or quick-frozen after coating with a preservative such as Tissue-Tek). One should determine appropriate sample processing beforehand by contacting the pathologist who will examine the biopsy samples.

Although renal biopsy results could provide useful diagnostic and prognostic information about the type of renal disease in horses with ARF (e.g., glomerulonephritis, tubular necrosis, interstitial nephritis), they have been used more often to document the presence of chronic disease in horses with CRF. In most cases of CRF, one cannot detect the inciting cause unless it can be associated with a historical event or immunofluorescence testing is pursued. This limitation can be attributed to the fact that significant renal disease develops before onset of azotemia. Pathologic lesions are widespread at this point, and involvement of all nephron segments and the interstitium often leads to the interpretation of end-stage kidney disease (ESKD). In occasional cases the results may help separate infectious (pyelonephritis) or congenital (renal dysplasia) causes from nonspecific causes of renal failure. Although such results could be useful in the therapeutic approach to these patients, one should consider the limitations and risks of renal biopsy before performing this technique in horses with CRF.

Urodynamic Procedures

Cystometrography and urethral pressure profiles are used to evaluate detrusor and urethral muscle function, respectively. Both techniques involve measurement of intraluminal pressure during inflation of the bladder or urethra. These techniques have been useful for diagnosis of myogenic and neurogenic disorders of the bladder and urethra in dogs and human beings.[171] The procedures have been performed experimentally in normal horses and ponies,[172-174] but little information is available about use of these techniques in clinical cases (see Urinary Incontinence and Bladder Dysfunction).

ACUTE RENAL FAILURE

Warwick M. Bayly

Acute renal failure is a clinical syndrome associated with abrupt reduction in GFR. Sustained reduction in GFR is associated with failure of the kidneys to excrete nitrogenous wastes causing azotemia and with disturbances in fluid, electrolyte, and acid-base homeostasis. The human medical literature is full of various terms and definitions for different forms of ARF. Veterinary medical definitions are simpler. Basically, ARF can result from decreased renal perfusion without associated cell injury (prerenal failure); obstruction or disruption of the urinary outflow tract (postrenal failure); or ischemic or toxic damage to the tubules, tubular obstruction, acute glomerulonephritis leading to a primary reduction in the filtering capacity of the glomeruli, or tubulointerstitial inflammation and edema. Any of these intrarenal causes can be associated with intrinsic renal failure. Prerenal azotemia and ischemic tubular insults or necrosis represent a continuum, the former resulting in the latter when perfusion is compromised sufficiently to result in death of tubule cells.[1] Classically, ARF has been associated with oliguria and occasionally with anuria, and these are certainly the most commonly noted clinical signs associated with this disease in horses; however, nonoliguric forms of ARF, particularly intrinsic renal failure, exist and are characterized by slower development of azotemia, lower peaks in Cr concentrations, more subtle increases in urinary sodium clearance, and a more rapid recovery of renal function in response to treatment. Nonoliguric renal failure seems to be diagnosed less commonly in horses, although it is not uncommon to recognize mildly azotemic horses that have apparently normal urine output. In some cases, localized proximal tubule damage and reduced solute reabsorption actually may lead to enhanced distal delivery of filtrate, which may result in polyuric ARF.

In horses, ARF is usually prerenal or renal in origin and most often is caused by hemodynamic or nephrotoxic insults.[2] With the exception of bladder rupture in the neonate, postrenal failure is uncommon in horses. Identification and correction of the cause of ARF is important, because in the early stages of failure renal dysfunction is frequently reversible, whereas established ARF often requires extensive supportive care and carries a guarded prognosis. By identifying patients at increased risk and attempting to interrupt the cycle of events leading to ARF, one possibly may reduce the incidence of this condition.

CAUSES

Prerenal failure is associated with conditions that result in decreased cardiac output or increased renal vascular resistance (or in both) and is the most common cause of reversible azotemia. In horses the most common causes of reduced cardiac output (and therefore reduced renal perfusion) are associated with diarrhea, endotoxemia, acute blood loss, septic shock, and prolonged exercise. The resultant reductions in RBF, GFR, and urine output usually result in azotemia and retention of water and electrolytes. Anesthesia also may decrease cardiac output enough to result in a degree of prerenal azotemia. NSAIDs also can precipitate prerenal azotemia in patients with decreased RBF.[3] Although prostaglandins play only a minor role in maintenance of RBF in the normal state, PGE_2 and PGI_2 are important vasodilatory mediators of RBF under conditions of reduced renal perfusion. Thus administration of NSAIDs to dehydrated or toxemic patients may contribute further to renal hypoperfusion by exacerbating a decrease in RBF. In some cases this also may be sufficient to produce ischemic renal parenchymal damage, thus causing intrinsic renal failure. Generally, the parenchymal lesion associated with NSAID toxicity is medullary crest or papillary necrosis. Such lesions develop because the renal medulla normally receives much less blood flow than the renal cortex and consequently is much more susceptible to NSAID-induced changes in RBF.

In human beings, intrinsic renal diseases that lead to ARF generally are categorized according to the primary site of injury: tubules, interstitium, glomeruli, or vessels.[1] Acute tubular necrosis (ATN) is the form of intrinsic renal failure recognized most often in horses (interstitial and primary glomerular disease being recognized occasionally, and vascular disease almost never). Ischemia, especially when associated with microvascular coagulation (which often leads to irreversible cortical necrosis[4]), and nephrotoxins probably are the most common causes of equine ATN. Important nephrotoxins include aminoglycoside antibiotics and NSAIDs. Less commonly, ATN develops after exposure to endogenous pigments (myoglobin or hemoglobin), heavy metals such as mercury (contained in some counterirritants), or vitamin D or K_3.[5-8] Use of aminoglycosides, particularly gentamicin, is a common cause of equine ATN.[9] Toxicity is a result of damage to proximal tubular epithelial cells that is mediated by impaired cell organelle function. Administration of potentially nephrotoxic agents such as NSAIDs or furosemide (which can exacerbate hypovolemia) can increase the risk of aminoglycoside nephrotoxicity.

Myoglobinuria and hemoglobinuria have been associated with development of ARF in horses (pigment nephropathy).[10] Myoglobinuric nephrosis can follow exertional rhabdomyolysis, heat stroke, or extensive crush injuries. Causes of intravascular hemolysis and hemoglobinuria include incompatible blood transfusions, immune-mediated hemolytic anemia, fulminant hepatic failure, and toxicosis from ingesting onions (*Allium* spp.) or withered red maple leaves (*Acer rubrum*). Although the mechanism of pigment-induced renal injury is still not well understood, increased hydroxyl radical formation associated with reduction of ferrous iron compounds and tubular obstruction by casts of heme proteins are likely contributing factors. The fact that pigment nephropathy is uncommon in well-hydrated horses suggests a possible link to renal perfusion. Myoglobin and hemoglobin have been suggested to induce renal vasoconstriction.

Acute interstitial nephritis often is not recognized but is believed usually to result from an allergic reaction to drugs such as the β-lactam and sulfa antibiotics. Autoimmune and embolic or ascending bacterial infections also may be associated with the condition, which is characterized by edema and inflammatory cell infiltration of the interstitium. Tubules frequently contain white and RBCs, which pass into the lumen through the disrupted tubular basement membrane.

Glomerulonephritis often is identified post mortem in aged horses[2,11] and apparently is most often immune mediated. Glomerulonephritis often results in subacute or nonoliguric renal failure. Although the condition is theoretically reversible with immunosuppressive agents, in horses such undertakings are usually impractical and rarely are tried for long.

Postrenal obstructive failure can develop after disease of the renal pelves, ureters, bladder, or urethra. The severity of the failure depends on the extent of the obstruction. Frequently, problems are not recognized in horses until urine output obviously is reduced or renal function is impaired to the point that systemic problems are manifested. Although a neurogenic bladder can cause a functional obstruction, postrenal failure in horses most often results from intraluminal blockage by uroliths, which can cause obstruction anywhere in the urinary outflow tract.[12,13] Other possible intraluminal causes include neoplasia or stricture formation. Extraluminal obstructive lesions such as retroperitoneal tumors or adhesions or bladder displacements also occasionally are associated with development of postrenal failure.

PATHOPHYSIOLOGY

The pathophysiology of equine ARF has received little study, and the mechanisms at work are assumed essentially to be the same as those identified in experimental studies of other animal species. Several mechanisms have been demonstrated to be involved in the development of ARF, the actual pathogenesis being complex and depending somewhat on the cause of the disease. Multiple factors probably operate in different combinations at different times and in different nephrons. These different mechanisms are discussed next in relation to the type of failure with which they are associated (i.e., prerenal, intrinsic, and postrenal failure).

The pathophysiology of prerenal failure and ischemic ARF tend to involve the same processes. Toxins that cause ATN also share many pathophysiologic features with ischemic ARF.[14] The heterogeneity of intra-RBF is an important factor in the development of this condition. The kidneys are particularly susceptible to ischemic and toxic injury because of their unique anatomic and physiologic features. Although they receive approximately 20% of the cardiac output, only about 10% to 20% of total RBF reaches the medulla via the vasa recta. This low medullary blood flow is necessary to ensure a functional countercurrent mechanism in this region of the kidney; however, low blood flow also creates a large corticomedullary oxygen gradient and renders the renal medulla hypoxic and highly susceptible to ischemic injury. Conversely, the renal cortex receives 80% to 90% of total RBF and is particularly susceptible to toxins.

Hypovolemia triggers compensatory systemic and renal responses. The systemic responses include activation of the autonomic nervous system and renin-angiotensin system and release of antidiuretic hormone. Peripheral vasoconstriction is one of the effects of these responses. Renal responses to decreases in circulating blood volume have several phases. Initially, tubular reabsorption of sodium and water increases and is mediated by nerves and hormones. Reabsorption usually is associated with reduced clearance of urea and an associated increase in serum urea nitrogen concentration in the face of preservation of GFR, which in turn maintains the plasma Cr concentration in the normal range. More severe hypovolemia overcomes renal autoregulation, RBF being redistributed from the cortex to the medulla and GFR thus declining. The renal circulatory changes further enhance tubule solute reabsorption in the face of the decreased GFR. The net effect is production of small amounts of concentrated urine, a high urine-to-plasma Cr ratio, and low fractional sodium clearance.[15]

A further reduction in RBF results in a syndrome considered intermediate between the prerenal and intrinsic ischemic forms of ARF. Urine concentrating ability apparently is disrupted earlier than is sodium reabsorptive capability, with the result that urine osmolality decreases and output increases, but fractional sodium clearance stays low. Patients may appear to be mildly polyuric.[16] With more severe or prolonged renal hypoperfusion and ischemic insult, urinary sodium and fractional sodium clearance start to increase and the animal develops nonoliguric, and then oliguric, ARF. These changes are associated with progressively more severe tubule necrosis as the ARF progresses from prerenal to renal. The more severe the insult is, the poorer is the prognosis.

Intrarenal vasoconstriction is caused by an imbalance between vasoconstrictive and vasodilating factors (systemic or local) that act on small renal vessels in particular. These mediators include the vasodilator nitric oxide and the constrictor endothelin. Hypercalcemia is associated with increases in free calcium in the vascular smooth muscle and leads to enhanced vascular tone. Vasopressin and angiotensin II also have been shown to induce significant vasoconstriction under certain experimental conditions, as have endotoxins and myoglobin. Some nephrotoxins—gentamicin, heavy metals, and radiographic contrast agents—can cause renal vasoconstriction in addition to having direct toxic effects on the proximal tubules.[17-19]

Prostaglandins E_2 and I_2 are potent mediators that are responsible for a critical vasodilating response in the face of reduced RBF when activation of the renin-angiotensin system alone would result in further vasoconstriction. Increases in circulatory concentrations of angiotensin II stimulate synthesis of these renal prostaglandins. Consequently, the vasoconstrictive effects of stimulating the renin-angiotensin system usually are blunted somewhat by concomitant increases in PGE_2 and PGI_2; however, in the face of increased angiotensin II and simultaneous inhibition of prostaglandin synthesis (e.g., because of an NSAID), a significant increase in renal vascular resistance results.[20]

The reduction in GFR associated with reduced renal perfusion is associated with a number of mechanisms involving the glomeruli, vasculature, and tubules. In the initial phases a reduction in glomerular capillary hydrostatic pressure is associated with a net drop in RBF and a rise in renal vascular resistance. The latter phenomenon usually is associated with afferent arteriolar vasoconstriction and efferent arteriolar vasodilation and initially is reversible with volume expansion. Later (2 days or more), restoration of RBF does not necessarily improve GFR, and a drop in RBF is associated with a disproportionately greater drop in GFR.[21] Even when vasoconstriction is reversed, GFR may not improve; this reflects loss of RBF autoregulation. This disproportionate reduction in GFR suggests a fall in the ultrafiltration coefficient of the glomeruli after a reduction in total filtering area. The mechanism for this is unclear but may be associated with increases in angiotensin II concentration, because this agent is known to induce mesangial contraction and a drop in the ultrafiltration coefficient.[22]

In addition to the aforementioned vascular changes that can affect GFR, the possible effects on GFR in the juxtamedullary region of even mild changes in RBF warrant specific mention. The glomeruli and adjacent straight portion of the proximal tubule and thick ascending limbs of the loops of Henle in this region are apparently particularly susceptible to hypoxia (i.e., ischemia) because of their high oxygen requirements. Swelling of endothelial and tubule cells after prolonged ischemia in this region results in increased vascular resistance and continued compromise of the medullary circulation, even when cortical RBF has been restored.[14,23]

GFR also can be compromised significantly by obstruction of tubular lumina by casts of cellular debris and inflammatory cells. Increased intratubular pressure decreases the net driving pressure for glomerular filtration in the same way that obstruction of the urinary outflow tract ultimately can lead to a lower GFR. One of the reasons that agents that accelerate the solute excretion rate (e.g., furosemide, mannitol) may be therapeutic adjuncts has been that they are believed to help disperse these luminal blockages.

Tubuloglomerular feedback is a regulatory mechanism that lowers GFR whenever solute (most notably NaCl) concentrations at the macula densa are increased. In ARF, impaired transport in the thick ascending limb of the loop of Henle in the context of preserved glomerular response to signals from the macula densa results in a decrease in GFR. This feedback is a normal protective mechanism mediated principally by the renin-angiotensin system, although prostaglandin, intracellular calcium, and adenosine may play a role in signal transmission or regulation. In essence the mechanism serves to prevent massive fluid losses associated with a reduction of tubular reabsorptive capacity; however, in cases of renal hypoperfusion and ischemia, the effect is the opposite, because basically the feedback mechanism exacerbates the effects of already reduced RBF.

Proximal tubule cells undergo morphologic changes early in cases of ischemia. They lose their brush borders and polarity, and the integrity of their tight junctions is disrupted, probably after alterations in the actin and microtubular cytoskeletons.[24,25] Under these conditions the glomerular filtrate is able to leap back to the peritubular circulation, thus reducing the net (or effective) GFR. This mechanism is thought to be an important source of GFR reduction only in more severe cases of ischemia or nephrotoxin exposure.

Tubule cells involved in solute reabsorption have a high metabolic rate and a high demand for oxygen. The existence of the corticomedullary oxygen gradient makes these cells vulnerable to the effects of hypoxia and ischemia, the thick ascending limb of the loop of Henle in the outer medulla being most susceptible.[26] Early in ischemic and toxic ARF, decreases in ATP and adenosine diphosphate tissue levels occur with associated elevations in adenosine monophosphate and inorganic phosphate concentrations. Much of the adenosine monophosphate is broken down further to adenosine and then to xanthine. Adenosine is a potent constrictor of cortical blood flow and probably enhances the effect of the tubuloglomerular feedback system. Depletion of ATP in tubular cells inhibits cell volume regulation, and the resultant swelling probably contributes to luminal obstruction and increased vascular resistance. Redistribution of Na^+,K^+-ATPase from the basolateral to the apical membrane of the tubule cells reduces the ability of the cells to extrude sodium into the peritubular fluid and circulation.[27] Redistribution of integrins to the apical surface contributes to the breakdown of tight junctions.[28] Depletion of ATP in tubule cells also leads to an increase in cytosolic calcium concentration. In addition to being a vasoconstrictor, calcium activates proteases and phospholipases, interferes with mitochondrial energy metabolism, and can break down the cytoskeleton.[1,29] Administration of calcium channel blockers has helped ameliorate ARF in some experimental situations.[30]

Reperfusion of renal tissue after a period of ischemia is associated with rapid production of oxygen free radicals and with significant tissue damage. Xanthines, neutrophils, phospholipase A_2, mixed-function oxidases, and mitochondrial electron transport are associated with the production of these oxidants.[31] Phospholipase A_2 hydrolyzes phospholipids in cell and mitochondrial membranes to free fatty acids and lysophospholipids and produces arachidonic acid. Arachidonate in turn is converted to eicosanoids that are vasoconstricting and chemotactic for neutrophils.[32] Cell membranes are particularly susceptible to phospholipase activity after reperfusion. Reperfusion injury is a major consideration in transplant surgery; however, the role it plays in the pathogenesis of prerenal and ischemic ARF is not clear.

Many of the cellular biochemical and structural changes that occur along with the ischemic form of ARF are also important parts of the pathogenesis of ATN associated with exposure to nephrotoxins. Toxin-associated dysfunction and necrosis of cells result in increased tubular pressure and a decreased glomerular capillary hydrostatic pressure gradient. Loss of reabsorptive capability triggers tubuloglomerular feedback and further reduces GFR by lowering RBF after vasoconstriction and a decrease in the glomerular ultrafiltration coefficient. Transepithelial backleak of solutes into the circulation further interferes with the excretory function of the kidneys.

Acute Tubular Necrosis

Many agents are recognized to have potential nephrotoxic effects. Aminoglycoside-induced renal toxicity results from accumulation of these agents within the renal cortex. Streptomycin is the least nephrotoxic of the aminoglycosides, whereas gentamicin and kanamycin are intermediate nephrotoxins. Neomycin is the most nephrotoxic. Most cases of aminoglycoside toxicity are associated with conditions that cause reduced renal perfusion because the healthy kidney usually can tolerate some degree of aminoglycoside overdosing. After filtration at the glomerulus, aminoglycosides bind to phospholipase on the brush border of proximal tubules and subsequently are reabsorbed by pinocytosis. Accumulation of these antibiotics interferes with lysosomal, mitochondrial, and Na^+,K^+-ATPase function by inhibiting phospholipase A activity. Binding to the brush border is saturable with the result that sustained exposure of the proximal cells to the drug (as with multiple daily-dosing) results in greater accumulation of the drug and increased nephrotoxicity. As a result, once-daily dosing may attenuate the risk of nephrotoxicosis while maintaining or improving therapeutic efficacy (because it results in higher peak concentrations).[33,34] Many mild cases of aminoglycoside toxicity notably are associated with nonoliguric ARF and therefore may go unrecognized in horses.

Some cephalosporins, such as cephaloridine, have considerable nephrotoxic potential. These agents cause necrosis because of mitochondrial toxicity after accumulation of the antibiotic in the cell.[35]

Not all cases of ATN are caused by direct toxic changes in tubule cells. For instance, whether myoglobin and hemoglobin are truly nephrotoxic is still debatable. The principal characteristics of pigment nephropathy caused by these agents are tubule obstruction and reduced RBF (caused by the direct vasoconstrictor effects of the pigment). Whether obstruction is physical, caused by pigment accumulation, or reflects aggregation of sloughed cells is not clear. Myoglobin tends to be associated with nephropathy more frequently than hemoglobin. Patients often quickly become oliguric, presumably because of the widespread tubule obstruction.

Acute Interstitial Nephritis

Distinguishing between drug-induced ATN and acute interstitial nephritis can be difficult, and the latter rarely is diagnosed in horses. Making a distinction may be a particular problem when continued use of antibiotics is indicated. With ATN one may alter the dosing regimen, whereas with interstitial nephritis, short-term corticosteroid therapy is often of benefit in human beings. Interstitial nephritis often is marked by eosinophiluria and eosinophilia and is more likely to be associated with the presence of red cells than is ATN. The exact immune mechanism by which interstitial nephritis develops is unclear, although it is thought most likely to be caused by delayed cell-mediated hypersensitivity or the presence of antitubule basement membrane antibodies.[36] The prognosis is usually grave in horses with acute interstitial nephritis.

Acute Glomerulonephritis

Acute glomerular nephropathy is rare in horses; however, when it occurs, it usually is manifested by the nephrotic syndrome, although hematuria and oliguria sometimes are apparent. Deposits of γ-globulin and complement are found along the basement membrane (global form) or in the mesangial area (mesangioproliferative form).[37] Group C streptococcal antigens have been identified along with equine glomerulonephritis, and equine infectious anemia (EIA) viral antigen-antibody complexes have been recognized in the glomeruli of horses that were not in renal failure.[11,38] Deposition of immune complexes activates the complement cascade. Formation of C_3b and C_5a causes platelet aggregation and attracts neutrophils. Tissue damage results from deposition of complement per se and from inflammation associated with neutrophil activation and release of reactive oxygen radicals, proteases, elastases, and other lysozymes. These enzymes, plus platelet-activating factor and leukotriene B_4, increase vascular permeability and upregulate expression of adhesion molecules, thus promoting further inflammation.[32] Severe reduction in GFR results from large drops in the glomerular permeability coefficient, which is associated with the widening of Bowman's spaces after inflammation and deposition of immune complexes.

Basically, increases in ureteral pressure for any reason result in GFR reduction because of a drop in the glomerular capillary hydrostatic pressure gradient, some tubular backleaking, a decrease in the glomerular permeability coefficient, and ultimately, a reduction in RBF. (See previous discussion of the pathophysiology of postrenal ARF.)

Clinical Signs

In most horses with hemodynamically mediated (i.e., prerenal, ischemic) ARF, clinical signs are usually referable to the primary problem, such as acute colic or enterocolitis, sepsis, coagulopathies, rhabdomyolysis, or heavy-metal poisoning, rather than to renal dysfunction. Therefore the predominant clinical signs are often dehydration (with or without diarrhea), depression, and anorexia. Other signs can include tachycardia, hyperemic mucous membranes, pyrexia, mild abdominal pain, and laminitis. Because clinical signs usually relate to the inciting problem, ARF may not be suspected or detected unless the veterinarian specifically evaluates renal function as part of the workup for a more obvious disease. In general, the clinical manifestations of ARF reflect the systemic effects of toxic substances usually excreted in the urine (i.e., uremia generally is reflected by anorexia and depression), urinary tract dysfunction, and derangements of fluid, electrolyte, and acid-base balance. One may observe signs of encephalopathy in horses with severe azotemia.

Although oliguria is considered the hallmark of ARF, urine production in horses varies. Oliguria frequently occurs in the early stages of hemodynamically mediated ARF and is the most frequently reported clinical sign that is related directly to urinary tract dysfunction. As outlined in the section on pathophysiology, however, nonoliguric and polyuric stages of prerenal and intrinsic ARF also can be associated with renal hypoperfusion. Anuria is rare. Nonoliguric or polyuric ARF also can be associated with exposure to nephrotoxins (ATN), and polyuria is common during the recovery phase of ARF, regardless of its cause. The magnitude of azotemia tends to be lower in nonoliguric than in oliguric ARF, possibly indicating less severe damage in the former condition. Similarly, nonoliguric ARF is associated with a more favorable prognosis.

Patients with ARF often are treated initially with large volumes of intravenous or oral fluids for the primary disease. In these cases, oliguria may progress to polyuria. When significant renal damage has been sustained, persistence of oliguria in the face of fluid administration usually is manifested as failure to produce a significant volume of urine in response to fluid therapy. The degree of change of azotemia also is minimal in the initial 24 to 36 hours of treatment. If one does not monitor these patients carefully, then fluid retention may lead to development of subcutaneous and pulmonary edema. Soft feces caused by fluid retention also may be apparent in patients with oliguric ARF.

Postrenal or obstructive uropathy usually is characterized by mild to severe abdominal pain and pollakiuria and stranguria (see Obstructive Disease of the Urinary Tract).

DIAGNOSIS

Increases in plasma urea nitrogen and Cr concentrations (i.e., azotemia) are frequently the initial findings that suggest compromised renal function. Azotemia simply reflects a reduction in GFR; it has almost no differential diagnostic value. After establishing recent development of azotemia, the equine internist must proceed systematically to differentiate between six possible syndromes associated with ARF: (1) prerenal ARF, (2) ischemic ARF, (3) ATN, (4) acute interstitial nephritis, (5) acute glomerulonephritis, and (6) obstructive (postrenal) ARF. A useful way to go about this is first to try to rule out pre- and postrenal ARF. If this is possible, then the patient must have a type of intrinsic ARF; therefore one can direct further diagnostic efforts to identifying the disease subtypes.

As described in greater detail later (see Urolithiasis), the diagnosis of postrenal obstructive disease usually is based on a combination of clinical signs, history, and the results of rectal palpation, ultrasonography, and urinary tract endoscopy. The frequency and volume of urination can vary with these cases, and total obstruction causes anuria. Salt and water reabsorption often are impaired as the problem persists, which results in hyponatremia (i.e., plasma sodium concentrations in the low-normal range). Although the mechanisms for this sodium wasting are not completely clear, the wasting apparently is related to impaired function of the ascending limb of the loop of Henle and an increased medullary blood flow after prostaglandin release. Both of these events greatly diminish the magnitude and effect of the medullary countercurrent concentrating mechanisms. Prostaglandin also directly inhibits the effect of antidiuretic hormone.[39]

Measurement of specific gravity in the azotemic horse is a commonly practiced means of detecting prerenal ARF. In these cases the value is usually greater than 1.025 and often as high as 1.055. In human beings, one can use a number of reliable indexes to differentiate renal azotemia from prerenal azotemia[40-42] that are based on urine osmolality and the ratio of urine-to-plasma osmolality (U/P_{osm}), urine sodium concentration and fractional sodium clearance, and ratios of urine-to-plasma urea concentrations (U/P_{UN}) and urine-to-plasma Cr concentrations (U/P_{Cr}). Fractional sodium clearance in particular is a good indicator of solute reabsorption and proximal tubule function, whereas U/P_{Cr}, and to a lesser extent U/P_{UN}, are useful indexes of the ability of the tubules to reabsorb water. The utility of these indexes in horses also has been investigated and has been shown to have considerable differential diagnostic value.[15] Although these tests are discriminatory, some degree of overlap occurs between them respecting prerenal and parenchymal or intrinsic problems. One also must bear in mind that these indexes do not allow differentiation between intrinsic and postrenal disease. A number of horses with prerenal (nonoliguric) ARF have urine osmolality less than 360 mOsm. A small percentage of horses in prerenal ARF have U/P_{Cr} less than 30 (usually >50) and fractional sodium clearance greater than 0.80% (usually <0.50%), most likely because of the unrecognized existence of tubule damage before volume depletion or because of a natriuretic effect of some treatments such as diuretics or intravenous fluids. Natriuresis is particularly likely to be induced along with bicarbonate administration because sodium cations are lost with unreabsorbed bicarbonate anions. In these cases the determination of the fractional chloride clearance may be a better indicator of the response of the kidney to hypoperfusion.

No parameter reliably differentiates between prerenal and ischemic ARF because of the pathophysiologic continuum between these diseases. At one end is reduced GFR with preserved tubule function and concentrating mechanisms. This form of disease is readily reversible with appropriate therapy. Additional or more prolonged decreases in GFR lead to disturbances in tubule function and slower reversal of damage until the other end of the spectrum is reached, in which complete and irreversible loss of renal function occurs. Assessment of urine specific gravity before initiation of fluid therapy is helpful in differentiating prerenal failure from renal failure. As normally functioning kidneys would preserve salt and water maximally in response to a transient decrease in RBF with prerenal failure, so urine specific gravity and osmolality are greater than the values associated with serum, whereas the urine produced by horses with intrinsic ARF is often isosthenuric (specific gravity <1.020). In a clinical situation, assessment of the response to fluid therapy is the most practical way to differentiate prerenal failure from intrinsic forms of ARF. Azotemia caused by prerenal problems should resolve quickly with replacement of fluid deficits and restoration of renal perfusion. In prerenal failure, volume repletion also should restore renal function, with the result that the magnitude of azotemia should decrease by 50% or more during the first day of therapy. In contrast, fluid therapy usually does not lead to prompt resolution of azotemia associated with intrinsic problems. Application of the measurement of U/P_{Cr} and U/P_{UN} ratios is limited to use on urine samples collected before initiation of fluid therapy or the first urine sample voided after fluid therapy has been started.

In prerenal ARF, electrolyte and acid-base abnormalities generally reflect problems caused by a primary disease (e.g., enterocolitis, colic, blood loss). Most frequently, horses are mildly acidotic, hyponatremic, and hypochloremic. Plasma concentrations of potassium and calcium vary according to what disease is causing renal hypoperfusion. Potassium concentration also is affected to some extent by urine output, hyperkalemia being most common in association with oliguria and anuria.

The technique for biopsy of the left kidney has been well described.[43] The main indication of kidney biopsy is to help differentiate between types of intrinsic renal disease when one thinks that this distinction will have therapeutic and prognostic relevance. One often can diagnose ischemic failure and ATN without biopsy. The primary complication associated with the biopsy procedure is renal hemorrhage, which can be severe. Ultrasonographic guidance and use of a spring-loaded biopsy instrument may reduce the risk of complications. Ultrasonography also allows biopsy of the right kidney. As the knowledge of equine renal physiology and pathology improves, and advances in molecular genetics lead to techniques that supplant or supplement standard histopathologic methods, the diagnostic usefulness of renal biopsy may increase. For example, biopsy results may dictate the use of immunosuppressive agents in the treatment of some forms of renal parenchymal disease (e.g., interstitial nephritis).

Identification of subtypes of intrinsic ARF often depends on analysis of urine and urine sediment. The availability of a history of exposure to ischemic insults or potential nephrotoxins such as aminoglycosides certainly helps in this regard, but determination of the severity of the condition and its prognosis still generally relies on the analysis of urine. Ischemic tubule disease is similar to ATN. In both cases a slight to moderate proteinuria with specific gravities usually less than 1.020 and urine osmolality less than 350 mOsm occurs. Fractional sodium clearance is nearly always greater than 1.0, regardless of urine output. Granular casts frequently are visible, particularly with ATN. Enzymuria and phosphaturia are frequently prominent early in the course of ATN.[44,45] Plasma sodium and chloride concentrations are usually low. Plasma concentrations of calcium and inorganic phosphate vary greatly: increases, decreases, and normal values are possible, depending on the diet of the horse, the nephrotoxin, and the location and severity of damage to the nephron.[38,44,45]

One must remember that GFR is reduced in cases of ATN and is most likely caused by the increase in presentation of sodium and chloride at the macula densa after dysfunction of proximal sodium reabsorption. Stimulation of the macula densa results in release of renin and local production of angiotensin II, thus increasing renal vascular resistance and lowering RBF. The low GFR may mask the absolute magnitude of the damage in tubule function; however, if one studies renal sodium reabsorption carefully over time in cases of ATN, then this defect appears to improve more rapidly than that of GFR.[46]

Acute interstitial nephritis often is not recognized in horses; however, in a study conducted about 20 years ago, the condition was diagnosed in approximately one eighth of all human patients who needed renal biopsy for diagnosis of unexplained ARF.[47]

Edema and diffuse or focal patches of interstitial inflammation characterize the disease. In human medicine, the number of drugs, toxins, and infectious agents known to induce this disease is growing. No reason exists to believe that similar agents are not capable of causing the same disease in equids. Inflammatory cells surround the tubules and can move between epithelial cells into tubule lumina. As a result, white blood cell casts are common. The leukocytes are also capable of disrupting the tubule basement membrane, making cell repair much less likely; this is an important distinguishing feature between ATN and interstitial nephritis. With the former disease the basement membrane usually stays intact. Reduction of GFR and azotemia probably result from the interstitial edema, intratubular obstruction, and release of vasoactive agents.

Acute interstitial nephritis and ATN have similar fractional sodium clearance, U/P_{Cr}, and U/P_{osm} values; however, the urine sediment may be different for each disease. Sterile pyuria and microscopic hematuria commonly occur with interstitial nephritis, although RBC casts are rare. Mild proteinuria and eosinophiluria are also common. Eosinophiluria generally seems to be limited to renal interstitial disease, mainly drug-induced interstitial nephritis but also chronic pyelonephritis and systemic lupus erythematosus.[48,49] Eosinophiluria may or may not be accompanied by eosinophilia. Eosinophils in equine urine should be easy to observe using Wright's stain, given the alkaline nature of the fluid. Occasionally, fevers are believed to be associated with the development of interstitial nephritis. This clinical sign is relatively nonspecific and might be misleading if the animal is being treated with antibiotics for an infection. What one might see with close monitoring of the patient is an initial reduction or resolution of the fever after the onset of antimicrobial therapy followed by recurrence of the fever and development of azotemia. If this happens, then acute interstitial nephritis should be on the rule-out list.

The nephrotic syndrome usually characterizes acute glomerulonephritis. Proteinuria is moderate to severe, and the urine usually is concentrated. Urine osmolality and U/P_{osm} are comparable with the values with prerenal ARF and are higher than those values normally seen in ATN. Urinary sodium concentration and fractional sodium clearance tend to be much lower than with other intrinsic renal and postrenal causes of ARF. The ratios of U/P_{UN} and U/P_{Cr} are often similar to those associated with prerenal failure and higher than those in ischemic, tubular, interstitial, or postrenal disease. Renal tubular secretion of Cr is increased in glomerulonephritis, with the result that Cr concentrations may not rise quickly and urea nitrogen-to-Cr ratios stay high, as they frequently do with prerenal problems. Therefore although urinary indexes should make possible differentiation of acute glomerulonephritis from other parenchymal and postrenal diseases, they overlap much with those associated with prerenal ARF. One is going to differentiate ARF caused by acute glomerulonephritis from that caused by hypoperfusion based on the significant proteinuria and red cell numbers usually associated with the former disease. Red cell casts are more common with glomerulonephritis than with other intrinsic causes of ARF. Some causes of postrenal ARF also may manifest red cell casts, but the proteinuria is not normally as great in those situations.

TREATMENT

Initially, treatment of horses with ARF should focus on reversing the inciting or underlying cause and correcting fluid and electrolyte imbalances. Early identification of patients at risk and prevention of problems by rapid restoration and accurate maintenance of intravascular fluid volume, glomerular filtration, and urine production (with fluids and possibly diuretics) is obviously preferable to treatment. The importance of prevention cannot be overstated. One should correct initial fluid deficits over the first 6 to 12 hours of treatment. Physiologic saline or a balanced electrolyte solution is the fluid of choice unless the patient is hypernatremic, as may be the case in prerenal ARF or acute glomerulonephritis. In the event of hypernatremia, solutions of 0.45% NaCl and 2.5% dextrose is recommended. The addition of 50 to 100 g of dextrose per liter of fluid to saline or polyionic fluids helps address the caloric needs of anorectic horses. If fluid administration is begun early in the course of the disease or if the problem is not severe, then diuresis should result. When this occurs, one should maintain intravenous fluid therapy at least at twice maintenance level (up to 100 ml/kg per day or more) until Cr concentration decreases dramatically. One then reduces the rate of fluid administration to 40 to 50 ml/kg per day until the Cr concentration is normal or the horse is eating and drinking adequately.

In the event that the horse remains oliguric 10 to 12 hours after starting fluid therapy, administration of dopamine in 5% dextrose slowly (3 to 5 μg/kg/min) may improve RBF and urine output. One should monitor blood pressure during dopamine infusion because the drug can induce significant hypertension. Administration of dopamine should be discontinued if blood pressure starts to rise. One can attempt to restart the infusion at a lower rate when pressure has returned to normal. Blood pressure also may increase because of overhydration of oliguric patients who are receiving isotonic fluids. Regular monitoring of body weight, hematocrit, and serum total protein concentration, central venous pressure, and lung sounds is important if one is to prevent problems caused by overhydration.

The use of diuretic agents such as mannitol and loop diuretics to treat ARF is controversial. Furosemide and ethacrynic acid are the loop diuretics most commonly used. Furosemide is a particularly potent short-acting agent that acts by blocking the $Na/K/2Cl^-$ co-transporter in the ascending limb of the loop of Henle. In addition to promoting diuresis, co-transporter inhibition also may protect these tubule cells by reducing their metabolic rate and thus oxygen demand in the face of limited oxygen availability after hypoperfusion. To be effective, loop diuretics must gain access to the tubule lumina. Therefore loop diuretics may be of limited value in prerenal or ischemic problems, although the potential protective effect of furosemide on the especially vulnerable cells of the thick ascending limb may warrant its administration. Loop diuretic administration also may exacerbate or induce volume depletion in cases of ARF that are characterized by isosthenuria or polyuria (e.g., early ATN), thus making the condition worse and rendering the patient more susceptible to the effects of nephrotoxins such as gentamicin. Loop diuretics appear to be most beneficial when used in cases characterized by tubule obstruction (e.g., pigmenturia) because the diuretic-induced increase in solute retention apparently helps flush these blockages and casts from the tubules.

Although loop diuretics have no direct effect on GFR, 20% mannitol (0.25 to 1.0 g/kg) given over 15 to 20 minutes may help combat oliguria by increasing RBF and GFR. The increase occurs after reductions in plasma protein concentration and oncotic pressure. These changes in turn result from the systemic effects of the increase in intravascular osmolality induced by the mannitol. Mannitol also may induce synthesis of the vasodilator PGE_2 and release of atrial natriuretic peptide, which also would increase RBF and GFR. Once filtered, the agent also acts as an osmotic diuretic, thus decreasing urine solute concentration and boosting urine volume. Consequently, mannitol also can be effective in treating conditions characterized by tubular obstruction and swelling of tubule cells.

Hyperkalemia is uncommon in equine ARF, except in some postrenal cases. When present, hyperkalemia is usually mild and responds to administration of potassium-free intravenous fluids. When hyperkalemia (>6.5 mEq/L) persists, correction of any associated acidosis with sodium bicarbonate or administration of glucose (up to 10% solution), or both, usually helps. In the worst or most refractory cases, insulin may be necessary. Potassium supplementation (KCl 20-40 mEq/L) may be necessary during the polyuric phase of recovery from ARF.

Calcium metabolism often is disrupted in cases of equine ARF, with hypocalcemia and hyperphosphatemia or hypercalcemia and hypophosphatemia having been reported variously. Hypercalcemia usually resolves with a switch to a grass or grass-hay diet and with time. Hypocalcemia probably occurs for a number of reasons, including skeletal resistance to parathyroid hormone during the early stages of ARF and deficiency of 1,25-dihydroxycholecalciferol, which results from downregulation of renal 1,25-hydroxylase by the hyperphosphatemia, dysfunction of this enzyme after renal parenchymal damage, or both.[45,50] Hypoalbuminemia and enhanced deposition of calcium in injured tissues, as can occur in cases of rhabdomyolysis, are other factors to consider. Administration of a calcium salt as part of the intravenous fluid therapy protocol is usually sufficient to correct this.

Severe uremia often decreases RBC life span and induces platelet dysfunction. Consequently, anemia (possibly also caused by decreased production of erythropoietin) and bleeding tendencies may be associated with ARF. These conditions may require treatment with transfusions, synthetic erythropoietin, or conjugated estrogens.

Because aminoglycoside toxicity is one of the more commonly recognized causes of equine ARF,[4,9,51] continued aminoglycoside use in horses with ARF warrants specific attention. Gentamicin and amikacin are the aminoglycoside antibiotics most often used in equine practice, and their pharmacokinetics have been well studied in healthy animals. Large interindividual and age variations occur in the volume of distribution and clearance of these drugs in normal horses, and this variability is even greater in diseased horses. Therefore when a patient with ARF requires aminoglycoside antibiotics, monitoring serum trough concentrations of the drug to adjust the dosing interval is strongly indicated, because it provides the best protection against exacerbating renal damage. Renal dysfunction associated with aminoglycoside toxicity usually is indicated by an increase of at least 0.3 mg/dl in Cr concentration. When this occurs, discontinuing therapy or increasing the dosing interval should be considered. One must remember that changes in urine sediment and development of enzymuria, mild proteinuria, glucosuria, and decreased urine-concentrating ability develop a number of days before Cr concentration increases and are good indicators of the development of aminoglycoside nephrotoxicity. One usually can address the problem successfully by maintaining or increasing intravenous fluid therapy to guard against renal hypoperfusion and by appropriately adjusting the dosing interval with the antibiotic.

PROGNOSIS

The prognosis for equine ARF depends on the underlying cause, the duration of renal failure, the response to initial treatment, and the development of secondary complications such as diarrhea, thrombophlebitis, and laminitis. Generally speaking, the duration of ARF before beginning therapy is the most important determinant of prognosis. Of the primary causes of ARF, severe ischemic failure and acute interstitial nephritis probably carry the worst prognosis in horses. ARF of any cause, however, should be associated with a reduced or poor prognosis in the event that early interruption of the pathophysiologic events leading to ARF is not achieved or that the animal displays prolonged oliguria or anuria (longer than 12 hours) after institution of vigorous therapy. Most cases of postrenal ARF carry a favorable prognosis, provided the initiating disease is treated successfully. When discussing prognosis with horse owners, practitioners always must bear in mind that a successful outcome is not always associated with complete return of normal function. Many horses live long after a bout of ARF but never fully regain the ability to concentrate urine as well as they did before the disease; in other cases they remain constantly polyuric. ATN, after nephrotoxicity in particular, carries a favorable prognosis when tubule basement membranes remain intact.

CHRONIC RENAL FAILURE

Harold C. Schott II

PREDISPOSING CONDITIONS

CRF is recognized infrequently in horses. For dogs and cats the prevalence of CRF has been reported to be 0.9% and 1.6%, respectively,[1] whereas the Veterinary Medical Data Base at Purdue University reported that only 515 of 442,535 horses admitted to participating veterinary teaching hospitals during the years 1964 through 1996 had CRF (prevalence of 0.12%). In actuality, this may be an underestimate, because when a diagnosis of CRF is established for a horse, the horse likely may be destroyed without presentation to a veterinary teaching hospital. As in dogs and cats, CRF appears to be a greater problem in older horses (the prevalence increased to 0.23% in horses older than 15 years). The 0.51% prevalence for intact males older than 15 years of age also suggests that stallions may be at greater risk.

Although the clinical syndrome of CRF is uncommon, one widely cited abattoir study revealed that 16% of 45 horses examined had glomerular lesions on light microscopic examination and 42% (22 of 53 horses examined) exhibited deposits of immunoglobulin or complement on immunofluorescence staining of tissue samples.[2] Although these findings suggest that as many as one third of horses may show microscopic evidence of renal disease, only one of the horses in this survey exhibited signs of CRF. This disparity can be attributed to a large renal reserve capacity, because clinical signs of renal failure do not become apparent until two thirds to three fourths of functional nephrons have been lost.[3] Although this rule of thumb is based on studies of partially nephrectomized laboratory animals, support for similar renal reserve capacity in horses is found in several clinical reports of unilateral nephrectomy used successfully to manage disorders of the upper urinary tract.[4-8] In addition, after experimental unilateral nephrectomy in ponies[9] and horses,[10] renal function remained within normal ranges and the animals maintained body weight.

Disorders of the kidneys leading to CRF may be congenital or acquired. In horses younger than 5 years with a history that includes no event that might have been complicated by ARF, one should suspect a congenital renal disorder: renal agenesis, hypoplasia, dysplasia, or PKD.[11-24] Although each of these congenital abnormalities occasionally is recognized, acquired disease consequent to glomerular or tubular injury is more often the cause of CRF in horses.[25-30] Acquired disease is usually insidious in onset, and renal injury may have been initiated years earlier. Thus identifying the cause of CRF is challenging because many horses have evidence of advanced glomerular and tubular disease, termed *ESKD,* by the time clinical signs of CRF develop. Nevertheless, knowing the various causes of CRF affords a better overall understanding of CRF in horses.

GLOMERULONEPHRITIS

Glomerular injury is a common precipitant of renal insufficiency and CRF in horses. Although immune-mediated glomerular injury is implicated most often in glomerulonephritis, glomerular integrity can be disrupted by a number of unrelated disease processes, including ischemia, toxic insults, and infection.[31] These mechanisms usually lead to significant vascular and tubulointerstitial changes in addition to glomerular injury. Thus the designation glomerulonephritis typically is reserved to denote renal disease of which immune-mediated glomerular damage is suspected to be the initiating factor in development of renal failure. Until the last decade, glomerulonephritis was considered a rare cause of CRF in domestic animals; interstitial nephritis was implicated more often.[32-34] Refinement of histologic examination with immunofluorescence staining techniques and electron microscopic examination of renal tissues has led to increased recognition of subclinical and clinically significant glomerulonephritis.[34]

A brief review of the subgross anatomy of the glomerulus sheds light on the pathophysiology of glomerulonephritis. The renal corpuscle, or glomerulus, is comprised of a tuft of glomerular capillaries surrounded by epithelial cells that line Bowman's capsule. The root that supports the pedicle of the glomerular capillary network is similar to the mesenteric root that supports the intestinal tract, and Bowman's capsule is analogous to the peritoneum (Figure 19-18-1, *A*). On a microscopic level, components of the glomerulus include capillary endothelial cells, mesangium (cells and matrix), GBM, and visceral epithelial cells. At the vascular pedicle, the latter become contiguous with parietal epithelial cells that line Bowman's space, much as mesothelial cells covering bowel serosa and mesentery become contiguous with the peritoneum at the mesenteric root.[31] Glomerular capillary endothelial cells are unique in that they are fenestrated with pores that represent the initial barrier for passage of blood components into the urinary space (Figure 19-18, *B*). The mesangium, which lies between endothelial and epithelial cells, is the support

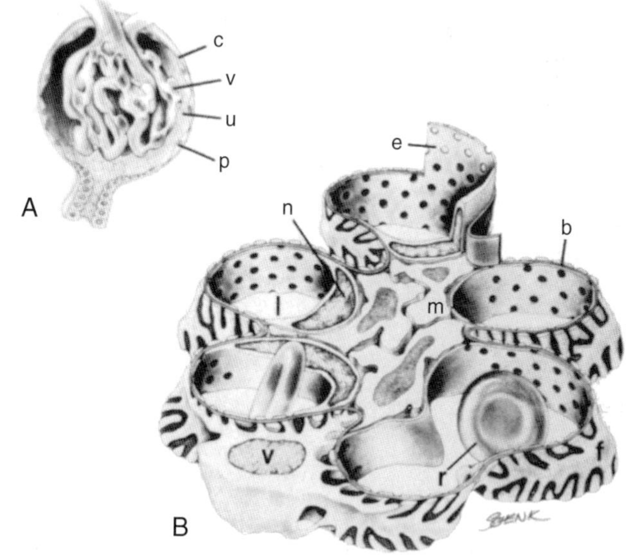

FIGURE 19-18 Subgross anatomy of a renal corpuscle. **A,** A renal corpuscle with a tuft of glomerular capillaries surrounded by Bowman's capsule (**c**) shows visceral (**v**) and parietal (**p**) epithelial cells separated by the urinary space (**u**). **B,** Cross-section of a portion of a glomerulus shows the nucleus (**n**) and fenestrations (**e**) of capillary endothelial cells, the glomerular basement membrane (GBM) (**b**), mesangial cells (**m**) separated by mesangial matrix, and the nucleus (**v**) of a visceral epithelial cell. A red blood cell (RBC) (**r**) is in the lumen (**l**) of one of the glomerular capillaries. (From Osborne CA, Hammer RF, Stevens JB et al: The glomerulus in health and disease: a comparative review of domestic animals and man, Adv Vet Sci Comp Med 21:207, 1977.)

structure of the glomerular capillaries and is analogous to the mesenteric tissue supporting bowel. Mesangial cells are a component of the reticuloendothelial system and phagocytize macromolecular substances, among them are fragments of old GBM or larger molecules that pass through endothelial cell pores but cannot pass subsequently through the GBM. In addition, mesangial cells have contractile elements that allow them to participate in regulation of glomerular hemodynamics. Furthermore, these cells proliferate in response to glomerular injury and can release a number of cytokines that modulate the glomerular inflammatory response.[35] The GBM lies between endothelial and epithelial cells and surrounds glomerular capillaries, except where mesangium is present (Figure 19-19, *A*). Returning to the abdominal cavity analogy, the GBM would lie beneath bowel serosa except in the area of mesenteric attachment, which would contain mesangial cells and matrix. The GBM consists of a central electron-dense layer, the lamina densa, and two thinner, more electron-lucent layers, the lamina rara externa and the lamina rara interna (Figure 19-19, *B*).[31,35] The main components of the GBM are collagen-like molecules and matrix glycoproteins that are produced principally by visceral epithelial cells. Normal GBM undergoes steady turnover with removal of debris by mesangial cells. The visceral epithelial cells, also called *podocytes,* cover the uriniferous duct side of the GBM and have many cytoplasmic extensions called *foot processes* that form extensive interdigitations with foot processes of adjacent epithelial cells. The narrow gap between foot processes—the filtration slit or slit pore—is bridged by a thin membrane, the slit pore diaphragm.[31,35]

The filtration barrier of the glomerulus consists of fenestrated endothelial cells, GBM, and slit pores between epithelial cell foot processes. These structures constitute a size-selective and charge-selective filtration barrier. Although all components of this barrier are anionic (i.e., they repel anionic macromolecules), the GBM is thought to be the principal agent of the permeability characteristics of the filtration barrier. The GBM is rich in glycosaminoglycans, containing heparin sulfate and sialic acid residues. These strongly anionic molecules are responsible for its negative charge barrier, which limits filtration of anionic macromolecules, predominantly albumin.[1,35]

Glomerulonephritis is initiated by deposition of circulating immune complexes along the GBM and in the mesangium, leading to complement activation and leukocyte infiltration and adherence. Release of oxidants and proteinases by neutrophils and macrophages; production of eicosanoids, cytokines, and growth factors by macrophages and mesangial cells; and platelet aggregation and activation of coagulation factors lead to endothelial and epithelial cell swelling (with fusion of foot processes), formation of microthrombi in glomerular capillaries, and mesangial cell proliferation.[1,31,36] Immune complexes can be deposited in a subendothelial, intra-GBM, or subepithelial site, depending on their size and charge properties, but most tend to be found in the subendothelial space. On electron microscopic examination these immune complexes appear as electron-dense granular deposits (Figure 19-20, *A*), and staining with anti-immunoglobulin G and anticomplement (C3) antibodies reveals an irregular (granular or "lumpy bumpy") immunofluorescence staining pattern (Figure 19-20, *B*).[1,2,31] The GBM proliferates to surround the immune deposits, leading to irregular thickening of the filtration barrier. Despite widening of the filtration barrier, the size-selective and charge-selective filtration properties are compromised, and microscopic hematuria and proteinuria result. In rare instances, glomerulonephritis may be attributed to a true autoimmune disorder in which autoantibodies directed against GBM components (e.g., type IV collagen) are produced. Electron

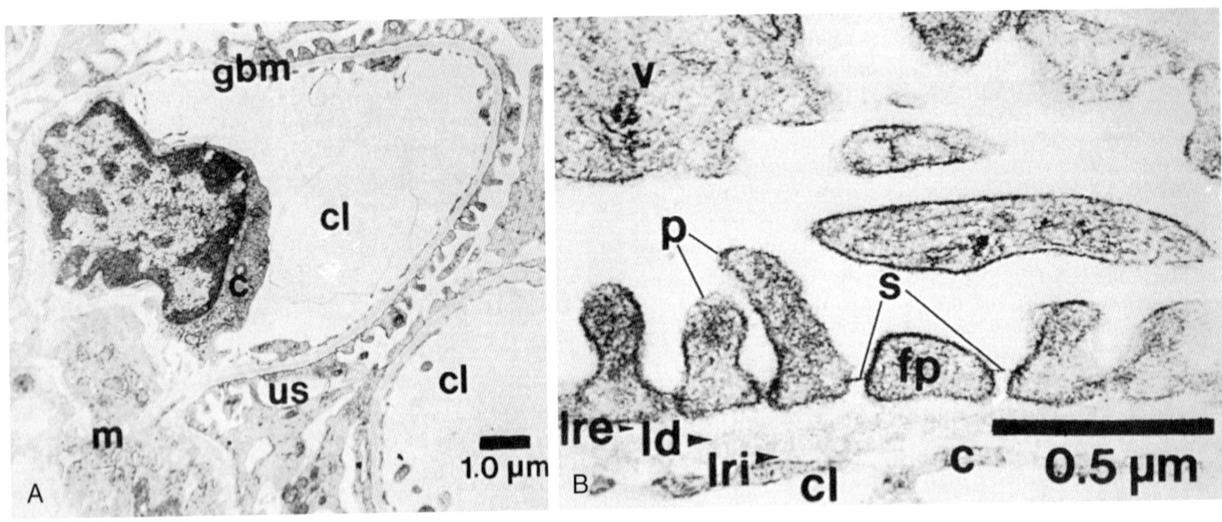

FIGURE 19-19 Electron micrograph of a normal glomerulus. **A,** Low-power magnification illustrates patent capillary lumens (**cl**) separated from the urinary space (**us**) by fenestrated endothelial cell cytoplasm (**c**), the glomerular basement membrane (GBM) (**gbm**), and foot processes of visceral epithelial cells. Mesangial cells and matrix (**m**) are also apparent (bar = 1.0 μm). **B,** Higher-power magnification reveals the ultrastructural features of the filtration barrier including, from bottom to top, the capillary lumen (**cl**) and endothelial cell cytoplasm (**c**); the lamina rara interna (**lri**), lamina densa (**ld**), and lamina rara externa (**lre**) of the GBM; and cytoplasm (**v**), foot processes (**fp**), and slit diaphragms (**s**) of the visceral epithelial cells. Deposits of glomerular polyanion or glycosaminoglycans (**p**) are visible on the foot processes (bar = 0.5 μm). (From Osborne CA, Hammer RF, Stevens JB et al: The glomerulus in health and disease: a comparative review of domestic animals and man, Adv Vet Sci Comp Med 21:207, 1977.)

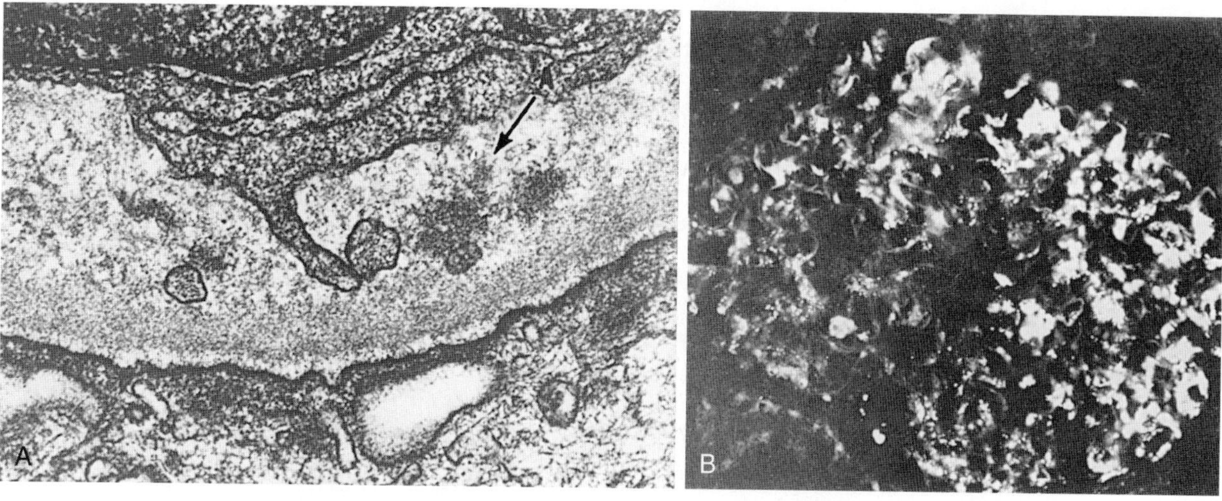

FIGURE 19-20 Immune-mediated glomerulonephritis in a horse 165 days after experimental infection with equine infectious anemia virus (EIAV). **A,** An electron micrograph (×32,500) shows endothelial cell swelling *(top)*, thickening of the glomerular basement membrane (GBM) with electron-dense immune deposits in a predominantly subendothelial location *(arrow)*, and fusion of foot processes of the visceral epithelial cells. **B,** Immunofluorescent staining with fluorescein-tagged antiequine immunoglobulin G antibody (×100) demonstrates granular or "lumpy bumpy" deposits of immunoglobulin G along the GBM and in the mesangium. (From Banks KL, Henson JB, McGuire TC: Immunologically mediated glomerulitis of horses. 1. Pathogenesis in persistent infection by equine infectious anemia virus, Lab Invest 26:701, 1972.)

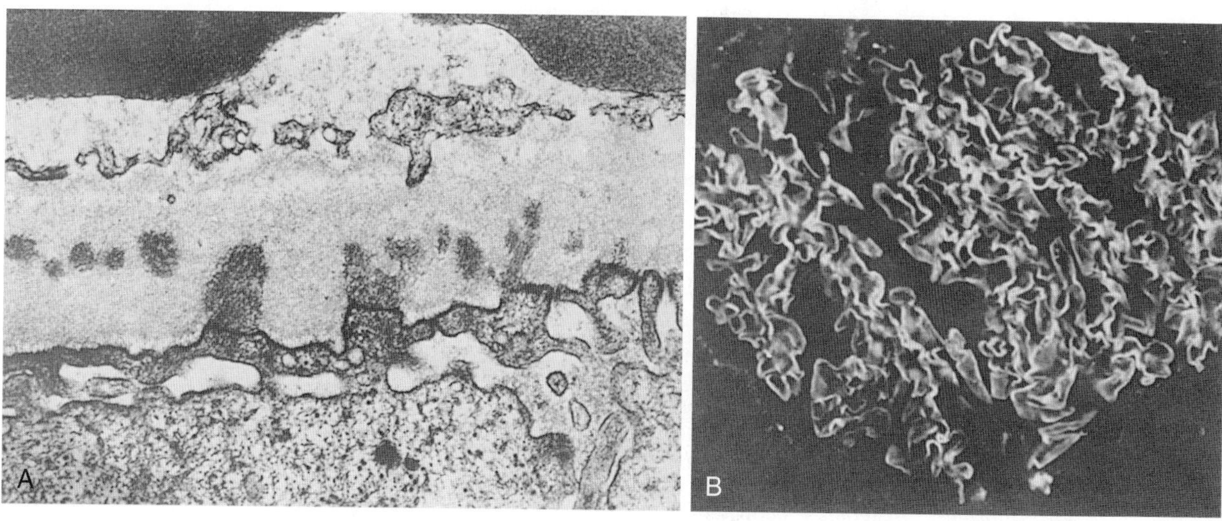

FIGURE 19-21 Spontaneous immune-mediated glomerulonephritis in a horse. **A,** An electron micrograph (×22,750) shows a RBC (RBC) in the capillary lumen *(top)*, relatively normal fenestrated endothelial cytoplasm, thickening of the glomerular basement membrane (GBM) with electron-dense immune deposits in a predominantly subepithelial location, and fusion of foot processes of the visceral epithelial cells. **B,** Immunofluorescent staining with fluorescein-tagged antiequine immunoglobulin G antibody (×160) demonstrates smooth, linear deposits of immunoglobulin G. (From Banks KL, Henson JB, McGuire TC: Immunologically mediated glomerulitis of horses. 2. Antiglomerular basement membrane antibody and other mechanisms of spontaneous disease, Lab Invest 26:708, 1972.)

microscopic examination in these cases also reveals GBM thickening with predominantly subepithelial electron-dense deposits (Figure 19-21, *A*), and immunofluorescence staining shows a more regular or smooth, linear pattern of immunofluorescence (Figure 19-21, *B*).[31,37,38] Autoimmune glomerulonephritis, accompanied by proteinuria, also has been described as one of the manifestations of systemic lupus erythematosus in horses.[39] Another immune mechanism of glomerulonephritis in horses is production of mixed or monoclonal cryoglobulins and deposition of antibody-antibody immune complexes along the glomerular GBM.[40,41] Cryoglobulinemia is associated with a number of diseases in human beings[35,40] but has been described in only a few horses.[41,42] Deposition of antibody-antibody immune complexes along the GBM may be a more

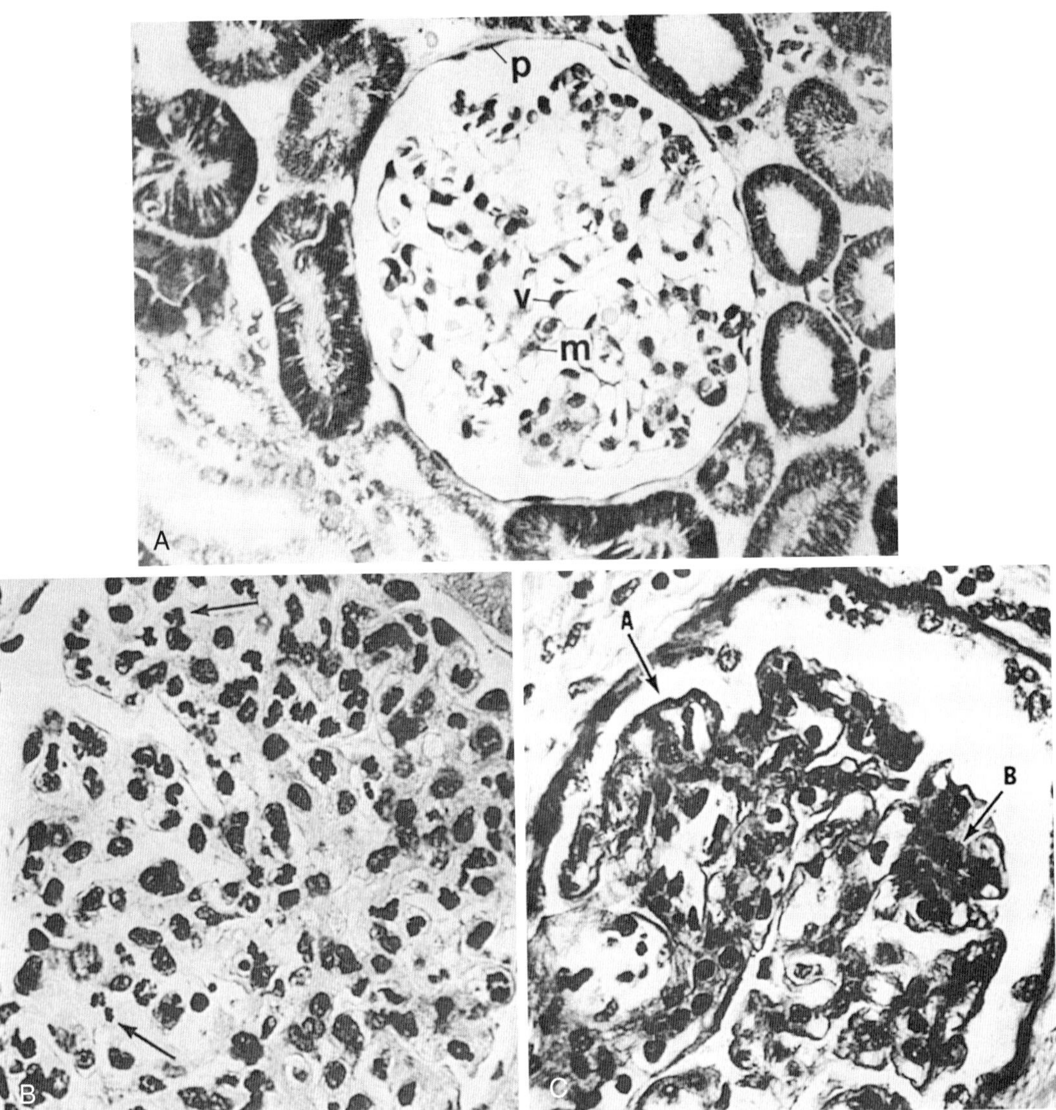

FIGURE 19-22 Histologic changes in equine glomerulonephritis. **A,** Photomicrograph of a normal glomerulus. Bowman's capsule is lined by flattened parietal epithelial cells (**p**). Visceral epithelial cells (**v**) are adjacent to the glomerular basement membrane (GBM), which is of uniform thickness. Mesangial cells (**m**) are surrounded entirely by glomerular capillaries (periodic acid–Schiff [PAS] stain, ×100). **B,** Photomicrograph demonstrates proliferative glomerulonephritis in a horse after experimental infection with equine infectious anemia virus (EIAV). A combination of neutrophil infiltration *(arrows)* and mesangial cell proliferation is apparent (hematoxylin-eosin stain, ×160). **C,** Photomicrograph demonstrates membranous glomerulonephritis in a horse after experimental infection with EIAV. The GBMs are thickened (**A**) and mesangial areas contain PAS-positive material (**B**) (PAS stain, ×160). (A from Osborne CA, Hammer RF, Stevens JB et al: The glomerulus in health and disease: a comparative review of domestic animals and man, Adv Vet Sci Comp Med 21:207, 1977; B and C from Banks KL, Henson JB, McGuire TC: Immunologically mediated glomerulitis of horses. 1. Pathogenesis in persistent infection by equine infectious anemia virus, Lab Invest 26:701, 1972.)

important precipitant of glomerulonephritis than was recognized previously because electron microscopic examination is required to demonstrate characteristic fibrillar or crystalline intracapillary and subendothelial deposits associated with the condition.[40] Regardless of what immune mechanism leads to glomerular injury, the end result is thickening of the filtration barrier, retarded GFR, and development of CRF in severe cases.

Although a number of terms are used to describe the specific morphologic changes associated with glomerular injury, glomerulonephritis is categorized most broadly histologically as *proliferative* or *membranous*.[1,31,34] Proliferative (or mesangioproliferative) glomerulonephritis describes glomerular injury associated with influx of inflammatory cells and proliferation of mesangial cells. The predominant histologic finding is increased cellularity in glomeruli (Figure 19-22, *A* and *B*). This lesion tends to be associated with the more acute stages of glomerulonephritis during which immune complexes are being deposited in a predominantly subendothelial site. Membranous glomerulonephritis describes glomerular injury accompanied by significant thickening of the capillary wall and GBM; with periodic acid–Schiff (PAS) staining, the predominant histologic finding is increased in the mesangial area and on the GBM (Figure 19-22, *C*). Methenamine silver stain further enhances visibility of the thickening of the GBM.[31,34] Membranous glomerulonephritis tends to be associated with more soluble immune complexes or autoantibodies that can pass through the GBM and localize in a predominantly subepithelial site, resulting in less infiltration of inflammatory cells. As would be expected, a spectrum of lesions is visible in naturally occurring glomerulonephritis, leading to varying histologic descriptions of the disease (membranoproliferative glomerulonephritis). As glomerular injury progresses, proliferation of the parietal epithelium also occurs, likely in response to filtration of macromolecules and cellular debris. Lesions associated with parietal cell proliferation can include layering of epithelial cells (termed *crescents*) on the inner aspect of Bowman's capsule (Figure 19-23, *A*), adhesion formation between the glomerular tuft and Bowman's capsule (Figure 19-23, *B*), and tuft collapse. Glomerulosclerosis describes the end stage of progressive, irreversible glomerular injury in which replacement of glomerular components with hyaline material is visible on histologic examination (Figure 19-23, *C*).[31]

Specific histologic categorization of glomerulonephritis provides causative and prognostic information for human beings with renal failure attributable to glomerular disease.[35] Subcategorization of glomerulopathies also has been done in a prospective study of naturally occurring chronic renal disease in canines. Although classifications—including focal glomerulonephritis, mesangioproliferative glomerulonephritis, endocapillary proliferative glomerulonephritis, crescentic glomerulonephritis, and sclerosing glomerulonephritis—could

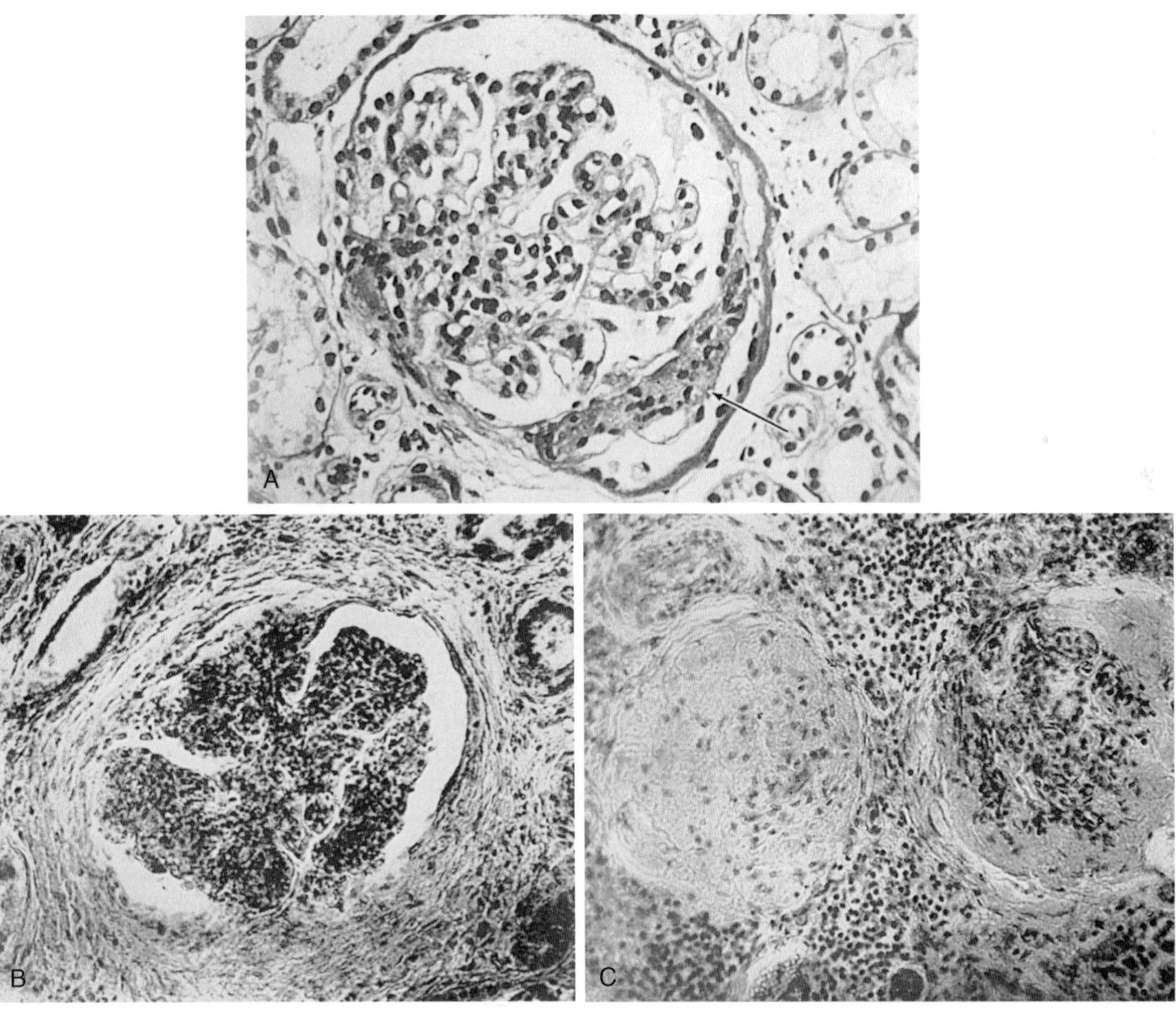

FIGURE 19-23 Progressive histologic changes in equine glomerulonephritis. **A,** Photomicrograph of a renal biopsy specimen illustrates membranoproliferative glomerulonephritis (an increase in cell numbers and thickening of the glomerular basement membrane [GBM]) and parietal epithelial cell proliferation resulting in crescent formation (*arrow;* periodic acid–Schiff stain [PAS], ×100). **B,** Photomicrograph demonstrates progressive glomerulonephritis resulting in adhesion formation between the capillary tuft and proliferating parietal epithelial cells. **C,** Photomicrograph of end-stage glomerulosclerosis shows replacement of glomerular components with hyaline material (more complete in glomerulus on the left). (A from Osborne CA, Hammer RF, Stevens JB et al: The glomerulus in health and disease: a comparative review of domestic animals and man, Adv Vet Sci Comp Med 21:207, 1977; B and C from Fincher MG, Olafson P: Chronic diffuse glomerulonephritis in a horse, Cornell Vet 24:356, 1934.)

be made, histologic findings were not prognostically useful.[43] This study also revealed that glomerular disease was responsible for 52% of canine CRF; however, an inciting disease (vegetative endocarditis) could be identified in only one of 31 dogs with glomerulonephritis.

Glomerulonephritis also appears to be an important cause of CRF in horses.[27] Of 60 reported cases of CRF attributable to acquired disease, glomerulonephritis was identified as the inciting cause of CRF in 32 (53%) (Table 19-8).[25-27, 36,40,41,44-56] Glomerulonephritis also may be the initiating disease process in cases of ESKD for which gross and histopathologic changes are so extensive that a primary mechanism of renal injury cannot be identified. A number of systemic inflammatory and infectious disease processes in horses may be accompanied by glomerulonephritis, but progression to CRF appears to be a rare sequela. For example, experimental *Leptospira pomona* infection produced subacute glomerulonephritis characterized by hypercellularity and edema of capillary tufts,[74] but leptospirosis appears to be a rare cause of clinical renal disease in horses.[75-77] Similarly, experimental infection with equine infectious anemia virus (EIAV) produced histologic and immunofluorescent evidence of glomerulonephritis in 75% and 87% of infected horses, respectively.[37] Immunoglobulins with anti–EIA activity were eluted from glomeruli collected from experimentally infected horses, but none of the horses showed clinical signs of renal disease. Poststreptococcal glomerulonephritis is a well-recognized cause of renal disease in human beings,[35,78] and Roberts and Kelly[79] speculated that glomerulonephritis in a horse with chronic pleuritis and purpura hemorrhagica likely resulted from circulating immune complexes involving streptococcal antigens. Divers et al.[56] provided support for this hypothesis by eluting group C streptococcal antigens from immune complex deposits in glomeruli collected from a horse with CRF. Finally, an occasional case of equine glomerulonephritis may result from true autoimmune disease, and in one instance, anti-GBM antibody was eluted from glomeruli with linear GBM immunofluorescent staining pattern isolated from a horse.[2] Little information is available about histopathologic subcategories of glomerulonephritis in horses, although several reports have attempted to make comparisons with glomerular lesions that have been better characterized in other species.[40,54,80] No reports have attempted to correlate histologic changes with the degree of renal failure in horses. Thus assessment of the severity of renal disease associated with glomerulonephritis in horses currently is based more on clinical findings (e.g., body condition, magnitude of azotemia) than on histologic changes in a renal biopsy sample.

Chronic Interstitial Nephritis

Tubulointerstitial disease usually results from ATN after ischemia, endotoxemia, sepsis, or exposure to nephrotoxic compounds. Hypovolemia associated with acute blood loss, colic, diarrhea, endotoxemia, or sepsis can lead to renal hypoperfusion and ischemic damage.[81] Severe localized infection (e.g., pleuritis, peritonitis) or septicemia also may be accompanied by tubule damage. Aminoglycoside antibiotics, NSAIDs, vitamin D, vitamin K_3, acorns, and heavy metals such as mercury are potentially nephrotoxic.[82] Intravascular hemolysis or rhabdomyolysis also can lead to acute tubular damage after the nephrotoxic effects of hemoglobin and myoglobin (see Acute Renal Failure). In horses tubulointerstitial disease culminating in CRF also can be caused by ascending UTI resulting in pyelonephritis[25,27,52,64-68,83] or bilateral obstructive disease caused by ureteroliths or nephroliths.[22,27,59-63,84] In other cases

TABLE 19-8

Causes of Chronic Renal Failure in Seventy-Five Horses (Excluding Reports of Congenital Renal Failure and Experimental Induction of Chronic Renal Failure)

Disorders	Number of Cases	References (Number of Cases)
CONGENITAL DISORDERS (15 OF 75 [20%])		
Renal agenesis/contralateral obstruction and hydronephrosis	1	11 (1)
Renal hypoplasia	4	13 (3), 24 (1)
Renal dysplasia	6	14 (1), 15 (1), 16 (2), 21 (1), 22 (1)
Polycystic kidney disease (PKD)	4	18 (1), 19 (1), 20 (1), 23 (1)
ACQUIRED DISORDERS (60 OF 75 [80%])*		
Glomerulonephritis	32	25 (1), 26 (2), 27 (1), 36 (1), 40 (7), 41 (1), 44 (1), 45 (1), 46 (1), 47 (1), 48 (1), 49 (1), 50 (1), 51 (1), 52 (5), 53 (2), 54 (1), 55 (2), 56 (1)
Chronic interstitial nephritis (CIN)	2	57 (1), 58 (1)
With obstructive nephrolithiasis and/or ureterolithiasis	11	59 (1), 60 (1), 61 (7), 62 (1), 63 (1)
With pyelonephritis	8	25 (1), 27 (1), 52 (1), 64 (1), 65 (1), 66 (1), 67 (1), 68 (1)
With papillary necrosis	2	27 (1), 69 (1)
End-stage kidney disease (ESKD)†	5	58 (1), 70 (1), 71 (1), 72 (1), 73 (1)

*In many reports of acquired renal disease leading to chronic renal failure (CRF), histopathologic changes involve glomeruli and interstitium. Categorization in this table is based on the authors' conclusions in these reports. When severe lesions involved glomeruli and interstitium, a categorization of ESKD was made.
†ESKD and reports of oxalate nephropathy.

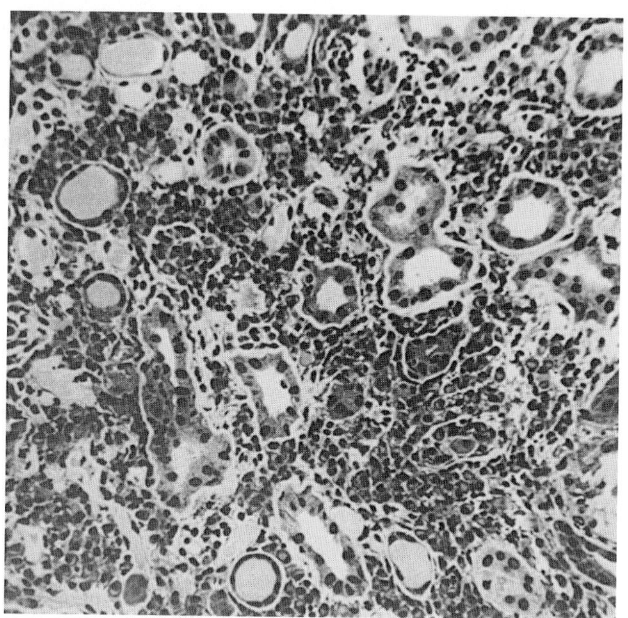

FIGURE 19-24 Histologic changes in interstitial nephritis. The interstitium contains dense infiltrates of lymphocytes and plasma cells superimposed on moderate interstitial fibrosis and tubular atrophy (hematoxylin-eosin stain, ×275). (From Brenner BM, editor: Brenner and Rector's the kidney, ed 8, 2008, Philadelphia, WB Saunders.)

a cause of the tubule disease may not be identified.[57,58] Finally, although this has not yet been described in horses, immune mechanisms, including anti-tubular basement membrane disease, can lead to chronic interstitial nephritis (CIN) in human beings.[35]

CIN is defined most strictly by clinical signs of renal disease associated with histologic changes of tubular damage and an interstitial inflammatory cell infiltrate (Figure 19-24). Inflammatory cells include lymphocytes, monocytes, and occasionally plasma cells. Neutrophils are uncommon; however, eosinophilic infiltrates suggest drug reactions in human patients.[35] Major glomerular and vascular lesions are not apparent. The hallmark that distinguishes CIN from acute tubular and interstitial disease is interstitial fibrosis.

Although CIN has a fairly strict histologic definition, a number of disease processes can lead to tubular damage. For all practical purposes, *CIN* is a catchall term for extraglomerular causes of CRF in horses. As a consequence, gross findings in horses with CIN can vary dramatically. For example, analgesic nephropathy (NSAID toxicity, of which phenylbutazone has the greatest nephrotoxic potential[85]) can produce papillary necrosis[69,86] manifested by hematuria[87] in the early stages of disease, whereas chronic disease may be associated with nephrolithiasis and hydronephrosis. The area of papillary necrosis serves as a nidus for stone formation, and subsequent obstructive disease leads to hydronephrosis.[61,84] Similarly, upper UTI can lead to minor or major changes in the architecture of the kidneys and to variable histologic changes.

Using CIN as a broad category for nonglomerulonephritis causes of CRF in horses, this group of tubulointerstitial diseases was responsible for 38% (23 of 60) of the previously reported cases of CRF in horses (see Table 19-8). Although in theory one would expect CIN to be accompanied by greater evidence of tubular dysfunction (e.g., enzymuria, glucosuria, increased fractional clearance of sodium), abnormal measures of tubule function have not been detected regularly. Similarly, microscopic hematuria and proteinuria, the hallmarks of glomerular disease, would not be expected.

End-Stage Kidney Disease

End-stage kidney disease describes the severe gross and histologic changes in kidneys collected from animals in the final stages of CRF. Grossly, the kidneys typically are pale, shrunken, and firm, and they may have an irregular surface and an adherent capsule. Histologically, severe glomerulosclerosis occurs along with hyalinization and extensive interstitial fibrosis. The end-stage lesions make determining the initiating cause of renal disease virtually impossible. In several cases with a pathologic description consistent with ESKD, the underlying cause of renal injury could not be established.[58,70-73]

Chronic Renal Failure of Other Causes

Several early cases of CRF in horses were attributed to oxalate poisoning because oxalate crystals were observed in renal tubules.[57,70] Horses appear to be more resistant than other domestic species to oxalate-induced renal damage[88]; however, experimental administration of various forms of oxalate (in large doses) produced hypocalcemia and gastrointestinal signs rather than renal failure.[89] In fact, the early reports of oxalate nephropathy in horses failed to demonstrate that the affected horses had been exposed to oxalates.[57,70] Furthermore, long-term ingestion of plants containing oxalate produces fibrous osteodystrophy (oxalates bind calcium in the intestinal tract, decreasing intestinal calcium absorption), but renal damage in affected horses has been minimal.[90] Formation of oxalate crystals in diseased equine kidneys now is recognized as a secondary change likely related to stasis of urine in damaged renal tubules.[50]

Amyloidosis is an unusual cause of CRF in horses.[88,91] Amyloid deposits associated with systemic disease typically are composed of aggregates of the amino-terminal fragment of serum amyloid A protein, an acute phase protein.[92-95] Concentrations of serum amyloid A increase with many inflammatory disease processes, and chronic elevations can result in amyloid deposition (AA type) in a variety of tissues, a condition termed *systemic reactive amyloidosis*.[96,97] Incidence and tissue localization of amyloid exhibit considerable species variation. Dogs appears to be affected most often, but the fact that the disease is familial in Abyssinian cats implies a genetic basis for the disease.[97] Amyloid deposits accumulate as stacks of protein in a β-pleated sheet conformation and are identified in tissue samples by their extracellular location and homogeneous, eosinophilic appearance when stained with hematoxylin and eosin. They are birefringent when viewed under polarized light, and staining with alkaline Congo red solution imparts a characteristic green color.[96,97] Amyloid deposition in the kidney is most common in dogs and cattle, and renal amyloidosis is a significant cause of CRF in dogs.[97] In horses, localized amyloidosis of the upper airway or skin is more common than systemic amyloidosis.[96] In the localized form, amyloid deposits are composed of immunoglobulin light chains (AL type). Although reports describe systemic reactive amyloidosis consequent to heavy parasite infestation in horses, renal involvement was minimal or not apparent.[98,99] Systemic amyloidosis has been recognized most often in horses hyperimmunized for antiserum production, and hepatic and splenic involvement may be more common than renal involvement in these horses.[88,91,93]

A final acquired cause of CRF, renal neoplasia, is discussed in greater detail elsewhere in this chapter. Although horses with renal neoplasia may have weight loss, the tumors are usually unilateral and development of CRF is uncommon.

UREMIC TOXINS AND THE UREMIC SYNDROME

Regardless of the underlying cause of nephron loss, the ensuing renal insufficiency leads to development of azotemia and its clinical manifestation, the uremic syndrome.[35,92-94,100] The uremic syndrome is a multisystemic disorder that develops as a result of the effects of uremic toxins on cell metabolism and function. Although the uremic syndrome originally was attributed to the effects of increased BUN concentration, a number of nitrogenous compounds now are known to accumulate in CRF and contribute to alterations of cell metabolism and function. In fact, the correlation between the severity of the uremic syndrome and the magnitude of azotemia is poor. For example, urea administered to human beings with normal renal function results simply in fluid shifts, osmotic diuresis, and increased thirst.[101] Urea toxicity also has been studied in nephrectomized dogs and in human patients with CRF sustained by dialysis. Increasing the urea concentrations of the dialysate to maintain BUN at artificially higher values has produced variable results. For example, BUN values up to about 150 mg/dl were associated with few clinical signs, whereas lethargy, weakness, anorexia, vomiting, and a bleeding diathesis (caused by platelet dysfunction) were produced when BUN was increased to values exceeding 175 to 200 mg/dl. Excess circulating urea also can degrade spontaneously to ammonia, carbonate, or cyanate. Cyanate can react with the N-terminal amino groups on a number of proteins and by altering tertiary structure can interfere with enzyme activity and structural integrity of cell membranes.[35] Thus accumulation of urea is likely responsible for some of the signs of uremic syndrome.

Cr and other guanidino compounds also accumulate in renal failure. These compounds are strong organic bases that contain an amidino group (N – C = NH).[35] With CRF, urinary excretion of Cr and other guanidino compounds actually may increase (because of tubular secretion) but not enough to prevent increases in blood concentrations. For example, the author has found that in naturally occurring cases of equine CRF (author's unpublished data), endogenous Cl_{Cr}, when measured simultaneously with Cl_{In}, overestimates GFR by 50% to 100%. These data indicate that tubular secretion of Cr, which Finco and Groves were unable to document in healthy ponies,[102] is initiated by or is quantitatively much greater with CRF. Although metabolic pathways have not been elucidated fully, guanidino compounds appear to be produced predominantly in the liver, and their concentration in blood and tissues increases with decreased renal function or increased dietary protein intake.[101] The relationship between guanidino compounds and the syndrome of uremia is also unclear. For example, administration of methylguanidine to healthy dogs resulted in weight loss, neurologic signs, and anemia, but only when blood concentrations were an order of magnitude greater than those in spontaneous cases of CRF.[35] In contrast, administration of another guanidino compound, guanidinopropionic acid, led to hemolysis by depleting erythrocyte glutathione concentrations (supporting a role for this uremic toxin in the anemia of CRF).

Products of intestinal bacterial metabolism—including secondary methylamines (from metabolism of choline and lecithin), aromatic amines (from metabolism of tyrosine and phenylalanine), polyamines (from metabolism of lysine and ornithine), and tryptophan breakdown products (indole, skatole, indoleacetic acid, and others)—can contribute to the clinical signs associated with the uremic syndrome. Some of these compounds have been studied thoroughly (e.g., the inhibitory effect of the polyamine spermine on erythropoiesis), whereas others are ill understood but likely contribute to altered neuromuscular and neurologic function.[35,100,101]

Another group of larger uremic toxins have been termed *middle molecules*.[35,101] These compounds are higher–molecular-weight compounds (500 to 3000 D) that are removed more readily from uremic patients by peritoneal dialysis than by hemodialysis. These compounds are not well characterized, and their existence is supported more by the difference in clinical response to peritoneal dialysis and hemodialysis in uremic human patients awaiting renal transplantation.

In addition to nitrogenous compounds, abnormal metabolism of hormones and trace minerals also accompanies the decline in renal function associated with acute and CRF. Secondary hyperparathyroidism (leading to osteodystrophy) and insulin insensitivity are well-recognized endocrine contributions to the uremic syndrome in human and small animal patients.[35,101,103,104] Endocrine dysfunction can be attributed to several factors: (1) decreased production of renal hormones (erythropoietin, vitamin D_3), (2) decreased hormone clearance prolonging plasma half-life (parathormone, gastrin), (3) decreased hormone production (testosterone), (4) tissue insensitivity (insulin, parathormone), and (5) hypersecretion to reestablish homeostasis (parathormone).[35] Regarding trace minerals, uremia may be accompanied by aluminum toxicity and zinc deficiency. Aluminum may contribute to some of the neurologic signs associated with azotemia (especially with ARF), whereas zinc has been implicated in testicular atrophy and abnormal taste in uremic human patients.[35,101] Presumed uremic encephalopathy has been reported in horses with CRF when neurologic dysfunction could not be attributed to other causes.[105] All five reported cases died or were euthanatized. Swollen astrocytes were observed histologically in all horses that were necropsied.

Clearly, because so many potential uremic toxins exert their effects as renal function declines, a single compound or even a few compounds likely will not ever be identified as the primary cause of the uremic syndrome in patients with CRF. Furthermore, these compounds together are more likely to impair basic cell function in a number of tissues, and the signs of uremia are more likely to reflect multisystemic organ dysfunction. Methylation of a number of membrane proteins recently has received considerable attention as one of the common mechanisms of cell dysfunction.[106] What is truly remarkable, however, is the tremendous adaptive capacity of the failing kidneys to maintain sodium and water balance within narrow ranges until GFR declines to 20% of the normal value or less.[107]

CLINICAL SIGNS

Horses with CRF present relatively late in the disease course, when their owners note lethargy, anorexia, and weight loss. A history of months to years of polydipsia and polyuria in some cases supports renal disease of long duration. In other animals, preexisting disease (e.g., colic, colitis, pleuropneumonia) or prolonged medication (e.g., aminoglycoside antibiotics, NSAIDs) may provide important information about the initiation and duration of renal failure. In most cases, however, the onset is insidious and identifying a precipitating event or gauging the duration of renal disease is not possible.

Chronic weight loss is the most common presenting complaint for horses with CRF.[25-30] Partial anorexia, ventral edema, polydipsia and polyuria, rough hair coat, lethargy, and poor athletic performance are other owner concerns. In addition, horses with advanced CRF may have a characteristic odor that likely reflects the combined effects of uremic halitosis and increased urea excretion in sweat. For the horses presented in Table 19-8, weight loss, ventral and peripheral edema, and polydipsia and polyuria, respectively, were reported in 53 of 63 (84%), 24 of 56 (43%), and 21 of 48 (44%) of the cases. Lethargy and weight loss can be attributed to several factors. An increase in the concentration of nitrogenous wastes in blood can have a direct central appetite-suppressant effect that can lead to partial or complete anorexia.[35,101] Next, as azotemia develops, excess urea diffuses across gastrointestinal epithelium and is metabolized to ammonia and carbon dioxide by bacterial urease. In the oral cavity, excess ammonia can lead to excessive dental tartar formation (Figure 19-25), gingivitis, and oral ulcers. In the gastrointestinal tract, excess urea and ammonia can lead to ulceration and mild to moderate protein-losing enteropathy, and severely uremic animals may produce soft feces.[1,35,101] The prolonged half-life of gastrin (eliminated through the kidneys) may contribute further to ulcer formation because of increased gastric acid secretion.[35] Finally, as the combined effects of uremic toxins render the affected patient catabolic, body mass declines as body reserves are tapped to meet basal energy requirements.[35,101]

Mild ventral edema with CRF may be attributable to three factors: (1) decreased oncotic pressure, (2) increased vascular permeability, and (3) increased hydrostatic pressure. Because albumin accounts for approximately 75% of plasma colloid oncotic pressure, decreases in albumin concentration (<2.0 g/dl) can decrease plasma oncotic pressure despite a normal total plasma protein concentration.[108,109] The effects of uremic toxins on endothelial cell membranes can alter vascular permeability, which contributes to edema.[35,101] Chronic renal insufficiency can lead to renal hypoxia and hypoperfusion, which stimulate renal juxtaglomerular cells to release renin. Activation of the renin-angiotensin system tends to elevate blood (and capillary hydrostatic) pressure and contributes to edema. Activation of the renin-angiotensin system also leads to increased sodium reabsorption in the proximal (direct effect of angiotensin II) and distal (effect of aldosterone) tubules.[109] Sodium retention leads to expansion of circulating volume, which is another factor in edema formation. Alterations in blood pressure in horses with CRF have not been evaluated routinely (as they have in small animal and human patients), and increased circulating concentrations of angiotensin II or aldosterone in horses have not been documented extensively. As a result the nephrotic syndrome (characterized by edema, hypoalbuminemia, and heavy proteinuria) is not as well documented in horses as in small animals and human beings with CRF. However, horses with CRF appear less at risk for the significant pleural effusion or ascites that can accompany the nephrotic syndrome in small animals.[1]

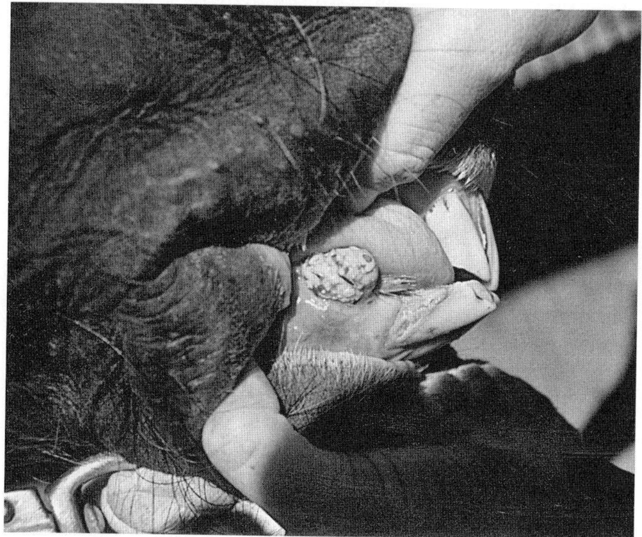

FIGURE 19-25 Excessive dental tartar on the canine tooth and lower corner incisor of a horse with chronic renal failure (CRF).

Polydipsia and polyuria are variable findings in horses with CRF. The magnitude of polydipsia and polyuria theoretically is related to the degree of tubulointerstitial damage; however, the degree of polyuria does not appear to correlate with the magnitude of azotemia in clinical cases. Typically, polyuria is not as severe with CRF as with diabetes insipidus or psychogenic water drinking and may not be noticed by an owner (see the Polyuria and Polydipsia section of this chapter). The wide variation in water intake in normal horses and common use of automatic waterers and large stock tanks also make observation of polydipsia more difficult. The mechanisms of polyuria with CRF can include (1) increased tubular flow rate in surviving nephrons, (2) decreased medullary hypertonicity, and (3) impaired response of collecting ducts to vasopressin (acquired nephrogenic diabetes insipidus). Although these mechanisms may contribute to the polyuria of CRF, which of them may be most important is not known.[1,110]

An early complaint for horses with CRF is poor performance, which may be related to mild anemia (PCV 25% to 30%) and lethargy. Although the anemia of CRF has been attributed to several factors—including blood loss, decreased erythrocyte survival time, nutritional deficiencies, and decreased erythropoietin activity—the latter clearly has emerged as the principal cause of anemia in human beings and small animals with CRF.[1,35,111] In fact, administration of recombinant human erythropoietin (rhEPO) to patients awaiting kidney transplant has been one of the most significant advances in management of human CRF because it has eliminated the need for blood transfusions, has improved exercise capacity, and has decreased morbidity associated with the uremic syndrome.[35,111] Administration of rhEPO has also benefited anemic dogs and cats with CRF, although both species may need iron supplementation to support erythropoiesis.[1,35] The response often has been only temporary because many small animal patients develop refractory anemia after production of anti-rhEPO antibodies within a few weeks to months after initiation of treatment.[1] Plasma concentrations of erythropoietin have been determined in normal horses,[112] and rhEPO administration (15 IU/kg IV, three doses per week for 3 weeks) has been reported to increase the hematocrit in splenectomized horses[113]; however, no reports describe rhEPO administration to horses with CRF. Furthermore, moderate to severe anemia that may be fatal has been reported to develop after repeated rhEPO administration to racehorses.[114-116] The risks of adverse reactions outweigh the potential benefits of rhEPO, and its use in horses should be avoided.

DIAGNOSIS AND LABORATORY EVALUATION

One establishes a diagnosis of CRF when persistent isosthenuria (specific gravity of 1.008-1.014) accompanies azotemia and typical clinical signs.[26-30,117] Rectal palpation of the left kidney may be normal or may reveal a kidney that is small or firm with an irregular surface. Less often, the kidneys and ureters may be enlarged if obstructed by uroliths or if infection or neoplasia is present. The ratio of BUN-to-Cr concentration (BUN-to-Cr ratio) in horses with CRF is typically greater than 10:1 (Table 19-9); that for horses with prerenal azotemia or ARF is often less than 10:1.[27] This difference can be attributed in part to different volumes of distribution for urea (all body fluids) and Cr (primarily the extracellular fluid space). As a consequence, with acute reductions in RBF, the increase in Cr concentration is usually greater, on a relative or percentage basis, than the increase in BUN. The point deserves emphasis, however, that BUN is influenced by dietary protein intake so that BUN-to-Cr values do not always distinguish ARF from CRF. In fact, one also can use the BUN-to-Cr ratio to assess adequacy of dietary protein intake in the management of horses with CRF because a value greater than 15:1 can reflect excessive protein intake.[29]

In addition to azotemia, further abnormal laboratory data accompanying CRF can include mild anemia, hypoalbuminemia, hyponatremia, hyperkalemia, hypochloremia, hypercalcemia, hypophosphatemia, and metabolic acidosis (see Table 19-9). A nonregenerative anemia is related largely to a deficient supply of the renally secreted glycoprotein erythropoietin; however, reduced erythrocyte life span may be another significant contributor to anemia. Normally, equine erythrocytes have a life span of 140 to 155 days.[115] With uremia, erythrocyte life span is shortened because excessive nitrogenous waste products alter the integrity of erythrocyte membranes and the function of ion channels, which regulate erythrocyte volume.[102] These less resilient erythrocytes are more likely to be removed from the circulation by the reticuloendothelial system.

The electrolyte alterations associated with CRF reflect loss of tubule function. Because sodium, chloride, bicarbonate, and phosphate are conserved by renal tubules, excessive urinary loss of these electrolytes accompanies CRF. Although fractional electrolyte clearance values (see Examination of the Urinary System) may remain within normal ranges or increase only slightly in horses with CRF, significant daily urinary loss of electrolytes still may occur. As an example, if a horse with CRF and Cr and sodium concentrations of 5.0 mg/dl and 130 mEq/L, respectively, is producing 20 L of urine daily with respective Cr and sodium concentrations of 50 mg/dl and 12.5 mEq/L, then the fractional clearance of sodium is 1.0% and daily urinary sodium loss is 250 mEq. An increase in urinary sodium concentration to 25 mEq/L after another decrease in tubular reabsorption would result in an increase in fractional sodium clearance to 2% but would represent an additional 250 mEq of daily sodium loss in the urine. The latter value would approach 1% to 2% of the exchangeable sodium in the body and would require an additional 15 g of salt intake daily to accommodate this loss. Hypercalcemia and hypophosphatemia (Williams-Smith syndrome) are fairly common findings in horses with CRF (see Table 19-9), and the degree of hypercalcemia appears to vary with the amount of calcium in the diet.[25,49,52,118] In human beings with ESKD, hypercalcemia is an occasional finding attributed to hyperparathyroidism, vitamin-D supplementation, or use of calcium-containing dialysate solutions. Furthermore, the osteodystrophy of CRF is associated with aluminum deposition in bone, which has been speculated to reduce skeletal buffering capacity for increases in serum calcium concentration and thereby contributes to hypercalcemia.[35] Because the equine kidney is an important route of calcium excretion (via $CaCO_3$ crystals), impaired tubular function in the face of continued intestinal absorption is the most common explanation for calcium accumulation in blood. This explanation is supported by the rapid development of hypercalcemia after experimental bilateral nephrectomy in ponies fed alfalfa hay (Figure 19-26).[9] In addition, parathormone concentrations have been found to be below the lower limit of detection in horses with CRF, indicating that hyperparathyroidism does not play a role in development of hypercalcemia.[23,58] However, parathormone clearance by the kidney also is reduced with CRF and may be associated with a change in the regulatory set point for serum calcium concentration in uremic human beings.[35] Whether hypercalcemia in horses with CRF leads to exacerbation of renal disease or tissue mineralization remains unknown. Nevertheless, one can demonstrate the effect of dietary calcium by changing the type of hay fed to horses with CRF. Horses with serum calcium concentrations exceeding 20 mg/dl on a diet of mostly alfalfa can have their serum calcium concentrations returned to the normal range within a few of days after changing the diet to

TABLE 19-9

Abnormal Laboratory Values Reported for Horses with Chronic Renal Failure

Parameter	Number*	Percentage
Blood urea nitrogen/serum creatinine concentrations (BUN/Cr) >10	29/34	85%
BUN/Cr >15	17/34	50%
Anemia (packed cell volume [PCV] <30%)	12/30	40%
Hypoalbuminemia (<2.5 g/dl)	12/14	86%
Hypoalbuminemia (<2.0 g/dl)	7/14	50%
Hyponatremia (Na^+ <135 mEq/L)	26/40	65%
Hyperkalemia (K^+ >5.0 mEq/L)	23/41	56%
Hypochloremia (Cl^- <95 mEq/L)	19/41	46%
Hypercalcemia (Ca^{2+} >13.5 mg/dl)	26/39	67%
Hypophosphatemia (P <1.5 mg/dl)	17/36	47%
Acidosis (pH <7.35)	3/5	60%

*Number of reports with this laboratory finding/total number of reports in which this laboratory parameter was reported.

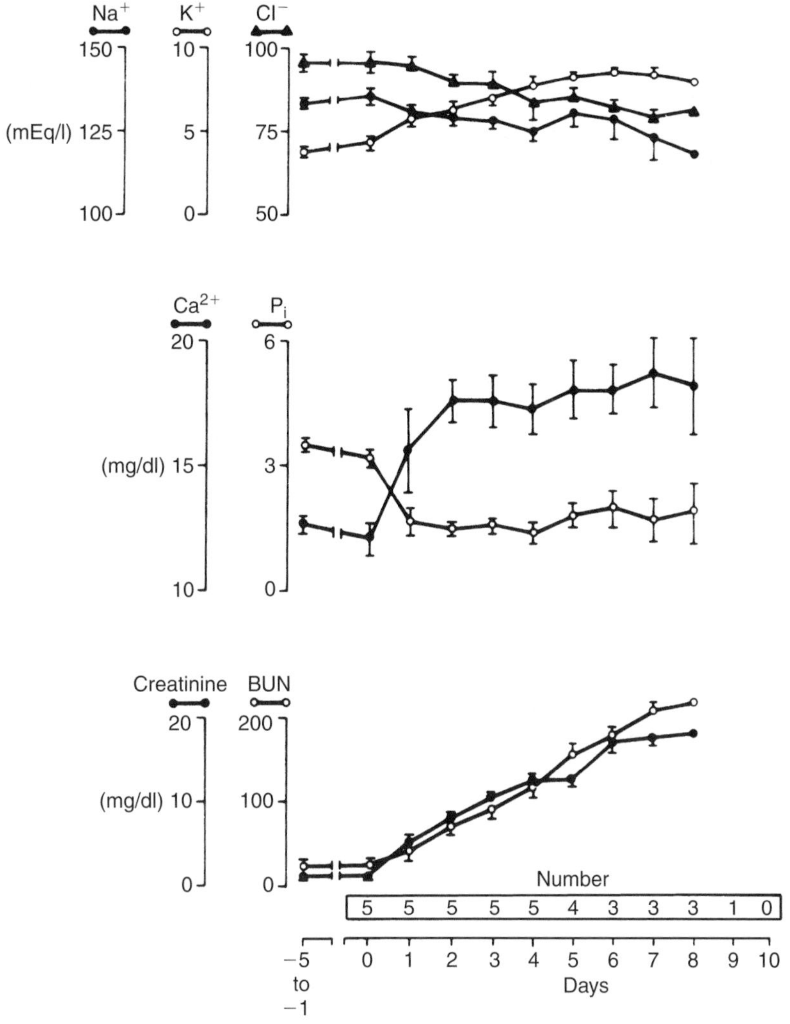

FIGURE 19-26 Changes in serum electrolyte concentrations, blood urea nitrogen (BUN) concentration, and serum creatinine (Cr) concentration after bilateral nephrectomy in Shetland ponies. (From Tennant B, Lowe JE, Tasker JB: Hypercalcemia and hypophosphatemia in ponies following bilateral nephrectomy, Proc Soc Exp Biol Med 167:365, 1981.)

grass hay.[20,27] Similarly, nephrectomized ponies fed grass hay did not become hypercalcemic.[27] The cause of hypophosphatemia in horses with CRF also remains undocumented, although it has been explained by the law of mass action, which leads to a decrease in serum phosphate concentration in association with hypercalcemia.[35,118] A similar response is not observable in horses that eat *Cestrum diurnum* (leading to a syndrome of hypervitaminosis D)—they develop hypercalcemia without hypophosphatemia.[119] Another possibility that has been suggested is that hypophosphatemia may result from long-standing anorexia associated with CRF.[58] Regardless of the cause, clinical problems associated with hypophosphatemia have not yet been recognized in horses with CRF.

A degree of metabolic acidosis accompanies CRF in human beings and small animals and is attributed to decreased ability of failing kidneys to excrete hydrogen ions and regenerate bicarbonate.[1,35] Normally, acid-base balance is maintained by reabsorption of filtered bicarbonate and excretion of hydrogen ions along with ammonia and phosphate. As renal function declines in the early stages of renal failure, hydrogen ion excretion via renal ammoniagenesis and ammonium excretion increases. As renal failure progresses, compromised renal ammoniagenesis and decreased medullary recycling of ammonia caused by structural renal damage likely contribute to impaired ammonium excretion. Because hepatic glutamine synthesis is required for renal ammoniagenesis, the earlier increase in ammonium excretion may contribute to protein malnutrition in patients with CRF.[1] Metabolic acidosis also contributes to a number of the clinical signs of the uremic syndrome and may exacerbate some of the electrolyte alterations (e.g., hyperkalemia) of CRF. Metabolic acidosis has been reported in a limited number of horses with CRF (see Table 19-9); however, in the author's experience and that of others,[26,58] most horses with CRF have normal acid-base status or are alkalotic until the terminal stages of the disease, when metabolic acidosis typically develops. Metabolic alkalosis has been attributed to enhanced bicarbonate reabsorption and production, in association with hypochloremia and increased renal ammoniagenesis, respectively. In some instances, hypochloremic metabolic alkalosis may be accompanied by paradoxical aciduria.[58] The mechanism of paradoxical aciduria is likely similar to that of hypochloremic metabolic alkalosis in ruminants with abomasal outflow obstruction.[120] Briefly, after all chloride has been reabsorbed from the glomerular filtrate, further sodium reabsorption occurs by exchange with (excretion of) potassium or hydrogen ions. Thus paradoxical aciduria is most likely to occur with concomitant hypokalemia or whole-body potassium depletion.

Horses with CRF also can develop hypercholesterolemia and hyperlipidemia (hypertriglyceridemia), and occasionally an animal has grossly lipemic plasma (hyperlipemia).[27,29,117] In fact, Naylor, Kronfeld, and Acland[121] reported a positive correlation between serum triglyceride and Cr concentrations in a group of azotemic horses. Twelve of 13 cases of hypertriglyceridemia in horses reviewed by Dunkel and McKenzie were azotemic.[122] With azotemia, hyperlipidemia can develop as a result of increased synthesis, decreased degradation, or increased mobilization of triglycerides from fat stores.[35] Lipoprotein lipase, which stimulates triglyceride uptake into cells, is inhibited by azotemia.[123] Heparin treatment (40 IU/kg subcutaneously every 8 hours) has been recommended to stimulate lipoprotein lipase in an attempt to clear the serum.[27,29] Hypercholesterolemia and hyperlipidemia increase the risk of atherosclerotic cardiovascular disease in human beings with CRF.[35] Furthermore, these conditions stimulate mesangial cell proliferation and matrix production in diseased glomeruli and thus accelerate progression to glomerulosclerosis.[124]

The failing kidneys have a tremendous adaptive capacity to maintain tubular function until GFR is low.[107] In the author's experience, tubular dysfunction resulting in significant sodium or phosphorous wasting (manifested by increased fractional clearance values), glucosuria, or enzymuria is more common with ARF than with CRF. When present, however, abnormal tubule function rarely leads to values for fractional sodium clearance in excess of 5%.[62,73,125] In contrast, loss of concentrating ability resulting in isosthenuria is a consistent feature of CRF that usually develops before azotemia. The associated polyuria may or may not be observed by the client, but the horse usually maintains water balance well through polydipsia. Polyuria typically results in urine that is clear and essentially devoid of crystals and mucus. Sediment examination is generally unremarkable, but increased numbers of red or white blood cells may occur with nephrolithiasis or ureterolithiasis or with pyelonephritis, respectively. Gross hematuria further supports lithiasis or neoplasia. One should include a quantitative urine culture in the diagnostic plan for all horses with CRF because bacteriuria may not always be accompanied by pyuria.

Alterations in the integrity of the highly anionic glomerular filtration barrier also can lead to loss of protein, predominantly albumin, in the urine. Few quantitative data are available on urinary protein loss in horses with CRF because in most previous reports proteinuria was assessed using urine reagent strips. Reagent strip results of +++ or ++++ correlate with protein concentrations of 100 to 300 and 1000 to 2000 mg/dl, respectively, depending on which reagent strip one uses. In a proteinuric horse that is producing 20 L of urine daily, these values would yield a wide range of urinary protein loss (20 to 400 g daily). The latter value would approach 25% of the total protein content of plasma and so is not realistic. In human beings with CRF, urinary protein loss exceeding 3.5 g per day (50 mg/kg per day for a 70-kg person) is classified as *nephrotic-range proteinuria,* and some patients with heavy proteinuria may lose in excess of 15 g per day (more than 200 mg/kg per day).[35] The upper limit of acceptable urinary protein excretion in dogs is 20 mg/kg per day.[126] Using these values, estimates for the upper acceptable limits for urinary protein loss and nephrotic-range proteinuria in a 500-kg horse would be 10 g and in excess of 25 g per day, respectively. These values agree well with a mean value of 3.2 mg/kg (1.6 g per day) and a range of 3.6 to 22.3 mg/kg (1.8 to 11.2 g) per day in normal mares reported by the Schott, Hodgson, and Bayly[127] and by Kohn and Strasser,[128] respectively.

Another method to document proteinuria is to determine the ratio of urinary protein to urinary Cr (in milligrams per deciliter). This technique is more practical because it avoids a timed urine collection period. Although a normal range has not yet been reported for horses, values in excess of 1.0:1 and 3.5:1 are considered above normal and indicate nephrotic-range proteinuria in dogs[126] and human beings,[35] respectively. Thus a urine protein-to-Cr ratio greater than 2.0:1 likely supports significant proteinuria in a horse with CRF. Finally, a horse with CRF and heavy proteinuria (more than 200 mg/kg per day) could excrete as much as 100 g of protein daily (5% to 7% of total plasma protein). Proteinuria of this magnitude can increase urine specific gravity to 1.020 or greater and certainly would be great enough to lead to a decline in serum albumin (and total protein) concentration, despite increased hepatic albumin production. In some horses with CRF and a normal total plasma protein concentration, increased globulin concentration offsets mild hypoalbuminemia, whereas in other cases hyperglobulinemia actually can result in an increase in total plasma protein concentration.

One can use ultrasonography to determine kidney size in horses with CRF and to evaluate for the presence of cysts or nephroliths. Horses with ESKD typically have small kidneys that are more echogenic than normal (because of sclerosis and possible tissue mineralization).[129-133] Cystoscopy also can be a useful diagnostic aid to assess urine production qualitatively in each kidney and is particularly useful when ultrasonographic imaging fails to identify a kidney.[131] Renal scintigraphy is another imaging option to detect functional renal tissue that may not be apparent by ultrasonography.[134] One can perform renal biopsy using ultrasonographic guidance to document renal disease. Unfortunately, because most horses are presented for evaluation in the later stages of disease, biopsy results typically reveal glomerular, tubular, and interstitial lesions consistent with ESKD. Rarely do the lesions provide information about the inciting cause of the renal disease unless immunofluorescence testing and electron microscopy are pursued. These require placing samples in special fixatives, in addition to the sample placed in formalin for routine histopathologic examination. In some cases, renal biopsy results supporting pyelonephritis or a congenital anomaly (dysplasia) as the cause of CRF are useful in developing a therapeutic plan or providing a prognosis.

One can assess the severity of CRF in affected horses using available sophisticated techniques. The magnitude of azotemia is the most readily available and practical parameter but is an insensitive one.[35] Azotemia becomes apparent only after 75% or more of renal function is lost. Furthermore, the degree of azotemia can vary with nonrenal factors such as diet, body mass, and hydration. In general, Cr concentration is a more reliable measure than BUN, and doubling of Cr roughly correlates to a 50% decline in GFR (see Figure 19-6). Cr concentrations in the range of 5 to 10 mg/dl indicate a significant decline in renal function, and values exceeding 15 mg/dl are consistent with a grave prognosis. In contrast,

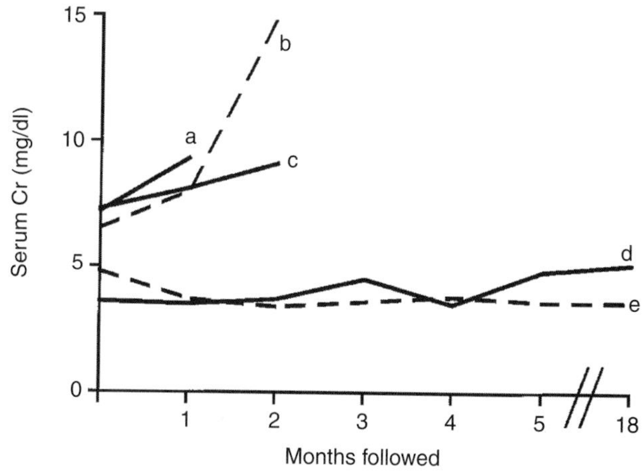

FIGURE 19-27 Serum creatinine (**Cr**) concentrations in five horses with chronic renal failure (CRF). The three horses with an initial Cr concentration greater than 5 mg/dl (**a** to **c**) had rapid progression of renal disease over a 1- to 2-month period, necessitating euthanasia, whereas the two horses with an initial Cr concentration less than 5 mg/dl (**d** and **e**) were maintained with supportive care for longer than 18 months.

horses with a Cr concentration below 5 mg/dl may exhibit few clinical signs and can be managed for months or years (Figure 19-27). Plotting the inverse of Cr concentration (1/Cr) over time also has been used to monitor progression of CRF in human beings [135,136] and in one horse[20] in an attempt to predict the end point of the disease process (Figure 19-28). Unfortunately, these plots are subject to considerable variation (because of changes in tubular secretion of Cr) and have not proved to be of any more value than monitoring Cr over time.[135,136]

Measurement of GFR provides the most accurate quantitative assessment of renal function but is pursued rarely because it is more time consuming and technically demanding than measurement of Cr concentration. Although a number of methods are available to measure GFR,[137] measurement of endogenous Cl_{Cr} or the plasma disappearance of exogenous Cr, sulfanilate,[2,138] or 99mTc-DTPA[139] are the most practical methods in a clinical setting. The former requires timed urine collections, whereas the latter may require special assays or nuclear medicine capabilities (see Examination of the Urinary System). Horses in the earlier stages of CRF can develop tubular Cr secretion, which could lead to overestimation of GFR measured by the Cl_{Cr} technique. As renal disease progresses, however, Cr excretion decreases faster than GFR declines

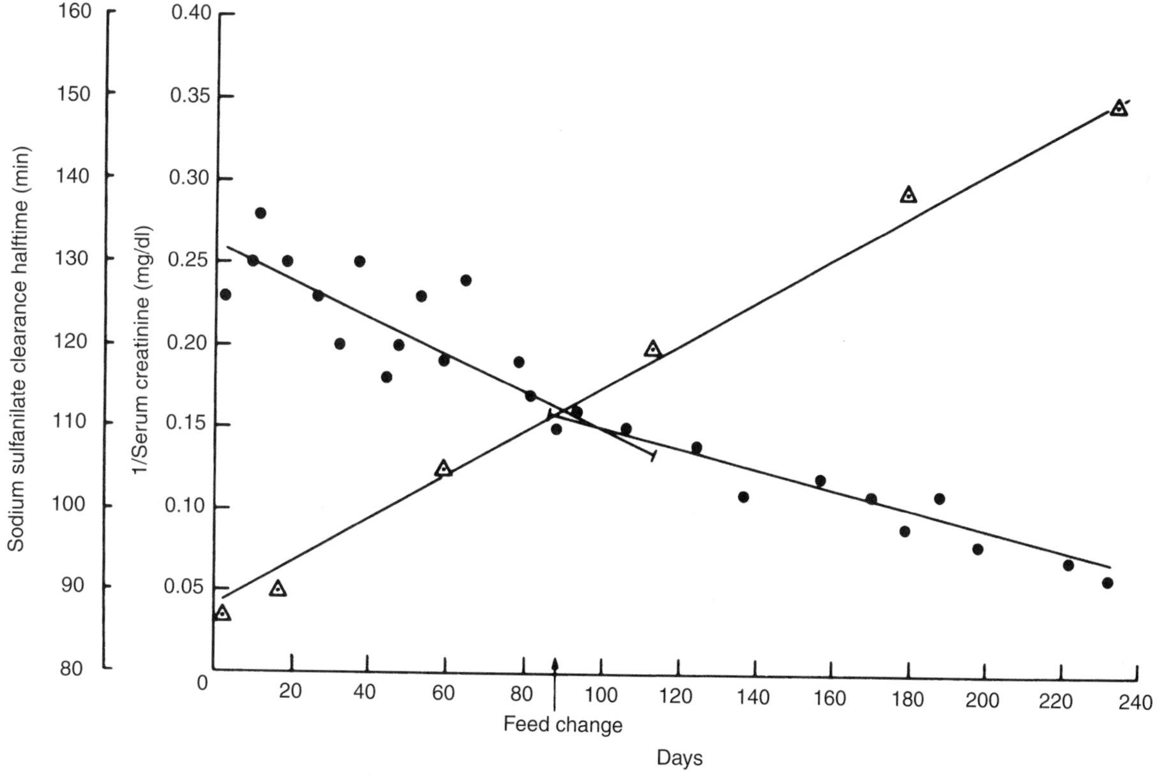

FIGURE 19-28 The inverse of the serum creatinine (Cr) concentration *(filled circles)* and the whole-blood sodium sulfanilate clearance half-time in a horse with chronic renal failure (CRF) associated with polycystic kidney disease (PKD). The slope of the line describing the reciprocals of Cr concentration from day 1 to day 98 was significantly different ($P < 0.05$) from that from day 99 to 235, and the slope change was associated with a change from alfalfa to grass hay. (From Bertone JJ, Traub-Dargatz JL, Fettman MJ et al: Monitoring the progression of renal failure in a horse with polycystic kidney disease: use of the reciprocal of serum creatinine concentration and sodium sulfanilate clearance half-time, J Am Vet Med Assoc 191:565, 1987.)

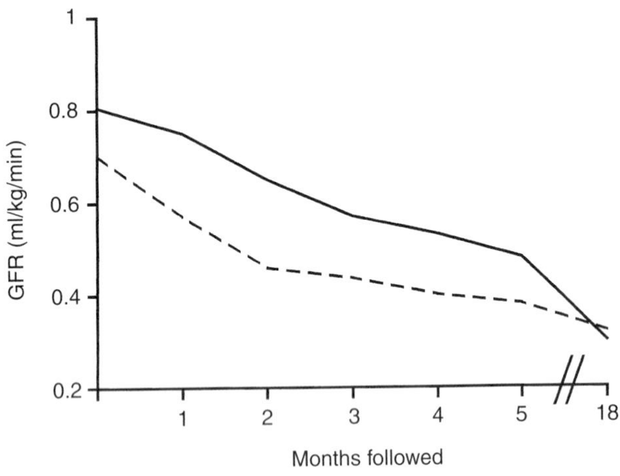

FIGURE 19-29 Glomerular filtration rate (GFR) as measured by endogenous creatinine clearance (Cl_{Cr}) *(solid line)* and inulin clearance (Cl_{In}) *(dashed line)* in a mare (see horse in Figure 19-28) with chronic renal failure (CRF). GFR declined steadily over the 18-month period, despite minimal change in serum creatinine (Cr) concentration. Compared with Cl_{In}, endogenous Cl_{Cr} overestimated GFR until the terminal stage of the disease process. This difference likely reflects tubule secretion of Cr in the earlier stages of CRF, which subsequently diminished during the final weeks of the disease course.

because of loss of compensatory secretion. Despite these limitations, repeated measurement of Cl_{Cr} in a single animal can be useful for monitoring progression of CRF over time (Figure 19-29).

DISEASE PROGRESSION

One of the hallmarks of CRF is the progressive nature of the disease,[140-142] and progression appears to be largely independent of the inciting cause because of the final common pathways of renal injury. The response to a decrease in renal functional mass is a compensatory increase in filtration (termed *single-nephron GFR*) and tubular function (e.g., Cr secretion, ammoniagenesis) by remaining nephrons. The increase in single-nephron GFR results from increased glomerular capillary blood flow and hydrostatic pressure leading to glomerular hyperfiltration. Hyperfiltration is associated with increased permeability of the GBM and proteinuria. Furthermore, increased filtration of macromolecules leads to activation and proliferation of mesangial and epithelial cells and eventually progression to glomerulosclerosis.[35,108,140-142] In addition to causing proteinuria, increased filtration of protein is accompanied by increased proximal tubular protein reabsorption. The latter leads to upregulation of genes encoding vasoactive and inflammatory mediators by tubular and interstitial cells and contributes substantially to injury of the renal interstitium.[142]

A number of studies investigating the mechanisms of glomerular hypertension have demonstrated that activation of the renin-angiotensin system and angiotensin II production are of considerable importance, because angiotensin II is a potent constrictor of glomerular efferent arterioles.[143-145] Activation of the intrarenal renin-angiotensin system can produce significant glomerular hypertension without producing increases in systemic angiotensin II concentration or blood pressure. In fact, administration of specific angiotensin II receptor antagonists or angiotensin-converting enzyme inhibitors has been demonstrated to decrease glomerular capillary hydrostatic pressure and the magnitude of proteinuria in experimental studies of renal disease.[143-146] Angiotensin-converting enzyme inhibitors have helped to control hypertension and proteinuria in small animals,[1,147] but no reports describe use of angiotensin-converting enzyme inhibitors in horses with CRF.

The role of dietary protein in the progression of CRF has been the subject of a number of investigations in human beings and small animals with a variety of renal diseases.[148-153] A well-established fact is that one can ameliorate clinical signs of uremia by decreasing dietary protein content; however, whether decreasing dietary protein slows progression of renal disease remains controversial. Increased dietary protein has been demonstrated to increase activation of the renin-angiotensin system; therefore decreasing dietary protein could be protective for the reasons discussed in the preceding paragraph. Next, a decrease in protein intake leads to production of smaller amounts of urea and other nitrogenous wastes. In theory, the workload on the kidneys is similarly decreased. Because all work (aerobic ATP production and use) is associated with a degree of free radical production, greater protein intake would generate more free radicals. Free radicals appear to be especially injurious to diseased kidneys because their scavenging mechanisms are compromised. Increased dietary protein also requires increased ammoniagenesis by renal tubules to excrete the associated proton load; however, ammoniagenesis can lead to noninflammatory, nonimmune complement activation in proximal tubule epithelial cells. One can ameliorate this proinflammatory consequence of ammoniagenesis by supplementation with sodium bicarbonate. In summary, excessive dietary protein leads to a greater degree of uremia and has the potential to exacerbate renal damage in CRF by several mechanisms.

In contrast, protein-calorie malnutrition is associated strongly with increased morbidity and mortality in human CRF patients and can be attributed to increased protein catabolism when dietary protein intake is marginal to low. In human beings a number of serum components, including prealbumin, cholesterol, and insulin-like growth factor; plasma and muscle amino acid profiles; and body composition measurements have been studied as potential indexes of nutritional status. However, serum albumin concentration is the most practical and most extensively studied nutritional index. In addition to heavy proteinuria, hypoalbuminemia also can be attributed to protein-calorie malnutrition. Furthermore, a BUN-to-Cr ratio less than 10:1 may be another indication of inadequate protein intake. Thus current dietary recommendations call for dietary protein and caloric intake at levels that meet or slightly exceed predicted requirements, which should render nitrogen balance neutral.[154] Finally, a critically important but often overlooked aspect of nutritional management of CRF patients is provision of a palatable diet.[1,154] Feeding smaller meals more frequently and varying the diet help to increase food intake in CRF patients of all species.

Experimental studies of CRF in horses are limited to reports that describe the effects of prolonged daily dosing of horses with mercurial compounds.[155-158] In these four reports, each involving a single horse, the subjects were destroyed between 85 and 191 days after mercury administration began. Anorexia, weight loss, and nonpruritic urticaria were the major clinical signs. The renal lesion was CIN, which was accompanied by a decrease in concentrating ability and an increase in water consumption. Additional tubular dysfunction included glucosuria in all four horses and a variable degree of proteinuria. Interestingly, the clinical signs and tubular dysfunction preceded the development of azotemia in all horses, and excretion of sodium or chloride did not increase. The final report focused principally on the effects on renal function, and azotemia did not develop until the final week of life; GFR (assessed by endogenous Cl_{Cr}) decreased to 35% of the highest measured value on the day before euthanasia.[158] Aciduria and increased phosphate excretion, in addition to glucosuria and proteinuria, also were detected during the final week of life.

TREATMENT

At the time of presentation most horses with CRF exhibit obvious weight loss and other clinical signs. Because of the progressive and irreversible nature of the renal disease, the long-term prognosis is grave. Specific corrective treatment for CRF (renal transplantation) is not available for horses, and maintenance by peritoneal dialysis or hemodialysis would only be practical for valuable breeding animals. Pyelonephritis could be considered an exception because antibiotic treatment in theory could lead to resolution of infection and improved renal function. Unfortunately, significant renal damage usually has occurred by the time the diagnosis is established in most cases of bilateral pyelonephritis, so the prognosis for a return to normal renal function is guarded to poor. In contrast, the short-term prognosis may be more favorable. Some horses with CRF may maintain Cr concentration of less than 5 mg/dl for months with minimal deterioration. To predict which patients will deteriorate more rapidly is difficult, but the recent history and initial ability to counteract weight loss with improved management are useful indicators. Laboratory analysis of blood samples at 2- to 4-week intervals to follow the degree of azotemia and serum electrolyte alterations may be useful in monitoring disease progression. In general, animals that are eating well and maintain reasonable body condition carry the best short-term prognosis and may still be able to perform some limited work. Their use as breeding animals may be reduced because azotemia and eventual weight loss would reduce the chance for normal conception and gestation. The goal in each case is to provide appropriate supportive care and to monitor the horse closely so as to provide humane euthanasia before the patient develops uremic decompensation.

As previously discussed, once significant renal disease is established, irreversible decline in GFR and progression of renal failure generally ensue.[35,140-142] Thus management of the equine patient afflicted with CRF involves palliative efforts to minimize further loss of renal function. The goals are to prevent complicating conditions (e.g., by providing plenty of water), to discontinue administration of nephrotoxic agents, and to provide a palatable diet to encourage appetite and minimize further weight loss.[27-30,159] Intravenous fluid therapy to promote diuresis, usually with 0.9% NaCl solution, is of much greater benefit in cases of acute, reversible renal failure but also may benefit patients that suffer a sudden exacerbation of CRF. One must administer intravenous fluid therapy cautiously because horses with CRF can develop significant peripheral or pulmonary edema.

Supportive care also can include supplementation of sodium bicarbonate (50 to 150 g per day) when serum bicarbonate concentration is consistently less than 20 mEq/L.[159] One may need to add supplemental bicarbonate to a bran mash. If sodium bicarbonate supplementation aggravates ventral edema, then one should limit or discontinue supplementation. Edema is not usually a significant problem, and the horse should tolerate mild edema (rather than being treated with diuretics that could be ineffective or lead to further electrolyte wastage) unless the edema interferes with ambulation. In a previous edition of this text, the author also recommended supplementation with NaCl to replace potential loss of these electrolytes in urine in horses with CRF. However, a recent study[160] found that supplementation with NaCl (used in an attempt to increase water intake) in cats with preexisting renal disease led to progression of renal disease that remained after salt supplementation was discontinued. Thus one should approach salt supplementation in horses with CRF with caution and should consider it only for patients with hyponatremia and hypochloremia.

Substituting high-calcium and high-protein feed sources such as alfalfa hay with good quality grass hay and carbohydrates (corn and oats) may help control hypercalcemia and the magnitude of azotemia. Ideally, the hay and grain should contain an adequate but not excessive amount of protein (<10% crude protein), which should maintain the BUN-to-Cr ratio in a target range between 10:1 and 15:1.[27] Providing unlimited access to fresh water and encouraging adequate energy intake by feeding a variety of palatable feeds are important. In fact, if appetite for grass hay deteriorates, then offering less ideal feeds (e.g., alfalfa hay, increased amounts of concentrate) to meet energy requirements and reduce the rate of weight loss is preferable. Often horses continue to graze at pasture when their appetite for hay is diminished. Administration of B vitamins or anabolic steroids for their touted appetite-stimulating effects may benefit some animals. Although dietary fat is calorie dense, one must approach supplementation judiciously in patients with hyperlipidemia and hypercholesterolemia.

Administration of corticosteroids or NSAIDs can limit the intrarenal inflammatory response associated with renal failure and also may attenuate renal injury. For example, administration of meclofenamate limited proteinuria in a group of human patients with severe manifestations of the nephrotic syndrome[161]; however, nonspecific blockade of prostaglandin production by corticosteroids and most available NSAIDs has the adverse effect of decreasing production of important renal vasodilating agents (prostaglandin E_2 and prostacyclin). Production of these prostanoids increases during periods of renal vasoconstriction or ischemia to maintain intra-RBF, particularly to the renal medulla. With excessive or long-term NSAID administration, renal papillary necrosis develops after medullary ischemia.[61,62,69,86] Thus the negative effects of corticosteroids and NSAIDs on RBF outweigh possible benefits, and they are not recommended routinely for the management of CRF in horses.

The progressive renal injury that occurs in CRF is associated with continued damage to glomerular and tubular membranes mediated by ongoing activation of the inflammatory cascade. In theory, treatment with antioxidant medications and free radical scavengers could be of benefit, but experimental data in horses do not bear this out. Similarly, interest in the role of dietary fatty acids as precursors of eicosanoids has been considerable. Specifically, dietary supplementation with sources rich in ω-3 fatty acids (linolenic acid) compared with ω-6 fatty acids (linoleic acid), appear to decrease generation of more damaging fatty acid metabolites during activation of the inflammatory cascade. In horses, dietary supplementation with ω-3 fatty acids (in the form of linseed oil) has been effective at ameliorating the effects of endotoxin in studies in vitro[162-164] and supplementation with fish oil (another rich source of ω-3 fatty acids) slowed the progression of renal failure in laboratory animals.[165,166] Unfortunately, the effects of endotoxin in vivo were not ameliorated by feeding linseed oil in preliminary equine studies,[167] and the possible benefits of feeding ω-3 fatty acids to horses with CRF are not known at this time.

Recently, control of hypertension and reduction of proteinuria have been recognized as the most successful interventions to limit progression of renal disease in human beings with CRF.[142] Thus monitoring the blood pressure and the level of proteinuria (urine protein-to-urine Cr ratio) in horses with CRF seems to be prudent. Treatment with angiotensin-converting enzyme inhibitors could be beneficial in horses with either of these problems but has not yet been pursued because of the expense of the available medications. Attention also has been directed to use of more specific anti-inflammatory or immunosuppressant medications to limit renal injury in immune-mediated glomerulonephritis. For example, inhibition of thromboxane synthetase activity (thromboxane A_2 is a potent vasoconstricting agent and platelet activator) was demonstrated to limit renal histologic and functional changes in a canine model of immune-mediated glomerulonephritis.[168] Similarly, cyclosporine was used as an adjunct treatment in a prospective study of naturally occurring canine glomerulonephritis. Unfortunately, renal function declined in cyclosporine-treated dogs, as it did in control dogs. The lack of any beneficial effect, along with the adverse reactions to cyclosporine, led to the conclusion that cyclosporine was of no use for treating CRF.[169] As these studies demonstrate, specific manipulation of the inflammatory or immune response can limit renal injury when one can administer medications before or early in the course of renal disease; however, with long-standing, naturally occurring disease, such treatments are much less likely to retard progression of renal failure significantly. Finally, other investigators are focusing on developing therapeutic strategies that may modulate or limit renal fibrosis. Their studies of the effects of cytokines, lymphokines, and proteoglycans on matrix synthesis and degradation by mesangial cells and on fibroblast activation in damaged glomeruli may lead to novel treatment options in the future.[170,171]

URINARY TRACT INFECTIONS

Harold C. Schott II

In human beings, bacterial UTIs are among the most common infections.[1] In contrast, bacterial UTIs appear to be uncommon in horses.[2-5] As in other species, ascending UTIs are more common, although septic nephritis may be an occasional consequence of septicemia, especially in neonatal foals.[6] Mares are at higher risk for UTIs than geldings or stallions because of their shorter urethra.

Development of a UTI requires initial urethral colonization with pathogenic bacteria, entry of pathogens into the bladder, and subsequent multiplication in the bladder.[1,9] Urethral colonization involves adherence to uroepithelial cells, typically by fecal bacteria that possess fimbrial adhesins (pili) that bind to specific glycolipid receptors on uroepithelial cells. Not surprisingly, pathogenic *Escherichia coli* are rich in these specific surface adhesins, whereas nonpathogenic *E. coli* have few specific surface adhesins. Further characterization of human pathogenic *E. coli* strains by their somatic (O), flagellar (H), and capsular (K) antigens has revealed that a small number of *E. coli* strains are responsible for a large percentage of UTIs.[1,8,9] Normal vulvar and preputial flora protect against urethral colonization by pathogenic bacteria, but any anatomic defect leading to turbulent urine flow compromises maintenance of normal flora and may increase the likelihood of colonization by pathogens.[10,11] Although broodmares have not been proved to be at greater risk, intercourse is a well-established risk factor for development of UTIs in women. In addition, human prostatic secretions contain a heat-stable cationic protein that has potent antibacterial activity.[1] Thus stallions may be at lower risk than geldings for UTIs.

Once a pathogen has colonized the distal urethra, rapid proliferation between micturitions allows invasion of the proximal urethra and bladder, which do not have a protective flora. Host defenses in the bladder include immunoglobulins in urine and a mucopolysaccharide layer rich in glycosaminoglycans covering the uroepithelial surface.[8,9] Production of protective glycosaminoglycans is under hormonal control by estrogen and progesterone in rabbits.[12] Thus lack of these hormonal effects has been suggested as an explanation for the increased risk for UTIs in prepubertal and postmenopausal women and in spayed dogs.[7] Furthermore, women with recurrent UTIs have been speculated to have decreased concentrations of secretory immunoglobulin A in their urine.[13] Although continued urine production dilutes proliferating bacteria, once pathogens have gained access to the bladder, the rate of replication far outweighs any dilution effect and allows the UTI to become established.[1] Although antibiotic therapy is highly effective in eliminating most UTIs, recurrent UTIs can be a challenge to manage. In addition to thorough evaluation to eliminate predisposing factors in these patients, one may consider additional approaches to prevention. For example, fimbrial vaccines are effective against experimental UTIs in monkeys.[8]

URETHRITIS

Bacterial urethritis has been described as a cause of hemospermia in stallions[14,15]; however, with the exception of traumatic, parasitic (habronemiasis), or neoplastic conditions of the penis or urethra that interfere with urine flow, the author is unaware of documented cases of primary bacterial urethritis resulting in dysuria.[16,17] Furthermore, hemospermia likely attributable to urethritis in a number of previous cases probably resulted from proximal urethral defects, which have become easier to identify with high-resolution videoendoscopy (see Hematuria).[18] Bacterial infections of accessory sex glands or the prepuce also may cause dysuria. Accessory sex gland infections generally are limited to intact males and are more likely to cause infertility or hemospermia than dysuria.[16,19] Preputial infections can occur after trauma, presence of a foreign body, habronemiasis, or neoplasia, and affected horses typically have a malodorous, swollen sheath. Examination of the sheath and penis, along with biopsy of abnormal tissue, allows diagnosis of the primary problem. Occasionally, an older gelding may develop recurrent sheath swelling or infection that cannot be attributed to a primary disease process. The pathogenesis of this problem is not known, although fat accumulation, poor hygiene, and inactivity may be contributing factors. Treatment involves repeated sheath cleaning, application of topical anti-inflammatory and antibacterial ointments, and when involvement is more severe, systemic antibiotic administration.

CYSTITIS

Primary cystitis is uncommon in horses, and a predisposing cause should be ruled out whenever cystitis is suspected. Bacterial cystitis is usually a secondary problem that may accompany alterations in urine flow caused by urolithiasis, bladder neoplasia, bladder paralysis, an anatomic defect of the bladder or urethra, or instrumentation of the urinary tract (e.g., catheterization, endoscopy).[2-5,10,11,20-24] Dysuria may be manifested by pollakiuria, stranguria, hematuria, or pyuria. One may observe scalding and accumulation of urine crystals on the perineum of affected mares or on the front of the hindlimbs of affected male horses. One should not confuse these findings with normal estrous activity in the mare. Although nosocomial UTIs are a well-documented problem in hospitalized human[1] and small animal patients,[25] this complication has not been well-recognized in equine patients except for ill neonatal foals. Diagnostic evaluation includes physical and rectal examinations and collection of a urine sample for urinalysis and quantitative bacterial culture. In the absence of uroliths or other bladder masses, transrectal palpation of the bladder is usually within normal limits; however, endoscopic and ultrasonographic examination of the bladder may be helpful in assessing mucosal damage and wall thickening in horses with cystitis.[26,27] Because normal equine urine is rich in mucus and crystals, gross examination may be unrewarding, but sediment examination may reveal increased numbers of white blood cells (more than 10 leukocytes per high-power field) and presence of bacteria in some cases of cystitis. Normal sediment examination results do not rule out UTI. A definitive diagnosis requires quantitative culture results exceeding 10,000 colony-forming units (CFUs) per milliliter in a urine sample collected by midstream catch or urethral catheterization.[3,5,28] For best results, one should evaluate urine sediment within 30 to 60 minutes of collection and should cool samples for culture during transport because bacterial numbers may increase in samples left at room temperature. Organisms that may be recovered on culture include *Escherichia coli*, *Proteus* spp., *Klebsiella* spp., *Enterobacter* spp., *Streptococcus* spp., *Staphylococcus* spp., *Pseudomonas aeruginosa*, and rarely *Corynebacterium renale*.[2-5,22] Isolation of more than one organism is common. *Salmonella* spp. occasionally have been isolated from the urine of apparently healthy horses, and *Candida* spp. infections of the lower urinary tract also have been documented in sick neonatal foals receiving broad spectrum antibiotics.[2,3]

Successful treatment of bacterial cystitis requires correction of predisposing problems such as urolithiasis and administration of systemic antibiotics. Ideally, selection of an antibiotic is based on the results of susceptibility testing of isolated organisms, and the initial recommended course of treatment traditionally has been at least 1 week.[2-5] A trimethoprim-sulfonamide combination, ampicillin, penicillin, and an aminoglycoside, or ceftiofur can be initial choices. In human beings with uncomplicated cystitis, single-dose antimicrobial therapy, which is less costly and is associated with fewer adverse effects, has a success rate comparable with that of longer-term conventional therapy (75% or greater). Furthermore, relapse after single-dose therapy is not accompanied by more severe clinical signs or more extensive urinary tract involvement[1]; however, if clinical signs recur after treatment is discontinued, then one should repeat urine culture along with additional diagnostic evaluation to determine a cause for altered urine flow or bacterial persistence.

Treatment of recurrent UTI usually requires long-term medication (4 to 6 weeks), and ease of administration and cost become additional considerations in antibiotic selection. Trimethoprim-sulfonamide combinations and the penicillins are excreted via the kidneys and concentrated in urine. Although results of in vitro susceptibility testing of isolated pathogens may reveal resistance, these drugs may have effective antimicrobial activity against the causative organisms because of the high concentrations achieved in urine.[5] Metabolism of the antibiotic is another consideration. For example, sulfamethoxazole is metabolized mostly to inactive products before urinary excretion, whereas sulfadiazine is excreted mostly unchanged in urine.[29]

Additional treatments for recurrent UTI can include supplementation with 50 to 75 g of loose salt to the diet[7] or provision of warm water during cold weather in an attempt to increase water intake and urine production. Administration of the urine-acidifying agent ammonium chloride (20 to 40 mg/kg PO daily) also has been recommended in cases of cystitis and urolithiasis.[20] Use of ammonium chloride at this dose, however, has not produced a consistent decrease in urine pH. Recently, use of larger oral doses of ammonium chloride (60 to 520 mg/kg/day),[30-32] methionine (1 g/kg every 24 hours), vitamin C (1 to 2 g/kg/day),[33] or ammonium sulfate (175 mg/kg/day)[34] were more successful in reducing urine pH to less than 6.0 in a limited number of horses; however, at these doses, medications were usually unpalatable and had to be administered by dose syringe or stomach tube. Adding grain to the diet is another simple way to decrease urine pH, although the decline is modest and urine pH typically remains greater than 7.0.[33] A final treatment aid is bladder lavage. This procedure most benefits horses with accumulations of large amounts of crystalloid material in the bladder, a condition that has been termed *sabulous urolithiasis*.[34] Whenever sabulous urolithiasis is present, neurologic control of bladder function should be assessed. Incomplete emptying of the bladder can result in excessive accumulation of urinary sediment. Although one can add a number of antiseptics to the sterile polyionic lavage fluid, the most important consideration is adequate volume to flush the crystalline debris completely from the bladder. Concurrent cystoscopy is a useful tool to assess the efficacy of bladder lavage.

One report of experimental induction of cystitis in equids exists.[35] After chemical irritation of the bladder mucosa, 2.5×10^{13} CFUs of *Proteus mirabilis* were instilled into the bladders of nine female ponies. Three days later all ponies demonstrated stranguria, and culture results yielded 20,000 to 100,000 CFUs/ml of *P. mirabilis*. Sediment examination revealed increased numbers of white blood cells (more than 10 per high-power field) in seven of nine ponies, and bacteria were observed in all samples (although in low numbers of one to three per high-power field). In two untreated ponies, the cystitis resolved spontaneously between 2 and 4 weeks after inoculation; however, resolution was complete within 3 to 6 days in ponies treated with a trimethoprim-sulfadiazine combination.

Epizootics of cystitis also have been reported in the Southwestern United States[22,36] and in Australia.[37] In the former reports a syndrome of ataxia and urinary incontinence was associated with ingestion of Sudan grass and Johnson grass (hybrids of *Sorghum* spp.). Both problems were attributed to sublethal intoxication with hydrocyanic acid in the plants, which resulted in demyelination of the lower spinal cord and bladder paralysis. Pyelonephritis was often the cause of death in affected horses.[36] Another outbreak of cystitis, manifested by hematuria more than incontinence, occurred in the Northern Territories and Western Australia in 1963.[37] The kidneys and ureters were not affected, and ataxia was not observed in these horses. The problem, which resulted in loss of more than 200 horses, began shortly after the end of the wet season. Affected horses were on range pasture and, although this was not proved, a fungal toxin was suspected because sporidesmin (a toxin produced by *Pithomyces chartarum*) was known to cause bladder lesions in sheep and cattle. An environmental cause was substantiated further when no additional cases developed in 1964, after a "dry" wet season.

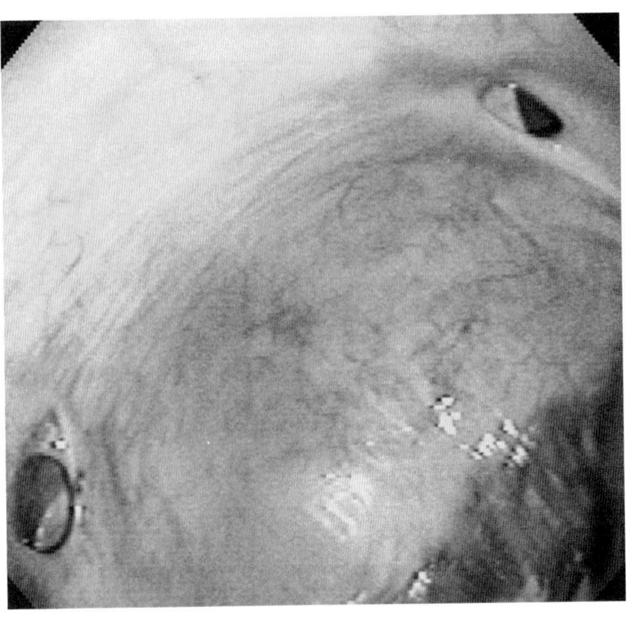

FIGURE 19-30 Endoscopic image of the bladder of a pony mare with recurrent cystitis and pyelonephritis. The ureteral openings were distended easily by insufflation of the bladder with air. Ureteral dilation resulted from long-term vesiculoureteral reflux.

PYELONEPHRITIS

Upper UTIs involving the kidneys and ureters are rare in horses.[2,3,5] The course of the distal segment of the ureters in the dorsal bladder wall creates a physical barrier or valve to prevent VUR, a prerequisite for ascending pyelonephritis. VUR is more common in children because the intramural portion of the distal ureter lengthens with growth. Furthermore, congenital VUR often occurs in families, which suggests a genetic tendency for the problem, which has been associated with developmental anomalies of the intramural insertion of one or both ureters.[1] More obvious problems that interfere with this barrier and increase the risk for VUR and associated upper UTIs include ectopic ureter or bladder distention, which may occur with bladder paralysis or urethral obstruction. Over time, VUR leads to progressive ureteral dilation and renal scarring (Figure 19-30). This effect explains the common finding of ureteral dilation in young horses with ectopic ureters and provides further support for unilateral nephrectomy, rather than reimplantation of the ureter, as the treatment of choice for ectopic ureter.[38,39] In addition to VUR, intrarenal reflux also is required to initiate renal damage predisposing the parenchyma to ascending infection. The renal papillae contain collections of papillary duct openings. These are typically conical structures that protrude into the renal pelvis. Similar to the protective nature of the intramural ureteral segment against VUR, this morphology protects against intrarenal reflux; however, in human infants and young pigs, a second type of large, concave, "refluxing" papillae also have been described in the areas of the renal pelvis most often affected with renal scarring.[1] Thus VUR and intrarenal reflux are important in development of pyelonephritis.

The role of recurrent lower UTI in the development of pyelonephritis is less clear. For example, pyelonephritic scarring (without infection) can develop after high-pressure urinary tract obstruction (urethrolithiasis) and can predispose to future upper UTI. In contrast, many cases of recurrent cystitis never proceed to involve the upper urinary tract.[1] Because the kidneys are densely vascular organs, septic nephritis may develop in association with septicemia in neonatal or adult horses.[6] Unless renal involvement is extensive, the upper UTI may go undetected but could lead to development of nephrolithiasis or CRF months to years later. As in the bladder, defense mechanisms within the normal kidney act to minimize bacterial colonization and proliferation. Efficacy of renal clearance varies with the species of bacteria entering the kidney. In addition, obstruction to urine flow (unilateral ureterolithiasis or nephrolithiasis) increases, rather than decreases, the risk of bacterial proliferation in the obstructed kidney.

Pyelonephritis in horses has been described in association with urolithiasis, recurrent cystitis, and bladder paralysis.[2,3,5,21,36] Other causes have included accidental amputation of the penis during castration,[40] foreign bodies in the bladder,[41] and lower urinary tract neoplasia.[23,42] With pyelonephritis, dysuria is manifested by hematuria or pyuria rather than stranguria and pollakiuria (as for cystitis). In addition, horses with upper UTIs generally have other clinical signs, including fever, weight loss, anorexia, or depression.[2,3,5,41-49] Upper UTIs also can be accompanied by nephrolithiasis or ureterolithiasis or both.[49] In such cases, whether lithiasis or infection develops first or whether both are consequences of VUR, intrarenal reflux, and renal parenchymal damage is unclear. In an occasional case, small uroliths may travel down the ureter and lead to recurrent urethral obstruction with renal colic as the presenting complaint.

As for cystitis, diagnostic evaluation includes physical and rectal examinations, urinalysis, and a quantitative urine culture. Careful palpation may allow detection of an enlarged ureter or kidney, although the kidney also may become shrunken in long-standing cases. In addition to the organisms causing cystitis, one also can isolate *Actinobacillus equuli, Streptococcus equi* subsp. *equi, Rhodococcus equi,* or *Salmonella* spp. from horses with hematogenous septic nephritis.[3,6] In horses with upper UTIs, one should perform a CBC and serum biochemistry profile to assess the systemic inflammatory response and renal function. Finally, cystoscopy (including watching for urine flow from each ureteral opening) and ultrasonographic imaging of the bladder, ureters, and kidneys are helpful adjunct diagnostic procedures.[26,27] Ureteral catheterization (by passing polyethylene tubing via the biopsy channel of the endoscope or by using a No. 8-10 French polypropylene catheter, which can be passed blind in mares) may allow collection of urine samples from each ureter to distinguish unilateral from bilateral disease.[50]

Treatment for upper UTIs includes a prolonged course of appropriate systemic antibiotics (selected based on susceptibility testing results on isolated pathogens). In select cases with unilateral disease, one may consider surgical removal of the affected kidney and ureter.[16,44,51] Prerequisites for a nephrectomy include documentation of unilateral disease by normal laboratory results for renal function (absence of azotemia), recovery of insignificant numbers of bacteria (fewer than 10,000 CFUs/ml) from urine collected from the ureter leading to the nonaffected kidney, and ultrasonographic evidence of abnormal structure (e.g., fluid-filled structures, nephrolithiasis) in the affected kidney. Alternatively, poor response to several weeks of appropriate antimicrobial therapy and recurrence of clinical signs of pyelonephritis are additional indications for nephrectomy. Unfortunately, successful treatment of bilateral pyelonephritis is rare, but the poor prognosis likely is related to failure to establish the diagnosis until late in the disease course.

PARASITIC INFECTIONS

One occasionally finds parasitic lesions associated with the nematodes *Strongylus vulgaris*, *Halicephalobus* (previously *Micronema*) *deletrix*, and *Dioctophyme renale* in equine kidneys.[52] Although larval migration of *S. vulgaris* in the renal artery and parenchyma is considered aberrant,[53] larval migration was found in more than 20% of horses in one abattoir survey. Passage through renal tissue may result in infarction or subcapsular or pelvic hemorrhage when parasites localize in these sites.[54] Although rare, *H. deletrix* infection is often life threatening because of CNS involvement leading to a variety of neurologic deficits that generally require euthanasia.[55-59] *Halicephalobus deletrix* has been suggested to be the most important cause of verminous meningoencephalomyelitis in horses.[60] Only the female parasite has been identified in equine tissues, typically in highly vascular organs. One usually finds large, granulomatous lesions that are full of the rhabditiform nematodes in the kidneys. The life cycle of *H. deletrix* is unknown, but the apparent saprophyte appears to have worldwide distribution. The finding of gingival lesions and oral granulomata in some horses suggests that ingestion is the likely route of infection. Attempts to find nematode larvae or eggs in urine have been unsuccessful, and whether the horse is an accidental host or is important for the life cycle of the parasite is unclear.[55] The free-living form is found in decaying organic debris (e.g., tree stumps) and also has been described to affect human beings.[59] Antemortem diagnosis has not been made, and CSF cytologic changes in affected horses cannot differentiate between nematodiasis and protozoal encephalomyelitis.[58] Renal involvement is typically inapparent, although one affected horse demonstrated a 2-week course of stranguria and polyuria before onset of neurologic deficits.[56] *Dioctophyme renale* is a large, bright-red nematode, and the female may reach 100 cm in length. The typical hosts are carnivorous species, but the parasite occasionally affects horses that ingest the intermediate host (annelid worm) while grazing or drinking from natural water sources.[61] Once localized in the kidney, the parasite may live 1 to 3 years; eggs are shed in the urine. The parasite completely destroys the renal parenchyma, and death of the parasite leads to shrinking of the host kidney into a fibrous mass. Occasionally, hydronephrosis or renal hemorrhage may be a serious complication of parasitic infection.[62,63]

In contrast to the nematodes, infection with the coccidian parasite *Klossiella equi* appears common, yet no reports describe clinical disease associated with this coccidial infection.[64-69] Although disorders accompanied by immunosuppression have been suggested to increase its likelihood, *K. equi* infection is still considered an incidental finding in affected horses. The life cycle has not been elucidated fully, but one proposal is that ingested sporocysts (or sporozoites) enter the bloodstream and undergo schizogony in endothelial cells of the glomeruli. Merozoites are released into the urinary space and undergo one or more additional rounds of schizogony in tubular epithelial cells. Eventually, a population of merozoites develops into microgametes and macrogametes. Little evidence of an inflammatory response to parasite replication in renal tissues is apparent. Sporogony follows with the subsequent release of sporocysts into the urine.[65,69] Although *K. equi* has not been associated with clinical disease, it warrants mention that the organism has been found worldwide in horses, ponies, donkeys, burros, and zebras, and a recent postmortem survey of 47 horses in Australia revealed that six (12.8%) were infected.[69]

OBSTRUCTIVE DISEASE OF THE URINARY TRACT

Harold C. Schott II

Most cases of obstructive urinary tract disease in horses are caused by urolithiasis. Urinary tract displacement, trauma, and neoplasia are other causes.[1-3] Urinary tract obstruction can result in a variety of clinical signs depending on the site and degree of obstruction. Incomplete obstruction can result in dysuria, incontinence, and mild abdominal pain, whereas complete obstruction usually results in moderate to severe pain termed *renal* or *kidney colic*. True "kidney colic" is an uncommon cause of abdominal pain, although horses may show signs of similar to signs of dysuria with gastrointestinal pain. Another complication of complete obstruction is rupture of the bladder or urethra. Signs of pain subside after rupture but are replaced by depression and inappetance, which accompany postrenal ARF. In some cases of disruption of the urinary tract, one also may observe progressive abdominal distention and enlargement of the penis and prepuce.

EPIDEMIOLOGY OF UROLITHIASIS

The epidemiology of urolithiasis varies with species.[4-7] Lower urinary tract stones predominate in veterinary species, whereas upper urinary tract stones are more common in human beings. Historically, lower urinary tract stones were a more substantial problem in human beings as well, and they remain the more common form of urolithiasis in underdeveloped countries. The shift in prevalence from lower to upper urinary tract stones appears to have accompanied industrialization, but the reasons for the shift are not entirely clear.[7]

From 1970 to 1989, urolithiasis was responsible for 0.11% of equine admissions to 22 veterinary teaching hospitals and accounted for 7.8% of the diagnoses of urinary tract disease.[4] Male horses, especially geldings, are predisposed to urolithiasis (75% of all cases), but a breed predisposition has not been described. This sex predilection has been attributed to the shorter, distensible urethra of the mare, which likely permits voiding of small calculi.[5] Urolithiasis is typically an adult disease, and the mean age of affected horses is about 10 years.[4] Nevertheless, young horses can be affected, and the author has seen bilateral nephrolithiasis in a weaning foal (likely a consequence of neonatal septicemia) and dysuria in a 3-month-old colt caused by multiple cystoliths that formed on sutures used for repair of a ruptured bladder as a neonate. Uroliths are most common in the urinary bladder (60%), although they also may develop in the kidneys (12%), ureters (4%), and urethra (24%).[4] Interestingly, as many as 10% of affected horses have had uroliths in multiple locations.[4] Uroliths can vary greatly in size. In one mare a cystolith weighing more than 6 kg was detected as an apparently incidental finding in a horse destroyed for a limb fracture.[8]

PATHOPHYSIOLOGY OF UROLITHIASIS

In general, two steps are required for calculus formation: (1) nucleation and (2) crystal growth.[9-12] Factors that contribute to precipitation of urinary crystals and nucleation include supersaturation of urine; prolonged urine retention; genetic tendencies to excrete larger amounts of calcium (hypercalciuria), uric acid (hyperuricosuria), or oxalates (hyperoxaluria); and inhibitors and promoters of crystal growth. For two or more ions in a solution to precipitate into a crystal, the product of their individual ion activities must exceed the equilibrium solubility product (K_{sp}). A supersaturated solution is one in which the ion activity product exceeds the K_{sp}. A mildly supersaturated solution is termed *metastable,* because crystals tend to precipitate and dissolve at similar rates, so that crystal growth does not occur and the solution remains clear. However, once the ion activity product exceeds a critical value (formation product ratio), precipitation outpaces dissolution, rapid crystal growth occurs, and the solution becomes cloudy.[9-12] Normal human urine typically is supersaturated with one or more ion activity products; however, the formation product ratios are considerably higher in urine (10 times greater than K_{sp}) than they are in an aqueous solution because of the presence of inhibitors of crystal growth.[9] This activity explains why observation of crystals in urine sediment examination is common, yet calculus formation is uncommon. Furthermore, although K_{sp} values are constant for each type of crystal, they vary with temperature and pH. Typically, cooling promotes crystal formation (as when samples are refrigerated), whereas effects of pH vary with the type of calculus (acidification leads to dissolution of calcium crystals but promotes crystallization of urate crystals).[10] Next, any problem resulting in urine retention or incomplete bladder emptying increases the chance of crystal growth. Although not described for horses, genetic variations in ion excretion rates are well-documented risk factors for human and canine urolithiasis. For example, hypercalciuria is inherited as an autosomal dominant trait in human beings and is responsible for 30% to 40% of nephroliths.[9] Similarly, dogs with cystine urolithiasis have an inherited defect in renal tubular transport of cystine, whereas Dalmatians are afflicted with urate stones because of a defect in uric acid metabolism in the breed.[6]

Normal urine is rich in a number of inhibitors of crystal growth, including pyrophosphate, citrate, magnesium ions, glycosaminoglycans, and several glycoproteins including nephrocalcin.[9,10,12] The degree of inhibitory activity varies with crystal type; for example, pyrophosphate is responsible for 50% of the inhibitory activity against calcium phosphate stone formation in human urine but has a much less inhibiting effect on calcium oxalate stone formation.[9] Although poorly documented, inhibitors of crystal growth in equine urine, including its high mucous content, likely play an important protective role against calculus formation, which would seem especially true in light of the substantial urinary excretion of $CaCO_3$ crystals by normal horses. Similar to the risk associated with increased ion excretion, one should not be surprised that defects in inhibitor activity also have been documented in syndromes of human urolithiasis.[9,10] Other urine components may act as promoters of crystal growth. These components principally include organic matrix components of calculi: matrix substance A, uromucoid, and a number of serum proteins.[10,11] Finally, some urine components may have inhibitor and promoter activity. For example, Tamm-Horsfall glycoprotein, a protein secreted in the ascending limb of the loop of Henle that forms the backbone of urine casts, has been shown to promote struvite crystal formation in feline urine.[13] In contrast, the glycoprotein also inhibits calcium oxalate crystal aggregation, and a group of human patients with calcium oxalate urolithiasis recently were demonstrated to have an abnormality in Tamm-Horsfall mucoprotein.[14]

Because normal urine of most species typically is supersaturated and is in balance between crystal precipitation and dissolution, spontaneous nucleation rarely initiates calculus growth. Rather nucleation generally requires stasis of urine flow, increasing the chance of contact between crystalloid material and uroepithelium (as occurs in areas of the renal pelvis) or a damaged uroepithelial surface.[10-13] The latter results in local activation of inflammatory and clotting pathways, producing a nidus for local crystal adherence.[15] In addition, desquamated epithelial cells, leukocytes, or necrotic debris may provide a nidus for crystal growth at more distal sites in the urinary tract. Tissue damage from a variety of causes is likely the most important factor for the development of uroliths in horses. For example, after urinary tract instrumentation (e.g., catheterization, endoscopy), areas of traumatized uroepithelium are covered rapidly with a fine layer of crystalline material. This material usually resolves spontaneously unless infection develops. Similarly, nephroliths may form in the renal medulla or pelvis after papillary necrosis accompanying phenylbutazone toxicity. Once crystal growth begins around a nidus, equine urine has the disadvantage of being highly alkaline, favoring crystallization of most urolith components, especially $CaCO_3$.

Horses develop two basic forms of uroliths, and both are composed primarily of $CaCO_3$.[5,16] More than 90% are yellow-green, spiculated stones that easily fragment (type I urolith) (Figure 19-31, *A*). Less commonly, uroliths are gray-white, smooth stones that are more resistant to fragmentation (type II urolith; Figure 19-31, *B*). The latter stones often contain phosphate in addition to $CaCO_3$. The crystalline composition of normal equine urine sediment ($CaCO_3$ crystals predominate, although calcium oxalate and phosphate crystals also occur) and uroliths is similar: $CaCO_3$ in the form of calcite

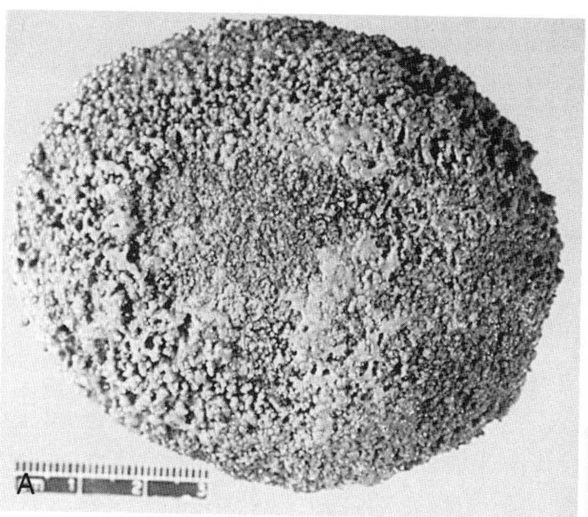

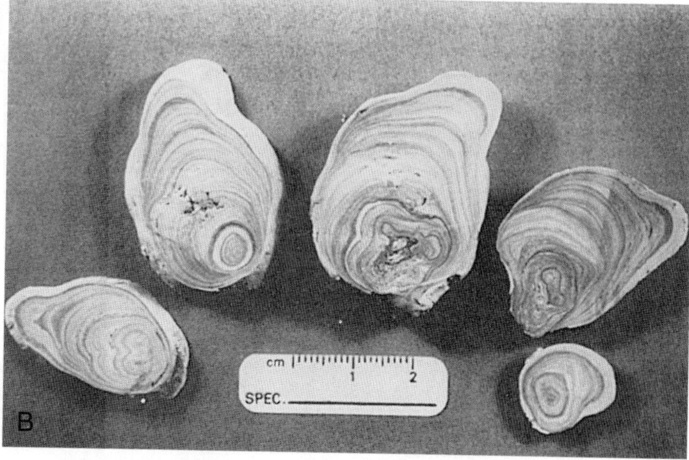

FIGURE 19-31 Equine cystic calculi. **A,** The more common flattened, spherical type of bladder calculus usually is spiculated. **B,** The less common form of gray, smooth-surfaced calculus may be more irregular in shape. (B from DeBowes RM: Surgical management of urolithiasis, Vet Clin North Am Equine Pract 4:461, 1988.)

TABLE 19-10

Published Results of Radiographic Crystallographic Analysis of Equine Urinary Calculi

	REFERENCE			
Type of Calculus	**17**	**18**	**19**	**16**
Total number of calculi	4	157	18	17
Calcite	2	58	2	11
Calcite/vaterite	1	11	9	5
Calcite/aragonite	1	—	—	1
Calcite/weddellite	—	63	4	—
Calcite/whewellite	—	2	—	—
Calcite/hydroxyapatite	—	8	—	—
Calcite/octacalcium phosphate	—	5	—	—
Calcite/struvite	—	3	—	—
Calcite/gypsum	—	2	—	—
Calcite/vaterite/weddellite	—	2	2	—
Calcite/whewellite/weddellite	—	3	—	—
Calcite/vaterite/sodium acid urate	—	—	1	—

(a hexagonal crystal form of $CaCO_3$) is most common, followed by vaterite (a metastable, hexagonal crystal form in which $CaCO_3$ is replaced partially by magnesium or to a lesser extent by manganese, strontium, and sulfur). Other less common components include aragonite (an orthorhombic crystal form of $CaCO_3$), weddellite (calcium oxalate dihydrate), struvite (magnesium ammonium phosphate hexahydrate), hydroxyapatite, and uric acid (Table 19-10).[16-21] Neumann et al.[16] examined the cut surface of a number of equine uroliths by scanning electron microscopy and described a pattern of irregular, concentric bands around the core (Figure 19-32, *A*) that were separated by small spherules of crystalline material (Figure 19-32, *B*). This pattern suggested that calculus growth occurs by accretion of preexisting microscopic spherules (the crystals already present in normal equine urine) on the surface of the growing urolith rather than by de novo crystal formation at the surface of the urolith. Furthermore, banding was speculated to represent growth through incorporation of organic matrix on the surface of the urolith at times when fewer spherules were present in urine. The gaps between adjacent spherules result in porosity to the urolith. Because precipitation and dissolution occur simultaneously during growth of urinary calculi, porosity allows exposure of inner aspects of the urolith to urine, which can lead to dissolution as urine composition changes. Neumann et al.[16] described two types of porosity observed by electron microscopy: (1) primary porosity, consisting of the original pores or gaps between spherules, and (2) secondary porosity, which developed after dissolution of inner areas of the uroliths. Greater dissolution or secondary porosity developed preferentially in areas of the urolith with higher magnesium content (vaterite). More extensive development of secondary porosity theoretically leads to increased urolith fragility, which has the therapeutic benefit of increasing the chance that the urolith can be crushed or fragmented before removal.

The role of UTI in the development of urolithiasis appears to vary with species.[6,9,11] Struvite urolithiasis in human beings and dogs appears to be almost exclusively a consequence of UTI, whereas most struvite uroliths in cats and sheep are not associated with infection.[11] In addition to contributing to uroepithelial injury and nidus formation, UTI with urease-positive bacteria (*Proteus* spp. and coagulase-positive staphylococci are most common) allows splitting of urea into two ammonia molecules, which are hydrolyzed rapidly to ammonium ions (a component of struvite crystals).[9,11,12] In a review of 68 horses with urolithiasis, Laverty et al.[4] reported positive urine culture results in only 2 of 19 horses in which urine culture was performed; however, culture of material from the centers of 30 calculi yielded positive results from 19 (63%), and a variety of different bacterial species were isolated. Only 1 of 28 calculi examined in this study contained struvite. The significance of finding bacteria in the center of equine $CaCO_3$ uroliths is not known, especially for isolates other than

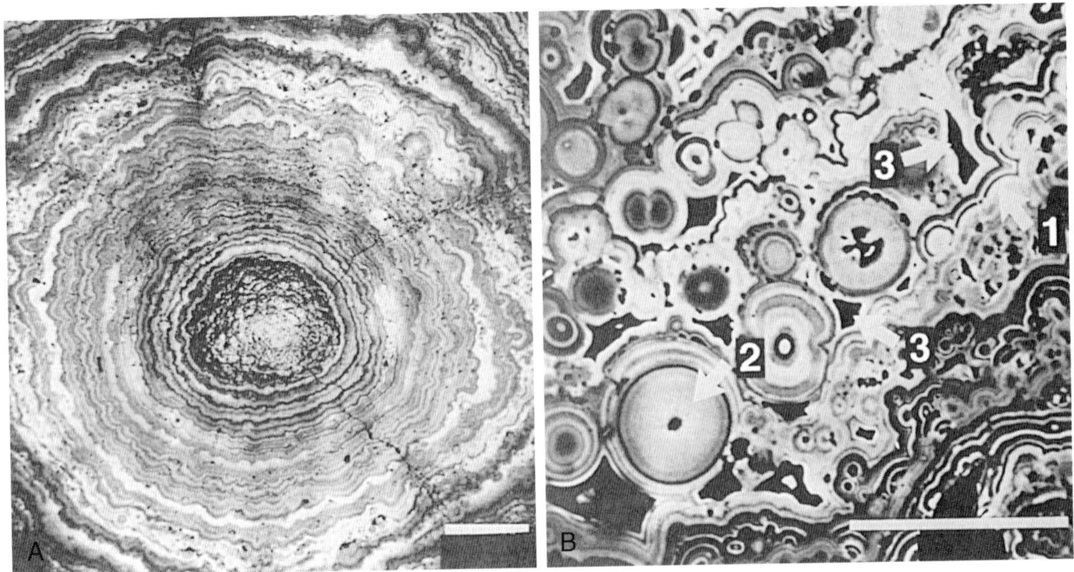

FIGURE 19-32 Scanning electron microscopic appearance of the cut surface of equine cystic calculi. **A,** Lower-power micrograph reveals the intricate pattern of concentric banding around the core (bar = 500 μm). **B,** Higher-power micrograph reveals the ultrastructural features, including bands (**1**), spherules (**2**), and primary porosity in black (**3**) (bar = 50 μm). (From Neumann RD, Ruby AL, Ling GV et al: Ultrastructure and mineral composition of urinary calculi from horses, Am J Vet Res 55:1357, 1994.)

coagulase-positive staphylococci and *Proteus* spp.; culture of an appropriately collected sample of urine always is preferred over culture of a calculus.[4,22] Nephroliths and ureteroliths also are found in some cases of pyelonephritis.[23-26] Laing et al.[26] described a 2-year-old colt with bilateral nephrolithiasis and CRF. They recovered a *Proteus* spp. from urine, and the nephroliths were composed principally of $CaCO_3$ but also contained lesser amounts of struvite. In contrast, Ehnen et al.[27] found evidence of infection in only one of eight horses with nephrolithiasis or ureterolithiasis (or with both) and CRF. In the author's experience, the presence of stones in the upper urinary tract or presence of multiple uroliths warrants concurrent evaluation for UTI, because the author has seen two horses with recurrent urinary tract obstruction with ureteroliths that were determined ultimately to be sequelae of unilateral pyelonephritis. Holt and Pearson[28] described a similar case in which a renal calculus and abscess were found 5 months after removal of a cystic calculus.

NEPHROLITHIASIS AND URETEROLITHIASIS

Renal or ureteral calculi rarely were described as a cause of equine urolithiasis before the last decade[29]; however, a number of recent reports [4,25-27,30-34] have described nephrolithiasis and ureterolithiasis in horses. In a review of 68 horses with urolithiasis by Laverty et al.,[4] 16% had uroliths in the kidneys and ureters and a few horses with cystic calculi also had calculi in the upper urinary tract. Interestingly, 9 of 15 horses with nephroliths in this review were stallions; 3 of 15 were geldings, and 3 of 15 were mares. Whether a true increase in prevalence of nephrolithiasis and ureterolithiasis has occurred, or whether these conditions have become easier to document with the simultaneous development of ultrasonographic imaging as a diagnostic tool for equine medicine, is not clear. An undocumented speculation is that young racehorses may be at greater risk of developing renal calculi because of the common use of NSAIDs (and risk for development of papillary necrosis) in these athletes.[27] The important point is that one should not overlook upper urinary tract lithiasis in horses.

Nephroliths may develop around a nidus associated with a variety of renal diseases, including PKD (see Figure 19-6), pyelonephritis (Figure 19-33, *A*), papillary necrosis (Figure 19-33, *B*), or neoplasia. At present, data on upper urinary tract stones in horses are insufficient to know whether they develop spontaneously (in the absence of tissue damage) as in human beings or whether they differ significantly in mineral composition from cystic calculi. Although nephrolithiasis and ureterolithiasis are painful conditions in human beings, horses with nephroliths or ureteroliths often remain asymptomatic until bilateral obstructive disease leads to development of acute or CRF. Upper urinary tract stones also may be an incidental finding at necropsy.[29] When clinical signs are present, nonspecific presenting complaints consistent with uremia (poor performance, lethargy, inappetance, and weight loss) are more common than signs of obstructive disease (colic, stranguria, hematuria). Occasionally in the horse, a stone or nidus may pass down the ureter and lead to urethral obstruction and signs of acute obstructive disease. Rectal palpation may reveal an enlarged kidney or ureter (or bladder with urethral obstruction), and ureteral calculi may be palpable in an enlarged ureter. Because normal ureters are not palpable on rectal examination, one should palpate the entire course of the ureters (retroperitoneally along the dorsal abdominal wall to the dorsolateral aspects of the pelvic canal to their insertion at the dorsal bladder neck) because an enlarged ureter is easy to overlook.

One usually diagnoses renal and ureteral calculi during rectal or ultrasonographic examination (Figure 19-34). Although ultrasonographic imaging may provide information on the presence, number, and location of calculi, one can miss stones smaller than 1 cm in diameter despite complete examination.

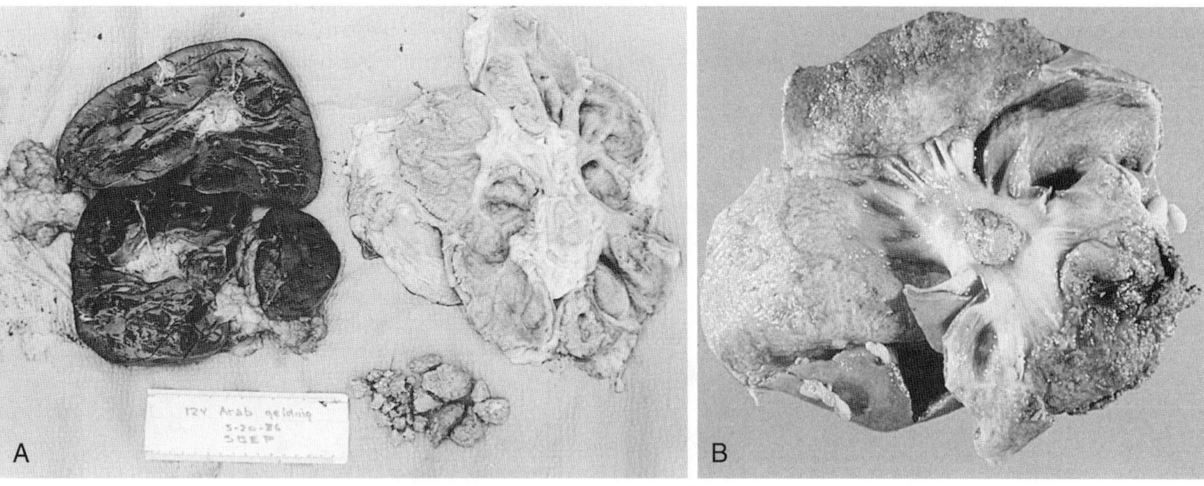

FIGURE 19-33 A, Multiple nephroliths developed in association with unilateral pyelonephritis in a gelding that was presented for repeated urethral obstruction. **B,** A small nephrolith lodged in the renal pelvis resulted in ureteral obstruction and development of hydronephrosis in a Standardbred gelding that had a 4-year history of phenylbutazone therapy.

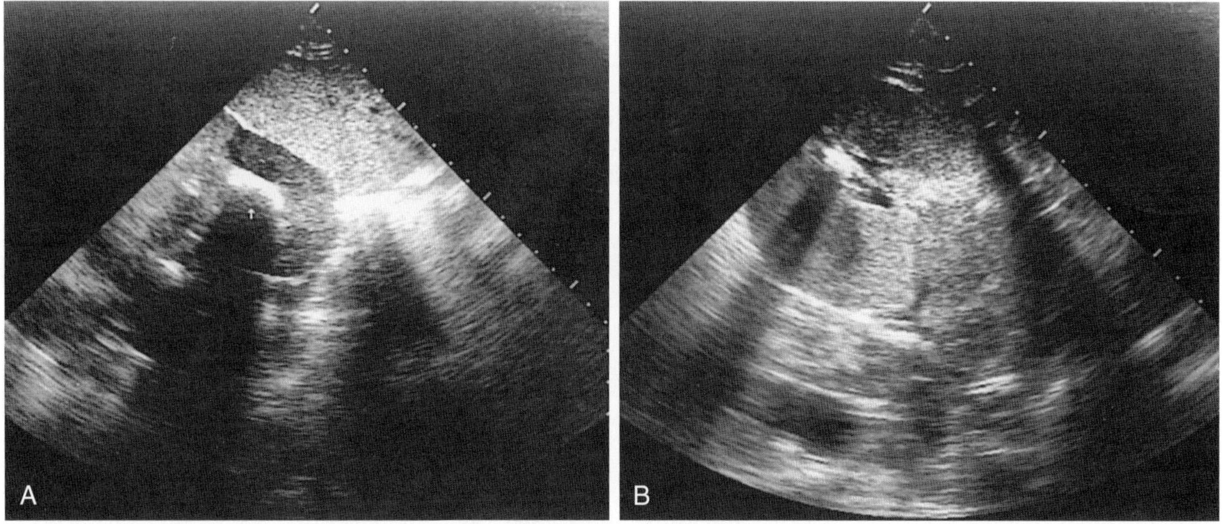

FIGURE 19-34 Ultrasonographic images of the left, **A,** and right, **B,** kidneys of a 10-month-old Arabian filly that developed bilateral nephrolithiasis and chronic renal failure (CRF) as sequelae of neonatal septicemia. The nephroliths are highly echogenic and cast acoustic shadows in both kidneys.

Other ultrasonographic findings to support upper tract lithiasis include dilation of the renal pelvis or proximal ureter and, in long-standing cases, hydronephrosis.[35,36] Although azotemia generally accompanies bilateral disease, horses with unilateral disease often maintain normal renal function. For reasons detailed previously, one should perform a quantitative urine culture in all horses with nephrolithiasis or ureterolithiasis to assess possible intercurrent UTI.

Because most horses with nephrolithiasis or ureterolithiasis are in CRF by the time the diagnosis is established,[27,37,38] few cases are amenable to treatment. Thus reports of successful management of horses with renal and ureteral calculi are few. Removal of the calculus, limited to horses with unilateral disease or mild azotemia, has been the only effective means of treatment.[30,32,34] In the absence of azotemia, nephrectomy is the preferred technique for management of unilateral renal calculi.[32] Furthermore, removal of the affected kidney and ureter should eliminate any associated upper UTI or chance of recurrence. The approach involves a dorsal flank incision, rib resection, and blunt retroperitoneal dissection to expose the kidney.[3,39,40] In one horse with mild azotemia, nephrotomy (via an approach similar to nephrectomy) was performed successfully to remove obstructing calculi in the renal pelvis and proximal ureter. Unfortunately, little improvement in azotemia occurred, and the horse was destroyed a few weeks later.[27] Ureteral calculi also have been removed by ureterolithectomy via ventral celiotomy and paralumbar approaches.[30,33] A basket stone dislodger (Dormia Stone Dislodger, V Mueller Co, McGow Park, Ill.), introduced through a vestibulourethral approach and guided by rectal palpation, also has been used for removal of distal ureteral calculi in the mare.[30] Medical management (antibiotics, grass hay, and salt to promote diuresis)

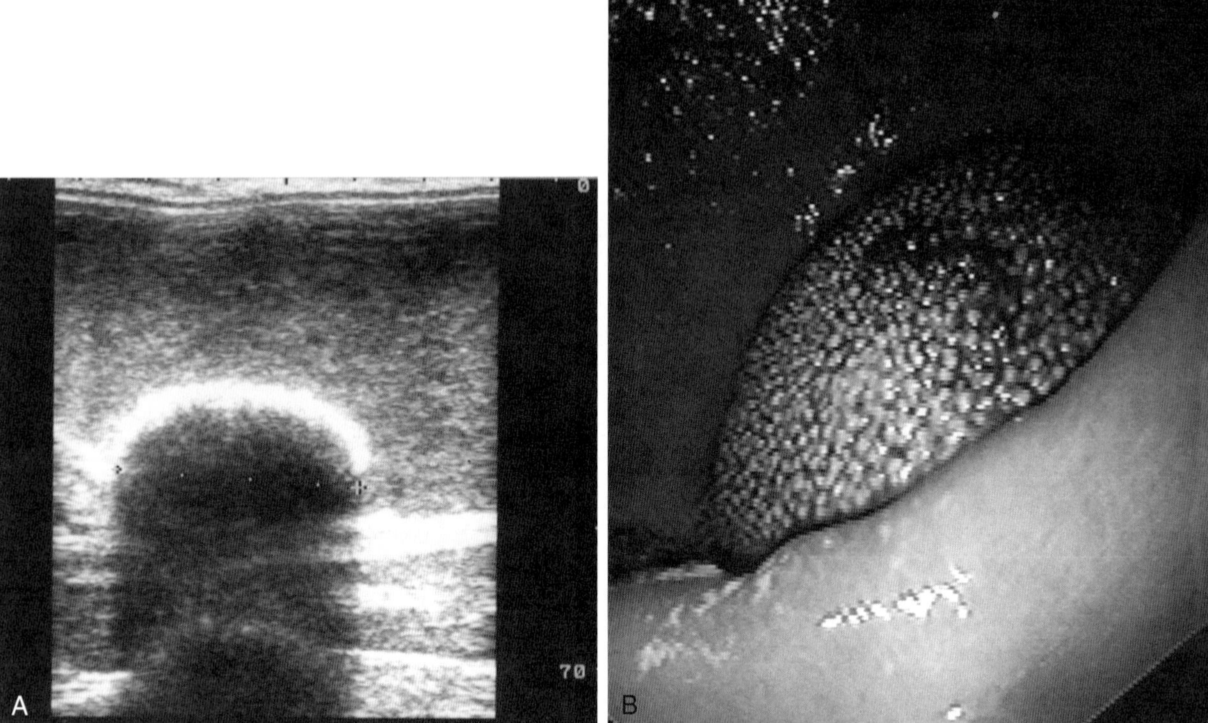

FIGURE 19-35 **A,** Transrectal ultrasound examination of the bladder using a 5 mHz linear array probe. A single large calculus is present with acoustic shadowing ventral to the urolith. **B,** A type I urolith within the bladder as seen during cystoscopy.

of bilateral ureterolithiasis was attempted in a 3-year-old Thoroughbred filly with incomplete ureteral obstruction and mild azotemia.[33] After 4 weeks, deterioration of clinical signs and more severe azotemia prompted ureterolithectomy to remove stones from the left ureter. Percutaneous nephrostomy was used successfully for placement of a catheter in the right renal pelvis (to establish percutaneous urine flow) for short-term management of azotemia in the postoperative period. Unfortunately, the filly was destroyed after developing cecal impaction 6 days later, and necropsy examination revealed a shrunken, nonfunctional left kidney and a previously undetected nephrolith in the right kidney. This case demonstrated the feasibility and potential benefits of accessing the renal pelvis of the horse via percutaneous nephrostomy.[41,42]

Rodger et al.[34] recently described the successful use of electrohydraulic lithotripsy through a ureteroscope to disintegrate a single, unilateral ureterolith in a horse with evidence of bilateral renal disease. Electrohydraulic lithotripsy is a means of converting electric energy into mechanical energy that can be directed to fragment the urolith.[34,43,44] Basically, the device produces an electric discharge arc (a spark) between two electrodes at the tip of the instrument. The heat associated with the discharge causes a small amount of the liquid medium (urine) to burst into gas bubbles, and the associated shock wave fractures the urolith. One must keep the end of the instrument adjacent to the urolith yet away from the mucosa, which could be disrupted by the same shock waves that destroy the calculus. Although the technique has not been highly successful for treatment of canine uroliths,[45] equine uroliths may be more amenable to its use because they are commonly porous (and fragile). Although electrohydraulic lithotripsy has been effective in treating selected equine cystoliths[43,44] and one ureterolith,[34] the expense of the equipment and availability of other surgical options likely will limit its use to selected cases that are not amenable to routine surgical treatments. A more recent development in upper tract stone removal for human beings and dogs is extracorporeal shock wave lithotripsy.[42] This noninvasive technology uses a reflector to focus the energy from a shock wave generated outside the body on a nephrolith in situ and has proved efficacious in treating human nephrolithiasis. Although extracorporeal shock wave lithotripsy and laser technology have not yet been attempted in horses, they provide future treatment options for equine nephrolithiasis and ureterolithiasis.

CYSTIC CALCULI

Cystic calculi are the most commonly recognized form of equine uroliths.[1-5,28] Cystoliths typically are flattened, spherical stones with a spiculated or smooth surface. Dysuria resulting from cystoliths may include hematuria, stranguria, pollakiuria, pyuria, or incontinence. Hematuria may be more apparent after exercise. An affected male horse may demonstrate stranguria by repeatedly dropping its penis and posturing to urinate but voiding little or no urine. An affected mare also may posture repeatedly to urinate and demonstrate winking, and these signs could be confused with estrous activity. Less common signs include an irritable attitude, recurrent colic, and loss of condition; one burro was presented for recurrent rectal prolapse.[46]

One usually diagnoses cystic calculi by palpation and ultrasound examination of the bladder per rectum (Figure 19-35). Bladder uroliths are usually large enough to be detected easily; however, if the bladder is distended, then one may need to

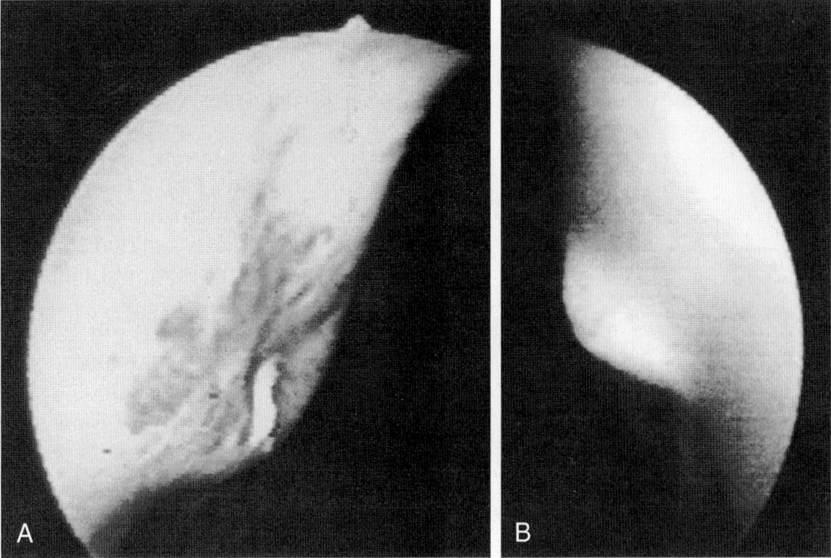

FIGURE 19-36 View of the abnormal left, **A,** and normal right, **B,** ureteral openings of a horse with unilateral pyelonephritis and recurrent cystic calculi. The diagnosis was confirmed by culture of urine samples collected from each ureter.

empty it by passing a catheter to facilitate palpation of the stone. Bladder catheterization also allows assessment of urethral patency and collection of samples for urinalysis and quantitative culture. One should perform a CBC and serum biochemical profile to document whether anemia, inflammation, or azotemia has developed. Cystoscopic examination is helpful in assessing the size and number of cystic calculi and the severity of damage to the bladder mucosa, as well as any asymmetry in appearance or function of the ureteral openings (Figure 19-36, *A* and *B*).[47,48] Because one may find calculi in multiple sites in the urinary tract, thorough evaluation of the upper urinary tract is warranted for all cases of cystic urolithiasis.

In contrast to upper urinary tract lithiasis, many reports[43,44,46,49-64] and several reviews detail the clinical signs and surgical options for management of cystic calculi.*

The size of the calculus, gender of the horse, and surgeon's preference play a role in treatment selection. The preferred technique in males, especially for larger stones, is laparocystotomy through a ventral midline or paramedian incision with the horse in dorsal recumbency under general anesthesia. Laproscopic-assisted cystotomy may also be used for urolith removal in geldings.[67] For removal of smaller cystoliths, one can perform a perineal urethrotomy in the standing male horse with the use of local or epidural anesthesia. One catheterizes the urethra to facilitate identification of the urethra and makes an incision at the level of the ischial arch. After incising the urethra, forceps are used to grasp and remove the calculus and the bladder is lavaged to remove remaining debris. One may attempt removal of larger calculi via this approach by using a lithotrite to crush the urolith into smaller fragments. The urethral incision can be closed, but it usually is allowed to heal by second intention. Although this approach can be performed less expensively and the risks associated with general anesthesia can be avoided, doing so increases the risk of complications, including urethral trauma and stricture formation,[28,68,69] urethrolith formation at the surgical site,[4,70] development of a urethral diverticulum,[70] and persistent urine passage through a fistula at the surgical site.[69,71] The distensible urethra of the mare allows retrieval of cystic calculi via this route in many cases. Using sedation and epidural anesthesia, one can remove the stone intact with forceps or by direct grasping if the surgeon has small hands. One may crush a spiculated urolith with a lithotrite to ease removal. Spiculated stones or urolith fragments can be manipulated further into a sterile plastic bag or palpation sleeve to minimize trauma to the urethral mucosa during removal. If necessary, then one also can enlarge the urethral lumen by performing sphincterotomy in the dorsal aspect of the urethra.[72] A pararectal (Gökels) approach for a dorsal cystotomy[39,64] and electrohydraulic lithotripsy,[43,44] as described for ureterolithiasis, also have been used in male and female horses to treat cystic calculi. Successful laser lithotripsy in horses depends on the composition of the urolith and type of laser.[73] Pulsed dye lasers may be more efficacious for fragmentation of equine uroliths. However, reports of laser lithotripsy in horses are limited, and it appears that certain lasers cannot be assumed to be uniformly successful against all types of equine uroliths.

After surgical removal of cystoliths, one administers systemic antibiotics and an anti-inflammatory agent for a minimum of 1 week. As for cystitis, antibiotic selection should be based on susceptibility testing of recovered isolates. If culture results are negative, then a sulfonamide-trimethoprim combination is an appropriate selection. An early report by Lowe[70] described excellent long-term results—and no recurrence—after removal of cystic calculi by laparocystotomy in four horses. Similar low rates of recurrence have been echoed in several reviews of equine urolithiasis.[5,28,39,65] In contrast to these favorable reports (most of which do not provide supporting data), Laverty et al.[4] reported that clinical signs of urolithiasis recurred in 12 of 29 horses (41%) for which follow-up data were available. The interval between episodes of recurrence was 1 to 32 months (mean: 13 months). As Lowe initially described in 1965,[70] Laverty et al.[4] also found greater recurrence of cystic calculi after treatment by perineal urethrotomy (7 of 15 horses)

*References 4, 5, 28, 39, 65, 66.

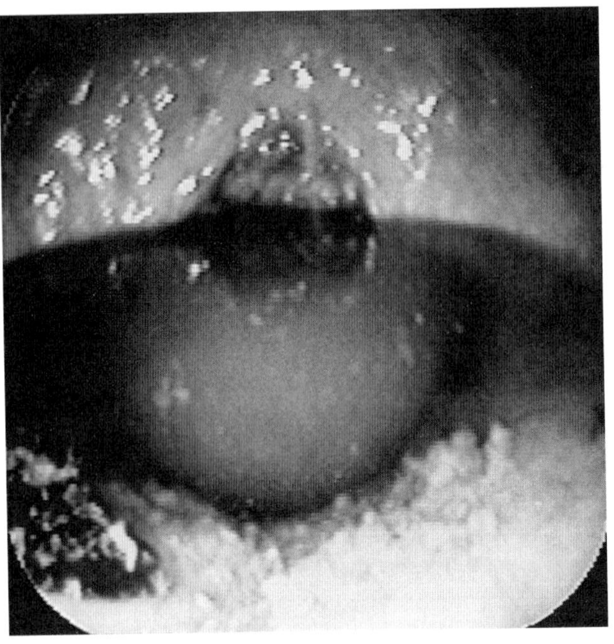

FIGURE 19-37 A large urolith is present in the bladder below the surface of the pool of urine. The cystolith was accompanied by bacterial cystitis and squamous cell carcinoma of the bladder.

compared with laparocystotomy. Other complications of cystic calculi unrelated to the surgical approach have included VUR and renal failure[74] and concurrent urolithiasis at other sites.[4] A more common complication of urethral obstruction,[68] bladder rupture, also may occur after cystic urolithiasis. The author also has seen a case of squamous cell carcinoma of the bladder that was associated with a large cystic calculus and development of uroperitoneum after bladder rupture (Figure 19-37).

Postoperative recommendations that may help prevent recurrence include control of UTI and use of urinary acidifiers, although the benefits of the latter are not well-documented (see Cystitis in the Urinary Tract Infections section of this chapter).[5,62,65,66,75] Other considerations for decreasing recurrence include dietary modifications to decrease calcium excretion and to promote diuresis. Changing the diet from a high-calcium hay (e.g., alfalfa) to grass or oat hay would decrease dietary calcium and thus should decrease urinary calcium excretion because fecal calcium excretion is relatively constant in horses.[76] This dietary change should decrease total calcium excretion and may decrease urinary nitrogen excretion and daily urine volume.[77] The latter changes could enhance supersaturation of urine. In theory, the addition of 50 to 75 g of loose salt daily to the concentrate portion of the diet should promote diuresis; however, in a study of ponies fed NaCl as 1%, 3%, or 5% of the total dry matter of the diet (1% approximates 75 g of NaCl for a 500-kg horse), no differences in water intake, urine production, or calcium excretion were observed.[78] Another factor that affects urine pH and urine calcium excretion is dietary cation-anion balance (DCAB = [Na + K] − [Cl + S]). A lower DCAB has been associated with a decrease in urine pH and an increase in urinary calcium excretion.[79-81] Increasing the amount of grain in the diet, changing to lower-quality hay, or adding one or more minerals to the diet (e.g., ammonium chloride, calcium chloride, ammonium sulfate) usually lowers DCAB. Not surprisingly, supplements that decrease DCAB are familiar as urinary acidifying agents. Because a diet low in calcium and DCAB could result in a negative calcium balance, a possible long-term effect could be decreased skeletal calcium content.

Despite the success of dietary management (low-protein, phosphorous, and magnesium) for medical dissolution of canine[82] and feline[83] uroliths, dietary management is unlikely to replace surgical treatment of cystic urolithiasis in horses. This problem can be attributed to the fact that dietary management for small animals has been directed at struvite urolithiasis and that such stones are not common in horses. Nevertheless, one should not overlook dietary management as one of the postoperative recommendations for urolithiasis, because it could decrease the risk of recurrence. At the least, legume hays and dietary supplements containing calcium should be avoided, and the diet could be supplemented with 50 to 75 g of loose salt daily. Remillard et al.[84] used these dietary manipulations effectively, along with administration of ammonium sulfate as a urine-acidifying agent, to manage one recurrent case of equine urolithiasis.

URETHRAL CALCULI

Urethral calculi are primarily a problem of male horses,[1-5,68,70,85,86] although they have been detected in a few mares.[4] In the absence of predisposing urethral damage or stricture formation, urethroliths are usually small cystoliths passed into the urethra. Thus most urethroliths initially lodge where the urethra narrows as it passes over the ischial arch. They may pass slowly farther down the urethra, until complete obstruction produces signs of renal colic. One should consider an obstructing urethral calculus when male horses show colic signs and frequently posture to urinate. Occasionally, one may see blood on the end of the urethra. Palpation of the penis may reveal repeated urethral contractions or a firm mass in the urethra. Rectal palpation reveals a distended bladder that is turgid, unlike the flaccid bladder distention of bladder paralysis. If the bladder ruptures, then colic signs are supplanted by progressive depression and anorexia after the development of postrenal ARF.[4,68,85,86] The diagnosis is confirmed by passage of a urinary catheter that is then obstructed by the urolith or by endoscopic examination of the urethra. One can confirm suspected bladder rupture by measuring a twofold or greater increase in peritoneal fluid Cr concentration compared with serum Cr concentration.

One can remove calculi lodged at the ischial arch through a perineal urethrotomy. Passage of a catheter into the bladder, if that is not achieved before surgery, is necessary to ensure a patent urinary tract after stone removal. The urethrotomy is allowed to heal by second intention, and temporary use of an indwelling bladder catheter usually is not necessary. One often can remove calculi lodged in the distal urethra from a sedated horse by gentle transurethral crushing of the urolith with a hand or forceps. For a calculus lodged distal to the ischial arch and unpalpable in the distal portion of the penis, general anesthesia and positioning the horse in dorsal recumbency are generally necessary for surgical removal of the stone. One may close the urethra or allow it to heal by second intention. Follow-up endoscopic examination of the urethra allows assessment of urethral healing and possible stricture formation (Figure 19-38). Further treatment includes administration of antibiotics and anti-inflammatory agents until dysuria resolves. Although initial treatment of urinary tract obstruction caused by a urethrolith is straightforward, the prognosis for affected horses should remain guarded because a number of potential complications of

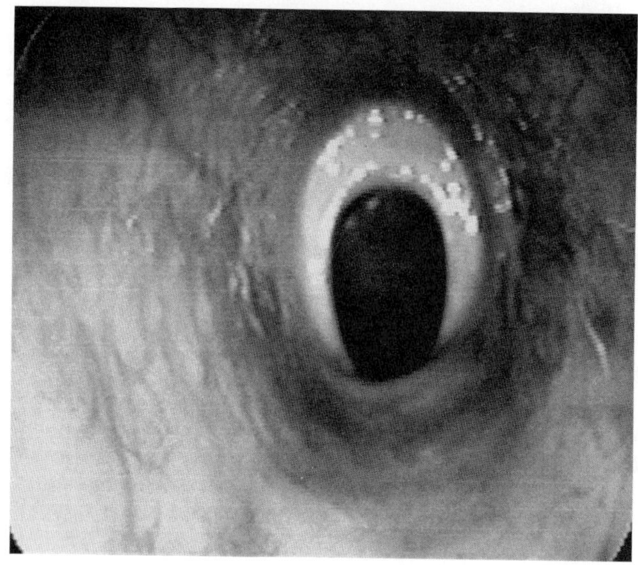

FIGURE 19-38 Stricture formation in the urethra at the level of the ischial arch formed as a complication of a perineal urethrotomy.

perineal urethrotomy (described previously) may occur. Furthermore, a substantial number of horses have had poor outcomes because of associated bladder rupture and peritonitis[4,68,85] or upper urinary tract lithiasis or pyelonephritis.[4,28]

SABULOUS UROLITHIASIS

Another form of equine urolithiasis termed *sabulous urolithiasis* also has been described in a limited number of horses.[28,87] *Sabulous* (Greek for *sand*) *urolithiasis* refers to the accumulation of large amounts of crystalloid urine sediment in the ventral aspect of the bladder. This condition is a secondary problem resulting from bladder paralysis or other physical or neurologic disorders interfering with complete bladder emptying.[88-90] Affected horses usually are presented for evaluation of urinary incontinence or hindlimb weakness and ataxia, and one may detect accumulation of urine sediment in a distended bladder during rectal palpation. A complete neurologic examination should be performed on horses with sabulous urolithiasis or bladder dysfunction. Common differential diagnoses for bladder paresis or paralysis include equine herpesvirus-1 (EHV-1), polyneuritis equi, illicit tail block, equine protozoal myeloencephalitis, and sacral fracture or osteomyelitis. Symptomatic treatment includes repeated bladder lavage, medications that promote bladder emptying, and broad spectrum antibiotics, but the condition carries a poor prognosis unless the primary problem resulting in bladder paralysis can be resolved (see Urinary Incontinence and Bladder Dysfunction).

BLADDER DISPLACEMENT

Displacement of the urinary bladder is a rare cause of obstruction and dysuria.[1,91-94] In mares, two types of bladder displacement can occur: (1) extrusion through a tear in the floor of the vagina or (2) true prolapse with eversion of the bladder.[95] Urethral obstruction also may occur with vaginal or uterine prolapse. In male horses, scrotal herniation of the bladder has been described, but this type of bladder displacement is rare.[96] Bladder displacements typically result from repeated abdominal contractions or straining. Thus they most often are associated with parturition and to a lesser extent with colic. Perineal lacerations after trauma or foaling may lead to extrusion, whereas excessive straining without laceration leads to prolapse and eversion. Because the bladder turns inside out with the latter problem, one establishes the diagnosis by recognizing the appearance of the bladder mucosa and ureteral openings. Eversion does not always result in obstruction.

With urethral obstruction, one should pass a catheter into the bladder before correction of the displacement. In the absence of obstruction, one corrects extrusions during repair of the perineal or vaginal laceration. One should institute a course of broad spectrum antibiotics and an anti-inflammatory agent because pelvic abscess and peritonitis are potential complications. Manual reduction of bladder eversions may be successful in some cases, but more often than not one may need to perform urethral sphincterotomy to replace the bladder.[94] In some cases, reduction via laparotomy may be necessary because the everted bladder may be filled with the pelvic flexure, complicating manual reduction.[93] A purse-string suture placed in the area of the external urethral sphincter may be of benefit to prevent recurrence of the prolapse, and medical treatment should include broad spectrum antibiotics and an anti-inflammatory agent because UTI is a potential complication.

PENILE TRAUMA

Urinary tract obstruction is an occasional complication of penile trauma or paraphimosis, and one should consider the patency of the urethra in all cases of penile injury. Causes may include blunt trauma, breeding injuries, use of stallion rings, sedation with phenothiazine tranquilizers, or laceration during castration.[1,97-99] In addition to preputial swelling, injury may result in a penile hematoma or possible paraphimosis.[100,101] In one report, hematoma formation in the corpus spongiosum penis (CSP) of a Quarter Horse stallion resulted in complete obstruction and bladder rupture.[102] In addition to ensuring patency of the urinary tract, treatment includes administration of antibiotics and anti-inflammatory agents until most of the swelling resolves. One may close lacerations of the urethra or leave them to heal by second intention depending on location and condition of the wound. Because stricture formation is a possible complication, some wounds may be treated better by phallectomy than by urethral repair.[98]

HEMATURIA

Harold C. Schott II

Hematuria can be a presenting complaint for a variety of disorders of the urinary tract, including vascular malformation, UTI, urolithiasis, and neoplasia.[1] In addition to these problems, which are discussed elsewhere in this chapter, several other specific causes of hematuria exist. These causes range from microscopic hematuria accompanying exercise to more severe conditions that can result in life-threatening urinary tract hemorrhage. In addition, normal equine urine may contain pyrocatechin, an oxidizing agent that can cause urine to turn red to brown after exposure to air, snow, or bedding (especially wood shavings).

Although values have not been determined in horses, normal human urine contains about 5000 (range: 2000-10,000) RBCs per milliliter.[2] This range of RBC excretion should yield negative results on reagent strip analysis and a report of not more than five RBCs per high-power field on sediment examination. Increases in RBC excretion may lead to microscopic or macroscopic hematuria. Microscopic hematuria, which implies an increase in RBC excretion that is not visible grossly, usually is associated with increases in the range of 10,000 to 2.5 million RBCs per milliliter of urine. On sediment examination at least 10 RBCs per high-power field should be apparent. Reagent strip analysis results can range from trace to +++. One must realize that reagent strip results, which use the peroxidase-like activity of hemoglobin and myoglobin to oxidize a chromogen in the test pad, do not differentiate between hemoglobin and myoglobin.[3] Thus positive results are not specific for hematuria and may be more appropriately termed *pigmenturia*. Despite this limitation, one can use reagent strips to differentiate hematuria from hemoglobinuria or myoglobinuria when the color change is limited to scattered spots on the test pad. This pattern implies that intact RBCs were adsorbed onto the pad, underwent lysis, and produced a localized color change caused by hemoglobin activity on the chromogenic substrates. Ability to differentiate hematuria from excretion of the heme pigments is limited to a threshold of 250,000 to 300,000 RBCs per milliliter of urine, unless urine samples are diluted with normal saline. Other limitations of reagent strip analysis include false-positive reactions when urine samples are contaminated with oxidizing agents (e.g., disinfectants) or false-negative reactions when urine samples contain vitamin C or have been preserved with formalin.[3]

Macroscopic or gross hematuria indicates RBC excretion in excess of 2.5 to 5 million RBCs per milliliter of urine (or about 0.5 ml of blood per liter of urine).[2-5] One can differentiate macroscopic hematuria from other causes of pigmenturia by centrifuging a sample of urine to produce a red cell pellet and yellow supernatant urine. Quantification of erythrocyte numbers in macroscopic hematuria is of little clinical value. In contrast, urinary RBC numbers may provide diagnostic and prognostic information in cases of microscopic hematuria in human beings.[2] However, variations in urine concentration complicate accurate counts. In concentrated urine (specific gravity >1.020), RBCs tend to become crenated because of the osmotic shift of water out of the cells. In urine with a specific gravity less than 1.010, osmotic swelling and dilution of hemoglobin lead to "ghost cell" formation.[2,6] Furthermore, many RBCs lyse in dilute urine (especially alkaline urine) so that RBC excretion is vastly underestimated. Reagent strip analysis can be useful in dilute urine samples to detect hemoglobin released from lysed erythrocytes.[5]

Microscopic examination of urine sediment in cases of hematuria is helpful in distinguishing glomerular from nonglomerular bleeding. The hallmark of glomerular bleeding is a substantial variation in RBC size, shape, and hemoglobin content (termed *dysmorphism*), whereas bleeding from other sites produces a more uniform population of urinary erythrocytes.[2,5,7] Dysmorphism is attributed to membrane deformation, which occurs as erythrocytes traverse the glomerular filtration barrier.[7] Urinary RBCs in normal persons are typically dysmorphic, indicating glomerular origin, but the excretion rate is low.[2] Thus one must interpret urinary RBC morphologic characteristics along with urinary RBC numbers to determine significance.[7,8] The volume of dysmorphic cells tends to be lower than that of erythrocytes of nonglomerular origin, so that measurement of mean corpuscular volume (MCV) also has been used to separate glomerular from nonglomerular bleeding.[9] The presence of RBCs or hemoglobin casts is also pathognomonic for glomerular bleeding.[2,5,7] These casts form when urinary RBCs and hemoglobin from the proximal portion of the nephron (glomerulus) combine with Tamm-Horsfall mucoprotein secreted in the ascending limb of the loop of Henle. Because urinary RBCs and casts deteriorate rapidly in urine samples, other methods of detecting glomerular hematuria, such as immunocytochemical staining for Tamm-Horsfall glycoprotein, have been developed but have not gained widespread use.[10]

Noting the timing of hematuria is usually a more practical means of initially localizing the site of urinary tract hemorrhage.[6] Hematuria throughout urination is consistent with hemorrhage from the kidneys, ureters, or bladder, whereas hematuria at the beginning of urination often is associated with lesions in the distal urethra. Hematuria at the end of urination usually results from hemorrhage from the proximal urethra or bladder neck. A thorough diagnostic evaluation, including physical examination, rectal palpation, analyses of blood and urine, endoscopy of the lower tract, and ultrasonography, usually is rewarding in establishing the source and cause of urinary tract hemorrhage.[1]

UTI, although uncommon in horses, may result in hematuria. With infection of the upper urinary tract, partial anorexia, weight loss, and fever may be additional presenting complaints, whereas horses with cystitis generally manifest stranguria and pollakiuria; however, hematuria has been the presenting complaint in several reports of cystitis and pyelonephritis.[11-15] The presence of uroliths at any level of the urinary tract may cause mucosal irritation and hemorrhage, resulting in hematuria.[16-18] Typically, affected horses also show signs of renal colic or painful urination (stranguria or pollakiuria), especially with uroliths in the bladder or urethra. Finally, neoplasia of the kidneys, ureters, bladder, or urethra may result in hematuria as the presenting complaint.[19-22] These conditions are discussed in detail in other sections in this chapter.

TOXICITIES

Nephrotoxicity, particularly after administration of NSAIDs (especially phenylbutazone), may result in microscopic or gross hematuria.[23-27] Historical or current use of nephrotoxic medications supports this diagnosis, and discontinuation of the nephrotoxic agent and supportive care are the appropriate treatments. Horses that consume alfalfa hay containing blister beetles (equine cantharidiasis) may void red urine. Cantharidin is excreted in urine and is very irritating to the lower urinary tract, resulting in cystitis and hemorrhage from the urinary bladder mucosa.[28]

URETHRAL DEFECTS

Although a recognized cause of hemospermia in stallions, rents or tears of the proximal urethra at the level of the ischial arch are a more recently described cause of hematuria in geldings.[1,29-31] Because the defects are difficult to detect without high-resolution videoendoscopic equipment, the lesions likely may have been missed in previous reports of urethral bleeding.[32,33] Consequently, hematuria has been attributed to urethritis or hemorrhage from "varicosities" of the urethral vasculature.[29,33] Because the vasculature underlying the urethral mucosa becomes prominent when the urethra is distended with air

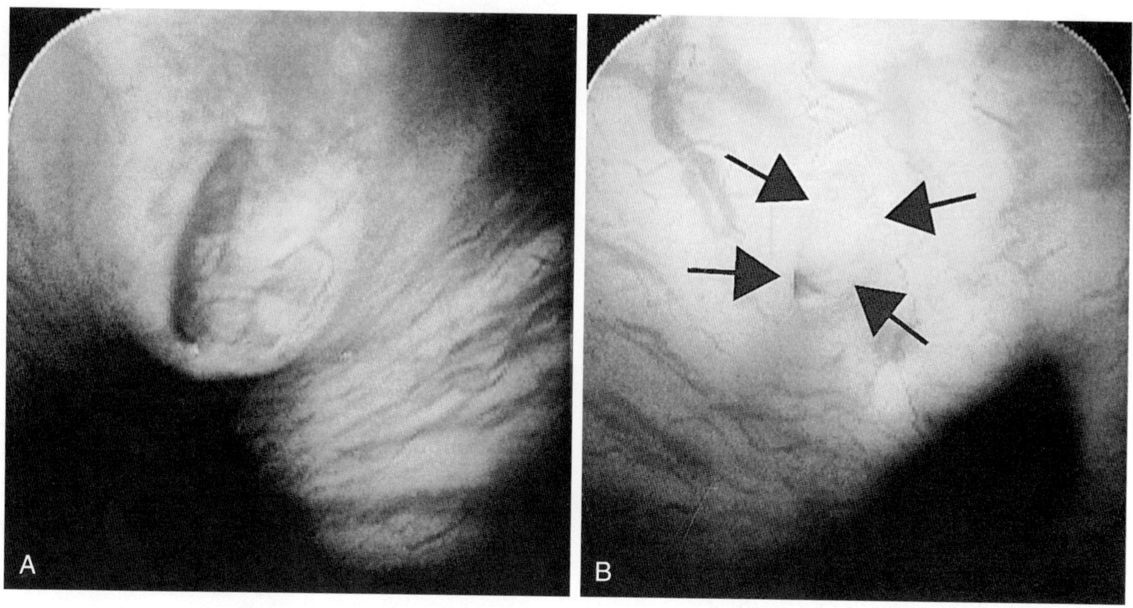

FIGURE 19-39 Endoscopic images of urethral defects or tears at the level of the ischial arch. **A,** A more acute lesion (hematuria for 2 weeks) is surrounded by a raised rim of tissue. **B,** A chronic lesion (hematuria for 6 months) is flat to recessed *(between arrows)*. Evidence of inflammation around both lesions is minimal.

during endoscopic examination, especially in the proximal urethra (to the point that blood can be seen flowing in the submucosal vasculature), one easily would suspect that hemorrhage could arise from apparent urethritis or urethral varicosity.

Urethral rents or tears in geldings typically result in hematuria at the end of urination in association with urethral contraction.[1,29,30] Affected horses generally void a normal volume of urine that is not discolored. At the end of urination, a series of urethral contractions results in squirts of bright-red blood. Occasionally, the horse may pass a smaller amount of darker blood at the start of urination. In most instances the condition does not appear painful or result in pollakiuria. Interestingly, most affected stallions with hemospermia and geldings with hematuria have been Quarter Horses or Quarter Horse crosses that have been free of other complaints.[30,33] Treatment with antibiotics for suspected cystitis or urethritis routinely has been unsuccessful, although hematuria has resolved spontaneously in approximately half of the cases seen by the author.

Examination of affected horses is often unremarkable. In comparison, horses with hematuria caused by neoplasms involving the distal urethra or penis usually have additional complaints such as pollakiuria, a foul odor to the sheath, or presence of a mass in the sheath or on the penis.[34] With urethral rents, laboratory analysis of blood reveals normal renal function, although mild anemia can be an occasional finding. Urine samples collected midstream or by bladder catheterization appear grossly normal. Urinalysis may have normal results, or the number of RBCs may be increased on sediment examination (a finding that also would result in a positive reagent strip result for blood). Bacterial culture of urine yields negative results.

One makes the diagnosis via endoscopic examination of the urethra, during which one typically sees a lesion along the dorsocaudal aspect of the urethra at the level of the ischial arch (Figure 19-39, *A*). With hematuria lasting several weeks, the lesion appears as a fistula communicating with the vasculature of the CSP (Figure 19-39, *B*). External palpation of the urethra in this area is usually unremarkable but can help localize the lesion, because external digital palpation is visible via the endoscope as movements of the urethra.

Although the complete pathophysiology of this condition remains unclear, the defect has been speculated to result from a "blowout" of the CSP into the urethral lumen (Figure 19-40).[30] Hemorrhage from urethral rents occurs with higher pressure within the CSP during urination in geldings and ejaculation in stallions.[31] Pressure in the CSP during urination is higher in geldings because of their smaller CSP diameter as compared with stallions. Hematuria at the end of urination in geldings with urethral rents is speculated to occur when a sudden decrease in intraluminal urethral pressure occurs while pressure in the CSP is still high. Once created, the lesion is maintained by bleeding at the end of each urination, and the surrounding mucosa heals by formation of a fistula into the overlying vascular tissue.[30]An explanation for the consistent location along the dorsocaudal aspect of the urethra at the level of the ischial arch has not been documented but may be related to the anatomy of the musculature supporting the base of the penis and an enlargement of the CSP in this area. Furthermore, a narrowing of the lumen of the urethra at the distal extent of the ampullar portion of the urethra occurs that also may contribute to the location of the defects. However, histologic studies in both geldings and stallions have shown that no differences exist in the urethral mucosa, lamina propria, or CSP between the ischial arch and other sites in the penis.[31] An anatomic predisposition in Quarter Horses has not been documented but could be speculated to be based on an apparently increased risk in this breed. In addition, some of the affected horses have asymmetry to the musculature under the tail in this area, supporting a possible developmental defect (Figure 19-41).

Because hematuria may resolve spontaneously, no treatment may be required initially. If hematuria persists longer than 1 month or if significant anemia develops, then a temporary subischial urethrotomy has been successful in a number of affected geldings. With sedation and epidural or local

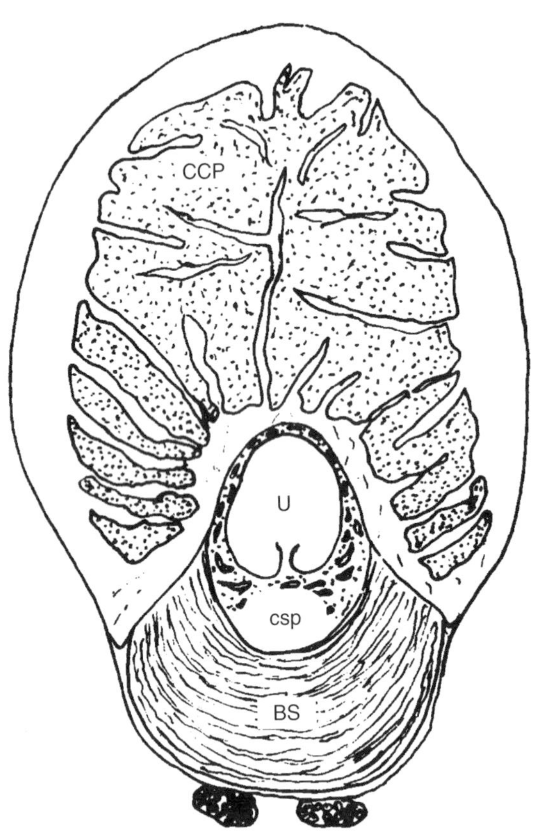

FIGURE 19-40 Cross-sectional diagram of the equine penis at the level of the ischial arch shows a defect between the corpus spongiosum penis (CSP) (**csp**) and the urethral lumen (**U**). The CSP is a cavernous tissue surrounding the urethra that is distinct from the corpus cavernosum penis (**CCP**); the CSP is also adjacent to the bulbospongiosus muscle (**BS**) caudally. (From Schumacher J, Varner DD, Schmitz DG et al: Urethral defects in geldings with hematuria and stallions with hemospermia, Vet Surg 24:250, 1995.)

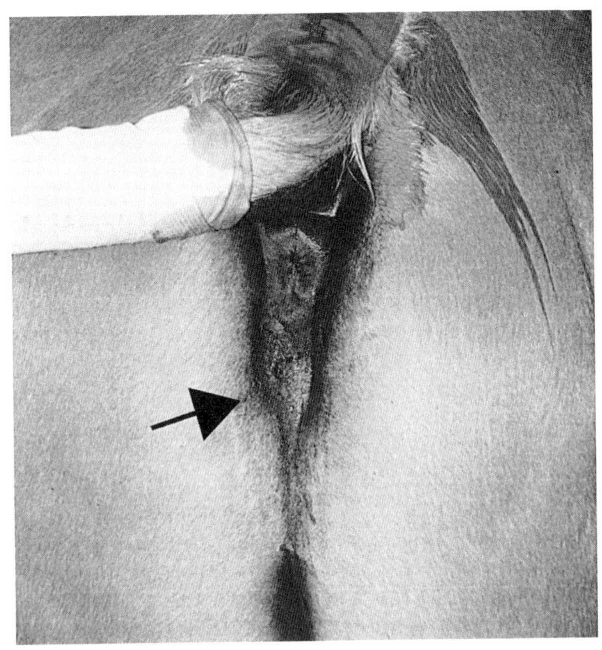

FIGURE 19-41 Perineum of Paint gelding with hematuria associated with a proximal urethral defect. The asymmetry of the perineal musculature is visible at the level of the ischial arch. (Arrow shows where asymmetry is more prominent on left side.)

anesthesia, one makes a vertical incision down to a catheter placed in the urethra. The surgical wound requires several weeks to heal, and moderate hemorrhage from the CSP is apparent for the first few days after surgery. Additional treatment consists of local wound care and prophylactic antibiotic treatment (typically a trimethoprim-sulfonamide combination) for 7 to 10 days. Hematuria should resolve within 1 week after this procedure. Limiting the incision to entry of the CSP but not into the urethral lumen also has been a successful treatment and is now the preferred surgical treatment.[30] This treatment option provides support for the blowout cause and lessens the risk of urethral stricture formation. Furthermore, the treatment decreases the chance of a permanent fistula forming at the site, a surgical complication that has occurred in geldings.

IDIOPATHIC RENAL HEMATURIA

Idiopathic renal hematuria is a syndrome characterized by sudden onset of gross, often life-threatening hematuria.[35,36] Hemorrhage arises from one or both kidneys and is manifested by passage of blood clots in urine. Endoscopic examination of the urethra and bladder usually reveals no abnormalities of these structures, but one may see blood clots exiting one or both ureteral orifices. Although a definitive cause of renal hemorrhage may be established in some horses (e.g., renal adenocarcinoma, arteriovenous or arterioureteral fistula),[37,38] the disorder is termed *idiopathic* when a primary disease process cannot be determined. Both sexes, a wide age range, and several breeds of horses (including a mammoth donkey and a mule) have been affected. However, more than 50% of animals with idiopathic renal hematuria have been Arabians.

Use of the term *idiopathic renal hematuria* to describe this syndrome of horses was adopted from its use in human patients and dogs with severe renal hemorrhage.[2,38-45] *Benign essential hematuria* and *benign primary hematuria* are other terms that describe less severe hematuria that is not associated with trauma or other obvious causes of hematuria. In the latter species, hematuria is more commonly a unilateral than a bilateral problem, similar to what has been observed in the few affected horses. The pathophysiology remains poorly understood, but macroscopic hematuria has been associated with immune-mediated glomerular damage (e.g., acute postinfectious glomerulonephritis, membranoproliferative glomerulonephritis, immunoglobulin A nephropathy, Berger's disease), thin basement membrane nephropathy, and the loin pain–hematuria syndrome in human patients.

Although hematuria and pigmenturia can accompany a number of systemic diseases in horses,[46-48] patients affected with idiopathic renal hematuria appear to have spontaneous, severe hematuria in the absence of other signs of disease. Although one report suggested that severe renal hemorrhage resulted from pyelonephritis,[15] supportive data were lacking. In cases managed by the author, neither UTI nor lithiasis has been detected; the magnitude of hematuria often resulted in the need for repeated blood transfusions. As with hemorrhage associated with guttural pouch mycosis, the syndrome may produce episodic hemorrhage. Initially, one notes hemorrhage by finding a large amount of clotted blood in stall bedding or in the pasture. However, other client complaints (e.g., depression, anorexia, weight loss) are typically absent. Examination

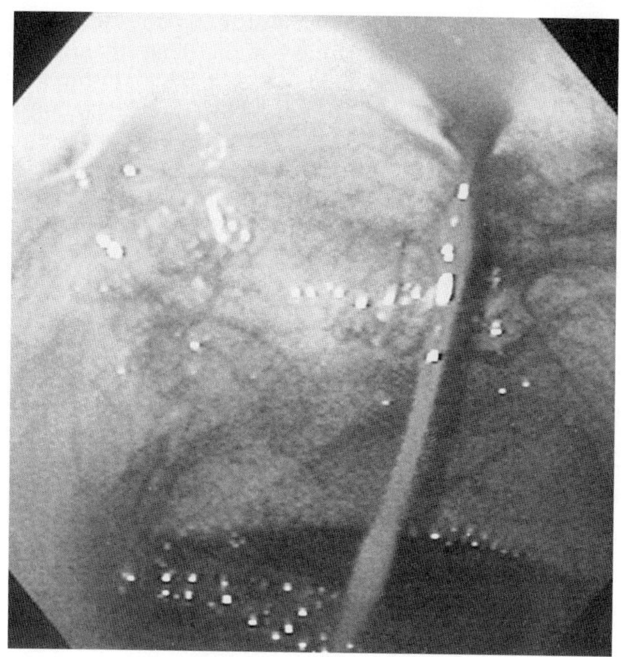

FIGURE 19-42 Endoscopic image of a large blood clot exiting the right ureteral opening of a gelding with idiopathic renal hematuria.

may reveal dried blood at the end of the penis or in the sheath of males or on the vulvar lips and between the hindlimbs of mares. In both sexes, neoplasia of the external genitalia or urinary tract is an important differential diagnosis, whereas in mares, one also must consider varicosities in the area of the vestibulovaginal sphincter, especially in multiparous mares. When blood is not detected in the sheath or vulvar areas, further evaluation may be unrewarding because the renal bleeding may cease spontaneously. Bleeding has been attributed anecdotally to cystitis and pyelonephritis in the absence of positive urine culture results, because hemorrhage stops during a course of antimicrobial therapy. More likely, spontaneous resolution has occurred. Furthermore, the magnitude of hematuria is considerably greater with idiopathic renal hematuria than with most UTIs, pyuria is absent, and urine culture results are negative. In the author's experience, one or two initial episodes of hemorrhage are followed by a more severe hemorrhagic crisis within months to several years after observation of the initial bleeding episode. Interestingly, renal colic has been notably absent in the history of affected horses.

One diagnoses idiopathic renal hematuria by exclusion of systemic disease, other causes of hematuria, and alterations in hemostasis. Physical examination may reveal tachycardia, tachypnea, and pale membranes consistent with acute blood loss. Rectal palpation may reveal an enlarged, irregular bladder because of the presence of blood clots. Azotemia is inconsistent. Endoscopic examination is important to document that hematuria is originating from the upper urinary tract and to determine whether hemorrhage is unilateral or bilateral (Figure 19-42). Repeated examinations may be required to answer the latter question. Ultrasonographic imaging is necessary to rule out nephrolithiasis or ureterolithiasis and occasionally may reveal a distended vascular space or renal vascular anomaly as the cause of hematuria. Renal scintigraphy can be a useful technique in affected horses because it may provide semiquantitative information about renal function when a nephrectomy is being considered. Renal biopsy and immunofluorescent staining may assist in documenting immune-mediated glomerular injury, but the significance of such results is not well understood at this time.

Treatment for idiopathic renal hematuria consists of supportive care for acute blood loss, including blood transfusions. Medications intended to promote hemostasis (e.g., aminocaproic acid, formalin) also have been administered, but their efficacy has not been validated. Treatment with corticosteroids may be useful in cases with potential immune-mediated mechanisms as the cause of bleeding. Because the condition may be self-limiting in some patients, supportive care is warranted. With severe and recurrent hematuria of unilateral renal origin, a nephrectomy may be indicated, but one should warn owners of the risk of hematuria developing in the contralateral kidney. In the author's experience, risk of contralateral renal bleeding appears to be greater in the Arabian breed.

EXERCISE-ASSOCIATED HEMATURIA

Exercise is accompanied by increased filtration of RBCs and protein across the glomerular barrier in a large percentage of human and equine athletes.[4,49] Typically the hematuria is microscopic, but occasionally one may observe gross discoloration of urine. Gross hematuria more often may result from bladder erosions, which may be induced traumatically by the abdominal contents pounding the bladder against the pelvis during exercise.[50] Detection of focal bladder erosions or ulcers with a contrecoup distribution and a history of emptying the bladder immediately before the exercise bout would be characteristic for this problem. A diagnosis of exercise-associated hematuria should be one of exclusion after diagnostic evaluation has ruled out other causes of hematuria such as presence of a cystolith.

PIGMENTURIA ASSOCIATED WITH SYSTEMIC DISEASE

With any systemic disease that may lead to hemolysis, thrombocytopenia, coagulopathy, or alterations in vascular permeability, hematuria or hemoglobinuria may develop. Discolored urine has the potential to be accompanied by a degree of nephrotoxicity because of interaction of iron ions of the heme molecules with surface molecules on proximal tubular epithelial cells. With transient pigmenturia (as with exercise-associated hematuria), changes in renal function may not be apparent, but with more severe disease processes, ARF may develop. In human beings, a syndrome of hemolytic anemia and thrombocytopenia leading to development of ARF has been termed the *hemolytic-uremic syndrome*.[51] The syndrome is recognized more commonly in children than in adults and is the most common cause of ARF in children. Similar syndromes have been described in a limited number of horses.[46-48] Furthermore, hemolysis and hemoglobinuria may be recognized with liver disease, medications, or intoxications (e.g., ingestion of red maple leaves). Finally, conditions accompanied by extensive rhabdomyolysis also may result in pigmenturia and ARF.[52] Assessment of muscle enzyme activity in these cases usually is rewarding in establishing myoglobin as the most likely cause of pigmenturia. In addition, one can use the Blondheim test (ammonium sulfate precipitation) to differentiate myoglobinuria from hemoglobinuria.[53]

POLYURIA AND POLYDIPSIA

Harold C. Schott II

For small animals, polyuria and polydipsia have been defined as urine output exceeding 50 ml/kg/day and fluid intake of more than 100 ml/kg/day.[1,2] These values would equate to 25 L of urine production and 50 L of water consumption for a 500-kg horse. Compared with normal values for daily urine production and water consumption of 5 to 15 L and 20 to 30 L, respectively,[3-10] these definitions of polyuria and polydipsia appear applicable to horses as well. One must remember that urine production and water consumption vary with age, diet, workload, environmental temperature, and gastrointestinal water absorption. For example, urine production increases by 50% to 100% when the diet is changed from a grass to a legume hay.[11] Although this increase in urine production has been associated with higher dietary protein intake and urinary nitrogen excretion,[12] increases in calcium intake and urinary calcium excretion may be another contributing factor. Similarly, horses that are exercised heavily, are stabled in hot climates, or have chronic diarrhea may have a water intake exceeding 100 L per day yet produce normal volumes of urine.[13]

A brief review of water turnover by the equine kidneys provides insight into how a small change in renal water reabsorption can lead to a dramatic increase in urine production (polyuria). In normal horses, GFR exceeds 1000 L per day, a volume that is 10 times greater than the total extracellular fluid volume; however, approximately 99% of this water is reabsorbed in the renal tubules and collecting ducts, resulting in production of between 5 and 15 L of urine daily. The result is urine that is three to four times more concentrated than plasma (urine osmolality of 900-1200 mOsm/kg and a specific gravity of 1.025 to 1.050). Furthermore, urea (in urine) has replaced sodium (in plasma) as the most important solute. If only 98% of water is reabsorbed, then urine volume would double and the additional water would result in more dilute urine (urine osmolality of 450 to 600 mOsm/kg and a specific gravity of 1.015 to 1.025). If water reabsorption decreased to 96% of filtered water, then the horse would produce approximately 40 L of urine with a urine osmolality of 225 to 300 mOsm/kg and a specific gravity of 1.005 to 1.010 (Table 19-11). In the latter case, urine is more dilute than plasma (hyposthenuria) and the kidneys are excreting or losing water actively. Under certain conditions, active water excretion by the kidneys is important for maintenance of plasma osmolality in the normal range. The best example is a neonatal foal that may ingest a volume of milk exceeding 20% of its body weight daily.[14] This ingestion equates to a fluid intake approaching 250 ml/kg/day, and failure to produce a large volume of hyposthenuric urine could result in water retention, decreased plasma osmolality, and clinical hyponatremia (manifested by neurologic signs).

Determining that a horse is producing more urine than normal is often difficult, especially in horses kept at pasture. Owners may report that a horse is polyuric when in fact the frequency of urination has increased (pollakiuria) rather than the volume. Pollakiuria occurs with conditions such as cystitis and urolithiasis or during estrus in the mare. Horses housed in stalls bedded with straw are difficult to evaluate because excessive urine may not be obvious to the casual observer. For those bedded on shavings or sawdust, excessively wet bedding may be easier to recognize, but this is a subjective impression. Occasionally in a horse the polyuria may be so severe that urine may flow from the stall into the barn aisle. When doubt exists as to whether a horse has polyuria and polydipsia, documentation of water consumption over one or more 24-hour periods may be necessary.[6] One can quantify urine production by collecting urine over a 12- or 24-hour period. For geldings and stallions, one can construct a collection device by cutting off the bottom of a large plastic bottle, padding it, and fitting it over the prepuce. One covers the opening of the bottle with a rubber tube and clip to allow removal of urine every few hours. In mares, one can place an indwelling Foley catheter in the bladder or apply a urine collection harness.[15-19] During the collection period, horses usually are tied to minimize interference with the collection device.

The major causes of polyuria in horses include renal failure, PPID (Cushing's disease), and primary or psychogenic polydipsia.[15,20] Less common causes include excessive salt consumption, central and nephrogenic diabetes insipidus, diabetes mellitus, sepsis and endotoxemia, and iatrogenic causes (sedation with α_2-agonists, corticosteroid therapy, or diuretic use).

TABLE 19-11

Relationship of the Percentage of Water Filtered that is Reabsorbed to Daily Urine Output and Renal Water Absorption

Glomerular Filtration Rate (GFR) (L/day)	Percentage of Filtered Water Reabsorbed	Urine Production (L/day)	Urine Osmole Excretion (mOsm)	Urine Osmolality (mOsm/kg)	Renal Water Reabsorption* (L/day)
1000	99%	10	10,000	1000	23.3
1000	98%	20	10,000	500	13.3
1000	96%	40	10,000	250	−6.7

*Renal water reabsorption (the inverse of free water clearance) is a calculated volume of water that is retained or lost by the kidney. Renal water reabsorption is calculated from actual urine volume and the calculated volume of urine required to excrete all osmoles in urine that is isosmotic with plasma. In this table a urine osmolality value of 300 mOsm/kg is assumed to be isosmotic to plasma, 1 kg of water is assumed to equal 1 L of water, and a total of 10,000 osm is assumed to be excreted daily. Thus when 98% of filtered water is reabsorbed, the 20 L of urine produced (if isosmotic) would contain 6000 mOsm. Because an additional 13.3 L of water would be needed to excrete the remaining 4000 mOsm (as isosmotic urine), the kidneys are considered to be actively reabsorbing 13.3 L of water.

RENAL FAILURE

Horses with ARF usually have a transient period of anuria or oliguria. If horses survive the acute phase of renal disease, then tubule damage results in a subsequent period during which impaired concentrating ability results in polyuria.[15,21] Urine is frequently hyposthenuric during this period of tubular repair. Owners should provide horses recovering from ARF with adequate water, salt, and a low-nitrogen (protein) and low-calcium diet. Such a diet consists of good quality grass hay or nonlegume pasture. Repair of tubules and return of concentrating ability may take several weeks. Although these animals appear to have normal renal function after this recovery period, a permanent reduction in total renal function likely persists because most animals can maintain apparently normal health with only about 30% to 50% of functioning nephrons.

CRF may develop after damage from nephrotoxins. In addition, immune-mediated mechanisms, chronic infection, and nephrolithiasis may give rise to CRF.[21-23] Horses that do not recover from the ischemic renal damage occurring with hypovolemic or endotoxic shock also may progress to CRF. Signs vary and include polyuria and polydipsia in some cases. When present, polyuria and polydipsia are usually moderate compared with the dramatic increases in urine production observed with primary polydipsia or diabetes insipidus. Most horses with CRF also exhibit other signs, including poor performance, weight loss, and ventral edema. A variable degree of azotemia is present, and urinalysis reveals isosthenuria (urine is isosmotic with plasma [260 to 300 mOsm/kg] with a specific gravity of 1.008 to 1.014).

The mechanisms of polyuria after acute and CRF are not entirely clear.[24] Increased tubular flow rate in surviving nephrons is one possible mechanism that would result in less time for water removal from tubular fluid. Next, medullary hypertonicity may decrease because of diminished transport of sodium and chloride out of tubular fluid passing through the ascending limb of the loop of Henle (diluting segment of the nephron) along with increased blood flow through the remaining medullary tissue. A third possibility is impaired response of collecting ducts to vasopressin (acquired nephrogenic diabetes insipidus). Although all these mechanisms may contribute to the polyuria of renal failure, which particular mechanism may be the most influential is not known. Furthermore, because the horse can produce hyposthenuric urine during the recovery phase of ARF, the mechanisms of polyuria differ somewhat for acute and CRF.

PITUITARY PARS INTERMEDIA DYSFUNCTION

PPID is a common disorder of older horses that is often referred to as *equine Cushing's disease* because of its similarity to Cushing's disease in dogs and humans.[20,25-32] The clinical syndrome of PPID in horses is associated with hirsutism, laminitis, weight loss, and polydipsia and polyuria. The disorder is discussed in detail elsewhere in this text.

In one review of 17 horses with PPID, polyuria and polydipsia were found in 13 (76%)[32]; however, in another series of 21 horses with PPID, polyuria and polydipsia were not a historical complaint in any of the affected horses.[31] Thus the polyuria and polydipsia associated with Cushing's disease are generally less severe than that observed with primary polydipsia or diabetes insipidus. PPID may lead to polyuria by several mechanisms. First, polyuria may result from actions of hormones derived from proopiomelanocortin, most specifically adrenocorticotropin. Hyperadrenocorticism resulting from excessive adrenocorticotropin activity on the adrenal cortex can lead to hyperglycemia, which may exceed the renal tubular threshold for reabsorption. The renal threshold for glucose in horses appears to be lower than in small animals (about 150 mg/dl).[33] When plasma glucose concentrations exceed this threshold value, the resultant glucosuria can lead to an osmotic diuresis. Although commonly implicated as the cause of polyuria in horses with PPID, glucosuria was found in only one of five affected horses in a recent clinical report.[31] Furthermore, horses with hyperglycemia and glucosuria still may be able to concentrate their urine in response to water deprivation.[28] A second mechanism implicated in the development of polyuria is cortisol antagonism of the action of vasopressin on the collecting ducts. Although frequently cited as the mechanism of polyuria in canine hyperadrenocorticism, experimental evidence to support this mechanism is lacking in dogs and horses. Furthermore, considerable species heterogeneity exists in the effects of corticoids on vasopressin activity, and in some species a primary dipsogenic effect may be more important. Next, growth of the pars intermedia may lead to impingement on the posterior pituitary and hypothalamic nuclei (located immediately dorsal to the pituitary gland), the sites of vasopressin storage and production, respectively. Decreased vasopressin production and release would result in a partial central diabetes insipidus as a third mechanism for polyuria.[25] Central diabetes insipidus, however, is not the cause of polyuria in all cases because some affected horses can concentrate their urine when deprived of water.[28] Consequently, polyuria and polydipsia seen in many horses with PPID is likely the combined result of several mechanisms.

PRIMARY POLYDIPSIA

Although rare, primary or psychogenic polydipsia is probably the most common cause of polyuria and polydipsia in adult horses for which clients have a primary complaint of excessive water consumption and urination.[15,20] Primary polydipsia can be attributed to the fact that horses that exhibit this problem are generally in good body condition and are not azotemic. Furthermore, the magnitude of polyuria typically is much greater than that observed with renal failure or PPID. Owners may report that horses with primary polydipsia drink two to three times more water than their stablemates and their stalls often are flooded with urine. In some instances, primary polydipsia appears to be a stable vice that reflects boredom in affected horses, whereas in other cases it may develop after a change in environmental conditions, stabling, diet, or medication administration. Anecdotally, primary polydipsia is reported to be more common in Southern states during periods of high temperature and humidity. In human beings, primary polydipsia can be a compulsive behavior associated with mental illness or may be caused by a primary abnormality in the osmoregulation of thirst, in which case it is referred to as *dipsogenic diabetes insipidus*.[34] The latter may be idiopathic or may occur after neurologic disease involving the hypothalamic osmoreceptors regulating thirst. Excessive water consumption causes expansion and dilution of body fluids, leading to a decrease in plasma osmolality and suppression of vasopressin release. With low plasma vasopressin concentrations, collecting ducts become impermeable to water and hyposthenuria is induced to allow rate of water excretion to balance intake. In human beings, the magnitude of polydipsia and resultant polyuria vary considerably between affected persons, and similar variation, although undocumented, likely occurs in affected horses as well.

One diagnoses primary polydipsia by exclusion of renal failure and hyperadrenocorticism. In addition, other factors, such as salt supplementation and medication administration, must be excluded. One excludes diabetes insipidus and confirms the diagnosis of primary polydipsia by demonstrating urine-concentrating ability after water deprivation.[7,9] Specific gravity should exceed 1.025 after water deprivation of sufficient duration (12-24 hours) to produce a 5% loss in body weight. In cases of long-standing polyuria, the osmotic gradient between the lumen of the collecting tubule and the medullary interstitium may be diminished (medullary washout). In these cases, vasopressin activity may not lead to an increase in urine specific gravity to values greater than 1.020. Consequently, horses with primary polydipsia lasting several weeks that fail to concentrate their urine after 24 hours of water deprivation may be given a modified water deprivation test. One performs the test by restricting water intake to approximately 40 ml/kg/day for 3 to 4 days. By the end of this time, urine specific gravity should exceed 1.025 in a horse that has had medullary washout. If the urine specific gravity remains in the isosthenuric range (1.008-1.014), then one should evaluate the polyuric horse further for early CRF, in which urine-concentrating ability may be compromised before the onset of significant azotemia. In theory, CRF could occur when between two thirds and three fourths of functional nephrons have been lost. Subtle signs of decreased performance and mild weight loss also would support early renal failure. Finally, horses with primary polydipsia typically produce hyposthenuric urine. Although such dilute urine would be an unlikely finding in the early stages of CRF, it could be found in the polyuric recovery phase after ARF. In the latter instance a thorough history should reveal whether any event that may have been complicated by ARF may have affected the horse recently.

Management of horses with primary polydipsia is empiric. Because the diagnosis is one of exclusion, once one establishes that the horse is not suffering from a significant renal disease, one may safely consider restricting water intake to meet maintenance, work, and environmental requirements of the horse. In addition, one should take steps to improve the attitude of the horse by reducing boredom. Increasing the amount of exercise or turning the horse out to pasture are possible options, as is providing a companion or toys in the stall. Increasing the frequency of feedings or the amount of roughage in the diet also may increase the time spent eating and thus reduce the habitual drinking.

EXCESSIVE SALT CONSUMPTION

In an occasional case of apparent primary polydipsia, polyuria and polydipsia may be attributed to excessive salt consumption and are manifested by increased fractional sodium clearance. Such psychogenic salt eaters appear to be less common than psychogenic water drinkers, because the former would have to consume a substantial amount of salt to develop polyuria. In fact, the authors are aware of only one well-documented report of psychogenic salt eating in which a yearling Paint filly drank in excess of 500 ml/kg/day and had excessive urination when provided free access to salt.[35] The fractional clearances of sodium (3.4%) and chloride (2.6%) were increased and supported excessive intake. Although salt intake was not quantified for this filly, it may have exceeded 10% of the dry matter intake and appeared to be associated causally with muscle fasciculations and a stilted gait. Such a high intake is suggested because no increases in water consumption or urine volume were detected in one study in which ponies were fed diets containing 1%, 3%, and 5% of NaCl.[36] The 5% NaCl diet contained 5 to 10 times the daily requirement of NaCl and was similar to feeding about 350 g NaCl daily to a 500-kg horse. Similar to cases of primary polydipsia, the filly described in this report was able to concentrate urine in response to water deprivation, and the problem was managed successfully by limiting water intake to 50 ml/kg/day and preventing access to salt.

DIABETES INSIPIDUS

Diabetes insipidus results in polyuria and polydipsia because of vasopressin deficiency or insensitivity of the renal collecting duct epithelial cells to vasopressin. In human beings, vasopressin deficiency, or neurogenic diabetes insipidus, is the more common form, with hereditary and acquired forms being described. The hereditary form appears to result from decreased numbers of neurosecretory neurons in the supraoptic nuclei of the hypothalamus and is inherited in an autosomal dominant fashion. However, polyuria and polydipsia do not develop until after the first few years of life in affected persons, suggesting progressive loss of neurosecretory tissue. The acquired form of neurogenic diabetes insipidus results from degeneration of neurons in the supraoptic nuclei after trauma, vascular abnormalities, infection, or a variety of tumors.[34,37,38] As with the hereditary form, polyuria and polydipsia usually are not manifested until 80% to 90% of the neurosecretory neurons are destroyed.

In equids, two well-documented cases of neurogenic diabetes insipidus have been described.[39,40] Neither animal could concentrate urine in response to water deprivation, but administration of exogenous vasopressin resulted in an increase in urine concentration and a decrease in urine volume. In a Welsh pony in which the condition was considered idiopathic, the absence of an increase in plasma vasopressin concentration after water deprivation (compared with control ponies) further supported a diagnosis of neurogenic diabetes insipidus.[39] Acquired neurogenic diabetes insipidus after encephalitis was confirmed histologically in the other horse.[40] Two other reports of diabetes insipidus in horses more likely described cases of primary polydipsia because both animals demonstrated an ability to concentrate urine during water deprivation or had random urine specific gravities greater than 1.020.[41,42]

Nephrogenic diabetes insipidus results from resistance of the cortical and medullary collecting ducts to the antidiuretic action of vasopressin.[34,37,38] In the absence of systemic disease, nephrogenic diabetes insipidus is most commonly a familial disorder in human beings with an X-linked semirecessive mode of inheritance. As such, the disorder is carried by females and expressed in male offspring.[43] Nephrogenic diabetes insipidus has been reported in three colts, two of which were sibling Thoroughbreds, suggesting that an inherited form of nephrogenic diabetes insipidus also may occur in horses.[44,45] Two of the three colts were underweight for their age. Affected colts could not increase urine concentration in response to water deprivation, although they did show appropriate increases in plasma vasopressin concentration. Furthermore, minimal response to exogenous vasopressin administration in all three colts confirmed resistance of the cortical and medullary collecting ducts to the antidiuretic action of vasopressin.

Nephrogenic diabetes insipidus also may be acquired after drug therapy or a variety of metabolic, infectious, or mechanical (postobstruction) disorders. Anomalous or neoplastic disorders resulting in structural deformation of the kidneys are another potential cause of nephrogenic diabetes insipidus.[34,37,38] Necropsy and histopathology revealed no lesions in one colt and few focal interstitial aggregates of lymphocytes, plasma cells, and rare areas of interstitial fibrosis in the kidneys with focal necrosis of the renal pelvis and ureteral epithelium in another.[44] Histopathologic lesions found in renal biopsies from one case[45] included severe vacuolization and intracytoplasmic eosinophilic granular changes in distal collecting duct epithelium and occasional slightly increased cellularity of glomeruli. However, these lesions were apparently reversible and not observed in repeat biopsies performed later, after dietary and supportive therapy for diabetes insipidus.

Neurogenic and nephrogenic forms of diabetes insipidus share some similarities in pathogenesis. Polyuria because of a lack of vasopressin activity results in net water loss and an increase in plasma osmolality. As plasma osmolality increases, stimulation of thirst results in a compensatory increase in water consumption. In normal individuals and those with nephrogenic diabetes insipidus, the osmoreceptors in the hypothalamus sense the increase in plasma osmolality and subsequently signal for vasopressin release. As little as a 1% increase in plasma osmolality (about 3 mOsm/kg) results in a 1 pg/ml increase in plasma vasopressin concentration. In normal individuals, this small change is substantial enough to increase urine osmolality and decrease urine flow. With greater increases in plasma osmolality, more vasopressin is secreted. In human beings, urine osmolality approaches a maximum after an increase in vasopressin concentration to about 5 pg/ml (from a resting value of about 1.0 pg/ml).[34,38]

Limited studies in ponies and horses suggest that a similar degree of vasopressin release occurs in response to minor increases in plasma osmolality[46-48]; however, vasopressin also appears to be a "stress hormone" in horses because substantially greater concentrations (tenfold higher than those induced by water deprivation) have been measured after application of a nose twitch, nasogastric intubation, or exercise.[49] Thus increases in plasma vasopressin concentration after water deprivation would be expected to vary in horses, and separating osmotic effects from stress effects in an individual horse may be difficult. A word of caution also is warranted about subjecting horses suspected of having diabetes insipidus to water deprivation. Because urine-concentrating ability may show minimal improvement with either form of diabetes insipidus, affected horses may continue to excrete excess water in the face of water deprivation. As a result, they may become substantially dehydrated (10% to 15%) within the first 12 hours of water deprivation. Thus one carefully should monitor horses suspected of having diabetes insipidus during the period of water deprivation to decrease the risk of inducing serious hypertonic dehydration.

The Hickey-Hare test to diagnose diabetes insipidus involves infusion of hypertonic (2.5%) saline (0.25 ml/min/kg IV for 45 minutes) to stimulate vasopressin release and water retention.[45] Normal animals will respond with concentrated urine and reduced urinary volume after sodium infusion. Horses with diabetes insipidus did not concentrate urine after hypertonic saline administration.[44,45]

In addition to assessing the effects of water deprivation on urine-concentrating ability and plasma vasopressin concentrations, the final diagnostic manipulation is often administration of exogenous vasopressin (2.5 mU/kg in 5% dextrose [5 U vasopressin/l] constant rate infusion over 60 minutes or 0.5 U/kg IM).[50] In normal horses, urine specific gravity should increase to at least 1.020 60 to 90 minutes after vasopressin administration. Alternatively, DDAVP, a synthetic vasopressin analog, may be used. DDAVP is available as a nasal solution (0.1 mg/ml) for humans with central diabetes insipidus. The nasal spray can be diluted in sterile water and administered (0.05 μg/kg IV) for the diagnosis of diabetes insipidus in horses. Normal horses that underwent experimentally induced diuresis by repeated dosing of water via nasogastric tube increased urine specific gravity to greater than 1.020 from 2 to 7 hours after administration of DDAVP.

The medullary interstitial osmotic gradient develops as a result of countercurrent exchange, and the magnitude of the gradient is related inversely to tubular flow. Medullary washout may occur with the high tubular flow rates that can accompany renal disease. Although partial medullary washout may contribute to the concentrating defect in diabetes insipidus, the rapid response to exogenous vasopressin administration in cases of neurogenic diabetes insipidus (increase in urine osmolality to 900 mOsm/kg or greater) indicates that the medullary concentration gradient is not severely compromised.[34,51] This response further explains why in some cases of diabetes insipidus urine osmolality can be greater than plasma osmolality after water deprivation. The mechanism for this response is thought to be a decrease in tubule flow rate that allows more time for passive water extraction from the hypo-osmotic tubular fluid. With nephrogenic diabetes insipidus, one also may observe mild improvement in urine-concentrating ability (an increase in urine osmolality up to 500 mOsm/kg) in response to exogenous vasopressin administration. This response has been attributed to partial sensitivity of the collecting ducts to vasopressin and to vasopressin activity at other portions of the renal tubule.[34,37]

Treatment of diabetes insipidus should aim to manage polydipsia and polyuria. With neurogenic diabetes insipidus, recovery of vasopressin secretion is rare once the secretory neurons have degenerated to the degree that polyuria and polydipsia become apparent. Consequently, treatment consists of hormone replacement. In the past, intramuscular injection of Pitressin tannate in oil every 2 to 3 days was successful in limiting polyuria; however, development of resistance or allergic reactions was an occasional problem, and long-acting vasopressin formulations are no longer available. Vasopressin has relatively short antidiuretic effects and a short plasma half-life, which makes replacement therapy in horses difficult.[52] With the development of potent vasopressin analogs (desmopressin), effective treatment by nasal insufflation is now available.[34] The use of desmopressin for diagnosis and treatment of neurogenic diabetes insipidus in small animals has been described.[51,53] Largely by chance, other oral medications, including chlorpropamide and clofibrate, have been found efficacious in treating neurogenic diabetes insipidus. The mechanism of action of these drugs is uncertain, but they are thought to potentiate the effect of vasopressin on the collecting ducts.[34,51]

With nephrogenic diabetes insipidus, replacement hormone therapy is ineffective, and the only practical form of treatment for many years has been to restrict sodium and water intake or to administer thiazide diuretics. The latter treatment may reduce polyuria by 50% in many cases.[34] Thiazide diuretics inhibit sodium reabsorption in the distal tubule (diluting segment of the nephron) and increase solute delivery to the collecting duct. The mechanism by which such therapy paradoxically benefits patients with nephrogenic diabetes insipidus is ill understood. Explanations include enhanced proximal tubular fluid reabsorption (via glomerulotubular balance) and decreased glomerular filtration and tubular flow (via a greater osmotic stimulus to the macula densa and subsequent tubuloglomerular feedback).[34,38] Recently, treatment with prostaglandin inhibitors or amiloride has decreased polyuria in patients with nephrogenic diabetes insipidus. The former agents probably work by decreasing RBF and glomerular filtration, whereas the latter drug, a sodium channel blocker, is thought to act in a manner similar to the thiazide diuretics.[34] One horse clinically improved with only dietary salt restriction (no additional salt other than what was contained in feed) and limited but regular access to water.[45]

DIABETES MELLITUS

Diabetes mellitus is a state of chronic hyperglycemia usually accompanied by glucosuria.[54,55] The resultant osmotic diuresis is an occasional cause of polyuria and polydipsia in horses that has been described to result in a water intake exceeding 80 L per day.[56,57] Type I (insulin dependent) diabetes mellitus results from a lack of insulin that in human beings is usually attributable to viral or autoimmune disease. Those with type II (noninsulin dependent) diabetes mellitus have normal to high insulin concentrations but their tissues are insulin insensitive. Thus the response to an oral carbohydrate load or an intravenous glucose challenge is impaired, resulting in prolonged hyperglycemia.[54] The mechanism of insulin resistance is not well documented for horses but may result from decreased numbers of insulin receptors or lack of insulin receptor activation in response to insulin binding. The most common causes of equine noninsulin-dependent diabetes mellitus are equine metabolic syndrome and PPID, both of which are discussed in detail elsewhere in this text.[26-30]

Although uncommon, a few reports describe insulin-dependent and noninsulin-dependent diabetes mellitus that were not caused by PPID or equine metabolic syndrome and that resulted in polyuria and polydipsia as one of the presenting complaints.[56-61] Diagnostic evaluation reveals consistent hyperglycemia but negative dexamethasone suppression test results (a normal decrease of plasma cortisol to low concentrations). Treatment in most instances is supportive, although replacement insulin therapy may be helpful in cases in which measured serum insulin concentrations are low (insulin-dependent diabetes mellitus). In one case of pancreatic β-cell failure,[57] treatment with glyburide (0.02 mg/kg) and metformin (1.9 mg/kg) lowered interstitial fluid glucose concentrations to normal ranges. Insulin therapy may be of some benefit in horses with elevated serum insulin concentrations because pharmacologic doses in part may overcome the insulin insensitivity. In such cases, synthetic insulin products may be preferable over protamine zinc insulin, because one horse with PPID and secondary diabetes mellitus developed anti-insulin antibodies and had a relapse in clinical signs after 7 weeks of insulin therapy.[30]

SEPSIS AND ENDOTOXEMIA

Polyuria and polydipsia also have been reported as clinical signs in horses with sepsis or endotoxemia, although other clinical signs such as fever, abdominal pain, and weight loss predominate.[62] The mechanism is unclear but may result from endotoxin-induced prostaglandin production. Prostaglandin E_2 is a potent renal vasodilating agent in laboratory animals, and it antagonizes the effects of antidiuretic hormone on the collecting ducts.[63] Some horses with chronic gram-negative bacterial infections (e.g., peritonitis, pleuritis) may have low-grade or intermittent endotoxemia as a mechanism for polyuria, similar to the polyuria observed with canine pyometra.[64]

IATROGENIC POLYURIA

Finally, polyuria can be iatrogenic, occurring after a number of management practices or medical treatments. The most obvious iatrogenic cause is fluid therapy, for which polyuria is a desired response. Polyuria also has been observed with exogenous corticoid administration, although as for PPID the mechanism remains unclear. Human beings and dogs appear to experience a potent thirst response to exogenous corticoids; thus polydipsia may be an important cause of the polyuria observed. In horses receiving long-term dexamethasone treatment for immune-mediated disorders, one may observe profound glucosuria (2 to 3 g/dl) that leads to osmotic diuresis in these patients. Finally, transient diuresis or polyuria accompanies sedation with the α_2-agonists xylazine and detomidine.[65,66] Although these agents cause hyperglycemia, and occasionally glucosuria, a more likely mechanism for the transient polyuria is the existence of α_2-adrenoreceptors on collecting duct epithelial cells. Activation of these receptors is another mechanism of vasopressin antagonism.[67]

RENAL TUBULAR ACIDOSIS

Warwick M. Bayly

The veterinary profession recognizes well that horses with acute or CRF are frequently acidotic. These animals are almost invariably azotemic, hypochloremic, and normo- or hyperkalemic and frequently have significant abnormalities on urinalysis. A less frequent renal disease associated with acidosis is renal tubular acidosis (RTA). RTA is a clinical syndrome of impaired renal acidification characterized by a hypokalemic, hyperchloremic acidosis without azotemia. Affected horses frequently have normal urinalysis. The condition has been well-described in human beings,[1-3] and several case reports documenting its existence in horses have appeared since the mid-1980s.[4-12]

The causes and pathogenic mechanisms responsible for the development of RTA are ill understood. In human beings RTA may be primary (genetic or idiopathic) or secondary, occurring after a variety of conditions, including hyperglobulinemia, various autoimmune disorders, kidney disease such as polynephritis and obstructive uropathy, cirrhosis, drug- or toxin-induced nephropathies (including amphotericin B toxicity), metabolic disorders involving nephrocalcinosis, and a number of genetically transmitted diseases. All reported equine cases apparently have been idiopathic, because no signs of primary renal, hepatic, or autoimmune disease or disturbance of calcium metabolism have been evident, and the horses have had no history of access to toxins. In some cases, however, low-grade renal tubular disease has been suspected because of mild proteinuria.

General agreement is that three types of RTA exist.[13] Type 1, also known as *distal* or *classic RTA,* arises from the inability of the cells of the distal tubule to establish a steep hydrogen ion gradient between the blood and the urine. This inability results from failure of normal H^+ from the distal tubules. In many cases, this gradient may be less than 10:1. Whether or not this low ratio is caused by an insufficient number of proton-secreting pumps in the distal nephron or by H^+ diffusing back across the lumenal membrane after being secreted is not clear. Accelerated K^+ secretion occurs because of the existing electrochemical driving forces in the distal nephron and the lack of protons to offset them. In addition to having high urinary K^+ clearances, patients may be hypercalciuric and hyperphosphaturic, although in horses this may be difficult to assess. Equine urinary concentrations of K^+ and Ca^{2+} in particular are high. In human beings, about 70% of adults with distal RTA develop some form of urolithiasis.[14] This condition has not been recognized in the few reported equine cases and may not be, given the significant differences between the two species.

Type 2, or proximal, RTA is caused by a failure of HCO_3^- resorption in the proximal tubule. This part of the nephron usually reabsorbs the bulk of the filtered HCO_3^- via Na^+ and H^+ exchange and the subsequent breakdown of carbonic acid to carbon dioxide and water under the influence of carbonic anhydrase. Disruption of normal Na^+ and H^+ exchange or carbonic anhydrase activity therefore results in excess flow of HCO_3^- to the distal tubule where the ability to resorb the anion is poor. This bicarbonaturia also results in accelerated K^+ secretion and hypokalemia. In human beings with this form of the disease, the suggestion is that a reduction occurs in the threshold concentration at which HCO_3^- is reabsorbed from the proximal nephron. As a result, reabsorption resumes once serum HCO_3^- concentration drops below this threshold, and a new steady state is said to develop. More likely because of the urinary HCO_3^- loss, plasma HCO_3^- concentration decreases, as does glomerular filtration of HCO_3^-. Eventually the distal tubule reaches a point at which it can handle the amount of HCO_3^- presented. Urine pH may start to decrease because of the lower amount of HCO_3^- being excreted. A new steady plasma HCO_3^- concentration is established, albeit considerably below the normal range, and acid-base homeostasis may return gradually. Consequently, the type 2 condition often appears to be self-limiting in human beings.[15] This form of the disease occurs rarely by itself in human beings and almost always is associated with other signs of proximal tubule dysfunction such as defective resorption of glucose, amino acids, and phosphate (Fanconi syndrome). Type 2 RTA has been reported in two horses.[4]

Type 4 RTA is characterized by hyperkalemic, hyperchloremic acidosis and is common in human beings, but it has not been reported in horses. Type 4 RTA apparently is associated with hypoaldosteronism or resistance of the distal nephron cells to the effects of aldosterone. As a result the renal clearance of K^+ and H^+ is reduced. The associated natriuresis ultimately may lead to a reduced ability to concentrate urine because of "washout" of the medullary concentrating gradient, if the condition becomes chronic. Another form of RTA (type 3), which formerly had been described as having characteristics of type 1 and type 2 RTA, now is considered to be a variation of type 1.[13]

Differentiating between the distal (H^+ retention) and proximal (HCO_3^--wasting) forms of RTA is theoretically important if the approach to the human form of the disease is any guide, because in human beings the two types differ with respect to clinical severity, treatment, and prognosis.[16] The ability to differentiate between the forms of the disease in horses appears to be less critical, because treatment does not seem to differ much according to the suspected type of RTA. Table 19-12 summarizes some differential characteristics of the two types of the disease. In human beings with type 2 RTA, plasma HCO_3^- concentrations tend to be higher than those associated with the distal form of the disease; but this does not appear to be the case in horses, because all the horses the author has seen, plus those that have been described in the literature, have been severely acidotic (HCO_3^- concentrations of 10 mmol/L or less). In horses, differentiation between the distal and proximal types of the condition has been based on measurement of the urine pH. Evaluation of urine ammonium excretion, urine net charge or anion gap, and urinary Pa_{CO_2} have not been reported in horses, although they are regarded as critical to the specific differentiation of RTA in human beings.[17-19] Because of the alkalinity of normal equine urine, measurement of urine Pa_{CO_2} is probably of little benefit. With type 1 RTA, urine pH tends to stay high (i.e., in the normal

TABLE 19-12

Features Used to Differentiate Type 1 and Type 2 Renal Tubular Acidosis

Variable	Type 1	Type 2
Acidosis	Severe	Less severe, self-limiting
Hypokalemia	Severe	Mild to moderate
Glycosuria, proteinuria	Absent	Often present
Urine pH during		
mild/moderate acidosis	Inappropriately high	Inappropriately high
Severe acidosis	Inappropriately high	Normal
Effect of alkali administration	Decreases or worsens hypokalemia, depending on stage of disease	Worsens hypokalemia
Amount of HCO_3^- needed to correct acidosis	Low	High
Ammonium chloride challenge	Failure to excrete acid (urine does not acidify)	Urine pH decreases
Bicarbonate loading	Filtered bicarbonate is reabsorbed	Bicarbonate is lost in the urine

to alkaline range). In type 2, urine pH is generally neutral or slightly acidic. A suggested way of making this differentiation is to assess the urinary response to the administration of the urine-acidifying agent ammonium chloride (0.1 g/kg). Typically, one gives this solution orally, and it should lower the urine pH to less than 7.0, which it supposedly does in normal horses and those with type 2 RTA. In cases of distal (type 1) RTA, the urine pH remains high in the face of the increased acid load. Because the administration of such acidifying agents potentially could worsen the degree of acidosis in cases of type 2 RTA (as a result of reduced buffering capacity), performance of this test is not recommended until one has attempted at least partial replacement of the HCO_3^- deficit. In the author's experience, the ammonium chloride challenge test has proved unreliable, having failed to acidify the urine of normal healthy horses even when given intravenously in a 4-L solution. The dose and rate of administration may need to be increased before the test can be considered worthwhile. A more suitable alternative may be to infuse sodium sulfate as is done sometimes in human beings.[1] The author could find no reports of the use of this test in horses.

Another diagnostic option that may be worthy of investigation in horses is calculation of the urine net charge. As in any body fluid, the sum of urinary cations must equal the sum of its anions. Therefore in urine,

$$Na^+ + K^+ + Ca^+ + Mg^{2+} + NH_4^+ = Cl^- + HPO^- + SO^- + \text{other urine buffers} + \text{organic anions}$$

In human beings, Ca^{2+} and Mg^{2+} tend to be present in urine in small, constant quantities. Excretion of HPO^-, SO^-, titratable buffers, and organic anions is also constant and exceeds the Ca^{2+} and Mg^{2+} by an amount that is referred to as the *urine anion gap* (AG_u). Thus

$$Na^+ + K^+ - Cl^+ = AG_u + NH_4^+$$

The expression ($Na^+ + K^+ - Cl^-$) is referred to as the *urine net charge* and reflects the excretion of NH_4^+.[18] Given the aforementioned plasma electrolyte and acid-base abnormalities, type 2 RTA has been shown likely to exist when the urine net charge is negative (i.e., $Cl^- > [Na^+ + K^+]$) because NH_4^+ is greater than AG_u. In other words, H^+ continues to be secreted normally from the distal tubule, and plenty of NH_4^+ is being produced. When ($Na^+ + K^+$) is greater than Cl^-, the net charge is positive, indicating that NH_4^+ excretion is low because of failure to excrete H^+ (i.e., type 1 or distal RTA exists).

No breed or sex predilection exists for RTA in horses, and the average age for 16 affected horses was 7 years.[11] The most common clinical signs in affected horses are depression, poor performance, weight loss, and anorexia. Various other signs such as chronic weight loss, ataxia, dysphagia, and periodic collapse also have been reported. The latter three signs may be manifestations of severe weakness, which probably is caused by the severe hypokalemia. The reduced K^+ concentration also may be associated with bradycardia.

On clinical examination, affected horses are usually afebrile. Mild icterus is common, presumably because of the anorexia, although significant indirect hyperbilirubinemia and increases in serum concentrations of GGT and ALP have been observed. Although cirrhosis of the liver has been associated with the development of RTA in human beings, the equine cases of which the author is aware have demonstrated no clinicopathologic changes compatible with severe liver disease. Sulfobromophthalein clearance half-time was normal in the one case in which it was measured.[5]

One should suspect RTA whenever a horse has a severe hyperchloremic metabolic acidosis in the absence of any obvious cause of extrarenal hypovolemia such as diarrhea or small intestinal ileus. In such cases the plasma anion gap usually is widened, whereas with RTA it remains normal. (However, hypoalbuminemia may mask widening of the anion gap because albumin is normally responsible for much of the normal anion gap.[20] Therefore the anion gap value should be smaller in hypoalbuminemic horses.) Azotemia has not been recognized in horses with RTA, although signs of tubular dysfunction, such as mild proteinuria and increases in fractional K^+ clearance and urine GGT activity, have been observed. The results from renal biopsy and ultrasonic examination of the kidneys are normal.

Definitive diagnosis of RTA is based on the demonstration of severe hypokalemia (2.3 mmol/L or less) and a urine pH that is generally neutral or alkaline in the face of a severe acidosis (venous blood pH <7.15), although theoretically one could observe a slight aciduria with type 2 RTA. Hypokalemia in the face of severe acidosis is uncommon. Classically, the reverse is expected because of intracellular buffering of H^+ and the reciprocal role of H^+ and K^+ in maintaining the electric neutrality of the extracellular fluid. Occasionally, serum chloride concentrations are in the high normal range rather than being increased. Blood gas measurement usually reveals some degree of compensatory respiratory alkalosis (Pa_{CO_2} = 25 to 35 torr).

The differential diagnosis of RTA includes those of any animal that has sudden weakness, depression, and possible collapse: cardiovascular failure, neurologic disease (including rabies), hypoglycemia, and peracute toxemia or endotoxemia. One usually can rule out all of these based on a thorough physical examination that finds nothing to support their possible existence. These findings, plus demonstration of the aforementioned electrolyte and acid-base abnormalities, suggest RTA. Conditions such as hypokalemic periodic paralysis, Addison's disease, PPID, and chronic corticosteroid or diuretic abuse could cause some of these clinicopathologic disturbances, but not the combination of hyperchloremia, acidosis, hypokalemia, and a normal plasma anion gap.

Prompt recognition of the disease and quick institution of therapy are important because the untreated condition is potentially fatal. All reported equine cases of RTA have responded satisfactorily to treatment, as have the cases the author has seen. Although the ability to differentiate between type 1 and type 2 RTA may be important in human beings from a therapeutic perspective, the distinction has not seemed to be essential in horses. Regardless of the suspected type of the disease, treatment of the condition in horses is associated with HCO_3^- and K^+ replacement therapy. Although the administration of $KHCO_3$ would seem to be ideal, the lack of ready availability of this substance and the need for prompt therapy means that treatment usually involves a combination of orally administered KCl and intravenously administered $NaHCO_3$ and KCl. That one should not give $NaHCO_3$ without some form of potassium supplementation deserves emphasis, to ensure that the hypokalemia does not get worse. Generally, a steady improvement in the condition of the patient occurs after 12 to 24 hours of treatment. Oral fluids usually are given four to six times per day for the first 48 hours, whereas intravenous fluids frequently are given at a slow but steady rate. Inclusion of glucose or dextrose in the latter helps to promote uptake of K^+ by the cells. The serum chloride concentration usually decreases as HCO_3^- concentration increases. In the author's experience, a steady improvement occurs in HCO_3^- values, and these tend to improve more rapidly than the K^+ concentrations. Serum concentrations of the latter appear to be slower to return to normal, possibly because intracellular stores are replaced first. Estimating the total potassium deficit before the onset of treatment is impossible because of the huge intracellular deficit these animals suffer. In the author's experience, total deficits of this cation frequently exceed 4000 mmol.

With the correction of the acid-base and electrolyte disturbances, muscle strength and appetite generally return within 48 hours of the onset of treatment. At this point, one usually can reduce potassium supplementation and subsequently discontinue it once the forage intake of the horse has returned to normal. Obviously, giving the horse a diet that includes ample amounts of good quality hay is important because of the high potassium content of this feedstuff. Bicarbonate therapy generally continues longer, although one usually discontinues intravenous assistance in the horse with return of the appetite. Long-term oral supplementation with sodium bicarbonate is often required for the maintenance of normal acid-base status. Periodic rechecking of the animal is advised until it becomes clear that its condition is stable. Long-term follow-up of cases the author has seen and those that have been reported in the literature suggest that the prognosis is favorable but horses with evidence of renal disease may be more likely to relapse.[11]

NEOPLASIA OF THE URINARY TRACT

Harold C. Schott II

Although neoplasia of the urinary tract is uncommon in horses,[1-6] reports exist of tumors involving the upper and lower urinary tract in this species. Renal neoplasms, which represent fewer than 1% of all equine tumors, include adenomata, renal cell carcinomata, and nephroblastomata.[7] Renal adenomata are small, well-circumscribed lesions in the renal cortex, that are usually incidental necropsy findings.[8] The best-described renal tumor in the horse is renal cell carcinoma or adenocarcinoma.[9-19] These lesions arise from epithelium of the proximal convoluted tubules in most cases. In human beings, renal cell carcinomata are known as the *internist's tumor* because of their diverse and often obscure presenting signs. Although a classic triad of symptoms including flank pain, gross hematuria, and palpable renal mass has been described, these symptoms occur in fewer than 10% of affected human beings at presentation.[20] Similarly, affected horses usually have nonspecific presenting complaints, including poor performance, depression, weight loss, and recurrent colic (Table 19-13). A paraneoplastic process leading to severe hypoglycemia has been reported in two cases of equine renal cell carcinoma, probably caused by production of an insulin-like factor, an abnormal variant of insulin-like growth factor II, or less likely from excessive glucose use by the tumor.[17,18] Signs that increase suspicion of a primary urinary tract problem include hematuria (7 of 15 cases in Table 19-13) and detection of a palpable mass on rectal examination (9 of 15 cases in Table 19-13). Renal cell carcinomata are typically unilateral, and the contralateral kidney maintains normal renal function. Therefore indices of renal function such as BUN and Cr concentration are usually normal. Although nephrectomy is the treatment of choice in human beings, tumors are typically large and adherent to surrounding organs by the time they are detected in horses. Thus surgical removal usually is not possible. Furthermore, frequent metastases (10 of 15 cases in Table 19-13) are another indication that renal adenocarcinoma is usually not a treatable disease. The poor prognosis can be attributed to the fact that clinical signs of intra-abdominal neoplasia in horses often are not apparent until the disease is advanced.[21] In one report of renal carcinoma, clinical signs of the tumor were absent until the horse was anesthetized for laryngeal surgery. After an uncomplicated surgery, the horse was repositioned for recovery but died shortly thereafter. Compression of the caudal vena cava by a large renal carcinoma was suspected to have led to a decrease in venous return as the cause of sudden death.[22] In another horse, clinical signs were not observed until bony metastasis to the olecranon caused lameness.[19] Other neoplastic diseases that may affect the kidneys include nephroblastoma,[23-25] transitional cell carcinoma,[21,26] and squamous cell carcinoma.[27] Nephroblastoma (Wilms' tumor) is an embryonal tumor that arises in primitive nephrogenic tissue or in foci of dysplastic renal tissue, whereas the latter tumor types arise from the uroepithelium of the renal pelvis or ureter.[8] Papillary renal adenoma of distal nephron differentiation has been described as an incidental finding during necropsy of an aged mare.[28] Neoplastic involvement of the upper urinary tract also may occur with dissemination of lymphosarcoma, hemangiosarcoma, melanoma, or adenocarcinoma arising from other tissues in the abdomen.[2,7,8,21,29] Finally, although they are not truly cancerous disease processes, mucinous hyperplasia of the renal pelvic and proximal ureteral uroepithelium or ureteropelvic polyp formation can lead to development of a tissue mass in either kidney, ureteral obstruction, and hydronephrosis.[30,31] Renal mucous gland cystadenomas have been found incidentally at necropsy.[32] Mucous gland hyperplasia of the renal pelvis or proximal urethra are differentiated from cystadenomas by their thin fibrous connective tissue capsule, compression of adjacent renal parenchyma, multiple proliferative intraluminal papillary projections, and large mucus-filled cystic lumens.

In addition to rectal palpation for a mass in the area of either kidney and examination of urine for RBCs (hematuria), ultrasonographic evidence of a tissue mass destroying the normal architecture of the kidney would support renal neoplasia. Unfortunately, attempts to establish a definitive antemortem diagnosis were successful in only two previous reports. In the first case, neoplastic cells were detected on analysis of a sample of peritoneal fluid,[12] whereas percutaneous biopsy of the tissue mass in a second horse demonstrated neoplastic tissue. Thus these procedures are warranted in all horses with a mass consistent with a renal neoplasm. In addition to analyzing urine for hematuria, cytologic examination of urine for neoplastic cells is also warranted.[33]

The most common presenting complaint for bladder neoplasia is hematuria.[33-35] Unlike dogs, in which transitional cell carcinoma is the most commonly described bladder neoplasm,

TABLE 19-13

Clinical Features of Fifteen Horses with Renal Cell Carcinoma

Breed	Age (Years)	Sex	Unilateral or Bilateral	Presenting Complaint	Weight Loss	Pain/ Colic	Hematuria	Palpable Mass on Rectal Examination	Azotemia	Postmortem Findings	Reference
American Saddlebred	15	G	Bilateral	Recurrent colic	Yes	Yes	No	Yes	No	25-cm diameter renal calculus, metastases to liver and other kidney	9
Albino	10	F	Unilateral, left	Abortion and ascites	No	No	No	Yes	Mild	75-cm diameter, 31-kg mass, metastases to peritoneum	11
Standard-bred	16	F	Unilateral, right	Weight loss, hematuria	Yes	No	Yes	Yes	No	30-cm diameter, 8-kg mass, adhesions to liver and bowel, no metastases	11
Thorough-bred	16	F	Unilateral, left	Weight loss	Yes	No	Yes	Yes	Mild	35-cm diameter, 20-kg mass, hemoperitoneum, no metastases	12
Thorough-bred	16	F	Unilateral, right	Weight loss, soft feces	Yes	No	No	No	Mild	Metastases to liver and lungs	13
Pony	15	G	Unilateral, left	Weight loss, hematuria	Yes	No	Yes	Yes	No	6.6-kg mass, metastases to liver and lungs	14
Pony	10	G	Unilateral, right	Weight loss, back pain, colic, polyuria/ polydipsia	Yes	Yes	Yes	No	No	6-cm diameter mass hemoperitoneum, no metastases	14
Thorough-bred	4	G	Unilateral, left	Respiratory noise	No	No	NR	NR	No	30-cm diameter mass, local invasion of sublumbar muscles	14
Grade	7	G	Unilateral, right	Hematuria, followed by weight loss and colic	Yes	Yes	Yes	No	Mild	40-cm diameter, 23-kg mass, hemothorax and hemoperi-toneum, metastases to liver and lungs	14

TABLE 19-13

Clinical Features of Fifteen Horses with Renal Cell Carcinoma*—cont'd

Breed	Age (Years)	Sex	Unilateral or Bilateral	Presenting Complaint	Weight Loss	Pain/ Colic	Hematuria	Palpable Mass on Rectal Examination	Azotemia	Postmortem Findings	Reference
Thoroughbred	9	F	Unilateral, right	Recurrent colic, weight loss	Yes	Yes	No	Yes	No	30-cm diameter mass, metastases to omentum and muscle	15
Shire	4	F	Unilateral, right	Hematuria, followed by weight loss	Yes	Yes	Yes	Yes	No	65-cm diameter, 47.7-kg mass, adhesions to liver and bowel, no metastases	16
Grade	14	F	Unilateral, left	Pyrexia, hematuria, diarrhea	Yes	No	Yes	Yes	No	5-kg mass; metastases to liver, pancreas, and lungs	17
Mustang*	14	G	Unilateral, right	Collapse Hypoglycemia Colic Anorexia Diarrhea	Yes	Yes	No	No	No		19
Thoroughbred*	6	G	Unilateral, right	Depression Head pressing Obtunded Weight loss Weakness	Yes	Yes	No	Yes	No	35-kg mass, duodenum and jejunum loosely adhered to mass, metastases to liver	18
Arabian	21	G	Unilateral, right	Forelimb lameness Poor appetite	No	Yes	No	NR	NR	2×5-cm extrarenal mass at cranial pole of kidney, single metastasis to lung	20

*Paraneoplastic syndrome (hypoglycemia).
G, Gelding; *F*, mare; *NR*, not reported.

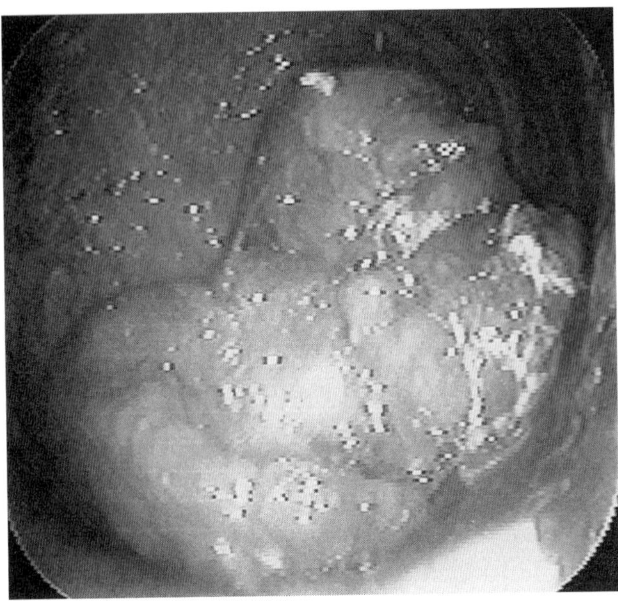

FIGURE 19-43 Leiomyosarcoma of the urinary bladder resulted in hematuria. (Courtesy R. MacKay, University of Florida.)

squamous cell carcinoma has been reported most frequently in horses.[33,34] Other types of bladder neoplasms affecting horses include transitional cell carcinoma, lymphosarcoma, leiomyosarcoma, and fibromatous polyps. In contrast to cattle, which develop bladder neoplasia in association with chronic ingestion of bracken fern and other plants (enzootic hematuria), dietary factors have not been incriminated in development of bladder cancer in horses.[8] One can establish diagnosis of bladder neoplasms by palpation or ultrasonographic imaging of a bladder mass, endoscopic examination and biopsy (Figure 19-43), and urine cytologic examination. Treatment has included partial bladder resection or intravesicular instillation of 5-fluorouracil, but successful outcomes have not been reported.[33] Doxorubicin (30 mg/m^2 IV) therapy was unsuccessful for the treatment of an extensive and poorly differentiated bladder leiomyosarcoma in one case.[36] Again, a poor prognosis likely is related to the extensive bladder involvement by the time clinical signs are apparent.

Tumors of the urethra and external genitalia are the most common urinary tract neoplasms of horses. Although reports describe a paraurethral lipoma[37] and fibrosarcomata[38] resulting in frequent urination or dribbling and UTI, respectively, tumors of the external genitalia are more common than urethral tumors.[39-41] Tumors affecting the external genitalia include squamous cell carcinoma, sarcoid, melanoma, mastocytoma, hemangioma, and papillomata or warts. Habronemiasis used to be a significant cause of genital lesions before the widespread use of ivermectin, and the disease should remain on the differential list because it can be distinguished from squamous cell carcinoma or sarcoid only by examination of a biopsy sample. Biopsy or simple impression smear of *Habronema* lesions will reveal extensive infiltration of eosinophils, which distinguishes habronemiasis from neoplasia. Breeds with nonpigmented genitalia (Appaloosas and Paints) appear to be predisposed to squamous cell carcinoma. Similarly, a predilection for geldings and stallions has been associated with a carcinogenic potential of smegma.[42] Affected horses may have a malodorous sheath or hematuria if the distal urethra is involved. Urinary tract obstruction is uncommon unless the tumors are large. Diagnosis is by visual examination and collection of a biopsy sample. Collection of the latter often is by complete excision of the lesion. In addition to surgical excision, a rather high rate of recurrence has led to use of a number of adjunct therapies, including immunotherapy, cryotherapy, hyperthermia, and radiation therapy. Some squamous cell carcinomas may respond well to adjunctive treatment with piroxicam (80 mg PO every 24 hours).[43] Tumor response is likely dependent on expression of cyclooxygenase-2 (COX-2) and not all equine squamous cell carcinomas produce COX-2 equally. Piroxicam is a selective COX-2 inhibitor in other species. Inhibition of COX-2 may induce apoptosis in neoplastic cells, inhibit angiogenesis, or act as an immunostimulant. Adverse gastrointestinal effects are possible during piroxicam therapy and may be avoided by administering every 48 to 72 hours. Piroxicam administration has also been recommended in the treatment of transitional cell carcinoma in small animals.[44] Because all treatment combinations have had variable success, some authors recommend aggressive surgical treatment early in the course of the disease.[45] Most recently, local injection of cisplatin, a cytotoxic antineoplastic agent, has been used with a high success rate to treat equine sarcoid and squamous cell carcinoma.[46,47] Topical 5% 5-fluorouracil cream (every 24 hours in mares; every 14 days in males) with or without surgical debulking may be effective for treatment of noninvasive squamous cell carcinoma of the external genitalia.[48]

URINARY INCONTINENCE AND BLADDER DYSFUNCTION

Warwick M. Bayly

Loss of control of bladder function is an infrequent problem in horses. When the condition is recognized, it is usually because a degree of incontinence develops, which by definition means that intravesicular pressure exceeds resting urethral pressure. Although a number of recognized abnormalities of bladder emptying can afflict human beings, dysfunctions of equine bladder control and micturition tend to fall into one of three categories, with the extent to which they are recognized depending on clinical signs. Basically, the three types of problems are (1) the reflex or upper motor neuron (UMN) bladder (also known as *spastic* or *autonomic bladder*), (2) paralytic or lower motor neuron (LMN) bladder, and (3) the myogenic or non-neurogenic bladder. Either of the last two conditions can be associated with the atonic bladder syndrome, which is probably appropriate given the similarity of clinical signs and subsequent treatment once either of the two types of conditions is recognized. In fact, although signs of UMN bladder problems are initially different from those of the other two groups, this condition in horses also usually is not recognized until a degree of incontinence develops. A final form of bladder neuropathy that has been described in human beings and dogs, but not in horses, is reflex dyssynergia. In this condition, loss of coordination of detrusor contraction and urethral relaxation occurs, with the result that the animal may make efforts to urinate but fail to do so. Such cases frequently appear similar to those of urethral obstruction, and one must distinguish between them.

Although treatment options are limited and tend to be the same, regardless of what type of condition is responsible for the incontinence, determining the origin of the problem is prognostically important. To accomplish this, the internist needs to have a good working knowledge of how micturition normally is controlled.

CONTROL OF MICTURITION

From a neurologic perspective, one can regard the bladder as having a body and an outlet, which can be divided further into the neck (or trigone) and the proximal urethra. Functionally, the bladder alternates between filling and storage and emptying and elimination phases.[1] Dysfunction in any of these areas or phases may result in clinical problems. Somatic innervation is primarily to the striated muscle of the urethra via a branch of the pudendal nerve, which originates from the sacral cord (S1 to S2). Other branches of this nerve go to the anal sphincter and perineum. The sympathetic nerve supply is provided via the hypogastric nerve, with the preganglionic fibers arriving from L1 to L4 and synapsing in the caudal mesenteric ganglion. From there, postganglionic fibers supply the bladder (β_2-receptors) and proximal urethra (primarily α_1- and some α_2-adrenergic receptors).[2] Parasympathetic innervation also originates in the sacral cord, with neurons combining to form the pelvic nerve. Many complex interneuronal connections exist between sympathetic and parasympathetic nerves in the wall of the bladder, as well as small adrenergic cells that facilitate contact between sympathetic and parasympathetic pathways.[3] As a result, complete denervation of the bladder is virtually impossible. During the filling phase, the tone of the smooth and striated muscles that together comprise the external and internal urethral sphincters increases. The pudendal nerve and the sympathetic nerves, respectively, innervate these muscles. Contraction of these muscles during filling maintains continence. Although the striated muscle forms a definite sphincter around the pelvic urethra, the anatomic existence of a bona fide internal sphincter is debatable.[4] However, the restriction to urine outflow that follows stimulation of the α-adrenergic receptors at the neck of the bladder has a sphincterlike effect. The smooth muscle of the bladder, referred to as the *detrusor muscle,* is innervated by the parasympathetic pelvic nerve and α_2-adrenergic postganglionic fibers.

The storage or filling phase is dominated by sympathetic nerve activity and provides an excellent example of the effects of reciprocal innervation.[5] During filling, the detrusor muscle relaxes because of α-receptor–mediated inhibition of pelvic nerve afferents and stimulation of sympathetic β_2-receptors in the smooth muscle of the bladder body. The latter is a reflex response that involves sensory input from bladder stretch and pressure receptors via the afferent pelvic nerve fibers to the sacral cord, interneurons in the cord, and pre- and postganglionic sympathetic axons in the hypogastric nerve. Relaxation of this muscle allows accumulation of large volumes of urine with little or no increase in intravesicular pressure.

Intravesicular pressure starts to rise once detrusor muscle fibers are stretched fully. Receptors in the bladder wall detect these increases, and impulses are transmitted via the pelvic nerve and ascending spinoreticular cord tracks to the pons, cerebrum, and cerebellum, where they are interpreted as the sensation of bladder fullness. Signals responsible for voluntary micturition originate in the cerebrum and exert their influence via the brainstem, from which UMNs descend in reticulospinal tracts to the sacral parasympathetic nuclei. This triggers the emptying phase. From these sacral segments, pelvic nerve impulses stimulate detrusor muscle contraction, action potentials traveling via parasympathetic ganglia in the pelvic plexus or bladder wall to postganglionic fibers that stimulate the smooth muscle. Depolarization waves spread throughout the bladder via tight junctions, resulting in a strong, coordinated, contractile process. Simultaneous inhibition of the pudendal nerve and hypogastric α- and β_2-sympathetic activity further facilitates detrusor muscle activity and relaxation of the external and internal urethral sphincters, respectively. Part of this inhibitory activity represents reflex neuronal activity linking pelvic and pudendal nerve axons in the sacral cord and inhibiting internuncial connections between sacral segments and the sympathetic neurons in the lumbar cord. Urethral sphincter relaxation also is coordinated centrally in a number of areas, including the cerebellum. Detrusor muscle contraction pulls the bladder neck open, and micturition occurs. The emptying phase ends when the bladder stretch receptors sense that the bladder is empty and afferent parasympathetic (pelvic nerve) impulses cease. Pelvic nerve efferent activity also stops, and pudendal motor and sympathetic nerve activity resumes (because it is no longer inhibited), with the result that the detrusor muscle relaxes, restoring external and internal urethral sphincter tone.

CLINICAL SIGNS OF BLADDER DYSFUNCTION

Control of bladder function obviously is complex, and many sites exist from which disruption of normal micturition could originate. In reality, problems are usually detectable in horses only when a degree of incontinence develops, which usually is manifested as constant or periodic dribbling of urine from the vulva or penis. In chronic cases, one frequently finds evidence of scalding and associated depilation of the perineum in mares and of the ventral abdomen in males, as well as the insides of the rear limbs in all animals. Any activity that results in increased intra-abdominal pressure, such as coughing or exercise, may exacerbate signs or else be associated with their initial observation. Adult horses develop these problems much more frequently than do foals.

Academically, being able to differentiate between the different neurogenic forms of bladder dysfunction and those of myogenic origin may seem important. In reality, the clinical signs and treatments tend to be the same, regardless of cause. UMN disease is characterized by increased urethral resistance, despite the presence of a full bladder, and may make catheterization or manual emptying of the bladder via rectal compression difficult. The condition usually occurs in association with broad, deep spinal cord lesions. In horses, these problems rarely are recognized in such cases because of the severe nature of associated clinical problems such as recumbency and myopathies. Frequently, such situations are deemed incompatible with life. (Possibly, a focal lesion caused by a disease such as equine protozoal myeloencephalopathy or an aberrant parasite migration could result in the development of spastic bladder without associated neurologic signs.)

If horses suffering from this type of problem are able to stand, are kept in a sling, or have an isolated problem, then in time they may develop the ability to urinate reflexively. This reflex develops because of the stimulation of pressure receptors connected to pelvic nerve afferents, which reflexively activate pelvic (parasympathetic) nerve efferents and the pudendal nerve. This activation results in detrusor muscle contraction and relaxation of the striated urethral muscle (external sphincter) leading to frequent urination, especially if the increases in abdominal pressure are regular, as may occur with any movement. These patients usually have some residual volume in the bladder after these voiding episodes. In such cases, urine dribbling usually is reported to occur intermittently, which is an important part of differentiating this type of dysfunction from paralytic (i.e., LMN) causes of incontinence.

As for the LMN bladder, lumbosacral trauma, EHV-1 myeloencephalitis, and cauda equina neuritis are probably the most common causes of this type of dysfunction, although in some parts of the world Sudan grass toxicity[6] and sorghum cystitis-ataxia (enzootic ataxia cystitis)[6,7] are major problems. Tumors of the lumbosacral spinal cord, such as lymphosarcoma and melanomas, are also capable of inducing paralytic bladder. Finally, iatrogenic paralysis after epidural administration of alcohol occasionally has been reported in show horses. Because this practice is taboo, how frequently the procedure leads to this problem is impossible to know.

With a paralytic (LMN) bladder, one usually sees other signs of LMN and lumbosacral dysfunction, including all or some of the following: loss of anal sphincter tone, tail paralysis, analgesia or hypalgesia over the perineum, atrophy of the muscles of the hip and hindlimb, and hindlimb weakness. Damage to the pudendal nerve and loss of external urethral sphincter integrity are therefore particularly important in the development of this problem. The bladder is atonic and distended with the urethral muscles relaxed, which results in urine dribbling because of overflow from the bladder. This incontinence may appear continuous, which helps to differentiate it from spastic (UMN) dysfunction. Sometimes the penis or vulva also may appear paralyzed. The prognosis is usually poor because of the development of secondary cystitis and general damage to the bladder wall and the detrusor muscle.

Myogenic problems occur mainly in geldings. Although myogenic problems can occur after the obstructive effects of cystic calculi and cystitis, the problem generally lacks a specific identifiable cause. The condition generally develops slowly, in association with the accumulation of large amounts of sabulous or mucoid urinary sediment or sludge in the bladder, which mainly is comprised of $CaCO_3$ crystals. In time, the weight and volume of this material, when coupled with that of normal urine accumulation, progressively stretch the detrusor muscle. Incontinence is not normally notable until the cranial aspect of the bladder begins to protrude over the edge of the pubis, which results in craniad and ventrad displacement of the sediment, with the result that the bladder muscle is stretched beyond its normal modulus of elasticity and normal contraction and micturition is no longer possible. Severe distention and stretching also lead to a breakdown in tight junctions that prevents depolarizing waves from passing from muscle fiber to muscle fiber. Eventually, overdistention becomes so significant that the ability to maintain sphincter function is lost and incontinence develops. These cases usually occur without any other signs of neurologic disease; however, because of the lack of any identifiable cause or specific pathophysiologic mechanism, specific focal lesions of a peripheral nerve such as the hypogastric nerve in fact could lead to a similar syndrome. Certainly, retention of urine in the bladder for any period results in the deposition of large quantities of sediment that in turn exacerbate the problem. One must recognize that part of the problem in cases of myogenic atony may stem from secondary cystitis, which develops after retention of urine for any period. The urea in retained urine breaks down to ammonia, which is irritating to the mucosal wall. Subsequent inflammation helps to damage the bladder musculature further.

Cystitis and chronic urethritis per se can be non-neurogenic, nonmyogenic causes of apparent incontinence. Irritation of stretch receptors in the bladder wall apparently causes regular stimulation of stretch receptors in parasympathetic afferents and stimulates detrusor contractions that cannot be inhibited voluntarily. This effect results in an apparent increase in the frequency of urination (pollakiuria) and an inability to control when it occurs. The condition frequently is referred to as *urge incontinence* and also may occur in association with a unilateral ectopic ureter in which the bladder is much smaller than usual (because of disuse) and incapable of storing a normal volume of urine. The frequency of micturition again is increased.

Hypoestrogenism also has been reported as a cause of non-neurogenic incontinence in an 18-year-old female Shetland pony.[8] A similar condition has been noted in older spayed bitches. The pathophysiologic mechanism of the condition is not known but probably is linked to a modulating effect of estrogen on the effects norepinephrine exerts on α-adrenergic receptor activity in the internal urethral sphincter.[9] In the documented case, the patient responded well to small doses (2 mg) of estradiol cypionate given intramuscularly every other day.

A transient postoperative condition that results in urine retention after abdominal or perineal operations has been noted in human beings.[10] The cause has not been explained, although the hypothesis is that a reflex depression of parasympathetic nerves may be responsible for detrusor muscle stimulation. This condition is distinct from that which may be associated with pain and reluctance to contract abdominal muscles after surgery. Whether such a condition exists in horses is unknown.

DIAGNOSIS

Careful general physical and neurologic examinations are the basis for characterization of the type of bladder dysfunction that exists in the equine patient and the basis for any efforts aimed at identifying a cause. Although never good, the prognosis appears to be most positive in cases in which the horse still can generate significant increases in intravesicular pressure. Therefore performance of tests aimed at evaluating bladder and urethral pressure–generating capacities may be diagnostically useful. Cystometry, which involves the inflation of the bladder with volumes of sterile water, isotonic saline, or carbon dioxide, has been described in horses and pony mares.[11,12] Briefly, one introduces a large-gauge (No. 30 French) catheter into the bladder and connects it via a three-way stopcock to an infusion pump and pressure transducer. The pressure transducer is connected to a chart recorder. One fills the bladder until micturition occurs. Intravesicular pressure is recorded continuously. Usually a gradual increase in pressure is related to the infusion of fluid until the pressure suddenly rises, reflecting the onset of detrusor muscle contraction. The pressure at the point of this sharp increase is regarded as the contraction threshold. In normal horses, this threshold is about 90 ± 20 cm H_2O.[11] One determines the urethral pressure profile in the same test by using a catheter with multiple side openings and positioning the tip at the urethral sphincter. One then fills the catheter with fluid and withdraws it at a constant rate while recording the intraurethral pressure. Normal values are usually greater than 50 cm H_2O. Pressures were significantly lower in recordings of three incontinent mares.[12] Although these tests have not been used widely, they have considerable prognostic potential. Put simply, the higher the pressures are, the better the prognosis is. One also can determine the distance over which high pressure is present in the urethra from these tests. Such determination also may be important, because it gives some further information on the integrity of the urethral sphincters.

TREATMENT

Some horses with UMN disease recover gradually, especially if one can determine and treat a specific cause. A major complication with paralytic and myogenic forms of bladder dysfunction is that cases often are not recognized until the atonia is irreversible. By that time the prognosis tends to be poor and identification of an initiating cause is difficult—and likely irrelevant. In such cases, the treatment is often futile; however, one often can determine this definitively only by assessing the response to attempted treatment. Regardless of whether dealing with UMN, LMN, or myogenic disorders, treatment tends to be the same concerning the bladder.

If a definitive cause such as EHV-1 myeloencephalitis or equine protozoal myeloencephalopathy is identified, then one should institute the specific treatment for that disease. Concerning bladder dysfunction, the basic aim is to provide support while hoping for spontaneous recovery, which may take a long time (e.g., months in cases of pelvic nerve damage). A basic aim of therapy is to prevent retention of urine because of the secondary problems that this entails. Therefore promotion of bladder emptying is an important goal that one may attempt to reach by regular catheterization or the use of an indwelling catheter. (In male patients, one normally inserts such catheters via a perineal urethrostomy.) Although facilitating drainage, intermittent or indwelling catheterization appears to predispose the horse to secondary bacterial cystitis and therefore should not be used without some forethought. Some horses that are chronically incontinent seem to survive comfortably without any catheterization.[7] Antimicrobial therapy is important for treating any incontinence cases but is especially critical when one uses indwelling or regular catheterization.

One may give the α-adrenergic blocker phenoxybenzamine (0.7 mg/kg PO every 6 hours) to eliminate any urethral resistance, thus facilitating emptying in the reflex UMN problem or in situations of great atonic overdistention. Bethanechol chloride is a parasympathomimetic agent resistant to the action of acetylcholinesterase and apparently has a selective effect on the smooth muscle of the gastrointestinal tract and bladder. The drug is used principally to stimulate detrusor muscle activity, and it acts by stimulating postganglionic parasympathetic effector cells rather than motor end plates. The recommended dosage ranges between 0.25 to 0.75 mg/kg subcutaneously three times a day. Starting the horse on the smallest dose is recommended. This drug reportedly has varying results.[13] Bethanechol has no effect when the bladder is completely atonic or areflexic. If the muscle is capable of generating weak contractions, then bethanechol may be useful. One could determine whether contractions are possible by cystometry. Although bethanechol can increase intravesicular pressure, whether it helps evacuate the bladder also depends on the status of the urethral sphincter and striated muscle. One must remember that drugs such as phenoxybenzamine and bethanechol can have undesired side effects on other body systems. The use of general muscle relaxants and an α-adrenergic blocker may be useful for achieving urethral muscle relaxation. Diazepam (0.2 to 0.5 mg/kg IV) and dantrolene are the most commonly used relaxants. Diazepam is effective in large doses, which also usually result in sedation. Dantrolene (10 mg/kg PO loading dose; 2.5 mg/kg PO maintenance every 6 hours) slows release of calcium from the sarcoplasmic reticulum and has been tried in dogs with varying effects.

Surgical removal of the sabulous sludge found in a number of these horses has been tried via perineal urethrostomy or cystotomy, with poor results.[14] Removal via cystotomy is not recommended because of difficulties in evacuating the material without contaminating the peritoneal cavity. Perineal urethrotomy, combined with irrigation with large volumes of fluid while the horse is anesthetized, seems to be the most effective way of removing this material. Five affected horses were managed for up to 3 years by repeatedly emptying the bladder through a urinary catheter and using saline lavage with cystoscopic guidance to remove residual sabulous material.[15] The cystitis was treated with antimicrobial and anti-inflammatory medications, and bethanechol chloride was also administered. Frequent catheterization resulted in a urethral stricture in one horse. Four horses returned to work and one was retired because of persistent incontinence.[15] The prognosis for most affected horses is poor because of chronic irreversible changes in the bladder wall, which seem to prohibit any possible return of normal detrusor muscle function.

REFERENCES

Anatomy and Development

1. Getty R, editor: *Sisson and Grossman's the anatomy of domestic animals*, ed 5, Philadelphia, 1975, WB Saunders.
2. Schummer A, Nickel F, Sack WO: *The viscera of the domestic animals*, ed 2, New York, 1979, Springer-Verlag.
3. Webb AI, Weaver BQM: Body composition of the horse, *Equine Vet J* 11:39–47, 1979.
4. Calhoun ML: Comparative histology of the ureters of domestic animals, *Anat Rec* 133:365, 1959.
5. Brenner BM, editor: *Brenner and Rector's the kidney*, ed 8, Philadelphia, 2008, WB Saunders.
6. Rytand DA: The number and size of mammalian glomeruli as related to kidney and to body weight, with methods for their enumeration and measurement, *Am J Anat* 62:507, 1938.
7. Beech DJ, Sibbons PD, Rossdale PD, et al: Organogenesis of lung and kidney in Thoroughbreds and ponies, *Equine Vet J* 33:438, 2001.
8. Yadava RP, Calhoun ML: Comparative histology of the kidney of domestic animals, *Am J Vet Res* 19:958, 1958.
9. DiBona GF: The function of renal nerves, *Rev Physiol Biochem Pharmacol* 94:75, 1982.
10. DiBona GF: Neural regulation of renal tubular sodium reabsorption and renin secretion, *Fed Proc* 44:2816, 1985.
11. Trim CM, Moore JN, Clark ES: Renal effects of dopamine infusion in conscious horses, *Equine Vet J Suppl* 7:124, 1989.
12. Denton MD, Chertow GM, Brady HR: Renal-dose dopamine for the treatment of acute renal failure: scientific rationale, experimental studies and clinical trials, *Kidney Int* 49:4, 1996.

13. Stone GW, Tumlin JA, Madyoon H, et al: Design and rationale of CONTRAST: a prospective, randomized, placebo-controlled trial of fenoldopam mesylate for the prevention of radiocontrast nephropathy, *Rev Cardiovasc Med* 2(Suppl 1): S31, 2001.
14. Thurmon JC, Steffey EP, Zinkl JG, et al: Xylazine causes transient dose-related hyperglycemia and increased urine volume in mares, *Am J Vet Res* 45:224, 1984.
15. Trim CM, Hanson RR: Effects of xylazine on renal function and plasma glucose in ponies, *Vet Rec* 118:65, 1986.
16. Gellai M: Modulation of vasopressin antidiuretic action by renal alpha 2-adrenoceptors, *Am J Physiol* 259:F1, 1990.
17. Prieto D, Hernandez M, Rivera L, et al: Catecholaminergic innervation of the equine ureter, *Res Vet Sci* 54:312, 1994.
18. Labadiáa A, Rivera L, Costa G, et al: Alpha and beta adrenergic receptors in the horse ureter, *Rev Esp Fisiol* 43:421, 1987.
19. Labadiáa A, Rivera L, Prieto D, et al: Influence of the autonomic nervous system in the horse urinary bladder, *Res Vet Sci* 44:282, 1988.
20. Prieto D, Benedito S, Rivera L, et al: Autonomic innervation of the equine urinary bladder, *Anat Histol Embryol* 19:276, 1990.
21. Prieto D, Benedito S, Rodrigo R, et al: Distribution and density of neuropeptide Y-immunoreactive nerve fibers and cells in the horse urinary bladder, *J Auton Nerv Syst* 27:173, 1989.
22. de Groat WC, Booth AM: Physiology of the urinary bladder and urethra, *Ann Intern Med* 92:312, 1980.
23. Carlson BM: *Patten's foundations of embryology*, ed 6, New York, 2003, McGraw-Hill.
24. Höflinger VH: Zur Kenntnis der kongenitalen unilateralen Nierenagenesie bei Haustieren II. Ihr Vorkommen bei den einzelnen Tierarten, *Schweiz Arch Tierheilkd* 13:330, 1971.
25. Jubb KVF, Kennedy PC, Palmer N, editors: ed 3, *Pathology of domestic animals* vol. 2, San Diego, 1985, Academic Press.
26. Huston R, Saperstein G, Leipold HW: Congenital defects in foals, *J Equine Med Surg* 1:146, 1977.
27. Johnson BD, Klingborg DJ, Heitman JM, et al: A horse with one kidney, partially obstructed ureter, and contralateral urogenital anomalies, *J Am Vet Med Assoc* 169:217, 1976.
28. Brown CM, Parks AH, Mullaney TP, et al: Bilateral renal dysplasia and hypoplasia in a foal with an imperforate anus, *Vet Rec* 122:91, 1988.
29. Schott HC, Papageorges M, Hodgson DR: Diagnosis of renal disease in the nonazotemic horse (abstract #15), *J Vet Intern Med* 3:116, 1989.
30. Jones TC, Hunt RD: *Veterinary pathology*, Philadelphia, 1983, Lea & Febiger.
31. Andrews FM, Rosol TJ, Kohn CW, et al: Bilateral renal hypoplasia in four young horses, *J Am Vet Med Assoc* 189:209, 1986.
32. Taxy JB: Renal dysplasia: a review, *Pathol Annu* 20:139, 1985.
33. Roberts MC, Kelly WR: Chronic renal failure in a young pony, *Aust Vet J* 56:599, 1980.
34. Anderson WI, Picut CA, King JM, et al: Renal dysplasia in a Standardbred colt, *Vet Pathol* 25:179, 1988.
35. Ronen N, van Amstel SR, Nesbit JW, et al: Renal dysplasia in two adult horses: clinical and pathological aspects, *Vet Rec* 132:269, 1993.
36. Ramirez S, Williams J, Seahorn TL, et al: Ultrasound-assisted diagnosis of renal dysplasia in a 3-month-old Quarter Horse colt, *Vet Radiol Ultrasound* 39:143, 1998.
37. Woolridge AA, Seahorn TL, Williams J, et al: Chronic renal failure associated with nephrolithiasis, ureterolithiasis, and renal dysplasia in a 2-year-old Quarter Horse gelding, *Vet Radiol Ultrasound* 40:361, 1999.
38. Gull T, Schmitz A, Bahr A, et al: Renal hypoplasia and dysplasia in an American Miniature foal, *Vet Rec* 149:199, 2001.
39. Zicker SC, Marty GD, Carlson GP, et al: Bilateral renal dysplasia with nephron hypoplasia in a foal, *J Am Vet Med Assoc* 196:1990, 2001.
40. Jones SL, Langer DL, Sterner-Kock A, et al: Renal dysplasia and benign ureteropelvic polyps associated with hydronephrosis in a foal, *J Am Vet Med Assoc* 204:1230, 1994.
41. Grantham JJ: Polycystic kidney disease: a predominance of giant nephrons, *Am J Physiol* 244:F3, 1983.
42. Gardner KD: Pathogenesis of human cystic renal disease, *Annu Rev Med* 39:185, 1988.
43. Zerres K, Eggermann T, Rudnik-Schoneborn S: DNA diagnosis in hereditary nephropathies, *Clin Nephrol* 56:181, 2001.
44. Cannon MJ, MacKay AD, Barr FJ, et al: Prevalence of polycystic kidney disease in Persian cats in the United Kingdom, *Vet Rec* 149:409, 2001.
45. Barrs VR, Gunew M, Beatty JA, et al: Prevalence of autosomal dominant polycystic kidney disease in Persian cats and related-breeds in Sydney and Brisbane, *Aust Vet J* 79:257, 2001.
46. O'Leary CA, Ghoddusi M, Huxtable CR: Renal pathology of polycystic kidney disease and concurrent hereditary nephritis in bull terriers, *Aust Vet J* 80:353, 2002.
47. Ramsey G, Rothwell TLW, Gibson KT, et al: Polycystic kidneys in an adult horse, *Equine Vet J* 19:243, 1987.
48. Scott PC, Vasey J: Progressive polycystic renal disease in an aged horse, *Aust Vet J* 63:92, 1986.
49. Bertone JJ, Traub-Dargatz JL, Fettman MJ, et al: Monitoring the progression of renal failure in a horse with polycystic kidney disease: use of the reciprocal of serum creatinine concentration and sodium sulfanilate clearance half-time, *J Am Vet Med Assoc* 191:565, 1987.
50. Aguilera-Tejero E, Estepa JC, Lopez I, et al: Polycystic kidneys as a cause of chronic renal failure and secondary hypoparathyroidism in a horse, *Equine Vet J* 32:167, 2000.
51. Ohba Y, Kitagawa H, Okura Y, et al: Clinical features of renal tubular dysplasia, a new hereditary disease in Japanese black cattle, *Vet Rec* 149:115, 2001.
52. Ohba Y, Kitagawa H, Kitoh K, et al: Inheritance of renal tubular dysplasia in Japanese black cattle, *Vet Rec* 149:153, 2001.
53. Sasaki Y, Kitagawa H, Kitoh K, et al: Pathological changes of renal tubular dysplasia in Japanese black cattle, *Vet Rec* 150:628, 2002.
54. Rhyan JC, Sartin EA, Powers RD, et al: Severe renal oxalosis in five young Beefmaster calves, *J Am Vet Med Assoc 201*:1992, 1907.
55. Schott HC, Bayly WM, Reed SM, et al: Nephrogenic diabetes insipidus in sibling colts, *J Vet Intern Med* 7:68, 1993.
56. Colahan PT, Mayhew IG, Merritt AM, et al: *Equine medicine and surgery*, ed 5, vol. 2, St Louis, 1999, Mosby.
57. Latimer FG, Magnus R, Duncan RB: Arterioureteral fistula in a colt, *Equine Vet J* 23:483, 1991.
58. Crotty KL, Orihuela E, Warren MM: Recent advances in the diagnosis and treatment of renal arteriovenous malformations and fistulas, *J Urol* 150:1355, 1993.
59. Takaha M, Matsumoto A, Ochi K, et al: Intrarenal arteriovenous malformation, *J Urol* 124:315, 1980.
60. Schott HC, Barbee DD, Hines MT, et al: Renal arteriovenous malformation in a Quarter Horse foal, *J Vet Intern Med* 10:204, 1996.
61. Schott HC, Hines MT: Severe urinary tract hemorrhage in two horses, *J Am Vet Med Assoc* 204:1320, 1994:letter.
62. Spiro I: Hematuria and a complex congential heart defect in a newborn foal, *Can Vet J* 43:375, 2002.
63. Wintzer HJ, editor: *Equine diseases: a textbook for students and practitioners*, New York, 1986, Springer-Verlag.
64. Baker JR, Ellis CE: A survey of post mortem findings in 480 horses 1958 to 1980: (1) causes of death, *Equine Vet J* 13:43, 1981.
65. Ordidge RM: Urinary incontinence due to unilateral ureteral ectopia in a foal, *Vet Rec* 98:384, 1976.
66. Rossdale PD, Ricketts SW: *Equine stud farm medicine*, ed 2, London, 1980, Baillière Tindall.

67. Christie B, Haywood N, Hilbert B, et al: Surgical correction of bilateral ureteral ectopia in a male Appaloosa foal, *Aust Vet J* 57:336, 1981.
68. Modransky PD, Wagner PC, Robinette JD, et al: Surgical correction of bilateral ectopic ureters in two foals, *Vet Surg* 12:141, 1983.
69. Robinson NE, editor: *Current therapy in equine medicine*, ed 6, St Louis, 2009, WB Saunders.
70. Richardson DW: Urogenital problems in the neonatal foal, *Vet Clin North Am Equine Pract* 1:179, 1985.
71. Robertson JT, Embertson RM: Surgical management of congenital and perinatal abnormalities of the urogenital tract, *Vet Clin North Am Equine Pract* 4:359, 1988.
72. Houlton JEF, Wright IM, Matic S, et al: Urinary incontinence in a Shire foal due to ureteral ectopia, *Equine Vet J* 19:244, 1987.
73. Sullins KE, McIlwraith CW, Yovich JV, et al: Ectopic ureter managed by unilateral nephrectomy in two female horses, *Equine Vet J* 20:463, 1988.
74. MacAllister CG, Perdue BD: Endoscopic diagnosis of unilateral ectopic ureter in a yearling filly, *J Am Vet Med Assoc* 197:617, 1990.
75. Pringle JK, Ducharme NG, Baird JD: Ectopic ureter in the horse: three cases and a review of the literature, *Can Vet J* 31:26, 1990.
76. Squire KRE, Adams SB: Bilateral ureterocystostomy in a 450-kg horse with ectopic ureters, *J Am Vet Med Assoc* 201:1213, 1992.
77. Blikslager AT, Green EM, MacFadden KE, et al: Excretory urography and ultrasonography in the diagnosis of bilateral ectopic ureters in a foal, *Vet Radiol Ultrasound* 33:41, 1992.
78. Blikslager AT, Green EM: Ectopic ureter in horses, *Compend Contin Educ Pract Vet* 14:802, 1992.
79. Odenkirchen S, Huskamp B, Scheidemann W: Two anomalies of the urinary tract of horses: ectopia ureteris and diverticulum vesicae, *Tierarztl Prax* 22:462, 1994.
80. Tech C, Weiler H: Ectopia ureteris: a contribution to diagnosis, therapy, and pathology, *Pferdeheilkunde* 12:843, 1996.
81. Jansson N, Thofner M: Ureterocystotomy for treatment of unilateral ureteral ectopia in a 300 kg horse, *Equine Vet Educ* 11:132, 1999.
82. Tomlinson JE, Farnsworth K, Sage AM, et al: Percutaneous ultrasound-guided pyelography aided diagnosis of ectopic ureter and hydronephrosis in a 3-week-old filly, *Vet Radiol Ultrasound* 42:349, 2001.
83. Holt PE, Thrusfield MV: Hotston Moore A: Breed predisposition to ureteral ectopia in bitches in the UK, *Vet Rec* 146:561, 2000.
84. Rossoff IS: *Handbook of veterinary drugs and chemicals*, ed 2, Taylorville, IL, 1994, Pharmatox Publishing.
85. Walker DF, Vaughan JT: *Bovine and equine urogenital surgery*, Philadelphia, 1980, Lea & Febiger.
86. Auer JA, Stick JA, editors: *Equine surgery*, ed 3, St Louis, 2006, WB Saunders.
87. Stickle RL, Wilcock BP, Huseman JL: Multiple ureteral defects in a Belgian foal, *Vet Med Small Anim Clin* 70:819, 1975.
88. Richardson DW, Kohn CW: Uroperitoneum in the foal, *J Am Vet Med Assoc* 182:267, 1983.
89. Robertson JT, Spurlock GH, Bramlage LR, et al: Repair of ureteral defect in a foal, *J Am Vet Med Assoc* 183:799, 1983.
90. Divers TJ, Byars TD, Spirito M: Correction of bilateral ureteral defects in a foal, *J Am Vet Med Assoc* 192:384, 1988.
91. Cutler TJ, MacKay RJ, Johnson CM, et al: Bilateral ureteral tears in a foal, *Aust Vet J* 75:413, 1997.
92. Jean D, Marcoux M, Louf CF: Congenital bilateral distal defect of the ureters in a foal, *Equine Vet Educ* 10:17, 1998.
93. Morisset S, Hawkins JF, Frank N, et al: Surgical management of a ureteral defect with ureterorrhaphy and of ureteritis with ureteroneocystostomy in a foal, *J Am Vet Med Assoc* 220:354, 2002.
94. Smith BP, editor: *Large animal internal medicine*, ed 4, St Louis, 2009, Mosby.
95. Kawashima A, Sandler CM, Corriere JN, et al: Ureteropelvic junction injuries secondary to blunt abdominal trauma, *Radiology* 205:487, 1997.
96. Chandler JC, MacPhail CM: Congenital urethrorectal fistulas, *Compend Contin Educ Pract Vet* 23:995, 2001.
97. Fuchsloser RK, Rusch K: Atresia recti bei einem Vollblutfohlen, *Dtsch Tierarztl Wochenschr* 78:519, 1971.
98. Gideon L: Anal agenesis with rectourethral fistula in a colt, *Vet Med* 72:238, 1977.
99. Chaudhry NI, Cheema NI: Atresia ani and rectovaginal fistula in an acaudate filly, *Vet Rec* 107:95, 1980.
100. Kingston RS, Park RD: Atresia ani with an associated urogenital tract anomaly in foals, *Vet Clin North Am Equine Pract* 4(1):32, 1982.
101. Furie WS: Persistent cloaca and atresia ani in a foal, *Vet Clin North Am Equine Pract* 5(1):30, 1983.
102. Jansson N: Anal atresia in a foal, *Compend Contin Educ Pract Vet* 24:888, 2002.
103. Cruz AM, Barber SM, Kaestner SBR, et al: Urethrorectal fistula in a horse, *Can Vet J* 40:122, 1999.
104. Rooney J: Rupture of the urinary bladder in the foal, *Vet Pathol* 8:445, 1971.
105. Adams RA, Koterba AM, Cudd TC, et al: Exploratory celiotomy for suspected urinary tract disruption in neonatal foals: a review of 18 cases, *Equine Vet J* 20:13, 1988.
106. Kablack KA, Embertson RM, Bernard WV, et al: Uroperitoneum in the hospitalized equine neonate: retrospective study of 31 cases, 1988–1997, *Equine Vet J* 32:505, 2000.
107. Wellington JKM: Bladder defects in newborn foals, *Aust Vet J* 48:426, 1972.
108. Bain AM: Diseases of foals, *Aust Vet J* 30:9, 1954.
109. Pascoe RR: Repair of a defect in the bladder of a foal, *Aust Vet J* 47:343, 1971.
110. Crowe MW, Swerczek TW: Equine congenital defects, *Am J Vet Res* 46:353, 1985.
111. Radostits OM, Blood DC, Gay CC: *Veterinary medicine: a textbook of the diseases of cattle, sheep, pigs, goats, and horses*, ed 9, Philadelphia, 2000, Baillière Tindall.
112. Dubs VB: Megavesica zufolge Urachusmangel bei einem neugeborenen Fohlen, *Schweiz Arch Tierheilkd* 118:395, 1976.
113. Dean PW, Robertson JT: Urachal remnant as a cause of pollakiuria and dysuria in a filly, *J Am Vet Med Assoc* 192:375, 1988.
114. Whitwell KE, Jeffcott LB: Morphological studies on the fetal membranes of the normal singleton foal at term, *Res Vet Sci* 19:44, 1975.
115. Rossdale PD, Greet TRC: Mega vesica in a newborn foal, *Int Soc Vet Perinatol Newsletter* 2(2):10, 1989.
116. Oikawa M, Yoshihara T, Katayama Y, et al: Ruptured bladder associated with smooth muscle atrophy of the bladder in a neonatal foal, *Vet Clin North Am Equine Pract* 15(7):38, 1993.
117. Whitwell KE: Morphology and pathology of the equine umbilical cord, *J Reprod Fertil Suppl* 23:599, 1975.
118. Britt B, Byars TD: Hagyard-Davidson-McGee: Proceedings, *Am Assoc Equine Pract* 43:170-177, 1997.
119. Turner TA, Fessler JF, Ewert KM: Patent urachus in foals, *Vet Clin North Am Equine Pract* 4(1):24, 1982.
120. Lavan RP, Madigan J, Walker R, et al: Effect of disinfectant treatments on the bacterial flora of the umbilicus of neonatal foals. In *Proceedings of the fortieth annual meeting of the American Association of Equine Practitioners*. Vancouver, Canada, 1994, 37.
121. Ford J, Lokai MD: Ruptured urachus in a foal, *Vet Med Small Anim Clin* 77:94, 1982.

122. Reef VB, Collatos C: Ultrasonographic examination of normal umbilical structures in the foal, *Am J Vet Res* 49(2143), 1988.
123. Reef VB, Collatos C, Spencer PA, et al: Clinical, ultrasonographic, and surgical findings in foals with umbilical remnant infections, *J Am Vet Med Assoc* 195:69, 1989.
124. Adams SB, Fessler JF: Umbilical cord remnant infections in foals: 16 cases (1975-1985), *J Am Vet Med Assoc* 190(316), 1987.
125. Lees MJ, Easley KJ, Sutherland JV, et al: Subcutaneous rupture of the urachus, its diagnosis and surgical management in three foals, *Equine Vet J* 21:462, 1989.
126. Textor JA, Goodrich L, Wion L: Umbilical evagination of the urinary bladder in a neonatal filly, *J Am Vet Med Assoc* 219:953, 2001.

Renal Physiology

1. Brenner BM, editor: *Brenner and Rector's the kidney*, ed 8, vol. 2, Philadelphia, 2008, WB Saunders.
2. Dimski DS: Ammonia metabolism and the urea cycle: function and clinical implications, *J Vet Intern Med* 8:73, 1994.
3. Kaneko JJ, editor: *Clinical biochemistry of domestic animals*, ed 3, New York, 1980, Academic Press.
4. Strombeck DR, Meyer DJ, Freedland RA: Hyperammonemia due to a urea cycle enzyme deficiency in two dogs, *J Am Vet Med Assoc* 166:1109, 1975.
5. Peek SF, Divers TJ, Jackson CJ: Hyperammonaemia associated with encephalopathy and abdominal pain without evidence of liver disease in four mature horses, *Equine Vet J* 29:70, 1997.
6. Hasel KM, Summers BA, De Lahunta A: Encephalopathy with idiopathic hyperammonaemia and Alzheimer type II astrocytes in equidae, *Equine Vet J* 31:478, 1999.
7. McConnico RS, Duckett WM, Wood PA: Persistent hyperammonemia in two related Morgan weanlings, *J Vet Intern Med* 11:264, 1997.
8. Koterba AM, Drummond WH, Kosch PC, editors: *Equine clinical neonatology*, Philadelphia, 1990, Lea & Febiger.
9. Prior RL, Hintz HF, Lowe JE, et al: Urea recycling and metabolism of ponies, *J Anim Sci* 38:565, 1974.
10. Hintz HF, Schryver HF: Nitrogen utilization in ponies, *J Anim Sci* 34:592, 1972.
11. Reitnour CM, Treece JM: Relationship of nitrogen source to certain blood components and nitrogen balance in the equine, *J Anim Sci* 32:487, 1971.
12. Landwehr K: *Untersuchungen über die Beeinflussung von Kreatinin und Harnstoff im Blutplasma des Pferdes durch extrarenale Faktoren, inaugural dissertation*, Hannover Germany, 1986, Tierärztliche Hochschule Hannover.
13. Miller PA, Lawrence LM: The effect of dietary protein level on exercising horses, *J Anim Sci* 66(2185), 1988.
14. Patterson PH, Coon CN, Hughes IM: Protein requirements of mature working horses, *J Anim Sci* 61:187, 1985.
15. Sticker LS, Thompson DL, Bunting LD, et al: Feed deprivation in mares: plasma metabolite and hormonal concentrations and responses to exercise, *J Anim Sci* 73:3696, 1995.
16. Baetz AL, Pearson JE: Blood constituent changes in fasted ponies, *Am J Vet Res* 33:1972, 1941.
17. Keenan DM: Changes of blood metabolites in horses after racing, with particular reference to uric acid, *Aust Vet J* 55:54, 1979.
18. Snow DH, Kerr MG, Nimmo MA, et al: Alterations in blood, sweat, urine and muscle composition during prolonged exercise in the horse, *Vet Rec* 110:377, 1982.
19. Rose RJ, Ilkiw JE, Arnold KS, et al: Plasma biochemistry in the horse during 3-day event competition, *Equine Vet J* 12:132, 1980.
20. Narayanan S, Appleton HD: Creatinine: a review, *Clin Chem* 26:1119, 1980.
21. Gärtner VK, Reulecke W, Hackbarth H, et al: Zur Abhängigkeit von Muskelmasse und Körpergröβe im Verleich von Maus, Ratte, Kaninchen, Hund, Mensch und Pferd, *Dtsch Tierarztl Wochenschr* 94:52, 1987.
22. Jones JD, Burnett PC: Creatinine metabolism in humans with decreased renal function: creatinine deficit, *Clin Chem* 20:1204, 1974.
23. Schott HC, Mansmann RA: Biochemical profiles of normal equine amniotic fluid at parturition, *Equine Vet J Suppl* 5:52, 1988.
24. Mascioli SR, Bantle JP, Freier EF, et al: Artifactual elevation of serum creatinine level due to fasting, *Arch Intern Med* 144:1575, 1984.
25. Morris DD, Divers TJ, Whitlock RH: Renal clearance and fractional excretion of electrolytes over a 24-hour period in horses, *Am J Vet Res* 45:2431, 1984.
26. Kohn CW, Strasser SL: 24-Hour renal clearance and excretion of endogenous substances in the mare, *Am J Vet Res* 47:1332, 1986.
27. Finco DR, Groves C: Mechanism of renal excretion of creatinine by the pony, *Am J Vet Res* 46:1625, 1985.
28. Rose BD, editor: *Clinical physiology of acid-base and electrolyte disorders*, ed 3, New York, 1989, McGraw-Hill.
29. Goldstein MB, Bear R, Richardson RMA, et al: The urine anion gap: a clinically useful index of ammonium excretion, *Am J Med Sci* 292:198, 1986.
30. Gronwall R, Brown MP: Probenicid infusion in mares: effect on para-aminohippuric acid clearance, *Am J Vet Res* 49:250, 1988.
31. Boveáe KC, editor: *Canine nephrology*, Media, PA, 1984, Harwal.
32. Carlson GP: *Thermoregulation and fluid balance in the exercising horse, Equine exercise physiology*, Cambridge, 1983, Granta Editions.
33. Carlson GP: Hematology and body fluids in the equine athlete: a review, *Equine exercise physiology*, ed 2, Davis, CA, 1987, ICEEP Publications.
34. Schott HC, Hinchcliff KW: Fluids, electrolytes, and bicarbonate, *Vet Clin North Am Equine Pract* 9:577, 1993.
35. Tasker JB: Fluid and electrolyte studies in the horse. III. Intake and output of water, sodium, and potassium in normal horses, *Cornell Vet* 57:649, 1967.
36. Carlson GP: Fluid and electrolyte dynamics in the horse, *Proc Annu Vet Med Forum Am Coll Vet Intern Med* 4:7–29, 1986.
37. Rose RJ: Electrolytes: clinical applications, *Vet Clin North Am Equine Pract* 6:281, 1990.
38. Groenendyk S, English PB, Abetz I: External balance of water and electrolytes in the horse, *Equine Vet J* 20:189, 1988.
39. Hinton M: On the watering of horses: a review, *Equine Vet J* 10:27, 1978.
40. Fonnesbeck PV: Consumption and excretion of water by horses receiving all hay and hay-grain diets, *J Anim Sci* 27:1350, 1968.
41. Cymbaluk NF: Water balance of horses fed various diets, *Vet Clin North Am Equine Pract* 11(1):19, 1989.
42. Martin RG, McMeniman NP, Dowsett KF: Milk and water intakes of foals sucking grazing mares, *Equine Vet J* 24:295, 1992.
43. Caljuk EA: Water metabolism and water requirements of horses, *Nutr Abstr Rev* 32:574, 1962.
44. Schryver HF, Parker MT, Daniluk PD, et al: Salt consumption and the effect of salt on mineral metabolism in horses, *Cornell Vet* 77:122, 1987.
45. Freeman DA, Cymbaluk NF, Schott HC, et al: Clinical, biochemical, and hygiene assessment of stabled horses provided continuous or intermittent access to drinking water, *Am J Vet Res* 60:1445, 1999.

46. Sufit E, Houpt KA, Sweeting M: Physiological stimuli of thirst and drinking patterns in ponies, *Equine Vet J* 17:12, 1985.
47. Keiper RR, Keenan MA: Nocturnal activity patterns of feral ponies, *J Mammal* 61:116, 1980.
48. Brenner BM, editor: ed 8, *Brenner and Rector's the kidney* vol. 1Philadelphia, 2008, WB Saunders.
49. Andersson B, Augustinsson O, Bademo E, et al: Systemic and centrally mediated angiotensin II effects in the horse, *Acta Physiol Scand* 129:143, 1987.
50. Fitzsimons JT: Angiotensin, thirst, and sodium appetite, *Physiol Rev* 78:583, 1998.
51. Houpt KA: Drinking: the behavioral sequelae of diuretic treatment, *Vet Clin North Am Equine Pract* 9(9):15, 1987.
52. Houpt KA, Thorton SN, Allen WR: Vasopressin in dehydrated and rehydrated ponies, *Physiol Behav* 45:659, 1989.
53. Jones NL, Houpt KA, Houpt TR: Stimuli of thirst in donkeys *(Equus asinus)*, *Physiol Behav* 46:661, 1989.
54. Houpt KA, Northrup A, Wheatley T, et al: Thirst and salt appetite in horses treated with furosemide, *J Appl Physiol* 71:2380, 1991.
55. Irvine CHG, Alexander SL, Donald RA: Effect of an osmotic stimulus on the secretion of arginine vasopressin and adrenocorticotropin in the horse, *Endocrinology* 124:3102, 1989.
56. Sneddon JC, van der Walt J, Mitchell G, et al: Effects of dehydration and rehydration on plasma vasopressin and aldosterone in horses, *Physiol Behav* 54:223, 1993.
57. McKeever KH, Hinchcliff KW, Schmall LM, et al: Plasma renin activity and aldosterone and vasopressin concentrations during incremental treadmill exercise in horses, *Am J Vet Res* 53:1290, 1992.
58. Nyman S, Hydbring E, Dahlborn K: Is vasopressin a "stress hormone" in the horse? *Pferdeheilkunde* 12:419, 1996.
59. Gellai M: Modulation of vasopressin antidiuretic action by renal α_2-adrenoceptors, *Am J Physiol* 259:F1, 1990.
60. Kinter LB, Huffman WF, Stassen FL: Antagonists of the antidiuretic activity of vasopressin, *Am J Physiol* 254:F165, 1988.
61. Thurmon JC, Steffey EP, Zinkl JG, et al: Xylazine causes transient dose-related hyperglycemia and increased urine volume in mares, *Am J Vet Res* 45:224, 1984.
62. Trim CM, Hanson RR: Effects of xylazine on renal function and plasma glucose in ponies, *Vet Rec* 118:65, 1986.
63. Clarke LL, Argenzio RA, Roberts MC: Effect of meal feeding on plasma volume and urinary electrolyte clearance in ponies, *Am J Vet Res* 51:571, 1990.
64. Youket RJ, Carnevale JM, Houpt KA, et al: Humoral, hormonal and behavioral correlates of feeding in ponies: the effects of meal frequency, *J Anim Sci* 61:1103, 1985.
65. Clarke LL, Ganjam VK, Fichtenbaum B, et al: Effect of feeding on renin-angiotensin-aldosterone system of the horse, *Am J Physiol* 254:R524, 1988.
66. Tasker JB: Fluid and electrolyte studies in the horse. IV. The effects of fasting and thirsting, *Cornell Vet* 57:658, 1967.
67. Yousef MK, Dill DB, Mayes MG: Shifts in body fluids during dehydration in the burro, *Equus asinus*, *J Appl Physiol* 29:345, 1970.
68. Maloiy GMO: Water economy of the Somali donkey, *Am J Physiol* 219:1522, 1970.
69. Carlson GP, Rumbaugh GE, Harrold D: Physiological alterations in the horse produced by food and water deprivation during periods of high environmental temperatures, *Am J Vet Res* 40:982, 1979.
70. Brobst DF, Bayly WM: Responses of horses to a water deprivation test, *J Equine Vet Sci* 2:51, 1982.
71. Genetzky RM, Lopanco FV, Ledet AE: Clinical pathologic alterations in horses during a water deprivation test, *Am J Vet Res* 48:1007, 1987.
72. Sneddon JC, van der Walt JG, Mitchell G: Water homeostasis in desert-dwelling horses, *J Appl Physiol* 71:112, 1991.
73. Sneddon JC: Physiological effects of hypertonic dehydration on body fluid pools in arid-adapted mammals: how do Arab-based mammals compare? *Comp Biochem Physiol* 104A:201, 1993.
74. Webb AI, Weaver BMQ: Body composition of the horse, *Equine Vet J* 11:39, 1979.
75. Meyer H, Coenen M: Influence of exercise on the water and electrolyte content of the alimentary tract, *Proc Equine Nutr Physiol Symp* 11:3, 1989.
76. Hubbard RW, Sandick BL, Matthew WT, et al: Voluntary dehydration and alliesthesia for water, *J Appl Physiol* 57:868, 1984.
77. Rumbaugh GE, Carlson GP, Harrold D: Urinary production in the healthy horse and in horses deprived of feed and water, *Am J Vet Res* 43:735, 1982.
78. Greenleaf JE: Problem: thirst, drinking behavior, and involuntary dehydration, *Med Sci Sports Exerc* 24:645, 1992.
79. Butudom P, Schott HC, Davis MW, et al: Drinking salt water enhances rehydration in horses dehydrated by furosemide administration and endurance exercise, *Equine Vet J Suppl* 34:513, 2002.
80. Parks CM, Manohar M: Distribution of blood flow during moderate and strenuous exercise in horses, *Am J Vet Res* 44:1983, 1861.
81. Staddon GE, Weaver BMQ, Webb AI: Distribution of cardiac output in anaesthetized horses, *Res Vet Sci* 27:38, 1979.
82. Brezis M, Rosen S: Hypoxia of the renal medulla: its implication for disease, *N Engl J Med* 332:647, 1995.
83. Epstein FH: Oxygen and renal metabolism, *Kidney Int* 51:381, 1997.
84. Heyman SN, Rosen S, Brezis M: The renal medulla: life at the edge of anoxia, *Blood Purif* 15:232, 1997.
85. Knudsen E: Renal clearance studies on the horse. I. Inulin, endogenous creatinine and urea, *Acta Vet Scand* 1:52, 1959.
86. Paul JW: *A comparative study of renal function in horses and ponies and a study of the pharmacokinetics of oxytetracycline in the horse, master's thesis*, Columbus, 1973, The Ohio State University.
87. Zatzman ML, Clarke L, Ray WJ, et al: Renal function of the pony and horse, *Am J Vet Res* 43:608, 1982.
88. Hood DM, Amoss MS, Gremmel SM, et al: Renovascular nuclear medicine in the equine: a feasibility study, *Southwest Vet* 35:19, 1982.
89. Manohar M, Goetz TE: Cerebral, renal, adrenal, intestinal, and pancreatic circulation in conscious ponies and during 1.0, 1.5, and 2.0 minimal alveolar concentrations of halothane-o_2 anesthesia, *Am J Vet Res* 46:2492, 1985.
90. Manohar M: Furosemide and systemic circulation during severe exercise, *Equine exercise physiology*, ed 2, Davis, CA, 1987, ICEEP Publications.
91. Brewer BD, Clement SF, Lotz WS, et al: A comparison of inulin, para-aminohippuric acid, and endogenous creatinine clearances as measures of renal function in neonatal foals, *J Vet Intern Med* 4:301, 1990.
92. Hinchcliff KW, McKeever KH, Schmall LM, et al: Renal and systemic hemodynamic responses to sustained submaximal exertion in horses, *Am J Physiol* 258:R1177, 1990.
93. Schott HC, Hodgson DR, Bayly WM, et al: Renal responses to high intensity exercise, *Equine exercise physiology*, ed 3, Davis, CA, 1991, ICEEP Publications.
94. Held JP, Daniel GB: Use of nonimaging nuclear medicine techniques to assess the effect of flunixin meglumine on effective renal plasma flow and effective renal blood flow in healthy horses, *Am J Vet Res* 52:1619, 1991.
95. Armstrong RB, Esseán-Gustavsson B, Hoppeler H et al: o2 delivery at $\dot{V}$ 2max and oxidative capacity in muscles of Standardbred horses, *J Appl Physiol* 73:2274, 1992.
96. Matthews HK, Andrews FM, Daniel GB, et al: Comparison of standard and radionuclide methods for measurement of glomerular filtration rate and effective renal blood flow in female horses, *Am J Vet Res* 53:1612, 1992.
97. Manohar M, Goetz TE, Saupe B, et al: Thyroid, renal, and splanchnic circulation in horses at rest and during short-term exercise, *Am J Vet Res* 56:1356, 1995.

98. Trim CM, Moore JN, Clark ES: Renal effects of dopamine infusion in conscious horses, *Equine Vet J Suppl* 7:124, 1989.
99. Holdstock NB, Ousey JC, Rossdale PD: Glomerular filtration rate, effective renal plasma flow, blood pressure and pulse rate in the equine neonate during the first 10 days postpartum, *Equine Vet J* 30:335, 1998.
100. Woods PR, Drost WT, Clarke CR, et al: Use of 99mTc-mercaptoacetyltriglycine to evaluate renal function in horses, *Vet Radiol Ultrasound* 41:85, 2000.
101. McConaghy FF, Hodgson DR, Hales JRS, et al: Thermoregulatory-induced compromise of muscle blood flow in ponies during intense exercise in the heat: a contributor to the onset of fatigue? *Equine Vet J Suppl* 34:491, 2002.
102. Rawlings CA, Bisgard GE: Renal clearance and excretion of endogenous substances in the small pony, *Am J Vet Res* 36:45–48, 1975.
103. Traver DS, Salem C, Coffman JR, et al: Renal metabolism of endogenous substances in the horse: volumetric vs clearance ratio methods, *J Equine Med Surg* 1:378, 1977.
104. Gelsa H: The renal clearance of inulin, creatinine, trimethoprim and sulphadoxine in horses, *J Vet Pharmacol Ther* 2:257, 1979.
105. Lane VM, Merritt AM: Reliability of single-sample phosphorous fractional excretion determination as a measure of daily phosphorous renal clearance in equids, *Am J Vet Res* 44:500, 1983.
106. Gronwall R: Effect of diuresis on urinary excretion and creatinine clearance in the horse, *Am J Vet Res* 46:1616, 1985.
107. Smith CM, Steffey EP, Baggott JD, et al: Effects of halothane anesthesia on the clearance of gentamicin sulfate in horses, *Am J Vet Res* 49:19, 1988.
108. McKeever KH, Hinchcliff KW, Schmall LM, et al: Renal tubular function in horses during sustained submaximal exercise, *Am J Physiol* 261:R553, 1991.
109. Walsh DM, Royal HD: Evaluation of 99mTc-labeled diethylenetriaminepentaacetic acid for measuring glomerular filtration rate in horses, *Am J Vet Res* 53:776, 1992.
110. Bickhardt K, Deegen E, Espelage W: Kidney function tests in horses: methods and reference values in healthy animals, *Dtsch Tierarztl Wochenschr* 103:117, 1996.
111. Gleadhill A, Marlin D, Harris PA, et al: Reduction of renal function in exercising horses, *Equine Vet J* 32:509, 2000.
112. McKenzie EC, Valberg SJ, Godden SM, et al: Comparison of volumetric urine collection versus single-sample urine collection in horses consuming diets varying in cation-anion balance, *Am J Vet Res* 64:284–291, 2003.
113. Matthews HK, Andrews FM, Daniel GB, et al: Measuring renal function in horses, *Vet Med* 88:349, 1993.
114. Driessen B, Zarucco L, Steffey EP, et al: Serum fluoride concentrations, biochemical and histopathological changes associated with prolonged sevoflurane anesthesia in horses, *J Vet Med A Physiol Pathol Clin Med* 49:337, 2002.
115. Dunn MJ, Zambraski EJ: Renal effects of drugs that inhibit prostaglandin synthesis, *Kidney Int* 18:609, 1980.
116. Gunson DE: Renal papillary necrosis in horses, *J Am Vet Med Assoc* 182:263, 1983.
117. Gunson DE, Soma LR: Renal papillary necrosis in horses after phenylbutazone and water deprivation, *Vet Pathol* 20:603, 1983.
118. Kanwar YS: Biology of disease: biophysiology of glomerular filtration and proteinuria, *Lab Invest* 51:7, 1984.
119. Snow DH, Munro CD, Nimmo MA: Effects of nandrolone phenylpropionate in the horse: (1) resting animal, *Equine Vet J* 14:219, 1982.
120. Gleadhill A, Marlin D, Harris PA, et al: Use of a three-blood-sample plasma clearance technique to measure GFR in horses, *Vet J* 158:204, 1999.
121. Steinhausen M, Endlich K, Wiegman DL: Glomerular blood flow, *Kidney Int* 38:769, 1990.
122. Lüscher TF, Bock HA, Yang Z, et al: Endothelium-derived relaxing and contracting factors: perspectives in nephrology, *Kidney Int* 39:575, 1991.
123. Molitoris BA, Finn WF, editors: *Acute renal failure: a companion to Brenner & Rector's the kidney*, Philadelphia, 2001, WB Saunders.
124. Breidenbach A, Schlumbohm C, Harmeyer J: Peculiarities of vitamin D and of the calcium and phosphate homeostatic system in horses, *Vet Res* 29:173, 1998.
125. Lakritz J, Madigan J, Carlson GP: Hypovolemic hyponatremia and signs of neurologic disease associated with diarrhea in a foal, *J Am Vet Med Assoc* 200:1114, 1992.

Examination of the Urinary System

1. Sneddon JC, Colyn P: A practical system for measuring water intake in stabled horses, *J Equine Vet Sci* 11:141, 1991.
2. Vander Noot GW, Fonnesbeck PV: Lydman RK: Equine metabolism stall and collection harness, *J Anim Sci* 24:691, 1965.
3. Warwick IS: Urine collection apparatus for male horses, *J Sci Technol* 12:181, 1966.
4. Tasker JB: Fluid and electrolyte studies in the horse. II. An apparatus for the collection of total daily urine and feces from horses, *Cornell Vet* 56:77, 1966.
5. Harris P: Collection of urine, *Equine Vet J* 20:86, 1988.
6. Brown CM, editor: *Problems in equine medicine*, Philadelphia, 1989, Lea & Febiger.
7. Kaneko JJ, editor: *Clinical biochemistry of domestic animals*, ed 3, New York, 1980, Academic Press.
8. Brenner BM, editor: *Brenner and Rector's the kidney*, ed 8, Philadelphia, 2008, WB Saunders.
9. Perrone RD, Madias NE, Levey AS: Serum creatinine as an index of renal function: new insights into old concepts, *Clin Chem* 38:1992, 1933.
10. Osborne CA, Polzin DJ: Azotemia: a review of what's old and what's new. I. Definition of terms and concepts, *Compend Contin Educ Pract Vet* 5:497, 1983.
11. Irwin DHG, Howell DW: Equine pyelonephritis and unilateral nephrectomy, *J S Afr Vet Assoc* 51:235, 1980.
12. Trotter GW, Brown CM, Ainsworth DM: Unilateral nephrectomy for treatment of a renal abscess in a foal, *J Am Vet Med Assoc* 184:1392, 1984.
13. Juzwiak JS, Bain FT, Slone DE, et al: Unilateral nephrectomy for treatment of chronic hematuria due to nephrolithiasis in a colt, *Can Vet J* 29:931, 1988.
14. Sullins KE, McIlwraith CW, Yovich JV, et al: Ectopic ureter managed by unilateral nephrectomy in two female horses, *Equine Vet J* 20:463, 1988.
15. Jones SL, Langer DL, Sterner-Kock A, et al: Renal dysplasia and benign ureteropelvic polyps associated with hydronephrosis in a foal, *J Am Vet Med Assoc* 204:1230, 1994.
16. Tennant B, Lowe JE, Tasker JB: Hypercalcemia and hypophosphatemia in ponies following bilateral nephrectomy, *Proc Soc Exp Biol Med* 167:365, 1981.
17. DeBowes R: Personal communication, 1991.
18. Landwehr K: *Untersuchungen über die Beeinflussung von Kreatinin und Harnstoff im Blutplasma des Pferdes durchextrarenale Faktoren, inaugural dissertation*, Hannover Germany, 1986, Tierärztliche Hochschule Hannover.
19. Koterba AM, Coffman JR: Acute and chronic renal disease in the horse, *Compend Contin Educ Pract Vet* 3:S461, 1981.
20. Finco DR, Duncan JR: Evaluation of blood urea nitrogen and serum creatinine concentrations as indicators of renal dysfunction: a study of 111 cases and a review of related literature, *J Am Vet Med Assoc* 168:593, 1976.
21. Osborne CA, Polzin DJ: Azotemia: a review of what's old and what's new. II. Localization, *Compend Contin Educ Pract Vet* 5:561, 1983.

22. Brobst DF, Grant BD, Hilbert BJ, et al: Blood biochemical changes in horses with prerenal and renal disease, *J Equine Med Surg* 1:171, 1977.
23. Bayly WM: A practitioner's approach to the diagnosis and treatment of renal failure in horses, *Vet Med* 86:632, 1991.
24. Divers TJ, Whitlock RH, Byars TD, et al: Acute renal failure in six horses resulting from haemodynamic causes, *Equine Vet J* 19:178, 1987.
25. Divers TJ: Chronic renal failure in horses, *Compend Contin Educ Pract Vet* 5:S310, 1983.
26. Tennant B, Dill SG, Rebhun WC, et al: Pathophysiology of renal failure in the horse, *Proceedings of the thirty-first annual meeting of the American Association of Equine Practitioners*, Toronto, Canada, 1985, p 627.
27. Grauer GF: Clinicopathologic evaluation of early renal disease in dogs, *Compend Contin Educ Pract Vet* 7:32, 1985.
28. Allen TA, Fettman MJ: Comparative aspects of nonoliguric renal failure, *Compend Contin Educ Pract Vet* 9:293, 1987.
29. Banks KL, Henson JB: Immunologically mediated glomerulitis of horses. IV. Antiglomerular basement membrane antibody and other mechanisms of spontaneous disease, *Lab Invest* 26:708, 1972.
30. Badr KF, Ichikawa I: Prerenal failure: a deleterious shift from renal compensation to decompensation, *N Engl J Med* 319:623, 1988.
31. Grossman BS, Brobst DF, Kramer JW, et al: Urinary indices for differentiation of prerenal azotemia and renal azotemia in horses, *J Am Vet Med Assoc* 180:284, 1982.
32. Roussel AJ, Cohen ND, Ruoff WW, et al: Urinary indices of horses after intravenous administration of crystalloid solutions, *J Vet Intern Med* 7:241, 1993.
33. Thurmon JC, Steffey EP, Zinkl JG, et al: Xylazine causes transient dose-related hyperglycemia and increased urine volume in mares, *Am J Vet Res* 45:224, 1984.
34. Trim CM, Hanson RR: Effects of xylazine on renal function and plasma glucose in ponies, *Vet Rec* 118:65, 1986.
35. Gellai M: Modulation of vasopressin antidiuretic action by renal α_2-adrenoceptors, *Am J Physiol* 259:F1, 1990.
36. Baek SM, Brown RS, Shoemaker WC: Early prediction of acute renal failure and recovery. I. Sequential measurements of free water clearance, *Ann Surg* 177:253, 1973.
37. Baek SM, Makabali GG, Brown RS, et al: Free-water clearance patterns as predictors and therapeutic guides in acute renal failure, *Surgery* 77:632, 1975.
38. Kosinski JP, Lucas CE, Ledgerwood AM: Meaning and value of free water clearance in injured patients, *J Surg Res* 33:184, 1982.
39. Taylor FGR, Hillyer MH: The differential diagnosis of hyperglycemia in horses, *Equine Vet Educ* 4:135, 1992.
40. Chapman DI, Haywood PE, Lloyd P: Occurrence of glycosuria in horses after strenuous exercise, *Equine Vet J* 13:259, 1981.
41. Kohn CW, Chew DJ: Laboratory diagnosis and characterization of renal disease in horses, *Vet Clin North Am Equine Pract* 3:585, 1987.
42. Edwards DJ, Brownlow MA, Hutchins DR: Indices of renal function: reference values in normal horses, *Aust Vet J* 66:60, 1989.
43. Rose BD, editor: *Clinical physiology of acid-base and electrolyte disorders*, ed 3, New York, 1989, McGraw-Hill.
44. Rumbaugh GE, Carlson GP, Harrold D: Urinary production in the healthy horse and in horses deprived of feed and water, *Am J Vet Res* 43:735, 1982.
45. Brobst DF, Bayly WM: Responses of horses to a water deprivation test, *J Equine Vet Sci* 2:51, 1982.
46. Genetzky RM, Lopanco FV, Ledet AE: Clinical pathologic alterations in horses during a water deprivation test, *Am J Vet Res* 48:1007, 1987.
47. Martin RG, McMeniman NP, Dowsett KF: Milk and water intakes of foals sucking grazing mares, *Equine Vet J* 24:295, 1992.
48. Wood T, Weckman TJ, Henry PA, et al: Equine urine pH: normal population distributions and methods of acidification, *Equine Vet J* 22:118, 1990.
49. Edwards DJ, Brownlow MA, Hutchins DR: Indices of renal function: values in eight normal foals from birth to 56 days, *Aust Vet J* 67:251, 1990.
50. Gingerich DA, Murdick PW: Paradoxic aciduria in bovine metabolic alkalosis, *J Am Vet Med Assoc* 166:227, 1975.
51. Bradford MM: A rapid and sensitive method for the quantification of microgram quantities of protein utilizing the principle of protein-dye binding, *Anal Biochem* 72:248, 1976.
52. Schott HC, Hodgson DR, Bayly WM: Haematuria, pigmenturia and proteinuria in exercising horses, *Equine Vet J* 27:67, 1995.
53. Kohn CW, Strasser SL: 24-Hour renal clearance and excretion of endogenous substances in the mare, *Am J Vet Res* 47:1332, 1986.
54. Grauer GF, Thomas CB, Eicker SW: Estimation of quantitative proteinuria in the dog, using the urine protein-to-creatinine ratio from a random, voided sample, *Am J Vet Res* 46(2116), 1985.
55. Link RP: Glucose tolerance in horses, *J Am Vet Med Assoc* 97:261, 1940.
56. Blondheim SH, Margoliash E, Shafrir E: A simple test for myohemoglobinuria (myoglobinuria), *J Am Med Assoc* 167:453, 1958.
57. Marcussen N, Schumann J, Campbell P, et al: Cytodiagnostic urinalysis is very useful in the differential diagnosis of acute renal failure and can predict the severity, *Ren Fail* 17:721, 1995.
58. Mair TS, Osborn RS: The crystalline composition of normal equine urine deposits, *Equine Vet J* 22:364, 1990.
59. Burchardt U, Peters JE, Neef L, et al: Der diagnostiche Wert von Enzymbestimmugen im Harn, *Z Med Lab Diagn* 18:190, 1977.
60. Raab WP: Diagnostic value of urinary enzyme determinations, *Clin Chem* 18:5, 1972.
61. Price RG: Urinary enzymes, nephrotoxicity and renal disease, *Toxicology* 23:99, 1982.
62. Stroo WE, Hook JB: Enzymes of renal origin in urine as indicators of nephrotoxicity, *Toxicol Appl Pharmacol* 39:423, 1977.
63. Bayly WM, Brobst DF, Elfers RS, et al: Serum and urine biochemistry and enzyme changes in ponies with acute renal failure, *Cornell Vet* 76:306, 1986.
64. Prescott LF: Assessment of nephrotoxicity, *Br J Clin Pharmacol* 13:303, 1982.
65. Mahrun D, Paar D, Bock KD: Lysosomal and brush-border enzymes in urine of patients with renal artery stenosis and with essential hypertension, *Clin Biochem* 12:228, 1978.
66. Adams R, McClure JJ, Gossett KA, et al: Evaluation of a technique for measurement of γ-glutamyltransferase in equine urine, *Am J Vet Res* 46:147, 1986.
67. Brobst DF, Carroll RJ, Bayly WM: Urinary enzyme concentrations in healthy horses, *Cornell Vet* 76:229, 1986.
68. Amend J, Nicholson R, King R, et al: Equine monensin toxicosis: useful ante-mortem and post-mortem clinicopathologic tests, *Proceedings of the thirty-first annual meeting of the American Association of Equine Practitioners*, Toronto, Canada, 1985, p 361.
69. Giusti EP, Sampaio AM, Michelacci YM, et al: Horse urinary kallikrein I: complete purification and characterization, *Biol Chem* 369:387, 1988.
70. Schmitz DG, Green RA: Effects of water deprivation and phenylbutazone administration on urinary enzyme concentrations in healthy horses, *Proceedings of the thirty-third annual meeting of the American Association of Equine Practitioners*, New Orleans, 1987, p 103.
71. Guder W, Ross B: Enzyme distribution along the nephron, *Kidney Int* 26:101, 1984.

72. Jung K, Pergande M, Schreiber G, et al: Stability of enzymes in urine at 37° C, *Clin Chim Acta* 131:185, 1983.
73. Goren M, Wright R, Osborne S, et al: Two automated procedures for N-acetyl-β-D-glucosaminidase determination evaluated for detection of drug-induced tubular nephrotoxicity, *Clin Chem* 32(2052), 1986.
74. Leaback D, Walker P: Studies on glucosaminidase. IV. The fluorometric assay of *N*-acetyl-β-d-glucosaminidase, *Biochem J* 78:151, 1961.
75. Irie A, Tabuchi A, Ura T: Influence of pH and temperature on the activities of the urinary enzymes, *Jpn J Clin Pathol* 13:441, 1985.
76. Vestergaard P, Leverett R: Constancy of urinary creatinine excretion, *J Lab Clin Med* 51:211, 1958.
77. Werner M, Heilbron DC, Mahrun D, et al: Patterns of urinary enzyme excretion in healthy subjects, *Clin Chim Acta* 29:437, 1970.
78. Mahrun D, Fuchs I, Mues G, et al: Normal limits of urinary excretion of eleven enzymes, *Clin Chem* 22:1567, 1976.
79. Akins JA: *Evaluation of equine urinary N-acetyl-β-d-glucosaminidase, gamma glutamyltransferase, and alkaline phosphatase as markers for early renal tubular damage,* master's thesis, Pullman, WA, 1989, Washington State University.
80. Mattenheimer H, Frolke W, Grotsch H, et al: Identification of inhibitors of urinary alanine aminopeptidase, *Clin Chim Acta* 160:125, 1986.
81. Reusch C, Vochezer R, Weschta E: Enzyme activities of alanine aminopeptidase (AAP) and *N*-acetyl-β-d-glucosaminidase (NAG) in healthy dogs, *Am J Vet Med* 38:90, 1991.
82. Werner A, Mahrun D, Atoba A: Use of gel filtration in the assay of urinary enzymes, *J Chromatogr* 40:234, 1969.
83. Hinchcliff KW, McGuirk SM, MacWilliams PS: Gentamicin nephrotoxicity. In *Proceedings of the thirty-third annual meeting of the American Association of Equine Practitioners*. New Orleans, 1987, 67.
84. Edwards DJ, Love DN, Rause J, et al: The nephrotoxic potential of neomycin in the horse, *Equine Vet J* 21:206, 1989.
85. Constable PD: Letter to the editor, *J Vet Intern Med* 5:357, 1991.
86. Rawlings CA, Bisgard GE: Renal clearance and excretion of endogenous substances in the small pony, *Am J Vet Res* 36:45–48, 1975.
87. Traver DS, Coffman JR, Moore JN, et al: Urine clearance ratios as a diagnostic aid in equine metabolic disease. In *Proceedings of the twenty-second annual meeting of the American Association of Equine Practitioners*, Dallas, 1976, p 177.
88. Traver DS, Salem C, Coffman JR, et al: Renal metabolism of endogenous substances in the horse: volumetric vs clearance ratio methods, *J Equine Med Surg* 1:378, 1977.
89. Morris DD, Divers TJ, Whitlock RH: Renal clearance and fractional excretion of electrolytes over a 24-hour period in horses, *Am J Vet Res* 45:2431, 1984.
90. Robinson NE, editor: *Current therapy in equine medicine*, ed 6, St Louis, 2009, WB Saunders.
91. Harris P, Colles C: The use of creatinine clearance ratios in the prevention of equine rhabdomyolysis: a report of four cases, *Equine Vet J* 20:459, 1988.
92. Lane VM, Merritt AM: Reliability of single-sample phosphorous fractional excretion determination as a measure of daily phosphorous renal clearance in equids, *Am J Vet Res* 44:500, 1983.
93. Caple IW, Doake PA, Ellis PG: Assessment of the calcium and phosphorous nutrition in horses by analysis of urine, *Aust Vet J* 58:125, 1982.
94. Cuddeford D, Woodhead A, Muirhead R: Potential of alfalfa as a source of calcium for calcium deficient horses, *Vet Rec* 126:425, 1990.
95. Brewer BD, Clement SF, Lotz WS, et al: Renal clearance, urinary excretion of endogenous substances, and urinary indices in healthy neonatal foals, *J Vet Intern Med* 5:28, 1991.
96. Coffman J: Percent creatinine clearance ratios, *Vet Med Small Anim Clin* 75:671, 1980.
97. King C: Practical use of urinary fractional excretion, *J Equine Vet Sci* 14:464, 1994.
98. McKenzie EC, Valberg SJ, Godden SM, et al: Plasma and urine electrolyte and mineral concentrations in Thoroughbred horses with recurrent exertional rhabdomyolysis after consumption of diets varying in cation-anion balance, *Am J Vet Res* 63:1053, 2002.
99. McKenzie EC, Valberg SJ, Godden SM, et al: Comparison of volumetric urine collection versus single-sample urine collection in horses consuming diets varying in cation-anion balance, *Am J Vet Res* 64:284, 2003.
100. Divers TJ, Whitlock RH, Byars TD, et al: Acute renal failure in six horses resulting from haemodynamic causes, *Equine Vet J* 19:178, 1987.
101. Bayly WM, Brobst DF, Elfers RS, et al: Serum and urine biochemistry and enzyme changes in ponies with acute renal failure, *Cornell Vet* 76:306, 1986.
102. Buntain BJ, Coffman JR: Polyuria and polydipsia in a horse induced by psychogenic salt consumption, *Equine Vet J* 13:266, 1981.
103. Schott HC, Bayly WM, Hodgson DR: Urinary excretory responses in exercising horses: effects on fractional excretion values. In *Proceedings of the eleventh annual meeting of the Association for Equine Sports Medicine*, Orlando, FL, 1992, p 23.
104. Caple IW, Bourke JM, Ellis PG: An examination of the calcium and phosphorous nutrition of Thoroughbred racehorses, *Aust Vet J* 58:132, 1982.
105. Mason DK, Watkins KL, McNie JT: Diagnosis, treatment and prevention of nutritional secondary hyperparathyroidism in Thoroughbred race horses in Hong Kong, *Vet Clin North Am Equine Pract* 10(3):10, 1988.
106. Ronen N, van Heerden J, van Amstel SR: Clinical and biochemistry findings, and parathyroid hormone concentrations in three horses with secondary hyperparathyroidism, *J S Afr Vet Assoc* 63:134, 1992.
107. Harris PA, Snow DH: Role of electrolyte imbalances in the pathophysiology of the equine rhabdomyolysis syndrome. In Persson SGB, Lindholm A, Jeffcott LB, editors: *Equine exercise physiology*, ed 3, Davis, CA, 1991, ICEEP Publications.
108. Beech J, Lindborg S: Potassium concentrations in muscle, plasma, and erythrocytes and urinary fractional excretion in normal horses and those with chronic intermittent exercise-associated rhabdomyolysis, *Res Vet Sci* 55:43, 1993.
109. Brooks CL, Garry F, Swartout MS: Effect of an interfering substance on determination of potassium by ion-specific potentiometry in animal urine, *Am J Vet Res* 49:710, 1988.
110. Traub-Dargatz JL, McKinnon AO: Adjunctive methods of examination of the urogenital tract, *Vet Clin North Am Equine Pract* 4:339, 1988.
111. Rantanen NW: Diseases of the kidneys, *Vet Clin North Am Equine Pract* 2:89, 1986.
112. Reef VB: Ultrasonic evaluation of large animal renal diseases, *Proc Annu Vet Med Forum Am Coll Vet Intern Med* 4:2–45, 1986.
113. Penninck DG, Eisenberg HM, Teuscher EE, et al: Equine renal ultrasonography: normal and abnormal, *Vet Radiol* 27:81, 1986.
114. Kiper ML, Traub-Dargatz JL, Wrigley RH: Renal ultrasonography in horses, *Compend Contin Educ Pract Vet* 12:993, 1990.
115. Hoffman KL, Wood AKW, McCarthy PH: Sonographic-anatomic correlation and imaging protocol for the kidneys of horses, *Am J Vet Res* 56:1403, 1995.
116. Divers TJ, Yeager AE: The value of ultrasonographic examination in the diagnosis and management of renal diseases in horses, *Equine Vet Educ* 7:334, 1997.
117. Reef VB: *Equine diagnostic ultrasound*, Philadelphia, 1998, WB Saunders.

118. Bayly WM, Elfers RS, Liggitt HD, et al: A reproducible means of studying acute renal failure in the horse, *Cornell Vet* 76:287, 1986.
119. Leveille R, Miyabayashi T, Weisbrode SE, et al: Ultrasonographic renal changes associated with phenylbutazone administration in three foals, *Can Vet J* 37:235, 1996.
120. Ramirez S, Seahorn TL, Williams J: Renal medullary rim sign in 2 adult Quarter horses, *Can Vet J* 39:647, 1998.
121. Jakovljeric S, Rivers WJ, Chun R, et al: Results of renal ultrasonography performed before and during administration of saline (0.9% NaCl) solution to induce diuresis in dogs without evidence of renal disease, *Am J Vet Res* 60:405, 1999.
122. Blikslager AT, Green EM, MacFadden KE, et al: Excretory urography and ultrasonography in the diagnosis of bilateral ectopic ureters in a foal, *Vet Radiol Ultrasound* 33:41, 1992.
123. Tomlinson JE, Farnsworth K, Sage AM, et al: Percutaneous ultrasound-guided pyelography aided diagnosis of ectopic ureter and hydronephrosis in a 3-week-old filly, *Vet Radiol Ultrasound* 42:349, 2001.
124. Rapp HJ, Tellhelm B, Spurlock SL: Die röntgenologische Darstellung der Harnableitenden wege der Stute mit Hilfe retrograder Kontrastmittelgabe, *Pferdeheilkunde* 3:309, 1987.
125. Konde LJ, Park RD, Wrigley RH, et al: Comparison of radiography and ultrasonography in the evaluation of renal lesions in the dog, *J Am Vet Med Assoc* 188:1420, 1986.
126. Tanagho EA, McAnninch JW, editors: *Smith's general urology*, ed 12, Norwalk, 1988, Appleton & Lange.
127. Blaufox MD: Procedures of choice in renal nuclear medicine, *J Nucl Med* 32:1301, 1991.
128. Twardock AR, Krawiec DR, Lamb CR: Kidney scintigraphy, *Semin Vet Med Surg (Small Anim)* 6:164, 1991.
129. Walsh DM, Royal HD: Evaluation of 99mTc-labeled diethylenetriaminepentaacetic acid for measuring glomerular filtration rate in horses, *Am J Vet Res* 53:776, 1992.
130. Schott HC, Roberts GD, Hines MT, et al: Nuclear scintigraphy as a diagnostic aid in the evaluation of renal disease in horses, In *Proceedings of the thirty-ninth annual meeting of the American Association of Equine Practitioners*, San Antonio, TX, 1993, p 251.
131. Schott HC: *Recurrent urolithiasis associated with unilateral pyelonephritis in five equids.* In *Proceedings of the forty-eighth annual meeting of the American Association of Equine Practitioners*, Orlando, FL, 2002, 136.
132. Sullins KE, Traub-Dargatz JL: Endoscopic anatomy of the equine urinary tract, *Compend Contin Educ Pract Vet* 11:S663, 1984.
133. Rapp HJ, Sernetz M: Urethroskopie und Ureterenkatheterisierung bei der Stute, *Pferdeheilkunde* 1:197, 1985.
134. Traub-Dargatz JL, Brown CM, editors: *Equine endoscopy*, ed 2, St Louis, 1997, CV Mosby.
135. Huffman JL, Bagley DH, Lyon ES: Extending cystoscopic techniques into the ureter and renal pelvis, *JAMA* 250:1983, 2002.
136. Ensor RD, Boyarksy S, Glenn JF: Cystoscopy and ureteral catheterization in the dog, *J Am Vet Med Assoc* 149:1067, 1966.
137. Senior DF, Newman RC: Retrograde ureteral catheterization in female dogs, *J Am Anim Hosp Assoc* 22:831, 1986.
138. Schott HC, Papageorges M, Hodgson DR: Diagnosis of renal disease in the nonazotemic horse, abstract #15, *J Vet Intern Med* 3:116, 1989.
139. MacHarg MA, Foerner JJ, Phillips TN, et al: Two methods for the treatment of ureterolithiasis in a mare, *Vet Surg* 13:95, 1984.
140. Rodger LD, Carlson GP, Moran ME, et al: Resolution of a left ureteral stone using electrohydraulic lithotripsy in a Thoroughbred colt, *J Vet Intern Med* 9:280, 1995.
141. Schott HC, Hodgson DR, Bayly WM: Ureteral catheterization in the horse, *Equine Vet Educ* 2:140, 1990.
142. Filar J, Ziolo T, Szalecki J: Diabetes insipidus in the course of encephalitis in the horse, *Med Weter* 27:205, 1971.
143. Breukink HJ, Van Wegen P, Schotman AJH: Idiopathic diabetes insipidus in a Welsh pony, *Equine Vet J* 15:284, 1983.
144. Schott HC, Bayly WM, Reed SM, et al: Nephrogenic diabetes insipidus in sibling colts, *J Vet Intern Med* 7:68, 1993.
145. Unpublished data
146. Irvine CHG, Alexander SL, Donald RA: Effect of an osmotic stimulus on the secretion of arginine vasopressin and adrenocorticotropin in the horse, *Endocrinology* 124:3102, 1989.
147. Houpt KA, Thorton SN, Allen WR: Vasopressin in dehydrated and rehydrated ponies, *Physiol Behav* 45:659, 1989.
148. Sneddon JC, van der Walt J, Mitchell G, et al: Effects of dehydration and rehydration on plasma vasopressin and aldosterone in horses, *Physiol Behav* 54:223, 1993.
149. Matthews HK, Andrews FM, Daniel GB, et al: Measuring renal function in horses, *Vet Med* 88:349, 1993.
150. Brobst DF, Bramwell K, Kramer JW: Sodium sulfanilate clearance as a method of determining renal function in the horse, *J Equine Med Surg* 2:500, 1978.
151. Hinchcliff KW, McGuirk SM, MacWilliams PS: Pharmacokinetics of phenolsulfonphthalein in horse and pony mares, *Am J Vet Res* 48:1256, 1987.
152. Hood DM, Amoss MS, Gremmel SM, et al: Renovascular nuclear medicine in the equine: a feasibility study, *Southwest Vet* 35:19, 1982.
153. Matthews HK, Andrews FM, Danile GB, et al: Comparison of standard and radionuclide methods for measurement of glomerular filtration rate and effective renal blood flow in female horses, *Am J Vet Res* 53:1612, 1992.
154. Brewer BD, Clement SF, Lotz WS, et al: A comparison of inulin, para-aminohippuric acid, and endogenous creatinine clearances as measures of renal function in neonatal foals, *J Vet Intern Med* 4:301, 1990.
155. Woods PR, Drost WT, Clarke CR, et al: Use of 99mTc-mercaptoacetyltriglycine to evaluate renal function in horses, *Vet Radiol Ultrasound* 41:85, 2000.
156. Bertone JJ, Traub-Dargatz JL, Fettman MJ, et al: Monitoring the progression of renal failure in a horse with polycystic kidney disease: use of the reciprocal of serum creatinine concentration and sodium sulfanilate clearance half-time, *J Am Vet Med Assoc* 191:565, 1987.
157. Knudsen E: Renal clearance studies on the horse. I. Inulin, endogenous creatinine and urea, *Acta Vet Scand* 1:52, 1959.
158. Gelsa H: The renal clearance of inulin, creatinine, trimethoprim and sulphadoxine in horses, *J Vet Pharmacol Ther* 2:257, 1979.
159. Zatzman ML, Clarke L, Ray WJ, et al: Renal function of the pony and the horse, *Am J Vet Res* 43:608, 1981.
160. Schott HC, Hodgson DR, Bayly WM, et al: Renal responses to high intensity exercise, *Equine exercise physiology*, ed 3, Davis, CA, 1991, ICEEP Publications.
161. Finco DR, Groves C: Mechanism of renal excretion of creatinine by the pony, *Am J Vet Res* 46:1625, 1985.
162. McKeever KH, Hinchcliff KW, Schmall LM, et al: Renal tubular function in horses during sustained submaximal exercise, *Am J Physiol* 261:R553, 1991.
163. Osborne CA, Fahning ML, Schultz RH, et al: Percutaneous renal biopsy in the cow and the horse, *J Am Vet Med Assoc* 153:563, 1968.
164. Bayly WM, Paradis MR, Reed SM: Equine renal biopsy: indications, technique, interpretation, and complications, *Mod Vet Pract* 61:763, 1980.
165. Modransky PD: *Comparative evaluation of ultrasound-directed biopsy techniques in the horse,* master's thesis, Pullman, WA, 1983, Washington State University.
166. Barratt-Boyes S, Spensley MS, Nyland TG, et al: Ultrasound localization and guidance for renal biopsy in the horse, *Vet Radiol* 32:121, 1991.
167. Striker GE: Controversy: the role of renal biopsy in modern medicine, *Am J Kidney Dis* 1:241, 1982.

168. Morel-Maroger L: The value of renal biopsy, *Am J Kidney Dis* 1:244, 1982.
169. Donadio JV: The limitations of renal biopsy, *Am J Kidney Dis* 1:249, 1982.
170. Turner MW, Hutchinson TA, Barre PE, et al: A prospective study on the impact of renal biopsy in clinical management, *Clin Nephrol* 26:217, 1986.
171. Gleason DM, Bottaccini MR, Drach GW: Urodynamics, *J Urol* 115:356, 1976.
172. Clark SE, Semrad SD, Bichsel P, et al: Cystometrography and urethral pressure profiles in healthy horse and pony mares, *Am J Vet Res* 48:552, 1987.
173. Kay AK, Lavoie JP: Urethral pressure profilometry in mares, *J Am Vet Med Assoc* 191:212, 1987.
174. Ronen N: Measurements of urethral pressure profiles in the male horse, *Equine Vet J* 26:55, 1994.

Acute Renal Failure

1. Thadhani R, Pascual M, Bonventre JV: Acute renal failure, *N Engl J Med* 334:1448, 1996.
2. Robinson NE, editor: *Current therapy in equine medicine*, ed 6, St Louis, 2009, WB Saunders.
3. Shankel SW, Johnson DC, Clark PS, et al: Acute renal failure and glomerulopathy caused by nonsteroidal anti-inflammatory drugs, *Arch Intern Med* 152:986, 1992.
4. Divers TJ, Whitlock RH, Byars TD, et al: Acute renal failure in six horses resulting from haemodynamic causes, *Equine Vet J* 19:178, 1987.
5. Schmitz DG: Toxic nephropathy in horses, *Compend Contin Educ Pract Vet* 10:104, 1988.
6. Markel MD, Dyer RM, Hattel AL: Acute renal failure associated with application of a mercuric blister in a horse, *J Am Vet Med Assoc* 185:92, 1984.
7. Harrington DD, Page EH: Acute vitamin D_3 toxicosis in horses: case reports and experimental studies of the comparative toxicity of vitamins D_2 and D_3, *J Am Vet Med Assoc* 182:1358, 1983.
8. Rebhun WC, Tennant BC, Dill SG, et al: Vitamin K_3-induced renal toxicosis in the horse, *J Am Vet Med Assoc* 184:1237, 1984.
9. Riviere JE, Traver DS, Coppoc GL: Gentamicin toxic nephropathy in horses with disseminated bacterial infection, *J Am Vet Med Assoc* 180:648, 1982.
10. Brown C: Equine nephrology, *Vet Annu* 26:1, 1986.
11. Banks KL, Henson JB: Immunologically mediated glomerulitis of horses. II. Antiglomerular basement membrane antibody and other mechanisms in spontaneous disease, *Lab Invest* 26:708, 1972.
12. Ehnen SJ, Divers TJ, Gillette D, et al: Obstructive nephrolithiasis and ureterolithiasis associated with chronic renal failure in horses, *J Am Vet Med Assoc* 197:249, 1990.
13. Laverty S, Pascoe JR, Ling GV, et al: Urolithiasis in 68 horses, *Vet Surg* 21:56, 1992.
14. Brezis M, Rosen F: Hypoxia of the renal medulla: its implications for disease, *N Engl J Med* 332:647, 1995.
15. Grossman BS, Brobst DF, Kramer JW, et al: Urinary indices for differentiation of prerenal azotemia and renal azotemia in horses, *J Am Vet Med Assoc* 180:284, 1982.
16. Miller PD, Krebs RA, Neal BJ, et al: Polyuric prerenal failure, *Arch Intern Med* 140:907, 1980.
17. Baylis C: The mechanism of the decline in glomerular filtration in gentamicin induced acute renal failure in the rat, *J Antimicrob Chemother* 6:381, 1980.
18. Flamenbaum W, McNeil JS, Kotchen TA, et al: Experimental acute renal failure induced by uranyl nitrate in the dog, *Circ Res* 31:682, 1972.
19. Katzberg RW, Morris TW, Schulman G, et al: Reactions to intravenous contrast media. II. Acute renal response in euvolemic and dehydrated dogs, *Radiology* 147:331, 1983.
20. Levenson DJ, Simmons CD Jr, Brenner BM: Arachidonic acid metabolism, prostaglandins, and the kidney, *Am J Med* 72:354, 1982.
21. Reineck HJ, O'Connor GJ, Lifschitz MD, et al: Sequential studies on the pathophysiology and glycerol-induced acute renal failure, *J Lab Clin Med* 96:356, 1980.
22. Dworkin LD, Ichikawa I, Brenner VN: Hormonal modulation of glomerular function, *Am J Physiol* 244:F95, 1983.
23. Frega NS, DiBona DR, Guertter B, et al: Ischemic renal injury, *Kidney Int* 10:517, 1976.
24. Molitoris BA: Ischemia-induced loss of epithelial polarity: potential role of the actin cytoskeleton, *Am J Physiol* 260:F769, 1991.
25. Abbate M, Bonventre JV, Brown D: The microtubule network of renal epithelial cells is disrupted by ischemia and reperfusion, *Am J Physiol* 267:F971, 1994.
26. Venkatachalam MA, Bernard DB, Donohoe DF, et al: Ischemic damage and repair in the rat proximal tubule: differences among the S1, S2, and S3 segments, *Kidney Int* 14:31, 1978.
27. Molitoris BA, Dahl R, Geerde SA: Cytoskeleton disruption and apical redistribution of proximal tubule Na^+/K^+ATPase during ischemia, *Am J Physiol* 263:F483, 1992.
28. Goligorsky MS, DiBona GF: Pathogenetic role of Arg-Gly-Asp-recognizing integrins in acute renal failure, *Proc Natl Acad Sci U S A* 90:5700, 1993.
29. Kribben A, Widder ED, Wetzels JFM, et al: Evidence for role of cytosolic free calcium in hypoxia-induced proximal tubule injury, *J Clin Invest* 93:1994, 1922.
30. Bonventre JV: Mechanisms of ischemic acute renal failure, *Kidney Int* 43:1160, 1993.
31. Johnson KJ, Weinberg JM: Postischemic renal injury due to oxygen radicals, *Curr Opin Nephrol Hypertens* 2:625, 1993.
32. Klausner JM, Paterson IS, Goldman G, et al: Postischemic renal injury is mediated by neutrophils and leukotrienes, *Am J Physiol* 256:F794, 1989.
33. Hinchcliff KW, McGuirk SM, MacWilliams TS: Gentamicin nephrotoxicity, *Proc Am Assoc Equine Pract* 33:67, 1988.
34. Hostetler K, Hall L: Aminoglycoside antibiotics inhibit lysosomal phospholipase A and C from rat liver in vitro, *Biochim Biophys Acta* 710:506, 1982.
35. Blantz RC: Intrinsic renal failure: acute. In Seldin DW, Giebsich G, editors: *The kidney: physiology and pathophysiology*, New York, 1985, Raven Press.
36. Galpin J, Shinaberger J, Stanley T, et al: Acute interstitial nephritis due to methicillin, *Am J Med* 17:756, 1978.
37. McCausland IP, Milestone BA: Diffuse mesangioproliferative glomerulonephritis in a horse, *N Z Vet J* 24:239, 1976.
38. Divers TJ, Timoney JF, Lewis RM, et al: Equine glomerulonephritis and renal failure associated with complexes of group-C streptococcal antigen and IgG antibody, *Vet Immunol Immunopathol* 32:93, 1992.
39. Shimizu K, Kurosawa T, Maeda T, et al: Free water excretion and washout of renal medullary urea by prostaglandin E_1, *Jpn Heart J* 10:437, 1969.
40. Eliahou HD, Bata A: The diagnosis of acute renal failure, *Nephron* 2:287, 1965.
41. Miller TR, Anderson RG, Linas SL, et al: Urinary diagnostic indices in acute renal failure, *Ann Intern Med* 89:47, 1978.
42. Espinel CH, Gregory AW: Differential diagnosis of acute renal failure, *Clin Nephrol* 13:73, 1980.
43. Bayly WM, Paradis MR, Reed SM: Equine renal biopsy: indications, technique, interpretations and complications, *Mod Vet Pract* 61:763, 1980.
44. Bayly WM, Brobst DF, Elfers RS, et al: Serum and urinary biochemistry and enzyme changes in ponies with acute renal failure, *Cornell Vet* 76:306, 1986.
45. Elfers RS, Bayly WM, Brobst DF, et al: Alterations in calcium, phosphorus, and C-terminal parathyroid hormone levels in equine acute renal disease, *Cornell Vet* 76:317, 1986.

46. Meroney WH, Rubini MD: Kidney function during acute tubular necrosis: clinical studies and a theory, *Metabolism* 8:1, 1959.
47. Wilson DM, Turner DR, Cameron JS, et al: Value of renal biopsy in acute intrinsic renal failure, *BMJ* 2:459, 1976.
48. Simenhoff NL, Guild WR, Gammin GJ: Acute diffuse interstitial nephritis, *Am J Med* 44:618, 1968.
49. Ruffing KA, Hoope SP, Blend D, et al: Eosinophils in urine revisited, *Clin Nephrol* 41:163, 1994.
50. Llach F, Felsenfeld AJ, Haussler MR: Pathophysiology of altered calcium metabolism in rhabdomyolysis-induced acute renal failure: interactions of parathyroid hormone, 25-hydroxycholecalciferol and 1,25-dihydroxycholecalciferol, *N Engl J Med* 305:117, 1981.
51. Sweeney RW, MacDonald M, Hall J, et al: Kinetics of gentamicin elimination in two horses with acute renal failure, *Equine Vet J* 20:182, 1988.

Chronic Renal Failure

1. Ettinger SJ, Feldman EC, editors: *Textbook of veterinary internal medicine*, ed 6, vol. 2, St Louis, 2005, WB Saunders.
2. Banks KL, Henson JB: Immunologically mediated glomerulitis of horses. II. Antiglomerular basement membrane antibody and other mechanisms of spontaneous disease, *Lab Invest* 26:708, 1972.
3. Osborne CA, Polzin DJ: Azotemia: a review of what's old and what's new. I. Definition of terms and concepts, *Compend Contin Educ Pract Vet* 5:497, 1983.
4. Irwin DHG, Howell DW: Equine pyelonephritis and unilateral nephrectomy, *J S Afr Vet Assoc* 51:235, 1980.
5. Trotter GW, Brown CM, Ainsworth DM: Unilateral nephrectomy for treatment of a renal abscess in a foal, *J Am Vet Med Assoc* 184:1392, 1984.
6. Juzwiak JS, Bain FT, Slone DE, et al: Unilateral nephrectomy for treatment of chronic hematuria due to nephrolithiasis in a colt, *Can Vet J* 29:931, 1988.
7. Sullins KE, McIlwraith CW, Yovich JV, et al: Ectopic ureter managed by unilateral nephrectomy in two female horses, *Equine Vet J* 20:463, 1988.
8. Jones SL, Langer DL, Sterner-Kock A, et al: Renal dysplasia and benign ureteropelvic polyps associated with hydronephrosis in a foal, *J Am Vet Med Assoc* 204:1230, 1994.
9. Tennant B, Lowe JE, Tasker JB: Hypercalcemia and hypophosphatemia in ponies following bilateral nephrectomy, *Proc Soc Exp Biol Med* 167:365, 1981.
10. DeBowes R: Personal communication, 1991.
11. Johnson BD, Klingborg DJ, Heitman JM, et al: A horse with one kidney, partially obstructed ureter, and contralateral urogenital anomalies, *J Am Vet Med Assoc* 169:217, 1976.
12. Brown CM, Parks AH, Mullaney TP, et al: Bilateral renal dysplasia and hypoplasia in a foal with an imperforate anus, *Vet Rec* 122:91, 1988.
13. Andrews FM, Rosol TJ, Kohn CW, et al: Bilateral renal hypoplasia in four young horses, *J Am Vet Med Assoc* 189:209, 1986.
14. Roberts MC, Kelly WR: Chronic renal failure in a young pony, *Aust Vet J* 56:599, 1980.
15. Anderson WI, Picut CA, King JM, et al: Renal dysplasia in a Standardbred colt, *Vet Pathol* 25:179, 1988.
16. Ronen N, van Amstel SR, Nesbit JW, et al: Renal dysplasia in two adult horses: clinical and pathological aspects, *Vet Rec* 132:269, 1993.
17. Zicker SC, Marty GD, Carlson GP, et al: Bilateral renal dysplasia with nephron hypoplasia in a foal, *J Am Vet Med Assoc* 196:1990, 2001.
18. Ramsey G, Rothwell TLW, Gibson KT, et al: Polycystic kidneys in an adult horse, *Equine Vet J* 19:243, 1987.
19. Scott PC, Vasey J: Progressive polycystic renal disease in an aged horse, *Aust Vet J* 63:92, 1986.
20. Bertone JJ, Traub-Dargatz JL, Fettman MJ, et al: Monitoring the progression of renal failure in a horse with polycystic kidney disease: use of the reciprocal of serum creatinine concentration and sodium sulfanilate clearance half-time, *J Am Vet Med Assoc* 191:565, 1987.
21. Ramirez S, Williams J, Seahorn TL, et al: Ultrasound-assisted diagnosis of renal dysplasia in a 3-month-old Quarter Horse colt, *Vet Radiol Ultrasound* 39:143, 1998.
22. Woolridge AA, Seahorn TL, Williams J, et al: Chronic renal failure associated with nephrolithiasis, ureterolithiasis, and renal dysplasia in a 2-year-old Quarter Horse gelding, *Vet Radiol Ultrasound* 40:361, 1999.
23. Aguilera-Tejero E, Estepa JC, Lopez I, et al: Polycystic kidneys as a cause of chronic renal failure and secondary hypoparathyroidism in a horse, *Equine Vet J* 32:167, 2000.
24. Gull T, Schmitz A, Bahr A, et al: Renal hypoplasia and dysplasia in an American Miniature foal, *Vet Rec* 149:199, 2001.
25. Tennant B, Kaneko JJ, Lowe JE, et al: Chronic renal failure in the horse, *Proceedings of the twenty-third annual meeting of the American Association of Equine Practitioners*, St Louis, 1978, p 293.
26. Koterba AM, Coffman JR: Acute and chronic renal disease in the horse, *Compend Contin Educ Pract Vet* 3:S461, 1981.
27. Divers TJ: Chronic renal failure in horses, *Compend Contin Educ Pract Vet* 5:S310, 1983.
28. Robinson NE, editor: *Current therapy in equine medicine*, ed 6, St Louis, 2009, WB Saunders.
29. Smith BP, editor: *Large animal internal medicine*, ed 4, St Louis, 2009, Mosby.
30. Kobluk CN, Ames TR, Geor RJ, editors: *The horse, diseases and clinical management*, Philadelphia, 1995, WB Saunders.
31. Osborne CA, Hammer RF, Stevens JB, et al: The glomerulus in health and disease: a comparative review of domestic animals and man, *Adv Vet Sci Comp Med* 21:207, 1977.
32. Langham RF, Hallman ET: The incidence of glomerulonephritis in domesticated animals, *J Am Vet Med Assoc* 49:471, 1949.
33. Slauson DO, Lewis RM: Comparative pathology of glomerulonephritis in animals, *Vet Pathol* 16:135, 1979.
34. Winter H, Majid NH: Glomerulonephritis: an emerging disease?, *Vet Bull* 54:327, 1984.
35. Brenner BM, editor: *Brenner and Rector's the kidney*, ed 8, Philadelphia, 2008, WB Saunders.
36. Van Biervliet J, Divers TJ, Porter B, et al: Glomerulonephritis in horses, *Compend Contin Educ Pract Vet* 24:892, 2002.
37. Banks KL, Henson JB, McGuire TC: Immunologically mediated glomerulitis of horses. I. Pathogenesis in persistent infection by equine infectious anemia virus, *Lab Invest* 26:701, 1972.
38. Banks KL: Animal model of human disease: antiglomerular basement antibody in horses, *Am J Pathol* 94:443, 1979.
39. Geor RJ, Clark EG, Haines DM, et al: Systemic lupus erythematosus in a filly, *J Am Vet Med Assoc* 197:1489, 1990.
40. Sabnis SG, Gunson DE, Antonovych TT: Some unusual features of mesangioproliferative glomerulonephritis in horses, *Vet Pathol* 21:574, 1984.
41. Maede Y, Inaba M, Amano Y, et al: Cryoglobulinemia in a horse, *J Vet Med Sci* 53:379, 1991.
42. Traub-Dargatz J, Bertone A, Bennett D, et al: Monoclonal aggregating immunoglobulin cryoglobulinaemia in a horse with malignant lymphoma, *Equine Vet J* 17:470, 1985.
43. MacDougall DF, Cook T, Steward AP, et al: Canine chronic renal disease: prevalence and types of glomerulonephritis in the dog, *Kidney Int* 29:1144, 1986.
44. Fincher MG, Olafson P: Chronic diffuse glomerulonephritis in a horse, *Cornell Vet* 24:356, 1934.
45. Frank ER, Dunlap GL: Chronic diffuse glomerulo-tubular nephritis in a horse, *North Am Vet* 16:20, 1935.
46. Kadaás I, Szaázados I: Membrano-proliferative diffuse glomerulonephritis in a horse, *Dtsch Tierarztl Wochenschr* 81:618, 1974.

47. McCausland IP, Milestone BA: Diffuse mesangioproliferative glomerulonephritis in a horse, *N Z Vet J* 24:239, 1976.
48. Brobst DF, Grant BD, Hilbert BJ, et al: Blood biochemical changes in horses with prerenal and renal disease, *J Equine Med Surg* 1:171, 1977.
49. Brobst DF, Lee HA, Spencer GR: Hypercalcemia and hypophosphotemia in a mare with renal insufficiency, *J Am Vet Med Assoc* 173:1370, 1978.
50. Roberts MC, Seiler RJ: Renal failure in a horse with chronic glomerulonephritis and renal oxalosis, *J Equine Med Surg* 3:278, 1979.
51. Dobos-Kovaács M: Chronic, diffuse, membrane-proliferative glomerulonephritis and its complications in a horse, *Magy Aállatorvosok Lapja* 36:533, 1981.
52. Tennant B, Bettleheim P, Kaneko JJ: Paradoxic hypercalcemia and hypophosphotemia associated with chronic renal failure in horses, *J Am Vet Med Assoc* 180:630, 1982.
53. Morris DD, Lee JW: Renal insufficiency due to chronic glomerulonephritis in two horses, *Vet Clin North Am Equine Pract* 4(8):21, 1982.
54. Waldvogel A, Wild P, Wegmann C: Membranoproliferative glomerulonephritis in a horse, *Vet Pathol* 20:500, 1983.
55. Scarratt WK, Sponenberg DP: Chronic glomerulonephritis in two horses, *J Equine Vet Sci* 4:252, 1984.
56. Divers TJ, Timoney JF, Lewis RM, et al: Equine glomerulonephritis and renal failure associated with complexes of group-C streptococcal antigen and IgG antibody, *Vet Immunol Immunopathol* 32:93, 1992.
57. Webb RF, Knight PR: Oxalate nephropathy in a horse, *Aust Vet J* 53:554, 1977.
58. Brobst DF, Bayly WM, Reed SM, et al: Parathyroid hormone evaluation in normal horses and horses with renal failure, *J Equine Vet Sci* 2:150, 1982.
59. Byars TD, Simpson JS, Divers TJ, et al: Percutaneous nephrostomy in short-term management of ureterolithiasis and renal dysfunction in a filly, *J Am Vet Med Assoc* 195:499, 1989.
60. Hope WD, Wilson JH, Hager DA, et al: Chronic renal failure associated with bilateral nephroliths and ureteroliths in a two-year-old Thoroughbred colt, *Equine Vet J* 21:228, 1989.
61. Ehnen SJ, Divers TJ, Gillette D, et al: Obstructive nephrolithiasis and ureterolithiasis associated with chronic renal failure in horses: eight cases (1981-1987), *J Am Vet Med Assoc* 197(249), 1990.
62. Hillyer MH, Mair TS, Lucke VM: Bilateral renal calculi in an adult horse, *Equine Vet Educ* 2:117, 1990.
63. Laing JA, Raisis AL, Rawlinson RJ, et al: Chronic renal failure and urolithiasis in a 2-year-old colt, *Aust Vet J* 69:199, 1992.
64. Held JP, Wright B, Henton JE: Pyelonephritis associated with renal failure in a horse, *J Am Vet Med Assoc* 189:688, 1986.
65. Carrick JB, Pollitt CC: Chronic pyelonephritis in a brood mare, *Aust Vet J* 64:252, 1987.
66. Sloet van Oldruitenborgh-Oosterbaan MM, Klabec HC: Ureteropyelonephritis in a Fresian mare, *Vet Rec* 122:609, 1988.
67. Mair TS, Taylor FGR, Pinsent PJN: Fever of unknown origin in the horse: a review of 63 cases, *Equine Vet J* 21:260, 1989.
68. Hamlen H: Pyelonephritis in a mature gelding with an unusual urinary bladder foreign body: a case report, *J Equine Vet Sci* 13:159, 1993.
69. Gunson DE: Renal papillary necrosis in horses, *J Am Vet Med Assoc* 182:263, 1983.
70. Andrews EJ: Oxalate nephropathy in a horse, *J Am Vet Med Assoc* 159:49, 1971.
71. Buntain B, Greig WA, Thompson H: Chronic nephritis in a pony, *Vet Rec* 104:307, 1979.
72. Alders RG, Hutchins DR: Chronic nephritis in a horse, *Aust Vet J* 64:151, 1987.
73. Snyder JR, Batista: de Cruz J: Chronic renal failure in a stallion, *Compend Contin Educ Pract Vet* 6:S134, 1984.
74. Morter RL, Williams RD, Bolte H, et al: Equine leptospirosis, *J Am Vet Med Assoc* 155:436, 1969.
75. Divers TJ, Byars TD, Shin SJ: Renal dysfunction associated with infection of *Leptospira interrogans* in a horse, *J Am Vet Med Assoc* 201:1391, 1992.
76. Hogan PM, Bernard WV, Kazakevicius PA, et al: Acute renal disease due to *Leptospira interrogans* in a weaning, *Equine Vet J* 28:331, 1996.
77. Frazer ML: Acute renal failure from leptospirosis in a foal, *Aust Vet J* 77:499, 1999.
78. Srivastava T, Warady BA, Alon US: Pneumonia-associated acute glomerulonephritis, *Clin Nephrol* 57:175, 2002.
79. Roberts MC, Kelly WR: Renal dysfunction in a case of purpura haemorrhagica in a horse, *Vet Rec* 110:144, 1982.
80. Wimberly HC, Antonovych TT, Lewis RM: Focal glomerulosclerosis-like disease with nephrotic syndrome in a horse, *Vet Pathol* 18:692, 1981.
81. Divers TJ, Whitlock RH, Byars TD, et al: Acute renal failure in six horses resulting from haemodynamic causes, *Equine Vet J* 19:178, 1987.
82. Schmitz DG: Toxic nephropathy in horses, *Compend Contin Educ Pract Vet* 10:104, 1988.
83. Boyd WL, Bishop LM: Pyelonephritis of horses and cattle, *J Am Vet Med Assoc* 90:154, 1937.
84. Divers TJ: Nephrolithiasis and ureterolithiasis in horses and their association with renal disease and failure, *Equine Vet J* 21:161, 1989:editorial.
85. MacAllister CG, Morgan SJ, Borne AT, et al: Comparison of adverse effects of phenylbutazone, flunixin meglumine, and ketoprofen in horses, *J Am Vet Med Assoc* 202:71, 1993.
86. Gunson DE, Soma LR: Renal papillary necrosis in horses after phenylbutazone and water deprivation, *Vet Pathol* 20:603, 1983.
87. Behm RJ, Berg IE: Hematuria caused by medullary crest necrosis in a horse, *Compend Contin Educ Pract Vet* 9:698, 1987.
88. Jubb KVF, Kennedy PC, Palmer N, editors: *Pathology of domestic animals*, ed 3, vol. 2, San Diego, 1985, Academic Press.
89. Stewart J, McCallum JW: The anhydraemia of oxalate poisoning in horses, *Vet Rec* 56:77, 1944.
90. Walthall JC, McKenzie RA: Osteodystrophia fibrosa in horses at pasture in Queensland: field and laboratory investigations, *Aust Vet J* 52:11, 1976.
91. Jakob W: Spontaneous amyloidosis of animals, *Vet Pathol* 8:292, 1971.
92. Nunokawa Y, Fujinaga T, Taira T, et al: Evaluation of serum amyloid A protein as an acute-phase reactive protein in horses, *J Vet Med Sci* 55:1011, 1993.
93. Husebekk A, Husby G, Sletten K, et al: Characterization of amyloid protein AA and its serum precursor SAA in the horse, *Scand J Immunol* 23:703, 1986.
94. Sletten K, Husebekk A, Husby G: The amino acid sequence of an amyloid fibril protein AA isolated from the horse, *Scand J Immunol* 26:79, 1987.
95. Sletten K, Husebekk A, Husby G: The primary structure of equine serum amyloid A (SAA) protein, *Scand J Immunol* 30:117, 1989.
96. van Andel ACJ, Gruys E, Kroneman J, et al: Amyloid in the horse: a report of nine cases, *Equine Vet J* 20:277, 1988.
97. DiBartola SP, Benson MD: The pathogenesis of reactive systemic amyloidosis, *J Vet Intern Med* 3:31, 1989.
98. Hayden DW, Johnson KH, Wolf CB, et al: AA amyloid-associated gastroenteropathy in a horse, *J Comp Pathol* 98:195, 1988.
99. Vanhooser SL, Reinemeyer CR, Held JP: Hepatic AA amyloidosis associated with severe strongylosis in a horse, *Equine Vet J* 20:274, 1988.
100. Bovée KC: The uremic syndrome, *J Am Anim Hosp Assoc* 12:189, 1976.
101. Wills MR: Uremic toxins, and their effect on intermediary metabolism, *Clin Chem* 31:5, 1985.

102. Finco DR, Groves C: Mechanism of renal excretion of creatinine by the pony, *Am J Vet Res* 46:1625, 1985.
103. Malluche H, Faugere MC: Renal bone disease 1990: an unmet challenge for the nephrologist, *Kidney Int* 38:193, 1990.
104. Nagode LA, Chew DJ: Nephrocalcinosis caused by hyperparathyroidism in progression of renal failure, *Semin Vet Med Surg (Small Anim)* 7:202, 1992.
105. Frye MA, Johnson JS, Traub-Dargatz JL, et al: Putative uremic encephalopathy in horses: five cases (1978-1998), *J Am Vet Med Assoc* 218:560–566, 2001.
106. Perna AF, Ingrosso D, Galletti P, et al: Membrane protein damage and methylation reactions in chronic renal failure, *Kidney Int* 50:358, 1996.
107. Hayslett JP: Functional adaptation to reduction in renal mass, *Physiol Rev* 59:137, 1979.
108. Pearson EG: Hypoalbuminemia in horses, *Compend Contin Educ Pract Vet* 12:555, 1990.
109. Rose BD, editor: *Clinical physiology of acid-base and electrolyte disorders*, ed 3, New York, 1989, McGraw-Hill.
110. Bovée KC: Functional responses to nephron loss. In Bovée KC, editor: *Canine nephrology*, Media, PA, 1984, Harwal.
111. Ersley AJ: Erythropoeitin, *N Engl J Med* 324:1339, 1991.
112. Jaussand P, Audran M, Gareau RL: Kinetics and haematological effects of erythropoietin in horses, *Vet Res* 25:568, 1994.
113. Effects of erythropoietin on plasma and red cell volume, V̇ 2max, and hemodynamics in exercising horses, *Med Sci Sports Exerc* 25:S25, 1993.
114. Geor RJ, Weiss DJ: Drugs affecting the hematologic system of the performance horse, *Vet Clin North Am Equine Pract* 9:649, 1993.
115. Piercy RJ, Swardson CJ, Hinchcliff KW: Erythroid hypoplasia and anemia following administration of recombinant human erythropoietin to two horses, *J Am Vet Med Assoc* 212:244, 1998.
116. Woods PR, Campbell G, Cowell RL: Nonregenerative anaemia associated with administration of recombinant human erythropoietin to a Thoroughbred racehorse, *Equine Vet J* 29:326–328, 1997.
117. Bayly WM: A practitioner's approach to the diagnosis and treatment of renal failure in horses, *Vet Med* 86:632, 1991.
118. Matthews HK, Kohn CW: Calcium and phosphorous homeostasis in horses with renal disease, *Proceedings of the eleventh annual Forum of the American College of Veterinary Internal Medicine*, San Diego, 1993, p 623.
119. Krook L, Wasserman RH, Shively JN, et al: Hypercalcemia and calcinosis in Florida horses: implication for the shrub *Cestrum diurnum* as the causative agent, *Cornell Vet* 65:26, 1975.
120. Gingerich DA, Murdick PW: Paradoxic aciduria in bovine metabolic alkalosis, *J Am Vet Med Assoc* 166:227, 1975.
121. Naylor JM, Kronfeld DS, Acland H: Hyperlipemia in horses: effects of undernutrition and disease, *Am J Vet Res* 41:899, 1980.
122. Dunkel B, McKenzie HC III: Severe hypertriglyceridaemia in clinically ill horses: diagnosis, treatment and outcome, *Equine Vet J* 35:590–595, 2003.
123. Mogg TD, Palmer JE: Hyperlipidemia, hyperlipemia, and hepatic lipidosis in American Miniature Horses: 23 cases (1990–1994), *J Am Vet Med Assoc* 207:604–607, 1995.
124. Gröne HJ, Hohbach J, Gröne EF: Modulation of glomerular sclerosis and interstitial fibrosis by native and modified lipoproteins, *Kidney Int* 49(Suppl 54):S18, 1996.
125. Grossman BS, Brobst DF, Kramer JW, et al: Urinary indices for differentiation of prerenal azotemia and renal azotemia in horses, *J Am Vet Med Assoc* 180:284, 1982.
126. Grauer GF, Thomas CB, Eicker SW: Estimation of quantitative proteinuria in the dog, using the urine protein-to-creatinine ratio from a random, voided sample, *Am J Vet Res* 46(2116), 1985.
127. Schott HC, Hodgson DR, Bayly WM: Haematuria, pigmenturia and proteinuria in exercising horses, *Equine Vet J* 27:67, 1995.
128. Kohn CW, Strasser SL: 24-Hour renal clearance and excretion of endogenous substances in the mare, *Am J Vet Res* 47:1332, 1986.
129. Rantanen NW: Diseases of the kidneys, *Vet Clin North Am Equine Pract* 2:89, 1986.
130. Kiper ML, Traub-Dargatz JL, Wrigley RH: Renal ultrasonography in horses, *Compend Contin Educ Pract Vet* 12:993, 1990.
131. Traub-Dargatz JL, McKinnon AO: Adjunctive methods of examination of the urogenital tract, *Vet Clin North Am Equine Pract* 4:339, 1988.
132. Divers TJ, Yeager AE: The value of ultrasonographic examination in the diagnosis and management of renal diseases in horses, *Equine Vet Educ* 7:334, 1997.
133. Reef VB: *Equine diagnostic ultrasound*, Philadelphia, 1998, WB Saunders.
134. Schott HC, Roberts GD, Hines MT, et al: Nuclear scintigraphy as a diagnostic aid in the evaluation of renal disease in horses. In *Proceedings of the thirty-ninth annual meeting of the American Association of Equine Practitioners*, San Antonio, TX, 1993, p 251.
135. Levey AS: Measurement of renal function in chronic renal disease, *Kidney Int* 38:167, 1990.
136. Walser M: Progression of chronic renal failure in man, *Kidney Int* 37:1195, 1990.
137. Matthews HK, Andrews FM, Daniel GB, et al: Measuring renal function in horses, *Vet Med* 88:349, 1993.
138. Brobst DF, Bramwell K, Kramer JW: Sodium sulfanilate clearance as a method of determining renal function in the horse, *J Equine Med Surg* 2:500, 1978.
139. Matthews HK, Andrews FM, Danile GB, et al: Comparison of standard and radionuclide methods for measurement of glomerular filtration rate and effective renal blood flow in female horses, *Am J Vet Res* 53:1612, 1992.
140. Klahr S, Schreiner G, Ichikawa I: The progression of renal disease, *N Engl J Med* 318:1657, 1988.
141. Remuzzi G, Bertani T: Pathophysiology of progressive nephropathies, *N Engl J Med* 339:1448, 1998.
142. Reggenenti P, Schieppati A, Remuzzi G: Progression, remission, regression of chronic renal diseases, *Lancet* 357:1601, 2001.
143. Yoshioka T, Mitarai T, Kon V, et al: Role for angiotensin II in an overt functional proteinuria, *Kidney Int* 30:538, 1986.
144. Heeg JE, de Jong PE, van der Hem GK, et al: Reduction of proteinuria by angiotensin converting enzyme inhibition, *Kidney Int* 32:78, 1987.
145. Keane WF, Anderson S, Aurell M, et al: Angiotensin converting enzyme inhibitors and progressive renal insufficiency: current experience and future directions, *Ann Intern Med* 111:503, 1989.
146. Taal MW, Brenner BM: Renoprotective effects of RAS inhibition: from ACEI to angiotensin II antagonists, *Kidney Int* 57:2000, 1803.
147. Brown SA, Walton C, Crawford P, et al: Long-term effects of antihypertensive regimens on renal hemodynamics and proteinuria in diabetic dogs, *Kidney Int* 43:1210, 1993.
148. Ihle BU, Becker GJ, Whitworth JA, et al: The effect of protein restriction on the progression of renal insufficiency, *N Engl J Med* 321:1773, 1989.
149. Mitch WE: Dietary protein restriction in patients with chronic renal failure, *Kidney Int* 40:326, 1991.
150. Fouque D, Laville M, Boissel JP, et al: Controlled low protein diets in chronic renal insufficiency: meta-analysis, *BMJ* 304:216, 1992.
151. Klahr S, Level AS, Beck GJ, et al: The effects of dietary protein restriction and blood-pressure control on the progression of chronic renal disease, *N Engl J Med* 330:877, 1994.

152. Polzin DJ, Osborne CA, Hayden DW, et al: Influence of reduced protein diets on morbidity, mortality, and renal function in dogs with induced chronic renal failure, *Am J Vet Res* 45:506, 1984.
153. Brown SA, Finco DR, Crowell WA et al: Dietary protein intake and the glomerular adaptations to partial nephrectomy in dogs, *J Nutr* 121:S125, 191.
154. Ikizler TA, Hakim RM: Nutrition in end-stage renal disease, *Kidney Int* 50:343, 1996.
155. Seawright AA, Roberts MC, Costigan P: Chronic methylmercurialism in a horse, *Vet Hum Toxicol* 20:6, 1978.
156. Roberts MC, Ng JC, Seawright AA: The effects of prolonged daily low level mercuric chloride dosing in a horse, *Vet Hum Toxicol* 20:410, 1978.
157. Roberts MC, Seawright AA, Ng JC: Chronic phenylmercuric acetate toxicity in a horse, *Vet Hum Toxicol* 21:321, 1979.
158. Roberts MC, Seawright AA, Ng JC, et al: Some effects of chronic mercuric chloride intoxication on renal function in a horse, *Vet Hum Toxicol* 24:415, 1982.
159. Divers TJ: Management of chronic renal failure in the horse, *Proceedings of the thirty-first annual meeting of the American Association of Equine Practitioners*, Toronto, Canada, 1985, p 1.
160. Kirk CA: Dietary salt and FLUTD: risk or benefit? *Proceedings of the twentieth annual forum of the American College of Veterinary Internal Medicine*, Toronto, Canada, 2002, p 553.
161. Velosa JA, Torres VE, Donadio JV: Treatment of severe nephrotic syndrome with meclofenamate: an uncontrolled pilot study, *Mayo Clin Proc* 60:586, 1985.
162. Morris DD, Henry MM, Moore JN, et al: Effect of dietary linolenic acid on endotoxin-induced thromboxane and prostacyclin production by equine peritoneal macrophages, *Circ Shock* 29:311, 1989.
163. Henry MM, Moore JN, Feldman EB: The effect of dietary alpha linolenic acid on equine monocyte procoagulant activity and eicosanoid synthesis, *Circ Shock* 32:173, 1990.
164. Morris DD, Henry MM, Moore JN, et al: Dietary alpha linolenic acid reduces endotoxin- induced production of tumor necrosis factor activity by peritoneal macrophages, *Am J Vet Res* 52:528, 1991.
165. Barcelli UO, Weiss M, Pollack VE: Effects of dietary prostaglandin precursor on the progression of experimentally induced chronic renal failure, *J Lab Clin Med* 100:786, 1982.
166. Scharschmidt LA, Gibbons NB, McGarry L, et al: Effects of dietary fish oil on renal insufficiency in rats with subtotal nephrectomy, *Kidney Int* 32:700, 1987.
167. Henry MM, Moore JN, Fischer JK: Influence of an omega-3 fatty acid-enriched ration on in vivo responses of horses to endotoxin, *Am J Vet Res* 52:523, 1991.
168. Longhofer SL, Frisbie DD, Johnson HC, et al: Effects of thromboxane synthetase inhibition on immune complex glomerulonephritis, *Am J Vet Res* 52:480, 1991.
169. Vaden SL, Breitschwerdt EB, Armstrong PJ, et al: The effects of cyclosporine versus standard care in dogs with naturally occurring glomerulonephritis, *J Vet Intern Med* 9:259, 1995.
170. Müller GA, Schettler V, Müller CA, et al: Prevention of progression of renal fibrosis: how far are we? *Kidney Int* 49(Suppl 5):S75, 1996.
171. Davies M, Kastner S, Thomas GJ: Proteoglycans: their possible role in renal fibrosis, *Kidney Int* 49(Suppl 54):S55, 1996.

Urinary Tract Infections

1. Brenner BM, editor: *Brenner and Rector's the kidney*, ed 8, Philadelphia, 2008, WB Saunders.
2. Robinson NE, editor: *Current therapy in equine medicine*, ed 6, St Louis, 2009, WB Saunders.
3. Smith BP, editor: *Large animal internal medicine*, ed 4, St Louis, 2009, Mosby.
4. Kobluk CN, Ames TR, Geor RJ, editors: *The horse, diseases and clinical management*, Philadelphia, 1995, WB Saunders.
5. Divers TJ: Diagnosis and management of urinary tract infections in the horse, *Proceedings of a symposium on trimethoprim/sulfadiazine, clinical application in equine medicine, Princeton Junction*, Yardley, PA, 1984, Veterinary Learning Systems.
6. Robinson JA, Allen GK, Green EM, et al: A prospective study of septicaemia in colostrum-deprived foals, *Equine Vet J* 25:214–219, 1993.
7. Senior DF: Bacterial urinary tract infections: invasion, host defenses, and new approaches to prevention, *Compend Contin Educ Pract Vet* 7:334, 1985.
8. Roberts JA: Bacterial adherence and urinary tract infection, *South Med J* 80:347, 1987.
9. Reid G, Sobel JD: Bacterial adherence in the pathogenesis of urinary tract infection: a review, *Rev Infect Dis* 9:470, 1987.
10. Johnson PJ, Goetz TE, Baker GJ, et al: Treatment of two mares with obstructive (vaginal) urinary outflow incontinence, *J Am Vet Med Assoc* 191:973, 1987.
11. Sertich PL, Hamir AN, Orsini P, et al: Paraurethral lipoma in a mare associated with frequent urination, *Equine Vet Educ* 2:121, 1990.
12. Mulholland SG, Qureshi SM, Fritz RW, et al: Effect of hormonal deprivation on the bladder defense mechanism, *J Urol* 127:1010, 1982.
13. Reidasch G, Heck P, Rauterberg E, et al: Does low urinary sIgA predispose to urinary tract infection? *Kidney Int* 23:759, 1983.
14. Voss JL, Pickett BW: Diagnosis and treatment of haemospermia in the stallion, *J Reprod Fertil Suppl* 23:151, 1975.
15. Sullins KE, Bertone JJ, Voss JL, et al: Treatment of hemospermia in stallions: a discussion of 18 cases, *Compend Contin Educ Pract Vet* 10:1396, 1988.
16. Auer JA, Stick JA, editors: *Equine surgery*, ed 3, St Louis, 2006, WB Saunders.
17. McKinnon AO, Voss JL, editors: *Equine reproduction*, Philadelphia, 1993, Lea & Febiger.
18. Schumacher J, Varner DD, Schmitz DG, et al: Urethral defects in geldings with hematuria and stallions with hemospermia, *Vet Surg* 24:250, 1995.
19. Blanchard TL, Varner DD, Hurtgen JP, et al: Bilateral seminal vesiculitis and ampullitis in a stallion, *J Am Vet Med Assoc* 192:525, 1988.
20. DeBowes RM, Nyrop KA, Boulton CH: Cystic calculi in the horse, *Compend Contin Educ Pract Vet* 6:S268, 1984.
21. Laverty S, Pascoe JR, Ling GV, et al: Urolithiasis in 68 horses, *Vet Surg* 21:56, 1992.
22. Adams LG, Dollahite JW, Romane WM, et al: Cystitis and ataxia associated with sorghum ingestion, *J Am Vet Med Assoc* 155:518, 1969.
23. Fischer AT, Spier S, Carlson GP, et al: Neoplasia of the urinary bladder as a cause of hematuria, *J Am Vet Med Assoc* 186:1294–1296, 1985.
24. Holt PE, Mair TS: Ten cases of bladder paralysis associated with sabulous urolithiasis in horses, *Vet Rec* 127:108, 1990.
25. Wise LA, Jones RL, Reif JS: Nosocomial canine urinary tract infections in a veterinary teaching hospital, *J Am Anim Hosp Assoc* 26(148):1990, 1983–1988.
26. Sullins KE, Traub-Dargatz JL: Endoscopic anatomy of the equine urinary tract, *Compend Contin Educ Pract Vet* 6:S663, 1984.
27. Traub-Dargatz JL, McKinnon AO: Adjunctive methods of examination of the urogenital tract, *Vet Clin North Am Equine Pract* 4:339, 1988.
28. Kohn CW, Chew DJ: Laboratory diagnosis and characterization of renal disease in horses, *Vet Clin North Am Equine Pract* 3:585, 1987.
29. Nouws JFM, Firth EC, Vree TB, et al: Pharmacokinetics and renal clearance of sulfamethazine, sulfamerazine, and sulfadiazine and their N_4-acetyl and hydroxy metabolites in horses, *Am J Vet Res* 48:392, 1987.

30. Johnson PJ, Crenshaw KL: The treatment of cystic and urethral calculi in a gelding, *Vet Med* 85:891, 1990.
31. White NA, Moore JN, editors: *Current practice of equine surgery*, Philadelphia, 1990, JB Lippincott.
32. Mair TS, Holt PE: The aetiology and treatment of equine urolithiasis, *Equine Vet Educ* 6:189, 1994.
33. Wood T, Weckman TJ, Henry PA, et al: Equine urine pH: normal population distributions and methods of acidification, *Equine Vet J* 22:118, 1990.
34. Remillard RL, Modransky PD, Welker FH, et al: Dietary management of cystic calculi in a horse, *J Equine Vet Sci* 12:359, 1992.
35. Divers TJ, Byars TD, Murch O, et al: Experimental induction of *Proteus mirabilis* cystitis in the pony and evaluation of therapy with trimethoprim-sulfadiazine, *Am J Vet Res* 42:1203, 1981.
36. Van Kempen KR: Sudan grass and sorghum poisoning of horses: a possible lathyrogenic disease, *J Am Vet Med Assoc* 156:629, 1970.
37. Hooper PT: Epizootic cystitis in horses, *Aust Vet J* 44:11, 1968.
38. Modransky PD, Wagner PC, Robinette JD, et al: Surgical correction of bilateral ectopic ureters in two foals, *Vet Surg* 12:141, 1983.
39. Pringle JK, Ducharme NG, Baird JD: Ectopic ureter in the horse: three cases and a review of the literature, *Can Vet J* 31:26, 1990.
40. Roberts MC: Ascending urinary tract infection in ponies, *Aust Vet J* 55:191, 1979.
41. Hamlen H: Pyelonephritis in a mature gelding with an unusual urinary bladder foreign body, *J Equine Vet Sci* 13:159, 1993.
42. Sloet van Oldruitenborgh-Oosterbaan MM, Klabec HC: Ureteropyelonephritis in a Fresian mare, *Vet Rec* 122:609, 1988.
43. Boyd WL, Bishop LM: Pyelonephritis of cattle and horses, *J Am Vet Med Assoc* 90:154, 1937.
44. Irwin DHG, Howell DW: Equine pyelonephritis and unilateral nephrectomy, *J S Afr Vet Assoc* 51:235, 1980.
45. Tennant B, Bettleheim P, Kaneko JJ: Paradoxic hypercalcemia and hypophosphotemia associated with chronic renal failure in horses, *J Am Vet Med Assoc* 180:630, 1982.
46. Held JP, Wright B, Henton JE: Pyelonephritis associated with renal failure in a horse, *J Am Vet Med Assoc* 189:688, 1986.
47. Carrick JB, Pollitt CC: Chronic pyelonephritis in a brood mare, *Aust Vet J* 64:252, 1987.
48. Mair TS, Taylor FGR, Pinsent PJN: Fever of unknown origin in the horse: a review of 63 cases, *Equine Vet J* 21:260, 1989.
49. Divers TJ: Chronic renal failure in horses, *Compend Contin Educ Pract Vet* 5:S310, 1983.
50. Schott HC, Hodgson DR, Bayly WM: Ureteral catheterization in the horse, *Equine Vet Educ* 2:140, 1990.
51. Trotter GW, Brown CM, Ainsworth DM: Unilateral nephrectomy for treatment of a renal abscess in a foal, *J Am Vet Med Assoc* 184:1392, 1984.
52. Wintzer HJ, editor: *Equine diseases: a textbook for students and practitioners*, New York, 1986, Springer-Verlag.
53. Cranley JJ, McCullagh KG: Ischaemic myocardial fibrosis and aortic strongylosis in the horse, *Equine Vet J* 13:35, 1981.
54. Poynter D: The arterial lesions produced by *Strongylus vulgaris* and their relationship to the migratory route of the parasite in its host, *Res Vet Sci* 1:205, 1960.
55. Rubin HL, Woodard JC: Equine infection with *Micronema deletrix*, *J Am Vet Med Assoc* 165:256, 1974.
56. Alstad AD, Berg JE, Samuel C: Disseminated *Micronema deletrix* infection in the horse, *J Am Vet Med Assoc* 174:264, 1979.
57. Blunden AS, Khalil LF, Webbon PM: *Halicephalobus deletrix* infection in a horse, *Equine Vet J* 19:255, 1987.
58. Darien BJ, Belknap J, Nietfeld J: Cerebrospinal fluid changes in two horses with central nervous system nematodiasis *(Micronema deletrix)*, *J Vet Intern Med* 2:201, 1988.
59. Angus KW, Roberts L, Archibald DRN, et al: *Halicephalobus deletrix* infection in a horse in Scotland, *Vet Rec* 131:495, 1992:letter.
60. Lester G: Parasitic encephalomyelitis in horses, *Compend Contin Educ Pract Vet* 14:1624, 1992.
61. Cheng TC: *General parasitology*, New York, 1973, Academic Press.
62. Smits GM, Misdorf W: Dioctophyma renale beim Hund in den Neiderlanden, *Zentralbl Veterinarmed B* 12:327, 1965.
63. Szwejkowski H: Sektionsbild der Dioctophymease der Hunde, *Arch Exp Veterinarmed* 14:1184, 1960.
64. Newberne JW, Robinson VB, Bowen NE: Histological aspects of *Klossiella equi* in the kidney of a zebra, *Am J Vet Res* 19:304, 1958.
65. Vetterling JM, Thompson DE: *Klossiella equi* Baumann, 1946 (Sporozoa: Eucoccidia: Adeleina) from equids, *J Parasitol* 58:589, 1972.
66. Todd KS, Gosser HS, Hamilton DP: *Klossiella equi* Baumann, 1946 (Sporozoa: Eucoccidiorida) from an Illinois horse, *Vet Med Small Anim Clin* 72:443, 1977.
67. Lee CG, Ross AD: Renal coccidiosis of the horse associated with *Klossiella equi*, *Aust Vet J* 53:287, 1977.
68. Austin RJ, Dies KH: *Klossiella equi* in the kidneys of a horse, *Can Vet J* 22:159, 1981.
69. Reppas GP, Collins GH: *Klossiella equi* infection in horses: sporocyst stage identified in urine, *Aust Vet J* 72:316, 1995.

Obstructive Disease of the Urinary Tract

1. Robinson NE, editor: *Current therapy in equine medicine*, ed 6, St Louis, 2009, WB Saunders.
2. Smith BP, editor: *Large animal internal medicine*, ed 4, St Louis, 2009, Mosby.
3. Kobluk CN, Ames TR, Geor RJ, editors: *The horse, diseases and clinical management*, Philadelphia, 1995, WB Saunders.
4. Laverty S, Pascoe JR, Ling GV, et al: Urolithiasis in 68 horses, *Vet Surg* 21:56, 1992.
5. DeBowes RM, Nyrop KA, Boulton CH: Cystic calculi in the horse, *Compend Contin Educ Pract Vet* 6:S268, 1984.
6. DiBartola Chew: DJ: Canine urolithiasis, *Compend Contin Educ Pract Vet* 3:226, 1981.
7. Sutor DJ, Wooley SE, Illingsworth JJ: A geographical and historical survey of the composition of urinary stones, *Br J Urol* 46:393, 1974.
8. Wharrier J: Cystic calculus in the horse, *Vet Rec* 76:187, 1964:(letter).
9. Brenner BM, editor: *Brenner and Rector's the kidney*, ed 8, Philadelphia, 2008, WB Saunders.
10. Smith LH: The medical aspects of urolithiasis: an overview, *J Urol* 141:707, 1989.
11. Osborne CA, Polzin DJ, Abdullahi SU, et al: Struvite urolithiasis in animals and man: formation, detection, and dissolution, *Adv Vet Sci Comp Med* 29:1, 1985.
12. Senior DF, Finlayson B: Initiation and growth of uroliths, *Vet Clin North Am Small Anim Pract* 16:19, 1986.
13. Buffington CA, Blaisdell JL, Sako T: Effects of Tamm-Horsfall glycoprotein and albumin on struvite crystal growth in urine of cats, *Am J Vet Res* 55:965, 1994.
14. Hess B, Nakagawa Y, Parks JH, et al: Molecular abnormality of Tamm-Horsfall glycoprotein in calcium oxalate nephrolithiasis, *Am J Physiol* 260:F569, 1991.
15. See WA, Williams RD: Urothelial injury and clotting cascade activation: common denominators in particulate adherence to urothelial surfaces, *J Urol* 147:541, 1992.
16. Neumann RD, Ruby AL, Ling GV, et al: Ultrastructure and mineral composition of urinary calculi from horses, *Am J Vet Res* 55:1357, 1994.

17. Sutor DJ, Wooley SE: Animal calculi: an x-ray diffraction study of their crystalline composition, *Res Vet Sci* 11:299, 1970.
18. Grünberg W: Carbonate urinary calculi in herbivorous domestic animals, *Zentralbl Veterinarmed A* 18:767, 1971.
19. Mair TS, Osborn RS: The crystalline composition of normal equine urine deposits, *Equine Vet J* 22:364, 1990.
20. Mair TS: Crystalline composition of equine urinary calculi, *Res Vet Sci* 40:288, 1986.
21. Osborne CA, Sanna JJ, Unger LK, et al: Analyzing the mineral composition of uroliths from dogs, cats, horses, cattle, sheep, goats, and pigs, *Vet Med* 84:750, 1989.
22. Ruby AL, Ling GV: Bacterial culture of uroliths: techniques and interpretation of results, *Vet Clin North Am Small Anim Pract* 16:325, 1986.
23. Boyd WL, Bishop LM: Pyelonephritis of cattle and horses, *J Am Vet Med Assoc* 90:154, 1937.
24. Held JP, Wright B, Henton JE: Pyelonephritis associated with renal failure in a horse, *J Am Vet Med Assoc* 189:688, 1986.
25. Hillyer MH, Mair TS, Lucke VM: Bilateral renal calculi in an adult horse, *Equine Vet Educ* 2:117, 1990.
26. Laing JA, Raisis AL, Rawlinson RJ, et al: Chronic renal failure and urolithiasis in a 2-year-old colt, *Aust Vet J* 69:199, 1992.
27. Ehnen SJ, Divers TJ, Gillette D, et al: Obstructive nephrolithiasis and ureterolithiasis associated with chronic renal failure in horses: eight cases (1981-1987), *J Am Vet Med Assoc* 197(249), 1990.
28. Holt PE, Pearson H: Urolithiasis in the horse: a review of 13 cases, *Equine Vet J* 16:31, 1984.
29. Jackson OE: Renal calculi in a horse, *Vet Rec* 91:7, 1972.
30. MacHarg MA, Foerner JJ, Phillips TN, et al: Two methods for the treatment of ureterolithiasis in a mare, *Vet Surg* 13:95, 1984.
31. Hope WD, Wilson JH, Hager DA, et al: Chronic renal failure associated with bilateral nephroliths and ureteroliths in a two-year-old Thoroughbred colt, *Equine Vet J* 21:228, 1989.
32. Juzwiak JS, Bain FT, Slone DE, et al: Unilateral nephrectomy for treatment of chronic hematuria due to nephrolithiasis in a colt, *Can Vet J* 29:931, 1988.
33. Byars TD, Simpson JS, Divers TJ, et al: Percutaneous nephrostomy in short-term management of ureterolithiasis and renal dysfunction in a filly, *J Am Vet Med Assoc* 195:499, 1989.
34. Rodger LD, Carlson GP, Moran ME, et al: Resolution of a left ureteral stone using electrohydraulic lithotripsy in a Thoroughbred colt, *J Vet Intern Med* 9:280, 1995.
35. Rantanen NW: Diseases of the kidney, *Vet Clin North Am Equine Pract* 2:89, 1986.
36. Kiper ML, Traub-Dargatz JL, Wrigley RH: Renal ultrasonography in horses, *Compend Contin Educ Pract Vet* 12:993, 1990.
37. Divers TJ: Chronic renal failure in horses, *Compend Contin Educ Pract Vet* 5:S310, 1983.
38. Divers TJ: Nephrolithiasis and ureterolithiasis in horses and their association with renal disease and failure, *Equine Vet J* 21:161, 1989:(editorial).
39. DeBowes RM: Surgical management of urolithiasis, *Vet Clin North Am Equine Pract* 4:461, 1988.
40. Auer JA, Stick JA, editors: *Equine surgery*, ed 3, St Louis, 2006, WB Saunders.
41. Donner GS, Ellison GW, Ackerman N, et al: Percutaneous nephrolithotomy in the dog: an experimental study, *Vet Surg* 16:411, 1987.
42. Mulley AG: Management of nephrolithiasis: new approaches to "surgical" kidney stones, *Annu Rev Med* 39:347, 1988.
43. MacHarg MA, Foerner JJ, Phillips TN, et al: Electrohydraulic lithotripsy for treatment of a cystic calculus in a mare, *Vet Surg* 14:325, 1985.
44. Eustace RA, Hunt JM: Electrohydraulic lithotripsy for treatment of cystic calculus in two geldings, *Equine Vet J* 20:221, 1988.
45. Senior DF: Electrohydraulic shock-wave lithotripsy in experimental canine struvite bladder stone disease, *Vet Surg* 13:143, 1984.
46. Snyder JR, Pascoe JR, Williams JW: Rectal prolapse and cystic calculus in a burro, *J Am Vet Med Assoc* 187:421, 1985.
47. Sullins KE, Traub-Dargatz JL: Endoscopic anatomy of the equine urinary tract, *Compend Contin Educ Pract Vet* 6:S663, 1984.
48. Traub-Dargatz JL, McKinnon AO: Adjunctive methods of examination of the urogenital tract, *Vet Clin North Am Equine Pract* 4:339, 1988.
49. Kendrick JW: Cystic calculi in a horse, *Cornell Vet* 40:187, 1950.
50. Usenik EA, Larson LL, Sauer F: Cystotomy and removal of a urolith in a Shetland mare, *J Am Vet Med Assoc* 128:453, 1956.
51. Menon MN, Lingam UM: Laparo-cystotomy in a horse, *Indian Vet J* 35:482, 1958.
52. Lowe JE: Suprapubic cystotomy in a gelding, *Cornell Vet* 50:510, 1960.
53. Furness TR: Cystic calculus in a three-year-old gelding, *Can Vet J* 1:221, 1960.
54. Wright JG, Neal PA: Laparo-cystotomy for urinary calculus in a gelding, *Vet Rec* 72:301, 1960.
55. Lowe JE: Surgical removal of equine uroliths via the laparocystotomy approach, *J Am Vet Med Assoc* 139:345, 1961.
56. Reed DG: Suprapubic cystotomy in a stallion, *Can J Comp Med Vet Sci* 28:95, 1964.
57. Williams KR: Laparo-cystotomy in a gelding, *Vet Rec* 76:83, 1964.
58. Williams PFB: Removal of an urinary calculus from a gelding, *N Z Vet J* 27:223, 1979.
59. Mair TS, McCaig J: Cystic calculus in a horse, *Equine Vet J* 15:173, 1983.
60. Belling TH: Equine laparocystotomy, *Vet Clin North Am Equine Pract* 5(1):16, 1983.
61. Kaneps AJ, Shires GMH, Watrous BJ: Cystic calculi in two horses, *J Am Vet Med Assoc* 187:737, 1985.
62. Johnson PJ, Crenshaw KL: The treatment of cystic and urethral calculi in a gelding, *Vet Med* 85:891, 1990.
63. Crabbe BG, Bohn AA, Grant BD: Equine urocystoliths, *Vet Clin North Am Equine Pract* 13(1):12, 1991.
64. van Dongen PL, Plenderleith RW: Equine urolithiasis: surgical treatment by Gökels pararectal cystotomy, *Equine Vet Educ* 6:186, 1994.
65. Mair TS, Holt PE: The aetiology and treatment of equine urolithiasis, *Equine Vet Educ* 6:189, 1994.
66. White NA, Moore JN, editors: *Current practice of equine surgery*, Philadelphia, 1990, JB Lippincott.
67. Röcken M, Stehle C, Mosel G, et al: Laparoscopic-assisted cystotomy for urolith removal in geldings, *Vet Surg* 35:394–397, 2006.
68. Sullins KE, Bertone JJ, Voss JL, et al: Treatment of hemospermia in stallions: a discussion of 18 cases, *Compend Contin Educ Pract Vet* 10:1396, 1988.
69. Dyke TM, Maclean AA: Urethral obstruction in a stallion with possible synchronous diaphragmatic flutter, *Vet Rec* 121:425, 1987.
70. Lowe JE: Long-term results of cystotomy for removal of uroliths from horses, *J Am Vet Med Assoc* 147:147, 1965.
71. Trotter GW, Bennett DG, Behm RJ: Urethral calculi in five horses, *Vet Surg* 10:159, 1981.
72. Firth EC: Urethral sphincterotomy for delivery of vesical calculus in the mare: a case report, *Equine Vet J* 8:99, 1976.
73. May KA, Pleasant RS, Howard RD, et al: Failure of holmium: yttrium-aluminum-garnet laser lithotripsy in two horses with calculi in the urinary bladder, *J Am Vet Med Assoc* 219: 957–961, 2001.

74. Crabbe BG, Grant BD: Complications secondary to a chronic urocystolith, *Vet Clin North Am Equine Pract* 13(3):8, 1991.
75. Wood T, Weckman TJ, Henry PA, et al: Equine urine pH: normal population distributions and methods of acidification, *Equine Vet J* 22:118, 1990.
76. Schryver HF, Hintz HF, Lowe JE: Calcium and phosphorous in the nutrition of the horse, *Cornell Vet* 64:493, 1974.
77. Cymbaluk NF: Water balance of horses fed various diets, *Vet Clin North Am Equine Pract* 11(1):19, 1989.
78. Schryver HF, Parker MT, Daniluk PD, et al: Salt consumption and the effect of salt on mineral metabolism in horses, *Cornell Vet* 77:122, 1987.
79. Hintz HF: Dietary cation-anion balance, *Vet Clin North Am Equine Pract* 13(10):6, 1991.
80. Wall DL, Topliff DR, Freeman DW, et al: Effects of dietary cation-anion balance on urinary mineral excretion in exercised horses, *J Equine Vet Sci* 12:168, 1992.
81. Cooper SR, Kline KH, Foreman JH, et al: Effects of dietary cation-anion balance on blood pH, acid-base parameters, serum and urine mineral levels, and parathyroid hormone (PTH) in weanling horses, *J Equine Vet Sci* 15:417, 1995.
82. Osborne CA, Polzin DJ, Kruger JM, et al: Medical dissolution of canine struvite urocystoliths, *Vet Clin North Am Small Anim Pract* 16:349, 1986.
83. Osborne CA, Lulich JP, Kruger JM, et al: Medical dissolution of feline struvite urocystoliths, *J Am Vet Med Assoc* 196:1053, 1990.
84. Remillard RL, Modransky PD, Welker FH, et al: Dietary management of cystic calculi in a horse, *J Equine Vet Sci* 12:359, 1992.
85. McCue PM, Brooks PA, Wilson WD: Urinary bladder rupture as a sequela to obstructive urethral calculi, *Vet Med* 84:912, 1989.
86. Gibson KT, Trotter GW, Gustafson SB: Conservative management of uroperitoneum in a gelding, *J Am Vet Med Assoc* 200:1692, 1992.
87. Holt PE, Mair TS: Ten cases of bladder paralysis associated with sabulous urolithiasis in horses, *Vet Rec* 127:108, 1990.
88. Hooper PT: Epizootic cystitis in horses, *Aust Vet J* 44:11, 1968.
89. Adams LG, Dollahite JW, Romane WM, et al: Cystitis and ataxia associated with sorghum ingestion, *J Am Vet Med Assoc* 155:518, 1969.
90. VanKempen KR: Sudan grass and sorghum poisoning of horses: a possible lathyrogenic disease, *J Am Vet Med Assoc* 156:629, 1970.
91. Pascoe JR, Pascoe RRR: Displacements, malpositions, and miscellaneous injuries of the mare's urogenital tract, *Vet Clin North Am Equine Pract* 4:439, 1988.
92. Donaldson RS: Eversion of the bladder in a mare, *Vet Rec* 92:409, 1973.
93. Haynes PF, McClure JR: Eversion of the urinary bladder: a sequel to third-degree perineal laceration in the mare, *Vet Surg* 9:66, 1980.
94. Alvarenga J, Oliveira CM: Correia da Silva LCL: Prolapse with eversion of the urinary bladder in a mare, *Vet Clin North Am Equine Pract* 17(8):8, 1995.
95. Jennings PB, editor: *The practice of large animal surgery*, vol. 2 Philadelphia, 1984, WB Saunders.
96. Noone JP: Scrotal herniation of the urinary bladder in the horse, *Ir Vet J* 20:11, 1966.
97. Wheat JD: Penile paralysis in stallions given propiopromazine, *J Am Vet Med Assoc* 148:405, 1966.
98. Yovich JV, Turner AS: Treatment of a postcastration urethral stricture by phallectomy in a gelding, *Compend Contin Educ Pract Vet* 8:S393, 1986.
99. Todhunter RJ, Parker JE: Surgical repair of urethral transection in a horse, *J Am Vet Med Assoc* 193:1085, 1988.
100. Gibbons WJ: Hematoma of penis, *Mod Vet Pract* 45:76, 1964.
101. Memon MA, McClure JJ, Usenik EA: Preputial hematoma in a stallion, *J Am Vet Med Assoc* 191:563, 1987.
102. Firth EC: Dissecting hematoma of corpus spongiosum and urinary bladder rupture in a stallion, *J Am Vet Med Assoc* 169:800, 1976.

Hematuria

1. Schumacher J, Schumacher J, Schmitz D: Macroscopic haematuria of horses, *Equine Vet Educ* 4:255, 2002.
2. Brenner BM, editor: *Brenner and Rector's the kidney*, ed 8, Philadelphia, 2008, WB Saunders.
3. Osborne CA, Stevens JB: *Handbook of canine and feline urinalysis*, St Louis, 1981, Ralston Purina Company.
4. Schott HC, Hodgson DR, Bayly WM: Haematuria, pigmenturia and proteinuria in exercising horses, *Equine Vet J* 27:67, 1995.
5. Fairley KF, Birch DF: Microscopic urinalysis in glomerulonephritis, *Kidney Int* 44(Suppl 42):S9, 1993.
6. Hitt ME: Hematuria of renal origin, *Compend Contin Educ Pract Vet* 8:14, 1986.
7. Pollock C, Pei-Ling L, Györy AZ, et al: Dysmorphisms of urinary red blood cells: value in diagnosis, *Kidney Int* 36:1045, 1989.
8. Jai-Trung L, Hiroyoshi W, Hiroshi M, et al: Mechanism of hematuria in glomerular disease: an electron microscopic study in a case of diffuse membranous glomerulonephritis, *Nephron* 35:68, 1983.
9. Gibbs DD, Lynn KL: Red cell volume distribution curves in the diagnosis of glomerular and non-glomerular hematuria, *Clin Nephrol* 33:143, 1990.
10. Janssens PMW: New markers for analyzing the cause of hematuria, *Kidney Int* 46(Suppl 47):S115, 1994.
11. Boyd WL, Bishop LM: Pyelonephritis of cattle and horses, *J Am Vet Med Assoc* 90:154, 1937.
12. Hooper PT: Epizootic cystitis in horses, *Aust Vet J* 44:11, 1968.
13. Johnson JK, Neely DP, Latterman SA: Hematuria caused by abdominal abscessation in a foal, *J Am Vet Med Assoc* 191:971, 1987.
14. Bernard WV, Williams D, Tuttle PA, et al: Hematuria and leptospiruria in a foal, *J Am Vet Med Assoc* 203:276, 1993.
15. Kisthardt KK, Schumacher J, Finn-Bodner ST, et al: Severe renal hemorrhage caused by pyelonephritis in 7 horses: clinical and ultrasonographic evaluation, *Can Vet J* 40:571, 1999.
16. DeBowes RM, Nyrop KA, Boulton CH: Cystic calculi in the horse, *Compend Contin Educ Pract Vet* 6:S268, 1984.
17. Laverty S, Pascoe JR, Ling GV, et al: Urolithiasis in 68 horses, *Vet Surg* 21:56, 1992.
18. Juzwiak JS, Bain FT, Slone DE, et al: Unilateral nephrectomy for treatment of chronic hematuria due to nephrolithiasis in a colt, *Can Vet J* 29:931, 1988.
19. Fischer AT, Spier S, Carlson GP, et al: Neoplasia of the urinary bladder as a cause of hematuria, *J Am Vet Med Assoc* 186:1294, 1985.
20. Owen RR, Haywood S, Kelly DF: Clinical course of renal adenocarcinoma associated with hypercupraemia in a horse, *Vet Rec* 119:291, 1986.
21. West HJ, Kelly DF, Ritchie HE: Renal carcinomatosis in a horse, *Equine Vet J* 19:548, 1987.
22. Patterson-Kane JC, Tramontin RR, Giles RC Jr, et al: Transitional cell carcinoma of the urinary bladder in a Thoroughbred, with intra-abdominal dissemination, *Vet Pathol* 37:692, 2000.
23. DiPiro JT, Talbert RL, Hayes PE, et al: *Pharmacotherapy: a pathophysiologic approach*, New York, 1989, Elsevier.
24. Gunson DE: Renal papillary necrosis in horses, *J Am Vet Med Assoc* 182:263, 1983.
25. Gunson DE, Soma LR: Renal papillary necrosis in horses after phenylbutazone and water deprivation, *Vet Pathol* 20:603, 1983.

26. Behm RJ, Berg IE: Hematuria caused by renal medullary crest necrosis in a horse, *Compend Contin Educ Pract Vet* 9:698, 1987.
27. Edwards JF, Carter GK: Severe renal pelvic necrosis and hematuria of Arabian horses associated with possible analgesic nephrosis, *Proceedings of the forty-second annual meeting of the American College of Veterinary Pathology*, 1991, p 45.
28. Helman RG, Edwards WC: Clinical features of blister beetle poisoning in equids: 70 cases (1983–1996), *J Am Vet Med Assoc* 211:1018–1021, 1997.
29. Lloyd KCK, Wheat JD, Ryan AM, et al: Ulceration in the proximal portion of the urethra as a cause of hematuria in horses: four cases (1978–1985), *J Am Vet Med Assoc* 194(1324), 1989.
30. Schumacher J, Varner DD, Schmitz DG, et al: Urethral defects in geldings with hematuria and stallions with hemospermia, *Vet Surg* 24:250, 1995.
31. Taintor J, Schumacher J, Schumacher J, et al: Comparison of pressure within the corpus spongiosum penis during urination between geldings and stallions, *Equine Vet J* 36:362–364, 2004.
32. Voss JL, Pickett BW: Diagnosis and treatment of haemospermia in the stallion, *J Reprod Fertil Suppl* 23:151, 1975.
33. Sullins KE, Bertone JJ, Voss JL, et al: Treatment of hemospermia in stallions: a discussion of 18 cases, *Compend Contin Educ Pract Vet* 10:1396, 1988.
34. Mair TS, Walmsley JP, Phillips TJ: Surgical treatment of 45 horses affected by squamous cell carcinoma of the penis and prepuce, *Equine Vet J* 32:406, 2000.
35. Schott HC, Hines MT: Severe urinary tract hemorrhage in two horses, *J Am Vet Med Assoc* 204:1320, 1994:letter.
36. Schott HC: Idiopathic renal hematuria. In *Proceedings of the eighteenth annual forum of the American College of Veterinary Internal Medicine*, Seattle, 2000, p 190.
37. Latimer FG, Magnus R, Duncan RB: Arterioureteral fistula in a colt, *Equine Vet J* 23:483, 1991.
38. Schott HC, Barbee DD, Hines MT, et al: Renal arteriovenous malformation in a Quarter Horse foal, *J Vet Intern Med* 10:204, 1996.
39. Pardo V, Berian MG, Levi DF, et al: Benign primary hematuria: clinicopathologic study of 65 patients, *Am J Med* 67:817, 1979.
40. Lano MD, Wagoner RD, Leary FJ: Unilateral essential hematuria, *Mayo Clin Proc* 54:88, 1979.
41. Aber GM, Higgins PM: The natural history and management of the loin pain/hematuria syndrome, *Br J Urol* 54:613, 1982.
42. Hughes JH, Stanisic TH, Buster D, et al: Massive nontraumatic hematuria: a challenging demand demanding immediate action, *Postgrad Med J* 67:97, 1990.
43. Stone EA, DeNovo RC, Rawlings CA: Massive hematuria of nontraumatic renal origin in dogs, *J Am Vet Med Assoc* 183:868, 1983.
44. Holt PE, Lucke VM, Pearson H: Idiopathic renal hemorrhage in the dog, *J Small Anim Pract* 28:253, 1987.
45. Kaufman AC, Barsanti JA, Selcer BA: Benign essential hematuria in dogs, *Compend Contin Educ Pract Vet* 16:1317, 1994.
46. Roberts MC, Kelly WR: Renal dysfunction in a case of purpura haemorrhagica in a horse, *Vet Rec* 110:144, 1982.
47. Morris CF, Robertson JL, Mann PC, et al: Hemolytic uremic-like syndrome in two horses, *J Am Vet Med Assoc* 191:1453, 1987.
48. Dolente BA, Seco OM, Lewis ML: Streptococcal toxic shock in a horse, *J Am Vet Med Assoc* 217:64, 2000.
49. Abarbanel J, Benet AE, Lask D, et al: Sports hematuria, *J Urol* 143:887, 1990.
50. Traub-Dargatz JL, Brown CM, editors: *Equine endoscopy*, ed 2, St Louis, 1997, Mosby.
51. Corrigan JJ Jr, Boineau FG: Hemolytic-uremic syndrome, *Pediatr Rev* 22:365, 2001.
52. Sprayberry K, Madigan J, LeCouteur RA, et al: Renal failure, laminitis, and colitis following severe rhabdomyolysis in a draft horse-cross with polysaccharide storage myopathy, *Can Vet J* 39:500, 1998.
53. Blondheim SH, Margoliash E, Shafrir E: A simple test for myohemoglobinuria (myoglobinuria), *J Am Med Assoc* 167:453, 1958.

Polyuria and Polydipsia

1. Grauer GF: The differential diagnosis of polyuric-polydipsic diseases, *Compend Contin Educ Pract Vet* 3:1079, 1981.
2. Hughes D: Polyuria and polydipsia, *Compend Contin Educ Pract Vet* 14:1161, 1992.
3. Tasker JB: Fluid and electrolyte studies in the horse. III. Intake and output of water, sodium, and potassium in normal horses, *Cornell Vet* 56:649, 1967.
4. Fonnesbeck PV: Consumption and excretion of water by horses receiving all hay and hay-grain diets, *J Anim Sci* 27:1350, 1968.
5. Groenendyk S, English PB, Abetz I: External balance of water and electrolytes in the horse, *Equine Vet J* 20:189, 1988.
6. Sneddon JC, Colyn P: A practical system for measuring water intake in stabled horses, *J Equine Vet Sci* 11:141, 1991.
7. Rumbaugh GE, Carlson GP, Harrold D: Urinary production in the healthy horse and in horses deprived of feed and water, *Am J Vet Res* 43:735, 1982.
8. Morris DD, Divers TJ, Whitlock RH: Renal clearance and fractional excretion of electrolytes over a 24-hour period in horses, *Am J Vet Res* 45:2431, 1984.
9. Brobst DF, Bayly WM: Responses of horses to a water deprivation test, *J Equine Vet Sci* 2:51, 1982.
10. Kohn CW, Strasser SL: 24 Hour renal clearance and excretion of endogenous substances in the mare, *Am J Vet Res* 47:1332, 1986.
11. Cymbaluk NF: Water balance of horses fed various diets, *Vet Clin North Am Equine Pract* 11(1):19, 1989.
12. Prior RL, Hintz HF, Lowe JE, et al: Urea recycling and metabolism of ponies, *J Anim Sci* 38:565, 1974.
13. Carlson GP: Fluid and electrolyte dynamics in the horse, *Proc Annu Vet Med Forum Am Coll Vet Intern Med* 5:7–29, 1987.
14. Martin RG, McMeniman NP, Dowsett KF: Milk and water intakes of foals sucking grazing mares, *Equine Vet J* 24:295, 1992.
15. Brown CM, editor: *Problems in equine medicine*, Philadelphia, 1989, Lea & Febiger.
16. Vander Noot GW, Fonnesbeck PV: Lydman RK: Equine metabolism stall and collection harness, *J Anim Sci* 24:691, 1965.
17. Warwick IS: Urine collection apparatus for male horses, *J Sci Technol* 12:181, 1966.
18. Tasker JB: Fluid and electrolyte studies in the horse. II. An apparatus for the collection of total daily urine and faeces from horses, *Cornell Vet* 56:77, 1966.
19. Harris P: Collection of urine, *Equine Vet J* 20:86, 1988.
20. Robinson NE, editor: *Current therapy in equine medicine*, ed 6, St Louis, 2009, WB Saunders.
21. Koterba AM, Coffman JR: Acute and chronic renal disease in the horse, *Compend Contin Educ Pract Vet* 3:S461, 1981.
22. Tennant B, Kaneko JJ, Lowe JE, et al: Chronic renal failure in the horse, *Proc Am Assoc Equine Pract* 23:293, 1978.
23. Divers TJ: Chronic renal failure in horses, *Compend Contin Educ Pract Vet* 5:S310, 1983.
24. Boveáe KC, editor: *Canine nephrology*, Media, PA, 1984, Harwal.
25. Love S: Equine Cushing's disease, *Br Vet J* 149:139, 1993.
26. King JM, Kavanaugh JF, Bentinck-Smith J: Diabetes mellitus with pituitary neoplasms in a horse and a dog, *Cornell Vet* 52:133, 1962.

27. Loeb WF, Capen CC, Johnson LE: Adenomas of the pars intermedia associated with hyperglycemia and glycosuria in two horses, *Cornell Vet* 56:623, 1966.
28. Green EM, Hunt EL: Hypophyseal neoplasia in a pony, *Compend Contin Educ Pract Vet* 7:S249, 1985.
29. Horvath CJ, Ames TR, Metz AL, et al: Adrenocorticotropin-containing neoplastic cells in a pars intermedia adenoma in a horse, *J Am Vet Med Assoc* 192:367, 1988.
30. Staempfli HR, Eigenmann EJ, Clarke LM: Insulin treatment and development of anti-insulin antibodies in a horse with diabetes mellitus associated with a functional pituitary adenoma, *Can Vet J* 29:934, 1988.
31. van der Kolk JH, Kalsbeek HC, van Garderen E, et al: Equine pituitary neoplasia: a clinical report of 21 cases (1990–1992), *Vet Rec* 133(594), 1993.
32. Hillyer MH, Taylor FGR, Mair TS: Diagnosis of hyperadrenocorticism in the horse, *Equine Vet Educ* 4:131, 1992.
33. Link RP: Glucose tolerance in horses, *J Am Vet Med Assoc* 97:261, 1940.
34. Brenner BM, editor: *Brenner and Rector's the kidney*, ed 8, Philadelphia, 2008, WB Saunders.
35. Buntain BJ, Coffman JR: Polyuria and polydipsia in a horse induced by psychogenic salt consumption, *Equine Vet J* 13:266, 1981.
36. Schryver HF, Parker MT, Daniluk PD, et al: Salt consumption and the effect of salt on mineral metabolism in horses, *Cornell Vet* 77:122, 1987.
37. Coggins CH, Leaf A: Diabetes insipidus, *Am J Med* 42:806, 1967.
38. Robertson GL: Differential diagnosis of polyuria, *Annu Rev Med* 39:425, 1988.
39. Breukink HJ, Van Wegen P, Schotman AJH: Idiopathic diabetes insipidus in a Welsh pony, *Equine Vet J* 15:284, 1983.
40. Filar J, Ziolo T, Szalecki J: Diabetes insipidus in the course of encephalitis in the horse, *Med Weter* 27:205, 1971.
41. Chenault L: Diabetes insipidus in the equine, *Southwest Vet* 22:321, 1969.
42. Satish C, Sastry KNV: Equine diabetes insipidus: a case report, *Indian Vet J* 55:584, 1978.
43. Forssman H: Two different mutations of the X-chromosome causing diabetes insipidus, *Am J Hum Genet* 7:21, 1955.
44. Schott HC, Bayly WM, Reed SM, et al: Nephrogenic diabetes insipidus in sibling colts, *J Vet Intern Med* 7:68, 1993.
45. Brashier M: Polydipsia and polyuria in a weanling colt caused by nephrogenic diabetes insipidus, *Vet Clin North Am Equine Pract* 22:219–227, 2006.
46. Houpt KA, Thorton SN, Allen WR: Vasopressin in dehydrated and rehydrated ponies, *Physiol Behav* 45:659, 1989.
47. Irvine CHG, Alexander SL, Donald RA: Effect of an osmotic stimulus on the secretion of arginine vasopressin and adrenocorticotropin in the horse, *Endocrinology* 124:3102, 1989.
48. Sneddon JC, van der Walt J, Mitchell G, et al: Effects of dehydration and rehydration on plasma vasopressin and aldosterone in horses, *Physiol Behav* 54:223, 1993.
49. Nyman S, Hydbring E, Dahlborn K: Is vasopressin a "stress hormone" in the horse?, *Pferdeheilkunde* 12:419, 1996.
50. Bertone JJ, Horspool LJ, editors: *Equine clinical pharmacology*, Philadelphia, 2004, WB Saunders.
51. Greene CE, Wong P, Finco DR: Diagnosis and treatment of diabetes insipidus in two dogs using two synthetic analogs of antidiuretic hormone, *J Am Anim Hosp Assoc* 15:371, 1979.
52. Plumb DC: *Plumb's veterinary drug handbook*, ed 6, Ames, IA, 2008, Blackwell.
53. Kraus KH: The use of desmopressin in diagnosis and treatment of diabetes insipidus in cats, *Compend Contin Educ Pract Vet* 9:752, 1987.
54. Corke MJ: Diabetes mellitus: the tip of the iceberg, *Equine Vet J* 18:87, 1986:editorial.
55. Taylor FGR, Hillyer MH: The differential diagnosis of hyperglycemia in horses, *Equine Vet Educ* 4:135, 1992.
56. Muylle E, van den Hende C, DePrez P, et al: Non-insulin dependent diabetes mellitus in a horse, *Equine Vet J* 18:143, 1986.
57. Johnson PJ, Scotty NC, Weidmeyer C, et al: Diabetes mellitus in a domesticated Spanish Mustang, *J Am Vet Med Assoc* 226:584–588, 2005.
58. Siegel ET: Diabetes mellitus in a horse, *J Am Vet Med Assoc* 149:1016, 1966.
59. Jeffrey JR: Diabetes mellitus secondary to chronic pancreatitis in a pony, *J Am Vet Med Assoc* 153:1168, 1968.
60. Baker JR, Richie HE: Diabetes mellitus in the horse: a case report and review of the literature, *Equine Vet J* 6:7, 1974.
61. Ruoff WW, Baker DC, Morgan SJ, et al: Type II diabetes mellitus in a horse, *Equine Vet J* 18:143, 1986.
62. Traver DS, Moore JN, Coffman JR, et al: Peritonitis in a horse: a cause of acute abdominal distress and polyuria-polydipsia, *J Equine Med Surg* 1:36, 1977.
63. Kinter LB, Huffman WF, Stassen FL: Antagonists of the antidiuretic activity of vasopressin, *Am J Physiol* 254:F165, 1988.
64. Hardy RM, Osborne CA: Canine pyometra: pathophysiology, diagnosis and treatment of uterine and extra-uterine lesions, *J Am Anim Hosp Assoc* 10:245, 1974.
65. Thurmon JC, Steffey EP, Zinkl JG, et al: Xylazine causes transient dose-related hyperglycemia and increased urine volume in mares, *Am J Vet Res* 45:224, 1984.
66. Trim CM, Hanson RR: Effects of xylazine on renal function and plasma glucose in ponies, *Vet Rec* 118:65, 1986.
67. Gellai M: Modulation of vasopressin antidiuretic action by renal alpha 2-adrenoceptors, *Am J Physiol* 259:F1, 1990.

Renal Tubular Acidosis

1. Gennari FJ, Cohen JJ: Renal tubular acidosis, *Annu Rev Med* 29:521, 1978.
2. Fauci AS, Braunwald E, Kasper DL, et al: *Harrison's principles of internal medicine*, ed 17, New York, 2008, McGraw-Hill.
3. Maxwell MM, Kleeman DR, Narins RG, editors: *Clinical disorders of fluid and electrolyte metabolism*, ed 4, New York, 1987, McGraw-Hill.
4. Trotter GW, Miller D, Parks A, et al: Type II renal tubular acidosis in a mare, *J Am Vet Med Assoc* 188:1050, 1986.
5. Hansen TO: Renal tubular acidosis in a mare, *Compend Contin Educ Pract Vet* 8:864, 1986.
6. Ziemer EL, Parker HR, Carlson GP, et al: Renal tubular acidosis in two horses: diagnostic studies, *J Am Vet Med Assoc* 190:289, 1987.
7. Van der Kolk JH, Kalsbeek HC: Renal tubular acidosis in a mare, *Vet Rec* 133:44, 1993.
8. Van der Kolk JH, de Graaf-Roelfsema E, Joles JA, et al: Mixed proximal and distal renal tubular acidosis without aminoaciduria in a mare, *J Vet Intern Med* 21:1121–1125, 2007.
9. Gull T, Type: 1 renal tubular acidosis in a broodmare, *Vet Clin North Am Equine Pract* 22:29–237, 2006.
10. Stewart AJ: Secondary renal tubular acidosis in a quarter horse gelding, *Vet Clin North Am Equine Pract* 22:e47–e61, 2006.
11. Aleman MR, Kuesis B, Schott HC: Renal tubular acidosis in horses (1980–1999), *J Vet Intern Med* 15:136–143, 2001.
12. MacLeay JM, Wilson JH: Type-II renal tubular acidosis and ventricular tachycardia in a horse, *J Am Vet Med Assoc* 212:1597–1599, 1998.
13. Rose BD: *Clinical physiology of acid-base and electrolyte disorders*, ed 3, New York, 1989, McGraw-Hill.
14. Van den Berg CJ, Harrington TM, Bunch TW, et al: Treatment of renal lithiasis associated with renal tubular acidosis, *Proc Eur Dial Transplant Assoc* 20:473, 1983.
15. Battle D: Renal tubular acidosis: symposium on acid-base disorders, *Med Clin North Am* 67:859, 1983.
16. Frolich ED, editor: *Pathophysiology: altered regulatory mechanisms in disease*, Philadelphia, 1984, JB Lippincott.

17. Halperin ML, Richardson RMA, Bear R, et al: Urine ammonium: the key to the diagnosis of distal renal tubular acidosis, *Nephron* 50:1, 1988.
18. Goldstein MB, Bear R, Richardson RMA, et al: The urine anion gap: a clinically useful index of ammonium excretion, *Am J Med Sci* 292:198, 1986.
19. Rodriguez-Soriano J, Vallo A: Renal tubular acidosis, *Pediatr Nephrol* 4:268, 1990.
20. van Leeuwen AM: Net cation equivalency (base-binding power) of the plasma proteins, *Acta Med Scand* 176 (Suppl 422):36, 1964.

Neoplasia of the Urinary Tract

1. Robinson NE, editor: *Current therapy in equine medicine*, ed 6, St Louis, 2009, WB Saunders.
2. Smith BP, editor: *Large animal internal medicine*, ed 4, St Louis, 2009, Mosby.
3. Wintzer HJ, editor: *Equine diseases: a textbook for students and practitioners*, New York, 1986, Springer-Verlag.
4. Brown CM: Equine nephrology, *Vet Annu* 26:1, 1986.
5. Sundberg JP, Burnstein T, Page EH, et al: Neoplasms of equidae, *J Am Vet Med Assoc* 170:150, 1977.
6. Cotchin E: A general survey of tumors in the horse, *Equine Vet J* 9:16, 1977.
7. Theilen GH, Madewell BR, editors: *Veterinary cancer medicine*, ed 2, Philadelphia, 1987, Lea & Febiger.
8. Jubb KVF, Kennedy PC, Palmer N, editors: *Pathology of domestic animals*, ed 3, vol. 2, San Diego, 1985, Academic Press.
9. Berggren PC: Renal adenocarcinoma in a horse, *J Am Vet Med Assoc* 176:1252, 1980.
10. Haschek WM, King JM, Tennant BC: Primary renal cell carcinoma in two horses, *J Am Vet Med Assoc* 179:992, 1981.
11. Pomroy W: Renal adenocarcinoma in a horse, *Equine Vet J* 13:198, 1981.
12. Van Amstel SR, Huchzermeyer D, Reyers F: Primary renal cell carcinoma in a horse, *J S Afr Vet Assoc* 55:35, 1984.
13. Brown PJ, Holt PE: Primary renal cell carcinoma in four horses, *Equine Vet J* 17:473, 1985.
14. Van Mol KAC, Fransen JLA: Renal carcinoma in a horse, *Vet Rec* 119:238, 1986.
15. Owen RR, Haywood S, Kelly DF: Clinical course of renal adenocarcinoma associated with hypercupraemia in a horse, *Vet Rec* 119:291, 1986.
16. West HJ, Kelly DF, Ritchie HE: Renal carcinomatosis in a horse, *Equine Vet J* 19:548, 1987.
17. Swain JM, Pirie RS, Hudson NPH, et al: Insulin-like growth factors and recurrent hypoglycemia associated with renal cell carcinoma in a horse, *J Vet Intern Med* 19:613–616, 2005.
18. Baker JL, Aleman M, Madigan J: Intermittent hypoglycemia in a horse with anaplastic carcinoma of the kidney, *J Am Vet Med Assoc* 218:235–237, 2001.
19. Rumbaugh ML, Latimer FG, Porthouse KP, et al: Renal carcinoma with osseous and pulmonary metastases in an Arabian gelding, *Equine Vet J* 35:107–109, 2003.
20. Brenner BM, editor: *Brenner and Rector's the kidney*, ed 8, Philadelphia, 2008, WB Saunders.
21. Traub JL, Bayly WM, Reed SM, et al: Intraabdominal neoplasia as a cause of chronic weight loss in the horse, *Compend Contin Educ Pract Vet* 5:S526, 1983.
22. Robertson SA, Waterman AE, Lane JG, et al: An unusual cause of anaesthetic death in a horse, *Equine Vet J* 17:403, 1985.
23. Nyka W: Sur une tumeur renal du cheval issue du blastème meátaneáphrique, *Bull Cancer* 17:241, 1928.
24. Köhler H: Nephroblastom in der Niere eines Pferds, *Dtsch Tierarztl Wochenschr* 84:400, 1977.
25. Jardine JE, Nesbit JW: Triphasic nephroblastoma in a horse, *J Comp Pathol* 114:193, 1996.
26. Servantie J, Magnol JP, Regnier A, et al: Carcinoma of the renal pelvis with bony metaplasia in a horse, *Equine Vet J* 18:236, 1986.
27. Vivotec J: Carcinomas of the renal pelvis in slaughter animals, *J Comp Pathol* 87:129, 1977.
28. Matsuda K, Kousaka Y, Nagamine N, et al: Papillary renal adenoma of distal nephron differentiation in a horse, *J Vet Med Sci* 69:763–765, 2007.
29. Carrick JB, Morris DD, Harmon BG, et al: Hematuria and weight loss in a mare with pancreatic adenocarcinoma, *Cornell Vet* 82:91, 1992.
30. Kim DY, Cho DY, Snider TG III: Mucinous hyperplasia in the kidney and ureter of horse, *J Comp Pathol* 110:309, 1994.
31. Jones SL, Langer DL, Sterner-Kock A, et al: Renal dysplasia and benign ureteropelvic polyps associated with hydronephrosis in a foal, *J Am Vet Med Assoc* 204:1230, 1994.
32. Loynachan AT, Bryant UK, Williams NM: Renal mucus gland cystadenomas in a horse, *J Vet Diagn Invest* 20:520–522, 2008.
33. Fischer AT, Spier S, Carlson GP, et al: Neoplasia of the urinary bladder as a cause of hematuria, *J Am Vet Med Assoc* 186:1294, 1985.
34. Lloyd KCK, Wheat JD, Ryan AM, et al: Ulceration in the proximal portion of the urethra as a cause of hematuria in horses: four cases (1978–1985), *J Am Vet Med Assoc* 194(1324), 1989.
35. Sweeney RW, Hamir AN, Fisher RR: Lymphosarcoma with urinary bladder infiltration in a horse, *J Am Vet Med Assoc* 199:1177, 1991.
36. Hurcombe SDA, Slovis NM, Kohn CW, et al: Poorly differentiated leiomyosarcoma of the urogenital tract in a horse, *J Am Vet Med Assoc* 233:1908–1912, 2008.
37. Sertich PL, Hamir AN, Orsini P, et al: Paraurethral lipoma in a mare associated with frequent urination, *Equine Vet Educ* 2:121, 1990.
38. Sloet van Oldruitenborgh-Oosterbaan MM, Klabec HC: Ureteropyelonephritis in a Fresian mare, *Vet Rec* 122:609, 1988.
39. Walker DF, Vaughan JT: *Bovine and equine urogential surgery*, Philadelphia, 1980, Lea & Febiger.
40. Auer JA, Stick JA, editors: *Equine surgery*, ed 3, St Louis, 2006, WB Saunders.
41. McKinnon AO, Voss JL, editors: *Equine reproduction*, Philadelphia, 1993, Lea & Febiger.
42. Plaut A, Kohn-Speyer AC: The carcinogenic action of smegma, *Science* 105:656, 1947.
43. Moore AS, Beam SL, Rassnick KM, et al: Long-term control of mucocutaneous squamous cell carcinoma and metastasis in a horse using piroxicam, *Equine Vet J* 35:715-718, 2003.
44. Plumb DC: *Plumb's veterinary drug handbook*, ed 6, Ames, IA, 2008, Blackwell.
45. Markel MD, Wheat JD, Jones K: Genital neoplasms treated by en bloc resection and penile retroversion in horses: 10 cases (1977-1986), *J Am Vet Med Assoc* 192(396), 1988.
46. Theáon AP, Pascoe JR, Carlson GP, et al: Intratumoral chemotherapy with cisplatin in oily emulsion in horses, *J Am Vet Med Assoc* 202:261, 1993.
47. Theáon AP, Pascoe JR, Meagher DM: Perioperative intratumoral administration of cisplatin for treatment of cutaneous tumors in Equidae, *J Am Vet Med Assoc* 205:1170, 1994.
48. Fortier LA, MacHarg MA: Topical use of 5-fluorouracil for treatment of squamous cell carcinoma of the external genitalia of horses: 11 cases (1988-1992), *J Am Vet Med Assoc* 205:1183-1185, 1994.

Urinary Incontinence and Bladder Dysfunction

1. Khanna OMP: Disorders of micturition, *Urology* 8:316, 1976.
2. Labadia A, Rivera L, Costa G, et al: Influence of the autonomic nervous system in the horse urinary bladder, *Res Vet Sci* 44:282, 1988.

3. de Groat WC, Booth AM: Physiology of the urinary bladder and urethra, *Ann Intern Med* 92:312, 1980.
4. Brorasmussen F, Sorensen AH, Bredahl E, et al: The structure and function of the urinary bladder, *Urol Int* 19:280, 1965.
5. Learmonth JR: Contribution to neurophysiology of urinary bladder in man, *Brain* 54:147, 1930.
6. VanKampen KR: Sudan grass and sorghum poisoning of horses: a possible lathyrogenic disease, *J Am Vet Med Assoc* 156:629, 1970.
7. Adams LG, Dollahite JW, Romaine WM, et al: Cystitis and ataxia associated with sorghum ingestion by horses, *J Am Vet Med Assoc* 155:518, 1969.
8. Madison JB: Estrogen-responsive urinary incontinence in an aged pony mare, *Compend Contin Educ Pract Vet* 6:S390, 1984.
9. Hodgson DJ, Dumas S, Bolling DR, et al: Effect of estrogen on sensitivity of the rabbit bladder and urethra to phenylephrine, *Invest Urol* 16:67, 1978.
10. Starr I, Ferguson LK: Beta-methylcholine-urethane: its action in various normal and abnormal conditions, especially post-operative urinary retention, *Am J Med Sci* 200:372, 1940.
11. Clark ES, Semrad SD, Bichsel T, et al: Cystometrography and urethral pressure profiles in healthy horse and pony mares, *Am J Vet Res* 48:552, 1987.
12. Kay AD, Lavoie JP: Urethral pressure profilometry in mares, *J Am Vet Med Assoc* 191:212, 1987.
13. Finkbeiner AE: Is bethanechol chloride clinically effective in promoting bladder emptying? A literature review, *J Urol* 134:443, 1985.
14. Holt PE, Mair TS: 10 Cases of bladder paralysis associated with sabulous urolithiasis in horses, *Vet Rec* 127:108, 1990.
15. Rendle DI, Durham AE, Hughes KJ, et al: Long-term management of sabulous cystitis in five horses, *Vet Rec* 162:783-788, 2008.

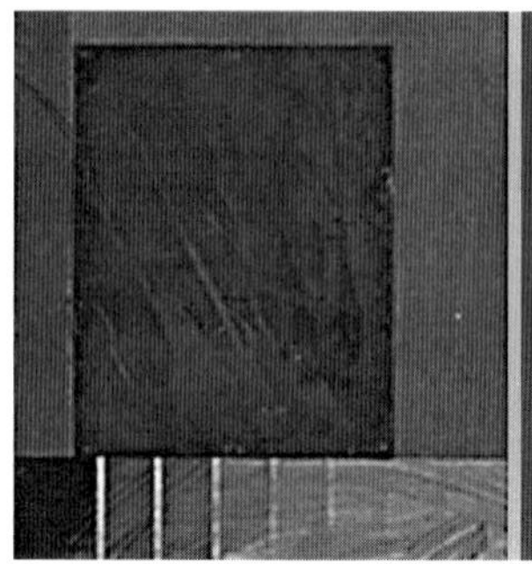

Disorders of the Endocrine System

CHAPTER
20

ADRENAL GLANDS

Ramiro E. Toribio

In horses, the adrenal glands lie retroperitoneally and embedded in the fat on the medial cranial pole of each kidney. They are red-brown, 7.0 to 8.0 × 3.0 to 3.5 cm, and weigh 15 to 20 g each. Blood supply to the adrenal gland is from the adrenal artery, which arises from either the aorta or the renal artery. Innervation involves sympathetic fibers from the splanchnic nerve. Accessory adrenal cortical tissue may be found in the adrenal gland capsule, periadrenal or perirenal adipose tissue, mesorchium, and in the vicinity of the equine testis.

The adrenal gland comprises two different organs, the *medulla* and the *adrenal cortex,* which differ in their embryologic origin, type of secretion, and function. The medulla is of neuroendocrine origin (neural crest), functionally related to the sympathetic nervous system, and secretes epinephrine and norepinephrine in response to sympathetic stimulation. The adrenal cortex derives from the mesoderm and secretes a different type of hormone, glucocorticoids, which are synthesized from cholesterol. The adrenal gland cortex consists of three zones: (1) the outermost zona glomerulosa, which secretes mineralocorticoids (aldosterone) in response to the renin-angiotensin system and changes in extracellular fluid osmolality; (2) the zona fasciculata, which secretes glucocorticoids (cortisol) in response to adrenocorticotropic hormone (ACTH, corticotrophin) stimulation; and (3) the zona reticularis, which secretes androgens.

Adrenocortical function (glucocorticoids) is controlled by the hypothalamus-pituitary-adrenal (HPA) axis. The hypothalamus secretes corticotrophin-releasing hormone (CRH) and arginine vasopressin (AVP) to stimulate pituitary ACTH secretion, which in turn stimulates the zona fasciculata to secrete cortisol. Subsequently, cortisol inhibits CRH and ACTH secretion as part of a negative-feedback control mechanism.

The adrenal gland cortex is involved in a wide variety of body functions, including maintenance of fluid and electrolyte balance, immunity, defense, and energy metabolism. Removal or destruction of the adrenal glands leads to death unless exogenous adrenocortical hormones are administered. Aldosterone increases renal sodium reabsorption and excretion of potassium. Hyperkalemia and increased activity of the renin-angiotensin system are the most important factors to stimulate aldosterone secretion. Hypernatremia decreases aldosterone secretion. Cortisol increases gluconeogenesis, causes mobilization of amino acids from extrahepatic tissues to enter the gluconeogenesis, decreases glucose use, increases glucose concentrations, and inhibits insulin actions on glucose uptake and lipogenesis. Cortisol increases fat and amino acid mobilization to make them available during stress. Endogenous glucocorticoids are anti-inflammatory and immunosupressors; increased cortisol concentrations result in eosinopenia and lymphopenia.

Unlike other species, maturation of the equine fetal adrenal glands occurs in late gestation and continues in the early postnatal period.[1] Diurnal variations in cortisol concentrations are noted in adult horses[2,3] and foals.[4]

ADRENAL INSUFFICIENCY

Adrenal insufficiency, also known as *adrenal exhaustion, hypoadrenocorticism, turnout,* or *steroid letdown syndrome,* is a poorly documented condition in horses. Horses with adrenal insufficiency have low cortisol concentrations and do not respond appropriately to the ACTH stimulation test. Adrenal insufficiency also occurs in critically ill horses (colic, enterocolitis, endotoxemia, sepsis) and septic foals because the adrenal gland is a shock organ, and adrenal hemorrhage, thrombosis, and cortical necrosis may lead to adrenal atrophy and dysfunction.

In adult horses, adrenal insufficiency is often associated with the discontinuation of glucocorticoids or anabolic steroid treatment.[5,6] The adrenal gland response to exogenous ACTH in Thoroughbred horses was not altered by training,[7] and low serum cortisol concentrations were not found in stressed racehorses with a history of poor performance.[8] High plasma cortisol and ACTH concentrations were found in horses after maximal exercise.[9-12] Endurance horses in a 160-km ride had significantly higher midride plasma cortisol concentrations than preride concentrations.[13] A sixfold increase in cortisol secretion rate and a threefold increase in plasma cortisol concentrations was also found in exercising horses.[14]

Horses are suspected of having adrenal insufficiency when they display a history of depression, anorexia, exercise intolerance, weight loss, poor hair coat, lameness, and serum electrolyte derangements. Therefore it is critical to obtain a complete history, including performance, previous diseases, drug administration, and stressing conditions.

Endogenous and exogenous glucocorticoids suppress the HPA axis and induce atrophy of the zona fasciculata. The zona glomerulosa is minimally affected, although electrolyte abnormalities may be present in some cases.

Clinical signs include depression, anorexia, exercise intolerance, weight loss, mild abdominal discomfort, poor hair coat, lameness, and seizures.[5,6,15,16] Serum biochemical analysis may be normal, or hyponatremia, hypochloremia, hyperkalemia, and hypoglycemia may be present.[5,6,15]

Some of the clinical features of equine hypoadrenocorticism (hyponatremia and hyperkalemia without evidence of renal disease) resemble Addison's disease in human beings and small animals; however, Addison's disease has not been documented in the horse.

Adrenal insufficiency is rarely diagnosed in equine practice; however, it should be suspected in any horse with a history of anorexia, lethargy, poor body condition, poor exercise performance, glucocorticoid administration, electrolyte imbalances (hyponatremia, hypochloremia, hyperkalemia), and hypoglycemia. Baseline cortisol and ACTH concentrations, as well as the ACTH stimulation test, are critical to achieve a diagnosis. Cortisol has daily fluctuations, and single measurements do not provide enough information to make a diagnosis of hypoadrenocorticism. Therefore the ACTH stimulation test is more useful in assessing adrenal gland function.[15,16] Horses with adrenal insufficiency have decreased cortisol concentrations and do not or minimally respond to the ACTH stimulation test.[15,17] In addition, measuring ACTH concentrations is important to determine other causes of hypoadrenocorticism (iatrogenic, adrenal, pituitary). It is anticipated that exogenous glucocorticoids decrease ACTH concentrations (secondary hypoadrenocorticism), whereas adrenal gland dysfunction (primary hypoadrenocorticism) is associated with increased ACTH concentrations from decreased endogenous glucocorticoid negative feedback. In horses with increased plasma ACTH concentrations, the clinician must rule out pars intermedia dysfunction.

To perform an ACTH stimulation test, one administers 1 IU/kg of natural ACTH gel intramuscularly between 8 and 10 AM.[17] Immediately before ACTH injection, a blood sample is obtained in heparinized or plain tubes. One obtains additional blood samples 2 and 4 hours after ACTH administration. Horses with a functional adrenal gland should have two- to threefold increases in plasma cortisol concentrations after ACTH stimulation as compared with baseline values.[6,17] To perform the cosyntropin stimulation test, one administers 100 IU (1 mg) of synthetic ACTH (cosyntropin; Cortrosyn) intravenously (IV) between 8 AM and noon.[18] One obtains a baseline, preinjection blood sample and a postinjection sample 2 hours later. As with the ACTH stimulation test, plasma cortisol concentrations should be at least twice baseline in the second sample. $ACTH_{1-24}$ (25 IU) can also increase cortisol concentrations to twice baseline in horses.[19]

Necropsy findings of horses with hypoadrenocorticism include adrenocortical hemorrhages and necrosis, as well as adrenal atrophy and fibrosis.

Treatment of hypoadrenocorticism involves rest and glucocorticoid supplementation. The duration and dosage of exogenous steroid treatment that induces adrenocortical atrophy in healthy horses is unknown. However, information on the doses that inhibit adrenocortical function in horses is available. Doses of dexamethasone as low as 4 mg suppress the HPA axis for up to 24 hours.[6] Dexamethasone dosages of 0.044 to 0.088 mg/kg every 5 days for six treatments reduced cortisol concentrations for up to 4 days but did not change the response to ACTH stimulation.[20] Toutain et al.[21] found that dexamethasone (50 µg/kg, IV or IM) suppressed adrenocortical function for up to 4 days, prednisolone sodium succinate (0.6 mg/kg, IV or IM) for less than 24 hours, and prednisolone acetate suspension (0.6 mg/kg, IM) for up to 21 days. Dexamethasone (0.044 mg/kg, IM) and triamcinolone (0.044 mg/kg, IM) produced HPA axis suppression for 7 and 14 days, respectively.[22] A single intra-articular dose of methylprednisolone acetate (200 mg) suppressed adrenocortical function for up to 10 days.[23] Based on this information, prednisolone sodium succinate (up to 300 mg daily) is the first choice to treat hypoadrenocorticism; low doses of dexamethasone are the second option (triamcinolone and prednisolone acetate must be avoided). Alternatively, oral prednisolone (200-400 mg/horse) can be used. A case of hypoadrenocorticism secondary to prolonged anabolic steroid administration was successfully treated with 300 mg of oral prednisone for 9 months.[5] Prednisone (40 mg, PO, b.i.d., or 50 mg, IV) was also used to treat a foal diagnosed with adrenal insufficiency.[15] The efficacy of prednisone as a therapeutic agent in horses is questionable because prednisone in poorly absorbed from the equine intestinal tract and the active metabolite, prednisolone, is rarely produced.[24] In contrast, oral prednisolone has excellent bioavailability and may be more useful as a therapeutic agent in horses. Like with any long-term glucocorticoid therapy, slow withdrawal is recommended.

ADRENAL INSUFFICIENCY IN CRITICALLY ILL FOALS

A substantial amount of information on the HPA axis of healthy and critically ill foals has been generated in recent years.[1,4,25-28] In foals, HPA axis dysfunction has been defined as an inappropriately low basal serum cortisol concentration (absolute adrenal insufficiency), an inadequate cortisol response to the ACTH stimulation test (low delta cortisol), and an abnormally high ACTH/cortisol ratio (relative adrenal insufficiency [RAI]).[4,25-27] For an accurate diagnosis of HPA dysfunction, results should be compared with values from healthy age-matched controls or to values generated in the same laboratory.

For many years it was proposed that adrenal insufficiency was a problem in premature and septic foals; however, not until recently was it demonstrated that dysfunction of the pituitary and adrenal glands is a frequent and serious problem in septic foals.[25-27] Hart et al.[26] found that 40% of septic foals had HPA axis dysfunction. Gold et al.[25] determined the ACTH/cortisol ratio in septic foals and found that RAI was common, with nonsurviving foals having the highest ratio. In a similar study, Hurcombe et al.[27] determined the AVP/ACTH and ACTH/cortisol ratios in septic foals and showed that HPA axis dysfunction at the pituitary and adrenal level was frequent in these foals. AVP is a major secretagogue for ACTH in the horse,[29] and a high AVP/ACTH ratio suggests a decreased ACTH response to AVP stimulation (pituitary insufficiency). Similarly, a high ACTH/cortisol ratio indicates decreased adrenal response to ACTH (RAI). The low cortisol concentrations observed in premature foals do not appear to be the result of ACTH insufficiency because high ACTH concentrations have been measured in these foals,[30] supporting adrenal insufficiency as a major problem in premature foals. A number of studies have found that septic foals with high baseline cortisol concentrations are more likely to die.[25-27]

To assess RAI in sick foals, a cosyntropin stimulation test was recently validated in healthy foals.[4] A baseline blood sample is obtained for cortisol analysis. One then administers 10 μg (low-dose protocol) or 100 μg (high-dose protocol) of IV cosyntropin, and additional blood samples are collected at 30, 60, 90, and 120 minutes. Blood samples for cortisol concentrations can be collected in heparinized tubes or in tubes with no additives. With the 10-μg test, cortisol should peak at a value twice baseline at 30 minutes; with the 100-μg test, cortisol should peak at 90 minutes at two to three times the baseline value. The time of the day did not affect the results of this test.[4] A simplified protocol would be to obtain a baseline blood sample, administer 100 μg of IV cosyntropin, and collect a second blood sample 90 minutes later. With this test it was found that a poor response to 100 μg of cosyntropin (0- and 90-minute samples) was associated with foal mortality.[26]

PHEOCHROMOCYTOMA

Pheochromocytomas are tumors that arise from the chromaffin cells of the adrenal medulla, which are part of the sympathochromaffin system (together with the sympathetic nervous system). During fetal life the chromaffin cells are associated with the sympathetic ganglia; after birth most of them degenerate, and the few remaining cells constitute the adrenal medulla. In human beings, approximately 90% of pheochromocytomas arise from the adrenal medulla, and often times are associated with a condition known as *multiple endocrine neoplasia* (MEN).[31] Extra-adrenal pheochromocytomas have been described in human beings but not in horses. In horses these tumors have a low incidence of malignancy and predominantly are unilateral.[32,33] Pheochromocytomas may be functional or nonfunctional. Functional pheochromocytomas secrete catecholamines at a rate sufficient to cause clinical signs.[33] Thus functional pheochromocytomas are diagnosed with more frequency than nonfunctional pheochromocytomas.[34] It is speculated that most equine pheochromocytomas are nonfunctional and go undiagnosed.[35] Both epinephrine and norepinephrine have been identified as the catecholamines produced by equine pheochromocytomas.[36]

Functional pheochromocytomas in horses have no breed or gender predilection[33] and have been described in horses older than 12 years.[34,37] Because clinical signs are of acute onset and of rapid progression from intense adrenergic stimulation, the clinical signs resemble those of colic, rhabdomyolysis, acute laminitis, enterocolitis, and hyperkalemic periodic paralysis. Clinical signs include abdominal pain from large hematomas or gastrointestinal distension secondary to ileus, anxiety, tachycardia, tachypnea, profuse sweating, muscle tremors, hyperthermia, dry and pale mucous membranes, increased capillary refill time, ataxia, and mydriasis.[33,34,37] Abortion has been documented. Clinical signs from nonfunctional pheochromocytomas in general are consistent with abdominal pain.[33,35,37]

Hematologic abnormalities of functional pheochromocytomas include hemoconcentration, stress leukogram (mature neutrophilia with lymphopenia),[37] and leukopenia with neutropenia.[34] Hemoconcentration likely results from epinephrine-induced splenic contraction rather than dehydration.[34,35,37] Epinephrine and epinephrine-induced steroid release may be responsible for the stress leukogram. Serum biochemical abnormalities are nonspecific and include azotemia, metabolic acidosis, hyperglycemia, hyponatremia, hyperkalemia, hypocalcemia, and hyperphosphatemia.[33,37] Hyperglycemia is likely a consequence of increased α- and ß-adrenergic activity.[31] Hyponatremia with hyperkalemia, hypocalcemia, and hyperphosphatemia suggests acute renal failure; however, renal function in most reported cases was normal.[34,35] Hyperkalemia, hypocalcemia, and hyperphosphatemia could be the result of prolonged muscle activity and ischemia.[33-35,37] Hyperkalemia is unlikely to be from increased catecholamine concentrations because catecholamines induce hypokalemia by shifting potassium to the intracellular compartment (ß-receptor mediated) and by increasing the activity of the renin-angiotensin system.[38] Glucosuria is also a frequent finding. Pheochromocytomas may secrete other hormones of neuroendocrine origin (calcitonin [CT], parathyroid hormone [PTH], ACTH, corticotropin-releasing hormone, somatostatin (SST), vasoactive intestinal peptide, leu-enkephalin);[34,39-41] however, this remains to be determined in horses.

The clinician should be aware that this condition carries a poor prognosis, and euthanasia may be a reasonable decision. Measurement of blood catecholamines or their metabolites in urine is valuable in establishing a diagnosis; however, this assessment can be a challenge, and most laboratories do not measure these hormones.[33,34,37,42] Ultrasonography and measurement of blood pressure (BP) can support the diagnosis.

If a diagnosis is reached, adrenalectomy can be attempted; however, the location of the adrenal glands, as well as the proximity of major blood vessels, tumor size, and arrhythmias (interaction between catecholamines and anesthetic agents),[35] make this a difficult decision.[33,35,37] Hypotensive α-adrenergic antagonists such as phentolamine, phenoxybenzamine hydrochloride, and prazosin hydrochloride are used in human beings with functional pheochromocytomas before surgery.

Functional pheochromocytomas in horses do not appear to metastasize, are unilateral, tend to bleed, and at necropsy the tumor is frequently found to be ruptured. Myocardial infarction and degeneration may be present, probably the result of increased concentrations of catecholamines.[33-35]

Malignant pheochromocytomas have been documented in young and old horses.[43,44] A malignant pheochromocytoma was reported in a 6-month-old filly with a history of hindlimb lameness and spinal cord disease.[44] Both adrenal glands had multiple and well-circumscribed yellow masses, and metastases were found in the liver, lungs, vertebral canal, left scapula, and azygous vein. A malignant pheochromocytoma was also diagnosed in a 22-year-old mare that died of massive intrauterine hemorrhage.[43] This mare also had a thyroid C cell medullary adenoma and bilateral nodular hyperplasia of the adrenal medulla, findings that were consistent with MEN. This was the first documented case of MEN in the horse, although previous reports have been consistent with MEN.[45]

HYPERADRENOCORTICISM

Hyperadrenocorticism from pituitary pars intermedia dysfunction (PPID; equine Cushing's disease) is discussed elsewhere in this text. Iatrogenic and adrenal hyperadrenocorticism are less common than pituitary-dependent hyperadrenocorticism (PDH) but have been described in horses.[46-48]

Iatrogenic hyperadrenocorticism was induced in a horse treated for a pruritic skin condition, after injecting 12 mg of triamcinolone acetonide followed by two injections of 200 mg of the same compound, all within 6 weeks.[46] Clinical signs included depression, polyuria-polydipsia, weight loss, and laminitis. Blood and urinalysis abnormalities (neutrophilia, lymphopenia, hyperglycemia, glucosuria) were similar to those of PPID. However, this horse also had increased serum activity of γ-glutamyltransferase (GGT), aspartate transaminase, and bile acid concentrations, indicating steroid-induced hepatopathy.

The diagnosis of iatrogenic hyperadrenocorticism is based on clinical history, low baseline ACTH and cortisol concentrations, and a low cortisol response to the ACTH stimulation test. Treatment consists of discontinuing exogenous steroids.

One case of pituitary-independent (adrenal dependent) hyperadrenocorticism has been documented in the literature.[48] In this case, a 12-year-old gelding displayed clinical signs of PDH. Baseline cortisol and ACTH concentrations were within the normal range, and the cortisol response to the ACTH stimulation test was normal. The horse was treated with bromocriptine with no improvement; over the next 11 months the clinical signs worsened. On necropsy, an adrenocortical adenoma associated with pituitary gland and contralateral adrenal gland atrophy was present.

ADRENOCORTICAL NEOPLASIA

Adrenocortical tumors are rare in horses,[19,48-50] and the few cases reported in the literature were nonfunctional tumors. One case of a 12-year-old Dutch Warmblood gelding with a functional adrenocortical adenoma and clinical signs consistent with Cushing's disease (hyperadrenocorticism) was recently reported.[48]

THYROID GLAND

Ramiro E. Toribio

The thyroid gland has two embryological origins: the *endoderm of the primitive larynx* that will give rise to the follicular cells that secrete thyroid hormones (THs) and the *ultimobranchial body of the fourth pharyngeal pouch* that contains neuroendocrine cells that will give rise to the C cells (parafollicular cells) that secrete CT.

In the horse, the thyroid glands are two discrete, firm lobes located in the dorsolateral aspect of the third to sixth tracheal rings.[1,2] The two lobes are connected by a narrow isthmus that contains fibrous tissue. In most healthy horses the thyroid glands are not visible but can be palpated as firm and movable structures. The weight of the thyroid glands relative to body weight is largest for fetuses and foals (mean, 0.28 g/kg; range, 0.12 to 0.67) and decreases with age; the ratio for adults is 0.08 g/kg (range, 0.01 to 0.15).[3] The normal total gland weight for newborn foals is around 15 g.[4] The glands are very vascular, receiving blood supply from two major arteries that arise from the external carotid and subclavian arteries. Thyroid gland blood supply is relatively greater (4 to 6 ml/min/g) than other highly vascular organs. Gland size does not parallel function, and functional tests must be used to establish an accurate diagnosis of thyroid dysfunction.

BOX 20-1

COMMON ABBREVIATIONS ASSOCIATED WITH THE THYROID GLAND

TH	Thyroid hormone
HPT axis	Hypothalamus-pituitary-thyroid axis
TSH	Thyroid-stimulating hormone
DA	Dopamine
SST	Somatostatin
NIS	Na^+/I^- symporter
MIT	Monoiodotyrosine
DIT	Diiodotyrosine
T_4	Thyroxine
T_3	Triiodothyronine
TBP	Thyroid-binding proteins
TBG	Thyroid-binding globulin
TBPA	Thyroid-binding prealbumin
NTIS	Nonthyroidal illness syndrome
MEN	Multiple endocrine neoplasia
TRH	Thyrotropin-releasing hormone

THYROID HORMONE FUNCTION

Understanding TH functions is important for the diagnosis and treatment of thyroidal and nonthyroidal diseases (Box 20-1). THs (triiodothyroidine-T_3, thyroxine-T_4) are important in cell growth, differentiation, and metabolism in nearly all tissues.

The synthesis and secretion of THs is regulated by a negative-feedback system that includes the hypothalamus, the pituitary gland, and the thyroid gland (hypothalamus-pituitary-thyroid [HPT] axis). TH synthesis and secretion is stimulated by thyroid-stimulating hormone (TSH, thyrotropin), which is a glycoprotein with two subunits (α and ß) secreted by the thyrotropes of the anterior pituitary gland. The α subunit of TSH is shared with other pituitary hormones (luteinizing hormone, follicle-stimulating hormone). TSH secretion is controlled by hypothalamic neurons that release a tripeptide, thyrotropin-releasing hormone (TRH).[5] TSH synthesis and secretion is also under the control of the negative feedback of THs.[6] The hypothalamus can also inhibit TSH secretion through dopamine (DA) and SST.[7] In the pituitary, T_3 decreases the TSH response to TRH stimulation, and in the hypothalamus, T_3 decreases the mRNA expression and secretion of TRH.[8-10] In the pituitary gland and central nervous system (CNS), a type II deiodinase converts T_4 to T_3. For T_4 to gain access to hypothalamic neurons it must be transported through the choroid plexus to the lateral ventricles bound to transthyretin (T_4-binding protein). In various species, including the horse, TRH induces prolactin release.[11-14]

Thyroid Hormone Metabolism

A major function of the thyroid gland is to actively trap and conserve iodine against a large concentration gradient.[1,7,15] Iodine can be absorbed in its soluble form, iodide (I^-), via the intestinal mucosa or any moist body surface or broken skin.[1] Iodide is actively transported and concentrated into the thyroid by a Na^+/ I^- symporter (NIS).[16] The trapped iodide is oxidized by a thyroid peroxidase and incorporated into the tyrosine residues of thyroglobulin to form the inactive precursors, monoiodotyrosine (MIT) and diiodotyrosine (DIT). Coupling of these precursors results in the synthesis of thyroxine (T_4) and triiodothyronine (T_3). The iodinated thyroglobulin containing MIT, DIT, T_3, and T_4 is stored as an extracellular polypeptide in the colloid of the thyroid follicles.[17] When needed, T_4 and T_3 are cleaved from the thyroglobulin, picked up by the follicular cells via endocytosis, and transported into the circulation.[1,7] Most of the TH released into circulation is T_4, because total serum T_4 concentrations are 20 times higher than serum T_3. Hormone synthesis and release are controlled by TSH and iodine availability. The feedback regulation of TSH secretion is closely related to the circulating concentrations of unbound (free) THs (fT_4 and fT_3).[1,7]

The circulating THs are T_4, T_3, and reverse T_3 (rT_3). Free T_4 and T_3 are the biologically active hormones. T_3 and rT_3 are both deiodination products of T_4. All of the circulating T_4 is directly derived from the thyroid gland, whereas only 10% to 20% of the circulating T_3 is directly secreted from the thyroid gland. The major pathway for the production of T_3 is the 5′-monodeiodination of T_4 by a type I deiodinase (a selenoprotein) in peripheral tissues. This is referred to as *T3 neogenesis*. In the fetus, type I deiodinase activity is delayed, so T_3 neogenesis is low, and most deiodinase activity results in high concentrations of rT_3. A switch in enzymatic activity near birth, partly the result of the influence of glucocorticoids, leads to high T_3 concentrations in newborns, including foals.[7,18-22] THs circulate bound to plasma proteins (thyroid-binding proteins [TBP]). Thyroxine-binding globulin (TBG) is the major protein (70% of T_4 and T_3 are bound to TBG); transthyretin (thyroid-binding prealbumin [TBPA]), and albumin bind to a lesser degree. In horses, the percentages of circulating T_4 bound to TBG, TBPA, and albumin is 61%, 22%, and 17%, respectively.[23] T_3 is bound to TBG and albumin but not to TBPA. Transthyretin is important to transport T_4 into the CNS. As THs are reversibly bound to transport proteins they act as TH reservoirs. T_4 has much greater protein-binding affinity and is considered a prohormone. Only free, unbound hormones cross the capillary endothelium to exert their biologic functions.[24] T_3 is much more potent than T_4, and it has a shorter half-life. The half-life of T_4 in horses is approximately 50 hours.[25] Because a large fraction of THs are bound to plasma proteins, changes in protein concentrations may change total TH concentrations.

The enzymes responsible for the production of T_3 and rT_3 are also responsible for their inactivation. Three classes of 5′-deiodoninases exist. *Type I deiodinase* is predominantly found in peripheral tissues such as thyroid, kidney, and liver, and is responsible for the conversion of most of T_4 to T_3 and rT_3, and is inhibited by propylthiouracil (PTU). Type I deiodinase activity is increased by TSH and T_3, and in hyperthyroidism, and it is decreased in hypothyroidism. *Type II deiodinase* is found in brown fat tissue, brain, and pituitary gland, is not affected by PTU,[7] and its primary function is to convert T_4 to T_3 in the intracellular compartment.[17] Type II deiodinase activity is increased in hypothyroidism, and is likely to sustain intracellular T_3 concentrations despite low peripheral T_4 concentrations, especially in the nervous system. *Type III deiodinase* is found in the placenta, developing brain, and skin, and its primary function is to inactivate T_4 and T_3 (converts T_4 to rT_3, inactivates T_3) to regulate T_3 availability during development. The generation of inactive rT_3 by type I and III deiodinases is essential in the regulation of TH function. Metabolites are excreted via the urine, and some are conjugated and enter the enterohepatic circulation. Most iodide is returned to the thyroid gland.

The thyroid gland is also the site of production of CT, secreted by the parafollicular cells (C cells). CT is involved in calcium homeostasis.[1,7,26]

Molecular Actions of Thyroid Hormones

The TH receptors belong to the superfamily of nuclear receptors that work as transcription factors. Two types of TH receptors exist (TR-α and TR-ß). T_3, directly transported into the cell or derived intercellularly from T_4, is the effector hormone. TH receptors interact with specific DNA sequences to regulate gene expression. Growth, thermogenesis, and energy metabolism depend on THs. T_3 stimulates thermogenesis, oxidative phosphorylation, oxygen consumption, protein synthesis, metabolic rate, carbohydrate absorption, glucose metabolism, lipid metabolism, lipoprotein lipase, lipolysis, and the conversion of cholesterol into bile salts. T_3 is also important for growth, maturation, and erythropoiesis, stimulation of heart rate, cardiac output, and blood flow, as well as critical for cerebral and neuronal development in young animals.[1,15] T_3 decreases the expression and synthesis of TSH and TRH.

FACTORS THAT AFFECT THYROID GLAND FUNCTION AND TESTING

Many endogenous and exogenous factors can affect thyroid function and test results. Being aware of these factors is important in the interpretation and establishment of an accurate diagnosis and treatment.

Age

Age-related differences exist in TH concentrations in horses. Late in gestation a powerful central drive exists to stimulate the HPT axis.[24] Serum concentrations of T_3 and T_4 in foals are very high at birth and decrease with age,[18-22,27,28] with most of the decline occurring in the first 3 to 4 months of life.[20,29] Total T_4, fT_4, total T_3, and fT_3 concentrations in the umbilical cord blood of newborn foals were found to be 14, 5, 7, and 3 times the adult concentrations, respectively.[24] At birth, plasma rT_3 declined rapidly as T_3 concentrations rose for the first 24 to 48 hours after birth.[24] Another study found that plasma T_3 concentrations decreased from 7.9 ng/ml at birth, to 0.9 ng/ml at 6 months, to 0.7 ng/ml at 9 months old.[22] Plasma T_3 concentration in mares was 0.5 ng/ml. In the same study, T_4 concentrations decreased from 233 ng/ml at birth to 49 ng/ml at 14 days and to 35 ng/ml at 6 months. Thus TH concentrations in newborn foals are ~10-fold higher than in adult horses, and TH concentrations in the range of adults may indicate a hypothyroid state.

Gender and Breed

A clear association does not exist between gender and TH concentrations. Various studies have found higher concentrations in male horses,[18,30,31] lower concentrations in stallions and geldings,[28,32] or lower concentrations in mares than in stallions,[30] whereas others have found no differences.[29,33-35] No evidence indicates that TH concentrations differ among breeds.[18,35]

Physiologic Status

Mares tested at all stages of the estrous cycle had no differences in TH concentrations.[34] T_4 concentrations, however, were lower after ovulation, which is the opposite pattern seen in other species. Higher TH concentrations have been reported in pregnant mares,[36] which is similar to other species.[7] This may be due in part to the increased TBG concentrations during gestation.[7] T_4 concentrations were statistically higher between days 49 and 55 of gestation as compared with mares in advanced pregnancy; however, T_3 did not vary with gestation.[37] Other studies found no differences between pregnant and nonpregnant mares.[25,32]

Hormones

Exogenous and endogenous glucocorticoids suppress pituitary TSH secretion, decrease the response of TSH to TRH, inhibit deiodination (except in the perinatal period where the conversion of T_4 to T_3 is enhanced), and decrease TH release.[7,38] Glucocorticoids decrease serum T_4 and T_3 concentrations, with the effect being more profound on T_3.[6] Dexamethasone administration to healthy horses for 5 days did not change total T_3 and total T_4 concentrations, but it increased serum rT_3 and fT_3 concentrations and blunted the fT_3 response to TSH stimulation.[39] Catecholamines enhance the rate of deiodination of T_4 to T_3, and have potentiating effects.[40] Estrogen enhances TBG production, whereas androgens tend to suppress it.[7] Oral administration of levothyroxine to healthy horses blunts the TSH and TH response to TRH stimulation.[41]

Season and Daily Rhythm

Cold temperatures stimulate and high temperatures inhibit the HPT axis.[25,42,43] A daily rhythm in TH concentrations has been identified in horses.[44,45] In geldings, T_4 peaked around 4 PM (2.4 ± 0.8 μg/dl), with the lowest T_4 values around 4 AM (1.8 ± 0.6 μg/dl). T_3 peaked between 8 AM and 4 PM (54 ± 13 ng/dl), with the lowest T_3 values around midnight (38.7 ± 10.8 ng/dl).[44] Higher T_4 concentrations between 5 and 8 PM, with lowest concentrations at 8 AM were reported in another study.[45] Diurnal variations in glucocorticoid concentrations appear to control the diurnal variations in TH by suppressing the pituitary response to TRH.[46]

Diseases: Nonthyroidal Illness Syndrome

Stress, illnesses, systemic inflammation, and starvation suppress the HPT axis. Because no clinical evidence indicates that low TH during disease is directly associated with hypothyroidism, this condition has been called the *low T3 syndrome* or the *euthyroid sick syndrome*. The designation *nonthyroidal illness syndrome* (*NTIS*) has been proposed because it does not presume the metabolic status of the patient.[47] In this syndrome, T_3 concentrations are decreased, whereas T_4 concentrations can be low, normal, or elevated. In critically ill human patients, a significant decrease in T_4 and T_3 or an increase in rT_3 concentrations is associated with increased mortality rate.[47] Low TH concentrations were found in premature and septic foals,[48] confirming that NTIS occurs in newborn foals. Low TH concentrations are a common finding in obese horses with insulin resistance (IR) (metabolic syndrome). Hypothalamic and pituitary dysfunction appears to be the proximal cause of NTIS,[47] because administration of TRH to patients with NTIS increases TSH, T_4, and T_3 release.[49] Although NTIS is a hypothyroid state, no evidence indicates that target tissues are chemically hypothyroid.[47]

Cytokines, glucocorticoids, and more recently, leptin are the key candidates in the pathogenesis of NTIS. Cytokines such as IL-1, IL-6, and TNF-α suppress TSH, T_4 and T_3 synthesis and secretion. IL-1 impairs TH synthesis, whereas IL-6 and TNF-α decrease T_4 and T_3 concentrations and increase rT_3 concentrations. Glucocorticoids are negative regulators of thyroid function; increased cortisol concentrations can be present in horses under different conditions, including stress, sepsis, obesity, IR, and pituitary gland dysfunction (Cushing's disease), and low TH concentrations can be measured in the same animals. The role of leptin in the pathogenesis of NTIS relates to caloric intake. A decline in energy intake decreases leptin concentrations, which reduces the hypothalamic synthesis of TRH.[50] No clear evidence indicates that TH replacement therapy in human beings or animals with NTIS is either beneficial or harmful. Some believe that replacement therapy may be harmful because exogenous TH may inhibit the HPT axis. The only clear indication for exogenous supplementation of THs in horses is to induce weight loss and enhance insulin sensitivity in obese animals, in particular those with metabolic syndrome.[51]

Activity

Several studies have found increased T_4 concentrations in horses in training.[19,52,53] Another investigator documented increases in T_4 within 30 minutes after exercise, with no differences in T_3.[33,36] Five minutes after a maximal speed race (1200 m), serum T_3 concentrations increased in Thoroughbred racehorses (from 55.6 ± 2.9 to 81.0 ± 3.7 ng/dl); however, T_4 concentrations did not change (0.67 ± 0.04 to 0.70 ± 0.05 μg/dl).[54] Significant increases in T_3 and T_4 concentrations were found 1 hour after swimming.[55]

Feeding

Feeding a high-energy and high-protein diet to weanlings stimulated TH secretion with a subsequent decrease 3 hours after each meal.[56] Soluble carbohydrates (glucose) rather than protein appear to be responsible for the TH increase in weanlings.[57] The conversion of T_4 to T_3 after a carbohydrate meal was associated with insulin release.[58] This response to carbohydrates is age dependent; by the time horses were 12 to 14 months old, feeding high-carbohydrate and protein diets had minimal effect on TH concentrations.[58] One study in ponies found greater T_3 concentrations when the animals were fed once a day rather than six times a day.[59]

Starvation in different species, including the horse, decreases T_3 and fT_3 concentrations.[47,60,61] Carbohydrate deprivation inhibits the deiodination of T_4 to T_3 (by the type I deiodinase) to decrease T_3 and increase rT_3 concentrations. Because starvation decreases the basal metabolic rate, the decrease in TH concentrations appears to be an adaptive process to conserve energy. In these animals, TSH concentrations are low or within the normal range despite low TH concentrations. When the effect of food deprivation on baseline TH concentrations was evaluated in euthyroid horses,[61] it was found that serum T_3, fT_3, and fT_4 concentrations decreased, whereas rT_3 concentrations increased after 1 day of food withdrawal. Serum T_3 concentrations were lowest after 2 days of deprivation, whereas T_4, fT_3, and fT_4 reached their lowest concentrations on day 4 of deprivation. Three days after the horses were placed on their normal ration, serum T_4 and fT_4 concentrations increased significantly, and rT_3 concentrations decreased.[61] Prolonged food restriction to Shetland ponies also decreased serum T_3 and fT_3 concentrations.[62] These studies provided valuable information in the interpretation of TH concentrations in anorectic and sick horses. If a decrease (>50%) in serum T_3 and T_4 concentrations can be present in 1 to 2 days of food deprivation, then the validity of measuring TH in diseased horses is questionable.

The mechanisms that regulate thyroid gland function during starvation remain unclear. The adipocyte-derived hormone leptin, which is the main regulator of hunger, is the critical neuroendocrine signal that regulates the HPT axis during fasting and disease.[63] Leptin concentrations decrease during starvation to increase appetite and conserve energy. Feed restriction decreases and excessive caloric intake increases leptin concentrations in horses,[64-66] with THs following similar patterns.[47,60,61] Even though information on leptin has been published in horses and foals,[64,67,68] its direct role on thyroid gland function is unknown.

Exogenous Compounds

Goitrogenic substances such as thiocyanate and perchlorate compete with iodide uptake. Iodide oxidation and coupling of iodotyrosines are inhibited by drugs such as sulfonamides, phenylbutazone, phenothiazines, thiouracils, thiopental, and methimazole. A recent study found no effect of trimethoprim-sulfadiazine on equine thyroid function.[69] Soybean meal, linseed meal, and plants of the Brassicaceae family. (i.e., rapeseed) contain goitrogenic substances.[1,15] Phenylbutazone administration decreases TH concentrations in horses,[45,70] and this effect can last up to 10 days after discontinuation of phenylbutazone administration.[70] The TSH stimulation test may be normal or exacerbated in horses receiving phenylbutazone.[45] High levels of nitrates in the water may induce thyroid gland hypertrophy,[71] because nitrates reduce the iodine transport into the thyroid gland.

PTU, in addition to affecting iodine metabolism, inhibits the peripheral conversion of T_4 to T_3. In human beings, aspirin competes for TH binding sites on transthyretin and TBG, decreasing T_4 and T_3, and increasing fT_4 and fT_3. This results in a hypermetabolic state from the increased free fractions of T_4 and T_3.[38] Anabolic steroids can decrease TBG concentrations[7]; however, short-term administration of anabolic steroids to horses did not affect thyroid function tests.[72] Exogenous compounds containing iodine or iodides are of particular interest. Iodine excess, as well as deficiency, can induce thyroid dysfunction and interfere with thyroid tests. Horses are exposed to iodine or iodide compounds in the form of feedstuffs, expectorants, leg paints, shampoos, injectable counterirritants, radiographic contrast media, and antiprotozoal drugs (iodochlorhydroxyquin). Animals can respond to excessive amounts of iodine by either suppressing or accelerating hormone production.

Iodine excess reduces iodine uptake and organification, decreases TH concentrations and the response to the TSH stimulation test, and inhibits the cleavage of T_4 and T_3; this phenomenon is known as the *Wolff-Chaikoff effect*. The end result of iodine excess may be hypothyroidism. The second way an animal can respond to large amounts of iodide is by elevating TH production. This is referred to as *Jod-Basedow phenomenon*, and in general it is seen in individuals with iodine deficiency.[7]

Newborn foals of mares grazing *Neotyphodium coenophialum*-infected fescue had lower T_3 concentrations than controls,[73] with no differences in T_4 and rT_3 concentrations. Endophyte alkaloids are dopaminergic D_2-receptor agonists, and DA is an inhibitor of TSH secretion. It is not clear whether the low TH concentrations in these foals is the direct effect of endophyte alkaloids on the fetal HPT axis or on placental and fetal development. Endophyte alkaloids do not appear to affect thyroid function in adult horses.[74]

DIAGNOSTIC TESTS

Unlike human practice in which a combination of functional and direct measurements of THs are often used, in equine medicine clinicians are far from assessing thyroid gland function in an organized manner. The traditional approach is to determine TH concentrations (compared with reference values) and make a diagnosis and specific recommendations, in many cases ignoring the underlying cause of abnormal TH concentrations. Normal TH concentrations have a wide range of values and vary among laboratories and measurement techniques (Tables 20-1 and 20-2). For consistent results the practitioner should use the same laboratory. Ratios of circulating hormones may be indicative of dysfunction.

Tests to assess thyroid gland function can be classified as *functional, causative,* and *anatomic*. Thyroid tests can be *direct* when serum TH concentrations or thyroid-regulating hormone concentrations are measured; they can be *indirect* when TH concentrations are calculated or when metabolites related to thyroid function are determined.

The T_4 secretion rate (TSR) is a functional test that calculates T_4 secretion after[83] iodide injection. This method is not clinically practical.[19]

Immunoassays are currently used to measure total T_4 and fT_4 concentrations. Equilibrium dialysis is the most accurate method to measure the free fractions of THs; however, it is being replaced by immunoassays. Several radioimmunoassays (RIAs) are validated for equine TH concentrations.[35,84] Quantification of T_4 and T_3 with RIA is not affected by hemolysis.[85] Enzyme-linked immunosorbent assays (ELISA) and immunoluminescence methods are also available. The unbound or free fractions of THs must be measured to determine available hormone to target tissues.[86]

Serum is the preferred sample to measure T_4 and T_3 concentrations, although heparin or EDTA plasma can be used. T_4 is stable in serum at 4° C for several weeks. The clinician should avoid using hemolyzed and lipemic samples, as well as samples from horses receiving "thyroid supplements" (a common practice).

TABLE 20-1

Thyroid Hormone Concentrations in Adult Horses

Investigators	Total T_4	Total T_3	fT_4	fT_3	TSH
McBride et al., 1985[43]	1.79 ± 0.17 μg/dl	62 ± 4.3 ng/dl			
Thomas and Adams, 1978[35]	1.57 ± 0.62 μg/dl (0.30-3.70 μg/dl)				
Anderson et al., 1988[31]	1.56 ± 0.081 μg/dl	67.7 ± 10.2 ng/dl	5.9 ± 0.39 pg/ml	3.22 ± 0.18 pg/ml	
Duckett et al., 1989[44]	2.13 ± 0.76 μg/dl	47.38 ± 13.66 ng			
Sojka et al., 1993[75]	6.2 to 25.1 ng/ml	0.21 to 0.80 ng/ml		0.07 to 0.47 ng/dl	
Breuhaus, 2002[76]	12.9 ± 5.6 nmol/L	0.99 ± 0.51 nmol/L	12.2 ± 3.5 pmol/L	2.07 ± 1.14 pmol/L	0.40 ± 0.29 ng/ml
Marcella, 1992[77]	2.57 ± 0.71 μg/dl	77.1 ± 45.75 ng/dl			
Wehr et al., 2002[78]	1.9 ± 0.4 μg/dl*	89.3 ± 26.2 ng/dl*			
Marcella, 1992[77]	0.25-3.70 μg/dl†	10.0-127.0 ng/dl†			
Frank et al., 2008[51]	1.7 ± 0.4 μg/dl	4.4 ± 1.6 ng/dl			
Rothschild et al., 2004[69]	1.1 ± 0.1 nmol/L			2.56 ± 0.35 pmol/L	
Johnson et al., 2003[79]	10.33 ± 6.92 nmol/L	0.92 ± 0.61 nmol/L			0.10 ± 0.06 ng/ml

*Ponies.
†Miniature horses.

TABLE 20-2

Thyroid Hormone Concentrations in Foals

Investigators	Age	Total T_4	Total T_3	fT_4	fT_3
Irvine and Evans, 1975[20]	1-10 hr	28.86 μg/dl	991 ng/dl	12.12 pg/ml	2.99 pg/ml
	4 day	11.2 μg/dl	935 ng/dl		
Murray and Luba, 1993[80]	4 day	231.7 ± 61.8 nmol/L	7.8 ± 4.2 nmol/L	1.2 ± 0.4 ng/dl	3.4 ± 1.1 pg/ml
	28 day	30.6 ± 17.4 nmol/L	3.1 ± 0.4 nmol/L		
Shaftoe et al., 1988[81]	1 day	4.4-25.1 μg/dl	26.0-732.7 ng/dl		
Chen and Riley, 1981[18]	1.5-4 mo	4.02-0.19μg/dl (2.9-5.25)	192.86 ± 8.54 ng/dl (135-270)		
Dudan et al., 1987[82]	5 min	29.3 μg/dl			
	48 hr	20.5 μg/dl			
Malinowski et al., 1996[22]	Birth	233.0 μg/dl	7.9 ng/ml		
	1	207.0 μg/dl	6.7 ng/ml		
	7	92.0 μg/dl	4.2 ng/ml		
	14	49.0 μg/dl	2.4 ng/ml		
	1 mo	26.0 μg/dl	1.6 ng/ml		
	6 mo	35.0 μg/dl	0.9 ng/ml		

Free THs circulate in blood in equilibrium with protein-bound THs, and changes in TBP (TBG, TBPA, albumin) can affect the total TH concentration. Immunoassays to determine human TBG concentrations are available but are not validated in horses.

In various species the ratio of circulating total T_4 to T_3 is 20:1. In horses, the T_4/T_3 ratio is 23:1 and the fT_4/fT_3 ratio is 1.83:1.[31] The concentrations of rT_3 are often increased in hyperthyroidism and NTIS.[7]

Commercial assays to determine TSH concentrations in human beings and dogs are available. The validity of human TSH assays to measure equine TSH is unknown; however, it is expected to be acceptable based on a 90% homology between human and equine TSH. Increased TSH concentrations are expected in hypothyroidism, and the opposite is expected in hyperthyroidism.[14,79] Equine TSH concentrations have been determined using customized assays.[48,68,69,76,79] Breuhaus[76] validated an equine-specific double-antibody TSH RIA in an equine model of hypothyroidism. In that study, hypothyroidism was induced in healthy horses by administering PTU for 6 weeks. Serum T_3 and fT_3 fell rapidly, whereas fT_4 and T_4 did not decrease until weeks 4 and 5, respectively.

TSH concentrations remained steady until week 5, increasing thereafter. The TSH response to TRH stimulation (1 and 5 mg) was exaggerated. Similar studies of PTU-induced primary hypothyroidism found a decrease in serum of T_3, T_4, and rT_3, as well as an increase in TSH concentrations.[14,79]

Increased cholesterol concentrations, hypothermia, bradycardia, and anemia are considered indirect indicators of hypothyroidism; however, they are not considered reliable.

Hormonal response tests are useful to differentiate primary from secondary thyroid dysfunction, and they remove the variability of endogenous and exogenous factors that could influence the results.

Thyroid-Stimulating Hormone Stimulation Test

The TSH stimulation test consists of injecting 2.5 to 5.0 IU of TSH, IV and comparing pre- and postinjection TH concentrations.[87,88] In normal horses, T_4 peaks 3 to 4 hours after injection at a concentration 2.4 times the preinjection value. T_3 doubles within 30 minutes and peaks at 2 hours at a concentration five times baseline.[89] Normal responses are characterized by a rise in T_3 that antedates the T_4. When 5 IU of TSH were given intramuscularly to horses, T_4 peaked at two times baseline value 3 to 12 hours after injection, and T_3 peaked in 1 to 3 hours.[45] No differences in T_4 concentrations were found between 2.5 and 5 IU of TSH.[87] The suggested protocol for the IV TSH response test is to measure TH concentrations at baseline and 3 to 4 hours after injection.[89] For the intramuscular protocol, hormone concentrations are measured at baseline and 3 and 6 hours after injection.[45] The protocol for 1-day-old foals is to measure T_3 concentrations at baseline and 1 and 3 hours after the IV injection of 5 IU of TSH. A normal response is a 50% increase by 3 hours. T_4 values after TSH stimulation are variable in foals.[81] An insufficient hormonal increase indicates primary hypothyroidism. The ability to perform a TSH stimulation test may be limited by the cost or availability of TSH.

Phenylbutazone decreases TH concentrations in horses, but it does not affect the response of the TSH stimulation test.[45] Dexamethasone blunts the TH response to the TSH stimulation test.[39] This information should be taken into account in the interpretation of the TSH stimulation test.[45,89] Treatment with DA agonists does not appear to affect serum T_3, T_4, rT_3, or TSH concentrations in horses.[79]

Thyrotropin-Releasing Hormone Stimulation Test

The TRH stimulation has become a widely used method to assess thyroid gland function and pituitary gland dysfunction in horses.[87,90-95] TRH is administered IV, 1 mg to horses and 0.5 mg to ponies and foals, with hormone measurements at baseline and 4 to 5 hours later. In a normal response both hormones should increase two- to threefold. An inadequate hormone response to TRH would occur in primary or secondary hypothyroidism. In normal animals, T_4 peaks at 4 hours[87,92] and T_3 at 2 hours after TRH administration.[92] Side effects of TRH administration include salivation, urination, defecation, vomiting, pupillary constriction, tachycardia, and tachypnea.[91] A low response to TRH administration suggests dysfunction at either the pituitary or the thyroid gland level. Additional tests (TSH concentrations, TSH stimulation test) may be necessary to differentiate thyroid from pituitary disease. Low TH and high TSH concentrations, and a low response to the TSH stimulation test suggest thyroid gland dysfunction. Low TH concentrations with low or normal TSH concentrations suggests hypothalamic or pituitary gland dysfunction. Low TH and TSH concentrations with a normal TSH and TH response to TRH stimulation indicates hypothalamic dysfunction. Levothyroxine administration blunts the response to the TRH stimulation test.[41]

Thyroid Suppression Test

TSH-independent secretion of THs can be demonstrated by the thyroid-suppression test. Exogenous administration of TH to suppress TSH secretion should also decrease TH secretion. The lack of TH suppression indicates primary hyperthyroidism. After T_3 administration, healthy horses are expected to have a decrease in T_4 concentrations, whereas no changes in T_4 concentrations are anticipated in hyperthyroid animals. This test was used to diagnose hyperthyroidism in a horse with a thyroid adenoma[96]; 2.5 mg of T_3 were administered intramuscularly, and serial sampling revealed no decrease in T_4 concentrations.

Imaging

Nuclear scintigraphy (technetium-99m) is useful in assessing equine thyroid gland function.[97]Abnormal uptake patterns have been seen with thyroid carcinoma in horses.[98-100] Ultrasonographic evaluation of the glands can differentiate solid structures from cystic ones.[7] Ultrasonography is the most commonly used imaging modality to assess equine thyroid gland morphology.[96,101]

Biopsy

Aspirate or biopsy sampling can help differentiate cysts, neoplasia, hyperplastic goiter, colloidal goiter, and inflammation.

HYPOTHYROIDISM

Hypothyroidism is defined as TH deficiency, a deficient thyroid activity, or disruption of the HPT axis. Hypothyroidism occurs from diseases that affect thyroid gland function, exogenous compounds that interfere with TH synthesis, and less frequent by disorders of the hypothalamus or pituitary gland. The liver, muscle, skeleton, kidney, heart, salivary glands, pancreas, and CNS during development are target organs for THs.[7] Hypothyroidism manifests in many ways, and the diagnosis can be a challenge because many nonthyroidal factors can lead to misinterpretation of the results. Hypothyroidism can be classified as *primary, secondary*, or *tertiary*. Primary hypothyroidism can be caused by iodine deficiency (endemic goiter) or excess (Wolff-Chaikoff effect), thyroiditis, neoplasia, biochemical defects, thyroid agenesis, or ingestion of goitrogenic compounds that block hormone synthesis. Of these, iodine excess, iodine deficiency, and neoplasia have been reported as causes of equine hypothyroidism. Histological lesions consistent with Hashimoto thyroiditis were recently described in horses.[102]

Horses with primary hypothyroidism have decreased T_4 and T_3 concentrations and increased TSH concentrations.[76] Secondary (central) hypothyroidism occurs from pituitary or hypothalamic dysfunction. Reports exist of low

TH concentrations in horses with pituitary adenoma.[90,103,104] *Tertiary hypothyroidism* denotes a defect in TH use, but it has not been reported in horses.

Hypothyroidism in Foals

The consequences of inadequate circulating TH can be devastating for the developing fetus and newborn foal. Chances for recovery are unlikely once critical developmental stages are passed. Tests to evaluate thyroid gland function may be within normal limits at the time of examination, making it difficult to confirm a previous transient or in utero TH deficiency.[24] The equine placenta is permeable to iodine, but impermeable to T_3 and T_4, and excessive ingestion of iodine may result in hyperplastic goiter (Figure 20-1, *A* and *B*).

SIGNS

Because decreased iodine intake is considered the main cause of neonatal hypothyroidism and goiter, pituitary gland function in these foals may be normal or increased. The lack of pituitary inhibition from low TH concentrations leads to excessive TSH secretion, thyroid follicular cell hyperplasia, and thyroid enlargement (goiter). The clinical signs reported in hypothyroid foals relate to the crucial role of THs in development and maturation of the nervous, respiratory, and musculoskeletal systems during the pre- and postnatal periods. Hypothyroid foals are often affected at birth. Clinical signs reported in hypothyroid foals include stillbirths, prematurity, weakness, and long hair coat[4,105]; weak suckle reflex[106]; respiratory insufficiency and distress[107,108]; incoordination[20]; lethargy, depression, and rough coat[109]; cold intolerance and hypothermia[24]; physeal dysgenesis[110]; defective ossification with tarsal bone collapse[110,111]; hypoplastic carpal bones, common digital extensor tendon rupture, forelimb contracture, and mandibular prognathism[112,113]; delayed incisor eruption, growth retardation, and death.[114] Foals can be born apparently normal but may develop skeletal lesions weeks later.[109]

CAUSE

The major cause of hypothyroidism in foals is nutritional. Congenital thyroid enlargement (congenital goiter) with decreased thyroid function is associated with both inadequate and excessive iodine intake by the mare. Several reports exist of goiter and hypothyroidism in foals associated with ingestion of excessive amounts of iodine in kelp-supplemented rations.[4,105,115-117] The dams of these foals may or may not be affected. Feeding 40 mg or more of iodine daily can produce this syndrome.[106]

DIAGNOSIS

Foals that exhibit any of the signs mentioned previously, with or without enlarged glands, are suspects. The mare and her nutrition should be examined. Because thyroid gland enlargement does not automatically imply hypo- or hyperthyroidism, functional tests (TSH and TRH stimulation tests) to confirm a diagnosis should be considered. When assessing TH concentrations in sick foals it is critical to compare results to age-matched healthy foals. Also crucial is to remember that high TH concentrations are normal in healthy foals (see Table 20-2). Premature and septic foals may have lower TH concentrations than controls, which does not necessarily mean hypothyroidism. Serum rT_3 concentrations in premature and septic foals may be lower than in term foals.[48,82] A foal with

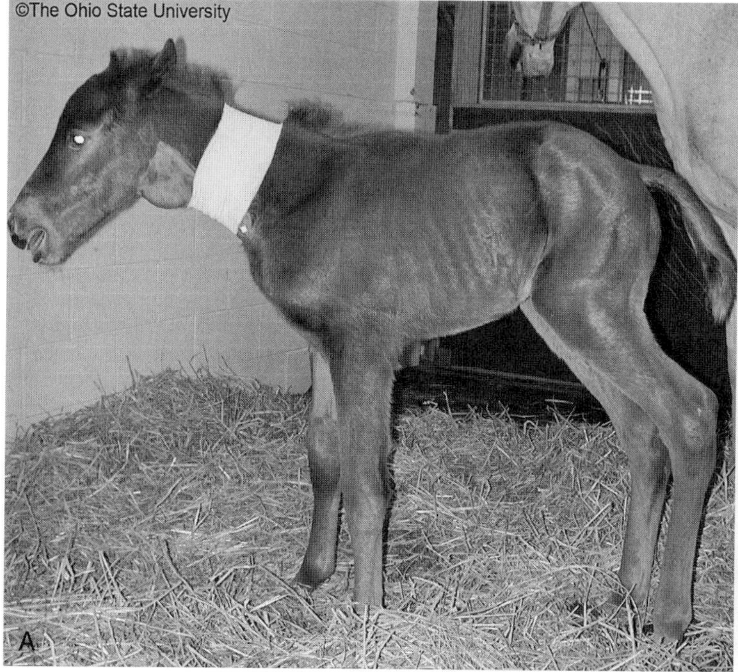

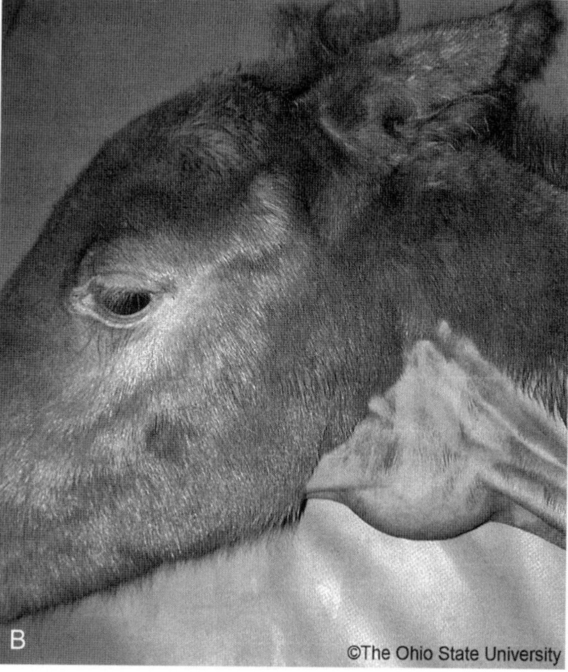

FIGURE 20-1 A, Newborn foal with respiratory distress and thyroid gland enlargement (congenital goiter). **B,** Thyroid hormone concentrations were normal but biopsy of the thyroid gland revealed follicular hyperplasia. (Courtesy The Ohio State University)

clinical evidence of hypothyroidism could have normal TH concentrations, suggesting that TH deficiency occurred during development. Hypothyroidism in foals carries a poor prognosis, even after thyroid supplement therapy.

Congenital Hypothyroidism and Dysmaturity Syndrome in Foals

A syndrome characterized by thyroid gland hyperplasia and multiple congenital musculoskeletal deformities has been described in neonatal foals in Western Canada and Northwestern region of the United States.[29,108,112,118-121] In some outbreaks, this disorder is reported to affect 30% to 100% of the newborn foals,[121] with no sex or breed predilection.[119] Abnormal musculoskeletal findings include prognathia, osteochondrosis and inappropriate ossification of carpal and tarsal bones, angular limb deformities, and rupture of the common digital extensor tendons (Figure 20-2, *A* to *C*).[121] These foals have signs of dysmaturity including a silky and short hair coat, floppy ears, tendon laxity, and incomplete closure of the abdominal wall.[121] Thyroid gland hyperplasia is associated with hypothyroidism.[120] This syndrome is referred to as *congenital hypothyroidism and dysmaturity* (CHD). The cause of this condition remains unknown. A case-control study found that foals with CHD had a longer gestation time and that mares grazing irrigated pastures, fed greenfeed, not receiving

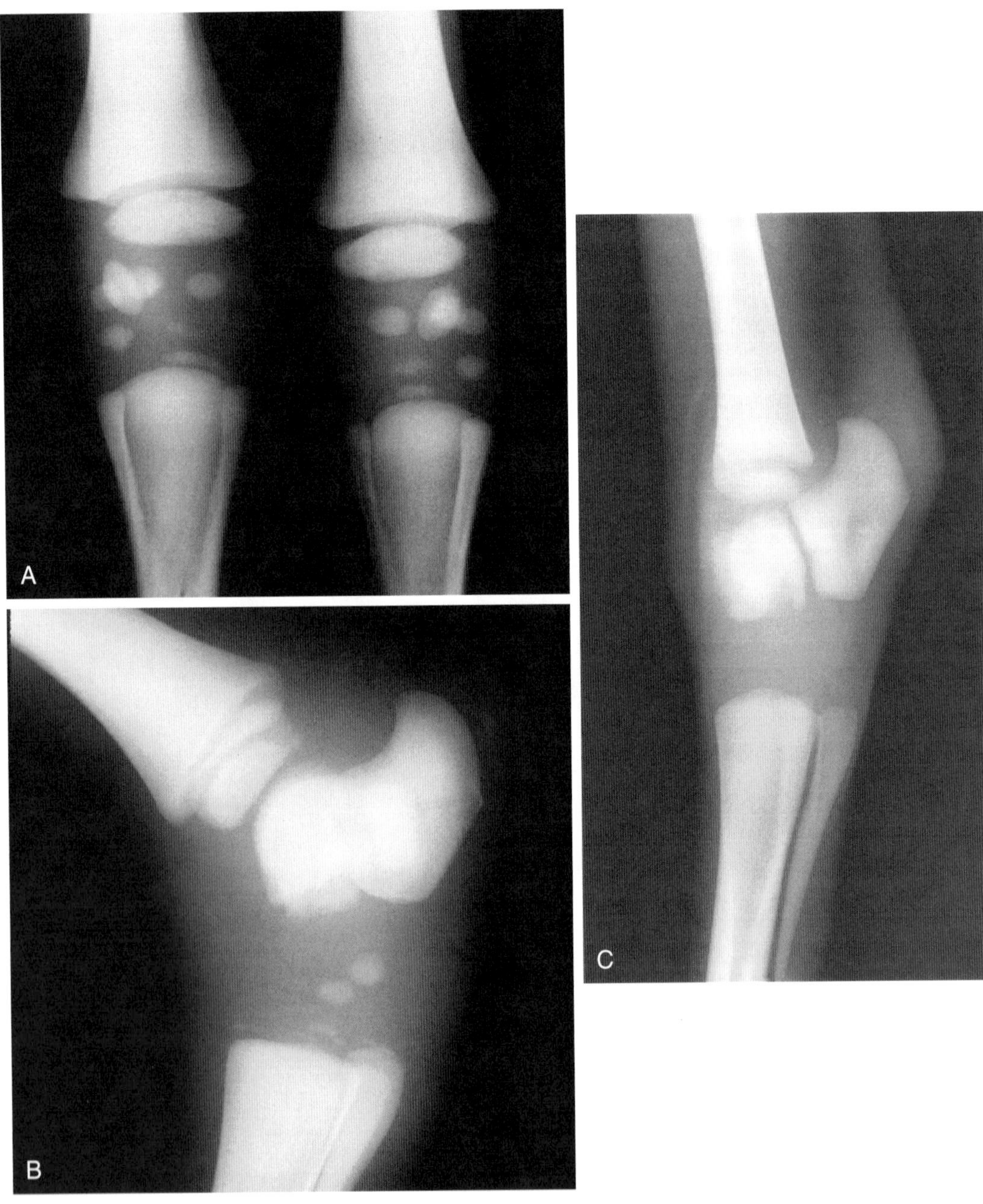

FIGURE 20-2 Radiographs from newborn foals with evidence of congenital hypothyroidism. Notice the, **A**, incomplete ossification of the cuboidal bones in the carpus and, **B**, **C**, tarsus. (Courtesy Dr. M.T. Hines [A,B] and the Ohio State University[C].)

mineral supplements, or that left their home farm were more likely to produce affected foals.[121] High nitrate intake has been proposed as the possible cause. Nitrates can cross the and impair thyroid gland function.[71] Greenfeed can concentrate high levels of nitrate and nitrite. Alfalfa, ryegrass, timothy, and cereal crops such as wheat, oats, rye, and barley also accumulate nitrate. In addition, these plants have low levels of iodine. Nitrates can also be in high concentrations in the water, in particular in areas with high use of fertilizers, feedlots, and dairies.[121]

Studies in the Northwestern United States have found an association between ingestion of pasture or hay contaminated with certain winter annuals of the mustard family (e.g., blue mustard, Jim Hill mustard, shepherdspurse, flixweed) and CHD. It has been postulated that glucosinolates in these plants may be broken down into compounds that are goitrogenic or act adversely on the thyroid gland of the developing fetus.

Hypothyroidism in Adult Horses

Hypothyroidism in adults is a rare condition, and unlike foals, is not life threatening. Low-grade anemia, decreased body temperature, heart rate, respiratory rate, and cardiac output have been reported in thyroidectomized horses.[104,122,123] Lethargy, rear limb edema, coarse hair coat, and decreased appetite were seen in thyroidectomized mares.[124] Reproductive problems in hypothyroid mares are irregular and absent estrus cycles.[4,122] Thyroidectomized mares could conceive and carry a foal to term.[124] Stallions exhibit decreased libido.[122,125] Thyroidectomized stallions had decreased total sperm count but normal semen characteristics and could sire foals.[114,124] Bradycardia, obesity, and lethargy were seen in mares with thyroid function that was suppressed from excessive iodine ingestion.[4] Alopecia attributed to iodinism and low circulating TH values were documented in a horse treated with an expectorant containing iodide and topical povidone iodine.[126] One report described low T_4 concentrations in agalactic mares.[12] Poor performance in racehorses in warm seasons could be related to low TH concentrations.[76] Hypothyroidism has been implicated as a cause of anhidrosis. Low or no differences in T_3 and T_4 concentrations have been found in anhidrotic horses.[127,128] Low TH concentrations may be present in horses with Cushing's disease and laminitis, but it remains to be documented that hypothyroidism is the cause of the laminitis in these animals.[129] TH concentrations are low, whereas TRH and TSH concentrations are elevated in hypothyroid horses.[130]

Treatment of Hypothyroidism

When hypothyroidism is suspected, it is important to determine if the animals are receiving appropriate amounts of iodine. Differentiating hypothyroidism from NTIS is critical because animals with NTIS may not require TH supplementation. Furthermore, TH therapy to euthyroid horses may be harmful, inhibiting the HPT axis and suppressing endogenous TH synthesis and secretion. The National Research Council recommends daily intakes of iodine of 1 to 5 mg per horse depending on age, physiologic status, and body weight.[4] The soil in some geographic areas (e.g., Great Lakes Region) has low or marginally low iodine content. Iodinated casein and thyroprotein (5 g/PO/day) have been used to reverse the effects of hypothyroidism.[114,131]

Hormone supplementation with T_4 should be effective unless a deiodination defect is noted. A starting oral dose of levothyroxine sodium of 20 μg/kg/day is recommended.[33] The animal should be monitored for clinical response to therapy, which can take at least 2 weeks. Periodical measurements of TH concentrations are recommended to adjust dosages. The use of thyroid supplements remains controversial; however, a clear indication for levothyroxine sodium is to induce weight loss in horses with obesity-associated laminitis and IR.

HYPERTHYROIDISM

Hyperthyroidism is a hypermetabolic disorder that is the result of high concentrations of fT_4 and fT_3. High TH concentrations can be found in physiologic states such as pregnancy, fetuses in late pregnancy, and in the first weeks of life.[18-22,24,27-29,37] Few documented cases of equine hyperthyroidism exist.[96,101] Tremors, excitability, tachycardia, sweating, and weight loss have been described in racehorses suspected of hyperthyroidism.[52,132] Horses with hyperthyroidism may improve with antithyroid therapy of potassium iodide (1 g/day, PO).[42,52] The use of thyroidectomy as a means of behavior modification for unmanageable horses had variable success.[114] No reports exist of hyperthyroidism associated with an autoimmune condition in the horse. Hyperthyroidism from a thyroid adenocarcinoma was documented in a horse.[101] After the T_3-suppression test, T_4 concentrations did not decrease in the affected horse compared with controls.

Horses are at risk for accelerated TH production when exposed to increased quantities of iodine-containing compounds such as expectorants, counterirritants, contrast media, drugs, leg paints, and povidone-based shampoos (Jod-Basedow phenomenon).[7] If severe distress from thyrotoxicosis is present, then administration of glucocorticoids should alleviate the signs.[7]

THYROID TUMORS

Tumors of the thyroid gland tend to occur more frequently in lightweight breeds than in draft-breed horses and more often in aged than in young horses.[83] Three cell types are noted in the equine thyroid gland: (1) undifferentiated cells, (2) parafollicular cells (secrete CT), and (3) follicular epithelial cells. A survey of aged horses found thyroid tumors in 30% of the animals,[133] with no tumors in horses younger than 18 years old. The majority of the tumors were microfollicular adenomas.

Adenoma

Adenoma is the most common neoplasia of the equine thyroid.[116,133-139] It is an age-related phenomenon, occurring mainly in horses older than 16 years. It is benign, usually unilateral, and is not associated with thyroid dysfunction. Occasionally its size may warrant surgical excision. Prognosis is good. A thyroid adenoma associated with hyperthyroidism was diagnosed in a 23-year-old gelding.[96] In this case the diagnosis was aided by percutaneous biopsy and the use of a T_3-suppression test, in which T_4 concentration was not suppressed after the administration of 2.5 mg of T_3, IM. Hemithyroidectomy of the affected gland restored TH concentrations.

ADENOCARCINOMA

Malignant neoplasia of the thyroid occurs less frequently. In four reported cases of thyroid adenocarcinomas, one horse was euthyroid, two were hypothyroid, and one was hyperthyroid.[98-101] One case of thyroid carcinoma with systemic metastasis and concurrent pituitary adenoma was reported.[140]

MEDULLARY CARCINOMA

Medullary carcinoma (C cell or parafollicular cell tumors) have been reported in horses.[2,141,142] In these cases, the youngest animal was 8 years old and the tumors were unilateral. In two horses, the complaint was constant gulping that was alleviated by surgical removal of the enlarged glands.[2] A C cell adenoma was reported in a 13-year-old horse with no clinical evidence of endocrine dysfunction.[143] In one horse a C cell adenoma associated with MEN was documented at necropsy.[141] C cell hyperplasia has been described in horses as young as 3 years old.[135] Immunohistochemistry or electron microscopy may be necessary to distinguish C cell tumors from other thyroid neoplasias.

MULTIPLE ENDOCRINE NEOPLASIA

MEN is a human syndrome characterized by multiple neoplasia of glands with a neuroendocrine origin. One case of a 22-year-old Thoroughbred mare with a C cell adenoma, a pheochromocytoma, and multicentric bilateral nodular hyperplasia of the adrenal medulla was reported.[141] A retrospective evaluation of endocrine tumors in horses that underwent necropsy suggested that hyperplasia and neoplasia of the thyroid and adrenal glands, as occurs in human beings with MEN, occurs in the horse.[140,141]

TREATMENT

In circumstances that warrant surgical excision, the prognosis is best when the condition is unilateral. Potential surgical complications include infection, hemorrhage, and laryngeal hemiplegia. As the equine parathyroid glands in general are not connected to the thyroid gland, hypocalcemia is not a complication.

ENDOCRINE PANCREAS

Ramiro E. Toribio

The islet of Langerhans is the endocrine functional unit of the pancreas. Important pancreatic hormones include insulin, glucagon, and SST. The pancreatic ß cells secrete insulin in response to glucose and glucagon, whereas SST inhibits insulin secretion. Blood glucose and amino acid concentrations are important regulators of glucagon and insulin secretion. Pancreatic endocrine function is also regulated by sympathetic and parasympathetic fibers that release norepinephrine, epinephrine, and acetylcholine. The sympathetic system inhibits insulin and stimulates glucagon secretion, whereas the parasympathetic system stimulates insulin secretion during food intake.[1,2]

Insulin is the primary hormone controlling the metabolism and storage of body fuels. Its actions involve three major fuels (carbohydrates, proteins, and fats) and three major tissues (liver, skeletal muscle, and adipose tissue). In the liver, insulin decreases glycogenolysis, gluconeogenesis, and ketogenesis, and stimulates gluconeogenesis and fatty acid synthesis. In adipose tissue, insulin decreases lipolysis and stimulates fatty acid uptake, synthesis, and esterification. In skeletal muscle, insulin decreases proteolysis and amino acid output and increases glucose and amino acid uptake, protein synthesis, and glycogen synthesis.[3] This information is relevant to understand the pathogenesis of equine diseases such as hyperlipemia, PPID, metabolic syndrome, and polysaccharide storage myopathy.

The equine endocrine pancreas is mature before birth. Pancreatic ß cell maturation in the equine fetus occurs in late gestation.[4] Before day 230, glucose has no effect on fetal insulin release; however, after day 290, glucose administration evokes a rapid insulin release.[4] Pancreatic maturation in foals is related to the increase in fetal cortisol concentrations; premature foals with low cortisol concentrations have a poor insulin response to glucose stimulation.[4,5] Immediately after birth the equine β cells are responsive to glucose administration; however, foals develop a physiologic IR in the first day of life that is related to the high cortisol concentrations around delivery.[6]

Glucagon has opposing effects of insulin on glucose metabolism. *Catecholamines* inhibit glucose-stimulated insulin secretion and increase glucose concentrations. *Growth hormone (GH)* counteracts insulin actions on lipid and glucose metabolism and is important in setting the basal glucose concentrations (glucostat).[3,7]

INSULIN RESISTANCE

IR is defined as a decreased response to endogenous insulin (hyperinsulinemia associated with normo- or hyperglycemia) or exogenous insulin administration. IR results from changes in insulin receptors, postreceptor effects, or both. Because a number of insulin receptors must be occupied to achieve a biologic action, when most receptors are nonfunctional, higher insulin concentrations are required to achieve a biologic effect, leading to *insulin insensitivity* or *resistance*. Clinically, this results in hyperinsulinemia with normoglycemia (compensated IR) or with hyperglycemia (noncompensated IR).

IR is reported in horses and ponies with pars intermedia dysfunction, equine metabolic syndrome (EMS), obesity, hyperlipemia, diabetes mellitus (DM), laminitis, endotoxemia, granulosa cell tumors, and osteochondrosis dissecans.[8-13] Carbohydrate-rich diets and glucocorticoids decrease insulin sensitivity in horses.[14,15] Increased insulin sensitivity has been documented in horses with polysaccharide storage myopathy and with equine motor neuron disease.[8,16]

Healthy ponies and Miniature Horses are less responsive than horses to endogenous and exogenous insulin, and obese ponies often develop IR.[10,17,18] Studies on insulin receptor or postreceptor signaling are lacking in equids. In human beings, decreased glucose transport 4 (GLUT4) activity is central to the development of IR; however, few studies assess GLUT4 and IR in the horse.[19,20] Physical activity increases muscular GLUT4 function and is the rationale for recommending exercise in human beings with IR.[21,22] Moderate exercise training in horses increased muscle GLUT4 content.[19] Exercise also increases insulin sensitivity in ponies.[23]

Glucocorticoids stimulate proteolysis, increase glycogen formation, stimulate gluconeogenesis, and decrease insulin sensitivity. Glucocorticoids also increase glycemia by decreasing the skeletal muscle and adipocytes response to insulin-stimulated glucose uptake. The anti-insulin effects of glucocorticoids are accompanied by hyperglycemia and hyperinsulinemia.[3] Increased glucocorticoid concentrations are associated with IR, and dexamethasone administration to healthy horses decreases insulin sensitivity.[15] One study found that GH induces IR in horses.[24]

DIABETES MELLITUS

DM is defined as persistent hyperglycemia and glucosuria from either hypoinsulinemia or IR. DM is a rare condition in horses[9,25] and is associated with disturbances in the secretion and sensitivity to hormones such as insulin, glucagon, catecholamines, GH, and glucocorticoids.[3] Most cases of IR in horses are associated with PPID, metabolic syndrome, and hyperlipemia.

Primary DM is a term used to describe pancreatic β cell dysfunction resulting in low insulin concentrations (insulin-dependent DM, type 1 DM) and hyperglycemia. This distinction is important to differentiate hyperglycemia associated with increased insulin concentrations (IR, type 2 DM). Horses suspected of having DM often have a history of depression, polyuria, polydipsia, polyphagia, progressive weight loss, and a rough hair coat. Similar clinical signs are observed in horses with PPID.

Hypoinsulinemia (primary DM) is an uncommon condition of horses that has been reported with pancreatitis from parasite migration, chronic pancreatitis, ovarian tumors, and pregnancy.[11,26-31] Few pancreatic β cells were present in a mustang diagnosed with DM.[9] Weight loss, depression, polyuria, polydipsia, polyphagia, hyperglycemia, glucosuria, and ketonuria were reported in a 7-year-old pony with chronic pancreatitis and primary DM.[27] Ketonemia, ketonuria, and ketone odor have been reported in diabetic ponies and horses.[26,27,30-32]

Because persistent hyperglycemia and glucosuria defines DM, factors that induce temporary hyperglycemia such as carbohydrate diets, stress, exercise, glucocorticoid treatment, and sedation with xylazine and detomidine must be avoided before testing.[33,34] Hyperglycemia may be present in horses with pheochromocytomas.[35]

Once a clinical diagnosis of DM has been made, diseases frequently associated with IR such as PPID and metabolic syndrome must be ruled out; many test protocols are available for the diagnosis of these conditions. Tests used for the diagnosis of IR in horses include the glucose tolerance test, the insulin tolerance test, the insulin suppression test, the combined glucose-insulin test (CGIT), the euglycemic-hyperinsulinemic clamp (EHC), and the minimal model analysis of a frequently sampled intravenous glucose tolerance test (FSIGT).[11,25,33,36] The EHC and the FSIGT are the most accurate methods to assess insulin sensitivity; however, they are tedious and rarely performed in the clinical setting.

Measurement of serum insulin and glucose concentrations should be the first step in the diagnosis of DM and IR. Insulin concentrations in healthy horses are less than 20 μU/ml, and concentrations higher than 30 μU/ml suggest IR. Hyperglycemia with hyperinsulinemia suggests IR, whereas hyperglycemia with hypoinsulinemia is consistent with insulin-dependent DM.

The *glucose tolerance test* is the most frequently used test because it is easy to perform and provides sufficient information for the diagnosis of IR. The test can be oral or IV. The IV test has fewer confounding factors (gastric emptying, glucose absorption, fasting, gastrointestinal motility) than the oral test.[37] In this test, the clinician places the IV catheter the day before testing to reduce stress. Glucose (0.2 to 0.5 g/kg/IV) is administered and serum concentrations of glucose and insulin determined every 30 minutes for 3 hours. In healthy horses, insulin is released immediately after glucose administration and serum glucose concentrations should return to baseline by 3 hours. In the case of insulin-dependent DM, insulin concentrations do not increase and glucose concentrations remain elevated (>3 hours). In horses with IR, insulin concentrations increase but the return of glucose concentration to baseline values is delayed (>3 hours). Handheld glucose meters can be used to determine glucose concentrations.

In the *insulin tolerance test*, soluble (regular) insulin (1 to 8 IU/kg/IV) is administered and glucose concentrations determined every 15 to 30 minutes for 3 hours.[11,26,27,29,31] Alternatively, crystalline insulin is administered (0.05 to 0.1 IU/kg/IV) and blood samples taken every 15 to 30 minutes for 3 hours. In healthy horses the clinician should expect a 30% to 50% decrease in glucose concentrations at 15 minutes, 60% at 30 minutes, and normal glucose concentrations at 2 hours. Failure of insulin to lower glucose concentrations by more than 30% baseline suggests insulin-resistant DM. When performing the insulin tolerance test it is important to have an injectable solution of dextrose available because insulin may induce hypoglycemic shock.[27,38] This test is being replaced by the CGIT.

In the CGIT, a dextrose solution (150 mg/kg/IV) is rapidly administered and immediately followed by an injection of regular insulin (0.1 IU/kg/IV). In this test the clinician places the IV catheter the day before testing to reduce stress. Blood samples are collected at times 0, 1, 5, 15, 25, 35, 45, 60, 75, 90, 105, 120, 135, and 150 minutes. For practical reasons this test can be limited to 90 minutes. The dextrose dose of 150 mg/kg is recommended because it increases blood glucose concentrations to approximately 200 mg/dl within 5 minutes of injection, which is close to the renal glucose threshold.[33] In healthy horses, glucose returns to baseline by 30 minutes, decreases by 50% baseline at 60 to 75 minutes, and is back to normal by 150 minutes after injection.[33] In horses with IR, glucose concentrations do not decrease below baseline for over 90 minutes. Horses with glucose concentrations above baseline for over 45 minutes are considered insulin resistant.[33] Xylazine interferes with the CGIT in healthy horses, with glucose remaining elevated for more than 75 minutes.[33] This is relevant to the clinician because α_2-adrenergic receptor agonists (xylazine, detomidine) can lead to the misdiagnosis of IR. Stressful conditions and the use of glucocorticoids should be avoided. In addition, grain and grass should be withheld for 24 hours, but water and grass hay do not appear to affect the results.[33] For additional information on testing, the reader is referred to the section on Equine Metabolic Syndrome.

The FSIGT (minimal model) is primarily used in research, in particular to assess IR in horses with metabolic syndrome. A baseline sample is collected and dextrose (0.5 g/kg/IV in a 50% solution) is administered. Blood samples are collected at 1, 2, 3, 4, 5, 6, 7, 8, 9, 10, 12, 14, 16, 18, 20, 30, 40, 50, 60, 70, 80, 90, 100, 120, 150, and 180 minutes after dextrose administration. Glucose concentrations are measured at all time points and insulin concentrations at 0, 2, 4, 6, 8, 10, 14, 18, 20, 30, 60, 90, 120, 150, and 180 minutes.[36] Data is analyzed by the minimal model method that provides information on the dynamics of glucose clearance, insulin release, and insulin effectiveness. The FSIGT is considered the only method that differentiates insulin-dependent and insulin-independent glucose clearance[13]; however, it is time-consuming, expensive, and can be impractical in clinical cases.

The treatment of DM depends on the primary cause. For obese ponies with IR, decreased caloric intake and increased physical activity are recommended. Treatment of IR associated with PPID and metabolic syndrome is discussed elsewhere. If a diagnosis of primary DM is reached, then treatment with insulin is indicated. During treatment it is important to monitor blood glucose concentrations to adjust insulin dosing. Treatment of DM with insulin has been attempted with variable results.[25] Improvement (in addition to deterioration including hyperglycemia, polyuria, and polydipsia; swelling at the injection sites; and development of antibodies against insulin) has been reported.[25,27] Recommended doses for insulin are 0.05 to 0.1 IU/kg/IV/b.i.d. to t.i.d. for regular insulin and 0.5 to 4.0 IU/kg/IM/b.i.d. for protamine zinc insulin (PZI). It is important to start with a low dose and adjust based on glycemia. Insulin administration can result in hypoglycemic shock, so having a dextrose solution available is suggested. The Somogyi effect is a paradoxical insulin-induced hyperglycemia that appears to be mediated by catecholamines, cortisol, and GH release after acute hypoglycemia.

Antihyperglycemic compounds such as biguanides (metformin) and sulfonylureas (glyburide) that are indicated to treat hyperglycemia and IR have been used in horses with promising results.[9,39] The thiazolidinediones is another group of drugs frequently used to treat type 2 DM; however, they have not been evaluated in the horse.

Evidence indicates that exercise increases insulin sensitivity and skeletal muscle glucose transport in horses and other species, thus physical activity is highly recommended.[19] Attention should be paid to laminitic horses in which physical activity can be detrimental.

HYPERINSULINEMIA AND HYPOGLYCEMIA

Hyperinsulinemia may result in hypoglycemic shock. Hyperinsulinemia with hypoglycemia may result from therapeutic[27] or fraudulent[38,40] injections of insulin, as well as from insulin-secreting pancreatic tumors.[41] Endogenous (pancreatic neoplasia) and exogenous (injected) insulin can be differentiated using high-pressure liquid chromatography.[40]

Depending on the degree of hypoglycemia, affected horses may show trembling, ataxia, hyperexcitability, tachycardia, tachypnea, mydriasis, nystagmus, profuse sweating, violent seizures, coma, and death. Hyperinsulinism secondary to a pancreatic adenoma (insulinoma) was documented in a 12-year-old Shetland pony broodmare.[41] The clinical signs, in particular seizures, were episodic and associated with feeding. During seizure episodes the pony was hypoglycemic.

The *glucagon tolerance* test has been used in dogs in the diagnosis of hyperinsulinemia. Glucagon administration increases glucose and insulin concentrations. The glucagon tolerance test was performed in a pony suspected of having hyperinsulinemia from a pancreatic adenoma.[41] Glucagon (1500 μg, IV) administration to the affected pony and a control pony resulted in a rapid increase in glucose and insulin concentrations in both animals; however, the affected pony had an exaggerated and sustained insulin response.[41] Major adverse effects of glucagon administration are cardiovascular.

During the second half of pregnancy, mares may develop hyperinsulinemia and can have an exaggerated β cell response to glucose infusion.[42]

NEOPLASIA

Exocrine pancreatic tumors (adenocarcinomas) are more frequently diagnosed than endocrine (islet cells) tumors. Pancreatic adenocarcinomas reported in the literature resulted in anemia, hyperammonemia, protein losing enteropathy, biliary obstruction, tachypnea, and pleural effusion.[43-46]

PITUITARY PARS INTERMEDIA DYSFUNCTION (EQUINE CUSHING'S DISEASE)

Dianne McFarlane and Ramiro E. Toribio

A clinical syndrome associated with hirsutism, laminitis, polyuria and polydipsia, and weight loss has been described in aged horses and ponies.[1-6] The syndrome was originally referred to as *equine Cushing's disease* because of similarities to Cushing's disease in human beings and dogs, in which excessive and autonomous secretion of proopiomelanocortin (POMC)-derived peptides occurs, including ACTH (corticotropin), resulting in secondary hyperadrenocorticism. However, in horses, pituitary adenomas arise from the pars intermedia (intermediate lobe) of the pituitary gland, unlike in human beings and dogs in which pituitary adenomas commonly arise from the anterior lobe (pars distalis, adenohypophysis). As a result, in the horse, hormones from the pars intermedia are excessively secreted as described following. PPID therefore seems to be more appropriate to describe the syndrome because, unlike human beings, adrenocortical hyperplasia and hypercortisolemia are not consistent findings in affected horses. Equine PPID has been described as equine Cushing's disease, equine Cushing's syndrome, pituitary adenoma, hypophyseal adenoma, chromophobe adenoma, pars intermedia adenoma, diffuse adenomatous hyperplasia of the pituitary, PDH, and pars intermedia hyperplasia.[1,3,6-23] However, PPID is used in this section.

CLINICAL SIGNS

PPID is a clinical syndrome of aged horses associated with hirsutism, poor hair coat, laminitis, polyuria and polydipsia, muscle wasting, weight loss, docility, lethargy, hyperhidrosis, narcolepsy, blindness, decreased responsiveness to painful stimuli, increased appetite, and recurrent infections.* Although many clinical signs are associated with PPID, only a subset of the signs typically manifest in the individual affected horse, perhaps because of differences in the secretion profile of

*References 1, 2, 16, 19, 21, 23.

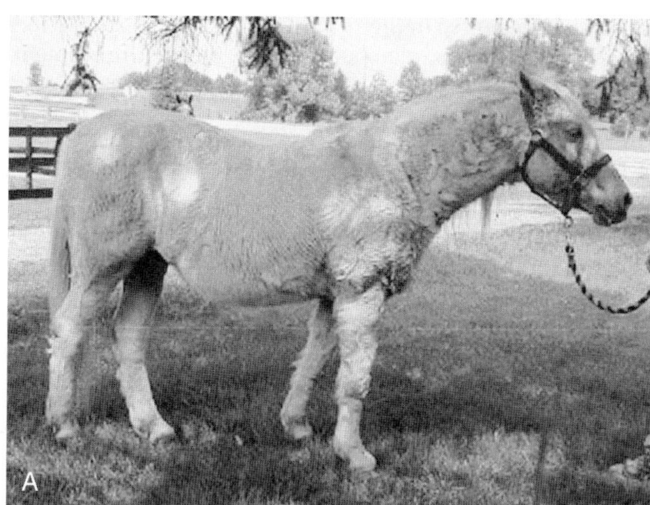

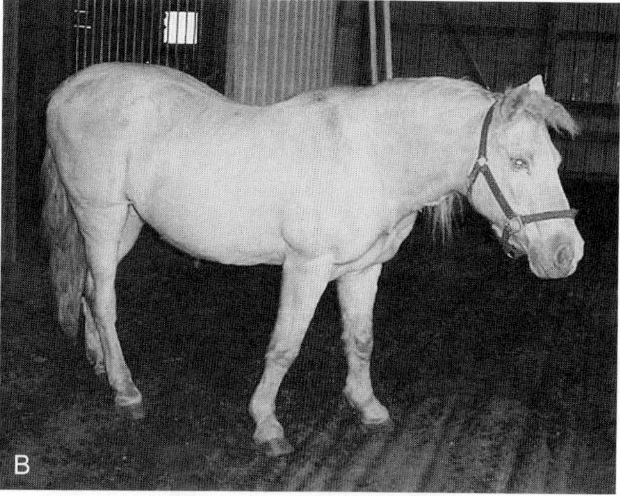

FIGURE 20-3 **A,** Horse diagnosed with pars intermedia dysfunction. **B,** The horse was treated with a combination of pergolide and cyproheptadine, and clinical signs improved by 8 weeks of treatment. (Courtesy The Ohio State University.)

POMC-derived peptides or the degree of compression of adjacent neuroendocrine tissues.

Hirsutism (55% to 80%) is considered the most frequent clinical sign in PPID horses, although these estimates may be biased because of the increased tendency to test aged horses with hair coat abnormalities for PPID* (Figure 20-3). Hirsute horses have a long, thick, often curly hair coat. Other hair coat abnormalities may include a failure to shed in a complete or timely manner. Some horses shed in late spring and grow a winter coat early in the fall; many develop a patchy coat with areas of alopecia. Retention of long hair in the jugular grove, on the legs, or along the ventral abdomen is also a frequent finding. The mechanisms underlying the abnormal hair coat and shedding process are not understood. The pathogenesis of hirsutism is unknown. Holscher et al.[8] suggested that hirsutism in horses with PPID may be the result of increased adrenal gland secretion of androgens, as occurs in women with Cushing's disease. It also has been suggested that hirsutism and hyperhidrosis may result from dysregulation of the thermoregulatory center of the hypothalamus, a consequence of pituitary compression.[7] Horses with adrenal exhaustion or insufficiency may also have an abnormal hair coat.[25]

Chronic laminitis is a frequent finding in horses with PPID.[24] The presentation of endocrinopathic laminitis is more insidious than laminitis as the result of other causes. It has been speculated that laminitis results from increased concentrations of glucocorticoids; however, more recent data suggests IR or hyperinsulinemia may have a role in inciting laminitis in horses with PPID. Laminitis-prone ponies were observed to have increased serum insulin concentrations compared with control ponies.[26] Maintenance of prolonged hyperinsulinemia in clinically normal ponies resulted in induction of laminitis within 72 hours of onset of hyperinsulinemia in all five ponies, suggesting increased serum insulin concentration in the absence of hyperglycemia or underlying IR can induce laminitis.[27] Regardless of the underlying cause of laminitis, PPID should be included in the differential diagnoses in any older horse with chronic laminitis, even if other clinical signs of PPID are not present.

Polyuria and polydipsia have been reported in up to 76% of horses diagnosed with PPID.[2] However, the pathogenesis behind the development of polyuria and polydipsia is unclear. It has been speculated that compression of the pars nervosa by a pars intermedia adenoma may result in decreased secretion of vasopressin (AVP; antidiuretic hormone [ADH]).[1,7] Hyperglycemia, which is a frequent laboratory finding in these horses, may result in osmotic diuresis. Glucocorticoids can increase GFR and may contribute to diuresis. It is important to rule out other differentials for polyuria and polydipsia, including neurogenic diabetes insipidus, nephrogenic diabetes insipidus, psychogenic polydipsia, and hyperglycemia of various origins (pancreatic disease, pheochromocytoma). Horses that are stalled are the ones most likely to have obvious polyuria and polydipsia.

Weight loss is reported in the majority of horses with PPID (up to 88%) and is often an early clinical sign.[2] However, some horses may be obese or in good body condition.[23] Affected horses often have a weak and pendulous abdomen, a sway back, and lose muscle mass along the dorsum of the back. The pot-bellied appearance is probably the result of lack of tone in the abdominal musculature. The muscle wasting along the dorsal midline and elsewhere results in prominence of the croup, tuber coxae, and tuber sacrale regions. It is unclear what the effect of different POMC-derived peptides is on equine energy metabolism or muscle atrophy. Weight loss in some horses may be the result of other conditions associated with aging (dental problems, disease because of immunosuppression and parasites) rather than the direct effect of an abnormally regulated HPA axis on body condition. Glucocorticoids, in addition to being immunosuppressive, have catabolic effects on skeletal muscle; however, the role of increased concentration of cortisol on weight loss in PPID is unclear. Muscle tissue from horses with PPID shows selective atrophy of type 2 muscle fibers,[28] consistent with what is observed in muscle atrophy associated with excessive cortisol in other species; however, the role of other POMC hormones on muscle atrophy has not been investigated. In horses with normal or

*References 1, 2, 5, 21, 23, 24.

low cortisol concentrations, other causes may be responsible for the weight loss.

Increased docility in affected horses is often reported by owners and clinicians. Horses with PPID have increased plasma and CSF concentrations of β-endorphin (β-END),[13] which may explain the docility and lethargy in some of these animals. Increased β-END concentrations may also explain the decreased responsiveness to painful stimuli.

Neurologic impairment, although uncommon, has been reported in horses with PPID and includes blindness, seizures, and narcolepsy. Blindness may be caused by compression of the overlying optic chiasm by the enlarged pituitary gland; however, blindness can occur in horses with PPID in the absence of postmortem evidence of optic nerve damage.[29] An increased occurrence of narcolepsy or sleep disorders has been suggested to occur in horses with PPID. The reason that some of these horses develop narcolepsy is unknown. One can speculate that the lack of dopaminergic control may be altering the sleep-wake cycle as occurs in human beings. Narcolepsy can result from decreased orexin activity in the hypothalamus. Orexins (hypocretins) are peptide neurotransmitters expressed in the lateral hypothalamus (orexinergic neurons) that are important in the sleep-wake cycle, and the absence of orexin effects results in narcolepsy.[30] Horses with PPID had decreased CSF concentrations of hypocretin (orexin).[31]

Excessive sweating (hyperhidrosis), and less commonly, lack of sweating (anhidrosis) are reported in horses with PPID, although the mechanisms underlying abnormal sweating have not been determined.

The bulging supraorbital fat pads often observed in horses with PPID are the result of fat redistribution.[2] These may be observed in horses that do not exhibit generalized obesity. Likewise, some horses in good body condition may have a "cresty neck" and fat accumulation around their tail.

Skin infections (dermatophilosis), sinusitis, pneumonia, dental disease, and abscess formation are common sequelae of PPID. The precise mechanism resulting in immune impairment is unknown, but the increased concentration of immunosuppressive hormones, including cortisol, α-melanocyte–stimulating hormone (α-MSH) or β-END is likely a contributing factor.

Abnormal estrus cycles and infertility have been reported in horses with PPID.[3] This may be a direct or indirect effect of PPID, or it may be an unrelated effect of advanced age. Compression of the pars distalis or hypothalamus could have a profound effect on reproductive hormones. In addition, a generalized decrease in DA output could directly affect release of reproductive hormones because many are under dopaminergic regulation, including gonadotropin-releasing hormone (GnRH) and prolactin. No controlled studies document the relationship between treated and untreated horses with PPID and fertility.

EPIDEMIOLOGY

Compared with other equine endocrine disorders, PPID is a common clinical syndrome. In two large-scale surveys, owners reported hair coat abnormalities consistent with PPID in 20% to 30% of aged horses.[32,33] In a study of more than 300 horses 15 years or older, horses were tested using plasma ACTH and α-MSH concentration, and 15% of horses were positive for PPID.[32] An incidence of 15% to 30% is markedly greater than originally reported in the 1970s (0.075%-0.15% of 4000 horses of all ages seen in an ambulatory practice).[6] At this time it is unclear whether this change reflects a true increase in prevalence of disease, a change in equine demographics with a larger aged population, or an increased awareness and recognition of disease because of changes in diagnostic testing methods or frequency.

PPID has been diagnosed in horses older than 7 years (range 7-40; average 19 to 21).[1,2,5,22,23] Although all breeds are susceptible, ponies and Morgan horses appear to be predisposed.[2,5,21,23,34] Despite earlier studies suggesting PPID to be more prevalent in female[1,11,13] or male[2] horses, there appears to be no sex preference.[2,5,23,32,34]

Pars intermedia adenomas and microadenomas are often identified at postmortem examination in older horses with no previous history or reported clinical signs of this condition.[35,36] The significance of these clinically silent histological findings is unknown.

PATHOGENESIS

Pars intermedia hyperplasia and hypertrophy are consistent findings in PPID,[15,21,35] and data suggest it is a lack of inhibitory control on pars intermedia cell function that triggers the excessive cell proliferation and the development of adenomas. The pars intermedia in horses and other species is inhibited by DA of hypothalamic origin.[37] Three neuroendocrine dopaminergic tracts exist: (1) the tuberoinfundibular, (2) the tuberohypophyseal, and (3) the periventricular dopaminergic neurons.[38] It is the periventricular neurons that appear most critical in regulating cell proliferation and hormone production and release in the pars intermedia.[39] The periventricular neurons originate in the periventricular nucleus, adjacent to the third ventricle, and project through the infundibular stack, terminating in the pars intermedia. In the pars intermedia the periventricular neurons directly innervate melanotropes where they release DA that interacts with dopaminergic D_2-type receptors on melanotropes. In the presence of DA, the D_2-receptors act to inhibit POMC mRNA expression and POMC-derived intermediate-lobe hormone release. In rodents, surgical disruption of the periventricular neurons results in increased α-MSH release, confirming a melanotropic inhibitory role for the periventricular neurons.[39] In contrast, prolactin release is regulated primarily by the tuberoinfundibular dopaminergic neurons. These originate in the arcuate nucleus and release DA at the median eminence. From there DA is transported to the anterior lobe through the hypophyseal portal system.[38]

In their study of the loss of dopaminergic inhibition in horses with PPID, Orth, Holscher, and Wilson et al.[9] found that D_2-receptor dopaminergic agonists (bromocriptine, pergolide) decreased POMC-derived peptide concentrations in horses with PPID. Millington et al.[13] found low concentrations of DA and DA metabolites in the pars intermedia of horses with PPID. This data suggested that although DA was lacking in the pars intermedia of horses with PPID, response to DA was intact.[9] This understanding has made it possible to recommend DA agonists (e.g., pergolide) in the palliative treatment of PPID. Several studies[25,27,40] have documented the efficacy of DA agonists in treatment of the PPID as described following. More recent studies[41] have suggested that the loss of dopaminergic input to the pars intermedia is a consequence of neurodegeneration of the periventricular neurons. A loss of

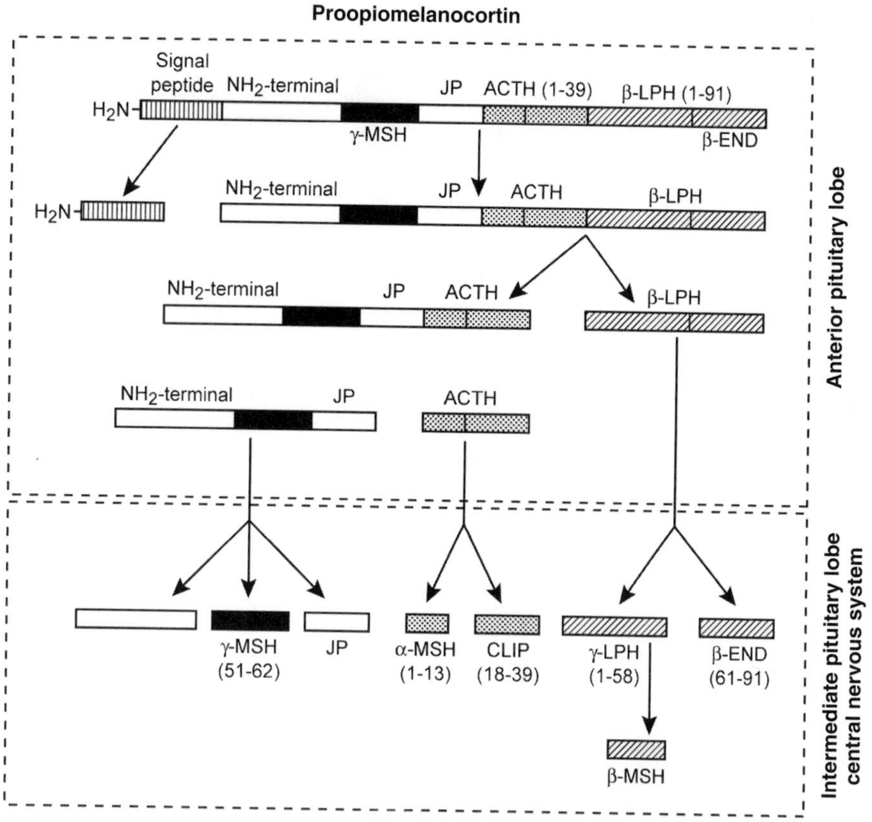

FIGURE 20-4 Processing of proopiomelanocortin (POMC) in the anterior pituitary lobe, the intermediate pituitary lobe, and the central nervous system (CNS). In the anterior lobe, adrenocorticotropic hormone (ACTH) and β-lipotropin (β-LPH) are the major products of POMC. In the intermediate lobe and in the CNS, ACTH is cleaved to produce α-melanocyte–stimulating hormone (α-MSH) and orticotropin-like intermediate lobe peptide (CLIP), and β-LPH is cleaved to produce β-endorphin (β-END). (Adapted from Castro MG, Morrison E: Post-translational processing of proopiomelanocortin in the pituitary and in the brain, Crit Rev Neurobiol 11:35–57, 1997.)

dopaminergic cell bodies in the periventricular nucleus of the hypothalamus and the nerve terminals in the pars intermedia was demonstrated in horses with PPID using immunohistochemistry.[41] In addition, in horses with PPID, dopaminergic nerve terminals showed evidence of oxidative stress damage, suggesting free radical damage may be a cause of periventricular neuronal damage and cell loss. Oxidative stress has been implicated as a contributing factor in the pathogenesis of many other neurodegenerative diseases.

Evidence from other species suggests additional hypothalamic factors, such as TRH, serotonin, and γ-aminobutyric acid (GABA) are important in regulating melanotrope function in the pars intermedia.[13,37,42] In horses a direct positive effect of TRH on melantropes has been shown.[43] When equine melanotropes were maintained in culture, treatment with TRH resulted in a release of α-MSH. In addition, horses administered TRH have a rapid and substantial increase in plasma α-MSH concentration.[43] In other species, serotonin is also a positive releasing factor for pars intermedia cells.[37] However, the role of serotonin on equine pars intermedia function is unclear, and Millington et al.[13] found no difference in serotonin concentrations in the pars intermedia of affected versus control horses. GABA has a tonic inhibitory effect on POMC synthesis in the pars intermedia of other species[42]; however, the role of GABA in the pathogenesis of equine PPID is unknown.

Both the anterior lobe (corticotropes) and the intermediate lobe (melanotropes) synthesize the identical hormone precursor molecule, POMC[9]; however, in the intermediate lobe the post-translational cleavage and processing of POMC is different from that in the anterior lobe.[13,44] In the anterior lobe, the major products of POMC are ACTH and β-lipotropin (β-LPH) (Figure 20-4). In the intermediate lobe, ACTH is further cleaved to produce α-MSH and corticotropin-like intermediate lobe peptide (CLIP), and β-LPH is processed to β-END.[44,45] Therefore in the pars intermedia, ACTH is a minor (2%) post-translational product of POMC.[10] It also appears that the POMC production and cleavage in the pars intermedia of the horse with PPID remains intact; however, postcleavage modification of the peptides is altered.[10,13] Millington et al.[13] found that the post-translational processing of β-END in normal tissues was different from that in equine pituitary adenomas, with significantly more of the active (agonist) form of β-END present in the pituitary of horses with PPID.

Although progress has been made in the understanding of the pathogenesis of PPID in horses, many questions remain unanswered. For example, why do a number of horses with PPID have low cortisol concentrations in spite of high ACTH concentrations? Cortisol concentrations are variable in affected horses,[14,16,46,47] and adrenocortical hyperplasia is not a consistent finding[1,14]; therefore it is difficult to explain hyperglycemia, neutrophilia, and lymphopenia, as well as other clinical signs such as laminitis and predisposition to infections such as those resulting from glucocorticoid excess. Cortisol may be responsible for some of the clinical signs associated with PPID; however, many studies have found that cortisol concentrations in horses with PPID may be within or below the normal range, suggesting that unidentified factors may be as or more important than hypercortisolemia in the pathogenesis of this condition. Furthermore, these findings are consistent with the low frequency (20%) of adrenocortical hyperplasia in horses diagnosed with Cushing's disease.[1,14] One explanation for the low cortisol concentration in some affected horses may be that glucocorticoid synthesis and secretion from the adrenal gland is downregulated from excessive and prolonged exposure to ACTH. Alternatively, ACTH secreted in horses with PPID may be immunologically active but biologically inert.

PATHOLOGIC FINDINGS

Horses with PPID have a grossly enlarged pituitary because of hypertrophy, hyperplasia, and adenoma formation in the pars intermedia. Adenomas of the pars intermedia are white to yellow, nodular or multinodular masses that can infiltrate or compress the pars distalis and pars nervosa.[1,14,35] In some horses, pituitary microadenomas (<1 cm) may be evident. Microscopically, these adenomas are comprised of a cellular pattern with large columnar, spindle-shaped, or polyhedral cells that form palisades and pseudoacini.[1,35] The tumor cells are slightly acidophilic with hematoxylin and eosin staining, and they are chromophobic with trichrome stain.[1] Pars intermedia adenomas may compress the overlying hypothalamus or optic chiasm, resulting in necrosis of nuclei that are important in endocrine and metabolic functions.

Adrenal cortical hyperplasia is not a consistent finding; 1 of 5 horses in one study[14] and 4 of 19 horses in another study[1] had adrenal cortical hyperplasia. The lack of cortical hyperplasia in most horses with PPID may indicate that the clinical signs in these horses are not the result of hyperadrenocorticism. The variability in response among affected horses to the ACTH stimulation test may be the result of variable adrenal hyperplasia.

Skin biopsies reveal normal hair follicles in anagen phase, normal epidermis and dermal collagen, and a lack of the characteristic lesions present in dogs with Cushing's disease from cortisol excess (C.C. Capen, personal communication, 2006). Although laminitis is a common finding in horses with PPID, the pathologic features in the lamina of these horses are nonspecific.

LABORATORY TESTING

The diagnosis of PPID in many cases can be suggested by history, clinical signs, and preliminary laboratory results. Initial testing should include a complete blood count (CBC), a serum chemistry profile, and urinalysis. Horses with PPID may have a normal CBC and serum chemistry profile. Clinicopathologic abnormalities reported in horses with PPID include anemia, neutrophilia, lymphopenia, eosinopenia, hyperglycemia, hyperlipemia, increased liver enzymes, and glucosuria.*

*References 2, 5, 12, 14, 23, 38, 48.

Persistent hyperglycemia is frequent in affected horses; more than 45% (94% in one study) of horses with PPID had hyperglycemia.[2,5,14,21,49] Many horses with PPID and hyperglycemia have IR (hyperglycemia and hyperinsulinemia).[11] Although insulin-resistant hyperglycemia can be present, it is also possible that hyperglycemia in some horses may result from stressing conditions. Glucosuria is a frequent finding (up to 77% in one study) in horses with PPID and hyperglycemia.[2] Hyperlipemia may be present in horses, but it is more frequent in ponies.[20,50]

Additional testing to help confirm the diagnosis might include determination of resting plasma cortisol and ACTH concentrations. Significant variability is noted in plasma cortisol concentration among horses with PPID,[14] and cortisol concentrations are affected by stress, exercise, and serum glucose concentrations. Therefore measurement of resting plasma cortisol concentrations is not diagnostic for PPID. Resting ACTH concentrations are considered to be more reliable in the diagnosis of PPID than resting cortisol concentrations.

DIAGNOSIS

Diagnostic testing for horses suspected of having PPID is based on history, clinical signs, and laboratory findings. Many tests for the diagnosis of PPID have been evaluated; however, based on the limited number of horses studied, as well as the variable results from some of these studies, it is difficult to recommend them without additional validation. One limitation in the diagnosis of PPID is establishing a gold standard; currently perhaps the only well-accepted gold standard is postmortem examination interpreted in conjunction with clinical signs. Another important consideration is the season during which the testing is performed. The equine pars intermedia is known to be more active in the fall; as a result, false-positive diagnostic tests may occur when testing is performed between August and October.

Baseline Cortisol Concentrations

Measurement of baseline plasma concentrations of cortisol has been proposed in the diagnosis of PPID. In horses with PPID, resting plasma concentrations of cortisol may be within the normal range,[14] mildly increased,[16] or decreased.[46,47] Therefore measuring baseline plasma cortisol concentrations to diagnose PPID is not recommended. Healthy horses have diurnal variations in plasma cortisol concentrations, with higher concentrations in the morning than in the late evening, although significant individual variation occurs.[16,51-53] No diurnal variations in cortisol concentrations are reported in horses with PPID.[16] Circadian cortisol variation may also be blunted in horses with other diseases or stress-related conditions,[54] thus limiting its usefulness as a diagnostic test.

In addition to plasma, cortisol concentrations have been determined in saliva and urine of healthy horses and horses with PPID.[16,49,51] van der Kolk et al.[52] measured salivary cortisol concentrations in healthy horses and found that there was a trend for higher salivary cortisol concentrations in the morning than in the evening; however, the differences were not statistically significant. They also found that plasma and salivary cortisol concentrations were correlated and that administration of dexamethasone decreased, and administration of ACTH increased, plasma and salivary cortisol concentrations.

Urinary Corticoid:Creatinine Ratio

The urinary corticoid/creatinine (c:c) ratio has been determined in ponies and horses suffering of PPID.[17,50] van der Kolk et al.[17] found that horses with PPID had higher urinary concentrations of corticoids and a higher c:c ratio than healthy horses; however, in their study there was overlap in the c:c ratio between healthy and diseased horses, resulting in a number of false-positive and false-negative results, thus limiting the value of this test alone for the diagnosis of PPID. In addition, horses were included in that study on the basis of the ACTH stimulation test, which itself has significant variability among horses with PPID and between healthy ponies and horses.[21] No ponies were included in the control group, and most of the affected animals were ponies. Additional studies comparing the c:c ratio to well-accepted and validated diagnostic procedures are necessary to recommend this test over other tests.

Dexamethasone Suppression Test

The dexamethasone suppression test (DST) has been a well-accepted and recommended test for the diagnosis of PPID in horses.[16,55,56] This test is based on the lack of suppression of plasma cortisol concentrations in horses with PPID at 19 to 24 hours after dexamethasone administration.[16] It has been suggested that plasma cortisol concentrations are not suppressed by dexamethasone administration in horses with PPID because of production of ACTH from melanotropes of the pars intermedia that, as described previously, are not responsive to cortisol feedback.[16] The most commonly used protocol for dexamethasone suppression is the overnight DST. A baseline blood sample is collected for serum cortisol measurement between 4 to 6 PM, after which dexamethasone is administered (40 μg/kg, IM). Blood samples are collected at 15 and 19 hours (8 AM and noon) after dexamethasone administration. Many clinicians will omit the 15-hour sample and collect only a single suppression cortisol sample at 19 hours postdexamethasone administration. Plasma cortisol concentrations should be less than 1 μg/dl in horses with an intact HPA axis. This test provides simplicity, is inexpensive, and is well accepted by clinicians. Although the test is useful in distinguishing horses with PPID from horses with an apparently functional HPA axis, both false positives and false negatives may occur. False positives are common when horses are tested during the fall. Donaldson et al.[57] reported a false-positive rate of 20% to 40% in healthy ponies and horses, respectively. False-negative test results most commonly are observed in the early course of the disease. Horses with clinical indicators of PPID and normal dexamethasone suppression should be monitored and retested after 4 to 6 months. Although many clinicians are concerned with steroid-induced laminitis results of the DST test, no adverse effects of this test were reported when a large number of horses with PPID were evaluated.[16,49]

Resting Adrenocorticotropic Hormone Concentrations

Increased plasma concentrations of ACTH and POMC-derived peptides have been reported in horses with PPID.* Couetil, Paradis, and Knoll[21] found that horses and ponies with PPID had significantly higher resting plasma concentrations of ACTH when compared with healthy horses and ponies. In this study, plasma ACTH concentrations for the diagnosis of PPID had a sensitivity of 90.9% in horses, 81.8% in ponies, and a specificity of 100% using dexamethasone suppression as the gold standard.[21] Other studies have reported false-positive and false-negative results.[34] Determination of resting ACTH concentrations is a good alternative when the results of the DST are nondiagnostic or when the DST is contraindicated. When determining baseline ACTH concentrations it is important to consider that stressful conditions may increase ACTH plasma concentrations. In addition, plasma ACTH concentrations are higher in the fall. In one study, greater than 90% of healthy animals with normal ACTH concentrations in May had concentrations above the laboratory normal reference range when tested in September and would be falsely considered positive for PPID.[57] Blood samples to determine ACTH concentrations should be collected in cold EDTA tubes, kept at 4° C, centrifuged within 8 hours, and plasma stored frozen until analysis.[21,40]

*References 9, 10, 13, 19, 21, 40, 58.

Adrenocorticotropic Hormone Stimulation Test

The administration of ACTH (1 IU/kg of natural ACTH gel, IM; 25 IU $ACTH_{1-24}$, IV; or 100 IU of synthetic ACTH [Cosyntropin], IV) has been used in different studies with different results.* A horse with PPID is expected to have an exaggerated (at least fourfold) cortisol response to ACTH stimulation, and when an increased response is present in a horse with elevated resting ACTH concentrations, a more accurate diagnosis of PPID can be made.[58] Dybdal et al.[16] failed to detect a statistical difference in cortisol concentrations between control horses and horses with PPID after administration of 1 IU/kg of natural ACTH gel, IM, between 8 and 10 AM, samples being collected in heparinized tubes before, and 2, 4, 8, and 12 hours post-ACTH administration. van der Kolk et al.[19] found a significantly greater increase in cortisol concentrations in horses with PPID after administration of 25 IU of synthetic $ACTH_{1-24}$, IV, at 9 AM, samples being collected in EDTA tubes just before and 2 hours post-ACTH administration. Although the ACTH stimulation test is useful in assessing adrenal gland function or exhaustion, it does not seem to be the test of choice to assess HPA axis function in horses suspected of having PPID. Combining the ACTH stimulation test with the DST failed to improve the tests' performance in distinguishing horses with PPID from control horses.[16]

*References 5, 16, 17, 19, 58, 59.

Thyrotropin-Releasing Hormone Stimulation Test

Beech and Garcia[46] evaluated the effect of TRH administration on plasma cortisol concentrations in healthy horses and in horses with PPID. They found that TRH administration (1 mg, IV) to horses with PPID, in addition to increasing T_3 and T_4 concentrations, also resulted in a significant increase in plasma concentrations of cortisol within 15 minutes post-TRH administration and that cortisol concentrations remained elevated for 90 minutes. No significant increases in plasma cortisol concentrations were present in healthy horses. Eiler et al.[47]

evaluated the TRH stimulation test in two horses suspected of having PPID and three healthy horses; they found that maximal cortisol concentrations overall were not statistically different between groups; however, too few horses were included to make any conclusion. Other studies have found increases in plasma cortisol concentrations after TRH administration to healthy horses.[18,43] TRH has been shown to be a direct releasing factor for equine melanotropes.[43] Therefore the increased cortisol response after TRH administration in horses with PPID is likely a result of greater POMC peptide release secondary to hyperplasia and hypertrophy of the melanotropes of the pars intermedia. Some clinicians have advocated the TRH stimulation test as an alternative method to the DST in horses with laminitis or at greater risk for developing steroid-induced laminitis.

Combined Dexamethasone Suppression Test and Thyrotropin-Releasing Hormone Test

The combination of a DST with the TRH stimulation test was evaluated as a diagnostic method for PPID in 42 horses.[36] After baseline sampling in EDTA-containing tubes, dexamethasone (40 μg/kg, IV) was administered (8 to 10 AM). A second sample was collected 3 hours later, and then TRH (1.1 mg, IV) was administered. Blood samples were collected at 3.5 (30 minutes after TRH administration) and 24 hours after dexamethasone administration. The test was considered positive if cortisol concentration was greater than 1 μg/dl at 24 hours or the 3 hour cortisol concentration increased by greater than or equal to 66% 30 minutes after TRH administration (Figure 20-5). Performance of the test was evaluated using postmortem diagnosis as the gold standard. The TRH component alone had a sensitivity of 41% and a specificity of 92%; the DST alone had a sensitivity of 65% and a specificity of 76%. When considered as a combined test, the sensitivity (88%) and specificity (76%) improved (see Figure 20-5). Based on the results of this study, it seems that the combined DST/TRH test is a promising method for the diagnosis of PPID. Disadvantages include expense and the need for multiple sample collections.

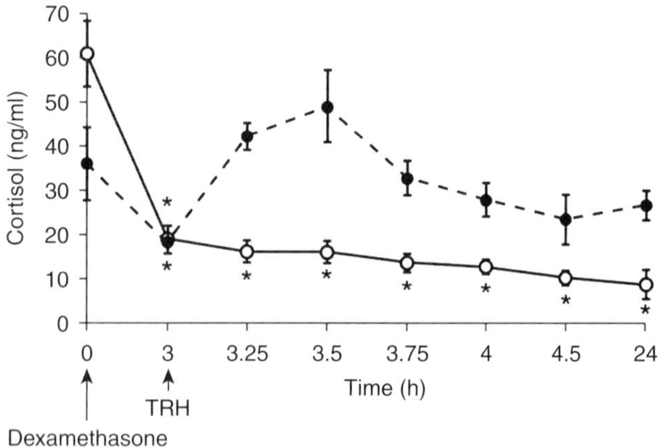

FIGURE 20-5 Combined dexamethasone suppression/thyrotropin-releasing hormone (TRH) stimulation test in healthy horses (n = 7; open circles) and in horses with pituitary pars intermedia dysfunction (PPID) (n = 5; closed circles). Plasma cortisol concentrations decreased 3 hours after dexamethasone administration in both groups; however, TRH administration resulted in a significant increase in cortisol concentrations in horses with PPID but not in healthy horses, and 21 hours after TRH administration cortisol concentrations were still less than baseline in healthy horses but were higher in horses with PPID. *Significant difference from baseline value at time 0. (Adapted from Eiler H, Oliver JW, Andrews FM, et al: *J Am Vet Med Assoc* 211:79–81, 1997.)

Resting Insulin Concentrations

In horses with hyperglycemia, measurement of fasting blood insulin concentrations together with glucose concentrations may be useful. Increased insulin concentration in the presence of persistent hyperglycemia is highly suggestive of IR (reported to occur in approximately 70% of horses with PPID[49]). Other conditions such as EMS and stress are also associated with IR; therefore the presence of IR alone is not diagnostic. Resting glucose and insulin concentrations are reported to have a sensitivity of 58% and 92% for the diagnosis of PPID, respectively.[19] Although IR alone is not diagnostic for PPID, IR does have prognostic value, because horses or ponies with IR are more likely to develop laminitis.[29,60] Therefore measurement of fasting insulin and glucose is recommended in horses suspected of having PPID. If resting insulin and glucose is not diagnostic but IR is suspected, then further tests may be useful to confirm IR, such as the CGIT, the glucose tolerance test, or the insulin tolerance test. Details on the CGIT can be found in the section on Equine Metabolic Syndrome.

Determination of Proopiomelanocortin Peptides

Based on the current knowledge of equine pars intermedia dysfunction, it would be reasonable to determine plasma concentrations of POMC-derived peptides (ACTH, α-MSH, β-END, CLIP) in horses suspected of having PPID. These peptides are increased in horses with PPID.* Determination of POMC-derived peptides in the clinical scenario has been limited to ACTH plasma concentrations, and the use of human immunoassays to determine equine ACTH concentrations has been validated.[21]

Plasma and CSF β-END concentrations are increased severalfold in horses with PPID.[13] Furthermore, pars intermedia POMC peptides (α-MSH, β-END, CLIP) are disproportionally higher when compared with ACTH plasma concentrations in affected horses.[9,10]

Domperidone Response Test

A new test being evaluated for diagnosis of PPID is the domperidone response test.[63] Domperidone is a DA receptor antagonist. In horses with PPID, administration of domperidone is suggested to exacerbate the loss of dopaminergic inhibition and result in release of ACTH from the pars intermedia. In a study of 33 horses, plasma ACTH concentration 8 hours after domperidone administration was positively correlated to histologic PPID severity score and morphometric analysis of pars intermedia size, although not all animals considered

*References 4, 9, 10, 13, 19, 21, 61, 62.

"positive" by histology and domperidone test exhibited clinical signs of disease. In the absence of any clinical signs it is difficult to determine if the relatively mild histologic changes (diffuse pars intermedia hyperplasia) were indicative of early disease or associated with an increased function of the intermediate lobe for other reasons. A greater number of animals will need to be assessed over time to determine the effect of season, disease, and other physiologic events on pituitary histology and pars intermedia domperidone response. Despite this, early indications suggest the domperidone response test warrants further study.

Radiographic Methods

Computed tomography has been used to diagnose PPID in horses, although measurements of the pituitary by this method have poor accuracy.[64-65] Levy, Blevins, and Janovitz[66] used ventral radiography and contrast venography to diagnose PPID in horses and ponies. Magnetic resonance imaging (MRI) is the preferred diagnostic imaging modality in human pituitary disease; however, no studies document the usefulness of MRI in diagnosis of PPID. A number of horses with PPID and neurologic signs had pituitary enlargement on MRI.[67] Although available to equine clinicians, these methods are far from being practical in the diagnosis of PPID; they require anesthesia and expensive equipment and are not cost-effective when compared with other diagnostic methods.

Treatment

Optimal treatment of PPID includes a combination of management and pharmaceutical interventions. PPID is observed primarily in older horses; therefore it is important to treat the dysfunctional HPA axis, as well as many of the pathologic conditions associated with aging. Special attention should be given to providing optimal management, including high-quality feed, dental care, deworming, and farrier care. It is also important to pay particular attention to the skin and hair coat. Many horses cannot properly shed their winter coats and as a result may develop hyperthermia. In addition, horses with PPID are prone to skin infections. The most difficult complication to manage is laminitis, which may be complicated by overfeeding of high-energy hay, grass, or grain. Therefore reducing the amount of soluble carbohydrates is advisable. In addition, in mildly affected horses exercise is recommended. Because of the insidious nature of the laminitis observed in horses with endocrinopathies, close monitoring of hoof growth and freedom of movement is desirable in all aged horses. Periodic radiographic assessment of the feet in horses at risk of PPID may be prudent.

As discussed earlier in this section, the regulation of POMC peptide synthesis and secretion is under the influence of the hypothalamic periventricular dopaminergic systems. Regulation of POMC synthesis and secretion by the pars intermedia of horses with PPID is under similar control as the pars intermedia from unaffected horses and other species.[9] Based on this information, the medical treatment of PPID involves the use of DA agonists or serotonin antagonists.

Bromocriptine and pergolide are the two most commonly used DA D_2-receptor agonists.[15,25,27,40,68-71] Bromocriptine can be given either orally or by subcutaneous injection (0.03-0.09 mg/kg/b.i.d.),[9,68,72] but its use in treatment of PPID is limited. Oral pergolide is widely used and has been shown to be beneficial in the treatment of horses and ponies with PPID, with lifelong treatment recommended.[25,27,40,49] Doses of pergolide from 0.2 mg up to 5 mg/horse per day, once a day, or divided twice daily have been used in ponies and horses, with treatment durations of greater than 5 years. Treatment typically should start with a total daily dose of 1.0 mg/day; if no clinical evidence of improvement is noted by 4 to 6 weeks, the dose should be increased gradually every 3 to 4 weeks by 0.5 mg.[23] Success of treatment should be assessed by both documenting improvement of clinical signs and normalization of either DST or plasma ACTH concentration. Most horses show improvement within 6 to 8 weeks of treatment with doses of 1.0 to 2.0 mg of pergolide per day. Failure to respond to pergolide treatment may occur in very advanced disease, if a poor-quality drug is obtained from a compounding pharmacy, or if the drug is not consumed completely by the patient; this may also indicate an incorrect diagnosis. Periodic reassessments of DST or ACTH are recommended as the dose required to control disease may change over time.[25] Some horses treated with pergolide may develop anorexia, which typically resolves by reducing the dose.[23] Although long-term pergolide therapy has been associated with fibrotic cardiac valvular lesions in human beings,[73] similar lesions have not been reported in horses.

A second drug suggested to be useful in treatment of PPID is cyproheptadine, although horses treated with pergolide show a better response than horses treated with cyproheptadine.[23,25,27] Cyproheptadine is a nonselective 5-hydroxytryptamine receptor blocking agent (serotonin antagonist) that reduces ACTH and β-END secretion from ACTH-producing tumors in human beings.[74] Limited information exists on serotonin functions in the hypothalamus and pituitary gland of the horse, and no difference in serotonin concentration was found between the pars intermedia of horses with PPID and control horses.[13] Serotonin is also a histamine receptor (H_1) antagonist with weak anticholinergic activity. Serotonin inhibits the release of prolactin from anterior pituitary cells in a nonserotonin receptor–dependent fashion by blocking calcium influx at the cell membrane.[75] Cyproheptadine has been used for many years to treat horses with PPID with variable results. It is estimated that one third of horses with PPID show improvement when treated with cyproheptadine.[23,27] This drug is recommended at 0.25 mg/kg, orally, once a day for 4 to 8 weeks.[23] If no clinical evidence exists of improvement and no reduction in plasma ACTH concentrations, then the dosage frequency should be increased to twice a day for 1 month, at which time ACTH concentrations should be determined or the DST repeated. In horses that fail to respond to high doses of cyproheptadine, switching to pergolide is recommended. A combination of cyproheptadine and pergolide has been suggested for horses that do not respond well to either drug alone.

Alternative therapeutic compounds have been suggested to treat horses with PPID. Aqueous extracts of *Vitex agnus-castus* (chasteberry, chaste tree, Evitex formally known as *Hormonise*) have been used to treat horses with PPID. *Vitex agnus-castus* extracts contain compounds (diterpenoids) that stimulate DA D_2-receptor activity and inhibit different opioid receptors.[76] Because of its dopaminergic effects, *Vitex agnus-castus* has been recommended as an alternative phytotherapeutic agent in the treatment of hyperprolactinemia and premenstrual syndrome in women.[77] In a blinded study there was no clinical improvement or improvement in diagnostic test results in

14 PPID-affected horses treated with *Vitex agnus-castus* extract.[78] Therefore although physiologic and pharmacologic rationale support the possible use of these extracts to increase dopaminergic activity in the equine pituitary, currently no evidence exists to recommend *Vitex agnus-castus* to treat horses with PPID.

Trilostane is an enzymatic inhibitor of 3β-hydroxysteroid dehydrogenase, an important enzyme in steroid synthesis. However, little information exists regarding the effects of trilostane in the equine steroid metabolism.[79] Trilostane has been proposed for the treatment of PPID, as well as in the treatment of EMS.[60,80] In a study of 20 horses or ponies treated over 1 to 2 years, improvement in clinical signs other than hirsutism was recorded; however, DST remained unimproved, suggesting an insufficient response to the drug.[80] Until the mid-1980s trilostane was recommended to treat Cushing's disease in human beings; however, because of its lack of potency in blocking cortisol synthesis, trilostane is no longer recommended to treat this condition.[81] In horses with PPID only a minority have evidence of adrenal hyperplasia; therefore treatments directed at restoring pars intermedia function and limiting expansion of the pituitary mass may be more appropriate than those that target cortisol synthesis inhibition.

PITUITARY INDEPENDENT CUSHING'S SYNDROME

Primary adrenocortical tumors are rare in horses,[5,72,82,83] and the few cases reported in the literature were nonfunctional tumors. Only one case of a functional adrenocortical tumor associated with clinical signs consistent with Cushing's disease has been reported.[72] A 12-year-old Dutch Warmblood gelding had a history of polyphagia, polydipsia, reduced muscle mass, hyperhydrosis, lethargy, and delayed shedding of the hair coat. The horse had persistent hyperglycemic and normal adrenocortical response to ACTH stimulation. After unsuccessful treatment with bromocriptine, the horse was euthanized and a unilateral adrenocortical adenoma was found.

ECTOPIC CUSHING'S SYNDROME

In human beings and small animals, Cushing's disease results from excessive secretion of ACTH from the pituitary gland, ectopic secretion of ACTH by nonpituitary tumors, ectopic secretion of CRH, or excessive and autonomous secretion of cortisol from adrenocortical tumors. The secretion of ACTH or CRH from nonpituitary tumors results in a condition known as *ectopic Cushing's syndrome* or *ectopic ACTH syndrome*. Ectopic production of ACTH or CRH has not been demonstrated in the horse.

INSULIN RESISTANCE AND EQUINE METABOLIC SYNDROME

Nicholas Frank

The two most common endocrine disorders affecting horses are PPID (also called *equine Cushing's disease*) and EMS. In general, PPID affects older horses, whereas EMS first develops in young and middle-aged animals. Many horses with EMS exhibit a predisposition toward obesity that first becomes evident when they reach maturity, and this problem is often exacerbated by environmental conditions that promote weight gain. IR is a key feature of EMS—and the reason for describing the condition as an *endocrine disorder*. However, IR also occurs in a subset of patients with PPID, so this can lead to confusion. For the following discussion, the author will consider EMS to be defined by the presence of IR that cannot be attributed to PPID (resulting instead from the metabolic condition of the animal). Laminitis is the most important clinical feature of EMS, and early recognition of this syndrome can lead to prevention of this painful disease.

DEFINITIONS

IR refers to the failure of tissues to respond normally to insulin. Skeletal muscle and adipose tissues are affected because they are two important sites for insulin-mediated glucose disposal. The liver also responds to insulin. Gluconeogenesis is inhibited and glycogen synthesis promoted as blood insulin levels rise after feeding. Up to 50% of the insulin secreted by the pancreas is cleared by the liver as blood circulates through this organ before entering the systemic circulation.[1] Hyperinsulinemia may therefore reflect increased production or reduced clearance of insulin.

Compensated IR is a term used when hyperinsulinemia is detected in an animal with reduced insulin sensitivity.[2] Insulin secretion from the pancreas increases to compensate for reduced tissue sensitivity and euglycemia is maintained. However, recent results from the author's laboratory show that resting hyperinsulinemia cannot be attributed to increased insulin secretion in all cases, which suggests that insulin clearance may be affected in some animals.

Uncompensated IR refers to reduced insulin sensitivity with hyperglycemia. Insulin concentrations may be elevated or within reference range, and it is assumed that uncompensated IR develops as a result of pancreatic insufficiency. Compensated IR is the most common form of IR in horses and ponies, but uncompensated IR should be considered when elevated blood glucose concentrations are detected. It is appropriate to use the term *type 2 DM* when hyperglycemia and glucosuria are present, and clinicians have recognized this condition in a few cases.

EMS is a term used to define a clinical syndrome recognized in horses. This is a controversial term because metabolic syndrome in human beings is a collection of risk factors used to predict the likelihood of coronary heart disease.[3] Critics therefore argue that the use of this term in equine medicine is inappropriate, because atherosclerosis and cardiac disease are not detected in affected horses. However, proponents of the term point out that herbivores are unlikely to develop atherosclerosis and laminitis is the manifestation of vascular disease seen in horses. This controversy can be resolved by accepting that EMS differs from the syndrome described in human beings.

EMS is characterized by (1) obesity or regional adiposity, (2) IR, and (3) subclinical or clinical laminitis.[4] Hypertriglyceridemia has also been associated with EMS, and blood leptin concentrations are often elevated in affected animals.[5,6] Leptin is a hormone released by adipose tissues that signals the hypothalamus to suppress appetite after feed consumption. Plasma leptin concentrations generally correlate with body condition score (BCS). However, elevated levels are sometimes detected in leaner horses, and this suggests a state of energy metabolism dysregulation.[5,7] Studies have been performed to compare horses with low- or high-plasma leptin concentrations, and a cutoff value of 7 ng/ml has been used to define groups.[8] Hypertension has also been associated with laminitis and IR in ponies kept on pasture.[9] Mean arterial blood pressure (ABP) was higher in laminitis-prone ponies when measured in the summer but did not differ from control ponies in the winter.

Obesity is defined as an increase in body weight as a result of excessive fat accumulation within the body. When the BCS system developed by Henneke et al.[10] is applied, obesity is defined by a BCS greater than or equal to 7 on at a 1 (poor) to 9 (extremely fat) scale. Obesity and IR are associated in horses and ponies.[5,11] It must be recognized, however, that body condition scoring systems are sometimes inadequate for assessing horses with endocrine disorders. Some horses with EMS and many with PPID are thin across the ribs, yet have pronounced adipose tissue deposits in the neck and tailhead regions. This accumulation of adipose tissue at specific locations is referred to as *regional adiposity*.

Laminitis is the most important component of EMS because of its negative effect on the welfare of the patient. It is the development of laminitis that often prompts the owner to seek veterinary attention for the horse, and this condition presents the greatest challenge with respect to management. Subclinical laminitis takes the form of divergent growth rings (also called *founder lines*) on the hooves or radiographic evidence of third phalanx rotation or sinking. This is sometimes referred to as *endocrinopathic laminitis* because of its association with EMS and PPID. The term *prelaminitic metabolic syndrome* has also been used to describe ponies that are at higher risk for developing pasture-associated laminitis because of IR.[6]

ROLE OF GENETICS

Genetic predisposition plays an important role in the development of obesity and IR in horses. Ponies tend to be more insulin resistant than horses,[11] and certain breeds and genetic lines of horses appear to more predisposed to obesity and IR.[4,5] Obesity can develop in horses of all breeds, but this problem is most common in Morgan horses, Paso Finos, Arabians, Saddlebreds, Quarter Horses, and Tennessee Walking Horses. Horses that are predisposed to obesity are sometimes referred to as *easy keepers* because they require fewer calories to maintain body weight.

Most horses or ponies with EMS are obese, and this syndrome begins with a genetic predisposition that affects metabolic efficiency. Affected animals seem to require fewer calories to maintain body weight and have an enhanced appetite. Owners often report that the horse spends more time grazing when turned out on pasture. The easy keeper concept is relevant to the issue of genetic susceptibility. Certain breeds or genetic lines may have undergone evolutionary adaptations to survive harsher environments, and these horses or ponies may be more efficient at converting poorer-quality forages into energy. Lack of exercise is also likely to play a role in the development of EMS because exercise increases insulin sensitivity.[12,13]

Genetics and environment interact when affected horses are given free access to pasture, particularly when a small number of animals are grazing on a large area. Carbohydrate intake on pasture is influenced by grazing time, the area grazed, geographic location, climate, soil quality, and season.[14] In many regions of the country, pasture grass is abundant and rich in nutrients. This is accentuated when certain types of grass are sown to improve pastures for cattle or when fertilizers are used. A second point of interaction occurs when susceptible horses are fed grain. This is unnecessary for metabolically efficient animals and promotes obesity and IR. Unfortunately, many horse owners feed grain to bring their horses in from pasture or because they perceive that their horses are unhappy if they are kept on a hay-only diet. It is a common mistake to feed grain to horses that are able to maintain their body condition on pasture or hay alone. Horses can also be overfed if they are fed as a group or if grain is used as a reward. Some horse owners deliberately feed their horses too much because they prefer a higher BCS, and these biases are sometimes reflected in the judging at horse shows. Other horse owners simply fail to recognize that obesity has developed in the animal.

Finally, human beings interfere with an important interaction between genetics and environment by feeding horses more grain in the winter to prevent weight loss. Seasonal weight loss is a natural occurrence in wild horses and is likely to correct problems with obesity that have developed during other times of the year.

CLINICAL SIGNS AND DIFFERENTIAL DIAGNOSES

Obesity is detected on physical examination of the horse and application of a BCS system. A horse suffering from EMS is shown in Figure 20-6. Regional adiposity is commonly detected in IR horses, and mean neck circumference has been negatively correlated with insulin sensitivity in obese horses with IR.[5] Neck circumference can be measured with a tape measure. One can make these measurements by dividing the distance along a line from the poll to the cranial aspect of the withers (x) by four and measuring the circumference of the neck at three equidistant points ($0.25x$, $0.50x$, and $0.75x$). Expansion of adipose tissues within the neck is commonly referred to as a *cresty neck* and, with the exception of stallions, this finding is suggestive of IR in horses.[5]

Enlarged fat deposits may also be found close to the tailhead or appear as randomly distributed subcutaneous swellings. Geldings are sometimes presented for evaluation of preputial swelling, and mares may show enlargement of the

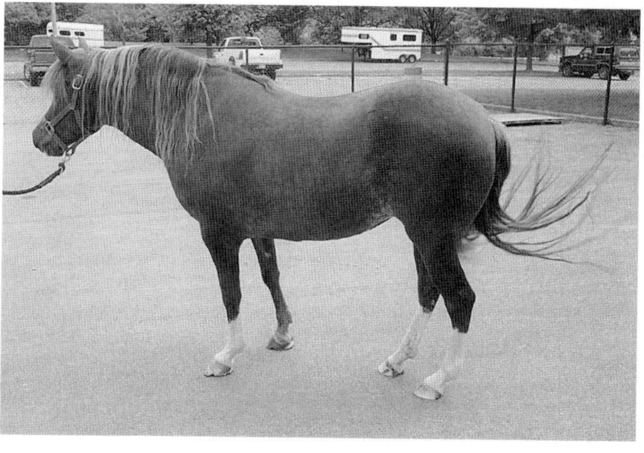

FIGURE 20-6 Photograph of a 7-year-old Morgan horse mixed breed mare that suffers from equine metabolic syndrome (EMS).

mammary glands. Both of these problems are related to adipose tissue accumulation, which can interfere with lymphatic return in these regions. Affected horses develop edema in these areas when they are left standing in a stall for too long; this problem improves with exercise. Supraorbital fat accumulation is also a frequent finding. EMS is sometimes recognized when horses develop other medical problems, including colic, hyperlipemia, and reproductive issues. The author has observed that horses with EMS develop pedunculated lipomas at a younger age, presumably because of additional fat surrounding the abdominal viscera. Obesity has also been associated with abnormal reproductive cycling in mares.[15]

Regional adiposity is a feature of EMS, but it must be recognized that fat redistribution is also seen in older horses with PPID. It is therefore necessary to examine the patient for clinical signs of PPID, including delayed hair coat shedding, hirsutism, loss of skeletal muscle mass, polyuria, polydipsia, or increased caloric demand.[16] Testing for PPID is recommended in middle-aged horses with EMS because these conditions overlap in some patients. Affected horses can enter a *transition state* when PPID develops in an animal with EMS. Delayed hair coat shedding is often the first sign of this transition, and owners should be advised to watch for this change. It is also hypothesized that horses with EMS are at greater risk for developing PPID at an earlier age, so treatment for pituitary dysfunction should be considered in middle-aged (10 to 20 years old) horses if clinical signs are recognized.

Horses with EMS commonly suffer from laminitis, which is recognized when lameness is detected or hoof testers are applied to the feet. Some horses are not lame on physical examination but have radiographic evidence of third phalanx rotation or sinking. Laminitis often first develops after the horse has been grazing on pasture grass that is rich in sugars and starches. This happens at times of the year when grass is abundant and growing rapidly or when responding to cooler temperatures in the fall. Owners of horses with recurrent laminitis also report that laminitis episodes occur after changes in season or with the onset of cold weather.

PATHOLOGY

Complete blood count and serum biochemical analysis results are usually unremarkable, with the exception of plasma glucose concentrations, which are discussed following. Hyperglycemia is more commonly associated with PPID and may be accompanied by mature neutrophilia and lymphopenia. Elevated serum triglyceride concentrations are sometimes detected in ponies[6] or horses[5] with obesity and IR, but this finding is inconsistent in horses with EMS. Mildly elevated GGT activity has been recognized in a small number of horses with chronic EMS; this may be a result of hepatic lipidosis.

Low resting total triiodothyronine (tT_3) and total thyroxine (tT_4) concentrations are sometimes detected in horses with EMS, but the significance of this finding has been overstated in the past. It is a common misconception that obese horses suffer from hypothyroidism because obesity is associated with hypothyroidism in dogs and human beings. However, serum TH concentrations rise appropriately when IV TRH is administered,[17] indicating that the HPT axis is functioning normally in these patients. It is therefore likely that low serum thyroid concentrations simply reflect responses to extrathyroidal changes in metabolism. Breuhaus et al.[18] detected markedly lower serum tT_4 and free thyroxine concentrations in horses with systemic illness. Phenylbutazone also significantly lowers serum tT_4 concentrations in horses,[19] and this drug is commonly used to treat laminitis in horses with EMS.

DIAGNOSTIC TESTING

The ease of testing procedures must be considered when diagnostic tests for IR are selected. Two tests for IR can be used in clinical practice: (1) resting blood measures and (2) the CGIT. The first procedure is straightforward because it is based on a single blood sample, whereas the CGIT is more involved and is therefore reserved for more challenging cases.

Resting Blood Measures

Currently clinicians use a measurement of blood insulin and glucose concentrations to diagnose IR in horses (Table 20-3), but it is hoped that a panel of tests for EMS will be developed in the future. Components of this panel might include connecting peptide (C-peptide), leptin, and adiponectin, as well as metabolites such as triglycerides and nonesterified fatty acids. Plasma triglyceride concentrations are currently available and can be requested as part of a plasma biochemistry analysis. Practitioners are also advised to measure plasma ACTH concentrations at the same time because EMS and PPID sometimes overlap in middle-aged animals.

RESTING INSULIN CONCENTRATIONS

Two important limitations must be considered when using this test for IR in horses. First, environmental conditions significantly affect results, so care must be taken to collect blood samples under standardized conditions. Second, insulin assays vary between laboratories, so different laboratories yield different results. This does not mean that laboratories are using inaccurate assays; it relates instead to the method used. It is therefore very important to interpret results according to the reference range provided by the laboratory. Clinicians are advised to send samples to a single laboratory and to select one that routinely handles equine serum or plasma. An insulin concentration above the reference range (for horses) provided by the laboratory defines hyperinsulinemia and therefore IR. In the author's laboratory, a resting insulin concentration greater than 20 μU/ml defines IR if the horse has been deprived of feed for approximately 6 hours before sample collection. If hay has been fed, then a cutoff value of 30 μU/ml can be used to define IR, but it is advisable to recheck the patient after feed deprivation. Note that some laboratories report insulin concentrations in pmol/L, and an approximate conversion factor of 7 is used to convert units from μU/ml to pmol/L (i.e., 30 μU/ml is approximately equal to 210 pmol/L).

Environmental conditions affect insulin concentrations. Stress raises insulin concentrations in horses because cortisol and epinephrine are released and these hormones induce IR. Glucose and insulin concentrations are therefore higher in a stressed animal, which increases the likelihood of hyperinsulinemia being detected. One of the most common confounding factors affecting results is laminitis because horses that are painful at the time of testing have higher insulin concentrations. It is therefore strongly recommended that testing be delayed until after the pain of laminitis has subsided. Housing and feeding conditions also affect insulin concentrations. Some recent results from the author's laboratory indicate that insulin sensitivity decreases when horses that have

TABLE 20-3

Guidelines for Interpreting Resting Glucose and Insulin Concentrations in Blood Samples Collected After Feed Deprivation

Glucose (mg/dl)	Insulin (μU/ml)	Interpretation*
<100	< 20 (Hay: <30)	No evidence of insulin resistance (IR) at this time Retest at another time of the year or perform the combined glucose-insulin test (CGIT) if equine metabolic syndrome (EMS) phenotype is recognized Address any problems with obesity
<100	>20	Normoglycemia with hyperinsulinemia Horse suffers from compensated IR; an increased risk of laminitis exists Recommend weight management plan, diet changes, and exercise
<100	>100	Normoglycemia with marked hyperinsulinemia Severe compensated IR; high risk of laminitis Strictly control diet and consider pharmacological intervention
>100	>20	Horse losing its ability to regulate glucose because pancreatic insufficiency is developing Transitioning from compensated to uncompensated IR; high risk of laminitis Test for pituitary pars intermedia dysfunction (PPID)
>120	<20	Glucose levels unregulated and pancreatic insufficiency has developed Horse suffers from uncompensated IR; high risk of laminitis Check urine glucose for evidence of diabetes mellitus and test for PPID

*Patient is not in pain or stressed; all feed withheld for 6 hours before sampling.

been housed on pasture in a herd are moved into the hospital. Horses are stressed by this change of environment, and insulin concentrations are higher in animals experiencing this transition. A patient that develops laminitis when grazing on pasture may experience this transition when it is moved into a stall to limit exercise.

Feeding conditions also affect insulin concentrations, and several issues must be considered before determining the sampling conditions for each patient. The author and colleagues have previously recommended that horses be fed hay the night before testing. This protocol was adopted after it was observed that horses with EMS became agitated when deprived of feed, resulting in stress-induced IR. However, results of a recent study revealed that horses with hyperinsulinemia had lower insulin concentrations when deprived of feed overnight. This suggests that hay, as well as pasture and grain, raises insulin concentrations in insulin-resistant horses. It is therefore the current recommendation to withhold all feed for approximately 6 hours before sample collection. One strategy is to leave a single flake of hay with the horse late at night and then delay the morning feeding until after the blood sample has been drawn. Unfortunately, some horses still become agitated when deprived of hay, and risks must be balanced in these cases. Owners can be asked to acclimatize their horses to feed deprivation by withholding hay on several occasions beforehand, or hay can be fed to these particular animals.

RESTING GLUCOSE CONCENTRATIONS

Most insulin-resistant horses maintain blood glucose concentrations within the reference ranges provided by laboratories because they are in a state of compensated IR. However, glucose concentrations tend to be toward the high end of reference range, and affected horses are likely to have exaggerated blood glucose responses to high-sugar feeds. It is therefore important to deprive horses of feed (preferred approach) for 6 hours or to feed only hay the night before blood collection. The reference range for glucose provided by the University of Tennessee Clinical Pathology Laboratory is 75 to 117 mg/dl, but feeding conditions were not controlled when this range was established. Therefore one should expect blood glucose concentrations to be below 100 mg/dl (5.5 mmol/L) in healthy horses if samples have been collected after feed deprivation, unless the animal is stressed at the time of blood collection. A blood glucose concentration above 120 mg/dl (6.5 mmol/L) indicates marked hyperglycemia. Glucose concentrations reported in mmol/L must be multiplied by 18 to convert to mg/dl.

It is important to measure blood glucose concentrations. A problem with only examining resting insulin concentrations is that horses with uncompensated IR or DM will escape detection. Insulin concentrations can return to reference range in these patients as insulin secretion decreases because of pancreatic insufficiency. However, blood glucose concentrations increase as a consequence of IR and reduced insulin output, so patients can be identified by the presence of hyperglycemia and sometimes glucosuria.

GLUCOSE/INSULIN RATIO

The glucose/insulin (G:I) ratio is calculated by dividing the glucose concentration in mg/dl by the insulin concentration in μU/ml (or mU/L). The correct units must be used, so insulin concentrations reported in pmol/L must be divided by 7 to provide values in μU/ml. Proponents of this test consider a ratio below 10 to be indicative of IR and refer to horses with ratios less than 4.5 as severely insulin resistant or decompensated. If one assumes a glucose concentration of 90 mg/dl, then these cutoff values are equivalent to serum insulin concentrations of 9 and 20 μU/ml, respectively.

The G:I ratio is not recommended because the values listed previously fall within the reference range for insulin in horses. Ratios below 10 are commonly detected in the author's clinic's herd of healthy Quarter Horse and Tennessee Walking Horse mares, and some fall below 4.5. Use of the G:I ratio therefore leads to the overdiagnosis of IR in horses. One other important limitation of the G:I ratio is that insulin results differ between laboratories, depending on the testing procedure used. However, most laboratories use the same colorimetric assay to measure glucose, so these results are more consistent. When resting insulin concentrations are interpreted independently, the reference range for the laboratory can be used to account for differences in methodology. However, this flexibility does not exist for the G:I ratio because set cutoff values have been established. It is therefore conceivable that insulin results from one laboratory will cause the ratio to be low, whereas results from another laboratory will give a ratio that falls within acceptable range.

It should also be noted that glucose concentrations decrease in blood samples if any delay exists between collection and centrifugation. Finally, a horse with uncompensated IR or DM will have a high glucose concentration with a low insulin concentration; this may result in a G:I ratio that exceeds 10 and will therefore be considered normal.

PROXY MEASUREMENTS

These values can be calculated from blood glucose and insulin concentrations to predict the risk of IR. The two proxies used are (1) the *reciprocal of the square root of insulin* (*RISQI*) and (2) the *modified insulin/glucose ratio* (*MIRG*).[2] The RISQI represents the degree of insulin sensitivity (a low number indicates IR) and the MIRG represents the ability of the pancreas to secrete insulin (most horses with IR have higher values). The RISQI value is more important and can be easily calculated. To do this, 1 is divided by the square root of the insulin concentration to obtain the RISQI value. A RISQI less than 0.29 indicates IR, which is equivalent to a serum insulin concentration of 12 μU/ml. However, this method of diagnosing IR is not recommended because values were established for a specific group of animals with the insulin assay used by the research laboratory. In the experience of the author and colleagues, a cutoff value of 12 μU/ml is too low and leads to the overdiagnosis of IR.

Combined Glucose-Insulin Test

This is a useful test that is likely more sensitive than resting glucose and insulin measurements.[5] Clinicians are therefore advised to consider this test when treating a horse or pony that exhibits the EMS phenotype but has resting glucose and insulin concentrations that fall within reference ranges. These patients may suffer from mild IR that gets worse at certain times of the year in response to changes in season, diet, or both. For instance, resting measures may be normal in a horse that is consuming hay in February, yet the same animal might develop pronounced IR in the summer when grazing on pasture. Two approaches can be taken in these situations. Resting insulin and glucose concentrations can be rechecked at another time of the year, or the CGIT can be performed on the same day to diagnose IR.

Stress induces false-positive results when the CGIT is used, so testing must be delayed until after laminitis has improved.[20] If testing is performed in a referral hospital, then it is advisable to give the patient several days to acclimate to the surroundings and place an IV catheter the night before testing. However, testing can also be performed on the farm, with the catheter inserted the same day if the horse remains calm throughout the procedure. Horses should be kept off pasture, and hay should be withheld for approximately 6 hours before the procedure. Sedatives such as xylazine can induce IR, so they should not be given within 12 hours of testing.[21]

A preinfusion blood sample is collected for baseline glucose and insulin measurements, and then 150 mg/kg of body weight 50% dextrose solution is infused IV, immediately followed by 0.10 U/kg of body weight of regular insulin (Humulin R; Eli Lilly, Indianapolis, Ind.) via the same route.[20] These dosages are equivalent to 150 ml of 500 mg/ml (50%) dextrose and 0.50 ml of 100 U/ml regular insulin for a horse weighing 500 kg. Insulin should be drawn into a tuberculin syringe and then transferred to a larger syringe containing 1.5-ml sterile saline (0.9% NaCl) before infusion. Blood glucose concentrations are measured using a handheld glucometer at 1, 5, 15, 25, 35, 45, 60, 75, 90, 105, 120, 135, and 150 minutes postinfusion. A blood sample is collected at 45 minutes and submitted for the second insulin measurement. The test can be shortened to 60 minutes when used in the field, but it is advisable to collect all of the measurements if IR is detected so that the response time can be recorded for future comparisons. Two 60-ml syringes containing 50% dextrose solution should be prepared in case clinical signs of hypoglycemia (sweating, weakness) are seen or if the glucose concentration drops below 40 mg/dl (2.2 mmol/L).

A handheld glucometer is used for this procedure and can be purchased at a drug store. The author's research group uses a Medisense Precision QID glucometer (Abbott Laboratories, Inc) that costs approximately $65. However, the AlphaTRAK (Abbott Laboratories, Inc., Princeton, N.J.) glucometer is now available for veterinary use. The start-up kit for this glucometer costs approximately $180. (NOTE: Products and manufacturers are accurate as of 2009.)

IR is diagnosed when either the glucose or insulin response is abnormal during the CGIT. For the glucose response, IR is defined by blood glucose concentrations remaining above the baseline (preinjection) value for 45 minutes or longer (Figure 20-7). The insulin response is evaluated by measuring insulin concentrations at 0 (preinjection) and 45 minutes. Resting

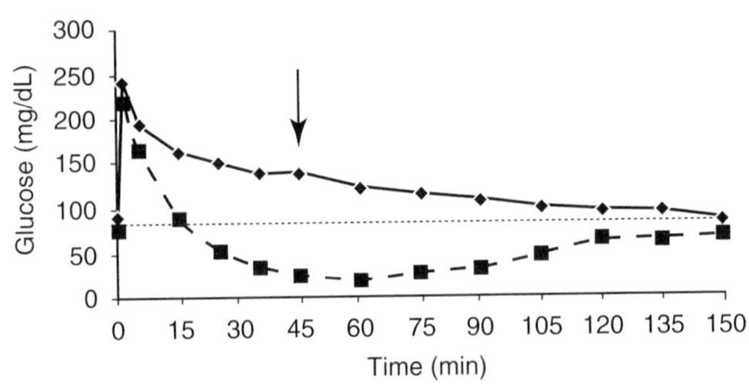

FIGURE 20-7 Blood glucose concentrations during the combined glucose-insulin test (CGIT) in a healthy nonobese mixed breed horse (*dashed line*) and an obese insulin resistant Morgan horse mare (*solid line*). The horizontal line represents the approximate baseline plasma glucose concentration, and the arrow indicates the time point (45 minutes postinjection) selected to define insulin resistance (IR) when the CGIT is used. Blood concentrations remain above the baseline value for 45 minutes or longer if the horse is insulin resistant.

hyperinsulinemia (>30 μU/ml) or detection of a serum or plasma insulin concentration above 100 μU/ml at 45 minutes indicates IR.

PATHOPHYSIOLOGY

Obese Horses with Equine Metabolic Syndrome

Relationships between obesity and IR are complex. It should be remembered that *not all obese horses are insulin resistant and IR is not always accompanied by obesity.*[6,15] However, these conditions are associated, and evidence indicates that IR predisposes ponies to laminitis.[6]

Adipose tissues expand as obesity develops through an increase in adipocyte size (hypertrophy), number (hyperplasia), or both. This is manifested as generalized obesity or regional adiposity, and either can be accompanied by IR. In horses, regional adiposity increases the size of adipose tissues within the nuchal crest, and neck circumference has been negatively correlated with insulin sensitivity in obese insulin-resistant horses.[5] Fat thickness over the rump has also been used as a measure of body fat mass in horses,[22] and some horses develop enlarged fat pads in this area.

Horses that are evolutionarily adapted to sparse forages and harsher conditions may be predisposed to obesity because lipid accumulates more readily when excessive calories are provided in the diet. This state of overnutrition is often induced when genetically predisposed horses are turned out on pasture. The natural equine diet contains little fat, but excess glucose can be converted into fat via de novo lipogenesis. Fats are used for energy or stored as triglyceride within cells. When the storage capacity of adipose tissues is exceeded, fats are directed toward nonadipose tissues (repartitioning). Skeletal muscle, liver, and pancreatic tissues attempt to use fats by increasing beta oxidation, but lipid can accumulate within these tissues and alter normal cellular functions. This pathophysiologic mechanism is sometimes referred to as *lipotoxicity*.[23]

Reactive oxygen species are also generated as oxidative pathways are upregulated. Oxidant damage contributes to lipotoxicity and lipid-induced programmed cell death (lipoapoptosis). Inflammation accompanies these events, resulting in the release of tumor necrosis factor-α (TNF-α) and interleukin-6 (IL-6) from adipose tissues. Adipocytes release these proinflammatory cytokines that act locally or enter the blood.[24] Hormones and cytokines released from adipose tissues are referred to as *adipokines*. Leptin is an adipokine that is involved in the satiety response within the brain. Obese and insulin-resistant horses often have higher plasma leptin concentrations. In contrast, the release of another adipokine (called *adiponectin*) decreases with obesity and IR, and this may serve as a marker for EMS in the future.[25] IR develops when insulin-sensitive adipose, liver, and skeletal muscle tissues fail to respond normally. Insulin receptors, downstream signaling pathways, and glucose transporters such as GLUT4 are potential sites of dysregulation. More insulin is released from pancreatic β cells to compensate for reduced tissue insulin sensitivity, which results in hyperinsulinemia. Pancreatic insufficiency develops as a result of chronic IR or the effects of lipid accumulation within pancreatic tissues. Uncompensated IR occurs when the pancreas fails to sustain the higher rate of insulin secretion necessary to compensate for reduced tissue insulin sensitivity, and hyperglycemia develops as a consequence.

All of the pieces of the puzzle must be assembled before one can fully understand the relationship between IR and laminitis in horses and ponies. At present, clinicians are limited to the knowledge that IR predisposes ponies to pasture-associated laminitis and that the disease can be experimentally induced by infusing IV insulin over several days.[6,26] Three broad mechanisms exist by which IR and obesity could predispose horses to laminitis: (1) altered blood flow or endothelial cell dysfunction within blood vessels of the foot, (2) impaired nutrient delivery to hoof tissues, or (3) a proinflammatory or pro-oxidative state induced by chronic obesity and IR. These processes are likely to contribute to the lower threshold for laminitis recognized in horses with EMS. Affected horses cannot withstand the laminitis-triggering events that are tolerated by healthy animals.

Lean Horses with Equine Metabolic Syndrome

The current understanding of chronic IR in the lean horse is very limited, but several explanations have been proposed. One explanation is that the liver responds differently to nutrients in affected animals. In one study, ponies with IR showed exaggerated insulin responses to a meal containing fructose, which suggests that the liver responds differently to certain nutrients in horses with EMS, and this may represent *hepatic IR*.[27] Another proposed cause of IR in leaner animals is the increased production of cortisol locally within adipose tissues surrounding the abdominal organs. This is thought to result from increased 11β-hydroxysteroid dehydrogenase 1 (11β-HSD1) activity within visceral adipose tissues, which increases local cortisol production and leads to the development of IR.[4] Johnson[4] referred to this condition as *peripheral Cushing's disease*, but this term is not recommended because it is easily confused with equine Cushing's disease, which results from PPID. Further studies are required to determine the activity of 11β-HSD1 in horses with EMS.

Finally, horses may suffer from pancreatic diseases, including neoplasia, pancreatic insufficiency, or pancreatitis. Horses and ponies with exceptionally high blood insulin level are occasionally encountered, and the presence of an insulinoma or GH-secreting tumor should be considered in these cases (although neither condition has been reported to date in the horse). Type 2 DM has been detected in a small number of horses with hyperglycemia and glucosuria, and pancreatic insufficiency is likely in these cases.[28,29] PPID should be considered when uncompensated IR is detected. Pancreatitis has also been reported in horses and may occur more frequently than previously thought.[30,31]

POSTMORTEM FINDINGS

On necropsy, horses are obese or exhibit regional adiposity and display evidence of laminitis. Hepatic lipidosis has been noted on some pathology reports, but it is unclear whether this simply reflects increased lipid storage or provides evidence of a pathologic process.

MANAGEMENT

Management of IR involves three approaches: (1) reducing the sugar and starch content of the feeds provided to the horse, (2) limiting or eliminating access to pasture until IR improves, and (3) increasing exercise. The first approach involves selection of hay with a lower sugar and starch content, which can be determined by submitting a sample for analysis. Equi-analytical Laboratories (or its partner company Dairy One Forage Laboratory) analyzes hay and provides starch, ethanol-soluble carbohydrate (ESC), and water-soluble carbohydrate (WSC) content. ESCs include simple sugars such as monosaccharides and disaccharides, whereas WSCs include fructans as well. The laboratory can be contacted at 1-877-819-4110 (or www.equi-analytical.com), and testing costs approximately $35 per sample. (Note: Products and manufacturers are accurate as of 2009.)

The nonstructural carbohydrate (NSC) content of the hay should be calculated from the values provided by the laboratory. Unfortunately, researchers disagree about the appropriate method of calculating NSC content. Some think that the WSC must be included, so NSC is calculated by adding WSC and starch values together. However, others argue that only ESC is relevant because fructans are primarily digested in the large intestine and do not therefore contribute to the rise in blood glucose concentrations after a meal. At present, it is recommended that NSC be calculated by adding starch and ESC together, and this level should ideally fall below 10% as fed in the hay. It is important to recognize that the relative importance of NSC intake varies with the severity of IR. Horses with severe IR (resting insulin concentration >100 μU/ml) must be maintained on a stringent diet with a NSC content less than 10%, whereas mildly affected animals can be fed hay with higher levels. If hay has already been purchased and the NSC level is between 10% and 12%, then soaking the hay in cold water for 60 minutes before feeding should lower the sugar content.

Leaner horses with EMS are challenging to manage from a dietary standpoint because more calories must be provided without exacerbating IR. This can be accomplished by feeding one of the commercial low-sugar/low-starch (low-NSC) pelleted feeds that are now available to horse owners. These feeds vary in their NSC content, so the severity of IR must be taken into account before one is selected. It is also better to divide the daily ration into multiple small meals and to feed hay beforehand to slow gastric emptying. These strategies are used to lower the glycemic response to the meal, which is the degree to which blood glucose concentrations rise in response to the feed. Individual horses may respond differently to the same feed, so it is advisable to recheck glucose and insulin concentrations 7 to 14 days after a new diet has been initiated. Severely insulin-resistant horses are particularly difficult to manage and may require individual diet formulation, with the help of a nutritionist. Rinsed and then soaked molasses-free beet pulp can be fed as lower-cost alternative to commercial feeds. This feed has a low glycemic response, yet provides calories through hindgut fermentation and volatile fatty acid production.

Weight loss should be induced in obese horses by restricting the total number of calories consumed. In horses that are being overfed, removal of all concentrates from the diet is often sufficient to achieve the ideal body weight. Total caloric intake should initially be met by feeding hay in amounts equivalent to 1.5% to 2.0% of current body weight (e.g., 18 to 24 lb of hay per day for a 1200-lb horse). If the horse does not lose weight, then the amount fed should be lowered over several weeks to 1.5% of ideal body weight (e.g., 15 lb of hay for an ideal weight of 1000 lb). These strategies are effective for horses kept in stalls or dirt paddocks, but weight loss is more difficult to achieve when horses are grazing on pasture. Strategies for limiting grass consumption on pasture include short (<1 hour) turnout periods; confinement in a small paddock, round pen, or area enclosed with electric fence; or use of a grazing muzzle. Appropriate vitamin and mineral supplements should be provided to horses confined to dirt paddocks or stalls. Pasture access must remain restricted or eliminated until insulin sensitivity has improved because carbohydrates consumed on pasture can trigger gastrointestinal events that lead to laminitis in susceptible horses. Grass is an unregulated source of starch and sugar, so these carbohydrates will continue to exacerbate IR, even when other aspects of the diet have been controlled.

Laminitis must be considered when managing horses with EMS, and horses with recurrent laminitis must be kept off pasture permanently. These patients should be housed in dirt paddocks so that they are able to exercise once hoof structures have stabilized. Mildly affected horses can be returned to pasture if IR can be controlled, but care should be taken to restrict pasture access when the grass is going through dynamic phases, such as rapid growth in the spring or preparation for cold weather in the fall. Measurement of pasture grass NSC content at different times of the day has revealed that grazing in the early morning is likely to be safer for horses with IR, except after a hard frost when grasses accumulate sugars.[32]

TREATMENT

Most horses or ponies with EMS can be effectively managed by lowering the sugar and starch content of the diet, reducing body fat mass if the animal is obese, instituting an exercise program, and limiting or eliminating access to pasture. However, it takes time for these management changes to take effect, so pharmacologic interventions can be considered to accelerate the improvement if the patient suffers from recurrent laminitis. Two options are currently available to clinicians, and each has its advantages and disadvantages. Levothyroxine sodium can be administered to accelerate weight loss and improve insulin sensitivity in obese horses, but its use should be avoided in leaner horses because of the reduction in body weight it produces.[33] Metformin is the other treatment option. This drug improves insulin sensitivity in insulin-resistant horses and ponies without affecting body weight.[34] However, the long-term effects of metformin on insulin sensitivity have not been determined, and the safety of this drug must be evaluated in horses.

Levothyroxine Sodium

Weight loss can be accelerated and insulin sensitivity improved in obese insulin-resistant horses when levothyroxine sodium is administered orally at a dosage of 48 mg (total per 500-kg horse)/day for 3 to 6 months.[33] Smaller ponies and Miniature Horses can be given 24 mg levothyroxine sodium per day for the same time period. Thyro L (Lloyd Inc; Shenandoah, Iowa) is recommended for this purpose, and 1 teaspoon (tsp) of powder provides 12 mg of levothyroxine sodium, so 4 tsp should be administered in the feed or by mouth once daily. When levothyroxine treatment is discontinued, horses should be weaned off the drug by lowering the dose to 24 mg (2 tsp)/day for 2 weeks and then 1 tsp (12 mg)/day for 2 weeks. The benefits of treating horses with levothyroxine at lower doses for longer periods have not been evaluated.

Measured serum tT_4 concentrations are elevated when levothyroxine is administered at a dosage of 48 mg (4 tsp)/day, but levels vary considerably within and between horses. Serum tT4 concentrations often range between 40 and 100 ng/ml in treated horses, indicating that levothyroxine sodium is being given at a supraphysiologic dose.[35] However, clinical signs of hyperthyroidism such as sweating or tachycardia have not been observed in treated horses.[36-38] It is important for horses to be placed on a controlled diet when levothyroxine sodium is administered because clinicians have subjectively observed that feed intake increases in response to treatment. Weight loss is unlikely to occur if the horse is given free access to pasture, and the owner will perceive this as a treatment failure.

Metformin

Metformin is a biguanide drug that enhances the action of insulin within tissues at the postreceptor level and inhibits gluconeogenesis within the liver.[34] This drug has been evaluated as a treatment for IR in horses and it is available as Glucophage (Merck Santé S.A.S.; Darmstadt, Germany), which is distributed in the United States by the Bristol-Myers Squibb Company.[15,34,39] When the effects of metformin on insulin sensitivity were assessed in horses and ponies with IR, a positive response was detected initially without hypoglycemia developing, but long-term results were variable.[34] Metformin was administered at a dosage of 15 mg/kg orally twice daily in the aforementioned study, but the pharmacokinetics of this drug have recently been examined and results suggest that the drug should be given every 8 hours.[40] Further studies are required to assess the safety and efficacy of this treatment for IR.

Numerous other treatments have been proposed for the management of IR in horses, including magnesium supplementation, chromium,[41] clenbuterol,[42] and cinnamon. Each of these therapies may be of some benefit, but further studies are required to establish their efficacy.

DISORDERS OF CALCIUM AND PHOSPHORUS

Ramiro E. Toribio

CALCIUM

Calcium is essential for physiologic processes such as muscle contraction, neuromuscular excitability, blood coagulation, enzyme activation, hormone secretion, cell division, and cell membrane stability.[1] Calcium also regulates processes that result in cell injury and cell death, including free radical production, cytokine release, protease activation, vasoconstriction, and apoptosis. Because of the importance of calcium in normal intracellular and extracellular processes, maintenance of a steady concentration of calcium is extremely important.[2]

Distribution and Physical Properties of Calcium

Calcium has structural and nonstructural functions, and it is found in three main compartments: (1) the skeleton, (2) the soft tissues, and (3) the extracellular fluid. The skeleton contains approximately 99% of the total body calcium as hydroxyapatite crystals. Calcium is a major component of the skeleton, providing support against gravity, protection of vital internal organs (brain, spinal cord, thoracic organs), and a niche for blood-forming elements. The skeleton also acts as a reservoir for calcium. The nonstructural functions are related to calcium as a regulatory ion. The remaining calcium is present in the cell membrane, mitochondria, endoplasmic reticulum (ER) (0.9%), and in the extracellular fluid (0.1%).[1] In blood, virtually all calcium is in plasma. In plasma, calcium exists as a free or ionized form (50% to 55%); bound to proteins (40% to 45%); and complexed to anions such as citrate, bicarbonate, phosphate, and lactate (5% to 10%; Figure 20-8).[1,3] In horses, serum ionized calcium represents 50% to 58% of the total serum calcium concentration.[4-6] Free or ionized calcium (Ca^{2+}) is the biologically active form of calcium. Of the protein-bound calcium, approximately 80% is associated with albumin and 20% with globulins.

Plasma Ca^{2+} binds to anionic proteins (albumin), and its affinity for anionic sites is pH dependent. During acidosis a decreased albumin Ca^{2+} binding occurs from increased H^+ concentrations, increasing Ca^{2+} concentrations, whereas in alkalosis Ca^{2+} concentrations are lower. Total calcium concentrations remain unchanged. Hypoalbuminemia results in total hypocalcemia (pseudohypocalcemia), with Ca^{2+} concentrations remaining within the normal range unless the primary cause of hypoabuminemia is also altering calcium homeostasis (sepsis, gastrointestinal disease). Plasma and serum calcium concentrations are lower in foals than in adult horses.[7]

Intracellular Calcium

Cytosolic Ca^{2+} (Ca^{2+}_i) concentrations are very low (10^{-6} to 10^{-7} *M*) when compared with extracellular Ca^{2+} concentrations (10^{-3} *M*; Box 20-2). This 10,000-fold Ca^{2+} gradient between the extracellular and intracellular fluid makes calcium an important cation in signal transduction. Approximately 95% of Ca^{2+}_i is in the ER and mitochondria (see Figure 20-8). Mechanisms that control changes in Ca^{2+}_i concentrations include Ca^{2+} channels in the plasma membrane (PM), the ER, and the sarcoplasmic reticulum (SR). Some of the mechanisms that remove Ca^{2+}_i from the cytosol include Ca^{2+}-ATPases and Na^+/Ca^{2+} in the PM, ER, and SR. The mitochondria are also important in regulating Ca^{2+}_i by providing energy for active calcium transport and by providing calcium storage.

The release of calcium from intracellular stores depends on messenger-activated channels present in the ER, SR, and mitochondria. For example, by interacting with specific cell membrane receptors, hormones may activate phospholipase C to hydrolyze phosphatidylinositol 4,5-biphosphate to inositol 1,4,5-triphosphate (IP_3) and diacylglycerol. IP_3 is highly diffusible and interacts with IP_3 receptors on the ER and SR, opening calcium channels, and increasing Ca^{2+}_i concentrations. The ryanodine receptors are intracellular calcium channels present in excitable cells (muscle, neurons), and their activation mediates calcium-induced calcium release (CICR) from the SR.

Ca^{2+} channels (slow channels) are slightly permeable to Na^+ and are abundant in cardiac and smooth muscle. Because Ca^{2+} channels are slow, depolarization in smooth muscle cells is slow and Ca^{2+}-dependent. In contrast, Na^+ channels (fast channels) are abundant in skeletal muscle and neurons. During hypocalcemia, fast Na^+ channels open with small changes in the membrane potential; nerve and muscle fibers become very excitable, causing hyperexcitability, muscle fasciculations, and tetany. Ca^{2+} binds to the exterior of the Na^+ channels to increase the depolarization threshold, thus stabilizing

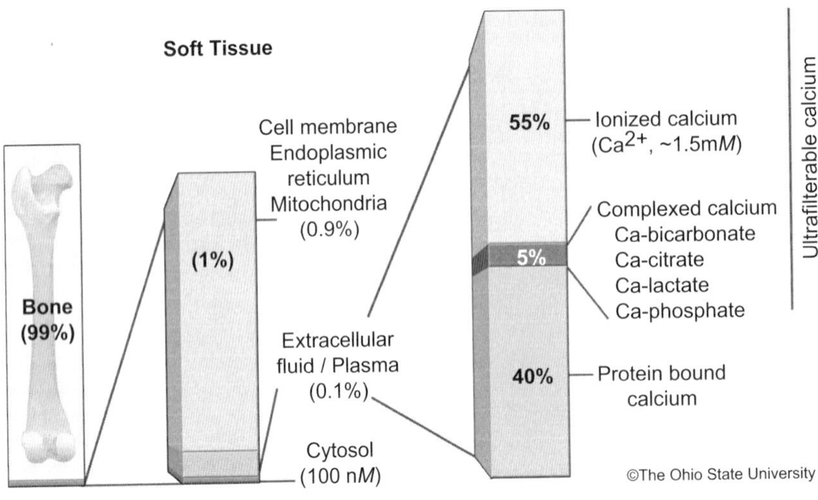

FIGURE 20-8 Calcium distribution in the body. The skeleton contains approximately 99% of the total body calcium. The remaining calcium is present in the cell membrane, mitochondria, endoplasmic reticulum (ER), and in the extracellular fluid. In blood, calcium exists as a free or ionized form (Ca^{2+}), bound to proteins, and complexed to anions such as citrate, bicarbonate, phosphate, and lactate. In horses, serum ionized calcium represent 50% to 58% of the total serum calcium concentration.[4-6] (Courtesy The Ohio State University.)

BOX 20-2

COMMON ABBREVIATIONS ASSOCIATED WITH DISORDERS OF CALCIUM AND PHOSPHORUS

Ca^{2+}_i	Cytosolic Ca^{2+}
PM	Plasma membrane
ER	Endoplasmic reticulum
SR	Sarcoplasmic reticulum
IP_3	Inositol 1,4,5-triphosphate
DOD	Developmental orthopedic disease
PTH	Parathyroid hormone
CT	Calcitonin
PTHrP	Parathyroid hormone-related protein
M-CSF	Macrophage colony-stimulating factor
RANK	Receptor activator of NF-κβ
RANKL	RANK ligand
OPG	Osteoprotegerin
C cells	Parafollicular cells
HHM	Humoral hypercalcemia of malignancy
PHPT	Primary hyperparathyroidism
NSHPT	Nutritional secondary hyperparathyroidism

the cell membrane. This is the mechanism by which Ca^{2+} antagonizes the effects of hyperkalemia.

In skeletal muscle almost all calcium ions required for excitation and contraction come from the SR. In contrast, in the smooth muscle cell the SR is rudimentary, and most of the Ca^{2+} required for contraction comes from the extracellular fluid. This has clinical implications because hypocalcemia may result in ileus.

Coagulation

Ca^{2+} (factor IV) is necessary for the coagulation process to occur. Ca^{2+} is a co-factor for factors II, VII, IX, X, XI, XII, and XIII, and without Ca^{2+} blood clotting does not occur. However, the Ca^{2+} concentration required for coagulation is minimal, and low Ca^{2+} concentrations do not seem to interfere with the clotting process.

Calcium and Phosphorus in the Horse

Requirements

Calcium and phosphorus requirements in horses and ponies depend on the age, physiologic status, and amount of work or exercise performed (Table 20-4). Horses do not have a nutritional drive to meet their calcium needs and are highly dependent on dietary calcium. However, there appears to be a nutritional drive for phosphorus because animals with phosphorus deficiency will eat or lick foreign materials (dirt, rocks, bones) in a condition known as *pica*. Because extracellular Ca^{2+} is under the homeostatic control of several factors, serum Ca^{2+} concentration is not a reliable indicator of dietary calcium intake. An acceptable diet for horses must have 0.15% to 1.5% of calcium in feed dry matter and 0.15% to 0.6% of phosphorus in feed dry matter (Table 20-5). Calcium/phosphorus ratio less than 1:1 may have negative effects on calcium absorption and skeletal development; however, calcium/phosphorus ratio as high as 6:1 for growing horses may not be detrimental if phosphorus intake is adequate.[8] Adult horses should receive approximately 40 mg of calcium/kg/day. These requirements depend on the physiologic status of the animal; pregnant mares require around 50 to 60 g of calcium/day, whereas lactating mares and growing horses may require 50 to 75 g of calcium/day.

The daily calcium requirements in the lactating mare at the onset of lactation are twice maintenance. Mare's milk calcium

TABLE 20-4

Calcium and Phosphorus Requirements in Horses

AGE GROUP	% IN DIET		DAILY (GRAMS)	
	Ca	P	Ca	P
Foals (<6 months)	0.80	0.55	33	20
Weanlings	0.60	0.45	34	25
Yearlings	0.50	0.35	31	22
Two-year-olds	0.40	0.30	25	17
Mares, late pregnancy	0.45	0.30	34	23
Mares, lactation	0.45	0.30	50	34
Mature horses	0.30	0.20	23	14

Adapted from Robinson NE, editor: *Current therapy in equine medicine*, ed 6, St Louis, 2009, WB Saunders.

TABLE 20-5

Acceptable Ranges of Minerals and Vitamins in Feed of Horses

MINERAL	In Dry Matter
Ca (%)	0.25-1.5
P (%)	0.15-0.6
Mg (%)	0.08-0.16 (14 mg/kg/body weight)
Vitamin D (IU/kg)	300-800

Data from Harrington DD: Influence of magnesium deficiency on horse foal tissue concentration of Mg, calcium and phosphorus, *Br J Nutr* 34:45–57, 1975; Hintz HF, Schryver HF: Magnesium metabolism in the horse, *J Anim Sci* 35:755–759, 1972; National Research Council: *Nutrient requirements of horses*, ed 5, Washington, DC, 1989, National Academic Press; Hintz HF, Schryver HF: Magnesium, calcium and phosphorus metabolism in ponies fed varying levels of magnesium, *J Anim Sci* 37:927–930, 1973; Meyer H, Ahlswede L: Magnesium metabolism in the horse, *Zentralbl Veterinarmed A* 24:128–139, 1977.

concentration ranges between 1.3 g/kg of fluid milk during the first 2 weeks of lactation to 0.8 g/kg of milk on weeks 15 to 17.[9,10] For a 500-kg mare producing 15 kg of milk/day, with a calcium concentration of 1.2 g/kg of milk, this represents a demand of 36 g of calcium (15 kg of milk × 1.2 g of calcium × 50% absorption) a day, in addition to maintenance.

It has been estimated that average horses must absorb 20 to 25 mg of calcium and 10 to 12 mg of phosphorus/kg/day to balance losses.[11-13] According to the National Research Council,[14] the maximum tolerable content of dietary phosphorus in horses fed adequate amounts of calcium is 1%. Calcium and phosphate content in some mineral supplements and equine feeds are presented in Tables 20-6 and 20-7.

Absorption

Horses absorb a large proportion of dietary calcium as compared with other species.[15] Horses absorb calcium and phosphorus with high efficiency and with little effect of age.[13,15]

TABLE 20-6

Calcium and Phosphorus Content (%) in Some Mineral Supplements

Calcium carbonate	34	0
Defluorinated phosphate	32	15
Bone meal	30	14
Dicalcium phosphate	27	21
Monocalcium phosphate	17	21
Monosodium phosphate	0	22
Calcium gluconate 23%	2.14*	0

Adapted from Robinson NE, editor: *Current therapy in equine medicine*, ed 6, St Louis, 2009, WB Saunders.
*Elemental calcium calculated on the basis of molecular weight of calcium gluconate hemicalcium salt. Each milliliter of the 23% solution contains 21.4 mg of elemental calcium.

TABLE 20-7

Mineral Composition of Some Equine Feeds on a Dry-Matter Basis

Source	Ca (%)	P (%)	Mg (%)
Alfalfa	1.71	0.30	0.36
Alfalfa hay	1.41	0.21	0.34
Timothy	0.40	0.26	0.16
Timothy hay	0.51	0.29	0.13
Bluegrass	0.50	0.4	0.18
Oat hay	0.32	0.25	0.29
Orchard grass	0.25	0.39	0.31
Barley	0.05	0.37	0.15
Corn	0.05	0.60	0.03
Oats	0.09	0.38	0.16
Wheat	0.05	0.42	0.14
Cottonseed meal	0.18	1.22	0.59
Linseed	0.43	0.90	0.67
Skim milk	1.36	1.09	0.13
Soybean meal	0.40	0.71	0.31
Molasses, cane	1.10	0.15	0.47
Wheat bran	0.14	1.27	0.63

Adapted from the National Academy of Sciences: *Nutrient requirements of horses*, ed 5, Washington, DC, 1989, National Research Council.

Horses fed diets with adequate amounts of calcium absorb 50% to 75% of the calcium and less than half the phosphorus present.[13,16] Calcium in most forages for horses is over 50% to 60% digestible (Table 20-8). The efficiency of calcium absorption is inversely related to the calcium content of the diet. The proximal half of the small intestine is the main site for calcium absorption in the horse, followed by the distal small intestine and the dorsal colon.[13,17] The amount of calcium

TABLE 20-8

Availability (%) of Calcium and Phosphorus in Some Equine Feeds and Supplements

Source	Calcium	Phosphorus
Corn	—	38
Timothy hay	70	42
Alfalfa hay	77	38
Milk products	77	57
Wheat bran	—	34
Limestone	67	—
Dicalcium phosphate	73	44
Bone meal	71	46
Monosodium phosphate	—	47

Adapted from Robinson NE, editor: *Current therapy in equine medicine*, ed 6, St Louis, 2009, WB Saunders.

TABLE 20-9

Plants Containing Harmful Amounts of Oxalate

Common Name	Scientific Name
Buffelgrass	*Cenchrus ciliaris*
Pangola	*Digitaria decumbens*
Setaria	*Setaria sphacelata*
Purple pigeon grass	*Setaria incrassate*
Foxtail grass	*Setaria* spp.
Kikuyu	*Pennisetum clandestinum*
Napier, mission grass	*Pennisetum* spp.
Rhubarb	*Rheum rhaponticum*
Halogeton	*Halogeton glomeratus*
Greasewood	*Sarcobatus vermiculatus*
Soursob, Shamrock	*Oxalis* spp.
Panic	*Panicum* spp.
Dallisgrass	*Paspalum* spp.
Bermuda grass	*Cynodon dactylon*
Para grass	*Brachiaria* spp.
Red-rooted pigweed	*Amaranthus* spp.
Purslane	*Portulaca oleraceae*
Sugar beet	*Beta vulgaris*
Sorrel	*Rumex* spp.
Lambsquarter	*Chenopodium* spp.
Russian thistle, tumbleweed	*Salsola* spp.

These plants have an oxalate content higher than 0.5% diabetes mellitus or have a calcium:oxalate ratio less than 0.5. Their ingestion can result in calcium deficiency and clinical signs consistent with nutritional secondary hyperparathyroidism (NSHPT). Some of these plants may also cause gastrointestinal irritation and diarrhea.

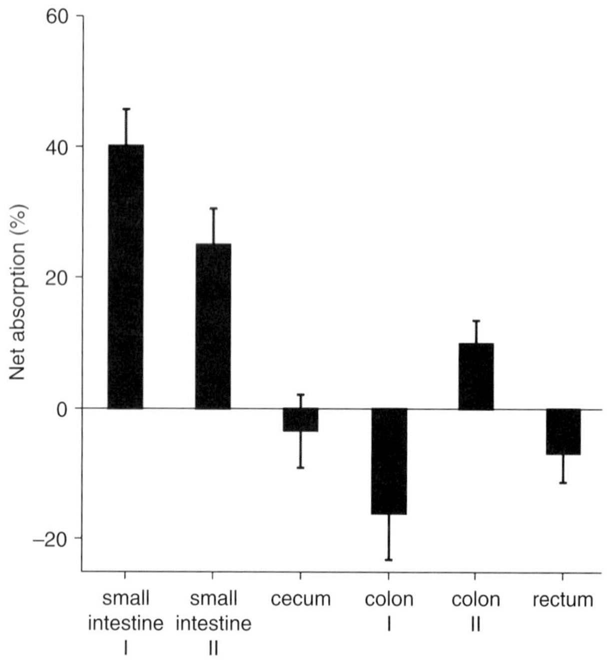

FIGURE 20-9 Net absorption of calcium from the intestine of the horse. The intestine was divided in six regions: proximal (small intestine I) and distal (small intestine II) halves of the small intestine, cecum, proximal (colon I) and distal (colon I) large colon, and transverse colon and rectum (rectum). (Adapted from Schryver HF, Craig PH, Hintz HF et al: The site of calcium absorption in the horse, J Nutr 100:1127–1131, 1970.)

absorbed in the dorsal colon is minimal, and the cecum and ventral colon are mainly secretory sites for calcium (Figure 20-9). High dietary phosphate (or phytate) content inhibits calcium absorption,[18] whereas a high calcium content has minimal effect on phosphorus absorption.[19] Oxalate reduces calcium absorption; a 1% oxalate content in an equine diet reduced calcium absorption by 66%.[20] Oxalate content in the diet higher than 0.5% or a calcium/oxalate ratio below 0.5 can result in a negative calcium balance.[21] Some plants containing harmful amounts of oxalate are listed in Table 20-9.

The dietary cation-anion balance (DCAB) affects Ca^{2+} absorption; anionic diets with a low DCAB increase intestinal Ca^{2+} absorption serum Ca^{2+} concentrations,[22] whereas a high DCAB has the opposite effect.

Glucocorticoids affect calcium metabolism in the horse. Dexamethasone decreases intestinal absorption of calcium, decreases bone resorption, and increases urinary excretion of calcium.[23,24]

Limited information exists on the effect of magnesium on calcium and phosphorus absorption in the horse.[25,26] No changes in serum calcium and phosphorus concentrations were detected in foals fed a magnesium-deficient diet; however, mineralization of the aorta was present.[25]

Elimination

Calcium is eliminated through the kidneys, milk, sweat, feces, and fetus. Because horses absorb a greater proportion of dietary calcium, fecal calcium content is lower than in ruminants when fed equivalent diets.[13,15] Endogenous losses of calcium in horses are estimated around 20 to 25 mg/kg/body weight/day.[11]

Assuming a 50% calcium digestibility, a 500-kg horse would require 20 g of calcium to replace losses, or 40 mg/kg/day; growing and lactating horses can double these requirements. Calcium elimination depends on physiologic status, amount of calcium ingested, presence of substances that interfere with calcium absorption (phosphates, oxalates, phytates), and diseases. The urinary fractional clearance of calcium and the ratio of urinary to serum calcium and phosphorus have been proposed as methods to estimate calcium intake.[27] However, interpretation of calcium clearance is difficult because of the large amounts of calcium eliminated in the equine urine.[28]

The fractional clearance of calcium or phosphorus can be calculated using the following formula:

$$\frac{\textit{Urine } Ca^{2+} \textit{or phosphorus}}{\textit{Serum } Ca^{2+} \textit{or phosphorus}} \times \frac{\textit{Serum creatinine}}{\textit{Urine creatinine}} \times 100$$

Deficiency

Calcium deficiency can be acute or chronic. Acute calcium deficiency is manifested with signs of neuromuscular excitability, whereas chronic calcium deficiency presents as abnormal cartilage and bone development, developmental orthopedic disease (DOD), and lameness. When calcium deficiency is suspected, feed analysis is recommended to determine if dietary calcium and phosphorus content are adequate.

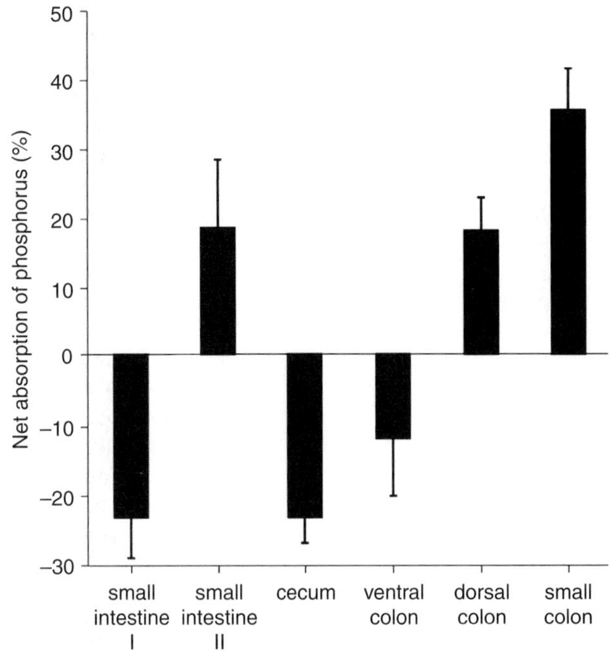

FIGURE 20-10 Net absorption of phosphorus from the intestine of ponies fed an alfalfa diet. (Adapted from Schryver HF, Hintz HF, Craig PH et al: Site of phosphorus absorption form the intestine of the horse, J Nutr 102:143–148, 1972.)

Phosphorus

Similar to calcium, most phosphorus (80%) in the skeleton is bound to calcium as hydroxyapatite crystals. In circulation phosphate is present in two forms: (1) organic phosphate (intracellular) and (2) inorganic (extracellular). Organic phosphate represents most of the phosphorus in circulation that is bound to lipids, proteins, and blood cells; however, only inorganic phosphate (PO_4) is measured. In plasma, phosphorus exists as ionized PO_4 (40%-50%; HPO_4^{2-}), complexed to cations (Na^+, Ca^{2+}, Mg^{2+}; 30%-40%), and bound to proteins (1%-15%). At physiologic pH, PO_4 exists as divalent (HPO_4^{2-}) and monovalent ($H_2PO_4^-$) anions in a 4:1 ratio. In acidosis this ratio is 1:1, and it can be as high as 9:1 during alkalosis.[29] Most phosphorus in soft tissues is organic, intracellular, and incorporated into phospholipids, nucleic acids, and energy compounds (ATP and creatine phosphate). Therefore phosphorus is important for nerve function; muscle contraction; electrolyte transport; oxygen transport (2,3-diphosphoglycerate); enzyme activity; gene transcription; metabolism of proteins, carbohydrates, and fats; and cell proliferation. PO_4 regulation is closely associated to Ca^{2+} homeostasis. Serum PO_4 concentrations and alkaline phosphatase activity are higher in foals than in adult horses because of increased bone osteoblastic activity and bone formation.

Phosphorus requirements depend on age, physiologic status, and amount of work or exercise performed (see Table 20-4). In horses, phosphorus absorption ranges between 30% to 55% and occurs in the small and large intestines (Figure 20-10).[13,30,31] High dietary aluminum and phytate reduce PO_4 absorption, and phytase activity in the equine large colon can enhance PO_4 absorption.[32] Most renal PO_4 reabsorption (>80%) occurs in the proximal tubules by Na^+-dependent mechanisms, with minimal reabsorption in the distal nephron, and the urinary fractional excretion of PO_4 in horses is low (<0.5%). Chronic excess of phosphorus is associated with clinical signs of calcium deficiency including lameness, abnormal cartilage and bone development, fractures, and osteodystrophia fibrosa (nutritional secondary hyperparathyroidism [NSHPT]). Chronic phosphorus deficiency is manifested as weight loss, weakness, depraved appetite (pica), lameness, and DOD. Serum PO_4 concentrations are more indicative of dietary phosphorus intake and status than serum calcium concentrations because the homeostatic control for PO_4 is not as precise as that of Ca^{2+}. Normal PO_4 concentrations are presented in Table 20-10 (mg/dl × 0.323 = mmol/L).

Acute renal failure and hypoparathyroidism are associated with hyperphosphatemia. PO_4 concentrations in horses with chronic renal failure (CRF) are variable.

Conditions that result in cell lysis such as hemolysis, rhabdomyolysis, and tumor necrosis may cause acute hyperphosphatemia. Conditions associated with hypophosphatemia include inadequate intake, decreased intestinal absorption, renal waste, hyperparathyroidism, sepsis, and PO_4 shift to the intracellular compartment. PO_4 shift to the intracellular compartment is a frequent cause of hypophosphatemia in critically ill human beings, and occasionally it occurs in horses with starvation, refeeding syndrome, parenteral nutrition (hyperglycemia, hyperinsulinemia), and hyperlipemia (personal communication, Toribio RE, 2008). Acute hypophosphatemia is associated with cell membrane fragility and lysis (hemolysis, rhabdomyolysis).

Treatment of hypophosphatemia should be based on the extracellular deficit; however, this deficit should be overestimated because phosphate is a major intracellular anion and cell depletion is likely to be present in animals with hypophosphatemia. A preferred parenteral treatment is potassium phosphate, although sodium phosphate is a good alternative. Critically ill horses can also be supplemented with oral

TABLE 20-10

Normal Serum Concentrations of Calcium, Phosphorus, Magnesium, Vitamin D, and Parathyroid Hormone in Healthy Horses

Total calcium (mg/dl)*	11.1-13.0
Ionized calcium (mg/dl)*	6.0-7.0
Phosphorus (mg/dl)†	1.2-4.8
Total magnesium (mmol/L)	0.53-0.91
Ionized magnesium (mmol/L)	0.46-0.66
PTH (pmol/L)	<4.0; (<40 pg/ml)
Calcitonin (pg/ml)	<20
25-Vitamin D_3	< 2.0 ng/ml[77] 4.7 ± 1.0 ng/ml[77] ‡ 1.90 ± 0.23 ng/ml—winter[74] 2.43 ± 0.09 ng/ml—summer[74] 4.2 ± 0.34 μg/L—winter[75] § 6.2 ± 0.36 μg/L—summer[75] § 11.42 ± 3.26 ng/ml[78]
1,25 Vitamin D_3	18.6 ± 7.3 ng/L—winter"bib75"[75] ‡ 18.7 ± 8.0 ng/L—summer[75] ‡ 55.0 ± 24.0 pmol/L[71]

Values from the chemistry laboratory at the College of Veterinary Medicine, The Ohio State University.
*Serum/plasma values are lower in foals than adults.
†Serum/plasma values are higher in foals.
‡D_2 metabolite.
§Includes D_2 and D_3 metabolites.
Calcium conversion: mg/d l= mmol/L × 4; mmol/L = mg/dl × 0.25.

potassium phosphate or monosodium phosphate. Hypokalemia and hypomagnesemia are frequent findings in horses with hypophosphatemia. For chronic phosphate deficiency, oral dicalcium phosphate is a good option (see Table 20-6).

Phosphorus homeostasis is discussed following in conjunction with calcium homeostasis.

CALCIUM HOMEOSTASIS

Regulation of extracellular ionized calcium (Ca^{2+}) concentration is controlled by a complex homeostatic system that includes three major hormones: PTH, CT, and 1,25-dihydroxyvitamin D_3 [1,25$(OH)_2D_3$, or calcitriol]).[3,5,33] PTH-related protein (PTHrP) shares considerable homology with PTH, binds and activates the PTH-1 receptor, and is important for calcium homeostasis in the fetus but not in the adult.[34,35] PTH increases during hypocalcemia, whereas CT increases during hypercalcemia.

PARATHYROID HORMONE

PTH is secreted by the chief cells of the parathyroid gland in response to small changes in extracellular Ca^{2+} concentrations. The biologic functions of PTH include stimulation of osteoclastic bone resorption, thereby increasing Ca^{2+} release into circulation, stimulation of Ca^{2+} reabsorption and inhibition of phosphate reabsorption in the renal tubules, and stimulation of calcitriol synthesis in the kidney. Calcitriol then increases intestinal Ca^{2+} and phosphate absorption and inhibits PTH secretion in the parathyroid gland.[1]

The relationship between serum Ca^{2+} concentrations and PTH secretion in horses is inverse and sigmoidal, which allows the parathyroid gland to rapidly respond to minimal changes in Ca^{2+} concentrations.[2,5,36-39] Changes in extracellular Ca^{2+} concentrations are detected by a Ca^{2+}-sensing G protein–linked cation receptor (CaR) in the parathyroid cells.[40]

Horses have four parathyroid glands. The parathyroid glands IV (cranial or upper) are usually located in the fat dorsolaterally to the cranial pole of the thyroid gland and along the thyroid artery; however, they can be found in any location around the thyroid gland. In the author's experience, a few horses may also have parathyroid gland tissue embedded within the thyroid tissue. The parathyroid glands III (lower, caudal) can be located at the bifurcation of the bicarotid trunk, at the cranial pole of the thymus, or embedded in the thymus (young horses). Generally they are twice the size of the upper parathyroids. The parathyroid gland consists of chief cells, oxyphil cells, and clear cells, which represents different morphologic and metabolic stages of the same parenchymal cells.

Mature equine intact PTH is a straight chain of 84 amino acids (molecular weight: 9393 daltons in the horse and 9500 daltons in human beings). Other forms of PTH (amino and carboxyterminal peptides) can be found in circulation after cleavage in different organs.[41] Around 50% to 90% of PTH immunoreactivity in blood is from carboxyterminal fragments.[42-44] The plasma half-life of PTH in various species is approximately 2 minutes[44-47]; however, equine PTH half-life has not been determined. The rapid metabolism of PTH, together with the rapid response of the parathyroid chief cells to changes in Ca^{2+} concentrations, ensures that PTH concentrations can rapidly adjust to changes in Ca^{2+}. Approximately 60% to 70% of PTH is removed in the liver (around 25% by the kidney) and the rest by other organs.[44,45,47]

PTH gene expression and secretion is under the influence of extracellular Ca^{2+}, phosphorus, and 1,25$(OH)_2D_3$ concentrations. Limited information exists on the role of vitamin-D metabolites on equine parathyroid gland function and calcium regulation; however, it is well accepted that 1,25$(OH)_2D_3$ decreases PTH gene expression and secretion.[48] This concept is important in understanding the role of the kidney in vitamin D metabolism and parathyroid gland physiology. In the chief cells, vitamin D binds to the vitamin D receptor (VDR) to decrease PTH gene transcription and secretion. Unlike vitamin D, the effects of Ca^{2+} and phosphorus regulating PTH secretion are not only mediated by gene transcription but also by altering PTH mRNA stability and translation.[49] Clinicians have shown that low Ca^{2+} concentrations increase PTH mRNA expression in equine parathyroid chief cells.[50]

PHYSIOLOGIC ACTIONS OF PARATHYROID HORMONE

Kidney The kidney is considered the main target organ for PTH, where it regulates Ca^{2+} and phosphate reabsorption, as well as 1,25$(OH)_2D_3$ synthesis. These effects are mediated by the PTH-1 receptor, which is widely distributed in different segments of the nephron.[43] The PTH-1 receptor is coupled to G proteins to activate adenylate cyclase and increase intracellular cyclic adenosine monophosphate (cAMP). PTH also activates phospholipases (A_2, C, D), protein kinase A, and protein kinase C.[43,51] The activation of these pathways depends on which segment of the nephron PTH is acting.

Effect on Ca^{2+} and Mg^{2+} reabsorption It has been estimated that 60% of filtered calcium and 20% of filtered magnesium are reabsorbed in the proximal tubules.[52,53] The reabsorption process in the proximal convoluted tubules (PCT) is passive and driven by high luminal concentrations of Ca^{2+} and Mg^{2+}.[52,53] In the PCT, Ca^{2+} and Mg^{2+} reabsorption is paracellular, and the difference between Ca^{2+} and Mg^{2+} reabsorption in this segment of the nephron results from differential permeability. In the cortical thick ascending loop of Henle (CTAL), Ca^{2+} and Mg^{2+} transport is paracellular, but more permeability exists in Mg^{2+} (60% for Mg^{2+} versus 20% for Ca^{2+}). The lumen in the CTAL is positively charged, and the driving force for Ca^{2+} and Mg^{2+} reabsorption is the transepithelial voltage gradient generated by the $Na^+/K^+/2Cl^-$ co-transporter.[54] PTH increases Ca^{2+} reabsorption in the CTAL by increasing the activity of the $Na^+/K^+/2Cl^-$ co-transporter.[53] Paracellin-1, a recently discovered protein, is essential for paracellular permeability of Ca^{2+} and Mg^{2+} in the CTAL.[55] PTH has minimal effect in the distal convoluted tubules (DCTs), where $1,25(OH)_2D_3$ is the main calcium-regulating hormone. Unlike the PCT and CTAL, where calcium transport is paracellular, calcium transport in the DCT is transcellular, mediated by epithelial calcium channels (ECaCs), calcium-binding proteins (calbindin), basolateral proteins, and regulated by $1,25(OH)_2D_3$ (Figure 20-11).[56,57]

Effects on Phosphorus PTH is central to renal phosphate regulation. The movement of phosphate in the PCT occurs against electrochemical and concentration gradients, and is mediated by Na^+/phosphate co-transporters. PTH lowers Na^+ and phosphate transport across the brush border by enhancing the degradation of the Na^+/phosphate co-transporters.[58,59] The end result is decreased phosphate reabsorption and phosphaturia. Low PTH concentrations result in hyperphosphatemia, whereas the opposite occurs with high PTH.

Effects on Vitamin D Metabolism PTH increases the synthesis of $1,25(OH)_2D_3$ by increasing gene expression and synthesis of 1α-hydroxylase and by decreasing synthesis of 24-hydroxylase, which inactivates $1,25(OH)_2D_3$. These effects are mediated by cAMP.[43]

Bone Bone is a very active organ that is in a continuous process of bone resorption and bone formation. Bone formation is mediated by osteoblasts, whereas bone resorption is mediated by osteoclasts. In adult vertebrates, the process of bone resorption is in equilibrium with bone formation. In growing animals, bone formation exceeds bone resorption, whereas in old animals and human beings the opposite occurs. No PTH receptors exist in the osteoclasts but rather in the osteoblasts. Thus the effect of PTH on osteoclast activation is indirect and mediated by the osteoblast. On PTH stimulation, the osteoblasts secrete a series of factors, including macrophage colony-stimulating factor (M-CSF) and receptor activator of NF-κβ ligand (RANKL).[60] These two factors (M-CSF and RANKL) are essential for osteoclast function (Figure 20-12). Osteoclasts express receptor activator of NF-κβ (RANK), which is a transmembrane receptor for RANKL. The interaction of RANKL with RANK and the interaction of M-CSF with its receptor result in osteoclast recruitment and activation. To keep a bone formation to resorption balance, the osteoblasts also release osteoprotegerin (OPG), which is a soluble decoy receptor for RANKL, interfering with RANKL action on the osteoclasts.[61] Other factors that stimulate osteoclast differentiation include $1,25(OH)_2D$ and IL-11.

Serum markers of bone formation in horses include osteocalcin, N-terminal peptide of type I procollagen, and bone-specific alkaline phosphatase.[62-64] Serum markers of bone

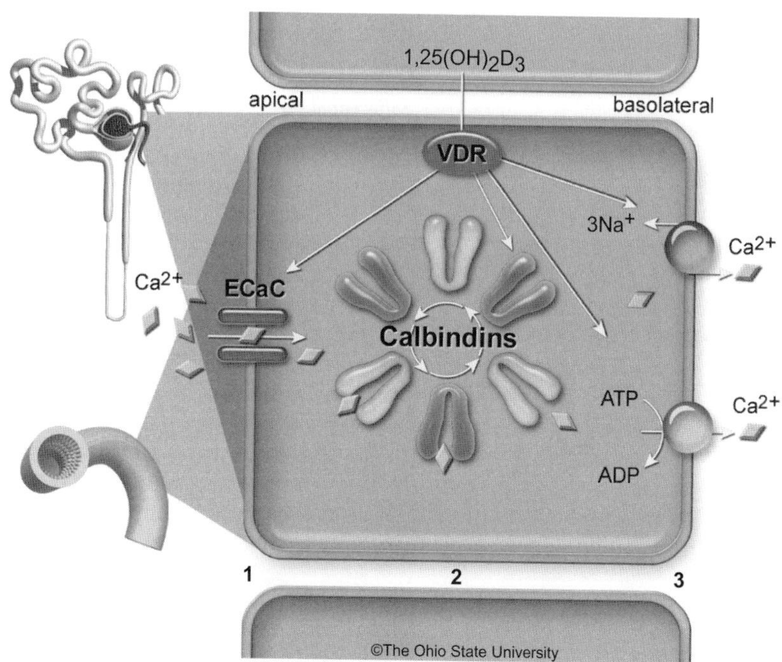

FIGURE 20-11 Schematic representation of the ECaC and the transcellular transport of calcium in the small intestine and kidney. The transcellular transport of Ca^{2+} is considered a three-step process in which calcium (1) enters the cell passively, (2) its diffusion through the cytosol is facilitated by calcium-binding proteins (calbindins), and (3) at the basolateral membrane calcium is extruded by a Ca^{2+}-ATPase and a Na^+-Ca^{2+} exchanger. $1,25(OH)_2D$ increases all three steps of transepithelial calcium transport.

resorption include the cross-linked carboxyterminal telopeptide of type I collagen and total deoxypyridinoline.[62,64]

Intestine PTH has minimal direct effect on intestinal calcium or phosphorus absorption. Indirect effects are mediated by renal synthesis of $1,25(OH)_2D$.

VITAMIN D

Vitamin D plays an important role in Ca^{2+} and phosphate homeostasis and to lesser extent in magnesium metabolism. Vitamin D derives from dietary sources (vitamin D_2 comes from yeasts and plants, and vitamin D_3 from animal-derived diets) and from activation of 7-dehydrocholesterol. In mammals, vitamin D_3 is produced in the skin by ultraviolet light (290-315 nm) photolytic cleavage of 7-dehydrocholecalciferol, producing previtamin D_3; after thermal isomerization, this forms vitamin D_3 (cholecalciferol).[65] From the skin, vitamin D_3 is translocated to the bloodstream by a vitamin D–binding protein (DBP). The next step in the formation of active vitamin D_3 is the hydroxylation of carbon 25, which occurs primarily in the liver, although other organs may also activate vitamin D_3 into 25-hydroxyvitamin D_3 $[25(OH)D_3]$. This reaction is catalyzed by a microsomal and mitochondrial mixed function P_{450} oxidase known as *25-α-hydroxylase*. The conversion of vitamin D_3 into $25(OH)D_3$ is a poorly regulated reaction, and therefore plasma concentrations of $25(OH)D_3$ are considered an indicator of the vitamin-D status.

25-Hydroxyvitamin D_3 is transported in blood bound to DBP, and at normal plasma concentrations this metabolite is considered inactive. The active metabolite of vitamin D_3, 1,25-dihydroxyvitamin D_3 $[1,25(OH)_2D_3]$, is produced in the kidney by another cytochrome P_{450} mixed-function oxidase, 25(OH)D-1α-hydroxylase (1α-hydroxylase). Under physiologic conditions, the kidney is considered the main site for $1,25(OH)_2D_3$ synthesis, although other organs (placenta, skin, monocytes) have 1α-hydroxylase activity. Unlike 25-hydroxylase, 1α-hydroxylase is a tightly regulated enzyme. Mutations of the 1α-hydroxylase gene in human beings and laboratory animals results in vitamin D–dependent type I rickets.[66] This chapter will refer to both vitamin-D active metabolites, $1,25(OH)_2D_2$ and $1,25(OH)_2D_3$, as 1,25-dihydroxyvitamin D $[1,25(OH)_2D]$. In blood, $1,25(OH)_2D$ concentrations are 1/1000 the concentrations of 25(OH)D. The half-life of 25(OH)D can be measured

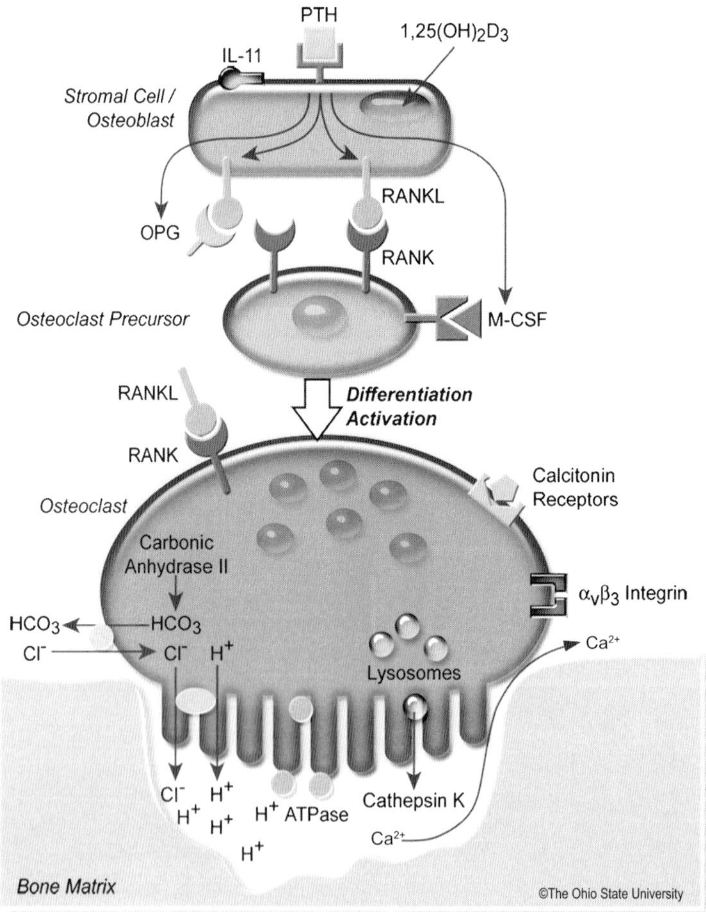

FIGURE 20-12 Representation of the cellular interactions responsible for osteoclastic activation and bone resorption. Factors that stimulate osteoclast differentiation include parathyroid hormone (PTH), $1,25(OH)_2D$, and IL-11. Calcitonin (CT) inhibits osteoclastic activity. Osteoblasts secrete macrophage colony-stimulating factor (M-CSF), as well as receptor activator of NF-κβ (RANK) and receptor activatitor of NF-κβ ligand (RANKL). Osteoclasts express RANK, which is a transmembrane receptor for RANKL. Osteoblasts also release osteoprotegerin (OPG), which is a soluble decoy receptor for RANKL. (Adapted from Rodan GA, Martin TJ: Therapeutic approaches to bone diseases, Science 289:1508–1514, 2000.)

in weeks, whereas the half-life of $1,25(OH)_2D$ is measured in few hours. Both 25(OH)D and $1,25(OH)_2D$ are inactivated at target organs by a D24 α-hydroxylase.

PTH and hypophosphatemia induce 1α-hydroxylase activity in the kidney, whereas increased Ca^{2+}, phosphate, and $1,25(OH)_2D$ inhibit 1α-hydroxylase and stimulate 24-hydroxylase, making this an effective self-regulatory mechanism. The synthesis of $1,25(OH)_2D$ in not related to calcium homeostasis.

REGULATION OF VITAMIN D METABOLISM

Blood concentrations of $1,25(OH)_2D$ are regulated by PTH, Ca^{2+}, phosphorus, and $1,25(OH)_2D$. The role of CT in vitamin-D metabolism remains unclear. Low extracellular Ca^{2+} concentrations stimulate PTH release, which increases renal 1α-hydroxylase activity and $1,25(OH)_2D$ synthesis. Hypophosphatemia also increases renal 1α-hydroxylase activity. An autoregulatory mechanism exists by which $1,25(OH)_2D$ inhibits 1α-hydroxylase.

ACTIONS OF VITAMIN D

Most of the biologic actions of vitamin D result from its active metabolite, $1,25(OH)_2D$, which stimulates intestinal Ca^{2+} and phosphate absorption, as well as renal Ca^{2+} and phosphate reabsorption. These actions are mediated by the VDR that is found in target organs (intestine, bone, kidney, parathyroid gland), as well as in organs not involved in Ca^{2+} homeostasis (skin, pancreas, immune system, and reproductive organs).[67]

In the intestine, as in the kidney, $1,25(OH)_2D$ regulates transcellular Ca^{2+} transport which occurs in three steps: (1) calcium entry by ECaC, (2) calcium diffusion across the cytosol that is facilitated by calcium-binding proteins (calbindins), and (3) calcium extrusion at the basolateral side by Ca^{2+}-ATPases and a Na^+-Ca^{2+} exchangers (see Figure 20-11).[68,69] Vitamin D increases the expression of these proteins. In addition to its effects on intestinal calcium transport, $1,25(OH)_2D$ increases phosphate transport by stimulating of the sodium phosphate co-transporter.

In the kidney, important effects of $1,25(OH)_2D$ include suppression of 1α-hydroxylase, stimulation of Ca^{2+} reabsorption in the DCT,[67] and phosphorus reabsorption in the PCT.

In bone, $1,25(OH)_2D$ is important for skeletal development and bone mineralization. Vitamin D deficiency in young animals results in rickets and osteomalacia in adults. No cases of rickets or osteomalacia have been documented in horses. Vitamin D ($1,25[OH]_2D$) induces osteoclast activity and bone resorption, which is important to maintain normocalcemia and normophosphatemia.

In the parathyroid gland, PTH synthesis is negatively regulated by $1,25(OH)_2D$. PTH increases 1α-hydroxylase activity in the kidney, increasing plasma concentrations of $1,25(OH)_2D$, which then inhibits PTH gene expression and synthesis and controls parathyroid gland chief cell growth and differentiation.[70] This is the explanation for the development of parathyroid hyperplasia in human beings and animals with CRF and vitamin D deficiency.

Vitamin D has nonclassical functions. Anemia, predisposition to infections from impaired immune system, skeletal muscle weakness, cardiomegaly, pancreatic glucose-mediated insulin secretion, and infertility are among conditions reported with vitamin D deficiency.[67] Vitamin D is important in skin and hair development, as well as in cell proliferation and differentiation. Because of these properties, several vitamin D-based compounds with antiproliferative and prodifferentiation properties have been developed to treat various pathologic conditions in human beings and small animals (seborrhea, psoriasis, secondary hyperparathyroidism, breast cancer, prostate cancer, leukemia).[67]

VITAMIN D METABOLISM IN THE HORSE

The amount of information on vitamin D in the horse is limited when compared with other species. Horses have unique features with regard to calcium metabolism, including high serum total and ionized calcium concentrations, poorly regulated intestinal calcium absorption, high urinary fractional clearance of calcium, a high Ca^{2+} set-point, and low serum concentrations of vitamin-D metabolites ($25[OH]_2D$ and $1,25[OH]_2D$).[5,13,50,71-78] As previously mentioned, 25(OH)D concentrations are considered an indicator of vitamin-D status. Plasma concentrations of 25(OH)D in the horse are approximately one tenth the plasma concentrations of 25(OH)D in other species.[75-77] In human beings and in most domestic animals, plasma concentrations of 25(OH)D range between 50 to 100 nmol/L,[72] with minimal differences between young animals and adults[73]; a plasma 25(OH)D concentration below 40 nmol/L is indicative of vitamin-D deficiency. In contrast, in the horse, plasma concentrations of $25(OH)D_3$ of 5 to 10 nmol/L or below are normal.[75-77] Despite the low vitamin-D concentrations, rickets or osteomalacia have not been documented in horses.[79] Horses with limited access to sunlight and fed a vitamin D–deficient diet had decreased growth, lameness, and lower bone density.[79] In northern latitudes, the synthesis of $25(OH)D_3$ and $1,25(OH)_2D_3$ in horses during winter months is low[74,75] (see Table 20-10). One study found that plasma 25(OH)D and $1,25(OH)_2D_3$ concentrations were very low or undetectable in healthy horses and ponies when compared with vitamin D metabolite concentrations from other species.[71] In the same study, renal 1α-hydroxylase activity could not be detected. Likewise, preliminary studies in the author and colleagues' laboratory did not detect 1α-hydroxylase mRNA expression in equine kidneys, indicating that equine 1α-hydroxylase activity is minimal.

CALCITONIN

Calcitonin (thyrocalcitonin) is a 32-amino acid peptide that inhibits osteoclast function during hypercalcemia. The parafollicular cells (C cells) of the thyroid gland secrete CT. Equine CT has 90% homology to human CT.[80] Secretion of CT is controlled by several factors, Ca^{2+} being the most important. The C cells of the thyroid gland sense changes in extracellular Ca^{2+} concentrations by the same calcium-sensing receptor present in parathyroid chief cells and renal tubular cells.[81] CT decreases plasma Ca^{2+} and phosphorus concentrations by inhibiting osteoclastic bone resorption—and to lesser extent by increasing urinary excretion of Ca^{2+} and phosphorus. Despite these effects on Ca^{2+} and phosphorus metabolism, the importance of CT on mammalian Ca^{2+} homeostasis remains unknown. Some authors have concluded that CT may be important in extreme hypercalcemia, but in the day-to-day Ca^{2+} variations, CT may not play a relevant role.[3,82] Based on recent research, the most important CT function in mammalians is to prevent excessive bone resorption during lactation.[83] Postprandial increases in serum CT concentrations are mediated by gastrin.

Unlike terrestrial vertebrates, CT plays a very important role in regulating Ca^{2+} concentrations in saltwater fish, where the ambient calcium concentrations are extremely high (10 mM; 40 mg/dl). Few studies have evaluated CT in the horse.[84-87] Equine osteoclasts are responsive to CT stimulation.[85] Serum concentrations of CT in horses have been measured using human CT RIAs.[88] However, defining the normal range of CT is a downside of these studies. The author and colleagues have evaluated serum CT concentrations in horses using different human CT immunoassays and have found a wide range of values among healthy horses.[89]

Parathyroid Hormone–Related Protein

PTHrP, first discovered as the factor responsible for humoral hypercalcemia of malignancy (HHM),[34] has important physiologic functions in skeletal development. PTH and PTHrP share homology in their first 13 amino acids and act through the same receptor (PTH-1 receptor). Although PTH is exclusively produced by the parathyroid glands, PTHrP is produced by almost every tissue in the body and has a broad range of functions.[33,35] Under physiologic conditions PTHrP functions are considered to be paracrine, autocrine, and intracrine (inside the cell), whereas the endocrine functions of PTHrP are considered pathologic (HHM). PTHrP is critical in fetal calcium regulation; however, in the adult, PTHrP has little effect on calcium homeostasis. Through different regions, PTHrP has different functions: the amino-terminus interacts with the PTH-1 receptor, initiating PTH-like actions (bone resorption, renal Ca^{2+} reabsorption); the midregion PTHrP is important for transplacental Ca^{2+} transport; and the carboxyterminal (osteostatin) inhibits osteoclastic bone resorption.[35] High concentrations of PTHrP (10,000-fold higher than plasma) are found in milk of lactating human beings and animals, including mares.[90] Although the functions of PTHrP in milk are unclear, PTHrP is important for Ca^{2+} transport into the milk, and perhaps for intestinal Ca^{2+} absorption in the newborn.

HHM, a paraneoplastic syndrome resulting from excessive secretion of PTHrP by some tumors, has been reported in horses with lymphoma, gastric and preputial squamous cell carcinoma, ameloblastoma, and multiple myeloma.[91-95]

CALCIUM DISORDERS IN THE HORSE

Calcium dysregulation in horses is associated with hypocalcemic or hypercalcemic disorders. Equine conditions associated with abnormal calcium homeostasis include hypocalcemia of foals,[96] hypoparathyroidism,[97,98] primary hyperparathyroidism (PHPT),[99] NSHPT,[100] hypercalcemia of malignancy,[93-95] vitamin-D toxicity,[101] renal failure,[102] exercise-induced hypocalcemia,[36,103] and sepsis.[5,104,105] Normal calcium concentrations of horses are presented in Table 20-10.

Hypocalcemia

Different pathologic concentrations are associated with hypocalcemia in the horse (Box 20-3). Clinical signs of hypocalcemia result from increased neuromuscular excitability and decreased smooth muscle cell contractility (Box 20-4). Extracellular Ca^{2+} concentrations affect the voltage at which the Na^+ channels in nerve and muscle fibers are activated; Ca^{2+} decreases Na^+ permeability and increases the depolarization threshold. Thus Ca^{2+} is a Na^+ channel antagonist. When Ca^{2+} concentrations are low Na^+ channels are easily activated, resulting in nerve and muscle fiber hyperexcitability, muscle fasciculations, tremors, and tetany. Tachycardia and cardiac arrhythmias may be present during hypocalcemia, although bradycardia may develop during severe hypocalcemia, probably from decreased cardiac muscle contractility.

SYNCHRONOUS DIAPHRAGMATIC FLUTTER

Synchronous diaphragmatic flutter (SDF) or *thumps* refers to a rhythmic movement on the flank as a result of diaphragmatic contractions that are synchronous with the heartbeat.

BOX 20-3

CLINICAL CONDITIONS IN THE HORSE IN WHICH HYPOCALCEMIA HAS BEEN REPORTED

Colic	Pancreatitis
Enterocolitis	Furosemide administration
Sepsis	Excessive administration of $NaHCO_3$
Endotoxemia	Oxalate ingestion
After endurance exercise	Primary hypoparathyroidism
Late pregnancy	Hypomagnesemia
During lactation (lactation tetany)	Cantharidin toxicosis
During transport (transit tetany)	Liver disease
Acute renal failure	Dystocia
Chronic renal failure (CRF)	Malignant hyperthermia
Rhabdomyolysis	Magnesium toxicosis
Pleuropneumonia	Retained placenta
Heat stroke	Postoperative myopathy

BOX 20-4

CLINICAL SIGNS REPORTED IN HORSES WITH HYPOCALCEMIA

Anxiety	Hypersalivation
Asphyxia	Hyperthermia
Ataxia	Ileus
Bruxism	Laryngeal spasm
Cardiac arrhythmias	Muscle fasciculation
Colic	Seizures
Convulsions	Stiff gait
Death	Synchronous diaphragmatic flutter (SDF)
Depression	Tachycardia
Dysphagia	Tachypnea
Dyspnea	Tetany
Excitation	Tremors
Hyperhidrosis	Trismus

SDF results from ionized hypocalcemia, hypomagnesemia, or both, and it has been reported in horses with gastrointestinal disease,[5,106] lactation tetany (eclampsia),[107] thoracic hematoma,[108] blister beetle toxicosis,[109] urethral obstruction,[110] endurance exercise,[111] hypoparathyroidism,[98,112] idiopathic hypocalcemia,[96] and sepsis.[5] Depolarization of the right atrium stimulates action potentials in the hyperexcitable phrenic nerve as it crosses over the heart.

This condition is frequent in horses after prolonged exercise, in which significant amounts of electrolytes (Ca^{2+}, Na^+, K^+, Mg^{2+}, Cl^-) are lost from excessive sweating.[113,114] During alkalosis, increased binding of Ca^{2+} and Mg^{2+} to plasma anions is noted, in particular albumin, resulting in ionized hypocalcemia and hypomagnesemia. Exercising horses often develop alkalosis from hyperventilation (respiratory alkalosis) and sweat loss of chloride (metabolic hypochloremic alkalosis).[108] Serum ionized magnesium (Mg^{2+}) concentrations are often low in horses with SDF, and as in hypocalcemia, hypomagnesemia also increases neuromuscular excitability. Hypomagnesemia should always be included in the differential diagnosis of hypocalcemia and SDF.

HYPOCALCEMIC TETANY

Low Ca^{2+} concentrations increase cell membrane excitability, and some horses may develop excessive and sustained skeletal muscular contractions or tetany. Lactation tetany occurs in mares from 2 weeks before foaling up to few days after weaning. The predisposing cause of lactation tetany is calcium loss in milk. Mares producing large amounts of milk, eating a low-calcium diet, and performing physical work (draft mares) are more at risk. Some horses transported for long distances may develop hypocalcemia and transit tetany.[107] Clinical signs may include anxiety, depression, ataxia, stiff gait, muscle fasciculations and tremors, tachypnea with flared nostrils, dyspnea, dysphagia, hypersalivation, hyperhidrosis, and seizures (see Box 20-3).

HYPOCALCEMIC SEIZURES

As occurs with peripheral nerves, decreased Ca^{2+} concentrations in the CNS increases neuroexcitability. Hypocalcemic seizures have been reported in foals and horses with hypocalcemia, sepsis, and hypoparathyroidism.[96] Clinical signs usually improve with calcium treatment, although some animals may require repeated treatments with calcium salts. Horses with hypocalcemic seizures have a poor prognosis for recovery.

ILEUS

Smooth muscle cells have more voltage-gated Ca^{2+} channels and fewer voltage-gated Na^+ channels than skeletal muscle fibers; therefore Na^+ is less important for the action potential and muscle contraction. This results in slower and prolonged contractions (Ca^{2+} channels are slow channels). Although in skeletal muscle almost all Ca^{2+} required for contraction comes from the SR, in smooth muscle cells the SR is a rudimentary organelle and cells depend on extracellular Ca^{2+} for contraction. Therefore any pathologic condition that reduces Ca^{2+} affects smooth muscle contractility. This is evident in horses that develop ileus and colic secondary to hypocalcemia (after exercise, transport, sepsis). Treatment with calcium gluconate may restore gastrointestinal motility.

RETAINED PLACENTA

Retained placenta in mares has been reported to occur in up to 10% of foalings.[115] Low serum total and ionized calcium concentrations are frequently seen in mares with retained placenta and acute endometritis. As for gastrointestinal motility, it is likely that decreased uterine tone and contractility results from a similar mechanism as ileus. One study found that Friesian mares with retained placenta had statistically lower serum total calcium concentrations than mares without retained placenta.[116] Furthermore, 64% of mares treated with a combination of oxytocin in a calcium-magnesium borogluconate solution responded to treatment compared with 44% of the mares treated with oxytocin in saline solution. No differences in serum magnesium concentrations were found in this study.

TREATMENT OF HYPOCALCEMIA

As for other electrolytes, when treating hypocalcemia, the clinician should consider calcium deficit, maintenance, losses, and sequestration. If parathyroid gland function is normal, then the amount of calcium required is minimal. Calcium therapy is more critical in horses that develop rapid hypocalcemia and in horses with impaired parathyroid gland function that cannot restore normocalcemia. The decision to treat horses with hypocalcemia should be based on the presence of hypocalcemia and not on the presence of clinical signs of hypocalcemia. In most cases, horses with ionized hypocalcemia do not show signs of hypocalcemia, or the signs are very subtle, and the lack of therapy may result in additional complications (ileus). Horses with mild hypocalcemia in general restore their normocalcemia without calcium administration; however, calcium administration should be considered. Horses with functional kidneys can rapidly eliminate large amounts of calcium, and hypercalcemia from excessive calcium administration is rare, in particular if the horse is receiving fluid therapy.

The use of standard formulas to calculate electrolyte deficits based on extracellular fluid and body weight do not apply to calcium. Calcium can rapidly be eliminated or sequestered in different compartments, and larger doses of calcium are often times required.

The following formula is used to calculate Ca^{2+} deficit:

$$\frac{(6.5\text{mg/dl} - Ca^{2+}) \times (0.3) \times (\text{body weight}) \times (10)}{Ca^{2+}\text{ ratio}} = Ca^{2+}\text{ deficit}$$

in which the difference between the measured Ca^{2+} and normal Ca^{2+} (6.5 mg/dl) is multiplied by the extracellular fluid volume, the body weight (kg), and a factor of 10 (Ca^{2+} is expressed in dl, but body weight is in kg = L), and then divided by the Ca^{2+} ratio (Ca^{2+}/total calcium). For a 450-kg horse with a serum Ca^{2+} concentration of 4.5 mg/dl and a total calcium of 10 mg/dl, the estimated Ca^{2+} deficit will be 6000 mg:

$$\frac{(6.5 - 4.5) \times (0.3) \times (450\,\text{kg}) \times (10)}{0.45} = 6000\,\text{mg}$$

This is a deficit of elemental calcium, and calcium gluconate or borogluconate are the salts of choice for parenteral treatment. Calcium gluconate contains 9.3% of elemental calcium; in other words, every 100 ml of calcium gluconate 23% solution contains 2.14 g of elemental calcium or 21.4 mg/ml. The horse in this example would require approximately 300 ml of calcium gluconate 23% solution over 24 hours to replace the Ca^{2+} deficit (Ca^{2+} conversion factors: mg/dl = mmol/L × 4; mmol/L = mg/dl × 0.25).

Total calcium concentration can be used to estimate calcium deficit; however, total calcium concentration has more variability than Ca^{2+} concentration. A horse may have total hypocalcemia, but serum Ca^{2+} concentrations may be within the normal range and calcium administration may not be necessary. Unfortunately, measurement of Ca^{2+} concentrations is not readily available for many practitioners. Replacing total calcium and normal total calcium (11.5 mg/dl) in the same formula, and dividing by a 0.5 Ca^{2+} ratio, gives a close approximation of calcium deficit.

Frequent monitoring of Ca^{2+} concentration is important to adjust dosage. Some horses with severe gastrointestinal disease and sepsis remain hypocalcemic despite aggressive calcium supplementation. Rapid administration of calcium may result in cardiovascular complications, in particular in septic horses, which may be more vulnerable to the cytotoxic effects of calcium. Horses can handle large calcium dosages.[117,118] Based on our experience treating critically ill horses, calcium doses of 2 mg/kg/hr are safe in horses. This represents approximately 50 ml of calcium gluconate 23% solution for a 500-kg horse in 1 hour, while receiving fluid therapy. A number of studies have found that calcium administration to septic patients may be detrimental.

Calcium chloride may be a good option to treat equine hypocalcemia; however, it is not available in large volumes and may cause irritation at the administration site. The clinician should not add calcium salts to fluid solutions containing bicarbonate because calcium carbonate complexes may form and precipitate.

Oral treatment with calcium salts is feasible in horses with nonlife-threatening hypocalcemia. Dicalcium phosphate and calcium carbonate (limestone) can be used safely (see Table 20-6).

Hypocalcemic Disorders

HYPOPARATHYROIDISM

Hypoparathyroidism is a condition characterized by hypocalcemia, hyperphosphatemia, and decreased serum PTH concentrations. Hypomagnesemia may be present. Primary hypoparathyroidism results from decreased synthesis and secretion of PTH, whereas secondary hypoparathyroidism most commonly results from hypomagnesemia or sepsis. Mg^{2+} has a permissive effect on PTH secretion, and low Mg^{2+} concentrations impair PTH release.

PRIMARY HYPOPARATHYROIDISM

This condition has been reported in horses.[98,112] Horses with clinical signs of hypocalcemia, including ataxia, seizures, hyperexcitability, SDF, tachycardia, tachypnea, muscle fasciculations, stiff gait, recumbency, ileus, and colic. The diagnosis in based on the determination of serum concentrations of Ca^{2+}, Mg^{2+}, phosphorus, and PTH. Hypocalcemia, hyperphosphatemia, hypomagnesemia, and low serum PTH concentrations are the features of primary hypoparathyroidism.[98,112] The low PTH leads to hypocalcemia, as well as decreased renal excretion of phosphorus, and it contributes to hypomagnesemia because PTH also stimulates Mg^{2+} reabsorption in the distal nephron. Horses with primary hypoparathyroidism may benefit from magnesium sulfate or chloride administration.

SECONDARY HYPOPARATHYROIDISM

Secondary hypoparathyroidism as a pathologic entity has not been described in horses; however, septic horses with hypocalcemia and impaired parathyroid gland function are most likely suffering a secondary hypoparathyroidism from hypomagnesemia and increased concentrations of inflammatory mediators. The author and colleagues have documented hypocalcemia, hypomagnesemia, and inappropriately low PTH concentrations in septic horses.[5] Moreover, studies have shown that inflammatory mediators that are increased in critically ill horses (IL-1, IL-6, TNF-α) impair PTH secretion.[5,119,120] Like others,[96] the author and colleagues have observed a number of critically ill foals with clinical evidence of hypocalcemia in which serum intact PTH concentrations are not increased, suggesting hypoparathyroidism. Secondary hypoparathyroidism with hypercalcemia was reported in an 11-year-old Andalusian gelding with CRF and polycystic kidney disease.[97]

SEPSIS

For reasons not yet understood, hypocalcemia is a frequent finding in human beings and animals with sepsis.[5,104,105,121-123] Sepsis is the most common cause of hypocalcemia in equine patients,[5,124] in particular those with severe gastrointestinal disease.[5,104,105,124] Hypocalcemia has been associated with equine mortality.[124]

In horses with enterocolitis admitted to Ohio State University Veterinary Hospital, 75% had total hypocalcemia, 80% had ionized hypocalcemia, and 70% had ionized hypomagnesemia.[5] Of interest, some horses with evidence of sepsis and hypocalcemia had inappropriately low serum PTH concentrations for the degree of hypocalcemia, indicating parathyroid gland dysfunction. Hypocalcemia is also frequent in septic foals. Increased endotoxin concentrations may be the trigger that leads to parathyroid gland dysfunction and hypocalcemia.[120] Horses with gastrointestinal disease may have detectable concentrations of endotoxin in plasma,[125-127] and parenteral administration of endotoxin to healthy horses results in hypocalcemia.[120,128]

The mechanisms responsible for the development of hypocalcemia during sepsis are poorly understood. Possible causes of hypocalcemia include renal loss of calcium,[129] calcium sequestration in the gastrointestinal lumen,[130] intracellular calcium accumulation,[131] impairment in calcium mobilization,[132-134] tissue sequestration,[121,129] impairment of calcium release by target tissues in response to PTH,[129] failure to synthesize $1,25(OH)_2D$,[122] and parathyroid gland dysfunction.[5] Renal loss of calcium as a cause of hypocalcemia in septic horses seems unlikely because horses were found with endotoxemia, enterocolitis, and hypocalcemia that had low fractional urinary clearance calcium.[5,120]

EXERCISE-INDUCED HYPOCALCEMIA

Horses under intense exercise develop electrolyte and acid-base abnormalities. Unlike human beings, who develop either ionized hypo- or hypercalcemia, ionized hypocalcemia seems to be a more consistent finding in exercising horses.[135] Common clinical signs in horses with exercise-induced hypocalcemia include SDF, muscle weakness, muscle fasciculation, ileus, colic, excitation, and cardiac arrhythmias. Hypocalcemia in exercising horses results from sweat losses of calcium,[113,136] calcium movement to the intracellular compartment,[137] and increased calcium binding to albumin because of alkalosis.[137] Exercising horses develop respiratory alkalosis from hyperventilation, metabolic alkalosis from sweat chloride losses (hypochloremic), or a combined alkalosis.

Information on exercise-associated hypocalcemia is lacking. A recent study in exercising horses found that serum Ca^{2+}

decreased while serum PTH increased, indicating parathyroid gland function as the cause of hypocalcemia was unlikely.[36] However, the PTH increase was not sufficient to restore normocalcemia. Another study in endurance horses[103] found that serum PTH concentrations did not increase in all horses that developed hypocalcemia, indicating parathyroid gland dysfunction. Renal loss of calcium as a cause of hypocalcemia during exercise is unlikely because urinary losses of calcium decrease in exercising horses.[114]

CANTHARIDIASIS

Equine cantharidiasis (blister beetle toxicosis) is a condition reported in the Southern and Midwestern United States and is produced by the ingestion of alfalfa contaminated with blister beetles (*Epicauta* spp.), which produce cantharidin (cantharidic acid) (see Chapter 22 for further discussion).[109,138] Horses are very susceptible to the irritant effects of this toxin over mucosal surfaces (gastrointestinal and urinary tracts). Cantharidin causes acute hypocalcemia and hypomagnesemia, SDF, muscle fasciculations, ataxia, dyspnea, laryngeal spasm, and cardiac arrhythmias.[138] Some horses with cantharidiasis develop myocardial necrosis.

ACUTE RENAL FAILURE

Hypocalcemia and hypomagnesemia are common findings in horses with acute renal failure (see Chapter 19 for further discussion). Reabsorption of Ca^{2+} and Mg^{2+} in the kidney is highly dependent on functional epithelial cells, and these cells are very susceptible to various insults (hypoxia, toxins). The loss of the epithelial cells and their absorptive capacity leads to increased urinary loss of Ca^{2+} and Mg^{2+}.

EXERTIONAL RHABDOMYOLYSIS

The pathogenesis of hypocalcemia in exertional rhadbomyolysis is unknown (see Musculoskeletal chapter for further discussion). Speculations are that muscle fiber damage during intense exercise results in Ca^{2+} influx and sequestration into the sarcoplasm and SR. A severalfold increase in sarcoplasmic $Ca^{2+}{}_i$ concentrations have been reported in horses with exertional rhabdomyolysis,[139] indicating that elevations in $Ca^{2+}{}_i$ concentrations may be important in the pathogenesis of ER.

Other causes of hypocalcemia include oxalate toxicity, tetracycline and furosemide administration, and bicarbonate overdose. Hypovitaminosis D remains to be documented as a cause of hypocalcemia in horses.

Hypercalcemic Disorders

Hypercalcemic disorders can be divided in two categories: (1) hypercalcemia associated with parathyroid gland dysfunction (parathyroid-dependent hypercalcemia), and (2) hypercalcemia independent of the parathyroid gland function (hypercalcemia develops despite parathyroid gland suppression). Parathyroid-dependent hypercalcemia in the horse is limited to PHPT, whereas parathyroid-independent hypercalcemia results from various conditions (secondary hyperparathyroidism, renal failure, cancer, vitamin-D intoxication).

PRIMARY HYPERPARATHYROIDISM

In PHPT the parathyroid gland chief cells secrete excessive and autonomous amounts of PTH and do not respond to the negative feedback of Ca^{2+}. In horses, PHPT results from parathyroid adenomas or parathyroid hyperplasia. Parathyroid carcinoma has not been reported in the horse. Elevated PTH concentrations lead to increased renal Ca^{2+} reabsorption (hypocalciuria), decreased phosphorus reabsorption (hyperphosphaturia), increased bone resorption, and increased $1,25(OH)_2D_3$ synthesis. Thus hypercalcemia, hypophosphatemia, hyperphosphaturia, and increased intact PTH concentrations are the laboratory findings of PHPT. The end result of PHPT is loss of cortical bone, and a condition known as *osteodystrophia fibrosa*. PHPT associated with osteodystrophia fibrosa has been reported in ponies and horses.[99,140-143] These horses may have enlargement of the facial bones, lameness, and a poor body condition. Radiographic findings include osseous proliferation of the maxilla and mandible, as well as loss of the lamina dura surrounding the molars.[99] Endoscopic examination may reveal narrowing of the nasal passages. Tests to rule out other conditions associated with hypercalcemia include assessment of renal function and measurement of PTHrP and vitamin-D metabolite concentrations.

Postmortem findings in horses affected with PHTP include enlargement of the maxilla and mandible, stenosis of the nasal passages, and loosening of premolars and molars. Histologic examination of the parathyroid gland is important to confirm the diagnosis of PHPT (hyperplasia); however, finding the parathyroid glands in horses may be a difficult task because of their small size and variable location.

SECONDARY HYPERPARATHYROIDISM

In secondary hyperparathyroidism, excessive PTH secretion is the response of the parathyroid gland to hypocalcemia, hyperphosphatemia, or both (as well as hypovitaminosis D) from renal disease or from nutritional imbalances.

RENAL SECONDARY HYPERPARATHYROIDISM

In the case of renal secondary hyperparathyroidism in small animals and human beings, phosphorus retention from renal disease and decreased $1,25(OH)_2D$ synthesis stimulate PTH secretion.[144] In addition, phosphorus lowers serum Ca^{2+} concentrations and inhibits 1α-hydroxylase, an enzyme required for $1,25(OH)_2D$ synthesis. Decreased concentrations of $1,25(OH)_2D$ also impair intestinal absorption of Ca^{2+}, contributing to hypocalcemia and PTH release. In contrast, horses with CRF have hypercalcemia, with variable phosphorus concentrations. Because equine intestinal calcium absorption is poorly regulated, the kidneys are important in eliminating the excess of calcium. The author and colleagues believe that calcium retention from abnormal renal function rather than increased PTH concentrations is the reason for the development of hypercalcemia in horses with CRF. Serum PTH concentrations in horses with CRF and hypercalcemia are often in the normal range.[97,145]

NUTRITIONAL SECONDARY HYPERPARATHYROIDISM

Horses fed a diet low in calcium, high in phosphorus, or both, may develop NSHPT. This condition, also known as *bran disease, Miller's disease, big head, osteodystrophia fibrosa, osteitis fibrosa,* and *equine osteoporosis,* can affect one or many animals in a herd. Diets containing a phosphorus/calcium ratio of 3:1 or higher may result in NSHPT.[100,146] NSHPT is relatively uncommon in developed countries; however, occasionally a young horse may display clinical signs consistent with NSHPT, including enlargement of facial bones, upper respiratory noise, and lameness. In older horses, facial bone enlargement may not be evident. In the past NSHPT was associated with grain-rich diets; however, with improvements in animal nutrition, NSHPT is rarely associated with excessive grain feeding. Rather it is associated with pastures containing large amounts of oxalates (see Table 20-9), which bind dietary calcium to form insoluble calcium oxalate [$Ca(COO)_2$].[147]

Excessive dietary phosphorus increases phosphorus and decreases calcium absorption, leading to hypocalcemia, hyperphosphatemia, and hyperparathyroidism in horses.[141] Hyperphosphatemia stimulates PTH secretion and inhibits renal $1,25(OH)_2D$ synthesis. Because $1,25(OH)_2D$ inhibits parathyroid cell function, low $1,25(OH)_2D$ concentrations contribute to parathyroid cell hyperplasia and PTH secretion. PTH increases osteoclastic activity, excessive bone resorption, and bone loss.[148] Facial bone loss and excessive accumulation of unmineralized bone matrix (osteodystrophia fibrosa) results in facial enlargement (big head) (Figure 20-13).

Because this is a condition of slow progression, the homeostatic mechanisms that regulate extracellular Ca^{2+} concentrations (PTH, vitamin D, CT) may be effective to maintain Ca^{2+} close to or within the normal range.

Clinical signs may include intermittent, shifting lameness, and a stiff gait.[149,150] In most cases swelling of the facial bones is noted. Younger animals may develop physeal enlargement and limb deformities.[146] The facial changes and the bone resorption around the *lamina dura* of the molars and premolars may result in masticatory problems. These horses are physically weak and may be in poor body condition. In severe cases, teeth may become loosened and spontaneous fractures may occur. Upper airway obstruction and dyspnea may be present.[151,152]

Clinical laboratory findings include mild hypocalcemia and hyperphosphatemia; however, these values may be within the reference ranges. Serum intact PTH concentrations are increased.[149] Urinary excretion of calcium is low and excretion of phosphorus is high. Serum alkaline phosphatase activity may be increased. Radiologic findings include decreased bone density;[149,153] however, bone density must be decreased 30% before radiographic evidence exists.[154] Resorption of the dental alveolar sockets may be present before any other radiographic changes.

Supplementation with calcium carbonate (limestone; $CaCO_3$) and dicalcium phosphate in the diet has resulted in clinical improvement.[100] The addition of alfalfa hay and decreasing the amount of grain may be helpful. An affected animal may require a total of 100 to 300 g/day, and the diet should have a calcium/phosphorus ratio of 3 or 4:1. Limestone may decrease feed palatability and adding molasses may be recommended. Confinement of severely affected horses is advised. The use of nonsteroidal anti-inflammatory drugs (NSAIDs) may be indicated in horses with severe pain. Supplementation with vitamin D has been proposed. Young horses may require up to 12 months for complete recovery. For horses consuming feeds with high oxalate content, an additional 20 mg of calcium/kg and 10 mg of phosphorus/kg of body weight per day may be necessary.[21]

HYPERVITAMINOSIS D

The ingestion or administration of ergocalciferol (vitamin D_2) or cholecalciferol (vitamin D_3) results in disturbances of the calcium and phosphorus metabolism in domestic animals.[101,155-162] Intoxication with both forms of vitamin D has been reported in horses.[101,156,162] Ingestion of plants containing $1,25(OH)_2D$-like compounds results in typical clinical signs of vitamin intoxication.[157,159-161] The ingestion of *Solanum glaucophyllum (S. malacoxylon)* results in a condition known as *enteque seco* in Argentina and *espichamento* in Brazil.[155,161] In Hawaii, the ingestion of *S. sodomaeum* results in hypercalcemia. The ingestion of day jessamine (*Cestrum diurnum*), a shrub widely distributed in the Southern United States (from Florida to California) may cause hypervitaminosis D.[157] In Europe,

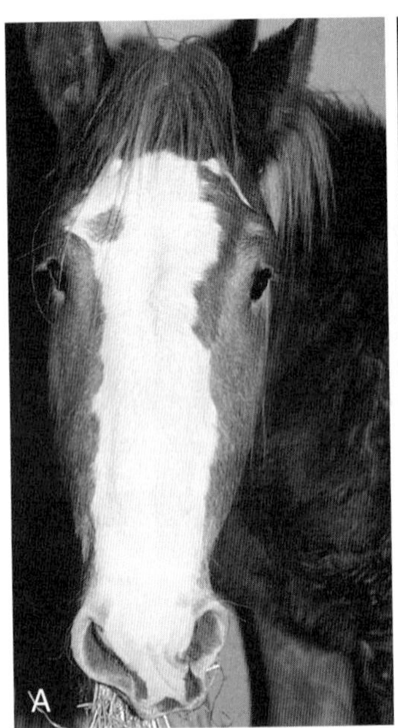

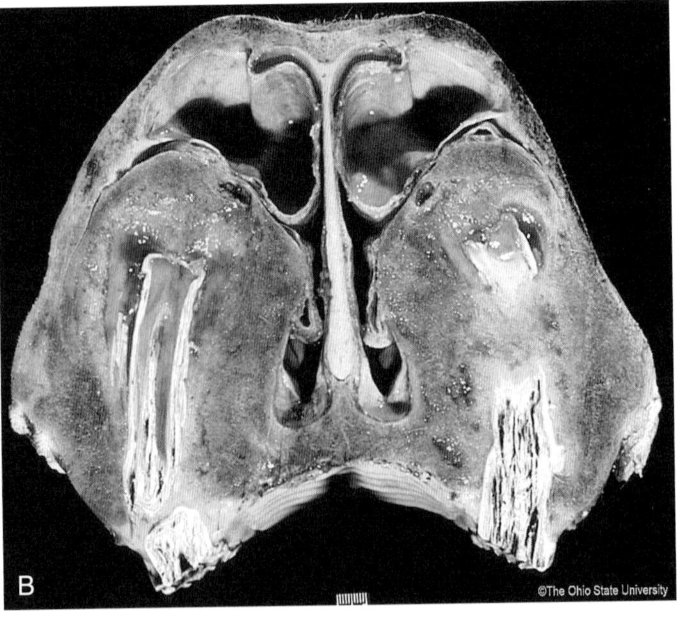

FIGURE 20-13 **A,** Belgiun yearling presented to the Ohio State University Veterinary Teaching Hospital with clinical signs consistent with nutritional secondary hyperparathyroidism (NSHPT), including enlargement of facial bones and upper respiratory noise. The horse was fed excessive amounts of grain. **B,** Narrowing of the nasal passages, loss of bone mass, and excessive accumulation unmineralized bone matrix (osteodystrophia fibrosa) was evident. (Courtesy The Ohio State University.)

the ingestion of *Trisetum flavescens* by horses results in a condition known as *enzootic calcinosis*. Hyperphosphatemia is the most consistent and early laboratory finding in horses with vitamin-D intoxication.[156] Serum calcium concentrations may be within the normal range or increased.[101,156,160,162] Because vitamin D is an important negative regulator of parathyroid cell proliferation, hypervitaminosis D causes parathyroid cell atrophy.[158]

Clinical signs include weight loss, poor appetite, lameness, painful stiffness, and reluctance to move.[156,162] Acute death from severe cardiovascular mineralization has been reported.[101] Renal mineral deposition may precede mineralization elsewhere, leading to renal failure, uremia, hyposthenuria, polyuria, and polydipsia.[101] Lameness is probably the result of calcification of ligaments and tendons.

Radiographically, these horses have increased bone density, decreased size of the medullary cavity, and increased calcification of soft tissues.

The prognosis for horses with hypervitaminosis D is poor. Treatment may include reducing dietary calcium intake. The use of calcium-binding agents such as sodium phytate, which is high in many cereals, has been proposed.[162] Glucocorticoids are used in human beings with hypervitaminosis D, with the rationale that they may inhibit the vitamin D–mediated calcium absorption in the intestine. Dexamethasone administration to pony foals results in decreased intestinal absorption of calcium, decreased bone resorption, and increased urinary excretion of calcium.[23,24] Dexamethasone has been administered to horses with hypervitaminosis D with inconclusive results.[162]

Postmortem examination may reveal mineralization of soft tissues. Extensive cardiovascular mineralization of the endothelium of the aorta and pulmonary vessels, as well as of the endocardium of the atrium and ventricles, is frequent. Mineralized plaques may be present in the endothelium and endocardium. Mineralization may be found in the kidney, liver, lymph nodes, lungs, ligaments, and tendons. Osteopetrosis of the epiphyses and metaphyses may be present. Atrophy of the parathyroid chief cells may be severe.[158]

PSEUDOHYPERPARATHYROIDISM

This term has been used to describe a paraneoplastic condition known as *HHM*. Tumors in human beings and animals may secrete PTHrP, resulting in hypercalcemia. HHM has been described in horses with gastric, vulvar, and preputial squamous cell carcinoma, adrenocortical carcinoma, lymphosarcoma, and ameloblastoma.[92-95,163,164]

NEONATAL HYPERCALCEMIA AND ASPHYXIA

Clinical observations indicate that a number of critically ill newborn foals develop hypercalcemia that is not associated with renal failure or excessive PTH secretion (personal communication, Toribio RE, 2008). Many of these foals have severe hypotension, somnolence, and often die of asphyxia. Factors to consider in the pathogenesis of this condition include PTHrP and 1,25(OH) cholecalciferol.

TREATMENT OF HYPERCALCEMIA

Hypercalcemia as an equine emergency is rarely presented; however, the differential diagnosis of hypercalcemia is important in the treatment of hypercalcemia. Mild to moderate hypercalcemia in general is not life threatening, and treatment should be directed to the primary cause (PHPT, CRF). Hypervitaminosis D can be fatal when mineralization of vital organs occurs. Surgical removal of epithelial tumors may be a successful treatment in some patients. In cases of severe hypercalcemia that require treatment, initial therapy should include the administration of 0.9% saline solution and loop diuretics. Furosemide is the diuretic of choice because it inhibits the $Na^+/K^+/2Cl^-$ co-transporter in the distal nephron, increasing urinary excretion of calcium. Thiazide diuretics are contraindicated because they stimulate calcium reabsorption. Glucocorticoid administration should be considered.

MAGNESIUM AND DISEASE

*Ramiro E. Toribio**

MAGNESIUM

Magnesium is an essential macroelement that participates in physiologic processes such as enzymatic activation, intermediary metabolism of carbohydrates, fats, and proteins, nucleic acid metabolism, regulation of membrane function, nerve function, muscle contraction, and cell proliferation.[1,2] Despite all these vital functions, magnesium is not under the tight control of a hormonal homeostatic system, and its extracellular concentrations depend on gastrointestinal absorption, renal excretion, and bone exchange.[1,2] However, various hormonal and nonhormonal factors influence extracellular magnesium concentrations.[1] Similar to total calcium and ionized calcium (Ca^{2+}), total magnesium (tMg) in biologic fluids exists bound to proteins, chelated to organic anions, and ionized or free (Mg^{2+}).

Mg concentrations are higher in the intracellular compartment, where it binds to negatively charged molecules (ATP, DNA, RNA), enzymes, and other proteins. Approximately 90% of intracellular magnesium is bound to ribosomes, polynucleotides, and to the phosphate backbone of nucleic acids to stabilize base pairing.[3] By interacting with various proteins, magnesium affects the cell cycle and stabilizes cell membranes.[3] Mg^{2+} interacts with Ca^{2+} in the intra- and extracellular compartments. Depending on the physiologic system or binding molecule, Mg^{2+} and Ca^{2+} interact in the following ways: (1) Mg^{2+} and Ca^{2+} can have similar biologic effects, (2) Mg^{2+} and Ca^{2+} can bind to molecules with different affinities resulting in synergy or antagonism, (3) they can be direct antagonists to each other, or (4) their effects can be dependent. The pathophysiology of magnesium-related disorders is often complicated by the Ca^{2+} status of the animal. Likewise, Ca^{2+}-related disorders can be complicated by the Mg^{2+} status. Hypomagnesemia exaggerates the effects of Ca^{2+}, whereas hypermagnesemia may antagonize the effects of Ca^{2+}.

Magnesium concentrations in body fluids are reported as mg/dl, mEq/L, or mmol/L. As the atomic weight of magnesium is 24.3 and its valence is 2^+; 1 mEq of magnesium equals 12.15 mg (0.5 mmol) of magnesium. Conversion factors are as follows: mmol/L = mg/dl × 0.41; mg/dl = mmol/L × 2.43; mg/dl = mEq/L × 1.21; mmol/L = mEq/L × 0.5. Dietary magnesium is reported as g/kg or parts per million (ppm; mg/kg).

The editors acknowledge and appreciate the contributions of Allison J. Stewart, a former author of this chapter. Her original work has been incorportated into this edition.

Magnesium Requirements in the Horse

Based on urinary and fecal losses of magnesium, it has been estimated that adult horses must absorb 5 mg/kg/body weight of magnesium to replace daily obligatory losses.[4] With an average absorption of 40%, dietary magnesium requirements for adult horses are around 12.5 mg/kg/body weight/day (7.5-12.0 g/horse/day).[4] A daily supply of 13 to 15 mg/kg/body weight/day should cover the requirements for most adult horses,[5] but these needs can be higher depending on the physiologic status. Growing, lactating, and exercising animals have higher demands; mares in early lactation and horses under intense exercise may require 15 to 30 mg/kg of magnesium (10-15 g/horse/day).[4] A daily magnesium intake of 5 to 6 mg/kg has been associated with hypomagnesemia.[6]

Distribution of Magnesium within the Body

Magnesium (molecular weight: 24.3) is the fourth most abundant cation in the body, being surpassed by Ca^{2+}, Na^+, and K^+, but is the second most abundant intracellular cation after K^+.[7] Magnesium distribution resembles that of K^+. The body of domestic animals contains 0.05% magnesium by weight, of which 60% is in the skeleton (0.5% to 1% bone ash), 38% in the soft tissue, and 1% to 2% in the extracellular fluid. Approximately 30% of bone Mg^{2+} is surface limited and readily available (thus serving as a reservoir to maintain extracellular Mg^{2+} concentrations), whereas the remaining 70% has structural functions as part of the hydroxyapatite lattice and its release depends on bone resorption. Cells with higher metabolic activity have higher magnesium content. Although most magnesium is in the intracellular compartment, intracellular and extracellular Mg^{2+} concentrations are similar, and the transmembrane gradient is small when compared with that of Ca^{2+}. Red blood cell (RBC) magnesium concentrations are around three times the serum magnesium concentrations.

In circulation, tMg is bound to proteins, chelated to organic anions (carbonate, sulfate, lactate, citrate), and ionized (Mg^{2+}). It is the ionized form of magnesium that is important for most biologic processes, in particular those related to neuromuscular excitability. When possible it is better to measure Mg^{2+} than tMg concentrations. In the horse, 60% of the serum magnesium is ionized, 30% is protein bound, and 10% is complexed to weak acids[8-13] (Figure 20-14). Serum tMg concentrations depend on protein concentrations (albumin), whereas Mg^{2+} concentrations depend on the acid-base status. Acidosis increases Mg^{2+}, and alkalosis does the opposite. This is clinically relevant as conditions associated with alkalosis (nasogastric reflux, duodenitis and jejunitis, exercise-associated alkalosis from hyperventilation and chloride loss) can lead to low Mg^{2+} concentrations, resulting in clinical signs of hypomagnesemia with normal tMg concentrations. Feeding an acidic diet with a low DCAB will increase the percentage of Mg^{2+}.[8]

Reported normal serum concentrations in horses are as follows: tMg = 1.4 to 2.2 mg/dl (0.6-0.9 mmol/L) [8,9,12-14], and Mg^{2+} = 0.45 to 0.6 mmol/L.[8-14] One study found higher tMg concentrations in donkeys.[11] Serum tMg and Mg^{2+} concentrations tend to be higher in foals.[13]

Magnesium Absorption

Mg is absorbed as a freely diffusing ion (Mg^{2+}) by paracellular (passive, nonsaturable, concentration dependent) and transcellular (saturable, active transport) mechanisms.[2,15] Magnesium absorption occurs in the distal small intestine and colon of monogastric animals.[2,16-18] In horses, most Mg^{2+} absorption occurs in the small intestine, with approximately 25% being absorbed in the proximal small intestine, 30% to 35% in the distal small intestine, and 5% to 10% in the large colon.[18] Intestinal magnesium absorption is proportional to its amount in the diet, but its absorptive efficiency decreases as dietary magnesium content increases.[2,16] Increased dietary

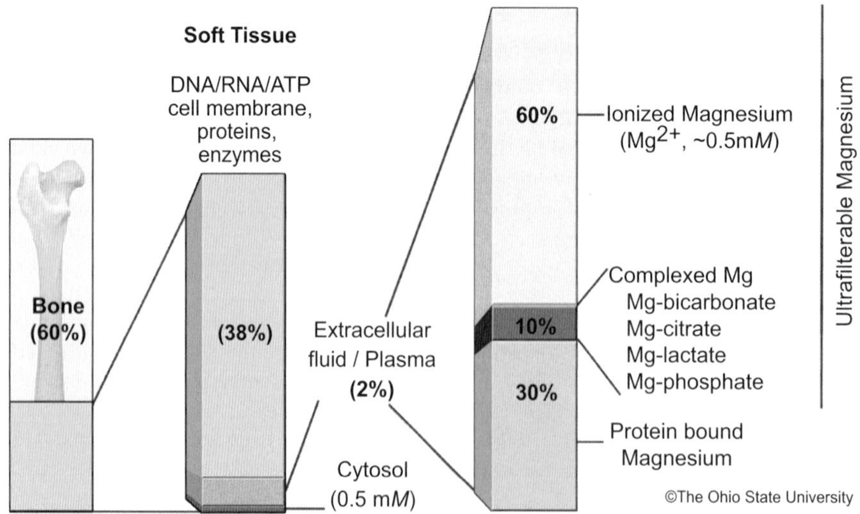

FIGURE 20-14 Magnesium (Mg) distribution in the body. Approximately 60% of the total body magnesium is in the skeleton, 38% is in soft tissue, and 2% in the extracellular fluid. Although most Mg is in the intracellular compartment bound to proteins and nucleotides, free cytosolic Mg^{2+} concentrations are similar to extracellular Mg^{2+} concentrations. In equine blood, 60% of magnesium exists as a free or ionized form (Mg^{2+}), 30% is bound to proteins, and 10% is complexed to anions such as citrate, bicarbonate, phosphate, and lactate.[8-13] (Courtesy The Ohio State University.)

magnesium leads to increased serum, erythrocyte, and tissue magnesium concentrations, especially in bone.[2,19] Dietary calcium content has minimal effect on magnesium absorption.[2] The digestibility of magnesium ranges between 30% to 50%, depending on diet, activity, and age. These values are higher in horses than other herbivores.[18] Alfalfa and alfalfa hay have the highest magnesium digestibility (50%) compared with pelleted feed and grain (20% ~ 30%).[20] Digestibility for oral supplements such as magnesium oxide (MgO), magnesium sulfate ($MgSO_4$), and magnesium carbonate ($MgCO_3$) is similar, ranging between 50% to 70%. Magnesium digestibility is higher in foals.[21] Excessive amounts of fatty acids, oxalates, phytates, phosphates, and fiber decrease intestinal Mg^{2+} absorption. High dietary phosphate content decreases magnesium absorption in horses; however, phytates, calcium, and aluminum content have a minimal effect.[18,22] Malabsorption syndromes and enteropathies decrease absorption.

Magnesium Excretion

The principal routes for magnesium excretion are (1) the gastrointestinal tract, (2) the kidneys, and (3) the mammary gland during lactation. In addition, magnesium can be lost in sweat and the developing fetus.

The kidneys play a major role in regulating magnesium balance and serum magnesium concentrations by controlling tubular reabsorption, mainly in the thick ascending limb of the loop of Henle (TAL).[1,12,23-25] Renal excretion of magnesium is tightly matched to gastrointestinal magnesium absorption; magnesium absorbed in excess is excreted by the kidneys. The tubular reabsorption rate is regulated by dietary availability of magnesium, serum Ca^{2+} and Mg^{2+} concentrations, certain hormones, and urinary Ca^{2+} excretion.[1,12,23,24]

Ionized and anion-bound magnesium (ultrafilterable magnesium) is filtered by the glomerulus, whereas protein bound magnesium is not. Approximately 70% of the blood Mg^{2+} is filtered by the glomeruli, with 70% to 90% being reabsorbed in different segments of the nephron.[12,24] Around 10% to 20% of the filtered magnesium is reabsorbed in the PCT, 50% to 70% is reabsorbed in the TAL, and the remaining 5% to 10% is reabsorbed in the DCT.[1] The DCT seems to be the site determining the final urinary excretion of Mg^{2+}.[12,15] Renal reabsorption of magnesium is paracellular and transcellular. Paracellular (passive, concentration dependent) reabsorption occurs in the PCT, whereas transcellular (active) reabsorption occurs in the DCT. Magnesium reabsorption in the TAL occurs by a voltage-dependent paracellular mechanism.[12]

The mammary gland actively secretes magnesium into milk. The output of magnesium into milk is 3 to 6 mg/kg/body weight/day and the magnesium requirements in lactating mares are 15 to 30 mg/kg.[4] In mare's milk, magnesium concentration is elevated during the first week of lactation (120-300 mg/L), then decreases and remains steady for 2 to 3 months (50 to 70 mg/L).[26,27] High-milk-producing mares are more likely to develop hypomagnesemia. Magnesium can also be lost in the sweat.[28]

Magnesium Homeostasis

No precise homeostatic system exists for Mg^{2+}, and its extracellular concentrations depend on gastrointestinal absorption, renal excretion, and bone exchange.[1,2] However, hormonal and nonhormonal factors influence magnesium absorption, excretion, and extracellular concentrations.[1,2] Hormones that *increase* renal reabsorption of Mg^{2+} include PTH, PTHrP, ADH (vasopressin), insulin, ß-adrenergic agonists, and aldosterone.[1,23,29-33] Activation of the calcium-sensing receptor in the TAL by hypercalcemia in various species, including the horse, increases the urinary excretion of Ca^{2+} and Mg^{2+}.[12,34] Impaired Mg^{2+} reabsorption occurs with osmotic diuresis (volume expansion, hyperglycemia), loop diuretics, hypercalciuria, hypercalcemia, hypermagnesemia, hypokalemia, hypophosphatemia, tubular acidosis, metabolic acidosis, and various toxicities (aminoglycosides, amphotericin B).[23,34-36] Furosemide and hypercalcemia in healthy horses decrease serum tMg and Mg^{2+} concentrations.[12,35] Of interest, both hypercalcemia and loop diuretics act by the same mechanism (inhibition of the $Na^+/K^+/2Cl^-$ co-transporter) in the TAL.[12,34] PTH indirectly increases Mg^{2+} release from bone during bone resorption.

MAGNESIUM AND EQUINE DISEASE

Although extensive data exists on the role of magnesium in inflammation and disease, information is limited in the horse. Magnesium plays essential roles in inflammation, protection against free radical injury, and neurotoxicity.[37,38] Hypomagnesemia has been associated with increased cytokine production and systemic inflammation.[37,38] A similar process is likely to occur in critically ill horses and foals where the same cytokines are elevated.[9,14,39,40] Horses and foals with gastrointestinal disease often have endotoxemia and hypomagnesemia,[9,14,40-42] and the induction of experimental endotoxemia in healthy horses decreases tMg and Mg^{2+}—supporting a role for magnesium in equine disease.[9]

One study in horses that had colic surgery found that serum tMg and Mg^{2+} concentrations were below the reference range in 17% and 54% of animals, respectively.[43] The same study found that nonsurvivor horses had significantly lower preoperative serum Mg^{2+} concentrations. Toribio et al.[14] found that 78% (50 of 64) of horses with severe gastrointestinal disease had ionized hypomagnesemia. In another study of hospitalized horses, 48.7% (401 of 823) of animals were hypomagnesemic; however, no association with mortality or length of hospitalization was found.[44] Although a clear association between hypomagnesemia, severity of disease, and mortality has been demonstrated in other species; minimal information exists in the horse.[9,14,43,44] Hurcombe et al.[42] did not find an association between serum Mg^{2+} concentrations and mortality in critically ill septic foals, although 15% of foals were hypomagnesemic.

Contrary to other species,[45] an association between IR and magnesium deficiency has not been shown in the horse. Mg^{2+} is important for insulin receptor signal transduction and glucose metabolism, and insulin increases intracellular Mg^{2+} transport.[45] Thus IR may lead to renal Mg^{2+} wasting from increased tubular flow (hyperglycemia) and decreased Mg^{2+} reabsorption.[45] Subsequently, magnesium depletion worsens IR to create a vicious cycle.

Magnesium and Hypocalcemia

An association between hypomagnesemia and hypocalcemia has been demonstrated in lactating mares, transported horses, and in horses with intestinal strangulation, ileus, enterocolitis, endotoxemia, SDF, and blister beetle poisoning.[9,14,43,46,47] Patients with hypocalcemia and hypomagnesemia often do not respond to calcium therapy until normomagnesemia is restored.[48] The mechanisms by which hypomagnesemia results in hypocalcemia are unclear; however, hypomagnesemia can impair PTH synthesis and secretion and induce target organ resistance to PTH.[49] This results in decreased renal reabsorption of Ca^{2+} and Mg^{2+} (waste), decreased bone resorption, and decreased renal synthesis of 1,25-dihydroxyvitamin D_3. Therefore hypocalcemia associated with magnesium deficiency may be attributed to a lack of PTH secretion (parathyroid gland dysfunction) associated with target organ refractoriness.

Magnesium and Other Electrolytes

Magnesium is a co-factor for the Na^+/K^+-ATPase that maintains the cell membrane potential. Hypomagnesemia leads to loss of intracellular K^+, intracellular Na^+ accumulation, lowering of the resting membrane potential, which causes hyperexcitability, seizures, arrhythmias, muscle weakness, muscle fasciculations, SDF, and cardiac arrhythmias. The link between hypomagnesemia and equine electrolytes remains unclear; however, the author and colleagues have found that hypomagnesemia in sick horses is often associated with hypokalemia, in particular in foals and ponies receiving parenteral nutrition (personal communication, Toribio RE, 2008). Of interest, hypophosphatemia is a frequent finding in these animals.

Magnesium and Brain Injury

Mg^{2+} is an essential regulator of neuroexcitability by blocking signal transmission via inhibition of Ca^{2+}-dependent, presynaptic excitation-secretion coupling.[16,50] Magnesium depletion contributes to tetany by increasing the release of acetylcholine at the neuromuscular junctions and delaying its degradation by acetylcholinesterase.[16,50] Although Mg^{2+} infusions are currently used in human beings with brain and spinal injury, the benefit of this treatment remains unclear.[51] The rationale for this treatment is that Mg^{2+} decreases free radical injury, modulates *N*-methyl-D-aspartate (NMDA) receptors, and antagonizes the cytotoxic effects of intracellular calcium. NMDA receptors' activation by glutamate allows intracellular Ca^{2+} influx that results in neuronal excitability and death; this process is blocked by cations such as Zn^{2+} and Mg^{2+}.[52,53] In addition, by blocking Ca^{2+} channels in vascular smooth muscle, Mg^{2+} prevents Ca^{2+} entry, resulting in vasodilation.[54] Under the same premise, Mg^{2+} has also been used to treat foals with hypoxic ischemic encephalopathy and horses with brain injury[55,56]; however, controlled studies on the benefits of Mg^{2+} therapy to equine adults or neonates are lacking. The clinical scenario appears to be different under experimental conditions of brain injury, where several studies have shown that $MgSO_4$ improves outcome.[57,58]

Clinical Signs of Magnesium Deficiency

Hypomagnesemia results from reduced magnesium intake (poor nutrition, low-magnesium diets), reduced absorption (chronic diarrhea, malabsorption, intestinal resection), redistribution (third-space and intracellular sequestration), and increased losses (renal tubular disorders, gentamicin, furosemide, hypercalcemia, gestation, lactation, and heavy exercise).

Magnesium depletion is associated with muscle weakness, tremors, seizures, hypokalemia, hypocalcemia, cardiac arrhythmias (ventricular arrhythmias, supraventricular tachycardia, atrial fibrillation), ileus, and SDF (thumps). Electrocardiographic changes from hypomagnesemia include prolonged P-R interval, widening of the QRS complex, depression of the ST segment, and tall T waves.[59] Hypocalcemic tetany has been reported in adult horses and ponies,[47,60] as well as in foals fed magnesium-deficient diets.[61] Affected foals exhibited nervousness, muscular tremors, ataxia, profuse sweating, hyperpnea, collapse, and convulsions.[61] On autopsy, all foals had severe mineralization of the elastic fibers of the aorta and pulmonary artery.[21,61] In one study of colic patients, nonsurviving horses had significantly lower preoperative serum Mg^{2+} concentrations.[43]

Diagnosis of Hypomagnesemia

The easiest way to assess the magnesium status of horses is by determining serum tMg and Mg^{2+} concentrations. Serum Mg^{2+} is more reliable because it is the active form of magnesium and is minimally affected by protein concentrations. In animals with respiratory or metabolic alkalosis (observed after prolonged exercise, proximal enteritis) serum Ca^{2+} and Mg^{2+} concentrations may be low from increased protein binding. Methods to assess total body magnesium status include 24-hour urinary magnesium excretion, percent of magnesium retention after parenteral magnesium loading, and RBC magnesium content. Of these, the 24-hour urinary excretion and the retention tests have been validated in horses.[8]

To assess renal excretion of magnesium, urine is collected over 24 hours (mg/kg/day). Urinary excretion of magnesium is useful to assess dietary intake. Magnesium excretion is low when dietary intake is decreased.[8] The fractional clearance of magnesium (FMg) can be determined by expressing the renal magnesium clearance relative to the creatinine clearance.[8,9,12] FMg in healthy horses ranges between 15% to 35%,[8,9,12] and values less than 6% indicate inadequate dietary magnesium intake.[8] Muscle magnesium content has been used to estimate total body stores in foals and horses.[8,62] One study evaluated magnesium muscle content and intracellular Mg^{2+} concentrations in horses fed a magnesium-deficient diet, with no differences found in muscle magnesium content compared with control horses; however, intracellular Mg^{2+} concentrations were lower in magnesium-deficient horses.[8]

The magnesium retention test to assess total body status has been evaluated in horses receiving magnesium-deficient diets.[8] $MgSO_4$ was given at a dose of 10 mg/kg/IV of elemental magnesium (100 mg/kg of $MgSO_4$). $MgSO_4$ (50% solution) was diluted to 10% before administration. The percent retention (%Ret) was calculated as follows[8]:

$$\%\text{Ret} = (1 - [\text{magnesium excretion in 24 hours}]/[\text{magnesium infused}]) \times 100$$

In this study the 24-hour magnesium excretion was a more sensitive indicator of reduced magnesium intake than the magnesium retention test, and the spot FMg reflected the 24-hour excretion of magnesium.[8] Thus the FMg can be used as a simpler way to assess magnesium status.

Treatment of Hypomagnesemia

Mg for oral administration is available as MgO, $MgCO_3$, and $MgSO_4$ (Epsom salt). $MgSO_4$ and $MgCl_2$ are available for IV administration. The type of salt and the route of administration are important when supplementing magnesium. For $MgSO_4$ (9.7% Mg^{2+}), a dose of 100 mg/kg will provide 9.7 mg/kg of elemental magnesium, whereas for $MgCl_2$ (25.5%) a dose of 100 mg/kg will provide 25.5 mg/kg of elemental magnesium. This is critical because overdosing can be fatal. Likewise, excessive oral (nasogastric) supplementation with $MgSO_4$ can be laxative and induce depression. Recommended dose rates for $MgSO_4$ in adult horses are 25 to 150 mg/kg/IV/day diluted in 0.9% NaCl, dextrose or polyionic isotonic solutions. Constant-rate infusion (CRI) of $MgSO_4$ at 100 to 150 mg/kg/day should meet the daily requirements of foals and adult horses (2-6 mg/kg/min/IV). $MgSO_4$ is used to treat ventricular arrhythmias, in particular quinidine intoxication (torsades de pointes), and should be considered in horses with refractory ileus and SDF. Doses of 50 to 100 mg/kg over 30 minutes are considered safe. This is equivalent to 25 to 50 g of $MgSO_4$ for an adult horse. In foals with ischemic encephalopathy, an initial $MgSO_4$ dose of 50 mg/kg in the first hour, followed by a CRI of 25 mg/kg/hr has been suggested.[55] This regimen can be continued for several days, adjusting the dose based on serum Mg^{2+} concentrations.[55]

Oral supplementation with MgO, $MgCO_3$, or $MgSO_4$ should be considered in animals with chronic hypomagnesemia, malabsorption, renal disease, and exercise-associated hypomagnesemia. Recommended doses are 30 to 50 mg/kg/day for MgO, 60 to 80 mg/kg/day for $MgCO_3$, or 80 to 100 mg/kg/day for $MgSO_4$. These doses are safe for horses, in particular when compared with the cathartic doses of $MgSO_4$ (0.5-1.0 g/kg).

HYPERMAGNESEMIA

Hypermagnesemia is rarely documented in horses and in general is iatrogenic from magnesium overdose, associated with renal failure, or in animals with extensive cellular damage (myonecrosis, cancer, hemolysis, severe sepsis). The presence of hyperkalemia and hyperphosphatemia is another indicator of cellular damage. Hypermagnesemia has been reported in horses treated with Epsom salt and dioctyl sodium sulfosuccinate for large colon impaction.[63] Clinical signs in these horses included sweating, hyperexcitability, muscle tremors, recumbency, flaccid paralysis, tachycardia, and tachypnea. Treatment of hypermagnesemia includes 0.9% NaCl, furosemide, and parenteral calcium administration. Sodium sulfate is considered a safer and more efficacious treatment for large colon impaction than $MgSO_4$.

ANHIDROSIS

Ramiro E. Toribio

Equine anhidrosis (dry coat) is defined as the inability of horses to sweat in response to appropriate stimulation. Anhidrosis is frequent in the tropics, as well as in areas with high temperatures and humidity, including the Southern United States. It is believed that anhidrosis results from a lack of adaptation to local conditions, in particular of horses from temperate climates; however, this does not appear to be the case because native horses in Southern states are as susceptible to anhidrosis as imported horses.[1-3] The prevalence of anhidrosis in the United States is unknown, although it has been estimated to range from 6% to 20% in Southern states.[1-4] Anhidrosis does not seem to be associated with exercise as previously suggested but rather to environmental conditions.[2] There is no association with sex or breed.[1-3] One study in Thoroughbred horses in central Florida found a prevalence of 6.1%, with horses in training and nonpregnant broodmares having the highest prevalence, but the disease was infrequent in young horses.[1] The role of genetics is unclear; however, based on experience the author believes that a genetic component exists in some animals. The influence of diet is controversial, with some authors claiming that anhidrosis is associated with high-protein diets and insufficient electrolyte intake.

PHYSIOLOGY

Similar to humans, sweating in the horse is the primary mechanism for heat loss, followed by respiratory evaporation. The efficiency of these thermoregulatory mechanisms is compromised by diseases, as well as environmental conditions. The equine sweat glands (400-1128/cm^2) are apocrine, associated with the hair follicle (epitrichial), and consist of a secretory portion and a serpentine duct that opens into the follicular canal.[5-7] An important feature of the equine sweat glands compared with other species is their rich capillary network.[6] Sweating in horses is controlled by endocrine and neural mechanisms. Endocrine mechanisms consist of ß-adrenergic stimulation by systemic catecholamines, whereas nervous mechanisms consist of sympathetic ß-adrenergic innervation.[8] Evidence indicates that in equidae the sympathetic neural control of sweating is indirect by controlling the local vascular beds, whereas the humoral control is direct to the glands.[6] This is evident in horses with Horner's syndrome in which sympathetic α-adrenergic denervation results in regional sweating that is believed to result from vasodilation.[9] Neural control appears to be more important in the horse. The equine sweat glands are primarily controlled by $ß_2$-adrenergic receptors.[4,6,7,10] The role of cholinergic, purinergic, and nitric oxide stimulation on equine sweating is unclear.[6,11,12]

PATHOPHYSIOLOGY

Even though a clear understanding of the pathogenesis of equine anhidrosis is lacking, proposed mechanisms include lack of β_2-adrenergic stimulation (β_2-adrenoreceptor agonist deficiency) or lack of sweat gland response to β_2-adrenergic stimulation (refractoriness).[2] With regard to neural control of sweating, it has been proposed that hypothalamic dysfunction from severe hyperthermia may be involved[4]; however, no evidence exists to substantiate this hypothesis. It seems that the pathogenesis of anhidrosis results from a combination of lack of neural and endocrine stimulation. Horses with skin denervation can sweat, although their response to thermal stimulation is impaired.[13,14] One study found that sweat gland innervation in horses with anhidrosis was normal,[15] making denervation unlikely in the pathogenesis of anhidrosis.[4,13]

With regard to the role of the adrenal medulla in the pathogenesis of equine anhidrosis, some studies have shown that medullary dysfunction is improbable in the development of this disease.[4,13,14,16] Likewise, vascular dysfunction to the sweat glands seems unlikely. Instead it has been proposed that abnormal dermal vascular perfusion could be relevant to anhidrosis.[6,11]

The fact that epinephrine concentrations in anhidrotic horses are normal or elevated[17] but the sweat glands have a decreased response to adrenergic stimulation suggests receptor downregulation.[16] Downregulation of β_2-adrenoreceptors have been demonstrated in anhidrotic horses.[18] It appears that this downregulation is the result of excessive or prolonged exposure to catecholamines. The presence of sweat gland atrophy, cell flattening, and ductal obstruction on histologic examination does not imply that these changes are the cause but rather the consequence of this disease.[11,19,20] No evidence indicates that inflammation or immune-mediated processes are central to the pathogenesis of anhidrosis. The low expression of the water channel aquaporin-5 in anhidrotic horses may be of clinical relevance to anhidrosis but does not imply that is the cause.[19]

The role of THs in the pathogenesis of anhidrosis is unclear. It is believed by some that anhidrosis is caused by hypothyroidism; however, no data indicate that this is the case. The fact that some horses may show improvement with L-thyroxine or iodinated casein supplementation indicates that THs may enhance adrenoreceptor sensitivity, as documented in other species.[21] It has been claimed that abnormal electrolyte concentrations are part of the pathogenesis of anhidrosis; however, in controlled studies no differences have been found between anhidrotic and healthy horses.[1]

Clinical Signs

Typical clinical signs include depression, poor performance, tachypnea, hyperthermia (in particular after exercise), lack or decreased sweating, alopecia, and dry coat. Initial signs are nonspecific and related to poor performance and respiratory problems. Early recognition of anhidrosis is important, in particular in hot climates where a delay in core temperature cooling can lead to heat stroke. In addition, anhidrosis represents a major stress to the animal, which can predispose to other diseases.

Diagnosis

In general the diagnosis of anhidrosis is based on clinical signs. The first specific method developed for the diagnosis of anhidrosis was the intradermal injection of epinephrine.[22] Horses with anhidrosis will have a delayed or lack of sweat response to this test. However, because epinephrine is not specific to β_2-receptors, α-adrenergic effects may mask the response of the sweat glands. Subsequently, tests based on β_2-receptor agonists (salbutamol, terbutaline) have been developed.[23,24] These methods are semiquantitative. Saline solution and serial dilutions of salbutamol or terbutaline (10^{-3} to 10^{-8} wt/vol) are injected intradermally over the side of the neck.[23,24] Sweating is evident by 10 minutes, but the final response is evaluated at 20 to 30 minutes. In the terbutaline test, 0.1-ml intradermal injections of terbutaline sulfate (diluted in 0.9% NaCl) in tenfold dilutions (0, 0.001, 0.01, 0.1, 1, 10, 100, 1000 mg/L) are injected intradermally with a 25-gauge needle at 5 cm apart.[23,24] Horses with anhidrosis have minimal or no response to any of the dilutions,[4,23,24] whereas normal horses have a sweat response to most dilutions.

Differential diagnoses are limited to the respiratory tract because most anhidrotic horses have tachypnea and an exaggerated respiratory response (tachypnea) after exercise. In addition, body temperature in these horses remains elevated for longer periods of time than healthy animals.

Treatment, Prevention, and Prognosis

No specific treatment exists for equine anhidrosis. Keeping these horses in a cool environment and reducing physical activity is central to the palliative treatment of anhidrosis. Measures that reduce environmental temperature or increase heat loss include shades, fans, air-conditioning, misting, and water cooling. Because many afflicted horses are used for various performance activities, unfortunately some of the management measures may not be practical or are not implemented. In hot weather, working these horses in the coolest part of the day is recommended. In severe cases, moving these animals to cooler climates should be considered. Dietary modifications and supplementation of minerals may help. The use of salts and electrolytes (KCl, $NaHCO_3$) may have some benefit, although they have not been critically evaluated. Dietary supplements containing ascorbic acid, L-tyrosine (catecholamine precursor), cobalt, vitamin E, and water-soluble vitamins have been claimed to improve clinical signs. Methyl-DOPA (3-4 g) to decrease central sympathetic activity has also been used, but information on the success of this treatment is lacking. It has been reported that daily oral administration of iodinated casein (10-15 g/day) or sodium levothyroxine (0.5 to 3.0 mg/lb; 1-6 mg/100 kg) may improve clinical signs.[4,11] Because information in other species indicates that THs enhance β2-adrenoreceptor sensitivity,[21] these supplements should be considered, keeping in mind potential complications (iatrogenic hyperthyroidism, weight loss).

The use of β_2-receptor agonists is controversial because available information indicates that β_2-receptor downregulation is the result of excessive adrenergic stimulation. However, some clinicians report that the use of clenbuterol in horses with mild anhidrosis or hypohidrosis when environmental temperature and humidity are elevated could ameliorate the severity of clinical signs.

No evidence indicates that anhidrosis is an immune-mediated process; however, glucocorticoids have been proposed in the treatment of this condition. Another combination that has been suggested is glucocorticoids with clenbuterol, with the idea that β_2-receptor agonists may potentiate the anti-inflammatory effects of corticoids. The rationale for this strategy is that glucocorticoids may enhance the ß$_2$-adrenoreceptors' response to agonists. Again, this approach remains unclear because excessive adrenergic stimulation seems to be part of the pathogenesis of anhidrosis. It is also important to avoid the use sedatives that may stimulate sweating in the horse (α_2-receptor agonists). The prognosis for horses with anhidrosis is guarded and dictated by the severity of this condition, response to therapy, and implementation of palliative measures.

REFERENCES

Adrenal Glands

1. O'Connor SJ, Gardner DS, Ousey JC, et al: Development of baroreflex and endocrine responses to hypotensive stress in newborn foals and lambs, *Pflugers Arch* 450:298-306, 2005.
2. Bottoms GD, Roesel OF, Rausch FD, et al: Circadian variation in plasma cortisol and corticosterone in pigs and mares, *Am J Vet Res* 33:785-790, 1972.
3. van der Kolk JH, Nachreiner RF, Schott HC, et al: Salivary and plasma concentration of cortisol in normal horses and horses with Cushing's disease, *Equine Vet J* 33:211-213, 2001.
4. Hart KA, Ferguson DC, Heusner GL, et al: Synthetic adrenocorticotropic hormone stimulation tests in healthy neonatal foals, *J Vet Intern Med* 21:314-321, 2007.

5. Dowling PM, Williams MA, Clark TP: Adrenal insufficiency associated with long-term anabolic steroid administration in a horse, *J Am Vet Med Assoc* 203:1166-1169, 1993.
6. Smith BP, editor: *Large animal internal medicine*, ed 4, St Louis, 2008, Mosby.
7. Wilson DW, Kingery S, Snow DH: The effect of training on adrenocortical function in Thoroughbred racehorses, *Equine exercise physiology*, ed 3, Davis, CA, 1991, ICEEP Publications, pp 482-489.
8. Baker HW, Baker ID, Epstein VM, et al: Effect of stress on steroid hormone levels in racehorses, *Aust Vet J* 58:70-71, 1982.
9. Church DB, Evans DL, Lewis DR, et al: The effect of exercise on plasma adrenocorticotropin, cortisol and insulin in the horse and adaptations with training. In Gillespie JR, Robinson NE, editors: *Equine exercise physiology*, Davis, CA, 1987, ICEEP Publications, pp 506-515.
10. Linden A, Art T, Amory H, et al: Comparison of the adrenocortical response to both pharmacological and physiological stresses in sport horses, *Zentralbl Veterinarmed A* 37:601-604, 1990.
11. Snow DH, Mackenzie G: Some metabolic effects of maximal exercise in the horse and adaptations with training, *Equine Vet J* 9:134-140, 1977.
12. Cayado P, Munoz-Escassi B, Dominguez C, et al: Hormone response to training and competition in athletic horses, *Equine Vet J* (Suppl):274-278, 2006.
13. Dybdal NO, Gribble D, Madigan JE, et al: Alterations in plasma corticosteroids, insulin and selected metabolites in horses used in endurance rides, *Equine Vet J* 12:137-140, 1980.
14. Lassourd V, Gayrard V, Laroute V, et al: Cortisol disposition and production rate in horses during rest and exercise, *Am J Physiol* 271:R25-R33, 1996.
15. Couetil LL, Hoffman AM: Adrenal insufficiency in a neonatal foal, *J Am Vet Med Assoc* 212:1594-1596, 1998.
16. Sojka JE, Levy M: Evaluation of endocrine function, *Vet Clin North Am Equine Pract* 11:415-435, 1995.
17. Dybdal NO, Hargreaves KM, Madigan JE, et al: Diagnostic testing for pituitary pars intermedia dysfunction in horses, *J Am Vet Med Assoc* 204:627-632, 1994.
18. Eiler H, Goble D, Oliver J: Adrenal gland function in the horse: effects of cosyntropin (synthetic) and corticotropin (natural) stimulation, *Am J Vet Res* 40:724-726, 1979.
19. van der Kolk JH, Kalsbeek HC, van Garderen E, et al: Equine pituitary neoplasia: a clinical report of 21 cases (1990-1992), *Vet Rec* 133:594-597, 1993.
20. MacHarg MA, Bottoms GD, Carter GK, et al: Effects of multiple intramuscular injections and doses of dexamethasone on plasma cortisol concentrations and adrenal responses to ACTH in horses, *Am J Vet Res* 46:2285-2287, 1985.
21. Toutain PL, Brandon RA, de Pomyers H, et al: Dexamethasone and prednisolone in the horse: pharmacokinetics and action on the adrenal gland, *Am J Vet Res* 45:1750-1756, 1984.
22. Slone DE, Purohit RC, Ganjam VK, et al: Sodium retention and cortisol (hydrocortisone) suppression caused by dexamethasone and triamcinolone in equids, *Am J Vet Res* 44: 280-283, 1983.
23. Soma LR, Uboh CE, Luo Y, et al: Pharmacokinetics of methylprednisolone acetate after intra-articular administration and its effect on endogenous hydrocortisone and cortisone secretion in horses, *Am J Vet Res* 67:654-662, 2006.
24. Peroni DL, Stanley S, Kollias-Baker C, et al: Prednisone per os is likely to have limited efficacy in horses, *Equine Vet J* 34: 283-287, 2002.
25. Gold JR, Divers TJ, Barton MH, et al: Plasma adrenocorticotropin, cortisol, and adrenocorticotropin/cortisol ratios in septic and normal-term foals, *J Vet Intern Med* 21:791-796, 2007.
26. Hart KA, Slovis NM, Barton MH: Hypothalamic-pituitary-adrenal axis dysfunction in critically ill neonatal foals. In *Proceedings of the twenty-sixth annual American College of Veterinary Internal Medicine forum*, San Antonio, TX, (June): 4-9, 2008, ACVIM.
27. Hurcombe SD, Toribio RE, Slovis N, et al: Blood arginine vasopressin, adrenocorticotropin hormone, and cortisol concentrations at admission in septic and critically ill foals and their association with survival, *J Vet Intern Med* 22:639-647, 2008.
28. Ousey JC, Rossdale PD, Fowden AL, et al: Effects of manipulating intrauterine growth on post natal adrenocortical development and other parameters of maturity in neonatal foals, *Equine Vet J* 36:616-621, 2004.
29. Livesey JH, Donald RA, Irvine CH, et al: The effects of cortisol, vasopressin (AVP), and corticotropin-releasing factor administration on pulsatile adrenocorticotropin, alpha-melanocyte-stimulating hormone, and AVP secretion in the pituitary venous effluent of the horse, *Endocrinology* 123:713-720, 1988.
30. Silver M, Ousey JC, Dudan FE, et al: Studies on equine prematurity. II. Post natal adrenocortical activity in relation to plasma adrenocorticotrophic hormone and catecholamine levels in term and premature foals, *Equine Vet J* 16:278-286, 1984.
31. Cryer PE: Diseases of the sympathochromaffin system. In Felig P, Baxter JD, Frohman LA, editors: *Endocrinology and metabolism*, New York, 1995, McGraw-Hill Inc, pp 713-748.
32. Buckingham JD: Case report. Pheochromocytoma in a mare, *Can Vet J* 11:205-208, 1970.
33. Yovich JV, Horney FD, Hardee GE: Pheochromocytoma in the horse and measurement of norepinephrine levels in horses, *Can Vet J* 25:21-25, 1984.
34. Duckett WM, Snyder JR, Harkema JR, et al: Functional pheochromocytoma in a horse, *Compend Contin Educ Equine Pract* 9:1118-1121, 1987.
35. Johnson PJ, Goetz TE, Foreman JH, et al: Pheochromocytoma in two horses, *J Am Vet Med Assoc* 206:837-841, 1995.
36. Gelberg H, Cockerell GL, Minor RR: A light and electron microscopic study of a normal adrenal medulla and a pheochromocytoma from a horse, *Vet Pathol* 16:395-404, 1979.
37. Yovich JV, Ducharme NG: Ruptured pheochromocytoma in a mare with colic, *J Am Vet Med Assoc* 183:462-464, 1983.
38. Kolloch RE, Kruse HJ, Friedrich R, et al: Role of epinephrine-induced hypokalemia in the regulation of renin and aldosterone in humans, *J Lab Clin Med* 127:50-56, 1996.
39. Ivanova RS, Dashev GI: Neuroendocrine features of adrenal pheochromocytomas: histological and immunocytochemical evaluation, *Neoplasma* 37:219-224, 1990.
40. Moreno AM, Castilla-Guerra L, Martinez-Torres MC, et al: Expression of neuropeptides and other neuroendocrine markers in human phaeochromocytomas, *Neuropeptides* 33: 159-163, 1999.
41. Wilson RB, Holscher MA, Kasselberg AG, et al: Leu-enkephalin and somatostatin immunoreactivities in canine and equine pheochromocytomas, *Vet Pathol* 23:96-98, 1986.
42. Hardee GE, Wang LJ, Semrad SD, et al: Catecholamines in equine and bovine plasmas, *J Vet Pharmacol Ther* 5:279-284, 1982.
43. De Cock HE, MacLachlan NJ: Simultaneous occurrence of multiple neoplasms and hyperplasias in the adrenal and thyroid gland of the horse resembling multiple endocrine neoplasia syndrome: case report and retrospective identification of additional cases, *Vet Pathol* 36:633-636, 1999.
44. Froscher BG, Power HT: Malignant pheochromocytoma in a foal, *J Am Vet Med Assoc* 181:494-496, 1982.
45. Chiba S, Okada K, Numakunai S, et al: A case of equine thyroid follicular carcinoma accompanied with adenohypophysial adenoma, *Nippon Juigaku Zasshi* 49:551-554, 1987.

46. Cohen ND, Carter GK: Steroid hepatopathy in a horse with glucocorticoid-induced hyperadrenocorticism, *J Am Vet Med Assoc* 200:1682-1684, 1992.
47. Traver DS, Bottoms GD: Adrenal dysfunction. In *Proceedings of the twenty-fourth annual American Association of Equine Practitioners*, 1981, AAEP, New Orleans, La., 499-514.
48. van der Kolk JH, Ijzer J, Overgaauw PA, et al: Pituitary-independent Cushing's syndrome in a horse, *Equine Vet J* 33: 110-112, 2001.
49. Fix AS, Miller LD: Equine adrenocortical carcinoma with hypercalcemia, *Vet Pathol* 24:190-192, 1987.
50. van der Kolk JH, Mars MH: van dG I: Adrenocortical carcinoma in a 12-year-old mare, *Vet Rec* 134:113-115, 1994.

Thyroid Gland

1. Kaneko JJ, Harvey JW, Bruss ML, editors: *Biochemistry of domestic animals*, ed 6, San Diego, 2009, Academic Press.
2. Lucke VM, Lane JG: C-cell tumours of the thyroid in the horse, *Equine Vet J* 16:28-30, 1984.
3. Dimock WW, Westerfield C, Doll ER: The equine thyroid in health and disease, *J Am Vet Med Assoc* 104:313, 1944.
4. Drew B, Barber WP, Williams DG: The effect of excess dietary iodine on pregnant mares and foals, *Vet Rec* 97:93-95, 1975.
5. Jackson IM: Thyrotropin-releasing hormone, *N Engl J Med* 306:145-155, 1982.
6. DeGroot LJ, Jameson JL, editors: *Endocrinology*, ed 5, Philadelphia, 2006, WB Saunders.
7. Kronenberg HM, Melmed S, Polonsky KS, et al: *Williams textbook of endocrinology*, ed 11, Philadelphia, 2008, WB Saunders.
8. Dahl GE, Evans NP, Thrun LA, et al: A central negative feedback action of thyroid hormones on thyrotropin-releasing hormone secretion, *Endocrinology* 135:2392-2397, 1994.
9. Dyess EM, Segerson TP, Liposits Z, et al: Triiodothyronine exerts direct cell-specific regulation of thyrotropin-releasing hormone gene expression in the hypothalamic paraventricular nucleus, *Endocrinology* 123:2291-2297, 1988.
10. Segerson TP, Kauer J, Wolfe HC, et al: Thyroid hormone regulates TRH biosynthesis in the paraventricular nucleus of the rat hypothalamus, *Science* 238:78-80, 1987.
11. Thompson DL, Nett TM: Thyroid stimulating hormone and prolactin secretion after thyrotropin releasing hormone administration to mares—dose-response during anestrus in winter and during estrus in summer, *Domest Anim Endocrinol* 1:263-268, 1984.
12. Thompson FN, Caudle AB, Kemppainen RJ, et al: Thyroidal and prolactin secretion in agalactic mares, *Theriogenology* 25:575-580, 1986.
13. Gentry LR, Thompson DL Jr, Stelzer AM: Responses of seasonally anovulatory mares to daily administration of thyrotropin-releasing hormone and (or) gonadotropin-releasing hormone analog, *J Anim Sci* 80:208-213, 2002.
14. Pruett HE, Thompson DL Jr, Cartmill JA, et al: Thyrotropin releasing hormone interactions with growth hormone secretion in horses, *J Anim Sci* 81:2343-2351, 2003.
15. Pineda M, Dooley MP, editors: *McDonald's veterinary endocrinology and reproduction*, ed 5, Philadelphia, 2003, Wiley Blackwell.
16. Dai G, Levy O, Carrasco N: Cloning and characterization of the thyroid iodide transporter, *Nature* 379:458-460, 1996.
17. Yen PM: Physiological and molecular basis of thyroid hormone action, *Physiol Rev* 81:1097-1142, 2001.
18. Chen CL, Riley AM: Serum thyroxine and triiodothyronine concentrations in neonatal foals and mature horses, *Am J Vet Res* 42:1415-1417, 1981.
19. Irvine CH: Thyroxine secretion rate in the horse in various physiological states, *J Endocrinol* 39:313-320, 1967.
20. Irvine CH, Evans MJ: Postnatal changes in total and free thyroxine and triiodothyronine in foal serum, *J Reprod Fertil* (Suppl (23)):709-715, October 1975.
21. Irvine CH, Evans MJ: Hypothyroidism in foals, *N Z Vet J* 25:354, 1977.
22. Malinowski K, Christensen RA, Hafs HD, et al: Age and breed differences in thyroid hormones, insulin-like growth factor (IGF)-I and IGF binding proteins in female horses, *J Anim Sci* 74:1936-1942, 1996.
23. Larsson M, Pettersson T, Carlstrom A: Thyroid hormone binding in serum of 15 vertebrate species: isolation of thyroxine-binding globulin and prealbumin analogs, *Gen Comp Endocrinol* 58:360-375, 1985.
24. Irvine CH: Hypothyroidism in the foal, *Equine Vet J* 16:302-306, 1984.
25. Katovich M, Evans JW, Sanchez O: Effects of season, pregnancy and lactation on thyroxine turnover in the mare, *J Anim Sci* 38:811-818, 1974.
26. Argenzio RA, Lowe JE, Hintz HF, et al: Calcium and phosphorus homeostasis in horses, *J Nutr* 104:18-27, 1974.
27. Khan VTS: Studies on thyroidal states in equines during normal and certain disturbed conditions of reproduction, *Mysore J Agr Sci* 14:1382, 1980.
28. Motley JS: Use of radioactive triiodothyronine in the study of thyroid function in normal horses, *Vet Med Small Anim Clin* 67:1225-1228, 1972.
29. McCall CA, Potter GD, Kreider JL, et al: Physiological-responses in foals weaned by abrupt or gradual methods, *J Equine Vet Sci* 7:368-374, 1987.
30. Reap M, Cass C, Hightower D: Thyroxine and triiodothyronine levels in ten species of animals, *Southwest Vet* 31:31, 1978.
31. Anderson RR, Nixon DA, Akasha MA: Total and free thyroxine and triiodothyronine in blood serum of mammals, *Comp Biochem Physiol A* 89:401-404, 1988.
32. Irvine CH: Protein bound iodine in the horse, *Am J Vet Res* 28:1687, 1967.
33. deMartin BW: Study on the thyroid function of thoroughbred horses by means of "in vitro" 125I-T3 modified and 125I-T4 tests, *Rev Fac Med Vet Univ Sao Paulo* 12:107, 1975.
34. Kelley ST, Oehme FW, Brandt GW: Measurement of thyroid gland function during the estrous cycle of nine mares, *Am J Vet Res* 35:657-660, 1974.
35. Thomas CL Jr, Adams JC: Radioimmunoassay of equine serum for thyroxine: reference values, *Am J Vet Res* 39:1239, 1978.
36. deMartin BW: Study on the thyroid function of male and female thoroughbred horses in different times after winning races at the Hippodrome Cidade Jardim, with the use of "in vitro" 125I-T3, and 125I-T4 tests, *Rev Fac Med Vet Univ Sao Paulo* 14:199, 1977.
37. deMartin BW: Study on the thyroid function of thoroughbred females in varying stages of pregnancy using "in vitro" tests 125I-T3 and 125I-T4, *Rev Fac Med Vet Univ Sao Paulo* 12:121, 1975.
38. Hershman JM: Use of thyrotropin-releasing hormone in clinical medicine, *Med Clin North Am* 62:313-325, 1978.
39. Messer NT, Ganjam VK, Nachreiner RF, et al: Effect of dexamethasone administration on serum thyroid hormone concentrations in clinically normal horses, *J Am Vet Med Assoc* 206:63-66, 1995.
40. Galton VA: Thyroid hormone-catecholamine interrelationships, *Endocrinology* 77:278-284, 1965.
41. Sommardahl CS, Frank N, Elliott SB, et al: Effects of oral administration of levothyroxine sodium on serum concentrations of thyroid gland hormones and responses to injections of thyrotropin-releasing hormone in healthy adult mares, *Am J Vet Res* 66:1025-1031, 2005.

42. Irvine CH: Thyroid function in the horse. In *Proceedings of the American Association of Equine Practitioners convention*, 1966, ACVIM, Los Angeles, Calif., p 197.
43. McBride GE, Christopherson RJ, Sauer W: Metabolic-rate and plasma thyroid-hormone concentrations of mature horses in response to changes in ambient-temperature, *Can J Anim Sci* 65:375-382, 1985.
44. Duckett WM, Manning JP, Weston PG: Thyroid hormone periodicity in healthy adult geldings, *Equine Vet J* 21:123-125, 1989.
45. Morris DD, Garcia M: Thyroid-stimulating hormone: response test in healthy horses, and effect of phenylbutazone on equine thyroid hormones, *Am J Vet Res* 44:503-507, 1983.
46. Brabant G, Brabant A, Ranft U, et al: Circadian and pulsatile thyrotropin secretion in euthyroid man under the influence of thyroid hormone and glucocorticoid administration, *J Clin Endocrinol Metab* 65:83-88, 1987.
47. De Groot LJ: Dangerous dogmas in medicine: the nonthyroidal illness syndrome, *J Clin Endocrinol Metab* 84:151-164, 1999.
48. Breuhaus BA, LaFevers DH: Thyroid function in normal, sick and premature foals. In *Proceedings of the twenty-third annual American College of Veterinary Internal Medicine forum*, Baltimore, MD, (June): 1-4, 2005, ACVIM.
49. Van den BG, de Zegher F, Baxter RC, et al: Neuroendocrinology of prolonged critical illness: effects of exogenous thyrotropin-releasing hormone and its combination with growth hormone secretagogues, *J Clin Endocrinol Metab* 83:309-319, 1998.
50. Flier JS, Harris M, Hollenberg AN: Leptin, nutrition, and the thyroid: the why, the wherefore, and the wiring, *J Clin Invest* 105:859-861, 2000.
51. Frank N, Buchanan BR, Elliott SB: Effects of long-term oral administration of levothyroxine sodium on serum thyroid hormone concentrations, clinicopathologic variables, and echocardiographic measurements in healthy adult horses, *Am J Vet Res* 69:68-75, 2008.
52. Snow DH, Persson SGB, Rose RJ, editors: *Equine exercise physiology*, Cambridge, 1983, Granta Editions.
53. Takagi S, Ito K, Shibata H: Effects of training on plasma fibrinogen concentration and thyroid hormone level in young race horses, *Exper Results Equine Health Lab* 11:94, 1974.
54. Gonzalez O, Gonzalez E, Sanchez C, et al: Effect of exercise on erythrocyte beta-adrenergic receptors and plasma concentrations of catecholamines and thyroid hormones in Thoroughbred horses, *Equine Vet J* 30:72-78, 1998.
55. Garcia MC, Beech J: Endocrinologic, hematologic, and heart rate changes in swimming horses, *Am J Vet Res* 47:2004-2006, 1986.
56. Gupta S, Glade MJ: Hormonal responses to high and low planes of nutrition in weanling Thoroughbreds, *Equine Vet Data* 4:170, 1983.
57. Biesik LM, Glade MJ: Changes in serum hormone concentrations in weanling horses following gastric infusion of sucrose or casein, *Nutr Rep Int* 33:651-658, 1986.
58. Glade MJ, Reimers TJ: Effects of dietary energy supply on serum thyroxine, tri-iodothyronine and insulin concentrations in young horses, *J Endocrinol* 104:93-98, 1985.
59. Youket RJ, Carnevale JM, Houpt KA, et al: Humoral, hormonal and behavioral correlates of feeding in ponies: the effects of meal frequency, *J Anim Sci* 61:1103-1110, 1985.
60. Christensen RA, Malinowski K, Massenzio AM, et al: Acute effects of short-term feed deprivation and refeeding on circulating concentrations of metabolites, insulin-like growth factor I, insulin-like growth factor binding proteins, somatotropin, and thyroid hormones in adult geldings, *J Anim Sci* 75:1351-1358, 1997.
61. Messer NT, Johnson PJ, Refsal KR, et al: Effect of food deprivation on baseline iodothyronine and cortisol concentrations in healthy, adult horses, *Am J Vet Res* 56:116-121, 1995.
62. Suwannachot P, Verkleij CB, Kocsis S, et al: Prolonged food restriction and mild exercise in Shetland ponies: effects on weight gain, thyroid hormone concentrations and muscle Na(+), K(+)-ATPase, *J Endocrinol* 167:321-329, 2000.
63. Boelen A, Wiersinga WM, Fliers E: Fasting-induced changes in the hypothalamus-pituitary-thyroid axis, *Thyroid* 18:123-129, 2008.
64. McManus CJ, Fitzgerald BP: Effects of a single day of feed restriction on changes in serum leptin, gonadotropins, prolactin, and metabolites in aged and young mares, *Domest Anim Endocrinol* 19:1-13, 2000.
65. Buff PR, Morrison CD, Ganjam VK, et al: Effects of short-term feed deprivation and melatonin implants on circadian patterns of leptin in the horse, *J Anim Sci* 83:1023-1032, 2005.
66. Steelman SM, Michael-Eller EM, Gibbs PG, et al: Meal size and feeding frequency influence serum leptin concentration in yearling horses, *J Anim Sci* 84:2391-2398, 2006.
67. Fitzgerald BP, McManus CJ: Photoperiodic versus metabolic signals as determinants of seasonal anestrus in the mare, *Biol Reprod* 63:335-340, 2000.
68. Berg EL, McNamara DL, Keisler DH: Endocrine profiles of periparturient mares and their foals, *J Anim Sci* 85:1660-1668, 2007.
69. Rothschild CM, Hines MT, Breuhaus B, et al: Effects of trimethoprim-sulfadiazine on thyroid function of horses, *J Vet Intern Med* 18:370-373, 2004.
70. Ramirez S, Wolfsheimer KJ, Moore RM, et al: Duration of effects of phenylbutazone on serum total thyroxine and free thyroxine concentrations in horses, *J Vet Intern Med* 11:371-374, 1997.
71. van Maanen JM, van Dijk A, Mulder K, et al: Consumption of drinking water with high nitrate levels causes hypertrophy of the thyroid, *Toxicol Lett* 72:365-374, 1994.
72. Morris DD, Garcia MC: Effects of phenylbutazone and anabolic steroids on adrenal and thyroid gland function tests in healthy horses, *Am J Vet Res* 46:359-364, 1985.
73. Boosinger TR, Brendemuehl JP, Bransby DL, et al: Prolonged gestation, decreased triiodothyronine concentration, and thyroid gland histomorphologic features in newborn foals of mares grazing *Acremonion coenophialum*-infected fescue, *Am J Vet Res* 56:66-69, 1995.
74. Breuhaus BA: Thyroid function in mature horses ingesting endophyte-infected fescue seed, *J Am Vet Med Assoc* 223:340-345, 2003.
75. Sojka JE, Johnson MA, Bottoms GD: Serum triiodothyronine, total thyroxine, and free thyroxine concentrations in horses, *Am J Vet Res* 54:52-55, 1993.
76. Breuhaus BA: Thyroid-stimulating hormone in adult euthyroid and hypothyroid horses, *J Vet Intern Med* 16:109-115, 2002.
77. Marcella KL: General care of miniature horses, *Vet Clin North Am Equine Pract* 14:26-28, 1992.
78. Wehr U, Englschalk B, Kienzle E, et al: Iodine balance in relation to iodine intake in ponies, *J Nutr* 132:1767S-1768S, 2002.
79. Johnson PJ, Messer NT, Ganjam VK, et al: Effects of propylthiouracil and bromocryptine on serum concentrations of thyrotrophin and thyroid hormones in normal female horses, *Equine Vet J* 35:296-301, 2003.
80. Murray MJ, Luba NK: Plasma gastrin and somatostatin, and serum thyroxine (T4), triiodothyronine (T3), reverse triiodothyronine (rT3) and cortisol concentrations in foals from birth to 28 days of age, *Equine Vet J* 25:237-239, 1993.
81. Shaftoe S, Schick MP, Chen CL: Thyroid-stimulating hormone response tests in one-day-old foals, *J Equine Vet Sci* 8:310-312, 1988.
82. Dudan FE, Ferguson DC, Little TV: Circulating serum thyroxine (T4), triiodothyronine (T3) and reverse T3 (RT3) in neonatal term and preterm foals. In *Proceedings of the fifth annual veterinary medical forum*, San Diego, 1987, p 881.

83. Tateyama S, Tanimura N, Moritomo Y, et al: The ultimobranchial remnant and its hyperplasia or adenoma in equine thyroid gland, *Nippon Juigaku Zasshi* 50:714-722, 1988.
84. Reimers TJ, Cowan RG, Davidson HP, et al: Validation of radioimmunoassay for triiodothyronine, thyroxine, and hydrocortisone (cortisol) in canine, feline, and equine sera, *Am J Vet Res* 42:2016-2021, 1981.
85. Reimers TJ, Lamb SV, Bartlett SA, et al: Effects of hemolysis and storage on quantification of hormones in blood samples from dogs, cattle, and horses, *Am J Vet Res* 52:1075-1080, 1991.
86. Stockigt JR, Nagatake S, editors: *Thyroid research VIII*, New York, 1980, Pergamon.
87. Harris P, Marlin D, Gray J: Equine thyroid-function tests—a preliminary investigation, *Br Vet J* 148:71-80, 1992.
88. Held JP, Oliver JW: A sampling protocol for the thyrotropin-stimulation test in the horse, *J Am Vet Med Assoc* 184:326-327, 1984.
89. Oliver JW, Held JP: Thyrotropin stimulation test—new perspective on value of monitoring triiodothyronine, *J Am Vet Med Assoc* 187:931-934, 1985.
90. Beech J, Garcia M: Hormonal response to thyrotropin-releasing hormone in healthy horses and in horses with pituitary adenoma, *Am J Vet Res* 46:1941-1943, 1985.
91. Chen CL, Li WI: Effect of thyrotropin releasing hormone (TRH) on serum levels of thyroid hormones in thoroughbred mares, *J Equine Sci* 6:58, 1986.
92. Lothrop CD Jr, Nolan HL: Equine thyroid function assessment with the thyrotropin-releasing hormone response test, *Am J Vet Res* 47:942-944, 1986.
93. Thompson DL Jr, Godke RA, Nett TM: Effects of melatonin and thyrotropin releasing hormone on mares during the nonbreeding season, *J Anim Sci* 56:668-677, 1983.
94. Beech J, Boston R, Lindborg S, et al: Adrenocorticotropin concentration following administration of thyrotropin-releasing hormone in healthy horses and those with pituitary pars intermedia dysfunction and pituitary gland hyperplasia, *J Am Vet Med Assoc* 231:417-426, 2007.
95. Frank N, Andrews FM, Sommardahl CS, et al: Evaluation of the combined dexamethasone suppression/thyrotropin-releasing hormone stimulation test for detection of pars intermedia pituitary adenomas in horses, *J Vet Intern Med* 20:987-993, 2006.
96. Alberts MK, McCann JP, Woods PR: Hemithyroidectomy in a horse with confirmed hyperthyroidism, *J Am Vet Med Assoc* 217:1051-1054, 2000.
97. Hillidge CJ, Theodorakis MC, Duckett WM: Scintigraphic evaluation of equine thyroid function. In *Proceedings of the twenty-seventh annual American Association of Equine Practitioners convention*, 1981, AAEP, New Orleans, p 477.
98. Held JP, Patton CS, Toal RL, et al: Work intolerance in a horse with thyroid carcinoma, *J Am Vet Med Assoc* 187:1044-1045, 1985.
99. Hillidge CJ, Sanecki RK, Theodorakis MC: Thyroid carcinoma in a horse, *J Am Vet Med Assoc* 181:711-714, 1982.
100. Joyce JR, Thompson RB, Kyzar JR, et al: Thyroid carcinoma in a horse, *J Am Vet Med Assoc* 168:610-612, 1976.
101. Ramirez S, McClure JJ, Moore RM, et al: Hyperthyroidism associated with a thyroid adenocarcinoma in a 21-year-old gelding, *J Vet Intern Med* 12:475-477, 1998.
102. Perillo A, Passantino G, Passantino L, et al: First observation of an Hashimoto thyroiditis-like disease in horses from Eastern Europe: histopathological and immunological findings, *Immunopharmacol Immunotoxicol* 27:241-253, 2005.
103. Green EM, Hunt EL: Hypophyseal neoplasia in a pony, *Compend Contin Educ Practic Vet* 7:S249, 1985.
104. Lowe JE, Kallfelz FA: Thyroidectomy and the T4 Test to Assess Thyroid Dysfunction in the Horse and Pony. In *Proceedings of the sixteenth annual American Association of Equine Practitioners Convention*, New Orleans, La., 1970, AAEP, p 135.
105. Conway DA, Cosgrove JS: Equine goiter, *Ir Vet J* 34:29-31, 1980.
106. Baker JR, Wyn-Jones G, Eley JL: Case of equine goiter, *Vet Rec* 112:407-408, 1983.
107. Murray MJ: Hypothyroidism and respiratory insufficiency in a neonatal foal, *J Am Vet Med Assoc* 197:1635-1638, 1990.
108. Doige CE, McLaughlin BG: Hyperplastic goitre in newborn foals in Western Canada, *Can Vet J* 22:42-45, 1981.
109. McLaughlin BG, Doige CE: A study of ossification of carpal and tarsal bones in normal and hypothyroid foals, *Can Vet J* 23:164-168, 1982.
110. Vivrette SL, Reimers TJ, Krook L: Skeletal disease in a hypothyroid foal, *Cornell Vet* 74:373-386, 1984.
111. Shaver JR, Fretz PB, Doige CE: Skeletal manifestations of suspected hypothyroidism in two foals, *J Equine Med Surg* 3:269, 1979.
112. McLaughlin BG, Doige CE: Congenital musculosketal lesions and hyperplastic goitre in foals, *Can Vet J* 22:130-133, 1981.
113. McLaughlin BG, Doige CE, McLaughlin PS: Thyroid-hormone levels in foals with congenital musculoskeletal lesions, *Can Vet J* 27:264-267, 1986.
114. Lowe JE, Baldwin BH, Foote RH, et al: Equine hypothyroidism: the long-term effects of thyroidectomy on metabolism and growth in mares and stallions, *Cornell Vet* 64:276-295, 1974.
115. Baker HJ, Lindsey JR: Equine goiter due to excess dietary iodide, *J Am Vet Med Assoc* 153:1618-1630, 1968.
116. Cubillos V, Norambuena L, Espinoza E: Cell growth and neoplasms of the thyroid gland in horses, *Zentralbl Veterinarmed A* 28:201-208, 1981.
117. Driscoll J, Hintz HF, Schryver HF: Goiter in foals caused by excessive iodine, *J Am Vet Med Assoc* 173:858-859, 1978.
118. McLaughlin BG, Doige CE, Fretz PB, et al: Carpal bone lesions associated with angular limb deformities in foals, *J Am Vet Med Assoc* 178:224-230, 1981.
119. Allen AL, Doige CE, Fretz PB, et al: Hyperplasia of the thyroid gland and concurrent musculoskeletal deformities in Western Canadian foals: reexamination of a previously described syndrome, *Can Vet J* 35:31-38, 1994.
120. Allen AL: Hyperplasia of the thyroid gland and musculoskeletal deformities in two equine abortuses, *Can Vet J* 36:234-236, 1995.
121. Allen AL, Townsend HG, Doige CE, et al: A case-control study of the congenital hypothyroidism and dysmaturity syndrome of foals, *Can Vet J* 37:349-351, 1996.
122. Lowe JE, Baldwin BH, Foote RH, et al: Semen characteristics in thyroidectomized stallions, *J Reprod Fertil* (Suppl (23)):81-86, October 1975.
123. Vischer CM, Foreman JH, Constable PD, et al: Hemodynamic effects of thyroidectomy in sedentary horses, *Am J Vet Res* 60:14-21, 1999.
124. Lowe JE, Foote RH, Baldwin BH, et al: Reproductive patterns in cyclic and pregnant thyroidectomized mares, *J Reprod Fertil Suppl* 35:281-288, 1987.
125. Stanley O, Hillidge CJ: Alopecia associated with hypothyroidism in a horse, *Equine Vet J* 14:165-167, 1982.
126. Fadok VA, Wild S: Suspected cutaneous iodism in a horse, *J Am Vet Med Assoc* 183:1104-1106, 1983.
127. Poomvises P, Gesmankit P, Tawatsin A: Studies on serum triiodothyronine and thyroxine in anhidrotic horses, *Centaur Lond Engl II* 139, 1986.
128. Mayhew IG, Ferguson HO: Clinical, clinicopathologic, and epidemiologic features of anhidrosis in central Florida Thoroughbred horses, *J Vet Intern Med* 1:136-141, 1987.
129. Hood DM, Hightower D, Amoss MS: Thyroid function in horses affected with laminitis, *Southwest Vet* 38:85, 1987.
130. Alexander SL, Irvine CH, Evans MJ: Inter-relationships between the secretory dynamics of thyrotrophin-releasing hormone, thyrotrophin and prolactin in periovulatory mares: effect of hypothyroidism, *J Neuroendocrinol* 16:906-915, 2004.

131. Waldron-Mease E: Hypothyroidism and myopathy in racing Thoroughbreds and Standardbreds, *J Equine Med Surg* 3:124, 1979.
132. deMartin BW: Study on the thyroid function of Thoroughbred horses using 131I-TBI, *Rev Fac Med Vet Univ Sao Paulo* 10:35, 1973.
133. Dalefield RR, Palmer DN: The frequent occurrence of thyroid tumours in aged horses, *J Comp Pathol* 110:57-64, 1994.
134. Damodaran S, Ramachandran PV: A survey of neoplasms in equidae, *Centaur Lond Engl* II:161, 1986.
135. Hopper LD, Kennedy GA, Taylor WA: Diagnosing and treating thyroid adenoma in a horse, *Vet Med* 82:1252, 1987.
136. Hovda LR, Shaftoe S, Rose ML, et al: Mediastinal squamous cell carcinoma and thyroid carcinoma in an aged horse, *J Am Vet Med Assoc* 197:1187-1189, 1990.
137. Ralston SL, Nockels CF, Squires EL: Differences in diagnostic test results and hematologic data between aged and young horses, *Am J Vet Res* 49:1387-1392, 1988.
138. Schlotthauer CF: The incidence and types of disease of the thyroid gland of adult horses, *J Am Vet Med Assoc* 78:211, 1931.
139. Yoshikawa T, Yoshikawa H, Oyamada T, et al: A follicular adenoma with C-cell hyperplasia in the equine thyroid, *Nippon Juigaku Zasshi* 46:615-623, 1984.
140. Chiba S, Okada K, Numakunai S, et al: A case of equine thyroid follicular carcinoma accompanied with adenohypophysial adenoma, *Nippon Juigaku Zasshi* 49:551-554, 1987.
141. De Cock HE, MacLachlan NJ: Simultaneous occurrence of multiple neoplasms and hyperplasias in the adrenal and thyroid gland of the horse resembling multiple endocrine neoplasia syndrome: case report and retrospective identification of additional cases, *Vet Pathol* 36:633-636, 1999.
142. van der Velden MA, Meulenaar H: Medullary thyroid carcinoma in a horse, *Vet Pathol* 23:622-624, 1986.
143. Kuwamura M, Shirota A, Yamate J, et al: C-cell adenoma containing variously sized thyroid follicles in a horse, *J Vet Med Sci* 60:387-389, 1998.

Endocrine Pancreas

1. Gilon P, Henquin JC: Mechanisms and physiological significance of the cholinergic control of pancreatic beta-cell function, *Endocr Rev* 22:565-604, 2001.
2. Conn PM, Melmed S, editors: *Basic and clinical principles*, Totowa, NJ, 1997, Humana Press, Endocrinology.
3. Felig P, Baxter JD, Frohman LA, editors: *Endocrinology and metabolism*, New York, 1995, McGraw-Hill Inc.
4. Fowden AL, Gardner DS, Ousey JC, et al: Maturation of pancreatic beta-cell function in the fetal horse during late gestation, *J Endocrinol* 186:467-473, 2005.
5. Fowden AL, Ellis L, Rossdale PD: Pancreatic beta cell function in the neonatal foal, *J Reprod Fertil Suppl* 32:529-535, 1982.
6. Holdstock NB, Allen VL, Bloomfield MR, et al: Development of insulin and proinsulin secretion in newborn pony foals, *J Endocrinol* 181:469-476, 2004.
7. Dominici FP, Turyn D: Growth hormone-induced alterations in the insulin-signaling system, *Exp Biol Med (Maywood)* 227:149-157, 2002.
8. Firshman AM, Valberg SJ: Factors affecting clinical assessment of insulin sensitivity in horses, *Equine Vet J* 39:567-575, 2007.
9. Johnson PJ, Scotty NC, Wiedmeyer C, et al: Diabetes mellitus in a domesticated Spanish mustang, *J Am Vet Med Assoc* 226(542):584-588, 2005.
10. Kronfeld DS, Treiber KH, Hess TM, et al: Metabolic syndrome in healthy ponies facilitates nutritional countermeasures against pasture laminitis, *J Nutr* 136:2090S-2093S, 2006.
11. McCoy DJ: Diabetes mellitus associated with bilateral granulosa cell tumors in a mare, *J Am Vet Med Assoc* 188:733-735, 1986.
12. Toth F, Frank N, Elliott SB, et al: Effects of an intravenous endotoxin challenge on glucose and insulin dynamics in horses, *Am J Vet Res* 69:82-88, 2008.
13. Treiber KH, Kronfeld DS, Geor RJ: Insulin resistance in equids: possible role in laminitis, *J Nutr* 136:2094S-2098S, 2006.
14. Treiber KH, Boston RC, Kronfeld DS, et al: Insulin resistance and compensation in Thoroughbred weanlings adapted to high-glycemic meals, *J Anim Sci* 83:2357-2364, 2005.
15. Tiley HA, Geor RJ, McCutcheon LJ: Effects of dexamethasone administration on insulin resistance and components of insulin signaling and glucose metabolism in equine skeletal muscle, *Am J Vet Res* 69:51-58, 2008.
16. Annandale EJ, Valberg SJ, Mickelson JR, et al: Insulin sensitivity and skeletal muscle glucose transport in horses with equine polysaccharide storage myopathy, *Neuromuscul Disord* 14:666-674, 2004.
17. Jeffcott LB, Field JR, McLean JG, et al: Glucose tolerance and insulin sensitivity in ponies and Standardbred horses, *Equine Vet J* 18:97-101, 1986.
18. Treiber KH, Kronfeld DS, Hess TM, et al: Evaluation of genetic and metabolic predispositions and nutritional risk factors for pasture-associated laminitis in ponies, *J Am Vet Med Assoc* 228:1538-1545, 2006.
19. McCutcheon LJ, Geor RJ, Hinchcliff KW: Changes in skeletal muscle GLUT4 content and muscle membrane glucose transport following 6 weeks of exercise training, *Equine Vet J* Suppl., 2002;34:199-204.
20. Pratt SE, Geor RJ, Spriet LL, et al: Time course of insulin sensitivity and skeletal muscle glycogen synthase activity after a single bout of exercise in horses, *J Appl Physiol* 103:1063-1069, 2007.
21. Daugaard JR, Richter EA: Relationship between muscle fibre composition, glucose transporter protein 4 and exercise training: possible consequences in non-insulin-dependent diabetes mellitus, *Acta Physiol Scand* 171:267-276, 2001.
22. Douen AG, Ramlal T, Rastogi S, et al: Exercise induces recruitment of the "insulin-responsive glucose transporter." Evidence for distinct intracellular insulin- and exercise-recruitable transporter pools in skeletal muscle, *J Biol Chem* 265:13427-13430, 1990.
23. Freestone JF, Beadle R, Shoemaker K, et al: Improved insulin sensitivity in hyperinsulinaemic ponies through physical conditioning and controlled feed intake, *Equine Vet J* 24:187-190, 1992.
24. de Graaf-Roelfsema E, Tharasanit T, van Dam KG, et al: Effects of short- and long-term recombinant equine growth hormone and short-term hydrocortisone administration on tissue sensitivity to insulin in horses, *Am J Vet Res* 66:1907-1913, 2005.
25. Staempfli HR, Eigenmann EJ, Clarke LM: Insulin treatment and development of anti-insulin antibodies in a horse with diabetes mellitus associated with a functional pituitary adenoma, *Can Vet J* 29:934-936, 1988.
26. Baker JR, Ritchie HE: Diabetes mellitus in the horse: a case report and review of the literature, *Equine Vet J* 6:7-11, 1974.
27. Jeffrey JR: Diabetes mellitus secondary to chronic pancreatitis in a pony, *J Am Vet Med Assoc* 153:1168-1175, 1968.
28. King JM, Kavanaugh JF, Bentinck-Smith J: Diabetes mellitus with pituitary neoplasms in a horse and dog, *Cornell Vet* 52:133-145, 1962.
29. Muylle E, Van den HC, Deprez P, et al: Non-insulin dependent diabetes mellitus in a horse, *Equine Vet J* 18:145-146, 1986.
30. Ruoff WW, Baker DC, Morgan SJ, et al: Type II diabetes mellitus in a horse, *Equine Vet J* 18:143-144, 1986.
31. Tasker JB, Whiteman CE, Martin BR: Diabetes mellitus in the horse, *J Am Vet Med Assoc* 149:393-399, 1966.
32. Bulgin MS, Anderson BC: Verminous arteritis and pancreatic necrosis with diabetes mellitus in a pony, *Comp Contin Educ Equine Pract* 5:482-485, 1983.
33. Eiler H, Frank N, Andrews FM, et al: Physiologic assessment of blood glucose homeostasis via combined intravenous glucose and insulin testing in horses, *Am J Vet Res* 66:1598-1604, 2005.

34. Stockham SL: Interpretation of equine serum biochemical profile results, *Vet Clin North Am Equine Pract* 11:391-414, 1995.
35. Yovich JV, Horney FD, Hardee GE: Pheochromocytoma in the horse and measurement of norepinephrine levels in horses, *Can Vet J* 25:21-25, 1984.
36. Pratt SE, Geor RJ, McCutcheon LJ: Repeatability of 2 methods for assessment of insulin sensitivity and glucose dynamics in horses, *J Vet Intern Med* 19:883-888, 2005.
37. Sojka JE, Levy M: Evaluation of endocrine function, *Vet Clin North Am Equine Pract* 11:415-435, 1995.
38. Meirs DA, Taylor BC: Insulin induced shock, *Vet Clin North Am Equine Pract* 2:47-49, 1980.
39. Durham AE, Rendle DI, Newton JE: The effect of metformin on measurements of insulin sensitivity and beta cell response in 18 horses and ponies with insulin resistance, *Equine Vet J* 40:493-500, 2008.
40. Given BD, Mostrom MS, Tully R, et al: Severe hypoglycemia attributable to surreptitious injection of insulin in a mare, *J Am Vet Med Assoc* 193:224-226, 1988.
41. Ross MW, Lowe JE, Cooper BJ, et al: Hypoglycemic seizures in a Shetland pony, *Cornell Vet* 73:151-169, 1983.
42. Fowden AL, Comline RS, Silver M: Insulin secretion and carbohydrate metabolism during pregnancy in the mare, *Equine Vet J* 16:239-246, 1984.
43. Carrick JB, Morris DD, Harmon BG, et al: Hematuria and weight loss in a mare with pancreatic adenocarcinoma, *Cornell Vet* 82:91-97, 1992.
44. Church S, West HJ, Baker JR: Two cases of pancreatic adenocarcinoma in horses, *Equine Vet J* 19:77-79, 1987.
45. Kerr OM, Pearson GR, Rice DA: Pancreatic adenocarcinoma in a donkey, *Equine Vet J* 14:338-339, 1982.
46. Rendle DI, Hewetson M, Barron R, et al: Tachypnoea and pleural effusion in a mare with metastatic pancreatic adenocarcinoma, *Vet Rec* 159:356-359, 2006.

Pituitary Pars Intermedia Dysfunction (Equine Cushing's Disease)

1. Heinrichs M, Baumgartner W, Capen CC: Immunocytochemical demonstration of proopiomelanocortin-derived peptides in pituitary adenomas of the pars intermedia in horses, *Vet Pathol* 27:419-425, 1990.
2. Hillyer MH, Taylor FGR, Mair TS, et al: Diagnosis of hyperadrenocorticism in the horse, *Equine Vet Educ* 4:121-134, 1992.
3. Love S: Equine Cushing's disease, *Br Vet J* 149:139-153, 1993.
4. Moore JN, Steiss J, Nicholson WE, et al: A case of pituitary adrenocorticotropin-dependent Cushing's syndrome in the horse, *Endocrinology* 104:576-582, 1979.
5. van der Kolk JH, Kalsbeek HC, van Garderen E, et al: Equine pituitary neoplasia: a clinical report of 21 cases (1990-1992), *Vet Rec* 133:594-597, 1993.
6. Evans DR: The recognition and diagnosis of a pituitary tumor in the horse, *Proc Am Assoc Equine Pract* 18:417-419, 1972, ACVIM.
7. Loeb WF, Capen CC, Johnson LE: Adenomas of the pars intermedia associated with hyperglycemia and glycosuria in two horses, *Cornell Vet* 56:623-639, 1966.
8. Holscher MA, Linnabary RL, Netsky MG, et al: Adenoma of the pars intermedia and hirsutism in a pony, *Vet Med Small Anim Clin* 73:1197-1200, 1978.
9. Orth DN, Holscher MA, Wilson MG, et al: Equine Cushing's disease: plasma immunoreactive proopiolipomelanocortin peptide and cortisol levels basally and in response to diagnostic tests, *Endocrinology* 110:1430-1441, 1982.
10. Wilson MG, Nicholson WE, Holscher MA, et al: Proopiolipomelanocortin peptides in normal pituitary, pituitary tumor, and plasma of normal and Cushing's horses, *Endocrinology* 110:941-954, 1982.
11. Garcia MC, Beech J: Equine intravenous glucose tolerance test: glucose and insulin responses of healthy horses fed grain or hay and of horses with pituitary adenoma, *Am J Vet Res* 47:570-572, 1986.
12. Robinson NE, editor: *Current therapy in equine medicine*, ed 6, St Louis, 2009, WB Saunders.
13. Millington WR, Dybdal NO, Dawson R Jr, et al: Equine Cushing's disease: differential regulation of beta-endorphin processing in tumors of the intermediate pituitary, *Endocrinology* 123:1598-1604, 1988.
14. Boujon CE, Bestetti GE, Meier HP, et al: Equine pituitary adenoma: a functional and morphological study, *J Comp Pathol* 109:163-178, 1993.
15. Beech J: Treatment of hypophyseal adenomas, *Compend Contin Educ Pract Vet* 4:119-121, 1994.
16. Dybdal NO, Hargreaves KM, Madigan JE, et al: Diagnostic testing for pituitary pars intermedia dysfunction in horses, *J Am Vet Med Assoc* 204:627-632, 1994.
17. van der Kolk JH, Kalsbeek HC, Wensing T, et al: Urinary concentration of corticoids in normal horses and horses with hyperadrenocorticism, *Res Vet Sci* 56:126-128, 1994.
18. Thompson JC, Ellison R, Gillet RBL: Problems in the diagnosis of pituitary adenoma (Cushing's syndrome) in horses, *N Z Vet J* 43:79-82, 1995.
19. van der Kolk JH, Wensing T, Kalsbeek HC, et al: Laboratory diagnosis of equine pituitary pars intermedia adenoma, *Domest Anim Endocrinol* 12:35-39, 1995.
20. van der Kolk JH, Wensing T, Kalsbeek HC, et al: Lipid metabolism in horses with hyperadrenocorticism, *J Am Vet Med Assoc* 206:1010-1012, 1995.
21. Couetil L, Paradis MR, Knoll J: Plasma adrenocorticotropin concentration in healthy horses and in horses with clinical signs of hyperadrenocorticism, *J Vet Intern Med* 10:1-6, 1996.
22. Colahan PT, Merritt AM, Moore JN, et al: *Equine medicine and surgery*, ed 5, St Louis, 1999, Mosby.
23. Schott HC: Pituitary pars intermedia dysfunction: equine Cushing's disease, *Vet Clin North Am Equine Pract* 18:237-270, 2002.
24. Donaldson MT, LaMonte BH, Morresey P, et al: Treatment with pergolide or cyproheptadine of pituitary pars intermedia dysfunction (equine Cushing's disease), *J Vet Intern Med* 16:742-746, 2002.
25. Dowling PM, Williams MA, Clark TP: Adrenal insufficiency associated with long-term anabolic steroid administration in a horse, *J Am Vet Med Assoc* 203:1166-1169, 1993.
26. Bailey SR, Habershon-Butcher JL, Ransom KJ, et al: Hypertension and insulin resistance in a mixed-breed population of ponies predisposed to laminitis, *Am J Vet Res* 9:122-129, 2008.
27. Asplin KE, Sillence MN, Pollitt CC, et al: Induction of laminitis by prolonged hyperinsulinaemia in clinically normal ponies, *Vet J* 174:530-535, 2007.
28. Aleman M, Watson JL, Williams DC, et al: Myopathy in horses with pituitary pars intermedia dysfunction (Cushing's disease), *Neuromuscul Disord* 16:737-744, 2006.
29. van der Kolk JH: Relation between relative pituitary weight in horses with Cushing's disease and some plasma and clinical parameters. In *Proceedings of the thirty-fifth Congress of the British Equine Veterinary Association* 47:82-83, 1996.
30. Chemelli RM, Willie JT, Sinton CM, et al: Narcolepsy in orexin knockout mice: molecular genetics of sleep regulation, *Cell* 98:437-451, 1999.
31. McFarlane D: Cerebrospinal fluid concentration of hypocretin-1 in horses with equine pituitary pars intermedia disease and its relationship to oxidative stress, *J Vet Intern Med* 21:602, 2007:abstract.
32. McGowan TW, Hodgson DR, McGowan CM: The prevalence of equine Cushing's syndrome in aged horses, *J Vet Intern Med* 21:603, 2007:abstract.
33. Brosnahan MM, Paradis MR: Assessment of clinical characteristics, management practices, and activities of geriatric horses, *J Am Vet Med Assoc* 223:99-103, 2003.

34. Schott HC, Coursen CL, Eberhart SW et al: The Michigan Cushing's Project. In *Proceedings of the forty-seventh annual convention of the American Association of Equine Practitioners* 47:22-24. 2001.
35. van der Kolk JH, Heinrichs M, van Amerongen JD, et al: Evaluation of pituitary gland anatomy and histopathologic findings in clinically normal horses and horses and ponies with pituitary pars intermedia adenoma, *Am J Vet Res* 65:1701-1707, 2004.
36. Frank N, Andrews FM, Sommardahl CS, et al: Evaluation of the combined dexamethasone suppression/thyrotropin-releasing hormone stimulation test for detection of pars intermedia pituitary adenomas in horses, *J Vet Intern Med* 20:987-993, 2006.
37. Saland LC: The mammalian pituitary intermediate lobe: an update on innervation and regulation, *Brain Res Bull* 54:587-593, 2001.
38. DeMaria JE, Lerant AA, Freeman ME: Prolactin activates all three populations of hypothalamic neuroendocrine dopaminergic neurons in ovariectomized rats, *Brain Res* 837:236-241, 1999.
39. Goudreau JL, Lindley SE, Lookingland KJ, et al: Evidence that hypothalamic periventricular dopamine neurons innervate the intermediate lobe of the rat pituitary, *Neuroendocrinology* 56:100-105, 1992.
40. Perkins GA, Lamb S, Erb HN, et al: Plasma adrenocorticotropin (ACTH) concentrations and clinical response in horses treated for equine Cushing's disease with cyproheptadine or pergolide, *Equine Vet J* 34:679-685, 2002.
41. McFarlane D, Dybdal N, Donaldson MT, et al: Nitration and increased alpha-synuclein expression associated with dopaminergic neurodegeneration in equine pituitary pars intermedia dysfunction, *J Neuroendocrinol* 17:73-80, 2005.
42. Garcia dY: Li S, Pelletier G: Regulation of proopiomelanocortin gene expression by endogenous ligands of the GABAA receptor complex as evaluated by in situ hybridization in the rat pars intermedia, *Brain Res* 750:277-284, 1997.
43. McFarlane D, Beech J, Cribb A: Alpha-melanocyte stimulating hormone release in response to thyrotropin releasing hormone in healthy horses, horses with pituitary pars intermedia dysfunction and equine pars intermedia explants, *Domest Anim Endocrinol* 30:276-288, 2006.
44. Orth DN, Nicholson WE: Bioactive and immunoreactive adrenocorticotropin in normal equine pituitary and in pituitary tumors of horses with Cushing's disease, *Endocrinology* 111:559-563, 1982.
45. Castro MG, Morrison E: Post-translational processing of proopiomelanocortin in the pituitary and in the brain, *Crit Rev Neurobiol* 11:35-57, 1997.
46. Beech J, Garcia M: Hormonal response to thyrotropin-releasing hormone in healthy horses and in horses with pituitary adenoma, *Am J Vet Res* 46:1941-1943, 1985.
47. Eiler H, Oliver JW, Andrews FM, et al: Results of a combined dexamethasone suppression/thyrotropin-releasing hormone stimulation test in healthy horses and horses suspected to have a pars intermedia pituitary adenoma, *J Am Vet Med Assoc* 211:79-81, 1997.
48. Cohen ND, Carter GK: Steroid hepatopathy in a horse with glucocorticoid-induced hyperadrenocorticism, *Am J Vet Res* 200:1682-1684, 1992.
49. Schott HC, Graves EA, Refsal KR, et al: Diagnosis and treatment of pituitary pars intermedia dysfunction (classical Cushing's disease) and metabolic syndrome (peripheral Cushing's syndrome) in horses, *Adv Vet Derm* 5:159-169, 2005.
50. van der Kolk JH, Wensing T: Urinary concentration of corticoids in ponies with hyperlipoproteinaemia or hyperadrenocorticism, *Vet Q* 22:55-57, 2000.
51. Bottoms GD, Roesel OF, Rausch FD, et al: Circadian variation in plasma cortisol and corticosterone in pigs and mares, *Am J Vet Res* 33:785-790, 1972.
52. van der Kolk JH, Nachreiner RF, Schott HC, et al: Salivary and plasma concentration of cortisol in normal horses and horses with Cushing's disease, *Equine Vet J* 33:211-213, 2001.
53. Haritou SJ, Zylstra R, Ralli C, et al: Seasonal changes in circadian peripheral plasma concentrations of melatonin, serotonin, dopamine and cortisol in aged horses with Cushing's disease under natural photoperiod, *J Neuroendocrinol* 20:988-996, 2008.
54. Douglas RH: Circadian cortisol rhythmicity and equine Cushing's-like disease, *J Equine Vet Sci* 19:684-686, 2000.
55. Sojka JE, Johnson MA, Bottoms GD: The effect of starting time on dexamethasone suppression test results in horses, *Domest Anim Endocrinol* 10:1-5, 1993.
56. Levy M, Sojka JE, Dybdal NO: Diagnosis and treatment of equine Cushing's disease, *Compend Contin Educ Pract Vet* 21:766-769, 1999.
57. Donaldson MT, McDonnell SM, Schanbacher BJ, et al: Variation in plasma adrenocorticotropic hormone concentration and dexamethasone suppression test results with season, age, and sex in healthy ponies and horses, *J Vet Intern Med* 19:217-222, 2005.
58. Sojka JE, Levy M: Evaluation of endocrine function, *Vet Clin North Am Equine Pract* 11:415-435, 1995.
59. Eiler H, Goble D, Oliver J: Adrenal gland function in the horse: effects of cosyntropin (synthetic) and corticotropin (natural) stimulation, *Am J Vet Res* 40:724-726, 1979.
60. McGowan CM, Frost R, Pfeiffer DU, et al: Serum insulin concentrations in horses with equine Cushing's syndrome: response to a cortisol inhibitor and prognostic value, *Equine Vet J* 36:295-298, 2004.
61. McFarlane D, Donaldson MT, McDonnell SM, et al: Effects of season and sample handling on measurement of plasma alpha-melanocyte-stimulating hormone concentrations in horses and ponies, *Am J Vet Res* 65:1463-1468, 2004.
62. Horowitz ML, Neal L, Watson JL: Characteristics of plasma adrenocorticotropin, β-endorphin, and α-melanocyte stimulating hormone as diagnostic tests for pituitary pars intermedia dysfunction in the horse, *J Vet Intern Med* 17:386, 2003:abstract.
63. Miller MA, Pardo ID, Jackson LP, et al: Correlation of pituitary histomorphometry with adrenocorticotrophic hormone response to domperidone administration in the diagnosis of equine pituitary pars intermedia dysfunction, *Vet Pathol* 45:26-38, 2008.
64. Allen JR, Barbee DD, Crisman MV: Diagnosis of pituitary tumors by computed tomography—part I, *Compend Contin Educ Pract Vet* 10:1103-1106, 1988.
65. McKlveen TL, Jones JC, Sponenberg DP, et al: Assessment of the accuracy of computed tomography for measurement of normal equine pituitary glands, *Am J Vet Res* 64:1387-1394, 2003.
66. Levy M, Blevins WE, Janovitz EB: Radiological diagnosis of pituitary adenoma in the horse. In *Proceedings of the Third Congress of the World Equine Veterinary Association* 18, 1993.
67. Reed SM: Personal communication, 2008.
68. Beck DJ: Effective long term treatment of a suspected pituitary adenoma with bromocriptine mesylate in a pony, *Am J Vet Res* 46:1941-1943, 1985.
69. Krieger DT, Amorosa L, Linick F: Cyproheptadine-induced remission of Cushing's disease, *N Engl J Med* 293:893-896, 1975.
70. Munoz MC, Doreste F, Ferrer O, et al: Pergolide treatment for Cushing's syndrome in a horse, *Vet Rec* 139:41-43, 1996.
71. Peters D: Low dose pergolide mesylate treatment for equine hypophyseal adenomas (Cushing's syndrome), *Proc Am Assoc Equine Pract* 41:154-155, 1995.
72. van der Kolk JH, Ijzer J, Overgaauw PA, et al: Pituitary-independent Cushing's syndrome in a horse, *Equine Vet J* 33:110-112, 2001.

73. Antonini A, Poewe W: Fibrotic heart-valve reactions to dopamine-agonist treatment in Parkinson's disease, *Lancet Neurol* 6:826-829, 2007.
74. Tanakol R, Alagol F, Azizlerli H, et al: Cyproheptadine treatment in Cushing's disease, *J Endocrinol Invest* 19:242-247, 1996.
75. Lamberts SW, Verleun T, Oosterom R: The mechanism of action of cyproheptadine on prolactin release by cultured anterior pituitary cells, *Life Sci* 36:2257-2262, 1985.
76. Meier B, Berger D, Hoberg E, et al: Pharmacological activities of *Vitex agnus-castus* extracts in vitro, *Phytomedicine* 7:373-381, 2000.
77. Berger D, Schaffner W, Schrader E, et al: Efficacy of *Vitex agnus castus* L. extract Ze 440 in patients with pre-menstrual syndrome (PMS), *Arch Gynecol Obstet* 264:150-153, 2000.
78. Beech J, Donaldson MT, Lindborg S: Comparison of *Vitex agnus castus* extract and pergolide in treatment of equine Cushing's syndrome, *Proc Am Assoc Equine Pract* 48:175-177, 2002.
79. Schutzer WE, Kerby JL, Holtan DW: Differential effect of trilostane on the progestin milieu in the pregnant mare, *J Reprod Fertil* 107:241-248, 1996.
80. McGowan CM, Neiger R: Efficacy of trilostane for the treatment of equine Cushing's syndrome, *Equine Vet J* 35:414-418, 2003.
81. Dewis P, Anderson DC, Bulock DE, et al: Experience with trilostane in the treatment of Cushing's syndrome, *Clin Endocrinol (Oxf)* 18:533-540, 1983.
82. Fix AS, Miller LD: Equine adrenocortical carcinoma with hypercalcemia, *Vet Pathol* 24:190-192, 1987.
83. van der Kolk JH, Mars MH, van dG I: Adrenocortical carcinoma in a 12–year-old mare, *Vet Rec* 134:113-115, 1994.

Insulin Resistance and Equine Metabolic Syndrome

1. Marques RG, Fontaine MJ, Rogers J: C-peptide: much more than a byproduct of insulin biosynthesis, *Pancreas* 29:231-238, 2004.
2. Treiber KH, Kronfeld DS, Hess TM, et al: Use of proxies and reference quintiles obtained from minimal model analysis for determination of insulin sensitivity and pancreatic beta-cell responsiveness in horses, *Am J Vet Res* 66:2114-2121, 2005.
3. Marchesini G, Forlani G, Cerrelli F, et al: WHO and ATPIII proposals for the definition of the metabolic syndrome in patients with Type 2 diabetes, *Diabet Med* 21:383-387, 2004.
4. Johnson PJ: The equine metabolic syndrome peripheral Cushing's syndrome, *Vet Clin North Am Equine Pract* 18:271-293, 2002.
5. Frank N, Elliott SB, Brandt LE, et al: Physical characteristics, blood hormone concentrations, and plasma lipid concentrations in obese horses with insulin resistance, *J Am Vet Med Assoc* 228:1383-1390, 2006.
6. Treiber KH, Kronfeld DS, Hess TM, et al: Evaluation of genetic and metabolic predispositions and nutritional risk factors for pasture-associated laminitis in ponies, *J Am Vet Med Assoc* 228:1538-1545, 2006.
7. Gentry LR, Thompson DL Jr, Gentry GT Jr, et al: The relationship between body condition, leptin, and reproductive and hormonal characteristics of mares during the seasonal anovulatory period, *J Anim Sci* 80:2695-2703, 2002.
8. Cartmill JA, Thompson DL Jr, Storer WA, et al: Endocrine responses in mares and geldings with high body condition scores grouped by high vs. low resting leptin concentrations, *J Anim Sci* 81:2311-2321, 2003.
9. Bailey SR, Habershon-Butcher JL, Ransom KJ, et al: Hypertension and insulin resistance in a mixed-breed population of ponies predisposed to laminitis, *Am J Vet Res* 69:122-129, 2008.
10. Henneke DR, Potter GD, Kreider JL, et al: Relationship between condition score, physical measurements and body fat percentage in mares, *Equine Vet J* 15:371-372, 1983.
11. Jeffcott LB, Field JR, McLean JG, et al: Glucose tolerance and insulin sensitivity in ponies and Standardbred horses, *Equine Vet J* 18:97-101, 1986.
12. Freestone JF, Beadle R, Shoemaker K, et al: Improved insulin sensitivity in hyperinsulinaemic ponies through physical conditioning and controlled feed intake, *Equine Vet J* 24:187-190, 1992.
13. Hawley JA: Exercise as a therapeutic intervention for the prevention and treatment of insulin resistance, *Diabetes Metab Res Rev* 20:383-393, 2004.
14. Vervuert I, Coenen M, Dahlhoff S, et al: Fructan concentrations in grass, silages and hay. In *Proceedings of the nineteenth Equine Science Society symposium* Tucson, Ariz. 309-310, 2005.
15. Vick MM, Sessions DR, Murphy BA, et al: Obesity is associated with altered metabolic and reproductive activity in the mare: effects of metformin on insulin sensitivity and reproductive cyclicity, *Reprod Fertil Dev* 18:609-617, 2006.
16. Reeves HJ, Lees R, McGowan CM: Measurement of basal serum insulin concentration in the diagnosis of Cushing's disease in ponies, *Vet Rec* 149:449-452, 2001.
17. Sojka JE, Levy M: Evaluation of endocrine function, *Vet Clin North Am Equine Pract* 11:415-435, 1995.
18. Breuhaus BA, Refsal KR, Beyerlein SL: Measurement of free thyroxine concentration in horses by equilibrium dialysis, *J Vet Intern Med* 20:371-376, 2006.
19. Ramirez S, Wolfsheimer KJ, Moore RM, et al: Duration of effects of phenylbutazone on serum total thyroxine and free thyroxine concentrations in horses, *J Vet Intern Med* 11:371-374, 1997.
20. Eiler H, Frank N, Andrews FM, et al: Physiologic assessment of blood glucose homeostasis via combined intravenous glucose and insulin testing in horses, *Am J Vet Res* 66:1598-1604, 2005.
21. Thurmon JC, Neff-Davis C, Davis LE, et al: Xylazine hydrochloride-induced hyperglycemia and hypoinsulinemia in Thoroughbred horses, *J Vet Pharmacol Ther* 5:241-245, 1982.
22. Kearns CF, McKeever KH, Kumagai K, et al: Fat-free mass is related to one-mile race performance in elite Standardbred horses, *Vet J* 163:260-266, 2002.
23. Slawik M, Vidal-Puig AJ: Lipotoxicity, overnutrition and energy metabolism in aging, *Ageing Res Rev* 5:144-164, 2006.
24. Vick MM, Murphy BA, Sessions DR, et al: Effects of systemic inflammation on insulin sensitivity in horses and inflammatory cytokine expression in adipose tissue, *Am J Vet Res* 69:130-139, 2008.
25. Kearns CF, McKeever KH, Roegner V, et al: Adiponectin and leptin are related to fat mass in horses, *Vet J* 172:460-465, 2006.
26. Asplin KE, Sillence MN, Pollitt CC, et al: Induction of laminitis by prolonged hyperinsulinaemia in clinically normal ponies, *Vet J* 174:530-535, 2007.
27. Bailey SR, Menzies-Gow NJ, Harris PA, et al: Effect of dietary fructans and dexamethasone administration on the insulin response of ponies predisposed to laminitis, *J Am Vet Med Assoc* 231:1365-1373, 2007.
28. Baker JR, Ritchie HE: Diabetes mellitus in the horse: a case report and review of the literature, *Equine Vet J* 6:7-11, 1974.
29. Johnson PJ, Scotty NC, Wiedmeyer C, et al: Diabetes mellitus in a domesticated Spanish mustang, *J Am Vet Med Assoc* 226:584-588, 2005.
30. Jeffrey JR: Diabetes mellitus secondary to chronic pancreatitis in a pony, *J Am Vet Med Assoc* 153:1168-1175, 1968.
31. Bakos Z, Krajcsovics L, Toth J: Successful medical treatment of acute pancreatitis in a horse, *Vet Rec* 162:95-96, 2008.
32. Allen EM, Meyer W, Ralston SL, et al: Variation in soluble sugar content of pasture and turf grasses. In *Proceedings of the nineteenth Equine Science Society symposium*, Tucson, Ariz. 321-323, 2005.

33. Frank N, Elliott SB, Boston RC: Effects of long-term oral administration of levothyroxine sodium on glucose dynamics in healthy adult horses, *Am J Vet Res* 69:76-81, 2008.
34. Durham AE, Rendle DI, Newton JE: The effect of metformin on measurements of insulin sensitivity and beta cell response in 18 horses and ponies with insulin resistance, *Equine Vet J* 40:493-500, 2008.
35. Frank N, Buchanan BR, Elliott SB: Effects of long-term oral administration of levothyroxine sodium on serum thyroid hormone concentrations, clinicopathologic variables, and echocardiographic measurements in healthy adult horses, *Am J Vet Res* 69:68-75, 2008.
36. Frank N, Sommardahl CS, Eiler H, et al: Effects of oral administration of levothyroxine sodium on concentrations of plasma lipids, concentration and composition of very-low-density lipoproteins, and glucose dynamics in healthy adult mares, *Am J Vet Res* 66:1032-1038, 2005.
37. Ramirez S, McClure JJ, Moore RM, et al: Hyperthyroidism associated with a thyroid adenocarcinoma in a 21-year-old gelding, *J Vet Intern Med* 12:475-477, 1998.
38. Alberts MK, McCann JP, Woods PR: Hemithyroidectomy in a horse with confirmed hyperthyroidism, *J Am Vet Med Assoc* 217:1051-1054, 2000.
39. Johnson PJ, Scotty NC, Wiedmeyer C, et al: Diabetes mellitus in a domesticated Spanish mustang, *J Am Vet Med Assoc* 226:584-588, 2005.
40. Firshman A: Personal communication, June 2008.
41. Ott EA, Kivipelto J: Influence of chromium tripicolinate on growth and glucose metabolism in yearling horses, *J Anim Sci* 77:3022-3030, 1999.
42. Kearns CF, McKeever KH, Malinowski K: Changes in adiponectin, leptin, and fat mass after clenbuterol treatment in horses, *Med Sci Sports Exerc* 38:262-267, 2006.

Disorders of Calcium and Phosphorus

1. Kaneko JJ, Harvey JW, Bruss ML, editors: *Biochemistry of domestic animals*, ed 6, San Diego, 2009, Academic Press.
2. Aguilera-Tejero E, Sanchez J, Almaden Y, et al: Hysteresis of the PTH-calcium curve during hypocalcemia in the dog: effect of the rate and linearity of calcium decrease and sequential episodes of hypocalcemia, *J Bone Miner Res* 11:1226-1233, 1996.
3. Hurwitz S: Homeostatic control of plasma calcium concentration, *Crit Rev Biochem Mol Biol* 31:41-100, 1996.
4. Kohn CW, Brooks CL: Failure of pH to predict ionized calcium percentage in healthy horses, *Am J Vet Res* 51:1206-1210, 1990.
5. Toribio RE, Kohn CW, Chew DJ, et al: Comparison of serum parathyroid hormone and ionized calcium and magnesium concentrations and fractional urinary clearance of calcium and phosphorus in healthy horses and horses with enterocolitis, *Am J Vet Res* 62:938-947, 2001.
6. Lopez I, Estepa JC, Mendoza FJ, et al: Fractionation of calcium and magnesium in equine serum, *Am J Vet Res* 67:463-466, 2006.
7. Berlin D, Aroch I: Concentrations of ionized and total magnesium and calcium in healthy horses: effects of age, pregnancy, lactation, pH and sample type, *Vet J* 181(3):305-311, 2008.
8. Jordan RM, Meyers VS, Yoho B, et al: Effect of calcium and phosphorus levels on growth, reproduction, and bone development of ponies, *J Anim Sci* 40:78, 1975.
9. Schryver HF, Oftedal OT, Williams J, et al: Lactation in the horse: the mineral composition of mare milk, *J Nutr* 116:2142-2147, 1986.
10. Schryver HF, Oftedal OT, Williams J, et al: A comparison of the mineral composition of milk of domestic and captive wild equids (*Equus przewalskii, E. zebra, E. burchelli, E. caballus, E. asinus*), *Comp Biochem Physiol A Comp Physiol* 85:233-235, 1986.
11. Schryver HF, Craig PH, Hintz HF: Calcium metabolism in ponies fed varying levels of calcium, *J Nutr* 100:955-964, 1970.
12. Schryver HF, Hintz HF, Craig PH: Phosphorus metabolism in ponies fed varying levels of phosphorus, *J Nutr* 101:1257-1263, 1971.
13. Schryver HF, Hintz HF, Lowe JE: Calcium and phosphorus in the nutrition of the horse, *Cornell Vet* 64:493-515, 1974.
14. National Research Council: *Mineral tolerance of domestic animals*, Washington, DC, 1980, National Academic Press.
15. Schryver HF, Foose TJ, Williams J, et al: Calcium excretion in feces of ungulates, *Comp Biochem Physiol A Comp Physiol* 74:375-379, 1983.
16. Meyer H, Stadermann B, Schnurpel B, et al: The influence of type of diet (roughage or concentrate) on the plasma level, renal excretion, and apparent digestibility of calcium and magnesium in resting and exercising horses, *J Equine Vet Sci* 12:233-239, 1992.
17. Schryver HF, Craig PH, Hintz HF, et al: The site of calcium absorption in the horse, *J Nutr* 100:1127-1131, 1970.
18. Schryver HF, Hintz HF, Craig PH: Calcium metabolism in ponies fed a high phosphorus diet, *J Nutr* 101:259-264, 1971.
19. Schryver HF, Hintz HF, Lowe JE: Calcium and phosphorus inter-relationships in horse nutrition, *Equine Vet J* 3:102-109, 1971.
20. Swartzman JA, Hintz HF, Schryver HF: Inhibition of calcium absorption in ponies fed diets containing oxalic acid, *Am J Vet Res* 39:1621-1623, 1978.
21. McKenzie RA, Gartner RJ, Blaney BJ, et al: Control of nutritional secondary hyperparathyroidism in grazing horses with calcium plus phosphorus supplementation, *Aust Vet J* 57:554-557, 1981.
22. McKenzie EC, Valberg SJ, Godden SM, et al: Plasma and urine electrolyte and mineral concentrations in Thoroughbred horses with recurrent exertional rhabdomyolysis after consumption of diets varying in cation-anion balance, *Am J Vet Res* 63:1053-1060, 2002.
23. Glade MJ, Krook L, Schryver HF, et al: Calcium metabolism in glucocorticoid-treated pony foals, *J Nutr* 112:77-86, 1982.
24. Glade MJ, Krook L: Glucocorticoid-induced inhibition of osteolysis and the development of osteopetrosis, osteonecrosis and osteoporosis, *Cornell Vet* 72:76-91, 1982.
25. Harrington DD: Influence of magnesium deficiency on horse foal tissue concentration of Mg, calcium and phosphorus, *Br J Nutr* 34:45-57, 1975.
26. Hintz HF, Schryver HF: Magnesium metabolism in the horse, *J Anim Sci* 35:755-759, 1972.
27. Caple IW, Doake PA, Ellis PG: Assessment of the calcium and phosphorus nutrition in horses by analysis of urine, *Aust Vet J* 58:125-131, 1982.
28. Coffman J: Percent creatinine clearance ratios, *Vet Med Small Anim Clin* 75:671-676, 1980.
29. Burtis CA, Ashwood ER, Bruns DE, editors: *Tietz textbook of clinical chemistry and molecular diagnostics*, St Louis, 2006, Elseiver Saunders.
30. Schryver HF, Hintz HF, Craig PH, et al: Site of phosphorus absorption from the intestine of the horse, *J Nutr* 102:143-147, 1972.
31. Schryver HF: Intestinal absorption of calcium and phosphorus by horses, *J S Afr Vet Assoc* 46:39-45, 1975.
32. Hintz HF, Williams AJ, Rogoff J, et al: Availability of phosphorus in wheatbran when fed to ponies, *J Anim Sci* 36:522, 1973.
33. Mundy GR, Guise TA: Hormonal control of calcium homeostasis, *Clin Chem* 45:1347-1352, 1999.
34. Suva LJ, Winslow GA, Wettenhall RE, et al: A parathyroid hormone-related protein implicated in malignant hypercalcemia: cloning and expression, *Science* 237:893-896, 1987.
35. Wysolmerski JJ, Stewart AF: The physiology of parathyroid hormone-related protein: an emerging role as a developmental factor, *Annu Rev Physiol* 60:431-460, 1998.

36. Aguilera-Tejero E, Garfia B, Estepa JC, et al: Effects of exercise and EDTA administration on blood ionized calcium and parathyroid hormone in horses, *Am J Vet Res* 59:1605-1607, 1998.
37. Brown EM: Four-parameter model of the sigmoidal relationship between parathyroid hormone release and extracellular calcium concentration in normal and abnormal parathyroid tissue, *J Clin Endocrinol Metab* 56:572-581, 1983.
38. Estepa JC, Aguilera-Tejero E, Mayer-Valor R, et al: Measurement of parathyroid hormone in horses, *Equine Vet J* 30:476-481, 1998.
39. Felsenfeld AJ, Llach F: Parathyroid gland function in chronic renal failure, *Kidney Int* 43:771-789, 1993.
40. Brown EM, Gamba G, Riccardi D, et al: Cloning and characterization of an extracellular $Ca^{(2+)}$–sensing receptor from bovine parathyroid, *Nature* 366:575-580, 1993.
41. LiVolsi VA, DeLellis RA, editors: *Pathobiology of the parathyroid and thyroid glands*, Baltimore, 1993, Williams & Wilkins.
42. Dambacher MA, Fischer JA, Hunziker WH, et al: Distribution of circulating immunoreactive components of parathyroid hormone in normal subjects and in patients with primary and secondary hyperparathyroidism: the role of the kidney and of the serum calcium concentration, *Clin Sci (Lond)* 57:435-443, 1979.
43. Bilezikian JP, Marcus R, Levine MA, editors: *The parathyroids: basic and clinical concepts*, San Diego, 2001, Academic Press.
44. Martin KJ, Hruska KA, Freitag JJ, et al: The peripheral metabolism of parathyroid hormone, *N Engl J Med* 301:1092-1098, 1979.
45. Bringhurst FR, Stern AM, Yotts M, et al: Peripheral metabolism of PTH: fate of biologically active amino terminus in vivo, *Am J Physiol* 255:E886-E893, 1988.
46. Fox J, Scott M, Nissenson RA, et al: Effect of plasma calcium concentration on the metabolic clearance rate of parathyroid hormone in the dog, *J Lab Clin Med* 102:70-77, 1983.
47. Segre GV, D'Amour P, Hultman A, et al: Effects of hepatectomy, nephrectomy, and nephrectomy/uremia on the metabolism of parathyroid hormone in the rat, *J Clin Invest* 67:439-448, 1981.
48. Silver J, Russell J, Sherwood LM: Regulation by vitamin D metabolites of messenger ribonucleic acid for preproparathyroid hormone in isolated bovine parathyroid cells, *Proc Natl Acad Sci U S A* 82:4270-4273, 1985.
49. Moallem E, Kilav R, Silver J, et al: RNA-protein binding and post–transcriptional regulation of parathyroid hormone gene expression by calcium and phosphate, *J Biol Chem* 273:5253-5259, 1998.
50. Toribio RE: *Parathyroid gland function and calcium regulation in healthy and septic horses*, Columbus, Ohio, 2001, The Ohio State University, pp 1-160.
51. Bellorin–Font E, Lopez C, Diaz K, et al: Role of protein kinase C on the acute desensitization of renal cortical adenylate cyclase to parathyroid hormone, *Kidney Int* 47:38-44, 1995.
52. de Rouffignac C, Quamme G: Renal magnesium handling and its hormonal control, *Physiol Rev* 74:305-322, 1994.
53. Friedman PA: Codependence of renal calcium and sodium transport, *Annu Rev Physiol* 60:179-197, 1998.
54. Brown EM: Physiology and pathophysiology of the extracellular calcium–sensing receptor, *Am J Med* 106:238-253, 1999.
55. Simon DB, Lu Y, Choate KA, et al: Paracellin-1, a renal tight junction protein required for paracellular Mg^{2+} resorption, *Science* 285:103-106, 1999.
56. HoenderopJG, van der KempAW, HartogA, et al: Molecular identification of the apical Ca^{2+} channel in 1, 25-dihydroxyvitamin D_3–responsive epithelia, *J Biol Chem* 274:8375-8378, 1999.
57. Hoenderop JG, Willems PH, Bindels RJ: Toward a comprehensive molecular model of active calcium reabsorption, *Am J Physiol Renal Physiol* 278:F352-F360, 2000.
58. Gmaj P, Murer H: Cellular mechanisms of inorganic phosphate transport in kidney, *Physiol Rev* 66:36-70, 1986.
59. Malmstrom K, Murer H: Parathyroid hormone regulates phosphate transport in OK cells via an irreversible inactivation of a membrane protein, *FEBS Lett* 216:257-260, 1987.
60. Teitelbaum SL: Bone resorption by osteoclasts, *Science* 289:1504-1508, 2000.
61. Simonet WS, Lacey DL, Dunstan CR, et al: Osteoprotegerin: a novel secreted protein involved in the regulation of bone density, *Cell* 89:309-319, 1997.
62. Lepage OM, Carstanjen B, Uebelhart D: Non-invasive assessment of equine bone: an update, *Vet J* 161:10-22, 2001.
63. Price JS: Biochemical markers of bone metabolism in horses: potentials and limitations?, *Vet J* 156:163-165, 1998.
64. Carstanjen B, Hoyle NR, Gabriel A, et al: Assessment of bone formation—and bone resorption—markers in horses, *J Bone Miner Res* 17:S319, 2002.
65. Holick MF, Frommer JE, McNeill SC, et al: Photometabolism of 7–dehydrocholesterol to previtamin D_3 in skin, *Biochem Biophys Res Commun* 76:107-114, 1977.
66. FuGK,LinD,ZhangMY,etal:Cloningofhuman25-hydroxyvitamin $D\text{-}_1$ alpha–hydroxylase and mutations causing vitamin D-dependent rickets type 1, *Mol Endocrinol* 11:1961-1970, 1997.
67. Brown AJ, Dusso A, Slatopolsky E: Vitamin D, *Am J Physiol* 277:F157-F175, 1999.
68. Friedman PA, Gesek FA: Cellular calcium transport in renal epithelia: measurement, mechanisms, and regulation, *Physiol Rev* 75:429-471, 1995.
69. Wasserman RH, Fullmer CS: Vitamin D and intestinal calcium transport: facts, speculations and hypotheses, *J Nutr* 125:1971S-1979S, 1995.
70. Szabo A, Merke J, Beier E, et al: 1,25$(OH)_2$ vitamin D_3 inhibits parathyroid cell proliferation in experimental uremia, *Kidney Int* 35:1049-1056, 1989.
71. Breidenbach A, Schlumbohm C, Harmeyer J: Peculiarities of vitamin D and of the calcium and phosphate homeostatic system in horses, *Vet Res* 29:173-186, 1998.
72. Horst RL, Littledike ET, Riley JL, et al: Quantitation of vitamin D and its metabolites and their plasma concentrations in five species of animals, *Anal Biochem* 116:189-203, 1981.
73. Horst RL, Littledike ET: Comparison of plasma concentrations of vitamin D and its metabolites in young and aged domestic animals, *Comp Biochem Physiol B* 73:485-489, 1982.
74. Maenpaa PH, Lappetelainen R, Virkkunen J: Serum retinol, 25–hydroxyvitamin D and alpha-tocopherol of racing trotters in Finland, *Equine Vet J* 19:237-240, 1987.
75. Maenpaa PH, Koskinen T, Koskinen E: Serum profiles of vitamins A, E and D in mares and foals during different seasons, *J Anim Sci* 66:1418-1423, 1988.
76. Maenpaa PH, Pirhonen A, Koskinen E: Vitamin A: E and D nutrition in mares and foals during the winter season: effect of feeding two different vitamin-mineral concentrates, *J Anim Sci* 66:1424-1429, 1988.
77. Smith BS, Wright H: 25–Hydroxyvitamin D concentrations in equine serum, *Vet Rec* 115:579, 1984.
78. Enbergs H, Karp HP, Schonherr U: Course of blood levels of calcium, inorganic phosphate, alkaline phosphatase, parathyroid hormone and calcidiol (25-OH- D_3) in one and two year old thoroughbred horses, *Dtsch Tierarztl Wochenschr* 103:491-493, 1996.
79. El Shorafa WM, Feaster JP, Ott EA, et al: Effect of vitamin D and sunlight on growth and bone development of young ponies, *J Anim Sci* 48:882-886, 1979.
80. Toribio RE, Kohn CW, Leone GW, et al: Molecular cloning and expression of equine calcitonin, calcitonin gene–related peptide–I, and calcitonin gene–related peptide-II, *Mol Cell Endocrinol* 199(1-2):119-128, 2003.

81. Garrett JE, Tamir H, Kifor O, et al: Calcitonin-secreting cells of the thyroid express an extracellular calcium receptor gene, *Endocrinology* 136:5202-5211, 1995.
82. Munson PL, Hirsch PF: Importance of calcitonin in physiology, clinical pharmacology, and medicine, *Bone Miner* 16:162-165, 1992.
83. Woodrow JP, Sharpe CJ, Fudge NJ, et al: Calcitonin plays a critical role in regulating skeletal mineral metabolism during lactation 1, *Endocrinology* 147:4010-4021, 2006.
84. Blahser S: Immunocytochemical demonstration of calcitonin-containing C-cells in the thyroid glands of different mammals, *Cell Tissue Res* 186:551-558, 1978.
85. Gray AW, Davies ME, Jeffcott LB: Generation and activity of equine osteoclasts in vitro: effects of the bisphosphonate pamidronate (APD), *Res Vet Sci* 72:105-113, 2002.
86. Garel JM, Martin-Rosset W, Barlet JP: Plasma immunoreactive calcitonin levels in pregnant mares and newborn foals, *Horm Metab Res* 7:429-432, 1975.
87. Sandusky GE Jr, Wightman KA: Application of the peroxidase–antiperoxidase procedure to the localization of pituitary hormones and calcitonin in various domestic animals and human beings, *Am J Vet Res* 46:739-741, 1985.
88. Chiba S, Kanematsu S, Murakami K, et al: Serum parathyroid hormone and calcitonin levels in racehorses with fracture, *J Vet Med Sci* 62:361-365, 2000.
89. Rourke KM, Kohn CW, Levine AL, et al: Rapid calcitonin response to experimental hypercalcemia in healthy horses. *Domest Anim Endocrinol.* 2009;36:197-201.
90. Care AD, Abbas SK, Ousey J, et al: The relationship between the concentration of ionized calcium and parathyroid hormone-related protein (PTHrP[1-34]) in the milk of mares, *Equine Vet J* 29:186-189, 1997.
91. Barton MH, Sharma P, LeRoy BE, et al: Hypercalcemia and high serum parathyroid hormone–related protein concentration in a horse with multiple myeloma 1, *J Am Vet Med Assoc* 225(376):409-413, 2004.
92. Karcher LF, Le Net JL, Turner BF, et al: Pseudohyperparathyroidism in a mare associated with squamous cell carcinoma of the vulva, *Cornell Vet* 80:153-162, 1990.
93. Marr CM, Love S, Pirie HM: Clinical, ultrasonographic and pathological findings in a horse with splenic lymphosarcoma and pseudohyperparathyroidism, *Equine Vet J* 21:221-226, 1989.
94. Meuten DJ, Price SM, Seiler RM, et al: Gastrict carcinoma with pseudohyperparathyroidism in a horse, *Cornell Vet* 68:179-195, 1978.
95. Rosol TJ, Nagode LA, Robertson JT, et al: Humoral hypercalcemia of malignancy associated with ameloblastoma in a horse, *J Am Vet Med Assoc* 204:1930-1933, 1994.
96. Beyer MJ, Freestone JF, Reimer JM, et al: Idiopathic hypocalcemia in foals, *J Vet Intern Med* 11:356-360, 1997.
97. Aguilera-Tejero E, Estepa JC, Lopez I, et al: Polycystic kidneys as a cause of chronic renal failure and secondary hypoparathyroidism in a horse, *Equine Vet J* 32:167-169, 2000.
98. Couetil LL, Sojka JE, Nachreiner RF: Primary hypoparathyroidism in a horse, *J Vet Intern Med* 12:45-49, 1998.
99. Frank N, Hawkins JF, Couetil LL, et al: Primary hyperparathyroidism with osteodystrophia fibrosa of the facial bones in a pony, *J Am Vet Med Assoc* 212:84-86, 1998.
100. Ronen N, Van Heerden J, van Amstel SR: Clinical and biochemistry findings, and parathyroid hormone concentrations in three horses with secondary hyperparathyroidism, *J S Afr Vet Assoc* 63:134-136, 1992.
101. Harrington DD, Page EH: Acute vitamin D_3 toxicosis in horses: case reports and experimental studies of the comparative toxicity of vitamins D_2 and D_3, *J Am Vet Med Assoc* 182:1358-1369, 1983.
102. Elfers RS, Bayly WM, Brobst DF, et al: Alterations in calcium, phosphorus and C-terminal parathyroid hormone levels in equine acute renal disease, *Cornell Vet* 76:317-329, 1986.
103. Aguilera-Tejero E, Estepa JC, Lopez I, et al: Plasma ionized calcium and parathyroid hormone concentrations in horses after endurance rides, *J Am Vet Med Assoc* 219:488-490, 2001.
104. Dart AJ, Snyder JR, Spier SJ, et al: Ionized calcium concentration in horses with surgically managed gastrointestinal disease: 147 cases (1988-1990), *J Am Vet Med Assoc* 201:1244-1248, 1992.
105. Garcia-Lopez JM, Provost PJ, Rush JE, et al: Prevalence and prognostic importance of hypomagnesemia and hypocalcemia in horses that have colic surgery, *Am J Vet Res* 62:7-12, 2001.
106. Kaneps AJ, Knight AP, Bennett DG: Synchronous diaphragmatic flutter associated with electrolyte imbalances in a mare with colic, *Vet Clin North Am Equine Pract* 2:18, 1980.
107. Baird JD: Lactation tetany (eclampsia) in a Shetland pony mare, *Aust Vet J* 47:402-404, 1971.
108. Mansmann RA, Carlson GP, White NA, et al: Synchronous diaphragmatic flutter in horses, *J Am Vet Med Assoc* 165:265-270, 1974.
109. Schoeb TR, Panciera RJ: Blister beetle poisoning in horses, *J Am Vet Med Assoc* 173:75-77, 1978.
110. Dyke TM, Maclean AA: Urethral obstruction in a stallion with possible synchronous diaphragmatic flutter, *Vet Rec* 121:425-426, 1987.
111. Carlson GP, Mansmann RA: Serum electrolyte and plasma protein alterations in horses used in endurance rides, *J Am Vet Med Assoc* 165:262-264, 1974.
112. Hudson NP, Church DB, Trevena J, et al: Primary hypoparathyroidism in two horses, *Aust Vet J* 77:504-508, 1999.
113. Kerr MG, Snow DH: Composition of sweat of the horse during prolonged epinephrine (adrenaline) infusion, heat exposure, and exercise, *Am J Vet Res* 44:1571-1577, 1983.
114. Schryver HF, Hintz HF, Lowe JE: Calcium metabolism, body composition, and sweat losses of exercised horses, *Am J Vet Res* 39:245-248, 1978.
115. Vandeplassche M, Spincemaille J, Bouters R: Aetiology, pathogenesis and treatment of retained placenta in the mare, *Equine Vet J* 3:144-147, 1971.
116. Sevinga M, Barkema HW, Hesselink JW: Serum calcium and magnesium concentrations and the use of a calcium-magnesium-borogluconate solution in the treatment of Friesian mares with retained placenta, *Theriogenology* 57:941-947, 2002.
117. Toribio RE, Kohn CW, Sams RA, et al: Hysteresis and calcium set-point for the calcium parathyroid hormone relationship in healthy horses, *Gen Comp Endocrinol;130:279-288*, 2003.
118. Toribio RE, Kohn CW, Rourke KM, et al: Effects of hypercalcemia on serum concentrations of magnesium, potassium, and phosphate and urinary excretion of electrolytes in horses, *Am J Vet Res* 68:543-554, 2007.
119. Toribio RE, Kohn CW, Capen CC, et al: Parathyroid hormone (PTH) secretion, PTH mRNA and calcium-sensing receptor mRNA expression in equine parathyroid cells, and effects of IL-1, IL-6, and TNF–alpha on equine parathyroid cell function, *J Mol Endocrinol* 31(3):609-620, 2003.
120. Toribio RE, Kohn CW, Hardy J, et al: Alterations in serum parathyroid hormone and electrolyte concentrations and urinary excretion of electrolytes in horses with induced endotoxemia, *J Vet Intern Med* 19:223-231, 2005.
121. Carlstedt F, Eriksson M, Kiiski R, et al: Hypocalcemia during porcine endotoxemic shock: effects of calcium administration, *Crit Care Med* 28, 2000:290-294.
122. Zaloga GP: Ionized hypocalcemia during sepsis, *Crit Care Med* 28:266-268, 2000.
123. Carlstedt F, Lind L, Rastad J, et al: Parathyroid hormone and ionized calcium levels are related to the severity of illness and survival in critically ill patients, *Eur J Clin Invest* 28:898-903, 1998.

124. Delesalle C, Dewulf J, Lefebvre RA, et al: Use of plasma ionized calcium levels and Ca^{2+} substitution response patterns as prognostic parameters for ileus and survival in colic horses, *Vet Q* 27:157-172, 2005.
125. King JN, Gerring EL: Detection of endotoxin in cases of equine colic, *Vet Rec* 123:269-271, 1988.
126. Meyers K, Reed S, Keck M, et al: Circulating endotoxin–like substance(s) and altered hemostasis in horses with gastrointestinal disorders: an interim report, *Am J Vet Res* 43:2233-2238, 1982.
127. Moore JN, White NA, Berg JN, et al: Endotoxemia following experimental intestinal strangulation obstruction in ponies, *Can J Comp Med* 45:330-332, 1981.
128. Pantaleon LG, Furr MO, McKenzie HC, et al: Effects of small– and large–volume resuscitation on coagulation and electrolytes during experimental endotoxemia in anesthetized horses, *J Vet Intern Med* 21:1374-1379, 2007.
129. Zaloga GP, Malcolm D, Chernow B, et al: Endotoxin–induced hypocalcemia results in defective calcium mobilization in rats, *Circ Shock* 24:143-148, 1988.
130. Nakamura T, Mimura Y, Uno K, et al: Parathyroid hormone activity increases during endotoxemia in conscious rats, *Horm Metab Res* 30:88-92, 1998.
131. Crouser ED, Dorinsky PM: Metabolic consequences of sepsis. Correlation with altered intracellular calcium homeostasis, *Clin Chest Med* 17:249-261, 1996.
132. Assicot M, Gendrel D, Carsin H, et al: High serum procalcitonin concentrations in patients with sepsis and infection, *Lancet* 341:515-518, 1993.
133. Dandona P, Nix D, Wilson MF, et al: Procalcitonin increase after endotoxin injection in normal subjects, *J Clin Endocrinol Metab* 79:1605-1608, 1994.
134. Sperber SJ, Blevins DD, Francis JB: Hypercalcitoninemia, hypocalcemia, and toxic shock syndrome, *Rev Infect Dis* 12:736-739, 1990.
135. Schott HC, Marlin DJ, Geor RJ, et al: Changes in selected physiological and laboratory measurements in elite horses competing in a 160 km endurance ride, *Equine Vet J* (Suppl):37-42, 2006.
136. McCutcheon LJ, Geor RJ, Hare MJ, et al: Sweating rate and sweat composition during exercise and recovery in ambient heat and humidity, *Equine Vet J* (Suppl 20):153-157, November 1995.
137. Geiser DR, Andrews FM, Rohrbach BW, et al: Blood ionized calcium concentrations in horses before and after the cross–country phase of three–day event competition, *Am J Vet Res* 56:1502-1505, 1995.
138. Gulick MA, MacAllister CG, Panciera R: Equine cantharidiasis, *Comp Cont Educ Equine Pract* 18:77-83, 1996.
139. Lopez JR, Linares N, Cordovez G, et al: Elevated myoplasmic calcium in exercise–induced equine rhabdomyolysis, *Pflugers Arch* 430:293-295, 1995.
140. Bienfet V, Dewaele A, Van Essch R: A primary parathyroid disorder. Osteofibrosis caused by a parathyroid adenoma in a Shetland pony, *Ann Med Vet* 108:252-256, 1964.
141. Krook L, Lowe JE: Nutritional secondary hyperparathyroidism in the horse, *Pathol Vet* 65:26-56, 1964.
142. Peauroi JR, Fisher DJ, Mohr FC, et al: Primary hyperparathyroidism caused by a functional parathyroid adenoma in a horse, *J Am Vet Med Assoc* 212:1915-1918, 1998.
143. Roussel AJ, Thatcher CD: Primary hyperparathyroidism in a pony mare, *Comp Cont Educ Equine Pract* 9:781-783, 1987.
144. Almaden Y, Canalejo A, Hernandez A, et al: Direct effect of phosphorus on PTH secretion from whole rat parathyroid glands in vitro, *J Bone Miner Res* 11:970-976, 1996.
145. Brobst DF, Bayly WM, Reed SM: Parathyroid hormone evaluation in normal horses and horses with renal failure, *J Equine Vet Sci* 2:150, 1982.
146. Joyce JR, Pierce KR, Romane WM, et al: Clinical study of nutritional secondary hyperparathyroidism in horses, *J Am Vet Med Assoc* 158:2033-2042, 1971.
147. Walthall JC, McKenzie RA: Osteodystrophia fibrosa in horses at pasture in Queensland: field and laboratory observations, *Aust Vet J* 52:11-16, 1976.
148. Argenzio RA, Lowe JE, Hintz HF, et al: Calcium and phosphorus homeostasis in horses, *J Nutr* 104:18-27, 1974.
149. Benders NA, Junker K, Wensing T, et al: Diagnosis of secondary hyperparathyroidism in a pony using intact parathyroid hormone radioimmunoassay, *Vet Rec* 149:185-187, 2001.
150. Hintz HF, Kallfelz FA: Some nutritional problems of horses, *Equine Vet J* 13:183-186, 1981.
151. Clarke CJ, Roeder PL, Dixon PM: Nasal obstruction caused by nutritional osteodystrophia fibrosa in a group of Ethiopian horses, *Vet Rec* 138:568-570, 1996.
152. Freestone JF, Seahorn TL: Miscellaneous conditions of the equine head, *Vet Clin North Am Equine Pract* 9:235-242, 1993.
153. Brook D: Osteoporosis in a six year old pony, *Equine Vet J* 7:46-48, 1975.
154. Robinson NE, editor: *Current therary in equine medicine*, ed 6, St Louis, 2009, WB Saunders.
155. Boland RL: Solanum malacoxylon: a toxic plant which affects animal calcium metabolism, *Biomed Environ Sci* 1:414-423, 1988.
156. Harrington DD: Acute vitamin D_2 (ergocalciferol) toxicosis in horses: case report and experimental studies, *J Am Vet Med Assoc* 180:867-873, 1982.
157. Hughes MR, McCain TA, Chang SY, et al: Presence of 1,25–dihydroxyvitamin D_3–glycoside in the calcinogenic plant *Cestrum diurnum*, *Nature* 268:347-349, 1977.
158. Kasali OB, Krook L, Pond WG, et al: *Cestrum diurnum* intoxication in normal and hyperparathyroid pigs, *Cornell Vet* 67, 1977:190-121.
159. Krook L, Wasserman RH, McEntee K, et al: *Cestrum diurnum* poisoning in Florida cattle, *Cornell Vet* 65:557-575, 1975.
160. Krook L, Wasserman RH, Shively JN, et al: Hypercalcemia and calcinosis in Florida horses: implication of the shrub, *Cestrum diurnum*, as the causative agent, *Cornell Vet* 65:26-56, 1975.
161. Worker NA, Carrillo BJ: "Enteque seco," calcification and wasting in grazing animals in the Argentine, *Nature* 215:72-74, 1967.
162. Muylle E, Oyaert W, de Roose P, et al: Hypercalcaemia and mineralization of non–osseous tissues in horses due to vitamin–D toxicity, *Zentralbl Veterinarmed A* 21:638-643, 1974.
163. Fix AS, Miller LD: Equine adrenocortical carcinoma with hypercalcemia, *Vet Pathol* 24:190-192, 1987.
164. Mair TS, Yeo SP, Lucke VM: Hypercalcaemia and soft tissue mineralisation associated with lymphosarcoma in two horses, *Vet Rec* 126:99-101, 1990.

Magnesium and Disease

1. Quamme GA: de RC: Epithelial magnesium transport and regulation by the kidney, *Front Biosci* 5:D694-D711, 2000.
2. Schweigel M, Martens H: Magnesium transport in the gastrointestinal tract, *Front Biosci* 5:D666-D677, 2000.
3. Wolf FI, Cittadini A: Chemistry and biochemistry of magnesium, *Mol Aspects Med* 24:3-9, 2003.
4. National Research Council Committee on Nutrient Requirements of Horses: *Nutrient requirements of horses*, rev ed 6, Washington, DC, 2007, National Academies Press.
5. Hintz HF, Schryver HF: Magnesium, calcium and phosphorus metabolism in ponies fed varying levels of magnesium, *J Anim Sci* 37:927-930, 1973.
6. Meyer H, Ahlswede L: Magnesium metabolism in the horse, *Zentralbl Veterinarmed A* 24:128-139, 1977.

7. Altura BM, Altura BT: Role of magnesium in patho-physiological processes and the clinical utility of magnesium ion selective electrodes, *Scand J Clin Lab Invest Suppl* 224:211-234, 1996.
8. Stewart AJ, Hardy J, Kohn CW, et al: Validation of diagnostic tests for determination of magnesium status in horses with reduced magnesium intake, *Am J Vet Res* 65:422-430, 2004.
9. Toribio RE, Kohn CW, Hardy J, et al: Alterations in serum parathyroid hormone and electrolyte concentrations and urinary excretion of electrolytes in horses with induced endotoxemia, *J Vet Intern Med* 19:223-231, 2005.
10. Lopez I, Estepa JC, Mendoza FJ, et al: Fractionation of calcium and magnesium in equine serum, *Am J Vet Res* 67:463-466, 2006.
11. Lopez I, Estepa JC, Mendoza FJ, et al: Serum concentrations of calcium, phosphorus, magnesium and calciotropic hormones in donkeys, *Am J Vet Res* 67:1333-1336, 2006.
12. Toribio RE, Kohn CW, Rourke KM, et al: Effects of hypercalcemia on serum concentrations of magnesium, potassium, and phosphate and urinary excretion of electrolytes in horses, *Am J Vet Res* 68:543-554, 2007.
13. Berlin D, Aroch I: Concentrations of ionized and total magnesium and calcium in healthy horses: effects of age, pregnancy, lactation, pH and sample type, *Vet J* 181(3):305-311, 2008.
14. Toribio RE, Kohn CW, Chew DJ, et al: Comparison of serum parathyroid hormone and ionized calcium and magnesium concentrations and fractional urinary clearance of calcium and phosphorus in healthy horses and horses with enterocolitis, *Am J Vet Res* 62:938-947, 2001.
15. Hoenderop JG, Bindels RJ: Epithelial Ca^{2+} and Mg^{2+} channels in health and disease, *J Am Soc Nephrol* 16:15-26, 2005.
16. Martens H, Schweigel M: Pathophysiology of grass tetany and other hypomagnesemias. Implications for clinical management, *Vet Clin North Am Food Anim Pract* 16:339-368, 2000.
17. Schweigel M, Park HS, Etschmann B, et al: Characterization of the Na^{+}-dependent Mg^{2+} transport in sheep ruminal epithelial cells, *Am J Physiol Gastrointest Liver Physiol* 290:G56-G65, 2006.
18. Hintz HF, Schryver HF: Magnesium metabolism in the horse, *J Anim Sci* 35:755-759, 1972.
19. Chester–Jones H, Fontenot JP, Veit HP: Physiological and pathological effects of feeding high levels of magnesium to steers, *J Anim Sci* 68:4400-4413, 1990.
20. Meyer H, Stadermann B, Schnurpel B: The influence of type of diet (roughage or concentrate) on the plasma-level, renal excretion, and apparent digestibility of calcium and magnesium in resting and exercising horses, *J Equine Vet Sci* 12:233-239, 1992.
21. Harrington DD: Influence of magnesium deficiency on horse foal tissue concentration of Mg, calcium and phosphorus, *Br J Nutr* 34:45-57, 1975.
22. Schryver HF, Millis DL, Soderholm LV, et al: Metabolism of some essential minerals in ponies fed high levels of aluminum, *Cornell Vet* 76:354-360, 1986.
23. Dai LJ, Ritchie G, Kerstan D, et al: Magnesium transport in the renal distal convoluted tubule, *Physiol Rev* 81:51-84, 2001.
24. Konrad M, Schlingmann KP, Gudermann T: Insights into the molecular nature of magnesium homeostasis, *Am J Physiol Renal Physiol* 286:F599-F605, 2004.
25. de RC, Quamme: G: Renal magnesium handling and its hormonal control, *Physiol Rev* 74:305-322, 1994.
26. Grace ND, Pearce SG, Firth EC, et al: Concentrations of macro– and micro–elements in the milk of pasture–fed thoroughbred mares, *Aust Vet J* 77:177-180, 1999.
27. Schryver HF, Oftedal OT, Williams J, et al: Lactation in the horse: the mineral composition of mare milk, *J Nutr* 116:2142-2147, 1986.
28. McConaghy FF, Hodgson DR, Evans DL, et al: Equine sweat composition: effects of adrenaline infusion, exercise and training, *Equine Vet J Suppl* (20):158-164, November 1995.
29. Dai LJ, Ritchie G, Bapty B, et al: Aldosterone potentiates hormone–stimulated Mg^{2+} uptake in distal convoluted tubule cells, *Am J Physiol* 274:F336-F341, 1998.
30. Dai LJ, Bapty B, Ritchie G, et al: Glucagon and arginine vasopressin stimulate Mg^{2+} uptake in mouse distal convoluted tubule cells, *Am J Physiol* 274:F328-F335, 1998.
31. de RC, Mandon B, Wittner M, et al: Hormonal control of renal magnesium handling, *Miner Electrolyte Metab* 19:226-231, 1993.
32. Kang HS, Kerstan D, Dai LJ, et al: β-Adrenergic agonists stimulate $Mg^{(2+)}$ uptake in mouse distal convoluted tubule cells, *Am J Physiol Renal Physiol* 279:F1116-F1123, 2000.
33. Dai LJ, Ritchie G, Bapty BW, et al: Insulin stimulates Mg^{2+} uptake in mouse distal convoluted tubule cells, *Am J Physiol* 277:F907-F913, 1999.
34. Brown EM, MacLeod RJ: Extracellular calcium sensing and extracellular calcium signaling, *Physiol Rev* 81:239-297, 2001.
35. Freestone JF, Gossett K, Carlson GP, et al: Exercise induced alterations in the serum muscle enzymes, erythrocyte potassium and plasma constituents following feed withdrawal or furosemide and sodium bicarbonate administration in the horse, *J Vet Intern Med* 5:40-46, 1991.
36. Norris CR, Nelson RW, Christopher MM: Serum total and ionized magnesium concentrations and urinary fractional excretion of magnesium in cats with diabetes mellitus and diabetic ketoacidosis, *J Am Vet Med Assoc* 215:1455-1459, 1999.
37. Weglicki WB, Phillips TM, Freedman AM, et al: Magnesium-deficiency elevates circulating levels of inflammatory cytokines and endothelin, *Mol Cell Biochem* 110:169-173, 1992.
38. Kramer JH, Misik V, Weglicki WB: Magnesium-deficiency potentiates free radical production associated with postischemic injury to rat hearts: vitamin E affords protection, *Free Radic Biol Med* 16:713-723, 1994.
39. Bueno AC, Seahorn TL, Cornick-Seahorn J, et al: Plasma and urine nitric oxide concentrations in horses given below a low dose of endotoxin, *Am J Vet Res* 60:969-976, 1999.
40. Seethanathan P, Bottoms GD, Schafer K: Characterization of release of tumor necrosis factor, interleukin-1, and superoxide anion from equine white blood cells in response to endotoxin, *Am J Vet Res* 51:1221-1225, 1990.
41. Barton MH, Morris DD, Norton N, et al: Hemostatic and fibrinolytic indices in neonatal foals with presumed septicemia, *J Vet Intern Med* 12:26-35, 1998.
42. Hurcombe SDA, Toribio RE, Slovis NM, et al: Calcium regulating hormones and serum calcium and magnesium concentrations in septic and critically ill foals and their association with survival, *J Vet Intern Med* 23(2):335-343, 2009.
43. Garcia-Lopez JM, Provost PJ, Rush JE, et al: Prevalence and prognostic importance of hypomagnesemia and hypocalcemia in horses that have colic surgery, *Am J Vet Res* 62:7-12, 2001.
44. Johansson AM, Gardner SY, Jones SL, et al: Hypomagnesemia in hospitalized horses, *J Vet Intern Med* 17:860-867, 2003.
45. Barbagallo M, Dominguez LJ, Galioto A, et al: Role of magnesium in insulin action, diabetes and cardio–metabolic syndrome X, *Mol Aspects Med* 24:39-52, 2003.
46. Helman RG, Edwards WC: Clinical features of blister beetle poisoning in equids: 70 cases (1983-1996), *J Am Vet Med Assoc* 211:1018-1021, 1997.
47. Meijer P: Two cases of tetany in the horse (author's translation), *Tijdschr Diergeneeskd* 107:329-332, 1982.
48. Fatemi S, Ryzen E, Flores J, et al: Effect of experimental human magnesium depletion on parathyroid hormone secretion and 1,25–dihydroxyvitamin D metabolism, *J Clin Endocrinol Metab* 73:1067-1072, 1991.
49. Abbott LG, Rude RK: Clinical manifestations of magnesium deficiency, *Miner Electrolyte Metab* 19:314-322, 1993.
50. Kaneko JJ, Harvey JW, Bruss ML, editors: *Biochemistry of domestic animals*, ed 6, San Diego, 2009, Academic Press.

51. Arango MF, Bainbridge D: Magnesium for acute traumatic brain injury, *Cochrane Database Syst Rev* 4(8), 2008:CD005400.
52. Mishra OP, Fritz KI, Ivoria-Papadopoulos M: NMDA receptor and neonatal hypoxic brain injury, *Ment Retard Dev Disabil Res Rev* 7:249-253, 2001.
53. Levenson CW: Regulation of the NMDA receptor: implications for neuropsychological development, *Nutr Rev* 64:428-432, 2006.
54. Seelig JM, Wei EP, Kontos HA, et al: Effect of changes in magnesium ion concentration on cat cerebral arterioles, *Am J Physiol* 245:H22-H26, 1983.
55. Wilkins PA: Magnesium infusion in hypoxic ischemic encephalopathy. In *Proceedings of the American College of Veterinary Internal Medicine nineteenth annual Veterinary Medical Forum*, Denver, 2001, ACVIM, 242-244.
56. MacKay RJ: Brain injury after head trauma: pathophysiology, diagnosis, and treatment, *Vet Clin North Am Equine Pract* 20:199-216, 2004.
57. Siemkowicz E: Magnesium sulfate solution dramatically improves immediate recovery of rats from hypoxia, *Resuscitation* 35:53-59, 1997.
58. Hallak M, Hotra JW, Kupsky WJ: Magnesium sulfate protection of fetal rat brain from severe maternal hypoxia, *Obstet Gynecol* 96:124-128, 2000.
59. Marr CM: *Arrhythmias. Cardiology of the horse*, London, 1999, WB Saunders, pp 190-205.
60. Green HH, Allcroft WM, Montgomerie RF: Hypomagnesemia in equine transit tetany, *J Comp Pathol Ther* 48:74-79, 1935.
61. Harrington DD: Pathological features of magnesium deficiency in young horses fed purified rations, *Am J Vet Res* 35:503, 1974.
62. Grace ND, Pearce SG, Firth EC, et al: Content and distribution of macro– and micro–elements in the body of pasture-fed young horses, *Aust Vet J* 77:172-176, 1999.
63. Henninger RW, Horst J: Magnesium toxicosis in two horses, *J Am Vet Med Assoc* 211:82-85, 1997.

Anhidrosis

1. Mayhew IG, Ferguson HO: Clinical, clinicopathologic, and epidemiologic features of anhidrosis in central Florida Thoroughbred horses, *J Vet Intern Med* 1:136-141, 1987.
2. Warner A, Mayhew IG: Equine anhidrosis: a review of pathophysiologic mechanisms, *Vet Res Commun* 6:249-264, 1983.
3. Warner AE, Mayhew IG: Equine anhidrosis: a survey of affected horses in Florida, *J Am Vet Med Assoc* 180:627-629, 1982.
4. Hubert JD, Beadle RE, Norwood G: Equine anhidrosis, *Vet Clin North Am Equine Pract* 18:355-369, 2002.
5. Watanabe A, Kanemaki N, Matsuura K: Distribution densities of hair follicles in racehorses, *Nippon Juigaku Zasshi* 4:55-60, 1993.
6. Jenkinson DM, Elder HY, Bovell DL: Equine sweating and anhidrosis. I. Equine sweating, *Vet Dermatol* 17:361-392, 2006.
7. Bijman J, Quinton PM: Predominantly beta–adrenergic control of equine sweating, *Am J Physiol* 246:R349-R353, 1984.
8. Hodgson DR, McCutcheon LJ, Byrd SK, et al: Dissipation of metabolic heat in the horse during exercise, *J Appl Physiol* 74:1161-1170, 1993.
9. DeLahunta A, Glass E, editors: *Veterinary neuroanatomy and clinical neurology*, ed 3, St Louis, 2009, WB Saunders.
10. Snow DH: Identification of the receptor involved in adrenaline mediated sweating in the horse, *Res Vet Sci* 23:246-247, 1977.
11. Jenkinson DM, Elder HY, Bovell DL: Equine sweating and anhidrosis. II. Anhidrosis, *Vet Dermatol* 18:2-11, 2007.
12. Wilson DC, Corbett AD, Steel C, et al: A preliminary study of the short circuit current (Isc) responses of sweat gland cells from normal and anhidrotic horses to purinergic and adrenergic agonists, *Vet Dermatol* 18:152-160, 2007.
13. Robertshaw D: Proceedings: neural and humoral control of apocrine glands, *J Invest Dermatol* 63:160-167, 1974.
14. Robertshaw D, Taylor CR: Sweat gland function of the donkey (*Equus asinus*), *J Physiol* 205:79-89, 1969.
15. Evans CL, Nisbet AM, Ross KA: A histological study of the sweat glands of normal and dry-coated horses, *J Comp Pathol* 67:397-405, 1957.
16. Beadle RE, Norwood GL, Brencick VA: Summertime plasma catecholamine concentrations in healthy and anhidrotic horses in Louisiana, *Am J Vet Res* 43:1446-1448, 1982.
17. Marlin DJ, Schroter RC, Scott CM, et al: Sweating and skin temperature responses of normal and anhidrotic horses to intravenous adrenaline, *Equine Vet J Suppl* 30:362-369, 1999.
18. Rakhit S, Murdoch R, Wilson SM: Persistent desensitization of the beta 2 adrenoceptors expressed by cultured equine sweat gland epithelial cells, *J Exp Biol* 201:259-266, 1998.
19. Bovell DL, Lindsay SL, Corbett AD, et al: Immunolocalization of aquaporin–5 expression in sweat gland cells from normal and anhidrotic horses, *Vet Dermatol* 17:17-23, 2006.
20. Jenkinson DM, Montgomery I, Elder HY, et al: Ultrastructural variations in the sweat glands of anhidrotic horses, *Equine Vet J* 17:287-291, 1985.
21. Bilezikian JP, Loeb JN: The influence of hyperthyroidism and hypothyroidism on alpha- and beta-adrenergic receptor systems and adrenergic responsiveness, *Endocr Rev* 4:378-388, 1983.
22. Evans CL: Physiological mechanisms that underlie sweating in the horse, *Br Vet J* 122:117-123, 1966.
23. Guthrie AJ, Van den Berg JS, Killeen VM, et al: Use of a semi–quantitative sweat test in Thoroughbred horses, *J S Afr Vet Assoc* 63:162-165, 1992.
24. MacKay RJ: Quantitative intradermal terbutaline sweat test in horses, *Equine Vet J* 40:518-520, 2008.

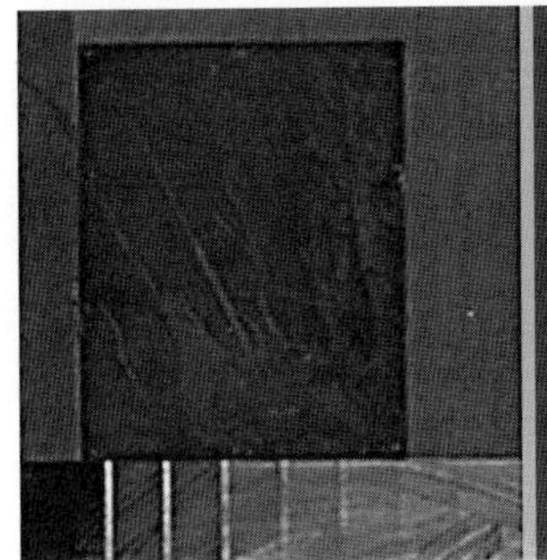

Disorders of Foals

CHAPTER 21

Pamela A. Wilkins

NEONATAL AND PERINATAL DISEASES

Pamela A. Wilkins

Before the 1980s intensive management of the compromised neonate was unusual and little was known regarding many of the problems of this special patient population. Although some specific conditions had been described by astute clinician-researchers, most notably the "dummy" foal syndrome[1] and respiratory distress syndrome caused by primary surfactant deficiency,[2] little information regarding the diagnosis and management of conditions of the foal during the neonatal period was available, although at least one active group was investigating fetal and neonatal physiology of the horse in Great Britain.[1-14] When treatment of compromised foals was undertaken, the approach usually resembled treating them as small adults, with little consideration given to the different physiology of the equine neonate. The advent of improved management of reproductive efficiency in mares led naturally to an increased interest in preservation of the conceptus to parturition and the foal thereafter. Interested clinicians, drawing on lessons from human perinatology and neonatology and sometimes collaborating with their counterparts in the human field, pioneered investigations of these small patients and created the fields of equine perinatology and equine neonatal intensive care.[1-19] Because of the foresight and energy of these early investigators, the field of veterinary perinatology-neonatology exploded in the 1980s, leading to the creation of equine neonatal intensive care units throughout the United States and the world. From these units information about the normal and abnormal physiology of foals, the medical conditions affecting them, and methods for treatment and management of these problems has been developed through observational, retrospective, and prospective studies. This veritable explosion of information over the last 20 years has greatly improved the ability of all practitioners to provide appropriate care for these patients, whether in the field or at an equine neonatal intensive care unit. The ability not only to save the lives of these patients but also to treat them in such a manner as to allow them to fulfill their purposes, whether as pleasure animals or racing athletes, has improved almost exponentially from those early days.[20-23] This section aims to provide the clinician with current information about the management of these patients, with the recognition that much still remains unknown and that advances will continue to be made in this dynamic field. The reader is cautioned that much of this chapter is flavored by the experiences of the authors and that variation in the approach to and treatment of specific problems exists among neonatal intensive care units (NICUs) and among clinicians in the same NICU; moreover, each year results in change. In some cases information that is presented has been gleaned from human NICU studies, essentially using the critically ill infant as the experimental model.

Many of the problems of the newborn foal have their genesis in utero. Identification of high-risk pregnancies is an important component of prenatal care of the foal, and some of the most commonly encountered problems of the dam that result in abnormal foals include previous or concurrent disease, poor reproductive history, poor perineal or pelvic conformation, poor general health, poor nutritional condition, prolonged transport, history of previous abnormal foals, placental abnormalities, and twins.[24]

Some of the more common causes of abortion can result in the birth of severely compromised foals of variable gestation lengths (Box 21-1). These include infectious causes such as equine herpesvirus (EHV) types 1 (most commonly) and 4 (rarely), equine infectious anemia, equine arteritis virus, bacterial and fungal placentitis, leptospirosis, equine ehrlichiosis, and septicemia-endotoxemia.[25-27] Noninfectious causes of abortion include twinning and noninfectious placental abnormalities such as extensive endometrial fibrosis, body pregnancy, and abnormal length (long or short) of the umbilical cord.[24,28]

To the equine neonatologist opportunities for intervention may appear limited, and in the case of many of the aforementioned causes of fetal loss, this is true. However, much can be done in the attempt to preserve the pregnancy and in effect treat the fetus. When confronted with a threatened pregnancy, the veterinarian has various ways of evaluating the fetus and its environment and may use many potential therapies.

PREPARTUM EVALUATION OF THE FETUS AND PLACENTA

Once a pregnancy has been established as high risk, the fetus should be evaluated for viability. Evaluation should include as thorough an evaluation as possible of the reproductive tract,

BOX 21-1

CONDITIONS ASSOCIATED WITH HIGH-RISK PREGNANCY

Maternal Conditions

Colic-endotoxemia
Abdominal hernia
Pelvic anatomic abnormalities
Malnutrition
Any debilitating disease
Uterine torsion
Uterine abnormalities
Mare reproductive loss syndrome
Hyperlipemia
Hypogalactia
History of previous abnormal foals

Conceptual Conditions

Placentitis
Twins
Hydrops
Prolonged gestation
Fetal abnormalities
Dystocia
Fescue toxicosis
Umbilical abnormalities
Congenital deformity

placenta, and fetal fluids. The details of this examination are described in Chapter 18. Prepartum disorders in the mare usually are readily recognizable, but disorders of the fetus and placenta can be more subtle and difficult to determine. The first step is to take a thorough history of the mare. Of particular interest is any history of previous abnormal foals, but the history taking should include questions regarding transportation; establishment of an accurate breeding date (sometimes more difficult than one would suspect); pertinent medical history, including any diagnostic testing performed for this pregnancy, such as culture, endometrial biopsy, and cytologic results; and any rectal and ultrasound examination results. Additionally, the clinician should obtain information regarding the possible ingestion of endophyte-infected fescue or exposure to potential infectious causes of abortion.[29,30] A complete vaccination and deworming history is requisite, as is a complete history of any medications and supplements administered during pregnancy.

After obtaining a history, the clinician performs a rectal examination, including palpation of the cervix, uterus, fetus, and all palpable abdominal contents. Any abnormalities should be noted. The cervix should be tight throughout gestation; the late-gestation uterus will be large and distended with fluid and usually pulled craniad in the abdomen. Palpation of the fetus frequently results in some fetal movement; however, lack of movement should be interpreted with caution insofar as some normal fetuses do not respond. Ultrasonographic evaluation of the uterus and conceptus by way of the rectum can provide valuable information, particularly regarding placental thickness if placentitis is a concern. The clinician may evaluate fetal fluids and estimate fetal size on the basis of the size of the eye later in gestation.[31] In some hospitals the practitioners choose not to perform vaginal or speculum examinations because of an association between these examinations and the subsequent development of placentitis. Unless placentitis is recognized with ultrasonographic evaluation by way of the rectum and culture is desirable, these types of examinations generally are not necessary.

After rectal examination a transabdominal ultrasonographic evaluation of the uterus and conceptus is performed.[28] The neonatologist can generate a biophysical profile of the fetus on the basis of this examination in the late-term fetus and readily determine viability.[32,33] It is also possible to determine the presence or absence of twins in the late pregnant mare in this manner. The sonogram is performed through the acoustic window from the udder to the xiphoid ventrally and laterally to the skin folds of the flank. Imaging of the fetus usually requires a low-frequency (3.5-MHz) probe, whereas examination of the placenta and endometrium requires a higher-frequency (7.5-MHz) probe. A complete description of this examination is beyond the scope of this chapter, but several complete descriptions of the technique and normal values for specific gestation lengths can be found by consulting the relevant veterinary literature.[33] The utility of this examination lies in its repeatability and low risk to the dam and fetus. Sequential examinations over time allow the clinician to follow the pregnancy and identify changes as they occur.

A companion to transabdominal ultrasonography is evaluation of the fetal electrocardiogram (ECG). Fetal ECGs can be measured continuously using telemetry or obtained through more conventional techniques several times throughout the day.[24,28,34] The operator places electrodes on the mare's skin in locations aimed at maximizing the magnitude of the fetal ECG. Because the fetus frequently changes position, multiple sites may be needed in any 24-hour period. To begin, one places an electrode dorsally in the area of the sacral prominence, with two electrodes placed bilaterally in a transverse plane in the region of the flank. The fetal ECG maximal amplitude is low, usually 0.05 to 0.1 mV, and can be lost in artifact or background noise, so it is often necessary to move electrodes to new positions to maximize the appearance of the fetal ECG. The normal fetal heart rate during the last months of gestation ranges between 65 to 115 beats/min, a fairly wide distribution. The range of heart rate of an individual fetus can be narrow, however. Bradycardia in the fetus is an adaptation to in utero stress, most commonly thought to be hypoxia. By slowing the heart rate, the fetus prolongs exposure of fetal blood to maternal blood, increasing the time for equilibration of dissolved gas across the placenta and improving the oxygen content of the fetal blood. The fetus also has altered the distribution of its cardiac output in response to hypoxia, centralizing blood distribution.[35,36] Tachycardia in the fetus can be associated with fetal movement, and brief periods of tachycardia should occur in the fetus in any 24-hour period. Persistent tachycardia is a sign of fetal distress and represents more severe fetal compromise than bradycardia. The author has recognized dysrhythmias in the challenged fetus, most commonly as atrial fibrillation but also as apparent runs of ventricular tachycardia.

The ability to monitor the fetus in a high-risk pregnancy inevitably has led to questions of whether, how, and when to intervene. Most equine neonatologists would agree that removal of the fetus from the uterus before it is ready for birth is not desirable. One of the difficulties in determining fetal preparedness for birth is that prediction of parturition is difficult in these mares. Many of the parameters used in normal mares are unreliable in the high-risk pregnant mare. One must have an accurate history of any previous gestation length in terms of days for the mare in question to allow a more accurate estimate of her usual gestational length. Evaluation of the usual mammary gland parameters, including size, the presence of "wax," and alteration of electrolyte concentrations, is not generally predictive in the high-risk mare; in the author's experience many of these mares have changes predictive of parturition for weeks before actual parturition.[37,38] This circumstance may be related to the observation that many high-risk pregnant mares, particularly those with placentitis, are presented for a primary complaint of early onset lactation. Although pulmonary system maturity in human beings can be assessed with some degree of accuracy using measurement of lecithin-sphingomyelin ratios, this measurement—along with sphingomyelin, cortisol, and creatinine concentrations in the amniotic fluid—has proved to be of no benefit in the horse.[39-41] Amniocentesis carries a high risk of abortion in the horse, even with ultrasound guidance, and is not a clinically useful technique at this time.[41] Currently, no clear-cut guidelines are available indicating the best time to intervene, but the presence of persistent fetal tachycardia or prolonged absence of fetal movements, including breathing movements, as determined by transabdominal ultrasound evaluation, should initiate discussion regarding the appropriateness of induction of parturition or elective cesarean section. The goal of induction or cesarean section is to remove a pregnancy that is threatening the survival of the dam, with no thought to fetal survival, or to remove the fetus from a threatening environment to improve its likelihood to survive. Preterm induction is ill advised if fetal survival is desirable because of the limited ability to treat severely immature neonates. Timing of intervention in these circumstances remains an art, not a science.

The approach to management of the high-risk pregnancy is dictated to some degree by the exact cause for concern, but for many mares therapy is similar. Many high-risk mares have placentitis, primarily caused by ascending bacterial or fungal infections originating in the region of the cervix. These infections can cause in utero sepsis or compromise the fetus by local elucidation of inflammatory mediators or altered placental function.[42,43] Premature udder development and vaginal discharge are common clinical signs. Treatment consists of administration of broad-spectrum antimicrobial agents and nonsteroidal anti-inflammatory drugs (Table 21-1). In some clinics trimethoprim-sulfonamide drugs have been the antimicrobial of choice because of unpublished studies that demonstrated an increased concentration of these agents in the fetal fluids compared with penicillin and gentamicin. However, if culture and sensitivity results are available, directed therapy should be instituted. Nonsteroidal anti-inflammatory agents such as flunixin meglumine are useful to combat alterations in prostaglandin balance that may be associated with infection and inflammation. Although the efficacy of these agents is best when administered before the development of clinical signs, to date no detrimental effects have been reported in the fetus or dam when chronically used at low doses in well-hydrated patients. Tocolytic agents and agents that promote

TABLE 21-1

Drugs Used to Treat High-Risk Pregnancy

Drug	Dose/Frequency/ Route	Reason
Trimethoprim-sulfonamide	25 mg/b.i.d.; PO	Antimicrobial
Flunixin meglumine	0.25 mg/kg t.i.d.; PO or IV	Anti-inflammatory
Altrenogest	0.44 mg/kg s.i.d.; PO	Tocolytic
Isoxuprine	0.4-0.6 mg/kg b.i.d.; IM* or PO	Tocolytic
Clenbuterol	0.8 μg/kg as needed PO*	Tocolytic
Vitamin E	6000-10,000 IU s.i.d.; PO	Antioxidant

b.i.d., Twice daily; *t.i.d.*, three times daily; *PO*, per os (by mouth); *IV*, intravenous; *s.i.d.*, once daily; *IM*, intramuscular
*Intravenous form currently not available in the United States.

uterine quiescence include altrenogest, isoxuprine, and clenbuterol.[44-48] Usually, altrenogest is administered, although its need in late gestation has been challenged. The efficacy of isoxuprine as a tocolytic in the horse is unproven, and the bioavailability of orally administered isoxuprine appears to be highly variable.[48] The long-term use of clenbuterol is inadvisable because of receptor population changes associated with chronic use and its unknown effects on the fetus at this time. Clenbuterol may be indicated during management of dystocia in preparation for assisted delivery or cesarean section.[46] The intravenous form of clenbuterol currently is not available in the United States.

Three additional strategies can be used in managing mares with high-risk pregnancies. In mares with evidence of placental dysfunction, with or without signs of fetal distress, the author provides intranasal oxygen supplementation in the hope of improving oxygen delivery to the fetus. Intranasal oxygen insufflation of 10 to 15 L/min to the mare significantly increases partial pressure of oxygen (Pa_{O_2}) and percent oxygen saturation of hemoglobin.[49,50] Because of the horse's placental vessel arrangement, improvement of these two arterial blood gas parameters should result in improved oxygen delivery to the fetus. Blood gas transport is largely independent of diffusion distance in the equine placenta, particularly in late gestation, and depends more on blood flow. Information from other species cannot be extrapolated to the equine placenta because of its diffuse epitheliochorial nature and the arrangement of the maternal and fetal blood vessels within the microcotyledons.[51,52] Umbilical venous pO_2 is 50 to 54 mm Hg in the horse fetus, compared with 30 to 34 mm Hg in the sheep, whereas the maternal uterine vein to umbilical vein pO_2 difference is near 0. Also unlike the sheep, the umbilical venous pO_2 values decrease 5 to 10 mm Hg in response to maternal hypoxemia and increase in response to maternal hyperoxia.[53-55]

Vitamin E (tocopherol) is administered orally to some high-risk mares as an antioxidant. Administration of large doses of vitamin E before traumatic brain injury improves neurologic outcome in experimental models and has been examined as possible prophylaxis for human neonatal encephalopathy.[56-58] Extrapolation of that information to the compromised equine fetus suggests that increased antioxidant concentrations in the fetus may mitigate some of the consequences of uterine and birth hypoxia, but no evidence is available to date demonstrating that protection occurs or that vitamin E accumulates in the fetus in response to supplementation of the mare. Finally, many high-risk mares are anorectic or restricted from feed because of their medical condition. These mares are at particularly great risk for fetal loss because of their lack of feed intake, which alters prostaglandin metabolism.[59] Therefore the clinician should administer 2.5% to 5% dextrose in 0.45% saline or water (5% dextrose) intravenously at maintenance fluid rates to these patients.

Perhaps the most important aspect of managing mares with high-risk pregnancies is frequent observation and development of a plan. These mares should be observed at least hourly for evidence of early-stage labor and should be under constant video surveillance if possible. Depending on the primary problem, the team managing the mare should develop a plan for handling the parturition once labor begins and for fetal resuscitation after delivery. Any equipment that may be needed should be readily available stallside, and a call sheet listing contact numbers for all involved should be posted on or near the stall. The plan should include a description of how a complicated dystocia would be handled, should it occur, with permission for general anesthesia and cesarean section obtained before the event so that time is not wasted. An important question to be posed to the owner at the outset is whether the mare or the foal is more important; this answer may dictate the direction of the decision tree once labor begins.[60,61]

EVALUATION OF THE NEWBORN FOAL

Bonnie Barr

Early recognition of abnormalities is of utmost importance for the successful management of critically ill foals. To recognize the abnormal, the normal must be known. Immediately after birth, several important physiologic and behavioral changes occur. Chief among these changes are the adaptation of the cardiovascular and respiratory systems to extrauterine life; thus persistent increases or decreases in heart or respiratory rates should alert the clinician to existing or impending problems. The normal transition of the respiratory tract involves opening closed alveoli and absorption of fluid from the airway, accomplished by a combination of breathing efforts, expiration against a closed glottis ("grunting"), and a change in sodium flux across the respiratory membrane from net secretion to net absorption.[1-5] The transition from fetal to neonatal circulatory patterns requires resolution of the pulmonary hypertension present in the fetus, normally shunting blood flow through the lower resistance ductus arteriosus in the fetal state, in order to direct cardiac output to the pulmonary vasculature for participation in gas exchange. This change is achieved by opening alveoli; decreasing airway resistance and providing radial support for pulmonary vessels; achieving functional closure of the ductus arteriosus; and increasing the oxygen tension in the lung, reversing pulmonary vasoconstriction mediated by hypoxia.[6,7] Pulmonary tree vasodilators (prostacyclin, nitric oxide [NO]) and vasoconstrictors (endothelin-1, leukotrienes) play apparently well-coordinated, but as yet not fully elucidated, roles. In the normal newborn this change is smooth and rapid. These critical events are undermined by factors such as inadequate lung development, surfactant deficiency (primary or secondary), viral or bacterial infection, placental abnormalities, in utero hypoxia, and meconium aspiration.

Spontaneous breathing should begin in the neonate within 1 minute of birth; many foals will attempt to breathe as their thorax clears the pelvic canal.[8,9] First breaths are normally triggered by the combination of removal of placental humoral inhibitory factor, cooling of the neonate, tactile stimulation, the catecholamine surge's induction of substances important for breathing (e.g., substance P) and increasing carbon dioxide. Apnea at birth can be caused by asphyxia, central nervous system (CNS) depression from maternal drugs, CNS injury, septicemia, anemia, primary muscular or neurologic disease, and obstructing congenital malformations or other mechanical obstruction of the airway. During the first hour of life, the respiratory rate of a healthy foal can be as high as 80 breaths per minute but should decrease to 30 to 40 breaths per minute within a few hours. Similarly, the heart rate of a healthy newborn foal will have a regular rhythm and be at least 60 beats per minute at the first minute.[8,9] By the time the foal is 1 day of age, the heart rate should range between 70 to 100 beats per minute. Persistent bradycardia can be caused by hypoxic damage, acid-base derangements, and sepsis and is an indication for rapid intervention. A continuous murmur can usually be ausculted over the left side of the heart, although its loudness may vary with position. This murmur is thought to be associated with some shunting through the ductus arteriosus. Variable systolic murmurs, thought to be flow murmurs, may be ausculted during the first week of life.[10] Murmurs that persist beyond the first week of life in an otherwise healthy foal should be more thoroughly investigated, as should any murmur associated with persistent hypoxia. Sinus arrhythmias can be noted relatively frequently during the immediate postpartum period. Various other arrhythmias (e.g., ventricular premature complexes, ventricular tachycardia, supraventricular tachycardia) occasionally can be observed in normal foals; however, all arrhythmias should disappear within 15 minutes post partum.[11] Physiologic changes associated with the adaptive period are probably the main factors contributing to these arrhythmias. The clinical significance of any unusual or abnormal arrhythmias should take into consideration clinical, metabolic, and homodynamic findings of the neonate.

Auscultation of the thorax shortly after birth will reveal a cacophony of sounds as airways are opened and fluid is cleared. End-expiratory crackles are consistently heard in the dependent lung during and after lateral recumbency. Changes in respiratory rate, effort, or breathing pattern are more appreciable than auscultable changes in neonates with respiratory disease. Premature and dysmature foals or foals subjected to peripartum hypoxia can demonstrate abnormal breathing patterns, especially when sleeping. Any sudden change in respiratory parameters should be investigated immediately because it may indicate deterioration in the foal's condition. It is not unusual for a normal newborn foal to appear slightly cyanotic during this initial adaptation period, but this should resolve within minutes of birth. The equine fetus, like all fetuses, exists in a moderately hypoxic environment, but the equine fetus has a greater partial pressure of oxygen, approximately 50 mm Hg.[12] Because the fetus is well adapted to low oxygen tensions, cyanosis is rarely present in newborn foals once adaption occurs, even those with low oxygen tensions. Although in many species the fetal blood oxygen affinity is greater than the maternal blood, in the equine fetus the O_2 affinity of its hemoglobin is only approximately 2 mm Hg greater than the maternal blood as a result of lower levels of 2,3 diphosphoglycerate (DPG) compared with other species.[13] The result is enhanced oxygen unloading in the equine fetus compared with others. DPG concentration increases after birth in the foal and reaches mature levels by 3 to 5 days of age. The major blood adaptation of the equine fetus to chronic hypoxia is an increase in PCV of up to 20%, increasing the oxygen content of the blood as compensation for decreased O_2 delivery at the placenta.[14] A higher than expected packed cell volume (PCV) in any newborn foal should alert the clinician to possible sequelae from chronic hypoxia. The presence of significant cyanosis that persists should prompt the clinician to thoroughly evaluate the foal for cardiac anomalies resulting in significant right to left shunting or separated circulations, such as transposition of the great vessels.

Within several minutes after birth, the mucous membranes should be moist and pink. The persistence of an abnormal color of the mucous membranes such as jaundice, cyanosis, injection, ulcerations, and petechial hemorrhages indicates problems to come. Jaundice can accompany a variety of neonatal diseases, such as neonatal isoerthrolysis, sepsis, and meconium retention. Other indications of sepsis include injection and petechial hemorrhages on the mucous membranes; petechiation of the pinnae of the ears, sclera, and vulva; depression; and, in an extreme case, recumbency. Peripheral pulses should be strong and can be detected at the facial artery, brachial artery, on the inside of the elbow joint, and at the great metatarsal artery. Distal extremities should be warm. Cold extremities result when blood is redirected away from them to other tissue, which most often occurs with sepsis. In this case the peripheral pulses may initially be strong and bounding, but as sepsis progresses, the pulses become weak.

The body temperature of the foal at birth is similar to the dam's temperature. Immediately after birth the healthy full-term neonate can effectively thermoregulate despite heat loss associated with wet hair coat and adverse environmental temperatures. Mechanisms of heat production in the healthy newborn foal include shivering, nonshivering thermogenesis, neuroendocrine stimulation, and behavioral processes.[15] Newborn foals shiver within a few minutes of birth and continue to shiver for several hours when exposed to low environmental temperatures. Thyroid hormones and catecholamines stimulate the onset of nonshivering thermogenesis, which involves the oxidation of brown adipose tissue to release energy as heat.[15] Behavioral thermoregulation involves the ability of the animal to modify its behavior to conserve or produce heat. Healthy foals maintain sternal recumbency to minimize heat loss but at the same time will increase heat production by physical activity, such as attempting to stand. A healthy foal should be nursing 1 to 2 hours after birth, thus relying on colostral fat, colostral glucose, and milk to provide sufficient energy to support metabolism such that fat stores are not seriously depleted. Premature foals are not able to maintain a steady rectal temperature because of inadequate heat production resulting from poor energy intake, diminished endogenous energy stores, lack of nonshivering thermogenesis associated with a lack of brown fat, and immaturity of the neuroendocrine system. Foals that suffer from a hypoxic insult, are septic, or are being treated with certain medications (e.g., phenobarbital) must be monitored and managed appropriately because they are unable to thermoregulate properly. In infants sedatives such as benzodiazepine affect the ability to thermoregulate; therefore sedation and general anesthesia used on the mare to correct a dystocia can have an impact on the newborn foal's ability to thermoregulate.

The abdomen should be visually examined and palpated for abnormalities. Congenital scrotal hernias are noted shortly after birth, are usually unilateral, and are easily reduced when the foal is rolled onto its back. Intestinal strangulation is rare with scrotal hernias, and resolution of the hernia usually occurs spontaneously in 3 to 6 months. Inguinal hernias are evident 4 to 48 hours after birth and cause intermittent colic, depression, severe scrotal and preputial swelling, and edema, with skin excoriation and splitting caused by abrasion against the inside of the thigh. Inguinal hernias are classified as either indirect or direct, as described in the human literature. In indirect herniation the herniated intestine is situated inside the vaginal tunic and occupies the same space as the testis.[16] Most indirect hernias are easily reduced and often resolve spontaneously as the foal ages and grows. In direct herniation the intestine herniates through a rent in the peritoneum and transverse fascia (and/or parietal vaginal tunic and scrotal fascia) and comes to lie subcutaneously (i.e., outside the common vaginal tunic, in the inguinal-scrotal region).[16] Surgical intervention is often necessary for direct herniation because of the risk of incarceration of bowel. The exact cause is unknown, but it seems probable that inguinal hernias are a result of an increased intra-abdominal pressure during birth in which the intestinal loops may be forced through the vaginal ring into the vaginal cavity. Tearing of the parietal vaginal tunic could be caused by the limited space in the vaginal cavity. Umbilical hernias are a common defect in neonates and may result from congenital malformations of the umbilical region; infection; traumatic parturition; or opening of the umbilicus caused by straining, which results in increased intra-abdominal pressure. Occasionally, the umbilical defect may be so large that small intestine will eviscerate into the hernia sac. Small umbilical hernias resolve spontaneously, whereas larger hernias may require surgery to correct the defect. Auscultation of the abdomen provides an assessment of gastrointestinal motility and should be performed from the paralumbar fossa to the ventral abdomen, on both the right and left sides. Decreases in motility suggest ileus, which may be due to inflammatory, ischemic, or obstructive lesions. Increased motility occurs during the early stages of enteritis or intestinal obstruction.

The development of the gastrointestinal tract appears to be mostly complete in the neonate. The presence and distribution of the interstitial cells of Cajal (ICC), which generate pacemaker activity, are complete in the small intestine at birth; however, the development in the large intestine and distal colon continues after birth.[17] This immaturity of the ICC at birth may contribute to retention of meconium in the distal colon and rectum in some neonatal foals. Other possible causes of meconium impaction include prematurity, sepsis, and asphyxia, or it can be secondary to prolonged recumbency, dehydration, or medications. Meconium, an accumulation of swallowed allantoic fluid, gastrointestinal secretions, and cellular debris, is generally black to brown and of firm to pasty consistency. Once meconium is passed, feces change to a lighter brown color and become softer. Evaluation of the quantity and quality of meconium is an important part of the physical examination, and the amount passed varies from foal to foal. Passage of meconium in utero is an indication of fetal distress during late gestation or parturition and should prompt a detailed assessment of the neonate. Aspiration of meconium results in severe pneumonia because of the caustic effect of the meconium on the respiratory epithelium.

Examination of the urogenital system includes evaluation of the external genitalia and the umbilicus. Many male foals have a persistent penile frenulum at birth, which resolves within a few days. When the cord is allowed to break naturally at birth, the umbilical vein and the urachus break at the navel stump and the umbilical arteries retract into their connective tissue sheath within the abdomen, closer to the bladder apex. Once the umbilical stump dries, it should remain dry. A moist stump or observation of urination from the umbilicus indicates a patent urachus, which is commonly found in foals that are recumbent for any reason. The neonate should be observed for the onset, frequency, and quantity of urine output. The mean time for first urination in the colt is 5.97 hours, and in the filly it is 10.77 hours; however, these times vary widely.[18] Evidence of urogenital disease includes depression, straining to urinate, pigmenturia, and decreased urine output (oliguria). When clinical signs of urinary tract disease exist, the foal's urine production should be monitored carefully and serum chemistries evaluated for azotemia and electrolyte disturbances, and a transabdominal ultrasound should be performed so that the clinician can examine the urogenital structures. The full-term neonatal foal has a glomerular filtration rate and effective renal plasma flow comparable with that of the adult.[18] The status of the premature foal's renal function has not been determined.

The musculoskeletal system should be closely evaluated for malformations or injuries secondary to the explosive nature of the equine birth. Congenital anomalies of the limbs include polydactylism, adactylia, defects in the hoof wall, and contractural deformities. Other congenital anomalies include brachygnathism, wry nose, cleft palate, torticollis, and scoliosis. Laxity in the neonate often manifests as weakness of the flexor tendons because of dysmaturity or prematurity, although full-term foals may exhibit a mild degree of fetlock laxity. In most foals the laxity will spontaneously resolve after a few days, but occasionally corrective trimming and shoeing are required. When the foal is malpositioned, injuries such as rib fractures and ruptures of the gastrocnemius muscle may occur. Rib fractures are common and occur even in apparently normal births. Rib fractures usually occur a few centimeters above the costochondral junction, with multiple fractures (4 to 12) commonly occurring in a straight line. Neonates with fractured ribs have soft tissue swelling over the fracture site, crepitus, and pain on palpation and occasionally respiratory distress resulting from pneumothorax or hemothorax. Rupture of the gastrocnemius muscle occurs during delivery if the hock is flexed and the stifle is forced into extension (i.e., the foal is "dog sitting").[19] This results in hyperflexion of the hock caused by tearing of the gastrocnemius muscle at the level of the femur. Most of the time these foals respond well to conservative management.

The righting reflex is present as the foal exits the birth canal, as is the withdrawl reflex. Cranial nerve responses are intact at birth, but the menace response may take as long as 2 weeks to fully develop. Lack of menace should not be considered diagnostic of visual deficits in the newborn foal. Within 1 hour of birth, the normal foal will demonstrate auditory orientation with unilateral pinna control. The normal pupillary angle is ventromedial in the newborn foal; this angle gradually becomes dorsomedial over the first month of life. Foals should begin attempting to stand shortly after birth and should be able to stand on their own within 2 hours of birth.[20] The normal newborn foal will have a suck reflex shortly after birth and should be searching for an udder even before it stands. A normal foal is expected to suck from the dam unaided by 3 hours post partum; many foals will suck well before this time.

The gait of the newborn foal is hypermetric, and the stance is base wide.[21] Extreme hypermetria of the forelimbs, usually bilateral but occasionally unilateral, has been observed in some foals and is associated with perinatal hypoxic-ischemic insults, but this gait abnormality usually resolves without specific therapy with a few days. Spinal reflexes tend to be exaggerated, while the crossed extensor reflex may not be fully present until 3 weeks of age.[22] Foals exhibit an exaggerated response to external stimuli (e.g., noise, sudden visual changes, touch) for the first few weeks of life. Foals are not strongly bonded to their mothers for the first few weeks of life and will follow any large moving object, including other horses and people. Until they are several months of age, orphan foals will bond with surrogate mothers; their primary motivation appears to be appetite. Conversely, mares strongly bond with their foals shortly after parturition: The process begins once the chorioallantois is ruptured, and is driven more by olfaction and taste rather than by vision or hearing. Interference with this process, by medical intervention or excessive owner manipulation of the foal, can disrupt normal bonding and cause the dam to reject the foal.[23]

NEONATAL RESUSCITATION

Pamela A. Wilkins

Most newborn foals make the transition to extrauterine life easily. However, for those in difficulty, immediate recognition of the condition and institution of appropriate resuscitation is of utmost importance. A modified Apgar scoring system has been developed as a guide for initiating resuscitation and assessing the probable level of fetal compromise (Table 21-2).[1] One also must at least perform a cursory physical examination before initiating resuscitation in case there are serious problems (e.g., limb contracture, microophthalmia, hydrocephalus) that would make resuscitation a less humane choice.

The initial assessment begins during presentation of the fetus. Although the following applies primarily to attending the birth of a foal from a high-risk pregnancy, quiet and rapid evaluation can be performed during any attended birth. The goal in a normal birth with a normal foal is to disturb the bonding process as little as possible. This goal also applies to high-risk parturitions, but some disruption of normal bonding is inevitable. The lead clinician should control tightly the number of persons attending, and the degree of activity surrounding, the birth.

One should evaluate the strength and rate of any palpable peripheral pulse and should evaluate the apical pulse as

TABLE 21-2

Apgar Score in the Foal

	ASSIGNED VALUE		
Parameter	**0**	**1**	**2**
Heart/pulse rate	Undetectable	<60 beats/min irregular	>60 beats/min regular
Respiratory rate/pattern	Undetectable	Slow, irregular	40-60 beats/min regular
Muscle tone	Limp/absent	Lateral, some tone	Sternal
Nasal mucosal stimulation	Unresponsive	Grimace, mild rejection	Cough or sneeze

From Mansmann RA, McAllister ES, Pratt PW, editors: *Equine medicine and surgery*, ed 3, vol 1, Santa Barbara, Calif, 1982, American Veterinary Publications.
One should determine the score at 1 and 5 minutes after birth. Scores of 7 to 8 generally indicate a normal foal; 4 to 6, mild to moderate asphyxia; and 0 to 3, severe asphyxia. A score of 4 to 6 should prompt stimulation, intranasal oxygen, or mechanical ventilation. For a score of 0 to 3, one should begin cardiopulmonary resuscitation.

soon as the chest clears the birth canal. Bradycardia (pulse <40 beats/min) is expected during forceful contractions, and the pulse rate should increase rapidly once the chest clears the birth canal. Persistent bradycardia is an indication for rapid intervention.

The fetus is normally hypoxemic compared with the newborn foal, and this hypoxemia is largely responsible for the maintenance of fetal circulation by generation of pulmonary hypertension. The fetus responds to conditions producing more severe in utero hypoxia by strengthening the fetal circulatory pattern, and the neonate responds to hypoxia by reverting to the fetal circulatory pattern.[2] During a normal parturition mild asphyxia occurs and results in fetal responses that pave the way for a successful transition to extrauterine life. If more than mild transient asphyxia occurs, the fetus is stimulated to breathe in utero; this is known as *primary asphyxia*.[3] If the initial breathing effort resulting from primary asphyxia does not correct the asphyxia, a second gasping period occurs in several minutes, known as the *secondary asphyxia response*. If no improvement in asphyxia occurs during this period, the foal enters secondary apnea, a state that cannot be reversed except by resuscitation.

Therefore the first priority of neonatal resuscitation is establishing an airway and breathing pattern. The clinician should assume that foals not spontaneously breathing are in secondary apnea and should clear the airway of membranes as soon as the nose is presented. If meconium staining is present, the airway should be suctioned before delivery of the foal is complete and before the foal breathes spontaneously. One should continue to suction the trachea if aspiration of the nasopharynx is productive. Overzealous suctioning worsens bradycardia as it worsens hypoxia. Suctioning should be stopped once the foal begins breathing spontaneously because hypoxia will worsen with continued suction. If the foal does not breathe or move spontaneously within seconds of birth, one should begin tactile stimulation. If tactile stimulation fails to result in spontaneous breathing, the foal should immediately be intubated and manually ventilated using an Ambu bag or equivalent. Mouth-to-nose ventilation can be used if nasotracheal tubes and an Ambu bag are not available. The goal of this therapy is to reverse fetal circulation, and hyperventilation with 100% oxygen is the best choice for this purpose. However, recent evidence suggests that no clinical disadvantages are apparent when room air is used for ventilation of asphyxiated human neonates rather than 100% oxygen.[4,5] Human infants resuscitated with room air recovered more quickly than those resuscitated with 100% oxygen in one study, as assessed by Apgar scores, time to the first cry, and the sustained pattern of breathing.[6] In addition, neonates resuscitated with 100% oxygen exhibited biochemical findings reflecting prolonged oxidative stress, present even after 4 weeks of postnatal life, which did not appear in the group resuscitated with room air. Thus the current accepted recommendations for using 100% oxygen in the resuscitation of asphyxiated neonates require further discussion and investigation.[7,8] Almost 90% of foals that need resuscitation respond to hyperventilation alone and require no additional therapy. One can initiate nasotracheal intubation while the foal is in the birth canal if the foal will not be delivered rapidly, such as with a difficult dystocia. This technique is "blind" and requires some practice but may be beneficial and lifesaving. Once spontaneous breathing is present, humidified oxygen should be administered by way of nasal insufflation at 8 to 10 L/min.

Cardiovascular support in the form of chest compression should be initiated if the foal remains bradycardic despite ventilation and a nonperfusing rhythm is present. The clinician should make sure that the foal is on a hard surface in right lateral recumbency with the topline against a wall or other support. Approximately 5% of foals are born with fractured ribs, and an assessment for the presence of rib fractures is in order before initiating chest compressions.[9] Palpation of the ribs identifies many of these fractures, which usually are multiple and consecutive on one side of the thorax and located in a relatively straight line along the part of the rib with the greatest curvature dorsal to the costochondral junction. Auscultation over the ribs during breathing results in a recognizable click, identifying rib fractures that may have escaped detection by palpation. Ultrasonography is the diagnostic modality of choice when evaluating for the presence or absence of rib fractures in foals.[10] Unfortunately, ribs 3 to 5 frequently are involved, and their location over the heart can make chest compression a potentially fatal exercise.[11]

Drug therapy should be initiated if a nonperfusing rhythm persists for more than 30 to 60 seconds in the face of chest compression. Epinephrine is the first drug of choice (Table 21-3). Practitioners pose various arguments regarding the best dose and the best frequency of administration for resuscitation. However, most of the data are derived from human cardiac arrest studies and are not strictly applicable to the equine neonate because the genesis of the cardiovascular failure is different.[12,13] Vasopressin is gaining attention as a cardiovascular resuscitation drug, and although the author has used this drug in resuscitation and as a pressor, experience is limited at this time and large doses of vasopressin may compromise gastrointestinal perfusion, according to some accounts.[14-16] The author does not use atropine in bradycardic newborn foals because the bradycardia usually is caused by hypoxia, and if

TABLE 21-3

Resuscitation Drugs Used for Cardiopulmonary Resuscitation of Foals*

				DOSE		
Drug	**How Supplied**	**Per Kg**	**ml/Kg**	**ml/30 Kg**	**ml/40 Kg**	**ml/50 Kg**
Epinephrine (low dose)	1 mg/ml (1:1000)	0.01-0.02 mg	0.01-0.02	0.3-0.6	0.4-0.8	0.5-1
				3-5 minutes		
Epinephrine (high dose)	1 mg/ml (1:1000)	0.1-0.2 mg	0.1-0.2	3-6	4-8	5-10
				3-5 minutes		
Lidocaine	2% (20 mg/ml)	1.5 mg	0.075	2.25	3	3.75
				Every 5 minutes for a maximum of 3 mg/kg		
Bretylium	50 mg/ml	5-10 mg	0.1-0.2	3-6	4-8	5-10
		(30-35 mg/kg maximum dose)		10 minutes		
Atropine	0.54 mg/ml	0.02 mg	0.037	1.1	1.5	1.8
				Maximum of 2 times		
CaCl	10% solution	0.5-1.0 mEq	0.2	6	8	10
$NaHCO_3$	1 mEq/ml	0.5-1 mEq	0.5-1	15-30	20-40	25-50
$MgSO_4$	50% (500 mg/ml)	14-28 mg	0.028-0.056	0.8-1.7	1.1-2.2	1.4-2.8

*Epinephrine is the most commonly used of the drugs.

the hypoxia is not corrected, atropine can increase myocardial oxygen debt.[17] The author also does not use doxapram in initial resuscitation because it does not reverse secondary apnea, the most common apnea in newborns. However, recent evidence suggests that doxapram may prove very useful for the treatment of persistent centrally mediated hypoventilation and deserves further study.[18,19]

Because birthing areas are generally cold, the foal should be dried and placed on dry bedding once resuscitation is complete. The fetus has some homeothermic mechanisms, but its size in relation to its mother and its position within her body means that it is in effect a poikilotherm. The body temperature of the foal generally reflects that of its environment, namely its dam, although the human fetal temperature directly measured at cesarean section, induction of labor, or during labor is approximately 0.5° C higher than the dam's.[20-22] Adaptation from poikilothermy to homeothermy normally takes place rapidly after birth. The fetus is capable of nonshivering thermogenesis, primarily through the oxidation of brown fat reserves, but this type of thermogenesis is inhibited in utero, probably by placental prostaglandin E_2 and adenosine.[22,23] Immediately after birth the foal must adapt to independent thermoregulation. Local physical factors, including ambient temperature and humidity, act to induce cold stress, and the newborn must produce heat by metabolic activity. In response to the catecholamine surge associated with birth, uncoupling of oxidative phosphorylation occurs within mitochondria, releasing energy as heat. This nonshivering thermogenesis is impaired in newborns undergoing hypoxia or asphyxiation and in those that are ill at birth. Infants born to mothers sedated with benzodiazepines are affected similarly, a consideration in the choice of sedative and preanesthetic medications in mares suffering dystocia or undergoing cesarean section.[24-26] Heat losses by convection, radiation, and evaporation are high in most areas where foals are delivered, resuscitated, and managed, and one must take care to minimize cold stress in the newborn and the critically ill foal. Supplementary heat, in the form of radiant heat lamps or warm air circulating blankets, may be required.

Fluid therapy should be used conservatively during postpartum resuscitation, because the neonate is not volume depleted unless excessive bleeding has occurred. Some compromised newborn foals are actually hypervolemic. Fluid therapy for the neonate is discussed in more detail later in this chapter. Because the renal function of the equine neonate is substantially different from the adult's, fluid therapy cannot simply be scaled down from adult therapy.[27-29] If intravenous fluids are required for resuscitation and blood loss is identified, administration of 20 ml/kg of a non-glucose-containing polyionic isotonic fluid over 20 minutes (about 1 L for a 50-kg foal)—once intravenous access is established—can be effective. The author stresses non-glucose-containing polyionic intravenous fluids because hyperglycemia, but not hypoglycemia, immediately after fetal or neonatal asphyxia interfered with the recovery of brain cell membrane function and energy metabolism in neonatal piglets in one recent study.[30] These findings suggest that post-hypoxic-ischemic hyperglycemia is not beneficial and might even be harmful in neonatal hypoxic-ischemic encephalopathy. Indications for this shock bolus therapy include poor mentation; poorly palpable peripheral pulses; and the development of cold distal extremities, compatible with septic or hemorrhagic shock (or both). The patient should be reassessed after the initial bolus, and additional boluses should be administered as necessary. Ideally, the clinician should follow up on blood pressures and ECG readings and initiate appropriate inopressor therapy if needed. Again, these procedures are discussed in detail later in the chapter.

Glucose-containing fluids can be administered after resuscitation at a rate of 4 to 8 mg/kg/min (about 250 ml/hr of 5% dextrose or 125 ml/hr of 10% dextrose) to the average

50-kg foal, particularly in the obviously compromised foal. This therapy is indicated to help resolve metabolic acidosis, to support cardiac output (because myocardial glycogen stores likely have been depleted), and to prevent postasphyxial hypoglycemia. Under normal conditions the fetal-to-maternal blood glucose concentration gradient is 50% to 60% in the horse, and glucose is the predominant source of energy during fetal development.[31,32] Glucose transport across the placenta is facilitated by carrier receptors (glucose transporter [GLUT] receptors), and a direct relationship exists between maternal and fetal blood glucose concentration when maternal glucose is in the normal range.[31] The GLUT receptors in the placenta are stereospecific, saturable, and energy independent.[33] Although the enzyme kinetics for GLUT isoform 1 suggest that they are not saturable under conditions of euglycemia, equine maternal hyperglycemia results in increased fetal glucose concentration to a plateau point, likely caused by GLUT saturation.

At term the net umbilical uptake of glucose is 4 to 7 mg/kg/min, with most of the glucose being used by the brain and skeletal muscle.[34-36] The fetus develops gluconeogenesis only under conditions of severe maternal starvation. A certain percentage of the delivered glucose is used to develop large glycogen stores in the fetal liver and cardiac muscle in preparation for birth, and at birth the foal liver produces glucose at a rate of 4 to 8 mg/kg/min by using these stores. Fetal glycogen stores also are built using the substrates lactate, pyruvate, and alanine; fetal uptake of lactate across the placenta is about half that of glucose.[31,37] The transition to gluconeogenesis, stimulated by increased circulating catecholamine concentration from birth and by stimulation of glucagon release at the time the umbilical cord breaks, takes 2 to 4 hours in the normal foal, and glycogenolysis supplies needed glucose until feeding and glucose production are accomplished.[38] In the challenged foal glycogen stores may have been depleted and gluconeogenesis delayed, so provision of glucose at rates similar to what the liver would normally produce during this period is requisite.

PERSISTENT PULMONARY HYPERTENSION

Pamela A. Wilkins

Persistent pulmonary hypertension (PPH) also is known as reversion to fetal circulation or persistent fetal circulation, and its genesis lies in the failure of the fetus to make the respiratory and cardiac transition to extrauterine life successfully or reversion of the newborn to fetal circulatory patterns in response to hypoxia or acidosis. Differentiating this problem from other causes of hypoxemia in the newborn requires some investigation, and multiple serial arterial blood gas analyses are necessary to confirm suspicion of this problem (see the section on arterial blood gas analysis, Respiratory Diseases Associated with Hypoxemia in the Neonate). However, the condition should be suspected in any neonate with hypercapnic hypoxemia that persists and worsens; these foals are in hypoxemic respiratory failure. The fetal circulatory pattern, with pulmonary hypertension and right-to-left shunting of blood through the patent foramen ovale and ductus arteriosus, is maintained in these cases.

Pulmonary vascular resistance falls at delivery to about 10% of fetal values, and pulmonary blood flow increases accordingly.[1] Early in the postnatal period these two changes balance each other, and mean pulmonary and systolic pressures remain increased for several hours. Systolic pulmonary pressures can remain equivalent to systemic pressure for up to 6 hours of age in human infants, although diastolic pulmonary pressures are well below systemic diastolic pressures by 1 hour.[2] Mean pulmonary artery pressures fall gradually over the first 48 hours.[3] The direct effects of lung expansion and increasing alveolar oxygen tension probably provide the initial stimulus for pulmonary arteriolar dilation and partly result from direct physical effects, but vasoactive substances are released in response to physical forces associated with ventilation (e.g., prostacyclin).[1] Other vasoactive mediators thought to play a role in regulating pulmonary arteriolar tone include NO, prostaglandins D_2 and E_2, bradykinin, histamine, endothelin-1, angiotensin II, and atrial natriuretic peptide. The increase in alveolar and arterial oxygen tensions at birth is required for completion of resolution of pulmonary hypertension. Much of this increase is thought to be mediated by NO, evidence for this being the parallel increase during gestation of the pulmonary vasodilation response to hyperoxia and the increase in NO synthesis.[4] However, inhibition of NO synthesis does not eliminate the initial decrease in pulmonary artery resistance occurring because of opening of the airways.[5]

When these mechanisms fail, PPH can be recognized. Right-to-left shunting within the lungs and through patent fetal conduits occurs and can result from many factors, including asphyxia and meconium aspiration, but in many cases the precipitating trigger is unknown. Inappropriately decreased levels of vasodilators (NO) and inappropriately increased levels of vasoconstrictors (endothelin-1) currently are being examined as potential mechanisms. One study of oxygen-dependent clone calves revealed increased neonatal and maternal endothelin concentrations.[6] Chronic in utero hypoxia and acidosis may result in hypertrophy of the pulmonary arteriolar smooth muscle.[7] In these cases reversal of PPH can be difficult and cannot be achieved rapidly.

Treatment of PPH is twofold: abolishment of hypoxia and correction of the acidosis, because both abnormalities only bolster the fetal circulatory pattern. Initial therapy is provision of oxygen intranasally at 8 to 10 L/min. Some foals respond to this therapy and establish neonatal circulatory patterns within a few hours. Failure to improve or worsening of hypoxemic respiratory failure after intranasal oxygen administration should prompt intubation and mechanical ventilation with 100% oxygen. This serves two purposes, one diagnostic and one therapeutic. Ventilation with 100% oxygen may resolve PPH and, if intrapulmonary shunt and altered ventilation-perfusion relationships are causing the hypoxic respiratory failure, arterial oxygen tension ($Pa{O_2}$) should exceed 100 mm Hg under these conditions. Failure to improve $Pa{O_2}$ suggests PPH or large right-to-left extrapulmonary shunt caused by congenital cardiac anomaly. The vasodilators prostacyclin and telazoline cause pulmonary vasodilation in human infants with PPH, but the effects on oxygenation vary and the adverse effects (e.g., tachycardia, severe systemic hypotension) are unacceptable.[8] Recognition of NO as a potent dilator of pulmonary vessels has created a significant step forward in the treatment of these patients, because inhaled NO dilates vessels in ventilated portions of the lung while having minimal effects on the systemic circulation.[9] According to presently available evidence, use of inhaled NO in an initial concentration of about 20 ppm in the ventilatory gas seems reasonable for term and near-term foals with hypoxic respiratory failure and PPH that fails to respond to mechanical ventilation using 100% oxygen alone.[9,10] The author has used this approach in the clinic, administering a range of 5 to 40 ppm NO with success.

NEONATAL NEUROLOGICAL EXAMINATION AND SELECTED DISORDERS

Peter R. Morresey

The goals of the neonatal neurologic examination are similar to those of the adult horse: neuroanatomic localization of any lesions present to suggest a diagnosis and thereby help formulate a rational treatment plan. Examination of the neonate should make allowances for the relative lack of maturity of many body systems.

NORMAL DEVELOPMENT

The neonatal foal has a strong desire to become sternally recumbent within minutes of birth.[1] Most foals stand within 1 hour of delivery, with pony foals standing sooner and larger breeds taking up to 2 hours. The reported range is 15 to 165 minutes.[1] Compromised neonates tend to remain recumbent longer. Initial attempts to stand are poorly coordinated, may be fleeting, and result in a wide-based stance. Once successful, the foal rapidly develops a more appropriate posture and the ability to ambulate freely in search of the mare.

The suckle reflex is present 5 to 10 minutes after birth. Foals actively suckle without the benefit of the udder. Even in the recumbent foal, extension of the tongue and suckling of air occurs. Although there are breed and size variations, most foals suckle the mare within 2 hours of birth, with greater than 3 hours considered an abnormal finding. The reported range of time until suckling is from 35 minutes to 7 hours.[1]

Foals tend to display a strong avoidance of handlers, seeking the shelter of the far side of the mare. If recumbent, they are easily roused, rise up, and seek the mare for suckling. When restrained within the first few hours of life, neonates become very relaxed (cataplectic).

Neurologic Examination

The neurologic examination is part of a more comprehensive assessment of the neonate. History taking and a thorough physical evaluation of the entire foal should precede assessment of any individual body system. Included in the process should be a complete assessment of the mare's medical and reproductive health. It is important to develop a comprehensive, systematic, and repeatable approach to examination. This should include observation from a distance, evaluating conformation, mentation, and behavior. More specific aspects of the examination assess cranial nerve function and spinal reflexes.

BEHAVIOR

General behavior of the neonate centers on feeding, investigating the surrounding environment, and evaluating its association with the mare. The degree of affinity for the mare is an important indicator of abnormal behavior. Loss of affinity for the mare, or lack of vigorous pursuit of nutrition, may be signs of hypoxic ischemic encephalopathy. Foals should struggle vigorously when first restrained; however, it is normal for them to become limp when compressed along their long axis and to display submissive behavior.

SUCKLE REFLEX

This reflex is present uniformly in normal foals. Loss of the suckle reflex may be the first indication of neurologic dysfunction and also be the last reflex to return once the foal recovers. Suckling is an instinctive process, although adequate cerebral function and an intact motor supply to the tongue (intact hypoglossal nerve) are necessary.

CRANIAL NERVE EXAMINATION

Evaluation of cranial nerve responses follows the familiar pattern of the adult, with allowance for the diminished strength of any reflex arcs. Care should be exercised by the examiner because vigorous head movements usually accompany any stimulus.

Pupillary light responses are sluggish at birth. In one study all foals had a positive pupillary light response on the first day post partum.[2] Pupil shape is rounded for the first 3 to 5 days of life, assuming a more adult-like shape after this period.[3] The pupillary light reflex arc is located in the brainstem and does not require a normal cerebral visual cortex.[4] Therefore the presence of an appropriate pupillary light response does not indicate the absence of a visual deficit.

Similar to that of mature horses, the pupillary light response in foals is biphasic, consisting of an initial rapid but small reduction in pupil diameter, followed by a slower and more complete constriction. Because of sympathetic stimulation from excitement or stress, the latter phase of this response can be overridden.[4]

The menace response may have to be learned or is due to an initial immaturity of the cerebellum.[3,4] The reflex is incompletely developed up to 2 weeks of age.

GAIT EVALUATION

Gait should be examined by observation at a short distance with the foal freely moving in the paddock or stall. Compared with those of adults, limb movements during ambulation of the neonatal foal can appear dysmetric, although this rapidly improves with exercise.[4] Foals that have undergone confinement have a delayed onset of an appropriate adult-like gait.

SPINAL REFLEXES

Spinal reflexes are assessed with the foal in lateral recumbency. The limbs respond to abrupt pressure on the sole of the hooves by rapidly extending. Although extensor tone predominates, continued gentle pressure will allow complete flexion of the limbs. Reflexes are hyperactive compared with adult responses. The crossed extensor reflex is brisk in response to withdrawal of the contralateral limb.

Spinal ataxia occurs in newborn foals but is less common than disease of cerebral origin. When diagnosed, it is most likely the result of congenital malformation, vascular accident, or trauma during the birth process.[4]

SEIZURE ACTIVITY

Recognition of seizure activity in the neonatal foal is problematic; however, it is essential to the successful management of neurologically compromised neonates. Subtle seizure signs include abnormal eye movement, tremors, excessive stretching when recumbent, excessive extensor tone, hyperaesthesia to touch and manipulation, and apneustic breathing.[1] Overt seizure activity is easier to discern, with rapid nystagmus, paddling, hyperextension, and excessive mouth movements ("chewing gum fits"). Unobserved episodes may result in signs of physical trauma (e.g., nasolabial and gingival excoriation). Seizure activity is an indication of central (cranial to the foramen magnum) neurologic dysfunction.

Differences from the Adult Examination

In summary, neurologic responses of foals tend to be exaggerated compared with adults.[5] Posture and movement of the foal's head is noticeably different from the adult's, the occipitoatlantal joint being more flexed, with jerking head movements resembling cerebellar dysfunction in the adult. Foals are much more sensitive to touch than are adults, with exaggerated responses to all tactile stimuli. Cranial nerve (CN) responses are similar to those of the adult but accompanied by head movements, as described above. The globe has a ventromedial deviation in the normal neonate, assuming an adult positioning within 1 month. Care should be taken not to misconstrue strabismus resulting from cerebral dysfunction. The menace response is absent at birth and may take up to 14 days of age to develop. Responses of the sensory CN V motor CN VII reflex arc appear comparatively weak compared with those of the adult. Extensor limb muscle tone predominates, most noticeably when in lateral recumbency. Limb reflexes, however, are exaggerated, with a brisk crossed-extensor reflex present in the forelimbs up to 3 weeks of age. When the foal is ambulating, its gait is stilted, with the predominant extensor tone giving the appearance of hypermetria.

Neuroanatomic Location of Lesions[6]

The most common neurologic problems of foals include depression, seizure activity, abnormal behavior, loss of affinity for the mare, and loss of the suckle reflex. All these signs are referable to dysfunction of the brain. Expression of neurologic lesions depends on the stage of development during which the inciting damage occurred (Table 21-4).

Diagnostic Aids

COMPLETE BLOOD COUNT AND SERUM CHEMISTRY

Assessment of the systemic health of foals with neurologic problems is essential. A complete blood count indicates the likelihood of systemic infection or potential for ongoing tissue hypoxia as a result of anemia. Serum chemistry evaluation gives insight into major organ system function. Assessment of immunoglobulin G (IgG) levels is a direct measure of the transfer of passive immunity from the mare, which is essential in the otherwise hypogammaglobulinemic neonatal foal. Blood gas evaluation assesses the integrity of pulmonary gas exchange and enables determination of acid-base status.

CEREOBROSPINAL FLUID ANALYSIS

Cytologic and microbiologic analysis of cerebrospinal fluid is essential in suspected cases of meningitis. Care should be taken to ensure that causes of increased intracranial pressure have been ruled out before aspiration from the atlanto-occipital space because herniation of the brain through the foramen magnum is possible.

IMAGING

Both radiography and magnetic resonance imaging have been reported in the diagnosis of neonatal neurologic disease. Characteristic bony changes are present with congenital malformations, and disruption of bony structures by trauma can be visualized. Both plain and contrast studies are possible. Magnetic resonance imaging is invaluable in the assessment of soft tissue or vascular disruption.[7,8]

PATHOPHYSIOLOGY OF NEUROLOGICAL DISEASE

Neonatal hypoxic-ischemic brain injury is the product of many biochemical cascades. Understanding of the mechanisms of this injury is largely derived from experimental studies involving neonatal laboratory and production animal species. Cerebral ischemia may result from systemic hypoxemia depressing myocardial performance. Reduced cerebral blood flow results in decreased delivery of oxygen and energy substrates to the brain, resulting in a combined hypoxic-ischemic insult. Anaerobic metabolism depletes the brain's stores of glucose and high energy phosphates (adenosine-5′-triphosphate [ATP] and phosphocreatine), with resulting accumulation of lactate and inorganic phosphate.[8] Energy failure impairs glutamate uptake, resulting in extracellular accumulation, which in turn leads to tonic overstimulation of postsynaptic excitotoxic amino acid receptors (excitotoxicity). Reperfusion and reoxygenation in the early postischemic recovery period after this insult are themselves harmful.

Maternal infection is strongly associated with neonatal brain injury.[9] Intrauterine infection may indirectly injure the brain through the induction of sepsis and poor perfusion or directly by the production of inflammatory mediators that devitalize neurons.[10]

The neonatal brain is highly susceptible to free radical-mediated injury.[11] Under normal conditions mitochondrial function generates low concentrations of superoxide anion and hydrogen peroxide. These are scavenged by multiple enzyme systems, including superoxide dismutase, catalase, and glutathione peroxidase. Other nonenzymatic antioxidants include α-tocopherol (vitamin E) and ascorbic acid (vitamin C). During reperfusion after ischemia, oxygen free radicals react with membrane phospholipids to form oxidized lipids with proinflammatory actions.[12]

Regardless of the inciting cause, neural injury results in an increased release of neurotransmitters that in turn generates an excess of second messengers, apoptosis, and increases in intracellular sodium and calcium.[12] Accumulation of sodium concurrent with failure of energy-dependent cell membrane ion pumps (e.g., Na+-K+ ATPase) leads rapidly to cell swelling. Accumulation of calcium caused by glutamate excess and mediated by *N*-methyl *D*-aspartate (NMDA) receptors can lead to activation of calcium-dependent phospholipases, NO synthase, and proteases. Increased activation of phospholipase A_2 (PLA_2) in postsynaptic neurons results in increased free arachidonic acid and platelet-activating factor (PAF), enhancing glutamate-mediated neurotransmission and further potentiating NMDA receptor activity, while decreasing glutamate reuptake. Cerebral ischemia induces cyclo-oxygenase-2 (COX-2) expression, facilitating metabolism of arachidonic acid to inflammatory lipid mediators. A self-reinforcing cycle is therefore initiated.[13,14]

TABLE 21-4

Neuroanatomic Localization Based on Results of Neurologic Examination

Evaluation	Pathways	Major Signs of Disorder
Behavior	Forebrain (mostly cerebrum)	Reduced affinity for dam, restlessness, head-pressing, compulsive walking
Alertness	All of brain	Lethargy, stupor, semicoma, coma
Avoidance, nasal	V,* pons, cerebral cortex II	Facial hypalgesia
Avoidance, visual	II, thalamus, cerebral cortex	Blindness
Head position	VIII, hindbrain	Head tilt, turn, body lean, walking in circles, ataxia, aystagmus
Eye position and movement	III, IV, VI, VIII, midbrain, hindbrain	Strabismus, nystagmus
Flick reflexes	V, VII, pons, hindbrain	Facial paralysis, facial hypalgesia, absent flick reflexes
Dazzle reflex	II, subcortex, midbrain, VII	Absent dazzle reflex
Pupillary light reflex	II, midbrain, III	Absent papillary light reflex
Suckle	V, VII, XII, pons, hindbrain, cerebrum	Weak or absent suckle
Swallow	IX, X, hindbrain	Flow of milk from the nose
Cervicofacial reflex	Cervical spinal nerves and spinal cord, VII, (hindbrain)	Diminished cervicofacial reflex
Cutaneous trunci reflex	Thoracic spinal nerves and spinal cord, brachial plexus, lateral thoracic nerve	Diminished reflex caudal to spinal cord lesion
Cutaneous sensation	Peripheral nerves, spinal cord, cerebral cortex	Cutaneous hypalgesia/anesthesia
Gait	VIII, cerebellum, hindbrain, spinal cord, peripheral nerves	Ataxia
Limb strength	Spinal cord, peripheral nerves	Limb weakness at or caudal to the level of the lesion
Flexor reflex (pelvic), patella, sciatic reflexes	Spinal cord, peripheral nerves (L3-S2)	Pelvic limb weakness, diminished or absent reflexes
Flexor reflex (thoracic), biceps, triceps reflexes	Spinal cord, peripheral nerves (C60T2)	Weakness of thoracic with or without pelvic limbs, diminished or absent reflexes
Anal/tail clamp reflex	Spinal cord, cauda equine, peripheral nerves (S2-Co)	Reduced or absent anal/tail clamp reflex

From MacKay RJ: Neurologic disorders of neonatal foals, *Vet Clin North Am Eq Pract* 21:387-406, 2005.
Co, coccygeal spinal cord segments.
*Roman numerals refer to cranial nerves.

A number of early equine neonatal studies have shown the presence of intracranial hemorrhage associated with neurologic compromise. Compared with a control group, convulsive foals that were receiving only treatments common at that time showed hemorrhage in various locations of the brain at necropsy in one early study.[15] Also present was necrosis of the cerebral cortex, diencephalon, and brainstem. Minimal hemorrhage occurred in the brains of control foals. In a second study CNS hemorrhage was found more frequently in premature foals compared with those born at full term, in foals born dead compared with live births, and in foals born after assisted delivery compared with foals born without intervention. Cerebral disease was associated with vascular accidents in the brain, and foals with spinal cord disease had hemorrhage restricted to that area.[16] In a third study, meningeal lesions were a common necropsy finding in foals dying perinatally.[17] There are no recent studies reporting similar findings, perhaps a reflection of improved treatment and fewer neonatal losses resulting from neurologic diseases.

Therapeutic Rationale for Treatment Agents

In addition to generalized supportive therapies, such as meeting metabolic requirements and fluid support, specific therapeutic agents are used in the treatment of neonatal neurologic disorders.

MAGNESIUM

Magnesium ions (Mg^{2+}) are essential for the function of a variety of cellular processes, including oxidative phosphorylation, glycolysis, cellular respiration, and synthesis of deoxyribonucleic acid (DNA), ribonucleic acid (RNA), and protein.[18] Magnesium ions also act as cofactors for many enzymes, including those involved in the maintenance of ion transport systems, DNA damage, and DNA repair. Alterations in magnesium ion homeostasis may therefore have significant physiologic consequences. Magnesium has been proposed as a pharmacologic intervention in brain injury that inhibits secondary injury factors, including glutamate release, activity of the NMDA receptor, calcium channels, lipid peroxidation, free radical production, edema formation, and alterations of mitochondrial permeability. Magnesium treatment also reduces apoptosis and expression of p53-related proteins.[19]

The use of magnesium supplementation is controversial, however, with one meta-analysis review showing neither benefit nor harm resulting from its use in traumatic brain injury in human adults.[20]

DIMETHYL SULFOXIDE

Dimethyl sulfoxide (DMSO) rapidly reduces increased intracranial pressure (ICP), increases cerebral perfusion pressure (CPP), and improves neurologic outcome without affecting systemic blood pressure and patient responsiveness.[21] Acting as a free radical scavenger agent, DMSO has a protective effect on the spinal cord during ischemic insult.[22] The production of free radicals has been implicated in neonatal brain injury.[23]

KETAMINE

NMDA-receptor antagonism, in addition to being the most important mechanism causing the analgesic effects of ketamine, is also thought responsible for its purported neuroprotective action.[24] Blockade of excitatory transmission at the NMDA receptor provides an approach to the initial treatment of cerebral ischemia.[25] Blockage of excessive NMDA receptor stimulation allows regulation of intracellular calcium levels and attenuated induction of NO, reducing neuronal degeneration and death. Cellular morphology is preserved, cellular energy status and ATP production is protected, and reduced cell swelling was noted subsequent to anoxia-hypoxia or excitatory neurotransmitter injury.[26]

CORTICOSTEROIDS

The use of anti-inflammatory corticosteroids during a CNS insult is controversial. Glucocorticoids increase expression of pro-apoptotic cell mediators and hypoxic-responsive genes, potentially enhancing a metabolic insult such as hypoxia.[27] A multicenter human medical trial showed an increase in mortality with corticosteroids, suggesting deleterious effects with traumatic head injury.[28]

OSMOTIC AGENTS

Mannitol and Hypertonic Saline The primary mechanism of action is to draw water out of the intracellular and interstitial spaces, resulting in temporary brain shrinkage. Cardiac and hemodynamic effects also occur. Mannitol and hypertonic saline appear to be equally effective at reducing ICP in brain-injured patients. Equiosmolar doses of 20% mannitol and 7.5% saline have produced similar changes in ICP.[29]

ANTIOXIDANTS

Acetylcysteine Free radical production (reactive oxygen species, reactive nitrogen species) is considered an important mediator of both inflammation and hypoxia-ischemia-induced perinatal brain injury. *N*-acetylcysteine has been shown to protect both gray and white matter during these events, likely the result of enhancement of antioxidative responses, attenuation of reactive oxygen species production, inhibition of apoptosis, and reduction of inflammation.[30]

Vitamin C Vitamin C (ascorbic acid) was shown to be neuroprotective when assessing damage percentage and macroscopic appearance of brain injury and cell death. The protective effect was not dose dependent.[31]

Vitamin E Oxygen radical-mediated lipid peroxidation is an important factor in neuronal degeneration, as shown by the beneficial effects of agents with lipid antioxidant activity (vitamin E, α-tocopherol) in models of spinal cord and brain injury. The slow CNS tissue uptake of vitamin E requires chronic dosing, making it an impractical agent for treatment of acute neural injury. The peroxyl radical scavenging chromanol portion of vitamin E is the neuroprotective agent.[32,33]

SELECTED CONGENITAL DISORDERS

Hydrocephalus

In one central Kentucky study, hydrocephalus was found to be present in 3% of deformed fetuses or newborn foals requiring euthanasia.[34] Detection by magnetic resonance imaging (MRI) has been reported.[7] Clinical signs were reported to be similar to hypoxic ischemic encephalopathy (HIE), with a depressed suckle reflex and failure to thrive. Marked dilation of the cerebral ventricles was present, with other intracranial structures reported as normal.

Occipitoatlantoaxial Malformation

Although isolated cases occur in other breeds, occipitoatlantoaxial malformation (OAAM) is predominantly a condition of newborn to juvenile Arabian foals.[35] Presenting signs include a progressive ataxia and tetraparesis, although stillbirth and sudden death have been reported. Physical findings include a palpably abnormal atlas and axis, with reduced flexion and audible clicking upon manipulation of the head. Confirmation requires radiologic evaluation, with the presence of occipitoatlantal fusion, hypoplasia of the dens, and inappropriate localized ossification.[7]

Narcolepsy and Cataplexy

Narcolepsy is the sudden uncontrollable onset of deep sleep. Cataplexy is the sudden loss of muscle tone and strength, often leading to collapse. Consciousness is not affected with cataplexy; however, cataplexy often occurs concurrently with narcolepsy.

Both narcolepsy and cataplexy may transiently occur in Thoroughbred and miniature foals. The application of compressive manual restraint over a wide area of a foal's body may induce a cataplectic state, thought to be an adaptation to the restrictive in utero environment of late pregnancy.[36] Diagnosis is made by differentiating the condition from syncope, the result of transient cerebral hypoxia caused by a cardiac abnormality, and seizure activity.

SELECTED ACQUIRED DISORDERS

Hypoxic Ischemic Encephalopathy

HIE is discussed in a preceding section and has been widely reviewed. Excitatory amino acids, calcium ions, free radicals, NO, pro-inflammatory cytokines, and products of lipid peroxidation are all thought to be involved in the syndrome. The immature brain is considered to have increased susceptibility to excitotoxicity and free radical injury and a greater tendency to undergo apoptotic cell death.[11,37]

In addition to the neurologic manifestations of HIE, respiratory compromise, renal insufficiency, and gastrointestinal ileus with or without mucosal compromise can occur. Aberrant pulmonary function can result in abnormal gas exchange, in particular decreased ventilation leading to retention of carbon dioxide. As a result, central depression and abnormal blood acid-base balance may result. Renal compromise leads to electrolyte and fluid balance derangements. With the loss of normal gastrointestinal function, diarrhea and sepsis can result from intestinal bacterial overgrowth.

Trauma

Traumatic injury should always be considered after the rapid onset of neurologic disease in the neonatal foal.[1,4] Overt signs of trauma may not be apparent and require diagnostic imaging to detect. The presence of blood at the nares or external auditory canal, palpable loss of symmetry of the skull, and the ability to elicit pain upon palpation of the cranium are strong evidence of trauma.

Bacterial Meningitis

Presenting symptoms of bacterial meningitis may be indistinguishable from those of HIE. Bacterial meningitis is an occasional result of sepsis.[38] Organisms recovered from meningitis cases are the same as those present in sepsis. Inflammation of the meninges is suggested by reluctance to move the neck, opisthotonus, proprioceptive deficits, or stupor. As inflammation progresses, cerebral blood flow decreases, leading to ischemic damage and further neurologic dysfunction.

Electrolyte Derangements

Abnormal electrolyte concentrations often result from systemic conditions such as sepsis, enteritis, rhabdomyolysis, acute renal failure, and ruptured urinary bladder. Acute adrenal insufficiency rarely occurs and can be confused with these conditions.[39] Disorders of sodium homeostasis disrupt osmotic equilibrium, leading to cell swelling (deficiency) or shrinkage (excess), with clinical signs ranging from depression to seizure activity.

Kernicterus

Elevated levels of unconjugated bilirubin have been demonstrated in neonatal liver disease, neonatal isoerythrolysis, glucose-6-phosphate dehydrogenase deficiency, and other causes of intravascular hemolysis.[40] Newborn foals are more susceptible to hyperbilirubinemia and bilirubin encephalopathy than are adults because of increased bilirubin production, decreased hepatic bilirubin uptake and conjugation, and an underdeveloped blood-brain barrier that unconjugated bilirubin can easily cross. Mitochondrial function and calcium homeostasis are disrupted, inducing neuronal degeneration, necrosis, and apoptosis.

Botulism

Botulism, caused by *Clostridium botulinum* (eight different toxins), is a progressive flaccid paralysis resulting from blocking of acetylcholine release at neuromuscular junctions (see Chapter 12). Diagnosis is aided by eliminating other causes of neurologic disease. Associated in adults with suspected spoiled feed ingestion, a toxicoinfectious form in the neonate is most commonly incriminated, similar to that seen in human infants with botulism, wherein the neonatal intestinal mileu allows germination of *C. botulinum* spores with subsequent liberation and local absorption of toxin.

Monovalent and polyvalent antitoxin preparations are available, but they are expensive. The antitoxin is most beneficial if used when foals first display suggestive signs. With antitoxin administration and intensive supportive care, recovery occurs in most cases, but severe intoxications may require mechanical ventilation; even so, the affected foal may succumb.[41,42] Death is generally due to respiratory failure secondary to paralysis of the muscles of respiration. Aspiration pneumonia and sepsis, resulting from prolonged recumbency, and decubital ulceration may occur if strict attention to prevention is not maintained.

PERINATAL ASPHYXIA SYNDROME

Pamela A. Wilkins

HIE, currently referred to as *neonatal encephalopathy* in human literature, is one systemic manifestation of a broader syndrome of perinatal asphyxia syndrome (PAS), and management of foals that exhibit signs consistent with a diagnosis of HIE requires the clinician to examine other body systems and provide therapy directed at treating other involved systems.[1] Although PAS primarily manifests as HIE, the gastrointestinal tract and kidneys frequently are affected by peripartum hypoxia-ischemia-asphyxia, and one should expect complications associated with these systems. HIE also may affect the cardiovascular and respiratory systems, and endocrine disorders may emerge in these patients.

HIE has been recognized as one of the most common diseases of the equine neonate for generations.[2-4] Typically, affected foals are normal at birth but show signs of CNS abnormalities within a few hours after birth. Some foals are obviously abnormal at birth, and some do not show signs until 24 hours of age. HIE commonly is associated with adverse peripartum events, including dystocia and premature placental separation, but a fair number of foals have no known peripartum period of hypoxia, which suggests that these foals result from unrecognized in utero hypoxia (Box 21-2). Severe maternal illness also may result in foals born with PAS. In human beings ascending placental infection now is suspected as a major contributor to neonatal encephalopathy in infants, and the incidence of neonatal encephalopathy increases with the presence of maternal fever, suggesting a role for maternal inflammatory mediators.[5]

Perinatal brain damage in the mature fetus usually results from severe uterine asphyxia caused by an acute reduction of uterine or umbilical circulation. The loss of oxygen results in a substantial decrease in oxidative phosphorylation in the brain with concomitant decreased energy production. The Na^+/K^+ pump at the cell membrane cannot maintain the ionic gradients, and the membrane potential is lost in the brain cells. In the absence of the membrane potential, calcium flows down its large extracellular-intracellular concentration gradient through voltage-dependent ion channels into the cell.

BOX 21-2

CAUSES OF HYPOXIA IN THE FETUS AND NEONATE

Maternal Causes

Reduced maternal oxygen delivery
- Maternal anemia
- Maternal pulmonary disease with hypoxemia
- Maternal cardiovascular disease

Reduced uterine blood flow
- Maternal hypotension (endotoxemia/colic)
- Maternal hypertension (laminitis/painful conditions)
- Abnormal uterine contractions
- Anything that increases uterine vascular resistance

Placental Causes
- Premature placental separation
- Placental insufficiency; for example, twins
- Placental dysfunction
  - Fescue toxicity
  - Postmaturity
  - Placentitis
  - Placenta edema

Reduced umbilical blood flow
- General anesthesia of the dam
- Congenital cardiovascular disease
- Inappropriate fetal blood distribution
- Fetal hypovolemia
- Excessive length of umbilical cord

Intrapartum Causes

Dystocia
Premature placental separation
Uterine inertia
Oxytocin induction of labor
Cesarean section
- General anesthesia
- Poor uterine blood flow because of maternal positioning
- Decreased maternal cardiac output
- Reduced umbilical blood flow
- Effects of anesthetic drugs on fetus

Anything that prolongs stage 2 labor

Neonatal Period Causes

Prematurity
Recumbency
- Musculoskeletal disease
- Sepsis
- Prematurity
- Mild hypoxic ischemic encephalopathy

Pulmonary disease
- Meconium aspiration
- Milk aspiration
- Persistent pulmonary hypertension
- Septic pneumonia
- Acute respiratory distress syndrome or acute lung injury

Severe disturbance in breathing pattern
Septic shock
Anemia
- Neonatal isoerythrolysis
- Excessive umbilical bleeding
- Fractured ribs(hemothorax) or long bone fracture

Congenital cardiovascular disease

Adapted from Palmer JE: Perinatal hypoxic-ischemic disease. *Proceedings of the International Veterinary Emergency Critical Care Symposium,* San Antonio, Tex, 1998, pp. 717-718.

This calcium overload of the neuron leads to cell damage by activation of calcium-dependent proteases, lipases, and endonucleases. Protein biosynthesis is halted. Calcium also enters the cells by glutamate-regulated ion channels as glutamate, an excitatory neurotransmitter, is released from presynaptic vesicles following anoxic cellular depolarization. Once the anoxic event is over, protein synthesis remains inhibited in specific areas of the brain and returns to normal in less vulnerable areas of the brain. Loss of protein synthesis appears to be an early indicator of cell death caused by the primary hypoxic-anoxic event.[6]

A second wave of neuronal cell death occurs during the reperfusion phase and is thought to be similar to classically described postischemic reperfusion injury in that damage is caused by production and release of oxygen radicals, synthesis of NO, and inflammatory reactions.[7] Additionally, an imbalance between excitatory and inhibitory neurotransmitters occurs.[6] Secondary cell death also is thought be caused by the neurotoxicity of glutamate and aspartate, resulting again from increased intracellular calcium levels.[8,9] In human infants the distribution of lesions with hypoxic-ischemic brain damage after prenatal, perinatal, or postnatal asphyxia falls into distinct patterns depending on the type of hypoxia-ischemia rather than on the postconceptual age at which the asphyxial event occurs.[9] Periventricular leukomalacia was associated with chronic hypoxia-ischemia, whereas the basal ganglia and thalamus were affected primarily in patients experiencing acute profound asphyxia, providing direct evidence that the nature of the event determines the severity and distribution of neurologic damage in human beings. This has important implications in the design of neuroprotective strategies and therapies for neonates experiencing hypoxic-ischemic-asphyxial events. Evidence is overwhelming that the excitotoxic cascade that evolves during HIE extends over several days from the time of insult and is modifiable.[8,9]

Excitatory amino acid neurotransmitters and magnesium are known to play at least a minimal role in secondary cell death after brain injury; a fair body of literature regarding these factors has been generated over the last 10 years. The activation of the NMDA subtype of glutamate receptors is implicated in the pathophysiology of traumatic brain injury and is suspected to play a role in HIE.[8-10] Mechanically injured neurons demonstrate a reduction of voltage-dependent Mg^{2+} blockade of NMDA current that can be restored partially by increasing extracellular Mg^{2+} concentration or by pretreatment with calphostin C, a protein kinase C inhibitor.[11] Clinical trials investigating the efficacy of magnesium treatment following hypoxia in infants are ongoing, with few reports currently in the medical literature.[12]

Therapy for the various manifestations of hypoxia-ischemia involves control of seizures; general cerebral support; correction of metabolic abnormalities; maintenance of normal arterial blood gas values; maintenance of tissue perfusion; maintenance of renal function; treatment of gastrointestinal dysfunction; prevention, recognition, and early treatment of secondary infections; and general supportive care. Control of seizures is important because cerebral oxygen consumption increases fivefold during seizures. Diazepam or midazolam can be administered for emergency control of seizures (Table 21-5). If a single-bolus administration of diazepam or midazolam does not readily stop seizures or more than two seizures are recognized, treatment with midazolam by constant-rate infusion may be of benefit.[11,13] For very refractory seizures phenobarbital may be combined with midazolam by constant-rate infusion or given singly to effect. The half-life of phenobarbital can be long in the foal (100 hours), and the clinician should keep this in mind when monitoring neurologic function in these cases after phenobarbital administration.[14,15] If phenobarbital fails to control seizures, phenytoin therapy may be attempted. In cases of HIE ketamine and xylazine should not be used because of their association with increased ICP. The foal must be protected from injury during a seizure, and the patency of the airway must be ensured to prevent the onset of negative pressure pulmonary edema[16] or aspiration pneumonia.

Probably the most important therapeutic interventions are aimed at maintaining cerebral perfusion, which is achieved by careful titration of intravenous fluid support, neither too much nor too little (see the section on fluid therapy in neonates) and judicious administration of inotropes and pressors to maintain adequate perfusion pressures (see the section on pressor and inotrope therapy). Cerebral interstitial edema is only truly present in the most severe cases;[17,18] in most cases the lesion is intracellular edema and most of the classic agents used to treat cerebral interstitial edema (e.g., mannitol and hypertonic saline) are minimally effective treating cellular edema. The author occasionally uses thiamine supplementation in the intravenous fluids to support metabolic processes, specifically mitochondrial metabolism and membrane Na^+,K^+-ATPases, involved in maintaining cellular fluid balance.[19,20] This therapy is rational and inexpensive, its efficacy is unproven. Only if cellular necrosis and vasogenic edema are present are drugs such as mannitol, hypertonic saline, or DMSO indicated, and again these cases are usually the most severely affected. The author has not used DMSO in neonates for the last decade and has not recognized a change in outcome by discontinuing its use. Naloxone has been advocated for treating HIE in human beings and in foals.[21-23] The use of naloxone in human neonatal resuscitation remains controversial; whether the effects are related to a reduction in acute neuronal swelling by osmotic effects or by a more direct receptor-mediated mechanism is currently unknown.[24] Some practitioners are using γ-aminobutyric acid adrenergic agonists to manage HIE in foals on the basis of evidence showing neuroprotection when used in ischemia alone and combined with NMDA antagonists.[25-27] The author currently has no experience with these compounds and cannot comment regarding their efficacy in foals. Regional hypothermia also is being investigated as a potential therapy for global hypoxia-ischemia; published data are consistent with the theory that cooling must be continued throughout the entire secondary phase of injury (about 3 days) to be effective.[28] Experimentally, this approach has resulted in dramatic decreases in cellular edema and neuronal loss; its practical application remains to be demonstrated.

Despite the lack of consensus regarding the use of magnesium to treat infants with HIE, the author has used magnesium sulfate infusion as part of the therapy for selected foals with HIE for the past several years. The rationale is based primarily on the evidence demonstrating protection in some studies and a failure of any one study to demonstrate significant detrimental effects. The clinical impressions of the author to date suggest that the therapy is safe and may decrease the incidence of seizure in patients. The author administers magnesium sulfate as a constant-rate infusion over 1 hour after giving a loading dose. The author has continued the infusion for up to 3 days without demonstrable negative effect beyond some possible trembling. Given the current evidence, a 24-hour course of treatment may be effective and sufficient in itself.

TABLE 21-5

Drugs Used to Control or Prevent Seizures in Foals

Drug	Dose	Route	Frequency	Comment
Diazepam	5-10 mg per foal	IV*	As needed	Short-term seizure control
Phenobarbital	2-3 mg/kg	IV	Bolus to effect	Bolus over 15-20 minutes; half-life can be prolonged; decreases thermoregulatory control, respiratory drive, and blood pressure
Phenytoin	5-10 mg/kg loading; 5 mg/kg maintenance	IV	Every 4 hr for first 24 hr; then b.i.d. (?)	Seizure control
Magnesium sulfate†	0.05 mg/kg/hr loading dose; 0.025 mg/kg/hr maintenance‡	IV	Constant-rate infusion for first hr and for maintenance	Discontinue if muscle tremors or hypotension occur; treat for 24-48 hours after hypoxic insult
Gabapentin	8 mg/kg	Oral	b.i.d. to t.i.d.	Seizure control

**IV*, Intravenous; *b.i.d.*, twice daily; *t.i.d.*, three times daily.
†To make 0.1 gm/ml solution, add 20 ml 50% $MgSO_4$ to 80 ml 0.9% NaCl.
‡Loading dose = 25 ml/hr of 0.1 gm/ml solution for 1 hour. Maintenance dose = 12 ml/hr of 0.1 gm/ml solution.

Foals with PAS often have a variety of metabolic problems, including hypoglycemia or hyperglycemia, hypocalcemia or hypercalcemia, hypokalemia or hyperkalemia, hypochloremia or hyperchloremia, hyperlactatemia, hyperphophatemia, and varying degrees of metabolic acidosis. Although these problems must be addressed, the clinician should not forget the normal period of hypoglycemia that occurs post partum and should not treat aggressively, which might worsen the neurologic injury. Foals suffering from PAS also have frequent recurrent bouts of hypoxemia and occasional bouts of hypercapnia. Intranasally administered oxygen generally is needed in these cases as a preventive therapy and as direct treatment because the appearance of the abnormalities can be sporadic and unpredictable. Additional respiratory support, particularly in foals with centrally mediated hypoventilation and periods of apnea or abnormal breathing patterns, include caffeine (10 mg/kg loading dose; 2.5 mg/kg as needed, administered orally or rectally[29]), doxapram constant-rate infusion [30,31] and positive pressure ventilation. Mechanical ventilation of these patients can be rewarding and generally is required for less than 48 hours.

Blood pH should be monitored and maintained within the normal range. Metabolic alkalosis can develop in some of these foals and requires that the clinician tolerate some degree of hypercapnia. The pH level is important in evaluation and consideration of alternatives for treatment. If respiratory acidosis is not so severe as to affect the patient adversely (generally PaO_2 >70 mm Hg) and pH is within normal limits, the foal may tolerate hypercapnia.[32] The goal is to normalize pH. Foals with respiratory acidosis as compensation for metabolic alkalosis do not respond to caffeine and may be adversely affected by doxapram infusion or mechanical hyperventilation. Metabolic alkalosis in critically ill foals frequently is associated with electrolyte abnormalities, creating differences in strong ion balance. This pH perturbation is best handled by correcting the underlying electrolyte problem.

Maintaining tissue perfusion and oxygen delivery to tissues is a cornerstone of therapy for PAS to prevent additional injury. The oxygen-carrying capacity of the blood should be maintained; some foals require transfusions to maintain a PCV greater than 20%. Adequate vascular volume is important, but the clinician should take care to prevent fluid overload in the foal. Early evidence of fluid overload is subtle accumulation of ventral edema between the front legs and over the distal limbs. Fluid overload can result in cerebral edema, pulmonary edema, and edema of other tissues, including the gastrointestinal tract, that interferes with normal organ function and worsens the condition of the patient. Perfusion is maintained by supporting cardiac output and blood pressure by judicious use of intravenous fluid support and inotrope-pressor support. For these patients to require inopressor therapy is not unusual, but in some cases the hypoxic damage is sufficiently severe to blunt the response of the patient to the drugs.

The kidney is a target for injury in patients with PPH, and for renal compromise to play a significant role in the demise of these foals is not unusual. Clinical signs of renal disease are generally referable to disruption of normal control of renal blood flow and tubular edema, leading to tubular necrosis and renal failure. These foals have signs of fluid overload and generalized edema. The clinician must balance urine output and fluid therapy in these cases to prevent additional organ dysfunction associated with edema. Although evidence has accumulated that neither dopamine nor furosemide play a role in protecting the kidney or reversing acute renal failure, these agents can be useful in managing volume overload in these cases.[33-35] The aim is not to drive oliguric renal failure into a high-output condition but rather to enhance urine output.

Overzealous use of diuretics and pressors in these cases can result in diuresis, requiring increased intravenous fluid support, and can be counterproductive. The author's approach is more conservative. Low doses of dopamine administered as a constant-rate infusion of 2 to 5 μg/kg/min are usually effective in establishing diuresis by natriuresis. Large doses of dopamine (>20 μg/kg/min) can produce systemic and pulmonary vasoconstriction, potentially exacerbating PPH.[36] One can administer a bolus (0.25 to 1.0 mg/kg) or constant-rate infusion (0.25 to 2.0 mg/kg/hr) of furosemide, but once furosemide diuresis is established, electrolyte concentrations and blood gas tensions must be frequently evaluated because potassium, chloride, and calcium losses can be considerable and because significant metabolic alkalosis can develop from strong ion imbalances. The author does not aim for urine production rates of 300 ml/hr, reported as a urine output goal for critically ill equine neonates, but rather looks for urine output that is appropriate for fluid intake.[37]Although the average urine output for a normal equine neonate is about 6 ml/kg/hr (~300 ml/hr for a 50-kg foal), these values were obtained from normal foals drinking a milk diet with a large free water component.[38-41] The urine of normal newborn foals is dilute, reflecting the large free water load they incur by their diet. Fluid therapy in the critically ill neonate is discussed later in this chapter.

One final caveat regarding renal dysfunction in PAS is that therapeutic drug monitoring should be performed when it is available. Many antimicrobial agents used to manage these cases, most notably the aminoglycosides, depend on renal clearance, and aminoglycoside toxicity occurs in the equine neonate and exacerbates or complicates the management of renal failure originally resulting from primary hemodynamic causes.

Foals with PAS suffer from a variety of problems associated with abnormalities within the gastrointestinal tract.[41] Commonly, they have ileus, recurrent excessive gastric reflux, and gas distention. These problems are exacerbated by constant feeding in the face of continued dysfunction and continued hypoxia. Frequently, enteral feeding cannot meet these foals' nutritional requirements, and partial or total parenteral nutrition is required. Special attention must be paid to passive transfer of immunity (see the section on failure of passive transfer) and glucose homeostasis in these cases. Appearance of damage to the gastrointestinal tract can be subtle and lag behind other clinical abnormalities for days to weeks. Low-grade colic, decreased gastrointestinal motility, decreased fecal output, and low weight gain are among the most common clinical signs of gastrointestinal dysfunction, but more severe problems, including necrotizing enterocolitis and intussusception, have been associated with these cases. The return to enteral feeding must be slow in many of these foods. A currently debated topic is constant versus pulsed enteral feeding.[42-44] The author uses pulsed feeding through an indwelling small-gauge feeding tube. In many foals these tubes stay in place for weeks and cause no problems as the foals are returned to their dams for sucking or are trained to drink from a bottle or bucket.

Foals with PAS are also susceptible to secondary infection. Treatment of recognized infection is covered in the same section of this chapter as sepsis. If infection is recognized in these patients after hospitalization, the clinician should consider the likelihood of nosocomial infection and should direct antimicrobial therapy on the basis of known nosocomial pathogens in the NICU and their susceptibility patterns until culture and sensitivity results become available. The clinician should make repeat determinations of immunoglobulin G (IgG) concentration; additional intravenous plasma therapy may be beneficial. Nosocomial infections are often rapidly overwhelming, and acute deterioration in the condition of a foal with PAS should prompt a search for nosocomial infection.

The prognosis for foals with PAS is good to excellent when the condition is recognized early and aggressively treated in term foals. Up to 80% of these neonates survive and go on to lead productive and useful athletic lives.[45-48] The prognosis decreases with delayed or insufficient treatment and concurrent problems such as prematurity and sepsis.

PREMATURITY, DYSMATURITY, AND POSTMATURITY

Pamela A. Wilkins

In human NICUs the survival rate for low-gestation-length infants has increased dramatically since the 1980s, coincident with improvements in obstetric and neonatal care. The now routine, well-validated use of antenatal steroid and artificial surfactant therapies has contributed greatly to the enhanced survival of this patient population, although the use of these particular therapies is not common or frequently indicated in the equine NICU.[1,2] However, with improved care, outcomes in the equine NICU population have improved also, with survival of premature patients in many NICUs exceeding 80%.[3] In the equine population gestation length is much more flexible than in the human population; however, the definition of the term *prematurity* requires re-examination. Traditionally, *prematurity* is defined as a preterm birth of less than 320 days of gestation in the horse. Given the variability of gestation length in the horse, ranging between 310 days to more than 370 days in some mares, a mare with a usual gestation length of 315 days possibly could have a term foal at 313 days, whereas a mare with a usual gestation length of 365 days may have a premature foal at 340 days, considered the normal gestation length. Foals that are born post term but are small are termed *dysmature;* a postmature foal is a post-term foal that has a normal axial skeletal size but is thin to emaciated. Dysmature foals may have been classified in the past as small for gestational age and are thought to have suffered placental insufficiency, whereas postmature foals usually are normal foals that have been retained too long in utero, perhaps because of an abnormal signaling of readiness for birth, and have outgrown their somewhat aged placenta. Postmature foals become more abnormal the longer they are maintained, may suffer from placental insufficiency, and are represented best by the classic foal born to a mare ingesting endophyte-infested fescue.[4] Box 21-3 compares the characteristics of premature and dysmature foals with those of postmature foals.

The causes of prematurity, dysmaturity, and postmaturity include the causes of high-risk pregnancy presented in Box 21-1. Iatrogenic causes include early elective induction of labor based on inaccurate breeding dates or misinterpretation of late-term colic or uterine bleeding as ineffective labor. Most causes remain in the category of idiopathic, with no discernible precipitating factor. Despite the lack of an obvious cause, premature labor and delivery does not just happen, and even if undetermined, the cause may continue to affect the foal in the postparturient period. All body systems may be affected by prematurity, dysmaturity, and postmaturity, and thorough evaluation of all body systems is necessary.

Respiratory failure is common in these foals, although the cause usually is not surfactant deficiency. Immaturity of the respiratory tract, poor control of respiratory vessel tone, and weak respiratory muscles combined with poorly compliant lungs and a greatly compliant chest wall contribute

BOX 21-3

CLINICAL CHARACTERISTICS OF PREMATURE/DYSMATURE AND POSTMATURE FOALS

Premature/Dysmature

Low birth weight
Small frame; thin
Poor muscle development possible
Flexor laxity common
Periarticular laxity
Hypotonia more common
High chest wall compliance
Low lung compliance
Short, silky hair coat
Domed forehead
Floppy ears; poor cartilage development
Weak suck reflex
Poor thermoregulation
Gastrointestinal tract dysfunction
Delayed maturation of renal function; low urine output
Entropion with secondary corneal ulcers
Poor glucose regulation

Postmature

Normal to high birth weight
Large frame; thin
Poor muscle development possible
Flexor contraction common
Hypertonia more common
Long hair coat
Fully erupted incisors
Weak suck reflex
Poor thermoregulation
Gastrointestinal tract dysfunction
Delayed maturation of renal function; low urine output
Poor glucose regulation
Delayed time to standing
Hyperreactive
Poor postural reflexes

Adapted from Palmer JE: Perinatal hypoxic-ischemic disease. *Proceedings of the International Veterinary Emergency Critical Care Symposium,* San Antonio, Tex, 1998, pp. 722-723.

to respiratory failure in these cases. Most require oxygen supplementation and positional support for optimal oxygenation and ventilation. One must extend effort to maintain these "floppy foals" in sternal recumbency. Some foals may require mechanical ventilation. These foals also require cardiovascular support but are frequently unresponsive to commonly used pressors and inotropes: dopamine, dobutamine, epinephrine, and vasopressin. Careful use of these drugs and judicious intravenous fluid therapy are necessary. The goal should not be one of achieving specific pressure values (e.g., mean arterial pressure of 60 mm Hg) but of adequate perfusion. Renal function, reflected in low urine output, is frequently poor initially in these cases because of the delay in making the transition from fetal to neonatal glomerular filtration rates.[5] The delay can result from true failure of transition or from hypoxic-ischemic insult. The clinician should approach fluid therapy cautiously in these cases; initial fluid restriction may be in order to avoid fluid overload. Many premature, dysmature, or postmature foals have suffered a hypoxic insult and have all of the disorders associated with PAS, including HIE. Treatment is similar to that of term foals with these problems. These foals also are predisposed to secondary bacterial infection and must be examined frequently for signs consistent with early sepsis or nosocomial infection.

The gastrointestinal system of these foals is not usually functionally mature, which may result from a primary lack of maturity or from hypoxia. Dysmotility and varying degrees of necrotizing enterocolitis are common, as are hyperglycemia and hypoglycemia. Hyperglycemia generally is related to stress, increased levels of circulating catecholamines, and rapid progression to gluconeogenesis, whereas hypoglycemia is associated with diminished glycogen stores, inability to engage gluconeongenesis, sepsis, and hypoxic damage.[6] Immature endocrine function is present in many of these foals, particularly regarding the hypothalamic-pituitary-adrenal axis, and contributes to metabolic derangements.[7,8] Enteral feeding should be delayed, when possible, until the foal has stable metabolic and cardiorespiratory parameters. On initiating enteral feeding, one should provide small volumes initially and slowly increase the volume over several days.

Musculoskeletal problems are common, particularly in premature foals, and include significant flexor laxity and decreased muscle tone. Postmature foals often are affected by flexure contracture deformities, most likely because of decreased intrauterine movement as they increase in size. Premature foals frequently exhibit decreased cuboidal bone ossification that predisposes them to crush injury of the carpal and tarsal bones if weight bearing is not strictly controlled. Physical therapy in the form of standing and exercise is indicated in the management of all these problems, but one should take care to ensure that the patient does not fatigue or stand in abnormal positions. Bandaging of the limbs is contraindicated because this only increases laxity, although light bandages over the fetlock may be necessary to prevent injury to that area if flexor laxity is severe. The foals are predisposed to angular limb deformity and must be observed closely and frequently for this problem as they mature.[9]

The overall prognosis for premature, dysmature, and postmature foals remains good with intensive care and good attention to detail. Many of these foals (up to 80%) survive and become productive athletes.[3] Complications associated with sepsis and musculoskeletal abnormalities are the most significant indicators of poor athletic outcome.

SEPSIS

Pamela A. Wilkins

The last 20 years have seen an explosion of new therapeutic agents purportedly useful for treating sepsis. Unfortunately, clinical trials investigating these new therapies have failed to demonstrate a positive effect, have shown negative results, or have resulted in diametrically opposed study results, one showing a benefit and another showing no benefit or a detrimental effect. On a positive note, the survival rate of foals being treated for sepsis has improved. Work was done regarding foal diseases and their treatment in the 1960s, but the field did not attract much serious attention until the 1980s. Since that time almost every major veterinary college and many large private referral practices have constructed NICUs or their equivalent. Next to hypoxic ischemic asphyxial syndromes, sepsis is the primary reason for presentation and treatment at these facilities. Neonatal septicemia of the horse has been the subject of five international workshops,[1-5] and a perinatology lecture covering some aspect of neonatal sepsis has been presented at almost every large continuing education meeting attended by equine veterinarians.

Consensus criteria conferences in the early 1990s defined *sepsis* and *septic shock* for human beings.[6,7] *Sepsis* was defined as the systemic response to infection manifested by two or more of the following conditions as a result of infection: (a) temperature greater than 38° C or less than 36°; (b) heart rate greater than 90 beats/min; (c) respiratory rate greater than 20 breaths per minute or $Paco_2$ less than 32 torr; and (d) white blood cell count greater than 12,000 cell/μl, less than 4000 cell/μl, or greater than 10% immature (band) forms. *Septic shock* was defined as sepsis-induced hypotension or the requirement for vasopressors-ionotropes to maintain blood pressure despite adequate fluid resuscitation along with the presence of perfusion abnormalities that may include lactic acidosis, oliguria, or acute alteration in mental status. These definitions, and several others, are broadly accepted and have been adapted to studies of neonatal sepsis in foals.[8,9] Many of the treatment modalities in human medicine have been applied in some manner to the equine neonatal patient. Additional definitions include the following: systemic inflammatory response system (SIRS), multiple organ system dysfunction (MODS), and multiple organ failure syndrome (MOFS). (SIRS is sick, MODS is sicker, and MOFS is dying.) The compensatory anti-inflammatory response syndrome (CARS) ideally balances SIRS and keeps it from reinforcing itself by way of positive feedback cytokine loops. If balance is achieved, recovery is possible. Imbalance progresses to septic shock, MODS, and MOFS. In horses MODS usually is manifested as respiratory (acute lung injury [ALI] and acute respiratory distress syndrome [ARDS]); renal, gastrointestinal, hepatic, and CNS dysfunction; and coagulopathy.[9-13] Managing the septic patient involves early recognition and support of the patient or intervening in the face of multiple clinical consequences, termed *CHAOS* (*c*ardiovascular compromise, *h*omeostasis, *a*poptosis, *o*rgan dysfunction, *s*uppression of the immune system).[14] Inflammatory mediators are involved in all these processes and can be beneficial or detrimental, depending on timing and opposing responses. Neutrophils, platelets, lymphocytes, macrophages, and endothelial cells are involved, and the number of implicated inflammatory molecules grows daily.

Sepsis in the foal initially can be subtle, and the onset of clinical signs varies depending on the pathogen involved and the immune status of the foal. For the purposes of this chapter, the discussion is limited to bacterial sepsis, but the foal also is susceptible to viral and fungal sepsis, which can resemble bacterial sepsis. Failure of passive transfer (FPT) of immunity can contribute to the development of sepsis in a foal at risk.[15,16] (See Chapter 1 for further discussion of FPT.) Testing for and treatment of FPT have received attention in the veterinary literature. It remains true, however, that foals brought to NICUs that have an ultimate diagnosis of sepsis usually have FPT.[17,18] The current recommendation is that foals have IgG levels greater than or equal to 800 mg/dl for passive transfer to be considered adequate. Other risk factors for the development of sepsis include any adverse events at the time of birth, maternal illness, or any abnormalities in the foal. Although the umbilicus frequently is implicated as a major portal of entry for infectious organisms in the foal, the gastrointestinal tract is the most likely primary portal of entry.[19] Other possible portals of entry include the respiratory tract and wounds.

Early signs of sepsis include depression, decreased suck reflex, increased recumbency, fever, hypothermia, weakness, dysphagia, failure to gain weight, increased respiratory rate, tachycardia, bradycardia, injected mucous membranes, decreased capillary refill time, shivering, lameness, aural petechia, and coronitis. If sepsis is recognized early, these patients may have a good outcome, depending on the pathogen involved. Gram negative sepsis remains the most commonly diagnosed, but increasingly gram positive septicemia is being recognized.[11-13,20,21] Foals in intensive care units and at referral hospitals have an additional risk of nosocomial infection. It is important to try to isolate the involved organism early in the course of the disease. If possible, the clinician should obtain blood cultures and, if localizing signs are present, samples as deemed appropriate.

Cultures should be aerobic and anaerobic. Recently, work has been done evaluating real-time polymerase chain reaction (PCR) technology in sepsis in the foal as a means of identifying causative organisms.[22-24] Until antimicrobial sensitivity patterns are obtained for the pathogen involved, broad spectrum antimicrobial therapy should be initiated (Table 21-6). Intravenously administered amikacin and penicillin are good first-line choices, but renal function should be closely monitored. Other first-line antimicrobial choices might include high-dose ceftiofur sodium or ticarcillin-clavulanic acid. The clinician should treat FPT if present. Intranasal oxygen insufflation at 3 to 10 L/min should be provided even if hypoxemia is not present, with caution taken to avoid hyperoxia, to decrease the work of breathing and provide support for the increased oxygen demands associated with sepsis.[25] Should arterial blood gas analysis reveal significant hypoventilation, caffeine

TABLE 21-6

Antimicrobial Drug Dosages Used in Foals in the Neonatal Intensive Care Unit

Drug	Dose	Route	Frequency	Comments
Amikacin sulfate	25-30 mg/kg	IV	s.i.d.	Requires therapeutic drug monitoring: peak >60; trough <2
Ampicillin trihydrate	20 mg/kg	Oral	t.i.d.	Poor absorption noted in foals >2-3 weeks of age
Sodium ampicillin	50-100 mg/kg	IV	q.i.d.	–
Amoxicillin trihydrate	20-30 mg/kg	Oral	t.i.d.	Poor absorption noted in foals >2-3 weeks of age
Cefotaxime	50-100 mg/kg	IV	q.i.d.	–
Cefuroxime (Ceftin)	30 mg/kg/day	Oral	b.i.d., t.i.d.	Total daily dose is divided into 10 mg/kg t.i.d. or 15 mg/kg b.i.d.
Cephalexin	10 mg/kg	Oral	q.i.d.	–
Ceftiofur (Naxcel)	10 mg/kg	IV	q.i.d.	Give slowly over 20 minutes as double-diluted volume in 0.9% saline
Chloramphenicol palmitate	50 mg/kg	Oral	q.i.d.	Public health concerns
Chloramphenicol succinate	10-25 mg/kg	IV	q.i.d.	Public health concerns
Enrofloxacin	2.5-10 mg/kg	IV, Oral	s.i.d.	Chondropathy and arthropathy reported in foals
Erythromycin stearate	20-30 mg/kg	Oral	t.i.d. to q.i.d.	Avoid warm temperatures and high humidity; colitis reported in dams of foals receiving this drug
Erythromycin lactiobionate	5 mg/kg	IV	Every 4-6 hours	–
Gentamicin sulfate	8.8 mg/kg	IV	s.i.d.	Requires therapeutic drug monitoring: peak >40; trough <2
Imipenem	10-20 mg/kg	IV	q.i.d.	Seizures reported as adverse reaction

TABLE 21-6

Antimicrobial Drug Dosages Used in Foals in the Neonatal Intensive Care Unit—cont'd

Drug	Dose	Route	Frequency	Comments
Metronidazole	15 mg/kg 25 mg/kg	Oral, as needed	q.i.d. b.i.d.	Anorexia can occur
Potassium penicillin Sodium penicillin	20,000-50,000 U/kg	IV	q.i.d.	Give potassium penicillin slowly over 5 to 10 minutes
Rifampin	5 mg/kg	Oral	b.i.d.	Always administer with second antimicrobial because of rapid development of resistance
Ticarcillin	50-100 mg/kg	IV	q.i.d.	–
Ticarcillin and clavulonic acid (Timentin)	50-100 mg/kg	IV	q.i.d.	–
Trimethoprim-sulfonamide	30 mg/kg	Oral	b.i.d.	–
Fluconazole	8 mg/kg loading; 4 mg/kg	Oral	b.i.d.	–

Adapted from Palmer JE: Neonatal drug doses. *Proceedings of the sixth International Veterinary Emergency Critical Care Symposium,* San Antonio, Tex., 2000.
IV, Intravenous; *s.i.d.,* once daily; *t.i.d.,* thrice daily; *q.i.d.,* 4 times daily; *b.i.d.,* twice daily.

TABLE 21-7

Inotrope and Pressor Medications Used in the Neonatal Intensive Care Unit*

Drug	Dose	Route	Comment
Dopamine	3-20 μg/kg/min	IV-CRI†	Follow the rule of 6: 6 × mass of foal (kg) = number of milligrams to add to 100 ml saline (1 ml/hr) = 1 μg/kg/min)
Dobutamine	3-40 μg/kg/min	IV-CRI	
Epinephrine‡	0.2-2 μg/kg/min	IV-CRI	
Norepinephrine‡	0.2-3 μg/kg/min	IV-CRI	

Data from Connoly Neonatal Intensive Care Unit, Kennet Square, Pa.
*One should use these medications to effect and should monitor blood pressure during their use.
†*IV-CRI,* Intravenously at constant-rate infusion.
‡For epinephrine and norepinephrine, apply a "rule of 0.6" where 0.6 × mass of foal (kg) = number of mg drug to add to 100 ml saline so 1 ml/hr = 0.1 μg/kg/min.

may be administered orally or rectally, or doxapram can be given by constant-rate infusion to increase central respiratory drive. Mechanical ventilation may be necessary in cases of severe respiratory involvement, such as with acute lung injury or ARDS. If the foal is hypotensive, the clinician may administer pressor agents or inotropes by constant-rate infusion (Table 21-7). Inotrope and pressor therapy generally is restricted to referral centers where these drugs can be given as constant-rate infusions and blood pressure can be monitored closely. Some practitioners use nonsteroidal anti-inflammatory agents and, in specific circumstances, corticosteroids. These drugs should be used judiciously because they may have several negative consequences for the foal, including renal failure and gastric or dunodenal ulceration.[26-28]

Recent work from several laboratories investigating possible functional decreased adrenal responsiveness in neonatal foals with sepsis may support the judicious use of corticosteroid therapy in selected cases, but a consensus is not yet established.[29,30]

Nursing care is one of the most important aspects of treating septic foals. Foals should be kept warm and dry. They should be turned at 2-hour intervals if they are recumbent. Feeding septic foals can be a challenge if gastrointestinal function is abnormal, and parenteral nutrition may be needed. If at all possible, foals should be weighed daily and blood glucose levels monitored frequently. Some foals become persistently hyperglycemic on small glucose infusion rates. These foals may benefit from constant-rate low-dose insulin infusions (Table 21-8). Recumbent foals must be examined frequently for the development of decubital sores, the appearance of corneal ulcers, and heat and swelling associated with joints and physes.

The prognosis for foals in the early stages of sepsis is fair to good. Once the disease has progressed to septic shock the prognosis decreases, although short-term survival rates are as good as those in human critical care units. Long-term survival and athletic outcomes are fair. Racing-breed foals that make it to the track perform similarly to their age-matched siblings.[31]

TABLE 21-8

Miscellaneous Drugs Used in the Neonatal Intensive Care Unit

Drug	Dose	Route	Frequency	Comments
Aminophylline	2-3 mg/kg	IV	b.i.d. to q.i.d.	Monitor theophylline levels. Therapeutic: 6-12 μg/l Toxic: >20 μg/l
Caffeine	10 mg/kg loading dose 2.5 mg/kg maintenance	Orally as needed	s.i.d., b.i.d.	Steady state level: 5-20 μg/l Toxic: >50-75 μg/l
Dimethyl sulfoxide	1 g/kg	IV	Once	Administer as 5% to 10% solution; dimethyl sulfoxide is hypertonic
Heparin	40-100 U/kg	SQ/IV	b.i.d.	–
Insulin (protamine zinc)	0.15 U/kg	IM/SQ	b.i.d.	–
Insulin (regular)	0.00125-0.2 U/kg/hr	IV	Constant-rate Infusion	Pretreat lines: insulin adsorbs to lines

Adapted from Palmer JE: Neonatal drug doses. Proceedings of the International Veterinary Emergency Critical Care Symposium, San Antonio, Tex., 2000.
IV, Intravenous; *b.i.d.*, twice daily; *q.i.d.*, 4 times daily; *s.i.d.*, once daily; *SQ*, subcutaneous; *IM*, intramuscular.

NUTRITIONAL MUSCULAR DYSTROPHY (WHITE MUSCLE DISEASE)

Pamela A. Wilkins

Nutritional muscular dystrophy or white muscle disease is a vitamin E/selenium–responsive muscle disease of horses of all ages that is probably caused by a dietary deficiency of selenium and vitamin E.[1] The condition occurs most commonly in geographic areas with low selenium levels in the soil, generally the northeastern, northwestern, Great Lakes, and mid-Atlantic regions of the United States.

Two forms of the disease are described in foals: the fulminant form, in which the foal is found acutely dead, and the subacute form. In the fulminant form death usually is attributed to myocardial lesions resulting in cardiovascular collapse. The subacute form is characterized by dysphagia and gait abnormalities primarily caused by stiffness of the muscles of locomotion. Paralysis, if present, is not flaccid as in botulism. Abnormal function of respiratory muscles may complicate the clinical situation. Aspiration pneumonia may be present because of problems associated with swallowing; the tongue and pharyngeal muscles frequently are affected in the early stages of disease.[1] Foals with severe disease may have widespread muscle necrosis leading to hyperkalemia, which can be severe and result in death of the foal. Serum activities of the muscle enzymes creatine kinase and aspartate aminotransferase may be greatly increased. Diagnosis is confirmed at necropsy or ante mortem by determination of decreased whole blood or serum selenium concentration or decreased glutathione peroxidase activity in the blood of the foal before supplementation. Myoglobinuria and acute renal failure are not uncommon in these foals.

Treatment of foals with nutritional muscular dystrophy is primarily supportive. The clinician should address all metabolic abnormalities. Some foals require intranasal oxygen tinsufflation. Affected foals are unable to suck effectively, and enteral (through an indwelling nasogastric tube) or parenteral nutritional support should be provided. Because of the high likelihood of aspiration pneumonia, broad spectrum antimicrobial therapy should be administered parenterally. The patient should be kept quiet and should be stimulated minimally. Affected foals should receive parenteral (intramuscular) vitamin E and selenium supplementation. Selenium is toxic in large doses. The prognosis for severely affected foals is guarded. For less severely affected foals, the prognosis is good with appropriate treatment. The disease can be prevented by ensuring that mares receive sufficient vitamin E and selenium while pregnant and by supplementing foals with parenteral injections of vitamin E and selenium at birth in endemic areas. A more complete discussion of the pathophysiology of this disease and the nutritional management is presented elsewhere in this text.

HEPATIC DISEASES OF FOALS

Bryan Waldridge

CLINICOPATHOLOGIC DIAGNOSIS

Activities of certain hepatic enzymes (alkaline phosphatase, γ-glutamyltransferase) and serum concentrations of some hepatic indices (bilirubin, bile acids, triglycerides) in clinically normal foals are significantly different from those of adult horses, especially during the neonatal period. For this reason absolute reference ranges used for adult horses cannot reliably be used to diagnose hepatic disease in foals.[1] The relatively greater ratio of hepatic mass to body weight and increased induction, production, or release of liver-specific enzymes in young animals may account for increased γ-glutamyltransferase (GGT) and other hepatic enzyme activity in foals.[1,2] Sorbitol dehydrogenase (SDH) and aspartate transaminase (AST) are more reliable clinicopathologic indicators of hepatocellular disease in foals.[1,3] These enzymes have more narrow standard deviations in foals, and their normal reference ranges are closer to those of adults. Therefore, if hepatic disease is suspected in a foal, further diagnostic procedures, such as clinical examination, ultrasonography and liver biopsy, are useful and often necessary to confirm the diagnosis.

Serum Alkaline Phosphatase

Several studies have reported significantly increased serum alkaline phosphatase (ALP) activity in foals compared with that of adult horses.[2,4,5] Serum ALP activity is highest in foals during the first 2 weeks of life.[2,4] Alkaline phosphatase activity in foals remains elevated for at least 90 days[6] and usually decreases to adult ranges by 1 year of age.[2] The normal wide individual variation and large standard deviation of ALP activity in foals limits its effectiveness to diagnose hepatobiliary disease.[1] Increased ALP activity in foals is mainly of hepatic origin.[252] However, some of the elevation of activity in young growing animals is due to increased osteoblastic activity and bone formation.[1,4,5]

γ-Glutamyltransferase

Foals also have significantly increased GGT activity compared with that of adult horses.[1-4,6] GGT activity in foals ranges from 1.5 to 3 times normal adult values for the first 3 to 4 weeks of life.[1,2] Increased GGT activity in foals is most different from that of adult horses between 7 to 21 days of age.[4] Similar to ALP activity, there is a normal wide individual variation in foal GGT activity, which restricts its diagnostic ability to identify hepatic disease.[1]

Unlike neonatal ruminants, the source of increased GGT activity in foals is endogenous and not secondary to ingestion of colostrum.[2,6] Colostral GGT activity is lower in mares than in ewes and cows.[6] In foals measurement of postsuckle GGT activity is not associated with serum IgG concentration[2] and cannot be used to determine colostrum intake.[6] Hepatic GGT activity in young animals is increased, and this may account for some of the increased GGT activity in foals.[1,2]

Serum Bile Acids

Serum bile acid (SBA) concentration in neonatal foals is significantly greater than normal reference ranges in adult horses.[3] SBA concentration is highest at birth and then gradually decreases. One study[3] reported that SBA concentrations remain elevated for at least 6 weeks post partum. Speculated mechanisms of increased SBA concentration in foals include increased hepatic production or decreased excretion into bile, gastrointestinal flora differences that affect the conjugation of bile acids, and enhanced intestinal absorption. Hepatic uptake of SBA and excretion into bile require active transport, which may not be fully functional in foals. Elevated serum concentrations of bilirubin or triglycerides can interfere with measurement of SBA. However, the degree of neonatal hyperbilirubinemia or hyperlipemia apparently is not correlated with increased SBA concentration in foals.

Bilirubin

Neonatal hyperbilirubinemia appears to be a normal transient event during the first 2 weeks of life.[3,4] Bilirubin concentrations are highest in young foals and drop to normal ranges for adult horses by 7 to 14 days of age.[3,4] One study[4] reported that both total and unconjugated bilirubin concentrations in foals were increased over adult values from birth through 7 to 14 days post partum. Neonatal hyperbilirubinemia may occur as a result of hemolysis of fetal erythrocytes or immature hepatic function. The fetal liver's ability to excrete bilirubin is also minimal. Bilirubin must be excreted across the placenta in fetuses, and conjugation may be delayed in neonates as the liver gains full function.

Triglycerides

Hyperlipidemia can be normal during the neonatal period. Triglyceride concentrations in foals tend to be highest during the first 2 weeks of life and moderately increased for up to 6 weeks of age.[3,4] Some authors have suggested that triglyceride concentrations in foals may decrease as hepatic function develops and triglycerides are used to synthesize other lipoproteins.[4]

PORTOSYSTEMIC SHUNTS

Portosystemic shunts (PSSs) are infrequently reported in foals. Most PSSs have been extrahepatic,[7-9] and there is a single case report of an intrahepatic PSS.[10] Another case report[11] describes an apparent arteriovenous anomaly of the portal vein that functioned as a PSS. Clinical signs of a PSS can be intermittent and are attributed to hepatoencephalopathy. These include abnormal behavior, depression or lethargy, ataxia, blindness, wandering or circling, head pressing, and being small for age.[7-11] Clinical signs often do not occur until the foal has been weaned.[9] Milk diets may have a protective effect against clinical signs until weaning, when the foal consumes solid feed with higher protein content.

Clinicopathologic findings with PSS include hyperammonemia and elevated SBA concentration with normal to mildly increased hepatic enzyme activity.[7,10] One case series of four PSSs in foals and calves[10] reported that blood ammonia concentrations in animals with PSSs were at least 7 times greater than matched controls. The authors considered elevated blood ammonia concentration more reliable than increased SBA in diagnosing PSS. Microcytic, normochromic erythrocytes have been reported in three foals,[9,10] one of which was anemic.[9] The exact pathogenesis of poikilocytosis with PSS is unknown but may be due to altered erythrocyte membranes or iron metabolism. [10] Leukocytosis with neutrophilia has also been reported in several cases.[11-13] Cerebrospinal fluid (CSF) with PSS is usually normal.[7,9,11] In one case[10] CSF was xanthochromic with increased nucleated cell count and total protein, suggestive of hemorrhage and inflammation.

Histopathologic lesions seen on a liver biopsy with PSS can include arteriolar proliferation in the area of the portal triad,[7,8] widespread hepatocyte atrophy,[7] bile duct hyperplasia, periportal fibrosis, poorly developed portal triads, and apparent absence of hepatic portal veins.[8]

Intraoperative contrast portography is the most reliable diagnostic technique to identify the location and extent of a PSS.[10] Jejunal mesenteric vein catheterization may be performed using a ventral midline,[8-10] flank,[7] or a right paracostal incision with resection of the eighteenth rib.[10] A right paracostal incision with resection of the eighteenth rib may provide better exposure and improve surgical access to the PSS, portal system, and liver.[10] A mesenteric vein is catheterized, and 50 to 80 ml of iodinated contrast media is injected.[7-10]

Images of the PSS can then be obtained using radiography or fluoroscopy. Radiographs taken near the end of contrast injection may provide better images than fluoroscopy in foals.[10] In normal foals contrast media should opacify the portal vein, intrahepatic portal system, and hepatic veins without opacifying the vena cava.[9] If a PSS is present, contrast media can be seen opacifying the portal vein and caudal vena cava by way of the PSS, without significant hepatic perfusion.[8-10]

Nuclear hepatic scintigraphy using intravenous ^{99m}technetium radiocolloid can be used to determine hepatic radiocolloid uptake and hepatic perfusion index.[7] The hepatic perfusion index of a normal foal was 0.8 and 2.3 in a PSS-affected foal, which suggested decreased portal circulation through the liver of the affected foal. Static images of the liver of the PSS-affected foal taken 15 minutes after injection of contrast showed that its liver was smaller than that of the normal foal. The major disadvantage of nuclear hepatic scintigraphy is that the type and location of the PSS cannot be determined.[7,9]

Ultrasound examination of a foal with PSS revealed no parenchymal abnormalities, but the liver appeared smaller than normal.[8] A large blood vessel that apparently communicated with the caudal vena (intrahepatic PSS) was identified in another foal.[10]

Surgical correction of PSS has been attempted with two extrahepatic PSSs[9,10] and one intrahepatic PSS.[10] One foal with a surgically corrected extrahepatic PSS is reported to have survived.[10] The filly was clinically healthy and neurologically normal 2 years postoperatively but was small for her breed (Belgian).

TYZZER'S DISEASE

Tyzzer's disease is a peracute rapidly fatal infectious hepatitis of foals 7 to 42 days of age.[11-13] The etiologic agent of Tyzzer's disease is *Clostridium piliforme*, a gram negative, spore-forming, obligate intracellular bacterium.[11,12] *C. piliforme* is found in soil and manure.[12] It is believed that foals are exposed through ingestion of contaminated soil or feces from infected adult horses.[11,12]

Clinical signs of Tyzzer's disease may include only acute death.[12] Other clinical signs include lethargy, recumbency, seizures, pyrexia, icterus, diarrhea, tachycardia, tachypnea, dehydration, and those associated with hepatoencephalopathy.[11-13] The mean survival time after appearance of clinical signs was 34.5 plus or minus 20.1 hours (range 16 to 62 hours) in a series of confirmed cases.[11] The mean age of affected foals was 18.7 plus or minus 12.1 days (range 6 to 45 days). Ultrasound examination of the liver may reveal hepatomegaly with increased echogenicity of the hepatic parenchyma or an increased vascular pattern.[11,13]

Clinicopathologic abnormalities include severe hypoglycemia, metabolic acidosis, increased hepatic enzyme activity, hemoconcentration, and hyperfibrinogenemia.[11,13] Cerebrospinal fluid in one case[13] was sterile and xanthochromic with normal protein concentration. Cytologic examination of CSF revealed erythrocytosis, mildly increased mononuclear cells, and rare nondegenerate neutrophils.

Definitive antemortem diagnosis of Tyzzer's disease is difficult. If available, *C. piliforme* can be detected using the PCR on liver biopsies.[11] Histopathologic lesions observed in liver biopsies include multifocal coagulative necrosis of hepatocytes surrounded by degenerate hepatocytes and inflammatory cells.[11,12] Filamentous, intracellular organisms near the periphery of lesions can be seen using silver-type (Warthin-Starry) stains.[11,13] Postmortem lesions include hepatomegaly with multifocal areas of light discoloration, generalized icterus, peritoneal effusion, petechiation, and abdominal lymphadenopathy.

Successful treatment of one liver biopsy PCR-confirmed case of Tyzzer's disease[11] and three suspected cases[12,13] have been reported. Treatment of Tyzzer's disease is largely supportive of hepatic failure. The PCR-confirmed case[11] was treated with intravenous balanced electrolyte solutions, dextrose and bicarbonate supplementation, intranasal oxygen, omeprazole (4 mg/kg/day, administered orally), vitamin E (20 U/kg/day, PO), total parenteral nutrition, and enteral feeding. A presumptive case of Tyzzer's disease[13] was successfully treated similarly with the addition of DMSO (1 g/kg/day, PO) and xylazine for seizure control. Antimicrobial therapy used in these cases included ampicillin (30 mg/kg, PO every 8 hours) and gentamicin (6.6 mg/kg/day, IV), followed by sulfamethoxazole-trimethoprim (30 mg/kg, PO every 12 hours)[13] or sodium penicillin (10,000 U/kg, IV every 6 hours) and sulfamethoxazole-trimethoprim (14 mg/kg, IV every 12 hours).

Cases of Tyzzer's disease on farms tend to be fairly isolated and sporadic, but clusters of cases may occur on a single farm.[13] A study investigating risk factors for Tyzzer's disease in foals associated with a Thoroughbred breeding farm in California[12] found that foals born between March 13 and April 13 were more than seven times more likely to develop *C. piliforme* infections than were foals born at any other time during foaling season. The reason for the increased risk may have been due to environmental and management conditions or that the number of horses arriving and leaving the farm was highest at this time. Although not statistically significant, foals born to visiting (nonresident) mares and mares younger than 6 years of age were approximately three times more likely to develop *C. piliforme* infections. This difference could be attributed to decreased colostral quality in younger mares or the arrival of mares that were naive to *C. piliforme*. Additionally, strain-specific antibody may be necessary to protect foals from multiple serotypes of *C. piliforme*.

CHOLANGIOHEPATITIS

Cholangiohepatitis occurs in foals despite intensive treatment and broad spectrum antimicrobial therapy. Bacteremic or septicemic foals also may have hepatocellular damage secondary to endotoxemia or hepatic abscessation. Ideally, suspected cholangiohepatitis is treated on the basis of a liver biopsy culture. However, in foals presumptive therapy can be based on blood culture and sensitivity results, if available. The addition of empiric therapy with sulfamethoxazole-trimethoprim (30 mg/kg, PO every 12 hours) often is helpful in foals that develop apparent cholangiohepatitis while receiving broad spectrum antimicrobials. Gastric and duodenal ulcers are an important etiology of reflux or ascending cholangiohepatitis in foals.[14] Duodenal ulceration, thickening, or spasm near the major duodenal papilla can cause reflux of ingesta, gastric acid, and bile salts through the common bile duct. It is important to include aggressive anti-ulcer prophylaxis and treatment whenever treating suspected cholangiohepatitis in foals.

NEONATAL ISOERYTHROLYSIS

Neonatal isoerythrolysis (NI) is the most common cause of icterus in foals and is discussed in detail later in this chapter.[15] Hepatic disease and elevated activities of hepatic enzymes are fairly common with NI in foals secondary to anemia and hypoxia. Hepatocellular injury caused by iron and bilirubin accumulation also may contribute to elevations in bilirubin and liver enzyme activity. Total and direct bilirubin, AST, ALP, and SDH activities may be increased in NI-affected foals. Foals with the lowest hematocrit concentrations tended to have the highest SDH activities in one study.[15] Liver biopsies of two very anemic (hematocrit ≤ 11%) NI-affected foals revealed hepatic necrosis, bile duct hyperplasia, diffuse hemosiderosis, and Kupffer's cell hyperplasia consistent with hepatic iron uptake.

GLYCOGEN BRANCHING ENZYME DEFICIENCY

Glycogen branching enzyme deficiency (GBED) in Quarter Horse foals is associated with neonatal mortality, flexural limb deformities, seizures, recumbency, and respiratory or cardiac failure (see Chapter 11).[16] Clinicopathologic abnormalities related to GBED are leucopenia; intermittent hypoglycemia; and elevated activities of creatine kinase, AST, and GGT. Accumulations of amylase-resistant, abnormal polysaccharide in liver and skeletal or cardiac muscle can be found on histopathologic examination after periodic acid Schiff's staining. The amount of abnormal polysaccharide in tissues is age-dependent and is more likely to be seen in older foals.

BOX 21-4

CAUSES OF FAILURE OF PASSIVE TRANSFER

Maternal Causes

- Premature lactation
  - Placentitis
  - Twins
  - Premature placental separation
- Poor colostral quality
  - Maiden mares
  - Older mares
- Failure of lactation
  - Aglactia
  - Fescue toxicosis

Foal Causes

- Failure to ingest colostrums
  - Weakness
  - Prematurity
  - Musculoskeletal deformity
  - Perinatal asphyxia syndrome
- Failure to absorb colostrums
  - Prematurity
  - Necrotizing enterocolitis

FAILURE OF PASSIVE TRANSFER

Debra C. Sellon, Pamela A. Wilkins

Causes, diagnosis, and treatment of FPT of immunity are discussed in detail in Chapter 1. FPT occurs when a foal fails to ingest a sufficient quantity of high-quality colostrum. FPT may result from the following: failure of the foal to suck from the dam for any reason and failure of the dam to produce sufficient quantity of high-quality colostrum. Box 21-4 presents causes of FPT. Several methods are available for measuring IgG concentration in blood; the most reliable are enzyme-linked immunosorbent assay and single radial immunodiffusion technology-based tests.[1-7] Foals usually are tested at 24 hours of age, but they can be tested earlier if colostrum ingestion has occurred and a concern exists regarding the passive transfer of immunity status of the foal, with the recognition that additional increases in IgG concentration may occur with additional time.[8,9] The concentration of IgG in the blood of the foal has been used as an indicator of the adequacy of passive transfer, but the actual blood concentration at which FPT is diagnosed has been challenged in recent years.[10-12] Foals with sepsis commonly have a serum IgG concentration of less than 800 mg/dl.[13,14] Foals with FPT are more likely to die from sepsis.[15,16,17-19] One should consider the IgG concentration only as a marker for adequacy of colostral absorption. All the measured IgG is unlikely to be directed against the specific pathogen affecting any particular neonate, and IgG is not the only immune protection afforded the foal by colostrum. Many factors that confer local and more general immunity to the newborn are present in colostrum; these include growth factors, cytokines, lactoferrins, CD14, leukocytes, and other yet to be described proteins.[20-27] By considering IgG a marker of adequacy for passive transfer, similar to GGT in calves, the clinician can choose a replacement that is more beneficial to the patient.[27] After FPT is identified, treatment depends on the current condition of the foal and its local environment. Foals not presently ill and on well-managed farms with low population density and low prevalence of disease may not require treatment if their IgG concentration is between 400 and 800 mg/dl. Critically ill neonates with FPT in an equine NICU are by definition ill and in an environment with high disease prevalence. These patients require immediate treatment of FPT and frequent reassessment of their passive immunity status. Critically ill foals often fail to demonstrate the expected increase in blood IgG concentration based on grams of IgG administered per kilogram of body mass compared with healthy, colostrum-deprived foals.[17,28,29] Sick foals also demonstrate a more rapid decline in IgG concentration than do healthy foals because they use and catabolize available protein.

Foals with FPT may be treated by oral or intravenous administration of various products containing IgG. One can attempt oral administration of additional colostrum or IgG-containing products such as plasma, serum, or lyophilized colostrum in foals younger than 12 to 24 hours of age.[30-32] Depending on the age of the foal and the maturity and function of the gastrointestinal tract, this treatment may be effective. Many NICUs and large breeding farms maintain colostrum banks for this purpose. Plasma should be administered intravenously if the foal is not expected to absorb additional colostrum or if the enteral route is unavailable. Commercially available hyperimmune plasma products designed for use in foals are available and can be stored frozen. Plasma and banked colostrum should be stored in a non–frost-free freezer to minimize protein loss associated with freeze-thaw cycling.[33] Plasma should be administered through special tubing with an inline filter, and clinicians should monitor patients closely for transfusion reactions.[34] Serum and concentrated IgG products may be used, but the practitioner should be aware that many of these products focus on IgG retention and not on other factors associated with passive transfer of immunity. IgG concentration should be measured after transfusion, and additional plasma should be provided as necessary. Administration of plasma to critically ill foals without FPT may be beneficial through provision of other factors present in the plasma. In these situations fresh frozen plasma or fresh plasma may be best, particularly if transfusion of clotting proteins is desired.

NEONATAL ISOERYTHROLYSIS

Debra C. Sellon, Pamela A. Wilkins

Neonatal isoerythrolysis is a hemolytic syndrome in newborn foals caused by a blood group incompatibility between the foal and dam and is mediated by maternal antibodies against foal erythrocytes (alloantibodies) absorbed from the colostrum. The disease most often affects foals born to multiparous mares and should be suspected in foals younger than 7 days of age with clinical signs of icterus, weakness, and tachycardia. A primiparous mare can produce a foal with NI if she has received a prior sensitizing blood transfusion or has developed placental abnormalities in early gestation that allowed leakage of fetal red blood cells into her circulation. Many are the causes of jaundice in newborn foals, including sepsis, meconium impaction, and liver failure, but these usually can be differentiated readily from NI by measuring the PCV, which is usually less than 20% in foals with neonatal NI.

Foals with NI are born clinically normal and then become depressed and weak and have a reduced suckle response within 12 to 72 hours of birth. The rapidity of onset and severity of disease are determined by the quantity and activity of absorbed alloantibodies. Affected foals have tachycardia, tachypnea, and dyspnea. The oral mucosa is initially pale and then becomes icteric in foals that survive 24 to 48 hours. Hemoglobinuria may occur. Seizures caused by cerebral hypoxia are a preterminal event.

The salient laboratory findings are anemia and hyperbilirubinemia. Most of the increased bilirubin is unconjugated, although the absolute concentration of conjugated bilirubin generally is increased well above normal. Urine may be red to brown and is positive for occult blood.

CAUSE AND PATHOGENESIS

The natural development of NI has several prerequisites. First the foal must inherit from the sire and express an erythrocyte antigen (alloantigen) that is not possessed by the mare. Blood group incompatibility between the foal and dam is not particularly uncommon, but most blood group factors are not strongly antigenic under the conditions of exposure through previous parturition or placental leakage. Factor Aa of the A system and factor Qa of the Q system are highly immunogenic, however, and nearly all cases of NI are caused by antibodies to these alloantigens. The exception is in the case of mule foals in which a specific donkey factor has been implicated.[1-3] Mares that are negative for Aa or Qa or both are considered to be at risk for producing a foal with NI. The risk involves approximately 19% and 17% of Thoroughbred and Standardbred mares, respectively. Second, and perhaps most important, the mare must become sensitized to the incompatible alloantigen and produce antibodies to it. The mechanism for this is not known in many instances but generally is believed to result from transplacental hemorrhage during a previous pregnancy involving a foal with the same incompatible blood factor.[3]

Sensitization through transplacental contamination with fetal erythrocytes earlier in the current pregnancy is possible, but an anamnestic response is generally necessary to induce a pathogenic quantity of alloantibodies.[4] Research shows that 10% of Thoroughbred mares and 20% of Standardbred mares have antibodies to the Ca blood group antigen without known exposure to erythrocytes.[3] Some common environmental antigen is postulated, possibly to lead to production of anti-Ca antibodies. Data suggest that these natural antibodies may suppress an immune response to other blood group antigens because mares negative for Aa that have anti-Ca antibodies often do not produce antibodies to Aa of the erythrocytes in their foals that also contain Ca antigen. This antibody-mediated immunosuppression is thought to result from the destruction of fetal cells before the dam mounts an immune response to other cell surface antigens. Natural alloantibodies have not been associated with NI in horses.

After the mare becomes sensitized to the erythrocytes of her foal, alloantibodies are concentrated in the colostrum during the last month of gestation. Unlike the human neonate, who acquires alloantibodies in utero and thus is born with hemolytic disease, the foal is protected from these antibodies before birth by the complex epitheliochorial placentation of the mare. Thus the final criterion for foal development of NI is ingestion in the first 24 hours of life of colostrum-containing alloantibodies specific for foal alloantigens. Immunoglobulin-coated foal erythrocytes are removed prematurely from circulation by the mononuclear phagocyte system or are lysed intravascularly by way of complement. The rapidity of development and severity of clinical signs are determined by the amount of alloantibodies that was absorbed and their innate activity. Alloantibodies against Aa are potent hemolysins and generally are associated with a more severe clinical syndrome than antibodies against Qa or other alloantigens. The highest alloantibody titers are likely to be produced by mares that were sensitized in a previous pregnancy and then subsequently re-exposed to the same erythrocyte antigen during the last trimester of the current pregnancy. Prior sensitization of a mare by blood transfusion or other exposure to equine blood products may predispose to NI.[4]

DIAGNOSIS

A tentative diagnosis of NI can be made in any foal that has lethargy, anemia, and icterus during the first 4 days of life. Blood loss anemia caused by birth trauma is attended by pallor. Icterus caused by sepsis or liver dysfunction would not be associated with anemia. The definitive diagnosis of NI must be based on demonstration of alloantibodies in the serum or colostrum of the dam that are directed against foal erythrocytes. The most reliable serodiagnostic test for neonatal NI is the hemolytic crossmatch using washed foal erythrocytes, mare serum, and an exogenous source of absorbed complement (usually from rabbits). Although this test is impractical in a practice setting, a number of qualified laboratories routinely perform this diagnostic service. The direct antiglobulin test (Coombs' test) may demonstrate the presence of antibodies on foal erythrocytes; however, false-negative results occur frequently. Most human or veterinary hematology laboratories can perform routine saline agglutination crossmatching between mare serum and foal cells. Because some equine alloantibodies act only as hemolysins, agglutination tests may yield false-negative results. Most field screening tests of colostrum have not proved to be reliable enough for practical use.

TREATMENT

If NI is recognized when the foal is younger than 24 hours old, the dam's milk must be withheld in favor of an alternative source of milk during the foal's first day of life. This can be accomplished by muzzling the foal and feeding it through a nasogastric tube. The minimum necessary amount of milk is 1% of body mass every 2 hours (e.g., a 50-kg foal should receive 500 ml or 1 pint of mare's milk or milk replacer every 2 hours). The udder of the mare should be stripped regularly (at least every 4 hours) and the milk discarded. In most instances clinical signs are not apparent until after the foal is 24 hours old, when colostral antibodies have been depleted or the absorptive capacity of the foal's intestine for immunoglobulin has diminished. Withholding milk at this point is of minimal benefit.

Supportive care to ensure adequate warmth and hydration is paramount. The foal should not be stressed, and exercise must be restricted. Confining the mare and foal to a box stall is best. Intravenous fluids are indicated to promote and minimize the nephrotoxic effects of hemoglobin and to correct any fluid deficits and electrolyte and acid-base imbalances. Antimicrobials may be necessary to prevent secondary infections.

One should monitor foals carefully for the necessity of blood transfusion, although transfusion should be used only as a lifesaving measure. When the PCV drops below 12%, blood transfusion is warranted to prevent life-threatening cerebral hypoxia. Erythrocytes from the dam are perfect in terms of nonreactivity with the blood of the foal; however, the fluid portion of the blood of the mare has to be removed completely from the cells to prevent administration of additional harmful alloantibodies to the foal. One can pellet the erythrocytes of the dam from blood collected in acid-citrate-dextrose solution by centrifugation or gravity and then aseptically draw off the plasma by suction apparatus or syringe and replace it with sterile isotonic (0.9%) saline. The cells are thoroughly mixed with the saline, and then the centrifugation or sedimentation is repeated, followed by aspiration and discarding of the saline. This washing process should be repeated at least three times. One then can suspend the packed erythrocytes in an equal volume of isotonic saline for administration. Erythrocyte washing by centrifugation is more desirable than gravity sedimentation because antibody removal is more complete and packed cell preparations can be prepared more quickly (each gravity sedimentation requires 1 to 2 hours). Packed red blood cells are advantageous in overcoming the problem of volume overload.

When equipment or conditions do not allow the safe use of dam erythrocytes, an alternative donor is necessary. Because the alloantibodies absorbed by the foal generally are directed against Aa or Qa and because the latter are highly prevalent among most breeds of horses, a compatible blood donor is difficult to identify. The odds of finding a donor without Aa or Qa are higher in Quarter Horses, Morgans, and Standardbreds than in Thoroughbreds and Arabians. Previously blood-typed individuals negative for Aa and Qa and free of alloantibodies are optimal. Between 2 and 4 L of blood or 1 to 2 L of packed erythrocytes should be given over 2 to 4 hours. These allogeneic cells have a short life span and represent a large burden to the neonatal mononuclear phagocyte system, which may cause increased susceptibility to infection. In addition, these cells sensitize the foal to future transfusion reactions. All potential harm must be measured against the benefit in each situation.

If a mule foal is the patient, blood from a female previously bred to a donkey should not be used. In cases in which transfusion will be delayed, a compatible donor cannot be identified, or the PCV is so low as to be life-threatening (hemoglobin <5 mg/dl), the clinician may administer polymerized bovine hemoglobin products, if available, at a dose of 5 to 15 ml/kg.[4] Dexamethasone (0.08 mg/kg) may be used to treat peracute NI if the PCV is less than 12% and transfusion may be delayed or is not fully compatible, but dexamethasone has detrimental effects on blood glucose regulation in the neonate, and because the antibody in question is of maternal origin, corticosteroid therapy in immunosuppressive doses probably is not indicated. Intranasal oxygen insufflation (5 to 10 L/min) may be beneficial. Most foals with NI have adequate passive transfer of immunity, but antimicrobial therapy is indicated to protect against secondary sepsis resulting from the compromised condition of the foal. Supportive care and good nursing care, which includes keeping the foal warm and quiet, are essential. The PCV is expected to decline again 4 to 7 days after transfusion.[5]

CLIENT EDUCATION

The prognosis for NI in foals depends on the quantity and activity of absorbed antibodies and is indirectly proportional to the rate of onset of signs. In peracute cases the foal may die before the problem is recognized, whereas foals with slowly progressive signs often live with appropriate supportive care.

Like most diseases, NI is much more effectively prevented than treated.[6] Any mare that has produced a foal with NI may well produce another affected foal; thus all subsequent foals should be provided with an alternative colostrum source and the colostrum of the dam discarded unless she is bred to a stallion with known blood type compatibility. Because mares negative for Aa and Qa alloantigens are most at risk of producing affected foals, they should be identified by blood typing. Subsequently, breeding of these mares may be restricted to Aa- and Qa-negative stallions, thus eliminating the possibility of producing an affected foal. In breeds with a high prevalence of Aa or Qa alloantigens (e.g., Thoroughbreds and Arabians), a stallion negative for these and suitable on the basis of other criteria may be difficult to identify. If these "at risk" mares are bred as desired, their serum should be screened in the last month of pregnancy for the presence of erythrocyte alloantibodies. Mares with low or equivocal titers must be tested closer to the time of parturition. If alloantibodies are detected, the colostrum of the dam should be withheld and the foal then should be provided with an alternative colostrum source. Maternal alloantibodies to Ca do not appear to mediate NI in foals and actually may be preventive by removing potentially sensitizing cells from the circulation; therefore foals should not be deprived of colostrum from mares possessing anti-Ca antibodies, even when Ca is present on their erythrocytes. Rarely, the antigens De, Ua, Pa, and Ab have been associated with NI in foals; however, to consider mares without these alloantigens to be at risk for NI is not practical.

IMMUNE-MEDIATED THROMBOCYTOPENIA AND NEUTROPENIA

Debra C. Sellon, Pamela A. Wilkins

Immune-mediated thrombocytopenia and neutropenia have only recently been described in foals, although they have been widely recognized in human neonates for many years.[1-5] In the first few days of life, affected foals have normal body condition with mild to moderate dehydration, depression, lethargy, and reluctance or inability to suckle. Petechia and ecchymoses of the mucous membranes are common. Some affected foals have crusting miliary dermatitis, especially in the pectoral and groin regions. Clinical pathologic evaluation reveals marked thrombocytopenia (frequently $<10,000/\mu l$) and neutropenia. The pathogenesis of this disorder is similar to that of NI. It is an alloimmune disorder resulting from ingestion of maternal antibody directed against the foal's platelets or neutrophils. Affected foals may be predisposed to sepsis. The diagnosis is confirmed by appropriate testing for platelet- and neutrophil-associated antibody.[6] Other causes of neonatal thrombocytopenia and neutropenia, particularly sepsis, must be ruled out. Future foals born to the mare seem likely to be at risk for developing similar problems, and these foals should be treated in the same manner as those with NI: prevented from sucking from the dam and provided with an alternative source of passive immunity in the form of banked colostrum or intravenous plasma. An alternative nutritional source, such as foal milk replacer, should be provided to the foal for the first 24 hours of life, and the foal should be muzzled while it is in the company of its dam for that period. Treatment is primarily supportive, but in the case of severe thrombocytopenia, transfusion of platelet-enriched fresh plasma may be indicated. Granulocyte colony-stimulating factor has been used in foals with neutropenia, but substantial efficacy has yet to be demonstrated. Broad spectrum antimicrobial therapy may be prudent in cases of alloantibody-associated neutropenia. Treatment with immunosuppressive doses of corticosteroids is probably unwarranted, given the increased risk of infection, because the antibody in question is of maternal origin. Corticosteroids occasionally may be warranted if the thrombocytopenia is considered to be life threatening.

Other specific diseases of the immune system of foals, severe combined immunodeficiency, selective IgM deficiency, transient hypogammaglobulinemia, agammaglobulinemia, and other unclassified immunodeficiencies are covered in detail elsewhere in this text.

DISEASES OF THE RESPIRATORY TRACT

Pamela A. Wilkins

RESPIRATORY DISTRESS

The neonate can experience respiratory distress immediately after birth because of several congenital respiratory tract or cardiac anomalies. Chief among these causes are bilateral choanal atresia, stenotic nares, dorsal displacement of the soft palate caused by anatomic deformity or neurologic impairment, accessory or ectopic lung lobes, lung lobe hypertrophy, lung lobe dysplasia, cardiac anomalies with right-to-left shunting, and miscellaneous causes such as subepiglotic cysts and severe edema of the larynx.[1-8] These situations must be evaluated and treated immediately, and they should be considered as true emergencies.

Foals with airway occlusion can be recognized by the lack of airflow through the nostrils despite obvious attempts to breathe and by respiratory stridor. These foals may demonstrate open-mouth breathing, and their cheeks may puff outward when they exhale. One foal with congenital bilateral choanal atresia was recognized during extrauterine intrapartum resusucitation because a nasotracheal tube could not be passed. Under most circumstances an effective airway can be established by orotracheal intubation, but some foals require an emergency tracheostomy. The clinician diagnoses the underlying problem by endoscopy or radiography in most cases. Treatment of choanal atresia and cystic structures is surgical, whereas severe laryngeal edema and laryngeal paralysis frequently respond to medical management. Until the underlying problem is resolved in these cases, broad spectrum antimicrobial therapy should be administered and the foal fed by intubation or total parenteral nutrition. Colostrum can be given, but because these foals frequently develop aspiration pneumonia if allowed to suck from their dams, intravenously administered plasma also may be necessary to provide sufficient passive immunity.

RESPIRATORY DISEASES ASSOCIATED WITH HYPOXEMIA IN THE NEONATE

Arterial blood gas determinations are the most sensitive indicator of respiratory function readily available to the clinician. The most convenient arteries for sampling are the metatarsal arteries and the brachial arteries. Portable arterial-venous blood gas analyzers now are making arterial blood gas analysis more practical in the field, and the technique is no longer reserved for large referral practices. Managing a critically ill equine neonate without knowledge of arterial blood gas parameters is nearly impossible. Pulse oximetry is useful, but these monitors only measure oxygen saturation of hemoglobin. Desaturation can occur rapidly in critically ill neonates. The utility of these monitors in the foal has yet to be demonstrated clearly, particularly in cases of poor peripheral perfusion.[9] The most common abnormalities recognized with arterial blood gas analysis are hypoxemia with normocapnia or hypocapnia and hypoxemia with hypercapnia. *Hypoxemia* is defined as decreased oxygen tension of the arterial blood (decreased Pa_{O_2}), and *hypoxia* is defined as decreased oxygen concentration at the level of the tissue, with or without hypoxemia. Hypoxia results from hypoxemia, decreased perfusion of the tissue bed in question, or decreased oxygen-carrying capacity of the blood resulting from anemia or hemoglobin alteration.

Five primary means by which hypoxemia may develop are (1) low concentration of oxygen in the inspired air, such as in high altitude or in an error mixing ventilator gas; (2) hypoventilation; (3) ventilation-perfusion mismatch; (4) diffusion limitation; and (5) intrapulmonary or intracardiac right-to-left shunting of blood. Hypoxemia is not an uncommon finding in neonates but must be evaluated in terms of the current age of the foal and its position.[10,11-14] One also must consider the

TABLE 21-9

Normal Arterial Blood Gas Values for Foals*

Gestational Age	Postnatal Age	Position	pH	Pa_{CO_2} (Mm Hg)	Pa_{O_2} (Mm Hg)
Term†	2 minutes	Lateral	7.31 ± 0.02	54.1 ± 2.0	56.4 ± 2.3
	15 minutes		7.32 ± 0.03	50.4 ± 2.7	57.5 ± 3.6
	30 minutes		7.35 ± 0.01	51.5 ± 1.5	57.0 ± 1.8
	60 minutes		7.36 ± 0.01	47.3 ± 2.2	60.9 ± 2.7
	2 hours		7.36 ± 0.01	47.7 ± 1.7	66.5 ± 2.3
	4 hours		7.35 ± 0.02	45.0 ± 1.9	75.7 ± 4.9
	12 hours		7.36 ± 0.02	44.3 ± 1.2	73.5 ± 3.0
	24 hours		7.39 ± 0.01	45.5 ± 1.5	67.6 ± 4.4
	48 hours		7.37 ± 0.01	46.1 ± 1.1	74.9 ± 3.3
	4 days		7.40 ± 0.01	45.8 ± 1.1	81.2 ± 3.1
Premature‡	0.5-11 hours	Lateral	7.21 ± 0.05	55.3 ± 3.6	53.7 ± 1.5

*Reported values are assumed to not be temperature corrected. Values are mean ± SEM.
†Data from Stewart JH, Rose RJ, Barko AM: Respiratory studies in foals from birth to seven days old, *Equine Vet J* 16:323, 1984.
‡Data from Rose RJ, Rossdale PD, Leadon DP: Blood gas and acid-base status in spontaneously delivered term-induced premature foals, *J Reprod Fert Suppl* 32:521, 1982.

difficulty encountered in obtaining the sample because severe struggling can affect the arterial blood gas results. Table 21-9 presents normal arterial blood gas parameters for varying ages of foals. The normal foal has a small shunt fraction (approximately 10%) that persists for the first few days of life and contributes slightly to a blunted response to breathing 100% oxygen compared with the adult. Hypoxemia frequently occurs in foals with prematurity, PAS, and sepsis, although other conditions also result in hypoxemia in the neonate. In the early stage of sepsis-associated hypoxemia, Pa_{CO_2} may be within normal limits or decreased if the foal is hyperventilating for any reason. If the lung is involved significantly in the underlying pathologic condition, such as with severe pneumonia, acute lung injury, or ARDS, increased Pa_{CO_2} may well be present, representing respiratory failure.[15,16]

Hypoxemia usually is treated with intranasal humidified oxygen insufflation at 4 to 10 L/min. Hypercapnia is not a simple matter to treat. The clinician must try to distinguish between acute and chronic hypercapnia. Acute hypercapnia usually is accompanied by a dramatic decrease in blood pH of 0.008 pH units for each 1 mm Hg increase in Pa_{CO_2}. This acidemia can promote circulatory collapse, particularly in the concurrently hypoxemic or hypovolemic patient. The effects of more chronic CO_2 retention are less obvious because the time course allows for adaptation. The pH change is less, about 0.003 pH units per 1 mm Hg increase in Pa_{CO_2}, because it is balanced by enhanced renal absorption of bicarbonate by the proximal renal tubule. Most foals with ARDS are in the acute stages of respiratory failure, but chronic adaptation begins to occur within 6 to 12 hours and is maximal in 3 to 5 days. An increase in bicarbonate is evident, particularly if the acidemia is primarily respiratory in origin. Intravenous administration of sodium bicarbonate to correct respiratory acidosis-acidemia should be done cautiously in these foals because CO_2 retention may only be increased. Also, it is important to remember that 1 mEq of sodium is administered with each mEq of bicarbonate, and hypernatremia has been seen in foals treated exuberantly with sodium bicarbonate. Foals with hypercapnia of several days' duration also may develop a blunted respiratory drive to increased CO_2. In these foals oxygen administration, although essential to treat hypoxemia, may further depress ventilation and further decrease pH. This effect is caused by a loss of hypoxic drive after oxygen therapy. These foals should be considered as candidates for mechanical ventilation if the Pa_{CO_2} is greater than 70 mm Hg or is contributing to the poor condition of the foal, such as causing significant pH changes.[15,16] If hypercapnia is caused by central depression of ventilation, as frequently occurs in foals with PAS, one can administer caffeine (10 mg/kg loading dose; then 2.5 mg/kg as needed) rectally or orally in foals with normal gastrointestinal function. Other clinicians may recommend constant-rate infusions of doxapram hydrochoride for these foals.[17,18] If this therapy fails, mechanical ventilation should be considered. Mechanical ventilation of foals with central respiratory depression is rewarding and may be necessary for only a few hours to days. A special category is the foal with botulism exhibiting respiratory failure caused by respiratory muscle paralysis. These foals do well with mechanical ventilation, although the duration of mechanical ventilation is more prolonged, frequently more than 1 week. Foals with primary metabolic alkalosis usually have compensatory respiratory acidosis. Treatment of hypercapnia is not necessary in these cases because it is in response to the metabolic condition. These foals do not respond to caffeine, and they should not be ventilated mechanically if this is the only disorder present.

BACTERIAL PNEUMONIA

In the neonate bacterial pneumonia usually results from sepsis or aspiration during sucking. Foals with sepsis can develop acute lung injury or ARDS as part of the systemic response to sepsis, and this frequently contributes to the demise of foals in septic shock.[19,20] The best way to diagnose bacterial pneumonia is by cytologic examination and culture of a transtracheal aspirate, but blood culture may aid in early identification of the causative organism and allow for early institution of directed antimicrobial therapy. A second frequent cause of bacterial pneumonia in the neonate is aspiration caused by a poor suck reflex or dysphagia associated with PAS, sepsis, or weakness. The clinician must take care to ensure that aspiration is not iatrogenic in foals being bottle fed. Auscultation over the trachea while the foal is sucking helps identify occult aspiration. Occult aspiration pneumonia should be suspected in any critically ill neonate that is being bottle fed or is sucking on its own and has unexplained fever, fails to gain weight, or has a persistently increased fibrinogen level.

Older foals develop bacterial pneumonia, frequently following an earlier viral infection.[21] Bacterial pneumonia is discussed in depth elsewhere in this text, but a few comments specific to the foal are necessary. The clinician should auscultate and percuss the thorax of the foal, but results may not correlate closely with the severity of disease. The most commonly isolated bacterial organism in foal pneumonia is *Streptococcus equi* subsp. *zooepidemicus,* and one may isolate it alone or as a component of a mixed infection.[21-23] Transtracheal aspirate for culture and cytologic examination is recommended because mixed gram positive and gram negative infections are common, and antimicrobial susceptibility patterns can be unpredictable. The obtained aspirate should be split and samples submitted for bacterial culture, virus isolation, and cytologic examination. Additional diagnostics include radiography, ultrasonography, and serial determination of white blood cell counts (with differential) and blood fibrinogen concentrations. Treatment includes administration of appropriate antimicrobial therapy. Some foals may benefit from nebulization with saline, antimicrobials, or other local products.[24] Ascarid larval migration through the lung can mimic bacterial pneumonia.[25] In these cases the foal may not respond to antimicrobial therapy and should be dewormed with ivermectin. Deworming the mare within 1 month of parturition and frequently deworming the foal prevent ascarid migration pneumonia in most foals.

A special category of bacterial pneumonia in foals is *Rhodococcus equi* bronchopneumonia. This pneumonia of young foals was described first in 1923.[26] The organism, originally known as *Corynebacterium equi,* is a gram positive pleomorphic coccobacillus usually less than 1 μm in diameter and 2 μm in length. *R. equi* has an acid-fast staining characteristic under some growing circumstances because of the presence of mycolic acid in its cell wall, similar to *Mycobacterium* and *Nocardia* species. Mycolic acid promotes granuloma formation. The organism is able to multiply in and destroy macrophages as it prevents phagosome lysosome fusion.[27,28] The organism is thought to be an opportunistic pathogen, and it lives in the soil of most geographic areas. Foals are affected most frequently between the ages of 1 and 6 months, when maternally derived immunity has begun to wane. The disease is insidious, and foals may have significant pulmonary involvement before developing noticeable clinical signs.

Phagocytosis of *R. equi* by equine macrophages is not associated with a functional respiratory burst and, at least in human beings, the L-arginine–NO pathway is not required for intracellular killing of this organism.[29,30] Optimal binding of *R. equi* to mouse macrophages in vitro requires complement and is mediated by Mac-1, a leukocyte complement receptor type 3 (CR3, CD11b/CD18).[31] Opsonization of *R. equi* with specific antibody is associated with increased phagosome-lysosome fusion and enhanced killing of *R. equi,* suggesting that the mechanism of cellular entry is important.[27] Neutrophils from foals and adult horses are fully bactericidal, and killing of *R. equi* is enhanced considerably by specific opsonizing antibody.[32]

The ability of *R. equi* to induce disease in foals likely depends on host and microbial factors. Knowledge of the virulence mechanisms of *R. equi* was speculative until the discovery of the virulence plasmid.[33] As opposed to most environmental *R. equi* organisms, isolates from clinically affected foals typically contain 85- to 90-kb plasmids encoding an immunogenic virulence-associated protein (VapA) that is expressed on the bacterial surface in a temperature-regulated manner.[34] Plasmid-cured bacteria lose their ability to replicate and survive in macrophages and are cleared from the lungs within 2 weeks of intrabronchial challenge without producing pneumonia.[35] However, expression of VapA alone is not sufficient to restore the virulence phenotype. Six other genes have approximately 40% overall amino acid identity with VapA, and the identification of multiple genes with considerable homology suggests that these genes constitute a virulence-associated gene family in *R. equi.*[36] Other candidates for virulence factors include capsular polysaccharides and cholesterol oxidase, choline phosphohydrolase, and phospholipase C exoenzymes ("equi factors"), but their roles have not been defined clearly.

The primary manifestation of disease caused by *R. equi* infection is severe bronchopneumonia with granuloma, abscess formation, or both. Up to 50% of foals diagnosed with bronchopneumonia also have extrapulmonary sites of infection.[37] As the pneumonia progresses, clinical signs may include decreased appetite, lethargy, fever, tachypnea, and increased effort of breathing characterized by nostril flaring and increased abdominal effort. Cough and bilateral nasal discharge are inconsistent findings. A smaller percentage of affected foals may have a more devastating, subacute form. These foals may be found dead or have acute respiratory distress with a high fever and no previous history of clinical respiratory disease.

Hyperfibrinogenemia is the most consistent laboratory abnormality in foals with *R. equi* pneumonia. Neutrophilic leukocytosis (>12,000 cells/μl), with or without monocytosis, is common.[38] Thoracic radiography is a useful diagnostic aid, frequently revealing a prominent alveolar pattern with poorly defined regional consolidation, abscessation, or both. Ultrasonography is a helpful diagnostic tool when the disease involves peripheral lung tissue.[39] Although a number of serologic tests have been described, serologic diagnosis of *R. equi* infections is controversial and difficult because exposure of foals to this organism at a young age leads to production of antibody without necessarily producing clinical disease.[40,41] Bacteriologic culture combined with cytologic examination of a tracheobronchial aspirate remains the most definitive method for accurate diagnosis of *R. equi* pneumonia. However, foals without clinical disease exposed to contaminated environments may have *R. equi* in their tracheae from inhalation of contaminated dust; therefore culture results should be interpreted in the context of the overall case presentation.[42] Culture results in one study were as sensitive as PCR-based assays and offered the advantage of allowing in vitro antimicrobial susceptibility testing.[43] However, PCR is likely to be a useful tool, and results from a second trial suggest that the assay is more sensitive and specific than culture of tracheobronchial aspirates for diagnosis.[44]

The combination of erythromycin and rifampin has long been considered the treatment of choice for *R. equi* infections in foals, and the combination reduces the likelihood of resistance to either drug. The recommended dosage regimen for rifampin is 5 mg/kg every 12 hours or 10 mg/kg every 24 hours orally. The recommended dose of estolate or ethylsuccinate esters of erythromycin is 25 mg/kg every 8 or 12 hours orally.[45] Recently, azithromycin has been recommended for treatment of *R. equi* infection at a dosage of 10 mg/kg orally every 24 hours for 5 to 7 days and then every other day.[46] Alternatively, clarithromycin at 7.5 mg/kg every 12 hours orally, in combination with rifampin, may be used. In a retrospective comparison of rifampin with either erythromycin, azithromycin, or clarithromycin, clarithromycin-rifampin was superior to other treatment options for treatment of pneumonia caused by *R. equi* in foals in a referral population.[47] Severely affected foals may require intranasal oxygen insufflation, intravenous fluid support, and nutritional support. Treatment generally continues for 4 to 10 weeks until all clinical and laboratory evidence of infection is resolved. Although well tolerated by most foals, erythromycin can result in soft feces. Although this diarrhea is generally self-limiting and does not require cessation of therapy, affected foals should be carefully monitored. An idiosyncratic reaction characterized by severe hyperthermia and tachypnea has been described in foals treated with erythromycin during periods of hot weather.[48] Affected foals should be moved to a colder environment and treated with antipyretic drugs and alcohol baths if necessary. *Clostridium difficile* enterocolitis has been reported in the dams of nursing foals given oral erythromycin.[49] The dam is exposed to active erythromycin by coprophagy or by drinking from a communal water source where the foal has rinsed its mouth.

Prevention of *R. equi* pneumonia on farms with recurrent problems is problematic. The most studied prophylactic measure to date has been the administration of plasma that is hyperimmune to *R. equi* to foals within the first week of life and then again when maternal immunity begins to wane, at approximately 30 days of age.[50-57] No effective vaccination protocols for the dam or foal have been described to date. Farm management is important in preventing disease, and control measures include frequent manure removal, avoidance of overcrowded conditions, and planting of dusty or sandy soils.[50]

The prognosis for *R. equi* bronchopneumonia is fair to good in foals with the more chronic form of the disease. Foals with acute respiratory distress have a more guarded prognosis, as do foals with sites of significant extrapulmonary infection. The long-term prognosis for survival for foals with *R. equi* bronchopneumonia is good, and many foals perform as expected as athletes.[58]

VIRAL PNEUMONIA

The most commonly identified causes of viral pneumonia in foals are EHV-1 and EHV-4, equine influenza, and equine arteritis virus (EVA). These infectious diseases are discussed in detail in Chapter 9. EHV-1 is probably the most clinically important viral respiratory disease of foals, but outbreaks of EVA in neonates have occurred and are devastating.[59-66] Adenovirus is reported sporadically and is a problem in Arabian foals with severe combined immunodeficiency.[67-69]

In the neonate infection with EHV-1 or EVA is almost uniformly fatal, and antemortem diagnosis is difficult, even once an outbreak on a particular farm is identified. Several factors appear common to foals with EHV-1, including icterus, leucopenia, neutropenia, and petechial hemorrhage, but these problems also are identified in foals with severe sepsis.[62,70,71] The antiviral drug acyclovir (10 to 16 mg/kg orally or rectally 4 to 5 times per day) has been used in cases of EHV-1 in neonates, with some evidence of efficacy in mildly affected foals or foals affected after birth.[71] Although acyclovir has poor oral bioavailability in adult horses, the pharmacokinetics remain unexamined in foals.[72] It is possible that valacylovir, an oral prodrug of acyclovir, may prove useful in the future.[73] If viral pneumonia is a possibility, blood and tracheal aspirates should be collected at presentation for bacterial and virus isolation. The lungs of foals with EHV-1 or EVA are noncompliant, and pulmonary edema may be present. Mechanical ventilation of these cases may prolong life, but death is generally inevitable because of the magnitude of damage to the lungs. Foals suspected of having EHV-1 or EVA should be isolated because they may be shedding large quantities of virus and pose a threat to other neonates and pregnant mares. Foals with EVA generally are born to seronegative mares, and intravenous treatment with plasma with a high titer against EVA may prove beneficial because passive immunity appears to have a significant role in protecting neonates against this disease.[66,74]

Older foals and weanlings may be affected by herpesviruses. Disease is usually mild, although a fatal pulmonary vasculotropic form of the disease has been described recently in young horses.[75,76] The clinical signs of disease are indistinguishable from influenza and include a dry cough, fever, and serous to mucopurulent nasal discharge, particularly if secondary bacterial infection occurs. Rhinitis, pharyngitis, and tracheitis may be present. Treatment of affected foals is primarily supportive. Foals also may become infected with EHV-2. The predominant clinical signs are fever and lymphoid hyperplasia with pharyngitis.[77,78] Diagnosis is by virus isolation.

OTHER CAUSES OF RESPIRATORY SIGNS IN FOALS

FRACTURED RIBS

Rib fractures have been recognized in 3% to 5% of all neonatal foals and can be associated with respiratory distress.[79,80] Potential complications of rib fractures include fatal myocardial puncture, hemothorax, and pneumothorax. Rib fractures frequently are found during physical examination by palpation of the ribs or by auscultation over the fracture sites. The diagnosis is confirmed by radiographic and ultrasonographic evaluation. Often, multiple ribs are affected on one side of the chest. Specific treatment generally is unnecessary, but direct pressure on the thorax is never recommended. Some patients may benefit from surgical stabilization of certain fractures, particularly those overlying the heart.[81]

PNEUMOTHORAX

Pneumothorax can occur spontaneously; as a complication of excessive positive pressure ventilation[80,82]; or after tracheostomy, surgery, or trauma. Any foal being ventilated mechanically that suddenly has respiratory distress and hypoxemia should be evaluated for pneumothorax. Diagnosis is by auscultation and percussion of the thorax, but one can confirm the diagnosis with radiographic and ultrasonographic evaluation of the thorax. Needle aspiration of air from the pleural space also confirms the diagnosis. Treatment is required when clinical signs are moderate to severe or progressive and involves closed suction of the pleural space. Subcutaneous emphysema can complicate treatment of this problem.

Idiopathic Tachypnea

Idiopathic or transient tachypnea has been observed in Clydesdale, Thoroughbred, and Arabian breed foals. In human infants transient tachypnea can be related to delayed absorption of fluid from the lung, perhaps because of immature sodium channels.[83] In foals tachypnea generally occurs when conditions are warm and humid and is thought to result from immature or dysfunctional thermoregulatory mechanisms. Clinical signs of increased respiratory rate and rectal temperature develop within a few days of birth and may persist for several weeks. Treatment involves moving the foal to a cooler environment, body clipping, and provision of cool water or alcohol baths. These foals frequently are treated with broad spectrum antimicrobial drugs until infectious pneumonia can be ruled out.

Atypical Interstitial Pneumonia

A syndrome of bronchointerstitial pneumonia and acute respiratory distress has been described in older foals and appears to be a distinct entity from ARDS in neonatal foals in association with sepsis.[19,20,84] The underlying cause has not been identified, but the genesis is probably multifactorial, with several potential pathogens being implicated. Affected foals have acute respiratory distress with significant tachypnea, dyspnea, nostril flare, and increased inspiratory and expiratory effort. Auscultation reveals a cacophony of abnormal sounds, including crackles and polyphonic wheezes in all lung fields. Loud bronchial sounds are audible over central airways, and bronchovesicular sounds are lost peripherally. Affected foals are cyanotic, febrile, and unwilling to move or eat. Foals may be found acutely dead. Laboratory abnormalities include leukocytosis, hyperfibrinogenemia, and hypoxemia with hypercapneic acidosis. Foals can be severely dehydrated and have coagulation changes consistent with disseminated intravascular coagulation. Hypoxic injury to other organs, primarily the kidneys and liver, can occur. Thoracic radiographs reveal a prominent interstitial pattern overlying a bronchoalveolar pattern that is distributed diffusely throughout the lung. This syndrome is a respiratory emergency. Treatment is broad based and includes administration of oxygen, nonsteroidal anti-inflammatory agents, broad spectrum antimicrobial therapy, nebulization, judicious intravenous fluid therapy, nutritional support, and corticosteroid therapy. Hyperthermia in the foal must be managed. Corticosteroid therapy appears to have been lifesaving in most of the reported surviving foals. Because this syndrome is associated with high environmental temperatures in some areas, prevention involves control of ambient temperatures, not transporting foals during hot weather, and keeping foals out of direct sun on hot days, particularly foals being treated with erythromycin for suspected or confirmed *R. equi* infection.[85]

DISEASES OF THE URINARY TRACT

Pamela A. Wilkins

UROPERITONEUM

Uroperitoneum has been recognized as a syndrome in foals for more than 50 years.[1,2] Classically, affected foals are 24 to 36 hours old when clinical signs are first recognized.[3] Previous reports had a proportionately larger affected male than female population.[4-6] The hypothesis was that colts were more at risk because their long, narrow, high-resistance urethra was less likely to allow bladder emptying, resulting in rupture of a full bladder during parturition when high pressures were applied focally or circumferentially around the bladder.[1] More recent reports suggest that such extreme sex bias may have been an artifact of small case numbers in the early reports.[6,7]

Rupture or disruption of any structure of the urinary tract can occur. The dorsal wall of the bladder has been reported as a frequent disruption site, with the ventral wall less likely to be involved.[3] The urachus appears to be the next most commonly affected structure. A few cases of ureteral and urethral defects have been reported.[3,6] Sepsis does not appear to favor one site over the others.[6,7]

The pathophysiology of uroperitoneum is not yet understood fully. The high pressure exerted on a full bladder during parturition once was thought to be the main cause. Full bladder and obstruction caused by a partial umbilical cord torsion at parturition, strenuous exercise, and external trauma have been reported as causes.[8] A few reports describe smooth and noninflamed edges of torn tissue, suggesting the possibility of congenital bladder wall defects.[6,9,10] Sepsis leading to urinary tract rupture and uroperitoneum may occur in foals hospitalized for a variety of unrelated problems. The onset of clinical signs of uroperitoneum may be insidious in these foals, and diagnosis may be less obvious.[6,7]

Clinical signs associated with uroperitoneum in the neonatal foal typically include straining to urinate, dribbling urine, and a stretched-out stance. Weakness, tachycardia, tachypnea, and not sucking well are also common. A distended abdomen may be evident, and one may feel a fluid wave on ballottement of the abdomen. Occasionally, urine accumulates in the scrotum and should not be confused with hernia. Foals also may show signs of sepsis, including fever, injected mucous membranes, diarrhea, and disease of other body systems.

Laboratory findings vary depending on the duration of the uroperitoneum and on the presence and severity of sepsis. Classic findings include hyperkalemia, hyponatremia, and hypochloremia arising from equilibration of urine electrolytes and water with blood across the peritoneal membrane.[3-5] The usual foal diet of milk, which is high in potassium and low in sodium, promotes the electrolyte abnormalities. Foals that develop uroperitoneum while receiving intravenous fluids may not have classic electrolyte imbalances at the time clinical signs are recognized.[6,7] Increased serum creatinine concentration is often present, whereas blood urea nitrogen concentrations occasionally, but not consistently, are increased.[3-5] Metabolic acidosis and hypoxemia may be present. Some patients also have serum hypo-osmolality.[4] Foals should be tested for FPT. One of the most sensitive laboratory tests for uroperitoneum is the ratio of peritoneal to serum creatinine. A ratio greater than or equal to 2:1 is considered diagnostic of uroperitoneum. Peritoneal fluid should be collected and tested for creatinine concentration, as well as for cytologic findings, bacteriologic culture, and sensitivity. Cytologic evaluation of peritoneal fluid is necessary to identify concurrent peritonitis or other gastrointestinal compromise. An electrocardiogram should be performed on initial evaluation of a foal with suspected uroperitoneum because hyperkalemia may result in bradycardia, increased duration of the QRS complex, a shortened Q-T interval, increased P-wave duration, prolonged P-R interval, or atrioventricular conduction disturbances. Other possible cardiac sequelae to hyperkalemia include cardiac arrest, third-degree atrioventricular block, ventricular premature contractions, and ventricular fibrillation.[3,8]

For any foal exhibiting signs of dypsnea, tachypnea, or hypoxemia, thoracic radiographs should be taken before induction of anesthesia to rule out pleural effusion, pneumonia, or ARDS, which could complicate ventilation and oxygenation during anesthesia and the postoperative period. Foals with uroperitoneum are frequently hypoxemic before surgical relief, particularly those in which the problem is the primary complaint, likely because of increased intra-abdominal pressure and the development of abdominal compartment syndrome.[11,12] Ultrasonography has become the tool of choice in the diagnosis of uroperitoneum and is a useful tool available to the practitioner.[13] Free peritoneal fluid is readily imaged, and tears in the bladder are readily visible. The empty bladder with a significant defect, in a fluid-filled abdomen, will collapse on itself and often have a U shape. Urachal and urethral lesions can also be visualized. Six of eight foals in one study had urinary tract lesions identified sonographically, and all 31 foals of another study underwent sonographic evaluation; a significant correlation between ultrasonographic findings and location of the lesion at surgery existed.[5,6]

Initial treatment aims to stabilize the patient and correct any electrolyte and acid-base abnormalities and provide fluid volume replacement. Until laboratory data are available, 0.9% or 0.45% saline with 5% dextrose should be used. A potassium concentration of greater than 5.5 mEq/L can be life threatening. Hyperkalemia can be managed by peritoneal drainage to decrease whole-body potassium stores using teat cannulae, Foley catheters, large-gauge (16 or 14) intravenous catheters, or human peritoneal dialysis catheters. Fluid replacement at least should equal the amount of fluid removed from the abdomen to prevent acute hypotension caused by expansion of previously collapsed capillary beds. Abdominal drainage also helps ventilation and decreases the work of breathing by decreasing pressure on the diaphragm. Calcium gluconate, glucose, sodium bicarbonate, or insulin may be administered intravenously to decrease serum potassium concentrations. These maneuvers do not correct the whole-body potassium overload, however, and once therapy is discontinued, hyperkalemia can reappear until the urine is removed from the abdomen. Hyponatremia should be corrected slowly. Because of the real possibility of concurrent sepsis, blood cultures should be obtained before preoperative administration of antimicrobials. Broad spectrum coverage (penicillin and amikacin or ceftiofur sodium) is recommended until culture results become available. Therapeutic drug monitoring should be perfomed when using aminoglycoside therapy. However, because the peak value may be depressed as a result of the increased volume of distribution represented by the volume of urine in the abdomen, the clinician should not adjust the dose on the basis of a low peak until a new peak is obtained after surgical correction of the uroperitoneum. Foals with FPT should be treated with adequate volumes of intravenously administered plasma.

After addressing the metabolic abnormalities, the clinician may consider surgical management. Medical management using an indwelling Foley catheter has been described.[14] Preoperative medical stabilization reduces anesthetic risk. Safer inhalant agents such as isoflurane also have decreased risk. Removal of the internal umbilical remnant at the time of surgery is usual. One should consider culturing any removed umbilical remnant and submitting the remnant for histopathologic evaluation. Urinary tract rupture can recur. Sepsis, hypoxemia, pneumonia, peritonitis, and ARDS complicate the management of uroperitoneum. Many affected foals are persistently oxygen dependent for several days after surgical correction, and serial arterial blood gas analyses should be performed before intranasal oxygen supplementation is discontinued.

Prognosis is associated closely with concurrent illness, especially septicemia. Uncomplicated uroperitoneum resulting from a defect in the bladder has a good prognosis. If the location of the lesion is other than the bladder, the prognosis is not as favorable.[6] Foals with septicemia have a much poorer prognosis.[6-8]

ACUTE RENAL FAILURE

Acute renal failure most often occurs as a complication of prenatal asphyxial syndrome, sepsis, or aminoglycoside therapy. Acute renal failure also has been reported after oxytetracycline administration in foals.[15] The dose of oxytetracycline commonly used to treat flexural deformities in foals is approximately 10 times the antimicrobial dose. Many foals treated in this manner also have suffered some degree of perinatal asphxia, which damages the kidney, because of prolonged parturition precipitated in part by the flexural deformity. Evaluation of renal function in these foals before the administration of the first dose of oxytetracycline and continued monitoring of serum creatinine concentrations before the administration of subsequent doses of this nephrotoxic compound would seem reasonable. Hemodialysis has been used as therapy in one of these cases, but prevention is important because these foals may fail to respond to usual therapy for oliguric renal failure and are euthanized.[15]

CONGENITAL RENAL DISEASE

The most commonly reported congenital deformity of the kidney of the foal is renal hypoplasia and dysplasia, which may have a heritable component.[16,17] Renal arteriovenous malformations also have been reported.[18] Ectopic ureters and fenestrated ureters have been described in the foal.[19-21] Congenital renal defects, among others, were reported in three weak, recumbent neonatal foals born to mares being treated for equine protozoal myeloencephalitis.[22] Mares received sulfadiazine or sulfamethoxazole-trimethoprim, pyrimethamine, folic acid, and vitamin E orally. The foals were anemic, leucopenic, azotemic, hyponatremic, and hyperkalemic. Serum folate concentrations were lower than those reported in the literature for clinically normal brood mares. Treatment was unsuccessful. Necropsy revealed lobulated kidneys with thin cortices and a pale medulla. The authors postulated that oral administration of sulfonamides, 2,4-diaminopyrimidines (pyrimethamine with or without trimethoprim), and folic acid to mares during pregnancy is related to congenital defects in newborn foals.

UMBILICAL DISORDERS

The umbilicus serves as the conduit for nutrition and gas exchange between the dam and the fetal foal. The urine from the foal is expelled through this structure into the allantoic cavity. The author has recognized cases of in utero bladder distention in the fetus that were associated with multiple twists decreasing urine flow or focal stenosis creating the same effect. Foals born with this condition did not have bladder rupture associated with parturition but did have other severe abnormalities that eventually resulted in their demise, primarily premature delivery with failure to adapt to extrauterine life.[23] At birth the umbilicus breaks, leaving a small external remnant and a large internal remnant. The umbilicus long has been regarded as the primary site of entry of pathogens into the neonate, although this has been challenged recently. Treatment of the umbilicus after birth involves dipping it (preferably just the most distal component) with various caustic compounds. The most current recommendation is to treat the umbilicus with dilute chlorhexidine, povidone-iodine, or dilute iodine solutions just a few times after birth. Exuberant treatment of the umbilical stump with caustic solutions can lead to scalding of the ventral abdomen and may promote patency of the urachus. The ultrasonographic appearance and measurements of the umbilical arteries, urachus, and umbilical vein of foals from 6 hours to 4 weeks of age have been described in detail.[24] A 7.5-MHz sector scanner transducer placed across the midline of the ventral portion of the abdominal wall of the foal works best because of the superficial location of these structures. The mean (± SD) diameter of the umbilical vein was 0.61 ±0.20 cm immediately cranial to the umbilical stalk, 0.52 ± 0.19 cm midway between the umbilicus and liver, and 0.6 ± 0.19 cm at the liver. The urachus and umbilical arteries of normal foals have a mean total diameter of 1.75 ± 0.37 cm at the bladder apex. The umbilical arteries scanned along either side of the bladder have a mean diameter of 0.85 ± 0.21 cm. These measurements and the ultrasonographic appearance of the internal umbilical structures from clinically normal foals can be used as references to diagnose abnormalities of the umbilical structures in neonatal foals.[24,25] The most common abnormalities of these structures are focal abscess formation, hematoma, and urachal tear.

HERNIA

Herniae traditionally have been thought to develop from failure of closure at the umbilical stump after birth. However, the closure of the body wall defect at the umbilicus was studied in relation to the development of umbilical herniae in a large group of normal foals followed from birth until 5 months of age or from birth until 11 months of age.[26] At birth approximately half of these foals had a defect in the body wall at the umbilicus that was termed a *palpable umbilical ring*. In 18 foals this defect disappeared within 4 days, but in one foal the ring did not close and a hernial sac with abdominal contents was palpable. This foal was considered to be the only foal to have a truly congenital umbilical hernia. Twelve foals developed an umbilical hernia between 5 and 8 weeks of age. The prevalence of umbilical herniae was much higher than in other studies, possibly because of the prospective nature of the study. On the basis of this study, the great majority of umbilical herniae would appear not to result from failure of closure but rather to be acquired after birth. One should consider the palpable ring structure within the body wall at the umbilicus a variant of normal in the foal and should not call it a hernia until the foal is at least 1 month of age.

In one study of 147 horses treated for umbilical herniae over a 13½-year period, only 8.8% developed complications in association with umbilical defects.[27] Six horses had intestinal incarceration; the incarceration was reduced manually in three horses before admission and resolved without treatment in two others. The hernia was surgically reduced in one horse. Herniorrhaphy was performed on four of the five horses in which the incarceration did not require surgical reduction, and the fifth was managed conservatively. The study confirmed that complications of umbilical herniae are rare in horses; however, when they do develop, they may be one of various forms, some of which are insidious in onset. The primary differential diagnosis for an external swelling in the umbilical stump region is an external abdominal abscess, which will be firm, variably painful, warm, and nonreducible. Ultrasonographic evaluation readily can confirm either possibility.

OTHER CONGENITAL ABNORMALITIES

One report describes a 3-day-old foal that died from intestinal strangulation caused by a remnant of vitelline vein that extended between the umbilicus and the portal vein.[28]

PATENT URACHUS

Patent urachus frequently is recognized in the abnormal neonate, probably because of the increased recumbency and decreased movement of these patients. Cauterization of a patent urachus is no longer recommended except in cases that persist for long periods of time (>1 month) after the foal becomes more active. Surgical resection may provide relief in some foals, but most cases resolve without treatment if given enough time. Foals with a patent urachus may posture and strain frequently to urinate; some of this may be associated with irritation or local infection of the urachus. These symptoms can be alleviated by administration of broad spectrum antimicrobial therapy that obtains high drug concentrations in the urine (e.g., trimethoprim-sulfa drug combinations) and by oral administration of phenazopyridine hydrochloride (Pyridium), a dye that anesthetizes the urinary tract epithelial surfaces (see Table 21-8). This dye turns the urine orange and stains everything yellow-orange that it or the urine touches but can provide a great deal of relief to foals with this problem.

UMBILICAL REMNANT INFECTION

The umbilicus has been considered the traditional point of entry of bacteria into the septic neonate, and septic foals were referred to as having "navel ill" and "joint ill" in the past. Although the gastrointestinal tract is now thought to be the route of entry in most septic neonates, infection of the umbilicus—termed *omphalitis,* or *omphalophlebitis* if the vessels are involved—still occurs as a single focus of infection or along with more generalized infection. External signs, such as swelling, heat, pain, ventral edema, or purulent discharge may be present in some foals, but usually external signs are minimal and infection is suspected because of infection in another site (e.g., an infected joint), fever, or otherwise unexplained increased blood fibrinogen concentration. The diagnosis is confirmed by ultrasonographic evaluation of the internal umbilical remnant. Any of the umbilical structures may be involved. A complete description of the evaluation is available in the relevant veterinary literature, but the examination is performed best using a 7.5-MHz probe with a standoff and with the foal standing. [24] The usual finding is that the affected structure is larger than expected. A fluid-filled core and echogeneic shadows consistent with gas may be apparent in some cases. Interpretation requires some experience, and the examiner should be familiar with variants of normal, such as gas shadows associated with a patent urachus and enlarged vessels caused by hematoma formation, so that treatment is not initiated inappropriately.

Two options for treatment are surgical and medical. Medical treatment is preferable in cases in which the lesion is well localized and small and in foals with a medical condition that is not amenable to anesthesia and surgical intervention. Broad spectrum antimicrobial therapy should be instituted and may need to be continued for 2 to 3 weeks. Most affected foals respond to medical therapy. Frequent reevaluation of the abnormality is necessary, every 5 to 7 days initially, and blood fibrinogen concentrations should be measured at re-evaluation because they should stabilize and decrease with effective treatment. Failure to respond to therapy in 10 days to 2 weeks suggests that an empiric change in the antimicrobial used may be necessary. In foals that are refractory to medical management or in which the lesion is large, surgical excision of the entire umbilical remnant may be desirable.

DISEASES OF THE GASTROINTESTINAL TRACT

Pamela A. Wilkins

COLIC IN THE NEONATE

Colic in the foal can be difficult to diagnose accurately because rectal examination is not possible. However, many diagnostic aids, the most important of which is ultrasonography, are available to help differentiate medical from surgical causes of abdominal discomfort in the foal.

OBSTRUCTION

Intestinal accidents of all types described in adult horses, with the possible exception of enteroliths, occur in foals. Intussusception, volvulus, displacement, diaphragmatic hernia, and intraluminal and extraluminal obstruction have been reported in foals. Abdominal ultrasonographic and radiographic evaluation greatly aids diagnosis. Treatment is primarily surgical. Foals with PAS and intestinal dysmotility are at increased risk of intussusception and displacement, and Miniature breed foals appear to be at increased risk for fecolith formation.

MECONIUM RETENTION AND IMPACTION

Meconium retention or impaction is a common cause of abdominal discomfort in newborn foals. Most foals defecate shortly after their first meal. The usual practice for most owners or veterinarians attending the birth of a foal is to administer an enema to aid this process. In the past phosphate-based commercially available enemas (e.g., Fleet) were used frequently, but if used excessively these types of enemas can create problems of their own, including rectal irritation and hyperphosphatemia. The best enema is warm soapy water made with a mild soap such as liquid Ivory soap that can be administered through soft rubber tubing using gravity flow. Foals with significant meconium retention become colicky within the first few hours of life as gas accumulates within the bowel. Frequently, the meconium can be palpated through the abdominal wall unless gas distention and abdominal tympany is advanced. Additional diagnostics can include abdominal ultrasonography and radiography, particularly if it is necessary to rule out other, more serious types of colic. These foals assume a classic stance with an arched back. The clinician must differentiate this stance from the stance assumed by foals with uroperitoneum, which is more extended. Foals with meconium retention may have simultaneous ruptured bladder, however, so the clinician must be sure to evaluate the foal fully for both problems. Foals that do not respond rapidly to enema administration need additional treatment, which can include giving mineral oil (2 to 4 ounces) by nasogastric tube. Persistent meconium retention resulting in significant abdominal distention is treated by muzzling the foal to prevent further milk intake and administering intravenous fluids at an appropriate maintenance rate. If constant-rate infusion is possible, 5% to 10% dextrose is the preferred fluid to use to provide some calories to the foal and approximate the free water needs of the foal. Dextrose should not be used as a bolus fluid. More aggressive treatment would include administration of retention enemas made using acetylcysteine, which serves as an irritant and increases secretion. A 4% acetylcysteine solution, pH 7.6, is made by adding 20 g of baking soda and 8 g of acetylcysteine to 200 ml of water. A 30-french Foley catheter is inserted approximately 2.5 to 5 cm into the rectum and the bulb is slowly inflated to occlude the rectum. Between 100 and 200 ml of the solution is administered by gravity flow and retained for 30 to 45 minutes by occluding the catheter.[1]

Extreme cases of meconium retention may require surgical intervention, but this is usually not necessary, and most cases resolve with medical management alone within 12 to 24 hours. Some foals require pain management. Nonsteroidal anti-inflammatory drugs should be used with caution in the neonate because of their effects on renal function and gastric mucosal blood flow (see the section on gastric ulcers). Many foals respond well to butorphanol administered intramuscularly at a dose of 0.05 to 0.1 mg/kg.[2] Intranasal oxygen insufflation is beneficial in foals with significant abdominal distention.[3]

One should evaluate foals with meconium impaction or retention for evidence of PAS because intestinal dysmotility is common with this condition. Colostrum is a laxative, and these foals also may suffer from FPT, with meconium retention resulting from the lack of adequate colostrum. These foals are also at risk of sepsis because the mucosal intestinal barrier probably has been disrupted and translocation of bacteria can occur. Blood cultures should be obtained, and the foals should be monitored closely for signs of sepsis.

CONGENITAL DEFECTS

Atresia within the gastrointestinal system of the foal occurs infrequently, but clinical signs are characteristic.[4] Acute colic occurs within the first few hours and is accompanied by abdominal distention similar to that produced by meconium retention. Three primary types of atresia are described in the foal: membrane atresia, cord atresia, and blind-end atresia. Antemortem diagnosis of atresia, short of abdominal exploratory surgery, is aided by the lack of meconium staining of the rectum or any administered enema fluids. Additional diagnostic tests may include administration of a barium enema for a radiographic study, colonoscopy, and abdominal ultrasonography. Abdominocentesis usually is normal until bowel rupture is imminent or has occurred. Affected foals may be made more comfortable by muzzling them to prevent further milk intake and by supplying them with fluids and nutrition intravenously. If surgical correction is attempted, broad spectrum antimicrobial therapy should be initiated and passive transfer status determined. Frequently, these foals are hypoxemic because of the abdominal distention, and oxygen supplementation is desirable.

LETHAL WHITE SYNDROME

Solid white foals born to overo-overo matings of American Paint Horses may suffer from congential aganglionosis of the ileum, cecum, and colon (see Chapter 15). These foals present similarly to foals with meconium impaction or atresia in that colic develops shortly after birth and involves progressive abdominal distention with feeding. The inherited defect is in the endothelin receptor gene.[5-8] No effective treatment exists, but the clinician should be aware that not all white foals of this mating are affected, and some simply may have meconium retention; therefore a short period of treatment may be warranted.

NECROTIZING ENTEROCOLITIS

Necrotizing enterocolitis is considered the most common acquired gastrointestinal emergency of human infants.[9,10] The 1500 to 2000 infants who die every year from this disease in the United States and the large number of infants who develop short gut syndrome from this disease represent only the tip of the iceberg of the problems necrotizing enterocolitis causes. The pathogenesis of necrotizing enterocolitis is unknown but may result from a disturbance of the delicate balance among gastrointestinal perfusion, enteric organisms, and enteral feeding. Risk factors for necrotizing enterocolitis in human infants include prematurity, hypoxic-ischemic insult, and formula or breast milk feedings. The clinical spectrum of necrotizing enterocolitis is multifactoral and ranges from temperature instability, apnea, lethargy, abdominal distention, bilious residuals, septic shock, disseminated intravascular coagulation, and death. Medical management is usually adequate treatment for necrotizing enterocolitis, although surgical resection and anastamosis may be required in the most severe cases. In the neonatal foal necrotizing enterocolitis is probably one of the most underrecognized causes of gastrointestinal dysfunction and in the past has been attributed only to infection with anaerobic organisms including *Clostridium perfringens* type C and *C. difficile*.[11] Although a specific form of enteritis in the foal is associated with intestinal infection by these organisms, most necrotizing enterocolitis is associated with prematurity or PAS in the infant and the foal.

Necrotizing enterocolitis should be suspected in any foal that is having difficulty tolerating oral feeding, demonstrating signs of ileus, or having episodes of colic and in any foal with occult blood, digested blood, or frank blood in the stool or reflux. Foals exhibiting any of these clinical signs should not be fed orally if possible and should receive parenteral nutrition until gastrointestinal function returns to near normal. The mucosal barrier of the intestine is unlikely to be fully intact, and these foals are at risk for sepsis resulting from bacterial translocation. These foals should receive broad spectrum antimicrobial therapy, and if any evidence of coordinated gastrointestinal motility is apparent, sucralfate should be administered orally as a protectant.

GASTRIC ULCERS

Gastric ulcer disease has been recognized in foals, and lesions vary in anatomic distribution, severity, and cause. In clinically normal neonatal foals (<30 days of age), gastric ulcers and mucosal desquamation have been documented (see Chapter 15).[12-15] Because of these reports and other early reports of death caused by ruptured clinically silent ulcers in neonatal foals, for years many clinicians believed prophylactic treatment of critically ill neonates with antiulcer medication was necessary.[16-18] Recently, this paradigm has been challenged.

The pathophysiology of gastric ulcer disease is described most reasonably as an imbalance in protective and aggressive factors.[19-21] These protective factors are responsible for maintaining a healthy gastrointestinal tract by promoting adequate mucosal blood flow, adequate mucus and bicarbonate production, prostaglandin E_2 production, epithelial growth factor production, gastric afferent innervation, epithelial cell restitution, and gastroduodenal motility. Probably the most important factor is maintenance of mucosal blood flow. Hypoxia, NO, prostaglandins, and gastric afferent innervation influence mucosal blood flow. The aggressive factors include gastric acid, bile salts, pepsin, and enzymes. Few specific causes have been found for gastric ulcer disease in foals. Excessive administration of nonsteroidal anti-inflammatory drugs can result in ulceration of the glandular and squamous epithelium because of an inhibition of prostaglandin production, which leads to a decrease in mucosal blood flow and an increase in acid production. Nonsteroidal anti-inflammatory drugs also can impair the healing of lesions and should be used with caution in neonatal equine medicine.[20,21]

In the critically ill neonate, the suspected cause of gastric ulcers has shifted away from an excessive amount of intraluminal gastric acid toward gastric mucosal ischemia caused by hypoxia, low blood flow conditions, or both.[22] Perforating gastric ulcers are more likely a manifestation of necrotizing enterocolitis than of excessive gastric acid. Shock, sepsis, or trauma can result in gastric mucosal ischemia, allowing for the disruption of epithelial cell integrity and permitting damage by aggressive factors or providing an environment suitable for the establishment of bacterial colonization.[22,23] Impairment of mucosal blood flow also may result in reperfusion injury, allowing the formation of gastric ulcers. In the sick neonatal foal (<7 days of age), a wide variability in the intragastric pH has been documented depending on the type of disease, severity, and milk intake frequency and volume, suggesting that in the critically ill equine neonate, ulcer prophylaxis using histamine antagonists or proton pump inhibitors is not only unnecessary but also unlikely to work.[24]

Clinically significant gastric ulcers can occur in the squamous, glandular, or both portions of the stomach as a primary problem or the result of another problem. Clinical signs include diarrhea, abdominal pain, restlessness, rolling, lying in dorsal recumbency, excessive salivation, and bruxism. In the neonatal foal the only clinical signs present may be depression or partial anorexia until a more catastrophic event, such as perforation, occurs. Some lesions in the gastric mucosa extend from the pylorus into the proximal duodenum and can result in stricture of the pylorus and proximal duodenum. These foals usually are older (>1 month of age) and have a greater volume of reflux. Bruxism and ptyalism also are more prominent in these older foals.

The most sensitive and specific method for diagnosing gastric ulcers is visualization by endoscopic examination.[12] Unfortunately, the use of gastric endoscopy has led to recognition of relative nonlesions and ulcers resulting from other problems and of clinically significant disease states. The clinician should not stop simply when ulceration of the stomach is recognized with endoscopy but should examine that patient fully for other potential sources of the clinical signs. Other diagnostic tests may help in determining the severity of the ulcers, including fecal occult blood or gastric blood assessments, contrast radiography, abdominal ultrasound, and abdominocentesis. Endoscopy of the foal stomach carries an additional risk of exacerbating colic in the short term, unless the examiner ensures that as much introduced air as possible is evacuated from the stomach at the end of the procedure.

The presence of a brown gastric reflux fluid may indicate the presence of bleeding ulcers or necrotizing enterocolitis. Blood in the feces of the neonate is more consistent with a diagnosis of necrotizing enterocolitis, which can be associated with gastric ulcers. Contrast radiography is useful if one suspects delayed gastric emptying or pyloric or duodenal stricture in older foals. If a stricture has occurred, a delay in complete emptying of barium from the stomach (>2 hours) will be apparent.[14] Abdominal ultrasound may be useful to visualize free abdominal fluid and gastric or small intestinal distention if a perforation is suspected. Portions of the descending duodenum can be visualized, and a thickened duodenum should increase the index of suspicion for duodenal stricture. Abdominocentesis also may confirm perforation.

Traditional therapy for gastric ulceration includes mucosal adherents, histamine type 2 receptor antagonists, proton pump inhibitors, and antacids.[25] The most widely used mucosal adherent is sucralfate, which is a hydroxy aluminum salt of sucrose. The main therapeutic action of sucralfate is to bind to the negatively charged particles in the ulcer crater.[25,26] At a pH less than 2, sucralfate is converted to a sticky viscous gel, which adheres to the ulcer crater and remains adhered for 6 hours, but at a higher pH sucralfate remains in a suspension. Sucralfate is still effective because it inhibits pepsin and buffers hydrogen ions. Other important actions of sucralfate include stimulating production of prostaglandin E, which maintains mucosal blood flow; increasing bicarbonate secretion; stimulating mucus secretion; decreasing peptic activity; and binding epidermal growth factor. The histamine type 2 receptor antagonists include cimetidine, ranitidine, and famotidine. These compounds block the interaction of histamine with the histamine type 2 receptor on the parietal cell, resulting in inhibition of gastric acid secretion. Clinically normal neonatal foals have a highly acidic gastric fluid that is influenced by sucking. Intravenous and oral administration of ranitidine increases intragastric pH in normal foals, but critically ill neonatal foals have a blunted response to ranitidine administration.[24,27] One possible conclusion reached from these studies is that in critically ill neonatal foals, gastric ulcers may not be caused by an increased intraluminal gastric acidity.

The most commonly used proton pump inhibitor is omeprazole. Omeprazole inhibits the secretion of hydrogen ions at the parietal cell by irreversibly binding to the H^+,K^+-ATPase proton pump of the cell. Most of the lesions in older foals were healed after daily administration of omeprazole for 28 days.[28] Omeprazole effectively increases intragastric pH in normal neonatal foals and in ill neonatal foals that have decreased pH before treatment, suggesting a functionally intact gastric mucosa in those foals.[29,30] The efficacy of omeprazole in treating very ill foals without the ability to generate gastric acid has not been demonstrated, but it is likely similar to that of ranitidine in critically ill foals.[27] Table 21-10 summarizes the therapeutic agents for treating gastric ulcers in foals.

Prophylactic treatment of critically ill neonates for gastric ulcers has been standard therapy for years because of the evidence of clinically silent ulcers. This approach may not be appropriate for several reasons. An increased incidence of nosocomial pneumonia and systemic sepsis is associated with high gastric pH in human patients in intensive care.[31-33] Patients in intensive care units treated prophylactically with histamine type 2 receptor antagonists are more likely to develop pneumonia during ventilation therapy and gastric colonization with potentially pathogenic bacteria or yeast.[31,34] An acidic environment appears to protect against airway colonization by bacteria of intestinal origin and bacteria translocated across the gastrointestinal tract. Pathogenesis of ulcers in the neonatal foal most likely does not involve increased intraluminal gastric acid but instead may be caused by decreased mucosal perfusion associated with shock, hypoxia, and hypoxic-ischemic insult to the gastric mucosa. One report revealed that gastric ulcer disease in equine NICU patients is independent of pharmacologic prophylaxis.[35] In this study the incidence of gastric ulcers found in these foals at necropsy had decreased significantly despite decreased treatment. The decrease was attributed to overall improvement in management of these cases. Similarly, in a human intensive care unit, the incidence of stress ulcers decreased independent of the use of prophylaxis.[22,36] Early treatment of sepsis, sufficient oxygenation, improved monitoring, institution of enteral feedings, and improved nursing care may contribute to the reduction in gastric ulcers in the neonatal patient. Use of histamine type 2 receptor antagonist and proton pump inhibitors apparently may not be necessary; however, in some instances sucralfate may be useful. Sucralfate reduced the rate of bacterial translocation in a rat model during hemorrhagic shock and also may prohibit the generation of acute gastric mucosal injury and progression to ulcer formation induced by ischemia-reperfusion.[37,38] In a human medical intensive care unit, airway colonization by new pathogens occurred more frequently in patients receiving agents that increased gastric pH than in those receiving sucralfate.[31,39] In the critically ill neonatal foal, risk factors for gastric ulceration

TABLE 21-10

Therapeutic Agents for Treating Gastric Ulcers in Foals

Drug Category	Drug	Dose	Route	Frequency
Mucosal protectant	Sucralfate	10-20 mg/kg	Oral	t.i.d. to q.i.d.
Histamine type 2	Cimetidine	10-20 mg/kg	Oral	every 4 hr
receptor antagonist	Ranitidine	6.6 mg/kg	IV*	every 4 hr
		5-10 mg/kg	Oral	b.i.d. to q.i.d.
		0.8-2.2mg/kg	IV	q.i.d.
Proton pump inhibitor	Omeprazole	4 mg/kg	Oral	s.i.d.
		1-2 mg/kg	Oral	s.i.d. (prophylaxis)
Antacids	Milk of Magnesia	2-4 oz	Oral	s.i.d. to b.i.d.
	Maalox	240 ml	Oral	every 4 hr

Adapted from Wilkins PA, Palmer JE, editors: *Recent advances in equine neonatal care,* Ithaca, NY, 2001, International Veterinary Information Service (A0413.1101).
**t.i.d.,* Three times daily; *q.i.d.,* four times daily; *IV,* intravenous; *b.i.d.,* twice daily; *s.i.d.,* once daily.

have not been identified clearly, although foals treated routinely with nonsteroidal anti-inflammatory drugs may be at increased risk for gastric lesions. Prophylactic treatment for gastric ulcers in critically ill neonates may not be necessary, and the clinician should consider carefully the pros and cons of their use before their administration.

DIARRHEAL DISEASES OF FOALS

Pamela A. Wilkins

FOAL HEAT DIARRHEA

Foal heat diarrhea is a mild, self-limiting form of diarrhea that occurs in foals between 5 and 14 days of age, about the time of the "foal heat" in the dam. The definitive cause of foal heat diarrhea has yet to be described, but the condition may be associated with dietary changes or changes in gastrointestinal function that occur around that time. This form of diarrhea is not caused by *Stongyloides westeri* infestation, as previously postulated.[1] Foals with foal heat diarrhea are not systemically ill and should not require therapy. Any foals with diarrhea should be evaluated fully at this time for other possible causes of diarrhea, particularly if they are unwell or exhibit anorexia or dehydration.

VIRAL DIARRHEA

Viral diarrhea usually occurs in large groups of mares and foals that are housed together. Rotavirus is an isolate from the feces of up to 40% of foals with diarrhea worldwide, alone or with another pathogen.[2,3] The virus infects and denudes the microvilli, resulting in increased secretion combined with decreased absorption. The virus interferes with disaccharidase function and alters the function of the intestinal sodium-glucose co-transport proteins. The initial clinical signs are anorexia and depression, with profuse watery diarrhea occurring shortly thereafter. Severely affected foals may become significantly dehydrated and have electrolyte abnormalities, primarily hyponatremia and hypochloremia with metabolic acidosis. These foals generally require intravenous fluid support, whereas less severely affected foals may require only symptomatic therapy. However, none of the available tests are particularly sensitive, and the virus also may be found with other intestinal pathogens. Definitive diagnosis is by detection of the virus in the feces of foals with diarrhea. Vaccination of pregnant mares has been suggested as a means of prevention, with preliminary results suggesting efficacy.[4,5] Although a definitive role for adenovirus has not been established in the foal, adenovirus is a common co-isolate from foals with rotaviral diarrhea.[6] An equine coronavirus has been isolated from an immunocompetent foal with diarrhea, and a second report of cornavirus diarrhea was published recently.[7,8] One case report suggests that a parvovirus caused diarrhea in the foal.[9]

Treatment of viral diarrhea in foals is primarily supportive. Intravenous fluid and parenteral nutritional support may be necessary in severe cases. Very young foals may benefit from intravenous plasma administration and broad spectrum antimicrobial coverage to limit bacterial translocation. Sucralfate can be administered orally in these cases as a gastrointestinal protectant and to discourage bacterial translocation. Foals with moderate to severe metabolic acidosis may benefit from sodium bicarbonate administration if their ventilatory function is normal. Nonspecific therapy of diarrhea is discussed elsewhere in this text.

BACTERIAL DIARRHEA

Because diarrhea frequently is the primary presenting complaint in foals with sepsis, this differential diagnosis should be ruled out in foals younger than 1 week of age. All neonatal foals with diarrhea should be evaluated for possible sepsis, and a blood culture should be included whenever possible.

C. perfringens and *C. difficile* are recognized increasingly as serious pathogens of the foal.[10-13] Foals with either pathogen generally have abdominal pain, dehydration, and profuse watery diarrhea. Some foals may have red-tinged or frankly bloody feces, which carries a poorer prognosis. Most foals with this type of diarrhea require intensive care or, at the minimum, intravenous fluid administration. Outbreaks of this type of diarrhea on farms occasionally occur, and the dam may have a role in transmission of the bacteria. Diagnosis is by recognition of the offending organism by Gram stain of the feces, by bacterial isolation from the feces, and by the presence of toxins associated with the organisms. Specific treatment includes oral administration of metronidazole and broad spectrum antimicrobial coverage as prophylaxis for bacterial translocation–associated sepsis in younger foals. Foals with severe blood loss in their feces may require transfusion of whole blood.

Salmonella spp., *Escherichia coli, Bacteroides fragilis,* and *Aeromonas hydrophila* have been implicated in diarrhea in foals. *Salmonella* organisms generally are associated with septicemia in foals, and although some convincing evidence exists for a role for *E. coli* in foal diarrheal disease, the extent of *E. coli* as a pathogen of the gastrointestinal tract in foals has yet to be described fully.[14-18] Approximately 50% of foals presenting with a complaint of diarrhea of any etiology will be bacteremic at the time of initial examination.[19]

Proliferative enteropathy is a transmissible enteric disease caused by *Lawsonia intracellulare*.[20,21] Most foals have been weaned before the appearance of clinical signs of depression, rapid and significant weight loss, subcutaneous edema, diarrhea, and colic. Poor body condition with a rough hair coat and a potbellied appearance are common in affected foals. Clinicopathologic abnormalities included hypoproteinemia, leukocytosis, anemia, and increased serum creatine kinase concentration. Postmortem examination reveals characteristic intracellular bacteria within the apical cytoplasm of proliferating crypt epithelial cells of the intestinal mucosa. Antemortem diagnosis of equine proliferative enteropathy is based on clinical signs, hypoproteinemia, and the exclusion of other common enteric pathogens. Fecal PCR analysis may be positive for the presence of *L. intracellulare,* and affected foals develop antibodies against *L. intracellulare*.[22] Treatment with erythromycin estolate alone or combined with rifampin for a minimum of 21 days is recommended, with additional symptomatic treatment when indicated.

PROTOZOAL DIARRHEA

Cryptosporidium spp. cause gastroenteritis and diarrhea in many animal species and are not host-specific. *Cryptosporidium* has been implicated as the causal agent of diarrhea in foals, but the organism is isolated from the feces of diarrheic foals and normal foals with the same frequency and concentration, making a clear role for the organism difficult to elucidate.[23-25] Diarrhea caused by *Cryptosporidium* in other species and that described for foals is generally self-limiting, with a clinical course of between 5 and 14 days. Immunosuppressed patients, including foals compromised by concurrent disease, are thought to be at increased risk for complications resulting from infection with this organism.[23,24] Treatment is symptomatic. Cryptosporidiosis is a disease with zoonotic potential, and appropriate precautions, including use of gloves and frequent hand washing, are necessary if organisms are identified in the feces of any patients so as to prevent spread to other patients and personnel. *Eimeria leukarti, Trichomonas equi,* and *Giardia equi* have been identified in the feces of normal horses and horses with diarrhea. Transmission studies have failed to produce reliable clinical signs, and the prevalence and significance of these organisms in the genesis of foal diarrhea remain unknown.

PARASITIC DIARRHEA

Strongyloides westeri is a common parasitic infection of foals.[2,26,27] Transmission is transmammary, and patent infection is recognizable in the foal by 8 to 12 days of age. This nematode previously was associated anecdotally with foal heat diarrhea, but the association has not been demonstrated clearly. The diarrhea is generally mild and is treated effectively by deworming with benzimidazole or ivermectin anthelmintics.[1]

Strongylus vulgaris fourth-stage larvae cause diarrhea in young foals during migration through the arterioles of the cecum and descending colon. Clinical signs may resemble those of thromboembolic colic.[26,27] The prepatent period is about 6 months, and diagnosis is based on clinical examination, clinicopathologic changes, and farm deworming history. Patients with diarrhea associated with this parasite may have peripheral leukocytosis, neutrophilia, eosinophilia, and hypoproteinemia. Appropriate deworming with ivermectin (label dose), fenbendazole (10 mg/kg/day orally for 5 days), or thiabendazole (440 mg/kg/day orally for 2 days) is recommended, with the last two drug dosages being larger than the label dose. Cyathostomiasis, or diarrhea resulting from the sudden emergence of encysted cyathostome larvae, is an unusual cause of diarrhea in the foal.

NEONATE THERAPY

Pamela A. Wilkins

FLUID THERAPY IN NEONATES

The clinician managing critically ill neonates must recognize that intravenous fluid therapy simply cannot be scaled down from adult management approaches. Fluid management of the ill neonate, particularly over the first few days of life, must take into consideration that the neonate is undergoing a large transition from the fetal to the neonatal state and that important physiologic changes are taking place.[1] These transitions include shifts in renal handling of free water and sodium and increased insensible losses because of evaporation from the body surface area and the respiratory tract. The newborn kidney has a limited ability to excrete excess free water and sodium, and the barrier between the vascular and interstitial space is more porous than that of adults. Water and sodium overload, particularly in the first few days of life, can have disastrous long-term consequences for the neonate.[2-4] In the ill equine neonate, excess fluid administration frequently manifests as generalized edema formation and excessive weight gain, frequently equivalent to the volume of excess fluid administered intravenously. In cases in which antidiuretic hormone secretion is inappropriate, as in some foals with PAS, generalized edema may not form, but the excess free water is maintained in the vascular space. This syndrome of inappropriate antidiuretic hormone secretion is recognized in the foal that gains excessive weight not manifested as edema generally, with decreased urine output and electrolyte abnormalities such as hyponatremia and hypochloremia.[5] The foal manifests neurologic abnormalities associated with hyponatremia. The plasma or serum creatinine concentration varies in these cases, but urine always is concentrated compared with the normally dilute, copious amounts of urine produced by foals more than

24 hours of age on a milk diet. If measured, serum osmolarity is less than urine osmolarity. The treatment for this disorder is fluid restriction until weight loss occurs, electrolyte abnormalities normalize, and urine concentration decreases. If unaware of this differential diagnosis, the clinician may assume mistakenly that the neonate is in renal failure, and the condition can be exacerbated by excessive intravenous fluid administration in an attempt to produce diuresis.

The problem of appropriate fluid management in critically ill neonates has been recognized by medical physicians for years and has resulted in changes in fluid management of these patients. The approach taken has been one of fluid restriction, in particular sodium restriction but also free water restriction, and has resulted in improved outcome and fewer complications, such as patent ductus arteriosus and necrotizing enterocolitis.[4,5] The calculations used for maintenance intravenous fluid support in these patients take into consideration the ratio of surface area to volume and partially compensates for insensible water losses. Maintenance fluids are provided as 5% dextrose to limit sodium overload and provide sufficient free water to restore intracellular and interstitial requirements. The calculation for maintenance fluid administration is shown in Table 21-11.[6]

As an example, the average 50-kg foal would receive 1000 ml/day for the first 10 kg of body mass, 500 ml/day for the next 10 kg of body mass, and 750 ml/day for the remaining 30 kg of body mass for a total of 2250 ml/day. This translates to an hourly fluid rate of about 94 ml/hr.

One should adjust the fluid and sodium requirements for ongoing losses exceeding the maintenance requirements. These losses can take the form of diarrheal losses and excessive urine output, such as those with glucose diuresis and renal damage resulting in an increased fractional excretion of sodium. The normal fractional excretion of sodium in neonatal foals is less than that of adult horses, usually less than 1%.[7] In the critically ill foal, the sodium requirement can be met with as little as 140 mEq of sodium per day, less than administered in a single liter of normal equine plasma. Sodium deficits can be addressed by separate infusion of sodium-containing fluids, although this may not be necessary if one considers the sodium being administered in other forms, including drugs administered as sodium salts and any constant-rate infusions (e.g., pressors, inotropes) that are being provided as solutions made with 0.9% sodium chloride.

The author has used this approach to fluid therapy for the last few years and believes that the percentage of foals suffering from generalized edema—and related problems—has decreased. If one takes this approach to fluid therapy, the weight of the patient should be taken once, or even twice, daily, and fluid intake and output should be monitored as closely as is practical. Any weight gains or losses that are larger than anticipated should be evaluated. Urine output should not be expected to approach the reported normal of 300 ml/hr for a 50-kg foal because the free water administered is limited, unless the patient is experiencing diuresis (glucosuria, resolution of the syndrome of inappropriate antidiuretic hormone secretion, resolution of previous edematous state, renal disease). The urine specific gravity should be obtained several times daily and the fractional excretion of sodium determined at regular intervals. If the volume of urine produced by the patient is measured accurately, the clinician can determine sodium losses accurately and obtain creatinine clearance values. Blood pressure measurements should be obtained at regular intervals throughout the day because hypotension can be a problem in these patients, particularly in septic foals and foals suffering from PAS, and it may be necessary to increase fluid therapy to maintain adequate vascular volume. Patients with hypotension may require inotrope and pressor support.

TABLE 21-11

Calculations for Maintenance Fluid Administration

Body Mass	Amount of fluid
First 10 kg body mass	100 ml/kg/day
Second 10 kg body mass	50 ml/kg/day
All additional kilograms of body mass	25 ml/kg/day

PRESSOR AND INOTROPE THERAPY IN NEONATES

Inotrope and pressor therapy generally is restricted to referral centers, where these drugs can be administered as constant-rate infusions and blood pressure can be monitored closely. Blood pressure can be monitored directly or indirectly by the use of cuffs placed on the base of the tail.[8] Both techniques have advantages and disadvantages. Although direct blood pressure measurements are considered the gold standard and are generally more accurate, the difficulty in placing and maintaining arterial catheters and lines in these patients severely restricts the utility of this method. Indirect techniques can be inaccurate and are affected by cuff size and placement. However, indirect techniques are easier to use in the NICU and can be useful if trained staff are using the equipment. Once the appropriate cuff size has been identified, that cuff should be dedicated to that patient for the duration of the hospitalization to decrease variability caused by use of different cuffs. The blood pressure of all recumbent patients should be monitored at regular intervals, and trends upward or downward should prompt the clinician to make necessary adjustments.

Foals suffering from PAS and sepsis are the patients most at risk for significant hypotension and perfusion abnormalities.[9-11] Perfusion is maintained by supporting cardiac output and blood pressure with judicious use of intravenous fluid support and inotrope-pressor support. The author does not aim for any specific target systolic, mean, or diastolic pressure. Instead, the author monitors urine output, mentation, limb perfusion, gastrointestinal function, and respiratory function as indicators that perfusion is acceptable. For NICU patients to require inotrope and pressor therapy is not unusual, but in some cases hypoxic and septic damage is sufficiently severe to blunt the response of the patient to the drugs. Each patient must be approached as an individual, and no single inotrope-pressor protocol will suffice for all patients.

Dobutamine is a β-adrenergic inotrope that is frequently used as first-choice therapy in NICU patients. Its effects are β_1 at the lower dose range. Neonates have a limited ability to increase stroke volume in an effort to maintain cardiac output, and tachycardia may be observed in these patients as heart rate increases to maintain cardiac output and vascular pressure. Dobutamine is useful after patients are volume replete for support of cardiac output. The dose range is between 2 to 20 μg/kg/min, provided as a constant-rate infusion, with best results generally obtained between 2 and 5 μg/kg/min. If larger doses are needed, a better approach might be to add a pressor to the treatment plan.

Dopamine has dopaminergic activity at low doses, β_1 and β_2 activity at moderate doses, and α_1 activity at high doses. Dopamine causes norepinephrine release, which has led to the suggestion that this is its major mode of action at higher doses. At doses greater than 20 μg/kg/min, intrapulmonary shunting, pulmonary venous vasoconstriction, and reduced splanchic perfusion may occur. Dopamine also produces natriuresis at lower doses through a direct effect on renal tubules. For these reasons dopamine has fallen out of favor in human critical care and at many veterinary referral institutions.[12,13]

Norepinephrine has α_1 and β_1 activity but variable β_2 activity, resulting in potent vasopressor effects; it has inotropic and chronotropic effects, but its chronotropic effect usually is blunted by vagal reflexes slowing the heart rate induced by the increase in blood pressure. In many critical care units, norepinephrine has become a pressor of choice and frequently is used along with dobutamine. Evidence suggests that splanchic perfusion is maintained better with norepinephrine than with some other pressors, and norepinephrine is frequently paired with dobutamine.[14] The dose range is 0.2 to 2.0 μg/kg/min, although larger doses have been used when necessary in certain patients.

Epinephrine has α_1, α_2, β_1, and β_2 activity; β activity predominates and results in increased cardiac output and decreased peripheral resistance at low doses. Epinephrine has been associated with hyperglycemia, hypokalemia, lipolysis, increased lactate concentration, and increased platelet aggregation. The effect on renal function is controversial. Use of epinephrine usually is limited to those patients not responding to other pressors.

Vasopressin (antidiuretic hormone) is a pressor gaining a great deal of attention in the critical care literature.[15-18] Vasopressin appears to be depleted from the neurohypophysis in septic shock,[16] and short-term administration of vasopressin spares conventional vasopressor use, in addition to improving some measures of renal function.[17] Low-dose vasopressin infusion (0.5-2.0 mU/kg/min) increases mean arterial pressure, systemic vascular resistance, and urine output in patients with vasodilatory septic shock that are hyporesponsive to catecholamines. These data indicate that low-dose vasopressin infusions may be useful in treating hypotension in patients with septic shock.[18] The author has been using low-dose vasopressin in patients in her NICU for the past few years and has the clinical impression that blood pressure is defended more readily using this agent in concert with other management strategies. The author will use low-dose vasopressin constant-rate infusion with dobutamine constant-rate infusion as an initial inotrope-pressor therapy in cases requiring pressure defense, although no prospective studies are available regarding this drug in veterinary medicine.

REFERENCES

Neonatal and Perinatal Diseases

1. Rossdale PD: Clinical studies on 4 newborn thoroughbred foals suffering from convulsions with special reference to blood gas chemistry and pulmonary ventilation, *Res Vet Sci* 10(3): 279–291, 1969.
2. Rossdale PD, Pattle RE, Mahaffey LW: Respiratory distress in a newborn foal with failure to form lung lining film, *Nature* 215(109):1498–1499, 1967.
3. Rossdale PD: Clinical studies on the newborn thoroughbred foal. 2. Heart rate, auscultation and electrocardiogram, *Br Vet J* 123(12):521–532, 1967.
4. Rossdale PD: Blood gas tensions and pH values in the normal thoroughbred foal at birth and in the following 42h, *Biol Neonat* 13(1):18–25, 1968.
5. Rossdale PD: Measurements of pulmonary ventilation in normal newborn thoroughbred foals during the first three days of life, *Br Vet J* 125(4):157–161, 1969.
6. Rossdale PD: Some parameters of respiratory function in normal and abnormal newborn foals with special reference to levels of paO2 during air and oxygen inhalation, *Res Vet Sci* 11(3):270–276, 1970.
7. Rossdale PD: Modern concepts of neonatal disease in foals, *Equine Vet J* 4(3):117–128, 1972.
8. Nathanielsz PW, Rossdale PD, Silver M, et al: Studies on fetal, neonatal and maternal cortisol metabolism in the mare, *J Reprod Fertil Suppl* 23:625–630, 1975.
9. Arvidson G, Astedt B, Ekelund L, et al: Surfactant studies in the fetal and neonatal foal, *J Reprod Fertil Suppl* 23:663–665, 1975.
10. Palmer AC, Rossdale PD: Neuropathology of the convulsive foal syndrome, *J Reprod Fertil Suppl* 23:691–694, 1975.
11. Kitchen H, Rossdale PD: Metabolic profiles of newborn foals, *J Reprod Fertil Suppl* 23:705–707, 1975.
12. Palmer AC, Rossdale PD: Neuropathological changes associated with the neonatal maladjustment syndrome in the thoroughbred foal, *Res Vet Sci* 20(3):267–275, 1976.
13. Rose RJ, Rossdale PD, Leadon DP: Blood gas and acid-base status in spontaneously delivered, term-induced and induced premature foals, *J Reprod Fertil Suppl* 32:521–528, 1982.
14. Rossdale PD, Ousey JC, Dudan FE, et al: Studies on equine prematurity. 1. Methodology, *Equine Vet J* 16(4):275–278, 1984.
15. Kosch PC, Koterba AM, Coons TJ, et al: Developments in management of the newborn foal in respiratory distress. 1. Evaluation, *Equine Vet J* 16(4):312–318, 1984.
16. Koterba AM, Brewer BD, Tarplee FA: Clinical and clinicopathological characteristics of the septicaemic neonatal foal: review of 38 cases, *Equine Vet J* 16(4):376–382, 1984.
17. Koterba AM, Drummond WH, Kosch P: Intensive care of the neonatal foal, *Vet Clin North Am Equine Pract* 1(1):3–34, 1985.
18. Koterba AM, Drummond WH: Nutritional support of the foal during intensive care, *Vet Clin North Am Equine Pract* 1(1): 35–40, 1985.
19. Brewer BD, Koterba AM, Carter RL, et al: Comparison of empirically developed sepsis score with a computer generated and weighted scoring system for the identification of sepsis in the equine neonate, *Equine Vet J* 20(1):23–24, 1988.
20. Baker SM, Drummond WH, Lane TJ, et al: Follow-up evaluation of horses after neonatal intensive care, *J Am Vet Med Assoc* 189(11):1454–1457, 1986.
21. Axon J, Palmer J, Wilkins PA: Short-term and long-term athletic outcome of neonatal intensive care unit survivors, *Proc Am Assoc Equine Pract* 45:224–225, 1999.
22. Freeman L, Paradis MR: Evaluating the effectiveness of equine neonatal intensive care, *Vet Med* 87:921–926, Sept 1992.
23. Lester GD: Short and long term evaluation of neonatal intensive care. In *Proceedings of the fourteenth annual meeting of the American College of Veterinary Internal Medicine*, San Antonio, 1996, Tex, pp 547–548.
24. LeBlanc MM: Identification and treatment of the compromised equine fetus: a clinical perspective, *Equine Vet J Suppl* 24:100–103, 1997.
25. Donahue JM, Williams NM: Emergent causes of placentitis and abortion, *Vet Clin North Am Equine Pract* 16(3):443–456, 2000.
26. Janosi S, Huszenicza G, Kulcsar M, et al: Endocrine and reproductive consequences of certain endotoxin-mediated diseases in farm mammals: a review, *Acta Vet Hung* 46(1):71–84, 1998.

27. Del Piero F: Equine viral arteriti, *Vet Pathol* 37(4):287–296, 2000.
28. Vaala WE, Sertich PL: Management strategies for mares at risk for periparturient complications, *Vet Clin North Am Equine Pract* 10(1):237–265, 1994.
29. Putnam MR, Bransby DI, Schumacher J, et al: Effects of the fungal endophyte Acremonium coenophialum in fescue on pregnant mares and foal viability, *Am J Vet Res* 52(12): 2071–2074, 1991.
30. Redmond LM, Cross DL, Strickland JR, et al: Efficacy of domperidone and sulpiride as treatments for fescue toxicosis in horses, *Am J Vet Res* 55(5):722–729, 1994.
31. Kahn W, Leidl W: [Ultrasonic biometry of horse fetuses in utero and sonographic representation of their organs], *Dtsch Tierarztl Wochenschr* 94(9):509–515, 1987.
32. Adams-Brendemuehl C, Pipers FS: Antepartum evaluations of the equine fetus, *J Reprod Fertil Suppl* 35:565–573, 1987.
33. Reef VB, editor: *Equine diagnostic ultrasound*, Philadelphia, 1998, Saunders.
34. Buss DD, Asbury AC, Chevalier L: Limitations in equine fetal electrocardiography, *Am Vet Med Assoc* 177(2):174–176, 1980.
35. Jensen A, Garnier Y, Berger R: Dynamics of fetal circulatory responses to hypoxia and asphyxia, *Eur J Obstet Gynecol Reprod Biol* 84(2):155–172, 1999.
36. Cohn HE, Piasecki GJ, Jackson BT: The effect of fetal heart rate on cardiovascular function during hypoxemia, *Am J Obstet Gynecol* 138(8):1190–1199, 1980.
37. Leadon DP, Jeffcott LB, Rossdale PD: Mammary secretions in normal spontaneous and induced premature parturition in the mare, *Equine Vet J* 16(4):256–259, 1984.
38. Ousey JC, Delclaux M, Rossdale PD: Evaluation of three strip tests for measuring electrolytes in mares' pre-partum mammary secretions and for predicting parturition, *Equine Vet J* 21(3):196–200, 1989.
39. Williams MA, Goyert NA, Goyert GL, et al: Preliminary report of transabdominal amniocentesis for the determination of pulmonary maturity in an equine population, *Equine Vet J* 20(6):457–458, 1988.
40. Williams MA, Schmidt AR, Carleton CL, et al: Amniotic fluid analysis for ante-partum foetal assessment in the horse, *Equine Vet J* 24(3):236–238, 1992.
41. Schmidt AR, Williams MA, Carleton CL, et al: Evaluation of transabdominal ultrasound-guided amniocentesis in the late gestational mare, *Equine Vet J* 23(4):261–265, 1991.
42. Cottrill CM, Jeffers-Lo J, Ousey JC, et al: The placenta as a determinant of fetal well-being in normal and abnormal equine pregnancies, *J Reprod Fertil Suppl* 44:591–601, 1991.
43. Giles RC, Donahue JM, Hong CB, et al: Causes of abortion, stillbirth, and perinatal death in horses: 3,527 cases (1986-1991), *J Am Vet Med Assoc* 203(8):1170–1175, 1993.
44. Daels PF, Stabenfeldt GH, Hughes JP, et al: Evaluation of progesterone deficiency as a cause of fetal death in mares with experimentally induced endotoxemia, *Am J Vet Res* 52(2): 282–288, 1991.
45. McKinnon AO, Lescun TB, Walker JH, et al: The inability of some synthetic progestagens to maintain pregnancy in the mare, *Equine Vet J* 32(1):83–85, 2000.
46. Gastal MO, Gastal EL, Torres CA, et al: Effect of oxytocin, prostaglandin F_2 alpha, and clenbuterol on uterine dynamics in mares, *Theriogenology* 50(4):521–534, 1998.
47. Niebyl JR, Johnson JW: Inhibition of preterm labor, *Clin Obstet Gynecol* 23(1):115–126, 1980.
48. Harkins JD, Mundy GD, Stanley S, et al: Absence of detectable pharmacological effects after oral administration of isoxsuprine, *Equine Vet J* 30(4):294–299, 1998.
49. Wilkins PA, Seahorn TL: Intranasal oxygen therapy in adult horses, *J Vet Emerg Crit Care* 10(3):221, 2000.
50. Wilson DV, Schott HC, Robinson NE, et al: Response to nasopharyngeal oxygen administration in horses with lung disease, *Equine Vet J* 38(3):219–223, 2006.
51. Samuel CA, Allen WR, Steven DH: Studies on the equine placenta. 1. Development of the microcotyledons, *J Reprod Fertil* 41(2):441–445, 1974.
52. Bjorkman N: Fine structure of the fetal-maternal area of exchange in the epitheliochorial and endotheliochorial types of placentation, *Acta Anat Suppl (Basel)* 61:1–22, 1973.
53. Comline RS, Silver M: pO2 levels in the placental circulation of the mare and ewe, *Nature* 217(123):76–77, 1968.
54. Silver M, Comline RS: Fetal and placental O_2 consumption and the uptake of different metabolites in the ruminant and horse during late gestation, *Adv Exp Med Biol* 75:731–736, 1976.
55. Fowden AL, Forhead AJ, White KL, et al: Equine uteroplacental metabolism at mid- and late gestation, *Exp Physiol* 85(5): 539–545, 2000.
56. Inci S, Ozcan OE, Kilinc K: Time-level relationship for lipid peroxidation and the protective effect of alpha-tocopherol in experimental mild and severe brain injury, *Neurosurgery* 43(2):330–335, 1998.
57. Clifton GL, Lyeth BG, Jenkins LW, et al: Effect of D, alpha-tocopheryl succinate and polyethylene glycol on performance tests after fluid percussion brain injury, *J Neurotrauma* 6(2): 71–81, 1989.
58. Daneyemez M, Kurt E, Cosar A, et al: Methylprednisolone and vitamin E therapy in perinatal hypoxic-ischemic brain damage in rats, *Neuroscience* 92(2):693–697, 1999.
59. Fowden AL, Ralph MM, Silver M: Nutritional regulation of uteroplacental prostaglandin production and metabolism in pregnant ewes and mares during late gestation, *Exp Clin Endocrinol* 102(3):212–221, 1994.
60. Freeman DE, Hungerford LL, Schaeffer D, et al: Caesarean section and other methods for assisted delivery: comparison of effects on mare mortality and complications, *Equine Vet J* 31(3):203–207, 1999.
61. Norton JL, Dallap BL, Johnston JK, et al: Retrospective study of dystocia in mares at a referral hospital, *Equine Vet J* 39(1): 37–41, 2007.

Evaluation of the Newborn Foal

1. Jain L: Alveolar fluid clearance in developing lungs and its role in neonatal transition, *Clin Perinatol* 26(3):585–599, 1999.
2. Folkesson HG, Norlin A, Baines DL: Salt and water transport across the alveolar epithelium in the developing lung: correlations between function and recent molecular biology advances, *Int J Mol Med* 2(5):515–531, 1998:review.
3. Dukarm RC, Steinhorn RH, Morin FC 3rd: The normal pulmonary vascular transition at birth, *Clin Perinatol* 23(4):711–726, 1996.
4. Tessier GJ, Lester GD, Langham MR, et al: Ion transport properties of fetal sheep alveolar epithelial cells in monolayer culture, *Am J Physiol* 270(6 pt 1):L1008–L1016, 1996.
5. Lakshminrusimha S, Steinhorn RH: Pulmonary vascular biology during neonatal transition, *Clin Perinatol* 26(3):601–619, 1999.
6. Shaul PW: Regulation of vasodilator synthesis during lung development, *Early Hum Dev* 54(3):271–294, 1999.
7. Steinhorn RH, Millard SL, Morin FC 3rd: Persistent pulmonary hypertension of the newborn: role of nitric oxide and endothelin in pathophysiology and treatment, *Clin Perinatol* 22(2):405–428, 1995.
8. Rossdale PD: Clinical studies on the newborn thoroughbred foal. 1. Perinatal behavior, *Br Vet J* 123(11):470–481, 1967.
9. Rossdale PD: The adaptive processes of the newborn foal, *Vet Rec* 87(2):37–38, 1970.
10. Lombard CW, Evans M, Martin L, et al: Blood pressure, electrocardiogram and echocardiogram measurements in the growing pony foal, *Equine Vet J* 16(4):342–347, 1984.
11. Yamamoto K, Yasuda J, Too K: Arrhythmias in newborn Thoroughbred foals, *Equine Vet J* 23(3):169–173, 1992.

12. Silver M, Comline RS: Transfer of gases and metabolites in the equine placenta: a comparison with other species, *J Reprod Fertil Suppl* 23:589–594, 1975.
13. Comline RS, Silver M: A comparative study of blood gas tensions, oxygen affinity and red cell 2,3 DPG concentrations in foetal and maternal blood in the mare, cow and sow, *J Physiol* 242(3):805–826, 1974.
14. Werner EJ: Neonatal polycythemia and hyperviscosity, *Clin Perinatol* 22(3):693–710, 1995.
15. Ousey JC: Thermoregulation and the energy requirement of the newborn foal, with reference to prematurity, *Equine Vet J Suppl* 24:104–108, 1997.
16. Van der Velden MA: Ruptured inguinal hernia in new-born colt foals: a review of 14 cases, *Equine Vet J* 20(3):178–181, 1988.
17. Fintl C, Pearson GT, Rickets SW, et al: The development and distribution of the interstitial cells of Cajal in the intestine of the equine fetus and neonate, *J Anat* 205:35–44, 2004.
18. Brewer BD, Clement SF, Lotz WS, et al: A comparison of inulin, paraaminohippuric acid, and endogenous creatinine clearances as measures of renal function in neonatal foals, *J Vet Intern Med* 4(6):301–305, 1990.
19. Jesty SA, Palmer JE, Parente EJ, et al: Rupture of the gastrocnemius muscle in six foals, *Journal of the American Veterinary Medical Association* 227(12):1965–1968, 2005.
20. Nathanielsz PW, Rossdale PD, Silver M, et al: Studies on fetal, neonatal and maternal cortisol metabolism in the mare, *J Reprod Fertil Suppl* 23:625–630, 1975.
21. Brewer BD, Koterba AM, Carter RL, et al: Comparison of empirically developed sepsis score with a computer generated and weighted scoring system for the identification of sepsis in the equine neonate, *Equine Vet J* 20(1):23–24, 1988.
22. Adams R, Mayhew IG: Neurological examination of newborn foals, *Equine Vet J* 16(4):306–312, 1984.
23. Crowell-Davis SL, Houpt KA: Maternal behavior, *Vet Clinic North Am Equine Pract* 2(3):557–571, 1986.

Neonatal Resuscitation

1. Martens RJ: Pediatrics. In Mannsmann RA, McCallister ES, Pratt PW, editors: ed 3, *Equine medicine and surgery* vol, 1 Santa Barbara, Calif, 1982, American Veterinary Publications.
2. Soifer SJ, Kaslow D, Roman C, et al: Umbilical cord compression produces pulmonary hypertension in newborn lambs: a model to study the pathophysiology of persistent pulmonary hypertension in the newborn, *J Dev Physiol* 9(3):239–252, 1987.
3. Gupta JM, Tizard JP: The sequence of events in neonatal apnoea, *Lancet* 2(7506):55–59, 1967.
4. Tarnow-Mordi WO: Room air or oxygen for asphyxiated babies? *Lancet* 352(9125):341–342, 1998.
5. Saugstad OD: Resuscitation with room-air or oxygen supplementation, *Clin Perinatol* 25(3):741–756, 1998.
6. Vento M, Asensi M, Sastre J, et al: Resuscitation with room air instead of 100% oxygen prevents oxidative stress in moderately asphyxiated term neonates, *Pediatrics* 107(4):642–647, 2001.
7. Vento M, Asensi M, Sastre J, et al: Six years of experience with the use of room air for the resuscitation of asphyxiated newly born term infants, *Biol Neonat* 79(3-4):261–267, 2001.
8. Saugstad OD: Resuscitation of newborn infants with room air or oxygen, *Semin Neonatol* 6(3):233–239, 2001.
9. Jean D, Laverty S, Halley J, et al: Thoracic trauma in newborn foals, *Equine Vet J* 31(2):149–152, 1999.
10. Jean D, Picandet V, Macieira S, et al: Detection of rib trauma in newborn foals in an equine critical care unit: a comparison of ultrasonography, radiography and physical examination, *Equine Vet J* 39(2):158–163, 2007.
11. Borchers A, van Eps A, Zedler S, et al: Thoracic trauma and postoperative lung injury in a neonatal foal, *Equine Vet Educ, accepted*, 21:186–191, 2009.
12. Kattwinkel J, Niermeyer S, Nadkarni V, et al: An advisory statement from the Pediatric Working Group of the International Liaison Committee on Resuscitation, *Middle East J Anesthesiol* 16(3):315–351, 2001.
13. Ushay HM, Notterman DA: Pharmacology of pediatric resuscitation, *Pediatr Clin North Am* 44(1):207–233, 1997.
14. Holland P, Hodge D: Vasopressin and epinephrine for cardiac arrest, *Lancet* 358(9298):2081–2082, 2001.
15. Walker D, Walker A, Wood C: Temperature of the human fetus, *J Obstet Gynaecol Br Commonw* 76(6):503–511, 1969.
16. Farand P, Hamel M, Lauzier F, et al: Review article: organ perfusion/permeability-related effects of norepinephrine and vasopressin in sepsis, *Can J Anaesth* 53(9):934–946, 2006.
17. Ushay HM, Notterman DA: Pharmacology of pediatric resuscitation, *Pediatr Clin North Am* 44(1):207–233, 1997.
18. Giguère S, Slade JK, Sanchez LC: Retrospective comparison of caffeine and doxapram for the treatment of hypercapnia in foals with hypoxic-ischemic encephalopathy, *J Vet Intern Med* 22(2):401–405, 2008.
19. Giguère S, Sanchez LC, Shih A, et al: Comparison of the effects of caffeine and doxapram on respiratory and cardiovascular function in foals with induced respiratory acidosis, *Am J Vet Res* 68(12):1407–1416, 2007.
20. Ousey JC: Thermoregulation and the energy requirement of the newborn foal, with reference to prematurity, *Equine Vet J Suppl* 24:104–108, 1997.
21. Macaulay JH, Randall NR, Bond K, et al: Continuous monitoring of fetal temperature by noninvasive probe and its relationship to maternal temperature, fetal heart rate, and cord arterial oxygen and pH, *Obstet Gynecol* 79(3):469–474, 1992.
22. Ball KT, Gunn TR, Gluckman PD, et al: Suppressive action of endogenous adenosine on ovine fetal nonshivering thermogenesis, *J Appl Physiol* 81(6):2393–2398, 1996.
23. Gunn TR, Gluckman PD: Perinatal thermogenesis, *Early Hum Dev* 42(3):169–183, 1995.
24. Gunn TR, Ball KT, Power GG, et al: Factors influencing the initiation of nonshivering thermogenesis, *Am J Obstet Gynecol* 164(1 pt 1):210–217, 1991.
25. Gunn TR, Ball KT, Gluckman PD: Reversible umbilical cord occlusion: effects on thermogenesis in utero, *Pediatr Res* 30(6):513–517, 1991.
26. Cree JE, Meyer J, Hailey DM: Diazepam in labour: its metabolism and effect on the clinical condition and thermogenesis of the newborn, *Br Med J* 4(5887):251–255, 1973.
27. Brewer BD, Clement SF, Lotz WS, et al: A comparison of inulin, paraaminohippuric acid, and endogenous creatinine clearances as measures of renal function in neonatal foals, *J Vet Intern Med* 4(6):301–305, 1990.
28. Edwards DJ, Brownlow MA, Hutchins DR: Indices of renal function: values in eight normal foals from birth to 56 days, *Aust Vet J* 67(7):251–254, 1990.
29. Buchanan BR, Sommardahl CS, Rohrbach BW, et al: Effect of a 24-hour infusion of an isotonic electrolyte replacement fluid on the renal clearance of electrolytes in healthy neonatal foals, *J Am Vet Med Assoc* 227(7):1123–1129, 2005.
30. Park WS, Chang YS, Lee M: Effects of hyperglycemia or hypoglycemia on brain cell membrane function and energy metabolism during the immediate reoxygenation-reperfusion period after acute transient global hypoxia-ischemia in the newborn piglet, *Brain Res* 901(1-2):102–108, 2001.
31. Fowden AL, Forhead AJ, White KL, et al: Equine uteroplacental metabolism at mid- and late gestation, *Exp Physiol* 85(5): 539–545, 2000.
32. Fowden AL, Silver M: Glucose and oxygen metabolism in the fetal foal during late gestation, *Am J Physiol* 269(6 pt 2): R1455–R1461, 1995.
33. Takata K, Hirano H: Mechanism of glucose transport across the human and rat placental barrier: a review, *Microsc Res Tech* 38(1-2):145–152, 1997.

34. Kalhan SC, D'Angelo LJ, Savin SM, et al: Glucose production in pregnant women at term gestation: sources of glucose for human fetus, *J Clin Invest* 63(3):388–394, 1979.
35. Kalhan SC, Bier DM, Savin SM, et al: Estimation of glucose turnover and 13C recycling in the human newborn by simultaneous [1-13C]glucose and [6,6-1H2]glucose tracers, *J Clin Endocrinol Metab* 50(3):456–460, 1980.
36. Cowett RM, Oh W, Pollak A, et al: Glucose disposal of low birth weight infants: steady state hyperglycemia produced by constant intravenous glucose infusion, *Pediatrics* 63(3): 389–396, 1979.
37. Levitsky LL, Paton JB, Fisher DE: Precursors to glycogen in ovine fetuses, *Am J Physiol* 255(5 pt 1):E743–E747, 1988.
38. Kawai Y, Arinze IJ: Activation of glycogenolysis in neonatal liver, *J Biol Chem* 256(2):853–858, 1981.

Persistent Pulmonary Hypertension

1. Leffler CW, Hessler JR, Green RS: The onset of breathing at birth stimulates pulmonary vascular prostacyclin synthesis, *Pediatr Res* 18(10):938–942, 1984.
2. Emmanouilides GC, Moss AJ, Duffie ER, et al: Pulmonary arterial pressure changes in human newborn infants from birth to 3 days of age, *J Pediatr* 65:327–333, 1964.
3. Evans NJ, Archer LN: Postnatal circulatory adaptation in healthy term and preterm neonates, *Arch Dis Child* 65(1 spec no):24–26, 1990.
4. Shaul PW, Farrar MA, Magness RR: Pulmonary endothelial nitric oxide production is developmentally regulated in the fetus and newborn, *Am J Physiol* 265(4 pt 2):H1056–H1063, 1993.
5. Fineman JR, Soifer SJ, Heymann MA: Regulation of pulmonary vascular tone in the perinatal period, *Annu Rev Physiol* 57: 115–134, 1995.
6. Wilkins PA, Boston R, Palmer JE, et al: Endothelin-1 concentrations in clone calves, their surrogate dams, and fetal fluids at birth: association with oxygen treatment, *J Vet Intern Med* 19(4):594–598, 2005.
7. Murphy JD, Rabinovitch M, Goldstein JD, et al: The structural basis of persistent pulmonary hypertension of the newborn infant, *J Pediatr* 98(6):962–967, 1981.
8. Noerr B: Tolazoline HCl (Priscoline), *Neonatal Netw* 7(3):74–75, 1988.
9. Finer NN, Barrington KJ: Nitric oxide for respiratory failure in infants born at or near term, *Cochrane Database Syst Rev* 4:CD000399, 2001.
10. Lester GD, DeMarco VG, Norman WM: Effect of inhaled nitric oxide on experimentally induced pulmonary hypertension in neonatal foals, *Am J Vet Res* 60(10):1207–1212, 1999.

Neonatal Neurological Examination and Selected Disorders

1. Koterba A, Drummond W, Kosch P, editors: *Equine clinical neonatology*, ed 1, Philadelphia, 1990, Lea &Febiger.
2. Enzerink E: The menace response and pupillary light reflex in neonatal foals, *Equine Vet J* 30:546–548, 1998.
3. McKinnon A, Voss J, editors: *Equine reproduction*, Philadelphia, 1993, Lea & Febiger.
4. Adams R, Mayhew IG: Neurologic diseases, *Vet Clin North Am Equine Pract* 1:209–234, 1985.
5. Robinson N, editor: *Current therapy in equine medicine*, ed 6, St Louis, 2009, Saunders.
6. MacKay RJ: Neurologic disorders of neonatal foals, *Vet Clin North Am Equine Pract* 21(2):387–406, 2005.
7. Mayhew IG, Watson AG, Heissan JA: Congenital occipitoatlantoaxial malformations in the horse, *Equine Vet J* 10:103–113, 1978.
8. Ferrell EA, Gavin PR, Tucker RL, et al: Magnetic resonance for evaluation of neurologic disease in 12 horses, *Vet Radiol Ultrasound* 43:510–516, 2002.
9. Yager JY, Brucklacher RM, Vannucci RC: Cerebral energy metabolism during hypoxia-ischemia and early recovery in immature rats, *Am J Physiol* 262:H672–H677, 1992.
10. Willoughby RE Jr, Nelson KB: Chorioamnionitis and brain injury, *Clin Perinatol* 29:603–621, 2002.
11. Eklind S, Mallard C, Leverin AL, et al: Bacterial endotoxin sensitizes the immature brain to hypoxic–ischaemic injury, *Eur J Neurosci* 13:1101–1106, 2001.
12. Edwards AD, Yue X, Cox P, et al: Apoptosis in the brains of infants suffering intrauterine cerebral injury, *Pediatr Res* 42:684–689, 1997.
13. Grow J, Barks JD: Pathogenesis of hypoxic-ischemic cerebral injury in the term infant: current concepts, *Clin Perinatol* 29:585–602, 2002.
14. Arundine M, Tymianski M: Molecular mechanisms of glutamate-dependent neurodegeneration in ischemia and traumatic brain injury, *Cell Mol Life Sci* 61:657–668, 2004.
15. Bazan NG, Rodriguez de Turco EB: Allan G: Mediators of injury in neurotrauma: intracellular signal transduction and gene expression, *J Neurotrauma* 12:791–814, 1995.
16. Palmer AC, Rossdale PD: Neuropathology of the convulsive foal syndrome, *J Reprod Fertil Suppl* :91–694, 1975.
17. Mayhew IG: Observations on vascular accidents in the central nervous system of neonatal foals, *J Reprod Fertil Suppl* 32: 569–575, 1982.
18. Haughey KG, Jones RT: Meningeal haemorrhage and congestion associated with the perinatal mortality of foals, *Vet Rec* 98:518–522, 1976.
19. Ebel H, Gunther T: Magnesium metabolism: a review, *J Clin Chem Clin Biochem* 18:257–270, 1980.
20. Lee JS, Han YM, Yoo DS, et al: A molecular basis for the efficacy of magnesium treatment following traumatic brain injury in rats, *J Neurotrauma* 21:549–561, 2004.
21. Arango MF, Mejia-Mantilla JH: Magnesium for acute traumatic brain injury, Cochrane Database Syst Rev CD005400, 2006
22. Kulah A, Akar M, Baykut L: Dimethyl sulfoxide in the management of patient with brain swelling and increased intracranial pressure after severe closed head injury, *Neurochirurgia (Stuttg)* 33:177–180, 1990.
23. Coles JC, Ahmed SN, Mehta HU, et al: Role of free radical scavenger in protection of spinal cord during ischemia, *Ann Thorac Surg* 41:551–556, 1986.
24. Bagenholm R, Nilsson UA, Gotborg CW, et al: Free radicals are formed in the brain of fetal sheep during reperfusion after cerebral ischemia, *Pediatr Res* 43:271–275, 1998.
25. Adams HA: [Mechanisms of action of ketamine], *Anaesthesiol Reanim* 23:60–63, 1998.
26. Meldrum BS, Evans MC, Swan JH, et al: Protection against hypoxic/ischaemic brain damage with excitatory amino acid antagonists, *Med Biol* 65:153–157, 1987.
27. Pfenninger E, Himmelseher S: [Neuroprotection by ketamine at the cellular level], *Anaesthesist* 46(Suppl 1):S47–S54, 1997.
28. Sandau US, Handa RJ: Glucocorticoids exacerbate hypoxia-induced expression of the pro-apoptotic gene Bnip3 in the developing cortex, *Neuroscience* 144:482–494, 2007.
29. Alderson P, Roberts I: Corticosteroids for acute traumatic brain injury, Cochrane Database Syst Rev CD000196, 2005.
30. Diringer MN, Zazulia AR: Osmotic therapy: fact and fiction, *Neurocrit Care* 1:219–233, 2004.
31. Wang X, Svedin P, Nie C, et al: N-acetylcysteine reduces lipopolysaccharide-sensitized hypoxic-ischemic brain injury, *Ann Neurol* 61:263–271, 2007.
32. Miura S, Ishida A, Nakajima W, et al: Intraventricular ascorbic acid administration decreases hypoxic-ischemic brain injury in newborn rats, *Brain Res* 1095:159–166, 2006.
33. Anderson DK, Waters TR, Means ED: Pretreatment with alpha tocopherol enhances neurologic recovery after experimental spinal cord compression injury, *J Neurotrauma* 5:61–67, 1988.

34. Hall ED, Yonkers PA, Andrus PK, et al: Biochemistry and pharmacology of lipid antioxidants in acute brain and spinal cord injury, *J Neurotrauma* 9(Suppl 2):S425–S442, 1992.
35. Crowe MW, Swerczek TW: Equine congenital defects, *Am J Vet Res* 46:353–358, 1985.
36. Wilson WD, Hughes SJ, Ghoshal NG, et al: Occipitoatlantoaxial malformation in two non-Arabian horses, *J Am Vet Med Assoc* 187:36–40, 1985.
37. Mayhew IG: Neurological and neuropathological observations on the equine neonate, *Equine Vet J Supplement* : 28–33, 1988.
38. Koterba AM, Brewer BD, Tarplee FA: Clinical and clinicopathological characteristics of the septicaemic neonatal foal: review of 38 cases, *Equine Vet J* 16:376–382, 1984.
39. Couetil LL, Hoffman AM: Adrenal insufficiency in a neonatal foal, *J Am Vet Med Assoc* 212:1594–1596, 1998.
40. Boyle AG, Magdesian KG, Ruby RE: Neonatal isoerythrolysis in horse foals and a mule foal: 18 cases (1988-2003), *J Am Vet Med Assoc* 227:1276–1283, 2005.
41. Wilkins PA, Palmer JE: Mechanical ventilation in foals with botulism: 9 cases (1989-2002), *J Vet Intern Med* 17(5):708–712, 2003.
42. Wilkins PA, Palmer JE: Botulism in foals less than 6 months of age: 30 cases (1989-2002), *J Vet Intern Med* 17(5):702–707, 2003.

Perinatal Asphyxia Syndrome

1. Whitelaw A: Systematic review of therapy after hypoxic-ischaemic brain injury in the perinatal period, *Semin Neonatol* 5(1):33–40, 2000.
2. Rossdale PD: Clinical studies on 4 newborn throughbred foals suffering from convulsions with special reference to blood gas chemistry and pulmonary ventilation, *Res Vet Sci* 10(3): 279–291, 1969.
3. Palmer AC, Rossdale PD: Neuropathology of the convulsive foal syndrome, *J Reprod Fertil Suppl* 23:691–694, 1975.
4. Palmer AC, Rossdale PD: Neuropathological changes associated with the neonatal maladjustment syndrome in the thoroughbred foal, *Res Vet Sci* 20(3):267–275, 1976.
5. Nelson KB, Willoughby RE: Infection, inflammation and the risk of cerebral palsy, *Curr Opin Neurol* 13(2):133–139, 2000.
6. Evrard P: Pathophysiology of perinatal brain damage, *Dev Neurosci* 23(3):171–174, 2001.
7. Andine P, Jacobson I, Hagberg H: Enhanced calcium uptake by CA1 pyramidal cell dendrites in the postischemic phase despite subnormal evoked field potentials: excitatory amino acid receptor dependency and relationship to neuronal damage, *J Cereb Blood Flow Metab* 12(5):773–783, 1992.
8. Sebastiao AM, de Mendonca A, Moreira T, et al: Activation of synaptic NMDA receptors by action potential-dependent release of transmitter during hypoxia impairs recovery of synaptic transmission on reoxygenation, *J Neurosci* 21(21): 8564–8571, 2001.
9. Vexler ZS, Ferriero DM: Molecular and biochemical mechanisms of perinatal brain injury, *Semin Neonatol* 6(2) :99–108, 2001.
10. D'Souza SW, McConnell SE, Slater P, et al: Glycine site of the excitatory amino acid N-methyl-D-aspartate receptor in neonatal and adult brain, *Arch Dis Child* 69(2): 212–215, 1993.
11. Zhang L, Rzigalinski BA, Ellis EF, et al: Reduction of voltage-dependent Mg2+ blockade of NMDA current in mechanically injured neurons, *Science* 274(5294):1921–1923, 1996.
12. Arango MF, Mejia-Mantilla JH: Magnesium for acute traumatic brain injury, Cochrane Database Syst Rev CD005400, 2006
13. Wilkins PA: How to use midazolam to control equine neonatal seizures, *Am Assoc Eq Pract Proceedings* 51:279–280, 2005.
14. JE Palmer, personal communication, 1998.
15. Spehar AM, Hill MR, Mayhew IG, et al: Preliminary study on the pharmacokinetics of phenobarbital in the neonatal foal, *Equine Vet J* 16(4):368–371, 1984.
16. Tute AS, Wilkins PA, Gleed RD, et al: Negative pressure pulmonary edema as a post-anesthetic complication associated with upper airway obstruction in a horse, *Vet Surg* 25(6):519–523, 1996.
17. Kortz GD, Madigan JE, Lakritz J, et al: Cerebral oedema and cerebellar herniation in four equine neonates, *Equine Vet J* 24(1):63–66, 1992.
18. Kempski O: Cerebral edema, *Semin Nephrol* 21(3):303–307, 2001.
19. Watanabe I, Tomita T, Hung KS, et al: Edematous necrosis in thiamine-deficient encephalopathy of the mouse, *J Neuropathol Exp Neurol* 40(4):454–471, 1981.
20. Wilkins PA, Vaala WE, Zivotofsky D, et al: A herd outbreak of equine leukoencephalomalacia, *Cornell Vet* 84(1):53–59, 1994.
21. Chernick V, Craig RJ: Naloxone reverses neonatal depression caused by fetal asphyxia, *Science* 216(4551):1252–1253, 1982.
22. Ting P, Pan Y: The effects of naloxone on the post-asphyxic cerebral pathophysiology of newborn lambs, *Neurol Res* 16(5):359–364, 1994.
23. Young RS, Hessert TR, Pritchard GA, et al: Naloxone exacerbates hypoxic-ischemic brain injury in the neonatal rat, *Am J Obstet Gynecol* 150(1):52–56, 1984.
24. Kattwinkel J, Niermeyer S, Nadkarni V, et al: Resuscitation of the newly born infant: an advisory statement from the Pediatric Working Group of the International Liaison Committee on Resuscitation, *Resuscitation* 40(2):71–88, 1999.
25. Bain FT: Neurologic disorders in foals other than hypoxic-ischemic encephalopathy. In *Proceedings of the International Veterinary Emergency Critical Care Symposium*, San Antonio, 1998, Tex, pp 691–692.
26. Lyden PD, Lonzo L: Combination therapy protects ischemic brain in rats: a glutamate antagonist plus a gamma-aminobutyric acid agonist, *Stroke* 25(1):189–196, 1994.
27. Madden KP: Effect of gamma-aminobutyric acid modulation on neuronal ischemia in rabbits, *Stroke* 25(11):2271–2274, 1994.
28. Gunn AJ: Cerebral hypothermia for prevention of brain injury following perinatal asphyxia, *Curr Opin Pediatr* 12(2):111–115, 2000.
29. Bhatia J: Current options in the management of apnea of prematurity, *Clin Pediatr (Phila)* 39(6):327–336, 2000.
30. Giguère S, Slade JK, Sanchez LC: Retrospective comparison of caffeine and doxapram for the treatment of hypercapnia in foals with hypoxic-ischemic encephalopathy, *J Vet Intern Med* 22(2):401–405, 2008.
31. Giguère S, Sanchez LC, Shih A, et al: Comparison of the effects of caffeine and doxapram on respiratory and cardiovascular function in foals with induced respiratory acidosis, *Am J Vet Res* 68(12):1407–1416, 2007.
32. Ambalavanan N, Carlo WA: Hypocapnia and hypercapnia in respiratory management of newborn infants, *Clin Perinatol* 28(3):517–531, 2001.
33. Filler G: Acute renal failure in children: aetiology and management, *Paediatr Drugs* 3(11):783–792, 2001.
34. Rudis MI: Low-dose dopamine in the intensive care unit: DNR or DNRx? *Crit Care Med* 29(8):1638–1639, 2001.
35. Kellum JA: M Decker J: Use of dopamine in acute renal failure: a meta-analysis, *Crit Care Med* 29(8):1526–1531, 2001.
36. Cheung PY, Barrington KJ: The effects of dopamine and epinephrine on hemodynamics and oxygen metabolism in hypoxic anesthetized piglets, *Crit Care* 5(3):158–166, 2001.
37. Corley KTT, McKenzie HC, Amoroso LM, et al: Initial experience with norepinephrine infusion in hypotensive critically ill foal, *J Vet Emerg Crit Care* 10:267–276, 2000.

38. Brewer BD, Clement SF, Lotz WS, et al: A comparison of inulin, paraaminohippuric acid, and endogenous creatinine clearances as measures of renal function in neonatal foals, *J Vet Intern Med* 4(6):301–305, 1990.
39. Buchanan BR, Sommardahl CS, Rohrbach BW, et al: Effect of a 24-hour infusion of an isotonic electrolyte replacement fluid on the renal clearance of electrolytes in healthy neonatal foals, *J Am Vet Med Assoc* 227(7):1123–1129, 2005.
40. Brewer BD, Clement SF, Lotz WS, et al: Renal clearance, urinary excretion of endogenous substances, and urinary diagnostic indices in healthy neonatal foals, *J Vet Intern Med* 5(1):28–33, 1991.
41. Martin-Ancel A, Garcia-Alix A, Gaya F, et al: Multiple organ involvement in perinatal asphyxia, *J Pediatr* 127(5):786–793, 1995.
42. Jawaheer G, Shaw NJ, Pierro A: Continuous enteral feeding impairs gallbladder emptying in infants, *J Pediatr* 138(6): 822–825, 2001.
43. McClure RJ: Trophic feeding of the preterm infant, *Acta Paediatr Suppl* 90(436):19–21, 2001.
44. Premji S, Chessell L: Continuous nasogastric milk feeding versus intermittent bolus milk feeding for premature infants less than 1500 grams, *Cochrane Database Syst Rev* 1:CD001819, 2001.
45. Baker SM, Drummond WH, Lane TJ, et al: Follow-up evaluation of horses after neonatal intensive care, *J Am Vet Med Assoc* 189(11):1454–1457, 1986.
46. Axon J, Palmer J, Wilkins PA: Short-term and long-term athletic outcome of neonatal intensive care unit survivors, *Proc Am Assoc Equine Pract* 45:224–225, 1999.
47. Freeman L, Paradis MR: Evaluating the effectiveness of equine neonatal intensive care, *Vet Med* 87:921–926, Sept 1992.
48. Lester GD: Short and long term evaluation of neonatal intensive care. In *Proceedings of the fourteenth annual meeting of the American College of Veterinary Internal Medicine*, San Antonio, 1996, Tex, pp 547–548.

Prematurity, Dysmaturity, Postmaturity

1. McEvoy C, Bowling S, Williamson K, et al: Functional residual capacity and passive compliance measurements after antenatal steroid therapy in preterm infants, *Pediatr Pulmonol* 31(6): 425–430, 2001.
2. Suresh GK, Soll RF: Current surfactant use in premature infants, *Clin Perinatol* 28(3):671–694, 2001.
3. Axon J, Palmer J, Wilkins PA: Short-term and long-term athletic outcome of neonatal intensive care unit survivors, *Proc Am Assoc Equine Pract* 45:224–225, 1999.
4. Putnam MR, Bransby DI, Schumacher J, et al: Effects of the fungal endophyte Acremonium coenophialum in fescue on pregnant mares and foal viability, *Am J Vet Res* 52(12): 2071–2074, 1991.
5. Berry LM, Ikegami M, Woods E, et al: Postnatal renal adaptation in preterm and term lambs, *Reprod Fertil Dev* 7(3):491–498, 1995.
6. Zanardo V, Cagdas S, Golin R, et al: Risk factors of hypoglycemia in premature infants, *Fetal Diagn Ther* 14(2):63–67, 1999.
7. Broughton Pipkin F, Ousey JC, Wallace CP, et al: Studies on equine prematurity. 4. Effect of salt and water loss on the renin-angiotensin-aldosterone system in the newborn foal, *Equine Vet J* 16(4):292–297, 1984.
8. Webb PD, Leadon DP, Rossdale PD, et al: Studies on equine prematurity. 5. Histology of the adrenal cortex of the premature newborn foal, *Equine Vet J* 16(4):297–299, 1984.
9. Livesay-Wilkins PA: Angular limb deformities in premature/dysmature foals, *Mod Vet Pract* 67:808–911, Oct-Nov 1986.

Sepsis

1. Neonatal Septicemia Workshop 1, Dorothy Havemeyer Foundation, Westminster, Massachussets, 1995.
2. Neonatal Septicemia Workshop 2, Dorothy Havemeyer Foundation, Boston, 1998.
3. Neonatal Septicemia Workshop 3, Dorothy Havemeyer Foundation, Talliores, France, 2001.
4. Neonatal Septicemia Workshop 4, Dorothy Havemeyer Foundation, Talliores, France, 2004.
5. Neonatal Septicemia Workshop 5, Dorothy Havemeyer Foundation, Salem, Mass, 2008.
6. Muckart DJ, Bhagwanjee S: American College of Chest Physicians/Society of Critical Care Medicine Consensus Conference definitions of the systemic inflammatory response syndrome and allied disorders in relation to critically injured patient, *Crit Care Med* 25(11):1789–1795, 1997.
7. Matot I, Sprung CL: Definition of sepsis, *Intensive Care Med* 27(suppl 1):S3–S9, 2001.
8. Corley KT, Donaldson LL, Furr MO: Arterial lactate concentration, hospital survival, sepsis and SIRS in critically ill neonatal foals, *Equine Vet J* 37(1):53–59, 2005.
9. Dallap Schaer BL, Bentz AI, Boston RC et al: Coagulation evaluation in critically ill neonatal foals: Comparison of viscoelastic analysis and standard coagulation profile, *J Vet Emerg Crit* Care 19:88–95, 2009.
10. Wilkins PA, Otto CM, Dunkel B, et al: Acute lung injury (ALI) and acute respiratory distress syndromes (ARDS) in veterinary medicine: consensus definitions, Special commentary, *J Vet Emerg Crit Care* 17(4):333–339, 2007.
11. Hollis AR, Wilkins PA, Palmer JE, et al: Bacteremia in equine neonatal diarrhea: a retrospective study (1990-2007), *J Vet Intern Med* 22(5):1203–1209, 2008.
12. Corley KT, Pearce G, Magdesian KG, et al: Bacteraemia in neonatal foals: clinicopathological differences between Gram-positive and Gram-negative infections, and single organism and mixed infections, *Equine Vet J* 39(1):84–89, 2007.
13. Wotman K, Wilkins PA, Palmer JE et al: Association of blood lactate concentration and outcome in foals. *J Vet Intern med* 23(3):598–605, 2009.
14. Dellinger RP, Bone RC: To SIRS with love, *Crit Care Med* 26(1):178–179, 1998.
15. Tyler-McGowan CM, Hodgson JL, Hodgson DR: Failure of passive transfer in foals: incidence and outcome on four studs in New South Wales, *Aust Vet J* 75(1):56–59, 1997.
16. Robinson JA, Allen GK, Green EM, et al: A prospective study of septicaemia in colostrum-deprived foals, *Equine Vet J* 25(3): 214–219, 1993.
17. Koterba AM, Brewer BD, Tarplee FA: Clinical and clinicopathological characteristics of the septicaemic neonatal foal: review of 38 cases, *Equine Vet J* 16(4):376–382, 1984.
18. Brewer BD, Koterba AM, Carter RL, et al: Comparison of empirically developed sepsis score with a computer generated and weighted scoring system for the identification of sepsis in the equine neonate, *Equine Vet J* 20(1):23–24, 1988.
19. Steinmetz OK, Meakins JL: Care of the gut in the surgical intensive care unit: fact or fashion? *Can J Surg* 34(3):207–215, 1991.
20. Marsh PS, Palmer JE: Bacterial isolates from blood and their susceptibility patterns in critically ill foals: 543 cases (1991-1998), *J Am Vet Med Assoc* 218(10):1608–1610, 2001.
21. Russell CM, Axon JE, Blishen A, et al: Blood culture isolates and antimicrobial sensitivities from 427 critically ill neonatal foals, *Aust Vet J* 86(7):266–271, 2008.
22. Madigan JE, Leutenegger CM: Development of real-time TaqMan PCR systems to facilitate the diagnosis and research of septicemia in foals. In *Proceedings of the Neonatal Septicemia Workshop 3*, Boston, 2001, pp 35–36.
23. Alcivar-Warren A, Pascual I, Dhar AK et al: Expressed sequence TAGS (ESTs) isolated from blood of a septic thoroughbred foal. In *Proceedings of the Neonatal Septicemia Workshop 3*, Boston, 2001, pp 37–40.
24. Pusterla N, Madigan JE, Leutenegger CM: Real-time polymerase chain reaction: a novel molecular diagnostic tool for equine infectious diseases, *J Vet Intern Med* 20(1):3–12, 2006.

25. Rivers E, Nguyen B, Havstad S, et al: Early goal-directed therapy in the treatment of severe sepsis and septic shock, *N Engl J Med* 345(19):1368–1377, 2001.
26. Traub-Dargatz JL, Bertone JJ, Gould DH, et al: Chronic flunixin meglumine therapy in foals, *Am J Vet Res* 49(1):7–12, 1988.
27. Carrick JB, Papich MG, Middleton DM, et al: Clinical and pathological effects of flunixin meglumine administration to neonatal foals, *Can J Vet Res* 53(2):195–201, 1989.
28. Rebhun WC, Dill SG, Power HT: Gastric ulcers in foals, *J Am Vet Med Assoc* 180(4):404–407, 1982.
29. Gold JR, Divers TJ, Barton MH, et al: Plasma adrenocorticotropin, cortisol, and adrenocorticotropin/cortisol ratios in septic and normal-term foals, *J Vet Intern Med* 21(4):791–796, 2007.
30. Hurcombe SD, Toribio RE, Slovis N, et al: Blood arginine vasopressin, adrenocorticotropin hormone, and cortisol concentrations at admission in septic and critically ill foals and their association with survival, *J Vet Intern Med* 22(3):639–647, 2008.
31. Axon J, Palmer J, Wilkins PA: Short-term and long-term athletic outcome of neonatal intensive care unit survivors, *Proc Am Assoc Equine Pract* 45:224–225, 1999.

Nutritional Muscular Dystrophy (White Muscle Disease)

1. Lofstedt J: White muscle disease of foals, *Vet Clin North Am Equine Pract* 13(1):169–185, 1997.

Hepatic Diseases of Foals

1. Gossett KA, French DD: Effect of age on liver enzyme activities in serum of healthy Quarter Horses, *Am J Vet Res* 45:354–356, 1984.
2. Patterson WH, Brown CM: Increase of serum γ-glutamyltransferase in neonatal Standardbred foals, *Am J Vet Res* 47:2461–2463, 1986.
3. Barton MH, LeRoy BE: Serum bile acids concentrations in healthy and clinically ill neonatal foals, *J Vet Intern Med* 21:508–513, 2007.
4. Bauer JE, Asquith RL, Kivipelto J: Serum biochemical indicators of liver function in neonatal foals, *Am J Vet Res* 50:2037–2041, 1989.
5. Dumas MB, Spano JS: Characterization of equine alkaline phosphatase isoenzymes based on their electrophoretic mobility by polyacrylamide gel disc electrophoresis, *Am J Vet Res* 41:2076–2081, 1980.
6. Braun JP, Tainturier D, Bézille P, et al: Transfer of gamma-glutamyltransferase from mother colostrum to newborn goat and foal, *Enzyme* 31:193–196, 1984.
7. Buonanno AM, Carlson GP, Kantrowitz B: Clinical and diagnostic features of portosystemic shunt in a foal, *J Am Vet Med Assoc* 192:387–389, 1988.
8. Hillyer MH, Holt PE, Barr FJ, et al: Clinical signs and radiographic diagnosis of a portosystemic shunt in a foal, *Vet Record* 132:457–460, 1993.
9. Lindsay WA, Ryder JK, Beck KA, et al: Hepatic encephalopathy caused by a portocaval shunt in a foal, *Vet Med* 83:798–805, 1988.
10. Fortier LA, Fubini SL, Flanders JA, et al: The diagnosis and surgical correction of congenital portosystemic vascular anomalies in two calves and two foals, *Vet Surg* 25:154–160, 1996.
11. Beech J, Dubielzig R, Bester R: Portal vein anomaly and hepatic encephalopathy in a horse, *J Am Vet Med Assoc* 170:164–166, 1977.
12. Borchers A, Magdesian KG, Halland S, et al: Successful treatment and polymerase chain reaction (PCR) confirmation of Tyzzer's disease in a foal and pathologic characteristics of 6 additional foals (1986-2005), *J Vet Intern Med* 20:1212–1218, 2006.
13. Fosgate GT, Hird DW, Read DH, et al: Risk factors for *Clostridium piliforme* infection in foals, *J Am Vet Med Assoc* 220:785–790, 2002.
14. Buote M: Cholangiohepatitis and pancreatitis secondary to severe gastroduodenal ulceration in a foal, *Can Vet J* 44:746–748, 2003.
15. Boyle AG, Magdesian KG, Ruby RE: Neonatal isoerythrolysis in horse foals and a mule foal: 18 cases (1988-2003), *J Am Vet Med Assoc* 227:1276–1283, 2005.
16. Valberg SJ, Ward TL, Rush B, et al: Glycogen branching enzyme deficiency in Quarter Horse foals, *J Vet Intern Med* 15:572–580, 2001.

Failure of Passive Transfer

1. Erhard MH, Luft C, Remler HP, et al: Assessment of colostral transfer and systemic availability of immunoglobulin G in new-born foals using a newly developed enzyme-linked immunosorbent assay (ELISA) system, *J Anim Physiol Anim Nutr (Berl)* 85(5-6):164–173, 2001.
2. Bertone JJ, Jones RL, Curtis CR: Evaluation of a test kit for determination of serum immunoglobulin G concentration in foals, *J Vet Intern Med* 2(4):181–183, 1988.
3. LeBlanc MM, McLaurin BI, Boswell R: Relationships among serum immunoglobulin concentration in foals, colostral specific gravity, and colostral immunoglobulin concentration, *J Am Vet Med Assoc* 189(1):57–60, 1986.
4. Kent JE, Blackmore DJ: Measurement of IgG in equine blood by immunoturbidimetry and latex agglutination, *Equine Vet J* 17(2):125–129, 1985.
5. Watson DL, Bennell MA, Griffiths JR: A rapid, specific test for detecting absorption of colostral IgG by the neonatal foal, *Aust Vet J* 56(11):513–516, 1980.
6. Buening GM, Perryman LE, McGuire TC: Practical methods of determining serum immunoglobulin M and immunoglobulin G concentrations in foals, *J Am Vet Med Assoc* 171(5):455–458, 1977.
7. McGuire TC, Crawford TB: Passive immunity in the foal: measurement of immunoglobulin classes and specific antibody, *Am J Vet Res* 34(10):1299–1303, 1973.
8. Jeffcott LB: Studies on passive immunity in the foal. 1. Gamma-globulin and antibody variations associated with the maternal transfer of immunity and the onset of active immunity, *J Comp Pathol* 84(1):93–101, 1974.
9. MacDougall DF: Immunoglobulin metabolism in the neonatal foal, *J Reprod Fertil Suppl* 23:739–742, 1975.
10. Baldwin JL, Cooper WL, Vanderwall DK, et al: Prevalence (treatment days) and severity of illness in hypogammaglobulinemic and normogammaglobulinemic foals, *J Am Vet Med Assoc* 198(3):423–428, 1991.
11. Clabough DL, Levine JF, Grant GL, et al: Factors associated with failure of passive transfer of colostral antibodies in standardbred foals, *J Vet Intern Med* 5(6):335–340, 1991.
12. Baldwin JL: Failure of passive transfer in foals, *J Vet Intern Med* 6(3):197–198, 1992.
13. Koterba AM, Brewer BD, Tarplee FA: Clinical and clinicopathological characteristics of the septicaemic neonatal foal: review of 38 cases, *Equine Vet J* 16(4):376–382, 1984.
14. Brewer BD, Koterba AM, Carter RL, et al: Comparison of empirically developed sepsis score with a computer generated and weighted scoring system for the identification of sepsis in the equine neonate, *Equine Vet J* 20(1):23–24, 1988.
15. Tyler-McGowan CM, Hodgson JL, Hodgson DR: Failure of passive transfer in foals: incidence and outcome on four studs in New South Wales, *Aust Vet J* 75(1):56–59, 1997.
16. Robinson JA, Allen GK, Green EM, et al: A prospective study of septicaemia in colostrum-deprived foals, *Equine Vet J* 25(3): 214–219, 1993.
17. Stoneham SJ, Digby NJ, Ricketts SW: Failure of passive transfer of colostral immunity in the foal: incidence, and the effect of stud management and plasma transfusions, *Vet Rec* 128(18):416–419, 1991.

18. Raidal SL: The incidence and consequences of failure of passive transfer of immunity on a thoroughbred breeding farm, *Aust Vet J* 73(6):201–206, 1996.
19. McGuire TC, Crawford TB, Hallowell AL, et al: Failure of colostral immunoglobulin transfer as an explanation for most infections and deaths of neonatal foals, *J Am Vet Med Assoc* 170(11):1302–1304, 1977.
20. Norcross NL: Secretion and composition of colostrum and milk, *J Am Vet Med Assoc* 181(10):1057–1060, 1982.
21. Sheoran AS, Timoney JF, Holmes MA, et al: Immunoglobulin isotypes in sera and nasal mucosal secretions and their neonatal transfer and distribution in horses, *Am J Vet Res* 61(9): 1099–1105, 2000.
22. Takahata Y, Takada H, Nomura A, et al: Interleukin-18 in human milk, *Pediatr Res* 50(2):268–272, 2001.
23. Hossner KL, Yemm RS: Improved recovery of insulin-like growth factors (IGFs) from bovine colostrum using alkaline diafiltration, *Biotechnol Appl Biochem* 32(pt 3):161–166, 2000.
24. Zablocka A, Janusz M, Rybka K, et al: Cytokine-inducing activity of a proline-rich polypeptide complex (PRP) from ovine colostrum and its active nonapeptide fragment analogs, *Eur Cytokine Netw* 12(3):462–467, 2001.
25. Bastian SE, Dunbar AJ, Priebe IK: Measurement of betacellulin levels in bovine serum, colostrum and milk, *J Endocrinol* 168(1):203–212, 2001.
26. van Hooijdonk AC, Kussendrager KD, Steijns JM: In vivo antimicrobial and antiviral activity of components in bovine milk and colostrum involved in non-specific defence, *Br J Nutr* 84(suppl 1):S127–S134, 2000.
27. Zanker IA, Hammon HM, Blum JW: Activities of γ-glutamyltransferase, alkaline phosphatase and aspartate-aminotransferase in colostrum, milk and blood plasma of calves fed first colostrum at 0-2, 6-7, 12-13 and 24-25 h after birth, *J Vet Med A Physiol Pathol Clin Med* 48(3):179–185, 2001.
28. Wilkins PA, Dewan-Mix S: Efficacy of intravenous plasma to transfer passive immunity in clinically healthy and clinically ill equine neonates with failure of passive transfer, *Cornell Vet* 84(1):7–14, 1994.
29. Liu IK, Brown C, Myers RC, et al: Evaluation of intravenous administration of concentrated immunoglobulin G to colostrum-deprived foals, *Am J Vet Res* 52(5):709–712, 1991.
30. Burton SC, Hintz HF, Kemen MJ, et al: Lyophilized hyperimmune equine serum as a source of antibodies for neonatal foals, *Am J Vet Res* 42(2):308–310, 1981.
31. Lavoie JP, Spensley MS, Smith BP, et al: Absorption of bovine colostral immunoglobulins G and M in newborn foals, *Am J Vet Res* 50(9):1598–1603, 1989.
32. Klobasa F, Goel MC, Werhahn E: Comparison of freezing and lyophilizing for preservation of colostrum as a source of immunoglobulins for calves, *J Anim Sci* 76(4):923–926, 1998.
33. O'Rielly JL: A comparison of the reduction in immunoglobulin (IgG) concentration of frozen equine plasma treated by three thawing techniques, *Aust Vet J* 70(12):442–444, 1993.
34. Hunt E, Wood B: Use of blood and blood products, *Vet Clin North Am Food Anim Pract* 15(3):641–662, 1999.

Neonatal Isoerythrolysis

1. McClure J, Koch C, Traub-Dargatz J: Characterization of a red blood cell antigen in donkeys and mules associated with neonatal isoerythrolysis, *Anim Genet* 25:119–120, 1994.
2. Bailey E: Prevalence of anti-red blood cell antibodies in the serum and colostrum of mares and its relationship to neonatal isoerythrolysis, *Am J Vet Res* 43:1917–1921, 1982.
3. Whiting J, David JB: Neonatal isoerythrolysis, *Compend Cont Educ Pract Vet* 22(10):968–976, 2000.
4. Perkins GA, Divers TJ: Polymerized hemoglobin therapy in a foal with neonatal isoerythrolysis, *J Vet Emerg Crit Care* 11(2):141–146, 2001.
5. Smith JE, Dever M, Smith J, et al: Post-transfusion survival of 50Cr-labeled erythrocytes in neonatal foals, *J Vet Intern Med* 6(3):183–187, 1992.
6. Hong CB: Congenital polyalveolar lobe in three foals, *J Comp Pathol* 115(1):85–88, 1996.

Immune-Mediated Thrombocytopenia and Neutropenia

1. Perkins GA, Miller WH, Divers TJ, et al: Ulcerative dermatitis, thrombocytopenia, and neutropenia in neonatal foals, *J Vet Intern Med* 19(2):211–216, 2005.
2. Ramirez S, Gaunt SD, McClure JJ, et al: Detection and effects on platelet function of anti-platelet antibody in mule foals with experimentally induced neonatal alloimmune thrombocytopenia, *J Vet Intern Med* 13(6):534–539, 1999.
3. Buechner-Maxwell V, Scott MA, Godber L, et al: Neonatal alloimmune thrombocytopenia in a Quarter horse foal, *J Vet Intern Med* 11(5):304–308, 1997.
4. Roberts IA, Murray NA: Neonatal thrombocytopenia: new insights into pathogenesis and implications for clinical management, *Curr Opin Pediatr* 13(1):16–21, 2001.
5. Sellon DC: Thrombocytopenia in horses, *Equine Vet Educ* 10:133–139, 1998.
6. Ramirez S, Gaunt SD, McClure JJ, et al: Detection and effects on platelet function of anti-platelet antibody in mule foals with experimentally induced neonatal alloimmune thrombocytopenia, *J Vet Intern Med* 13(6):534–539, 1999.

Diseases of the Respiratory Tract

1. James FM, Parente EJ, Palmer JE: Management of bilateral choanal atresia in a foal, *J Am Vet Med Assoc* 229(11):1784–1789, 2006.
2. Reef VB: Cardiovascular disease in the equine neonate, *Vet Clin North Am Equine Pract* 1(1):117–129, 1985.
3. Hong CB: Congenital polyalveolar lobe in three foals, *J Comp Pathol* 115(1):85–88, 1996.
4. Hinchcliff KW, Adams WM: Critical pulmonary stenosis in a newborn foal, *Equine Vet J* 23(4):318–320, 1991.
5. Riley CB, Yovich JV, Bolton JR: Bilateral hypoplasia of the soft palate in a foal, *Aust Vet J* 68(5):178–179, 1991.
6. Hultgren BD: Pulmonary lobar hypertrophy in a foal, *J Am Vet Med Assoc* 188(4):422–423, 1986.
7. Crowe MW, Swerczek TW: Equine congenital defects, *Am J Vet Res* 46(2):353–358, 1985.
8. Aylor MK, Campbell ML, Goring RL, et al: Congenital bilateral choanal atresia in a standardbred foal, *Equine Vet J* 16(4): 396–398, 1984.
9. Chaffin MK, Matthews NS, Cohen ND, et al: Evaluation of pulse oximetry in anaesthetised foals using multiple combinations of transducer type and transducer attachment site, *Equine Vet J* 28(6):437–445, 1996.
10. Kosch PC, Koterba AM, Coons TJ, et al: Developments in management of the newborn foal in respiratory distress. 1. Evaluation, *Equine Vet J* 16(4):312–318, 1984.
11. Yamamoto K, Yasuda J, Too K: Electrocardiographic findings during parturition and blood gas tensions immediately after birth in thoroughbred foals, *Jpn J Vet Res* 39(2-4):143–157, 1991.
12. Hodgson DR: Blood gas and acid-base changes in the neonatal foal, *Vet Clin North Am Equine Pract* 3(3):617–629, 1987.
13. Rossdale PD: Blood gas tensions and pH values in the normal thoroughbred foal at birth and in the following 42h, *Biol Neonat* 13(1):18–25, 1968.
14. Madigan JE, Thomas WP, Backus KQ, et al: Mixed venous blood gases in recumbent and upright positions in foals from birth to 14 days of age, *Equine Vet J* 24(5):399–401, 1992.
15. Palmer JE: Ventilatory support of the neonatal foal, *Vet Clin North Am Equine Pract* 10(1):167–185, 1994.
16. Palmer JE: Ventilatory support of the critically ill foal, *Vet Clin North Am Equine Pract* 21(2):457–486, 2005.

17. Giguère S, Slade JK, Sanchez LC: Retrospective comparison of caffeine and doxapram for the treatment of hypercapnia in foals with hypoxic-ischemic encephalopathy, *J Vet Intern Med* 22(2):401–405, 2008.
18. Giguère S, Sanchez LC, Shih A, et al: Comparison of the effects of caffeine and doxapram on respiratory and cardiovascular function in foals with induced respiratory acidosis, *Am J Vet Res* 68(12):1407–1416, 2007.
19. Wilkins PA, Otto CM, Dunkel B, et al: Acute lung injury (ALI) and acute respiratory distress syndromes (ARDS) in veterinary medicine: consensus definitions (special commentary), *J Vet Emerg Crit Care* 17(4):333–339, 2007.
20. Dunkel B, Dolente B, Boston RC: Acute lung injury/acute respiratory distress syndrome in 15 foals, *Equine Vet J* 37(5): 435–440, 2005.
21. Report of foal pneumonia panel, *AAEP Newslett* 2:76, 1978.
22. Hoffman AM, Viel L, Prescott JF, et al: Association of microbiologic flora with clinical, endoscopic, and pulmonary cytologic findings in foals with distal respiratory tract infection, *Am J Vet Res* 54(10):1615–1622, 1993.
23. Hoffman AM, Viel L, Prescott JF: Microbiologic changes during antimicrobial treatment and rate of relapse of distal respiratory tract infections in foals, *Am J Vet Res* 54(10):1608–1614, 1993.
24. McKenzie HC: Characterization of antimicrobial aerosols for administration to horses, *Vet Ther* 4(2):110–119, 2003.
25. Srihakim S, Swerczek TW: Pathologic changes and pathogenesis of Parascaris equorum infection in parasite-free pony foals, *Am J Vet Res* 39(7):1155–1160, 1978.
26. Magnusson H: Spezifische infektiose Pneumonie beim Fohlen, Ein neuer Eiterreger beim Pferd, *Arch Wiss Prakt Tierheilkd* 50:22, 1923.
27. Hietala SK, Ardans AA: Interaction of Rhodococcus equi with phagocytic cells from Rhodococcus equi-exposed and non-exposed foals, *Vet Microbiol* 14:307–320, 1987.
28. Zink MC, Yager JA, Prescott JF, et al: Electron microscopic investigation of intracellular events after ingestion of Rhodococcus equi by foal alveolar macrophages, *Vet Microbiol* 14:295–305, 1987.
29. Brumbaugh GW, Davis LE, Thurmon JC, et al: Influence of *Rhodococcus equi* on the respiratory burst of resident alveolar macrophages from adult horses, *Am J Vet Res* 51:766–771, 1990.
30. Vullo V, Mastroianni CM, Lichtner M, et al: Rhodococcus equi infection of monocytes/macrophages from human immunodeficiency (HIV)-infected patients and healthy individuals: evaluation of intracellular killing and nitric oxide production, *FEMS Immunol Med Microbiol* 21:11–17, 1998.
31. Hondalus MK, Diamond MS, Rosenthal LA, et al: The intracellular bacterium Rhodococcus equi requires Mac-1 to bind to mammalian cells, *Infect Immun* 61:2919–2929, 1993.
32. Martens RJ, Martens JG, Renshaw HW: Rhodococcus (Corynebacterium) equi: bactericidal capacity of neutrophils from neonatal and adult horses, *Am J Vet Res* 49:295–299, 1988.
33. Takai S, Koike K, Ohbushi S, et al: Identification of 15- to 17-kilodalton antigens associated with virulent Rhodococcus equi, *J Clin Microbiol* 29:439–443, 1991.
34. Takai S, Iie M, Watanabe Y, et al: Virulence-associated 15- to 17 kilodalton antigens in Rhodococcus equi: temperature-dependent expression and location of the antigens, *Infect Immun* 60:2995–2997, 1992.
35. Giguère S, Hondalus MK, Yager JA, et al: Role of the 85-kilobase plasmid and plasmid-encoded virulence-associated protein A in intracellular survival and virulence of Rhodococcus equi, *Infect Immun* 67:3548–3557, 1999.
36. Wernery U, Wade JF, Mumford JA, Kaaden OR, editors: *Equine infectious diseases VIII,* Newmarket, England, 1999, R & W Publications.
37. Zink MC, Yager JA, Smart NL: Corynebacterium equi infections in horses, 1958–1984: a review of 131 cases, *Can J Vet Res* 27:213–217, 1986.
38. Giguere S, Prescott JF: Clinical manifestations, diagnosis, treatment, and prevention of Rhodococcus equi infections in foals, *Vet Microbiol* 56(3-4):313–334, 1997.
39. Ramirez S, Lester GD, Roberts GR: Diagnostic contribution of thoracic ultrasonography in 17 foals with Rhodococcus equi pneumonia, *Vet Radiol Ultrasound* 45(2):172–176, 2004.
40. Hietala SK, Ardans AA, Sansome A: Detection of Corynebacterium equi-specific antibody in horses by enzyme-linked immunosorbent assay, *Am J Vet Res* 46:13–15, 1985.
41. Wilkins PA, Lesser FR, Gaskin JM: Rhodococcus equi pneumonia in foals: comparison of ELISA and AGID serology on a commercial thoroughbred breeding farm. In *Proceedings of the eleventh ACVIM Forum,* Washington, DC, 1993, p 957.
42. Ardans AA, Hietala SK, Spensley MS, et al: Studies of naturally occurring and experimental Rhodococcus equi (Corynebacterium equi) pneumonia in foals, *Proc Am Assoc Equine Pract* 32:129–144, 1986.
43. Takai S, Vigo G, Ikushima H, et al: Detection of virulent Rhodococcus equi in tracheal aspirate samples by polymerase chain reaction for rapid diagnosis of *R. equi* pneumonia in foals, *Vet Microbiol* 61:59–69, 1998.
44. Sellon DC, Besser TE, Vivrette SL, et al: Comparison of nucleic acid amplification, serology, and microbiologic culture for diagnosis of *Rhodococcus equi* pneumonia in foals, *J Clin Microbiol* 39(4):1289–1293, 2001.
45. Hillidge CJ: Use of erythromycin-rifampin combination in treatment of *Rhodococcus equi* pneumonia, *Vet Microbiol* 14:337–342, 1987.
46. Jacks S, Giguere S, Gronwall PR, et al: Pharmacokinetics of azithromycin and concentration in body fluids and bronchoalveolar cells in foals, *Am J Vet Res* 62(12):1870–1875, 2001.
47. Giguère S, Jacks S, Roberts GD, et al: Retrospective comparison of azithromycin, clrithromycin, and erythromycin for the treatment of foals with *Rhodococcus equi* pneumonia, *J Vet Intern Med* 18:568–573, 2004.
48. Traub-Dargatz J, Wilson WD, Conboy HS, et al: Hyperthermia in foals treated with erythromycin alone or in combination with rifampin for respiratory disease during hot environmental conditions, *Proc Am Assoc Equine Pract* 42:243–244, 1996.
49. Baverud V, Franklin A, Gunnarsson A, et al: Clostridium difficile associated with acute colitis in mares when their foals are treated with erythromycin and rifampicin for Rhodococcus equi pneumonia, *Equine Vet J* 30:482–488, 1998.
50. Giguère S, Prescott JF: Strategies for the control of Rhodococcus equi infections on enzootic farms, *Proc Am Assoc Equine Pract* 43:65–70, 1997.
51. Becu T, Polledo G, Gaskin JM: Immunoprophylaxis of Rhodococcus equi pneumonia in foals, *Vet Microbiol* 56:193–204, 1997.
52. Hurley JR, Begg AP: Failure of hyperimmune plasma to prevent pneumonia caused by Rhodococcus equi in foals, *Aust Vet J* 72:418–420, 1995.
53. Martens RJ, Martens JG, Fiske RA, et al: Rhodococcus equi foal pneumonia: protective effects of immune plasma in experimentally infected foals, *Equine Vet J* 21:249–255, 1989.
54. Madigan JE, Hietala S, Muller N: Protection against naturally acquired Rhodococcus equi pneumonia in foals by administration of hyperimmune plasma, *J Reprod Fert Suppl* 44:571–578, 1991.
55. Muller NS, Madigan JE: Methods of implementation of an immunoprophylaxis program for the prevention of Rhodococcus equi pneumonia: results of a 5-year field study, *Proc Am Assoc Equine Pract* 38:193–201, 1992.
56. Higuchi T, Arakawa T, Hashikura S, et al: Effect of prophylactic administration of hyperimmune plasma to prevent *Rhodococcus equi* infection on foals from endemically affected farms, *Zentralbl Veterinarmed B* 46:641–648, 1999.

57. Hooper-McGrevy KE, Giguere S, Wilkie BN, et al: Valuation of equine immunoglobulin specific for Rhodococcus equi virulence-associated proteins A and C for use in protecting foals against Rhodococcus equi-induced pneumonia, *Am J Vet Res* 62(8):1307–1313, 2001.
58. Ainsworth DM, Eicker SW, Yeager AE, et al: Associations between physical examination, laboratory, and radiographic findings and outcome and subsequent racing performance of foals with Rhodococcus equi infection: 115 cases (1984-1992), *J Am Vet Med Assoc* 213:510–515, 1998.
59. Del Piero F: Equine viral arteriti, *Vet Pathol* 37(4):287–296, 2000.
60. Burrell MH: Endoscopic and virological observations on respiratory disease in a group of young thoroughbred horses in training, *Equine Vet J* 17(2):99–103, 1985.
61. Gilkerson JR, Whalley JM, Drummer HE, et al: Epidemiology of EHV-1 and EHV-4 in the mare and foal populations on a Hunter Valley stud farm: are mares the source of EHV-1 for unweaned foals? *Vet Microbiol* 68(1-2):27–34, 1999.
62. McCartan CG, Russell MM, Wood JL, et al: Clinical, serological and virological characteristics of an outbreak of paresis and neonatal foal disease due to equine herpesvirus-1 on a stud farm, *Vet Rec* 136(1):7–12, 1995.
63. Frymus T, Kita J, Woyciechowska S, et al: Foetal and neonatal foal losses on equine herpesvirus type 1(EHV-1) infected farms before and after EHV-1 vaccination was introduced, *Pol Arch Weter* 26(3-4):7–14, 1986.
64. Hartley WJ, Dixon RJ: An outbreak of foal perinatal mortality due to equid herpesvirus type 1: pathological observations, *Equine Vet J* 11(4):215–218, 1979.
65. Del Piero F, Wilkins PA, Lopez JW, et al: Equine viral arteritis in newborn foals: clinical, pathological, serological, microbiological and immunohistochemical observations, *Equine Vet J* 29(3):178–185, 1997.
66. Peek SF, Landolt G, Karasin AI, et al: Acute respiratory distress syndrome and fatal interstitial pneumonia associated with equine influenza in a neonatal foal, *J Vet Intern Med* 18(1): 132–134, 2004.
67. Webb RF, Knight PR, Walker KH: Involvement of adenovirus in pneumonia in a thoroughbred foal, *Aust Vet J* 57(3): 142–143, 1981.
68. Moorthy AR, Spradbrow PB: Adenoviral infection of Arab foals with respiratory tract disease, *Zentralbl Veterinarmed B* 25(6):469–477, 1978.
69. Thompson DB, Spradborw PB, Studdert M: Isolation of an adenovirus from an Arab foal with a combined immunodeficiency disease, *Aust Vet J* 52(10):435–437, 1976.
70. Perkins G, Ainsworth DM, Erb HN, et al: Clinical, haematological and biochemical findings in foals with neonatal equine herpesvirus-1 infection compared with septic and premature foals, *Equine Vet J* 31(5):422–426, 1999.
71. Murray MJ, del Piero F, Jeffrey SC, et al: Neonatal equine herpesvirus type 1 infection on a thoroughbred breeding farm, *J Vet Intern Med* 12(1):36–41, 1998.
72. Wilkins PA, Papich M, Sweeney RW: Acyclovir pharmacokinetics in adult horses, *J Vet Emerg Crit Care* 15(3):174–178, 2005.
73. Garré B, Shebany K, Gryspeerdt A, et al: Pharmacokinetics of acyclovir after intravenous infusion of acyclovir and after oral administration of acyclovir and its prodrug valacyclovir in healthy adult horses, *Antimicrob Agents Chemother* 51(12): 4308–4314, 2007.
74. Hullinger PJ, Wilson WD, Rossitto PV, et al: Passive transfer, rate of decay, and protein specificity of antibodies against equine arteritis virus in horses from a standardbred herd with high seroprevalence, *J Am Vet Med Assoc* 213(6):839–842, 1998.
75. Del Piero F, Wilkins PA, Timoney PJ, et al: Fatal nonneurological EHV-1 infection in a yearling filly, *Vet Pathol* 37(6): 672–676, 2000.
76. Del Piero F, Wilkins PA: Pulmonary vasculotropic EHV-1 infection in equids, *Vet Pathol* 38(4):474, 2001.
77. Borchers K, Wolfinger U, Ludwig H, et al: Virological and molecular biological investigations into equine herpes virus type 2 (EHV-2) experimental infections, *Virus Res* 55(1): 101–106, 1998.
78. Murray MJ, Eichorn ES, Dubovi EJ, et al: Equine herpesvirus type 2: prevalence and seroepidemiology in foals, *Equine Vet J* 28(6):432–436, 1996.
79. Jean D, Laverty S, Halley J, et al: Thoracic trauma in newborn foals, *Equine Vet J* 31(2):149–152, 1999.
80. Borchers A, van Eps A, Zedler S, et al: Thoracic trauma and postoperative lung injury in a neonatal foal, *Equine Vet Educ, accepted* 21: 186–191, 2009.
81. Marble SL, Edens LM, Shiroma JT, et al: Subcutaneous emphysema in a neonatal foal, *J Am Vet Med Assoc* 208(1):97–99, 1996.
82. Kraus BM, Richardson DW, Sheridan G, et al: Multiple rib fracture repair in a neonatal foal using nylon strand suture repair technique, *Vet Surg* 34(4):399–404, 2005.
83. O'Brodovich HM: Immature epithelial Na+ channel expression is one of the pathogenetic mechanisms leading to human neonatal respiratory distress syndrome, *Proc Assoc Am Physicians* 108(5):345–355, 1996.
84. Lakritz J, Wilson WD, Berry CR, et al: Bronchointerstitial pneumonia and respiratory distress in young horses: clinical, clinicopathologic, radiographic, and pathological findings in 23 cases (1984-1989), *J Vet Intern Med* 7(5):277–288, 1993.
85. Stratton-Phelps M, Wilson WD, Gardner IA: Risk of adverse effects in pneumonic foals treated with erythromycin versus other antibiotics: 143 cases (1986-1996), *J Am Vet Med Assoc* 217(1):68–73, 2000.

Diseases of the Urinary Tract

1. Bain AM: Disease of foals, *Aust Vet J* 30:9–12, 1954.
2. Du Plessis JL: Rupture of the bladder in the newborn foal and its surgical correction, *J S Afr Vet Assoc* 29:261–263, 1958.
3. Behr MJ, Hackett RP, Bentinick-Smith J, et al: Metabolic abnormalities associated with rupture of the urinary bladder in neonatal foals, *J Am Vet Med Assoc* 178:263–266, 1981.
4. Adams R, Koterba AM, Cudd TC, et al: Exploratory celiotomy for suspected urinary tract disruption in neonatal foals: a review of 18 cases, *Equine Vet J* 20:13–17, 1988.
5. Richardson DW, Kohn CW: Uroperitoneum in the foal, *J Am Vet Med Assoc* 182:267–271, 1983.
6. Kablack KA, Embertson RM, Bernard WV, et al: Uroperitoneum in the hospitalized equine neonate: retrospective study of 31 cases, 1988-1997, *Equine Vet J* 32:505–508, 2000.
7. Dunkel B, Palmer JE, Olson KN, et al: Uroperitoneum in 32 foals: influence of intravenous fluid therapy, infection, and sepsis, *J Vet Intern Med* 19(6):889–893, 2005.
8. Pascoe RR: Repair of a defect in the bladder of a foal, *Aust Vet J* 47:343–344, 1971.
9. Hackett RP: Rupture of the urinary bladder in neonatal foals, *Compend Cont Educ Pract Vet* 6:S488–S492, 1984.
10. Wellington JKM: Bladder defects in newborn foals, *Aust Vet J* 48:426, 1972:letter.
11. Wong DM, Leger LC, Scarratt WK, et al: Uroperitoneum and pleural effusion in an American Paint filly, *Equine Vet Educ* 16(6):290–293, 2004.
12. Wilkins PA: Respiratory distress in foals with uroperitoneum: possible mechanisms, *Equine Vet Educ* 16(6):293–295, 2004.
13. Reef VB, editor: *Equine diagnostic ultrasound*, Philadelphia, 1998, Saunders.
14. Lavoie JP, Harnagel SH: Nonsurgical management of ruptured urinary bladder in a critically ill foal, *J Am Vet Med Assoc* 192:1577–1580, 1988.

15. Vivrette S, Cowgill LD, Pascoe J, et al: Hemodialysis for treatment of oxytetracycline-induced acute renal failure in a neonatal foal, *J Am Vet Med Assoc* 203(1):105–107, 1993.
16. Andrews FM, Rosol TJ, Kohn CW, et al: Bilateral renal hypoplasia in four young horses, *J Am Vet Med Assoc* 189(2): 209–212, 1986.
17. Brown CM, Parks AH, Mullaney TP, et al: Bilateral renal dysplasia and hypoplasia in a foal with an imperforate anus, *Vet Rec* 122(4):91–92, 1988.
18. Schott HC 2nd, Barbee DD, Hines MT, et al: Clinical vignette: renal arteriovenous malformation in a Quarter horse foal, *J Vet Intern Med* 10(4):204–206, 1996.
19. Tomlinson JE, Farnsworth K, Sage AM, et al: Percutaneous ultrasound-guided pyelography aided diagnosis of ectopic ureter and hydronephrosis in a 3-week-old filly, *Vet Radiol Ultrasound* 42(4):349–351, 2001.
20. Cutler TJ, Mackay RJ, Johnson CM, et al: Bilateral ureteral tears in a foal, *Aust Vet J* 75(6):413–415, 1997.
21. Stickle RL, Wilcock BP, Huseman JL: Multiple ureteral defects in a Belgian foal, *Vet Med Small Anim Clin* 70(7):819–821, 1975.
22. Toribio RE, Bain FT, Mrad DR, et al: Congenital defects in newborn foals of mares treated for equine protozoal myeloencephalitis during pregnancy, *J Am Vet Med Assoc* 212(5):697–701, 1998.
23. PA Wilkins, JE Palmer, FT Bain, unpublished data,
24. Reef VB, Collatos C: Ultrasonography of umbilical structures in clinically normal foals, *Am J Vet Res* 49(12):2143–2146, 1988.
25. Reef VB, Collatos C, Spencer PA, et al: Clinical, ultrasonographic, and surgical findings in foals with umbilical remnant infections, *J Am Vet Med Assoc* 195(1):69–72, 1989.
26. Enzerink E, van Weeren PR, van der Velden MA: Closure of the abdominal wall at the umbilicus and the development of umbilical hernias in a group of foals from birth to 11 months of age, *Vet Rec* 147(2):37–39, 2000.
27. Freeman DE, Orsini JA, Harrison IW, et al: Complications of umbilical hernias in horses: 13 cases (1972-1986), *J Am Vet Med Assoc* 192(6):804–807, 1988.
28. De Bosschere H, Simoens P, Ducatelle R: Persistent vitelline vein in a foal, *Vet Rec* 145(3):75–77, 1999.

Diseases of the Gastrointestinal Tract

1. Pusterla N, Magdesian K, Maleski K, et al: Retrospective evaluation of the use of acetylcystein enemas in the treatment of meconium retention in foals: 44 cases (1987-2002), *Equine Vet Educ* (6):170–174, 2004.
2. Arguedas MG, Hines MT, Papich MG, et al: Pharmacokinetics of butorphanol and evaluation of physiologic and behavioral effects after intravenous and intramuscular administration to neonatal foals, *J Vet Intern Med* 22(6):1417–1426, 2008.
3. Wilkins PA: Respiratory distress in foals with uroperitoneum: possible mechanisms, *Equine Vet Educ* 16(6):293–295, 2004.
4. Young RL, Linford RL, Olander HJ: Atresia coli in the foal: a review of six cases, *Equine Vet J* 24(1):60–62, 1992.
5. Santschi EM, Purdy AK, Valberg SJ: Endothelin receptor B polymorphism associated with lethal white foal syndrome in horses, *Mamm Genome* 9(4):306–309, 1998.
6. Yang GC, Croaker D, Zhang AL, et al: A dinucleotide mutation in the endothelin-B receptor gene is associated with lethal white foal syndrome (LWFS): a horse variant of Hirschsprung disease, *Hum Mol Genet* 7(6):1047–1052, 1998.
7. Metallinos DL, Bowling AT, Rine J: A missense mutation in the endothelin-B receptor gene is associated with lethal white foal syndrome: an equine version of Hirschsprung disease, *Mamm Genome* 9(6):426–431, 1998.
8. Santschi EM, Vrotsos PD, Purdy AK, et al: Incidence of the endothelin receptor B mutation that causes lethal white foal syndrome in white-patterned horses, *Am J Vet Res* 62(1): 97–103, 2001.
9. Hostetler MA, Schulman M: Necrotizing enterocolitis presenting in the emergency department: case report and review of differential considerations for vomiting in the neonate, *J Emerg Med* 21(2):165–170, 2001.
10. Caplan MS, Jilling T: New concepts in necrotizing enterocolitis, *Curr Opin Pediatr* 13(2):111–115, 2001.
11. Jones RL, Adney WS, Alexander AF, et al: Hemorrhagic necrotizing enterocolitis associated with Clostridium difficile infection in four foals, *J Am Vet Med Assoc* 193(1):76–79, 1988.
12. Murray MJ: Endoscopic appearance of gastric lesions in foals: 94 cases (1987-1988), *J Am Vet Med Assoc* 195:1135–1141, 1989.
13. Murray MJ, Grodinsky BS, Cowles RR, et al: Endoscopic evaluation of changes in gastric lesions of thoroughbred foals, *J Am Vet Med Assoc* 196:1623–1627, 1990.
14. Murray MJ: Gastroduodenal ulceration in foals, *Equine Vet Educ* 11:199–207, 1999.
15. Murray MJ, Murray CM, Sweeney HJ, et al: Prevalence of gastric lesions in foals without signs of gastric disease: an endoscopic survey, *Equine Vet J* 22:6–8, 1990.
16. Rebhun WC, Dill SG, Power HT: Gastric ulcers in foals, *J Am Vet Med Assoc* 180(4):404–407, 1982.
17. Traub-Dagartz J, Bayly W, Riggs M, et al: Exsanguination due to gastric ulceration in a foal, *J Am Vet Med Assoc* 186(3): 280–281, 1985.
18. Palmer JE: Gastrointestinal diseases of foals, *Vet Clin North Am Equine Pract* 1(1):151–168, 1985.
19. Murray MJ: Pathophysiology of peptic disorders in foals and horses: a review, *Equine Vet J Suppl* 29:14–18, 1999.
20. Andrews FM, Nadeau JA: Clinical syndromes of gastric ulceration in foals and mature horses, *Equine Vet J Suppl* 29:30–33, 1999.
21. Becht JL, Byars TD: Gastroduodenal ulceration in foals, *Equine Vet J* 18:307–312, 1986.
22. Navab F, Steingrub J: Stress ulcer: is routine prophylaxis necessary? *Am J Gastroenterol* 90:708–712, 1995.
23. Mertz HR, Walsh TH: Peptic ulcer pathophysiology, *Med Clin North Am* 75:799–814, 1990.
24. Sanchez LC, Lester GD, Merritt AM: Intragastric pH in critically ill neonatal foals and the effect of ranitidine, *J Am Vet Med Assoc* 218:907–911, 2001.
25. MacAllister CG: A review of medical treatment for peptic ulcer disease, *Equine Vet J Suppl* 29:45–49, 1999.
26. Borne AT, MacAllister CG: Effect of sucralfate on healing of subclinical gastric ulcers in foals, *J Am Vet Med Assoc* 202: 1465–1468, 1993.
27. Sanchez LC, Lester GD, Merritt AM: Effect of ranitidine on intragastric pH in clinically normal neonatal foals, *J Am Vet Med Assoc* 212:1407–1412, 1998.
28. MacAllister CG, Sifferman RL, McClure SR, et al: Effects of omeprazole paste on healing of spontaneous gastric ulcers in horses and foals: a field trial, *Equine Vet J Suppl* 29:77–80, 1999.
29. Sanchez LC, Murray MJ, Merritt AM: Effect of omeprazole paste on intragastric pH in clinically normal neonatal foals, *Am J Vet Res* 65(8):1039–1041, 2004.
30. Javsicas LH, Sanchez LC: The effect of omeprazole paste on intragastric pH in clinically ill neonatal foals, *Equine Vet J* 40(1):41–44, 2008.
31. Kappstein I, Schulgen G, Frienrich T, et al: Incidence of pneumonia in mechanically ventilated patients treated with sucralfate or cimetidine as prophylaxis for stress bleeding: bacterial colonization of the stomach, *Am J Med* 91:125S–131S, 1991.
32. Dinsmore JE, Jackson RJ, Smith SD: The protective role of gastric acidity in neonatal bacterial translocation, *J Pediatr Surg* 32:1014–1016, 1997.
33. Crill CM, Hak EB: Upper gastrointestinal tract bleeding in critically ill pediatric patients, *Pharmacotherapy* 19:162–180, 1999.

34. Ortiz JE, Sottile FD, Sigel P, et al: Gastric colonization as a consequence of stress ulcer prophylaxis: a prospective, randomized trial, *Pharmacotherapy* 18:486–491, 1998.
35. Barr BS, Wilkins PA, DelPiero F, et al: Is prophylaxis for gastric ulcers necessary in critically ill equine neonates? A retrospective study of necropsy cases 1995-1999. In *Proceedings of the eighteenth annual meeting of the Veterinary Medical Forum*, Seattle, 2000, Wash, p 705.
36. Devlin JW, Ben-Menachem T, Ulep SK, et al: Stress ulcer prophylaxis in medical ICU patients: annual utilization in relation to the incidence of endoscopically proven stress ulceration, *Ann Pharmacother* 32:869–874, 1998.
37. Georgopoulos A, Feistauer SM, Makristathis A, et al: Influence of stress ulcer prophylaxis on translocation of bacteria from the intestinal tract in rats, *Wien Klin Wochenschr* 108:321–325, 1996.
38. Wada K, Kamisaki Y, Kitano M, et al: Effects of sucralfate on acute gastric mucosal injury and gastric ulcer induced by ischemia-reperfusion in rats, *Pharmacology* 54:57–63, 1997.
39. Devlin JW, Ben-Menachem T, Ulep SK, et al: Stress ulcer prophylaxis in medical ICU patients: annual utilization in relation to the incidence of endoscopically proven stress ulceration, *Ann Pharmacother* 32:869–874, 1998.

Diarrheal Diseases of Foals

1. Ludwig KG, Craig TM, Bowen JM, et al: Efficacy of ivermectin in controlling Strongyloides westeri infections in foals, *Am J Vet Res* 44(2):314–316, 1983.
2. Netherwood T, Wood JL, Townsend HG, et al: Foal diarrhoea between 1991 and 1994 in the United Kingdom associated with Clostridium perfringens, rotavirus, Strongyloides westeri and Cryptosporidium spp, *Epidemiol Infect* 117(2):375–383, 1996.
3. Dwyer RM: Rotaviral diarrhea, *Vet Clin North Am Equine Pract* 9(2):311–319, 1993.
4. Powell DG, Dwyer RM, Traub-Dargatz JL, et al: Field study of the safety, immunogenicity, and efficacy of an inactivated equine rotavirus vaccine, *J Am Vet Med Assoc* 211(2):193–198, 1997.
5. Barrandeguy M, Parreno V, Lagos Marmol M, et al: Prevention of rotavirus diarrhoea in foals by parenteral vaccination of the mares: field trial, *Dev Biol Stand* 92:253–257, 1998.
6. Corrier DE, Montgomery D, Scutchfield WL: Adenovirus in the intestinal epithelium of a foal with prolonged diarrhea, *Vet Pathol* 19(5):564–567, 1982.
7. Guy JS, Breslin JJ, Breuhaus B, et al: Characterization of a coronavirus isolated from a diarrheic foal, *J Clin Microbiol* 38(12):4523–4526, 2000.
8. Davis E, Rush BR, Cox J, et al: Neonatal enterocolitis associated with coronavirus infection in a foal: a case report, *J Vet Diagn Invest* 12(2):153–156, 2000.
9. Baker JC, Ames TR: Total parenteral nutritional therapy of a foal with diarrhoea from which parvovirus-like particles were identified, *Equine Vet J* 19(4):342–344, 1987.
10. Jones RL: Clostridial enterocolitis, *Vet Clin North Am Equine Pract* 16(3):471–485, 2000.
11. East LM, Savage CJ, Traub-Dargatz JL, et al: Enterocolitis associated with Clostridium perfringens infection in neonatal foals: 54 cases (1988-1997), *J Am Vet Med Assoc* 212(11):1751–1756, 1998.
12. Netherwood T, Binns M, Townsend H, et al: The Clostridium perfringens enterotoxin from equine isolates: its characterization, sequence and role in foal diarrhoea, *Epidemiol Infect* 120(2):193–200, 1998.
13. Jones RL, Adney WS, Shideler RK: Isolation of Clostridium difficile and detection of cytotoxin in the feces of diarrheic foals in the absence of antimicrobial treatment, *J Clin Microbiol* 25(7):1225–1227, 1987.
14. Palmer JE: Gastrointestinal diseases of foals, *Vet Clin North Am Equine Pract* 1(1):151–168, 1985.
15. Browning GF, Chalmers RM, Snodgrass DR, et al: The prevalence of enteric pathogens in diarrhoeic thoroughbred foals in Britain and Ireland, *Equine Vet J* 23(6):405–409, 1991.
16. Walker RL, Madigan JE, Hird DW, et al: An outbreak of equine neonatal salmonellosis, *J Vet Diagn Invest* 3(3):223–227, 1991.
17. Eugster AK, Whitford HW, Mehr LE: Concurrent rotavirus and Salmonella infections in foals, *J Am Vet Med Assoc* 173(7): 857–858, 1978.
18. Ward AC, Sriranganathan N, Evermann JF, et al: Isolation of piliated Escherichia coli from diarrheic foals, *Vet Microbiol* 12(3):221–228, 1986.
19. Hollis AR, Wilkins PA, Palmer JE, et al: Bacteremia in equine neonatal diarrhea: a retrospective study (1990-2007), *J Vet Intern Med* 22(5):1203–1209, 2008.
20. Lavoie JP, Drolet R, Parsons D, et al: Equine proliferative enteropathy: a cause of weight loss, colic, diarrhoea and hypoproteinaemia in foals on three breeding farms in Canada, *Equine Vet J* 32(5):418–425, 2000.
21. Williams NM, Harrison LR, Gebhart CJ: Proliferative enteropathy in a foal caused by Lawsonia intracellularis-like bacterium, *J Vet Diagn Invest* 8(2):254–256, 1996.
22. Cooper DM, Swanson DL, Gebhart CJ: Diagnosis of proliferative enteritis in frozen and formalin-fixed, paraffin-embedded tissues from a hamster, horse, deer and ostrich using a Lawsonia intracellularis-specific multiplex PCR assay, *Vet Microbiol* 54(1):47–62, 1997.
23. Mair TS, Taylor FG, Harbour DA, et al: Concurrent cryptosporidium and coronavirus infections in an Arabian foal with combined immunodeficiency syndrome, *Vet Rec* 126(6): 127–130, 1990.
24. Snyder SP, England JJ, McChesney AE: Cryptosporidiosis in immunodeficient Arabian foals, *Vet Pathol* 15(1):12–17, 1978.
25. Cole DJ, Cohen ND, Snowden K, et al: Prevalence of and risk factors for fecal shedding of Cryptosporidium parvum oocysts in horses, *J Am Vet Med Assoc* 213(9):1296–1302, 1998.
26. Brown CA, MacKay RJ, Chandra S, et al: Overwhelming strongyloidosis in a foal, *J Am Vet Med Assoc* 211(3):333–334, 1997.
27. DeLay J, Peregrine AS, Parsons DA: Verminous arteritis in a 3-month-old thoroughbred foal, *Can Vet J* 42(4):289–291, 2001.

Neonate Therapy

1. Berry LM, Ikegami M, Woods E, et al: Postnatal renal adaptation in preterm and term lambs, *Reprod Fertil Dev* 7(3):491–498, 1995.
2. Buchanan BR, Sommardahl CS, Rohrbach BW, et al: Effect of a 24-hour infusion of an isotonic electrolyte replacement fluid on the renal clearance of electrolytes in healthy neonatal foals, *J Am Vet Med Assoc* 227(7):1123–1129, 2005.
3. Kavvadia V, Greenough A, Dimitriou G, et al: Randomised trial of fluid restriction in ventilated very low birthweight infants, *Arch Dis Child Fetal Neonatal Ed* 83(2):F91–F96, 2000.
4. Bell EF, Acarregui MJ: Restricted versus liberal water intake for preventing morbidity and mortality in preterm infants, Cochrane Database Syst Rev 2:CD000503, 2000, and 3: CD000503, 2001 (update).
5. Bussmann C, Bast T, Rating D: Hyponatraemia in children with acute CNS disease: SIADH or cerebral salt wasting? Childs Nerv Syst 17(1-2):58–62, 2001 (discussion 63); erratum in Childs Nerv Syst 17(9):575, 2001.
6. Palmer JE: Fluid therapy in the neonate: not your mother's fluid space, *Vet Clin North Am Equine Pract* 20(1):63–75, 2004.
7. Palmer JE, unpublished data,
8. Giguère S, Knowles HA Jr, Valverde A, et al: Accuracy of indirect measurement of blood pressure in neonatal foals, *J Vet Intern Med* 19(4):571–576, 2005.

9. Corley KTT, McKenzie HC, Amoroso LM, et al: Initial experience with norepinephrine infusion in hypotensive critically ill foal, *J Vet Emerg Crit Care* 10:267–276, 2000.
10. Corley KT, Donaldson LL, Furr MO: Arterial lactate concentration, hospital survival, sepsis and SIRS in critically ill neonatal foals, *Equine Vet J* 37(1):53–59, 2005.
11. Corley KT, Pearce G, Magdesian KG, et al: Bacteraemia in neonatal foals: clinicopathological differences between Gram-positive and Gram-negative infections, and single organism and mixed infections, *Equine Vet J* 39(1):84–89, 2007.
12. Yang Y, Qiu HB, Zhou SX, et al: Comparison of norepinephrine-dobutamine to dopamine alone for splanchnic perfusion in sheep with septic shock, *Acta Pharmacol Sin* 23(2):133–137, 2002.
13. Bellomo R, Wan L, May C: Vasoactive drugs and acute kidney injury, *Crit Care Med* 36(4 Suppl):S179–S186, 2008.
14. Sharshar T, Carlier R, Blanchard A, et al: Depletion of neurohypophyseal content of vasopressin in septic shock, *Crit Care Med* 30(3):497–500, 2002.
15. Hurcombe SD, Toribio RE, Slovis N, et al: Blood arginine vasopressin, adrenocorticotropin hormone, and cortisol concentrations at admission in septic and critically ill foals and their association with survival, *J Vet Intern Med* 22(3):639–647, 2008.
16. Tsuneyoshi I, Yamada H, Kakihana Y, et al: Hemodynamic and metabolic effects of low-dose vasopressin infusions in vasodilatory septic shock, *Crit Care Med* 29(3):487–493, 2001.
17. Patel BM, Chittock DR, Russell JA, et al: Beneficial effects of short-term vasopressin infusion during severe septic shock, *Anesthesiology* 96(3):576–582, 2002.

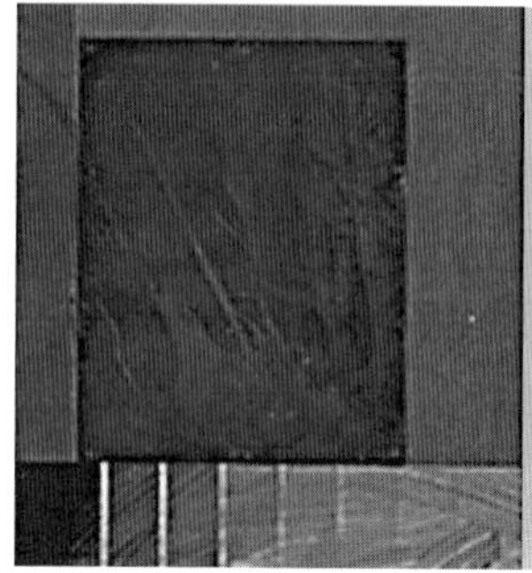

Toxicologic Problems

CHAPTER 22

*Patricia Talcott**

In today's world any list of substances that are toxic or potentially toxic is probably incomplete. Industrial societies continue to produce new and different compounds that are potentially hazardous or fatal to human beings and many species of animals. Knowledge of toxic compounds and the mechanisms whereby they produce disease also is changing constantly, so certain substances that previously were thought to be inert now are known to affect the health of animals or human beings. As the saying goes, almost everything is toxic in the right dose.

It behooves the veterinary clinician to be as informed as possible about the potentially toxic substances found in an animal's environment. Not all toxins are distributed uniformly in nature (this is particularly true of toxic plants), so another reasonable assumption would be that in any given geographic area, certain toxicities are much more common than others.

Many factors influence the toxicity of a given substance, and a detailed discussion is not within the scope of this chapter. Books cover the specific aspects of toxicity and all the different mechanisms that come into play when a specific substance causes harm to a specific animal at a specific point in time. The reader is referred to other sources for information regarding general toxicologic principles and measurements and quantification. It is important to note that age, species of animal, reproductive status, nutritional status, management, diet, and numerous other factors relating to the animal can influence the toxicity of a given substance. Other factors related to the compound itself—such as its bioavailability, its chemical form or structure, its concentration—also can influence the toxicity of a substance at any point.

Most toxins do not damage a solitary tissue, organ, or organ system preferentially but frequently affect several organs or body systems at the same time. Although for clinical signs to be related predominantly to a single organ system is not unusual, multiple organ involvement is the rule rather than the exception. This fact necessitates a thorough physical examination and evaluation of any animal presented for diagnosis of possible toxicosis. The clinician should evaluate all body systems horses that are suspected of having a toxicity.

The clinical manifestations of many toxicologic problems do not occur immediately but rather some time after initial exposure to the toxin. This delay can make diagnosis and treatment difficult. For this reason many cases of suspected toxicity are treated empirically. If a specific antidote is available or indicated, however, it should be used in the treatment regimen (Box 22-1).

In this chapter the toxins have been divided into broad categories of general clinical signs. A toxin is discussed most completely under the system to which the major clinical signs are referable. One must remember, however, that most toxins involve more than one organ system, so a number of toxins can be found in several categories.

BOX 22-1

GENERAL RULES REGARDING TREATMENT OF SUSPECTED TOXICOSES

1. Removal of the toxicant or animal from the environment
2. Removal of the toxin from the body of the animal, if possible
3. Cleaning of the skin or contact surface with suitable agents if the route of exposure is dermal
4. Evacuation of the gastrointestinal tract by appropriate means if contamination resulted from ingestion of the toxin
5. Maintenance of normal body functions and physiologic processes by means of basic supportive care measures, such as fluid administration and blood pH and electrolyte modification
6. Elimination of the toxin from the system of the animal as expeditiously as possible
7. Measures to prevent reexposure or recontamination of the animal by the toxic substance

*The authors wish to acknowledge David G. Schmitz, whose original work has been incorporated into this chapter.

TOXICOSES DISPLAYING SIGNS RELATING TO THE GASTROINTESTINAL SYSTEM

There is a wide range of toxic agents capable of inducing signs of gastrointestinal disease. Signs vary from mild to peracute and life threatening. Determination that a toxicosis is the cause of a problem such as diarrhea or colic sometimes is difficult, time consuming, and relatively costly.

PLANTS

Oak (*Quercus* species)

CLINICAL SIGNS

Oak blossoms, buds, leaves, stems, and acorns can be toxic to most animals. Most reports of toxicosis in livestock involve cattle and sheep, with a rare occurrence in the horse. Clinical signs attributed to acorn toxicosis in horses are acute onset of severe abdominal pain, rectal straining, hemorrhagic diarrhea, and pronounced intestinal borborygmi. Acorn parts may be apparent in feces. Occasionally, horses are found dead; other signs are hemoglobinuria and elevated heart and respiratory rates.

PATHOPHYSIOLOGY

The toxicity of oak is attributed to a group of structurally similar compounds called *gallotannins* and their metabolites. Digallic acid is the major active metabolite produced by oak tannins. After bacterial fermentation digallic acid is converted to gallic acid and pyrogallol, both of which are considered toxic.[1] Pyrogallol and gallic acid are toxic to renal tubules and result in acute tubular necrosis, anuria, electrolyte abnormalities, and uremia.[1,2] Pyrogallol is also responsible for causing hemorrhagic gastroenteritis, subcutaneous hemorrhage, and hemolysis. Tannic acid itself is thought to result in increased vascular permeability, hemorrhage, and subsequent fluid loss into body spaces.[1]

DIAGNOSIS

The diagnosis of oak toxicity is based on clinical signs and a history of potential exposure to the plant. Under adequate forage conditions horses would seem to find large quantities of oak leaves and acorns distasteful; therefore most horses with oak trees in their environment do not develop toxicity. Toxicosis is more likely to result when abnormal conditions coupled with environmental factors (e.g., lack of access to normal forage or feed) result in large numbers of oak leaves and acorns becoming accessible to horses.

Laboratory findings compatible with oak toxicosis include dehydration or hemoconcentration to varying degrees, azotemia, hyperphosphatemia, hypocalcemia, and hypoproteinemia. Abnormal urine findings might include occult blood, proteinuria, and casts. An increase in gallic acid equivalent content in urine also has been used to support exposure to oak trees.[1] However, oak trees are not the only plant that can contain these tannins, and normal and toxic ranges of gallic acid in urine have not been well established in livestock.

Necropsy findings suggestive of oak toxicosis include pericardial, thoracic, and peritoneal effusion; gastrointestinal and mesenteric edema; and pale and swollen kidneys that may bulge on cut surface. The intestinal tract may contain large quantities of acorn parts, and colonic ulceration has been reported.[1]

SPECIFIC TREATMENT AND MANAGEMENT

No specific antidote for oak toxicity is available. Animals should be allowed no further access to oak. Treatment of the acutely affected animal aims to maintain fluid and acid-base balance and to correct any electrolyte abnormalities. Balanced polyionic fluids given intravenously to promote diuresis are the basic therapy. This therapy should be supplemented with calcium, bicarbonate, and other electrolytes as necessary. Anuric animals may gain additional benefit from furosemide at 1 mg/kg intravenously or dimethyl sulfoxide (DMSO) at 1 g/kg given intravenously as a 10% solution in addition to fluid therapy. The clinician should attempt evacuation of the intestinal tract using mineral oil or another suitable laxative.

The prognosis for affected horses is guarded. A paucity of information exists regarding mortality rates in affected horses, but death caused by ingestion of acorns has been reported.[1]

Castor Bean (*Ricinus communis*)

CLINICAL SIGNS

Castor beans contain ricin, a protein phytotoxin that acts as a potent proteolytic enzyme with significant antigenic qualities.[2] A latent period ranging from hours to several days usually occurs before the onset of clinical signs in affected horses. The bean is apparently distasteful to horses, and intoxication most likely occurs when the bean inadvertently is mixed into the feed source. To cause problems, the bean must be broken apart by chewing; beans swallowed intact are thought to pass through the gastrointestintal tract uneventfully.

The most commonly reported clinical signs of castor bean toxicosis described in the literature are varying degrees of abdominal pain, diarrhea, depression, incoordination, profuse sweating, and increased body temperature. Muscle twitching, convulsions, and prominent cardiac contractions occasionally are observed. If the horse absorbs enough ricin, signs of shock and anaphylaxis predominate.[2,3] Death may ensue as soon as 24 to 36 hours after ingestion.

Ricin is reported to be toxic to horses. One reference cites a ricin dosage of 0.1 μg/kg as a lethal dose,[2] and a second source indicates 25 g of castor beans is lethal.[3] A published report in 1945 describes seven deaths attributed to castor bean toxicosis from a stable of 48 horses in London in 1931.[4] The exact number of affected horses was not reported. A review of the literature suggests that castor bean (ricin) toxicosis in human beings and dogs is not nearly as lethal as reported in the literature of the early twentieth century.[5,6] Whether this holds true for horses is open to speculation.

PATHOPHYSIOLOGY

The oil extract of the bean contains ricinoleic acid. Within the small intestine ricinoleate acts to reduce net absorption of fluid and electrolytes and stimulates peristalsis.[7] The fibrous residue of the seed contains the water-soluble toxalbumin ricin. Ricin is absorbed from the gastrointestinal tract and is a potent inhibitor of protein synthesis. Ricin contains two polypeptide chains. Chain B, a lectin, binds to the cell surface to facilitate toxin entry into the cell. Chain A disrupts protein synthesis by activating the 60S ribosomal subunit. The red blood cell–agglutinating properties of ricin are independent of these toxic effects.[8]

DIAGNOSIS

Diagnosis is made by a combination of history of exposure to the plant; clinical signs; and the identification of seeds in feed material, gastric contents, or feces. Analyses for ricin content in urine, as well as other samples, are available from certain laboratories.[8]

TREATMENT

Ricin has no specific antidote. Initial therapy aims to combat shock, alleviating abdominal pain and evacuating the bowel. Maintenance of fluid and electrolyte balance is important. Various sedatives and analgesics may be useful to control abdominal pain, if present. Oral administration of laxatives and protectants such as mineral oil and charcoal may be warranted. Antihistamines also have been recommended.[2]

POKEWEED (*PHYTOLACCA AMERICANA*)

CLINICAL SIGNS

Pokeweed intoxication in horses is an uncommon occurrence. However, one text reports that horses show signs of gastrointestinal irritation and abdominal discomfort as the primary clinical signs. The plant also produces a burning sensation of the oral mucous membranes and may cause a hemolytic crisis. Fatalities caused by pokeweed ingestion are said to result from respiratory failure and convulsions.[2]

PATHOPHYSIOLOGY

The plant contains phytolaccine, a powerful gastrointestinal irritant that in human beings causes symptoms ranging from a burning sensation of the alimentary tract to severe hemorrhagic gastritis. Five nonspecific mitogens that have hemagglutinating and mitotic activity have been isolated. These substances vary in concentration in the plant throughout the growing season. Noncardiac steroids and triterpenoid glycosides (saponins) also are present in significant quantities, but their role in pokeweed toxicity is unknown.[8] Saponins may potentiate gastrointestinal toxicity and produce vasodilation when given parenterally.

DIAGNOSIS AND TREATMENT

No specific diagnostic test is available. Horses suspected of having toxicosis must be treated symptomatically. The clinician should attempt to evacuate the gastrointestinal tract using laxatives. Adsorbents such as charcoal and protectants may be useful. If the horse develops a hemolytic crisis, ancillary therapy such as whole-blood transfusions may be lifesaving. Fluid and electrolyte balance must be maintained in these horses in an attempt to prevent or minimize hemoglobin- or hypoxic-induced nephrosis.[2]

NIGHTSHADE (*SOLANUM* SPP.)

CLINICAL SIGNS

A number of species of *Solanum* spp. have been incriminated in causing toxicity in horses. However, these plants rarely are a source of natural intoxication to horses. Reported clinical signs are referable to the gastrointestinal and central nervous systems. The primary gastrointestinal signs observed are salivation, abdominal pain, increased borborygmi, and diarrhea. Signs of central nervous system (CNS) dysfunction include mydriasis, dullness, depression, weakness, and progressive paralysis, which can lead to prostration and death.[2,9,10]

PATHOPHYSIOLOGY

Solanine is a toxic substance found in *Solanum* species; it is a water-soluble glycoalkaloid capable of producing local irritation[2,3,8] and is absorbed poorly from the gastrointestinal tract. Intravenous doses caused ventricular fibrillation in rabbits, and intraperitoneal doses caused mild to moderate inhibition of specific and nonspecific cholinesterase activity.[8] It has been shown that exposure to *Solanum* plants can potentiate the effects of ivermectin in horses.[11]

DIAGNOSIS AND TREATMENT

No specific diagnostic test is available to confirm a diagnosis of *Solanum* toxicosis. Animals suspected of having toxicosis should be treated symptomatically. Evacuation of the gastrointestinal tract using laxatives and protectants may be indicated. Charcoal also has been recommended for treatment of toxicosis in human beings.[8] The clinician should monitor the fluid, electrolyte, and acid-base status of affected animals and make corrections as needed.

JIMSONWEED, THORNAPPLE (*DATURA* SPP.)

CLINICAL SIGNS

Several species of *Datura* grow throughout North America, all of which can produce signs of toxicosis in livestock. However, these plants are rarely a source of natural intoxication in horses, probably because of the unpalatability of the plant.[9,10] One report of equine acute toxicosis resulted when ingested feed was contaminated heavily with jimsonweed seeds. According to this report, one horse was affected acutely and died because of gastric rupture and gas-filled intestinal loops. A second horse was treated for several days before being euthanized. Clinical signs observed in the treated horse included abdominal distention with gas-filled intestinal loops, prolonged ileus, mydriasis, tachycardia, hyperpnea, and dry mucous membranes.[12]

PATHOPHYSIOLOGY

The toxic substances found in *Datura* spp. are the tropane alkaloids atropine (a racemic mixture of D- and L-hyoscyamine) and scopolamine (L-hyoscine).[9,10,12] These substances exert an antimuscarinic effect by competitive inhibition with acetylcholine for receptor sites, resulting in attenuation of the physiologic response of neuroeffector junctions to parasympathetic nerve impulses. Blockade of the muscarinic receptors of different tissues accounts for the various clinical signs observed.

DIAGNOSIS AND TREATMENT

Toxicity is suspected when animals exhibit signs compatible with atropine overdose. Identification of seeds or plant material in ingesta, gastric lavage contents, or feedstuffs may support a diagnosis. Treatment is largely symptomatic and includes immediate removal of the offending feed or plants, evacuation of the gastrointestinal tract, and supportive care. The use of pilocarpine and physostigmine to counteract the atropine-like effects of these alkaloids has been recommended by some, but this treatment is considered controversial.[9,10]

MISCELLANEOUS AGENTS

Dioctyl Sodium Sulfosuccinate

Dioctyl sodium sulfosuccinate (DSS) is an anionic surface active agent commonly used to treat constipation and intestinal impaction in horses. The recommended dose of DSS is 17 to 66 mg/kg, with a maximum dose of 200 mg/kg.[2,13]

CLINICAL SIGNS

Signs of overdose commence within 60 to 120 minutes in affected horses. Initial signs are restlessness and increased intestinal sounds accompanied by steadily increasing heart and respiratory rates. Abdominal pain, watery diarrhea, and dehydration become apparent soon afterward, and horses gradually deteriorate to lateral recumbency and death in 14 to 72 hours.

PATHOPHYSIOLOGY

Much information about the pharmacologic action of DSS remains uncertain.[7] The primary organ of involvement is the small intestine, where epithelial denudation, villous atrophy, and submucosal edema and congestion occur. DSS has been suggested possibly to cause epithelial detachment by lowering the surface tension on the basement membranes of intestinal epithelial cells.[13] Once detachment occurs, loss of fluid and electrolytes into the intestinal lumen is possible. The absorptive capacity of the epithelium is lost, and the osmotic effect of intestinal content causes further loss of fluid into the lumen. With extensive mucosal damage, the horse also becomes much more susceptible to endotoxemia. The rapid death in affected animals is caused by hypovolemic shock, endotoxemia, and circulatory collapse resulting from the loss of fluids and electrolytes into the intestinal lumen.

DIAGNOSIS AND TREATMENT

Diagnosis of DSS toxicity depends on observation of the aforementioned clinical signs along with oral DSS administration. No specific antidote for DSS exists, and once clinical signs commence, treatment is aimed at supporting circulation and combating the effects of systemic endotoxin. Specific treatment for circulatory collapse and endotoxemia is covered elsewhere, but medications that might be useful include polyionic electrolyte solutions, electrolyte supplementation, corticosteroids, nonsteroidal anti-inflammatory drugs (NSAIDs), bicarbonate, and orally administered gastrointestinal protectants.

Inorganic Arsenic

Arsenic is found in a number of products, including insecticides, herbicides, defoliants, rodenticides, livestock dips, medications, wood preservatives, paint pigments, detergents, and certain insulation materials.[14,15] Horses are most likely to be exposed to arsenic by eating contaminated or treated forage being exposed accidentally to stored or improperly discarded pesticides.[15] Horses cannot receive a significant exposure through cribbing on arsenic-treated wood. However, if arsenic-treated lumber is burned, ingestion of the arsenic-laced ash could be problematic.

CLINICAL SIGNS

The clinical signs associated with arsenic toxicity are essentially those of a severe gastrointestinal irritant. Most toxicities result from inorganic forms of arsenic, and signs are similar in several animal species.

In peracute cases the animals may be found dead with no premonitory signs. Acute signs of toxicity include severe colic, staggering, weakness, salivation, diarrhea that may contain blood or shreds of mucosa, and signs of shock that indicate cardiovascular collapse. Death usually occurs in 1 to 3 days.[14-16] In subacute poisoning animals may live for several days, exhibiting signs of depression, anorexia, colic, diarrhea that may contain blood and mucus, polyuria followed by anuria, and subsequent shock before death. Horses that are poisoned by topical application of arsenic can show signs of blistering and edema of the skin.[14] Chronic arsenic poisoning rarely occurs in domestic animals.

PATHOPHYSIOLOGY

Many factors play a role in the development of arsenic toxicosis in horses. In general, horses that are debilitated, weak, or dehydrated are more susceptible to toxicosis than normal animals. The formulation of the compound (trivalent arsenicals are more toxic than pentavalent forms), the solubility of the compound, the route of exposure, the rate of absorption from the gastrointestinal tract, and the rate of metabolism and excretion by the individual animal are factors that can influence the toxicity of the various arsenic formulations.[14] The most hazardous preparations are products in which the arsenical is in a highly soluble trivalent form, usually trioxide or arsenite. Sodium arsenite is 3 to 10 times more toxic than arsenic trioxide. The average total oral lethal doses of these compounds for the horse are 10 to 45 g arsenic trioxide and 1 to 3 g sodium arsenite.[14,15]

Soluble forms of arsenic are absorbed from all body surfaces. Less soluble arsenicals are absorbed poorly from the gastrointestinal tract and essentially are excreted unchanged in the feces. After absorption trivalent arsenic is excreted readily by way of the bile into the intestine, and pentavalent arsenic is excreted by the kidney. Regardless of whether an introduced arsenical is in the trivalent or pentavalent form, all the major actions can be attributed to the trivalent form.[14]

All arsenicals are thought to exert their effects by reacting with sulfhydryl groups in cells. Trivalent arsenic acts primarily by combining with the two sulfhydryl groups of lipoic acid, thereby inactivating this essential cofactor necessary for the enzymatic decarboxylation of the keto acids pyruvate, ketoglutarate, and ketobutyrate. By inactivating lipoic acid, arsenic inhibits the formation of acetyl, succinyl, and propionyl coenzymes A. The net effect is the blocking of fat and carbohydrate metabolism and cellular respiration.[14,15] Trivalent arsenic may inactivate sulfhydryl groups of oxidative enzymes and the sulfhydryl group of glutathione and other essential monothiols and dithiols. Arsenic also causes a local corrosive action on the intestine.[15]

Arsenic seems to prefer tissues rich in oxidative enzymes such as the liver, kidney, and intestine. The capillary endothelial cells in these organs appear sensitive to arsenic because it relaxes capillaries and increases capillary permeability. Blood vessels with smooth muscle in their walls also dilate. In the intestinal tract the mucosa easily sloughs away because of the accumulation of fluid in the submucosa. In the kidney renal tubular degeneration occurs.[15]

DIAGNOSIS

The clinical signs described previously should cause the practitioner to consider inorganic arsenic poisoning. Antemortem laboratory findings are consistent with gastrointestinal, hepatic, and renal damage. Feces may contain blood, mucus, and increased numbers of white blood cells. The liver enzymes sorbitol dehydrogenase, lactate dehydrogenase (LDH), AST, and γ-glutamyltransferase (GGT) may be increased in serum, and urine might contain protein, red blood cells, and casts. Urine arsenic concentration in affected animals often exceeds 2 ppm.[14]

Postmortem findings are characteristic of severe gastroenteritis and may include hepatic lipidosis and necrosis. In horses in which arsenic poisoning is suspected, the liver, kidneys, stomach, intestinal contents, milk, blood, and urine should be evaluated.

TREATMENT

Specific therapy for arsenic toxicity is dimercaprol (or British antiLewisite [BAL]). This chelating agent forms a nontoxic and easily excretable complex with arsenic. However, BAL may mobilize stored arsenic in tissues and cause an initial exacerbation of clinical signs by allowing more arsenic to circulate to the intestine and liver. BAL also can be toxic in sufficient doses. Signs of overdose include tremors, convulsions, coma, and death. In horses the recommended dose is 3 mg/kg intramuscularly as a 5% solution in a 10% solution of benzyl benzoate in peanut oil. This dose is administered every 4 hours for the first 2 days, every 6 hours on the third day, and twice daily for the next 10 days until recovery.[15]

Sodium thiosulfate also has been advocated for treatment of arsenic toxicosis, but its efficacy is questionable. The recommended dose for horses is 20 to 30 g orally in 300 ml of water, plus 8 to 10 g intravenously in a 10% to 20% solution.[15]

Symptomatic care of affected animals includes evacuation of the gastrointestinal tract with laxatives and oral demulcents to coat the intestinal tract. The clinician should evaluate fluid, acid-base, and electrolyte indices and provide support if necessary. Aggressive intravenous fluid diuresis is advocated by many to maintain adequate hydration and enhance urinary arsenic excretion. Because endotoxemia may develop as a result of the intestinal and liver lesions, prophylactic administration of flunixin meglumine at a dosage of 0.25 mg/kg every 8 hours may be beneficial. Other therapy to prevent shock and cardiovascular collapse also may be indicated.

ALUMINUM

One report describes an unexpectedly high incidence of horses on the same farm showing clinical signs compatible with granulomatous enteritis and the presence of abnormally high levels of aluminum in various body organs and tissues of the affected horses.[17] Clinical signs included weight loss with or without diarrhea, hyperkeratosis, ulcerative coronitis, and neurologic deficits compatible with cervical stenotic myelopathy. Laboratory abnormalities included hypoalbuminemia and elevated serum concentration of alkaline phosphatase in some horses. All horses had histologic evidence of granulomatous inflammation of the gastrointestinal tract in varying degrees of severity and distribution. Granulomas occurred in the mucosa, submucosa, and serosa of the small and large intestines and in the abdominal lymph nodes, portal areas of the liver, and pancreas. Aluminum was found within granulomas, and elevated aluminum levels were present in kidney and liver tissue.

Chronic environmental exposure to aluminum was postulated as a cause for the condition. Environmental factors (e.g., soil pH, moisture content, plants) may have an effect on the bioavailability of aluminum, and it has been suggested that repeated exposure may induce hypersensitivity to aluminum in these horses. In human beings aluminum is known to induce nonimmunologic (foreign body) and immunologic granulomas after administration of aluminum-containing vaccines and hyposensitization products.[18] The association between high environmental concentrations of aluminum and increased incidence of generalized granulomatous inflammation in horses warrants further investigation.

PETROLEUM DISTILLATES

Horses can be exposed to excessive amounts of crude oil or petroleum distillates through contamination of rangeland with by-products of the oil industry or by iatrogenic application, because petroleum distillates commonly are used as carrier agents for many insecticides.

CLINICAL SIGNS

The most frequently noted signs associated with ingestion of petroleum products are essentially those of gastrointestinal and respiratory dysfunction. Petroleum products are irritating to mucous membranes, and hence prominent signs of gastrointestinal dysfunction might include salivation and fluid feces. The feces actually may contain oil or oily substances. Chronically affected animals also may exhibit anorexia and weight loss over several days to weeks.

Signs of respiratory dysfunction are a common manifestation of excessive petroleum exposure. Aspiration of the oil or fumes is irritating to pulmonary tissue, and aspiration pneumonia is probably the most serious consequence of petroleum toxicity.[14] Signs of toxicity include increased respirations, anorexia, depression, weight loss, a variable degree of fever, and possibly increased nasal discharge.

Products that are applied inadvertently to the skin might cause some degree of respiratory embarrassment, but they are more likely to cause signs related to the absorption of excessive hydrocarbons.[15] Topically applied agents also may cause signs associated with a contact irritant.

PATHOPHYSIOLOGY

The toxicity of crude oil is correlated with the gasoline, naphtha, and kerosene content in the oil. Crude oil rich in these low-temperature distillates is more toxic than petroleum containing a great deal of sulfur but less of the low-temperature distillates.[15] Petroleum products are irritating to mucous membranes, and their oiliness makes them difficult to remove from skin and mucous membranes and virtually impossible to remove from the respiratory epithelium. Once aspirated, they serve as a focus for foreign body pneumonia that may progress to abscessing pneumonia, pleuritis and pleural effusion, and death.

DIAGNOSIS

History of possible exposure, clinical signs, and pathophysiologic signs are important in establishing a diagnosis. Suspected contents (i.e., gastrointestinal content or feces) may be mixed with water, and any oil that is present will float to the surface and be readily visible. Analytic chemistry methods sometimes can be used to establish the identity of an oil.[14]

TREATMENT

Treatment is supportive. The clinician should evacuate and protect the gastrointestinal tract by using laxatives and demulcents. Products applied to the skin can be removed with warm soapy water followed by thorough rinsing. Products such as mechanic's hand degreasers can be tried first to remove fat-soluble compounds. Aspiration pneumonia may be frustrating to treat, and supportive care such as fluids and electrolytes, NSAIDs, and broad spectrum antimicrobial therapy is potentially helpful.

Slaframine

Slaframine is an indole alkaloid produced by *Rhizoctonia leguminicola*, a mold that infects red clover, alfalfa, and other legumes.[14,15,19] *R. leguminicola* is a ubiquitous soil fungus that infects certain legumes during conditions of high rainfall or humidity.[19] The toxin can survive and persist in dried and baled hay.[14]

CLINICAL SIGNS

The most consistently reported clinical sign is excessive salivation characterized by profuse, viscous, clear saliva.[19] Salivation may begin 30 to 60 minutes after eating the affected feed, and response from one feeding may persist for up to 24 hours. Other, less commonly reported clinical signs include anorexia, polyuria, and sometimes watery diarrhea.[14] One case of abortion in an affected mare has been reported.[19] Clinical signs generally abate 48 to 96 hours after the infected feed is removed from the diet.[14]

PATHOPHYSIOLOGY

Slaframine apparently is activated by liver microsomes after absorption. The active compound seems to have direct histaminergic effects or possibly a histamine-releasing effect, which is borne out in laboratory animal studies in which clinical signs responded better to antihistamines than to atropine.[15]

DIAGNOSIS

The combination of acute clinical signs of excessive salivation coupled with digestive disturbances and identification of *R. leguminicola* in forage generally is adequate to establish a diagnosis. It is possible to analyze slaframine in feeds, but usually such tests are unnecessary.[14]

TREATMENT

No specific treatment usually is necessary. Animals generally recover uneventfully 48 to 96 hours after withdrawal of the contaminated forage.[14] Atropine and antihistaminic therapies have been suggested to help control clinical signs,[14,15] but their efficacy is questionable.

Pentachlorophenol

Documented instances of horses becoming intoxicated with pentachlorophenol are rare. However, because pentachlorophenol was used routinely as a wood preservative and because other domestic animals, including cattle and swine, have been poisoned, some aspects of this toxin require description. Exposure potentially occurs as a result of the horse drinking from a container containing pentachlorophenol or lying on recently treated lumber or contaminated soil.

The chlorophenols (which include pentachlorophenol) generally are not water soluble but are soluble in oils and organic solvents.[15,20] Pentachlorophenol is volatile and can give off toxic vapors.[15] The chlorophenols are absorbed readily from the gastrointestinal tract, by inhalation, and from intact skin and are excreted rapidly by the kidney.[15,20]

Several factors affect the toxicity of chlorophenols. High ambient temperature, physical activity, poor body condition, oily or organic solvent vehicles, prior exposure, and hyperthyroid states serve to enhance toxicity in human beings and other animal species. Cold temperatures, antithyroid drugs, and increased amounts of body fat help diminish the toxicity.[15]

The mechanism whereby the chlorophenols exert their toxicity involves the energy production sites of mitochondria, where they uncouple oxidative phosphorylation. The chlorophenols act at sites of adenosine triphosphate (ATP) production to decrease or block their production without blocking the electron transport chain. Free energy from the electron transport chain then is converted to body heat. As the body temperature is increased, the heat-dissipating mechanisms are overcome and metabolism is increased. The electron transport chain responds by using more oxygen in an effort to produce ATP, but much of the free energy is liberated as more body heat. Eventually, the oxygen demand overcomes the oxygen supply, and energy reserves become depleted.[15]

CLINICAL SIGNS

Clinical signs, if observed, may include fever, tachycardia, dyspnea, sweating, lethargy, incoordination, weakness, cyanosis, collapse, and death. Less severely affected animals may primarily manifest signs of hyperthermia and oxygen deficiency.[15] Pentachlorophenol in high doses to pregnant animals also is reported to cause embryonic and fetal deaths but is not teratogenic.[14]

DIAGNOSIS AND TREATMENT

Pentachlorophenol toxicity is associated with the combination of clinical signs and blood pentachlorophenol levels greater than 40 ppm. No specific treatment is available, but saline diuresis has been suggested to be helpful in certain instances of human toxicosis.[14]

Chlorates

Chlorate salts (sodium chlorate or potassium chlorate) are used as herbicides and defoliants. Horses may become exposed by grazing in recently sprayed areas or by ingesting sodium chlorate when it is mistakenly substituted for sodium chloride as a feed additive.

CLINICAL SIGNS

Initial signs are those of gastrointestinal irritation and include colic and diarrhea. Hematuria and hemoglobinuria also are present early in the disease course. Within hours the horse shows dyspnea, cyanosis, and increased respiratory effort. Death can occur suddenly, without obvious signs.[14]

PATHOPHYSIOLOGY

Chlorates are absorbed readily from the intestine, and once absorbed they continue to exert their damaging effects as long as they are present.[14,15] A dose of 250 g is reported to be lethal to horses.[14]

Chlorates cause toxic changes by three different mechanisms of action:

1. Direct irritation of the gastrointestinal tract
2. Oxidation of hemoglobin to methemoglobin
3. Inducement of hemolysis

The net effect of methemoglobinemia and hemolysis is a severe compromise in the oxygen-carrying capacity of blood, and animals may be so severely affected that they die as a result of anoxia.[15]

DIAGNOSIS

The prolonged, extensive methemoglobinemia found in affected animals should alert the veterinarian to the possibility of chlorate poisoning. A history of exposure to chlorates also should accompany these clinical signs before a presumptive diagnosis is made. Analysis of blood, urine, or ocular fluid can help determine chlorate concentration, and because chlorates normally are not found in animals, their presence in a sample would confirm poisoning if clinical signs, history, lesions, and response to therapy also suggest this diagnosis.[15]

TREATMENT

After making the diagnosis, the clinician should immediately seek out the chlorate source and remove it from the horse's environment. Methemoglobinemia is treated with methylene blue at a dose of 4.4 mg/kg given as a 1% solution by intravenous drip. This dose may be repeated in 15 to 30 minutes if a clinical response is not obtained.[2,15] Other recommended therapeutic measures include gastric lavage with 1% sodium thiosulfate and the oral administration of intestinal protectants and demulcents.[2,14] Blood transfusion and oxygen supplementation may be beneficial in certain instances.[15]

PYRIMINIL (VACOR)

Pyriminil currently is not commercially available, but in previous years it was marketed as a rodenticide. Reports of toxicosis in horses are rare,[21] and no deaths caused by pyriminil ingestion have been reported.[21,22]

CLINICAL SIGNS

Reported signs in affected horses include severe muscular fasciculation, profuse sweating, dehydration, and mydriasis with a weak pupillary response. Hindlimb weakness, ataxia, persistent inappetence, and abdominal pain also have been reported.[21] Hyperglycemia is a fairly consistent laboratory finding.[14,21]

PATHOPHYSIOLOGY

Pyriminil is absorbed from the gastrointestinal tract and excreted in the urine. Pyriminil acts as a nicotinamide antagonist, but its exact mechanism of action is unknown.[2,14,22] Pyriminil also has been shown to damage the pancreatic β-cells and to depress glucose uptake by erythrocytes.

DIAGNOSIS

A presumptive diagnosis is based on compatible clinical signs and history of exposure to the rodenticide.

TREATMENT

Specific therapy for pyriminil toxicity is reported to be nicotinamide. However, the use of this drug in human beings appears to be effective only when given within 1 hour of ingestion of pyriminil. The reported dosage is 50 to 100 mg nicotinamide intramuscularly every 4 hours for up to eight injections. This dosage is followed by 25 to 50 mg orally 3 to 5 times daily for 7 to 10 days.[14] Other therapies that may be beneficial include gastric lavage and the oral administration of mineral oil and activated charcoal.[14,22] Apparently, affected horses recover because no deaths caused by pyriminil toxicosis have been recorded.

TETRACHLORODIBENZODIOXIN

The polychlorinated dibenzodioxins include a large number of isomers that differ chemically only in the number and location of chlorine atoms on the dioxin nucleus but that vary greatly in their toxic potential to various animal species. Of the 75 possible isomers of polychlorinated dibenzodioxin, the specific isomer designated 2,3,7,8-tetrachlorodibenzodioxin (TCDD; dioxin) is most toxic and generally is considered the most toxic synthetic molecule known. TCDD was once a contaminant of certain herbicides and is a by-product of certain chemical manufacturing and combustion processes.[14] It can also be found in soil as a naturally occurring compound or as a result of contamination by industrial waste. As recently as a few years ago, dioxins have been found in ball clay that had been used as a binding agent for livestock feed. Currently, dioxins are more of a tissue residue issue for production animals rather than a toxicologic hazard for livestock.The chemical is a highly stable contaminant in the environment, with a half-life in soil of approximately 1 year.[23]

CLINICAL SIGNS

In one reported outbreak the initial signs began 4 days after exposure and included abdominal pain, polydipsia, anorexia, severe weight loss, alopecia, skin and oral ulcers, conjunctivitis, dependent edema, joint stiffness, and laminitis. A total of 85 horses were exposed, 58 became ill, and 43 subsequently died. The length of illness varied from 4 to 132 weeks in the terminally ill horses, with those having a heavier exposure exhibiting a shorter disease course (average of 32 weeks) than others (average of 74 weeks). In addition, abortions occurred in pregnant mares, and many foals that were exposed only in utero died at birth or shortly thereafter.[23] Other reported signs in animals included gastrointestinal hemorrhage with necrosis and ulceration of the gastrointestinal mucosa, cerebrovascular hemorrhage, hepatotoxicity, and thymic and peripheral lymph node atrophy.[14,23]

PATHOPHYSIOLOGY

Tetrachlorodibenzodioxin is absorbed readily by oral and dermal routes, and following absorption appears to be retained primarily by liver and adipose tissue. The mechanism of action of TCDD in various organs in not well defined. TCDD is known to induce microsomal mixed function oxidases in liver and kidney, and hepatic δ-aminolevulinic acid synthetase and aryl hydrocarbon hydroxylase, but the role of these processes in the induction of toxicity of TCDD remains to be elucidated.[14] TCDD also induces immunosuppression by causing thymic and peripheral lymph node atrophy.

DIAGNOSIS

A combination of the described clinical signs and possible exposure to industrial waste oil products should alert the veterinarian to the possibility of TCDD toxicity. Dioxin content is confirmed in various tissues by means of gas-liquid chromatography and mass spectroscopy, but few laboratories offer this service, and the analysis is generally expensive.[14]

A characteristic liver lesion seen at necropsy in a number of horses was microscopic evidence of bile stasis, hepatocyte necrosis, bile duct proliferation, and extensive fibrosis that was pronounced around the central veins but minimal in the peripheral liver lobules. Other microscopic changes noted were thickened vascular walls and endothelial proliferation in the smaller blood vessels of several different organs.[23]

TREATMENT

No known antidote exists for TCDD toxicity once clinical signs develop. After their onset, the clinician can offer only symptomatic and supportive care, and one should use every precaution to prevent laminitis. Soil and activated charcoal appear to bind strongly to TCDD and inhibit its absorption, so if known ingestion has occurred, immediate oral administration of activated charcoal may have beneficial effects by reducing the amount absorbed.[14]

Cantharidin Toxicosis (Blister Beetle Toxicosis)

Cantharidin toxicosis results from ingestion of dead blister beetles that become entrapped in hay during harvesting. Essentially all reports are of horses being fed alfalfa hay or alfalfa products, but anecdotal reports exist of horses intoxicated by ingesting grass hay. More than 200 species of blister beetles inhabit the continental United States, but toxicity results primarily from beetles of the genus *Epicauta*.[24] Depending on the species of beetle, as few as a half dozen ingested beetles can be problematic. The liquid form of cantharidin is suspected in the malicious poisoning of horses.

Cantharidin is the sole toxic principle and is contained in the hemolymph, genitalia, and possibly other tissues of the beetle. Cantharidin is a highly irritating substance that causes acantholysis and vesicle formation when in contact with skin or mucous membranes, and the substance is absorbed from the gastrointestinal tract and rapidly excreted by the kidney. Storage of hay does not reduce the toxicity of cantharidin.[24]

CLINICAL SIGNS

The signs associated with toxicosis are many, varied, and dose dependent. Horses affected with a minimal dose may show only signs of depression, anorexia, and occasionally polyuria, whereas horses ingesting a lethal dose may show signs of profound shock, gastrointestinal and urinary tract irritation, myocardial dysfunction, and hypocalcemia.[24,25] The onset and duration of clinical signs vary from hours to days, but horses that succumb to cantharidin generally die within 48 hours of onset of signs. Horses that live longer than 48 hours have a better prognosis for recovery if no complications arise.

The most commonly observed clinical signs include varying degrees of abdominal pain, anorexia, depression, and repeatedly submerging the muzzle in water or frequently drinking small amounts of water. The respiratory and cardiac rates are elevated, and cardiac contractions are occasionally forceful enough to be observed through the thoracic wall. Mucous membranes are congested and cyanotic, and capillary refill time is prolonged. The feces may be watery in consistency but rarely contain blood or mucus. Profuse sweating is typical of more severely affected horses and may be a sign of severe abdominal pain. Affected horses often make frequent attempts to void urine. The urine is grossly normal early in the disease course but later may become tinged with blood or contain clots of blood. Gross hematuria, if it occurs, is usually in the later stages of the disease process. Less commonly observed signs include synchronous diaphragmatic flutter; erosions of the gingival and oral mucous membranes; and occasionally a stiff, short-strided gait similar to that seen in acute myositis. Sudden death also has been reported.[24]

PATHOPHYSIOLOGY

The mechanism of action of cantharidin at the cellular level has not been elucidated fully. Acantholysis and vesicle formation result from disrupted cell membranes. Cantharidin does not have a direct effect on membranes but is thought to interfere with oxidative enzymes bound to mitochondria. These enzyme systems are involved directly in active transport across the plasma membrane, and their failure results in cell death caused by significant permeability changes in the cell membrane.[24]

Hypovolemic shock and pain develop rapidly in more severely affected horses. The normal transfer of fluid, nutrients, and electrolytes across the intestinal mucosa is disrupted because of the morphologic changes induced by cantharidin. Although renal tubular damage is not severe enough to cause death, changes in the renal tubular epithelium also may be related to the development of fluid, acid-base, and electrolyte abnormalities.[24,25]

Hypoproteinemia develops later in the disease course, probably as a result of protein loss across the damaged intestinal mucosa. Protein also is lost into the peritoneal space, and a minor amount may be lost through the urine.[24]

The profound hypocalcemia and hypomagnesemia that may occur in many horses have not been explained fully. Calcium loss, derangement of calcium homeostasis, or a combination of both is the most likely explanation because the acute onset of the disease eliminates reduced intake as a possible cause. Calcium can be lost through urine and sweat and as protein-bound calcium through the damaged intestinal wall. An influx of intracellular calcium also may occur in certain tissues. Whether cantharidin has an effect on calcium-binding sites on proteins or in cells is unknown.[24]

The low urine specific gravity in most horses may be caused by decreased permeability of the collecting ducts to water. Other findings, however, point to a mild pathologic insult as a cause of the low urine specific gravity. These findings include the facts that a low specific gravity occurs suddenly within hours of toxin exposure; specific gravity returns to normal in 2 to 4 days in surviving horses; only mild to moderate changes are noted in other renal function tests; and the histologic renal lesions are mild, and neither acute nor chronic renal failure is associated with cantharidin toxicosis in horses.[24]

Myocardial necrosis is a common finding in affected horses and may be caused by the direct effect of cantharidin on cardiac muscle. Dose-related intracellular changes involving the mitochondria, cristae, nuclear chromatin, sarcoplasmic reticulum, and myofibrils have been observed in the cardiac muscle of rabbits that were given cantharidin. A proposed mechanism for these changes suggests that an excessive transport of calcium into the myocardial cells occurs, leading to an intracellular calcium overload. This overload may result in a high-energy phosphate deficiency within the cell, leading to necrosis and cell death.[24]

DIAGNOSIS

The clinician should consider cantharidin toxicosis when horses exhibit signs of abdominal pain, depression, or polyuria, and their diet contains alfalfa hay or alfalfa products. The diagnosis can be made when horses have clinical signs and laboratory findings compatible with cantharidin toxicosis and beetles are found in the hay. Because the beetles can be difficult to identify in hay, it should be thoroughly searched. Cantharidin can be assayed using high-pressure liquid chromatography and gas chromatography–mass spectrometry techniques.[24,26] Samples to be tested are serum, urine, kidney, and stomach content from horses in which cantharidin toxicosis is suspected.

Laboratory findings are nonpathognomonic, but several abnormalities typically are noted. Packed cell volume (PCV) and serum protein concentrations are elevated early, but hypoproteinemia frequently develops after about 24 hours. Mild hypokalemia can occur but is not a striking feature of this disease. Blood urea nitrogen (BUN) concentration may be elevated moderately, and hyperglycemia is almost always present initially.[24]

Serum calcium and magnesium concentrations are significantly decreased in most horses and remain low for longer than 48 hours if untreated. The urine generally contains red blood cells and has a low specific gravity, even in the face of clinical dehydration. Abnormal peritoneal fluid findings include increased protein concentration but relatively normal fibrinogen and white blood cell values. Feces are often positive for occult blood. Serum creatine kinase (CK) activity may be elevated in more severely affected horses and augurs a poor prognosis.[24] Although not diagnostic, laboratory findings of prolonged hypocalcemia and hypomagnesemia and elevated CK concentration may help differentiate cantharidin toxicosis from other causes of acute abdominal crisis.

TREATMENT

No specific antidote is available for cantharidin. Once the diagnosis is suspected, all suspect feed should be removed from the horse's environment and all hay carefully examined for the presence of beetles.

Horses suspected of having cantharidin toxicosis should be given mineral oil as soon as possible. The oil helps evacuate the bowel and also may help reduce the amount of cantharidin available for absorption because cantharidin is lipid soluble. Activated charcoal given through a nasogastric tube also may have beneficial effects.[24]

Polyionic fluids should be administered intravenously throughout the disease course to correct dehydration and promote diuresis. Diuretics also may be given once the horse is volume loaded. Analgesics usually are required because of the severity of the abdominal pain, and glucocorticoids may be necessary to aid in treating shock. Calcium gluconate should be administered to elevate the serum calcium concentration, and calculated deficits of magnesium should be replaced by slow intravenous infusion.[24]

PHOSPHORUS

Elemental phosphorus can be available in red and white forms. Red phosphorus is used in manufacturing fertilizers and safety matches and is considered inert and relatively nontoxic. White phosphorus was used as a rodenticide and can be found in pastes containing from 1.5% to 5% phosphorus. The reported toxic dose for horses is 0.5 to 2. g.[14]

CLINICAL SIGNS

The toxic manifestations of phosphorus poisoning are generally threefold: Toxic signs commence within hours of ingestion; are followed by a latent period of 48 hours to several days, when the animal may appear to have recovered; and finally recur with greater severity.

The initial signs are characterized by severe abdominal pain, and gastrointestinal irritation, with occasional episodes of diarrhea. Blood may be present in feces. Cardiac arrhythmias may occur during this phase, and if the dose is sufficiently large, cyanosis, shock, incoordination, and coma can develop, and the animal may die before the second and third stages develop.[14]

The latent period may occur from 48 to 96 hours after the onset of clinical signs, and during this time the animal may appear normal. The third stage is characterized as a recurrence of severe abdominal pain, and signs of liver dysfunction may become evident. Icterus and a tendency to bleed from the gingiva, stomach, intestine, or kidney may be evident.[14]

PATHOPHYSIOLOGY

Phosphorus is absorbed from the gastrointestinal and respiratory tracts. Although dermal exposure may cause skin irritation or burning, absorption does not occur by this route. The mechanism of action of phosphorus is unknown but is noted for causing irritation and necrosis of affected tissue. Phosphorus is also known to cause peripheral vasodilation.[14]

DIAGNOSIS AND TREATMENT

Clinicopathologic abnormalities reflect hepatic and renal damage. Hypoglycemia may be pronounced, and liver enzymes such as AST, lactate dehydrogenase (LDH), and sorbitol dehydrogenase are elevated. Renal damage is reflected by increased BUN and creatinine concentrations. Albumin, blood, and increased concentrations of amino acids may be present in the urine. The phosphorus concentration in blood is usually normal. Although elemental phosphorus in tissues can be assayed, in time a large portion may be oxidized to phosphates, thereby making confirmation of poisoning difficult by chemical means.[14]

No specific antidote is available for phosphorus in toxication. Therapy is essentially symptomatic and supportive.

THALLIUM

Thallium is toxic to all animals, including human beings, but clinical reports of toxicity are extremely rare. However, an oral dose of thallous acetate 27 mg/kg has been suggested as potentially lethal to horses.[15] Thallium has been used historically as a rodenticide, but its use now is limited and restricted only to government agencies.

CLINICAL SIGNS

Thallium ingestion can result in acute, subacute, or chronic syndromes. In the acute form clinical signs in animals usually begin within 1 to 4 days of ingestion. Initial signs are those of severe gastrointestinal insult and include vomiting or regurgitation, severe hemorrhagic diarrhea, abdominal pain, and anorexia. Labored breathing is apparent early in the disease course, and motor paralysis and trembling may occur. Signs suggesting renal dysfunction also may occur.[14]

The subacute form generally manifests signs in 3 to 7 days after ingestion. Signs of gastric distress and motor disturbances are less marked than in the acute form, but they persist for a longer time. In this form reddening of the skin and pustule formation occur. A pronounced reddening of the oral mucous membranes also seems to be unique to this particular toxicosis. Other clinical signs observed include conjunctivitis, hair loss, and crusty skin lesions. Secondary bacterial infections also may develop in affected animals.[14]

The chronic stage requires 7 to 10 days to appear. Signs of gastrointestinal and nervous system dysfunction are mild, but hair loss and dry, scaly skin become pronounced.[14]

PATHOPHYSIOLOGY

Thallium is absorbed readily from the intestinal tract or through the skin; is distributed to all body tissues, although higher levels accumulate in the kidneys and liver; and is excreted principally in feces and to a lesser extent in urine; and undergoes an enterohepatic cycle for resorption and excretion.[15]

Thallium is thought to combine with mitochondrial sulfhydryl enzymes at a specific yet unknown place in the scheme of sulfur metabolism. Thallium therefore interferes with oxidative phosphorylation within cells. Recent evidence suggests that thallium exchanges for potassium in muscle and nerve cells primarily and also has a necrotizing effect on the intestinal tract, kidney, and occasionally the brain.[14,15]

DIAGNOSIS

Thallium toxicosis is suspected on the basis of clinical signs, and urine can be assayed for thallium content. The finding of thallium in tissue in any amount is diagnostic, but liver and kidney levels tend to be higher than in other tissues.

TREATMENT

Chelation therapy using diphenylthiocarbazone (dithizon) at a dosage of 70 mg/kg administered orally thrice daily has been recommended for use in dogs.[14] However, cats react adversely to this agent. Its effect in horses is unknown.

Potassium chloride may aid in the elimination of thallium and can be given intravenously or orally, but the oral route is contraindicated in animals that also are being treated with an ion exchange agent.

One can attempt to trap thallium in the intestine with the ion exchange agent potassium ferric cyanoferrate-II (potassium–prussian blue). Experimentally, potassium–prussian blue is not absorbed from the intestinal tract and acts to immobilize the thallus ion by exchanging with the potassium of potassium–prussian blue. Once trapped, thallium is not released readily from potassium–prussian blue, and fecal excretion of thallium increases.[15,38]

Other forms of symptomatic therapy include intestinal protectants and demulcents, fluid and electrolyte support, analgesics, oral activated charcoal, and general nursing care.[15]

TOXICOSES CAUSING SIGNS OF CENTRAL NERVOUS SYSTEM STIMULATION

Dealing with horses showing signs of CNS stimulation can be one of the most difficult and challenging situations faced by the equine internist. Signs can be hard to control, and clients' emotions often run high at the sight of a horse showing severe or uncontrollable signs such as hyperexcitability, exaggerated gait abnormalities, and seizures. The immediate clinical emphasis is usually on minimizing the risk or severity of self-induced trauma. Etiologic diagnosis may be difficult and protracted.

PLANTS

Locoweed

A nervous syndrome in horses, cattle, and sheep has long been associated with eating plants of the genera *Astragalus, Swainsona,* and *Oxytropis*. This group of plants is large. The *Astragalus* species that grow in North America number more than 300. Not all species of *Astragalus* and *Oxytropis* are toxic, however, and some species make nutritious forage for livestock.[1] Some debate still exists regarding the taxonomy of these species, but because the clinical signs that they induce are essentially the same, they are discussed together.

The toxic species of locoweed produce three different syndromes in livestock. Some species contain nitroglycosides, which cause methemoglobinemia and competitive inhibition of certain cellular enzymes; others accumulate toxic levels of selenium; and a third group contains alkaloids that cause locoism.[1,2] The first group of plants is of minor importance to the horse, and the selenium concentrators are discussed in the section on selenium toxicosis. A discussion of the clinical syndrome locoism follows.

The species of locoweed that have been associated with locoism include *Astragalus lentiginosus* (36 varieties); *Astragalus mollissimus* (11 varieties); *Astragalus wootonii* (2 varieties); *Astragalus thurberi; Astragalus nothoxys; Oxytropis sericea; Oxytropis lambertii;* and *Oxytropis saximontana*.[1] Additional *Astragalus* species incriminated in causing disease include *Astragalus argillophilus, Astragalusbisulcatus,* and *Astragalus earlei*.[60] Geographically, locoweeds are found from western Canada southward to include the western United States and northern Mexico.[1]

CLINICAL SIGNS

Locoweeds cause a number of problems in livestock, including neurologic and reproductive dysfunction, emaciation, and habituation.[1] Typical signs exhibited by affected horses include a slow, staggering gait; depression; an unthrifty appearance; emaciation; muscular incoordination; and nervousness, especially when the animal is under stress. The affected horse may become solitary and hard to manage and may have difficulty eating and drinking. In some animals sexual activity may become suppressed. Visual impairment also occurs in some horses, and mares ingesting locoweed during pregnancy have been known to abort or produce foals with various limb deformities.[2,3] Horses that are affected chronically are generally useless for riding or draft purposes because their behavior is so unpredictable.[1]

The onset of clinical signs varies from as short as 2 weeks to as long as 2 months after the horse starts to graze the plant. The plants generally are considered unpalatable to horses, but once they start to ingest the plant, they seem to become addicted to it and will search it out.[1] The addiction can extend to subsequent growing seasons, so clinical signs can worsen progressively in successive years if animals continue to graze the plant.[2] Affected horses can recover if feeding or grazing is discontinued before they become too emaciated and if nutritious forage is provided.[1] However, the syndrome eventually may lead to death in chronically affected horses.[2]

PATHOPHYSIOLOGY

The indolizidine alkaloids swainsonine and swainsonine N-oxide have been suggested as the toxic principles in locoweeds.[2] These alkaloids were first recovered from *Swainsona* species in Australia.[1,2] Evidence suggests that these alkaloids are actually mycotoxins, or toxins produced by endophytes located within the plant. Swainsonine inhibits α-mannosidase, a lysosomal enzyme essential in the cellular metabolism of oligosaccharides. As a result, mannose-rich oligosaccharides accumulate in lysosomes and disrupt cellular function. These accumulations are visible microscopically as intracytoplasmic vacuoles. Vacuolization of the renal cortical tubular cells can occur as early as 4 days after ingestion of locoweed begins, and neurons of the CNS, including Purkinje cells, may show vacuolization by 8 days. The vacuoles disappear shortly after consumption ceases in the early stages of disease, but if grazing is prolonged, permanent cellular damage occurs. Continuous feeding of the plant for 30 days or longer results in vacuolization of almost all tissues of the body except skeletal and cardiac muscle.[2]

Neurologic signs result from vacuolization of the axons, glial cells, and Purkinje cells of the cerebellum and cerebral cortex. The weight loss and emaciation result from impairment of the liver, pancreas, thyroid, and parathyroid glands. Vacuolization of cells of the retina and decreased lacrimation are responsible for impaired vision in some animals. Vacuoles also occur in lymph nodes, placenta, testicles, and lymphocytes.[1,2] The pathogenesis and lesions of locoism are similar to mannosidosis, a heritable lysosomal storage disease of Angus and Murray Grey cattle.[2]

DIAGNOSIS AND TREATMENT

A few laboratories test for swainsonine and mannosidase activity in a variety of biologic specimens. The diagnosis is suspected when horses show clinical signs compatible with locoism and have a history of exposure to the plant. Laboratory testing is nonspecific, and test results are expected to be consistent with multiple organ dysfunction. Microscopic lesions of intracytoplasmic vacuolization in various organs, including the CNS, are compatible with a diagnosis of locoism.[1,2] Peripheral lymphocytes that contain intracytoplasmic vacuoles also are considered indicative of locoism, if clinical signs are present.[2]

No effective cure exists for horses with chronic locoism that have had clinical signs for some time. Mild cases usually resolve in 1 to 2 weeks once ingestion ceases, so successful recovery from locoism depends on early recognition of the disease syndrome and prevention of further consumption. Reserpine has been suggested to be helpful in relieving some of the clinical signs of locoism in horses.[2]

Nervous Ergotism

Two forms of ergotism are observed in domestic animals, a nervous or convulsive form and a gangrenous form. Horses appear rarely to be affected with ergotism, but the nervous form is reported to occur much more frequently in horses than the gangrenous form.[4,5] Ergotism is caused by a number of alkaloids contained in *Claviceps purpurea*, a fungus infecting grains such as wheat, barley, rye, and oats and wild grasses such as quackgrass, smooth bromegrass, wheatgrass, bluegrasses, and wild rye. The fungal mass, or sclerotium, replaces the seed or kernel of the plant and may have the same general configuration as the seed but is usually larger, dark colored, and hard. Ergotism is rarely of concern in dry seasons, but abundant fungal growth can occur during wet periods.[4] Although well-documented cases of ergotism caused by *C. purpurea* in horses are absent in the literature, a nervous syndrome typical of *Claviceps paspali* poisoning has been observed in horses in Australia. However, the cause of the clinical signs in these horses was suggested to have been the tremorogenic mycotoxins in *C. paspali* rather than the alkaloids found in ergot.[6]

CLINICAL SIGNS

The first sign of nervous ergotism in animals is reported to be dizziness or an unsteady gait. This phase may be interrupted by convulsions and temporary posterior paralysis and drowsiness.[4] Other behavioral effects that have been described include incoordination, lameness, difficulty in breathing, excessive salivation, and diarrhea.[5]

PATHOPHYSIOLOGY

Approximately 40 different alkaloids have been isolated from *C. purpurea*. All of these alkaloids are derivatives of the tetracyclic compound 6-methylergoline, a lysergic acid base structurally similar to a number of biogenic amines such as dopamine, serotonin, and norepinephrine.[4,7] The most pharmacologically potent alkaloids in ergot are ergonovine, ergotamine, ergotsine, ergocristine, ergocryptine, and ergocornine.[4] Additionally, tyrosine, tryptophan, tyramine, histamine, histidine, choline, and acetylcholine have been isolated from ergot sclerotia, but their clinical significance is uncertain.[7]

The mechanism whereby ergot alkaloids induce CNS signs in horses has not been elucidated. Of the ergot alkaloids known to affect the CNS in human beings, bromocriptine is the prototype. Bromocriptine is a long-acting dopamine agonist that has central stimulating effects and may cause hypotension. Another ergot alkaloid, isoergine (lysergic acid amide), has one tenth the mind-altering potency of the structurally related compound lysergic acid diethylamide (LSD). LSD is thought to produce hallucinations by a series of complex agonist and antagonist actions on several central monoamine neurotransmitters, particularly serotonin.[7]

DIAGNOSIS AND TREATMENT

The diagnosis of nervous ergotism in horses is based primarily on clinical signs and eliminating other causes of CNS stimulation. One can assay the ergot alkaloid content of feed.[4]

No specific antidote exists for ergot alkaloid toxicity. Treatment of affected horses is largely symptomatic. Recommendations for control include using ergot-free feed, rotating crops, plowing deeply (because shallow cultivation and seeding leave the sclerotia near the soil surface, where they can germinate more readily), and mowing surrounding grasses to limit the spread of fungus into the cultivated crop.[5] Pasture grasses that may be infested with ergot should be mowed before the development of seedheads because *Claviceps* replaces the seed or kernel of the plant.

Blue-Green Algae (Cyanobacteria)

The occurrence of cyanobacterial poisoning in livestock is not uncommon in many areas. Most cases of toxicity involve other grazing animals, principally cattle and sheep, but horses are reported to be susceptible.[8] Toxicity may occur during times that favor algal growth in surface water. The most important factors that favor rapid algal growth are a nutrient source (e.g., nitrogen, phosphate); quiet, calm weather conditions; and warm water temperature. Therefore toxicosis is most likely to occur during periods of warm weather (i.e., late spring through fall), when surface water may be contaminated with fertilizer runoff or organic waste high in nitrogen, such as that from feedlots.[8,9] However, it is important to note that livestock toxicities caused by cyanobacteria have been reported in the winter months in the Northern hemisphere. In more temperate areas cyanobacterial blooms can be a year-round occurrence.

At least eight genera of cyanobacteria are known to be toxic: *Anabaena, Aphanizomenon, Microcystis (Anacystis), Coelosphaerium, Gloeotrichia, Lyngbya, Nodularia,* and *Nostoc,* but the first three are of most concern in veterinary medicine. Toxins produced by cyanobacteria are either neurotoxic or hepatotoxic; therefore signs of poisoning are typically neurologic or hepatic, but rarely both are observed in an animal (even though some blooms are mixed). Most blooms are composed of one predominant cyanobacterial organism. *Microcystin (Anacystin)* organisms produce the hepatotoxin microcystin; and *Anabaena* and *Aphanizomenon* produce the neurotoxins anatoxin-a and anatoxin-a(s).

CLINICAL SIGNS

Common signs of cyanobacterial poisoning associated with microcystins may include rapid appearance of abdominal pain, diarrhea, muscle tremors, dyspnea and cyanosis, prostration, and death. Animals surviving several days may exhibit hemorrhagic diarrhea, muscle tremors, signs of liver damage, and secondary photosensitization.[8,9] Animals exposed to neurotoxic blooms frequently develop signs within a few minutes (<1 hour) of ingestion and may show rapid onset of CNS dysfunction with seizures, prostration, and death.

PATHOPHYSIOLOGY

Anabaena and *Aphanizomenon* species may contain the low-molecular-weight alkaloid anatoxin-a. This toxin produces a potent postsynaptic depolarizing neuromuscular-blocking action that has a curare-like effect. Death results from respiratory arrest. Blooms of some *Aphanizomenon* species may produce small amounts of the neurotoxin (saxitoxin) and at least three related toxic compounds of unknown structure.[7,8] Saxitoxin blocks sodium conductance through excitable membranes, which subsequently stops nerve action potential. Death resulting from saxitoxin is caused by respiratory neuromuscular paralysis.[8] Anatoxin-a(s) can also be produced by these organism, whose action is to inhibit acetylcholinesterase activity. *Microcystis* species of cyanobacteria can produce the cyclic hepatotoxin microcystin.[7,8] The immediate cause of death is hemorrhagic shock resulting from massive hepatocellular necrosis and collapse of the hepatic parenchyma.[10]

DIAGNOSIS AND TREATMENT

Analytic methods are now available that can isolate and identify the cyanobacteria organism and the toxins from affected animals (gastric contents, liver) or suspect water. Because the concentrations of cyanobacteria and toxins can vary tremendously over a short time, recovery of the organism or toxin from water may not be possible when clinical signs are noted in exposed animals. A diagnosis can be based on history of exposure to a water source when conditions favoring cyanobacterial overgrowth are present, coupled with onset of compatible clinical signs and analysis of tissues and water for the toxin. One can analyze water samples to identify specific blue-green algae, the presence of which may help support a diagnosis of algal toxicity if toxin testing is not feasible.[8]

No specific antidote is available, and animals often are found dead before treatment can be initiated.[8] Algal growth in surface water can be controlled by a variety of herbicides and copper sulfate. When water is treated with these compounds, it is important to ensure that the compounds are being used in a safe manner for all susceptible livestock.

PESTICIDES

ACETYLCHOLINESTERASE-INHIBITING INSECTICIDES

The carbamate pesticides are composed of cyclic or aliphatic derivatives of carbamic acid, and numerous ones are commercially available.[8,11] A partial list of these compounds is carbaryl, aldicarb, carbofuran, methiocarb, methomyl, and oxamyl. Carbamates are absorbed readily through the lungs, gastrointestinal tract, and skin. Carbamates do not accumulate in any particular tissue but do cross the rat placenta and depress fetal acetylcholinesterase; they are not metabolized readily in the fetus.[11] In human beings the carbamates generally penetrate the blood-brain barrier poorly and therefore may produce few CNS signs.[7] Carbamates do not require activation by liver enzymes to exert their effect. Toxicity data are not complete for several domestic animals, but lethal doses of the different compounds vary from less than 1 mg up to several hundred mg per kg of body weight. Carbamates are not stable in the environment and are fairly insoluble in water, but organic solvents and oils can carry the compounds across cell barriers.[11] It is important to note that not all so-called carbamate pesticides inhibit acetylcholinesterase activity, so the clinician must determine exactly which carbamate compound the animal is exposed to and determine its mechanism of action.

CLINICAL SIGNS

Clinical signs can commence a few minutes to several hours after exposure but are short-lived. The clinical episode frequently is less than 36 to 48 hours in duration, with the animal succumbing or recovering during this time.[8,11]

Signs of toxicity in horses reflect muscarinic and nicotinic cholinergic overstimulation. The signs suggestive of muscarinic cholinergic overstimulation include profuse salivation, severe gastrointestinal disturbances characterized by hypermotility, severe pain, abdominal cramps and diarrhea, excessive lacrimation, miosis, sweating, dyspnea, cyanosis, and urinary and fecal incontinence. Affected animals also may cough frequently as a sign of excessive accumulation of respiratory tract secretions. The signs reflected by nicotinic overstimulation include excessive stimulation of the skeletal muscles. The muscles of the face, eyelids, and tongue, in addition to the general musculature, may twitch. Some animals exhibit signs of generalized tetany that causes them to walk in a stiff-legged fashion. This hyperactivity may be followed by weakness and paralysis of the skeletal muscles.[8]

Signs of CNS involvement in domestic food-producing animals may include hyperactivity reflecting excessive stimulation of the CNS, but domestic animals rarely exhibit convulsive seizures (however, this can occur at high dose exposures). CNS depression is reported to be more common than CNS stimulation.[8]

PATHOPHYSIOLOGY

Carbamates induce excessive stimulation of the parasympathetic nervous system by inhibiting acetylcholinesterase and pseudocholinesterase. The carbamate pesticides occupy the anionic and esteratic sites of acetylcholinesterase, with the esteratic site being carbamylated. Acetylcholinesterase can hydrolyze carbamate pesticides but at a slower rate than that for acetylcholine. Therefore carbamates are reversible inhibitors of acetylcholinesterase, but toxicosis occurs when the amount of pesticide is large enough that the rate of carbamylation of acetylcholinesterase exceeds the rate of hydrolysis of pesticide by the enzyme.[11] As a result, acetylcholine accumulates in neuroeffector and synaptic regions, resulting in the observed clinical signs of parasympathetic overstimulation.

The continuous stimulation of secretory glands leads to excessive salivation and accumulation of fluid within the respiratory tract and within the lumen of the bowel. Extensive pulmonary edema may occur and, along with bronchoconstriction, can lead to death in affected animals.[8]

Carbamates are removed from the circulation largely by spontaneous hydrolysis of the carbamate-cholinesterase complex. In addition, blood esterases can inactivate a portion of the circulating carbamate, and certain liver microsomal enzymes break down the compounds within hours of exposure.[7,11] The clinical signs associated with carbamate toxicity are generally rather short-lived, with recovery occurring in less than 36 to 48 hours in most animals.

DIAGNOSIS AND TREATMENT

The clinician is most likely to make a diagnosis on the basis of a history of possible exposure, clinical signs, and response to atropine treatment. Chemical analyses of biologic samples for carbamate residues can be rewarding; finding the pesticide in stomach contents, the liver, or feed samples may confirm the diagnosis.[8]

Cholinesterase activity in blood and brain tissue can also be used as a screening tool to determine exposure to this group of compounds. However, discretion must be used when interpreting these results because recommended therapeutic levels of carbamates applied to animals can result in some depression of blood cholinesterase activity. In one author's opinion, clinical signs of acute carbamate toxicity are associated with blood cholinesterase activity of less than 50% to 75% of normal values. Because the inactivation of cholinesterase by carbamates involves a much weaker and less stable binding than that by organophosphates, one should not dilute blood samples from suspect animals and should refrigerate them and analyze them as soon as possible.[8]

Affected animals should be treated as quickly as possible. Initial therapy should consist of atropine sulfate at 0.2 mg per kg of body weight. This initial dose should be divided, with approximately one fourth of the dose administered intravenously and the remainder given subcutaneously or intramuscularly. Repeated doses of atropine may be required but should be used only to counteract the parasympathetic signs. The skeletal muscle tremors may not respond to atropine therapy.[8]

Orally administered adsorbents such as activated charcoal may be useful in binding ingested pesticide, and aqueous cathartics may further aid in evacuation of the intestinal tract. Mineral oil probably should not be given orally in suspect cases because organic solvents and oils can carry the compound across cell barriers. Dermally exposed animals should be washed with soap and water and rinsed thoroughly to prevent further exposure. Oximes such as pralidoxime are of questional benefit in treating carbamate toxicosis, and their use may worsen the condition of the animals.[8,11] The cost of this drug may be a prohibiting factor in their use in horses.

ORGANOPHOSPHATES

The organophosphate pesticides are being used increasingly in a variety of ways. Some of the typical uses for these compounds include animal insecticides and parasiticides; plant insecticides, soil nematocides, fungicides, herbicides, and defoliants; insect repellents; and chemosterilants.[11] Horses can become intoxicated in several ways because these products are used so commonly in their environment.

A wide variety of organophosphorus compounds have been developed, and their toxicity varies greatly among compounds and among animal species. Osweiler, Carson, Buck, et al. have tabulated a good list of various organophosphorus compounds and their relative toxicities.[8] In addition to variations in compound toxicity, a number of physicochemical factors also can affect the toxicity of organophosphorus compounds. The toxicity of these compounds decreases as they are degraded by sun, water, microbes, alkali, or metal ions such as iron or copper. An increase in toxicity may occur by storage activation, a process in which highly toxic isomers of certain pesticides are formed spontaneously in polar solvents or water. This reaction is speeded by heat. Parathion, malathion, fenthion, chlorpyrifos, diazinon, and coumaphos are some of the compounds that can undergo this type of storage activation.[11] The storage activation phenomena provide good reasons to use only freshly prepared preparations of organophosphate compounds on horses.

Other factors that can influence the toxicity of a particular organophosphorus compound are ambient temperature (higher temperatures may increase the toxicity of certain compounds); the vehicle in which the pesticide is dispersed; the age and sex of the animal; and the presence of other chemicals that may alter organophosphate toxicity. The combined effects of two organophosphates may be synergistic or antagonistic, and drugs that compete with organophosphates for target esterases, such as succinylcholine, phenothiazine, and procaine, may enhance organophosphate toxicity. In addition, drugs that have neuromuscular-blocking properties (e.g., inhalant anesthetics, magnesium ions, certain aminoglycoside antibiotics, and the depolarizing and nondepolarizing neuromuscular-blocking agents) also may enhance organophosphate toxicity. The organophosphates are poorly soluble in water but are soluble in organic solvents, fats, and oils. Oily vehicles or organic solvents also can facilitate passage of the organophosphates through the skin.[11]

CLINICAL SIGNS

Clinical signs of organophosphate toxicity are similar to those of carbamate toxicity and essentially are those of overstimulation of the parasympathetic nervous system, skeletal muscles, and CNS.

Overstimulation of muscarinic cholinergic sites results in profuse salivation and lacrimation; serous or seromucous nasal discharge; increased respiratory sounds and coughing resulting from bronchoconstriction and excessive bronchial secretions; profound gastrointestinal disturbances of increased motility, abdominal pain, and diarrhea; bradycardia; miosis; sweating; and frequent urination. Signs of nicotinic cholinergic overstimulation include muscle fasciculations, tremors, twitching, spasms, and a stiff or rigid gait. CNS signs frequently include anxiety, restlessness, and hyperactivity.[8,11] If the exposure is not severe enough to result in the death of the horse, the horse may require several days to recover completely; compounds that are more chlorinated can be stored in fat reserves and therefore have a longer half-life.[11]

PATHOPHYSIOLOGY

Organophosphates can be absorbed from the gastrointestinal tract and lungs and through the skin. After absorption, they are distributed throughout the body, but most do not accumulate in any particular tissue. Most of the organophosphates must be activated by hepatic microsomal oxidative enzymes before they become potent esterase inhibitors. Phosphorothiolate and the phosphate class of organophosphates do not require activation and can inhibit esterases immediately after entering the bloodstream.[11]

Organophosphates act as irreversible inhibitors of true cholinesterase and pseudocholinesterase in mammals. They irreversibly phosphorylate the esteratic site of cholinesterases throughout the body. As a result, endogenous acetylcholine is not inactivated. Therefore acetylcholine accumulates in neuromuscular junctions; in parasympathetic postganglionic sites in smooth muscle, cardiac muscle, and glands; in all autonomic ganglia; and in cholinergic synapses within the CNS. The result is overstimulation of these sites, leading to clinical signs of toxicosis.[8,11]

Lethal amounts of organophosphates cause death by the combined effects of nicotinic, muscarinic, and central cholinergic overstimulation or receptor paralysis. These effects include hypotension, bradycardia, bronchoconstriction and excessive bronchial secretion, inability of the respiratory muscles to work properly, cyanosis, and central respiratory depression. The animal actually dies of asphyxia.[11]

Detoxification of organophosphates is accomplished mostly by serum and liver esterases. However, other enzymes in the liver and other tissues may attack the pesticides at rates dependent on the class of pesticide, the species, and the age of the animal. Water-soluble metabolites may be formed rapidly and the pesticide excreted quickly in the urine.[8,11]

DIAGNOSIS AND TREATMENT

The clinician should suspect organophosphate toxicosis when the horse has a history of possible exposure within the past 48 hours, along with characteristic signs of parasympathetic overstimulation. One can analytically test for organophosphate residues in body tissues or specimens and in other suspect materials. Some tissue specimens analyzed for organophosphate content yield negative results because some of the compounds do not stay in tissues long after the animal has been exposed.[8,11]

A test for cholinesterase activity in blood or brain tissue is a rapid screening tool that can assist in determining if an animal has been exposed to excessive amounts of a cholinesterase inhibitor. Blood or brain cholinesterase activity values of less than 50% to 75% of normal can be compatible with exposure of the animal to excess organophosphates or other cholinesterase inhibitors (false inhibition can be observed if the patient is anemic). It should be noted that some depression of blood cholinesterase activity occurs when therapeutic levels of organophosphates or carbamates are used, so these results should be considered with discretion.[8,11]

Treatment to help control the muscarinic overstimulation should involve immediate use of atropine sulfate at 0.2 mg per kg of body weight. Approximately one fourth of this dose should be given intravenously, and the remainder should be given subcutaneously or intramuscularly. It may be necessary to repeat this dose at 3- to 6-hour intervals. Because atropine does not block the nicotinic cholinergic effects, the horse may continue to show signs of muscle fasciculation or tremors.[8,11] Atropine should be used with great discretion in the horse so as not to cause further complications, such as gut stasis with atropine overdosage (see the section on atropine).

The oximes, such as pralidoxime and pralidoxime chloride, act specifically on the organophosphorus-enzyme complex to free the enzyme and also react directly with the organophosphate to form a nontoxic complex that is excreted in urine. However, the use of these products in horses may not be economically feasible. The recommended dose varies between 20 mg/kg[98] and 25 to 50 mg/kg given as a 20% solution intravenously, slowly, over several minutes. Oximes are reported to work best in the presence of atropine, so they should be given to the animal after atropine administration. Treatment with the oximes can be repeated if signs reappear.[11]

Other treatment measures include removal of the source, if possible; use of orally administered activated charcoal; laxatives to aid in evacuation of the bowel; washing with soap and water and thorough rinsing if dermal exposure has occurred; and supportive therapy such as fluids and electrolyte administration, if necessary. Drugs that should not be used when treating organophosphate toxicosis include phenothiazine tranquilizers, succinylcholine, and morphine.[8,11]

Chlorinated Hydrocarbons

The current use of chlorinated hydrocarbon pesticides is limited and severely restricted because of their persistence in the environment and their incorporation into the food chain. However, certain agents still are being used, primarily as contact insecticides and as ectoparasiticides.[8,11,12] A partial list of compounds includes lindane, aldrin, dieldrin, endosulfan, endrin, and methoxychlor.

The chlorinated hydrocarbon insecticides are poorly soluble in water but are soluble in organic solvents and oils. Oily vehicles or organic solvents can facilitate penetration of the insecticide through intact skin. Because this group of compounds also is characterized by volatility, exposure to the pesticide can occur through inhalation of the vaporized compound.[11] Because these compounds accumulate in body tissues, primarily adipose tissue, signs of toxicosis can result from repeated exposure to lesser amounts or after a single excessive dose.[12] Toxicity varies greatly among the different compounds, and Osweiler, Carson, Buck, et al.[8] have tabulated the toxicity of a number of these compounds for various animal species.

CLINICAL SIGNS

The chlorinated hydrocarbons generally act as diffuse stimulants (less commonly as depressants) of the CNS, with the onset of signs ranging from several minutes to several days after exposure. The signs displayed may be progressively severe or explosive and fulminating.[8] Initially, the animal may be hypersensitive, apprehensive, or belligerent. These behavioral aberrations may progress to abnormal posturing or frenzied or maniacal behavior. Nervous signs can begin with hypersensitivity and muscle fasciculations beginning around the head and facial area and proceeding caudally eventually to include the hind quarters. These muscle spasms can occur intermittently or continuously. Clonic-tonic seizures often follow and may result in death or be followed by intermittent periods of CNS depression. Autonomic manifestations of profuse salivation, mydriasis, diarrhea, urination, and bradycardia or tachycardia with arrhythmias may occur. Some animals may lose coordination and stumble while walking, walk aimlessly, or move in circles. Other notable signs may include increased rate and depth of respiration and fluid sounds in the lungs. Death may occur within minutes, hours, or days or not at all. [8,11,12]

PATHOPHYSIOLOGY

Chlorinated hydrocarbon pesticides gain entry into the body by way of the gastrointestinal and respiratory tracts and absorption through the skin. Once they enter the bloodstream, they are thought to bind to serum lipoproteins and are distributed throughout the body. Eventually, an equilibrium is reached in which the pesticide concentration varies among different body compartments. Most of the absorbed pesticide is stored in fat, but brain and fetus also can accumulate significant amounts.[8,11]

Adipose tissue is the main storage tissue for chlorinated hydrocarbons and as such can retain some of these compounds for an extended period. The pesticide is mobilized slowly from fat, which can account for its presence in blood and milk for weeks to months after a single exposure.[11]

The chlorinated hydrocarbons are broken down by liver microsomal enzymes, and the pesticide and its metabolites are excreted in urine, bile, milk, and feces. This first stage of elimination is fairly rapid and may account for 40% to 50% of the compound being eliminated during the first 3 to 4 days after exposure.[11]

The exact mechanism of action of all of the chlorinated hydrocarbons is unknown, but they act as nonspecific stimulants of the CNS. A suggested mechanism is that some of these compounds easily enter neural membranes and prolong the time during which some of the sodium channels in the membrane are open during depolarization. In addition, potassium efflux from the cell is hindered. The net effect of these ion imbalances is a decreased transmembrane resting potential that causes a decreased firing threshold and an increased neuronal excitability.[11]

An increase in whole-brain free ammonia concentration and brain glutamine also occurs, but whether these changes are a cause or an effect of the sodium-potassium flux defect is unknown. However, the onset and disappearance of convulsions in animals is correlated with an increase and decrease of brain ammonia concentration.[11]

The depression produced by some chlorinated hydrocarbons may result from rapid depolarizing blockade of neurons of the reticular activating system. Excessive depolarization of the medullary neurons may be responsible for respiratory failure, which is the usual cause of death in chlorinated hydrocarbon pesticide toxicosis. The muscle tremors in chlorinated hydrocarbon toxicosis are thought to be partly central in origin and partly caused by direct depolarizing effects on peripheral motor nerves.[11]

DIAGNOSIS AND TREATMENT

The clinician can make a tentative diagnosis when animals are known to have been exposed to an insecticide and are exhibiting compatible signs of toxicosis. Tissue samples may be assayed for residues of the specific compound, but it is important to exercise caution when interpreting results because some of the compounds may be found in the fat of normal animals as a result of exposure to small concentrations in the environment. However, ppm concentrations may have diagnostic significance if history and clinical signs are consistent with chlorinated hydrocarbon poisoning. Brain and liver concentrations of this category of pesticides are reported to be better correlated with toxicosis than are concentrations in body fat.[11] Other suitable tissue specimens include blood, milk, kidney, and gastrointestinal contents.[8]

Because no specific antidote is available for the chlorinated hydrocarbons, treatment is symptomatic. For animals exhibiting convulsive seizures or neuromuscular hyperactivity, intravenous chloral hydrate or pentobarbital can be administered carefully to effect. Sedative doses of these two agents should control most of the behavioral, nervous, and locomotor signs. Sedation usually can be discontinued after 24 to 48 hours.

Oral exposure should be treated with saline cathartics and an adsorbent such as activated charcoal. If exposure was by the dermal route, the animal requires a thorough bathing with soap and water, followed by a thorough rinsing. As in all cases of pesticide toxicity, the source of contamination should be eliminated if possible.[8,11]

STRYCHNINE

The present-day use of strychnine is primarily as a rodenticide. Although strychnine is available to the public through many retail outlets, instances of horses becoming intoxicated by strychnine are not common.[8,11,13] The approximate oral lethal dose for horses is 0.5 mg/kg.[8]

CLINICAL SIGNS

The clinical manifestation of strychnine toxicosis can appear as rapidly as 10 minutes to 2 hours after ingestion. Initial signs include apprehension, nervousness, and muscle stiffness. These signs are followed by stiffness and tetanic spasms that may appear spontaneously or may be initiated by stimuli such as sound, touch, or light. These tetanic spasms may vary from a few seconds to a minute or more and are characterized by extreme extensor muscle rigidity. Apnea frequently occurs during the spasms. Sometimes, intermittent periods of relaxation occur between seizures but become less frequent as the clinical episode progresses. In lethal cases the convulsive spasms become more frequent until death eventually occurs during a seizure or as a result of exhaustion and anoxia. The entire clinical episode typicallys lasts less than 2 hours.[8,11] Additional signs that are reported in horses include sweating, incoordination, prostration, convulsions, and death within approximately 2 hours.[11]

PATHOPHYSIOLOGY

Strychnine is absorbed rapidly from the intestinal tract but not from the stomach. The alkaloid nature of the compound promotes its ionization within an acid medium; hence minimal absorption occurs from the stomach.[8] Once absorbed, strychnine is distributed readily throughout the body. Strychnine does not accumulate in any given tissue, but detectable concentrations can be found in the blood, urine, liver, and kidney.[8,11] Strychnine is metabolized in the liver by hepatic microsomal enzymes, and it and its metabolites are excreted in urine.[8] Excretion of strychnine is rapid, with most of a lethal dose being eliminated within 24 hours.[11]

Glycine is an inhibitory neurotransmitter in the spinal cord and medulla that serves to dampen or modulate efferent motor neuron activity. The purpose of this modulating effect is to provide smooth, coordinated muscle contraction and activity that are appropriate and consistent with the requirements for locomotion and respiration. Strychnine acts competitively to antagonize glycine by blocking its uptake at postsynaptic sites on receptors in the spinal cord and brainstem. The result of this blockade is hyperexcitation of muscle groups caused by lack of normal inhibition. Muscle reflex activity is allowed to proceed in basically an uncontrolled manner. All striated muscles are affected, but the more powerful extensor muscles tend to predominate and produce generalized rigidity and tonic seizures.[8,11]

DIAGNOSIS AND TREATMENT

A tentative diagnosis of strychnine poisoning can be made on the basis of a history of possible exposure, characteristic limb rigidity, and a rapid recovery (i.e., less than 24 hours in many cases) in animals aggressively treated in time. To confirm the diagnosis, the clinician may submit tissue samples for evaluation. Stomach content is the most suitable specimen for analysis.[8,11] Many commercial strychnine baits contain grain (e.g., wheat, oat, barley, sorghum) dyed red or green; seeing this in the stomach contents allows the clinician to pursue strychnine poisoning as a differential diagnosis.

Treatment of strychnine poisoning is symptomatic because no specific antidote is available. The horse should be kept in a quiet environment with minimal stimulation. Of primary importance is maintenance of relaxation and prevention of asphyxia. Pentobarbital or chloral hydrate solutions should be given intravenously to produce effective sedation. Complete anesthetization of the horse usually is not necessary or desired. Other medications have been recommended for use in dogs and should be effective in horses as well. These medications include the centrally acting muscle relaxants methocarbamol (150 mg/kg intravenously) and guaifenesin (110 mg/kg intravenously), repeated as needed; diazepam and xylazine to control seizures; and inhalation anesthetics if necessary.[8] Oxygen therapy and assisted ventilation may be necessary in some animals.

Additional agents that are beneficial are activated charcoal given orally and followed by a laxative to evacuate the bowel. Acidification of urine with oral ammonium chloride at 132 mg/kg also may enhance excretion of strychnine, but the efficacy of this treatment is not well documented. Although toxic doses of strychnine may be depleted from the body in a short time, it may be necessary to maintain relaxation and sedation in the horse for 24 to 48 hours.[8]

METALDEHYDE

Metaldehyde is used primarily as a molluscicide in snail and slug baits in coastal and low-lying areas. The baits are generally in the form of meal or pellets and are placed around crops or ornamental plants.[8,11] Horses can become poisoned through inadvertent exposure to bags of bait. No specific toxicity studies could be found regarding horses, but reports indicate that horses may be more susceptible to toxicosis than dogs, in which the acute oral LD_{50} may be as little as 60 to 100 mg/kg.[11] In two separate reports, horses died after ingestion of as little as 60 mg/kg[67] and 120 mg/kg. Experimentally, a parasitized yearling colt died after exposure to 0.1 mg/kg.[15]

CLINICAL SIGNS

The clinical signs reported in horses include acute onset of signs within 1 hour after exposure; excessive sweating, profuse salivation, restlessness, hyperesthesia, incoordination, and tachycardia can be observed. One horse exhibited violent muscle spasms just before death.[14] Other signs include muscle fasciculations, clonic spasms, and rapid and deep respiratory movements.[15] Death occurs rapidly (3 to 5 hours) in horses exposed to a lethal amount of metaldehyde[14,15] and is thought to result from acute respiratory failure.[11] Dogs also are reported to exhibit signs of convulsions and elevated body temperature (often refered to as "shake and bake").[8,11]

PATHOPHYSIOLOGY

Metaldehyde is absorbed readily from the gastrointestinal tract. Gastric hydrochloric acid enhances its decomposition to acetaldehyde, and metaldehyde and acetaldehyde are absorbed and readily cross the blood-brain barrier. The exact mechanism of action of metaldehyde is yet to be elucidated.[11]

DIAGNOSIS AND TREATMENT

A history of possible exposure to a molluscicide coupled with the appropriate clinical signs can lead to a tentative diagnosis of metaldehyde toxicity. Stomach contents can be analyzed to detect metaldehyde or acetaldehyde, and a formaldehyde-like odor may be present in the stomach contents.[8,11]

No antidote is available for metaldehyde. Treatment is symptomatic and aimed at sedation; removing the compound from the stomach; and supportive therapy such as maintaining proper fluid, electrolyte, and acid-base indexes. Sedatives such as xylazine, acepromazine, and diazepam may be useful to control convulsive behavior. Methocarbamol may help control muscle spasms and fasciculations, and mineral oil can be given orally to aid evacuation of the gastrointestinal tract.[8,11]

METHIOCARB

This molluscicide has been reported to cause toxicity in two horses: one died, and the other fully recovered.[16,17] In each instance the amount ingested was estimated to be from 100 to 125 g of a 4% weight per volume preparation.

CLINICAL SIGNS

The onset of signs was rapid, beginning within a few minutes of ingestion. Muscle tremors, which became severe, and profuse sweating and salivation were noted. Both horses had increased heart and respiratory rates, and the surviving horse also exhibited signs of abdominal discomfort. Clinical signs gradually lessened until they became absent approximately 12 hours after onset in the surviving horse.[17] The horse that was fatally intoxicated died approximately 12 hours after initially showing signs. Postmortem findings included severe generalized pulmonary congestion with froth accumulation in the airways and a number of large hemorrhagic areas scattered throughout the intestinal tract.[16] Methiocarb is an acetylcholinesterase-inhibiting carbamate compound; readers may wish to consult the section on carbamate and organophosphate pesticides for more information.

TREATMENT

The specific antidote for methiocarb is atropine sulfate.[16,17] Repeated dosing may be necessary. Other suggested remedies include supportive therapy consisting of sedatives, calcium solutions, and mineral oil.[17]

4-Aminopyridine

4-Aminopyridine is used commercially as a bird repellent and often is mixed with grain before its distribution. In the one reported instance of 4-aminopyridine toxicity, affected horses were exposed to corn that contained the substance.[18]

CLINICAL SIGNS

The two affected horses began showing signs of profuse sweating, severe convulsions, behavioral abnormalities, and rapid fluttering of the third eyelid. Both horses died within 2 hours of the onset of clinical signs and approximately 8 hours after ingesting the contaminated corn. No specific lesions were noted at necropsy. The estimated lethal dose of 4-aminopyridine for these two horses was 2 to 3 mg per kg of body weight.[18]

PATHOPHYSIOLOGY

The mechanism whereby 4-aminopyridine causes death has not been elucidated. However, this substance readily crosses the blood-brain barrier and may enhance the release of acetylcholine and other neurotransmitters from prejunctional nerve endings.[11,19] The result is a stimulatory effect on the CNS.

DIAGNOSIS AND TREATMENT

A diagnosis of suspected toxicity is confirmed by testing the suspect material and stomach contents of affected horses.[18] No specific antidote for 4-aminopyridine toxicity is suggested, but the clinician can give affected horses supportive therapy and mineral oil orally to enhance evacuation of the intestinal tract. Given the known mechanism of action of this compound, CNS depressants such as phenobarbital would seem to have some value in treating the CNS signs of affected horses. However, the efficacy of this treatment.

Levamisole

Levamisole has not gained widespread use as an equine anthelmintic, principally because of its limited efficacy in destroying strongyles and because its toxic dose is close to its therapeutic dose. Levamisole is effective, however, in eliminating lungworms, ascarids, and adult pinworms from horses. The drug also has been used in human beings and other animal species in an attempt to enhance immune system function.

CLINICAL SIGNS

Clinical signs associated with levamisole toxicity occur within 1 hour of administration and include hyperexcitability, muscle tremors, hyperactivity, excessive sweating, and lacrimation. Recumbency may follow these signs, but animals that recover generally appear normal within 12 hours after exposure.[20-22] Adverse effects are more likely after subcutaneous injection than oral drenching.[22] The toxic dose of 20 mg/kg is close to the therapeutic dose of 15 mg/kg, and 20 mg/kg may cause death in some horses.[11]

DIAGNOSIS AND TREATMENT

The diagnosis is suspected when horses exhibit clinical signs suggesting levamisole toxicosis and exposure is known to have occurred. No specific antidote is available, so therapy includes supportive care. Most animals recover uneventfully if a sublethal dose has been given.

Carbon Disulfide

Carbon disulfide is seldom used as an anthelmintic in present times but has enjoyed widespread use in the past for treatment of infestation caused by *Parascaris equorum* and *Gastrophilus* species.[23] Carbon disulfide is a manufactured product used as a solvent for resins, pesticides, and waxes and as an agent to remove greases. The chemical is used widely as a fumigant to control insects in stored grain.[8] Carbon disulfide is an exceptional fat solvent and in the pure state is a clear, colorless volatile liquid with a sweet, aromatic odor resembling that of decaying cabbage. The chemical is well absorbed through the skin and lungs and after ingestion.[7,8]

CLINICAL SIGNS

Reported signs of acute toxicity in animals include dyspnea and cyanosis, spasmodic tremors, vascular collapse, prostration, convulsions, coma, and death.[8] Signs referable to local irritation following inhalation might include salivation and coughing. A combination product of piperazine–carbon disulfide and phenothiazine caused transitory signs of overtranquilization and unsteady gait when dosed at 8 oz per 45 kg of body weight.[23] Whether any of these effects were related directly to carbon disulfide was not determined. Chronic exposure causes neuropsychiatric changes, peripheral neuropathies, and cranial nerve dysfunction in human beings,[7] but chronic exposure in horses is unlikely.

PATHOPHYSIOLOGY

Because carbon disulfide is a potent fat solvent, local skin contact results in erythema and pain, and prolonged contact produces chemical burns and vesiculation.[7] The chemical is irritating to mucous membranes when inhaled or ingested.[7,78]

At the cellular level carbon disulfide acts to block enzymatic processes by reacting with nucleophilic compounds, including pyridoxamine, monoamine oxidase in the cerebrum, and dopamine decarboxylase. Carbon disulfide binds to microsomal enzymes, thereby reducing their activity, and produces a centrilobular hepatic necrosis. In addition, carbon disulfide chelates copper and zinc and therefore can produce disturbances in tract mineral balance.[7]

DIAGNOSIS AND TREATMENT

No specific diagnostic test is available for use in animals suspected of suffering from carbon disulfide toxicosis. In one report affected animals had increased BUN and bilirubin concentrations, increased serum activities of AST and alanine aminotransferase, and increased serum cholesterol concentration. Affected horses also had depressed serum concentrations of protein-bound iodine and magnesium.[23]

In human beings the iodine-azide test is useful to identify carbon disulfide metabolites in urine,[7] but the efficacy of this procedure for diagnostic use in horses is unknown. Treatment of toxicosis primarily involves removal of the source and symptomatic care.

MISCELLANEOUS AGENTS

NICOTINE

Nicotine is an alkaloid contained in tobacco leaves. Although toxicosis might result from ingestion of excessive amounts of tobacco leaves or cured tobacco in cigarettes or cigars, this route of toxicosis probably is rare in horses. Horses are more likely to be intoxicated by ingestion or exposure to the salt nicotine sulfate.[8,11] A concentrated solution of nicotine sulfate (Blackleaf 40) has been used to control leaf-eating insects and occasionally as a premises spray to control certain ectoparasites.[8,12] Horses may ingest this substance from spills of the solution, from open containers, or from foliage that has been sprayed with the product.[11] Topical exposure may result when horses are housed in stables where this product has been used for mite control.[24] The lethal dose of nicotine in the horse is 100 to 300 mg.[8]

CLINICAL SIGNS

The signs of nicotine toxicity are rapid in onset, often occurring within a few minutes after exposure. Initially, the signs noted are those of cholinergic overstimulation (i.e., excitement, increased respiration, and salivation). Increased peristalsis and diarrhea also can occur.[8,12] These signs are transitory and are followed rapidly by depression, muscle weakness and ataxia, slow and shallow respiration, and an increased heart rate. Convulsions also can occur. In fatal cases these signs progress to collapse, coma, and death within minutes to hours after the onset of clinical signs.[8,11,12]

PATHOPHYSIOLOGY

Nicotine is absorbed readily from the oral mucosa, respiratory tract, and gastrointestinal tract (excluding the stomach) and through intact skin.[7,8] If ingested, nicotine also can exert a direct, rapid caustic action on the mucosa of the mouth and throat, esophagus, and stomach.[8] The substance is metabolized primarily in the liver, and nicotine and its metabolites are excreted in urine. In human beings urinary acidification greatly enhances clearance of nicotine and its metabolites.[7]

Initially, and only for a short time, nicotine stimulates the autonomic nervous system ganglia, neuromuscular junctions, and some synapses in the CNS by depolarization of the postsynaptic membrane.[7,8] With toxicosis, however, the stimulation is followed rapidly by a depolarizing-type blockade of all these nicotinic cholinergic receptors.[7,8,11] Large doses result in a descending paralysis of the CNS, and death results from respiratory failure caused by paralysis of the diaphragm and chest muscles.[8,11] The effects of a sublethal dose should diminish in a few hours.[11]

DIAGNOSIS AND TREATMENT

No diagnostic lesions are present at necropsy. However, the distinct odor of nicotine may be present in stomach contents.[8,11] One can evaluate urine, blood, liver, kidney, and other tissues for nicotine content in suspect cases.[8]

Treatment often is ineffective because of the rapid course of the toxicosis. However, because no specific antidote exists for nicotine toxicity, affected horses should be treated symptomatically. If exposure has been through the skin, washing with soap and water, followed by thorough rinsing, is indicated.[8] After oral exposure, affected horses can be treated with oral laxatives, tannic acid, or potassium permanganate in an attempt to reduce absorption of the toxin. Activated charcoal also may be beneficial in adsorbing residual nicotine in the intestinal tract.[8,12] Atropine sulfate is reported to be without value in affected horses because it does not protect vital nicotinic receptors in the respiratory muscles and the CNS from the effects of nicotine.[11] Artificial respiration becomes the only means of maintaining life once the respiratory depression reaches a critical level. This last-ditch effort usually fails.[11]

AMMONIA

Ammonia toxicosis in the horse can occur in two ways: by primary exposure to ammonia gas or by secondary metabolism of urea to ammonia within the body (see the section on urea and nonprotein nitrogen substances).[7,8] Primary exposure to toxic concentrations of ammonia gas probably is rare in horses, even though ammonia is the air pollutant most frequently found in high concentrations in animal facilities. The concentrations of ammonia found in stables may be irritating to horses but probably will never reach lethal concentrations. Another source of ammonia toxicosis to horses might be compressed anhydrous ammonia, which is used as an agricultural fertilizer. An accidental spill or spray of anhydrous ammonia near a horse or livestock facility could have disastrous and possibly lethal results.[8] Human beings can detect the odor of ammonia at a concentration of 30 ppm, eye and nasal irritation occurs near 50 ppm, and severe pulmonary dysfunction results from concentrations greater than 1000 ppm. Immediate death occurs at concentrations nearing 1500 ppm.[7]

CLINICAL SIGNS

Signs associated with low concentrations of aerial ammonia are those of irritation to the eyes and respiratory tract. Excessive tearing, shallow breathing, coughing, and nasal discharge are common findings. Higher concentrations can induce laryngospasm and pulmonary edema.[7] Exposure to anhydrous ammonia can result in impairment of eyesight, permanent loss of eyesight, respiratory disease, and skin burns.[8]

PATHOPHYSIOLOGY

Ammonia is a highly water-soluble, irritating alkaline gas that causes liquefactive necrosis at high concentrations.[7] Because ammonia is so highly water-soluble, it readily reacts with the mucous membranes of the eye and the respiratory tract.[8]

DIAGNOSIS AND TREATMENT

A diagnosis of aerial ammonia toxicosis is based primarily on history and physical examination findings. Laboratory evaluation is of little value in establishing a diagnosis of inhalation exposure,[8] but laboratory evaluation can be useful to assess the degree of damage to the respiratory tract and evaluate the effectiveness of therapy.

Treatment involves removing the horse from the source of exposure. If exposure has been severe enough to result in ophthalmic or respiratory tract disease, these conditions should be treated accordingly.

UREA AND NONPROTEIN NITROGEN SUBSTANCES

Urea and other nonprotein nitrogen substances, including various ammonium salts, are added to ruminant rations as a source of nonprotein nitrogen because ruminants can use these compounds to provide a large percentage of their protein nitrogen requirements. Urea has additional uses as a fertilizer and as a substitute for salt in melting snow and ice in metropolitan areas.[8,11] Horses are only mildly susceptible to urea toxicosis, and it is highly unlikely that horses would ingest urea or urea-containing feedstuffs in amounts sufficient to cause clinical signs.[8,12] However, horses are more susceptible to toxicosis caused by ingestion of ammonium salts,[8] which may occur after accidental exposure to these substances. In horses urea is lethal when ingested at a rate of 4 g per kg of body weight, and ammonium salts are lethal at a dose of 1.5 g per kg of body weight.[11] Urea and other nonprotein nitrogen formulations are toxic to animals simply because they are hydrolyzed to ammonia, which is responsible for causing the derangements associated with toxicosis.

CLINICAL SIGNS

The spectrum and intensity of signs in ruminants with urea toxicosis vary, and the same is probably true for horses. The clinical course is usually acute and rapid, often occurring from a few minutes to a few hours after consumption.[8] Occasionally, animals are found dead, or they may die quickly after exhibiting signs of weakness, dyspnea, colic, and terminal tonic convulsions. Other varied signs can be present. Behavioral abnormalities such as restlessness and dullness may be present. Excitement and even belligerency may follow these signs. Nervous signs such as hyperesthesia, tremors, and muscle twitching and spasms can occur. Autonomic nervous system derangements may include salivation, bradycardia, hypertension, and severe colic. More terminal signs may include increased and labored respirations, cardiac arrhythmias, frothing at the mouth, and cyanosis. Intermittent tonic-opisthotonic seizures also can be elicited near death. The onset of signs may range from 10 minutes to 4 hours, and death typically occurs within a few hours after exposure.[11]

PATHOPHYSIOLOGY

Urea is hydrolyzed to ammonia by the action of the enzyme urease. This reaction is hastened by an alkaline pH, and in the horse these requirements are found in the cecum. In horses urea is absorbed from the small intestine and excreted in the urine. The only urea that might contribute to toxicity in the horse would be that excessive amount that reaches the cecum and is available for hydrolysis.[12]

In normal animals ammonia liberated from nonprotein nitrogen sources can be in the form of the ammonium ion. This ion is soluble, but its charge prevents it from being efficiently absorbed across membranes. Ammonia is also soluble; however, because it lacks an ionic charge, it can be absorbed readily across membranes to enter the bloodstream.[11] Ammonia is a normal by-product of tissue metabolism, and in hepatocytes it is converted to urea by the urea cycle or is incorporated into glutamic acid in the synthesis of glutamine. Toxicosis occurs when the amount of ammonia absorbed into the bloodstream exceeds the ability of the horse to detoxify it.[11]

The primary mechanism of ammonia toxicosis is thought to be inhibition of the citric acid cycle, but the exact mechanism by which this occurs is not known.[11] Ammonia saturation of the glutamine-synthesizing system has been suggested to have an inhibitory effect on the citrate cycle, creating a decrease in its intermediates and a subsequent decrease in cellular energy production and respiration. As the citrate cycle fails, cells begin to malfunction. Cellular energy and respiration deficits may cause ultrastructural damage leading to degenerative changes and eventual cell death. The role of ammonia in causing signs of encephalopathy is controversial and not well understood.[24]

Laboratory abnormalities associated with ammonia toxicosis include elevated serum ammonia, potassium, phosphorus, lactic acid, glucose, and serum activity of the liver enzyme AST. Urine output decreases, and PCV increases as impending cardiac failure and shock ensue.[11]

The ultimate cause of death is inconsistent in urea toxicosis and poisoning by ammonium compounds. Cardiac failure may be induced by hyperkalemia, or ventricular fibrillation may result from the myocardial effects of ammonia itself. Convulsions may be prolonged and responsible for fatal anoxia. Pulmonary edema may be a complicating factor in some cases. Death also has been postulated to result from asphyxiation.[11]

DIAGNOSIS AND TREATMENT

Animals that die of ammonia toxicosis exhibit no characteristic lesions. Generalized venous stasis and congestion of organs may be present, along with pulmonary edema and scattered petechiation and ecchymoses. A strong odor of ammonia may be present, but this is probably much more characteristic of ruminants than of monogastric animals.[11]

Clinical signs and history can be helpful in establishing a diagnosis. Blood and ocular fluid ammonia can be evaluated in the laboratory, but the results must be interpreted with caution.[11] Storage of the sample, length of time between death and time of sampling, and length of time between sampling and analysis can influence the blood ammonia concentration. Tissue specimens must be frozen immediately if they are to be analyzed.[8] Suspect feeds can also be analyzed for urea or total nitrogen content.

Treatment is often unrewarding because of the rapidity of onset. No specific antidote is available for ammonia, so therapy is mostly symptomatic. Orally administered laxatives such as mineral oil may be beneficial. The clinician should correct any deficits in fluid volume or abnormalities in acid-base or electrolyte concentrations. Horses that are convulsing can be controlled with pentobarbital, and a patent airway should always be maintained. Assisted ventilation, if necessary, is usually futile because of the poor survival rate of severely affected animals.[11]

TOXICOSES CAUSING SIGNS RELATING TO CENTRAL NERVOUS SYSTEM DEPRESSION

As with toxic problems associated with other primary clinical signs, it can be difficult to determine the source of CNS depression. The principal task is to rule out the existence of primary cranial disease. Even with the availability of advanced imaging equipment, this can be difficult. Unless the clinical signs or history is definitive, the diagnosis of a toxic problem is often presumptive.

PLANTS

BLACK LOCUST (*ROBINIA PSEUDOACACIA*)

The black locust tree has been described as toxic to horses.[1,2]

The toxic principle is classified as a lectin, which is present in seeds, sap, roots, wood, leaves, and bark of the plant. Lectin has been used in cytologic research because of its ability to stimulate glycoprotein biosynthesis and cell proliferation in lymphocytes of various animal species.[3] Horses may become intoxicated by ingesting the bark. Only small amounts of lectin are reported to precipitate clinical disease.[2]

The clinical signs reported are mental depression, weakness, posterior paralysis, irregular heart rate, pale mucous membranes, and anorexia. Abdominal discomfort and diarrhea of varying degrees also may be evident.[1,2]

No definitive diagnostic test is available. Treatment of suspected toxicosis is mostly symptomatic and should include removal of the source; evacuation of the intestinal tract; and maintenance of normal fluid, electrolyte, and acid-base indexes.

Bracken Fern (*Pteridium aquilinum*)

Bracken fern is found most commonly in forested areas, burns, or abandoned fields in the northern and western United States.[2] Toxicity can occur at any time of year, but horses are more likely to consume the plant in late summer and fall, when other forage is scarce. However, horses also might acquire a taste for the plant in pastures or when it is incorporated in bedding. Horses also can become intoxicated from hay contaminated with large amounts of bracken fern. The entire plant is considered to be toxic.[1]

CLINICAL SIGNS

Signs of toxicosis occur after the horse has been consuming the plant for 30 to 60 days. Horses also can exhibit signs even if they have not ingested bracken fern for 2 to 3 weeks.[1] The signs most frequently reported are incoordination, which may progress to severe ataxia; postural abnormalities, including arching of the back, crouching, and a base-wide stance; muscle fasciculations, which can progress to severe tremors; and bradycardia with cardiac arrhythmias early in the disease course, although tachycardia is most prevalent terminally. Terminal stages of the disease are characterized by signs of opisthotonus and clonic convulsions.[1,2] One report also describes an affected horse showing signs of colic and acute hemolytic anemia.[4]

PATHOPHYSIOLOGY

The agent in bracken fern that is toxic to horses is thiaminase.[1,2] Bracken fern also is reported to contain ptaquiloside,[5] which is capable of inducing bone marrow suppression, and a β-glucopyranoside, which may enhance the release of endogenous histamine.[2] The significance of these last two compounds in the development of toxicity in horses is unknown. Thiamine plays an integral role in carbohydrate, fat, and protein metabolism and acts as a cofactor in enzymatic pathways responsible for energy production. Thiamine is an important cofactor in the decarboxylation of pyruvate to acetyl coenzyme A, which subsequently enters the tricarboxylic acid cycle.

Thiamine deficiency acts to interrupt these cellular energy processes and also limits certain metabolic pathways available for pyruvate metabolism, resulting in the systemic accumulation of a variety of metabolites, including pyruvate and lactate.

DIAGNOSIS AND TREATMENT

History and clinical signs are helpful in arriving at a diagnosis. No pathognomonic lesions or laboratory abnormalities occur, but some laboratory findings may include elevated blood pyruvate concentration and decreased plasma thiamine and red blood cell transketolase concentrations.[2]

Thiamine should be administered daily to affected horses at a dose of 0.25 to 0.5 mg per kg of body weight intravenously, subcutaneously, or intramuscularly for several days. Initially, thiamine can be given at a dose of 5 to 10 mg/kg intravenously, but this dose should be diluted in fluids and administered slowly because of the frequency of adverse reactions when thiamine is given intravenously. Thiamine deficiency usually can be prevented by dietary supplementation of yeast or cereal grains.[2]

Equisetum (*Equisetum arvense*)

Equisetum, commonly called *horsetail, marestail,* or *scouring rush,* has a geographic distribution similar to that of bracken fern. Like bracken fern, *Equisetum* is unpalatable to horses, and toxicosis usually results from hay contaminated with the plant.[1,2] Thiaminase is the toxic principle found in *Equisetum,* and the clinical signs, pathogenesis, and treatment are virtually identical to those of bracken fern.[1,2] Large amounts in the diet are necessary to induce clinical problems.

Milkweed (*Asclepias* species)

Several species of *Asclepias* have been reported to be toxic to large animals.[2,6] The plants are reported to be distasteful to animals and not commonly grazed, but the plant may become incorporated into hay. Affected animals are reported to have a weak, rapid pulse; dyspnea; loss of muscular control; and muscular spasms. Salivation, bloating, and convulsions also may occur.[2,6] Most animals that reach the convulsive stage die.[6] Numerous compounds have been isolated from *Asclepias* species, including resinoids and cardioactive glycosides. One resinoid produces smooth muscle spasms of the gastrointestinal tract.[2] The mechanism of action of the other toxins has not been elucidated. No specific antidote is available,[2] but supportive care, including evacuation of the gastrointestinal tract, is indicated.

Yellow Starthistle (*Centaurea solstitialis*) and Russian Knapweed (*Acroptilon repens*)

Both yellow starthistle and Russian knapweed cause nigropallidal encephalomalacia in horses. These plants are found scattered over much of the western United States and are most abundant in nonirrigated pastures during the dry seasons of summer and fall. Both plants have a minimal moisture requirement and so may be the only green plants remaining in a dry season. Consequently, most poisonings occur during the summer or fall months.[2,7,8]

Horses apparently reject the plants when more suitable vegetation is available; the disease does not commonly occur in horses grazing improved pastures or grassland range.[8] However, some horses are reported to develop a craving for the plant and selectively seek it out.[2] Horses may eat the weeds, occasionally or frequently, without becoming ill, and continuous and protracted exposure to the plants is necessary for toxicosis to develop under experimental conditions. Feeding trials have shown that horses must consume an amount of weed equivalent to 59% to 200% of their body weight of yellow starthistle and 59% to 63% of their body weight of Russian knapweed for 3 to 11 weeks of continuous feeding before clinical signs develop. The plants retain their toxicity when dried and incorporated into hay. All ages may be affected, but younger horses generally seem more prone to the disease. One study reported a median age of about 2 years in affected horses.[8] Equids appear to be the only animals that develop nigropallidal encephalomalacia when exposed to these plants.

CLINICAL SIGNS

The onset of signs is always sudden, beginning with variable degrees of impairment of eating and drinking. Coordinated movements of prehension, mastication, and deglutition are often lacking. Affected horses are unable to chew adequately and propel the food to the back of the mouth. Some horses may show only faulty prehension, whereas others are unable to eat at all. Most horses, however, appear to be able to swallow if feed or water gains access to the posterior pharynx. More severely affected horses may attempt to drink by immersing their muzzles deeply into the water in an attempt to force water into the posterior pharynx.[2,8-10]

Hypertonicity of the facial muscles is a characteristic sign, particularly when feed is offered.[2] The horse often holds the mouth partially open with the lips retracted, resulting in a fixed facial expression. The tongue may protrude from the mouth, and many horses display constant chewing movements—hence the name "chewing disease."[2,10]

Other characteristic signs include weight loss, mild to moderate depression, and yawning. Most horses can be roused readily from somnolence by mild stimulation. Few animals may show aimless, slow walking or circling early in the disease course. The gait is usually normal, but occasional deficits are apparent, including stiffness, slowness, ataxia, tetraparesis, and conscious proprioceptive deficits.[2,10] In cases of prolonged exposure, a wobbly, shuffling gait may occur because of weakness. Sensation and reflexes appear normal, and the animals are afebrile.[10]

Horses less severely affected may adopt unusual means of eating by scooping feed into the mouth. These animals may survive for months, but complete recovery has not been observed in confirmed cases of the disease. In some instances, however, residual signs may become almost undetectable.[8] Death of affected horses is from starvation and dehydration.

PATHOPHYSIOLOGY

The pathogenesis of the necrotic brain lesions is unknown, but these plants have been postulated possibly to contain a specifically toxic substance or to lack some nutritional component necessary for the health and well-being of the horse.[9,10] Several sesquiterpene lactones and polyacetylenes have been isolated from these plants, but their significance remains undetermined.[11] Dipyrone has been postulated to be the inciting agent.

DIAGNOSIS AND TREATMENT

The antemortem diagnosis of nigropallidal encephalomalacia is based largely on observation of clinical signs and prolonged exposure of the horse to the plants by grazing or by severely contaminated hay. If available, magnetic resonance imaging can identify characteristic lesions on T1-weighted, T2-weighted, and proton density images. These lesions do not contrast enhance after gadolinium-diethylenetriaminepentaacetic acid administration.[12] Characteristic necropsy findings include unilaterally or, more commonly, bilaterally symmetric softening and necrosis in areas of the globus pallidus and substantia nigra. These areas usually are sharply defined and may be cavitary.[2,10]

No known treatment exists for affected horses. Prevention requires keeping horses from the plant and providing adequate, suitable forage.

Milkvetch and Timber Milkvetch (*Astragalus* species)

Most of the variants of *Astragalus miser* are referred to as *timber milkvetch* or *milkvetch*. These plants are found primarily in the western United States from northern Mexico to Canada and are essentially a cause of toxicosis to ruminants. Horses are reported to be poisoned by this group of plants, but there are no reports of the lesions.[13]

The disease in ruminants is characterized primarily by general depression, mental dullness, incoordination, and eventual hindlimb paralysis. Respiratory distress, cyanosis, and acute collapse also may occur. Acute and chronic forms of the syndrome are reported.[13]

The toxic principle, referred to as *miserotoxin,* is a β-D-glucoside of 3-nitro-1-propanol, which is metabolized in the intestinal tract to the highly toxic compound 3-nitro-1-propanol. Miserotoxin is broken down into inorganic nitrite and a three-carbon side chain. The nitrite is responsible for producing methemoglobinemia in animals but is not the primary cause of death.[13]

No specific antidote is recommended. Poisoning is prevented by controlling the plants with herbicides and preventing livestock from grazing the plant.

MISCELLANEOUS AGENTS

PROPYLENE GLYCOL

Propylene glycol is used commercially as a diluent for injectable drugs and as a glucose precursor in the treatment of hypoglycemia in ruminants. Horses may become intoxicated by the inadvertent use of propylene glycol if it is mistaken for a similar-appearing liquid paraffin preparation. Reports of toxicosis in horses are rare.[14,15]

Propylene glycol has a low oral toxicity in human beings. Approximately 45% of the absorbed dose is excreted unchanged by the kidney, whereas the remainder is metabolized by hepatic alcohol dehydrogenase to acetate, pyruvate, and lactate.[16]

CLINICAL SIGNS

Adverse signs occur within 10 to 30 minutes after a toxic dose of propylene glycol. Initial findings include salivation and profuse sweating, ataxia, depression, and tachypnea. Additional signs can include cyanosis, seizures, and coma.[14] Diarrhea also has been reported in one horse experimentally given a large dose of propylene glycol.[15] Death has occurred 1 to 3 days after ingestion of excessive amounts of the product.[14,15]

PATHOPHYSIOLOGY

Propylene glycol is metabolized by hepatic alcohol dehydrogenase to form acetate, lactate, and pyruvate. After a large exposure, excessive amounts of these products accumulate, resulting in severe systemic lactic acidosis.[16] The clinical signs and toxicologic findings result from the effects of this severe acidemia on various body organs and tissues.

The acute oral LD_{50} for horses has not been established, but the doses for rats, rabbits, and dogs are 32, 18, and 9 ml/kg, respectively. One 450-kg horse died after intubation with 3.8 L (7.6 ml/kg) of propylene glycol,[14] but other horses have survived this dose. Toxic signs were reported in horses receiving 1.9 to 7.6 L of propylene glycol, but the only death occurred in the horse getting 7.6 L.[15]

DIAGNOSIS AND TREATMENT

Exposure to propylene glycol is confirmed by chemical analysis of serum and urine. Necropsy findings associated with propylene glycol toxicosis may be minimal.[14] The horse given 7.6 L exhibited sloughing of the gastric mucosa, diffuse enterocolitis, renal congestion, and brain edema.[15] Histopathologic findings typically include hepatic necrosis, renal tubular necrosis and infarcts, myocardial perivascular edema, and pulmonary edema.[14,15]

Because no specific antidote is available, treatment of propylene glycol toxicosis aims at alleviating the severe acidemia that develops and providing supportive care for the other organs and tissues that may become compromised. Sodium bicarbonate solutions should be given to treat the acidosis. When possible, the clinician should monitor blood pH and adjust bicarbonate administration according to need. Intravenous fluids should be given to aid diuresis and maintain normal fluid volume. Pulmonary and renal function should be thoroughly evaluated in affected horses, and precautions should be taken to prevent the development of further pulmonary edema. Such precautions may require the use of diuretics and careful monitoring of the fluid administration rate.

Serum electrolyte concentrations should be maintained in normal ranges, and oxygen therapy may be beneficial in horses exhibiting tachypnea and cyanosis. Activated charcoal has been recommended in treating human toxicosis.[16]

TRICLOPYR

Triclopyr is a herbicide used to control hardwood species on road rights-of-way, industrial sites, and forest planting sites. Horses may become exposed to the herbicide by grazing areas that have were inappropriately treated with the product in the past.

An experimental study was conducted to determine the toxic level of triclopyr to ponies. Ponies given 60 mg/kg/day for 4 days did not show any clinical sign of illness. Ponies given 300 mg/kg/day for 4 days did develop clinical signs. This study indicated that the toxic dosage in ponies was 5 times the estimated maximal intake for the highest recommended usage rate as a herbicide.[17] Therefore poisoning from the proper use of this herbicide is unlikely.

CLINICAL SIGNS

Initial signs of depression and decreased gastrointestinal motility were first noticed on the fourth day of the trial. Additional signs that developed were ataxia, weakness, muscle tremors, increased respiratory rate, cyanotic mucous membranes, and normal to slightly elevated body temperature. Some ponies became recumbent as clinical signs progressed. Two ponies died on the fifth and sixth days of the trial, and two other ponies were euthanized on the fifth day. The remaining two ponies were only mildly affected and recovered.

No significant changes were apparent in clinical chemistry values. Gross necropsy lesions consisted of pale livers and pale swollen kidneys, and a few horses had excessive intestinal fluid contents. Microscopic changes were mild and were those of nonspecific hepatosis and nephrosis.[17]

PATHOPHYSIOLOGY

The mechanism whereby triclopyr produces clinical disease in horses has not been elucidated.

DIAGNOSIS AND TREATMENT

Toxicosis caused by triclopyr appears highly unlikely under natural circumstances.[17,18] Diagnosis of suspect cases is based on clinical signs and a history of exposure to the herbicide. No specific antidote is available. Affected individuals require supportive and symptomatic care.

LEUKOENCEPHALOMALACIA

Equine leukoencephalomalacia, a sporadically occurring disease of horses, ponies, donkeys, and mules, has a worldwide distribution. The disease usually is seasonal, with most cases occurring from late fall through early spring, and most outbreaks have been associated with a dry growing period followed by a wet period.[19,20]

This malady is caused by the mycotoxin fumonisin B1, a metabolite of *Fusarium moniliforme*. Equidae become affected usually by ingesting *F. moniliforme*–infected corn or corn screenings, but the problem also has been associated with the consumption of commercially prepared diets.[19-22] Infected kernels often have a pink to reddish-brown discoloration, and damaged kernels and cob parts may have a much greater concentration of fumonisin B1 than do undamaged kernels.[20,22] Feeds containing less than 10 ppm fumonisin B1 have not been associated with disease, but concentrations of greater than 10 ppm can be lethal to horses.[23]

CLINICAL SIGNS

Two clinical syndromes are associated with fumonisin B1 intoxication. The more common is the classic neurotoxic syndrome, but hepatotoxicosis also occurs in some horses. Older animals may be more susceptible than younger animals, and clinical signs become evident approximately 3 to 4 weeks after daily ingestion of contaminated feed. Onset of signs is typically abrupt, and death usually occurs in 2 to 3 days.[19,20] Occasionally, horses that showed few to no premonitory signs are found dead.[19]

The neurologic syndrome is characterized initially by incoordination, aimless walking, intermittent anorexia, lethargy, depression, blindness, and head pressing. These signs may be followed by hyperexcitability, belligerence, extreme agitation, profuse sweating, and delirium.[19,20] Recumbency and clonic-tetanic convulsions may occur before death. Recovery from acute episodes has been reported, but some horses retain neurologic deficits.[20]

Clinical signs associated with the hepatotoxic syndrome are swelling of the lips and nose, somnolence, severe icterus and petechiae of mucous membranes, abdominal breathing, and cyanosis. Affected horses also have acute onset of clinical signs with death occurring within a few hours to days.[19,20]

PATHOPHYSIOLOGY

The gross lesions typical of equine leukoencephalomalacia include liquefactive necrosis and degeneration of the cerebral hemispheres, but degenerative changes also can occur in the brainstem, cerebellum, and spinal cord.[19-22] Necrotic areas can vary in size, and regions adjacent to the necrosis often are edematous and rarefied.[20,21]

Gross hepatic lesions in affected horses generally are not pronounced. The liver may be slightly swollen, have a yellowish-brown discoloration, and contain irregular foci or nodules scattered throughout the parenchyma. Histologic abnormalities noted in the liver may include centrilobular necrosis and fibrosis, fatty infiltration of hepatocytes, portal fibrosis, biliary stasis, and bile duct proliferation.[19-21]

The mechanism whereby these changes occur has not been well elucidated. The brain lesions may be induced by ingesting smaller quantities of infected corn over a long period of time, whereby ingestion of higher quantities may produce fatal hepatotoxicosis over a shorter time interval.[20,24]

Several metabolites of *F. moniliforme* have been identified in feeds associated with outbreaks of equine leukoencephalomalacia. These include fusarin C, moniliformin, fusaric acid, 2-methoxy-4-ethylphenol, fumonisin B1, and fumonisin B2.[21,22] Toxicity information about fumonisin B2 is unknown, but moniliformin, fusaric acid, and 2-methoxy-4-ethylphenol do not produce leukoencephalomalacia when injected intravenously into donkeys. Their role in the pathogenesis of the liver lesions in equine leukoencephalomalacia is likewise unknown. However, the neurologic and hepatotoxic syndromes can be produced by oral and intravenous administration of fumonisin B1.[21]

DIAGNOSIS AND TREATMENT

The diagnosis of equine leukoencephalomalacia has been based mostly on observation of clinical signs coupled with a history of exposure to moldy corn. Typical postmortem lesions, when available, help confirm the diagnosis.

Clinicopathologic abnormalities are nonspecific and usually indicate some degree of liver dysfunction. Increased serum concentrations of bilirubin, AST, GGT, and LDH have been reported.[19,21,24] Cerebrospinal fluid abnormalities may include increased protein and total nucleated cell counts and an increased concentration of myelin basic protein.[20,24]

With identification of fumonisin B1 as the causative agent, analytic methods have been developed to assay this toxic metabolite in feed material. Feed containing greater than 10 ppm fumonisin B1 is not safe to feed to horses.[23] Because the disease requires a fairly prolonged exposure to infected corn, representative feed samples should be submitted for analysis. Feed currently being ingested may not be contaminated with the mold.

Treatment of equine leukoencephalomalacia is largely supportive. Horses that are hyperexcitable should be sedated to minimize injury to themselves and their handlers. Supportive therapy for hepatic dysfunction should be initiated if liver damage is evident, and some horses may require forced feeding and watering if they become unable to eat and drink. Mannitol or DMSO may be administered to aid resolution of cerebral edema, and laxatives and activated charcoal may be given to eliminate toxins already in the digestive tract, although their usefulness is probably minimal because this disease is not an acute intoxication. Contaminated feed should be removed immediately from all exposed horses, and pastured horses should be moved to pastures without access to corn. Preventive measures include providing suitable feed material to horses and storing grains, particularly corn, under conditions that discourage mold growth.

TRICHOTHECENES

The trichothecenes are a group of compounds elaborated primarily by *Fusarium tricinctum* and other *Fusarium* species. Only four of approximately 40 trichothecene derivatives have been found to occur naturally in feedstuffs. These four include T-2 toxin, deoxynivalenol, diacetoxyscirpenol, and nivalenol.[25,26] Of these, only one reported episode of T-2 intoxication in horses was found in the literature.[26] This group of mycotoxins more commonly causes gastrointestinal problems in other animals.

In the reported outbreak horses showed clinical signs and laboratory abnormalities similar to those of equine leukoencephalomalacia caused by fumonisin B1. Gross lesions in necropsied horses were also similar to those of equine leukoencephalomalacia. *F. tricinctum* was isolated from all suspect feed samples, and T-2 toxin was detected in varying concentrations in all examined feed samples. Other *Fusarium* metabolites detected in this outbreak included HT-2, verrucarin A and J, and roridin A. The toxicity of these metabolites in farm animals is not yet determined.[26]

LEAD

Lead is reported to be one of the more common toxicants found in veterinary practice, but it rarely is a cause of poisoning for horses now. Materials that can serve as a source of lead toxicity to animals include lead-based paints, putty and caulking materials, used crankcase oil, greases, linoleum, leaded gasoline, solid lead solder, roofing materials, asphalt, and industrial effluents contaminating streams or forage. Discarded automobile batteries and water from lead plumbing also might serve as a source of toxicity.[2,25]

Acute and chronic forms of toxicosis can occur depending on the amount of lead ingested and the time frame in which ingestion occurs. Lead toxicosis in horses is usually chronic and is associated with some type of forage contamination.[27,28] Foliage near lead smelters often contains excessive lead, and grasses located near busy highways have been reported to contain high lead concentrations.[2,28] Horses appear to be much more sensitive than cattle to prolonged, low-dose exposure to lead, yet they are much less sensitive than cattle to short-term exposure of large doses.[25,27] The acute oral lethal dose of lead acetate in horses is 500 to 750 g total dose, but chronic toxicosis can arise when 1 to 7 mg/kg/day is ingested over a period of days, weeks, or months.[25]

Numerous factors can influence the toxicity of lead in horses. Young animals and malnourished animals are reported to be more susceptible than older animals; solid lead is not as toxic as the more soluble salts, which are absorbed more readily; and concurrent exposure to lead and cadmium results in increased severity of clinical signs of lead poisoning. In addition, lead may interact with other minerals to affect toxicity. High levels of dietary calcium cause decreased gastrointestinal absorption of lead.[2,25,28]

CLINICAL SIGNS

The clinical signs of lead toxicity in horses are caused primarily by peripheral nerve dysfunction. The motor nerves are at greater risk, with minimal sensory perception loss in affected horses. Initially, affected horses may appear weak or have slight incoordination. Depression and weight loss become apparent and worsen over the disease course. Laryngeal and pharyngeal paralysis, dysphagia, dysphonia, and proprioceptive deficits occur. As the disease progresses, horses may exhibit flaccidity of the rectal sphincter; paresis of the lower lip; and difficulty in prehension, mastication, and deglutition. Aspiration pneumonia resulting from dysphagia and regurgitation of food is common, and fine muscle tremors may occur intermittently. Terminally, horses may show severe incoordination, anorexia, emaciation, and almost complete pharyngeal and esophageal paralysis with inability to swallow food or water. Seizures also may occur terminally. Colic and diarrhea may be apparent, but they are not common signs.[2,27,28] Progression of these disease signs may require weeks.

Dietary lead crosses the placental barrier, and mares chronically exposed to lead in late pregnancy may deliver premature or small, weak foals. These foals are at greater risk of developing secondary disease complications.[27]

PATHOPHYSIOLOGY

Lead enters the body primarily through ingestion. Inorganic lead cannot readily penetrate the skin, but organic forms such as tetraethyl lead and tetramethyl lead are absorbed through the skin. However, exposure of horses to organic lead compounds would seem to be a rare occurrence. Metallic lead shot or bullets lodged in tissues do not dissolve because tissue pH is too high.[25]

Metallic lead and lead sulfide are less absorbed than the acetate, carbonate, hydroxide, oxide, and phosphate salts. Less than 10% of ingested lead is absorbed across the gastrointestinal tract in adults, but if sufficient quantities of soluble salts are ingested, a significantly greater amount of lead can cross into blood. Even though intestinal absorption is inefficient, increases in blood lead concentrations can occur within 3 hours of dosing.[2,25]

Once absorbed, a large portion of lead is carried on erythrocyte membranes, where it is bound irreversibly to erythrocyte proteins. Much of the remaining lead becomes bound to albumin, and only a small proportion of the absorbed lead actually is free in serum. Unbound lead is in equilibrium with lead bound to erythrocytes and albumin, and distribution to various tissues takes place from the unbound fraction.

Much of the blood lead is removed in the liver. Within the liver, cellular trapping of lead is thought to occur by lead binding to cytoplasmic proteins called *metallothioneins*. Lead also accumulates within the renal cortex, where it becomes trapped as intranuclear lead proteinate inclusions in tubular epithelial cells. Unbound lead is excreted into milk, and it readily passes membrane barriers such as the placenta and the blood-brain barrier to become distributed in many body tissues.[25]

Unbound lead becomes immobilized and bound to bone substance, particularly in the physeal region, by an unknown mechanism. However, bone is considered to be the "sink" for lead and eventually may contain greater than 90% of the total body burden of lead. Deposition of lead into bone is a slow, gradual process, entailing redistribution of lead from other soft tissues. In this manner, bone serves as a detoxification mechanism under conditions of chronic exposure to small concentrations. Bone cannot hold an infinite amount of lead, however, and when saturation occurs, signs of toxicosis may appear suddenly because of rising blood and soft tissue concentrations after continued exposure.[25]

Bile and feces are thought to be the primary pathways of lead excretion, and feces may contain unabsorbed lead and lead that has undergone enterohepatic circulation. Gastrointestinal secretions, including pancreatic secretions, also might be involved in elimination of lead from the body.[2,25]

The mechanism of action of lead at the cellular level is still under scrutiny. The known toxic effects of lead include inhibition of sulfhydryl groups of enzymes essential to cellular metabolism and inhibition of heme synthesis. Lead also is known to cause a decrease in local concentrations of the essential trace metals copper, iron, and zinc. These metals have important functions in mitochondrial enzymes, and interference by lead with these may adversely affect cellular respiration, oxidative phosphorylation, and the ATP synthetase complex.[25]

The peripheral neuropathy associated with lead toxicosis in horses is thought to be caused by peripheral nerve segmental demyelination, which impedes nerve impulse conduction and contributes to the clinical signs observed. The metabolic inhibitory effects of lead are speculated to cause the demyelination.[25,27]

Lead is known to damage the blood-brain barrier and capillary endothelial cells, resulting in cerebral edema and hemorrhage. Additionally, the damaged blood-brain barrier may allow cytotoxic solutes normally excluded from the brain to enter the brain substance.[25] Whether these mechanisms have any appreciable effect on the development of clinical signs observed in the horse is unknown.

Inhibition of heme synthesis is an important aspect of lead toxicosis in several animal species. This pathologic mechanism also occurs in the horse, but its significance to the overall disease course is limited. The result of heme metabolism interference and altered function of other erythrocyte proteins is a shortened erythrocyte half-life that can produce a normochromic, normocytic anemia, which is generally marginal in affected horses (PCV of 25% to 30%).[27,28] The anemia also may be accompanied by nucleated red blood cells and Howell-Jolly bodies in peripheral blood.[28]

Two enzymes in the heme synthesis pathway that are particularly susceptible to lead are δ-aminolevulinic acid dehydratase (ALA dehydratase) and ferrochelatase. Inhibition of ALA dehydratase results in reduced levels of porphobilinogen in erythrocytes and an accumulation of ALA dehydratase, which is excreted in urine. Interference with ALA dehydratase also may be partly responsible for brain damage associated with lead toxicity in some species. Inhibition of ferrochelatase limits the formation of heme from protoporphyrin, resulting in an accumulation of unmetabolized porphyrins. These include protoporphyrin I, which is retained in the erythrocyte; uroporphyrins, which are excreted in urine; and coproporphyrins, which are excreted in feces. Lead also interferes with pyrimidine-specific 5′-nucleotidase activity, resulting in basophilic stippling of affected erythrocytes.[2]

Another important implication of lead toxicity is the suggestion that lead may be immunosuppressive by way of its interference with humoral and cell-mediated immune responses.[2,25]

DIAGNOSIS AND TREATMENT

Confirmation of suspected lead poisoning often is based on determination of blood or tissue lead concentrations. Blood levels of 0.30 ppm or greater are diagnostic if horses are showing clinical signs, but blood lead concentrations do not reflect the severity of poisoning.[27,28] Lead concentrations greater than 5 ppm in liver and kidney and 30 ppm in bone are considered diagnostic of lead intoxication in horses.[25]

In instances of chronic toxicity, however, blood lead values may be within the normal reference range. In such instances diagnosis of toxicity may be aided by administration of calcium disodium EDTA, which chelates lead in bone stores and increases the lead concentration in blood. The soluble lead complexes then are excreted in urine, with a resultant manyfold increase in urinary lead concentration within a few hours of EDTA administration.[2,25,26] The recommended dose of calcium disodium EDTA is 75 mg/kg intravenously.[2]

Clinicopathologic aberrations include increased concentrations of erythrocyte ALA and erythrocyte porphyrins and decreased activity of erythrocyte ALA dehydratase. Increased amounts of coproporphyrins, uroporphyrins, and aminolevulinic acid are found in urine, but measurement of erythrocytic ALA dehydratase is considered more diagnostic than measurement of urinary ALA dehydratase content.[2,25,27] Increased blood concentration of zinc protoporphyrin also has been documented in an affected horse.[29] These analyses generally are not routinely run by veterinary diagnostic laboratories.

Hematologic abnormalities in affected horses include a marginal anemia frequently accompanied by metarubricytes and Howell-Jolly bodies in peripheral blood.[2,28] Anisocytosis, poikilocytosis, hypochromasia, polychromasia, and basophilic stippling also can occur. These changes are suggestive but not pathognomonic of lead toxicity in horses.[2] One also can measure the concentration of lead in soil and in forages. Poisoning in horses has been reported when grazed forage contains lead levels in excess of 300 ppm.[2,27]

Treatment of affected horses should include immediate elimination of the lead source, if possible, and prompt initiation of chelation therapy. Calcium disodium EDTA is the chelator of choice; it chelates osseous lead but not tissue-bound lead. The chelated lead then becomes soluble and is excreted by the kidney. The unsaturated bone stores then re-equilibrate with the lead in soft tissues. Calcium disodium EDTA can be administered by slow intravenous infusion at a dosage of 75 mg per kg of body weight daily for 3 to 5 days. A 2-day nontreatment period may follow to allow re-equilibration of soft tissue and bone and then an additional 5-day treatment regimen if needed. An alternative dosage schedule is 110 mg/kg intravenously twice daily for 2 days. After a 2-day nontreatment period, this same regimen may be repeated. The clinician should base the decision to continue therapy with EDTA on post-treatment blood lead concentrations and renal function tests.[2]

Additional therapy should include fluid and nutritional support. Although thiamine administration has been advocated along with chelation therapy in small animal and ruminant lead toxicosis,[2] its efficacy in treating horses with lead poisoning has not been investigated. Dietary calcium supplementation or sodium-magnesium sulfate, may have some beneficial effect by helping to reduce further gastrointestinal absorption of lead.

Methods aimed at reducing exposure to lead and preventing intoxication include appropriate cutting and disposal of contaminated forage, tilling or burning of the stubble, and addition of lime to the soil.[27] Use of alfalfa as a roughage also might be beneficial, possibly because of the high calcium content in alfalfa, because intoxication is more difficult to produce experimentally in horses when alfalfa is being fed and because increased dietary calcium decreases the gastrointestinal absorption of lead.[2,27]

TOXICOSES CAUSING SIGNS RELATING TO THE CARDIOVASCULAR AND HEMOLYMPHATIC SYSTEMS

Certain plants and ionophores are the most frequently encountered causes of cardiac problems in horses. Manifestations associated with hemolysis and anemia also are possible.

PLANTS

Oleander (*Nerium oleander*)

CLINICAL SIGNS

According to most research, sudden death is the most common sign attributed to oleander poisoning. Some reports suggest that affected horses exhibit lethargy, inappetence, and occasional signs of abdominal pain.[1,2] Profuse, watery, catarrhal, or bloody diarrhea also may occur within a few hours of ingestion.[3] Cardiac irregularities, including alternating bradycardia and tachycardia, may be accompanied by a variety of arrhythmias.[3,4] The extremities of the horse may feel cold to the touch, and mucous membranes may appear blanched. Profuse sweating and muscle twitching are followed by weakness and death. Death may occur less than 12 hours after ingestion.

The green plant apparently is unpalatable to horses. Most toxicities occur when leaves have been incorporated into lawn clippings and offered to horses. Drying does not affect the toxicity of the leaves; therefore leaves incorporated into hay also may be toxic. According to reports, 0.005% of an animal's body weight of green oleander is lethal.[1]

PATHOPHYSIOLOGY

Common oleander contains at least five cardiac glycosides that are found in all parts of the plant.[1,3,5] These glycosides (i.e., oleandrin, digitoxigenin, neriin, folinerin, rosagenin) inhibit the Na^+,K^+ -ATPase (adenosine triphosphatase) system, resulting in hyperkalemia, conduction abnormalities, and ventricular arrhythmias. Which glycosides or metabolites cause specific abnormalities is unclear because of the undefined pharmacokinetics of the individual glycosides.[5]

DIAGNOSIS AND TREATMENT

Exposure to the plant along with the aforementioned clinical signs should alert the clinician to the possibility of oleander toxicity. The rapidity of onset of clinical signs or the finding of dead animals may preclude any effective treatment. Symptomatic therapy should be initiated in those animals in which toxicosis is suspected. Decontamination measures, such as evacuation of the intestinal tract by laxatives and enemas, may be useful. Atropine and propranolol have been advocated, but they must be used with extreme caution.[3,4] Fluids containing calcium should not be used because they may augment the effects of the glycoside on the myocardium.[1]

White Snakeroot (*Eupatorium rugosum*) and Rayless Goldenrod (*Isocoma wrightii*)

Cases of white snakeroot intoxication have been reported primarily in the eastern half of the United States, from Michigan south to Alabama and eastward.[6] The toxic principle is tremetol, which has been described as a fat-soluble, high-molecular-weight alcohol.[7,8] Tremetol poisoning is reported to be most prevalent in dry years or in circumstances in which animals are subjected to inadequate pasturage. The toxin is excreted slowly and therefore tends to accumulate in animals grazing the plant. Because of this cumulative effect, repeated small doses can result in toxicosis as well as a single, larger exposure to the plant. A total amount of green plant varying between 1% to 10% of body weight may be lethal to horses.[6] The toxic principle remains in the dried plant after freezing.[8] In the southwestern United States, rayless goldenrod is the source of tremetol, and ingestion of this plant produces the same clinical syndrome as that of white snakeroot intoxication.

CLINICAL SIGNS

Depression; a stiff gait with frequent crossing of the hindlimbs; and patchy, profuse sweating seem to be the most profound signs of tremetol toxicity. Other, less frequently noted findings include muscle tremors, particularly of the shoulders and limbs; labored or shallow respirations; normal to subnormal body temperature; pupillary dilation; cardiac arrhythmias; and darkly discolored urine.[6,8]

The time of onset of signs varies considerably, from less than 2 days to as long as 3 weeks after the last exposure to the plant. Most horses showing clinical signs die. Recovery is reported to be rare and usually is prolonged and often incomplete. However, a recent report describes two horses that apparently fully recovered from suspected tremetol toxicity.[8] Death often follows within 1 to 3 days of the appearance of clinical signs.[6]

Routinely noted laboratory abnormalities include hematuria, hemoglobinuria and proteinuria, mild elevations in serum alkaline phosphatase activity, elevated AST concentration, and significant elevation of serum CK activity. Acidosis, hyperglycemia, and glucosuria also have been documented.[6,8]

Postmortem findings primarily consist of mild renal tubular degeneration and necrosis; nonsuppurative colitis; pulmonary congestion; increased amounts of pleural and peritoneal fluid; and moderate to severe centrolobular vacuolar changes in the liver. Other significant findings include pericarditis and extensive, patchy myocardial degeneration and necrosis. Extensive, minute epicardial hemorrhage also has been reported.[6,8] One reported case also exhibited moderate, multifocal degeneration of skeletal muscle.[6]

PATHOPHYSIOLOGY

The mechanism whereby tremetol causes the aforementioned lesions and signs remains unknown.

DIAGNOSIS AND TREATMENT

Diagnosis of tremetol toxicity is based on observation of the described clinical signs and concurrent clinicopathologic abnormalities. Additionally, evidence that the affected horses have been exposed to either plant should be present, and, when available, necropsy findings should be compatible with those described for tremetol toxicity. Analysis for tremetol from suspect samples is not readily available.[6]

Treatment is symptomatic. The primary goal of therapy is promptly removing the horse from exposure to the plants and providing supportive care. The clinician should attempt to evacuate the horse's gastrointestinal tract with laxatives such as mineral oil. Activated charcoal also has been suggested as being beneficial in removing the toxin.[8] Based on observed histopathologic abnormalities, volume diuresis of affected animals seems appropriate, and the clinician should attempt to maintain normal acid-base and serum electrolyte concentrations. All affected horses and herdmates should receive adequate and suitable forage and ample fresh water.

Maple (*Acer* spp.)

Several species of maple have been documented as causing hemolysis in horses; however, because of its widespread distribution, red maple is the most commonly identified species. All maples should be considered a potential risk to equines. Intoxication of the horse by leaves of the red maple tree is a seasonal disorder that occurs during the summer and fall months, primarily in the eastern United States.[9,10] Fresh leaves appear to present no problem to the horse, but wilted or dried leaves are toxic, and overnight freezing and storage of dried leaves for 30 days does not alter their toxicity.[11] Experimentally, dried leaves are toxic when administered at a dose of 1.5 mg per kg of body weight.[10,11] The toxin present in red maple leaves is unknown, but the clinical syndrome produced is one of acute hemolytic anemia with methemoglobinemia and Heinz body production.[9-12] Red maple toxicity has been recognized in horses[12] and Grevy's zebras,[13] and horses electively ingest the leaves when other suitable forage is available. Donkeys and mules should be considered potentially susceptible to maple's toxic effects.

CLINICAL SIGNS

Signs of toxicity generally commence within 48 hours of ingestion. Affected horses show acute onset of lethargy, anorexia, weakness, and depression. Increased heart and respiratory rates are typical, and the animals are afebrile. Two outstanding characteristics of most affected horses are the obvious presence of icteric, pale, or brown mucous membranes and a brownish discoloration of blood and urine. Many horses appear cyanotic, and petechiae on mucous membranes have been reported. Signs of secondary acute renal failure also have been documented.[12] Death, when it occurs, generally happens 3 to 7 days after ingestion.[9-12] The mortality rate in naturally occurring and experimental cases is approximately 60%.[14]

The aforementioned signs are representative of naturally occurring instances of toxicity. In an experimental study, however, two patterns of toxicity were recognized. One group of ponies given dried leaves accumulated before September 15 exhibited signs of the typical hemolytic syndrome and died 3 to 5 days later. Ponies given leaves collected after September 15 died within 18 hours of dosing and exhibited clinical signs only of cyanosis and depression.[11] The reason for this disparity of signs was not offered.

PATHOPHYSIOLOGY

Although the toxin in wilted or dried red maple leaves has not been well characterized, it produces an acute hemolytic anemia with methemoglobinemia and Heinz body production in affected horses. The mechanism of erythrocyte damage has not been determined, but these hematologic abnormalities are characteristic of an oxidant.[10-12]

Heinz bodies are intracellular precipitates of oxidized hemoglobin that result from oxidant injury to erythrocytes. They damage the erythrocyte membrane and produce intravascular and extravascular hemolysis. Intravascular hemolysis results when erythrocyte membrane functions involving active and passive ion transport become impaired. The hyperpermeability changes that then occur alter the osmotic gradient of the erythrocyte and cause rupture of the affected red blood cell. Extravascular hemolysis occurs when the red blood cell remains intact, but the damaged erythrocyte is removed from circulation by cells of the reticuloendothelial system.[9,10,12]

Methemoglobin is formed when hemoglobin is oxidized from the ferrous to the ferric form of iron. A certain amount of direct oxidation of hemoglobin to methemoglobin occurs naturally, but erythrocytes are able to reduce methemoglobin back to hemoglobin. Excessive production of methemoglobin occurs under conditions of excessive oxidative stress or when methemoglobin reduction is impaired.[9,11] Although methemoglobin itself does not produce hemolysis, it is incapable of transporting oxygen and therefore contributes to hypoxia. When present in sufficient quantities, methemoglobin imparts a brown discoloration to peripheral blood and mucous membranes.

DIAGNOSIS AND TREATMENT

Maple leaf toxicosis occurs under rather specific conditions but is characterized by an acute onset of hemolytic anemia with methemoglobinemia and Heinz body production. The typical clinical signs and conditions supporting maple leaf intoxication should be in evidence before making a diagnosis. Because the toxic principle is yet unidentified, no specific assay of feed or tissue specimens is available.

Hematologic abnormalities noted in affected horses include moderate to severe anemia (PCV often <10% in severely affected horses), hemoglobinemia, methemoglobinemia, Heinz bodies, anisocytosis, hyperbilirubinemia, and increased erythrocyte fragility. Blood chemistry analysis may reveal depletion of erythrocyte-reduced glutathione and increased serum concentrations of LDH, creatine phosphokinase, AST, and sorbitol dehydrogenase.[9-12] Transient hypercalcemia has been recorded in some horses,[9] and increases in BUN and creatinine concentrations are expected in horses undergoing significant renal insult secondary to hemolysis.[12] Urine analysis may indicate varying degrees of hemoglobinuria, hematuria, bilirubinuria, and proteinuria.[9-11]

Treatment of affected horses is primarily symptomatic. Exposure to red maple leaves should be eliminated immediately, and affected horses should be kept in a quiet, calm environment. Oxygen therapy may be beneficial in selected cases, and blood transfusions can be administered to severely affected individuals.

Balanced, polyionic fluid administration is important to maintain renal function and to aid in diuresis because affected horses may be at great risk of developing hemoglobin nephrosis and acute renal failure. Blood electrolyte and acid-base parameters should be monitored and abnormalities corrected as needed. Acute renal failure should be treated appropriately if it develops.

Other symptomatic therapies that have been suggested include nasogastric intubation with activated charcoal to aid in binding toxin; dexamethasone to aid in stabilizing red blood cell membranes and decrease phagocytosis of damaged red blood cells; and ascorbic acid (30 mg/kg) given in intravenous fluids twice daily, which may reduce oxidative damage to red blood cells. Whether dexamethasone increases the risk of laminitis in affected horses is unknown, and the efficacy of ascorbic acid is questionable.[14]

Prevention of the disease is accomplished by preventing exposure of horses to dried maple leaves.

ONION (*ALLIUM* SPP.)

Onion toxicosis in horses is a rare event and occurs when horses are fed large amounts of culled onions (from commercial onion farms) or are forced to eat wild onions because of inadequate available forage. Horses appear to avoid these plants when suitable forage is available.[15,16] The toxic principles in onions, n-propyl disulfide and sulfoxide, affect only circulating erythrocytes and cause oxidant injury to the red blood cell, with resultant Heinz body formation and subsequent hemolytic anemia. Severely affected horses succumb to onion toxicosis because of severe anemia or secondary renal failure caused by hemoglobin nephropathy.

The clinical signs, laboratory values and pathogenesis of the anemia are all similar to those of maple leaf toxicosis, with the exception that methemoglobin formation does not seem to be nearly as pronounced in onion toxicity as in the former. The carcasses of horses that die as a result of onion toxicosis may have an onion odor at necropsy.[15]

Affected horses may recover from onion toxicity if they are removed from the onion source soon enough and if anemia is not severe. Treatment is largely symptomatic and should include removal of the onion source and provision of adequate, suitable forage. Hematinics are of little value, but oxygen therapy and blood transfusions may be indicated in more severely affected animals.

Maintenance of renal function is of primary concern because affected horses are at risk of developing secondary hemoglobin nephropathy. The clinician should give balanced, polyionic fluids to promote diuresis and should correct electrolyte and acid-base abnormalities. Diuretics should be used with caution, but they may be of value in the volume-loaded horse.

MISCELLANEOUS AGENTS

COUMARIN DERIVATIVES

Coumarin normally is present in some species of sweet clover and has no anticoagulant action. However, certain molds present within the plant can convert coumarin to dicoumarol; hence the term *moldy sweet clover poisoning*. Dicoumarol also has been detected in sweet vernal grass. Coumarin derivatives are used widely as anticoagulants, with bishydroxycoumarin (dicoumarol) and 3-(α-acetonylbenzyl)-4-hydroxycoumarin (warfarin sodium) being the first oral anticoagulants developed from coumarin.[7] These first-generation compounds are used therapeutically as anticoagulants and as rodenticides. There are currently 11 anticoagulants on the market, representing both first- and second-generation compounds. In horses warfarin has been used therapeutically to treat thrombotic disorders such as thrombophlebitis and navicular disease.[17,18] Horses may exhibit signs of toxicity while being medicated with warfarin if a therapeutic concentration is exceeded. Rarely are horses exposed to anticoagulants used as rodenticides around buildings or feed storage areas. Second-generation anticoagulant rodenticides (e.g., brodifacoum and bromadiolone) have been developed because of acquired rodent resistance to the first-generation compounds. Because no indications exist for human or veterinary medicinal use of brodifacoum, toxicity associated with this compound is caused by accidental ingestion.[19]

CLINICAL SIGNS

The clinical signs of toxicity noted with anticoagulants are largely those of a hemorrhagic diathesis. Onset of signs usually is acute and may include hematoma formation, epistaxis, anemia, weakness, pale mucous membranes, or ecchymoses of mucous membranes. Hematuria and melena can occur, and hemorrhage into various body compartments may result in secondary signs caused by malfunction of the involved organ or tissue. Occasionally, affected animals are found dead.[20] Multiple fractional doses of first-generation compounds given over several days may be more toxic to horses than a single larger dose.[17] Brodifacoum, however, differs from warfarin in that a single oral dose has the potential of causing illness and may even be lethal (estimated LD_{50} of 1 to 2 kg per adult horse).[19,21]

The onset of clinical signs is delayed from the time of ingestion. In an experimental model the hypothrombogenic effect of warfarin anticoagulation was noticed 60 hours after an acute dose.[22] This effect persisted for approximately 30 hours. The effect of brodifacoum, however, is much longer and may persist for weeks, despite its half-life of 1.22 days.[19] In an experimental study horses given a single dose of brodifacoum (0.125 mg/kg body mass) showed increased partial thromboplastin time (PTT) at 24 hours and one-stage prothrombin time (PT) at 48 hours after exposure. These values returned to pretreatment levels by day 12. However, two horses required 23 days for clotting times to return to normal. In these horses peak plasma concentration of brodifacoum occurred 2 to 3 hours after oral administration. Additionally, four of the six experimental horses showed clinical signs of depression, anorexia, and weight loss.[21]

PATHOPHYSIOLOGY

Warfarin is absorbed readily from the gastrointestinal tract but also may be administered intravenously for therapeutic purposes.[7,17] Once absorbed, warfarin is highly bound (>90%) to plasma proteins, and some is stored in the liver.[7,17,22] The degree of anticoagulant protein binding in horses is not known but may be similar.[19] Warfarin is hydroxylated by hepatic enzymes to inactive compounds that are eliminated by the kidney. The metabolites have no anticoagulant effect,[7] and the biologic half-life of warfarin in the horse is approximately 13 hours.[22] Coumarins also cross the placenta and are secreted in milk.[7]

Protein binding of warfarin is reversible, and the protein-bound, pharmacologically inactive warfarin serves as a reservoir. The unbound portion remains fairly constant in plasma.[7,17]

A number of factors can influence the amount of unbound free warfarin in serum. Protein-bound drugs such as phenylbutazone, chloral hydrate, and sulfonamides may enhance the toxicity of warfarin by displacing warfarin from protein-binding sites. This allows a greater proportion of the drug to be in the free form and thus able to exert its pharmacologic effect.[7,20] Corticosteroids and thyroxine may lower the therapeutic dose of warfarin by increasing clotting factor catabolism and receptor site affinity.[17]

Certain physiologic factors also may enhance the toxicity of warfarin. Hypoalbuminemia may result in fewer binding sites available, thereby increasing the amount of free drug. Hepatic dysfunction may impede metabolism of the anticoagulants, and reduced amounts of vitamin K in the diet may predispose to toxicity.[7]

Some drugs reduce the therapeutic response to a given dose of warfarin. Barbiturates, rifampin, and chloramphenicol induce hepatic microsomal enzyme activity, thereby accelerating the metabolism of warfarin. If these drugs are withdrawn during warfarin therapy, toxicosis may result.[7,17] Likewise, excessive dietary intake of vitamin K or vitamin K administration can reduce or inhibit the anticoagulant effects of warfarin.[17]

Warfarin acts as an anticoagulant by inhibiting production of the vitamin K–dependent clotting factors II, VII, IX, and X. Vitamin K is a cofactor in the synthesis of clotting factors II, VII, IX, and X and also acts on all clotting factor precursors to convert glutamyl residues to γ-carboxyglutamyl residues. During this carboxylation process vitamin K_1 is converted to vitamin K_1 2,3- epoxide, an inactive metabolite. This epoxide returns to active vitamin K_1 by the action of the microsomal enzyme vitamin K_1 epoxide reductase. The coumarin anticoagulants inhibit vitamin K_1 epoxide reductase, thereby creating a vitamin K_1 deficiency. The result is decreased production and subsequent deficiency of the vitamin K–dependent clotting factors.[5] The delayed onset of action of the coumarin derivative anticoagulants results from this impediment to clotting factor synthesis rather than from a direct effect on the clotting mechanism per se.

The various blood clotting factors have different plasma half-lives. Factor VII has a shorter half-life than the other clotting factors, so the earliest laboratory indication of anticoagulant toxicity is a prolonged PT. As the other clotting factors become depleted, activated PTT also increases as toxicity continues.[17] The clinician should monitor horses given warfarin therapeutically for clotting abnormalities. Prolongation of PT by 1.5 to 2 times the baseline value has been suggested as the effective range of anticoagulation. However, some horses maintained in this range may show signs of hemorrhage.[18] In fact, reports in horses suggest that factor IX may be depleted from circulation more rapidly than factor VII, indicating that the PTT would be the more sensitive clotting assay to assess in horses after exposure to anticoagulants.[19]

DIAGNOSIS AND TREATMENT

The diagnosis of warfarin or other coumarin-derivative anticoagulant intoxication is based on evidence of exposure to the compound, presence of a bleeding diathesis, and prolongation of PTT and PT. The platelet count, fibrinogen concentration, fibrin degradation product concentration, and antithrombin III activity remain within their respective normal ranges of activity.[17,18] However, in dogs exposed to toxic doses of anticoagulant rodenticides, fibrinogen and fibrinogen degradation products (FDPs) have been found to be elevated 50% of the time.

Blood, liver, stomach and intestinal contents, and feces can be submitted for analytic testing for the anticoagulant residues. Specimens should be frozen for transportation to the laboratory.[20,22]

In horses intoxicated by warfarin, discontinuance of warfarin therapy or removal of the product from the environment is of primary importance. Mineral oil may be used to enhance fecal excretion of any orally ingested warfarin products. Vitamin K_1 should be given at a dosage of 300 to 500 mg subcutaneously every 4 to 6 hours until PTT and PT return to their baseline values (5 to 7 days is generally sufficient). PTT and PT should be monitored daily for 3 to 4 days thereafter to ensure stability. The subcutaneous route of vitamin K_1 administration is preferable because of the possibility of adverse reactions if the product is given intravenously or intramuscularly. Intravenous injection of vitamin K_1 may result in transient restlessness, tachypnea, tachycardia, sweating, and anaphylactic reactions.[23,24] Intramuscular administration of vitamin K_1 results in erratic response times and therefore may be inappropriate for a hemorrhaging patient.[23] Alternative doses for vitamin K_1 administration are 0.3 to 0.5 mg/kg intravenously, and a dosage of greater than 0.5 mg/kg intravenously has been suggested to inhibit coumarin activity for several days.[17] If the intravenous route is chosen, vitamin K_1 should be diluted in 5% dextrose or saline and administered slowly.[20]

In horses intoxicated with long-acting anticoagulant rodenticides, treatment with vitamin K_1 may be required for 2 to 4 weeks or until coagulation status is normal 2 to 3 days after the last dose of vitamin K_1. Affected horses were given vitamin K_1 (2.5 mg/kg) subcutaneously every 12 hours for 36 hours and then orally twice daily for the duration of treatment.[19]

If bleeding is serious, fresh blood or fresh plasma given intravenously may be necessary to control hemorrhage and help correct hypovolemia. Other supportive measures such as bandaging and keeping the animal in a quiet environment may be helpful. Alfalfa hay added to the diet may provide a natural source of vitamin K_1.[19] Organ dysfunction induced by hemorrhage and hypoxia should be treated appropriately. The prognosis for horses intoxicated with anticoagulant compounds is good if the disorder is recognized early and appropriate therapy is instituted. For symptomatic patients the prognosis is highly dependent on the severity, site, and extent of blood loss.

To prevent warfarin toxicosis, the clinician should strive to minimize exposure to the product and carefully monitor the therapeutic use of the drug in the horse. Contraindications to its use include any clinical or laboratory suggestion of hepatic disease, hypoproteinemia, or other condition that might increase the risk of toxicity. The practitioner should evalute the concurrent use of other medications, because they may affect the potential for toxicosis to develop, and re-evaluate the dosage of warfarin administered if other concurrent medications are changed. Additionally, the potential for traumatic injury in horses undergoing warfarin therapy should be minimized.

Dimethyl Sulfoxide

Dimethyl sulfoxide, a by-product of the papermaking industry, is a colorless liquid originally used as an industrial solvent. The chemical is a polar compound that readily mixes with ethyl alcohol and many organic solvents; it is extremely hygroscopic and can absorb more than 70% of its weight of water from air. DMSO possesses some antimicrobial and antifungal activity, but its primary medical use has been as an anti-inflammatory agent and a transdermal transport agent.[25] More recently, DMSO has been used as a diuretic and has shown promising results when used to treat acute cranial and spinal cord trauma.[25,26]

The systemic toxicity of DMSO is considered to be low, and its greatest toxic potential appears to result from its combination with other agents.[27] However, in an experimental study rapid infusion of DMSO in 20% and 40% concentrations caused hemolysis, hemoglobinuria, diarrhea, muscle tremors, and signs of colic in some horses.[28] The LD_{50} of DMSO has not been established for horses, but ranges between 2.5 to 9.0 g/kg as a single intravenous dose have been reported in a number of animal species.[27] A dose of 1 g/kg intravenously has been suggested for use in horses. This dose should be diluted to a 10% to 20% solution and administered slowly intravenously.[26,27]

DMSO produces hemolysis when given intravenously in concentrations of 20% to 50% or greater.[25-27] If hemolysis is severe, affected horses may be at increased risk of developing hemoglobin nephrosis. Concentrations of 10% or less are considered suitable for intravenous injection in horses.[25,26,28] Additionally, increased white blood cell adherence and fibrinogen precipitation have been reported when concentrations greater than 50% were administered.[25]

DMSO is a mild cholinesterase inhibitor, and its concurrent use with organophosphates or other cholinesterase inhibitors is not recommended.[25,27] DMSO also is known to induce histamine release from mast cells, but the significance of this phenomenon is uncertain.[27]

Skin reactions to topically applied DMSO sometimes occur. Varying degrees of erythema, pruritus, drying, hardening, and desquamation of normal skin may be evident. These reactions are usually self-limiting and typically diminish with repeated applications.[27]

The greatest risk of toxicity resulting from DMSO is probably a consequence of its concomitant use with other toxic or potentially toxic agents. DMSO may aid transport of a variety of toxic compounds across skin, thereby inducing toxicosis from the transported agent. For example, mercury toxicity has been reported in a horse that had a blister after DMSO and mercury were applied topically to a leg.[29] In such instances, the clinician should treat the specific toxic reaction (or reactions) appropriately. No specific antidote is recognized for DMSO, and it should always be used judiciously and conscientiously. The practitioner should heed the aforementioned precautions when administering the drug.

Bicarbonate

Sodium bicarbonate is one of the most common alkalizing agents used in animals, including horses. Sodium bicarbonate is indicated specifically to treat acute, severe metabolic acidosis because of its rapid effect on blood pH when given intravenously.[30] Sodium bicarbonate also has been used in performance horses to treat exertional myopathies and in attempts to prevent rhabdomyolysis. More recently, sodium bicarbonate administration in performance horses has been investigated because of its suggested role in limiting or preventing systemic lactic acidosis, thereby enhancing performance level.[31,32] The adverse effects of bicarbonate administration occur when it is given too rapidly or in excessive quantities or when it is given in the presence of certain systemic abnormalities.

CLINICAL SIGNS

Animals, including horses, that suffer from an acute overdose of bicarbonate may exhibit signs of delirium, depression, and coma. Rapidly induced alkalosis also has been associated with cardiac dysrhythmias.[30]

Horses such as endurance horses or racehorses that are volume depleted and have sustained excessive electrolyte loss through sweat often have clinicopathologic changes of hypokalemia, hypochloremia, hypocalcemia, and metabolic alkalosis. When such horses are given bicarbonate, dramatic deleterious effects occur. These animals may exhibit signs of muscle fasciculation, synchronous diaphragmatic flutter, bruxism, and decreased respiratory rate. One also may note clinical evidence of further dehydration, such as increased capillary refill time, delayed jugular distensibility, diminished skin turgor, and decreased arterial pulse.[32]

PATHOPHYSIOLOGY

The rapid administration or overdose of sodium bicarbonate has been associated with extracellular hyperosmolality, intracranial hemorrhage, and cerebrospinal fluid (CSF) acidosis. Hyperosmolality results from hypernatremia because sodium bicarbonate dissociates into sodium ions and bicarbonate ions. An abrupt increase in serum osmolality can lead to intracranial hemorrhage as intracellular water moves into the extracellular space. This extracellular fluid accumulation may result in engorgement of perivascular spaces, with subsequent tearing of bridge veins and resultant hemorrhage. The CSF acidosis results from the rapid diffusion of generated carbon dioxide into the CSF. Carbon dioxide enters the CSF almost instantaneously, establishing new steady-state levels within minutes. Bicarbonate ion, however, is slow to enter the CSF and requires hours to days to achieve new steady-state levels. With sodium bicarbonate administration the increasing amount of carbon dioxide generated readily enters the CSF disproportionately more than does the bicarbonate ion. As a consequence, the CSF becomes acidic.[33] These mechanisms, individually or collectively, are thought to be responsible for development of the clinical signs observed with rapid or excessive administration of sodium bicarbonate solution.

Another effect of alkalosis is a shift to the left of the oxyhemoglobin dissociation curve. This left shift indicates an increased affinity of hemoglobin for oxygen, with a resultant decrease in the amount of oxygen available for cellular use. This change in hemoglobin affinity for oxygen has been associated with cardiac dysrhythmias following rapidly induced alkalosis.[30]

Horses undergoing extensive exercise or horses that are treated with furosemide (primarily as prerace medication for exercise-induced pulmonary hemorrhage) are at risk of developing hypochloremic, hypokalemic metabolic alkalosis. When sodium bicarbonate is given to these volume-depleted horses with electrolyte loss and concurrent metabolic alkalosis, another deleterious series of events can result. Further reduction of the circulating fluid volume may occur, along with development of serum hyperosmolality, electrolyte abnormalities of hypernatremia, hypokalemia, hypochloremia, and hypocalcemia and further development of metabolic alkalosis.[32]

Excessive sodium bicarbonate produces hyperosmolality caused by hypernatremia because sodium bicarbonate dissociates into sodium and bicarbonate ions. The hypokalemia is explained partially by the intracellular shift of potassium in response to metabolic alkalosis, and the bicarbonate ion adds to the alkalosis already present. Furosemide administration causes urinary loss of potassium, chloride, and calcium, and sweating also can result in significant loss of chloride and calcium. Additionally, rapid intravenous infusion of 5% sodium bicarbonate in normal horses results in hypochloremia.[34]

The muscle fasciculations and diaphragmatic flutter noted in some horses likely result from hypocalcemia.[32] The total serum calcium concentration may be within a normal range, but alkalosis causes a reduction in the amount of circulating ionized calcium. Because ionized calcium is responsible for neuromuscular function, reduction in this fraction can cause clinical signs of hypocalcemia.

DIAGNOSIS AND TREATMENT

Horses being treated with sodium bicarbonate solutions should be monitored closely for clinical signs of alkalosis. Blood pH obviously is elevated, but rapid infusion of sodium bicarbonate or excessive use in horses already sustaining fluid and electrolyte loss can result in a number of clinicopathologic alterations. Affected horses typically exhibit increases in PCV, total serum protein, and serum bicarbonate and sodium concentrations. Additional findings of hypokalemia, hypochloremia, and hypocalcemia usually are present.

Treatment of affected horses involves cessation of bicarbonate administration and correction of the alkalosis and electrolyte abnormalities. Potassium chloride administration is indicated in horses with hypokalemic, hypochloremic metabolic alkalosis and is much more effective in correcting these electrolyte abnormalities than is sodium chloride. Potassium chloride also has been shown to cause a prompt, significant decline in venous blood pH in these horses.[32]

Apparently, hypertonic sodium bicarbonate solutions should not be used in dehydrated horses. The concurrent use of furosemide and sodium bicarbonate also appears to be contraindicated; if this is necessary, they must be used with extreme caution and close observation with laboratory assessment. Sodium bicarbonate should not be mixed with fluids containing calcium because insoluble complexes may form. The use of sodium bicarbonate orally in horses subjected to short-term intense exercise remains controversial.

MONENSIN

Monensin is one of several biologically active compounds categorized as ionophore antibiotics (others include lasalocid, salinomycin, narasin, laidlomycin, maduramycin, and virginiamycin) because they can form lipid-soluble complexes with specific metal cations and transport them across biologic membranes. Monensin is produced by the fungus *Streptomyces cinnamonensis* and is selective in transporting sodium and potassium ions between intracellular and extracellular spaces.[20,35,36] Monensin is used routinely as a poultry coccidiostat and as a feed additive to improve feed efficiency in pasture and feedlot cattle. Horses are the domestic animals most sensitive to monensin toxicosis. The LD_{50} and possibly a single acute toxic dose of monensin for the horse is 1 to 2 mg/kg.[20]

CLINICAL SIGNS

Several syndromes of toxicity occur and seem to be dose related. Peracute toxicity may manifest as progressive, severe hemoconcentration; hypovolemic shock; and death within a few hours of ingestion. The acute form of the disorder is characterized by partial to complete feed aversion, abdominal pain, occasional watery diarrhea, intermittent profuse sweating, stiffness, progressive muscle weakness (especially in the hindquarters), progressive ataxia, tachycardia, hypotension, dyspnea, and polyuria. Affected horses may show clinical signs for 1 to 4 days before death.[36-38] Horses surviving sublethal doses of monensin exhibit signs of reduced athletic performance, unthriftiness, and cardiac failure. Cardiac arrhythmias, including atrial fibrillation and tachycardia; a prominent jugular pulse; and pleural and pericardial effusion are apparent.[20] Intravascular hemolysis also may occur to a limited degree.[35]

PATHOPHYSIOLOGY

The primary action of monensin is the selective transport of sodium and potassium ions between the intracellular and extracellular spaces. Two mechanisms have been suggested to explain the toxic action.

According to one theory, monensin interacts with the mechanism regulating potassium entry into cell organelles, especially the mitochondria.[20] Low concentrations of monensin lead to a net accumulation of potassium within the cell, whereas higher doses cause a net loss of potassium from the cell.[35] Because potassium is required for ATP hydrolysis by the mitochondria, the effect of monensin might be to inhibit ATP hydrolysis in mitochondria. As a result, cell energy production is decreased and can result in loss of cell function and death.[20,35]

The second hypothesis suggests that increased intracellular calcium concentration is the mechanism responsible for cell death. When the intracellular calcium concentration is increased, the mitochondria are forced to maintain calcium homeostasis by sequestering the excess calcium. This requires energy, which could take priority over ATP production. When the mitochondria become overloaded with calcium, oxidative phosphorylation is inhibited and less energy is produced to pump calcium out of the cell. When intracellular calcium levels reach a critical level, degradative enzymes are released, swelling of the mitochondria and sarcoplasmic reticulum occur, and cell necrosis and death follow.[20,35]

The heart is the primary target organ of monensin toxicosis, and electron microscopic studies of acute monensin toxicosis in ponies have shown structural changes in myocardial cells consistent with severe mitochondrial damage.[39] In horses ingesting a sublethal dose of monensin, the myocardial sarcolemma is damaged and is replaced by fibrous tissue in the healing process. Myocardial lesions are characterized microscopically by pale myofibers, loss of fiber striation, multifocal vacuolar degeneration, and scattered areas of necrosis. The result is a structurally weakened heart that can succumb to stress and cause acute collapse of the horse. Other lesions that may be present in affected horses include pericardial, pleural, and peritoneal effusions; hemopericardium; and epicardial hemorrhage. Chronically affected horses also may have hepatic congestion with centrilobular necrosis and hydropic degeneration of the renal tubules.[20,35]

DIAGNOSIS

Monensin toxicosis is suspected when horses show clinical signs of feed refusal, abdominal discomfort, muscle weakness, and heart failure and when a possible exposure to contaminated feed has occurred. The practitioner can evaluate feeds, serum, liver, gastrointestinal content, and feces for the presence of monensin.

Clinicopathologic abnormalities are nonpathognomonic but include early signs of severe hemoconcentration and dehydration in horses affected peracutely. Serum potassium and calcium may be decreased moderately in the first 12 to 16 hours but then tend to come back to normal levels. BUN and creatinine concentrations are elevated in horses acutely affected but return to normal in surviving animals. Other enzymes that show elevated serum activity include CK, AST, and LDH isoenzyme fractions 1 (cardiac muscle) and 2 (red blood cell origin). Total serum bilirubin also may be elevated.[20,35]

Abnormal findings in urine can include a progressive decrease in urine osmolality during the initial few hours of the disease course.[20] One also might expect elevations in urinary activity of renal tubular enzymes such as γ-glutamyl transferase and N-acetylglucosaminidase. Urinalysis abnormalities tend to correlate well with the degree of renal insult and are nonspecific indicators of renal damage.

TREATMENT

No specific antidote exists for monensin. Horses that have ingested a large amount should be treated early and aggressively with polyionic fluids to combat hemoconcentration and hypovolemic shock. Electrolyte and acid-base analysis should be performed, if possible, and any deficiencies corrected. The clinician should attempt to evacuate the bowel of the horse using orally administered laxatives such as mineral oil; activated charcoal may help decrease the absorption of monensin. Affected horses should be kept as quiet and nonstressed as possible for weeks after exposure to allow the damaged myocardium to heal.[20,35] Administration of selenium and vitamin E should be considered; these compounds have been shown to be somewhat protective against the toxic effects of monensin in swine.

Digitalis glycosides should never be used in acutely affected horses because they and monensin have been shown to be synergistic and immediately fatal to cardiac muscle cells. Digitalis glycosides should be used only with great caution in the weeks after recovery from the toxic episode. Likewise, calcium should not be given to acutely affected horses for two reasons. First, serum hypocalcemia is transitory, and serum calcium usually recovers to normal by 24 hours. Second, calcium can be dangerously irritating to an already injured myocardium.[35]

It is important to note that affected horses are susceptible to cardiac damage, which is often permanent. A critical evaluation of cardiac function and the integrity of any previously intoxicated horse that is destined to return to some form of athletic endeavor is judicious.

LASALOCID

Lasalocid, another carboxylic ionophore antibiotic, is a fermentation product of the mold *Streptomyces lasaliensis* that is used commercially as a poultry coccidiostat and as a feed additive to improve feed efficiency in ruminants.

CLINICAL SIGNS

The signs observed in horses given toxic amounts of lasalocid are similar to those of monensin toxicosis. Affected horses exhibit depression, ataxia, paresis, and paralysis with partial to complete feed aversion. Once recumbent, some horses rise when given assistance. Most horses that survive appear normal 2 to 3 days after exposure. The lowest dose that has been reported to cause fatality was 15 mg per kg of body weight, but the LD_{50} for a single oral dose of lasalocid was estimated to be 21.5 mg/kg. Death occurred between 31 and 96 hours after oral dosing in the nonsurvivors.[40]

Results of a toxic feeding study indicated that poultry rations containing approved concentrations of lasalocid (75 to 125 g per metric ton) are not toxic or lethal to horses. This study revealed that horses voluntarily reduced their feed intake with increasing amounts of lasalocid in the ration and refused to eat the commercial premix when it was offered in place of their normal ration.[40]

PATHOPHYSIOLOGY

The mechanism of action of lasalocid is thought to be similar to that of monensin. Lasalocid is the least toxic of the ionophores and differs from monensin in that it accepts divalent as well as monovalent cations.[7]

DIAGNOSIS

No signs or laboratory findings are pathognomonic for lasalocid toxicity. In horses in which it is suspected, feedstuffs, stomach contents, serum, liver, and feces can be analyzed for lasalocid content.

Abnormal laboratory findings in affected horses may include hypocalcemia, hypophosphatemia, and hypokalemia early in the disease course (within 24 hours of exposure), but these values return to normal ranges by 120 hours after ingestion. Serum activity of AST frequently is increased, as is total serum bilirubin and glucose concentrations. Occasionally, the BUN concentration is increased.[40]

TREATMENT

Initial treatment should include removal of all suspected feed sources and the oral administration of laxatives to enhance evacuation of the gastrointestinal tract. Other nonspecific supportive care may be helpful, but horses receiving a sublethal dose probably will recover with minimal assistance. If a lethal dose is forced into an animal inadvertently, oral laxatives and adsorbents such as activated charcoal may help bind lasalocid and reduce the amount absorbed. Administration of selenium and vitamin E before the onset of signs may help alleviate the severity of the clinical signs once they occur.

SALINOMYCIN

Salinomycin is an ionophore, also marketed as a coccidiostat, that is related more closely to monensin than is lasalocid. The ionic affinity of salinomycin is predominantly to sodium and potassium ions, and its mode of action and cellular effects are similar to those of monensin.[7]

In one report of affected horses, the clinical signs were similar to those of the other ionophore toxicoses. The range of clinical signs included partial to complete feed aversion, depression, occasional sweating, colic, dyspnea, weakness, ataxia, and recumbency. Occasionally, horses showed reduced performance for several weeks after exposure, but many horses that became recumbent were destroyed humanely. The clinicopathologic abnormalities exhibited by affected horses included elevated serum activities of CK, AST, and alkaline phosphatase.[41]

The diagnosis of salinomycin toxicity is hampered by the fact that none of the clinical signs are pathognomonic. However, one may assay suspect feed, gastrointestinal content, serum, liver, and feces for the presence and quantity of salinomycin.

Treatment of affected horses is mostly symptomatic because no specific antidote is available. Evacuation of the bowel by laxatives may be helpful in reducing the amount of toxic material available for absorption. Fluid balance and electrolyte and acid-base indices should be maintained within normal ranges. Administration of selenium and vitamin E should be considered. Affected horses generally require an extended convalescence, and the clinician should consider the possibility of a persistent cardiomyopathy.[41] Affected horses should undergo a rigorous cardiac examination before returning to performance events.

NITRATES AND NITRITES

Nitrates are an important component in the naturally occurring nitrogen cycle and as such are present in soils, groundwater, forages, row crops, weeds, animal tissues, and excreta. Nitrates also are used widely in fertilizers. Toxicity problems can arise when animals consume plants, feed, or water containing excessive amounts of nitrates or nitrites or when they ingest nitrate fertilizers. Nitrates naturally undergo microbial decomposition to nitrites, so nitrite toxicity can occur when animals ingest feed or water in which the nitrates have decomposed to yield large amounts of nitrites. This decomposition can occur in moist haystacks, water troughs, farm ponds, silages, and pig swills. Nitrite also is administered intravenously to treat cyanide poisoning, and overzealous use of this therapy can result in toxicity.[7]

The primary exposure to nitrate or nitrite for most animals is the plants they consume. Many plants and forages are known to be nitrate accumulators, and a number of factors influence the uptake of nitrates in plants. Nitrate concentration by plants is enhanced by low soil pH; low soil molybdenum, sulfur, or phosphorus content; low soil temperature; drought; soil aeration; decreased light; and use of phenoxyacetic acid herbicides such as 2,4-dichlorophenoxyacetic acid. Nitrate and nitrite accumulation in ponds and groundwater is caused by water runoff from nitrate-rich soils or by direct contamination with nitrates and nitrites.[7,20] Nitrates and nitrites are water soluble and are carried easily from feedlots, pigpens, and fertilized areas into the soil and subsequently into plants, wells, and ponds.

The most important aspect of nitrates is their ease of microbial conversion to nitrites. Nitrite is responsible for the primary signs associated with toxicity in nitrate poisoning.

CLINICAL SIGNS

Although apparently rare, horses are reported to be susceptible to nitrate intoxication. Experimentally, an oral dose of 1 g/kg potassium nitrate caused illness but not death in horses. However, nitrites have been associated with death of horses under field conditions.

In monogastric animals nitrate ingestion is reported to produce gastrointestinal irritation with resulting emesis or enteritis. Salivation, diarrhea, colic, and frequent urination may be evident if the nitrate is sufficiently concentrated.

Signs of acute poisoning with nitrites usually begin 30 minutes to 4 hours after ingestion of high-nitrite feed or water. The most characteristic signs are those referable to respiratory insufficiency and include dyspnea, cyanosis, rapid and weak pulse, and anxiety. Exertion may exacerbate these signs and induce muscle tremors and collapse. The horse may have terminal clonic convulsions. The blood of affected animals is usually brown or chocolate-colored and this imparts a cyanotic or pale appearance to mucous membranes. Death may occur in several hours or be delayed until 12 to 24 hours after ingestion.[20,7]

PATHOPHYSIOLOGY

Nitrites are absorbed rapidly from the gastrointestinal tract into the bloodstream. The nitrite ion acts directly on vascular smooth muscle to cause relaxation and easily enters erythrocytes in exchange for chloride ion. Nitrite also can pass the placenta to enter fetal erythrocytes, which are especially sensitive to nitrite. The biologic half-life of blood nitrate in horses is 4.8 hours. Only small amounts of nitrate or nitrite are bound to plasma proteins.[7,42]

Nitrite causes acute poisoning by two mechanisms. The primary action of nitrite is to interact with hemoglobin to form methemoglobin. One molecule of nitrite interacts with two molecules of hemoglobin, causing the oxidation of normal ferrous hemoglobin to ferric hemoglobin, which is called *methemoglobin*. Methemoglobin is incapable of transporting oxygen to tissues, and if sufficient quantities are formed, severe oxygen deficiency can occur. Clinical signs become evident when methemoglobin levels approach 30% to 40%, and death occurs when 80% to 90% of hemoglobin is oxidized to methemoglobin.[7,20] However, death can occur in active animals with only 50% to 60% methemoglobin.[7]

Normally, methemoglobin is converted back to ferrous hemoglobin by two reducing enzyme systems. This conversion occurs slowly, and in instances of nitrate toxicity, methemoglobin formation far exceeds the ability of these enzyme systems to regenerate hemoglobin.[7]

The second action of nitrite is to cause direct relaxation of smooth muscle, particularly vascular smooth muscle. The mechanism by which this occurs is unknown, but the physiologic changes brought about by the vasodilating action of nitrite include pulmonary arterial, central venous, and systemic arterial hypotension and decreased cardiac output. These changes may contribute to tissue anoxia and act to enhance tissue oxygen starvation already initiated by methemoglobin.[7]

DIAGNOSIS AND TREATMENT

The diagnosis of nitrate or nitrite toxicity is based on compatible clinical signs; methemoglobinemia; history of exposure to potential nitrate- or nitrite-containing plants, water, or fertilizers; and nitrate quantitation in blood. One should perform blood methemoglobin determinations soon after collection because methemoglobin is not stable in refrigerated, heparinized blood for more than a few hours. However, blood mixed with a phosphate buffer preserves the methemoglobin and allows shipment to a diagnostic laboratory. Forage, hay, and water samples can be analyzed for nitrate or nitrite content, as well as other body fluids such as ocular fluid collected post mortem.[20]

Treatment aims to reduce methemoglobin back to hemoglobin. Mildly affected animals may recover spontaneously if the toxic source is removed and if they are given sufficient time for normal methemoglobin reduction processes to occur. Intravenous methylene blue may be used to treat more severely affected horses at a suggested dosage of 4.4 mg/kg, given slowly as a 1% solution in isotonic saline. The dose may be repeated in 30 minutes if clinical response is unsatisfactory. Caution is necessary, however, because excessive amounts of methylene blue may directly oxidize hemoglobin to methemoglobin. Methylene blue is converted to leukomethylene blue by an $NADPH_2$-dependent system. Leukomethylene then reduces methemoglobin to hemoglobin. In this reaction leukomethylene blue is oxidized back to methylene blue but can be reconverted to leukomethylene blue as long as sufficient $NADPH_2$ is available. If this $NADPH_2$ system becomes saturated with methylene blue, excessive methylene blue may oxidize hemoglobin directly to more methemoglobin.[7] Because methylene blue is difficult to obtain, ascorbic acid has been suggested as a less effective alternative.

Other nonspecific therapies include blood transfusion, oxygen therapy, and laxatives such as mineral oil to aid evacuation of the gastrointestinal tract.[7]

CYANIDE

Hydrogen cyanide, cyanide, hydrocyanic acid, and *prussic acid* are terms that refer to the same toxic substance. Horses become exposed primarily through ingestion of certain plants that contain cyanogenic glycosides, but compounds containing cyanide also have been used as fumigants, rodenticides, and fertilizers.[7,20]

Numerous plants or plant parts may accumulate large quantities of cyanide or cyanogenic glycosides, and a more complete description of them can be found elsewhere.[43] When these cyanogenic glycosides undergo hydrolysis, free HCN is formed. Plant cells contain degradative enzymes that can hydrolyze these glycosides, but under natural conditions the enzymes are kept separated spatially from the glycosides in intact cells. Damage to the plant cells by wilting, freezing, or stunting allows enzymatic degradation of the glycoside.[20] Rapid hydrolysis and release of HCN occur only when the plant cell structure is disrupted. When the glycoside is exposed to an acid medium, or when maceration of the plant occurs within the intestinal tract, hydrolysis and subsequent formation of HCN also occur.

A number of factors can influence the toxic potential of cyanogenic plants. Because plant cyanogenic glycosides and degradative enzymes are controlled genetically by a dominant gene, selectively breeding plants with low cyanogenic potential is possible. Therefore different species and varieties of forage contain varying cyanogenic content. The ability to genetically remove plants with high cyanogenic potential is one reason that plant-related cyanide toxicity is an uncommon event. Sudan and Johnson grass historically have been problematic forages for livestock. High-nitrogen fertilization, nitrogen and phosphorus imbalance in soil, and drought conditions also can influence cyanide potential in plants.[20]

Most of the cyanogenic activity in the plant is located in the leaves and seeds, and immature and rapidly growing plants have the greatest potential for high glycoside levels. Conditions that damage the plant, such as drought, wilting, or freezing, may allow for more rapid combination of glycoside and enzyme, thereby enhancing plant toxicity. Other factors that may affect toxicity are the size of the animal, speed of ingestion, the type of food ingested along with the cyanogen, and the presence of active degradative enzymes in the plant and in the digestive tract of the horse.[20]

CLINICAL SIGNS

Because cyanide is such a potent, rapidly acting poison, affected animals commonly are found dead. On observation clinical signs may range from mild tachypnea and anxiousness to severe panting, gasping, and behavioral excitement.

Salivation, lacrimation, muscle tremors, defecation, urination, and mydriasis may be evident. These signs are followed by prostration, clonic convulsions, and death. The mucous membranes may have a bright red appearance, and blood color may be bright cherry red, although this is not commonly reported in cases. Clinical signs may last from only a few minutes to a few hours, but horses that survive longer than 90 to 120 minutes after exposure usually survive.[4,7,20,43]

PATHOPHYSIOLOGY

HCN is absorbed rapidly from the gastrointestinal tract or from the lungs. After absorption, endogenous thiosulfate combines with the cyanide ion to form thiocyanate, which is relatively harmless. This reaction occurs in the liver and other tissues, and the generated thiocyanate is excreted in urine. Another inherent detoxification mechanism involves inactivation of HCN in the bloodstream by combining with the ferric iron of methemoglobin. However, because a small amount of methemoglobin normally is present in blood and endogenous stores of thiosulfate can be depleted rapidly, these two endogenous mechanisms of detoxification are overcome rapidly in cases of clinical toxicity.[20]

Excessive cyanide ion reacts readily with the trivalent (ferric) iron of cytochrome oxidase to form a stable cyanide–cytochrome oxidase complex. When iron is maintained in the ferric form, electron transport can no longer occur, and the chain of cellular respiration is brought to a halt. As a consequence, hemoglobin is unable to release its oxygen to the electron transport system, and cellular hypoxia results. This action occurs despite a large concentration of oxygen in the bloodstream. Cytochrome oxidase is most concentrated in tissues that have a high oxidative metabolic rate, such as the CNS and cardiac muscle. All tissues can be affected from this lack of usable oxygen, but death primarily is caused by anoxia in the brain.[7,20] The acute oral LD_{50} of HCN is 2 to 2.3 mg/kg, and rapid intake of plant material equivalent to about 4 mg/kg is thought to be a lethal amount.[7]

DIAGNOSIS AND TREATMENT

Cyanide poisoning should be considered when animals consuming cyanogenic plants are affected with acute signs of oxygen starvation and bright red blood. The presence of cyanide is confirmed chemically, and samples of forage, blood, liver, muscle, brain, and heart may be submitted. All samples should be frozen as soon as possible and shipped.[7,20] Plant materials containing greater than 200 ppm HCN and concentrations in brain and ventricular myocardium greater than 100 mg/100 g wet weight are considered significant.[7]

Treatment aims at splitting the cyanide–cytochrome oxidase complex, with subsequent removal of the cyanide complex, and augmenting available thiosulfate in the bloodstream. Sodium nitrite displaces the cyanide molecule from the cytochrome enzyme and changes some of the hemoglobin to methemoglobin, which then competes with cytochrome oxidase for the cyanide ion. In this process methemoglobin and the cyanide ion form cyanomethemoglobin, and cytochrome oxidase subsequently is regenerated. Sodium nitrite should be used cautiously because of the possible danger of producing nitrite toxicosis, but it can be administered intravenously at dosages ranging from 6 mg/kg, given as a 20% solution,[44] to 15 to 25 mg/kg.[7]

Sodium thiosulfate reacts with the cyanide ion in the blood or liberated from cyanomethemoglobin and forms thiocyanate, which is essentially harmless and is excreted in urine. Sodium thiosulfate also can be given intravenously at dosages ranging from 60 to 660 mg/kg, as a 20% solution,[4] to 1.25 g/kg. Sodium nitrite and thiosulfate are not easy to obtain; thus these compounds rarely are used to treat clinically affected animals. In small animals a commercially available kit containing a vitamin B_{12} precursor, hydroxocobalamin, is currently recommended. An additional recommended therapy includes large doses of mineral oil. The cobalt in the vitamin B_{12} preparation may bind additional cyanide in the circulation, and mineral oil aids evacuation of the gastrointestinal tract. Animals that survive 24 hours usually do not require further treatment.[7]

Sodium Fluoroacetate (1080)

Sodium fluoroacetate and fluoroacetamide are highly toxic to many animal species. They have been used as rodenticides and in predator control, and because of their toxicity, their use in the United States is highly restricted. The compounds are odorless, tasteless, and water soluble and typically are incorporated into baits composed of carrot chunks, bread, bran, or meats. In the United States these compounds often are mixed with a dye before being placed in baits. Horses may become intoxicated by inadvertent exposure to these baits.[7,20]

CLINICAL SIGNS

Sodium fluoroacetate causes signs primarily related to cardiac dysfunction in herbivores. The onset of signs usually occurs from 30 minutes to 2 hours after ingestion. When signs begin, they usually have an acute onset and follow a rapid, usually violent course. Significant cardiac arrhythmias with rapid, weak pulse and eventual ventricular fibrillation are typical findings. Horses may exhibit staggering, trembling, restlessness, urination, and defecation. Moaning and bruxism may occur along with profuse sweating and signs of colic. Terminal convulsions also may occur. Ventricular fibrillation is the cause of death, and some horses may be found dead with no outward signs of struggle.[7,20]

PATHOPHYSIOLOGY

Fluoroacetate is absorbed readily from the gastrointestinal tract, lungs, or open wounds but not through intact skin. After absorption, fluoroacetate is distributed throughout the body and does not accumulate in any specific tissue. The acute oral LD_{50} of fluoroacetate in horses is 0.35 to 0.55 mg/kg.[7]

After entry into cells, fluoroacetate can replace acetyl coenzyme A, combining with oxaloacetate to form fluorocitrate. Fluorocitrate then competes with citrate for the active site of aconitase, a Krebs cycle enzyme, and also inhibits succinate dehydrogenase, which catalyzes succinate metabolism. The inhibition of these two enzymes and the subsequent accumulation of citrate block the Krebs cycle, leading to decreased glucose metabolism, energy stores, and cellular respiration. These actions occur in all cells, but organs with high metabolic rates (e.g., brain, gastrointestinal tract, and heart) are affected most severely.[5,7,20]

The short latent period between ingestion and onset of signs occurs because fluoroacetate must be converted to the more toxic fluorocitrate. The accumulation of toxic levels of fluorocitrate therefore requires some time.[20]

DIAGNOSIS AND TREATMENT

Diagnosis of fluoroacetate toxicity must rely heavily on history of potential exposure, compatible clinical signs, and absence of other pathologic findings. Laboratory detection of these compounds can be difficult, but suspect baits, stomach contents, liver, kidney, and urine are the best samples to submit for evaluation.[7,20] Significantly increased kidney citrate levels suggest 1080 toxicity.[7]

Laboratory abnormalities in affected animals might include hyperglycemia and lactic acidemia.[20] However, these findings are inconclusive and accompany many disease states in the horse.

Therapy is largely supportive and apparently unrewarding in horses already showing signs of toxicity. The practitioner may attempt intestinal decontamination using orally administered mineral oil and activated charcoal. If hypocalcemia develops, calcium gluconate or calcium chloride may be administered. Glycerol monoacetate at 0.1 to 0.5 mg/kg, administered intramuscularly with treatments repeated hourly, has been suggested but may not be effective after onset of clinical signs.[4,20]

TOXICOSES CAUSING SIGNS RELATING TO THE EPITHELIUM, SKELETAL SYSTEM, AND GENERAL BODY CONDITION

Toxicoses causing these clinical signs can be among the most difficult to diagnose. Signs often are mild or moderate and quite nonspecific. In some cases the history is nonspecific, and the possibility of exposure to a toxin is difficult to evaluate.

PLANTS

Black Walnut (*Juglans nigra*)

Ingestion of shavings and aqueous extracts from black walnut trees is responsible for a toxic syndrome in horses characterized by acute onset of laminitis and variable degrees of limb edema.[1-3]

CLINICAL SIGNS

Horses begin showing signs of toxicity within 10 to 12 hours of being bedded with black walnut shavings. The primary signs are those of laminitis and include reluctance to move, shifting weight from limb to limb, increased digital pulse and temperature of the hoof, and positive response to hoof testers. The laminitis may vary from mild to severe.[1-3] Another characteristic finding is that of limb edema, which can become pronounced. Additional signs noted may include increased respiratory rate with flared nostrils, anorexia and lethargy, and abdominal pain.[2] Horses removed from the bedding after clinical signs have developed have a good prognosis for full recovery.[1,2]

PATHOPHYSIOLOGY

The toxic principle involved in this toxicosis is unidentified. Juglone, a naphthoquinone found in roots, bark, and nuts of black walnut trees, was suggested in the past to be the causative agent.[1-3] Further work has shown, however, that an aqueous soluble toxin other than juglone that is found in the heartwood is more likely to be responsible for generation of clinical signs.[3] The mechanism of action of this soluble toxin has not been elucidated fully, but it has been shown to reversibly enhance vasoconstriction of isolated digital vessels in vitro induced by administration of epinephrine potentiated with hydrocortisone.[4]

DIAGNOSIS AND TREATMENT

Diagnosis of black walnut–induced laminitis is based primarily on known exposure to shavings containing the plant and subsequent development of clinical signs. The treatment of laminitis is covered elsewhere in this text, but horses have a good prognosis for recovery if they are removed from the offending bedding. Black walnut shavings should not be used as bedding for horses.

Wild Jasmine (*Cestrum diurnum*)

Cestrum diurnum (wild jasmine, day cestrum, day-blooming jessamine, king-of-the-day, Chinese inkberry) is a tropical to subtropical plant native to the West Indies that has been introduced and cultivated widely as an ornamental in warmer parts of the United States, including Florida, Texas, and southern California. The plant grows rapidly from seeds, and birds may contribute to its spread because of their appetite for ripe berries that contain seeds. The plant is naturalized in Hawaii and India. It also tends to multiply along fence rows, on roadsides, and in neglected pastures and fields. Horses show signs of disease after ingestion of the plant for several weeks to months.[5]

CLINICAL SIGNS

Affected horses show signs primarily of weight loss and lameness. Weight loss occurs over several weeks to months in spite of normal appetite. Lameness usually is of increasing severity and may begin with signs of generalized stiffness. Eventually, the fetlock joints may become overextended, and horses may exhibit kyphosis. The flexor tendons and particularly the suspensory ligament become sensitive to palpation. The lameness may grow so severe that euthanasia becomes necessary.[5] Signs of renal failure also may become evident in isolated cases.

PATHOPHYSIOLOGY

Cestrum diurnum and certain other members of the Solanaceae family contain a potent steroid glycoside with vitamin D–like activity. The toxic agent is a 1,25-dihydroxycholecalciferol ($1,25[OH]_2D_3$) glycoside found in the leaves of the plant.[6,7] Normally, vitamin D_3 is acquired from the diet or is produced in the skin by a reaction dependent on ultraviolet light. Vitamin D_3 is hydroxylated in the liver to yield 25-hydroxycholecalciferol, which subsequently is hydroxylated in the kidney to $1,25(OH)_2D_3$. This compound is the most active form of the vitamin and acts to increase calcium absorption and stimulate production of calcium-binding protein in the intestine.[6]

The normal rate of production of $1,25(OH)_2D_3$ is regulated by a negative feedback mechanism. Calcium or phosphorus deprivation stimulates the production of $1,25(OH)_2D_3$, and a decreased rate of production occurs when calcium or phosphorus is present in adequate amounts.[6]

This natural feedback mechanism is bypassed when $1,25(OH)_2D_3$ is supplied exogenously, as in the case of ingestion of *C. diurnum*. As a consequence, excessive calcium-binding protein is synthesized in the intestine, and excessive amounts of calcium and phosphorus are absorbed. If the calcium load exceeds the capacity of the kidney to excrete it, soft tissue mineralization (dystrophic calcification) and osteopetrosis occur.[6]

In horses that have ingested toxic amounts of *C. diurnum*, calcification of the flexor tendons, suspensory ligament, and other elastic tissues appears to predominate over deposition of calcium into other soft tissues. Osteopetrosis is thought to result from sustained hypercalcemia and secondary elevation of calcitonin.[5]

DIAGNOSIS AND TREATMENT

A diagnosis of toxicosis is suspected when horses exhibit signs of weight loss and lameness and they are known to have had prolonged access to *C. diurnum*. Affected horses typically are hypercalcemic, but serum phosphorus concentration usually is within a normal range. Renal dysfunction, if present, may be characterized by elevations in BUN and creatinine concentrations. Urine analysis may indicate an increased fractional excretion of sodium, potassium, and phosphorus, along with other laboratory findings associated with renal failure. Horses should be denied access to *C. diurnum* plants.

Hairy Vetch (*Vicia villosa*)

One report of toxicosis suspected to result from ingestion of hairy vetch is described.[8] The affected horse was a 1-year-old crossbred female that required euthanasia because of severe weight loss and bilateral corneal ulceration with perforation.

The clinical signs reported were weight loss despite good appetite, fluctuating body temperature, subcutaneous swelling that started around the lips and spread to involve the rest of the body, and bilateral corneal ulceration with eventual perforation.

The only recorded abnormal laboratory findings consisted of elevated serum concentrations of LDH and AST measured 2 weeks after onset of clinical signs. Histologic lesions consisted of multifocal to diffuse granulomatous inflammation of the heart, lungs, kidneys, skin, lymph nodes, ileum, colon, skeletal muscle, and choroid.

The toxic substance has not been identified, and no specific therapy has been recommended. A similar toxic condition occasionally occurs in other livestock grazing hairy vetch, with most cases of toxicosis occurring between April and July.

Photosensitizing Plants

Many plants can cause photosensitive reactions in horses. Some plants contain photodynamic substances that are absorbed from the gastrointestinal tract intact or in a form metabolically altered into an active compound (primary photosensitizing plants). Other plants may cause photodermatitis after liver dysfunction, in which the photodynamic toxin is a metabolite normally excreted in bile (secondary photosensitivity). Because of hepatic damage induced by the plant, these metabolites enter the circulation, and subsequent interaction with light results in clinical manifestation of disease. Box 22-2 lists plants[9-11] known to induce photosensitization in herbivores.

BOX 22-2

PLANTS INDUCING PHOTOSENSITIZATION IN HERBIVORES

Primary Photosensitizers

Ammi majus (bishop's weed): contains furocoumarins
Avena fatua (oatgrass)
Brassica (rape)
Cooperia pedunculata
Cymopterus watsonii (spring parsley): contains furocoumarins
Erodium (trefoil)
Fagopyrum sagittatum (buckwheat): contains the naphthodi-anthrone derivative fagopyrin
Hypericum perforatum (St. John's wort, Klamath weed): contains the naphthodianthrone derivative hypericin
Perennial ryegrass
Ricinus communis (castor bean)
Rutaceae
Trifolium (clover)
Umbelliferae

Secondary or Hepatogenous Photosensitizers

Agave lecheguilla (lecheguilla)
Blue-green algae
Brachiaria brizantha
Brassia hyssopifolia
Brassica napus (cultivated rape)
Holocalyx glaziovii
Lantana spp.
Lippia rehmanni
Myoporum laetum (ngaio)
Narthecium ossifragum (bog asphodel)
Nolina texana (sacahuiste)
Panicum spp. (panic grass, kleingrass)
Pithomyces chartarum and *Periconia minutissima*
Senecio spp. (ragwort, groundsel)
Tetradymia canescens (gray horsebrush)
Tetradymia glabrata (spineless horsebrush)
Tribulus terrestris (puncturevine)

Other Photosensitizers

Avena (oats)
Euphorbia maculata (milk purslane)
Kochia scoparia (summer cyprus, fireweed)
Medicago (alfalfa)
Polygonum spp. (smartweed)
Sorghum vulgare (Sudan grass)
Trifolium (clover)
Vicia spp. (vetches)

CLINICAL SIGNS

Signs of photosensitization are similar, regardless of the cause, and vary in degree. Factors that influence the severity of signs include the amount of reactive pigment present in the skin at a given time; the degree of exposure to light of appropriate wavelength; and the severity of hepatic damage, if hepatogenous photosensitization is the cause.[11]

Restlessness and discomfort usually are the first evident signs. Erythema may be apparent, followed by edema of affected areas. Blister formation and subsequent serum exudation and scab formation occur as the condition progresses. Affected sites usually are painful when touched, and animals often attempt to protect themselves from direct sunlight.[9,11]

The light-colored or nonpigmented areas of skin are affected most severely, particularly the face, nose, back, escutcheon, and coronary band. Severely affected animals also may have involvement of pigmented areas of skin, and secondary self-trauma and bacterial infection may arise from attempts to rub the affected areas. Horses may lose patches of skin that slough in large, leathery plaques.[9,11]

PATHOPHYSIOLOGY

Plants causing primary photosensitization contain a photodynamic agent that is absorbed from the gastrointestinal tract intact or that is later metabolically altered into an active compound. Secondary photosensitizing plants induce hepatic damage of sufficient magnitude to inhibit adequate clearance of photodynamic agents. Normally, these photodynamic toxins are metabolites excreted in bile. When the liver is damaged sufficiently or bile flow is hindered, these metabolites enter the circulation. Phylloerythrin, a normal chlorophyll breakdown product, is considered the only important photodynamic substance in instances of secondary photosensitization.[12] These photodynamic agents then are circulated throughout the body, eventually reaching the dermal capillaries.

Interaction of long-wave ultraviolet light with these photodynamic agents circulating in the skin capillaries results in chemical excitement of these substances. As a consequence, free radicals form that are highly inflammatory and cause degradation of cell phospholipid membranes, polypeptide proteins, and nucleic acids.[9,13] These processes disrupt the cells and ultimately result in the dermal lesions noted with this toxicity.

DIAGNOSIS AND TREATMENT

Clinical signs of photosensitivity are fairly typical and seldom are confused with other afflictions of skin. When clinical signs become evident, the horse should be evaluated thoroughly for evidence of hepatopathy because primary and secondary photosensitivity produce the same clinical signs. If hepatic disease is present, the clinician should ascertain the cause and institute appropriate therapy.

Primary photodynamic agents can be identified with several biologic assay systems, but this is rarely done. A mouse assay system and a microbial assay using *Candida albicans* are available for this purpose.[9]

Specific therapy for photodermatitis is not available. Horses should be removed from direct sunlight until skin lesions are healed and the offending plant is removed from the environment. Various topical agents may be used to facilitate skin healing. Superficial bacterial dermatitis should be treated with appropriate antibiotics, and NSAID therapy may be beneficial during the initial stages of the disease process.

TALL FESCUE (*FESTUCA ARUNDINACEA*)

The causative agent of the disorder associated with grazing tall fescue is *Neotyphodium coenophialum*[14] (formerly identified as *Acremonium coenophialum*), a fungal endophyte that grows within the stem, leaf sheaths, and seeds of tall fescue.[15,16] This endophyte is highly indigenous to many areas of the United States and may contaminate as much as 90% of fescue pastures in certain geographic areas.[15]

CLINICAL SIGNS

Horses grazing or being fed tall fescue hay preparations may develop a condition termed *summer slump* or *summer syndrome*.[9,17] The disorder is characterized by anorexia, weight loss, poor hair quality, pyrexia, and hypersalivation. Additionally, mares may sustain a variety of pregnancy- and reproduction-related disorders. Typical findings include the presence of a thick, tough placenta; prolonged gestation; abortion; birth of dead or weak foals; and high perinatal foal mortality.[18] Mares frequently are affected with agalactia, retained placenta, and rebreeding difficulties as well.[9,13,15]

PATHOPHYSIOLOGY

The fungus produces multiple toxins, including peramines, lolines, and ergopeptine alkaloids. Peramines have no apparent effect on animal health, but the lolines (N-acetyl loline and N-formyl loline) present in *Neotyphodium* are pyrrolizidine alkaloids. However, the hepatotoxicity characteristic of pyrrolizidine alkaloids has not been observed with tall fescue toxicosis in any species.[16]

The ergopeptine alkaloids appear to be responsible for most of the abnormalities associated with fescue toxicosis. Ergotamine, ergosine, ergovaline, ergoine, ergocristine, ergocryptine, and ergocornine have been isolated, but ergovaline and ergosine are most prominent. Ergovaline is thought to account for 84% to 97% of the ergopeptine concentration of infected tall fescue. The concentration of ergot alkaloids in tall fescue tends to increase with nitrogen fertilization and drought stress, and toxicity varies from season to season and year to year depending on the percentage of endophyte present, drought stress, nitrogen fertilization, and probably other factors.[16]

Agalactia occurs for a variety of reasons. First, ergopeptines are dopamine D_2-receptor agonists, and dopamine is thought to be the major inhibitor of prolactin secretion in the body. Second, ergot alkaloids inhibit adrenocorticotropic hormone secretion, resulting in reduced fetal cortisol concentration that subsequently causes reduced progesterone secretion by the placenta. Third, these alkaloids decrease tissue binding of estradiol, which can lead to an elevated serum concentration of estradiol-17β[16] (normally, serum estradiol concentrations decline near parturition). The interaction of appropriate levels of prolactin, progesterone, and estradiol-17β plays a major role in preparing the mammary gland for lactation. The combination of reduced concentrations of prolactin and progesterone and elevated concentration of estradiol-17β likely is the major cause of the agalactia and impaired udder development in affected mares.

The gestation period may be prolonged because ergopeptines have been hypothesized to block corticotropin-releasing hormone activity in the foal, which results in a lack of fetal production of adrenocorticotropic hormone and cortisol. Because increased fetal cortisol concentration acts to signal the mare for parturition, lack of fetal production of corticotropin-releasing hormone, adrenocorticotropic hormone, and cortisol may contribute to extended gestation periods in affected mares.[16]

The placental abnormalities frequently noted have been suspected to be associated with vasoconstriction. Edema, fibrosis, and mucoid degeneration of arteries in placentae from affected mares have been observed.[17] These changes were thought to be consistent with anoxia, which was hypothesized to be associated with vasoconstriction. Ergovaline and N-acetylloline, which are present in infected fescue, have vasoconstrictive properties.[16]

Ergot alkaloids also may have a negative effect on fertilized ovum implantation in the endometrium, resulting in reduced reproductive efficiency of affected mares. In the mare the effects of ergopeptines on implantation are inconclusive, but ergocryptine, ergocornine, ergosine, and ergovaline are capable of interrupting early pregnancy in the rat.[16]

Foals born alive to affected mares may be hypothyroid, although the mechanism responsible for this is unknown.[18] High perinatal foal mortality probably also is influenced by agalactia and poor colostral antibody production by the mare, resulting in failure of passive transfer with associated septicemia and failure of the foal to thrive.[16]

DIAGNOSIS AND TREATMENT

Diagnosis often is empiric, based on clinical signs and access to fescue pasture or hay during late gestation. Affected mares typically have reduced serum concentrations of prolactin and progesterone and elevated levels of estradiol-17β. Reduced-serum concentrations of triiodothyronine, adrenocorticotropic hormone, cortisol, and total progestogens may be present in affected foals. Hay and pasture samples also may be evaluated for the presence of endophytes and ergovaline.[16]

Treatment of gravid mares past their foaling date should include removal from fescue as quickly as possible. Domperidone given orally once daily at 1.1 mg/kg during the last 15 days of gestation may be efficacious in helping establish udder development and lactation. Postfoaling mares may benefit from domperidone (1.1 mg/kg orally) administered once daily for several days in an attempt to stimulate milk production.

Prevention requires removing mares from fescue pasture or hay during late gestation. In one study fescue removed from the diet at 300 days of gestation was not associated with any problems in mares.[17] Thus the most critical time for exposure to infected fescue in pregnant mares seems to be during the last 30 days of pregnancy. Local or regional authorities can provide important information regarding current methods of managing infected pastures.

Hoary Alyssum (*Berteroa incana*)

Toxicosis in horses related to ingestion of hoary alyssum was first reported in 1992.[19,20] This plant is a member of the Cruciferae (mustard) family and can behave as an annual, biannual, or perennial. Hoary alyssum grows primarily in the northeastern and northcentral United States and Canada but also is reported in the states of Oklahoma, Washington, Oregon, Idaho, and California and in Europe. The plant tends to flourish under conditions of drought, frost, and overgrazing and in areas of poor soil.[20,21] Toxicity has been reported in horses grazing contaminated pasture, eating plant-contaminated hay, and being fed oats containing hoary alyssum seed.[19-22] Reported cases are more prevalent during summer months after ingestion of recently cut hay, but toxicosis has resulted from feeding hay stored for 9 months.[20]

CLINICAL SIGNS

Not all horses exposed to hoary alyssum develop clinical signs of toxicosis. An estimated 45% of horses exposed to the plant under field conditions did not develop any signs of illness. However, the most common clinical signs observed under field and experimental conditions were varying degrees of fever, edema of one to four limbs, and laminitis. Horses affected with laminitis rarely are reported to develop rotation of the distal phalanges. These signs typically commence within 24 hours of ingestion (although this varies depending on the amount of plant material ingested) and in most cases subside within 2 to 4 days after removal of the source.[20] Other signs noted have been lethargy, short-term diarrhea, and abdominal discomfort.[21] Early parturition and abortion are rare occurrences in pregnant mares.[19,21] Rarely, individual horses are affected more severely and exhibit clinical signs of endotoxemia, hypovolemic shock, acute renal failure, and ventral rotation of the distal phalanges. Death can occur in these horses.[20,22]

Pregnant mares may be more susceptible to toxicity and develop more severe clinical signs, however. In one report 23 of 29 broodmares developed signs of fever, tachycardia, tachypnea, distal limb edema, and mild to severe laminitis.[21] Of these mares 15 subsequently developed moderate to profuse bloody diarrhea, dehydration, abdominal pain, hematuria, and oliguria. Four of these mares were euthanized, and two had necropsy findings of hemoperitoneum, hemothorax, and ventral rotation of distal phalanges. Three of the mares aborted spontaneously, but no abnormalities were noted in the placentae or fetuses.

PATHOPHYSIOLOGY

The toxic agent in hoary alyssum remains unknown,[20] as does the mechanism of action of the toxic substance (or substances). However, red blood cell destruction appears to occur by way of hemolysis or some other mechanism.[20,21] No consistent laboratory abnormalities have been noted in an experimental feeding trial and in most field cases.[20] However, laboratory findings in more severely affected horses include significant red blood cell hemolysis; elevations in serum concentrations of creatinine, urea nitrogen, phosphorus, alkaline phosphatase, AST, CK, sorbitol dehydrogenase, and total bilirubin; neutropenia; proteinuria; hematuria; hemoglobinuria; and occult blood in feces and gastric fluid.[20-22] Which of these abnormalities are the direct result of the toxin and which result from physiologic deterioration of various organs is unknown.

DIAGNOSIS AND TREATMENT

A diagnosis is suspected on the basis of history of exposure to the plant and clinical signs. No specific therapy is indicated, but horses immediately should be denied access to the plant, and all contaminated hay and grain should be removed. One should initiate symptomatic treatment with fluids, NSAIDs, and gastrointestinal tract evacuation. Activated charcoal (1 to 3 g/kg administered through a nasogastric tube) has been suggested to help prevent absorption of the unknown toxin.[22] Intravenous DMSO should be used with caution because it has the potential to cause intravascular hemolysis, thereby compounding the red blood cell destruction caused by the toxin.[20,22] Most horses recover uneventfully in 2 to 4 days after removal of the plant and provision of supportive care.

MISCELLANEOUS AGENTS

Iodine

Iodine toxicosis or iodism is a rarely reported cause of toxicosis in horses. When iodism occurs, it most likely is caused by iatrogenic administration of iodine-containing substances. Many rations contain iodine in the form of various iodized salts, and sodium iodide and potassium iodide, along with the organic iodide compound ethylenediamine dihydroiodide, are used to treat various medical conditions.[9,23]

CLINICAL SIGNS

Nonpruritic generalized alopecia and diffuse scaliness of the skin were reported in a horse given 45 g of ethylenediamine dihydroiodide twice daily for 14 days.[24] Other reported clinical signs include goiter after excessive iodine intake, increased secretions of the respiratory tract, nasal discharge, intermittent nonproductive cough, and excessive lacrimation.[9,12,24] Pregnant mares receiving excessive amounts of iodine may produce weak foals with enlarged thyroid glands. Such foals have a high mortality rate.[9]

PATHOPHYSIOLOGY

Organic and inorganic forms of iodine are absorbed rapidly and almost completely from the gastrointestinal tract in the ionic form and are distributed throughout the body. Iodine is excreted primarily in the urine, but smaller amounts are present in feces, sweat, and milk.[12,23] The only known metabolic role of iodine is involvement in synthesis of the thyroid hormones thyroxine and triiodothyronine.[12]

Oral iodine salts, whether organic or inorganic, taken in higher doses stimulate nerve receptors in the stomach wall. Subsequently, the vagus nerve becomes stimulated and causes reflex secretion by cells in the upper respiratory tract.[12,25] Excessive iodine intake causes thyroidal organic iodine formation to increase to a maximal amount, and then a sharp decline in organic iodine formation occurs. Excessive iodine also inhibits release of organic iodine from the thyroid gland if the gland is stimulated by thyroid-stimulating hormone. The net results are clinical signs of increased amount and viscosity of respiratory tract secretions and occasional goiter development.[25] The mechanism underlying the development of the dermal lesions associated with iodism is unknown.[24]

DIAGNOSIS AND TREATMENT

Diagnosis of iodism is based on a history of exposure to high levels of iodine for a prolonged time coupled with compatible clinical signs of nasal discharge and excessive lacrimation, intermittent nonproductive cough, and nonpruritic generalized alopecia and scaling. Serum iodine concentrations, which are elevated in cases of iodism, can be measured, but blood levels decrease rapidly to near background levels within a few days if iodine exposure ceases.[12] Serum concentrations of thyroxine and triiodothyronine may be below normal reference values in affected horses.[24]

Treatment consists of removing the source of the iodine. Because iodine is mobilized rapidly and excreted from tissues, clinical signs usually subside rapidly when excessive iodine is removed.[12,23,24]

SNAKE VENOM

The venomous snakes in North America belong to the families Crotalidae (pit vipers), Elapidae (cobra), and Viperidae (true vipers). Most poisonous snakebites reported in human beings are inflicted by members of the Crotalidae family, and the same is probably true for horses as well. Of this family *Crotalus* (rattlesnakes), *Agkistrodon* (copperhead, cottonmouth), and *Sistrurus* (pigmy rattlesnake, massasauga) are the three genera most commonly involved in snakebites of livestock. The eastern coral snake *(Micrurus fulvius)* and the Arizona coral snake *(Micruroides euryxanthus)* are two members of the Elapidae family indigenous to the United States, but they account for only about 3% of poisonous bites reported in human beings.[9,26]

Venom injected into prey is an aid to digestion and greatly reduces the time for complete digestion to occur in the snake. The amount of venom injected at a given time is under voluntary control, and larger amounts are injected into larger prey or when the snake strikes for defensive purposes. Not all bites result in envenomation, and rattlesnakes are estimated to fail to inject venom in up to 20% of bites.[9,26]

Snake venom is a highly complex mixture of enzymes, lipids, biogenic amines, free amino acids, metal ions, proteins, and polypeptides. Most snake venoms contain up to 25 different fractions, yet many of them are not yet identified. Venom composition and toxic properties vary among *Crotalus* species and among individuals of the same species. Factors influencing venom composition include age, time from last feeding, and seasonal influences related to changes in feeding patterns or physiologic responses such as hibernation. The LD_{50} in mice exposed to venom of *Crotalus* species ranges from 0.23 mg/kg for the Mojave rattlesnake *(Crotalus scutulatus)* to 3.77 mg/kg for the red diamond rattlesnake *(Crotalus ruber ruber)*. The LD_{50} for mice for the copperhead *(Agkistrodon contortrix)* and cottonmouth *(Agkistrodon piscivorus)* is 10.92 mg/kg and 4.17 mg/kg, respectively.[26] This large variation in dose and chemical composition of venom accounts for the extreme amount of variation in the physiologic responses of animals to these substances.

CLINICAL SIGNS

Snakebites in horses are most common on or near the muzzle, but bites also may occur on the limbs or other parts of the body. The classic signs noted in most horses are acute onset of swelling and edema at the bite site. The muzzle and nasal passages may become swollen to the extent that respiration can become extremely labored, necessitating a tracheotomy. Epistaxis also may be apparent. Initially, fang marks may be evident, but they soon disappear with the onset of extensive swelling. Skin discoloration at the injection site is a common occurrence with many rattlesnakes but rarely occurs with copperhead and Mojave rattlesnake bites.[9] Varying degrees of necrosis of local tissue may occur, as well as secondary bacterial infections at the wound site. In the author's experience, bites involving the distal extremities of horses frequently have a prolonged convalescent period that may be accompanied by residual lameness.

Systemic manifestations of snake envenomation may be apparent when venom is injected intravascularly or perivascularly. In a retrospective study of rattlesnake venom poisoning in 32 horses, manifestations included fever, tachycardia, tachypnea, cardiac arrhythmia, hemolytic anemia, thrombocytopenia, hemorrhage, thrombosis of venipuncture sites, colic, diarrhea, and prehensile and masticatory dysfunction. Chronic problems included cardiac disease, pneumonia, laminitis, pharyngeal paralysis, and wound complications. The most common chronic problem observed in these horses was cardiac disease.[27] Labored respiration may result from pulmonary edema caused by passive congestion after vascular hypotension or precipitation of pulmonary emboli. Muscle fasciculation may be evident.[9] The venom of the Mojave rattlesnake produces respiratory paralysis that may result in death in human beings.[26] The overall mortality rate in 32 horses acutely affected with bites of prairie rattlesnake was 25%.[27]

The venom of coral snakes produces neurologic signs in affected human beings, with death occurring within 24 hours as a result of respiratory depression, hypotension, and cardiovascular collapse.[26] However, the coral snake requires prolonged contact (30 seconds or longer) to work the venom into the skin of its prey. Therefore it seems improbable that horses would become exposed to coral snake venom except under extremely unusual circumstances.

PATHOPHYSIOLOGY

The venoms of Crotalidae are rich in enzymes. Proteases cause severe tissue damage by digesting tissue proteins and peptides, and hyaluronidase allows rapid spread of venom through tissue by hydrolyzing connective tissue hyaluronic acid. L-Amino acid oxidase, L-arginine ester hydrolases, and 5′-nucleotidase also may contribute to tissue destruction. Phospholipases A, B, C, and D hydrolyze lipids and cause hemolysis by destroying lecithin in the red blood cell membranes. They also disrupt neurotransmission at the presynaptic and postsynaptic junctions. Other enzymes present in crotalid venom include ribonuclease, deoxyribonuclease, transaminase, phosphomonoesterase, phosphodiesterase, ATPase, DNAase, alkaline phosphatase, acid phosphatase, and endonuclease.[26]

Crotalid venom contains a number of polypeptides in addition to the enzymes. These polypeptides are low-molecular-weight proteins that are 5 to 20 times more lethal than crude venom in animal models, and they do not have enzymatic activity. They are present in higher concentrations in cobra venom than in rattlesnake venom and are mainly responsible for blood dyscrasias and coagulopathies. Small peptides are partly responsible for the generation of disseminated intravascular coagulation, and a venom fraction of the timber rattlesnake *(Crotalus horridus horridus)* causes platelet aggregation with resultant thrombocytopenia. Additionally, the venoms of the Mojave and Southern Pacific rattlesnakes contain a direct cardiotoxin.[26]

Rattlesnake venom contains substances with anticoagulant, procoagulant, and plasminogen-induced fibrinogenolytic properties. The coagulopathy that occurs in a given instance varies and depends on the content of the various venom components and on the dose of venom injected. The anticoagulant activity of crotalid venom appears to result from reversible binding of venom to prothrombin. Thrombinlike enzymes produce hypofibrinogenemia and increased concentration of FDPs. They also are capable of directly converting fibrinogen to fibrin, which may result in excessive fibrin formation and rapid disseminated intravascular coagulation. The fibrinolytic characteristics of crotalid venom occur directly or indirectly through the activation of endogenous plasminogen.[9,26]

DIAGNOSIS AND TREATMENT

Diagnosis of snakebite usually depends on clinical signs and accessibility to poisonous snakes. Laboratory abnormalities that may be present in affected horses include thrombocytopenia, hypofibrinogenemia, anemia, prolonged PT and PTT, hematuria, proteinuria, and myoglobinuria.[9,26]

Affected horses should be kept calm and quiet. Incision over the fang marks and suction are rarely indicated and probably of minimal value except in the immediate time frame of the bite, because the venom is absorbed almost immediately into the surrounding tissues. Tracheotomy is indicated in those horses that develop excessive edema and swelling of the head and external nares to the point that respiration becomes impaired. Topical cold therapy may have some beneficial effect if applied early and for short periods. Prolonged or excessive cold application, however, may enhance further tissue necrosis. Antivenom therapy commonly is used in instances of human snakebite but often is considered unnecessary in horses because of the low mortality rate, financial considerations, and availability of other therapies. An exception may be the horse or foal that is extremely valuable.

The clinician should initiate tetanus prophylaxis and systemic antibiotic therapy. Broad spectrum antimicrobial drugs should be used because gram positive and gram negative organisms are found in the mouth of North American pit vipers. The most common organisms isolated include *Proteus vulgaris, Escherichia coli, Corynebacterium* spp., *Streptococcus* spp., and Enterobacteriaceae.[26]

NSAIDs should not be used during the early stages of the bite wound because they may enhance the defects in primary hemostasis frequently induced by snake venom. NSAIDs may be used in the later stages of the disease to help reduce pain, swelling, and inflammation. Corticosteroids should be used with caution because they may diminish the clearance of FDPs from the peripheral vasculature by the reticuloendothelial system, and they may increase susceptibility to wound infection at the site. Corticosteroids may be beneficial, however, in treating severe hypotensive shock in young animals or in patients with intravenous envenomation. Heparin therapy also has been suggested to be helpful in instances of thrombus formation.[9]

Animals affected with systemic hypotension and cardiac dysrhythmias should be treated appropriately. Treatment may include the administration of intravenous fluids and plasma and the use of specific antiarrhythmic medications.

FLUORIDE

Fluoride toxicosis in horses appears to be a rare event.[28] Although acute and chronic fluoride toxicosis have been described in various animals, chronic fluorosis appears more common. Common sources of fluoride in chronic fluorosis include forages subjected to airborne contamination from nearby industrial plants such as aluminum smelters, steel mills, or fertilizer plants that heat fluorine-containing materials and discharge fluorides; drinking water containing excessive fluoride; feed supplements and vitamin and mineral additives with high fluoride concentration; and vegetation grown on soils containing high fluoride levels.[12]

Animals normally ingest small amounts of fluoride throughout their lives, and it accumulates in the body as long as constant or increasing amounts are ingested. Chronic toxicosis can result from prolonged ingestion of sufficiently high levels. The long-term dietary tolerance for fluoride in the horse is reported to be 40 to 60 ppm dietary fluoride.

Fluoride is absorbed almost totally from the gastrointestinal tract. Once absorbed, approximately half is excreted rapidly in urine, with the remaining half being stored in bone and teeth. Fluoride accumulates in calcified tissues, but once exposure ceases, bone fluoride is depleted slowly over months to years.

CLINICAL SIGNS

Chronic fluorosis in the horse is a rare event. In one suspected case the affected horse exhibited chronic weight loss of months' duration; poor growth; difficulty in mastication; and deformed, discolored, and absent deciduous incisors. The horse also was missing some deciduous premolars and molars.[28] Classic dental abnormalities reported in other species include mottled, hypoplastic enamel and brown discoloration with uneven wear of teeth.[12] Additional signs associated with chronic fluorosis in other animals include hyperostosis, enlargement and roughening of involved bones, intermittent lameness and generalized stiffness, dry and roughened hair coat, and decreased weight and milk production.[28] Because of the insidious nature of chronic fluorosis, it is important to remember that a time lag may occur between ingestion of excessive fluoride and the appearance of clinical signs.

PATHOPHYSIOLOGY

Excessive fluoride produces dental abnormalities by affecting the teeth during development. The primary effect of fluorine is thought to be a delaying and alteration of normal mineralization of the pre-enamel, predentine, and precementum. High fluoride levels appear to cause specific ameloblastic and odontoblastic damage. The matrix laid down by these damaged cells fails to accept minerals normally, resulting in faulty mineralization of the tooth bud. Once the tooth is formed fully, the ameloblasts have lost their constructive ability and the enamel lesions cannot be repaired. However, odontoblasts can produce secondary dentine to compensate for deficiencies brought about by excessive fluoride.[12] The brown to black discoloration of affected teeth results from oxidation of organic material in the teeth.

The pathogenesis of bone lesions associated with fluoride toxicosis is still undecided. One theory is that high fluoride levels lead to inadequate matrix and defective, irregular mineralization of bone. Another theory is that hydroxyl radicals in the hydroxyapatite crystal structure are replaced by fluoride ions, resulting in a decrease in crystal lattice dimensions. The pathologic results of skeletal fluorosis include dissociation of normal sequences of osteogenesis, production of abnormal bone, accelerated remodeling of bone, and occasional accelerated bone resorption.[12]

DIAGNOSIS AND TREATMENT

Diagnosis of chronic fluorosis is based primarily on clinical findings and history of possible exposure to fluorides. Fluorosis usually is confirmed by analysis of skeletal or dental tissues for fluoride content and evaluation of fluoride concentration in urine. Water and feed consumed by the animals also should be analyzed for fluoride content.

Treatment of chronic fluorosis aims mainly at dietary restriction of fluoride-containing substances. Aluminum sulfate, aluminum chloride, calcium aluminate, calcium carbonate, and defluorinated phosphate have been used to reduce the toxic effects of fluoride, but no substance completely prevents the toxic effects of ingesting excessive amounts of fluorides.

ZINC

Excessive exposure to dietary zinc can be a problem for young, growing horses. Sources of excessive zinc usually are soil and forage contamination from nearby smelters and pastures that were topdressed with zinc oxide.[29,30] Classic signs of copper deficiency associated with excessive zinc ingestion have been produced by experimental feeding of excessive zinc to young foals.[31,32] Skeletally mature horses do not appear to be susceptible to the effects of zinc-contaminated pastures.[32]

CLINICAL SIGNS

Signs associated with zinc-induced copper deficiency include swelling at the physeal region of long bones, gradual onset of lameness and stiffness that may become so severe that affected animals are reluctant to rise from lateral recumbency, swollen joints resulting from synovial effusion, unthriftiness, and weight loss despite normal appetite.[29-31] Anemia also may develop in more chronically affected individuals.[31] The joint swellings in affected horses are typical of those of osteochondrosis desiccans, and severe generalized osteochondrosis also develops in copper deficient horses.[29,30,32]

PATHOPHYSIOLOGY

In horses this disease actually appears to be a manifestation of copper deficiency and the subsequent development of hypocupremia-induced articular cartilage disease.[29,32] Copper is an essential cofactor for lysyl oxidase, an enzyme involved in the formation of collagen cross-links. Copper deficiency interferes with collagen metabolism and results in production of weak connective tissue. This allows articular cartilage fractures and growth physeal fractures to occur in the zone of hypertrophic cells, producing the clinical syndrome of osteochondrosis desiccans.

The mechanism of zinc-induced copper deficiency is not totally understood. Experimentally, affected foals at necropsy had high hepatic copper content despite low serum copper concentration, suggesting that the hepatic copper was not readily available for production of ceruloplasmin or could not be mobilized rapidly enough for use by other tissues.[32] Excessive zinc stimulates production of metallothionein, an intestinal cell protein that binds to excessive zinc, copper, and other divalent metal ions and facilitates their excretion in bile, feces, and saliva. Copper has a higher affinity for metallothionein than does zinc, and increased production of metallothionein, with subsequent binding to copper, may lead to copper deficiency through increased copper excretion.[33]

DIAGNOSIS AND TREATMENT

Once signs of osteochondrosis develop, the condition should be appropriately treated. Diagnosis of excessive zinc intake may be difficult in that zinc is excreted rapidly after absorption, and blood and tissue zinc concentrations tend to decline quickly to normal levels with cessation of intake. Liver, kidney, and serum zinc concentrations can be measured, but fecal samples collected from affected horses may be more suitable. Feed and water supplies also can be evaluated for zinc content.[34]

Treatment of affected horses aims to restore proper copper concentration in the diet and remove the source of excessive zinc. Diets containing 7.7 mg copper per kilogram and 250 mg zinc per kilogram of dry weight were sufficient to maintain normal serum copper and zinc concentrations and did not induce disease in treated foals. Diets containing 1000 mg/kg or greater of zinc caused hypocupremia and subsequent osteochondrosis desiccans when fed to foals over a period of several weeks.[32] Osteochondrosis desiccans is treated surgically.

SELENIUM

Selenium toxicity in horses usually results from prolonged ingestion of plants containing excessive amounts of selenium. Intoxication can result from horses foraging on soil with high levels of selenium and ingesting selenium-accumulating plants growing on soils with minimal amounts of selenium.[34-37] Acute toxicosis also can occur through inadvertent overdosing of selenium supplements added to rations or given by parenteral injection.[38] The acute single oral toxic dosage of selenium given as sodium selenite is between 3.3 and 6 mg/kg for the horse.[34,39]

CLINICAL SIGNS

Three different syndromes are attributed to selenium intoxication: acute toxicity and two chronic forms described as "blind staggers" and "alkali disease." Signs of acute toxicity develop within 6 hours of ingestion and include sweating, diarrhea, tachycardia, tachypnea, mild pyrexia, lethargy, and mild to severe colic. Death may occur within 24 hours, and some horses exhibit a dumb attitude before death. Head pressing before death is suggested as a classic sign of acute selenosis.[34,39]

Chronic selenium intoxication described as blind staggers results from frequent ingestion of plants over weeks to months. Signs associated with this syndrome include aimless wandering or circling, muscle weakness, incoordination, respiratory difficulty, and decreased vision. In classic cases blindness eventually develops and is followed by paralysis and death.[40] Some have hypothesized that blind staggers is not due to selenium at all but is actually polioencephalomalacia associated with excess sulfur intake.

Alkali disease, the more common presentation of selenosis in horses, results from ingestion of seleniferous plants, and signs may develop weeks to months after exposure. Initially, lameness and swelling of the coronary band regions are apparent, along with anorexia and mild depression. These signs progress to transverse cracking of the hoof wall distal to the coronary band with associated lameness. The hooves eventually may be sloughed. Loss of hair from the mane and tail occurs because the hairs become brittle and are broken easily. Compromised reproductive and immune function also may develop in affected horses.[35-38]

PATHOPHYSIOLOGY

Selenium is absorbed readily from the gastrointestinal tract, but organic forms of selenium generally are retained in greater amounts than are inorganic forms. Elimination occurs rapidly through urine, sweat, feces, and exhaled air. The clinician also must recognize hoof and hair as routes of excretion because excess selenium is deposited in these structures.[38] This latter fact has important diagnostic implications.

Selenium functions in a number of enzymatic and physiologic processes. The toxic effects of selenium have been associated with its affinity for reacting with sulfur-containing amino acid residues such as cystine that are incorporated synthetically into biologically active glycoproteins and polypeptides. As a result, various selenosulfides are formed as a substitute for disulfide bonds.[41]

DIAGNOSIS AND TREATMENT

A presumptive diagnosis of selenium intoxication can be made on the basis of typical clinical signs and history of possible exposure to selenium iatrogenically in the form of selenium supplementation or through ingestion of appropriate plants. The clinician can attempt to make a definitive diagnosis by assaying blood, serum, hair, and hoof material for selenium content. In acute fatal selenosis serum selenium concentration may exceed 1 ppm.[34,39] A selenium concentration greater than 5 ppm in hair and hoof wall is considered diagnostic of selenosis.[34,35,37] It also is possible to measure selenium concentration in liver and kidney samples.

Treatment of affected horses involves removal of the selenium source, symptomatic treatment of lesions, and provision of good nursing care. Oral dosing of naphthalene at 4.5 g/day for 5 days, waiting 5 days, and then repeating the dose for an additional 5 days has been suggested for treatment of adult horses; however, this is not commonly done, and its efficacy is questionable.[34,35] Prevention of selenosis has been attempted by adding copper,[38] methionine,[42] or sodium arsenite[34,35] to the diet of at-risk animals.

Gangrenous Ergotism (*Claviceps purpurea*)

Claviceps purpurea is a fungal parasite that invades the developing ovary of the grass flower and cereal grains. This fungus commonly parasitizes rye, oats, wheat, and Kentucky bluegrass, which are associated most often with outbreaks of gangrenous ergotism. The fungus replaces the seed ovary with a dark brown to purple oblong body called a *sclerotium.* Sclerotia are slightly larger than the original whole grain seed, and their growth is promoted by warm, moist conditions. Horses rarely are affected by this condition, in part because of the distasteful nature of affected feedstuffs and because most fungal elements are removed during commercial grain processing procedures.[12,13]

CLINICAL SIGNS

Signs of intoxication may become apparent if infected feeds are ingested over several days to weeks. Dry gangrene of the extremities is the classic sign associated with *C. purpurea* toxicosis and can affect the limbs, nose, ears, and tail. Early signs of toxicosis are lameness and cool extremities. The hindlimbs often are affected first, with swelling and tenderness in the fetlock area. The involved tissues become dark and discolored, and a transverse line of demarcation may occur between normal skin and the distal parts of the limb. Eventually, the hoof and associated bones and tissue may slough. This same sequence may involve the nose, ears, and tail. Gangrenous signs may be preceded by colic and constipation or diarrhea. Possible subacute effects include depression, partial anorexia, general unthriftiness, and increased pulse and respiratory rates.[12,13] Abortions also occur.

PATHOPHYSIOLOGY

The major toxic alkaloids in ergot are a group of structurally similar ergopeptides. They are absorbed slowly and incompletely from the gastrointestinal tract, reaching peak plasma concentrations in approximately 2 hours. The liver is the primary site of metabolism, and approximately 90% of metabolites are excreted in bile. Small amounts of unmetabolized alkaloids are excreted in urine. The total concentration and proportions of alkaloids present in ergot sclerotia may vary with species and environmental conditions.[12,13]

Ergotamine, the most abundant of the alkaloids, is a polypeptide derivative of lysergic acid. The varied physiologic effects of ergot are caused primarily by mixtures of levoisomers of ergotamine, coupled with smaller amounts of acetylcholine, histamine, and tyramine.[12]

Ergotamine is a vasoactive substance that causes arterial and venous constriction. Ergotamine also may damage capillary endothelium. The combined effects of vasoconstriction and endothelial damage produce increased blood pressure, decreased blood flow through the extremities, vascular stasis, thrombosis, and eventually gangrene.[12,13]

The ergotoxine group of alkaloids produce α-adrenergic blockade and antagonize 5-hydroxytryptamine. This produces an increase in blood pressure as a result of peripheral vasoconstriction, particularly in postcapillary vessels.[12]

DIAGNOSIS AND TREATMENT

A tentative diagnosis of ergotism is based on clinical signs and exclusion of other disease processes. An experienced person can readily identify ergot sclerotia in grains. However, once grinding or pelleting of feed has occurred, ergot can be recognized only by microscopic examination or chemical analysis for ergot alkaloids. Ergot alkaloids can be identified and quantitated by chromatographic methods, and a sample of the individual grain components should be obtained for analysis whenever possible.[12]

No specific treatment exists for gangrenous ergotism. The offending grain should be removed, and affected animals should be kept warm to avoid cold-induced vasoconstriction in the extremities. Supportive therapy in the form of antibiotics and analgesics may be indicated. The use of anti-α-adrenergic pharmaceuticals to effect vasodilation also may be helpful. Such agents might include acepromazine, isoxsuprine, phenoxybenzamine, and similar products.[12,13]

TOXICOSES CAUSING SIGNS RELATING TO LIVER DISEASE OR DYSFUNCTION

PLANTS

Pyrrolizidine Alkaloids

Pyrrolizidine alkaloid toxicity results from consumption of plants that contain various pyrrolizidine alkaloids. Horses can become intoxicated after ingesting fresh plants and dried plants incorporated into hay. As with many toxic plants, however, these plants are frequently unpalatable to most horses, although certain conditions may render them more appetizing. This toxicity is characterized by a chronic, progressive disorder manifested by signs of liver failure. The more common plants that cause toxicosis in horses include *Senecio jacobaea* (tansy ragwort), *Senecio vulgaris* (common groundsel), *Senecio longilobus* (groundsel), and *Cynoglossum officinale* (houndstongue).[1,2] Other plants that contain pyrrolizidine alkaloids but are not commonly associated with clinical disease in horses include *Amsinckia intermedia* (fiddleneck tarweed), *Crotalaria* spp. (rattlebox), *Echium plantagineum* (Viper's bugloss), and *Heliotropium europaeum* (common heliotrope).

CLINICAL SIGNS

Signs of pyrrolizidine alkaloid intoxication in horses are essentially those of liver failure. The most frequently noted signs include weight loss of weeks to months in duration, icterus, and behavioral abnormalities. The behavioral changes indicate hepatoencephalopathy and may include aimless pacing or wandering, ataxia, licking inanimate objects, blindness, head pressing, and uncharacteristic aggression. Convulsions and coma may precede death. Clinical signs of abnormal behavior usually are a terminal event in the disease process and typically have an acute onset.[2,3] Other signs less frequently reported include diarrhea, photosensitization of nonpigmented areas of skin, hemoglobinuria, and inspiratory dyspnea.[2,4] Abortion and poor exercise tolerance (reduced athletic performance) also have been observed in horses after ingestion of sublethal amounts.[5] Because toxicity of these plants is related to liver dysfunction, clinical signs of disease may not become apparent for weeks to months after ingestion.

PATHOPHYSIOLOGY

A number of pyrrolizidine alkaloids are present in various plant species, and some plants may contain multiple alkaloids. These substances are absorbed from the gastrointestinal tract and carried to the liver, where they are metabolized by hepatic microsomal enzymes to pyrroles. These pyrroles then can cross-link double-stranded deoxyribonucleic acid (DNA) and bind to proteins and nucleic acid within hepatocytes.[1,2]

The cross-linking of DNA has an antimitotic effect on hepatocytes. The hepatocytes are unable to divide and subsequently become megalocytes. As these cells die, they are replaced by fibrous tissue rather than normal hepatocytes. Binding of protein and nucleic acid results in inhibition of cytoplasmic protein synthesis. These changes may lead to more rapid death of hepatocytes and cause centrilobular necrosis. Eventually, liver function begins to fail because of progressive hepatocellular death and subsequent fibrosis.[1,2] As the disease progresses, generalized fibrosis develops. Once connective tissue bridges form between portal areas, the disease is fatal.[1]

Variation in the dosage and frequency of administration of alkaloids results in a wide spectrum of hepatic lesions. Acute toxicosis resulting from massive doses is more likely to produce centrilobular necrosis with hemorrhage; however, this type of exposure is extremely rare. Chronic doses tend to produce hepatocellular death in the portal areas, along with megalocytosis, fibrosis, biliary hyperplasia, and occlusion of hepatic veins.[1,2] Liver failure is thought to be ultimately responsible for the clinical signs observed in pyrrolizidine alkaloid toxicosis.

The toxic dose of dried *Senecio* is estimated to be 5% of the body weight of the horse. This amount does not need to be ingested all at once, however, because the effects are cumulative. The total dose of alkaloids consumed determines the toxic effect, regardless of the amount of time in which the alkaloids were consumed.[1,2]

DIAGNOSIS AND TREATMENT

Most cases of pyrrolizidine alkaloid toxicosis are diagnosed on the basis of history, compatible clinical signs, serum liver enzyme activities, and liver biopsy findings. When active hepatocellular damage is occurring early in the disease process, sorbitol dehydrogenase and LDH usually are elevated, but they often decline to normal values by the time the horse is showing clinical signs. Serum GGT, alkaline phosphatase, and AST activities tend to be elevated throughout the disease course. Serum concentration of bile acids also is reported to be elevated in affected horses. Serum bilirubin concentration tends to be elevated in later stages of the disease, and hypoglycemia and hypoalbuminemia rarely are seen except in cases of severe hepatic disease.[1,2,4,5]

Other diagnostic aids that may be useful from a diagnostic and prognostic standpoint include measurement of the ratio of branched-chain amino acids to aromatic amino acids in serum. The branched-chain amino acids isoleucine, leucine, and valine are catabolized primarily in muscle, and the aromatic amino acids phenylalanine and tyrosine are catabolized mainly in the liver. The ratio of the sums of these amino acids (branched-chain to aromatic) decreases progressively from normal in horses affected with pyrrolizidine alkaloid toxicosis. If the ratio is below normal range and the horses are exposed continually to alkaloid-containing plants, they have a poor chance of survival. Some affected horses also showed a dramatic decrease in this ratio just before death.[6] Liver biopsy findings of a triad of fibrosis, bile duct proliferation, and megalocytosis are highly suggestive of pyrrolizidine alkaloid toxicosis. Liver biopsy samples also can help in establishing prognosis because the presence of advanced or generalized hepatic fibrosis warrants a grave prognosis.[1,2]

Feed samples may be analyzed for pyrrolizidine alkaloid content, but the process is often time consuming and unnecessary.[1] Pyrrole testing of liver tissue can be helpful in confirming exposure to the plant in the early stages of the disease; however, this analysis is offered by only a few laboratories.

No specific treatment for pyrrolizidine alkaloid toxicity exists. Affected horses may survive if they are denied further exposure to alkaloid-containing plants and are fed a suitable diet. However, some horses still may show signs of liver disease even though they have not had exposure to the plant for some time. Specific treatment of acute and chronic liver failure is discussed elsewhere.

Prevention entails keeping horses away from pasture or feed contaminated with pyrrolizidine alkaloid–containing plants.

Mushroom (*Amanita* spp.)

One report describes fatal intoxication of a horse by ingestion of mushrooms *(Amanita* spp.*)*.[7] Mushrooms apparently are unpalatable to livestock species, but the described horse also suffered from meningioangiomatosis, a rare benign tumor of the meninges and brain. The authors speculated that the presence of the tumor may have resulted in abnormal mentation and altered the normal eating behavior of the horse, resulting in mushroom consumption.

CLINICAL SIGNS

The described horse had acute onset of depression, head pressing, ataxia, and repeated recumbency with difficulty in rising. Before the onset of liver disease, many poisoned animals display signs of gastrointestinal distress. Clinical signs of shock, including hypothermia, poor capillary perfusion, and weak pulse, also were apparent. The horse was euthanized because of continued deterioration and lack of response to supportive therapy.

PATHOPHYSIOLOGY

Some species of *Amanita* mushrooms contain a number of biologically active cyclic peptides such as amatoxins, phallotoxins, phallolysin, and antaminide. Some of these peptides affect actin polymerization and cause hepatocytes to lose their cytoskeletal organization and cellular attachments, resulting in hepatocellular dissociation and necrosis. Amanitins are peptides that inhibit ribonucleic acid (RNA) polymerase II within the nucleus, thereby preventing DNA transcription and subsequent protein synthesis. The result is acute submassive hepatic necrosis, which was present in the described horse.

DIAGNOSIS AND TREATMENT

Diagnosis in the described horse was based on histologic findings of submassive hepatic necrosis, acute onset of clinical signs, and presence of partially digested mushrooms in stomach contents. No specific therapy is recommended, although prompt evacuation of the gastrointestinal tract coupled with supportive care would seem prudent. The quantity of mushrooms ingested appears to be the primary prognostic indicator. If sufficient amounts of toxin are absorbed, the prognosis is grave. Hepatic coma often ensues in other species.

MISCELLANEOUS AGENTS

Iron

Iron toxicosis in horses is rare and can result from iatrogenic overdose of injected or oral products given to foals or from accidental consumption of iron-containing supplements. Supplemental iron is available in injectable and oral formulations, and presently more than 120 iron preparations are on the market.[8] Iron dextrin, iron polysaccharide, iron sorbitol, and ferric ammonium citrate are available injectable preparations. Oral formulations include iron salts such as ferris sulfate, citrate, and ammonium citrate; ferrous sulfate, chloride, glutamate, lactate, fumarate, and carbonate; and ferric phosphate with sodium citrate. Chelated iron compounds are about one fourth as toxic as other compounds. Some forms of iron are more bioavailable than others.

The toxicity of iron is least by the oral route, with intramuscular and intravenous routes being increasingly more toxic. Because most animals do not have a mechanism for iron excretion, the toxicity of iron depends on the amount of iron already present in the body.

CLINICAL SIGNS

Two syndromes of iron toxicosis in animals are reported. A peracute syndrome is represented by sudden death a few minutes to hours after injection. This syndrome may resemble an anaphylactic reaction, but the triggering mechanism is unknown. A subacute reaction characterized by progressive depression, icterus, and disorientation leading to coma and death seems to be the more typical syndrome seen in horses.[8-10]

PATHOPHYSIOLOGY

Experimentally, 5% to 10% of some forms of oral iron is absorbed in the small intestine, primarily from the duodenum and jejunum, by a rate-limited mucosal transfer system. The ferrous forms are absorbed to a greater extent than the ferric forms, but both can be absorbed if they are in the ionized state. Phosphates reduce the absorption of iron, and a high-sugar diet increases absorption. Once absorbed, iron is bound in serum by transferrin.[8]

Toxic doses of orally administered iron overwhelm the mechanism controlling absorption of iron from the intestine, resulting in massive iron absorption. Toxicity occurs when serum iron levels exceed the iron-binding capacity of transferrin. Free circulating iron then damages blood vessels, may cause erosion and ulceration of the stomach and intestine, causes hepatocellular necrosis and fatty degeneration of the myocardium, and can produce cerebral edema.[8,11] In horses hepatic failure appears to be the cause of death.[9]

At the cellular level, excessive iron causes extensive peroxidation of lipids in biologic membranes. A resulting decline in the ratio of unsaturated to saturated fatty acids leads to increased membrane rigidity, reduction of membrane potential, and increased permeability to various ions, leading to rupture of the membrane. The intracellular organelles adversely affected include the mitochondria and the lysosomal and sarcoplasmic membranes.[12] Elevated serum iron also inhibits the thrombin-induced conversion of fibrinogen to fibrin, thereby adversely affecting coagulation and enhancing any hemorrhagic process.[10] Histologically, affected livers are characterized by small size and have prominent bile duct proliferation, periportal fibrosis, and hepatocellular necrosis.[11]

DIAGNOSIS

Measurement of serum iron concentration is the best method of confirming a diagnosis of iron toxicity.[8] In addition, a history of iron administration coupled with clinical signs and laboratory evidence of hepatocellular damage and cardiovascular collapse is highly suggestive of toxicity.

Abnormal laboratory findings include prolonged PTT and PT, high concentrations of aromatic amino acids (tyrosine, phenylalanine, tryptophan, methionine), elevated plasma ammonia concentration, and increased activities of the liver-derived enzymes alkaline phosphatase and GGT. In addition, a high ratio of aromatic to branched-chain amino acids and an elevated total serum bilirubin content can be found.[9]

TREATMENT

Treatment of peracute iron toxicosis usually is unrewarding. Once clinical signs become evident, major organ damage usually is present. No specific treatment for horses affected with iron toxicity is known. Treatment of affected dogs has included supportive therapy with glucose and norepinephrine and magnesium oxide given orally to help complex the ingested iron. Experimentally, a specific chelator of ferric iron, deferoxamine, has been used at 0.75 mg/kg/min intravenously to chelate the circulating iron in dogs. This drug should be administered slowly by intravenous drip because it can cause a sharp decline in blood pressure. Plasma extenders and intravenous fluids also have been used to counteract cardiovascular shock present in some dogs.[8]

In cases of human toxicosis, gastric lavage, chelating agents, and cathartics (sodium sulfate and magnesium sulfate) have been used. The use of oral bicarbonate solutions to decrease iron absorption is controversial, and activated charcoal is given orally to absorb the iron-deferoxamine complex, even though charcoal does not effectively bind free iron.[11]

The chelator of choice in human toxicosis is deferoxamine. Deferoxamine is administered intravenously for maximum effect; the drug has a plasma half-life of about 1 hour. Deferoxamine is detoxified by the liver, but the iron-deferoxamine complex is excreted by the kidneys.[11]

AFLATOXIN

Aflatoxicosis is a rarely documented disorder of horses, as demonstrated by the paucity of clinical cases reported in the literature.[13-15] In reported instances toxicosis developed in horses being fed contaminated feedstuffs, but horses also have been affected experimentally by forced feeding of aflatoxin-contaminated material.[16,17]

Aflatoxins are toxic metabolites primarily produced by the fungi *Aspergillus flavus* and *Aspergillus parasiticus*. These molds are ubiquitous and normally can be found in stored feeds. The molds are not inherently toxigenic, but they can grow rapidly and produce large amounts of aflatoxin under environmental conditions of adequate temperature and humidity. Many feedstuffs can support the growth of these molds, but cereal grains, cottonseed meal and cake, and peanuts seem to be affected most commonly.[18]

These molds produce five major aflatoxins: B1 and B2, which fluoresce blue under long-wave ultraviolet light; G1 and G2, which fluoresce green; and M1 aflatoxin, which is present in milk. B1 is the most important of these because of its toxicity and it abundance under natural conditions.[18]

Aflatoxins are a group of polycyclic, unsaturated compounds that have a coumarin nucleus coupled to a reactive bifuran system and a pentenone or lactone. These toxins are insoluble in water and are heat resistant; they are absorbed rapidly from the gastrointestinal tract and bound to serum albumin. Most of the toxins are removed from the bloodstream in the liver, where aflatoxins bind to macromolecules such as DNA, endoplasmic steroid-binding sites, and certain enzymes within the hepatocytes. In the liver a variety of metabolites are produced at rates that vary among species. The metabolites may be lipid-soluble or water-soluble conjugates and are excreted in bile. At least some of the metabolites undergo an enterohepatic cycle of absorption and excretion. The aflatoxins and their metabolites are excreted in urine and feces, and complete elimination may take several days. The aflatoxins are not known to be stored in any particular tissue.[18]

Acute and chronic aflatoxicoses are reported in a variety of animal species, including human beings. However, clinical reports of equine disease are concerned primarily with acute intoxication. The acute oral LD_{50} of aflatoxin B1 in horses is reported to be 2 mg/kg or greater. One author reported signs of toxic hepatopathy and gastrointestinal upset in horses that consumed feed containing 2 to 50 ppb of aflatoxin B1. Toxicity of aflatoxins also is reported to be enhanced by riboflavin; exposure to light; and a diet low in protein, choline, and vitamin B_{12}.[18]

CLINICAL SIGNS

Clinical signs associated with acute aflatoxicosis include anorexia, elevated temperature, increased heart and respiratory rates, ataxia, depression, lethargy, convulsions, icterus, colic and abdominal straining, bloody feces, and death. These signs were exhibited by horses experimentally intoxicated with aflatoxin at dosages of 2 to 5 mg/kg. Onset of signs began as early as 4 hours after dosing, and deaths occurred from 68 hours to 32 days after intoxication.[14,16,17] An additional sign observed in a naturally occurring instance of toxicosis was subcutaneous hemorrhages.[14]

The feed concentration of aflatoxin B1 necessary to cause signs of chronic aflatoxicosis in horses has not been established, and reports of chronic aflatoxicosis were not found in the literature. Signs of chronic aflatoxicosis in other species have included reduced feed efficiency, rough hair coats, anemia, anorexia, depression, mild jaundice, and occasionally abortion.[18] It should be noted that experimental trials have indicated that some horses refuse mold-contaminated grain and well-fleshed animals may be at lesser risk of developing aflatoxicosis than unthrifty animals.[14,16]

PATHOPHYSIOLOGY

The hepatic cytotoxicity of aflatoxins is thought to be related to their binding to intracellular macromolecules. Aflatoxin B1 binds to nuclear DNA to inhibit RNA synthesis, which subsequently inhibits synthesis of intracellular enzymes and other proteins. Aflatoxin also binds to endoplasmic steroidal ribosome-binding sites, resulting in ribosomal disaggregation. Metabolites of aflatoxin B1 also can bind to cellular macromolecules, and most of the cytotoxicity of aflatoxin B1 appears to result from binding of certain of these metabolites rather than from aflatoxin B1 itself. This impairment of protein synthesis and the related ability to mobilize fats is thought to cause the early lesions of hepatic necrosis and fatty degeneration of the liver in aflatoxicosis.[8]

The possibility of other mechanisms being responsible for the other signs and lesions noted with aflatoxicosis has been suggested. Aflatoxins are known to be carcinogenic, they can be immunosuppressive, and they also can inhibit synthesis of clotting proteins. The mechanisms whereby these changes take place have not been well described.[18]

DIAGNOSIS AND TREATMENT

Definitive diagnosis of aflatoxicosis can be difficult because of the nonspecificity of many clinical signs and because the disease can mimic many other conditions. Experimentally intoxicated horses have elevations in serum concentrations of AST, alanine aminotransferase, GGT, iditol dehydrogenase, and arginase.[14,16,17] Other laboratory abnormalities include hypoglycemia, hyperlipidemia, lymphopenia, and elevated PT.[13,14,17]

Gross necropsy lesions typically consist of variable degrees of hepatic degeneration and necrosis, visceral petechial hemorrhages, and hemorrhagic enteritis.[13,14,17] Other lesions noted at necropsy include encephalomalacia of the cerebral hemispheres, myocardial degeneration, fatty infiltration of the kidney, and subcutaneous and intramuscular hemorrhage.[13,14] Histopathologic abnormalities may include fatty degeneration and necrosis of hepatocytes, bile duct hyperplasia, periportal fibrosis, and inflammatory cell infiltration into the liver. Renal lesions have included lipid accumulation in the tubular epithelial cells of the proximal tubules and protein precipitation in the tubular lumen.[13,17]

Although metabolites of *Aspergillus* species fluoresce under ultraviolet light, the presence of fluorescence in suspect feed samples is not pathognomonic for aflatoxin. Aflatoxin can be assayed definitively in feed samples by a variety of analytical methods.[14] It also is possible to quantitate aflatoxin in animal tissues, although this test is not routinely available through diagnostic laboratories.[13,17] Tissue residue testing can come up negative because of the long delay between time of exposure and demise of the patient. Mold culture is nondiagnostic.[18]

Treatment is largely symptomatic and must include removal of the offending feed material, if it still is being fed. An easily digested, low-fat diet containing appropriate protein has been recommended. Multiple vitamin supplementation might be beneficial, and treatment of specific organ dysfunction should be initiated. In acutely intoxicated horses orally administered charcoal has been recommended.[18] Prevention of the condition requires storing feeds in a suitable environment that discourages mold growth and the feeding of noncontaminated feedstuffs.

TOXICOSES CAUSING SIGNS RELATING TO THE URINARY SYSTEM

Detection of renal disease can be difficult, regardless of cause. Whereas nephrotoxicity associated with equine administration of medications is well established and usually recognized, that linked to ingestion of plants is less commonly detected, which makes it more difficult to make a definitive diagnosis. Although heavy metals such as cadmium and mercury have long been known for their nephrotoxic effects, clinical signs are nonspecific, and the diagnosis will be made only if the clinician performs diagnostic tests to specifically rule these problems in or out.

PLANTS

Oxalate Toxicosis

The most common source of oxalates for livestock is plants, particularly those of the Chenopodiaceae family. These plants contain varied amounts of soluble oxalates, usually in the form of sodium or potassium salts. However, because plants containing oxalates (Box 22-3) are generally unpalatable to horses, plant-associated oxalate intoxication is rare.

Of the plants listed in Box 22-3, *Halogeton* and *Sarcobatus* seem to be the primary offenders in range animals in the western United States.[1]

Because oxalates accumulate in the plants throughout the growing season, the incidence of toxicosis may be highest in the fall and winter months.[2] The oxalate content is highest in the leaves, with a lesser amount in seeds and a minimal amount present in the stems. The nonfatal toxic dosage of sodium oxalate for adult horses is approximately 200 g/day for 8 days.[1]

CLINICAL SIGNS

Affected horses may begin to show signs of depression, mild to moderate colic, muscular weakness, and irregular gait 2 to 6 hours after ingestion. Weakness may proceed to lateral recumbency, unconsciousness, and death in 10 to 12 hours. Some animals may exhibit convulsions before succumbing.[1] The observed clinical signs of acute toxicity are typical of those of hypocalcemia.

PATHOPHYSIOLOGY

Oxalates combine with serum calcium ions to form insoluble calcium oxalate. The result is a functional hypocalcemia in acute cases, with associated signs of altered behavior and neuromuscular abnormalities.

BOX 22-3

PLANTS THAT CONTAIN LARGE AMOUNTS OF SOLUBLE OXALATES

Amaranthus spp.	Pigweed
Beta vulgaris	Beet, mangold
Chenopodium album	Lambsquarters
Halogeton glomeratus	Halogeton
Oxalis spp.	Wood sorrel, soursob
Portulaca oleracea	Purslane
Rheum rhaponticum	Rhubarb
Rumex spp.	Sorrel, dock
Salsola kali	Russian thistle
Sarcobatus vermiculatus	Black greasewood

Chronic ingestion of oxalates can result in renal failure. Insoluble calcium oxalate crystals can lodge in the renal tubules, producing tubular blockage and necrosis. Oxalates also may crystallize in the vasculature and infiltrate blood vessel walls, producing necrosis and hemorrhage.[1]

DIAGNOSIS AND TREATMENT

In instances of acute toxicosis, consistent clinicopathologic abnormalities include moderate to significant hypocalcemia and varied electrolyte alterations. In chronic toxicity urinalysis may reveal the presence of characteristic calcium oxalate crystals on microscopic examination. Impending renal failure also is characterized by increases in BUN and creatinine concentrations.[1]

Treatment usually is of little value once clinical signs have appeared. Calcium gluconate can be administered intravenously, but usually it provides only temporary relief of signs. Balanced electrolyte solutions are indicated to aid diuresis, and diuretics also may have benefit in the volume-loaded patient. Prevention primarily entails keeping horses from the plants by providing adequate suitable sources of feed.[1]

SORGHUM

Ingestion of *Sorghum* species and certain hybrid Sudan grasses has been associated with the development of an ataxia-cystitis syndrome.[3,4] The toxicity occurs when horses graze the plants. More cases occur when the plant is young and rapidly growing, but mature and second-growth plants also have been incriminated. Horses being fed well-cured *Sorghum* species hay have not developed signs of toxicity. Occurrence of toxicity may increase during seasons of medium to high rainfall, but no cases have been recognized following the date of the first frost. Signs of toxicity may develop following a grazing period of 1 week to several months.[3]

CLINICAL SIGNS

The primary clinical signs are those of posterior ataxia and urinary incontinence or cystitis. The neurologic signs usually develop first and begin as posterior ataxia and incoordination. Affected horses may sway from side to side if forced to move, and signs tend to worsen on backing the animal. Occasionally, the rearquarters may drop almost to the ground, and flaccid paralysis of the tail and the rear legs may develop within 24 hours of the onset of neurologic signs. Affected horses remain alert and afebrile and have a normal appetite and pulse and respiratory rates. Mares frequently exhibit continual opening and closing of the vulva and relaxation of the perineal muscles. Males typically have a relaxed and extended penis.[3,4]

Urinary incontinence exhibited by continual urine dribbling is prominent in both sexes, and urine scalding on dependent skin becomes pronounced. The urinary bladder typically is distended and atonic, resulting in moderate to severe cystitis. Urethritis and ureteritis also may develop, and in horses that die because of the disease, ascending pyelonephritis usually is the cause of death. Other clinical signs include abortion and birth of foals with arthrogryposis.[3,4]

PATHOPHYSIOLOGY

The clinical signs result from axonal degeneration and demyelination of nerve fibers in the spinal cord, particularly in the lumbar and sacral segments. The toxic substance in *Sorghum* species responsible for causing this change is unknown. Most *Sorghum* species are cyanogenic plants and contain various amounts of HCN. Exposure to multiple sublethal doses of HCN has been suggested to induce axonal degeneration and demyelination.[3] Another hypothesis is that sorghum plants contain lathrogenic precursors and that this toxicosis may be caused by the ingestion of lathrogenic nitriles present in rapidly growing plants.[1,4]

DIAGNOSIS AND TREATMENT

Diagnosis of sorghum ataxia-cystitis is based primarily on approriate clinical signs, history of grazing the plants, and exclusion of other known causes of posterior ataxia or paresis. No specific diagnostic tests are available. Cystitis and pyelonephritis are diagnosed by standard laboratory methods.

No specific treatment is available. The offending feed should be removed immediately. Once the feed is removed, affected horses usually show gradual improvement over several weeks to months, but complete recovery may not occur. Supportive and symptomatic therapy should include appropriate antibiotic treatment of bacterial urinary tract infections and topical treatment of urine scald dermatitis. Periodic manual decompression of the urinary bladder may be helpful. Catheterization and frequent aspiration of bladder contents may be necessary to aid resolution of cystitis.

MISCELLANEOUS AGENTS

VITAMINS D2 AND D3

Horses are capable of meeting their requirement for vitamin D if they are exposed to sunlight or have access to sun-cured forages. Although dietary requirements for the horse have not been established, a maximum safe level of 44 IU per kg of body mass daily has been proposed for long-term feeding (>60 days).[5] Most cases of vitamin D intoxication are iatrogenic, resulting from overzealous use of vitamin supplements or improperly formulated vitamin D–supplemented feeds. Ingestion of *C. diurnum* (wild jasmine) also can result in vitamin D toxicosis because this plant contains a metabolically active glycoside of 1,25-dihydroxycholecalciferol (see the section on wild jasmine [*Cestrum diurnum*]).

Vitamins D_2 (ergocalciferol) and D_3 (cholecalciferol) are potentially toxic, but vitamin D_3 is much more active and results in more severe lesions with wider tissue distribution than does an equivalent dose of vitamin D_2.[6,7] Other variables that may affect toxicosis include duration of treatment and route of administration. High concentrations of dietary calcium also might enhance the effects of excessive amounts of vitamin D. The effect of vitamin D supplementation is cumulative, and signs of toxicity may occur weeks after supplementation has begun.

CLINICAL SIGNS

The clinical signs associated with vitamin D toxicosis are associated with impairment of the renal, cardiovascular, and musculoskeletal systems. Signs may include depression, anorexia, weakness, polyuria and polydipsia, cardiac murmurs and tachycardia, limb stiffness with impaired mobility, and recumbency. Calcification of tendons, ligaments, and other soft tissue structures may be palpable on physical examination.[6] Ultrasonographic examination of these structures also may demonstrate abnormal mineralization within the tissues.

The toxicity of excessive amounts of vitamin D_3 results from extensive dystrophic mineralization rather than from any inherent toxicity of vitamin D itself. Soft tissue sites most frequently affected include the kidneys, the endocardium and walls of large blood vessels, and tendons and ligaments.[6,7]

Laboratory findings associated with toxicosis vary with the organ system affected, but generally include persistent hypercalcemia and hyperphosphatemia, although the latter may not be especially pronounced. Serum calcium concentration may remain within a normal range in some horses. Other laboratory evidence of chronic renal failure may become evident with progression of toxicosis. A definitive diagnosis is made by measuring serum concentrations of vitamins D_2 and D_3 and 1,25-dihydroxycholecalciferol.[7]

TREATMENT

Treatment of vitamin D intoxication should include removal of all exogenous sources of vitamin D. A cation chelator such as sodium phytate may be helpful in reducing intestinal absorption of calcium, but the efficacy of this product has not been determined. If necessary, symptomatic therapy for renal insufficiency and failure should be instituted. Recovery may take months in less severely affected horses,[7] but treatment usually is unrewarding if excessive mineralization has occurred.

Menadione Sodium Bisulfite (Vitamin K3)

Vitamin K_3 is a reported cause of acute renal failure in horses, but the product has been withdrawn from the U.S. market. When the product was given at the manufacturer's recommended dosage of 2.2 to 11 mg/kg intravenously or intramuscularly, signs of toxicity became evident 6 to 48 hours after injection in affected horses.[8] Clinical signs included depression, anorexia, colic, hematuria, and stranguria. Azotemia, electrolyte abnormalities, proteinuria, and isosthenuria also were apparent. Pathologic lesions noted at necropsy were those of acute tubular necrosis. Interstitial fibrosis and chronic renal failure also were present in one horse.[8] Treatment of affected horses is symptomatic for acute or chronic renal failure.

Cadmium

Intoxication with cadmium rarely is reported in horses but has been seen in animals raised near smelting operations.[9] Environmental contamination of soil and forage by cadmium and zinc was the cause of excessive intake.

Affected horses exhibited signs of unthriftiness, lameness, and swollen joints. Some of these signs were attributed to excess zinc in the diet, but the horses also had pronounced osteoporosis and nephrocalcinosis, which along with proteinuria are typical findings of cadmium toxicosis in human beings.[9]

Serum concentrations of zinc and potassium were elevated in these horses, and the serum magnesium concentration was low in one foal. Sodium, calcium, chloride, and bicarbonate concentrations also were decreased. Extensive nephrocalcinosis was characterized by multifocal loss of cortical tubules, which were replaced by dense deposits of calcium phosphate crystals.

Cadmium induces changes in proximal renal tubular cells by an unknown mechanism. However, increased numbers of lysosomes and mitochondrial swelling in the proximal tubular cells are early changes. Proteinuria usually is the first abnormality noted in human beings and laboratory animals. With continued chronic exposure, fibrosis and atrophy resulting from interstitial nephritis may ensue, leading to chronic renal failure.[10] Cadmium exposure can be confirmed by analyzing blood and various biologic tissues, including liver and kidney.

In human beings treatment essentially is supportive, with elimination of exposure to cadmium being imperative. Research data suggest a possible beneficial role of zinc, vitamin B complex, and nickel preparations, but their clinical efficacy is unproven.[10]

Mercury

Mercury exists in a variety of organic and inorganic forms. Both forms can be toxic to horses, but more recently reported cases involve acute toxicity resulting from inorganic mercury-containing blistering agents topically applied to skin.[11,12] Ingestion of feed or seed grain contaminated with organic mercurial seed preservatives has been a source of contamination in previous years.

Acute and chronic forms of toxicosis can occur in horses. The acute toxic dose of inorganic mercury in adults is 5 to 10 g.[1] Experimentally, chronic toxicity from inorganic mercury has been produced by ingestion of mercuric chloride, 0.8 mg/kg/day, over a 14-week period.[13] Chronic organic mercury toxicosis also has been produced experimentally by feeding methylmercury at 0.4 mg/kg/day for 10 weeks.[14]

CLINICAL SIGNS

Signs associated with toxicity of the various mercurial compounds differ, but they all include some degree of renal dysfunction. Acute toxicity resulting from inorganic mercury can cause signs of acute renal failure, including oliguria and depression, and signs of gastrointestinal irritation. Ulcerative stomatitis, excessive salivation, colic, and diarrhea are common findings associated with gastrointestinal tract disturbances.[11,12] Chronic intoxication with inorganic mercury can result in signs of oral ulceration, reduced appetite and weight loss, alopecia, progressive respiratory difficulty, gradually increasing urine production, and terminal azotemia.[13] Signs reported with chronic organic mercury toxicity include development of neurologic dysfunction characterized by proprioceptive deficits, exudative dermatitis, reluctance to move, reduced appetite and weight loss, dullness, and renal changes exhibited by a steadily increasing BUN concentration and glucosuria.[14]

PATHOPHYSIOLOGY

Inorganic mercury compounds are absorbed from the lungs and gastrointestinal tract and absorbed poorly through the skin. After ingestion and absorption, accumulation in the liver and particularly the kidney occurs. Some forms of organic mercury are degraded in the body to inorganic forms, which then also accumulate in the kidney before excretion.[1]

Inorganic mercury is concentrated to high levels within the proximal renal tubular cells. Metallothionein, a low-molecular-weight metal-binding protein is synthesized within 48 hours after exposure to heavy metals. This protein binds mercuric ions within the endoplasmic reticulum of the tubular epithelial cells and then slowly releases mercury. This slow release of sequestered mercury can cause continuing damage to tubular cells after the source of mercury is removed.[15] Hence the development of mercury nephropathy appears to be a function of the amount of protein-bound mercury concentrated in the renal tubules. Bound mercury can persist in the kidneys for several weeks after exposure.[250] Acute toxicity results in massive tubular necrosis and acute renal failure, and chronic exposure may cause renal interstitial fibrosis leading to chronic renal failure.

Methylmercury can be biotransformed in the body to inorganic mercury, but methylmercury also accumulates in the brain to a much greater extent than do other forms of mercury.[1] The exact mechanism whereby methylmercury and other alkylmercurials damage the nervous system is not understood.[14]

At the cellular level mercury combines with sulfhydryl groups within cells. As a result, sulfhydryl enzyme systems essential to cellular metabolism and respiration are inhibited, resulting in cell death.

DIAGNOSIS AND TREATMENT

Mercury intoxication is suspected when horses show compatible clinical signs and have a history of exposure. Laboratory abnormalities are similar to those of other causes of acute or chronic renal failure and irritative gastrointestinal diseases. Definitive diagnosis usually is based on measurement of mercury concentrations in blood, kidney, and liver.[1] Stomach and intestine samples also may be submitted for analysis in acute cases.

Treatment of mercury intoxication initially involves removal of the source. In acute toxicity evacuation of the bowel with a mild laxative may be helpful. The oral administration of 500 g of activated charcoal might help block absorption of mercury, but its efficacy has not been demonstrated. Dimercaprol (used to inactivate circulating mercury) can be given at a dosage of 3 mg/kg intramuscularly every 4 hours for the first 2 days, 4 times on the third day, and twice daily for the next 10 days until recovery is complete.[11] The clinician also should follow other principles of therapy for acute or chronic renal failure. Treatment of chronic mercury intoxication usually is unrewarding.

REFERENCES

Toxicoses Displaying Signs Relating to the Gastrointestinal System

1. Anderson GA, Mount ME, Vrins AA, et al: Fatal acorn poisoning in a horse: pathologic findings and diagnostic considerations, *J Am Vet Med Assoc* 182:1105-1110, 1983.
2. Smith BP, editor: *Large animal internal medicine*, ed 4, St Louis, 2009, Mosby.
3. Robinson NE, editor: *Current therapy in equine medicine*, ed 6, St Louis, 2009, Saunders.
4. McCunn J: Castor bean poisoning in horses, *Vet J* 101:136, 1945.
5. Rauber A, Heard J: Castor bean toxicity re-examined: a new perspective, *Vet Hum Toxicol* 27:498-502, 1985.
6. Albretsen JC, Gwaltney-Brant SM, Khan SA: Evaluation of castor bean toxicosis in dogs: 98 cases, *J Am Anim Hosp Assoc* 36:229-233, 2000.
7. Gilman AG, Rall TW, Nies AS, et al: *Goodman and Gilman's the pharmacological basis of therapeutics*, ed 8, Elmsford, NY, 1990, Pergamon Press.
8. Ellenhorn MJ, Schonwald S, Ordog G, et al: *Ellenhorn's medical toxicology: diagnosis and treatment of human poisoning*, ed 2, Philadelphia, 1997, Lippincott Williams & Wilkins.
9. Hart CR, Garland T, Barr AC, et al: *Toxic plants of Texas, College Station, Texas, Texas Agricultural Extension Service*, 2001, Texas A&M University System.
10. Knight AP, Walter RG: *A guide to plant poisoning of animals in North America*, Jackson, Wyo, 2001, Teton NewMedia.
11. Garland T, Barr AC, editors: *Toxic plants and other natural toxicants*, New York, 1998, CAB International.
12. Schulman ML, Bolton LA: Datura seed intoxication in two horses, *J S Afr Vet Assoc* 69:27-29, 1998.
13. Moffatt RE, Kramer LL, Lerner D, et al: Studies on dioctyl sodium sulfosuccinate toxicity: clinical, gross and microscopic pathology in the horse and guinea pig, *Can J Comp Med* 39:434-441, 1975.
14. Osweiler GD, Carson TL, Buck WB, et al: *Clinical and diagnostic veterinary toxicology*, ed 3, Dubuque, Iowa, 1985, Kendall/Hunt.
15. Riviere JE, Papich MG, editors: *Veterinary pharmacology and therapeutics*, ed 9, Philadelphia, 2010, Wiley-Blackwell.
16. Pace LW, Turnquist SE, Casteel SW, et al: Acute arsenic toxicosis in five horses, *Vet Pathol* 34:160-164, 1997.
17. Fogarty U, Perl D, Good BS, et al: A cluster of equine granulomatous enteritis cases: the link with aluminum, *Vet Hum Toxicol* 40(5):297-305, 1998.
18. Garcia-Patos V, Pujol RM, Alomar A, et al: Persistent subcutaneous nodules in patients hypersensitized with aluminum-containing allergen extracts, *Arch Dermatol* 131:1421-1424, 1995.
19. Sockett DC, Baker JC, Stowe CM: Slaframine (Rhizoctonia leguminicola) intoxication in horses, *J Am Vet Med Assoc* 181:606, 1982.
20. Exon JH: A review of chlorinated phenols, *Vet Hum Toxicol* 26:508-520, 1984.
21. Russel SH, Monin T, Edwards WC: Rodenticide toxicosis in a horse, *J Am Vet Med Assoc* 172:270-271, 1978.
22. Peoples SA, Maddy KT: Poisoning of man and animals due to ingestion of the rodent poison, vacor, *Vet Hum Toxicol* 21:266-268, 1979.
23. Kimbrough RD, Carter CD, Liddle JA, et al: Epidemiology and pathology of a tetrachlorodibenzodioxin poisoning episode, *Arch Environ Health* 32:77-86, 1977.
24. Schmitz DG: Cantharidin toxicosis in horses, *J Vet Intern Med* 3:208-215, 1989.
25. Schoeb TR, Panciera RJ: Blister beetle poisoning in horses, *J Am Vet Med Assoc* 173:75-77, 1978.
26. Ray AC, Kyle ALG, Murphy MJ, et al: Etiologic agents, incidence, and improved diagnostic methods of cantharidin toxicosis in horses, *Am J Vet Res* 50:187-191, 1989.

Toxicoses Causing Signs of Centeral Nervous System Stimulation

1. James LF, Hartley WJ, Van Kampen KR: Syndromes of Astragalus poisoning in livestock, *J Am Vet Med Assoc* 178:146-150, 1981.
2. Knight AP: Locoweed poisoning, *Compend Cont Educ Pract Vet* 9:F418, 1987.
3. McIlwraith CW, James LF: Limb deformities in foals associated with ingestion of locoweed by mares, *J Am Vet Med Assoc* 181:255-258, 1982.
4. Burfening PJ: Ergotism, *J Am Vet Med Assoc* 163:1288-1290, 1973.
5. Hintz HF: Ergotism, *Equine Pract* 10:6, 1988.
6. Wyllie TD, editor: *Mycotoxic fungi, mycotoxins, mycotoxicoses*, New York, 1978, LG Moorehouse.
7. Ellenhorn MJ, Schonwald S, Ordog G, et al: *Ellenhorn's medical toxicology: diagnosis and treatment of human poisoning*, ed 2, Philadelphia, 1997, Lippincott Williams & Wilkins.

8. Osweiler GD, Carson TL, Buck WB, et al: *Clinical and diagnostic veterinary toxicology*, ed 3, Dubuque, Iowa, 1985, Kendall/Hunt.
9. Zin LL, Edwards WC: Toxicity of blue-green algae in livestock, *Bovine Pract* 14:151, 1979.
10. Steyn PS, Vleggaar R, editors: *Mycotoxins and phycotoxins: a collection of invited papers presented at the sixth International IUPAC Symposium on Mycotoxins and Phycotoxins*, Amsterdam, 1986, Elsevier Science.
11. Riviere JE, Papich MG, editors: *Veterinary pharmacology and therapeutics*, ed 9, Philadelphia, 2010, Wiley-Blackwell.
12. Smith BP, editor: *Large animal internal medicine*, ed 4, St Louis, 2009, Mosby.
13. Lilley CW: Strychnine poisoning in a horse, *Equine Pract* 7:7, 1985.
14. Sutherland C: Metaldehyde poisoning in horses, *Vet Rec* 112:64-65, 1983.
15. Harris WF: Metaldehyde poisoning in three horses, *Mod Vet Pract* 56:336-337, 1975.
16. Edwards HG: Methiocarb poisoning in a horse, *Vet Rec* 119:556, 1986.
17. Alexander KA: Methiocarb poisoning in a horse, *Vet Rec* 120:47, 1987.
18. Ray AC, Dwyer JN, Fambro GW, et al: Clinical signs and chemical confirmation of 4-aminopyridine poisoning in horses, *Am J Vet Res* 39:329-331, 1978.
19. Kitzman JV, Wilson RC, Hatch RC, et al: Antagonism of xylazine and ketamine anesthesia by 4-aminopyridine and yohimbine in geldings, *Am J Vet Res* 45:875-879, 1984.
20. Drudge JH, Lyons ET, Swerczek TW: Critical tests and safety studies on a levamisole-piperazine mixture as an anthelmintic in the horse, *Am J Vet Res* 35:67-72, 1974.
21. DiPietro JA, Todd KS: Anthelmintics used in treatment of parasitic infections of horses, *Vet Clin North Am Equine Pract* 3:1-14, 1987.
22. Marriner S: Anthelmintic drugs, *Vet Rec* 118:181-184, 1986.
23. Glenn MW, Burr WM: Toxicity of a piperazine-carbon disulfide-phenothiazine preparation in the horse, *J Am Vet Med Assoc* 160:988-992, 1972.
24. Morris DD, Henry MM: Hepatic encephalopathy, *Compend Cont Educ Pract Vet* 13:1153, 1991.

Toxicoses Causing Signs Relating to Central Nervous System Depression

1. Robinson NE, editor: *Current therapy in equine medicine*, ed 6, St Louis, 2009, Saunders.
2. Smith BP, editor: *Large animal internal medicine*, ed 4, St Louis, 2009, Saunders.
3. Fleischmann G, Rudiger H: Isolation, resolution and partial characterization of two Robinia pseudoacacia seed lectins, *Biol Chem Hoppe Seyler* 367:27-32, 1986.
4. Kelleway RA, Geovjian L: Acute bracken fern poisoning in a 14-month-old horse, *Vet Med Small Anim Clin* 73:295-296, 1978.
5. Hintz HF: Bracken fern, *Equine Pract* 12:6, 1990.
6. Sperry OE, Dollahite JW, Hoffman GO, et al: Texas plants poisonous to livestock, Texas Agricultural Experiment Station Pub No B-1028, College Station, Texas, Agricultural Extension Service.
7. Farrell RK, Sande RD, Lincoln SD: Nigropallidal encephalomalacia in a horse, *J Am Vet Med Assoc* 158:1201-1204, 1971.
8. Young S, Brown WW, Klinger B: Nigropallidal encephalomalacia in horses caused by ingestion of weeds of the genus Centaurea, *J Am Vet Med Assoc* 157:1602-1605, 1970.
9. Mettler FA, Stern GM: Observations on the toxic effects of yellow star thistle, *J Neuropathol Exp Neurol* 22:164-169, 1963.
10. Cordy DR: Nigropallidal encephalomalacia in horses associated with ingestion of yellow star thistle, *J Neuropathol Exp Neurol* 13:330-342, 1954.
11. Stevens KL, Wong RY: Structure of chlororepdiolide, a new sesquiterpene lactone from Centaurea repens, *J Nat Prod* 49:833, 1986.
12. Sanders SG, Tucker RL, Bagley RS, et al: Magnetic resonance imaging features of equine nigropallidal encephalomalacia, *Vet Radiol Ultrasound* 42:291-296, 2001.
13. James LF, Hartley WJ, Van Kampen KR: Syndromes of Astragalus poisoning in livestock, *J Am Vet Med Assoc* 178:146-150, 1981.
14. Dorman DC, Haschek WM: Fatal propylene glycol toxicosis in a horse, *J Am Vet Med Assoc* 198:1643-1644, 1991.
15. Myers VS, Usenik EA: Propylene glycol intoxication of horses, *J Am Vet Med Assoc* 155:1841, 1969.
16. Ellenhorn MJ, Schonwald S, Ordog G, et al: *Ellenhorn's medical toxicology: diagnosis and treatment of human poisoning*, ed 2, Philadelphia, 1997, Lippincott Williams & Wilkins.
17. Osweiler GD: Toxicology of triclopyr herbicide in the equine, *Proc Am Assoc Vet Lab Diagn* 26:193, 1983.
18. Whisenant SG, McArthur ED: Triclopyr persistence in northern Idaho forest vegetation, *Bull Environ Contam Toxicol* 42:660, 1989.
19. Buck WB, Haliburton JC, Thilsted JP, et al: Equine encephalomalacia: comparative pathology of naturally occurring and experimental cases, *Proc Am Assoc Vet Lab Diagn* 22:239, 1979.
20. McCue PM: Equine leukoencephalomalacia, *Compend Cont Educ Pract Vet* 11:646, 1989.
21. Marasas WFO, Kellerman TS, Gelderblom WCA, et al: Leukoencephalomalacia in a horse induced by fumonisin B1 isolated from Fusarium moniliforme, *Onderstepoort J Vet Res* 55:197-203, 1988.
22. Wilson TM, Ross PF, Rice LG, et al: Fumonisin B1 levels associated with an epizootic of equine leukoencephalomalacia, *J Vet Diagn Invest* 2:213-216, 1990.
23. Ross PF, Rice LG, Reagor JC, et al: Fumonisin B1 concentrations in feeds from 45 confirmed equine leukoencephalomalacia cases, *J Vet Diagn Invest* 3:238-241, 1991.
24. Brownie CF, Cullen J: Characterization of experimentally induced equine leukoencephalomalacia (ELEM) in ponies (Equus caballus): preliminary report, *Vet Hum Toxicol* 29:34-38, 1987.
25. Riviere JE, Papich MG, editors: *Veterinary pharmacology and therapeutics*, ed 9, Philadelphia, 2010, Wiley-Blackwell.
26. Gabal MA, Awad YL, Morcos MB, et al: Fusariotoxicoses of farm animals and mycotoxic leucoencephalomalacia of the equine associated with the finding of trichothecenes in feedstuffs, *Vet Hum Toxicol* 28:207-212, 1986.
27. Burrows GE: Lead poisoning in the horse, *Equine Pract* 4:30, 1982.
28. Burrows GE, Borchard RE: Experimental lead toxicosis in ponies: comparison of the effects of smelter effluent–contaminated hay and lead acetate, *Am J Vet Res* 43:2129-2133, 1982.
29. Kowalczyk DF, Naylor JM, Gunson D: The value of zinc protoporphyrin in equine lead poisoning: a case report, *Vet Hum Toxicol* 23:12-15, 1981.

Toxicoses Causing Signs Relating to the Cardiovascular and Hemolymphatic Systems

1. Knight AP: Oleander poisoning, *Compend Cont Educ Pract Vet* 10:262, 1988.
2. Oleander poisoning in equines, *J R Army Vet Corps* 42:8, 1971.
3. Robinson NE, editor: *Current therapy in equine medicine*, ed 6, St Louis, 2009, Saunders.
4. Smith BP, editor: *Large animal internal medicine*, ed 4, St Louis, 2009, Mosby.
5. Ellenhorn MJ, Schonwald S, Ordog G, et al: *Ellenhorn's medical toxicology: diagnosis and treatment of human poisoning*, ed 2, Philadelphia, 1997, Lippincott Williams & Wilkins.

6. Olson CT, Keller WC, Gerken DF, et al: Suspected tremetol poisoning in horses, *J Am Vet Med Assoc* 185:1001, 1984.
7. Riviere JE, Papich MG, editors: *Veterinary pharmacology and therapeutics*, ed 9, Philadelphia, 2010, Wiley-Blackwell.
8. Smetzer DL, Coppock RW, Ely RW, et al: Cardiac effects of white snakeroot intoxication in horses, *Equine Pract* 5:26, 1983.
9. Tennant B, Dill SG, Glickman LT, et al: Acute hemolytic anemia, methemoglobinemia, and Heinz body formation associated with ingestion of red maple leaves by horses, *J Am Vet Med Assoc* 179:143-150, 1981.
10. Divers TJ, George LW, George JW: Hemolytic anemia in horses after the ingestion of red maple leaves, *J Am Vet Med Assoc* 180:300-302, 1982.
11. George LW, Divers TJ, Mahaffey EA, et al: Heinz body anemia and methemoglobinemia in ponies given red maple (Acer rubrum L.) leaves, *Vet Pathol* 19:521-523, 1982.
12. Plumlee KH: Red maple toxicity in a horse, *Vet Hum Toxicol* 33:66-67, 1991.
13. Weber M, Miller RE: Presumptive red maple (Acer rubrum) toxicosis in Grevy's zebra (Equus greyvi), *J Zoo Wildl Med* 28:105-108, 1997.
14. Corriher CA, Parviainen AKJ, Gibbons DS, et al: Equine red maple leg toxicosis, *Compend Cont Educ Pract Vet* 21:74-80, 1999.
15. Pierce KR, Joyce JR, England RB, et al: Acute hemolytic anemia caused by wild onion poisoning in horse, *J Am Vet Med Assoc* 160:323-327, 1972.
16. Hutchison TWS: Onion toxicosis, *J Am Vet Med Assoc* 172:1440, 1978.
17. Vrins A, Carlson G, Feldman B: Warfarin: a review with emphasis on its use in the horse, *Can Vet J* 24:211-213, 1983.
18. Scott EA, Byars TD, Lamar AM: Warfarin anticoagulation in the horse, *J Am Vet Med Assoc* 177:1146-1151, 1980.
19. McConnico RS, Copedge K, Bischoff KL: Brodifacoum toxicosis in two horses, *J Am Vet Med Assoc* 211:882-886, 1997.
20. Osweiler GD, Carson TL, Buck WB, et al: *Clinical and diagnostic veterinary toxicology*, ed 3, Dubuque, Iowa, 1985, Kendall/Hunt.
21. Boermans HJ, Johnstone I, Black WD, et al: Clinical signs, laboratory changes and toxicokinetics of brodifacoum in the horse, *Can J Vet Res* :21-27, 1991.
22. Thijssen HHW, van den Bogaard AEJM, Wetzel JM, et al: Warfarin pharmacokinetics in the horse, *Am J Vet Res* 44:1192-1196, 1983.
23. Byars TD, Greene CE, Kemp DT: Antidotal effect of vitamin K_1 against warfarin-induced anticoagulation in horses, *Am J Vet Res* 47:2309-2312, 1986.
24. Mount ME, Feldman BF, Buffington T: Vitamin K and its therapeutic importance, *J Am Vet Med Assoc* 180:1354-1356, 1982.
25. Alsup EM, DeBowes RM: Dimethyl sulfoxide, *J Am Vet Med Assoc* 185:1011-1014, 1984.
26. Blythe LL, Craig AM, Appell LH, et al: Intravenous use of dimethyl sulfoxide (DMSO) in horses: clinical and physiologic effects, *Proc Am Assoc Equine Pract* 32:441-446, 1986.
27. Brayton CF: Dimethyl sulfoxide (DMSO): a review, *Cornell Vet* 76:61-90, 1986.
28. Blythe LL, Craig AM, Christensen JM, et al: Pharmacokinetic disposition of dimethyl sulfoxide administered intravenously to horses, *Am J Vet Res* 47:1739-1743, 1986.
29. Schuh JCL, Ross C, Meschter C: Concurrent mercuric blister and dimethyl sulfoxide (DMSO) application as a cause of mercury toxicity in two horses, *Equine Vet J* 20:68-71, 1988.
30. Hartsfield SM, Thurmon JC, Benson GJ: Sodium bicarbonate and bicarbonate precursors for treatment of metabolic acidosis, *J Am Vet Med Assoc* 179:914-916, 1981.
31. Lawrence L, Kline K, Miller-Graber P, et al: Effect of sodium bicarbonate on racing standardbreds, *J Anim Sci* 68:673, 1990.
32. Freestone JF, Carlson GP, Harrold DR, et al: Furosemide and sodium bicarbonate–induced alkalosis in the horse and response to oral KCl or NaCl therapy, *Am J Vet Res* 50:1334-1339, 1989.
33. Posner JB, Swanson AG, Plum F: Acid-base balance in cerebrospinal fluid, *Arch Neurol* 12:479-496, 1965.
34. Rumbaugh GE, Carlson GP, Harrold D: Clinicopathologic effects of rapid infusion of 5% sodium bicarbonate in 5% dextrose in the horse, *J Am Vet Med Assoc* 178:267-271, 1981.
35. Amend JF, Mallon FM, Wren WB, et al: Equine monensin toxicosis: some experimental clinicopathologic observations, *Compend Cont Educ Pract Vet* 11:S173, 1980.
36. Matsuoka T: Evaluation of monensin toxicity in the horse, *J Am Vet Med Assoc* 169:1098-1100, 1976.
37. Blomme EAG, La Perle KMD, Wilkins PA, et al: Ionophore toxicity in horses, *Equine Vet Educ* 11:153-158, 1999.
38. Bila CG, Perreira CL, Gruys E: Accidental monensin toxicosis in horses in Mozambique, *J S Afr Vet Assoc* 72:163-164, 2001.
39. Mollenhauer HH, Rowe LD, Cysewski SJ, et al: Ultrastructural observations in ponies after treatment with monensin, *Am J Vet Res* 42:35-40, 1981.
40. Hanson LJ, Eisenbeis HG, Givens SV: Toxic effects of lasalocid in horses, *Am J Vet Res* 42:456-461, 1981.
41. Rollinson J, Taylor FGR, Chesney J: Salinomycin poisoning in horses, *Vet Rec* 121:126-128, 1987.
42. Schneider NR, Yeary RA: Nitrite and nitrate pharmacokinetics in the dog, sheep, and pony, *Am J Vet Res* 36:941-947, 1975.
43. Kingsbury JM: *Poisonous plants of the United States and Canada*, Englewood Cliffs, NJ, 1964, Prentice-Hall.
44. Baggot JD, Davis LE: Plasma protein binding of digitoxin and digoxin in several mammalian species, *Res Vet Sci* 15:81-87, 1973.

Toxicoses Causing Signs Relating to the Epithelium, Skeletal System, and General Body Condition

1. Ralston SL, Rich VA: Black walnut toxicosis in horses, *J Am Vet Med Assoc* 183:1095, 1983.
2. Uhlinger C: Black walnut toxicosis in ten horses, *J Am Vet Med Assoc* 195:343-344, 1989.
3. Minnick PD, Brown CM, Braselton WE, et al: The induction of equine laminitis with an aqueous extract of the heartwood of black walnut (Juglans nigra), *Vet Hum Toxicol* 29:230-233, 1987.
4. Galey FD, Beasley VR, Schaeffer D, et al: Effect of an aqueous extract of black walnut (Juglans nigra) on isolated equine digital vessels, *Am J Vet Res* 51:83-88, 1990.
5. Krook L, Wasserman RH, Shively JN, et al: Hypercalcemia and calcinosis in Florida horses: implication of the shrub, Cestrum diurnum, as the causative agent, *Cornell Vet* 65:26-56, 1975.
6. Keeler RF, Van Kampen KR, James LF, editors: *Effects of poisonous plants on livestock*, New York, 1978, Academic Press.
7. Hughes MR, McCain TA, Chang SY, et al: Presence of 1,25-dihydroxy-vitamin D_3-glycoside in the calcinogenic plant Cestrum diurnum, *Nature* 268:347-349, 1977.
8. Anderson CA, Divers TJ: Systemic granulomatous inflammation in a horse grazing hairy vetch, *J Am Vet Med Assoc* 183:569-570, 1983.
9. Smith BP, editor: *Large animal internal medicine*, ed 4, St Louis, 2009, Mosby.
10. Osweiler GD, Carson TL, Buck WB, et al: *Clinical and diagnostic veterinary toxicology*, ed 3, Dubuque, Iowa, 1985, Kendall/Hunt.
11. Kingsbury JM: *Poisonous plants of the United States and Canada*, Englewood Cliffs, NJ, 1964, Prentice-Hall.
12. Johnson AE: Toxicologic aspects of photosensitization in livestock, *J Natl Cancer Inst* 69:253-258, 1982.
13. Riviere JE, Papich MG, editors: *Veterinary pharmacology and therapeutics*, ed 9, Philadelphia, 2010, Wiley-Blackwell.

14. Glenn AE, Bacon CW, Price R, et al: Molecular phylogeny of Acromonium and its taxonomic implications, *Mycologia* 88:369-383, 1996.
15. Putnam MR, Bransby DI, Schumacher J, et al: Effects of the fungal endophyte Acremonium coenophialum in fescue on pregnant mares and foal viability, *Am J Vet Res* 52:2071-2074, 1991.
16. Blodgett DJ: Fescue toxicosis, *Vet Clin North Am Equine Pract* 17(3):567-577, 2001.
17. Poppenga RH, Mostrom MS, Haschek WM, et al: Mare agalactia, placental thickening, and high foal mortality associated with the grazing of tall fescue: a case report. In *Proceedings of the twenty-seventh annual meeting of the American Association of Veterinary Laboratory Diagnosticians*, Fort Worth, 1984, Texas, pp 325-336.
18. Boosinger TM, Brendemuehl JP, Bransby DL, et al: Prolonged gestation, decreased triiodothyronine concentration, and thyroid gland histomorphologic features in newborn foals of mares grazing Acremonium coenophialum-infected fescue, *Am J Vet Res* 56:66-69, 1995.
19. Ellison SP: Possible toxicity caused by hoary alyssum (Berteroa incana), *Vet Med* 87(5):472-475, 1992.
20. Goer RJ, Becker RL, Kanara EW, et al: Toxicosis in horses after ingestion of hoary alyssum, *J Am Vet Med Assoc* 201(1):63-67, 1992.
21. Hovda LR, Rose ML: Hoary alyssum (Berteroa incana) toxicity in a herd of broodmard horses, *Vet Hum Toxicol* 35(1):39-40, 1993.
22. Kanara EW, Murphy MJ: Ingestion of hoary alyssum as a cause of laminitis in horses. In *Proceedings of the thirteenth annual meeting of the American College of Veterinary Internal Medicine,* Lake Buena Vista, Fla, 1995, pp 571-573.
23. Stowe CM: Iodine, iodides, and iodism, *J Am Vet Med Assoc* 179:334-336, 1981.
24. Fadok VA, Wild S: Suspected cutaneous iodism in a horse, *J Am Vet Med Assoc* 183:1104-1106, 1983.
25. Schwink AL: Toxicology of ethylenediamine dihydriodide, *J Am Vet Med Assoc* 178:996-997, 1981.
26. Ellenhorn MJ, Schonwald S, Ordog G, et al: *Ellenhorn's medical toxicology: diagnosis and treatment of human poisoning*, ed 2, Philadelphia, 1997, Lippincott Williams & Wilkins.
27. Dickinson CE, Traub-Gargatz JL, Dargatz DA, et al: Rattlesnake venom poisoning in horses: 32 cases (1973-1993), *J Am Vet Med Assoc* 208:1866-1871, 1996.
28. Stewart KA, Genetzky RM: Odontodysplasia in a horse, *Mod Vet Pract* 65:87, 1984.
29. Gunson DE, Kowalczyk DF, Shoop CR, et al: Environmental zinc and cadmium pollution associated with generalized osteochondrosis, osteoporosis, and nephrocalcinosis in horses, *J Am Vet Med Assoc* 180:295-299, 1982.
30. Messer NT: Tibiotarsal effusioin associated with chronic zinc intoxication in three horses, *J Am Vet Med Assoc* 178:294-297, 1981.
31. Willoughby RA, MacDonald E, McSherry BJ, et al: Lead and zinc poisoning and the interaction between Pb and Zn poisoning in the foal, *Can J Comp Med* 36:348-359, 1972.
32. Bridges CH, Moffitt PG: Influence of variable content of dietary zinc on copper metabolism of weanling foals, *Am J Vet Res* 51:275-280, 1990.
33. Ringenberg QS, Doll DC, Patterson WP, et al: Hematologic effects of heavy metal poisoning, *South Med J* 81:1132-1139, 1988.
34. Ruckebusch Y, Toutain PL, Koritz GD, editors: *Veterinary pharmacology and toxicology*, Lancaster, England, 1983, MTP Press.
35. Hultine JD, Mount ME, Easley KJ, et al: Selenium toxicosis in the horse, *Equine Pract* 1:57, 1979.
36. Crinion RAP, O'Connor JP: Selenium intoxication in horses, *Ir Vet J* 32:81, 1978.
37. Traub-Dargatz JL, Knight AP, Hamar DW: Selenium toxicity in horses, *Compend Cont Educ Pract Vet* 8:771, 1986.
38. Dewes HF, Lowe MD: Suspected selenium poisoning in a horse, *N Z Vet J* 35:53-54, 1987.
39. Stowe HD: Effects of copper pretreatment upon the toxicity of selenium in ponies, *Am J Vet Res* 41:1925-1928, 1980.
40. James LF, Van Kampen KV, Hartley WJ: Astragalus fisulcatus: a cause of selenium or locoweed poisoning, *Vet Hum Toxicol* 25:86-89, 1983.
41. Painter EP: The chemistry and toxicity of selenium compounds, with special reference to the selenium problem, *Chem Rev* 28:179, 1941.
42. Sellers EA, Vou RW, Lucas CC: Lipotropic agents in liver damage produced by selenium or carbon tetrachloride, *Proc Soc Exp Biol Med* 75:118-121, 1950.

Toxicoses Causing Signs Relating to Liver Disease or Dysfunction

1. Smith BP, editor: *Large animal internal medicine*, ed 4, St Louis, 2009, Mosby.
2. Knight AP, Kimberling CV, Stermitz FR, et al: Cynoglossum officinale (hound's-tongue): a cause of pyrrolizidine alkaloid poisoning in horses, *J Am Vet Med Assoc* 185:647-650, 1984.
3. Giles CJ: Outbreak of ragwort (Senecio jacobea) poisoning in horses, *Equine Vet J* 15:248-250, 1983.
4. Pearson EG: Liver failure attributable to pyrrolizidine alkaloid toxicosis and associated with inspiratory dyspnea in ponies: three cases (1982-1988), *J Am Vet Med Assoc* 198:1651-1654, 1991.
5. Lessard P, Wilson WD, Olander HJ, et al: Clinicopathologic study of horses surviving pyrrolizidine alkaloid (Senecio vulgaris) toxicosis, *Am J Vet Res* 47:1776-1780, 1986.
6. Gulick BA, Liu IKM, Qualls CW, et al: Effect of pyrrolizidine alkaloid-induced hepatic disease on plasma amino acid patterns in the horse, *Am J Vet Res* 41:1894-1898, 1980.
7. Frazier K, Liggett A, Hines M, et al: Mushroom toxicity in a horse with meningioangiomatosis, *Vet Hum Toxicol* 42(3): 166-167, 2000.
8. Osweiler GD, Carson TL, Buck WB, et al: *Clinical and diagnostic veterinary toxicology*, ed 3, Dubuque, Iowa, 1985, Kendall/Hunt.
9. Divers TJ, Warner A, Vaala WE, et al: Toxic hepatic failure in newborn foals, *J Am Vet Med Assoc* 183:1407, 1983.
10. Arnbjerg J: Poisoning in animals due to oral application of iron with description of a case in a horse, *Nord Vet Med* 33:71, 1981.
11. Ellenhorn MJ, Schonwald S, Ordog G, et al: *Ellenhorn's medical toxicology: diagnosis and treatment of human poisoning*, ed 2, Philadelphia, 1997, Lippincott Williams & Wilkins.
12. Hershko C: Mechanism of iron toxicity and its possible role in red cell membrane damage, *Semin Hematol* 26:277-285, 1989.
13. Angsubhakorn S, Poomvises P, Romruen K, et al: Aflatoxicosis in horses, *J Am Vet Med Assoc* 178:274-278, 1981.
14. Asquith RL, Edds GT: Investigations in equine aflatoxicosis, *Proc Am Assoc Equine Pract* 26:193-200, 1980.
15. Greene HJ, Oehme FW: A possible case of equine aflatoxicosis, *Vet Toxicol* 17:76, 1975.
16. Aller WW, Edds GT, Asquith RL: Effects of aflatoxins in young ponies, *Am J Vet Res* 42:2162-2164, 1981.
17. Bortell R, Asquith RL, Edds GT, et al: Acute experimentally induced aflatoxicosis in the weanling pony, *Am J Vet Res* 44:2110-2114, 1983.
18. Riviere JE, Papich MG, editors: *Veterinary pharmacology and therapeutics*, ed 9, Philadelphia, 2010, Wiley-Blackwell.

Toxicoses Causing Signs Relating to the Urinary System

1. Osweiler GD, Carson TL, Buck WB, et al: *Clinical and diagnostic veterinary toxicology*, ed 3, Dubuque, Iowa, 1985, Kendall/Hunt.
2. Hulbert LC, Oehme FW: *Plants poisonous to livestock*, ed 3, Manhattan, Kan, 1968, Kansas State University.

3. Adams LG, Dollahite JW, Romane WM, et al: Cystitis and ataxia associated with sorghum ingestion by horses, *J Am Vet Med Assoc* 155:518-524, 1969.
4. Van Kampen KR: Sudan grass and sorghum poisoning of horses: a possible lathyrogenic disease, *J Am Vet Med Assoc* 156:629-630, 1970.
5. Nutrient requirements of horses, Washington, DC, 1989, National Academy of Sciences.
6. Harrington DD: Acute vitamin D_2 (ergocalciferol) toxicosis in horses: case report and experimental studies, *J Am Vet Med Assoc* 180:867-873, 1982.
7. Harrington DD, Page EH: Acute vitamin D_3 toxicosis in horses: case reports and experimental studies of the comparative toxicity of vitamins D_2 and D_3, *J Am Vet Med Assoc* 182:1358-1369, 1983.
8. Rebhun WC, Tennant BC, Dill SG, et al: Vitamin K_3–induced renal toxicosis in the horse, *J Am Vet Med Assoc* 184:1237-1239, 1984.
9. Gunson DE, Kowalczyk DF, Shoop CR, et al: Environmental zinc and cadmium pollution associated with generalized osteochondrosis, osteoporosis, and nephrocalcinosis in horses, *J Am Vet Med Assoc* 180:295-299, 1982.
10. Roxe DM, Krumlovsky FA: Toxic interstitial nephropathy from metals, metabolites, and radiation, *Semin Nephrol* 8:72-81, 1988.
11. Schuh JCL, Ross C, Meschter C: Concurrent mercuric blister and dimethyl sulfoxide (DMSO) application as a cause of mercury toxicity in two horses, *Equine Vet J* 20:68-71, 1988.
12. Markel MD, Dyer RM, Hattel AL: Acute renal failure associated with application of a mercuric blister in a horse, *J Am Vet Med Assoc* 185:92-94, 1984.
13. Roberts MC, Seawright AA, Ng JC, et al: Some effects of chronic mercuric chloride intoxication on renal function in a horse, *Vet Hum Toxicol* 24:415-420, 1982.
14. Seawright AA, Roberts MC, Costigan P: Chronic methylmercurialism in a horse, *Vet Hum Toxicol* 20:6, 1978.
15. Massry SG, Glassock RJ, editors: *Massry and Glassock's textbook of nephrology*, ed 4, Baltimore, 2001, Lippincott Williams & Wilkins.

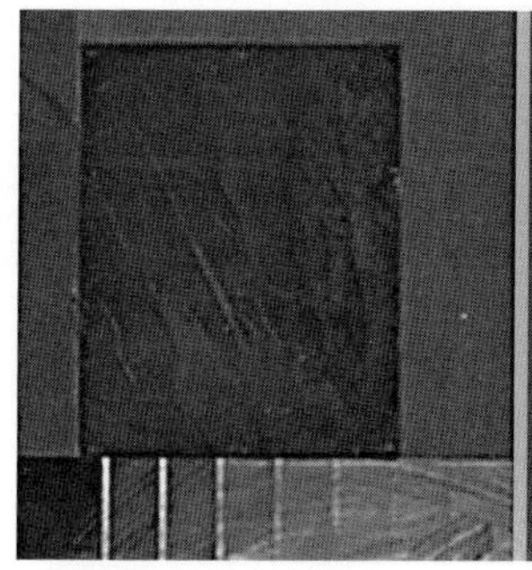

Index

Page numbers followed by f indicate figures; t, tables; b, boxes.

E

G